W9-ASW-667

Infectious Diseases

OF THE DOG AND CAT

Infectious Diseases

OF THE DOG AND CAT

THIRD EDITION

Craig E. Greene, DVM, MS, DACVIM

Professor Emeritus and Josiah Meigs Distinguished Teaching Professor
Department of Infectious Diseases and Department of Small Animal Medicine
College of Veterinary Medicine
The University of Georgia
Athens, Georgia

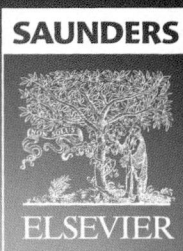

SAUNDERS

ELSEVIER

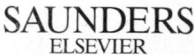

SAUNDERS
ELSEVIER

11830 Westline Industrial Drive
St. Louis, Missouri 63146

Previous editions copyrighted 1990 and 1998.

ISBN-13: 978-1-4160-3600-5
ISBN-10: 1-4160-3600-8

Publishing Director: Linda Duncan
Acquisitions Editor: Anthony Winkel
Developmental Editor: Shelly Stringer
Publishing Services Manager: Julie Eddy
Project Manager: JoAnn Amore
Designer: Julia Dummitt

Printed in Canada

Last digit is the print number: 9   8   7   6   5   4   3   2   1

Contributors

Diane D. Addie, PhD, BVMS, MRCVS
Senior Lecturer in Veterinary Virology
Institute of Comparative Medicine
University of Glasgow
Scotland, United Kingdom
Feline Parvovirus Infections
Feline Coronavirus Infections

Xavier Alvarez, PhD
Assistant Professor
Pathology
Tulane National Primate Research Center
Covington, Louisiana
Microsporidiosis

Max J. Appel, DVM, PhD
Professor of Virology
James A. Baker Institute for Animal Health
College of Veterinary Medicine
Cornell University
Ithaca, New York
Canine Distemper

P. Jane Armstrong, DVM, MS, MBA, DACVIM
Professor
Veterinary Clinical Sciences Department
University of Minnesota
College of Veterinary Medicine
St. Paul, Minnesota
Canine Granulocytotropic Ehrlichiosis (E. ewingii *Infection*)
Canine Granulocytotropic Anaplasmosis
   (A. phagocytophilum *Infection*)

Ashley Ayoob, DVM
Small Animal Resident
Department of Small Animal Medicine and Surgery
The Ohio State University
Columbus, Ohio
Laboratory Testing for Infectious Diseases of Dogs and Cats

Charles A. Baldwin, DVM, MS, PhD, DACVM
Director and Virologist
Veterinary Diagnostic and Investigational Laboratory
The University of Georgia
Tifton, Georgia
Mosquito and Gnat-Borne Infections

Gad Baneth, DVM, PhD, DECVCP
School of Veterinary Medicine
Hebrew University
Rehovot, Israel
Leishmaniasis
Canine and Feline American Tegumentary Leishmaniasis
Hepatozoon canis *Infection*
Feline Hepatozoonosis

Stephen C. Barr, BVSc, MVS, PhD, DACVIM (Small Animals)
Professor of Medicine
Department of Clinical Sciences
Cornell University
Ithaca, New York
American Trypanosomiasis
Giardiasis
Amebiasis
Balantidiasis
Cryptosporidiosis and Cyclosporiasis

Jeanne A. Barsanti, DVM, MS, DACVIM (Internal Medicine)
Professor and Head
Small Animal Medicine and Surgery
Internist
The University of Georgia Teaching Hospital
The University of Georgia
Athens, Georgia
Botulism
Genitourinary Infections

Derrick Baxby, BSc, PhD, FRCPath
Honorary Senior Research Fellow
Department of Medical Microbiology
University of Liverpool
Liverpool, United Kingdom
Poxvirus Infection

Malcolm Bennett, BVSc, PhD, MRCVS, FRCPath, DECVPH
Professor of Veterinary Pathology
Department of Veterinary Pathology
University of Liverpool
Liverpool, United Kingdom
Poxvirus Infection

Anna-Lena Berg, DVM, PhD
Associate Professor
Associate Director, Experimental Morphology
Safety Assessment, R&D Södertälje
AstraZeneca R&D Södertälje
Södertälje, Sweden
Hantavirus Infection
Borna Disease Meningoencephalomyelitis

Anneli Bjöersdorff, DVM, PhD
Consultant in Medical Microbiology
Department of Clinical Microbiology
Research Institute for Zoonotic Ecology and
   Epidemiology
Kalmar, Sweden
Feline Granulocytotropic Anaplamosis

Ross Bond, BVMS, PhD, DVD, MRCVS, DECVD
Senior Lecturer in Veterinary Dermatology
Department of Veterinary Clinical Sciences
Royal Veterinary College
North Mymms, Hertsfordshire, United Kingdom
Malassezia *Dermatitis*

Edward B. Breitschwerdt, DVM, DACVIM
Professor of Medicine and Infectious Diseases
Department of Clinical Sciences
College of Veterinary Medicine
North Carolina State University
Raleigh, North Carolina
Canine Granulocytotropic Ehrlichiosis (E. ewingii *Infection*)
Feline Mononuclear Ehrlichiosis
Feline Granulocytotropic Anaplamosis
Rocky Mountain Spotted Fever, Murine Typhuslike Disease, Rickettsialpox, Typhus, and Q Fever
Canine Bartonellosis
Canine Visceral Leishmaniasis in North America
Rhinosporidiosis

Cathy A. Brown, VMD, PhD, DACVP
Athens Diagnostic Laboratory
College of Veterinary Medicine
The University of Georgia
Athens, Georgia
Leptospirosis

Steven C. Budsberg, DVM, MS, DACVS
Professor, Clinical Research Coordinator
Department of Small Animal Medicine and Surgery
The University of Georgia
Athens, Georgia
Musculoskeletal Infections

Janet Calpin, BS, LATg
Laboratory Animal Technician
Animal Resources
College of Veterinary Medicine
The University of Georgia
Athens, Georgia
Recommendations for Core and Noncore Vaccinations of Dogs
Recommendations for Core and Noncore Vaccinations of Cats
Antimicrobial Drug Formulary

Clay A. Calvert, DVM, DACVIM
Professor
Department of Small Animal Medicine
College of Veterinary Medicine
The University of Georgia
Athens, Georgia
Canine Viral Papillomatosis
Cardiovascular Infections

Leland E. Carmichael, DVM, PhD, Dhc
The John M. Olin Professor of Virology
James A. Baker Institute for Animal Health
College of Veterinary Medicine
Cornell University
Ithaca, New York
Canine Herpesvirus Infection
Canine Brucellosis

M. Cecilia Castellano, DVM
Associate Professor
Small Animal Clinics
Facultad de Ciencias Veterinarias
Universidad Nacional de La Plata
La Plata, Argentina
Rhinosporidiosis

Sharon A. Center, DVM
Professor
Department of Clinical Sciences
College of Veterinary Medicine
Cornell University
Ithaca, New York
Hepatobiliary Infections

Francis W. Chandler, DVM, PhD, DACVP
Professor Emeritus of Pathology
Department of Pathology
Medical College of Georgia
Augusta, Georgia
Candidiasis and Rhodotorulosis
Trichosporonosis
Pneumocystosis

Bruno B. Chomel, DVM, PhD
Professor
Population Health and Reproduction
School of Veterinary Medicine
University of California, Davis
Davis, California
Hantavirus Infection
Canine Bartonellosis

Hollis Utah Cox, DVM, PhD, DACVM
Professor of Veterinary Bacteriology
Department of Pathobiological Sciences
School of Veterinary Medicine
Louisiana State University
Baton Rouge, Lousiana
Staphylococcal Infections

Thomas M. Craig, DVM, PhD
Professor
Department of Veterinary Pathobiology
Texas A&M University
College Station, Texas
Hepatozoon americanum *Infection*

Susan Dawson, BVMS, PhD, MRCVS
Senior Lecturer
Veterinary Clinical Science
University of Liverpool
Liverpool, United Kingdom
Feline Respiratory Disease

Michael J. Day, BSc, BVMS (Hons), PhD, FASM, DECVP, MRCPath, FRCVS
Professor of Veterinary Pathology
School of Clinical Veterinary Science
University of Bristol
Langford, North Somerset, United Kingdom
Canine Disseminated Aspergillosis
Feline Disseminated Aspergillosis

Michael G. Dearmin, DVM, MS
Resident, Small Animal Surgery
Department of Small Animal Medicine and Surgery
College of Veterinary Medicine
The University of Georgia
Athens, Georgia
Surgical and Traumatic Wound Infections

Brad M. DeBey, DVM, PhD
Associate Professor
Department of Diagnostic Medicine/Pathobiology
Kansas State University
Manhattan, Kansas
Tularemia

Douglas J. DeBoer, DVM
Associate Professor
Department of Medical Sciences
School of Veterinary Medicine
University of Wisconsin-Madison
Madison, Wisconsin
Dermatophytosis

Elizabeth S. Didier, PhD
Research Scientist
Division of Microbiology and Immunology
Tulane National Primate Research Center
Tulane University Health Sciences Center
Covington, Louisiana
Microsporidiosis

Peter J. Didier, DVM, PhD
Veterinary Pathologist
Department of Comparative Pathology
Tulane National Primate Research Center
Covington, Louisiana
Microsporidiosis

J. P. Dubey, BVSc AH, MVSc, PhD
Senior Scientist
Animal Parasitic Diseases Laboratory
ARS, NRI, USDA
Beltsville Agricultural Research Center
Beltsville, Maryland
Toxoplasmosis and Neosporosis
Enteric Coccidiosis

Robert W. Dunstan, DVM, MS, DACVP
Pfizer Global Research and Development
Ann Arbor, Michigan
Sporotrichosis

David F. Edwards, DVM, DACVIM, DACVP
Professor
Department of Pathobiology
College of Veterinary Medicine
University of Tennessee
Knoxville, Tennessee
Actinomycosis and Nocardiosis

Herman F. Egberink, DVM, PhD
Associate Professor
Department of Infectious Diseases and Immunology
Virology Division
Faculty of Veterinary Medicine
Utrecht University
Utrecht, The Netherlands
Feline Viral Papillomatosis

James F. Evermann, MS, PhD
Professor of Infectious Diseases
Department of Veterinary Clinical Sciences
Washington Animal Disease Diagnostic Laboratory
College of Veterinary Medicine
Washington State University
Pullman, Washington
Laboratory Diagnosis of Viral and Rickettsial Infections and Epidemiology of Infectious Disease

Sidney A. Ewing, DVM, PhD
Wendell H. and Nellie G. Krull Professor of Veterinary Parasitology, Emeritus
Department of Veterinary Pathobiology
College of Veterinary Medicine
Oklahoma State University
Stillwater, Oklahoma
Antiprotozoal Chemotherapy

Carol S. Foil, MS, DVM, DACVD
Professor
Department of Veterinary Clinical Sciences
School of Veterinary Medicine
Louisiana State University
Baton Rouge, Louisiana
Miscellaneous Fungal Infections

Janet Foley, DVM, PhD
Assistant Professor
Department of Medicine and Epidemiology
School of Veterinary Medicine
University of California, Davis
Davis, California
Prevention and Management of Infectious Diseases in Multiple-Cat Environments

Richard B. Ford, DVM, MS
Professor of Medicine
Department of Clinical Sciences
North Carolina State University
Raleigh, North Carolina
Canine Infectious Tracheobronchitis

William J. Foreyt, MS, PhD
Professor
Veterinary Microbiology and Pathology
Washington State University
Pullman, Washington
Salmon Poisoning Disease

Sue Foster, BVSc, MVetClinStud, FACVSc
Adjunct Senior Lecturer
School of Veterinary and Biomedical Sciences
Murdoch University
Murdoch, Australia
Medical Consultant
Mayne Health Vetnostics
Sydney, Australia
Infections Caused by Rapidly Growing Mycobacteria

James G. Fox, DVM
Professor and Director
Division of Comparative Medicine
Massachusetts Institute of Technology
Cambridge, Massachusetts
Adjunct Professor
School of Veterinary Medicine
University of Pennsylvania
Philadelphia, Pennsylvania
Adjunct Professor
School of Veterinary Medicine
Tufts University
North Grafton, Massachusetts
Campylobacter *Infections*
Gastric Helicobacter *Infections*
Intestinal and Hepatic Helicobacter *Infections*

Rosalind M. Gaskell, BVSc, PhD, MRCVS
Professor
Department of Veterinary Pathology
University of Liverpool
South Wirral, United Kingdom

Feline Respiratory Disease
Poxvirus Infection

Urs Giger, PhD, DMV, MS, FHV, DACVIM, DECVIM
Charlotte Newton Sheppard Professor and Chief of
　Medical Genetics
Section of Medical Genetics
School of Veterinary Medicine
Ryan Veterinary Hospital
University of Pennsylvania
Philadelphia, Pennsylvania
Immunodeficiencies and Infectious Diseases

Ellie J. C. Goldstein, MD
Clinical Professor
School of Medicine
University of California, Los Angeles
Los Angeles, California
Director
R. M. Alden Research Laboratory
Santa Monica, California
Bite Wound Infections

Jody L. Gookin, DVM, PhD, DACVIM (Internal Medicine)
Assistant Professor
Department of Molecular Biomedical Sciences
College of Veterinary Medicine
North Carolina State University
Raleigh, North Carolina
Trichomoniasis

John R. Gorham, DVM, PhD
Department of Veterinary Microbiology and Pathology
Washington State University
Pullman, Washington
Salmon Poisoning Disease

Craig E. Greene, DVM, MS, DACVIM
Professor Emeritus and Josiah Meigs Distinguished
　Teaching Professor
Department of Infectious Diseases and Department of
　Small Animal Medicine
College of Veterinary Medicine
The University of Georgia
Athens, Georgia
Canine Distemper
Infectious Canine Hepatitis and Canine Acidophil Cell
　Hepatitis
Canine Herpesvirus Infection
Nonrespiratory Parainfluenza Virus Infection of Dogs
Feline Parvovirus Infections
Feline Enteric Viral Infections
Feline Foamy (Syncytium-Forming) Virus Infection
Feline Paramyxovirus Infections
Hantavirus Infection
Foot-and-Mouth Disease
Vesicular Exanthema
Hepatitis E Virus Infection
Rabbit Hemorrhagic Disease
Lymphocytic Choriomeningitis
Borna Disease Meningoencephalomyelitis
Rabies and Other Lyssavirus Infections
Enterovirus Infections
Mumps and Influenza Virus Infections
Mosquito and Gnat-Borne Infections
West Nile Virus Infection
Wolbachia Infection
Rocky Mountain Spotted Fever, Murine Typhuslike Disease,
　Rickettsialpox, Typhus, and Q Fever

Chlamydial Infections
Mycoplasmal, Ureaplasmal, and L-Form Infections
Antibacterial Chemotherapy
Streptococcal Infections
Enterococcal Infections
Rhodococcus equi Infection
Corynebacterium Infections
Listeriosis
Anthrax
Erysipelothrix Infections
Anaerobiospirillum Infection
Salmonellosis
Shigellosis
Yersiniosis
Plesiomonas shigelloides Infection
Tyzzer's Disease
Canine Brucellosis
Anaerobic Infections
Tetanus
Leptospirosis
Borreliosis
Miscellaneous Bacterial Infections
Tularemia
Infections Caused by Slow-Growing Mycobacteria
Dermatophilosis
Abscesses and Pyogranulomatous Inflammation Caused by
　Bacteria
Bite Wound Infections
Surgical and Traumatic Wound Infections
Antifungal Chemotherapy
Histoplasmosis
Candidiasis and Rhodotorulosis
Trichosporonosis
Pneumocystosis
Protothecosis
Antiprotozoal Chemotherapy
African Trypanosomiasis
Cytauxzoonosis
Blastocystosis
Nonenteric Amebiasis: Acanthamebiasis, Hartmannelliasis, and
　Balamuthiasis
Enteric Coccidiosis
Prion Diseases and Feline Spongiform Encephalopathy
Otitis Externa
Musculoskeletal Infections
Bacterial Respiratory Infections
Gastrointestinal and Intraabdominal Infections
Environmental Factors in Infectious Disease
Immunodeficiencies and Infectious Diseases
Immunocompromised People and Shared Human and Animal
　Infections: Zoonosis, Sapronoses, and Anthroponoses
Immunoprophylaxis
Recommendations for Core and Noncore Vaccinations of
　Dogs
Recommendations for Core and Noncore Vaccinations of
　Cats
Canine and Feline Biologics Manufacturers and Products
　Available Worldwide
Laboratory Testing for Infectious Diseases of Dogs and Cats
Manufacturers of Diagnostic Test Kits and Their Products
Disease Rule-Outs for Medical Problems
Antimicrobial Drug Formulary

Russell T. Greene, DVM, PhD, DACVIM, DACVM
President
Phoenix Veterinary Internal Medicine Services, Inc.
Phoenix, Arizona
Miscellaneous Bacterial Infections
Coccidioidomycosis and Paracoccidioidomycosis

Barbara Greig, DVM, DACVP
Veterinary Pathologist
Laboratories—Veterinary Diagnostic Services
Marshfield Clinic
Marshfield, Wisconsin
Canine Granulocytotropic Ehrlichiosis (E. ewingii Infection)
Canine Granulocytotropic Anaplasmosis (A. phagocytophilum Infection)

Amy M. Grooters, DVM, DACVIM
Associate Professor, Companion Animal Medicine
Department of Veterinary Clinical Sciences
Chief, Companion Animal Medicine
Veterinary Teaching Hospital
Louisiana State University
Baton Rouge, Louisiana
Miscellaneous Fungal Infections

Danielle A. Gunn-Moore, BSc, BVM&S, PhD, MACVSc, MRCVS, RCVS Specialist in Feline Medicine
Nestlé Purina Senior Lecturer in Feline Medicine
Head of Feline Clinic
R(D)SVS Hospital for Small Animals
Department of Clinical Veterinary Science
University of Edinburgh
Edinburgh, United Kingdom
Easter Bush Veterinary Centre, Roslin
Midlothian, Scotland, United Kingdom
Infections Caused by Slow-Growing Mycobacteria

Lynn Guptill-Yoran, DVM, PhD, DACVIM
Associate Professor
Department of Veterinary Clinical Sciences
Purdue University
West Lafayette, Indiana
Feline Bartonellosis

Gerryll Gae Hall, DVM
Companion Animal Technical Services
Schering-Plough Animal Health
Union, New Jersey
Recommendations for Core and Noncore Vaccinations of Dogs
Recommendations for Core and Noncore Vaccinations of Cats
Canine and Feline Biologics Manufacturers and Products Available Worldwide

Shimon Harrus, DVM, PhD, DECVCP
Senior Lecturer of Veterinary Internal Medicine
Department of Small Animal Internal Medicine
School of Veterinary Medicine
Hebrew University
Rehovot, Israel
Canine Monocytotropic Ehrlichiosis and Neorickettsiosis (E. canis, E. chaffeensis, E. ruminatium, N. sennetsu, and N. risticii Infections)

Katrin Hartmann, DMV, DMV habil, DECVIM-CA
Professor
Department of Small Animal Medicine
Ludwig Maximilian University
Munich, Germany
Antiviral and Immunodulatory Chemotherapy
Feline Leukemia Virus Infection
Feline Immunodeficiency Virus Infection
Leptospirosis
Antimicrobial Drug Formulary

John W. Harvey, DVM, PhD, DACVP
Professor and Chair
Department of Physiological Sciences
College of Veterinary Medicine
Veterinary Medical Teaching Hospital
Clinical Pathology Service
University of Florida
Gainesville, Florida
Thrombocytotropic Anaplasmosis (A. platys [E. platys] Infection)
Hemotrophic Mycoplasmosis (Hemobartonellosis)

Marian C. Horzinek, Prof.emer., Dr.Dr.h.c.mult.
The Netherlands
Feline Viral Papillomatosis

Johnny D. Hoskins, DVM, PhD
Professor Emeritus
Department of Veterinary Clinical Sciences
School of Veterinary Medicine
Louisiana State University
Baton Rouge, Louisiana
Canine Viral Enteritis

Geoff Houser, Cand. Med. Vet
Hospital Administrator
Department of Small Animal Clinical Sciences
The Royal Veterinary and Agricultural University
Frederiksberg, Denmark
Laboratory Testing for Infectious Diseases of Dogs and Cats

Elizabeth W. Howerth, DVM, PhD
Professor
Department of Pathology
College of Veterinary Medicine
The University of Georgia
Athens, Georgia
Nonenteric Amebiasis: Acanthamebiasis, Hartmannelliasis, and Balamuthiasis

M. Siobhan Hughes, BSc, PhD
Senior Scientific Officer
Veterinary Sciences Division
Department of Agriculture and Rural Development for Northern Ireland
Belfast, Northern Ireland
Feline Leprosy Syndromes
Canine Leproid Granuloma Syndrome (Canine Leprosy)

Peter J. Ihrke, VMD, DACVD
Professor of Dermatology
Department of Medicine and Epidemiology
Chief, Dermatology Service
Veterinary Medical Teaching Hospital
School of Veterinary Medicine
University of California, Davis
Davis, California
Bacterial Infections of the Skin

Spencer S. Jang, BA
Clinical Laboratory Scientist Supervisor
Microbiology Service, Veterinary Medical Teaching Hospital
School of Veterinary Medicine
University of California, Davis
Davis, California
Anaerobic Infections
Laboratory Diagnosis of Fungal and Algal Infections

Oswald Jarrett, PhD, BVMS, MRCVS, FRSE
Honorary Senior Research Fellow
Institute of Comparative Medicine
University of Glasgow
Glasgow, United Kingdom
Feline Coronavirus Infections

Deborah Joiner, BS, DVM
Pruyn Veterinary Hospital
Missoula, Montana
Manufacturers of Diagnostic Test Kits and Their Products

Boyd R. Jones, BVSc, FACVSc, DECVIM-Ca, MRCVS
Professor and Dean
Department of Small Animal Clinical Studies
University College, Dublin
Dublin, Ireland
Tyzzer's Disease

Robert L. Jones, DVM, PhD, DACVM
Professor
Department of Microbiology, Immunology and Pathology
Colorado State University
Fort Collins, Colorado
Laboratory Diagnosis of Bacterial Infections

Elizabeth J. Kather
University of California, Davis
Davis, California
Clostridium perfringens– and Clostridium
  difficile*–Associated Diarrhea*

Frances A. Kennedy, DVM, MS
Specialist
Diagnostic Center for Population and Animal Health
Michigan State University
East Lansing, Michigan
Feline Adenovirus Infection

Marc Kent, BA, DVM
Assistant Professor
Department of Small Animal Medicine and Surgery
Veterinary Teaching Hospital
College of Veterinary Medicine
The University of Georgia
Athens, Georgia
Bacterial Infections of the Central Nervous System

A. Alan Kocan, PhD†
Professor
Department of Veterinary Pathobiology
Oklahoma State University
Stillwater, Oklahoma
Cytauxzoonosis

Mark Krockenberger, BSc(vet), BVSc, PhD, MACVSc
Lecturer in Veterinary Pathology
Faculty of Veterinary Science
University of Sydney
Sydney, Australia
Cryptococcosis

**Stephen A. Kruth, DVM, DACVIM
  (Internal Medicine)**
Professor
Department of Clinical Studies
University of Guelph
Guelph, Ontario, Canada

†Deceased.

Gram-Negative Bacterial Infections
Endotoxemia

Michael R. Lappin, DVM, PhD, DACVIM
Kenneth W. Smith Professor in Small Animal Clinical
  Veterinary Medicine
Department of Clinical Sciences
Colorado State University
Fort Collins, Colorado
Feline Mononuclear Ehrlichiosis
Feline Granulocytotropic Anaplasmosis
Toxoplasmosis and Neosporosis

Kenneth S. Latimer, DVM, PhD, DACVP
Professor
Director, Clinical Pathology Laboratory
Department of Pathology
College of Veterinary Medicine
The University of Georgia
Athens, Georgia
Protothecosis

Dennis F. Lawler, DVM
Veterinary Research Scientist
Nestle Research Center—St. Louis
Nestle Purina Pet Care Company
St. Louis, Missouri
Prevention and Management of Infection in Kennels

Alfred M. Legendre, DVM, MS
Professor of Medicine and Oncology
Department of Small Animal Clinical Sciences
University of Tennessee
Knoxville, Tennessee
Blastomycosis

Julie K. Levy, DVM, PhD, DACVIM
Associate Professor
Department of Small Animal Clinical Sciences
College of Veterinary Medicine
University of Florida
Gainesville, Florida
*Immunocompromised People and Shared Human and Animal
  Infections: Zoonoses, Sapronoses, and Anthroponoses*

Carol A. Lichtensteiger, DVM, PhD
Assistant Professor
Department of Pathobiology
Veterinary Diagnostic Laboratory
University of Illinois at Urbana-Champaign
Urbana, Illinois
West Nile Virus Infection

Susan E. Little, DVM, PhD
Associate Professor
Department of Veterinary Pathobiology
Oklahoma State University
Stillwater, Oklahoma
Laboratory Diagnosis of Protozoal Infections

**Remo Lobetti, BVSc (Hons), MMed Vet (Med), DECVIM
  (Internal Medicine)**
Professor
Department of Companion Animal Clinical Studies
Faculty of Veterinary Science
University of Pretoria
Onderstepoort, South Africa
Internist
Bryanston Veterinary Hospital
Bryanston, South Africa

Pneumocystosis
Babesiosis

Katharine F. Lunn, BVMS, MS, PhD, MRCVS, DACVIM
Assistant Professor
Department of Clinical Sciences
Colorado State University
Fort Collins, Colorado
Fever

Hans Lutz, DMV
Professor
Director, Clinical Laboratory
Veterinärmedizinisches Labor
Universität Zürich
Zürich, Switzerland
Feline Paramyxovirus Infections

Douglass K. Macintire, DVM, MS, DACVIM, DACVECC
Professor, Acute Medicine and Critical Care
Department of Clinical Studies
College of Veterinary Medicine
Auburn University
Auburn, Alabama
Hepatozoon americanum *Infection*

Dennis Macy, DVM, MS
Professor of Medicine and Oncology
Department of Clinical Sciences
College of Veterinary Medicine and Biomedical Science
Colorado State University
Fort Collins, Colorado
Plague

Richard Malik, BVSc, DipVetAn, MvetClinStud, PhD, FACVSc, MASM
Post Graduate Foundation in Veterinary Science
The University of Sydney
Sydney, New South Wales, Australia
Feline Leprosy Syndromes
Canine Leproid Granuloma Syndrome (Canine Leprosy)
Infection Caused by Rapidly Growing Mycobacteria
Cryptococcosis

Stanley L. Marks, BVSc, PhD, DACVIM (Internal Medicine, Oncology), DACVN
Professor
Department of Medicine and Epidemiology
School of Veterinary Medicine
Professor
Veterinary Medical Teaching Hospital
University of California, Davis
Davis, California
Clostridium perfringens– *and* Clostridium difficile–*Associated Diarrhea*

Patricia Martin, BVSc, MVSc
Faculty of Veterinary Science
The University of Sydney
Sydney, New South Wales, Australia
Feline Leprosy Syndromes
Canine Leproid Granuloma Syndrome (Canine Leprosy)
Infection Caused by Rapidly Growing Mycobacteria
Cryptococcosis

George Matete, BVM, MSc, Vet Pathol & Micobiol, UoN
Veterinary Research Officer
Trypanosomiasis Research Centre
Kenya Agricultural Research Institute

Muguga, Kenya
Expatriate Field Veterinary Trainer
Itinerant Training Programme Phase III
Terra Nuova
Nairobi, Kenya
African Trypanosomiasis

Kyle G. Mathews, DVM, MS, DACVS
Associate Professor
Department of Clinical Sciences
College of Veterinary Medicine
North Carolina State University
Raleigh, North Carolina
Canine Nasal Aspergillosis-Penicilliosis
Feline Nasal Aspergillosis-Penicilliosis

Christie Mayo
Veterinary Student (Class of 2006)
The University of Georgia
Athens, Georgia
Disease Rule-Outs for Medical Problems

Dudley L. McCaw, DVM
Associate Professor
Veterinary Medicine and Surgery
College of Veterinary Medicine
University of Missouri at Columbia
Columbia, Missouri
Canine Viral Enteritis

Linda Medleau, DVM, MS, DACVD
Professor of Veterinary Dermatology
Department of Small Animal Medicine and Surgery
The University of Georgia
Athens, Georgia
Cryptococcosis

James Meinkoth, DVM, PhD, DACVP
Professor
Department of Veterinary Pathobiology
Oklahoma State University
Stillwater, Oklahoma
Cytauxzoonosis

George E. Moore, DVM, MD, DACVPM, DACVIM
Research Assistant in Epidemiology
Department of Veterinary Pathobiology
College of Veterinary Medicine
Purdue University
West Lafayette, Indiana
Anthrax

Karen A. Moriello, DVM, DACVD
Professor of Dermatology
Department of Medical Sciences
School of Veterinary Medicine
University of Wisconsin at Madison
Madison, Wisconsin
Dermatophytosis

T. Mark Neer, DVM, DACVIM (Internal Medicine)
Professor of Medicine
Department of Veterinary Clinical Sciences
Small Animal Medicine Section Head
Veterinary Teaching Hospital and Clinics
Louisiana State University
Baton Rouge, Louisiana
Canine Monocytotropic Ehrlichiosis and Neorickettsiosis
 (E. canis, E. chaffeensis, E. ruminatium, N. sennetsu, and
 N. risticii Infections)

Carolyn R. O'Brien, BVSc, M.Vet.Clin.Stud., MACVSc
Senior Registrar in Small Animal Medicine
University Veterinary Centre Sydney
University of Sydney
Sydney, New South Wales, Australia
Miscellaneous Bacterial Infections
Cryptococcosis

John F. Prescott, MA, VetMD, PhD
Professor
Department of Pathobiology
University of Guelph
Guelph, Ontario, Canada
Streptococcal Infections
Enterococcal Infections

Alan Radford, BVSc, BSc, PhD, MRCVS
Lecturer
Veterinary Clinical Science
University of Liverpool
Liverpool, United Kingdom
Feline Respiratory Disease

Pauline M. Rakich, DVM, PhD, DACVP
Associate Professor
Athens Veterinary Diagnostic Laboratory
College of Veterinary Medicine
The University of Georgia
Athens, Georgia
Protothecosis

Hugh W. Reid, MBE, BVMS, DipTVM, PhD, MRCVS
TSE Research Coordinator
Virology
Moredun Research Institute
Midlothian, Scotland, United Kingdom
Louping-Ill

Carol Norris Reinero, DVM, DACVIM, PhD
Assistant Professor
Department of Veterinary Medicine and Surgery
University of Missouri at Columbia
Columbia, Missouri
Bacterial Respiratory Infections

Edmund J. Rosser, Jr., DVM, DACVD
Professor of Dermatology
Department of Small Animal Clinical Sciences
College of Veterinary Medicine
Michigan State University
East Lansing, Michigan
Sporotrichosis

Charles E. Rupprecht, VMD, MS, PhD
Chief, Rabies Section
Viral & Rickettsial Zoonoses Branch
Centers for Disease Control and Prevention
Atlanta, Georgia
Rabies and Other Lyssavirus Infections

Peter M. Schantz, VMD, PhD
Epidemiologist
Division of Parasitic Diseases, NCID
Centers for Disease Control and Prevention
Atlanta, Georgia
Canine Visceral Leishmaniasis in North America

Ron D. Schultz, MS, PhD, DACVM
Professor and Chair
Department of Pathobiological Sciences
School of Veterinary Medicine
University of Wisconsin at Madison
Madison, Wisconsin
Immunoprophylaxis

Rance K. Sellon, DVM, PhD
Associate Professor
Department of Veterinary Clinical Sciences
College of Veterinary Medicine
Washington State University
Pullman, Washington
Laboratory Diagnosis of Viral and Rickettsial Infections and Epidemiology of Infectious Disease
Feline Immunodeficiency Virus Infection

Nick J. H. Sharp, BVM, PhD, DACVS, DECVS, DACVIM (Neurology)
Adjunct Associate Professor of Neurology
Department of Clinical Sciences
College of Veterinary Medicine
North Carolina State University
Raleigh, North Carolina
Clinical Neurologist
Animal Critical Care Group
Vancouver, British Columbia, Canada
Canine Nasal Aspergillosis-Penicilliosis

Karen Snowden, DVM, PhD
Associate Professor
Department of Veterinary Pathobiology
Texas A&M University
College Station, Texas
Microsporidiosis

Reinhard K. Straubinger, PhD, Priv.-Doz. Dr. habil.med.vet.
Head, Junior Research Group, Molecular Medicine of Infectious Diseases
Biotechnological-Biomedical Center (BBZ) and Institute for Immunology of the College of Veterinary Medicine
University of Leipzig
Leipzig, Germany
Borreliosis

Jean Stiles, DVM, MS, DACVO
Associate Professor, Ophthalmology
Veterinary Clinical Sciences
Purdue University
West Lafayette, Indiana
Ocular Infections
Concentrations and Dosages of Locally Used Ocular Antibacterial Agents

Jane E. Sykes, BVSc(Hons), PhD, DACVIM (Small Animal Internal Medicine)
Assistant Professor
Department of Medicine and Epidemiology
University of California, Davis
Davis, California
Laboratory Diagnosis of Viral and Rickettsial Infections and Epidemiology of Infectious Disease
Chlamydial Infections Leptospirosis

Joseph Taboada, DVM, DACVIM (Small Animal Internal Medicine)
Associate Dean
Office of Student and Academic Affairs
Professor of Small Animal Internal Medicine
Department of Veterinary Clinical Sciences

School of Veterinary Medicine
Louisiana State University
Baton Rouge, Louisiana
Babesiosis

Andrea Tipold, DECVN
Department of Small Animal Medicine and Surgery
University of Veterinary Medicine, Hannover
Hannover, Germany
Central European Tick-Borne Encephalitis
Granulomatous Meningoencephalitis
Encephalitis in Pug and Maltese Dogs
Encephalitis in Yorkshire Terriers
Hydrocephalus with Periventricular Encephalitis in Dogs
Nonsuppurative Meningoencephalitis in Greyhounds
Feline Poliomyelitis
Steroid-Responsive Meningitis-Arteritis

Kamil Tomsa, DMV, DECVIM-CA (Internal Medicine)
Kleintierklinik Rigiplatz
Cham, Switzerland
Feline Nasal Aspergillosis-Penicilliosis

Marc Vandevelde, DMV, DECVN
Professor and Chairman
Clinical Veterinary Medicine
University of Berne
Berne, Switzerland
Pseudorabies
Central European Tick-Borne Encephalitis
Granulomatous Meningoencephalitis
Encephalitis in Pug and Maltese Dogs
Encephalitis in Yorkshire Terriers
Hydrocephalus with Periventricular Encephalitis in Dogs
Nonsuppurative Meningoencephalitis in Greyhounds
Feline Poliomyelitis
Steroid-Responsive Meningitis-Arteritis
Prion Diseases and Feline Spongiform Encephalopathy

Nancy A. Vincent-Johnson, DVM, MS, DACVIM, DACVAM
Lieutenant Colonel
United States Army Veterinary Corps
Commander
National Capital District Veterinary Command
Fort Belvoir, Virginia
Hepatozoon americanum Infection

Richard L. Walker, DVM, PhD, MPVM
Professor
Department of Clinical Microbiology
California Animal Health and Food Safety Laboratory
School of Veterinary Medicine
University of California, Davis
Davis, California
Laboratory Diagnosis of Fungal and Algal Infections

Michelle Wall, DVM, DACVIM
Resident, Medical Oncology
Department of Small Animal Medicine
College of Veterinary Medicine
The University of Georgia
Athens, Georgia
Canine Viral Papillomatosis
Cardiovascular Infections

A. D. J. Watson, BVSc, PhD, MACVSc, FRCVS, FAAVPT, DECVPT
Glebe, Australia
Antibacterial Chemotherapy

Denise Wigney, BVSc, DVP, MASM
Faculty of Veterinary Science
The University of Sydney
Sydney, New South Wales, Australia
Feline Leprosy Syndromes
Canine Leproid Granuloma Syndrome (Canine Leprosy)
Infection Caused by Rapidly Growing Mycobacteria
Cryptococcosis

This book is dedicated...

To Jeanne, Casey, and Anna
for their personal sacrifice during its writing.

To the book's contributors
and to researchers in the field who have advanced our knowledge.

To my unsung heroes, Janet Calpin, Kip Carter, Mamie Watson,
the staff of the Department of Educational Resources,
and the many other current and former faculty, staff,
and students of the College of Veterinary Medicine,
University of Georgia, without whose dedication and assistance
this book would not have been possible.

To my memory of a former mentor and friend, Oscar W. Schalm,
who inspired me to consider an academic career.

Preface

The first edition of this book, published in 1990, was a sequel to the text *Clinical Microbiology and Infectious Diseases of the Dog and Cat*, which I edited in 1984. With the advent of molecular technology, considerable new information and updates were made in the second edition (1998). From that time to the present, and with the further application of genetic technology, there has been an exponential increase in the body of new information concerning existing and emerging infections of dogs and cats. Genetic analysis has further established the lineage of pathogenic microorganisms; facilitated our detection of disease-causing agents in the host; and in certain infections, assisted in determining the efficacy of treatment in eliminating persistent pathogens. Molecular diagnostic methods such as the polymerase chain reaction have moved from research to reference laboratories, and in some instances, such as hemotrophic mycoplasmosis, babesiosis, and bartonellosis in the nonreservoir host, have become indispensable clinical diagnostic tools. Genetic methodologies have also been employed to produce recombinant proteins for development of diagnostic immunoassays, cytokine chemotherapeutics, and vaccines.

The entire third edition has been extensively updated due to the vast number of discoveries in the past 7 years. Exceptional additions or modifications have been made in expanding coverage of certain diseases for which more information is available or for those caused by newly discovered or taxonomically reclassified agents. More extensive coverage was made for SARS viral infection (Chapter 11), hepatitis E viral infection (Chapter 21), rabbit hemorrhagic disease (Chapter 21), foot and mouth disease (Chapter 21), vesicular exanthema (Chapter 21), lymphocytic choriomeningitis (Chapter 21), lyssaviral infections (Chapter 22), West Nile viral infection (Chapter 26), anaplasmosis, neorickettsiosis, and *Wolbachia* infection (Chapter 28), *Rickettsia felis* infection (Chapter 29), hemotrophic mycoplasmosis (Chapter 31), *Plesiomonas shigelloides* infection (Chapter 39), *Anaerobiospirillum* infection (Chapter 39), *Clostridium perfringens*— and *Clostridium difficile*—associated diarrhea (Chapter 39), melioidosis (Chapter 46), canine leproid granuloma syndrome (Chapter 50), pyogranulomatous inflammation caused by bacteria (Chapter 52), *Malassezia* Dermatitis (Chapter 58), new diseases under Miscellaneous Fungal Infections (Chapter 67), African trypanosomiasis (Chapter 72), canine tegumentary leishmaniasis (Chapter 73), canine visceral leishmaniasis in North America (Chapter 73), *Hepatozoon americanum* infection (Chapter 74), new diseases under Microsporidiosis (Chapter 75), blastocystosis (Chapter 78), trichomoniasis (Chapter 78), hartmannelliasis and balamuthiasis (Chapter 79), transmissible spongiform encephalopathies (Chapter 84), nonsuppurative meningoencephalitis in greyhounds (Chapter 84), newly recognized immunodeficiencies under Immunodeficiencies and Infection (Chapter 95), and new diseases such as Ebola virus infection in dogs, under Immunocompromised People and Shared Human and Animal Infections (Chapter 99). In addition, discussions of bioterroristic risks have been included in chapters on anthrax (35), botulism (42), and plague (47).

The goal of this book has been to provide a comprehensive reference while at the same time serving as a clinically useful source of information for diagnosis and treatment of canine and feline infections. The first four sections (I to IV) include current information on diseases caused by viruses, rickettsiae, and chlamydia (Chapters 1 to 30); mycoplasmas and bacteria (Chapters 31 to 55); fungi and algae (Chapters 56 to 69); and protozoa and prions (Chapters 70 to 84), respectively. Rhinosporidiosis has been placed with the protozoa; however, recent genetic classification considers it a fungal infection. This was an oversight as it was substituted with Pneumocystosis, which also has been reclassified genetically as a fungal infection. This error, which was detected too close to publication, should be corrected in subsequent editions. Each of these major sections is introduced by a chapter concerning diagnostic testing for the type of microorganisms covered in that section. The aim of these diagnostic chapters is to help the clinician determine indications and methods for sample collection and submission to the laboratory, interpretation of results, and when applicable, performance of in-office diagnostic procedures. The therapy chapter follows the diagnostic chapter and covers indications and pharmacologic considerations of antimicrobials used to treat various infections discussed in the respective section. Section V involves principles of diagnosis and therapy of infections in various body organ systems (Chapters 85 to 93) and clinical problems concerning infectious diseases, such as environmental control of infections, fever immunodeficiency disorders, prevention of infection in communal environments, immunocompromised people and pets, and immunization (Chapters 94 to 100).

Modifications have been made to maximize the information presented in this text while preserving the readability and clinical usefulness of the book. Drug dosage tables have been furnished for most diseases, and those used in the prior edition have been updated to give complete and consistent prescribing information in each applicable chapter. The appendices have followed the format and content of prior editions of the book with extensive updating. Topics covered include vaccines (Appendices 1 to 4), diagnostic test kits and laboratories (Appendices 5 and 6), clinical problems associated with the various infectious diseases (Appendix 7), and a comprehensive drug formulary (Appendix 8). The drug formulary is referred to throughout the book. This formulary is cross-referenced in each chapter and refers the reader to references and tabulated dosage information found in the applicable disease coverage located elsewhere in the book.

Because of space limitations, appendices on staining and microscopic techniques and environmental survival of infectious agents have not been listed. The reader should consult the first edition of this book (1990) as this information has changed relatively little during this time interval. An appendix on required infectious disease testing and vaccination for travel requirements was not included in this edition because these regulations are constantly changing and the most current information can be obtained by contacting respective state offices or consulates. Such information is also readily available on the Internet. The reference listings, which in the past were restricted to only those published since the prior edition, have been made cumulative. We have compiled a comprehensive list of references on each subject that were published in the previous editions. These complete reference listings are accessible with the accompanying CD-ROM, which also provides network links to accessible citations. A supplemental reading list, which incorporates a select few of these references, is provided at the end of each chapter. Websites have also been provided throughout the book to allow ready access to pertinent reference information that supplements the text. All listed references for each chapter have been reviewed in the preparation of this and previous editions of the book but are not necessarily cited in the chapter. The references cited in the Drug Formulary (Appendix 8) appear in the respective antimicrobial therapy chapters and elsewhere in the text. These are labeled by chapter number followed by the specific reference number.

As the editor, I am ultimately responsible for coordinating the delivery of this book; however, the task was only possible with the assistance of many other people. My contributors were commendable in their commitment to add yet another task to their already busy schedules. I certainly could not have done the work or provided the needed expertise without their assistance. The amount of time they spend compared to the remuneration they receive means that they have made an unselfish contribution to our education. I dedicate this book to them. I know we will all miss our colleague Dr. A. Alan Kocan; he died suddenly and unexpectedly during the production of this book. He provided me with many references on a variety of vector-borne diseases and was an invaluable contributor on the chapter on Cytauxzoonosis. The other people involved in the logistics of this book are my unsung heroes to whom I dedicate it. The efforts of their hard work made this edition possible. First and foremost, I must thank my loyal and dedicated editorial assistant, Janet Calpin, a technician in Animal Resources at the University of Georgia. As in previous editions of this text, she was involved in all phases of this book, from inception to completion. I don't think I would have considered working on another edition of this book without her commitment. Anyone who uses this reference has her to thank for its existence. She is one of the people to whom I dedicate this book because of her concern for details, accuracy, and extensive knowledge of the science and technology of veterinary medicine. As an exceptional veterinary technician, she is truly one of the pillars that keep us veterinarians productive in our jobs. Another person whose efforts went beyond the call of duty was Kip Carter, an award-winning medical illustrator, who fortunately has been the primary illustrator for this and most of the previous editions of the book. His heart and soul were devoted to developing the best possible and most scientifically accurate presentation of the material at hand with artistic perfection. His drawings are a dominating aspect of the full-color edition of this book, and the life-cycle and technical illustrations come to life on the page. Kip has exceptional medical knowledge, pays close attention to all details, and has amazing artistic talent. It was primarily at his prompting that we decided to consider color for this edition of the book; it was originally contracted for black and white illustrations, similar to previous editions. I also dedicate this book to Kip and the entire staff of the department of Educational Resources, headed by Dr. Lari Cowgill. Many of the individuals in this department helped me at one point or another in compiling the illustrative material used in this book. For this edition, I relied heavily on the artistic talents of Brad Gilleand. He is an accomplished medical illustrator and was responsible for a number of new life cycle and technical images. His excellent artistic ability, attention to detail, and scientific knowledge have allowed many complex concepts to be displayed in colorful, comprehensible drawings. Thel Melton reigned as map-master supreme in this edition. He, with the assistance of Harsh Jain, provided novel renditions or updated revisions of known geographic prevalence data of the infectious diseases. These maps permit the reader to correlate insect or tick vector distribution with that of the disease. A number of images created by Dan Beisel, previously in this department, were used again but transformed by the current illustrators into full-color format. Photographic assistance was handled entirely by Chris Herron. His mastery of computer photographic skills were invaluable in the complete transition to color images. He was involved in converting much of my teaching file of photographs into suitable format for inclusion in this book. Susan Brinkley was the administrative secretary who kept projects on track. Vivian Freeman and Ladonna Beasley helped with duplicating.

Library assistance of Linda Tumlin, Wendy Simmons, and Lucy M. Rowland was of great benefit in obtaining many of the publications needed and tracking down omissions in bibliographic listings. Lucy was also an invaluable assistant in reading many of the finished page proofs for accuracy and content. This was well suited as her background and degrees are in medical microbiology and the library sciences. Debbie Joiner and Lisa Harvey, recent veterinary graduates, were also very helpful in reviewing the page proofs.

I was fortunate to have Mamie Watson, who was also involved with the last edition, type all the manuscripts submitted to the publisher. Her close attention to details and excellent background in computer skills and medical transcription were invaluable. She took material in all types of formats and produced the finished product. She is one of the few people who can read my scrawl, even in the smallest perceptible dimensions. She is meticulous and accurate in her keyboard skills, and her knowledge of medical vocabulary helped us to view and submit the manuscript and tabular material in a format that echoed the final published work. I have also chosen to dedicate the book to her for her meticulous accuracy and invaluable assistance throughout the entire manuscript. Many other people were helpful in the preparation of this edition. Debbie Joiner collected and formulated much of the data used in constructing many of the maps. Christie Mayo helped me label and collate many illustrations. Brandon Pogue also helped in organizing the figures. By being "good mothers," the secretaries of the Department of Small Animal Medicine, Fran Cantrell, Laura Ansley, and April Fowler helped me meet all my other obligations so that I could retain my sanity—whatever might be left of it. I could not have met all my research, teaching, and service obligations without the additional help of our departmental technicians, Lynn Reece, Tanya Cooper, and Melinda Pethel, as well as all the technical staff in the veterinary teaching hospital. Heather Fitzsimmons was very helpful in locating drug information for the formulary.

Many people helped me with their expertise in reviewing particular sections of the book or providing me with materials for publication. Pat Conrad of the University of California, Davis, reviewed the chapter on babesiosis. I also greatly appreciate the lending of photographic material by many persons throughout the world. They are acknowledged in the respective figure legends. Practitioners have also contributed to this book in their determination in managing cases. A number of veterinarians and pet owners have also been helpful in drawing my attention to new topics or inaccuracies in the previous edition. I am appreciative of the biologics manufacturers listed in Appendix 3 for providing the information needed to compile the detailed international information on the available biologics. Laboratories listed in Appendices 5 and 6 were very helpful in providing the information on their testing services and test kits, respectively, where information online was either not available or incomplete.

I am indebted to those who have provided me research and clinical support on infectious diseases over the years. Some of the graduate students I have worked with since the last edition include Laura Ridge, David Drum, and Matt Chenoweth. They have worked on various infectious disease problems in my research laboratory. Richard Moyer, and his late wife

Joanne, formerly of Crozet, Virginia, have provided financial support through the Memorial Fund of Edward Gunst, Richmond, Virginia, and established the Gunst Professorship at the University of Georgia, College of Veterinary Medicine. I was fortunate enough to be in this position for many years, and the funds helped me to develop many teaching illustrations that have become the foundation of those used in this edition. I also appreciate the private support for my efforts in teaching and research that have been funded by Walter Ringger and Tracy French.

I would also like to thank Dr. Keith Prasse, former Dean of the College of Veterinary Medicine; Dr. Fred Quinn, Head of the Department of Infectious Diseases; the entire Faculty of the Department of Small Animal Medicine; and the present and former faculty, staff, and students of The University of Georgia College of Veterinary Medicine for their hard work in making it a respected veterinary institution as well as an enjoyable place to work.

The people at Elsevier have done a commendable job in their efforts with this book. Tony Winkel has been my editor who allowed this book to transform into a full-color reference at the lowest cost to the reader. He placed me in the very competent hands of his developmental editor, Shelly Stringer, who answered all my questions and put me in touch with all the necessary people to proceed. She provided me with the guidance and nagging needed to complete the work in a timely fashion. Jennifer Hong was extremely helpful and assisted me in many tasks involved with completing the manuscript. Ellen Kunkelmann was in charge of the production of the book and all the details involved in transforming the manuscript and illustrations into the final printed format. She and her associates had a challenging job because of the large number of new large tables and color figures. The book should be relatively current at the time of publication because the current literature and reference lists were updated during the editing process. Approximately 6 months elapsed from the time of the final submission of the manuscript until publication.

I would like to thank all of those over the years who have complimented the value of this text to their work or recreation in the animal health field. This is what drives me to continue to compile references in the field of infectious diseases. Comments on the text, ideas for future editions, or identifying errors or omissions are appreciated in any format. For consultation, I can be reached through the University of Georgia or at *www.craiggreene.com*.

CRAIG E. GREENE
Athens, Georgia
June 2005

Contents

Section II:
Bacterial Diseases

Section III:
Fungal Diseases

Section IV:
Protozoal Diseases

Section V:
Clinical Problems

Infectious
Diseases
OF THE DOG AND CAT

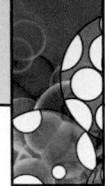

CHAPTER • 1

Laboratory Diagnosis of Viral and Rickettsial Infections and Epidemiology of Infectious Disease

James F. Evermann, Rance K. Sellon, and Jane E. Sykes

Clinical diagnosis of viral and rickettsial infections is of utmost importance as the range of clinical inquiry expands. Veterinarians are under increasing pressure to assist with and develop testing strategies to accurately determine the infection status of dogs and cats. Clinical inquiry generates information that not only clarifies the disease status of an animal but also determines whether an infectious microbe is present. Once its presence is confirmed, additional considerations include the infectious agent's potential to be shed and infect other susceptible animals and humans, its potential to be carried as an asymptomatic infection, and its risk of causing disease (Table 1-1).

Various technologies exist for detecting viral and rickettsial infections of dogs and cats. In some cases, diagnosing disease is the veterinarian's paramount goal so that the correct course of action can be determined (e.g., diagnosing canine distemper virus [CDV] in a dog with neurologic symptoms). In other situations, it may be important to determine the *infection* status of a dog, such as during a prebreeding screen for canine herpesvirus (CHV) and *Brucella canis*. As testing strategies have evolved, so have applications of different assays to address these issues.[12] Such assays include the more recent use of serologic assays to monitor immune competence and the evaluation of serum antibody titers to assess frequency of vaccination boosters.[47] Other areas important to companion animal veterinarians include clinical epidemiology as it relates to multiple animal households, population-based preventative veterinary medicine in humane facilities,[13,21,37] interspecies spread of infections between dogs and cats, and zoonotic potential of infections.[4,25]

DIAGNOSIS OF DISEASE VERSUS DETECTION OF INFECTION

Clinicians use diagnostic testing for two main reasons: (1) to diagnose an acute or chronic infectious disease process and (2) to detect a preclinical infection when susceptible animals or humans may be vulnerable to disease or shedding of infection.[1,7,32] As expectations of preventative medicine have increased, so has the demand for early detection of infectious diseases.[11,12,40] Although the majority of diagnostic assays have been designed to assist in making a disease diagnosis (e.g., the canine parvovirus [CPV] antigen enzyme-linked immunosorbent assay [ELISA] for fecal samples), more clinicians are using nucleic acid detection assays that use the polymerase chain reaction (PCR) for amplification of minute quantities of microbial RNA or DNA (see Molecular Diagnostics). This technology has uncovered the latent phases of herpesviral and retroviral infections, such as CHV, feline leukemia virus (FeLV), and feline immunodeficiency virus (FIV) infections.[1,12,21,32] It has also allowed clinicians to recognize the importance of carrier animals in the population, which harbor low levels of certain microbes as infections, such as CDV as upper respiratory infections and canine coronavirus as gastrointestinal infections.[13,36] Early detection of infections has added a new dimension to diagnostic testing and has assisted the veterinarian in making decisions at the individual level (e.g., whether to give medication or vaccinate a particular animal) or at a population level (whether to segregate or depopulate).[17,20,40]

Diagnostic tests in nonclinical areas of veterinary practice are used in surveillance, monitoring or screening for unusual clinical presentations, estimating infection prevalence in a practice area, and performing risk factor analysis.[20,22,41] Preclinical testing of animals is also being performed more frequently before show, sale, adoption, breeding, or placement in high-risk human environments (such as children's classrooms and convalescent care centers), which may require an animal to be certified not only as "disease free" but also as "infection free."[4,12,16]

DIAGNOSTIC ASSAY INTERPRETATION

Although the goal of a diagnostic assay is 100% accuracy, it is important to recognize that laboratory tests have varying degrees of sensitivity and specificity[20,39,41] (Fig. 1-1). *Test sensitivity* is the likelihood that an animal known to have a particular disease or infection with a particular microbe will be identified with a positive test result. A test with high sensitivity has few false-negative results.[41] The limits of test sensitivity can extend to an animal with a preclinical infection (i.e., an animal with a latent infection, that is an asymptomatic carrier, or that is in the incubatory phase of disease), therefore the values vary for either disease or infection. One assay may yield false-positive results for disease but true-positive results for infection, such as a PCR for CPV (Fig. 1-2). Conversely, the CPV antigen ELISA is an excellent way to detect CPV-associated disease but not sensitive enough to detect CPV in an asymptomatic carrier.

Test specificity is the likelihood that an animal known to be free of disease, infection, or both will have a negative test result. A highly specific test has few false-positive results. Knowing the specificity of a diagnostic test is very important because more false-positive results occur with a test of low specificity.[41]

Table • 1-1

Interpretation of Laboratory Analysis of a Suspect Case of Canine Parvoviral Enteritis

CLINICAL INQUIRY	TEST	LEVEL OF INTERPRETATION
Is the dog infected with CPV?	ELISA for antigen	Yes/no
When was the dog exposed?	IgM serology	7–10 days
Is the CPV a new strain or variant?	Virus isolation, neutralization with monoclonal antibody	Strains 2, 2a, or 2b
Are other infectious agents present?	EM, virus isolation	Rotavirus, coronavirus, calicivirus
	ELISA for antigen	Rotavirus
	Bacteriology	*Salmonella* sp., *Campylobacter* sp., *Escherichia coli*
	Parasitology	*Giardia* sp.
Is the dog protected?	IgG serology, HI serology	≥1 : 100 (IgG) or ≥1:80 (HI)
Is the dog shedding low levels of virus subclinically?	Nucleic acid-based (PCR) assays	Yes/no
What are the risks of infection in susceptible dogs and cats?	IgG serology, risk analysis	≥1 : 100 (IgG)
What are the risks of disease in susceptible dogs and cats?	IgG serology, concurrent CCV infection, risk analysis	≥1 : 100 (IgG)

CPV, Canine parvovirus; *CCV,* canine coronavirus; *EM,* electron microscopy; *HI,* hemagglutination-inhibition; *PCR,* polymerase chain reaction; *ELISA,* enzyme-linked immunosorbent assay.
A case in which canine parvoviral enteritis was suspected or being monitored based on clinical signs or at-risk category. Interpretation depends on the level of clinical inquiry and types of laboratory tests used.

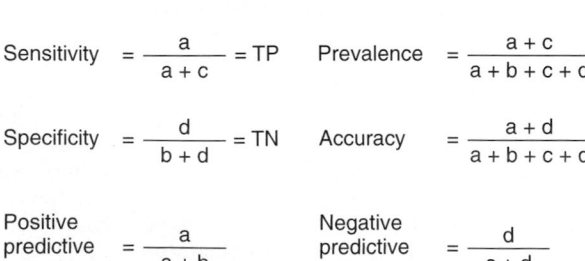

INFECTION (DISEASE)

$$\text{Sensitivity} = \frac{a}{a+c} = TP$$

$$\text{Prevalence} = \frac{a+c}{a+b+c+d}$$

$$\text{Specificity} = \frac{d}{b+d} = TN$$

$$\text{Accuracy} = \frac{a+d}{a+b+c+d}$$

$$\text{Positive predictive value} = \frac{a}{a+b}$$

$$\text{Negative predictive value} = \frac{d}{c+d}$$

Fig 1-1 Calculation of sensitivity, specificity, and predictive values using a two-by-two table.

Because an assay may not be able to distinguish an animal that is a preclinical carrier of infection status from an animal with the actual disease, a test's predictive value is very important to the veterinarian (see Fig. 1-1).[41] Classically, a positive predictive value is the probability that an animal with a positive test result has the disease. A negative predictive value is the probability that an animal with a negative test result does

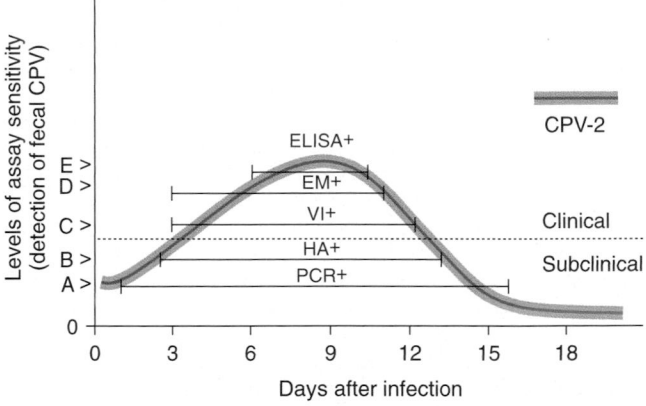

Fig 1-2 The various levels of assay sensitivity, with canine parvovirus (CPV-2) as an example. Note the five different assays (*A through E*) and the assays that would be of greatest value for clinical diagnosis versus subclinical detection of infection.

not have the disease. The predictive values depend on the prevalence of the disease in the regional population.

SAMPLE SELECTION AND PRESERVATION

Laboratory diagnosis of viral and rickettsial infections requires proper sample selection, collection, and submission.[42] A disease-causing organism is best detected when an animal is in the acute phase of the disease.[32,44] During this phase the microbe is in its highest concentrations in areas such as body fluids, excretions, secretions, and blood. Postmortem samples may be valuable in the management of other animals in the susceptible population; however, the degree of diagnostic accuracy is generally reduced because of protein and nucleic acid degradation of live microbes or their antigens or genomes.[1,11,32] Fresh samples should be promptly refrigerated for short-term shipment (24 to 36 hours) to a laboratory close to the clinic or by overnight carrier service. For long-term shipments (2 to 4 days), samples should be frozen and shipped on wet ice to the laboratory. Tissues for histopathology and immunohistochemistry (IHC) should be promptly fixed in buffered formalin. Serology may be of diagnostic value if acute and convalescent sera samples are available for IgG analysis or single samples are available for IgM analysis.[23,49] Table 1-2 and Appendix 5 list collection samples used to make a laboratory diagnosis of viral and rickettsial diseases. As mentioned, of equal importance is specimen preservation and shipment to the testing laboratory. As more diagnostic test kits become available for use in clinics, long-term sample preservation becomes less important than appropriate sample collection. Table 1-3 gives guidelines for specimen collection, processing, and shipment for laboratory diagnosis. Because of the changing nature of diagnostic assays and the ability to detect some infections earlier, it is recommended that the laboratory be contacted for updated guidelines on sample collection, processing, and shipment.

LABORATORY ANALYSIS

Viral Infections

Table 1-3 presents the five primary methods used in diagnostic virology.[11,32,44] Veterinary hospitals have the ability to perform in their clinics ELISA assays for detection of FeLV and CPV antigens and FIV antibody. Specialized laboratories should be consulted for more in-depth analysis of specimens from a particular case if the number of clinically ill animals significantly increases, unusual clinical signs are found, or new variants of preexisting viruses such as CPV and CDV are suspected. Veterinarians should be on the alert for first-line detection of emerging infections in primary and secondary hosts.[13] The main methods of viral detection are electron microscopy (EM); immunologic detection of viral-coded proteins through immunofluorescence, ELISA, and immunoperoxidase-IHC; virus isolation in cell cultures or embryonating eggs; serologic assays that detect antibodies to specific viral-coded proteins; and nucleic acid-based detection using PCR for amplification of viral nucleic acid.[42] Isolation and PCR are the techniques of choice for detection of unknown or new strains of viruses and rickettsia.[32] See the respective chapters (Chapters 3 to 32) for additional information on viral infections of dogs and cats.

Rickettsial Infections

Rickettsiae are small, obligate, intracellular gram-negative bacteria that are often included with viruses in diagnostic discussions because common methods are used to diagnose them.[16,23,26] Rickettsiae generally require living cells for propagation and are usually cultured in embryonating chicken eggs or in cell culture. Because of their fastidious nature, serology has been extremely valuable in the diagnosis of rickettsial infections.[3,23] More recently, PCR assays have been used for detection of some rickettsial infections.[2,14,16,38] Rickettsiae of veterinary importance and commonly used diagnostic assays are listed in Table 1-4. See the respective chapters (Chapters 27 to 30) for additional information on rickettsial and chlamydial infections of dogs and cats.

Recognition of Newly Emerging Viral and Rickettsial Infections

The observation of unusual clinical manifestations in dogs and cats can serve as an initial clue that an infection is emerging from a new disease-producing agent.[13] Emerging infections may be caused by interspecies spread of infectious microorganisms such as the transmission of feline calicivirus to dogs, West Nile virus (WNV) from insects to accidental dead-end hosts (e.g., dogs, horses, humans), and *Rickettsia felis* from cat fleas to dogs and humans.[5,13,38] Emerging infections may also be caused by intraspecies mutations in which the microorganism becomes more virulent within a host species or in

Table • 1-2

Sample Collection for Laboratory Diagnosis of Viral and Rickettsial Diseases

SITES OR CLINICAL SIGNS	ANTEMORTEM SAMPLES[a]	POSTMORTEM SAMPLES[b]
Respiratory and ocular tissues	Nasal, ocular, pharyngeal swabs; conjunctival scraping; serum; whole blood[c]; transtracheal wash	Selected tissues[d] and bronchiolar lymph nodes
Gastrointestinal tract	Feces, vomitus, serum, whole blood[c]	Selected small intestine sections, intestinal contents, mesenteric lymph nodes
Skin and mucous membranes	Vesicle fluid, swabs, scrapings of lesions, serum, whole blood[c]	Selected tissues[d] and regional lymph nodes
Central nervous system[a,e]	Cerebrospinal fluid, serum, whole blood[c], feces	Selected brain sections
Genitourinary tract	Urogenital swabs, vaginal mucus, urine, serum, whole blood[c]	Selected sections from placenta, fetal lung, liver, kidney, and spleen
Immunosuppression, hematologic abnormalities, blood dyscrasias	Whole blood[c], serum, bone marrow	Selected tissues[d] and lymph nodes

Modified from Murphy F, Gibbs EPJ, Horzinek MC, et al. 1999. *Veterinary virology*, 3rd ed, pp 193–224. New York, Academic Press.
[a]Samples should be kept moist and chilled.
[b]Fresh samples should be fixed (in 10% buffered formalin) for histologic and immunohistochemistry analysis.
[c]Sample should be collected in ethylenediaminetetraacetic acid (EDTA) and kept refrigerated.
[d]Hematogenous organs: lung, liver, kidney, bone marrow, and spleen.
[e]An animal with neurologic signs should be handled with extreme caution; before further diagnostic testing is performed, a public health laboratory should state the animal is free of rabies virus (see Chapter 22).

Table • 1-3

Specimen Collection, Processing, and Shipment for Diagnosis of Viral and Rickettsial Diseases

PROCEDURE AND SPECIMEN	COLLECTION AND PROCESSING	SHIPMENT
Organism isolation, nucleic acid-based testing, ELISA for antigen *Specimens:* Tissue, excretions, secretions	Collect aseptically to prevent bacterial contamination, and store at ≤10° C to prevent inactivation; do not freeze or fix.	Use whole blood,[a] tissue biopsy, feces, swabs,[b] commercial transport media, or sterile minimal essential medium 10% FBS with penicillin (100 U/ml) and gentamicin (50 µg/ml) to inhibit bacterial growth; double bag for shipment; pack on wet ice to last 48–72 hr.
Serology *Specimens:* Serum, cerebrospinal fluid, synovial fluid	Collect aseptically to prevent contamination, and handle gently to prevent hemolysis; remove needle from syringe before dispensing; allow to clot at room temperature; rim clot and centrifuge at 650 g for 20 min; pipette serum fraction into clean tube; although paired samples (10–14 days apart) are preferred, single samples may be diagnostic (e.g., CDV IgM).	Refrigerate until shipping; double bag for shipment; use leak-proof vial.
Histology, immunohistochemistry *Specimens:* Tissue	Collect aseptically to prevent contamination, 5 mm thick; fix in 10% buffered formalin (10 × volume).	Double bag for shipment; ship in leak-proof container with adequate fixative.
Direct FA testing *Specimens:* Tissue, tissue impression	Make tissue impression on clean, dry microscope slide and air dry; fix in alcohol for cytology or in acetone for direct FA.[c]	Pack on wet ice and ship as for isolation; smears can be shipped unrefrigerated.
Electron microscopy *Specimens:* Tissue	Collect aseptically, 1 × 2 mm thick; fix in 2%–4% glutaraldehyde (10 × volume) for 24 hr at 20° C.	Double bag for shipment; ship in leak-proof container with adequate fixative.
Feces or body fluids	Collect fresh; do not freeze or fix.	Refrigerate until shipping; double bag for shipment; pack on wet ice to last 48–72 hr.

ELISA, Enzyme-linked immunosorbent assay; *FA,* fluorescent antibody; *FBS,* fetal bovine serum; *CDV,* canine distemper virus
[a]Collected in ethylenediaminetetraacetic acid (EDTA) and kept refrigerated.
[b]Use Culturettes (Becton Dickinson, Cockeysville, Md).
[c]Use Michel's fixative to preserve tissue specimens for antibody testing by indirect FA. For antigen detection, other fixatives may be used.

an immunocompromised host.[13] Detection strategies initially using culture and broad-based PCR identify these microorganisms. This is followed by the development of new serologic assays, which enables surveillance and eventual control.[32,40]

SERODIAGNOSIS AND SEROSURVEILLANCE

Serology, the measure of antibodies in serum or other body secretions or excretions, has maintained a valuable presence in the diagnosis of viral and rickettsial infections.[42] Its value is due in part to the development of more specific assays that incorporate purified antigen substrates for capturing specific antibodies and to increased sensitivity from Western blot and ELISA technology. Serologic assays are the foundation for serodiagnosis and serosurveillance. Serodiagnosis is the use of a serologic assay to assist in the diagnosis of current disease,[32]

such as the use of IgM (early antibody) assay with indirect fluorescent antibody to detect acute CDV-associated disease. Serosurveillance is the use of a serologic assay for determining whether an individual animal has been infected or exposed to an infection, or if multiple animal serums are analyzed, the prevalence of infection in a population. Serosurveillance has expanded during the past decade and can now be used to assess an individual animal's level of protection against certain infections and determine the need for booster vaccination (see Serologic Testing, Chapter 100).[30,31] Dogs with CDV titers of defined levels are generally considered protected against CDV-induced disease. However, additional studies must be conducted by laboratories to determine whether this antibody level can be used with multiple breeds of dogs under varying degrees of CDV challenge. Comparisons can also be made by sending duplicate samples to laboratories that have completed this reference standardization.

Table • 1-4

Rickettsial Infections of Veterinary Importance

AGENT	HOST	DISEASE	DIAGNOSIS[a]
Neorickettsia helminthoeca and Elokomin fluke fever agents (see Chapter 27)	Dogs, coyotes, foxes, ferrets	Salmon poisoning and salmon fever	Observation of fluke eggs (Nanophyetus salmincola) in feces Demonstration of the agent in lymph node aspirates
Ehrlichia spp. (see Chapter 28)	Humans; dogs, cats, and other domestic animals	Ehrlichiosis	Indirect FA test for antibody in serum Giemsa-stained blood smears or marrow PCR on whole blood
Rickettsia spp. (see Chapter 29)	Humans, dogs, cats	Rocky Mountain spotted fever	Indirect FA test for antibody in serum Giemsa-stained blood smears PCR on whole blood
Mycoplasma haemofelis (see Chapter 31)	Cats	Feline infectious anemia	Giemsa- or FA-stained blood or tissue smears; presence of agent on red blood cells inconsistent

[a]FA, Fluorescent antibody; PCR, polymerase chain reaction.

Table • 1-5

Discrepancies in Polymerase Chain Reactions

False Positive
Contaminated sample or reagents
Nonspecific primers
Inactive nucleic acid detected
Immunization with suspected antigen

False Negative
Nucleic acid inactivation
Nucleases
Desiccation
Heating
Formalin fixation

MOLECULAR DIAGNOSTICS

Nucleic acid-based assays such as PCR have been developed for the detection of viral and rickettsial infections such as CDV, FeLV, feline rhinotracheitis virus, WNV, and Ehrlichia canis.* Partly because of the higher costs associated with establishing and maintaining PCR assays, selected laboratories have adopted multilayered testing techniques in which animals may be screened initially by a less expensive assay such as serology or antigen ELISA. If initial tests results are positive, PCR may help clarify issues such as the quantity of microbial shedding. Similarly, if screening assays are negative, then questions regarding latent conditions (such as FeLV in a valuable kitten) may arise, so PCR analysis could be recommended because of its increased sensitivity.[8,27]

PCR can also be used to assess animals in the acute stages of disease, which are likely to have low antibody titers or have antigen levels too low to permit early detection by ELISA.[39,40] PCR is not confounded by the presence of vaccination-induced or maternal antibodies, which may interfere with interpretation of serologic results. Tissues submitted for histologic examination may have characteristic pathologic lesions but not contain enough infectious agents or antigens to be detectable by virus isolation or IHC.[40] Occasionally, definitive documentation of the presence of some agents may be impaired because of the existence of similar but nonpathogenic organisms in the sample (e.g., coronavirus-like particles in feces prepared for EM). Molecular diagnostics have the potential to overcome these shortcomings.

The application of techniques to detect nucleic acids by PCR and reverse transcriptase (RT) PCR (RT-PCR) is increasingly useful in veterinary clinics.[40] PCR detects DNA and thus is appropriate for documenting the presence of DNA viruses and rickettsial organisms (Fig. 1-3). RT-PCR detects RNA—either messenger RNA (mRNA) or ribosomal RNA (rRNA)—after the enzyme RT has made a copy of DNA (cDNA) complementary to the RNA sequence. RT-PCR is appropriate for detection of RNA viruses such as feline caliciviruses (FCV). RT-PCR can also be used to detect organism-specific RNA of any infectious agent, including DNA viruses and rickettsial agents. Because RNA is usually quickly degraded in living organisms, the detection of RNA is more suggestive than DNA of active infection. Therefore RT-PCR may be advantageous because it does not detect DNA in animals recovering from viral and rickettsial infections.[40]

The strength of PCR and RT-PCR as tools in the diagnosis of infectious disease is their increased sensitivity compared with the other diagnostic assays listed in Table 1-4. Studies that have examined the sensitivity of PCR and RT-PCR have been performed primarily in experimentally infected animals, but some reports on naturally occurring disease support the conclusion that these molecular assays are more sensitive than most routine diagnostic tests.[40] Sensitivity is inherent in these assays, which amplify a few copies of nucleic acid (e.g., in an animal with a very few infectious microorganisms) to millions of copies that are readily detectable. Detection of the amplified product is usually accomplished by gel electrophoresis or nucleic acid hybridization techniques. RT-PCR using rRNA as the template has been suggested as being even more sensitive than PCR because rickettsial organisms typically have more copies of rRNA than DNA, increasing the number

*References 1, 5, 11, 18, 21, 40.

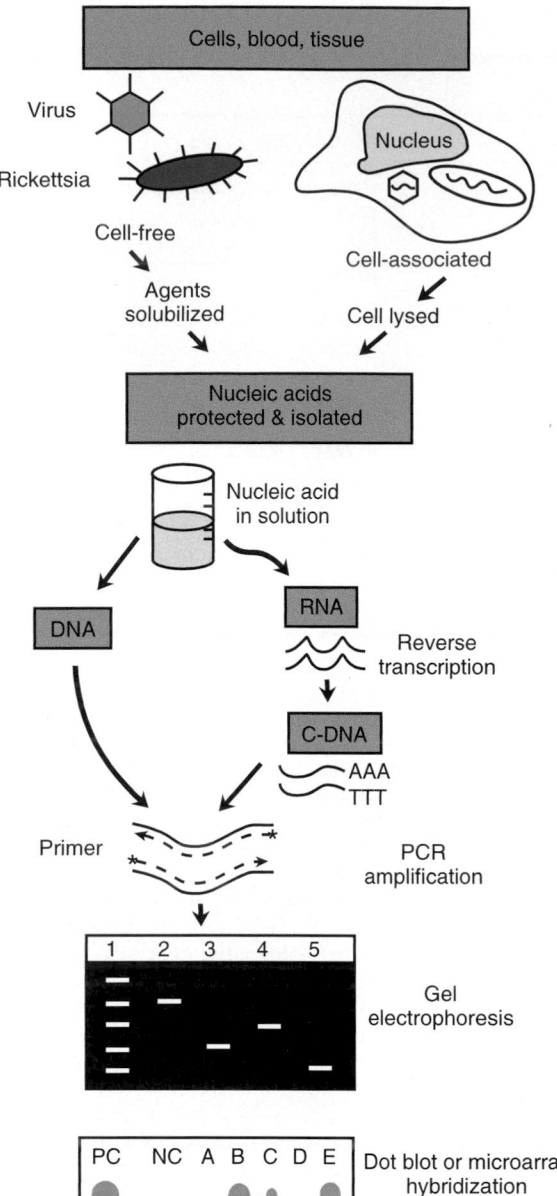

Fig 1-3 The principles of nucleic acid extraction, amplification by PCR, separation and identification by gel electrophoresis, and dot blot or microarray hybridization with specific oligonucleotide probes. Dot blot: *PC*, Positive control; *NC*, Negative control. Blots *A* and *D* show a negative result for viral or rickettsial nucleic acid, and blots *B*, *C*, and *E* show a positive result. (Modified from Evermann JF. 1998. *Infectious diseases of the dog and cat*, 2nd ed, pp 1–6. Philadelphia, WB Saunders.)

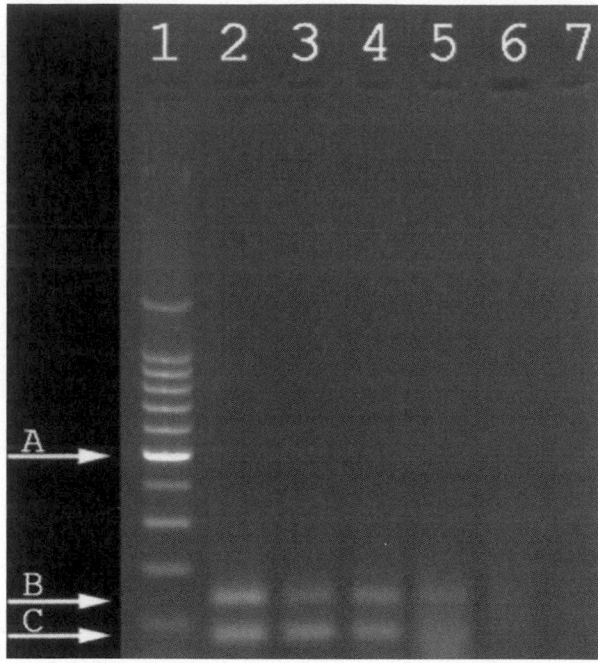

Fig 1-4 Gel electrophoresis (2% agarose) of PCR-amplified CDV from archival canine brain (formalin fixed, paraffin embedded). Lane *1* is the molecular marker control; lanes *2, 3, 4,* and *5* show positive reactions for CDV; lane *6* is the negative control; and lane *7* is the water-only negative control. *A*, 500-Base-pair band; *B* and *C*, expected PCR products specific for CDV. (From Stanton JB, Poet S, Frasca Jr S, et al. Development of a semi-nested reverse transcription polymerase chain reaction assay for the retrospective diagnosis of canine distemper virus, *J Vet Diagn Pract* 14:47–52.)

of templates and therefore the number of amplified sequences. Specificity of the assays may also be increased by the sequence of the primers—short DNA segments that are complementary to specific DNA sequences in the target microorganisms.[39,40]

PCR and RT-PCR also provide the clinician the ability to make retrospective diagnoses of viral and rickettsial infections because the assays can be performed on archived samples (tissue blocks, frozen serum, blood, or other fluid samples).[40,43] Viral or rickettsial infection may not be a clinician's chief consideration but may become suspect after histopathology on biopsies or necropsy tissues. The PCR and RT-PCR can prove

useful in such instances because DNA and occasionally RNA can be extracted from samples for the assays (Fig. 1-4).

Another advantage of PCR and RT-PCR in the diagnosis of viral and rickettsial infections (and infections of other etiologies) is that primers can be designed to detect broad groups of organisms (e.g., all members of the genus *Ehrlichia*) rather than single species.[10] Such an approach was used to indicate that a clinical illness in certain dogs was caused by *Ehrlichia ruminatium* even though their symptoms were consistent with infection by *Ehrlichia canis*, and their *E. canis* serologic and PCR results were negative.[2] Although more study is needed to define *E. ruminatium* as a cause of clinical disease in dogs, the approach indicates the power of the nucleic acid-based assays to detect agents that are not yet described as pathogens but are related to known pathogens.[22]

As useful as PCR and RT-PCR can be for diagnosing infectious disease, like other assays they have their limitations (Table 1-5).[39,40] The greatest strength of the assays—their sensitivity—is also one of their weaknesses; contamination of the reactions with mere traces of DNA or RNA molecules can create false-positive results. Accredited laboratories follow quality control measures to prevent contamination of the reactions and use controls in the assays designed to help detect potential contamination. False-positive results may also result if an animal has been very recently vaccinated with modified live virus vaccines against the infection being evaluated. Compared with DNA, RNA is a less stable molecule and subject to degradation, thus RT-PCR results could be falsely negative if the RNA in the sample has denatured during storage or handling.

Unfortunately PCR and RT-PCR methods do not definitively document the presence of viable organisms, thus posi-

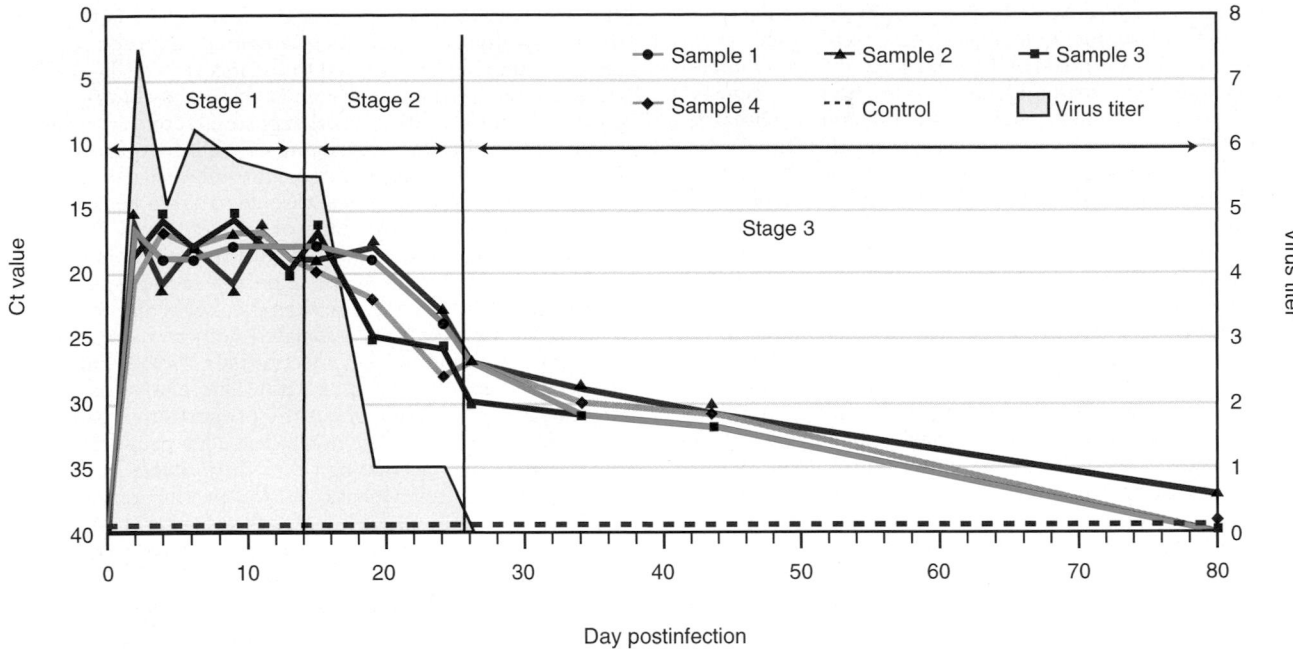

Fig 1-5 Graphic presentation of feline herpesvirus (FHV) shedding after an experimental inoculation (oronasal and ocular); shedding is measured by virus isolation in CrFK cells (virus titer) and PCR amplification of FHV-specific DNA sequences by cycle threshold (ct). Note the presence of infectious virus peaks 1 to 2 days postinfection, which are sustained until days 18 to 19 after infection and are undetectable by day 26. The presence of FHV-specific DNA was detected until more than 80 days after infection. (From Vogtlin A, Fraefel C, Albini S, et al. 2002. Quantification of feline herpesvirus 1 DNA in ocular fluid samples of clinically diseased cats by real-time Tag man PCR. *J Clin Microbiol* 40:519–523.)

tive results need to be assessed in light of other available information about the patient (Fig. 1-5). History, clinical signs, physical examination, and results of diagnostic testing should also link the presence of a given microbe in a patient with the clinical illness before concluding that the result of a PCR or RT-PCR is diagnostic of the disease.[17,45,48]

CLINICAL EPIDEMIOLOGY

Epidemiology is the study of the distribution and frequency of an event within a defined population, as well as the factors governing the occurrence of the event within the population.[37] An understanding of epidemiologic features of a particular infectious disease facilitates the identification of outbreaks or decreases of the disease's occurrence and increases understanding of the spectrum of signs observed; it is essential for development, implementation, and monitoring of prevention and control strategies. For example, worldwide, rabies virus is maintained in nature in wild and feral animal reservoirs; however, the dog is the most important source of rabies virus infection in people.[7,25] Widespread vaccination of the dog population has reduced the incidence of human rabies in the United States, and most human cases are now associated with rabies virus variants of wild animals, especially bats.[25]

The terms *incidence* and *prevalence* are often used to describe the frequency of a disease's occurrence in a population, and it is important to differentiate between them. *Incidence* refers to the number of new cases occurring in a population over a defined sequential time.[41] *Prevalence* refers to the number of current cases of a disease within a population at a given point in time. If a disease has an acute course, such as CPV enteritis, its incidence is generally greater than its prevalence. In contrast, the prevalence of a disease such as FIV infection is greater than its incidence because cats may live for years after becoming infected.

Accurate descriptions of the epidemiology of a disease require precise definition of the population being sampled.[15,22,41] For example, the incidence of FeLV infection is considerably higher in young cats than older cats because older cats develop an age-related resistance to infection with this pathogen. The incidence of FeLV-related myeloproliferative *disease* is lower than the incidence of FeLV *infection* because the majority of infected cats develop subclinical infections without developing FeLV-related disease. Accurate epidemiologic descriptions of infection and disease require data gathered from diagnostic assays with high sensitivity and specificity. Use of an assay that generates numerous false-negative results (i.e., an assay with low sensitivity) causes numerous cases to be excluded from a survey. In contrast, use of assays that generate numerous false-positive results (i.e., assays with low specificity) cause incorporation of irrelevant cases. Both of these situations lead to erroneous conclusions regarding the epidemiology of infections and diseases.[41] When the prevalence of infection is low, the test used must also have a high positive predictive value (see Diagnostic Assay Interpretation in this chapter).

The epidemiology of infectious disease depends on factors associated with the microorganism itself (microbial ecology) and factors associated with the host. Important microorganism factors include the ability of the microorganism to survive in the environment, the ability of the microorganism to infect the primary host and secondary host (interspecies transmission) and cause disease, the resistance of the microorganism to antimicrobial drugs, and the microorganism's ability to evade host immune defenses (i.e., escape mutants).[12,13,17,41] Numerous host factors have the potential to influence exposure and disease. Age and immune status are considered the most critical of these factors.

Epidemiology also encompasses the analysis of contact patterns in the population. For example, the incidence of feline infectious peritonitis (FIP) in catteries can reach 5%, whereas in single- or two-cat households it is 0.02%.[35] This increased incidence in catteries reflects heightened levels of infectious virus in the environment, increased viral replication from acquired immune suppression (caused by concurrent infections and stress of crowding), as well as host cat genetic factors (see Immunodeficiencies and Infectious Diseases, Chapter 95). To replicate successfully, a highly infectious virus that causes a strong protective immune response needs a steady influx of susceptible hosts. For example, the ability of CPV-2 to persist well in the environment allows the virus to encounter susceptible canine and feline hosts.[13,33] In contrast, pathogens that persist within the host for months or years depend less on frequent contact with susceptible individuals. *E. canis* establishes a chronic, subclinical infection in dogs, providing a reservoir for infection of new ticks that feed on the infected host.[16] Analysis of contact patterns also provides insight into the origin of a pathogen (Fig. 1-6). For example, a recent outbreak of feline hemorrhagic disease caused by FCV was traced back to a shelter kitten with upper respiratory tract disease that was brought into a veterinary hospital in Southern California.[34,37]

After identifying factors that might contribute to an animal's susceptibility to infection or disease, the importance of those factors in the animal's risk is often presented in terms of a relative risk or an odds ratio.[41] *Relative risk* is the ratio of the rate of disease or infection in animals exposed to the risk factor to animals not exposed to the risk factor (Fig. 1-7). Relative risk is determined through analysis of a cohort, in which groups of animals with defined exposure factors are monitored prospectively for the development of infection or disease. *Odds ratios*, which approximate the relative risk, are determined through retrospective, case-control studies (see Fig. 1-7). A relative risk or odds ratio of greater than 1 implies that the exposure factor is associated with the infection or disease. If the ratio is less than 1, the exposure factor is related to a decreased risk of disease. For example, FeLV and rabies vaccinations in cats have been associated with an increased risk of sarcoma formation at the injection site (see Feline Vaccine Associated Sarcomas, Chapter 100). The relative risk does not provide any information about the proportion of cases resulting from exposure to that risk factor. This proportion can be determined by calculating the *attributable risk*, which accounts for the relative risk and the proportion of the population exposed to the risk factor (see Fig. 1-7). When more than one factor is statistically associated with infection or disease, confounding must be considered. Confounding occurs in situations in which an association with one factor might

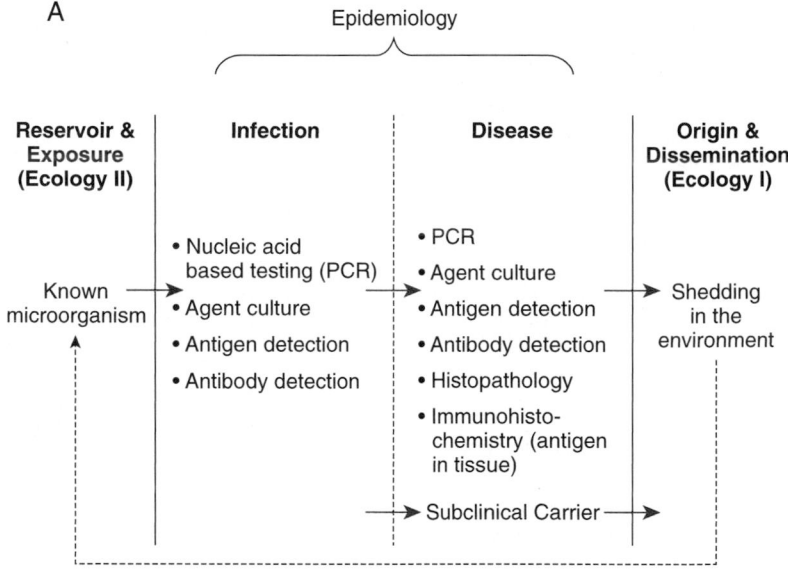

Fig 1-6 A, Schematic of the continuum between epidemiologic and ecologic movement of microorganisms. Note how the areas of infection and disease are flanked by origin and dissemination of an infectious agent and the connection with reservoirs and exposure. The various testing strategies are listed for detection of infection and diagnosis of disease. **B,** An example of an emerging infection via strain variation and infection of a new host species, such as occurs with canine calicivirus and *Rickettsia felis*.

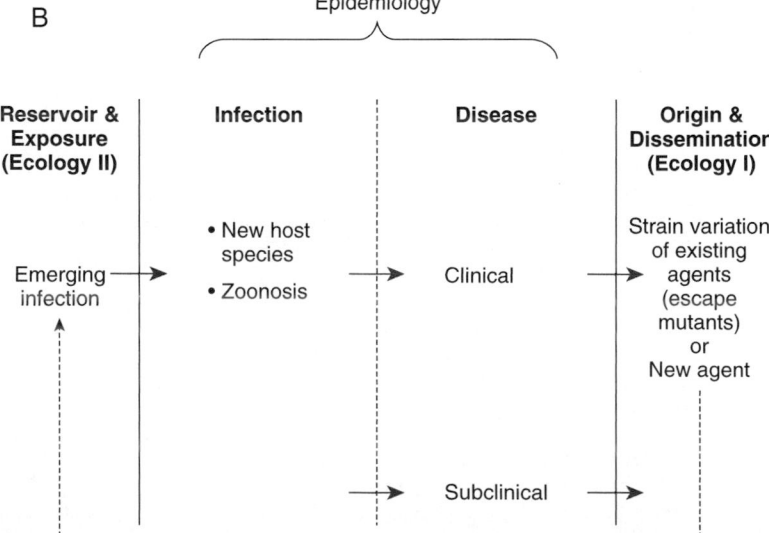

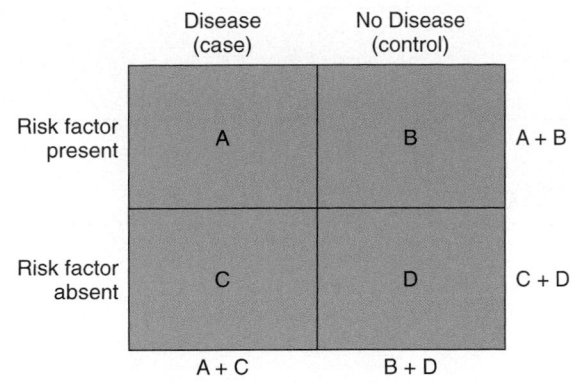

	Disease (case)	No Disease (control)	
Risk factor present	A	B	A + B
Risk factor absent	C	D	C + D
	A + C	B + D	

$$\text{Relative risk (RR)} = \frac{A}{A+B} \div \frac{C}{C+D}$$

$$\text{Odds ratio (OR)} = \frac{AD}{BC}$$

$$\text{Attributable risk (AR)} \% = P(RR-1) \div [1+P(RR-1)] \times 100$$
$$(P = \text{prevalence of exposure})$$

Fig 1-7 Calculation of relative risk, odds ratio, and attributable risk using a two-by-two table.

lead to an apparent association with another factor, such as a coinfection with a virus and secondary bacteria.[24] Use of computer software that performs multiple logistic regression analysis allows the investigator to control for multiple factors and simultaneously determine the effect of individual factors on infection or disease.

Although the pattern of spread can be approximated through comparisons of clinical signs and exposure factors, precise reconstruction of the network through which a pathogen is spread often requires the use of applied molecular diagnostics,* such as the aforementioned PCR and RT-PCR and microarrays, which allow subtyping of viruses and rickettsia.[46,50] Most methods now rely on analyzing the DNA or RNA of the pathogen by either sequencing a section of the organism's nucleic acid or analyzing DNA banding patterns. DNA banding patterns are most commonly generated using *restriction enzymes*, which are enzymes that always cleave DNA at a certain point within a specific short sequence (an area known as a *restriction site*). For example, the enzyme *Eco*RI cleaves DNA to the right of the guanine (G) residue in the DNA sequence GAATTC. Every time this sequence is present within an organism's DNA, the enzyme cuts the DNA after the guanine, generating numerous DNA fragments. The DNA is then processed in a gel matrix using electrophoresis, which separates the fragments on the basis of size and creates a banding pattern. Two identical isolates would have the same number of restriction sites in the same locations on their DNA, therefore their DNA banding patterns would be identical (see Fig. 1-4). An identical banding pattern would indi-

cate that it is likely both DNA samples came from the same organism. Organisms that differ have *restriction fragment length polymorphisms*, and their DNA banding patterns are different.[51]

Numerous other PCR-based molecular typing methods have been developed. PCR-based methods eliminate the requirement for culture before typing, which for viral and rickettsial pathogens may be difficult because of their fastidious growth requirements or public health concerns.[10,11,38,39,40] The amplified DNA can subsequently be sequenced so that strains can be compared, or the DNA can treated with restriction enzymes and then subjected to electrophoresis (PCR-RFLP) to generate patterns unique to the strain or species of organism. Other PCR-based typing methods include *repetitive element PCR*, or *rep-PCR*, which uses PCR to amplify regions between known genes that have multiple copies spaced throughout the genome. Amplification of sections of DNA between the repeats generates a range of fragment lengths that is unique to a particular strain. Rep-PCR has been used to type ehrlichial pathogens. *Arbitrarily primed PCR* involves using primers of low specificity that bind to multiple sites in an organism's genome, generating multiple PCR products that can be separated using agarose gel electrophoresis and subsequently used for typing.[57]

Many viruses are being typed using serologic techniques such as virus neutralization, but these methods are gradually being replaced by molecular approaches because they are better able to detect subgenotypes.[50] For example, PCR-based typing methods are being used increasingly for investigation of the epidemiology of CDV, FCV, and feline enteric coronavirus/FIP.[1] The knowledge of infectious disease ecology and epidemiology has greatly increased because of these methods and is providing evidence for the field of predictive microbiology.[46] As additional detection methods become available and existing methods become more standardized, the ability to rapidly identify and type microorganisms will improve. This improvement will increase understanding of microbial epidemiology, resulting in more successful control and prevention strategies.

SUGGESTED READINGS*

1. Addie D, Ramsey I. 2001. The laboratory diagnosis of infectious diseases, pp 1-17. *In* Ramsey IK, Tennant BJ, (eds): *Manual of canine and feline infectious diseases*, British Small Animal Veterinary Association, Glouchester, England.

12. Evermann JF, Eriks IS. 1999. Diagnostic medicine: the challenge of differentiating infection from disease and making sense for the veterinary clinician. *Adv Vet Med* 41:25-38.

17. Foxman B, Riley L. 2001. Molecular epidemiology: focus on infection. *Am J Epidemiol* 153:1135-1141.

39. Sachse K. 2003. Specificity and performance of diagnostic PCR assays, pp 3-29. *In* Sachse K, Frey J, (eds): *PCR detection of microbial pathogens*, Totowa, NJ, Humana Press.

*References 29, 33, 34, 37, 38, 40.

*See the CD-ROM for a complete list of references.

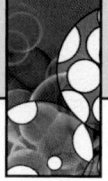

CHAPTER • 2

Antiviral and Immunomodulatory Chemotherapy

Katrin Hartmann

ANTIVIRALS

Clinical use of antiviral drugs is still not very common in veterinary medicine, and the number of controlled studies about their usefulness is limited. Unlike with antibacterial therapy, complete elimination of the agent is usually not achieved with antivirals, mainly because viruses are inhibited only during their replicative cycle and are not susceptible to antivirals during their latent or nonreplicative phases. Furthermore, achieving selective interference by antiviral chemotherapy is difficult because viral replication is more dependent on host cell metabolism than is bacterial replication. Treatment of acute viral infections is problematic primarily because diagnosis is often made after the replicative phase of infection is complete. Thus antiviral agents are useful mainly in treating chronic viral infections and in preventing reactivation of latent infections.

Many antiviral drugs that have been experimentally tested never appear on the market because they are too toxic. With the exception of the new feline interferon (IFN)-ω and some immunomodulatory substances, no antiviral drugs are licensed for veterinary medicine, and drugs licensed for humans have to be used in animals. Most antivirals are specifically intended for treatment of human immunodeficiency virus (HIV) infection. Therefore retroviral infection in cats, and more specifically feline immunodeficiency virus (FIV) infection, is the most important indication in veterinary medicine. Many compounds have been shown to be active against FIV, in cell culture and in cats. However, many FIV treatment studies were conducted to screen new compounds in the FIV model to document a potential benefit for HIV-infected patients. Most of these compounds are in an experimental state and will never appear on the market or be accessible to veterinarians, even if some have good efficacy against FIV.

Some of the anti-HIV drugs on the market have been used to treat naturally FIV- or feline leukemia virus (FeLV)–infected cats, and improvement of clinical signs and prolongation of life can be achieved in some of these cats using antiviral therapy. Furthermore, feline herpesvirus (FHV)–1 infection can be treated with antiviral compounds, either systemically or topically (mainly eye infections). Attempts to treat feline infectious peritonitis (FIP) with antiviral compounds have not been successful. In canine viral infections, antiviral chemotherapy plays only a minor role so far. Overall, antiviral drugs that are available and useful for cats and dogs are limited, and few controlled studies have been performed to support their use. In this chapter, only drugs will be addressed that are available on the market and have been used clinically or experimentally against feline or canine viral infections. Other drugs used to treat human infections may be found in the Drug Formulary, Appendix 8.

"True" antivirals are compounds that interfere with one step (or several steps) in the viral replication cycle. Closer scrutiny of the relationship of the virus to the cell reveals several points at which the viral cycle can be interrupted, including adsorption to and penetration of the cell, uncoating of the viral nucleic acid, the various stages of nucleic acid replication, assembly of new viral particles, and release of infectious virions, if the cell is not destroyed (Table 2-1).

The most common antiretroviral drugs are inhibitors of the reverse transcription inhibiting the retroviral enzyme reverse transcriptase (RT) (e.g., nucleoside analogues). Drugs with a broader spectrum inhibit other viral enzymes such as DNA or RNA polymerases and thus interfere with virus genome replication (e.g., phosphonoformate, acyclovir) or by inhibiting proteinases (e.g., proteinase inhibitors) that are important for the splitting of precursor proteins during viral assembly. Other drugs target the viral entry by binding to specific receptors that the virus uses for adsorption (e.g., bicyclams, a new class that inhibits the CXCR4 receptor, which is important for HIV and FIV entry), by acting as fusion inhibitors preventing the conformational changes of the virus necessary for the fusion process, or by interfering with uncoating (e.g., amantadine). Currently used inhibitors of the viral replication cycle can be divided into five classes of compounds: nucleoside analogues, cycloalkylamine derivatives, phosphonic acid derivatives, trypan red derivatives, and amino acids (Table 2-2).

Nucleoside Analogues

In the event of viral replication, the process of nucleic acid replication, which is extremely rapid relative to most mammalian cells, has proved to be the most vulnerable point of attack. The most clinically useful antiviral agents are nucleoside analogues interacting with this specific step. These nucleoside analogues are derivatives of nucleosides, so-called "antimetabolites." A nucleoside consists of a nitrogenous base covalently attached to a sugar (ribose in RNA, 2-deoxyribose in DNA); a nucleotide consists of a nitrogenous base, a sugar, and a phosphate group. A nucleic acid (RNA and DNA) contains a chain of nucleotides covalently linked together to form a sugar-phosphate backbone with protruding nitrogenous bases. For integration of these nucleotides (or monophosphates) into the nucleic acid, three phosphate groups have to be bound to the nucleoside first (triphosphates), two of which are removed, releasing energy during elongation of the nucleic acid chain.

Nucleoside analogues are similar molecules to the "true" nucleoside; they have to be equally phosphorylated intracellularly to become active compounds. Because of their structural similarities, they can bind to the active center of enzymes (e.g., RT, other polymerases) and block enzyme activity. Many of these analogues also can be integrated in developing DNA or RNA strands, but because of differences in the molecular structure of the next nucleotide, they cannot be attached. This leads to chain termination or nonfunctional nucleic acids.

Nucleoside analogues can be divided into antimetabolites with "wrong" base (e.g., ribavirin, idoxuridine, trifluridine), antimetabolites with "wrong" sugar (e.g., zidovudine, acyclovir, vidarabine), and antimetabolites with "wrong" base and "wrong" sugar (e.g., didanosine). Nucleoside analogues are not

Table • 2-1

Effects of Antivirals on Stages of Viral Replication Cycle

STAGE OF REPLICATION	SPECIFIC STAGE AFFECTED	ANTIVIRAL DRUGS
Virus entry	Adsorption Binding to cellular receptor Penetration Virus cell fusion Uncoating	Cycloalkylamine derivatives
Virus replication	Reverse transcription (retroviruses) Integration (retroviruses) Synthesis of viral RNA/DNA	Nucleoside analogues
Synthesis of viral proteins	Translation Processing Splitting of precursor proteins	Proteinase inhibitors Phosphonoformate acid derivatives L-lysine
Release of virus particles	Assembly Budding	Interferons

only accepted as false substrates by viral enzymes, but also by cellular enzymes, and this is the major cause of their toxicity. Selectivity, however, results from differences in DNA synthesis of infected and noninfected cells; in noninfected cells, DNA synthesis is intermittent, although it is continuous and fast in infected cells.

Zidovudine

Zidovudine (3'-azido-2',3'-dideoxythymidine [AZT]) was the first drug to be approved for treatment of HIV infection. AZT inhibits replication of retroviruses and has a mild inhibitory effect in the replication of herpesviruses. The inhibitory effect of zidovudine is 100 times higher against HIV-RT than mammalian cell DNA polymerases.[43] AZT is the most thoroughly studied antiviral drug in veterinary medicine; it has been used in experimental and in clinical trials in FIV- and in FeLV-infected cats.

The mechanism of AZT of inhibiting nucleoside phosphorylation explains its antiherpesviral activity, as well as its side effects. It is converted to zidovudine triphosphate, which blocks the retroviral RT. AZT inhibits FIV replication in vitro and in vivo[43]; it reduces plasma viral load, improves the immunologic and clinical status of FIV-infected cats, increases quality of life, and prolongs life expectancy.

In a placebo-controlled trial, AZT improved stomatitis and increased the CD4/CD8 ratio in naturally FIV-infected cats.[53-55] Neurologic abnormalities also tend to respond favorably to treatment with AZT. In some cats with FIV-associated neurologic signs, a marked improvement occurs within the first days of therapy. As is the case in HIV, evidence exists that FIV can become resistant to nucleoside analogues. AZT-resistant mutants of FIV can arise after only 6 months' use. A single-point mutation in the FIV gene was identified that can create resistance to AZT.[135] In humans, resistance to AZT frequently develops, but the addition of lamivudine to a therapeutic protocol can cause AZT-resistant strains to revert to AZT-sensitive strains. A combination of these two drugs might be a promising approach in FIV-infected cats to prevent resistance development.

AZT is effective against FeLV in vitro.[151] It has also been shown to be somewhat effective in treating cats experimentally infected with FeLV when treatment is initiated less than 3 weeks after infection. When treated less than 1 week after challenge, cats were protected from bone marrow infection

and persistent viremia.[43] In a study in naturally FeLV-infected cats that were treated with AZT and high dose subcutaneous human IFN-α for 6 weeks, however, treatment with AZT or human IFN-α, or both, did not lead to a statistically significant improvement of clinical, laboratory, immunologic, or virologic parameters.[58] In general, therapeutic efficacy of AZT in FeLV-infected cats seems to be less promising than in FIV-infected cats. For AZT dosage and handling instructions, see the Drug Formulary, Appendix 8.

Pregnancy of FIV-infected queens is a potential indication for AZT treatment if the owner wants the kittens to be delivered, although in utero transmission occurs infrequently in natural FIV infection. During AZT treatment, regular blood cell counts are necessary because nonregenerative anemia is a common side effect, especially if the higher dose is used. A complete blood count should be performed weekly for the first month. If values are stable after the first 4 weeks, a monthly recheck is recommended. Cats with bone marrow suppression should not be treated because of the risk of life-threatening anemia. In cats with concurrent chronic renal failure, the dosage should be reduced to avoid toxicity. Studies in which cats were treated with AZT for 2 years showed that the drug is well tolerated in most FIV-infected cats. Hematocrit declines within 3 weeks of initiating treatment to approximately 60% of baseline but comes back up afterwards in most cases, even without discontinuation of treatment. If hematocrit drops below 20%, discontinuation is recommended, and anemia usually resolves within a few days.[54] Neutropenia is less frequent than anemia. Neutropenia may be prevented or treated with filgrastim in FeLV- but not in FIV-infected cats, which may lead to increased viral loads. Other side effects in cats, including vomiting or anorexia, rarely develop. One side effect that is sometimes positively noted by owners is the development of a fuller and shiny hair coat. AZT should not be combined with drugs that are myelosuppressive. Concurrent use of nonsteroidal antiphlogistics has to be monitored carefully because it can delay AZT metabolism, result in kidney toxicity, or lead to neutropenia.

Stavudine

Stavudine (2',3'-didehydro-2',3'-dideoxythymidine, [d4T]) is a thymidine-based nucleoside analogue and was the fourth drug to receive U.S. Food and Drug Administration (FDA) approval for use against HIV infection. d4T is closely related

Table • 2-2

Classes of Antiviral Drugs That Inhibit the Viral Replication Cycle

DRUG	INFECTION	EFFICACY IN VITRO?	CONTROLLED STUDY IN VIVO?	EFFICACY IN VIVO?	COMMENTS
ANTIVIRALS					
Nucleoside Analogues					
Zidovudine	FIV	yes	yes	yes	Effective in some cats
	FeLV	yes	yes	no	Not very effective
Stavudine	FIV	yes	no	n.d.	Possibly effective
	FeLV	n.d.	no	n.d.	Possibly effective
Didanosine	FIV, FeLV	yes	no	n.d.	Possibly effective
Zalcitabine	FIV	yes	no	n.d.	Possibly effective
	FeLV	yes	yes	no	Toxic in high dosages
Lamivudine	FIV	yes	yes	no	Toxic in high dosages
	FeLV	no	no	n.d.	Toxic in high dosages
Ribavirin	FIV, FeLV	yes	no	n.d.	Toxic in cats
	FCV	yes	yes	no	Possibly as aerosol
	FIPV	yes	yes	no	Toxic in cats
	BDV	yes	no	n.d.	Toxic in cats
	CHV	n.d.	no	n.d.	Possibly as aerosol
	FHV-1, CPiV	yes	no	n.d.	Possibly as aerosol
Acyclovir	FHV-1	yes	yes	+/−	Not very effective
	CHV	n.d.	no	n.d.	Unknown
Valacyclovir	FHV-1	yes	yes	no	Toxic in high dosages
	CHV	n.d.	no	n.d.	Unknown
Idoxuridine	FHV-1	yes	no	n.d.	Toxic; topical use only
	CHV	n.d.	no	no	Unknown
Trifluridine	FHV-1	yes	no	n.d.	Toxic; topical use only
	CHV	n.d.	no	n.d.	Unknown
Vidarabine	FHV-1	yes	no	n.d.	Toxic; topical use only
	FIPV	yes	no	n.d.	Likely ineffective
	CHV	n.d.	no	n.d.	Possibly effective
Phosphonic Acid Derivatives					
Foscarnet	FIV, FeLV	yes	no	n.d.	Toxic
	FHV-1, CHV	n.d.	no	n.d.	Toxic
Cycloalkylamine Derivatives					
Amantadine	BDV	+/−	no	n.d.	Unknown
	CPiV	no	no	n.d.	Possibly effective
Trypan Red Derivatives					
Suramin	FIV, FeLV	no	no	n.d.	Likely ineffective
Amino Acids					
L-lysine	FHV-1	yes	yes	+/−	Possibly effective
	CHV	n.d.	no	n.d.	Possibly effective

FIV, Feline immunodeficiency virus; *FeLV,* feline leukemia virus; *n.d.,* not determined; *FCV,* feline calicivirus; *FIPV,* feline infectious peritonitis virus; *BDV,* Borna disease virus; *CHV,* canine herpesvirus; *FHV-1,* feline herpes virus 1; *CPiV,* canine parainfluenza virus; *n.d.,* no data.

Table • 2-3

Immune-Enhancing Drugs for Treatment of Viral Infections

DRUG	INFECTION	EFFICACY IN VITRO?	CONTROLLED STUDY IN VIVO?	EFFICACY IN VIVO?	COMMENTS
IMMUNOGLOBULINS					
Commercial products	FHV-1, FCV, FPV,	n.d.	no	n.d.	Likely effective
	CDV, CPV	n.d.	yes	yes	Likely effective
Hyperimmune or	FIV, FeLV	n.d.	no	n.d.	Likely ineffective
immune sera	FHV-1, FCV, FPV,	n.d.	no	n.d.	Likely effective
	CHV, CPiV, CPV,				
	CDV				
	FIPV	n.d.	no	n.d.	Contraindicated
Immunomodulators					
Interferons					
Human interferon-α	FIV	yes	no	n.d.	Likely ineffective
SC high dose	FHV-1	yes	yes	yes	Possibly effective
	FCV	yes	no	n.d.	Possibly effective
	FeLV, FIPV	yes	yes	no	Ineffective
	FPV, CHV, CPiV,	n.d.	no	n.d.	Possibly effective
	CPV, CDV				
	Papillomatosis	n.d.	no	n.d.	Possibly effective intralesionally
PO low dose	FeLV	yes	yes	no	Ineffective
	FHV-1, FCV	yes	no	n.d.	Likely ineffective
	FIV, FIPV	yes	no	n.d.	Contraindicated
	FPV, CHV, CPiV,	n.d.	no	n.d.	Likely ineffective
	CPV, CDV,				
	papillomatosis				
Feline interferon-ω	FIV	n.d.	yes	no	Short term ineffective
	FeLV	yes	yes	+/−	Short term likely ineffective
	FHV-1, FCV, FIPV	yes	no	n.d.	Possibly effective
	FPV	n.d.	no	n.d.	Likely effective
	CPV	yes	yes	yes	Effective
	CDV	n.d.	no	n.d.	Likely ineffective
	CHV, CPiV,	n.d.	no	n.d.	Possibly effective
	papillomatosis				
Growth Factors					
Filgrastim	FIV, FPV, CPV	—	yes	no	Contraindicated
	FeLV	—	yes	no	Likely ineffective
Erythropoietin	FIV	—	yes	+/−	Possibly effective[a]
	FeLV	—	no	n.d.	Possibly effective[a]
Insulinlike growth	FIV	—	yes	+/−	Possibly effective in young cats
factor-1		—			
	FeLV	—	no	n.d.	Likely ineffective
Interferon Inducers					
Polyriboinosinic-	FIV, FIPV	n.d.	no	n.d.	Contraindicated
polyribocytidylic	FeLV, FCV	n.d.	no	n.d.	Likely ineffective
acid	FHV-1, CHV	n.d.	no	n.d.	Possibly effective
	ICH		yes	no	Ineffective
PIND-AVI	FeLV	n.d.	yes	no	Ineffective
PIND-ORF	FHV-1, FCV	n.d.	no	n.d.	Likely ineffective
	FIV, FIPV	n.d.	no	n.d.	Contraindicated

Continued

Table • 2-3

Continued

DRUG	INFECTION	EFFICACY IN VITRO?	CONTROLLED STUDY IN VIVO?	EFFICACY IN VIVO?	COMMENTS
Bacteria-Derived Immunostimulants					
Acemannan	FIV, FIPV	n.d.	no	n.d.	Contraindicated
	FeLV, papillomatosis	n.d.	no	n.d.	Likely ineffective
Staphylococcus protein A	FIV, FIPV	n.d.	no	n.d.	Contraindicated
	FeLV	n.d.	yes	+/−	Possibly effective
Propionibacterium acnes	FIV	n.d.	no	n.d.	Contraindicated
	FeLV	n.d.	no	n.d.	Likely ineffective
	FIPV	n.d.	yes	no	Contraindicated
Bacille Calmette-	FIV, FIPV	n.d.	no	n.d.	Contraindicated
Guérin	FeLV	n.d.	yes	no	Ineffective
Serratia marcescens	FIV, FIPV	n.d.	no	n.d.	Contraindicated
	FeLV	n.d.	yes	no	Ineffective
Other Drugs with Immunomodulatory Activity					
Levamisole	FIV, FIPV	n.d.	no	n.d.	Contraindicated
	FeLV	n.d.	no	n.d.	Likely ineffective
Diethylcarbamazine	FIV, FIPV	n.d.	no	n.d.	Contraindicated
	FeLV	n.d.	yes	no	Ineffective
Lactoferrin	FIV	n.d.	yes	+/−	Possibly in stomatitis
	FeLV	n.d.	no	n.d.	Possibly in stomatitis
	FCV	n.d.	no	+/−	Possibly stomatitis
Nosodes	FIV	n.d.	no	n.d.	Contraindicated
	FeLV	n.d.	no	n.d.	Very likely ineffective
	FIPV	n.d.	no	n.d.	Contraindicated
	CPV	n.d.	yes	no	Ineffective

FIV, Feline immunodeficiency virus; *FeLV,* feline leukemia virus; *n.d.,* not determined; *FCV,* feline calicivirus; *FIPV,* feline infectious peritonitis virus; *CHV,* canine herpesvirus; *FHV-1,* feline herpes virus 1; *CPiV,* canine parainfluenza virus; *FPV,* feline parvovirus; *CDV,* canine distemper virus; *CPV,* canine parvovirus; *SC,* subcutaneous; *PO,* by mouth; *PIND-AVI,* parapoxvirus avis; *PIND-ORF,* parapoxvirus ovis; *+/−,* partial.
[a]In cats with anemia or neutropenia.

in mode of action to AZT because both are thymidine analogues. d4T is active against FIV in vitro.[7,182] Mutants of FIV that are resistant to d4T and cross resistant to several other antivirals, including AZT, didanosine, and foscarnet, have been found. A single-point mutation in the RT-encoding region of the pol gene that is responsible for the resistance was identified.[182] No in vivo data in FIV-infected cats are published. d4T activity against FeLV is unknown.

Stampidine
This experimentally nucleoside RT inhibitor has been used to treat cats that are chronically infected with FIV.[156] A single oral bolus of 50 to 100 mg/kg resulted in a decrease in FIV in peripheral blood mononuclear cells. A 4-week course of 50 to 100 mg/kg was well tolerated, and cumulative doses as high as 8.4 g/kg were given. Further studies may be needed to evaluate the safety and toxicity of this drug.

Didanosine
Didanosine (2′,3′-dideoxyinosine [ddI]) is also used to treat HIV infection in humans (second anti-HIV drug approved by the FDA). ddI is an inosine analogue, an antimetabolite containing a "wrong" base and a "wrong" sugar molecule. It is intracellularly converted to the active substance dideoxyadenosine

triphosphate that competitively inhibits RT. Additionally, ddI is less bone marrow suppressive in humans but is less active against HIV than AZT and is active against FIV[39] and FeLV[151] in vitro. Controlled in vivo studies confirming the efficacy in cats with retroviral infections are not available to date.

Zalcitabine
Similar to AZT, zalcitabine (2′,3′-dideoxycytidine [ddC]) was originally developed as an antitumor agent; and 20 years later, its antiretroviral activity was detected. Currently, ddC is used to treat HIV infection in humans (the third drug approved by the FDA). ddC is an analogue of the nucleoside 2′-desoxycytidine. The active compound is the intracellularly produced 2′,3′-dideoxycytidine-5′-triphosphate that acts as an RT inhibitor.

In vitro, antiviral efficacy has been demonstrated against FIV,[103] but no in vivo data exist demonstrating its efficacy in FIV-infected cats. A mutant of FIV that is resistant to ddC was selected in cell culture that showed cross resistance to other antiviral compounds (e.g., ddI, foscarnet).[103] ddC is effective against FeLV in vitro[62,119,151] and has been used in experimental studies to treat FeLV-infected cats. It has a very short half-life (clearance and half-life values for ddC in cats are 6.5 ml/min/kg and 54.7 min, respectively)[119] and therefore was administered in these studies either via intravenous (IV) bolus dosage or via controlled-release subcutaneous implants. Controlled-release delivery of ddC inhibited de novo FeLV replication and delayed onset of viremia; however, when therapy was discontinued (after 3 weeks), an equivalent incidence and level of viremia were established rapidly.[62] In a study evaluating the prophylactic antiviral activity against FeLV, ddC was administered by continuous IV infusion for 28 days. Doses of 22 and 15 mg/kg/hr were extremely toxic, causing death in 8 of 10 cats. A dose of 10 mg/kg caused thrombocytopenia, and only 1 of 10 cats receiving 5 or 10 mg/kg remained antigen-negative, although onset of viremia was delayed for several weeks.[119]

Therefore ddC should not be used in concentrations over 5 mg/kg/hr continuous infusion in feline patients. In humans, ddC is used orally (with greater than 80% bioavailability), but no data exist on oral application in cats.

Lamivudine

This compound, (2R,cis)-4-amino-1-(2-hydroxymethyl-1,3-oxathiolan-5-yl)-(1H)-pyrimidin-2-one, 3TC, the newest of the approved HIV drugs, is the (-)enantiomer of a dideoxy analogue of cytidine with activity against HIV and hepatitis B virus (HBV). Intracellularly, 3TC is phosphorylated to its active triphosphate metabolite, 3TC triphosphate. The principal mode of its antiretroviral action is the inhibition the RT via DNA chain termination after incorporation into the viral DNA. 3TC triphosphate is also a weak inhibitor of mammalian DNA polymerases α and β and mitochondrial DNA polymerase, which explains its anti-HBV activity. 3TC is often combined with AZT in HIV-infected patients, given that both drugs show a synergistic effect. However, HIV mutants exist that are resistant to both 3TC and AZT.

3TC is active against FIV in vitro.[4,12] Combination of AZT and 3TC had synergistic anti-FIV activities in primary peripheral blood mononuclear cell cultures.[4] FIV mutants resistant to 3TC containing a point mutation in the RT gene were selected in vitro and showed cross resistance to AZT.[135] One in vivo study was performed in experimentally FIV-infected cats that were treated with a high-dose AZT-3TC combination (100 or 150 mg/kg/day for each drug). The combination protected some cats when the treatment was started before experimental infection. However, AZT-3TC treatment had no anti-FIV activity in chronically infected cats. Severe side effects that included fever, anorexia, and marked hematologic changes were observed in some of the cats with such high-dose dual-drug treatment.[4] Data on the anti-FeLV activity of 3TC are not available.

The pharmacokinetic of 3TC in cats shows considerable similarity to AZT pharmacokinetics in cats and to that of 3TC in humans.[69] Thus in naturally infected cats, 3TC doses similar to AZT are probably recommended.

Ribavirin

Ribavirin (1-β-D-ribofuranosyl-1H-1,2,4-triazole-3-carboxamide [RTCA]) is a broad-spectrum triazole nucleoside that has marked in vitro antiviral activity against a variety of DNA and RNA viruses. The strongest antiviral activity is against RNA respiratory viruses and herpesviruses. RTCA has been effective in HIV infection, Lassa fever (a human adenovirus infection), and in Hantavirus infections.[43] Systemic use, however, is limited because of the development of dose-dependant hemolytic anemia in humans. Thus RTCA is currently used by aerosol route to treat only people with respiratory syncytial viral infection. If used as an aerosol, only low concentrations appear in the systemic circulation, and side effects are tolerable.[43]

RTCA is active against a significant number of feline and canine viruses in vitro, including FIV,[137] FeLV,[43] FHV-1,[121] feline calicivirus (FCV),[121] feline coronavirus (FCoV),[9,170] Borna disease virus (BDV),[109] and canine parainfluenzavirus (CPiV).[121] In vivo, however, therapeutic concentrations are difficult to achieve because of toxicity, and cats are extremely sensitive to side effects.

In a study investigating its anti-FCV activity in cats, RTCA administered (25 mg/kg orally [PO] every 8 hours for 10 days) beginning either 1 or 4 days after aerosol exposure failed to have any beneficial effect on the clinical course of the disease or to reduce viral excretion. In contrast, enhanced severity of the clinical findings occurred in the treated group.[120]

Although active against FCoV in vitro, ribavirin was not effective in treating cats with FIP. RTCA was administered (16.5 mg/kg, PO, intramuscular [IM], or IV, every 24 hours for 10 to 14 days) to specific-pathogen–free (SPF) kittens 18 hours after experimental challenge exposure with a FIP-causing virus. All kittens, including RTCA-treated and untreated kittens, succumbed to FIP. Clinical signs of disease were even more severe in the RTCA-treated kittens, and their mean survival times were shortened.[167]

The most common side effect in cats described in several studies (using low doses of 11 mg/kg) is hemolysis that develops as a result of sequestration of the drug in erythrocytes.[120,166] In addition, there is a dose-related toxic effect on bone marrow, primarily on megakaryocytes (resulting in thrombocytopenia and hemorrhage) and erythroid precursors. In longer treatment or higher doses, the drug suppresses the number of neutrophilic granulocytes. Liver toxicity also occurs. Weiss and co-workers[167] tried to decrease the toxicity of RTCA by incorporating it into lecithin-containing liposomes and giving it at lower doses (5 mg/kg) IV to cats challenged with a FIP-causing virus. The drug, however, was not able to reach therapeutic concentration with this therapeutic regimen.

Overall, side effects have limited the systemic use of RTCA in veterinary practice. It may be used as an aerosol in cats or dogs with respiratory virus infections as it is currently used in people. For further information, see the Drug Formulary, Appendix 8.

Acyclovir

Acyclovir (acycloguanosine, 9-[2-hydroxyethoxymethyl] guanine, AZV) is a nucleoside analogue that only interferes with actively replicating but not latent herpesviruses. AZV is given parenterally, orally, and topically in people to treat mucocutaneous and genital herpesviral infections and parenterally against herpesviral encephalitis. Resistance of human herpesviruses to AZV occurs. AZV is the only antiherpesviral drug that has been used systemically in cats.

AZV is effective against FHV-1 infection[112]; however, it is less effective against human herpes simplex virus (HSV). AZV was used in several studies in FHV-1-infected cats, but the results of these studies were not conclusive about the antiviral efficacy.[49,61,111] When AZV is combined with human IFN-α, however, synergistic antiviral effects were found[164] resulting from the different mechanisms of action of the two drugs; AZV inhibits viral DNA polymerase, and IFN-α interacts mainly with translation of viral proteins. The synergy observed also may result from AZV blocking the synthesis of an IFN-α inhibitor produced by the virus.

Oral and IV administration is less frequently recommended. If used topically in eye infections, frequent application (every 4 to 6 hours) is recommended. In cats, AZV should be combined with human IFN-α or feline IFN-ω because these drugs can potentially increase the antiviral effect of AZV.

AZV has a relatively low toxicity because uninfected cells do not activate it. When given in higher doses, when maximal solubility of acyclovir (2.5 mg/ml at 37° C) is exceeded, systemically, however, the drug itself (not the triphosphate) may precipitate in the renal tubules, causing obstructive nephropathy if diuresis is inadequate. In these cases, needle-shaped AZV crystals can be detected in the urine sediment. Urinalysis should be performed regularly in long-term AZV treatment. Renal failure is reversible with adequate rehydration. In a toxicity study in healthy dogs, a shorter high-dose regimen (210 mg/kg/day via constant infusion for 43 hours), which maintained AZV plasma concentrations, was more detrimental to the kidneys than a longer exposure to a lower dose of the drug given intermittently (15 mg/kg via intermittent infusion every 8 hours for 28 days).[71]

Accidental ingestion of AZV in dogs seems to be a problem as it was recently presented in a retrospective study of 105 cases reported to the National Animal Poison Control Center.[126] The most common signs of toxicity included vomiting, diarrhea, anorexia, and lethargy; polyuria and polydipsia was reported in only one dog.

Valacyclovir

Valacyclovir (2-[[(2-amino-1,6-dihydro-6-oxo-9H-purin-9-yl)methoxy]ethyl L-valinate hydrochloride, VAZV) is a prodrug for AZV. It is the L-valine ester of AZV and has the same antiviral spectrum but has a much higher (three to five times) oral bioavailability than acyclovir. In humans, it is mainly indicated for treatment of herpes zoster, treatment or suppression of genital herpes, and cytomegalovirus (CMV) prophylaxis in kidney transplant recipients.

In a placebo-controlled, experimental study to determine whether orally administered VAZV can be used safely and effectively, cats with FHV-1 infection were treated with high-dose VAZV (60 mg/kg orally). Cats appeared to be uniquely sensitive to the toxic effects (renal tubular epithelium and hepatocellular necrosis, severe bone marrow suppression), and even high doses appeared not to suppress FHV-1 replication in these acutely infected cats.[113]

Pharmacokinetics of VAZV in cats is unknown, but in humans, it is rapidly absorbed orally and hydrolyzed to AZV and L-valine. Its oral bioavailability (as AZV) is 54%. Approximately 50% is excreted in the urine (mainly as AZV) and 50% in the feces. VAZV should probably be used at the same dose as AZV (10 mg/kg every 8 hours) the low bioavailability makes it less effective. Combination with human IFN-α or feline IFN-ω should be considered. Use of higher doses of VAZV is not recommended because of toxicity.

Idoxuridine

Idoxuridine (5-iodo-2'deoxyuridine, [IDU]) was developed in 1954 and was the first clinically used drug for treatment of HSV infection. IDU is a halogenized thymidine analogue that acts as a pyrimidine antagonist after being phosphorylated by cellular enzymes to the active triphosphate, which inhibits DNA synthesis of virus and host. Latent virus infections are unaffected. Its clinical use is topical in human medicine, with the main indication of HSV keratitis and dermatitis. IDU is highly toxic when given systemically; this is mainly because of bone marrow suppression.

IDU is active against FHV-1 in vitro[112] and is used topically in cats with ocular FHV-1 infection.[96,141] Experimentally, systemic use in cats was not effective and caused severe toxicity (e.g., gastrointestinal [GI] disorders, bone marrow suppression).[140] Treatment of systemic canine herpesvirus (CHV) infections with IDU was not successful.[17] Therefore only topical treatment with IDU is recommended in cats with ocular FHV-1 infection. Frequent application (every 4 hours) is important. Prolonged topical use may cause irritation or nonhealing corneal ulcers.

Trifluridine

Trifluridine (5-trifluoromethyl-2'-deoxyuridine, trifluorothymidine, [TFT]) is a halogenized thymidine analogue similar to IDU that acts as pyrimidine antagonist. TFT is phosphorylated either by viral or by cellular thymidine kinases and inhibits cellular thymidilate synthase, causing a reduction in thymidine building and thus increasing the phosphorylation of TFT. Given that noninfected cells are also inhibited in their DNA synthesis, side effects are comparable to IDU if the drug is given systemically (GI and bone marrow toxicity); thus TFT is used only topically to treat ocular herpesvirus infections.

TFT is active against FHV-1 in vitro[112] and is used topically in FHV-1 eye infections.[96,141] It has a better cornea penetration than IDU. Frequent application (every 4 hours) is necessary.

Vidarabine

Vidarabine (9-β-D-arabinofuranosyladenine monohydrate, adenine arabinoside, Ara-A), a purine nucleoside, also inhibits DNA synthesis by incorporating into nucleic acids and inhibiting DNA-synthesizing enzymes. It is effective in vitro against herpesviruses, poxviruses, and retroviruses, but its clinical use in humans has been restricted to treatment of smallpox and HSV keratitis, dermatitis, and encephalitis.[43] Ara-A is phosphorylated intracellularly to Ara-A triphosphate that is incorporated into the DNA of virus and host where it terminates elongation. It inhibits DNA polymerase of DNA viruses approximately 40 times more than those of the host.

Ara-A is active against FHV-1 in vitro[112] and is used topically in FHV-1 eye infections.[96,141] Case reports indicate that a beneficial effect may occur in dogs with CHV infection. In one case, Ara-A was given to five littermates (two puppies had died from CHV infection), and all five survived.[17] Ara-A also shows activity against FIP-causing FCoV strains in vitro,[9] but no data have been found to demonstrate efficacy in vivo.

The major disadvantage of Ara-A is its poor solubility; therefore, if it is given systemically, Ara-A must be administered IV and in large volumes of fluid over extended periods. Ara-A is rapidly deaminated by adenosine deaminase to hypoxanthine arabinoside. Toxic effects include local irritation at infusion sites, nausea, vomiting, and diarrhea. The drug also causes bone marrow suppression, resulting in anemia, neutropenia, and thrombocytopenia. Systemic toxicity restricts its use in veterinary practice mainly to topical ophthalmic treatment, with frequent applications (every 4 hours) being necessary.

Phosphonic Acid Derivatives

The main compound of the phosphonic acid derivatives is foscarnet, the salt of phosphonoformate acid.

Foscarnet

Foscarnet (trisodium phosphonoformate hexahydrate [phosphonoformic acid (PFA)]) is a pyrophosphate analogue that inhibits virus-specific DNA and RNA polymerase and RT. It has a wide spectrum of activity against DNA and RNA viruses, including herpesviruses and retroviruses. Some AZV-resistant herpesvirus infections in people have been treated successfully with PFA. It also has been administered to treat HIV infection, especially if co-infection with CMV is present, but significant nephrotoxicity has limited its use. Renal dysfunction is evident in most people after 2 weeks of therapy.[43] PFA is only virustatic, and after treatment is stopped, viral replication is activated.

In vitro, PFA has been shown to be active against FIV[39] and FeLV.[145] As for HIV, PFA-resistant FIV strains can develop.[39] No reliable data exist on its efficacy in cats and dogs in vivo, and its use in veterinary medicine is limited because of toxicity. For dosages, toxicity, and further information on PFA, see the Drug Formulary, Appendix 8.

Cycloalkylamine Derivatives

Cycloalkylamine derivatives are used in human medicine mainly against influenza virus infections. Amantadine is the most important example of cycloalkylamine derivatives and the only one that has been used in veterinary medicine. Rimantadine, a closely related analogue, has equal or greater efficacy with reduced central nervous system (CNS) side effects but more GI irritation. No experience exists in veterinary medicine. Tromantadin, another related substance, is used locally in human herpesvirus infection, but no data exist in animals.

Amantadine

Amantadine (tricyclo[3,3,1,13,7]dec-1-ylamine hydrochloride, L-adamantanamine) is a highly stable cyclic amine that acts against enveloped RNA viruses. As an antiviral drug, amantadine is administered mainly for prophylaxis of human influenza and is most efficacious when administered before or during early infection. As a dopaminergic drug, amantadine has been used to treat Parkinson's disease, cocaine dependence, and apathy in multiple sclerosis. It has mild antidepressive effects; however, marked antidepressive effects occur in some patients attributed to antiviral activity against human BDV infection (see Chapter 21). Some investigators have linked BDV to patients with depressive episodes and psychiatric disorders. Experimental BDV infections of rats show virus-induced behavioral changes and emotional and learning deficits.[87] Amantadine was effective against BDV in vitro,[87] and other authors found no effect in cell culture in concentrations that were effective against influenzavirus.[48] In one study involving patients with BDV receiving amantadine, peripheral viral antigen was cleared, and a significant antidepressive response was described.[35]

Data on the usefulness of amantadine in dogs and cats are limited. Anecdotal reports exist from cats with BDV infection in Northern Europe that benefit from treatment with amantadine. Potentially beneficial effects might be expected in CPiV outbreaks.

Trypan Red Derivatives

Suramin

This 1-(3-benzamido-4-methylbenzamido)naphthalene 4,6,8-trisulfonic acid sym-3′-urea sodium salt, a sulfated naphthylamine and trypan red derivative, is one of the oldest known antimicrobial agents. It is still used in the treatment of African trypanosomiasis (see Chapter 72) and river blindness (onchocerciasis). It also inhibits angiogenesis, and recent interest has been found in suramin as a therapy for patients with advanced prostate cancer because of its effects on growth factors involved in prostate cancer cell growth. It exerts an inhibitory effect on the RT activity of several retroviruses. Suramin has been used for treating patients with HIV infection; it has, however, only minor clinical value.

Suramin was used to treat FeLV-infected cats, although only a limited number of cats have been evaluated. In one study, serum viral infectivity ceased transiently in two cats with naturally acquired FeLV infection during suramin treatment but returned to high levels approximately 14 days after treatment was stopped.[19] In another study, six anemic cats received suramin (10 to 20 mg/kg as 10% solution over 3 minutes every 7 days for 7 to 9 weeks), and within 4 to 14 days, erythropoiesis improved. However, progenitor cells remained infected.[1] No studies on the efficacy of suramin against FIV have been conducted.

Although effective, suramin is associated with a significant number of severe side effects, and the lack of studies involving larger numbers of animals limit its use in veterinary medicine. For further information, see the Drug Formulary, Appendix 8.

Amino Acids

L-lysine

This amino acid suppresses clinical manifestation of herpesviral infection.[47] Oral administration of L-lysine in cats has been adopted from human medicine. Inhibition of FHV-1 in vitro is similar to the data obtained for HSV.[94] In an experimental placebo-controlled, double-blind study including eight cats, oral administration of L-lysine (500 mg per cat every 12 hours) was well tolerated and resulted in less severe manifestation of conjunctivitis caused by acute FHV-1 infection compared with cats that received placebo.[142] The effects of L-lysine (400 mg PO per cat every 24 hours) on clinical signs and ocular shedding of FHV-1 in latently infected cats was studied after reactivation of a latent infection. Significantly fewer viral shedding episodes were identified after a stress event of rehousing in the treatment group cats compared with the control group cats. Fewer cats and eyes were affected by conjunctivitis, and onset of clinical signs of infection was delayed in cats receiving L-lysine.[95]

In conclusion, L-lysine may be beneficial in cats with FHV-1 infection but should be used as early as possible after infection is established. It also can be recommended as long-term treatment in cats with recurring clinical signs of FHV-1 infection to prevent reactivation of latent infection. For further information, see the Drug Formulary, Appendix 8.

IMMUNOMODULATORS

In general, immunotherapy includes any form of treatment that alters the immune system. This discussion is limited to nonspecific means of stimulating the immune system in an attempt to restore immunocompetence and control or treat infectious diseases (Table 2-3). Immunomodulators have been used to treat more than viral diseases for which the first part of this chapter covered. Nonspecific immunotherapy has been used to treat infections caused by facultative intracellular bacteria, viruses, fungal agents, or metazoan parasites for which vaccination or specific forms of chemotherapy are unavailable.

Immunomodulators or immunostimulatory agents or biologic response modifiers are probably the most widely used medications in feline and canine viral infections, especially in FIV and FeLV infections (Table 2-4). Theories suggest that these agents benefit infected animals by restoring compromised immune function, thereby allowing the patient to control viral burden and recover from associated clinical syndromes. These substances modify the responses of immunocompetent cells through cytokines or other mechanisms. Immunomodulators are used against viruses and other infectious agents. Some of them have an effect on the immune system and a true antiviral activity (e.g., some interferons, acemannan).

Microorganisms

Microorganisms and their extracts have been classically used as nonspecific immunostimulators. Freund's complete adjuvant is a water-in-oil emulsion containing inactivated whole mycobacteria. The antigen is contained in the aqueous phase, and the mycobacteria are in the oil phase. Injection of this mixture induces cell-mediated immune (CMI) response and humoral antibody formation. It produces a severe reaction of local inflammation and large granuloma formation. The adjuvant, which is the active ingredient in Freund's, is N-acetyl-muramyl-L-alanyl-D-isoglutamine (muramyl dipeptide). Purified, it can produce a response without side effects. Bacille Calmette-Guérin (BCG) is a nonpathogenic strain of *Mycobacterium bovis* that has been used in treating neoplasia in dogs and cats and in cats infected with FeLV. Ribigen-B and

Table • 2-4

Immunomodulators Used in Dogs and Cats

EXAMPLE OR SOURCE	MODE OF ACTION	TYPE OF IMMUNE RESPONSE	DISEASE SPECIFIC	SPECIES SPECIFIC
Microorganisms				
Bacteria				
BCG, Freund's complete adjuvant (muramyl dipeptide) *Salmonella, Serratia, Bordetella pertussis,*	Cell wall components: enhances phagocytosis and intracellular killing, increases macrophage chemotaxis and T-cell response	Cell mediated Humoral: primarily IgG	No	No
Staphylococcal protein A	Humoral immune interference, T-cell responses	Humoral and cell mediated	No	No
Propionibacterium acnes	Stimulate cytokine release	Cell mediated1	No	No
Viruses				
Newcastle disease virus, avian poxvirus	Interferon inducer	Interferon	No	Variable
Cytokines				
Interferons α, β, γ, ω	Antiviral or immunostimulatory	Interferon effect	No	No[a]
Filgrastim (G-CSF)	Stimulates granulocytopoiesis	Granulocyte phagocytes enhanced	Granulocytopenia	No[a]
Sargramostim (GM-CSF)	Stimulates leukopoiesis	All phagocytes enhanced	Leukopenia	No[a]
Insulinlike growth factor	Stimulates lymphoid system	Cell mediated immunity	No	No[a]
Macromolecules That Induce Cytokines				
RNA, poly-IC, poly-AU	Interferon inducer, can enhance cellular and antibody response	Interferon Cell mediated	No	Variable
Acemannan	Carbohydrate polymer stimulates cytokines	Cell mediated	No	No
Small Chemicals				
Organic: vitamin A, fatty acid, lipids, LPS, Freund's incomplete adjuvant, glycosides (Quil A), Liposomes	Delays antigen absorption, alters antigen presentation	Humoral and cellular	No	No
Inorganic: beryllium, alum, silica	Prolongs release of antigen	Humoral: primarily IgE	No	No
Pharmacologic agents: Levamisole	Similar to thymic hormone: stimulates macrophage phagocytosis, immune killing, and chemotaxis	Cell mediated: enhances T-cell activity	No	No

BCG, Bacille Calmette-Guérin; *IgG*, immunoglobulin G; *G-CSF*, granulocyte colony-stimulation factor; *GM-CSF*, granulocyte-macrophage colony-stimulating factor; *poly IC*, polyriboinosinic-polyribocytidylic acid; *poly AU*, polyadenylic-polyuridylic acid; *LPS*, lipopolysaccharides; *IgE*, immunoglobulin E.

[a]Repeated parenteral use of these recombinant products made for people may stimulate antibodies, which make them ineffective and potentially detrimental.

Table • 2-5

Immunomodulators Licensed for Use in Dogs or Cats

PRIVATE PRODUCT	MANUFACTURER	ACTIVE PRINCIPLE	LICENSED INDICATIONS
Acemannan Immunostimulant	Carrington Labs	Complex carbohydrate from Aloe vera	Adjunctive therapy for canine and feline fibrosarcomas
ImmunoRegulin	Immunovet (Vetoquinol)	Killed *Propionibacterium acnes*	Adjunctive therapy with antibacterials for canine pyoderma
Regressin-V	Vetrepharm	Mycobacterial cell wall fraction	Treatment of canine mammary tumors
Nomagen[a]	Fort Dodge	Mycobacterial cell wall fraction	Treatment of equine sarcoid or bovine ocular carcinoma
Staphage Lysate	Delmont Labs	*Staphylococcus aureus* components with bacteriophage	Treatment of canine pyoderma
Rubeola virus[b]	Eudaemonic Corp	Inactivated rubeola virus	Treatment of ossifying spondylitis in dogs

[a]Same as Regressin-V, which is no longer available.
[b]Conditional license.

Ribigen-E (Ribi, Immunochem Research, Hamilton, Mass.) are mycobacterial cell wall fractions that are given as adjuvants. Facultative intracellular organisms such as mycobacteria that are immunostimulators have a marked affinity for localizing in and stimulating mononuclear-phagocyte clearance mechanisms.

An emulsion of the cell wall from a nonpathogenic species of mycobacteria (Regressin-V, Vetrepharm Inc., Athens, Ga.; Nomagen, Fort Dodge Labs, Fort Dodge, Iowa), which has been modified to decrease toxicity and antigenicity while retaining antineoplastic activity, has been licensed as a CMI stimulant for treating equine sarcoids. It has been recommended for immunotherapy for other neoplasms, such as canine mammary tumors, lymphomas, and sarcomas, although studies demonstrating its efficacy for this purpose are not available at this time (Table 2-5). Various other bacteria, including *Propionibacterium acnes (Corynebacterium parvum)* and certain species of *Staphylococcus* and *Salmonella*, have also been proposed as immunostimulants. Immuno Regulin (ImmunoVet Inc, Tampa, Fla.) is a preparation of *P. acnes* that acts as a nonspecific immunostimulant. Clinical studies have involved the treatment of cats with FeLV infection, FHV infection, and canine staphylococcal pyoderma (see the Drug Formulary, Appendix 8).

Modified inactivated, rubeola virus immunomodulator (Eudaemonic Corp., Omaha, Neb.) has been licensed as an immunomodulator to decrease the inflammatory reaction generated by activated T lymphocytes. It has not been adequately evaluated in controlled studies but has received conditional licensing for treatment of navicular disease in horses and ossifying spondylitis in dogs.[161]

Staphylococcus aureus phage lysate is a sterile preparation containing cell wall components of this bacteria. It has been licensed for the treatment of staphylococcal or polymicrobial pyoderma in dogs. It is thought to act through the stimulation of cytokine production. Local or systemic allergic reactions are potential side effects.

Staphylococcal protein A

Staphylococcal protein A (SPA) is a bacterial polypeptide product purified from cell walls of *S. aureus* Cowan I. It may combine with immune complexes at the Fc (non–antigen-binding) region of certain IgG subclasses and stimulate complement activation, as well as induce T-cell activation, natural killer cells stimulation, and IFN-γ production. Antitumor activity has been described.[13,75]

A variety of SPA sources and treatments have been used in FeLV-infected cats. Interest was first generated when plasma from FeLV-infected lymphoma-bearing cats was passed over SPA or *S. aureus* columns to remove circulating immune complexes and then returned to the cats. More than 100 cats were treated in this manner, generally undergoing treatments twice a week for 10 to 20 weeks.* In some studies, a high rate of tumor remission and conversion to FeLV-negative status was observed; in others, responses were less dramatic and short-lived. Subsequently, it was determined that SPA and other products may have leached from the filters and columns used for immunosorption and been returned to the cats as contaminants in the treated plasma.[50] The possibility that these products exerted a positive immunomodulatory effect caused investigators to treat cats with small doses of SPA. In such a study including kittens with experimental FeLV infection, treatment with SPA (7.3 mg/kg IP twice weekly for 8 weeks) did not correct anemia or improve humoral immune function. In a placebo-controlled study, treatment of ill client-owned FeLV-infected cats with SPA (10 mg/kg intraperitoneally [IP], twice per weekly for up to 10 weeks) did not cause a statistically significant difference in the FeLV status, survival time, or clinical and hematologic parameters when compared with a placebo group, but it caused a significant improvement in the owners' subjective impressions on the health of their pets. When SPA was combined with low dose (30 U/day) oral IFN-α on alternate weekly intervals, the effect was less than with SPA alone.[102] For further information on use of this drug, see the Drug Formulary, Appendix 8.

Propionibacterium acnes

P. acnes, formerly *Corynebacterium parvum* (ImmunoRegulin, ImmunoVet) is available for veterinary use and consists of a killed bacterial product that has been shown to stimulate macrophages resulting in release of various cytokines and IFNs and to enhance T-cell and natural killer cell activity in mice. It was effective in preventing development of rabies in some mice after challenge.[104] In cats and dogs, it has been used for the treatment of certain tumors (e.g., malignant melanoma).[91,152] It was effectively used as adjunct treatment to antibiotic therapy against chronic recurrent canine pyoderma.[10] As an antiviral, *P. acnes* has been given to cats with FeLV infection, FHV-1 infection, and FIP.

*References 26, 33, 68, 83, 84, 138, 163.

P. acnes has been used in FeLV-infected cats, but no prospective studies have been performed. Clinical experience has been documented in roundtable discussions and in two anecdotal reports.[80,82] In one report, a practitioner reported treating 76 clinically ill cats with natural FeLV infection with *P. acnes* (0.1 to 0.2 mg/cat IV twice weekly, then every other week for 16 weeks) and supportive care. Although no specific clinical and laboratory evaluations were discussed, 72% of the cats became FeLV test-negative and survived for an unspecified period. In the other report, 700 cats with natural FeLV infection were treated with *P. acnes* (0.2 mg/cat IV every 3 days, then every week for 6 or more weeks) in conjunction with supportive care. Approximately 50% of the cats clinically improved, although conversion to a FeLV-negative status was rare.

P. acnes treatment was used in 74 cats with experimentally induced FIP that received either *P. acnes*, high-dose subcutaneous (SC) human IFN-α, a combination, or placebo.[168] Although *P. acnes* alone was ineffective, some indication showed that a combination of *P. acnes* and high doses of IFN-α was more effective than IFN-α alone in prolonging the mean survival time in the treated cats for a few days.

Bacille Calmette-Guérin

BCG (Tice BCG, Organon, West Orange, N.J.) is a cell wall extract of a nonpathogenic strain of *Mycobacterium bovis* that was originally developed in 1908 by Calmette and Guérin as a "vaccine" against tuberculosis in humans. Facultative intracellular organisms such as mycobacteria are immunostimulators that have a marked affinity for localizing in and stimulating mononuclear-phagocyte clearance mechanisms.[44] Severely immunodeficient animals or those on immunosuppressive therapy might develop infection rather than stimulation by this vaccine. BCG has been used in treating neoplasia in cats and dogs.[89] Other mycobacterial cell wall preparations, used as adjuvants in vaccines, have been modified (decreasing toxicity and antigenicity while retaining antineoplastic activity) and licensed as CMI stimulants for treating equine sarcoid (Regressin-V, Vetrefarm, Athens, Ga.).

Feline sarcoma virus (FeSV) is a recombinant virus that can develop in a cat after FeLV infection. Kittens experimentally infected with FeSV were inoculated with BCG SC, either at the same time and site as the FeSV inoculation, or at the same site but 1 week after FeSV inoculation, or with a mixture of viable autochthonous neoplastic cells approximately 35 days after FeSV inoculation. The BCG treatment was not able to prevent tumor development or increase survival rate.[6]

Serratia marcescens

A commercially available orphan biological extract of *S. marcescens* (BESM) (ImuVert, Cell Technology, Boulder, Colo.) containing DNA and membrane components of *S. marcescens* is used as immunomodulatory substance. *S. marcescens* is a motile facultative anaerobic gram-negative bacillus that occurs naturally in soil and water, as well as the intestines and produces a red pigment at room temperature. It can cause nosocomial infections associated with urinary and respiratory tract infections, endocarditis, osteomyelitis, septicemia, wound and eye infections, and meningitis in humans; systemic infections in cats and dogs are also described.[5] BESM stimulates normal feline bone marrow-derived macrophages to release maximal concentrations of interleukin (IL)-6, tumor necrosis factor, and IL-1, leading to elevations in rectal temperature and neutrophil counts.[32] In one study in dogs, BESM (0.08 mg/kg SC every 24 hours beginning the day after administration of doxorubicin) was effectively used to reduce the duration and severity of doxorubicin-induced myelosuppression.[116] In a study with FeLV-infected cats, weekly treatment with BESM, however, failed to prevent or reverse viremia in cats when initiated before or 6 weeks after inoculation with FeLV.[32]

Interferons

IFNs are polypeptide molecules produced by vertebrate cells in response to viral infections or certain inert substances, such as double-stranded RNA, and other microbial agents. In people, at least three types can be found: IFN-α (formerly leukocyte IFN), IFN-β (formerly fibroblast IFN), and IFN-γ. IFN-α and IFN-β are structurally similar, being produced in response to viral infection or polyribonucleotide administration. IFN-γ is structurally distinct and is produced by T lymphocytes in response to a specific antigenic stimulus. Human IFNs have been manufactured by recombinant DNA technology and are available commercially. IFNs are not strictly species-specific in their effects, although their biologic activity and toleration are greater in cells of genetically related species. For more information on each human IFN, see the Drug Formulary, Appendix 8.

Human IFN-α

Recombinant human (rHu) IFN-α has immunomodulatory and antiviral activity. IFN-α is active against many DNA and RNA viruses, although in vitro sensitivity varies (e.g., myxoviruses are susceptible, whereas adenoviruses are not). In people, high-dose parenteral IFN-α administration has shown some efficacy against influenza viruses, rhinoviruses, herpesviruses, and papillomaviruses. IFN-α has also been shown to inhibit oncogenic transformation induced by retroviruses. It has been licensed for the treatment of people with myelogenous leukemia, papillomatosis, and HIV infection. IFN-α is applied topically, intranasally, ocularly, and intralesionally (e.g., in papillomavirus infections). Human IFN-α has been used in cats with FIV, FeLV, FHV-1, and FCV infections, and with FIP, as well as in papillomatosis in cats and dogs. IFN-α acts as a cytokine having immunomodulatory effects, but it also has direct antiviral effects. It is not virucidal but merely inhibits viral nucleic acid and protein synthesis.

There are two common treatment regimens for use of rHuIFN- in cats, SC injection of high-dose (10^4 to 10^6 IU/kg every 24 hours) IFN-α or oral application of low-dose (1 to 50 IU/kg every 24 hours) IFN-α. When given parenterally to cats (or dogs), it becomes ineffective after 3 to 7 weeks because of development of neutralizing antibodies that limit its activity. In one study, cats that were treated with human IFN-α SC became refractory to therapy after 3 or 7 weeks, respectively, depending on whether the high parenteral (1.6×10^6 IU/kg) or the low parenteral (1.6×10^4 IU/kg) dosage was used.[179]

It can be given orally for a longer period as no antibodies develop. It has also been used in this manner to treat FIV and FeLV infections. With oral use, antiviral effects are unlikely but immunomodulatory activity occurs. The rational behind the use of low doses (versus high doses) orally is to mimic natural defense processes. In studies comparing low-doses oral IFN-α with higher concentrations, increasing the dose did not improve the effect.[24]

Human IFN-α is active against FIV in vitro.[148] It is frequently used in the field for treating FIV-infected cats. However, no placebo-controlled studies that evaluate the effect of either low-dose oral or high-dose parenteral use of human IFN-α in FIV-infected cats have been conducted. However, use of oral human IFN-α should be considered critically because of the expected immunomodulatory activities but lack of antiviral activity after oral use. As in HIV infection, nonspecific stimulation of the immune system in FIV infection can lead to increased viral replication and activation of latently infected lymphocytes and macrophages and potential progression of disease. In cell culture, stimulation of FIV-infected cells is consistently associated with enhanced production of FIV.

Several studies have been conducted on the use of human IFN-α in FeLV-infected cats. In vitro, FeLV replication is inhibited by human IFN-α.[67] Another study[180] compared the therapeutic efficacy of either high-dose human IFN-α (1.6×10^4 IU/kg to 1.6×10^6 IU/kg SC) or AZT, or IFN-α plus AZT in experimentally FeLV-infected presymptomatic cats with high levels of persistent antigenemia. Treatment with IFN-α, either alone or in combination with AZT, resulted in significant decreases in circulating FeLV p27 antigen beginning 2 weeks after the initiation of therapy. However, because of anti-IFN-α antibody development, cats became refractory to therapy 3 or 7 weeks after the beginning of treatment. In naturally FeLV-infected cats using a similar high dose treatment regimen, however, treatment with human IFN-α (1×10^5 IU/kg SC every 24 hours for 6 weeks) with or without AZT did not lead to a statistically significant improvement of clinical, laboratory, immunologic, or virologic parameters.[58] Low-dose oral IFN-α was used in a placebo-controlled study in experimentally induced FeLV infection; 0.5 IU/cat (eight cats) or 5 IU/cat (five cats) was given orally (following experimental challenge) on 7 consecutive days on alternate weeks for a period of 1 month.[25] No difference was found in the development of viremia between groups; however, treated cats had significantly fewer clinical signs and longer survival times when compared with the placebo group (with a better response in the cats given 0.5 IU/cat). Several uncontrolled studies reported a beneficial response in cats when treated with low-dose oral IFN,[139,153,169] but they only include a limited number of cats and are difficult to interpret without control groups. In a larger study, outcome of 69 FeLV-infected cats with clinical signs that were treated with low-dose oral IFN (30 IU/kg for 7 consecutive days on a 1-week-on–1-week-off schedule) was compared with historical controls, and significant longer survival times were reported in the treated cats.[169] In a placebo-controlled study, treatment of ill client-owned FeLV-infected cats with low-dose oral IFN-α (30 IU/cat for 7 consecutive days on a 1-week-on–1-week-off schedule) either alone or in combination with SPA did not result in any statistically significant difference in FeLV status, survival time, clinical or hematologic parameters, or subjective improvement in the owners' impression when compared to a placebo group.[102]

In vitro, FHV-1 replication can be inhibited when cells are treated with human IFN-α.[38] Weiss[164] demonstrated a synergistic effect of IFN-α when combined with AZV against FHV-1 in cell culture. In one experimental in vivo study, 12 kittens infected with FHV-1 received either 10^8 IU/kg human IFN-α SC every 12 hours for 2 consecutive days starting 1 day before the challenge or placebo. IFN-α was effective in reducing the clinical signs in the cats over a 14-day period.[18] In practice, IFN-α is commonly used topically in FHV-1–induced keratoconjunctivitis. Topical use is preferred over systemic use because an antiviral effect can develop directly at the application site; however, frequent application is important. Combination with a nucleoside analogue (e.g., AZV) is recommended owing to the synergistic effects. However, no controlled studies have been conducted using this combination in naturally infected animals.

FCV replication can also be reduced in vitro when cell cultures are treated with human IFN-α.[38] In vivo studies are lacking.

Antiviral activity of human IFN-α against an FIP-causing FCoV strain was demonstrated in vitro. Combination of IFN-α with RTCA in vitro resulted in antiviral effects significantly greater than the sum of the observed effects from either RTCA or IFN-α alone.[170] In one study, 74 cats (52 treated, 22 controls) with experimentally induced FIP received IFN-α, *P. acnes*, a combination, or placebo. Prophylactic and therapeutic administration of high-dose (10^4 or 10^6 IU/kg) IFN-α did not significantly reduce mortality in treated versus untreated cats; only the mean survival time in cats treated with 10^6 IU/kg IFN-α and *P. acnes* was significantly prolonged for a few days.[168]

In dogs, knowledge about efficacy of human IFN-α is limited. It has been used in dogs with viral papillomatosis, but controlled studies are lacking. In people with papillomatosis, IFN-α is used at 10^6 IU/person parenterally until regression occurs; a similar treatment regimen, or oral low-dose treatment, might be effective in dogs as well.[15] Intralesional injection, however, might be more beneficial.

In cats with ocular manifestation of FHV-1 infection, topical use of human IFN-α every 4 to 6 hours for a duration of 1 week beyond clinical resolution has been recommended. Combination with topical nucleoside analogues (e.g., AZV) is recommended to exacerbate synergistic effects.[96] For further information on this and other available human IFNs such as IFN-β and IFN-γ, see the Drug Formulary, Appendix 8.

Feline IFN-ω

IFNs are species-specific and the feline IFN is less antigenic and has greater antiviral activity in feline cells than the human recombinant IFNs. IFNs of dogs and cats are closely related, and feline IFN-ω is almost as effective in canine cells as it is in feline cells. Besides antiviral activity, it has antitumor effects against canine neoplastic cells, including antiproliferation and anti–colony-forming activities. It might be useful for treatment of some feline and canine neoplastic conditions,[122,150] but in vivo studies are lacking.

In one placebo-controlled, multi-center study, 62 cats naturally infected with FIV were treated with IFN-ω at 10^6 IU/kg SC every 24 hours on 5 consecutive days. No significant changes in survival rate were reported; however, some clinical improvement was noted.[100] The treatment regimen used, however, was probably too short to treat a chronic FIV infection.

Feline IFN-ω inhibits FeLV replication in vitro.[128] In a placebo-controlled field study involving 48 cats with FeLV infection, treatment was IFN-ω at 10^6 IU/kg SC every 24 hours on 5 consecutive days. A statistically significant prolongation of the survival time was found in treated versus untreated cats in a 2-month follow-up period.[100] Virologic parameters were not measured throughout the study to support the hypothesis that the IFN actually had an anti-FeLV effect rather than inhibited secondary infections.

Feline IFN-ω has an antiviral effect on FHV-1 in vitro.[38,155] No in vivo data have been conducted to support its efficacy in FHV-1 infected cats. Because human IFN-α seems to have a beneficial effect when it is applied topically in the eye of cats with FHV-1–induced ocular change, similar effects of feline IFN-ω might be considered.

Feline IFN-ω also inhibits FCV replication in vitro,[38,110,155] although the antiviral effect was less prominent than against other feline viruses when tested in the same cell culture system.[155] In a noncontrolled field study, cats with clinical signs (e.g., stomatitis) that were suspected to have acute FCV infection were treated with 2.5×10^6 IU/kg IFN-ω IV every 48 hours (three times) and showed improvement of clinical signs.[157] Controlled studies, however, are not available.

Data on the efficacy of feline IFA-ω in cats with FIP are limited. FCoV replication is inhibited by feline IFN-ω in vitro.[110,155] In one uncontrolled study, involving 12 cats suspected of having FIP, IFN-ω (10^6 IU/kg) was given SC every 48 hours in combination with glucocorticoids and supportive care. Dexamethasone (1 mg/kg intrathoracic or IP) or prednisolone (2 mg/kg PO every 24 hours) was continued until clinical improvement was demonstrated, and then the prednisolone was gradually tapered to 0.5 mg/kg every 48 hours. Although most cats died, four cats survived over a period of 2 years; all of them had initially presented with effusions.[65] Although no control group was in this study and FIP was not confirmed in the four surviving cats, these results suggest either another disease or therapeutic success. Cats with chronic effusions from FIP or other causes usually do not survive for 2 years without proper treatment.

Feline panleukopenia virus (FPV) replication can be inhibited by feline IFN-ω in vitro.[110,155] No data are found in cats with panleukopenia; however, a large number of studies have been done that prove the efficacy of feline IFN-ω in dogs with canine parvovirus (CPV) infection, and thus beneficial effect would also be expected in cats with panleukopenia. Feline IFN-ω has the best efficacy in feline cells compared with cells of dogs or other species.

Feline IFN-ω also inhibits CPV replication in vitro.[155] The effect of feline IFN-ω on the outcome of experimental parvovirus infection was examined in 29 beagle puppies of 3 to 4 months of age in a placebo-controlled study. Although the number of dogs that developed clinical signs did not differ significantly between the treated dogs and the placebo group, clinical signs were less severe in dogs treated with IFN-ω.[66] In a placebo-controlled, double-blind challenge, 10 beagle puppies of 8 to 9 weeks of age, inoculated with CPV, developed clinical illness. One half was treated with saline placebo, and the other received IFN-ω 2.5×10^6 IU/kg IV every 24 hours for 3 consecutive days starting 4 days after challenge. All five dogs in the placebo-group died within 10 days postinoculation. In the treated group, one animal died on day 2 after the treatment was started, whereas the other four dogs survived the challenge and recovered gradually.[97] Efficacy of feline IFN-ω was also evaluated under field conditions for treating dogs with CPV infection in a multi-center, placebo-controlled, double-blind trial. Ninety-two dogs from 1 to 28 months of age were randomly assigned to two groups (43 IFN-ω, 49 placebo) and were treated IV with either feline IFN-ω (2.5×10^6 IU/kg, every 24 hours for 3 consecutive days) or placebo. Clinical signs of the treated animals improved significantly, and mortality was lower, in comparison with control animals. In the IFN-ω group, three dogs died compared with 14 in the placebo group.[29] In a similar field study including 93 dogs with CPV infection in Japan, mortality was also significantly reduced in the dogs treated with IFN-ω (14/72) when compared to the control group (13/21).[107] These data suggest that the feline IFN-ω can be beneficial in treating dogs with parvovirus infections by improving clinical signs and reducing mortality. See the Drug Formulary, Appendix 8, for dosages.

Growth Factors and Cytokines

Besides IFNs, other cytokines have been used in some viral infections. They do not have a direct antiviral effect but may alter bone marrow function and interfere with viral infections that disrupt hematopoiesis. Hematopoietic growth factors are glycoproteins that affect growth and differentiation of blood cells, including erythrocytes, platelets, monocytes, granulocytes, and lymphocytes. Several feline and canine hematopoietic growth factors have been cloned but are not commercially available. Human factors must be used instead; however, cats and dogs develop antibodies against them, limiting the length of treatment.

Filgrastim

Filgrastim, granulocyte colony-stimulation factor (G-CSF), is on the market as recombinant human product (rHuG-CSF). Potential uses in viral infections are neutropenias associated with FIV, FeLV, or parvovirus infections or concurrent with antiviral chemotherapy to avoid neutropenic side effects. See the Drug Formulary, Appendix 8 or further information.

Filgrastim has been used in FIV-infected cats. In one study, a small number of naturally FIV-infected cats were treated, but no significant changes were seen when compared with untreated cats.[77]

Data on the use of filgrastim in FeLV infection are limited. In one study involving treatment of a few naturally FeLV-infected cats, no significant changes in neutrophil counts were found.[77] Filgrastim was also used in cats with severe neutropenia caused by FPV infection. Differences in numbers of

neutrophils were not observed in the cats with panleukopenia when compared with control cats, but the number of cases in this study was limited.[77] Furthermore, use of filgrastim in parvovirus-infected animals may be contraindicated because the virus replicates in actively dividing cells.

In dogs, filgrastim has been used to treat gray collies with cyclic hematopoiesis (see Chapter 95). In other instances, it has been recommended to treat CPV infection (see Chapter 8). Use of filgrastim in this disease, however, is questionable. In one uncontrolled study including profoundly neutropenic dogs, an improvement of neutrophil count was observed 24 hours after treatment.[37] In a randomized, placebo-controlled, clinical trial including 23 puppies with confirmed parvoviral infection and neutropenia (less than 1000 neutrophils/μl); however, treatment did not cause significant differences between the treatment and placebo group regarding duration of hospitalization, lowest neutrophil count, or time until neutrophil count increased.[125] Similar results were found in another clinical double-blind study including 43 dogs.[108] These disappointing results might be explained by the fact that endogenous G-CSF is already increased in dogs with CPV infection. G-CSF was not detectable in plasma of experimentally infected dogs before the onset of neutropenia, but became detectable just after it, and reached very high concentrations throughout the remaining infection,[20] making the necessity of filgrastim treatment questionable. As in cats with FPV infection, use of filgrastim in CPV-infected dogs may exacerbate the disease because the virus replicates in actively dividing cells. Increasing the proportion of cycling neutrophil precursors may actually prolong the neutropenic period, owing to viral infection and destruction of these cells.[86] Extended use of this drug in dogs and cats may result in antibody formation to the drug and resultant neutropenia. See the Drug Formulary, Appendix 8 for further information on this drug.

Sargramostim

Also known as granulocyte-macrophage colony-stimulating factor (GM-CSF), sargramostim controls the differentiation and proliferation of bone marrow precursors of granulocyte and monocyte lineages. GM-CSF also induces the proliferation of myeloid and erythroid progenitors. Cats may show increases in neutrophils, eosinophils, lymphocytes, and monocytes in varying combinations. Sargramostim (5 mg/kg every 12 hours for 14 days) was used in treating clinically healthy cats (control group) and those that were chronically infected with FIV.[3] Side effects of treatment in some cats were irritation of the injection site and low-grade fever. All cats developed neutrophilia; however, only FIV-infected cats developed a significant increase in viral load of FIV in peripheral blood mononuclear cells during treatment. Enhancement of the viremia may relate to increased replication in or enhanced expression of the virus by infected lymphocytes. Therefore use of sargramostim in FIV-infected cats is contraindicated. High-dose treatment (150 μg/kg) of dogs with rHuGM-CSF induces neutralizing antibodies to the drug beginning 10 days after treatment and presumably resulted in a subsequent decline in the observed leukocytosis during treatment.[99] Cats treated with rHuGM-CSF had a similar inducement of antibodies; however, their leukocytosis was maintained suggesting another mechanism for the transient response in the dog.

Erythropoietin

Erythropoietin (EPO) is on the market as recombinant human erythropoietin (rHuEPO) and is effectively used in cats and dogs with nonregenerative anemia caused by endogenous EPO deficiency in chronic renal failure. EPO treatment increases not only erythrocyte counts, but also platelet and megakaryocyte numbers in animals and humans with clinical disease.[115] Human EPO also increases leukocyte counts in cats.[3]

In one study, FIV-infected cats were treated with human EPO (100 IU/kg SC three times a week for 2 weeks). All treated cats had a gradual increase in erythrocytes and either neutrophils or lymphocytes, or both. In contrast to treatment with filgrastim, no increased viral loads were observed, and thus human EPO can be used safely in FIV-infected cats with cytopenias.[3]

Interleukin-2 and interleukin-8

This lymphokine is produced by activated helper T cells and is responsible for stimulating specific cell-B–mediated cytotoxicity. It has been synthesized in large quantities through recombinant DNA technology; however, it may cause toxicity. Potential applications include treatment of neoplastic and viral diseases. IL-2 in low doses has been shown to increase the immune response to concurrent vaccination when it was given to immunodeficient people.[105] IL-8, a cytokine produced by monocytes and a variety of other tissue cells, has a role in activating neutrophils and has been given to dogs to potentiate neutrophil chemotaxis.[181]

Insulinlike growth factor-1

Insulinlike growth factor-1 (IGF-1) is on the market as recombinant human product (rHuIGF-1) and it acts as an immunostimulant of thymic tissue and T lymphocytes. In HIV infection, thymus inhibition and limited T-cell maturation result in depletion the peripheral lymphoid pool. Therapeutic modulation to protect or enhance thymus function may ameliorate peripheral lymphopenia and retard disease progression in lentivirus infections.

In experimental FIV-infected cats, treatment with rHuIGF-1 resulted in a significant increase in thymus size and weight and evidence of thymic cortical regeneration and a reduction in B cells.[45,174] Although T-cell stimulation was observed, viral load was not increased during treatment, and no data have yet been found for naturally FIV-infected cats. The drug is administered by continuous infusion (see the Drug Formulary, Appendix 8).

Interferon and Other Cytokine Inducers

Nonspecific immunostimulants, which induce synthesis of IFNs and other cytokines, are widely used medications in virus-infected cats and dogs. Several macromolecules and certain microorganisms (viruses) are known to produce antiviral and other antimicrobial activities in the host. Most of the substances known to have this effect have a structure similar to double-stranded nucleic acid that can be of microbial origin or new synthetic nucleic acid polymers.

Therapy and prophylaxis with IFN inducers have become more attractive in treating infections in veterinary practice because they provide a more natural means of restoring compromised immune function, thereby allowing the patient to control the viral burden and recover from the disease. Their effect is generally transient, lasting for approximately 1 week; thus they must be given repeatedly to be clinically helpful. However, administration at an interval shorter than every 2 weeks can cause pronounced interference with IFN induction. Effects of these compounds on nonspecific defense functions are difficult to test, and in vitro test results cannot simply be transferred to in vivo situations. Most reports are difficult to interpret because of unclear diagnostic criteria, lack of clinical staging or follow-up, the natural variability of the course of disease, the lack of placebo-control groups, the small number of animals used, and concurrent supportive treatments given. Although reports of uncontrolled studies frequently suggest clinical improvement or increased survival times, these effects have not always been supported by subsequent controlled studies. In some cases, nonspecific stimulation of the immune system in already infected animals might be detrimental. In people, and perhaps cats with retroviral infection, these drugs can lead to an increased viral replication caused by activation of latently infected lymphocytes and macrophages and can therefore cause progression of disease. In cell culture, stimulation of FIV-infected cells is consistently associated with enhanced production of FIV. These compounds should also be avoided in cats with FIP because clinical signs develop as a result of an immune-mediated response to the mutated FCoV.

Polyriboinosinic-polyribocytidylic acid

Polyriboinosinic-polyribocytidylic acid (poly-IC) is a chemical IFN inducer that was used to treat cats and dogs. It only induced minimal IFN induction in dogs,[134] but it was reported to be effective in protecting dogs from infectious canine hepatitis (ICH).[42] In a controlled experimental study, however, mortality in dogs with ICH was not decreased, and survival time was prolonged only for a few days.[175] In one report, poly-IC was helpful in preventing CHV infections in newborn puppies.[42]

The recommended dose of poly-IC is 0.2 mg/kg SC once. The concentration of IFNs generally peaks 8 hours after administering poly-IC but declines gradually by 24 hours. Inhibition of IFN production is pronounced if poly-IC is readministered at a frequency greater than every 2 weeks. The duration of the effect of IFNs is less than 2 weeks; thus a continuous effect cannot be maintained. Side effects in cats and dogs include lymphopenia, lymphoid necrosis, CNS depression, hemorrhagic gastroenteritis, and coagulation disorders.[42]

Parapoxvirus avis and parapoxvirus ovis

Parapoxvirus avis (PIND-AVI) and parapoxvirus ovis (PIND-ORF) (Baypamun®, Bayer, Mijdrecht, Netherlands) are γ-ray inactivated poxviruses that are so-called "paramunity inducers." Their proposed mode of action is through induction of IFNs and colony-stimulating factors, and activation of natural killer cells. They are available in some European countries and have been used to treat a variety of viral infections in animals, both prophylactically and therapeutically. However, most reports on their efficacy are anecdotal or lack control animals. In all placebo-controlled, double-blind studies published thus far, no beneficial effect have been documented. Paramunity inducers may be contraindicated in already immunosuppressed cats with FIV infection because nonspecific immunostimulation may lead to progression of infection.

PIND-AVI and PIND-ORF were reported to cure 80% to 100% of FeLV-infected cats[63] when they were administered at a dose of 1 ml SC one to three times a week for 4 to 30 weeks. However, two placebo-controlled, double-blind trials in naturally FeLV-infected cats under controlled conditions were not able to repeat these results.[56,57] In 120 cats treated with either compound or placebo, no significant difference was found in eliminating viremia during the 6-week treatment period (12% in the treated cats, 7% in the control group). In the second study, 30 naturally infected cats were treated in a placebo-controlled, double-blind trial, and 20 immunologic, clinical, laboratory, and virologic parameters were examined (including FeLV p27 antigen concentration, clinical signs, lymphocyte subsets, and survival time), but no statistically significant differences were demonstrated between paramunity inducer and placebo application in any of these parameters.

Similar to other immunomodulators that produce nonspecific stimulation of the immune system, PIND-AVI and PIND-ORF are probably contraindicated in cats with FIP. No controlled studies have been conducted supporting an effect in any other viral infections in cats and dogs.

Acemannan

Acemannan (Carrisyn, Carrington Labs, Irving, Tex.) is a water-soluble, long-chained complex carbohydrate (mannan) polymer derived from the aloe vera plant and licensed for veterinary use. Acemannan may be taken up by macrophages, which stimulate release of cytokines, producing cell-mediated immune responses, including cytotoxicity. Acemannan has been used as an adjuvant in vaccines or intralesional, by itself, to enhance regression of tumors, such as in the management of postvaccinal injection-site sarcomas in cats.[51,72]

Acemannan has been used in clinically ill FIV-infected cats that received acemannan for 12 weeks, either by IV or SC injection once weekly or by daily oral administration.[178] The reported beneficial effects observed in this study are not clear because cats were concurrently treated with antibiotics and other symptomatic or supportive therapies and the study did not contain a control group. Presently, acemannan should be used with caution in FIV-infected cats because of its immunostimulatory effects, which can stress an already impaired immune system.

In one noncontrolled, open-label trial, 50 cats with natural FeLV infection were treated with acemannan (2 mg/kg IP every 7 days for 6 weeks).[133] Use of concurrent supportive care was not described. At 12 weeks, 71% of the cats were alive, and results for FeLV antigen were positive. No significant change in clinical signs or hematologic parameters was found. No control group or clinical and laboratory evaluations were available to document improvement from pretreatment evaluations.

In dogs, data on the effect of acemannan in viral infections are limited. Intralesional injection of acemannan have been recommended as treatment for dogs with papillomatosis.[15] For specific information on its use, see the Drug Formulary, Appendix 8.

Other Drugs with Immunomodulatory Activity

A significant number of drugs used for different other reasons in animals also have immunomodulatory activity. Some of these drugs have been used to treat virus infections in dogs and cats.

Levamisole

This broad-spectrum anthelmintic, used for example for heartworm treatment in cats and dogs,[30,123] nonspecifically stimulates cell-mediated immunity in a variety of species. Levamisole was detected as immunomodulatory substance when treatment applied against nematode infection not only killed the parasites, but also improved clinical signs of other infections. Levamisole influences phosphodiesterase activity, leading to increased cyclic guanosin-3',5'-monophosphate and decreased cyclic adenosine monophosphate. Increased cyclic guanosin-3',5'-monophosphate in lymphocytes stimulates proliferative and secretory responses. It also potentiates mononuclear cells in phagocytosis, chemotaxis, and intracellular destruction of bacteria. Levamisole has been used in cats with mammary tumors but has had no significant effect.[90]

Levamisole has been given to FIV- and in FeLV-infected cats,[22] but its effect has never been substantiated by controlled studies; it remains investigational.

Toxicity of levamisole is relatively high; hypersalivation, vomiting, diarrhea, and CNS signs have been observed similar to signs observed in nicotine poisoning.[64] Morphologic lesions, characterized by perivascular, nonsuppurative, or granulomatous meningoencephalitis, were described in the CNS of treated dogs.[144,160] Potential facilitation of the cell-mediated immune system may produce the lesions in the CNS by causing the body to react against latent agents (e.g., canine distemper virus).[42]

Cimetidine

The H2-receptor antagonist cimetidine has been shown to be effective in potentiating CMI in people with common immunodeficiencies. It appears to block receptors on suppressor T cells. Controlled studies in dogs or cats are not available.

Diethylcarbamazine

Diethylcarbamazine (N,N-diethyl-4-methyl-1-piperazine carboxamide [DEC]) is an antiparasitic agent widely used, especially in tropical regions, to prevent and treat filariasis in humans and that has been used as heartworm preventative in cats and dogs. The antifilarial effect of this drug has been attributed to immunomodulation.

Some evidence indicates that DEC might mitigate the course of FeLV infection in cats. Uncontrolled studies have suggested that continuous oral DEC treatment given shortly after evidence of FeLV infection prevents or delays FeLV-associated lymphopenia and prolongs survival.[73,74] In one controlled study, its therapeutic effect against FeLV infection was investigated in 24 SPF kittens experimentally infected with a lymphoma-causing strain of FeLV. The kittens were divided into four groups and were orally administered a high dose of DEC (12 mg/kg, every 24 hours), a low dose of DEC (3 mg/kg, every 24 hours), AZT (15 mg/kg every 12 hours), or a placebo for 10 weeks. Although AZT was effective in preventing persistent viremia, DEC in either dose was not effective; however, both doses of DEC, as well as AZT, prevented lymphoma development.[114] DEC has potentially severe side effects, including hepatic injury.[14]

Lactoferrin

Lactoferrin is a protein of bovine origin that binds iron, reducing its availability for bacteria. It has been used for its local immunomodulatory effect in the oral cavity, and it has been shown to increase phagocytic activity of neutrophils.[131] A protective effect of lactoferrin during lethal bacteremia has been reported in mice. In a study in healthy humans, orally administered lactoferrin increased the phagocytic activity of peripheral mononuclear cells in some but not all individuals.[177] In vitro studies suggest activity against canine herpesvirus (see Chapter 5).

Lactoferrin has been used in cats with FIV infection and stomatitis. It was applied topically (40 mg/kg every 24 hours for 14 days) to the oral mucosa of the cats with intractable stomatitis (FIV-infected cats and FIV-negative control cats) and improved clinical signs of disease (pain-related response, salivation, appetite, and oral inflammation) in all cats independent of their FIV status.[131]

Recently, a cat with stomatitis and FCV infection was treated with lactoferrin powder (200 mg) applied directly to the lesions. Clinical signs began to resolve after 11 months, and resolution of clinical signs coincided with the cessation of FCV shedding.[2] However, the cat also received other medications, and further studies are necessary to investigate beneficial effects of lactoferrin. The studies suggest, however, that lactoferrin might be beneficial for local treatment of stomatitis in cats because many of these inflammatory reactions are probably caused or triggered by viral infections. For further information, see the Drug Formulary, Appendix 8.

Liposomes

These synthetic microscopic structures are composed of multiple concentric lipid bilayers surrounding an equal number of aqueous layers. The lipid layers are relatively impermeable to aqueous substances trapped within. Immunologic mediators, antigenic substances, and drugs have been placed within the aqueous compartment of liposomes to facilitate delivery of these substances to selected tissues in the body. Liposomes themselves are relatively nonantigenic, nontoxic, and biodegradable because they are prepared from lipids normally found in cell membranes. As with microspheres, alterations in their physical properties can be used to modify antigen release. Liposomes may have potential to act as carriers of immunogens for purposes of vaccination. Adding adjuvants within the liposomal membrane can increase immunogenicity. Liposomal antigens, which normally stimulate only humoral immunity, can stimulate CMI if bacterial wall substances such as lipid A or muramyl dipeptide are added in the membrane. Liposomes also have been employed for selective in vivo delivery of drugs to cells of the mononuclear phagocyte system, which preferentially removes these compounds from the circulation. Intracellular parasites (e.g., systemic fungi, mycobacteria, *Babesia canis*, *Ehrlichia canis*, *Trypanosoma cruzi*, *Leishmania donovani*) that reside in these cells may be more susceptible to chemotherapeutic agents delivered in liposomes (see also Lipid-Based Amphotericin B in Chapter 57 and the Drug Formulary, Appendix 8).

Nosodes

Nosodes are homeopathic preparations of tissues from animals with the disease for which they are intended to prevent. Recommendations are that nosodes be given immediately after exposure to an infectious agent. These alternative medical therapeutic preparations have been claimed to protect animals as specific immunomodulators against a variety of infectious diseases, including viral infections. Preparations consist of serial dilutions with intervening agitation (succession, potentiation, vortexing) of tissues, discharges, or excretions from animals with corresponding diseases; they are administered orally. Clinical trials involving nosodes to prevent infectious diseases have usually not been controlled, and information about their usefulness or toxicity is limited. In one controlled CPV challenge of puppies, nosodes were not protective.[176]

SUGGESTED READINGS*

3. Arai M, Darman J, Lewis A, et al. 2000. The use of human hematopoietic growth factors (rhGM-CSF and rhEPO) as a supportive therapy for FIV-infected cats, *Vet Immunol Immunopathol* 77:71-92.

20. Cohn LA, Rewerts JM, McCaw D, et al. 1999. Plasma granulocyte colony-stimulating factor concentrations in neutropenic, parvoviral enteritis-infected puppies, *J Vet Intern Med* 13:581-586.

24. Cummins JM, Beilharz MW, Krakowka S. 1999. Oral use of interferon, *J Interferon Cytokine Res* 19:853-857.

29. De Mari K, Maynard L, Eun HM, et al. 2003. Treatment of canine parvoviral enteritis with interferon-omega in a placebo-controlled field trial, *Vet Rec* 152:105-108.

29a. DeMari K, Maynard L, Sanquer A, et al. 2004. Therapeutic effects of recombinant feline interferon-ω on feline leukemia virus (FeLV)-infected and FeLV-feline immunodeficiency virus (FIV)-coinfected cats, *J Vet Intern Med* 18:477-482.

56. Hartmann K, Block A, Ferk G, et al. 1998. Treatment of feline leukemia virus-infected cats with paramunity inducer, *Vet Immunol Immunopathol* 65:267-275.

102. McCaw DL, Boon GD, Jergens AE, et al. 2001. Immunomodulation therapy for feline leukemia virus infection, *J Am Anim Hosp Assoc* 37:356-363.

142. Stiles J, Townsend WM, Rogers QR, et al. 2002. Effect of oral administration of L-lysine on conjunctivitis caused by feline herpesvirus in cats, *Am J Vet Res* 63:99-103.

165. Weiss RC. 1995. Treatment of feline infectious peritonitis with immunomodulating agents and antiviral drugs—a review, *Feline Pract* 23:103-106.

*See the CD-ROM for a complete list of references.

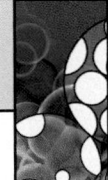

CHAPTER • 3

Canine Distemper

Craig E. Greene and Max J. Appel

ETIOLOGY

Canine distemper virus (CDV) is a member of the genus *Morbillivirus* of the family Paramyxoviridae and is closely related to other viruses (Table 3-1). CDV has a relatively large, variable diameter (150–250 nm) with single negative-stranded RNA enclosed in a nucleocapsid of helical symmetry. It is surrounded by a lipoprotein envelope derived from virus glycoproteins incorporated into the cell membrane (Fig. 3-1 and Table 3-2). Viruses such as CDV that code for proteins capable of integrating in the cell membrane make infected cells susceptible to damage by immune-mediated cytolysis. CDV also may induce cellular fusion as a means of direct intercellular spread. Genetic analysis of a 388-bp P gene fragment and of the H-protein encoding region has been used to separate the genotypes of wild and vaccine types.[75]

CDV is susceptible to ultraviolet light, although protein or antioxidants help protect it from inactivation. Extremely susceptible to heat and drying, CDV is destroyed by temperatures greater than 50° C to 60° C for 30 minutes. In excised tissues or secretions, it survives for at least an hour at 37° C and for 3 hours at 20° C (room temperature). In warm climates, CDV does not persist in kennels after infected dogs have been removed. Storage and survival times of CDV are longer at colder temperatures. At near-freezing (0° C to 4° C), it survives in the environment for weeks. Below freezing the virus is stable, surviving at −65° C for at least 7 years. Lyophilization reduces the lability of the virus and is an excellent means of preserving it for commercial vaccine and laboratory use. CDV remains viable between pH 4.5 and 9.0. As an enveloped virus, it is susceptible to ether and chloroform, dilute (<0.5%) formalin solution, phenol (0.75%), and qua-

Table • 3-1

Host Susceptibility to Morbilliviruses

DISEASE (VIRUS ABBREVIATION)	NATURAL HOSTS	EXPERIMENTAL INFECTION
Measles (MV)	Domestic: human Wild: nonhuman primate	Macaque, marmoset, mouse, hamster, rat

Rinderpest (RPV)	Domestic: cattle, pig, goat, sheep
	Wild: buffalo, eland, giraffe, kudu,
	    warthog, wildebeest, banteng,
	    black buck, gaur, nilgai, sambhar
		Rabbit, mouse, hamster, dog, ferret, rat, suslik

Peste des petits ruminants (PPRV)	Domestic: goat, sheep Wild: gazelle, ibex, gemsbok	Goat, cattle, pig, deer
Phocine distemper (PDV)	Seal	Dog, mink, seal

Canine distemper (CDV)	Seal (previously PDV-2)
	Canidae (e.g., dog, fox, wolf, coyote)
	Mustelidae (e.g., weasel, mink, skunk,
	    badger, ferret)
	Procyonidae (e.g., kinkajou, coati, red
	    panda, raccoon)
	Felidae (e.g., cat, lion, leopard, tiger)
	Suidae (peccary)
		Dog, mouse, rat, hamster, mink, pig, cat,
		    nonhuman primate, ferret

Dolphin morbillivirus (DMV)	Dolphin	Cattle, sheep, goat, dog
Porpoise morbillivirus (PMV)	Porpoise	Cattle, sheep, goat, dog
Equine morbillivirus (EMV; Hendra virus)	Domestic: horse, human Wild: Pteropus bat	Cat
Porcine morbillivirus (Menangle virus)	Domestic: pig, human Wild: Pteropus bat	No data

Modified from Osterhaus ADME, de Swart RL, Vos HW, et al. 1995. Morbillivirus infections of aquatic mammals: newly identified members of the genus. *Vet Microbiol* 44:219–227.

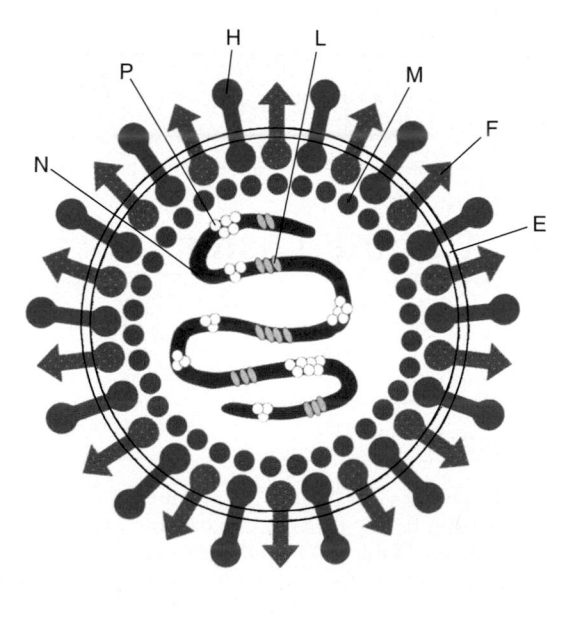

Fig 3-1 Structure of canine distemper virus. (*H,* Hemaglutinin [neuraminidase]; *F,* fusion protein; *M,* matrix protein; *E,* lipoprotein envelope; *L,* large protein; *P,* polymerase protein; *N,* nucleocapsid.) (Courtesy University of Georgia, Athens, Ga.)

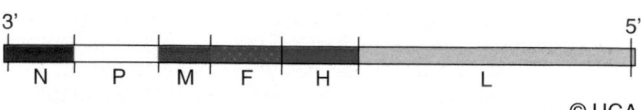

© UGA

Table • 3-2

Structure of Canine Distemper Virus

COMPONENTS	ABBREVIATION	MOLECULAR WEIGHT (kDa)	FUNCTION
Envelope			
Hemagglutinin	H	76	Structural: viral attachment
Matrix protein	M	34	Structural: penetration
Fusion 1 protein	F_1	40	Structural: penetration
Fusion 2 protein	F_2	20–23	Structural: penetration
Nuclear			
Large protein	L	180–200	Functional: polymerase complex
Polymerase	P	66	Functional: polymerase complex
Nucleocapsid	N	58	Structural: protects genome

Table • 3-3

Order Carnivora Susceptible to Canine Distemper

ORDER	DESCRIPTION
Ailuridae	Lesser panda
Canidae	Coyote, dingo, raccoon dog, wolf, fox
Mustelidae	Ferret, marten, mink, otter, skunk, wolverine, badger
Procyonidae	Coati, kinkajou, raccoon
Ursidae	Bear, giant panda
Viverridae	Binturong, fossa, linsang, civet
Herpestidae	Mongoose, meerkat
Felidae	Cheetah, lion, jaguar, margay, ocelot

From Appel MJG, Summers BA. 1995. Pathogenicity of morbilliviruses for terrestrial carnivores. *Vet Microbiol* 44:187-191.

ternary ammonium disinfectant (0.3%). Routine disinfection procedures are usually effective in destroying CDV in a kennel or hospital.

The disease and natural host ranges of CDV include certain species of terrestrial carnivores (see Tables 3-1 and 3-3), and other species can be infected experimentally with varying degrees of susceptibility.[13] Central nervous system (CNS) signs have been produced in mice and hamsters by intracerebral inoculation. Rabbits and rats are resistant to parenteral inoculation. Inapparent, self-limiting infections, produced in domestic cats, nonhuman primates, and humans by parenteral inoculation of virulent CDV, resemble those in dogs that have been given modified live virus (MLV) vaccines. In recent years the host range of this disease appears to have widened as interspecies transmissions occurred, leading to epizootics with high mortality.[75] Despite the wide host range, dogs are the principal reservoir host for CDV, and they likely act as reservoirs of infection for wildlife.[40,75] Certain wildlife species such as raccoons may serve as a reservoir of infection for susceptible dog populations. CNS infections in captive and wild, large, exotic Felidae have been attributed to infection with CDV[14,110,135,147,171] (see Feline Paramyxovirus Infections, Chapter 18). Pigs are subclinically infected, and peccaries *(Tayassu tajacu)* that have been naturally infected develop encephalitis.[14] Encephalitis was documented in a naturally infected monkey.[176] Phocine distemper virus, *Morbillivirus* most closely related to CDV, and some wild strains of CDV

have caused severe morbidity in Baikal *(Phoca sibirica)* and Caspian *(Phoca caspica)* seals (see Tables 3-1 and 3-4).[50,87] It may have spread to the seals from dogs or other susceptible terrestrial carnivores. Genetic analysis of strains causing outbreaks shows that CDV does not become more virulent and spread to new host species in a region, but the same strain circulates among susceptible animals of several host species in a given geographic area.[28,34,75] Other closely related but distinct morbilliviruses cause illness in other aquatic mammals (dolphins and porpoises), and they are more closely related to ruminant morbilliviruses.

EPIDEMIOLOGY

Viral shedding occurs by 7 days postinfection. CDV, most abundant in respiratory exudates, is commonly spread by aerosol or droplet exposure; however, it can be isolated from most other body tissues and secretions, including urine. Transplacental infection can occur from viremic dams. Virus can be excreted up to 60 to 90 days after infection, although shorter periods of shedding are more typical. Contact among recently infected (subclinical or diseased) animals maintains the virus in a population, and a constant supply of puppies helps provide a susceptible population for infection. Although immunity to virulent canine distemper is prolonged or lifelong, it is not as absolute after vaccination. Dogs that do not receive periodic immunizations may lose their protection and become infected after stress, immunosuppression, or contact with diseased individuals. The infection rate is higher than the disease rate, which reflects a certain degree of natural and vaccine-induced immunity in the general dog population. Estimates are that 25% to 75% of susceptible dogs become subclinically infected but clear the virus from the body without showing signs of illness. Although most dogs that recover clear the virus completely, some may harbor virus in their CNS.

The prevalence rate of spontaneous distemper in cosmopolitan dogs is greatest between 3 and 6 months of age, correlating with the loss of maternal antibodies in puppies after weaning. In contrast, in susceptible, isolated populations of dogs, the disease is severe and widespread, affecting all ages. Increased susceptibility among breeds has been suspected but not proved. Brachiocephalic dogs have been reported to have a lower prevalence of disease, mortality, and sequelae compared with dolichocephalic breeds.

Despite minor genetic variation, CDV isolates are serologically homogeneous. However, different strains differ in their pathogenicity, which may affect the severity and extent or

Table • 3-4

Aquatic Morbillivirus Infections

VIRUS	DATE	SPECIES	LOCATION
Dolphin morbillivirus (DMV)	1990s	Striped dolphin	Mediterranean
Porpoise morbillivirus (PMV)	Late 1980s	Harbour porpoise	Northwestern Europe
Phocine distemper virus (PDV)	Late 1980s	Harbour seal, grey seal	Northwestern Europe
Canine distemper virus (CDV)	Late 1980s	Baikal seal	Siberia

Data from Osterhaus ADME, De Swart RL, Vos HW, et al. 1995. Morbillivirus infections of aquatic mammals: newly identified members of the genus. *Vet Microbiol* 44:219-227. Used with permission.

type of clinical disease. Certain isolates, such as Snyder Hill, A75/17, and R252 strain, are highly virulent and neurotropic. The first causes polioencephalomyelitis, whereas the other two cause demyelination. Others vary in their ability to cause CNS lesions. Properties of the N and M-genes contain the determinants of viral persistence.[150]

PATHOGENESIS

Systemic Infection

During natural exposure, CDV spreads by aerosol droplets and contacts epithelium of the upper respiratory tract (Fig. 3-2). Within 24 hours, it multiplies in tissue macrophages and spreads in these cells via local lymphatics to tonsils and bronchial lymph nodes. By 2 to 4 days postinfection, virus numbers increase in tonsils and retropharyngeal and bronchial lymph nodes, but low numbers of CDV-infected mononuclear cells are found in other lymphoid organs.[9] By days 4 to 6 postinfection, virus multiplication occurs within lymphoid follicles in the spleen, the lamina propria of the stomach and small intestines, the mesenteric lymph nodes, and the Kupffer's cells in the liver. Widespread virus proliferation in lymphoid organs corresponds to an initial rise in body temperature and leukopenia between days 3 to 6 postinfection. The leukopenia is primarily a lymphopenia caused by viral damage to lymphoid cells, affecting both T and B cells.

Further spread of CDV to epithelial and CNS tissues on days 8 to 9 postinfection probably occurs hematogenously as a cell-associated and plasma-phase viremia and depends on the dog's humoral and cell-mediated immune status. Shedding of virus begins at the time of epithelial colonization and occurs from all body excretions, even in dogs with subclinical infections. By day 14, animals with adequate CDV antibody titers and cell-mediated cytotoxicity clear the virus from most tissues and show no clinical signs of illness. Specific IgG-CDV antibody is effective in neutralizing extracellular CDV and inhibiting its intercellular spread.

Dogs with intermediate levels of cell-mediated immunoresponsiveness with delayed antibody titers by days 9 to 14 postinfection have virus spread to their epithelial tissues. Clinical signs that develop may eventually resolve as antibody titer increases. Virus is cleared from most body tissues as antibody titers increase but may persist for extended periods as complete virus in uveal tissues and neurons and in integument such as footpads. Recovery from CDV infection is associated with long-term immunity and cessation of viral shedding. Protection may be compromised if the dog is exposed to a highly virulent or large quantity of virus or if it becomes immuno-compromised or stressed.

Dogs with poor immune status by days 9 to 14 postinfection undergo virus spread to many tissues, including skin, exocrine and endocrine glands, and epithelium of the gastrointestinal (GI), respiratory, and genitourinary tracts. Clinical signs of disease in these dogs are usually dramatic and severe, and virus usually persists in their tissues until death. The sequence of pathogenic events depends on the virus strain and may be delayed by 1 to 2 weeks.[152] Secondary bacterial infections increase the severity of clinical illness.

Studies on serologic response to CDV in gnotobiotic dogs confirm that serum antibody titers vary inversely with the severity of the disease. Antibody response in dogs has been separated into envelope and core determinants of the virus. Only dogs producing antienvelope antibodies appear to be able to prevent persistent viral infection of the CNS. The outcome of CNS infection seems to depend on the appearance of circulating IgG antibodies to the H glycoprotein.[134] Mortality in gnotobiotic dogs approaches that of naturally infected animals, deemphasizing the role of secondary bacterial infection in influencing the severity of CNS disease. However, bacteria are probably important in complicating the signs of disease in the respiratory and GI tracts.

Studies have documented the occurrence of cell-mediated immunosuppression after CDV infection. Lymphocyte transformation testing of experimentally infected neonates has shown profound depression of lymphocyte response to phytomitogens at a time corresponding to acute viremia and lymphopenia. This depressed response persisted for more than 10 weeks in convalescing puppies and never returned to baseline values in those that died of acute causes.[92a] Prenatal and neonatal distemper infections are causes of immunodeficiency in surviving puppies and may make concurrent infections with other viruses such as parvovirus more severe.

Central Nervous System Infection

As previously discussed, the spread of virus to the CNS depends on the degree of systemic immune responses mounted by the host. Virus probably enters the nervous system of many viremic CDV-infected dogs whether neurologic signs are observed or not. Antiviral antibody and resultant immune complex deposition may facilitate the spread of virus to the CNS. Virus (free, platelet- or mononuclear cell–associated) may enter the perivascular spaces in the meninges, the choroid plexus epithelial cells of the fourth ventricle, and the ependymal cells lining the ventricular system. Viral antigen is first detected in CNS perivascular astrocytic foot processes and then neurons. The infection of choroid plexus epithelium is productive throughout the course of infection because virus is continually being produced. Primary spread of CDV to the CNS is hematogenous. From the choroid plexus, free or lymphocyte-associated virus may enter the cerebrospinal fluid (CSF), where it spreads to periventricular and subpial structures. Spread of virus through CSF pathways might explain the early distribution of lesions in subependymal areas, such as the cerebral cortex (primarily archicortex and paleocortex), optic tracts

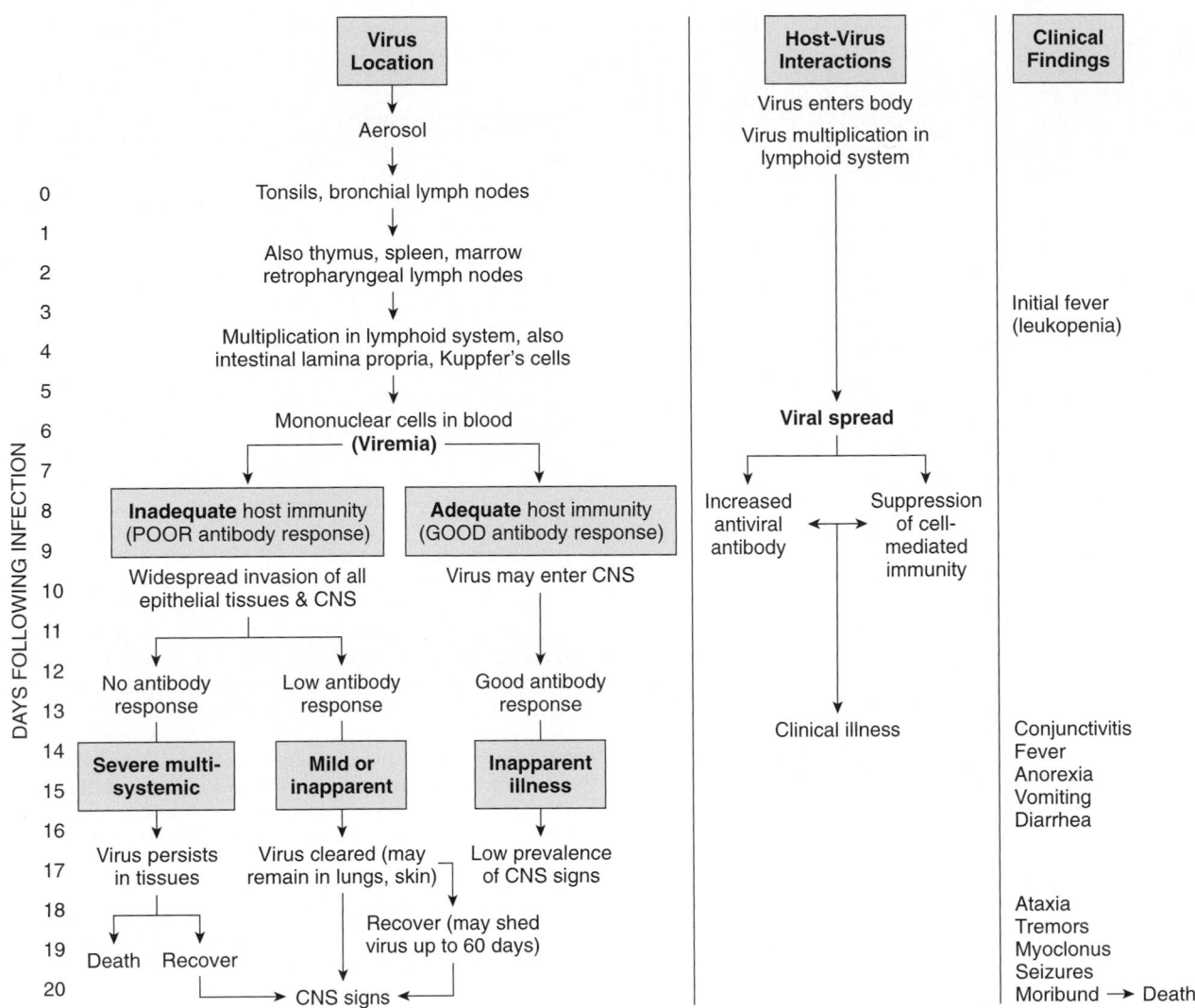

Fig 3-2 Sequential pathogenesis of canine distemper.

and nerves, rostral medullary velum, cerebral peduncles, and spinal cord.

The type of lesion produced and the course of infection within the CNS depend on numerous factors, including the age and immunocompetence of the host at the time of exposure, the neurotropic and immunosuppressive properties of the virus, and the time at which lesions are examined. Either acute or chronic encephalitis can occur independently, or acute-phase lesions may progress to the chronic form in animals that survive.[22]

Acute CDV encephalitis, which occurs early in the course of infection in young or immunosuppressed animals, is characterized by direct viral replication and injury. CDV antigen and messenger RNA (mRNA) are detected in lesions, whereas inflammatory cells and class II major histocompatibility complex (MHC) antigen expression are minimal or absent. These animals have lymphoid depletion, and CDV is found concurrently in lymphoid cells and macrophages throughout the body.[173] Virus causes multifocal lesions in the gray and white matter. Gray matter lesions are the result of neuronal infection and necrosis and may lead to predominant polioencephalomalacia. However, neuronal infection can also occur with minimal evidence of cytolysis. Early in the clinical illness, inflammatory changes are minimal, and theories for the lack of inflammation have included immunodeficiency resulting

from the physiologic immaturity of the immune system and virus-induced immunosuppression.

Light and electron microscopy (EM) reveal noninflammatory demyelination in acute lesions to be associated with viral infection of microglial and astroglial cells rather than oligodendroglial cells, the myelin-producing cells.[33,56,113] Despite the lack of viral replication in oligodendroglial cells, their function has been impaired when observed in primary canine brain cell cultures, where CDV causes a slow-spreading, noncytolytic infection. CDV viral proteins and nucleocapsids are difficult to detect in oligodendroglia by immunocytochemical or ultrastructural methods. However, the use of in situ hybridization shows that the complete viral genome is present.[182] The restricted infection likely leads to metabolic dysfunction and morphologic degeneration of oligodendroglial cells[62] and results in demyelination via a down-regulation of myelin gene expression.[179]

In the normal brain, expression of class II MHC antigen is low. As effector cells, microglia express class II MHC when activated, presumably through increases in interferon (IFN), a T-cell cytokine. Elevated levels of IFN-γ are seen in the CNS during viral infection and in human multiple sclerosis (MS). Class II MHC is up-regulated in demyelinating diseases such as experimental allergic encephalomyelitis and MS. In a study of acute CDV encephalitis in dogs, virus was present in a diffuse or multifocal distribution, and class II MHC was up-regulated throughout the white matter and in CDV-infected foci.[7] Despite the visible absence of an inflammatory response in the CNS and an apparent lack of systemic immune response, entry of CD3+ lymphocytes occurs in the CNS in response to the presence of CDV nucleocapsid protein and increased interleukin (IL)-8 activity.[156] CD8+ lymphocytes dominated the infiltrates during all states of distemper encephalitis.[172] In the CNS, up-regulation of proinflammatory cytokines such as IL-6 and tumor necrosis factor is balanced by increased IL-10 and transforming growth factor, which help temper the immune response.[52]

In contrast to acute CDV encephalitis, subacute to chronic CDV encephalitis is characterized by reduced expression of CDV antigen and mRNA and a strong up-regulation of class II MHC expression. This results in perivascular mononuclear cell infiltrations and a virus-independent immunopathologic process. These animals have no evidence of lymphoid depletion throughout the body, and they have a significant increase in T- and B-lymphocyte populations compared with dogs with acute CDV encephalitis. Virus is found predominantly in follicular dendritic cells of the lymphoid system, suggesting a change in cell tropism for viral persistence.[173] Perivascular infiltrates in subacute and chronic distemper encephalitis consists of CD4+ and B cells. These cells result in a strong humoral immune response, and increased intrathecal virus-neutralizing antibodies are present.[109,172] Antimyelin antibodies are thought to be a secondary reaction to the inflammatory process. Antibodies to CDV appear to interact with infected macrophages in CNS lesions, causing their activation with the release of reactive oxygen radicals. This activity can lead to destruction of oligodendroglial cells and myelin through an "innocent bystander" mechanism.[29,33] The reaction of the immune system, not viral interference, is the pathogenic mechanism for demyelination in this phase.

In surviving animals, CDV is cleared from the inflammatory lesions but can persist in brain tissue in unaffected sites.[112] If the spread through the CNS has been extensive by the time the host responds to the virus, widespread damage occurs. Some unaffected areas of virally infected brain tissue are spared the inflammatory process and immune recognition, presumably because of noncytolytic infections.[164,177,181] Reduced expression of CDV proteins on the surface of inflammatory cells has also been implicated as a means of immune avoidance.[5,6,112]

Old dog encephalitis (ODE) is a rare, chronic, active progressive inflammatory disease of the gray matter of the cerebral hemispheres and brainstem of the CNS, which may result from neural persistence of virus after acute CDV infection. This form of infection occurs in infected animals that are immunocompetent and have virus persisting in their nervous tissue. ODE is a unique variant of CDV-CNS infection in which persistent virus exists strictly in neurons in a replication-defective form.[15] Transmission of infection using brain homogenates of dogs with ODE was unsuccessful; however, reisolation of infectious virus required prolonged cocultivation of brain explant cells with susceptible Vero cells.[15] Similar observations have been made with persistent measles virus in humans with subacute sclerosing panencephalitis.

Inclusion body polioencephalitis is a variant form of encephalitis with lesions and pathogenesis similar to ODE. It can occur after vaccination[116] or in dogs with a sudden onset of only neurologic manifestations of distemper.[117] Multifocal gray matter necrosis, perivascular lymphocytic inflammation, and cytoplasmic and intranuclear inclusions are observed. The immune response is dominated by T-cell infiltration and class II MHC up-regulation. Abundant expression of all viral protein mRNAs and reduced or lacking protein expression, especially of matrix and fusion proteins, are evident. Low viral protein antigen levels may be a means by which CDV persists by evading immune recognition.

CLINICAL FINDINGS

Systemic Signs

Clinical signs of canine distemper vary depending on virulence of the virus strain, environmental conditions, and host age and immune status. More than 50% of CDV infections are probably subclinical. Mild forms of clinical illness are also common, and signs include listlessness, decreased appetite, fever, and upper respiratory tract infection. Bilateral serous oculonasal discharge can become mucopurulent with coughing and dyspnea. Many mildly infected dogs develop clinical signs that are indistinguishable from those of other causes of "kennel cough" (see Chapter 6). Keratoconjunctivitis sicca may develop after systemic or subclinical infections in dogs. Persistent anosmia was reported as a sequela in dogs that had recovered from canine distemper.[66]

Severe generalized distemper is the commonly recognized form of the disease. It can occur in dogs of any age, but it most commonly affects unvaccinated, exposed puppies 12 to 16 weeks of age that have lost their maternal immunity or younger puppies that have received inadequate concentrations of maternal antibody. The initial febrile response in natural infections is probably unnoticed. The first sign of infection is a mild, serous-to-mucopurulent conjunctivitis, which is followed within a few days by a dry cough that rapidly becomes moist and productive. Increased lower respiratory sounds from the thorax can be heard on auscultation. Depression and anorexia are followed by vomiting, which is commonly unrelated to eating. Diarrhea subsequently develops, varying in consistency from fluid to frank blood and mucus. Tenesmus can be present, and intussusceptions may occur. Severe dehydration and emaciation can result from adipsia and fluid loss. Animals can die suddenly from systemic illness, but adequate therapy can decrease the risk in many cases.

Skin Lesions

Vesicular and pustular dermatitis in puppies is rarely associated with CNS disease (Fig. 3-3), whereas dogs developing

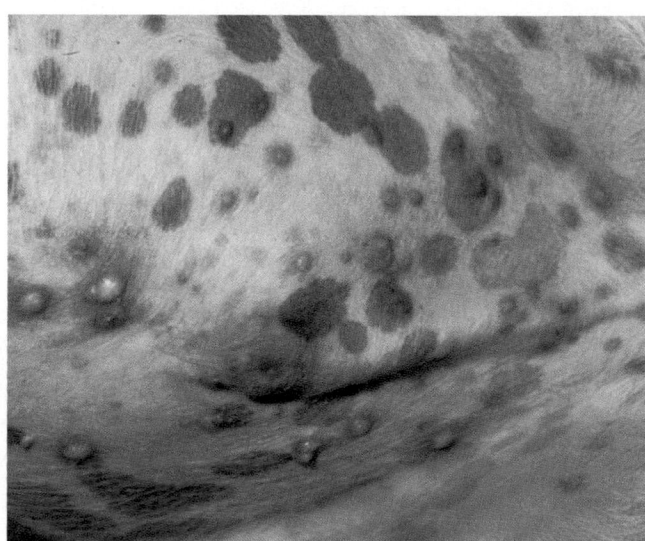

Fig 3-3 Pustular dermatitis in a puppy with canine distemper. Rarely associated with neurologic complications, this is usually a favorable prognostic sign. (Courtesy University of Georgia, Athens, Ga.)

nasal and digital hyperkeratosis usually have various neurologic complications (Figs. 3-4 and 3-5). Viral invasion of these tissues has been demonstrated.[97] Lesions consist of hyperkeratosis and parakeratosis with vesicles and pustule formation.[123] Virus has entered the footpad keratinocytes as it causes the observed hyperkeratosis; however, neither the virus nor its nucleic acid appear to persist indefinitely.[68,70]

Neurologic Signs

Neurologic manifestations usually begin 1 to 3 weeks after recovery from systemic illness; however, no way is known to predict which dogs will develop neurologic disorders. Neurologic signs can also coincide with multisystemic illness or less commonly, they can occur weeks to months later. Neurologic signs frequently develop in the presence of nonexistent or very

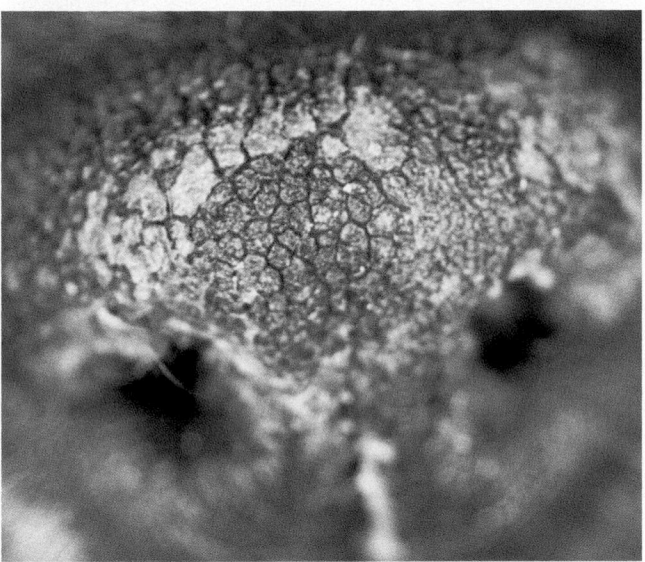

Fig 3-4 Nasal hyperkeratosis in a dog with systemic distemper. (Courtesy University of Georgia, Athens, Ga.)

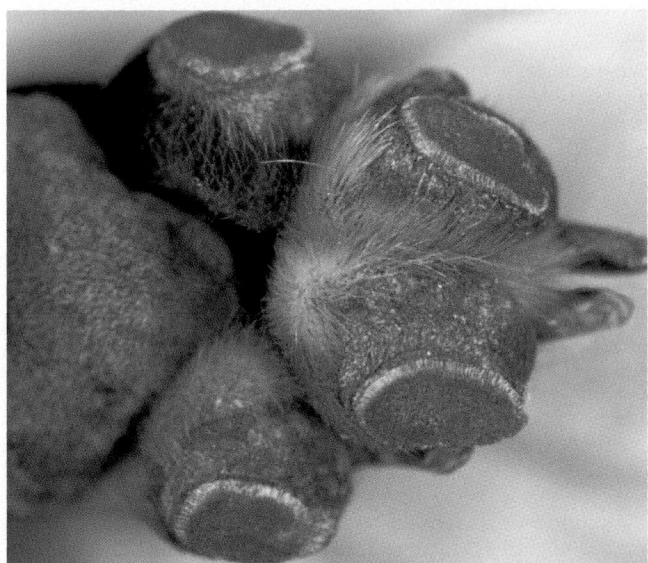

Fig 3-5 Digital hyperkeratosis ("hard pads") in a dog dying of distemper encephalomyelitis. (Courtesy University of Georgia, Athens, Ga.)

mild extraneural signs.[158] Empirically, certain features of systemic disease can be predictive of the incidence of neurologic sequelae. Mature or partially immune dogs that have been previously vaccinated and have no history of systemic disease can suddenly develop neurologic signs.[129] Neurologic signs, whether acute or chronic, are typically progressive. Chronic relapsing neurologic deterioration with an intermittent recovery and a later, superimposed acute episode of neurologic dysfunction can occur. ODE is characterized by this type of progressive history.

Neurologic complications of canine distemper are the most significant factors affecting prognosis and recovery from infection. Neurologic signs vary according to the area of the CNS involved. Hyperesthesia and cervical or paraspinal rigidity can be found in some dogs as a result of meningeal inflammation, although parenchymal rather than meningeal signs usually predominate. Seizures, cerebellar and vestibular signs, paraparesis or tetraparesis with sensory ataxia, and myoclonus are common. Seizures can be of any type, depending on the region of the forebrain that is damaged by the virus. The "chewing-gum" type of seizures, classically associated with CDV infection, often occurs in dogs developing polioencephalomalacia of the temporal lobes. However, lesions in these lobes from other causes can produce similar seizures.

Myoclonus, the involuntary twitching of muscles in a forceful simultaneous contraction, can be present without other neurologic signs. With more extensive spinal cord damage, the dog may have upper motor neuron paresis of the affected limb associated with myoclonus. The rhythmic contractions can be present while the dog is awake, although they more commonly occur while it is sleeping. The neural mechanisms for myoclonus originate with local irritation of the lower motor neurons of the spinal cord or cranial nerve nuclei. Although considered specific for CDV infection, myoclonus can also be seen in other paramyxovirus infections of dogs and cats (see Chapters 7 and 18) and less commonly, in other inflammatory conditions of the CNS.[155]

Transplacental Infection

Young puppies infected transplacentally may develop neurologic signs during the first 4 to 6 weeks of life.[92] Mild or inapparent infections are seen in the bitch. Depending on the stage of gestation at which infection occurred, abortions, stillbirths, or the births of weak puppies may occur. Puppies infected in utero that survive such infections may suffer from permanent immunodeficiencies because of damage to primordial lymphoid elements.

Neonatal Infections

Young puppies infected with CDV before the eruption of permanent dentition may have severe damage to the enamel, dentin, or roots of their teeth.[23] The puppies may have enamel or dentin with an irregular appearance (Fig. 3-6), in addition to partial eruption, oligodontia, or impaction of teeth. Enamel hypoplasia with or without neurologic signs may be an incidental finding in an older dog and is relatively pathognomonic for prior infection with CDV.

Neonatal (<7 days old) gnotobiotic puppies have developed virus-induced cardiomyopathy after experimental infection with CDV. Clinical signs including dyspnea, depression, anorexia, collapse, and prostration develop from 14 to 18 days postinfection. Lesions are characterized by multifocal myocardial degeneration, necrosis, and mineralization, with minimal inflammatory cell infiltration. The clinical significance of this process after natural infection is uncertain, and whether it has a relationship with onset of adult cardiomyopathy in dogs remains to be determined. Other viruses such as CPV-1 and CPV-2 can produce similar lesions (see Canine Enteric Viral Infections, Chapter 8).

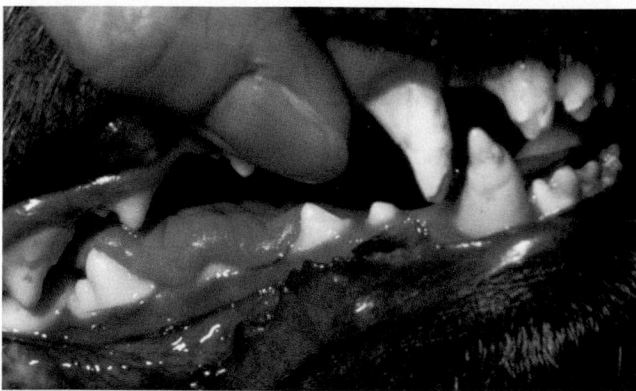

Fig 3-6 Enamel hypoplasia characterized by irregularities in the dental surface in an older dog that survived neonatal distemper. (Courtesy University of Georgia, Athens, Ga.)

Bone Lesions

Young, growing dogs with experimentally and naturally induced CDV infection develop metaphyseal osteosclerosis of the long bones.[2,19,51,96,104] Large-breed dogs between 3 and 6 months of age are most commonly affected. Studies have not shown animals with systemic distemper to develop overt clinical signs related to these long bone lesions. However, CDV RNA transcripts have been seen in the bone cells of young dogs with hypertrophic osteodystrophy (HOD), a metaphyseal bone disease which can be similar to and confused with metaphysical osteomyelitis (see Musculoskeletal Infections, Chapter 86).[106,108] Juvenile cellulitis, HOD, or both have developed in some puppies in association with MLV distemper vaccination (see Chapter 100 and Modified-Live Virus Vaccines in this chapter).[100] Morbilliviral RNA transcripts have also been detected in the bony lesions of people with Paget's disease (see Public Health Considerations in this chapter).

Rheumatoid Arthritis

Dogs with rheumatoid arthritis had high levels of antibodies to CDV in sera and synovial fluid compared with dogs with inflammatory and degenerative arthritis.[21] CDV antigens were found in immune complexes from synovial fluid of dogs with rheumatoid arthritis but were not found in synovial fluid from dogs with inflammatory or degenerative arthropathies.

Ocular Signs

Dogs with CDV encephalomyelitis often have a mild anterior uveitis that is clinically asymptomatic. More obvious ophthalmologic lesions in canine distemper have been attributed to an effect of the virus on the optic nerve and the retina (see Canine Distemper, Chapter 93). Optic neuritis can be characterized by a sudden onset of blindness, with dilated unresponsive pupils. Degeneration and necrosis of the retina produce gray-to-pink irregular densities on the tapetal or nontapetal fundus or both. Bullous or complete retinal detachment can occur where exudates dissect between the retina and choroid. Chronic, inactive fundic lesions are associated with retinal atrophy and scarring. These circumscribed, hyperreflective areas are called *gold medallion lesions* and are considered characteristic of previous canine distemper infection.

Combined Infections

Immunosuppression caused by or responsible for systemic CDV infection can be associated with combined opportunistic infections. Salmonellosis has been a common complication, causing protracted or fatal hemorrhagic diarrhea or sepsis in

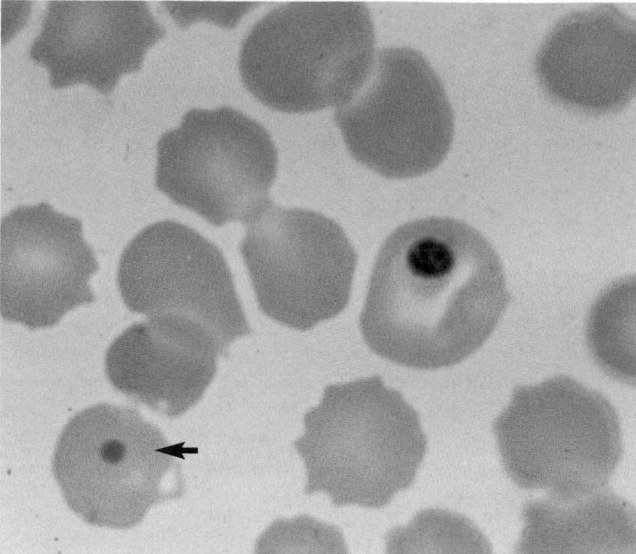

Fig 3-7 Distemper inclusion in an erythrocyte from a peripheral blood film *(arrow)*. Compare its appearance with that of a Howell-Jolly body (Wright stain, ×1000). (Courtesy O.W. Schalm, Davis, Calif.)

affected dogs. Combined infections with *Toxoplasma gondii* or *Neospora caninum* have produced lower motor neuron dysfunction from myositis and radiculoneuritis (see Chapter 80). *Pneumocystis carinii* pneumonia has also been associated with CDV infection (see Chapter 68).[151]

DIAGNOSIS

Practical diagnosis of canine distemper is primarily based on clinical suspicion. A characteristic history of a 3- to 6-month-old unvaccinated puppy with a compatible illness supports the diagnosis. Most dogs with severe disease have clinical signs distinctive enough to make a presumptive diagnosis, but upper respiratory infections in older dogs are often incorrectly diagnosed as infectious tracheobronchitis (see Chapter 6). Specific laboratory tests are not always available to confirm the suspicion of CDV infections, so the practicing veterinarian must rely on nonspecific findings of routine laboratory procedures.

Clinical Laboratory Findings

Abnormal hematologic findings include an absolute lymphopenia caused by lymphoid depletion. This frequently persists in very young dogs with rapidly progressive systemic or neurologic signs. Thrombocytopenia (as low as 30,000 cells/µl) and regenerative anemia have been found in experimentally infected neonates (<3 weeks) but have not been consistently recognized in older or spontaneously infected dogs. Distemper inclusions can be detected in the early phase of disease by examination of stained peripheral blood films, in low numbers in circulating lymphocytes, and with even less frequency in monocytes, neutrophils, and erythrocytes. Wright-Leishman–stained inclusions in lymphocytes are large (up to 3 µm), single, oval, gray structures, whereas erythrocytic inclusions (which are most numerous in polychromatophilic cells) are round and eccentrically placed and appear light blue (Fig. 3-7). The sizes of erythrocytic inclusions are between those of metarubricyte nuclei and Howell-Jolly bodies. Buffy coat and bone marrow examination and use of phloxinophilic stains can improve the chances of detecting inclusions. EM has confirmed that these inclusions consist of paramyxovirus-like nucleocapsids.

The magnitude and type of serum biochemistry changes in acute systemic infections are nonspecific. Total protein analysis includes decreased albumin and increased α- and γ-globulin concentrations in nonneonates. Some puppies infected prenatally or neonatally with CDV have marked hypoglobulinemia from persistent immunosuppression caused by the virus.

Radiology

Thoracic radiography demonstrates an interstitial lung pattern in early cases of distemper. An alveolar pattern is seen with secondary bacterial infection and more severe bronchopneumonia (Fig. 3-8).

Cerebrospinal Fluid Analysis

Abnormalities are detectable in dogs with neurologic signs of distemper; however, false-negative results can be anticipated. Dogs with acute noninflammatory demyelinating encephalomyelitis may have normal CSF analysis results. Increases in protein (>25 mg/dl) and cell count (>10 cells/μl with a predominance of lymphocytes) are characteristic of subacute to more chronic, inflammatory forms of CDV encephalomyelitis. Intracytoplasmic inclusions may be found in CSF cells.[1] When increased protein is present in CSF, it is primarily IgG with specific anti-CDV activity. IFN levels are also increased in the CSF of dogs with acute and chronic distemper encephalitis.[160] Differences in the humoral immune response in CSF and sera to the H and F envelope proteins (see Table 3-2) have been noted between some dogs with chronic progressive encephalitis and those with other forms of distemper encephalitis.[134]

Increased anti-CDV antibody in CSF offers definitive evidence of distemper encephalitis because antibody is locally produced; these increases have not been found in vaccinated dogs or those with systemic distemper without CNS disease. CSF antibody may be increased from traumatic collection procedures causing contamination by whole blood. An antibody ratio can help identify the effect of nonspecific leakage of distemper-specific IgG into the CSF from serum. Divide the concentration of distemper-specific IgG in CSF by that of IgG in serum. Compare the result with a corresponding CSF-serum antibody ratio for another infectious agent for which serum antibody titers are expected, such as canine adenovirus (CAV) or canine parvovirus (CPV). If the ratio for CDV is higher than that for CAV or CPV, then de novo local production of CSF antibody caused by CNS infection with distemper is expected. Ideally the titer determination for both diseases should use the same methodology (e.g., neutralization, enzyme-linked immunosorbent assay [ELISA], indirect fluorescent antibody [FA]). Alternatives are to compare the CDV-specific CSF-serum ratio with the ratio of IgG or albumin in CSF and serum,[157] but this approach is less accurate because of the differences in methodology used in their determinations. The CSF IgG antibody concentration is more likely to be increased in dogs with inflammatory demyelinating encephalitis than in younger or immunosuppressed dogs with acute polioencephalitis and noninflammatory virus-induced cellular injury.[145,158] Although the test for CSF antibodies is sensitive and specific for CDV, it can be performed only by properly equipped diagnostic or research laboratory personnel (see Appendix 5). In acute CNS infections, some mononuclear cells may contain large (15 to 10 μm), oval homogenous eosinophilic intracytoplasmic inclusions.[8]

Immunocytology

Immunofluorescent techniques can facilitate a specific diagnosis of canine distemper; however, these tests also require special equipment and are usually handled by regional diagnostic laboratories. In clinically affected dogs, immunofluorescence is usually performed on cytologic smears prepared from conjunctival, tonsillar, genital, and respiratory epithelium. The technique also can be performed on cells in CSF, blood (buffy coat), urine sediment, and bone marrow (Fig. 3-9). Smears should be made on precleaned slides, air-dried thoroughly, and preferably fixed in acetone for 5 minutes before transport to the laboratory. At the laboratory, they are stained directly or indirectly with fluorescein-conjugated CDV antibody and examined by fluorescent microscopy.

Antigen, first detected in buffy coat smears from 2 to 5 days postinfection decreases as antibody titer increases by 8 to 9 days postinfection. Clinical signs become apparent shortly

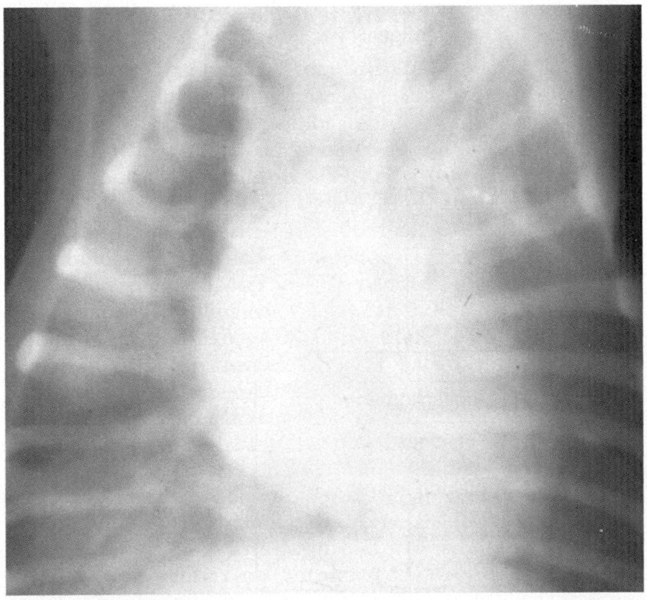

Fig 3-8 Dorsoventral thoracic radiograph from a puppy with canine distemper bronchopneumonia. (Courtesy University of Georgia, Athens, Ga.)

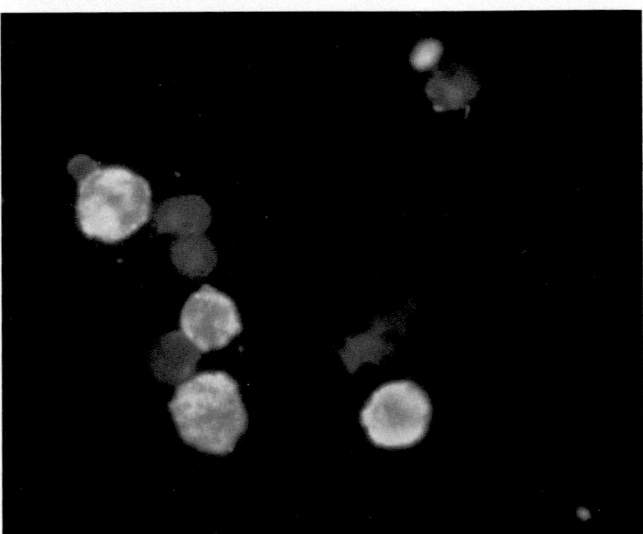

Fig 3-9 Immunofluorescence confirming CDV in a buffy coat smear of a dog with acute distemper.

after this time (day 14), and positive results are not recognized except in dogs that do not mount a sufficient immune response and succumb to infection. Positive fluorescence in conjunctival and genital epithelium is usually detected only within the first 3 weeks postinfection, when systemic illness is apparent. Virus also disappears in these tissues after the first 1 to 2 weeks of clinical illness (21 to 28 days postinfection) as antibody titers rise in association with clinical recovery. Beginning with the recovery stage, antibody may bind and mask antigen in infected cells, resulting in false-negative results. Virus may be detected for longer periods in epithelial cells and macrophages from the lower respiratory tract, and transtracheal washings can be obtained for diagnosis. Virus also persists for at least 60 days in the skin, uveal tissue, footpad, and CNS. Direct FA examination of cells in conjunctival scrapings, CSF, or blood films is helpful in acute phases of illness. In chronic cases, it is usually unrewarding because antibody coating or elimination of viral antigen yields negative results with diagnostic immunofluorescence. ELISA has been used to detect viral antigen in serum and CSF of naturally and experimentally infected dogs.[60,82,144] A test based on this methodology would be extremely valuable to the practitioner. In one study, MLV vaccination produced a false-positive result in testing for serum antigen.[144] Viral antigen detected by FA or ELISA is difficult to find in body fluid specimens from dogs with neurologic distemper that lack or have recovered from systemic signs. More sensitive tests such as the polymerase chain reaction (PCR) might be more valuable in such instances.

Immunohistochemistry

CDV antigen detected in the nasal mucosa, footpad epithelium, and haired skin of the dorsal neck has been used consistently for the antemortem diagnosis of infection.[72] FA techniques can also be performed on frozen sections of biopsy or necropsy specimens. Tissues collected from dogs that died from distemper should include spleen, tonsils, lymph nodes, stomach, lung, duodenum, bladder, and brain. Animals dying of generalized infection frequently have abundant quantities of virus in these tissues. FA techniques can also be adapted to paraffin-embedded sections if special cold (4° C) ethanol (95%) fixation is used. Footpad biopsy has been recommended as an antemortem diagnostic technique (Fig. 3-10).

Other immunochemical techniques have been developed for histologic detection of distemper antigen in formalin-fixed and paraffin-embedded tissues and cell culture.[20,59] Immuno-

histochemical demonstration of CDV antigen is superior to reliance on inclusion bodies in brain tissue to confirm distemper encephalitis (Fig. 3-11).[124] Results are more likely to be positive in acute than chronic infections in which viral antigens may not be expressed. Monoclonal antibodies are available to detect CDV by immunohistochemical methods (VMRD Inc., Pullman, Wash.).

Nucleic Acid Detection

Reverse transcription has been used to detect CDV RNA in buffy coat cells from dogs with acute CDV infection[167] and the serum, whole blood, and CSF from dogs with systemic or neurologic distemper.[53] Regardless of the duration and form of distemper, a positive result was highly specific for diagnosis. This test is very valuable for premortem diagnosis; however, it is not widely available. As with FA methods, viral mRNA was detected in footpad specimens from infected dogs.[68,70] Similarly, PCR and nucleic acid hybridization studies using single-stranded RNA probes have been performed to detect virulent virus in tissue culture and histologic sections.[178] Seminested PCR was also efficient in detecting CDV in paraffin-embedded nervous tissue.[148] In general, a positive PCR result is indicative of infection, whereas a negative one can result from many factors including improper sample handling. During an outbreak of distemper in Alaska, PCR was used to detect the infection and trace the origin of the responsible strain to Siberia.[99]

Serum Antibody Testing

The neutralization test is still considered the gold standard for measuring protection against infection, and serum titers correlate well with the level of protection.[12] Neutralizing antibodies are directed against the membrane proteins (H and F) of the virus, appear beginning 10 to 20 days postinfection, and may persist for the life of a recovered animal. A microneu-

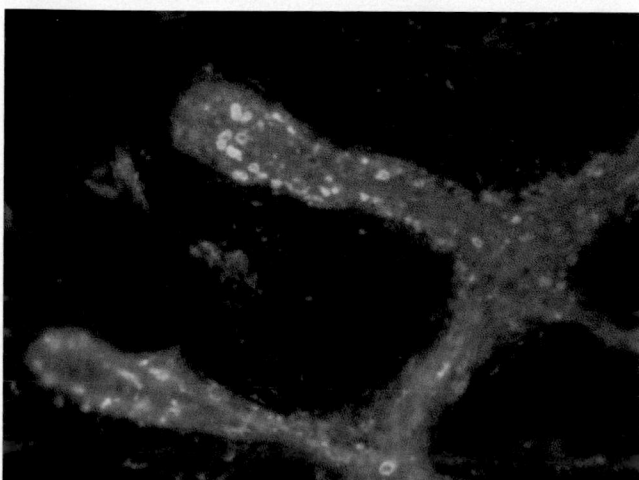

Fig 3-10 Immunofluorescence confirming CDV in a footpad biopsy of an infected dog.

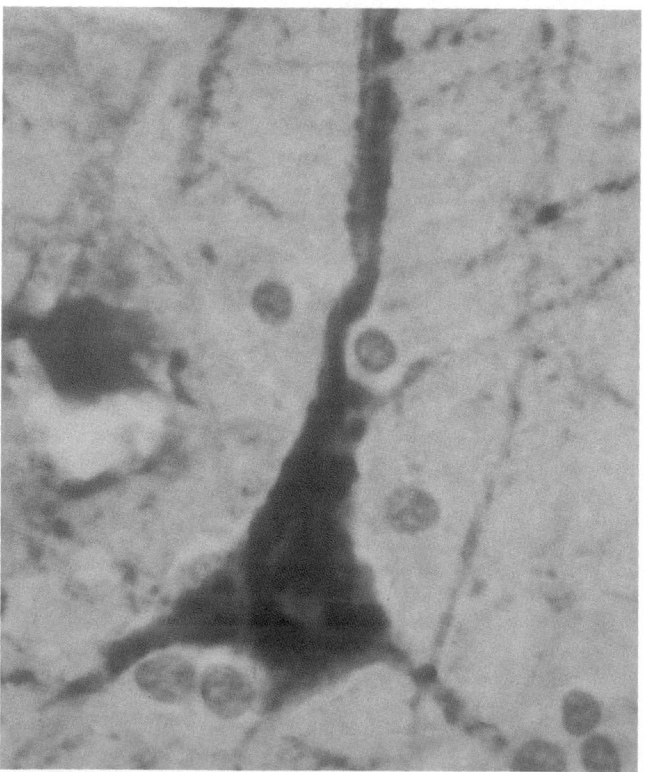

Fig 3-11 Immunocytochemical demonstration of CDV antigen within the cell body and processes of neurons.

tralization method has further simplified neutralizing antibody testing in diagnostic laboratories. A plaque-staining method has been shown to be more sensitive than the neutralization assay.[143] Indirect FA testing has also been used to measure postvaccination titers and gives results comparable to those of neutralization.[161] Although sometimes less specific, whole-virus ELISA has been used to detect serum IgG and IgM antibodies to CDV. Increased specificity has been achieved using recombinant N protein–based ELISA in dogs.[16,167] Antibody to N and P proteins may appear 6 to 8 days postinoculation when measured by ELISA. Increased titers of serum IgM-neutralizing antibody can be measured in dogs that survive the acute phase of infection and usually disappear by 3 months. High serum IgM titers have been more accurate in detecting acute clinical distemper cases (81%) compared with chronic progressive inflammatory encephalitis (60%). Transient IgM increases can also be seen for up to 3 weeks after first immunization with CDV vaccine. Unlike increases in serum IgM titers, high IgG titers are ambiguous and can indicate either past or present infection with CDV or past vaccination for CDV. Analyzing CSF-specific IgG levels and determining a CSF-serum ratio may be more reliable uses of antibody measurements in detecting chronic CDV infections of the nervous system (see Cerebrospinal Fluid Analysis in this chapter).

Viral Isolation

Virulent CDV can be readily cultured in macrophages or activated lymphocytes, but it grows only with adaptation in epithelial or fibroblast cell lines. As a result, isolation of virulent CDV has been difficult in routine cell cultures. The most successful viral replication occurs during direct cultivation of target tissues from the infected host. Buffy coat specimens taken during the early course of illness provide the best opportunity. Alveolar macrophage cultures detect the virus in 24 to 48 hours. Giant cell (syncytia) formation, a characteristic cytopathic effect of CDV in many tissue cultures, is detected within 2 to 5 days, at which time the virus can be isolated by overlays made on other cells. Macrophage cultures have been replaced by dog lymphocyte cultures for isolation of CDV.[10] Buffy coat cells or tissues from infected animals can be cultivated with mitogen-stimulated canine blood lymphocytes, and cultures are examined 72 to 144 hours later by immunofluorescence.[10] A marmoset lymphoid cell line (B95a) has also been used.[86]

Growth in pulmonary macrophages or lymphocytes was once considered an essential feature of virulent CDV isolates, although virulent CDV has occasionally been isolated in Vero cells or primary dog kidney and bladder epithelial cell cultures without the need for adaptation or loss of virulence of the virus. However, the success rate is low. In general, titers of vaccine viruses are high in macrophage, lymphocyte, kidney cell, and epithelial cell lines, whereas virulent field strains grow better in macrophages[48] and lymphocytes.[10] Cultures can be examined with FA for virus when cytopathic effects are not observed. Because of defective viral replication, specimens from dogs with chronic or vaccine-induced encephalitis do not yield successful cultures.

PATHOLOGIC FINDINGS

Young dogs prenatally or neonatally infected with CDV have thymic atrophy. Pneumonia and catarrhal enteritis are present in infected puppies with systemic disease. Upper respiratory tract lesions include conjunctivitis, rhinitis, and inflammation of the tracheobronchial tree. Hyperkeratosis of the nose and footpads may be seen in dogs with neurologic disease. Gross lesions in the CNS are not often found except for occasional

meningeal congestion, ventricular dilation, and increased CSF pressure resulting from brain edema in acute encephalitis. Necrosis and cavitation may develop in the white matter in chronic inflammatory lesions.

Lymphoid depletion is a typical histologic finding in a dog with systemic illness. Diffuse interstitial pneumonia is characterized by thickened alveolar septa and proliferation of alveolar epithelium. Alveoli contain desquamated epithelial cells and macrophages; transitional epithelium of the urinary system may contain cytoplasmic inclusions. Puppies developing distemper may have defects in dental enamel, and necrosis and cystic degeneration of ameloblastic epithelium are usually present. (See Chapter 93 for a description of ophthalmic lesions.) Mild interstitial epididymitis and orchitis are commonly seen in dogs with canine distemper, an observation that may help explain the transient decrease in spermatogenesis, prostate fluid, and testosterone that occurs in recovering animals.

With acute fatal encephalitis of neonates, neuronal and myelin degeneration or primary demyelination can occur without significant perivascular inflammation (Fig. 3-12). In surviving animals, patchy areas of necrosis are replaced by hypertrophic astrocytes that form a network for macrophages ingesting myelin. The most severe white matter changes in the CNS can be found in the predilection sites of lateral cerebellar peduncles, the dorsolateral medulla adjacent to the fourth ventricle, and the deep cerebellar white matter. Lesions are also present in the midbrain, basal nuclei, and pyriform lobes of the cerebral cortex. Superficial areas such as the optic tracts, crus cerebri, central components of cranial nerve pathways, and infundibulum also can be affected. Noninflammatory polioencephalomyelitis in some dogs can predominantly affect the cerebrum and thalamus.[154] Acute noninflammatory lesions include demyelination with spongy vacuolation of white matter and reactive gliosis. Intracytoplasmic or intranuclear inclusions can be found predominantly in astrocytes and neurons.

Older or more immunocompetent dogs tend to develop leukoencephalomyelitis with a predominance of lesions in the caudal brainstem and spinal cord. These lesions are usually associated with signs of ataxia and vestibular involvement. Lesions are characterized by widespread perivascular lymphoplasmacytic infiltration with areas of demyelination and neuronal degeneration (Fig. 3-13). They can be more wide-

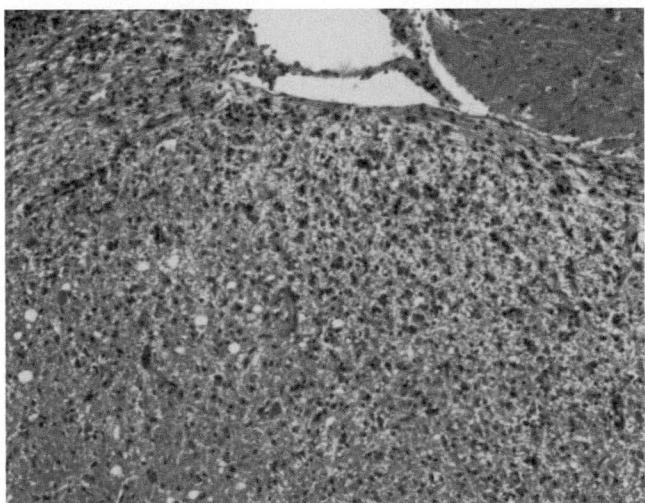

Fig 3-12 Large zone of noninflammatory demyelination in the cerebellar white matter of a dog with acute distemper encephalitis hematoxylin and eosin (H and E stain).

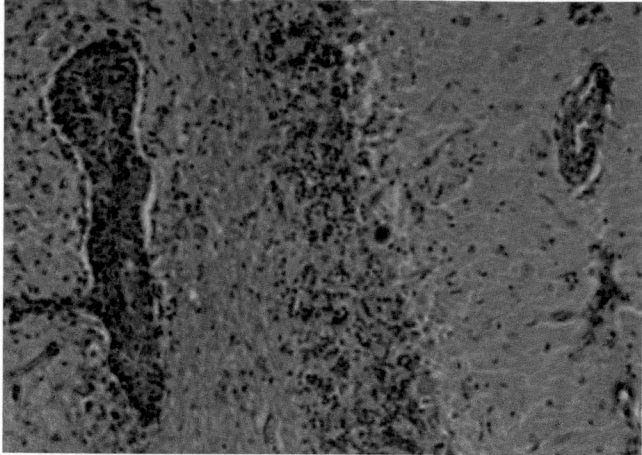

Fig 3-13 Chronic inflammatory lesions with prominent perivascular cuffing in the cerebellar white matter with mild meningitis in a dog with inflammatory distemper encephalitis. (H and E stain.)

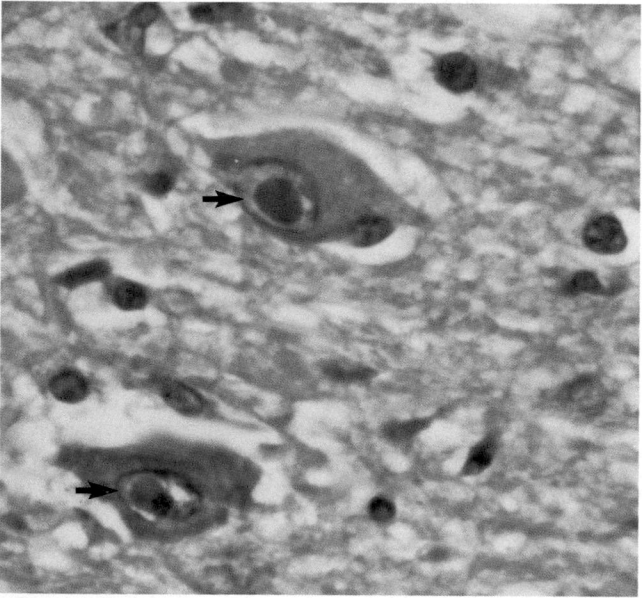

Fig 3-14 Postvaccinal form of CDV with numerous inclusion bodies in brainstem neurons.

spread and severe than lesions in dogs with acute encephalitis. In more chronic cases the lesion may develop into sclerosing panencephalitis characterized by infiltration and replacement of nervous tissue by a dense astrocytic network.

In contrast, lesions of vaccine-induced distemper are typically those of a necrotizing polioencephalitis of the caudal brainstem with preference for the ventral pontine nuclei (see previous section Neurologic Signs in this chapter and Postvaccinal Complications in Chapter 100).[163,169] Inclusions can be found in the nucleus or cytoplasm of astrocytes and neurons (Fig. 3-14).

Histologic examination reveals that CDV inclusions are most commonly cytoplasmic and acidophilic staining. They are 1 to 5 μm in diameter and can be found in epithelial cells of the mucous membranes, reticulum cells, leukocytes, glia, and neurons. Inclusions can be found up to 5 to 6 weeks

postinfection in the lymphoid system and urinary tract. Intranuclear inclusions are most common in lining or glandular epithelium and ganglion cells.

The morphologic significance of distemper inclusions is not completely understood. Histochemically, they are composed of aggregates of viral nucleocapsids and cellular debris as a result of viral infection. Intranuclear inclusions contain viral nucleocapsid and heat shock protein.[119] Caution must be used when absolutely confirming a diagnosis of canine distemper based solely on the presence of inclusions. Cytoplasmic inclusions typical for CDV infection have been identified in the urinary bladder of normal dogs. Unfortunately, inclusion bodies are not only nonspecific but also may appear too late in the disease to be routinely useful. In contrast, using only the presence of inclusion bodies to detect CDV infection can lead to a false-negative diagnosis in dogs, whereas immunocytochemical and in situ hybridization methods are more sensitive for CDV detection in tissues (see previous sections Immunohistochemistry and Nucleic Acid Detection).

Formation of giant cells primarily in CNS white matter and anterior uvea of the eye and secondarily in lymph nodes, lung, and leptomeninges is specific to paramyxoviruses such as CDV. This finding can be used to substantiate CDV infection.

THERAPY

Despite vast advances in research on canine distemper, only minor changes have been made in therapeutic recommendations. Although supportive and nonspecific, aims in treatment are frequently beneficial because they reduce mortality. The only reason for refusing to initiate treatment at an owner's insistence is the presence of neurologic signs that are incompatible with life. Even in the absence of neurologic signs, owners should always be warned that such sequelae may develop at a later time. The spontaneous improvement seen in many dogs with symptomatic management of nonneurologic systemic distemper can be inappropriately credited to the success of certain treatment regimens. However, unlike the systemic signs, neurologic signs themselves are not usually reversible unless they are caused by vaccine strains and frequently are progressive.

Dogs with upper respiratory infections should be kept in environments that are clean, warm, and free of drafts. Oculonasal discharges should be cleaned from the face. Pneumonia is frequently complicated by secondary bacterial infection, usually with *Bordetella bronchiseptica*, which requires broad-spectrum antibiotic therapy and expectorants or nebulization and coupage. Good initial antibiotic choices for bronchopneumonia include ampicillin, tetracycline, and chloramphenicol (Table 3-5). However, because of dental staining, tetracycline use must be avoided in puppies, and chloramphenicol is less desirable because of its public health risks. Newer parenteral florfenicol should be considered (see Drug Formulary, Appendix 8). Parenteral therapy is essential when GI signs are present. Antimicrobial therapy should be altered when indicated by susceptibility testing based on transtracheal washing or by lack of response to the initial antibiotics.

Food and water and oral medications or fluids should be discontinued if vomiting and diarrhea are present. Parenteral antiemetics may be required. Supplementation with polyionic isotonic fluids such as lactated Ringer's solution should be given intravenously (IV) or subcutaneously (SC), depending on the hydration status of the patient. B vitamins should be administered as nonspecific therapy to replace vitamins lost from anorexia and diuresis and to stimulate the appetite. Historically, IV administration of ascorbic acid has been beneficial; however, this treatment is controversial, and its

Table • 3-5

Drug Therapy for Canine Distemper

DRUG[a]	DOSE[b] (mg/kg)	ROUTE	INTERVAL (HOURS)	DURATION (DAYS)
Antimicrobial				
Ampicillin, amoxicillin	20	PO, IV, SC	8	7
Doxycycline[c]	5—10	PO, IV	12	7
Chloramphenicol	15—25	PO, SC	8	7
Florfenicol	25—50	SC, IM	8	3—5
Cephapirin	10—30	IM, IV, SC	6—8	3—5
Anticonvulsive				
Phenobarbital	2	PO, IV, IM	12	prn
Antiinflammatory				
Dexamethasone				
CNS edema	1—2	IV	24	1
Optic neuritis[d]	0.1	PO, IV, SC	24	3—5

PO, By mouth; *IV*, intravenous; *SC*, subcutaneous; *IM*, intramuscular; *prn*, as needed; *CNS*, central nervous system.
[a]See Appendix 8, Drug Formulary, for more detailed information on these drugs.
[b]Dose per administration at specified interval.
[c]In dogs younger than 6 months of age, dental staining is less of a problem with doxycycline than with tetracycline..
[d]Equivalent glucocorticoid dosage of prednisolone in mg/kg is 5 times this dose.

effectiveness remains unproven. Controlled studies have documented a decrease in morbidity and mortality in children with measles who received two 200,000-IU (60-mg) doses of vitamin A within 5 days of the onset of systemic illness.[79] Although its effectiveness in treating distemper is unproven, a similar regimen could be tried for puppies with acute systemic infection.

Therapy for neurologic disturbances in canine distemper is less rewarding. Progressive multifocal encephalitis usually leads to tetraplegia, semicoma, and incapacitation so great that euthanasia should be recommended. Despite ineffective therapy, dogs should not be euthanized unless the neurologic disturbances are progressive or incompatible with life. Variable or temporary success in halting neurologic signs in some dogs may result from a single anti-CNS edema dose (2.2 mg/kg IV) of dexamethasone. Subsequent maintenance therapy with antiinflammatory doses may be needed, and this treatment can be tapered with time.

Seizures, myoclonus, or optic neuritis are three neurologic manifestations in dogs that can be tolerated by many owners. Myoclonus is usually untreatable and irreversible; many forms of therapy have been attempted without success. Recommendations have been made to administer anticonvulsants after the onset of systemic disease but before the development of seizures. No evidence shows that anticonvulsants prevent entry of the virus into the CNS; however, they may suppress irritable foci from causing seizures, which may prevent seizure circuits from becoming established. Seizures are best treated with parenteral diazepam (5- to 10-mg dose rectally or slow IV) for status epilepticus and phenobarbital for maintenance prevention. Primidone or potassium bromide are alternative choices, and combinations or higher doses may be needed in refractory cases. Glucocorticoid therapy in antiinflammatory to anti-CNS edema dosages may have variable success in controlling the blindness or papillary dilation from optic neuritis or the other neurologic signs associated with vaccine-induced or chronic inflammatory forms of encephalitis.

PREVENTION

The following discussion describes features that are unique to CDV protection; see Chapter 100 and Appendix 1 for overall recommendations on vaccination for canine distemper. Immunity to natural CDV infection is considered long term, and lasting immunity and immunologic homogeneity of the virus have made disease prevention possible through vaccination. Maternal antibody, received in utero and in colostrum from the dam, blocks adequate immunization in puppies for a period after birth and a period after weaning. Maternal antibody to CDV decreases with a half-life of 8.4 days. Three percent of antibody transfer for CDV occurs in utero, and 97% occurs in the colostrum, resulting in an initial titer in nursing newborn puppies that is usually equal to 77% of that in the bitch. A puppy that has not had colostrum is probably protected for at least 1 to 4 weeks. In nursing puppies, nomograms based on the bitch's titer can be used to determine when immunization should be done, although this is not routinely practical. Maternal antibodies are usually absent by 12 to 14 weeks of age. Vaccines for CDV are generally given every 3 to 4 weeks between 6 and 16 weeks of age in puppies that have received colostrum.

After recovery from natural infection or booster vaccination, immunity can persist for years. This protection may be adequate unless the dog is exposed to a highly virulent strain of virus or large quantities of virus or becomes stressed or immunocompromised. After a single distemper vaccination, naive puppies do not generally develop immunity that lasts at least 1 year. Therefore despite the lack of maternal antibody interference, at least two distemper vaccines should be given at 2- to 4-week intervals when first vaccinating colostrum-deprived neonates and in dogs older than 16 weeks. Similarly, and because older vaccinated dogs can still develop distemper, periodic boosters are recommended for this disease, despite the relatively long-lived immunity afforded by vaccination.

Humoral immune mechanisms do not totally explain resistance to CDV. Vaccination with attenuated virus appears to protect previously unvaccinated dogs when it is given IV at least 2 days before exposure to virulent distemper virus, as compared with at least 5 days with SC vaccination.[39] Because of allergic reactions that may develop, CAV-1 and leptospiral antigens should be avoided with IV vaccination. IV or intramuscular (IM) administration should be reserved to protect exposed, unvaccinated dogs. This rapid protection against distemper may be related to immune interference, IFN, or cell-mediated immune mechanisms. Despite a decrease in antibody titer, immunity to distemper after booster or anamnestic vaccination is known to last as long as 7 years, as demonstrated in somewhat isolated, virus-challenged dogs. The duration of protection is much greater than that predicted from antibody titer alone and demonstrates that challenge with virulent organisms is more meaningful than neutralizing antibody titer for predicting the duration of immunity. However, the neutralizing antibody titer is the best indicator of protection against infection.

Nonliving Antigen Vaccines

Inactivated canine distemper whole-virus vaccines do not produce sufficient immunity to prevent infection after challenge exposure (sterile immunity), but vaccinated dogs show an anamnestic immune response and less severe disease than unvaccinated controls. Inactivated vaccines are not available in the United States. They were discontinued when MLV vaccines became available. Inactivated or recombinant products produce shorter immunity that is often bolstered by natural exposure. With improved adjuvants, some animals such as exotic species may be given some protection without any associated risk. Inactivated or recombinant CDV vaccines are recommended in vaccine virus-susceptible wild or exotic species such as ferrets or red pandas. Whereas inactivated whole-virus vaccines have provided inconsistent protection, purified surface glycoproteins (F) of CDV (see Table 3-2) have been used to protect dogs against subsequent experimental challenge with virulent virus.[118,149] Similarly, an inactivated subunit vaccine containing membrane F antigen and H glycoprotein modified into immune-stimulating complexes has been effective in protecting dogs from challenge by virulent virus.[44] Vaccination of puppies born to immune dams with a CAV-2 vector vaccine expressing the F antigen and H glycoprotein was effective against virulent CDV challenge.[49] A vaccine produced by expressing measles virus H protein in Vaccinia virus has been effective in producing neutralizing antibody and protecting dogs against challenge with virulent CDV.[153] Experimental vaccines of recombinant pox or canarypox viruses expressing genes for H proteins of measles or CDV have been tested in mice and dogs.[39,168] A commercial recombinant canarypox-based CDV vaccine is available for dogs (see Chapter 100).[125] A DNA plasmid vaccine containing genes for H and F proteins induced persistent humoral immune responses in mice and protected them against intracerebral challenge.[142] Recombinant vaccines may fail when the interval of booster vaccinations extends beyond 1 year or the vaccines are being used to protect naive pups entering an endemic environment. Protection does not occur until 2 to 3 weeks after the second immunization.

Modified Live-Virus Vaccines

Vaccination with MLV vaccines offers superior protection against CDV infection. Vaccine-induced immunity is never as long lasting as the immune response that occurs after natural or experimental infection with virulent virus. However, despite changes in the H protein of wild-type CDV strains, it is unlikely that virulent CDV strains can break through solid MLV vaccine-induced immunity. Not all MLV distemper vaccines produce the same level of protection.[133] Often, increased potency of protection means higher vaccine virulence. Unfortunately the most potent vaccines have been associated with induced illness, especially in certain wild or immunocompromised domestic carnivores.

Use of MLV vaccines for distemper has led to questions concerning vaccine stability and safety. Efficacy and safety of MLV distemper vaccination in dogs with compromised immune systems are important considerations. Unlike virulent virus, MLV itself does not appear to suppress measurable cell-mediated immunity. However, when CDV has been combined with CAV-1 or CAV-2 antigens, significant suppression in lymphocyte transformation testing response occurred.[67,127] The clinical significance of this suppression is self-limiting and mild.

MLV viruses have not reverted to virulence under natural conditions and do not spread to other dogs. However, reversion to virulence has been experimentally demonstrated in attenuated vaccine virus passed serially in dogs and ferrets or in pulmonary macrophages in tissue culture. Two major types of MLV distemper vaccines exist. The Onderstepoort strain was adapted to chicken embryos and chicken cells. This vaccine strain may produce lower measured levels of humoral immunity[121] but no postvaccinal disease. The canine-cell–adapted Rockborn strain, grown in canine kidney cells, induces high titers of neutralizing antibody and longer term protection. The Snyder Hill strain is indistinguishable from the Rockborn strain. Unfortunately the Rockborn strain occasionally produces a postvaccinal encephalitis in dogs and more commonly in exotic carnivores. Red pandas (*Ailurus fulgens*), black footed ferrets (*Mustela nigripes*), European mink (*Mustela lutreola*), gray foxes (*Urocyon cinereoargenteus*), and African wild dogs (*Lyacon pictus*) are highly susceptible to vaccine-induced illness with MLV vaccines. However, vaccination with an MLV strain provided no untoward effects and good protection in African wild dogs, whereas inactivated vaccine failed to provide adequate immunity.[165] Postvaccinal distemper can be prevented in ferrets by using inactivated virus or recombinant vector vaccines rather than canine-cell–propagated vaccines. Domestic ferrets and lions are less susceptible to vaccine-induced illness and have been successfully vaccinated with MLV Onderstepoort strain vaccines.[89,170]

Encephalitis has been reported in dogs after vaccination with MLV distemper vaccines[41,98,116] (see Postvaccinal Encephalomyelitis, Chapter 100). The Rockborn strains have been the most common cause, although they generally provide very strong protection against the disease. Onderstepoort strain vaccines, which have been adapted to chick embryo or avian cell cultures vaccines, appear safer. The recombinant poxvirus-vectored vaccine is the safest.

MLV vaccination of dams in whelp or during the first few days postpartum has resulted in systemic infection, encephalitis, or both in their puppies.[30,101] CDV vaccine-induced encephalomyelitis has been documented in 3-week-old puppies simultaneously infected with virulent canine parvovirus; however, similar findings were not reported in 11- to 15-week-old puppies.[66] CDV vaccine-induced disease is usually encephalitis, although immunosuppression or neonatal or prenatal infections can result in systemic manifestations. The neurologic signs typically begin 3 to 20 days[41,42,169] after receiving an MLV canine distemper vaccine. The clinical signs vary but often consist of an acute onset of "chewing-gum" or generalized motor seizures, paraparesis, tetraparesis, and vestibular or sensory ataxia. The seizure form is often progressive and difficult to control with anticonvulsants. The ataxic form can be progressive but may improve in some dogs. Unlike naturally acquired infections from virulent virus, the neurologic signs of vaccine-induced illness may stabilize, improve, or disappear with time or antiinflammatory or supportive therapy. Lesions in the CNS may be multifocal and typically involve the gray matter or white matter but are usually most severe in the pontomedullary gray matter (see Pathologic Findings in this chapter). CSF findings are indistinguishable from those of virulent CDV infections. If it could be isolated, vaccine virus could be distinguished by the ease with which it propagates in tissue culture (see Viral Isolation in this chapter) or by genetic analysis of very minor differences of the N gene (see Table 3-2) that have been detected.[98,178] Vaccine virus replication is incomplete in that viral protein mRNAs are expressed, but protein translation is reduced or absent.[116] This makes culture of virus or demonstration by routine histochemistry difficult.

HOD and juvenile cellulitis has also been associated with distemper vaccination in young, growing dogs (see Vaccine-Associated Hypertrophic Osteodystrophy and Juvenile Cellulitis, Chapter 100).[2,76,96,104] Signs usually develop within 10 days of MLV vaccination, but the range has been from 4 days to 3 weeks. All MLV vaccine strains have been associated with this phenomenon. Lesions typical of HOD are detected in the metaphyseal regions of many long bones and sometimes the phalynges (Fig. 3-15). These lesions must be differentiated from metaphyseal osteomyelitis caused by systemic bacteremia in young puppies (see Hematogenous Osteomyelitis, Chapter 86). Weimaraners are the most frequently affected breed, probably because of an immunodeficiency (see Immunodeficiency in Weimaraners, Chapter 95), and some dogs have an associated hypoglobulinemia.[2] Additional laboratory abnormalities include increased activity of serum alkaline phosphatase and neutrophilic leukocytosis. Many dogs have systemic signs including an increased rectal temperature, anorexia, a reluctance to walk, and limb hyperesthesia, especially on palpation of the long bones. In some dogs, especially Weimaraners, multisystemic signs of GI, respiratory, or neurologic disease have been reported.[2] Treatment with restricted activity and nonsteroidal analgesics generally offers temporary or no improvement, and antiinflammatory to immunosuppressive doses of glucocorticoids are often needed for up to 1 week. Dogs that are not treated early may have an extended course of recovery or develop relapses after treatment is discontinued; treatment must be extended for 4 to 6 weeks in these animals. Use of recombinant distemper vaccine in young Weimaraners is suggested, especially if a familial tendency for this syndrome exists. Subsequent vaccination with MLV vaccines after growth is complete does not cause problems in previously affected dogs.

Measles Vaccines

CDV and human measles virus are antigenically related, and experimental infection of dogs with measles virus protected the dogs from subsequent infection with CDV. Distemper virus antibody titers are minimally elevated after measles vaccination despite the adequate protection provided. Cell-mediated immunity and other factors are thought to be the primary elements involved in the protective response. Measles vaccine virus produces a self-limiting, noncontagious infection in the lymphoid system of dogs, an infection similar to that of MLV-CDV vaccines. Danger of reversion to virulence is likely minimal, as is the danger to humans, when proper vaccination procedures are followed. Only measles vaccines licensed for use in dogs (not human products) should be administered by veterinarians. Higher antigen mass in canine products is required because of the heterologous nature of the product.

Theoretically, measles vaccination protects young puppies that have high concentrations of maternal antibodies to distemper. It should only be used as a replacement for the first vaccination in 6- to 12-week-old puppies. Dogs younger than 6 weeks with very high maternal antibody concentrations (serum-neutralizing antibody titer > 1:300) do not respond well to either distemper or measles vaccination. If female puppies are vaccinated with measles vaccine after 12 weeks of age, they will passively transfer measles antibody to their offspring, especially if they are bred during the first heat cycle.

Immunity to distemper acquired from measles vaccination is not only transient but also weaker than that derived from successful vaccination with MLV distemper vaccine. Sterile immunity is not produced after challenge with virulent CDV. SC inoculation of measles vaccine is not as effective as the initially recommended IM route. However, puppies older than 6 weeks immunized with measles virus vaccine are protected within 72 hours of challenge with CDV, despite the lack of increase in distemper virus antibody titer.[38] During an initial vaccination series, measles vaccination alone or in combination with distemper vaccination should be followed by at least two distemper vaccinations to produce adequate long-term immunity of at least 12 months.

Vaccine Failures

Viability of MLV canine distemper vaccines is an important factor in vaccination failures. Lyophilized tissue culture vaccines are stable for 16 months under refrigeration (0° C to 4° C), 7 weeks at 20° C, and 7 days when exposed to sunlight at 47° C. When reconstituted, tissue culture virus remains stable for 3 days at 4° C and 24 hours at 20° C. Vaccine should be used immediately once it is reconstituted for injection, or it

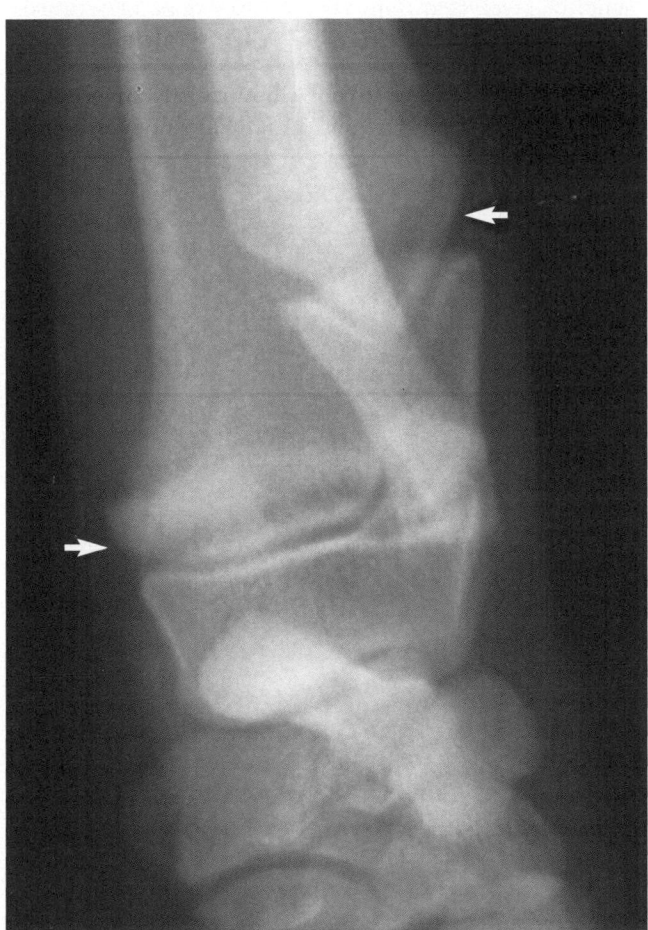

Fig 3-15 Forelimb radiographs from a dog with vaccine-associated HOD. Periosteal reaction can be noted at arrows. (Courtesy University of Georgia, Athens, Ga.)

should be refrigerated if the delay until usage will be longer than 1 hour.

Adverse environmental influences can affect the response to distemper vaccination in dogs. High humidity (85% to 90%) and high temperatures that cause dogs to have rectal temperatures averaging 39.8° C (103.6° F) reduce the immune response after distemper vaccination.[66]

Dogs that received anesthesia (barbiturate induction with halothane maintenance) and underwent surgery were studied for their response to distemper vaccination.[66] The humoral antibody response to vaccination had no demonstrable impairment, although challenge studies were not performed. Some depression of the peripheral blood lymphocyte response to phytohemagglutinin did occur.

Glucocorticoid therapy given at immunosuppressive doses for 3 weeks did not suppress the normal humoral response to distemper vaccine, although treated dogs developed depressed responses to phytohemagglutinin stimulation of lymphocytes.[66] These dogs also survived subsequent challenge with virulent CDV.

Concurrent parvoviral infection has been suspected of reducing the antibody response of dogs vaccinated against canine distemper. Simultaneous vaccination against parvoviral infection was suspected of inhibiting dogs' response to vaccination against CDV infection, although adequate control data were lacking; this finding has not been substantiated in older dogs.[66] (See Chapters 8 and 100 for an additional discussion of canine parvovirus-induced immunologic interference with CDV vaccination.)

Antigenic drift of wild-type CDV strains might cause distemper outbreaks in domestic dog and wild animal populations. Serologic studies of H protein antigens have confirmed recognizable differences in epitopes, as expected from genetic analyses.[75] Because heterotypic vaccination with measles and rinderpest virus offers at least partial protection, it is unlikely that currently available CDV vaccines are ineffective. Unfortunately the current vaccination programs, low vaccination rates, use of less virulent or nonliving vaccines, lapses in booster frequency, and presence of largely unvaccinated, highly susceptible feral or wild canids or other carnivores may contribute to the outbreaks that have been reported. Outbreaks in Europe have been related to reduced population immunity caused by lapses in booster vaccination with concurrent use of chick-embryo–adapted CDV vaccine that produced less immunity than vaccines adapted to canine cell cultures.[47] Outbreaks have occurred in animal shelters where dogs were not vaccinated with an MLV vaccine immediately on entry before being exposed to an endemically infected population of animals.

The broad host range of potential reservoirs makes eradication of this disease difficult. Several measures can be instituted to help control the disease in carnivores. First, every attempt should be made to achieve the highest vaccination rate possible in domestic dogs, especially in areas where they cohabitate or live near feral or wild animal populations. The most potent vaccines that can be tolerated without producing vaccine-induced illness should be used. Use of recombinant products must be considered for exotic carnivores with a high susceptibility to vaccine strains. Unfortunately the shorter duration of immunity of these products necessitates more consistent booster administration and likely chemical restraint. Perhaps after being exposed to products of lesser or no virulence, these animals might better tolerate vaccination with some of the more virulent products. Research is needed to substantiate this possibility. Because of the emerging host range of CDV, exposure to a vaccine strain may be preferred to an epidemic from virulent wild virus. Vaccination of captive and free-ranging wild carnivores should be seriously considered.

Serum Antibody Monitoring and Duration of Immunity

Immunity to MLV canine distemper vaccines is longer than 1 year, despite vaccine label recommendations that annual vaccination of dogs be performed. The American Veterinary Medical Association and American Animal Hospital Association recommendations are for 3-year intervals after the initial series and a 1-year later booster. The clinician decides whether to provide more frequent vaccination based on the animal and environmental considerations. Serum-neutralizing antibody titers are most accurate for withstanding infection, and a serum-neutralizing antibody titer of 1:100 or greater is considered protective when the dog has received maternal antibodies. A serum-neutralizing antibody titer of 1:20 is considered protective when measuring a vaccination response. ELISA-based test kits for use in the clinic are available to determine this response (see Appendix 6). In a study of dogs brought to a veterinary hospital for vaccination, titers decreased with older age and number of years since boosters had been given (see Immunoprophylaxis in Chapter 100).[102] Overall, 25% of all dogs examined required a booster based on marginal titer values; 17% that had received a booster in fewer than 400 days, 24% of those that had received one in 461 to 476 days, and 44% of those receiving one in 787 to 1665 days required boosters.[102] Dogs with prior mean vaccination intervals of 5 years show lower antibody titers.[120]

Environmental Control

CDV is extremely susceptible to common disinfectants. Infected animals are the primary source of the virus, so they should be segregated from other healthy dogs. Dogs usually shed the virus in secretions for 1 to 2 weeks after the acute systemic illness. Those recovering from systemic illness or that are developing later neurologic signs (without systemic disease) may still be shedding some virus.

PUBLIC HEALTH CONSIDERATIONS

Multiple sclerosis (MS) is a neurologic affliction of humans that is similar to subacute sclerosing panencephalitis (SSPE), an encephalitis of humans thought to be caused by a chronic infection with defective or latent measles virus, and chronic progressive distemper encephalitis in dogs. SSPE and chronic progressive distemper encephalitis have similar pathologic findings, with demyelination, glial proliferation, and other findings characteristics of a chronic, persistent nonsuppurative encephalitis. The cause of MS is still uncertain, but no substantial evidence for human measles virus or CDV involvement exists.[77] The evidence for the role of CDV is indirect, and examination of the case control data for reported associations reveals that the existing evidence is weak.[77] Human measles and paramyxovirus are still likely candidates for MS involvement, and herpesviruses have also been implicated.[137] Furthermore, the incidence of MS has not decreased since before 1960, despite the widespread reduction of measles and distemper through effective vaccines.

Some have suggested that Paget's disease, an inflammatory bone disorder in humans, might be related to CDV acquired from exposure to dogs. Paget's disease is a chronic disease that leads to progressive destruction, remodeling, and deformity of bone. Evidence shows that the disease may be caused by chronic paramyxovirus infection of osteoclasts. Nuclei and cytosol of pagetic osteoclasts contain viral-like inclusions. Erythroid and osteoclast cells from patients with Paget's disease express paramyxoviral mRNA.[130] Using in situ hybridization, CDV genetic sequences have been found in the bone of 63.5% of untreated humans with Paget's disease.[37,63,64,65] In a study using in situ hybridization, CDV RNA was detected in 100%

of lesions from pagetic patients but in none of the control specimens, including uninvolved sites of pagetic patients, normal bone, and active remodeling bone.[105] Owning a dog was found to be highly correlated with Paget's disease, but this indirect relationship should not be overstated because a similar correlation was found between Paget's disease and ownership of cats and birds. Other studies have implicated other paramyxoviruses such as measles virus variants.[131,132,136,141] Until such viruses are isolated and completely sequenced, CDV's role if any in such infections is questionable.

SUGGESTED READINGS*

9. Appel MJG. 1969. Pathogenesis of canine distemper. *Am J Vet Res* 30:1167-1182.

13. Appel MJG, Summers BA. 1995. Pathogenicity of morbilliviruses for terrestrial carnivores. *Vet Microbiol* 44:187-191.

39. Chappuis G. 1995. Control of canine distemper. *Vet Microbiol* 44:351-358.

53. Frisk AL, König M, Moritz A, et al. 1999. Detection of canine distemper virus nucleoprotein RNA by reverse transcription-PCR using serum, whole blood, and cerebrospinal fluid from dogs with distemper. *J Clin Microbiol* 37:3634-3643.

72. Haines DM, Martin CAL, Chelack BJ, et al. 1999. Immunohistochemical detection of canine distemper virus in haired skin, nasal mucosa, and footpad epithelium: a method for antemortem diagnosis of infection. *J Vet Diagn Invest* 11:396-399.

92a. Kuehn BM. 2004. Multidisciplinary task force tackles Chicago distemper outbreak. Questions raised about vaccinations. *J Am Vet Med Assoc* 225:1315-1317.

102. McCaw DL, Thompson M, Tate D, et al. 1998. Serum distemper virus and parvovirus antibody titers among dogs brought to a veterinary hospital for revaccination. *J Am Vet Med Assoc* 213:72-75.

111. Moritz A, Frisk AF, Baumgartner W. 2000. The evaluation of diagnostic procedures for the detection of canine distemper virus. *Eur J Comp Anim Pract* 10:37-47.

144. Soma T, Ishii H, Hara M, et al. 2003. Detection of canine distemper virus antigen in canine serum and its application to diagnosis. *Vet Rec* 153:499-501.

*See the CD-ROM for a complete list of references.

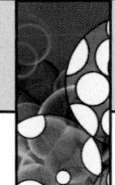

CHAPTER • 4

Infectious Canine Hepatitis and Canine Acidophil Cell Hepatitis

Craig E. Greene

INFECTIOUS CANINE HEPATITIS

Etiology

Infectious canine hepatitis (ICH), caused by canine adenovirus (CAV)-1, has worldwide serologic homogeneity, as well as immunologic similarities to human adenoviruses. It is antigenically and genetically distinct from CAV-2, which produces respiratory disease in the dog (see Etiology and Pathogenesis, Chapter 6). Genetic variants of CAV-2 have been isolated from the intestine of a puppy with hemorrhagic diarrhea and from kenneled dogs with diarrhea. Human adenoviruses have been used as vectors for recombinant vaccine testing in dogs.[16]

As with other adenoviruses, CAV-1 is resistant to environmental inactivation, surviving disinfection with various chemicals such as chloroform, ether, acid, and formalin and is stable when exposed to certain frequencies of ultraviolet radiation. CAV-1 survives for days at room temperature on soiled fomites and remains viable for months at temperatures below 4° C. CAV-1 is inactivated after 5 minutes at 50° to 60° C, which makes steam cleaning a plausible means of disinfection. Chemical disinfection has also been successful when iodine, phenol, and sodium hydroxide are used.

CAV-1 causes clinical disease in dogs, coyotes, foxes, and other Canidae and in Ursidae (bears). The high incidence of naturally occurring neutralizing antibodies in the unvaccinated feral and wildlife dog population suggests that subclinical infection is widespread.[5,7] CAV-1 has been isolated from all body tissues and secretions of dogs during the acute stages of the disease. By 10 to 14 days postinfection (PI), the virus can be found only in the kidneys and is excreted in the urine for at least 6 to 9 months. Aerosol transmission of the virus via the urine is unlikely insofar as susceptible dogs housed 6 inches apart from virus shedders do not become infected. Viral spread can occur by contact with fomites, including feeding utensils and hands. Ectoparasites can harbor CAV-1 and may be involved in the natural transmission of the disease.

Pathogenesis

After natural oronasal exposure, the virus initially localizes in the tonsils (Fig. 4-1) where it spreads to regional lymph nodes and lymphatics before reaching the blood through the thoracic duct. Viremia, which lasts 4 to 8 days PI, results in rapid dissemination of the virus to other tissues and body secretions, including saliva, urine, and feces. Hepatic parenchymal cells and vascular endothelial cells of many tissues are prime targets of viral localization and injury.

Initial cellular injury of the liver, kidney, and eye is associated with cytotoxic effects of the virus. A sufficient antibody response by day 7 PI clears the virus from the blood and liver and restricts the extent of hepatic damage. Widespread centrilobular to panlobular hepatic necrosis is often fatal in experimentally infected dogs, with a persistently low (less than 1:4)

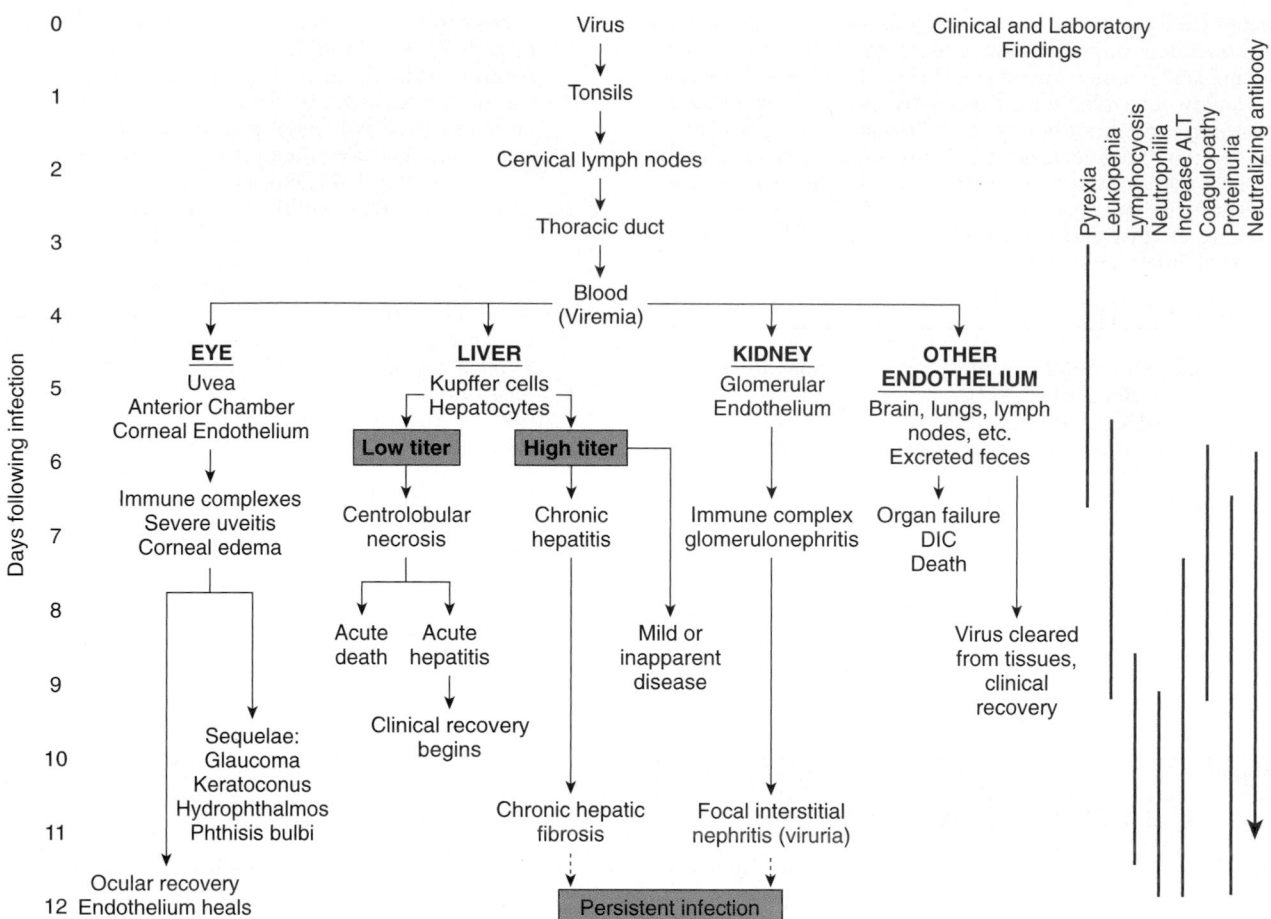

Fig 4-1 Sequential pathogenesis of ICH. Solid vertical bars on the right correspond to the chronologic occurrence and duration of the respective clinical or laboratory findings associated with ICH.

antibody titer. Acute hepatic necrosis can be self-limiting and centrilobularly restricted such that hepatic regeneration occurs in dogs that survive this phase of the disease. Dogs demonstrating a partial neutralizing antibody titer (greater than 1:16, less than 1:500) by day 4 or 5 PI develop chronic active hepatitis and hepatic fibrosis. Persistent hepatic inflammation continues, probably as a result of chronic latent hepatic infection with virus. Dogs with sufficient antibody titers (1:500 or greater) on the day of infection usually show little clinical evidence of disease. Dogs immune to parenteral challenge with CAV-1 are still susceptible to respiratory disease via aerosolized viral particles.

Both virulent and modified live strains of CAV-1 produce renal lesions. Virus detected by positive immunofluorescence and ultrastructural evaluation initially localizes in the glomerular endothelium in the viremic phase of disease and produces initial glomerular injury. An increase in neutralizing antibody at approximately 7 days PI is associated with the glomerular deposition of circulating immune complexes (CICs) and transient proteinuria. CAV-1 is not detected in the glomerulus after 14 days PI; however, it persists in renal tubular epithelium. Tubular localization of the virus is primarily associated with viruria, and only a transient proteinuria is noted. A mild focal interstitial nephritis is found in recovered dogs; however, unlike the liver disease, evidence that chronic progressive renal disease results from ICH cannot be found.

Clinical complications of ocular localization of virulent CAV-1 occur in approximately 20% of naturally infected dogs

and in less than 1% of dogs after subcutaneous–modified live virus (SC-MLV) CAV-1 vaccination. The development of ocular lesions begins during viremia, which develops 4 to 6 days PI; the virus enters the aqueous humor from the blood and replicates in corneal endothelial cells.

Severe anterior uveitis and corneal edema develop 7 days PI, a period corresponding to an increase in neutralizing antibody titer. CIC deposition with complement fixation (CF) results in chemotaxis of inflammatory cells into the anterior chamber and extensive corneal endothelial damage. Disruption of the intact corneal endothelium causes accumulation of edematous fluid within the corneal stroma.

Uveitis and edema are usually self-limiting unless additional complications or massive endothelial destruction occurs. Clearing of corneal edema coincides with endothelial regeneration and restoration of the hydrostatic gradient between the corneal stroma and aqueous humor. Normal recovery of the eye is usually apparent by 21 days PI. If the inflammatory changes are severe enough to block the filtration angle, increased intraocular pressure may result in glaucoma and hydrophthalmos.

Complications are often associated with the pathogenesis of ICH. Dogs are more prone to develop pyelonephritis as a result of renal damage after ICH infection. Disseminated intravascular coagulation (DIC), a frequent complication of ICH, begins in the early viremic phase of the disease and may be triggered by endothelial cell damage, with widespread activation of the clotting mechanism, or by the inability of the diseased liver to remove activated clotting factors. Decreased hepatic synthesis of clotting factors in the face of excessive consumption compounds the bleeding defect.

Although the cause of death in ICH is uncertain, the liver is a primary site of viral injury. Hepatic insufficiency and hepatoencephalopathy may result in a semicomatose state and death. Some dogs die so suddenly that liver damage with resulting hepatic failure does not have time to occur. Death in these dogs may result from damage to the brain, lungs, and other vital parenchymal organs or from the development of DIC.

Clinical Findings

ICH is most frequently seen in dogs younger than 1 year, although unvaccinated dogs of all ages can be affected. Severely affected dogs become moribund and die within a few hours after the onset of clinical signs. Owners frequently believe that their dog was poisoned. Clinical signs in dogs that survive the acute viremic period include vomiting, abdominal pain, and diarrhea with or without evidence of hemorrhage.

Abnormal physical findings in the early phase of infection include increased rectal temperature (39.4° C to 41.1° C [103° F to 106° F]) and accelerated pulse and respiratory rates. Fever may be transient or biphasic early in the course of the disease. Tonsillar enlargement, usually associated with pharyngitis and laryngitis, is common. Coughing and auscultated harsh lower respiratory sounds are manifestations of pneumonia. Cervical lymphadenomegaly is frequently found with SC edema of the head, neck, and dependent portions of the trunk. Abdominal tenderness and hepatomegaly are usually apparent in the acutely ill dog. A hemorrhagic diathesis that is demonstrated by widespread petechial and ecchymotic hemorrhages, epistaxis, and bleeding from venipuncture sites may occur. Icterus is uncommon in acute ICH, but it is found in some dogs that survive the acute fulminant phase of the disease. Abdominal distention is caused by accumulation of serosanguineous fluid or hemorrhage. Central nervous system (CNS) signs, including depression, disorientation, seizures, or terminal coma, may develop at any time after infection.

Clinical signs of uncomplicated ICH frequently last 5 to 7 days before improvement. Persistent signs may be found in dogs with a concurrent viral infection such as canine distemper or in dogs that develop chronic active hepatitis.

Corneal edema and anterior uveitis usually occur when clinical recovery begins and may be the only clinical abnormalities seen in dogs with inapparent infection (also see ICH in Chapter 93). Dogs with corneal edema show blepharospasm, photophobia, and serous ocular discharge. Clouding of the cornea usually begins at the limbus and spreads centrally (Fig. 4-2) (see Fig. 93-12). Ocular pain, present during the early stages of infection, usually subsides when the cornea becomes completely clouded. However, pain may return with the development of glaucoma or corneal ulceration and perforation. In uncomplicated cases, clearing of the cornea begins at the limbus and spreads centrally.

Diagnosis

Early hematologic findings in ICH include leukopenia with lymphopenia and neutropenia. Neutrophilia and lymphocytosis occur later in dogs with uncomplicated clinical recovery. An increased number of dark staining (activated) lymphocytes and nucleated erythrocytes may be found. Serum protein alterations, detectable only on serum electrophoresis, are a transient increase in α_2-globulin by 7 days PI and by a delayed increase in γ-globulin, which peaks 21 days PI.

The degree of increased activities of alanine aminotransferase (ALT), aspartate aminotransferase, and serum alkaline phosphatase (ALP) depends on the time of sampling and the magnitude of hepatic necrosis. These enzyme increases continue until day 14 PI, after which they decline, although

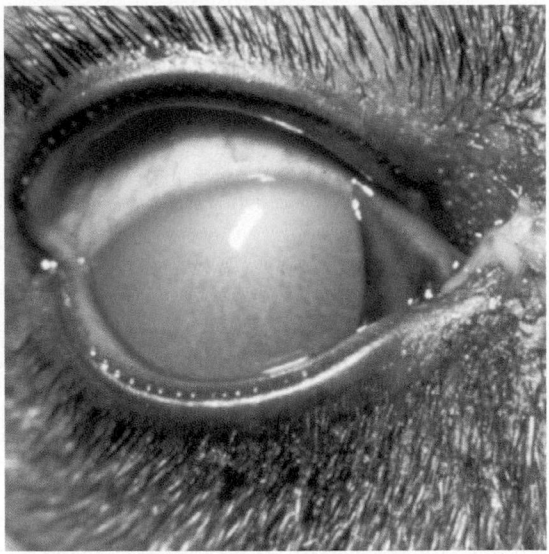

Fig 4-2 Blue eye characteristic of ICH being caused by viral and subsequent immunologic damage to the corneal endothelium. (Courtesy University of Georgia, Athens, Ga.)

persistent or recurrent elevations may be found in dogs that develop chronic active hepatitis. Moderate to marked bilirubinuria is frequently found owing to the low renal threshold for conjugated bilirubin in the dog; hyperbilirubinemia is uncommon. Bromsulphalein retention at 30 minutes may be increased during the acute course of ICH or later in dogs that develop chronic hepatic fibrosis. Hypoglycemia may be found in dogs in the terminal phases of the disease.

Coagulation abnormalities characteristic of DIC are most pronounced during the viremic stages of the disease. Thrombocytopenia with or without altered platelet function is usually apparent. One-stage prothrombin time (PT), activated partial prothrombin time (aPTT), and thrombin time (TT) are variably prolonged. Early prolongation of the aPTT probably results from factor VIII consumption. Factor VIII activity is decreased, and fibrin or fibrinogen degradation products (FDPs) are increased. Platelet dysfunction and later prolongation of the aPTT probably result from increased FDPs. Prolongation of the PT is usually less noticeable.

Proteinuria (primarily albuminuria) is a reflection of the renal damage caused by the virus and can usually be detected on random urinalysis because the concentration is greater than 50 mg/dl. The increase in glomerular permeability can result from localization of the virus in initial stages of infection. Alternatively, as the disease progresses, glomeruli become damaged by CICs or as an effect of DIC. Abdominal paracentesis yields a fluid that varies in color from clear yellow to bright red, depending on the amount of blood present. It is usually an exudate with a protein content ranging from 5.29 to 9.3 g/dl (specific gravity from 1.020 to 1.030).

Bone marrow cytology reflects the dramatic change in leukocytes in the peripheral circulation. Megakaryocytes are absent or decreased during the viremic stage of the disease, and those that are present may have altered morphology.

Cerebrospinal fluid (CSF) is normal in dogs with neurologic signs caused by hepatoencephalopathy; it is usually abnormal in dogs that develop nonsuppurative encephalitis from localization of the virus within the brain. Protein concentration (greater than 30 mg/dl) increases with mononuclear pleocytosis (more than 10 cells/mm³). The aqueous humor also has increased concentrations of protein and cells associated with anterior uveitis.

Results of laboratory procedures previously discussed are suggestive of ICH and are the primary means of making a diagnosis in clinical practice. Antemortem confirmation, although not essential for appropriate therapy, can be obtained by serologic testing, virus isolation, and immunofluorescent evaluation. Serologic tests include indirect hemagglutination assay, CF, immunodiffusion, and enzyme-linked immunosorbent assay. These tests usually show higher titers after infection with virulent virus in contrast with MLV vaccines.

CAV-1 can be isolated because it readily replicates in cell cultures of several species, including dogs. Typical adenovirus-induced cytopathology includes clustering of host cells and detachment from the monolayers with the formation of intranuclear inclusions. When viremia begins, on day 5 PI, CAV-1 can be cultured from any body tissue or secretion. The virus is isolated in the anterior chamber during the mild phase of uveitis before antibody infiltration and immune complex formation. Culturing the virus from the liver of dogs is often difficult because hepatic arginase inhibits viral nucleic acid replication. The virus has not been isolated from the liver later than 10 days PI, even in dogs with chronic active hepatitis, perhaps because viral latency develops. The kidney is the most persistent site of virus localization, and CAV-1 can be isolated from the urine for at least 6 to 9 months after the initial infection.

Immunofluorescent techniques are used experimentally to confirm the presence of virus within various tissues. This method has helped locate the sites of viral replication, the spread of the virus within the cells, and the presence of viral antigen in inclusion bodies. Immunoperoxidase procedures, applied to formalin-fixed, paraffin-embedded tissues, have detected virus in liver tissues stored for up to 6 years. Polymerase chain reaction (PCR) techniques have been developed to detect CAV-1 in biologic specimens and to separate the virus from CAV-2 in clinical specimens without resorting to hemagglutination and neutralization tests.[3,10]

Pathologic Findings

Findings on necropsy or biopsy examination of tissues from dogs can usually confirm a diagnosis of ICH. Dogs that die during the acute phase of the disease are often in good flesh, with edema and hemorrhage of superficial lymph nodes and cervical SC tissue. Icterus is not usually apparent. The abdominal cavity may contain fluid that varies from clear to bright red in color. Petechial and ecchymotic hemorrhages are present on all serosal surfaces. The liver is enlarged, dark, and mottled in appearance, and a prominent fibrinous exudate is usually present on the liver surface and in the interlobar fissures (Fig. 4-3). The gallbladder is thickened and edematous and has a bluish-white opaque appearance. Fibrin may be deposited on other abdominal serosal surfaces, giving them a ground glasslike appearance. Intraluminal gastrointestinal (GI) hemorrhage is a frequent finding. The spleen is enlarged and bulges on the cut surface.

Variable gross lesions in other organs include multifocal hemorrhagic renal cortical infarcts. The lungs have multiple, patchy, gray-to-red areas of consolidation. Hemorrhagic and edematous bronchial lymph nodes are found. Scattered hemorrhagic areas, present on coronal section of the brain, are primarily located in the midbrain and caudal brain stem. Ocular lesions, when present, are characterized by corneal opacification and aqueous humor clouding.

Dogs surviving the acute phase of the disease may have lesions that can be found on subsequent necropsy examination. The liver of those with chronic hepatic fibrosis may be small, firm, and nodular. The kidneys of many dogs that

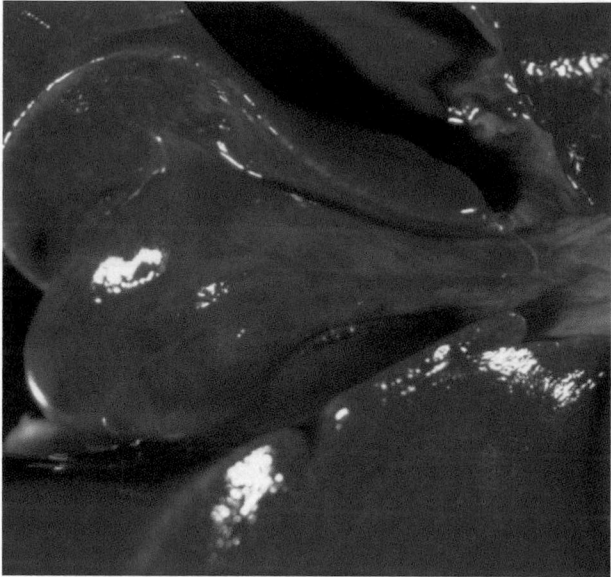

Fig 4-3 Swollen, mottled liver with rounded lobar edges and gallbladder edema characteristic of ICH. (Courtesy University of Georgia, Athens, Ga.)

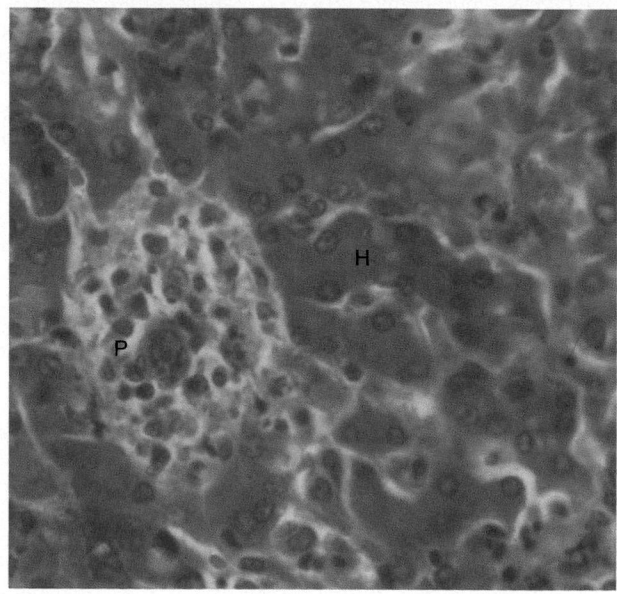

Fig 4-4 Histologic appearance of massive centrolobular necrosis in a fatal case of ICH, which shows a few remaining viable hepatocytes *(H)* around a portal vein *(P)* in the peripheral lobular area (H and E stain, ×250). (Courtesy University of Georgia, Athens, Ga.)

recover are studded with multiple white foci (0.5 cm diameter) extending from the renal pelvis to the outer cortex. Ocular sequelae from the acute disease can include either glaucoma or phthisis bulbi.

Histologic changes in the liver of dogs that die of acute hepatitis include widespread centrilobular to panlobular necroses. In dogs with mild hepatocellular necrosis, the margin between necrotic and viable hepatocytes is sharply defined within the liver lobule (Fig. 4-4). The preservation of the underlying support stroma allows for eventual hepatic regeneration. Only in severe cases does coagulation necrosis of entire hepatic lobules prevent regeneration of the liver. Neutrophilic and mononuclear cell infiltrates are associated with the removal of underlying necrotic tissue. Bile pigment rarely accumulates in most cases because of the transient nature of hepatocellular necrosis and the frequent lack of peripheral lobular involvement of portal radicles. Intranuclear inclusions are initially found in Kupffer's cells and later in viable hepatic parenchymal cells. Subacute to chronic hepatic disease is marked by sporadic foci of necrosis with neutrophilic, mononuclear, and plasma cell infiltration and is found in dogs with partial immunity that survive initial stages of infection.

Historically, CAV-1 has been observed with direct fluorescent antibody in hepatocytes of recovered dogs with chronic hepatic inflammation. PCR and histochemical staining of tissues was used to examine for CAV-1 in the livers of dogs with naturally occurring ICH, chronic active hepatitis, and hepatic fibrosis.[3] Although the ICH cases had positive test results, viral DNA or antigens were not detected in specimens from the other animals.

Widespread histologic alterations occur in other organs as a result of endothelial injury caused by the virus. The gallbladder has marked subserosal edema, but the epithelium remains intact. Viral inclusions are first found in the renal glomeruli but are later found in renal tubular vascular endothelium. Focal interstitial accumulations of neutrophils and mononuclear cells are found in the renal cortex and medulla. These mild changes often progress to focal interstitial fibrosis. Lymphoid organs, including the lymph nodes, tonsils, and spleen, are congested with neutrophilic and mononuclear cell infiltrates. Lymphoid follicles are dispersed with central areas of necrotic foci. Intranuclear inclusions are present in vascular endothelial cells and histiocytes. The lungs have thickened alveoli with septal cell and peribronchial lymphoid accumulations. Alveoli in consolidated areas are filled with an exudate consisting of erythrocytes, fibrin, and fluid. Mucosal and submucosal edema with focal subserosal hemorrhage is found in the intestinal tract. Widespread vascular degeneration and tissue hemorrhage and necrosis are associated with the presence of intravascular fibrin thrombi.

Swollen, desquamated endothelial cells in meningeal vessels contain intranuclear inclusions. Mononuclear cuffing is present around small vessels throughout the parenchyma of the CNS. Mild endothelial proliferation and mononuclear perivascular infiltration persist for at least 3 weeks after clinical recovery.

Ocular changes are characterized by granulomatous iridocyclitis with corneal endothelial disruption and corneal edema. Iridial and ciliary vessels are congested with inflammatory cells that are also present in the iris and filtration angle.

The **inclusion bodies** seen in ICH have been classified as Cowdry type A and are present in both ectodermal and mesodermal tissues. That they are abundant in the liver makes this the most logical tissue for impression smears obtained by biopsy or at necropsy (Fig. 4-5). Initial hypertrophy of the cell nucleus is followed by peripheral margination of the chromatin network and nucleolus, which forms a central, dark-staining nuclear remnant surrounded by a halo of chromatin. The initial inclusions are acidophilic but become basophilic as the chromatin marginates. Care must be taken to distinguish inclusions from faintly staining hepatocyte nucleoli.

Therapy

Clinical management of dogs that develop ICH is primarily symptomatic and supportive. Fulminant hepatic failure from hepatocellular necrosis is a common cause of death in dogs that do not survive the acute stages of the disease. In the absence of complicating factors, clinical recovery and hepatocellular regeneration can occur with centrilobular necrosis. Therapy is supportive until adequate time is available for hepatocellular repair. Because the dogs are frequently semi-

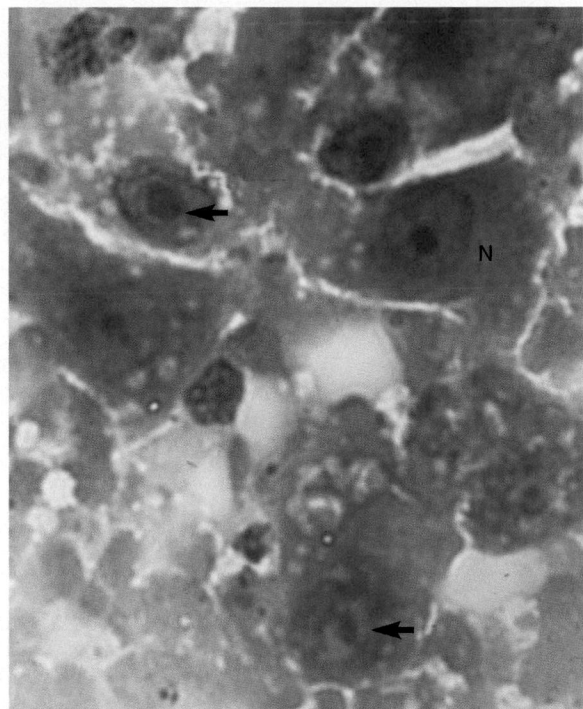

Fig 4-5 Cytologic appearance of intranuclear inclusions in hepatocytes *(arrows)* from an impression smear of liver tissue at necropsy (Wright stain, ×400) from a pup that died of ICH. Compare to hepatocyte nucleolus *(N)*. (Courtesy University of Georgia, Athens, Ga.)

comatose, predicting whether the neurologic signs are related to hepatoencephalopathy or viral encephalitis is impossible. However, this issue can be partially resolved by evaluating blood glucose or ammonia concentrations when therapy is instituted.

Immediate placement of an indwelling intravenous (IV) catheter is a necessity in severely affected dogs; however, because of incoagulability, care must be taken to avoid excessive hemorrhage. Fluid therapy with a polyionic isotonic fluid such as Ringer's solution will correct losses from vomiting and diarrhea and assist in lowering the body temperature. Animals that are too depressed to drink or that continue to vomit must be given daily maintenance fluid requirements (45 ml/kg) by parenteral route.

Treatment of DIC depends on the stage of the clotting deficit. Removal of the inciting stimulus is the initial aim of therapy, but this is not possible in viral diseases. Because of insufficient hepatic synthesis, replacement of clotting factors and platelets by fresh plasma or whole blood may be necessary in conjunction with anticoagulant therapy when marked incoagulability is present.

Because the possibility exists that hypoglycemia is responsible for the comatose state, an IV bolus of 50% glucose (0.5 ml/kg) should be given over a 5-minute period. Hypoglycemia is likely to recur if continuous infusion of hypertonic glucose is not maintained. Hypertonic glucose infusion should be continued at a rate not greater than 0.5 to 0.9 g/kg/hr for efficient utilization. Therapy to decrease the blood ammonia concentration is directed at reducing protein catabolism by colonic bacteria and ammonia resorption in the renal tubules. Ammonia production from protein degradation in the bowel can be reduced by decreasing the quantity of protein intake and by stopping GI hemorrhage. The colon can be evacuated by cleansing and acidifying enemas that relieve bowel stasis and retard ammonia absorption. Nonabsorbable oral antibiotics such as neomycin have been advocated to reduce ammonia-producing bacteria in the intestine, but their effectiveness is questionable. Acidification of the colonic contents can also be achieved by feeding oral lactulose to nonvomiting animals. Renal resorption of ammonia can be reduced by administration of parenteral or oral potassium and correction of the metabolic alkalosis. Urinary acidification with a nontoxic acidifier such as ascorbic acid may greatly reduce ammonia reabsorption by the kidney.

Polyinosinic-polycytidylic acid, an interferon inducer, has been used experimentally to reduce the mortality of dogs experimentally infected with ICH virus, but its clinical application is impractical (see Interferon Inducers, Chapter 100).

Prevention

Maternal Immunity

The duration of passively acquired immunity in the pup is dependent on the antibody concentration of the bitch. The half-life of ICH antibodies is 8.6 days compared with 8.4 days for antibodies to distemper virus, and these values correlate well with the half-life for canine globulin (see Maternal Immunity, Chapter 100). Immunization for ICH is usually successful when maternal antibody titers decrease below 100, which may occur beginning at 5 to 7 weeks of age. The level of ICH maternal antibodies in the newborn pup declines to negligible concentrations by 14 to 16 weeks.

Vaccination

Canine hepatitis caused by CAV-1 has been effectively controlled and practically eliminated from the domestic dog population because of vaccination. Sporadic cases are still seen in which dogs do not get adequate vaccination during puppyhood. Because the virus is environmentally resistant and has a reservoir in wild carnivore, vaccination must be continued as a core antigen for all dogs. Inactivated CAV-1 vaccines do not produce any lesions in vaccinated dogs, but they must be given frequently to equal the protection afforded by MLV vaccines. MLV vaccines can be given every 3 to 5 years because they provide long-term protection, and infections are never reported in adult animals that received an adequate puppyhood series. Adjuvants must be added to inactivated products to make them more immunogenic; however, this also makes them potentially more allergenic than MLV vaccines. Annual revaccination against ICH with an inactivated CAV-1 vaccine provides continuous protection against infection. These products are not available in the United States.

An inactivated CAV-2 vaccine was tested for use in dogs against challenge infection with CAV-2 infection. Dogs received two doses of vaccine at a 14-day interval and were challenged 14 days after the second dose. All dogs became seropositive after vaccination but had mild clinical signs of infection compared with challenged unvaccinated dogs. The clinical usefulness of this vaccine remains to be determined, and long-term protection studies are needed.

In contrast to inactivated vaccines, modified live CAV-1 vaccines can produce lifelong immunity with a single dose. A potential disadvantage of MLV vaccines, however, has been that vaccine virus localizes in the kidney and causes mild subclinical interstitial nephritis and persistent shedding of vaccine virus. Increased passage of the virus in cell culture can reduce the incidence of urinary shedding. Ocular localization with associated anterior uveitis occurs in approximately 0.4% of dogs after IV and SC injection. IV CAV-1 vaccination produces a transient systemic illness characterized by pyrexia and tonsillar enlargement and a 20% incidence of anterior uveitis. A summary of the pathogenicity of modified live CAV-1

Table • 4-1

Comparison of Pathogenicity of Modified Live Canine Adenovirus Vaccines

ROUTE ADMINISTERED	CLINICAL SIGNS OBSERVED	
	CAV-1[a]	CAV-2[b]
Intravenous	Fever Uveitis (20%) Urinary shedding	Fever Mild respiratory disease Tonsillitis
Intranasal	None	Mild respiratory disease
Intraocular (anterior chamber)	Uveitis (100%)	Uveitis (100%)
Intramuscular or subcutaneous	Uveitis rare (0.4%), urinary shedding (some strains)	None

[a]Canine adenovirus 1.
[b]Canine adenovirus 2.

vaccine and a comparison with that for CAV-2 vaccine are listed in Table 4-1.

Some CAV-1 and CAV-2 strains are known to be oncogenic in hamsters, but those in commercial vaccines do not appear to produce this side effect. Oncogenic reactions in dogs have not been reported in more than 20 years of field use of these products.

CAV-2 vaccines have been developed as an alternative in the prevention of ICH. Modified live CAV-2 vaccine rarely, if ever, produces ocular or renal disease when given intramuscularly or SC, although the vaccine virus may localize in and be shed from the upper respiratory tract. The vaccine produces ocular lesions only when experimentally injected into the anterior chamber. Given IV and intranasally (IN), modified live CAV-2 vaccine may produce a mild respiratory disease with associated coughing and tonsillar enlargement, although such an infection has been shown to be subclinical and self-limiting. More severe respiratory signs might develop with CAV-2 vaccine with secondary bacterial infections. Care should be taken to avoid aerosolizing the vaccine when it is given by the IM or SC routes. Dogs are adequately protected by the heterotypic antibody titer against CAV-1 infection if CAV-2 vaccine is used; however, the homotypic antibody response is usually greater. CAV-2 vaccine was experimentally given to 3- to 4-week-old pups in an attempt to break through the heterotypic maternal antibodies to ICH virus. Although parenteral vaccination at this age was ineffective, IN vaccination produced a delayed antibody response to CAV-2 and a weak response to CAV-1, 4 to 8 weeks later. Modified live CAV-2 probably localized in the respiratory tract until maternal antibody declined and then spread systemically, stimulating an immune response.

The recommended schedule with any vaccine for ICH involves at least two vaccinations 3 to 4 weeks apart at 8 to 10 and 12 to 14 weeks of age. This is most commonly accomplished through the combination of this antigen with the canine distemper virus vaccination protocol (see Immunoprophylaxis, Chapter 100, and Appendix 1). Earlier and more frequent vaccination may be advised in areas of high prevalence. Sporadic ICH infection will be noted in puppies when their vaccinations are delayed. Annual vaccination is often recommended but is probably not essential because of the long-standing immunity produced by MLV vaccines.

CANINE ACIDOPHIL CELL HEPATITIS

A hepatitis distinct from ICH and characterized by acute, persistent, or chronic forms was described in Great Britain.[11] Evidence implying that this syndrome has an infectious nature came from the high prevalence of hepatocellular carcinoma in dogs. The agent, suspected to be a virus, has not been identified, although the disease can be reproduced by inoculating bacteriologically sterile liver homogenates not containing CAV-1 and CAV-2 from spontaneously affected animals into experimental dogs. Presumably, acute infections with this agent lead to acute to chronic hepatitis; cirrhosis with multilobular hyperplasia; and, in some cases, hepatocellular carcinoma.[12]

Clinical findings in the early phase of the illness can be vague and include variable fever, inappetence, vomiting, and abdominal pain, but fever is usually lacking. Terminal clinical signs include abdominal distention with ascites, episodes of seizures, mental status abnormalities, and semicoma.

The only consistent laboratory abnormalities include episodic increased ALT and ALP activities. Diagnosis involves gross and microscopic examination of liver tissue. Gross biopsy or necropsy findings include hepatomegaly with rounded lobe edges and enlarged tonsils, regional lymph nodes, and Peyer's patches. Chronically affected dogs may have reduced hepatic size with exaggerated delineation of the portal radicles or nodular proliferation. Increased fibrous tissue is apparent histologically, both centrally and peripherally. Acidophil cells are scattered throughout hepatic lesions and are characterized by angular cytoplasm with acidophil cytoplasm and hyperchromatic nucleus.

Therapy for this condition is uncertain, and it appears to progress with time. Prevention would not seem plausible until the nature of the suspected infectious agent is determined. Although reported only in Great Britain, the disease may be more widespread. It should be suspected when a high frequency of chronic active hepatitis or hepatic fibrous, hepatocellular carcinoma is reported.

SUGGESTED READINGS*

3. Chouinard L, Martineau D, Forget C, et al. 1998. Use of polymerase chain reaction and immunohistochemistry for detection of canine adenovirus type 1 in formalin-fixed, paraffin-embedded liver of dogs with chronic hepatitis or cirrhosis, *J Vet Diagn Invest* 10:320-325.
11. Jarrett WFH, O'Neil BW. 1985. A new transmissible agent causing acute hepatitis, chronic hepatitis and cirrhosis in dogs. *Vet Rec* 116:629-635.
19. Pratelli A, Martella V, Elia G, et al. 2001. Severe enteric disease in an animal shelter associated with dual infections by canine adenovirus type 1 and canine coronavirus, *Vet Med B Infect Dis Vet Public Health* 48:385-392.

*See the CD-ROM for a complete list of references.

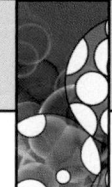

CHAPTER • 5

Canine Herpesvirus Infection

Craig E. Greene and Leland E. Carmichael

ETIOLOGY

Canine herpesvirus (CHV) has a worldwide distribution, with biologic and pathogenic properties similar to α-herpesviruses affecting other species. α-Herpesviruses are cytocidal, causing tissue necrosis and localized mucosal or generalized systemic infection in young or immunosuppressed animals. Recovery is associated with a lifelong latent infection, usually localized to nerve ganglia. CHV has a relatively narrow host specificity compared with other members of the α-herpesviruses. CHV only infects dogs or canine tissue cells. Specific receptors on the cell surface have been identified that contribute to this specificity.[14] Although an antigenic relationship to human herpes simplex virus has not been confirmed, CHV shares approximately 51% genetic homology with feline herpesvirus type 1 (FHV-1).[25] An antigenic relationship between the canine and feline herpesviruses has also been confirmed in immunoblots with polyvalent or monoclonal antibodies (MAB).[8,32] One differentiating feature between these viruses is their glycoprotein D hemagglutinins, which offer selective adherence to cells from their like species and may partially explain the species specificity of these viruses.[11] Less defined immunologic relationships exist between CHV and herpesviruses isolated from harbor seals *(Phoca vitulina)*.[7] Analysis of CHV isolates by restriction endonuclease cleavage of viral DNA revealed differences in the viruses isolated from unrelated individuals, but cleavage patterns of isolates derived from members of the same litter were indistinguishable.[33]

CHV, as an enveloped virus, is readily inactivated by exposure to most disinfectants, to lipid solvents (e.g., ether, chloroform), and to heat above 40° C (56° C for 5 to 10 minutes, 37° C for 22 hours, and longer at 34° C to 35° C). Like other herpesviruses, CHV is readily inactivated at −20° C unless stabilizing solutions are added, when it is stable at −70° C. It is stable at a pH between 6.5 and 7.6 but is rapidly destroyed below pH 5.0 or above pH 8.0.

CHV has a restricted host range and appears to infect only domestic and wild Canidae or canine cell cultures, especially primary or secondary kidney or testicular cells. The virus causes a rapidly spreading, highly destructive cytopathic clear plaque effects in cell cultures with formation of type A intranuclear inclusions; some isolates induce syncytial cell formation (see Viral Isolation in this chapter). Although CHV has not been reported in cats, it is unclear whether an FHV-1 isolate from a pup with a distemper-like syndrome and pancreatic atrophy causes canine infections. Young pups given large (>10[6]) doses of this FHV-1 virus by multiple routes failed to develop clinical illness or histopathologic changes.[8] Cross-species infections with herpesviruses may be established in unnatural hosts through artificial means. A nonpathogenic strain of human herpes simplex virus 1 was injected into the brain of normal dogs, establishing a latent infection with no pathologic changes.[28]

The replication of CHV is similar to that of other α-herpesviruses. Synthesis of viral DNA and nucleocapsids occurs within the host cell nucleus, with the viral envelope being acquired at the nuclear membrane. Virus is transported through the endoplasmic reticulum and Golgi apparatus to the cell surface and released, although most of the virus remains intracellular.

Equine herpesvirus 9 (EHV-9) is a neurotropic virus that infects horses. Dogs challenged intranasally with EHV-9 developed a fulminant nonsuppurative encephalitis.[36] The forebrain was predominantly affected, and virus was detected in neurons. Dogs also had bronchopneumonia and clinical signs of weight loss, fever, anorexia, and neurologic symptoms. The clinical significance of natural infections is unknown.

EPIDEMIOLOGY

CHV is not stable in the environment, but it is maintained in nature by persistence in its canine host. CHV is a temperature-sensitive virus, with optimal replication at temperatures less than 37° C. It persists in the ganglionic and lymphoid tissues of the oronasal and genital mucosae. As with other herpesviruses, lifelong latent infections are typical. When infections reactivate, CHV replicates in the cooler temperatures of the mucous membranes, and shedding occurs. Virus reshedding occurs sporadically, usually when animals are stressed, such as those in high population densities, those being transported, those that are pregnant, or those that are receiving immunosuppressive therapy. Transmission occurs through direct contact with mucosal secretions from the respiratory or genital tract of infected animals. Serologic surveys in dogs have ranged from 30% to as high as 100% in some kennels.[21,5] Despite these high rates of exposure, clinical disease may not be evident. Pups that are born in these environments are exposed at birth but have no symptoms. Factors that predispose neonatal pups to generalized infection are hypothermia and poorly developed immune systems.

PATHOGENESIS

Newborn puppies can acquire CHV infection in utero, from passage through the birth canal, from contact with infected littermates, from oronasal secretions of the dam, or from fomites (although this is rare). A systemic cell-associated viremia is possible in immunoincompetent or immunosuppressed hosts. Neonatal puppies experimentally infected when they are younger than 1 week are particularly susceptible to fatal generalized infections; dogs older than 2 weeks at the time of infection are relatively resistant and generally develop mild or inapparent clinical illness. Virus replication in older dogs is restricted to the nasopharynx, genital tract, tonsils, retropharyngeal lymph nodes, bronchial lymph nodes, and occasionally lungs. Virus may be harbored in the tonsils and parotid salivary gland.[3] The breed of dog may play an important role in immunity. Adult European red foxes (*Vulpes vulpes*) developed systemic and respiratory illness after exper-

imental intravenous (IV) challenge that produced mild signs in adult domestic dogs.[22] Mucosal immune mechanisms are likely important in natural infection because adult foxes given the same challenge by mouth (per os) had no clinical disease but seroconverted.[22] In experimental studies, route of inoculation has also been shown to be important in the spread and tissue localization of virus. Dogs given CHV intranasally (IN) or both IN and IV had virus isolated from nasal secretions.[12] Dogs given an intravaginal inoculation had virus isolated in both nasal and vaginal secretions. Two to 4 months after inoculation, necropsies were performed on the animals, and CHV could not be cultured from any tissues. However, using the polymerase chain reaction (PCR), the CHV genome was found in trigeminal ganglia and retropharyngeal lymph nodes, regardless of the inoculation route. Convalescent dogs also had the viral genome in the lumbosacral ganglia, tonsils, and mediastinal and hypogastric lymph nodes.[12] However, the CHV genome could not be detected in peripheral blood mononuclear cells. Within the trigeminal and lumbosacral ganglia and associated lymph nodes, virus is localized in the neurons or intranuclear in lymphocytes during this quiescent period. These are likely sites for latency, and recrudescence results in virus replicating and shedding from the respiratory and genital mucosae.

In Utero Infection

Although neonatal infection usually is acquired at or soon after birth, transplacental transmission may also occur. The effects of transplacental infection with CHV depend on the stage of gestation at which infection occurs (Fig. 5-1). Infer-

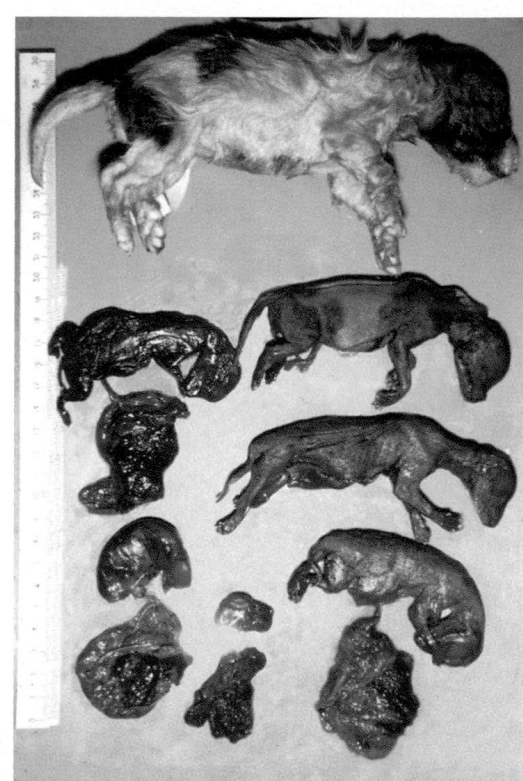

Fig 5-1 Pups delivered by cesarean section from pregnant bitch 31 days after experimental IV infection with CHV. Two fetuses are partially mummified. (From Hashimoto A, Hirai K, Suzuki Y, et al. 1983. Experimental transplacental transmission of canine herpesvirus in pregnant bitches during the second trimester of gestation. *Am J Vet Res* 44:610–614.)

tility and abortion of stillborn or weak pups with no clinical signs in the dam have been reported. Although some puppies may survive such in utero infections and appear normal after delivery by cesarean section, others harbor the virus inapparently in their tissues. However, most pups develop systemic herpesvirus infection within 9 days of birth.

Systemic Neonatal Infection

After oronasal exposure, CHV is first detected in the nasal epithelium and pharyngeal tonsils (Fig. 5-2). Primary replication occurs in epithelial cells and mucosa within 24 hours postinoculation. The virus then enters the blood stream by way of macrophages. Intracellular viremia results in viral spread throughout the body within 3 to 4 days after inoculation. Localization in the mononuclear phagocytic cells of the lymph nodes and spleen results in cell-to-cell spread and lymphoid hyperplasia and necrosis. Progressive multifocal hemorrhagic necrosis occurs in several organs; the highest concentrations of virus are found in the adrenal glands, kidneys, lungs, spleen, and liver. Multifocal hemorrhage associated with necrotic lesions may be related to the vasculitis and marked thrombocytopenia that occurs during infection. Thrombocytopenia may result from disseminated intravascular coagulation associated with widespread vascular endothelial damage and tissue necrosis.

Ganglioneuritis of the trigeminal nerve is a frequent lesion in puppies infected by oronasal exposure. CHV may travel up the nerve axons to the central nervous system (CNS), as does herpes simplex virus in humans. Meningoencephalitis commonly occurs in oronasally infected neonatal puppies, but CNS signs are not always apparent. Under normal circumstances, puppies usually die from systemic illness before neurologic signs are manifest.

Several factors, including temperature regulation and immune status, are involved in the abrupt development of resistance to infection that occurs between 1 and 2 weeks of age. Optimal growth of CHV in cell cultures has been shown to occur between 35° C and 36° C. The normal rectal temperature of adult dogs, 38.4° C to 39.5° C (101° F to 103° F), is above the critical range. Temperature regulation of the newborn pup is not developed until 2 to 3 weeks of age, and rectal temperature is usually 1° C to 1.5° C (2° F to 3° F) lower than that of the adult dog. In addition to having a reduced capacity for temperature regulation, neonatal pups are incapable of adequate fever production. Cell-mediated immune functions are also suppressed at temperatures lower than 39° C, rendering hypothermic pups more susceptible not only to CHV but also to vaccinal distemper and canine adenovirus infection. Puppies 4 to 8 weeks of age are normally clinically asymptomatic after infection, but they develop systemic CHV infection if their body temperatures are artificially reduced. Conversely, elevation of the environmental temperature and consequently the body temperature of CHV-infected puppies younger than 1 week results in reduction of the severity of infection; it does not eliminate the infection.

Immunity acquired from the dam also appears to be important in the survival of infected puppies. Pups nursing seronegative bitches develop a fatal multisystemic illness when they are infected with CHV. In contrast, puppies suckling seropositive bitches become infected but remain asymptomatic, and the virus is recovered primarily from their oropharyngeal region. Maternal antibody or immune lymphocytes acquired through the milk may explain why naturally infected bitches that give birth to diseased puppies, with rare exception subsequently give birth to healthy litters. Serum antibody titers in previously infected pregnant bitches may also suppress viremia and spread of infection to the fetus.

Adult Genital Infection

Occasionally herpesviruses have been isolated from papulovesicular lesions of the canine genital tract; such lesions may be recurrent episodes in previously infected bitches. With CHV, localized genital or respiratory infections and viral shedding can occur in the presence of circulating antibodies. Infection of the genital tract generally appears to be asymptomatic or limited to vaginal hyperemia with hyperplastic lymphoid

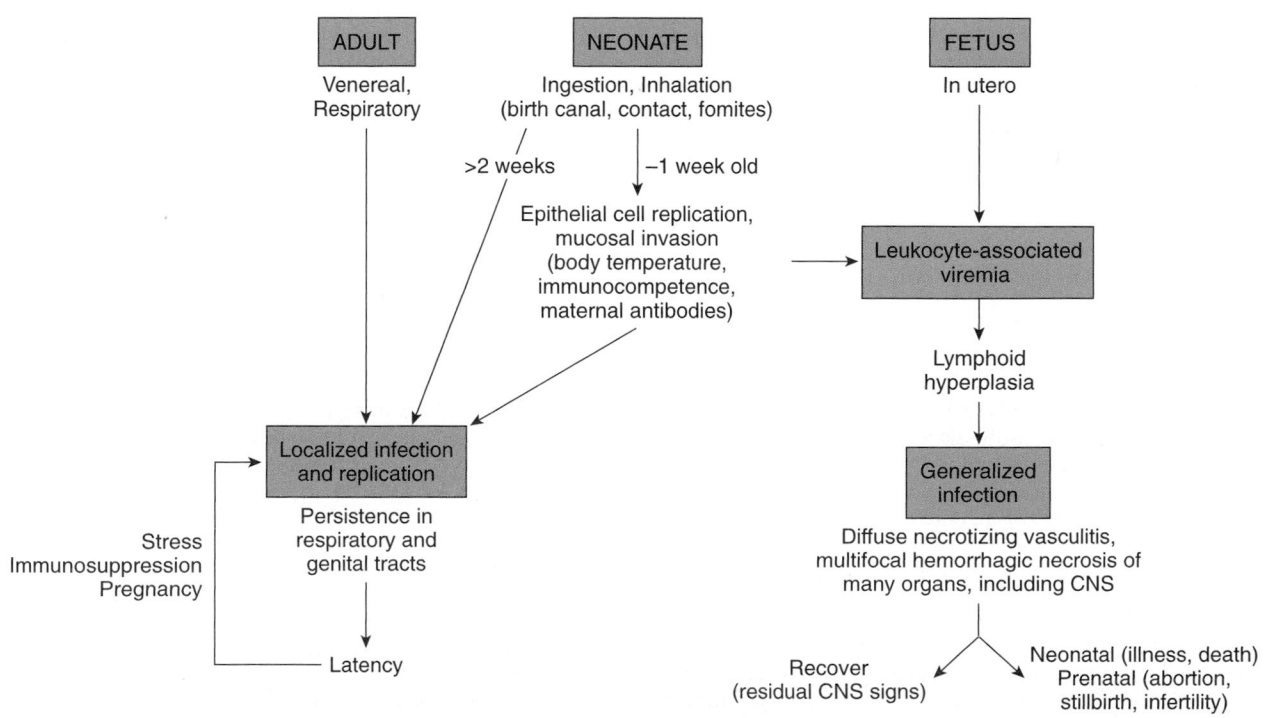

Fig 5-2 Pathogenesis of CHV infection.

follicles. Genital localization of the virus in adult dogs may be a means of venereal transmission of the virus, but it is most important as a source of infection for pups at birth. Spread of CHV from seropositive males to susceptible females at the time of breeding does not appear to be a significant mode of transmission, although such a mechanism is believed to occur. PCR has shown persistence of the virus in the lumbosacral ganglion, with presumed recrudescence and mucosal replication with subsequent shedding.[3,12]

Adult Respiratory Infection

Field evidence suggests that CHV might be a cause of respiratory disease, but studies have failed to incriminate CHV as a primary cause of respiratory illness. Although of uncertain significance, CHV has been recovered from the lungs of dogs with distemper and from dogs with acute conjunctivitis. Neonates that recover from CHV infections or older dogs that have subclinical infections have periodic episodes of viral recrudescence in their oronasal secretions. Viral latency has been demonstrated in intranasally infected dogs for as long as 6 months after infection, with recrudescence occurring within 1 week after treatment with glucocorticoids or antilymphocyte serum. Recrudescence of latent virus also has been demonstrated in seropositive adults after being exposed to seronegative juveniles, suggesting a stress mechanism for CHV transmission that is similar to that of FHV infection. Reactivation of latent infections with asymptomatic shedding of virus from nasal, oral, ocular, and vaginal secretions occurred in most bitches given repeated high immunosuppressive doses of glucocorticoids.[18] Recrudescence is a plausible explanation for subclinical persistence and the rare recurrences of abortions, fetal infections, or neonatal illnesses. It also serves as a mode of viral transmission to susceptible dams, especially when they are in a kennel for breeding.

CLINICAL FINDINGS

Neonatal Puppies

No premonitory signs of illness or history of neonatal mortality is seen in bitches with litters of puppies that die of CHV. Transplacental infections may occur at mid to late gestation and can result in abortion of mummified or dead fetuses, premature or stillborn pups, or weak or runt newborn puppies. Death of neonatal puppies younger than 1 week appears to be less common and probably indicates in utero infection. Among puppies born alive within a litter, some may not be affected, and the gestational age when illness occurs may vary among those that are affected.

CHV infection in postnatally infected puppies is associated with an acute and fatal illness, primarily occurring between 1 and 3 weeks of age. If affected when older than 3 weeks, pups have disseminated CHV infection that is believed to be exacerbated by concurrent infection or immunosuppression. Infected puppies appear dull and depressed, lose interest in nursing, lose body weight, and pass soft, yellow-green feces. They cry persistently and show discomfort during abdominal palpation. Despite the continued muscular activity associated with crying, restlessness, and shivering, the pups have no elevation in body temperature. Rhinitis is frequently manifest by serous to mucopurulent or, although rare, hemorrhagic nasal discharges. Petechial hemorrhages are widespread on the mucous membranes. An erythematous rash consisting of papules or vesicles and subcutaneous edema of the ventral abdominal and inguinal region are occasionally noted. Vesicles are occasionally present in the vulva and vagina of the female puppies, prepuce of the males, and the buccal cavity. Puppies lose consciousness and may have opisthotonos and seizures just before death. Rectal temperatures become subnormal

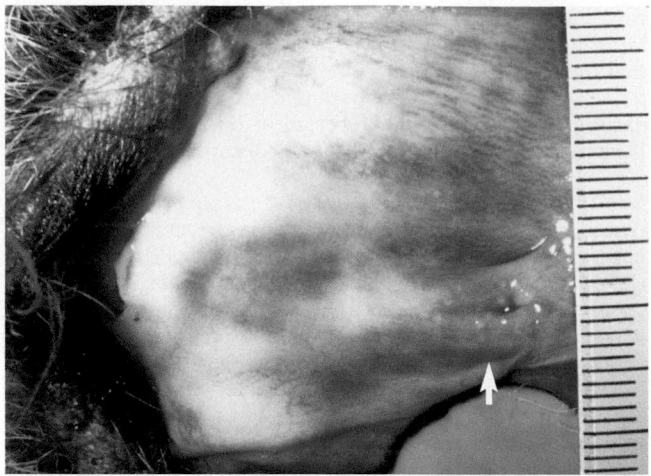

Fig 5-3 CHV vaginitis. *Arrow* points to vesicular lesion. (Courtesy Akira Hashimoto, Hokkaido University, Sapporo, Japan.)

before death, which usually occurs within 24 to 48 hours after the onset of clinical illness.

Some puppies develop mild clinical disease with subsequent recovery. Animals that survive the systemic infection are likely to have persistent neurologic signs. Ataxia, blindness, and cerebellar vestibular deficits are most common.

Older Puppies and Adult Dogs

Dogs older than 3 to 5 weeks develop a mild or inapparent upper respiratory infection as a result of CHV. Signs of systemic infection are rare in older pups; however, vomiting, anorexia, depression, serous ocular discharge, hepatomegaly, and sudden death have been reported in naturally infected 8- to 10-week-old coyote pups (see Chapter 93 for a discussion of ocular lesions).

Primary genital infections in older female dogs are characterized by lymphofollicular lesions, variable degrees of vaginal hyperemia, and occasionally petechial or ecchymotic submucosal hemorrhage (Fig. 5-3). No discomfort or vaginal discharge is noted in affected pregnant dogs, even in those who had abortions or stillbirths. Vesicular lesions have been noted during the onset of proestrus and regress during anestrus. Male dogs with similar lesions over the base of the penis and preputial reflection may have a preputial discharge.

DIAGNOSIS

Clinical Laboratory Findings

The determination of CHV infection in neonatal pups usually depends on information obtained from the clinical history, physical examination, and characteristic pathologic changes seen in affected puppies. Hematologic and biochemical abnormalities are nonspecific, but marked thrombocytopenia may be observed. A marked increase in the alanine aminotransferase activity can be found in infected neonates.

Viral Isolation

CHV can be isolated from several parenchymal organs of puppies dying of acute systemic infection but are most commonly obtained from the adrenal glands, kidneys, lungs, spleen, lymph nodes, and liver. In animals that have recovered or are older, growth of CHV is usually restricted to the oral mucosa, upper respiratory tract, and external genitalia. Viral isolation has not been demonstrated later than 2 to 3 weeks after infection. As noted, viral recrudescence may be provoked by immunosuppressive doses of glucocorticoids and may also be caused by stressful situations, such as the introduction of unfamiliar dogs into a kennel.

CHV grows only in cultured cells of canine origin, primarily in dog kidney cells at an optimal temperature range of 35° C to 37° C. Infected cells become rounded and detach from the glass surfaces, leaving clear plaques surrounded by necrotic cells. Plaque formation is best observed by overlaying monolayers with semisolid media such as agar or methylcellulose. Plaque morphology has been used as a marker for virus pathogenicity. CHV produces Cowdry type A intranuclear inclusions, which can be difficult to demonstrate and are best revealed in tissues that have been fixed in Bouin's fluid. Multinucleation of infected cells is unusual with CHV, but it has been observed with one isolate from the canine genital tract. Fluorescent antibody techniques, electron microscopy, and PCR can be used to detect CHV in tissues and cell cultures (Fig. 5-4). Although not routine, screening animals for infection is best done by viral detection during recrudescence with respiratory or genital signs. PCR has shown that latent herpesvirus infections are prevalent in asymptomatic dogs.[3]

Serologic Testing

Serologic testing for CHV antibodies has been based on virus neutralization (VN) tests, which rely on reduction in cytopathogenicity or plaque formation. An enzyme-linked immunosorbent assay and an hemagglutination inhibition assay also have been developed.[15,23,30,33] Neutralizing antibodies increase after infection and may remain high for only 1 to 2 months; low titers may be detected for at least 2 years. Seropositivity merely indicates exposure, not necessarily active infection, although viral persistence and latent infection might be presumed. Serum neutralization titers increase after treatment of convalescent animals with dexamethasone, presumably because of reactivation of latent infection.[12] Because serologic tests are not standardized, variations in the level and prevalence of positive results can be expected among laboratories.

Organism Detection

Virus can be isolated from tissues of fatally infected pups using primary canine lung or kidney cells. Nucleic acid detection has been evaluated in suspected cases of spontaneous CHV infection and is the most reliable means of detecting latent infection in older animals. Nested PCR and in situ hybridization was used to detect virus in formalin-fixed, paraffin-embedded tissues from naturally infected puppies.[26] Viral nucleic acid has been found within nuclei adjacent to and within hemorrhagic lesions in pups. Many epithelial cells, neurons, fibrocytes, cardiac myocytes, and hepatocytes contain virus. Nucleic acid testing for CHV is offered by at least one commercial laboratory (see Appendix 5, HealthGene, Inc., Toronto, Can.).

PATHOLOGIC FINDINGS

Gross lesions of fatal CHV infection in neonates include diffuse multifocal hemorrhage and gray discoloration in various parenchymal organs, especially the kidney, liver, and lungs (Figs. 5-5 and 5-6). On cut surface, the kidney lesions consist of wedge-shape hemorrhages radiating outward from the renal pelvis. These wedge-shape renal lesions are caused by CHV-induced fibrinoid necrosis of interlobular arteries.[35] Serous to hemorrhagic fluid is usually present in the pleural and peritoneal cavities. The lungs are usually firm and edematous with pronounced hyperemia and focal areas of hemorrhage; the bronchial lymph nodes are markedly enlarged. Splenomegaly and generalized lymphadenomegaly are consistent findings. Petechial hemorrhages are often distributed throughout the serosal surfaces of the intestinal tract. Icterus has been rarely reported.

Histologic findings in disseminated infections of neonates are characterized by foci of perivascular necrosis with mild cellular infiltration in the lung, liver, kidney, spleen, small intestine, and brain. Less severe lesions develop in the stomach, pancreas, adrenal glands, omentum, retina, and myocardium. The lymph nodes and spleen show reactive hyperplasia of mononuclear phagocyte elements. Multifocal necrotizing lesions have been described in the placentas of pregnant bitches and the pups that acquired infection in utero. Cutaneous or mucosal lesions, which may be seen as the primary lesions in older infected animals, consist of various sizes of vesicles produced by profound degeneration of the

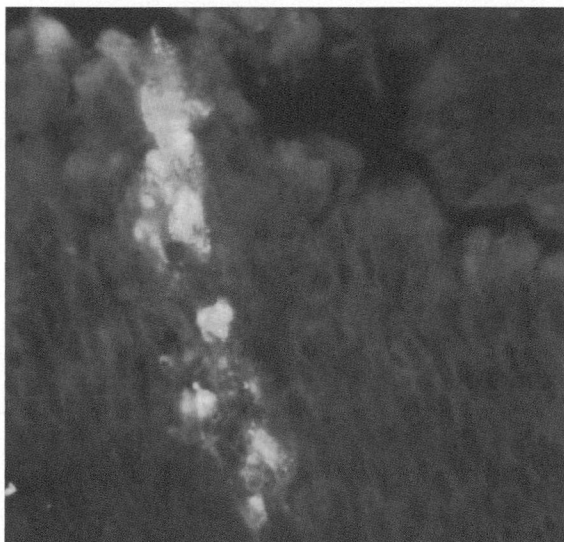

Fig 5-4 Focus of herpesvirus-infected cells in nasal turbinate epithelium from a 12-week-old pup inoculated with CHV (fluorescent antibody method, ×125). (From Appel MJG, Menegus M, Parsonson IM, et al. 1969. Pathogenesis of canine herpesvirus in specific-pathogen–free dogs: 5- to 12-week-old pups. *Am J Vet Res* 30:2067–2073.)

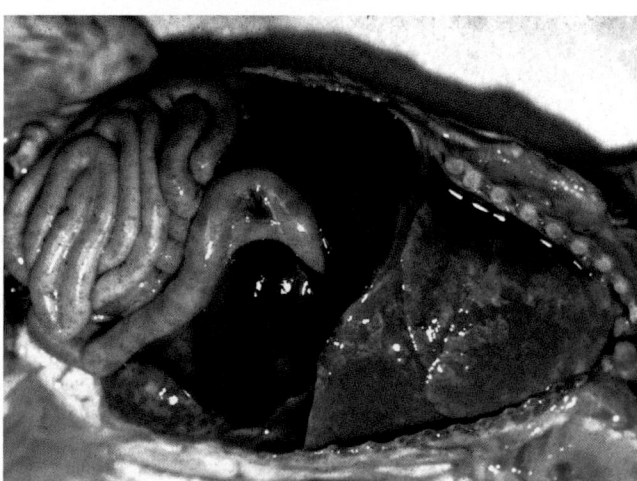

Fig 5-5 Gross CHV lesions of a pup that died 11 days after birth. Note prominent necrotic lesions in lung and liver. Typical kidney lesions are not clearly revealed.

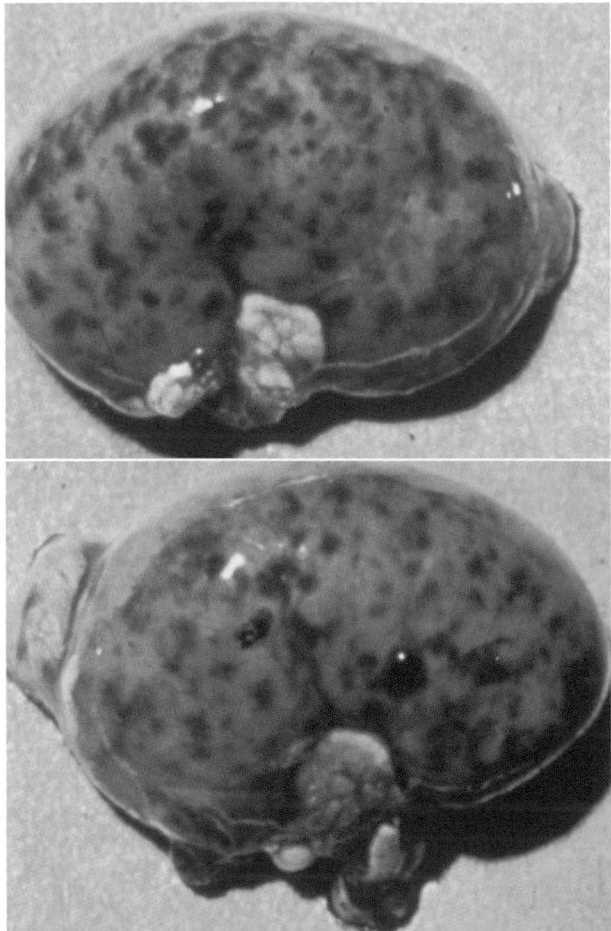

Fig 5-6 Kidney from a puppy inoculated with CHV. Hemorrhagic areas consist of necrotic foci packed with erythrocytes. (Courtesy University of Georgia, Athens, Ga.)

epithelial cells, resulting in marked acantholysis. Depending on the stage of cellular infection and method of fixation, basophilic or acidophilic inclusions may be noted, but they are less common than those caused by other herpesvirus infections. Inclusions are more readily seen in the nasal epithelium or kidney than in areas of widespread necrosis, such as the lung or liver. Renal dysplasias may be present in surviving animals.

Lesions in the CNS of recovered puppies are nonsuppurative ganglioneuritis and meningoencephalitis. The parenchymal lesions are multifocal and granulomatous, characterized by increased pericapillary cellular proliferation, and they occur primarily in the brainstem and cerebellum. Cerebellar and retinal dysplasias are frequent findings.

THERAPY

Once a diagnosis has been made, treatment of puppies with signs of systemic CHV infection is unrewarding because of the rapid and fatal progression of the disease. In some cases, mortality may be reduced during an epizootic episode by injecting each pup intraperitoneally with 1 to 2 ml of immune sera. Immune sera can be obtained by pooling sera from bitches that had recently given birth to litters of puppies that died of CHV infection. Only one injection is required because of the short susceptibility period. This empirical treatment seems to help reduce losses within an exposed litter, but its success

Table • 5-1

Therapy for Herpesvirus Infection of Puppies[a]

DRUG	DOSE[b]	ROUTE	INTERVAL (HOURS)	DURATION
Acyclovir[c]	10 mg total	Oral	6	Until 3.5 weeks old

IM, Intramuscular; *SC*, subcutaneous; *PO*, oral.
[a]See Drug Formulary, Appendix 8 for specific information on each drug. Because of the small size of neonates, fluids or plasma therapy may have to be given intraperitoneally, intramedullarly, or subcutaneously rather than the preferred intravenous route. Additional warming of the animals is essential.
[b]Dose per administration at specified interval.
[c]Available as 200-mg capsules. Contents of capsule are added to 10 ml of warm water. The powder does not dissolve; however, each pup receives 0.5 ml (10 mg) of the suspension orally every 6 hours.

depends on the presence of adequate levels of serum antibodies and administration of the sera *before* the full development of systemic disease. If neurologic signs have already developed, they will likely persist.

Elevating the environmental temperature of already affected puppies is ineffective. Newborn puppies in experimental conditions maintained at 36.6° C to 37.7° C (98° F to 100° F) and 45% to 55% humidity have been able to maintain rectal temperatures of 38.4° C to 39.5° C (101° F to 103° F). Under experimental conditions in which body temperatures were elevated artificially before exposure to virus, puppies had reduced mortality, less severe clinical signs, and minimal pathologic changes. At elevated temperatures, viral growth in tissues was restricted compared with growth in conventionally reared pups. Pretreatment by raising ambient temperature is obviously not possible for puppies with natural CHV infections; however, it could be tried for remaining unaffected puppies in a litter.

Treatment of systemic CHV infection with antiviral drugs such as 5-iodo-2-deoxyuridine has been unsuccessful, and few studies have been performed on newer antiviral agents that are effective in treating localized and CNS infections of herpes simplex virus in humans and laboratory animals. In one such study, two 15-day-old pups died of confirmed CHV. Five littermates were given a course of vidarabine as soon as the cause of the deaths was identified, and they all survived. The surviving pups had high (>1:64) neutralizing antibody titers 2 months later, indicating that they had been infected.[4] A 10-mg dose of acyclovir was given to one litter of 1- to 1.5-kg pups every 6 hours until they were 3.5 weeks old[2] (Table 5-1). Antiviral treatment may spare the pups, but residual damage to the CNS and myocardium may occur. This possibility must be discussed with owners before considering antiviral treatment of an infected litter. Lactoferrin, an iron-binding protein found in milk and other mammalian secretions, inhibits the replication of CHV in cell culture. Lactoferrin has been used topically to treat other mucosal viral infections (see Chapter 2 and Drug Formulary, Appendix 8). Lactoferrin could be administered orally on an empirical basis to protect exposed, clinically healthy pups when peroral transmission of virus is suspected or anticipated.[29]

PREVENTION

The low frequency of clinical outbreaks and poor immunogenicity of CHV reduce the incentive to produce a commercial vaccine for this disease. Reports from Europe and the United States have demonstrated a prevalence of anti-CHV antibodies in 6% of the random dog population, whereas it may be as high as 100% in some kennels.

Vaccination and Immunotherapy

Because CHV infects pups in utero or as neonates, active immunization can only be considered in the dam. Passive immunization has been shown to reduce mortality in affected or exposed pups, so the used of vaccines seems logical. Live virus vaccines, although presumably attenuated, could establish a latent infection. Immunization with a commercially inactivated vaccine in Europe has been shown to provoke fourfold increases in VN titers in most vaccinated dogs, but it did not appear to provide long-term protection.[4] An attenuated, cold-adapted CHV mutant virus vaccine has been used on an experimental basis. Also experimentally, neutralizing antibodies to CHV have been produced in mice by immunization with antiidiotypic antibodies.[32] A lyophilized, inactivated, purified CHV-1 strain F205 vaccine prepared with enriched glycoproteins was used to vaccinate bitches 10 days postcoitus and 6 weeks later near the end of gestation.[20] The near-term booster was used to enhance the short-live humoral response. As analyzed by PCR, 100% of vaccinated pups challenged oronasally with virulent CHV-1 at 3 days of age were protected against clinical illness and in most instances (93.5% of 31 pups) against viral infection. In contrast a majority of challenged control pups (81% of 31 pups) died of generalized CHV disease between 6 and 14 days after challenge. A vaccine using this inactivated strain is licensed for use in some European countries (EURICANHerpes205, Merial, Lyons, France). The low prevalence of illness and the paucity of clinical signs in adult animals make such a vaccine justifiable primarily in problematic kennels with valuable breeding stock.

CHV has also been evaluated as a vector for genetically engineered vaccines against other infections in dogs. Recombinant vaccines incorporating genes for *Neospora caninum*, pseudorabies virus, and rabies virus have all been produced.[16,17,31] The low virulence and species specificity of CHV make it an ideal candidate for a recombinant vector to protect dogs against other pathogens.

If a problem exists in a kennel, prevention of disease in exposed puppies may be achieved with the administration of immune serum or globulin during the first few days of life. Other methods have been of little value, although administration of an interferon inducer (avian poxvirus) to bitches before breeding and whelping and to newborn puppies in problem kennels was claimed to induce nonspecific protection against fatal CHV infection.[4] This treatment needs additional evaluation in controlled studies.

Husbandry

On a practical basis, eradication of CHV from a kennel is impossible. Screening for infected animals also is impractical (see Diagnosis in this chapter), and owners should be advised that subsequent litters from an affected bitch have a very low risk of developing clinical illness. Accordingly, cesarean delivery or artificial insemination (AI) is not justified to reduce spread of infection. AI could be used when a male that is known or suspected to be infected is bred to a primiparous bitch, but the benefit of such a practice has not been studied.

As a preventive practice, care should be taken to ensure that the environmental temperature of newborn puppies is kept warm with heated whelping boxes, heat lamps, or other warming devices that do not cause excessive dehydration. Viral shedding for 1 week generally ensues with introduction of new dogs in a kennel, during concurrent illnesses, or in a dog with drug-induced immunosuppression.

Inapparent infections are common in dogs that have recovered from CHV-infection, with occasional mild rhinitis, vaginitis, or balanoposthitis as the only clinical sign. Such dogs may act as reservoirs of infection for neonates and should be separated from new litters. Clinically affected puppies shed large quantities of virus in their secretions for 2 to 3 weeks after recovery. Virus persists for only short periods in respiratory or vaginal secretions, so its spread is most common through immediate direct contact with infected animals or through fomites.

PUBLIC HEALTH CONSIDERATIONS

Herpesviruses are generally highly species specific; the dog does not become naturally infected with the human strains, and the canine organisms do not infect people. In one study, human herpesvirus type 1 was inoculated into the brain of normal dogs, and it established a latent infection without causing clinical illness or pathologic changes.[28]

SUGGESTED READINGS*

12. Miyoshi M, Ishii Y, Takiguchi M, et al. 1999. Detection of canine herpesvirus DNA in the ganglionic neurons and the lymph node lymphocytes of latently infected dogs. *J Vet Med Sci* 61:375-379.
13a. Morresey P. 2004. Reproductive effects of canine herpesvirus. *Compend Cont Educ Pract Vet* 26:804-811.
20. Poulet H, Guigal PM, Soulier M, et al. 2001. Protection of puppies against canine herpesvirus by vaccination of the dams. *Vet Rec* 148:691-695.
26. Schulze C, Baumgärtner W. 1998. Nested polymerase chain reaction and in situ hybridization for diagnosis of canine herpesvirus infection in puppies. *Vet Pathol* 35:209-217.

*See the CD-ROM for a complete list of references.

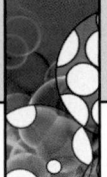

CHAPTER • 6

Canine Infectious Tracheobronchitis

Richard B. Ford

ETIOLOGY

Infectious tracheobronchitis ([ITB] synonyms: "kennel cough," "canine cough," "canine croup") describes an acute, highly contagious respiratory infection of dogs characterized by sudden-onset, paroxysmal cough with variable expectoration and nasoocular discharge. The cough is typically described as "hoarse" or a loud "honking" sound. Clinical signs are attributed to infection by one or a combination of bacterial or viral agents (or both) that colonize the epithelium of the nasal cavity, larynx, and trachea, as well as bronchi, bronchioles, and the pulmonary interstitium (Table 6-1).[55] Vaccines are available for most of the organisms known to be associated with canine ITB, and immunoprophylaxis of puppies and adult dogs is recommended for those considered to be at risk of exposure. Although uncommon, *Bordetella bronchiseptica* infections have been reported in people as a zoonosis (see Public Health Considerations in this chapter).

Respiratory signs of ITB in dogs known to have single-agent infections are generally mild and frequently self-limiting. The prognosis for recovery from uncomplicated infections is excellent, although the duration of postinfection immunity may be short-lived (months). In the clinical setting, the high prevalence of multiple-agent infections complicates the clinical presentation. Canine parainfluenza virus (CPiV) and *B. bronchiseptica* are the most common organisms isolated from dogs with signs of ITB. However, several other viruses and bacteria are known to influence the clinical course and outcome of infection. Compared with adults, puppies appear more vulnerable to life-threatening *B. bronchiseptica* pneumonia.

Viruses

For several years, CPiV-2 has been reported as the most common virus isolated from the respiratory tract of dogs with ITB. Distribution is apparently worldwide. CPiV-2 is a single-stranded RNA virus belonging to the family Paramyxoviridae and is closely related to simian virus 5.[5] Infection generally results in self-limiting, short-lived cough, with minimal systemic effects. Although natural infection may result in detectable serum antibody for periods of up to 3 years, antibody titer to CPiV-2 does not correlate well with protection from clinical disease.[43]

Canine adenovirus type 2 ([CAV-2]; cause of infectious laryngotracheitis) and, to a lesser extent, CAV type 1 ([CAV-1]; infectious canine hepatitis virus) are reported to cause mild, self-limiting acute upper respiratory disease, characterized by cough, in dogs. These viruses are antigenically related DNA viruses of the family Adenoviridae (see Chapter 4).[4]

Depending on virus strain, canine distemper virus (CDV) can cause acute to subacute systemic infections associated with a high mortality rate among infected dogs. Infections are known to occur in dogs worldwide. CDV is also known to cause lower respiratory tract disease in dogs independent of other systemic signs. Although CDV does act synergistically with CPiV-2 and *B. bronchiseptica*, it is not regarded as a primary pathogen in the cause of ITB (also see Chapter 3).

Other viruses, such as canine herpesvirus (CHV; see Chapter 5) and reovirus-1, -2, and -3, have occasionally been isolated from coughing dogs. However, none of these viruses is regarded as being primarily responsible for the clinical syndrome described as ITB.[6]

Bacteria and Mycoplasmas

B. bronchiseptica is a gram-negative bacterium and a principal etiologic agent of ITB in dogs.* Hundreds of isolates of *B. bronchiseptica*, with variable virulence patterns and pathogenicity, have been recovered from dogs. Several other domestic and wild animal species may become infected with *B. bronchiseptica*, and it may play an important role in kittens with acute herpesvirus-1 or calicivirus infection (see Chapter 16).[27] Of the hundreds of isolates, considerable variation exists among individual clones with respect to host distribution and virulence potential.[30,38,42]

Other bacteria recovered from the respiratory tract of dogs with ITB include *Streptococcus* sp., *Pasteurella* sp., *Pseudomonas*, and various coliforms.[49] Although these bacteria are regarded as opportunistic invaders, secondary bacterial infections are the cause of serious, life-threatening complications (pneumonia and sepsis) in the patient with ITB. *Streptococcus equi* subsp. *zooepidemicus* has been associated with increased severity of ITB in kenneled dogs with endemic respiratory disease[10]; it is also considered a cause of pneumonia in dogs as a primary pathogen (see Streptococcal Infections, Chapter 35).

Mycoplasmas are fastidious, prokaryotic microbes that are distinguished from bacteria by the fact that they are enclosed in a cytoplasmic membrane but lack a distinct cell wall.[7,32,41] Nonetheless, unclassified groups of mycoplasmas, acholeplasmas, and ureaplasmas are commonly recovered in specimens collected from the nasopharyngeal and laryngeal mucosa of healthy dogs and cats. The presence of *Mycoplasma* in specimens collected from the lower respiratory tract of dogs (especially *M. cynos*) and cats (*M. felis*) is usually associated with pneumonia (see Chapters 32 and 88).[7,41,44]

EPIDEMIOLOGY

Canine ITB is considered to be among the most prevalent infectious respiratory diseases of dogs. Outbreaks of canine ITB are relatively common. Clinical infections can reach epizootic proportions when dogs are housed in high-density population environments such as pet shops, boarding facilities, commercial kennels,[6,7] and veterinary hospitals.[15,23] Despite their apparent synergism in producing disease, *B. bronchiseptica* and CPiV–2 the two pathogens appear to spread independently in the dog population.[17] The host range of *B. bronchiseptica* includes wildlife, rodents, and cats;

*References 7, 20, 21, 38, 56.

however, most outbreaks are the result of direct dog-to-dog or airborne contact with infectious respiratory secretions. Theories suggest that *B. bronchiseptica* can be transmitted from dogs to cats. *B. bronchiseptica* has been shown to survive in unsupplemented lake water for up to 24 weeks and replicate in natural waters for at least 3 weeks at 37° C.[39] Both CPiV-2 and *B. bronchiseptica* are spread from mixing older carrier animals with younger or otherwise naïve dogs, allowing for outbreaks of clinical disease and more rapid spread of infection.

The common viral agents of ITB are transmitted for up to 2 weeks postinfection. For *Mycoplasma* sp. and *B. bronchiseptica*, however, shedding may occur for 3 months or longer.[5,6] Although infections are transmitted rapidly and efficiently in high-density populations with high morbidity, death associated with complicated respiratory infection is uncommon, particularly in adult dogs.

PATHOGENESIS

Viruses

Because CPiV does not replicate in macrophages, infections with CPiV are typically restricted to the upper respiratory tract in dogs. CPiV infection of the larynx can cause edema of the vocal folds resulting in the high-pitched, honking cough commonly associated with canine ITB. Damage to the tracheal epithelium allows for secondary infection by other pathogens (Figs. 6-1, *A*, and 6-1, *B*). Animals 2 weeks of age and older

Table • 6-1	
Agents Associated with Infectious Tracheobronchitis in Dogs	
Viruses	Canine parainfluenza virus
	Canine adenovirus-2
	Canine distemper virus
	Canine herpesvirus
Bacteria	*Mycoplasma*
	Bordetella bronchiseptica
	Streptococcus spp.

are susceptible.[6] Transmission occurs predominantly by aerosolized microdroplets. After a 3- to 10-day incubation period, viral shedding can occur for 6 to 8 days postinfection.[5] In single-agent infections, signs are limited to a dry, hacking cough and serous nasal discharge. After recovery, a CPiV carrier state does not appear to exist. Cats are capable of becoming subclinically infected and shedding the virus. Whether this is a significant source of infection for dogs is unknown.

Infection with CAV-2 occurs after oronasal contact. The virus replicates in the epithelium of the nasal mucosa, pharynx, tonsillar crypts, trachea, and bronchi and in nonciliated bronchiolar epithelium. Replication peaks by day 3 to 6 after inoculation corresponding to a peak in serum antibody titer.[4] In immunocompetent dogs, infection is typically short-lived; virus usually cannot be isolated beyond day 9 of infection. Infection of type-2 alveolar cells has been associated with interstitial pneumonia.[4] Single-agent infections may be associated with tonsillitis or lung consolidation, or both.[6] In other dogs, overt clinical signs may not be apparent.

Bacteria and Mycoplasmas

B. bronchiseptica has been associated with respiratory infections in dogs and cats (see Chapter 16).[29] *B. bronchiseptica* is a gram-negative, aerobic coccobacillus regarded as one of the principal causative agents of canine ITB. Although either CPiV or CAV-2 may cause mild clinical infections, clinical disease is expected to be more severe in dogs co-infected with *B. bronchiseptica* than with any these agents alone. Transmission most likely occurs after direct contact with infected dogs or contact with aerosolized microdroplets either from infected dogs or through contaminated dishware, human hands, and other fomites.

During an incubation period of approximately 6 days, *B. bronchiseptica* preferentially attaches to, and replicates on, the cilia of respiratory epithelium. *Bordetella* attach to the surface of ciliated respiratory mucosae by means of adhesin molecules (Fig. 6-2). Once they colonize the respiratory tract, *Bordetella* produce a variety of potent toxins that impair phagocytic function and induce ciliostasis. *B. bronchiseptica* is uniquely capable of facilitating co-colonization of the respiratory tract by other opportunistic organisms. *B. bronchiseptica* possesses several intrinsic mechanisms for evading host defenses.[4,15,40,60] It is well recognized for its role as a significant complicating factor in dogs with multiple-agent respiratory infections. For example,

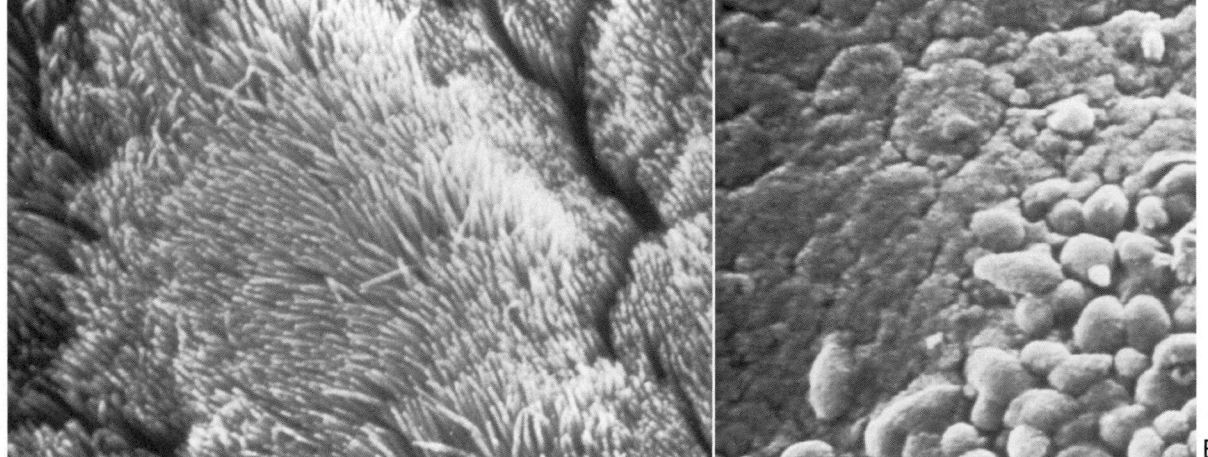

Fig 6-1 **A,** Electron microscopic (EM) scan of normal canine tracheal epithelium. **B,** EM scan shows mucous hypersecretion and the tracheal epithelium completely denuded of cilia only 72 hours after experimental infection with CPiV. (Courtesy Pfizer Laboratories, New York, N.Y.)

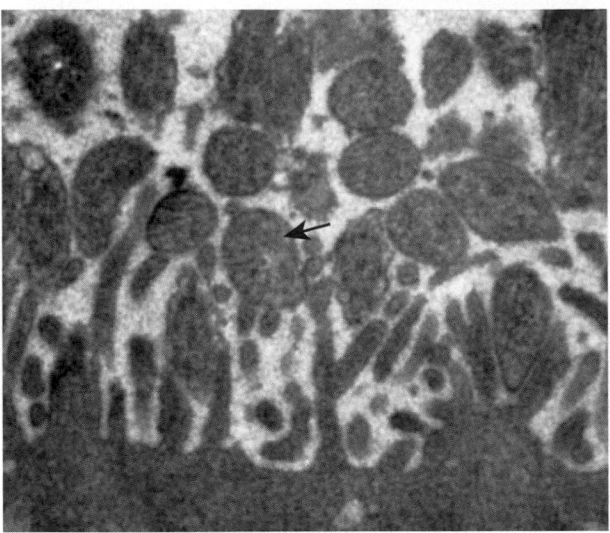

Fig 6-2 Transmission EM scan of tracheal mucosa showing ciliated epithelial cells with adherent *B. bronchiseptica (arrow)*. (Courtesy EM Laboratory, College of Veterinary Medicine, University of Georgia, Athens, Ga.)

fimbriae (hairlike appendages extending from the cell membrane of *B. bronchiseptica*) recognize specific receptors within the respiratory tract.[8] This allows *B. bronchiseptica* to colonize specific tissues where it then releases various exotoxins and endotoxins that impair the function and integrity of the respiratory epithelium and compromise the ability of the infected host to eliminate the infection.[15,23] Additionally, although *B. bronchiseptica* has been regarded as an extracellular pathogen, it has the unique ability to invade host cells. Once contained within the intracellular environment, bacteria are able to avoid immunologic defense mechanisms and establish a persistent infection or carrier state. The pathogenesis of *B. bronchiseptica* has recently been reviewed.*

Despite the fact that infection elicits production of local antibody, the organisms are not completely cleared from the respiratory tract for an average of 3 months. Although by itself *B. bronchiseptica* can cause rhinitis, mucous nasal discharge, and cough, the most naturally occurring illness is associated with viruses or other bacteria. The organism has been isolated primarily from the upper respiratory tract of clinical healthy dogs. In combined infections with CPiV, tracheal mucosal injury is associated with clinically apparent pneumonia.

In addition to *B. bronchiseptica*, several species of *Mycoplasma* and *Ureaplasma* have been associated with pneumonia in dogs.[7,32,41,44] Although endogenous to the nasopharynx of dogs and cats, mycoplasmas are not typically found in the lower respiratory tract. Unlike *B. bronchiseptica*, mycoplasmas colonize both ciliated and nonciliated epithelia. Both natural and experimental infections are characterized by purulent bronchitis and bronchiolitis. Epithelial and lymphoid hyperplasia and interstitial pneumonia may develop. Systemic infection is rare. Once bacteria colonize the lower respiratory epithelium, chronic bacterial shedding of several months' duration is likely.[7]

*References 4, 20, 21, 38, 56.

CLINICAL FINDINGS

B. bronchiseptica and CPiV are among the most common agents isolated from dogs affected with ITB. Because multiple agents cause most natural infections of ITB, associating a distinct set of clinical signs with a particular bacterium or virus is difficult.[7,49]

Acute-onset, paroxysmal coughing episodes, typically associated with retching, in an otherwise healthy, active dog characterizes the clinical presentation. Swollen vocal folds, associated with laryngitis, restrict airflow through the glottis during a cough. This results in a loud, high-pitched cough described as a honking sound. Cough is likely to be productive. However, expelled secretions are not consistently observed because of the small volume and the tendency for dogs to swallow expectorated secretions. Although dogs are affected most commonly during summer and fall, the high density of dogs living in shelters or kennels can be expected to result in infections at any time of year. Dogs that have received prior vaccination against CDV and CAV-2 may still develop signs.[4,6,43,49] The time between exposure and onset of signs of canine ITB ranges from 3 to 10 days, regardless of the agents involved in the primary infection.[4-6,38] A history of exposure to other dogs, particularly in kennel or shelter settings, although common, not a prerequisite. Expectoration of mucus, described as retching or hacking, may occur after a coughing episode and is commonly misinterpreted by owners as vomiting. Physical examination is usually unremarkable, although cough may be easily elicited on manipulation of the trachea, particularly at the thoracic inlet. The ability to elicit a cough on manipulation of the trachea is an inconsistent clinical finding that should not be used exclusively to rule canine ITB in or out. Although secondary bacterial pneumonia can develop in affected dogs, most infections are self-limiting and may resolve without treatment.

A second more severe syndrome is described in dogs with no prior natural or vaccine exposure to the various agents that cause ITB or complicating bacterial infection.[6] Affected dogs are more likely to have a history of recent stays in a pet shop, boarding facility, kennel, or shelter. ITB may be associated with or without rhinitis and accompanying mucoid to mucopurulent nasal and ocular discharges. Complications associated with bronchopneumonia may become life threatening, particularly in puppies. On physical examination, affected dogs are usually febrile and may be lethargic, anorexic, or dyspneic. Affected dogs are difficult to distinguish from those with CDV infections or other pneumonias. Outbreaks of ITB may affect more than 50% of dogs in a densely populated environment.

DIAGNOSIS

Clinical diagnosis is based on a history of recent exposure to other dogs, signs, and response to empiric therapy. An uncertain vaccination history can be helpful in determining susceptibility. However, a history of recent vaccination (within 6 months) in a dog with characteristic respiratory signs does not exclude a diagnosis of ITB. Routine hematology and biochemistry profiles are not diagnostic but do serve to establish and monitor the health status of affected dogs. A stress leukogram characterized by mature neutrophilia, lymphopenia, and eosinopenia may be evident. An inflammatory leukogram with significant leukocytosis or left shift may be present in dogs with complicating bacterial pneumonia. Fluid obtained from transtracheal aspirates may provide evidence of a neutrophilic exudate. Neutrophils are often degenerate in the presence of numerous extracellular and intracellular bacteria. Bacterial culture of aspirated fluid may be particularly helpful in confirming bacterial pneumonia and prescribing appropriate therapy.[26]

Because of indigenous microflora, bacterial isolates obtained from swabs of the nasal and oral cavities, oropharynx, and nasopharynx do not necessarily represent primary or secondary pathogens. However, bacteria cultured from transtracheal aspiration fluid, endotracheal or bronchoalveolar lavage, or sterile swabs of tracheal epithelium are more likely to represent disease-causing organisms. In collecting specimens for *Bordetella* isolation, nasopharyngeal swab collections yield fewer bacteria than does aspiration of lavage fluids because these bacteria adhere to fiber-tipped swabs made of Dacron, alginate, or cotton.[25] The best results are improved if a transport medium intended for *Bordetella* is used.

Thoracic radiographic findings are typically unremarkable in animals with uncomplicated ITB. Dogs with complications associated with ITB may have radiographic signs of pulmonary hyperinflation and segmental atelectasis. Dogs with combined *B. bronchiseptica* and CPiV infections may develop lobar consolidation evident on thoracic radiographs.

Although uncommonly performed on clinical patients, viral isolation of CPiV or CAV-2 can be accomplished on swabs taken from the nasal, pharyngeal, or tracheal epithelium. The ability to inhibit virus growth, cytopathic effect, or hemadsorption with a standardized antiserum confirms the diagnosis.[6] Acute and convalescent serum neutralizing or hemagglutination inhibition antibody titers can be used to establish exposure to any of the viral agents involved in canine ITB. The ability to demonstrate a rising titer, however, has little clinical application because of the relatively short duration of viral infection. Antibody titers to lipopolysaccharide (LPS) antigens of *B. bronchiseptica* had no predictive value in determining which animals will contract respiratory disease, how severe the disease will be, or which dogs have colonization of their lungs.[11]

Nested polymerase chain reaction has been shown to be most sensitive in detecting *B. pertussis* in human patients.[25]

THERAPY

Antimicrobials

In uncomplicated cases of ITB, the value of antimicrobial therapy appears limited. However, in at least one study,[50] administration of an oral or a parenteral antibacterial agent reduced the duration of coughing in affected dogs. Drugs found to be particularly effective were trimethoprim-sulfonamide and amoxicillin. Because dogs with clinical signs of ITB may be at increased risk for bacterial bronchopneumonia, administration of empiric antimicrobial therapy is justified even when infections are not complicated by overt bacterial pneumonia.[54]

Systemic antimicrobial therapy is indicated if deeper respiratory or systemic bacterial infection develops, particularly bacterial bronchopneumonia or interstitial pneumonia. Although the antimicrobial prescribed should be ideally based on results of bacterial culture and susceptibility results, in the clinical setting empiric antimicrobial therapy may be most appropriate.[21,54] Table 6-2 lists appropriate antimicrobials in the empiric treatment of dogs with signs consistent with ITB. With increasing antimicrobial use, more recent isolates of *B. bronchiseptica* from cats in California and Liverpool have been resistant to a large number of antibiotics, including some cephalosporins, fluoroquinolones, and sulfonamides.[18,45] Isolates from dogs in Liverpool and California were

Table • 6-2

Treatment Options for Canine Infectious Tracheobronchitis

DRUG	DOSE[a] (mg/kg)	ROUTE	INTERVAL (HOURS)	DURATION (DAYS)
Antimicrobials				
Amoxicillin-clavulanate	12.5–25.0	PO	12	10–14 (minimum)
Azithromycin	5.0	PO	24	5–7
Trimethoprim-sulfonamide[b]	15	PO	12	10–14 (minimum)
Doxycycline[c]	2.5–5.0	PO	12	10 (minimum)
Enrofloxacin[d]	5.0	PO	24	10
Chloramphenicol[e]	15–25	PO	12	10
Antitussives				
Hydrocodone	0.22	PO	8–12	prn
Butorphanol	0.55	PO, SC	8–12	prn
Glucocorticoids				
Prednisolone	0.25–0.50	PO	12	3–5 days
Bronchodilators				
Aminophylline	10	PO	8–12	prn
Terbutaline	2.5	PO, SC	8–12	prn

PO, By mouth; *SC*, subcutaneous; *prn*, as needed.
[a]Dose per administration at specified interval. For additional information on antimicrobials, see formulary, Appendix 8.
[b]In vitro susceptibility is higher than clinical efficacy since resistance develops rapidly.
[c]Dental staining is possible in young (under 16 weeks) animals, although this is less likely than with tetracycline.
[d]Adverse effects on cartilage of young growing animals; susceptibility of *Bordetella* isolates (40%–60%) is not as high as with others gram-negative bacteria.
[e]High susceptibility of isolates; however causes idiosyncratic aplastic anemia in people and reversible myelosuppression in dogs.

sensitive to doxycycline, amoxicillin-clavulanate, and enrofloxacin.[3,46]

Glucocorticoids

Antiinflammatory doses (see Table 6-2) of orally administered glucocorticoids are effective in ameliorating the cough associated with uncomplicated cases of ITB. Orally administered prednisolone can be used as needed to suppress coughing for periods of up to 5 to 7 days. However, glucocorticoids do not significantly shorten the clinical course.[50] In contrast to previous claims,[52] no controlled studies substantiating the value of intratracheal administration of glucocorticoids over oral administration have been conducted.

Antitussives

Antitussives, alone and in combination with bronchodilators, have been recommended in the treatment of canine ITB. Objectively, these drugs are intended to interrupt the cough cycle; however, certain limitations to antitussive therapy should be noted. Over-the-counter cough suppressant drugs appear to offer little or no relief from the cough associated with ITB. Narcotic cough suppressants, such as hydrocodone, are generally effective in suppressing cough frequency and intensity. However, excessive or prolonged use of these drugs can lead to compromised ventilation and reduced expectoration, with subsequent retention of respiratory secretions and diminished clearance of bacteria.[6,49,50] In cases of ITB that are complicated by bacterial pneumonia, administration of narcotic antitussives is not recommended.

Bronchodilators

The methylxanthine bronchodilators, theophylline and aminophylline (theophylline-ethylenediamine), prevent bronchospasm and may therefore be effective cough suppressants in selected conditions, such as occurs in human asthma. However, dogs with signs of ITB are not expected to derive significant benefit from bronchodilator therapy alone.

Aerosol Therapy

Aerosol therapy (or nebulization) refers to the production of a liquid particulate suspension within a carrier gas, usually oxygen. Patients with ITB that derive the most benefit from aerosol therapy are those with excessive accumulations of bronchial and tracheal secretions and those with secondary bronchial or pulmonary infections, particularly with *B. bronchiseptica*. Small, disposable, hand-held jet nebulizers are inexpensive and available through hospital supply retailers. From 6 to 10 ml of sterile saline can be nebulized over 15 to 20 minutes one to four times daily. Oxygen is delivered at flow rates of 3 to 5 L/min to nebulize the solution. Aerosol therapy must be administered in the hospital. Most patients tolerate aerosol therapy well and generally do not require physical restraint after the first treatment.

There is no value in nebulizing mucolytic agents, for example, acetylcysteine, which can be irritating and induce bronchospasm. Furthermore, liquefying tenacious respiratory secretions may not be an effective means of facilitating airway clearance. Nebulization of glucocorticoid solutions, such as methylprednisolone sodium succinate, has not been critically studied in veterinary medicine. However, in acute paroxysms of cough that may lead to or predispose the animal to airway obstruction, such therapy may provide short-term benefits.

Dogs that are unresponsive to oral or parenteral administration of antibiotics may respond to nebulized antibiotics. Aerosolized nonabsorbable antibiotics, such as kanamycin, gentamicin, and polymyxin B, have been shown to be effective in reducing the population of *B. bronchiseptica* in the trachea and bronchi of infected dogs for up to 3 days after discontinuation of treatment.[7] Although clinical signs are not eliminated, the severity of signs may be significantly reduced.

Supportive Care

Supportive treatment of the individual dog with ITB is directed at maintaining adequate caloric and fluid intake during the acute infection; preventing secondary or opportunistic bacterial infections, especially pneumonia; suppressing the cough; and reducing exposure to other dogs. When practical, this treatment is better accomplished in the owner's home rather than in a kennel or veterinary hospital. This approach can reduce the potential spread of infection by separating affected dogs from susceptible ones.

TREATMENTS NOT RECOMMENDED

Considering the fact that canine ITB represents a significant percentage of the total cases of infectious upper respiratory disease in dogs, it is not unusual that creative therapeutic modalities have been administered in an attempt to shorten the course of disease and minimize the clinical signs. The treatments listed in this chapter are largely anecdotal, have not been subjected to scientific scrutiny, and at this time are *not* recommended in the treatment of canine ITB.

Antiviral Therapy

Given that at least three agents associated with canine ITB are viruses (CPiV, CAV-2, and CDV), the administration of various antiviral drugs approved for use in humans has been suggested for use in dogs with ITB. However, antiviral therapy is highly specific and is generally targeted at specific viruses. In veterinary medicine, antiviral therapies for use against viruses associated with canine ITB are not available. At this time, no human antiviral therapy is recommended for use in either the dog or the cat.

Intranasal Vaccination

Unpublished and anecdotal reports from veterinarians have suggested that some dogs with ITB may derive therapeutic benefit from administration of a single dose of an intranasal (IN) *B. bronchiseptica* vaccine. Experience with this treatment modality in outbreaks of canine ITB within a shelter environment have not been shown to diminish the intensity of clinical signs or to shorten the course of disease. Also suggested is that dogs experiencing chronic or persistent cough beyond the expected recovery time for acute ITB may benefit from *therapeutic* vaccination. To date, no controlled studies have been done to support this recommendation. Because attenuated *B. bronchiseptica* vaccines in themselves produce mild respiratory signs, vaccination of already ill animals may cause more severe respiratory illness.

Expectorants

A variety of over-the-counter expectorants have been used in canine ITB to facilitate the clearance of mucous secretions within the trachea and bronchi. Saline expectorants, guaifenesin, and volatile oils that can be inhaled as a vapor are intended to stimulate secretion of the less viscous bronchial mucus and, thereby, enhance clearance of viscous respiratory secretions. However, the value of expectorant therapy in dogs with ITB has not been established and is not currently recommended. Numerous over-the-counter cough suppressant medications are available and are occasionally administered to coughing dogs. The author's experience with these products suggests that they offer little to no physical benefit in ameliorating the clinical signs associated with ITB.

PREVENTION

Maternal Immunity

Maternal immunity to the viruses known to cause canine ITB provides variable degrees of protection. Maternally derived CPiV antibody does not appear to interfere with parenteral vaccination of puppies that are 6 weeks of age and older.[5] In contrast, maternal antibody interference to parenteral CAV-2 vaccination can persist for as long as 12 to 16 weeks, but it does not protect against infection.[4]

Natural Immunity

The duration of immunity after recovery from CPiV and CAV-2 infection has not been studied, although one unpublished study documented CPiV neutralizing antibody 2 years after infection in dogs that were not reexposed to virus.[6] However, enzyme-linked immunosorbent assay–based antibody titers to LPS did not correlate to the degree of protection in infected dogs in one outbreak.[11] Dogs that have recovered from B. bronchiseptica infection are highly resistant to reinfection for at least 6 months.[7] However, the level of protection derived from infection should be expected to vary, depending on the age and health status of the individual animal, the viruses and bacteria involved, and the opportunity for reexposure.

Vaccination

Both viral and bacterial vaccines are available against most of the agents having a known pathogenic role in canine ITB. Various B. bronchiseptica, CAV-2, and CPiV vaccines are licensed for parenteral administration or for IN administration to dogs. Intranasal vaccines are attenuated and those for parenteral use are inactive whole cell or cellular antigenic extracts (Table 6-3). Vaccines must be administered only by the route indicated on the package label (vaccine insert). Cur-

rently, no vaccine has been approved for administration by both routes. CDV, CAV-2, and CPiV vaccines are commonly incorporated into routine vaccine protocols recommended for all dogs (see Table 6-3). B. bronchiseptica bacterins are in widespread use throughout the United States; no commercial vaccine is currently in use for protecting dogs against Mycoplasma sp. For a listing of some currently available vaccines, see Table 6-4 and Appendix 3. For further recommendations on vaccination for ITB, see Chapter 100 and Appendix 1.

Despite the numerous monovalent and combined canine vaccines on the market today, only B. bronchiseptica vaccination has been recently evaluated for efficacy against a defined challenge.[12,15,16] Studies support the fact that B. bronchiseptica vaccines, whether administered by the parenteral or IN route, are effective in providing substantial reduction in clinical signs associated with ITB in puppies challenged under laboratory conditions. Vaccinating seronegative puppies by both routes sequentially appears to provide a greater degree of protection compared with puppies vaccinated by either the parenteral or IN route alone (compare Figs. 6-3 and 6-4).[15] When the disease prevalence is high in an environment, current protocols should be modified to use at least two parenteral and one intranasal vaccine during the primary vaccination series. For adult dogs, annual vaccination with parenterally administered products can be used in addition to intranasal vaccination before anticipated exposure.

On the other hand, administering B. bronchiseptica vaccine sequentially by the parenteral and IN routes to adult, seropositive (previously vaccinated) dogs does not appear to effectively boost systemic antibody titers. In fact, administration of IN vaccines to adult, seropositive dogs may not be effective as a booster inoculation.[16] Parenterally administered (subcutaneous) B. bronchiseptica vaccine, on the other hand, has been shown to boost antibody levels in previously vaccinated or

Table • 6-3

Types of Licensed Vaccine for Protection of Dogs Against Bordetella bronchiseptica, Canine Parainfluenza Virus, and Canine Adenovirus-2

VACCINE	VOLUME/ROUTE[a]	MINIMUM AGE AT FIRST DOSE	INITIAL SERIES
B. bronchiseptica (killed-extracted cellular antigens)	1 ml parenteral (SC only)	8 weeks	2 doses, 2–4 weeks apart
B. bronchiseptica (a virulent live culture) plus MLV CPiV, CAV-2, CDV	1 ml parenteral SC or IM	Not stipulated (8 weeks recommended)	2 doses, 2–4 weeks apart. Dogs vaccinated before the age of 4 months should receive a single dose on reaching 4 months of age.
B. bronchiseptica (avirulent live culture) plus MLV CPiV	0.4 or 1.0 ml, depending on manufacturer IN	2 or 3 weeks, depending on manufacturer	1 dose (NOTE: some manufacturers stipulate a second dose at 6 weeks of age in puppies that receive the first dose between 3 and 6 weeks of age.)
B. bronchiseptica (avirulent live culture) plus MLV CPiV, CAV-2	0.4 or 1.0 ml, depending on manufacturer IN	3 or 8 weeks, depending on manufacturer	1 dose

CPiV, Canine parainfluenza virus, CAV-2, canine adenovirus-2; CDV, canine distemper virus; IM, intramuscular; SC, subcutaneous; IN, intranasal.
[a]When the vaccine manufacturer stipulates the route of administration for a particular vaccine, optional routes are not indicated.

Table • 6-4

Vaccines Available for Canine Infectious Tracheobronchitis[a]

VACCINE NAME	MANUFACTURER	TYPE	ANTIGENS	ROUTE
Bronchi-Shield III	Fort Dodge	Attenuated	Bb, CAV-2, CPiV	IN
Intra-Trac-II ADT	Schering Plough	Attenuated	Bb, CPiV	IN
Intra-Trac-II	Schering Plough	Attenuated	Bb, CPiV	IN
Naramune-2	Bio-Ceutic	Attenuated	Bb, CPiV	IN
Progard-KC	Intervet	Attenuated	Bb, CPiV	IN
Nasaguard-B	Pfizer	Attenuated	Bb	IN
Cough Guard B	Pfizer	Whole cell	Bb	SC
Vanguard-5B	Pfizer	Whole cell	Bb, CPiV and others	SC
Bronchicine	Bayer	Antigen extract	Bb	SC
Camune B	Bayer	Antigen extract	Bb	SC
Performer Borde-Vac	Agri Labs	Antigen extract	Bb	SC

Bb, Bordatella bronchiseptica; CAV-2, canine adenovirus-2; CPiV, canine parainfluenza virus; IN, intranasal; SC, subcutaneous.
[a]See Appendix 3 for further information on these products and manufacturers.

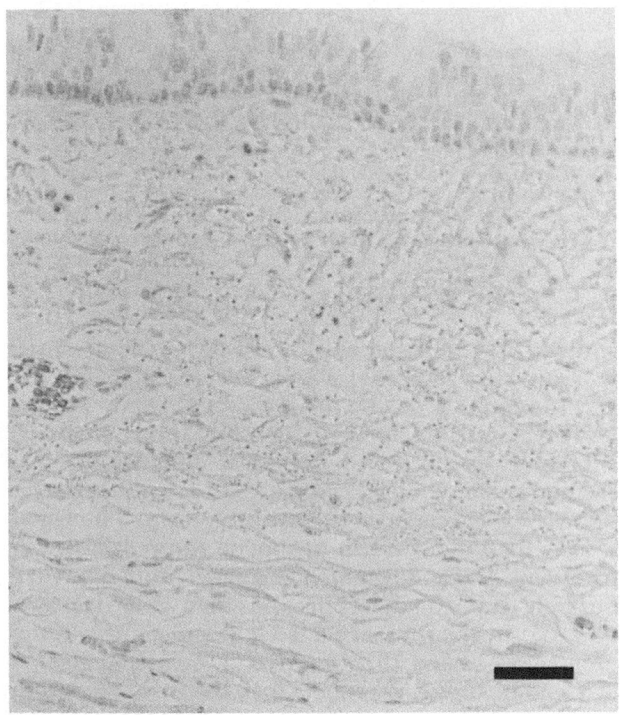

Fig 6-3 Photomicrograph of a section of trachea from a pup that was vaccinated IN with modified-live, and intramuscularly with inactivated *B. bronchiseptica* and was euthanatized 10 days after challenge exposure. The absence of bacterial colonies is noted on the epithelium. Bar, 100 μm. (From Ellis JA, Haines DM, West KH, et al. 2001. Effect of vaccination on experimental infection *Bordetella* bronchiseptica in dogs, *J Am Vet Med Assoc* 218:367–375, with permission.)

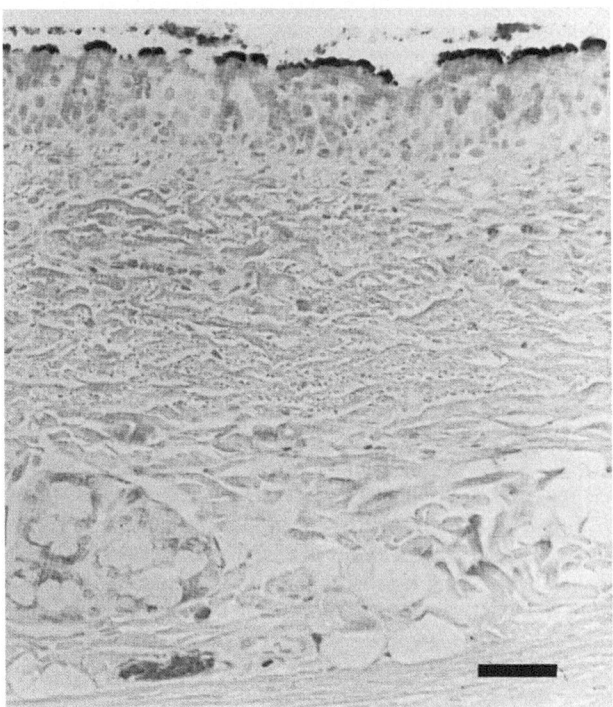

Fig 6-4 Photomicrograph of a section of trachea from an unvaccinated control pup that was euthanatized 10 days after challenge exposure with *B. bronchiseptica*. Numerous brown-stained bacterial colonies are noted on the epithelium. Immuno-histochemical stain; Bar, 100 μm. (From Ellis JA, Haines DM, West LK et al. 2001. Effect of vaccination on experimental infection *Bordetella* bronchiseptica in dogs, *J Am Vet Med Assoc* 218:367–375, with permission.)

exposed dogs.[16] These findings are in contrast to previous reports suggesting that vaccine administered by the IN route induce both local and systemic immunity and protect against challenge more rapidly than parenterally administered vaccines.[7,26,48] Depending on the vaccine, puppies inoculated by the IN route can be immunized as early as 2 to 3 weeks of age.

Many parallels can be drawn between *B. bronchiseptica* vaccination for kennel cough for dogs and *B. pertussis* vaccination for whooping cough in people. Vaccines for *B. bronchiseptica* were originally developed based on the genetic homogeneity of the bacteriocin. As for *B. pertussis*, antigenic divergence of strains is one reason for outbreaks that have occurred following vaccination.[37] Similarly, in a genetic study of more recent

B. bronchiseptica isolates from dogs, the genotypic polymorphism of encoding for outer membrane proteins were much more heterogeneous than the original licensed vaccine strains.[28] Another problem in people is that primary vaccination has been restricted to children, and waning immunity has occurred beginning in adolescence and an increasing exposure.[31] The problem of immune senescence may be overcome by broadening recommendations to use boosters in adults at risk with newly developed parenteral acellular products that are less reactogenic. In animals, vaccine development shifted to the use of IN-attenuated products. In the future, purified acellular vaccines may solve the dilemma of being highly immunogenic for extended immunity with little risk of postvaccinal illness.

Annual revaccination is recommended for dogs considered at risk for exposure. Before known or potential exposure to other dogs (e.g., boarding), a single booster vaccination, administered IN, is recommended at least 5 days before exposure in dogs that have not been vaccinated within the preceding 6 months.[7,16] Vaccination has not been proven to provide any therapeutic effect in dogs with active infection.

The occurrence of adverse reactions after administration of parenteral vaccine for canine ITB is rare and typically is limited to local irritation at the injection site. In contrast, IN vaccines can be associated with development of a cough or nasal discharge (or both) 2 to 5 days after inoculation, sometimes longer. Postvaccinal signs will rarely be sufficiently severe or persistent that administration of an antimicrobial will be indicated. Occurrence of postvaccinal cough in dogs inoculated by the IN route can have significant implications in animal shelters because it may be difficult to distinguish vaccinates from clinically affected dogs. Inadvertent subcutaneous inoculation of an attenuated IN CPiV-2 and *B. bronchiseptica* vaccine resulted in local inflammation and acute nonseptic hepatocellular degeneration and necrosis.[51]

An experimental IN vaccine against *B. bronchiseptica* has been developed by selective inactivation of the aroA gene a known virulence gene in *Bordetella* that enables colonization of the respiratory tract.[47] The vaccine induced higher antibody titers and resulted in lower bacterial counts in the respiratory tract of experimentally challenged mice. Clinical signs were avoided in vaccinates in this rationally attenuated vaccine.

Management of Outbreaks

Environments in which transient dogs are housed in adjoining kennels are conducive to efficient and rapid transmission of the agents capable of causing canine ITB. Although important in preventing infections, vaccination may not guarantee protection against development of signs, particularly in high-density populations. Because airborne transmission is common, dogs suspected of having contagious respiratory disease should be isolated when signs first develop in an effort to limit exposure to susceptible dogs. Thorough, routine cleaning of housing facilities, preferably using fresh sodium hypochlorite, chlorhexidine, or benzalkonium solution, is necessary to control the spread of ITB. Disinfection of surfaces is important to remove pathogenic viruses and bacteria; however, airborne spread from respiratory discharges of infected animals poses the greatest risk for exposure. Adequate ventilation, from 12 to 20 air exchanges per hour,[6,26] is recommended in kennel or shelter facilities. To further limit exposure, relative humidity should be maintained between 50% and 65%, with ambient temperature between 21° C and 23.8° C. No evidence exists that IN vaccination, administered when clinical signs are exhibited, will alter the course of an outbreak.

Once an outbreak has developed, isolating or depopulating the entire facility for up to 2 weeks may be the only reasonable and most efficacious method of containing infections.

This measure is necessary because clinically healthy previously infected dogs can be shedding organisms in low numbers. In addition to extensive cleaning, individual dogs are treated as necessary to manage clinical signs.

Animal facilities that maintain a large number of dogs, especially transient populations, are at considerable risk for canine ITB outbreaks. A reduction in the incidence of ITB has been observed in dogs whose vaccinations for all infections were current. However, attempts to prevent outbreaks through routine, widespread IN vaccines may be ineffective if vaccination and exposure are likely to occur within the same day. Furthermore, postvaccinal coughing or nasal discharge may preclude adoption of otherwise healthy dogs from impoundment facilities. In addition to vaccination, adequate housing, proper cleaning, and adequate ventilation are critical factors in preventing outbreaks of ITB whenever dogs are housed within crowded environments. For further information, see Chapter 98.

PUBLIC HEALTH CONSIDERATIONS

The zoonotic potential of canine *B. bronchiseptica* infection has been reviewed.[16,19,58,59] Over the last several years, reports of human respiratory infections caused by *B. bronchiseptica* continue to appear in the human literature. At greatest risk are individuals who are immunosuppressed resulting from conditions related to alcoholic malnutrition, hematologic malignancy, long-term glucocorticoid therapy, concurrent human immunodeficiency virus infection, splenectomy, and pregnancy. As expected, individuals subjected to tracheostomy or endotracheal tube intubation are also at risk for infection. Humans with preexisting respiratory disease, such as chronic bronchitis, bronchiectasis, and pneumonia, are particularly susceptible. Although human bordetellosis has been associated with a variety of domestic and wildlife animal species, transmission of disease from pets to humans is largely circumstantial. In one instance, infection associated with exposure to rabbits was found to persist in a person with bronchopneumonia for at least 2.5 years.[24]

Estimates suggest that up to 40% of immunocompromised adults living in the United States today have pets.[2] A logical assumption therefore is that, as pet owners, these individuals may be at increased risk of acquiring opportunistic zoonotic infections.* The risk of a child or immunocompromised adult becoming infected with pet-associated *B. bronchiseptica* infection must be considered small, particularly when exposure to a large number of dogs in kennels and animal shelters can be avoided. For further discussion concerning immunocompromised people and pets, see Chapter 99.

SUGGESTED READINGS†

15. Ellis JA, Haines DM, West KH, et al. 2001. Effect of vaccination on experimental infection with Bordetella bronchiseptica in dogs, *J Am Vet Med Assoc* 218:367-375.

16. Ellis JA, Krakowka SG, Dayton AD, et al. 2002. Comparative efficacy of an injectable vaccine and an intranasal vaccine in stimulating Bordetella bronchiseptica-reactive antibody responses in seropositive dogs, *J Am Vet Med Assoc* 220:43-48.

---

*References 1, 14, 33, 35, 36.
†See the CD-ROM for a complete list of references.

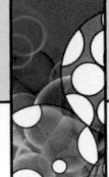

CHAPTER • 7

Nonrespiratory Parainfluenza Virus Infection of Dogs

Craig E. Greene

ETIOLOGY

Canine parainfluenza virus (CPiV) is a member of the family *Paramyxoviridae*, which includes canine distemper virus, simian virus 5 (SV-5), and human measles and mumps viruses. Human, simian, and canine type 2 parainfluenza viruses have all been called *SV-5-like viruses* because of their close antigenic relationship. Monoclonal antibody studies have shown minor antigenic differences between SV-5 isolates.[11] Whether different SV-5 isolates are transmitted among people, nonhuman primates, and dogs remains to be established. The virus associated with respiratory disease in dogs is CpiV,[5] which causes an acute, self-limiting cough in the syndrome of canine infectious tracheobronchitis (ITB, see Chapter 6) and is recognized worldwide as an important cause of respiratory disease in dogs.[1,10] Serologic studies indicate that the overall prevalence of CPiV in the canine population is high but variable. Experimental inoculation of CPiV in newborn pups can cause viral spread to internal tissues. Evidence shows that related but distinct paramyxoviruses may cause systemic or nonrespiratory infections in older dogs.[6] In addition, parainfluenza virus was consistently isolated from the prostatic fluid of a dog.[12]

CLINICAL FINDINGS

A parainfluenza virus variant was isolated from the cerebrospinal fluid (CSF) of a 7-month-old dog with ataxia and paraparesis lasting 3 to 4 days.[7] The dog had been vaccinated against canine distemper at 7.5 weeks of age. Gnotobiotic puppies inoculated intracerebrally with this virus isolate developed two forms of clinical illness.[3,4] Some developed acute encephalitis characterized by seizures, myoclonus (involuntary rhythmic muscle contractions), and progressive neurologic signs within a few days after inoculation. Five of six inoculated dogs observed for 6 months after inoculation developed internal hydrocephalus, although clinical signs were not noted at the time. The hydrocephalus was thought to result from ependymitis with decreased absorption of CSF, with or without aqueductal obstruction (see Chapter 84 for an additional discussion about this type of hydrocephalus from suspected infectious causes). Seven-week-old seronegative ferrets intracerebrally inoculated with this CPiV isolate have also been found to develop a self-limiting nonsuppurative ependymitis and choroiditis.[2] A 6-week-old puppy was found in extremis as a result of acute hemorrhagic enteritis.[4] Although a paramyxovirus variant was isolated, it has not been confirmed that it was responsible for the clinical illness.

At present, it is uncertain whether the central nervous system or gastrointestinal forms of disease caused by paramyxoviral variants occur with any frequency under natural circumstances. Neurologic illness has been more commonly recognized as a complication of other paramyxovirus infections, such as with canine distemper in dogs (see Chapter 3) and in people with measles and mumps viruses (see Chapter 25). In laboratory rodents, other paramyxoviruses have been shown to produce encephalitis and hydrocephalus that are very similar to those that result when the paramyxoviral variant is injected into dogs. Naturally occurring encephalitis, periventriculitis, and hydrocephalus of a suspected bacterial origin have been described in young dogs (see Periventricular Encephalitis, Chapter 84).

DIAGNOSIS

Paramyxovirus-induced encephalitis or hydrocephalus may be confirmed serologically by the hemagglutination inhibition assay; however, because of the high prevalence of antibody in canine populations and the routine use of a vaccine for CPiV, confirmation requires demonstration of a rising serum antibody titer. CSF antibody titer to this variant virus was shown to remain persistently high in dogs after experimental infection.[7] Viral isolation can be performed using CSF or brain tissue of infected dogs. In addition, direct fluorescent antibody methods can be used to detect viruses in nervous tissue. For cases of enteritis, virus isolation and electron microcopy of feces would be most valuable. Serologic techniques such as virus neutralization or HI must be used to distinguish these variant paramyxoviral strains from CPiV.

PATHOLOGIC FINDINGS

Gross pathologic findings have been identified only in experimentally infected dogs that became hydrocephalic. Moderately enlarged lateral and third ventricles are present. Microscopically, acute meningoencephalitis was characterized by multifocal neuronal necrosis, lymphoplasmacytic cellular infiltrates, and reactive gliosis. Focal ependymitis was also apparent. Flattening and discontinuities of the ependymal cells lining the ventricles were seen in dogs developing hydrocephalus. Ultrastructurally, the virus could not be found in the brains of dogs developing hydrocephalus and encephalitis that were examined 1 to 6 months after experimental infection. In the previously mentioned puppy with enteritis, the intestinal and gastric contents were blood tinged. Atrophy of small intestinal villi, mucosal congestion, and lymphoid necrosis were noted.

THERAPY AND PREVENTION

The prevalence of paramyxoviral variant diseases is unknown at present, and they have no known treatment. It is possible that the CPiV vaccine, which was developed for ITB (see Chapter 6), may help to prevent these other paramyxoviral diseases.

SUGGESTED READINGS*

6. Evermann J. 1985. Paramyxovirus infections of dogs. *Vet Rec* 117:450-451.
9. Macartney L, Cornwell HJ, McCandlish IA, et al. 1985. Isolation of a novel paramyxovirus from a dog with enteric disease, *Vet Rec* 117:205-207.

12. Vieler E, Herbst W, Baumgartner W, et al. 1994. Isolation of a parainfluenza virus type 2 from the prostatic fluid of a dog, *Vet Rec* 135:384-385.

*See the CD-ROM for a complete list of references.

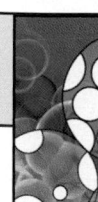

CHAPTER • 8

Canine Viral Enteritis

Dudley L. McCaw and Johnny D. Hoskins

Since the late 1970s, viral enteritis has become recognized as one of the most common causes of infectious diarrhea in dogs younger than 6 months. Canine parvovirus (CPV)–1 and –2), canine coronavirus (CCV), and canine rotaviruses (CRVs) have been incriminated as primary pathogens. Astrovirus, herpesvirus, enteroviruses, calicivirus, parainfluenza viruses, and viruslike particles have been isolated from or identified in feces from dogs with diarrhea, but their pathogenicity is uncertain.[21,29,51]

CANINE PARVOVIRAL ENTERITIS

Etiology

CPVs are small, nonenveloped, DNA–containing viruses that require rapidly dividing cells for replication (Fig. 8-1). As is the case with all parvoviruses, CPV-2 and -1 are extremely stable and are resistant to adverse environmental influences. CPV-2 is known to persist on inanimate objects, such as clothing, food pans, and cage floors, for 5 months or longer.

Most common detergents and disinfectants fail to inactivate CPVs. A noteworthy exception is sodium hypochlorite (1 part common household bleach to 30 parts water), which is an effective and inexpensive disinfectant. It is important that exposure to this disinfectant be prolonged (at least 10 minutes) and thorough.

Canine parvoviral enteritis is probably one of the most common infectious disorders of dogs. This highly contagious, often fatal disease is caused by CPV-2. Since its emergence in the late 1970s, CPV-2 has undergone genetic alterations in the dog, with development of new strains of the virus.[90,91,93] In 1980, the original strain of CPV-2 evolved into type 2a (CPV-2a); and in 1984, another variant designated type 2b (CPV-2b) appeared. These CPV-2 alterations were associated with a genetic adaptation, enabling the parvovirus to replicate and spread more effectively in susceptible dogs. In the United States and Japan, CPV-2b has largely replaced those previously isolated strains, whereas in the Far East[10,68] and Europe,[17,26] both CPV-2a and -2b predominate.[24] In 2000, another strain was reported (CPV-2c), which was an adaptation that allowed infection of cats.[44] Although CPV-2c has been isolated only from leopard cats, infection in domestic cats and dogs is likely.[44] Genetic mutations in the structure of the surface transferrin receptor (TfR) of the virus has resulted in structural alterations that control the host adaptation of CPV strains.[41] For a further discussion of CPV strains in cats, see Canine Parvovirus Infection of Cats in Chapter 10.

Epidemiology

Natural CPV-2 infections have been reported in domestic dogs, bush dogs *(Speothos venaticus)*, coyotes *(Canis latrans)*, crab-eating foxes *(Cerdocyon thous)*, and maned wolves *(Chrysocyon brachyurus)*; and most if not all *Canidae* are susceptible. Experimental infections can be produced in domestic ferrets, mink, and cats; however, the infection is generally self-limiting. The original CPV-2 isolates produced only systemic and intestinal infections in dogs,[128] whereas the newer type 2a and 2b strains may infect felines under experimental[68,73,131] and natural[71,127] circumstances (see Chapter 10). In domestic dogs, CPV-2 infection does not necessarily result in apparent disease; many dogs that become naturally infected never develop overt clinical signs. When the disease occurs, clinical illness is most severe in young, rapidly growing pups that harbor intestinal helminths, protozoa, and certain enteric bacteria such as *Clostridium perfringens*, *Campylobacter* spp., and *Salmonella* spp. In susceptible animals, the incidence of severe disease and death can be very high.

CPV-2 is highly contagious, and most infections occur as a result of contact with contaminated feces in the environment. In addition, people, instruments (equipment in veterinary facilities or grooming operations), insects, and rodents can serve as vectors. Dogs may carry the virus on their hair coat for extended periods. The incubation period of CPV-2 in the field is 7 to 14 days; experimentally, the incubation period has been found to be 4 to 5 days. With CPV-2a and -2b strains, the incubation period in the field can be as brief as 4 to 6 days.

Acute CPV-2 enteritis can be seen in dogs of any breed, age, or sex. Nevertheless, pups between 6 weeks and 6 months of age, and Rottweilers, Doberman pinschers, Labrador retrievers, American Staffordshire terriers, German shepherds, and Alaskan sled dogs seem to have an increased risk.[25,39]

Pathogenesis

CPV-2 spreads rapidly from dog to dog via oronasal exposure to contaminated feces (Fig. 8-2). Virus replication begins in lymphoid tissue of the oropharynx, mesenteric lymph nodes, and thymus and is disseminated to the intestinal crypts of the small intestine by means of viremia. Marked plasma viremia is observed 1 to 5 days after infection. Subsequent to the viremia, CPV-2 localizes predominantly in the gastrointestinal (GI) epithelium lining the tongue, oral and esophageal mucosae, and small intestine and lymphoid tissue, such as thymus, lymph nodes, and bone marrow. It may also be isolated from the lungs, spleen, liver, kidney, and myocardium.[138]

Normally, intestinal crypt epithelial cells mature in the small intestine and then migrate from the germinal epithelium

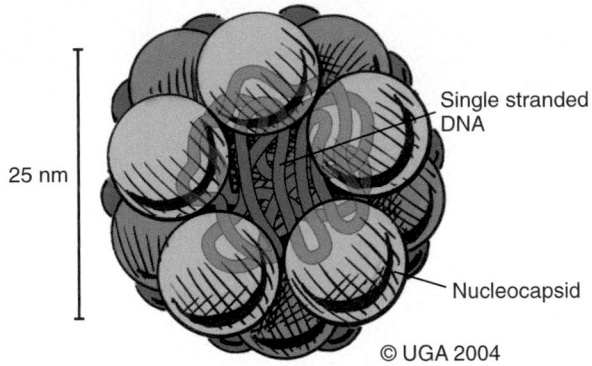

Fig 8-1 Structure of parvovirus. (Courtesy University of Georgia, Athens, Ga.)

of the intestinal crypts to the tips of the villi (Fig. 8-3, *A*). After reaching the villous tips, the intestinal epithelial cells acquire their absorptive capability and aid in assimilating nutrients. Parvovirus infects the germinal epithelium of the intestinal crypts, causing destruction and collapse of the epithelium (see Fig. 8-3, *B*). As a result, normal cell turnover (usually between 1 and 3 days in the small intestine) is impaired, and the villi become shortened. CPV-2 also destroys mitotically active precursors of circulating leukocytes and lymphoid cells. In severe infections, the results are often neutropenia and lymphopenia. Secondary bacterial infections from gram-negative and anaerobic microflora cause additional complications related to intestinal damage, bacteremia and endotoxemia, and disseminated intravascular coagulation (DIC).[84,129,130] Active excretion of CPV-2 begins on the third or fourth day after exposure, generally before overt clinical signs appear. CPV-2 is shed extensively in the feces for a maximum of 7 to 10 days. Development of local intestinal antibody is most likely important in the termination of fecal excretion of parvovirus. Serum antibody titers can be detected as early as 3 to 4 days after infection and may remain fairly constant for at least 1 year.

Clinical Findings

CPV-2 infection has been associated with two main tissues—GI tract and myocardium—but the skin and nervous tissue can also be affected. In addition, other clinical complications of secondary infection or thrombosis can occur. A marked vari-

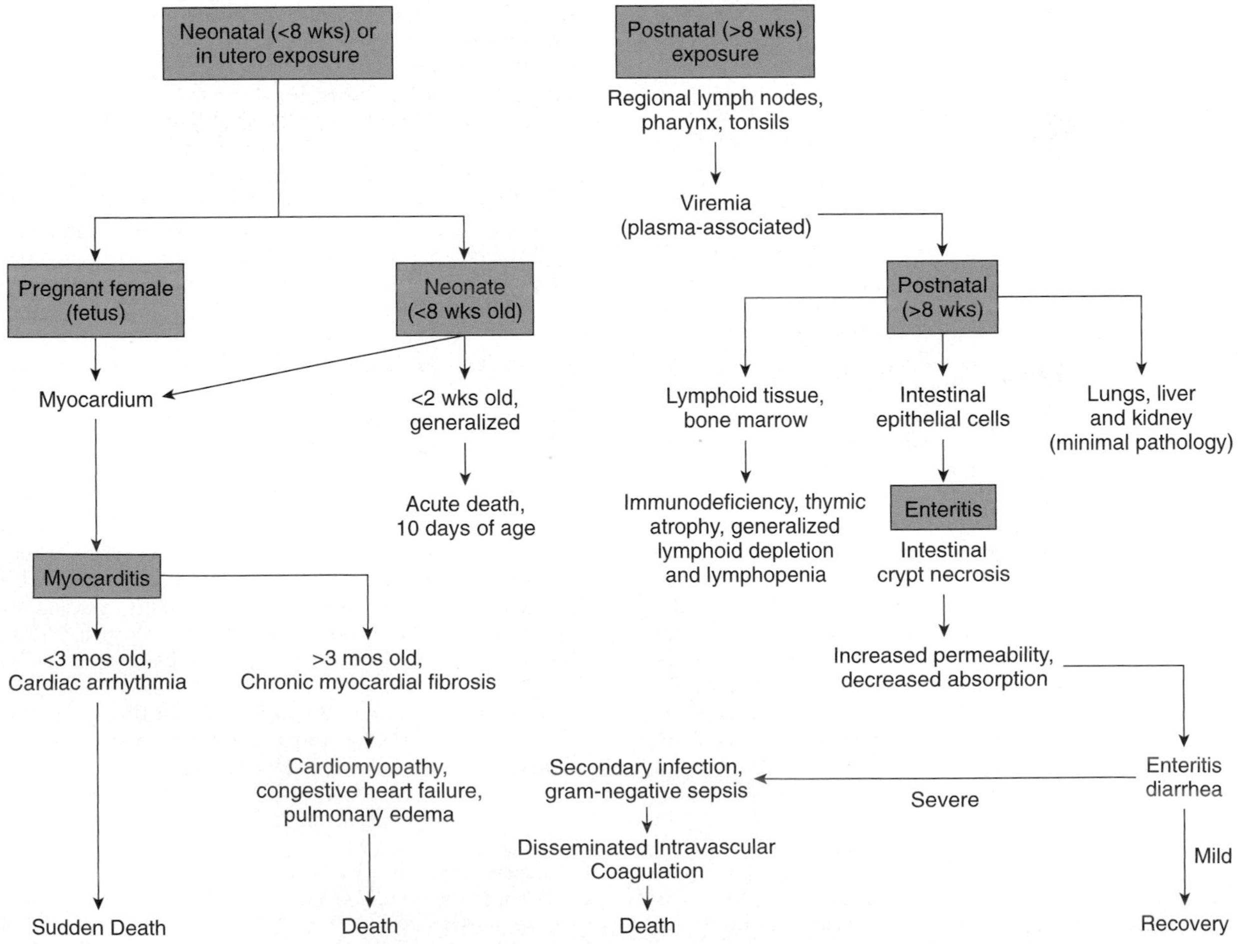

Fig 8-2 Sequential pathogenesis of CPV-2 infection.

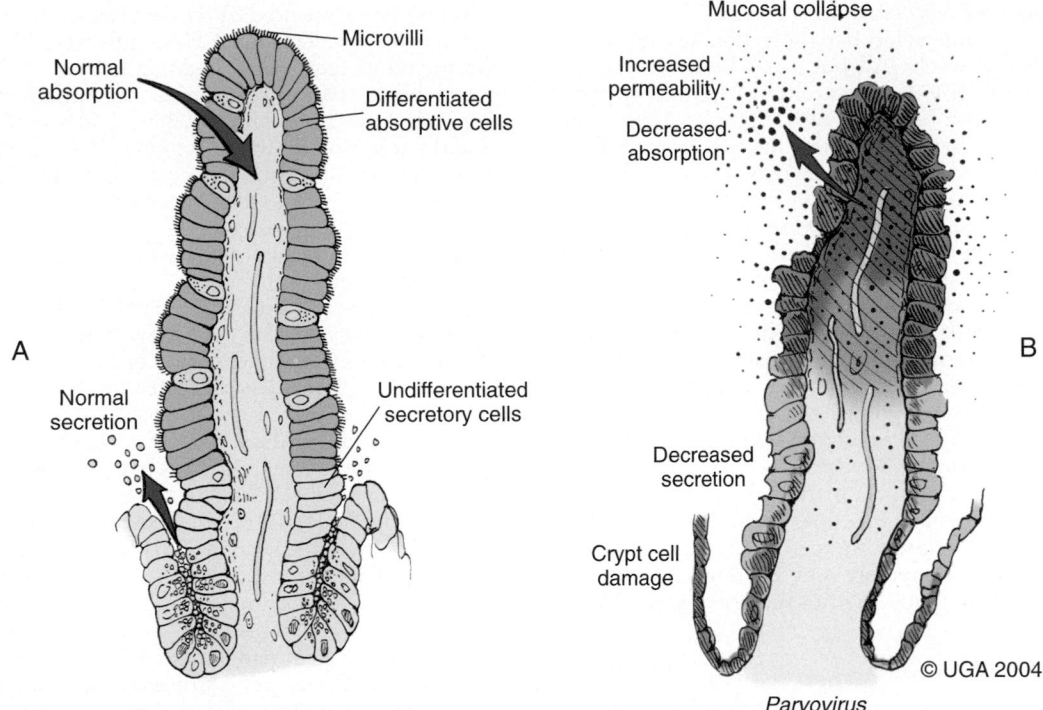

Fig 8-3 A, Normal intestinal villus showing cellular differentiation along the villus. B, Parvovirus-infected villus showing collapse and necrosis of intestinal villus. (Courtesy University of Georgia, Athens, Ga.)

ation is found in the clinical response of dogs to intestinal infection with CPV-2, ranging from inapparent infection to acute fatal disease. Inapparent, or subclinical, infection occurs in most dogs. Severity of the CPV-2 enteritis depends on the animal's age, stress level, breed, and immune status. The most severe infections are usually in pups younger than 12 weeks because these pups lack protective immunity and have an increased number of growing, dividing cells.

Parvoviral Enteritis

CPV-2 enteritis may progress rapidly, especially with the newer strains of CPV-2. Vomiting is often severe and is followed by diarrhea, anorexia, and rapid onset of dehydration. The feces appear yellow-gray and are streaked or darkened by blood (Fig. 8-4). Elevated rectal temperature (40° to 41° C [104° to 105° F]) and leukopenia may be present, especially in severe cases. Death can occur as early as 2 days after the onset of illness and is often associated with gram-negative sepsis or DIC, or both. Younger age, neutropenia, and Rottweiler breed have been associated with a poorer chance of survival (unpublished data).[31]

Neurologic Disease

Primary neurologic disease may be caused by CPV-2 but more commonly occurs as a result of hemorrhage into the central nervous system (CNS) from DIC or from hypoglycemia during the disease process, sepsis, or acid-base-electrolyte disturbances.[1] Concurrent infection with viruses such as canine distemper virus is also possible. Cerebellar hypoplasia, common in kittens prenatally or neonatally infected with feline panleukopenia virus, has not been adequately reported in pups with CPV-2 infection. CPV DNA was amplified using polymerase chain reaction (PCR) from brain tissue of two dogs with cerebellar hypoplasia, but time of exposure to CPV was not mentioned.[114] CPV-2 has been identified in the

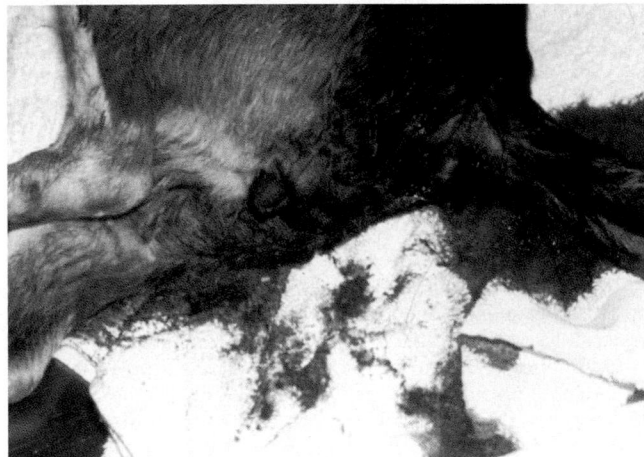

Fig 8-4 Dog with severe bloody diarrhea characteristic of severe parvoviral enteritis. (Courtesy University of Georgia, Athens, Ga.)

CNS of cats (see Central Nervous System Infection in Chapter 10).

Cutaneous Disease

Erythema multiforme was diagnosed in a dog with parvoviral enteritis.[20] Skin lesions included ulceration of the footpads, pressure points, and mouth and vaginal mucosa. Vesicles in the oral cavity and erythematous patches on the abdomen and perivulvar skin were also present. Parvovirus was confirmed in the affected cells by immunohistochemistry.

Canine parvovirus–2 Myocarditis

CPV-2 myocarditis can develop from infection in utero or in pups younger than 8 weeks. All pups in a litter are usually affected. Pups with CPV-2 myocarditis often die, or they succumb after a short episode of dyspnea, crying, and retching. Signs of cardiac dysfunction may be preceded by the enteric form of the disease or may occur suddenly, without apparent previous illness. The spectrum of myocardial disease in individuals is wide and may include any of the following: acute diarrhea and death, without cardiac signs; diarrhea and apparent recovery followed by death, which occurs weeks or months later as a result of congestive heart failure; or sudden onset of congestive heart failure, which occurs in apparently normal pups at 6 weeks to 6 months of age. Myocarditis is still occasionally found in pups born to isolated, unvaccinated bitches[135] in contrast to its frequent occurrence during the widespread epizootic outbreaks of the late 1970s in CPV-naive dogs.[1] Myocarditis, with or without enteritis, has been associated with natural CPV-2a and -2b infections in 6- to 14-week-old dogs from Korea.[139] CPV infection appears not to be a common cause of heart disease because PCR analysis at necropsy of 27 dogs with either dilated cardiomyopathy or myocarditis did not detect CPV in any of the samples.[63]

Thrombosis

Dogs with naturally occurring CPV-2 infections have clinical and laboratory evidence of hypercoagulability.[86] These dogs may develop thrombosis or phlebitis with catheters or visceral thrombi.

Bacteriuria

Asymptomatic urinary tract infection has been detected in approximately 25% of pups following CPV-2 enteritis.[50] This predisposition was attributed to fecal contamination of the external genitalia in association with neutropenia. Untreated subclinical urinary tract infection may lead to chronic urinary infection as an undesirable consequence.

Intravenous Catheter Infection

Bacteria from GI or environmental origin have been isolated from the intravenous (IV) catheters removed from dogs being treated for suspected parvoviral infections.[55] Most of these organisms were gram-negative types (Serratia, Acinobacter, Citrobacter, Klebsiella, and Escherichia). Most organisms were resistant to penicillins, first-generation cephalosporins, and macrolides while being susceptible to aminoglycosides, fluoroquinolones, chloramphenicol, potentiated sulfonamides, and clavulanate-potentiated penicillins. Despite the positive culture results of the catheter tips, none of the dogs showed systemic clinical signs of infection, and only one developed local phlebitis.

Diagnosis

The sudden onset of foul-smelling, bloody diarrhea in a young (under 2 years) dog is often considered indicative of CPV-2 infection. However, all dogs with bloody diarrhea (with or without vomiting) are not infected necessarily with CPV-2. Other enteropathogenic bacterial infections should also be considered (see Chapter 39). All clinical signs characteristic of CPV-2 infection are seldom present at any one time. Leukopenia, although not found in all dogs, is usually proportional to the severity of illness and the stage of disease at the time the blood is taken. Abnormal coagulation test results may include prolongation of the activated partial thromboplastin time, increased thromboelastogram amplitude, and decreased antithrombin III activity.[86]

Fecal enzyme-linked immunosorbent assay (ELISA) antigen tests are available for in-hospital testing for CPV-2 infection (see Appendix 6). These tests are relatively sensitive and specific for detecting CPV-2 infection.[38,44,45,52] However, the period of fecal virus shedding is brief; CPV-2 is seldom detectable by 10 to 12 days after natural infection. This corresponds to 5 to 7 days of clinical illness. Positive results confirm infection or may be induced by all attenuated live CPV-2 vaccines (vaccine virus can yield a false-positive result in dogs 5 to 12 days after vaccination); negative results do not eliminate the possibility of CPV-2 infection. Generally, vaccine-induced reactions are weak positive compared with natural infection.

CPV-2 typically produces lesions in the jejunum, ileum, mesenteric lymph nodes, and other lymphoid tissues. CPV-2 can be isolated from these tissues or feces using tissue culture systems, if performed early. Later in the course of disease, virions become coated by antibodies and cleared. In most tissues, intranuclear inclusions are observed. In the glossal epithelium, these may appear as being within the cytoplasm, when in fact they originate in the nuclear space.[42] Immunochemical methods can also be used to detect virus in tissue culture, electron microscopy (EM) scan of feces or tissues (see Pathologic Findings in this chapter). PCR has been used as a specific and sensitive means of detecting CPV in feces of infected dogs.[68,73,132] This method can also help to differentiate between virulent and vaccine CPV strains.[118]

As a general rule, parvoviruses cause hemagglutination of erythrocytes. Inhibition of hemagglutination by CPV-2 antisera can be used to demonstrate serum antibody. The presence of high hemagglutination inhibition (HI) titer in a single serum sample collected after the dog has been clinically ill for 3 or more days is diagnostic for CPV-2 infection. Rising titers (seroconversion) can also be demonstrated when acute and 10- to 14-day convalescent serum samples are compared using either canine or feline parvovirus in HI and virus neutralization (VN) tests. ELISA tests are also available that permit distinction between IgG and IgM.[111] In-office ELISA test kits are commercially available for semiquantitative IgG and IgM measurements (Immunocomb, Biogal Labs, Megiddo, Israel)[137,136] and for determining adequate IgG titers for vaccination (CPV/CDV Test Kit, Synbiotics, San Diego, Calif.). See Appendix 6 for further information on these products.

Pathologic Findings

Early lesions are most pronounced in the distal duodenum; later, the jejunum is more severely affected. The intestinal wall is generally thickened and segmentally discolored, with denudation of intestinal mucosa and the presence of dark, sometimes bloody, watery material within the stomach and intestinal lumen (Fig. 8-5). In mild cases, the lesions are not easy to distinguish from those of nonspecific enteritis. Enlargement and edema of thoracic or abdominal lymph nodes have been observed.

The intestinal lesions are characterized by necrosis of the crypt epithelium in the small intestine. Intranuclear viral inclusion bodies may be seen in these epithelial cells and throughout the squamous epithelia of the upper GI tract.[62] The pathologic changes may range from mild inflammation to diffuse hemorrhagic enteritis. The villi are shortened or obliterated, owing to lack of epithelial replacement by maturing crypt cells, resulting in collapse of the lamina propria (Fig. 8-6). Necrosis and depletion of the lymphoid tissue (e.g., Peyer's patches; mesenteric lymph nodes, thymus, and spleen) are present. Pulmonary edema or alveolitis may be observed in dogs dying of complicating septicemia.[130] Histologic examination is usually definitive; however, specific identification of parvovirus in tissue specimens can be done by immunofluorescence or other immunochemical methods. Using indirect fluorescent antibody (FA) testing, antigen in dogs with

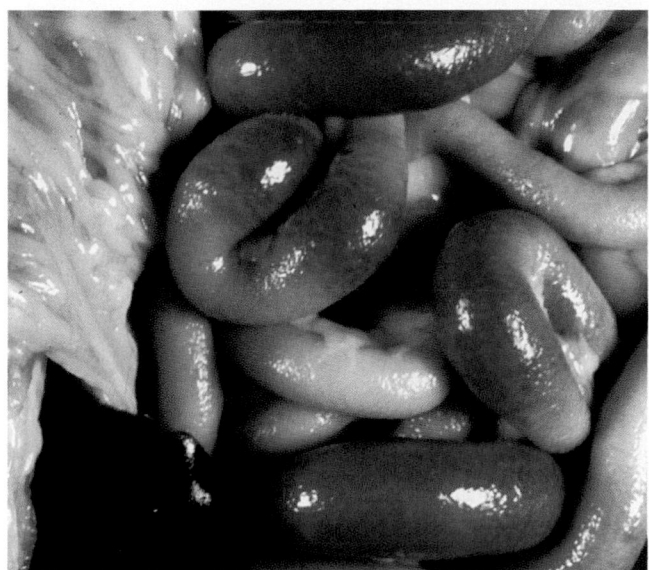

Fig 8-5 Small intestine at necropsy from a dog that died suddenly of parvoviral enteritis. Note the discoloration of the intestinal wall and fibrin on the serosal surfaces. (Courtesy Veterinary Pathology, University of Georgia, Athens, Ga.)

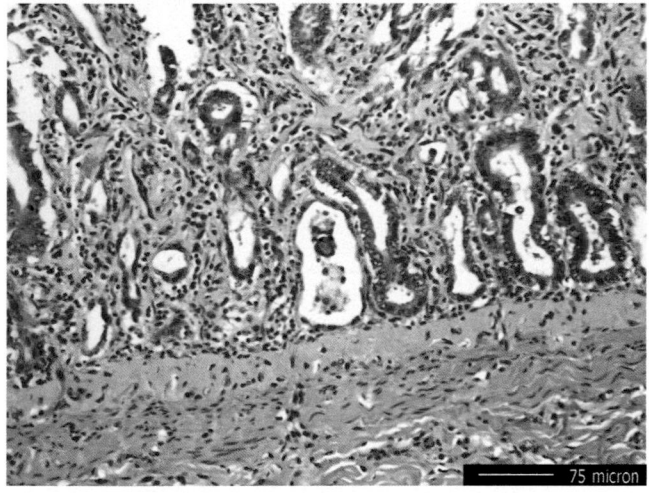

Fig 8-6 Photomicrograph of the small intestine of a dog that died of parvoviral enteritis. Villi are collapsed, and crypt lumina are dilated and filled with necrotic debris (H and E stain, ×100). (Courtesy Barry Harmon, University of Georgia, Athens, Ga.)

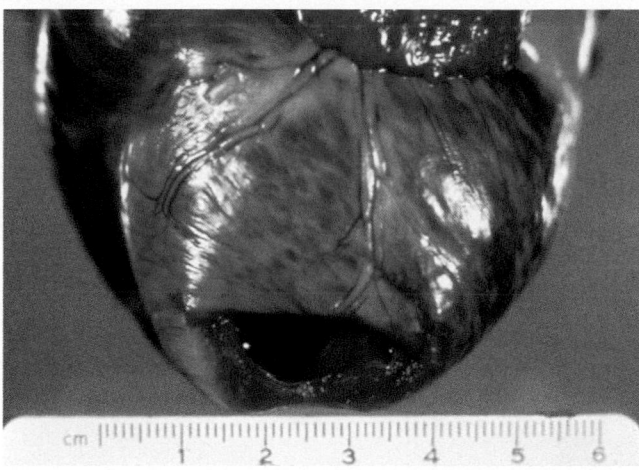

Fig 8-7 Heart from a dog that died of the myocardial form of CPV-2 infection. Pale streaking of the myocardium is apparent. A similar lesion will be noted with CPV-1 infection in puppies younger than 3 weeks. (Courtesy Pfizer Animal Health, Lincoln, Neb.)

virus particles have been demonstrated by EM and by in situ hybridization[135] in the inclusion bodies.

Therapy

The primary goals of symptomatic treatment for CPV-2 enteritis are restoration of fluid and electrolyte balance and preventing secondary bacterial infections. Antimicrobial agents, motility modifiers, and antiemetic agents are given in Table 8-1. Fluid therapy is probably the single most important aspect of clinical management and should be continued for as long as vomiting or diarrhea (or both) persists. Hypoglycemia and hypokalemia are common and should be corrected through additions to the IV fluids. Antimicrobial agents are recommended because the combination of severe disruption of the intestinal epithelium allowing bacteria into the blood and peripheral neutropenia increases the risk of sepsis.[108] The most common bacteria appear to be *Escherichia coli* and *Clostridium perfringens*.[129,130] The best antibacterial spectrum is provided by combination of a penicillin and an aminoglycoside. Before a nephrotoxic drug such as an aminoglycoside is administered, the patient should be fully hydrated. Antiemetic drugs are helpful to reduce fluid loss and decrease patient distress and allows for enteral nutrition. Metoclopramide hydrochloride and prochlorperazine have proved helpful in most dogs with persistent vomiting. The serotonin receptor antagonists are the most efficacious antiemetics.[57,83] Ondansetron and dolasetron have both been used in dogs. Drug therapy to alter gut motility is seldom recommended in the treatment of CPV-2 enteritis. If needed, narcotic antispasmodics (e.g., diphenoxylate hydrochloride, loperamide hydrochloride) are preferred when motility modifiers are needed.

Although withholding food and water are general recommendations in treating GI diseases, including parvovirus enteritis, recent information suggests this is not necessary. When dogs with parvovirus enteritis were fed beginning on the first day of treatment (via nasoesophageal tube), their recovery time was shortened, and they maintained body weight when compared with dogs that were treated the conventional method of withholding food until signs had ceased for 12 hours.[75]

After GI signs abate, a broad-spectrum dewormer and treatment for *Giardia* infection should be given. During the

lethal CPV enteritis can be found in the dorsal side of the tongue (96.3%), pharynx (81%), esophagus (50%), ventral tongue (20.4%), planum nasale (5.6%), small intestinal mucosa (85.2%), bone marrow (81.6%), spleen (79.6%), thymus (66.7%), mesenteric nodes (50.4%), palatine tonsils (58.5%), and myocardium (1.9%).[138] In situ hybridization is a valuable specific tool for virus identification in formalin-fixed or wax-embedded tissue specimen.[134]

Parvoviral myocarditis, when present, is recognized grossly as pale streaks in the myocardium (Fig. 8-7). The myocardial lesions consist of a nonsuppurative myocarditis with multifocal infiltration of lymphocytes and plasma cells within the myocardium. Basophilic intranuclear inclusion bodies have been observed in cardiac muscle fibers, and parvolike

Table • 8-1

Drug Therapy for Canine Viral Enteritis

DRUG	DOSAGE[a] (mg/kg)	ROUTE	INTERVAL (HR)	DURATION (DAYS)
Antiemetic Agents				
Chlorpromazine	0.5	IM	8	prn
	1.0	Rectally	8	prn
	0.05	IV	8	prn
Metoclopramide	0.2–0.4	SC	8	prn
	1–2	IV[b]	24	prn
Prochlorperazine	0.1	IM	6–8	prn
Ondansetron	0.1–0.15	IV	6–12	prn
Dolasetron	1	IV, PO	24	prn
Antimicrobial Agents				
Ampicillin	10–20	IV, IM, SC	6–8	3–5
Cefazolin	22	IV, IM	8	3–5
Ceftiofur	2.2–4.4	SC	12	3–5
Gentamicin[c]	2	IM, SC	8	3–5
Interferon-ω	2.5×10^6 units/kg	IV	24	3
Gastric Protectants				
Cimetidine	5–10	IM, IV	6–8	prn
Ranitidine	2–4	SC, IV	6–8	prn
Miscellaneous Therapy				
Whole blood	10–20 ml/kg	IV[d]		prn
Plasma	10–20 ml/kg	IV[d]		prn
Dexamethasone sodium phosphate[c]	2–4	IV		Do not repeat
Flunixin meglamine[c]	1	IV		Do not repeat
Antiendotoxin serum[e]	4.4 (diluted in equal amount crystalloid fluid)	IV		Do not repeat
Colloid fluid[c,f]	20 ml/kg	IV	24	prn

IM, Intramuscular; *IV*, intravenous; *SC*, subcutaneous; *PO*, by mouth, *prn*, as needed.
[a]Dose per administration at specified interval. For additional information on these drugs, see Drug Formulary, Appendix 8.
[b]Slow infusion can be used for severe vomiting.
[c]Administered after correction of dehydration.
[d]Administered over 4 hours.
[e]SEPTI-SERUM; Immvac Inc., Columbia, MO.
[f]Hetastarch or Dextran 70.

initial stage of CPV-2 enteritis, recommended adjunctive therapy has included transfusion of specific hyperimmune plasma or administration of antiendotoxin sera[18] (see Passive Immunization, Chapter 100, and Drug Formulary, Appendix 8). These adjuncts reportedly decrease mortality and the length of hospitalization[18] but are expensive. A recombinant bactericidal-permeability–increasing (BPI) protein, which counteracts endotoxin, did not alter clinical outcome or survival in dogs naturally infected with CPV-2.[85] This result is despite increases in plasma endotoxin in affected animals.

Recombinant human granulocyte colony-stimulating factor (G-CSF) has been advocated for the treatment of severe neutropenias induced by CPV-2 infection.[22] However, supplementing recombinant human G-CSF to neutropenic pups with CPV-2 infection did not change any aspect of their clinical outcome.[67,109,110] The lack of efficacy of exogenous G-CSF is probably the result of already existent high levels of endogenous G-CSF that are maximally stimulating the production of neutrophils.[11]

Dogs with experimental and natural parvovirus infection have been treated with recombinant feline IFN-ω in high IV dosages (2.5×10^6 units/kg) beginning early (4 days or less after infection) in the course of parvoviral infection.[15, 45,60,66] Reduced signs of clinical illness and mortality were observed in treated dogs. See Drug Formulary, Appendix 8 for further information on its availability and usage.

Several therapies have been recommended and empirically would seem of benefit, but they have not been examined well enough to indicate that they are efficacious.[56] Some puppies are severely anemic, which may be the result of GI loss of blood caused by the parvovirus enteritis, or it might be unrelated to parvovirus such as parasitism. Transfusion of whole blood might benefit these puppies. Hypoproteinemia is present in some puppies. A whole blood transfusion will help resolve the problem, but if erythrocytes are not needed, a more appropriate therapy is plasma transfusion. Ideally, serum albumin concentration should be maintained at 2.0 g/dl or greater. If edema is present as a result of decreased proteins and is not corrected by a plasma transfusion, then synthetic colloid such as hetastarch should be considered. Colloids should not be given until dehydration is corrected. Glucocorticoids and flunixin meglumine may have beneficial effects in treating early sepsis or endotoxemia. These agents should not be used until dehydration is corrected, and repeated doses should not be given.

The use of hyperimmune plasma might be questioned because, at the time of clinical signs, the levels of antibodies are generally increased. However, pups that had a delayed or lower response are often more severely affected. Canine lyophilized IgG has been beneficial in treatment of dogs with naturally occurring CPV-2 infection.[58] Compared with control dogs, those receiving IgG as adjunctive therapy had reduced severity of disease, reduced cost of treatment, and reduced hospitalization time.

Pups that survive the first 3 to 4 days of CPV-2 enteritis usually make a rapid recovery, generally within 1 week in uncomplicated cases. Severely ill pups that develop secondary sepsis or other complications may require prolonged hospitalization.

Prevention

Immunity After Infection

A puppy that recovers from CPV-2 enteritis is immune to reinfection for at least 20 months and possibly for life. On reexposure to the various strains of CPV-2, protected pups will not have increased serologic titers, show overt signs of illness, or shed virus in the feces. In general, a good correlation exists between serum antibody titer, determined by either HI or VN testing, and resistance to infection. Serum antibody titers remain high for a prolonged period after CPV-2 enteritis, even if reexposure does not occur. If serum antibody titers become low, a localized infection is possible, but viremia and generalized illness are unlikely to develop. Although it may help in protection against entry of CPV-2, intestinal secretory IgA probably does not play a role in the longevity of protective immunity because intestinally derived antibody titers do not persist for longer than 15 days after infection.

Immunization and Duration of Immunity

Inactivated CPV-2 vaccines of sufficient antigenic mass protect dogs against wild-type CPV-2 exposure. If protective immunity is defined as complete resistance to subclinical infection, then that produced by most inactivated CPV-2 vaccines is short lived. Dogs vaccinated with inactivated CPV-2 vaccine can become subclinically infected as early as 2 weeks after vaccination. If a dog is given sequential doses of inactivated CPV-2 vaccine, however, a rapid secondary immune response is mounted, and the dog is protected for as long as 15 months.

Commercially prepared attenuated live and inactivated CPV-2 vaccines are available. These vaccines produce varying levels of protective immunity and are safe either alone or in combination with other vaccine components. Transient lymphopenia occurs 4 to 6 days after the administration of some attenuated live CPV vaccines. Most attenuated live CPV vaccine strains replicate in the intestinal tract and are briefly shed in the feces. Although concern has been expressed about the possibility of attenuated CPV-2 vaccine undergoing reversion of virulence and causing apparent disease, experimental studies have shown that modified live virus (MLV) CPV-2 vaccines are safe.[49] The events following administration of attenuated live CPV-2 vaccines parallel those following wild-type CPV-2 infection. On day 2 after subcutaneous (SC) administration of vaccine, viremia and systemic distribution occur with shedding from GI tract on days 3 to 10. One difference between vaccine-induced and wild-type infections is that lower quantities of virus are shed after vaccination. Humoral immune responses to attenuated live vaccines that have been studied are similar to those observed with wild-type infection.

Serum antibody is usually detectable 3 days after vaccination, with levels rising rapidly to those observed after subsequent natural infection. Even if reexposure does not occur, protective antibody titers may persist for at least 2 years, and dogs exposed during this time should not become infected. Vaccination with potentiated attenuated CPV-2 vaccine has been shown to protect dogs on subsequent experimental challenge exposure.[115] On the basis of serum antibody titers, in a veterinary hospital setting, 27% of the dogs being evaluated for revaccination had titers below the protective level for CPV-2.[65] Although serum antibody titers are not absolute indicators of protection, they have a good correlation with protection against CPV-2 infection (see also Canine Parvoviral Infection, Chapter 100). Even systemic chemotherapy for neoplasia in dogs did not affect serum CPV-2 antibody titers.[33]

Attenuated Live CPV-2 Immunization

Contrary to publicized information, vaccination failure is not related to strain differences between field and vaccine strains. The primary causes of failure of vaccines are interfering levels of maternal antibody to CPV-2[82,96] and lack of sufficient seroconversion to the CPV-2 vaccine administered. The age at which pups can be successfully immunized is proportional to the antibody titer of the bitch, effectiveness of colostral transfer of maternal antibody within the first 24 hours of life, and immunogenicity and antigen titer of the CPV-2 vaccine. Pups from a bitch with low protective titer of antibody to CPV-2 can be successfully immunized by 6 weeks of age, but in pups from a bitch with a very high titer to CPV-2, maternal antibody may persist longer.[96]

Without knowledge of the antibody status of each puppy, recommending a practical vaccination schedule that will protect all of them is difficult. In addition, pups become susceptible to wild-type CPV-2 infection 2 to 3 weeks before they can be immunized. No vaccines are available that completely eliminate this window of susceptibility before pups become immunized.[96] With the *potentiated* vaccines presently available, which are more immunogenic than the original or *conventional* CPV vaccines, low levels of maternal antibody will not prevent successful response. Pups of unknown immune status can be vaccinated with a high-titer–attenuated live CPV-2 vaccine at 6, 9, and 12 weeks of age and then revaccinated annually.[37] A check for serum antibody level or an additional vaccination might be done at 15 to 16 weeks of age, especially in breeds that are at increased risk for CPV-2 enteritis.[13] See discussion of parvoviral infection in Chapter 100 for additional information.

Attenuated Live Canine Parvovirus–2b Immunization

Although not currently commercially available, experimental use of a modified live vaccine derived from CPV-2b produced higher antibody titers to CPV-2b and CPV-2 than did a vaccine derived from CPV-2.[102] In addition, the CPV-2b vaccine was able to produce a titer increase in puppies with higher maternal antibody levels.[101]

Experimental Vaccines

A large number of genetically engineered vaccines have been developed in an attempt to improve the protection afforded by inactivated products while reducing the antigenicity of the potentiated vaccines. A DNA vaccine containing a plasmid encoding the full length of the viral protein (VP)1 region of CPV-2 protected 9-month-old pups from clinical signs and fecal shedding of virus experimental challenge-infection.[48] A vaccine based on a recombinant plant virus expressing the VP2 peptide, coded by a subset of the VP1 gene, protected against clinical disease, with limited fecal shedding following challenge.[53] Neither of these vaccines produced sterile immunity as follows attenuated CPV-2 vaccination. Intranasal or SC vaccination of mice with a plant virus expressing a CPV-2 peptide elicited systemic and mucosal antibody responses.[79,80]

Husbandry

CPV is one of the most resistant viruses to infect dogs. As a result, the hair coat and environment of the ill dog become contaminated. Diluted household bleach (1:30) with water should be applied to tolerable surfaces or used as a dip for animals leaving isolation facilities. Bleach should be added to washing of all utensils and bedding. The solutions require a 10-minute minimum exposure time. The shedding period is so short (under 4 to 5 days following the onset of illness) that the environment is of major concern. The virus can persist for months to years away from sunlight and disinfectants. Steam cleaning can be used for instantaneous disinfection of surfaces that do not tolerate hypochlorite. For further information on disinfection, see Chapter 94.

Public Health Considerations

Studies have failed to find any evidence of human infection by CPV-2, even among kennel workers in heavily contaminated premises, although people apparently can act as passive transport vehicles for the virus between dogs. Although CPV-2 is not itself a human pathogen, extra care should always be practiced in handling fecal materials from diarrheic animals.

CANINE PARVOVIRUS-1 INFECTION

Etiology

In 1967, CPV-1 (also referred to as minute virus of canines [MVC]) was first isolated from the feces of military dogs. Physical and chemical properties of CPV-1 are typical of parvoviruses. CPV-1 is distinctly differentiated from CPV-2 by its host cell range, spectra of hemagglutination, genomic properties, and antigenicity.[7] Using genetic analysis, it is most closely related to bovine parvovirus.[117]

CPV-1 can be propagated on the Walter Reed canine (WRC) cell line. By HI tests, CPV-1 is serologically distinct from parvoviruses of a number of other species. Apparently, CPV-1 and CPV-2 are different viruses; no homology in DNA-restriction sites between the two viruses has been demonstrated using several restriction enzymes.

Epidemiology

The domestic dog is the only proven host, although other *Canidae* are likely susceptible. Before 1985, CPV-1 was considered a nonpathogenic parvovirus of dogs. Since that time, clinical infections of CPV-1 in neonatal pups have been encountered by practicing veterinarians and diagnostic laboratory personnel. Serologic evidence indicates that its distribution is widespread in the dog population but is usually restricted to causing clinical disease in pups younger than 3 weeks,[8] but disease has been reported in pups 5 weeks of age.[100] A reasonable assumption is that the spread is similar to that of CPV-2. Although it was first identified in the United States, isolations have been made worldwide,[69] and similar to CPV-2, it is likely ubiquitous.

Pathogenesis

The virulence of CPV-1 for dogs is uncertain; however, it has been identified by immunoelectron microscopy in the feces of pups and dogs with mild diarrhea. Between 4 and 6 days after oral exposure, CPV-1 can be recovered from the small intestine, spleen, mesenteric lymph nodes, and thymus. Histologic changes in lymphoid tissue are similar to those observed in

pups infected with CPV-2 but less severe. In addition, CPV-1 is capable of crossing the placenta and producing early fetal death and birth defects.[7] Experimental oronasal infection of neonatal specific pathogen-free (SPF) pups, with laboratory isolates from pups dying of enteric illness, produced only mild respiratory disease.[8] Naturally induced disease in young pups has been characterized by enteritis, pneumonia, and myocarditis.[47] Naturally infected dogs have been shown to have a reduction in both numbers and killing activity of phagocytes.[14]

Clinical Findings

CPV-1 has been observed infrequently in field dogs with mild diarrhea, as well as in the feces of clinically healthy animals. Primarily, CPV-1 infection is a cause of enteritis, pneumonitis, myocarditis, and lymphadenitis in pups between 5 and 21 days of age.[31] Many of these pups have mild or vague symptoms and eventually die, being classified as "fading pups." Affected pups usually have diarrhea, vomiting, and dyspnea and are constantly crying. Some puppies have respiratory disease with no enteric signs.[100] Sudden death with few premonitory signs has also been observed. Because of transplacental infections, this virus can cause failure to conceive or fetal death or abortion.

Diagnosis

CPV-1 infection should be considered in young (under 8-week-old) pups with mild diarrhea that clinically or histologically resemble CPV-2 disease but are serologically CPV-2 negative, or in unexplained fetal abnormalities, in abortions, or in fading pups. CPV-1 will not cross react with any of the serologic or fecal detection methods for CPV-2. EM has observed CPV-1 in fecal and rectal swab samples from field dogs. Immunoelectron microscopy is necessary to distinguish CPV-1 from CPV-2. Inhibition of hemagglutinating activity in stool suspensions by specific antiserum is also diagnostic for CPV-1. To determine exposure, sera can be tested for specific antibody with VN or HI tests. Because only the WRC cell line supports growth of CPV-1, the availability of virus isolation and serum VN tests is limited.

Pathologic Findings

Pathologic changes in nursing pups have included thymic edema and atrophy, enlarged lymph nodes, pasty soft stool in the intestinal tract, and pale gray streaks and irregular areas deep within the myocardium as found with CPV-2 (see Fig. 8-7). Histopathologic lesions are predominantly restricted to large intranuclear epithelial inclusions at the tips of the villi in the duodenum and jejunum. These inclusions are eosinophilic and often fill the nuclei. Other intestinal changes noted include crypt epithelial hyperplasia and single-cell necrosis of crypt epithelial cells. Lesions seen in other tissue include moderate to marked depletion or necrosis (or both) of lymphoid cells of Peyer's patches and thymus, severe pneumonitis with exudate in airways, and mineralized focal to diffuse areas of myocardial necrosis with cellular infiltration.

Therapy and Prevention

Once a diagnosis has been made, treatment of pups suffering CPV-1 infection is unrewarding because of the rapid progression of the disease. However, mortality may be reduced by ensuring that the environmental temperature of newborn pups is kept warm and by adequate nutrition and hydration. No vaccine is available at present.

Public Health Considerations

No known public health concern exists; however, extra care should always be practiced in handling sick pups and fecal material from diarrheic animals because other enteropathogens may be present.

CANINE CORONAVIRAL ENTERITIS

Etiology

CCV is a member of the virus family *Coronaviridae* belonging to the order *Nidovirales* (Fig. 8-8). Different coronaviruses of this family infect a large number of species, including humans, cattle, swine, dogs, cats, horses, poultry, rats, and mice (see Table 11-1). To date, several strains of CCV have been isolated from outbreaks of diarrheal disease in dogs. The virus genome is composed of a single-stranded RNA chain; replication occurs in the cell cytoplasm of the host. Coronaviruses are fairly resistant and can remain infectious for longer periods outdoors at frozen temperatures. The virus loses infectivity in feces after approximately 40 hours at room temperature (20° C) and 60 hours when refrigerated (4° C).[123] Coronaviruses can be inactivated by most commercial detergents and disinfectants.

Epidemiology

In 1971, a CCV was isolated from feces of military dogs that were suffering from suspected infectious enteritis. Since then, several outbreaks of contagious enteritis have occurred and a similar coronavirus has been isolated. The true importance of CCV as a cause of infectious enteritis in dogs is unknown; however, CCV was genetically detected[3] or isolated[70] from 16% or 57%, respectively, of dogs with diarrhea in Japan. Serologic testing of Australian dogs showing signs of diarrhea revealed that 85% were positive for CCV–IgM antibodies, which indicates recent infection.[78] Serologic information suggests that CCV has been present indefinitely in the dog population and is an infrequent cause of infectious enteritis. CCV is highly contagious and spreads rapidly through groups of susceptible dogs. Neonatal pups are more severely affected than those of weaning age and adult dogs. CCV is shed in the feces of infected dogs for weeks to months or longer, and fecal contamination of the environment is the primary source for its transmission via ingestion.[124]

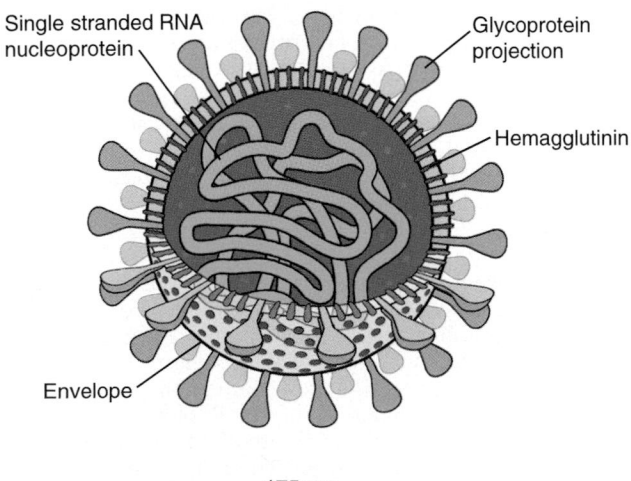

Single stranded RNA nucleoprotein

Glycoprotein projection

Hemagglutinin

Envelope

175 nm

Fig 8-8 Structure of coronavirus. (Courtesy University of Georgia, Athens, Ga.)

Pathogenesis

The incubation period is short: 1 to 4 days in the field and only 24 to 48 hours experimentally. CCV can generally be isolated from the feces of infected dogs between 3 and approximately 14 days after infection.

After ingestion, CCV goes to the mature epithelial cells of the villi of the small intestine.[124,125] After uptake of CCV by M cells in the dome epithelium of Peyer's patches virus and viral antigen is transported to the underlying lymphoid tissue. Uptake in the gut lymphoid tissue suggests that CCV may persist or become latent in dogs, similar to the situation for feline coronavirus. Genetic analysis suggested that nucleotide substitutions occurred in the transmembrane protein M gene during the time of clinical illness.[104] The virus also rapidly reproduces within epithelial cells and accumulates within cytoplasmic vacuoles. Virions from these vacuoles may be released directly into the external environment via the apical plasmalemma or may be released after lysis of the apical cytoplasm of infected cells. After production of mature virus, infected cells develop severe cytoplasmic changes, and the microvilli of the brush border become short, distorted, and lost. The overall result is that infected cells become lost from the villi at an accelerated rate and are replaced by increased replication rate of immature cells in the crypts of the mucosa. Crypt epithelium is not destroyed; on the contrary, hyperplasia develops. Affected villi become covered by low columnar to cuboidal epithelium, show variable levels of villous atrophy and fusion, and become infiltrated by mononuclear cells in the lamina propria. Unlike CPV infection, villius necrosis and hemorrhage are rare.

Dogs can have CCV and CPV infections simultaneously, and some studies suggest that CCV infection enhances the severity of CPV infection. Conversely, three of four puppies in a litter died from CCV enteritis 2 weeks after surviving CPV enteritis.[107] Concurrent infections with canine adenovirus-1 and CCV was suspected as the cause of severe enteric disease in an animal shelter.[104] Other enteropathogens such as *Clostridium perfringens*, *Campylobacter* spp., *Helicobacter* spp., and *Salmonella* spp. may increase the severity of CCV illness (see Chapter 39).

Clinical Findings

Differentiating CCV from other infectious causes of enteritis is difficult. Theories suggest that CCV infection is usually less dramatic than CPV-2 infection. The clinical signs can vary greatly, and dogs of any breed, age, and sex are affected. This finding contrasts with CPV infections in which affected dogs are usually younger than 2 years. Infected dogs usually have a sudden onset of diarrhea preceded sometimes by vomiting. Feces are characteristically orange in color, very malodorous, and infrequently contain blood. Loss of appetite and lethargy are also common signs. Unlike CPV-2 infection, fever is not constant, and leukopenia is not a recognized feature.

In severe cases, diarrhea can become watery, and dehydration and electrolyte imbalances can follow. Concurrent ocular and nasal discharges have been noted, but their relationship to the primary infection is unknown. Most of the dogs affected recover spontaneously after 8 to 10 days. When secondary complicating factors are present (parasites, bacteria, or other viruses), the disease can be significantly prolonged.

Diagnosis

Making a definitive diagnosis of CCV-induced disease is difficult. EM can detect CCV in fresh feces. Approximately 1 × 10^6 virions are needed in unconcentrated fecal samples for identification of CCV by EM; thus false-negative findings are possible. Viral isolation is difficult because CCV does not grow well in tissue or cell culture systems. A highly sensitive reverse transcriptase PCR has been developed to detect CCV in fecal specimens.[28,99,106] Serum VN and ELISA tests for CCV antibody have been developed.[111] Positive CCV serum titers of affected dogs can only confirm exposure to CCV, and serum IgG titers have no relationship to protection as do intestinal secretory IgA titers.

Pathologic Findings

Mild infections are grossly unremarkable. In severe cases, the intestinal loops are dilated and filled with thin, watery, green-yellow fecal material. Mesenteric lymph nodes are commonly enlarged and edematous.

Atrophy and fusion of intestinal villi and a deepening of the crypts characterize the intestinal lesions of CCV. Also present are an increase in cellularity of the lamina propria, flattening of surface epithelial cells, and discharge of goblet cells. With well-preserved tissues, FA staining can enable specific detection of virus in the intestinal lesions.

Therapy

Deaths associated with diarrheal disease are uncommon but occur in pups as a result of electrolyte and water loss with subsequent dehydration, acidosis, and shock. Management must emphasize supportive treatment to maintain fluid and electrolyte balance as described for CPV-2 infection. Although rarely indicated, broad-spectrum antimicrobial agents can be given to treat secondary bacterial infections. Good nursing care, including keeping the dogs quiet and warm, is certainly essential.

Prevention

Inactivated and MLV vaccines are available for protection against CCV infection.[23,87] Two doses 3 to 4 weeks apart and annual revaccination are recommended for immunization of dogs regardless of age. These vaccines are relatively safe but provide incomplete protection in that they reduce but do not completely eliminate replication of CCV in the intestinal tract after challenge.[88,89] Assessing the role of the CCV vaccines in protection against disease is difficult because CCV infections are usually inapparent or cause only mild signs of disease. For additional information on vaccination, see Coronaviral Infection in Chapter 100.

Public Health Considerations

CCV is not believed to infect people. Coronaviruses are not strictly host specific; thus the possibility of human infection cannot be excluded. For this reason, extra care should always be practiced in handling sick pups and fecal material from diarrheic animals.

CANINE ROTAVIRAL INFECTION

Etiology

Rotaviruses are recognized as important enteric pathogens in many animal species and in people. They are sometimes referred to as duovirus, reovirus-like, and rotalike virus agents. Currently, rotaviruses are classified as distinct members of the family *Reoviridae*. CRV is a double-stranded RNA, nonenveloped virus that is approximately 60 to 75 nm in diameter (Fig. 8-9). CRV is resistant to most environmental conditions outside the host.

Rotaviruses have been isolated in tissue cultures or observed by EM of specimens from many species, including mice, monkeys, calves, pigs, foals, lambs, humans, rabbits, deer, cats, and dogs.

Epidemiology

Rotaviruses are transmitted by fecal-oral contamination. The viruses are well adapted for survival outside the host and for

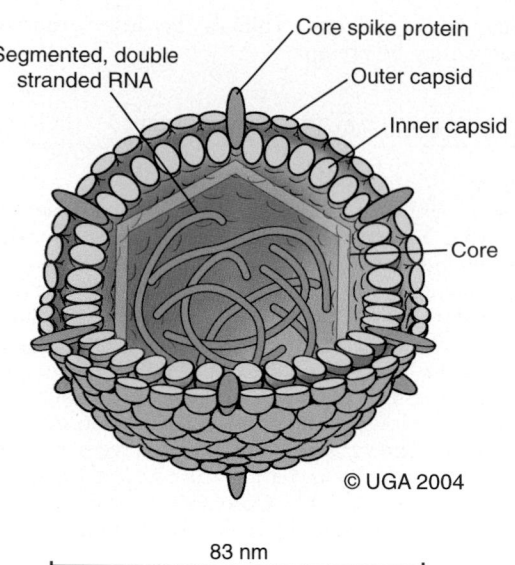

Fig 8-9 Structure of rotavirus. (Courtesy University of Georgia, Athens, Ga.)

passage through the upper GI tract. Serum antibodies to rotavirus have been identified in dogs and cats of all ages.

Pathogenesis

Rotaviruses infect the most mature epithelial cells on the luminal tips of the small intestinal villi, leading to mild-to-moderate villous atrophy. Infected cells swell, degenerate, and desquamate into the intestinal lumen, where they release a large number of virions that become sources of infection for lower intestinal segments and for other animals. Necrosis of rotavirus-infected cells is most pronounced 18 to 48 hours after oral infection. Necrotic cells are rapidly replaced by immature crypt epithelium. Clinical signs result primarily from the villous atrophy, leading to mild to moderate maldigestion and malabsorption and osmotic diarrhea.

Clinical Findings

Most clinical rotaviral infections have been demonstrated in the feces of pups younger than 12 weeks, with mild diarrhea. Some cases of severe fatal enteritis associated with CRV have been reported to occur in pups as young as 2 weeks. The clinical signs are usually not as severe as those for the other canine enteric viruses (CPV-2 and CCV). A watery to mucoid diarrhea is usual, and this lasts for 8 to 10 days. The pups usually remain afebrile. CRV may contribute to enteric disease in mixed viral infections.

Diagnosis

Most pathogenic rotaviruses share common group-specific internal capsid antigens that can be detected by many methods, including commercial fecal ELISA (Rotazyme, Abbott Labs, N. Chicago, Ill.; Enzygnost, Behring Inst., Marburg, Germany) and latex agglutination (Rotalex, Orion Diag, Helsinki, Finland; Slidex Rota-kit, Biomerieux, Marcy-1'Etoile, France) tests used to diagnose human rotavirus infection (see also Appendix 6).[111] Rotaviruses can also be identified in fecal specimens by EM, although care must be taken to differentiate rotaviruses from the apparently nonpathogenic reoviruses occasionally present in dog feces. EM improves specificity of the test. Testing for seroconversion is possible but not widely available.

Pathologic Findings

Pathologic changes are limited to the small intestine, consisting of mild to moderate villous blunting. The virus can be detected in frozen sections by fluorescent antibody techniques.

Therapy and Prevention

Most dogs recover naturally from their infection. Treatment, if needed, consists solely of symptomatic therapy as described for CPV-2 enteritis. No vaccines are available for CRV, and current estimates of the frequency and severity of the disease do not appear to justify vaccine development.

Public Health Considerations

Rotaviruses are generally host specific; however, the various strains cannot be easily distinguished, and the possibility of human infection cannot be eliminated. Rotaviral infections in people usually occur in young infants and children (younger than 4 years). Poor sanitation and hygiene, as exist in developing countries, increase the prevalence of infection. Persons handling feces from diarrheic dogs should take routine precautions.

OTHER VIRAL ENTERITIDES

A large number of other viruses have been identified in feces of dogs both with and without diarrhea. For the most part, the pathogenicity and importance of these viruses as causes of infectious enteritis remain unknown. Based on work in other species, some viruses may be true enteric pathogens, whereas others are most likely incidental findings.

Astrovirus-like particles have been reported in the stools of clinically healthy and diarrheic dogs. Astroviruses are known to cause enteritis in other species, such as swine, but whether this is either true or common in the dog is unknown. The viruses have also been identified in diarrheic cats (see Chapter 12).

A herpesvirus antigenically related to feline herpesvirus has been isolated from a dog with diarrhea, but Koch's postulates have not been fulfilled.[51] Similarly, the importance of serologic reactivity of some dogs to human echoviruses and coxsackieviruses is unclear (see also Enteroviral Infections, Chapter 24).

An apparently specific canine calicivirus has been isolated on several occasions from the feces of dogs with enteritis, sometimes alone and sometimes in conjunction with other known enteric pathogens.[72,113] Similarly, an antigenically distinct parainfluenza virus, isolated from a dog with bloody diarrhea, was believed to be causal (see Chapter 7).

The study of viral enteritis in dogs is in its infancy. Undoubtedly, there are other viruses that affect the GI tract of dogs, but they remain to be discovered and characterized.

SUGGESTED READINGS*

15. DeMari K, Maynard L, Eun HM, et al. 2003. Treatment of canine parvoviral enteritis with interferon-omega in a placebo-controlled field trial, *Vet Rec* 152:105-108.
31. Harrington DP, McCaw DL, Jones BD. 1996. A retrospective study of canine parvovirus gastroenteritis: 89 cases, *J Am Coll Vet Intern Med* 10:157.
32. Harrison LR, Styer EL, Pursell AR, et al. 1992. Fatal disease in nursing puppies associated with minute virus of canines, *J Vet Diagn Invest* 4:19-22.
54. Larson LJ, Schultz RD. 1996. High-titer canine parvovirus vaccine: serologic response and challenge-of-immunity study, *Vet Med* 90:210-218.
75. Mohr AJ, Leiswitz AL, Jacobson LS, et al. 2003. Effect of early enteral nutrition on intestinal permeability, intestinal protein loss,, and outcome in dogs with severe parvoviral enteritis, *J Vet Intern Med* 17:791-798.
92. Parrish CR. 1999. Host range relationships and the evolution of canine parvovirus, *Vet Microbiol* 69:29-40.
115. Schultz, RD, Larson LJ. 1996. The new generation of parvovirus vaccines. A comparison study, *Compend Cont Educ Pract Vet* 18:640-641.

*See the CD-ROM for a complete list of references.

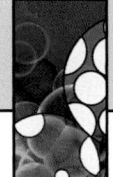

CHAPTER • 9

Canine Viral Papillomatosis

Michelle Wall and Clay A. Calvert

ETIOLOGY

The papillomavirus was first described in 1933 when Shope discovered the agent responsible for cutaneous papillomas in the cottontail rabbit.[19] Multiple canine papillomas in dogs are uncommon, comprising less than 12.5% of canine skin tumors.[20] Benign mucocutaneous tumors of epithelial origin are caused by infectious papillomavirus of the *Papovaviridae* family. The papilloma viruses are categorized with the polyomaviruses to form the papovaviruses. Members of this family are small (33 to 60 nm), naked, ether-resistant, double-stranded circular DNA tumor viruses, similar in structure to but larger than parvoviruses; they form crystalline structures within the nuclei of infected cells.[22,34] These viruses lack a lipid envelope and are acid stable and relatively thermostable, which may explain much of their inherent resistance.[34] Papillomaviruses are naturally oncogenic, producing benign warts, and are usually species and site specific. Cross-species infection of horses by bovine papillomaviruses type 1 and type 2 have been reported.[13] Most isolated viruses lack serologic cross-reactivity. Although antigenically distinct, papillomaviruses of humans, cattle, horses, dogs, and cats share at least one group-specific determinant. Inoculation of canine oral papillomavirus (COPV) into kittens, mice, rats, guinea pigs, rabbits, and nonhuman primates has failed to produce papillomas. Tumors can be transmitted experimentally within the species of origin by scarification with whole cells or cell-free filtrates. A distinct papillomavirus has been identified in cutaneous papillomas of cats (see Chapter 20) and dogs.[26,41] The close genetic relationship between feline and canine papillomas compared with those of other species supports the hypothesis that papillomaviruses have coevolved with vertebrates during host evolution.[49,52]

EPIDEMIOLOGY

Papillomas (also referred to as *warts, verruca vulgaris squamous cell papillomas,* or *cutaneous papillomatosis*) may be either (1) naturally occurring noninfectious or virus-induced solitary tumors or (2) transmissible virus-induced multiple tumors. The virus is transmitted by direct and indirect contact, but damaged epithelial surfaces may be necessary for successful inoculation.[3,16] The papillomavirus must overcome the host's immune response to replicate and produce clinical infection, so the significance of these warts is greater in immunocompromised patients.[13,34] Four or more separate papillomaviruses may infect dogs, usually without papilloma development. Numerous clinical syndromes and symptoms have been described in dogs with papillomavirus: oral papillomatosis, venereal papillomas, cutaneous papillomas, cutaneous inverted papillomas, multiple papillomas of the footpad, and papillomavirus-associated canine-pigmented plaques.

Most infectious papillomas undergo spontaneous regression, but occasionally papillomavirus infections persist or lesions recur, especially when the host is immunocompromised and the immune system cannot eliminate the virus (e.g., in a dog with concurrent infections). Dogs with granulocytic ehrlichiosis had remission of oral papillomatosis after treatment.[50] Malignant transformation into squamous cell carcinoma has been reported in various species, especially cattle. Progression to sarcoid tumors has also been reported in horses, donkeys, and mules as a result of bovine papillomavirus infection.[18]

The association of human papillomavirus and bladder cancer remains unresolved,[24,37] but strong evidence supports the role of human papillomavirus in cancer of the anogenital tract.[22] The human papillomavirus is a critical factor in the development of cervical cancer.[4] Progression of the papillomavirus to carcinoma can occur in dogs, although malignant transformation is uncommon. Reports have been made of a beagle with oral papillomatosis and a collie with an oral and a corneal papilloma that experienced malignant transformation.[1,54] The interaction of certain chemicals, genetic background, or other carcinogens with papillomavirus-infected cells is believed to produce the potential for malignant transformation; for example, human laryngeal papillomas exposed to irradiation and bladder tumors in cattle exposed to bracken fern create the potential for transformation.[8,13]

PATHOGENESIS

The life cycle of the papillomavirus is closely associated with the differentiating epithelial cell, and infections with papillomavirus are usually confined to the epidermis and epithelium.[39] Papillomavirus infects basal keratinocytes of the stratum germinativum; the basal cell is the only cell in the squamous epithelium that is capable of undergoing division.[55] Once it has infected the basal layer, the virus expresses itself in the basal and suprabasal layers, undergoes genome replica-

tion in the granular and spinous layers, packages its DNA in the squamous layers, and releases a new infectious virus with the keratinized squames.[13] The first tissue response to COPV infection is an increase in mitotic activity, resulting in acanthosis and hyperkeratosis. As the disease progresses, some infected cells begin producing virus. These cells develop inclusion material but do not undergo cytoplasmic differentiation. Cytoplasmic degeneration and cell death ensue with viral persistence in strands of keratin; however, the majority of basal layer cells differentiate into keratogenetic normal cells. Spontaneous tumor regression is the usual course. The virus is latent in the basal layers, although complete viral particles may be identified at the granular level.

The incubation period of COPV is usually 4 to 8 weeks postinoculation. Concentration of COPV in the inoculum may influence subsequent tumor growth and regression in various ways. Papillomavirus infection delays the activation of the host's immune system. The virus targets end-stage differentiating cells and is often protected from systemic immune defenses, and the production of papillomavirus is not accompanied by inflammation.[34] Dogs given small doses of virus develop more papillomas and have delayed regression compared with dogs given larger doses of virus. Antibodies to papillomavirus are produced, but they do not correlate with growth or regression. Once regression occurs, subsequent immunity develops.

The mechanisms resulting in spontaneous regression or spread of papillomas are unknown. Papilloma regression is thought to be associated with the presence of CD4+ and CD8+ lymphocytes. These cells, especially the CD4+ cells, activate macrophages, inhibit viruses via cytokines, kill keratinocytes, or all of these.[34] Virus-neutralizing antibody inactivates COPV in sensitized animals but does not inhibit established virus or papillomas. Serum from dogs whose papillomas have undergone spontaneous regression usually not only fails to produce tumor regression but also can enhance tumor growth in naive dogs. Passive transfer of serum immunoglobulins from immune dogs may occasionally protect naive dogs.[34,48] Failure of protection by serum immunoglobulins from dogs that have undergone spontaneous regression may be the result of the induction of blocking antigen-antibody factors that impede cytotoxic lymphocyte action on target cells. Severe oral papillomatosis occurs in beagles with IgA deficiency.[47] Cellular immune mechanisms may be more important in inhibiting the development of early papillomas in dogs. Regression is enhanced by the injection of immune lymphocytes from dogs in which COPV has regressed. In contrast, COPV papillomatosis spread from the oral cavity throughout the haired skin of a Shar-pei dog given glucocorticoids.[47] Multiple cutaneous papillomas caused by a new papillomavirus developed in a boxer dog receiving long-term glucocorticoid therapy, and similar associations were recognized in dogs with hypogammaglobulinemia, IgM deficiency, impaired T-cell responses, and high dose, long-term cyclosporine administration.[7,9,26,40] In humans, increased prevalence of papillomatosis is associated with defects in the cell-mediated or humoral immune system as well.

Puppies inoculated with COPV develop hyperplastic and neoplastic lesions at sites other than the oropharyngeal mucosa. Lesions have included epidermal hyperplasia, epidermal cysts, squamous papilloma, basal cell epithelioma, and squamous cell carcinoma; however, very few inoculations were associated with these extraoral lesions.

CLINICAL FINDINGS

Oral papillomas occur on the oral, labial, and pharyngeal mucosa, as well as on the tongue, on the hard palate, and on the epiglottis; it rarely occurs in the esophagus (Fig. 9-1). Oral

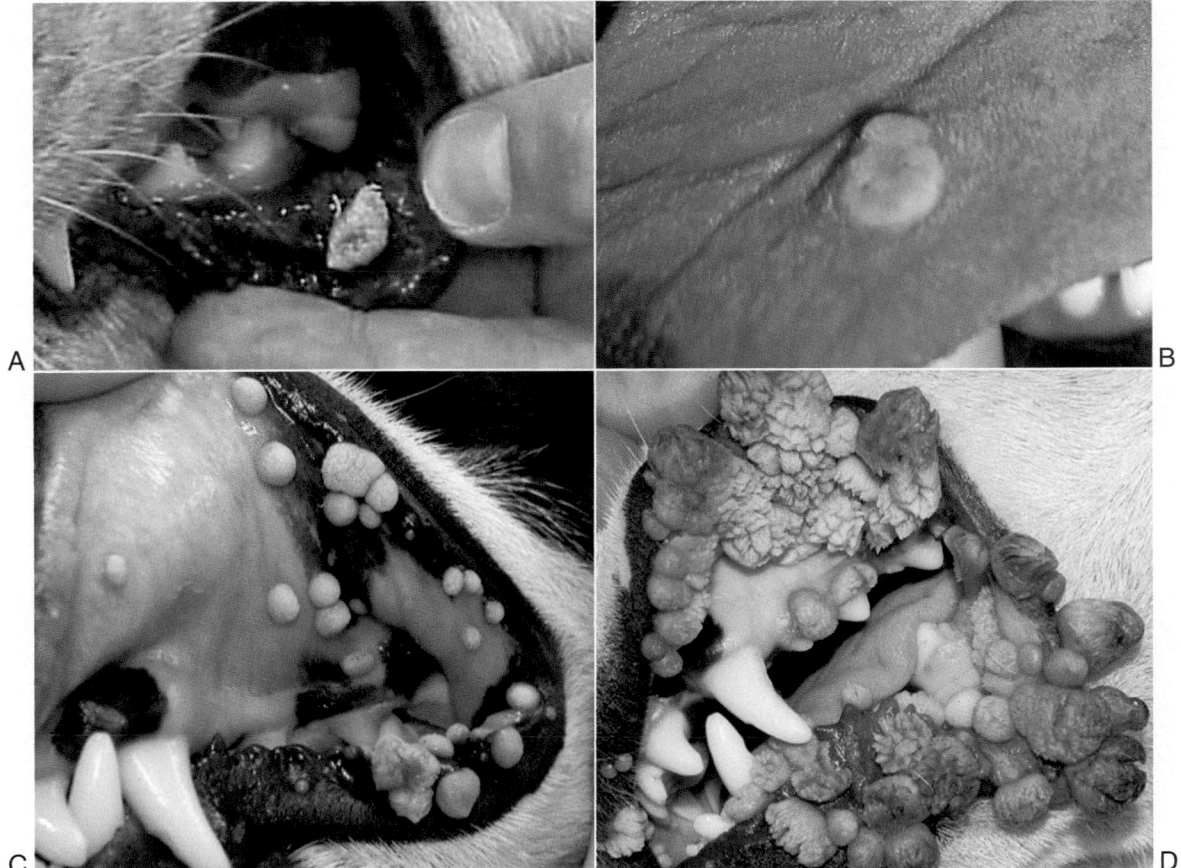

Fig 9-1 Typical canine oral papillomatosis in young dogs. **A,** Single labial papilloma. **B,** Papillomas on the tongue, hard palate, and labial surface. **C,** Multiple labial papillomas. **D,** Extensive oral papillomatosis. (Courtesy Patrick Hensel and Tracy Gieger, University of Georgia, Athens, Ga.)

papillomatosis of young dogs (with a median age of 1 year) is a contagious viral disease.[27] The lesions typically begin as white, smooth, flat, shiny plaques that progress, usually 4 to 8 weeks postinfection, to pedunculated or cauliflower-like masses.[13,27] The oral form is usually a self-limiting disease, although the lesions may persist without spontaneous regression or spread to other areas of the body.[39]

Ocular papillomas can occur on the conjunctivae, cornea, and eyelid margins (Fig. 9-2). Ocular papillomas are less common than oral papillomas and are caused by a virus that is similar in structure to the oral papillomavirus.

Virus-induced cutaneous papillomas are uncommon and usually solitary lesions caused by a subtype of the canine papillomavirus; they are not associated with the papovavirus. Although usually solitary, the cutaneous lesions may be multifocal and are often found elsewhere on the body (Fig. 9-3). COPV inoculated into the skin of the face may produce a papilloma, but attempts to produce a tumor by inoculating the skin of the abdomen or back with COPV have usually failed.

Dogs older than 2 years of age seldom develop oral papillomas, and older dogs appear to be resistant to COPV infection. Ocular papillomas occur most often in dogs 6 months to 4 years of age but have been reported in dogs as old as 9 years. The susceptible age range of dogs with cutaneous papillomas is broader. Cutaneous papillomas occur in older dogs and appear to be more common in males.[39] The Kerry blue terrier and the cocker spaniel have been reported to be overrepresented.[39,41] The cutaneous warts are distinct from the oral

form and usually occur on the head, feet, and eyelids. In Australia, cutaneous papillomas of the distal limbs and interdigital pad area in racing greyhounds occur in dogs 12 to 18 months of age.[14]

Cutaneous inverted papillomas usually occur on the ventrum and inguinal regions.[11] They have been reported to occur in dogs from 8 months to 7 years of age.[11,41] These small, firm, raised masses appear as cup-shape lesions with a central core of keratin that have a small pore opening to the skin surface.[27] Their surface is similar to that of an intracutaneous cornifying epithelioma, but they have a papillary projection of epidermis into the lumen that epitheliomas do not possess.[11] Single or multiple lesions may develop, and they are covered by skin with a central pore opening to the surface.

Multiple papillomas affecting the footpads have been described in adult dogs.[39] The lesions are very firm and hyperkeratotic. They can occur on more than one foot and often cause lameness (Fig. 9-4). They do not seem to be associated with a virus.

Papillomavirus-associated canine-pigmented plaques have been documented in several miniature schnauzers and pugs during young adulthood.[32] These lesions often progress over time and do not regress. Potential for malignant transformation exists.

Although oral papillomatosis is the most common clinically relevant disease, other forms are recognized. Oral papillomatosis is a contagious, usually self-limiting disease affecting the oral mucosa, labial margins, tongue, palate, pharynx, and epiglottis. Initially, oral papillomas are pale, smooth, elevated lesions, but they soon become cauliflower-like, with fine, white, stringy projections. Early tumors appear to "seed" the rest of the susceptible oral tissues. Recognition of the lesions usually occurs while the numbers of tumors are still increasing. Halitosis, ptyalism, hemorrhage, and oral discomfort are clinical signs observed by the owners of affected dogs. These lesions often bleed when traumatized. As many as 50 to 100 tumors are often present at the time of diagnosis (see Fig. 9-1, C and D).

Papillomavirus infections usually regress spontaneously, but the time to regression varies from weeks to years. Regres-

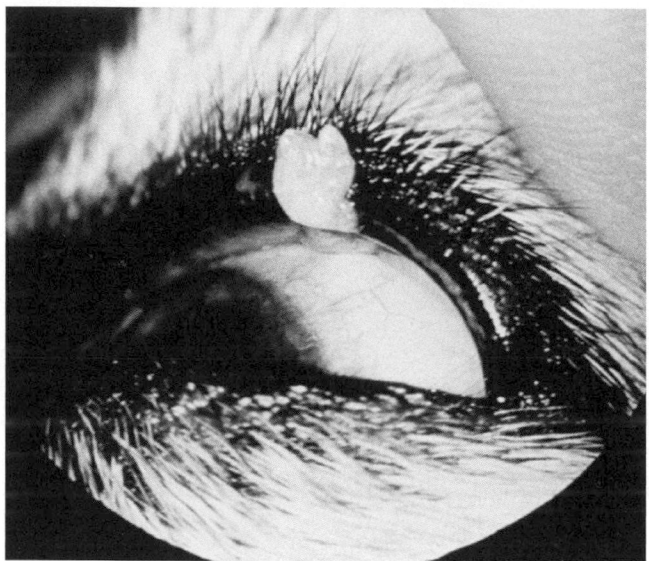

Fig   9-2   Eyelid papilloma in a dog.

sion typically occurs within 4 to 8 weeks. Oral papillomas usually regress after 4 to 8 weeks, although they may persist for up to 24 months. Cutaneous papillomas may persist for 6 to 12 months before undergoing spontaneous regression. Occasionally, incomplete regression occurs, and a few papillomas persist indefinitely. Dogs affected by persistent papillomas often have many large tumors and may become malnourished. Secondary bacterial infection of large, persistent, and ulcerated tumors is common and characterized by a mucopurulent discharge.

Ocular papillomas tend to persist longer than oral papillomas and are usually less numerous. When COPV was inoculated into the eyelids of dogs, only 50% of the dogs developed papillomas, the incubation period was longer than it is in the oral cavity, and the tumors persisted longer than they do in the oral cavity.[53] Experimentally papillomavirus isolated from ocular lesions can produce oral papillomatosis, but it has not been proven that this occurs naturally.[27]

DIAGNOSIS

The diagnosis of papillomatosis is based on the epidemiology and gross appearance of the tumors. Ocular papillomas are usually biopsied and examined histologically because they are not as morphologically distinct as oral papillomas. Microscopic features of papillomas include marked epidermal hyperplasia on fibrovascular stalks. Small, intranuclear, basophilic inclusions may be noted and in some cases, keratinocytes within the papillomas may contain large eosinophilic cytoplasmic inclusions.[15] Cutaneous papillomas, usually morphologically distinct, are often excised for aesthetic reasons and examined microscopically. Cutaneous papillomas can occur at many sites, most often on the lower extremities, often in the interdigital areas and footpads, and occasionally subungually. The viral cause can be confirmed by immunohistochemistry staining for viral antigen, electron microscopy findings demon-

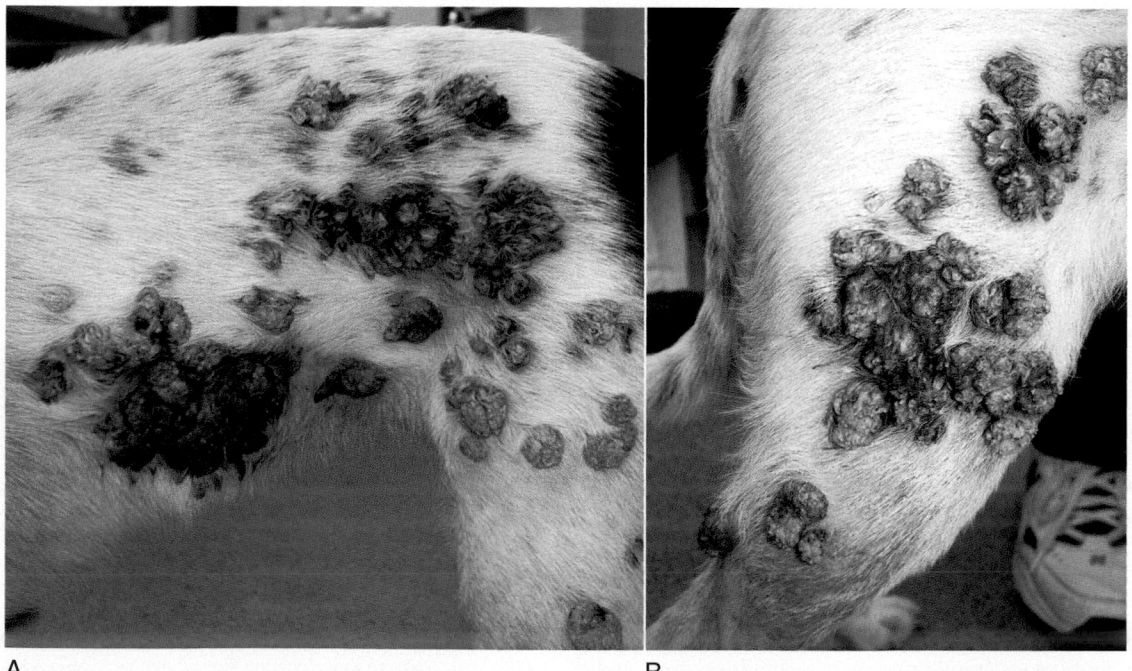

A   B

Fig   9-3   Multiple papillomas on the **(A)** lateral flank and **(B)** caudal thigh of two different dogs. (Courtesy Patrick Hensel, University of Georgia, Athens, Ga.)

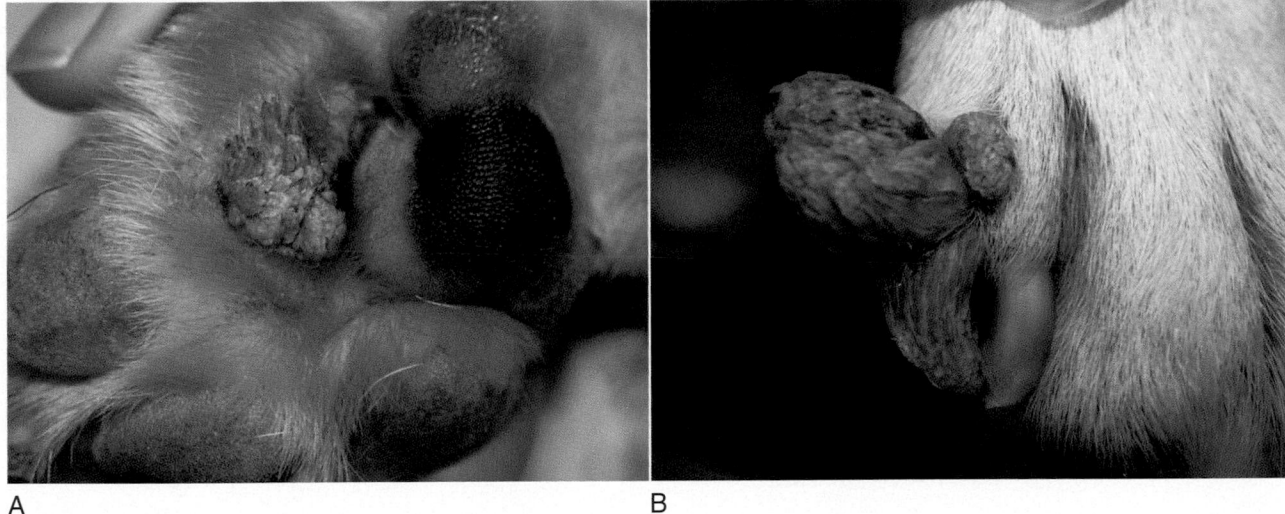

A   B

Fig 9-4 Footpad papilloma in a young dog. **A,** Papilloma near the metacarpal pad. **B,** Papilloma at the nail bed. (Courtesy Patrick Hensel, University of Georgia, Athens, Ga.)

strating the virus, or polymerase chain reaction and in situ hybridization techniques to detect papillomavirus DNA.*

THERAPY

Treatment is not indicated if only a few papillomas are present because they are usually self-limiting, and afterward dogs are immune to reinfection.[39] However, the patient should be frequently monitored to determine whether the tumor numbers are increasing. Spontaneous regression is the usual course, but treatment may be indicated when tumors persist; when large, multiple tumors produce pharyngeal obstruction; when problems eating occur; and for aesthetic reasons. Treatment efficacy is often difficult to determine because of the high incidence of spontaneous regression.

The ideal therapy remains unknown because of the lack of sufficient knowledge regarding papillomavirus. Surgical excision, cryosurgery, and electrosurgery are acceptable modes of oral tumor treatment. Surgical removal, freezing, or simply crushing 5 to 15 of the tumors may induce spontaneous regression, presumably a result of antigenic stimulation. Laser therapy has been effective in the treatment of several resistant human warts and has been described for human recurrent respiratory papillomatosis.[17] Oral papillomatosis has been unsuccessfully treated with a CO_2 laser.[25] Although autogenous vaccines are commonly recommended, their efficacy in dogs is questionable, and they are often not effective against persistent papillomatosis. Recombinant vaccines have been shown to induce regression in several species including the dog and can be used prophylactically to prevent mucosal infections with COPV.[3,23,25,47] It has been demonstrated that systemic immunization with COPV L1 protein can induce a humoral response that will provide protection against oral papillomatosis.[48] The vaccines may also play a role in decreasing the development of squamous cell carcinomas. In a case report of a 16-month-old Siberian husky that did not respond to surgical therapy, an autogenous vaccine appeared to induce regression of the resistant oral papillomas, and high circulating neutralizing antibodies against COPV were produced.[25] The titers appeared to be correlated with regression of the oral

papillomas.[25] Anecdotal reports have been made of success with the use of autogenous vaccines. Additional studies should be performed regarding the effectiveness of recombinant COPV vaccines because the development of neoplasms has been reported to occur at the injection site of live COPV vaccines in dogs.[8,28,45] Cutaneous papillomas that arise as a result of glucocorticoid-induced immunosuppression may regress once this therapy is discontinued.

Surgical excision or cryosurgery is effective for papillomas of the conjunctiva or eyelid. Cryosurgery is not recommended for corneal papillomas. Care should be taken to prevent spread of the virus to adjacent ocular tissues, and cryosurgery or possibly laser therapy may offer an advantage in this regard.

Systemic and intralesional (bleomycin) chemotherapy using single-agent vincristine, cyclophosphamide, or doxorubicin has been ineffective in the majority of dogs treated. Topical application of 5-fluorouracil (0.5% solution) has been used successfully in humans with numerous cutaneous warts, a treatment that may be useful for cutaneous lesions in dogs. However, ingestion of 5-fluorouracil can result in local irritation and severe systemic toxicity. The retinoid etretinate has been useful in the treatment of a few dogs with cutaneous papillomatosis. Widespread papillomavirus-associated canine-pigmented plaques have been effectively treated with etretinate (1 mg/kg orally every 24 hours).[32,33] Possible retinoid toxicity can include conjunctivitis, pruritis, vomiting, diarrhea, joint stiffness, pedal and mucocutaneous erythema, hyperactivity, and teratogenicity. Interferons (IFNs) have been administered parenterally and intralesionally to affected humans until regression occurs. Low doses of oral IFNs rather than high doses of parenteral IFNs are more commonly used in pets and less expensive, but not likely to be effective. In vitro studies of IFN therapy have shown a reduction in the papillomavirus in mouse cells transformed by bovine papillomavirus-1.[32] The immune modulator Acemannan (*Acemman Immunostimulant,* Carrington Labs, Irving, Tex.) has been administered intralesionally to cause regression of fibrosarcomas and might be an alternative to IFN therapy. Photodynamic therapy has induced good responses for several types of skin cancer and may play a role in future treatment of canine papillomas. Dogs recovering from oral papillomatosis are immune, as are most dogs older than 2 years (see Interferons, Chapters 2 and 100; Acemannan, Chapter 100; and

*References 7,15,39,42,47,51.

Drug Formulary, Appendix 8 for additional information on administration and precautions of these drugs).

PREVENTION

Protection against viral challenge with COPV has been achieved by sequential immunization doses via DNA delivery of a plasmid encoding COPV major capsid L1 protein or oncoproteins E1 or E2 to cutaneous and oral mucosal sites in beagles.[31,43,44] Codon-optimized E1 gene sequences (but not wild-type gene sequences) provided complete protection after DNA vaccination of beagle dogs with COPV.[31] Both cell-mediated and humoral immune responses were detected. No vaccine is commercially available.

SUGGESTED READINGS*

12. Campo MS. 2002. Animal models of papillomavirus pathogenesis. *Virus Res* 89:249-261.
31. Moore RA, Walcott S, White KL, et al. 2003. Therapeutic immunization with COPV early genes by epithelial DNA delivery. *Virology* 314:630-535.
32. Nagata M. 2000. Canine papillomatosis, pp 569-571. *In* Bonagura JD (ed), *Kirk's current veterinary therapy XIII.* WB Saunders, Philadelphia, PA.
36. Nicholls PK, Stanley MA. 1999. Canine papillomavirus—a centenary review, *J Comp Pathol* 120:219-233.

*See the CD-ROM for a complete list of references.

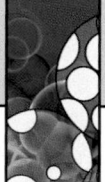

CHAPTER • 10

Feline Parvovirus Infections

Craig E. Greene and Diane D. Addie

ETIOLOGY

Feline panleukopenia is caused by a small, serologically homogeneous parvovirus (feline panleukopenia virus [FPV]), with single-stranded DNA. Genetically, structurally, and antigenically, it is closely related to blue fox parvovirus (BFPV), mink enteritis virus (MEV), and canine parvovirus (CPV) (Table 10-1).[38] In addition, CPV strains 2a and 2b have been isolated from healthy cats[39] and from those with signs of feline panleukopenia (see later discussion, Canine Parvoviral Infection, and Chapter 8).[40,59] In contrast, FPV has limited replication in dogs after experimental inoculation.[61] FPV is very stable, able to survive for 1 year at room temperature in organic material on solid fomites. It resists heating to 56° C for 30 minutes and remains viable for longer periods at lower temperatures. The virus survives disinfection with 70% alcohol and various dilutions of organic iodines, phenolics, and quaternary ammonium compounds. FPV is inactivated by bleach (6% sodium hypochlorite), 4% formaldehyde, and 1% glutaraldehyde in 10 minutes at room temperature.

EPIDEMIOLOGY

FPV can cause disease in all members of the family Felidae. Some Viverridae, Procyonidae, and Mustelidae, including the binturong, raccoon, coatimundi, ring-tailed cat, and mink, are also susceptible (see Table 100-20). The virus is ubiquitous because of its contagious nature and capacity for persistence in the environment. Virtually all susceptible cats are exposed and infected within the first year of life. Unvaccinated kittens that acquire maternally derived antibody (MDA) through colostrum are usually protected for up to 3 months of age (though longer duration of MDA to 20 weeks sufficient to

interfere with vaccination has been reported).[2] Most infections are subclinical, inasmuch as 75% of unvaccinated, clinically healthy cats have demonstrable antibody titers by 1 year of age. Seasonal variations in the incidence of panleukopenia and disease outbreaks presumably parallel increases in the number of susceptible newborn kittens. Although panleukopenia is regarded as a condition of unvaccinated random-source cats, infection has been reported in kittens born into pedigree breeding cats from well-vaccinated queens.[1,2,7]

A perception exists among veterinary practitioners that the prevalence of FPV infection in cats has diminished over the last two decades. Reasons for this decrease may be the more widespread vaccination of cats and the use of modified live virus (MLV) vaccines, which may cause virus shedding, thereby immunizing exposed cats. Secondly, the newly emerging CPV-2 strains infecting cats may offer some cross-protection against FPV infection. FPV may be more adapted to its host; however, other prenatal or neonatally acquired forms of disease such as neurologic or cardiac manifestations are occurring (see later discussion under Pathogenesis).

Because of its short shedding period, but long environmental survival, FPV is most commonly transmitted by indirect contact of susceptible animals with contaminated premises. It is shed from all body secretions during active stages of disease but is most consistently recovered from the intestine and feces. Virus shedding usually lasts 1 to 2 days, but cats can shed virus in their urine and feces for a maximum of 6 weeks after recovery.[9] FPV is maintained in the population by its environmental persistence rather than by prolonged viral shedding. In utero transmission occurs. The virus has been isolated for a maximum of 1 year from the kidneys of neonatally infected kittens, but shedding does not occur.

Table • 10-1

Comparison of Parvoviral Isolates

VIRUS	YEAR OF ORIGIN	NATURAL HOST	EXPERIMENTAL HOST-TISSUE OF REPLICATION	CELL CULTURE LINES	A3B10	B6D5	B2C11	B4E1	A4E3	C1D1	B4A2	P2-215	239	246	259	279	308	699	871	889	899	913	967	1038	1167	1276	1623	1691	1703
FPV/MEV-1	<1900 1940	Cat, mink, raccoon	Dog—only thymus, marrow	Feline only	++	++	++	++	−	−	++	++	A	A	A	A	A	T	T	C	T	C	G	A	T	A	A	A	C
BFPV/MEV-2	1983	Blue fox, mink, raccoon		Feline only	−	++	−	−	−	−	++	++	A	A	A	A	T	T	C	C	T	G	G	G	G	A	A	A	C
CPV-2	1978	Dog, raccoon dog	Cat—no replication	Feline, canine	++	++	+	++	++	−	++	−	G	G	A	C	C	C	C	C	C	C	A	G	G	A	A	A	G
CPV-2a	1981	Dog, cat	Cat—, lymphoid intestinal	Feline, canine	++	++	−	−	++	++	++	−	G	G	T	C	C	C	C	C	G	T	G	G	G	C	C	A	G
CPV-2b	1985	Dog, cat	Cat—, lymphoid intestinal	Feline, canine	++	++	−	−	++	++	−	−	G	G	T	C	C	C	C	C	G	G	A	G	G	C	C	G	G
CPV-2c (a)	1997	Leopard cat	Cat? Dog?	Feline, canine	−	−	−	−	++	−	++	−	G	G	T	C	C	C	C	C	A	T	A	G	G	A	C	C	G
CPV-2c (b)	1997	Leopard cat	Cat? Dog?	Feline, canine	−	−	−	−	++	−	−	−	G	G	T	C	C	C	C	C	A	T	A	G	G	A	C	C	G

Column group headers: HOSTS (YEAR OF ORIGIN, NATURAL HOST, EXPERIMENTAL HOST-TISSUE OF REPLICATION); MONOCLONAL ANTIBODY REACTIVITY (A3B10, B6D5, B2C11, B4E1, A4E3, C1D1, B4A2, P2-215); NUCLEOTIDE POSITION VP2 GENE (239–1703).

FPV, Feline panleukopenia virus; *MEV,* mink enteritis virus-1; *BFPV,* blue fox parvovirus; *CPV,* canine parvovirus; *MAB,* monoclonal antibody; ++, strong; +, weak; −, negative; *A,* adenine; *T,* thymidine; *C,* cytosine; *G,* guanidine; *?,* unknown.

Owners who lose a kitten to feline panleukopenia should *not* introduce a new kitten into the household without having it vaccinated.

Fomites play a relatively important role in disease transmission because of prolonged survival of the virus on contaminated surfaces. Vehicles for exposure include contaminated litter trays, clothing, shoes, hands, food dishes, bedding, and infected cages. Transmission also probably occurs via flies and other insect vectors during warm periods.

PATHOGENESIS

As a parvovirus, FPV requires rapidly multiplying cells for successful infection, and the distribution of lesions within a prospective feline host occurs in tissues with the greatest rate of mitotic activity (Fig. 10-1). Lymphoid tissue, bone marrow, and intestinal mucosal crypts (intestinal glands) are most commonly invaded in adult animals. Late prenatal and early neonatal infections in cats result in some lymphoid and bone marrow lesions, but the central nervous system (CNS), including the cerebrum, the cerebellum, the retina, and optic nerves, can be affected.

Systemic Infections

Experimental infections have been produced in specific pathogen-free (SPF) and germ-free kittens. Clinical severity of infection is milder in these animals compared with that in field cases and in experimentally infected conventional cats, suggesting that co-pathogenic factors may play a role in the natural disease. The virus undergoes replication in lymphoid tissues of the oropharynx 18 to 24 hours after intranasal (IN) or oral infection. A plasma-phase viremia, occurring between 2 and 7 days, disseminates the virus to all body tissues, although pathologic lesions primarily occur in tissues with the highest mitotic activity. Lymphoid tissue undergoes initial necrosis followed by lymphoid proliferation. Thymic involution and degeneration are found in germ-free and SPF cats infected up to 9 weeks of age. Decreased T–cell responsiveness has been reported in FPV-infected cats, but no interference in humoral immune responses occurs. Cats surviving infection have a decrease in viremia corresponding to a rapidly rising virus neutralization (VN) serum antibody titer by 7 days postinoculation (PI).

During intestinal infection, the virus selectively damages replicating cells deep in the crypts of the intestinal mucosa. Differentiated absorptive cells on the surface of the villi are nondividing and are not affected. Shortening of the intestinal villi results from damage to the crypt cells, which normally migrate up the villi, replacing absorptive cells. Damage to the intestinal villi results in diarrhea caused by malabsorption and increased permeability (see Fig. 89-6, C).

SPF kittens have more severe intestinal lesions compared with germ-free kittens. The proliferation rate of crypt epithelium is faster in SPF kittens as a result of indigenous microflora or their metabolic by-products, which stimulate the turnover rate of intestinal epithelial cells. The extent of damage throughout the intestinal tract parallels the presence of FPV, and lesions are milder in the colon, where epithelial mitotic rates are slower than they are in the small intestine. The jejunum and ileum are more affected than the duodenal segment, which may reflect lower number of indigenous microorganisms in the proximal small bowel.

SPF and conventional cats with panleukopenia are also susceptible to secondary bacterial infections with enteric

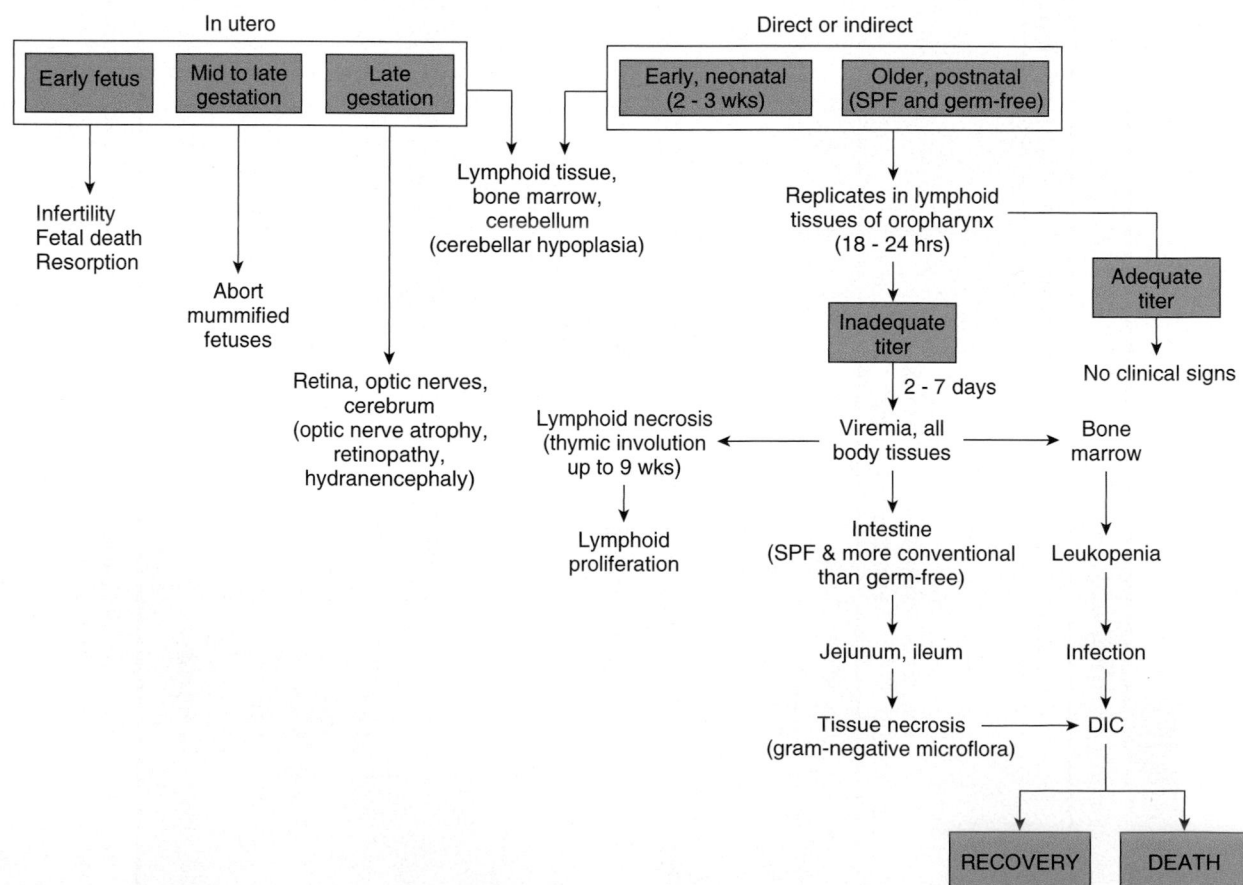

Fig 10-1 Pathogenesis of feline panleukopenia. *SPF*, specific pathogen–free; *DIC*, disseminated intravascular coagulation.

microflora. Gram-negative endotoxemia, with or without bacteremia, is a common complication of systemic FPV infection. Disseminated intravascular coagulation (DIC), a frequent complication of endotoxemia, can also develop with feline panleukopenia.

Co-infections

Concurrent infections with co-pathogens can increase the severity of FPV infections in cats, similar to the situation in dogs with parvoviral infection. Intestinal cell replication increases during insults to the bowel mucosa, which can increase the virulence of parvoviruses that infect rapidly dividing cells. Dual infection with *Clostridium piliforme*, the causative agent of Tyzzer's disease, was found in kittens (see also Chapter 39).[32] Co-infections with salmonellae and FPV have also been described in purebred catteries, with severe mortality.[14] FPV may be an immunosuppressive agent in these enteric bacterial co-infections given that it causes both leukopenia and bowel injury, which allows bacterial proliferation.

In Utero Infection

Early in utero infection can produce a spectrum of reproductive disorders in the pregnant queen, including early fetal death and resorption with infertility, abortions, or the birth of mummified fetuses. Closer to the end of gestation, infections will result in birth of live kittens with varying degrees of damage to the late-developing neural tissues. FPV produces variable effects on animals from the same litter. Some kittens are apparently unaffected owing to either innate resistance or the acquisition of maternal antibody, but they may harbor virus subclinically for up or 8 to 9 weeks in some cases.[9]

Central Nervous System Infection

The CNS, optic nerve, and retina are susceptible to injury by virulent or vaccine strains of FPV during prenatal or early neonatal development, and, of CNS lesions, cerebellar damage has been most commonly reported. This predilection for cerebellar disease may be explained by the fact that in cats the cerebellum develops during late gestation and early neonatal periods. FPV interferes with cerebellar cortical development, resulting in reduced and distorted cell layers. The cerebellum can be affected by infections occurring as late as 9 days of age. Polymerase chain reaction (PCR) has confirmed that parvoviral DNA can be found in the cerebellum of cats with cerebellar hypoplasia.[48] Other CNS lesions can be produced by earlier prenatal infections. Lesions of the spinal cord and cerebrum, including hydrocephalus, hydranencephaly, and optic nerve and retinal abnormalities, can occur (see Clinical Findings later in this chapter).[19,53] Purkinje's cell degeneration in the cerebellum was described in one adult feral cat with systemic FPV infection.[13] Unexpectedly, parvoviruses appear to be capable of replicating in neurons, which are considered to be terminally differentiated cells. Cats that had died of various diseases including panleukopenia had parvovirus detected histochemically in their brains.[62] These cats did not have the clinical signs of cerebellar hypoplasia nor were they of that susceptible age group. Viral nucleic acid was found by in situ hybridization to be in brain nuclei, especially in the diencephalic areas. Some of the virus appeared to be CPV-2 of the old antigenic type. The clinical significance of this neuronal infection is unknown.

Myocarditis and Cardiomyopathy

Myocarditis in people and animals can be induced by a large number of viruses. Myocarditis was one of the early-recognized features of CPV-2 infections in dogs, and it continues to be a feature of CPV-1 infection in dogs (see Chapter 8). With CPV-2, a lack of maternal immunity, during the early epidemic period of the late 1970s and before the advent of

available vaccines, resulted in increased susceptibility of the fetus to infection. FPV likely infects kittens born to queens that were exposed to the virus during pregnancy. Hearts from cats dying of idiopathic hypertrophic, dilated, and restrictive forms of cardiomyopathy were examined by PCR for genomic evidence of FPV, feline calicivirus (FCV), feline herpes virus (FHV)-1 and feline coronavirus (FCoV).[36] Only FPV was identified in a significant number of the hearts. These data suggest that FPV is important in the pathogenesis of this disease in cats.

CLINICAL FINDINGS

The frequency with which cats show evidence of clinical disease with FPV is much less than the number of cats infected with the virus. This fact is supported by the high prevalence of FPV antibodies in the cat population. Subclinical cases, more common in older susceptible cats, remain unrecognized. Severe clinical illness is the rule in young unvaccinated kittens; the highest morbidity and mortality occurs between 3 and 5 months of age. Sudden neonatal or adolescent death (fading kittens) has been observed in kittens of 4 weeks to 12 months of age from households of vaccinated pedigree cats.[2] In one study in the United Kingdom, FPV was the cause of 25% of kitten mortality.[7]

The disease has an acute self-limiting course, and other diseases probably cause chronic leukopenia or diarrhea. In the most peracute form, cats may die within 12 hours, as if poisoned, with little or no premonitory signs. They may be found in terminal stages of septic shock, being profoundly dehydrated, hypothermic, and comatose.

The acute form is most common, with fever (40° to 41.6° C [104° to 107° F]), depression, and anorexia occurring within 3 to 4 days before presentation. Vomiting, which develops during the illness in most cats, is frequently bile-tinged and occurs unrelated to eating. Extreme dehydration, sometimes exhibited by the cat crouching with its head over the water dish, may occur as a nonspecific feature of this disease (Fig. 10-2). Diarrhea occurs with less frequency. When it is present, the diarrhea usually occurs somewhat later in the course of illness.

On abdominal palpation, the intestinal loops may have a thickened, ropelike consistency, and discomfort is commonly noted. Mesenteric lymphadenomegaly is usually present, whereas peripheral lymph nodes are not enlarged. Oral ulceration, bloody diarrhea, or icterus may be noted in complicated infections. Petechial and ecchymotic hemorrhages may be found in cats with complicating DIC, although cats do not

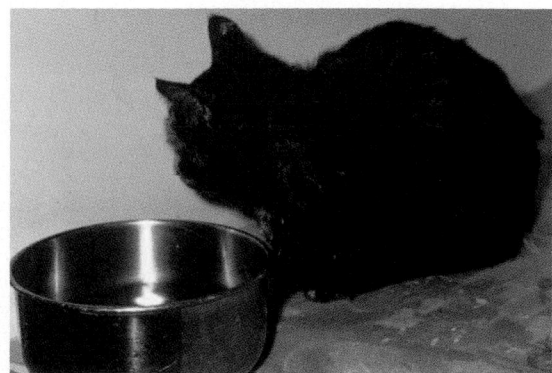

Fig 10-2 Cat with head hanging over water bowl, a frequent but nonspecific finding in panleukopenia and other acute causes of gastroenteritis. (Courtesy University of Georgia, Athens, Ga.)

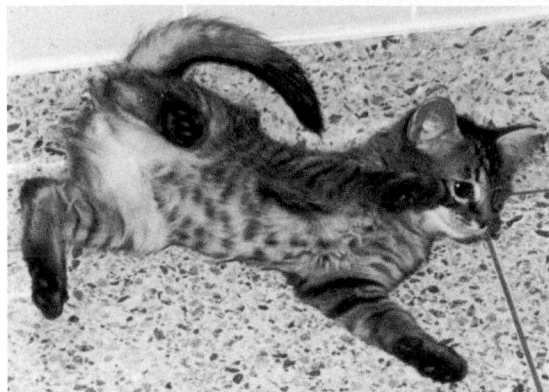

Fig 10-3 Kitten with congenital feline panleukopenia and cerebellar hypoplasia showing marked ataxia. (Courtesy University of Georgia, Athens, Ga.)

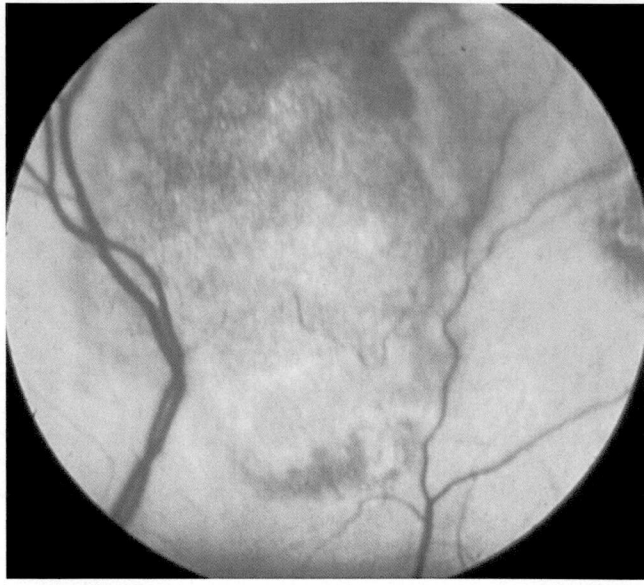

Fig 10-4 Dark foci in the retina from a kitten with hydranencephaly and optic nerve hypoplasia as a result of in utero FPV infection. (Courtesy Charles Martin, Athens, Ga.)

frequently show overt signs of hemorrhage, even with marked thrombocytopenia.

Severe dehydration associated with anorexia, vomiting, and diarrhea can lead to progressive weakness, depression, and semicoma. Cats become hypothermic during the terminal stages of the illness. They can die suddenly from complications associated with secondary bacterial infection, dehydration, and DIC. Animals that survive infection for longer than 5 days without developing fatal complications usually recover, although recovery frequently takes several weeks.

Queens infected or vaccinated during pregnancy may show infertility or abortion of dead or mummified fetuses, but clinical signs are never exhibited in the aborting female. Some kittens in a litter may be born with ataxia, incoordination, tremors, and normal mental status typical of cerebellar disease (Fig. 10-3). They walk with a broad-based stance with hypermetric movements, and they frequently show intention tremors of the head. Tremors and incoordination are absent when kittens are at rest. Not all kittens in a litter are affected or have the same degree of neurologic deficits.[53] Signs of forebrain damage include seizures, behavioral changes, and relatively normal gait despite postural reaction deficits. Affected kittens with minimal cerebellar dysfunction can compensate to a degree with time and may make suitable pets with subtle residual deficits.

Retinal lesions may be visible on fundic examination of kittens affected with neurologic signs or as an incidental finding in clinically normal cats. These areas of retinal degeneration appear as discrete, gray foci with darkened margins, and retinal folding or streaking may be seen (Fig. 10-4).

DIAGNOSIS

Clinical Laboratory Findings

A presumptive diagnosis of systemic feline panleukopenia is usually made based on clinical signs and the presence of leukopenia. Leukocyte counts during the height of severe infection (days 4 to 6 of infection) are usually between 50 and 3000 cells/µl. Less affected animals have counts between 3000 and 7000 cells/µl. Leukopenia, from which the disease derives its name, is not pathognomonic for FPV infection alone and may not occur in all cases. The severity of leukopenia usually parallels that of clinical illness, and leukopenia also develops in infected germ-free and SPF cats. In FPV, neutropenia develops first, as neutrophils exude into the infected gut, then followed by leukopenia from bone marrow sup-

pression, a resurgence of leukopoiesis characterized by neutrophilia with a left shift follows in cats that recover. As in dogs, CPV infection of cats leads to lymphopenia. Subsequent examination of the leukocyte count in 24 to 48 hours in recovering FPV-infected cats will show a rebound in leukocyte numbers.

Feline salmonellosis with overwhelming septicemia may mimic feline panleukopenia with the presence of leukopenia and acute gastrointestinal (GI) illness. Fecal culture may be helpful under these circumstances (see Chapter 39).

A transient decrease in absolute reticulocyte count and a mild (5% to 10%) decrease in hematocrit have been found during the viremic period in experimentally infected kittens. Because of the sudden onset of the disease and relatively long life span of erythrocytes, marked anemia is also less common in panleukopenia unless intestinal blood loss is severe. A persistent, nonregenerative anemia and leukopenia are more suggestive of feline leukemia virus (FeLV) infection (see Diagnosis, Chapter 13).

Thrombocytopenia is a variable feature of feline panleukopenia and may be found with other coagulation abnormalities in cats that develop DIC. Thrombocytopenia, resulting from direct bone marrow injury, can also occur in association with leukopenia early in the course of infection.

Biochemical findings in FPV infections are usually nonspecific. Increases in alanine aminotransferase (ALT) and aspartate aminotransferase (AST) activities or bilirubin can reflect hepatic involvement, but elevations are mild to moderate and icterus is rare. Azotemia is frequently present from prerenal or nonrenal causes such as dehydration, although the virus can produce minimal renal pathologic effects.

Magnetic resonance imaging or computed tomographic scanning can be used to visualize cerebral or cerebellar cortical defects in cats with neurologic signs resulting from in utero infections.[53]

Serologic Testing

These procedures are available for the properly equipped diagnostic and research laboratory, although they are rarely indicated for clinical practice. Serum VN is the most common method. Twofold serial dilutions of antisera are performed against precalculated amounts of FPV. Virus and sera are incubated before inoculation of the cell culture. Cultures can be examined for specific cytopathic changes and inclusion bodies produced by the virus. The first sample is taken as soon as possible during the illness, and the second is taken 2 weeks later. A fourfold rise in VN titer is indicative of acute infection. Complement fixation (CF) titers also can be performed. Hemagglutination inhibition (HI) and hemagglutination tests can be performed using some strains of FPV, which, as with CPV, will variably agglutinate porcine erythrocytes at 0° C but at pH 6.4 rather than 7.2. The variation is usually related to individual variation among pig erythrocytes in the test. A fourfold rising titer is considered indicative of active infection. VN and HI titers have been used as the reference standards for protection against infection.[34,51] Minimum titers (greater than 1:10) that correlate with resistance to challenge infection have been determined in these studies. The highest titers are consistent with natural exposure to virus, as few cats mount these titer responses after vaccination. In one study,[34] the enzyme-linked immunosorbent assay (ELISA) method was too sensitive in that positive titer results were detected in a low number of unvaccinated cats that were not protected following challenge infection.

Fecal Enzyme-Linked Immunosorbent Testing

ELISA for CPV antigen, in feces or intestinal contents, is a sensitive and practical indicator of FPV infection in kittens.[1,2,12] Commercially available kits are available for this purpose (see Appendix 6). Results using fecal ELISA kits for CPV have varied between these commercial assays[2] so that preliminary evaluation is advisable. Assays have also been performed on tissue specimens taken at necropsy. These are homogenized, and the supernatant has been applied directly on the test strip.[2] However, it must be borne in mind that FPV may be detectable only in the feces by ELISA kits for 24 to 48 hours PI and that by the time clinical signs occur, the virus is no longer detectable. The virus can be detected for longer periods using viral isolation; however, this method is not clinically practical. For these reasons, antibody testing or histology (or both) is also recommended.

Viral Isolation

Feline cells are required to support viral replication in cell cultures, and frequent mitosis is needed to ensure a continuing infection, although FPV has been shown to replicate in cells in which DNA synthesis has been blocked. Cytopathic effects, required to substantiate the presence of the virus, are more easily demonstrated in young, rapidly multiplying cells. Plaque-detection methods are possible when certain cell types and cell synchronization are used. Virus can be isolated from the urine and feces of kittens surviving experimental in utero inoculation at 3 and 6 weeks after birth, respectively. Using PCR, attenuated FPV has been detected in tissues for at least 19 days after vaccination.[8] Direct culture from trypsinized lung and kidney tissues allows improved isolation of the virus for up to 70 days. Virus has been isolated by direct culture for up to 1 year from the lungs and kidneys of prenatally infected kittens, despite a high level of circulating antibody. Virus can be found in the CNS for at least 22 days after neonatal infection and thereafter persists in Purkinje's cells. Direct fluorescent antibody (FA) testing can be used to detect virus in cell cultures and from tissues (usually intestine) of infected cats within 2 days after infection. Monoclonal antibodies can be used to distinguish FPV from CPV strains, as can PCR followed by restriction enzyme digestion analysis.[2,22,50]

Genetic Detection

PCR has been used to identify FPV in intestinal and tissue samples from cats.[14,33,36,53] This technique is especially valuable in localized tissue infections, given that viral quantities are low. It also can be used on formalin-fixed, paraffin-embedded tissues. Because carnivore parvoviruses can cross-infect multiple species, genetic detection permits specific identification of the viral strain.

PATHOLOGIC FINDINGS

Gross pathologic changes in naturally infected cats are usually minimal. The intestinal tract is obviously dilated; the bowel loops are firm and may be hyperemic (Fig. 10-5) with petechial and ecchymotic hemorrhages on the serosal surfaces. The feces frequently have a fetid odor when blood is present. Prenatally infected cats may have a small cerebellum, hydrocephalus, or hydranencephaly (Fig. 10-6). Thymic atrophy, present in all infected neonates, is the only gross finding in germ-free kittens.

Histologic abnormalities in the intestine include dilated crypts, with sloughing of epithelial cells and necrotic debris into the lumen (Fig. 10-7). Crypt-lining cells may slough completely in some cases so that only the basement membrane remains. Shortening of villi occurs secondary to the necrosis of crypt cells. The most severe histologic lesions are found in the jejunum and ileum; the duodenum and colon are less severely affected. Focal damage is most prominent around lymphoid follicles in the submucosa of the small intestine. Lymphocytic infiltrations are conspicuously absent from all tissues, and lymphocyte depletion is present in the follicles of lymph nodes, Peyer's patches, and spleen. Lymphoid atrophy is present with concomitant mononuclear phagocyte hyperplasia. FeLV-associated enteritis has been confused with FPV enteritis, being described as a panleukopenia-like syndrome. In cats with FPV infection, mucosal infiltration is mild, caused by the absence of leukocytes, and T cells predominate.[33] In contrast, cats with FeLV-associated enteritis have marked mucosal infiltrates associated with mononuclear and T cells.

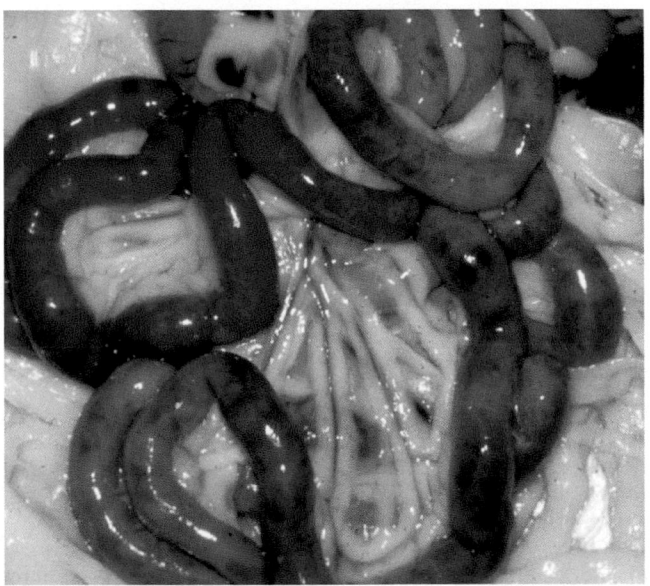

Fig 10-5 Segmental hyperemia of the intestine seen at necropsy of a cat with feline panleukopenia. (Courtesy Diane Addie, University of Glasgow, Glasgow, Scotland.)

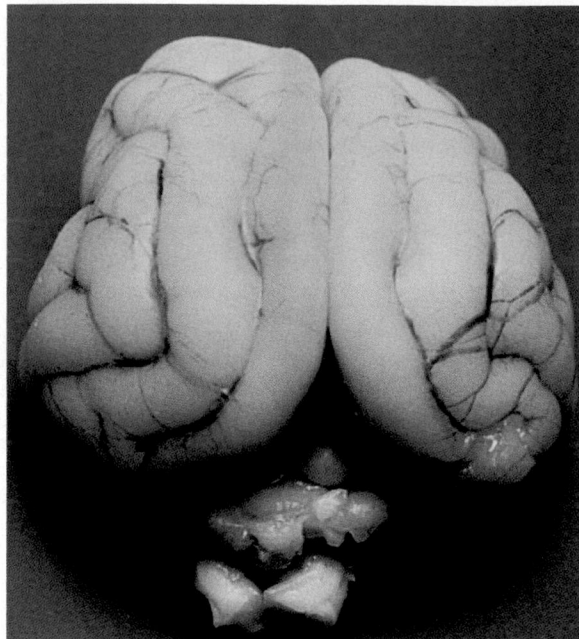

Fig   10-6   Cerebellar hypoplasia in a brain from a cat with in utero FPV infection.

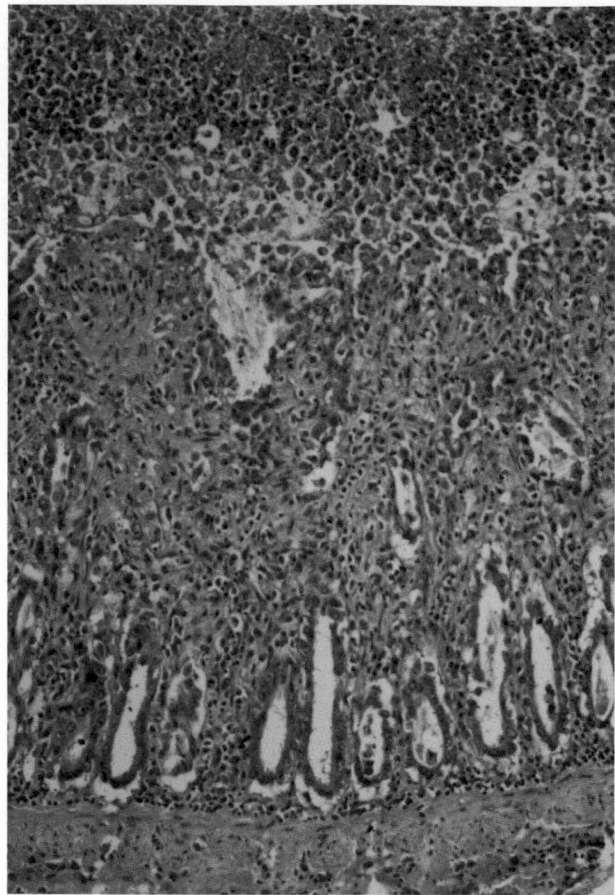

Fig   10-7   Microscopic appearance of the jejunum from a cat with FPV infection. Dilated crypt lumina and collapsed villi are visible in the lower part of the figure; there is sloughing of epithelial cells. Necrotic debris and overlying inflammatory exudate are present in the intestinal lumen in the upper part of the figure (H and E stain, ×100). (Courtesy University of Georgia Athens, Ga.)

Histologic abnormalities in the cerebrum of prenatally or neonatally infected kittens can include dilation of the ventricles and disruption of the ependymal cells with malacia of subcortical white matter. Cerebellar degeneration is marked by disorientation and reduced population of the granular and Purkinje's cell layers. Myelin degeneration can be found predominantly in the lateral funiculi of the spinal cord.

Eosinophilic intranuclear inclusions can be found in FPV infection, although they are transient and are frequently absent with routine formalin fixation. Bouin's or Zenker's fixatives must be used. Electron microscopic (EM) findings indicate that the inclusions correspond with sites of virus replication. As with CPV infection, EM can detect viral particles in intestine and fecal specimens. Immunohistochemical staining can be used to detect virus in tissue specimens.

THERAPY

Mortality caused by FPV infection can be avoided with appropriate symptomatic therapy and nursing care. Cats that can be kept alive for several days with supportive measures usually develop adequate immune defense mechanisms to overcome the infection. Parenteral fluid therapy is employed to replace lost electrolytes, counteract dehydration, and replace daily maintenance needs. Oral intake of food and water should be withheld during this time to lessen vomiting and slow the bowel mitotic activity that is necessary for viral replication. Fluid volumes that must be replaced as a result of vomiting and diarrhea can be calculated by evaluating the cat's state of hydration. Additional maintenance needs from insensible losses are administered at a rate of 44 ml/kg/day. Balanced isotonic fluid replacement with lactated Ringer's solution is desirable, and potassium supplementation may be beneficial. Fluids can be administered subcutaneously (SC) unless severe dehydration associated with reduced peripheral vascular circulation occurs for which intravenous (IV) therapy is required.

Antiemetics may be required to control persistent vomiting (Table 10-2). The use of anticholinergic medications is controversial and is contraindicated because they produce sustained ileus of the bowel. Metoclopramide given parenterally works best. GI protectants such as kaolin-pectin and bismuth subsalicylate have been recommended to coat the bowel but cannot be given to vomiting animals. Bismuth compounds have the added a theoretic advantage of reducing increased intestinal secretion and resulting diarrhea. Glucocorticoid therapy should not be selected routinely at antiinflammatory or higher dosages because of its immunosuppressive effects.

Plasma or blood transfusion therapy may be required in cats that develop severe anemia, hypotension, or hypoproteinemia (plasma protein less than 5.0 g/dl). A platelet count and activated coagulation time should be evaluated before administration of blood products in cases of ongoing DIC. Low-dose SC heparin therapy (50 to 100 U/kg given every 8 hours) can be administered simultaneously with transfusion if thrombocytopenia and severe incoagulability are present. Antiserum or high-titer parvoviral antiserum from vaccinated or recovered cats is beneficial if given after exposure and before clinical signs are noted. After signs are observed, it is too late.

Table • 10-2

Drug Therapy for Feline Panleukopenia

DRUG	DOSAGE[a] (mg/kg)	ROUTE	INTERVAL (HOURS)	DURATION (DAYS)
Antiemetics				
Metoclopramide	0.2—0.4[b]	PO, SC	6—8	prn
	1—2	IV	24[c]	prn
Thiethylperazine	0.5—5.0	IM, SC	8	prn
Trimethobenzamide	3.0	IM, SC	8	prn
Antimicrobials				
Ampicillin, amoxicillin	15—20	IV, SC	6—8	prn
Cephapirin	10—30	IV, SC, IM	6—8	prn
Gentamicin	2	IV, SC, IM	8	prn[d]
Interferon-ω	2.5×10^6 units/kg	IV	24	prn

PO, By mouth; SC, subcutaneous; IV, intravenous; IM, intramuscular; prn, as needed.
[a]Dose per administration at specified interval. For additional information on these drugs, see Drug Formulary, Appendix 8.
[b]Should not be given in conjunction with other motility modifiers.
[c]Total dose IV not to exceed 1 to 2 mg/kg/day; this dose may be divided as multiple bolus infusions throughout the day.
[d]Renal function (blood [serum] urea nitrogen [BUN], urine casts) should be closely evaluated, and the drug should not be continued for longer than 7 to 10 days at this dosage.

Broad-spectrum antibiotics, such as ampicillin or cephalosporin, are administered to control secondary bacterial infection resulting from virus injury to the intestinal mucosa (see Table 10-2). Parenteral therapy is preferred because of continued vomiting. A combination of a penicillin or cephalosporin derivative with parenteral aminoglycosides may be required for cats that are septic or moribund. Caution must be taken with aminoglycosides, because of their nephrotoxic potential, and with quinolones, because of cartilaginous toxicity in growing animals and retinal toxicity, especially in cats (see Antibacterial Chemotherapy, Chapter 34, and Drug Formulary, Appendix 8). One rationale for antibiotic therapy in this disease is to reduce the mitotic activity of the bowel epithelium by decreasing intestinal microflora, because germ-free animals have been shown to have a mild form of disease.

Combination B-vitamin therapy should be given parenterally to all cats with feline panleukopenia because of decreased food intake from anorexia, high requirements for B vitamins, and loss in diuresis to prevent development of thiamine deficiency. Low-dose oral or parenteral diazepam (2.5 mg total) can be used intermittently, a few minutes before feeding, to stimulate the appetite of anorectic cats that are not vomiting. IV recombinant feline interferon used to treat CPV reduced mortality 6.4-fold,[11] and no reason can be found to think that it would not be equally effective in feline parvovirus infections.

Response to therapy can be followed by monitoring the total and differential leukocyte counts because a resurgence of leukopoiesis occurs within 24 to 48 hours. Bizarre forms of leukocytes can be detected in the blood and bone marrow.

After the nursing period, the cat can be started on oral alimentation by frequent feedings of small quantities of bland baby food, broth, or blended food. Eventually, the cat may be fed larger quantities of solid foods. Semimoist foods have lower residue and help firm the feces of cats with persistent diarrhea. On rare occasions, cats that refuse to eat after several days should be force-fed by mouth or by pharyngostomy or gastrostomy tube or given diazepam, as indicated previously.

PREVENTION

Maternal and Passive Immunity

Colostral antibodies to feline panleukopenia have a half-life of 9.5 days (see Tables 100-2 and 100-4). MLV vaccines and inactivated tissue culture (TC)–origin vaccines are both ineffective when maternal-derived antibody VN titers, as measured by some laboratories, are greater than 1:10. Successful vaccination without maternal antibody interference can be achieved by 12 to 14 weeks of age in most cases (range is 6.8 to 18.8 weeks), depending on the antibody titer in the queen. Kittens with VN titers from 1:10 to 1:30 cannot be successfully vaccinated but are susceptible to infection with FPV. Similar to pups infected with CPV, kittens can still be infected with FPV before the time they are immunized, although this problem has not been as widely recognized. Recovery from natural infection with virulent virus probably results in lifelong immunity.

Therapeutic passive immunity has been used to prevent panleukopenia. Homologous antisera from cats with a high titer to infection will provide immunity according to the titer of the product and the amount administered. The recommended dose is 2 ml per kitten given SC or intraperitoneally (IP). Because administered immunoglobulins persist for up to 2 to 4 weeks, the neonatal vaccination series must be delayed. Passive administration of antisera is recommended for use *only in exposed susceptible* (unvaccinated) cats that require immediate protection or in colostrum-deprived kittens, with subsequent vaccinations at 2 to 3 or 4 to 5 weeks of age with inactivated or MLV vaccines, respectively. Newborn kittens are immunologically competent to FPV and can respond with neutralizing antibodies at 7 to 12 days of age.

Active Immunization

Active immunization has been the most important factor in reducing the incidence of the disease. Both inactivated and MLV products have been effective in preventing this disease. TC-origin-inactivated products can break through maternal immunity as early as MLV vaccines. Unlike MLV products, they have the advantage of being safe in pregnant queens and in kittens younger than 4 weeks. Inactivated vaccines may be given to febrile kittens when an effective immune response is doubtful. No danger exists of postvaccinal virus spread or clinical illness as a result of reversion to virulence, although the suspicion is that inactivated products can contain live virus. The major disadvantage of these products is that, in the absence of maternal antibody, two injections are required to achieve a titer that can be obtained from one injection of MLV product. Protection with inactivated vaccines does not consistently occur until 3 to 7 days after the second vaccination. Antibody titers to inactivated vaccine have been adequate for protection by 2 weeks after the first vaccination but have been greatly boosted by the second injection. Cell-mediated immune (CMI) responses to FPV were stimulated as early as 3 days after the second of two doses of adjuvant inactivated FPV vaccine. Long-term duration of immunity studies show protection against challenge infection after 7.5 years in cats that were vaccinated as kittens.[52] The inactivating agents used in some of these vaccines are also irritating to cats. With cloning of FPV into bacterial plasmids, developing a more purified subunit vaccine against this infection may be possible. A raccoon poxvirus-vector, recombinant FPV vaccine has protected cats against challenge infection.[23]

MLV vaccines produce more rapid and effective immunity than do inactivated virus vaccines. In the absence of maternal antibodies, one injection of any of the currently available MLV products for panleukopenia will produce a protective titer or HI or serum neutralizing titers greater than 1:8 to $1:10^{34,52}$ in a previously unvaccinated cat; however, a second vaccination is recommended. Oral vaccination with MLV vaccine is ineffective, whereas IN or aerosol exposure to vaccine produces an active immune response. MLV vaccines are recommended in contaminated areas such as shelters and infected catteries or in outbreaks to provide faster protection. MLV vaccines should be avoided in immunosuppressed cats because of the risk of vaccine-induced disease (see Chapter 100).

Colostrum-deprived kittens can be vaccinated regardless of age, but MLV products should be avoided in kittens younger than 4 weeks because of the danger of producing cerebellar degeneration. Colostrum-deprived kittens younger than 4 weeks at first presentation should receive at least two inactivated FPV vaccines 2 to 3 weeks apart. If 4 weeks or older, these kittens can receive one MLV-FPV vaccine with an optional one given 2 to 3 weeks later.

Initial vaccinations for nursing kittens are generally begun at 8 to 9 weeks of age and are followed by at least one more MLV product or two more inactivated vaccines, depending on which type of antigen is used. Subsequent vaccines should be given 2 to 4 weeks thereafter; the last vaccine is given at 12 to 20 weeks of age. In situations of apparent vaccine breaks or kitten mortality, prior or subsequent vaccinations in the initial series might be considered.[2] Panleukopenia vaccines are usually given SC. Combined vaccines that contain FPV and rabies or feline respiratory viruses have been marketed. See Feline Panleukopenia in Chapter 100 and Appendix 2 for overall vaccination recommendations for prevention of this disease.

Annual vaccination against panleukopenia is recommended and performed by most veterinarians, although it is probably not essential. Actually, one MLV product or two inactivated vaccines may produce lifelong immunity. Two inactivated vaccines given at 8 and 12 weeks to SPF kittens isolated in a barrier-maintained research facility produced high persistent VN antibody titers for at least 6 years.[50-52] In all likelihood, revaccination produces an anamnestic response and presumably is not harmful. After the kitten series, and a first booster 1 year later, triennial vaccination in conjunction with the rabies vaccine offers adequate protection.[50]

Proper disinfection procedures are essential to prevent or control an outbreak owing to the high resistance of FPV. Household bleach diluted 1:32 (1 oz/gallon) should be used on all cages, feeding dishes, floors, and holding areas, in addition to general cleansing. In cat holding facilities, all new cats should be vaccinated on arrival with MLV products and kept in disinfected cages separate from the resident cats for several days.

Control of Outbreaks

Disease clusters of FPV infection in cats have been described in recent years. In some cases, this incidence has been in catteries with currently vaccinated pedigree cats.[2,7] Such outbreaks can develop because of inherent immunodeficiency associated with young age, inbreeding, maternal antibody interference, or a highly contaminated environment. Some of the kittens were infected before they could be successfully immunized as a result of maternal antibody blockade, coupled with a highly contaminated environment. An early vaccination of kittens beginning at 6 weeks of age, instead of the conventional 8- to 9-week age period, was shown to induce a response in a significant proportion of kittens by 9 weeks of age. It did not interfere with subsequent response to vaccination at 9 and 12 weeks.[10] Furthermore, cases in which outbreaks are noted in older kittens, vaccination should be continued beyond 12 weeks, with an additional dose at 18 to 20 weeks to obtain seroconversion.[2] Other outbreaks have occurred in large congregations of cats in humane society or animal control facilities.[7] These outbreaks usually occur in young cats that have been born or brought into these facilities. Use of inactivated vaccines has been one contributing factor to outbreaks in these highly contaminated environments. Protection with inactivated vaccines is generally delayed for 2 to 3 weeks after the second vaccine in naïve kittens. These cats are generally exposed and infected before immunity can develop. Use of MLV vaccines at the time of entry, and before exposure, may help control such outbreaks. In some instances, these outbreaks might relate to infection with CPV-2 variants (see later discussion) because these may infect cats with preexisting immunity to FPV. Generally, infections with these strains are mild, even in naïve cats; however, laboratory challenge studies with CPV-2 strains may not always reflect natural circumstances.

IN vaccination for parvoviral infections are not as effective as parenterally administered vaccines. Parvoviruses cause a systemic viremia in their host, and circulating antibody has a major role in immunity and clearing the virus from the body. During viremia, parvoviruses cause cytolysis and subsequently spread extracellularly and must escape to new dividing cells, thereby becoming exposed to circulating antibody. An outbreak of salmonellosis and panleukopenia was reported in a purebred cattery where IN trivalent vaccine was used.[14]

CANINE PARVOVIRAL INFECTION IN CATS

Etiology

Parvoviruses as a group are relatively stable. Viruses isolated for many decades appear to be homogeneous. The basic parvoviral gene sequence has a common ancestral sequence; however, viruses isolated from particular carnivore hosts are very closely related and have only minor differences. This relationship suggests that host adaptations have been constant and evolving with time. FPV was the only type parvovirus recognized to infect cats until the mid 1940s. An outbreak of enteritis and mortality in mink was ascribed to a virulent closely related mutant MEV. Both FPV and MEV are closely related and are divided into at least three subtypes; the first two are commonly isolated from mink. The original CPV-2 strain, detected in the mid to late 1970s, was thought to have originated from an FPV or closely related parvoviral strain of mink or other carnivore. CPV-2 differed in two specific epitopes on it cell surface and its ability to cause hemagglutination (HA) of feline erythrocytes at specific pH. The HA specificity is determined by binding of a specific viral epitope to N-glycolylneuraminic acid, a sialic acid present on feline blood group-A erythrocytes, but not on dog erythrocytes. In cell culture, feline and canine parvoviruses replicate in most feline cells; however, only CPV-2 and its variants replicate in dog cells. FPV can replicate in dog thymus and bone marrow cells, but no other canine tissues. Therefore infections of dogs with FPV are self-limiting and do not spread. The CPV-2 mutation was associated with the ability of this virus to replicate in the canine gut and associated lymphoid tissues, with transmission to other hosts via excreta. The ability to infect and spread in cats was lost.

Since its evolution and host adaptation to dogs, CPV-2 in domestic and wild dog populations spread throughout the world between 1974 and 1978. Genetic analysis indicated that alterations in four sequences in the viral capsid protein gene were responsible for this change in host specificity. Since that occurrence, CPV has undergone several changes in the ancestral sequence with the origination of three new variants to date. CPV-2a was recognized, as the predominant isolate between 1979 and 1981. It had five to six amino acid differences on the nucleocapsid surface, which can be detected by monoclonal antibody and later by genetic analysis (see Table 10-1). CPV-2b was first detected beginning in 1984, and, although all three strains co-exist, it is currently the predominant worldwide isolate from dogs.[46] Unlike CPV-2, CPV-2a and CPV-2b strains readily replicate in feline ileum and lymphoid tissues. A new CPV-2c variant having two subtypes (a and b) was isolated from leopard cats in southeast Asia.[28,29] These subtypes have not been isolated from naturally infected cats or dogs and may represent an offshoot mutation.

One of the confusions with the parvoviral nomenclature for carnivores is that viruses have been named according to the host from which they were isolated, rather than their genetic relatedness. Because of the close genetic relationship, and spread of many of these isolates between hosts, a newer designation must be devised. With the present system, CPV-2a and CPV-2b might be termed as variants of FPV in their behavior, even though they cannot be distinguished from identical isolates made from dogs. Therefore the designated terms as listed in Table 10-1 should be used to describe certain genetic, antigenic, and host range differences between various isolates.

The nature of host specificity has been elucidated through genetic analysis and x-ray crystallography. Regions in the capsid structure located around VP2 residues can influence canine transferrin receptor and affect the host cell species of infectivity.[17,25,26] Mutations in the genes controlling these capsid moieties and selective pressures allow the parvoviruses to evolve and infect new hosts.[24]

Epidemiology

CPV-2 and its newer strains are actually host range variants of FPV. CPV-2 does not replicate in cats, but CPV-2a and -2b do so very efficiently. CPV-2a and -2b have been isolated from between 10% and 20% of domestic cats with naturally occurring parvoviral disease from Germany.[59] In such areas, FPV is still the major parvovirus infecting cats. In southeast Asia, CPV-2a, -2b, and -2c strains predominate in isolations from

large exotic cats.[42,56] One supposition is that large felids are more susceptible to CPV than they are to canine distemper virus.[56] Another theory is that these large cats were not vaccinated and that the subtypes 2a and 2b can spread more effectively because of the wider reservoir host range. Under these conditions, domestic and exotic cats likely acquire their CPV-2a and -2b infections from an environment that is contaminated by dog feces. Isolations from domestic and exotic cats have varied between these two strains, according to the predominant strain in the local dog population. Levels of CPV-2 strain shedding by cats (0.5 to 2.0 $\log_{10}$) are lower than those found with similar infections in dogs (6 to 9 $\log_{10}$), although they are sufficient to infect susceptible in contact cats. Nevertheless, infected dogs are more likely to disseminate virus in the environment and be reservoirs for feline infection. A prediction for the future is that CPV-2a and -2b will replace FPV and CPV-2 as the predominant carnivore parvoviruses worldwide.[30]

Clinical Signs

CPV strains 2a and 2b can induce disease in infected cats with signs similar to those of feline panleukopenia.[8,37,43,47] The natural infection has often been asymptomatic as have the experimental infections of SPF cats.[40,59] However, the development of clinical illness may relate to the general condition of the cats involved at the time of exposure. Laboratory experiments with parvoviruses in SPF animals do not always match corresponding disease in conventional animals or in those animals that acquire infection in nature. Host factors are likely important because infections with CPV-2a, -2b, and -2c have been clinically significant in exotic felids.[29,43,56]

Given that clinical signs are milder or unapparent in CPV-2a or -2b–infected cats as compared with those with FPV infection, the suspicion was that CPV-2 strains were less virulent. Of the new strains, CPV-2c appears to be relatively the most pathogenic.[29] In SPF cats, those inoculated with CPV-2c became clinically ill with leukopenia and diarrhea.[43] Correspondingly, more severe signs were noted in FPV-infected cats while signs were milder or absent in CPV-2a–infected cats.

Diagnosis

Pronounced lymphopenia and mild leukopenia have been observed in cats challenged with CPV, similar to the leukocyte alterations with this infection in dogs.[8] This condition contrasted to the marked leukopenia and mild lymphopenia observed in corresponding cats challenged with FPV.

Antibody titers in serum to CPV-2a, -2b, and -2c cross react with those to FPV. Titers would be lower between the heterologous agents; however, this would not be clinically detectable unless multiple viruses were used as antigen simultaneously. Parvo-ELISA test kits can be used to detect parvoviruses; however, the levels of virus in stool using one kit was 2.76 $\log_{10}$ lower than those found with corresponding FPV infection in cats.[8]

Carnivores that recover from parvoviral infections generally stop shedding virus once high levels of serum antibodies are present. Although they may persist for variable periods, tissues and secretions of recovered animals are cleared of virus. Surprisingly, CPV-2a and -2b strains have been isolated from the peripheral blood mononuclear cells of clinically healthy cats with high VN antibody titers against FPV.[28,29,37] Whether these infections are associated with intermittent or chronic virus shedding is uncertain.

Therapy

CPV infections in cats have been reported to be milder than those associated with FPV infection. Treatment would be identical with that for treating feline panleukopenia (see the previous section on Therapy).

Prevention

CPV and FPV viruses cross-react with VN and HI antibody titers. Lower cross-reactivity of these antibodies are observed against CPV strains in cats experimentally inoculated with FPV or vaccinated with inactive FPV vaccines, as compared with cats being challenged with CPV strains.[42] Vaccination of large cats in zoos against feline parvovirus is recommended to produce immunity against that infection and protect against heterologous infection with CPV-2a and -2b. FPV vaccines may have a short duration and partial protection against CPV-2 strain infections.

Attenuated FPV vaccines have protected domestic cats from clinical illness and virus shedding following challenge with CPV-2b isolates at 2 weeks after vaccination.[8] Similar challenge studies have not been performed with inactivated vaccines, and longer-term challenge studies are not available. Cheetahs have been infected with CPV strains despite FPV vaccination.[56] In vitro, a cross-neutralization study following inactivated FPV vaccination indicated antibodies developed against FPV, CPV-2a, -2b, and -2c.[42] However, the antibody titers against the CPV strains were considerably lower. CPV-2c had the lowest degree of cross-reactivity with FPV, which may explain the higher degree of virulence of this CPV-2 strain for cats. Interestingly, cats infected with CPV-2c have had high cross-reactive titers against CPV-2a and -2b. Specific vaccines against CPV-2 strains may be needed to protect domestic and exotic cats in the future. A CPV-2c strain would be a logical candidate for the antigen.

SUGGESTED READINGS*

1. Addie DD, Jarett O, Simpson J, et al. 1996. Feline parvovirus in pedigree kittens, *Vet Rec* 138:119.
8. Chalmers WSK, Truyen U, Greenwood NM, et al. 1999. Efficacy of feline panleukopenia vaccine to prevent infection with an isolate of CPV-2b obtained from a cat, *Vet Microbiol* 69:41-45.
14. Foley JE, Orgadu, Hirsh DC, et al. 1999. Outbreak of fatal salmonellosis in cats following use of a high-titer modified-live panleukopenia virus vaccine, *J Am Vet Med Assoc* 214:67-70.
30. Ikeda Y, Nakamura K, Miyazawa T, et al. 2002. Feline host range of canine parvovirus: Recent emergence of new antigenic types in cats, *Emerg Infect Dis* 8:341-346.
34. Lappin MR, Andrews J, Simpson D, et al. 2002. Use of serologic tests to predict resistance to feline herpesvirus-1 feline calicivirus, and feline parvovirus infection in cats, *J Am Vet Med Assoc* 220:38-42,.
52. Scott FW, Geissinger CM. 1999. Long-term immunity in cats vaccinated with an inactivated trivalent vaccine, *Am J Vet Res* 60:652-658.

*See the CD-ROM for a complete list of references.

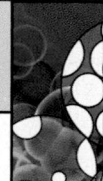

CHAPTER • 11

Feline Coronavirus Infections

Diane D. Addie and Oswald Jarrett

The clinical condition of feline infectious peritonitis (FIP) was first described in the 1960s.[82] Subsequent studies of the lesions of FIP by electron microscopy (EM) incriminated a coronavirus. FIP is the major infectious cause of mortality in cats.[184] A possible explanation for an apparent increase in the prevalence of FIP is that management of the domestic cat has changed.[141,143] With the introduction of cat litter, more cats have been kept permanently indoors, exposing them to large doses of feline coronavirus (FCoV) in the feces, which would previously have been buried outdoors. More and more cats are spending part of their lives in multi-cat crowded environments such as at cat breeders or shelters, which increases their stress and chance of exposure to pathogens while in such an environment.

ETIOLOGY

FCoVs belong to the order Nidovirales and family *Coronaviridae*. The coronaviruses are large, enveloped, positive-stranded RNA viruses. The major viral proteins are the spike (S), nucleocapsid (N), and membrane (M). Until the emergence of the severe acute respiratory syndrome (SARS) caused by SARS coronavirus (SARS-CoV), coronaviruses were divided into three groups. It has been debated whether SARS-CoV belongs to the second group or forms a different, fourth group.[54,110,156,169] Rota et al[156] found no genetic similarities between SARS-CoV and FCoV, but Stavrinides and Guttman[169] demonstrated that SARS-CoV S protein is a mosaic of group I CoVs and an avian CoV. They found many similarities between the S of type II FCoV strain 79-1146[28] and the Urbani SCoV strain (except for a 200-base-pair region that was similar to an avian sequence). At the time of writing, the SARS-CoV is thought to have originated from the masked palm civet cat *(Paguma larvata)*, which is not a feline but is a member of the mongoose family (Viverridae). Nevertheless, cats may become infected with SARS-CoV experimentally[119] and naturally; a single cat from a household of infected people seroconverted (though remained healthy). The consensus is that people cannot get SARS from their pet cats *(Felis catus)*.

FCoVs are in group I of *Coronaviridae*, the same group as transmissible gastroenteritis virus (TGEV), porcine respiratory coronavirus canine coronavirus (CCV),[75,121,127] and human bronchitis, coronavirus serotype 229E (HCV 229E).[17] A comparison of these viruses and their pathogenicity for cats is summarized in Table 11-1.

Types I and II Feline Coronaviruses

The isolation of FCoV in cell culture is very difficult.[68] Laboratory strains of FCoV can be classified into types I and II according to their growth characteristics in cell culture, cytopathogenicity, and comparative degree of neutralization by antisera to canine coronavirus.[84,143,185] Type I is wholly feline, whereas type II FCoVs are genetically more closely related to CCV than are type I FCoVs.[67,127,185] Type II FCoVs have arisen by recombination between type I FCoV and CCV.[67,68,127,185] Most of the spike of the type II FCoV is CCV spike.[67] Type I is the more prevalent type in field infections.[9,68,74] Each type is capable of causing a spectrum of clinical signs in cats, ranging from asymptomatic infections to diarrhea to FIP.

Biotypes Feline Enteric Coronavirus and Feline Infectious Peritonitis Virus

Laboratory strains of FCoV vary in their ability to cause disease when administered to cats.[17] Some laboratory isolates are unable to cause FIP when inoculated intraperitoneally (IP) into cats and are named feline enteric coronavirus (FECV). It was once thought that these viral strains did not leave the gut, but it is now known that they can. It was previously believed that in nature two biotypes of FCoV existed: feline infectious peritonitis virus (FIPV) and FECV, with differing potential for causing disease. In fact, it is now believed that all natural FCoV infections have the potential to cause FIP, although they do so in only approximately 10% of infected cats.

Differing cell tropism of either enteritis- or peritonitis-producing viruses has been suggested as a possible explanation of different manifestations of disease: FECV replicates in enterocytes, causing diarrhea or asymptomatic infection, whereas FIPV replicates in macrophages, leading to systemic

Table • 11-1

Features of Coronaviruses That Infect Cats

VIRUS	HOST	VIRUS INFECTS CATS	CATS DEVELOP FIP	SEROCONVERTS CATS	COMMENTS AND REFERENCES
FCoV	Cat	+	±[a]	+	Designation for coronaviruses that cause asymptomatic infections, diarrhea, or FIP in cats; previously called "FECV" and "FIPV"; can infect newborn pigs, producing lesions similar to mild TGEV.[145]
CVLP	Cat	+	–[b]	–	Observed in feces of cats[26,85]; not cross reactive with FCoV; not believed to cause disease in cats[85,145] but has been associated with diarrhea[12b]; may be excreted for 12 months after infection.[85]
CCV	Dog	+	–[c]	+	Causes diarrhea in dogs; infected cats seroconvert but are clinically normal after oronasal exposure[9]; cats develop effusive FIP after IM or IP inoculation[121]; shed from oropharynx but not not feces of experimentally infected cats for 1 week;[9] vaccines given IM can cause ADE in cats,[83,121] and one caused FIP-like signs in dogs.
TGEV	Pig	+	–	+[d]	Causes vomiting and diarrhea in piglets younger than 1 month; replicates in villous tip epithelium of SI; mutation in 1980 caused new variant—porcine respiratory coronavirus[84]; can subclinically infect cats but no ADE with subsequent FCoV infection[18]; serologic cross-reactive with CCV and FCoV.
SCoV	Human	+	–	+	No clinical signs in cats; seroconversion by 28 days after infection; virus detected in oropharyngeal and nasal swabs 4 and 6 days after infection, respectively, but not in rectal swabs.[119]
HCV-229E	Human	+	–	+	Causes common cold in people and nonsymptomatic feline infection with minimal viral replication and no ADE.[9]

FCoV, Feline coronavirus; *CVLP*, coronavirus-like particles; *CCV*, canine coronavirus; *TGEV*, transmissible gastroenteritis virus; *SCoV*, severe acute respiratory syndrome coronavirus; *HCV-229E*, human coronavirus-229E; *ADE*, antibody-dependent enhancement; +, occurs; ±, variable occurrence; –, = does not occur.
[a]Diarrhea or FIP.
[b]Nonsymptomatic or diarrhea. Virus may be excreted in feces for up to 12 months.
[c]Oronasal infection. Virus is shed from oropharynx but not feces for 1 week although asymptomatic virus can cause FIP if given parenterally.
[d]Diarrhea and lesions indistinguishable from mild TGEV infection. In the 1980s a new TGEV variant called porcine respiratory coronavirus was developed.

infection and FIP. One theory is that for FIP to occur, a mutation must occur in an FECV to permit replication in macrophages.[170,184] Detection of messenger RNA (mRNA) in circulating monocytes is evidence that the virus is infecting cats systemically and is replicating. A reverse transcriptase polymerase chain reaction (RT-PCR) that detects mRNA was positive in 94% of 49 confirmed cases of FIP and in none of 12 cats with histologically confirmed non-FIP disease. However, 6% of 326 clinically healthy cats had positive test results.[164] Whether detection of mRNA is predictive of development of FIP in the healthy cat remains to be seen.

Comparison of the genomes of FIPV and FECV laboratory strains WSU 79-1146 and WSU 79-1683 revealed a deletion of the 7b open reading frame (ORF) in FECV strain 79-1683, which was postulated to account for the FECV's lack of virulence.[68] However, ORF7b deletions readily arise during in vitro passage,[68] and intact 7b genes have been found in most FECV isolates,[68,184] indicating that deletions in ORF7b are not a universal distinguishing property of FECVs.[68] Deletions, or nonsense mutations, in the ORF3c of FIPVs are more consistently found in pathogenic strains, having been found in 11 of 13 laboratory strains of FIPV that were compared with the corresponding FECVs from which they had arisen.[184] Deletions turning FECVs into FIPVs make more sense as frequent naturally occurring events than insertions, which would be required to turn FECVs into FIPVs if the 7b theory had been correct. The 7b protein is a secreted, nonstructural glycoprotein whose function is unknown.[184] However, deletions in the 7b gene do seem to correlate with attenuation of virulence, and it has been postulated that it modulates the inflammatory or immune response.[68]

If the mutation hypothesis of FCoV to FIPV is correct, no two cases of FIP are caused by genetically identical viruses. An alternative to the mutation theory is that kittens developing FIP do so because they are subjected to a large viral dose at a time in life when their still undeveloped immune systems are also coping with other infections and the stress of vaccination, rehoming, and neutering.[12,41,68] Furthermore, pedigree kittens and certain large cats (cheetahs[19]) may also be genetically predisposed to developing FIP.[39] Preliminary studies failed to show any association of FIP or resistance to FCoV infection with the class II feline leukocyte antigen DRB.[7] Researchers will explore other genetic markers for susceptibility in attempts to help cat breeders develop dines not susceptible to FIP.

Clearly, wherever natural FCoV infection exists, so does the potential for the development of FIP.[12] In accordance with the guidelines set forth in the Fifth International Symposium on Coronaviruses,[113] the generic term *feline coronavirus (FCoV)* is used when discussing the virus, unless it is meaningful to differentiate FECV and FIPV. *Feline infectious peritonitis (FIP)* is used to denote the multisystemic disease state associated with viral dissemination.

PATHOGENESIS

Cats become infected with FCoV by ingestion and possibly by inhalation of virus. The receptor for the type II FCoV is an enzyme, aminopeptidase-N, found in the intestinal brush border.[18] The type I FCoV receptor is unknown.[71] Type II FCoV probably replicates in the small intestinal epithelial cells. The main site of type I FCoV viral replication is unknown but is likely to be in the ileum and colon.[66] Virus is shed in feces from 2 days postinfection.[11,65,171] In early infection, virus may replicate in the tonsils[145,171] and oropharynx[140] and is shed in the saliva[117] for only a few hours or days.[6]

Although the etiology of FIP is still uncertain, it is an immune-mediated disease involving virus or viral antigen,

antiviral antibodies, and complement. A more appropriate name would be *feline coronaviral vasculitis*. Cats that have no anti-FCoV antibodies do not develop FIP, and if FCoV-seropositive cats are decomplemented using cobra-venom factor, FIP does not ensue. Complement fixation leads to the release of vasoactive amines, which cause endothelial cell retraction and thus increased vascular permeability. Retraction of capillary endothelial cells allows exudation of plasma proteins, hence the characteristic protein-rich exudate that develops in effusive FIP.[17]

Two possible explanations describe the development of FIP once virus has become systemic. The first is that FCoV is distributed throughout the body by infected monocytes/macrophages; the second is that FIP is an immune complex disease. FCoV-infected monocytes attach to the endothelium of affected blood vessels, extravasate,[100,104] and enable virus to enter the tissues.[143] The virus attracts antibodies, complement is fixed, and more macrophages and neutrophils are attracted to the lesion.[143] Circulating immune complexes have been demonstrated in cats with FIP,[60] but FIP is atypical of an immune complex disease in that joints and skin are rarely affected.

Effusive FIP is the acute form, usually occurring 4 to 8 weeks after infection or a stressful event, although it can occur terminally in cases of noneffusive FIP, the chronic form of the disease, which occurs weeks to months postinfection. Cats that develop effusive FIP may have a large quantity of virus, leading to the destruction of many blood vessels and the formation of many pyogranulomata. Noneffusive FIP may result from a partially successful cell-mediated immune (CMI) response[143] or from fewer but often larger pyogranulomata.

The clinical and pathologic signs that occur in FIP are direct consequences of the vasculitis and organ damage that result from damage to the blood vessels that supply them. In effusive FIP, many blood vessels are affected, hence the exudation of fluid and plasma proteins into the body cavities. In noneffusive FIP, the clinical presentation depends on which organs are damaged by the FIP pyogranulomata.

Some viruses have immunomodulating effects on their hosts, which moderate the body's attempts to eliminate the virus. Cats with FIP are lymphopenic, and lymphoid depletion is evident in spleen and lymph nodes. In particular, the number of CD4+ lymphocytes in tissues decreases during the evolution of FIP lesions, most likely because of an increased lymphocyte apoptotic rate. In contrast, cats who survive FCoV infection develop follicular hyperplasia in the peripheral lymph nodes.[137] Haagmans et al[57] showed that FCoV-infected cells released a substance that caused apoptosis in bystander T lymphocytes in lymph nodes. The nature and function of this protein has not yet been defined. Possible candidates are the proteins of the FCoV genes 3a-c and 7a-b because these genes are rapidly lost from viruses grown in cell culture with no loss of ability to replicate, indicating that their function is in the cat's body, perhaps as a virokine.

Protective Immune Response to Feline Coronavirus Infection

The mechanism by which cats are protected against developing FIP is not understood. It is generally assumed cats do not develop FIP because of a successful CMI response and that a humoral response is harmful. Evidence from experimental infections show that cats surviving a challenge mount a greater CMI response than those who succumb.[31] However, clearance of natural infections also correlated with the presence of a humoral immune response to the FCoV spike protein,[53] and it is known that kittens are protected by maternally derived antibody.[4] Therefore it is possible that some antibody protection also occurs. Humoral immunity associated with secretory IgA is suspected to be important in preventing initial infection of epithelial cells.[4] In exposed cats, seroconversion occurs within 18 to 21 days after infection.

The role of other biologic substances in protecting cats against FIP is also unknown: four surviving cats had a transient rise in serum amyloid A (SAA); whether this increase and the decrease in α_1-acid glycoprotein (AGP) seen in these cats had some protective role has been questioned.[47] The biologic function of AGP is not completely known. AGP is a natural antiinflammatory and immunomodulatory agent. The immunomodulatory function of AGP is affected by its carbohydrate composition.[16,43] The Sialyl Lewis X form of AGP is induced during inflammation and ameliorates complement and neutrophil-mediated injuries, whereas the non-Sialyl Lewis X form does not.[43] Moreover, Sialyl Lewis X is the ligand for the cell adhesion molecules involved in adherence of monocytes to endothelial cells,[43] and one of the earliest stages of the pathogenesis of FIP is the adhesion of FCoV-infected monocytes to the endothelium in FIP vasculitis. It is possible that development of FIP has little to do with the virus and everything to do with the AGP response of the cat.[1]

Antibody-Dependent Enhancement of Feline Infectious Peritonitis

Antibody-dependent enhancement (ADE) is a phenomenon that has foiled many attempts to find a successful FIP vaccine.[132,143,161,180] A greater proportion of cats that had been vaccinated with trial vaccines developed FIP than cats in the unvaccinated control group also exposed to a laboratory strain of FCoV—usually the very virulent 79-1146 type II strain. The proposed mechanism is that antibody facilitates the uptake of FCoV into macrophages.* Cats with ADE develop disease in fewer than 12 days, whereas controls take 28 days or more.[161] By contrast, field studies have shown that seropositive pet cats that were naturally reinfected by FCoV showed no evidence of ADE.[9] Indeed the opposite occurred, because many of the cats that had become seropositive after natural infection appeared to be immune.[12] The mortality rate of cats that were in contact at the time of initial FCoV infection was 14%, compared with about 8% at the time of reinfection.[12] In practical terms a seronegative cat introduced into a household in which FCoV is endemic has a 1 in 6 chance of developing FIP, whereas a seropositive cat has a 1 in 12 chance. Cats are at greatest risk of developing FIP in the first 6 to 18 months after infection, and the risk decreases to about 4% 36 months after infection.[12] Olsen provided an excellent review of ADE of FIP.[132]

Viral Shedding

It is likely that when naive cats in a multicat household first encounter FCoV, most become infected because they seroconvert. FCoV is shed mainly in the feces. In early stages of infection, it may be found in saliva for hours or days[6] and possibly in the respiratory secretions and urine.[65,171] It is possible that viral shedding of types I and II are different; laboratory strains, which are typically type II, are shed for only a couple weeks,[171] whereas in natural infection, type I virus is shed by 65% of cats for 2 to 3 months and longer by many cats. Thirteen percent of naturally infected cats become lifelong carriers.[6] A curious feature of lifelong carrier cats is that they shed the same strain of virus continuously in the feces until death, and they rarely develop FIP.[9] Detection of carrier cats requires positive fecal RT-PCR test results for 9 months (Table 11-2). Cats that are eliminating FCoV may shed virus intermittently or at undetectable levels toward the end of infection.[66] Virus is maintained in the cat population by chronic carrier cats and through reinfection of transiently infected cats.[9]

*References 23, 24, 29, 73, 131, 133, 134.

The stress of entering a rescue shelter increases viral shedding 10^1- to 10^6-fold.[147] However, the stress of pregnancy and lactation did not cause infected queens to shed more virus.[40] Of cats with naturally occurring FIP, 42% to 75% shed virus.[11] Because RT-PCR cannot measure the viability of the detected organism, the infectivity of the shed virus cannot be absolutely ascertained. However, a correlation between strong RT-PCR results and infectivity has been made.[40]

Although serologic testing has limitations, it is clear that seronegative cats, as determined by a *reliable* diagnostic test, do not shed FCoV,[4,40] whereas approximately one in three FCoV-seropositive cats do shed virus.[4] Cats with higher antibody titers are more likely to shed virus,[6,140] although cats with relatively low indirect fluorescent antibody (FA) titers of 1:40 to 1:80 have a 26% to 39% chance of shedding FCoV.[4,5,6,65] Evidence of viral shedding is never a good reason to euthanize a cat because most FCoV shedders stop within a few months, and less than 10% develop FIP.[5] In addition, if a cat has survived one exposure to FCoV, it may be better to use it for breeding rather than introduce new susceptible animals that may not be resistant, because a genetic element may play a role in susceptibility to FCoV infection.[39]

Transmission

Transmission is primarily indirect through contact with virus-containing feces or fomites. The major sources of FCoV for uninfected cats are litter trays shared with infected cats.[144] In new infections, transmission through sneezed droplets, sharing food bowls, and mutual grooming are also possibilities but only for a matter of hours. FCoV is a relatively fragile virus, but in dry conditions it has been shown to survive for up to 7 weeks outside the cat.[160] Transmission through lice or fleas is considered unlikely.[17] Although documented, transplacental transmission is extremely uncommon because most kittens that are removed from contact with adult virus-shedding cats at 5 to 6 weeks of age do not undergo seroconversion.[4]

Whether FCoV transmission is significant at cat shows is unknown. In one survey, showing cats appeared to be of minor significance in FIP incidence,[90] whereas in another survey 84% of cats at shows in the United Kingdom were found to be seropositive.[167]

CLINICAL FINDINGS

Initial Feline Coronavirus Infection

Most FCoV infections are subclinical. When FCoV first infects cats, they may have a brief episode of upper respiratory tract signs or diarrhea, although these signs are usually not severe enough to warrant veterinary attention. Kittens infected with FCoV generally have a history of diarrhea and occasionally of stunted growth and upper respiratory tract signs.[4]

Coronaviral Enteritis

FCoV can cause transient and clinically mild diarrhea,[143] vomiting, or both in cats. However, occasionally the virus can be responsible for a severe acute or chronic course of vomiting or diarrhea with weight loss, which may be unresponsive to treatment and continue for months.[103]

Feline Infectious Peritonitis

Two basic forms of FIP—effusive (wet) and noneffusive (dry)—have been characterized. Approximately half the cats with FIP are younger than 2 years,[61,70] but cats of any age can be affected. Evaluation of the history of cats with FIP typically reveals that they lived in a multicat environment in the previous year, usually in cat breeders or rescue facilities. Occasionally, they have been to a boarding cattery, cat show, or veterinary clinic. Cats that have spent several years in a

Table • 11-2

Feline Coronavirus Elimination Using Sequential FA and RT-PCR Testing[a]

Cat	SEQUENTIAL TITERS						
	March 1996	May 1996	July 1996	October 1996	August 1997	January 1998	August 2000
Todd	1:1280	1:1280	1:320	1:640	1:20	1:10	
	−	+	+	−	−	−	
Teafa	1:1280	1:1280	1:640	1:1280	1:640	1:160	
	−	+	+	+	−	−	
Garfield	1:640	1:640	1:640	1:640	1:160	1:20	
	+	+	+	+	−	−	
Geordie	1:640	1:320	1:160	1:80	N/D	0	
	+	+	+	−		−	
Skully	1:80	1:80	1:40	1:20	1:20	0	0
	+	−	−	+	−	N/D	N/D
Cassey	1:160	1:40	1:20	1:40	1:20	0	0
	+	−	+	−	−	−	N/D
Rosie	1:40	1:20	1:10	0	1:10	1:10	0
	+	−	−	−	−	−	N/D
Holly	1:1280	1:320	1:160	1:160	1:80	1:80	
	−	−	−	−	−	−	
Sedgeley	1:1280	1:1280	1:1280	1:1280	1:1280	1:160	
	+	+	+	+			
Sooty	1:640	1:640	1:640	1:1280	1:1280	1:1280	>1:1280
	+	+	+	+	+	+	+
Elsa	1:10	1:20	0	1:20			
	−	−	−	−			N/D
Brewster	0	0	0	0			
	−	−	−	−			N/D
Tabby				0			
				−			
Ginger				0			
				−			

FA, Fluorescent antibody; *RT-PCR*, reverse transcription polymerase chain reaction; +, positive RT-PCR result from feces or rectal swabs; −, negative RT-PCR result from feces or rectal swabs; *N/D*, not done.

[a]Author's (DDA) data from a household of cats in which FCoV was successfully eradicated by isolating cats that had eliminated FCoV infection from those who were still shedding virus. The shaded boxes indicate when a cat was moved to another household. By August 1997 the carrier cat was identified as Sooty, and in April 1998 she was rehomed. Note that occasionally cats with antibody titers of less than 100 were shedding FCoV. Newcomers Tabby and Ginger were prevented from becoming infected by being isolated from infectious cats.

single-cat environment are extremely unlikely to have FIP. Nevertheless, FIP, especially the noneffusive form, can incubate for months or even years.[175] Cats with FIP usually have a history of stress in the previous few months.[117,153] Those with effusive FIP are usually taken to their veterinarians within 4 to 6 weeks of arriving in a new home, elective surgery, or a similar stressful situation, whereas cats with noneffusive FIP develop disease after a greater interval. Clinical signs may reflect the specific organ systems involved.

Effusive Feline Infectious Peritonitis

Cats with effusive FIP have ascites (although very few owners notice the abdominal distension [Fig. 11-1]),[153] thoracic effusion (Fig. 11-2), or both. The cat may be bright or dull, anorexic, or eating normally. Abdominal swelling with a fluid wave, mild pyrexia (39° C to 39.5° C), weight loss, dyspnea, tachypnea, scrotal enlargement, muffled heart sounds, and mucosal pallor or icterus may be noted. In one survey, FIP accounted for 14% of cats with pericardial effusion, second only to congestive heart failure (28%).[158] Abdominal masses may be palpated, reflecting omental and visceral adhesion, and the mesenteric lymph node may be enlarged.

Noneffusive Feline Infectious Peritonitis

Signs of noneffusive FIP are often vague and include mild pyrexia, weight loss, dullness, and depressed appetite. Cats may be icteric. Abdominal palpation usually reveals enlarged mesenteric lymph nodes[101] and may also reveal irregular kidneys or nodular irregularities in other viscera. If the lungs are involved, the cat may be dyspneic, and thoracic radiographs may reveal patchy densities in the lungs.[177]

Cats with noneffusive FIP frequently have ocular lesions. The most common ocular sign in FIP is iritis, manifest by color change of the iris. Usually all or part of the iris becomes brown, although occasionally blue eyes appear green. Iritis may also manifest as aqueous flare, with cloudiness of the anterior chamber, which in some cases can be detected only in a darkened room using focal illumination. Large numbers of inflammatory cells in the anterior chamber settle out on the back of the cornea and cause keratic precipitates, which may be hidden by the nictitating membrane (Fig. 11-3). Some cats hemorrhage into the anterior chamber. If the cat has no sign of iritis, the retina should be checked because FIP can cause cuffing of the retinal vasculature, which appears as fuzzy grayish lines on either side of the blood vessel (Fig. 11-4).

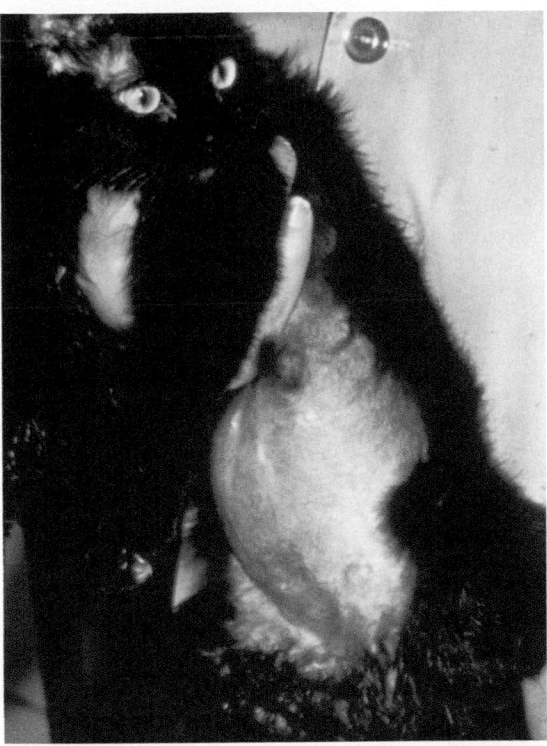

Fig 11-1 Abdominal distention from FIP effusion. (Courtesy University of Georgia, Athens, Ga.)

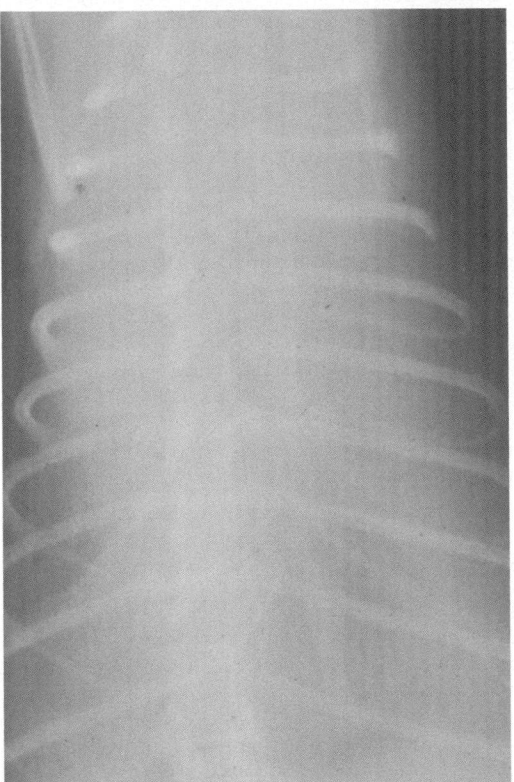

Fig 11-2 Radiograph of a cat with FIP and thoracic effusion.

Occasionally, pyogranulomata are seen on the retina, or the vitreous appears cloudy. Retinal hemorrhage or detachment may also occur[173] but is more commonly a sign of hypertension. Similar ocular signs can also be caused by infections with *Toxoplasma* organisms, feline immunodeficiency virus (FIV),

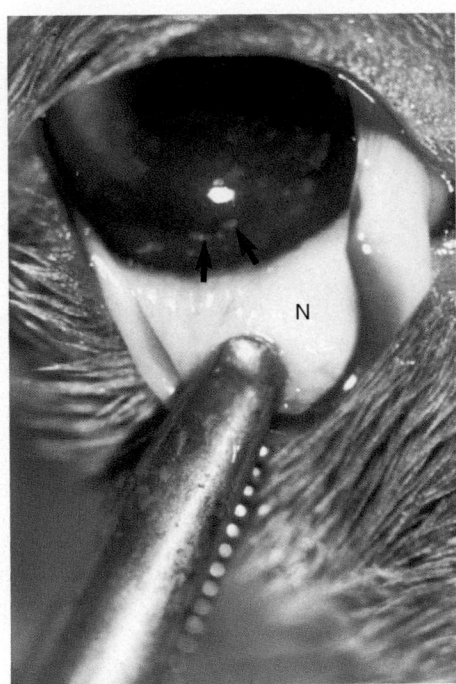

Fig 11-3 Keratic precipitates on the cornea *(arrows)* in noneffusive FIP. The nictitating membrane *(N)* has been deflected down to enable visualization of the precipitates. (Courtesy Diane Addie, University of Glasgow, Glasgow, Scotland.)

feline leukemia virus (FeLV), or systemic fungi (see Chapter 93).[112,173]

Of cats with FIP, 12.5% have neurologic signs[153]; signs are variable and reflect the area of central nervous system (CNS) involvement. With noneffusive FIP, 25% to 33% of cats have neurologic abnormalities.[37] The most common clinical sign is ataxia followed by nystagmus and then seizures.[108] When FIP causes meningitis, the signs reflect damage to the underlying nervous tissue: incoordination, intention tremors, hyperesthesia, behavioral changes, seizures, cranial nerve defects, and unexplained fever. When the FIP lesion is a pyogranuloma on a peripheral nerve or the spinal column, lameness, progressive ataxia, or paresis (tetraparesis, hemiparesis, or paraparesis) may be observed. Cranial nerves may be involved, causing symptoms such as visual deficits and loss of menace reflex,[108] depending on which cranial nerve is damaged.

In a study of 24 cats with FIP and neurologic involvement, 75% were found to have hydrocephalus on gross or histologic postmortem examination.[108] Because other diseases such as cryptococcosis, toxoplasmosis, and lymphoma have not been reported to cause hydrocephalus, detecting it on a computed tomography scan is highly suggestive of a diagnosis of neurologic FIP.[108,37] Meningeal and periventricular contrast enhancement may also be observed.

Colonic or Intestinal Feline Infectious Peritonitis

Occasionally, the primary or only organ affected by FIP granulomas is the intestine. Lesions are most commonly found in the colon or ileocecocolic junction but may also be in the small intestine.[61,178] Cats may have various clinical signs as a result of this lesion—usually constipation, chronic diarrhea, or vomiting.[61,178] Palpation of the abdomen often reveals a thickened intestine. A hematologic finding may be increased numbers of Heinz bodies.

Clinical Signs in Neonatal and Prenatal Kittens

FIP is the second most common infectious cause of death in kittens after weaning[20] but causes no deaths from birth to

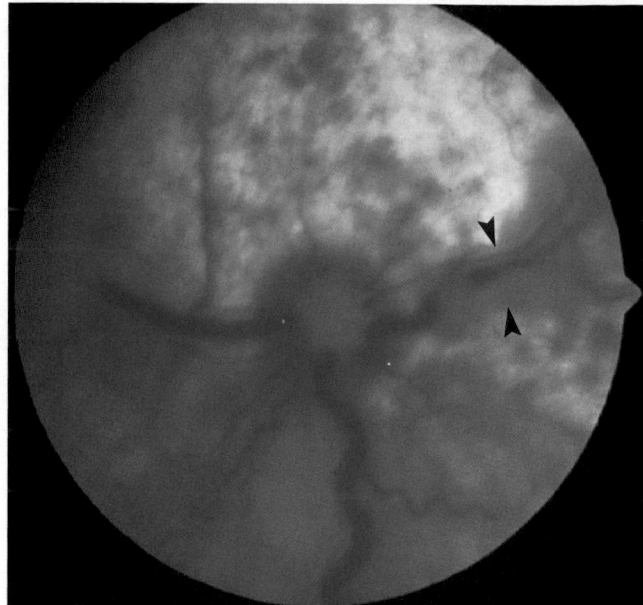

Fig 11-4 The retina of a cat with noneffusive FIP. The photograph is in focus but appears cloudy because of the high-protein exudate into the vitreous. Cuffing of the retinal blood vessels appears as grayish lines on either side *(arrowheads)*. Retinal blood vessels can be seen disappearing into pyogranulomata *(P)*. (Courtesy John Mould, Herefordshire, U.K.)

weaning ("fading kittens"). However, FCoV infection does result in stunting of kittens, increased incidence of diarrhea, and upper respiratory signs. FCoV does not cause infertility.

Nondomestic Felidae

FCoV can be an important pathogen for domestic and exotic Felidae. Enteric coronavirus infections have produced chronic weight loss, diarrhea, and anorexia. In a survey of captive felids, more than 50% had positive test results for infection based on fecal PCR and serologic testing for type I and type II coronavirus.[92] Mortality from FIP has been observed among captive exotic felids, with cheetahs *(Acinonyx jubatus)* having the highest risk for clinical illness. Necrotizing colitis caused by FCoV is a major health problem in these cats.[92]

DIAGNOSIS

Coronaviral Enteritis

No specific tests exist for coronaviral enteritis, and FCoV can only be assumed to be the cause of diarrhea in FCoV-seropositive or RT-PCR fecal-positive cats in which other infectious or dietary causes have been eliminated. Even biopsy is of limited use because the histopathologic features of villous tip ulceration, stunting, and fusion are nonspecific. FCoV infection may only be confirmed if immunohistochemical or immunofluorescent staining of gut biopsies is available.

Feline Infectious Peritonitis

Good clinical skills are more important for diagnosing FIP than for diagnosing any other disease. Positive predictive value (PPV) and negative predictive value (NPV) rises in populations in which the prevalence of a disease is higher; therefore available tests are more valuable for clinicians who have already narrowed down the diagnosis to FIP and a few other conditions by a thorough clinical examination and patient history.

At the time of writing and despite what manufacturers may claim, no single diagnostic test for FIP is commercially available; histopathology is still the gold standard. However, two tests are promising. One involves detection of mRNA in circulating monocytes,[164] and another is detection of FCoV in macrophages in effusions, although a negative result does not rule out FIP.[60,139]

It is often helpful to consider effusive and noneffusive FIP in different ways, although they do not overlap and each may progress to the other. Various schemes and algorithms have been devised that give high PPVs of an FIP diagnosis.[117,153,163] An algorithm for the diagnosis of FIP is presented in Table 11-3 and is used in the rest of this section.

Clinical Laboratory Findings

The typical hematologic changes in effusive and noneffusive FIP are lymphopenia[135] and neutrophilia with a left shift. In noneffusive FIP, cats have a nonregenerative anemia (hematocrit [HCT] < 30%) associated with chronic inflammation; cats that are constipated from granulomatous colitis have an increase in Heinz bodies in the erythrocytes.

An important feature of FIP is hyperglobulinemia (Fig 11-5). The albumin-globulin (A:G) ratio is a useful diagnostic tool, especially when measured in the effusion. Total protein in the effusion should be greater than 3.5 g/dl, and an A:G ratio less than 0.4 indicates that FIP is very likely.[163] The serum A:G ratio decreases in FIP because the albumin level remains normal or falls slightly and globulin levels increase, possibly through stimulation of B cells by interleukin-6, which is produced as part of the disease process.[50] Thus the total serum protein level is often high. FIP should be suspected when serum protein electrophoresis reveals a polyclonal hypergammaglobulinemia. (Differential diagnoses include lymphosarcoma, multiple myeloma or other plasma cell neoplasm, chronic infection, or FIV.[108,118])

Measurement of AGP is helpful in the diagnosis of FIP.[32] It is an acute-phase protein that exists in higher levels in several infectious diseases of cats and is therefore not specific for FIP. However, AGP levels in the plasma or effusions are usually greater than 1500 μg/ml in FIP, a level that helps distinguish FIP from other clinically similar but noninflammatory conditions such as cardiomyopathy and neoplasia. Cats with FIP have a tenfold increase in SAA compared with FCoV-exposed cats.[47] Reference concentrations are less than 20 μg/ml; in cats with FIP, they can increase to 80 μg/ml.

Other biochemical alterations reflect damage to the organs containing FIP lesions and are not specifically useful for diagnosing FIP. However, they may help the clinician determine whether treatment is worthwhile. Hyperbilirubinemia may be observed and frequently is a reflection of hepatic necrosis. Despite this fact, the alkaline phosphatase and alanine transaminase activities are often not increased as dramatically as they are with cholestatic disorders such as cholangiohepatitis and hepatic lipidosis. Analysis of cerebrospinal fluid (CSF) from cats with neurologic signs may reveal elevated protein levels (56 to 348 mg/dl, with normal being less than 25 mg/dl)[108] and pleocytosis (100 to 10,000 nucleated cells/ml—neutrophils, lymphocytes, and macrophages).[108] Similar findings may be apparent in aqueous humor of cats with uveitis. CSF may be difficult or impossible to withdraw as a result of inflammatory cell accumulation.[108]

Effusion

The next most useful step in diagnosis is to sample the fluid, which in FIP may be clear, straw colored, and viscous and because of the high protein content may froth when shaken (Fig. 11-6). The effusion may clot when refrigerated. If the sample is bloody, pus filled, chylous, or foul smelling, then FIP is unlikely,[153] although in rare cases it can appear pink and

Table • 11-3

Algorithm for the Diagnosis of Feline Infectious Peritonitis

PARAMETER	LIKELIHOOD[a]	PROCEED TO
A. Presenting Signs		
1. Nonspecific illness, anorexia, chronic recurrent, antibiotic-unresponsive pyrexia, with or without weight loss	>3	>B
2. Abdominal distention or dyspnea	>3	>B
B. Environment		
1. Single-cat household more than 1 year	>1	>C,H
2. Multicat household, cat breeder, humane shelter, in previous 6–12 months	>3	>C
3. Stressed in previous 1–12 months (e.g., was rehomed, was neutered, gave birth, visited veterinarian)	>3	>C
C. Clinical Signs		
1. Ascites with or without thoracic or pericardial effusion	>3	>D3,D4,D5
2. No effusion		
a. Systemic: depression, icterus, renal failure, diarrhea or constipation; neurologic or ocular signs	>3	>D1,D2
b. Neurologic: ataxia, nystagmus, seizures, tremor, paresis or paralysis, circling, menace deficit, behavioral changes, head tilt, magnetic resonance imaging suggesting periventricular contrast enhancement, ventricular dilatation, and hydrocephalus	>3	>D1,D2,E2
c. Ocular: iritis, uveitis, keratic precipitates, aqueous flare, retinal vascular cuffing, nystagmus, blindness	>4	>D1,D2
d. No ocular findings	>1	>E1,H2
e. Computed tomography scan: hydrocephalus	>5	>G
D. Laboratory Findings		
1. Hematologic findings		
a. Lymphopenia, nonregenerative anemia, left shift neutrophilia	>3	>D2,E1,F3a
2. Blood biochemistry		
a. A : G ratio <0.45	>5	>E1,F3a
High globulin (≥35 g/L or ≥3.5 g/dl)		
High α_1-acid glycoprotein (>1500 µg/ml)		
b. A : G ratio 0.45–0.8	>3	>E1,F3a
Moderate globulin (25–35 g/L or 2.5–3.5 g/dl)		
c. A : G ratio >0.8	>0,1	>H
Low globulin (<25 g/L or ≤2.5 g/dl)		
d. Normal α_1-acid glycoprotein (<500 µg/ml)	>0	>H
3. Effusion		
a. Clear, straw colored, clots on standing, froths if shaken	>4	>D4,D5
b. Pus, chyle (milky), or blood	>1	>H, ±F2
4. Cytology of effusion		
a. Low cellularity (<5000 nucleated cells/µl); cells mostly macrophages and neutrophils	>5	>E,F2
b. High cellularity, bacteria present, mitotic figures present, or mainly lymphocytes	>0	>H
5. Biochemistry of effusion		
a. High total protein (>3.5 g/dl)	>5	>E,F2
A : G ratio <0.45		
α_1-acid glycoprotein >1500 µg/ml		
b. A : G ratio 0.45–0.8	>3	>E
c. Albumin >48%, low globulins (<32%)	>1	>H
d. Albumin-globulin ratio >0.8	0	>H
6. a. Rivalta test positive	>2	>D7
b. Rivalta test negative	>0	>H
7. Immunofluorescence of macrophages in effusion		
a. Positive	>5	>G
b. Negative	>3	>E,H

Continued

Table • 11-3

Continued

PARAMETER	LIKELIHOOD[a]	PROCEED TO
E. Serologic Testing		
1. Antibody titer blood or effusion		
a. High antibody titer	>5	>G
b. Medium to low antibody titer	>2,0	>F
c. Absent antibody titer	>2,0	>F2,F3,H
2. Antibody titer cerebrospinal fluid		
a. Positive	>5	>G
b. Negative	>2,0	>H
F. Organism-Specific Identification		
1. Histopathologic findings compatible on tissue biopsy	>4,5	>F2,F3
2. Immunohistochemistry: fluid or tissues		
a. Immunofluoresence or immunoperoxidase positive	>5	>G
b. Immunofluoresence or immunoperoxidase negative	>1	>H
3. Virus detection		
a. mRNA positive	>5	>G
b. Effusion RT-PCR positive	>5	>G
G. Final Diagnosis FIP		Done
H. Consideration of Similar-Appearing Diseases[b]		
1. *Cardiomyopathy:* thoracic radiographs, echocardiography; *toxoplasmosis, lymphoma:* FeLV test, radiography, ultrasound, laparotomy, biopsy; *liver disease:* hepatic function testing, laparotomy, biopsy; *lymphocytic cholangitis*	>1	>H2
2. *Diagnosis uncertain:* evaluate for diseases not listed above		Done

RT-PCR, Reverse transcriptase polymerase chain reaction.
[a]*0,* FIP very unlikely; *1,* FIP less likely; *2,* FIP suspected; *3,* FIP possible; *4,* FIP likely; *5,* FIP very likely.
[b]Refer to specific chapters for discussion of diagnostic tests for other diseases.

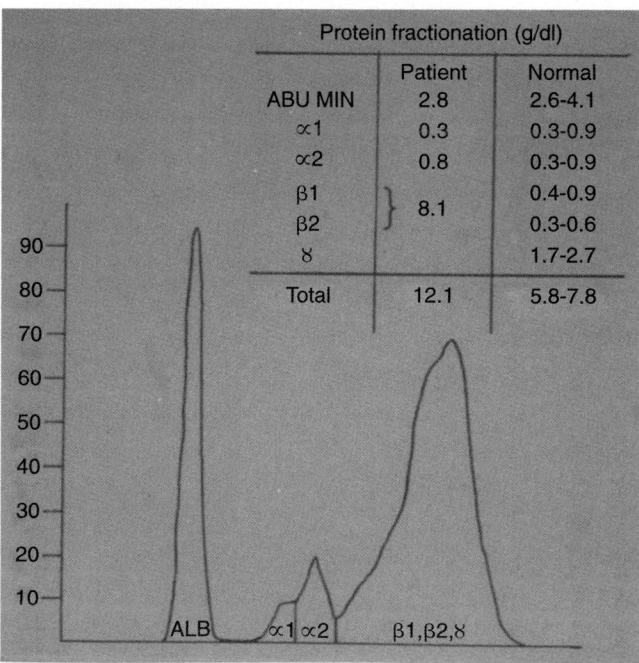

Fig 11-5 Serum electrophoretic pattern from a cat with FIP hyper β and γ globulinemia. (Courtesy University of Georgia, Athens, Ga.)

chylous.[159] The effusion in FIP is classified as a modified transudate in that the protein content is usually very high (>3.5 g/dl), reflecting the composition of the serum, whereas the cellular content approaches that of a transudate (<5000 nucleated cells/ml).[124] The protein content of the effusion is high because of the increased levels of gamma globulins, thus a low A:G ratio in an effusion is highly predictive of FIP. An A:G ratio of more than 0.8 almost certainly excludes FIP,[163] and with values between 0.45 and 0.8, FIP remains a possibility.[117,165] An A:G ratio of less than 0.45[166] in an effusion with greater than 3.5 g/dl of total protein and low cellularity, consisting of predominantly neutrophils and macrophages, is diagnostic of effusive FIP.[153] The main diseases with similar fluids are lymphocytic cholangitis and occasional tumors, usually of the liver. Cytology of the effusion, as well as radiographic and ultrasonographic findings, may help to differentiate neoplasia, which in addition to cardiomyopathy and liver disease is the condition most often mistaken for effusive FIP.[70,163] Adding a small drop of fluid to a 98% acetic acid solution can cause a precipitate because of the high protein content, and the procedure is easily performed in the veterinary office. A negative result is useful in ruling out FIP.[60]

Positive staining of FCoV-infected macrophages from an effusion is diagnostic of FIP, but a negative result does not rule it out (Fig. 11-7).[60,139] One difficulty with this test is that often the effusion has few macrophages.

Serologic Testing

Serologic testing for diagnosis of FIP has been frequently criticized. However, it has an important role in the diagnosis and management of FIP when certain methodologies are used and results are properly interpreted. Serologic testing for FIP can be

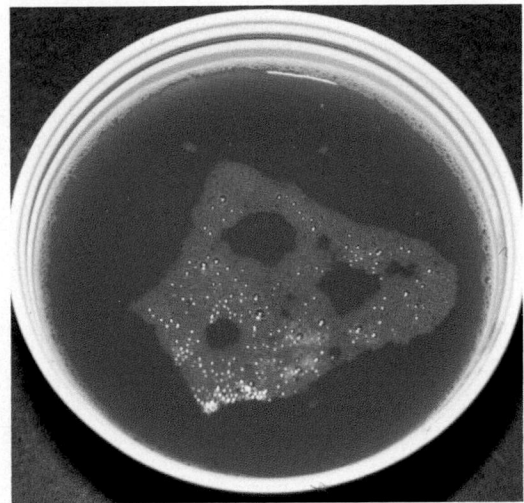

Fig 11-6 Body cavity effusion from a cat with FIP. Note froth and opacity from high protein content. (Courtesy University of Georgia, Athens, Ga.)

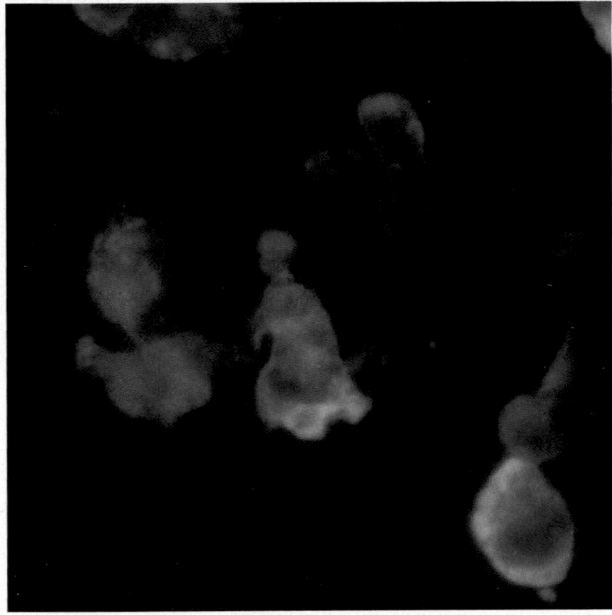

Fig 11-7 Direct immunofluorescent staining of abdominal effusion showing intracellular coronavirus in a cat with FIP. (Courtesy Wayne Roberts, University of Georgia, Athens, Ga.)

useful if the laboratory is reliable and consistent and the test results have been correlated with clinical findings. However, in one study a single serum sample was divided and sent to five different laboratories in the United States and yielded five different results.[149] Methodologies and antibody titer results may vary among laboratories, but each should have established two levels. One is the least significant level of reactivity (or *low* positive titer value) and another is the *high* antibody titer value. High titers have been correlated with a greater chance of FCoV shedding. (Antibody titers expressed in this chapter are those established by the authors' laboratory in Glasgow, Scotland.) When searching for a reliable laboratory, repeat samples from the same animal should be sent without warning to the same laboratory and an FCoV-referenced laboratory for comparison. Serum or plasma samples store well at −20° C without loss of antibody titer. An in-house test—the FCoV Immunocomb (Biogal Galed

Laboratories Kibbutz Galed, M.P. Megido Israel)—compared favorably with the gold standard immunofluorescent antibody test.[8] (See Appendix 5 for a listing of some established laboratories for the immunofluorescent antibody test.)

It has been said that more cats have died of FCoV-antibody test results than of FIP.[142] At times, clinicians have mistakenly equated a positive antibody titer result with a diagnosis of FIP, which is partly the fault of kit manufacturers who specifically call their tests "FIP tests," when in fact they actually detect FCoV or FCoV antibodies. In addition, FCoV tests are often requested for inappropriate reasons. Five major indications for FCoV antibody testing exist as outlined below.

Diagnosis of Feline Infectious Peritonitis or Coronaviral Enteritis

Serologic tests are very useful for cats with suspected FIP, but clinicians should be aware of their limitations. First, many healthy cats and cats with conditions other than FIP are seropositive. Second, some cats with effusive FIP appear to have low titers or be seronegative because large amounts of virus in their bodies are binding to antibody, making them unavailable to bind the antigen in the serologic test. Although exceptions have been reported,[108,168] cats with noneffusive FIP usually have a high FCoV-antibody titer and are rarely seronegative, thus coronavirus serology can usually be used to rule out a diagnosis of FIP in suspected noneffusive cases. The presence of a high FCoV-antibody titer in a sick cat from a low-risk, one- or two-cat household is also unusual; it is a stronger indicator of a diagnosis of FIP than the same antibody titer in a cat from a multicat household in which FCoV is likely to be endemic.

Serologic testing should only be performed to diagnose FIP in conjunction with a compatible history, clinical signs, and examination of the effusions or blood for high globulins and a low A:G ratio (see Table 11-3). Serologic tests performed on ascites or thoracic effusions yield the same results as when done on blood samples provided they have high protein concentrations that approximate blood. Seronegative cats with suspected effusive FIP can be examined further for the presence of virus by RT-PCR[33] when available.

Occasionally, healthy cats are considered to have noneffusive FIP simply because they are seropositive and have no ascites. This assumption is incorrect because cats with noneffusive FIP are clinically ill.

Cats with neurologic FIP had higher antibody titers but lower FCoV loads than cats with generalized FIP.[42] Measurement of antibodies to FCoV in CSF has been reported to assist in the diagnosis of neurologic FIP.[37] The ratios of serum protein to CSF protein and serum FCoV antibody to CSF-FCoV antibody were always equal to or greater than one. None of eight controls cats with nonneurologic FIP had anti-FCoV antibodies in the CSF. Unfortunately, these control cats were experimentally infected and had relatively low serum antibody titers to FCoV. Nonspecific leakage of serum proteins into CSF cannot be eliminated. It can only be controlled by (1) considering the CSF titer in light of increased CSF cellularity that suggests nonspecific leakage or (2) comparing a ratio of the CSF-serum titers to another infectious agent (antibody indexing). Seronegativity in diarrheic cats rules out FCoV as a cause; however, FCoV may or may not be a cause of diarrhea in seropositive cats.

Contact with Suspected or Known Viral Excretor

Testing of a cat that may have been exposed to FCoV is usually done for one of two reasons. First, the owner wants to know the prognosis for an exposed cat. Second, the owner wants to obtain another cat and needs to know whether the exposed cat is shedding FCoV. In either case, it is very likely that the cat will be seropositive because 95% to 100% of cats exposed to FCoV become infected and seroconvert approximately 18 to 21 days after exposure. The owner should be advised of this possibility and reassured that it does not necessarily indicate a poor prognosis. Most cats infected with FCoV do not develop FIP, and many in households of less than 10 cats eventually clear their infection and become seronegative within a few months or years. Adult cats can be retested using the same laboratory every 3 to 6 months until the antibody titer falls threefold to fourfold. Kittens and adults that have been exposed only once often have a quicker reduction in antibodies and may be tested every 1 to 2 months. Some cats remain seropositive for years but are not necessarily virus shedders. A rise in antibody titer or maintenance at a high level does not necessarily indicate a poor prognosis for the cat. Of 50 cats tested by the authors, antibody titers remained at 1:640 or greater on at least three occasions, yet only four cats died of FIP. However, in an endemic infection, a constant low titer of 1:20 or less is highly indicative that a cat will not develop FIP.

The aim of serotesting and segregating cats is to prevent exposure of cats that have eliminated infection to chronic virus-shedding cats. The lowest dilution of sample that a laboratory considers *positive* (the least significant level of reactivity [LSLR]) in its diagnostic test should be ascertained. Laboratories have different techniques, and the LSLR level can vary from 1:10 to 1:100. If a laboratory uses an LSLR serum dilution of less than 1:100 as negative, some cats that are excreting FCoV will not be identified—FCoV excretors with indirect FA titers as low as 1:40 have been found.[4-6,65] Cats with sera that are nonreactive at lower dilutions by the indirect FA test (i.e., dilution of less than 1:10) are unlikely to shed FCoV. Approximately one third of seropositive cats excrete virus,[4,5] so if a cat is seropositive, it is unwise to obtain another cat unless it also has antibodies. After 3 to 6 months, the antibody titer can be rechecked to determine whether it has become negative. In a stable, isolated population of fewer than 10 cats that are mixing together, in which half remain seronegative, it is reasonable to infer that the other cats are probably not excreting virus.

Cat Breeder Requests Testing

Cat breeders often request that their cats be screened for FCoV antibodies before mating. Such testing is worthwhile only if a reliable test is used and the laboratory's negative LSLR is low (i.e., less than a titer of 1:10 or 1:20). If the cat is seronegative, it can be safely mated with another seronegative cat. If the cat is seropositive, it can be mated with a seropositive cat; isolation and early weaning should prevent the resulting kittens from becoming infected.[3,4,69] Alternatively, a breeder may prefer to isolate a seropositive cat, wait 3 to 6 months, and retest in the hope that it will have become seronegative.

Screening a Cattery for Feline Coronavirus

FCoV infection is highly contagious. If many cats are housed in a group, then a random sampling of three to four cats indicates whether FCoV is endemic. If cats are housed individually, it may be necessary to test them all. Cats in households with fewer than 10 cats (that do not take in any new cats) and in those in which the cats are isolated from each other in groups of three or less often eventually lose their FCoV infection.[52] Retesting is worthwhile *only* if the cats are kept in these small groups and not commingled. Testing every 3 to 16 months establishes the loss of infection because antibody titers fall, and an increasing proportion of cats become seronegative if not reexposed to infection (see Table 11-2).

Screening a Cat for Introduction into a Feline Coronavirus-Free Cattery

Once a cattery has been established as FCoV seronegative, it can be maintained FCoV free by testing and isolating new cats before they are introduced. Seropositive cats should never be

introduced; for the safety of other cats, it should be assumed that they are shedding FCoV.

RT-PCR Testing

PCR is a highly sensitive technique for amplifying and detecting small amounts of DNA (see Molecular Diagnosis, Chapter 1, and Fig. 1-3). Because FCoV is an RNA virus, a DNA copy must first be made using the enzyme RT.

Viral detection is clinically useful to veterinarians in two areas: (1) confirming the presence of FCoV in cats that appear to have FIP but are seronegative and (2) detecting viral shedding for epidemiologic purposes.[6,9,40,66] Viral detection in body tissues or fluids is not a useful prognostic indicator in the healthy cat because FCoV has been detected in the blood of healthy FCoV-seropositive cats.[65] However, virus was detected in 13 brains of 17 cats with neurologic FIP,[42] so a positive result was useful but a negative result did not rule out FIP. In addition, the absence of FCoV in the blood stream does not mean a cat is not going to develop FIP.[36] False-negative results can also be generated in the laboratory by accidental introduction of (or not inhibiting) enzymes that destroy RNA (ribonucleases, or RNases). Detection or absence of FCoV in the feces or saliva is not helpful as a prognostic test but is a useful research tool. Cats that are chronic FCoV shedders are not at special risk of developing FIP,[9,40] but they make it difficult to contain infections in a cattery. However, lifelong FCoV shedders can only be identified by nine consecutive monthly positive RT-PCR fecal tests.[6]

Antigen Detection in Tissues

Viral detection by direct FA and immunohistochemistry can be applied to effusion, cytologic, or biopsy specimens but requires a specialized laboratory. Immunofluorescence can confirm the presence of FCoV in macrophages in the effusions of cats with wet FIP.[139] Both tests are commercially available (see Appendix 6) and are confirmatory tests in cases in which the histologic findings are not typical of FIP.[174,187] FCoV antigen has been detected in swabs made from the nictitating membranes of cats with FIP[80]; however, these results have not been confirmed by other laboratories.[174]

PATHOLOGIC FINDINGS

The essential lesion of FIP is the pyogranuloma. In effusive FIP, all the surfaces of the abdominal contents, thoracic contents, or both can be covered in small (1- to 2-mm) white plaques (Figs. 11-8 and 11-9). Few other diseases have similar lesions, although occasionally miliary tumors or systemic mycoses can appear. In noneffusive FIP, gross pathologic lesions can be much more variable; however, the kidney is frequently affected and should be examined carefully for pyogranulomata in the cortex (Fig. 11-10). In colonic FIP the colon may be thickened and have a gross appearance that is similar to alimentary lymphosarcoma.[61] In some cats, abnormalities are minimal, and a diagnosis can be made only by histologic examination. In the meninges, gross changes are often minimal or consist of hyperemia of the surfaces; however, histologic lesions are characterized by diffuse meningeal infiltration with pyogranulomatous inflammation (Fig. 11-11). To diagnose FIP definitively, vasculitis must be demonstrated. The lesion consists of an arteriole or venule bordered by a central area of necrosis that is surrounded by a perivascular infiltration of mononuclear cells, proliferating macrophages and lymphocytes, plasma cells, and neutrophils. Immunohistochemistry used to demonstrate the presence of virus in the lesions is the absolute gold standard.

In cats with coronaviral diarrhea, FCoV can infect the mature columnar epithelium of the tips of the villi of the alimentary tract, resulting in sloughing of the villous tips. FCoV can be demonstrated in the epithelial cells by immunohisto-

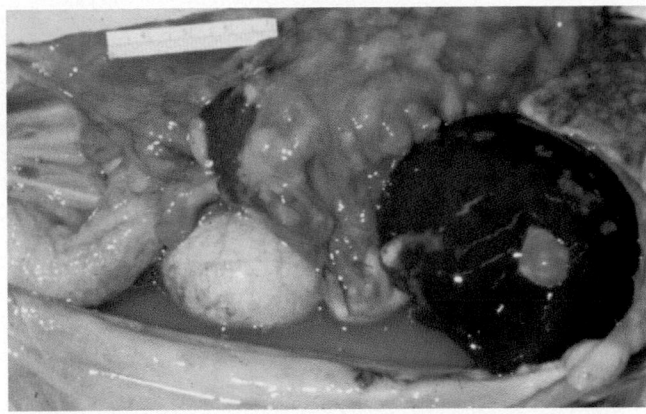

Fig 11-8 Abdominal cavity of a cat with effusive FIP at necropsy. Note multifocal granulomas on the serosal surfaces of many organs.

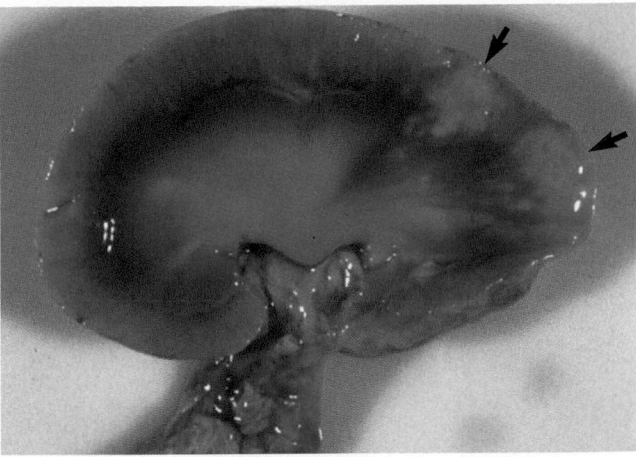

Fig 11-10 Bisected kidney of a cat with noneffusive FIP showing pyogranulomata *(arrows)*.

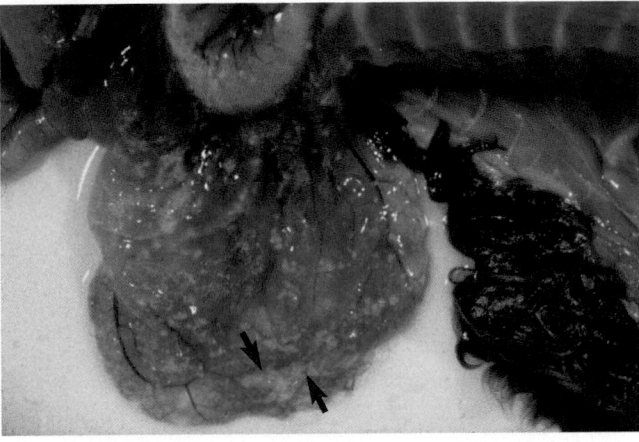

Fig 11-9 Omentum of a cat with effusive FIP. Note gelatinous appearance and small, white perivascular pyogranulomata *(arrows)* typical of effusive FIP on gross postmortem examination.

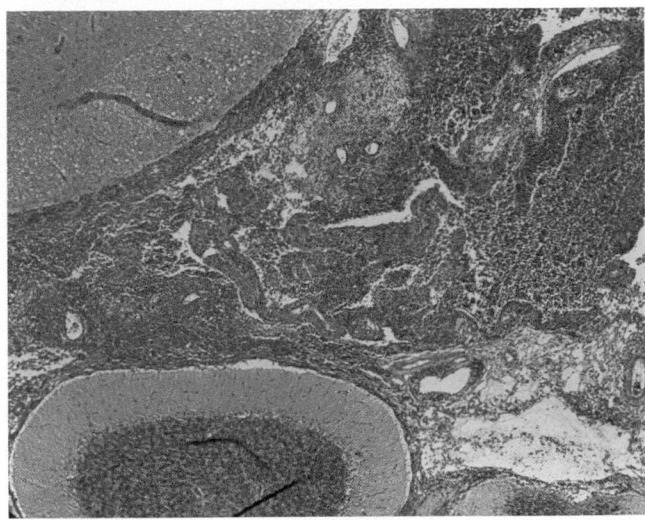

Fig 11-11 Histopathologic section of surface of cerebellar cortex from a cat with meningeal inflammation from dry FIP (H and E stain, ×100). (Courtesy University of Georgia, Athens, Ga.)

chemical staining or immunofluorescence.[140] Mild to moderate villous atrophy may be seen, and villi may be fused.[140]

THERAPY

Various drugs are available for treatment of FIP (Table 11-4). For additional information, an excellent review of therapy by Richard Weiss has been written.[188] No antiviral drugs targets FCoV; however, much work has been done on the viral enzyme 3C-like protease of the coronavirus,[13,14,62,64] and anticoronaviral drugs are being developed for use in people with SARS.

Clinical Category
Healthy Feline Coronavirus-Seropositive Cat
No evidence suggests that any treatment of a healthy seropositive cat could prevent development of FIP. Treatment with glucocorticoids could conceivably prevent clinical signs from occurring, but immunosuppression might have the opposite effect and precipitate onset of clinical FIP. However, because stress is a common factor in the development of FIP in infected cats,[153] avoiding unnecessary stress such as rehoming, elective surgery, or placement in a boarding cattery may be beneficial.

Coronaviral Enteritis
Most cases of coronaviral diarrhea are self-limiting. Cats with chronic diarrhea in which other possible causes have been

eliminated, that are seropositive for FCoV, or in which FCoV has been detected in the feces can only be treated supportively using fluid-electrolyte replacement and restricted caloric oral diet with living natural yogurt or with probiotics (see Chapter 89), as appropriate.[143] No specific antiviral treatment has yet been demonstrated to cure this condition. Some cats respond to low doses of prednisolone (0.5 to 1 mg/day per cat).

Clinical Feline Infectious Peritonitis
Because FIP is an immune-mediated disease, treatment is aimed at controlling the immune response to FCoV, and the most successful treatments consist of relatively high doses of immunosuppressive and antiinflammatory drugs and feline interferon–ω. Rest, avoidance of stressful situations, and a high-protein diet may also help cats with mild clinical signs.[143]

Prednisolone
Prednisolone is the main immunosuppressant used in the treatment of FIP. It is safe, tends to make the cat feel better, and stimulates the cat's appetite. Prednisolone suppresses the humoral and CMI response. One cat with noneffusive FIP treated with prednisolone alone survived for 10 months. Prednisolone has the advantage of also being the treatment

Table • 11-4

Drug Therapy for Feline Infectious Peritonitis

DRUG	DOSAGE	ROUTE
Antiinflammatory Drugs[a]		
Prednisolone	2—4 mg/kg/day, reducing by half every 10 days until stabilization or remission	PO
Feline interferon-ω (Virbagen Omega, Carros, France)	1×10^6 U every other day for five injections then once or twice weekly or 50,000 U daily until total remission of clinical signs	SC PO
Human interferon-α (Roferon, Roche Pharmaceuticals, Nutley, N.J.)	*Effusive FIP:* 2×10^6 IU/kg/day *Noneffusive FIP:* 30 IU/day for 7 days at alternate weeks	IM PO
Thromboxane synthetase inhibitor (ozagrel hydrochloride)	5 mg/kg twice daily	SC
Supportive Drugs[b]		
Aspirin	10 mg/kg every 48—72 hr	PO
Ampicillin	50 mg three times daily	PO
Anabolic steroids	Routine dosage	IM, PO
Ascorbic acid	125 mg twice daily	PO
Vitamin A (not beta-carotene form)	200 IU/kg/day	PO
Vitamin B$_1$ (thiamine)	100 µg/day	PO

[a]Use either prednisolone and interferon or thromboxane synthetase inhibitor from Antiinflammatory Dugs and any or all of the drugs Supportive Drugs.
[b]Use of all or a combination of these drugs is recommended. (See Drug Formulary, Appendix 8 for additional information on each drug. See also Weiss R: *In* August JR (ed): *Consultations in feline internal medicine.* WB Saunders, 1994, pp 3–12.)[188]

for lymphocytic cholangitis, which can be mistaken for FIP; when the diagnosis is in doubt, prednisolone can be given. A cat with lymphocytic cholangitis has a good chance of recovery, whereas a cat with FIP will die.

Prednisolone should never be used in cats with septic peritonitis or pleurisy, which is why cytology is a very important part of FIP diagnosis. The effusion of a cat with sepsis has many more leukocytes, and an attentive cytologist can detect the bacteria or fungi.

The dosage is 2 to 4 mg/kg/day given orally, with a gradually reducing dose every 10 to 14 days until the optimal dosage for the cat is determined by continued response to treatment. Cats on immunosuppressive drugs should also be given broad-spectrum antibiotics if secondary bacterial infections arise and possibly given L-lysine (see Chapters 16 and 93) to prevent recrudescence of latent herpesvirus.

Thalidomide

The rationale of using thalidomide in the treatment of FIP is to reduce inflammation and the humoral immune response to FCoV while leaving the CMI (antiviral) response intact. Only four cats with FIP have been treated with thalidomide, and all died. However, one with a thoracic effusion did eliminate his effusion and was in remission for 3 months. To be effective, thalidomide needs to be used very early in the disease before too many blood vessels became damaged.

The owner's consent must be obtained for treatment with this drug because it is not licensed for use in cats. The dose is 50 to 100 mg and should be given at night. It should *not* be given to pregnant cats because it is teratogenic.

Interferon

Feline Interferon-ω

Recombinant feline IFN-ω (Virbagen Omega, Virbac SAs Carros, France) is available in some countries and has been used in treatment of FIP.[87] Because it is a homologous protein,

it is likely to have a more sustained effect than the human recombinant proteins.

IFN-ω initially was given subcutaneously at 1×10^6 MU/kg every other day and then once weekly or 50,000 U orally per cat for variable period if remission was seen. Cats were also treated with glucocorticoids: (1) 1 mg/kg dexamethasone administered intrathoracically or by IP injection or (2) prednisolone. Oral prednisolone was initially given at 2 mg/kg once daily, and the dosage was gradually tapered to 0.5 mg/kg every other day after remission.[87]

Using this combined drug protocol, 4 cats of 12 completely recovered, and 2 survived for 4 and 5 months, respectively. All cats that recovered completely had the effusive form and were relatively older cats (older than 4 years). Unfortunately, this study did not have a control group (i.e., a group of cats that had similar presenting signs and were treated conventionally), so the efficacy of the treatment cannot be wholly evaluated. However, histologic examination showed the cats that did succumb had FIP, and the same diagnostic criteria were used for all cats.

At the time of writing, data are being collated about the effectiveness of feline IFN-ω in the treatment of FIP. It seems to helps approximately one third of FIP cases treated.

Human Interferon-α

For noneffusive FIP, 30 IU/day of human interferon-α (IFN-α) for 7 days at alternate weeks is given by mouth. In effusive FIP, the same oral dosage can be used, or larger doses of IFN (10^4 to 10^6 IU/day) can be given by intramuscular (IM) injection. After 6 to 7 weeks, if the cat is still alive, IFN no longer works at this dose because the cat makes antibodies against it (see Drug Formulary, Appendix 8).

Vitamins and Antioxidants

- **Vitamin A,** an antioxidant, is given at a dosage of 200 IU/day orally (by mouth or in food). Cats cannot metabolize the β-carotene form, so it must be given as fish oil (e.g., halibut liver oil). Too much vitamin A can cause excessive deposition of bone at the joints, so this supplement should not be used for more than 4 to 6 weeks.

- **Vitamin B$_1$ (thiamine)** has been used at a dosage of 100 µg/day orally (by mouth or in food).
- **Vitamin B complex** is a good appetite stimulant and can be obtained from health food shops or pharmacists. The dosage that is recommended by the manufacturer for children can be used for cats.
- **Vitamin C (ascorbic acid),** at a dosage of 125 mg twice daily, can be given by mouth or in food. Vitamin C is an antioxidant. Given over a long period, vitamin C can cause a predisposition for developing oxalate crystals in the urine.
- **Vitamin E,** at a dosage of 25 to 75 IU per cat twice daily, is given orally (by mouth or in food). Vitamin E is an antioxidant.
- **Anabolic steroids** are used for appetite enhancement and anticatabolism, especially if evidence of renal failure exists.
- **Thromboxane synthetase inhibitors** have been used in two cats with abdominal effusions. Ozagrel hydrochloride (5 to 10/mg/kg twice daily) and prednisolone (2 mg/kg/day) were used with success.[186]

Monitoring Treatment and Prognosis

Regardless of the treatment chosen, it is important to monitor each cat's progress. Regular checks every 7 to 14 days of the HCT, globulins, A:G, AGP, and the cat's weight serve as indicators of the cat's progress. Later, examinations could be performed only monthly if the cat is improving. It is not worthwhile to measure the FCoV-antibody titer more often than every month because no discernible difference within a shorter period can be detected. The AGP should be the first to decrease if treatment is having a positive effect because AGP is a measure of inflammation. Positive signs also include decreasing globulin levels, increasing A:G and HCT, the appearance of reticulocytes in blood smears, and weight gain. Negative signs are AGP remaining high, globulins staying high or increasing, A:G decreasing, and weight loss. When the HCT becomes less than 20% and is nonregenerative (i.e., no reticulocytes are seen on blood smear examination), the cat should probably be humanely euthanized if its quality of life is impaired. Clearly, if the cat is distressed at any point in the treatment, euthanasia should be considered. Cats with effusive FIP usually only survive a few days—weeks at best. Cats with noneffusive FIP can survive many weeks or months, although after neurologic signs begin, death usually ensues fairly rapidly.

PREVENTION

More than any other factor, management of kittens determines whether they become infected with FCoV.[3,4,41,69] Kittens of FCoV-shedding queens should be protected from infection by maternally derived antibody until they are at least 5 to 6 weeks old. A protocol for the prevention of FCoV infection in kittens is presented in Table 11-5. When reliable serologic tests are available, kittens should be tested when older than 10 weeks to ensure that isolation and early weaning have been effective. Infected kittens younger than 10 weeks may not yet have seroconverted.[4] A protocol for minimizing the spread of FCoV in catteries is presented in Table 11-6.

Many attempts have been made to develop effective vaccines, but unfortunately most have failed because of ADE.[161,180] However, a vaccine, Primucell, was produced (Pfizer Animal Health, New York, N.Y.) incorporating a tem-

perature-sensitive mutant of the FCoV strain DF2-FIPV, which could replicate in the cool lining of the upper respiratory tract but not at the higher internal body temperature.[22,44-46] This vaccine, administered intranasally, produces local immunity at the site where FCoV first enters the body—the oropharynx—and also induces a long-lasting CMI response. The vaccine has been available in the United States since 1991 and has been introduced in some European countries.[36] The two concerns about this vaccine are its safety and efficacy.

The safety concern is whether the vaccine can cause ADE. Although some experimental vaccine trials have recorded ADE on challenge,[122,162] the overwhelming evidence from field studies is that Primucell is safe.[36,150] In two double-blind trials (one of 609 cats and one of 500 cats), the animals were vaccinated with either Primucell or a placebo, and in both trials fewer FIP deaths occurred in the Primucell-vaccinated group than the placebo group.[36,150] Clearly, Primucell afforded protection from FIP and did not cause ADE. Furthermore, immediate side effects from vaccination such as sneezing, vomiting, or diarrhea were not statistically different between the vaccinated group and the placebo group.[36]

Primucell vaccination causes seroconversion, and although it may be at a lower level than that caused by natural infection, it can still cause low positive antibody titers. Cats shed

Table • 11-5

Protocol for Prevention of Feline Coronavirus Infection in Kittens

STEP	DESCRIPTION
Prepare kitten room.	1. Remove all cats and kittens 1 week before introducing new queen.
	2. Disinfect room using 1:32 dilution of sodium hypochlorite (bleach).
	3. Dedicate separate litter trays and food and water bowls to this room, and disinfect with sodium hypochlorite.
	4. Introduce single queen 1–2 weeks before parturition.
Practice barrier nursing.	1. Work in the kitten room before tending other cats.
	2. Clean hands with disinfectant before going into kitten room.
	3. Have shoes and coveralls dedicated to the kitten room.
Wean and isolate kittens early.	1. Test queen for FCoV antibodies either before or after she gives birth.
	2. If queen is seropositive, she should be removed from the kitten room when the kittens are 5–6 weeks old.
	3. If the queen is seronegative, she can remain with the kittens until they are older.
Test kittens.	1. Test kittens for FCoV antibodies after 10 weeks of age.

vaccine virus oronasally for up to 4 days.[22] The recommendation for vaccination is to give two doses 3 weeks apart from 16 weeks onward. Although Primucell is recommended to be given to cats at least 16 weeks old, it has also been administered to 9-week-old kittens and found to be safe. In these kittens the vaccine did not prevent infection; however, the amount of FCoV isolated from the gut and mesenteric lymph nodes was significantly reduced.[86,154] Primucell seems to be safe to administer to pregnant cats and does not affect kitten mortality or reproductive capability in breeding colonies.[44,154] Primucell is also safe to administer simultaneously with other vaccines or to FeLV-infected cats.[44] Annual boosters are recommended. Because mucosal immunity is involved, the duration of protection after natural exposure or vaccination is short lived in most cats after virus is cleared, and reinfection is possible. Vaccine must be given periodically to maintain this immunity.

The efficacy has been questioned because the vaccine strain is a serotype II coronavirus, and the serotype I coronavirus is more prevalent in field isolates. A double-blind trial of 609 16- to 53-week-old vaccinated pet cats was conducted in Switzerland.[36,116] At the start of the trial, 358 cats were seropositive. Up to 150 days after vaccination, the number of cats that developed FIP was not significantly different. However, after 150 days, only one FIP-associated death in the vaccinated group of cats (0.4%) occurred, compared with seven FIP deaths in the placebo group (2.7%).[36] RT-PCR of blood from all of the vaccinated cats that developed FIP showed that virus was present in the cats before the vaccine was administered. Thus many of the cats in which Primucell appeared ineffective had been vaccinated when they were already incubating FIP.[116] Because the vaccine works partly by stimulating local immunity, it is less effective if virus has already crossed the mucous membranes. Obviously, it follows that Primucell is more efficacious in cats that have not been exposed to FCoV (or are seronegative) than in seropositive cats. Clearly, an attempt must be made to prevent kittens from becoming infected with FCoV—by early weaning and isolation—before they are vaccinated.

The efficacy of Primucell, based on preventable fraction (see Vaccine Efficacy, Chapter 100) has been reported to be 50% to 75%.[143] In a survey of 138 cats from 15 cat breeders, in which virtually all of the cats were seropositive, no difference in FIP-associated deaths was found between the vaccinated group and the placebo group.[36] The manufacturers do not specify that FCoV antibody testing should precede vaccination. However, because Primucell does not work in a cat that is incubating the disease, FCoV antibody testing is beneficial. Because Primucell causes seroconversion and low antibody titers, testing before vaccination is advisable.

USEFUL WEB SITES

www.catvirus.com
www.felinecoronavirus.com
www.orionfoundation.com

SUGGESTED READINGS*

36. Fehr D, Holznagel E, Bolla S, et al. 1995. Evaluation of the safety and efficacy of a modified live FIPV vaccine under field conditions, *Feline Pract* 23:83-88.
42. Foley JE, Rand C, Leutenegger C. 2003. Inflammation and changes in cytokine levels in neurological feline infectious peritonitis, *J Feline Med Surg* 5:313-322.
101. Kipar A, Koehler K, Bellmann S, et al. 1996b. Feline infectious peritonitis presenting as a tumour in the abdominal cavity, *Vel Rec* 144:118-122.
165. Sparkes AH, Gruffydd-Jones TJ, Harbour DA. 1991. Feline infectious peritonitis: a review of clinicopathological changes in 65 cases, and a critical assessment of their diagnostic value, *Vet Rec* 129:202-212.

*See the CD-ROM for a complete list of references.

Table • 11-6

Protocol for Minimizing Feline Coronavirus Introduction or Spread in a Cattery[144]

PROTOCOL	DESCRIPTION
Reducing fecal contamination of the environment	Have adequate numbers of litter trays (one tray for every one or two cats).
	Declump litter trays at least daily.
	Remove all litter, and disinfect litter trays at least weekly.
	Keep litter trays away from the food area.
	Vacuum around litter trays regularly.
	Clip fur of hindquarters of longhaired cats.
Cat numbers	Ordinary households should have no more than 8—10 cats.
	Cats should be kept in stable groups of up to three or four.
	In rescue facilities, each cat should be kept in single quarters and not commingling with other cats.
	In a FCoV eradication program, cats should be kept in small groups according to their antibody or virus shedding status: seronegative or nonshedding cats together and seropositive or virus-shedding cats together.
Antibody or virus testing	Incumbent cats should be tested before introducing new cats or breeding.
	Only seronegative or virus-negative cats should be introduced into FCoV-free catteries.
	It is safer to introduce seropositive cats than seronegative cats into infected households, but the newcomer and the incumbent cats are still at risk for developing FIP.
Isolation and early weaning	Cat breeders and rescuers of pregnant cats should follow the protocol outlined in Table 11-5.
Vaccination with Primucell	If new cats must be introduced into a household with endemic infection, they should be vaccinated with Primucell (Pfizer Animal Health, New York, NY) before introduction.

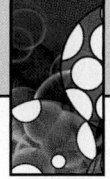

CHAPTER 12

Feline Enteric Viral Infections

Craig E. Greene

FELINE ASTROVIRAL INFECTIONS

Etiology and Epidemiology

Astroviruses were first described in feces from cases of human infantile gastroenteritis. These viruses have since been identified in several other species, including cats. When negatively stained and examined by transmission electron microscopy (EM), astroviruses appear as unenveloped, spherical particles approximately 28 to 30 nm in diameter, with a characteristic five- or six-point, star-shaped surface pattern, depending on the orientation (Fig. 12-1).

A limited serologic and virologic survey of diarrheic cats from the United Kingdom suggests that the infection is not very common; less than 10% of animals tested have antibody to the Bristol isolate. However, more than one serotype may exist, as in humans, in whom seven serotypes are known.[12]

Clinical Findings

Only two cases of a natural astrovirus infection in cats have been reported in detail. In both cases, the illness was characterized by persistent green, watery diarrhea; dehydration; and anorexia. No hematologic abnormalities were noted, and the only biochemical abnormalities were mild acidosis and hypokalemia in one of the cats. Other variable signs were gas-distended loops of the small intestine, pyrexia, depression, poor body condition, and vomiting. Vomiting and diarrhea have been reported in another infected cat, although no further clinical details were given.

In an outbreak of diarrhea in a breeding colony, EM revealed astrovirus in the feces of 25% of affected kittens. Initial signs in these kittens were inappetence, depression, and prolapse of the third eyelid. Other litters in the colony previously had developed a similar syndrome, with diarrhea that persisted 4 to 14 days. A significant number of adult cats were also affected. Sera from several of these animals had antibody to astrovirus.

Experimental oral administration of an astroviral isolate to specific pathogen-free (SPF) kittens resulted in mild diarrhea 11 to 12 days later. This condition coincided with a period of pyrexia and virus shedding with subsequent seroconversion. The kittens remained otherwise well.

Diagnosis

EM most conveniently diagnoses astrovirus infection of negatively stained preparations of diarrheic stools. Growing some isolates in cell culture is possible, although no cytopathic effect is produced, and virus-infected cells must be located by specific immunofluorescence. Other isolates cannot be grown in cell culture at the present time; therefore this method of diagnosis is not viable. Information on the sequence of the viral RNA is becoming available and should lead to improved methods of diagnosis based on molecular techniques, such as polymerase chain reaction (PCR).[2]

Therapy, Prevention, and Public Health Considerations

Treatment of affected animals is probably not necessary other than to replace lost fluids and electrolytes if the diarrhea is severe or prolonged. No vaccine is available.

Human serum can contain antibody to feline astrovirus, but whether this finding reflects zoonotic infection or a serologic relationship between human and feline astroviruses is unknown. Molecular evidence suggests that, in recent evolutionary history, feline and porcine rotaviruses have become established in the human population.[1]

FELINE ROTAVIRAL INFECTIONS

Etiology and Epidemiology

Rotaviruses are classified as a genus within the family *Reoviridae* and are of worldwide distribution. They can be distinguished from reoviruses and orbiviruses, when viewed by negative-stain EM, by the characteristic morphology of the 70 nm–diameter intact virion. This virion appears as a wheel with the core in the center forming a hub, the inner layer of capsomeres radiating outward as spokes, and the outer layer giving a sharply defined rim.

Rotaviruses are classified into various serogroups (A through G) based on genetic and immunologic similarities. They have been isolated from many species of animals and are the major enteric viral pathogens in humans and the main species in domestic livestock, causing significant economic losses. By contrast, although infection of cats is common, with up to 100% of populations being seropositive, clinical disease is rare.

Analysis of the capsid encoding genes (VP4, VP6, and VP7) by restriction endonuclease assay allows the differentiation among the strains of different origin. The VP7 profiles differentiate strains of animal and human origin more efficiently.[16]

Nonstructural glycoprotein NSP4 of group A rotaviruses from mice has been identified as a viral enterotoxin. The amino acid sequence of this protein from rotaviruses isolated from diarrheal and asymptomatic kittens were similar; however, no consistent difference was found between these isolates from clinically healthy or ill cats.[13] Group C rotaviruses, similar to those from pigs, have been isolated from dogs in Germany.[14]

Clinical Findings and Diagnosis

Feline rotavirus was first described in 1979 in kittens of 6 weeks and 8 months of age that passed semiformed to liquid stools. The virus isolated from the 6-week-old kitten induced anorexia and diarrhea when given to a 3-day-old, colostrum-deprived kitten. Subsequently, feline rotavirus has been recognized more frequently in the stools of normal cats, and a transmission study using a strain isolated from a diarrheic

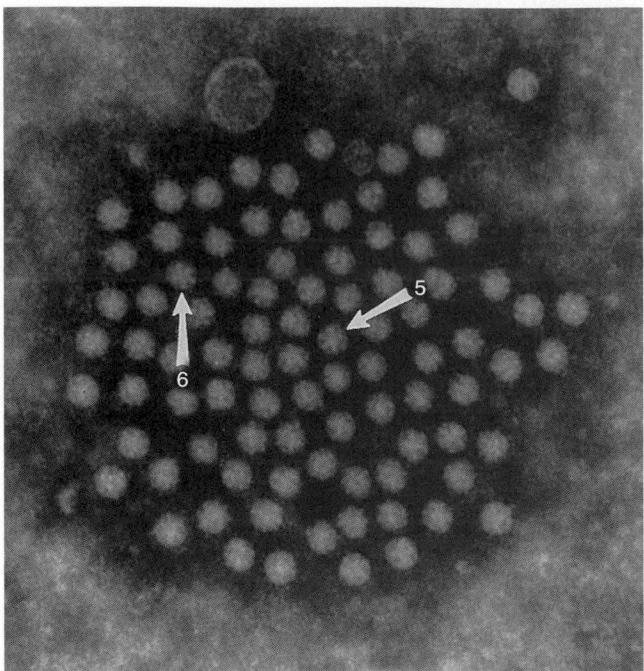

Fig 12-1 Negatively stained astrovirus particles. *Arrows* indicate particles with five- and six-pointed, star-shaped surface patterns. (Courtesy Charles Ashley, Bristol Public Health Laboratory, Bristol, United Kingdom.)

cat failed to produce disease in adult cats or kittens as young as 10 days.

Rotavirus may be readily demonstrated in feces by negative-stain EM or by polyacrylamide gel electrophoresis and silver staining of RNA extracted directly from feces. The latter method is more suitable for screening large numbers of specimens. A PCR method has been described that is considerably more sensitive than either of the other two methods.[19] Other methods, such as enzyme-linked immunosorbent assay or latex agglutination, have been used, but they have been developed for group A viruses, whereas many feline isolates belong to other groups. Some, but not all, isolates can be grown in cell culture, but this is time consuming.

Pathologic Findings
Histologic findings include swollen intestinal villi with mild infiltration by macrophages and neutrophils. Viral antigen can be detected by fluorescent antibodies, and virions by EM, in epithelial cells.

Therapy, Prevention, and Public Health Considerations
Treatment is symptomatic for diarrhea. Signs are mild and transient, and mucosal integrity is not impaired. Fluid therapy can be given intravenously or subcutaneously, depending on the severity of dehydration. No vaccine is currently available for cats.

Genetic characterization of group G3 canine rotavirus strains in Italy, the United States, and Japan, and human and simian rotavirus isolates have shown highly conserved genetic sequences in the VP4 and VP7 genes, suggesting close genetic homogeneity.[3,4] Rotaviruses of different hosts can infect other

species when inoculated experimentally, but these cross infections generally are asymptomatic. Human rotavirus strain HCR3, which was isolated from a healthy infant in 1984, has close genetic homologies with feline rotavirus strain FRV64 and canine rotavirus strains CU-1 and K9, but not with other rotaviruses more commonly isolated from people.[11] Evidence from molecular studies[6,10] suggests that feline rotaviruses may have infected people in Japan. Similarly, in Thailand, a human isolate from an infected infant with diarrhea showed close genetic and phenotypic homologies to other human and feline strains.[15]

OTHER VIRAL ENTERITIDES

Torovirus-Like Agent
During the course of a microbiologic survey of cats with the syndrome of protruding nictitating membranes and diarrhea, a novel virus was detected that hemagglutinated rat erythrocytes.[8] Hemagglutination-inhibition (HI) testing and immune EM suggested that the virus was torovirus-like, but PCR and thin-section EM failed to confirm this finding. The virus could not be grown in cultured cells. Experimental inoculation of SPF kittens induced mild, intermittent diarrhea and pyrexia with hematologic changes (principally neutrophilia, but one kitten also developed lymphocytosis). The agent appears to be ubiquitous, because the majority of cats have antibody against it, but its significance as an enteric pathogen is unclear. In another study, torovirus particles were not detected in the feces of cats with protruding nictitating membranes.[17]

Feline Reovirus
All mammalian reoviruses belong to three serotypes, and all three of these have been isolated from cats. Feline reoviruses have generally been considered to be minor respiratory or ocular pathogens, although they can readily be isolated from both respiratory and enteric tracts. Experimental inoculation of kittens with serotype-2 isolates, however, has resulted in the development of mild diarrhea.[7,9] Feline reoviruses are widespread in nature as judged by serosurveys.

Other Viruses
A large number of other viruses have been detected in the stools of normal and diarrheic cats, but their role as pathogens is unclear. These viruses include parvovirus-like particles (serologically unrelated to feline panleukopenia virus), picornavirus-like particles, coronavirus-like particles (morphologically distinct from feline infectious peritonitis viruses and feline enteric coronavirus), calicivirus, "togavirus-like particles," and "thorn apple-like particles."

SUGGESTED READINGS*

9. Muir P, Harbour DA, Gruffydd-Jones TJ. 1992. Reovirus type 2 in domestic cats: isolation and experimental transmission, *Vet Microbiol* 30:309-316.

16. Santos N, Clark HF, Hoshino Y, et al. 1998. Relationship among serotype G3P5A rotavirus strains isolated from different host species, *Mol Cell Probes* 12:379-386.

19. Xu L, Harbour D, McCrae MA. 1990. The application of polymerase chain reaction to the detection of rotaviruses in feces, *J Virol Methods* 27:29-38.

*See the CD-ROM for a complete list of references.

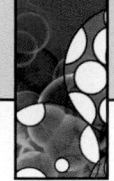

CHAPTER 13

Feline Leukemia Virus Infection

Katrin Hartmann

Feline leukemia virus (FeLV) was first described in 1964 by William Jarrett and co-workers when virus particles were seen budding from the membrane of malignant lymphoblasts from a cat with naturally occurring lymphoma.[156,157] The virus was shown to produce a similar malignancy when experimentally injected into healthy cats and thus was proven to be capable of transmitting lymphocytic neoplasia. Although household clusters of lymphoma cases had been observed among cats for many years, it was not until the discovery of FeLV that an infectious etiology was considered likely. However, following this discovery, it was assumed that all hematopoietic tumors in cats were caused by FeLV independent of whether the cats remained FeLV positive.[96] It is currently accepted that tumor-causing factors other than FeLV play more important roles, specifically in older cats.

FeLV infection occurs globally.[38] For many years after its discovery, FeLV was considered to (1) be the principal scourge in cats, (2) account for most disease-related deaths in pet cats, and (3) be responsible for more clinical syndromes than any other single agent.[268] It had been estimated that approximately one third of all cancer deaths in cats were caused by FeLV, and an even greater number of infected cats died of anemia and infectious diseases caused by suppressive effects of the virus on bone marrow and the immune system.[38] However, today these assumptions are changing because the prevalence and importance of FeLV as a pathogen in cats are decreasing, primarily because of testing and eradication programs and routine use of FeLV vaccines.

ETIOLOGY

FeLV, a γ-retrovirus of domestic cats, is a member of the Oncornavirus subfamily of retroviruses and contains a protein core with single-stranded RNA protected by an envelope. FeLV is an exogenous agent that replicates within many tissues, including bone marrow, salivary glands, and respiratory epithelium. The virus is noncytopathic and escapes from the cell by budding from the cell membrane (Figs. 13-1 and 13-2). It can cause clinical illness related to the hematopoietic and immune systems and neoplasia. After initial infection, if the immune response does not intervene, FeLV spreads to the bone marrow and infects hematopoietic precursor cells. In infected cells, DNA copies of the viral RNA are transcribed, and it is these copies that are inserted randomly into the host DNA (Fig. 13-3). Once this provirus is integrated, cell division results in daughter cells that also contain the viral DNA. This ability of the virus to become part of the host's own DNA is the most important factor in the lifelong presence of the virus after bone marrow infection. Consequently, every infected cell has to be recognized and destroyed to "cure" an infection. Once the pool of hematologic and immune stem cells becomes infected, true elimination of the virus becomes unlikely.[184]

Virus Origin

Both, exogenous (foreign, "pathogenic") and endogenous (inherited, "nonpathogenic") retroviruses are present in cats. Pathogenic exogenous viruses that can be transmitted horizontally from cat to cat include FeLV, feline immunodeficiency virus (FIV, see Chapter 14), and feline syncytium-forming virus (FeSFV, see Chapter 17), which is widespread but has a low pathogenicity.

On the basis of similarities in nucleotide sequences, it has been determined that FeLV evolved from a virus in an ancestor of the rat. It is likely that this event took place in the late Pleistocene up to 10 million years ago in the North African desert. Ancestral rats and cats roamed freely, and the virus was transmitted to cats through ingestion or a rat bite. The initial spread of FeLV among cats might have been inhibited by the aridity of the North African desert.[18]

FeLV is divided into several subgroups (based on the genetic map), but only subgroup FeLV-A is infectious and transmitted from cat to cat. The other subgroups (e.g., FeLV-B, FeLV-C, FeLV-*myc*) are not transmitted from cat to cat under natural circumstances but can be generated de novo in an FeLV-A-infected cat by mutation and recombination of the FeLV-A genome with cellular genes or genes from endogenous retroviruses in the cat's genome. In addition, feline sarcoma virus (FeSV) is a recombination of the FeLV-A genome with cancer-associated cellular genes (proto-oncogenes) and is generated de novo in an FeLV-A–infected cat.

Certain endogenous, nonpathogenic retroviruses (e.g., RD-114 virus, enFeLV, MAC-1 virus) are normally present in the genome of the cat population and inherited by transmission from cat to kitten through germline. These endogenous fractions of proviral DNA (also called *proviral sin*) cannot be induced to produce infectious virus particles. They are present but not replicating in every feline cell. Their main importance is based on the fact that these DNA fractions can potentially recombine with FeLV-A DNA in case of FeLV-A infection and thus increase the pathogenicity of FeLV-A. RD-114 is the most studied endogenous feline retrovirus. Although no evidence shows pathogenicity of or any immune response to RD-114 virus in cats, it may play some role in normal fetal differentiation. RD114 is most closely related to an endogenous baboon retrovirus and only distantly related to FeLV.[34,38,310]

FeLV Genome and Proteins

FeLV is a typical retrovirus, containing single-stranded RNA that is transcribed by the enzyme reverse transcriptase (RT) into DNA, the so-called *provirus* that is subsequently integrated into the cellular genome. The gene sequence contains long terminal repeats (LTRs), which are repeated sequences that have regulatory function and control expression of the other viral genes but generally do not code for a protein product. From the 5' to the 3' end the gene order is LTR-*gag-pol-env*-LTR (Table 13-1). Within the LTRs, recurrent

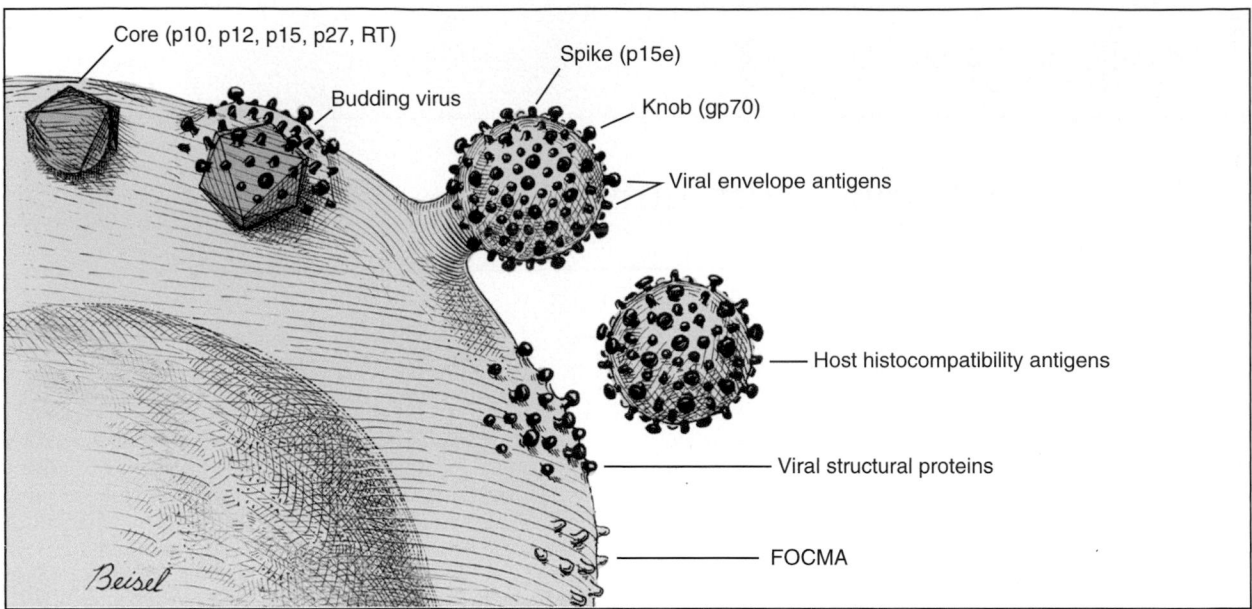

Fig 13-1 Production and release of virus from a feline malignant cell. Viral envelope antigens can have a spike or knob shape. Host histocompatibility antigens may appear on the virus as the virus buds from the cell membrane. Viral structural proteins may appear on the host cell. Virus replication can also occur in nonmalignant cells. *FOCMA,* Feline oncornavirus membrane antigen. (Courtesy University of Georgia, Athens, Ga.)

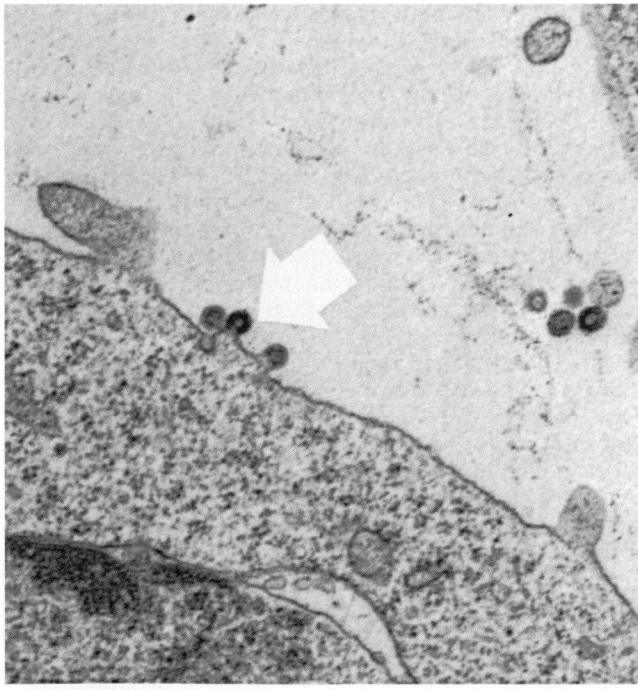

Fig 13-2 Ultrastructural view of FeLV budding from cell surface *(arrow).* (Courtesy SmithKline Beecham Animal Health, Exton, Pa.)

Table • 13-1

Summary of Genetic Map and Function of FeLV Proteins[a]

GENE	LOCATION	TYPE	FUNCTION
gag	Core		Basis for indirect FA and ELISA tests, immune complex disease, and cytotoxic effects
		p15c	Matrix protein
		p12	Unknown
		p27	Capsid protein commonly used for testing
		p10	Nucleocapsid protein
pol	Core	RT	Copies viral protein into complementary DNA strand
env	Envelope	gp70	External surface unit; type-specific antigens A, B, C; responsible for neutralizing or protective antibody against viral infection
		p15e	Transmembrane protein; viral immunosuppression

P, Protein (number is molecular weight in kilodaltons); *gp,* glycoprotein; *gag,* group-associated antigen gene; *pol,* polymerase; *env,* envelope; *RT,* reverse transcriptase; *FA,* fluorescent antibody; *ELISA,* enzyme-linked immunosorbent assay.
[a]As listed in chart, genes are located from the 5′ to the 3′ end with long terminal repeat (LTR) sequences at each end.

enhancer sequences (UREs) are frequently found in myeloid leukemias of cats and thought to be associated with oncogenesis.[209,230] The *gag* (group-associated antigen) gene encodes the internal structural proteins, including p15c, p12, p27, and p10. The *gag* protein p27, which is used for clinical detection of FeLV, is produced in virus-infected cells in amounts exceeding what is necessary for assembly of new virus particles. Thus it is abundant in the cytoplasm of individual infected cells and also in the plasma of infected cats, which is why most avail-

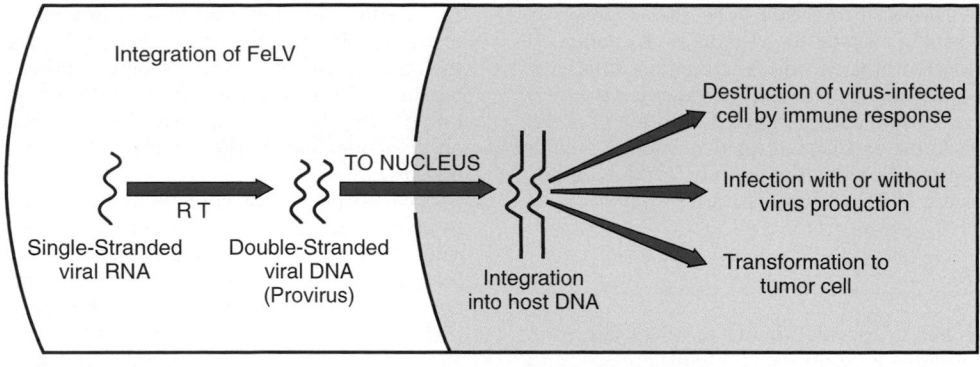

Fig 13-3 Formation of FeLV and integration into cells. (*RT*, Reverse transcriptase.)

Table • 13-2

FeLV Subgroups[a]

VIRAL SUBGROUPS	FREQUENCY OF ISOLATION IN FeLV-POSITIVE CATS	ASSOCIATED DISEASE	COMPARISON BY SPECIES OF IN VITRO REPLICATION
A	100% viremic cats, mildly pathogenic but highly contagious, mildly cytopathogenic	Hematopoietic neoplasia, experimentally may cause hemolysis	Cat, rabbit, pig, mink, human
B	Occurs with subgroup A in 50% or more of cats with neoplastic disease (lymphoma)	Not pathogenic alone, virulent in recombination with subgroup A, noncontagious	Cat, dog, cow, hamster, pig, human
C	Rarely isolated, arises by mutation from FeLV subgroup A	Nonregenerative anemia and erythremic myelosis, nonreplicating and noncontagious	Cat, dog, guinea pig, human
T[b]	Highly cytopathic, T-cell tropic virus; affinity for two host cell proteins: Pit1 and FeLIX; evolved from FeLV subgroup A	Lymphopenia, neutropenia, fever, diarrhea	Cat

[a]Modified from Jarrett O. 1990. Feline leukemia virus subgroups, pp 473–479. *In* Hardy WD, Essex M, McClelland AJ (eds), *Feline leukemia virus*. Elsevier, New York, NY; Nakata R, Myiazawa T, Shin YS, et al. 2003. Reevaluation of host ranges of feline leukemia virus subgroups, *Microbes Infect* 5:947–950.
[b]Subgroup T is a variant of subgroup A. Changes in the envelope protein result in increased cytopathogenicity of T strains.

able immunochromatographic tests such as the enzyme-linked immunofluorescent assay (ELISA) or fluorescent antibody (FA) assays are designed to detect this protein. Free p27 not only circulates in plasma but is also shed in tears and saliva, where it also can be detected. The *pol* (polymerase) gene specifies the viral enzyme RT, which is responsible for synthesis of DNA on the RNA template. The *env* (envelope) gene encodes the envelope components gp70 and p15e. The *env* protein gp70 defines the virus subgroup and appears to be important for inducing immunity. Antibodies to gp70 are subgroup specific and result in neutralization of the virus and immunity to reinfection. Thus gp70 is important in natural resistance and as a target for vaccine production. The transmembrane protein p15e is thought to interfere with host cell immune responses, thus facilitating viral persistence.

FeLV Subgroups

The three most important FeLV subgroups (FeLV-A, FeLV-B, FeLV-C) have been classified on the basis of interference testing, virus neutralization, and ability to replicate in nonfeline tissues (Table 13-2). Only FeLV-A is contagious and passed horizontally from cat to cat in nature. Subgroups B and C evolve de novo in an FeLV-A–infected cat by mutation and

recombination between FeLV-A and cellular or endogenous retroviral sequences contained in normal feline DNA. Replication of FeLV-B and FeLV-C is only possible with the help of FeLV-A because important genomic sequences are replaced in these recombinant viruses. Proposed FeLV-A helper functions include enhanced replication efficiency, immune evasion, and replication rescue for defective FeLV-B and FeLV-C virions. However, in certain experiments, it was possible to induce replication without FeLV-A. In newborn specific-pathogen–free (SPF) kittens an experimental FeLV-B or FeLV-C infection has been established without FeLV-A.[17,276] However, all naturally infected cats carry subgroup A either alone or in combination with subgroup B, subgroup C, or both. Thus if antibodies against subgroup A are produced, the cat is protected. Pathogenicity of subgroup B and C is higher than of subgroup A.[267] Different properties of the envelope proteins in the different subgroups have been shown to be the major pathogenic determinant, but the mechanisms by which envelope differences influence pathogenesis are not well understood.[224] Subgroup B is commonly associated with malignancies. Subgroup C is rare and is mainly associated with nonregenerative anemia. In experimental infections a subgroup B strain (Rickard strain) caused lymphoma in nearly

100% of kittens by 1 year of infection, whereas subgroup C isolates repeatedly produced fatal nonregenerative anemia.[242] Simultaneous inoculation of subgroup A in combination with subgroup B in cats was associated with an attenuated infection compared to infection with subgroup A alone.[246] Thus subgroup B may be acting as an attenuated vaccine. A fourth FeLV subgroup, subgroup T, is highly cytolytic for T lymphocytes and causes severe immunosuppression.[15,177,178]

EPIDEMIOLOGY

In nature, FeLV has been reported mainly to infect domestic cats. Case reports of FeLV in nondomestic felids are few, and FeLV does not appear to be enzootic in wild felids other than European wildcats *(Felis silvestris)* in France and Scotland.[45] Some evidence shows that other wild felids may be susceptible. A multicentric T-cell lymphoma associated with FeLV infection was found in a captive Namibian cheetah *(Acinonyx jubatus).*[206] FeLV was also detected in an 11-month-old captive-bred male neutered bobcat *(Felis rufus)* showing signs of lethargy, anorexia, neutropenia, lymphopenia, and non-regenerative anemia.[289] Introduction of FeLV into free-living and captive nondomestic felid populations could have serious consequences for their health and survival.

Some evidence shows that FeLV might replicate in non-felid tissue (see Table 13-2). For example, FeLV-B replicates in cells of cats, dogs, cows, pigs, hamsters, monkeys, and humans; FeLV-C replicates in cells of cats, dogs, guinea pigs, and humans.[152,155,275] Although malignant transformations do not occur in nonfelid cell cultures,[191] experimental FeLV infection with development of lymphomas could be induced in young dogs and marmosets[260]; in experimental infections with FeSV, fibrosarcomas could be produced in nonfelids in vivo. It was thought that FeLV-A only replicates in cat cells in vitro, and that infection in vivo that always requires FeLV-A, cannot happen in nonfelids. However, it has been found that two independent FeLV-A isolates from United Kingdom and United States also have infected various nonfeline cell lines including cells from humans, rabbits, pigs, and minks.[227] However, no reports have been made on natural transmission of FeLV to nonfelids.

Prevalence
FeLV infection exists in domestic cats worldwide. In contrast to FIV infection, in which the prevalence varies significantly, the FeLV infection rate of free-roaming cats is similar throughout the world, ranging from 1% to 8% in healthy cats. Infection rates of up to 21% have been reported from large studies of sick cats.[184] Originally, certain diseases such as lymphoma and leukemia were associated with very high rates (up to 75%) of FeLV infection or feline infectious peritonitis (FIP; up to 32%). In recent years, cats that test negative for FeLV but have these diseases have become more common because the overall prevalence of FeLV has decreased.[37]

Clear evidence shows that the overall rate of FeLV infection is decreasing. For example, the Tufts Veterinary Diagnostic Laboratory annually evaluates 1500 to 2400 FeLV test results submitted by practitioners from healthy and ill cats. A gradual but significant decline from 8% in 1989 to 4% in 1995 occurred in the number of positive test results.[36-38] An overall seroprevalence rate of infection in Japan was 2.9%, with higher rates of infection in southern and urban sites than in northern and suburban sites.[207] Germany has had a clear decrease in prevalence over the last 20 years from 5% to 2.5%.[114] The decreased infection rate is particularly true in catteries. The availability of testing in these closed facilities made it possible to remove all infected animals. Likewise, the current practice of testing cats in animal shelters and testing new pets entering a household has contributed to the decline in prevalence. Vaccination also contributes to the decrease, but epidemiologic studies suggest that the testing and removal practice is more effective than vaccination.[272] The first vaccine was introduced in 1985, but the observed decline in the overall infection rate began before this time.[184]

The prevalence of FeLV is higher in cats that are allowed to go outside because direct contact is required for transmission. In a study in the United States, antibody prevalence (which predicts exposure) was clearly related to the time spent outdoors and the degree of exposure to other cats. Cats in a study in Boston and Detroit, of which many were allowed to roam outside, had 63% and 47% positive antibodies rates, respectively, whereas only 5% of New York cats that were primarily confined to high-rise apartments had antibodies.[242]

Risk groups for FIV and FeLV infections are different. Whereas fighting, free-roaming, intact male cats are at highest risk for acquiring FIV infection, FeLV infection is the infection of "social cats" because it is mostly spread through social contacts. Thus in contrast to FIV infection, which is transmitted primarily through biting—behavior common among male cats because of their propensity for fighting—FeLV infection is found almost equally in male and female cats, with a slightly higher rate in male cats. This may be a result of the wandering behavior that is more common in male cats and the subsequent increased number of cat contacts. In one study, 733 unowned free-roaming cats in Raleigh, North Carolina, and 1143 unowned free-roaming cats in Gainesville, Florida, were tested for FIV and FeLV infection, and prevalence of FeLV infection was not significantly different between males (4.9%) and females (3.8%).[179]

Although no breeds are predisposed to being infected with FeLV, infection is less commonly found in purebred cats today, mainly because they are usually kept indoors. In addition, awareness in the cat breeder community of FeLV infection leads to frequent testing and avoidance of bringing an infected cat into a closed cat population.

Transmission
FeLV is contagious and spreads through close contact between viral shedding cats and susceptible cats. Transmission of FeLV occurs primarily via saliva, where the concentration of virus is higher than in plasma. Viremic cats constantly shed millions of virus particles in the saliva. The concentration of virus in saliva and blood of healthy viremic cats is as high as it is in those with signs of illness. FeLV is passed effectively horizontally among communal cats that have prolonged close contact. Social behavior such as sharing food and water dishes, mutual grooming, and using common litter areas are the most effective means of transmission. Although the virus may enter many tissues, body fluids, and secretions, it is less likely to spread via urine and feces. Fleas have been considered a potential source of transmission because FeLV RNA has been detected in fleas and their feces.[319,320] Iatrogenic transmission can occur via contaminated needles, instruments, fomites, or blood transfusions.

The viral envelope is lipid soluble and susceptible to disinfectants, soaps, heating, and drying. Virus is readily inactivated in the environment within a few seconds. Therefore close contact among cats is required for spread of infection, and indirect transmission (e.g., via human beings) is not possible. Single cats strictly kept indoors are not at risk for acquiring infection. It is only because of latency and potential reactivation that viremia is occasionally detected in middle-age cats that have lived alone indoors since they were adopted as kittens. Because of the viral lability, a waiting period is not needed before introducing a new cat into a household after removal of an infected cat. FeLV is not a hazard in a veterinary hospital or boarding kennel as long as cats are housed separately and routine cage disinfection and hand washing are performed between handling cats. FeLV is maintained in nature because infected cats may live and shed virus for several years.

Vertical transmission from mother to kittens occurs in FeLV-viremic cats. Neonatal kittens can be infected transplacentally or when the queen licks and nurses them. Transmission also can occur in queens that are latently infected (and therefore have a negative result on routine tests) because a latent infection may be reactivated during pregnancy. In addition, isolated FeLV infection of the mammary glands of FeLV-negative cats with transmission of FeLV via milk has been described. If in utero infection occurs, reproductive failure in the form of fetal resorption, abortion, and neonatal death is common, although up to 20% of vertically infected kittens may survive the neonatal period to become persistently infected adults.[184] It is possible to observe that newborn kittens from infected queens have negative FeLV antigen test results at the time of birth but may become positive over the following weeks to months once the virus starts replicating. Thus if the queen or any kitten in her litter is infected, the entire family should be treated as if infected and isolated from uninfected cats.

Susceptibility to FeLV infection is highest in young kittens. Studies in a household with many FeLV-infected cats showed that 7 of 10 kittens placed there at 3 months of age became viremic within 5 months, whereas only 3 of 17 adults in the same household became viremic over 7 years.[34,38] Experimental infection is difficult if not impossible in healthy adult cats. Depending on the FeLV strains used, experimental infection can even be difficult to achieve in kittens older than 16 weeks of age.[134] This age resistance is independent of immunity from previous contact or vaccination. An explanation for the age resistance is that the number of cellular receptors necessary for FeLV-A to enter target cells seems to decrease in older cats, thus establishment of infection becomes more difficult. The cellular receptors are not fully identified, and strain-dependent differences seem to exist. For example, T-cell–tropic FeLV cannot infect cells unless a classic multiple membrane-spanning receptor molecule and a second co-receptor or entry factor are present. This cellular protein can function either as a transmembrane protein or a soluble component to facilitate infection.[7] Age resistance to FeLV also may be related to maturation of macrophage function.[131] In addition, age resistance seems to exist in nature; the prevalence of anti-FeLV antibodies increases steadily over time, indicating an increased exposure to the virus throughout life. In a survey in Scotland, only 6% of kittens younger than 5 months had anti-FeLV antibodies. The percentage increased to 55% at 1 to 2 years of age and to 74% by 3 years.[242] Despite the evidence for increased exposure to FeLV throughout life, the cumulative rate of persistent viremia is opposite that of antibody production. Of 8642 cases of FeLV reported by North American veterinary teaching hospitals since 1973, the highest rate of viremia was reported in cats younger than 2 years of age.[184] Although FeLV infection was reported in cats of all ages, the rate declined steadily as cats aged. Considering these results in addition to the antibody surveys, this suggests that although exposure to FeLV accumulates with age, susceptibility to develop persistent viremia after infection simultaneously decreases. However, the age-related resistance is not absolute and depends on the infection pressure. Risk of developing persistent viremia increases also in adult cats when they are housed together with FeLV-shedding cats. This is shown by the increased rate of viremic cats in households with endemic FeLV infection and by natural exposure studies in which a certain percentage of cats becomes FeLV-positive over years when they are housed together with infected cats. However, the risk of an adult cat becoming persistently viremic after one short contact with a FeLV-shedding cat is certainly very low and probably lower than the risk of developing vaccine-associated sarcomas after FeLV vaccination. Therefore use of FeLV vaccination should be considered carefully in adult cats.

PATHOGENESIS

The outcome of FeLV infection is very different in each cat. Although it mainly depends on immune status and age of the cat, it is also affected by pathogenicity of the virus, infection pressure, and virus concentration.

Stages of FeLV Viremia

Different courses, outcomes, and classifications of FeLV infection are described in Figs. 13-4 and 13-5 and Table 13-3. After initial infection, which most commonly occurs via oronasal routes, virus replicates in the local lymphoid tissue in the oropharyngeal area. In many immunocompetent cats, viral replication is stopped by an effective cell-mediated immune (CMI) response, and virus is completely eliminated from the body. These cats usually have high levels of neutralizing antibody and are called *regressor cats*. In these cats, virus never spreads systemically, and infection remains undetected because they never react positively with antigen testing methods. This explains why the majority of cats in a population show evidence of exposure by the presence of anti-FeLV antibodies after contact with FeLV, but only a small proportion actually become viremic. These regressor cats build a very effective immunity and are protected against new viral challenges, probably for several years. Protective immunity is partly humoral and partly cellular, and antibody production is not necessarily required for protection; about 2% are effectively protected without detectable antibodies.

If the immune response does not intervene adequately, replicating FeLV spreads systemically within mononuclear cells (lymphocytes and monocytes). During this first viremic episode, free FeLV-p27 antigen is detectable, and cats have positive results on tests that detect free antigen in plasma (e.g., ELISA). The initial viremia may be characterized by malaise, fever, or lymphadenomegaly resulting from lymphocytic hyperplasia. The virus spreads to target tissue including thymus, spleen, lymph nodes, and salivary glands. If the viremia can be terminated within weeks or months, it is called *transient viremia*. In most cats, transient viremia only lasts 3 to 6 weeks (with a maximum of 16 weeks). During this time, cats shed virus and are infectious. Many cats are able to clear viremia very early before bone marrow becomes infected. These cats not only terminate the viremia, they also completely eliminate the virus from the body. These cats also develop a very effective immunity and are protected against new exposures to virus. They have a low risk of developing FeLV-related illnesses.

After about 3 weeks of viremia, bone marrow cells become involved and affected hematopoietic precursor cells produce infected granulocytes and platelets that circulate in the body. At this time, a high level of viremia has developed, and lymphoid organs and salivary glands become infected with up to 1 million viruses per milliliter of saliva. From this time point on, viral antigen is also detectable in platelets and granulocytes by tests such as direct FA that detect intracellular antigen. In contrast to antigen tests (e.g., ELISA) that detect free p27 antigen and become positive during the first viremia, direct FA test results become positive later and only after infection is established in bone marrow. This explains discordant ELISA and direct FA results.

FeLV Infection

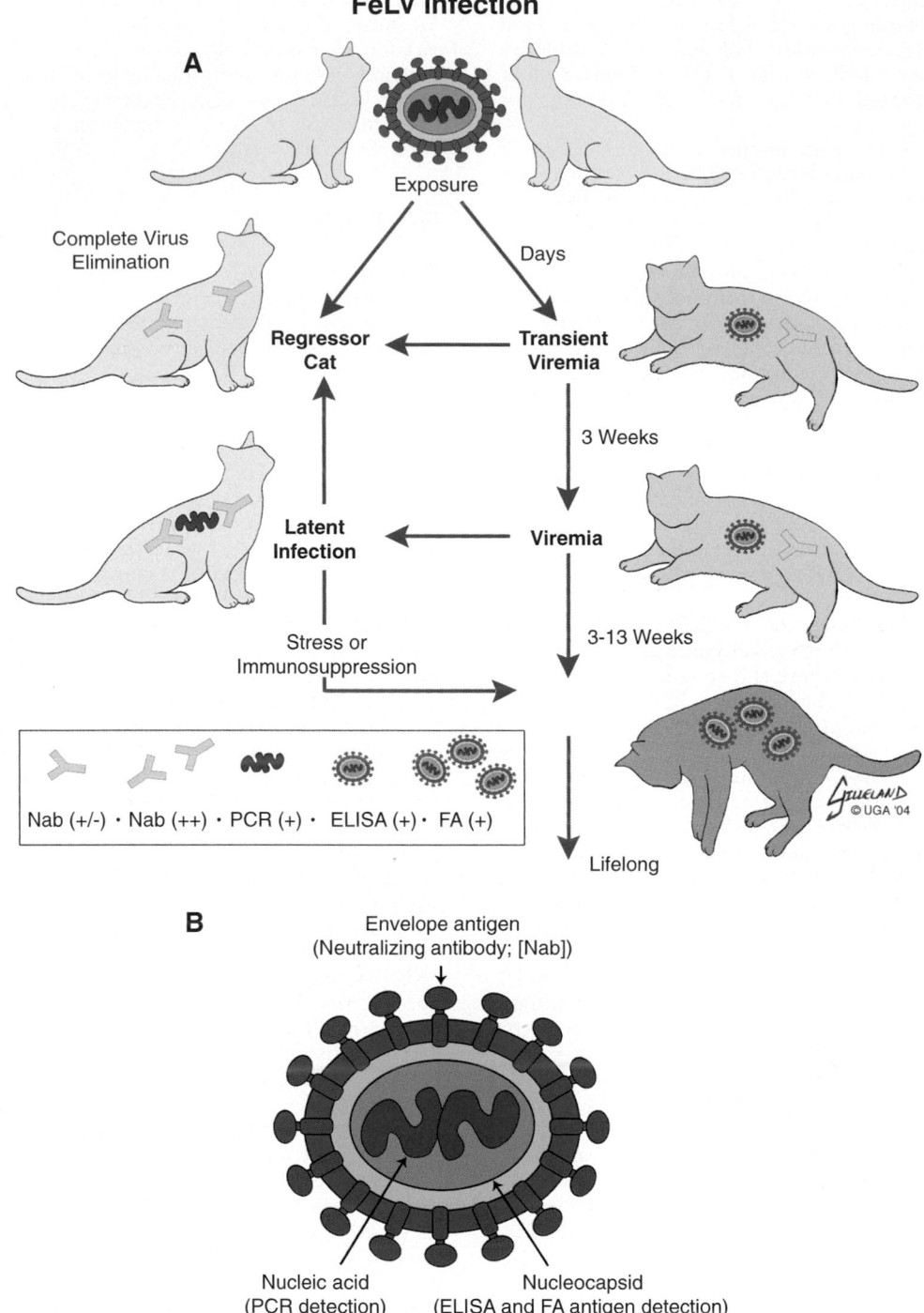

Fig 13-4 **A,** Time course of FeLV infection. **B,** Components of FeLV from part **A.** (Courtesy University of Georgia, Athens, Ga.) *PCR*, polymerase chain reaction; *ELISA*, enzyme linked immunosorbent assay; *FA*, fluorescent antibody.

Even if bone marrow becomes infected, a certain percentage of cats can clear the viremia; the longer the viremia lasts, the less likely it is that these cats can clear it. However, once bone marrow cells are infected (after 3 weeks of viremia), cats cannot completely eliminate the virus from the body even if they terminate the viremia because the information to build the virus (its proviral DNA) is present in bone marrow stem cells—it is a *latent infection.* Although proviral DNA remains, no virus is actively produced, and cats with latent infection have negative results from routine tests that detect FeLV antigen. Latent infection can only be diagnosed by culturing

bone marrow samples or with the polymerase chain reaction (PCR).

Latent infection can be reactivated spontaneously or in response to immune suppression, and cats can become viremic and show positive results again in antigen tests. Latent infections may reactivate in pregnancy, which also may explain the reemergence of FeLV infection in kittens. Mammary glands of latently infected queens may begin producing infectious viral particles during the induction of lactation.[239]

If the immune response of the cat is not strong enough and viremia persists longer than 16 weeks, chances are very high

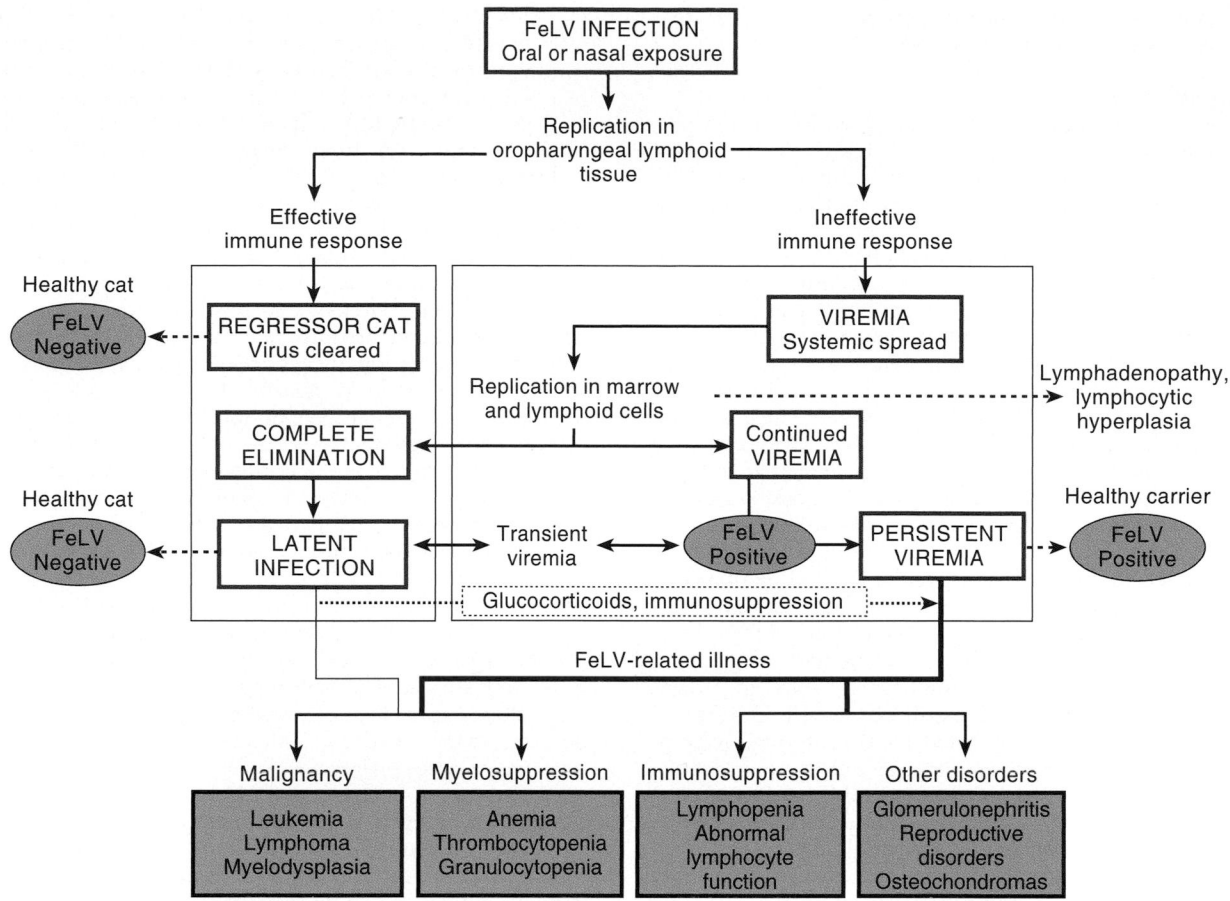

Fig 13-5 Interactions of FeLV with host cells and immune system leading to various clinical problems in cats with ineffective immune responses.

Table • 13-3

Classification of FeLV Infection Based on Viral and Immune Testing

FeLV STATUS	FeLV ANTIGENS TEST RESULTS			VIRUS-POSITIVE BONE MARROW CULTIVATION OR PCR[a]	ELEVATED SERUM NEUTRALIZING ANTIBODY	ELEVATED SERUM FOCMA ANTIBODY
	BLOOD ELISA	DIRECT FA	BONE MARROW DIRECT FA			
Never exposed	–	–	–	–	–	–
Recovered	–	–	–	–	±	±
Latent	–	–	–	+	+	±
Immune carrier	+	–	–	+	+	±
Persistently viremic	+	+	+	+	–	±

+, Results positive; –, results negative ; ±, results variable, *ELISA*, enzyme-linked immunosorbent assay; *FA*, Fluorescent antibody; *PCR*, polymerase chain reaction; *FOCMA*, feline oncornavirus membrance antigens.
[a]PCR can be performed on bone marrow, blood, or tumors.

that the cat will remain persistently viremic and infectious to other cats for the remainder of its life—a condition called *persistent viremia*. Persistently viremic cats have low levels of neutralizing antibody, and virus persistently replicates in bone marrow, spleen, lymph nodes, and salivary glands. These cats develop FeLV-associated diseases, and most of them die within 3 years. The risk for the development of a fatal persistent viremia primarily depends on immune status and age of the cat but also on the infection pressure. Young and immunosuppressed cats are at higher risk for developing persistent viremia. In a cat with a first-time single contact with a FeLV-shedding cat, the risk of developing persistent viremia averages only 3%. However, if an FeLV-shedding cat is introduced to a naive group of cats and the cats are housed together for an extended period, the risk for a cat to develop persistent viremia increases to an average of 30%.[131]

Latent Infection

Cats that are viremic for longer than 3 weeks develop persistent infection of the bone marrow. High levels of circulating FeLV-specific effector cytotoxic T lymphocytes (CTLs) appear before neutralizing antibodies in cats that recover from infection after primary exposure to FeLV.[74,75] Neutralizing antibodies, which develop after infection but not vaccination, are markers for a protective immune response. In previously exposed immune cats, neutralizing antibody may be helpful in protecting against subsequent challenge exposure by preventing viral expression. Although latency is a sequel to FeLV infection, the majority of cats completely eliminate the viral genes from their cells by 9 to 16 months after infection, and all but 10% have done so after 30 months.[239] Once the bone marrow has been infected, virus can remain integrated in a small number of cells for a long time, kept in check by a partial immune response. As antibody concentration increases, virus production decreases.

The molecular basis of latency is the integration of a copy of the viral genome (provirus) into cellular chromosomal DNA. During the replication cycle, the enzyme RT produces a DNA copy using the viral RNA as a template. The copy is integrated into the cellular chromosomal DNA and maintained as a provirus for the lifespan of the cell. During cell division, proviral DNA is replicated and the information given to the daughter cells. Thus complete cell lineages may contain FeLV proviral DNA. However, the proviral DNA is not translated into proteins, and no infectious virus particles are produced. Therefore latently infected cats do not shed FeLV and are not infectious to others; however, as an exception, latently infected queens stressed by pregnancy have reverted to overt viremia and transmitted FeLV to their kittens. No harmful virus is produced during latent infections, and clinical signs (with few exceptions such as neoplasia or myelodysplasia) do not occur. Because no virus replicates, no FeLV antigen is produced, and the cats have negative results by routine tests that detect viral antigen (such as ELISA, direct FA, or viral culture of blood cells). However, the presence of latent virus can be demonstrated by bone marrow PCR or when bone marrow cells are cultured in vitro, thereby bypassing the effects of the immune system. Growth can be facilitated by adding glucocorticoids to the culture.

Latent infection can be reactivated because the information for producing complete viral particles is present and can potentially be reused when antibody production decreases (e.g., after immune suppression). This usually occurs after stress and can be experimentally induced in cats by administration of high doses of glucocorticoids.[269] Reactivation is more likely the earlier the stress factor occurs after the viremic phase. In the first weeks after viremia, viral replication can be experimentally reactivated in most cats. As the time passes, latent infections become more difficult to reactivate, even with high doses of glucocorticoids. By 1 year after infection, reactivation is considered unlikely and is almost impossible after 2 years. This may be explained by genetic code-reading mistakes that may occur if the information is frequently reproduced in these fast-dividing cells. Thus information to produce infectious viral particles gets lost, and reactivation becomes more and more unlikely over time. It has been demonstrated experimentally that the proportion of experimentally infected cats that had latent FeLV infections in their bone marrow decreased with time following disappearance of viremia.[244] In the first 3 months after recovery from viremia, integrated virus could be isolated from the bone marrow of approximately 50% of experimentally infected cats. A pronounced decrease in the incidence of latent infections occurred 190 days after

the viremia.[239,244] More than 1 year later, only 5 of 19 previously challenge-exposed cats that were FeLV negative according to ELISA still had FeLV detectable in several tissues (e.g., bone marrow, spleen, lymph node, small intestine).[118] At 3 years postviremia, only about 8% of cats still harbored latent infections in bone marrow, myelomonocytic cells, and stromal fibroblast cells.[129,203,239,244,269] Latency is probably a stage in the elimination process of the virus. Most latent infections are not clinically significant because viral reactivation is unusual under natural circumstances. As long as the infection remains latent, the cats are not contagious.

However, viral latency explains relapsing viremias, protracted incubation periods, and persistent high titers of antibodies. A question always arises regarding whether latent FeLV infection can be responsible for clinical signs. However, for the majority of pathogenic mechanisms by which FeLV causes clinical signs, active virus replication is necessary; this is not the case in latent FeLV infections, in which the virus is harbored in a "dormant" and nonproductive form. However, latent infections may explain how myelosupression or hematopoietic malignancy could be FeLV related in FeLV-negative cats. FeLV provirus can be inserted at many different sites in the host's genome, carrying potent regulatory signals. In the development of myelosuppressive disorders or tumors, integrated FeLV provirus may interrupt or inactivate cellular genes in the infected cells, or regulatory features of viral DNA may alter expression of neighboring genes. In addition, because bone marrow microenvironment cells (e.g., myelomonocytic progenitor cells and stromal fibroblasts) provide a reservoir of latent FeLV infections, it seems possible that the integrated provirus may alter cellular functions and contribute to the pathogenesis of myelosuppressive disorders. Finally, FeLV not only contributes its genes to the host, it also has been shown to appropriate cellular genes; several such transducted genes that are also in latently infected cells have been implicated in viral oncogenesis.[259,266,281]

Atypical Infection

Only a few cats (in experimental studies, up to 10%) have persistent atypical local viral replication (e.g., in mammary glands, bladder, and eyes).[131] This can lead to intermittent or low-grade production of p24 antigen. Therefore these cats may have weakly positive or discordant results in antigen tests, or positive and negative results may alternate. Queens with atypical infection of their mammary glands may transmit the virus to their kittens via milk but not have positive test results.

A particular FeLV feline acquired immunodeficiency syndrome (FAIDS) is composed of subgroup A virus and highly immunopathogenic variants that infect CD4+ and CD8+ T lymphocytes and IgG+ B lymphocytes in blood, lymph nodes, and myeloid cells.[252] This widespread proliferation greatly impairs the immune response.

CLINICAL FINDINGS

FeLV can cause variable clinical signs. The prevalence of hematopoietic malignancy, myelosuppression, and infectious diseases is higher in FeLV-infected multicat households than in the general population. The death rate of persistently viremic cats in multicat households is approximately 50% in 2 years and 80% in 3 years.[38,184] Survival rates for persistently viremic cats kept indoors in single-cat households are higher. In closed households with endemic feline coronavirus (FCoV), FeLV, FIV, or all of these infections, FeLV infection has the greatest impact on mortality.[2]

Although the virus was named after the contagious malignancy that first garnered its attention, most infected cats are brought to the veterinarian for anemia or immune suppression. Of 8642 FeLV-infected cats examined at North American veterinary teaching hospitals, various coinfections (including FIP, upper respiratory infection, FIV infection, hemotrophic mycoplasmosis, and stomatitis) were the most frequent findings (15%), followed by anemias (11%), lymphoma (6%), leukopenia or thrombocytopenia (5%), or leukemia or myeloproliferative disease (4%).[35]

The exact mechanisms for the varied clinical responses of persistently viremic cats are poorly understood. It is clear that the clinical course is determined by a combination of viral and host factors. Some of these differences can be traced to properties of the virus itself, such as the subgroup that determines differences in the clinical picture. (For example, FeLV-B is primarily associated with tumors, and FeLV-C is primarily associated with nonregenerative anemia.) A study tried to define dominant host immune effector mechanisms responsible for the outcome of infection by using longitudinal changes in FeLV-specific CTLs. As mentioned previously, high levels of circulating FeLV-specific effector CTLs appear before virus neutralizing antibodies in cats that have recovered from exposure to FeLV. In contrast, persistent viremia has been associated with a silencing of virus-specific humoral and CMI host effector mechanisms. These results suggest an important role for FeLV-specific CTLs in immunity to FeLV.[74] Probably the most important host factor that determines the clinical outcome of cats persistently infected with FeLV is the age of the cat at the time of infection.[134] Neonatal kittens develop marked thymic atrophy after infection ("fading kitten syndrome"), resulting in severe immunosuppression, wasting, and early death. As cats mature, they acquire a progressive resistance. When older cats become infected, they tend to have milder signs and a more protracted period of apparent good health.[184] Clinical signs that are associated with FeLV infection can be classified as tumors induced by FeLV, bone marrow suppression syndromes, immunosuppression, immune-mediated diseases, and other syndromes (including reproductive disorders, fading kitten syndrome, and neuropathy).

Tumors

FeLV is a major oncogene that causes different tumors in cats, most commonly malignant lymphoma and leukemia and less commonly other hematopoietic tumors. Lymphomas also occur in the absence of detectable FeLV.[322] In addition, other tumors including osteochondromas, olfactory neuroblastoma, and cutaneous horns have been described in FeLV-infected cats.

The mechanism by which FeLV causes malignancy may be explained by insertion of the FeLV genome into the cellular genome near a cellular oncogene (most commonly *myc*), resulting in activation and overexpression of that gene. This effect leads to uncontrolled proliferation of that cell (clone). A malignancy results in absence of an appropriate immune response. FeLV-A may also incorporate the oncogene to form a recombinant virus (e.g., FeLV-B, FeSV) containing cellular oncogene sequences that are then rearranged and activated. When they enter a cell, these recombinant viruses are oncogenic. In a study of 119 cats with lymphomas, transduction or insertion of the *myc* locus had occurred in 38 cats (32%).[312]

Feline oncornavirus cell membrane antigen (FOCMA), an antigen present on the surface of transformed cells, was detected in 1973 but remains a subject of discussion and confusion among researchers. Its value as clinical tool (either diagnostic or preventative) is certainly limited. FOCMA was first detected on the surface of cultured lymphoma cells incubated with serum of cats that did not develop tumors, although they were infected with FeSV—a recombinant of FeLV with an oncogenic potential.[67,291] FOCMA can be found on the surface of feline lymphoma cells and FeSV-induced fibrosarcomas but not on the surface of normal feline lymphocytes.[104,318] FOCMA was first considered to be a cellular antigen that is expressed after FeLV infection or tumor transformation.[65,104,291] It has also been proposed that FOCMA is a viral antigen of FeLV-C.[318] However, in other studies, it was shown that FOCMA and FeLV-C-gp70 are similar but not completely homologous.[292] Some authors believed that development of large amounts of antibodies against FOCMA could protect against the development of FeLV-induced lymphomas by complement-dependent lysis of tumor cells.[39,63,65,85] Evidence for this was provided when experimentally FeLV-infected kittens did not develop neoplasia if they produced or passively received sufficient amounts of antibodies against FOCMA.[64,67] Many cats with FeLV in cluster households have antibody titers to FOCMA. Those with the highest titers are most likely to remain free of malignancies. However, in cluster households, some cats that were initially viremic with a high FOCMA antibody titer developed lymphoma or leukemia months or years later after the titer declined.[38] Opinions about identity and importance of FOCMA are still diverse. FOCMA can be considered a nonhomogenous group of viral antigens that may, although not always, be present on the surface of FeLV-infected cells. At the least, FOCMA antibodies indicate exposure to FeLV but may not mean more than this. Alternatively, FOCMA antibodies may provide a protective mechanism against tumor development.

Lymphoma and Lymphoid Leukemia

Association with FeLV In the 1960s, studies found that the most common primary feline malignancies are hematopoetic tumors, of which about 90% are malignant lymphomas. Malignant lymphomas and leukemias account for about 30% of all feline tumors, which is the highest proportion recorded in any animal species.[42,56,57,95,96] The estimated incidence of feline lymphoma and leukemia in the 1960s was 200 cases per 100,000 cats per year.[38] Feline lymphomas are most commonly high grade with an immunoblastic or a lymphoblastic morphology, but they may be mixed lymphoblastic and lymphocytic or occasionally low-grade lymphocytic.[316,317]

The association between FeLV and lymphomas has been clearly established in several ways. First, these malignancies could be induced in kittens by experimental FeLV infection.[100,153,261] Second, cats naturally infected with FeLV had a higher risk of developing malignant lymphoma than uninfected cats.[63,100] Third, most cats with malignant lymphoma were FeLV-positive in tests that detected infectious virus or FeLV antigens. Previously, up to 80% of feline lymphomas and leukemias were reported to be FeLV related*; however, this is no longer considered to be the case. Since the 1980s a dramatic reduction in the prevalence of viremia has been noted in cats with lymphoma.[114,210,221] The decrease in prevalence of FeLV infection in cats with lymphoma or leukemia also indicates a shift in tumor causation in recent years. Whereas 59% of all cats with malignant lymphoma or leukemia were FeLV positive in one German study from 1980 to 1995, only 20% of the cats were FeLV positive in the years 1996 to 1999 in the same institution.[114] In 1975 a survey of 74 Boston area cats with lymphoma or leukemia showed that 70% were FeLV positive, but only 3 cats had the alimentary form.[34] Between 1988 and 1994, 72% of all feline lymphomas treated at the Animal Medical Center in New York were of the alimentary form, and only 8% of affected cats were FeLV positive.[38] In a recent study in the Netherlands, only 4 of 71 cats with lymphoma were FeLV positive, although 22 of these cats had

*References 39, 77, 78, 102, 107, 255, 282.

mediastinal lymphoma, which was previously highly associated with FeLV infection.[306] A greater prevalence of lymphoma in older-age cats has been observed. One major reason seems to be the decreased prevalence of FeLV infection in the overall cat population as a result of FeLV vaccination, as well as testing and elimination programs. Of the purebred cat breeds, Siamese cats may be predisposed to lymphosarcoma.[40]

Overall, the proportion of cats with lymphomas that test negative for the FeLV antigen (versus cats with lymphomas that test positive) has increased significantly during the last 20 years, and the prevalence of FeLV infection is decreasing. However, prevalence of lymphomas caused by FeLV may be higher than indicated by conventional antigen testing of blood specimens. Cats from FeLV cluster households had a fortyfold higher rate of development of FeLV-negative lymphomas than did those from the general population. FeLV-negative lymphomas have also occurred in laboratory cats known to have been infected previously with FeLV.[266] FeLV proviral DNA was detected in malignant lymphomas of older cats that tested negative for FeLV antigen, also suggesting that the virus may be associated with a larger proportion of lymphomas than previously thought. PCR detected proviral DNA in formalin-fixed, paraffin-embedded tumor tissue in 7 of 11 FeLV-negative cats with lymphoma.[142] However, other groups found evidence of provirus in only 1 of 22[281] and in 0 of 50 FeLV-negative lymphomas.[114] FeLV-negative lymphomas that are induced by FeLV can be explained by different ways. First, latent FeLV infection may be responsible for the tumor development. Second, FeLV could be responsible for the development of the tumor, inducing a malignant cell clone, but not be persistently integrated into the genome of the neoplastic cell and therefore be eliminated while the tumor grows to a detectable size. Third, FeLV infection could be present in other cells (and not been detected) and induce oncogenesis via mechanisms such as cytokine release or chronic immune stimulation.

The FeLV status of cats with lymphomas varies depending on the type and locations of tumors. FeLV-positive lymphomas are mainly of a T-cell origin; FeLV-negative lymphomas are mainly of a B-cell origin.[77,96,104,228] FeLV transforms mature T cells and immature or prothymocytes, null cells, and possibly monocytes. Transformation of mature B cells does not occur, because feline lymphoma cell lines and primary tumors lack surface immunoglobulin expression.[271]

Classification Lymphomas can be classified according to their location—in mediastinal (thymic), alimentary (intestinal), and multicentric lymphomas. *Mediastinal lymphoma,* frequently associated with FeLV infection and seen mainly in cats younger than 3 years, was previously the most prevalent site in cats but is now seen less frequently. Of cats with mediastinal lymphoma, 80% to 90% have been reported as FeLV positive,[37] but this rate has also seemed to decrease according to the study of Teske and coworkers.[306] The tumor arises in the area of the thymus and eventually causes a malignant pleural effusion (Figs. 13-6 and 13-7). The fluid-nucleated cell count is usually greater than 8000/µl; the majority are large, immature lymphocytes. The most common presenting sign is dyspnea, but occasionally regurgitation from pressure on the esophagus or Horner syndrome from pressure on sympathetic nerves at the thoracic inlet is present.[38]

Alimentary lymphoma occurs primarily in older cats that are usually FeLV negative. Clinical signs of alimentary lymphoma include vomiting or diarrhea, but many cats have anorexia and weight loss only.[204] Tumors of the stomach and intestines may be focal or diffuse, and mesenteric lymph nodes are usually involved. Estimates of the prevalence of FeLV antigenemia in cats with alimentary lymphomas range from 25% to 30%.[38] However, in another study, only 6% of the cats with intestinal lymphomas were FeLV positive, which is about twice the prevalence of gastrointestinal (GI) lymphoma in the general population.[114] These data suggest that other stimuli (such as food components or inflammatory bowel disease) in the GI tract of older cats may be more important predisposing factors for tumor development.

Multicentric lymphoma is described with major involvement of several sites. About half of the cats with multicentric lymphoma are FeLV positive. Any organ may be involved, such as the retrobulbar area, nasal cavity, gingiva, skin, liver, kidneys, urinary bladder, brain, and lungs. Renal lymphoma is usually bilateral and does not cause signs of illness until the kidneys are so extensively infiltrated that renal failure occurs. Kidneys are enlarged and usually irregular. Epidural lymphoma may cause sudden or gradual onset of posterior paralysis (Fig. 13-8). The bone marrow is involved in about

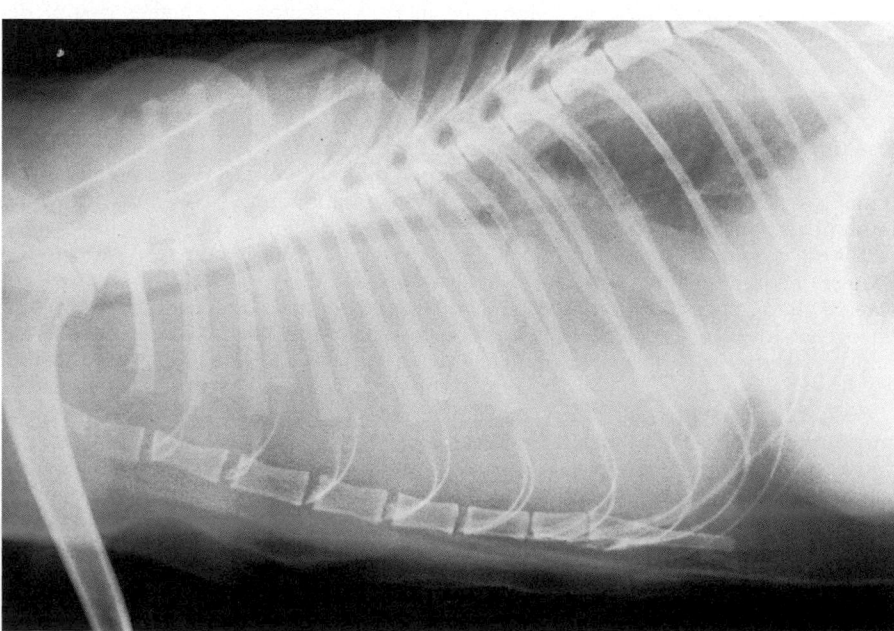

Fig 13-6 Lateral thoracic radiograph of a cat with severe pleural effusion and mediastinal mass. The trachea is displaced dorsally, and the cardiac shadow is not shown.

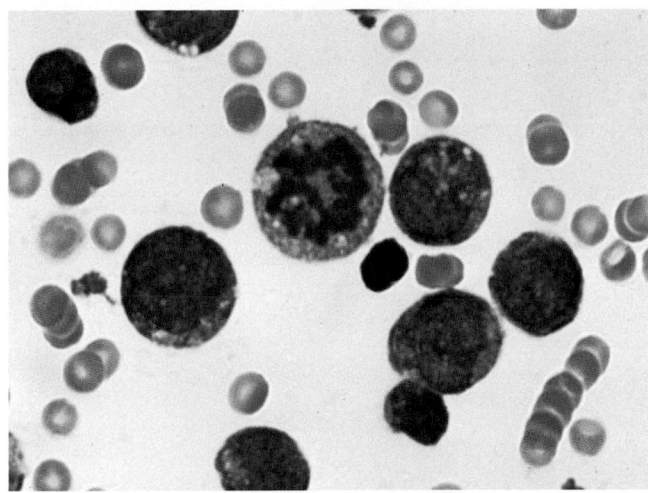

Fig 13-7 Examination of thoracic fluid aspirated from a cat showing a pleomorphic lymphoid population composed of blasts, a mitotic figure, and a small lymphocyte. Diagnosis of lymphoma was made (Wright stain, ×1000). (Courtesy Ken Latimer, Athens, Ga.)

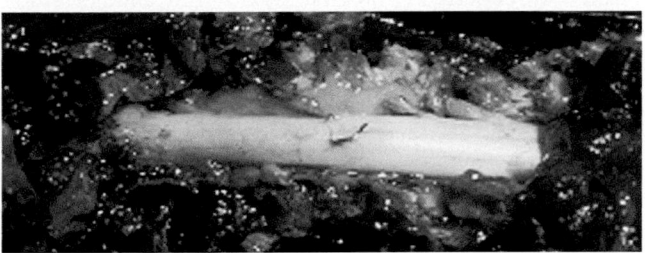

Fig 13-8 Postmortem dissection of spinal canal reveals a cream-color gelatinous mass in the epidural space. Histologic findings were diagnostic of lymphoma. (Courtesy University of Georgia, Athens, Ga.)

70% of these cats even though complete blood cell count (CBC) may be normal.[175,294]

Hematopoietic Neoplasia (Myeloproliferative Disorders)

Leukemias

More than half of the cats with nonlymphoid leukemia are FeLV positive. All hematopoietic cell lines are susceptible to transformation by FeLV, resulting in myeloproliferative disease or myelodysplastic syndrome (MDS; Figs. 13-9 and 13-10). Thus lymphoid and myeloid (including granulocytic, erythroid, and megakaryocytic) types occur. In erythremic myelosis, proliferation of erythrocyte precursors is usually associated with FeLV subgroup C, and most have positive test results for FeLV. Cats with this disorder have low hematocrit (HCT) levels (12% to 15%) with normal leukocytes and variable thrombocytopenia. The anemia is usually nonregenerative or poorly regenerative, and with time the HCT level does not increase. Despite the lack of regeneration, the mean corpuscular volume (MCV) and numbers of nucleated erythrocytes are usually higher. Abnormal erythrocyte stages are found in bone marrow and often in peripheral blood. MDS may result as a clonal proliferation of hematopoietic cells that is a preleukemic state of acute myeloid leukemia.[125,286] In acute leukemia or MDS of any type, the bone marrow is filled with blast cells, and normal hematopoiesis is suppressed.[126] Clinical signs with acute leukemia are related to the loss of

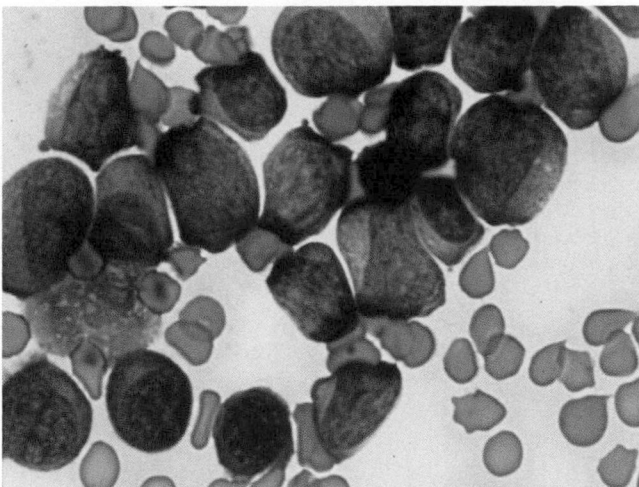

Fig 13-9 Peripheral blood film of a cat with erythroleukemia. Cat had severe anemia without reticulocytosis. More than 95% of circulating nucleated cells were erythroid precursors of varying degrees of maturity. Severe granulocytopenia was noted (Wright stain, ×1000). (Courtesy Ken Latimer, Athens, Ga.)

normal hematopoietic cells and include lethargy from anemia, signs of sepsis with granulocytopenia, and bleeding with thrombocytopenia. Hepatomegaly with icterus and splenomegaly are frequently present because of malignant infiltration or extramedullary hematopoiesis. Diagnosis of acute leukemia is made by CBC and bone marrow examinations. Bone marrow cytologic studies show increased cellularity, megaloblastic maturation, increased myelofibrosis, and immature blast cells.[283] In cats with large numbers of circulating blast cells, the CBC may in itself be diagnostic. Although classifications have been proposed for the acute leukemias, the predominant cell type may be difficult to identify even with histochemical stains. Transformation, especially for the nonlymphoid leukemias, usually occurs at or very close to the stem cell level, so more than one cell line may be affected. Chronic leukemias are rare in cats and rarely associated with FeLV. They include well-differentiated chronic lymphocytic leukemia (CLL), chronic myelogenous leukemia (CML), polycythemia vera, and thrombocythemia. Eosinophilic leukemia may be a subtype of CML and has been described in association with FeLV. The differentiation between severe reactive eosinophilia (hypereosinophilic syndrome [HES]) and malignancy is difficult because both have been associated with large numbers of morphologically normal eosinophils in the marrow, peripheral blood, and other organs.[38] The prognosis for cats with myeloproliferative diseases is poor.

Myelofibrosis

Abnormal proliferation of fibroblasts results from chronic stimulation of the bone marrow, such as chronic bone marrow activity from hyperplastic or neoplastic regeneration caused by FeLV. In severe cases the entire endosteum within the medullary cavity can be obliterated. Bone marrow involvement may require a core biopsy instead of needle aspiration to confirm the diagnosis.

Fibrosarcoma

Fibrosarcomas that are associated with FeLV are caused by FeSV, a recombinant virus that develops de novo in FeLV-A-infected cats by recombination of the FeLV-A genome with cellular oncogenes. Through a process of genetic recombination, FeSV acquires one of several oncogenes such as *fes*, *fms*,

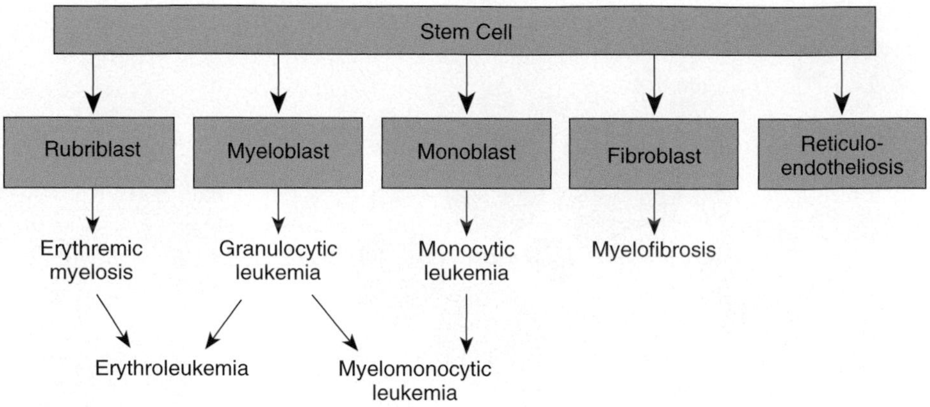

Fig 13-10 Origin of cell lines in myeloproliferative disease. (Modified from Morrison JA. 2001. Erythemic myelosis. *Compend Cont Educ Pract Vet* 23: 880-885; with permission.)

or *fgr*. As a result, FeSV is an acutely transforming (tumor-causing) virus, causing a polyclonal malignancy with multi-focal tumors arising simultaneously after a short incubation period. With the decrease in FeLV prevalence, FeSV also becomes less common. FeSV-induced fibrosarcomas are multicentric and usually occur in young cats. Several strains of FeSV that have been identified from naturally occurring tumors are defective. They are unable to replicate without the presence of FeLV as a helper virus that supplies proteins (such as those coded by the *env* gene) to FeSV. The host range for FeSV depends on the helper FeLV-A. By manipulation of the helper virus in the laboratory, FeSV can enter cells of species not naturally infected. Experimental inoculation of FeSV has produced tumors in cats, rabbits, dogs, sheep, rats, and non-human primates.[307] Many of these tumors regress spontaneously, even after reaching a large size.[38]

Fibrosarcomas caused by various strains of FeSV tend to grow rapidly, often with multiple cutaneous or subcutaneous nodules that are locally invasive and metastasize to the lung and other sites. Solitary fibrosarcomas in old cats are not caused by FeSV. These tumors are slower growing, locally invasive, slower metastasizing, and occasionally curable by excision. The tumors are caused by the granulomatous inflammatory reaction at the injection site after inoculation of adjuvant-containing vaccines. It has been demonstrated that neither FeSV nor FeLV play any role in vaccine-induced sarcomas.[60]

In addition to fibrosarcomas, FeSV has experimentally caused melanomas, showing that FeSV can transform cells of ectodermal as well as of mesodermal origin.[34] Intradermal or intraocular inoculation of FeSV into kittens produced melanomas in the skin or anterior chamber of the eye.[38] However, FeSV has not yet been associated with naturally occurring melanomas of cats.

Fibrosarcoma cells express FOCMA just as lymphoma cells do. Experimental infection with FeSV causes tumors that progress in some cats and regress in others. Those in which the tumors regress have high FOCMA antibody titers.

Other Tumors

Multiple *osteochondromas* (cartilaginous exostoses on flat bones) have been described with increased prevalence in FeLV-infected cats. Although histologically benign, they may cause significant morbidity if they occur in an area such as a vertebra and put pressure on the spinal cord or nerve roots. The pathogenesis of these tumors is unknown.[195,250]

Spontaneous feline *olfactory neuroblastomas* are aggressive, histologically inhomogenous tumors of the tasting and smelling epithelium of nose and pharynx, and have high metastasis rates. Budding FeLV particles were found in the tumors and lymph node metastases, and FeLV PCR was pos-

itive in tumor tissue.[278] Two of the three cats described had positive antigen test results. The exact role of FeLV in the genesis of these tumors is uncertain.

Cutaneous horns are a benign hyperplasia of keratinocytes that have been described in FeLV-infected cats.[243] The exact role of FeLV in the pathogenesis is unclear.

Iris melanomas are *not* associated with retroviral infections as once believed. In one study, 3 of 18 eyes had positive test results for FeLV-FeSV proviral DNA.[297] In another study, immunohistochemical staining and PCR did not reveal FeLV or FeSV in the ocular tissues of any cats with this disorder.[43]

Nonneoplastic Hematologic Dysfunction

Hematopoietic disorders, particularly cytopenias caused by bone marrow suppression, are a common finding in cats infected with FeLV. According to past literature, anemia is a major nonneoplastic complication that occurs in a majority of symptomatic FeLV-infected cats. In turn, it has been cited that more than two thirds of all nonregenerative anemias in cats are the result of FeLV infection. Currently, as is the case with all FeLV-associated syndromes, this is clearly an overestimation because of the decrease in FeLV prevalence. Bone marrow suppression syndromes described in association with FeLV have included anemia (nonregenerative or regenerative), persistent, transient, or cyclic neutropenias, panleukopenia-like syndrome, platelet abnormalities (thrombocytopenia and platelet function abnormalities), and aplastic anemia (pancytopenia). For the majority of pathogenic mechanisms in which FeLV causes bone marrow suppression, active virus replication is necessary. However, it has been demonstrated that in some FeLV-negative cats, latent FeLV infection may be responsible for bone marrow suppression. Provirus may interrupt or inactivate cellular genes in the infected cells, or regulatory features of viral DNA may alter expression of neighboring genes. Additionally, cell function of latently infected myelomonocytic progenitor and stromal fibroblasts that provide bone marrow microenvironment may be altered. Alternatively, FeLV provirus may cause bone marrow disorders by inducing the expression of antigens on the cell surface, resulting in an immune-mediated destruction of the cell.

Anemia

Various causes of anemia associated with feline leukemia infection are summarized in Table 13-4 and the following sections.

Hemolytic Anemia   Approximately 10% of FeLV-associated anemias are regenerative, indicated by a high reticulocyte count, high MCV, and presence of anisocytosis, nucleated erythrocytes, and polychromasia.[283] They are caused by FeLV-induced immune-mediated hemolysis, secondary *Mycoplasma*

Table • 13-4

Comparison of Hematologic Disorders Related to FeLV Infection

CAUSES	MECHANISM	HEMATOLOGIC FINDINGS AND TREATMENT
Regenerative Anemia		
Immune-mediated hemolysis	Virus-induced expression of foreign antigens on erythrocyte surface	*Findings:* Regenerative anemia (macrocytosis and reticulocytosis), variable icterus and hemoglobinemia, plasma proteins within reference ranges *Treatment:* Immunosuppression, which is generally effective
Hemotrophic *Mycoplasma* infection (hemobartonellosis)	Virus-induced immunosuppression that allows hemopathogen proliferation	*Findings:* Regenerative anemia, variable icterus and hemoglobinemia, plasma proteins within reference ranges, organisms observed or PCR positive for *Mycoplasma hemofelis* *Treatment:* Doxycycline
Blood loss from thrombocytopenia	Virus-induced suppression of platelet production by bone marrow	*Findings:* Regenerative anemia, thrombocytopenia (<50,000 platelets), low serum protein level *Treatment:* Transfusion and treatment of cause of thrombocytopenia
Nonregenerative Anemia		
Myelosuppression: pancytopenia	Virus-induced alteration of hematopoietic gene expression that affects early marrow precursor; affects multiple cell lines	*Findings:* Nonregenerative anemia, thrombocytopenia, leukopenia, often FeLV positive; may note more advanced myeloid effect of subgroup C infection *Treatment:* Poor response to bone marrow stimulants or immunosuppressive therapy
Myelodestruction: panleukopenia-like syndrome	Virus-induced replication and destruction of myeloid and lymphoid precursors and intestinal epithelium	*Findings:* Pancytopenia, leukopenia, vomiting, diarrhea *Treatment:* Poor response to bone marrow stimulation or treatment of overwhelming sepsis
Myelosuppression: pure erythrocyte aplasia	Virus-induced alteration of hematopoietic gene expression that is selective for red blood cell precursors	*Findings:* Nonregenerative anemia, other cell lines within reference ranges; if viral-induced, often subgroup C infection *Treatment:* Responsive to immunosuppression
Anemia of chronic inflammatory disease	Virus or secondary bacterial stimulation of inflammatory cytokines that sequester iron	*Findings:* Nonregenerative anemia, usually with normocytosis *Treatment:* Removal or treatment of coexisting inflammatory disease if present; no response to erythropoietin
Anemia of chronic disease	Virus-induced neoplastic disease or immunosuppression-induced secondary debilitating illness	*Findings:* Nonregenerative normochromic, normocytic anemia *Treatment:* Treatment of secondary disease
Myeloproliferative disease: erythroleukemia (erythremic myelosis), reticuloendotheliosis, various leukemias	Virus-induced neoplastic transformation of erythrocyte precursors, leukocyte precursors or stem cells, or all of these	*Findings:* Nonregenerative anemia with macrocytosis and variable numbers and types of nucleated erythrocytes; often FeLV positive *Treatment:* Poor response to cytotoxic chemotherapy
Myelophthisis: lymphoma, lymphocytic or granulocytic leukemia, or other bone marrow proliferative syndrome	Virus-induced neoplastic process that crowds bone marrow, causing suppression of erythrogenesis	*Findings:* Nonregenerative anemia and may affect other cell lines; may detect abnormal nucleated cells in peripheral blood *Treatment:* Cytotoxic chemotherapy

Continued

Table • 13-4

Continued

CAUSES	MECHANISM	HEMATOLOGIC FINDINGS AND TREATMENT
Pure Leukocyte and Platelet Abnormalities		
Leukemia	Virus-induced neoplastic process involving leukocytes of myeloid or lymphoid cell lines	*Findings:* Nonregenerative anemia with large increase in leukocyte or precursors in peripheral blood; often FeLV positive *Treatment:* Poor response to chemotherapy
Neutropenia	Virus-induced immune-mediated or idiopathic neutropenia, often follows stressful episode	*Findings:* Pure neutropenia, usually without a left shift; normal findings with all other cell lines *Treatment:* Glucocorticoid therapy
Thrombocytopenia	Virus-induced immune-mediated thrombocytopenia	*Findings:* Pure thrombocytopenia *Treatment:* Glucocorticoid therapy
Thrombocytosis	Virus-induced neoplastic proliferation of megakaryocytes	*Findings:* Marked thrombocytosis (>600,000 platelets) *Treatment:* Poor response to cytotoxic chemotherapy

haemofelis infection (hemobartonellosis; see Chapter 31), or hemorrhage from FeLV-induced thrombocytopenia. Clinical signs are lethargy, anorexia, depression, pale mucous membranes, icterus, dehydration, and splenomegaly associated with anemia. It is suspected that FeLV can induce an immune-mediated response leading to secondary autoimmune hemolytic anemia with positive Coombs' test, autoagglutination, and spherocytosis. Hemotropic *Mycoplasma* organisms are not always observed on peripheral blood smears; however, diagnosis is possible with PCR techniques. Clinical manifestation of *M. haemofelis* infection is commonly found secondary to FeLV-induced immunosuppression (see Chapter 31).[82,107] Regardless of the cause, regenerative FeLV anemias usually have a favorable response to treatment (see Therapy in this chapter).

Anemia from Inflammatory Cytokines Most FeLV-associated anemias are nonregenerative and caused by the bone marrow suppressive effect of the virus, resulting from primary infection of hematopoietic stem cells and infection of stroma cells that constitute the supporting environment for hematopoietic cells. In vitro exposure of normal feline bone marrow to some strains of FeLV causes suppression of erythrogenesis.[38] The exact mechanisms of the way FeLV causes this bone marrow suppression is not completely known; however, these cats have normocytosis or macrocytosis without evidence of reticulocyte response. Whenever macrocytic anemia (MCV > 60 fl) occurs in a cat in absence of reticulocytosis, FeLV infection should be suspected. These cats do not have folate or vitamin B_{12} deficiencies. Iron is present in macrophages but not erythrocyte precursors; however, iron kinetics are normal. This anemia contrasts with anemia of chronic inflammatory disease caused by bacterial infection in which iron sequestration causes microcytosis. As in many FeLV-associated nonregenerative anemias, suppression of erythrogenesis results in markedly increased serum erythropoietin levels.

Macrocytosis in chronic FeLV infection is believed to represent an FeLV-induced defect by skipped mitoses in cell division during erythropoiesis. It is usually associated with normocellular bone marrow; hypocellularity may be found with an increased myeloid-erythroid ratio.[38,184]

Pure Erythrocyte Aplasia Severe isolated anemia (HCT <15%) without regeneration (pure erythrocyte aplasia) suggests infection with FeLV-C.[283] FeLV-C causes pure erythrocyte aplasia that likely occurs through interactions of the cell surface receptor.[254,302] The cell-surface receptor interactions block the differentiation of erythroid progenitors between burst-forming units and colony-forming units by interfering with signal transduction pathways essential for erythropoiesis.[253,283,329] Bone marrow examination shows an almost complete lack of erythroid precursors with normal myeloid and megakaryocytic precursors. In this case, serum erythropoietin levels are also markedly increased, indicating that anemia is not caused by an erythropoietin deficiency.[184] It is not a neoplastic or immune-mediated process because it is resistant to therapy. Treatment with immunosuppressive drugs (glucocorticoids and cyclophosphamide or cyclosporin) resulted in resolution of anemia within 3 to 5 weeks; however, relapse occurred when treatment was discontinued.[299]

Pancytopenia Severe pancytopenia or aplastic anemia may be present in FeLV-infected cats and involves all cell lines. Bone marrow cytology is usually hypocellular or may show necrosis.[287] Cats with pancytopenia often test positive for FeLV. The virus probably affects precursors near the stem cell level. In some cats, cyclic hematopoiesis with periodic fluctuation in reticulocytes, granulocytes, and platelets may be noted. Alteration of accessory cells within the bone marrow microenvironment providing the structural framework, cytoadhesive molecules, and growth-regulatory cytokines necessary for normal hematopoiesis may be the cause. FeLV can affect bone marrow accessory cell viability, growth, production, or all of these of hematopoietic progenitor growth-regulating substances by altering cytokine messenger RNA levels in general and strain-specific patterns.[186-188] During a bone marrow evaluation, few if any precursors may be found with cytologic methods, and core biopsy specimens may be needed. The aplastic marrow may represent a more advanced stage of myelosuppression than pure erythrocyte aplasia. Bone marrow transplantation or immunosuppression has been used to treat people; however, it has not been successful in cats.

Anemia of Chronic Disease In addition to the direct effect of the virus on erythropoiesis, other factors can cause nonregenerative anemia in FeLV-infected cats. Lymphoma or leukemia, as well as secondary infectious diseases such as systemic mycosis or mycobacteriosis, may cause severe anemia by "crowding out" bone marrow cells. Some FeLV-infected cats develop a mild anemia (HCT of 20% to 30%) referred to as *anemia of chronic disease* caused by systemic infection or stress. The HCT often increases spontaneously if the underlying problem is treated successfully, even if the cat continues to test positive for FeLV.

Platelet Abnormalities

Thrombocytopenia may occur secondary to decreased platelet production from FeLV-induced bone marrow suppression or leukemic infiltration. Platelet abnormalities in FeLV-infected cats may involve changes in quantity, size, shape, and function. The lifespan of platelets is shortened in some FeLV-infected cats. Platelets harbor FeLV proteins as a result of infection, and giant platelets and thrombocytosis have been observed in some persistently viremic cats.[283] In addition, megakaryocytes, the marrow precursors of blood platelets, are frequent targets of productive FeLV infection. Immune-mediated thrombocytopenia, which rarely occurs as a single disease entity in cats, often accompanies immune-mediated hemolytic anemia in cats with underlying FeLV infection. Platelet abnormalities may result in bleeding tendencies.

Leukocyte Abnormalities

FeLV-infected cats may have reductions in granulocyte or lymphocyte counts. Lymphopenia is primarily a result of direct replication of the virus in lymphocytes. Neutropenia is also common[23] and generally occurs alone or in conjunction with other cytopenias. In some cases, myeloid hypoplasia of all granulocytic stages is observed, suggesting direct cytopathic infection of neutrophil precursors by FeLV. In some neutropenic FeLV-infected cats, an arrest in bone marrow maturation may occur at the myelocyte and metamyelocyte stages.

Glucocorticoid-Responsive Neutropenia

It has been hypothesized that an immune-mediated mechanism is responsible for cases in which neutrophil counts recover with glucocorticoid treatment. Cyclic neutropenia also has been reported in cats with FeLV infection and usually is effectively treated with glucocorticoids, suggesting that immune-mediated mechanisms are likely to be involved in this syndrome. The cycles are usually regular, ranging from 8 to 14 days. Bone marrow cytology during the neutropenic phase may indicate either granulocytic hyperplasia or hypoplasia, with a disproportionate number of cells in the promyelocytic stage. Similar bone marrow findings could result from inflammatory or immune-mediated diseases, myelodysplasia, or granulocytic leukemia. Cats with neutropenia usually have recurrent fever or persistent bacterial infections. Some cats show persistent gingivitis, occasionally without the usual signs of inflammation such as hyperemia and purulent exudate because granulocytes are necessary for the inflammatory response.[38]

Feline Panleukopenia-Like Syndrome

Feline panleukopenia-like syndrome (FPLS), also known as *myeloblastopenia*, consists of severe leukopenia (<3000 cells/µl) with enteritis and destruction of intestinal crypt epithelium that mimics feline panleukopenia (FPV) infection (see Chapter 10). Unlike panleukopenia, anemia is also usually present in FeLV-infected cats. Recently, FPV antigen has been demonstrated by direct FA in intestinal sections of cats that died with this syndrome after being experimentally infected with FeLV.[196] FPV was also demonstrated by electron microscopy (EM) despite negative ELISA test results for FPV. It appears that this syndrome is actually not caused by FeLV itself as previously thought but by coinfection with FPV. FPLS has many clinical similarities to FeLV-associated enteritis (FAE) and FeLV-FAIDS, which results in replication in many lymphoid, myeloid, and intestinal cells.

Immune Suppression

Diseases associated with immune suppression account for a large portion of the morbidity and mortality of FeLV-infected cats.[53,235,241] FeLV-infected cats are predisposed to secondary infections primarily because of immune suppression similar to that in human patients infected with the human immunodeficiency virus (HIV), but it is more severe than the immune suppression caused by FIV infection. Evaluation of the immune status of FeLV-infected cats is hampered by the lack of well-characterized tests. Thus clinicians primarily depend on CBC and clinical presentation for diagnosing immune dysfunction. Some commercial laboratories offer selective counts of CD4+ and CD8+ cells, but the value of these parameters rarely has been evaluated in naturally infected cats (see Appendix 5).[127]

The exact mechanisms of the way the virus damages the immune system is poorly understood, as is why different animals have such varying degrees of immune suppression in response to the same virus. Immune suppression is occasionally associated with unintegrated viral DNA from replication-defective viral variants.[238] These pathogenic immunosuppressive variants, such as FeLV subgroup T, require a membrane-spanning receptor molecule (Pit1) and a second coreceptor protein (FeLIX) to infect T lymphocytes.[178] The latter protein is an endogenously expressed protein encoded by an endogenous provirus arising from FeLV subgroup A, which is similar to the FeLV receptor-binding protein of FeLV subgroup B.[15] Affected cats may develop thymic atrophy and depletion of lymph node paracortical zones following infection. Lymphopenia and neutropenia are common. In addition, neutrophils of viremic cats have decreased chemotactic and phagocytic function compared with those of normal cats. This abnormality persists for an unknown period, even if viremia is transient. In some cats, lymphopenia may be characterized by preferential loss of CD4+ helper T cells, resulting in an inverted CD4+-CD8+ ratio (which is more typical of FIV infection).[253] More commonly, substantial losses of helper cells and cytotoxic suppressor cells (CD8+ cells) occurs.[127] Many immune function tests of naturally FeLV-infected cats have been reported to be abnormal, including poor response to T-cell mitogens, prolonged allograft reaction, reduced immunoglobulin production, depressed neutrophil function, and complement depletion. Interleukin-2 (IL-2) and interleukin-4 (IL-4) are decreased in some cats.[184,187] However, studies disagree on whether interferon-γ (IFN-γ) is deficient or increased. FeLV does not appear to suppress interleukin-1 (IL-1) production from infected macrophages. Increased tumor necrosis factor-α (TNF-α) has been observed in serum of infected cats and infected cells in culture. Although each cytokine plays a vital role in the generation of a healthy immune response, the excess production of certain cytokines such as TNF-α can also cause illness.

Primary and secondary humoral antibody responses to specific antigens are delayed and decreased in FeLV-infected cats. In vaccination studies, FeLV-infected cats have not been consistently able to mount an adequate immune response to vaccines such as rabies. Therefore protection in an FeLV-infected cat after vaccination is not comparable to that in a healthy cat, and more frequent vaccinations have to be considered. T cells of FeLV-infected cats produce significantly lower levels of B-cell stimulatory factors than do those of normal cats.[53] This defect becomes progressively more severe over time. However, when B cells of FeLV-infected cats are stimulated in vitro by uninfected T cells, their function in FeLV-infected cats is normal. Although humoral immunity to specific stimulation decreases, nonspecific increases of IgG and IgM have been noted.

Many reports have been made of FeLV-infected cats having concurrent bacterial, viral, protozoal, and fungal infections, but few studies exist proving these cats have a higher rate of infection than do FeLV-negative cats or that they have a less favorable response to therapy. Thus although FeLV is well known to suppress immune function, it should not be assumed that all concurrent infections are a result of FeLV infection. Secondary infections most commonly associated with FeLV include FIP, hemobartonellosis, coccidiosis, and upper respiratory infections.[184,256,257] From a clinical standpoint, it is important to realize that many of these secondary diseases are treatable.

Skin Disease

Infections associated with dermatologic conditions are usually caused by immunodeficiency.[247] Retrovirus-infected cats have a greater diversity of cutaneous and mucosal microflora compared with uninfected cats.[288] Traumatic injuries are complicated by secondary bacterial infections or abscesses. Otitis externa and miliary dermatitis may develop from ectoparasites or allergies but persist because of secondary bacterial infections.

Immune-Mediated Diseases

In addition to immune suppression, FeLV-infected cats are subject to various immune-mediated diseases caused by an overactive or dysregulated immune response to the virus. FeLV-associated immune-mediated diseases including autoimmune hemolytic anemia, glomerulonephritis,[6] uveitis with immune complex deposition in iris and ciliary body,[21] and polyarthritis. Chronic progressive polyarthritis can be triggered by FeLV; in about 20% of cats with polyarthritis, FeLV seems to be an associated agent.[243]

The loss of T-suppressor cell activity and the formation of antigen-antibody complexes contribute to these immune-mediated diseases.[242] Measurement of FeLV antigens has shown that cats with glomerulonephritis have more circulating viral proteins that do other FeLV-infected cats. Proteins that can lead to antigen-antibody complex formation include not only whole virus particles but also free gp70, p27, or p15E.[48,313] Circulating immune complexes have also been observed after experimental treatment of persistent viremia with monoclonal antibodies to gp70 and in studies of inoculation of complement-depleting factors.

Other Syndromes
FeLV-Associated Enteritis (FAE)

FAE has been observed in cats with chronic FeLV viremia.[167,168] Clinical GI signs most frequently observed were hemorrhagic diarrhea, vomiting, oral ulceration or gingivitis, anorexia, and weight loss. Other systemic signs were nonspecific or included rhinitis, dyspnea, or apathy. Cats often die or are euthanized for an illness other than the one affecting the GI tract. FAE is associated with degeneration of intestinal epithelial cells and crypt necrosis, symptoms that are similar to those caused by FPV infection. Unlike cats with FPV infection, cats with FAE have normal or hyperplastic intestinal lymphoid tissue and no lymphoid depletion. FAE differs in a similar way from the panleukopenia-like syndrome reported with coinfection of FPV and FeLV.[196] In contrast to FeLV-infected cats without enteritis, those with FAE have large quantities of FeLV gp70 and p15E proteins in their intestinal crypt epithelial cells.

FeLV-Feline Acquired Immunodeficiency Syndrome

Enteritis with proliferation of FeLV-antigen within the enterocytes is also seen when cats have been experimentally infected with FeLV-FAIDS variants of FeLV. FAIDS begins with a prodromal period of lymphoid hyperplasia associated with viral replication in lymphoid follicles, followed by lymphoid depletion associated with extinction of viral replication. When affected by FAIDS, cats develop enterocolitis with crypt necrosis and villous atrophy.[133] Intractable diarrhea and weight loss are associated with an immunodeficiency syndrome characterized by lymphopenia, suppressed lymphocyte stimulation, impaired cutaneous allograft rejection, hypogammaglobulinemia, and opportunistic infections such as respiratory disease or stomatitis. These observations suggest that the development of FAE may be FeLV-strain dependent.

Reproductive Disorders

FeLV-infected queens can transmit the virus transplacentally. Reproductive failure in the form of fetal resorption, abortion, and neonatal death is common if in utero infection occurs. The apparent infertility might actually be early resorption of fetuses. Abortions usually occur late in gestation, with expulsion of normal-appearing fetuses. Bacterial endometritis may accompany these abortions, particularly in cats with leukopenia.[38]

Fading Kitten Syndrome

Kittens born to an infected queen may become exposed to FeLV transplacentally, but heavy exposure also occurs at birth and throughout the nursing period. Some kittens become immune, but most become viremic and die at an early age of the so-called fading kitten syndrome, characterized by failure to nurse, dehydration, hypothermia, and thymic atrophy within the first 2 weeks of life.[184]

Neuronopathy

Neurologic dysfunction has been described in FeLV-infected cats. Although most neurologic signs seen in FeLV-infected cats are caused by lymphoma and lymphocytic infiltrations in brain or spinal cord leading to compression, in some cases no tumor is detectable with diagnostic imaging methods or by necropsy. Anisocoria, mydriasis, central blindness, or Horner's syndrome have been seen without morphologic changes. In some regions (such as the southeastern United States), urinary incontinence caused by neuropathies in FeLV-infected cats has been described.[27] Direct neurotoxic effects of FeLV have been discussed as pathogenetic mechanisms. The ability of the HIV envelope glycoprotein gp120 to produce increased intracellular free calcium leading to neuronal death has been observed in infected humans. Envelope glycoproteins of other retroviruses including FeLV may have similar calcium-increasing effects. A polypeptide of the FeLV envelope was found to cause dose-dependent neurotoxicity associated with alterations in intracellular calcium ion concentration, neuronal survival, and neurite outgrowth. The polypeptide from an FeLV-C strain was significantly more neurotoxic than the same peptide derived from an FeLV-A strain.[69,217]

Clinical signs in 16 cats with chronic FeLV infection consisted of abnormal vocalization, hyperesthesia, and paresis progressing to paralysis. Some cats developed anisocoria or urinary incontinence during the course of their illness. Others had concurrent FeLV-related illnesses such as myelodysplastic disease. The clinical course of affected cats involved gradually progressive neurologic dysfunction. Microscopically, white-matter degeneration with dilation of myelin sheaths and swollen axons was identified in the spinal cord and brain stem of affected animals.[27] Immunohistochemical staining of affected tissues revealed consistent expression of FeLV p27 antigens in neurons, endothelial cells, and glial cells. Furthermore, proviral DNA was amplified from multiple sections of spinal cord.[27] These findings suggest that in some FeLV-infected cats, the virus may cytopathically affect cells in the CNS.

Hepatopathy

Feline leukemia was associated with icterus and various inflammatory and degenerative liver diseases.[256,257] Hepatic lipidosis is a major complicating factor that can explain some of these cases; however, unexplained focal liver necrosis was also observed.

DIAGNOSIS

FeLV Testing

General Guidelines

Testing for FeLV and consequently preventing exposure of healthy cats to FeLV-infected cats is the most effective way to prevent the spread of infection. Testing to identify infected cats is the mainstay of preventing transmission, and FeLV vaccination should not be considered a substitute for testing. The American Association of Feline Practitioners (AAFP) in conjunction with the Academy of Feline Medicine (AFM) has established guidelines for testing cats for FeLV (Table 13-5).[182] All sick cats (regardless of any prior test results), new cats being brought into a household, cats with unknown FeLV status, cats exposed to the virus, and cats at high risk of infection should be tested. Identifying infected cats before other cats are exposed provides the best opportunity to prevent spread of the disease. The AAFP also recommends retesting all cats that show clinical signs because symptoms might be associated with an underlying infection, and a positive FeLV test result significantly alters prognosis and influences the choice of treatment. In addition, all cats should be tested before receiving a vaccination. Cats can be tested at any age. Because the screening tests detect antigen and not antibodies, neither maternal antibodies nor antibodies from vaccination or previous viral exposure interfere with testing. To completely eliminate any risk to an established household when bringing in a new cat, a follow-up test should be performed at least 90 days after the initial test or after a possible exposure to FeLV because cats may be in the early stage of infection at the time of the first test; the test should be performed before bringing the cat into the home.[182] General principles for FeLV testing are outlined in Table 13-6.

Methodology

Routine screening for FeLV became available with the development of direct FA testing for virus in 1973.[100] When ELISA methods were developed a few years later, clinicians gained the ability to perform rapid and reliable in-house testing. In 1979 the first commercial ELISA came on the market. It was very sensitive in detecting low concentrations of antigen in serum of infected cats,[193] but it was not very specific. Lutz and others[1983] developed an ELISA containing monoclonal antibodies against three different epitopes of p27 antigen that do not cross-react with proteins of other retroviruses, so the resulting test was more specific. Today, several ELISA and other immunochromatographic assays (ICGAs) or rapid immunomigration (RIM) assays are in use. These newly developed, membrane-fixed ICGAs are based on a principle similar to ELISA in which color is generated as a result of an immunologic reaction, but the assays have a slightly different design than ELISA. These tests are available for use as rapid in-house tests.[264]

FA and ELISA/ICGA have remained the mainstay of clinical testing.[103] FA and ELISA/ICGA detect FeLV core protein p27, which is produced abundantly in most infected cats;

Table • 13-5

Recommendations for FeLV Testing[a]

General Considerations

Indications for Testing

General health screening, at least once for all cats

Illness, regardless of prior negative test results or vaccination

Disorders associated with FeLV infection (hematologic, neoplastic, or immunosuppressive)

Adoption (regardless of age): prevents exposure, serves as baseline for future problems

Potential exposure: test at least 28 days from exposure or retest again

Test Selection

ELISA for screening: better on serum or plasma than whole blood

Saliva or tears testing: highly inaccurate and should not be used

Direct FA tests for cell-associated antigen: usually present with high viral loads

PCR: detects latent infection, only indicated if other tests results negative, has false-negative results, widely varied and nonstandardized methods, best on bone marrow

Direct Fluorescent Antibody Testing

Interpretation

Not 100% accurate test

Positive result: (1) only indicates viral infection and does not indicate current illness, (2) should be confirmed by another method or test system, (3) has no bearing on predicting morbidity or mortality

Discordant Results

Defined as conflicting results with various test methods

If two ELISA methods differ: perform direct FA

Positive ELISA and direct FA: suggest persistent viremia and true positive status

Positive ELISA and negative direct FA: suggest repeated assay in 6 to 8 weeks

Recommend annual retesting after any discordant test result until agreement

Negative FeLV results in young (younger than 12 weeks old) kittens: requires retesting in 4 to 6 weeks

[a]Modified from American Association of Feline Practitioners and Academy of Feline Medicine: Advisory panel report on feline retrovirus testing and management, 2001.[183]

however, ELISA/ICGA detects free soluble FeLV p27 in plasma or serum, whereas direct FA detects p27 antigen within the cytoplasm of infected blood cells.

Some ELISAs have been developed for tear and saliva samples in place of blood.[116] In general, these tests are not as accurate as blood testing because viral shedding is intermittent and the tests are subject to more technical errors[12,116]; they are not recommended because the consequences for false-negative and false-positive results can be disastrous for individual cats or multiple-cat populations.[184]

ELISA/ICGA ELISA/ICGA methods detect free soluble FeLV-p27 in plasma or serum and are the recommended screening tests. A positive whole blood, serum, or plasma

Table • 13-6

Summary of General Principles for FeLV Testing[182]

1. All cats should be tested for infection with FeLV.
2. FeLV-infected cats may live for many years. A decision for euthanasia should never be made solely on the basis of whether a cat is infected.
3. A confirmed positive test result should be considered only an indication of retrovirus infection, not clinical disease. Disease in FeLV-infected cats may not necessarily be a result of retrovirus infection.
4. No test is 100% accurate under all conditions, therefore all results should be interpreted in light of the patient's health and prior exposure to FeLV.

ELISA/ICGA result means that the cat is viremic. These tests become positive in the first phase of viremia within the first weeks after infection, before the bone marrow is affected. Thus positive results may be reflective of transient or persistent viremia.[16] In experimental settings, most cats have positive results within 28 days after exposure.[150]

Even the new improved ELISA/ICGAs can have false-positive results for numerous reasons. They can be performed on serum, plasma, or whole blood. In some studies, higher rates of false-positive results were recorded when whole blood samples were used, particularly when the samples were hemolyzed. Thus ELISA should only be performed with plasma or serum. However, the newer ICGA contains a filtering membrane, so whole blood and serum and plasma do not produce different results.[115] False-positive results were also a problem in some test systems that used murine-derived reagents in cats that had naturally occurring antimouse antibodies,[193] which are present in about 1% to 2% of all cats. Newer tests have solved that problem by including additional control steps. Technical and user errors contribute to false-positive results as well.[103,198] These errors are most likely to occur during the washing steps of kits using microwell or plate formats. Membrane-based tests eliminate separate washing steps and include positive and negative controls for each test sample. Because many new ELISA/ICGA tests have come on the market, especially in Europe, comparative studies are necessary. In two studies, specificities of commercially available ELISA/ICGA were comparable, and positive predictive values (PPVs) of most tests were about 80%.[88,115] False-positive results are more important today because the decreasing prevalence of FeLV is leading to lower predictive values of the available tests. The reliability of a test (its predictive value) depends on the rate of infection within a cat population. For example, FeLV is present in most cats with thymic lymphoma, so a positive test result is likely to be accurate in this situation. In a lower-risk population, such as a closed cattery known to be free of FeLV, a positive test should be viewed with more suspicion, and confirmatory tests should be performed.[184] False-negative results are rare in all tests and PPVs are very high (close to 99%).[88,115] Therefore positive results have to be interpreted carefully, and confirmatory tests have to be considered after a positive result. If confirmatory tests (e.g., virus isolation, PCR) are not available or too expensive to perform, at the very least a second in-house test should be performed to rule out a false-positive result. If the second test is positive, it significantly increases the predictive value. Retesting should be performed immediately and has nothing to do with the dif-

ferent stages of viremia; it is only used to compensate for the weaknesses of the test systems. Confirmation tests should at least be performed in low-risk cats before any decisions are made that have major consequences for cat and owner.

Direct Fluorescent Antibody Testing Direct FA was the first method developed for routine testing for FeLV infection.[100] Direct FA detects cell-associated p27 antigen primarily in neutrophils and platelets in the peripheral blood and only becomes positive after infection of the bone marrow (after at least 3 weeks of viremia). Positive results are likely to reflect persistent viremia,[97,99,184] therefore direct FA is not recommended as a screening test because cats that are in the first weeks of viremia and still infectious to others are not detected. Direct FA can be used for prognostic reasons or to confirm positive and suspicious samples. Because direct FA requires special processing and fluorescent microscopy, it must be performed by a qualified reference laboratory (see Appendix 5). Generally, two or more quality blood smears should be air dried and mailed, unfixed, to the laboratory. Because the antigen is present at highest concentrations in neutrophils and platelets, false-negative results may occur when these two cell lines are deficient. False-positive results occur when smears are too thick, background fluorescence is high, and the test is prepared and interpreted by inexperienced personnel. Using anticoagulated blood rather than fresh blood for making smears can also cause errors.[147,324] Variations in quality control among facilities has been reported, and careful attention should be paid to the selection of the reference laboratory.[184]

Sequential Testing ELISA/ICGA and direct FA are useful clinically. Cats that only have positive ELISA/ICGA results are more likely to convert and have negative results than are cats with positive results on ELISA/ICGA and direct FA. To distinguish between transient and persistent viremia, cats should be retested with ELISA 6 weeks after the first positive test result. If a cat still has a positive result, it should be retested after another 10 weeks. If at this time the cat still has a positive result, it is most likely persistently viremic and will have positive results for the rest of its life. Another rapid method without the retesting delay is to immediately test a cat with a positive ELISA/ICGA result with direct FA. If the direct FA result is positive, the likelihood of a transient viremia is small. Only 3% to 9% of cats with positive direct FA results have a transient viremia.[96,103,150,154,197] A small number of cats with discordant test results that develop persistently ELISA-positive and direct FA-negative results may have focal infections that are kept localized by their immune systems.[154] A negative ELISA result but positive direct FA result is always a false result—either a false-negative ELISA result (which is very unlikely) or a false-positive direct FA result.

Virus Isolation

The virus isolation test is the test that was originally developed to identify FeLV-infected cats.[51,151] It is not practicable for routine diagnosis because it is difficult and time consuming to perform and requires special facilities. It can be used for the confirmation of positive test results and suspicious samples.

Nucleic Acid Detection

PCR has been adapted to clinical use for the diagnosis of FeLV infection. However, current reagents and testing protocols are neither standardized nor validated.[334] This test differs from direct FA and ELISA/ICGA methods in that it does not detect viral antigen (protein) but rather detects viral nucleic acid sequences (RNA or proviral DNA). It is sensitive because the process involves amplification of FeLV sequences to enhance detection. PCR must be performed by well-equipped and well-trained laboratories because minor alterations in sample handling can destroy the delicate nucleic acid material or introduce minute amounts of cross-contamination, leading to either false-negative or false-positive results, respectively (see Appendix 5).[184] In addition, PCR is highly strain specific. As a retrovirus, mutations in FeLV occur naturally. Minor strain variations may prevent binding of the primers, a step necessary to amplify the viral genome. Cats infected with mutated FeLV react negatively with a specific PCR. A negative result does not necessarily mean they are uninfected. PCR is only diagnostic if it has a positive result and is performed by a reputable laboratory so that contamination can be excluded. With this in mind, PCR has greatly enhanced the possibilities to detect FeLV infection in blood, cultures, solid tissue, and fixed specimens. Most FeLV-PCR tests detect proviral DNA, the viral genome sequence that is integrated into the host genome. The main indications for PCR are the suspicion of a latent infection in cats with lymphomas, chronically inflamed oral gingival lesions, and bone marrow suppressive syndromes.[118,142,314] In latent infection, no or minimal replication virus is present, thus tests such as ELISA that detect viral antigen are negative. Using quantitative PCR, viral loads in experimentally infected cats with negative ELISA test results (i.e., that were latently infected) that mount an effective immune response were much lower (300-fold less) than in cats with positive ELISA test results (i.e., that were transiently or persistently viremic).[129] Furthermore viral antigen (as detected by ELISA) is often not produced because of host immunity. However, proviral DNA may be integrated in the cellular genome and can be detected by PCR. PCR of peripheral blood may not yield more accurate results than ELISA testing,[144,219] probably because of the low levels of viral genome present in latently infected cats and the difficulty associated with extracting nucleic acid from whole blood. However, using nested and real-time quantitative PCR, proviral genome could be detected in 10% of experimentally and naturally exposed cats with negative ELISA test results.[129] PCR of bone marrow samples in cats with myelosuppression and of tumor tissue samples from cats with lymphoma have demonstrated in latent FeLV infection in FeLV-antigen-negative cats.[142] PCR was also better than immunohistochemical methods in detecting virus in lymphomas.[142,144] Positive PCR results on peripheral blood from cats with lymphosarcoma were low (2%), whereas those from cats with corresponding lymphogenous tumors were much higher (26%).[81] Rates of detection are similarly greater on bone marrow versus blood from latently infected cats that test negative by other methods. PCR may also be useful in determining the true status of cats with discordant results from other testing techniques. Ideally, samples should be taken from bone marrow, lymph node aspirates, or neoplasms rather than peripheral blood. The combination of routine screening testing combined with confirmatory tests accurately determines the FeLV infection status of most cats. However, some animals have repeatedly discordant results. Presently, approximately 10% of cats suspected to be FeLV infected that have antigen-negative blood results have been found by PCR on blood or bone marrow to latently harbor FeLV. Improvements in PCR extraction, methods, and primer selection may improve its level of detection in the future.

THERAPY

Despite the fact that persistent FeLV viremia is associated with a decreased life expectancy, many owners elect to provide treatment for the myriad clinical syndromes that accompany infection. Although some older studies suggested that FeLV-infected cats only live a maximum of 3 years after diagnosis, the studies involved group-housed cats in multiple-cat, FeLV-endemic environments. With proper care, FeLV-infected cats may live many more than 3 years and in fact may die at an older age from causes completely unrelated to their retroviral infection. As mentioned, decisions about treatment or euthanasia should never be based solely on the presence of FeLV infection. It is important to realize that FeLV-infected cats are subject to the same diseases that befall uninfected cats, and the mere presence of an FeLV-related disease may or may not be caused by FeLV.

Management of FeLV-Infected Cats
FeLV-Infected Households
Shedding of virus generally occurs through salivary glands, and cat to cat transmission can occur by allogrooming and sharing of food and water bowls and litter boxes. In a household with an FeLV-infected cat, all cats should be tested so that their status is known. If one or more FeLV-positive cats are identified in an otherwise negative household, the owner must be informed of the potential danger to other cats in the house. They should be told that the best method of preventing the spread of infection is to isolate the infected individuals in other rooms to keep the infected cats from interacting with other housemates. The risk of transmission is not very high because the cats that have lived together with the FeLV-shedding cats have already been infected and are more likely to be immune to new infection. However, studies in cluster households have shown that virus neutralization is not lifelong, therefore a previously immune cat can become viremic. In a household with few cats, an owner may elect to keep all the cats. The risk of infection in adult FeLV-negative cats is approximately 10% to 15% if they have lived with a viremic cat for more than several months.[35] If owners refuse to separate housemates, the uninfected cats should receive an FeLV vaccination in an attempt to enhance their natural level of immunity in this environment of high viral exposure. However, vaccination does not provide high levels of protection under these circumstances. If the household is closed to new cats, the FeLV-negative cats will tend to outlive the infected cats, so after months or years all remaining cats will be immune.

Individual Cats
FeLV-infected cats should be confined indoors not only to prevent spread to other cats in the neighborhood but also to protect the vulnerable immunosuppressed cats from other infectious agents carried by other animals. Good nutrition and husbandry are essential to maintaining good health. FeLV-infected cats should be fed a high-quality, commercial feline diet. Raw meat, eggs, and unpasteurized milk should be avoided because the risk of acquiring foodborne bacterial or parasitic infections is greater in immunosuppressed individuals.[182]

Wellness visits to the veterinary clinic should occur at least semiannually to promptly detect changes in health status. A detailed history should be obtained to assist the veterinarian in identifying possible problems requiring more intensive investigation. A thorough physical examination should be performed at each visit. Special attention should be paid to the oral cavity to detect the frequently occurring dental and gum diseases. Lymph nodes should be palpated and carefully evaluated for changes in size or shape. The anterior and posterior segments of both eyes should be thoroughly examined. The skin should be examined closely for evidence of external parasite infestation or fungal disease. The body weight should be accurately measured and recorded because weight loss is often the first sign of deterioration in the cat's condition. A CBC should be performed at each visit. Biochemistry profiles and urinalyses should be performed yearly. Urine should be collected by cystocentesis so cultures can be performed if necessary. Fecal examinations should be considered for cats with a possible exposure to internal parasites or a history of GI disease. A routine program should be used for control of GI parasites, ectoparasites, and heartworms if applicable. Intact males and females should be neutered to reduce stress associated with estrus, mating behaviors, or both. Neutered animals are also less likely to roam outside the house. Surgery is generally well tolerated by asymptomatic FeLV-infected cats. Perioperative antibiotic administration should be used during dental procedures and invasive surgeries.[182]

Vaccination programs to prevent common serious infectious diseases should be maintained. Although no scientific evidence proves that FeLV-infected cats are at increased risk from modified live virus (MLV) vaccines, attenuated viral vaccines to prevent other infections should not be given to FeLV-infected cats because MLV vaccines may regain their pathogenicity. Although FeLV vaccines are nonliving, they are not recommended because they have no effect on the viremia, carrier state or elimination, or clinical FeLV disease in already infected cats. If an owner cannot be convinced to keep an FeLV-positive cat inside, a rabies vaccination should be given in accordance with state and local regulations. In vaccination studies, it was demonstrated that FeLV-infected cats may not be able to mount an adequate immune response to vaccines. This has been proven for rabies but is likely to be true for other vaccines as well. Therefore protection in an FeLV-infected cat after vaccination is not comparable with that in a healthy cat, so more frequent vaccinations have to be considered in these cats, especially in areas with high rabies prevalence.

Treatment of FeLV-Associated Diseases and Drug Precautions

For the most part, secondary diseases in FeLV-infected cats are treated in the same way they are treated in uninfected cats. However, more intensive diagnostic testing should proceed as soon as possible in the course of illness for FeLV-infected patients. Secondary infectious conditions in infected cats may require more intensive and prolonged therapy than in uninfected cats. The owner should be forewarned, and the clinician should not be discouraged if the response to treatment takes longer than expected.

Cats with FeLV infection may have a fever. FeLV itself does not cause fever, so a search for a concurrent infection must be made in febrile cats. Fevers of unknown origin that are unresponsive to antibiotics may be caused by a coinfecting virus, protozoa, or fungus.

Glucocorticoids and other immune suppressive drugs should be avoided whenever possible unless clearly indicated for a specific problem. They interfere with granulocyte chemotaxis, phagocytosis, and the killing of bacteria, thus compounding the risk of infection.[38] In FeLV-negative cats living in a household with FeLV-positive cats, glucocorticoid treatment should be avoided because it increases the risk of reactivation of a latent infection. All myelosuppressive drugs should be avoided in FeLV-infected cats because they potentiate the myelosuppressive syndromes caused by FeLV.

Bone Marrow Suppression Syndromes

In FeLV-infected cats with anemia, blood transfusion is a very important part of the treatment, especially if the anemia is nonregenerative. Most cats respond after the first transfusion. Of 29 anemic (HCT < 20%) FeLV-infected cats treated with blood transfusions for more than 2 weeks, the HCT returned to normal ranges in eight cats. This may be explained by the cyclic cytopenias that are occasionally seen in FeLV-infected cats. Prednisone may increase the life span of erythrocytes if

any component of the anemia is immune mediated, but it should be used only if there is proof of an immune-mediated reaction. Occasionally secondary infections (e.g., erythrocytic mycoplasmal infections) are responsible for the anemia. Because this type of anemia (which is regenerative) has the best prognosis of the FeLV-induced anemias, the possibility of an animal having such infectious diseases should always be examined. Deficiencies of iron, folate, or vitamin B_{12} are rare, therefore replacement therapy is not likely to be helpful.[38] Even though erythropoietin concentrations are often elevated in cats with FeLV-related anemia, treatment with human recombinant erythropoietin (rHuEPO) may be helpful. rHuEPO treatment not only increases erythrocyte counts but also increases platelet and megakaryocte numbers in animals and humans with clinical disease.[233] In one study, rHuEPO also increased leukocyte counts in cats.[9] No study has been performed involving FeLV-infected cats but in a study in FIV-infected cats, all treated cats had a gradual increase in erythrocyte counts, hemoglobin concentrations, and HCT levels, as well as increased leukocyte counts consisting of either increased numbers of neutrophils, lymphocytes, or a combination of these.[9] The recommended dosage is 100 IU/kg given subcutaneously (SC) every 48 hours until the desired HCT (usually 30%) is reached and then as needed to maintain the HCT. A response may not be seen for 3 to 4 weeks and if it does not occur, iron supplementation may be required. Iron should not be given to cats that have received transfusions because whole blood contains 0.5 mg/ml of iron, and hemosiderosis may occur in the liver. Antierythropoietin antibodies may develop in 25% to 30% of treated animals after 6 to 12 months. Binding of these antibodies to the rHuEPO and the native erythropoietin nullifies their physiologic actions on erythroid progenitor cells, causing bone marrow failure and refractory anemia. However, antierythropoietin antibodies dissipate after discontinuation of treatment.

Some FeLV-infected cats do not respond to rHuEPO treatment. Reasons for resistance to erythropoietin, other than development of antierythropoietin antibodies and iron deficiency, include concurrent infection with FeLV and other infectious agents of bone marrow stromal cells. In some nonresponsive cats, repeated blood transfusions may be the only treatment possible.

In some FeLV-infected cats with neutropenia, an immune-mediated mechanism is suspected of leading to a maturation arrest in the bone marrow at myelocyte and metamyelocyte stages. Neutrophil counts can be corrected in many of these cats by immune suppressive doses of glucocorticoids.

In animals with myeloid hypoplasia and in the absence of myeloid precursors, direct effects of FeLV are suspected and glucocorticoids should not be used. Treatment with filgrastim, a granulocyte colony-stimulating factor (G-CSF) that is marketed as recombinant human product (rHuG-CSF) for treatment of neutropenia in humans, has caused transient responses. Filgrastim is used in cats at 5 µg/kg SC every 24 hours for up to 21 days. Potential side effects include bone discomfort, splenomegaly, allergic reactions, and fever.[9,86] Short-term increases in neutrophil counts may be followed by neutropenia with continued use of filgrastim because of development of dose-dependent neutralizing antibodies to this heterologous product after 10 days to 7 weeks; treatment should not be used for more than 3 weeks.[9,86] Another potential risk is the development of persistent antibodies against endogenous feline G-CSF after 10 days (at higher dosages) to 7 weeks, resulting in rebound neutropenia. One study suggests that filgrastim is contraindicated in FIV-infected cats because it led to an increased viral load,[9] but data on the use of filgrastim in FeLV infection are limited. In one study, a small number of naturally FeLV-infected cats were treated with filgrastim; however, treatment did not result in significant changes in neutrophil counts.[172] Other authors reported that it has been used in FeLV-infected cats with cyclic neutropenia with some success.[184]

Lymphoma and Leukemia

Although untreated lymphoma is usually fatal within 1 to 2 months, many cats can be helped with chemotherapy, and a few will have remissions that may last several years. Although the prognosis is worse when lymphomas are associated with FeLV,[68,173,306,315] some cats greatly benefit from a treatment. Before treatment is considered, a diagnosis of lymphoma must be confirmed by cytologic or histologic studies and the condition of the cat evaluated to determine its prognosis (Table 13-7). Staging of lymphoma in cats is more difficult than in dogs because cats are more likely to have visceral involvement. For example, cats with alimentary lymphoma generally have a poorer prognosis than cats with lymphoma at other sites because anorexia and debilitation are often present. However, cats with a resectable intestinal mass or well-differentiated histologic features have extended survival times after treatment with chemotherapy. Cats with mediastinal lymphoma have a generally favorable response to chemotherapy.[205,306] Nasal lymphoma seems to remain localized longer than lymphomas in other sites, and radiation alone has significantly prolonged survival. A staging system recommended by Mooney and co-workers is of value in cats with less advanced disease because these cats have a better rate of remission and longer survival.[220]

Combinations of chemotherapeutic drugs offer the best chance for complete remission (Tables 13-8 and 13-9). Single-agent glucocorticoids are minimally effective and should be considered for palliation only after clients have rejected the option of combination chemotherapy. The drugs most frequently administered in combination include cyclophosphamide, vincristine, and prednisone, a combination called COP. This combination has been effective in achieving remission rates of up to 75%.[306] The drugs are occasionally combined with doxorubicin, a combination called COPA. Less commonly, L-asparaginase, cytosine arabinoside, and methotrexate are included in feline protocols. In a report of 38 cats treated with COP, approximately 75% achieved complete remission, with a median remission duration of 150 days and a 1-year remission rate of 20%.[33,34] Most cats in this group were FeLV infected, and the most frequent tumor site was the mediastinum. Years later, the same number of cats that were from the same geographic area and treated with the same protocol had a complete remission rate of only 47%, with a median remission duration of 86 days. In the latter group, few cats were FeLV infected, and the alimentary form was the most frequent.[221] Therefore FeLV infection should not be a reason not to treat lymphoma in a cat. At this time, COP is still a reasonable protocol for induction of remission. For maintenance of remission, adding doxorubicin (a combination called COPA) has been more successful than continued COP, with a median complete remission of 243 days.[221] In contrast, doxorubicin alone was not effective for induction of remission.[36,38] Therefore if doxorubicin is used for treatment of feline lymphoma, it should be combined with other effective chemotherapeutic drugs in a combination protocol.[173]

All these drugs are immunosuppressive and some are myelosuppressive, so they could lead to production of other FeLV-associated diseases. Owners must be advised to watch for signs of illness. Infections must be treated quickly and aggressively, especially if they occur at the time of the granulocyte nadir. The point at which therapy may safely be

Table • 13-7

Prognostic Indicators in Feline Lymphoma

PROGNOSTIC INDICATORS	DESCRIPTION
Good	Small tumor burden
	Peripheral lymph nodes, nasal cavity, or mediastinum as primary site
	Normal major organ function
	Good appetite, minimal weight loss
Adverse	Anemia, neutropenia, or thrombocytopenia
	Bone marrow involvement
	Prolonged paralysis with spinal lymphoma
	Fever, sepsis, or focal infection (e.g., gingivitis, chronic rhinitis)
	Skin or alimentary involvement
	Emaciation or anorexia
Factors with minimal ramifications	FeLV status
	Age, gender
	Histopathologic findings (lymphoblastic vs. immunoblastic): not known to affect cat prognosis, but immunoblastic more favorable in dogs

Table • 13-8

COPA Therapy Protocol for Treatment of Feline Lymphoma

	WEEK NUMBER															
	1	2	3	4	5	6	7	8	9	10	11	12	13	16	19	22
THERAPY COPA																
Cyclophosphamide	1			1												
Vincristine	1	1	1	1												
Prednisone	1	. . . .														
Doxorubicin							1			1			1	1	1	1

Outline of the COPA protocol: *cyclophosphamide*–300 mg/m² PO, round off dose to nearest 25 mg on low side of dose; *vincristine*–0.75 mg/m² IV; *prednisone*–2 mg/kg PO daily. Beginning on week 7, substitute *doxorubicin* (25 mg/m² IV) for cyclophosphamide and vincristine. Continue treatment every 3 weeks until relapse or until week 22 of continuous remission. Stop treatment, and taper prednisone over 3 weeks.

Table • 13-9

Sequential Multiagent Chemotherapy Protocol for Cats with Lymphoma[205]

Therapy[a]	|								WEEK NUMBER													
	1	2	3	4	5	6	7	8	9	10	11	12	13	14	15	16	17	19	20	21	22	23
Cyclophosphamide		1				1				1				1				1				
Vincristine	1				1				1		1		1				1					
L-Asparaginase	1							1														
Prednisolone	1...0		1						...0													
Doxorubicin			1				1								1							
Methotrexate																						1

[a]Outline of the multiagent protocol: *cyclophosphamide*–10 mg/kg PO; *vincristine*–week 1, 0.025 mg/kg IV; weeks 5, 9, 11, 13, and 17, 0.03 mg/kg IV; *l-asparaginase*–450 IU/kg SC; *prednisolone*–week 1, 4 mg/kg PO daily; week 3. 3 mg/kg PO daily; weeks 4 and 5, 2 mg/kg PO daily; weeks 6 and 7, 1 mg/kg PO daily; *doxorubicin*–week 3, 20 mg/m² (1 mg/kg) IV; weeks 7 and 15, 25 mg/m² (1.1 mg/kg) IV; *methotrexate*–0.8 mg/kg PO. Give treatment once a week as indicated, but give prednisolone daily for the first week and weeks 3 through 8.

discontinued is controversial, but the trend is toward shorter treatment times for cats in continuous complete remission. Previously, most protocols continued for a year or more; now many stop after 6 months of continuous complete remission. Some cats can be expected to relapse when treatment ends, so owner awareness and periodic checkups are important.

Cats with acute leukemia are difficult to treat because the bone marrow becomes filled with neoplastic blast cells, which must be cleared before the normal hematopoietic precursors can repopulate. This process may take 3 to 4 weeks, therefore neutropenia and anemia may not be immediately reversible. Although prophylactic antibiotics are not given routinely in the treatment of feline leukemia or lymphoma, broad-spectrum bactericidal antibiotics should be given to FeLV-infected cats, especially if fever or other signs of infection occur. The remission rate for cats with acute lymphatic leukemia treated initially with vincristine and prednisone is approximately 25%, whereas the rate for cats with acute myelocytic leukemia (treated with doxorubicin or cytosine arabinoside) is close to zero. The reason for the extremely poor response may be that a very early stem cell is involved, and nearly total ablation of the bone marrow is necessary to clear the malignant clone.[38]

Antiviral Chemotherapy

In numerous studies, naturally or experimentally FeLV-infected cats have been treated with various substances. More antiviral or immunomodulatory treatment trials are published for FeLV infection than any other infectious disease. Unfortunately, many results are difficult to interpret, and evaluation of these data is hampered by the lack of well-controlled clinical trials in which new treatments are compared against a standard care or placebo. Currently, no treatment has been proved effective in clearing FeLV infection. To be effective in treatment of FeLV infection, an agent must inhibit viral replication effectively and allow for recovery of the immune system. Lifelong treatment may be required, thus the agent should be effective when given orally and should be relatively nontoxic and inexpensive. So far, no such agent has been found to treat cats with FeLV infection (see Chapter 2 and Appendix 8 for additional information on the drugs in the following section).

Zidovudine

Zidovudine (AZT) has been used in experimental and clinical trials in FeLV-infected cats. It is effective against FeLV in vitro.[305] It has been shown to be somewhat effective in treating cats experimentally infected with FeLV when treatment is initiated less than 3 weeks after infection. When treated less than 1 week after challenge, cats were protected from bone marrow infection and persistent viremia.[87] However, in a study involving naturally FeLV-infected cats that were treated with AZT and high-dose SC human IFN-α for 6 weeks, treatment with AZT, human IFN-α, or both did not lead to a statistically significant improvement of clinical, laboratory, immunologic, or virologic parameters.[112] In general, therapeutic efficacy of AZT in FeLV-infected cats seems to be less promising than in FIV-infected cats. AZT should only be used at a low dosage of 5 mg/kg every 12 hours orally (PO) or SC in FeLV-infected cats. For SC injection, the lyophilized product (marketed for intravenous [IV] injection in humans) should be diluted in isotonic sodium chloride solution (5 ml) to prevent local irritation. For PO administration, syrup (raspberry flavor) or gelatin capsules (compounded individually for every cat) can be given. AZT is rapidly and completely absorbed from the GI tract, and absorption is unaffected by the presence of food. During treatment, routine CBCs are necessary because nonregenerative anemia is a common side effect, especially if FeLV-associated bone marrow suppression is already present. CBCs should be performed weekly for the first month. If values are stable after the first 4 weeks, it is recommended that a CBC be done monthly for monitoring. Cats with severe bone marrow suppression should not be treated because of the risk of a life-threatening anemia. In cats with concurrent chronic renal failure, the dosage should be reduced to avoid toxicity. HCT declines within 3 weeks of initiating treatment to about 60% of baseline but rebounds afterward in most cases, even without discontinuation of treatment. If HCT drops below 20%, discontinuation is recommended and anemia usually resolves within a few days.[108,109,113] Neutropenia occurs less frequently than anemia and may be prevented or treated with filgrastim. Other side effects in cats, including vomiting or anorexia, rarely develop. One side effect occasionally noted by owners is the development of a fuller and shinier hair coat. AZT should not be combined with other myelosuppressive drugs. Concurrent use of nonsteroidal antiphlogistics has to be monitored carefully because it can delay AZT metabolism, result in kidney toxicity, or lead to neutropenia.

Didanosine

Didanosine (ddI) is also used to treat HIV infection in human beings (see Chapter 2). The drug treats FeLV in vitro[305];

however, controlled in vivo studies confirming the efficacy of ddI in cats with FeLV infection are not available.

Zalcitabine

Like AZT, zalcitabine (ddC) is currently used to treat HIV infection in humans. It is effective against FeLV in vitro[136,248,305] and has been used in experimental studies to treat FeLV-infected cats. It has a very short half-life (see Chapter 2) and therefore has been administered via IV bolus dose or controlled-release SC implants. Controlled-release administration of ddC inhibited de novo FeLV replication and delayed onset of viremia. However, when therapy was discontinued after 3 weeks, an equivalent incidence and level of viremia were established rapidly.[136] In a study evaluating the prophylactic antiviral activity against FeLV, dosages were toxic, although in some cats onset of viremia was delayed for several weeks.[248] In humans, the drug is used orally; however, no data exist on PO administration in cats.

Ribavirin

Use of ribavirin (RTCA) is limited because of the development of dose-dependant hemolytic anemia in humans. RTCA is also a nucleoside analog but in contrast to other anti-HIV compounds that act primarily to inhibit RT activity, RTCA allows DNA synthesis to occur but prevents the formation of viral proteins, probably by interfering with capping of viral mRNA. RTCA is active against FeLV in vitro.[87] However, in vivo therapeutic concentrations are difficult to achieve because of toxicity, and cats are extremely sensitive to the side effects (see Chapter 2 and Drug Formulary, Appendix 8). Therefore it cannot be recommended for use in feline patients.

Foscarnet

Foscarnet (PFA) is a pyrophosphate that has a wide spectrum of activity against DNA and RNA viruses including retroviruses (see Chapter 2). It has in vitro activity against FeLV,[301] but no reliable data exist on its efficacy in cats in vivo. Toxicity limits its use, and renal dysfunction is evident in most people after 2 weeks of therapy. As it does in humans, it causes nephrotoxicity and myelosupression in cats.

Suramin

Although suramin has been used for the treatment of patients with HIV infection, it has only minor clinical value. Suramin was used to treat FeLV-infected cats, although a limited number of cats was used (see Chapter 2 and Appendix 8).

Antibody Therapy

Antibody therapy has been used in an attempt to treat FeLV. Antibodies were derived from immune cats or were obtained as murine monoclonal antibodies (MABs) to epitopes of gp70. Antibodies have successfully treated experimentally infected cats only when given within 3 weeks of infection. Naturally infected cats showed no response, even though the MABs persisted longer in viremic cats than in normal control animals. FeLV-infected cats also developed residual circulating immune complexes that could cause adverse reactions.[38]

Immune Modulatory Therapy

Immune modulators or cytokine inducers have been used in the treatment of FeLV-infected cats. Attempts to stimulate the immune response have been used more extensively in FeLV infection than in any other infectious disease in veterinary medicine. However, controlled studies including large numbers of naturally infected cats do not exist for most of these agents.

Interferon-α

IFN-α has immunomodulatory and antiviral activity. Two common treatment regimens have been created for use of recombinant human IFN-α in cats: high-dosage SC injection (10^4 to 10^6 IU/kg every 24 hours) or low-dosage PO administration (1 to 50 IU/kg every 24 hours; see Chapter 2 and Appendix 8). Parenteral administration of IFN-α leads to the development of neutralizing antibodies that limit its activity. Several studies have been performed on the use of human IFN-α in FeLV-infected cats. In vitro, FeLV replication is inhibited by human IFN-α. Treatment with high-dose IFN-α, either alone or in combination with AZT, resulted in significant decreases in circulating FeLV p27 antigen; however, because of anti–IFN-α antibody development, cats became refractory to therapy.[333] In another study in naturally FeLV-infected cats using high-dose parenteral treatment, IFN-α with or without AZT did not lead to a statistically significant improvement of clinical, laboratory, immunologic, or virologic parameters.[112] Low-dose oral IFN-α was used in a placebo-controlled study in cats with experimentally induced FeLV infection.[44] Cats were given IFN-α orally either 0.5 IU or 5 IU once daily following experimental challenge on 7 consecutive days on alternate weeks for 1 month. No difference was noted in the development of viremia; however, treated cats had significantly fewer clinical signs of illness and longer survival times when compared with the placebo group. The cats given 0.5 IU had a better response. Several uncontrolled studies have reported a beneficial response in cats when treated with low-dose oral IFN,[295,311,326] but they only included a limited number of cats and have been difficult to interpret without control groups. In a larger study, prognostic outcomes of 69 FeLV-infected cats with clinical signs that had been treated with low-dose oral IFN (30 IU/kg for 7 consecutive days on a 1-week-on, 1-week-off schedule) were compared with historical controls. Significantly longer survival times were reported in the treated cats.[326] Alternate-week treatment is continued until the cat is considered clinically healthy, and treatment may be reinstituted if clinical signs recur.[326] In another placebo-controlled study, treatment of client-owned, ill FeLV-infected cats given oral low doses of IFN-α (30 IU per cat for 7 consecutive days on a 1-week-on, 1-week-off schedule) either alone or in combination with Staphylococcus protein A did not result in any statistically significant difference in FeLV status, survival time, clinical or hematologic parameters, or subjective improvement in the owners' impressions when compared with a placebo group.[214]

Interferon-ω

Feline IFN-ω has been licensed for use in veterinary medicine in some European countries and Japan (see Chapter 2 and Appendix 8). Cats will not develop antibodies to IFN-ω because of it homologous origin. Feline IFN-ω inhibits FeLV replication in vitro.[265] In a placebo-controlled field study, 48 cats with FeLV infection were treated with IFN-ω in a dosage of 10^6 IU/kg every 24 hours SC on 5 consecutive days. The survival times of treated versus untreated cats in a 2-month follow-up period showed a statistically significant difference.[211] The same investigators studied a similar regimen of three 5-day series of IFN-ω beginning on days 0, 14, and 60 in FeLV-FIV coinfected cats.[49a] Cats (39 were treated and 42 received placebo) were monitored for up to 1 year, and supportive therapies were used in both groups. There was greater clinical illness during the initial 4 months and higher mortality at the 9-month (1.7 times the risk) and 12-month (1.4 times the risk) periods in the control group compared with the treated group. However, no virologic parameters were measured throughout these studies to support the hypothesis that the IFN actually had an anti-FeLV effect rather than an inhibitory effect on secondary infections. Additional studies are needed. A treatment protocol of 10^6 IU/kg IFN-ω every 24 hours SC on 5 consecutive days is suggested but may be modified in the future. No side effects have been reported in cats.

Parapox Virus Avis and Parapox Virus Ovis

Parapox virus avis (PIND-AVI) and parapox virus ovis (PIND-ORF) are attenuated poxviruses that induce IFN and colony-stimulating factors and activate natural killer cells. Initial reports suggested that these compounds were able to cure 80% to 100% of FeLV-infected cats.[137] However, two placebo-controlled double-blind trials using the same treatment protocol were not able to repeat these striking results.[110,111] More than 20 immunologic, clinical, laboratory, and virologic parameters were examined (including FeLV p27 antigen concentration, clinical signs, lymphocyte subsets, and survival time), but no statistically significant differences could be demonstrated between paramunity inducer and placebo administration.

Acemannan

Acemannan, is a water-soluble, long-chain complex carbohydrate (mannan) polymer derived from the aloe vera plant (see Chapter 2 and Appendix 8). In one noncontrolled open-label trial, 50 cats with natural FeLV infection were treated with acemannan (2 mg/kg intraperitoneally [IP] every 7 days for 6 weeks). At the end of the 12-week study, 71% of the cats were known to be alive.[280] All cats remained FeLV-antigen positive, and no significant change was detected in clinical signs or hematologic parameters. The fact that the study did not include a control group and clinical and laboratory evaluations failed to document improvement from pretreatment evaluations makes it difficult to determine whether the use of acemannan improved the outcome of infection.

Staphylococcus Protein A

Staphylococcus protein A (SPA) is a bacterial polypeptide that has been used in various modalities to treat FeLV-infected cats (see Chapter 2). In a study, kittens with experimental FeLV infection were treated with SPA (7.3 µg/kg IP twice per week for 8 weeks); however, neither anemia nor humoral immune function improved.[214] In a placebo-controlled study, treatment of client-owned ill FeLV-infected cats with SPA (10 µg/kg twice per week for up to 10 weeks) did not cause a statistically significant difference in the FeLV status, survival time, or clinical and hematologic parameters when compared with a placebo group, but it caused a significant improvement in the owners' subjective impressions of the health of their pets. Interestingly, a combination of SPA with low-dose oral IFN-α was less effective than SPA alone.[214]

Propionibacterium acnes

P. acnes, formerly *Corynebacterium parvum*, is available for veterinary use and has been used in treating FeLV-infected cats, but no prospective studies have been performed. Veterinarians have described their clinical experience in round-table discussions and anecdotal reports (see Chapter 2).[184,185]

Bacille Calmette-Guérin

Bacille Calmette-Guérin (BCG) is a cell wall extract of a nonpathogenic strain of *Mycobacterium bovis* that has been used to treat kittens experimentally infected with FeSV (see Chapter 2). However, BCG was not able to prevent tumor development or increase the survival rate in any setting.[13]

Serratia marcescens

A commercially available biologic extract of *Serratia marcescens* (BESM) stimulates normal feline macrophages derived from bone marrow to release maximum concentrations of IL-6, TNF-α, and IL-1, leading to elevations in rectal temperature and neutrophil counts (see Chapter 2). In a study with FeLV-infected cats, weekly treatment with BESM preparations failed to prevent or reverse viremia in cats when initiated before or 6 weeks after inoculation with FeLV.[60]

Levamisole

Levamisole (see Chapter 2) is a broad-spectrum anthelmintic that has been given to FeLV-infected cats,[35] but its effect has never been substantiated by controlled studies. Levamisole remains an investigational therapy.

Diethylcarbamazine

Diethylcarbamazine (DEC) may mitigate the course of FeLV infection in cats. Uncontrolled studies have suggested that continuous oral DEC treatment given shortly after evidence of FeLV infection prevents or delays FeLV-associated lymphopenia and prolongs survival.[169,170] In one controlled study, its therapeutic effect against FeLV infection was investigated in 24 SPF kittens experimentally infected with a lymphoma-causing strain of FeLV. The kittens were divided into four groups and received either a high dosage of DEC (12 mg/kg every 24 hours), a low dosage of DEC (3 mg/kg every 24 hours), AZT (15 mg/kg every 12 hours), or a placebo orally for 10 weeks. Although AZT was effective in preventing persistent viremia, neither dosage of DEC was effective. However, AZT and both dosage levels of DEC prevented lymphoma development.[229] DEC has severe side effects including hepatic injury.[24]

Treatment of Viral-Induced Feline Sarcomas

Treatment of FeSV-induced fibrosarcoma is early, wide, and deep surgical excision. If no metastases are present and microscopic tumors remain after surgery, radiation can be successful in delaying recurrence. Experimentally FeSV-induced fibrosarcomas in kittens occasionally regress after treatment with anti-FOCMA serum, but this is unlikely to translate into clinical efficacy.[38]

PREVENTION

General Considerations

Because FeLV is prevalent in body excretions such as saliva, cats with viremic infections pose an immediate risk to other cats in their environment. Because of the environmental lability of retroviruses such as FeLV, direct contact among cats and immediate fomite transfer are the major risk factors. Viremic cats should be physically separated from other cats in the environment. In a veterinary clinic, FeLV-infected cats can be housed in the same ward as other hospitalized patients as long as certain precautionary measures are taken. FeLV is very fragile, surviving only seconds at most outside the host animal. The virus is susceptible to all disinfectants including common soap, so simple precautions and routine cleaning procedures can prevent transmission in the hospital setting. FeLV-infected patients should be housed in individual cages and confined to them throughout their hospitalization. They should *never* be placed in a "contagious ward" with cats that have other infections such as viral respiratory disease. Animal caretakers and other hospital staff members should be advised to wash their hands between direct contacts with patients and after cleaning cages. (These measures are taken primarily to protect FeLV-infected, immune suppressed cats.) Dental and surgical instruments, endotracheal tubes, and other items potentially contaminated with body fluids of a FeLV-infected cat should be thoroughly cleaned and sterilized between uses. Fluid lines, multidose medication containers, and food can become contaminated with body fluids (especially blood or saliva) and should not be shared among patients. FeLV can be transmitted hematogenously, therefore all feline blood donors should be screened and confirmed to be free of infection before donating blood.[182] Because FeLV was detected in the corneal tissues of cats by PCR and immunohistochemistry,[122] screening potential corneal donors for FeLV infection is also generally warranted.

Preventative methods, including testing and removal strategies and vaccination, have been very successful in significantly decreasing the prevalence of FeLV infection in the last 20 years.

Test and Removal Strategy

When FeLV was first described in the mid 1960s, the highest rate of infection was found in large multiple-cat households and catteries. In contrast, free-roaming cats had lower rates of infection, and those housed in single-cat households were only rarely infected. Convenient and reliable testing became available in the mid-1970s. Very quickly, cat breeders implemented test and removal programs, which proved to be extremely effective for eliminating the virus from catteries. The most dramatic example was a mandatory test and removal program in the Netherlands in 1974 that was imposed on all cat breeders.[323] When testing was first implemented, the prevalence of FeLV in purebred catteries was 11%. Within 4 years, the rate was reduced to less than 2%, and no infected cat has been reported since 1984. FeLV should be considered an abnormality in a well-run cattery. Many stray-cat shelters also implement testing in their conditioning protocols, thus further reducing the rate of FeLV infection.[184] Epidemiologic studies suggest that the testing and removal strategies have more influence on the decrease in prevalence than vaccination.[272]

Vaccination

History and Efficacy

Because most naturally exposed cats produce antibodies to virus and become immune, it is theoretically possible to produce an effective vaccine. However, accomplishing the task proved to be more difficult than anticipated. The mechanism of protection against FeLV, and especially the role of CMI, is not completely understood. Neutralizing antibody to subgroup A virus is probably most important because it is the only subgroup that is transmitted naturally. The other subgroups arise by recombinant events only after a cat is infected.

Development of a safe and effective vaccine against FeLV presented a special challenge that other infections did not. Early vaccines carried a higher risk of anaphylaxis than did other feline vaccines. Original prototypes of inactivated-virus vaccines were not only ineffective but also increased the severity of the immunosuppression. Live-virus vaccines produced immunity, but some vaccinated kittens developed clinical disease from "attenuated" virus. Researchers were also concerned that the vaccine virus could integrate into the host genome and later cause FeLV-negative lymphomas, thus most vaccine research focused on the use of whole killed-virus preparations or subunit vaccines.

The first anti-FeLV vaccine was licensed in 1985. Since that time, the original vaccine has undergone modifications, and several other products have appeared on the market. Licensed vaccines use whole killed virus, and most contain adjuvant or genetically engineered recombinant parts of the virus. Vaccination does not interfere with testing for FeLV. Currently, recommendations for most vaccines are for two SC doses for initial protection followed by annual boosters; some are licensed for a 3-year booster. It is not necessary to administer vaccine from the same manufacturer for boosters (see Chapter 100 and Appendixes 2 and 3 for additional information on FeLV vaccination recommendations).

The relative efficacy of the vaccines is the subject of much controversy. Many of the published vaccine efficacy trials were performed or funded by the manufacturers, without having simultaneous evaluation of more than one vaccine. Furthermore, testing protocols vary widely among studies, making meaningful comparison rather difficult. Because of the natural resistance of cats (especially older cats) to FeLV infection, investigators often use artificial immune suppression (e.g., glucocorticoids) and administration of large viral doses to increase the challenge virulence in FeLV vaccine studies. Some have immunosuppressed vaccinated and control cats before intranasal (IN) challenge with virulent virus, and others have performed parenteral challenge with large doses of virus without immune suppression. The relationship of these challenges to natural exposure has been questioned,[31,124,131,180,181] making it difficult to know what the vaccine's actual effect in a natural exposure environment would be. Some studies have involved natural challenges when vaccinated and control cats lived together with FeLV-shedding cats.[89,174] This type of challenge is preferable, but no standard challenge protocol has been accepted by vaccine manufacturers. This type of natural exposure challenge experiment, in which naive cats are housed together with an FeLV-shedding cat and that are most comparable to multiple-cat household situations, provide an environment with a very high infection pressure. In this high-pressure situation, none of the licensed vaccines proved to be 100% effective. Therefore it is not safe to bring an FeLV-shedding cat into a household with FeLV-negative cats, even if these cats are vaccinated.

No accurate postvaccination measure exists that can determine whether cats are protected after vaccination. Neutralizing antibody titers develop in few vaccinated cats despite their being protected against challenge infection.[148] The immune mechanism protecting cats from persistent viremia is CMI through the effects of CTLs.[75,93] Neutralizing antibody titers do not predict postvaccinal protection; however, they can indicate which cats are protected after recovery from natural infection. Although ELISA and other antibody assays against envelope antigens exist, only neutralizing antibody titers are predictive of protection. Unfortunately, commercially available testing for neutralizing antibody is not available.

Vaccine-Associated Sarcomas

A clear epidemiologic association exists between rabies and FeLV vaccinations and later development of soft tissue sarcomas at the injection site (sarcomas referred to as *injection site sarcomas*, *vaccine-associated sarcomas*, and *vaccine site-associated sarcomas*).[119,120,162,163,199] The most frequently occurring type of these soft tissue sarcomas are fibrosarcomas, but undifferentiated sarcomas, rhabdomyosarcomas, chondrosarcomas, osteosarcomas, and malignant fibrous histiocytomas are also found. The estimated incidence ranges from 1 tumor per 1,000 vaccines to 1 tumor per 10,000 vaccines.[199] Reported rates of reactions were 0.32 vaccine-associated sarcomas per 10,000 vaccines and 11.8 postvaccinal inflammation reactions per 10,000 vaccines in cats.[84] If inflammatory reactions are a necessary prelude to sarcoma, then these rates suggest that 1 in 35 to 40 reportable inflammatory reactions transition to sarcomas. These tumors may occur as soon as 4 months or as long as 2 years after vaccination, with a median of approximately 1 year.[162] They are derived from the granulomatous inflammation at the injection site. In addition to FeLV vaccination, every SC, intradermal (ID), or IM injection can cause these tumors in cats, and certain long-acting injectable medications may also be associated with sarcoma formation.[163] However, an apparent association exists between inflammation or injury at an injection site and the risk of tumor development. Cats seem to have a unique response to adjuvants in vaccines.[28] Usually in attenuated vaccines, adjuvant is added to enhance the inflammation that is necessary in a killed product to provide necessary immunity. However, this inflammation promotes malignant transformation. Traces of adjuvants can be seen in the inflammatory reaction and later in histologic sections of tumors in the transformed fibroblast.[119] Intracellular crystalline particulate material was found in an ultrastructural study in 5 of 20 investigated tumors and in one case was identified as aluminum based.[202] Although no specific vaccine or adjuvant has been incriminated,[163] local irritation from adjuvants might stimulate fibroblasts to the point that malignant transformation occurs.[180] FeLV and FeSV themselves are not involved in the tumor development.[60] Also, replication or expression of endogenous retroviruses is obviously not involved.[166]

The recognition of the malignancies associated with widespread annual vaccination has led the AAFP to revise vaccination recommendation for cats[4] and create new guidelines for testing of feline retrovirus infections.[182] Until the safety of vaccines improves, care should be taken to weigh the risk of FeLV infection against the risk of receiving the vaccine. The AAFP questions the automatic annual revaccination in cats and recommends tailoring vaccine protocols for each feline patient. Only cats at risk of contracting the disease should be vaccinated. Cats living in closed households that have no risk should not be vaccinated. New cats in multicat households or in shelters should be tested before being introduced. Testing is recommended before every FeLV vaccination so that only FeLV-negative cats undergo vaccination. FeLV vaccination of FeLV-positive cats is not beneficial, although it is probably not harmful either. Vaccination of a latently infected cat does not prevent reactivation and is not beneficial, although again, it is probably not harmful either. Adult cats have an age resistance, and in an older cat the risk of developing a vaccine-associated sarcoma is most likely higher than the risk of developing a persistent FeLV viremia. Unfortunately, no studies provide data on the age at which vaccination should be stopped.

The AAFP recommends administering any vaccine with an FeLV component SC in the left rear leg, whereas the rabies vaccination is given in the right rear leg ("left for leukemia, right for rabies") as far distally as possible. The vaccination locations aid in the treatment of subsequent sarcomas (by amputation of the leg) because these tumors are very difficult to completely excise and often recur after resection.[199] Administration of the vaccine between the scapulae is contraindicated because tumor resection is almost impossible in this location. IM injection is also contraindicated because the tumors develop with the same frequency but are more difficult to detect early. Any nodule that is present longer than 3 months at an injection site should be removed and examined histologically. FeLV vaccines that are licensed for 3-year boosters should be used if available. Vaccines that do not contain adjuvant should be used instead of adjuvant-containing vaccines. In Europe a licensed recombinant vaccine containing all three genes of FeLV was cloned in a canarypox vector. The advantage of this new technology is that it does not need inflammation at the injection site because it is distributed in the body by the canarypox and exposed to the immune system by other mechanisms. Genetic information of certain FeLV proteins is integrated into the canarypox genome with which it enters the cell. It is here that the FeLV proteins are produced leading to antibody production and reaction of the cellular immunity. Safety of this type of vaccine has been proven. Very good, immediate, and long-term efficacy in this vaccine has been established.[251,304] In a natural challenge experiment, vaccinated cats were housed together with FeLV-shedding cats for 27 weeks; the canarypox vaccine was equally as effective as commercially available vaccines.[89] This vaccine is commercially available for use in cats and is administered by a needle-less air injection system (see Chapter 100 and Appendix 3). In one study in rats, inflammation at the injection site was less with recombinant canarypox vaccines compared with conventional vaccines.[200,201] In a limited experiment in cats, the typical granulomatous inflammation did not develop at the injection site when using this vaccine.[52] A DNA vaccine has also been developed for FeLV that contains all FeLV genes and the feline IL-

18 gene as an adjuvant. It has been highly protective in challenge experiments with kittens by producing FeLV-specific CTLs and protection against challenge infection.[75,93,149]

PUBLIC HEALTH CONSIDERATIONS

Because FeLV is known to be contagious, concern arose about the possible danger of FeLV to people. Numerous facts suggest that human infection is not impossible. The virus does grow in human bone marrow cells in culture.[222] Lymphoma has been experimentally induced by injection of large doses of virus into neonatal pups and marmosets.[260] One epidemiologic study linked prior contact with sick cats to subsequent development of childhood leukemia. The contact between FeLV-infected cats and children with leukemia was double that of contact between healthy children and healthy cats.[22,245] Cell-bound antibody believed to be directed toward FeLV-RT has been found on malignant cells of people with chronic myelocytic leukemia in blast cell crisis. Veterinarians were shown to have a higher death rate from leukemia than a control population of physicians and dentists.[19,31,34,71,91] However, the increased death rate could also be explained by their higher exposure rate to radiation.

Epidemiologic studies searching for FeLV or antibody to any of its components in people have been confusing and inconclusive. Some investigators have found antibodies to FeLV in humans with leukemia and owners of viremic cats,[25,72,146,236] whereas others using more specific radioimmune assays have obtained negative results. No person has ever been found to be viremic with FeLV. PCR was used unsuccessfully to find FeLV sequences in blood and bone marrow of young and adult humans with leukemia but with no success.[231] One explanation for the discrepancy between culture of the virus in human cells and the absence of proof of human infection may be related to the lytic action of human complement on the virus. No case of human leukemia has ever been traced to FeLV. Although it is almost impossible to prove a negative hypothesis, it appears that FeLV is not a human health hazard. A potential risk to immunosuppressed people that live in close contact with FeLV-infected cats cannot be completely excluded and should be discussed with such owners. However, the risk involved is mainly from secondary zoonotic infections that an immunosuppressed cat might acquire and potentially transmit to an immune suppressed person.

SUGGESTED READINGS*

5. American Association of Feline Practitioners/Academy of Feline Medicine (AAFP/AFM) Advisory Panel on Feline Retrovirus Testing and Management. 2001. Feline retrovirus testing and management, *Compend Contin Educ Pract Vet* 23:652-657, 692.

49a. de Mari K, Maynard L, Sanquer A, et al. 2004. Therapeutic effect of recombinant feline interferon-omega on feline leukemia virus (FeLV)-infected and FeLV/feline immunodeficiency virus (FIV)-coinfected symptomatic cats, *J Vet Intern Med* 18:477-482.

68. Ettinger SN. 2003. Principles of treatment for feline lymphoma, *Clin Tech Small Anim Pract* 18:98-102.

81. Gabor LJ, Jackson ML, Trask B, et al. 2001. Feline leukaemia virus status of Australian cats with lymphosarcoma, *Aust Vet J* 79:476-481.

111. Hartmann K, Block A, Ferk G, et al. 1999. Treatment of feline leukemia virus (FeLV) infection, *Vet Microbiol* 69:111-113.

115. Hartmann K, Werner RM, Egberink H, et al. 2001. Comparison of six in-house tests for the rapid diagnosis

of feline immunodeficiency and feline leukaemia virus infections, *Vet Rec* 149:317-320.

129. Hofmann-Lehmann R, Huder JB, Gruber S, et al. 2001. Feline leukaemia provirus load during the course of experimental infection and in naturally infected cats, *J Gen Virol* 82:1589-1596.

168. Kipar A, Kremendahl J, Jackson ML, et al. 2001. Comparative examination of cats with feline leukemia virus-associated enteritis and other relevant forms of feline enteritis, *Vet Pathol* 38:359-371.

200. Macy DW. 1999. Current understanding of vaccination site-associated sarcomas in the cat, *J Feline Med Surg* 1:15-21.

205. Malik R, Gabor LJ, Foster SF, et al. 2001. Therapy for Australian cats with lymphosarcoma, *Aust Vet J* 79:808-817.

306. Teske E, van Straten G, van Noort R, et al. 2002. Chemotherapy with cyclophosphamide, vincristine, and prednisolone (COP) in cats with malignant lymphoma: new results with an old protocol, *J Vet Intern Med* 16:179-186.

*See the CD-ROM for a complete list of references.

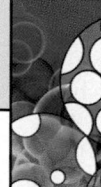

CHAPTER • 14

Feline Immunodeficiency Virus Infection

Rance K. Sellon and Katrin Hartmann

ETIOLOGY

Feline immunodeficiency virus (FIV) is a lentivirus that shares many properties characteristic of other lentiviruses, such as human immunodeficiency virus (HIV). FIV has remained the object of intense investigation as a model of lentiviral pathogenesis and prevention. The amount of knowledge generated with regard to FIV continues to increase in many arenas. Acquainting the reader with all of the information that exists is beyond the scope of this chapter; rather, the object is to familiarize the reader with current concepts of FIV that are clinically relevant. Readers interested in a review of the basic genetic organization and life cycle of FIV, function of FIV genes and gene products, and its comparisons to other lentiviruses are referred to other sources.*

Although discussion of the FIV genome and its products is not the focus of this chapter, several FIV genes have clinically important aspects. For example, regions in the viral integrase enzyme determine the site of binding and integration of FIV provirus into the host cell DNA, which can influence host cell function.[568,569]

Of the FIV genes, the envelope *(env)* gene and its proteins[471] provide the best examples of the clinical importance of FIV gene structure and function. Field isolates of FIV are divided into several subtypes based on sequence differences in a hypervariable region of the *env* gene.[469,640] Worldwide, five different subtypes (or clades) have been recognized, subtypes A, B, C, D, and E.[443,477] Extensive analysis of field subtypes in the United States and Canada has yet to be conducted. However, some studies suggest that subtypes A and B predominate in the United States, with occasional cats infected

with subtype C.[21,667] These studies also suggest regional differences in subtype distribution, with subtype A common in the western United States and subtype B predominant in the eastern United States. In Australia and Africa, subtype A has been described, and in South America, subtypes B and E have been found. European cats are infected with subtypes A, B, C, and D, with subtype A being the major subtype in the northern countries (e.g., Germany, The Netherlands), and subtype B being more important in southern countries (e.g., Italy).[155,488,597] Subtypes B, C, and D predominate in Japan and other Asian countries, although subtypes A, B, C, and E have also been observed.* Analysis of European FIV subtypes has suggested that subgroupings within a given subtype are also possible, reflecting the genetic plasticity of FIV.[597]

As demonstrated by seroprevalence studies, naturally infected cats can harbor multiple subtypes,[332,456] and superinfection indicates a lack of cross-protection among some subtypes, a finding that has bearing on FIV vaccine success (see Prevention).[101,332,456] Evidence suggests that exchange of gene segments encoding the *env* protein from different subtypes can occur between isolates in superinfected cats.[101]

Env properties are clinically relevant because they determine cell tropism[†] and influence pathogenicity.[‡] Interactions of FIV *env* proteins with host cell ligands are critical initial steps during host cell infection.[263,657] *Env* proteins are targets of immune responses,[§] and differences in, or conservation of, *env* sequences may reflect selection pressures exerted by the immune response of the infected cat.[¶]

Differences in *env* antigenic determinants still represent potential obstacles in the development of FIV vaccines pro-

*References 8, 9, 15, 41, 46, 51, 78, 79, 80, 103, 104, 138, 163, 164, 200, 204, 228, 280, 283, 284, 315, 334, 335, 345, 365, 370, 376, 415, 433, 441, 476, 491, 512, 562, 590, 606, 618, 632, 653, 666, 670, 677, 678, 689.

*References 254, 331, 439, 443, 629.
†References 252, 324, 351, 469, 575, 633.
‡References 294, 298, 324, 469, 640.
§References 86, 142, 188, 268, 399, 574.
¶References 45, 218, 470, 472, 532.

tective against widely prevalent, and different, isolates of FIV[250,573,576] (see Prevention).

EPIDEMIOLOGY

Prevalence

FIV is common worldwide, and its prevalence varies among geographic locations. Across the United States, the seroprevalence of FIV in cats at high risk of exposure and in clinically ill cats ranges from approximately 4% to 24%, with few apparent regional differences.[108,346,451] Seroprevalence outside the United States varies. Some countries report few infected cats, and others, such as Italy and Japan, with large populations of free-roaming cats have prevalence rates that can approach 30%.* Pockets of high prevalence, such as 47% reported in one group of feral cats in the United Kingdom, can also be seen.[101] The prevalence of FIV in healthy cats is usually lower than in sick cats,[391,435,679] with rates commonly at 2% to 5%,[46,590] and foci of higher prevalence reflecting local cat population dynamics.[18] Seroprevalence in nearly all surveys is higher in male cats than it is in female cats, which is considered the result of higher rates of virus transmission among biting and fighting cats.[†] Adult cats are found infected more often than adolescent cats and kittens are,[435] which again likely reflects aggressive behavior between cats as the predominant means of natural transmission. In serologic surveys, it is uncommon for enzyme-linked immunosorbent assay (ELISA)-positive results to be confirmed by Western blotting; thus true infection prevalence may be overestimated, especially in the healthy cat population, because of false positive results.

Evidence from retrospective serosurveys suggests that FIV has been present in the domestic feline population since at least 1966.[564] Infection with lentiviruses related to FIV has been reported in Florida panthers and many other nondomestic feline species in United States zoos, as well as in free-roaming nondomestic felids in the United States, Europe, Africa, Saudi Arabia, and Asia.[‡] The greater diversity of viral nucleic acid sequences and the decreased pathogenicity of the nondomestic felid isolates, compared with those that affect domestic cats, suggest that nondomestic felids have been living with the virus for a longer time and that the domestic cat strains may have emerged more recently from nondomestic strains.[457] Domestic cats are susceptible to persistent infection with isolates from nondomestic felids, but the clinical and immunologic abnormalities that develop in FIV-infected domestic cats are typically not observed when domestic cats are infected with nondomestic feline lentiviruses.[638] Furthermore, cross-infection studies suggest that infection with a nondomestic feline lentivirus (lion or puma lentivirus) may blunt the immunologic and virologic responses to subsequent FIV infection.[635,636] Probable transmission of an FIV isolate from domestic cats to an exotic cat species has also been documented.[444]

Transmission

In natural settings, FIV is transmitted primarily by parenteral inoculation of virus present in saliva or blood, presumably by bite and fight wounds, accounting for the higher prevalence in male cats. Experimentally induced bites are effective at transmitting virus from infected to naïve cats. Additional evidence supporting the importance of this route of transmission is the observation that FIV can be found in salivary gland epithelium[402,474] during acute infection, as well as in saliva, blood lymphocytes, and plasma or serum.[402] Experimentally,

FIV is easily transmitted by all parenteral routes (intravenous [IV], subcutaneous [SC], intramuscular [IM], intraperitoneal [IP]) using cell-free or cell-associated virus.

In experimental settings, high rates of transmission (over 50%), both in utero and postparturition via milk, have been documented in queens with acute and chronic FIV infections.* The presence of greater viral loads in milk than milk secreting cells or plasma suggests that virus can be concentrated in milk.[6] Available evidence suggests that, in a given litter, some kittens can acquire infection in utero, and others will not.[539] Transmission has also been reported after oral,[425,560] intrarectal, and intravaginal inoculation with cell-free or cell-associated virus.[81,322,448-450] The feline female reproductive tract has CD4 and CD8 T cells, B cells, macrophages, and dendritic cells, all known targets of FIV infection. Systemic spread following mucosal routes of inoculation can occur within days.[91,450]

Despite the experimental evidence of transmission via the mucosal routes, no evidence suggests that these routes have an important role in maintaining natural infections. Available epidemiologic and serologic surveys do not, however, exclude the possibility of occasional transmission by these routes. High kitten mortality in FIV-positive neonates or rapidly progressive infections, as observed in some experimental studies,[†] may lead to underestimates of in utero and neonatal transmission in natural settings. Additionally, the observation that kittens born to FIV-infected mothers can have FIV provirus detected in tissues, but not necessarily blood, in the absence of detectable antibodies further complicates the understanding of congenital transmission rates under natural conditions.[5]

Infectious virus has been documented in both cell-free and cell-associated fractions of semen from acutely and chronically infected male cats.[300,304] Infection can be established following laparoscopic insemination of queens with semen from infected male cats.[301,303] Although contribution of seminal transmission to maintenance of natural infections is unknown, it is likely low.

Horizontal transmission of FIV in multiple-cat households is an arguably infrequent event, with some studies suggesting it rarely occurs and others suggesting that horizontal transmission may be common.[3,478] FIV DNA-positive but antibody-negative cats have been detected in situations in which the DNA-positive cats had been housed in experimental colonies for long periods (months to years) with FIV-infected cats. Despite being DNA-positive, the cats were asymptomatic and did not develop typical immunologic abnormalities observed in antibody-positive cats.[125] Similar cases of DNA-positive but antibody-negative cats have been observed in other studies.[5,449] The clinical consequences, if any, of this latent type of infection remain unknown at present.

Experimentally, miscellaneous modes of transmission, such as using suture contaminated with blood from an FIV-positive cat, have been documented.[154] Inoculation of proviral DNA has also produced infection.[486,533,591] Although infection has been established with these modes, natural infections are unlikely to occur through these routes.

PATHOGENESIS

The picture emerging from recent studies of FIV pathogenesis suggests that the events that follow infection, such as differences in viral kinetics, clinical features and progression of FIV infection, and the character of immune responses to FIV following infection, are likely the result of an interplay of a

*References 18, 24, 150, 212, 344, 396, 420, 435, 438, 482, 590, 629.
†References 112, 150, 201, 262, 321, 346, 435, 665.
‡References 34, 49, 74, 83, 173, 198, 457, 466, 500.

*References 95, 458, 459, 538, 539, 560, 650.
†References 5, 6, 448, 449, 458, 459.

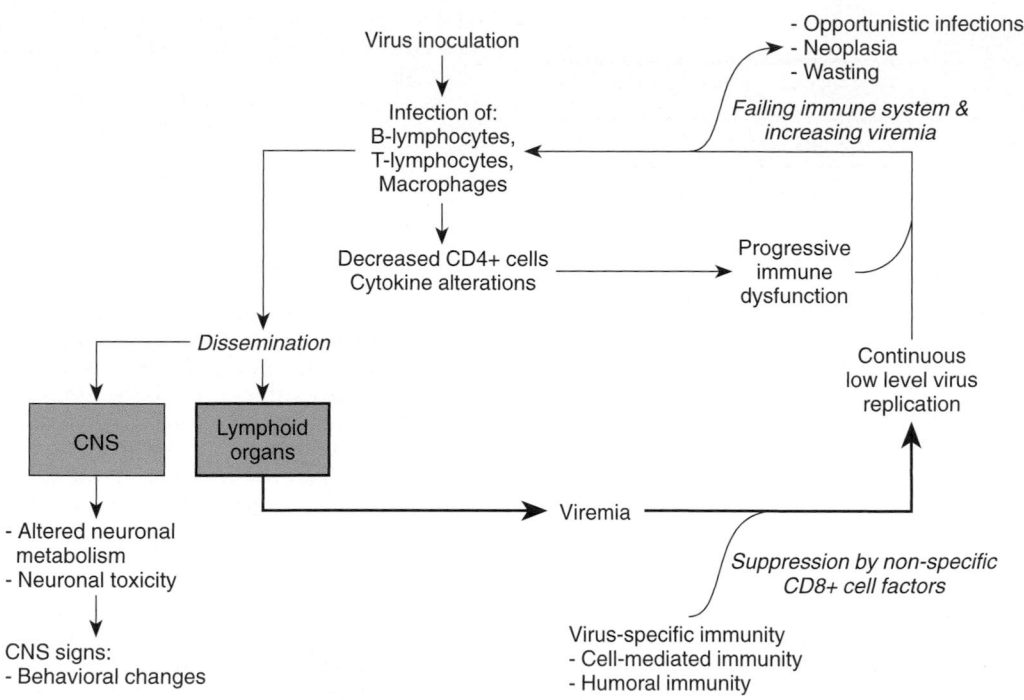

Fig 14-1 Pathogenesis of FIV infection.

large number of factors. Such factors include the age of the animal at the time of infection (young animals developing clinical signs faster), properties of the FIV isolate, the amount of virus used for infection, the route of infection (parenteral versus mucosal or other route), and whether the inoculum is in the form of cell-free or cell-associated (i.e., infected cells) virus.*

After experimental inoculation, viral particles are cleared by tissues rich in macrophages, and viral replication then occurs in target cells of lymphoid organs (thymus, spleen, lymph nodes), and other tissues rich in macrophages and lymphoid cells.† Viremia peaks within several weeks postinoculation (PI).[42,130] Using polymerase chain reaction (PCR) or viral culture, the virus is easily detected in plasma or peripheral blood lymphocytes by 2 weeks PI or earlier.[402] FIV also spreads to mononuclear cells (lymphocytes, monocytes, and macrophages) in organs such as the bone marrow, lung, intestinal tract, brain, and kidney.[42,540,547] Virus-infected follicular dendritic cells in lymph nodes may infect naïve T cells migrating through the lymph node.[20,624]

After peak viremia, circulating virus decreases to low levels as the host mounts an immune response to FIV. A vigorous, but ultimately ineffective, humoral immune response is mounted against the virus (Fig. 14-1). Generally, anti-FIV antibodies first become detectable in experimentally infected cats 2 to 4 weeks PI, although exposure to lesser amounts of virus may delay the appearance of detectable responses.[46] Antibodies are produced against many FIV proteins,[162,176,268,534] especially those of the viral envelope, capsid, and transmembrane proteins.[399] Virus-neutralizing antibodies can be detected with in vitro assays,[23,464,625] but the role that neutralizing antibodies play in suppression of FIV viremia in vivo is not clear.‡ Some studies suggest that the humoral immune response in infected cats is responsible for driving the emergence of FIV variants that are resistant to in vitro

neutralization.[211] As noted previously, occasional cats will be provirus (DNA) positive, but remain antibody negative.

Although a robust humoral immune response is mounted, current evidence suggests that CD8+ T-cell-mediated immunity (CMI) is responsible for suppressing early virus production after initial infection.[81,82,114,203] Suppression of virus production has been demonstrated in vitro through mechanisms involving both cell-cell interactions and secretion of soluble factors, perhaps interleukin(IL)-16 or others.[356] One interesting feature of the antiviral activity of the soluble factor is that it is not restricted to a specific FIV isolate.* The mechanism behind this nonspecific, noncytolytic, T-cell–mediated, viral-suppressive activity may be inhibition of viral mRNA transcription.[253,258] Inhibitory activity can be detected in some cats approximately 1 week PI and before detection of a humoral immune response, with virus-specific cytolytic T-cell activity detected later.[190] T-cell–suppressive activity can be maintained through the asymptomatic period, but as infection progresses into the chronic phase, suppressor activity may wane in infected cats.[189,259] Virus-specific cytotoxic T-cell activity emerges in the weeks after infection and also plays a role in virus control.[86]

Following acute infection and suppression of viremia, cats enter a clinically asymptomatic period of variable duration. This period is not one of true viral latency because FIV production continues in infected cells in tissues, and virus can still be recovered from blood lymphocytes, serum or plasma, cerebral spinal fluid (CSF), semen, and lymphoid tissues.† Plasma levels of virus and viral RNA can increase again during the terminal phases of infection (see Fig. 14-1).[145,216,325]

FIV infects a wide range of cell types in vitro and in vivo (Table 14-1), but cell tropism is isolate dependent.[131,152] Unlike HIV, FIV does not use the feline CD4 molecule as a cellular receptor to infect target cells.[272,445] A molecule with receptor function for FIV has been identified as a chemokine

*References 86, 87, 260, 449, 450, 479.
†References 54, 292, 386, 446, 449, 540, 669.
‡References 136, 207, 282, 403, 407.

*References 106, 114, 189, 256, 356.
†References 20, 46, 153, 169, 302, 585.

Table • 14-1

In Vivo and in Vitro Cell Tropism of FIV

IN VIVO	IN VITRO
Lymphocytes (CD4+, CD8+, B cells)[25,37,51,540]	Brain endothelial cells[543]
Monocytes/ macrophages[44,152,603,450,540]	Brain microglial cells[151,153]
Follicular dendritic cells[20,624,450,540]	Astrocytes[151,153]
Thymic epithelial cells[540]	Macrophages[395,67]
Astrocytes[386]	
Bone marrow fibroblasts[603]	
Megakaryocytes[44]	
Salivary gland epithelium[474]	

receptor designated CXCR4.* Expression of CXCR4 mRNA or antigen can be demonstrated in a large number of cell types known to be susceptible to FIV infection, including lymphocytes and astrocytes, and intraepithelial mononuclear cells and epithelial cells of the rectum, colon, and female reproductive tract, perhaps accounting for some degree of transmucosal transmission observed in experimental studies.† However, not all cell types susceptible to infection express CXCR4. Some cells that express CXCR4 are not susceptible to infection with all FIV isolates, especially primary field isolates, and not all viral isolates display evidence of using CXCR4 as a pathway to cell infection.[197,263,351] Thus other, or additional, receptor molecules or modes of cell entry may likely be important in establishing productive infections in target cells.[263,296] Potential candidates include heparan,[139] immunoglobulin-mediated entry into cells bearing the immunoglobulin Fc receptor (macrophages, B cells), or intercellular infection through contact of infected and uninfected cells. The hypothesis holds that for some FIV isolates and cell targets, CXCR4 acts as primary receptor for FIV and the CCR5 receptor, another type of chemokine receptor, influences FIV infection by modulating the expression of CXCR4, or serves as another FIV receptor.[328,656]

The hallmark of FIV pathogenesis is progressive disruption of normal immune function, some of the mechanisms of which have been elucidated. Early and persistent immunologic abnormalities that occur after experimental[2,26,621] and natural[248,447] infection in both domestic and nondomestic felids are decreases in both the number and relative proportions of CD4+ cells (see Fig. 14-1) in the peripheral blood, as well as in most primary lymphoid tissues examined.[84] Causes of CD4+-cell loss may include decreased production secondary to bone marrow or thymic infection, lysis of infected cells induced by FIV itself (cytopathic effects), destruction of virally infected cells by the immune system, or death by apoptosis.‡ Apoptosis is a form of cell death that follows receipt of a membrane signal initiating a series of programmed intracellular events that ultimately lead to cell death. Apoptosis of CD4+, CD8+, and B cells has been documented in lymph nodes, spleen, and thymus of FIV infected cats[261,548,620]; the degree of apoptosis has correlated inversely with CD4+ numbers and the CD4+/CD8+ ratio.[261] Ultimately, loss of

CD4+ cells impairs immune responses because CD4+ cells have critical roles in promoting and maintaining both humoral and CMI.

As is seen with HIV infection in people, loss of CD4+ cells leads to inversion of the CD4+/CD8+ ratio (see Fig. 14-1). The inversion may occur weeks to months after infection, depending on the viral isolate studied.[2,621] Contributing to the inverted ratio in some cases is an increase in the proportion of CD8+ cells (cytotoxic or T lymphocytes),[2,248,658] in particular a population referred to as CD8+ alpha-hi, beta-low cells,[570,571] a subset of CD8+ cells that arguably may contribute to suppression of viremia in FIV-infected cats. Although inversion of the CD4+/CD8+ ratio is a consistent feature of both natural and experimental infections, its use as a prognostic tool for cats is questionable, as has been demonstrated with HIV-infected people.[59,644] FIV-infected cats may show severe inversion for prolonged periods without developing clinical signs, and available work demonstrates no correlation of the ratio with clinical stage of infection or plasma viremia.[217,248] Despite being a target of viral infection, no reported changes have been found in numbers or proportions of B cells after FIV infection.

Other immunologic abnormalities occur with FIV infection. Over time, lymphocytes from infected cats lose the ability to proliferate in response to stimulation with B- and T-cell mitogens, and have impaired priming of T cells by T-cell–dependent immunogens in vitro.* Lymphocyte function may also be impaired by reduced or altered expression of cell surface molecules, such as CD4, major histocompatibility complex II antigens or other co-stimulatory molecules, and cytokine receptors,† each of which has a critical role in antigen presentation, or amplification and control of immune responses.

FIV infection is associated with disrupted production of cytokines, molecules essential to normal immune function. Cytokine patterns detected from cultures of FIV-infected lymphocytes are dependent to some extent on the FIV isolate and tissue compartment studied.[132,373] Reported changes in cytokine production in FIV-infected cats, as compared with noninfected cats, have included increased production of interferon (IFN)-γ, tumor necrosis factor (TNF)-α, IL-4, IL-6, IL-10, and IL-12.[352,366,462,536] Increased IL-10/IL-12 ratios have been observed in FIV-infected cats also infected with *Toxoplasma gondii*,[363] a pattern that would impair the development of CMI responses to *T. gondii*. Similarly, increased IL-10 has been documented in FIV-infected cats infected with *Listeria monocytogenes*, with FIV-infected cats exhibiting delayed clearance and more severe clinical signs of infection as compared with FIV-negative cats.[130]

Alterations in function of nonspecific defenses such as neutrophils have also been described in FIV-infected cats.[225,330] Natural killer cell activity has been reported as diminished[681] or increased[687] in FIV-infected cats, depending on whether the cats were acutely or asymptomatically infected, respectively.

Another manifestation of the immunologic dysregulation observed in many FIV-infected cats is hypergammaglobulinemia, primarily from increases in IgG.[2,186] Hypergammaglobulinemia reflects polyclonal B-cell stimulation because the IgG produced is not FIV specific. It is a direct consequence of FIV infection because healthy FIV-positive, specific pathogen-free (SPF) cats are also hypergammaglobulinemic.[186] In addition to increased IgG, increased circulating immune complexes have been detected in FIV-infected cats.[400] FIV has also been incriminated as causing a delay in the class shift of antibody

---

*References 69, 139, 161, 197, 273, 497, 529, 655, 656, 657.
†References 99, 202, 327, 328, 437.
‡References 55, 222, 223, 290, 421, 423, 424, 430, 432, 453, 454, 487, 620.

*References 26, 58, 59, 226, 268, 604, 605, 622.
†References 107, 422, 455, 531, 659.

isotypes from IgM to IgG based on work in cats infected with both FIV and *T. gondii*.[341]

Abnormal neurologic function has been described in FIV-infected cats with varying degrees of central nervous system (CNS) inflammation. Although occasional studies have linked neurologic dysfunction and neuronal injury with the amount of virus present in the brain of infected cats,[297] many studies support the hypothesis that neurologic dysfunction and histologic changes in the CNS are indirect events and not an immediate consequence of CNS-cell infection or viral replication within the CNS.[410,475,506,542] Experimental infections in vivo have caused brain lesions in the absence of massive CNS infection.[542] Neurotoxins such as glutamate have been implicated as one cause of neuronal loss.* Other work has incriminated a role for matrix metalloproteinases, which can break down collagen and alter properties of the blood-brain barrier, or altered neuronal cytoskeletal properties in the pathogenesis of neurologic dysfunction in FIV-infected cats.[287,294,298] In vitro and, occasionally, in vivo studies suggest that infection of cells in the CNS, in particular the astrocyte and macrophage, may impair normal CNS-cell metabolism.† Documented abnormalities of astrocyte and macrophage functions include altered intercellular communication, abnormal glutathione reductase activity that may render cells more susceptible to oxidative injury, alterations in mitochondrial membrane potential that disrupt energy-producing capacities of the cell, and impaired maintenance of intracellular calcium concentrations.[65] Some studies suggest that sequences in the viral envelope protein are important in neurovirulence properties,‡ and others indicate that neurologic cell dysfunction does not necessarily correlate with envelope-mediated replicative capacity.[53,294] Interestingly, purified FIV gp120, an envelope protein, caused neurologic abnormalities when administered to rats.[515,545]

The pathogenesis of some clinical features of FIV remains unexplained but, similar to neurologic disease, may result from abnormal function of, or inflammation in, affected organs. Wasting disease has been observed in the absence of obvious causes such as diarrhea or neoplasia. Abnormal renal function and nephritis have also been reported in FIV-infected cats.[362] Some aspects of clinical FIV will reflect the pathogenesis of the secondary diseases such as infections and neoplasms to which FIV-infected cats are considered susceptible.

CLINICAL FINDINGS

FIV infection progresses through several stages, similar to HIV-1 infection in people. Recognized clinical stages in cats include an acute phase, a clinically asymptomatic phase of variable duration, and a terminal phase of infection often referred to as feline acquired immunodeficiency syndrome (AIDS).[169,217] Some investigators note two other phases in keeping with the terminology for HIV infection: progressive generalized lymphadenomegaly, which follows the asymptomatic phase, followed by AIDS-related complex (ARC).[217,285,286,478] Still other researchers describe a sixth category to encompass miscellaneous diseases such as neoplastic, ocular, and immune-mediated diseases that are observed in some infected cats.[478]

Although division of FIV infection into these clinical stages may prove useful from the standpoint of gauging prognosis, no sharp distinction exists between them, and not all stages will be apparent in some infected cats. Furthermore, no readily available predictor has been found of the transition from the asymptomatic phase to the ARC or AIDS phase, although one study found that higher levels of viremia during the acute stage of infection were associated with more rapid progression to the terminal phases of the disease.[146] In a study of naturally infected cats, a trend was noted for increasing viremia with progression of clinical signs, with cats in the AIDS category of infection exhibiting higher viral loads than cats in the ARC or asymptomatic phase of infection.[217]

Clinical signs of FIV infection are nonspecific (Table 14-2). Clinical signs attributed directly to FIV infection likely go unobserved in many naturally infected cats. During acute experimental infection, clinical signs may be transient and so mild as to go unnoticed. Some cats exhibit fever and malaise. Signs of acute enteritis, stomatitis, dermatitis, conjunctivitis, and respiratory tract disease can be seen. Generalized lymph node enlargement is common during acute experimental infection.[449] The acute phase may last several days to a few weeks, after which cats will enter a period in which they appear clinically healthy. The duration of the asymptomatic phase varies and likely depends on factors such as the pathogenic potential of the infecting isolate and the exposure of the infected cats to other pathogens but can last for years. One experimentally infected cat, kept isolated from other cats, had FIV-infection for over 8 years without developing clinical signs.[325] The age of the cat at the time of infection may also influence the length of the asymptomatic stage and the severity of clinical disease, depending on the isolate studied.[479,493] During the later stages of infection, clinical signs are often a reflection of opportunistic infections, neoplasia, myelosuppression, and neurologic disease.

Infections with a significant number of opportunistic pathogens of viral, bacterial (Fig. 14-2), protozoal, and fungal origin have been reported in FIV-infected cats (Table 14-3). Few studies, however, have compared the prevalence of most of these infections in FIV-infected and noninfected cats. No correlation was found between FIV infection and infection with *Cryptococcus* or *Cryptosporidium*.[434,646] Another study reported a higher number of fungal genera isolated from the skin, oropharynx, and rectum of FIV-infected cats compared with noninfected cats, but FIV-infected cats had no symptoms of fungal infections at the time of examination,[392] and no correlation was found between FIV infection and the presence of *Cryptococcus neoformans* or dermatophytes.[578] In one study, seroprevalence of *T. gondii* was similar in both FIV-infected and noninfected cats, and FIV-infected cats did not have detectable oocyst shedding.[601] In another study, the prevalence of FIV was higher in *T. gondii* antibody–positive cats.[150] The prevalence of *Bartonella henselae*, the agent of cat scratch disease, or *B. clarridgeiae* has not been positively associated with FIV infection.[213,245,396,397] An increased prevalence of FIV

*References 62, 68, 511, 579, 680.
†References 53, 67, 124, 326, 685.
‡References 68, 221, 244, 294, 296.

Table • 14-2

Clinical Signs in Cats with Naturally Acquired Infection[a]

Fever	Weight loss, emaciation
Dermatitis, otitis	Enteritis, diarrhea
Lymph node enlargement	Abscesses
Stomatitis, gingivitis	Chronic renal insufficiency
Neurologic signs	Respiratory tract infection
Uveitis, pars planitis, conjunctivitis	

[a]References 76, 170, 229, 503, 530, 566, 590, 592.

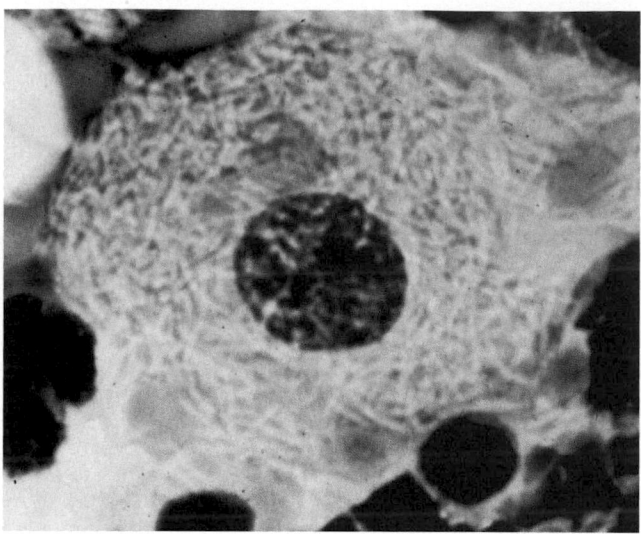

Fig 14-2 Mycobacteria in a blood macrophage in an FIV-infected cat with disseminated mycobacterial infection. (Courtesy Julie Levy, University of Florida, Gainesville, Fla)

Table • 14-3

Concurrent Infections and Neoplasms Reported in Cats with Naturally Acquired FIV Infection

INFECTIONS	NEOPLASMS
Feline leukemia virus[451,564] (Chapter 13)	Lymphoma, leukemia[279]
Calicivirus[651] (Chapter 16)	Myeloproliferative disease[564,590]
Feline foamy (syncytium-forming) virus[684] (Chapter 17)	Squamous cell carcinoma[279,194]
Poxvirus[73] (Chapter 19)	Mammary gland adenocarcinoma[566]
Papilloma virus[160] (Chapter 20)	Mast cell tumor[30]
Mycoplasma haemofelis (Haemobartonella felis)[567] (Chapter 31)	Bronchoalveolar carcinoma[532]
Mycoplasma spp.[115] (Chapter 32)	
Mycobacterium spp.[275] (Chapter 50)	
Dermatophytes[590] (Chapter 58)	
Cryptococcus[92,175] (Chapter 61)	
Sporothrix schenckii[558] (Chapter 63)	
Hepatozoon sp.[25] (Chapter 74)	
Theileria annae[115] (Chapter 77)	
Babesia felis[557] (Chapter 77)	
B. canis[115] (Chapter 77)	
Toxoplasma gondii[241,461] (Chapter 80)	
Cryptosporidium[434] (Chapter 82)	

infection has also been reported in cats that were antibody-positive for *Bornavirus*,[274] a virus detected in cats in eastern and northern European countries, and cats with orthopoxvirus.[626] No significant association between FIV infection in cats with *Mycoplasma haemofelis/M. haemominutum (Haemobartonella felis)* has been found.[227]

Stomatitis is a common condition of FIV-infected cats and can occur during any stage of infection. The cause of stomatitis is uncertain, although the histologic findings of lymphocytes, plasma cells, and variable degrees of neutrophilic and eosinophilic infiltrates suggest either an immune response to chronic antigenic stimulation or immune dysregulation. Stomatitis is not often seen in SPF cats, suggesting that exposure to infectious agents may also play a role.[362] Experimental and naturally occurring co-infection of FIV-infected cats with calicivirus resulted in more severe disease.[524,609] Odontoclastic resorptive lesions have been reported with higher prevalence in experimentally infected cats as compared with noninfected cats; such lesions have been speculated to be a consequence of gingivitis or stomatitis present in the cats.[249]

Diarrhea has been seen in experimentally infected cats in the absence of detectable enteric pathogens. Bacterial overgrowth and inflammatory lesions have been proposed as a cause in such cases but are not always evident.[473]

FIV-positive cats can develop ocular disease,[170,340,461,664] and abnormalities may be found in both anterior and posterior segments. Anterior uveitis may result from secondary infections such as toxoplasmosis or may be directly related to FIV infection.[170,461,664] Glaucoma, with and without uveitis, has also been described.[170,461,664] Posterior segment changes that may be seen include pars planitis (an infiltration of leukocytes, mainly plasma cells, into the vitreous behind the lens), focal retinal degeneration, and inner retinal hemorrhages.[170,664]

Respiratory disease may be observed in FIV-positive cats and can result from bacterial, fungal, protozoal, or parasitic infections.[35] Experimentally, FIV infection worsened the respiratory disease observed in an experimental model of acute toxoplasmosis.[127]

Neoplasia is a common reason that FIV-infected cats are brought to a veterinary clinic. Lymphomas, leukemias, and a variety of other tumor types (see Table 14-3) have been reported in association with FIV infection.* Statistically, FIV-infected cats are much more likely to develop lymphoma or leukemia compared with noninfected cats.[96,499] Most lymphomas in FIV-infected cats are B-cell tumors.[96,201,499,610] FIV provirus is only occasionally detected in tumor cells,[39,38,37,649] suggesting an indirect role for FIV in lymphoma formation, such as decreased CMI surveillance or chronic B-cell hyperplasia.[39,166] However, clonally integrated FIV DNA was recently found in lymphoma cells from one cat that had been experimentally infected 6 years earlier,[37,38] raising the possibility of an occasional direct oncogenic role of FIV in some animals. The prevalence of FIV infection in one cohort of cats with lymphosarcoma was 50%,[201] much higher than the FIV prevalence in the population of cats without lymphosarcoma, which is supportive of a cause and effect relationship between FIV and feline lymphosarcoma.

Neurologic signs have been described in both natural and experimental, and acute and terminal, FIV infections.† Neurologic impairment following FIV infection appears to be isolate dependent.[510] The most common neurologic sign observed is behavioral change. Other deficits that have been described include seizures, paresis, multifocal motor abnormalities, impaired learning, and disrupted sleep patterns.[224,514,594] Neurologic signs may improve if they occur during the acute stage of infection, although residual deficits are possible. Abnormal

---

*References 30, 85, 97, 113, 183, 279, 499.
†References 1, 151, 153, 172, 484, 496.

forebrain electrical activity and abnormal visual and auditory-evoked potentials have also been documented in cats that appeared otherwise normal.[32,486,493,495] Less commonly, secondary infections such as feline infectious peritonitis, toxoplasmosis, or cryptococcosis cause neurologic deficits.

In the terminal phase of infection, a wasting syndrome may occur. If experimentally infected with some particularly pathogenic FIV isolates, SPF cats have developed a terminal wasting syndrome within 6 to 8 weeks PI.[144,146]

DIAGNOSIS

Clinical Laboratory Findings

A large number of clinicopathologic abnormalities have been described in FIV-infected cats, but none are specific or pathognomonic for infection. During the acute phase of infection, cats may exhibit neutropenia and lymphopenia, which resolve as the cat progresses to the asymptomatic phase of infection.[371,393] During the asymptomatic phase of infection, results of complete blood count (CBC) and biochemical analyses are often normal,[371,374,393,567] but leukopenia may be encountered.[18,567] Clinically ill FIV-infected cats may have a variety of cytopenias. Lymphopenia, caused mainly by decreases in CD4+ cells, is most common. Anemia and neutropenia may also be seen,[75,565,566,592] although these abnormalities may be as much a reflection of concurrent disease as direct effects of FIV infection itself. Anemia, leukopenia, and less commonly thrombocytopenia[229] have been observed in FIV-infected cats in the absence of other identifiable causes.[18,479] Soluble factors have been shown to inhibit bone marrow function in FIV-infected cats, and bone marrow infection has been associated with decreased ability to support hematopoietic potential in vitro.[603]

Abnormalities of the biochemical profile of FIV-infected cats typically are few. Some cats have an increase in total protein caused by hyperglobulinemia. Azotemia has been reported in FIV-infected cats in the absence of other detectable causes of renal disease,[362,503,611] but FIV as a definitive cause of renal disease awaits clarification. Other biochemical abnormalities, when found, will usually reflect concurrent disease. When compared with control cats, after 9 months of FIV infection, experimentally infected cats had increased serum globulin, glucose, triglyceride, urea, and creatinine concentrations and reduced serum cholesterol levels.[250] The mechanism of such changes may include altered energy metabolism, subclinical hypercortisolemia, and release of cytokines in infected cats. Prolongations of the activated partial thromboplastin time have been reported in FIV-infected cats in the absence of other obvious causes of coagulopathy, although the prolongations were mild and not clinically apparent.[229]

Few descriptions of CSF changes have been provided in FIV-infected cats with neurologic disease. Cellular pleocytosis and increases in concentrations of IgG in the CSF have been reported,[153] expecting increases in cell number and total protein in CSF is not unreasonable. Viral RNA can be found in the CSF of some cats and suggests parenchymal infection.[542]

Serologic Testing

A definitive diagnosis of FIV infection is made most commonly by detection of FIV-specific antibodies in blood by either ELISA or rapid immunomigration-type assays, which are widely available and easy to use (see Appendix 6).[505] These assays are reasonably sensitive and specific, although reported sensitivity and specificity can be quite variable, and both false-positive and false-negative results can be obtained with any of these "in-house" assays.[201,238,537] Technical error in a specific test kit, and use of whole blood rather than serum, have been incriminated as causes of false-positive test results performed with in-house assays.[238] Variability in sensitivity and specificity, in conjunction with differences in infection prevalence, affects the predictive values of these assays. One comparison of six in-house assays found positive predictive values that ranged from 83% on the high end to only 51% on the low end, while negative predictive values ranged from 96% to 99%.[238] Such results emphasize the importance of confirmatory testing. Cats that have positive results by an in-house test should be retested, ideally by Western blot (see Chapter 1), to confirm the diagnosis.

Because FIV produces a persistent infection from which cats do not recover and infected cats usually develop high amounts of FIV-specific antibodies, detection of antibody has historically been synonymous with infection. However, the introduction of a commercial vaccine in the United States has the potential to complicate interpretation of antibody tests. Currently available assays, including Western blots, are incapable of distinguishing antibody responses induced by infection from vaccinal antibodies. In patients that are known with certainty to not have been vaccinated, antibody tests are still reliable to diagnose FIV infection. Misdiagnosis of FIV in uninfected cats (e.g., positive results in vaccinated cats) may lead to the inappropriate euthanasia of vaccinated cats or of kittens born to vaccinated queens. This issue is especially problematic in shelter medicine, given that confirmatory testing is frequently impractical. Experimental evidence also suggests that superinfection with different subtypes is possible (i.e., inconsistent cross-protection), and thus a cat vaccinated with a dual subtype vaccine may be susceptible to infection with a subtype not included in the vaccine. Serologic assays would not be helpful in determining the infection status of such cats.

Antibody tests also have to be interpreted carefully in kittens less than 6 months of age. Kittens up to 12 weeks of age can have passively acquired anti-FIV antibodies from mothers that are infected or have been vaccinated.[386a] Rarely do kittens become infected from their mothers under natural circumstances; therefore most kittens that initially test positive will eventually turn negative when maternal antibodies wane. Retesting these kittens after 6 months of age is advised. If the second test is negative, the earlier positive result was likely the result of maternal antibody. If still positive, the kitten is likely infected. A kitten of unknown background that is initially antibody negative is likely to be truly negative, but a small chance exists that the kitten has not had time to develop a detectable antibody response. These kittens should be retested after 8 to 12 weeks. If still negative, the kitten is unlikely to be infected. If positive, the kitten is probably infected.

Cats in the acute phase of infection may be antibody negative, and retesting suspect cats in 6 to 8 weeks is warranted to establish a diagnosis in cats with a recent history that puts them at risk of exposure. Most cats develop a detectable antibody response within 8 weeks of initial infection; however, in some experimental studies, antibody development has not been observed until 10 weeks after inoculation and in occasional animals has required 6 months or longer.[253,478] Antibody development may not occur in rapidly progressive infections.[460] These observations from experimental infections suggest that a single negative test result may, in some instances, be insufficient to discriminate recently infected animals from true negative animals.

FIV-specific antibodies are readily detected in blood of most cats throughout the asymptomatic phase of infection. Asymptomatic kittens with regressive infections (i.e., infections associated with very low or no antibody titers) have been observed after experimental infection, and evidence of FIV infection can be only demonstrated by culture or PCR.[449,460] Because of debilitation of the immune system, some cats entering the terminal phase of infection may lose detectable antibody.[145] For such cats, Western blots may show FIV-specific antibodies not detected by some ELISAs. Flow cytometric analysis of peripheral blood lymphocytes may demonstrate inverted CD4+/CD8+ ratios in antibody-negative cats and is available at many veterinary teaching hospitals. Inverted CD4+/CD8+ ratios are only consistent with, but not diagnostic of, FIV infection.

With the introduction of the FIV vaccine and the associated problems of interpreting serologic test results in vaccinated animals, attention has turned to other methods of confirming FIV infection in suspect cats. Detecting infection by virus isolation or PCR-based assays has been suggested as an alternative to serologic testing.[630] Although classical virus detection by blood cell culture and virus isolation from plasma is possible over the whole infection period, it is time consuming, expensive, and requires expertise. Therefore this method is not practical for routine diagnosis. PCR is a very sensitive and specific method currently used in research cats. If appropriately inactivated, the current vaccine should not result in provirus production and thus would not interfere with PCR assays that detect viral DNA.[630] However, potential conflicts may arise in the future with PCR tests, depending on the level of attenuation of a vaccine. PCR requires specialized equipment and thus is presently performed only by specialized laboratories. Current PCR tests are not standardized across laboratories, and little is known about sensitivity, specificity, and overall diagnostic performance in naturally infected cats.[50a] False-positive results are possible with FIV PCR as with any other PCR assay (see Chapter 1). The marked variability of the viral genome has raised concerns about the ability of the PCR to detect all FIV variants. False-negative rates of up to 50% have been reported.[597] PCR reagents, including primer and probe sequences, are often selected based on genetic sequences of a few well-characterized FIV strains and so may not detect all isolates. Additionally, some laboratory cats with documented FIV infection have insufficient circulating provirus copies for detection by conventional PCR.[5,362] Failure to identify infected cats (e.g., PCR-negative results caused by strain variations) may lead to inadvertent exposure and transmission of FIV to uninfected cats.

The American Association of Feline Practitioners, in conjunction with the Academy of Feline Medicine, has established guidelines for testing cats for FIV (Table 14-4). Although these guidelines were developed before the introduction of the FIV vaccine, the guidelines are still appropriate.

PATHOLOGIC FINDINGS

Numerous pathologic changes may occur after FIV infection. The lymph nodes of FIV-infected cats may be hyperplastic during the acute phase of infection and, in the terminal phase of infection, may have disruption of normal architecture with loss of follicles and cellular depletion.[168,449,675] Dysplastic changes have been reported in the bone marrow of FIV-infected cats, along with the appearance of granulocytic hyperplasia and the formation of marrow lymphoid aggregates.[70] Inflammation in the respiratory and gastrointestinal (GI) tracts has also been seen. Infected cats can develop lymphoid interstitial pneumonitis, characteristic of lentiviral infections in other species.[93] Recent studies have also documented the existence of an FIV-associated myopathy characterized by infiltrates of lymphocytes and plasma cells in perivascular and pericapillary areas, and myofiber infiltrates of skeletal muscles in conjunction with myofiber necrosis. Affected animals, however, did not exhibit clinical signs of myopathy.[492]

Experimentally infected cats that develop neurologic disease may have lymphocytic infiltration of perivascular areas

Table • 14-4

Guidelines for FIV Testing in Cats

Testing cats for FIV is recommended for the following circumstances:

All cats that are sick.

All cats that are to be adopted.

All cats that are of unknown status.

All cats that have risk factors for recent exposure, or suspected or known to have been recently exposed (retesting of negative cats may be needed to allow time for seroconversion).

Bite or fight wounds

Unsupervised outdoor activity

Resides with a cat whose FIV status is unknown

Resides with an FIV positive cat (annual testing recommended)

All cats that have been vaccinated for FIV (negative test results advised before vaccination).

Modified from Richards J. 2003. Report of the American Association of Feline Practitioners and Academy of Feline Medicine Advisory Panel on Feline Retrovirus Testing and Management, *J Feline Med Surg* 5:3–10; American Association of Feline Practitioners. 2002. Information Brief in response to inquiries regarding Fel-O-Vax FIV, *J Am Vet Med Assoc* 221:1233–1234.

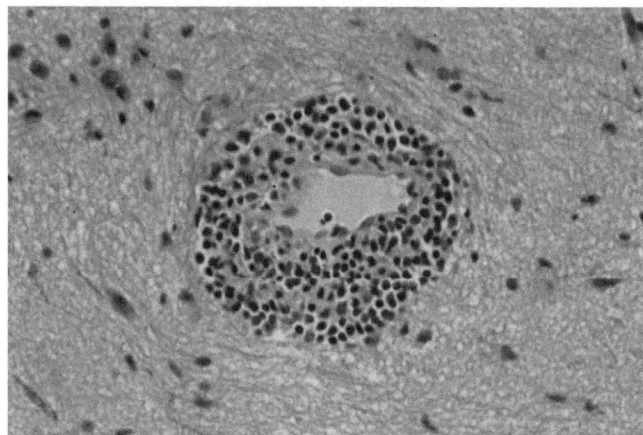

Fig 14-3 Perivascular inflammation in the CNS from a cat with FIV infection and polioencephalomyelitis (H and E stain, ×100). (Courtesy Bob English, North Carolina State University, Raleigh, N.C.)

(Fig. 14-3).[1] Loss and reorganization of neurons, axonal sprouting, and gliosis are described in FIV-infected cats; many of these changes can be found in cats without obvious evidence of clinical signs of infection.[411,416,417,501] Giant cell formation has also been reported.[224] Renal lesions found in FIV-infected cats include glomerulosclerosis and tubulointerstitial infiltrates.[362,503] Some of the common pathologic abnormalities observed in FIV-infected cats are listed in Table 14-5.

THERAPY

In many naturally infected cats, FIV does not directly cause a severe clinical disease. With proper care, FIV-infected cats can live many years with a high quality of life and, in fact, may

Table • 14-5

Pathologic Abnormalities Described in FIV-Positive Cats[a]

AREA	ABNORMALITY
Lymph node	Follicular involution
	Follicular hyperplasia
	Follicular plasmacytosis
Thymus	Cortical involution, atrophy
	Lymphoid follicular hyperplasia and germinal center formation
Intestinal tract	Villous blunting
	Pyogranulomatous colitis
	Lymphoplasmacytic stomatitis
Liver	Periportal hepatitis
Bone marrow	Myeloid hyperplasia, lymphoid aggregates
Kidney	Interstitial nephritis
	Glomerulosclerosis
Central nervous system	Perivascular cuffing
	Gliosis
	Myelitis
	Decreased neuron density, axonal sprouting, vacuolar myelinopathy
Lung	Interstitial pneumonitis, alveolitis
Skeletal muscle	Lymphocytic myositis
	Myofiber necrosis
	Perivascular cuffing

[a]From references 42, 44, 76, 98, 133, 144, 153, 174, 278, 401, 503, 504, 530, 70, 93, 292, 386, 411, 416, 417, 492, 501, 675.

die in older age from causes unrelated to FIV infection. Nonetheless, treatment of FIV has been an area of investigation not only for the potential of helping FIV-infected cats, but also for the potential benefits of HIV-infected people. Approaches to treatment fall broadly into antiviral chemotherapy, immune modulatory therapy, and husbandry and supportive care.

Antiviral Chemotherapy

Most antivirals developed for lentivirus infections are specifically intended for treatment of HIV infection, but several can be used to treat FIV infection because many enzymes of FIV and HIV have similar sensitivities to various inhibitors. In cell culture, many compounds have activity against FIV. However, many FIV treatment studies screen new compounds in vitro or in vivo to document a potential benefit for HIV-infected people. Most of these compounds will not appear on the market and will not be accessible to veterinarians even if some had very good efficacy against FIV. Thus the drugs available for cats are limited, and few controlled studies have been performed to support their clinical use. Refer to Appendix 8 and Chapter 2 for more information on drugs discussed in this section.

Treatment with nucleoside analogues such as zidovudine (3'-azido-2',3'-dideoxythymidine [AZT]) alone or in combination with other drugs, and phosphonylmethoxyethyladenine (PMEA) has been investigated in vitro and in vivo.* AZT blocks lentivirus–reverse transcriptase (RT) activity and is the

most thoroughly studied anti-FIV drug. AZT is integrated into the developing DNA strand, thus inhibiting infection of new cells, but not replication of virus already present in infected cells. AZT reduces plasma virus load, improves the immunologic and clinical status of FIV-infected cats, increases quality of life, and prolongs life expectancy.[231,232] Depending on the study, treatment with AZT or PMEA before inoculation with FIV does not prevent infection or accumulation of provirus in target tissues but delays the onset of detectable viremia and some of the immunologic changes.* AZT improves neurologic abnormalities in FIV-infected cats.[362] Regression of stomatitis and increased CD4+/CD8+ ratios have been observed in placebo-controlled studies of naturally infected cats treated with AZT, PMEA, or related compounds.[159,235,237] As is the case with HIV, evidence from in vitro studies suggests that FIV can become resistant to nucleoside analogs.[214,520,521] In fact, a single point mutation in the FIV gene can create resistance to one or more of the nucleoside analogs.[408,583]

During treatment with AZT, regularly performed CBCs are necessary because nonregenerative anemia is a common side effect, especially if the higher dosage is used.[159,584] CBCs should be performed weekly for the first month. Some cats may develop a mild decrease of hematocrit (HCT) initially in the first 3 weeks that resolves even if treatment is continued. If the HCT drops below 20%, discontinuation of treatment is recommended, and anemia usually resolves within a few days. If values are stable after the first month, a monthly CBC is sufficient. Cats with bone marrow suppression should not be treated because of the risk of life-threatening anemia. In cats with concurrent chronic renal failure, the dose should be reduced to avoid toxicity from accumulation of the compound. Studies in cats treated with AZT for 2 years showed that AZT is well tolerated in most FIV-infected cats. A dosage regimen for AZT is listed in Table 14-6.

Type 1 IFNs have both immunomodulatory and direct antiviral effects. Human IFN-α has been used in cats with FIV infection.[535] Parenteral administration of IFN-α is more likely to produce an antiviral effect than is oral administration.[555] Human IFN-α can be given in high doses (10^5 to 10^6 IU/kg) parenterally for a maximum of 6 to 7 weeks, after which cats are likely to develop antibodies.[682] Human IFN-α given orally, as is used by many veterinarians to treat retrovirus infections, is likely not absorbed but rather destroyed in the GI tract so measurable serum levels do not develop. Oral IFN-α may have an effect by stimulation of local lymphoid tissue in the oral cavity. However, no placebo-controlled studies have been done that have shown a positive effect of low-dose oral human IFN-α in FIV-infected cats. Feline IFN-ω was licensed for use in veterinary medicine in some European countries and Japan. Feline IFN-ω effectively inhibits FIV replication in vitro[602] but has yet to show antiviral benefit in FIV-infected asymptomatic cats.[100] One study of symptomatic cats co-infected with FeLV and FIV has been reported.[136a] (See Interferon-ω, Chapter 13.) IFN-τ has shown some efficacy against FIV in vitro, but in vivo studies have not been reported.[508]

Additional compounds, including other nucleoside analogs, protease inhibitors, fluoroquinolone derivates, cyclosporine A and tacrolimus, androgenic steroids, quassinoids, N-acetylcysteine, ascorbic acid, peptides derived from the FIV-env and transmembrane regions, and bacterial-derived protein peptides with natural antimicrobial activity, DNA-binding polyamides, and algal extracts, have been investigated with some promising results from in vitro or in vivo studies. However, their clinical efficacy has not been established.[†]

*References 61, 159, 230, 231, 235, 236, 408, 485, 584, 631.

*References 159, 235, 236, 239, 240, 412, 485.
†References 61, 143, 158, 208, 208, 236, 313, 314, 347, 384, 388, 389, 398, 409, 429, 430, 431, 442, 480, 563.

Table • 14-6

Drug Therapy for FIV Infection

DRUG	DOSE[a] (MG/KG)	ROUTE	INTERVAL (HOURS)	DURATION (WEEKS)
Antiviral				
AZT[b]	5 mg/kg	PO, SC[c]	12	prn
Cytopenias				
Erythropoietin	100 IU/kg	SC	48	2[d]
Granulocyte colony-stimulating factor	5 µg/kg	SC	12	1—2
Stomatitis				
Metronidazole	5 mg/kg	PO	8	2—4
Clindamycin	12.5 mg/kg	PO	8	2—4
Prednisone	5 mg/cat	PO	12	2—4
Bovine lactoferrin	40 mg/kg	Topically to oral cavity	24	prn

PO, By mouth; *SC*, subcutaneously; *prn*, as needed; *AZT*, zidovadine.
[a]Dose per administration at specified intervals. See Drug Formulary, Appendix 8, for additional information.
[b]Monitor CBC regularly for Heinz body anemia.
[c]For PO, administer in gelatin capsules with specific calculated dose; for SC, dilute lyophilate in 5 ml sodium chloride.
[d]Until desired hematocrit is reached.

Given the identification of the role of the CXCR4 molecule in viral transmission, CXCR4 ligands such as stromal derived factor-1 have been developed and investigated for their anti-FIV potential, but inhibitory activity has been inconsistent, reflecting the likely existence of other molecules that play a role in cell infection.[167,263] Bicyclams, a new class of compounds, selectively block CXCR4 receptors on feline and human cells. The prototype bicyclam, 1,1'-bis-1,4,8,11-tetraaza cyclotetradekan (AMD3100), effectively inhibited FIV replication in vitro[161] and significantly reduced the virus load of naturally FIV-infected cats.[598]

Proteinase inhibitors, which have been used to successfully control illness in HIV-infected people, are retroviral specific. An experimental drug developed for FIV, known as TL-3, was effective in prevention and resolution of FIV-induced CNS disease.[277a] Treatment had to be continued to maintain remission. In cats with specific clinical signs, such as stomatitis or disorders of the CNS, antiviral therapy such as AZT treatment may be a valid treatment consideration until protease inhibitors are available. For further information see Drug Formulary, Appendix 8.

Immune Modulatory Therapy

Immunostimulatory agents such as acemannan, staphylococcus protein A, and *Propionibacterium acnes* have been advocated for use in retrovirus-infected cats to restore compromised immune function, thereby allowing the patient to control viral burden and recover from associated clinical syndromes. Most reports that appear in the veterinary literature are difficult to interpret because of unclear diagnostic criteria, absence of clinical staging or follow-up, the natural variability in the progression of infection, the lack of placebo-control groups, the small number of cats used, and concurrent administration of other supportive treatments.[362] Thus no conclusive evidence from controlled studies has been found that immunomodulator or alternative drugs have any beneficial effects on the health or survival of asymptomatic or symptomatic FIV-infected cats.

Management of FIV-Infected Cats

In all cats, FIV status should be known because FIV infection affects long-term management. Management of FIV-infected cats should differ from that of noninfected cats. The strategy most likely to prolong the life of an FIV-infected cat is keeping the cat strictly indoors.[3] Such a strategy prevents both exposure of the immunosuppressed cat to infectious agents carried by other animals and spread of FIV to other cats. Secondary diseases cause the majority of health problems in FIV-infected cats. Secondary infections cause clinical signs in FIV-infected cats, influence the clinical course of cats infected with FIV, and play a role in the progression of FIV infection.

If FIV infection is diagnosed, regular veterinary examinations should be encouraged at least semi-annually to promptly detect changes in health status. Annual evaluation of a CBC, biochemistry profile, and urinalysis have also been recommended.[525] If FIV-infected cats are sick, prompt and accurate identification of the secondary illness is essential to allow early therapeutic intervention and a successful treatment outcome. Therefore intensive diagnostic testing should occur earlier in the course of illness for an FIV-positive cat than might be recommended for an uninfected cat. In addition to a thorough physical examination and laboratory database, thoracic and abdominal radiographs or abdominal ultrasonography may be required to identify disease. Consideration should be given to cytology and culture of pertinent samples (e.g. urine, blood, effusions, tracheal wash) as additional diagnostic tests and as guides to pharmacologic choices. Cats with cytopenias may require bone marrow aspiration or biopsy to identify underlying causes.

When underlying infections are identified in FIV-infected cats, treatment with appropriate antibiotics or antifungals is encouraged because no evidence suggests that the FIV-infected cat is incapable of responding to treatment. More prolonged courses of treatment may be required in some animals. Systemic fungal infections in FIV-infected cats should be treated the same as in noninfected cats. Itraconazole is useful for cryptococcal infections and is effective for treatment of dermatophytosis. FIV-infected cats with dermatophyte infections should not be treated with griseofulvin because this drug has been associated with the development of severe neutropenia in cats with naturally acquired FIV infection (see Drug Formulary, Appendix 8).

Treatment of FIV-associated stomatitis is often difficult. Repeated treatment with dental cleaning and antibiotics may offer palliative relief but is rarely sufficient to resolve the lesions. Although the pathogenesis of stomatitis is considered to be immune mediated, glucocorticoids should be avoided in FIV-associated stomatitis. In some cases, treatment with AZT can be beneficial (see Table 14-6). Topical bovine lactoferrin has also been beneficial for FIV-related stomatitis (see also Chapter 100 and Appendix 8).[552] An effective treatment can be extraction of all teeth, paying careful attention to removal of all of the roots of the teeth (Figs. 14-4, A, and 14-4, B). In many cases, long-term resolution of inflammation is achieved, and cats return to eating a normal diet.

In those cats in which underlying causes of anemia are not found, consideration may be given to treating with erythropoietin (100 IU/kg, SC every other day until desired HCT is reached, then as needed to maintain the HCT). In one study of the use of hematopoietic factors, administration of recombinant human granulocyte macrophage colony–stimulating factor (rhGM-CSF), but not erythropoietin, was associated with increases in virus production both in vitro and in vivo,[16] and therefore potential benefits of administration of rhGM-CSF to neutropenic cats should be weighed carefully against potential risks. See Chapter 2 and Appendix 8 for further information.

Glucocorticoids have been administered to cats with acute and chronic experimental FIV infections, and although increases in plasma viremia and decreased CD8+ suppressor-cell activity were noted afterwards in acutely infected cats, beneficial effects have included delays in the onset of brain stem auditory-evoked potentials (BAEPs) abnormalities, or normalization of BAEPs in chronically infected cats.[32] Because of the effects on viremia, indiscriminate treatment with glucocorticoids or other immunosuppressive drugs should be avoided unless a compelling indication for their use exists.[11,361]

Intact male and female FIV-infected cats should be neutered to reduce stress associated with estrus and mating behavior and the desire to roam outside the house or interact aggressively with other cats. Surgery is generally well tolerated by asymptomatic FIV-infected cats, although perioperative antibiotic administration should be considered. Because the virus lives only minutes outside the host, and is susceptible to all disinfectants, including common soap, simple precautions and routine cleaning procedures will prevent transmission while in the hospital. FIV-infected patients should be kept in individual cages and can be maintained in this manner in the general hospital population.[11,361,525]

Opinions about general vaccination of FIV-infected cats differ. Experimental evidence shows that FIV-infected cats are able to mount immune responses to administered antigens,[128,343] but responses may be impaired during the terminal phase of infection.[193] FIV-infected cats have developed illness with modified live virus (MLV) feline panleukopenia vaccine (see Postvaccinal Complications, Systemic Illness, Chapter 100) so that inactivated boosters should be considered. Other studies suggest that immune stimulation helps stabilize CD4+ cell numbers.[522] In contrast, stimulation of FIV-infected lymphocytes is also known to promote virus production in vitro. In vivo, vaccination of chronically infected FIV-infected cats with a synthetic peptide was associated with a decrease in the CD4+/CD8+ ratio.[350] Thus vaccination and antigenic stimulation may potentially be disadvantageous with a potential tradeoff of protection from infection for progression of FIV infection secondary to increased virus production, although this has never been proven in experimental studies. If FIV-infected cats are kept strictly indoors, the risk of being infected with other pathogens may be lower than the possible harmful effect of vaccination. If potential exposure to parvovirus, herpesvirus, or calicivirus cannot be excluded, only core vaccines (against panleukopenia and upper respiratory infection) and inactivated vaccines should be considered. The

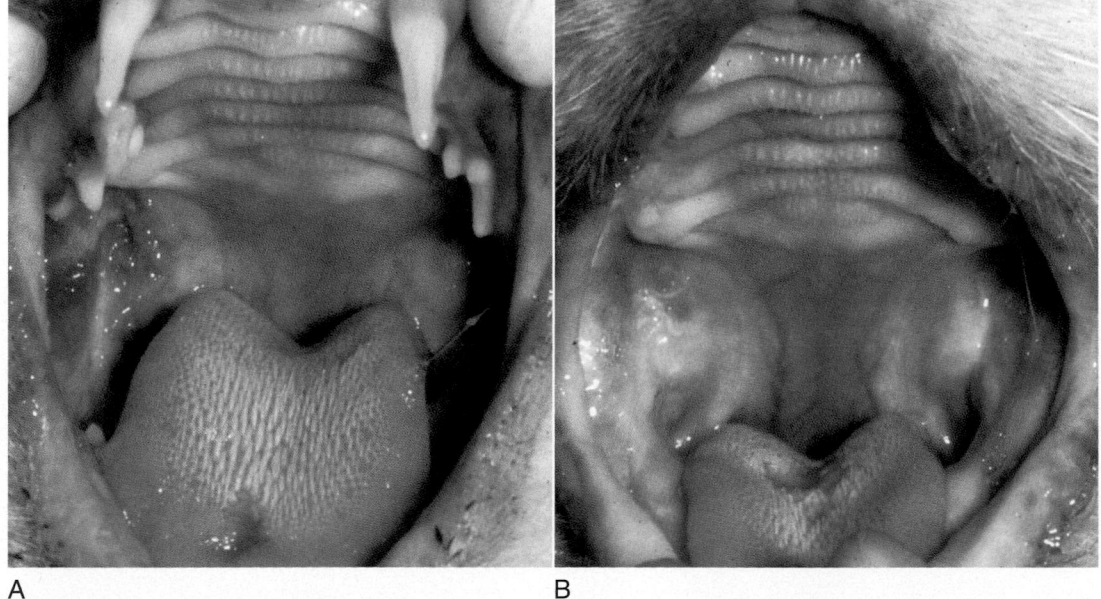

A   B

Fig 14-4 **A,** Stomatitis in the glossopharyngeal fauces in an FIV-infected cat before dental extraction. (Courtesy Julie Levy, University of Florida, Gainesuille, Fla.) **B,** Stomatitis with less inflammation following dental extraction from the cat in Fig. 14-4.

duration of immunity following vaccination of FIV-infected cats with inactivated products is unknown.

PREVENTION

One of the more prolific areas of FIV study has been in the area of vaccine development, spurred by use of the FIV model for development of HIV vaccines. A large number of different approaches have been taken in attempts to create FIV vaccines,[165,215,614,641] including DNA and subunit vaccines with or without adjuvants such as cytokines,* peptide or recombinant vector vaccines using various elements of the FIV virion,† mutant viruses,[323,375] and fixed infected cells or inactivated or attenuated virus.‡ Various routes of vaccine administration, including mucosal application and injection directly into a lymph node, have also been explored.[179,180,600] One result of this work has been the introduction of an FIV vaccine marketed in the United States (Fel-O-Vax, Ft. Dodge, Fort Dodge, IA). The marketing of this vaccine has been met with controversy regarding its use, the interpretation of currently used FIV tests, and the extent of protection afforded by the vaccine.[109,247,306,426] Using available serologic tests including immuno (Western) blotting, antibodies detected following vaccination cannot be distinguished from those caused by natural infection.[220] In one study, vaccination of cats with a recombinant or the commercial vaccine caused a greater level of viremia and salivary shedding of virus in vaccinates as compared to the control animals.[48]

One of the major obstacles in design of a widely effective vaccine against FIV infection is the large genetic diversity among viral isolates. Five known subtypes of FIV have been discovered, and sequence divergence within a subtype ranges from 2% to 15%, and that between subtypes ranges up to 26%. Single-strain vaccines have only provided adequate protection against homologous and closely related strains but not against moderately to greatly heterologous strains. Fel-O-Vax FIV®, the first vaccine licensed in the United States, is a dual-subtype vaccine containing inactivated FIV subtype A and subtype D with an adjuvant.[516,630] The combination of two genetically distinct subtypes elicits strong anti-FIV cellular immunity and broad spectrum virus-neutralizing antibodies. So far, this vaccine has not been field tested against natural FIV infection, and the extent of protection against B subtype viruses, frequently found in the United States, is uncertain. Because the vaccine contains whole virus, cats respond to vaccination by producing antibodies that are indistinguishable from those produced during natural infection.[630]

The existing literature on FIV vaccines gives some reasons for scrutiny when using any FIV vaccine. First, although many vaccine studies have shown protection against FIV infection following challenge with either homologous, or in some instances, heterologous isolates, the results have been quite inconsistent. In a particularly telling study, cats vaccinated with inactivated whole virus were not protected against challenge with a heterologous isolate even though the isolates used in the study were within the same subtype (subtype A) as the vaccine isolate.[264] The isolates of this study were all of different pathogenicity, emphasizing the importance of understanding the challenge inocula and the vaccine strategy employed. The difficulties in developing FIV vaccines need to be understood by the clinician when evaluating vaccine claims, and for FIV, perhaps more facets need to be considered than with other infectious agents (Table 14-7). Although not demonstrated with the commercially available vaccine, in

some instances, concern still exists that vaccination against FIV may enhance infection.[209,310,311,527] For all the reasons previously noted, the best prevention of FIV infection remains segregation of FIV-infected from noninfected cats.[3]

Other strategies for preventing infection have been explored. Protection against homologous isolates has been achieved by passive immunization and adoptive transfer of lymphocytes from vaccinated cats.[518] Kittens may be protected from infection if the queen has a high concentration of FIV-specific antibody, suggesting that stimulation of humoral immunity has a role in protection.[257,517] Detection of cytotoxic T-lymphocyte activity after vaccination implicates a role for CMI in protection.[192,518,608]

PUBLIC HEALTH AND OTHER CONSIDERATIONS

FIV is a feline pathogen, and no demonstrated evidence has been found that it can infect people, even those such as veterinarians who are at greater risk of exposure.[90] However, infection of human peripheral blood mononuclear cells has been accomplished in vitro with a laboratory-maintained FIV isolate,[296,299] and clinical disease was induced in cynomolgus monkeys after autologous transfusion with peripheral blood mononuclear cells infected in vitro.[295] However, no evidence has been found to link FIV infection to any human disease, including AIDS. Investigations have failed to identify antibodies in people that have been bitten by infected cats or that have inadvertently injected themselves with virus-containing material.[673] A large number of studies have investigated the potential of FIV to serve as a gene-delivery system with the ultimate goal of treating nonlentiviral diseases. Genetically manipulated isolates of FIV have shown some promise as a vector for gene transfer in a number of systems involving cell lines derived from people and other species.*

Table • 14-7

Factors to be Considered in the Evaluation of FIV Vaccine Efficacy

Vaccine type: DNA vaccine, subunit vaccine, inactivated vaccine

Route of vaccination: parenteral, mucosal

Origin of challenge isolates: homologous or heterologous, relatedness of challenge homologous isolates to vaccine strain, cell-culture adapted or field isolates

Type: cell-free versus cell-associated virus

Amount of challenge inoculum

Interval between vaccination and challenge

Route of challenge: parenteral, mucosal

Methods of detecting evidence of infection following challenge: PCR/RT-PCR, viral cultures

Tissues sampled for virus detection following challenge: peripheral blood cells, tissues

Sampling intervals

Duration of study or immunity

Number and relatedness of animals in challenge studies

PCR, Polymerase chain reaction; *RT-PCR*, reverse transcriptase polymerase chain reaction.

---

*References 118, 156, 191, 256, 277.
†References 63, 87, 117, 179, 187, 353, 354, 528, 607, 613.
‡References 180, 209, 255, 264, 310, 311, 404, 406, 407, 489, 490.

*References 4, 64, 72, 80, 116, 119, 120, 121, 122, 141, 147, 199, 276, 293, 308, 333, 377, 378, 379, 380, 382, 440, 497, 513, 553, 554, 580, 581, 587, 595, 596, 647.

SUGGESTED READINGS*

10. Association of Feline Practitioners. 2002. Information brief in response to inquiries regarding Fel-o-Vax FIV, *J Am Vet Med Assoc* 221:1233-1234.
50a. Bienzle D, Reggeti F, Win X, et al. 2004. The variability of serological and molecular diagnosis of feline immunodeficiency virus infection, *Can Vet J* 45:753-757.
136a. de Mari K, Maynard L, Sanquer A, et al. 2004. Therapeutic effects of recombinant feline interferon-omega on feline leukemia virus (FeLV) and feline immunodeficiency virus (FIV)-coinfected symptomatic cats, *J Vet Intern Med* 18:477-482.
386a. MacDonald K, Levy J, Tucker SJ, et al. 2004. Effects of passive transfer of immunity on results of diagnostic tests for antibodies against feline immunodeficiency virus in kittens born to vaccinated queens, *J Am Vet Med Assoc* 225:1554-1557.
525. Richards J. 2003a. 2001 Report of the American Association of Feline Practitioners and Academy of Feline Medicine Advisory Panel on Feline Retrovirus testing and management, *J Feline Med Surg* 5:3-10.
630. Uhl EW, Heaton-Jones TG, Pu R, et al. 2002. FIV vaccine development and its importance to veterinary and human medicine: a review. FIV vaccine 2002 update and review, *Vet Immunol Immunopathol* 90:113-132.

*See the CD-ROM for a complete list of references.

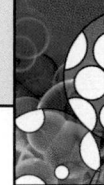

CHAPTER • 15

Feline Adenovirus Infection

Frances A. Kennedy

Clinically apparent disease caused by systemic adenoviral infection is most common in immunologically compromised animals.[1,2] In studies of cats in Hungary, Scotland, the Netherlands, the Czech Republic, and the United States, serologic findings confirmed adenovirus in 15%, 10%, 20%, 25%, and 26% of cats, respectively.[6,7,10] However, only one case of confirmed disseminated adenovirus infection in a cat has been reported.[5] Inclusion body hepatitis reported in a black panther[3] was suggestive of adenovirus infection; however, the causative agent could not be confirmed by electron microscopy (EM) or by virologic identification.

In the confirmed case of disseminated adenovirus infection, a comatose, 8-year-old, spayed, female, domestic shorthair cat had petechiae on the oral mucous membranes. Abnormal hematologic findings included leukopenia (2,100 cells/μl) and thrombocytopenia (73,000/μl). Treatment with intravenous (IV) lactated Ringer's solution, dexamethasone, and vitamin K produced no response. The cat died 4 hours after presentation.

Necropsy revealed that the abdominal cavity and pericardial sac were filled with serous fluid. Serosal and mucosal surfaces of the small and large intestines were diffusely dark red with scattered serosal petechiae, and the intestinal contents were fluid and dark red. The liver and kidneys were swollen, and the liver had an accentuated lobular pattern.

An undiluted sample of serous abdominal fluid gave a positive test result for the group-specific antigen (p27) of the feline leukemia virus (FeLV) and a negative result for antibody to the feline immunodeficiency virus (FIV). A specimen of ileum was positive for feline coronavirus by direct fluorescent antibody (FA) testing. An enzyme-linked immunosorbent assay (ELISA) test for feline panleukopenia virus was negative on specimens of liver, kidney, ileum, mesenteric lymph node, and spleen. An adenovirus particle was identified by EM examination of the intestinal contents.

Histologic examination showed that the endothelial cells were detached from the intramyocardial arteries, and the sloughed cells were large and spindle shaped, with occasional multinucleated cells (Fig. 15-1). Nuclei of these cells were large and pleomorphic, with intranuclear inclusion bodies. Multiple round eosinophilic inclusions were present in some nuclei, with amphophilic granular inclusions filling other nuclei. Some nuclei were almost filled with well-delineated basophilic inclusions, with margination of the small amount of surrounding chromatin. Some of the basophilic nuclei had indistinct borders, resulting in the appearance of "smudge cells." Their cytoplasm was eosinophilic. Minimal perivascular infiltrates of lymphocytes were present in the myocardium.

The stomach had diffuse, submucosal edema. Diffuse superficial necrotizing and hemorrhagic enteritis with submucosal edema was present in the small intestine. Necrosis was more severe in the ileum, with full-thickness mucosal necrosis over Peyer's patches. Moderate lymphoid depletion and peripheral hemorrhage in submucosal lymphoid tissue was noted. Sections of colon were comparably affected, with submucosal edema and particularly severe mucosal necrosis overlying areas of prominent submucosal lymphoid tissue. Submucosal and mesenteric blood vessels at all levels of the gastrointestinal (GI) tract had endothelial lesions as described in the heart. Similar vascular lesions were seen in small hepatic arteries, pulmonary arteries, trachea, thymic remnant, urinary bladder, thyroid gland, adrenal gland, bone marrow, spleen, lymph node, and kidney. Depletion of lymphoid follicles in the spleen and lymph nodes was noted.

EM examination of detached endothelial cells revealed intranuclear aggregates of viral particles measuring approximately 65 nm in diameter (Fig. 15-2). Some of these particles were roughly icosahedral, with dense central cores. In some areas, viral particles formed loose crystalline arrays.

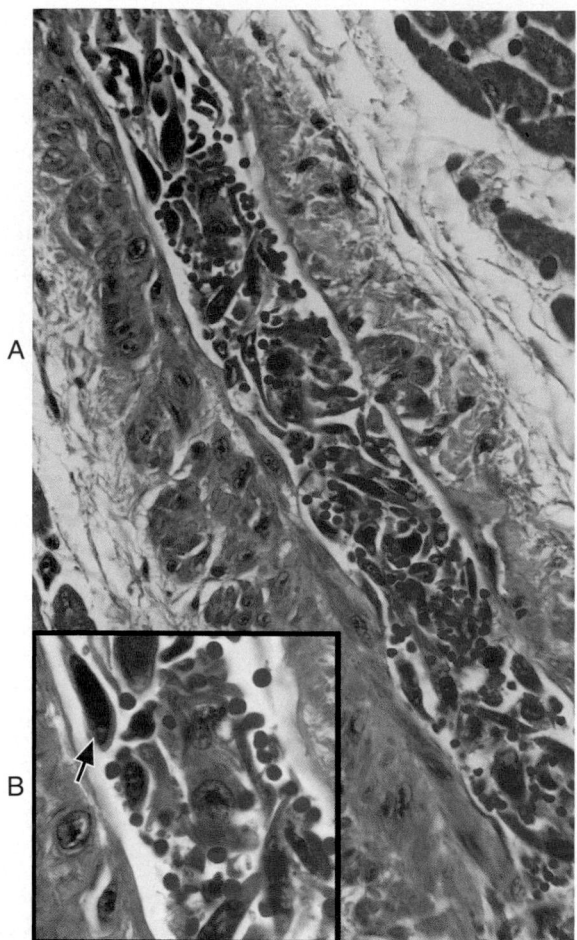

Fig 15-1 A, Photomicrograph of an intramyocardial artery with sloughed endothelial cells. Spindle-shape cells within the arterial lumen have large, pleomorphic nuclei and intranuclear inclusion bodies (H and E stain, ×400). **B,** Intranuclear inclusion bodies (*arrow;* H and E stain, ×1000). (Courtesy Frances Kennedy, Michigan State University, East Lansing, Mich.)

Because adenoviruses have relatively narrow ranges of host specificity, the horses, dogs, and goat on the property of the infected cat (all of which were clinically normal) were considered to be unlikely sources of infection in this cat. Other cats on the property were clinically normal. It is possible that FeLV infection produced an immunodeficient state in the affected cat, predisposing it to develop disseminated adenovirus infection. Leukopenia may have been a consequence of FeLV infection, terminal endotoxemia, or both. The cat's thrombocytopenia was most likely associated with consumption secondary to vascular lesions, because the bone marrow had adequate numbers of megakaryocytes.

The positive direct FA test for feline coronavirus probably indicated a subclinical infection with feline enteric coron-

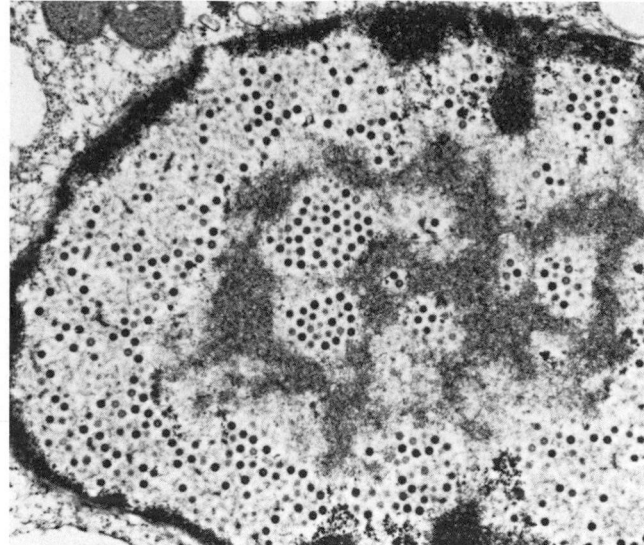

Fig 15-2 Electron micrograph of an endothelial cell with intranuclear viral particles. Moderate autolytic change is responsible for disruption of adenoviral arrays (×17,900). (From Kennedy FA, Mullaney TP. 1993. *J Vet Diagn Invest* 5:273-276.)

avirus. No gross or histologic lesions typical of feline infectious peritonitis were found.

Serologic studies have suggested that persistent, subclinical adenovirus infection exists in the feline population. Significant increases in rates of positive titers were found with increasing age and among cats with signs of respiratory or GI disease.[10] In a group of five FIV-positive laboratory cats in Italy, serologic testing revealed that four were positive for adenovirus.[7] However, to date, only one case of adenovirus infection in a cat has been confirmed by the polymerase chain reaction.[8,9] The affected cat had a period of transient hepatic failure, and serologic testing confirmed adenovirus infection. Adenovirus hexon capsid nucleic acid was detected in two rectal swabs taken at a 1-year interval and a pharyngeal swab taken at the second sampling from this cat. This finding suggests that in addition to persistent subclinical infections, cats may be a source of persistent adenovirus shedding.

SUGGESTED READINGS*

5. Kennedy FA, Mullaney TP. 1993. Disseminated adenovirus infection in a cat, *J Vet Diagn Invest* 5:273-276.
7. Lakatos B, Farkas J, Adam E, et al. 2000. Serologic evidence of adenovirus infection in cats, *Arch Virol* 145:1029-1033.

*See the CD-ROM for a complete list of references.

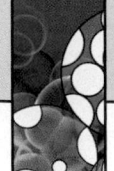

CHAPTER 16

Feline Respiratory Disease

Rosalind M. Gaskell, Susan Dawson, and Alan Radford

ETIOLOGY

Feline infectious respiratory disease is most commonly seen in cats that are grouped together, as in multicat households, boarding catteries, and breeding establishments. The disease is multifactorial, with several etiologic agents involved and a significant number of other risk factors identified.[3,4,94]

The majority of cases of infectious respiratory disease are caused by one of two viruses: feline herpesvirus-1 (FHV-1, or feline rhinotracheitis virus) and feline calicivirus (FCV). FHV-1 generally induces more severe disease than FCV does, but FCV appears to be relatively more common.[7,27,60] This prevalence may relate to the antigenic diversity of the virus and the inability of current vaccines to protect equally well against all FCV strains.[47,60]

Increasingly apparent is that *Bordetella bronchiseptica* is also a primary pathogen of the feline respiratory tract, although its precise contribution to disease in the field is not yet fully established.[3,24,89] Interestingly, transmission of the organism between dogs and cats may occur, which has implications for disease control in both species.[3,5,15,24]

Chlamydophila felis (previously *Chlamydia psittaci* var. felis) is also involved in feline respiratory disease, although it is considered predominantly a conjunctival pathogen (see also Chapter 30). Other agents that have been implicated in the syndrome include mycoplasmas and other bacteria, feline reovirus, and cowpox virus.[27]

Feline Herpesvirus-1

FHV-1 is a typical α-herpesvirus containing double-stranded DNA, with a glycoprotein-lipid envelope. As in most herpesviruses, FHV-1 is relatively fragile in the external environment and is highly susceptible to the effects of common disinfectants. It can survive for only up to 18 hours in a damp environment, less in dry conditions. It is also relatively unstable as an aerosol.

As well as infecting domestic cats, FHV-1 has been shown to infect several other members of the Felidae.[13,70,104] The virus is also very closely related genetically and antigenically to canine herpesvirus-1 and phocine (seal) herpesvirus-1 (PhV-1), and cross-protection between feline and PhV-1 has been reported.[55,110]

FHV-1 has little strain variation. Most isolates produce a relatively uniform disease, although some show reduced or increased virulence. Antigenically, all strains belong to one serotype, and apart from some minor differences, they are relatively homogeneous on restriction enzyme analysis of their DNA. Therefore no easy method is currently available to study the role of individual FHV-1 isolates in disease.

Feline Calicivirus

FCV is a small, unenveloped, single-stranded RNA virus, a member of the *Vesivirus* genus of the calicivirus family. Both domestic cats and other members of the Felidae family can be infected, and a similar virus has also been isolated from lions.[13,45] Although dogs have their own genetically distinct calicivirus,[56,82] caliciviruses antigenically and genetically related to FCV have also been detected in dogs (see Chapter 8),[35,54,83] and some epidemiologic evidence suggests a link between the two.[4]

FCV is slightly more resistant than is FHV-1, surviving for up to a week in the external environment or possibly longer if conditions are damp. The virus is not as susceptible to the effects of disinfectants as FHV-1,[20] but a useful disinfectant for both viruses is bleach diluted 1 part in 32 in water with added detergent.

A large number of different strains of FCV exists, which vary slightly in antigenicity and pathogenicity, although they are all sufficiently cross-reactive to be classified as one serotype. Genetically, these strains appear to represent one large group or genogroup, although again, considerable variability may be seen between isolates, particularly in immunogenic regions of the viral capsid gene.* This genetic diversity is useful epidemiologically in that it allows differentiation between FCV strains.[71,73-75,96]

Most strains of FCV are closely related enough to induce some degree of cross-protection, but cats can still be sequentially infected with different viruses and show varying degrees of clinical illness. Some isolates appear to be more immunogenic and cross-reactive than do others, and several such strains (e.g., the original vaccine strain F9 and strain 255) have been widely used in vaccines. However, no single strain is likely to protect equally well against all field isolates, and some evidence indicates that the percentage of isolates neutralized by such strains may be decreasing, possibly caused by immune selection pressures from widespread vaccine use.[8,27,47,60] Routine monitoring of vaccine efficacy against current isolates would be useful.

B. bronchiseptica

B. bronchiseptica is an aerobic, gram-negative coccobacillus that is a well-known respiratory pathogen in dogs, swine, and rodents. It also causes occasional opportunistic infection in people: indeed, a case has been reported in a veterinary student.[24] (See Public Health Considerations, Chapter 6, for further information on this risk.) In the past, *B. bronchiseptica* was thought to play only a secondary role in feline respiratory disease, but it is now established as a primary pathogen in cats. Respiratory disease has been reproduced in *Bordetella*-free, specific-pathogen–free (SPF) cats after aerosol or nasal challenge,[12,42,44,109] and a large number of field cases have been reported.† However, a significant number of factors likely play a role in whether disease occurs in the field, and various risk factors for *B. bronchiseptica* infection in cats have been identified in epidemiologic studies.[3]

*References 1, 30, 31, 40, 46, 72.
†References 41, 48, 89, 101, 108.

Other Organisms

C. felis causes acute to chronic conjunctivitis in cats, although respiratory signs may also be seen. The prevalence of *C. felis* in cats with conjunctival or upper respiratory tract disease has been reported in studies using polymerase chain reaction (PCR) to range between 14.3%[94] and 59%.[7] The disease is discussed in more detail in Chapter 30.

Reoviruses have been occasionally isolated from cats, and conjunctival and respiratory signs have been induced after experimental inoculation. However, no evidence has been found that reoviruses are important as respiratory pathogens in cats in the field.

Cowpox virus infection in cats causes primarily skin lesions, but occasionally respiratory or ocular signs may also be seen (see Chapter 19). The reservoir hosts of cowpox virus in Europe are small wild mammals, and cats occasionally become infected by contact through hunting. Other orthopoxviruses, that may infect cats, exist in other parts of the world.

The role of mycoplasmas in feline respiratory disease is not clear. Undoubtedly, they can be important as secondary pathogens, but their role as primary agents is more equivocal (see Chapter 32). Infection is common in both colony cats and household pets, and mycoplasmas have been isolated from both diseased and healthy animals. Increasing evidence indicates that mycoplasmas may be associated with disease in the lower respiratory tract; however, their role in upper respiratory tract disease is less clear.[10,32,76] Mycoplasmas have been isolated in pure culture from cases of bronchopneumonia, which have responded to antimycoplasmal therapy.[25] Other bacteria such as *Staphylococcus* spp., *Streptococcus* spp., *Pasteurella multocida*, and *Escherichia coli* are thought to play a role as secondary invaders in feline respiratory disease.

EPIDEMIOLOGY

Feline Herpesvirus-1 and Feline Calicivirus Infections

FHV-1 and FCV are fairly widespread in the general cat population, with a higher prevalence in multicat households. The viruses are mainly shed in ocular, nasal, and oral secretions, and spread is largely by direct contact with an infected cat. Acutely infected animals are clearly one of the most important sources of virus, but infection also commonly occurs from clinically recovered carrier cats. In some situations, particularly within a cattery, indirect transmission may also occur. Contaminated secretions may be present on cages, feeding and cleaning utensils, and on personnel. However, because the viruses are relatively short lived outside the cat, the environment is usually not a long-term source of infection.

Aerosols are not thought to be of major importance for the spread of FHV-1 and FCV. Cats do not appear to produce an infectious aerosol for these agents during normal respiration, although sneezed macrodroplets may transmit infection over a distance of 1 to 2 meters.

Despite vaccination, carriers are widespread in the population and are probably the main reason why these viruses are so successful. An understanding of the FHV-1 and FCV carrier states is important to help determine strategies for control.

Carrier State for Feline Herpesvirus-1

As with other α-herpesviruses, virtually all recovered cats become latently infected carriers. However, intermittent episodes of detectable virus shedding (reactivation) may occur, particularly after periods of stress (Fig. 16-1). During such episodes, infectious virus is present in oronasal and conjunctival secretions, and cats may infect other cats. The epidemiologic significance of PCR-positive cats, which are negative by traditional virus culture, is not clear, but they are likely to be less infectious.[6,95,107]

Virus reactivation may occur spontaneously but is most likely after stress, for example, going into a boarding cattery, to a cat show, or to stud. Glucocorticoid treatment can also induce shedding, but using this drug to detect carriers is inadvisable because severe disease may occasionally result. Some carrier cats appear to shed virus more frequently than do others and therefore are of greater epidemiologic importance.

Shedding does not occur immediately after the stress; a lag period of approximately 1 week occurs, followed by a shedding episode of from 1 to 2 weeks. Thus carrier cats are most likely to be infectious for up to 3 weeks after a stress factor. In some cases, carriers show recrudescence of mild clinical signs while they are shedding, which can be a useful indicator that they are likely to be infectious.

The stress of parturition and lactation may also precipitate virus shedding in latently infected queens, but whether or not the kittens develop disease depends on their levels of maternally derived antibody (MDA). On some occasions, kittens with low levels of MDA may become subclinically infected and become latent carriers without showing clinical signs. Such a mechanism is obviously ideal for the virus because it can spread to the next generation without harming its host.

As with some other herpesviruses, FHV-1 remains latent in carriers in the trigeminal ganglia, although virus has also been detected by PCR in a large number of other tissues.[81,107] The latent carrier state is almost certainly lifelong, but a refractory phase of several months occurs after a period of virus shedding when animals are less likely to experience another reactivation episode.

Carrier State for Feline Calicivirus

Unlike FHV-1 carriers, FCV carriers shed virus more or less continuously and are mostly therefore always infectious to other cats (Fig. 16-2). The virus persists in tonsillar and other oropharyngeal tissues. In some cats, the carrier state appears to be lifelong, but most animals at some point spontaneously recover and appear to eliminate virus. In some experimental studies, most cats were shedding FCV 30 days after infection, and by 75 days, approximately 50% of cats were still shedding. This proportion continues to decline, with only a minority of animals becoming long-term carriers. In other studies, carrier states have been difficult to reproduce, suggesting that virus strain differences or other factors may be involved. Some evidence indicates that preexisting feline immunodeficiency virus (FIV) infection may potentiate FCV shedding from carriers, either in terms of duration or titer of virus.[16,79]

FCV carriers have been arbitrarily divided into high, medium, and low level, each shedding a fairly constant amount of virus that fluctuates around a mean for that individual cat. High-level shedders are very infectious and easily detected by oropharyngeal swabbing; low-level shedders are less infectious, and a series of swabs taken over several weeks may be necessary to identify them.

FCV carriers are very common, and prevalence rates are still similar to those reported some years ago, before the introduction of vaccination. Surveys have shown that approximately 20% to 30% of cats, depending on the population studied, are shedding FCV.[4,27,74] Although many of these cats will be carriers, some may be undergoing reinfection, and others may be undergoing primary infection with an nonpathogenic strain. Vaccination protects against disease but not infection or the carrier state, and mathematical modeling studies suggest that a reduction in FCV prevalence is unlikely with the current levels of vaccine efficacy.[77]

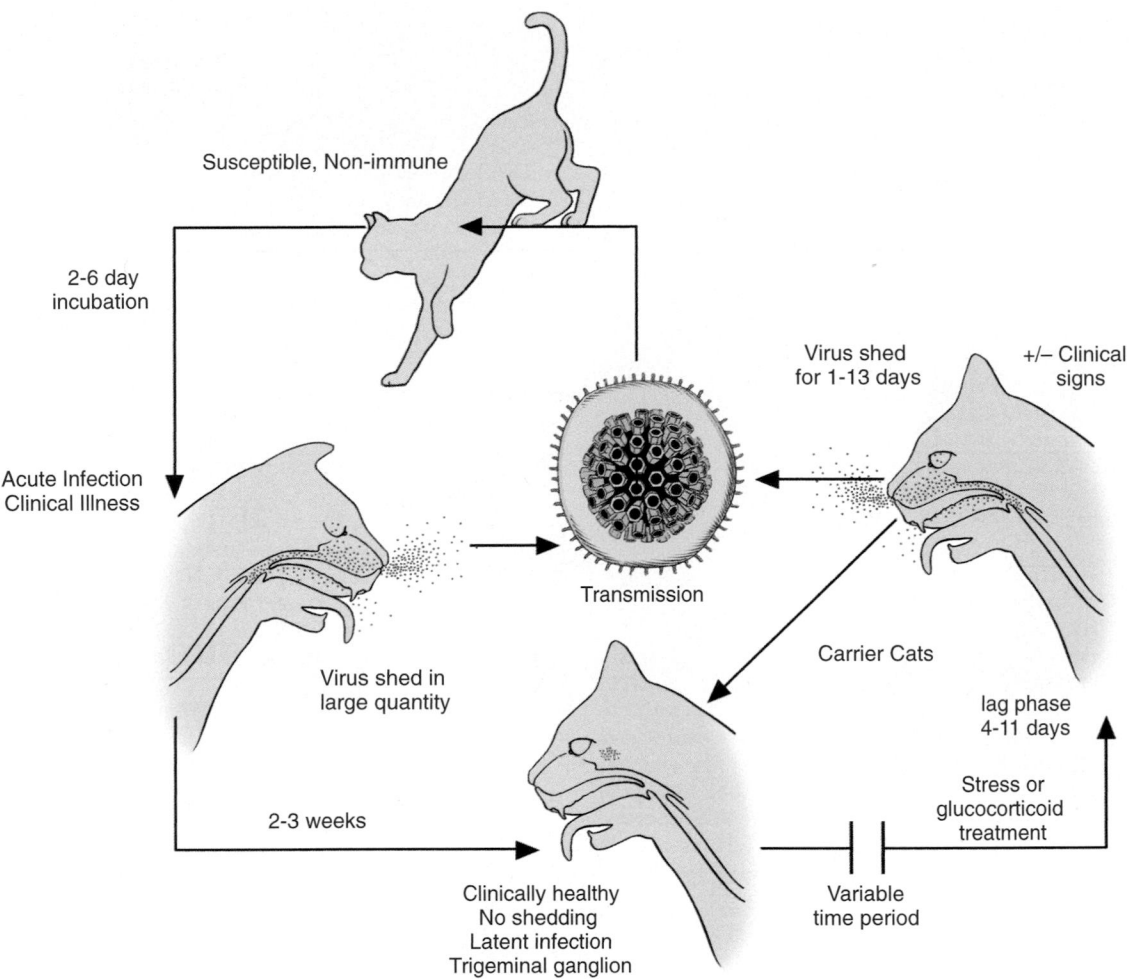

Fig 16-1 FHV-1 carrier state: epidemiology. (From Gaskell RM, Radford AD, Dawson S. 2004. Feline infectious respiratory disease, p 583. *In* Chandler EA, Gaskell CJ, Gaskell RM [eds], *Feline medicine and therapeutics*, ed 3, Blackwell Publishing, Oxford. Used with permission.)

B. bronchiseptica Infection

Serosurveys have shown that *B. bronchiseptica* is widespread in the cat population. Seroprevalence of between 24% and 79% and isolation rates of up to 47% have been reported, depending on the type and clinical status of the population tested.* In a large-scale epidemiologic survey of cats in the United Kingdom with and without respiratory disease, 11% of 740 cats were found to be shedding *B. bronchiseptica* from the oropharynx, with a higher positive number in rescue catteries and in households with larger numbers of cats.[3] An association between *B. bronchiseptica* infection and respiratory disease was found in the rescue cattery population, which fits with previous empirical observations that the organism is more likely to cause disease in stressful, crowded situations.

Also apparent is that transmission of this bacterium may occur between dogs and cats, which clearly has implications for control, especially where dogs and cats are housed on the same premises. Epidemiologic studies have shown that contact with dogs with recent respiratory disease was found to be a risk factor for *B. bronchiseptica* infection in cats.[3] In addition, typing of isolates from dogs and cats using pulsed-field gel electrophoresis (PFGE) has shown that isolates from both species on the same premises are likely to be similar.[5,24] Another report showed two cats developing respiratory

disease following contact with two dogs with kennel cough, and *B. bronchiseptica* isolated from all four animals were found to be the same using PFGE.[15] Interestingly, Foley and colleagues[24] noted that the majority of isolates circulating in dogs and cats in two shelters in the United States appeared to be similar to a canine and feline vaccine strain.

Epidemiologic evidence suggests that a carrier state may exist in cats with *Bordetella* infection, with 9% of clinically healthy cats shedding the organism.[3] Experimental work has shown that *B. bronchiseptica* is shed in both oropharyngeal and nasal secretions, in some cases for at least 19 weeks after infection.[12] In the same study, *B. bronchiseptica* was detected in two seropositive queens after parturition despite being negative beforehand, suggesting the stress of parturition may have initiated shedding.

PATHOGENESIS

Feline Herpesvirus-1 Infection

The natural routes of infection for FHV-1 are nasal, oral, and conjunctival, and virus replication takes place predominantly in the mucosae of the nasal septum, turbinates, nasopharynx, and tonsils. Virus shedding can be detected in oropharyngeal and nasal swabs as early as 24 hours after infection and generally persists for 1 to 3 weeks.

*References 2, 3, 24, 42, 89.

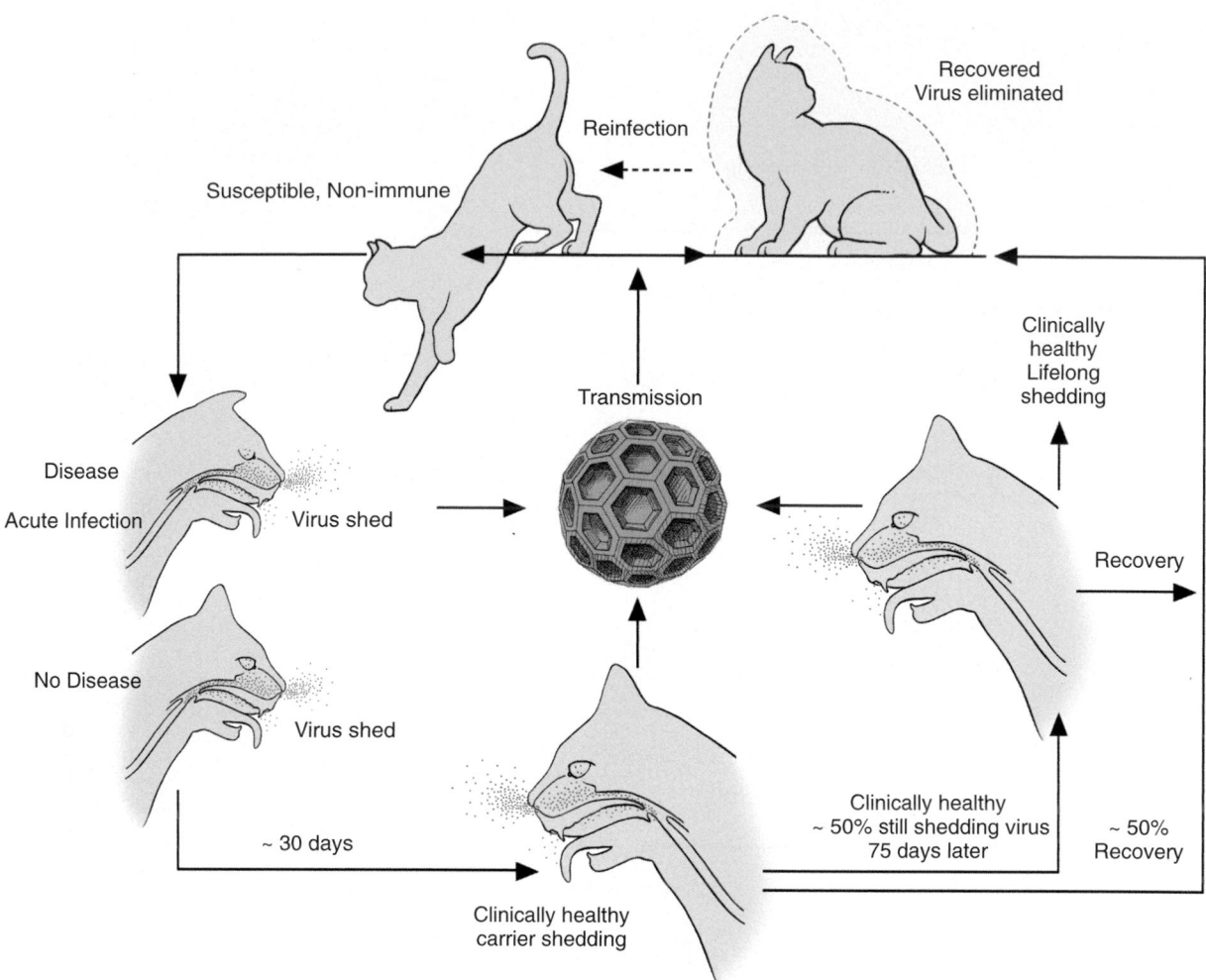

Fig 16-2 FCV carrier state: epidemiology. (Flow diagram from Gaskell RM, Radford AD, Dawson S. 2004. Feline infectious respiratory disease, p 584. *In* Chandler EA, Gaskell CJ, Gaskell RM [eds], *Feline medicine and therapeutics*, ed 3, Blackwell Publishing, Oxford. Used with permission. Virus drawing courtesy of University of Georgia, Athens, Ga.)

Viremia is rare because virus replication is normally restricted to areas of lower body temperature, such as the respiratory tract. However, viremia has occasionally been reported, and generalized disease may be seen, particularly in debilitated animals or in neonatal kittens.

Infection leads to areas of multifocal epithelial necrosis, with neutrophilic infiltration and exudation with fibrin. In early infections, intranuclear inclusion bodies may be seen. Viral damage can also lead to osteolytic changes in the turbinate bones. Lesions normally take between 2 and 3 weeks to resolve, although bone damage to the turbinates may be permanent. Primary lung involvement may occur but is rare. Secondary bacterial infection can enhance the pathogenic effect of FHV-1; thus bacterial sinusitis or pneumonia is possible.

Feline Calicivirus Infection

Similar to FHV-1, the natural routes of infection for FCV are nasal, oral, and conjunctival. Virus replication mainly occurs in the oral and respiratory tissues, although some differences between strains can be found. Some strains have a predilection for the lung, and others have been found in the macrophages within the synovial membrane of joints.[14,100] Virus may also be found in visceral tissues and feces and occasionally in the urine.

Oral ulcers are the most prominent pathologic feature of FCV infection. These ulcers begin as vesicles, which sub-sequently rupture, with necrosis of the overlying epithelium and infiltration of neutrophils at the periphery and the base. Healing takes place over 2 to 3 weeks.

Pulmonary lesions appear to result from an initial focal alveolitis, which leads to areas of acute exudative pneumonia and then to the development of a proliferative, interstitial pneumonia. Although primary interstitial pneumonia can occur in FCV infection, particularly with more virulent strains, it has probably been overemphasized in the past as a result of experimental studies using aerosol challenge rather than the more natural oronasal routes.

Lesions seen in FCV-infected joints consist of an acute synovitis with thickening of the synovial membrane and an increased amount of synovial fluid within the joint.

B. bronchiseptica Infection

In most species, the primary route of infection with *B. bronchiseptica* appears to be via the oronasal cavity where the organism colonizes mucosal surfaces. The bacterium uses several virulence factors to adhere to the cilia of the respiratory epithelium. Once attached, ciliostasis and destruction of the cilia occur, resulting in the failure of the mucociliary clearance mechanism and facilitating further colonization and persistence of bacteria. The release of toxins from *B. bronchiseptica* following colonization is responsible for local and systemic inflammatory damage.

In dogs, the organism appears to target mainly the mucosa of the trachea and bronchi, leading to tracheobronchitis. Although the precise pathogenesis of the disease in cats is unclear, upper respiratory tract involvement appears to be more common. However, clearly in some instances, the lower respiratory tract may also be targeted, given that bronchopneumonia and coughing may occur.

Although *B. bronchiseptica* may appear to be a primary pathogen in cats, undoubtedly other factors such as combined infections with the respiratory viruses and stress factors such as weaning, overcrowding, and poor hygiene and ventilation all play roles. Such factors may account for the severe cases of bronchopneumonia that have been reported in the field.

CLINICAL FINDINGS

Whatever the respiratory pathogen, the observed clinical signs will depend on a large number of factors, such as the infecting dose and strain of the agent, the general health and husbandry conditions of the cat, the nature of its microbial flora, and any preexisting immunity (Table 16-1). Concurrent infection with immunosuppressive viruses such as FIV and feline leukemia virus may lead to more severe disease.[16,78,79]

Feline Herpesvirus-1 Infection

In susceptible animals, FHV-1 infection generally causes a severe upper respiratory disease. The incubation period is usually 2 to 6 days but may be longer with lower levels of challenge virus.

Early signs include depression, marked sneezing, inappetence, and pyrexia, followed rapidly by serous ocular and nasal discharges (Fig. 16-3). These initial clinical signs may be accompanied by excessive salivation with drooling. Conjunctivitis, sometimes with severe hyperemia and chemosis, typically develops, and copious oculonasal discharges occur. These discharges gradually become mucopurulent, and crusting of the external nares and eyelids can occur (Fig. 16-4). In severe cases, dyspnea and coughing may also develop. Oral ulceration can occur with FHV-1 infection, but it is rare. Occasionally, generalized infections and primary viral pneumonia may occur, particularly in young or debilitated animals.

Other manifestations of FHV-1 infection include ulcerative and interstitial keratitis and corneal sequestration; a possible association with uveitis has also been reported (Fig. 16-5).[51] Improved diagnosis, for example, using PCR, has lead to greater recognition of such conditions.[64,91] Skin ulcers and dermatitis syndrome in domestic cats and cheetahs[33,34,62a] and nervous signs have been described, but these are likely to be rare sequels to infection.

Although abortion is a feature of some other α-herpesvirus infections, experimental studies have suggested that, in FHV-1, the severe systemic effects of the illness, rather than a direct effect of the virus itself, are most likely the cause of abortion. Indeed, in an investigation of a natural outbreak of FHV-1 in SPF cats, no cases of abortion were seen, even in severely affected pregnant queens.[37]

In very young kittens or immunosuppressed cats, the mortality rate may be high, but on the whole, mortality with FHV-1 is low. Clinical signs generally resolve within 10 to 20 days.

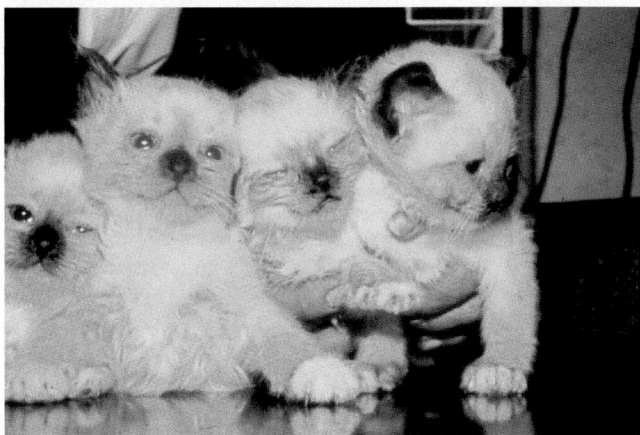

Fig 16-3 A litter of kittens with early FHV-1 infection. (From Gaskell RM, Radford AD, Dawson S. 2004. Feline infectious respiratory disease, p 588. *In* Chandler EA, Gaskell CJ, Gaskell RM [eds], *Feline medicine and therapeutics*, ed 3, Blackwell Publishing, Oxford. Used with permission.)

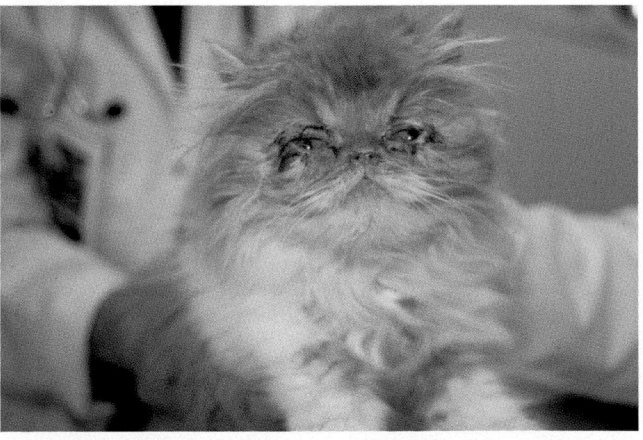

Fig 16-4 Kitten with FHV-1 infection showing mucopurulent discharges typical of the later stages of the disease. (Courtesy Susan Dawson, University of Liverpool.)

Table • 16-1

Essential Features of Clinical Respiratory Disease Related to the Pathogen Involved

FEATURE	FHV-1	FCV[a]	Bb	ChF
Lethargy	+++	+	+	+
Sneezing	+++	+	++	+
Conjunctivitis	++	+	–	+++[b]
Hypersalivation	++	–[c]	–	–
Ocular discharge	+++	+	(+)	+++
Nasal discharge	+++	+	++	+
Oral ulceration	(+)	+++	–	–
Keratitis	+	–	–	–
Coughing	(+)	–	++	–
Pneumonia	(+)	(+)	+	+/–
Lameness	–	+	–	–

FHV-1, Feline herpesvirus; *FCV*, feline calicivirus; *Bb*, *Bordetella bronchiseptica*; *ChF*, *Chlamydophila felis*; +++, marked; ++, moderate; +, mild; (+), less common; +/–, subclinical; –, absent.
Adapted from Gaskell RM, Radford AD, Dawson S. 2004. Feline infectious respiratory disease, p 580. In Chandler EA, Gaskell CJ, Gaskell RM (eds), *Feline medicine and therapeutics*, ed 3, Blackwell Publishing, Oxford. Used with permission.
[a]Strain variation.
[b]Often persistent.
[c]Slight wetness may be seen around the mouth if ulcers present.

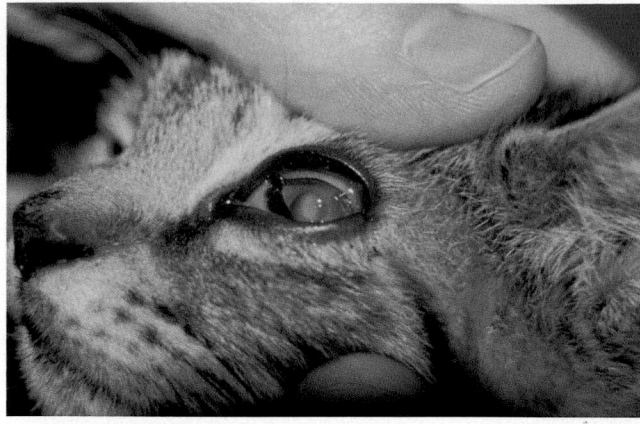

Fig 16-5 Cat with ulcerative keratitis caused by FHV-1 infection. (Courtesy Susan Dawson, University of Liverpool.)

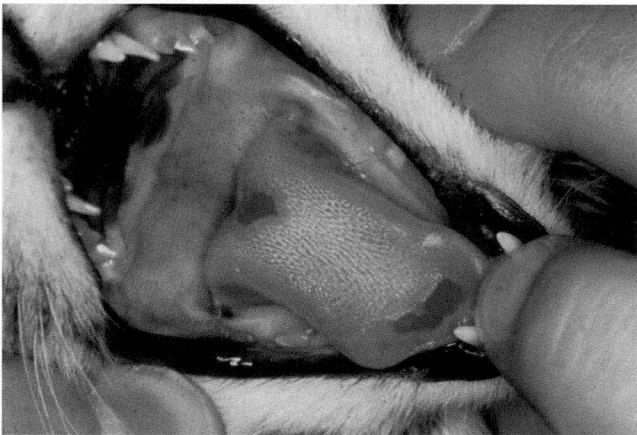

Fig 16-6 Two lingual ulcers on the tongue of a cat infected with FCV. (From Gaskell RM, Radford AD, Dawson S. 2004. Feline infectious respiratory disease, p 588. *In* Chandler EA, Gaskell CJ, Gaskell RM [eds], *Feline medicine and therapeutics*, ed 3, Blackwell Publishing, Oxford. Used with permission.)

However, in some cats the acute damage may have been severe enough to lead to permanent damage to the mucosae and turbinates, leaving individual cats prone to chronic bacterial rhinitis, turbinate osteomyelitis, sinusitis, and conjunctivitis. Short-nosed purebred cats such as Persians or Himalayans appear to have an increased tendency to develop chronic upper respiratory complications, although the reasons for this are not yet clear.

Feline Calicivirus Infection

Strains of FCV can differ in tropism and virulence; therefore a wide range of clinical signs may be seen. Most strains induce a fairly characteristic, mild syndrome characterized by pyrexia, oral ulceration, and mild respiratory and conjunctival signs. Some strains of FCV, however, are nonpathogenic; others are more virulent and may induce more severe systemic disease. Several outbreaks of a severe acute systemic febrile disease with high mortality have been described, caused by particularly virulent strains of FCV.[23,43,66,84]

In a typical case of FCV infection, early signs include depression and pyrexia, although cats typically stay brighter than with FHV-1 infection. Oral ulceration is the most characteristic feature of FCV infection and may be the only clinical sign present (Fig. 16-6). Ulceration is usually on the tongue but can occur elsewhere in the mouth, on the lips, and on the nose. Skin ulceration on other parts of the body occurs rarely.

Sneezing, conjunctivitis, and ocular and nasal discharges typically occur but are generally much less prominent compared with FHV-1 infection. Cats with oral ulcers may show hypersalivation with moisture on the fur around the mouth, but generally, no drooling of saliva occurs. Some of the more virulent strains can cause pneumonia with associated dyspnea.

Some FCV strains produce lameness and pyrexia.[27,100] The lameness may or may not be associated with oral and respiratory signs, and it is likely that considerable overlap exists between the conditions.[99] Affected cats are often dull and anorexic. In most cases, full recovery occurs within 24 to 48 hours, and so far, no evidence can be found of any long-term effects on the joints. Acute lameness has also been observed after vaccination, and in some of these cases, viruses originating from live vaccines may be involved.[71]

Several outbreaks of the recently reported severe systemic syndrome have been described.[23,43,66,84] Affected cats variably show facial and paw edema (approximately 50%), pyrexia (90%), classic signs of upper respiratory infection (50%), icterus (20%) and hemorrhages from the nose and in the feces (30% to 40%). Necropsy findings included pneumonia, hepatomegaly, pancreatitis, and pericarditis. Many of the affected cats were fully vaccinated, suggesting that, as with more typical strains of FCV, vaccines may not completely protect against these virulent systemic disease-producing isolates. The outbreaks were relatively well controlled with strict quarantine and isolation, but given that FCV is an inherently variable pathogen, clinicians must remain vigilant in the event of such viruses appearing again.

The chronic oral disease, lymphoplasmacytic gingivitis stomatitis complex (LPGS) has also been associated with FCV infection. In some studies, more than 80% of cats with chronic oral disease have been found to shed FCV compared with approximately 20% of controls,[27] but these figures probably depend on the criteria used to select clinical cases.[98] FCV infection has been associated with acute faucitis,[80] and in one colony of cats chronic stomatitis developed after the accidental introduction of FCV.[106] However, other agents, in particular FIV, and various host factors appear to be involved in the condition, and the pathogenesis is not yet fully understood (see Stomatitis, Chapter 89).

B. bronchiseptica Infection

In naturally occurring disease, a wide range of clinical signs have been reported in cats infected with *B. bronchiseptica*, varying from upper respiratory tract signs of sneezing, oculonasal discharge, and coughing to severe dyspnea, cyanosis, and death caused by bronchopneumonia.* In general, coughing appears to be less marked in cats than it is in dogs infected with *B. bronchiseptica*. Young kittens appear to be most susceptible to disease, particularly bronchopneumonia.

In experimental studies using SPF cats, the main clinical signs of *B. bronchiseptica* infection were pyrexia, lethargy, coughing, sneezing, oculonasal discharge, and submandibular lymphadenopathy, which resolved after approximately 10 days.[12,42,44,109]

DIAGNOSIS

Diagnosis may be attempted based on clinical signs alone. For example, predominantly oral ulceration might indicate FCV, whereas marked sneezing with more severe respiratory and conjunctival signs might suggest FHV-1 (see Table 16-1). With

*References 3, 15, 89, 101, 108.

Table • 16-2

Therapy of Feline Respiratory Infections

DRUG	DOSE[a]	ROUTE	INTERVAL (HOURS)	DURATION (DAYS)	INDICATIONS
Idoxuridine (0.1% solution)	One drop	Topical in eye	4–6	21	FHV-1 ulcerative keratitis
Interferon-α	30 U	PO	24	7[b]	Acute respiratory and ocular herpesvirus infections
Interferon-α (25–50 U/ml solution)[c]	One drop	Topical in eye	4–6	prn	Ocular herpesvirus infections
L-lysine	200–500 mg	PO	12	prn	Acute and latent FHV-1 infections
Tetracycline	15–22 mg/kg	PO[d]	8	14–21	Bordetellosis, *Chlamydophila* infection
Doxycycline	5 mg/kg	PO[d]	12	14–21	Bordetellosis, *Chlamydophila* infection
Trimethoprim-sulfonamides	15 mg/kg	PO	12	7–14[e]	Bordetellosis
Enrofloxacin	5 mg/kg	PO	24	7–14[f]	Bordetellosis, *Chlamydophila* infection
Phenylephrine 2.5% solution	1 drop	Topical in each nostril	12	7	Nasal decongestion

FHV-1, Feline herpesvirus-1; *U*, units; *PO*, by mouth; *prn*, as needed.

[a]Dose per administration at specified interval. For additional information on antimicrobial drugs, see Drug Formulary, Appendix 8.

[b]Drug is given on and off on 7 day cycles for an indefinite period.

[c]Note: use of IFN-ω topically has not been studied.

[d]Tetracyclines, especially as the hydrochloride salts, can cause esophagitis unless precautions are taken. See Drug Formulary, Appendix 8.

[e]This drug can be myelosuppressive or have nephrotoxicity in cats. Monitoring of complete blood count and renal function should be done with repeated or longer treatment intervals. See Drug Formulary, Appendix 8.

[f]This drug can cause retinal toxicity and blindness in cats when used at higher doses or for longer periods. See Drug Formulary, Appendix 8.

Chlamydophila infection, the main clinical sign is a marked persistent conjunctivitis (see Chapter 30).

Confirmatory diagnosis of FHV-1 and FCV can be made from oropharyngeal or conjunctival swabs by virus isolation in feline cell cultures, by immunofluorescence or enzyme-linked immunosorbent assay (ELISA) techniques, or by PCR.* PCR is more sensitive than virus isolation is for detection of FHV-1, although the significance of PCR-positive, isolation-negative cats are unclear. For FCV, reverse transcriptase polymerase chain reaction is not currently routinely used for diagnosis, but PCR and sequencing are useful for distinguishing between FCV isolates in investigating the epidemiology of the disease.[71,73–75] Serology is generally not helpful in the diagnosis of FHV-1 and FCV infection because of widespread antibody from vaccination.

For diagnosis of *B. bronchiseptica* infection, oropharyngeal or nasal swabs should be taken and placed into charcoal Amies transport medium (Beckton Dickenson, Cockeysville, Md.) before plating at the laboratory on appropriate selective medium that prevents overgrowth by other respiratory flora.[89] Transtracheal wash specimens can also be used for the isolation of *B. bronchiseptica* from clinical cases. Serology is not widely available, and many healthy cats are seropositive in any case.

Diagnosis of *C. felis* infection is described in Chapter 30. *C. felis* infection should be considered when conjunctivitis is the predominant clinical sign.

When an organism is isolated from an animal with respiratory disease, a reasonable assumption is that the agent has been involved in the disease process. However, especially for FCV and *Bordetella*, a relatively large number of clinically healthy cats will also be shedding the organisms. Isolation may therefore be a coincidental finding.

*References 36, 51, 71, 91, 92, 95, 97, 105, 107.

THERAPY

No antiviral drugs are in widespread use for the treatment of FHV-1 and FCV. Drugs such as acyclovir, given in human herpesvirus infections, do not seem to have good activity against FHV-1, and others are either toxic or awaiting evaluation.[63] However, in cases of ulcerative keratitis associated with FHV-1 infection, other antivirals have been used with some success, largely based on their efficacy in human ocular herpesvirus infections.[11,90] See Chapter 93 for further information of antiviral treatment of ocular viral infections. Interferon may also be useful for cats with acute respiratory viral infections, and for ocular herpes infections, although evidence for its success is limited.[61,90] Some data from both in vitro and in vivo studies suggest that orally administered lysine may be useful in treating acutely and latently FHV-1-infected cats.[50,53,93] For FCV, ribavirin has been shown to be effective in cell culture but was too toxic for in vivo use.[68,69] For additional information on the use of these drugs, see Table 16-2, Antiviral Chemotherapy, Chapter 2, and Drug Formulary, Appendix 8.

In viral respiratory disease, broad-spectrum antibiotic therapy should be given to help control secondary bacterial infection. Because swallowing solid tablets may be painful for cats, antibiotics can be given as pediatric syrups or long-acting injections. Cats should be reexamined after 4 to 5 days and, if necessary, bacterial culture and susceptibility tests performed.

In vitro studies have suggested that tetracyclines, and in particular doxycycline with its longer half-life, are the antibiotics of choice for the treatment of feline bordetellosis, although occasional resistance has been observed.[24,88] However, limited experimental evidence suggests that treatment with doxycycline may not eliminate the organism from the cat during the later stages of infection. Notably, systemic tetracyclines are theoretically contraindicated in pregnant cats or young kittens in which dental development is occurring. This is potentially less of a problem with doxycycline, although other side effects associated with its use may occur, such as esophagitis.[58,59] Also see Drug Formulary, Appendix 8. Other antibacterials that have shown good in vitro activity against *B. bronchiseptica* include trimethoprim-sulfamethoxazole and enrofloxacin.[9,24,88] Newer erythromycin derivatives such as azithromycin and clarithromycin have been effective against human *Bordetella* isolates[39] and might be effective against feline *B. bronchiseptica* that is resistant to the previously mentioned antimicrobials. However, these are not licensed for feline use in European Union counties.

Good nursing care is essential in cases of feline respiratory disease and, in milder cases, is generally best given at home by the owner. The cat should be encouraged to eat by offering strongly flavored aromatic foods. If eating is painful, baby foods or specialized proprietary or blended food may be helpful. Severe cases may require hospitalization and fluid therapy, and when anorexia is prolonged, a nasogastric or gastrotomy tube may be indicated. Nasal decongestants (e.g., phenylephrine) in the acute phase and mucolytic drugs (e.g., bromhexine hydrochloride) in the more chronic phase have been suggested to help clear airways, but conventional steam inhalation (e.g., placing the cat in steamy room) or nebulizing saline may also be useful.

PREVENTION

Immunity

For both FHV-1 and FCV, immunity has generally been measured by serum virus neutralizing (VN) antibody levels, although for FHV-1 cell-mediated immunity (CMI) is likely to be a better reflection of immune status. VN antibody has always been considered the hallmark of immunity for FCV and is certainly important in protection, as recent studies using mouse-cat chimeric antibodies have also shown.[102,103] However, some cats with no detectable VN antibody have demonstrated immunity to rechallenge with a heterologous strain, and several types of CMI responses have been reported.[27] For both viruses, local immune responses are also likely to be important. The ultimate test of immunity is, of course, response to challenge.

In FHV-1 infection, just after the primary disease, cats are generally resistant to challenge, although VN antibody titers are generally low and in some cases undetectable. After 6 months or more, protection may be only partial, and indeed, carrier cats may develop recrudescent disease. After either reactivation or field challenge, VN antibody titers rise to more moderate levels and thereafter remain reasonably stable, independent of virus shedding episodes.

Most cats are protected following the use of modified live or inactivated FHV-1 vaccines. However, immunity is not necessarily complete in all animals, even if challenge takes place within 3 months of the initial vaccination.[28] Similar levels of protection have been reported after a year. More studies have shown that the relative efficacy of an inactivated vaccine decreased from 83% shortly after primary vaccination to 52% after 7.5 years.[86]

With FCV infection, VN antibody titers are higher than those in FHV-1, and immunity is generally longer lived. However, some variation exists, depending on the virus strain involved and whether homologous or heterologous protection is being considered. Reinfection with a second strain will generally boost responses to both strains.

After vaccination against FCV, reasonable protection has been reported to last 10 to 12 months.[29] VN antibody levels tend to be higher compared with those in FHV-1, and in general, a better correlation exists with protection. In more studies, moderate levels of VN antibody have been shown to persist in a group of vaccinated cats for at least 4 years, although after 7.5 years, titers had declined to low or nondetectable levels.[85,86] Protection against a homologous FCV challenge decreased from 85% 3 weeks after vaccination to 63% after 7.5 years.

MDAs (i.e., essentially colostral) in kittens may persist for 2 to 10 weeks for FHV-1, with mean levels falling below detectable levels (less than 1:2) by 9 weeks of age. For FCV, in most kittens, MDAs persist for 10 to 14 weeks. However, for both viruses, low levels of MDAs do not necessarily protect against subclinical infection. Interestingly, some animals with no detectable FHV-1 antibody appeared to be protected against disease but not infection.

Studies on immunity in *B. bronchiseptica* infection have concentrated on the measurement of IgG levels in serum as measured by ELISA. After primary infection, antibody levels rise by 4 weeks to reasonably high titers. Experimental studies with an intranasal (IN) feline *B. bronchiseptica* vaccine showed that protection against challenge was present within 72 hours of vaccination and lasted for at least a year.[109] MDAs for *Bordetella* have been detected in experimental cats, although these appear to be fairly short lived, lasting for only 2 to 6 weeks.[27]

Vaccination

Vaccination has been available for many years against the two respiratory viruses and has been relatively successful in controlling disease. However, disease can still be a problem, especially when cats are kept grouped together and when kittens lose their MDAs before vaccination. Both viruses are very widespread in the cat population and carriers are common, ensuring plenty of exposure. Prevention and control therefore often require a combined approach of vaccination and management.

Three types of FHV-1 and FCV vaccines are commercially available: modified live virus (MLV) vaccines administered parenterally or IN and inactivated adjuvanted virus vaccines given parenterally. In addition, a significant number of genetically engineered vaccines for both FHV-1 and FCV have been reported.*

For routine FHV-1 and FCV vaccination programs, all types of vaccine appear to be suitable. In previously unexposed cats, all vaccines induce reasonable protection against disease but generally do not protect against infection or the development of the carrier state.

Several FCV strains are used in commercial vaccines, including strains F9 and 255. Most of these strains seem to protect against the majority of FCV isolates but not as well against all. Some evidence suggests that multivalent vaccines may increase the proportion of strains neutralized.[38]

Parenteral MLV vaccines should be administered carefully because clinical signs can be induced if the vaccine virus reaches the oral-respiratory mucosa (i.e., if the cat licks the injection site or if an aerosol is made with the syringe). Vaccine virus should not generalize, but spread of the MLV-FCV component within the cat after parenteral inoculation may sometimes occur, possibly leading to disease in the individual cat and possibly spreading to other cats.[67,71] However, genetic typing has shown that, although some cases of disease following vaccination may be caused by the vaccine virus, the majority are associated with coincidental field virus infection.[71,73]

IN-MLV vaccine induces better protection but often induces slight side effects, such as sneezing and ocular and nasal discharges. IN vaccines, however, are useful for rapid (2 to 4 days) onset of protection. IN vaccines used in conjunction with parenteral vaccine on entry have reduced the severity of upper respiratory disease in cats maintained at contaminated shelters for 3 or more days.[19]

*References 18, 26, 57, 87, 111.

Inactivated adjuvanted vaccines can be reasonably effective, and modern adjuvants have led to improvements in immunogenicity (see Chapter 100). However, adjuvants can sometimes cause local or systemic reactions. Very rarely, feline vaccine–associated sarcomas may develop at the site of injection, particularly following the use of aluminium-based adjuvants.[28,49,62] Inactivated vaccines are helpful in virus-free colonies because no risk of spread or reversion to virulence is present. Some inactivated vaccines are licensed for use in pregnant queens, and vaccination during pregnancy can help protect kittens by prolonging MDAs.

Boosters for FCV and FHV-1 vaccines are traditionally recommended every year, although evidence indicates that immunity may last longer in some cases.[85,86] In view of this finding, and because of concerns over vaccine site reactions, it has been suggested that after the first annual booster, revaccination intervals may be extended up to 3 years.[21,22] In addition, an individual risk-benefit assessment is proposed to determine the most appropriate vaccination strategy for a particular animal.[28,29]

For B. bronchiseptica, an IN-MLV vaccine is available, which has been shown to have a duration of immunity of at least a year.[109] The vaccine is similar to IN products available for dogs. Mild respiratory signs such as sneezing and nasal discharge may occur following vaccination, as for the IN viral vaccines. The vaccine is indicated in cases in which cats are at specific risk of acquiring Bordetella infection, for example, in rescue shelters or boarding catteries, or where bordetellosis is known to be a problem.

An inactivated, fimbrial subunit–based vaccine has also been marketed in some countries, but the IN vaccine will likely replace this.

Disease Control

The following measures apply in general to both viral respiratory disease and B. bronchiseptica infection. Routine vaccination for the respiratory viruses is indicated, but B. bronchiseptica vaccination is probably best recommended primarily for high-risk situations, such as in boarding and shelter facilities. The possibility of transmission of B. bronchiseptica between dogs and cats should also be considered.

Household Cats

Pets should be vaccinated regularly. If the cat goes into a boarding cattery or other high-risk situations, it should be boosted every year. From the point of view of infectious disease, ideally, a friend or neighbor should feed the cat while the owner is on vacation. Individual cats should be protected from stress and social contact as much as possible to avoid exposure.

Boarding Catteries

All cats entering the cattery should have an up-to-date vaccination record, with annual boosters. When rapid protection is required, IN vaccine may be given. Clients should be aware that such vaccines themselves may induce mild clinical signs.

Cattery owners should not rely on vaccination alone for disease control because pathogens will inevitably be present either from the occasional cat incubating disease or from carriers. Thus measures should be taken to prevent spread of infection and reduce the concentration of infectious agents in the environment (Table 16-3). Such measures may appear complicated, but in practice, they are not difficult to implement and, in the authors' (RG, SD, AR) experience, can actually increase the efficiency within a cattery.

Shelter Facilities

In general, the same management measures apply as those with boarding catteries. Although this practice may be more difficult to achieve, molecular typing studies have demon-

strated that limiting the spread of individual FCV isolates within a shelter is possible if good hygiene measures are used.[74] Because the immune status of the cats in a rescue shelter is often unknown, incoming animals should be quarantined and isolated from others. Those with clinical signs should be kept apart. Unless animals can be isolated on arrival for 3 to 4 weeks, parenteral vaccines may not have time to become effective. In these circumstances, using the IN vaccines may be advisable if available. Infected dogs, which can act as a source of B. bronchiseptica infection in cats, should be housed separately where possible, especially if an outbreak of canine infectious tracheobronchitis occurs.

Breeding Catteries

In disease-free colonies, cats should be vaccinated regularly if any contact, direct or indirect, occurs with other cats. Inactivated vaccines are preferable. Care should be taken to avoid bringing virus into the colony; any cat with a history of or contact with oral or respiratory disease may be a carrier. Vaccinated cats can be carriers, and kittens can be infected subclinically because of MDAs. Thus stud cats and new breeding stock should be from a respiratory disease–free colony. The risk of infection from cat shows is possible, but the greatest risk of infection to disease-free households is from stud cats and new breeding stock when exposure is prolonged.

Table • 16-3

Recommendations to Prevent the Spread of the Respiratory Viruses in a Boarding Cattery

Admit only fully vaccinated cats.

House cats individually with solid partitions between pens, unless cats are from same household.

Ensure that frontages are at least 1 meter apart.

Put known carriers or cats with history of respiratory disease in a separate section or at least at one end of the cattery; and feed last.

Ensure that surfaces of pen are easily washable and that food and litter bowls can be easily removed without entering the pen (i.e., do not handle cats more than necessary).

Feed cats in same order each day and attend to each pen completely before moving on to the next.

Either disinfect hands between each pen or have individual rubber gloves for each pen, for use only with that pen. Disinfect gloves thoroughly before use with a new boarder. Alternatively use disposable gloves.

Wear rubber boots and step into a disinfectant bath if it is necessary to enter a pen.

Either use disposable food trays or have two sets of food bowls used on alternate days. Soak used set in a 1 : 32 bleach solution with detergent for several hours and then rinse and allow to dry until reuse 24 hours later.

Prepare food in a central area.

Use similar system to food bowls for litter trays.

When a cat goes home, thoroughly disinfect cage, allow to dry, and preferably leave empty for 2 days before reusing.

Reduce concentration of virus in the environment by providing adequate ventilation, low relative humidity, and optimal environmental temperatures.

Adapted from Gaskell RM, Radford AD, Dawson S. 2004. Feline infectious respiratory disease, p 590. In Chandler EA, Gaskell CJ, Gaskell RM (eds), *Feline medicine and therapeutics*, ed 3, Blackwell Publishing, Oxford. Used with permission.

Table • 16-4

Feline Respiratory Disease Control Program in a Breeding Cattery with Endemic Disease

Provide regular vaccination programs.

Give booster vaccinations to queens either before mating or during pregnancy (inactivated vaccine only).

Keep cats as stress free as possible, and use good management practices to reduce spread of viruses within the colony.

Avoid breeding from queens with a history of oral or respiratory disease in their kittens.

Move queens into isolation at least 3 weeks before term so that the kittens are not exposed to carriers in the colony and that any shedding episode from the queen, as a result of the move, will end before parturition.

Wean kittens into isolation away from the queen as soon as feasible (ideally at 4 to 5 weeks before MDAs wane if it is likely she is a carrier).

Vaccinate all kittens as soon as MDAs are at a noninterfering level (normally 9 or more weeks), and keep them in strict isolation until a week after the second dose (normally at 12 weeks).

Earlier FHV-1 and FCV vaccination schedules with IN or parenteral vaccines may be used, although these are not always licensed for early use and should be used with care. Parenteral vaccines can be given from 6 weeks of age, at 3 week intervals until 12 weeks of age. IN vaccination should be carried out 7 to 10 days or so before disease has been occurring and then again at 12 weeks. Some evidence indicates that multiple doses are not necessary, although they were originally advocated.

MDAs, Maternally derived antibodies; *FHV-1,* feline herpesvirus-1; *FCV,* feline calicivirus; *IN,* intranasal.

Cats entering the disease-free colony should be quarantined for 3 weeks to identify animals incubating the disease. Cats should be swabbed for virus detection at least twice a week during this time. This practice increases the probability of detecting FHV-1 excretion and low-level shedding FCV carriers. Even so, the risk still exists of importing a latent FHV-1 carrier or a low-level FCV carrier that may be a source of infection. Oropharyngeal swabs may also be tested for *B. bronchiseptica* infection.

In breeding colonies where the disease is endemic, achieving or maintaining virus-free or *Bordetella*-free status is difficult. For both respiratory viruses and *B. bronchiseptica,* carriers are common providing a frequent source of infection. For most situations, the only reasonable course is to attempt disease control (Table 16-4).

SUGGESTED READINGS*

3. Binns SH, Dawson S, Speakman AJ, et al. 1999. Prevalence and risk factors for feline *Bordetella bronchiseptica* infection, *Vet Rec* 144:575-580.
17. Dawson S, Willoughby K, Gaskell RM, et al. 2001. A field trial to assess the effect of vaccination against feline herpesvirus, feline calicivirus and feline panleukopenia virus in 6-week-old kittens, *J Feline Med Surg* 3:17-22.
21. Elston T, Rodan H, Flemming D, et al. 1998. 1998 report of the American Association of Feline Practitioners and Academy of Feline Medicine Advisory Panel on Feline Vaccines, *J Am Vet Med Assoc* 212:227-241.
29. Gaskell RM, Gettinby G, Graham SJ, et al. 2002. Veterinary Products Committee working group report on feline and canine vaccination, *Vet Rec* 150:126-134.
43. Hurley KF, Pesavento PA, Pedersen NC, et al. 2004. An outbreak of virulent systemic feline calicivirus disease. *J Am Vet Med Assoc* 224:241-249.
51. Maggs DJ, Lappin MR, Nasisse MP. 1999. Detection of feline herpesvirus-specific antibodies and DNA in aqueous humor from cats with or without uveitis, *Am J Vet Res* 60:932-936.
66. Pedersen NC, Elliott JB, Glasgow A, et al. 2000. An isolated epizootic of hemorrhagic-like fever in cats caused by a novel and highly virulent strain of feline calicivirus, *Vet Microbiol* 73:281-300.
75. Radford AD, Sommerville L, Ryvar R, et al. 2001. Endemic infection of a cat colony with a feline calicivirus closely related to an isolate used in live attenuated vaccines, *Vaccine* 19:4358-4362.
86. Scott FW, Geissinger CM. 1999. Long-term immunity in cats vaccinated with an inactivated trivalent vaccine, *Am J Vet Res* 60:652-658.

*See the CD-ROM for a complete list of references.

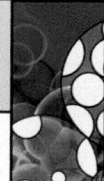

CHAPTER • 17

Feline Foamy (Syncytium-Forming) Virus Infection

Craig E. Greene

ETIOLOGY

Feline foamy virus (FeFV), previously known as "feline syncytium-forming virus," has been classified in the family *Retroviridae,* subfamily *Spumavirinae.* Host-specific viruses of this genus have been isolated from many other mammals. The prevalence of FeFV infection is high in normal and diseased cats. Virus has been isolated from primary cultures of tissue and body secretions in up to 90% of a population of cats.[6] More typically the prevalence of infection in a cat population varies between 4% and 50%, depending on the age, geographic location, and local environment of the cats.[11,13] Fifty percent or more of kittens born to FeFV-infected queens are infected at birth,[13] and 15% of cultures of fetal cats are positive for the virus, suggesting that it can be transmitted vertically.[5] In utero infection probably occurs by the transfer of infected maternal leukocytes across the placenta, but infection is not transmitted through milk of lactating animals.[13]

In contrast to most feline infectious diseases, the FeFV infection rate in cat colonies is actually lower than that in the random cat population. Roaming or outdoor cats have the highest prevalence, suggesting transmission through bite wounds.

FeFV is a nuisance to virologists and manufacturers of feline vaccines because it is found in many normal feline tissues and cell cultures that have been subjected to multiple passages. In vitro, it is not host specific; in addition to cat cells, it infects cells of dogs, chickens, humans, and bats.[16] It is not usually present in primary cell cultures.[10] FeFV is difficult to distinguish morphologically from feline leukemia virus (FeLV), which is visualized only as it buds from the cell. FeFV forms a recognizable nucleocapsid within the cytoplasm before budding. The suitability of FeFV as a vector for feline vaccine antigens has been studied.[21]

FeFV was given its prior name of syncytium-forming virus because it produces multinucleated syncytia within 1 to 2 weeks of growth in certain rapidly multiplying tissue cultures. Cell lysis is rarely if ever noted, and intranuclear inclusions are never seen. Only in some instances has malignant transformation been noted in tissue culture. Syncytium formation in cell culture is not unique to this feline virus; it has also been associated with a variant of FeLV.[17] A genetic insertion in the envelope glycoprotein gene was responsible for this cytopathic effect.

PATHOGENESIS

FeFV has not been associated with any disease; many cats have been infected naturally and experimentally and had no clinical illness. This scenario is typical of host adaptation because these viruses are apathogenic in their respective hosts.[19] Virus replication appears to be moderated by the infected cat. Reports about its pathogenicity are controversial and confusing. The presence of the virus in 100% of cats affected with chronic progressive polyarthritis has been reported.[15] Concurrent FeLV infection was found in 70% of these cats. The prevalence of infection with both viruses was 2 to 10 times greater than that in age-matched cats not having chronic progressive polyarthritis. By altering the host immune system, FeLV may potentiate the ability of FeFV to produce disease. Therefore one of Koch's postulates has not been fulfilled. Other factors must be involved as well because the disease cannot be induced by inoculation of FeFV alone. Combined infections with FeFV and feline immunodeficiency virus (FIV) are also frequently found. Coinfection with FeFV and FIV did not increase the severity of FIV-induced illness in the early stages of the disease.[23] A combined infection is most likely a result of a common mode of transmission rather than a mutual pathogenic mechanism. In vitro FeFV strains infect lymphoblastoid cells, producing altered replication, syncytia formation, and fragmentation of cellular DNA.[8] These features of apoptosis may be responsible for independent immune alterations in infected cats.

Arthritis, which is thought to result from chronic antigenic stimulation and immune complex deposition, is characterized histologically by lymphoplasmacytic infiltrates and is temporarily responsive to immunosuppressive therapy. An inherent genetic tendency may explain the reason certain male cats are more prone to developing disease despite the high prevalence of these viral infections in the general population.

CLINICAL FINDINGS

Most infected cats are asymptomatic. Chronic progressive polyarthritis of cats generally affects males between 1.5 and 5 years of age.[12,14,15,22] Two forms of the disease have been described: one with osteoporosis and periarticular periosteal proliferation, the other with periarticular erosions, collapse of the joint space, and joint deformities. Lymphadenomegaly, swollen joints, and stiff gait are caused by both types.

DIAGNOSIS

Joint fluid abnormalities consist of increased numbers of neutrophils and large mononuclear cells. That FeFV stimulates antibody production in infected hosts has been used as the basis for immunodiffusion and indirect fluorescent antibody testing for antibody.[1,15] Serology can be performed in addition to blood cultures to screen cats for infection. Infected kittens can be detected at birth by culturing buffy coat cells from their peripheral blood. Animals are infected for life and develop persistent, nonprotective antibody titers to the virus. For this reason, cats showing a serologic response to the virus are presumed to be infected. Several strains may exist, and the actual prevalence of infection may be higher than indicated by seropositivity. Neonatal kittens born to infected queens lose their maternal antibody by 6 to 8 weeks of age if they are not infected. Serum antibody titers increase after this time if they become infected.[5]

Virus can be isolated from most tissues but requires one to four passages in vitro. Actually, FeFV is detected only in vivo in cells and secretions of the oropharynx. Despite genetic material being supplied by the host, viral replication is suppressed. Latency can be expressed by cocultivating buffy coat white blood cells with fetal cat cells or by exposing cells to oropharyngeal secretions.

THERAPY AND PREVENTION

Chronic progressive polyarthritis has no known cure, and the clinical and pathologic changes it causes usually are temporarily responsive for weeks to months to immunosuppressive therapy such as prednisolone (10 to 15 mg/day per cat) and cyclophosphamide (Cytoxan, Bristol-Myers Squibb, Princeton, N.J.; 7.5 mg/day per cat for 4 days each week). Cats identified as having polyarthritis should be eliminated from research projects and removed from vaccine production and specific-pathogen–free colonies.

SUGGESTED READINGS*

15. Pedersen NC, Pool RR, O'Brien T. 1980. Feline chronic progressive polyarthritis, *Am J Vet Res* 41:522-535.
19. Saib A. 2003. Non-primate foamy viruses. *Curr Top Microbiol Immunol* 277:197-211.
23. Zenger E, Brown WC, Song W, et al. 1983. Evaluation of cofactor effect of feline syncytium-forming virus on feline immunodeficiency virus infection, *Am J Vet Res* 54:713-718.

*See the CD-ROM for a complete list of references.

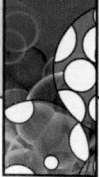

CHAPTER 18

Feline Paramyxovirus Infections

Craig E. Greene and Hans Lutz

Viruses of the family *Paramyxoviridae* (genera *Paramyxovirus*, *Morbillivirus*, and *Hendra* virus) have been shown to cause infections in the central nervous system (CNS) of domestic and large exotic Felidae, although none of the viruses in this group are known to be primarily feline viruses.

AVIAN NEWCASTLE VIRUS INFECTION

Avian Newcastle disease virus *(Paramyxovirus)* has been experimentally inoculated into the CNS of domestic adult cats and kittens, producing disseminated encephalomyelitis.[12,17] Neonatal kittens can also be infected by intraocular or intranasal exposure to large quantities of virus. The incubation period of oculonasally administered virus was relatively long (11 to 17 days) compared with that following direct CNS inoculation (3 to 4 days). Clinical signs of encephalomyelitis were seizures, head tilt, and myoclonus. Progressive lower motor neuron paralysis developed in limbs and cranial nerve musculature. In some affected animals, behavioral alterations were present. A disseminated nonsuppurative meningoencephalitis was found histologically; virus appeared to spread throughout the nervous system along descending and ascending neuronal pathways.

UNTYPED PARAMYXOVIRUS INFECTION

A paramyxovirus-like agent has also been isolated from the CNS of naturally infected cats that had focal demyelinating encephalitis and inclusion body formation.[9] The virus was isolated from affected cats by co-cultivating CNS tissue with fetal feline kidney cell lines. The isolated virus, serologically unrelated to known paramyxoviruses, was inoculated into the CNS of neonatal mice that developed a similar encephalitis 5 months later.

Paramyxovirus-like nucleocapsids have also been observed by electron microscopy (EM) in explant cultures of CNS tissue from clinically healthy cats or those with demyelinating optic nerve lesions that were co-cultured with feline kidney or Vero cell lines.[34] The significance of these ultrastructural findings is uncertain.

Nonsuppurative encephalitis has been reported in an adult Siberian tiger *(Panthera tigris)*, in which intranuclear inclusion bodies detected on light microscopy and nucleocapsid material detected on EM were found to be similar to those of viruses of the family *Paramyxoviridae*.[11] These observations could represent infections with canine distemper virus (CDV) or a variant, but definitive information is unavailable.

CANINE DISTEMPER VIRUS INFECTION

CDV, a *Morbillivirus*, has been shown to infect a wide variety of terrestrial carnivores. Domestic cats were experimentally inoculated, but clinical signs were absent (see Epidemiology, Chapter 3). In contrast to domestic cats, large exotic Felidae appear to be more susceptible to infection with CDV. Isolates appear to be immunologically similar to virulent isolates from other carnivores, but this finding does not exclude differences in viral biotypes.[5] Mutant viral strains, originating from wildlife and domestic dogs in close proximity to the large cats, are the most likely explanation for outbreaks of CDV infection in large cats.[8] A chronic, progressive, nonsuppurative meningoencephalitis, clinically and pathologically similar to that caused by CDV in dogs, has been described in a Bengal tiger *(P. tigris)*.[12] Marked increases in serum and cerebral spinal fluid (CSF) antibodies against CDV were found. Myoclonus was similar to that seen in other paramyxovirus-type infections in dogs and cats. CDV was suspected as the cause of respiratory and neurologic disease in two snow leopards *(Uncia uncia)* that had simultaneous feline panleukopenia.[10] CDV was not isolated; however, histologic lesions, intranuclear inclusions, virus ultrastructure, immunofluorescence, and serologic testing were all positive for CDV infection. Feline panleukopenia virus (FPV)-induced immunosuppression was presumed to have allowed development of CDV infection.

Canine distemper outbreaks have occurred in captive leopards *(P. pardus)*, tigers, lions *(P. leo)*, and a jaguar *(P. onca)* in North America.[5,36] Initial illness was manifest systemically by anorexia, gastrointestinal or respiratory signs (or both), followed by CNS signs of ataxia, myoclonus, seizures, and coma. The source of infection for one epizootic was CDV-infected raccoons and skunks having a concurrent outbreak. Viruses isolated from the affected cats were identified as CDV by monoclonal antibody testing and genetic analysis. The isolates were linked to strains from the feral nonfelid hosts and not vaccine virus.[15] CNS lesions were focal and mild, consisting of nonsuppurative polioencephalitis, lymphocytic meningitis, and mild microgliosis in white matter. These lesions were less extensive and severe and did not have the demyelination and perivascular cuffing as typically observed in infected dogs. These features are more typical of acute CDV infection in susceptible carnivores (see Chapter 3).[31]

In 1994, an outbreak of CDV infection occurred in lions in the Serengeti in Tanzania.[20,26,29] Clinical signs included seizures, myoclonus, and other neurologic symptoms. Pathology revealed encephalitis and pneumonia. Histopathology typical for CDV infection was seen in 18 of 19 lions examined. Inclusion bodies immunologically cross-reacting with CDV proteins were identified in 14 of 19 lion samples that were available for examination. Of 83 serum samples tested for anti-CDV antibodies, 71 were found to be positive for CDV.[26] To determine the genetic relationship of the virus involved in the disease outbreak with other *Morbilliviruses*, buffy coat cells collected from two lions with neurologic signs were subjected to reverse transcriptase-polymerase chain reaction (RT-PCR), and the nucleotide sequence of the conserved P gene was determined.[26] These tests suggested that the lion CDV isolate was closely related to the Onderstepoort strain of CDV. The belief holds that the lion distemper outbreak originated from distemper infections in domestic dogs living around the Serengeti parks. However, for transmission between dogs and lions, hyenas were probably responsible. Based on neurologic signs, several hyenas were found to be affected and were also proved to be infected with CDV. In addition, hyenas, in contrast to lions, are known to roam into the villages of the local inhabitants, where they may have come into contact with domestic dogs. Natural exposure or infections with CDV have been shown in wild canids in Africa.[1,28] To determine whether the presence of other lion viruses may have favored the susceptibility to CDV, serum samples were tested for presence of antibodies to feline immunodeficiency virus (FIV), feline herpesvirus (FHV-1), feline rhinotracheitis virus (FRV), feline calicivirus (FCV), FPV, and feline coronaviruses. No relationship between the occurrence of CDV and antibodies to these other pathogens was found. Despite the apparent recent appearance of outbreaks of CDV infection in exotic Felidae, retrospective analysis of cases indicated infections as far back as 1972.[23]

To reduce the probability of future outbreaks of CDV in these lions, a program to vaccinate the domestic dogs living around the parks has been initiated and is recommended for all captive large Felidae. Inactivated distemper virus vaccine has been recommended to protect large exotic Felidae against infection with this virus.[5] However, the efficacy of inactivated vaccines in dogs and other exotic carnivores, not to mention cats, has not been documented. Because chick embryo-adapted (Onderstepoort strain) vaccines are generally safer than tissue culture-adapted (Rockborn strain) ones, they should be considered for evaluation in large Felidae.[4,5]

HENDRA VIRUS (EQUINE MORBILLIVIRUS) INFECTION

In September 1994, an outbreak of acute respiratory disease in horses occurred in Hendra, a suburb of Brisbane, Queensland, Australia.[21] The horses developed pneumonia that was clinically characterized by anorexia, depression, pyrexia, tachypnea, and ataxia. Terminally, head pressing and a frothy nasal discharge occurred. A stable hand and horse trainer became ill with an influenza-like illness. The stable hand was ill for 6 weeks, and the trainer died of respiratory distress. A novel virus, closely related but distinct from *Morbillivirus*, was isolated from both the horses and the people. Another episode was retrospectively identified in Mckay, a town in North Coastal Queensland in a farmer who developed an acute progressive encephalitis.[27] The farmer had assisted with treatment and subsequent necropsy of the affected horses. Most interestingly, the horses developed myoclonic twitches similar to those observed in dogs with canine distemper. Meningoencephalitis has subsequently been documented in experimentally infected horses.[35]

The predominant pathologic lesions in horses from the Hendra outbreak were in the lungs, which were congested and edematous. Histologically, interstitial pneumonia with pneumocyte and capillary degeneration was apparent. Virus was immunologically detected in the endothelial cells by direct fluorescent antibodies. In the Mckay episode, virus was detected by positive PCR in CSF and in the Hendra episode, in brain tissue and serum.[24]

The equine *Morbillivirus* (EMV) was unusual in its ability to grow in cell cultures originating from a significant number of animal species, including submammalian vertebrates. A large number of laboratory animal species, including dogs and cats, were experimentally inoculated subcutaneously with the virus.[33] The dogs and cats were vaccinated for common viral diseases but notably the dogs for CDV. The dogs did not become ill, but the cats developed inappetence and tachypnea by the fifth day postinoculation (PI) and died on the sixth and seventh days PI. The cats had gross lesions of pulmonary edema, hilar lymphadenomegaly, pneumonia, and pleural effusion. Histologic lesions of vasculitis matched those in affected horses. The virus was isolated from the lungs, spleen, kidney, and brain. Surviving cats did not develop specific serum viral neutralizing antibody. Cats have also been experimentally infected via intranasal and oral exposure to virus and by direct contact with previously infected cats.[16] Because EMV is so genetically distinct from other *Morbilliviruses*, it is suspected to have existed for a long time and to have been acquired from a mammalian reservoir host. Of all laboratory species inoculated, cats were most susceptible and developed an illness that matched that in horses and in people.

A limited serosurvey of cats in the metropolitan Brisbane area did not reveal detectable antibody to the virus.[33] Subsequent studies in cats have shown that they can be infected by nonparenteral routes and that the virus can spread naturally among cats.[32] Of many wildlife species tested, *Pteropus* bats have serum antibodies to the virus and may be the reservoir species.[37] Transmission from bats to another species, such as the horse, may be required for human exposure.

In contact, transmission studies have shown that the virus is not highly contagious. Horses in direct contact with experimentally infected cats and infected horses in contact with other horses or cats did not transmit infection.[35] Similarly experimentally infected cats did not transmit the infection to horses. In experimentally infected animals, regardless of species, organisms were most prevalent in the kidney and urine, which suggests urinary transmission as the means of spread.[35] The organism was isolated for up to 3 weeks following infection of a horse and 14 months in a human developing infection, suggesting viral persistence and a carrier state.

NIPAH VIRUS INFECTION

An outbreak of fatal human encephalitis during 1998 and 1999 was attributed to a newly recognized paramyxovirus acquired from swine. Pigs, people who were predominantly pig farmers, dogs, and cats were infected. Although illness resulted in the other species, the disease in pigs was self-limiting and, in some cases, subclinical. Human infection was attributed to close contact with pigs. The role of dogs or cats as secondary sources of infection could not be excluded. In cats, Nipah virus was very similar in its behavior to that of closely related *Hendravirus*. Two cats were oronasally infected with Nipah virus from an outbreak in pigs that caused respiratory and neurologic signs.[18] Respiratory and neurologic disease was observed in the cats, and virus was found in secretions of the oropharynx and excreted in urine. The virus causes a widespread vasculitis in many organs, especially the respiratory tract and CNS. Eosinophilic, predominantly cytoplasmic, inclusions are seen within neurons. Pulmonary lesions are giant cell pneumonia, and the secretions and tissues contain large amounts of virus.

SUGGESTED READINGS*

4. Appel MJG, Summers BA. 1995. Pathogenicity of *Morbilliviruses* for terrestrial carnivores, *Vet Microbiol* 44:187-191.
7. Chua KB, Bellini WJ, Rota PA, et al. 2000. Nipah virus: a recently emergent deadly paramyxovirus, *Science* 288:1432-1435.
8. Cleaveland S, Appel MGJ, Chalmers WSK, et al. 2000. Serological and demographic evidence for domestic dogs as a source of canine distemper virus infection for Serengeti wildlife, *Vet Microbiol* 72:217-227.
16. Hooper PT, Westbury HA, Russell GM. 1997. The lesions of experimental equine *Morbillivirus* disease in cats and guinea pigs, *Vet Pathol* 34:323-329.
19. Spencer LM. 1995. CDV infection in large exotic cats not expected to affect domestic cats, *J Am Vet Med Assoc* 206:579-580.

*See the CD-ROM for a complete list of references.

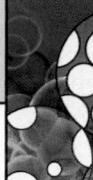

CHAPTER • 19

Poxvirus Infection

Malcolm Bennett, Rosalind M. Gaskell, and Derrick Baxby

ETIOLOGY AND EPIDEMIOLOGY

The best described and most common poxvirus infection of cats is cowpox, caused by an *Orthopoxvirus* organism,[2] but infections with *Parapoxvirus*[16] organisms and uncharacterized poxviruses in India and North America[28] have been reported. Poxviruses are relatively environmentally stable and can remain infective in dry conditions for several months to years. However, they are readily inactivated by many disinfectants, especially hypochlorites.

Cowpox virus is found only in Eurasia.[2] In western and northern Europe, the reservoir hosts are voles (*Clethrionomys* spp. and *Microtus* spp.) and wood mice (*Apodemus* spp.),* whereas in Turkmenia and Georgia the reservoir hosts are ground squirrels *(Citellus fulvus)* and gerbils *(Rhombomys opimus* and *Meriones libicus).*[2]

Although the domestic cat is the most frequently recognized incidental host,[6,7,23,25] cowpox virus can also infect humans,[3,14] cattle, and various captive exotic mammals.[2] A small number of cases have also been reported in domestic dogs.[7] Rats *(Rattus norvegicus)* and house mice *(Mus musculus)* also may be rare incidental hosts.

Feline cowpox is seen primarily in rural cats that hunt rodents, and most cases are seen in summer and autumn[5,7] when the opportunities for infection from the wildlife hosts are greatest. No sex or age predisposition to infection exists. Occasional cat-to-cat transmission occurs, as does cat-to-human transmission.[3]

Reports of natural orthopoxvirus infection in wild or domestic dogs are rare, although specific antibodies were found 6% to 20% of foxes in Germany.[19,23] Intradermal inoculation of 2×10^5 PFU of cowpox virus into red foxes *(Vulpes vulpes)* produced mild skin lesions with minimal viral replication.[8] No lesions were found after oral inoculation of virus. Another orthopoxvirus, murine ectromelia, has caused congenital disease in farm-raised silver foxes (*Vulpes vulpes* winter coat), blue foxes (*Alopex lagopus* winter coat), and mink *(Mustela vison)* in the Czech Republic.[22] Orthopoxvirus infec-

tion was identified in a dog, a cat, and the owner in a household in Germany.[35] The infection was presumed to have spread from the cat, with lesions in the dog healing after 1 to 4 months. A natural orthopoxvirus infection, characterized by ulcerative dermatitis at the site of a suspected rat bite, was identified in a domestic dog in the United Kingdom.[33] This infection was likely caused by cowpox because this has been the only orthopoxvirus in the United Kingdom since smallpox was eradicated. The natural reservoir of ectromelia virus is not known.

PATHOGENESIS

The usual route of cowpox infection in cats is skin inoculation, probably through a bite or other skin wound, although oronasal infection is also possible. Local viral replication produces a primary skin lesion, and spread to the draining lymph nodes and a leukocyte-associated viremia give rise to widespread secondary skin lesions. During the viremic period, virus can be isolated from the respiratory tract.

CLINICAL FINDINGS

Cats

Feline cowpox usually causes widespread skin lesions, but most cats have a history of a single primary skin lesion, generally on the head, neck, or forelimb. Primary lesions often are accompanied by a concurrent bacterial infection and may vary in appearance from a small, superficial scabbed-over wound to a large abscess or area of cellulitis.

Although some cats may have only a single, primary lesion, most develop secondary skin lesions within 1 to 3 weeks. First apparent as randomly distributed, small epidermal nodules, the lesions increase in size (1-cm diameter) over 3 to 5 days to form well-circumscribed ulcers, which soon become scabbed (Figs. 19-1, *A* and *B*). These gradually dry and after 4 to 5 weeks, they exfoliate (Fig. 19-1, *C*). New hair growth soon occurs, although some lesions may result in small, permanently bald patches.[6,7,24,27]

*References 4, 9, 12, 13, 18, 20.

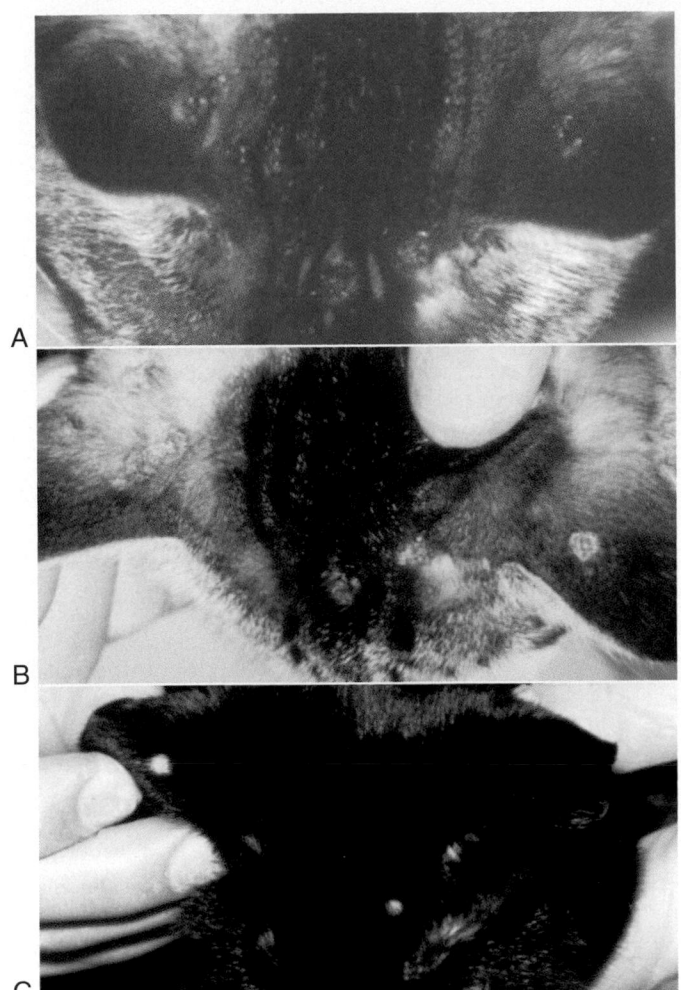

Fig 19-1 Various stages of cowpox lesions on the heads of three cats. **A,** Secondary papules. **B,** Scabbed secondary lesions. **C,** Healing lesions after scabs dropped off. (Courtesy Malcolm Bennett, University of Liverpool, Liverpool, England.)

Many cats show no clinical signs other than skin lesions. Signs of systemic illness are usually mild and occur during the viremic period just before development of secondary skin lesions. Cats may be pyrexic, inappetent, or depressed; a few may have coryza or transient diarrhea. More severe disease is rare in domestic cats and is often associated with severe bacterial infection or immune dysfunction often resulting from feline leukemia virus or feline immunodeficiency virus infection or from glucocorticoid treatment.[6] However, in exotic felids (e.g., cheetahs) a rapidly fatal pneumonia frequently develops. Severely ill cats have a poor prognosis, and euthanasia may be advised.

Feline parapoxvirus infection, probably from sheep or goats, also causes multiple crusty skin lesions, which heal over a few weeks. Anecdotal accounts of similar conditions exist in North America.

Dogs
Infection in dogs is similar to the cat infection, except that in the few cases seen only a small number of lesions develop. Orthopoxvirus infections should be suspected in animals with ulcerative skin lesions, especially if they have had contact with rodents.

Humans
In humans, a single painful skin lesion develops at the site of inoculation, although more severe and widespread lesions may develop in those with preexisting skin diseases or who are immunosuppressed in some way.

No clinical signs are usually seen in rodent hosts, although infection may be associated with reduced fecundity and survival.[34]

DIAGNOSIS

Dried scab material can be sent in a sealed container without transport medium to a laboratory by mail. Cowpox virus can be readily isolated in various cell cultures, and virions often can be seen in scab homogenates by electron microscopy (EM). EM is the easiest way to recognize parapoxviruses because of their characteristic morphology and because they are difficult to grow in cell culture. Some laboratories now use the polymerase chain reaction routinely to diagnose cowpox virus infection.[30] Serum antibodies can be detected by various methods; we routinely use an immunofluorescent assay for cowpox (see Appendix 5).[13]

PATHOLOGIC FINDINGS

The histologic appearance of feline cowpox includes epithelial hyperplasia and hypertrophy, with multilocular vesicle formation and ulceration. Many infected cells contain intracytoplasmic, eosinophilic inclusion bodies.[4] Immunostaining is a useful aid to histologic diagnosis.

THERAPY AND PREVENTION

Broad-spectrum antibiotics are recommended to control secondary bacterial infections, and general supportive therapy, including fluids, may be necessary. Glucocorticoids are contraindicated because they may exacerbate the condition. Cidofovir has been shown active against cowpox virus in cell culture and some animal systems[10,32]; however, the authors (MB, RMG, DB) are unaware of any reports of its use in cats. The drug had to be given early in the course of experimental infection and to immunocompetent animals to be most effective.

No vaccines are available, but vaccinia virus may be considered for valuable zoo collections at risk for cowpox infection. Vaccinia virus appears to be of low infectivity and pathogenicity for cats and cheetahs, but its ability to provoke a protective immune response is unknown.

PUBLIC HEALTH CONSIDERATIONS

Cowpox
Cowpox is a zoonotic virus. In addition to a painful skin lesion, it usually causes systemic illness, which may require hospitalization but rarely causes death.[3,14] People with a preexisting skin condition or immune deficiency seem particularly at risk of more severe disease. Human cowpox is rare (with one or two cases occurring each year in the United Kingdom), but cats are thought to be the source of more than 50% of these cases.[3] The risk of cat-to-human transmission is small if basic hygienic precautions are taken. With few exceptions the illness does not warrant euthanasia of the cat. Even a recent smallpox vaccination is unlikely to provide protection for humans against the primary cowpox lesions, although it might help prevent more severe disease.[1]

Vaccinia

Vaccinia is an orthopoxvirus that originally infected cattle and was later developed as a vaccine strain for smallpox in humans. It has no natural reservoir host. Most mammals, including domestic species, are susceptible to vaccinia virus. With the advent of widespread vaccination for smallpox, there is concern that domestic pets might become infected from people and act as transport hosts. Interspecies transmission from vaccinated people to dogs and cats can be minimized if lesions are protected and dressings disposed of properly.[29] Secondary generalized vaccinia infections, especially in children, may occur after vaccinia vaccination. This condition, known as *eczema vaccinatum*, is characterized by diffuse dermatitis with open vesicles, fever, lymphadenomegaly, and rarely encephalitis.[31] Vesicles contain large amounts of virus that may contaminate the environment and put humans and pets at risk. This risk is extreme for humans with immunosuppression, such as those infected with human immunodeficiency virus. Experimental and epidemiologic evidence show that infections in pets are self-limiting.

Vaccinia has been used as a vector for rabies virus glycoprotein in the oral bait programs being used to control wildlife rabies throughout the world. A human developed a localized and self-limiting infection after inadvertent self-inoculation with the oral bait vaccine (see Oral Vaccination of Wildlife, Rabies, Chapter 22). A similar problem was experienced by a laboratory worker preparing vaccine virus.[25] Humans who are immunocompromised develop more progressive and disseminated lesions.[11]

Canarypox

Canarypox has been used as a vector in a number of new vaccines available for dogs and cats, including a rabies vaccine (Purevax, Merial, Duluth, Ga.) in cats and distemper vaccine (Recombitek, Merial, Duluth, Ga.) in dogs. The canarypox virus is not associated with any known public health risk.

Monkey Pox

Monkey pox is found in the tropical rain forests of countries in western and central Africa. The reservoir is arboreal squirrels. Monkey pox developed in a young child within 2 weeks of a bite from a pet prairie dog (*Cynomys* spp.). The prairie dog was sold from a pet shop where it may have come in contact with a Gambian pouched rat (*Cricetomys gambianus*) from Africa. The family contacts became systemically ill and developed multifocal skin lesions. One family member developed vesiculation around a scratch from a household cat; however, this vesicle may have been incidental to the systemic infection acquired from the child. For more information see *http://research.marshfieldclinic.org/crc/files/MonkeyPox_MarshfieldWI_ClinicalPhotos_v3.pdf*. Dogs and cats are not considered hosts for this disease, but various rodents are cause for concern.

Other Poxvirus Infections

Other poxviruses, including many parapoxviruses, may also be zoonotic, but the risk of animal-to-human transmission of these viruses is unknown.

SUGGESTED READINGS*

3. Baxby D, Bennett M, Getty B. 1994. Human cowpox: a review based on 54 cases, 1969-93, *Br J Dermatol* 131:598-607.
12. Chantrey J, Meyer H, Baxby D, et al. 1999. Cowpox: reservoir hosts and geographic range, *Epidemiol Infect* 122:455-460.
17. Hawranek T, Tritscher M, Muss WH, et al. 2003. Feline orthopoxvirus infection transmitted from cat to human. *J Am Acad Derm* 49:513-518.
33. Smith KC, Bennett M, Garrett DC. 1999. Skin lesions caused by orthopoxvirus infection in a dog, *J Small Anim Pract* 40:495-497.

*See the CD-ROM for a complete list of references.

CHAPTER • 20

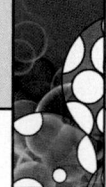

Feline Viral Papillomatosis

Herman F. Egberink and Marian C. Horzinek

ETIOLOGY AND EPIDEMIOLOGY

Papillomavirus (PV), a genus of the *Papovaviridae* family, contains small nonenveloped viruses with icosahedral symmetry and double-stranded circular DNA genome. They are widespread in nature and infect many species of mammals and birds.[14] These viruses also cause benign cutaneous and mucosal proliferations that are usually self-limiting and only rarely progress to malignant tumors.[1,18] All members of the genus share at least one antigenic determinant.[15] PVs are highly species specific, transmission having so far been reported only within a single animal species or between closely related hosts. In one isolate that had its genome completely sequenced, the virus was closely related to the canine

PV.[20,22] In several studies of papillomatous and hyperplastic lesions in cats, papillomaviral antigen was not demonstrated in the lesions, and only a few reports indicate that papillomavirus infection was proven.[2-4,9] This sparse occurrence may be the result of the inconspicuous nature and uncharacteristic morphology of the lesions, which preclude a clinical diagnosis by analogy. Besides a few case reports of individual cats with papillomas, a series of papillomatous lesions was published.[19] PV infection has been confirmed by immunohistochemical staining of lesions in six species of felids: the domestic cat, mountain lion (*Felis concolor*), Florida panther (*Puma concolor coryi*), bobcat (*Felis rufus*), Asian lion (*Panthera leo persica*), snow leopard (*Uncia uncia*), and clouded leopard (*Neofelis nebulosa*).[12,19] In most of these animals, the lesions were localized in the oral cavity, especially on the tongue.

PVs may be involved in the development of other feline tumors. A novel PV was cloned from hyperkeratotic cutaneous lesions of a Persian cat.[20] PVs were also identified in squamous cell carcinomas in situ. PV antigen could be demonstrated in skin biopsies in 30 out of 63 cats showing these skin lesions.[7] Cutaneous PV infections were also demonstrated in association with fibropapillomas.[11,21] Using polymerase chain reaction (PCR), investigators in these two studies found PV in 17 out of 19 and 9 out of 12 feline tumors with clinicopathologic features similar to equine sarcoids. Although the DNA was detected, PV antigen was not expressed suggesting a nonproductive viral infection of connective tissue.[21] This strong association suggests a causal relationship. However, also reports on fibropapillomas in cats are rare,[5] and evidence of a viral origin is mostly not provided.

Serologic studies to determine the prevalence of subclinical infections in the feline population have not been reported. A spill-over from another reservoir species (e.g., from a prey animal, similar to the epidemiology of poxviruses) cannot be excluded but is unlikely. In the case of equine sarcoids, an association with bovine papillomavirus (BPV) types 1 and 2 has been suggested.[1] A similar association was suggested for the feline fibropapillomas, given that 11 of the 20 cats in that study had known exposure to cattle and all but one were living in an area known for its dairy farms.[11] Additionally, in the case of feline cutaneous fibropapillomas, the nucleotide sequence of the amplified DNA from the feline tumor was distinct from, but similar to, BPV type 1.

Although the feline papovavirus has not been fully characterized, it was shown to be different from other PVs. A unique staining pattern using a panel of monoclonal antibodies against papillomavirus capsid protein epitopes may be demonstrated.[7,8] Interestingly, genetic and antigenic studies of the papillomas of exotic cats revealed that each species was infected with a different virus, underlining the high species specificity of PVs.

PATHOGENESIS

In general, papillomas will develop after introduction of virus through lesions or abrasions of the skin. Experimental infection of healthy cats with material from wartlike lesions of affected cats did not result in papilloma development. PVs have a specific tropism for squamous epithelial cells. The basal layer of the epithelium is infected, and early gene expression can be detected there. However, protein synthesis and virion assembly are restricted to the most terminally differentiated keratinocytes at the surface of the papilloma. After infection, hyperplasia in the stratum spinosum occurs, and proliferation of the epithelium becomes clinically evident 4 to 6 weeks postinoculation.

Host immunity is important in the development of viral papillomas. Age resistance is unknown. Lesions in 6- to 7-month-old kittens have been reported, but most cases were in cats 6 to 13 years of age.[4,19] Papillomas are more prevalent in animals and humans under conditions that impair T-cell functions.[4,10,18] Immunodeficiency seems to be a factor, increasing the chance of clinical manifestation; indeed, the first reports of papillomas in cats concerned animals under immunosuppressive therapy or infected with feline immunodeficiency virus.[2-4]

CLINICAL FINDINGS

The macroscopic appearance of feline lesions is not typical of papillomas seen in other domestic animals.[2-4,19] Although the

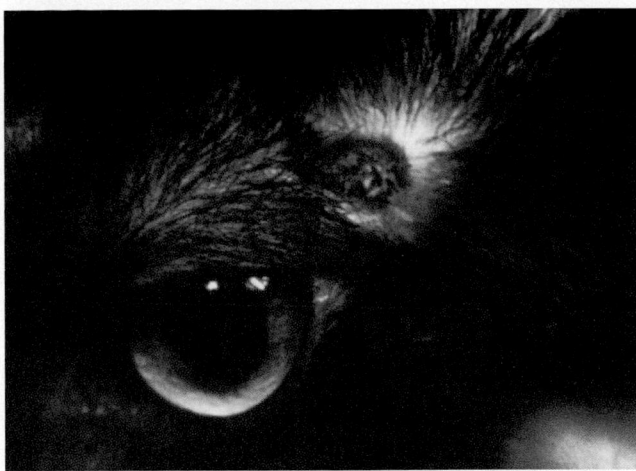

Fig 20-1 A papilloma plaque dorsolateral to the eye of a cat. (Courtesy University of Georgia, Athens, Ga.)

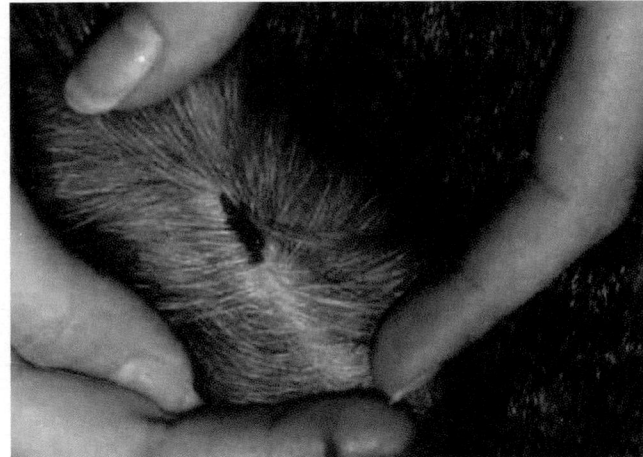

Fig 20-2 An elongated papillomatous growth on the ear margin of a cat. (Courtesy University of Georgia, Athens, Ga.)

surface of the lesions is verrucous, they appear as slightly raised plaques rather than warts (Fig. 20-1). The plaques are several millimeters in diameter; elongated lesions can sometimes be noticed. Plaques can be white or pigmented, scaly and greasy to the touch (Fig. 20-2). The wartlike lesions are located on the head, neck, dorsal part of the thorax, and abdomen. The oral papillomas seen in exotic felids are as multifocal, small, soft, light-pink, oval, slightly raised flat, sessile lesions. They are localized mainly on the ventral lingual surfaces. In some animals (snow leopards), lesions are also present on the tip and dorsal surface of the tongue, as well as the buccal mucosa.[19] The signs of systemic illness are not induced by the PV infection but are the consequence of a concurrent immunodeficiency.

DIAGNOSIS

A full-thickness biopsy of an entire lesion with adjacent normal tissue should be taken and processed for histopathologic, immunohistochemical, or electron microscopy (EM) examinations.

Histologic examination of cutaneous squamous papillomas reveals pigmented, hyperplastic epidermal plaques with defined boundaries. Proliferation of all layers is evident. The epidermal hyperplasia is characterized by acanthosis and hypergranulocytosis with hyperkeratosis. No inflammatory cells are observed in either the plaques or the adjacent stroma. Ballooning degeneration of cells in the stratum spinosum and stratum granulosum with nuclear changes can be observed. In the upper part of the former and in the stratum granulosum, solitary cells with large, irregularly shaped amphophilic inclusion-like structures occur. These are found in the cytoplasm, but ill-defined, probably intranuclear inclusions have also been reported. By EM, intranuclear papillomavirus-like particles are demonstrated in keratinized cells in the superficial epithelial strata of the plaques. The cytoplasmic inclusions appear as keratohyalin-like granules. The histology of feline fibropapillomas is virtually identical to that of equine sarcoids and is characterized by fibroblastic proliferation, hyperplasia of the overlying epidermis and rete ridges.[11]

For definite identification, immunohistochemical staining can be performed on sections through selected skin lesions using a broad-reactive, genus-specific antiserum (see Appendix 5). Staining of PV group-specific antigens is found mainly in the stratum granulosum and stratum corneum of the papilloma; some cells in the stratum spinosum also retain stain. Immunoreactivity predominates in the nuclei; however, weak staining of the cytoplasm is sometimes noticed, possibly after injury of the nuclear membrane. Besides the detection of PV antigen, a PCR can be performed to demonstrate the presence of PV DNA in the lesions. PCR can also be used for specific identification of the viral strains.

THERAPY

No specific treatment is known. The location and the number of papillomas will often not warrant surgical excision. In analogy with papillomas in other species such as dogs, spontaneous regression can be expected (see Chapter 9).

SUGGESTED READINGS*

7. LeClerc SM, Clark EG, Haines DM. 1997. Papillomavirus infection in association with feline cutaneous squamous cell carcinoma in situ, *Proc Am Assoc Vet Derm Am Coll Vet Derm* 13:125-126.
11. Schulman FY, Krafft AE, Janczewski T. 2001. Feline cutaneous fibropapillomas: clinicopathologic findings and association with papillomavirus infection, *Vet Pathol* 38: 291-296.
19. Sundberg JP, Van Ranst M, Montali R, et al. 2000. Feline papillomas and papillomaviruses, *Vet Pathol* 37:1-10.

*See the CD-ROM for a complete list of references.

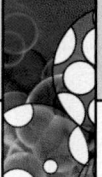

CHAPTER • 21

Miscellaneous Viral Infections

HANTAVIRUS INFECTION

Craig E. Greene, Anna-Lena Berg, and Bruno B. Chomel

Etiology

Hantaviruses are enveloped spherical RNA viruses in the family *Bunyaviridae*, which contains three other major genera that can be distinguished genetically, morphologically, and antigenically. Unlike other members of the *Bunyaviridae*, transmission of hantaviruses does not require arthropod vectors (for comparison, see *Bunyaviridae*, Chapter 26, Arboviral Infections). Each strain of *Hantavirus* is uniquely adapted to its respective subclinically infected rodent reservoir. This evolutionary relationship is a product of millions of years of coadaptation. The genus *Hantavirus* comprises many strains that are pathogenic for humans. In the Old World, Hantaan, Seoul, Dobrava, and Puumala viruses are associated with hemorrhagic fever with renal syndrome, whereas in the New World, Sin Nombre virus (SNV) is the main virus involved in human cases of hantavirus pulmonary syndrome in North America. However, Monongahela, New York, Bayou, and Black Creek Canal viruses also cause HPS and are found in eastern Canada and the eastern and southeastern regions of the United States. In South and Central America, several hantaviruses have been identified as causing HPS, including Andes virus in Argentina and Chile; Andes-like viruses such as Oran, Lechiguanas, and Hu39694 in Argentina; Laguna Negra virus in Bolivia and Paraguay; Bermejo virus in Argentina; Juquitiba virus in Brazil; and Choclo virus in Panama (Table 21-1).[72]

Epidemiology

Aerosol transmission from excreta of infected rodents is the principal means by which hantaviruses are transmitted; however, bite transmission between rodents and inadvertent transmission to humans has been documented. Aerosolized virus is the likely means of spread of infection between rodents and humans. Direct physical contact with the rodents is not required. Hantavirus infections of domestic and wild rodents are subclinical. Species differences exist among rodents in the length of salivary excretion, with times ranging up to 1 year. Infected rodents are thought to harbor the virus in their lungs and kidneys for life. The disease peaks during seasons and years when population densities of rodent colonies are highest and have the greatest chance of contacting human populations. The greatest incidence of infection in humans occurs when their work or recreational activities expose them to rodents. Infections occur on farms, in suburbs, and in residential areas, depending on the habitat of the reservoir host. In laboratory rats in the United States, the disease

Table • 21-1

Comparison of Features of Some Zoonotic Hantavirus Infections

DISEASE	VIRAL STRAIN	GEOGRAPHIC DISTRIBUTION	RESERVOIR HOST	USUAL CONTACT
Hemorrhagic fever with renal syndrome (HFRS)	Hantaan	Korea, China, eastern Soviet Republics, Balkans	*Apodemus agrarius* (Striped field mouse)	Agricultural activities
Nephropathia epidemica (milder HFRS)	Puumala	Scandinavia, western Soviet Republics, Europe,	*Clethrionomys glariolus* (Bank vole)	Forests and agricultural hedge rows, rural and suburban gardens, high forest crop
	Dobrava/Belgrade	Germany, Balkans, Russia, Estonia	*Apodemus agrariu* (Striped field mouse) *Apodemus flavicollis* (Yellow-necked field mouse)	Outdoor activities
Milder HFRS, chronic hypertensive renal failure	Seoul	Worldwide	*Rattus norvegicus* (Norway rat) and *Rattus rattus* (Roof rat)	Farms and residential areas, laboratory rats outside U.S.
Hantavirus pulmonary syndrome	Sin Nombre[a]	Western and southwestern United States, Canada	*Peromyscus maniculatus* (Deer mouse)	Human dwellings and outbuilding
Acute cardiopulmonary syndrome	Andes[b]	Argentina, Chile,	*Oligoryzomys longicaudatus* (long-tailed pygmy rice rat)	Rodent contact, person-to-person
	Laguna Negra	Paraguay, Bolivia	*Calomys laucha* (Vesper mouse)	Rodent contact
	Juquitiba	Brazil	Unknown	Unknown

HFRS = hemorrhagic fever with renal syndrome.
[a]Closely related strains are New York, *Peromyscus leucopus* (white-footed mouse) (*Eastern US*); Monongahela, *Peromyscus maniculatus* (deer mouse) (*Eastern US and Canada*); Black Creek Canal, *Sigmodon hispidus* (cotton rat) (*Florida*); Bayou, *Oryzomys palustris* (rice rat) (*Southeastern US*).
[b]Closely related strains are: Oran, *Oligoryzomys longicaudatus* (*Northwestern Argentina*); Lechiguanas, *O. flavescens*, (*Central Argentina*) HU39694, unknown reservoir (*central Argentina*).

has been controlled by serologic testing and by producing rodents from cesarean-derived stock maintained under strict barrier conditions.

Although hantavirus infections in humans receive the most attention, the viruses have a wide potential host range among other mammals. Any role of the cat or dog in the transmission of hantaviruses from rodents to humans is quite unlikely as indicated by a relatively low seroprevalence rate. The possibility of cats being a risk for hantavirus infection was initially raised by an epidemiologic study in China that indicated an increased risk factor of cat ownership for humans who developed hantavirus infection.[77] Several studies conducted in Europe showed the presence of hantavirus antibodies in domestic cats. Five percent of outdoor cats in Austria were found to be seropositive, with higher titers against Puumala than the Hantaan strain.[55] Similarly, serologic studies with cats in Great Britain showed an overall positive rate of 9.6%.[5] The seropositive rate was much higher (23%) for cats with various chronic illnesses. Cats that are allowed to roam or hunt outdoors have the highest seroprevalence. Among 100 such cats, immunofluorescent detection of hantavirus antigen (using three different polyclonal anti-Puumala serum specimens) in lungs and kidneys showed the virus in specimens of lung from

two cats.[58] A serosurvey of rural cats and dogs from the southwestern Canadian prairie found a 2.9% seroprevalence rate for cats, whereas virus-specific antibodies were not found in dogs.[40] In the United States the Four Corners states (Arizona, Colorado, New Mexico, and Utah) have been the location of the majority of the human infections. In a serosurvey for hantavirus infection in Arizona, dogs and cats had a low prevalence (3.5% and 2.8%, respectively) of seroreactivity to nucleocapsid proteins of SNV.[49] Polymerase chain reaction (PCR) testing of a few animals failed to amplify any hantavirus sequences. Neither coyotes nor dogs or cats appear to have a major role in the maintenance and transmission of SNV. Like humans, they likely acquire their infection from rodents and rodent excreta.

Pathogenesis

Different strains of the virus worldwide are associated with pulmonary or renal dysfunction or both. In infected humans the pulmonary syndrome is a result of acute pulmonary edema and shock. Viral antigens in pulmonary capillaries cause a sudden onset of interstitial pulmonary edema, cardiopulmonary compromise, and death. Renal insufficiency also has been found in patients.

Clinical Findings

No clinical signs have been attributed to hantavirus infection in cats. It is likely that their infection is asymptomatic because of the low carriage and quantities of virus.[58]

Clinical signs in humans vary according to the strain causing infection. Signs of Hantaan, Seoul, and Puumala infections are fever, headache, abdominal pain, renal dysfunction, and hemorrhagic diathesis. The pulmonary syndrome of SNV begins with fever and flulike symptoms that progress to signs of pulmonary edema and shock. Radiographs reveal acute bilateral pulmonary interstitial infiltrates, which have been attributed to pulmonary vasculitis. Most deaths associated with HPS are related to cardiac failure rather than pulmonary failure, therefore the term *Hantavirus acute cardiopulmonary syndrome* is more appropriate than *Hantavirus pulmonary syndrome*.[72]

Diagnosis

The diagnosis in humans is made by serologic demonstration of antiviral IgM and IgG in serum and cerebrospinal fluid (CSF). Diagnosis in rodents and carnivores (cats, dogs) is made by serologic testing (IgG). Culture can be performed because rodents excrete virus in their saliva, urine, and feces. Some excrete virus in the saliva for short periods, and others excrete it in the urine for up to 1 year.

Therapy

Intravenous ribavirin, the RNA-inhibitory antiviral drug (see Chapter 2), has been effective in the treatment of human hantavirus infections when used early in the illness. Excessive fluid administration must be avoided because it may lead to severe edema and increase the severity of the pulmonary edema.

Public Health Considerations

Most humans become infected by the aerosol route when inhaling dust after disturbing nests or closed spaces inhabited by infected mice. A few cases have been documented in which infection resulted from contact with urine-contaminated garbage and/or rodent bites. Avoiding contact with rodents and their excreta or insect vectors are the most effective ways to reduce the prevalence of disease. Rodent-infested structures and soil contaminated with feces must be avoided because harmful aerosols can spread infection. Masks, and in some cases respirators, should always be worn by people cleaning rodent-infested areas. Feral rodents should not be kept in captivity, and care should be taken when entering or cleaning closed buildings infested with rodents. Areas to be cleaned should be thoroughly soaked with disinfectants such as dilute sodium hypochlorite before they are mopped. Vacuuming and sweeping should be avoided to minimize dust. Although cats have been found to be subclinically infected and test seropositive for exposure, it is unlikely that cat-to-cat or cat-to-human transmission occurs. An epidemiologic link between cat ownership and hantaviral disease has not been suspected in North America or Europe.[58] Serologic studies in coyotes and domestic cats and dogs in the southwestern United States indicated seropositive rates of 0%, 2.8%, and 4.7%, respectively.[49] The data suggest that these animals are not important in viral maintenance or in transmission of the infection to humans.

FOOT-AND-MOUTH DISEASE

Craig E. Greene

Foot-and-mouth disease is a highly contagious illness of wild and domestic cloven-hoofed animals and is caused by strains of an *Aphthovirus* organism in the family *Picornaviridae*. It occurs worldwide; however, eradication has been variably successful in Australia, New Zealand, Japan, the British Isles, and North America. Carnivorous animals are relatively resistant to infection and do not play a major role in spreading or harboring the disease under conditions of natural exposure. The virus has been propagated in canine cell cultures.[67] Dogs and cats can be experimentally infected[27]; however, no epizootics have been found among carnivores. These animals may become incidentally infected during outbreaks in herbivores by contacting these animals or their offal. Reports have been made of dogs that became infected by scavenging remains of dead animals.[35,64]

As a result of epizootics, guidelines have been established for dog owners in areas known to have infected animals.[3] Dogs must be kept under control—on a leash or within an enclosure—at all times. Dogs should not be walked across farmland and should have minimal contact with livestock and wild animals. Certain sporting activities involving dogs should not be allowed in quarantined areas. Minimal restrictions have been placed on cats, although they should be kept indoors as much as possible. Disinfectants suitable for inactivating the virus are 4% sodium carbonate, 0.5% citric acid, 2% formalin, or 2% sodium hydroxide.[62] Phenolic disinfectants, quaternary ammonium compounds, and biguanides are not effective. Halogens such as sodium hypochlorite or iodine are less effective because of inactivation by organic matter.

VESICULAR EXANTHEMA

Craig E. Greene

A calicivirus that causes vesicular exanthema of swine produces lesions on the mouth, lips, snout, and feet is often confused with foot-and-mouth disease. Dogs have developed clinical signs of illness characterized by vesicular eruptions when outbreaks of vesicular exanthema virus infection have occurred in swine.[4] Virus was not definitely isolated in these cases. However, in other studies, experimentally infected dogs developed fever within 24 hours after inoculation and vesicular eruptions on their tongue and in their oral cavity.[4] These lesions healed within a few days. Virus was isolated from the spleen of a dog that became febrile after inoculation.

HEPATITIS E VIRUS INFECTION

Craig E. Greene

Hepatitis E virus (HEV) is an unclassified virus that causes an acute self-limiting hepatitis in humans. It is the most common form of acute hepatitis in adults in regions of Asia. It has been reported in developing countries in southeast and central Asia, the Middle East, and North Africa. More sporadic outbreaks have occurred in Mexico and the United States and other countries in the Western Hemisphere. The virus is spherical and nonenveloped, ranging from 30 to 32 nm in diameter, with its nucleic acid in a single-stranded positive sense RNA molecule. Although its structure resembles that of a calicivirus, its genome is closest to that of rubella virus, a member of the *Togaviridae* family. The strains found worldwide can be classified into three major genotypes.

Experimentally the virus has a broad host range. Chimpanzees, Old World and New World monkeys, pigs, rodents, and sheep have been experimentally infected. One swine isolate has been shown to have the broadest host range. In one report a person from Japan with hepatitis E had not traveled and was suspected to have become infected in the home environment.[39] Fever, malaise, icterus, and brown-colored urine were observed in the family members. They were seronegative; however, the patient's cat had a high HEV IgG titer.

Anti-HEV globulins have been detected in species of wild and domestic animals. The virus is shed in feces and can be detected by genomic methods. The epidemics of HEV infection in humans have generally been foodborne or waterborne. For prevention, animal feces must be handled with care in endemic areas. General sanitation helps prevent the infection.

RABBIT HEMORRHAGIC DISEASE

Craig E. Greene

Rabbit hemorrhagic disease (RHD) is an acute fatal disease of European rabbits (Oryctolagus cuniculus) caused by an RHD virus of the family Caliciviridae. The disease has been reported in Asia, Europe, Africa, and Americas. Feral cats in New Zealand have antibodies to RHD virus, and nested reverse transcriptase PCR (RT-PCR) has identified virus in the liver of one seropositive cat.[79] Cats fed rabbit livers infected with RHD virus developed serologic titers to the virus, and RHD viral RNA was detected in the tonsils, mesenteric lymph nodes, spleen, and liver. Even though large amounts of virus were found, clinical disease was not observed. Active replication of RHD virus was not demonstrated.

LYMPHOCYTIC CHORIOMENINGITIS

Craig E. Greene

Lymphocytic choriomeningitis (LCM) virus is an arenavirus of mice that is transmitted in utero or at birth and persists for life in high concentrations in various tissues. Outbreaks of rodent LCM infections have prompted concern that domestic dogs or cats might serve as reservoirs or vectors of the virus. Puppies (8 to 12 weeks old) did not develop clinical illness after parenteral or cerebral inoculation.[20] Challenged animals had increased neutralizing antibody titers to the virus, and infection was transmitted from infected to noninfected puppies. Except for intranuclear inclusions in the adrenal cortex, pathologic changes were not observed in the animals indicating the infection was subclinical. It is unlikely that dogs or cats become infected or spread the virus by natural exposure, because most human infections have resulted from direct contact with rodents.

BORNA DISEASE MENINGOENCEPHALOMYELITIS

Craig E. Greene and Anna-Lena Berg

Etiology and Epidemiology
Borna disease virus (BDV) is an enveloped, nonsegmented, negative-stranded RNA virus of the family Bornaviridae in the order Mononegavirales.[22] Other members of this order include Paramyxoviridae and Rhabdoviridae. BDV persistently infects the central nervous system (CNS) after experimental infection of various animal species, ranging from birds to primates. BDV naturally infects horses, cats, sheep, cattle, rabbits, ostriches, and numerous other species, probably including humans.[42,65] Cases of classic BDV encephalomyelitis, known as Borna disease (BD), in horses, sheep, and cattle are restricted to endemic regions in Germany, Switzerland, and Austria. Naturally occurring feline BD, characterized by behavioral and motor dysfunction (staggering disease), was first described in Sweden.[30,47] Although BDV infection has been reported in cats with ataxia and other neurologic signs in the United Kingdom[63] and Japan,[53,60] a direct etiologic role of BDV has not been established in these cases. One case of feline BD, verified by immunohistochemistry, has been reported from Switzerland.[13] Two dogs have been reported as having BD, one from Austria and the other from Japan.[59,75] A large wild cat (Lynx lynx) in Sweden was also diagnosed with classic BD.[21]

Specific BDV antibodies have been detected in horses and cats in various regions of the world. The disease in horses may be largely subclinical because the prevalence of antibodies in sera is much greater than clinical illness.[69] Based on serologic and nucleic acid screening, many feline infections are also subclinical.[54] Serologic studies indicate that in addition to Europe, cats have been subclinically exposed in the Philippines, Indonesia, Iran, Turkey, and Japan.[31,32] BDV antibodies have also been detected in cats with a wide variety of clinical signs.[31] Although the clinical manifestations may not be directly caused by BDV, they may indicate that the virus is an opportunistic pathogen. In two studies, twice as many FIV-positive cats had antibody titers to BDV as did cats with negative FIV test results.[31,33] In one of these instances, domestic cats kept indoors had twice the infection rate (57%) of feral cats (26%).[31]

Disease associated with BDV occurs most frequently in spring and summer and thus arthropod transmission has been suspected. Viral nucleic acid has been detected in salivary, nasal, and conjunctival secretions of horses and sheep; animals may become infected by direct contact with these secretions or fomites such as contaminated food or water.[65,74] A definitive reservoir host has not been documented, but rodents and birds are suspected.[9,69] Infection does not appear to spread readily between cats. Epidemiologic studies suggest that risk factors for infection in cats are highest for intact males that hunt mice in rural woodland environments.[8]

Pathogenesis
The virus is highly neurotropic and probably gains access to the CNS by transmucosal entry into nerve endings terminating in the olfactory, oropharyngeal, or gastrointestinal mucosae.[65] Similar to rabies virus, BDV spreads to and throughout the CNS by intraaxonal transport and from there spreads centrifugally into peripheral nerves.[28] Unlike rabies virus the replication rate of BDV is slow. The immune response to viral antigens is not protective but incites an immunopathologic response. Neutralizing antibodies appear in the serum and CSF. This response fails to clear the infection; the inflammation subsides, and BDV persists at low levels in the CNS of the host.[41] BDV infects neurons, astrocytes, oligodendrocytes, and ependymal cells.[70] Infection of feline astrocytes has been shown to impair their glutamate uptake function, a proposed mechanism for additional neuronal injury.[10]

In experimentally infected rats, acute phase immunity is cellular, with T cells as the predominant cell infiltrate. With chronic infection, plasma cell infiltrates and antibody titers increase and may magnify the inflammatory reaction.[70] These findings are similar to those found with naturally infected cats with staggering disease-feline BD, in which T cells predominate in the CNS and peripheral circulation.[7] Cytotoxic CD8+ T cells are thought to induce this immune response against the virus. Antibody titers increase with persistent infection of the CNS. Vaccination of rats before infection reduces the viral load in the CNS but increases their inflammatory reaction to the virus and resultant degree of neurologic impairment.[41]

Experimentally and naturally infected cats develop humoral immune responses to the BDV proteins p24 and p40. A Japanese group also reported serum antibodies to another BDV protein, p10, in cats with ataxia.[60] In addition to the systemic humoral response, BDV-specific antibodies are produced intracerebrally in naturally and experimentally infected cats.[36] Intracerebral inoculation of BDV produces high antibody titers against the immunodominant proteins in CSF; however, natural infections induce a weak humoral immune response in cats, primarily directed against BDV p24.[36]

Clinical Findings
Clinical signs of staggering disease-feline BD include paraparesis and ataxia, mental alteration, anorexia, hypersalivation, hypersensitivity to light and sound, visual impairment,

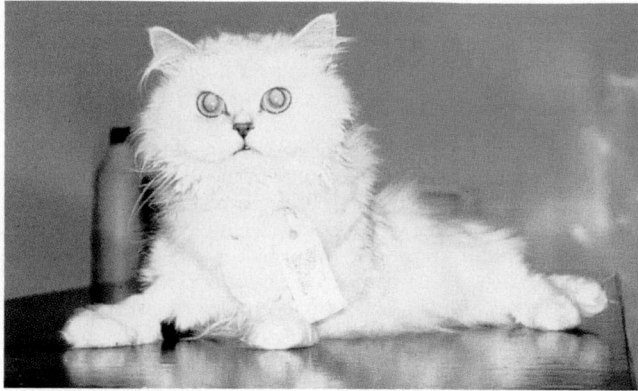

Fig 21-1 Cat with Borna disease showing posterior paresis. (Courtesy Anna-Lena Berg, AstraZeneca R&D, Södertälje, Sweden.)

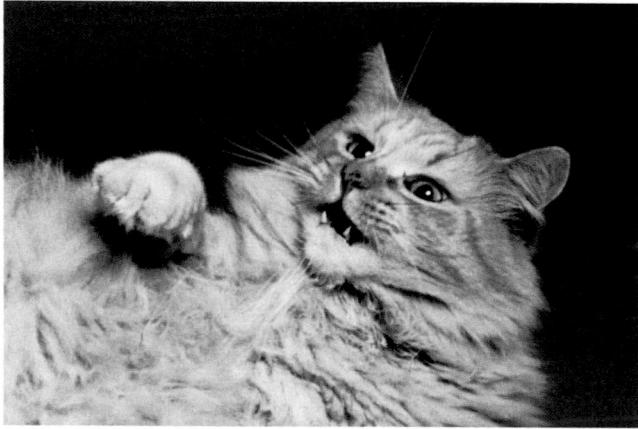

Fig 21-2 Cat with Borna disease with a "star gazing" disoriented appearance. (Courtesy Anna-Lena Berg, AstraZeneca R&D, Södertälje, Sweden.)

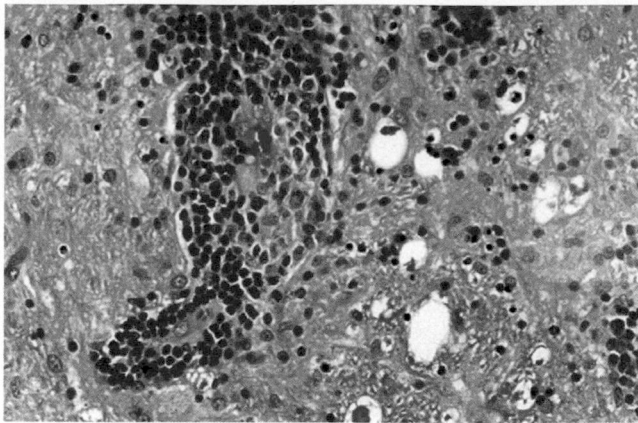

Fig 21-3 Histopathologic findings showing characteristic nonsuppurative perivascular cuffs in gray matter of the CNS (H and E stain, ×200). (Courtesy Anna-Lena Berg, AstraZeneca R&D, Södertälje, Sweden.)

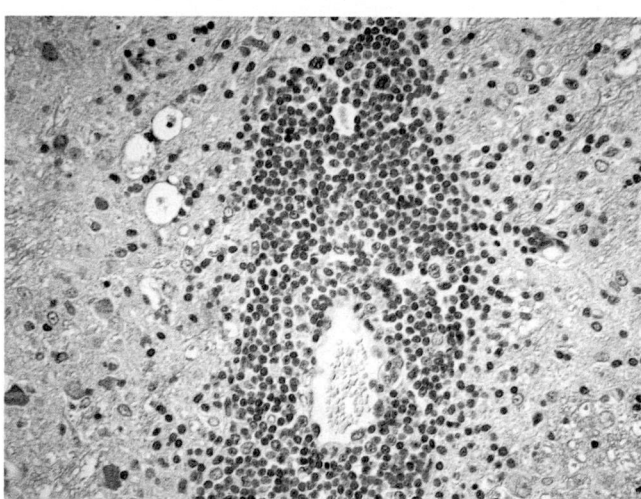

Fig 21-4 Immunohistochemistry with BDV antigen (brown staining) within astrocytes. Anti-BDV p24 antibody staining. (Courtesy Anna-Lena Berg, AstraZeneca R&D, Södertälje, Sweden.)

and seizures. The signs progress within 1 to 4 weeks until the clinical condition either deteriorates to complete paralysis and death or stabilizes, leaving most cats permanently afflicted with motor dysfunction, personality changes, or both (Figs. 21-1 and 21-2). Leukopenia is the only hematologic abnormality, and mononuclear pleocytosis and increased protein typical of viral inflammation are noted with CSF analysis. Treatment with glucocorticoids, especially when initiated at an early stage of disease, is sometimes beneficial.

Pathologic Findings
The inflammatory reaction in the CNS is characterized by a nonsuppurative meningoencephalitis in the gray matter of the olfactory bulb, cerebral cortex, hippocampus, basal ganglia, and brainstem. The spinal cord is affected to a lesser degree. Perivascular mononuclear cell infiltrates consisting of lymphocytes and macrophages accompany neuronal degeneration (Fig. 21-3). BDV antigen and nucleic acid persist in brain tissue of cats, particularly within astrocytes, causing chronic inflammatory lesions (Fig. 21-4). In one cat, large amounts of virus but no inflammation were found within neurons, presumably from viral persistence by infection at an early age.[1]

BD in dogs has been characterized by a rapid onset of progressive intracranial CNS deficits that are similar to canine distemper.[59,75] Histopathologic lesions, which predominated in the forebrain and midbrain, were a nonsuppurative menin-

goencephalitis with perivascular cuffing and diffuse mononuclear cell infiltrates of adjacent neuropil. Viral antigen was present in neurons as demonstrated by immunohistochemistry. In situ hybridization detected BDV RNA in the nucleus and cytoplasm of neurons. Inflammatory cells in the cuffs largely comprised CD3+ T cells.

Diagnosis
Controversy exists regarding the diagnosis and relative significance of BDV infection in animals.[69] There is little doubt that BDV can be pathogenic because isolates have been inoculated intracerebrally into specific-pathogen–free cats, resulting in neurologic signs and encephalitis.[44] However, the mere presence of BDV in an animal is not sufficient to confirm that clinical disease is a result of BDV infection because many animals may have subclinical infections. Presence of antibody titers in sera merely suggests exposure, and nucleic acid detection by RT-PCR in peripheral blood mononuclear cells or nonneurologic tissues may represent a carrier state. The extremely high sensitivity of nested PCR can also result in laboratory con-

tamination. Another problem is the possibility of false-negative results with RT-PCR because of sequence differences of target genes.[56] For this reason, detection in the CNS of BDV antigen by immunohistochemistry, of BDV RNA by in situ hybridization, or both in combination with neurohistopathologic alterations is considered the most reliable method of confirming active CNS disease (classical BD). The virus can be isolated in cell culture and by inoculation of rats.[30]

Although some investigators have suggested that lesions of feline BD resemble those of feline polioencephalomyelitis, no evidence suggests that these disorders are related. The histologic and clinical features of BD should be contrasted with feline polioencephalomyelitis, which predominantly affects the spinal cord, causing progressive lower motor neuron dysfunction with milder brainstem involvement (see Chapter 84, Neurologic Disease of Suspected Infectious Origin).

Public Health Considerations

BDV has been examined as a cause of human neuropsychiatric illnesses.[15,23] Antibodies to the virus have been detected in sera of patients with psychiatric disorders in Germany, Japan, and the United States. Similar to cats with FIV infection, humans with HIV infection have an increased risk of acquiring opportunistic infections. The prevalence of BDV-specific antibodies is fourfold higher in patients with HIV infection as compared with control patients.[12]

As with some aspects of the diagnosis in animals, findings regarding the significance of BDV infection in humans are controversial.[66] The potential contamination risks when using nested RT-PCR applies to humans as well as to animals. Isolation and immunologic detection of BDV in seropositive patients has been inconsistent. In the most definitive work, BDV-specific antigen and RNA were found in the brain of humans with hippocampal sclerosis.[19,24] The modes of transmission of BDV to humans are unknown. Although no formal proof of direct cross-species transmission exists, the potential of BDV as a zoonotic agent should be taken into consideration.

SUGGESTED READINGS*

3. Anonymous. 2001. Foot and mouth disease: implications for dogs, *J Small Anim Pract* 42:206.
14. Calisher CH, Mills JN, Root JJ, et al. 2003. Hantaviruses: etiologic agents of rare, but potentially life-threatening zoonotic diseases. *J Am Vet Med Assoc* 222:163-166.
33. Huebner J, Bode L, Ludwig H. 2001. Borna disease virus infection in FIV-positive cats in Germany, *Vet Rec* 149:152.
59. Okamoto M, Kagawa Y, Kamitani W, et al. 2002. Borna disease in a dog in Japan, *J Comp Pathol* 126:312-317.
61. Peters CJ, Khan AS. 2002. Hantavirus pulmonary syndrome: the new American hemorrhagic fever, *Clin Infect Dis* 34:1224-1231.
62. Quinn JP, Markey BK. 2001. A review of foot-and-mouth disease, *Irish Vet J* 54:183-190.
63. Reeves NA, Helps CR, Gunn-Moore DA, et al. 1998. Natural Borna disease virus infection in cats in the United Kingdom, *Vet Rec* 143:523-526.

*See the CD-ROM for a complete list of references.

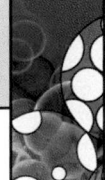

CHAPTER • 22

Rabies and Other Lyssavirus Infections

Craig E. Greene and Charles E. Rupprecht

ETIOLOGY

Rabies virus is the prototype of the genus *Lyssavirus* in the family *Rhabdoviridae*.[55] The agents are enveloped, bullet-shaped RNA viruses that usually measure 75 × 180 nm (Fig. 22-1). The single strand of nonsegmented RNA (negative-sense) encodes five structural proteins: a nucleocapsid (N) protein, a phosphoprotein (P), a matrix (M) protein, a glycoprotein (G), and a RNA-dependent RNA polymerase (L). These viruses have been isolated worldwide and were originally considered to belong to one common antigenic type. However, techniques using monoclonal antibodies (MABs) produced against viral proteins and gene-sequencing techniques have provided evidence for antigenic and genetic differences (variants) among various isolates from major wildlife and domestic animal hosts within a given geographic region. Analysis of sequences from the nucleoprotein gene of worldwide virus isolates supports studies of MAB typing, which suggest that rabies may have spread to the Americas, Asia, and Africa from European colonization.[203,204] Infection in imported domestic dogs may have contributed to sylvatic species spread, with establishment of enzootic foci in these areas.

Rabies virus replicates by budding from the host cell membranes, and viral nucleocapsid develops in the cytoplasm. Complete viral particles may be formed at the cell surface, but, more commonly, they bud from intracytoplasmic membranes. Free virus particles infect new or adjacent cells by fusing their envelopes with the host cell membrane, which allows direct entry of viral genetic material.

As an enveloped virus, rabies is inactivated by various concentrations of formalin, phenol, alcohol, halogens, mercurials, mineral acids, and other disinfectants. The virus is extremely labile when exposed to ultraviolet (UV) light and heat.

Rabies virus can remain viable in a carcass for several days at 20° C, although it may survive much longer when the body of the victim is refrigerated.[143] Immunofluorescent testing, commonly used for rabies diagnosis, does not depend on the presence of viable viral particles. Viral antigen may be detected at times beyond the presence of viable virus. Virus

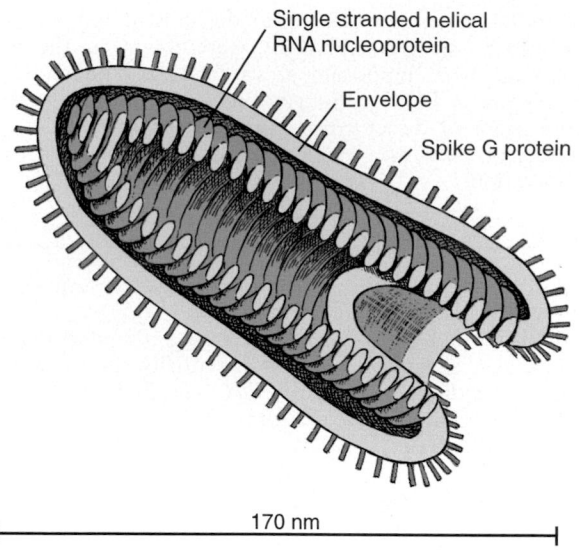

Single stranded helical RNA nucleoprotein

Envelope

Spike G protein

170 nm

Fig 22-1 The bullet-shaped rhabdovirus. (Courtesy University of Georgia, Athens, Ga.)

survival for isolation by mouse inoculation can be greatly increased in unrefrigerated tissue by storing it in 50% glycerol in phosphate-buffered saline at room temperature (20° C). Preservation can also be enhanced if a 20% suspension of infected tissue or virus culture is made with a solution that is high in protein or amino acids. Storage at ultra-low temperatures (−30° to −80° C) prolongs viral activity for years in untreated fresh-frozen tissue. However, freezing samples in a household-type freezer with subsequent defrosting cycles will damage the tissue and destroy the virus for subsequent detection. Inactivation of specimens may also be possible for diagnostic purposes using genetic detection (see later discussion, Submission of Specimens). A modified-live Evelyn-Rokitniki-Abelseth (ERA) strain oral rabies virus vaccine was found to be stable for 28 days under field conditions; however, the product life was maintained at −30° C before use.[140]

Besides rabies virus, at least six other *Lyssavirus* genotypes have been described, with more to follow as surveillance is enhanced, particularly among bats.[16]

EPIDEMIOLOGY

Susceptibility

All warm-blooded animals are vulnerable to infection with rabies virus, but mammals are the only known vectors and reservoirs in nature. Factors such as the viral variant, the quantity of virus inoculated, and the bite site affects susceptibility. In addition, the degree of species susceptibility varies considerably. Foxes, coyotes, jackals, wolves, and certain rodents are among the most susceptible animal groups. Skunks, raccoons, bats, rabbits, cattle, and some members of the families Felidae and Viverridae have a high susceptibility. Groups with only moderate susceptibility include domestic dogs, sheep, goats, horses, and nonhuman primates. Birds and primitive mammals such as the opossum may have low susceptibility. Cats are actually more resistant than dogs are to experimental infection with some canine rabies virus isolates but are much more prone to develop infection with some field isolates from wildlife and with vaccine virus. Younger animals are usually more susceptible to rabies infection than are older ones.

Transmission

The disease is nearly always caused by the bite of an infected animal that has rabies virus in its saliva. Other modes of transmission are infrequently involved in infections of the dog and cat but may serve to maintain infection in wildlife. Transmission from exhaled or excreted virus has been suggested for spread between animals in extremely large colonies of cave-dwelling bats and by infections following laboratory exposures.[74,105] Such airborne infections probably involve large quantities of aerosolized virus under conditions of poor ventilation and a susceptible exposed host. Rabies can occasionally result from ingesting infected tissue or secretions.[82] Suspected transplacental rabies infections in skunks, bats, and a cow have been reported.[57] Environmental transmission by fomites is rarely, if ever, involved. Human rabies is usually caused by a bite but has been acquired by corneal transplantation. The disturbing number of human cryptic rabies cases in which no obvious source of exposure can be determined argues against complacency with this disease. Infections with salivary shedding of virus before obvious clinical signs have been observed so that the absence of dramatic neurologic abnormalities cannot be used to rule out absolutely the possibility of rabies infection.

Hosts and Range

More than 27,000 cases of animal rabies are reported yearly in the world. The estimated actual number of cases is many times greater. The World Health Organization (WHO) reported 31,223 cases of human rabies for 1993, with additional cases from nonreporting countries. Total estimates are closer to 50,000 deaths annually.[179] Reports suggest that more than 25,000 human rabies deaths may occur in India alone. Most affected regions are tropical countries in Africa, Asia, and South America. Many island or peninsular nations, such as Antarctica, New Zealand, Taiwan, some of the Caribbean islands, Ireland, Norway, Finland, Sweden, Iceland, Hawaii, and Japan, are reportedly free of rabies. In Western Europe, countries such as Spain, Portugal, Italy, and Greece have become free of terrestrial rabies at considerable cost through oral vaccination of wildlife, especially the red fox (*Vulpes vulpes*), with a continual risk of importation. Compulsory parenteral vaccination and serologic testing for imported domestic animals have also been instituted in some areas to help maintain this status. Rabieslike European bat *Lyssavirus* (EBLV) strains still exist in these regions and occasionally infect terrestrial mammals as a "spill-over." No evidence has been found that these infections have resulted in adaptation to these inadvertent hosts. Although once boasting a rabies-free status, some isolated nations such as Great Britain and Australia have *Lyssavirus* strains in bats.[70,118,229] The role of these rabieslike bat *Lyssavirus* strain in the spread of infection to people is thought by some researchers to be marginal.[232] However, a fatal human rabies caused by EBLV type 2a was reported in the United Kingdom in an unvaccinated bat handler.[161] This was the first indigenous classical case of rabies in a person within the United Kingdom in over 100 years.

Seven genotypes of *Lyssavirus* are known (Table 22-1): rabies virus, Lagos bat virus, Mokola virus, Duvenhage virus, and two EBLVs.[212] The seventh *Lyssavirus* has been identified in fruit bats ("flying foxes") in Australia,[71] and it has been identified in all species of wild and some captive Australian bats.[68,226] It has been termed Australian bat *Lyssavirus* (ABLV) or *Ballina* virus. Fatal infections in two people have been reported.[6] Serologic evidence suggests a closely related virus exists in the Philippines.[18] Because of the close antigenic relationship of ABLV with rabies virus, cross-protection from vaccination is presumed effective.[212] EBLV type 2 (EBLV-2) occurs in mainland Europe; however, it has been identified

Table • 22-1

Classification of the Genus Lyssavirus

GENOTYPE	PHYLOGROUP	SEROTYPE	DESCRIPTION OF STRAINS
1	I	1	Classical rabies virus, including street and fixed varieties
2	II	2	Lagos bat viruses 1, 2, and 3
3	II	3	Mokola 1, 2, 3, and 5
4	I	4	Duvenhage 1, 2, and 3
5 and 6	I	5	European bat *Lyssavirus* types 1 and 2
7	I	6	Australian bat *Lyssavirus*

Modified from Woldehiwet Z. 2002. Rabies: recent developments,, *Res Vet Sci* 73:17–25.

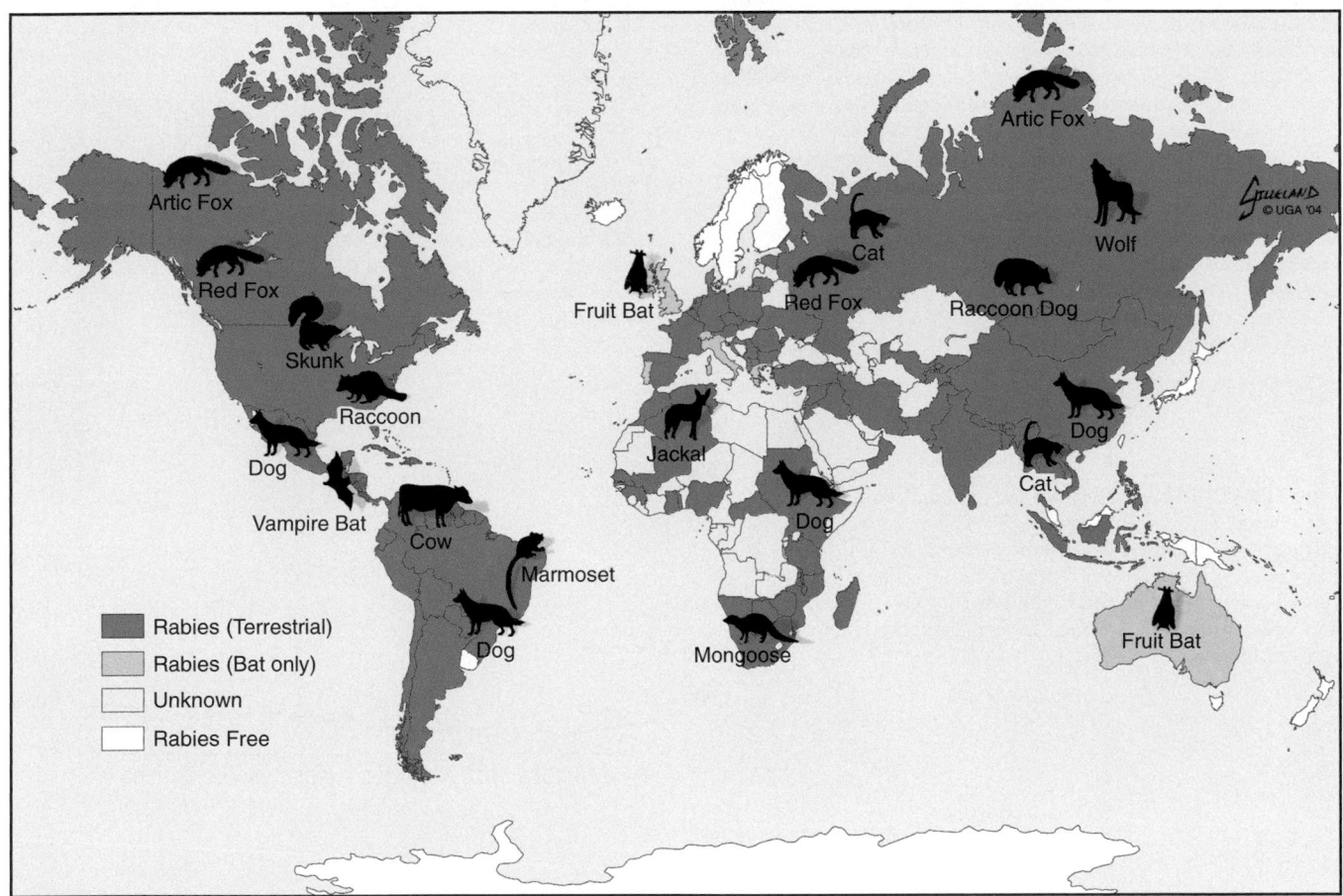

Fig 22-2 Principal animal vectors of rabies for major regions of the world. Some countries are reportedly free of rabies (see Hosts and Range in text). (Courtesy University of Georgia, Athens, Ga.)

from four Daubenton's bats *(Myotis daubentonii)* in England.[70,118,229] Transmission of EBLV-2 to terrestrial mammals is rare. However, an infection occurred in a person handling a Daubenton's bat (see previous discussion). A sero-survey conducted on Daubenton's bats in Scotland indicated between 6% and 19% of the bat sera had positive test results for antibodies to *Lyssavirus*,[15] indicating an endemic reservoir.

Although all mammals are susceptible to rabies virus, members of Canidae, Viverridae, and chiropteran species are the most capable vectors of the disease. Throughout the world, in most of the Northern Hemisphere, rabies is predominately a sylvatic disease of wildlife, whereas in the Southern Hemisphere, the feral dog in urban areas is the primary

species involved in the transmission of the disease (Fig. 22-2). Turkey is the only country in Europe where dog rabies exceeds that in wildlife species.[146] Despite the fact that all warm-blooded animals are susceptible, rabies virus in a given enzootic area is usually a distinct variant that adapts itself to a single dominant reservoir host. Therefore independent host-specific enzootic cycles of infection exist among individual host species. For example, wildlife reservoir species in various geographic areas of the United States are raccoons, skunks, foxes, coyotes, and insectivorous bats (Fig. 22-3). In Europe and parts of Asia, the primary species are foxes and raccoon dogs *(Nyctereutes procyonoides)*, whereas in South Africa and certain Caribbean nations jackals *(Canis adustus* and *C.*

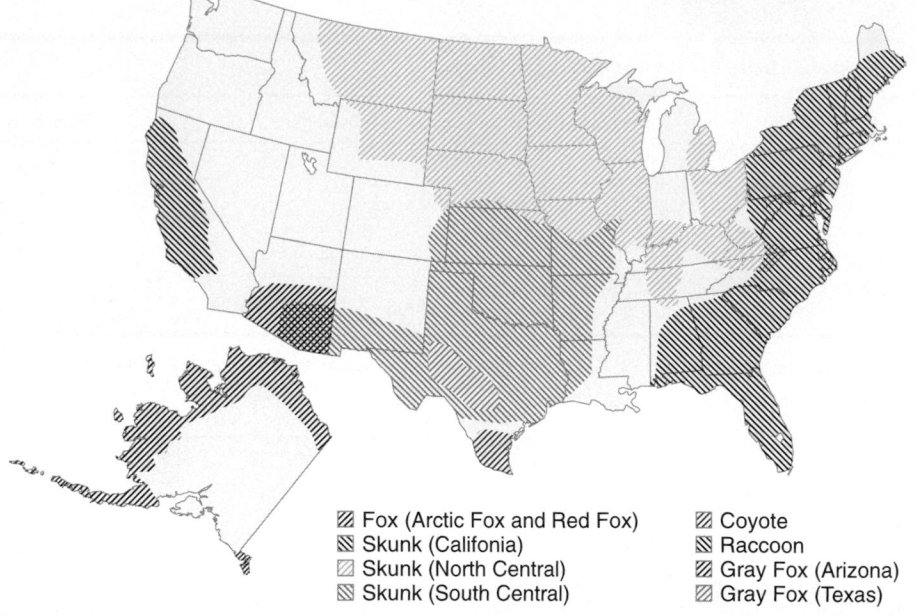

Fig 22-3 Currently recognized areas of endemic rabies in wild terrestrial animals in the United States. (Data adapted from maps provided by the Centers for Disease Control and Prevention, Atlanta, Ga.; map courtesy University of Georgia, Athens, Ga.)

Fox (Arctic Fox and Red Fox)   Coyote
Skunk (Califonia)   Raccoon
Skunk (North Central)   Gray Fox (Arizona)
Skunk (South Central)   Gray Fox (Texas)

CDC data

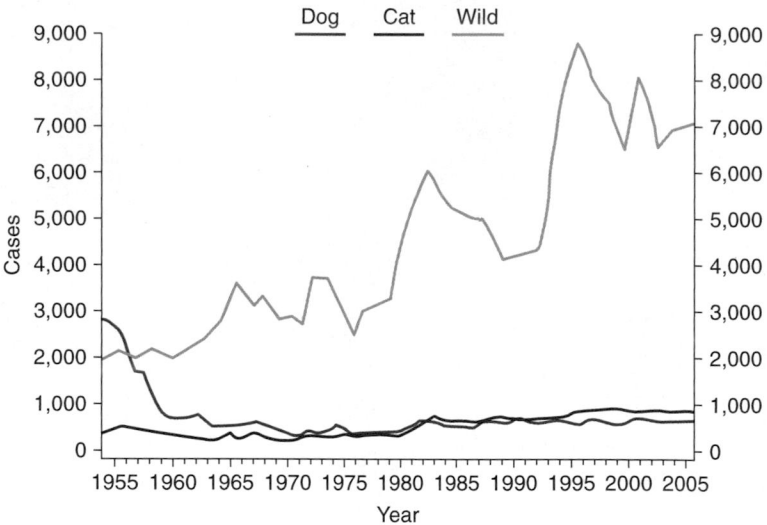

Fig 22-4 Rabies cases in dogs, cats, and wildlife in the United States from 1955 to 2005. The prevalence in dogs has decreased because of vaccination, and cats now have a greater occurrence of rabies. (Data from records maintained at the Centers for Disease Control and Prevention, Atlanta, Ga.; Drawn courtesy University of Georgia, Athens, Ga.)

mesomelas) and mongooses *(Suricata suricata)* predominate, respectively. Although bats can transmit their infection to terrestrial carnivores, the genotypes affecting bats or carnivores also remain distinct.

Rabies in enzootic areas appears to be cyclic. It spreads into unexposed, susceptible wildlife populations in a region; subsequent decreases and increases in the prevalence of disease are caused by population mortality and immunity, which periodically cycles in the wildlife population. These wild animals serve as maintenance hosts for virus transmission to dogs, cats, cattle, and horses. Most human exposures result from contact with these domestic species.

Dogs and Cats
The highest occurrence of dog and cat rabies in the United States generally occurs in areas where wildlife rabies is endemic. Most dogs and cats are infected with the predicted terrestrial rabies virus variant associated with the dominant wildlife reservoir host in their respective geographic region.[150]

Although the prevalence of wildlife rabies has been on the increase, cases of rabies in dogs and farm animals have been decreasing (Fig. 22-4). Vaccination of dogs and animal control programs has been the main factors responsible for this decline. Although cases of dog rabies have declined, dogs account for the majority of reported animal bites in the United States (see Bite Infections, Chapter 53). Many of these bites result in people seeking antirabies prophylaxis. In the United States, Texas had the greatest occurrence of dog rabies in recent years because of the problem with rabies in coyotes *(Canis latrans)* (Fig. 22-5).[136] Worldwide, domestic and feral dogs account for most of human rabies deaths and postexposure prophylaxis.[44] In less developed nations, where dog rabies has not been controlled, the prevalence of canine and human rabies is quite high. Adequate vaccination of at least 50% to 70% of dogs in a given population may be necessary to block the occurrence of rabies epidemics.[50]

An increase in cases of rabies in cats usually is related to spill-over of infection from wildlife because no specific virus

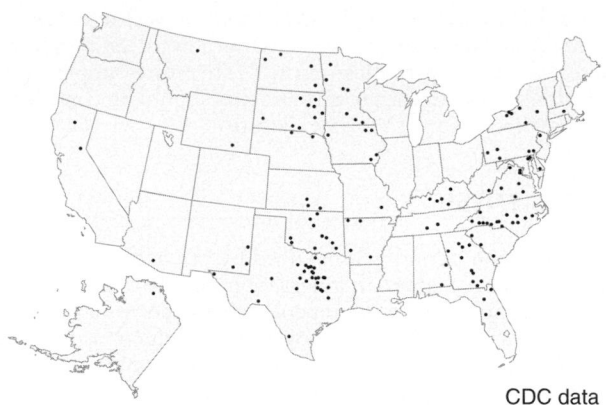

CDC data

Fig 22-5 Reported cases of rabies in dogs in the United States for 2002. (Data courtesy the Centers for Disease Control and Prevention, Atlanta, Ga.; map courtesy University of Georgia, Athens, Ga.)

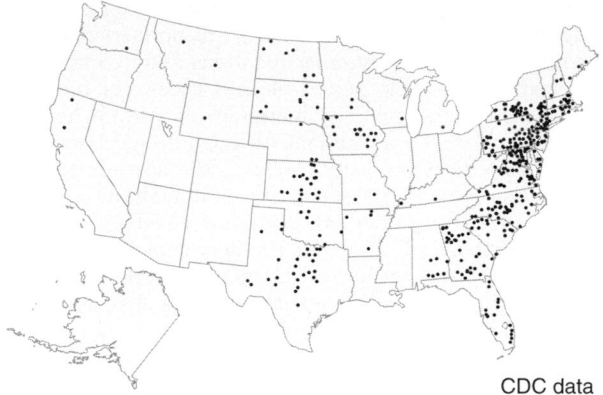

CDC data

Fig 22-6 Reported cases of rabies in cats in the United States for 2002. (Data courtesy the Centers for Disease Control and Prevention, Atlanta, Ga; map courtesy University of Georgia; Athens, Ga.)

variant attributed to cats has been reported. The relative importance of rabies in cats as a source for human exposure in a given geographic area depends on whether canine rabies is being controlled by vaccination. In the United States, since 1979, rabies in cats has shown a slight increase over the previous 7-year period. Beginning in 1981, more cases of rabies in cats than in dogs have been reported annually. This increase probably reflects the low number of cats vaccinated for rabies and the epidemics of wildlife rabies in the mid-Atlantic and Northeast regions of the United States (Fig. 22-6). Numerically, cats have been the most important domestic animal affected since 1992.[191] Most cases of rabies in cats are from states where the raccoon variant of virus is present. The frequency of human rabies exposures attributed to rabid cats is now increasing at a greater rate than those from dogs. Rabid cats, which usually are reclusive, often become aggressive and may attack humans and other animals when disturbed.[60]

Wild Carnivores

The striped skunk (*Mephitis mephitis*), the most common skunk in the United States, is one of the most important species in perpetuating wildlife rabies in the United States. Studies based on antigenic typing have demonstrated the existence of at least three distinct variants in skunks: one in the south central states, another in the north central states, and another in California, extending into Canada. Although the spotted skunk (*Spilogale* sp.) presented a serious rabies threat in the western United States during the 1800s, the involvement of this small, secretive animal is relatively minor today.

The threat to people from rabid skunks is based on the animal's susceptibility to the virus, the high prevalence of rabies infection in the population, their ability to live in proximity to humans, and the excretion of relatively large quantities of virus in their saliva during the prolonged period of clinical illness. Rabid skunks often attack anything that moves with extreme fury and frequently roam during daylight hours, which is unusual behavior for this nocturnal animal.

Foxes are important reservoirs in the ecology of wildlife rabies throughout the Northern Hemisphere, although they account for relatively few human exposures. In North America, fox rabies occurs throughout the range of the red fox, the gray fox *(Urocyon cinereoargenteus)*, and the Arctic fox *(Alopex lagopus)*. An outbreak occurring among red foxes in 1990 in upstate New York was probably an extension of a Canadian fox epidemic. Coyotes have a role in the maintenance of the disease in southern Texas. A focus of another variant of rabies virus in gray foxes has been found in Arizona and Texas. The prevalence of the disease seems to decline when fox populations are reduced to levels in balance with available resources through either natural mortality or fox population–reduction programs. Oral vaccination programs, using modified live virus (MLV) or recombinant vaccine placed in bait, had considerable success in control of red fox rabies in Europe and Ontario, Canada, and are now being used to control gray fox and coyote rabies in Texas. Despite wildlife vaccination in Europe, the nidus of infected foxes from Eastern Europe maintains the infection cycle.[176]

Rabid foxes may exhibit either furious or paralytic forms of the disease; however, regardless of form, the disease is invariably fatal. Despite the shorter course of clinical illness, foxes can effectively transmit the virus to other species, but the need for human postexposure prophylaxis from direct exposure to rabid foxes has been extremely low.

Before the mid-1950s, rabies was not a serious problem among raccoons in the United States. However, from 1950 to 1970, the occurrence of rabid raccoons began to rise dramatically in Florida and Georgia and soon spread to Alabama and northward to South Carolina.

In the mid-Atlantic Coast states, a major epidemic began in the late 1970s caused by the apparent translocation of infected animals from the Southeast. The mid-Atlantic outbreak spread throughout the northeastern states and southward into North Carolina by the mid-1990s. Foci from this and the Florida-Georgia-Alabama epidemic have now merged. The epidemic had spread west into Ohio from Pennsylvania.[10] Raccoons have adapted well to suburban and semiurban environments; thus the number of rabies cases in cats and dogs and other domestic animals in the Northeast has dramatically increased.[34] The danger of human exposure to rabid raccoons has also increased, and at least one human death directly associated with rabid raccoons has been confirmed in Virginia. Exposure of people to rabid domestic animals such as the cat, which commonly become infected by raccoon attacks, has resulted in the greatest public health risk. Oral bait vaccination of raccoons in these regions has been shown to be effective in reducing the spread of rabies within the zone of immunization.[181] Occasionally, raccoons may be co-infected with canine distemper virus, which may alter the immune response within the nervous system and confuse the diagnosis as to the cause of neurologic dysfunction.[84]

Bats

Lyssaviruses have been identified in bats in the Americas, Africa, Australia, and Eurasia. Because of their mobility and the opportunity for bats to infect new areas, no geographic region can be truly considered free of Lyssaviruses.[33] Rabies in North American insectivorous bats was first recognized in the early 1950s, but studies suggest that rabid bats were in this region much earlier. The range of bat rabies is widespread throughout North America. In the United States, less then 1% of randomly caught bats are infected, and 5% to 15% of dead or ill bats submitted for examination may have rabies.[22] Bats that interact with humans are more likely to have rabies than those avoiding people; bats that bite people have the highest prevalence.[173] Rabid bats may develop paresis or paralysis. They may be disoriented and fly into obstacles. Aggression has been observed in some cases. In the United States, most wild bats are insectivorous. Subclinical infection has been suggested in fruit bats in zoological gardens in Europe, but additional investigation is needed.[185,196]

Although multiple co-circulating variants of rabies virus can be found in insectivorous bats, most submissions and rabid bats are from only a few of the common species (primarily *Eptesicus fuscus, Myotis lucifugus, Lasiurus borealis,* and *Tadarida brasiliensis*). Phylogenetic studies have shown that bat rabies virus variants found in terrestrial animals are distinct, and variants identified in different bat species are also quite distinct. From 1970 to 2002, 66 persons have died from rabies in the United States. Brain tissues from most of them have been examined by MAB or gene-sequencing techniques, or both. Variants associated with insectivorous bats were identified most frequently, usually associated with the silver haired bat *(Lasionycteris noctivagans)* or eastern pipistrelle *(Pipistrellus subflavus)*, but victims had no history of bite. Bats are small and cause tiny lesions, and people may not realize that exposure has occurred.[74,154,155,202] Therefore reported infection of people from nonbite exposure is higher for bats as compared with terrestrial carnivores, not the least related to public education and perceived greater concern and prophylaxis associated with bite lesions. Despite these reports in people, few authenticated cases of rabies transmission have been reported from insectivorous bats *(E. fuscus)* to cats and even fewer cases of transmission to dogs.[171] Rabid bats seldom attack; bat bites usually occur from bats found paralyzed or semiparalyzed or from normal-appearing bats found in buildings.

Vampire bats, which feed exclusively on blood, are a major rabies threat to people and animals in Mexico, Central America, and parts of South America. More than 100,000 cases of rabies in cattle attributed to vampire bats occur annually in Latin America. The routine nightly feeding of vampires makes them extremely effective in transmitting rabies virus, and the presence of rabies in vampire bats parallels that seen in insectivorous bats and terrestrial animals. The vampire bat is not found in North America, except for Mexico. Use of the same cave by vampires and other species of bat may be a source of transmission between species. Genetic characterization of rabies isolates from vampire bats and dogs in Brazil indicated two independently maintained cycles of infection.[106] A focus in Colombia in domestic dogs and people was found to be caused by virus variants found in insectivorous bats.[171] In addition, an independent focus in marmosets *(Callithrix jacchus jacchus)* has been associated with human infections.[64]

Rodents and Lagomorphs

The prevalence of clinical rabies among rats, mice, squirrels, and rabbits and hares is virtually nonexistent. Rodents and rabbits account for a high percentage of animal bites to people, but no cases of human rabies have ever been associated with these species, probably because they are extremely susceptible to infection and generally will not survive the attack by a rabid carnivore. For such reasons, these species are not routinely examined for rabies in public health laboratories. In the United States, rabies has been reported among large rodents such as woodchucks *(Marmota monax)* and beavers *(Castor canadensis);* most cases have been in the eastern states where raccoon epizootics exist.[14] Therefore unprovoked encounters with large aggressive rodents should be considered as a possible source of rabies exposure.

PATHOGENESIS

The incubation period is influenced by the age of the bitten individual, the degree of innervation of the bite site, the distance from the point of inoculation to the spinal cord or brain, the variant and amount of virus introduced, postexposure prophylaxis, and other factors. The virus may be undetectable in local tissues following the bite, and it does not enter the blood. Rabies is unique in that the incubation period, which is relatively prolonged compared with that of other infectious diseases, is primarily a result of the route of virus entry into and spread within the central nervous system (CNS) (Fig. 22-7).

Entry of Virus

After intramuscular (IM) inoculation, virus may enter peripheral nerves directly or replicate locally in nonnervous tissue. Virus may enter neuromuscular junctions and neurotendinal spindles after a variable period of days, weeks, or months.[41] Rabies virus glycoprotein has homology to certain neurotoxins and attach to axon terminals through lipoprotein receptors, including those for acetylcholine. Virus spreads passively by intraaxonal flow in peripheral nerves at a rate of up to 100 (range, 10 to 400) mm per day. Both motor and sensory fibers may transport virus. The greater the degree of innervation at the site of the bite, the shorter the incubation period. In naturally occurring cases of rabies, ranges of incubation periods

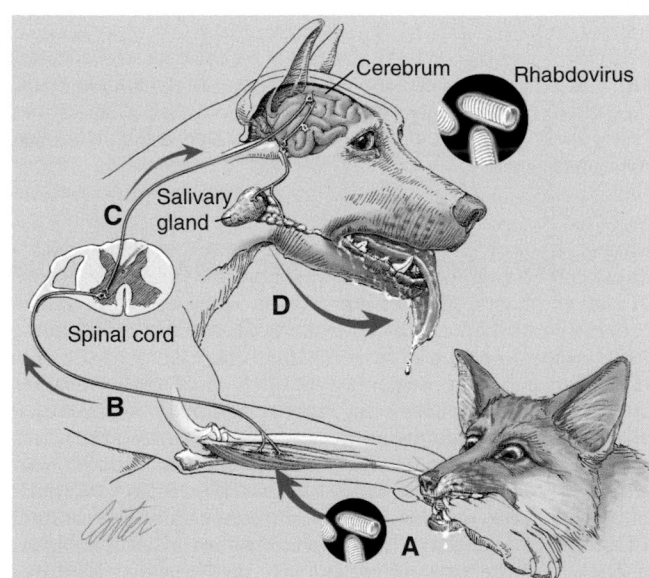

Fig 22-7 Pathogenesis of rabies virus infection. Rabies virus enters peripheral nerves, or may replicate in myocytes and spread to motor nerve endings *(A)*. Retrograde intra-axonal (centripetal) spread to the CNS occurs in peripheral nerves *(B)*. Virus replicates in spinal cord neurons and spreads rapidly throughout the nervous system, causing progressive lower motor neuron paralysis *(C)*. Virus enters the brain, causing cranial nerve deficits and behavioral changes. Virus spreads centrifugally in peripheral and cranial nerves, from which it enters the salivary glands and saliva *(D)* and other tissues. (Courtesy University of Georgia, Athens, Ga.)

before CNS signs have been reported to be 3 to 24 weeks (average, 3 to 8 weeks) in dogs, 2 to 24 weeks (average, 4 to 6 weeks) in cats, and 3 weeks to 1 year or more (average, 3 to 6 weeks) in people.

Although uncommon, infection by routes other than by bite is possible. After intranasal (IN) exposure, virus enters the trigeminal nerves and ganglia in its course to the CNS. The cribriform plate and olfactory bulbs have been suggested as a route of spread, but this is not well documented. After ingestion, the virus can infect cells of the oral mucosa, taste buds, pulmonary system (by aspiration), and intestinal mucosa. From these sites, virus migrates up branches of the cranial nerves and spreads to the brain stem.

Rabies virus variants may vary in their ability to be transmitted by nonbite means. In comparing the dog and coyote strains with silver-haired bat viruses, the latter was better able to infect epithelial cells, replicate at lower temperatures, and have neuroinvasive tendencies.[72,92,158]

Spread in the Central Nervous System

Interneuronal spread of virus corresponds to the progression of clinical signs that are noted. The virus enters the spinal cord or brain stem ipsilateral to the site of initial virus inoculation by retrograde axoplasmic flow. Once in the CNS, virus spreads by intraaxonal means to involve the contralateral neurons and ascends rapidly and bilaterally, in the spinal cord or brain stem to the forebrain. Damage to the motor neurons causes progressive lower motor neuron (LMN) disease, which, in turn, produces the typical ascending flaccid paralysis of rabies. Damage to the CNS caused by rabies virus has mainly been attributed to direct viral invasion of the nervous system. Damage to neural tissue is visibly limited for the degree of paralysis; inhibition of function or synthesis of neural transmitters is suspected. Apoptosis, or genetically induced premature cell death, may be important in the limited amount of observed neuronal necrosis.[109] Host immune responses to rabies virus may accentuate the inflammation and degeneration of nervous tissue. Interference with cardiorespiratory control results in death.

Spread from the Central Nervous System

After replication within the CNS, the virus moves outward to other body tissues via the peripheral, sensory, and motor nerves at a rate of 100 to 400 mm per day. Both visceral and somatic portions of cranial and spinal cord nerves become involved, including the autonomic nervous system. Virus also spreads via cranial nerves to the acinar cells of the salivary glands at this time. The presence of virus in saliva demonstrates that the brain has already been infected. Although virtually every tissue may be infected, outward spread in the peripheral nervous system does not occur in all cases. The rate (20% to 88% positive) of salivary gland infection also varies, depending in part on the species infected and the virus variant. Death may occur before salivary gland involvement.

Recovery

Recovery from rabies has been exceedingly rare.[110] In many instances, demonstrating the presence of virus may be difficult. During the early incubation period, rabies virus may be sequestered at the site of inoculation while replicating in myocytes and nerves. The long period between exposure and clinical signs may be the result of local replication and has been associated with high titers of antirabies virus antibody in the cerebrospinal fluid (CSF) and CNS tissue. Adequate serum titers of antirabies virus antibody, acquired by active or passive immunization, have been correlated with protection against infection and restricted viral replication. Effective cell-mediated immunity is essential to the eventual elimination of rabies virus. Recovery should be regarded as of extremely minor importance in the epidemiology of the disease and not relevant in public health considerations.

Excretion of Virus

Typically, virus excretion occurs for a brief period before the onset of neurologic signs and continues until the animal dies within a few days. Most public health laws require a 10-day observation period after a bite from a suspected dog or cat because the period of virus shedding before onset of neurologic signs in naturally infected animals is generally between 1 and 5 days. Dogs that develop neurologic signs and die suddenly actually may have lower concentrations of virus in their brains and salivary glands than do those that live longer. Typically, excretion of virus in experimentally infected cats has started from 1 to 2 days before to 3 days after the onset of clinical signs.

CLINICAL FINDINGS

Rabies virus infection has classically been divided into two major types: furious and paralytic. The classification and progression of infection is artificial because rabies can be quite variable in its presentation, and atypical signs are commonly seen. Not all animals progress through all the clinical stages. The initial history may reveal that the pet has a wound history. Because of the severity of wounds, signs may not always be suspected as coming from a bite.

Dogs and Cats

During the prodromal phase in dogs, which usually lasts 2 to 3 days, apprehension, nervousness, anxiety, solitude, and variable fever may be noted. Friendly animals may become shy or irritable and may snap, whereas fractious ones may become more docile and affectionate. Pupillary dilation with or without sluggish palpebral or corneal reflexes may become apparent. Most animals will constantly lick the site of viral inoculation. Some dogs may develop pruritus at the site of exposure and claw and chew at the area until it is ulcerated. The behavior of cats during the prodromal period is similar to that of dogs; however, cats more typically show fever spikes and unusual or erratic behavior for only 1 or 2 days.

The furious or psychotic type of the disease in dogs usually lasts for 1 to 7 days and is associated with forebrain involvement. Animals become restless and irritable and have increased responses to auditory and visual stimuli. They frequently become excitable, photophobic, and hyperesthetic and bark or snap at imaginary objects. As they become more restless, they begin to roam, usually becoming more irritable and vicious. Dogs may eat unusual objects (pica), especially wood, that become gastrointestinal foreign bodies. They may avoid contact with people and prefer to hide in dark or quiet places. When caged or confined, dogs often try to bite or attack their enclosure. They usually develop muscular incoordination, disorientation, or generalized grand mal seizures during this phase. If they do not die during a seizure, they may experience a short paralytic stage and then die (Fig. 22-8).

Cats may develop more consistently the furious phase of the disease, showing erratic and unusual behavior. These cats are described as having anxious, staring, wild, spooky, or blank looks in their eyes.[69] When confined in cages, they may make vicious, striking movements and attempt to bite or scratch at moving objects. In addition, they may have muscular tremors and weakness or incoordination. Some cats may run continuously until they seem to die of exhaustion.

The paralytic or dumb type of rabies usually develops within 2 to 4 days (range, 1 to 10 days) after the first clinical signs are noted. LMN paralysis usually progresses from the site of injury until the entire CNS is involved. Cranial nerve paral-

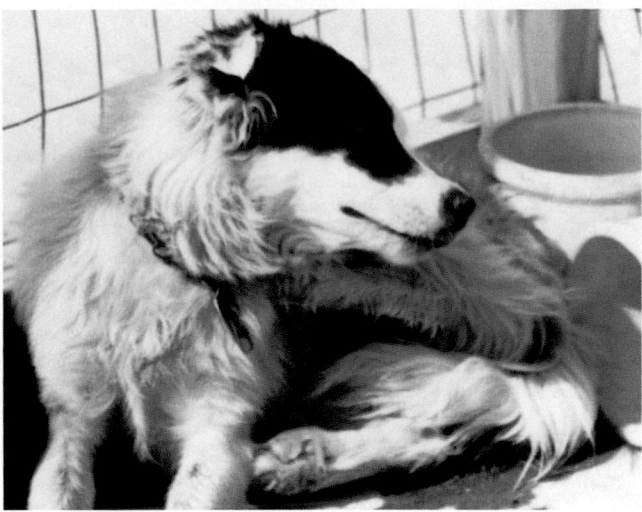

Fig   22-8   Dog with paralytic stage of rabies in sternal recumbency with torticollis. (Courtesy CDC, Atlanta, Ga.)

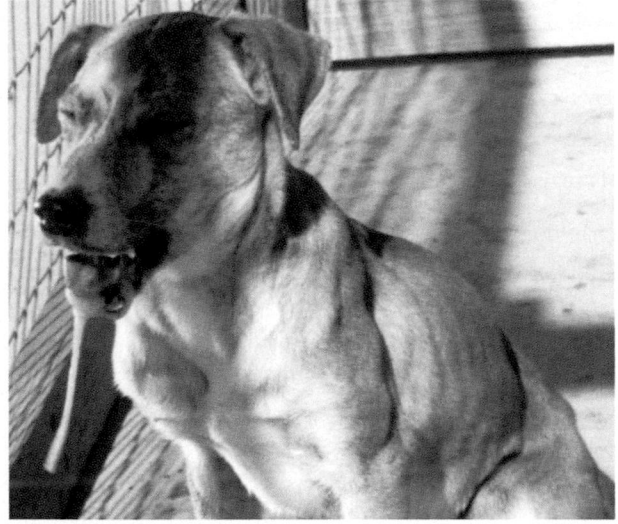

Fig   22-9   Dog with rabies. Note open jaw and visible tongue with excessive salivary secretions resulting from the inability to swallow. (Courtesy CDC, Atlanta, Ga.)

ysis may be the first recognizable clinical syndrome if the bite occurs on the face. When the brain stem becomes affected, a change in the tone of the bark, resulting from laryngeal paralysis, may be observed. Dogs, which more commonly show this type of disease, may begin to salivate or froth excessively as a result of the inability to swallow and the deep labored respiration that occurs. A "dropped jaw" develops as a result of paralysis of the masticatory muscles (Fig. 22-9). Dogs may make a choking sound, which convinces an owner that something is caught in the animal's throat. Owners or veterinarians may then become exposed to the virus in the saliva while attempting to remove a suspected foreign object. The course of the paralytic phase usually lasts 2 to 4 days. The animal often goes into a coma and dies of respiratory failure.

The paralytic disease in cats often follows the furious form of the disease and begins around day 5 of clinical illness. Although the total course of illness may last 10 days, rabid cats often die after 3 to 4 days.[191] As in dogs, initial paralysis

of the bitten extremity can progress to paraparesis, incoordination, and ascending or generalized paralysis, terminating in coma and death. Mandibular and laryngeal paralysis is less common in cats. Increased frequency of vocalization is a commonly reported sign in cats, and owners often recognize a change in the pitch of the cat's voice.[69] Cats occasionally develop the paralytic form directly after the prodromal phase with little or no signs of excitement.

Atypical, abortive forms of rabies virus infection with recovery may occur but are considered very rare phenomena. Experimentally infected dogs that developed acute progressive LMN paralysis have shown clinical improvement a few days to months later. Survival with chronic infection has been reported to rarely occur after experimental rabies infection in cats, but clinical recovery from paralysis has not been observed.

People
The clinical syndrome of rabies in people is similar in duration and variability to that in dogs and cats. Genetic studies of viral isolates from human rabies indicate that clinical manifestations such as encephalitic or paralytic rabies are not determined by different virus variants but by other factors such as the site of the inoculation and spread of virus within the nervous system.[97] Fever, headache, anxiety, nervousness, and hyperesthesia at the bite site have been reported. As the syndrome progresses to the excitable phase, clinical signs consist of excitability, restlessness, hyperkinesis, and violent behavior. Humans salivate incessantly and may refuse to drink water. They experience painful pharyngeal spasms when attempting to swallow fluids, which gives rise to the term hydrophobia. As disorientation and excitability continue, some patients die in convulsive episodes, whereas others develop generalized LMN paralysis and respiratory arrest. Although the rare instance of recovery has been reported after extraordinary efforts, the disease is considered to be invariably fatal after the onset of clinical signs.

DIAGNOSIS

Rabies is often suspected because of neurologic abnormalities in an affected animal. However, because of the atypical nature of the clinical signs now recognized, rabies should be considered in any animal that suddenly develops profound behavioral changes or features of LMN paralysis, or both.

For a review of the diagnosis of rabies, also see the Centers for Disease Control and Prevention (CDC) web site at www.cdc.gov/ncidod/dvrd/rabies/. The definitive diagnostic test is the demonstration of rabies virus antigen by the direct fluorescent antibody (FA) test in suitable brain tissue.[30] No premortem diagnostic tests are sensitive enough to be consistently reliable for rabies diagnosis in animals. Nevertheless, there may be some limited indications for testing serum, CSF, or biopsy specimens before the death of the animal. No hematologic or serum biochemical changes are characteristic or specific for rabies. Biochemical changes in CSF have been minimal in experimentally infected dogs and have been rarely reported in natural infections. Increased CSF protein (110 to 150 mg/dl) and leukocytes (120 to 1140 cells/μl), with small lymphocytes predominating, have been reported in dogs with postvaccinal rabies encephalomyelitis.[25a] Cats with postvaccinal rabies also have had increased CSF protein (55 to 80 mg/dl) and increased CSF lymphocyte count (5 to 17 cells/μl).

Direct Fluorescent Antibody Testing of Dermal Tissues
This method has been predominantly used to diagnose rabies antemortem in people. Because virus enters extraneural tissues via outward spread from the CNS, it arrives at nerve

endings in the skin and at the salivary glands simultaneously. Because of the heavy sensory innervation, the skin at the nape of the neck (in humans) and the sensory vibrissae on the maxillary areas (in animals) may be selected for direct FA testing. Direct FA testing of a skin biopsy has a 25% to 50% probability of being positive about the time that clinical rabies develops; accuracy is increased as the disease progresses. Of all dogs and cats tested that were confirmed to be rabid by positive results of brain immunofluorescence, neurologic signs developed within 10 days of the biting incident.[209a] Inactivated or recombinant rabies vaccines commonly used in dogs and cats do not give false-positive results. The skin biopsy technique should never be substituted for brain examination of an unvaccinated animal with suspect neurologic signs. This test appears to be accurate if the virus is present, but a negative test result does not rule out the possibility that the animal is infected. Use of this method is restricted at present to human diagnostics and has not been approved for routine laboratory diagnosis of rabies in animals.

Testing of Saliva for Virus

Salivary tests for rabies virus have been used as one test to diagnose rabies in people. Rabies virus has been detected in dog saliva by slide agglutination using latex particles coated with polyclonal immunoglobulin.[121] The load of viral particles in saliva is lower than it is in brain tissue, and negative results must be confirmed by more reliable means such as the direct FA procedure on brain. Increased sensitivity and specificity can be achieved by using virus isolation or genetic detection methods (see later discussion).

Serologic Testing

Serologic tests are rarely used for epidemiologic surveys or for diagnosis because of the low percentage of animals surviving that have time to develop postinoculation antibody. Serologic tests are used to determine vaccine immunogenicity. Some countries require a positive antibody titer for importation.[9] Mouse inoculation was performed historically for serologic testing but has been replaced by cell culture methods. The rapid fluorescent-focus inhibition test (RFFIT), can quantify concentrations of specific rabies virus antibody in serum. Other tests for rabies virus antibodies, based on enzyme-linked immunosorbent assay (ELISA, or fluorescent antibody virus neutralization [FAVN] test), have been proposed to augment the RFFIT for serodiagnosis or support of immunization.*

During incubation, antibody responses are not usually observed, and the virus may be hidden from the immune system. After neurologic signs develop, antibodies appear in serum and later in the CSF.[179] Testing dogs or cats for serum antibodies to rabies virus to determine recent exposure to rabies virus can be ambiguous because elevated titers can result from vaccination or from past or recent exposure to virus. Therefore a serologic response can in no way be definitively differentiated from vaccination or infection. Testing for rabies virus antibody in CSF is a possible means of documenting rabies infection because antibody is locally produced, and CSF titers may increase 2 to 3 weeks or more after the onset of clinical rabies. Because of this delay, a negative titer result does not eliminate rabies infection as a possibility.

Documentation of Rabies Immunization with Antibody Titers

The WHO and the Office International des Epizooties have developed minimum guidelines as supportive evidence of rabies immunization in animals. This measurement has been adopted as one requirement for importation of animals into rabies quarantine areas (see later discussion, Quarantine and Shipment of Animals). In an update of these guidelines, the RFFIT test has been augmented by the FAVN test.[8] This latter test has become another international standard for shipment of animals. No difference has been observed in sensitivity or specificity for either method in comparing sera of vaccinated or unvaccinated animals.[36,199] Modification of the FAVN using MABs and peroxidase conjugates has allowed automation of the procedure for dogs.[104] A titer of 0.5 IU/ml has been used as the standard level expected for an adequate titer in people and animals. Although parenteral vaccination may more readily achieve this level, oral vaccination with the SAG2 strain did not always induce this level of seroconversion.[192] Nevertheless, dogs showing any measurable titer after vaccination were protected. A titer of 0.5 IU/ml is required for animals exported to most rabies-free areas. No "protective" titer has been found in animals. Individual interpretation is the responsibility of the veterinarian submitting the specimen and the agency requesting the test be done. See Appendix 5 for laboratories that perform these assays.

PATHOLOGIC FINDINGS

Submission of Specimens

Selection and submission of proper specimens are critical for accurate rabies diagnosis. Handling live, suspected rabid animals must be done with extreme care. Heavy protective gloves must be worn, and catchpoles, cages, and other equipment often facilitate capture and transport of such animals. The animal must be euthanized by a humane method, and the brain must be protected from damage. The use of an ax or power saw should be discouraged when opening the skull, because these may create hazardous aerosols. A procedure to remove the brain of a suspected rabid animal has been published.[213] Small specimens such as mice and kittens may be submitted whole. A technique for retroorbital removal of brain specimens for collection of material for epidemiologic studies has been described.[156] Complete brain removal is still indicated when human exposure has occurred. When brain tissue has been inadvertently damaged or destroyed, the spinal cord is an alternative but less desirable substitute.

The head (or body) of an animal suspected of having rabies that has died or been euthanized should be cooled immediately and maintained chilled (wet ice) or refrigerated until examined. The head or brain should not be frozen because this delays examination, and the thawing process causes brain tissue damage. A complete history should accompany each specimen. Various approved shipping containers are available from public health or animal control facilities and must protect the specimen, as well as those handling the container. The container should always indicate that hazardous laboratory specimens are enclosed.

Specimens must be sent to the laboratory as quickly as possible. Postexposure treatment is often delayed while awaiting laboratory results. Recommendations are that specimens be delivered personally or by courier whenever possible to minimize delay or potential loss.

A method of submitting brain tissue, dried on filter paper, has been described that permits submission of specimens without refrigeration.[222] Brains from rabid and control dogs were spotted on filter paper which was dried and stored for up to 222 days. Analysis was performed by nucleic acid sequence-based amplification and reverse transcriptase-polymerase chain reaction (RT-PCR).

Gross and Microscopic Lesions

No gross lesions are detectable in the CNS with rabies infection. Despite the dramatic neurologic signs and high mortal-

---

*References 26, 48, 63, 73, and 151.

ity, neuropathologic changes are mild. Pathologic changes depend on the severity and duration of infection at the time of examination. Acute polioencephalitis characterized by minimal neuronophagia, neuronal degeneration, and nonsuppurative inflammation is seen very early in the course of the disease. Necrotizing encephalitis is seen in the next phase of infection and corresponds to a gradually increasing titer in the serum and CSF. Chronic infections are characterized by focal or widespread lymphocytic and plasmacytic perivascular cuffing and focal mononuclear cell infiltrates in the CNS. Ganglioneuritis is usually present. The longer the course of illness, the more pronounced is the nonsuppurative inflammatory response in the brain and spinal cord. In some cats, spongiform lesions appear as vacuolation in the neutropil of the gray matter, most commonly in the thalamus and inner layers of the cerebral cortex.

Direct Fluorescent Antibody and Immunohistochemical Testing of Nervous Tissue

This postmortem test is both rapid and sensitive and is currently the most widely used and preferred and reliable method of diagnosing potential rabies infection in animals.[91] False-negative results are rare with this test when compared with those of mouse inoculation.[209] Thin touch impressions of the medulla, cerebellum, or hippocampus are used for this test. In decomposing canine brains at room temperature of 25° to 29° C, the direct FA test result remains positive in most cases for up to 96 hours; the corresponding mouse inoculation test usually becomes negative by 48 hours.[5] Unless it is completely decomposed, the head should be submitted because specific fluorescence may still be detected. Rabies virus has also been detected by immunoperoxidase techniques on formalin-fixed, partially autolyzed and paraffin-embedded tissue.[19a,83,139,224] Animals need not show neurologic signs at the time of examination, and all animals excreting virus in the saliva will have detectable virus in the CNS by immunohistochemical examination.

Genetic Detection of Virus and Genetic Sequencing

Rabies virus RNA has been detected in nervous tissue by RT-PCR.* Amplified sequences have included the phosphoprotein, nucleoprotein, and glycoprotein genes. PCR has been used as a confirmatory test in direct FA-negative samples or in decomposed brain tissue that is difficult to evaluate with direct FA methods or virus culture,[54,94] but the predictive ability of a negative result has not been discussed. In situ hybridization can detect rabies virus genomic RNA in paraffin-embedded brain tissues.[111,224] For detection of rabies in living human patients, RT-PCR has been used on saliva, CSF, and urine[53,164,220,221]; however, it is not considered a desirable alternative in animals, in which the brain tissue is preferred. In people, RT-PCR analysis of saliva has been the most accurate means of antemortem diagnosis of rabies when compared with other detection methods and is as accurate as is brain biopsy.[164] Direct sequencing of PCR products along with automated gene sequencing can also help distinguish between virus variants to determine the most probable wildlife reservoir for an isolate from human or animal infection.

Intracellular Inclusions

The classic test for the presence of rabies is to examine the brain for the presence of intracytoplasmic inclusions, known as Negri bodies, in larger neurons (Fig. 22-10).[137] They are most commonly found in the thalamus, hypothalamus, pons, cerebral cortex, and dorsal horns of the spinal cord. Negri bodies are most common in neurons of the hippocampus in

*References 81, 95, 107, 120, and 224.

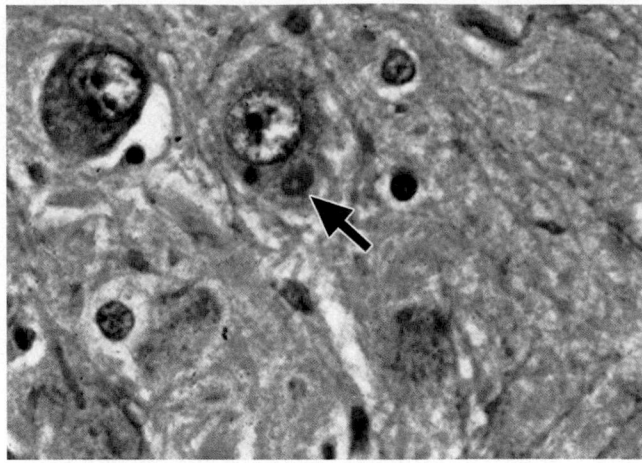

Fig 22-10 Negri body *(arrow)* in a neuron within the CNS. (Courtesy Elizabeth Howerth, University of Georgia, Athens, Ga.)

carnivores and in Purkinje's cells of herbivores. Negri bodies in tissue sections or impressions of brain tissue are best demonstrated with Seller's or van Gieson's stains, in which they stain magenta. Unfortunately, Negri bodies take time to develop and cannot be found during all stages of infection and in all infected cats. They usually cannot be detected until neurologic signs are apparent; therefore premature killing of the animal may reduce the chances of finding these inclusions. Negri bodies may be found in approximately 50% of the samples that test positive by direct FA. In some cases, nonrabid tissues have displayed inclusions that resemble Negri bodies. Cytoplasmic inclusions that are confused with Negri bodies can be found in the brain of healthy cats.[37,38] They occur in the pyramidal cells of the hippocampus and in neurons of the dorsal part of the lateral geniculate nucleus. This test is no longer used in most developed nations for routine diagnostic confirmation.

Mouse Inoculation and Virus Isolation

Intracerebral inoculation of laboratory mice with fresh or fresh-frozen homogenized tissue is a confirmatory test for rabies but is not widely conducted for routine diagnosis of suspected rabies cases in the United States. Specific neutralizing antibody is incubated with extracted tissue before its inoculation to confirm that rabies virus is responsible for the observed neurologic signs. Brain tissues from infected mice are examined for virus by direct FA. This test does not distinguish between virulent and vaccine viruses because, regardless of attenuation, many of the virus strains produce a similar illness in mice. Replacement of mouse inoculation by viral inoculation into tissue culture (TC) is now feasible because virulent virus can now be grown in various cell lines.[187]

Monoclonal Antibody

MABs produced against specific rabies virus nucleocapsid and glycoprotein moieties are able to distinguish various antigenic variants. Strains of virus to be tested are grown in TC or are found in tissue sections and are tested by direct FA to determine the antigenic composition of the virus. The pattern of staining with different MABs is compared with that of reference strains of virus. This technique is extremely valuable in distinguishing between vaccine and virulent strains of rabies virus, especially in cases of human exposure to animals with postvaccinal neurologic disease.

THERAPY

Supportive care for rabies-infected animals is not recommended because no therapy has proved effective in this fatal encephalitis. An asymptomatic dog or cat suspected of contracting rabies should be quarantined as recommended (see Compendium of Animal Rabies Vaccines, Appendix 4)[116] or, as for all other species, appropriately euthanized and the brain submitted for examination.

PREVENTION

For control of rabies in dog populations, vaccinating a minimum of 50% to 70% of dogs is theoretically necessary.[50,153] Eliminating unvaccinated feral dog populations alone has not proved effective and is expensive. Eliminating wildlife populations is nearly impossible and is expensive. Therefore the control measures centered on vaccination of dogs and cats are most appealing and effective.

Vaccine Types
Parenteral Modified Live Vaccines
No measure has helped reduce the incidence of human rabies as effectively as the widespread vaccination of the domestic dog population. Early vaccines were developed from virus grown in nervous tissue and later in avian embryos. Low egg passage vaccine virus was produced by approximately 50 serial passages of the virus in chicken embryos (CEOs). The virus lost its viscerotropic properties but retained some of its neurotropic traits. Vaccine-induced rabies was occasionally reported if the product was given to cats. High egg passage CEO vaccine was produced by approximately 180 passages of the virus. It no longer caused neurologic signs in laboratory mice, except when neonates were injected intracerebrally. The vaccine was safe for dogs and only occasionally caused encephalomyelitis in more susceptible species such as cats and cattle. Newer MLV vaccines were produced in TC. These products produced fewer allergic reactions compared with CEO vaccines. Despite better immunity produced by MLV vaccines compared with inactivated vaccines, occasional post-vaccinal rabies is still a distinct disadvantage. No MLV rabies vaccines are currently available in the United States. They are still being used to control rabies epidemics in countries in which domestic dogs are rabies reservoirs, and financial resources for more expensive products are limited.[28,29,141,167]

Oral Modified Live Vaccines
Although they are uncommonly used for parenteral vaccination, several modified-live strains are being used for oral vaccination of feral or wild animals. The SAD B19 strain has been used for many years. In fox cubs less than 8 weeks of age, maternally derived antibody (MDA) inhibited the immune response to oral SAD B19 strain vaccine.[159] A newer SAG2 strain, isolated as an escape mutant by selection with MABs, is derived from the SAD strain.[138] The SAG2 strain is avirulent following intracerebral inoculation of immunocompetent mice. This strain protected a majority of vaccinated dogs against challenge that killed all unvaccinated controls.[85,168,192] It also has been useful in the protection of African wild dogs (Lycaon pictus), which have been problematic because of their high susceptibility to the disease.[124] The SAG2 vaccine produces no clinical illness in vaccinates and is difficult to isolate from the oral cavity, even within the first 24 hours of administration.[67,168] This virus will not likely be transmitted to other hosts.

Parenteral Inactivated Cell Culture Vaccines
To develop effective inactivated rabies virus vaccines, the virus had to be produced in high concentrations, which was initially done by growing it in the nervous system of suckling mice. Neonatal mice were chosen because they lacked the antigenic myelin responsible for allergic encephalomyelitis produced by early nervous tissue origin vaccines. An important advance in the development of inactivated rabies vaccines has been the production of less allergenic but more immunogenic products by their production in TC cells, thereby producing large quantities of virus. Newer adjuvants have increased the immune response to the antigen in these products but have also caused some problems with allergenicity and oncogenicity (see Vaccine-Induced Complications, Chapter 100).

Oral or Parenteral Recombinant Vaccines
A Vaccinia virus—rabies virus glycoprotein recombinant (V-RG), capable of expressing the glycoprotein of rabies virus, has immunized most major carnivore reservoirs. For example, the V-RG vaccine was effective in producing a serologic response in captive fox cubs (V. vulpes)[32] and some control of infection in wild coyotes (C. latrans).[65] MDA did not interfere with oral vaccination in fox cubs. Purified subunit rabies vaccines may be the recommended vaccines in the future. With purified glycoprotein vaccines, 5 to 50 times the quantity of purified glycoprotein alone is required to produce an immune response compared with intact virion vaccines. Some theories suggest that incorporating glycoprotein on lipid complexes would greatly increase the potency of subunit vaccines. Recombinant vaccines, using other poxviruses or adenoviruses as vectors, have been developed. After oral use, these vaccines induce the synthesis of rabies virus glycoprotein in infected cells, virus neutralizing (VN) antibodies, and protection in susceptible animals.[56,237] Transgenic plants have also been made, which express rabies virus antigens.

A replication-defective recombinant adenovirus expressing rabies virus glycoprotein was effective in inducing increased VN titers against rabies virus by 10 days after parenteral vaccination.[214] Titers following a recombinant herpesvirus-vectored vaccine expressing glycoprotein were higher compared with those with a commercial inactivated vaccine.[236] In some countries, recombinant parenteral rabies virus vaccine using a canarypox virus–vector is commercially available for cats.[39,208] (See also Rabies, Chapter 100 and Appendices 2, 3, and 4.)

Nucleic Acid Vaccines
IM immunization with bacterial plasmid DNA vectors encoding rabies virus glycoprotein has protected dogs against a lethal challenge with a wild-type dog rabies virus variant.[178] Neutralizing antibodies were detected against rabies virus and EBLVs; however, the titers to the latter viruses were low. In other studies, the serologic response of dogs was higher by IM immunization; cats had a greater response by the intradermal (ID) route.[169] However, sera passively administered to mice from dogs vaccinated ID in the ear pinnae elicited elevated and long-lasting levels of neutralizing antibody that protected mice to challenge following passive transfer of immune sera.[144] In mice, a single dose of DNA vaccine was shown to be as effective as five injections of cell culture-derived vaccine.[25] The versatility of DNA recombinant methods makes it possible to generate chimeric Lyssavirus glycoproteins to protect against the many strains in the wild, and these products may be licensed in the near future, particularly if a single dose is needed for efficacy.

Antirabies Virus-Specific Agents
Certain oligodeoxynucleotides complimentary to rabies virus genomic or messenger RNA have been shown to interfere with rabies virus replication in cultures.[72] These in vitro studies are promising; however, treatment of active infections is a distant possibility, especially for people.[110]

Vaccine Recommendations
Preexposure Prophylaxis

Many vaccines are currently marketed in the United States for preexposure rabies prophylaxis in dogs and cats. All currently licensed products must protect at least 88% of animals vaccinates against challenge with virulent virus, whereas at least 80% of those not vaccinated are challenged and develop rabies. In preventing rabies epizootics, the WHO recommends that 70% of dogs in a population should be effectively immunized.[50] Currently available inactivated vaccines have been shown to be safe and effective when administered in neonatal puppies and kittens. However, because of the potential interference by MDA blockade and a relatively poor immune response in the young, the first rabies vaccination is given at a minimum of 3 months of age and then repeated 1 year later (Table 22-2).[2] Subsequent vaccinations are repeated every 1 or 3 years, depending on the product and local public health regulations. The total dose should be given to each animal, regardless of its size, in a route as recommended by the manufacturer. The current Compendium of Animal Rabies Vaccines (Appendix 4) and Appendices 1 and 2 and Chapter 100 should be consulted for canine and feline rabies vaccination protocols.[116] The latest compendium can be found online at www.avma.org/pubhlth/rabcont.asp. Studies have shown that one injection of inactivated rabies vaccine to a naive animal does not produce a lasting antibody titer in a significant proportion of dogs.[194,210] However, serum antibody titers can be misleading as a measure of protection because previously vaccinated dogs usually show an anamnestic response to boosters, even when antibodies are no longer detectable in their sera. Nevertheless, the second vaccination 1 year after the primary inoculation is extremely important. A multiple-dose primary canine rabies vaccination schedule with annual boosters may be considered for dogs in rabies endemic countries in which the disease has been a high risk for people. Booster vaccinations are recommended for dogs and cats whenever vaccination history cannot be established because of the potential for vaccine failures.[51,69,114] A very small proportion of dogs and cats identified with rabies have had at least one rabies vaccination during their lifetime. No available vaccine is 100% effective; therefore an immediate booster dose is recommended to the previously immunized dog or cat after a known rabies exposure. However, current vaccines in one country may not help protect against imported rabies virus variants from abroad. Therefore vigilance in monitoring is essential. Fortunately, current veterinary vaccines are cross-protective against some newly identified strains such as the *Lyssavirus* reported from Australia.[189] Fortunately, current veterinary vaccines are cross-protective against the *Lyssavirus* identified in Australia.[75]

Oral Vaccination of Feral and Wild Animals

Despite the widespread reservoir of rabies in wildlife, rabies in domestic, feral, or wild dogs is the greatest single human health

Table • 22-2

Recommendations for Rabies Vaccination of Animals and People in the United States[a]

ANIMAL EXPOSED	RECOMMENDATION
Preexposure	
Dogs and cats	Vaccinate at 3 months of age; revaccinate 1 year later and every 1 or 3 years thereafter, depending on product recommendations
Ferrets	May be vaccinated at 3 months of age and revaccinated annually with an approved vaccine
Wildlife	Discourage ownership; no parenteral vaccine is approved for use; oral vaccination in government programs
People	Three doses of an FDA-approved vaccine given as 1 ml IM, based on manufacturer's recommendation, in the upper deltoid on days 0, 7, and 28; booster based on risk group
Postexposure	
Dogs and cats	*Previously unvaccinated:* euthanize immediately or quarantine in secure enclosure for 6 months; vaccinate 1 month before release
	Vaccination not current: evaluate on case-by-case basis
	Vaccination current: revaccinate immediately and keep under owners' control for 45 days
Ferrets	Euthanize if not vaccinated; if vaccinated with an approved vaccine and vaccine is current, revaccinate immediately and place in strict isolation for 45 days
Wildlife	Regard as rabid and euthanize for examination
People	*Previously unvaccinated:* H-RIG[b], 20 IU/kg, infiltrated at site of bite once on day 0–7; FDA-approved vaccine[c] given at recommended dose IM in the upper deltoid on days 0, 3, 7, 14, and 28; ID use not appropriate
	Previously vaccinated: two doses of an approved vaccine at recommended dose IM in upper deltoid on days 0 and 3; no H-RIG

FDA, U.S. Food and Drug Administration; *IM*, intramuscular; *ID*, intradermal; *H-RIG*, human rabies immune globulin.
[a]For most current preexposure information for people, consult the Advisory Committee on Immunization Practices (ACIP) recommendations online at www.avma.org/pubhlth/rabprev.asp. For most current pre- and postexposure information for animals, consult Compendium of Animal Rabies Vaccines, Appendix 4 or online at www.avma.org/pubhlth/rabcont.asp.
[b]Imogam®RabiesHT (Connaught Laboratories, a subsidiary of Pasteur-Merieux Serum et Vaccins, Marnes La Coquette, France); BayRab™, (Bayer Corp, Research Triangle Park, N.C.).
[c]Approved rabies products are: (1) human diploid cell rabies vaccine (HDCV), IM (Imovax® Rabies, Pasteur-Merieux Serum et Vaccins, Connaught Laboratories); (2) rabies vaccine adsorbed (RVA), IM (Rabies Vaccine Adsorbed, Bioport Corporation); (3) purified chick embryo cell vaccine (PCEC), IM, (RabAvert™, Chiron Corporation).

risk. Parenteral vaccination of dogs has helped reduce the threat of rabies for humans; however, it is financially and practically difficult in many countries. Oral ingestion of rabies virus might result in infection; however, it often stimulates an immune response. Using an attenuated strain of rabies virus, a protective immune response is more certain. Oral vaccination via dispersion of safe and effective baits has been beneficial in reducing the threat from wildlife and various dog populations.[166] Vaccines for this purpose must be living so as to penetrate the mucosae. The modified live SAD B19 strain, the V-RG recombinant, and SAG2 vaccines have been employed for this purpose.[23] Contact of people with V-RG containing bait-vaccine units does not pose a major public health risk for Vaccinia virus exposure.[149] However, infection with vaccine virus has occurred and such exposures should be reported.[190] For additional information on the concern of vaccinia poxvirus transmission to people, see Poxvirus Infections, Chapter 19.

Postvaccinal Complications

For additional information on the complications discussed next, the reader should consult Postvaccinal Complications, Chapter 100. Encephalomyelitis in cats and dogs, caused by rabies MLV vaccine, has been observed in the past. As a result, such vaccines are no longer available in many countries. The most frequent nonneurologic complications associated with rabies virus vaccine are local soreness, lameness, and regional lymphadenomegaly in the injected limb. Fever and systemic signs or anaphylaxis are sometimes noted. These signs have been more frequently observed with the newer inactivated TC rabies vaccines because of the need for higher antigenic mass and adjuvants to produce an immune response equal to that of the older MLV products. Focal cutaneous vasculitis and granulomas have been described in dogs, occurring within 3 to 6 months after inoculation. They consist of well-circumscribed, subcutaneous inflammatory reactions that involve the overlying dermis. Similar reactions result in palpable nodules in cats that can be detected by clients or veterinarians.[197]

Sustained inflammatory reactions that develop at vaccination sites are considered to be precursors of sarcoma, which may develop months to years later.[59,102,122] Postvaccinal sarcomas can develop in dogs and cats but have been more frequently documented in cats. Sarcomas that develop after vaccination are often aggressive and invasive. For a further discussion, see Vaccine Site–Associated Sarcomas in Cats, Chapter 100.

Autoimmune polyradiculoneuritis has been observed with inactivated suckling mouse brain–origin rabies vaccines and theoretically can result following any type vaccination. A small proportion of dogs that were vaccinated with these products developed acute diffuse LMN paralysis with intact pain sensation and hyperesthesia (see Chapter 100).

Control of Epizootics

Where rabies epizootics have occurred, vaccination programs have been shown to reduce greatly the spread of an outbreak. Management of stray and unwanted cats and dogs is essential, and unclaimed animals should be humanely euthanized. Leash laws must be enforced. Reduction in the population of wildlife vectors has been used on a limited scale when epidemics of rabies in dogs and cats have been traced to a particular wildlife reservoir species, but this has been largely ineffective. Control through trapping and poison baits not only is difficult, but may also cause public resentment, as well as ecologic repercussions. As previously described, oral vaccination of wild carnivores has worked on a limited basis worldwide and may be expanded in the future.

Postexposure Management for Dogs and Cats

Management of a dog or cat that has been bitten or scratched by a potentially rabid mammal is difficult when the biting animal is not available for testing, because the dog or cat must be considered as having been exposed to a rabid animal (see Table 22-2 and Compendium, Appendix 4). Differences in management depend on whether the exposed animal has been previously immunized and local public health laws. The final decision concerning the management of exposed animals generally is made by local or state public health authorities. The current Compendium of Animal Rabies Control (Appendix 4) and local public health officials should be consulted when such circumstances arise.

Postexposure Vaccination

The National Association of State Public Health Veterinarians recommends euthanasia or 6 months confinement for unvaccinated dogs and cats exposed to a rabid animal, with rabies vaccination 1 month before release (see Compendium, Appendix 4). Although not widely accepted for animals, postexposure prophylaxis (PEP) has been instituted in Texas because of adverse emotional and monetary consequences if an animal must be euthanized.[231] In that protocol, immediate vaccination against rabies was followed by a strict isolation period of 90 days with rabies boosters during the third and eighth weeks of the isolation period. With such measures, four failures were observed out of 830 animals, including 621 dogs and 71 cats, given PEP. Experimental PEP of dogs has been less than ideal.[87] In contrast, immediate vaccination combined with MABs against rabies virus glycoprotein provided protection to the dogs. Unfortunately, such immunoglobulin is not available commercially.

Disposition of Animals That Bite Humans

Dogs and cats with current rabies vaccinations are of less concern as a transmission risk, although current vaccination status does not eliminate the need for follow-up (Table 22-3). Any illness or neurologic disease in quarantined animals must be immediately reported to local public health authorities. Management of potentially rabid animals other than dogs or cats depends on the species, the circumstances of the bite, and the epidemiology of rabies in the area.

Quarantine and Shipment of Animals

The current standard for shipment of animals into "rabies-free" areas involves a four part plan of identification, health examination, vaccination, and blood testing (Table 22-4). Embassies should be consulted regarding the latest requirements for rabies.

PUBLIC HEALTH CONSIDERATIONS

Prevention in Dogs and Cats

Worldwide, more than 30,000 people die from rabies each year, with many more undocumented cases, and 10 to 12 million receive postexposure treatment.[58] These statistics have been reduced through the years by public health practices. Parenteral vaccination of dogs has been the single most important means of controlling rabies in people throughout the world. In addition, rabies incidents involving dog or cat bites or scratches monopolize scarce public health resources. Efforts of large-scale vaccination of dogs by inoculation or distribution of vaccine in oral baits may offer other solutions. Having animals well vaccinated for rabies minimizes the postexposure recommendations for involved people. Cats have now replaced dogs in the United States as the most commonly rabid domestic animal. Increased awareness and vaccination of cats will help reduce the need for PEP, especially in states involved with raccoon rabies epizootics.[162] Restricting the free-ranging behavior of dogs and cats that are too young for vaccination will reduce their chance of becoming infected. As vaccination for

Table • 22-3

Postexposure Recommendations for Rabies Exposure of People in the United States[a]

POTENTIAL SOURCE OF INFECTION	SITUATION	ANIMAL DISPOSITION	POSTEXPOSURE PROPHYLAXIS FOR PEOPLE
Dog, cat, or ferret[b]	All bites; healthy, owned	Confine; observe for at least 10 days, especially if unprovoked attack	None or consider, if unprovoked; yes, if CNS signs develop in animal
	All bites; healthy, stray (available or escaped)	If available, euthanize immediately; submit head for examination	Yes; stop if laboratory results negative, or continue if animal unavailable
	All bites; CNS signs or illness	Euthanize immediately; submit head for examination	Yes; if negative FA result, stop
Bat	Bite, scratch, mucous membrane exposure, or reasonable probability of close direct contact (e.g., in same room indoors)	Safely collect bat; submit for examination	Yes; if negative FA result, stop
Wild carnivore	All bites	If captured, euthanize immediately; submit head for examination	Yes, if positive or animal at large; if negative FA result, stop
Small rodents[c]	All bites	Usually not examined	None, but consult public health officials if circumstances of bite warrant
Inoculation of attenuated vaccine[d]	Any episode	Not applicable	No postexposure prophylaxis required

CNS, Central nervous system; FA, fluorescent antibodies.

Data, in part, from Human Rabies Prevention—United States, 1999. Recommendations of the Advisory Committee on Immunization Practices (ACIP), *MMWR* 48:RR-1.

Bite: any penetration of skin by teeth; injuries by bats can be small and undetected. **Nonbite**: contamination of open wounds, abrasions, mucous membranes or scratches with saliva or neural tissue of a rabid animal.

Nonexposure: petting, contact with blood, urine, or feces (e.g., guano) of rabid animal, especially if dry or exposed to sunlight, virus is inactivated.

[a]Other countries have different guidelines.

[b]Vaccination status of animal *should not* be used to make a decision on outcome for prophylaxis. An unprovoked attack by an animal is more likely than a provoked attack to indicate rabies. Bites from a healthy dog, cat, or ferret during feeding or handling should be considered as being provoked. Offspring of wild animals crossbred to domestic dogs and cats are considered wild carnivores and are handled in that category. In the United States, the likelihood of rabies transmission occurs by region. Dog rabies occurs predominantly along the Mexican border. Rabies in cats is more prevalent and is primarily associated with raccoon rabies in the eastern regions. In many developing countries, dogs are the major vectors of rabies; thus an increased risk of transmission exists and prophylaxis would be more likely.

[c]Squirrels, hamsters, guinea pigs, gerbils, chipmunks, rats, and mice. Lagomorphs are also included. Larger rodents such as woodchucks and beavers have been infected in areas where raccoon rabies is endemic and should be tested.

[d]Accidental inoculation.

dogs and cats becomes more uniform and oral vaccination of terrestrial carnivores becomes more widespread, the relative risk of infection from bats may be more prominent.

Postexposure Prophylaxis for People

The most common source of infection for people is untreated animal bites, although in areas in which bats are a source, the bite exposure may not be recognized. Once the infection develops, it is incurable; thus prompt postexposure management at the earliest indication is critical.[110] Although less than five human cases of rabies occur each year in the United States, approximately 20,000 to 40,000 people annually are given antirabies PEP. In less developed countries, the cost of prophylaxis is prohibitive and so many cases are not prevented.

Wound Care

In cases of known bites, therapy of wounds should be aggressive because immediate, thorough washing of the wound has been shown to be effective in reducing the chance of rabies

virus infection. Ethanol (43% or stronger) or commercial povidone-iodine solutions can be applied locally to open wounds. Bites should also be irrigated with large quantities of a 20% aqueous soap solution or quaternary ammonium compound (QUAT) under pressure. The optimal concentration of benzalkonium chloride, a QUAT, has been shown to be 1% to 4%; however, most commercial hospital disinfectants have a 0.13% concentration. Deep puncture wounds can be effectively cleaned by irrigation using a 15-ml syringe fitted with a blunted 19-gauge needle that is filled with a sterile saline solution. This provides 20 pounds per square inch of pressure, sufficient for cleaning but not so excessive as to cause further tissue damage.

Immunoglobulin

Specific prophylaxis in people has been most successful in reducing the number of deaths caused by rabies when active immunization is combined with human rabies immune globulin (H-RIG) (see Table 22-2). H-RIG is preferable to unpurified γ-globulin because of its greater potency and lesser

Table • 22-4

General Guidelines for Importation of Dogs and Cats into "Rabies Free" Areas[a]

1. Rabies certification and animal's health status
   a. Owner name, address, telephone number
   b. Identifying name of dog, cat, or ferret
   c. Species, breed, sex, markings, age
   d. Date of vaccination
   e. Date of vaccination expiration
   f. Rabies vaccination tag number
   g. Vaccine producer and product name
   h. Manufacturer's serial or lot number
   i. Confirmation that animal found in good health
   j. Veterinarian's signature
   k. Veterinarian's address and license number
   l. Owner retains original copy
   m. Owner places tag securely on animal's collar
2. Identification
   a. Electronic Microchip Implantation
   b. Readable with ISO compatible reader (AVID®, Trovan®, Home Again®, or Destron®)
   c. Implanted at time of blood serology
   d. Microchip number must be on laboratory submission forms
3. Vaccination for Hawaii, United States of America[b]
   a. Previously unvaccinated: need 3 or more months between at least two vaccinations
   b. Pups vaccinated at greater than 3 months of age for first vaccine
   c. Kittens vaccinated at greater than 2 months (recombinant) or 3 months (inactivated) of age for first vaccine
   d. Previously vaccinated: need a booster between 90 days and 12 months of arrival
   e. The most recent vaccination is valid for 12 months to qualify for 30-day quarantine
   f. No rabies vaccine within immediate 90 days before arrival
4. Blood testing
   a. Done by Office International des Epizooties (OIE) Standards
   b. FAVN test or RFFIT used
   c. Passing result is 0.5 IU/ml or greater
   d. Results are reported directly to veterinarians
   e. Collect blood at least 10 to 14 days after vaccination
   f. Cannot enter until at least 90 days have passed from the time laboratory receives sample

FAVN, Fluorescent antibody virus neutralization; *RFFIT*, rapid fluorescent-focus inhibition test.
For Hawaii: 30 days' quarantine if above qualifications are met; otherwise 120-day quarantine.
For United Kingdom: Quarantine period is 6 months with the following exceptions, whereby the quarantine is waived for commercially traded animals: (1) The animal must be born on a registered holding facility where it has remained with no contact to wild animals susceptible to rabies. (2) It has been vaccinated with a one unit (WHO standard) inactivated product when at least 6 months of age and at least 6 months before export. (3) It must have a certified blood test and veterinary health certificate, vaccination record, and implanted microchip as outlined above. (4) Agriculture Department, United Kingdom, must be notified of entry within 24 hours of arrival.
For Australia: The minimum quarantine is generally 30 to 60 days if the above guidelines are met and is variable depending on the country of origin and time interval between blood titer testing and arrival. A period of 180 days between the time of the titer and travel is maintained because this is the maximum incubation period for dogs and cats.[142] Only a single vaccination is required, preferably within 6 to 12 months of entry. (1) Animals must be more than 6 months of age, not pregnant, or not of certain banned breeds. (2) If a first vaccination, it must be given at least 3 months of age and for boosters within 3 to 12 months of entry. (3) Animals must be accompanied by a health and rabies certificate, have an implanted microchip or unique tattoo and have an approved rabies viral neutralizing antibody test result as outlined above. In addition to some other parasite screenings, dogs must have seronegative test results to *Ehrlichia canis* and *Brucella canis* within 45 days and *Leptospira canicola* within 21 days of travel. If residing in Africa, dogs must be treated prophylactically for babesiosis.
[a]Information from the World Health Organization and Office International des Epizooties and the regulating authorities of the various countries below.
[b]Guidelines may vary and respective consulate for the country of interest should be contacted for the latest information. Some exceptions to the above guidelines are listed for the indicated geographic area.

allergenicity. H-RIG is given one time, simultaneously with the initial dose of vaccine, or up to 7 days later. However, the dose is not repeated because it may interfere with the active immune response to subsequent vaccinations. If feasible, the H-RIG is infiltrated in the area around the wounds. Remaining volumes are given IM at a site away from the vaccination. Worldwide, H-RIG is in short supply and, in many countries,

equine rabies immunoglobulin (E-RIG) is used.[230] Unfortunately, the production of E-RIG has been discontinued in many countries.

Vaccination
Rabies human diploid cell vaccine (HDCV) is highly effective and safe for pre- and postexposure immunizations; however,

it is too expensive for use in many developing countries. Two additional vaccines are rabies vaccine adsorbed (RVA), a fetal rhesus monkey lung cell culture rabies vaccine that is in very limited supply, and a purified chick embryo cell (PCEC) vaccine. These are the only commercial rabies vaccines currently available in the United States (see footnotes, Table 22-2). They are more immunogenic and less allergenic than previously available human rabies vaccines.[219] Five doses of 1.0 ml each are given IM. Postexposure therapy with HDCV, PCEC, or RVA and H-RIG must begin as soon as possible, preferably within 24 hours or less (see Table 22-2, Postexposure, People). Postexposure failures have been noted when the vaccine has been given in the gluteal rather than the deltoid muscle. If previously immunized people are exposed to potentially rabid animals, IM boosters are administered on days 0 and 3. In some regions, 0.1 ml ID booster doses have been substituted for some of the standard IM doses as a safe, convenient, and more economical solution, such as in developing countries.[207] The ID route is not recommended for PEP in the United States. Veterinarians and other animal health care professionals should not receive boosters unless tests show no detectable titer. Based on serologic evidence from biennial testing, approximately 80% of vaccinated veterinarians will continue to sustain protective titers; they should be given boosters when an exposure is identified.

Exposure Incident

The decision to administer PEP in people is a medical urgency and is based on a large number of factors concerning the bite incident. The species of animal that inflicts the bite wound is important because dogs, cats, and especially wild carnivores and bats are more likely to transmit the virus. Many people might have been spared the concern and inconvenience of prophylactic therapy had cats been routinely vaccinated. Bites of rodents such as squirrels, chipmunks, rats, mice, and lagomorphs seldom if ever result in human PEP (see Table 22-3, Rodents). Despite this fact, PEP has often been performed unnecessarily.

The type of exposure is important in determining if PEP should be used. Canids are the most important vector for rabies transmission to people of Asia, Africa, and Latin America. In other areas of the world, with more extensive canine vaccination programs, wild mammals, especially bats, predominate as vectors. Exposure to rabies is via a bite, scratch, or other situation in which saliva or CNS tissue of a potentially rabid animal enters an open or a fresh wound or comes in contact with mucous membrane of the eye, nose, or mouth. Nearly all cases of human rabies have been acquired by exposure to saliva in bite wounds or, very rarely, on abraded or scratched skin. Nonbite exposures rarely result in rabies virus infection. Indirect nonbite exposure has never resulted in a human infection. This situation might occur if a rabid animal had bitten a dog and the owner cleaned the wounds. Handling of blood or urine in carcasses of infected dogs did not appear to be of risk.[200] Live rabies virus could not be isolated from blood or urine although viral RNA was found in the urine samples and urinary tissues, especially the urinary bladder. In many human infections with bat rabies variants, the type of exposure is often not evident[164] but is believed to be caused by an unrecognized bite. The lack of a demonstrable bite or scratch, and therefore clinical suspicion, often delays a diagnosis and potential early prophylaxis. Therefore a new recommendation, although often controversial and expensive to implement, has been to consider PEP if a reasonable chance of exposure exists when bats are involved.[11,87] Unfortunately, the tendency to err on the side of caution means that PEP is often administered without confirmation.[164,235] PEP is always indicated in people with compromised immune systems such as those with AIDS.[1] The use of PEP may be associated with potential adverse effects such as local swelling, myalgia, pyrexia, vomiting, or systemic allergic reactions.

The epidemiology of the biting incident is also important in determining the need to initiate prophylaxis before laboratory confirmation (see Table 22-3). Bites from rabies-infected

Table • 22-5

Recommendations for Preexposure Rabies Prophylaxis in Researchers, Animal Health Professionals, and the Population at Large

EXPOSURE	POPULATION	NATURE OF EXPOSURE	ROUTE OF EXPOSURE	RECOMMENDED PROPHYLAXIS
Continuous	Rabies research laboratory staff, biologics production staff	High concentration of virus	Aerosol, mucosal, bite, etc.	Primary series; serologic test at 6-month intervals, booster when level not adequate
Frequent	Rabies diagnostic laboratory staff, spelunker, veterinarians and staff, wildlife workers, travelers visiting enzootic areas (over 30 days)	Episodic exposure, recognized source	Bite or nonbite	Primary series; serologic test every 2 years; consider booster when level not adequate; antibody titers are surrogate markers for continuing immunity
Infrequent	Veterinarians, animal control and wildlife workers in low rabies enzootic areas, veterinary students	Episodic, recognized source	Bite or nonbite	Primary series; no serologic testing or booster vaccination
Rare	U.S. population at large, including people in enzootic areas for rabies	Episodic	Bite with recognized source	No vaccination

Modified from: Human Rabies Prevention—United States, 1999, Recommendations of the Advisory Committee on Immunization Practices (ACIP). *MMWR* 1999:48{No. RR-1}
Minimum acceptable antibody titer complete neutralization at a 1:5 serum dilution with rapid fluorescent focus inhibition test.

animals usually occur without provocation. Animals that show neurologic signs at the time of the bite or soon after should be considered rabid. Bite exposures are much more likely to result in rabies infection than scratches, unless the scratches were contaminated by the animal's saliva. The prevalence of rabies in the geographic area is also important. People accidentally injected with inactivated animal rabies vaccines do not require PEP. For additional information on rabies in exposed people, consult the CDC rabies web page (http://www.cdc.gov/ncidod/dvrd/rabies).

Preexposure Prophylaxis for People

Preexposure prophylaxis is warranted in people with a high vocational or recreational risk of contacting rabid animals (see Table 22-2 and Table 22-5). An initial three-dose series (days 0, 7, and 21 or 28) has provided superior protection, when followed for 10 years, as compared with the two-dose (days 0 and 28) primary immunization sequence.[205] Veterinarians, animal health technicians and caretakers, animal control officers, wildlife biologists, bat handlers, laboratory workers, and spelunkers in rabies-endemic and epidemic areas should receive preexposure vaccination. Disaster response personnel should also consider preexposure vaccination because of packs of dogs that create risk under these circumstances.[93] Despite CDC recommendations for vaccination of animal health workers, a large proportion of at-risk staff in these areas have not received vaccination.[215] Cost or short-term employment may be barriers to uniform compliance. Unfortunately, many rabies endemic countries do not have the means to administer rabies vaccines for people in the quantities desired.

Substitution of 0.1 ml dose of ID HDCV is also effective for primary immunization and is cost-effective alternative in underdeveloped countries to the less costly but often used nervous tissue–derived vaccines.[207] More frequent boosters are needed with ID as compared with IM use because of a shorter duration of immunity.[17] Concerns have surfaced about the consistency of the vaccines used for ID procedure and immune response that results.[225] The use of ID rabies vaccine has been discontinued in the United States as a business decision but not for public health reasons. Hypersensitivity reactions have been the main side effects noted in approximately 6% of those receiving booster vaccinations with HDCV after having received the primary series. Local and systemic immune complex–mediated allergic reaction have developed with the use of HDCV, although the reactions are less than those with previously available products. Hives, urticaria, arthralgia, fever, nausea, and vomiting can develop within 1 week of booster vaccinations.

The risk of veterinarians being exposed to rabid animals is more than 300 times greater than that of the general population.[78] In one study, most (230) of the 380 exposures occurred to veterinarians during nonbite contact while they examined rabid animals. Seventy-nine exposures were the result of an animal bite.[78] Seventeen were the result of exposures at necropsy. Many of these potential exposures resulted from contact with infected cattle, although a summary claimed only 13 known confirmed instances of rabies transmission from cattle to people worldwide. No human rabies has been documented after preexposure vaccine administration by the IM route.

SUGGESTED READINGS*

13. Anonymous. 1999. Rabies, quarantine and the veterinary profession: the BVA's position, *Vet Rec* 146:396-397.
36. Briggs DJ, Smith JS, Mueller FL, et al. 1998. A comparison of two serological methods for detecting the immune response after rabies vaccination in dogs and cats being exported to rabies-free areas, *Biologicals* 26:347-355.
69. Fogelman V, Fischman HR, Horman JT, et al. 1993. Epidemiologic and clinical characteristics of rabies in cats, *J Am Vet Med Assoc* 202:1829-1838.
74. Gibbons RV. 2002. Cryptogenic rabies, bats, and the question of aerosol transmission, *Ann Emerg Med* 39:528-536.
220. Wacharapluesadee S, Hemachudha T. 2001. Nucleic acid sequence based amplification in the rapid diagnosis of rabies, *Lancet* 358:892-893.

*See the CD-ROM for a complete list of references.

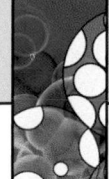

CHAPTER • 23

Pseudorabies

Marc Vandevelde

ETIOLOGY

Pseudorabies virus (PRV) is an enveloped DNA virus and an alpha-herpesvirus. As with other herpesviruses, PRV can cause latent infection, with viral DNA being incorporated into the host cell genome. The virus is relatively resistant to environmental factors and can survive outside the host for several months under favorable climatic conditions. Survival of PRV depends on temperature (10 days at 37° C, 40 days at 25° C) and pH (optimum, 7), and it is quickly inactivated by drying and exposure to ultraviolet light.[4] The genes of PRV have been cloned and sequenced, and its genetic relationship to other animal herpesviruses has been studied.

EPIDEMIOLOGY

PRV infection (known as *Aujeszky's disease, mad itch,* and *infectious bulbar paralysis*) occurs in most countries of the world with the exception of Australia and has been responsible for massive economic losses. Although many mammalian species are susceptible to infection with PRV, it is predominantly a problem in pigs, the main reservoir of the virus. However, cattle, fur-bearing animals, dogs, and cats are sporadically affected.[15,20] It does not appear to affect humans; most reports have been circumstantial and have not been documented. Infection frequently is subclinical in pigs because they have become well adapted to the virus. The disease is spread by commercial movement of infected pigs or contaminated pork products. Venereal transmission occurs when infected boars shed PRV in semen. Although wild animals such as raccoons, panthers,[10] and rats may act as transient reservoirs, they are not important in maintaining the disease in nature. Their role is limited to temporary local spread of virus within enzootic areas. Similarly, PRV infection in dogs and cats only occurs in areas where the disease is enzootic in pigs. Such epidemiologic interaction among species has been documented by molecular biological studies on viral isolates.[11] In fact, the occurrence of typical pseudorabies signs in pets can be the first indication that the disease is enzootic in the local pig population. Pets almost invariably are infected as a result of consuming contaminated raw pork. Dogs also have developed pseudorabies after having bitten infected pigs. Direct spread from dog to dog has not been shown to occur.[27]

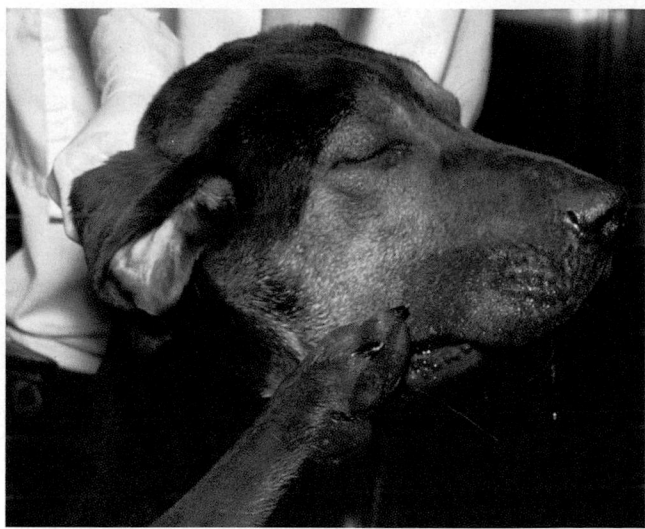

Fig 23-1 Dog with pseudorabies and self-mutilation injuries. (Courtesy Daniel Harrington, Purdue University, West Lafayette, Ind.)

PATHOGENESIS

Naturally acquired infection in dogs and cats occurs after ingestion of the virus, although a similar sequence of events occurs after parenteral inoculation of virus. PRV enters the nerve endings at the inoculation site and travels in retrograde fashion via the axoplasm of the nerve fibers to the brain.[7] The incubation time in dogs and cats, regardless of inoculation sites, is 3 to 6 days. Experimental studies in orally infected cats have shown that PRV replicates in the tonsils and travels from the oral mucosa via the sensory branches of the ninth and tenth cranial nerves to the nucleus, tractus solitarius, and area postrema in the medulla oblongata.[14] The fifth cranial nerve has been less frequently involved. Experimental infections in rats have shown that PRV spreads in a highly specific manner through synaptic connections.[3,7] Apart from visible damage to the brain tissue associated with inflammatory changes, the virus can cause considerable functional alterations of the nerve cells.[5]

CLINICAL FINDINGS

The majority of dogs and cats that become infected develop severe clinical signs. The onset of clinical illness is hyperacute, and signs progress rapidly until death occurs; the total course rarely lasts longer than 48 hours. With very few exceptions, pseudorabies is always fatal in dogs. Cats may be somewhat more resistant but have rarely recovered from the disease.

The initial sign often noted by the owner is a change in behavior, such as inactivity, lethargy, and indifference, although some animals become aggressive or restless. Dyspnea, diarrhea, and vomiting are occasionally seen. The dyspnea is often caused by severe pulmonary edema. Body temperature may be normal or abnormal, and hypersalivation is common. However, the most characteristic sign is intense pruritus, which usually occurs in the head region and rarely occurs in other areas such as the neck and shoulders. The animals violently scratch their faces and ears and rub their heads against the floor or walls. One side of the head and neck may become swollen. Self-mutilation results in erythema, excoriation, and ulceration of the skin and underlying tissues (Fig. 23-1). The scratching becomes increasingly more frantic

and may end in generalized convulsions. Most of the other neurologic signs that are observed in PRV infection refer to lesions in the lower brainstem and consist of one or several deficits in cranial nerve function. These deficits are usually unilateral and include anisocoria, mydriasis, lack of direct or consensual pupillary light reflexes, trismus, paresis and paralysis of the facial muscles, head tilt, inability to swallow, and vocal changes. Anisocoria and a hoarse voice are considered to be highly consistent signs in the cat.[24] Less commonly observed neurologic signs include behavioral abnormalities such as aggressiveness, generalized hyperesthesia, head pressing, and generalized convulsions. The latter often occur as sequelae to frantic scratching. Paresis and paralysis of the limbs are sometimes noted shortly before death. Although less common, in some cats death has been preceded predominantly by acute GI signs.[35] Arrhythmias may manifest by an irregular pulse and dropped beats as a result of myocarditis.[32]

An atypical course of the disease has also been observed in cats that died suddenly without developing neurologic signs.[18] Pruritus has been absent in some cases of spontaneous PRV infection in dogs[37] and in experimental oral infection in cats.[14] gastrointestinal signs have been the predominant feature of some infected dogs.[9]

DIAGNOSIS

Hematologic or biochemical abnormalities are not found in pseudorabies. Cerebrospinal fluid may show increased protein concentration and mononuclear pleocytosis. This finding is strongly indicative of viral encephalitis but is not specific for pseudorabies. Electrocardiographic findings may include cardiac arrhythmias.[23,32]

Traditionally, the diagnosis of pseudorabies consisted of cutaneous inoculation of infected tissue (usually brain) into a rabbit. Scratching and automutilation of the inoculation site occurred after an incubation of 5 to 6 days, followed by the rapid death of the animal. Virus can also be propagated in the brains of mice after intracranial inoculation.[31] Pruritus can occur in some mice at the site of inoculation. Newer diagnostic methods such as direct fluorescent antibody examination for virus have made animal inoculation studies obsolete. This procedure can detect virus in smears or frozen sections of various tissues. The brain and tonsils are the tissues of choice in such studies. Polymerase chain reaction (PCR) has been used to detect PRV.[30] PCR has been used successfully to detect the virus in a cat in Japan.[16]

Virus can be isolated in tissue culture from lung and spleen and especially from brain and tonsils of animals with pseudorabies. Although many cell lines have been used, most laboratories use pig kidney epithelial cells. A definite cytopathic effect consisting of syncytial formation is visible after 12 to 24 hours. Virus isolation is not always easy in dogs, even in well-substantiated cases.[2] Pharyngeal washings, tonsillar swabs, and saliva are unsuitable for viral isolation in dogs.[19]

Virus neutralization, immunodiffusion, and enzyme-linked immunosorbent assay (ELISA) methods commonly are used to detect serum antibody to PRV in pigs. Serologic studies have been valuable in determining the incidence of disease in pig populations from an epizootiologic and a disease prevention point of view. PCR has been able to detect latency in the porcine population.[30] Virus neutralizing antibodies have not been found in sera from dogs tested during an outbreak of PRV infection.[19]

PATHOLOGIC FINDINGS

No gross lesions are diagnostic of pseudorabies, with the exception of the skin lesions that result from intense pruritus. In some cases, abnormal stomach contents have been noted because of pica. Pulmonary edema and congestion have been consistent findings. Focal myocarditis has been found in dogs and cats. Lesions in the central nervous system are almost exclusively located in the brainstem and primarily involve cranial nerve nuclei.[8] They may be unilateral and consist of perivascular cuffing with mononuclear cells and pronounced proliferation of astrocytes and microglial cells (Fig. 23-2, A). The areas of focal gliosis often show degeneration (karyorrhexis) in the center and may progress to the formation of microabscesses (Fig. 23-2, B and C). Severe changes occur in neurons, with chromatolysis and disintegration of the nucleus. The most significant finding is the presence of weak eosinophilic viral inclusion bodies in the nuclei of astrocytes and neurons (Fig. 23-2, D). Viral antigen can be specifically demonstrated in formalin-fixed, paraffin-embedded tissues with immunocytochemical methods[6] or in situ hybridization.[28,34] Inflammatory changes can also be found in the nerves and ganglia associated with the site of viral entry. Severe inflammation of the myenteric plexus in the alimentary canal of dogs naturally infected with PRV has also been reported.[9,13] Experimentally infected dogs had ganglioneuritis of autonomic nerves of the heart.[23]

THERAPY

Treatment of pseudorabies is generally futile because the disease is almost always fatal. Heavy sedation and anesthesia may lessen or relieve the itching and convulsions; however,

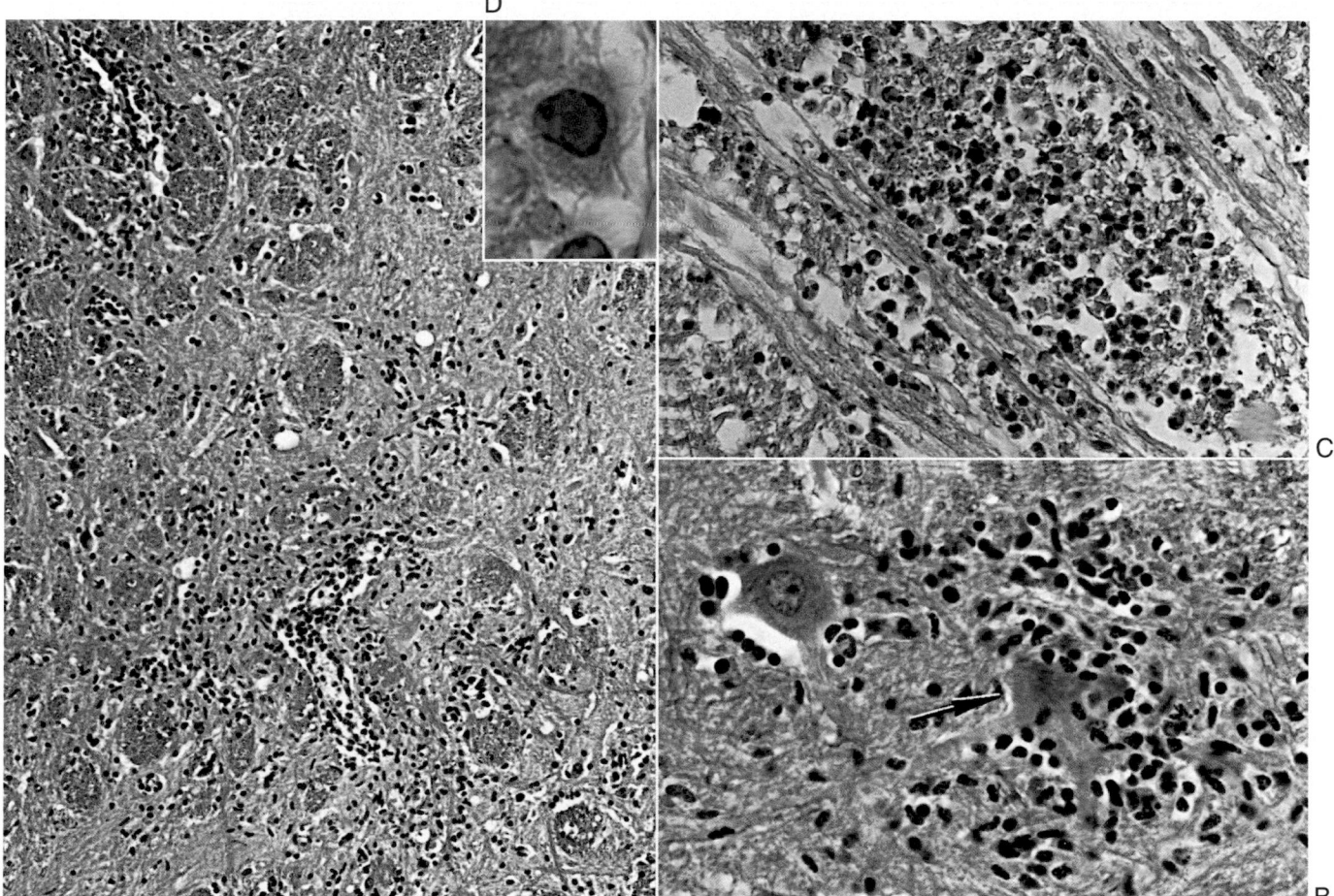

Fig   23-2   Histologic findings of pseudorabies encephalitis. **A,** Disseminated perivascular cuffing and gliosis in the medulla oblongata (H and E stain, ×100). **B,** Neuronal degeneration *(arrow)* with nodular gliosis (H and E stain, ×250). **C,** Microabscess (H and E stain, ×250). **D,** PRV inclusion body in glial cell nucleus (H and E stain, ×400).

nothing can alter the outcome of the disease. Treatment with anti-PRV serum did not improve the condition of a dog with Aujeszky's disease[29] and is considered to be ineffective in the prevention of infection.[27]

PREVENTION

Prevention is the most important means of control of PRV infection in dogs and cats. Contact with pigs and especially the use of raw pork from endemic areas as animal food should be avoided. It is possible to vaccinate small animals against PRV, although this is indicated only in endemic areas, where exposure to infected pigs may occur. Natural infection with PRV has not been observed in vaccinated dogs and cats.[1] However, experimental vaccination challenge studies showed that it may be difficult to protect dogs with an inactivated vaccine, although most animals develop serum neutralizing antibodies to PRV.[27] Attenuated PRV vaccines may cause postvaccinal reactions that may be as lethal as the natural infection. PRV deletion mutants have been developed for vaccination of pigs.[21,22,25] Such vaccines are safe and very useful for controlling the disease because serologic surveys can distinguish between vaccine-induced and natural anti-PRV antibodies. Deletion vaccines have been tested in raccoons, albeit with limited success.[36] DNA vaccines have also been developed.[17] Human adenoviruses have been used as vectors for experimental immunization of cats against PRV antigens.[12] To the author's knowledge, none of these modern vaccines have been systematically tested or applied in dogs and cats. In recent years, considerable progress has been made in the eradication of PRV infection in swine in many areas of the world.[26] As a result, Aujeszky's disease is becoming a very rare condition in dogs and cats, and the development and application of PRV vaccines in small animals have remained insignificant.

SUGGESTED READINGS*

10. Glass CM, McLean RG, Katz JB, et al. 1994. Isolation of pseudorabies (Aujeszky's disease) virus from a Florida panther, *J Wildl Dis* 30:180-184.
17. Hong W, Xiao S, Zhou R, et al. 2002. Protection induced by intramuscular immunization with DNA vaccines of pseudorabies in mice, rabbits and piglets, *Vaccine* 20:1205-1214.
20. Matsuoka T, Iijima Y, Sakurai K, et al. 1988. Aujeszky's disease in a dog, *Jpn J Vet Sci* 50:277-278.
22. Mettenleiter TC. 2000. Aujeszky's disease (pseudorabies) virus: the virus and molecular pathogenesis-state of the art, June 1999, *Vet Res* 31:99-115.

*See the CD-ROM for a complete list of references.

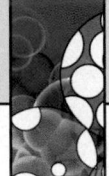

CHAPTER • 24

Enterovirus Infections

Craig E. Greene

Picornaviridae, the family of the smallest RNA viruses, contains the genus *Enterovirus*. Species in this genus commonly infect humans and have classically been separated into polioviruses, coxsackieviruses, enteric cytopathogenic human orphan (echo) viruses, and as yet unclassified enteroviruses. Newer members of the genus are called enteroviruses and are designated by a sequential numbering system. Enteroviruses are environmentally resistant and infect people primarily via the fecal-oral route. After replication in submucosal lymphatic tissues, the viruses may spread systemically to various other tissues.

Dogs have been tested to determine whether they harbor a variety of human enteroviruses because of the possible zoonotic potential (Table 24-1). Similar information is not available for cats. Dogs have been shown to be exposed to and to chronically shed human enteroviruses; however, serologic evidence of infection does not always correlate with shedding of the viruses. Although dogs appear to become infected with these viruses, clinical signs have not been apparent. The viruses can be found in the stools for a period of months, but whether the extended shedding represents reexposure is uncertain. Enteroviruses recovered from nasopharyngeal or fecal cultures of dogs have been grown and cause cytopathogenic effects, primarily in monkey kidney but not canine cell lines, supporting the fact that they are human viruses. Furthermore, neutralization tests have shown them to be indistinguishable from the human isolates.[8,9] In some

Table • 24-1

Human Enteroviruses Recovered from Asymptomatic Dogs

VIRUS	SPECIMEN SOURCE	GEOGRAPHIC LOCATION
Poliovirus 1	Feces	West Bengal[2]
	Feces	Costa Rica[5]
Echovirus 6	Feces	California[1]
	Nasopharynx, feces	New Mexico[1,6,10]
Echovirus 7	Feces	West Bengal[2]
Coxsackievirus A9, A20	Feces	Costa Rica[5]
Coxsackievirus B₁	Nasopharynx, feces	Texas, New Mexico[1,6]
Coxsackievirus B₃	Nasopharynx, feces	New Mexico[6]
Coxsackievirus B₅	Nasopharynx, feces	New Mexico[6]
Unclassified enteroviruses	Feces	Philippines[12]

instances, enteroviruses were found in canine feces that were "just passing through," not causing infection. These viruses may have been obtained from sources contaminated by human feces. Alternatively, they may be enteroviruses antigenically related to human enteroviruses or other viruses neutralized by nonspecific substances in the testing sera. Newer techniques to determine viral homogeneity by genetic analysis must be performed on isolates to resolve this issue.

Feeding of echovirus 6 or coxsackievirus B1 to dogs produced minimal signs suggestive of enteric disease. Although the virus could be isolated from the feces, seroconversion could not be demonstrated.[7,11] Infection seems to be limited to the alimentary tract of dogs and does not spread systemically as such infections do in people. Although dogs shed these viruses in low amounts, viral spread to susceptible dogs has resulted in infection.[11] Whether infected dogs can be a source of human infection is uncertain.

SUGGESTED READINGS*

5. Grew N, Gohd RS, Arguedas J, et al. 1970. Enteroviruses in rural families and their domestic animals, *Am J Epidemiol* 91:518-526.
13. Waldman EA, Moreira RC, Saez SG, et al. 1996. Human enterovirus in stray dogs. Some aspects of interest to public health, *Rev Inst Med Trop Sao Paulo* 38:157-161.

*See the CD-ROM for a complete list of references.

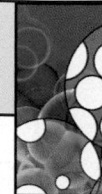

CHAPTER 25

Mumps and Influenza Virus Infections

Craig E. Greene

MUMPS

Mumps virus is a member of the family *Paramyxoviridae* and genus *Paramyxovirus*. The virus causes illness in humans—its primary natural hosts; however, nonhuman primates and other laboratory animals have been experimentally infected. Clinical signs in affected humans include fever, anorexia, and progressive, independent enlargement of the parotid salivary glands. Meningitis, the main complication of infection that sometimes develops, results in headache and nuchal rigidity. Encephalitis, polyarthritis, and pancreatitis may develop, although they are uncommon. Vaccination programs have greatly reduced the prevalence and severity of this infectious disease throughout the world.

Mumps viral antibodies have been identified in the sera of healthy dogs; however, dogs can be infected with canine parainfluenza viruses (similar to but distinct from simian virus 5 of nonhuman primates; see Chapters 6 and 7), which may cross-react with some mumps viral antigens. Interpretation of prior serologic studies may be misleading for this reason. Nevertheless, reports have been made of parotid salivary gland enlargement in dogs from households in which children in the family have had concurrent or recent mumpslike infections.[1,9,13] Antibody to mumps viral antigen was detected in the serum of some affected dogs.[9,13] A virus that had been neutralized by mumps viral antisera was found in one dog.[9] Early experimental attempts to produce mumps in dogs or cats by inoculation of virus directly in the gland were inconclusive.[9] Although in vivo transmission studies are inconclusive, mumps virus does grow well in primary dog kidney cell culture and has been a source of attenuated vaccine for human use.[8,14] Veterinarians in practice should be aware of the possible association between mumps in children and pets, although definitive evidence for animal infection is lacking.

INFLUENZA

Influenza viruses are in the family *Orthomyxoviridae*. Almost every winter, two genera—types A and B—produce episodic outbreaks of an acute self-limiting febrile illness in susceptible humans. Type C influenza viruses are less closely related but produce a similar disease. Fever, myalgia, and signs of upper or lower respiratory tract infections are the most common manifestations. Mortality is the result of pulmonary complications. Pandemic spread of influenza may result periodically when genetic alterations of surface glycoproteins results in a new viral strain to which the world population has no immunity.

Influenza virus spreads through the transfer of virus-containing respiratory secretions from an infected to a susceptible human. Transfer through small (<10 μm) aerosols is the primary mode of spread.

Because of the close association of pets with humans, concern has been raised that dogs and cats may be important in the spread or maintenance of influenza infection. Many reports exist of serologic evidence of infection of dogs and cats with influenza virus. Experimental intranasal or intravenous infection of dogs[7,11,12,15] and cats[11,12] with influenza virus A strains, of dogs[15] and cats[11] with type B strains, and of dogs[10] with type C strains has provided convincing evidence that they are susceptible to these infections. Clinical signs in infected animals either were absent or consisted of a mild conjunctivitis, serous nasal discharge, and variable fever. Serologic responses have been inconsistent, although viruses could be recovered from the respiratory secretions. Cats and dogs were also infected in some instances by contact with animals that were infected.

Spontaneous influenza viral infections of dogs and cats have been associated with human populations that are experiencing epidemics of the disease.[2,12] No evidence suggests that the virus spreads from infected pets back to humans. This finding is in contrast to the situation in which the virus spreads between species, from humans and birds and back ("mixing vessel hypothesis") probably occurs, with genetic recombination and evolution of new viral strains.[18] Pigs have played an important role in the emergence of pandemic human influenza viral strains in the past.

In the avian influenza virus outbreak of 2004 caused by A H5N1 strain, a household of cats and some captive exotic cats in Thailand died in association with the death of some chickens. The possibility that this was caused by influenza virus has not yet been substantiated.[19] Numerous other mammalian species such as seals, whales, mink, and ferrets are also susceptible to avian influenza viruses; however, viral replication in most of these animals, as it is in cats, is self-limiting. Only the pig appears important in the amplification of the virus between chickens and humans.

In Florida, a strain of equine influenza virus that had been isolated in Wisconsin in 2003 jumped the species barrier and infected racing greyhounds.[16] It is likely the strain that is spreading through the horse population. Virus isolation and serum antibody titers were used to confirm the viral cause. Past outbreaks of fatal respiratory disease in greyhounds have been attributed to streptococcal infections (see Chapter 35); however, this may have been responsible in the past.

SUGGESTED READINGS*

1. Chandler E. 1975. Mumps in the dog, *Vet Rec* 96:365-366.
2. Chang CP, New AG, Taylor JF, et al. 1976. Influenza virus isolations from dogs during a human epidemic in Taiwan, *Int J Zoon* 3:61-64.
16. University of Florida Online News Release. URL:// www.sciencedaily.com/releases/2004/04/040429055247 .htm

*See the CD-ROM for a complete list of references.

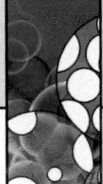

CHAPTER • 26

Arthropod-Borne Viral Infections

All arthropod-borne (Arbo-) viruses known to infect dogs and cats belong to the families *Togaviridae, Flaviviridae, Bunyaviridae,* or *Reoviridae* (Table 26-1). These RNA viruses are usually maintained in nature by a sylvan cycle involving an arthropod vector and a vertebrate reservoir host (Fig. 26-1). The worldwide distribution of the mosquito-borne infections is presented in Fig. 26-2. Arboviruses usually replicate within their insect vectors, causing minimal or no cell injury. In contrast, vertebrate hosts' cells are often damaged by cytolysis. Although domesticated animals are usually incidental hosts for these infections, in some cases, they serve as reservoirs. As unnatural hosts, domesticated animals may be subclinically affected or show signs of disease (usually nonsuppurative, neurotropic encephalitis, abortion, or teratology). The clinical susceptibility of people, dogs, and cats for each disease also varies. Results of serologic testing indicate that a large number of dogs and cats may be exposed to these viruses; however, clinical illness is uncommon. Because serologic cross-reactivity between certain viruses can occur, and because dogs and cats can be subclinically infected, the following discussion emphasizes instances in which virus isolation and consistent pathologic findings have been present or experimental inoculation of dogs or cats has been performed.

Classical methods of diagnosing arboviral infections have included isolation and replication of virus, production of antigen extracts, and preparation of polyclonal or monoclonal antisera. Newer techniques, which involve RNA fingerprinting, immunohistochemistry, nucleic acid hybridization, polymerase chain reaction (PCR), and nucleic acid sequencing, have replaced some of the classical testing. These latter genetic techniques have now replaced viral isolation and serotyping as the initial screening procedures. Genotypic and phenotypic information should be complementary; however, in most cases, deducing the phenotype of these viruses from the known genomic sequences is not yet possible. Although genomics have been epidemiologically used to track virus strains, pathogenicity and cross-protectivity are difficult to assess without isolates.

MOSQUITO AND GNAT-BORNE INFECTIONS

Craig E. Greene and Charles A. Baldwin

Togaviridae

Alphaviruses in this family are grouped into seven antigenic complexes, and three of these (see Table 26-1) occur in the New World, causing sporadic equine, human, canine, and feline infections. Natural and experimental susceptibility of dogs to Venezuelan equine encephalitis (VEE) virus has been well described.[50] In both natural and experimental infections involving mosquitoes, viremia and seroconversion occur without clinical illness. For this reason, dogs have been considered good sentinel hosts for human VEE infection. Dogs also have been used to monitor the spread of infection into geographic areas. Parenteral inoculation of VEE in dogs has produced fever, leukopenia, and neurologic deficits at the peak of the febrile response. Cerebrovascular hemorrhage and infarction were detected. Naturally occurring VEE was also suspected as causing encephalitis in a puppy.[50] Eastern equine encephalitis (EEE) has been diagnosed in naturally infected dogs from south-central Georgia.[10] All of these pups were younger than 6 weeks, with signs of diffuse encephalitis exhibited by ataxia, tremor, excessive salivation, and seizure.

Petechial hemorrhages have been grossly evident on the surface of the brain at necropsy. Histologic lesions in the brain were inflammation with macrophage infiltration and perivascular cuffing, edema, gliosis, hemorrhage, and multifocal necrosis (Fig. 26-3). Mononuclear and neutrophilic infiltrates have been present in the meninges. Foci of myocardial degeneration and necrosis with mononuclear infiltration have been found in the heart. The viral association has been confirmed by use of an oligonucleotide probe and viral isolation. EEE has also been isolated from the central nervous system (CNS) of a litter of dying 6-week-old puppies in which no microscopic lesions could be demonstrated.[11] The infection may have been coincidental. Experimentally, dogs have developed diffuse encephalitis after intracerebral or parenteral inoculation of western equine encephalitis virus.[50]

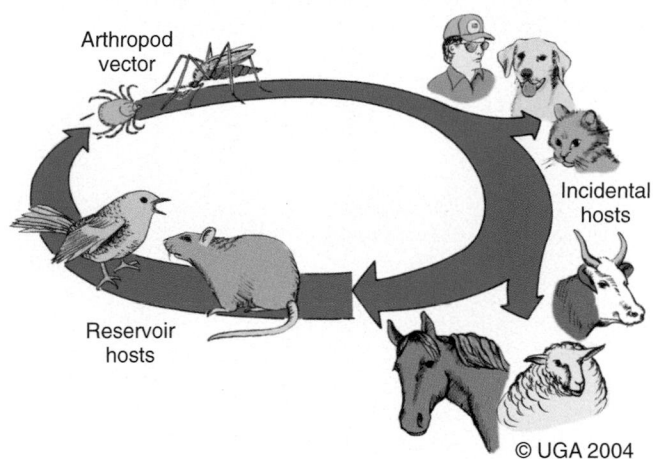

Fig 26-1 Arthropod-borne viral infections have a sylvan cycle involving arthropod vectors that feed on reservoir hosts. Domestic animals and people are usually incidental hosts, but they may serve as reservoirs in some instances (see Table 26-1). (Courtesy University of Georgia, Athens, Ga.)

Ross River and Barmah Forest viruses are endemic in Australia, primarily with kangaroos and wallabies (family Macropodidae) acting as major mammalian reservoirs. Serum neutralizing antibodies are widespread in human and mammalian populations, and some dogs and cats have neutralizing antibodies to these viruses. Dogs and cats experimentally infected by feeding mosquitoes were relatively resistant to both viral infections.[20] Only a few animals seroconverted, and none developed viremia or clinical signs. Although these animals are naturally exposed, they are not likely to be important reservoirs of these viruses.

Bunyaviridae

Tenshaw virus inoculated into dogs and cats produced asymptomatic viremia.[50] Mosquito transmission from infected dogs was also demonstrated. Rift Valley fever virus (RVFV) has produced viremia, severe hepatic necrosis, myocarditis, splenic congestion, meningitis, diffuse petechiae, and death in puppies and kittens younger than 3 weeks.[50] Virus can also be transmitted from puppies to their mother and to other puppies. Older puppies do not succumb to infection but do develop viremias. The virus can cause abortions and stillbirths in pregnant bitches. Inhalation or ingestion of the virus from infected carcasses may occur under natural circumstances. (For a complete discussion of RVFV infection, see below.) La Crosse virus infection is remarkable in adaptation to at least one of its vectors, *Aedes triseriatus*. Vector infection is life long, and the virus is transmitted transovarially to subsequent generations of mosquitoes. It is the primary cause of arboviral encephalitis in the United States. Two litters of puppies younger than 3 weeks developed a sudden onset of seizures and neurologic dysfunction after infection with La Crosse virus.[17] An adult dog from Florida developed CNS signs of forebrain disease that responded to simultaneous treatment with antibacterials and glucocorticoids; however, it then developed seizures.[112] Severe diffuse necrotizing to granulomatous meningoencephalitis (GME) affecting primarily the cerebral cortex was noted in the affected dogs described previously (Figs. 26-4 and 26-5). Immunohistochemical testing demonstrated La Crosse virus within the affected brain tissue.

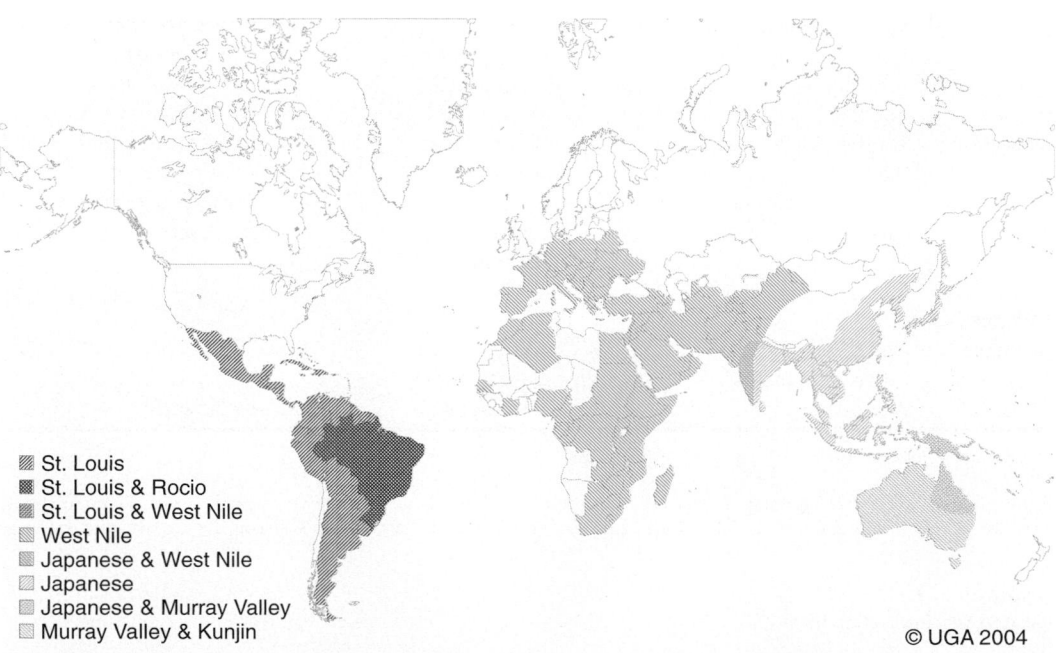

St. Louis
St. Louis & Rocio
St. Louis & West Nile
West Nile
Japanese & West Nile
Japanese
Japanese & Murray Valley
Murray Valley & Kunjin

© UGA 2004

Fig 26-2 Worldwide distribution of arboviral infections from the World Health Organization. (Map drawn courtesy University of Georgia, Athens, Ga.)

Table • 26-1

Arthropod-Borne Viral Infections Affecting Dogs and Cats

DISEASE	GEOGRAPHIC DISTRIBUTION	ARTHROPOD VECTOR	USUAL HOSTS: RESERVOIR (DOMESTIC)	SUSCEPTIBILITY OF HUMANS, DOGS, AND CATS
Togaviridae (Alphaviruses)				
Eastern equine encephalitis	Eastern United States, Central America, Caribbean islands, Brazil, Guyana, Argentina	*Culiseta melanura Aedes* spp., *Culex* spp.	Birds (horses, quail, pheasants, cows, sheep)	H, D
Western equine encephalitis	United States, Canada, Central America, Guyana, Brazil, Argentina	*Culiseta melanura, Culex* spp.	Birds, small mammals, snakes (horses)	H, D
Venezuelan equine encephalitis	Florida, Texas, northern South America, Central America	*Psorophora confinnis, Aedes* spp., *Culex* spp.	Rodents (horses)	H, D, C
Ross River and Barmah Forest virus infections	Australia, from Tasmania to Queensland	*Ochlerotatus vigilax*	Wallabies, kangaroos	H, D,[a] C[a]
Flaviviridae[b]				
St. Louis encephalitis	United States, Canada, Central America, Caribbean Islands, Colombia, Brazil, Argentina	*Culex* spp.	Birds (usually inapparent)	H, D,[a] C[a]
Japanese encephalitis	Siberia, Japan, China, many Far East countries	*Culex* spp.	Birds (pigs, horses)	H, D, C[a]
West Nile virus infection	Africa, Asia, Middle East, Europe, United States	*Culex* spp.	Birds	H, D, C
Powassan virus infection	United States, Canada	*Ixodes cookei, Ixodes marxil.*	Rodents (sheep)	H, D[a]
Louping-ill	Scotland, Ireland	*Ixodes ricinus*	Sheep(?), red grouse (sheep, cattle)	H, D
Tick-borne encephalitis	Europe, Soviet Republics	*Ixodes* spp., *Dermacentor* spp.	Rodents, birds (sheep, goats, cattle)	H, D
Wesselsbron disease	South Africa	*Aedes* spp.	Ungulates, sheep (sheep)	D
Yellow fever	South America, Africa	*Aedes* spp.	Nonhuman primates, humans (none)	H, C[a]
Bunyaviridae[c]				
Tenshaw virus infection	Southeastern United States	*Anopheles* spp.	Rodents (cattle, dogs)	D, C
La Crosse virus infection	Midwestern, eastern, and southern United States	*Aedes* spp.	Small mammals (chipmunks)	D[d]
Rift Valley fever	East Africa	*Culex theileri, Aedes caballus*	Ungulates (sheep)	H, D,[d] C[e]
Reoviridae (Orbiviruses)				
African horse sickness	Africa, Middle East, Mediterranean	*Culicoides* spp., mosquitoes(?)	Equidae (horse)	D[f]
Bluetongue	Worldwide	*Culicoides* spp.	Ovidae (sheep)	D[g]

H, Human; *D*, dog; *C*, cat; *?*, uncertain.
[a]Subclinical.
[b]Also includes Kunjin, Alfuy, Kokobera, Koutango (West Nile virus subtypes) and Murray Valley encephalitis viruses in Australia.
[c]Sixteen serogroups are in this family. Members of the California serogroup include Jamestown Canyon, La Crosse, and Tahyna viruses.
[d]Puppies.
[e]Kittens.
[f]Subclinical, carnivorism.
[g]Parenterally inoculated vaccine contaminant.

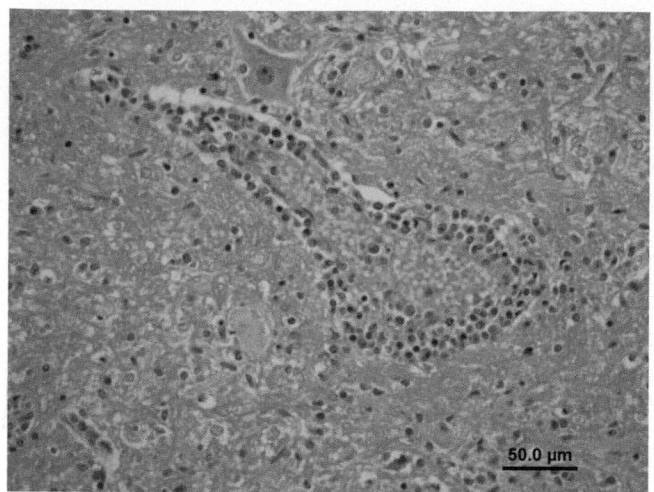

Fig 26-3 Perivascular cuff in the brain from a dog with EEE infection (H and E stain, ×40). (Courtesy Charles A. Baldwin, University of Georgia, Athens, Ga.)

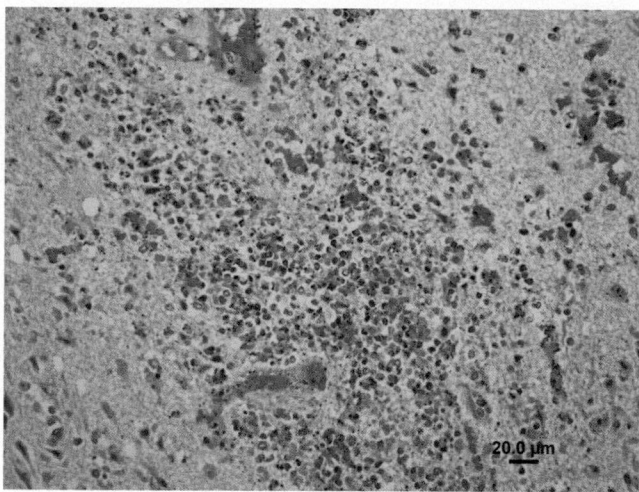

Fig 26-5 Perivascular necrosis in the brain from a pup with La Crosse virus infection (H and E stain, ×40). (Courtesy Charles A. Baldwin, University of Georgia, Athens, Ga.)

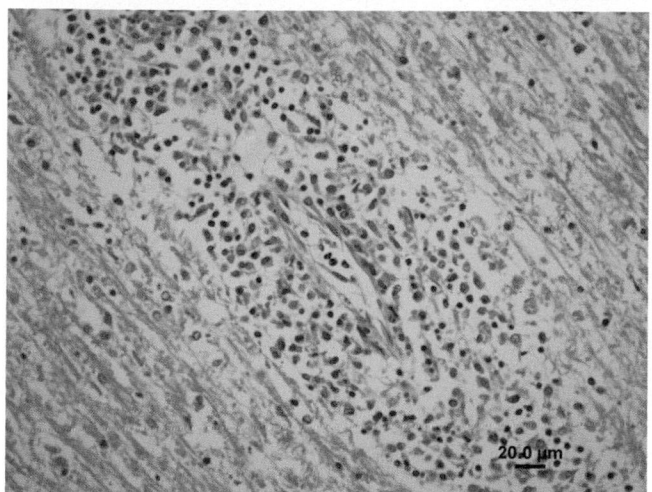

Fig 26-4 Perivascular cuff in the brain from a pup with La Crosse virus infection (H and E stain, ×40). (Courtesy Charles A. Baldwin, University of Georgia, Athens, Ga.)

Whether La Crosse virus is cause of idiopathic GME in dogs is uncertain (see Chapter 84, Neurologic Diseases of Uncertain Causes).

Rift Valley Fever

RVFV, a *Phlebovirus* infection of Africa and the Middle East, is capable of being transmitted by many species of mosquitoes. Among domestic species, RVFV affects predominantly sheep, cattle, and goats, and occasionally human beings. In people, the disease is characterized by hepatocellular failure, acute renal failure, and hemorrhagic manifestations.[2] Sera from wild and domestic dogs and cats in endemic regions have had positive test results. However, in a study using the more specific plaque reduction neutralization test, only lions from areas of three prior outbreaks had positive test results.[55] The mammalian reservoir for infection may exist in exotic carnivores such as the lion; however, domestic dogs and cats can be experimentally infected and maintain a viremia sufficient to infect mosquitoes.

Clinical illness in inoculated dogs is seen only in the first few weeks of life.[123] Some pups became hyperthermic during infec-

tion, while all died in a terminal hypothermic state. Some of the animals showed signs of CNS dysfunction near death. In older animals, 50% develop viremia and a corresponding increase in serum neutralization titer. Clinical signs in older animals were unapparent; however, transmission of infection from pup to mother and from pup to pup was demonstrated.

High mortality has been observed when kittens less than 3 weeks of age were inoculated with virus.[124] Certain strains of feline panleukopenia virus vaccine used in the challenged kittens may have partially protected them against challenge with RVFV. A transient febrile response was followed by terminal hypothermia. Neurologic signs were ataxia followed by recumbency and paddling movements within 24 hours before death. As with pups, evidence indicated that the virus spread to other kittens and adults.

On gross necropsy of dying pups and kittens, the liver and spleen were enlarged and soft in consistency.[86] In the liver, faint gray to yellow foci, 1 mm in diameter, are surrounded by thin hyperemic borders. Petechial and ecchymotic hemorrhages were found on the serosal surfaces of the heart, abdominal lymph nodes, and mucosal surfaces of the gastrointestinal tract. Histologically, hepatocellular necrosis has been the most consistent finding. In less severe areas, foci of necrosis are evident, whereas in the most severe cases, the entire liver is necrotic with little normal parenchyma. Multifocal inflammation and necrosis have been evident in the myocardium. Perivascular nonsuppurative meningoencephalitis, characteristic of other arboviral infections, was found in the CNS. Lesions in experimentally infected dogs and cats did not show characteristic eosinophilic intranuclear inclusions or Councilman-like bodies observed in other hosts.[86]

Reoviridae

Orbiviruses are one of nine genera in the family *Reoviridae*. Dogs, which can be infected subclinically with African horse sickness virus, develop a serologic response and a viremia enabling them to transmit the infection.[50] They are thought to acquire infection naturally and suffer illness and death from eating infected horse meat or from the tick *Rhipicephalus sanguineus*.[56] Abortion in pregnant bitches and their subsequent death have occurred 7 to 9 days after vaccination with a bluetongue virus–contaminated, modified live virus combination canine vaccine.[1,39,133] Lesions in the dam consisted of interstitial pneumonia, myocardial degeneration, hepatic vasculitis, and renal glomerulitis.[39] Natural disease with this virus in dogs is unlikely based on the observed low seropositivity of dogs tested in endemic areas.[57]

Flaviviridae

Flaviviruses are small, icosahedral, enveloped virions (45 to 60 nm diameter; 45 nm for West Nile virus [WNV]) with a single-stranded, positive-sense RNA genome.[89] The genus type species is the yellow fever virus (*flavi*, Latin for yellow); the genus also includes the St. Louis encephalitis (SLE) virus, which serologically cross-reacts with WNV.

SLE, Murray Valley encephalitis, and Kunjin viruses, along with other closely related viruses, belong to the Japanese encephalitis serocomplex. Infections caused by these viruses are maintained in nature by cycles involving birds as vertebrate hosts and predominantly *Culex* mosquitoes as vectors. Although dogs have been more resistant to SLE, serosurveys have demonstrated that they develop titers during human epidemics. Parenteral inoculation of Japanese encephalitis virus has resulted in subclinical infection, but intracranial inoculation resulted in encephalitis with corresponding neurologic deficits.[50] Louping-ill is described in a separate section of this chapter. Dogs have developed fever, viremia, and serologic response to Powassan virus.[50] Wesselsbron virus was isolated from the CNS of a dog with encephalitis.[50] Inoculation of brain tissue from this animal into naïve dogs produced seroconversion, viremia, and transient paralysis in one dog. Yellow fever virus has produced a transient viremia in cats after inoculation; however, puppies, even when splenectomized, could not be infected. European tick-borne encephalitis and louping-ill—two tick-transmitted flavivirus infections that can infect dogs—are discussed later in this chapter.

Cats have been reported to be refractory to SLE virus because they do not develop a humoral immune response after experimental infection and have not shown measurable antibody levels in field serosurveys.[69] Cats do develop antibodies to Powassan virus.[69]

WEST NILE VIRUS INFECTION

Carol A. Lichtensteiger and Craig E. Greene

Etiology

WNV is a mosquito-borne arbovirus of the family *Flaviviridae*, genus *Flavivirus*, and serocomplex group of Japanese encephalitis virus. WNV was originally isolated in 1937 from a febrile woman in the West Nile area of Uganda, Africa (see Reviews).* The virus has two lineages; only linage 1 has been associated with disease in mammals.[16,23] Based on genome sequence, the WNV isolate circulating in the novel outbreak in the United States is relatively stable and is most closely related to an isolate from a goose from a 1998 outbreak in Israel.[†]

Epidemiology

Historically, WNV has had a bird-mosquito-bird sylvatic cycle in Africa (endemic), parts of Asia, Australia (Kunjan variant), and Southern Europe, with only occasional small outbreaks of mild febrile illness in people and rare human or equine neurologic disease.[‡] In the 1990s, several outbreaks with neurologic disease in people and horses occurred in Europe and the Middle East, and a 1998 outbreak in Israel was the first reported outbreak with avian mortality.[§] WNV was not

---

Table • 26-2

Spread of West Nile Virus Activity Across the United States

YEAR	STATES[a]	PEOPLE[b]		EQUINE CASES	CANINE CASES
		CASES	DEATHS		
1999	4[c]	63	7	25	—
2000	7	21	4	65	—
2001	27	66	9	733	—
2002	44	4156	284	14,539	7
2003	46[d]	9122	223	~4105[e]	27[e]

[a]Number of states with activity; the activity remained in affected states with new states added each year. Human disease usually occurred in a few less states than viral activity in birds, mosquitoes, and horses; activity in birds can be a harbinger of human disease.[49] In addition to the states listed, starting in 2000, Washington, D.C. has also had viral activity.
[b]Recognized humans cases in the first 3 years were essentially all neurologic disease. In 2003, many of the reported patients were febrile, not neurologic. Recognition of the milder disease likely explains the decreased fatality rate.
[c]New York, New Jersey, Maryland, and Connecticut.
[d]States spared are Oregon, Nevada, Alaska, and Hawaii.
[e]As of November 20, 2003.

recognized in the Western Hemisphere before its emergence in New York City in 1999.[74] In the following 3 years, viral activity and disease spread nationwide in the United States (Table 26-2).*

Before the United States outbreak, one dog and no cats had been reported ill with WNV. The affected dog died over 35 years ago in Botswana, Africa, after being diagnosed with a neurologic disease; the isolated virus was originally identified as Wesselbron; however, with subsequent sequence data, it was identified as WNV.[23,107] Serologic surveys for prevalence indicated dogs seroconvert without clinical disease in areas with WNV activity: 37% in Africa in 1988; 24% in India in early 1990s; 5% in New York City in 1999; and 2.4% in Missouri in 2002.[18,21,68,79]

The WNV outbreak in the United States has been the largest ever recorded arbovirus epidemic. It deviated from historic outbreaks by its marked avian mortality and increased diversity of affected host species. Mortality in covids (crows and blue jays) was especially high. Deaths associated with WNV have been reported (including nonrefereed reports) in over 150 avian species.[†] Birds were a direct source of virus spread, as virus is shed in saliva and cloacal excretions, and carnivores may ingest carcasses.[8,12,67] In the United States outbreak, in addition to widespread disease in birds, people, and horses, published reports document WNV disease in squirrels, two dogs, a wolf, two sheep, an alpaca, and several hundred farmed alligators.[‡] Other animals reported as infected in a surveillance survey included three cats, 27 dogs, a skunk, and a few bats, raccoons, and rabbits (ArboNET, CDC Reporting Service www.cdc.gov/mmwr/preview/mmwrthml/mm5322a9.htm).[5,26,52,70]

Mosquitoes are the major transmission vectors of WNV, although other ectoparasites such ticks can be viable vectors,[58]

---

and birds are the major vertebrate reservoir host. Although most of the natural transmission in the United States has been associated with two *Culex* subspecies, WNV has been isolated from at least 37 mosquito species. Most WNV disease is associated with the mosquito season, and disease usually peaks in late summer. However, the means by which the virus overwinters has not been established, and disease can occur in mid winter.[12]

In general, mammals are considered incidental or dead end hosts. The viremia is thought to be too low for transmission to mosquitoes; at most, rare inefficient transmission might occur.[8,18,22,66] In experimental infections in cats and dogs, cats developed higher virus serum titers (10^3 to 10^4 pfu/ml, 0.5 to 8 days postinoculation) than did dogs ($10^{1.6}$ to $10^{2.2}$ pfu/ml between 0.5 and 3.5 days postinoculation).[8] However, the titers in the cats were still low and transient compared with those found in birds; therefore even cats are unlikely to be efficient reservoirs for mosquito infection. The viral titer needed for transmission varies with mosquito species and is not precisely defined; however, transmission to mosquitoes can occur with titers in the range of at least 10^2 Vero cell pfu/ml of blood.

With the WNV outbreak in the United States, new natural routes of infection were suspected: ingestion (predation, milk consumption by nursing), blood transfusion, organ transplantation, and transplacental transfer.[28,31] Rare laboratory transmission to people occurred via local trauma while working with carcasses of infected birds and rodents.[27,103] Oral transmission was documented experimentally in cats and is the likely route of a large outbreak in farmed alligators fed tissues from infected horses.[8,85] Summer of 2002 was the first time that WNV disease was recognized in canids in the United States outbreak; details have been reported on three occasions (two adult dogs and a juvenile captive wolf). Thirty-one other dogs and three cats have been reported to surveillance databases as possible affected.

Pathogenesis

WNV causes high viremia in birds and low viremia in other vertebrate hosts. The virus infects parenchymal cells of multiple organs and causes cell necrosis. From studies in mice, both the B-cell and T-cell components of the immune system control WNV infection.[35,126] The generation of IgM is critical for host protection.[36] However, the T-cell limb may also be immunopathogenic in the CNS.[126]

Clinical Findings

Dogs

When experimentally infected by mosquito, dogs have remained clinically healthy.[8] They developed a viremia of low magnitude and short duration and showed no clinical manifestations of illness except for transient pyrexia in one dog. Virus was not detected in the saliva of any dogs during the course of their infections.

Natural infections do occur. Based on the four published canid cases (two adult dogs and a captive juvenile wolf), fever, central neurologic disease (especially ataxia), and possibly heart disease are expected.[21,76,98a] In addition, one dog had unspecified renal disease and marked granulomatous inflammation (possibly a preexisting disease).[21] Another dog had pulmonary edema and arrhythmias from heart disease. This patient also had immune-mediated thrombocytopenia and hemolytic anemia, also likely a preexisting condition. Common neurologic findings in the canids include lethargy, weakness, and ataxia; some also had conscious proprioceptive defects, head tilt, head bobbing, stupor, and blindness. Dogs can seroconvert with no clinical signs.* No reports have been

published of canids surviving natural WNV disease. All the reported dogs had encephalitis, myelitis, and myocarditis.[21,76] In canids, virus is found in multiple organs and is not restricted to inflamed organs.

Cats

Experimentally infected cats remained clinically healthy when they were infected via consumption of infected mice.[8] However, the cats that were experimentally inoculated by mosquito feeding develop mild transient fever, inappetence, and lethargy. As with dogs, virus was not detected in saliva of the cats; however, viremia was greater and more sustained than that of correspondingly infected dogs. The three cats reported to surveillance databases, and the experimentally infected dogs and cats lack histopathology data.[8,18]

People

The incubation period in human infections is 2 to 15 days (usually 2 to 6 days).[103] Of the people infected in the United States outbreak, the infection was asymptomatic in approximately 80% and a mild febrile illness in approximately 20% of infected people. In people who become ill, approximately 1 in 150 develop neurologic disease.[87] Most of the neurologically affected patients had meningoencephalitis, although a few developed severe myelitis and flaccid paralysis.[63] Mortality was up to 10%, and approximately 35% of recovered patients had residual neurologic deficits.[97] The disease is not age restricted; however, older people are more susceptible, likely caused by waning immune competence. Besides the fever and meningoencephalomyelitis in people, pancreatitis (one United States patient), rare myocarditis, and, in endemic Africa, hepatitis has been associated with WNV disease.

Other Animals

Similar to people, encephalomyelitis is the major disease in horses.[25,95,98,129] Mortality in neurologically affected horses is approximately 40%.[98,129] Many birds, especially covids, develop copious antigen in multiple organs and die without histopathologic changes, apparently resulting from rapidity of death. In birds, viral antigen is most abundant in the heart and kidney and is often also detectable in the spleen and brain. Other birds, especially raptors, tend to have an encephalitis and myocarditis at the time of death.[41,110] Similar to dogs, horses and squirrels have encephalitis and myelitis, and squirrels have myocarditis.*

Diagnosis

Detection of virus specific antibodies in serum confirms exposure to WNV. Options for serologic testing include serum neutralization (plaque reduction neutralization), IgG–enzyme-linked immunosorbent assay (IgG-ELISA), and capture assays for IgG or IgM.[21,22,67,95] Compared with antiviral IgG, IgM has minimal cross-reactivity with other arboviruses.[78] The duration of antibody titers is undocumented; IgM titers are thought to be short lived.[95] However, serum IgM titers persist in people up to 500 days and therefore may not be a specific marker for acute active infection.[103] Antiviral IgM in the cerebrospinal fluid (CSF) does indicate intrathecal production. A fourfold or greater rise in plaque reduction neutralization titer is evidence of an active infection.[95]

At necropsy, diagnosis is based on lesions (encephalitis, myelitis, and myocarditis) and documentation of virus in tissues: viral antigen by immunohistochemistry, viral genome by reverse transcriptase polymerase chain reaction (RT-PCR), or viable virions by virus isolation.†

---

*References 8, 18, 21, 68, 79.

*References 25, 53, 64, 95, 98, 129.
†References 8, 21, 22, 60, 75, 76.

For immunohistochemistry, both polyclonal rabbit antibody and polyclonal and monoclonal mouse antibody preparations have been used to label WNV antigen in fixed tissues. However, the labeling by different antibodies is not necessarily congruent.[21] In the three published canid cases, viral antigen has been documented (number positive/number tested) in brain (1/3), heart (3/3), kidney (2/3), and adrenal glands (2/2).[21,76] The two spleens that were tested did not show any presence of antigen.

Viral genome is detected by RT-PCR with amplicon detection by resolution in a gel or by 5' nuclease fluorogenic real time PCR.[21,76] The published cases of diseased canids are too few to validate the optimal tissue collection. Viral genome has been documented (number positive/number tested) in brain (2/2), kidney (2/2), liver (1/2), and the heart, lung, and spleen (each 1/1).[21,76] Although the published canid PCR studies used fresh or cryopreserved tissues, formalin-fixed tissue should also be adequate.[64]

WNV is usually isolated using Vero cells, a cell line that develops a cytopathic effect 3 to 5 days following inoculation.[8,22,108] Virus identification can be confirmed by serum neutralization or PCR assays. However, virus isolation is not readily available because a biosafety level-3 laboratory is required. In addition, virus isolation is not a sensitive method to document presence of virus in infected mammals, likely because of the low transient viral titer.[60,98,103]

Pathologic Findings

Three cases of natural disease in canids and two cases of experimental infections in dogs and one in cats have been published, although the experimental studies lack histopathologic data.[8,18,21,76] No specific changes are seen in serum chemistry or on complete blood counts, and generally no gross necropsy findings are produced, although the myocarditis may be grossly visible. Histologically, both encephalomyelitis and myocarditis are expected.

The encephalomyelitis is of variable intensity and characterized by gliosis, lymphocytic infiltrate, and neuronal necrosis (Fig. 26-6). The inflammation affects the gray matter more intensely than it does the white matter and includes glial nodules and mild vascular cuffing. To date, meningitis has not been recognized as a disease component in canids. The intensity of the myocarditis among canine patients varies from minimal to severe. In areas of myocarditis, myocytes are degenerative and necrotic, and lymphocytes predominate in the infiltrate with a few contributing neutrophils (Fig. 26-7). Two of the three published canid cases had scattered small foci of necrosis and lymphoid infiltrate in the adrenal gland cortex, these foci correspond to areas of immunolabeling for virus (Fig. 26-8, A and B). Viral antigen has been identified by immunohistochemistry in neurons (the wolf pup), myocytes (Fig. 26-9), renal tubular cells, and adrenal glands (see Fig. 26-8, B). One dog had unspecified clinical renal disease and a granulomatous nephritis with viral antigen. Although the kidney of this dog had a 1000-fold more viral genome than the heart, brain, or spleen,[21] the nephritis may have been a preexisting renal disease given the nature of the inflammation and the fact that canids and other host species have West Nile antigen in the kidney without lesions. However, in Africa, rare unspecified renal disease has been associated with human cases.[62] Dogs and cats experimentally infected with the NY99 West Nile isolate had no gross lesions, and the published studies did not include histopathologic data.[8]

Therapy

No specific therapy is available for affected dogs or cats; treatment is limited to supportive care for the patient and treatment of any underlying immunosuppressive disease. Some immunosuppressed human patients have improved following treatment with specific immune globulin transfusions.[106] Experimentally infected animals have been treated with pentoxifylline, gentamicin, or glucorticoids.[66] The efficacy of the antiviral drugs and glucocorticoid therapy used in humans or horses is unknown.[91]

Prevention

No vaccine is available for any species other than horses. Two experimental vaccines for people are in early first-phase clinical trials.[91] In dogs and cats, as in people, the main means of prevention is protection from mosquitoes.

Because transmission in people has occurred via blood transfusions,[31] blood donor dogs should be protected from

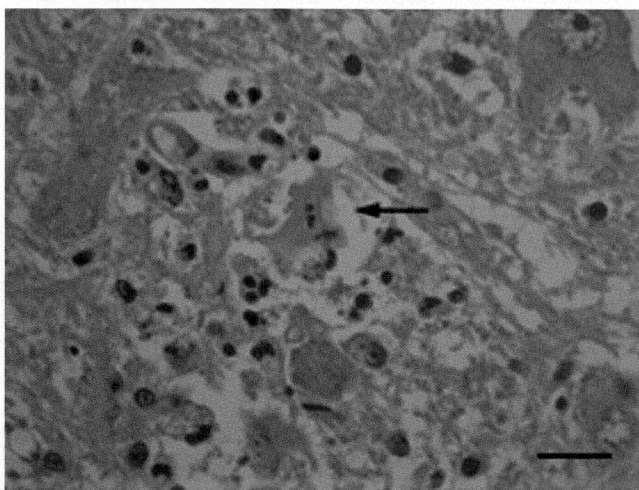

Fig 26-6 West Nile virus encephalitis in the brain stem of a dog. Glial cells and a few lymphocytes form the infiltrate. *Arrow*, necrotic neuron. Of the three reported canids, the wolf had more marked encephalitis and was the only brain to label with immunohistochemistry for viral antigen (H and E stain, bars, 20 microns). (Courtesy Veterinary Pathology, University of Illinois, Urbana, Ill.)

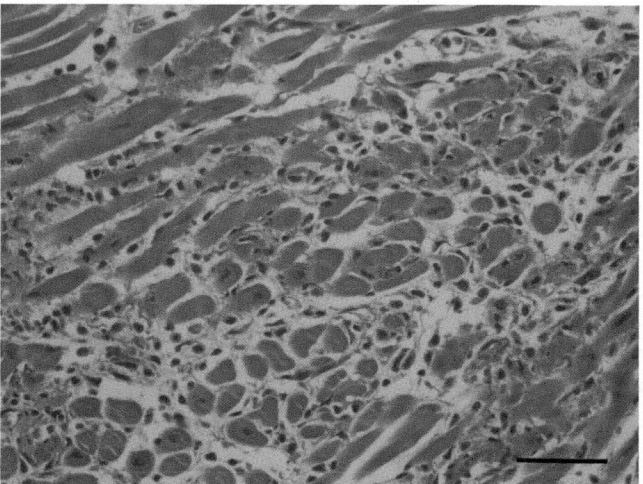

Fig 26-7 West Nile virus myocarditis in atrium of a dog. Marked myocarditis with an infiltrate of lymphocytes and a few neutrophils and necrosis of myocytes (H and E stain, bars, 50 microns). (Courtesy Veterinary Pathology, University of Illinois, Urbana, Ill.)

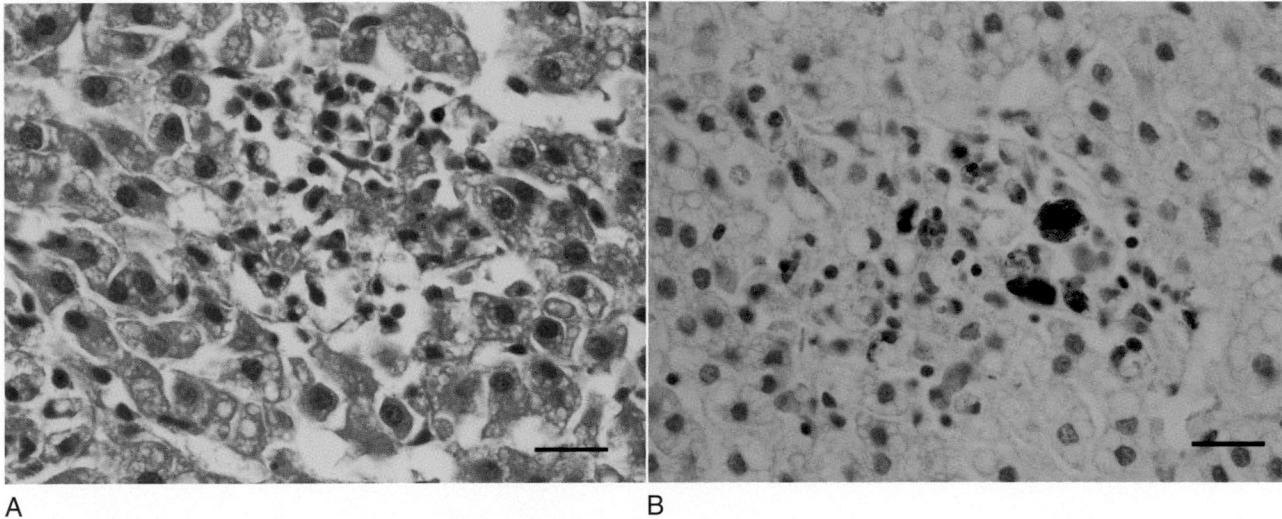

A   B

Fig 26-8 West Nile virus adrenalitis, adrenal cortex of a dog. **A,** Focus of necrosis with a lymphocytic infiltration (H and E stain). **B,** Viral antigen labeling is associated with the necrotic focus. West Nile virus immunohistochemistry (Bars, 50 microns). (Courtesy Veterinary Pathology, University of Illinois, Urbana, Ill.)

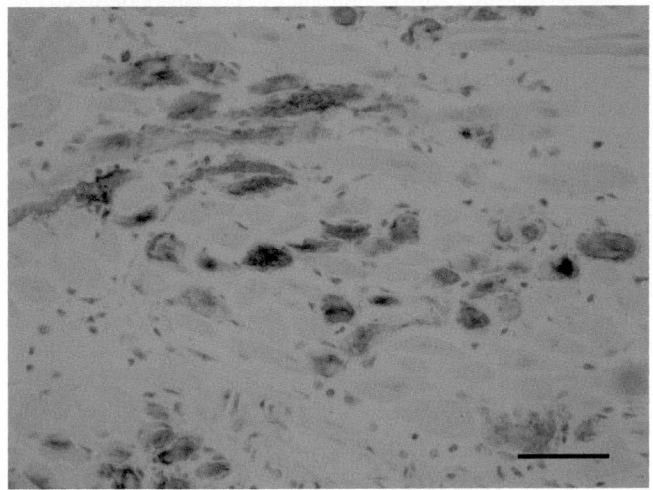

Fig 26-9 Copious viral antigen labeled in the myocytes of dog in Fig. 26-7. West Nile virus immunohistochemistry (Bars, 50 microns). (Courtesy Veterinary Pathology, University of Illinois, Urbana, Ill.)

mosquito exposure. Although its role in the natural epidemiology is undefined, oral transmission can occur; hence preventing predation or carcass consumption, especially of squirrels, horses, and birds may be warranted.[8]

TICK-BORNE INFECTIONS

CENTRAL EUROPEAN TICK-BORNE ENCEPHALITIS
Andrea Tipold and Marc Vandevelde

Etiology
Central European tick-borne encephalitis is caused by a flavivirus and transmitted by ticks *(Ixodes ricinus)*.[46] The disease has been described in people, dogs, horses, monkeys, and wild ruminants, but not in cats. The disease has been observed in

dogs, in central Europe (Switzerland, Austria, Germany, the Czech Republic), and in Sweden, Norway, Italy, and Greece; it tends to be endemic in focal areas.[34a,114] The central disease is in the overlap region between the eastern and western forms of the disease, which follows the distribution of the respective vectors, *I. ricinus* and *I. persulcatus* (Fig. 26-10, *A* and *B*).

Clinical Findings
In the dog, three different courses of the disease are observed.[65,102,115] Dogs may be asymptomatic[40,65] or develop severe encephalitis[46,115] from which they either recover or die. Severe cases exhibit fever (over 39° C [102.5° F]) and multifocal neurologic signs consisting of myoclonus, convulsions, hemiparesis to tetraparesis, stupor, hyperesthesia, and multiple deficits of the cranial nerves. Spinal reflexes may be reduced (polioencephalomyelitis).[115] Rottweilers are overrepresented in the literature (8 Rottweilers from 22 described cases).[114] The signs are usually progressive and dogs die within 4 to 7 days or are euthanized. Some dogs may recover showing a rising antibody titer.[65]

Diagnosis
As in other viral infections of the CNS, mononuclear pleocytosis is found in CSF.[115] Antibodies against the virus can be measured in serum and CSF.[40,65] However, because of a high seroprevalence in endemic areas, clinically healthy dogs, as well as dogs with other CNS diseases, may also exhibit significant antibody titers.[34a,40] Therefore a firm clinical diagnosis remains difficult. Only rising antibody titers can confirm the diagnosis. In view of the rapid progression of the disease in many cases, only postmortem histopathology will allow a definitive diagnosis.

Pathologic Findings
A nonsuppurative meningoencephalomyelitis with predominant lesions in the gray matter of the brain stem and cerebellum is found.[82,115,129,130] Immunohistochemical staining revealed central European tick-borne encephalitis virus in Purkinje cells, neurons of brain stem nuclei, neuronal cell processes, and cytoplasm of macrophages.[130] Rapid clearance of the virus apparently occurs given that viral antigen is not easily found in advanced cases.

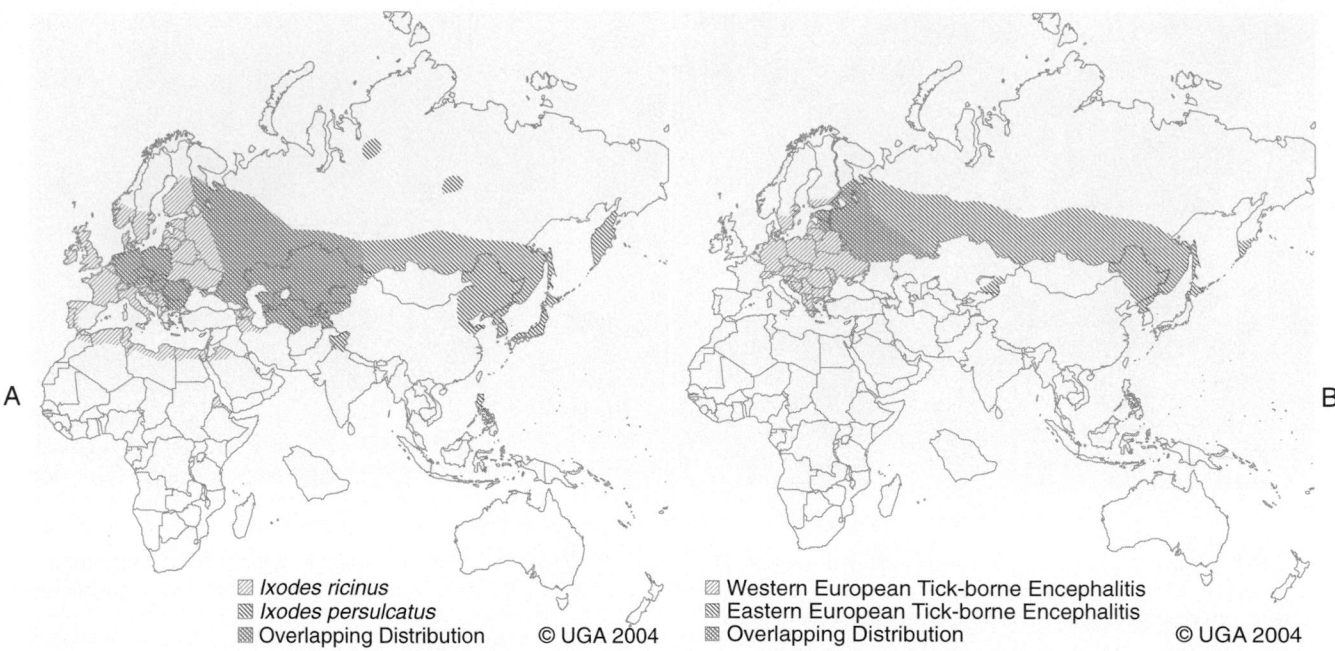

Fig   26-10 **A,** Map of distribution of *Ixodes ricinus* and *Ixodes persulcatus* ticks in the Western Hemisphere. **B,** Map of distribution of Western and Eastern tick-borne encephalitis virus infection in people showing corresponding distribution and overlap. (Courtesy University of Georgia, Athens, Ga.)

Therapy and Prevention

Treatment can only be supportive; glucocorticoids may worsen the disease process. Neither specific vaccines nor vaccination schedules exist for the dog; although human vaccines have been used in dogs in endemic areas. Antibody production may be shown in such dogs; however, until recently, no proof has been found for the efficacy of such vaccines in animals. In some endemic areas, the measurement of serum antibody titers against the central European tick-borne encephalitis virus is used to examine the spread of infected ticks.[65]

LOUPING-ILL
Hugh W. Reid

Etiology
Louping-ill is an acute viral encephalomyelitis transmitted by the sheep tick *Ixodes ricinus*. Although louping-ill occurs most frequently in sheep, it has been reported in people, horses, pigs, cattle, goats, farm-raised deer, and dogs but not in cats.[54,77]

The causal virus is a member of an antigenically closely related complex of arthropod transmitted viruses (family *Flaviviridae*) known as the tick-borne encephalitides (TBE) as described in the previous section. These viruses, present throughout the northern temperate latitudes, are primarily associated with disease in people. Infection in domestic animals has been recognized on a regular basis only in the British Isles in areas of rough pastures where sheep ticks are prevalent. However, encephalomyelitis in sheep resulting from infection by either louping-ill virus or closely related viruses has occurred also in Bulgaria, Turkey, Spain, and Norway, suggesting that the disease may be more widespread.[99]

In addition, meningoencephalitis caused by TBE viruses affecting dogs has been reported from Austria, Germany, and Switzerland,[101,132] suggesting that disease in dogs caused by this complex of viruses has a wide distribution in Europe.

Risk of infection is generally restricted to the periods of tick activity, mainly in the spring and early summer, with a recrudescence in some areas in the fall. However, the precise periods of tick activity vary with latitude and altitude. In dogs, infection has been diagnosed most frequently in working sheepdogs and gun dogs, but any animal visiting enzootic areas during periods of tick activity may become infected.

Infection is assumed to be via the bite of the tick. Alternative routes of transmission should not be overlooked because disease in people is encountered in abattoir workers. Young goats and pigs can become infected by the ingestion of virus-infected milk and carcasses, respectively.

Clinical Findings
The initial systemic phase after infection generally is not associated with clinical signs, but during this period, the animal is viremic. The virus invades the CNS, and the subsequent course of disease is variable. Many infections are not recognized clinically because virus is eliminated by the immune response that subsequently maintains protection and detectable serum antibody titers, probably for the life of the animals. In animals that do develop clinical disease, initial signs, which are primarily caused by cerebellar dysfunction, include mild paresis, ataxia, and tremors that are sometimes associated with difficulty in eating. Within 24 hours, severe incoordination develops. The affected animal is usually in lateral recumbency, paddling its limbs, but this may progress to complete tetraplegia or opisthotonos.

Death may occur at any time, but in dogs that survive, recovery is slow, and locomotor dysfunction may persist for months. On recovery, temperamental and physical changes may be present, the animal being nervous, exercise intolerant, and less tractable.

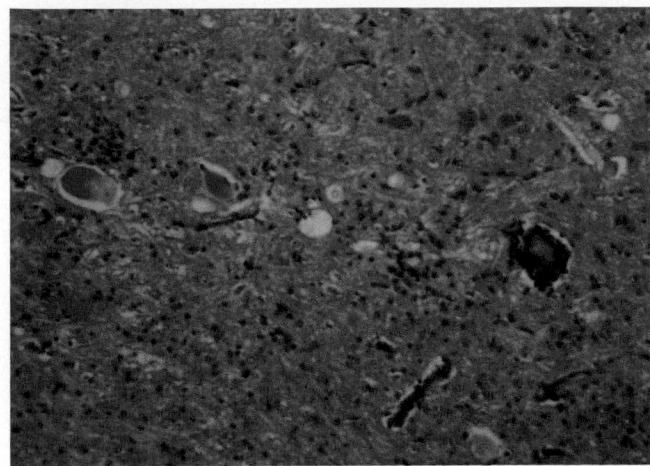

Fig 26-11 Brain stem from an animal clinically affected with louping-ill, showing neurononecrosis, gliosis, and lymphocytic perivascular cuffing (H and E stain, ×1000). (Courtesy D. Buxton, Moredun Research Institute, Edinburgh, Scotland.)

Diagnosis

Diagnosis relies on the detection of a rising serum antibody response to louping-ill virus during the course of the infection. In fatal cases, histologic examination of the brain accompanied by virus isolation can confirm the disease. Histologic changes include neuronal necrosis and perivascular lymphoid cell accumulations that are particularly prominent in the spinal cord and cerebellum (Fig. 26-11). Immunohistochemical staining for virus in tissue specimens has been used but may give false negative results in the more protracted cases.[72] Virus may be isolated from a homogenate of brain tissue by intracerebral inoculation of 3-week-old mice or in tissue culture cells.

Therapy and Prevention

Supportive therapy during the acute phase is beneficial, but no specific therapy is available. An inactivated, tissue culture–propagated vaccine incorporated in an oil adjuvant is available for protection of cattle, sheep, and goats and has been used in dogs. However, dogs appear to require at least two injections to elicit a detectable serum antibody response, and a proportion of them develop painless, fluid-filled swellings at the site of injection that may require surgical drainage.[113]

The ecology of louping-ill virus depends largely on a sheep-tick cycle, with little involvement of the native fauna. Systematic vaccination of sheep may reduce the prevalence of virus and may therefore reduce the risk of infecting other incidental hosts such as dogs. In continental Europe the virus is mainly maintained in a cycle involving ticks and woodland rodents and control is largely limited to vaccination of people.

SUGGESTED READINGS*

7. Asnis DS, Conetta R, Waldman G, et al. 2001. The West Nile virus encephalitis outbreak in the United States (1999-2000), *Ann NY Acad Sci* 951:161-171.
8. Austgen LE, Bowen RA, Bunning ML, et al. 2004. Experimental infection of cats and dogs with West Nile virus, *Emerg Infect Dis* 10:82-86.
21. Buckweitz S, Kleiboeker S, Marioni K, et al. 2003. Serological reverse transcriptase-polymerase chain reaction, and immunohistochemical detection of West Nile virus in a clinically affected dog, *J Vet Diagn Invest* 15:324-329.
37. Dumpis U, Crook D, Oksi J. 1999. Tick-borne encephalitis, *Clin Infect Dis* 28:882-890.
55. House C, Alexander KA, Kat PW, et al. 1996. Serum antibody to Rift Valley fever virus in African carnivores, *Ann N Y Acad Sci* 791:345-349.
57. Howerth EW, Dorminy M, Dreesen DW, et al. 1995. Low prevalence of antibodies to bluetongue and epizootic hemorrhagic disease viruses in dog from southern Georgia, *J Vet Diagn Invest* 7:393-394.
76. Lichtensteiger CA, Heinz-Taheny K, Osborne TS, et al. 2003. West Nile virus encephalitis and myocarditis in a dog, *Emerg Infect Dis* 9:1303-1306.
98a. Read RW, Rodriquez DB, Summers BA. 2005. West Nile virus encephalitis in a dog, *Vet Pathol* 42:219-222.
102. Reiner B, Fischer A, Goedde T, et al. 1999. Clinical diagnosis of canine tick-borne encephalitis (TBE): contribution of cerebrospinal fluid (CSF) analysis and CSF antibody titers, *Zentrabl Bakteriol* 289:605-609.
113. Thomson JR, Reid HW, Pow I. 1987. Louping-ill vaccination of dogs, *Vet Rec* 120-94.
114. Tipold A. 2002. Central European tick-borne encephalitis—a review, *Tieraerztl Praxis* 30:106-110.

*See the CD-ROM for a complete list of references.

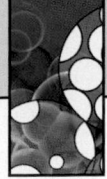

CHAPTER • 27

Salmon Poisoning Disease

John R. Gorham and William J. Foreyt

ETIOLOGY

Salmon poisoning disease (SPD), or salmon disease, is a highly fatal, helminth-transmitted rickettsial disease of domestic and wild Canidae that occurs on the western slopes of the Cascade Mountains from northern California to central Washington (Fig. 27-1). Occasionally, cases of SPD occur outside the indigenous range of the disease in areas where infected fish migrate or are transported. The presence of cases in British Columbia may indicate that the indigenous range of the disease is greater than previously reported.[1] A similar disease has been reported in Brazil.[18a]

Salmon Disease Agent

The etiologic agent of SPD is *Neorickettsia helminthoeca*, a coccoid or coccobacillary rickettsia that is approximately 0.3 μm.[4,22] Pleomorphic rods up to 2 μm long, sometimes bent in rings or crescents, have been observed. The gram-negative rickettsial organisms appear purple with Giemsa stain, red with Macchiavello's stain, black or dark brown with Levaditi's method, and pale blue with hematoxylin and eosin stain. The rickettsiae almost fill the cytoplasm of cells of the mononuclear phagocyte system (MPS) that they primarily infect (Fig. 27-2). The rickettsiae have been grown in canine monocytes,[12] canine leukocytes and sarcoma cells, mouse lymphoblasts, and a macrophage cell line.[21,24] Antigenically and genetically, *N. helminthoeca* is closely related to *Ehrlichia* spp. Based on 16SrRNA gene sequences, *N. helminthoeca* is most closely related to *Neorickettsia (Ehrlichia) risticii*, the agent of Potomac horse fever, and *Neorickettsia (Ehrlichia) sennetsu*, the agent of human sennetsu fever in Japan (see Table 28-1).[5]

In dead fish, rickettsiae in metacercariae (encysted trematode larvae) of *Nanophyetus salmincola* do not survive 30 days at 4° C.[11] In lymph nodes, organisms resist freezing at −20° C for 31 to 158 days;[23] they remain viable in leukocytes at 4.5° C and 52.5° C for 48 hours and 2 minutes, respectively, but not at 60° C for 5 minutes.[27] At −80° C the agent can be maintained in cell culture fluid for up to 3 months.[3]

Elokomin Fluke Fever Agent

It is highly likely that the Elokomin fluke fever (EFF) agent[6] is another strain of *N. helminthoeca*.[12,13] The disease in dogs associated with the EFF agent results in high morbidity but a lower mortality than SPD. It appears that metacercariae can harbor EFF and SPD agents simultaneously. EFF is rarely recognized as a distinct entity in naturally occurring disease. Histologically, EFF infections in dogs are similar to but less severe than those seen with SPD. In a survey of 331 practitioners in endemic areas, 35% reported that they had diagnosed SPD in dogs that had been treated previously for SPD.[14] Although it has been generally accepted that dogs surviving SPD infection had a solid immunity, the data now suggest that other strains such as EFF may be pathogenic under field conditions,[1] or the initial SPD infection failed to evoke a durable immunity.[2]

EPIDEMIOLOGY

The vector of SPD is a trematode, *N. salmincola*, which harbors the rickettsiae throughout its life cycle stages from egg to adult.[19] Three different hosts are required for the completion of the trematode life cycle—snails, fish, and mammals or birds (Fig. 27-3). Lists of intermediate and definitive hosts of the fluke can be found elsewhere.[19] The snail intermediate host, *Oxytrema silicula*, is a pleurocerid that inhabits fresh or brackish stream water in coastal areas of Washington, Oregon, and northern California. Areas of trematode infection therefore depend on the distribution of *O. silicula*. Cercariae (free-swimming trematode larvae) leave the snail and penetrate the second intermediate host, which is usually a salmonid fish, certain species of nonsalmonid fish, or the Pacific giant salamander *(Dicamptodon ensatus)*. The metacercariae usually localize in the kidneys of fish (Fig. 27-4) but can be found in any tissue, as well as slime on the skin of the fish. Fish are infected in freshwater and retain the trematode and the rickettsial infection throughout their ocean migration before returning to fresh water up to 3 years later.[28]

Adult trematodes develop in the intestine approximately 6 days after the ingestion of metacercariae-infected fish by dogs and certain other fish-eating mammals that serve as definitive hosts, such as bears and raccoons, and certain birds. Clinical signs of rickettsial disease occur in Canidae, primarily dogs, foxes, and coyotes. However, two captive polar bears receiving long-term glucocorticoid therapy for skin conditions succumbed to an SPD-like disease after eating inadequately frozen salmon.[26] Cats are not susceptible to SPD, but trematodes develop when infected fish are ingested.[19]

SPD also has been transmitted by parenteral injection of infected blood, spleen and lymph suspensions, adult flukes, helminth-infected snail livers, and helminth eggs. Partial transmission success was obtained by allowing ticks (*Haemaphysalis leachi* and *Rhipicephalus sanguineus*) that had fed on infected dogs to subsequently feed on susceptible dogs and by parenteral injection of suspensions of *R. sanguineus* into dogs.[22] Susceptible dogs also have been experimentally infected with cell-cultured *Neorickettsia* organisms[24] and aerosolized lymph node suspensions from infected dogs; on rare occasions, direct transmission of infection between dogs has been suspected.[2]

PATHOGENESIS

After ingestion of raw, metacercariae-infected salmonid fish by a susceptible dog, the fluke matures, and the adult stage attaches to the mucosa of the intestine and by some unknown mechanism inoculates the rickettsiae (Fig. 27-5). Initial replication of rickettsiae probably takes place in the epithelial cells of the villi or the intestinal lymphoid tissue. Inflammation of the solitary lymphoid follicles and Peyer's patches along the intestinal tract contributes to enteritis. Mild enteritis may be

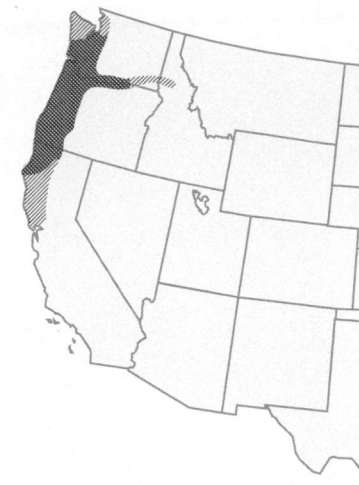

☒ Occasional cases of salmon poisoning

☒ Oxytrema silicula distribution and usual distribution of salmon poisoning

© UGA 2004

Fig 27-1 Distribution of indigenous salmon poisoning disease. Area with *slashed lines* represents the distribution of O. *silicula* and the usual distribution of salmon poisoning disease. Area with *dots* represents occasional cases of salmon poisoning disease usually resulting from infected migrating fish. (Courtesy University of Georgia, Athens, Ga.)

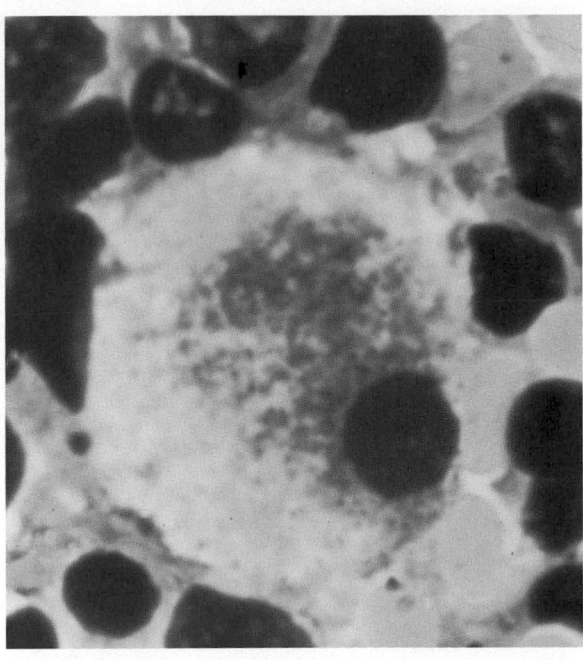

Fig 27-2 *N. helminthoeca* in a lymph node smear (Giemsa stain, ×400).

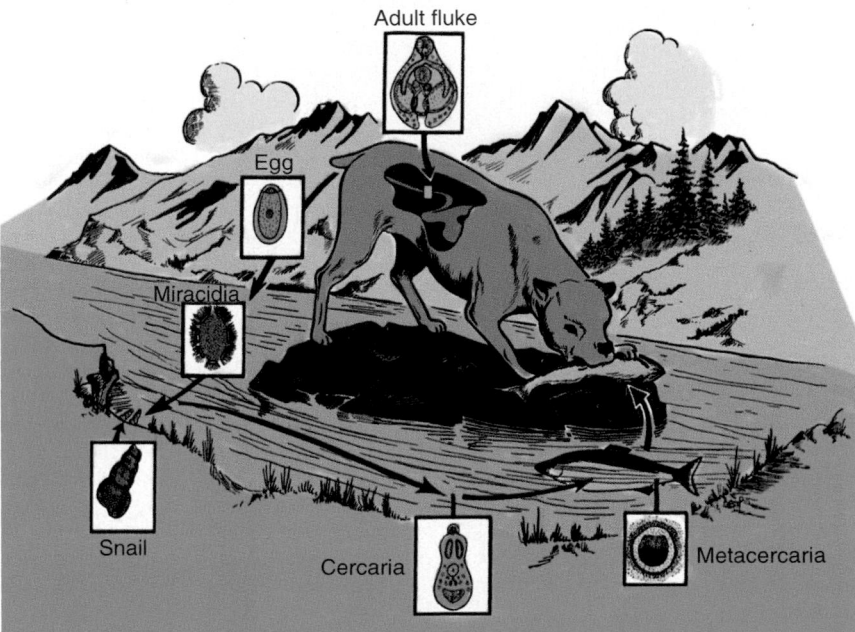

Fig 27-3 Life cycle of *N. salmincola*.

Fig 27-4 Squash preparation of salmon kidney containing numerous metacercariae of *N. salmincola* (×200).

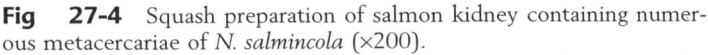
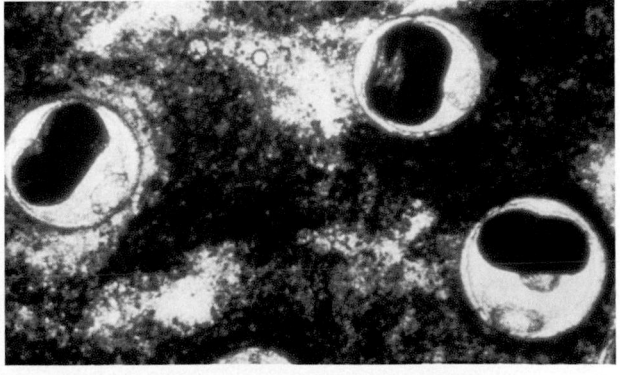

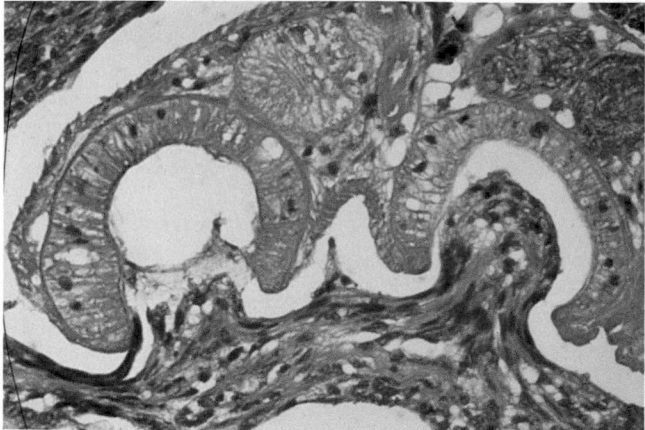

Fig 27-5 *N. salmincola* ingesting intestinal mucosa and initiating *N. helminthoeca* infection in a dog (H and E stain, ×300).

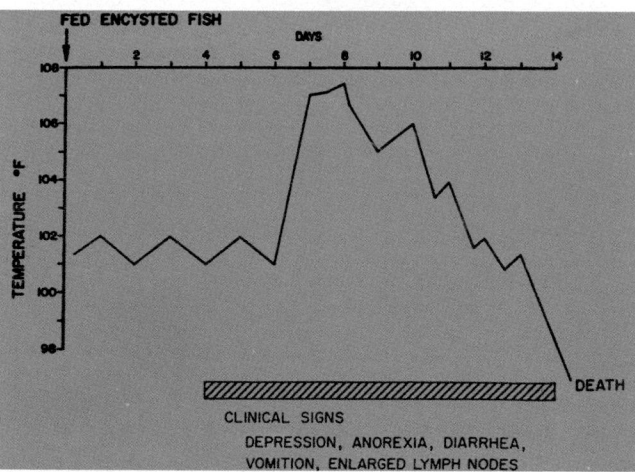

Fig 27-6 Clinical course of salmon poisoning disease in a dog. (University of Georgia, Athens, Ga.)

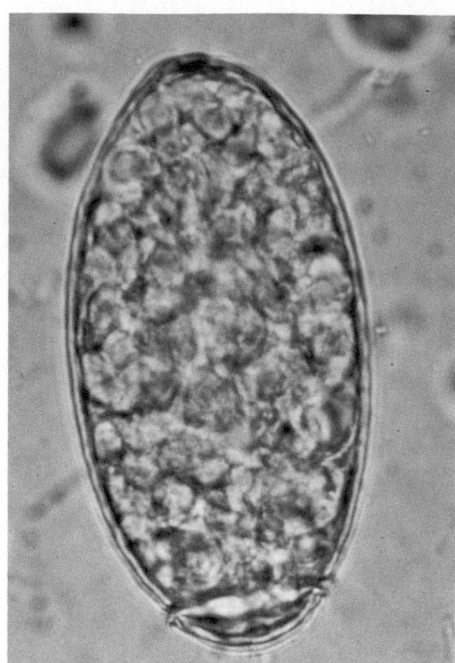

Fig 27-7 Egg of *N. salmincola* (×480).

observed in dogs infected only with the flukes but without rickettsiae.

Rickettsiae enter the blood early in the course of the disease and spread to the lymph nodes, spleen, tonsils, thymus, liver, lungs, and brain.[13] Although secondary bacterial infections often occur, the exact cause of death in SPD is unknown. Investigations to demonstrate a toxin have been limited.

CLINICAL FINDINGS

Salmon Poisoning Disease

The signs of SPD are consistent in all Canidae. The usual incubation period after the ingestion of parasitized fish is 5 to 7 days, although some dogs have incubation periods as long as 19 to 33 days. The first sign usually is a sudden febrile response, which typically reaches a peak of 40° C to 42° C (104° F to 107.6° F; Fig. 27-6). The temperature gradually decreases to normal or below normal over the next 4 to 8 days. Dogs are frequently hypothermic when death occurs 7 to 10 days after the initial clinical evidence of infection. Some animals show only a slight increase in temperature or a short-

ened febrile period; however, they may still die if left untreated.

Anorexia frequently accompanies or follows the onset of fever and may be marked and complete. Affected animals often continue to have inappetence throughout the course of the disease. Marked weight loss, weakness, and depression usually follow. Within 14 days of eating infected fish, coyotes on a controlled experiment lost approximately 58% of their body weight when compared with uninfected coyotes.[11] Diarrhea and vomiting may occur, with the diarrhea becoming progressively worse and often consisting primarily of blood at the time of death. The animal occasionally exhibits extreme thirst and drinks copious quantities of water. A serous nasal discharge may develop early in the febrile period. Later, a mucopurulent conjunctival exudate may be seen. Enlarged cervical and prescapular lymph nodes can be palpated as early as 5 days after infection.

SPD-infected dogs may show severe gastrointestinal signs, which are often clinically indistinguishable from canine parvoviral enteritis (see Chapter 8). Distemper and SPD can also occur concurrently, and appropriate laboratory tests can be conducted to determine which agent is involved in a particular animal (see Appendix 5, Laboratory Testing for Infectious Diseases of Dogs and Cats).

Elokomin Fluke Fever

The incubation period for EFF is generally 5 to 12 days. The febrile period, which differs from that of SPD, is marked by an elevated temperature plateau lasting 4 to 7 days, followed by a decline, usually to a subnormal temperature.[6] Other signs are similar to those of SPD.

DIAGNOSIS

Operculated trematode eggs appear in dog feces 5 to 8 days after the ingestion of infected fish. The light brown eggs are approximately 87 to 97 μm long and 35 to 55 μm wide, with a small, blunt point on the end opposite the indistinct operculum (Fig. 27-7). Eggs can be detected on direct smears or by a washing-sedimentation technique.[7] In addition, the authors of this chapter have routinely recovered *N. salmincola* eggs with the standard sugar flotation technique (specific gravity, 1.27). Eggs recovered by this method are somewhat deformed but easily recognizable.[9] Diagnosis of the rickettsial disease cannot be made entirely on the presence of trematode eggs in feces, because trematode infection does not necessarily indicate rickettsial infection. In addition, animals that have recovered from the rickettsial disease may continue to shed eggs in feces or can be reinfected with the trematode. The trematode infection can remain patent for 60 to 250 days.[11]

Fluid aspirated from enlarged lymph nodes can be air dried on a microscope slide, fixed, defatted for 1 minute with a mixture of equal parts of ether and absolute alcohol, and then stained by Giemsa or Macchiavello's stain. In addition, a rapid-staining Giemsa technique can be used that involves staining the fixed smears for 2 minutes with equal parts of stock Giemsa and buffered water at pH 7.2 and then flushing the slides with tap water.[7] Typical intracytoplasmic rickettsial bodies are characteristically seen in MPS cells (see Fig. 27-2). Extracellular organisms are not easily separated from artifacts and should not be considered diagnostic for SPD.

Table • 27-1

Results of Initial Laboratory Tests in Dogs with Salmon Poisoning[a,20]

	NORMAL RANGE	MAXIMUM	MINIMUM	MEAN	SD	NUMBER OF DOGS ABOVE NR	NUMBER OF DOGS BELOW NR	NUMBER OF DOGS TESTED
Leukocytes (/μl)	6000–17,000	66,000	4200	12,800	10,600	6	6	44
Mature neutrophils	3000–11,500	62,604	1792	10,908	10,296	13	1	44
Band neutrophils	0–300	2548	0	168	430	8	0	44
Lymphocytes	1000–4800	3776	92	791	667	0	34	44
Eosinophils	100–1250	891	0	77	202	0	34	44
Monocytes	150–1350	4137	0	824	811	10	0	44
Packed cell volume (%)	37–55	54	25	43	7	1	8	43
Platelet counts (×10³/dl)	200–500	377	16	113	108	0	14	16
Fibrinogen (mg/dl)	200–400	700	100	400	160	14	3	38
Serum sodium (meq/L)	145–154	159	126	141	8	1	13	16
Serum potassium (meq/L)	4.1–5.3	5.3	3.4	4.4	0.5	0	3	16
Serum chloride (meq/L)	105–116	134	84	106	12	1	4	14
Total CO_2	16–26	24	15	18	3	0	4	10
Serum calcium (mg/dl)	9.9–11.4	10.8	7.3	9.1	0.9	0	30	37
Serum phosphorus (mg/dl)	3.0–6.2	7.9	3.0	4.8	1.5	7	0	36
Creatinine (mg/dl)	0.8–1.6	1.7	0.5	1.1	0.5	2	2	17
Blood urea nitrogen (mg/dl)	8–31	90	9	22	19	6	0	37
Serum glucose (mg/dl)	70–118	133	44	92	17	4	2	37
ALT (IU/L)	19–102	499	21	92	83	9	0	37
AST (IU/L)	15–66	274	24	90	60	17	0	35
Alkaline phosphatase (IU/L)	15–150	2098	60	254	339	23	0	36
Total protein (g/dl)	5.4–7.4	8.2	3.9	5.9	1.1	4	11	37
Albumin (g/dl)	2.5–3.5	3.3	1.6	2.5	0.4	0	18	37
Total bilirubin (mg/dl)	0–0.4	2.0	0	0.4	0.6	4	0	37
Globulins (mg/dl)	2.9–3.9	5.8	1.9	3.4	0.9	9	10	37
Cholesterol (mg/dl)	135–300	408	99	215	85	8	6	37
Age (years)		12	0.3	5	3.7	NA	NA	45

SD, standard deviation; *NR,* normal range; *ALT,* alanine transaminase; *AST,* aspartate transaminase; *NA,* not available.
[a]*n,* 45.

Table • **27-2**

Drug Therapy for Salmon Poisoning Disease

DRUG[a]	DOSE[b] (mg/kg)	ROUTE	INTERVAL (HOURS)	DURATION (DAYS)
Oxytetracycline[c]	7	IV[d]	8	3—5
Doxycycline[c]	10	IV[d]	12	7
Tetracycline[c]	22	PO	8	3—5
Praziquantel[e]	10—30	PO, SC	Once	3—5

IV, Intravenous; *PO*, by mouth; *SC*, subcutaneous.
[a]See Appendix 8, Drug Formulary, for additional information.
[b]Dose per administration at specified interval.
[c]For rickettsial infection.
[d]Parenteral therapy preferred because of gastrointestinal signs.
[e]For fluke infection.

Hematologic and biochemical findings of SPD-infected domestic dogs are often nonspecific, and total leukocyte counts have ranged from leukopenia to leukocytosis.[25] Laboratory results of 45 dogs representing 17 breeds and various mixed breeds that were naturally infected with SPD are listed in Table 27-1.[20] Thrombocytopenia in 88% of the dogs tested, lymphopenia (77%) eosinophilia (77%), increased alkaline phosphatase (ALP) values (64%), and reduced serum albumin values (49%) were the consistent findings.[20] In experimentally infected coyotes, significantly higher numbers of band cells, lower numbers of eosinophils, and lower concentrations of creatinine, glucose, calcium, inorganic phosphorus, albumin, and ALP were detected when compared with uninfected coyotes.[11]

PATHOLOGIC FINDINGS

The principal gross findings at necropsy are changes in lymphoid tissues. The tonsils, thymus, and visceral and somatic nodes are markedly enlarged. The most pronounced swelling occurs in the ileocecal, colic, mesenteric, portal, and lumbar nodes. The nodes are usually yellowish, with prominent white foci representing the cortical follicles. Occasionally, nodes show diffuse petechiae, and edema is often observed.

The spleen frequently ranges from slightly swollen to nearly twice the normal size. Splenic follicles, which often appear as grayish-white nodules in foxes, are unaffected in dogs. The spleens of animals that die of SPD are typically a dark bluish red, smooth, soft, and blood filled. Livers of dogs are usually normal, although those of foxes are usually soft and a pale yellowish brown. Hemorrhages may appear in the gallbladder wall. Petechiae may be the only change in the pancreas. The kidneys of dogs are grossly normal, whereas those of foxes may have a slight color change and become a pale yellowish brown. The mucosa of the urinary bladder may show petechiae.

Along the intestinal tract, petechiae may be apparent in the mucosae of the lower esophagus, large intestine, ileocolic valve, distal colon, rectum, and gastric serosa. Bleeding ulcers may be found in the pylorus. Intussusception of the ileum in the colon may also occur. The intestinal contents frequently contain free blood. Some blood may also appear in the colon and rectum. The intestines are typically empty except for some bile-stained mucus. Flukes in the intestinal tissue, primarily found in the duodenum, cause some tissue damage but are usually not pathogenic.

Microscopically, a characteristic pattern is observed in lymphocytic tissues. The lymph nodes show a marked and consistent depletion in the number of mature lymphocytes, with hyperplasia of the MPS cells in the cortex and medulla. Most foxes and dogs have foci of necrosis in the MPS cells. The central nervous system is usually involved with nonsuppurative meningitis or meningoencephalitis.[18]

THERAPY

All patients should be hospitalized so that they receive adequate monitoring and nursing care. Control of the infectious agent, *N. helminthoeca*, can be achieved with oral or parenteral sulfonamides, penicillin, chlortetracycline, chloramphenicol, doxycycline, or oxytetracycline. Aminoglycosides are ineffective. The preferred treatment schedule is oxytetracycline given for at least 3 days (Table 27-2). Oral tetracycline therapy, used for most rickettsial disease, may be difficult and may not be indicated because of the severe vomiting and diarrhea that is usually present.

Relief of dehydration, emesis, and diarrhea is also important. Fluid therapy with appropriate electrolytes should be administered intravenously. In cases of hemorrhagic diarrhea, transfusion of whole blood may be necessary. Other antidiarrheal treatments include fasting followed by gradual introduction of a bland, high-calorie diet. In addition, the most supportive treatment consists of keeping the dog dry, clean, and warm.

Praziquantel, when given as one dose at appropriate dosages (see Table 27-2), is highly effective against *N. salmincola* in coyotes and dogs.[10] Elimination of *N. salmincola* from infected animals minimizes the diarrhea associated with fluke infections alone and minimizes or eliminates fluke eggs from feces.

PREVENTION

Vaccines have not been developed against SPD, therefore keeping dogs from feeding on infected fish is the best means of preventing infection. Because metacercariae can remain viable for months in rotting fish carcasses, dogs become infected with the fluke if they eat decomposed fish; however, they may not develop SPD. In addition, in many areas, metacercariae apparently contain nonpathogenic rickettsiae.[17] Freezing fish at −20° C for 24 hours or thoroughly cooking infected fish kills the metacercariae and rickettsiae.[8] Supplemental prevention methods include isolation of dogs with SPD and sterilization of equipment used around infected dogs.

Infection of fish in hatcheries can be prevented by using water that is not inhabited by snails. However, this is not possible in most hatcheries other than those that use drilled well water rather than stream water. Other control techniques such as snail elimination are impractical.

SUGGESTED READINGS*

1. Booth AJ, Stogdale L, Grigor JA. 1984. Salmon poisoning disease in dogs on southern Vancouver Island, *Can Vet J* 25:2-6.

18a. Headley SA, Vidotto D, Scorpio D, et al. 2004. Suspected cases of *Neorickettsia*-like organisms in Brazilian dogs, *Ann NY Acad Sci* 1026:79-83.

20. Mack RE, Becovitch MG, Ling GV, et al. 1990. Salmon disease complex in dogs—A review of 45 cases, *Calif Vet* 44:42-45.

*See the CD-ROM for a complete list of references.

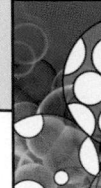

CHAPTER • 28

Ehrlichiosis, Neorickettsiosis, Anaplasmosis, and *Wolbachia* Infection

Bacteria within the families *Rickettsiaceae* and *Anaplasmataceae* of the order *Rickettsiales* underwent reclassification in 2001. Reclassification was indicated after the molecular analyses of bacterial 16S rRNA and groESL gene sequences were elucidated.[146] The genera *Ehrlichia* and *Wolbachia* were moved from the family *Rickettsiaceae* and are now in the family *Anaplasmataceae*. The genera *Rickettsia* and *Orientia* remain in the family *Rickettsiaceae*. In addition, species within the genus *Ehrlichia* were reorganized: *E. phagocytophila*, *E. equi*, and *E. platys* now reside in the genus *Anaplasma*, and *E. risticii* and *E. sennetsu* are now in the genus *Neorickettsia*. The diseases caused by all of these organisms, despite their new genetic groupings, are intracellular parasitisms of mammalian leukocytes and are characterized as being monocytotropic (organisms predominantly residing in monocytes and macrophages), granulocytotropic (organisms predominantly in neutrophils and eosinophils), or thrombocytotropic (Table 28-1).

The genus *Ehrlichia* consists of tick-transmitted gram-negative obligate intracellular bacteria that infect primarily leukocytes (monocytes, macrophages, granulocytes). These acid-sensitive, pleomorphic coccobacilli of approximately 0.5 μm diameter are aerobes that lack a glycolytic pathway.[406] *E. canis*, *E. chaffeensis*, *E. ewingii*, and *E. muris* remain members of the genus *Ehrlichia*. *E. (Cowdria) ruminantium*, the cause of heartwater of cattle in Africa, has been added to this genus.

N. sennetsu and *N. risticii* were reclassified because of their close relationship with *N. helminthoeca*, the cause of salmon poisoning disease (see Chapter 27). These agents are transmitted by invertebrate intermediate hosts, rather than tick vectors. *N. risticii* has been determined to be acquired by ingestion of infected snails. The vector of *N. sennetsu* has not been determined, but as with *N. helminthoeca*, transmission may involve the ingestion of raw fish that contains the pathogenic organism that was acquired by the fish from the snail.

The family *Anaplasmataceae* is composed of obligatory gram-negative intracellular organisms that parasitize leukocytes, erythrocytes, endothelial cells, or platelets. These agents are naturally transmitted to people and domestic animals from specific ticks that acquire their infections by feeding on mammalian wildlife reservoirs. The designation of *Anaplasma phagocytophilum* as a species group now comprises all strains

of human granulocytotropic *Ehrlichia* (HGE) described worldwide; *E. equi* in the Western United States; and the European agent infecting ruminants, *E. phagocytophila*. They appear genetically and biologically indistinguishable, except for geographic, host, and pathogenic adaptations. *A. (E.) bovis*, *A. (E.) platys*, and *A. phagocytophilum* have all been classified within the genus *Anaplasma* because of their close genetic relationship to *A. marginale*. This chapter will discuss canine and feline diseases caused by these organisms that preferentially infect monocytic cell, granulocytic cell, or thrombocytic cells.

Wolbachia, and its sole species *W. pipientis*, is an obligate intracellular bacterium residing in the cytoplasmic vacuoles of the ovaries and other tissues of arthropods and helminths.[146] This genus is genetically intermediate to organisms in the two tick-transmitted genera of *Ehrlichia* and *Anaplasma*. However, it had not generally been considered a vertebrate pathogen until isolations were made from people and dogs (see later discussion of *Wolbachia* infection).

CANINE MONOCYTOTROPIC EHRLICHIOSIS AND NEORICKETTSIOSIS (*E. CANIS, E. CHAFFEENSIS, E. RUMINATIUM, N. SENNETSU,* AND *N. RISTICII* INFECTIONS)

T. Mark Neer and Shimon Harrus

Etiology and Epidemiology

Canine monocytic ehrlichiosis and neorickettsiosis are caused by obligate intracellular parasites of the genera *Ehrlichia* and *Neorickettsia*, respectively.[146] These small pleomorphic gram-negative coccoid bacteria appear intracytoplasmically in clusters of organisms called morulae (Figs. 28-1 and 28-2). Table 28-1 summarizes the monocytotropic ehrlichial species known to cause disease in animals throughout the world. Three members of the *E. canis* genogroup I, *E. canis*, *E. chaffeensis*, and *E. ruminantium*, infect monocytes of dogs. *N. risticii* (genogroup III) naturally infects horses, although dogs can be experimentally infected and an atypical strain infects dogs naturally. The following discussion concentrates on canine monocytotropic ehrlichiosis (CME) caused by *E. canis*, the principal member of the *E. canis* genogroup, for which the

Table • 28-1

Ehrlichia, Neorickettsia, and Anaplasma Species Infecting People and Domestic or Laboratory Animals

SPECIES (DISEASES)	GEOGRAPHIC DISTRIBUTION	INFECTED CELL TYPE	VECTOR	INFECTED ANIMAL HOSTS[b]		
				RESERVOIR	NATURAL, DOMESTIC	EXPERIMENTAL
Monocytotropic, Geno/Serogroup I						
Ehrlichia canis (Canine monocytotropic ehrlichiosis)	Worldwide, tropical and temperate	Mono, macro, lymph?	*Rhipicephalus sanguineus, Dermacentor variabilis*	Wild and domestic canids	Canids, cat?	None
E. chaffeensis (Human monocytotropic ehrlichiosis)	United States (primarily southern), Missouri	Mono, macro, neut, lymph	*Amblyomma americanum, Amblyomma testudinarium, D. variabilis, Ixodes ovatus, Haemaphysalis yeni, Haemophysalis flava Ixodes persulcatus*	White-tailed deer, coyotes, opossums, raccoons, voles	People, dogs, goats, lemurs in captivity	White-footed mice, red foxes
	Asia					
(*E. canis*) (Venezuelan ehrlichiosis agent)	Venezuela	Mono, macro	*R. sanguineus*	?	People, dogs	Mice
E. ruminantium[c] (Heartwater)	Sub-Saharan Africa	Endothel, mono, macro, neut	*Amblyomma hebraeum*	Wild ungulates?	Cattle, sheep, goats, dogs	Dogs
Monocytotropic, Geno/Serogroup III						
Neorickettsia sennetsu (Sennetsu fever)	Western Japan, Malaysia	Mono, macro	?	Fish?	People	Mice, dogs, nonhuman primates
N. risticii (Equine monocytotropic ehrlichiosis)	United States, Canada	Mono, entero	Trematode larvae	Snails[d]: *Elimia livescens, Juga yrekaensis*	Horses	Dogs, cats, mice, nonhuman primates
N. risticii (subsp. *atypicalis*)	United States	Mono, mast, entero	?	?	Dogs	?
N. helminthoeca (Salmon poisoning disease, see Chapter 27)	Northwest coastal United States	Mono, macro	Trematodes: *Nanophytes salmincola*	Fish	Dogs	?
Monocytotropic, Geno/Serogroup II						
Anaplasma bovis (Bovine ehrlichiosis)	Middle East, Africa	Mono, macro, eryth	*Hyalomma* spp., *Boophilus* spp., *Rhipicephalus* spp.	Wild ungulates?	Cattle	?
Granulocytotropic, Geno/Serogroup I						
E. ewingi (Canine granulocytotropic ehrlichiosis)	United States (primarily southern, Missouri)	Neut, eos	*A. americanum, D. variabilis?, R. sanguineus?, Otobius megnini?*	White-tailed deer	Dogs	?

Table • 28-1

Continued

SPECIES (DISEASES)	GEOGRAPHIC DISTRIBUTION	INFECTED CELL TYPE	VECTOR	INFECTED ANIMAL HOSTS[b]		
				RESERVOIR	NATURAL, DOMESTIC	EXPERIMENTAL
Granulocytotropic, Geno/Serogroup II						
A. phagocytophilum (HGE strain)	United States (upper Midwest, Northeast)	Neut, eos	*Ixodes scapularis (northern)*	White-footed mouse, white-tailed deer, wood rat, coyotes, cotton mice, llamas, meadow voles	People, dogs, cats, horses	Mice?, sheep (cattle seroconvert only)
	Europe (including United Kingdom)	Neut, eos	*Ixodes ricinus, I. persulcatus,*	Roe deer, red deer, bank voles, yellow-necked mice	People, dogs, cats, sheep, horses, goats, cattle?	Splenectomized mice, guinea pigs, reindeer, lambs
E. equi strain	United States, Canadian West Coast?	Neut, eos	*Ixodes pacificus*	Horses, cervids (deer and elk), dusky-footed wood rat	People, dogs, horses	Donkeys, goats, nonhuman primates, mice, guinea pigs (cattle seroconvert only)
E. phagocytophila strain	Northern & Eastern Europe, Africa, Asia	Neut, eos	*I. ricinus, Ixodes. trianguliceps, I. persulcatus ?*	Wild ruminants	Sheep, cattle	
	Asia	Neut, eos	*I. persulcatus, Ixodes turdus Hyalomma longicornis ?*	?	?	?
Thrombocytotropic, Geno/Serogroup II						
A. platys (Infectious canine cyclic thrombocytopenia)	Southern United States, Australia	Platelets	*R. sanguineus?*	?	Dogs	Dogs
	Southern Europe (Mediterranean), South America, Asia, Middle East, Africa	Platelets	*Dermacentor auratus?*		Dogs	Dogs

Mono, monocytes; *macro*, macrophages; *lymph*, lymphocytes; *neut*, neutrophils; *endothel*, endothelial cells; *enter*, enterocytes; *mast*, mast cells; *eryth*, erythrocytes; *HGE*, human granulocytotropic ehrlichiosis; *?*, uncertain.
[a]Sero/genogroups I = *Ehrlichia*, II = *Anaplasma*, III = *Neorickettsia*.
[b]Naturally infected hosts have also been experimentally infected; however, they are not also listed in this column. Some of these experimental infections are subclinical or transient.
[c]Genetic relatedness to *E. canis* indicates reconsidered classification in the tribe *Ehrlichiae*.
[d]Trematode infected snails; Pleuroceridae (*Elimia livescens, Juga yrekaensis*), mayflies, caddflies.

majority of the information is present. Where indicated, the other infections are described in more detail.

E. canis

E. canis was first identified by Donatien and Lestoquard in Algeria in 1935.[139] CME gained considerable attention when hundreds of American military dogs, many of which were German shepherds, died from the disease during the Vietnam War. *E. canis* received further attention in the late 1980s when the rickettsia was erroneously suspected to infect people. However, in 1991, a new species of the *Ehrlichia* genus, *E. chaffeensis*, was found to be the cause of human monocytotropic ehrlichiosis.

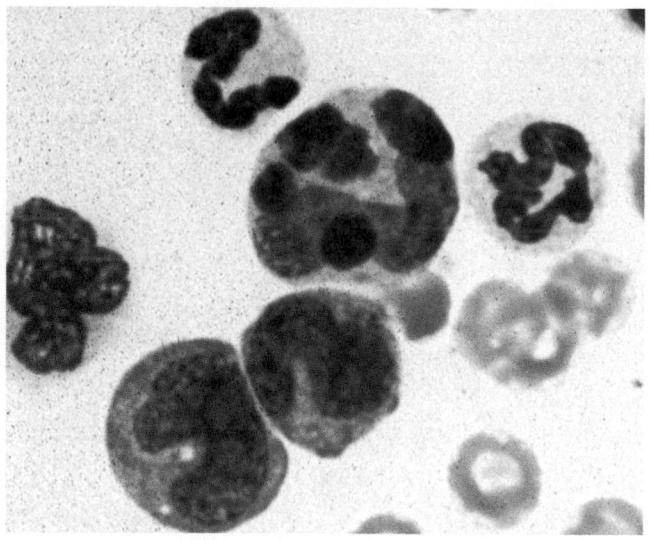

Fig 28-1 A mononuclear leukocyte containing a compact *E. canis* morula in the cytoplasm. (Courtesy Ken Latimer, University of Georgia, Athens, Ga.)

E. canis has a worldwide distribution (Asia, Africa, Europe, and the Americas). Despite the presence of suitable vectors, oceanic or island areas that have maintained quarantine, such as Australia and the United Kingdom, appear to be free of *E. canis* infection.[252,335] Only recently has the first case been reported in a dog imported to Japan.[501] Although, in a recent epidemiologic survey of ticks collected from dogs in Japan, no positive polymerase chain reaction (PCR) results were found for *E. canis* in 1211 ticks examined.[239] Vertebrate hosts for *E. canis* include members of the family Canidae. The coyote, fox, and jackal, in addition to the domestic dog, are considered reservoir hosts (see Fig. 28-2). New information suggests that *E. canis* or a closely related organism might also infect cats (see later discussion on Feline Monocytotropic Ehrlichiosis).[70] The arthropod vector of *E. canis* is the brown dog tick, *Rhipicephalus sanguineus*. This one-host tick preferentially feeds on dogs in all three stages of its life cycle and can live indoors in domiciled environments in which dogs are housed. Experimentally, infection has also been transmitted by *Dermacentor variabilis*, the American dog tick.[257] The mode of transmission is transstadial. Because transovarial spread does not occur, the vector tick cannot be a true reservoir. Ticks acquire *E. canis* as either larvae or nymphs by feeding on rickettsemic dogs. They transmit infection to susceptible dogs for at least 155 days after infection.[201] This permits the pathogen to overwinter in the tick and then in the following spring allows the tick to infest and infect susceptible dogs. Most CME cases occur during the warm season when the vector ticks are abundant; however, unlike the other rickettsiae that depend on outdoor vectors, *E. canis*–induced disease has a more even seasonal distribution. This may also be a result of the prolonged subclinical period in chronically infected animals. The minimal time required of tick attachment to transmit *E. canis* infection has yet to be determined, as it is known for some other tick-borne diseases.[272] Dogs living in or traveling to endemic regions are candidates for the disease.

E. chaffeensis

E. chaffeensis, the etiologic agent of human monocytotropic ehrlichiosis (HME) has been convincingly identified from people, deer, dogs, coyotes, one domestic goat, and one captive lemur, and from ticks only in the United States, mainly the south-central, southeastern, mid-Atlantic states, and from

California (Fig. 28-3). White-tailed deer (*Odocoileus virginianus*) serve as excellent natural sentinels for both *E. chaffeensis* and *A. phagocytophilum*.[562] Detection of *E. chaffeensis* DNA by PCR amplification provided evidence for natural canine *E. chaffeensis* infection in southeastern Virginia, Oklahoma, and North Carolina.[74,368,383,562] In the eastern United States, the rickettsia is transmitted by *Amblyomma americanum* (Lone Star tick) and to lesser extent by *D. variabilis*. Persistently infected white-tailed deer and possibly dogs or other carnivores, serve as reservoir hosts. Serologic evidence of *E. chaffeensis* has been reported from people residing in countries in Africa, South America, and Asia, as well as from Mexico and Russia. However, other closely related monocytotropic *Ehrlichia* such as *E. muris* are likely responsible for cross-reactive antibodies.[383] PCR has been used to document the presence of *E. chaffeensis* DNA in ticks from southern China and South America, but more evidence is needed to determine if in fact the organism and disease is present outside North America.[383]

N. risticii

N. risticii, the etiologic agent of Potomac horse fever, was reported to cause monocytotropic ehrlichiosis in dogs, a disease described as atypical ehrlichiosis (see Table 28-1). Its significance in cats under natural conditions is uncertain. However, cats can be experimentally infected with *N. risticii* (see later discussion on Feline Monocytotropic Ehrlichiosis). This organism is closely related to *N. helminthoeca* and *N. sennetsu*, the etiologic agents of salmon poisoning disease and human Sennetsu fever, respectively.[146] The mode of transmission of *N. risticii* is unknown; however, *N. risticii* DNA was found in trematodes (virgulate cercariae from freshwater *Juga* snails from California and in virgulate xiphidiocercariae from *Elimia* snails in Ohio)[38,262,434] and in various aquatic insects.[100] These findings suggest that they play an important role in the transmission of the rickettsia.

E. ruminantium

E. ruminantium, or a closely related organism, was genetically detected in the blood of clinically healthy and ill dogs from Kenya, Uganda, Ethiopia, and Mali.[8] The organism was not isolated in culture or tested for its infectivity; therefore its virulence, potential vectors, and definitive classification are uncertain. Several closely related organisms comprise the clade of organisms in this group.

N. helminthoeca

N. helminthoeca, the cause of salmon poisoning disease, is more thoroughly covered in Chapter 27 and will not be discussed further in the present chapter.

Pathogenesis

A wide variety of factors, including the *E. canis* inoculum size, can influence the course and outcome of infection. The severity of the disease is greater with certain strains of the organism. An immunoblot analysis of the IgG response to *E. canis* has shown that antigenic diversity may exist among *E. canis* organisms from different parts of the world and has suggested that this may affect the severity of the disease.[371] Concomitant disease with other tick-borne parasites or other pathogens may also affect the severity and manifestation of the disease. Immunodeficient animals may develop more severe manifestations of disease and are more likely to have large numbers of circulating morulae. No age or sex predilection exists for CME; however, German shepherd dogs seem to be more susceptible than other breeds. Moreover, the disease in this breed is more severe and has a poorer prognosis than in other breeds.[377] Variation in breed susceptibility can be attributed to breed differences in the ability to mount adequate cellular

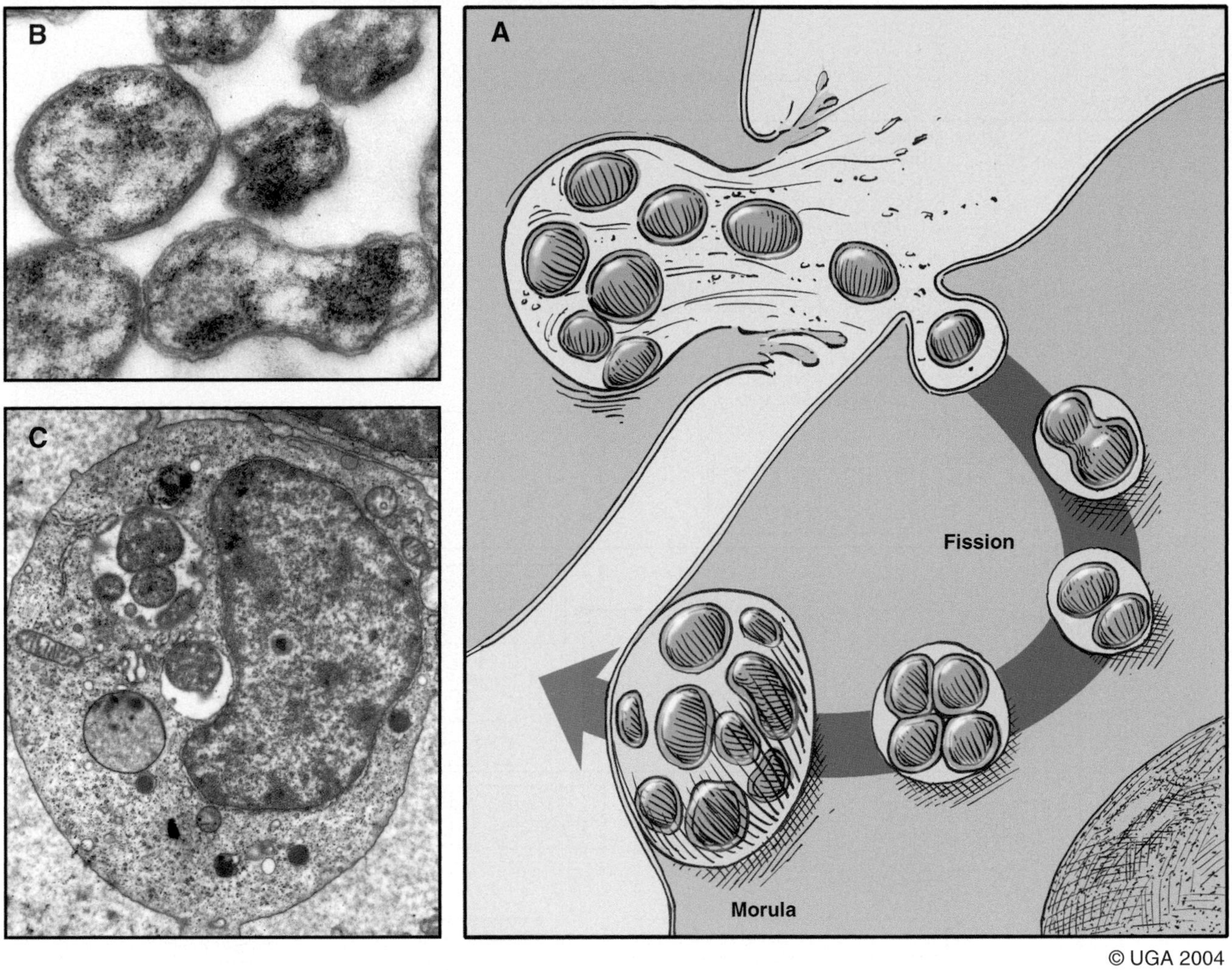

© UGA 2004

Fig 28-2 **A,** Developmental cycle of *E. canis* in dog cells. **B,** Mononuclear cell containing *E. canis* inclusions, ×12,000. (From Simpson CF. 1974. Relationship of *Ehrlichia canis*-infected mononuclear cells to blood vessels of the lungs, *Infect Immun* 10:590-596. Reprinted with permission.) **C,** *E. canis* organisms within canine monocyte have a pleomorphic shape and double membrane. (University of Georgia, Athens, Ga.)

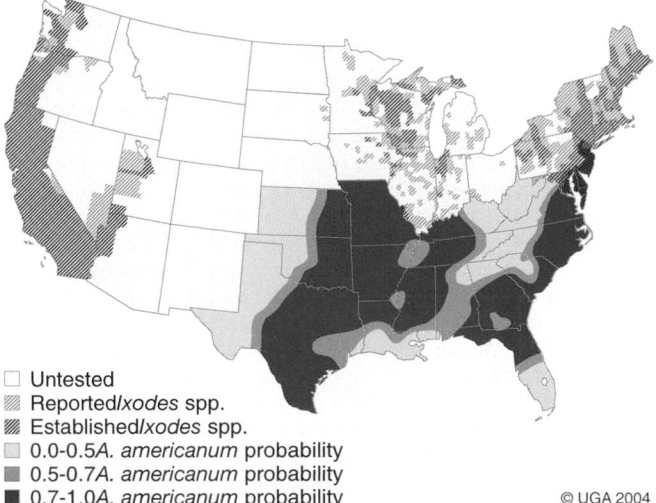

☐ Untested
▨ Reported *Ixodes* spp.
▨ Established *Ixodes* spp.
☐ 0.0-0.5 *A. americanum* probability
▨ 0.5-0.7 *A. americanum* probability
■ 0.7-1.0 *A. americanum* probability

© UGA 2004

Fig 28-3 Map of distribution of some tick vectors of ehrlichiosis (*Amblyomma* spp.) and anaplasmosis (*Ixodes* spp.) in the United States. (Courtesy University of Georgia, Athens, Ga.)

or humoral immune response, or both. The cellular immune response to *E. canis* infection is depressed in German shepherd dogs compared with beagle dogs, while no significant differences were recorded in the humoral response between the two breeds.[377]

Natural infection of the vertebrate host occurs when an infected tick ingests a blood meal and salivary secretions contaminate the feeding site. Iatrogenic spread can occur with blood transfusions from infected donors. During the incubation period of 8 to 20 days, organisms multiply in macrophages of the mononuclear-phagocyte system, by binary fission, spreading throughout the body (Fig. 28-4). The subsequent course of ehrlichiosis has been divided into three phases—acute, subclinical, and chronic—based on clinical signs and clinicopathologic abnormalities following experimental inoculation. However, with naturally occurring infection, accurate staging of the disease is difficult. The acute phase lasts 2 to 4 weeks during which signs such as fever, oculonasal discharge, anorexia, depression, petechiae, ecchymoses, lymphadenomegaly, and splenomegaly may be seen. Typical laboratory abnormalities in this phase include thrombocytopenia, mild leukopenia, and mild anemia. Most dogs recover from the acute disease with adequate treatment. Untreated and inappropriately treated dogs may enter the subclinical phase. During this phase, the dog's weight normalizes and the

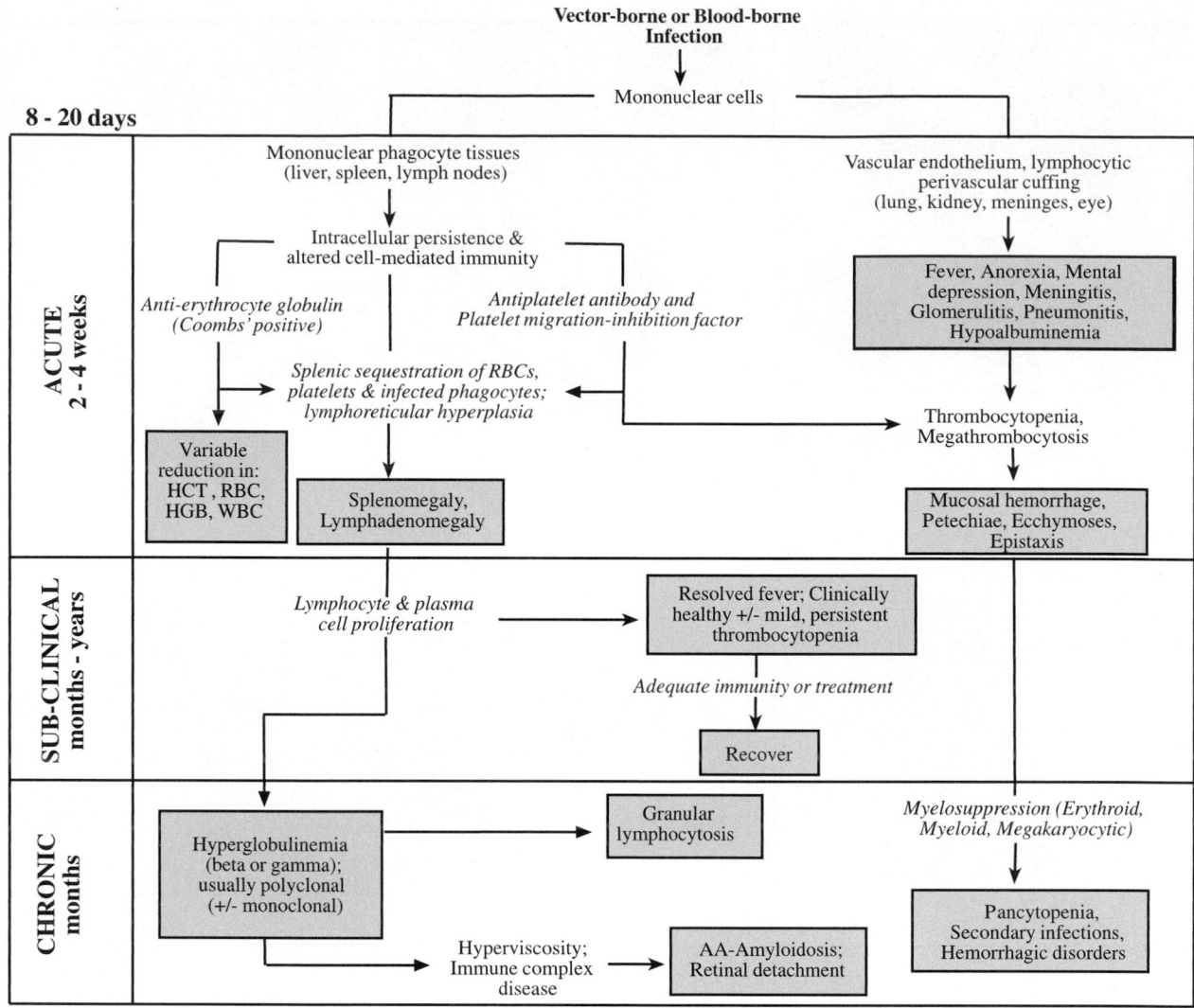

Fig   28-4   Pathogenesis of *E. canis* infection in dogs.

pyrexia resolves. Clinically, dogs appear healthy; however, their platelet counts may remain below reference ranges.[533,534] Dogs in the subclinical phase have the potential to remain persistent carriers for years as described in one 3-year follow-up study.[212] Results of experimental infections indicate that the spleen is most likely to harbor *E. canis* organisms during the subclinical phase of CME and the last organ to accommodate the parasite before elimination. The spleen is believed to have an important role in the pathogenesis and expression of the disease. Splenectomized dogs, experimentally infected with *E. canis*, had mild clinical illness compared with nonsplenectomized dogs.[219] During the course of infection, repeated recombinations occur in the outer membrane major antigenic protein-genes of ehrlichiae leading to the generation of variations in immunogenic epitopes.[432] In this manner, the organisms may evade host defense mechanisms resulting in persistent infections. Immunocompetent dogs may eliminate rickettsiae; otherwise, they may remain carriers for life or may enter the chronic phase of infection. The chronic phase, in its severe form, is characterized by impaired bone marrow production of blood elements, resulting in pancytopenia. The prognosis for dogs with the chronic severe form is grave. Dogs in this phase may eventually die of secondary infections or uncontrollable bleeding, or both. Therefore identifying the disease before dogs enter the chronic phase of CME is of utmost importance.

Survival and multiplication of ehrlichial organisms in infected cells rely on the organism's ability to inhibit phagosome-lysosome fusion, as shown for *N. risticii* and *N. sennetsu*.[371] Doxycycline was shown to restore the host's phagocytic ability, probably by inhibiting the synthesis of a bacterial fusion-hindering protein.[544] Apparently, T cell–induced immunity and interferon (IFN)-γ secretion play a predominant role in recovery from and immunity to ehrlichial infections.[78,535] The generation of nitric oxide accompanied by limited access of iron is the mechanism by which IFN-γ inhibits *N. risticii* in vitro.[390] IFN-γ–activated human monocytes have been shown to inhibit *E. chaffeensis* infection by downregulation of surface transferrin receptors that lead to the limitation of available cytoplasmic iron.[40] Evasion of the immune response may be another means by which *E. canis* may establish chronic infection in its canine host. In vitro studies in mononuclear cell cultures have indicated downregulated expression of major histocompatibility complex class II receptors.[218] Lymphocyte subset alterations have been characterized by decreased CD4+:CD8+ ratio.[224]

Infection with *E. canis* results in the development of specific antibodies. IgM and IgA appear 4 to 7 days after infection; IgG generally increases beginning 15 days postinfection.[535] The hypergammaglobulinemia is usually polyclonal; however, some dogs may develop monoclonal gammopathy.[214,522] The role of antibody response in eliminating persistent intracellular ehrlichial infections is minimal. High *E. canis*–antibody titers do not provide protection when animals are challenged.[40,446] Moreover, they may have a detrimental effect on progression of the disease because of their immunopathologic consequences.[446] Increasing evidence supports the assumption that hyperimmune mechanisms are involved in the pathogenesis of CME. These include extensive plasma cell infiltration of the bone marrow and parenchymal organs; the occurrence of polyclonal hypergammaglobulinemia that does not correlate with specific *E. canis*-antibody titers; positive Coombs' and autoagglutination test results; the induction of antiplatelet antibody production following natural and experimental infection; and the recent detection of circulating immune complexes in dogs naturally and artificially infected with *E. canis*.[199,209,215] The latter finding suggests that some pathologic and clinical manifestations in CME are immune-complex mediated. No antinuclear antibodies were found in dogs naturally or experimentally infected with *E. canis*, suggesting other mechanisms in the pathogenesis of CME.[209] Dogs with monoclonal gammopathy may develop hyperviscosity with associated clinical signs and pathologic lesions. Cases of sudden blindness caused by subretinal hemorrhage associated with hyperviscosity have been documented.[211,371] Reactive AA amyloidosis associated with proteinuria and glomerulopathy has been implicated as a pathologic complication of chronic *E. canis* infection.[318]

Hematologic changes in CME are associated with inflammatory and immune processes triggered by the infection. Thrombocytopenia, the most common hematologic abnormality of dogs infected with *E. canis*, occurs in all phases of disease.[183,215,221] Various mechanisms are involved in the pathogenesis of thrombocytopenia; these mechanisms include increased platelet consumption and decreased platelet half-life, probably as a result of splenic sequestration and immune-mediated destruction. Platelet-bound and circulating antiplatelet antibodies have been detected in whole blood and serum, respectively, of dogs in the acute phase after artificial and following natural infections with *E. canis*.[371,537] In addition, a serum cytokine, platelet migration–inhibition factor (PMIF), has been found to exist in dogs with ehrlichiosis, and its level is related inversely to the platelet count.[1] Higher levels of PMIF are associated with more virulent strains of *E. canis* (Fig. 28-5). PMIF inhibits platelet migration and is produced by lymphocytes when they are exposed to infected monocytes. Decreased production of platelets as a result of hypoplastic bone marrow is considered to be the mechanism responsible for the thrombocytopenia in the chronic phase.[215] Platelet function, as measured by aggregation responses, is decreased in *E. canis*–infected dogs. This, in conjunction with the low platelet count, contributes to the hemorrhages seen with CME.[216,217,221]

Clinical Findings

Canine ehrlichiosis is a multisystemic disorder that is now known to be caused by a variety of ehrlichial species. In the past, all clinical reports of this disease confirmed by cytologic or serologic means have been attributed to *E. canis* infections. In the United States, previously reported cases diagnosed cytologically as "granulocytotropic strain" infections may have been caused by *A. phagocytophilum* or by *E. ewingii* (see later discussion). Because of cross-reactivity with *E. canis*, serologically confirmed cases using only *E. canis* as antigen could have also been caused by *E. chaffeensis* or *E. ewingii*. The following discussion categorizes previously published clinical features based on body systems and primarily focuses on *E. canis* infection and other monocytotropic ehrlichial species. For discussion of clinical features of the granulocytotropic ehrlichias, see later discussion on Canine Granulocytotropic Ehrlichiosis.

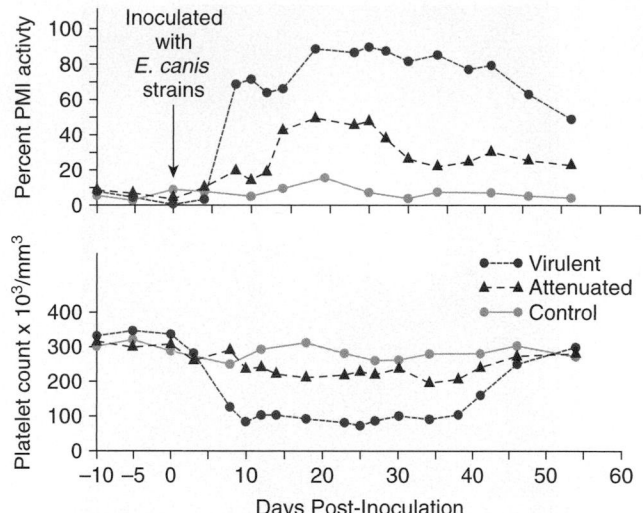

Fig 28-5 Graphs showing the temporal relationship between platelet counts and platelet migration inhibition (PMI) activity after infection with different strains of *E. canis*. (From Abeygunawardena I, Kakoma I, Smith RD. 1990. Pathophysiology of canine ehrlichiosis, pp 78–92. *In* Williams JC, Kakoma I [eds], *Ehrlichiosis*, Dordrecht, Netherlands. Reprinted with permission from Kluwer Academic Publishers.)

Multisystemic Signs

A common presentation is depression, lethargy, mild weight loss, and anorexia, with or without hemorrhagic tendencies. If present, the bleeding is usually exhibited by dermal petechiae or ecchymoses, or both. Although bleeding can occur from any mucosal surface, epistaxis is most frequent. Physical examination may also reveal lymphadenomegaly and splenomegaly in 20% and 25% of the patients, respectively.[561] Another point all clinicians should keep in mind when considering tick-borne disease as a cause for multisystemic signs is the issue of co-infection with multiple tick-borne pathogens.[286] This concern is increasing and adds confusion in interpreting previously published reports (see later discussion on Concurrent or Secondary Infections).

Ocular Signs

Dogs may show changes in eye color or appearance or may develop blindness. Anterior uveitis and retinal disease, such as chorioretinitis, papilledema, retinal hemorrhage, retinal perivascular infiltrates, and bullous retinal detachment (Fig. 28-6), are the more common findings and may result in acute blindness.[192] Uveitis has also been associated with *A. platys* infection in the dog (see Canine Thrombocytotropic Ehrlichiosis).

Neuromuscular Signs

The neurologic signs of ehrlichiosis are the result primarily of meningitis from inflammation or bleeding, or both. Neurologic dysfunction occurs with damage to the adjacent central or peripheral nervous tissue. Infections with *E. canis* and granulocytotropic strains have been most common,[331,515] and signs are indistinguishable from those of Rocky Mountain spotted fever (RMSF) (see Chapter 29). Seizures, stupor, ataxia with upper or lower motor neuron dysfunction, acute central or peripheral vestibular dysfunction, anisocoria, cerebellar dysfunction, intention tremors, and generalized or localized hyperesthesia have been observed. Morulae have been found in cells from the cerebrospinal fluid (CSF) in some instances.[331,356] Two dogs that were seropositive for *E. canis* had polymyositis, and the signs consisted of acute-onset progressive tetraparesis, hyporeflexia, and muscle wasting.[89] Skeletal muscles were atrophic and characterized histologically by lymphoplasmacytic and immature lymphoreticular

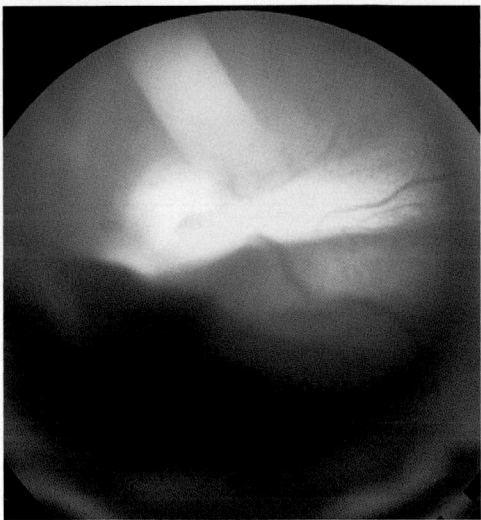

Fig 28-6 Retinal detachment caused by subretinal hemorrhage in a dog with *E. canis* infection. (Courtesy University of Georgia, Athens, Ga.)

cellular infiltrates within areas of necrosis. Unfortunately, the histopathology of peripheral nerves was not reported.

Polyarthritis

Dogs with ehrlichiosis may develop lameness with a stiff gait secondary to polyarthropathy. Joint disease may occur from hemarthrosis or immune complex deposition with resultant arthritis and neutrophilic effusion into the joint. Most instances of polyarthritis have been associated with infection by granulocytotropic strains (*A. phagocytophilum* or *E. ewingii*) or *N. risticii*.[119,488,489] When titers have been determined, approximately 81% of the dogs with the granulocytotropic strain had titers to *E. canis*, which cross-reacts with *E. ewingii*, and 8% had titers to *E. equi*.[488]

Concurrent or Secondary Infections

Ticks can harbor multiple pathogenic organisms resulting in co-infections in the infected dog.[113,286] Positive results for antibody reactivity or nucleic acid detection methods should be interpreted with caution with regard to *Ehrlichia* being the sole cause of clinical illness unless a wide variety of potential pathogens have been evaluated. In addition, dogs with ehrlichiosis can become secondarily infected with opportunistic bacterial, fungal, or protozoal diseases.[140] Ehrlichial testing should be considered as an evaluation of host immunocompetence in dogs that are diagnosed with opportunistic infections.

Ehrlichial Species–Specific Signs

Table 28-2 summarizes the clinical and laboratory findings of monocytotropic ehrlichial infections in dogs.

E. canis   *E. canis* infections can be acute or chronic in dogs. The dog acts as the reservoir host for this infection, and chronic persistent infections can result in pancytopenia or hyperglobulinemia. The hyperglobulinemia is usually polyclonal; however, on occasion, monoclonal gammopathy has been observed. Granular lymphocytosis, which has been confused with well-differentiated lymphocytic leukemia, has been observed in some dogs.

N. risticii   *N. risticii* (previously *E. risticii*) infection can be experimentally established in dogs and cats, producing minimal clinical illness.[126,129,445] Of eight cats inoculated with *N. risticii*, one cat had mild, self-limiting disease consisting of intermittent diarrhea, and another cat had lymphade-

nomegaly, acute depression, and anorexia.[126] Even though this ehrlichial species appears to cause little, if any, clinical disease in experimentally infected dogs and cats, it has yet to be determined whether this is the case with natural infections.

In 100 cases of serologically atypical canine ehrlichiosis, with three deaths, the indirect fluorescent antibody (FA) test was negative for *E. canis* and *N. sennetsu* but positive for *N. risticii*.[260] Subsequent genetic sequencing techniques characterized an isolated agent to be *N. risticii*. Clinicopathologic findings included vomiting, lethargy, anemia, thrombocytopenia, polyarthropathy, fever, or any combination. The 100 cases were distributed geographically as follows: California (32), Texas (26), Arizona (16), Illinois (10), Washington State (9), Florida (5), and Michigan (2). A new species name, *N. risticii* subsp. *atypicalis*, was proposed.[260] If typical signs of ehrlichiosis are present in a dog and it is seronegative for *E. canis*, evaluation for the presence of antibody titers to *N. risticii* should be considered.

E. chaffeensis   *E. chaffeensis* has been experimentally inoculated into pups, and signs were mild compared with corresponding *E. canis*–inoculated animals.[129] Only fever was apparent. This finding, which may be related to species differences or attenuation of the agent in cell culture, contrasts to the clinical syndrome observed in people infected with *E. chaffeensis*. The clinical significance of natural infections in dogs or cats is still being defined. Dogs experimentally infected with *E. chaffeensis* developed thrombocytopenia without other systemic manifestations of disease.[575] Organisms could be cultured from the blood for up to 102 days following infection and DNA was found for up to 117 days. High antibody titers were maintained for up to 6 months of observation, suggesting that the dogs became chronic inapparent carriers and therefore possible reservoirs of disease. Serologic and PCR testing has suggested that dogs in animal shelters and kennels in southeastern Virginia are naturally infected.[128] Three dogs had naturally occurring clinical disease secondary to *E. chaffeensis* infection.[74] These dogs had signs very similar to classic *E. canis* infection consisting of anterior uveitis, epistaxis, and lymphadenopathy. In people, *E. chaffeensis*–induced illness is more severe in immunocompromised individuals[453]; similar findings might be expected in dogs.

E. ruminantium   *E. ruminantium* or a closely-related organism was detected in subsaharan Africa in the blood of clinically healthy dogs and in those with clinical illness typical of *E. canis* infection.[8] Whether the signs were caused by or incidental to the infection with this organism is uncertain.

Diagnosis

The diagnosis of ehrlichiosis is usually made based on a combination of clinical signs, hematologic abnormalities, thrombocytopenias, and serologic findings. PCR and immunoblotting techniques are now being used more in the clinical setting to obtain a diagnosis, and specific comments regarding their use will also be addressed.

Clinical Laboratory Findings

Hematologic changes are best documented for infections caused by *E. canis* and include thrombocytopenia (82%), anemia (82%), which is usually nonregenerative, and leukopenia (32%, of which 20% had neutropenia).[515,526] Pancytopenia is usually a result of hypoplasia of all bone marrow precursor cells and occurs in the severe chronic phase (18% of cases) and more often in German shepherd dogs.[561]

Thrombocytopenia has been consistently reported in all stages of *E. canis* infection; because it is often a screening test for ehrlichiosis, this proportion may be overestimated.[85a] In one study in an endemic area of Brazil, there was a general correlation between positive blood PCR results for *E. canis* and the presence of marked (<100,000 platelets/µl) throm-

Table • 28-2

Comparison of Naturally Occurring Canine Disease Caused by Ehrlichia *spp.,* Neorickettsia risticii, *and* Anaplasma *spp.*

SPECIES	CLINICAL FEATURES	LABORATORY ABNORMALITIES	REFERENCES
Monocytotropic			
E. canis	Fever, anorexia, weight loss, hemorrhagic diathesis, CNS signs, lymphadenomegaly	Anemia, leukopenia, marked thrombocytopenia, hyperglobulinemia, pancytopenia, proteinuria, mononuclear pleocytosis	208, 210, 514, 371
N. risticii (subsp. atypicalis)	Fever, lethargy, hemorrhagic diathesis, polyarthritis, periarticular joint swelling	Anemia, thrombocytopenia	260, 259
E. chaffeensis	Anterior uveitis, vomiting, epistaxis, erythema multiforme, lymphadenomegaly	Thrombocytopenia, lymphocytic pleocytosis	74, 371
E. ruminantium	Asymptomatic	No data	8
Granulocytotropic			
E. ewingii	Fever, anorexia, lameness, joint swelling, CNS signs	Mild thrombocytopenia Mild nonregenerative anemia, neutrophilic polyarthritis, neutrophilic CSF pleocytosis	488, 489, 187
A. phagocytophilum	Fever, anorexia, lethargy, splenomegaly, hepatomegaly, CNS signs, lameness, joint swelling	Thrombocytopenia, mild hypoalbuminemia, high serum ALP activity, occasional neutropenia or regenerative left shift, neutrophilic polyarthritis, predominantly neutrophilic CSF pleocytosis	198, 256
Thrombocytotropic			
A. platys	Mild fever, uveitis, petechia and ecchymoses, often asymptomatic	Thrombocytopenia	207, 222

CNS, central nervous system; *CSF,* cerebrospinal fluid; *ALP,* alkaline phosphatase.

bocytopenia.[85a] However, ehrlichiosis should never be eliminated from consideration because the platelet count is normal. Serology should be performed if other clinical signs are compatible. In another study involving hospitalized dogs from Brazil, anemia was more of an epidemiologic risk factor for ehrlichiosis than thrombocytopenia.[137]

Granular lymphocytosis has been observed with *E. canis* infection.[224,543] Affected dogs had absolute lymphocyte counts ranging from 5200 to 17,200 cells/µl with granularity to their cytoplasm typical of well-differentiated lymphocytic leukemia. Some of these dogs had monoclonal gammopathies, which may further lead to a misdiagnosis of lymphocytic leukemia. Therefore ehrlichial testing should be performed on dogs when well-differentiated lymphocytosis is observed.

The most frequent serum chemistry abnormalities have included hyperproteinemia (33%), hyperglobulinemia (39%), hypoalbuminemia (43%), and elevated alanine aminotransferase (ALT) and alkaline phosphatase (ALP) activities (43%

and 31%, respectively).[371] The hyperproteinemia results from elevated globulin levels, but no direct correlation exists between the levels of serum globulins and serum *E. canis* antibodies. Serum electrophoresis generally shows a polyclonal hyperglobulinemia,[210] although monoclonal gammopathies can occur. An *E. canis*–antibody titer should be measured in all dogs in which a diagnosis of benign monoclonal gammopathy is contemplated or in which definitive evidence of myeloma, leukemia, or macroglobulinemia is lacking. Infected dogs with pancytopenia generally have lower serum γ-globulin concentrations compared with nonpancytopenic dogs.[210] Dogs with *E. canis* often have plasmacytosis in the bone marrow or sometimes other tissues, which can be confused with plasma cell myeloma.[371]

Other clinicopathologic findings include positive antinuclear antibody test results,[479a] proteinuria, hematuria, prolonged bleeding time (even in some dogs that have normal platelet counts), and pulmonary interstitial radiopacity

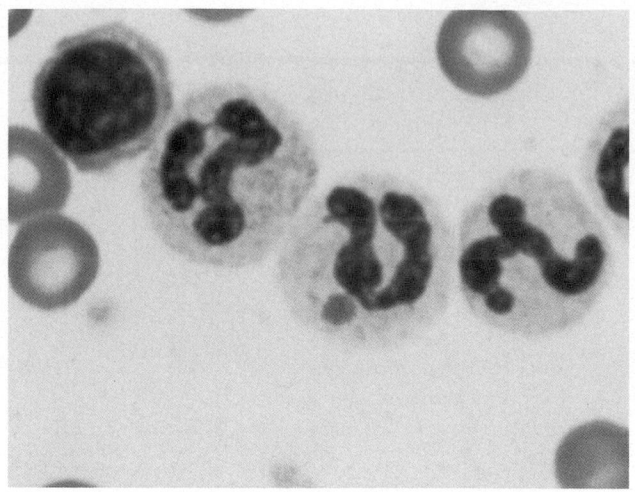

Fig 28-7 A segmented neutrophil from a dog that contains a morula of a granulocytic species of *Ehrlichia*. (Courtesy University of Georgia, Athens, Ga.)

ranging from a mild linear pattern to marked interstitial infiltration with peribronchial opacities. Experimentally, peak urine protein loss, consisting principally of albumin, is observed 2.5 to 3.5 weeks after inoculation and resolves by 6 weeks after infection.[114,115] During the peak loss, urine protein/creatinine ratios ranged from 4.5 to 23.2 (reference ratio less than 1.0). A corresponding drop in serum albumin concentrations was noted (mean 2.1 g/dl). CSF analysis in dogs with signs of central nervous system (CNS) disease has revealed increased protein level and predominant lymphocytic pleocytosis similar to that found in viral infections.[429] Comparable CSF findings have been noted in human monocytotropic ehrlichiosis.

Cytology

A definitive diagnosis of ehrlichial disease can be made by demonstration of morulae in leukocytes from blood smears or tissue aspirates such as spleen, lung, and lymph node. The finding of morulae is difficult and time consuming but may be optimized by performing buffy coat smears or examining thin blood smears made from a peripheral capillary bed of the ear margin. Morulae may be visualized within monocytes present in peripheral blood smears or within synovial fluid (or both) or rarely CSF (Fig. 28-7). Cytologic studies of peripheral blood, buffy coat, lymph node aspirates, bone marrow aspirates, and short-term culture of blood specimens have shown highest sensitivity in detecting the organisms in buffy coat and lymph node aspirates.[369] Morulae were more often found in lymphocytes than monocytes. Platelets, lymphocytic azurophilic granules, lymphoglandular bodies, and phagocytosed nuclear material can all be confused with ehrlichial inclusions.

Serologic Testing

A diagnosis of ehrlichiosis is usually based on positive results of an indirect FA test. This test detects serum antibodies as early as 7 days after initial infection, although some dogs may not become seropositive until 28 days after infection begins. Therefore a dog may be acutely infected and have no demonstrable serum antibody titer. When *E. canis* antibody titer results are negative, a follow-up examination in 2 to 3 weeks or serotesting for other agents is recommended. Serum antibody levels in untreated dogs peak at 80 days after infection. During the first 7 days postinfection, the titer consists of IgA and IgM, and by 20 days, the majority is IgG. Most laboratories measure this antibody. Methodology and reporting differ among laboratories; thus no consensus concerning an absolute

level of reactivity has been reached. An IgG titer of 1:80 or greater is generally considered to be evidence of infection or exposure, or both, but this finding may vary with each laboratory's methods. Conversely, because of measurable titer persistence after treatment or potential recovery, a positive titer result does not necessarily mean that the animal's disease or clinical symptoms are strictly the result of ehrlichiosis, especially in endemic areas inhabited by asymptomatic animals with titers to *E. canis*.

In one study, 20.3% of healthy kenneled dogs had antibody titers to *E. canis*.[233] We have dealt with at least 30 dogs during the last 14 years in which platelet counts were less than 50,000/µl, each had positive titers to *E. canis* with no concurrent increase in platelet numbers following tetracycline therapy. However, all dogs had dramatic platelet count increases in response to immunosuppressive doses of glucocorticoids. These dogs most likely had immune-mediated thrombocytopenia coincidentally or as a result of exposure to *E. canis*. They developed antiplatelet antibodies but at the time were not clinically affected by the *Ehrlichia* infection.

After treatment, in most dogs, the titer progressively declines and generally becomes negative in 6 to 9 months. Some dogs may become asymptomatic after therapy but yet retain very high titers to *E. canis* for years.[41,397] Whether the organism is persisting cannot always be determined.[41] Treated dogs are assumed to have eliminated the organism if thrombocytopenia, hyperglobulinemia, and other clinical and laboratory abnormalities resolve progressively after treatment.

Antigenic cross-reactivity exists with *E. canis* and other organisms in different regions of the world.[225] Differences can be detected in serologic response by Western immunoblotting. Some cross-reactivity also occurs between ehrlichial species, which may pose problems in the interpretation of indirect FA serology in certain geographic areas. A shift in reactivity to various antigenic determinants of *E. canis* has been detected in dogs during the course of infection.[350] For information on cross-reactivity among *Ehrlichia*, *Neorickettsia*, and *Anaplasma*, see Table 28-3. Little, if any, cross-reactivity occurs between *E. canis* and *Rickettsia rickettsii*, the etiologic agent of RMSF. Because the clinical presentation of these two diseases is similar, dogs with clinical signs of ehrlichiosis in the absence of a titer to *E. canis* should be tested for RMSF by collecting serum for paired IgG titers, acute and 2-week convalescent sera (see Chapter 29). *N. helminthoeca* will cause cross-reactions to *E. canis*, *N. risticii*, and *N. sennetsu* (see Chapter 27).[437] Titers to other *Ehrlichia* should be examined depending on the geographic area and compatible clinical signs. Antibodies to *E. ewingii* cross-react with *E. canis* and *E. chaffeensis*, and the use of one of these antigens will detect infection with either of the three, while *E. canis* sera can cross-react with *A. phagocytophilum* antigens.[495,538]

E. ewingii cannot be cultured in vitro beyond isolation in primary cells; therefore a specific serologic test is not available. Cross-reactive antigens are also present between *E. chaffeensis* and HGE agent using human but not dog sera.[352,444] *E. equi* will detect infection with HGE agent or *A. phagocytophilum*, and some cross-reactivity exists between *N. risticii* and *N. sennetsu*. In addition to indirect FA, enzyme-linked immunosorbent assay (ELISA) can be used to detect antibodies in dogs to *E. canis* and circulating antigen.[180] A "point of care" ELISA test using recombinant proteins has been developed for in-clinic testing for *E. canis* antibodies (Snap Canine Combo or Snap3Dx, IDDEXX laboratories Inc., Westbrook, Me.). This test was initially marketed to have positive results at a dilution of 1:100 or greater; however, this level was subsequently increased to a dilution of 1:500 or greater. Another ELISA-based point of care test, the Dip-S-Ticks (PanBio InDx, Inc., Baltimore, Md.) has been found to have higher sensitivity but lower specificity than the Snap Canine Combo and lower accuracy than the Snap3Dx test

Table • 28-3

Cross-Reactivity with Ehrlichial Antigens in Indirect FA Testing of Canine Sera[a]

Antigen Used in Test (Genogroup)[a]	SERA FROM DOGS WITH NATURAL OR EXPERIMENTAL INFECTIONS							
	E. canis	E. chaffeensis	E. ewingii	E. ruminantium	A. platys	A. phagocytophilum	N. risticii	N. helminthoeca
Ehrlichia canis (I)[340,437,442]	++++	+++	+++	++	0	0	0	++
E. chaffeensis (I)[144,396,442,557]	++	++++	++	(?)	0	0	(?)	(?)
E. ruminantium (I)[149,268]	+++	(?)	(?)	++++	(?)	(?)	(?)	(?)
Anaplasma phagocytophilum (II)	+[b]	0	+[c]	(?)	++	++++	0	(?)
Neorickettsia risticii (III)[80,437]	++	(?)	(?)	(?)	(?)	(?)	++++	+++
N. helminthoeca (III)[437]	++	(?)	(?)	(?)	(?)	(?)	+++	++++

Reactivity is: *0*, none; *+*, weak; *++*, low; *+++*, high; *++++*, strong; *(?)*, no data.
[a]Known seroreactivity based on data and references cited in Table 28-3 in Neer, 1998.
[b]Reactivity increases with time during the course of infection.[533]
[c]Occasional low cross reactivity noted in some dog sera.[34]

when these were compared with the indirect FA assay.[53] An ELISA in-house test using whole rickettsiae has also been developed in Israel (Immunocomb, Biogal, Kibbutz Gal'ed, Israel) that is clearly able to differentiate *E. canis* seronegative samples from those with titers of *at least* 1:320.[539] Titers in the range of 1:80 to 1:160 were not adequately evaluated with a large number of samples; however, a positive reaction was set at 1:80. Both test kits have been able to differentiate *E. canis* seronegative samples from those with titers of over 1:320.[206] In cases in which low titers are involved, repeating the serologic test after several weeks may give a positive result. For further information on these test kits, see Appendix 6.

With the advent of readily available screening tests, clinically healthy animals have been found to have increased serum antibody titers to *Ehrlichia* or *Anaplasma*. Some of these results may be falsely positive in that they are caused by exposure to cross-reacting, less pathogenic rickettsiae. When recombinant protein–based tests are used, clinically significant infections with other rickettsiae may not be detected, and in some cases, true infections may be missed. Western blotting or PCR may be needed to resolve some of these issues. Treatment of seropositive asymptomatic dogs is therefore a controversial matter. Clinically healthy infected animals might serve as a reservoir for *E. canis*, although this risk can be overcome by more intensive vector control. Whether all subclinically infected animals will progress to the phase of chronic illness is uncertain. Some animals may never develop permanent immunity, and with reexposure in their environment, infection may recur. Indiscriminant treatment of all seropositive animals may theoretically lead to future resistance of these organisms to tetracyclines; however, such resistance has not been reported to date.

Immunoblotting

On a research basis, Western immunoblotting and PCR have been used to characterize and distinguish between infection with different organisms causing ehrlichiosis, anaplasmosis, or neorickettsiosis and may prove clinically helpful in the future.* The immunoblots for *E. canis* show a large number

*References 80, 128, 225, 248, 249, 260, 343, 437, 442, 580.

of reacting antigens, the most prominent being those separating in a broad band at 22 to 30 kDa.[225,343] A 30-kDa protein is the major antigen recognized by both naturally and experimentally infected dog sera.[380] The major antigenic protein 2, a 27-kDa protein was recently characterized and suggested to serve as a diagnostic tool for CME.[7,53] More recently, the 120-kDa protein (p 120) and the rP43 protein have been shown to be very specific for *E. canis* and may be a potential antigen for the serodiagnosis of canine ehrlichiosis.[348,570] Western immunoblotting will detect *E. canis* antibodies as early as 2 to 8 days after exposure, and PCR tests have positive results as early as 4 to 10 days after exposure to *E. canis* in experimental studies.[248,547] The indirect FA test also becomes positive within a similar time frame. From a practical clinical standpoint, the indirect FA test will continue to be the initial screening test of choice. Western immunoblotting has also been useful in distinguishing between infections with *E. canis* and *E. ewingii*.[442] This characteristic is beneficial because most dogs with *E. ewingii* infection will have positive indirect FA titers to *E. canis*. No indirect FA test is available for *E. ewingii*.

Organism Cultivation

Blood cultures may take up to 8 weeks to yield growth. This method is expensive, not routinely available, and is highly specific for the organism causing infection; however, it is considered a research tool.

Nucleic Acid Detection

PCR has been shown to be a sensitive method for detecting acute experimental *E. canis* infection in dogs,[160,349] often within 4 to 10 days postinoculation and before seroconversion occurs. The sensitivity of blood PCR in the naturally infected dog is not as clear. False negative results that will occur are caused by difficulties in extracting the organism, inherent problems in technique, and with inappropriate sample selection. The principal reason for false positive results is nonspecific amplification or sample contamination during handling or testing. Current laboratory techniques and reagents have not been standardized. Few reports have surfaced on the use of blood PCR for the initial diagnosis of naturally occurring canine ehrlichiosis, when the blood PCR result was compared with an indirect FA result. In one study, poor correlation between indirect FA titers and PCR results was noted.[497] In this study, only 13 of 49 (27%) had a positive blood-PCR result, while the indirect FA test results for antibody to *E. canis* were positive in all dogs. Poor correlation of blood-PCR results compared with indirect FA results was also found in a recent study in Tennessee, where 10 of 90 dogs had positive indirect FA test results and none were found to be blood-PCR positive.[464] This lack of correlation, which may indicate either insensitivity of the blood-PCR method or exposure with clearance of the organism, has also been reported in people with HGE.[27] In this study, convalescent indirect FA titers were more sensitive than blood-PCR for diagnostic confirmation of HGE. Insensitivity of blood-PCR is evident in that ehrlichial DNA could be amplified from the spleen, while it could not be amplified from corresponding blood specimens.[212] Appropriate selection of tissue or body fluid specimens is therefore important for a positive diagnosis by amplification of ehrlichial DNA. The sensitivity of blood-PCR for the initial confirmation of ehrlichial infections is not consistently high enough to recommend it as the only test for diagnosing ehrlichiosis. It should be used in conjunction with serology to detect acutely infected animals before seroconversion. PCR of splenic aspirates can be considered as a more sensitive alternative than blood-PCR, especially in follow-up treatment.[210a] With localized infections, assays on joint fluid, CSF, or aqueous humor might be more beneficial. In addition, as PCR becomes more refined, it may prove useful in distinguishing treated animals with persistent *E. canis* infection from those that retain persistent high indirect FA titers after successful treatment.[250,547] Other than organism cultivation, PCR is the most specific means of determining which rickettsial species is infecting an animal. Furthermore, primers can be constructed for genus-specific screening to minimize the number of specific reactions that must be performed. A real-time PCR assay has been developed for detecting *E. chaffeensis*.[316]

Pathologic Findings

Gross pathologic findings of *E. canis*–infected dogs include petechial and ecchymotic hemorrhages on the serosal and mucosal surfaces of most organs, including the nasal cavity, lung, kidney, urinary bladder, gastrointestinal (GI) tract, and subcutaneous tissue. Generalized lymphadenomegaly, splenomegaly, and hepatomegaly are present most often during the acute phase.[195,135] All lymph nodes may be enlarged and have a brownish discoloration. Emaciation with loss of overall body condition is an additional finding in chronic cases. Bone marrow is hypercellular and red in color in the acute phase but, with chronic disease, becomes hypoplastic and pale caused by fatty discoloration.

One of the more characteristic histopathologic findings is a perivascular plasma cell infiltrate in numerous organs, including the lungs, brain, meninges, kidneys, lymph nodes, bone marrow, spleen, and sometimes skin or mucosa. The degree of lymphoid and plasma cell infiltrates appears to increase in chronically affected dogs.[514] Ehrlichial organisms are difficult to detect histologically in tissues fixed in either formalin or Bouin's solution. Morulae are infrequently observed in mononuclear phagocytic cells of tissues stained with hematoxylin and eosin.[195] The difficulty with which organisms are found histologically may explain why the disease is not frequently diagnosed at necropsy.

In the CNS, a multifocal, nonsuppurative meningoencephalitis involving the brain stem, midbrain, and cerebral cortex is noted. Most lesions are located ventrally in the brain stem and around the periventricular gray and white matter.[514] Only a very mild encephalitis of the cerebellum occurs. Mild neuroparenchymal vascular cuffing and gliosis often accompany the meningitis in CME. The meningeal inflammatory cell infiltrate may be monocytic or lymphoplasmacytic, or both.[371,388] Microscopic meningeal lesions are present in nearly all dogs at necropsy, yet few dogs demonstrate clinical signs of meningitis.

Ocular signs have been reported to involve nearly every structure of the eye. These signs include conjunctivitis, conjunctival or iridal petechiae and ecchymoses, corneal edema, uveitis, and hyphema. Subretinal hemorrhage and retinal detachment may also occur. In a study, the eyes of dogs experimentally infected with *E. canis* were histologically examined.[388] Uveitis occurred in each of the dogs infected with the organism (see Fig. 93-13). The inflammatory infiltrate was predominately lymphocytic, monocytic, and plasmacytic. Ocular inflammation was most common in the ciliary body, becoming less intense in the choroid, iris, and retina, respectively.

Pulmonary changes in ehrlichiosis are consistent with interstitial pneumonia. Initially, subendothelial accumulation of mononuclear cells occurs, and interstitial and alveolar hemorrhages may be present. *E. canis* organisms may be found in septal mononuclear cells and macrophages of the pulmonary vascular endothelium.

Glomerulonephritis and interstitial plasmacytosis may occur in dogs with ehrlichiosis and may account for the proteinuria of some cases. Minimal histologic changes were noticed in the kidneys of dogs experimentally infected with *E. canis*. However, ultrastructural examination showed fusion of podocyte processes that coincided with the development of proteinuria.[114]

Therapy

Specific Drug Therapy

The treatment of canine ehrlichiosis consists of antirickettsial agents and supportive care. Efficacious drugs have included tetracyclines, chloramphenicol, imidocarb dipropionate, and amicarbalide (Table 28-4). Generally, the earlier treatment is initiated in the disease process, the more favorable the prognosis and outcome because dogs in the severe chronic stage are difficult to cure.[369a] In these dogs, multisystemic inflammatory changes and myelosuppression may be difficult to resolve.

Tetracycline and oxytetracycline have been considered the initial drugs of choice in the past and still work well, but doxycycline and minocycline are used more frequently now. Doxycycline and minocycline are semisynthetic, lipid-soluble tetracyclines that are readily absorbed to produce high blood, tissue, and intracellular concentrations. Given that ehrlichiae may persist intracellularly, drug penetration in the cell is important in eliminating infection. Therefore lipid-soluble tetracyclines can be given for shorter duration and at a lower dose than tetracycline and still be effective. The suggested duration of therapy with doxycycline is 7 to 10 days, although one study found that doxycycline (10 mg/kg daily) for 7 days was ineffective in eliminating experimentally induced *E. canis* infection from 3 to 5 dogs.[249] In other studies, doxycycline (5 mg/kg twice daily) used for 10 or 14 days was effective in eliminating experimentally induced *E. canis* from 8 of 8 and 13 of 13 acutely infected dogs, respectively.[72,73,370,373] Whether these shorter treatment times are adequate in naturally occurring cases is still in question. Some authors have found that even a 6-week course of doxycycline may not be sufficient to clear *E. canis* parasites from all subclinically infected dogs.[213] The standard length of therapy in natural infection is 21 to 28 days, and the Ehrlichial consensus statement from the American College of Veterinary Internal Medicine recommends a minimum of 10 mg/kg daily for 28 days.[372] The dosage regimens for tetracyclines and other drugs are summarized in Table 28-4.

Table • 28-4

Antimicrobial Therapy for Canine Monocytotropic Ehrlichiosis and Neorickettsiosis

DRUG[a]	DOSE[b] (mg/kg)	ROUTE PREFERRED (ALTERNATIVE)	INTERVAL[c] (HOURS)	DURATION[d] (DAYS)
Doxycycline	10	PO (IV)	12—24	28
Minocycline	10	PO (IV)	12	28
Tetracycline	22	PO	8	28
Oxytetracycline	25	PO (IV)	8	28
Chloramphenicol	15—25	PO (IV, SC)	8	28
Imidocarb dipropionate[e]	5	IM	Once	Repeat in 2—3 wks
Amicarbalide	5—6	IM	Once	Repeat in 2—3 wks

PO, By mouth; *IV*, intravenously; *SC*, subcutaneously; *IM*, intramuscularly.
[a]See Drug Formulary, Appendix 8, for additional information.
[b]Dose per administration at specified interval.
[c]Expressed in hours unless otherwise stated.
[d]For *E. canis* infection, current recommendations are for at least 28 days. Other monocytotropic rickettsiae may require shorter intervals.
[e]The effectiveness of imidocarb over doxycycline has been questioned.[372]

Dramatic clinical improvement generally occurs within 24 to 48 hours after initiation of tetracycline therapy in dogs with acute-phase or mild chronic–phase disease. The platelet count correspondingly begins to increase during this time and is usually in the normal range by 14 days after treatment. Recovery is not equated with permanent immunity, and dogs can become reinfected with *E. canis* after a previously effective treatment. Partial immunity does develop given that experimental reinfection with heterologous strains has caused more severe disease manifestations than those with homologous strains.[72] Intramuscular (IM) administration of long-acting repositol oxytetracycline can be considered when oral administration of drug is difficult because of GI or neurologic signs or when poor compliance of drug administration is anticipated.[273]

Chloramphenicol has been recommended for puppies younger than 5 months to avoid the yellow discoloration of erupting teeth from tetracyclines. However, doxycycline is less likely to produce this effect (see Drug Formulary, Appendix 8). Chloramphenicol should be used in dogs that have persistent infections despite therapy with tetracyclines.[514] However, because of the public health risks associated with chloramphenicol and because it directly interferes with heme and bone marrow synthesis, its administration in anemic or pancytopenic dogs should be avoided whenever possible.

Other antibacterial agents that are ineffective against monocytotropic *Ehrlichia* spp. in people are erythromycin, new macrolides (azithromycin, clarithromycin, and telithromycin), penicillins, and aminoglycosides. The efficacy of quinolones is variable according to the drug used and organism involved. *N. sennetsu* is susceptible to ciprofloxacin in vitro.[81] Enrofloxacin has been shown to be effective for the treatment of experimental RMSF in dogs (see Chapter 29).[71] In contrast, *E. chaffeensis* was resistant to ciprofloxacin but sensitive to doxycycline and rifampin in vitro.[82] In addition to doxycycline, rifampin, and fluoroquinolones have in vitro activity against *E. phagocytophilum*.[278] The effectiveness of enrofloxacin for treatment of experimentally induced *E. canis* infection has been evaluated.[370] At a dose of 5 mg/kg twice daily and 10 mg/kg orally (PO) twice daily for 21 days, 6 of 7 and 5 of 5 dogs, respectively, remained blood culture-positive and thrombocytopenic after each treatment regimen. Three of the latter five dogs had improved platelet counts at the end of enrofloxacin treatment, but all dogs had recurrence of thrombocytopenia 14 days after completion of enrofloxacin therapy. All 12 dogs were then treated with doxycycline (5 mg/kg twice daily, PO, for 10 days) and had culture negative blood results and platelet counts returned to normal. Based on these results, enrofloxacin would not appear to be effective against *E. canis*. Authors in another study treated six dogs with enrofloxacin (5 mg/kg once daily for 15 days) and found clinical and laboratory improvement in all six dogs on day 15 of the treatment period.[284] Whether the platelet counts would have dropped several weeks posttreatment is unknown. It is interesting to note that recently, the effectiveness of enrofloxacin against *E. canis*, or lack thereof, has been evaluated with an in vitro study that showed that the *E. canis* genogroup had a natural gyrase-mediated resistance to fluoroquinolones.[346]

Imidocarb, an antiprotozoal drug, has been successful in treating resistant *E. canis* infections (see also Chapter 71 and Drug Formulary, Appendix 8).[342] This drug persists in the tissues for up to 1 month following one dose. When imidocarb was given as a single IM injection, 83.9% of dogs with ehrlichiosis recovered. Apparently, the successful treatment of *E. canis* with imidocarb results from prolonged exposure of the organism to the drug, given that in vitro growth of *E. canis* is unaffected by short-term (3 days) exposure to apparently low or high levels of imidocarb.[267] Transient, dose-dependent side effects of imidocarb dipropionate include excessive salivation, serous nasal discharge, diarrhea, and dyspnea. These signs may be the result of an anticholinesterase effect. In a three-way comparison of the efficacy of doxycycline (10 mg/kg for 28 days) versus imidocarb dipropionate (5 mg/kg IM, twice, 2 to 3 weeks apart) versus doxycycline-imidocarb combination treatment (with the same dosage regimen) in naturally occurring ehrlichiosis, no statistically significant difference among treatment groups was found.[459] Approximately 93% to 94% of dogs were considered responders in this study regardless of which treatment group they were assigned. Based on these and other findings, the clinical effectiveness of imidocarb dipropionate over doxycycline has been questioned.[279] Amicarbalide is a closely related carbanilide that has been used to treat ehrlichiosis.

In addition to antimicrobial therapy, supportive therapy with fluids for dehydration or blood transfusions may be justified if the dog is severely anemic. Blood transfusions will not significantly increase platelet numbers; therefore platelet-rich plasma may be needed in an emergency situation. Data are lacking to support the use of growth factors such as erythropoietin (Epogen, Amgen, Thousand Oaks, Calif.) and granulocyte colony-stimulating factor (Neupogen, Amgen, Thousand Oaks, Calif.). However, results from a single case report suggest that they might be useful for treating severe chronic ehrlichiosis.[17] See Drug Formulary, Appendix 8 for more information on these drugs.

Short-term (2 to 7 days) therapy with immunosuppressive doses of glucocorticoids (2 mg/kg prednisolone) may be beneficial early in the treatment period when severe or life-threatening thrombocytopenia is present. An immune-mediated mechanism is partially responsible for the thrombocytopenia and decreased platelet function. The rationale for prednisone therapy has some scientific basis. Some clinicians prefer to use glucocorticoids and tetracycline in combination initially because of the difficulty in distinguishing between canine ehrlichiosis and immune-mediated thrombocytopenia and because of the lag time before serologic test results are available. When serologic testing will not be performed, using tetracyclines alone initially allows for a therapeutic diagnosis by clinical improvement in 24 to 48 hours. Glucocorticoids should not be excluded in these situations if the hemorrhage is life threatening because they help reduce the tendency for hemorrhage in various causes of primary thrombocytopenic disorders. Glucocorticoids may also be helpful in the treatment of other immune-mediated conditions associated with ehrlichiosis such as polyarthritis, vasculitis, and meningitis. In one dog with meningitis secondary to granulocytotropic ehrlichiosis, glucocorticoids were required in addition to doxycycline before clinical resolution of signs was achieved.[331]

Monitoring Therapy

Monitoring response to treatment of ehrlichial infections is important because some species can cause persistent infections. Resolution of thrombocytopenia is the most rapid development that may occur within a 7- to 10-day period following treatment. Because infection can recrudesce after treatment is stopped, platelet counts should be evaluated at least 1 to 3 months after treatment is discontinued. Changes in serum proteins caused by hyperglobulinemia can take up to 6 to 12 months to resolve. Specific *Ehrlichia* antibody titers of high magnitude are very difficult to follow because most laboratories report a maximum value rather than an endpoint dilution, and the decline of such high levels is often not linear with time. Some dogs have a resolution of all clinical and laboratory abnormalities; however, they may have a persistently high antibody titer. In these instances, evaluation of PCR, perhaps of a splenic aspirate, may be warranted. In some of these instances, as with other infectious diseases, serum antibody titers may remain increased after elimination of the organism; however, all clinical and laboratory abnormalities should resolve in drawing this conclusion. Dogs can also become reinfected after recovery, especially when they reside in highly endemic environments. Therefore proving elimination of infection following treatment can be difficult. If an animal does not show clinical improvement following recommended treatment regimens, then another or compounding cause of illness should be considered. Most dogs with ehrlichial infections show some resolution of clinical illness within 24 to 48 hours following institution of treatment, even if clinical laboratory parameters remain abnormal. Although experimentally infected dogs can be predictably cleared of infection with appropriate regimens, anecdotal concern exists that natural infections in some areas of the world are more resistant to therapy. In addition, in one instance in which dogs with various ehrlichial infections were treated, *E. chaffeensis* appeared to be more resistant to doxycycline.[74] Possibly, this apparent resistance to treatment may really involve reinfection under natural conditions in tick-infested environments.

Prevention

A vaccine is not currently available; therefore chemotherapy, chemoprophylaxis, and tick-control measures are the primary means of prevention. Compared with untreated dogs, seroconversion was reduced in dogs entering an area endemic for *E. canis* infection if they were treated with once monthly fipronil application.[124] For *E. canis* infections in kenneled dogs, tetracycline has been shown to be an effective prophylactic drug against initial infection or reinfection when administered PO at 6.6 mg/kg/day. Indiscriminant use of this drug to all dogs might theoretically lead to drug resistance.

Control in endemic areas can be accomplished by maintaining strict tick-control programs for dogs and premises, by using the indirect FA test to identify exposed and infected dogs, and by treating all infected dogs with the therapeutic regimen of tetracycline. All newly introduced animals into a kennel should be serotested, treated for ticks, and isolated until the results are available. When these measures fail, maintenance of all dogs (susceptible and successfully treated) on prophylactic levels of tetracycline may be the only recourse. If these guidelines are followed, the cycle of *E. canis* infection in the tick should be broken, because transovarian transmission of *E. canis* does not occur in the *Rhipicephalus* tick. Being a domiciled tick, and having the preference of all stages feeding on dogs, *R. sanguineus* is important in the maintenance of *E. canis* infections in kennel environments. Importation of *E. canis*–infected dogs or infected *R. sanguineus* ticks is a continual risk for countries such as the United Kingdom where canine ehrlichiosis is not endemic.[473] Precautions must be taken to screen incoming dogs for ehrlichiosis using serologic methods. For the other ehrlichial, anaplasmal, and neorickettsial species, outdoor ticks are potential sources of infection in conjunction with multiple, as yet unidentified wildlife reservoir hosts. Tick-control measures on the susceptible dog are the only solution.

Public Health Considerations

Before 1986, the only ehrlichial species recognized as infecting people was *N. sennetsu* (see Table 28-1). This agent, first isolated in Japan, is responsible for a mild mononucleosis-like syndrome. Two new ehrlichial agents have since been reported to cause disease in people in the United States. The first is *E. chaffeensis*, the causative agent for HME,[12,462,483] which is exhibited as an acute influenza-like illness characterized by fever, headache, malaise, and sometimes death in severely affected people. *E. chaffeensis* is closely related to *E. canis*, and although dogs can be experimentally infected, they do not develop clinical disease.[129] Natural infections in dogs may develop a different course (see previous discussion on Clinical Signs). HME, which is predominant in the south-central and southeastern United States, likely involves a sylvan cycle in nature, with deer or rodents, or both, as reservoir hosts, and *A. americanum* (or possibly *D. variabilis*) being the most likely vectors. Although wildlife reservoirs are most important, dogs might be carriers of *E. chaffeensis* in endemic geographic regions. Dogs may be involved in transporting ticks in closer proximity to people, and the role of handling ticks or their excretions or body fluids might be a possible risk. See later discussion for further information on zoonotic aspects of *Anaplasma* infections. In addition, the Venezuelan human ehrlichiosis agent has been suggested to be a variant of or a subspecies of *E. canis* transmitted by *R. sanguineus* ticks.[371,518] Therefore, in South America, dogs may serve as a reservoir for Venezuelan human ehrlichiosis, and *R. sanguineus* may serve as the vector. The potential risk of transmission of ehrlichiosis to dogs via blood transfusions has been known for years, and this is also becoming an increasing concern in human transplantation medicine.*

*References 306, 353, 452, 453, 504.

CANINE GRANULOCYTOTROPIC EHRLICHIOSIS (*E. EWINGII* INFECTION)

Barbara Greig, Edward B. Breitschwerdt, and P. Jane Armstrong

Etiology and Epidemiology

E. ewingii is the causative agent of one of a pair of zoonotic diseases that have each previously been given the name "granulocytic (meaning, granulocytotropic) ehrlichiosis" (GE). In mammalian hosts, morulae of *E. ewingii* can be seen in peripheral blood neutrophils, eosinophils, and rarely monocytes, and in neutrophils in synovial fluid.[86,185,385,488]

When canine *E. ewingii*–GE was first described in 1971, the etiologic agent was believed to be a granulocytic form of *E. canis*.[163] In 1992, after amplifying and sequencing the bacterial 16S rRNA gene from the blood of a dog with GE, *E. ewingii* was identified as a distinct species, separate from, but closely related to *E. canis* and *E. chaffeensis*.[13] The 16S rRNA genes of all bacteria of the genus *Ehrlichia* are at least 97.7% homologous (i.e., nearly 98% of the 1400 nucleotides are identical). *E. ewingii* is 98.0% similar to *E. canis* and 98.1% similar to *E. chaffeensis*.[13,146]

To date, *E. ewingii* infection has been found only in the United States and almost exclusively in the southern and southeastern sections, except for one case of an infected dog from New York state that had traveled multiple times to Boston but had not visited southern or southeastern sections.* Disease attributed to this organism has been reported in domestic and wild canids and people.† *E. ewingii* infection has been diagnosed in dogs from Missouri, Arkansas, Oklahoma, Tennessee, Virginia, North Carolina, Mississippi, and New York.[185,187,488,563] Human cases have been diagnosed in Missouri, Oklahoma, and Tennessee.[86,385] The only tick proven to be a competent vector of *E. ewingii* is the ixodid tick, *A. americanum*, the Lone Star tick. In an experimental study, *A. americanum* successfully transmitted *E. ewingii* transstadially between dogs, while *D. variabilis* did not succeed.[16] However, *E. ewingii* DNA has been found in field-collected *A. americanum*, *D. variabilis*, and *R. sanguineus* ticks from Oklahoma.[368] No published report has been produced of successful transmission using *R. sanguineus* or *Ixodes scapularis*. In North Carolina, *E. ewingii* DNA has been found in field-collected *A. americanum* ticks, but not *D. variabilis* or *I. scapularis* ticks.[556] *E. ewingii*-PCR-positive–*A. americanum* ticks have also been found in Arkansas, Georgia, Kentucky, and South Carolina.[556] *A. americanum* is commonly found throughout much of the southeastern United States, including Texas, Oklahoma, Arkansas, Missouri, and the Atlantic coast states. White-tailed deer are an important reservoir for *E. ewingii*.[563]

Pathogenesis

E. ewingii reside within phagosomes in vertebrate leukocytes after they have been internalized via endocytosis.[406] Within the phagosome they evade phagosome-lysosome fusion by an unknown mechanism. After intracellular invasion, ehrlichiae proceed to replicate for 2 to 3 days by binary fission. Replication within the vacuole can produce up to 50 organisms,[406] forming the classic morula ("mulberries") seen with light microscopy, a hallmark of acute ehrlichial infections (Fig. 28-8). Host cell mitochondria and endoplasmic reticulum aggregate around the ehrlichial-laden phagosome, and these organelles tend to remain in close contact with the morulae.[406] The phagosomal membrane and the host cell plasma membrane eventually rupture, releasing organisms into circulation to infect new cells. Incubation for ehrlichial diseases is 1 to 2 weeks.[488] The actual length of feeding time required for ticks

*References 13, 86, 185, 187, 286, 368, 385, 488, 563.
†References 86, 185, 187, 385, 488.

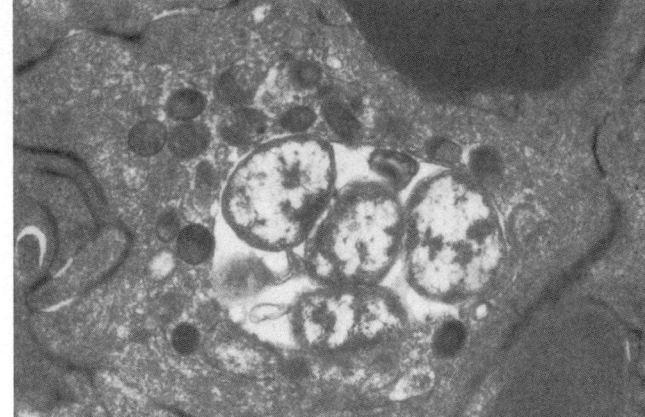

Fig 28-8 Ultrastructure of *E. canis* morula in a monocyte showing a "mulberry appearance" because the intracytoplasmic inclusion is made up of numerous organisms.

to transmit ehrlichial agents to a susceptible mammalian host is unknown. In mammals, ehrlichial organisms tend to be most abundant in tissues of the mononuclear-phagocyte system (bone marrow, spleen, liver, and lymph node),[142] but the mechanisms by which the organisms cause disease are poorly understood.

Clinical Findings

Disease caused by *E. ewingii* was originally described as an acute polyarthritis syndrome.[488] Although polyarthritis is a common feature of *E. ewingii* infection,[185,187,488] dogs may have nonspecific signs of illness, including fever, depression, and lethargy (see Table 28-2).[185,187] Dogs having neurologic manifestations frequently display ataxia, paresis, proprioceptive deficits, anisocoria, intention tremors, or vestibular dysfunction.[187] Vomiting and diarrhea have been reported infrequently.[185,187] Clinical and hematologic abnormalities found with *E. ewingii* and *E. canis* infections are often similar, but clinical disease caused by *E. ewingii* appears to be milder than that of *E. canis*. To date, no reported canine or human deaths have been attributed to *E. ewingii*.* *E. ewingii* infection has also been documented in clinically healthy dogs, presumably reflecting chronic subclinical ehrlichemia.[187] Dogs with immune-mediated, inflammatory, endocrine, or other diseases have been diagnosed with concurrent *E. ewingii* asymptomatic infection or clinical disease.[185,187]

Diagnosis

E. ewingii causes a seasonal and regional disease that depends on the activity and geographic range of its tick vector, *A. americanum*. These ticks are active feeders (i.e., are actively seeking hosts) from spring to late autumn. Large tick populations have been found in forested areas frequented by deer. Acute disease caused by *E. ewingii* is less likely to be seen during the winter because disease incubation is 1 to 2 weeks following a tick bite; however, chronic asymptomatic canine infections have been documented in winter months.[187] In addition, weather does influence tick activity (i.e., long warm autumn months may result in cases being diagnosed into the winter months). Travel histories are important to identify dogs that have recently traveled to, but do not live in, *A. americanum*–endemic regions. *E. ewingii* infection should be high on a disease differential list for dogs in southern, southeastern, and Atlantic coastal states of the United States that have acute fever, lameness, or neurologic abnormalities in the spring through autumn. History, clinical signs, hematologic findings,

*References 86, 185, 187, 385, 488.

presence of morulae in granulocytes of blood or synovial fluid, and serologic findings can all be used to help make a presumptive diagnosis of *E. ewingii* infection, but definitive diagnosis currently relies on microbial DNA analysis via PCR.

Clinical Laboratory Findings

The only consistent hematologic abnormality is mild-to-moderate thrombocytopenia with or without large platelets.[185,187,488] Normochromic normocytic nonregenerative anemia may be present.[185,187,488] Neutrophil and lymphocyte counts vary and reactive lymphocytes are frequently present.[187,488] Ehrlichial morulae have been seen in 1% to 26% of neutrophils and occasional eosinophils of peripheral blood.[86,385,488] In experimental *E. ewingii* infections, ehrlichial morulae are evident in circulation for up to 6 days maximum[16]; therefore the lack of morulae in circulating granulocytes does not preclude a diagnosis of *E ewingii* infection. Dogs treated with glucocorticoids for thrombocytopenia, immune-mediated anemia, or polyarthritis are more likely to have morulae present in neutrophils of peripheral blood.[187] No consistent serum chemistry abnormalities have been associated with *E. ewingii* infection. Mild increases in serum ALP or ALT activities are present in less than one half of dogs diagnosed with *E. ewingii* infection.[185,187] *E. ewingii* infection frequently causes neutrophilic polysynovitis in dogs.[185,187,488] The synovial fluid from dogs with polyarthritis should be examined for neutrophils containing morulae. Morulae are found in 1% to 7% of neutrophils from affected joints.[185]

Serologic Testing

No specific serologic test has been produced for *E. ewingii* because this organism has yet to be cultivated in vitro. Because bacteria within the genus *Ehrlichia* are closely related, polyclonal antibodies to one species within the genus frequently cross-react to antigens of the other species within the genus (see Table 28-3).[202] *E. canis* indirect FA is recommended as a preliminary screening tool for *E. ewingii* infection.[185,187,488] As with most infectious diseases, the usefulness of serologic testing relies on acute to convalescent seroconversion to diagnose active ehrlichial disease. Because no serologic test is specific for *E. ewingii*, *E. canis* seroconversion in dogs simply indicates potential infection with *E. canis*, *E. ewingii*, or *E. chaffeensis*. Sera from *E. ewingii*–infected dogs also occasionally display low-level indirect FA cross-reactivity to *A. phagocytophilum* antigens.[142]

Serologic cross-reactivity is caused by cross-reactive immunodominant surface proteins that are of similar molecular size, particularly those of the family of immunodominant outer membrane proteins of 27 to 32 kDa present in *E. canis*, *E. ewingii*, *E. chaffeensis*, *E. ruminatum*, and *E. muris* (see Table 28-3).[202] Additionally, a similar family of proteins in *A. phagocytophilum* are likely responsible for the occasional low-grade serologic cross-reactivity between *E. ewingii* or *E. canis* and *A. phagocytophilum*.[577] Because *E. canis* and *E. chaffeensis* can be cultivated in vitro, expressed recombinant *E. canis* and *E. chaffeensis* genes of this family are used to make Western and dot blot immunoassays for species-specific serodiagnosis; monoclonal antibodies made to expressed proteins usually do not cross-react with the related proteins of another species.[80] Positive *E. canis*–indirect FA seroconversion can be followed up by *E. canis*-specific and *E. chaffeensis*-specific Western blot or dot blot assays to confirm infections with one of these two agents. However, because of the possibility that dogs can be co-infected with two or more of these ehrlichial species, *E. ewingii*-PCR may be necessary to determine if *E. ewingii* infection is present. Species differentiation among these organisms is of greater academic and zoonotic importance than of clinical relevance to the infected dog. Therapy for all three of these agents is identical, as well as all identified members of genera *Ehrlichia* and *Anaplasma*, is the same: all of these agents are susceptible to doxycycline.

Nucleic Acid Detection

PCR assays that amplify 16S rRNA, groESL, and p28 genes specific for *E. ewingii* have been developed.[13,202] PCR testing of blood using 16S rRNA was used to identify *E. ewingii* infected symptomatic and nonsymptomatic naturally infected dogs in Missouri.[305] A single positive PCR test implies active infection. Commercial veterinary 16S rRNA PCR assays are available from a small number of diagnostic laboratories (see Appendix 6). Optimally, ethylenediaminetetraacetic acid (EDTA)-anticoagulated peripheral blood, obtained before antibiotic administration, should be submitted for PCR testing.

Organism Cultivation

Currently, this diagnostic method is not available because cell lines that can support *E. ewingii* growth in vitro have not been identified.

Pathologic Findings

E. ewingii infection is not considered a life-threatening disease in dogs or people. No postmortem or surgical biopsy findings have been published.

Therapy

The tetracyclines are almost exclusively recommended for treating canine ehrlichial diseases (Table 28-5). Tetracycline (22 mg/kg, PO, every 8 hours for 14 to 21 days) or doxycycline (5 to 10 mg/kg, PO, every 12 to 24 hours for 10 days)

Table • 28-5

Antimicrobial Therapy for Canine Granulocytotropic Ehrlichiosis and Anaplasmosis

DRUG[a]	DOSE[b] (mg/kg)	ROUTE PREFERRED (ALTERNATIVE)	INTERVAL (HOURS)	DURATION[c] (DAYS)
Tetracycline	22	PO	8	14—21
Doxycycline	5—10	PO (IV)	12—24	10
Minocycline	10	PO (IV)	12	10
Chloramphenicol	15—25	PO (IV, SC)	8	14—21

PO, Orally; *IV*, intravenously; *SC*, subcutaneously.
[a]See Drug Formulary, Appendix 8, for additional information.
[b]Dose per administration at specified interval.
[c]For *E. canis* infection, current recommendations are for at least 28 days; however, shorter intervals are effective with other rickettsiae.

is the recommended treatment protocol. Minocycline has been substituted at an equivalent dose. For puppies younger than 1 year, chloramphenicol has been recommended to avoid yellowing of teeth (Table 28-5).[371] No proof has been produced that long-term treatment beyond the recommended intervals is beneficial for *E. ewingii* infection. Although evidence for persistent *E. canis* infection exists, despite treatment, persistent *E. ewingii* infection has not been documented.[371] Dogs exhibiting acute polyarthritis respond rapidly to treatment and frequently are clinically normal 24 to 48 hours after initiation of therapy.[185,488] Dogs with other clinical signs or with concurrent diseases may require weeks of therapy for complete resolution of clinical or laboratory abnormalities.[185] Concurrent illnesses should be treated appropriately. If response to tetracycline antibiotics is poor, the probability that the dog has a concurrent disease is high.

Prevention

At present, no vaccine is available to prevent *E. ewingii* infection or any other ehrlichial infection. Prevention relies on (1) avoiding exposure to the tick vector, *A. americanum*, during its active feeding season, spring through fall; (2) using antiacaricides; or (3) administering prophylactic tetracycline–doxycycline when visiting *A. americanum* tick–endemic regions.

Public Health Considerations

Human *E. ewingii* GE was first reported in 1999 in four male residents of Missouri.[86] Since then, the disease has been diagnosed in people from Tennessee and Oklahoma.[385] Most patients have been male and most have been immunocompromised.[86,385] Human *E. ewingii* GE cannot be distinguished clinically from monocytotropic ehrlichiosis caused by *E. chaffeensis* or GE caused by *A. phagocytophilum*.[86,385] The most consistent physical examination and laboratory findings in human *E. ewingii* infections are fever, headache, malaise, leukopenia, and thrombocytopenia.[86,385] Peripheral blood neutrophils containing morulae were found in only one half of reported cases.[86,385] Diagnosis relies on *E. ewingii*–specific PCR.[86,385] The potential for dogs to be a zoonotic risk factor for human *E. ewingii* infection is not known. Both dogs and people are likely incidental hosts for this infection.

CANINE GRANULOCYTOTROPIC ANAPLASMOSIS (*A. PHAGOCYTOPHILUM* INFECTION)

Barbara Greig and P. Jane Armstrong

Etiology and Epidemiology

A. phagocytophilum is the causative agent of one of a pair of tick-transmitted zoonotic diseases that have each previously been given the name "granulocytotropic ehrlichiosis" (see Table 28-1). See previous discussion on Canine Granulocytotropic Infection. The term *granulocytotropic ehrlichiosis* is now a misnomer for *A. phagocytophilum* infections because the causative agent has been removed from the genus *Ehrlichia* and placed into the genus *Anaplasma* (see previous discussion, introduction of chapter).[146] The disease caused by *A. phagocytophilum* is appropriately termed *canine granulocytotropic anaplasmosis*.

Bacteria of the family *Anaplasmataceae* are gram-negative, nonmotile, coccoid to ellipsoid organisms, varying in size from 0.2 to 2.0 μm diameter. They are obligate aerobes, lacking a glycolytic pathway, and all are obligate intracellular parasites. All species in the genus *Anaplasma* inhabit membrane-lined vacuoles in immature or mature hematopoietic cells of mammalian hosts.[146] *A. phagocytophilum* infects neutrophils and the term *granulocytotropic* refers to infected neutrophils. Rarely, organisms have been found in eosinophils.

The geographic distribution of the disease in people and domestic animals worldwide follows that of its *Ixodes* spp. vectors that feed on larger mammals. As a result of a common vector, the distribution of this disease follows that caused by *Borrelia burgdorferi sensu lato* (see Fig. 45-2,*B*). Co-infections with these two organisms are common among these ticks, and an onset of illness within 20 days following exposure to these ticks is more likely caused by *A. phagocytophilum* rather than *B. burgdorferi*, which has a longer incubation period of up to 60 to 90 days. Although these ticks are co-infected, their reservoir hosts and maintenance cycles in nature are likely different. Studies comparing larval and nymphal ticks have shown markedly different carriage rates of the two organisms in a given geographic region.[290,301] In North America, *A. phagocytophilum* is found in upper midwestern and northeastern regions of the United States, and the western coastal regions from California to British Columbia. In South America, a single *A. phagocytophilum*-PCR-positive dog has been found in Venezuela.[496] In the European region, reports have been from the United Kingdom, Norway, Sweden, Switzerland, Germany, Netherlands, and Slovenia.* In Korea, *A. phagocytophilum* has been genetically detected in *I. persulcatus* and *Haemaphysalis longicornis* ticks that were field collected or found on domestic animals.[274] Additionally in Asia, an *A. phagocytophilum*-PCR-positive dog has been identified in Thailand, and PCR-positive *I. persulcatus* ticks have been identified in western Siberia, Russia[497,360]; the disease potential of these organisms is uncertain. In upper midwestern and northeastern United States, human and canine disease caused by *A. phagocytophilum* is diagnosed in spring to early summer and again in the fall; few cases are diagnosed midsummer and in the winter months.[26,29,197] In Sweden, canine cases have been diagnosed midsummer through autumn.[158] The seasonality and the geographic distribution of *A. phagocytophilum* infections are determined by the feeding habits and ranges of its particular tick vectors. Several ixodid ticks of the genus *Ixodes* are vectors of *A. phagocytophilum*. *I. scapularis* is the vector in upper midwestern and northeastern United States; *I. pacificus* is the vector in California and British Columbia; and *I. ricinus* is the vector in Europe and the United Kingdom.† *Ixodes* ticks are three-host ticks. Because *A. phagocytophilum* is transferred transstadially only between ticks, only nymph and adult stages are potential disease carriers.[146] A significant number of small mammals and deer have been implicated as natural reservoirs of *A. phagocytophilum*. In the United States, the white-footed mouse, eastern chipmunk, dusky-footed wood rat, southern red-backed vole, and white-tailed deer are all considered reservoirs.[57,387,482,531] In Europe, the bank vole, wood mouse, yellow-necked mouse, common shrew, and roe and red deer are likely natural reservoirs.[312,400] In addition to terrestrial mammals, birds may be important in the geographic distribution or spread of infection. Larval *I. ricinus* feeding on migratory birds in Sweden have been shown to be infected with *A. phagocytophilum*.[61] These birds have wintering grounds in continental Europe and Africa. Similarly, birds in North America have been infected, and evidence suggests that, in addition to spreading infection, they also can act as reservoirs by transmitting infection to tick larvae that co-feed with infected nymphs.[120]

Although tick-transmission is the predominant means of infection, perinatal transmission has been documented in people[232] and transplacental infection has been documented

---

*References 44, 260, 197, 494, 565.
†References 35, 36, 111, 138, 164, 197, 258, 312, 328, 387, 402, 421, 436, 508, 525, 565.

in cows.[413] Infections with these organisms can cause abortions in cows and sheep, and the organism has been found in milk from infected cows; therefore the risk of spread of these infections directly to newborns should be considered.

A. phagocytophilum sensu lato causes infection and potential clinical illness in domestic dogs; horses; in European cattle, sheep, and goats; and in llamas, cats, and people.* Within this newly combined species, *A. phagocytophilum*, the strains derived from *E. phagocytophila*, *E. equi*, and HGE agent display genetic and biologic differences. Disease caused by the *E. phagocytophila* strain was the first ever described "granulocytic ehrlichial disease" in 1932 in Scottish sheep.[189] Not until 1969 was equine *E. equi*–"granulocytic ehrlichiosis" reported in horses from California.[321] *E. phagocytophila* and *E. equi* were originally determined to be separate species based on ultrastructural morphology and phenotypic expression, the previously established tools for microbial phylogenetic classification. In the early 1990s, 16S rRNA gene sequencing became available for microbial phylogenetic classification. This process coincided with the emergence of HGE in 1990 in Minnesota and Wisconsin patients. When a 1433 nucleotide sequence of the 16S rRNA genes of the HGE agent, *E. phagocytophila*, and *E. equi* were compared, these three agents were found to be very closely related but not genetically identical. The 1433 nucleotide sequence differs by two nucleotides between *E. phagocytophila* and *E. equi* and by two and three nucleotides between the agent of HGE and *E. phagocytophila* and *E. equi*, respectively.[108,146,197] Because of the speculation that these three differently named agents actually were of the same species, the causative agent of HGE was not initially given a species designation but was simply called "the human granulocytic ehrlichiosis agent." In 2001, when the order Rickettsiales was reorganized, the HGE agent was brought together with *E. phagocytophila* and *E. equi* into the single *A. phagocytophilum* species (see previous discussion, introduction to chapter).[146]

Despite their genetic similarities, the three strains of *A. phagocytophilum* are dissimilar in the mammalian species in which they cause disease and in their geographic distributions (see Table 28-1). The *E. phagocytophila* strain causes disease only in domestic ruminants of many European countries (Sweden, Norway, Finland, Great Britain, Ireland, Holland, Switzerland, France, Austria, Germany, and Spain).† No strain of *A. phagocytophilum* has ever been isolated from domestic or wild North American ruminants. All European isolates from people, dogs, and cats are of the HGE strain.[62,158,401,418] All United States isolates from dogs and cats are of the HGE strain, and all human isolates are identical to the HGE strain, except for isolates from several patients in California that differ by one nucleotide base.‡ All equine isolates from midwestern and northeastern United States are of the HGE strain, but horses from California have either the *E. equi* strain or the HGE strain with one nucleotide difference.§ Cattle and sheep do not become ill when infected with the HGE strain, but they do seroconvert.[411,425] Experimental *E. phagocytophila*–strain infection in horses and *E. equi*–strain infection in cattle produce asymptomatic infections with seroconversion that provide cross-protection against subsequent infections with *E. equi*–strain and *E. phagocytophila*–strain, respectively.[411,425] Experimental cross-infections have shown the strong antigenic relatedness among these three strains.

In addition to the previously mentioned genetic and biologic differences, other less well-defined genetic variations of *A. phagocytophilum* have been revealed. Sequence analyses of the ankyrin gene from various animal and human isolates have identified conserved genetic sequences that differ between isolates from different regions in the United States and between isolates from the United States and from Europe.[337,524] Clinicians have isolated 16S rRNA HGE-strain variants from ticks and deer but none have been found in dogs or people. The potential pathogenicity of these variants is not known.[57,336,329] A variety of minor nucleotide differences in the *E. phagocytophila*–strain 16S rRNA gene have been identified between different Norwegian sheep isolates from the same flock and between isolates from different flocks; and these differences are associated with discordant serologic responses.[494] Antigenic diversity among *A. phagocytophilum* isolates exists also, denoted by the occurrence of variable serologic reactions to isolate-specific *A. phagocytophilum* immunoblot assays among sera from infected animals of different geographic regions.[22] The investigation to identify additional genetic and phenotypic variations and to determine their significance is ongoing.

Although genetic and phenotypic differences do exist among the *E. phagocytophila*, *E. equi*, and HGE strains, all three share 99.1% 16S rRNA gene sequence homology and display strong antigenic serologic cross-reactivity.[146] By comparison, *A. phagocytophilum* has only 94.1% 16S rRNA gene sequence homology with any species in the newly organized *Ehrlichia* genus, and serologic cross-reactivity between *A. phagocytophilum* and *E. canis*, *E. chaffeensis*, and *E. ewingii* is uncommon to rare.[146]

The first published report of canine *A. phagocytophilum* infection came from Sweden in 1995, but cases were likely seen in Sweden as early as 1989.[256] *A. phagocytophilum* was identified in Minnesota and Wisconsin dogs in 1990, simultaneous with the discovery of human infections in Minnesota and Wisconsin.[26,197] Canine *A. phagocytophilum* infection has been reported in dogs from Minnesota, Wisconsin, Rhode Island, California, Sweden, Switzerland, and Slovenia. HGE caused by *A. phagocytophilum* has been identified in Minnesota, Wisconsin, New York, Massachusetts, Connecticut, California, Slovenia, Sweden, Norway, Netherlands, and Switzerland.*

Pathogenesis

A minimum feeding time of 24 hours and up to 48 hours or more is required for *Ixodes* spp. ticks to transmit *A. phagocytophilum* to susceptible mammalian hosts.[138,263] Disease incubation following a tick bite is 1 to 2 weeks. The average disease incubation period for horses in experimental tick-transmission of *A. phagocytophilum* is 10.5 days.[421] In vitro, *A. phagocytophilum* infects both granulocytic and monocytic bone marrow progenitor cells, but the more differentiated cells of the neutrophil lineage are most susceptible to infection.[275] P-selectin ligand-1 is one known neutrophil surface receptor for *A. phagocytophilum*; this cell surface glycoprotein is rich on the surface of neutrophils.[205,275] After binding to the cell surface receptor, *A. phagocytophilum* bacteria enter neutrophils via endocytosis and are incorporated into phagosomes. The organisms prevent phago-lysosome fusion, block the cellular oxidative respiratory burst activity of the nicotinamide adenine dinucleotide phosphate (NADPH) oxidase enzyme complex, and inhibit cellular apoptosis.[30,176,363,540] By these mechanisms, *A. phagocytophilum* bacteria prevent their destruction by cells designed to kill microbes. Inside the phagosome, the bacteria proceed to multiply by binary fission. Replication produces twenty or more organisms, forming the classic "morula" (mulberry) seen with light microscopy, a hallmark of ehrlichial diseases (see Fig. 28-7).[406] The bacteria-laden phagosome and the host cell plasma membrane eventually rupture, releasing

---

*References 2, 26, 35, 37, 58, 158, 160, 189, 197, 494.
†References 189, 258, 412, 413, 425, 494.
‡References 26, 171, 197, 235, 566.
§References 35, 87, 171, 256, 320, 421.

*References 2, 26, 56, 58, 145, 167, 176, 197, 231, 401, 509.

organisms to infect new cells. Cells infected with *A. phagocytophilum* are found in neutrophils in peripheral blood and in tissues of the mononuclear phagocytic system (spleen, liver, and bone marrow).[146,155,157]

Exactly how *A. phagocytophilum* causes disease remains unknown. The cytokine alterations in the host are not typical in that the organism does not possess endotoxin, and the classic proinflammatory cytokines, interleukin (IL)-1, IL-6, or tumor-necrosis factor-α are not released by infected cells. Other mechanisms have been found to cause thrombocytopenia, leukopenia, and anemia in infected hosts. In vitro, *A. phagocytophilum*–infected neutrophils stimulate increased production of IL-8 and other cytokines (MIP-1α, MIP-1β, MCP-1, and RANTES). MIP-1α, MIP-1β and IL-8 inhibit hematopoiesis in vitro.[275,276] IL-8 is chemotactic to neutrophils and naïve T lymphocytes, enhances phagocytosis, enhances the neutrophil cellular respiratory burst activity, and enhances angiogenesis.[63,85] MIP-1α and MIP-1β are chemoattractant to monocytes, macrophages, and T lymphocytes.[63,85] MCP-1 and RANTES activate monocytes, macrophages, and T lymphocytes.[63,85] The production of these leukocyte attractants, which are also capable of suppressing hematopoiesis, results in myelosuppression. Thrombocytopenia may be compounded by additional mechanisms. In a mouse model of *A. phagocytophilum*–induced thrombocytopenia, immune-mediated splenic removal and decreased platelet production were shown to be unlikely mechanisms for the thrombocytopenia that occurs in acute infection.[64] Increased production of monocyte tissue procoagulant activity in peripheral blood mononuclear cells has been documented in vitro.[52] Therefore increased coagulatory consumption of platelets is suspected. Serum levels of IFN-γ rise early in *A. phagocytophilum* infections, during the initial 8 to 10 days.[4] This increase in IFN-γ appears to be important for early control of the degree of bacteremia.[4] After the initial 8 to 10 days of infection, cellular and humoral immunity is believed to be responsible for infection control.[4,334]

Sheep infected with *E. phagocytophila* strains are predisposed to opportunistic and secondary infections that can be fatal.[494] No canine deaths have been associated with *A. phagocytophilum* infection.[158,196,197] Human deaths have occurred but were attributed to opportunistic infections or concurrent immunocompromising diseases.[26]

Clinical Findings
Natural Infection
All reported natural cases of canine *A. phagocytophilum* infection were identified by finding morulae in circulating neutrophils.[158,196,197] In each published study of natural cases, *A. phagocytophilum* infection was confirmed by the sequencing of the microbial 16S rRNA gene from only a proportion of the dogs. The other genetically unconfirmed canine cases came from *A. phagocytophilum*–endemic regions that were outside the range of *E. ewingii* or its vector tick, *A. americanum*, and infection with *A. phagocytophilum* had been presumed.[158,196,197] Reported clinical findings are almost exclusively from acute disease, during the bacteremic phase. Chronic *A. phagocytophilum* natural disease has not been documented, although at least one Swedish dog was ill for 30 days before the diagnosis was made.[158] Given that the dog is an unnatural host for this infection, self-limiting infection would be expected.

No sex predisposition for canine *A. phagocytophilum* infections has been found.[158,196,197] Although breed predilection may be established in the future, documented cases are currently too few to draw any conclusions. Of 178 Minnesota and Wisconsin dogs with *A. phagocytophilum* infection, 28% have been Labrador retrievers, 18% golden retrievers, 14% mixed breed, 9% cocker spaniel, 6% Samoyed, 4% shih tzu, 3% Brit-

tany spaniel, 3% chow-chow, and 3% springer spaniel. Of these 178 dogs, there were two Doberman pinschers, two Vizslas, two Pomeranians, two pugs, and one each of 11 other breeds.[196,197] Of the 14 Swedish dogs reported to have *A. phagocytophilum* infections, six were golden retrievers, two Samoyed, and one each of six other breeds.[158] Golden and Labrador retrievers are very popular dogs, and the high number of infections in these two breeds may represent only their popularity.

Age may be a susceptibility factor for *A. phagocytophilum* infection. Thirty-seven percent of Minnesota and Wisconsin dogs diagnosed with *A. phagocytophilum* infection were age 8 to 10 years; 56% were at least age 8 years.[196,197] One-third of reported cases of Swedish canine infections were over 9 years of age.[158] Only 3% of Minnesota and Wisconsin dogs were less than 1 year, and no Swedish cases were less than 1 year.[158,196,197] Of interest, human patients tend to be in their fifth and sixth decades, and infection is rare in children.[26,28,56] The canine age data need to be compared with canine population demographics before conclusions can be made about age-related susceptibility.

The majority of dogs with *A. phagocytophilum* infections have nonspecific signs of illness (see Table 28-2). Fever (at or above 39.2° C [102.6° F]), lethargy or depression, and anorexia are the most consistent findings, occurring in over 75% of dogs.* Musculoskeletal pain or discomfort is evident in over one half of dogs, characterized by reluctance to move, stiffness, weakness, soreness, and lameness.[158,196,197] Fewer than 10% of dogs display overt joint pain.[158,196,197] Neutrophilic synovitis was documented in one Minnesota dog at the same time the dog had circulating morulae in neutrophils; the dog had positive *E. equi* and *Borrelia burdorferi* (Lyme) indirect FA results and a negative *E. canis* indirect FA result (no convalescent sample was tested).[196] These results indicate that dogs infected with *A. phagocytophilum* may exhibit inflammatory arthritis. A low number of dogs have vomiting or diarrhea (or both) or respiratory signs of coughing or labored breathing.[158,196,197,418] Dogs may also exhibit lymphadenomegaly, splenomegaly, hepatomegaly, and CNS signs (seizures, ataxia, and so forth).† Unlike manifestations associated with *E. canis* or *A. platys*, dogs do not show signs of a bleeding disorder. Concurrent diagnoses of malignant lymphoma, phosphofructokinase deficiency, systemic lupus erythematosus, cardiomyopathy, and epilepsy have been documented, but major concurrent systemic diseases are unusual.[197,418]

Dogs appear to be susceptible to reinfection with *A. phagocytophilum*. Individual dogs have been diagnosed as having *A. phagocytophilum* infections twice, with 5 months or more of disease-free intervals occurring between documented infections.[158,196] Serum antibody levels in treated dogs revert to low or negative levels by 7 to 8 months posttreatment, which would likely leave them susceptible to reinfection.[158]

Experimental Infection
Experimental canine *A. phagocytophilum* infections have been carried out in Sweden. All dogs were infected with Swedish isolates of *A. phagocytophilum*. All infected dogs developed fevers, and some became depressed and anorectic for several days; one dog displayed lameness and one displayed staggering.[155,157,307] In one study, spontaneously recovered dogs were administered glucocorticoids at immunosuppressive dosages at least 1 month after they had recovered from clinical illness and had eliminated bacteria from circulation, as evidenced by lack of circulating morulae and negative *A. phagocytophilum*

---

*References 158, 196, 197, 418, 512.
†References 158, 194, 196, 197, 331.

PCR. Following immunosuppression, the dogs became bacteremic again, although all remained asymptomatic for disease. This condition was seen even when immunosuppression occurred 6 months after initial infection.[157] This study reveals that dogs have the potential to become chronic asymptomatic carriers, which has significance because of recrudescence of latent infection, as well as the potential for disease transmission. Whether treated dogs also remain subclinical carriers is unknown. Chronic experimental canine *A. phagocytophilum* infections with clinical illness, have not been documented.[157]

DIAGNOSIS

A. phagocytophilum causes seasonal and regional disease, depending on the activity of its particular tick vector (*I. scapularis* in upper midwestern and northeastern United States, *I. pacificus* in California and British Columbia, and *I. ricinus* in Europe). In midwestern and northeastern United States, *I. scapularis* ticks actively feed in early spring into early summer and again in the fall. This seasonal tick activity corresponds with the incidence of human and canine *A. phagocytophilum* infections diagnosed in Minnesota and Wisconsin.[26,28,197] Eighty percent of canine infections in Minnesota and Wisconsin are diagnosed in May, June, October, and November.[196,197] In contrast, Swedish canine *A. phagocytophilum* infections have been diagnosed continuously midsummer through autumn.[158] Infections are rare to none in midwinter, midsummer, and early autumn in Minnesota and Wisconsin.[196] Weather does influence tick activity (i.e., early spring or warm falls and winters can result in cases occurring at unexpected times). Season, history, clinical signs, hematologic (particularly seeing morulae in neutrophils) and clinical chemistry data, and serology can all assist in making a strong presumptive diagnosis of *A. phagocytophilum* infection, but definitive diagnosis relies on microbial DNA analysis via PCR.

Clinical Laboratory Findings
Natural Infection

All reported natural cases of canine *A. phagocytophilum* infection were identified by finding morulae in circulating neutrophils using light microscopy with routine hematologic stains. The morulae of *A. phagocytophilum* cannot be differentiated from the morulae of *E. ewingii* using light microscopy. At the time of diagnosis, 7% to 37% of neutrophils contained *A. phagocytophilum* morulae.[158,197,418] Almost all reported clinical laboratory findings are from samples collected during the bacteremic phase, which can be short lived, lasting for 1 to 9 days in experimental infections.[155,157,307]

Excluding the presence of morulae, the most diagnostically helpful laboratory finding is mild to severe thrombocytopenia, present in more than 80% of cases.[158,196,197,418] Additionally, over 90% of infected dogs from Minnesota and Wisconsin are lymphopenic, many severely so.[196,197] Dogs from Sweden and Switzerland have also been lymphopenic.[158,418] Most dogs are eosinopenic.[196] Neutrophil counts are almost always within reference range, with no significant increase in the number of band neutrophils.[158,196,197,418] Less than 50% of dogs have a mild to moderate nonregenerative normochromic normocytic anemia.[158,196,197] One half of dogs from Minnesota and Wisconsin have mild to moderate hypoalbuminemia.[196,197] Serum ALP activity is mildly to moderately increased in 65% or more of dogs from Minnesota and Wisconsin, but this abnormality is rarely reported in Swedish dogs.[158,196,197] Proteinuria has been documented, but only a small number of dogs were sampled, and significant proteinuria was confirmed in only one Swedish dog.[158,197] Serum amylase activity was examined in a small number of dogs and was increased in 50% of them.[197]

Experimental Infection

Dogs experimentally infected with the Swedish strain of *A. phagocytophila* developed thrombocytopenia with increased mean platelet volume, a lymphopenia of 1 to 3 days' duration followed by a lymphocytosis with the presence of blast-stimulated erythrocytes, a mild nonregenerative normochromic normocytic anemia, and morulae in 3% to 34% of circulating neutrophils.[155,157] Morulae were seen in neutrophils for 4 to 9 days.[155,157,307] Eosinopenia occurred while the dogs were bacteremic.[307] Decreased serum iron and decreased total iron-binding capacity developed during bacteremia, but levels returned to normal 1 week after the disappearance of morulae.[307] Hypoalbuminemia and hyperfibrinogenemia occurred when dogs were febrile, and values returned to reference range levels 1 week after fevers abated.[155]

Nucleic Acid Detection

PCR is a more sensitive diagnostic tool than finding circulating morulae and provides a reliable species-specific diagnosis. A genogroup-specific PCR has been developed for *A. phagocytophilum*.[414] PCR allows for a specific diagnosis whereas serologic testing can be hampered by cross-reactivity to closely related rickettsial bacteria. Experimentally infected dogs are *A. phagocytophilum*-PCR-positive 6 to 8 days earlier than the first appearance of morulae in peripheral blood.[155] PCR testing for the 16S rRNA gene of *A. phagocytophilum* is available from a small number of state diagnostic or private diagnostic veterinary laboratories (see Appendix 5). Submitting EDTA-anticoagulated peripheral blood for PCR testing is optimal. Samples need to be taken before antibiotic administration.

Serologic Testing

Experimental studies in horses and dogs have documented that seroconversion to *A. phagocytophilum* occurs 2 to 5 days after the first appearance of morulae in peripheral blood.[155,421] Antibody titers to *A. phagocytophilum* can revert to nondetectable (negative) levels by 7 to 8 months postacute experimental canine infection or can remain detectable at low levels for at least 7 to 8 months.[158] Diagnosis of *A. phagocytophilum* infection may require serologic testing if no morulae are found in peripheral blood neutrophils and if a PCR assay is not available. Both polyclonal indirect FA and Western immunoblot serologic assays have been developed, but most veterinary laboratories only offer indirect FA testing. Using indirect FA, acute to convalescent fourfold seroconversion to *A. phagocytophilum* is necessary to diagnose active infection confidently because up to 40% of acutely ill, morulae-positive dogs can be seronegative at the time of presentation and because dogs may have detectable levels of antibody from previous exposure.[158,196,197] This latter point is important to consider when interpreting a single titer in a sick or healthy dog that is negative for circulating morulae. Strain differences are enough among isolates of *A. phagocytophilum* that titers may vary on the same sera sent to different laboratories.[326] Therefore using the same laboratory is especially important when serial assays are being used to determine a changing titer for diagnosis or a reduction in titer in response to treatment.

For antibody determination, the immunoblot assays are more species-specific, but cross-reactivities to other related species can occur with immunoblotting as with indirect FA testing. Serologic cross-reactivity is caused by immunodominant surface proteins that are of similar molecular size, particularly those of the family of immunodominant outer membrane proteins present on both *Ehrlichia* spp. and *A. phagocytophilum*.[146] Serologic cross-reactivity between *A. phagocytophilum* and other microbes, particularly other tick-transmitted agents, has been evaluated. Serologic cross-reactivity is strong between the strains of *A. phagocytophilum*, is uncommon between *A. phagocytophilum* and ehrlichial agents (*E. canis*, *E. ewingii*, or *E. chaffeensis*) (see Table 28-3), and is nonexistent between *A. phagocytophilum* and *B. burgdorferi*, *Bartonella* sp., or *R. rickettsii*.* The immunodominant outer surface membrane 44-kDa protein (p44) on *A. phagocytophilum* used in Western immunoblotting has been identified as a consistent marker for *A. phagocytophilum* seroconversion, with minimal cross-reactivity with *Ehrlichia* and other *Anaplasma* species.[237,238,327] Acute and convalescent antisera, from dogs naturally infected with *A. phagocytophilum* in Minnesota and Wisconsin, did not cross-react to *E. canis* antigens.[196,197] No cross-reactivity occurred between *E. canis*–positive antisera and *A. phagocytophilum*–positive antisera from dogs from New York and Connecticut using both indirect FA and Western immunoblotting.[325] In contrast, in a report of natural canine *A. phagocytophilum* infections in Sweden, all acute phase sera were indirect FA seronegative to *E. canis*, but one half of convalescent phase sera were seropositive to *E. canis*.[158] Additionally, two dogs from North Carolina and Virginia with PCR-confirmed *E. ewingii* infections seroconverted to *A. phagocytophilum* antigen using indirect FA.[185]

In spite of cross-reactivity, serologic testing still remains the most common method of diagnosing *A. phagocytophilum* infection if morulae are not present or if it is desirable to differentiate between *E. ewingii* and *A. phagocytophilum* infections. In the upper midwestern United States, canine *E. ewingii* and *E. canis* infections are rare to nonexistent, and a positive seroconversion to *A. phagocytophilum* predictably confers a diagnosis of *A. phagocytophilum* infection. Because all *Ehrlichia* spp. and *Anaplasma* spp. infections are tetracycline-responsive, differentiating between infections with these different organisms is usually of more zoonotic or academic importance than it is of clinical relevance to the ill dog. Ruling out *E. canis* infection is the exception because *E. canis* does have the potential to cause life-threatening chronic disease.

Organism Cultivation

All strains of *A. phagocytophilum* can be cultivated in vitro in a human leukemic cell line, HL-60 cells.[186] This method has been used extensively in the laboratory for the study of this disease; however, it is not available commercially.

Pathologic Findings

Pathologic lesions of *A. phagocytophilum* infections from human patients and experimental infections of dogs, monkeys, mice, horses, and sheep are mild.† Splenic lymphoid depletion or hyperplasia occurs with histiocytosis and erythrophagocytosis. Lymph nodes exhibit benign histiocytosis with either lymphopenia or benign mild paracortical hyperplasia. The liver displays scattered hepatocellular apoptosis, mild periportal or peribiliary lymphohistiocytic infiltrates, mild lobular hepatitis, and mild benign sinusoidal histiocytosis. Throughout many tissues, mild lymphohistiocytic perivascular infiltrates can be found. The bone marrow is of normal cellularity or is hypercellular and may exhibit mild plasmacytosis and mild benign histiocytosis.‡ A human patient in the recovery phase of disease developed bone marrow plasmacytosis with intramedullary lymphoid follicles. Pulmonary interstitial infiltration is also observed in some human patients.[433] In one equine study, vasculitis and marked perivascular mixed inflammatory cell populations within skeletal muscle and tendons were reported.[300]

Therapy

Susceptibility testing of *A. phagocytophilum* shows doxycycline, rifampin, and levofloxacin to be most effective.[347] Tetracyclines are almost exclusively recommended for treating *A. phagocytophilum* infections. For puppies under 1 year of age, chloramphenicol can be used to avoid yellowing of teeth. (see Table 28-5) Doxycycline (5 to 10 mg/kg, PO, every 12 to 24 hours for 10 days) or tetracycline (22 mg/kg, PO, every 8 hours for 14 to 21 days) is the recommended treatment protocol. No proof has been produced that long-term treatment beyond the previously recommended interval is beneficial because no evidence exists of chronic disease. Although evidence does exist of chronic subclinical infections from Swedish studies, no clinical signs were seen, and whether antibiotics will eliminate this carrier state are unknown. Most dogs respond rapidly to treatment and are frequently clinically normal 24 to 48 hours after initiation of therapy, but owners occasionally report that weeks or years are needed for their dogs to completely recover.[158,196] Concurrent illnesses should be treated appropriately. If response to tetracycline antibiotics is poor, the probability that the dog has a concurrent disease is high.

Prevention

No vaccine is available to prevent *A. phagocytophilum* infection. Prevention relies on (1) avoiding exposure to the tick vectors (*I. scapularis*, *I. pacificus*, *I. ricinus*) from spring through fall, (2) prophylactic use of antiacaricides, and (3) prophylactic use of doxycycline or tetracycline when visiting *I. scapularis*, *I. pacificus*, or *I. ricinus* tick–endemic regions.

Public Health Considerations

Human *A. phagocytophilum* infection was first reported in 1994 in residents of Minnesota and Wisconsin.[26] Since then, human infections have been diagnosed in Massachusetts, California, Rhode Island, Connecticut, New York, and Slovenia.* Clinical disease is indistinguishable from that seen with *E. chaffeensis* and *E. ewingii* infections and from many other systemic infectious diseases. The most frequent clinical signs are fever, malaise, headache, and myalgia.[26,28,528] Less frequently exhibited, but still common signs, are arthralgia, vomiting, diarrhea, coughing, a stiff neck, and confusion. Rarely, a rash is present.[26,28,528] The most consistent laboratory findings are thrombocytopenia, leukopenia, and mild increases in serum ALT and aspartate aminotransferase activities.[26,28,528] Peripheral blood neutrophils containing morulae are present in only 80% of cases, and even when morulae are present, only a low number of neutrophils may be infected.[28] Patients with *A. phagocytophilum* infections have died, but all deaths have been caused by complications resulting from opportunistic infections.[528] A small proportion of recovered patients complain of persistent symptoms of illness for 1 to 3 years after treatment.[428] The potential for dogs, horses, sheep, and other domestic animals to be zoonotic risks for human *A. phagocytophilum* infection is not known. Wildlife hosts such as rodents are probably the maintenance reservoirs, with immature tick stages as vectors; deer may become infected or involved in vector maintenance. The vectors are *Ixodes* spp. ticks, which also transmit *Borrelia* spp. (see Chapter 45) explaining the superimposed worldwide geographic distribution of these diseases. Co-infections with *Borrelia* and *Ehrlichia* spp. may result in more severe disease in infected hosts. The suspicion holds that people have become infected while handling deer blood or carcasses or engorged infected ticks.[28,507] The affected individuals had butchered a large number of deer carcasses and sustained numerous cuts during the process. An electric saw,

---

*References 144, 146, 158, 325, 328, 495, 529.
†References 64, 155, 174, 230, 231, 300, 334.
‡References 64, 174, 230, 231, 300, 307, 334.

*References 2, 167, 197, 231, 334, 400, 509, 565.

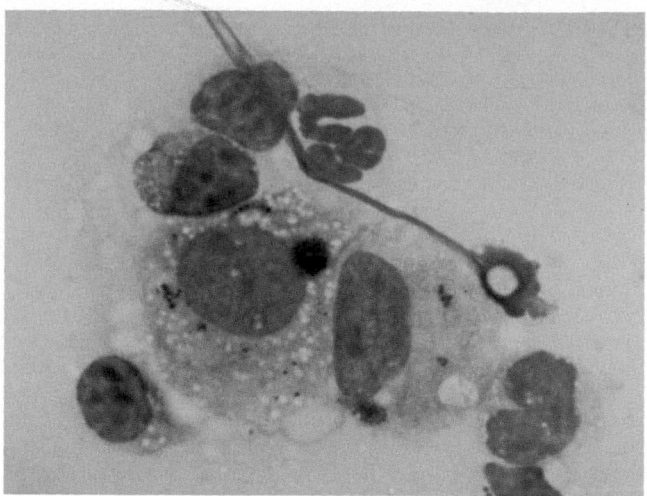

Fig 28-9 *Ehrlichia* inclusion in the mononuclear cell of a cat. (Courtesy Mike Lappin, Colorado State University, Fort Collins, Colo.)

which produces aerosolized blood particles, was also used. Precautions should always be taken when necropsies are performed on animals suspected of harboring this infection.

FELINE MONONUCLEAR EHRLICHIOSIS

Michael R. Lappin and Edward B. Breitschwerdt

Etiology and Epidemiology

The species of *Ehrlichia* that infect cats after natural exposure have not been fully determined (Table 28-6). To date, only two studies of naturally infected cats have confirmed DNA from a strain of *Ehrlichia* generally found in mononuclear cells.[47,70] In the North American report,[70] DNA most consistent with *E. canis* was documented in the blood of three clinically ill cats. In the French report,[47] the 16S rDNA *Ehrlichia* sequences obtained from two cats were identical to those obtained from North American cats. In other reports, *Ehrlichia*-like bodies or morulae have been detected in peripheral lymphocytes or monocytes of naturally exposed cats in the United States (Fig. 28-9),[66] Kenya,[88,90] France,[46,49-51,107] Brazil,[10] and Thailand.[255] Electron microscopic (EM) assessment of an isolate from feline mononuclear cells revealed organisms from 0.54 to 1.3 μm, intermediate in size between *E. canis* and *N. sennetsu*.[88]

To the authors' (MRL and EB) knowledge, only two experimental inoculation studies of cats with *Ehrlichia* spp. have been conducted.[126,291] Morulae of *N. risticii*[146] were detected in mononuclear cells from two of six cats inoculated intravenously (IV) (but not subcutaneously [SC]); diarrhea developed in one cat, and depression, anorexia, and lymphadenomegaly developed in the other.[126] When cats were inoculated SC with an *E. canis* strain (North Carolina State University canine isolate) maintained in cell culture, organismal DNA or antibodies that reacted to *E. canis* morulae were not detected in an 8-week follow-up period.[291] These results can be interpreted in the following manner: the *E. canis*-like DNA amplified from naturally infected cats may be a different *Ehrlichia* sp. more infective to cats (not all *E. canis* strains will infect cats, and not all cats are susceptible to infection by *E. canis*) or SC inoculation is not an effective method for infecting cats with *E. canis*.[70]

Sera from cats have been assessed for *Ehrlichia* spp. antibodies using indirect FA or Western immunoblot. However, standardization of methodologies between laboratories has not been performed, and the most appropriate cutoff values have not been determined. Results of serologic tests performed by different laboratories have not had 100% concordance.[70] Additionally, variable serologic cross-reactivity occurs among *Ehrlichia* spp., *Neorickettsia* spp., and *Anaplasma* spp.; therefore seroreactivity to a specific test antigen does not definitely document exposure to the *Ehrlichia* spp. morulae used for testing.[80,144,372,490] Thus results of antibody-based surveys should be interpreted with caution until such time as laboratories can correlate serologic results with feline *Ehrlichia* spp. isolates or PCR assay findings.

By the use of indirect FA, serum antibodies that react with *E. canis* morulae have been detected in cats from multiple states of the United States,[66,490] France,[50,51] Italy,[154] and Kenya.[345] By use of immunofluorescence, antibodies to *N. risticii* were detected in serum of 26.4% and 16.6% of the cats tested in Maryland[126] and Virginia,[398] respectively. Antibodies to *N. risticii* were detected by indirect FA and Western immunoblot in five cats in a household in California.[394] In a neighborhood in Colorado from which a cat with a mononuclear form of *Ehrlichia* was identified, 14 of 17 cats (82.4%) and 9 of 17 cats (52.9%) had serum antibodies against *E. canis* and *N. risticii*, respectively, detected by indirect FA.[66] Cats with antibodies against both species generally had higher titers to *E. canis* antigens.

The way in which the clinically ill, naturally exposed cats with ehrlichiosis described in the literature were infected is unknown. Documentation of arthropod exposure in proven cases has been variable. However, *Haemaphysalis leachi* was found on each of four cats with clinical ehrlichiosis in Kenya.[88,90]

Pathogenesis

Pathogenesis of disease associated with ehrlichiosis in cats is unknown. Based on clinical, laboratory, and radiographic findings, pathogenesis of disease is likely similar to that for *E. canis* infection of dogs. In the three cats with *E. canis*–like DNA in blood, antinuclear antibodies were detected, similar to results reported for infected dogs.[70]

Clinical Findings

Clinical manifestations of ehrlichiosis have been described in 22 cats with suspected morulae in mononuclear cells* and in three cats with *E. canis*–like DNA in blood[70] (see Table 28-6). Ehrlichiosis has also been suspected in 33 reported feline cases in which the diagnosis was presumptively based on the combination of positive *E. canis* or *N. risticii* serology, clinical or laboratory findings consistent with ehrlichial infection, and response to known antiehrlichial drugs.† Thus at least 55 cases have been reported in which feline ehrlichiosis was implicated.

Most cats for which age was reported were older than 1 year and were domestic shorthaired. Both male and female cats have been affected. Fever and the nonspecific signs of lethargy, inappetence, and weight loss are common clinical manifestations and have been exhibited by most cats. Hyperesthesia, joint pain, and irritable disposition were also common. Dyspnea, vomiting, diarrhea, and weight loss also occurred in some cats. Splenomegaly, lymphadenomegaly, dyspnea, petechiae, retinal detachments, vitreous hemorrhages, and pale mucous membranes were reported physical examination abnormalities. Concurrent diseases detected in some cats included *Haemobartonella felis* (now *Mycoplasma haemofelis* and *Candidatus Mycoplasma haemominutum*), *Cryptococcus neoformans*, feline

*References 10, 46, 50, 66, 88, 107.
†References 46, 50, 51, 66, 394.

Table • 28-6

Summary of Clinical Mononuclear Ehrlichiosis in Cats

SIGNALMENT (COUNTRY)	CLINICAL FINDINGS	LABORATORY FINDINGS	DIAGNOSIS	TREATMENT/ RESPONSE	REFERENCE
10 yr, FS, DSH (United States)	Fever, anorexia, hyperesthesia	Nonregenerative anemia, hyperglobulinemia	Morulae in mononuclear cells; *E. canis* and *N. risticii* seropositive	Doxycycline/ excellent	66
10 yr, M, DSH (Kenya)	Fever, anorexia, dyspnea, splenomegaly, pale mucous membranes	Nonregenerative anemia, hyperglobulinemia, interstitial lung disease	Morulae in mononuclear cells, rarely in neutrophils	Tetracycline/ excellent	88
4 yr, M, DSH (Kenya)	Fever, anorexia, splenomegaly, pale mucous membranes	Nonregenerative anemia	Morulae in mononuclear cells, rarely in neutrophils	Imidocarb/ excellent	88
2 yr, F, DSH (Kenya)	Fever, anorexia, dyspnea, splenomegaly, pale mucous membranes, lymphadenomegaly	Nonregenerative anemia, neutropenia, interstitial lung disease	Morulae in mononuclear cells, rarely in neutrophils	Imidocarb/ excellent	88
Adult lioness (Kenya)	Lethargy, emaciation, lymphadenomegaly	Neutrophilic leukocytosis	Morulae in mononuclear cells	Not treated	91
6 yr, MC, DSH (France)	Fever, anorexia, pale mucous membranes, depression	Regenerative anemia, *Mycoplasma haemofelis* leukocytosis, lymphocytosis, monocytosis, hyperbilirubinemia	Morulae in mononuclear cells	Tetracycline/ Groulade,	107
11 yr, FS, DSH (France)	Fever, weight loss, anorexia, depression, joint pain	Nonregenerative anemia, leukopenia, hypoalbuminemia, hyperglobulinemia	Morulae in lymphocytes, *E. canis* seropositive	Doxycycline/ glucocorticoids/ euthanasia	49
9 yr, MC, DSH (France)	Anorexia, gingivitis, pale mucous membranes, polyuria, polydipsia, weight loss	Anemia, FeLV positive, FIV positive, hyperglobulinemia	Morulae in lymphocytes, *E. canis* seropositive	Euthanasia	49
14 yr, MC, DSH (France)	Dyspnea, pale mucous membranes, weight loss, lethargy	Pleural effusion, hyperglobulinemia	Morulae in lymphocytes, *E. canis* seropositive	Euthanasia/ lymphosarcoma	49

M, Male; *DSH*, domestic shorthair; *F*, female; *MC*, male, castrated; *FS*, female, spayed; *FeLV*, feline leukemia virus; *FIV*, feline immunodeficiency virus.

leukemia virus and feline immunodeficiency virus infections, and lymphosarcoma.

Diagnosis
Hematology
Complete or partial blood cell evaluations were available for many of the cats. Anemia was most commonly nonregenerative and occurred in cats with chronic disease histories. One cat with regenerative anemia was co-infected with a hemotropic *Mycoplasma* species (previously *H. felis*).[107] Leukopenia, leukocytosis, neutrophilia, neutropenia, lymphocytosis, monocytosis, and thrombocytopenia occur in some cats; alone or in combinations. Bone marrow evaluation of cats with cytopenias revealed primarily hypoplasia of the effected cell line. However, one cat had bone marrow cytologic characteristics consistent with myeloid leukemia.[70] Based on the cases reported to date, ehrlichiosis should be considered on the differential list for cats with unexplained leukocytosis or cytopenias.

Biochemistry
Biochemical abnormalities were infrequently reported in cats with suspected clinical ehrlichiosis and were apparently nonspecific. Hyperproteinemia is the most consistent abnormality; polyclonal gammopathy was detected in four of the cats assayed by protein electrophoresis.[46,49] In a separate study, an epidemiologic association was made between monoclonal gammopathy and cats seropositive for *E. canis* antibodies.[490] Based on these results, ehrlichiosis should be on the differential list for cats with hyperglobulinemia.

Radiographic Findings
Of the cats with historical or physical examination findings consistent with respiratory disease, interstitial lung patterns were the only abnormalities that were reported in association with feline ehrlichiosis. Thoracic and abdominal radiographs were commonly considered within normal limits.

Serologic Testing
Not all cats with ehrlichiosis reported to date were tested with the same antibody methodology, and comparison studies of indirect FA tests between laboratories do not show 100% concordance.[70] Standardized serologic tests for detection of antibodies against ehrlichial species in cats are needed.

Most of the cats with morulae documented in mononuclear cells have had antibodies in serum that react with *E. canis* morulae. However, some cats with clinical ehrlichiosis are seronegative on initial evaluation, and thus clinicians may have to perform more than one serologic assessment to document seroconversion. Of the three cats with *E. canis*–like DNA in blood, none had antibodies that reacted with *E. canis* morulae in two different laboratories.[70] Five cats with presumed ehrlichiosis had serum antibodies that reacted with *N. risticii* morulae but not to *E. canis* morulae.[394] In addition, *A. phagocytophilum* causes similar clinical signs in cats and usually does not induce antibodies that cross-react with *E. canis* antigens.[62,292] Thus ehrlichiosis cannot be excluded in cats based on failure to detect seroreactivity to *E. canis* morulae by indirect FA testing.

Many healthy cats have serum antibodies that react with *E. canis* or *N. risticii* antigens; however, similar serologic cross-reactivity may occur among ehrlichial species as observed for dogs (see Table 28-3).[490] A diagnosis of clinical ehrlichiosis therefore should never be based on positive serologic test results alone. Clinicians should always exclude other potential causes of the clinical syndrome.

Other Testing
Antinuclear antibody tests results were positive in some cats.[70] Coombs' test results were usually negative. Neutrophilic poly-

arthritis and increased CSF protein concentrations were confirmed in one cat.[70] Lymph node aspirates, when performed, showed lymphoid or plasma cell hyperplasia.

Organism Detection
The presence of morulae can be used to strengthen the diagnosis of ehrlichiosis in cats. Infected cells were reported to be more common in blood collected from an ear vein than a large vein.[49] However, false-positive and false-negative results can occur. In addition, documentation of morulae cannot be used to determine the *Ehrlichia* spp. involved. For example in four cats with presumed *E. canis* infection, neutrophils and mononuclear cells were infected.[11,88]

Organism Cultivation and Nucleic Acid Detection
Infection by *Ehrlichia* spp. can be confirmed by cell culture or PCR. The organism was isolated from whole blood on monocyte cultures in the domestic cat cases[88] but not from a lioness from Kenya.[90] Monocyte cultures failed to document *N. risticii* infection in the seropositive cats from California, but morulae were not seen in circulating blood of these cats.[394] Although results of PCR assays will likely be used to help further define feline ehrlichiosis, clinicians should assist research laboratories in efforts to obtain feline *Ehrlichia* spp. isolates for comparative microbiologic studies. PCR assays should be used that amplify *Ehrlichia*, *Anaplasma*, and *Neorickettsia* genus DNA, (i.e., these PCR primers should amplify all members of the genus), subsequently, a species-specific PCR assay, DNA sequencing, or both, can be used to determine which organism is involved. However, further information concerning the diagnostic sensitivity of species-specific PCR testing is needed. Although PCR testing has been used successfully in some feline cases,[70,292] PCR of blood using *N. risticii*–specific primers proved negative in the seropositive cats tested in California.[21,394]

In summary, until diagnostic testing of cats for ehrlichiosis is better defined, clinicians will need to combine PCR assay results with those of serum antibody testing against multiple *Ehrlichia* spp. so as to confirm or exclude these organisms from the differential list for clinically ill cats.[372]

Pathologic Findings
Before treatment, pyogranulomatous lymphadenitis was detected in a mesenteric lymph node from a cat from Colorado with antibodies against *E. canis* and *N. risticii*.[66] Perivascular plasma cell and lymphocyte infiltrates were detected in the lungs, kidneys, and liver of the untreated lioness in Kenya.[90] After doxycycline treatment in one cat, an acute respiratory distress syndrome developed that resulted in death.[70] Neutrophilic and histiocytic myocarditis and pneumonia, multifocal lymphoplasmacytic nephritis, and multifocal lymphoplasmacytic pancreatitis were the predominant findings. However, *Ehrlichia* spp. or other infectious causes were not identified after death.

Therapy
Therapy with tetracycline, doxycycline, or imidocarb dipropionate was attempted in most of the cases with suspected clinical feline mononuclear ehrlichiosis (Table 28-7). Administration of doxycycline at 5 mg/kg, twice daily, PO, for 21 days resulted in resolution of clinical signs of disease in three cats.[66] One cat was seropositive 180 days after discharge but seronegative 1365 days after discharge. Serologic follow-up was available for multiple presumptive cases in France[50,51]; the majority became seronegative with time. However, increasing or persistent titers can occur as reported for the dog.[41] Recurrence of disease and serum antibodies were reported in the five *N. risticii*–seropositive cats in California treated with a lower dose of doxycycline, but these cats appeared to respond

Table • 28-7

Antimicrobial Therapy for Feline Monocytotropic Ehrlichiosis and Granulocytotropic Anaplasmosis

DRUG[a]	DOSE[b] (mg/kg)	ROUTE PREFERRED (ALTERNATIVE)	INTERVAL[c] (HOURS)	DURATION (DAYS)
Tetracycline	22	PO	8	21
Doxycycline	10	PO[d]	24	28
Doxycycline	5–10	PO[d]	12–24	10–28
Chloramphenicol	25	PO (IV, SC)	12	≤ 14[e]
Imidocarb dipropionate[f]	5	IM	once	Repeat day 14

PO, By mouth; *IV,* intravenously; *SC,* subcutaneously; *IM,* intramuscularly.
[a]See Drug Formulary, Appendix 8, for additional information.
[b]Dose per administration at specified interval.
[c]Expressed in hours unless otherwise stated.
[d]Doxycycline tablets or powder can cause esophagitis so they should be dosed to the nearest whole size of tablet or capsule and water should be given after each dose.
[e]Myelosuppression is a concern and repeat blood counts should be done at the conclusion of therapy.
[f]The effectiveness of imidocarb is uncertain in infected cats.

when administered doxycycline at 10 mg/kg, PO, twice daily for 21 days.[394] Imidocarb dipropionate administered at 5 mg/kg, IM, and repeated in 14 days resulted in clinical resolution of disease of two cats in Kenya.[88] This drug has been used for the treatment of infected dogs[342] and has been shown to be safe when administered to cats with chronic haemoplasmosis.[294] Enrofloxacin was used to treat two cats with presumed mononuclear ehrlichiosis.[51] However, this drug is considered to be inferior to tetracyclines for the treatment of ehrlichiosis in dogs.[372,373] The Infectious Disease Study Group of the American College of Veterinary Internal Medicine currently recommends treating cats with suspected clinical ehrlichiosis with doxycycline at 10 mg/kg, PO, every 24 hours for a minimum of 28 days.[372] Whether the treatment protocols used to date eliminate the organism is currently unknown.[249,548]

Euthanasia was chosen for two cats with documented morulae in mononuclear cells because of treatment failures with tetracycline[107] or doxycycline[49] and because one cat died.[70] Some cats with suspected ehrlichiosis based on clinical signs and positive serologic test results failed to respond to doxycycline administration.[46] However, because ehrlichiosis was not definitively diagnosed by culture or PCR, whether these cases represent treatment failures is also unknown. For a summary of the drugs and dosages recommended for treatment of feline ehrlichiosis, see Table 28-7.

Prevention

Because routes of transmission for naturally infected cats are unknown, definitive statements concerning prevention cannot be made. In addition, further studies are needed to determine whether *E. muris* infection of rodents can be transmitted to cats.[264,546] Exposure of cats to potential arthropod vectors and ingestion of rodents should be avoided. Apparently, *Ehrlichia* spp. can be transmitted by blood; therefore cats used as blood donors should be screened for infection, ideally using both serologic and PCR testing. Cats with positive results should be excluded as donors.

Public Health Consideration

Although *Ehrlichia* spp. might infect both people and cats, human infection has never been associated with cat contact. If cats are housed indoors and arthropod control is maintained, the risk to people should be minimal.

FELINE GRANULOCYTOTROPIC ANAPLASMOSIS

Michael R. Lappin, Anneli Björsdorff, and Edward B. Breitschwerdt

Etiology and Epidemiology

A. phagocytophilum (previously *E. equi, E. phagocytophila,* canine granulocytotropic *Ehrlichia,* and HGE agent)[146] is known to infect a variety of animals, including small mammals,[67,531] mountain lions,[172] coyotes,[416] sheep,[378] cattle,[425] deer,[57] dogs,[157,286] horses,[21,415,425] and people (Table 28-8).

Susceptibility of cats to *A. phagocytophilum* infection was first documented in an experimental inoculation study.[302] Although clinical abnormalities were not reported, two of five cats inoculated with *E. equi* developed morulae in eosinophils and eosinophilia. More recently, cats with and without FIV were inoculated with *A. phagocytophilum* and developed clinical signs of disease.[175]

DNA consistent with *A. phagocytophilum* has been detected in blood from naturally infected cats in Sweden,[62,502] Denmark,[470] Ireland,[469] and the United States.[292] Morulae consistent with *A. phagocytophilum* have been detected cytologically in neutrophils of naturally infected cats in Sweden,[62,502] Brazil,[10,11] Kenya,[88] and Italy.[505] With the exception of the cases in Sweden, whether the morulae-like structures were *A. phagocytophilum* or another organism is unknown.

A. phagocytophilum is transmitted by *Ixodes* ticks.* Of the six naturally infected, clinically ill cats with *A. phagocytophilum* DNA in blood, all lived in an *I. scapularis, I. pacificus,* or *I. ricinus*–endemic region, all were allowed to roam outdoors, and four were known to be infested by *Ixodes* spp. at the time of initial examination.[62,292] Therefore this genus of ticks can also likely serve as the vector for transmission of *A. phagocytophilum* to cats. Although rodents are commonly infected with *A. phagocytophilum,* whether ingestion or direct contact with rodents plays a role in *A. phagocytophilum* infection of cats is currently unknown.[67,531]

Pathogenesis

Pathogenesis of disease associated with *A. phagocytophilum* in cats is unknown. Based on clinical, laboratory, and radiographic findings, pathogenesis of disease is likely similar to that for

*References 36, 67, 162, 378, 415, 386.

Table • 28-8

Clinical and Laboratory Findings from Six Cats with Molecular and Serologic Evidence of Anaplasma phagocytophilum **Infection in North America and Sweden**

CAT[a]	SIGNALMENT	UNITED STATES OR OTHER COUNTRY	PRIMARY ABNORMALITIES	DAY	MORULAE	PCR[b]	RECIPROCAL INDIRECT FA TITERS[c]
1	9 mo, MC, DSH	Massachusetts	Fever, lethargy, anorexia	0	neg	pos	>1:640
				25	neg	neg	1:160
				139	neg	neg	1:20
2	3 yr, FS, DSH	Massachusetts	Fever, anorexia, *Ixodes*	0	neg	pos	NT
				37	neg	pos	>1:640
				139	neg	neg	1:160
3	13 mo, MC, DSH	Massachusetts	Fever, lethargy	0	neg	pos	NT
				120	neg	pos	1:160
4	1 yr, FS, DSH	Massachusetts	Fever, anorexia, *Ixodes*	0	neg	pos	NT
				27	neg	neg	NT
				62	neg	neg	1:40
5	1 yr, MC, DSH	Connecticut	Fever, anorexia, lethargy, *Ixodes*	0	neg	pos	neg
				30	neg	neg	>1:640
				70	neg	neg	1:20
				136	neg	neg	1:640
6	14 mo, MC, European shorthair	Sweden	Fever, lethargy, anorexia, tachypnea, *Ixodes*	0	pos	pos	neg
				15	neg	neg	1:640
				29	neg	neg	1:2,560
				263	neg	neg	1:5,120

NT, Not tested; *pos*, positive; *neg*, negative; *DSH*, domestic shorthair; *MC*, male, neutered, *FS*, female, spayed.
[a]Cats 1–5, see reference 291; cat 6, see reference 62 on the CD.
[b]The PCR assays and sequencing used for Cats 1–5 are discussed in reference 291, and for cat 6 in reference 62.
[c]Cats 1–5 were tested for antibodies using indirect FA slides coated with *A. phagocytophilum (E. equi)* infected cells; cat 6 had equivalent results with indirect FA with *E. equi*, *E. phagocytophilum* and a Swedish isolate of granulocytotropic *Ehrlichia*-infected cells.

infection of other species. Some cats experimentally inoculated with *A. phagocytophilum* developed antinuclear antibodies and increased IFN-γ mRNA suggested that an immune pathogenesis of disease may contribute to the clinical findings.[175]

Clinical Findings

The cats with morulae in neutrophils that came from Brazil[10] and Kenya[88] had larger numbers of morulae in mononuclear cells. Thus the following information, which is summarized in Table 28-8, comes from the six animals with documented *A. phagocytophilum* infections based on positive PCR testing and gene sequencing.[62,292] Fever, anorexia, and lethargy were the most common clinical abnormalities. The cat from Sweden was also tachypneic. *Ixodes* ticks were detected on 4 to 6 cats. Overall, clinical signs associated with *A. phagocytophilum* infection in these cats were mild and resolved quickly after initiating tetracycline therapy.

Diagnosis
Clinical Laboratory Findings

Each of the cats listed in Table 28-8 had erythrocyte counts within reference limits. Thrombocytopenia (reference range of 175,000 to 500,000/μl) was detected in cat 3 (118,000/μl), cat 4 (84,000 μl), and cat 5 (66,000/μl), but platelet clumps were reported for cat 5. Neutrophilia with a left shift and lymphopenia were detected in cat 6. Morulae were detected in 24% of the neutrophils in cat 6.[62] The abnormalities resolved quickly after doxycycline treatment was initiated.

Mild hyperglycemia detected in cats 2 and 6 was attributed to stress. No other serum biochemical abnormalities were detected in the cats.

In cat 5, urinalysis was normal and aerobic urine culture failed to grow bacteria. Each cat was negative for FeLV p27 antigen and antibodies against FIV in serum (Snap Combo, IDEXX Laboratories, Portland, Md.; see Appendix 6).

Serologic Findings

On day 0, two of three cats tested for antibodies against *A. phagocytophilum* were seronegative, but all six cats ultimately seroconverted (see Table 28-8). None of the six cats developed antibodies that reacted with *E. canis* morulae. Thus diagnostic laboratories providing serologic test results to veterinarians that practice in *Ixodes* spp.–endemic areas must offer assays that detect antibodies against *A. phagocytophilum*, not just *N. risticii* and *E. canis*. In three cats with molecular evidence of infection by an *E. canis*–like organism, antibodies that reacted with *E. canis* morulae were not detected by two research laboratories, even though chronic disease existed.[70] These results suggest that not all cats seroconvert when infected with *Ehrlichia* spp. or that another organism molecularly similar to *E. canis* that does not induce cross-reacting antibodies is present. Thus, in addition to serologic testing, also recommended is that blood of cats with suspected clinical ehrlichiosis or anaplasmosis also be evaluated with a PCR assay that amplifies all sequenced *Ehrlichia* spp. and

Anaplasma spp. Because animals can be infected with more than one organism concurrently, sequencing of the PCR products or additional PCR testing with species-specific primers can be used to define the *Ehrlichia* spp. or *Anaplasma* spp.–causing infection.[62,70,292,500]

As with canine ehrlichiosis, clinical illness apparently can develop before seroconversion in cats (see Table 28-8, cats 5 and 6), and thus a single negative antibody result in an acutely infected cat does not exclude infection. *A. phagocytophilum* DNA was amplified from the blood of eight mountain lions that did not have serum antibodies that reacted with the organism in indirect FA tests.[172] Therefore, when confronted with an acute illness consistent with feline anaplasmosis, both acute and convalescent serum samples should be examined or PCR testing should be used to document infection. Reevaluation of antibody titer results from cats 5 and 6 also suggested that administration of antibiotics during the acute phase of infection did not completely attenuate seroconversion (see Table 28-8).

Organism and Nucleic Acid Detection
In the six cats with *A. phagocytophilum* DNA in blood, only one had detectable morulae (see Table 28-8). This cat (cat 6) was cytologically negative on all subsequent test dates. DNA of *A. phagocytophilum* was detected in all six cats on Day 0, and therefore PCR testing may be more sensitive than antibodies for diagnosing acute anaplasmosis.

Pathologic Findings
None of the cats with naturally occurring *A. phagocytophilum* infections have had tissue biopsies or necropsies performed; thus pathologic findings are unknown. No gross or microscopic lesions attributed to *A. phagocytophilum* infection could be found in experimentally inoculated cats.[302]

Therapy
Supportive care consisting of SC or IV administration of balanced electrolyte solutions was provided to all six cats with molecular evidence of *A. phagocytophilum* infection.[62,292] Antimicrobial therapy was also administered to the cats listed in Table 28-8. Enrofloxacin (cats 1 and 2), penicillin and gentamycin (cat 3), or chloramphenicol (cat 4), was administered parenterally for 1 day before administering doxycycline at approximately 5 mg/kg, PO, for 28 to 30 days. Cat 5 was treated with two doses of doxycycline IV but developed phlebitis at the catheter site. Ampicillin was administered for 1 day, and the cat was discharged with amoxicillin plus clavulanate to be administered at 13.75 mg/kg for 10 days. Lethargy and inappetence recurred after discontinuing the antibiotic.[292] Given that the *A. phagocytophilum* results were known to be positive at that time, the referring veterinarian prescribed tetracycline at 22 mg/kg, PO, every 8 hours for 21 days. Cat 6 was initially treated with doxycycline at 10 mg/kg, IV, once and then doxycycline at 10 mg/kg, PO, daily for 20 days. All cats (cat 5 after recurrence of clinical signs) became normal within 24 to 48 hours after initiation of tetracycline administration, and recurrence was not reported. The clinical and hematologic abnormalities in these six cats might have resolved without treatment. Clinically ill cats with serologic or molecular evidence of *E. canis*–like infections have generally had more severe cytopenias and have been more refractory to treatment than the cats described here.[70] In dogs, infection with *E. canis* also seemingly induces a more severe disease than infection with *A. phagocytophilum* or *E. ewingii*.[372]

After 21 to 30 days of tetracycline treatment, serum from all cats in Table 28-8 still had antibodies that seroreacted with *A. phagocytophilum* when tested 32 to 242 days after cessation of therapy. These results are similar to those that occur in *E. canis*–infected dogs, which frequently have persistence

of antibody titers after treatment.[41] Cats 2 and 3 were still PCR positive 17 days and 90 days after treatment (see Table 28-8); experimentally infected dogs can also be infected for months.[157,212] These results, when combined with the persistence of antibody titers, suggest that treatment with tetracyclines for 21 to 30 days may be inadequate for eliminating the organism from the body. The four cats that became PCR-negative may have been persistently infected despite treatment with the organism sequestered in low numbers in tissues such as the spleen, as has been reported for dogs.[249] At this time, whether cats can be reinfected is unknown.

Prevention
A. phagocytophilum is apparently transmitted to people and cats by *Ixodes* spp. Thus exposure of cats to potential arthropod vectors should be avoided or tick control maintained with acaricidal products that are approved for use on cats. *A. phagocytophilum* can likely be transmitted by blood; therefore cats used as blood donors should be screened for infection by using serum antibody tests or PCR assay, and positive cats should be excluded as donors.

Public Health Considerations
Although *A. phagocytophilum* is known to infect both people and cats, no association has ever been exhibited between human infection and cat contact. If cats are housed indoors and arthropod control is maintained, the risk to people should be minimal.

THROMBOCYTOTROPIC ANAPLASMOSIS (*A. PLATYS [E. PLATYS]* INFECTION)

John W. Harvey

Etiology
Dogs
Infectious cyclic thrombocytopenia of dogs is caused by a small rickettsial parasite of platelets originally classified as *E. platys*.[178,223] Based on comparisons of the sequences of the 16S rRNA gene, this organism is more closely related to *Anaplasma* organisms than it is to *Ehrlichia* organisms. Consequently, *E. platys* has been reclassified as *A. platys*.[146] This classification as an *Anaplasma* species is further substantiated based on nucleotide sequences determined for the groEL heat shock protein gene, groESL heat shock operon, and the gltA citrate synthase gene.[242,572] *A. platys* was first reported in the United States in 1978[223] and has subsequently been reported in Western Europe,[285,456,481] Asia,* South America,[19,496] the Middle East,[207] Australia,[84] and Africa.[460]

A. platys organisms appear as blue inclusions in platelets when blood films are stained with Giemsa or new methylene blue (Fig. 28-10). Ultrastructurally, organisms range from 350 to 1250 nm in diameter, are round, oval, or bean shaped, and are surrounded by a double membrane. Infected platelets may contain one to three single membrane–lined vacuoles with 1 to 15 organisms per vacuole (Fig. 28-11).[19,223,340] Organisms appear to enter platelets by adhering to the platelet surface followed by endocytosis. Therefore the vacuolar membrane probably is derived from the external platelet membrane. Repeated binary fission of organisms within the vacuole results in the formation of a morula.

Megakaryocytes in bone marrow have not been observed to contain organisms, either before or during parasitemia. *A. platys* antigen has been identified in macrophages using immunofluorescent staining of frozen tissues 14 days after

---

*References 102, 234, 239, 241, 244, 361, 497.

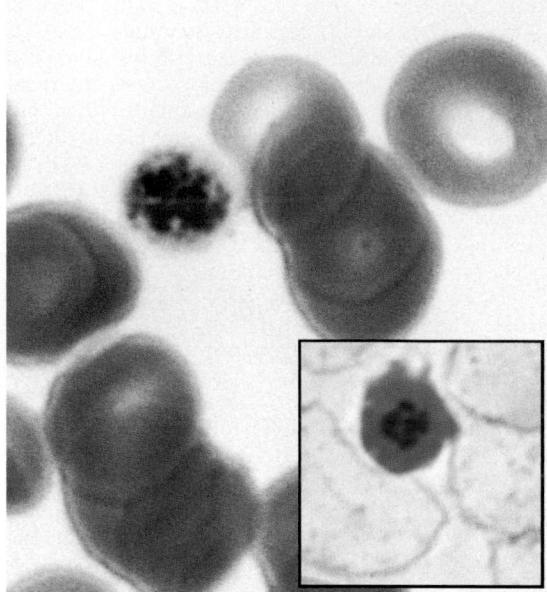

Fig 28-10 *A. platys* morula in a platelet from a dog with thrombocytic anaplasmosis (Giesma stain, original magnification ×2500). *Inset,* Platelet containing morula of *A. platys* (new methylene blue, ×2300).

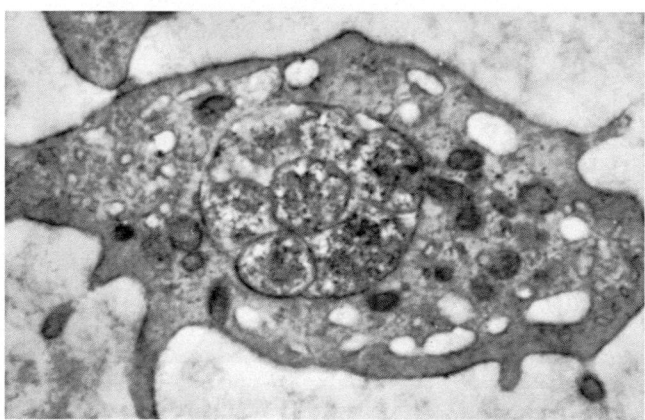

Fig 28-11 Ultrastructure of *A. platys*. Platelet with a membrane-lined vacuole containing seven visible organisms. (From Harvey JW et al. 1978. Cyclic thrombocytopenia induced by a *Rickettsia*-like agent in dogs, *J Infect Dis* 137:182–188. Reprinted with permission from the University of Chicago.)

experimental infection, but this may represent the fate of infected platelets rather than a site of replication. Attempts to culture the organism have been unsuccessful.

Cats and Other Animals
Inclusions that appeared identical to *A. platys* have been seen in platelets in a stained blood film from a cat in Brazil[461] but an attempt to infect a cat by IV inoculation with the canine isolate from Florida was unsuccessful. Transmission electron micrographs prepared from the blood of seven South African impala revealed similar organisms in platelets.[150] In addition, 16S rRNA gene sequences have been identified in blood from South African sheep that were 99.5% identical to *A. platys*; however, the morphology of these parasites and the cells they infect have not been identified. Infection with *A. platys* was suspected in people from Venezuela based on the

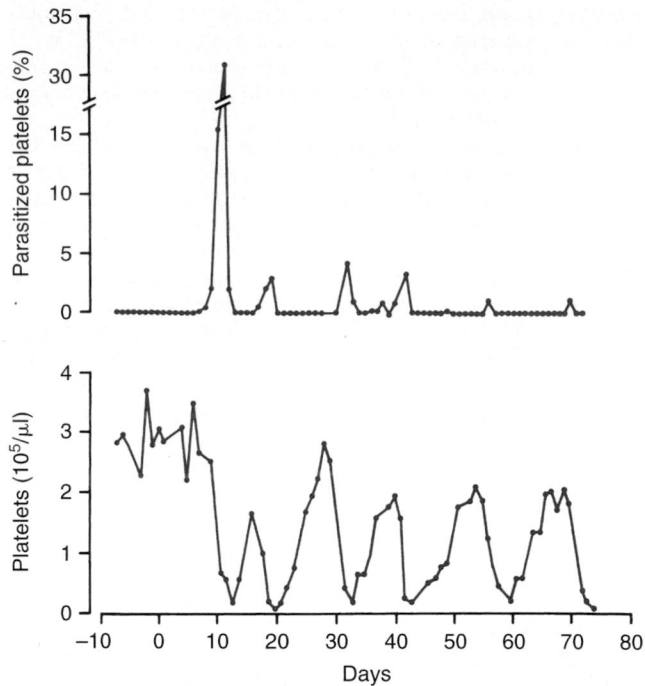

Fig 28-12 Percentage of parasitized platelets and platelet counts from a dog inoculated IV with *A. platys*; 0 on the abscissa represents the day of inoculation. (From Harvey JW et al. 1978. Cyclic thrombocytopenia induced by a *Rickettsia*-like agent in dogs, *J Infect Dis* 137:182–188. Reprinted with permission from the University of Chicago.)

appearance of inclusions in platelets in stained blood films. However, the morphology of these inclusions visualized using transmission electron microscopy was not consistent with *A. platys*, and patients were seronegative against *A. platys* antigens.[18]

Pathogenesis
The natural mode of transmission has not been demonstrated conclusively, but it likely involves a tick vector. Although attempts to transmit the agent with *R. sanguineus* ticks were not successful,[478] *A. platys* has been detected by PCR in *R. sanguineus* ticks in Okinawa, Japan,[247,361] and the Democratic Republic of the Congo, Africa.[460] The sequences of the amplified 16S rRNA gene fragments from these ticks were identical to sequences obtained from dogs infested by the ticks. *A. platys* have also been detected in *Dermacentor auratus* ticks collected from dogs in Thailand.[391]

The incubation period following experimental IV infection in dogs is 8 to 15 days. The highest percentage of parasitized platelets occurs during the initial parasitemic episode (Fig. 28-12). Within a few days after the appearance of parasitized platelets, platelet count decreases precipitously, and organisms are usually no longer seen. Platelet counts generally drop below 20,000/µl in association with parasitemic episodes. After the disappearance of microorganisms, platelet counts increase rapidly, reaching normal values within 3 to 4 days.

Parasitemias and subsequent thrombocytopenic episodes recur at 1- to 2-week intervals (see Fig. 28-12). Although the percentage of infected platelets decreases to as low as 1% or less with subsequent parasitemias, thrombocytopenic episodes are as severe as those following the initial parasitemia. Whereas initial thrombocytopenia may develop primarily as a consequence of direct injury to platelets by replicating organisms, immune-mediated mechanisms of platelet removal may be more important during subsequent thrombocytopenic episodes.[178] The cyclic nature of the parasitemias and thrombocytopenic episodes diminishes with time, resulting in mild, slowly resolving thrombocytopenia in association with sporadically occurring organisms in blood platelets.

In some instances, transient decreases in total leukocyte counts have occurred concomitantly with parasitemias, but values usually do not fall below the reference interval for dogs. Mild normocytic normochromic anemias may occur during the first month of infection. Based on serum iron and bone marrow studies, decreases in hematocrit may be attributed to the anemia of inflammation syndrome. Slight to moderate increases in acute phase proteins and immunoglobulins and slightly decreased albumin may be present in serum samples.

Clinical Findings

Minimal clinical signs have been recognized in experimentally infected dogs in the United States. A slight increase in rectal temperature has sometimes been noted during initial parasitemias, and slight hematochezia has been recognized in some thrombocytopenic dogs. Splenectomy before experimental infection results in higher preinoculation platelet counts, but it does not alter the periodicity of the parasitemias or the severity of disease. The age of the animal does not appear to have a significant effect on the course of infection; clinical and hematologic findings in a group of three weanling pups were similar to that in mature dogs.[178] Minimal clinical signs appear in most naturally infected dogs as well,[68] but more severe clinical signs, including fever and uveitis in one dog and petechial and ecchymotic hemorrhages and epistaxis in another dog, have been reported in natural cases in the United States.[551]

More pathogenic strains of *A. platys* are reported to occur outside the United States.[207,285] Clinical signs, including fever, lethargy, pale mucous membranes, petechial hemorrhages of skin and oral mucosae, decreased appetite, weight loss, purulent nasal discharges, and lymphadenomegaly, have been reported in both experimental and natural studies of dogs infected with a Greek strain of *A. platys*[285] and in natural cases of dogs infected with *A. platys* in Israel.[207] Although *E. canis* serology was negative in some of these ill, *A. platys*–positive dogs, PCR-based assays were not done to determine whether the dogs were also infected with other tick-transmitted diseases. Co-infection with as many as six tick-borne pathogens has been reported in dogs using PCR-based assays[286]; consequently, infection with one or more additional agents may have contributed to the clinical signs that have been reported in dogs with *A. platys* infections.

The occurrence of *A. platys* with other infectious agents (e.g., *E. canis*, *Babesia canis*) may potentiate the clinical disease produced by these agents alone. As with *E. canis*, certain breeds of dogs or individual animals may be more severely affected compared with the dogs studied experimentally. Dogs with thrombocytopenia may bleed following trauma or surgery. Finally, even if *A. platys* infection seldom produces clinical illness as a single agent in the United States, it must be considered in the differential diagnosis of thrombocytopenia in dogs.

Diagnosis

A diagnosis of *A. platys* infection may be made by finding organisms within platelets on stained blood films. In most instances, this method of diagnosis is not reliable because the parasites are either absent or present in very low numbers. An avidin-biotin immunocytochemical staining procedure has been described that can specifically identify *A. platys* morulae in platelets and can help differentiate organisms from large platelet granules or remnants of megakaryocyte nuclei.[477] In addition, inclusions in platelets stained positively in an indirect FA test using mouse anti-*A. phagocytophilum* serum.[241]

An indirect FA test for detection of serum antibodies to *A. platys* is commercially available. Using indirect FA tests, serologic cross-reactivity between *A. platys* and *E. canis* does not appear to occur, but serologic cross-reactivity between *A. platys* and closely related *A. phagocytophilum* organisms is likely.[241] Sera of dogs experimentally infected with *A. platys* change from negative to positive coincident with or shortly after the peak of the first parasitemia.[134,178] Based on serologic studies, *A. platys* infection is apparently widely distributed in the United States. As many as one-third of thrombocytopenic dogs in Florida and Louisiana have positive titers, and over 50% of dogs seropositive for *E. canis* also have positive titers to *A. platys*. Evidence for positive serologic reactions to both organisms in serum samples from some dogs probably represents combined infections, because other dogs have positive titers to either agent alone.[456] Combined infections with *A. platys* and *E. canis* have been confirmed using PCR and 16S rRNA gene sequence analyses.[234,286,496] PCR has also documented infection in dogs and their associated *R. sanguineus* ticks.[481]

PCR-based assays have been used to detect *A. platys* infected dogs.* Selection of appropriate primers for PCR-based assays is critical. A primer combination believed to be specific for *A. phagocytophilum* was found to also amplify *A. platys*.[204] Nearly 28% of free-roaming dogs in subtropical Okinawa Prefecture, Japan, were positive for *A. platys* infection using PCR.[244]

Pathologic Findings

Generalized lymph node enlargement was the only gross finding at necropsy in an experimental study of dogs euthanized during the early weeks of infection.[25] Histologic lesions were generally mild and included lymphoid hyperplasia and plasmacytosis in lymph nodes and the spleen, crescent-shaped perifollicular hemorrhages in the spleen, and multifocal Kupffer cell hyperplasia in the liver. Megakaryocyte numbers in the bone marrow were normal or increased.

Therapy and Prevention

Based on preliminary studies, tetracyclines and enrofloxacin at dosages recommended for *E. canis* infections are apparently effective against *A. platys* (Table 28-9).[178,284] Because ticks (and possibly other arthropods) are undoubtedly responsible for natural transmission of this disease, adequate vector control is recommended to prevent its spread.

WOLBACHIA INFECTION

Craig E. Greene

Organisms of the genus *Wolbachia* have been identified as endosymbionts living within filarial parasites. *Wolbachia* spp. have been identified in the filarial parasite *Onchocerca volvulus*, a cause of human filariasis. One hypothesis asserts that the microorganism may have a role in the pathogenesis of the inflammatory reaction caused by the filarid.[454] A *Wolbachia* sp. was detected in the blood of a dog from Japan suspected to be infected with *Ehrlichia*.[519] The *Wolbachia* sp. had the closest genetic identity to one previously identified in *Dirofilaria immitis*. These findings suggest that *Wolbachia* sp. might have a role in canine febrile illnesses or heartworm disease. *Wolbachia pipientis* is also found as a symbiont in insects and it was found in 17.8% of cat fleas from France and the United States.[448,190] The potential or frequency of this infection spreading to dogs and cats from infected fleas, and any clinical significance of such infections, is unknown.

*References 102, 103, 204, 241, 332a, 340.

Table • 28-9

Antimicrobial Therapy for Canine and Feline Thrombocytic Anaplasmosis

DRUG[a]	SPECIES	DOSE[b] (mg/kg)	ROUTE PREFERRED (ALTERNATIVE)	INTERVAL (HOURS)	DURATION (DAYS)
Tetracycline	D	22	PO	8	14–21
Oxytetracycline	D	25	PO (IV)	8	14–21
Doxycycline	D	5–10	PO	12	10
	C	10	PO	12	10
Minocycline	D	10	PO (IV)	12	10
Enrofloxacin	D	5	PO (IV, SC)	12	14–21

D, Dog; *C*, cat; *PO*, by mouth; *IV*, intravenously; *SC*, subcutaneously.
[a]See Drug Formulary, Appendix 8, for additional information.
[b]Dose per administration at specified interval.

SUGGESTED READINGS*

73. Breitschwerdt EB, Hegarty BC, Hancock SI. 1998a. Doxycycline hyclate treatment of experimental canine ehrlichiosis followed by challenge inoculation with two *Ehrlichia canis* strains, *Antimicrob Agents Chemother* 42:362-368.
74. Breitschwerdt EB, Hegarty BC, Hancock SI. 1998b. Sequential evaluation of dogs naturally infected with *Ehrlichia canis, Ehrlichia chaffeensis, Ehrlichia equi, Ehrlichia ewingii,* or *Bartonella vinsonii, J Clin Microbiol* 36:2645-2651.
213. Harrus S, Waner T, Aizenberg I, et al. 1998c. Therapeutic effect of doxycycline in experimental subclinical canine monocytic ehrlichiosis: evaluation of a 6-week course, *J Clin Microbiol* 36:2140-2142.
219. Harrus S, Waner T, Keysary A, et al. 1998d. Investigation of splenic function in canine monocytic ehrlichiosis, *Vet Immunol Immunopathol* 62:15-27.
353a. McQuiston JH, McCall CL, Nicholson WL, et al. 2003. Ehrlichiosis and related infections, *J Am Vet Med Assoc* 223:1750-1756.

434. Reubel GH, Barlough JE, Madigan JE. 1998a. Production and characterization of *Ehrlichia risticii,* the agent of Potomac horse fever, from snails (Pleuroceridae: *Juga* spp.) in aquarium culture and genetic comparison to equine strains, *J Clin Microbiol* 36:1501-1511.
459. Sainz A, Tesouro MA, Amusategui I, et al. 2000b. Prospective comparative study of 3 treatment protocols using doxycycline or imidocarb dipropionate in dogs with naturally occurring ehrlichiosis, *J Vet Intern Med* 14:134-139.
497. Suksawat J, Xuejie Y, Hancock SI, et al. 2001c. Serologic and molecular evidence of coinfection with multiple vector-borne pathogens in dogs from Thailand, *J Vet Intern Med* 15:453-462.
537. Waner T, Leykin I, Shinitsky M, et al. 2000a. Detection of platelet-bound antibodies in beagle dogs after artificial infection with *Ehrlichia canis, Vet Immunol Immunopathol* 77:145-150.

*See the CD-ROM for a complete list of references.

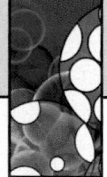

CHAPTER • 29

Rocky Mountain Spotted Fever, Murine Typhuslike Disease, Rickettsialpox, Typhus, and Q Fever

Craig E. Greene and Edward B. Breitschwerdt

ROCKY MOUNTAIN SPOTTED FEVER

Etiology and Epidemiology

Rocky Mountain spotted fever (RMSF) is a tickborne, rickettsial disease of the Americas that affects dogs and people. RMSF was first recognized in the western United States before 1930. RMSF is now known to occur throughout the contiguous United States with the exception of Maine. Overall, the reported prevalence of human disease appears to have increased since its discovery; the highest yearly incidence is now reported to be from the eastern United States (Fig. 29-1). Presumably, this increase reflects better recognition and reporting rather than true geographic spread of the disease.

The disease has been reported in people living in western Canada, Mexico, Panama, Costa Rica, Honduras, Nicaragua, Colombia, Argentina, and Brazil.[43] Deciduous forests,

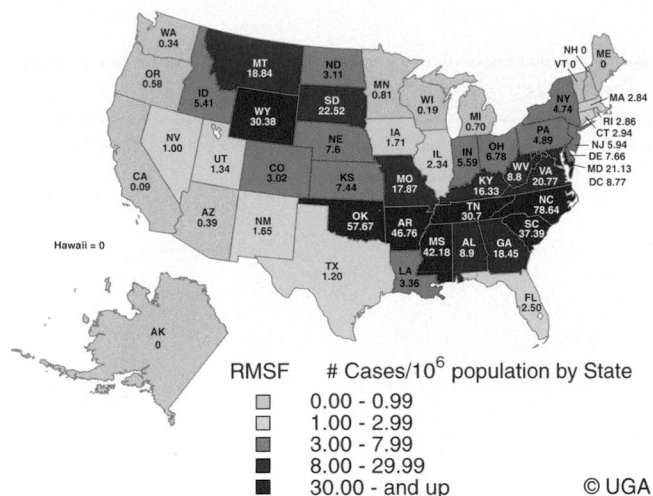

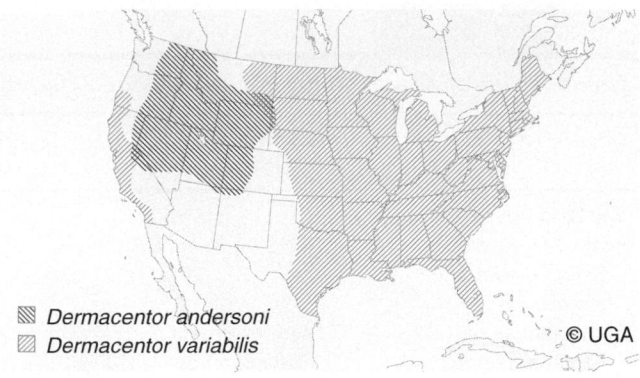

Fig 29-1 Distribution of RMSF cases in people in United States from 1981 to 2002 reported as average yearly incidence per million population. (Data from Dalton MJ, et al. 1995. *Am J Trop Med Hyg* 52:405-413 and subsequent reports from the Centers for Disease Control and Prevention, Atlanta, Ga. Map courtesy University of Georgia, Athens, Ga.)

Fig 29-3 Geographic range of two primary ticks that transmit RMSF. (Courtesy University of Georgia, Athens, Ga.)

In addition, the role of nonpathogenic SFG rickettsiae in immunocompromised individuals has not been clarified.

Diseases similar to RMSF and caused by SFG rickettsiae have been described in people the Eastern Hemisphere. *Rickettsia conorii*—the etiologic agent of boutonneuse, or Mediterranean spotted fever—is an analogous organism transmitted by dog ticks of the genus *Rhipicephalus*.[65-67,129] Dogs and rodents have a transient rickettsemia with *R. conorii* and are subclinically infected. Their role in MSF is as carriers of ticks and occasional reservoirs.[83,128] Queensland tick typhus *(Rickettsia australis)*, Flinder's Island spotted fever *(Rickettsia honei)*, African tick bite fever *(Rickettsia africae)*, Astrakhan fever (Astrakhan fever rickettsia), Japanese spotted fever *(Rickettsia japonica)*, North Asian tick typhus *(Rickettsia sibirica)*, and European tickborne lymphadenopathy *(Rickettsia helvetica, Rickettsia mongolotimonae, Rickettsia slovaca)*, are analogous diseases of people caused by other SFG rickettsiae and transmitted by arthropods in geographically distinct regions.[11,63,108] The clinical significance or reservoir status of dogs or cats for these infections in the Eastern Hemisphere has not been determined. In this chapter, RMSF as it occurs in the United States is emphasized as the model disease for SFG rickettsiosis in dogs. Although cats and other domestic animals can be seropositive, knowledge concerning the occurrence of disease in these other animals is minimal.[90]

The natural history and distribution of RMSF in the United States appears to center primarily on the distribution of two ticks, *Dermacentor andersoni* and *Dermacentor variabilis*, which serve as natural hosts, reservoirs, and vectors for *R. rickettsii*. *D. andersoni* (the wood tick) is a three-host tick that is found in the region from the Cascade Mountains to the Rocky Mountains (Fig. 29-3). It is the principal vector of RMSF in the western United States and is also present in Canada in the provinces of southern British Columbia, Alberta, and Saskatchewan. *D. variabilis* (the American dog tick) is a three-host tick found from the Great Plains region eastward to the Atlantic coast of the United States and southern Canada. It has also been reported in California, southwestern Oregon, southern Washington, and Idaho.

Three other ticks have been incriminated in the United States in the transmission of RMSF to animals and people, but their significance is uncertain. The Lone Star tick *(Amblyomma americanum)* is found in the United States from Texas eastward to the Atlantic Coast. The brown dog tick, *Rhipicephalus sanguineus*, is found throughout the United States, southern Canada, Mexico, and South America. Unlike the other vector ticks, *R. sanguineus* feeds on dogs during all three stages and has rarely been reported to feed on people. *Haemaphysalis leporispalustris*, the rabbit tick, resides throughout the Western Hemisphere. Although some rickettsiae recovered

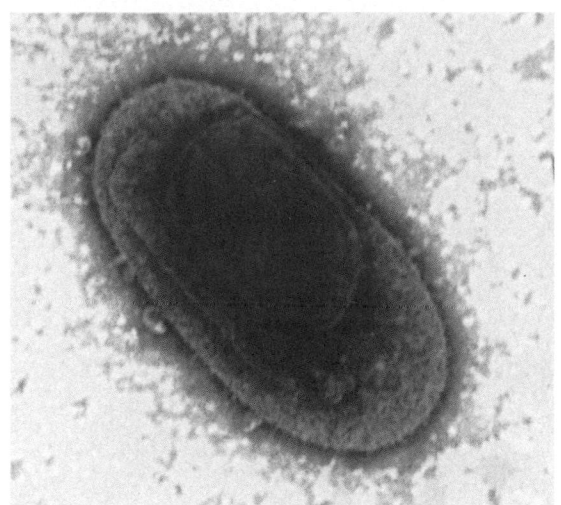

Fig 29-2 *R. rickettsii* in yolk sac culture (×15,000).

increased humidity, and warmer temperatures are factors associated with the high prevalence of this tick-transmitted disease in these areas. Infections in people have even been acquired in urban foci such as in the South Bronx, N.Y., and Philadelphia, Penn.

Rickettsia rickettsii, the etiologic agent of RMSF, is an obligate intracellular bacterium in the family Rickettsiaceae (Fig. 29-2). Members of the spotted fever group (SFG), such as *R. rickettsii*, are most closely related to the typhus group of rickettsiae (Table 29-1) but are distinct from other rickettsial genera. Serologically, genetically, and pathogenically distinct strains of SFG rickettsiae have been described throughout the world.[29,39] Four main SFG species—*R. rickettsii, Rickettsia montana, Rickettsia rhipicephali,* and *Rickettsia bellii*—are isolated from ticks on dogs in the United States.[29] *R. rickettsii* is the only SFG species in the Western Hemisphere known to be pathogenic for people and animals. However, serologic evidence supports potential infection with *Rickettsia canada* or other as yet uncharacterized rickettsiae in dogs and people.[17]

Table • 29-1

Comparison of Some Pathogenic Rickettsiae Affecting Dogs and Cats[a]

DISEASE (AGENT)	GEOGRAPHIC LOCATION	ARTHROPOD VECTOR	INCIDENTAL HOST	RESERVOIR HOST
Spotted Fever Group[b]				
Rocky Mountain spotted fever (*Rickettsia rickettsii*)	North and South America	Ticks (*Dermacentor, Amblyomma, Rhipicephalus*)	People, dogs, cats	Rodents, small mammals, birds
Boutonneuse or Mediterranean spotted fever, Israeli spotted fever (*R. conorii*)	Mediterranean and Caspian Sea littorals, Middle East, Indian subcontinent, Africa	Ticks (*Rhipicephalus*)	People	Rodents, dogs
Japanese spotted fever (*R. japonica*)	Japan	Ticks (*Dermacentor taiwanensis?*)	People	Rodents, dogs
Cat flea typhuslike infection (*Rickettsia felis*)	North and South America, Europe, Africa, Asia	Cat fleas (*Ctenocephalides*)	People	Opossum, cats
	France, Spain, Brazil, Germany, U.K., Japan[c]	Cat fleas (*Ctenocephalides*)	People	Dogs, cats
Rickettsialpox (*R. akari*)	Worldwide	Mites (*Liponyssoides*)	People, dogs	House mice, rats
Typhus Group				
Epidemic typhus (*R. prowazekii*)	South America, Africa, Asia	Body lice (*Pediculus*)	Domestic animals	People
Recrudescent typhus (*R. prowazekii*)	Eastern United States, Mexico, Guatemala	Lice and fleas	People	Flying squirrels
Murine (endemic) typhus (*R. typhi*)	Worldwide, tropical and subtropical	Rat fleas (*Xenopsylla*)	People	Rats, cats
	Texas, California	Cat fleas (*Ctenocephalides*)	People	Cats, opossum
Scrub Typhus (*Orientia tsutsugamushi*)	Asia, India, Australia	Mites (*Leptotrombidium*)	People, dogs (subclinical)	Rats, birds
Other				
Q fever (*Coxiella burnetii*)	Worldwide	Aerosols, ticks	People, dogs	Cattle, sheep, goats, cats
Salmon poisoning disease (see Chapter 27) (*Neorickettsia helminthoeca*)	Pacific northwestern United States	Flukes	People (rare)	Dogs, foxes

[a]For ehrlichiosis and other related rickettsiae, see Table 28-1.
[b]Also includes spotted fever group (SFG)-rickettsiae causing recognized human illnesses: Queensland tick typhus (*Rickettsia australis*: Queensland and New South Wales, Australia), North Asian tick typhus (*Rickettsia sibirica*: Siberia, Mongolia), African tick bite fever (*Rickettsia africae*: Africa, West Indies; *Rickettsia aeschlimannii*: Mediterranean region, Africa), European tickborne lymphadenopathy (*Rickettsia slovaca*: Hungary, France; *Rickettsia helvetica*: Switzerland, France, Slovenia, Sweden; *Rickettsia mongolotimonae*: Europe), and Flinders Island spotted fever and Indian and Thai tick typhus (*Rickettsia honei*: southeastern Victoria, Flinders Island and Tasmania, Australia; India; Thailand). Astrakhan fever *Rickettsia* is closely related to Israel tick typhus *Rickettsia*, and both are genotypes in the *Rickettsia conorii* complex. *R. parkeri*, which was previously thought to be nonpathogenic, is carried by *Amblyomma maculatum* ticks, and was identified as a cause of SFG rickettsial infection in the southern United States.[105a]
[c]In Japan, *Rickettsia felis* has been also identified in ticks.

from this tick have been antigenically similar to *R. rickettsii*, they do not produce disease in laboratory animals. *R. sanguineus* and *Amblyomma cajennense* are the most commonly implicated ticks in transmission of *R. rickettsii* to people in Mexico or Central America and South America, respectively.

Ticks become infected by two means (Fig. 29-4). First, horizontal transmission can occur as noninfected ticks feed on certain small mammals, including chipmunks, voles, and ground squirrels, that develop sufficient rickettsemia during acute infection. The primary sylvan cycle, which maintains the transmission cycle in nature, occurs among these small rodents and immature (larval and nymphal) tick stages, and it is possible that medium-size mammals such as raccoons, opossums, and foxes are additional sources for infecting ticks. Although of minor importance, birds are a means by which infected ticks can be transported into new areas. Second, ticks can be infected transstadially and also vertically by transovarial passage between generations. Venereal transmission of *R. rick-*

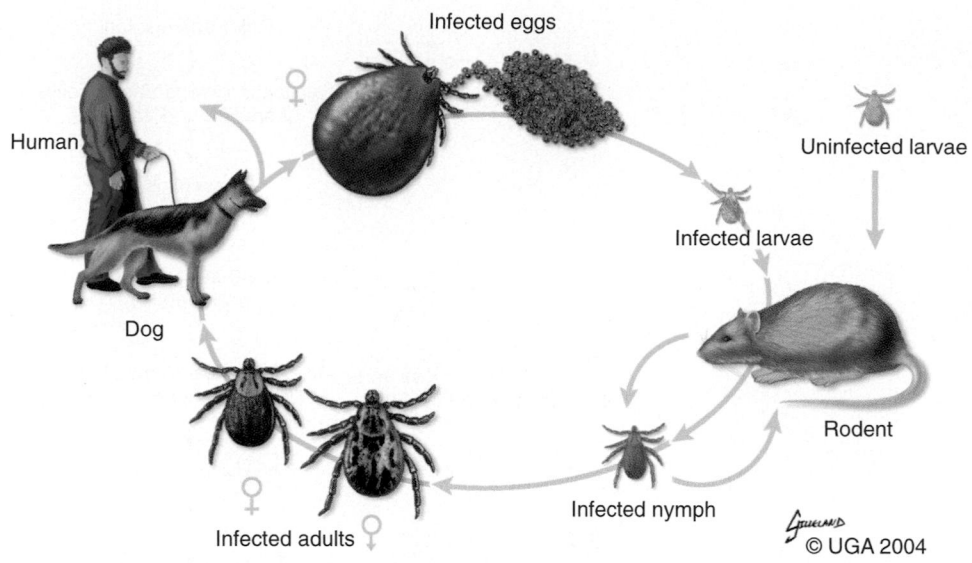

Fig 29-4 Relationship of tick and hosts in RMSF transmission. (Courtesy University of Georgia, Athens, Ga.)

ettsii can also occur when adult ticks copulate.[132] *R. rickettsii* initially replicates in the epithelial cells of the tick midgut, enters the hemocoel, and from there spreads to and multiplies in other tick tissues, including the salivary glands and ovaries. Ticks must ingest numerous rickettsiae for successful transovarial transmission, which is the primary means by which *R. rickettsii* is maintained in nature.

Several restrictions may explain the reason RMSF is limited to geographic islands in the Americas. The overall low prevalence of infection in ticks, less than 2% even in areas with a high prevalence of RMSF, suggests that most mammalian hosts of adult ticks, such as dogs, rarely develop rickettsemia of sufficient magnitude and duration to infect large numbers of ticks. Furthermore, rickettsial infection of ticks is not an ideal symbiotic relationship; it can impair tick reproduction or cause death. Last, resistance to infection with *R. rickettsii* develops in ticks and possibly mammalian hosts as a result of infection with the other common nonpathogenic SFG rickettsiae. In endemic areas, less than 10% of the ticks contain *R. rickettsii*.[146]

For reasons that are not completely understood, ticks do not usually infect a new host until they have been attached for a minimum of 5 to 20 hours. A reactivation period within the tick with an apparent increased rickettsial virulence is thought to occur after ticks reattach and take their first blood meal of the season. A period of feeding also may be needed for the continued replication of infective rickettsiae in the salivary glands. Delayed transmission may also relate to the ticks' need to produce a cement collar around their mouth parts before they begin feeding. Although infections that people acquire from tick bites require extended attachment, those acquired from contact of mucous membranes with feces or hemolymph from preengorged ticks on animals or contact with laboratory-infected cultures or mammalian blood do not appear to involve extended contact periods.

Pathogenesis

R. rickettsii usually enter the body through the bite of infected ticks (Fig. 29-5). Rickettsiae are disseminated via the circulatory system and invade and replicate in endothelial cells of smaller arteries and venules. Phospholipase and proteases have been incriminated as mechanisms for rickettsial damage to cell membranes. Subsequent endothelial cell damage initiates a vasculitis with platelet activation and activation of the coagulation system accompanied by decreased plasma levels of antithrombin III and plasminogen and increased fibrinogen degradation products (FDPs). These hematologic changes are consistent with simultaneous activation of the fibrinolytic and coagulation systems. Coagulation factor consumption is not usually extensive enough to cause hypofibrinogenemia or overt disseminated intravascular coagulation (DIC).[145] Results of coagulation factor analysis suggest activation of the extrinsic and intrinsic pathways. Elevated platelet-associated immunoglobulin in dogs with experimentally and naturally induced RMSF suggests an immune-mediated cause of the thrombocytopenia.[49] Progressive necrotizing vasculitis may be caused sequentially by complement activation, cellular chemotaxis, and subsequent vascular necrosis and extravasation of blood. Organs with endarterial circulation, such as the skin, brain, heart, and kidneys, are most adversely affected.

Significantly increased plasma and extracellular fluid volume have been described in experimental infections of nonhuman primates. Accumulation of extracellular fluid and electrolytes, renal water retention, and edema were correlated with increased concentrations of aldosterone and antidiuretic hormone (ADH) in people. Hyponatremia, which occurs in dogs and people, may be related to the syndrome of inappropriate ADH release. Fluid overload in the circulation and edema of the medulla oblongata in experimental animals suggest that intravenous fluid therapy be used sparingly in the management of dogs with RMSF. Central nervous system (CNS) signs and death may relate to cardiorespiratory depression through edema involving medullary centers. Fulminant infection may result in peripheral vascular collapse and death in the first week of infection, before proliferative and thrombotic lesions occur. Acute renal failure, a fatal complication of RMSF in people, has not been frequently reported in dogs.

Clinical Findings

Clinical and subclinical illnesses have been reported in dogs with naturally occurring and experimentally produced RMSF. Naturally acquired immunity has an important role in pro-

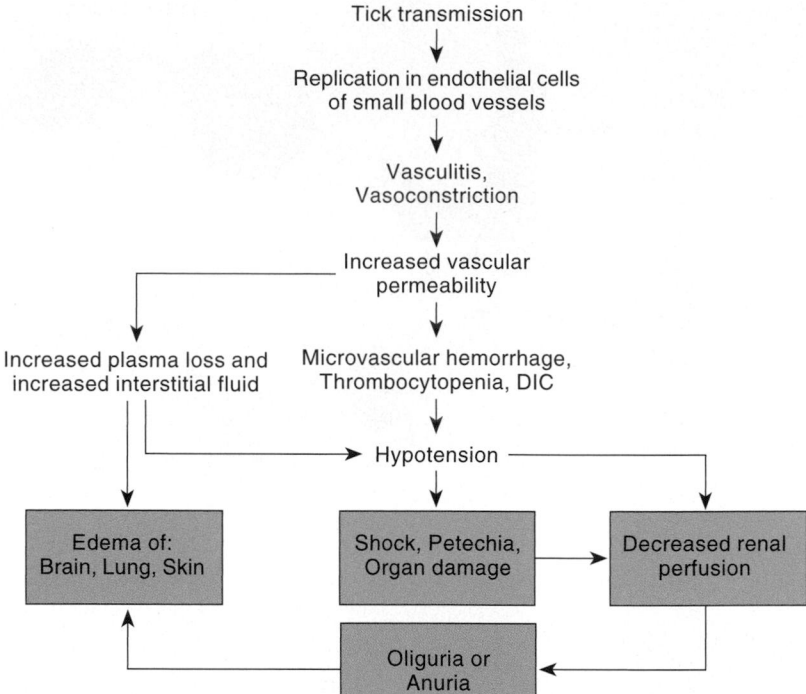

Fig 29-5 Pathogenesis of RMSF.

tection against clinical illness. Anti-SFG rickettsial antibodies can be found in the healthy canine population in endemic areas. This observation may be a consequence of subclinical infections or the result of exposure to nonpathogenic SFG rickettsiae in ticks. Immunogenic contact with *R. rickettsii* induces a protective response in experimental dogs to reinfection for at least up to 3 years.[18] Most dogs are examined for illness during the months of March to October. Purebred dogs appear to be more prone to develop clinical illness than mixed breed dogs, and the German shepherd dog has a particularly high prevalence of disease. People with glucose-6-phosphate dehydrogenase deficiency and English springer spaniels with suspected phosphofructokinase deficiency have a more fulminant course of illness and are more likely to develop dermal necrosis,[151] as are animals in which treatment is delayed. Clinical signs of illness in dogs are similar to those of naturally infected people (Tables 29-2 and 29-3).

Fever, one of the first and most consistent findings, can occur within 2 to 3 days after tick attachment. The range of the incubation period is 2 to 14 days. Early cutaneous lesions in some dogs consist of edema and hyperemia of the lips, penile sheath, scrotum, pinna, other extremities (Fig. 29-6), and rarely the ventral abdomen. Discrete clear vesicles and focal erythematous macules have been observed on the buccal mucosa. Male dogs that develop scrotal edema or epididymal swelling often have a stiff gait and are reluctant to walk. Gait abnormalities are a result of inflammation of joints, muscles, and meninges.

Petechial and ecchymotic hemorrhages may develop subsequent to the acute illness in some dogs and if present occur on ocular, oral, and genital mucous membranes rather than the skin (Fig. 29-7). Funduscopic examination provides a more sensitive means of detecting these hemorrhagic lesions (see Fig. 93-14).[32] Epistaxis, melena, and hematuria may be noted in severely affected animals.

Neurologic signs of generalized cerebral and spinal cord involvement have been found (see Table 29-2). More severe neurologic abnormalities caused by meningitis progressing to encephalomyelitis are found in dogs and people in which the

Table • 29-2

Medical Problems Associated with Rocky Mountain Spotted Fever

History
Lethargy, anorexia, weight loss, vomiting, diarrhea, seasonal (warm months)

Physical Examination
Fever, ocular signs (e.g., scleral congestion, conjunctivitis, anterior uveitis, iridal hemorrhage, retinitis), lymphadenomegaly, edema, hyperemia, tachycardia, tachypnea, dyspnea, cutaneous necrosis, subcutaneous edema, icterus, hepatomegaly, petechiae, ecchymoses, myalgia, arthralgia, joint swelling and stiffness, neurologic signs (e.g., hyperesthesia, tetraparesis, ataxia, vestibular signs, seizures)

Ancillary Diagnostics
Hematologic tests: Thrombocytopenia, leukocytosis with shift, hypoalbuminemia, elevated serum ALP activity, hyperbilirubinemia, hyponatremia, artifactual hypocalcemia, prolonged coagulation times
Cytologic examination: Suppurative polyarthritis, suppurative meningitis, lymph node hyperplasia
Radiography: Interstitial pneumonia

ALP, Alkaline phosphatase.

diagnosis and treatment are delayed. Focal or localizing neurologic signs, such as vestibular disease, are common in the early phases of illness and are often the reason the animal is taken to the veterinarian.

Infected dogs may make a rapid and complete recovery if they are mildly affected or antimicrobial therapy is instituted

Table • **29-3**

Frequency of Clinical Findings in People and Dogs with RMSF

CLINICAL FINDINGS	PEOPLE[a] (N = 262)	DOGS[b] (N = 79)	DOGS[c] (N = 30)
Low fever	99 (> 37.8°C)	67 (> 39.2°C)	70[d]
High fever	90 (> 38.9°C)	54 (> 40°C)	NR
Headache	91	NR	NR
Rash, petechiae	88	19	12
Myalgia, arthralgia	83	49	27
Anorexia	NR	51	70
Known tick exposure	67	52	17
Nausea, vomiting	60	18	NR
Abdominal or lumbar pain	52	30	NR
Conjunctivitis, scleral congestion	30	34	52[e]
Lymphadenomegaly	27	43	50
CNS signs	26	83	67
Vestibular deficits[f]	18	41	33
Cervical pain, nuchal rigidity	18	8	20
Coma, unconsciousness	9	4	NR
Seizures	8	10	20
Diarrhea	19	16	NR
Edema of face, extremities	18	25	32
Polydipsia, polyuria	NR	5	NR
Splenomegaly	16	3	NR
Hepatomegaly	12	3	12
Pneumonitis, dyspnea, cough	12	39	20
Jaundice	9	4	12
Cardiac arrhythmias	7	8	NR
Death	4	3	0

NR, Not reported or not stated as such; *CNS*, central nervous system.
[a]Data from Helmick CG, et al. *J Infect Dis* 150:480–488, 1984
[b]Data from Greene CE. 1987. *J Am Vet Med Assoc* 19:666–671; Greene CE. 1989. Unpublished observations. University of Georgia, Athens, Ga.
[c]Data from Gasser AM, et al. 2001. *J Am Anim Hosp Assoc* 37:41–48, 2001.
[d]Temperature > 39.5°C
[e]Include vestibular signs of nystagmus, head tilt, circling, and incoordination.
[f]Includes ocular discharge, scleral and conjunctival congestion, scleral and conjunctival hemorrhage, conjunctivitis, scleral petechiae, anterior uveitis, hyphema, iridal hemorrhage, and retinitis.

early. Permanent organ damage, particularly resulting in residual neurologic dysfunction, may occur within 1 to 2 weeks of onset of clinical signs in severely affected dogs that survive the acute stages of illness. Necrosis of the extremities and previously hyperemic or edematous portions of the body may occur at this time (Fig. 29-8). Dogs may die in the acute stages of illness as a result of hemorrhagic diathesis or from thrombosis of vital organs. Cardiovascular, neurologic, and renal damage are the most consistent causes of death or permanent organ dysfunction. Death in some severely affected dogs has been caused by disseminated, rapidly progressing meningoencephalitis. Shock, cardiovascular collapse, and oliguria become apparent in the terminal stages of illness.

Diagnosis
Clinical Laboratory Findings
Mild leukopenia, which may develop early in the course of illness, is followed by a moderate leukocytosis generally characterized by a stress leukogram or accompanied by a minimal left shift and toxic granulation of neutrophils. The longer the duration of clinical signs before diagnosis, the more pronounced the leukocytosis. A normocytic normochromic

anemia and elevated erythrocyte sedimentation rate are nonspecific hematologic changes. Fibrinogen concentration, which increases as a result of an acute-phase reaction in mildly to moderately affected dogs, may be decreased in severely affected dogs as a result of rapid consumption secondary to vasculitis.

Thrombocytopenia is one of the most consistent hematologic abnormalities in infected dogs. Platelet counts generally range from 23,000/μl to 220,000/μl. Megathrombocytosis is usually detectable in a majority of cases. Thrombocytopenia in RMSF is often not less than 75,000/μl; however, lower trends have been reported.[44] Electronic counting of thrombocytopenic specimens below this level generally gives lower counts than hemocytometer methods on the same specimen when correlations are made. A mild prolongation of the activated clotting time may be the only coagulation abnormality.[30,31] Rarely, overt DIC characterized by prolongation of the activated coagulation time, prothrombin time, activated partial thromboplastin time, and thrombin time with elevated FDPs occurs in dogs.[32]

Biochemical abnormalities may include mildly increased serum glucose concentration and elevated serum alkaline

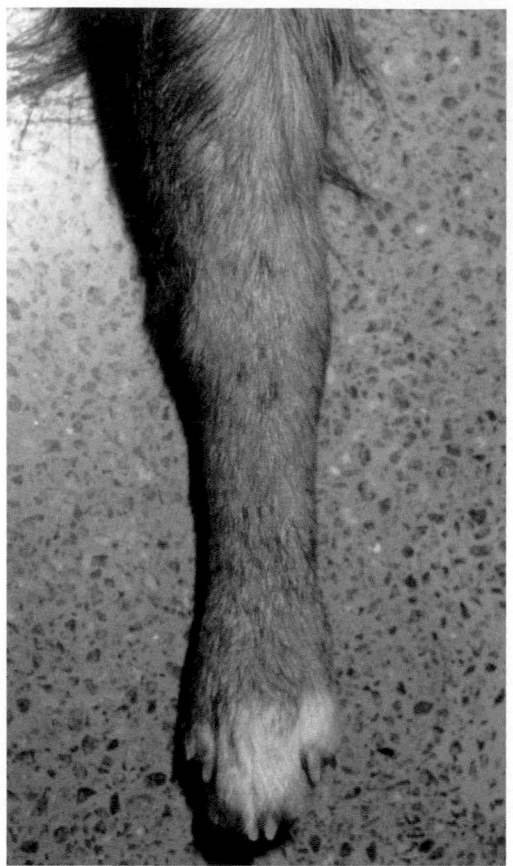

Fig 29-6 Pelvic limb edema in dog with RMSF. (Courtesy University of Georgia, Athens, Ga.)

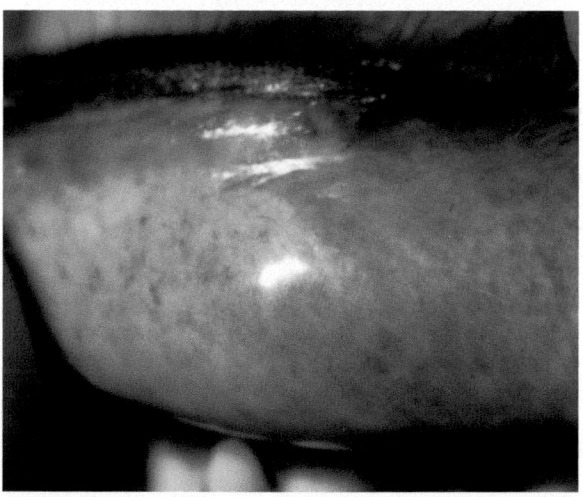

Fig 29-7 Petechiae on oral mucosa of dog with RMSF. (Courtesy University of Georgia, Athens, Ga.)

phosphatase, alanine transferase, and aspartate transferase activities. Hypercholesterolemia has been one of the more consistent findings in affected dogs. Hypoalbuminemia is often observed and probably caused by leakage associated with generalized vascular endothelial damage. Hyponatremia, hypochloremia, and metabolic acidosis are variable findings.

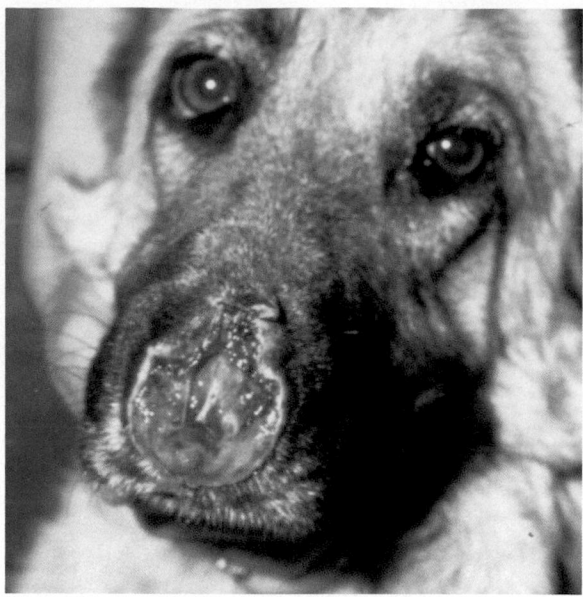

Fig 29-8 Necrosis of planum nasale in dog with RMSF. (Courtesy University of Georgia, Athens, Ga.)

The serum urea nitrogen may increase in terminal stages of the disease corresponding with oliguria and renal failure. Proteinuria and hematuria occur as a result of incoagulability or glomerular and tubular injury. Bilirubinuria and hyperbilirubinemia occur in some dogs, but these are usually mild. Serum creatine kinase has been mildly to moderately increased in some dogs. Cerebrospinal fluid analysis is frequently normal; however, mildly increased protein (greater than 25 mg/μl but less than 100 mg/μl) and polymorphonuclear or mononuclear cells may be found. Analysis of synovial fluid in dogs with accompanying polyarthritis has shown inflammatory changes, with a predominant increase in neutrophils. Results of lupus erythematosus cell, rheumatoid factor, antinuclear antibody, platelet autoantibody, and Coombs' testing and of bacterial blood culture are usually negative. The presence of co-infections with other tickborne agents such as *Ehrlichia* or *Babesia* organisms may cause positive Coombs' test results (see Chapters 28 and 77, respectively).

If present, electrocardiographic abnormalities consist of sinoatrial node dysfunction, ST-segment and T-wave depressions, and premature ventricular contractions. Thoracic radiography reveals diffuse increased interstitial density, especially in dogs having dyspnea and coughing.[34]

Serologic Testing
Measurement of *R. rickettsii* serum antibodies is the primary method of confirmation of RMSF in clinical practice. Mammalian hosts differ in regard to the specificity of their immune response to rickettsiae. Well-adapted hosts, such as mice, develop highly specific antibody titers against each species of organism. Human serologic responses generally react strongly with group-reactive antibodies but do not consistently distinguish between typhus group and SFG rickettsiae. Seroreactivity of dogs appears to be between that of rodents and people. Cross-reactions in dog sera develop between SFG antigens; however, the titer is generally highest to the specific rickettsial species causing infection. Generally, minimal reactions to typhus group or other rickettsiae occur. Clinically healthy dogs on the Atlantic seaboard have between 5% and 15% seropositivity to SFG rickettsiae, indicating infection by anti-

genically related avirulent rickettsiae or subclinical infection. Some ill dogs have shown stronger reactivity to nonpathogenic *R. bellii* and typhus group antigens than *R. rickettsii*, suggesting that another yet unidentified *Rickettsia* organism may be pathogenic.[17]

Several serologic tests have been developed to detect antibodies to RMSF in people, including Weil-Felix, complement fixation, microscopic immunofluorescence (Micro-IF), microagglutination, indirect hemagglutination, enzyme-linked immunosorbent assay (ELISA), and latex agglutination (LA).[62] The Micro-IF, ELISA, and LA tests appear to be the best suited to examine canine sera.[47]

An increased IgM titer or fourfold increase in IgG titer is needed to confirm active infection with *R. rickettsii*. The Micro-IF test, an indirect fluorescent antibody (FA) test, and the ELISA have the advantages of requiring small amounts of sera and reagents, having high sensitivity, and classifying antibodies to *R. rickettsii* as IgM or IgG. Measurement of IgG antibodies to *R. rickettsii* using the Micro-IF method is used by most diagnostic laboratories that test canine sera (see Appendix 5). Acute and convalescent IgG titers have been generally less than 1:64 in uninfected dogs and in those with ehrlichiosis, although titers vary among laboratories. Actively infected dogs may or may not have increased titers ≥1:64 by the time clinical signs are apparent and the first sample is taken. IgG titers in experimentally infected dogs with disease manifestations by 3 to 6 days after infection have not increased until 2 to 3 weeks after infection. Therefore seronegative results do not discount the possibility of RMSF, and a convalescent sample should be tested at a later date. An IgG titer increase of fourfold or greater is required to document active infection definitively. High IgG titers that develop in actively infected dogs generally decrease after 3 to 5 months, although some may remain elevated (1:128) for at least 10 months.[40,48] Thus unless single titers are markedly increased (1:1024), active infection cannot be absolutely ascertained, and paired samples must be obtained. Differences can be found among laboratories performing the test and within laboratories testing the same sample at a later date. Therefore it is recommended that acute and convalescent serum samples be submitted together. Simultaneous assessment of IgM and IgG titers can provide more accurate assessment as to the time course of infection when evaluating a single serum sample. Seroconversion to *R. rickettsii* antigen is suppressed by administration of antimicrobials early in the disease.[19]

A modification of the test that allows for measurement of IgM has advantages in permitting more specific diagnosis of recent infection with a single convalescent titer, and IgM titers can be increased before increases in IgG titers. The IgM titers in naturally and experimentally infected dogs only increase (≥1:8) during the first week after infection and decrease after 4 to 8 weeks or less. The maximum measured titers are generally two to four dilutions lower in magnitude than the corresponding IgG titers in the same animal.

The LA test appears to be a rapid and specific assay for recent *R. rickettsii* infection in dogs.[48] Because the sensitivity is lower than the Micro-IF test, false-negative results occur, although a single increased titer (1:32) appears to be diagnostic for RMSF in dogs.

Direct Immunodetection

Direct FA staining of infected tissues has been used in the past for rapid clinical or postmortem diagnosis of RMSF. Direct FA procedures have also been used to detect organisms in embryonated eggs or tissue culture, tissues at necropsy, ticks, and skin biopsies from acutely infected people and dogs. Full-thickness skin biopsies should be surgically removed from visible lesions on the skin or mucosae and placed in isotonic saline on melting ice or in formalin at room temperature until they are processed. Formalin fixation causes some decrease in sensitivity of rickettsial detection. Rickettsiae can be found in approximately 75% of specimens taken from affected lesions and are rarely found in unaffected skin. Trypsin digestion and deparaffinization are needed to examine specimens that have been processed for light microscopy. Tissue sections are stained by fluorescein-conjugated antibody to *R. rickettsii* for the presence of coccobacillary organisms in endothelial cells and vascular walls of the dermis.

The advantages of the direct FA procedure on tissue are that it may be able to confirm the diagnosis on a single sample as early as the third or fourth day of disease. Direct FA procedures can be performed by veterinary or human laboratories without regard to host species differences. Few false-positive results are found with the direct FA test, but many (30% to 40%) false-negative reactions can occur and are usually a result of prior therapy with chloramphenicol or tetracycline or failure to obtain a sample through an area of vasculitis. Specimens should be obtained early in the course of infection because organisms are eliminated from the tissue within a few days, especially after institution of antimicrobial therapy. Because of the usual absence of cutaneous petechiae in dogs, biopsy specimens could be obtained from mucosal hemorrhages or from vesicles that may develop in the buccal mucosa. Adaptation of this method using immunoperoxidase staining increases the test sensitivity and specificity.[77] Immunohistochemical methods have been used to substantiate infection in people dying of RMSF that was not detected by serologic means.[105]

Genetic Detection

The polymerase chain reaction (PCR) has made it possible to detect DNA from low numbers of rickettsiae in whole blood or tissue specimens and for comparison of isolates.[131,144] Amplification of a unique region of the 16S rRNA gene sequence of *R. rickettsii* facilitates acute-phase diagnosis of RMSF, but with current techniques it has not been highly sensitive. A nested PCR is more sensitive than culture in detecting rickettsial DNA in dogs after treatment and may remain positive for longer periods because of the persistence of nonviable nucleic acid.[19] PCR has documented that many dogs infected with *R. rickettsii* may be coinfected with various *Ehrlichia*, *Bartonella*, *Babesia*, other *Rickettsia* species, or all of these, making a specific diagnosis uncertain and causing higher morbidity than with a single-agent infection.[72]

Rickettsial Isolation

Bioassays involving isolation of *R. rickettsii* in susceptible species of laboratory animals have been a means of diagnosing RMSF in the research laboratory.[29] Fresh- or deep-frozen (−80° C) tissue such as liver, spleen, or brain or clotted blood from biopsy or necropsy specimens can be inoculated into meadow voles or guinea pigs. Their serum may be tested for the presence of antibody to *R. rickettsii*. Tissues or blood of the affected or laboratory animal may be inoculated into embryonated chicken eggs or tissue culture to isolate and purify the agent. A described shell vial method which involves using concentrated inoculum to infect a small number of cells permits detection in cell culture in as few as 24 to 48 hours.[106] A staining technique using carbol basic fuchsin is widely used for the identification of SFG and typhus group rickettsiae. Rickettsiae may replicate sufficiently within several days within in vitro isolation procedures, whereas bioassays often require a month to complete. Isolation of *R. rickettsii* requires an appropriate tissue culture system and a biosafety level 3 laboratory and could infect laboratory workers by inadvertent parenteral or aerosol inoculation.

Pathologic Findings

When RMSF proves fatal, gross lesions (if present) consist of widespread petechial and ecchymotic hemorrhages in all tissues. Generalized hemorrhagic lymphadenomegaly and splenomegaly are usually found.

Microscopic findings consist of necrotizing vasculitis with perivascular polymorphonuclear and lymphoreticular cell infiltrations. Vascular lesions are most prominent in the skin, epididymis, testicle, gastrointestinal tract, pancreas, kidneys, urinary bladder, myocardium, meninges, retina, and skeletal muscle. Acute meningoencephalitis with vasculitis and small focal nodular gliosis is found in brain parenchyma of dogs with acute infections (Fig. 29-9). Focal myocardial and hepatic necrosis and acute interstitial pneumonia are common lesions. Rickettsiae can be detected in many tissues by previously described staining and isolation procedures but not by routine histologic methods.

Therapy

Mortality in dogs with RMSF is usually associated with incorrect diagnosis and treatment or rapidly progressive shock or severe CNS infections. Antibody titers are generally not available when the dog is admitted and even then, results from the first sample may not be diagnostic because it may take 1 to 3 weeks for maximal IgG response. For this reason a response to therapy is used to increase the index of suspicion. It is judicious to begin treatment immediately after obtaining samples for diagnostic testing. Presumptive diagnosis of RMSF can be made based on the seasonal occurrence and clinical and laboratory abnormalities. The antibiotics used to treat RMSF are considered to be rickettsiostatic (Table 29-4). Although they slightly prolong the duration of rickettsemia, antiinflammatory and immunosuppressive doses of glucocorticoids do not increase the severity of disease in experimentally infected dogs.[16] They may help avert the signs of the concurrent immune-mediated thrombocytopenia[49]; however, their use is not generally recommended because appropriate antimicrobial therapy is curative. Tetracyclines are the antibiotics of choice to treat RMSF.[57]

Tetracycline or oxytetracycline should be given for at least 7 days. Lipid-soluble tetracyclines, such as minocycline or doxycycline, have been shown to be as effective in treating rickettsial infections in people when they have been used for fewer than 7 days. Their use early in the course of illness may attenuate the serologic response to infection but in most instances, it does not interfere with serologic confirmation (a fourfold change in antibody titer) of RMSF. Chloramphenicol is also effective and might be considered for pregnant animals or in young (younger than 6 months old) puppies to avoid dental staining; however, use of doxycycline has minimal effects on dental color and has been more effective than chloramphenicol.[81,110] Fluoroquinolones such as enrofloxacin or trovafloxacin are also effective;[15,19] however, because they can cause cartilaginous injury, their use must be restricted to older animals. Josamycin, a newer macrolide antimicrobial with activity similar to erythromycin, has been used successfully in treating pregnant women with *R. conorii* infection.[33] Azithromycin and clarithromycin, newer erythromycin derivatives, have been used effectively to treat SFG rickettsioses in people, especially children in whom tetracyclines are contraindicated.[22,127] Azithromycin was less effective in clearing RMSF rickettsemia in dogs as compared with doxycycline or trovafloxacin[19] and therefore is not recommended. Parenteral administration of antimicrobial drugs may be required in patients that are semicomatose or have nausea or are vomiting. Dogs treated early in the course of illness have rapid clinical improvement, generally within 24 to 48 hours after therapy is instituted. Defervescence within 12 hours is not unusual. Delayed or incomplete recovery is associated with organ failure or CNS damage. Some dogs treated with chloramphenicol and although less common, with tetracycline, develop depression, nausea, and vomiting, which can appear to delay their clinical recovery. Antibiotics are only effective in reducing the severity of the illness if they are given before the development of advanced pathologic changes, such as thrombosis and tissue necrosis. The extremities of dogs that develop acryl gangrene and recover

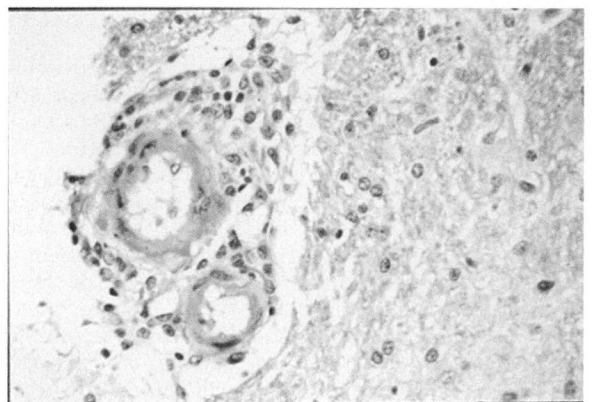

Fig 29-9 Perivascular cuffing of meninges from dog that died of rapidly progressive RMSF associated with meningoencephalitis (H and E stain, ×400). (Courtesy University of Georgia, Athens, Ga.)

Table • 29-4

Therapy for Rocky Mountain Spotted Fever

DRUG[a]	DOSE[b] (mg/kg)	PREFERRED ROUTE (ALTERNATE ROUTE)	INTERVAL (HOURS)	DURATION (WEEKS)
Tetracycline	22–30	PO (IV)	8	1
Chloramphenicol	15–30	PO (IV, SC, IM)	8	1
Doxycycline	10–20	PO (IV)	12	1
Enrofloxacin	3	PO (SC)	12	1

PO, By mouth; *IV*, intravenous; *SC*, subcutaneous; *IM*, intramuscular.
[a]For additional information on each drug, see Appendix 8.
[b]Dose per administration at specified interval.

eventually heal but have permanent scarring or disfigurement.

Supportive care must be used in dogs with shock, coagulation disorders, and clinical or laboratory evidence of organ failure. IV fluid therapy must be used with caution because increased vascular permeability and expanded extracellular fluid volume can give rise to pulmonary and cerebral edema.

Prevention

Dogs recovering from infection with *R. rickettsii* have been immune to reinfection when challenged 6 to 36 months later. Experimentally, infection with nonpathogenic rickettsiae such as *R. montana* does not seem to protect dogs from subsequent infection with the more virulent *R. rickettsii*. Naturally infected dogs that recover from RMSF have never been shown to be reinfected.

No vaccines are available for use in dogs or people. Challenge infection in people after vaccination with inactivated products has been associated with a prolonged incubation period, a shorter and milder course of illness, and reduced prevalence of relapses, but reinfection is not prevented. Experimental, inactivated, tissue-culture origin vaccines appear to offer protection against infection in experimental animals. Specific antigenic components of *R. rickettsii* responsible for producing protective antibody response were identified. Vaccines containing recombinant outer membrane proteins A of *R. rickettsii* or *R. conorii* have been shown to be immunoprotective in rodents.[4,27,142]

The best means of prevention of RMSF in dogs is avoidance of tick-infested areas and rapid, safe removal of attached ticks. Pets should be protected with an insecticide-impregnated collar or topical or systemic acaricides if they frequent areas inhabited by ticks. Tick eradication in the environment is impossible because of the maintenance of the life cycle by rodents and other reservoir hosts. Elimination of small ground rodents is difficult if not impossible to achieve. Some reduction in tick numbers has been achieved locally in the eastern and southern United States through insecticide application to surrounding vegetation in the form of aqueous suspension or dust.

Public Health Considerations

SFG rickettsial infections are important zoonotic diseases because of their endemic nature, high prevalence, and severity when mistreated or misdiagnosed. Of the more than 1000 cases of rickettsial diseases reported each year in the United States, approximately 90% are RMSF. The mortality rate in people, which is highest among the tickborne illnesses, remains between 2% and 10%.[28,89] The yearly incidence rate probably reflects a summation of factors, including encroachment of people on undeveloped wooded areas, improved recognition and reporting of disease, and a periodic cyclicity of infection. The prevalence of seropositive reactions in dogs within a given area usually parallels risk of human infection.

The seasonal occurrence of RMSF in people parallels that in dogs.[28] The rate of infection is highest in children and young adults and is higher in males than females. Patients from rural areas have a greater proportion of confirmed diagnoses than those from suburban and urban areas. Approximately 60% of infected people have reported a tick bite, and an additional 30% said that they were in a wooded area just before the clinical illness developed. The lack of known exposure does not eliminate tick involvement in infection, especially because small larval and nymphal stages can feed transiently and remain undetected. Most exposures in the eastern United States occur at the place of residence, but a number have been related to an outdoor recreational activity. Approximately 10% of reported human cases occur only after known expo-

sure to dogs or their ticks, but this should not imply an absolute association; common exposure to the same tick population is a more likely source of infection. The high mortality of the human disease in large part is a result of its severe manifestations; however, the diagnosis of many cases is delayed because of the broad geographic region and sporadic nature of its occurrence and its diverse clinical manifestations. Veterinarians can play an important role in recognition of the human illness because dogs in a household have often been ill in association with or before their human counterparts.[36,104] Veterinarians should be proactive by educating their clients and contacting human health caregivers should the human form of the illness be observed in association with a dog with SFG rickettsial infection.

In addition to common exposure to ticks, dogs are also a potential source for human infections because they carry infected ticks into nonendemic environs or closer to people. Unattached ticks may move from the dogs and attach to people. More frequently, people expose their abraded skin or conjunctivae to an engorged tick's hemolymph or excreta during tick removal.[129] It is not the secretions from infected dogs but the effluents from engorged, infected ticks that pose the greatest danger. Aerosol exposure from an infected dog's secretions is unlikely under natural conditions because the organism does not survive outside host or tick cells. Aerosol exposure has only occurred in the laboratory, where inadvertent inoculation of infected tissues may also occur.

The clinical manifestations in affected people closely parallel the signs seen in dogs (see Table 29-2). Early signs in people are vague and may mimic an upper respiratory tract infection. Although the rash is considered typical of RMSF, it never develops in up to 12% of people and when it does develop, it is seen in less than 50% of the cases within the first 3 days of illness. Not all people develop all manifestations of RMSF, although fever and headache are most consistent. Neurologic signs usually develop later in the course of illness. Death appears to be more of a problem in people who develop severe hepatomegaly, jaundice, stupor, and azotemia (serum urea > 25 mg/dl). Cardiac arrhythmias from myocarditis, meningoencephalitis, and DIC often are detected in terminal patients. Subclinical infections in people have been suspected, but the role of nonpathogenic rickettsiae in causing the observed serologic responses has not been determined. Primary infection or coinfection with *Ehrlichia* organisms can confound the diagnosis of RMSF in people. Manifestations of RMSF and *Ehrlichia chaffeensis* or *Anaplasma phagocytophilum* infections (see Chapter 28) are clinically indistinguishable and occur in overlapping geographic locations. Broad serologic testing must be incorporated to determine the cause of illness in most instances.

Ticks should be removed by applying constant traction with curved forceps or (although less desirable) with tweezers or fingers protected with facial tissue placed as close as possible to the point of insertion. Ticks should not be squeezed or crushed with bare fingers because the organism can be transmitted via tick feces or hemolymph. Hands should be washed thoroughly with soap and water after removal of the tick.

The most effective measures to prevent tick-induced infections have been to wear permethrin-treated clothing and tuck trouser legs into boots when spending time in tick-infested areas.[156] Wearing clothing that is tight around the ankles and wrists when walking through wooded areas is advised. After outdoor activities the skin along the hairline and clothing around the cuffs and collars should be examined. Bathing in a tub of water with a cup of added bleach is recommended after leaving tick-infested areas (see Chapter 45, Lyme Borreliosis, for additional information on tick control).

CAT-FLEA TYPHUSLIKE ILLNESS (*RICKETTSIA FELIS* INFECTION)

In North America a typhuslike illness caused by *Rickettsia felis* has been reported in people in southern Texas,[35] California,[138] and Mexico.[157] Opossums *(Didelphis virginiana)* have been implicated as reservoir hosts in these areas, and the vector is the cat flea *(Ctenocephalides felis)*. The disease in southern Texas and California overlaps that of human murine typhus caused by *Rickettsia typhi*, and opossums and fleas have been found to be coinfected with both rickettsiae in these areas.[13] In these areas, cat flea infection with *R. felis* is more common than with *R. typhi*.[124,125,155] An infection cycle in people with *R. felis* and *C. felis* has been found in France, Germany, and Brazil.[113,118] *R. felis* has been found in *C. felis* on dogs and cats in France,[119] Spain,[84] Mexico,[159] the United Kingdom,[67a,69] and Brazil[102] and in ticks from Japan.[61] Affected people develop cutaneous flea bite reactions, fever, hyperesthesia, myalgia, and a maculopapular rash.[118,157] The infection probably exists worldwide in areas where cat fleas are prevalent. The rickettsial agent *R. felis* (previously "ELB agent")[54] is ultrastructurally and serologically indistinguishable from *R. typhi* and *Rickettsia prowazekii* and has been identified by PCR in infected fleas, opossums, and people in the same area of the United States reported to be endemic for *R. typhi*.[124,125] Despite these morphologic and serologic similarities, genetic analysis with phylogenetic comparison has placed *R. felis* in the SFG rickettsiae.[14] PCR and restriction fragment length polymorphism identified *R. typhi* in four of five people from Texas who had typhus, and *R. felis* was found in the remaining person.[124] In addition to opossums, cats (but not dogs or rats) have been seropositive to *R. typhi* antigen in these areas.[125,138] The newly recognized *R. felis* agent is the predominant rickettsiae (rather than *R. typhi*) in cat fleas found feeding on opossums in these endemic regions.[125,155] It has not been cultured, although molecular techniques have been used to demonstrate its presence. *R. felis* is transmitted transovarially and transstadially in successive generations of *C. felis*.[6,55] Infection can be maintained in cat fleas for up to 12 generations without the fleas having fed on an infected host.[150] Infection has also been transmitted among cats by infected fleas.[149] Cats may be likely hosts that transport infected fleas into human habitats. The reservoir potential of cats for *R. felis* and its pathogenicity for cats has not been determined. Experimental infection of cats has produced subclinical infection with seroconversion between 2 to 4 months.[149] In the United States, *R. felis* has been detected in cat fleas from California, Florida, Georgia, Louisiana, New York, North Carolina, Oklahoma, Tennessee, and Texas and is probably even more widespread.[5] Although *R. typhi* and *R. felis* have never been found in the same fleas in these regions, experimental infections have produced coinfected fleas.[99]

RICKETTSIALPOX

Rickettsialpox, a nonfatal febrile zoonotic illness caused by *Rickettsia akari*, predominantly affects people in urban areas. Serum antibodies to *R. akari* were found in dogs examined during routine veterinary care in New York City.[24] Approximately 7% of the results of an ELISA screening test for antibody to *R. rickettsii* were positive, and seroprevalence increased with advancing age and a history of tick infestation. The dogs also had seropsositve results to *R. rickettsii;* however, cross-absorption studies indicated a stronger reaction to *R. akari*. The only possible source of exposure for a person in North Carolina developing rickettsialpox was to captured mice brought in by a pet cat.[73] The maintenance of *R. akari*

involves horizontal transmission between the house mouse *(Mus musculus)* and its mite *(Liponyssoides sanguineus)*. Transovarial and transstadial transmission occurs in the mite. Seropositivity in dogs indicates that an alternative form of this cycle must exist. It is presumed that mites feed on dogs, *R. sanguineus* has a broader host range than dogs under some circumstances, or other as yet unknown tick vectors are responsible for infecting dogs.

TYPHUS

Humans are the primary reservoirs of *louseborne typhus*, or *epidemic typhus*, a sporadic illness caused by *Rickettsia prowazekii* (see Table 29-1). It occurs when events favor proliferation and spread of lice, such as unsanitary conditions and natural disasters. Human cases of recrudescent or recently introduced typhus are thought to initiate outbreaks. The organism infects the louse's alimentary tract and is excreted in its feces. Irritation from biting lice causes the person to scratch their skin, thereby contaminating the abraded site with infected louse feces. Infection can also occur after rubbing contaminated hands on mucosal surfaces. Lice affected by *R. prowazekii* die within 1 to 3 weeks after ingestion of infected blood. Lice do not transmit the infection transovarially to their progeny. Another reservoir for this infection in people in the United States appears to be the southern flying squirrel. The clinical signs of disease in people are generally similar to those of RMSF. Antibody reactivity to typhus group rickettsiae has been observed in the sera of dogs suspected of having rickettsial disease.[17] Rabbits have been experimentally infected by inoculation in attempts to transmit infection to lice.[58] *R. prowazekii* caused no illness or sustained infection in experimentally inoculated immunocompetent dogs.[17] No information clarifies whether this organism infects cats.

Murine typhus, or *endemic typhus*, has a more worldwide distribution and is caused by *Rickettsia typhi*, which is transmitted by fleas (see Table 29-1). It is most prevalent in the temperate and subtropical climates where the reservoir rodent hosts and their fleas are found. The disease is transmitted by scratching of infected flea feces into a pruritic bite wound. Some transovarial transmission occurs, so direct bites from fleas can also produce illness. The clinical signs in people are very similar to those of RMSF. In the United States, murine typhus is endemic in southern California and South Texas. The natural host and vector system is the opossum and cat flea. Dog and cat owners were no more seropositive than nonowners, indicating that pet contact is not a risk factor for exposure.[152]

Scrub typhus is a rickettsial disease of people caused by *Orientia* (previously *Rickettsia*) *tsutsugamushi* in southeastern Asia, the South Pacific, and Australia. It is transmitted by the chigger mite, and wild rodents and birds are reservoir hosts. Clinical signs are similar to those of RMSF. Dogs have been experimentally infected with *O. tsutsugamushi* without signs of clinical illness. The organism has been susceptible to tetracyclines and chloramphenicol; however, resistant strains of infection have been treated with fluoroquinolones.

Q FEVER

Etiology and Epidemiology

Query fever (Q fever) is caused by the obligate intracellular gram-negative bacteria *Coxiella burnetii* (see Table 29-1). The organism is not stained by the Gram technique, so the

Gimenez method is used. It has been classified in the gamma subdivision of *Proteobacteria*, which also includes *Francisella*. The organism has two distinct life cycle stages that are morphologically and functionally different. The large-cell form is the metabolically active intracellular vegetative stage. The small-cell extracellular variant is thought to be metabolically inactive and is the environmentally resistant stage. Considerable genetic heterogeneity exists in geographically diverse isolates. Q fever is an endemic zoonosis worldwide except in geographically isolated countries such as Sweden, Norway, Iceland, and New Zealand, where reports of the disease are rare. In the United States, most of the reported cases are from the western region (Fig. 29-10). Reservoir hosts vary depending on the geographic location and include domestic and wild animals and their ectoparasites. Approximately 40 species of ticks and many other arthropods are naturally infected with *C. burnetii*. The tick facilitates a sylvan cycle with reservoir animals. Resultant infection of people and domestic animals may occur when infected ticks feed on them. However, domestic animals and people are more commonly infected by inhalation or ingestion of environmentally resistant organisms. Cattle, sheep, and goats are the most common domestic animal reservoirs for human infection. Wildlife and farm animal species may be the reservoir hosts for domestic pets. Birds may also serve as reservoirs, and one outbreak was associated with exposure to aerosols of pigeon feces and bites from ticks feeding on these birds. Typically, animals are subclinically infected and shed environmentally resistant organisms in their urine, feces, milk, and parturient discharges. The female's uterus and mammary glands are the main sites of chronic infection and reactivation of infection occurs during pregnancy, so shedding mainly occurs during parturition. The placenta in late gestation may contain the greatest concentration of C. burnetii organisms (10^9 per g of tissue). Within the herd, infection is probably maintained by inhalation of infected dust and aerosols or by fomites.

C. burnetii sporulates and is highly resistant, maintaining viability in spite of elevated temperatures, desiccation, osmotic shock, ultraviolet light, and chemicals.[126] Hypochlorite (0.5%), phenolics (15%), formalin (5%), and quaternary ammonium compounds (2%) are not completely effective in killing the organism after 24 hours. After 30 minutes, solutions of alcohol (70%) or chloroform (5%) are effective in destroying C. burnetii.

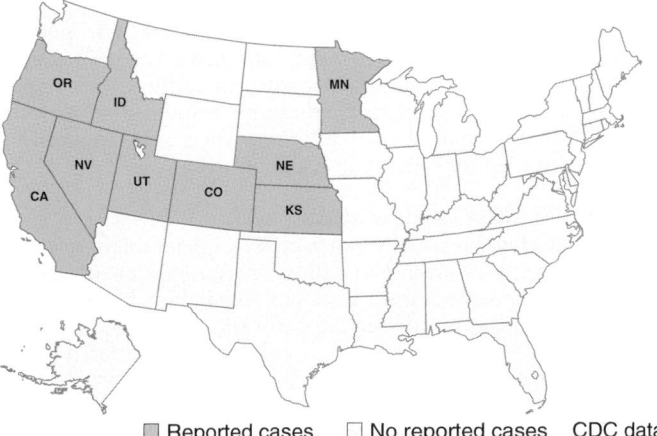

■ Reported cases ☐ No reported cases CDC data

Fig 29-10 Reported cases of Q fever in United States and U.S. territories in 2000. (Data from Centers for Disease Control and Prevention, Atlanta, Ga. Map courtesy University of Georgia, Athens, Ga.)

Serologic and organism isolation studies indicate that dogs and cats can be infected (Table 29-5). Dogs and cats may acquire infection under natural circumstances by tick bites or ingestion or inhalation of organisms while feeding on infected body tissues, milk, placentas, or carcasses. The prevalence of infection in dogs having contact with sheep is much higher than in those with no contact.[12] Inhalation of infected aerosols is also possible in contaminated environments. In one study, dogs had a higher prevalence of antibody (>50%) than cats (9%).[153] Data from seroprevalence studies in Japan show higher positive rates among stray cats than among pet cats.[71] C. burnetii has been found in the blood of experimentally infected cats for 1 month and in their urine for 2 months. It has been isolated from vaginal swabs of clinically healthy or ill cats at veterinary clinics[97] and from the uteri of postpartum cats and dogs.[91] Bitches can shed coxiellae in their milk for 1 month and in urine for at least 70 days. Infected dogs and cats, especially those that are parturient, can be a source of infection for people. The organism was isolated from dogs on farms where human outbreaks of Q fever occurred and from *R. sanguineus* ticks that were feeding on the dogs. People have become infected via contact with pets that have acquired their infections from exposure to herbivores. Reports have described people becoming infected after exposure to aerosols from environments or fomites contaminated with parturient or aborted tissues from infected cats[75,86-88,107] and a dog.[20]

Pathogenesis

Studies of the time course and progression of illness have been established for people, and it is likely similar in animals. After inhaling organisms from infected fomites, the lungs appear to be the main portal of entry for the organism into the systemic circulation, and an atypical pneumonia develops. If the organism is ingested, the liver is prone to develop more severe lesions with resultant granulomatous hepatitis. The incubation period is shorter and severity of disease is greater when people are exposed to increasing numbers of organisms, after exposure to highly virulent strains, or when the organism is inhaled rather than ingested. This bacterium has a predilection for entry, replication, and persistence in macrophages; however, in the host, injured tissues include vascular endothelium and respiratory, renal tubular, and serosal epithelia. Widespread vasculitis causes focal necrotizing hemorrhagic pneumonitis and necrosis and hemorrhage of many other organs, including the liver, CNS, and mononuclear phagocyte system. After recovery, the virulent organism can persist in mononuclear phagocytes, and people can be latently infected with C. burnetii for extended periods. During chronic infection, immune complex phenomena can develop in many organs. During replication in the cell, highly resistant small-cell variants of the organism are produced. In chronically infected people and subclinically infected animals, the organism remains latent until parturition, at which time large numbers enter the placenta, parturient fluids, feces, urine, and milk. The highly resistant small-cell variants are dispersed in the environment. Chronically infected animals may continue to shed organisms in their urine and feces.

Clinical Findings

Infections in dogs and cats are usually subclinical. Splenomegaly is usually the only clinical finding in infected dogs. Fever, anorexia, and lethargy beginning 2 days after inoculation and lasting for 3 days occur in experimentally infected cats. Abortion has occurred in some of the cats and has also been associated with human outbreaks, but the organism has also been isolated from cats having normal parturition. A dog that transmitted the infection to people delivered pups that died within 24 hours of birth.[20] Animals do not usually

Table • 29-5

Prevalence of Serum Antibodies to Coxiellia burnetii in Dogs and Cats

ANIMAL	GEOGRAPHIC LOCATION	SEROPOSITIVITY (%)	REFERENCE
Pound cats	Southern California, United States	20	111
Dogs	Northern California	48	74
Stray dogs	Northern California	66	74
Cats	Maritime Canada	20	53
Dogs	Japan	15	59
Cats	Japan	16	59
Dogs	Egypt	15.9	74
Pet dogs	Bologna, Italy	0.87	8
Stray dogs	Sicily, Italy	32	74
Dogs	Central Italy	24.5	74
Stray dogs	Czechoslovakia	23.7	70
Farm dogs	Czechoslovakia	13.6	70
Dogs	Switzerland	31.4	74
Dogs	West Germany	13	74

develop the endocarditis and chronic infections found in people.

Diagnosis

Lymphocytosis and thrombocytopenia are the main non-specific hematologic changes in infected people. Definitive diagnosis of Q fever is made by serologic testing or isolation of the organism. Isolation must be made in cell culture of macrophage or fibroblast lines, embryonated eggs, or laboratory rodents. All isolations must be made in biosafety level 3 laboratories. The Micro-IF test is the preferred method for measuring antibodies. Although information concerning human exposure can be obtained by examining a single serum sample, it is recommended that a second sample be submitted 4 weeks later. A fourfold increase in C. burnetii-specific IgG titer is diagnostic. Cross-reactions to organisms in closely related genera such as Bartonella occur. More than 50% of chronic Q fever patients have sera that cross-react at measurable but lower levels with Bartonella henselae, another zoonotic agent of cats (see Chapter 54).[76]

Coxiella organisms undergo a phase variation in their outer surface proteins during the course of infection in people. Two separate phase antigens are used in detecting antibodies. Phase I antigens are isolated from organisms taken directly from animals or their parasites. This natural phase is highly infectious, contains large amounts of lipopolysaccharide (LPS), and forms smooth colonies in culture. Phase II antigens are found in organisms that have been passed serially in embryonated eggs, have a truncated LPS, and lack some cell surface antigens. During acute illness, antibody to phase II antigen increases, whereas antibody to phase I antigen is low. In chronic infections, antibody to phase I antigen equals or is greater than that of the phase II type.[37] Titers from cats involved in outbreaks have shown a similar pattern of reactivity to phase I and phase II antigens. Newer diagnostic tests that can provide a convincing diagnosis on a single sample involve measurement of specific IgM to phase II antigen or of IgA to phase I antigen using immunofluorescent or ELISA methods.[26,137] Organism isolation is usually performed by inoculation of tissue samples into laboratory rodents whose serum and lymphoid tissues are examined for evidence of infection. PCR or immunohistochemical methods can be used for detection of C. burnetii in tissue culture or tissue specimens derived from patients.[139]

Therapy

Rickettsiostatic drugs such as tetracyclines and chloramphenicol are as effective in the treatment of Q fever as in the treatment of RMSF; however, chronic infections in people are more difficult to resolve (see Table 29-4). Dosages that achieve higher serum concentrations (>5 ug/ml) of doxycycline are more effective in treating endocarditis.[119] Use of erythromycin and trimethoprim-sulfonamide has been variably successful in treating infected people. Quinolones vary, with sparfloxacin being most effective in vitro;[91] however, clinical use in people is accompanied by relapses. Newer erythromycin derivatives such as clarithromycin may be more effective.[20] Because many affected people recover spontaneously from their acute illness, interpretation of recovery is difficult without an untreated control population. The most successful in vitro combinations have included rifampin combined with doxycycline or trimethoprim. Chronic infections in people with endocarditis have been treated effectively with a combination of quinolones and doxycycline for 3 years[79]; however, relapses are usual.

Prevention

Q fever vaccines are not available for animals or people. Experimentally, dogs have been vaccinated with formalin-inactivated phase I and phase II antigens and have developed humoral and cell-mediated immunity responses to C. burnetii.[154] Unfortunately, the vaccines or their adjuvants caused significant reactions at the inoculation sites.

Public Health Considerations

Human Q fever is usually contracted by inhalation of infected aerosols, such as after parturition or by ingestion of raw or poorly cooked food from livestock. Inhalation has been the suspected means of infection in outbreaks associated with parturient cats[75,86-88] and a dog.[20] Because of occupational exposure, abattoir workers, wool sorters, tanners, farm workers (shepherds, dairy workers), and veterinary and laboratory personnel are particularly susceptible to infection from livestock. Investigational inactivated vaccines are available in the United States for such high-risk exposure groups. Acute infections in people are usually subclinical or are associated with a mild, flulike illness and spontaneous recovery. In some people, more persistent pneumonitis, myocarditis, hepatitis, meningitis, or other syndromes may develop from vasculitis throughout the body. People most at risk include those with previous cardiac valve defects, pregnancy, or immunosuppression. Chronic infections are associated with a delayed onset of endocarditis and include myocarditis or meningoencephalitis. Children, who are commonly infected after the ingestion of raw milk, are usually nonsymptomatic, regardless of the source of infection. Venereal transmission can occur among infected people, and females may transmit infection transplacentally.

Dogs have been reported to transmit infection to people on a few occasions. These have usually been rural exposures associated with farm dogs that have had exposure to sheep or their offal. Some of the previously reported outbreaks of Q fever in urban settings have related to exposure to environments contaminated by infected cats. In cat-associated Q fever, the incubation period, from time of contact until the first signs of illness, ranges from 4 to 30 days. The radiographic appearance of pneumonia in people infected from cats is more often associated with rounded pulmonary opacities.[88] Common source exposure is likely under such circumstances because the organism can be spread on clothing, dust, and other fomites to other people. Direct person-to-person transmission is uncommon but can occur because the organism is present in the body secretions of infected people. Direct transmission between people has been most common in situations in which infected pregnant females deliver or abort their fetus.

After a prolonged incubation period (14 to 39 days), acute systemic manifestations consist of headache, fever (≥40° C [104° F]), chills, and myalgia. Less commonly, nausea, vomiting, diarrhea, arthralgia, or erythematous macules are noted. Although the respiratory tract is the usual source of infection and clinical or radiographic findings of interstitial pneumonitis may develop, respiratory signs occur infrequently. Signs of acute hepatitis may also occur. The acute illness generally lasts 15 days, and mortality rates are low, except in older or immunosuppressed individuals. A diagnosis is often made in infected people by measuring serum antibodies (see Diagnosis in this chapter).

Only a small number (<1%) of patients with acute Q fever develop chronic illness. Chronic Q fever is a potentially fatal, multisystemic disorder that may develop up to 20 years after an acute episode. Signs of chronic endocarditis or hepatitis, such as fever, lethargy, dyspnea, cardiac murmurs, hepatomegaly, thrombocytopenia, and occasional thromboembolism or jaundice, occur.

Biohazard Potential
The environmental resistance, low infectious dose, spread by inhalation, and high environmental resistance of *C. burnetii* makes it a potential agent of bioterrorism.[3]

SUGGESTED READINGS*

49. Grindem CB, Breitschwerdt EB, Perkins PC, et al. 1999. Platelet-associated immunoglobulin (antiplatelet antibody) in canine Rocky Mountain spotted fever and ehrlichiosis, *J Am Anim Hosp Assoc* 35:56-61.
93. McQuiston JH, Childs JE, Thompson HA. 2002. Q Fever, *J Am Vet Med Assoc* 221:796-799.
103. Olson JG, Paddock CD. 1999. Emerging rickettsioses, *Inf Dis Rev* 1:113-114.
104. Paddock CD, Breener O, Vaid C, et al. 2002. Short report: concurrent Rocky Mountain spotted fever in a dog and its owner, *Am J Trop Med Hyg* 66:197-199.
115. Raoult D, La Scola B, Enea M, et al. 2001. A flea associated *Rickettsia* pathogenic for humans, *Emerg Infect Dis* 7:73-81.
148. Warner RD, Marsh WW. 2002. Rocky Mountain spotted fever, *J Am Vet Med Assoc* 221:1413-1417.
159. Zavala-Velazquez JE, Zavala-Castro JE, Vado-Solis I, et al. 2002. Identification of *Ctenocephalides felis* fleas as a host of *Rickettsia felis*, the agent of a spotted fever rickettsiosis in Yucatan, Mexico, *Vector Borne Zoon Dis* 2:69-75.

*See the CD-ROM for a complete list of references.

CHAPTER • 30

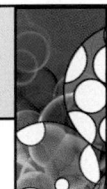

Chlamydial Infections

Craig E. Greene and Jane E. Sykes

ETIOLOGY

The genus *Chlamydophila* is a member of the class *Microtatobiotes*, order Chlamydiales, and family *Chlamydiaceae*. Chlamydophilae are obligate, generally gram-negative, intracellular parasites that, similar to bacteria, have a cell wall, DNA, and RNA but lack the metabolic machinery required for autonomous survival and replication. They multiply by binary fission within membrane-bound cytoplasmic vacuoles of host cells. They have an unusual developmental cycle that involves both extracellular (elementary body) and intracellular (reticulate body) forms (Fig. 30-1).

Elementary bodies are small (0.2 to 0.6 μm), resistant, metabolically inactive, infectious particles with rigid cell walls. They undergo a transient extracellular migration to infect new cells, where within vacuolar inclusions, they transform into larger vegetative replicating forms. These larger forms (0.5 to 1.5 μm), the reticulate bodies, lack cell walls and are noninfectious. The reticulate bodies proliferate by means of budding and fission within the cytoplasmic vesicle, or phagosome, of the host cell. This proliferation is followed by a phase of rapid division during which the initial bodies transform to become a large, membrane-bound population of elementary bodies. This cycle takes approximately 2 days. Elementary bodies are released from the cell after lysis and are able to infect new host cells.

Chlamydophilae persist on the ocular, respiratory, gastrointestinal (GI), and genitourinary mucosae. They produce

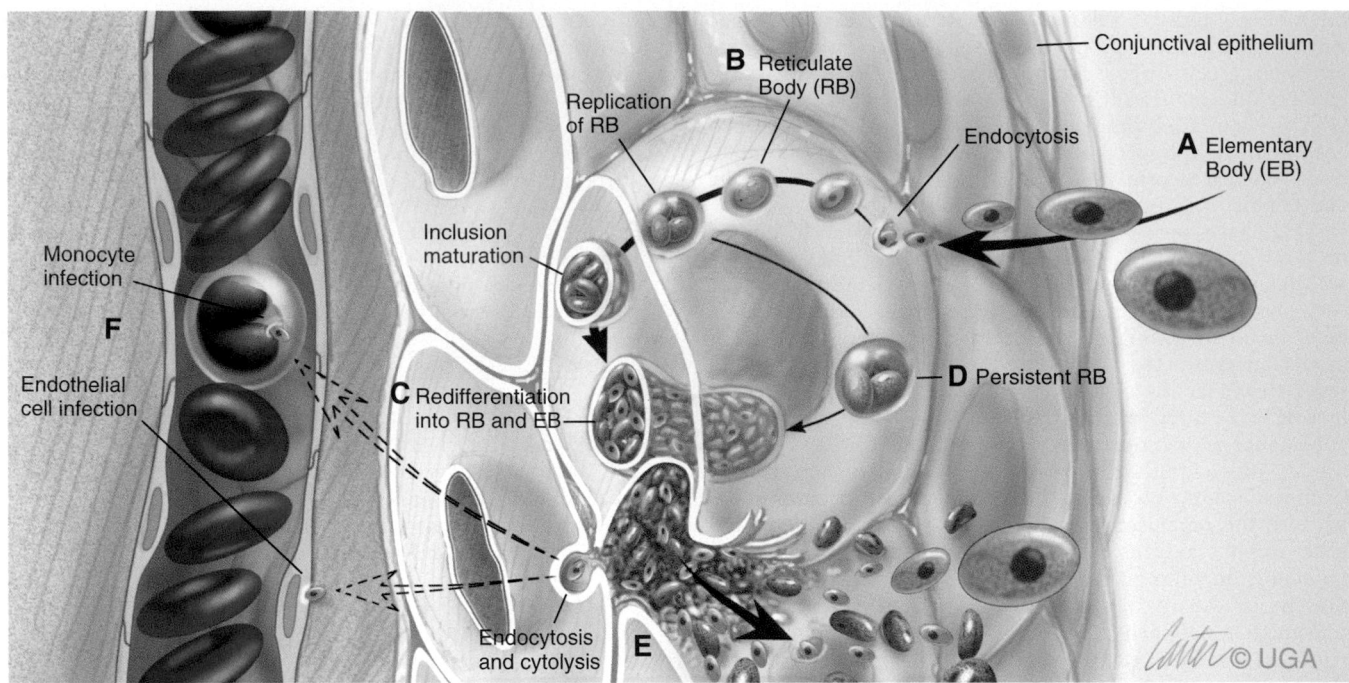

Fig 30-1 Sequential steps in the reproduction and development of *Chlamydia*. Two forms exist, the infectious elementary body (EB) and the replicative reticulate body (RB). In steps *A-B*, the EB transforms to the RB and replicates. Some RBs differentiate into EB *(C)*, and the host cell lyses *(E)* resulting in infection of adjacent host cells and dissemination (rarely) to other tissues *(F)* via phagocytes. In cases when the body's immune response contains the infection, some RBs persist intercellularly *(D)* without replication. (Courtesy University of Georgia, Athens, Ga.)

Table • 30-1

Comparison of Classification of Chlamydophila *and* Chlamydia

HOSTS	PREFERENTIAL TISSUES	BEFORE 1999	AFTER 1999
Chlamydophila			
Birds	Genital, lung, internal organs	*Chlamydia psittaci*	*psittaci*
Cattle, sheep	Brain, eye, joints	*Chlamydia percorum*	*percorum*
People, koala, horses	Lung, joints, endothelial	*Chlamydia pneumoniae*	*pneumoniae*
Sheep, mammals	Intestines, placenta	*Chlamydia psittaci*	*abortus*
Guinea pigs	Bladder, eye, spleen	*Chlamydia psittaci*	*caviae*
Cats	Eye, genital, joints, lung	*Chlamydia psittaci*	*felis*
Chlamydia			
People	Ocular and urogenital, neonatal lung	*Chlamydia trachomatis*	*trachomatis*
Rodents	Many internal organs	*Chlamydia trachomatis*	*muridarum*
Swine	Eye, intestines, lung	Novel species	*suis*

inapparent-to-overt infections in a variety of hosts. The hosts provide a natural reservoir for these environmentally susceptible organisms. They spread directly between hosts via contact or aerosols, surviving only a few days in the environment at room temperature. Immunity to these organisms involves cellular and hormonal mechanisms. Their tendency to cause chronic, relapsing, or latent infections indicates that only a partial host immune response is evoked.

The genomic classification has undergone major revisions since 1999, and the family *Chlamydiaceae* has been divided into two genera, *Chlamydia* and *Chlamydophila* (Table 30-1).[14] Previously, this family consisted only of the genus *Chlamydia*, composed of the species *C. trachomatis, C. pneumoniae, C. pecorum*, and *C. psittaci*.[32] The genus *Chlamydia* now contains *C. trachomatis*, which causes ocular and urogen-

ital disease in people, *C. muridarum*, which infects rodents, and *C. suis*, which infects swine. The genus *Chlamydophila* contains *C. percorum*, previously *Chlamydia pecorum*, which infects cattle and sheep, *C. pneumoniae*, as well as four new species: *C. psittaci, C. abortus, C. caviae*, and *C. felis*, each derived from the formerly named species *Chlamydia psittaci*.[14] *C. psittaci* is the type species for this genus and is the causative agent of psittacosis in birds. *C. felis* (previously *Chlamydia psittaci* var. *felis*) is the predominant organism of cats; *C. abortus* and *C. caviae* infect sheep and guinea pigs, respectively. *C. pneumoniae* is a human pathogen producing respiratory infections and has also been linked to coronary artery disease, asthma, cerebrovascular disease, sarcoidosis, and reactive arthritis.

In addition to genetic differences, the different species can be differentiated phenotypically by their monoclonal antibody

(MABs) reactivity, and to a certain extent, morphologically and by their staining properties. The morphology of *C. psittaci* and *Chlamydia trachomatis* are virtually identical, but *C. pneumoniae* forms pear-shaped elementary bodies.[16] *Chlamydia trachomatis* forms compact rigid cell wall inclusions, containing glycogen, that stain with iodine, a characteristic distinguishing it from *C. psittaci*. Generally, each *Chlamydophila* species has a preferred host range, often of a few or single host animal species, sometimes producing respiratory, genital, and systemic illness. Isolates from cats worldwide are genetically similar with at least two subtypes.[48,59] Serologic relationships may be more diverse.[27,47] The following discussion concentrates on *Chlamydophila* infections in dogs and cats.

EPIDEMIOLOGY

Dogs

Little information is available about the epidemiology of chlamydial infections in dogs.

Cats

Positive antibody titers to chlamydiae have been detected in as many as 9% of healthy, laboratory-reared cats and 45% of farm cats. Despite this high prevalence of seropositivity, *Chlamydophila* were isolated from conjunctival or rectal swabs from only 6% and 4%, respectively, of clinically healthy cats. Isolation rates of up to 30% of household cats with conjunctivitis were reported.[68] Serologic studies in cats coupled with organism culture or genetic detection indicate that the chance of exposure and increasing immunity are greater with advancing age.[49,58,68] Cats 2 to 6 months of age are likely to be infected with *C. felis*, as are cats up to 1 year of age. Thereafter, the prevalence of infection decreases, and cats older than 5 years of age are very unlikely to be infected with *C. felis*. Cats less than 8 weeks of age are less likely to be infected, presumably from passive immunity from nursing.

A primary mode of transmission of infection for neonatal kittens is thought to be from the genital mucosae of the dam during parturition. In older cats, transmission occurs from close direct or aerosol contact. Venereal transmission, as described in other hosts, has not yet been confirmed in cats. In epidemiologic surveys for respiratory disease, the prevalence of detection depends on the method used, geographic location, presence of clinical illness, and age of cats (Table 30-2). Cats over 1 year of age have progressively lower isolation rates as they continue to age, which likely relates to natural immunity and clearing of infection with advancing age. Conjunctivitis is more likely associated with *Chlamydophila* infection, while sneezing is more likely in feline herpes virus type 1 (FHV-1) infections.[58] *Chlamydophila* prevalence rates have been higher in the summer months.[58]

Non–*C. felis* chlamydial DNA was detected in conjunctival specimens that was 99% homologous to the sequence of *Neochlamydia hartmannellae*, an amebic endosymbiont.[66] These chlamydiae were found in association with their obligate ameboid host, *Hartmannella vermiformis*. These organisms were not observed cytologically and such detection often involves tissue biopsy and confocal microscopy. This free-living amoeba has been identified as a cause of ocular surface infection in people and may have some role in feline ocular infections (see Chapter 93).

PATHOGENESIS

Dogs

Little is known about the course or genospecies of chlamydial infection in dogs. Presumably, it is similar to that of other host species; however, respiratory and genital infections have not been recognized and may be asymptomatic. Disease in the dog may reflect dissemination and persistence in deeper host tissues. Research in human infections, using polymerase chain reaction (PCR), shows that these organisms may enter a latent, noncultivable phase during which the host's immune reaction induces chronic immunopathologic lesions. Such has been shown with *C. trachomatis*, inducing Reiter's arthritis, and *C. pneumoniae*, causing atherosclerotic disease. Organisms likely spread to internal tissues during acute illness or immunosuppression. Using immunohistochemistry with MABs and PCR, chlamydiae have been detected in atheromatous lesions of the aorta, coronary, and splenic arteries of dogs.[52]

Cats

Cats infected with *C. felis* develop upper respiratory signs, including fever, ocular discharge, and sneezing. The appearance of conjunctivitis parallels the ocular shedding of chlamydiae. The predominant feature is inflammation of the conjunctiva or nictitating membrane. A low dose produces unilateral signs, and higher doses produce bilateral illness.[61] Organisms spread internally to colonize many tissues, including the tonsil, lung, liver, spleen, and kidney.[33] Infections often become chronic and insidious. Cats may become asymptomatic but harbor the organism in the conjunctiva for 2 months or longer. Organisms have been isolated from the conjunctiva for up to 215 days after experimental infection.[45,67] Whether chronic disease is the result of repeated reinfection or the presence of persistent chlamydiae is unclear. Persistent chlamydiae in the form of atypical reticulate bodies have been identified in the joints of people with reactive arthritis. Localization of persistent chlamydiae to deeper tissues, such as the subsynovial layer in human patients with arthritis, may afford protection from the continual rapid turnover characteristic of epithelial tissues. Shedding from the reproductive tract has not been documented in kittens younger than 13 weeks, even though they shed organisms from the ocular discharges.[61] When they are infected at 4 to 6 months or older, most of the animals shed organisms from the reproductive tract within a week after ocular inoculation. Reactivation of shedding may occur in late pregnancy. These factors suggest that the hormonal influence on reproductive tissues or immune system may be important for the replication of organisms in the reproductive tract. Long-term infections have been described as a sequel to some chlamydial infections in people and animals. The intestinal tract is a potential site of persistent infection in cats as has been seen in other species. Cell-mediated immune clearance is required to eliminate persistent intracellular pathogens. Co-infections with other agents such as feline coronavirus (FCV), FHV-1, *Bordetella*, or *Mycoplasma* may increase the clinical severity of infection and duration of shedding. Other bacteria, including those that normally colonize the healthy conjunctival sac, can also act as secondary invaders and worsen disease.

The febrile response in chlamydiosis is associated with chlamydemia, an acute phase reaction in which a release of interleukin (IL)-1, IL-6, tumor necrosis factor, and interferons occurs. Acute phase reactants and IL-6 are increased in plasma of experimentally infected cats.[61]

CLINICAL FINDINGS

Dogs

Chlamydiosis has not been well documented as a spontaneously occurring entity in dogs. Serologic surveys have detected antibodies to chlamydiae in up to 50% of healthy dogs. Chlamydiae have been suggested as a cause of chronic superficial keratitis in dogs; however, they can be found as

Table • 30-2

Prevalence of Chlamydophila *Infection in Naturally Infected Domestic Cats Based on Culture or Genetic Detection Methods*[a]

COUNTRY/SAMPLES COLLECTED	CAT DEMOGRAPHICS	METHOD	NUMBER POSITIVE/ NUMBER TESTED	PERCENT POSITIVE
Australia[58]—conjunctival swabs	Conjunctivitis, rhinitis, keratitis	PCR	82/578	14.2%
	< 8 weeks of age		5/19	26.3%
	9 weeks to 6 months of age		22/79	27.8%
	1 to 11 months of age		6/22	27.3%
	1 to 5 years of age		21/142	14.8%
	5 to 10 years of age		4/87	4.6%
	> 10 years of age		3/46	6.5%
	Clinically healthy cats, various ages	PCR	1/95	1.1%
Japan[5]—conjunctival, some nasal swabs	Conjunctivitis, respiratory disease	PCR	39/66	59.1%
		Isolation-yolk sac	11/66	16.7%
Japan[41]—conjunctival swabs	Conjunctivitis, rhinitis	PCR	7/26	26.9%
Japan[23]—conjunctival, nasal, oral swabs	Conjunctivitis, respiratory disease, stomatitis	PCR	7/52	13.5%
		Isolation-cell culture	6/52	11.6%
Italy[49]	Conjunctivitis	PCR	14/70	20%
	Clinically healthy cats	PCR	0/35	0%
Switzerland[66]	Conjunctivtis	PCR	114/226	50%
	Clinically healthy cats	PCR	7/30	23%
United Kingdom[68]	Conjunctivitis	Isolation-cell culture	226/753	30%
Scotland[39]—conjunctival swabs	Clinical health status:	PCR		
	Ocular discharge		5/20	25%
	Recurrent or chronic conjunctivitis		7/39	18%
	Conjunctivitis and upper respiratory disease		6/33	18%
	Acute conjunctivitis		2/21	10%
	Upper respiratory tract signs only		3/43	7%
	Healthy in-contact cats		2/2	100%
	Healthy cats		0/6	0%
	Other disease		1/7	14%
	Unknown reason		5/45	11%
	Serologic indirect FA titer results:			
	< 1:20		0/24	0%
	1:20—1:40		0/10	0%
	1:80—1:160		3/15	20%
	> 1:320		9/22	41%

PCR, Polymerase chain reaction; *FA,* fluorescent antibody.
[a]Numerous serosurveys show a higher prevalence of positive results, indicating that exposure to *Chlamydophila* infection in cats is higher than the actual infection rate.

ocular flora in clinically healthy animals. Although never established as the cause, chlamydiae were isolated from dogs with encephalitis and systemic illness. *Chlamydophila* isolated from a sheep with polyarthritis produced fever, anorexia, depression, pneumonia, joint pain, and diarrhea when experimentally inoculated into dogs.[72] The organism has been reisolated from parenchymal tissues, the intestinal tract, and synovial fluid; lesions were focal hepatitis, lymphoid hyperplasia, fibrinopurulent polyarthritis, and meningitis. Chlamydiosis was diagnosed in a febrile dog with shifting leg lameness.[1] The organisms were demonstrated in the cytoplasm of macrophages in thoracic fluid, which had positive culture results for an avian strain, and the dog seroconverted. Systemic signs including lymphadenomegaly and arthritis were also described in a dog.[28] *Chlamydophila*-like organisms were detected by direct fluorescent antibody (FA) testing and PCR for *Chlamydophila* antigen in its joint fluid.

Cats

Chlamydiae have been recognized as a cause of ocular, nasal, and lower respiratory tract infections of cats (see Chapters 16 and 93); however, ocular signs are predominant. Typically acute, chronic, or recurrent conjunctivitis occur, and only sometimes are additional respiratory signs seen. Clinical signs are conjunctival hyperemia, chemosis, blepharospasm, and mucopurulent to serous ocular discharge (Fig. 30-2). Corneal disease is rare, and if present, is likely caused by other or co-infecting pathogens such as FHV-1 or bacteria. Most cats remain well and continue to eat. Pneumonia is generally subclinical; thus signs of coughing or dyspnea are rarely, if ever, seen. The strain and route of infection may influence the extent of respiratory involvement. Some cats develop nasal discharge and sneezing; however, signs of rhinitis such as sneezing or nasal discharge, without ocular involvement, are unlikely caused by *C. felis* infection.[58] *C. felis* has occasionally been isolated from neonatal conjunctivitis in kittens, although most kittens appear to be protected by maternal antibody.[56] Whether such cases are associated with genital infection in the queen, as occurs in people infected with *Chlamydia trachomatis*, is unclear.

Experimental infection of cats results in a systemic phase of disease that has been less commonly reported in natural infections. Following ocular inoculation, *C. felis* colonizes the GI and genital mucosae, resulting in persistent infection in some cats. In other studies, systemic signs of fever, lethargy, lameness, and weight loss have developed.[61] These signs can develop within 2 weeks after those of conjunctivitis in cats infected by intraocular instillation of virulent organisms. Lameness has been observed in association with the febrile

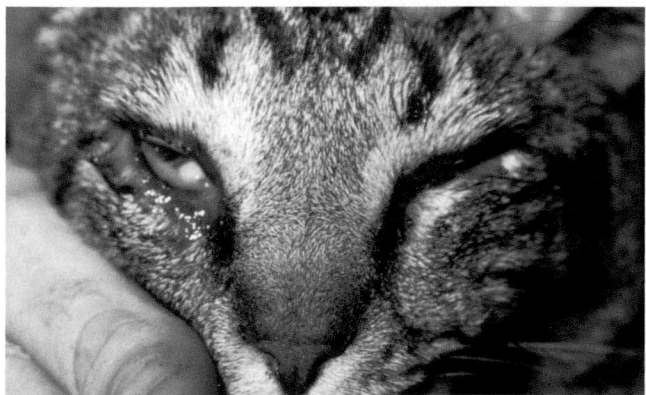

Fig 30-2 Marked chemosis and conjunctival inflammation in a cat with ocular *Chlamydophila* infection. (Courtesy University of Georgia, Athens, Ga.)

response in experimental infections of cats, [61] and it may be similar to Reiter's syndrome, which follows human *Chlamydia trachomatis* infections. Although polyarthritis is the proposed mechanism, further study such as synovial fluid analysis is needed.

Chlamydiae were isolated from the superficial mucus–producing cells of the gastric mucosa in some cats.[20] No consistent association could be found of GI-infected cats with GI or respiratory signs, which may represent subclinical carrier infection. Chlamydiae were isolated from the gastric mucosa of young cats in research colonies with signs of weight loss. Experimental inoculation of the gastric isolates into the respiratory tract produced upper respiratory tract infection similar to that caused by respiratory isolates and only mild gastritis in some cats.

Reproductive shedding of organisms and vaginal discharge occur following experimental conjunctival inoculation; however, clinical signs of reproductive dysfunction have not been substantiated with experimental or natural infections. Intravaginal and intraurethral inoculation has produced vaginal discharge and bleeding in female cats, urethritis and urethral discharge in male cats, and proctitis in both sexes. Instillation of organisms directly in the fallopian tubes resulted in 2 months of shedding, and suspected infertility from inflammation, resulting in scars and adhesions. Placental infection was documented in a cat experimentally infected by intraocular exposure during gestation. No histologic evidence of inflammation was found in the placental tissues or infection of the neonate; however, vaginal shedding commenced in the queen after parturition. Although the valvular structures in the feline reproductive tract may prevent chlamydial infection ascending from the vagina, hematogenous dissemination may allow the agent to relocate to the reproductive tract. Although *C. felis* DNA could not be detected using the PCR in serial blood samples collected from experimentally infected cats,[60] infection has been transmitted experimentally by blood transfusion, with subsequent development of systemic signs and conjunctivitis.[61] Whether chlamydiae are responsible for reproductive disorders in cats is uncertain. Possibly, for *C. felis* to cause infertility or abortion, certain criteria may need to be met. The stage of pregnancy at which infection occurs, co-infection with other organisms, concurrent immunosuppression, route of infection, and the strain involved may be important. Genital infections are likely a means by which the organism is spread from queens to their kittens. FHV-1 may be responsible for a large number of suspected cases of *C. felis*–induced genital and perinatal disease.

Concurrent feline immunodeficiency virus (FIV) infection in cats prolonged the duration of conjunctivitis and clinical signs noted after ocular inoculation of *C. psittaci*.[45] Prolonged (270 days) excretion of *Chlamydophila* was noted in FIV infected cats compared with control cats (70 days). Peritonitis also was attributed to *Chlamydophila* infection in one cat.[8]

DIAGNOSIS

Cultivation

Culture of the organism is the most definitive diagnostic test. Isolations from cats are usually highest from conjunctival swabs, although nasal and pharyngeal isolations have been used. Culture of rectal and vaginal swabs may also yield organisms. The organism is occasionally isolated from aspirations or specimens of deeper tissues, such as the spleen, liver, or peritoneum. Vigorous swabbing of mucosal surfaces is essential to obtain enough epithelial cells that contain the organism. Cotton swabs are best; Dacron swabs or those with wooden sticks should not be used. To enhance organism survival, swabs should be placed immediately in a chlamydial transport medium such as 2SP (0.2 M sucrose and 0.02 M phosphate). Routine viral transport media containing antibiotics will inactivate the organisms. The sample should be refrigerated (4° C) if it is not immediately sent to the laboratory and ideally should reach the laboratory within 24 hours of sample collection. Specimens can also be frozen at −70° C, but this may result in the loss of some organisms and consequent false negatives.[29] Organisms can be cultured from swabs for up to 8 days at 22° C and 30 days when in tissues.[39] In the laboratory, organisms can be grown in the yolk sac of embryonating eggs or in monolayers of mouse, monkey, or human cells.[13] Isolates are generally differentiated using genetic typing methods.

Microscopic and Enzyme-Linked Immunosorbent Assay Detection

For cytology, swabs or conjunctival spatulas are swiped across the inferior cul-de-sac, and cells are smeared on glass slides. The slides are air dried and fixed in acetone. Intracytoplasmic inclusions composed of clusters of coccoid (0.5-μm diameter) bodies are usually 10 μm in diameter in phagocytes or epithelial cells and stain basophilic (Fig. 30-3). Giemsa is the traditional stain for demonstrating *Chlamydiaceae*, but artifacts in the cytoplasm may stain similarly. Inclusions are generally visible only early, if at all, during the course of infection. Melanin granules in the cytoplasm of conjunctival epithelial cells can yield false-positive results. Direct FA techniques using MABs make identification more specific.

Enzyme-linked immunosorbent assay (ELISA) methodology can detect antigen directly in patient specimens. A variety of commercial antigen detection kits are available (see Appendix 6). Cross-reaction with all the members of the genera *Chlamydia* and *Chlamydophila* occurs with these tests as currently used commercially (Chlamydiazyme, Abbott Labs, Chicago, Ill.; IDEIA Chlamydia Test, Boots-Celltech Diagnostics Inc., East Hanover, N.J.). Unfortunately, these kits vary in their sensitivity and specificity. In general, ELISA methods have lower sensitivity and specificity as compared with cell culture or direct FA methods in detecting feline infections. See Appendix 6 for further information on test kits.

Genetic Detection

Until the development of DNA-based detection, the gold standard for diagnosis was cultivation as previously described. Currently, PCR and other DNA-based identification methods make speciation of isolates from culture or infected tissues

routine. Furthermore, because the organism does not need to be viable for PCR testing, special transport conditions are not as critical as for culture. PCR followed by restriction digestion can distinguish all species of chlamydiae.[13] *C. felis* strains worldwide appear similar to each other based on these restriction digests of the ompA gene.[5,59] Real time quantitative PCR has been used to detect *C. felis* in cats.[22] PCR has been used to detect *Chlamydophila* in atheromas of canine blood vessels.[52] Variation in PCR methods can be traced to differences in nucleic acid extraction and primer selection. PCR methods are usually more sensitive compared with cultural isolation in which comparisons have been made in naturally infected cats (see Table 30-2). In experimental studies, PCR was more sensitive than was culture (PCR 85.7%, culture 72.9%) in untreated cats with or without clinical illness.[60] PCR and culture had equivalent sensitivity (100%) during the first month of infection in clinically ill cats; however, PCR was more sensitive during the second month (PCR 72.9%, culture 47.9%). During treatment of infected cats, culture results are positive for 1 day after treatment is initiated, and PCR results are positive for up to 5 days.[60] Presumably, this difference reflects the greater sensitivity of PCR and its ability to detect nonviable organisms. Discrepancy in viability occurs with death of organisms on transit to the laboratory or persistence of nucleic acid when organisms die in the host. Chlamydial DNA has been detected in samples placed in the environment up to 10 weeks at 22° C, well beyond its viability based on culture.[39] A multiplex PCR procedure has been developed to simultaneously detect three feline respiratory pathogens, chlamydiae, FCV, and FHV-1, in mucosal swabs.[57]

Serologic Testing

Serologic testing can be used to distinguish the various species of chlamydiae. Unfortunately, testing for serum antibodies to chlamydiae is of limited diagnostic benefit in determining active infection because the IgG antibody titer increase is variable or prolonged, and IgM antibody titers are inconsistently elevated. However, the highest antibody titers are generally associated with symptomatic cats.[68] Chlamydial infections persist in the presence of high serum antibody levels; therefore serologic testing documents only exposure and cannot be used to evaluate protection afforded by vaccines. Higher indirect FA antibody titers correlate with recent infection and may correspond with the isolation of *Chlamydophila* in the clinically healthy animal.[39] Seronegative animals are less likely to be carriers. Unfortunately, serologic tests are not widely available. Serial titers may be needed to document active infections, and recent vaccination may interfere with interpretation of positive titer results.

THERAPY

Treatment of chlamydial infections has involved primarily antimicrobial therapy. In evaluating the response to treatment, also important to consider is concurrent presence of the viral causes of feline upper respiratory tract disease (see Chapter 16). Treatment of co-infected cats may result only in temporary improvement caused by resolution of secondary bacterial and *Chlamydophila* infections.

Recommended dosages for all drugs are in Table 30-3. Most of the information on therapeutic efficacy involves cats. Oral administration of tetracycline is usually preferred at a dosage of 22 mg/kg three times daily for 3 to 4 weeks or doxycycline at 5 to 10 mg/kg twice daily for the same period. A dose of 10 to 15 mg/kg once daily can also be used.[53,55] Higher dosage rates of doxycycline are used for cats to avoid giving partial tablets. Crushed or broken tablets are not recommended because of the risk of causing esophagitis; administration of

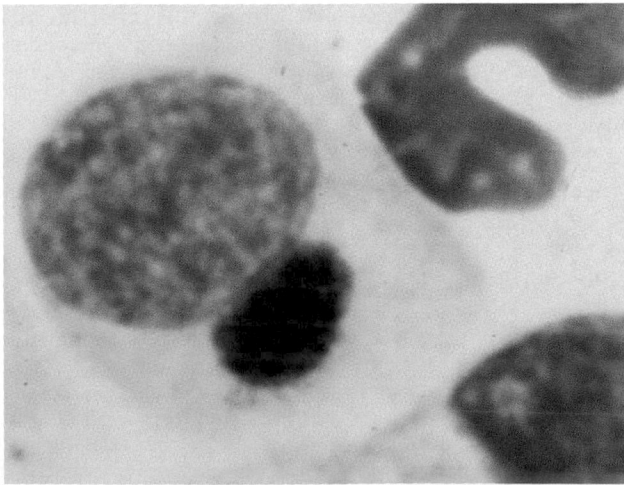

Fig 30-3 Chlamydial inclusion in an epithelial cell from a conjunctival scraping of a cat. (Courtesy University of Georgia, Athens, Ga.)

Table • 30-3

Recommended Therapy for Chlamydiosis

DRUG[a]	SPECIES	DOSE[b] (mg/kg)	ROUTE	INTERVAL (HOURS)	DURATION (WEEKS)
Amoxicillin-clavulanate	B	12.5—25	PO, SC, IV	12	4
Doxycycline	B	5—10	PO, IV	12	3—4
	C	10—15[c]	PO	24	3—4
Tetracycline	B	22	PO	8	4

B, Dog and cat; C, cat; PO, by mouth; SC, subcutaneous; IV, intravenous.
[a]For additional information, see Drug Formulary, Appendix 8.
[b]Dose per administration at specified interval.
[c]The dose should be rounded off to the nearest whole- or half-tablet size to help prevent esophagitis. In addition, small amounts of food or water should be administered after each dose to help rinse the tablet into the stomach.

doxycycline suspension is least likely to be associated with this problem. Tetracyclines have also been associated with toxic hepatitis or dental staining. However, doxycycline is less likely to stain the teeth because of its reduced calcium-binding avidity (see Drug Formulary, Appendix 8). Ocular infections alone may respond to tetracycline eye ointment applied three times daily, although the likely systemic nature of the infection must be considered.

Experimentally infected cats, treated with oral doxycycline, have shown clinical improvement beginning 24 to 48 hours after treatment was instituted compared with placebo-treated cats or those treated with topical antimicrobial therapy.[53,60] Three weeks' duration has been effective.[60] In cat colonies with chlamydial infection, treatment may have to be continued for up to 6 to 8 weeks to ensure that all cats have been successfully treated. The entire population may have to be treated simultaneously. Treatment should always continue for at least 2 weeks after the resolution of clinical signs.

In other studies, experimentally infected cats were treated with amoxicillin-clavulanate, doxycycline, or placebo for 19 days.[55] Both treated groups had a reduction in isolation rates and improvement in clinical signs, with slightly better initial efficacy at 2 to 4 days with the amoxicillin-clavulanate. However, a majority of the cats treated with amoxicillin-clavulanate had a relapse of infection 14 to 20 days after treatment was discontinued. These cats had to be retreated for 4 weeks, and recovery was complete when monitored for 6 months. Treatment with amoxicillin-clavulanate has less risk of potential side effects as compared with tetracyclines. In addition, some cats will eat amoxicillin-clavulanate but not doxycycline tablets voluntarily.[55] Both doxycycline and amoxicillin-clavulanate can be considered as effective treatment for chlamydiosis. Drugs such as sulfonamides or chloramphenicol are ineffective, and penicillin is only inhibitory in vitro at higher doses.[56]

Infections with *Chlamydia trachomatis* in people are susceptible to treatment with other drugs such as erythromycin and its newer derivative, azithromycin, and with fluoroquinolones and rifampin. Controlled studies have not been conducted in *C. felis*–infected cats with many of these other drugs; however, azithromycin has been recommended on an empirical basis to treat cats on a once-daily or once-weekly dosage regimen.[51] In other studies with *C. felis*–experimentally infected, specific-pathogen–free cats, azithromycin suspension was given at 10 to 15 mg/kg, orally, daily for 3 days and then twice weekly thereafter for a total treatment period of 4 weeks.[46] This regimen produced rapid resolution of clinical signs, and organisms were no longer able to be isolated after 6 days. However, *C. felis* was subsequently isolated beginning 14 days after institution of treatment. Even daily administration of azithromycin for a similar period was ineffective in clearing the infection. In comparison, cats receiving doxycycline tablets at 10 to 15 mg/kg once daily for 4 weeks had a clearing of their infection after 6 days for the duration of the observation period. Because of these findings, azithromycin is not recommended for treatment of *C. felis* infections.

Most of the treatment studies in infected cats have relied on culture to determine the efficacy of therapy in eliminating *C. felis*. In cats with natural disease that tested positive using PCR, recent treatment with antichlamydial drugs or glucocorticoids was not associated with a lower prevalence of infection.[60] This finding may indicate a lack of efficacy of currently used drugs or the increased sensitivity of PCR to detect latent infections. Nucleic acid detected using PCR may also be nonviable. Further studies may be needed using PCR to determine if the carrier state is eliminated.

PREVENTION

Kittens acquire maternal antibodies to *C. felis* that usually protect them from infection until 7 to 9 weeks of age. Both inactivated and modified live vaccines have been available to protect cats from chlamydial respiratory disease (see Prevention, Chapter 16, and Feline Viral Respiratory Disease, Chapter 100). Even modified live vaccines, which provide the best protection, do not entirely prevent colonization of mucosae and shedding of chlamydiae after challenge. They minimize the replication of the organism and hence reduce the clinical signs in subsequently infected cats. A delayed postvaccinal reaction of transient fever, anorexia, lethargy, and occasional limb soreness 7 to 21 days after use of combined vaccines containing modified live *Chlamydophila* has been reported in a low percentage of cats (see Postvaccinal Complications, Chapter 100).[59] These vaccines are indicated only for cats with a high risk of acquiring infection, such as those in catteries with endemic chlamydiosis. Transmission of the organism will also be minimized by good hygiene, quarantine, and disinfection practices in cattery situations. The organism is readily inactivated by detergents.

PUBLIC HEALTH CONSIDERATIONS

Chlamydophila of feline origin has been suspected as the cause of human conjunctivitis on several occasions. Many of these associations have never been substantiated, because of the lack of valid scientific tests to identify specific species and isolates. Relatively crude methods, such as serologic similarities or biochemical features, have been used to characterize the isolates. Many of the reports of human chlamydiosis from cats before the advent of genetic typing cannot be substantiated. For example, *Chlamydophila* has been associated with cat scratch disease in people; but recent studies suggest that this association was inaccurate because of cross-reactivity between some species of *Chlamydophila* and *Bartonella* on serologic tests.[35,36,64]

With the new focus on genetic detection, many of these concerns of identifying particular Chlamydophila species can be addressed. *C. felis* was isolated from the conjunctiva of a person with nontrachomatous *Chlamydia* infection.[21] This organism was genetically indistinguishable from an isolate later recovered from the patient's cat. Although these associations have been difficult to document, people should take precautions in medicating cats with conjunctivitis, and infected cats may have to be treated with systemic antimicrobials simultaneously with people in households in which people develop chlamydial conjunctivitis.

The interspecies transmission of avian chlamydiosis (psittacosis, ornithosis, *C. psittaci*) from birds to people is a better-substantiated veterinary and public health problem.[12] *Chlamydophila* causing conjunctivitis in a cat was suspected to have been acquired from a pet macaw in the same household.[30] The *C. psittaci* strain causing infection in birds is known to cause human psittacosis. In another household, three humans and three dogs developed infection attributed to psittacosis from a cockatiel.[19] Although the bird was euthanized, the affected people and dogs had clinical recovery with treatment.

C. pneumoniae is a ubiquitous pathogen that causes acute respiratory disease in people and has been incriminated as a cause of coronary and cerebral vascular disease.[6,17] People appear to be the reservoir host for this agent, and it is not known to infect dogs or cats. However, similar vascular lesions have been attributed to chlamydial infection in dogs (see previous discussion on Pathogenesis). Rabbits and mice can be experimentally infected with this organism. Veterinarians should have knowledge of this relationship because they may be questioned regarding the risk of pets for this infection in people. Virtually all people are infected with *C. pneumoniae*,

and many become reinfected. Antibody prevalence to this organism increases with advancing age. Following treatment, the organism can be detected with PCR in tissues of people, even after it can no longer be cultured. The metabolically inactive elementary bodies are not affected by antibiotics and may persist in the body for indefinite periods. Morphologic studies have shown this organism in atheromatous plaques of coronary and large blood vessels. The definitive relationship between their presence and vascular disease remains to be established.

SUGGESTED READINGS*

3. Bart M, Guscetti F, Zurbriggen A, et al. 2000. Feline infectious pneumonia: a short literature review and a retrospective immunohistological study on the involvement of *Chlamydia* spp. and distemper virus, *Vet J* 159:220-230.
14. Everett KD, Bush RM, Andersen AA. 1999. Emended description of the order Chlamydiales, proposal of *Parachlamydiaceae* fam. Nov. and *Simkaniaceae* fam. Nov., each containing one monotypic genus, revised taxonomy of the family Chlamydiaceae, including a new genus and five new species, and standards for the identification of organisms, *Int J Syst Bacteriol* 49:415-440.
58. Sykes JE, Anderson GA, Studdert VP, Browning GF. 1999a. Prevalence of feline *Chlamydia psittaci* and feline herpesvirus 1 in cats with upper respiratory disease as determined by duplex polymerase chain reaction, *J Vet Intern Med* 13:153-162.
60. Sykes JE, Studdert VP, Browning GF. 1999b. Comparison of the polymerase chain reaction and culture for the detection of feline *Chlamydia psittaci* in untreated and doxycycline-treated experimentally infected cats, *J Vet Intern Med* 13:146-152.
61. Ter Wee J, Sabara M, Kokjohn K, et al. 1998. Characterization of the systemic disease and ocular signs induced by experimental infection with *Chlamydia psittaci* in cats, *Vet Microbiol* 59:259-281.

*See the CD-ROM for a complete list of references.

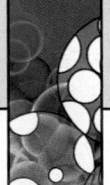

CHAPTER • 31

Hemotrophic Mycoplasmosis (Hemobartonellosis)

John W. Harvey

ETIOLOGY

Hemotrophic mycoplasmas are gram-negative, nonacid-fast, epicellular parasites of erythrocytes. These organisms were classified as rickettsia in the genera *Haemobartonella* and *Eperythrozoon* for many years; however, results from recent sequencing of the 16S rRNA gene indicate that they are mycoplasmas.[15,42,51] Consequently, *Haemobartonella* and *Eperythrozoon* genera are being discarded and these hemotrophic parasites being moved to the genus *Mycoplasma*. Species names often include the prefix "haemo-" (e.g., *Mycoplasma haemofelis*) to identify these unique mycoplasmas

that attach to erythrocytes. Haemoplasmas has been proposed as a general name for these hemotrophic mycoplasmas.[47]

Hemotrophic mycoplasmas contain DNA and RNA and replicate by binary fission. These organisms have not been cultivated outside their hosts. Hemotrophic mycoplasmas are distinctly different from *Bartonella* organisms, which are bacteria that can be cultured in cell-free media.

Hemotrophic Mycoplasmas in Cats

Two distinctly different hemotrophic mycoplasmas have been identified in cats based on 16S rRNA gene sequences. The similarities of gene sequences between these organisms is only about 83%.[16] One organism was previously referred to as the *Haemobartonella felis* large (Hflg) variant because the organism appeared larger than the second organism, which was referred to as the *H. felis* small (Hfsm) variant.[15] The Hflg organism is now classified as *M. haemofelis*,[48] and the Hfsm organism is now classified as *Mycoplasma haemominutum*.[16] Organisms previously classified as Florida, Ohio, Oklahoma, and Illinois isolates of *H. felis* are now classified as *M. haemofelis* isolates, and organisms previously classified as California and Birmingham isolates of *H. felis* are now classified as isolates of *M. haemominutum* based on similarities in the sequence of the 16S rRNA gene (Table 31-1).[55] An Australian strain of *M. haemofelis* has been reported with a 16S rRNA gene sequence identical to the Ohio and Florida isolates.[11]

In polychrome-stained blood films, hemotrophic mycoplasmas appear as small (0.3 to 0.8 µm), blue-staining cocci, rings, or rods that are usually attached to erythrocytes (Fig. 31-1). The genome size of *M. haemofelis* is about 1200 kb.[2] In thick blood films or thick areas of thin films, nearly all organisms appear as cocci. Ring- and rod-shape organisms are seen more readily in thin blood films or the feathered edges of thick blood films. *M. haemominutum* organisms are rarely observed in stained blood films from infected cats. When seen, *M. haemominutum* appear as small rods, rings, or coccoid organisms that are reported to stain less densely and measure about half the size of *M. haemofelis*.[15-17] However, this reported size difference has been challenged by the finding of a *M. haemominutum* isolate in Great Britain that is about 0.6 µm in diameter.[55] Morphologic appearance is not reliable in distinguishing isolates, and genetic analysis is needed for specific identification.

The epicellular nature of *M. haemofelis* on erythrocytes is readily apparent by scanning electron microscopy (EM) examinations (Fig. 31-2). Organisms appear to be partially buried in indented foci on the surface of the erythrocytes. Discoid, conical, coccoid, rod-shape, and doughnut-shape organisms have been observed. Parasitized erythrocytes generally lose the normal biconcave shape and become spherocytes or stomatospherocytes.

The epicellular nature of *M. haemofelis* parasites is also readily apparent by transmission EM (Fig. 31-3).[53] A single membrane surrounds the organisms. The cytoplasm of organisms is composed of granules that vary in size and density. No cytoplasmic organelles have been recognized. Electron-lucent areas (vacuoles) appear to be present in some organisms. Organisms appear to adhere to the erythrocyte membrane by intermittent contact points. Although smudging of the erythrocytic membrane in association with organism attachment

has been reported, complete erosion of the membrane has not been documented.

Hemotrophic *Mycoplasma* Organisms in Dogs

Mycoplasma haemocanis (formerly *Haemobartonella canis*)[39,44] is considered to be the causative agent of hemotrophic mycoplasmosis in dogs; however, the sequence of the 16S rRNA gene of *M. haemocanis* was remarkably similar (99% homology) to that of *M. haemofelis*, suggesting that these agents might be different strains of the same organism.[8] Other

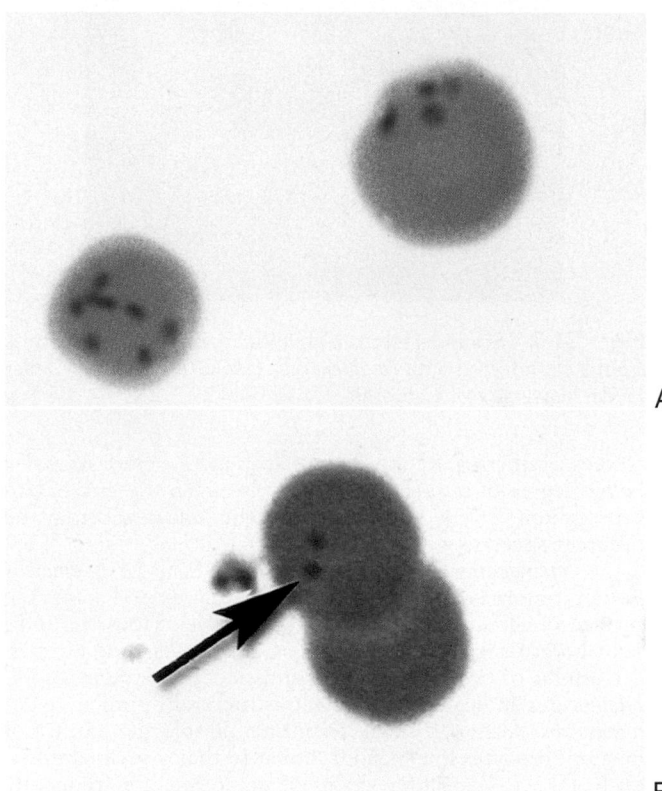

Fig 31-1 *M. haemofelis* (**A**) and *M. haemominutum* (**B**; *arrow*) in blood films from infected cats (Wright stain, ×1600). (**B**, Courtesy Janet Foley, University of California, Davis, Calif.)

Table • 31-1

Comparison of Hemotrophic Mycoplasmas of Cats

SPECIES	MYCOPLASMA HAEMOFELIS	MYCOPLASMA HAEMOMINUTUM
Synonyms	Large variant *Haemobartonella felis* Ohio strain Florida strain Oklahoma strain Illinois strain	Small variant *Haemobartonella felis* California strain Birmingham strain
Morphologic findings	Common in blood films Coccoid in thick smear Ring and rod in thin areas	Rare in blood films, stain lightly Small rods, rings, or coccoid
Clinical illness	Mental depression, fever, anemia, dehydration, hepatosplenomegaly, lymphadenomegaly, icterus, dyspnea	Minimal or absent

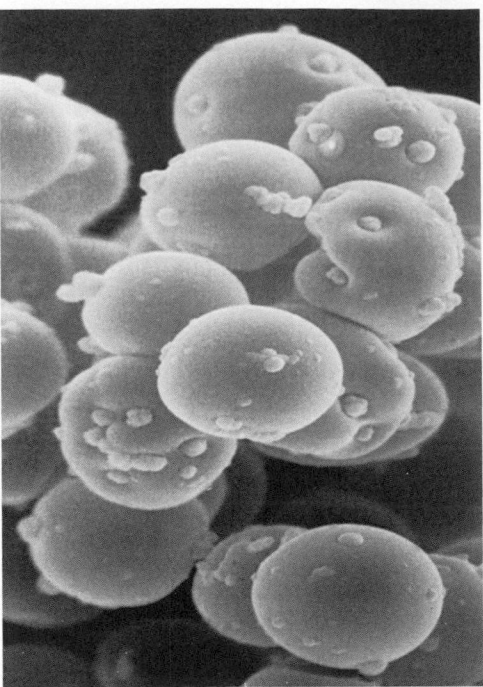

Fig 31-2 Scanning electron photomicrograph of erythrocytes from a cat infected with *M. haemofelis* (×5000). (Courtesy Dallas Hyde, University of California, Davis, Calif.)

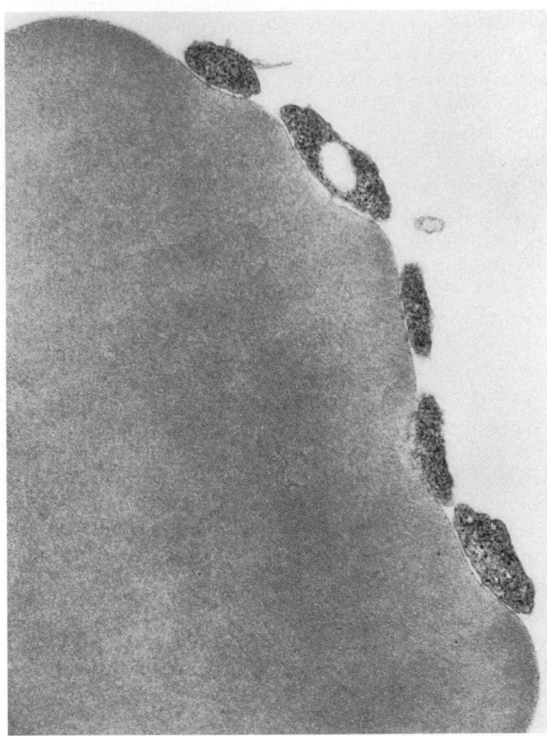

Fig 31-3 Transmission electron photomicrograph of five *M. haemofelis* organisms in intermittent contact with the plasmalemma of a parasitized erythrocyte (×17,000). (From Simpson CF, et al. 1978. Ultrastructure of erythrocytes parasitized by *Haemobartonella felis, J Parasitol* 64:504-511.)

studies evaluating RNase P gene sequences demonstrated a lower degree of sequence homology between the two organisms (about 95%), indicating that the organisms may be different species.[6]

M. haemocanis differs morphologically from *M. haemofelis* in that it more commonly forms chains that extend across the surface of affected erythrocytes (Fig. 31-4). However, individual organisms may also appear as small cocci, rods, or rings.

Results of scanning and transmission EM studies of *M. haemocanis* indicate that it is ultrastructurally similar to *M. haemofelis*. Although single organisms dimple the surface of host erythrocytes in a manner similar to that described previously for *M. haemofelis*, chains of organisms are frequently found in grooves or deep folds, which can markedly distort the erythrocyte shape.

A novel small haemoplasma, '*Candidatus mycoplasma Mycoplasma haematoparvum*,' which is genetically more closely related to M. haemominitum than M. haemofelis, was isolated from the blood of a splenectomized dog with hematopoietic neoplasia.[53a] In a study involving PCR of blood from dogs in France, this novel organism was more prevalent than *M. haemocanis*.[30c]

EPIDEMIOLOGY AND PATHOGENESIS

Cats

Based on the morphologic appearance of the organisms, clinical signs, and laboratory findings, it appears that most publications concerning feline hemotrophic mycoplasmal infections published before 1998 involved *M. haemofelis*. The Florida and Ohio strains of the organism used in experimental studies cited in this chapter were shown to be *M. haemofelis* by the polymerase chain reaction (PCR) and sequencing of the 16S rRNA gene.[51] Reports to date indicate that *M. haemofelis* often produces anemia and clinical signs of disease, whereas *M. haemominutum* generally results in inapparent infections and a minimal change in hematocrit (HCT), unless complicated by feline leukemia virus (FeLV)

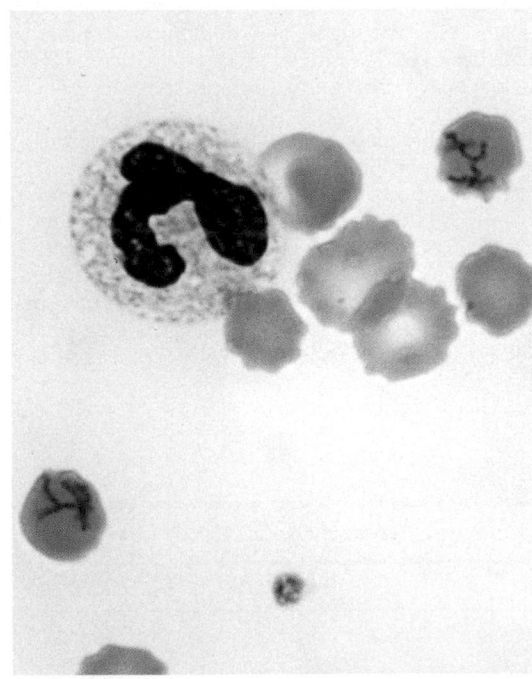

Fig 31-4 Two erythrocytes parasitized by *M. haemocanis* organisms (Wright-Giemsa stain, ×1800).

infections.[15-17,54,61] The following discussion focuses on the pathogenesis of disease associated with *M. haemofelis* infection.

Experimentally, *M. haemofelis* infection has been transmitted by intraperitoneal and intravenous (IV) injection and oral (PO) administration of infected blood. Dissemination of infection by blood-sucking arthropods such as fleas is considered by many to be the primary mode of transmission, although such transmission has not been established experimentally in cats. *M. haemofelis* can be transmitted from queens with clinical disease to their newborn offspring in the absence of arthropod vectors. It is not known whether transmission occurs in utero, during parturition, or via nursing. Iatrogenic transmission of *M. haemofelis* can occur by the transfusion of blood from normal-appearing carrier cats.

The severity of disease produced by *M. haemofelis* varies, with some cats having mild anemia and no clinical signs and some cats having marked depression and severe anemia leading to death.

To facilitate the understanding of feline hemotrophic mycoplasmosis caused by *M. haemofelis*, the disease has been divided into preparasitemic, acute, recovery, and carrier phases, or stages (Fig. 31-5).[26] The preparasitemic phase is generally about 1 to 3 weeks after IV injection. The acute phase of disease represents the time from the first to the last major parasitemia. This phase often lasts a month or more, but occasionally cats die quickly from massive parasitemias and precipitous decreases in HCT early in the course of the disease. Parasites generally appear in the blood in a cyclic manner within discrete parasitemic episodes (see Fig. 31-5). The number of parasites generally increases to a peak value over 1 to 5 days, followed by a rapid decline. The synchronized disappearance of organisms from the blood can occur in 2 hours or less. Few if any parasites are seen in blood films for several days following parasitemic episodes, although low numbers of organisms can still be detected in blood using PCR.[3,56]

In many instances a rapid decrease in HCT followed by a rapid increase occurs in association with the appearance and disappearance of large numbers of organisms from the blood. These fluctuations in HCT appear to be associated with splenic sequestration of parasitized erythrocytes and with later release of nonparasitized erythrocytes. In other instances the HCT remains lower or continues to decline for 1 or more days after a parasitemic episode, probably as a result of erythrocyte destruction.

Repetitive parasitemic episodes appear to cause progressive erythrocyte damage and shortened erythrocyte life spans. Some damage to erythrocytes may be caused directly by the parasite, but immune-mediated injury appears to be more important. Coombs' (direct antiglobulin) tests (37° C) may have positive results within a week following the first parasitemia, and Coombs' test results generally remain positive during the acute stage of disease, regardless of whether parasites are present. It is postulated that the attachment of organisms to erythrocytes either exposes hidden erythrocyte antigens or results in altered erythrocyte antigens, and the host responds by producing antierythrocyte antibodies. Specific antibodies against *M. haemofelis* antigens have been detected in serum within 14 days after experimental infections.[1] Consequently, another possible mechanism of immune-mediated injury should also be considered. If antibody-mediated complement fixation occurs, the erythrocytic membrane may be damaged as an "innocent bystander." However, minimal intravascular hemolysis occurs in this disorder. The anemia occurs primarily as a result of extravascular erythrophagocytosis by macrophages in the spleen, liver, lungs, and bone marrow.

As a lymphocyte- and macrophage-rich blood filter, the spleen is of primary importance in the clearance of blood-

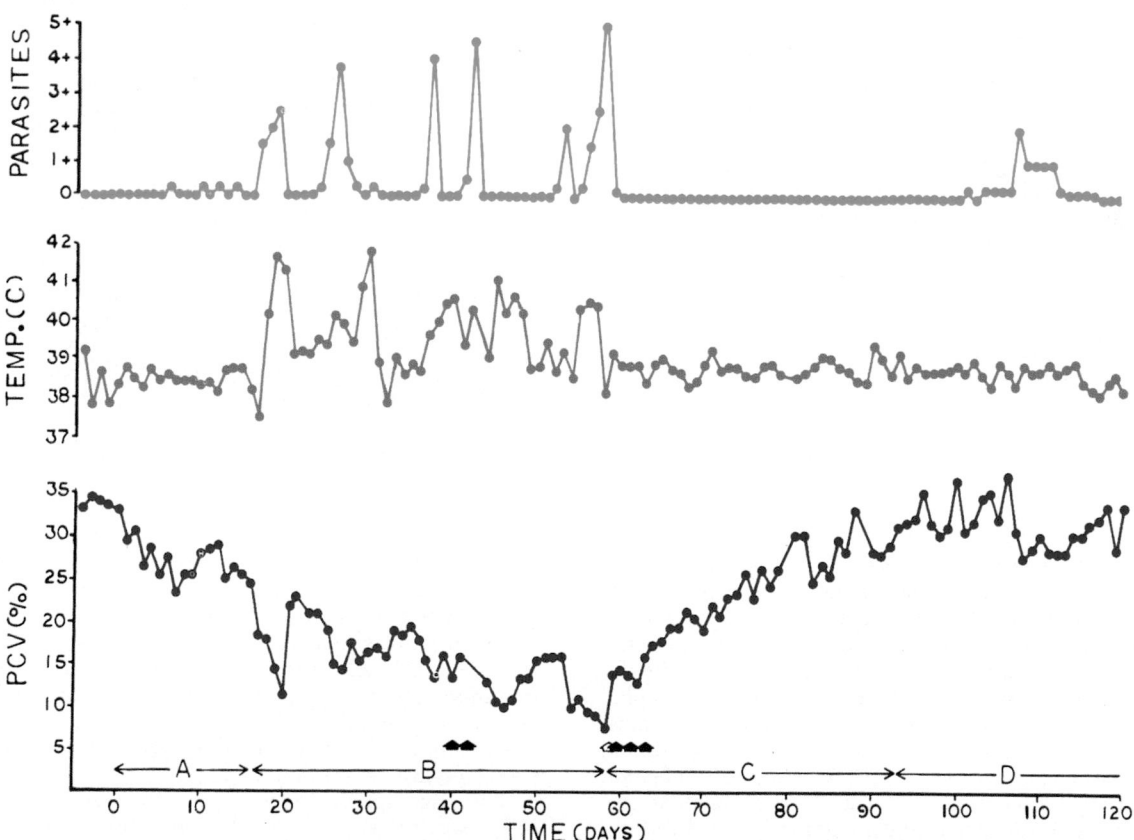

Fig 31-5 Daily measurements of hematocrit (HCT, or packed cell volume [PCV]), rectal temperature, and blood parasite value in a cat after IV inoculation with *M. haemofelis*-infected blood on day 0. *Closed arrows* indicate intravenous administration of thiacetarsamide sodium (1 mg/kg). *Open arrow* at day 60 indicates a 25-ml IV whole blood transfusion. Phases of disease are indicated by letter and shading, with *A* being the preparasitemic phase, *B* the acute phase, *C* the recovery phase, and *D* the carrier phase. (From Harvey JW, Gaskin JM. 1977. Experimental feline haemobartonellosis, *J Am Anim Hosp Assoc* 13:28-38.)

borne particulate antigens and the elaboration of specific immune responses to these antigens. In animals other than the cat, splenectomy is generally required before clinical disease is produced by the various species-specific hemotrophic mycoplasmal organisms. *M. haemofelis* organisms are removed less readily in splenectomized cats, resulting in parasitemias that last about twice as long as those in intact cats. However, splenectomy performed before infection does not appear to affect the incubation period or severity of disease in cats. Splenectomy after cats have recovered results in transient reappearance of blood parasites, but in most animals the HCT does not drop to a clinically significant level.

Without therapy, up to one third of the cats with uncomplicated acute *M. haemofelis* infection die as a result of severe anemia. Cats that mount a sufficient immune response to the organism and a regenerative bone marrow response that compensates for the erythrocyte destruction recover from the disease. The recovery phase—the time from the last major parasitemia until the HCT has stabilized within or close to the reference range—often takes a month or more. In untreated cats, organisms are commonly observed in low numbers in the blood during the recovery phase but do not usually occur as discrete parasitemic episodes.

Cats that recover from acute infections with *M. haemofelis* remain chronically infected for months to years, if not for life. Although an extracellular parasite should be eliminated by immune mechanisms, intact organisms have been reported within phagocytic vacuoles of splenic and pulmonary macrophages. Some organisms may survive within these cells, which would account for the indefinite, chronically infected state (although in situ hybridization studies of an infected cat using a specific DNA probe only demonstrated organisms on erythrocytes).[5] Carrier cats (those with latent infections) appear clinically normal. They may have a normal HCT or mild regenerative anemia. Low numbers of organisms are regularly observed in some cats, but in others no organisms are visible in blood films for weeks. Carrier cats appear to be in a balanced state in which replication of organisms is balanced by phagocytosis and removal of organisms.

M. haemofelis may be an opportunistic agent that exists commonly in healthy cats and produces disease when the cat is stressed by other diseases or surgical procedures; however, some cats with hemotrophic mycoplasmosis do not have identifiable predisposing disease or stress conditions. Cat-bite abscesses appear to be the most frequent disorder recognized to precede hemotrophic mycoplasmosis by a few weeks. Although an abscess is undoubtedly stressful, the possibility of transmission of the disease through a cat bite should be considered. Other factors associated with an increased likelihood of finding *M. haemofelis* organisms in stained blood films include male sex, lack of vaccinations, outdoor roaming, and positive FeLV and feline immunodeficiency virus (FIV) tests.[18,21]

Of particular interest is the possible interrelationship between *M. haemofelis* and FeLV-produced disease. About 40% to 50% of cats with clinical hemotrophic mycoplasmosis are FeLV positive.[18,21,59] Because FeLV can suppress the normal immune response to unrelated antigens, this viral infection might increase the susceptibility of cats to hemotrophic mycoplasmosis or convert a latent hemotrophic mycoplasmal infection into a patent infection with clinical disease. However, experimental studies have demonstrated that the opposite can also occur (i.e., *M. haemofelis* infection can increase the susceptibility of cats to FeLV infection).[31] Regardless of how the concurrent infections occur, infection with *M. haemofelis* and FeLV generally results in more severe anemia and clinical signs than occurs with infection by either agent alone.[7,21,31] In contrast, concurrent infection with FIV and *M. haemofelis* does not appear to cause more severe anemia than does *M. haemofelis* infection alone.[21,50]

Limited information is available concerning the pathogenesis of *M. haemominutum* infections. Substantial parasitemias can occur in blood with little change in HCT,[55,56] a finding that has been reported in nonsplenectomized cattle infected with a similar hemotrophic mycoplasma.[58] However, a mild regenerative anemia can occur in some cats infected only with *M. haemominutum*. As in *M. haemofelis*-infected cats discussed previously, cats co-infected with FeLV and *M. haemominutum* have more severe anemia than cats only infected with *M. haemominutum*.[17] In addition, the stress of infection with *M. haemominutum* may induce the development of myeloproliferative disease in FeLV-infected cats.[17]

Although some investigators indicate that infection with *M. haemominutum* is protective against challenge with the virulent *M. haemofelis*,[16] other investigators report that cats chronically infected with *M. haemominutum* are not protected against *M. haemofelis* infection.[61] This latter group of investigators provides evidence that the anemia occurring with combined infections is more severe than the anemia occurring in cats only infected with *M. haemofelis*. Prior infection with one strain might predispose cats to having heightened immune-mediated responses when they become infected with a second strain.[57]

Dogs

Transmission of *M. haemocanis* by the brown dog tick *(Rhipicephalus sanguineus)* has been demonstrated experimentally.[52] Transstadial and transovarial transmission in ticks has also been described, indicating that the tick may be an important reservoir as well as a vector of infection. Iatrogenic transmission of *M. haemocanis* organisms by blood transfusions from clinically normal carrier dogs can also occur but is of less concern than it is in cats, because the recipient dog generally must be splenectomized before clinically significant disease occurs. Hemotrophic mycoplasmosis resulting in the death of two animals from a litter of 4-week-old pups was reported.[24] Experimental studies to demonstrate transmission to puppies in utero or through nursing have not been successful, but indirect evidence for in utero transmission has been found.[34] Transmission by PO administration of infected blood has also been reported.[38]

In contrast to *M. haemofelis* infection in cats, most nonsplenectomized dogs infected with *M. haemocanis* do not develop clinical evidence of disease. They probably do not become anemic or have sufficient numbers of organisms present in the blood to be recognized during routine blood film examination.

The prepatent period following IV injection of infected blood into splenectomized dogs has been reported to range from 1 or 2 days to 2 weeks or more. Some cases have been characterized by a rapidly progressive anemia associated with nearly constant parasitemia. In these dogs, death generally occurs within a month following inoculation. In other dogs the development of anemia is more gradual, occurring as a result of repetitive parasitemic episodes. Parasites are generally observed in large numbers in the blood for a week or more, with a few intervening days when organisms are not observed. Approximately 1 to 2 months are generally required for the HCT and hemoglobin concentration to drop to minimum values, and an equal time is required for them to return to normal. Although immunologic evaluation of infected dogs has been limited, it appears that antibodies are produced against erythrocytes.

Although splenectomy is generally required before clinically significant hemotrophic mycoplasmosis occurs in dogs,[30a,b,33,37,46] cases have been described in nonsplenectomized dogs with concurrent *Ehrlichia*, *Babesia*, bacterial, and viral infections.[28] Hemotrophic mycoplasmosis has also occurred in dogs given immunosuppressive drugs[20] and in dogs with pathologic splenic symptoms. Rare cases have occurred in spleen-intact dogs in which no evidence for immunosuppression was found.

CLINICAL FINDINGS

Cats

Acute hemotrophic mycoplasmosis occurs in cats of all ages. Several studies have reported an increased incidence in adult males and attributed it to their increased roaming and fighting behavior, resulting in greater exposure to cats infected with *M. haemofelis*.[18,21] Feline hemotrophic mycoplasmosis is usually a disease of individual cats, although multiple infections in multicat households have been reported.[46]

No clinical signs may be recognized in cats with subclinical infections and mild anemia.[46] The most common clinical signs in ill cats are tachypnea, depression, weakness, anorexia, weight loss, pale mucous membranes, dehydration, icterus, and splenomegaly.[15,21] Clinical signs depend on the stage of disease and the rapidity with which anemia develops. If anemia develops gradually, a cat may exhibit weight loss but remain bright and alert. In contrast, a precipitous drop in HCT early in the disease in association with a severe parasitemia causes little weight loss, but marked mental depression and other clinical signs of anemia occur.

The rectal temperature generally is normal except during the acute phase of disease, when it is increased approximately 50% of the time. Subnormal temperatures may be present in moribund cats.

Clinical signs are mild or absent in cats experimentally infected only with *M. haemominutum*.[15] Mild fever may occur at times.[61] *M. haemominutum* infection has been demonstrated more often in sick cats than in healthy cats, but it is unclear whether the clinical signs present were related to the *M. haemominutum* infection or to other accompanying disease processes.[54]

Dogs

Unless other diseases are also present, clinical signs are rarely apparent in nonsplenectomized dogs infected with *M. haemocanis*. Splenectomized experimental dogs infected with *M. haemocanis* become listless and develop pale mucous membranes as the anemia progresses but generally have normal rectal temperatures and appetites.

DIAGNOSIS

Clinical Laboratory Findings

Cats

M. haemofelis organisms are only present in sufficient numbers to be easily recognized in stained blood films about 50% of the time during the acute phase of disease. The HCT is usually below 20% and frequently below 10% before clinical signs of disease are apparent to the client. The HCT is not always a good indicator of total erythrocyte mass in cats with hemotrophic mycoplasmosis. Parasitized erythrocytes that are primarily sequestered in the spleen and other organs may return to the general circulation following the removal of organisms from their surface.

If the HCT decreases rapidly, the mean cell volume (MCV) may be normal with few reticulocytes present. In most instances, by the time clinical signs of disease are apparent, the cat has a regenerative anemia with polychromasia and reticulocytosis. Erythrocytes are usually macrocytic, with an MCV greater than 50 fl, and frequently hypochromic, with a mean cell hemoglobin concentration (MCHC) less than 31 g/dl. Although anisocytosis, nucleated erythrocytes, and increased numbers of Howell-Jolly bodies are consistently observed in the circulation during the acute phase of feline hemotrophic mycoplasmosis, these findings are not reliable indicators of a regenerative response to anemia in the cat. Howell-Jolly bodies are often observed in normal cats, nucleated erythrocytes may appear in a wide variety of feline diseases, and marked anisocytosis without polychromasia has been reported in cats with myeloproliferative disease. Cats with latent infections (carriers) occasionally have low numbers of parasites visible in the blood. Their HCT fluctuates over time; it may be normal or slightly to moderately decreased, although not below 20%. Slight reticulocytosis with polychromasia and increased MCV are present at times.

Because two morphologic forms of reticulocytes have been described in cats, it is important to know which criteria a reference laboratory uses to count reticulocytes. Aggregate reticulocytes occur as a low proportion (0 to 0.4%) of the erythrocytes in blood from normal cats. The percentage of this form correlates well with the percentage of polychromatophilic erythrocytes. A greater proportion (up to 10%) of circulating erythrocytes in normal cats are punctate reticulocytes, which contain punctate inclusions of precipitated ribosomes. Reticulocyte counts are not valid in blood heavily parasitized with *M. haemofelis*, because organisms also stain as blue inclusions with reticulocyte stains.

Total and differential leukocyte counts are quite variable and of limited diagnostic assistance, although increased monocyte reactivity may be observed.[15,21,59] Erythrophagocytosis by monocytes or macrophages may be observed if blood films are scanned at low magnification. Platelet counts are usually normal.

Phagocytosis of erythrocytes by mononuclear cells in the circulation appears to occur as a result of antibodies, complement, or both on erythrocyte surfaces. Autoagglutination is frequently observed in refrigerated blood samples during early stages of acute hemotrophic mycoplasmosis,[63] but the clinical significance of these IgM cold agglutinins is unclear.[9] The Coombs' test (37° C) is often positive by the time a patient is presented for diagnostic evaluation.

Ratios of bone marrow myeloid to erythroid (M:E) are normal in the early stages of disease but are generally decreased later in the disease. Erythroid hyperplasia is manifested not only by an increase in the total number of erythroid cells but also by an increased proportion of immature stages. Slight to marked erythrophagocytosis by macrophages is often present.

Icteric plasma is not consistently observed in feline hemotrophic mycoplasmosis, but it may be present within 1 to 2 days after a rapid decrease in HCT. Icterus index values and plasma bilirubin concentration are not always increased subsequent to rapid decreases in HCT, probably because of the fact that erythrocytes can be sequestered in capillaries and vascular spaces within the spleen without being destroyed. Plasma protein concentrations are usually in the reference range (6 to 8 g) but may be increased in some cats. Serum alanine transferase and aspartate transferase activities are often mildly increased.[21] These increases may be attributed to hepatic hypoxia secondary to anemia or hepatic lipidosis secondary to anorexia. Serum urea concentrations may be slightly to moderately increased without an accompanying increase in serum creatinine concentration.[21] Increased serum urea concentrations are believed to be prerenal secondary to dehydration. Moribund cats may be hypoglycemic.

Cats infected with *M. haemominutum* may have a slight regenerative anemia or have normal hematologic findings.

Dogs

M. haemocanis organisms are usually present when clinical evidence of anemia caused by hemotrophic mycoplasmosis is recognized in dogs. Although the anemia has varied from mild to severe in studies of splenectomized experimental dogs, the HCT has generally been below 20% before clinical signs of hemotrophic mycoplasmosis were observed. Organisms may be found incidentally during hematologic screening, when an animal is examined early in the disease because of clinical signs attributable to other concurrent disorders.

In most cases, sufficient time has elapsed between the development of anemia and initial recognition of the disease for there to be peripheral blood evidence of a regenerative bone marrow response to the anemia. Hematologic findings include reticulocytosis with increased polychromasia and anisocytosis, circulating nucleated erythrocytes, and frequent Howell-Jolly bodies. Macrocytosis takes more time to develop and therefore may not be present when animals are initially seen by a veterinarian.

No consistent leukogram abnormalities are recognized in canine hemotropic mycoplasmosis. Neither icteric plasma nor hemoglobinemia is generally recognized in uncomplicated cases, but substantial bilirubinuria may occur.[46] Spherocytosis and positive Coombs' test results occur in some animals. Dogs with latent infections generally have normal hemograms.

Organism and Nucleic Acid Detection
Cats

Thin, well-stained blood films, without artifacts caused by improper drying or fixation or by precipitated stain, are required to identify hemotrophic mycoplasmas. Numerous Romanowsky-type blood stains (e.g., Wright-Giemsa) may be used, although low numbers of organisms are difficult to recognize using the Diff-Quik stain (Dade Behring, Deerfield, Ill.). Blood films must be examined before therapy begins because organisms are absent while cats are being treated with tetracycline antibiotics. Organisms may detach from erythrocytes during storage in ethylenediaminetetraacetic acid (EDTA), so it is advisable to make blood smears as soon as possible after sample collection.[1] The clinician must be able to differentiate hemotrophic mycoplasmas from stain precipitate, drying artifacts, Howell-Jolly bodies, basophilic stippling, siderotic inclusions, and *Cytauxzoon* parasites, which are small protozoa with a nucleus and cytoplasm (Table 31-2; see Chapter 76).[25] New methylene blue wet preparations and reticulocyte stains should not be used to diagnose hemotrophic mycoplasmal infections, because even normal cats have up to 10% punctate reticulocytes, and precipitated ribosomal material in reticulocytes cannot be accurately differentiated from hemotrophic mycoplasmas.

Because of the cyclic nature of the parasitemias, the absence of *M. haemofelis* organisms in blood films does not rule out a diagnosis of hemotrophic mycoplasmosis. A regenerative anemia with a positive Coombs' test result, the presence of autoagglutination in refrigerated blood samples, or erythrophagocytosis by blood monocytes is suggestive of hemotrophic mycoplasmosis. However, other diseases such as primary autoimmune hemolytic anemia or FeLV-induced hemolytic anemia should also be considered.

M. haemominutum organisms are rarely seen in blood and when present are difficult to identify with certainty because they are so small.[17,61]

Highly sensitive feline PCR-based assays have been developed that can detect hemotrophic mycoplasmas in blood when too few organisms are present to make a diagnosis using stained blood films.[29,42,58]

Using competitive, quantitative PCR, it has been determined that about 50 *M. haemofelis* organisms can be detected by PCR.[12] Specific PCR primers have been developed to differentiate between *M. haemofelis* and *M. haemominutum* infections in cats based on amplified DNA products.[15,29,61] PCR results were positive 4 to 15 days after experimental infections with hemotrophic mycoplasmas, and results remained positive until appropriate antibiotic therapy was initiated.[14,15,61] PCR results were generally negative during antibiotic therapy, but most cats showed positive results again between 3 days and 5 weeks after therapy was discontinued, although low numbers of animals had negative results up to 6 months after treatment.[3,7a,14,15] Using quantitative PCR, the concentration of *M. haemofelis* DNA in blood was forced to be inversely proportional to the hematocrit of infected cats.[54a,37a]

Whether diagnosed by identification of parasites in blood films or PCR-based assays, the significance of hemotrophic mycoplasmal infections must be interpreted in light of hematologic and clinical findings. The mere presence of hemotrophic mycoplasmas in the blood does not necessarily indicate that the clinical illness present was produced by this agent, because parasites may be incidentally observed in carrier cats with other diseases. On the other hand, even if the anemia appears nonregenerative the clinician should not automatically discount the significance of organisms in cats. If the HCT drops precipitously after infection, a cat can be depressed and anemic for several days before a substantial regenerative bone marrow response is evident in the peripheral blood. However, a persistent nonregenerative anemia should make the clinician investigate other causes of anemia, such as FeLV infection.

PCR testing has been beneficial in testing clinically healthy cats being screened as blood donors or for entry into specific pathogen–free colonies. It has also been valuable in epidemiologic studies evaluating the variety and prevalence of infection in cat populations. Community shelter-source cats,

Table • 31-2

Cytologic Inaccuracies for Detection of Hemotrophic Mycoplasmas of Cats

REASONS	APPEARANCE	REMEDY
False Positive		
Stain precipitate	Above focal plane, larger and denser-staining consistency, variable size	Use fresh-filtered stains
Drying artifacts	Irregular borders, refractile on focusing	Make thin smears, dry rapidly
Howell-Jolly bodies	Larger size (1–2 μm) nuclear remnants	None
Siderotic inclusions	Focal fine, blue-staining granules	Positive with Prussian blue stain
False Negative		
Transient parasitemia	No organisms seen despite regenerative anemia	PCR assay
Excess amount or exposure time to EDTA	No organisms seen despite regenerative anemia	New blood specimen, fresh smears, heparin or no anticoagulant

outside cats, and those with flea exposure, which were screened for blood donation by PCR, had the highest prevalence of infection.[19]

Dogs

Based on current information, it appears that *M. haemocanis* can generally be identified in blood of dogs with clinically significant hemotrophic mycoplasmosis, although organisms may be few and difficult to find. As in cats, the clinician must be able to differentiate between organisms and staining artifacts, basophilic stippling, and Howell-Jolly bodies. The most useful criterion is the tendency of *M. haemocanis* to form chains of organisms across the erythrocyte surface. Blood films should be inspected closely if an anemia develops or becomes worse in a dog after splenectomy.

PCR-based assays have been developed to identify *M. haemocanis* infections.[6,8] Although not evaluated, it is assumed that these assays are sensitive enough to identify animals with subclinical infections.

Prevalence of Infections

Using PCR-based assays, investigators in the United States[29] and Spain[13] reported finding about 30% of anemic cats suspected of having hemotrophic mycoplasmosis to be positive for hemotrophic mycoplasmas by PCR, with a majority of cats being positive for *M. haemofelis* alone or in combination with *M. haemominutum*. Additionally, about 14% of healthy control cats in the United States study were PCR positive for hemotrophic mycoplasmas. Of these PCR-positive healthy cats, 19 were infected only with *M. haemominutum* and 1 was infected with both variants.[29] Some caution is needed in interpreting these results, because only one variant was subsequently identified by PCR in some cats experimentally infected with both variants.[61]

A lower prevalence of *M. haemofelis* infections was found in a survey of British cats.[54] Less than 2% of ill cats (anemic or nonanemic) and less than 2% of healthy cats were infected with *M. haemofelis*. In contrast, about 20% of ill cats (anemic or nonanemic) and 8% of healthy cats were infected with *M. haemominutum*. A survey of feral cats in northern Florida revealed that 8% were PCR positive for *M. haemofelis* and 12% were PCR positive for *M. haemominutum*.[40] As in other reports, males were more commonly infected than females, and a positive correlation was found between hemotrophic mycoplasmal infections and FeLV and FIV infections.[40] In a survey identifying infected domestic cats in Japan, 67% had positive PCR results for *M. haemofelis*, 22% were positive for *M. haemominitum*, and 11% were coinfected.[60]

PATHOLOGIC FINDINGS

Gross necropsy findings in cats include pale tissue in all cases, emaciation in approximately 75% of the cats, slight to marked splenomegaly in approximately 50%, and slight to moderate icterus in some cats.

Abnormal histologic findings are variable and include erythroid and at times myeloid hyperplasia of bone marrow and passive congestion, extramedullary hematopoiesis, follicular hyperplasia, erythrophagocytosis, and increased hemosiderin in the spleen. In some cases, fatty degeneration and centrilobular necrosis of the liver is recognized.

Necropsy findings in canine hemotrophic mycoplasmosis have not been thoroughly reported. The blood appears watery and tissues appear pale. The bone marrow is red and gelatinous. Hyperplasia of the mononuclear phagocyte system may be present.

THERAPY

Cats

Doxycycline or tetracycline/oxytetracycline antibiotics should be given for 3 weeks (Table 31-3). Unfortunately, tetracycline antibiotics may produce fever, evidence of GI disease (e.g., esophageal stricture), or both in cats.[41] Preliminary findings indicate that enrofloxacin (10 mg/kg, PO, once daily) may be an efficacious alternative for cats that do not tolerate tetracycline antibiotics.[14,56a,62] Glucocorticoids, such as prednisolone (1 to 2 mg/kg, PO, every 12 hours), may be given to severely anemic animals to decrease erythrophagocytosis. The glucocorticoid dosage should be gradually decreased as the HCT increases. Blood transfusions are required when the anemia is considered life-threatening. IV fluid containing glucose is recommended for moribund animals.

Treated and untreated animals that recover from *M. haemofelis* infections generally remain carriers but seldom relapse with clinical disease once the HCT returns to normal.[3,17,27] Following immunosuppression with glucocorticoids, organisms can still be detected by PCR.[3] Azithromycin or imidocarb dipropionate are not effective in treating hemotrophic mycoplasmal infections in cats.[35,61] Chloramphenicol has previously been recommended for the treatment of *M. haemofelis* infections, but it should not be used for this purpose, because it causes dose-dependent erythroid hypoplasia in the bone marrow of cats.[25] Antimicrobial treatment reduces or eliminates visible parasitemia, but it does not clear the parasite from the body.

Table • 31-3

Drug Dosages for Canine and Feline Hemotrophic Mycoplasmosis

DRUG[a]	SPECIES	DOSE[b] (mg/kg)	ROUTE	INTERVAL (HOURS)	DURATION (DAYS)
Tetracycline	Dog, cat	20	PO, IV	8	21
Oxytetracycline	Dog, cat	20	PO, IV	8	21
Doxycycline	Dog, cat	10	PO	24	21
Doxycycline	Dog, cat	5	PO	12	21
Enrofloxacin	Cat	5–10[c]	PO	24	14
Prednisolone[d]	Dog, cat	1–2	PO	12	prn

PO, By mouth; *IV*, intravenous; *prn*, as needed.
[a]See Drug Formulary, Appendix 8, for additional information on these drugs.
[b]Dose per administration at specified interval.
[c]Recommendation based on efficacy study of *Mycoplasma haemofelis* infection in cats.[36,56a] However, dosages at a level of > 5 mg/kg/day may cause retinotoxicity in cats and should be used with caution or substituted with other drugs.
[d]Value of glucocorticoids is not substantiated. Cats with experimental disease have responded to therapy with tetracyclines alone.

Dogs

Experimental studies evaluating therapy for canine hemotrophic mycoplasmosis have been limited. Blood transfusions should be administered when the anemia is considered life-threatening. Orally administered oxytetracycline is reported to be effective in treating *M. haemocanis* infections (see Table 31-3). Dogs that recover from hemotrophic mycoplasmosis probably have latent infections. Data is not available for the need or efficacy of treatment of 'Candidatus M. haematoparvum' infection in dogs.

PREVENTION

Elimination of blood-sucking arthropods from dogs and cats is recommended because they may transmit infectious diseases, including hemotrophic mycoplasmosis. Iatrogenic transmission of *M. haemocanis* in dogs is usually of concern only if the recipient has been splenectomized. Iatrogenic transmission can likely be prevented in cats and dogs by testing blood donors using PCR-based tests.

SUGGESTED READINGS*

29. Jensen WA, Lappin MR, Kamkar S, et al. 2001. Use of a polymerase chain reaction assay to detect and differentiate two strains of *Haemobartonella felis* in naturally infected cats, *Am J Vet Res* 62:604-608.

30c. Kenny MJ, Shaw SE, Beugnet F, et al. Demonstration of two distinct hemotropic mycoplasmas in French dogs. *J Clin Microbiol* 42:5397-5399.

35. Lappin MR, Brewer M, Radecki S. 2002. Effects of imidocarb dipropionate in cats with chronic haemobartonellosis, *Vet Therap* 2:149.

42. Messick JB, Berent LM, Cooper SK. 1998. Development and evaluation of a PCR-based assay for detection of *Haemobartonella felis* in cats and differentiation of *H. felis* from related bacteria by restriction fragment length polymorphism analysis, *J Clin Microbiol* 36:462-466.

54. Tasker S, Binns SH, Day MJ, et al. 2003. Use of a PCR assay to assess the prevalence and risk factors for *Mycoplasma haemofelis* and 'Candidatus Mycoplasma haemominutum' in cats in the United Kingdom, *Vet Rec* 152:193-198.

57. Tasker S, Lappin MR. 2002. *Haemobartonella felis*: recent developments in diagnosis and treatment, *J Feline Med Surg* 4:3-11.

*See the CD-ROM for a complete list of references.

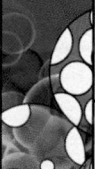

CHAPTER 32

Mycoplasmal, Ureaplasmal, and L-Form Infections

Craig E. Greene

MYCOPLASMAL AND UREAPLASMAL INFECTIONS

Etiology

Mycoplasmas, the smallest free-living microorganisms, are prokaryotes within the class Mollicutes. Mycoplasmas are currently divided into hemotrophic and nonhemotrophic types. Only the nonhemotrophic types will be described here; hemotrophic organisms are discussed in Chapter 31, Hemotrophic Mycoplasmosis. Mycoplasmas have the smallest of genomes, with replicating cells as small as 300 nm and a DNA molecule expressing as few as 700 genes (Fig. 32-1). Although this molecule is large enough for an extracellular existence, its size restricts its metabolic capacity. Mycoplasmas therefore depend on nourishment from a rich environment, which they find on mucosal membranes of the respiratory and urogenital tracts of their warm-blooded hosts. The lack of a rigid, protective cell wall makes mycoplasmas rather fragile outside the host but resistant to lysozyme and cell wall–inhibiting antibiotics such as penicillin, cephalosporin, vancomycin, and bacitracin. Animal mycoplasmas survive for variable time periods outside the host, depending on the species, amount of moisture, and temperature.[53] Under dry conditions, most mycoplasmas are stable at 4° C, but many are unstable at higher temperatures. Stability is influenced by pH, being more stable at 7.5 than 6.5. The presence of organic material such as host tissues or body fluids helps their preservation. Survival times vary between species but generally range from 50 to 150 days at 4° C in liquid media to 7 to 14 days under dry conditions at 30° C.[53]

Despite their limited genome, mycoplasmas have marked genetic alterability, which allows them to vary the expression of major surface antigenic proteins as a means of avoiding host immune surveillance. Genetic studies of mycoplasmas of animals and people have shown that host preference does not derive from bacterial phylogenetic closeness.[7] This finding suggests that switching to new hosts from genetic alterations may have occurred at several times during their evolution.

Mycoplasmas of the genera *Mycoplasma*, *Ureaplasma*, and *Acholeplasma* are represented in the natural mucosal flora of dogs and cats (Table 32-1). The term *Mycoplasma* in this chapter refers to any of these organisms. Ureaplasmas are organisms with an adaptive preference for the genitourinary mucosae. Many species may have a role in diseases by virtue of being isolated from disease processes, but few have been conclusively proved to be pathogenic. Table 32-1 also contains a list of diseases of dogs and cats in which mycoplasmas may be causal factors. These diseases most often involve inflammation of mucosal or serosal surfaces of the respiratory tract, urogenital tract, joints, mammary glands, and conjunctiva.

Studies in experimental mycoplasmal infections of mice have shown that IgA response is a primary factor in resistance to respiratory tract infections.[28] Generation of this response was best induced by intrarespiratory, but not parenteral,

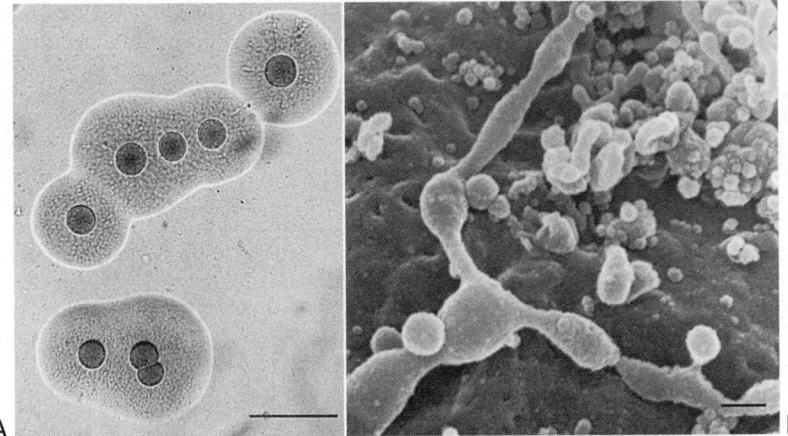

Fig 32-1 A, Colonies of mycoplasmas grown for 4 days on solid substrate and viewed in a dissecting microscope (bar, 1 mm). **B,** Scanning electron micrograph of mycoplasmas colonizing the surface of epithelial cells (bar, 200 μm). (Courtesy V. Bermudez, Ontario Veterinary College, Guelph, Ontario, Canada.)

Table • 32-1

Species of Mycoplasma, Acholeplasma, *and* Ureaplasma *Isolated From Dogs and Cats*

SITUATION	DOGS	CATS
Upper respiratory tract (oropharynx, nasopharynx, larynx) of clinically healthy animals	Three unclassified, *M. canis, M. spumans, M. maculosum, M. opalescens, M. edwardii, M. cynos, M. molare, M. feliminutum, M. gateae, M. arginini, M. bovigenitalium, Acholeplasma laidlawii, Ureaplasma* spp., *Mycoplasma* spp.[59]	*M. felis, M. gateae, M. feliminutum, M. arginini, Acholeplasma* spp., *Ureaplasma* spp., *M. pulmonis, M. arthritidis, M. allisepticum*[58]
Lower respiratory tract (lung and tracheobronchial secretions) of healthy animals	Rarely isolated[59]	Usually more, *M. felis, M. gateae*[56,58]
Lower respiratory tract of pneumonic animals	*M. canis, M. spumans, M. cynos, M. edwardii, M. gateae, M. feliminutum, M. bovigenitalium, Mycoplasma* spp., *Ureaplasma* spp.[31, 39,59]	*M. felis, M. arginini*[52,13]
Pleuropulmonary abscesses	NR	*Mycoplasma* spp.[46,24]
Conjunctiva of healthy animals	NR	None[25]
Conjunctivitis	NR	*M. felis*[25,54]
Peritoneal cavity	NR	NR
Genital tract	*M. canis, M. cynos, M. felis, Ureaplasma* spp., *Mycoplasma* spp.[45,42]	*M. felis, M. gateae*[9]
Urinary tract	*M. canis, M. spumans, M. cynos*[42,32]	NR
Epididymoorchitis	*M. canis*[42]	NR
Abscesses	NR	*Mycoplasma*-like organisms: cat bites,[a] *M. canis, M. spumans*: dog bite[69]

NR, Not reported.
[a]These may represent L-form infections.

administration of *Mycoplasma* antigen. Addition of cholera toxin as an adjuvant was beneficial in producing a protective immunity. *Mycoplasma* may also induce T-cell responses, which cause both beneficial and adverse immunologic consequences. Increased cytokines promote antimicrobial clearance and increased tissue injury. Mycoplasmal products may act as superantigens, which may stimulate chronic immune-mediated diseases such as rheumatoid arthritis. In addition, some mycoplasmas may become intracellular, resulting in chronic persistent infections.

Mycoplasma DNA has been identified by polymerase chain reaction (PCR) methods in live virus veterinary vaccines; however, no viable organisms could be cultivated.[40] Presumably, contamination during their production was the cause. Further work is needed to clarify this finding.

Clinical Findings
Ocular
Mycoplasma felis is considered to be a significant pathogen in conjunctivitis of cats. Experimental inoculation of *Myco-*

plasma has produced conjunctivitis only when cats are young or when a large amount of inoculum is used. Spontaneously observed conjunctivitis usually occurs when infected cats are housed in groups and develops soon after weaning with loss of maternal immunity. The incidence of *M. felis* in cats with conjunctivitis is 25%; it is not isolated from clinically healthy cats, although it may be present in levels below the sensitivity of culture.[25] The clinical signs of mycoplasmal conjunctivitis have been described as serous discharge followed by mucoid and sticky exudate. The conjunctiva is initially hyperemic and edematous and later becomes indurated. Untreated cats may show signs as long as 60 days, but the cornea is usually not involved.

Respiratory

Most *Mycoplasma* spp. normally appear in the upper respiratory tract. They have also been isolated at necropsy from lungs of dogs and cats with various types of pneumonia but are not generally present in the lungs of healthy animals, especially cats.[56,58] Isolation of *Mycoplasma* from tracheobronchial lavage specimens of clinically healthy animals was 0% for cats and 25% for dogs, whereas animals with pulmonary disease had a 21% isolation rate.[58,59] Ureaplasmas are rarely, if ever, isolated from the respiratory tract of healthy or diseased animals.[58,59] In animals with impaired pulmonary clearance resulting from viral infection, mycoplasmas inhaled from the upper respiratory tract may establish an infection in the lung or pleural cavity, or both, as a secondary opportunistic pathogen.[17,52]

Chronic pulmonary mycoplasmosis has been observed in dogs with primary ciliary dyskinesia.[3] These bacteria have the tendency to produce prolonged suppurative infection of the conducting airways.[3] Histopathologic features consist of purulent bronchitis and bronchiolitis with bronchiectasis early, followed by bronchial and bronchiolar epithelial hyperplasia, mononuclear infiltration, lymphoid hyperplasia, interstitial pneumonia, and bronchiolitis obliterans.[39] When a large number of mycoplasmal species isolated from lungs of dogs with distemper pneumonia were evaluated for virulence by experimental exposure of healthy puppies, only one strain of *Mycoplasma cynos* induced pulmonary disease. Although it is not likely to play a primary role, *M. cynos* undoubtedly contributes to the multifactorial cause of canine pneumonia.[12a] For example, mycoplasmas have been isolated, alone and in combination with other bacteria, from the airway washings of dogs with lower respiratory diseases.[13] Common but variable anatomic changes in these dogs included collapsing trachea and interstitial, bronchointerstitial, and alveolar pulmonary disease. Whether these isolations represent contamination of upper airway microflora during retrograde collection methods is uncertain because these organisms have been isolated from the respiratory tract of clinically healthy dogs.

Because isolation of *Mycoplasma* from the respiratory tract washings of clinically healthy cats is uncommon, culturing these organisms may have clinical significance. *M. felis* is likely a primary pathogen in the cat because pneumonia has developed after experimental challenge of kittens. A kitten with congenital mitral valve dysplasia developed pneumonia and pyothorax associated with *M. felis* infection.[46] *Mycoplasma* spp. were isolated in pure culture from bronchoalveolar lavage specimens from three cats with either suppurative bronchitis or bronchopneumonia.[21] *Mycoplasma* and *Arcanobacterium* (*Corynebacterium*) *pyogenes* were isolated from pyothorax in a kitten.[24] Cats with pleural effusion show minimal signs of dyspnea compared with dogs. Nonodorous fluid is expected with uncomplicated mycoplasma pyothorax.

Genitourinary

Isolating mycoplasmas in large numbers from the urine of dogs with urinary tract infection (UTI) is not uncommon. Although in most situations the mycoplasmas are in mixed culture with bacteria, they are also occasionally isolated.[32,42] The same conditions such as tumors and urinary calculi, predisposing the animal to bacterial infection, may promote *Mycoplasma* infection. The source of the mycoplasmas in the urinary tract is undoubtedly the abundant microflora in the distal urogenital tract. More credibility exists for their role in infection when urine is collected by cystocentesis and no other bacteria are isolated. Collection of urine by voiding or catheterization will result in contamination of the urine specimen. Conditions causing obstruction and urine stasis of the urethra will allow ascending contamination of the urinary system so that they may be isolated with cystocentesis. *M. felis* and *Mycoplasma gateae* have not been able to survive under osmotic conditions present in normal feline urine,[9] indicating that mycoplasmas are unlikely candidates for urinary disorders of cats. *Ureaplasma* spp. are more resistant to osmotic damage by urine and are more likely candidates for UTIs in dogs and cats.[9] No features can be used to distinguish mycoplasmal UTI from other bacterial urinary infections. Studies in cats with feline lower urinary tract disease have not implicated either mycoplasmas or ureaplasmas.[64]

Mycoplasmas of the reproductive tract are currently considered to be opportunistic. *M. canis* has been isolated from dogs with endometritis. The assumed opportunistic role of mycoplasmas in endometritis is probably overlooked in many cases of mixed infection when conventional bacteria are cultured. Alternatively, opportunistic bacterial infections may be responsible for the reproductive disorders in kennels where both mycoplasmas and bacteria are found. Vaginal and preputial swabs and semen samples are often submitted for mycoplasmal culture in dogs with infertility problems. Very often, these samples give positive results; however, their significance as pathogens is uncertain. Weighing the culture results in relation to other diagnostic findings and judging whether antibiotic treatment for mycoplasmas will solve the infertility problem are important. Deep vaginal or semen cultures are the most accurate means of determining the presence of the organisms.

A survey showed that infertile dogs had ureaplasmas in vaginal and preputial samples more often than fertile dogs. This difference was statistically significant in male dogs but not in female dogs.[18] Because ureaplasmas are associated with infertility in other animals, research work is urgently needed to evaluate the role of these organisms in dogs and cats. The percentages of dogs with positive culture results for *Mycoplasma* from the vagina or semen have not been statistically different between fertile and infertile dogs.[19]

Systemic

The general assumption holds that microorganisms from the natural flora cross the mucosal barrier with regularity, but healthy individuals eliminate these invaders by specific and nonspecific defense reactions. Mycoplasmas originating from the natural flora may therefore occasionally be isolated from parenchymatous organs of dogs and cats with debilitating diseases such as malignancies and immunosuppression.

Musculoskeletal

Dysgammaglobulinemia has been a predisposing cause of mycoplasmal polyarthritis and sepsis in people.[43] Naturally occurring mycoplasmal arthritis has occurred in cats.[20] Cats injected intravenously with *M. gatae* developed polyarthritis, thus confirming the potential virulence of this organism. Predisposing conditions were not identified in a young greyhound with polyarthritis caused by *Mycoplasma spumans*.[2]

Gastrointestinal

Mycoplasmas are occasionally isolated from rectum and colon biopsy samples of dogs with colitis, but conclusive evidence for their etiologic role in the inflammatory condition has not been found.

Abscesses

Organisms with the characteristics of mycoplasmas have been isolated from cats with abscesses, most likely introduced by bite-inflicted wounds.[36] Unfortunately, the isolates have been difficult to adapt to in vitro conditions and therefore have been impossible to classify. In some cases, these isolates may represent L-form infections (see later discussion). In one cat with multiple abscess wounds from a dog bite, *M. canis* and *M. spumans* were isolated.[69] In one report, three cats had mycoplasmal abscesses in subcutaneous and muscle tissue, and another cat was diagnosed with a cervical and a pulmonary abscess. Mycoplasmal abscesses are characterized by nonodorous, nondegenerate, neutrophilic exudates in which bacteria cannot be visualized with gram-stained smears. In all situations, the abscesses did not respond to surgical débridement or to cell wall–inhibiting antibacterials, but they did respond to treatment with tetracycline or tylosin (see also L-Form Infections).

Diagnosis

Mycoplasmas are often recovered as commensals from mucosal surfaces. To determine whether mycoplasmas are causative agents, they should be isolated from animals with disease in greater frequency than in healthy animals. Antibody responses should also be more prevalent in diseased animals, and clinical improvement should occur with *Mycoplasma*-susceptible antibiotics.

Exudates from draining lesions, inflamed mucosae, or body cavity effusions usually contain intact nondegenerate neutrophils, but no bacteria are noted. Organisms can be visualized by examining exudate or colony cultures by negative staining with transmission electron microscopy (EM). The clinician should be aware of the fragile nature of mycoplasmas. Special requests should be made of the laboratory if mycoplasmosis is suspected. Cotton swabs placed in Hayflicks broth medium or commercially available swabs with either Amies medium (without charcoal) or modified Stuart bacterial-transport medium can be submitted to the diagnostic laboratory for *Mycoplasma* culture. The specimens should be cooled and shipped with an ice pack if transport time is less than 24 hours but must be frozen and shipped with dry ice if longer transport time is expected. Urine sediment is cultured following centrifugation at 3000 × g for 10 minutes. Mycoplasmas from dogs and cats grow best on special media prepared according to Hayflicks formula and can be identified quite easily, provided specific reference antisera are available. Incubation at 37° C in 5% carbon dioxide is followed by anaerobic conditions for 48 hours.

Colonies have a characteristic "fried egg" appearance. They do not revert to parent cell wall–containing bacteria when they are grown on antibiotic-free media.

Mycoplasmas can be characterized by their biochemical features[48]; however, this does not always follow consistent patterns among species. An immunobinding assay using polyclonal antisera has been used to distinguish *M. felis* and *M. gateae* isolated from cats and from other species.[4,8] Mycoplasmas have also been identified by dot immunobinding and direct fluorescent antibody (FA) techniques. Molecular methods have included nucleic acid hybridization and random amplified polymorphic methods. PCR methods can help detect and differentiate *Mycoplasma* in cell culture[70] and clinical specimens.[22,34,12a] Bacteria such as *Fusobacterium necrophorum* cross-react with certain PCR reactions intended to detect a wide range of *Mycoplasma* species.[33]

Therapy and Prevention

Susceptibility testing to antimicrobial agents is not available for mycoplasmas on a routine basis. They are generally susceptible to the macrolides (tylosin, erythromycin, azithromycin, clarithromycin), pleuromutilins (valnemulin, tiamulin), tetracyclines, chloramphenicol, spiramycin, lincomycin, clindamycin, fluoroquinolones, nitrofurantoin, and aminoglycoside in vitro. Given that no agents are bactericidal, animals must be treated for an extended period (Table 32-2; also refer to the Drug Formulary, Appendix 8, for dosages). The immune system must be competent to eradicate the infection. Because tetracycline and chloramphenicol should not be used in pregnant animals, erythromycin and lincomycin, although less effective, are safer. Azithromycin causes less gastrointestinal side effects compared with erythromycin. The fluoroquinolones have been shown to be effective against mycoplasmas in vitro and in vivo.[15,35,71] Drug-resistant systemic mycoplasmal meningitis and arthritis in immunocompromised people have been treated successfully with pleuromutilins, a new class of antibiotic.[26]

No vaccines are available to prevent mycoplasmal infections in dogs and cats or other species. Attempts to protect animals against challenge with these agents have been discouraging. Studies in the respiratory tract indicate IgA is crit-

Table • 32-2

Therapy for Mycoplasma *and L-Form Infections*

DRUG[a]	SPECIES	DOSE[b] (mg/kg)	ROUTE PREFERRED (ALTERNATE)	INTERVAL (HOURS)	DURATION (WEEKS)
Doxycycline	B	10—20	PO (IV)	12	1
Tetracycline	B	22—30	PO	8	1
Chloramphenicol	D	25—50	PO (IV, SC, IM)	8	1
	C	25	PO	12	1
Clindamycin	B	5—11	PO	12	1
Enrofloxacin	B	5	PO (SC)	24	1

D, Dog; *C*, cat; *B*, both dog and cat; *PO*, by mouth; *IV*, intravenous; *SC*, subcutaneous; *IM*, intramuscular.
[a]See Appendix 8 for additional information.
[b]Dose per administration at specified interval.

ical in providing immunity against these agents. Intranasal immunization has been most effective in experimental studies; however, inclusion of mucosal adjuvants such as cholera toxin was required.[28]

Public Health Considerations

Mycoplasmal infections of dogs and cats have not been considered as major public health risks. A veterinarian developed suppurative tenosynovitis 1 week after being scratched on a finger by a cat being treated for colitis.[47] The infection was resistant to erythromycin, cloxacillin, and penicillin but was cured with doxycycline. This report was the first of mycoplasmal infection as a zoonosis and of *Mycoplasma* producing an abscess in people. Subsequently, *M. felis* has produced septic arthritis of the hip and knee in a person with common variable immunodeficiency syndrome who was receiving glucocorticoid therapy.[5]

L-FORM INFECTIONS

Etiology

L forms of bacteria represent cell wall–deficient forms and are morphologically similar to *Mycoplasma*. They are distinguishable from the latter by their variable size (1- to 4-μm diameter), their greater pleomorphism, and their penicillin-binding affinities. Cell wall deficiencies can be induced in vitro or in vivo in many bacteria by exposing them to cell wall–damaging chemicals or antimicrobials (e.g., β-lactam drugs) or host immune responses.

Clinical Findings

Cell wall–deficient bacteria have been isolated from cats with a syndrome of fever and persistently draining, spreading cellulitis and synovitis that often involve the extremities.[12,36,57] The usual source of infection has been contamination of penetrating bite wounds or surgical incisions. Cats have also presumably been infected from wound exudates from other cats. Infection begins at the point of inoculation, and lesions spread, drain, dehisce, and do not permanently heal (Fig. 32-2). Bacteremic spread of infection can occur, and polyarthritis or distant abscess formation may develop as a sequela. Progressive polyarthritis, unresponsive to antibiotics and glucocorticoids, occurred in a dog infected with an L form of *Nocardia asteroides*.[10]

Diagnosis
Laboratory Findings

Clinical laboratory abnormalities in cats with polyarthritis may include leukocytosis (over 25,000 cells/μl) with a mature neutrophilia and monocytosis, lymphocytosis, and eosinophilia.[12] Hyperfibrinogenemia and hyperglobulinemia may be found. The exudates contain predominantly macrophages and neutrophils with a few lymphocytes. Erythrophagia may be present; organisms *cannot* be detected by numerous cytologic stains. Radiographic abnormalities include periarticular soft tissue swelling and periosteal proliferation.[12] In severe cases, damage occurs to the articular cartilage and subchondral bone.

Organism Isolation

Diagnosis is difficult because these organisms are difficult to demonstrate by light microscopy. The organisms are also difficult to culture on bacterial or mycoplasmal media. Infection has been transmitted experimentally by subcutaneous inoculation with cell-free material from tissues or exudates of affected cats. EM evaluation of tissues may show the characteristically pleomorphic, cell wall–deficient organisms in phagocytes (Fig. 32-3).[57]

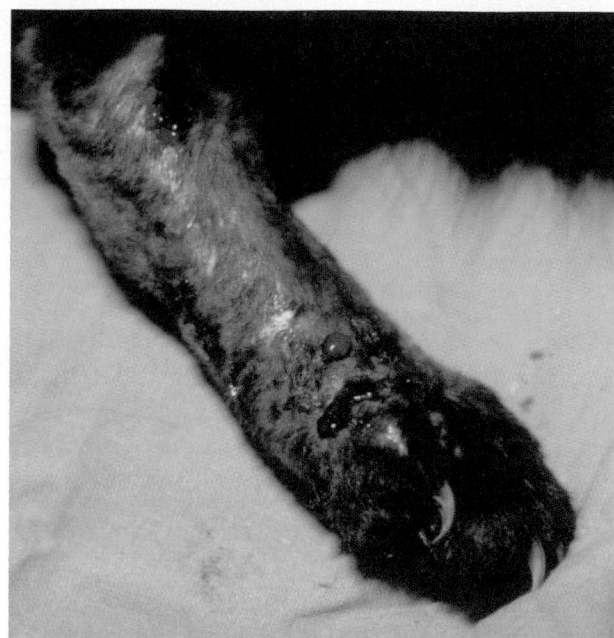

Fig 32-2 Distal pelvic limb from a cat with L-form infection with multiple fistulas draining purulent exudates. (Courtesy University of Georgia, Athens, Ga.)

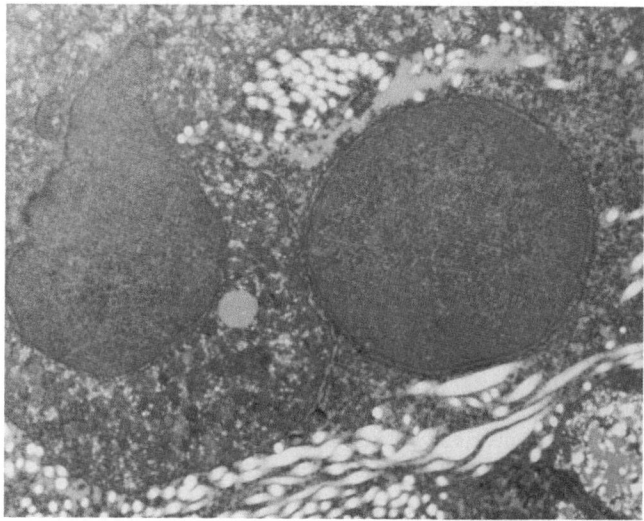

Fig 32-3 Transmission electron microphotograph of cell wall–deficient bacteria from draining lesions of the cat in Fig. 32-2. (Courtesy University of Georgia, Athens, Ga.)

Therapy

Cell wall–deficient organisms found in cats have been most responsive to tetracyclines. (For dosages, see Table 32-2.) Erythromycin and chloramphenicol have been used in canine infections, but these infections do not respond to most antimicrobials. They are characteristically resistant to cell wall–synthesis inhibitors such as the β-lactam antibiotics or many other broad-spectrum antimicrobials often chosen for persistent multifocal infections. Response to therapy should occur within 2 days, and therapy should continue for at least 1 week after discharges have stopped.[12,36,57]

Public Health Considerations

The public health risk of L-form infections in dogs and cats is uncertain because all of the cell wall–deficient organisms have not been adequately characterized. Instances of L-form infections in people are rare. In one report, a person developed an L-form infection at the site of a permanent indwelling catheter used for hemodialysis.[14] The L-form isolate was characterized as *Streptococcus sanguis* of animal origin. The same strain of this organism was also isolated from the person's pet dog.

SUGGESTED READINGS*

13. Chandler JC, Lappin MR. 2002. Mycoplasmal respiratory infections in small animals: 17 cases (1998-1999), *J Am Anim Hosp Assoc* 38:111-119.

20. Ernst S, Goggin JM. 1999. What is your diagnosis? Mycoplasma arthritis in a cat, *J Am Vet Med Assoc* 215:19-20.

21. Foster SF, Barrs VR, Martin P, et al. 1998. Pneumonia associated with *Mycoplasma* spp. in three cats, *Aust Vet J* 76:460-464.

37. Kirchhoff H, Runge M. 1998. 100 years of Mycoplasma pathogenicity for domestic and farm animals, *Tierarztl Wochenschr* 111:387-392.

50. Minion FC. 2002. Molecular pathogenesis of mycoplasma animal respiratory pathogens, *Front Biosci* 7:1410-1422.

*See the CD-ROM for a complete list of references.

SECTION II
Bacterial Diseases

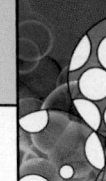

CHAPTER • 33

Laboratory Diagnosis of Bacterial Infections

Robert L. Jones

The purpose of clinical bacteriology is to provide information rapidly and accurately concerning the presence or absence of a bacterial agent in an infectious disease process. It usually requires at least 24 to 72 hours for bacteria to be isolated, but the clinician can seldom wait that long to institute therapy. Knowledge of the prevalence of specific pathogens responsible for defined clinical syndromes and trends in antimicrobial susceptibility patterns provides the basis for making early rational treatment decisions and selecting the antimicrobial agent most likely to be effective. This knowledge can only be developed and updated by submission of specimens to the laboratory for isolation, identification, and antimicrobial susceptibility testing. Therefore the use of the laboratory builds a database that can guide the design of treatment plans for future as well as current patients.

Use of the microbiology laboratory is subject to unique pitfalls posed by the diversity of bacterial agents, each with unique requirements for identification: multiple and often poorly accessible sites for collection of specimens, contamination of specimens with indigenous flora, and the necessity for subjective interpretation of results. Problems in communication may occur between the microbiology laboratory and the clinician regarding the suitability of the specimen for laboratory examination, uncertainty of the significance of bacterial isolates, interpretation of reports, and length of delay between the submission of the specimen and the production of needed information. Special efforts by the clinician to provide history and signalment information along with the specimen assist the laboratory in recognizing and reporting significant results.

Major technologic advances have changed the way microbiology laboratories function. Bacterial identification is now achieved largely through the use of miniaturized packaged systems, many of which are automated. Antimicrobial susceptibility testing is commonly accomplished with a commercial microdilution system or some form of instrumentation. Immunodiagnostic methods for antigen and antibody detection have benefited greatly from radioimmunoassay, direct and indirect fluorescent antibody (FA) testing, enzyme-linked immunosorbent assay, latex agglutination, and immunoblotting, as well as the development of monoclonal antibody technology. Nucleic acid technology is leading the clinical microbiology laboratory into a new era of molecular diagnostics for detecting and identifying microorganisms. Cost constraints for all this new technology increasingly limit the scope of services that can reasonably be provided by any one laboratory. Therefore it is unreasonable to expect equal diagnostic capabilities from all microbiology laboratories for all microorganisms. With increasing frequency, specimens must be sent to reference laboratories that perform specialized diagnostic tests. Appendix 5 lists commercial, state, and federal diagnostic laboratories that provide specific microbiologic testing for infectious diseases of dogs and cats.

DIAGNOSTIC METHODS

Microbiologic tests complement clinical judgment, enhance the clinician's ability to select specific antimicrobial drugs, and ultimately improve patient care through detection and identification of the etiologic agents.

Direct Microscopic Examination

Direct microscopic examination of exudates or infected body fluids is the single most important and cost-effective laboratory procedure that can be done for diagnosis and management of bacterial infections. Evaluations can be done in various clinical settings to obtain immediate information on the number, morphologic characteristics, and Gram-staining properties of microorganisms (Table 33-1) and the host cellular response. Purulent inflammatory responses are most suggestive of bacterial infection. Microscopic examination also gives an indication of the suitability of the specimen for culture, the likelihood of the presence of infection, the likely pathogens, and the predominant organisms in a mixed infection. This information may be used as a basis for interpretation of the significance of subsequent culture results.

Bacteria are readily observed in a smear from a specimen when they occur in a concentration of about 10^4 to 10^5 per ml. Examination of specimens such as blood or cerebrospinal fluid (CSF) for bacteria is usually unrewarding because even when present, the bacteria are too few in number to be detected. Some bacteria, such as spirochetes and mycoplasmas, do not stain well with Gram stain. Dark-field microscopy allows visualization of spirochetes, but mycoplasmas are too small for observation by light microscopy. Background material and artifacts can interfere with interpretation. Mucus or other proteinaceous matter that stains gram negative may cause slender, weakly staining bacilli to blend into the background, making them difficult to visualize. Differential staining techniques that enhance visualization of gram-negative bacteria include methylene blue, Giemsa, and Wright stains.

Isolation and Identification

Whether isolation and identification are attempted depend on many factors—the most important of which are the source of

the specimen and whether or not a presumptive diagnosis can be made microscopically. Most commonly encountered pyogenic bacteria readily grow on routinely inoculated blood agar plates. Liquid media provide enrichment for recovery of organisms present in small numbers and facilitate isolation of fastidious organisms. In some cases, selective media must be used to suppress growth of contaminants and normal flora while allowing growth of the pathogen.

Certain infectious diseases may be more efficiently diagnosed by direct detection of antigens, nucleic acids, or toxins. For diagnosis of some clostridial diseases, such as botulism (see Chapter 42), tetanus (see Chapter 43), and enterocolitis (see Chapter 39), it is imperative to identify the toxin rather than rely solely on isolation of the bacteria. Direct or indirect FA stains are extremely helpful for the rapid presumptive diagnosis of infection with some bacteria. Because *Yersinia pestis* (see Chapter 47) and *Francisella tularensis* (see Chapter 48) are hazardous to laboratory personnel, antigen detection by direct FA staining of exudate or tissue is the best tool for their rapid and specific identification. DNA probes and nucleic acid amplification techniques are useful for identification of microorganisms for which culture and serologic methods are difficult, extremely expensive, or unavailable.

Specimen Collection

Specimens must be collected from the actual site of infection with a minimum of contamination from adjacent tissues, organs, or secretions (Fig. 33-1). They must then be transported to the laboratory without further contamination or change in the relative numbers of bacteria. Some specimens are likely to become contaminated with indigenous flora during the collection process. Great care must be taken to use aseptic technique when collecting specimens to reduce the amount and likelihood of contamination. Some specimens are simply inaccessible except by aspiration or biopsy of deeper tissues. For all specimens obtained by biopsy or fine-needle aspiration, skin decontamination should be performed as it is before surgery. Specimens should be collected as early in the course of the disease process as possible. As the disease progresses and necrosis of tissue occurs, some microorganisms may die or be overgrown by other bacteria.

Whenever possible, specimens should be obtained before the administration of antimicrobials. However, their use does not necessarily preclude the recovery of bacteria from selected tissues in which low antimicrobial concentrations are achieved or from those animals infected with antimicrobial-resistant bacteria. If it is not possible to collect the specimen before any antimicrobials are administered, the specimen should be collected just before the next dose is given. If antimicrobials are concentrated at the sampling site, such as during urine collection, it is best to wait 48 hours after the last dose before collecting a specimen.

An adequate (several millimeters or grams) quantity of material should be obtained for appropriate laboratory tests. All too frequently, an inadequate amount of material is obtained with a swab, making it nearly impossible for the laboratory to make appropriate smears and inoculate adequate culture media. A swab should *never* be submitted in lieu of curettings, biopsy material, fluid (especially urine), or surgically removed tissue.

Multiple specimens should be submitted when lesions are present at several sites or when more than one laboratory procedure is requested. Multiple blood samples are necessary for detection of bacteremia. Multiple fecal samples are

Table • 33-1	
Appearance of Clinical Material in Gram-Stained Preparations	
COMPONENT	**STAINING REACTION**
Gram-positive bacteria	Organisms retain the crystal-violet iodine complex and appear dark blue or purple.
Gram-negative bacteria	Organisms lose the primary complex, take up the secondary dye safranin, and appear red.
Fungi (yeasts)	Organisms appear gram positive.
Inflammatory cells	Organisms appear gram negative. Epithelial cells may appear gram positive, gram negative, or both depending on the thickness of the smear.
Backgrounds	Organisms usually appear gram negative but may appear gram positive. Fibrin, mucus, and erythrocytes often stain gram negative.

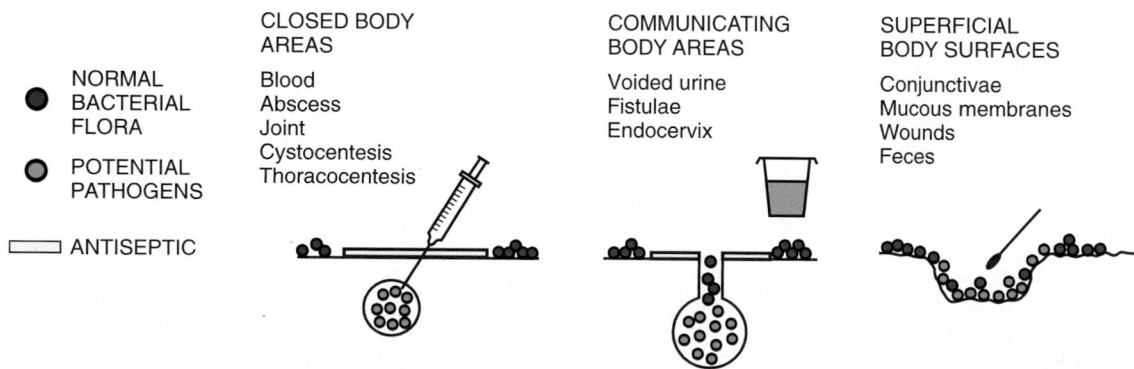

Fig 33-1   Collection of bacterial culture specimens from various sites, illustrating approaches used to prevent excessive contamination of specimen and probable sources of contamination. (From Jones RL 1985 Laboratory diagnosis of bacterial infections, pp 110-147. *In* McCurnin DM (ed), *Clinical textbook for veterinary technicians.* WB Saunders, Philadelphia, PA.)

also indicated for detection of enteric pathogens such as salmonellae.

Collection Devices and Transport

Appropriate collection devices and specimen transport systems are needed to ensure survival of the microorganism without overgrowth and for optimal isolation and identification. Various containers are commercially available, ranging from simple swab and plastic tube combinations to complicated specimen collection devices (Fig. 33-2). Swabs must be made of noninhibitory materials and transported in a sterile container. Many bacteria are susceptible to desiccation during transport. Swabs are only acceptable for transport of specimens when provided with a humidified transporting chamber or placed in transport medium. Several swab-transport medium systems exist and are often available from the clinical laboratory. Tissue, exudate, feces, or fluid should be submitted in an appropriate closed (leak-proof), sterile container. Self-sealing plastic food storage bags and blood collection tubes that do not contain anticoagulants or preservatives are examples of recommended specimen containers. Each tissue or specimen must be placed in a separate container. Direct aspiration into a syringe is often a convenient and satisfactory means for of tissue and fluid collection. However, the needle must be removed for transport to avoid injuries, and the syringe should be capped.

Various types of media may be used for transporting specimens to the laboratory. Transport media such as Stuart's, Cary-Blair, Amies, and anaerobic devices (frequently available from the microbiology laboratory) are buffered non-nutritive formulations that preserve the viability of fastidious organisms in the specimen as well as minimize overgrowth by rapidly-growing bacteria that may be present. Use of transport media eliminates the need to refrigerate or chill most specimens for shipment to the laboratory. The ordinary nutrient type of broth such as that in blood culture bottles may be used only when swabs or aspirates are collected from normally sterile body sites (e.g., CSF, synovia) and when great care has been taken to avoid any contamination. Special anaerobic transport devices must be used to prevent exposure of obligate anaerobes to lethal concentrations of oxygen (see Chapter 41). Because reduced oxygen is not lethal for the aerobes and facultative anaerobes, they can be transported in the same anaerobic transport devices. Tissue in formalin, dry swabs, urine

collected several hours earlier and not refrigerated, and selective swabs for isolation of mycobacteria are unsuitable for bacterial culture.

Blood

Successful isolation of microorganisms from blood requires an understanding of the intermittence and low order of magnitude of most bacteremias (see Blood Culture, Chapter 87, for the appropriate technique). Several specimens must be collected for culture over a period of time. If possible the first blood culture specimen should be drawn at the onset of fever. Another suggestion is to take three or four cultures within 1.5 to 3 hours; if more than one culture yields the same organism, it is probably significant.

Urine

The collection, transport, and storage of urine specimens are important adjuncts to the reliability of culture results. Urine is an excellent growth medium for some organisms; unless proper precautions are taken, urine allows small, insignificant numbers of bacteria to multiply rapidly. Culture results from a voided specimen taken without cleansing the genitalia are useful only if no bacterial growth exists; for example, growth may be from urethral contamination, infection, or both. Contamination of a midstream-voided sample must be considered when less than 10^5 colony-forming units (CFU) per milliliter are isolated, although total counts of viable bacteria may be reduced in some infections. Gram staining of a drop (allowed to dry without spreading) of well-mixed urine not only provides a means of determining the adequacy of collection but also provides the findings for the diagnosis of significant bacteriuria ($>10^5$ CFU/ml) when at least two bacteria per oil immersion ($\times1000$) field are found. Gram-positive bacteria are much more readily observed in smears than gram-negative bacteria, so caution must be exercised to avoid overlooking gram-negative bacilli.

Urine collection for culture by urethral catheterization is seldom indicated except in those animals in which catheterization must otherwise be performed for diagnostic or therapeutic reasons. Urine contamination by urethral flora is best prevented by cystocentesis, a relatively safe and simple procedure if performed by an experienced technician (see Chapter 91). This procedure solves the problem of equivocal

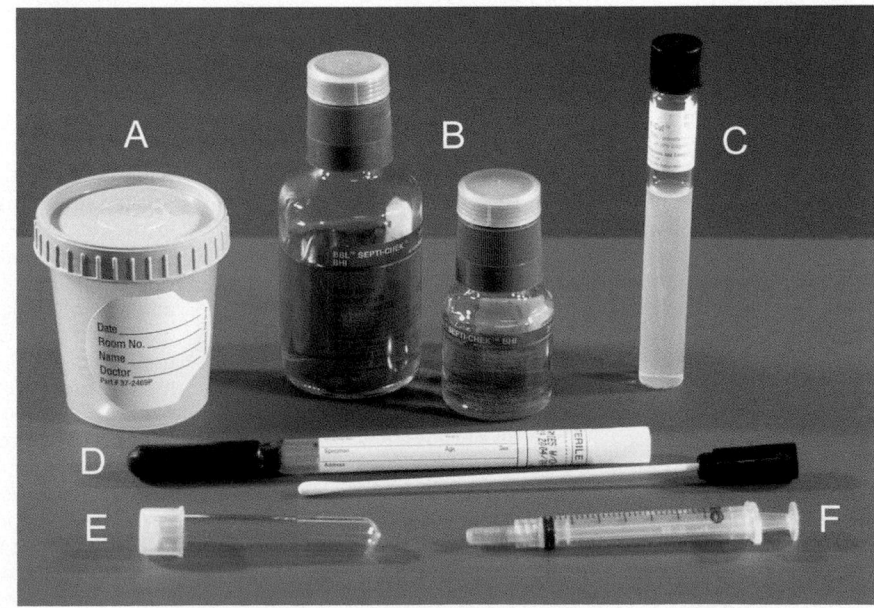

Fig 33-2 Specimen collection devices include fecal cups, blood culture bottles, transport media and swabs, tubes, and syringes. Fecal specimens should be transported in screw-top cups *(A)*. Blood and aseptically drawn body fluids such as joint taps should be collected and transported in blood culture bottles *(B)*. Swabbed specimens can be transported in anaerobic transport media *(C)* or special chambers *(D)*. Fluid specimens can be transported in tubes *(E)* or capped syringes *(F)*. (Courtesy Robert L. Jones, Colorado State University, Fort Collins, Colo.)

counts and the risk of nosocomial urinary tract infections associated with catheterization.

Urine must be collected and stored in a sterile capped syringe or a capped container or tube, not collected merely by a "clean" cup or swab. If urine cannot be cultured within 1 to 2 hours after its collection, it must be refrigerated for a maximum of 8 hours. For longer storage or transport and storage, a urine preservation tube (VACUTAINER Brand Urine Transport System, Becton-Dickinson, Franklin Lakes, N.J.) allows for analysis and culture of specimens held for up to 48 hours at room temperature and for quantitative culture for up to 72 hours at refrigerated (4° C) temperatures.

Transudates and Exudates

A sterile syringe and needle should be used to collect a generous quantity of liquid material from unopened abscesses and body cavities after an antiseptic has been applied to the surface. After aspiration, air remaining in the syringe should be expelled and the end capped or the specimen transferred immediately into an anaerobic transport device. When a wash solution is used to aid in collection of a specimen such as a tracheal aspirate, it is imperative to have a solution that does not contain a bacteriostatic preservative. Best results can be expected when a buffered solution such as lactated Ringer's solution is used instead of isotonic saline solutions, which tend to be acidic.

Feces

Proper collection and preservation of feces are frequently neglected but important requirements for the isolation of pathogenic bacteria contributing to intestinal disease. Unless the specimen can be taken immediately to the laboratory and properly handled on delivery, salmonellae may not survive because of the pH changes that occur with a reduction from body temperature. A small quantity of feces (2 to 3 g) is the preferred specimen; a rectal swab specimen is less satisfactory, yielding fewer positive results. Portions of the feces containing mucus and blood may harbor a larger number of the pathogenic organisms than the customary-appearing samples. Fecal specimens should be collected in clean, sealed, leak-proof containers for transport to the laboratory.

Repeated cultures are often required for screening fecal specimens, because some pathogens may be shed only several days after onset of diarrhea, whereas other organisms may be few or absent later in the disease. Although performing three cultures is not absolutely required, repeated cultures are indicated if the clinical picture suggests gastrointestinal (GI) infection by pathogenic bacteria and the first cultures are unrewarding. For some enteropathogenic strains, toxin analysis may be more beneficial than culture.[3]

Tissue Samples

Surgical biopsy specimens are of considerable importance for culture and may represent the entire pathologic process. They are usually obtained at considerable expense and some risk to the patient. Therefore they should be handled carefully to avoid contamination or desiccation, which would reduce their diagnostic value. A portion of the tissue rather than a swabbed specimen should be submitted. When the lesion is large or the individual has several lesions, multiple specimens from different sites should be collected. Samples from an abscess should include pus and a portion of the abscess wall. When collecting necropsy specimens, it is best to anticipate which specimens will be needed for microbiologic analysis before starting the necropsy and then to collect these first, before excessive tissue handling and exposure cause additional contamination. Samples from the GI tract should be taken last to avoid contaminating other tissues. When collecting fluid from a body compartment (e.g., joints, CSF, pericardial fluid), a syringe and needle should be used rather than a swab. The fluid sample should be aseptically aspirated. Tissue specimens should be placed (unfixed and without preservative) in sealed, leak-proof sterile containers to prevent contamination or desiccation. If the delivery of specimens to the laboratory is delayed, they should be refrigerated.

Specimen Submission, History, and Signalment

Specimen management is the one process in clinical microbiology that has the most influence on accurate laboratory results. Specimens that are improperly selected, collected, transported, or stored will very likely provide information that is misleading and could result in inaccurate diagnosis and inappropriate treatment. Ideally, the microbiology laboratory should provide the clinician with directions for collecting and transporting specimens and guidance in ordering tests. In turn, the clinician should provide the laboratory with sufficient history and signalment from the animal and description of the specimen source for proper processing of the specimen and interpretation of the results. Information about the animal aids in the selection of appropriate media to be inoculated and additional tests to be performed and increases the probability of significant results being recognized, properly interpreted, and reported to the clinician. Spending extra time and effort to submit adequate information to the laboratory is the best way to ensure better quality results and prevent the necessity for repeat specimen collection.

In most cases of infection with an unknown cause that do not yield results after initial culturing attempts, consultation between the microbiologist and clinician is recommended. Simply repeating culture after culture is expensive and often unsuccessful.

INTERPRETATION OF CULTURE RESULTS

Specimens that have been properly collected, carefully transported to the laboratory, and processed for bacteriologic culture and antimicrobial susceptibility testing frequently yield important information about the cause of the infection and the antimicrobials expected to be most effective. However, laboratory identification of a bacterium is not necessarily indisputable evidence of disease. The findings must be interpreted by evaluating the clinical signs or lesion, the collection site of the specimen, the presence of normal flora or other contaminants, the method of handling and transporting the specimen to the laboratory, and the number of different bacteria isolated and quantitative recovery of the agents.

Normal Flora

All mucous membranes and external body surfaces can be colonized with bacteria as part of the normal flora. These bacteria may be pathogenic if they are invading the tissue and causing inflammation, or they may be just colonizing the surfaces. Therefore culture results must be correlated with clinical signs. Quantitation of culture results is often an aid to evaluating the significance of the findings. Isolation of a mixture of four or more aerobic microorganisms in light or moderate numbers is typical of normal flora. Frequently, the number of species of bacteria isolated from a specimen is indirectly proportional to the patient care value of the report.

Quantitation of Growth

The amount of bacterial growth can aid in interpreting the significance of isolates, although the number of bacteria can be related to the vigor of swabbing to collect the specimen and subsequent handling. The laboratory report should indicate whether growth is light, moderate, or heavy. Finding large numbers of a single microorganism in nearly pure culture is a strong indication of significance. Light growth, including growth from broth enrichment alone, is often typical of normal flora, insignificant contaminants, or suppression of growth by antimicrobials. Such culture results usually have limited significance unless the sample was taken from a normally sterile body site and knowledge exists that the specimen was properly collected.

Absence of Specified Pathogens

Sometimes it is more important to know that the laboratory sought to isolate specific pathogens but was unable to find them rather than to receive a report identifying the microorganisms that were present. For example, a culture report on a fecal sample stating that no *Salmonella* or *Campylobacter* organisms were isolated is much more useful than a report naming several species of normal fecal flora, because it indicates that a specifically directed effort was made to identify particular pathogens in the specimen.

No-Growth Cultures

Failure to isolate bacteria may be a false-negative result for numerous reasons, including sampling and transporting mistakes, such as desiccation or inappropriate transport media; previous antimicrobial therapy; and infections caused by fastidious microorganisms for which proper culture procedures were not performed, such as mycoplasmas, obligate anaerobes, spirochetes, and rickettsias. If microscopic examination of the specimen reveals microorganisms but comparable microorganisms are not isolated, transporting and culturing procedures should be evaluated during a consultation with the clinical microbiologist. Innovative techniques of molecular detection and immunochemistry are now being developed for direct application to specimens to identify microorganisms that are difficult to cultivate.

MOLECULAR DETECTION AND IDENTIFICATION

Direct nucleic acid hybridization probe and gene amplification protocols have a tremendous potential for detecting microbial pathogens, and significant progress has been made in the development of these assays.[9,12] Many improvements have occurred in specificity and sensitivity as well as in protocols for processing samples. DNA probe assays are particularly well suited for in situ hybridization in tissue in which the location and distribution of the organisms must be ascertained, for identification of slow-growing bacterial cultures (e.g., *Mycobacterium* sp. and *Leptospira* sp.), and for identification of toxicogenic strains of bacteria that cannot be differentiated from nontoxicogenic strains by conventional methods (e.g., enteropathogenic genotypes of *Escherichia coli* and *Clostridium perfringens*.[4]) Nucleic acid amplification assays that can be performed in situ or on specimens employ primers and the polymerase chain reaction (PCR) to provide enough specificity and sensitivity to detect even a single organism or up to 10 copies of a specific gene sequence (see Chapter 1). In addition to being specific enough to detect a single genotype based on the selection of the primer, strategies are now emerging for using universal primers for large groups of related infectious agents or multiplex assays using a selected set of primers. Microarrays of synthetic nucleotides (detection probes) placed on a silicon matrix (chip) enable automated searching of hundreds to thousands of sequences for identification of specific genotypes (strains) through amplification of a single specimen.

Ultimately, the goal of these molecular techniques is the direct determination of identities of microorganisms in clinical specimens and prediction of their antimicrobial susceptibility patterns. As the technology for nucleic acid amplification currently stands, application of the procedure is limited to referral and research laboratories. Partial or full automation and improved technology are reducing costs and increasing access to these assays. Specimen handling and preparation remain the most critical limiting steps. Specimen preparation must release the nucleic acids from the target organism, prevent degradation of the free nucleic acids, remove any substances inhibitory to nucleic acid amplification or hybridization, concentrate the nucleic acids into a small volume, place the nucleic acids in amplification or hybridization buffer, and prevent false-positive results caused by contaminating nucleic acids. Various samples have to be processed differently to extract the nucleic acids from their matrix. Therefore to obtain useful results, clinicians must consult with the laboratory when collecting specimens.

Despite their sensitivity and specificity, molecular detection procedures will never totally replace conventional cultural and serologic procedures because the results of nucleic acid amplification procedures and the results of culture or serology have different purposes. Nucleic acid detection procedures determine whether DNA or RNA from a particular organism is present in the specimen. They cannot determine whether the organism is involved in an infectious process, and they reveal nothing about the viability of the organism because they can detect DNA from dead organisms. Culture, by comparison, clearly demonstrates the viability of the organism, and a rise in titer of antibody to a specific organism strongly suggests active infection. Undoubtedly, the greatest asset of molecular diagnostics is the sensitivity to detect very small amounts of signal. However, the author (RLJ) must continue to recognize the potential for contamination of samples and asymptomatic carriage of small numbers of microorganisms, perhaps in sites previously considered sterile by conventional cultural procedures. These tools hold the power to enhance detection of new agents and enable clinicians to recognize new disease associations, but they require continued vigilance in evaluating disease causation. In some cases, epidemiologic characterization of disease may require different approaches. For example, the serovars of *Leptospira* organisms do not correlate precisely with genotypes that can be identified by nucleic acid analysis, yet serovars continue to be the best correlate of epidemiologic patterns of disease (see Chapter 44). See Chapter 1 for additional discussion on molecular diagnostic methods.

ANTIMICROBIAL SUSCEPTIBILITY TESTS

Testing bacteria for their susceptibility to antimicrobials is one of laboratory procedures that has a significant impact on the prescribing of antimicrobials. To improve the predictive value of susceptibility tests, the indications for these tests and their limitations must be understood. *Susceptible* and *resistant* are relative terms (and somewhat arbitrarily defined) because a microorganism within the animal may be susceptible in one location as a result of attainable antimicrobial concentrations but resistant in another. Susceptibility tests measure the lowest concentration of antimicrobial required to macroscopically inhibit growth of the microorganism, a level called the *minimum inhibitory concentration* (MIC). The concentration of antimicrobial that inhibits the infectious agent, either by killing it outright or by slowing its growth sufficiently so that normal body defense mechanisms can take over, is assumed to be similar to the in vitro MIC. Comparison of the MIC with the concentration of antimicrobial that can be attained in various body compartments allows prediction of the susceptibility or resistance of the organism to the drug at the infection site.

Indications

Some microorganisms are known to be susceptible to a particular highly effective antimicrobial, so testing is unnecessary. Susceptibility testing is indicated for any microorganism contributing to an infectious process if its susceptibility cannot be reliably predicted or resistance is anticipated based on knowledge of the organism's identity. Generally, isolates from normally sterile body sites should be tested, although questions have been raised about the cost effectiveness of routine testing of all urinary tract isolates. Susceptibility testing of multiple bacterial isolates from abscesses and wounds or normal flora is meaningless. Testing the susceptibility of anaerobes remains a technical problem and an unsettled issue; most anaerobes except those that produce β-lactamases are predictably susceptible.

Test Methods

The reference method of antimicrobial susceptibility testing measures the MIC in micrograms per ml by incorporating serial twofold dilutions of antimicrobials in a bacteriologic growth medium (Fig. 33-3). These dilutions can be made in microdilution wells, a procedure used by many larger laboratories. The clinical significance is determined by interpreting the results according to the criteria in Table 33-2.

In contrast to the dilution method, the most common antimicrobial susceptibility test performed in small laboratories and veterinary practices is the agar diffusion test. This method uses antimicrobial-impregnated paper disks applied to the surface of agar that have been inoculated with pure cultures of the test organism (Fig. 33-4). The diameter of the zone of inhibition of growth around the disk correlates inversely with the MIC. The disk diffusion technique is not difficult to perform; however, strict guidelines must be followed to use the standard zone size interpretive chart for each drug. Any variation in technique changes the relationship between the zone size and the MIC, leading to possible misinterpretation of the test result.

Conventional susceptibility testing methods assess the in vitro effects of antimicrobial agents on the growth of microorganisms under laboratory-defined conditions. In some cases,

clinical response is better predicted by directly determining the production of antimicrobial-modifying enzymes even at very low levels (e.g., β-lactamases by *Staphylococcus* sp. and *Bacteroides fragilis*).

Genetic susceptibility test methods that have the potential to provide more rapid and reliable assessment of antimicro-

Table • 33-2

Interpretation Categories for Antimicrobial Susceptibility Tests

CATEGORY	DEFINITION
Susceptible	Infection caused by a strain that can be appropriately treated with the standard dosage of antimicrobial recommended for that type of infection and infecting species unless otherwise contraindicated.
Intermediate	Infection caused by a strain with antimicrobial MICs approaching blood and tissue levels that are usually attainable; therapeutic response rates may be lower than for susceptible isolates; selected drugs should be physiologically concentrated (e.g., quinolones and β-lactams in urine) or given at a high dosage without toxicity (e.g., β-lactams).
Resistant	Infection caused by a strain not inhibited by the usually achievable systemic concentrations of the antimicrobial at usual dosages; specific microbial resistance mechanisms are likely, and clinical efficacy has not been reliable in treatment studies.

MIC, Minimum inhibitory concentration.

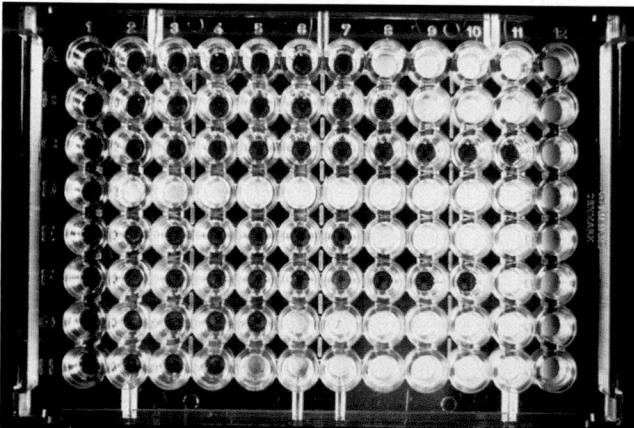

Fig 33-3 Antimicrobial susceptibility testing by the microdilution method. Each row of microwells contains serial twofold dilutions of an antimicrobial. The lowest concentration of drug that inhibits growth of the bacteria is defined as the MIC. For example, the first row contains ampicillin (256 µg/ml in well A1, decreasing to 0.25 µg/ml in well A11). The pellet of bacteria in the lower four wells (A8 to A11) indicates that 4 µg/ml (well A7) is the MIC. Susceptibility to seven other drugs has also been tested in this microwell plate. (Courtesy Robert L. Jones, Colorado State University, Fort Collins, Colo.)

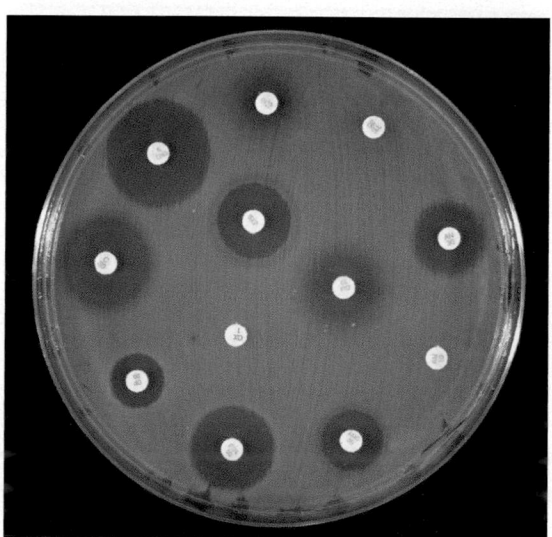

Fig 33-4 Antimicrobial susceptibility testing by the agar diffusion method using disks containing antimicrobials. The diameter of the zone of inhibited microbial growth correlates inversely with the susceptibility of the microorganism. (Courtesy Robert L. Jones, Colorado State University, Fort Collins, Colo.)

bial resistance in comparison with growth (phenotypic) methods have emerged in the past decade. Genetic tests can be performed directly on clinical specimens, eliminating the need to isolate an organism when it is not readily cultivatable. Most genotypic methods include amplification of the resistance gene through the use of PCR and subsequent confirmation methods similar to those used for microbial identification. The genetic presence of resistance can now be detected for vancomycin-resistant *Enterococcus*, methicillin-resistant *Staphylococcus aureus*, extended-spectrum β-lactamase resistance in the Enterobacteriaceae family, and resistance genotypes of *Helicobacter* sp. and *Mycobacterium* sp. that are difficult or slow growing.

Interpretations

In general, in vitro susceptibility testing is useful and reliably applied only to common, rapidly growing microorganisms such as staphylococci, enterococci, Enterobacteriaceae, and *Pseudomonas aeruginosa*. Infections caused by fastidious bacteria are usually treated more reliably on the basis of published guidelines. A helpful guide to empiric therapy can be compiled by monitoring susceptibility trends of microorganisms recently isolated from animals within the practice region.

Susceptibility test results are a prediction of the expected response to treatment, not a guarantee. Most susceptibility tests use class-representative drugs rather than each possible antimicrobial. Furthermore, the interpretive criteria are based on the average blood levels of antimicrobials that can be achieved with a standard, fixed dose. Extralabel drug use in patients of other species, ages, and body sizes or modified dosages (flexible-label dosages) may significantly alter drug distribution. Levels of drug in tissues usually differ from levels in serum (e.g., low levels in CSF, high levels in urine). Although in vitro susceptibility testing predicts effectiveness, the drug may not be able to penetrate to the site of infection. In addition the pharmocodynamics of bacterial killing (time dependent versus concentration dependent) must be considered in the interpretation of susceptibility tests and subsequent dosage design. Therefore the predictive value of susceptibility tests for a favorable response is moderate at best. The MIC's value in predicting failure is much better but still not totally accurate. For example, a technician who interprets an MIC result as resistant according to blood levels may not have taken into account that the organism was recovered from urine, where the drug is concentrated, or that a topical treatment is being applied with drug concentrations of milligrams per milliliter rather than micrograms per milliliter.

SEROLOGIC TESTING

Detection of specific antibodies in the serum of an animal can be an indication of previous exposure, ongoing infection, vaccination, or passively acquired antibody. It is not always easy to discern the origin of these antibodies. Therefore serology is most effective as a diagnostic tool when the prevalence of antibodies in a population is low or when paired serum samples are collected to evaluate changes in antibody titers. The more common bacterial infections for which serologic tests are useful include brucellosis (see Chapter 40), leptospirosis (see Chapter 44), borreliosis (see Chapter 45), and rickettsial and ehrlichial infections (see Chapters 27 to 29).

For best results from serologic tests, serum should be transferred to a sterile tube as soon as possible after complete clotting and centrifugation to separate it from cellular elements. Excessive hemolysis interferes with some tests. Bacterial growth in serum may alter the immunoglobulin molecules. Once separated, serum samples should be refrigerated until testing begins if it starts within 72 hours. For longer periods of storage, serum may be preserved for extended periods by storage in a freezer (−20° C). Frozen serum samples should be packaged and shipped with adequate insulation and ice to prevent thawing before arrival at the laboratory.

SUGGESTED READINGS*

1. Brooks MB, Morley PS, Dargatz DA, et al. 2003. Survey of antimicrobial susceptibility testing practices of veterinary diagnostic laboratories in the United States, *J Am Vet Med Assoc* 222:168-173.
3. Hines J, Nachamkin I. 1996. Effective use of the clinical microbiology laboratory for diagnosing diarrheal diseases, *Clin Infect Dis* 23:1292-1301.
4. Houpikian P, Raoult D. 2002. Traditional and molecular techniques for the study of emerging bacterial diseases: One laboratory's perspective, *Emerg Infect Dis* 8:122-131.
7. Murray PR (ed). 1999. *Manual of clinical microbiology*, ed 7, American Society for Microbiology, Washington, DC.
8. National Committee for Clinical Laboratory Standards. 1999. Performance standards for antimicrobial disk and dilution susceptibility tests for bacteria isolated from animals: approved standard (NCCLS document M31-A). NCCLS, Villanova, PA.
10. Quinn PJ, Markey BK, Carter ME, et al. 2002. *Veterinary microbiology and microbial disease*, Iowa State University Press, Ames, IA.

*See the CD-ROM for a complete list of references.

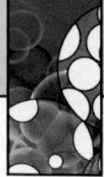

CHAPTER • 34

Antibacterial Chemotherapy

Craig E. Greene and A. D. J. Watson

Antibacterials, among the most widely used drugs in veterinary practice, are often administered without adequate documentation that an infection exists. Although this practice may not immediately harm the patient, routine and irrational use of antimicrobials may have several undesirable consequences. Unrestricted use encourages the selection of resistant strains of bacteria, which subsequently limits the choice of effective agents. Long-term treatment with antimicrobials may suppress the animal's resident microflora, thereby allowing overgrowth of more resistant microorganisms.

The increase in antimicrobial resistance worldwide has paralleled the use of drugs to combat microbial infections in people and animals.[284] For example, increases in multiresistant *Enterobacter*, *Enterococcus*, and *Pseudomonas* spp. were observed in canine urinary tract infections (UTIs) from 1994 to 1998.[305] However, other studies have not shown this trend.[277] Once resistance emerges, selection pressure forces it to remain if antimicrobial usage is continued. Therefore veterinary hospitals must develop protocols that minimize inappropriate and indiscriminate antibacterial usage.

Selection of bacterial subpopulations with greater antimicrobial resistance than the original population is an inevitable consequence of antibacterial treatment. Selection pressures are highest when bacteria are exposed to suboptimal dosage regimens (i.e., concentrations of drug below the minimum inhibitory concentration [MIC]).

Antibiotics can be divided into two groups based on their patterns of bactericidal activity: concentration-dependent drugs and time-dependent drugs.[80] For the *concentration-dependent drugs*, optimal activity is achieved with high peak-drug concentration and area under the concentration time (AUC) curve; this group comprises aminoglycosides, fluoroquinolones, azithromycin, tetracyclines, vancomycin, quinupristin-dalfopristin, and metronidazole. The highest safe, achievable drug concentration is the most important factor for aminoglycosides and quinolones. Pulse infusion or once-daily dosing is likely to maximize the efficacy of these agents and induce the least amount of bacterial resistance. Most of the remaining antimicrobials are the *time-dependent drugs*, which show optimal activity when plasma concentrations of approximately four times the MIC are maintained for 50% to 80% of the dosage interval.[377] Drugs of this type are the β-lactams (penicillins, cephalosporins, monobactams, carbapenems), clindamycin, and most macrolides. Administration of these drugs by continuous infusion or multiple daily doses would be most efficacious.

A postantibacterial effect (PAE) refers to persistent suppression of bacterial growth following exposure to an antimicrobial agent. All antibacterials appear to have this effect with susceptible gram-positive bacteria. With gram-negative bacteria, this effect is noted only with inhibitors of protein or nucleic acid synthesis, such as aminoglycosides, quinolones, tetracyclines, macrolides, chloramphenicol, and rifampin. In some instances, as with quinolones and aminoglycosides, the PAE is longer in vivo because they achieve higher concentration in leukocytes at sites of inflammation.

Antimicrobial combinations are used widely in veterinary practice, but few instances have occurred in which a synergistic outcome is documented; in many cases, combined use might reduce efficacy or enhance toxicity. However, several potentially effective combinations exist. β-Lactams act on bacterial cell walls and increase the uptake of aminoglycosides. Cell wall–active agents such as penicillins, cephalosporins, imipenem, and vancomycin have been synergistic with the aminoglycosides streptomycin, gentamicin, and amikacin.[2] Agents acting sequentially in a pathway, for example, sulfonamides and diaminopyrimidines (see later discussion), have also been effective and more bactericidal than either drug by itself. Combinations of agents acting on the cell wall, such as aminopenicillin (ampicillin, amoxicillin) together with a cephalosporin (cefotaxime, ceftriaxone) have been more effective against bacteria in vitro and in vivo, presumably because they attach to different binding proteins on the bacterial cell wall. The streptogramins (see later discussion) consist of two components that act synergistically to inhibit protein synthesis in bacteria. β-lactamase inhibitors (see later discussion) increase the activity and spectrum of β-lactams against various bacteria. Other synergistic antimicrobial combinations include quinolones, macrolides, or tetracyclines with rifampin, especially against persistent intracellular microorganisms in difficult to reach areas such as pyogranulomatous lesions or meninges. Presumably rifampin facilitates intracellular penetration of the other drugs. Combinations of quinolones with β-lactams or aminoglycosides may also be beneficial.[335] Clinical applications that justify combination therapy include bacterial endocarditis, resistant *Pseudomonas* infections, meningitis, febrile neutropenia, and *Brucella*, *Helicobacter*, and *Mycobacterium* infections.

Antimicrobial antagonism that is possible in certain circumstances can be avoided. The general advice is that cell wall–inhibiting drugs such as the β-lactams should not be used with bacteriostatic agents such as tetracyclines or chloramphenicol because rapid replication is needed for the cell wall–acting drugs to be effective. Macrolides should not be combined with lincosamides because complete antibacterial cross-resistance develops.

The prophylactic use of antimicrobials to prevent anticipated infections is controversial because of the increased risk of selecting for resistant microorganisms. Indiscriminant use of antibacterials may alter the patient's microbial flora and allow colonization by resistant bacteria. Several instances have occurred in which prophylactic administration were beneficial, as when infection is anticipated from contamination of otherwise sterile tissues. These cases include contaminated wounds following trauma, surgical procedures when contamination is expected, surgery in immunosuppressed patients, and during surgical procedures involving prolonged exposure of healthy tissue to air. Antibiotics may also be indicated prophylactically before major dental procedures and high-risk medical conditions, including diabetes mellitus, hyperadrenocorticism, immunosuppressive or cancer chemotherapy, and chronic bronchopulmonary disease. For further discussion of antimicrobials in traumatic and surgical wounds, see Traumatic and Surgical Infections, Chapter 55.

This chapter presents a review of the general properties of antibacterial drugs by pharmacologic groups. Information on specific antibacterial drugs used in dogs and cats can be found in the Drug Formulary (Appendix 8) at the end of this book. Because of space limitations, a discussion of general principles of antibacterial chemotherapy has been omitted here. Antibacterial drug resistance and prophylaxis are discussed in Chapter 94. The administration of antibacterial drugs in treating bacterial infections of various organ systems is covered in Chapters 85 through 93. Dosage charts are listed in each of these chapters. In addition, Appendix 8 also contains a list of appropriate antibacterial drugs for particular infection types and locations.

β-LACTAM DRUGS

This group of drugs, which includes penicillins, cephalosporins, monobactams, and carbapenems, acts by disrupting bacterial cell wall synthesis. These drugs are most effective when organisms are reproducing rapidly because of the high rate of cell wall formation. The most common mechanism of bacterial resistance to β-lactams is production of β-lactamase, which damages the β-lactam ring of these compounds. Genes for β-lactamase, encoded on chromosomes or plasmids, may spread within and among populations of bacteria. An increasing number of staphylococci have a modified penicillin-binding protein in their cell wall with a reduced affinity for all β-lactam drugs. These organisms have been classified as methicillin-resistant types and comprise a majority of nosocomial isolates from human hospitals. β-Lactam drugs act synergistically with aminoglycosides by facilitating their entry into bacterial cells; however, they should never be premixed before administration because the aminoglycoside can damage the β-lactam ring. Synergism has been noted when a β-lactam such as ticarcillin has been combined with a quinolone for treating *Pseudomonas* infections.

Penicillins
Natural Penicillins
Penicillin G (benzyl penicillin) is a naturally occurring bactericidal antibiotic produced by certain molds of the genus *Penicillium*. It primarily inhibits synthesis of the gram-positive bacterial cell wall, causing osmotic fragility of susceptible bacteria. Penicillin G has three significant therapeutic limitations: it is degraded by gastric acid, which reduces systemic availability after oral administration; it is inactivated by β-lactamases produced by certain staphylococci and many gram-negative organisms; and at usual therapeutic dosages, it is active mainly against gram-positive aerobic and facultative anaerobic organisms (Table 34-1). Newer semisynthetic penicillins have been produced to overcome these disadvantages. Penicillins are believed generally to work synergistically with aminoglycosides in vivo.

Despite the production of newer derivatives, penicillin G remains the most active drug against many gram-positive aerobic bacteria. Most streptococci, except for enterococci (see Chapter 35), are susceptible. Many gram-positive bacilli and anaerobic bacteria, with the exception of β-lactamase–producing *Bacteroides fragilis*, are susceptible. Staphylococci are frequently resistant because of β-lactamase production. Procaine penicillin and benzathine penicillin are poorly soluble compounds that slowly dissolve at the site of injection, liberating penicillin G.

Penicillin V (phenoxymethyl penicillin) is an acid-stable derivative that is better absorbed from the alimentary tract, although resulting blood concentrations are much lower than that produced by parenteral administration of the same dose of penicillin G. Therapeutic effects equivalent to those obtained with penicillin V may be achieved at less expense by giving oral penicillin G to fasting animals at four times the usual parenteral dosage.

β-Lactamase–Resistant Penicillins
Methicillin, the first semisynthetic penicillin developed, resists β-lactamase but is inactivated by gastric acid and must be administered parenterally, limiting its clinical usefulness. Similarly, nafcillin has poor systemic availability after oral administration and is usually administered parenterally. The isoxazolyl derivatives (cloxacillin, dicloxacillin, flucloxacillin, oxacillin) can be administered orally with reasonable absorption from the gut and are resistant to staphylococcal β-lactamase but are less active compared with penicillin G against other penicillin G–sensitive organisms. These substances are highly protein-bound drugs, which delays their elimination and maintains high plasma-drug concentrations. However, this protein binding limits penetration of the drug into tissues. Possible indications for these drugs include infections caused by β-lactamase–producing staphylococci, as in pyoderma or osteomyelitis.

Aminopenicillins
Although ampicillin, amoxicillin, and hetacillin are susceptible to β-lactamase, they can be given orally or parenterally. They are slightly less active than penicillin G against gram-positive and anaerobic pathogens but have wider activity against gram-negative aerobic bacteria such as *Escherichia*, *Proteus*, and *Salmonella*. Amoxicillin has antibacterial spectrum identical to ampicillin but is better absorbed orally and has more rapid and longer action compared with ampicillin. Hetacillin is an inactive derivative of ampicillin, is more stable in gastric acid than ampicillin, and is hydrolyzed rapidly to ampicillin in vivo. Bacampicillin, pivampicillin, and talampicillin are similar derivatives.

Carboxypenicillins
Carbenicillin and ticarcillin have increased activity against gram-negative aerobes, including *Acinetobacter*, *Proteus*, *Enterobacter*, some *Klebsiella*, and some anaerobes. Ticarcillin is especially active against *Pseudomonas*. Carboxypenicillins are destroyed by β-lactamase and are less effective against gram-positive organisms. These drugs are generally not well absorbed orally and must be given parenterally for systemic activity, but carindacillin and carfecillin are two esters of carbenicillin that are available for oral administration. The MICs for susceptible organisms are relatively high; therefore large doses must be administered. Co-administration with an aminoglycoside improves efficacy against *Pseudomonas* and reduces development of drug resistance. Ticarcillin and ticarcillin-clavulanate have been used successfully in managing canine otitis externa caused by *Pseudomonas aeruginosa* (see Drug Formulary, Appendix 8, and Chapter 85, Otitis Externa).[280] Expense generally limits systemic use of carboxypenicillins.

Ureidopenicillins
Azlocillin, mezlocillin, and piperacillin have acid instability and β-lactamase resistance similar to those of the carboxypenicillins but have greater activity against gram-negative aerobes, including *Pseudomonas*, and less activity against some anaerobes. The main area of interest is their antipseudomonal activity, but piperacillin is one of few drugs consistently effective against enterococci and *B. fragilis*. Cost

Table • 34-1

Properties of Penicillins and Associated β-Lactam Derivatives[a]

GENERIC NAME (TRADE NAME)	ROUTE OF ADMINISTRATION	ANTIMICROBIAL SPECTRUM						
		GASTRIC ACID STABILITY	STAPHYLOCOCCAL β-LACTAMASE RESISTANCE	GRAM POSITIVE	GRAM NEGATIVE	ANAEROBIC	*PSEUDOMONAS*
Natural Penicillins							
Penicillin G (many)	IM, IV	−	−	+	−	+	−
Penicillin V (many)	PO[b]	+	−	+	−	+	−
β-Lactamase—Resistant Penicillins							
Methicillin (Staphcillin, Celbenin)	IM, IV	−	+	+	−	−	−
Nafcillin (Unipen, Nafcil)	IM, IV	±	+	+	−	−	−
Cloxacillin (Tegopen)	PO[b]	+	+	+	−	−	−
Dicloxacillin (Veracillin, Pathocil, Dynapen)	PO	+	+	+	−	−	−
Flucloxacillin (Flopen, Floxapen)	PO	+	+	+	−	−	−
Oxacillin (Prostap-hy lin, Bactocil)	PO, IM, IV	+	+	+	−	−	−
Aminopenicillins[c]							
Ampicillin (many)	PO,[b] SC, IM, IV	+	−	+	±	±	−
Amoxicillin (Omnipen)	PO,[b] IM	+	−	+	±	±	−
Hetacillin (Hetacin)	PO	+	−	+	±	±	−
Extended-Spectrum Carboxypenicillins							
Carbenicillin (Pyopen, Geopen)	IM, SC, IV	−	−	±	+	+	+
Ticarcillin (Ticar)	IM, SC, IV	−	−	±	+	+	+
Ureidopenicillins[d]							
Mezlocillin (Mezlin)	IM, IV	−	−	+	++	±	++
Piperacillin (Pipracil, Pipril)	IM, IV	−	−	+	++	±	++

Table • 34-1

Continued

GENERIC NAME (TRADE NAME)[a]	ROUTE OF ADMINISTRATION	ANTIMICROBIAL SPECTRUM						
		GASTRIC ACID STABILITY	STAPHYLOCOCCAL β-LACTAMASE RESISTANCE	GRAM POSITIVE	GRAM NEGATIVE	ANAEROBIC	*PSEUDOMONAS*
Other β-Lactams							
Aztreonam (Azactam)	IM, IV	–	++	–	++	–	++
Imipenem-cilastatin (Primaxin)	IV	–	++	++	++	++	++
β-Lactamase Inhibitors							
Clavulanate [CA][e]	PO, IV	+	++	–	–	–	–
CA + amoxicillin (Clavulox, Clavamox, Augmentin)	PO[b]	+	++	++	++	+	–
CA + ticarcillin (Timentin)	IV	–	++	±	+	+	+
Sulbactam [SB][e]	IV	–	++	+	±	±	–
SB + ampicillin (Unasyn, Synergistin)	IV	–	++	+	+	+	+
Tazobactam [TZ][e]	IV	–	++	+	+	±	±
TZ + piperacillin (Zosyn)	IV	–	++	+	++	±	++

IM, Intramuscular; *IV*, intravenous; *PO*, by mouth; *SC*, subcutaneous; –, none; ±, variable; +, good; ++, excellent.
[a]See Appendix 8 for dosages.
[b]For best results, administer on empty stomach.
[c]Also includes bacampicillin (Spectrobid), cyclacillin (Cyclapen), epicillin, pivampicillin, and talampicillin.
[d]Also includes azlocillin (Azlin).
[e]Susceptibility data indicate efficacy of inhibitor alone, although the drug is not available by itself.

is a limiting factor with these drugs, but co-administration with a cephalosporin or quinolone might be considered when managing difficult-to-treat gram-negative aerobic bacterial infections.

Pharmacokinetics

Absorption and duration of activity of penicillins depend on the dose administered, the vehicle containing the drug, and the solubility of the salt formulation. The potassium and sodium salts are soluble and can be given by the oral (PO), intramuscular (IM), subcutaneous (SC), intravenous (IV), and topical routes, whereas insoluble trihydrates are absorbed less rapidly by PO, IM, and SC routes. Soluble penicillin derivatives are absorbed from serous and mucosal surfaces but not through unbroken skin. Food in the stomach can adversely affect bioavailability of orally administered penicillins. All penicillins are eliminated by the kidney through active tubular secretion. As a result, soluble penicillin derivatives must be given at least every 4 hours to maintain therapeutic blood concentrations. Probenecid inhibits this rapid elimination. Activity can also be prolonged by delaying release of penicillins from injection sites by placing them in water-insoluble vehicles or combining them with organic salts. Examples are procaine penicillin and benzathine penicillin.

In general, penicillins are widely distributed into most highly perfused tissues, body fluids, and bone. Brain and cerebrospinal fluid (CSF) are exceptions, but concentrations in CSF are higher when meninges are inflamed. Penetration of body fluids and tissues by the highly protein-bound isoxazolyl derivatives is more limited. Dose reduction may not be necessary in patients with renal failure, despite impaired elimination, because of low inherent toxicity and the increased biliary secretion obtained with the semisynthetic penicillins. Potassium-containing penicillins should not be given IV to oliguric patients because of the risk of hyperkalemia.

Most aqueous solutions of penicillins are unstable, especially at higher temperatures. They should be maintained at a pH of 5.5 to 7.5 and not added to solutions containing bicarbonate or other alkalinizing ingredients. Oral suspensions of penicillins must be kept refrigerated after reconstitution. They generally remain stable for only 1 week. IV solutions should be used within 24 hours of preparation.

Penicillins should never be mixed with blood, plasma, or other proteinaceous fluids or with other antibiotics before administration. They might display in vivo antagonism with tetracycline and chloramphenicol; variable interactions with erythromycin, novobiocin, and lincomycin; no antagonism with sulfonamides; and possible synergism with aminoglycosides, cephalosporins, and polymyxins. Penicillins should not be mixed in the same syringe with aminoglycosides because of potential inactivation of both drugs.

Pharmacodynamics

Dosing schedules for β-lactams have been based on maintenance of blood levels above MIC for all or most of the dosing interval.[386] Unlike the aminoglycosides and quinolones, β-lactams do not exhibit concentration-dependent killing. Their efficacy is time dependent; and for optimal effect, plasma drug concentrations should exceed the MIC for 50% to, at, or above 80% of the treatment interval so that bacterial cell walls can be disrupted as they form. A bactericidal effect is usually achieved at between one and four times the MIC. Higher doses of β-lactams have often been used for more severe infections, but reaching the MIC may be all that is necessary, and impairment of excretory mechanisms in septic animals may permit use of lower doses.[237] Because of their low toxicity, β-lactams may have been given in overdoses. Additional studies on bioactivity and pharmacokinetics in ill and organ-impaired animals will be needed to resolve the dosing schedules for these drugs. Unlike aminoglycosides and quinolones, penicillins and cephalosporins have no PAE on gram-negative bacteria at clinically achievable concentrations. A PAE for certain gram-positive organisms, such as some staphylococci, has occurred. The PAE allows antibiotic concentrations to fall below the MIC for a portion of the treatment interval without impairing efficacy. Nevertheless, for most infections, β-lactams should be administered at a dose and interval sufficient to maintain plasma concentrations high enough to affect the target organism in the tissues of concern. In severe infections with resistant organisms, this action may necessitate constant IV infusions.

Toxicity

Toxic reactions are relatively rare with penicillins, and they generally have a high margin of safety. Rapid IV infusion or occasional IM injections may cause neurologic signs and convulsions. Hypersensitivity reactions such as hives, fever, joint pain, and acute anaphylaxis have been noted immediately after administration to dogs and cats. Administration of any penicillin derivatives should be avoided in known sensitized animals because of cross-reactivity.

Bleeding has been an important side effect in human patients treated with antipseudomonal and extended-spectrum penicillins. This effect has been attributed to various factors, including delayed fibrin polymerization, suppression of vitamin K–dependent procoagulants, and platelet dysfunction. Acute postoperative (within 5 days) azotemia has been ascribed to administration of nafcillin to dogs during surgery.[296]

Other β-Lactam Drugs
Monobactams

Aztreonam, the only clinically available member of this group, is resistant to β-lactamase and active against a wide range of aerobic and facultative gram-negative bacteria, including many strains resistant to other drugs. However, it has no useful activity against gram-positive or anaerobic pathogens. Aztreonam is given parenterally and enters many body tissues and fluids of dogs, including the CSF. Adverse effects are minimal and include diarrhea and vomiting. Primary use has been to treat patients with serious gram-negative infections in which resistance or toxicity to aminoglycosides is anticipated.

Carbapenems

This group includes imipenem, panipenem, biapenem, meropenem, and ertapenem. Imipenem is active against very many gram-positive and gram-negative aerobes and anaerobes. It is primarily indicated for treatment of infections caused by cephalosporin-resistant members of the family Enterobacteriaceae and some anaerobes. Resistant *Pseudomonas* isolates have emerged during therapy. Breakdown of imipenem by dehydropeptidase-1 in the kidney and other tissues produces nephrotoxic metabolites and decreases urine concentrations of active drug. Co-administration of cilastatin, a metabolic inhibitor of dehydropeptidase-1, increases urine drug concentrations and decreases potential nephrotoxicity. Panipenem is combined with betamipron for the same reason. Biapenem and meropenem are more stable and do not require any inhibitor be given concurrently. Meropenem pharmacokinetics have been studied in dogs.[27] The protein binding of meropenem is such that plasma concentrations parallel those in interstitial fluid.[28] Ertapenem has a narrower spectrum of activity than others in this class. Parenteral administration of imipenem-cilastatin is necessary because neither is absorbed orally. The dose should be reduced in renal failure. Adverse effects include nausea, vomiting, diarrhea, phlebitis at the infusion site, fever, and seizures. See Drug Formulary (Appendix 8) for further information on each of these drugs.

β-Lactamase Inhibitors

Some naturally occurring β-lactam drugs have low antibacterial activity by themselves but bind irreversibly to and inactivate bacterial β-lactamase. Concurrent administration of these agents increases the activity of penicillins and decreases the in vitro MIC required to inactivate many β-lactamase–producing organisms, such as staphylococci, *Escherichia*, *Capnocytophaga canimorsus*, some *Proteus* and *Klebsiella*, *B. fragilis*, *Salmonella*, and *Campylobacter* (Table 34-2). Organisms such as *Enterobacter*, *Serratia*, *Citrobacter*, and *Pseudomonas* remain resistant.

Clavulanate

Clavulanate has weak antibacterial activity against a wide range of organisms but is a potent inhibitor of β-lactamase. It is rapidly absorbed, unaffected by food, and widely distributed in extravascular sites with the exception of the central nervous system (CNS). Clavulanate is excreted rapidly in unchanged form in urine.

An orally administered product combining amoxicillin with potassium clavulanate is licensed for small animal use. A parenteral formulation of ticarcillin with potassium clavulanate is licensed for human and equine use. This combination is best suited to treat resistant infections caused by members of the family Enterobacteriaceae (except some *Pseudomonas* spp.) and anaerobes. It is given commonly to treat infections of the skin, lower respiratory tract, soft tissue, middle ear, and sinuses. The primary side effect has been diarrhea. Studies over a 9-year period on bacteria isolated from

Table • 34-2

Comparison of Antibacterial Activity of Selected β-Lactam and β-Lactamase Inhibitor Combinations[a]

| | | BACTERIAL SUSCEPTIBILITY | | | |
PENICILLIN	INHIBITOR	GRAM POSITIVE	GRAM NEGATIVE	ANAEROBES	*PSEUDOMONAS*
Amoxicillin	Clavulanate	+	+	+	−
Ticarcillin	Clavulanate	++	++	+++	+
Ampicillin	Sulbactam	+	+	+	−
Piperacillin	Tazobactam	++	+++	++	++

+++, Excellent; ++, very good; +, good; −, poor.
[a]See Appendix 8 for further drug information and dosages.

Table • 34-3

Comparison of Antimicrobial Activity of Cephalosporins

| | BACTERIAL SUSCEPTIBILITY | | | | |
GENERATION	GRAM POSITIVE	GRAM NEGATIVE	ANAEROBES	β-LACTAMASE RESISTANT	SELECTED SUSCEPTIBLE ORGANISMS
First[a]	+++	+	++	+	*Staphylococcus*
Second[b]	++	++	++	+	*Proteus*
Third[c]	+	+++	+	++	*Pseudomonas*
Fourth[d]	+	+++	+	+++	Enterobacteriaceae

+++, Excellent; ++, very good; +, good; −, poor.
[a]**First generation:** primarily active against gram-positive aerobes and facultative anaerobes; resistant to staphylococcal β-lactamase, which is responsible for penicillin ineffectiveness, but is less effective on a weight basis than penicillin G against obligate anaerobes.
[b]**Second generation:** similar attributes to first generation but (as with aminopenicillins) is also active against some gram-negative aerobes and facultative anaerobes; second best cephalosporin group against anaerobes.
[c]**Third generation:** enhanced activity against gram-negative aerobes and facultative anaerobes, low activity against obligate anaerobes, but less active against gram-positive aerobes and facultative anaerobes; variable activity against *Pseudomonas*; see Table 34-4 for antipseudomonal efficacy of selected cephalosporins.
[d]**Fourth generation:** very active against Enterobacteriaceae and *Staphylococcus* (including methicillin-resistant strains); moderate antipseudomonal activity.

dogs and cats showed little decrease in relative susceptibility to this drug combination.[393]

Sulbactam

This drug, an irreversible β-lactamase inhibitor, has weak intrinsic antibacterial activity against most gram-positive and some gram-negative organisms, with best activity against *Neisseria* and *Bacteroides*. It extends the bacterial spectrum of ampicillin to include *Staphylococcus*, *Bacteroides*, and most *Escherichia*. Sulbactam has been given with ampicillin to treat resistant bacterial meningitis in people and to treat those with intraabdominal, pelvic, skin, soft-tissue, bone, and joint infections.

Tazobactam

This β-lactamase inhibitor has been added to enhance the antibacterial spectrum of piperacillin. It is active against many resistant Enterobacteriaceae, *Staphylococcus*, and *Bacteroides*.

CEPHALOSPORINS

The cephalosporins are a group of antibiotics derived chemically from a substance produced by the fungus *Cephalosporium acremonium*. Several related compounds can also be considered in the cephalosporin group because they have

similar antibacterial activity, pharmacology, and indications. This group includes cefoxitin and cefotetan (both cephamycins), loracarbef (a carbacephem), and latamoxef (an oxacephem).

Similar to penicillins, cephalosporins are bactericidal β-lactam antibiotics that inhibit bacterial cell wall synthesis, resulting in osmotic fragility. These drugs are generally more effective than penicillin in penetrating the outer cell wall of gram-negative bacteria and are less susceptible to inactivation by bacterial β-lactamases.

Cephalosporins have been separated into four generations or classes, based on the chronology of discovery, chemical structure, and therapeutic activity. The characteristics of the classes are compared in Table 34-3, and important features of common cephalosporins are presented in Table 34-4. For further information on specific drugs and dosage, see the Drug Formulary (Appendix 8).

First Generation

The first-generation cephalosporins are primarily active against gram-positive bacteria, with the exception of some resistant *Staphylococcus*, and some gram-negative aerobes, such as *Escherichia*, *Klebsiella*, and *Proteus mirabilis*. The activity of these drugs against susceptible aerobes and facultative anaerobes is not as strong as that of penicillin G. They are not as effective against anaerobes, including *Bacteroides*. First-

Table • 34-4

Properties of Cephalosporins[a]

GENERIC NAME (TRADE NAME)	ROUTE OF ADMINISTRATION	COMMENTS
First Generation[b]		
Cephalexin (Keflex)	PO	Less active against *Staphylococcus*
Cefazolin (Ancef, Kefzol)	IV, IM	Achieves greatest blood concentration; longest half-life; most protein-bound; more active against *Escherichia, Klebsiella, Enterobacter* than others in its class
Cephapirin (Cefadyl)	IV, IM	Resists β-lactamase; high doses for life-threatening infections when causative organism shows susceptibility to first-generation drugs
Cefadroxil (Duricef, Cefa-Tabs)	PO	Rapid and complete oral absorption even with food; enters prostate
Cephradine (Velosef, Anspor)	IV, IM, PO	Spectrum similar to cephalexin; less active against some gram-negative organisms
Second Generation[c]		
Cefaclor (Ceclor)	PO	Similar spectrum but more active than first generation against *Proteus, Escherichia, Enterobacter,* and *Klebsiella;* adequate soft-tissue concentrations; minor amount excreted in urine unchanged
Cefotetan (Cefotan)[d]	IV, IM	Similar indications to cefoxitin, but may be less expensive
Cefoxitin (Mefoxin)[d]	IV, IM	Pain on IM injection; active against *Bacteroides fragilis* and *Serratia;* particularly effective against most anaerobes
Cefuroxime (Zinacef, Kefurox)	IV, IM	Crosses blood-brain barrier; good for lower respiratory tract and central nervous system infections
Third Generation[e]		
Cefixime (Suprax)	PO	High bioavailability and long half-life in dogs; for urinary tract and respiratory infections caused by resistant bacteria; not active against *Pseudomonas* or *Bordetella*
Ceftiofur (Naxcel)	IV, IM	Licensed for treatment of bovine respiratory disease; good for broad-spectrum treatment of systemic infections; low activity against *Staphylococcus*
Cefotaxime (Claforan)	IV	Active against *Leptospira* and gram-negative aerobes except *Pseudomonas;* metabolized in liver to active drug; good central nervous system penetration
Ceftriaxone (Recephin)	IV, IM	Longest duration for once-daily dosing; active against resistant gram negatives except *Pseudomonas;* good against *Borrelia*
Antipseudomonal Third Generation[f]		
Ceftazidime (Fortaz, Tazidime, Tazicef)	IV	Primarily active against gram-negative aerobes and best of cephalosporins against *Pseudomonas*
Cefoperazone (Cefobid)	IV	Less active than other third-generation drugs against gram-positive and -negative aerobes; second best of its class against *Pseudomonas;* can produce coagulation deficiencies; erratic central nervous system penetration; predominant (80%) biliary excretion
Fourth Generation[g]		
Cefepime (Maxipime)	IV	High blood levels and widely distributed in tissues; good against *Pseudomonas* and *Mycobacterium avium-intracellulare;* variable activity against gram positives and anaerobes

IM, Intramuscular; *IV,* intravenous; *PO,* by mouth.
[a]See Drug Formulary (Appendix 8) for further information on pharmacokinetics and appropriate dosages for each drug.
[b]Also includes cephaloglycin, cephalothin, and cephaloridine.
[c]Also includes cefuroxime axetil (Ceftin), cefmetazole, cefonicid (Monocid), and three more (given orally): cefprozil, cefpodoxime (Vantin), and loracarbef.
[d]Cefoxitin and cefotetan are cephamycins.
[e]Also includes ceftriaxone (Rocephin), ceftizoxime (Cefizox), flomoxef, ceftibuten (Cedax), cefmenoxime, and latamoxef (Moxam, Latoxacef [an oxacephem]).
[f]Also includes cefsulodin and cefpiramide.
[g]Also includes cefpirome.

generation cephalosporins can be administered orally or parenterally, depending on the drug, and they have variable protein binding with wide distribution into pleural, pericardial, peritoneal, and synovial fluids and most soft tissues. They enter the CSF only in the presence of meningeal inflammation. Most are excreted unchanged in the urine. Cephalosporins may give atypical or false-positive reactions with copper reduction methods for determining urine glucose (e.g., Clinitest tablets).

Two members of this group are of historic significance but are no longer used. Cephalothin is found in susceptibility disks, but it is of limited use because of pain and sterile abscesses produced on IM injection. Cephaloridine produces similar complications and is nephrotoxic. Cephalothin is the only first-generation drug to penetrate CSF well. First-generation agents available for parenteral use include cefazolin, cephapirin, and cephradine. Oral drugs include cefadroxil and cephalexin, which have both been marketed for veterinary use. These two oral drugs have uses for treating gram-negative urinary and gram-positive skin infections in dogs and skin and soft-tissue infections in cats. Both agents reach effective blood plasma concentrations after oral dosing of dogs and cats.

Second Generation
Second-generation cephalosporins have a broader spectrum of antibacterial activity and greater efficacy against gram-negative aerobic bacteria and anaerobes than does the first generation (see Table 34-3). This activity is largely the result of the greater resistance of these drugs to β-lactamases. They are more effective than first-generation drugs against *Proteus* (other than *P. mirabilis*), *Escherichia*, *Klebsiella*, *Enterobacter*, and anaerobic bacteria. As with first-generation drugs, second- and third-generation cephalosporins are relatively ineffective against *Bacteroides*. Exceptions are cefoxitin, and cefotetan, which are effective against most obligate anaerobes. Cefoxitin is also effective against *Serratia*. Second-generation drugs are generally given parenterally, but drugs effective orally include cefaclor, cefuroxime axetil (a pro-drug), cefprozil, cefpodoxime, and loracarbef.

Third Generation
The third-generation cephalosporins have longer duration of activity compared with the other two classes. Excretion in either urine or bile is variable, depending on the drug, although most undergo some inactivation and excretion by the liver. Third-generation drugs—except for latamoxef, ceftriaxone, and cefotaxime—do not penetrate CSF well in the absence of inflammation. Third-generation cephalosporins have marked activity against aerobic gram-negative organisms and less effectiveness against aerobic gram-positive organisms and anaerobes than the preceding classes (see Table 34-3). They are more active than second-generation drugs against *Citrobacter*, *Acinetobacter*, *Pseudomonas*, and *Serratia*. Most third-generation drugs are given parenterally, but a few oral drugs such as cefixime and cefpodoxime proxetil (a pro-drug) are available. Unfortunately, these oral preparations are not always as effective as the other members of this class against difficult organisms. Third-generation cephalosporins have been recommended for IV use in septicemia, bacteremia, intraabdominal infection, and endocarditis. Second- and third-generation drugs have had good efficacy against drug-resistant *Salmonella* isolated from people.

Antipseudomonal Cephalosporins
Unlike other cephalosporins, cefoperazone and ceftazidime are among the most effective drugs against *P. aeruginosa*. However, most third-generation cephalosporins are not as effective against *Pseudomonas* as are the newer extended-spectrum penicillins.

Fourth Generation
Fourth-generation cephalosporins are not affected by some chromosome-mediated and many plasmid-mediated β-lactamases. Cefepime and cefpirome are members of this class. They have good activity against *Staphylococcus*, Enterobacteriaceae, and *Pseudomonas* but, as with third-generation drugs, are not reliable against anaerobes (see Table 34-3).

Indications
The varied indications for use of cephalosporins include treatment of bacterial infections of respiratory, urinary, and genital tracts, as well as soft tissues, bones and joints, and skin. Cephalosporins are effective when given prophylactically for polymicrobial intraabdominal infections after bowel surgery. In addition, cephalosporins have also been recommended for prophylactic purposes in biliary surgery and for treating biliary infections because many are excreted unchanged in bile. However, they do not enter the biliary tract when complete biliary obstruction and jaundice are present. Failure of cephalosporins to prevent postoperative staphylococcal infections has been associated with strains that hydrolyze cephalosporins.[192] Cefotaxime, latamoxef, and ceftriaxone are effective for meningitis caused by drug-resistant bacteria. None of the cephalosporins are effective against methicillin-resistant staphylococci or enterococci.

Most oral cephalosporins administered in small animal practice are first-generation drugs but oral second- and third-generation products are available (see Table 34-4). Cefazolin and cephapirin are the most commonly used parenteral first-generation cephalosporins. The second-generation drugs, such as cefoxitin, have increased efficacy against anaerobic infections. Of the second-generation drugs, cefuroxime has a high degree of penetration into the CNS and CSF for treatment of meningitis. Some concern has surfaced of the increasing use of third-generation drugs in animal patients.[20] This concern stems from the risk of producing antimicrobial-resistant strains that might spread to people.

Toxicity
The toxicity of cephalosporins is minimal compared with that of other antibiotics. In this regard, the cephalosporins are similar to the penicillin derivatives.[272] Allergic skin reactions have been reported with cephalosporins in dogs. A greater prevalence of diarrhea is associated with agents undergoing biliary excretion. Cephaloridine is nephrotoxic, but this is not characteristic of the newer drugs. Because the kidney excretes most cephalosporins, plasma concentrations are increased and half-lives prolonged in renal failure or when probenecid, loop diuretics, or aminoglycosides are used. All parenteral formulations of cephalosporins may cause phlebitis and myositis after IV and IM administration, respectively. Gut irritation may cause vomiting and diarrhea with oral administration. Bleeding disorders in people resulting from vitamin K antagonism, platelet dysfunction, and immune-mediated thrombocytopenia have been associated with third-generation cephalosporins, most frequently cefamandole, cefoperazone, and latamoxef. Cephalosporin-induced blood dyscrasias, a result of immune-mediated destruction of blood cells and direct marrow toxicity, have occurred in dogs given high-dose, long-term cephalosporins.[89] Myelosuppression resolves when therapy is withdrawn. For individual drug characteristics, consult the Drug Formulary (Appendix 8).

AMINOGLYCOSIDES

These bactericidal antibiotics interfere with the synthesis of bacterial protein. Aminoglycosides (AGs) are relatively small, primarily basic, water-soluble molecules that are active against certain gram-negative and gram-positive aerobic and facultative anaerobic bacteria, including many staphylococci and some mycobacteria. They are particularly effective against aerobic gram-negative bacilli such as *Escherichia, Klebsiella, Proteus,* and *Enterobacter,* and some are effective against *Pseudomonas.* AGs are not active against fungi or obligate anaerobic bacteria and should not be used to treat abscesses or granulomatous infections. Their uptake across bacterial cell membranes requires the presence of oxygen. For this reason, AGs demonstrate poor activity against anaerobes and have decreased ability to penetrate bacteria within abscesses with limited oxygen tension. When used alone, AGs are relatively ineffective against *Streptococcus* but are effective against *Staphylococcus intermedius.* Co-administration with β-lactams increases their activity against some gram-positive aerobes including *Enterococcus* spp. In serious systemic infections, in which mixed organisms are anticipated, an aminoglycoside given with a β-lactam plus a β-lactamase–inhibitor combination acts against a broad spectrum of organisms. The properties and indications for various AGs are summarized in Table 34-5.

Dihydrostreptomycin, streptomycin, neomycin, and kanamycin have been used extensively for many years. However, with such frequency of use, extensive bacterial resistance has developed. The first two drugs listed are no longer commercially available in many countries. Amikacin and gentamicin are more effective and routinely given. Amikacin is generally more effective compared with gentam-

Table • 34-5

Properties of Aminoglycosides[a]

GENERIC NAME (TRADE NAME)	ROUTE OF ADMINISTRATION	COMMENTS
Streptomycin (many)	IM, SC	Occasional IM use for bacteremias, *Brucella canis, Leptospira* carriers; limited availability
Dihydrostreptomycin (many)	IM, SC	Same as streptomycin; many resistant strains; limited availability
Neomycin (Biosol, Mycifradin)	PO, topical	PO for local gastrointestinal effect; topical use in solutions, ointments, and so forth; spectrum similar to kanamycin; absorbed and toxic if bowel wall damaged
Kanamycin (Kantrim, Kantrex, Klebcil)	PO, IM, SC	PO for local gastrointestinal effect; useful in urinary tract infection, injections, and superficial and systemic infections; spectrum similar to gentamicin but resistant strains much more common; effective against *Staphylococcus*
Gentamicin (Gentocin, Garamycin, Apogen, Bristagen, U-Gencin)	IM, SC, IV, aerosol, topical	For bacteremia; in aerosol for respiratory infections caused by *Escherichia, Pasteurella, Pseudomonas, Proteus, Staphylococcus, Enterobacter, Serratia, Klebsiella, Bordetella*
Paromomycin (Humatin)	PO	PO for local gastrointestinal effect; for susceptible *Staphylococcus, Escherichia, Salmonella,* and protozoa (*Entamoeba, Balantidium, Cryptosporidium*)
Tobramycin (Nebcin)	IM, SC	Gram-negative spectrum similar to gentamicin; effective against some *Pseudomonas* resistant to gentamicin; less nephrotoxic than gentamicin
Amikacin (Amikin, Amiglyde)	IM, SC	Widest antibacterial spectrum aminoglycoside; effective against *Pseudomonas* and many gram-negative bacilli resistant to gentamicin and tobramycin (e.g., *Klebsiella*)
Sisomicin (Sisomin)	IM, SC	More active than gentamicin against many bacteria, especially *Pseudomonas* and *Escherichia;* not effective against organisms resistant to gentamicin; toxicity parallels gentamicin
Netilmicin (Netromycin)	IM, SC	*Staphylococcus* highly susceptible; active against some organisms resistant to gentamicin; more active than sisomicin or tobramycin; slightly less active than amikacin against *Pseudomonas;* less toxic than tobramycin
Framycetin (Soframycin, Neomycin B)	PO, topical	PO for local gastrointestinal effect; topical in ointment, drops, and so forth; gram-negative spectrum similar to neomycin
Dactinomycin[b]	IM, SC	Intraabdominal infections; wide activity against gram-positive and gram-negative aerobes; may be combined with metronidazole for anaerobic spectrum; most active aminoglycoside against *Acinetobacter* and *Staphylococcus*
Isepamicin[b]	IV, IM, SC	Exceptional activity against Enterobacteriaceae and *Pseudomonas*

IM, Intramuscular; *SC,* subcutaneous; *PO,* by mouth; *IV,* intravenous.
[a]See Drug Formulary, Appendix 8, for appropriate dosages.
[b]Not available commercially.

icin against resistant strains. Tobramycin and netilmicin have been developed to increase antibacterial activity and reduce toxicity. Sisomicin, isepamicin, and dactimicin are newer AGs being evaluated for clinical purposes. The latter two drugs have broad-spectrum activity against gram-positive and gram-negative aerobes.

Antimicrobial synergy is often observed when AGs are combined with β-lactam drugs. The β-lactams may also enhance AG activity under conditions of reduced oxygen tension. β-Lactams are indicated to treat gram-negative bacterial infections but must be given parenterally for systemic infections. β-Lactams are used in combination with other antibiotics to treat difficult infections, such as enterococcal endocarditis.

Pharmacokinetics

The pharmacokinetics of many AGs have been studied in dogs and cats. AGs are poorly absorbed from the gastrointestinal (GI) tract and must be administered parenterally to achieve therapeutic plasma concentrations; however, some AGs such as neomycin and paromomycin are administered orally for local treatment of bacterial or protozoal enteritis or to suppress enteric microflora in hepatic coma. They are poorly absorbed through intact skin but may cross-damage squamous, mucosal, or visceral epithelium, resulting in potential toxicity. Topical AG creams and solutions can help control bacterial growth and facilitate healing of open wounds. They are absorbed following IM or SC administration,[424] although more slowly with the latter. IV administration is best for immediate effects. Following intraoperative IV administration, AGs enter surgical wounds on a time course that parallels plasma concentrations. They are minimally bound to plasma proteins but are poorly lipid soluble and highly ionized; thus they penetrate little beyond extracellular fluid compartments, including synovial, peritoneal, and pleural spaces. They also diffuse poorly into the CNS, prostate, amniotic fluid, and eyes, even in the presence of inflammation. Obese cats have smaller volumes of distribution of AGs than lean cats, warranting dose reductions in obese animals.[429] Little excretion into bile and feces occurs, but unchanged AG is eliminated rapidly in urine by glomerular filtration and tubular excretion. Within 1 hour after administration, urine AG concentrations are 25 to 100 times greater than peak blood plasma concentrations and remain above therapeutic levels for several days. These drugs may accumulate in renal tubular cells and are eliminated slowly from renal tissue; once-daily dosing produces less renal accumulation than thrice-daily dosing with higher peak tissue concentrations. The pH at which optimal antibacterial activity occurs is 7.5 to 8.0. AGs such as gentamicin have been effective in treating canine bronchopulmonary infections when administered as aerosols: drug concentration in airways is increased and toxicity is reduced because of poor absorption from this site.

Individual variability in distribution and elimination of AGs accounts for unpredictable variability in blood and tissue concentrations. Consequently, the monitoring of blood plasma concentration is common in human medicine. Liposomal encapsulation of AGs has been used in an attempt to increase therapeutic efficacy and decrease toxicity.[363]

Pharmacodynamics

AGs, in contrast to some other antibiotics, show marked concentration-dependent killing of bacteria, after which a distinct PAE, a bacteriostatic phase without regrowth, is observed. With concentration-dependent antibacterial activity, the rate and efficacy of bacterial killing increases with higher drug concentrations: all the organisms may die if concentrations are sufficiently high. When the peak blood plasma concentration is less than approximately 10 times the MIC, the time of exposure to the antibiotic concentration may still be important, and the entire AUC must be considered in these cases. Because of the peak concentration requirement, once-daily AG therapy has been considered superior to multidosing in producing higher concentrations and, incidentally, lower toxicity. Nevertheless, a reduction in toxicity by less frequent administration has not been well substantiated.[210] Gentamicin has been given to dogs once daily for 5 days with minimal or no nephrotoxicity.[4] AGs are thought to have a PAE after exposure of some gram-negative or gram-positive organisms to an antibiotic. Drug-induced nonlethal damage from bacteriostatic suppression of infecting strains has been seen against both gram-positive and gram-negative bacterial strains.

Bacteria are likely to develop resistance to AGs by one of three mechanisms: alteration of receptor sites on bacterial ribosomes, decreased bacterial cell penetrability, or plasmid-associated production of enzymes that inactivate AGs. Bacterial resistance to AGs is greater with the older drugs and less with newer compounds. Cross-resistance is not uniform among all members of the class. For example, although many *Klebsiella* are resistant to kanamycin and gentamicin, they are susceptible to amikacin, a derivative of kanamycin. In general, the degree of cross-resistance between gentamicin and other AGs is high, except for amikacin and tobramycin.

Toxicity

Toxicities with AG antibiotics are relatively common and depend on the individual drug and dosage, duration of therapy, state of patient hydration, presence of upper UTI, and pretreatment of renal function. Nephrotoxicity can be attributed to the uptake of AGs by proximal renal tubular cells and drug retention in lysosomes of these cells in the cortex. Above a certain concentration, cell necrosis occurs. Although species differences exist, nephrotoxicity in decreasing order is as follows: neomycin, kanamycin, gentamicin, tobramycin, amikacin, and streptomycin. Nephrotoxicity has been associated with high trough plasma concentrations (greater than 2.0 µg/ml for gentamicin and 5.0 µg/ml for amikacin). Frequent administration of small doses to maintain constant plasma AG concentrations is considered more toxic than less frequent administration of larger dosages. Frequent (three to four times daily) dosing has been recommended for treatment of systemic infections in animals, but renal function must be monitored closely with such protocols. AGs may be given at higher doses and less frequent intervals than commonly recommended. Pulse administration of large (10 mg/kg) doses of gentamicin at 5-day intervals has been shown to maintain effective tissue concentrations in dogs. Pulse administration should be less nephrotoxic than frequent dosing because plasma concentrations decrease sufficiently between administrations; however, further documentation of the efficacy of such regimens is needed.[127] Renal proximal tubular dysfunction is the most common and serious side effect of AG administration. Higher protein diets have protected dogs against development of gentamicin-induced nephrotoxicity.[136] Inadvertent absorption of gentamicin administered topically when lavaging an abscess produced nephrotoxicity in a cat.[251] Use of AGs should be restricted in puppies and kittens because these animals may be more prone to develop renal failure than older animals.

The best method of detecting early renal tubular dysfunction in practice is to examine the urine for casts and proteinuria. Although mainly a research tool, the most sensitive way to detect AG toxicity in dogs and cats is to measure urinary concentrating ability and urinary enzyme activities.[137] Serum urea and creatinine concentrations are primarily measures of glomerular filtration and are less sensitive indications of AG nephrotoxicity. Acute renal failure typically develops several days after therapy is initiated but may develop several days after the drug is discontinued. Because AGs accumulate in renal tubular cells, the insult persists after administration ceases. The prognosis for recovery from AG-induced renal failure is poor in dogs and cats. In human patients, AG concentrations are monitored to avoid toxicity; dosages are modified so that plasma concentrations are high enough 1 hour after administration to be bactericidal but are below toxic threshold levels 30 minutes later.

Clinical reports from human hospitals have noted increased nephrotoxicity when AGs are given with cephalosporins, although studies in rats indicated the combination may actually be protective. Similarly, combinations of piperacillin with gentamicin or cephaloridine were shown to have reduced nephrotoxicity. Furosemide may enhance nephrotoxicity and ototoxicity of AGs, probably because of decreased extracellular fluid volume and decreased drug excretion causing increased plasma AG concentration. Other diuretics may have similar effects and should be avoided in combination with AGs. Cats and dogs should be well hydrated whenever AG therapy is instituted. Other nephrotoxic drugs such as amphotericin B and cisplatin should be avoided because they may potentiate nephrotoxicity.

Gentamicin-impregnated methyl methacrylate beads and methyl methacrylate cement have been applied successfully for prophylaxis in orthopedic surgery.[362] Local release of the gentamicin into surrounding bone, soft tissue, and synovial fluid allowed for long-term therapy, effective cure, and no side effects. AGs have also been incorporated into liposomes to reduce systemic toxicity.

Irreversible ototoxicity has been a problem with AG therapy; both vestibular and auditory impairment from damage to sensory end-organs have been reported. High concentrations of AGs remain in the perilymph fluid of the ear for extended periods compared with plasma. AGs are potentially ototoxic when instilled directly into the external ear canal of dogs and cats, especially if the tympanic membrane has been ruptured. However, ototoxicity has not been found at concentrations present in commercial otic preparations.[356] Table 34-6 summarizes relative otic and renal toxicities of AGs for dogs and cats. In cats, the ototoxicity of AGs in decreasing order is streptomycin, dihydrostreptomycin, gentamicin, tobramycin, and netilmicin, with vestibular damage more likely than auditory damage. As with nephrotoxicity,

ototoxicity is more likely with higher doses, with longer treatment durations, and with animals that are dehydrated or have poor renal perfusion.

AGs, associated with underlying risk factors, may produce neuromuscular blockade by competitive antagonism of acetylcholine at the myoneural junction. In addition to their own neuromuscular blocking effects, they enhance the actions of other neuromuscular blocking agents and general anesthetics.[116] Therefore irrigation of body cavities or parenteral administration of AGs should be avoided during surgery that requires general anesthesia.

Circulatory depression, exhibited by decreased systemic blood pressure and heart rate, has been found in cats, dogs, and nonhuman primates given AGs during pentobarbital anesthesia. Cardiac arrest has been reported in people overdosed with kanamycin. If possible, AG administration should be avoided in animals in shock or with cardiovascular insufficiency. Calcium gluconate, given IV, may reverse AG-induced neuromuscular blockade or myocardial depression and restore blood pressure.

Prolonged high oral doses of neomycin or paromomycin may produce diarrhea and malabsorption caused by overgrowth of resistant indigenous intestinal flora. Hypersensitivity and allergic reactions have been reported rarely in people receiving AGs. AGs should not be administered to pregnant animals because they can cross the placenta and may produce fetal intoxication. Penicillins and AGs should never be mixed in the same solution before administration—depending on the type and concentration of penicillin, mixing can inactivate the AGs. They should not be administered IV with solutions containing calcium, other antimicrobials, heparin, or sodium bicarbonate. For individual drug characteristics and dosages, consult the Drug Formulary (Appendix 8).

SPECTINOMYCIN

Aminocyclitol antibiotics, composed of a basic cyclic structure with an amino group, include the AGs along with spectinomycin and its derivatives. Spectinomycin shares many properties with the AGs, including low plasma protein binding, high water solubility, poor GI absorption, primary renal excretion, inhibition of bacterial ribosomal protein synthesis, and optimal antibacterial activity at pH 8.

Spectinomycin has bacteriostatic activity, mainly against gram-negative aerobic pathogens such as *Escherichia*, *Klebsiella*, *Salmonella*, *Enterobacter*, and *Proteus*, as well as mycoplasmas. Efficacy is low against gram-positive aerobes, most pseudomonads, and chlamydiae. Obligate anaerobes are resistant. Parenteral administration of spectinomycin may be useful to treat bacteremia associated with infectious gastroenteritis caused by susceptible enteropathogenic bacteria and for intraabdominal sepsis (see Intraabdominal Infections, Chapter 89). As with some AGs, development of resistant bacteria is a problem with spectinomycin. Trospectomycin is an analog with similar activity against enterobacteria but increased activity against gram-positive aerobes.

PEPTIDES

Vancomycin

This complex glycopeptide molecule has bactericidal activity, inhibits cell wall formation and RNA production, and alters cytoplasmic membranes in susceptible replicating bacteria. Vancomycin is active primarily against gram-positive organisms, mainly *Staphylococcus* (including methicillin-resistant strains), *Streptococcus*, and *Clostridium*. Most gram-negative bacteria are resistant.

Table • 34-6

Relative Toxicity of Aminoglycosides

DRUG[a]	RENAL	VESTIBULAR	AUDITORY
Streptomycin	−	+	−
Dihydrostreptomycin	?	−	+
Neomycin	+	−	+
Gentamicin	+	+	±
Kanamycin	+	−	+
Tobramycin	+	+	+
Amikacin	±	−	+
Netilmicin	±	±	±

−, Lesions have not been detected; +, lesions have been detected; ?, information concerning lesions is lacking; ±, milder lesions than +. Adapted from data from Conzelman GM. 1980.
Pharmacotherapeutics of aminoglycoside antibiotics, *J Am Vet Med Assoc* 176:1078–1080; McCormick GC et al. 1985., *Toxicol Appl Pharmacol* 77:478–489; Pickrell JA et al. 1993. Ototoxicity in dogs and cats, *Semin Vet Med Surg Small Anim* 8:42–49.
[a]See Drug Formulary, Appendix 8, for appropriate dosages.

Vancomycin can be administered orally to treat enteric infections. It is absorbed poorly from the GI tract and must be given IV for systemic infections. The drug is distributed well into body cavities and across inflamed meninges. Excretion is largely by glomerular filtration, with small amounts entering the bile.[436]

The most frequent side effects with vancomycin in people have been fever, chills, and phlebitis at injection sites. These effects can be reduced if the drug is administered slowly in a large volume of fluid. Leukopenia and eosinopenia have been reported.

Possible uses for vancomycin in animals are limited but may be considered for treating severe, persistent staphylococcal infections and colitis associated with overgrowth of *Clostridium difficile*. At present, antimicrobial resistance to vancomycin does not appear to be as much a problem in fecal microflora of dogs and cats as to other more routinely used antimicrobials.[315] This status might change subsequent to indiscriminate use of this drug. See the Drug Formulary (Appendix 8) for further information. In some countries, such as the United States, restrictions have been placed on the use of glycopeptides in food-producing animals.[11]

Teicoplanin and Dalbavancin
Teicoplanin is a complex glycopeptide whose structure, activity, and other properties are similar to those of vancomycin. It is primarily active against aerobic and some anaerobic gram-positive organisms. Teicoplanin is more protein bound and lipophilic than vancomycin. The half-life in plasma is much longer, which may allow once daily administration. Possible indications for veterinary use are as for vancomycin. Further information is given in the Drug Formulary (Appendix 8). Dalbavancin is a novel glycopeptide under clinical development with a long elimination half-life but minimal cross-resistance with other compounds in this group. It has a similar spectrum and is generally more bactericidal as compared with vancomycin or teicoplanin.[342]

POLYMYXINS

These agents form a group of closely related, cationic, cyclic peptides. Of the types A through E, polymyxin B and polymyxin E (colistin) are therapeutically most important. Polymyxins appear to exert their bactericidal effects as cationic detergents by binding to cell membrane phospholipids and increasing cell permeability of gram-negative bacteria. Most gram-negative organisms such as *Pasteurella*, *Escherichia*, *Shigella*, *Salmonella*, *Bordetella*, and some *Klebsiella* and *Pseudomonas* are susceptible, whereas *Brucella* and *Proteus* are frequently resistant. Resistance is also a factor of increased usage, and although emergent strains develop during usage, they become susceptible again once polymyxin therapy is stopped.

Polymyxins are poorly absorbed when given orally and topically. They do not produce high plasma concentrations after parenteral administration, presumably because of high affinity for host cell membranes. Polymyxins diffuse poorly through biologic membranes and are excreted unchanged in urine.

These drugs are provided chiefly as topical preparations for treating localized infections in the ear canal, eye, bowel, and urinary tract. Respiratory therapy may be achieved by means of nebulization. Intrathecal administration has been performed with aqueous preparations, but they are highly irritating. For topical use, polymyxins have been combined with neomycin and bacitracin or tetracycline to widen antibacterial activity.

Polymyxins have been given systemically (IM) to treat infections that are resistant to AGs and have shown some synergism with sulfonamide and trimethoprim. Colistin sulfomethate (sodium colistimethate) is the least toxic parenteral preparation. The major side effect of polymyxins is nephrotoxicity, although pain at the injection site, CNS signs, and neuromuscular blockade have also been noted. Toxicity has limited the usefulness of these drugs for systemic therapy.

CHLORAMPHENICOL, FLORFENICOL, AND THIAMPHENICOL

Chloramphenicol is a highly lipid-soluble, broad-spectrum antibiotic that is predominantly bacteriostatic and inhibits microbial protein synthesis. It is effective against a variety of pathogens, including *Mycoplasma*, *Rickettsia*, *Ehrlichia*, *Anaplasma*, *Neorickettsia*, *Chlamydia*, *Staphylococcus*, *Streptococcus*, *Pasteurella*, *Bordetella*, *Haemophilus*, and Enterobacteriaceae, including many *Escherichia*, *Proteus*, and *Salmonella*. This antibiotic has good activity against most obligate anaerobic bacterial pathogens. Thiamphenicol and florfenicol, closely related drugs, have been marketed for use in food-producing animals.

Administration
Chloramphenicol can be administered orally or parenterally, and absorption depends on formulation. The drug is usually given orally in capsular form but can be bitter tasting, causing salivation and anorexia if capsules are not swallowed intact. Oral film-coated tablets may overcome this problem. Chloramphenicol palmitate is an oral suspension that requires hydrolysis by digestive enzymes before absorption can occur. Plasma concentrations are lower initially with this dosage form in cats and poor in those that are not eating. Capsules or tablets therefore may be preferable in cats. Chloramphenicol sodium succinate, a water-soluble ester, is recommended for systemic use. Otic, ophthalmic, and topical preparations are also available.

Pharmacokinetics
Less than 50% of the drug is bound to plasma protein. In dogs and cats, most of the drug is metabolized by the liver to inactive metabolites excreted in urine, and a minor amount is excreted in bile, from where it undergoes enterohepatic circulation. Chloramphenicol diffuses rapidly and well into most tissues. Highest concentrations are found in liver, kidney, bile, spleen, lung, pancreas, and urine, and it penetrates all body fluids. Several hours are required for the brain concentration to approximate that of the plasma concentration; however, brain tissue concentration remains adequate for up to 12 hours, although plasma concentration diminishes before that time. The concentration of active chloramphenicol in urine is usually sufficient to be effective against susceptible bacteria. Thiamphenicol is also poorly protein bound, is not acted on to any great extent by the liver, and is mostly excreted unchanged in the urine.

Indications
Chloramphenicol is effective against most aerobic and anaerobic bacterial pathogens in dogs and cats. It is a preferred antibiotic for treating *Salmonella* and *Escherichia* infections in the GI tract. Chloramphenicol has been recommended for prophylaxis before intestinal surgery or dental procedures but is contraindicated with pentobarbital anesthesia. Chloramphenicol can be considered for treatment of UTIs in dogs with subnormal renal function because the drug is unlikely to accumulate in dogs unless renal failure is advanced.

Chloramphenicol penetrates the cornea well because it is lipid soluble and has low molecular weight. Systemic administration is required to treat intraocular and orbital infections and deep corneal lesions.

Toxicity

The most common side effects of chloramphenicol administration in dogs and cats are depression, anorexia, dysphagia, salivation, nausea, vomiting, and sporadic diarrhea. Reversible bone marrow suppression and severe irreversible bone marrow failure have been reported in people. The persistent pancytopenia is idiosyncratic and not dose related. However, only reversible bone marrow changes have been demonstrated in dogs and cats, with variable suppression of erythropoiesis and granulopoiesis. Chloramphenicol is more toxic to cats than it is to dogs, perhaps because of relatively poor hepatic glucuronidation capacity, which is important in elimination of chloramphenicol in other species. Bone marrow changes in cats can occur after only 1 week of therapy. Toxic changes do not develop if cats are given the drug on an intermittent basis or at low doses. Clinical improvement and resolution of hematologic changes usually occur within several days after cessation of therapy. A normal hemogram does not rule out toxicosis because bone marrow changes precede those in peripheral blood.

The small public health hazard associated with inadvertent contact with chloramphenicol has limited its use in food-producing species and may increase the veterinarian's liability to owners handling the drug intended for pets. Thiamphenicol, an analog of chloramphenicol, has been widely provided in Europe as a substitute. It has similar antibacterial properties, is associated with enhanced renal excretion of active drug, and is said not to cause irreversible marrow failure in people. Another drug related to thiamphenicol, florfenicol, is licensed for cattle and has not been reported to cause aplastic anemia in people. For further information on chloramphenicol, thiamphenicol, florfenicol, and dosage regimens, consult the Drug Formulary (Appendix 8).

TETRACYCLINES

Tetracycline antibiotics are bacteriostatic and interfere with protein synthesis of bacterial RNA in a concentration-dependent manner. They have a similar but weaker effect on eukaryotic cells. As a group, tetracyclines have broad-spectrum activity that includes certain aerobic and anaerobic gram-positive and gram-negative bacteria, mycobacteria, spirochetes, mycoplasmas, rickettsiae, chlamydiae, and some protozoa (Table 34-7). Being more lipid-soluble tetracyclines, doxycycline, and minocycline have increased activity against anaerobes and several facultative intracellular bacteria such as *Brucella canis*, presumably because of their ability to better penetrate bacterial cell walls. These two drugs are most commonly prescribed of the group because of a reduction in their dosing frequency and side effects and increased intracellular penetration. Newer glycylcycline derivatives are under clinical development and are administered parentrally.[314] For additional information on susceptibility of pathogens to individual tetracyclines, consult the Drug Formulary (Appendix 8).

Bacterial resistance to tetracyclines is present among various genera of bacteria and can relate to the usage level of these drugs. Resistance is usually plasmid mediated, although it may occur following genetic mutation. Resistance has been a major problem with some tetracyclines but occurs less often with doxycycline and minocycline. Resistance has been less of a problem among obligate intracellular pathogens such as *Chlamydophila* and *Rickettsia*. However, tetracycline-resistant

Table • 34-7

Properties of Tetracyclines[a]

GENERIC NAME (TRADE NAME)	ROUTE OF ADMINISTRATION	COMMENTS AND SPECIFIC INDICATIONS
Short Acting, Water Soluble		
Tetracycline (Panmycin, Achromycin, Tetracyn)	PO, IV, IM	Therapeutic or prophylactic use for *Ehrlichia;* IM injections painful; do not inject intraarticularly
Oxytetracycline (Terramycin)	PO, IV, IM	Reaches high concentration in lung liver, kidney, and mononuclear phagocyte system; better tolerated orally by cats
Chlortetracycline (Aureomycin)	PO	pH is very important for activity
Intermediate Acting[b]		
Demeclocycline[c] (Declomycin)	PO	Photosensitivity may occur; dosage-dependent nephrogenic diabetes insipidus
Long Acting, Lipid Soluble		
Minocycline (Minocin, Vectrin)	PO, IV	More effective against *Ehrlichia, Babesia, Brucella;* greater activity against *Nocardia, Staphylococcus,* anaerobes; wide distribution in tissues
Doxycycline (Vibramycin, Doxychel)	PO, IV	Same as for minocycline; tetracycline of choice for extrarenal infections with concurrent renal failure; more active against *Bacteroides;* prophylaxis for bowel surgery; used to treat chronic prostatitis

PO, By mouth; *IV,* intravenous; *IM,* intramuscular.
[a]See Appendix 8 for appropriate dosages.
[b]Also includes methacycline.
[c]Formerly demethylchlortetracycline.

strains of *Chlamydia suis* have been isolated from swine that had been given low-dose tetracyclines in their feed.[219]

Pharmacokinetics

All the tetracyclines can be given orally. They vary markedly in lipid solubility, a factor that determines their relative enteral absorption and tissue penetration. Highly lipid-soluble doxycycline and minocycline show better absorption and wider tissue distribution, although they are more protein bound. Absorption, a passive process that occurs primarily in the duodenum, is impeded by sodium bicarbonate and by divalent and trivalent cations in food, milk, aluminum hydroxide gels, calcium and magnesium salts, and iron preparations. Because absorption of doxycycline and minocycline is affected somewhat less by food or cations, these two agents are often given with meals to reduce GI irritation. However, tetracyclines undergo enterohepatic circulation, and intraintestinal multivalent cations can still chelate and reduce the bioavailability of parenterally administered drug.

The less lipid-soluble agents, tetracycline and oxytetracycline, are primarily excreted in urine: 60% is recovered as unchanged drug in urine, whereas 40% is excreted by the liver and found in feces. In contrast, lipid-soluble minocycline is eliminated primarily by hepatic metabolism, and only 10% enters the urine. The excretion of doxycycline is not controlled by hepatic or renal excretion; this drug is unique in that the major means of elimination appears to be diffusion across the intestinal wall. Doxycycline is highly protein bound in dogs so that plasma concentrations are higher than in interstitial fluid during constant IV infusion.[28] Minocycline and doxycycline may not reach high enough concentrations in the urine to be effective against some pathogens, although doxycycline has been given to eliminate the renal carrier state of *Leptospira*.

Indications

Tetracyclines enter most tissues, including the eye and CNS of dogs. They even penetrate well into the paranasal sinuses and secretions and are therefore useful for treating bacterial sinusitis. Tetracyclines are less active in alkaline media, especially in the case of chlortetracycline. Doxycycline and minocycline are better able to penetrate bacterial cell walls, as they do tissues, thereby being more effective against persistent intracellular pathogens such as species of *Brucella*, *Ehrlichia*, and *Mycobacterium*. Tetracyclines have been effective, especially topically, in reducing the progression of periodontal disease in dogs (see Chapter 89).[437]

Tetracyclines inhibit the activity of neutral matrix metalloproteinases, perhaps related to their chelation of multivalent cations. These enzymes are involved in the progression of cartilage degeneration in osteoarthritis. Dogs with experimentally induced anterior cruciate ligament injuries had less severe osteoarthritis when treated with doxycycline.[435] This nonspecific protective effect should be considered in dogs that improve with tetracycline-responsive polyarthritis, which is often considered to have an infectious cause.

Tetracyclines also appear to have antiinflammatory activity in nonskeletal diseases, presumably also by inhibiting metalloproteinase enzyme inhibitors. In combination with niacinamide, tetracyclines have been useful in treating some immune-mediated skin diseases such as discoid lupus erythematosus, pemphigus foliaceus, sterile pyogranulomatous dermatitis, and feline lymphoplasmacytic pododermatitis.[25,267] Despite this immunosuppressive effect, treatment does not interfere with humoral immune response to vaccination.[267]

Toxicity

Numerous side effects have been associated with tetracyclines and are covered in detail with individual drugs in the Drug Formulary (Appendix 8). GI disturbances result from esophageal, gastric, and intestinal irritation and changes in enteric microflora. Esophagitis has been problematic, especially in cats given doxycycline. Because doxycycline and minocycline are well absorbed in the upper GI tract, they are less likely to alter lower intestinal flora. Orally administered tetracyclines frequently produce fever in cats with or without severe GI upsets from local irritation. As with chloramphenicol, tetracyclines inhibit hepatic microsomal enzymes and may delay elimination of hepatically metabolized drugs. Hepatotoxicity (including increased serum alanine aminotransferase activity) has been found in cats receiving tetracyclines.[189]

Except for doxycycline, tetracyclines should be avoided in patients with renal failure because drug excretion is delayed and azotemia may worsen. The use of tetracyclines in dogs has been associated with direct nephrotoxicity from acute tubular necrosis. In people, the use of outdated tetracyclines or the drug's breakdown products has produced a Fanconi's syndrome–like disorder with reversible renal tubular dysfunction. Findings on urinalysis have included glucosuria, phosphaturia, and aminoaciduria with or without proteinuria. The nephrotoxicity occasionally produced by methoxyflurane anesthesia is accentuated by tetracyclines given before surgery. Demeclocycline has been shown to induce acute reversible nephrogenic diabetes insipidus in people.

Anaphylactic reactions to parenterally administered tetracyclines or their vehicles have occasionally been noted in dogs and cats. Phototoxic reactions, characterized by erythema and edema of the skin, have been associated with certain tetracyclines after exposure to ultraviolet (UV) light.

Tetracyclines become fixed in growing osseous structures. Staining of deciduous teeth of neonates and enamel hypoplasia may occur when tetracyclines are given to a bitch or queen during the last 2 or 3 weeks of pregnancy. The deciduous teeth of puppies or kittens may also be affected if these drugs are given during the first months of life. Doxycycline is less likely to cause this problem (see Drug Formulary, Appendix 8).

Thrombophlebitis frequently occurs after IV injections of tetracyclines and is seen more often with the less lipid-soluble agents. IM administration of soluble tetracyclines is discouraged because it causes pain and necrosis.

Tetracyclines may cause false-positive urine test results for glucose if copper sulfate reagents are employed (Clinitest, Ames Laboratories, Elkhart, Ind.), and false-negative test results may occur with glucose oxidase reagents. Leukocytosis, atypical lymphocytes, toxic granulation, and immune-mediated hemolytic anemia have been reported with tetracyclines in people. Interference of tetracycline with coagulation factors has also been noted.

MACROLIDES AND LINCOSAMIDES

Macrolides inhibit peptide formation by the 50s ribosomal subunit. Erythromycin is the parent drug of the macrolides. Oleandomycin and troleandomycin, two older members of the group, are less active and more toxic and are rarely administered now. Rosamicin is similar to erythromycin in antibacterial spectrum and usage. Josamycin is better absorbed and less toxic and is less likely to lead to bacterial resistance than erythromycin. Rokitamycin achieves higher plasma concentrations after oral administration and causes fewer GI side effects than erythromycin. Dirithromycin is a potent derivative that has been shown to produce higher and longer lasting plasma concentrations than erythromycin base. This pro-drug is hydrolyzed during intestinal absorption to the active moiety erythromycylamine.

Macrolides are effective primarily against gram-positive bacteria, *Chlamydophila*, *Mycoplasma*, *Helicobacter*, *Campylobacter*, and some rickettsiae. The efficacy of macrolides against extracellular pathogens depends on the concentration of free drug and the organism's susceptibility. Macrolides are slowly bactericidal, with a poor relation between increasing concentration and rapidity of bacterial killing.

All macrolides accumulate intracellularly, primarily in neutrophils and macrophages. Several macrolides, namely erythromycin, azithromycin, clarithromycin, and tylosin, are discussed briefly here and more extensively in the Drug Formulary (Appendix 8). Because of its antiprotozoal efficacy, spiramycin is discussed in Chapter 71.

The lincosamide antibiotics are structurally unrelated to macrolides but have similar antibacterial and pharmacokinetic attributes. Lincomycin and clindamycin are discussed later, and additional information is given in the Drug Formulary (Appendix 8).

Erythromycin

Erythromycin inhibits protein synthesis in bacterial cells and is bacteriostatic for susceptible organisms at usual dosages. Because its mechanism of action resembles that of chloramphenicol and lincosamides, erythromycin can compete with these drugs for binding sites.

Erythromycin is a weak base and is unstable in the presence of gastric acid, which reduces systemic availability after oral administration. Different formulations of erythromycin have been made to circumvent this effect, incorporating enteric coating, acid-stable salts (stearate), esters (ethylsuccinate), and salts of esters (estolate) (Table 34-8). GI absorption of erythromycin base and stearate is impaired by ingesta and gastric acid. The lactobionate and gluceptate esters can be administered parenterally but are relatively expensive. Topical preparations are also available for general use and as ophthalmic ointments to treat chlamydial and mycoplasmal conjunctivitis.

Erythromycin diffuses readily into most tissues and extracellular fluids, and therapeutic concentrations are reached within 2 to 3 hours. It is concentrated by the liver and excreted in bile in high concentration, undergoing enterohepatic circulation and final excretion in feces. High concentrations are found in most body fluids and secretions, with the exception of CSF and urine.

Erythromycin has a primarily gram-positive spectrum and is most effective against *Streptococcus*, *Staphylococcus*, *Erysipelothrix*, *Clostridium*, *Bacteroides*, *Borrelia*, and *Fusobacterium*. It is also effective against a few gram-negative organisms, such as *Pasteurella* and *Bordetella*, but not against aerobic enteric bacteria unless the environmental pH is alkaline (~ 8.0). Erythromycin has exceptional activity against *Campylobacter*, *Legionella*, *Mycoplasma*, chlamydiae, rickettsiae, spirochetes, some atypical mycobacteria, *Leptospira*, and amebae. Resistance in some bacteria has developed with increased usage. Erythromycin is rarely selected as a first-choice drug, except for treating *Campylobacter* or *Legionella* infections, and is used more often as an alternative to penicillin G or a lincosamide.

Erythromycin has relatively low toxicity; the most frequent side effect is GI irritation resulting in nausea, vomiting, and diarrhea. Water or dilute antacid solution, given with the drug, may decrease irritation and facilitate absorption. Erythromycin estolate and occasionally erythromycin ethylsuccinate have been associated with increased risk of cholestasis and hepatotoxicity, which may cause increased blood bilirubin concentration and hepatic enzyme activity. All parenteral preparations are irritating at injection sites.

Azithromycin and Clarithromycin

These azalides are derivatives of erythromycin with better enteral absorption and increased resistance to destruction by gastric acid. After oral administration, they are distributed widely to tissues in high concentrations except for the brain and eye.[396] Azithromycin produces low extracellular concentrations but has high intracellular penetration, whereas clarithromycin produces high concentrations in both extracellular fluid and intracellular sites. They reach high concentrations in phagocytic cells throughout the body and are slowly released

Table • 34-8

Comparison of Erythromycin Formulations for Oral Use[a]

GENERIC NAME (TRADE NAME)	ABSORBED AS FREE BASE	ABSORPTION AFFECTED BY GASTRIC ACID/INGESTA	FORMULATION	COMMENTS
Erythromycin base (Erythromycin, Ilotycin, Robimycin, E-Mycin, Eryc)	+	+/±	Tablets	Enteric coating reduces irritation
Erythromycin stearate (Erythrocin, Ethril, Erypar, Wyamycin)	+	±/+	Tablets	Absorption increased by drinking large amounts of water
Erythromycin estolate (Ilosone)	−	−/−	Drops, tablets, suspension	Associated with increased risks of cholestasis and hepatotoxicity
Erythromycin ethylsuccinate (Pediamycin, Eryped, E.E.S.)	−	±/±	Drops, capsules, tablets, suspension	Milk enhances absorption

+, Yes; ±, variable; −, no.
[a]See text for properties and indications for each product. See Drug Formulary (Appendix 8) for appropriate dosages.

over several days after a single dose. These drugs are less active than erythromycin against gram-positive bacteria but more active against gram-negative aerobes and anaerobes. Azithromycin and clarithromycin have strong activity against *Mycoplasma*, *Borrelia*, and *Leptospira*. Clarithromycin has been suggested as an alternative treatment against *Toxoplasma* and atypical *Mycobacterium*. For further information on these drugs, see the Drug Formulary (Appendix 8).

Tylosin

Similar to other macrolides, tylosin is generally bacteriostatic against susceptible bacteria. Gram-positive bacteria, *Campylobacter*, and *Mycoplasma* are particularly susceptible to its effects, as are most organisms that are susceptible to erythromycin. Oral absorption of tylosin is variable, depending on the product formulation. The drug is metabolized by the liver and excreted in both urine and bile. Tylosin has been suggested also for the management of clostridial enteritis (see Chapter 39), inflammatory bowel disease, and chronic colitis in dogs and cats and in the supportive treatment of systemic coronaviral diseases in cats. Proof of efficacy in the latter disorder, however, is lacking. The drug is effective in the treatment of staphylococcal pyoderma in dogs.[337,338] For additional information consult the Drug Formulary, Appendix 8.

Lincomycin and Clindamycin

Lincosamides bind to 50s ribosomal subunits and inhibit protein synthesis in susceptible bacteria. The mode of action resembles that of chloramphenicol and the macrolides. Depending on the concentrations achieved, lincomycin is bacteriostatic to bactericidal. Clindamycin, a chlorosubstituted lincomycin, has increased bactericidal activity and rate of absorption and has shown less toxicity in animals than lincomycin.

Lincomycin and clindamycin are widely distributed in body tissues and fluids, including bile, peritoneal and pleural fluids, milk, placenta, prostatic fluid, and bone. For example, mean levels of clindamycin in canine mandibular bone were 8.18 μg/g following 5 days of treatment at 11 mg/kg.[438] Neither drug enters the CSF or ocular structures unless inflammation is present. Both drugs accumulate in neutrophils, macrophages, and abscesses, making them useful in treating infections caused by anaerobic or persistent intracellular pathogens.

Both agents are primarily indicated to treat infections caused by gram-positive aerobes and obligate anaerobes. Lincomycin has been recommended for use in a variety of skin, respiratory, GI, soft-tissue, and bone infections, especially when gram-positive organisms are involved. Clindamycin is effective against a greater variety of organisms, including anaerobic bacteria and protozoa such as *Toxoplasma* and *Neospora* (see Therapy, Chapter 41 and Therapy, Chapter 80, respectively; and the Drug Formulary, Appendix 8). Clindamycin has been beneficial in treating oropharyngeal infections, including periodontal disease associated with anaerobic bacteria.[274]

Toxicity of these drugs has been relatively low in dogs that received supratherapeutic doses for relatively long periods. GI irritation, vomiting, and diarrhea may occur with oral administration.

Pseudomembranous colitis, a complication in some people treated with either drug, is exhibited by abdominal pain, fever, and mucus or blood in the stools. Overgrowth of resistant, toxin-producing strains of *C. difficile* is believed responsible. Diarrhea in treated dogs and cats does not seem to be caused by *C. difficile* toxin.[142] If this side effect occurs, the practitioner should discontinue the drug and substitute vancomycin or metronidazole.

METRONIDAZOLE

For a discussion of this antimicrobial against anaerobic bacterial and protozoal infections, see Antiprotozoal Chemotherapy, Chapter 71, and Drug Formulary, Appendix 8.

NOVOBIOCIN

This antibiotic has a spectrum of activity similar to, but not as consistent as, that of penicillin G. Many gram-positive aerobic bacteria, including *Streptococcus* and *Staphylococcus*, are susceptible, whereas effectiveness against *Proteus* and *Pasteurella* is variable. Novobiocin inhibits bacterial DNA and subsequent RNA and protein synthesis, and antibacterial resistance to this drug does not transfer to other antibiotics.

Novobiocin is absorbed well after oral administration and is predominantly excreted in bile and feces. The antibiotic has been marketed mainly in fixed combination with tetracycline. In vitro studies have suggested possible inhibition reactions between these compounds. However, a subjective evaluation reported more clinical improvement in upper respiratory tract infections in dogs treated with novobiocin plus tetracycline than in dogs treated with either drug alone.[244]

NITROFURANS

These synthetic antibacterial compounds are chemical derivatives of 5-nitrofuraldehyde. The exact mechanism of action is uncertain, although they are known to interfere with many cellular enzymes. Nitrofurans are bacteriostatic or bactericidal, depending on the organisms and the amount of drug at the infection site. The nitrofurans have a relatively broad spectrum of activity but generally are more effective against gram-negative organisms. *Escherichia*, *Salmonella*, *Staphylococcus*, and *Streptococcus* are usually susceptible, whereas *Pseudomonas* and some *Proteus* and *Klebsiella* are resistant. *Pseudomonas* can actually grow in many preparations of nitrofurazone, which may lead to nosocomial wound infection. Resistance develops rarely during therapy with nitrofurans. Table 34-9 summarizes the uses of nitrofurans in veterinary practice.

Nitrofurantoin is absorbed rapidly after oral administration, but the low plasma concentrations are insufficient to treat systemic infections. Most of the drug is excreted rapidly in urine, which makes it helpful in UTIs. However, treatment with nitrofurantoin is probably not warranted if other drugs have failed. Nitrofurantoin in urine may cause positive test results for glucose when copper sulfate reduction method is used. Alkalinization of the urine, which increases the amount of nitrofurantoin excreted, should be avoided because the drug is more effective at acid pH. A macrocrystalline formulation is absorbed more slowly, reducing GI irritation and prolonging its effect. Nifuratel, an analog with a similar pattern of absorption, is unaffected by urine pH and has a wider spectrum of activity, including efficacy against *Candida*.

Furazolidone is not absorbed after oral administration and has been administered to treat local infections caused by enteric pathogens. Nitrofurazone is applied topically as powder, cream, or spray solution and is not absorbed. Evidence exists that the spray preparation may be carcinogenic. Nitrofurazone is frequently incorporated in an oil-base rather than a water-soluble cream, but this practice reduces its antibacterial efficacy and can delay healing by causing maceration of tissues.

Adverse reactions to nitrofurans are not uncommon. Nitrofurantoin frequently causes nausea and emesis in dogs and cats. The authors (CEG and AJDW) have observed acute

Table • 34-9

Properties of Nitrofurans[a]

GENERIC NAME (TRADE NAME)	ROUTE OF ADMINISTRATION (FORMULATION)	USES/COMMENTS
Nitrofurantoin (Furadantin, Macrodantin)	PO (tablet, suspension), IM (solution)	UTI; avoid in renal failure; macrocrystalline is absorbed slower and is less toxic
Nifuratel (Magmilor)	PO (tablet)	UTI; also effective against *Candida* at any urine pH
Furazolidone (Furoxone)	PO (tablet, suspension)	For enteric pathogens; not absorbed PO; used for *Salmonella* and coccidia
Nitrofurazone (Furacin)	Topical (ointment, powder, solution, cream, suppository)	For skin and mucosal infections; *Pseudomonas* can contaminate
Nifuroxime (numerous)	Topical (suppository, cream)	Antifungal properties; used together with other nitrofurans

PO, By mouth; *IM*, intramuscular; *UTI*, urinary tract infection.
[a]See Drug Formulary (Appendix 8) for dosages of systemically administered drugs.

polyneuropathy and myopathy in a dog given nitrofurantoin. For more information on nitrofurantoin and furazolidone, consult the Drug Formulary (Appendix 8).

SULFONAMIDES

Sulfonamides were developed early in the era of antibacterial chemotherapy and have been superseded by many of the newer antimicrobial agents. However, resurgence has occurred in sulfonamide therapy since the introduction of diaminopyrimidine compounds that enhance their antimicrobial efficacy. Sulfonamides are derivatives of sulfanilamide and act by interfering with bacterial synthesis of folic acid from para-aminobenzoic acid (PABA). They are bacteriostatic and ineffective in the presence of pus, necrotic tissue, or blood containing PABA. Bacteria that are highly susceptible to sulfonamides include *Streptococcus, Bacillus, Corynebacterium, Nocardia, Campylobacter, Pasteurella,* and chlamydiae. However, *Bacteroides, Enterococcus, Pseudomonas, Serratia,* and *Klebsiella* are generally resistant. Caution must be exercised in interpreting disk susceptibility test results with these drugs because they frequently do not correlate with in vivo susceptibility. An increasing number of organisms are becoming resistant to sulfonamides. Resistance appears to develop more commonly with long-term therapy.

With few exceptions, sulfonamides are readily and rapidly absorbed and reach bacteriostatic plasma concentrations. Levels attained depend on the drug, route of administration, and dose. Sulfonamides are variably bound to plasma protein and distributed widely to all tissues and pleural, peritoneal, synovial, and ocular fluids. They cross the placenta and readily enter CSF. Sulfonamides generally undergo hepatic metabolism, with metabolites excreted mainly in urine, with smaller amounts in the bile. Sulfonamides have been used alone to treat a variety of human infections, but the combination of sulfonamides with a diaminopyrimidine (see later discussion) is now mostly used in dogs and cats. The orally absorbed sulfonamides can be divided into four groups (Table 34-10). The short-acting drugs, rapidly absorbed and excreted, require doses at 8-hour intervals. These drugs are given for systemic infections and UTIs. The intermediate-acting sulfonamides are excreted more slowly, administered every 12 to 24 hours, and are used mainly to treat UTIs; sulfisoxazole is often provided for this purpose. Long-acting sulfonamides, such as sulfadoxine, are excreted slowly and require administration every few days.

Some sulfonamides, poorly absorbed from the GI tract, will alter enteric microflora but will not disrupt the balance of microflora and rarely cause superinfection. Phthalylsulfathiazole has been administered to reduce coliform flora, stool bulk, and gas before colonic surgery.

Although marketed for topical application, sulfonamides are relatively ineffective in the presence of exudates. Mafenide, the only exception, is helpful for prophylaxis in burn patients because of its ability to inhibit *Pseudomonas*.

Certain sulfonamides have been administered for specific indications. Sulfapyridine, which is relatively toxic, is given only for treating dermatitis herpetiformis. Sulfasalazine (salicyl-azosulfapyridine) is used to treat colitis in dogs. Sulfasalazine is hydrolyzed by colonic microflora to sulfapyridine and 5-aminosalicylate.

Toxic reactions to sulfonamides are relatively common in dogs and cats. Acute hemolytic complications and precipitation of sulfonamide metabolites in renal tubules seen in people have not been seen in dogs. Failure of insoluble acetylated metabolites to cause renal problems in dogs may be explained by the fact that deacetylation of metabolites occurs more rapidly than their formation. Dogs given high doses of sulfonamides can develop cystic sulfonamide uroliths. Sulfonamide crystalluria and neurologic signs, including convulsions, occurred in a dog ingesting sulfonamide cream.[118] However, cats may develop azotemia and renal failure during sulfonamide or trimethoprim-sulfonamide (T-S) therapy. Keratitis sicca can develop in dogs on acute or long-term treatment.[94] Schirmer's tear tests should be performed on dogs before administering these drugs, and sulfonamides should be avoided if tear production is low. The prognosis for return of lacrimation is poor, but topical cyclosporine appears to be effective in some cases.[94] For additional information, refer to the following discussion of T-S and the Drug Formulary (Appendix 8).

DIAMINOPYRIMIDINES-SULFONAMIDES

Sulfonamides inhibit bacterial synthesis of dihydrofolic acid. Trimethoprim and related pyrimidine-like compounds (ormetoprim, baquiloprim) interfere with dihydrofolate reductase, an enzyme that prevents the conversion of dihydrofolic acid (folic acid) to tetrahydrofolic acid (folinic acid), which is essential for synthesis of purines and pyrimidines and thus of DNA. Mammals, unlike microorganisms, acquire most folic acid preformed in the diet, which explains the selective

Table • 34-10

Properties of Sulfonamides Commonly Used in Small Animal Practice[a]

GENERIC NAME (TRADE NAME)	ROUTE OF ADMINISTRATION	INDICATIONS AND COMMENTS
Short Acting[b]		
Sulfadiazine (Suladyne, Debenal)	PO, IM	Systemic and urinary infections and nocardiosis; frequently combined as triple sulfa to minimize renal tubular precipitation; may be combined with trimethoprim (see below)
Sulfamethazine (Sulmet)	PO, IM	As above
Sulfamethoxazole (Gantanol, Methoxal)	PO, IM	As above
Intermediate Acting[c]		
Sulfisoxazole (Gantrisin, Soxisol, Sulfasox)	PO	UTI
Sulfadimethoxine (Sudine, Bactrovet, Albon, Madribon)	PO	UTI
Gastrointestinal Preparations[d]		
Succinylsulfathiazole (Sulfasuxidine)	PO	Local antibacterial effects on gastrointestinal tract; administer with kaolin-pectin
Phthalylsulfathiazole (Sulfathalidine)	PO	*Shigella* enteritis, preoperative prophylaxis for gastrointestinal surgery; mineral oil, laxatives, and purgatives interfere with action
Special/Combination		
Sulfasalazine (Azulfidine)	PO	Colitis; salicylate component may help in therapy
Mafenide (Sulfamylon cream)	Topical	Burns; prophylaxis only
Trimethoprim and sulfamethoxazole (Septra, Bactrim)	PO	Systemic, respiratory, and urinary infections, *Pneumocystis* pneumonia, *Brucella*; must be given to dogs at least twice daily for systemic infections; effective once daily for urinary infections and coccidiosis
Trimethoprim and sulfadiazine (Tribrissen, Di-Trim)	PO, IM	As for trimethoprim-sulfamethoxazole
Ormetoprim and sulfadimethoxine (Primor)	PO	Skin and UTI, wounds, coccidiosis
Baquiloprim and sulfadimethoxine (Zaquilan)	PO, IM	Skin, respiratory, urogenital, gastrointestinal, and soft-tissue infections

PO, By mouth; *IM*, intramuscular; *UTI*, urinary tract infection.
[a]Most of these drugs are licensed for human use. See the Drug Formulary (Appendix 8) for specific information and dosages.
[b]Rapidly absorbed and rapidly excreted.
[c]Rapidly absorbed and slowly excreted.
[d]Poorly absorbed.

action of sulfonamides against microbes. Increased production of dihydrofolate reductase by enteric bacteria makes them more resistant to the effects of this drug. Trimethoprim has less affinity for dihydrofolate reductase in mammals than it does in microorganisms, which accounts for the reduced toxicity of the drug for mammalian cells. Each drug alone is generally bacteriostatic, but synergistic interaction is expected when trimethoprim and sulfonamide are co-administered in a 1:5 ratio, with bactericidal activity whenever the optimum in vivo ratio of 1:2 is achieved.

Trimethoprim and its co-administered sulfonamides are rapidly and completely absorbed and widely distributed after oral administration. Therapeutic concentrations are achieved in CSF, brain, eye, prostate, bone, and joints. CSF concentrations can range up to 80% of plasma concentrations. Reducing the dosage is unnecessary in renal failure unless it is severe. Sulfadiazine has been chosen for administration with trime-

thoprim in dogs. Sulfamethoxazole is used in human preparations. Trimethoprim is available by itself in some countries but offers little advantage because it is less active and just as toxic as the combined product.

T-S has been recommended for treatment of respiratory infections and UTIs caused by *Escherichia, Streptococcus, Proteus, Salmonella,* and *Pasteurella*. Lesser and more variable activity is noted against *Staphylococcus, Klebsiella, Corynebacterium, Clostridium,* and *Bordetella. Moraxella, Nocardia,* and *Brucella* are moderately susceptible. T-S has been administered simultaneously with AGs to enhance activity against gram-negative organisms. Bacterial resistance has developed with continued usage. Because of good CNS penetrability, the combination is an excellent choice for gram-negative pathogens producing meningitis.

All the side effects noted previously with sulfonamides can be seen with the drug combination (see trimethoprim-sulfonamide, adverse reactions, in the Drug Formulary, Appendix 8). T-S causes greater adverse reactions and has less margin of safety in cats, which are more likely to develop anorexia, vomiting, azotemia, anemia, and leukopenia.

Other toxicities have been reported in dogs and cats. Ataxia has sometimes been observed when higher therapeutic doses are given. Reversible cholestatic hepatitis has been observed in dogs with preexisting hepatic disease.[141] Fatal hepatic necrosis and hepatic failure have been reported as an idiosyncratic reaction in dogs,[370,387] unrelated to dose and duration of therapy. The hepatotoxic substance from sulfamethoxazole metabolism is thought to be a metabolite that concentrates in the periportal hepatobiliary areas and induces a cytotoxic response.[129] Aplastic anemia was associated with trimethoprim-sulfadiazine and fenbendazole administration in a dog.[414] Anemia resolved after withdrawal of the drugs and may have reflected drug idiosyncrasy or immune hypersensitivity rather than inhibited folate metabolism. Thyroid hormone synthesis is also impaired resulting in reduced levels in dogs treated with T-S for 10 weeks or longer.[422] See Drug Formulary, Appendix 8, for further information.

Treatment with the trimethoprim-sulfadiazine combination has been associated with allergic immune complex reactions in dogs specifically as a result of the sulfonamide. Fever, polyarthritis, lymphadenomegaly, polymyositis, glomerulonephritis (proteinuria), urticaria, eosinophilic pneumonitis, pancreatitis, focal retinitis, suspected meningitis, hemolytic anemia, facial palsy, leukopenia (neutropenia), and thrombocytopenia have been noted.[143,379] Doberman pinschers may be predisposed to these reactions. In a review of 40 dogs with potentiated sulfonamide hypersensitivity, Samoyeds (8%) and miniature Schnauzers (13%) were also overrepresented.[379] Immune-mediated, cutaneous drug eruptions have occurred in dogs treated with trimethoprim-sulfamethoxazole (see Drug Formulary, Appendix 8). A presumed immune-mediated meningitis has been described in people given trimethoprim-sulfamethoxazole. An association exists between hypersensitivity after the receipt of sulfonamides and a subsequent reaction to sulfonamide nonantibiotics, but this appears to be a predisposition to allergic reactions because these individuals also have a higher reaction rate to penicillins.[358] People have developed increased serum potassium and creatinine concentrations in some instances.[238] See the Drug Formulary (Appendix 8) for a summary of the adverse reactions associated with T-S.

QUINOLONES

Pharmacokinetics

The quinolones (fluoroquinolones) are a diverse group of bactericidal naphthyridine derivatives that prevent bacterial DNA synthesis by partly inhibiting bacterial topoisomerase (TP)-II (DNA gyrase) and TP-IV. Quinolones affect primarily TP-II in gram-negative organisms and TP-IV in some gram-positive organisms. They have less activity against mammalian TPs. The lower susceptibility of TP-IV to quinolones may partly explain the higher MICs for many gram-positive organisms. Compared with some rarely used first- and second-generation compounds (nalidixic acid, flumequine, pipemidic acid), the third-generation quinolones, such as ciprofloxacin, marbofloxacin, difloxacin, orbifloxacin, ibafloxacin, and enrofloxacin (Table 34-11), have improved antibacterial spectrum, increased bioavailability, favorable pharmacokinetics, and less toxicity and bacterial resistance. The last five drugs named are marketed for use in small animals; danofloxacin has been licensed for use in cattle and sarafloxacin for poultry. Third-generation quinolones have limited plasma protein

binding and differ with respect to extent and rate of biotransformation, elimination rate, and route of excretion. Enrofloxacin is converted to ciprofloxacin, and then approximately 50% of the administered amount is excreted in urine as ciprofloxacin and its metabolites. Difloxacin is largely metabolized and excreted in bile, with minimal amounts in urine, while approximately 40% of orbifloxacin is excreted in urine. Approximately 50% of marbofloxacin is excreted unchanged in urine with equal amounts excreted unchanged in bile.

Fourth-generation quinolones licensed in human medicine have included levofloxacin, cilinafloxacin, sparfloxacin, gatifloxacin, gemifloxacin, grepafloxacin, trovafloxacin, and moxifloxacin and have enhanced pharmacokinetics and increased spectrum of activity against important pathogens. In people, these drugs are generally well absorbed orally and have longer half-lives, supporting once-daily dosing. Although levofloxacin is excreted primarily by the kidneys, the others are predominantly eliminated in the bile. The dose of levofloxacin must be reduced in renal failure, while that of the others must be reduced in patients with hepatic dysfunction. Additional studies are needed to show whether findings are similar for animals.

Variable GI absorption occurs with quinolones. Food and antacids inhibit their absorption. Absorption of all quinolones is impaired by concurrent administration of preparations containing multivalent cations (magnesium, bismuth, iron, zinc, aluminum) such as antacids and by sucralfate-containing preparations. To improve plasma concentrations in dogs and cats in these circumstances, giving the quinolone at least 2 hours before these preparations or using parenteral administration might be preferable.

Quinolones have high bioavailability, low ionization, and low protein binding and are lipophilic. Consequently, concentrations attained in tissues and body fluids often equal or exceed those in plasma. High levels are achieved in prostate, kidney, liver, and lung, with lower but therapeutic concentrations in respiratory secretions, saliva, and prostatic fluid. Urine concentrations are well above the MICs of most urinary pathogens, and CSF concentrations are adequate if inflammation is present. Fecal levels are adequate to inhibit most GI enteropathogens. Quinolones exhibit concentration-dependent killing of bacteria. High peak concentration reached in vivo and persistence of good concentrations, which together contribute to the AUC, are important in determining a dosage regimen to treat a particular infection.[228,377] The total amount of drug given daily, rather than the dosing regimen, primarily determines the in vivo potency of these drugs.[9] However, once-daily dosing achieves higher maximum fluid and tissue concentrations than divided dosing, and better owner compliance is anticipated. Marbofloxacin and difloxacin have half-lives that are twice that of enrofloxacin; hence the dose rate is somewhat lower for susceptible pathogens. When the maximum concentration of quinolone achieved exceeds twice the pathogen's MIC, a favorable response is expected. When the concentration of quinolone in a body fluid or tissue is eight or more times higher than the MIC, bacterial regrowth from selection of resistant subpopulations can be prevented. Higher plasma concentrations enhance penetration of quinolones into body fluids, secretions, and other harder-to-enter tissues, including CSF, prostate, and bone. Concentrations of quinolones in bile or urine may be hundreds of times greater than the MIC for susceptible bacteria. The drugs also enter skin and may accumulate there, especially with inflammation. High concentrations are achieved in phagocytic cells, exceeding plasma concentrations by a factor of 100. Coadministration with probenecid, furosemide, and nonsteroidal antiinflammatory drugs increases plasma concentrations of quinolones. For resistant organisms, the lowest recommended

Table • 34-11

Quinolones Licensed for Human and Veterinary Use[a]

GENERIC NAME (TRADE NAME [Mfgr])		ORAL BIOAVAILABILITY (%)	FORMULATIONS
First and Second Generation[b]			
Nalidixic acid (NegGram [Sandofi])		95	Tablets: 500 mg
Cinoxacin (Cinobac [Oclassen])		95	Tablets: 250 mg, 500 mg
Third Generation[c]			
Human	Norfloxacin (Noroxin [Merck])	30—50	Tablets: 400 mg
	Ciprofloxacin (Cipro [Bayer])	75—80	Tablets: 250 mg, 500 mg, 750 mg Injection: 200-mg and 400-mg vials
	Ofloxacin (Floxin [Ortho])	>95	Tablets: 200 mg, 300 mg, 400 mg Injection: 200-mg and 400-mg vials
	Lomafloxacin (Maxaguin [Searle])	>95	Tablets: 400 mg
	Enoxacin (Penetrex [Rhone-Poulenc])	90	Tablets: 200 mg, 400 mg
	Fleroxacin (Megalone [Roche], Quinodis [Roche])	>80	Tablets: 200 mg, 400 mg
	Amifloxacin (Investigational [Sterling Winthrop])	>90	200 mg
Veterinary[a]	Enrofloxacin[d] (Baytril [Bayer])	>80	Tablets 5.7 mg, 22.7 mg, 68 mg Injection: 22.7 mg/ml
	Marbofloxacin (Marbocyl [Vetoquinol], Zeniquin [Pfizer])	>90	Tablets: 5 mg, 20 mg, 80 mg
	Orbifloxacin (Orbax [Schering-Plough])	97	Tablets: 5.7 mg, 22.7 mg, 68 mg
	Difloxacin (Dicural [Fort Dodge])	>80	Tablets: 11.4 mg, 45.4 mg, 136 mg
	Ibafloxacin (Ibaflin [Intervet])	69—81	Tablets: 30 mg, 150 mg, 300 mg, 900 mg
Fourth Generation[e]			
Levofloxacin (Levaquin [Ortho-McNeil])		~100	Tablets: 250 mg, 500 mg Injection: 250-mg and 500-mg vials
Moxifloxacin (Avelox [Bayer])		>90	Tablets: 400 mg Injection: 400-mg bags
Gatifloxacin (Tequin [Bristol-Myers])		>90	Tablets: 200 and 400 mg Injection: 200- and 400-mg vials
Gemifloxacin (Factive [GeneSoft])		~61	Tablets: 320 mg

[a]Only third-generation drugs are licensed for veterinary purposes. The listed veterinary preparations are licensed for dogs and cats. In some countries, sarafloxacin, benofloxacin, enrofloxacin, and ofloxacin are licensed for poultry; enrofloxacin, danofloxacin, and orbifloxacin are licensed for cattle and swine. See Drug Formulary (Appendix 8) for more specific information and dosages.
[b]Restricted to use in gram-negative urinary tract infections; not recommended because of high toxicity.
[c]Primarily active against gram-negative aerobic bacteria, *Mycoplasma*, chlamydiae, some *Mycobacterium*, and rickettsiae.
[d]Metabolized to ciprofloxacin. Bioavailability is extrapolated from absorption of ciprofloxacin.
[e]Similar to third generation but more active against staphylococci, streptococci, and obligate anaerobes. Grepafloxacin, temafloxacin, trovafloxacin, and sparfloxacin have been withdrawn or have restricted use in people because of adverse effects such as cardiac arrhythmias, hepatic necrosis, or hemolytic-uremic syndrome.

label dosages may not be suitable, and higher or twice daily dosing may be necessary. Current labeling for quinolones in the United States requires flexible dosing. Knowing the concentration likely to be achieved at the site of infection and the MIC data for the intended pathogen is helpful in making this determination. Achievable concentrations in tissues following intended dosages are listed in quinolone product inserts and the Drug Formulary (Appendix 8).

Quinolones kill bacteria at concentrations close to MIC values and have marked PAE, which account for their ability to inhibit bacterial growth up to 4 to 8 hours after drug is eliminated from the body. The high drug concentrations in phagocytes means they reach higher concentrations at inflammatory sites.[30] They are partially metabolized by the liver and excreted in bile or urine as parent drug or metabolites, or both, most of which have antibacterial activity. Concentrations achieved in bile and urine are 10 to 20 times higher than that in plasma. Urine recovery varies from 30% to 70%, depending on the drug. The biliary excreted fraction of some quinolones undergoes enterohepatic circulation. At recommended dosages in dogs, levels of enrofloxacin were adequate to kill most pathogens; however, higher levels were needed to achieve levels for resistant organisms such as *P. aeruginosa.*[37]

Use of quinolones in neonates and cats is restricted, because of their potential toxicity to growing cartilage and retinal tissue (see Toxicity later in this text). Pharmacokinetics of enrofloxacin in nursing kittens has been compared with that of young and adult cats.[341] The half-life and elimination of enrofloxacin administered IV or SC to 2-, 6-, and 8-week-old kittens was shorter than that in adults resulting in lower peak plasma concentrations. SC administration resulted in poor uptake by the 2- to 4-week-old kittens. Oral administration to all age kittens resulted in poor bioavailability and inadequate therapeutic concentrations. See Drug Formulary, Appendix 8, for further information.

Indications

The third-generation quinolones are active primarily against gram-negative aerobic and facultative anaerobic bacteria and are more effective in alkaline pH (above 7.4). Although many gram-positive bacterial pathogens are susceptible, MIC ranges usually are higher than those for gram-negative organisms. Third-generation quinolones are not ideal for treating infections caused by obligate anaerobes or *Streptococcus*, and other drugs should be considered first. Activity against *Staphylococcus* is variable, but some staphylococci resistant to many other drugs may be susceptible to quinolones. Fourth-generation quinolones are broad-spectrum antimicrobials with excellent in vitro activity against gram-positive and gram-negative bacteria, including activity against intracellular pathogens. Although these quinolones have better activity against gram-positive organisms, they have less efficacy against gram-negative bacteria. For example, gatifloxacin, moxifloxacin, and gemifloxacin have enhanced activity against gram-positive bacteria, especially against streptococci; and although their efficacy against gram-negative bacteres is preserved, it is often less than the earlier generation quinolones.[328] This lower activity is particularly true for *P. aeruginosa.* The activity of fourth-generation drugs against anaerobes is variable and not as strong as other first-choice drugs that offer better alternatives. Some rickettsiae are susceptible to quinolones. Some of the drugs have activity against chlamydiae, *Mycoplasma, Bartonella,* and some mycobacteria.[360] Enrofloxacin was effective in treating *Mycoplasma haemofelis* infection in cats (see Chapter 31) but only at a higher dose that had a risk of retinal toxicity.[105] However, enrofloxacin was not effective in treating *Ehrlichia canis* infection in experimentally infected dogs.[271] Ciprofloxacin, enrofloxacin, and ofloxacin are active against *Mycobacterium tuberculosis* and some atypical mycobacteria but not against *Mycobacterium avium* complex. Quinolones have good activity against bacterial enteropathogens, such as *Salmonella, Shigella, Campylobacter, Yersinia enterocolitica,* and *Escherichia.* Third-generation drugs have some activity against some anaerobes such as *Bacteroides, Clostridium, Fusobacterium, Porphyromonas, Bilophila,* and *Prevotella.* However, activity against these anaerobic bacteria is weakest.

The primary indications for quinolones are recurrent UTIs caused by organisms that are difficult to eliminate, such as *Pseudomonas, Proteus,* and *Klebsiella.* They are very effective in the treatment of bacterial prostatitis. In treating *Brucella,* quinolones must be used in combination with another drug, such as doxycycline, to reduce risk of relapse. Quinolones have also been used to treat enteric and respiratory infections caused by organisms resistant to other agents. Marbofloxacin, enrofloxacin, ciprofloxacin, and difloxacin have been shown to be effective, at varying levels, against *Bordetella bronchiseptica* in vitro.[59] Bone concentrations of quinolones are adequate to treat osteomyelitis if the pathogen is susceptible. Oral administration is advantageous for long-term therapy. When mixed flora are present in intraabdominal infections, quinolones have been effective against aerobic or facultative bacteria when given in combination with a drug effective against anaerobes, such as clindamycin or metronidazole. Gatifloxacin, gemifloxacin, and moxifloxacin have been licensed for use in respiratory tract infections in people. See Tables 34-12 and 34-13 for summaries of information on quinolones used in dogs and cats.

Drug Resistance

Quinolones are now being used frequently in small animal practice. Unfortunately, this trend has led to increasing bacterial resistance of isolates from dogs and cats, as has been observed in human medicine.[334] In essence, quinolones should only be prescribed when these drugs are expected to have optimal activity against the pathogen in a given organ system and other more empirically used drugs have expected or known resistance. A common misconception is that bacteria do not become resistant during treatment with quinolones. Resistance, which most often occurs during treatment of infections caused by *Pseudomonas, Klebsiella, Enterobacter, Acinetobacter, Serratia, Enterococcus,* and *Staphylococcus,* is chromosomal rather than plasmid mediated.[226,227] Bacteria may become cross-resistant to several quinolones at one time but not necessarily to antimicrobials in other classes. The quinolones have been restricted from use in food-producing animals in hopes of preventing development of drug-resistant strains of zoonotic pathogens.[11] Multidrug- and quinolone-resistant *Escherichia* have been isolated with increasing frequency from companion animals under veterinary care.[76,404] A significant increasing resistance was noted to canine urinary isolates such as *Proteus mirabilis, Staphylococcus intermedius,* and *E. coli* between the years of 1992 and 2001 for either ciprofloxacin or enrofloxacin.[73] A cause for concern is that these organisms, which can be isolated from many areas in the hospital environment, develop resistance from frequent exposure to a variety of broad-spectrum antimicrobials.[327] To avoid increasing resistance, quinolones should be used prudently and carefully and not as drugs for first-time treatments or for infections that will likely respond to other drugs. One example would be in treatment of anaerobic infections or pyodermas in which other drugs should be tried first. Dosing for infections should always be adequate enough to prevent the induction of antimicrobial resistance as subinhibitory concentrations of enrofloxacin have caused a selection for drug-resistant mutants of *S. intermedius* in culture.[121] In vitro studies with canine bacterial isolates from otitis externa and urinary infection showed that *Pseudomonas aeruginosa* and *Enterococcus* spp. develop resistance more rapidly and more consistently than *Klebsiella, Proteus,* and *Streptococcus* when exposed to enrofloxacin.[46]

Toxicity

See Table 34-14 for a summary of toxic effects of quinolones.

Gastrointestinal

The most common adverse events induced by quinolones are vomiting, diarrhea, abdominal discomfort, and taste disturbances. These effects are usually mild or moderate and can be alleviated by temporarily reducing or discontinuing therapy. Alimentary reactions associated with quinolones are product and dose related. The mechanism is uncertain but presumably relates to direct irritation of the GI tract and to CNS stimulation because it can occur with both PO and parenteral administration. Dogs inadvertently or experimentally given high doses of quinolones have often vomited and therefore may not develop other acute toxic manifestations.

Cardiovascular

Quinolones are relatively safe at routine oral and parenteral dosages. Prokaryotic DNA gyrase is partially affected by these

Table • 34-12

Relative Activity of Selected Veterinary Quinolones Against Bacteria Isolated from Animals, as Determined by MIC90[a]

	CONCENTRATIONS (µg/ml)			
ORGANISM	DIFLOXACIN	ENROFLOXACIN	MARBOFLOXACIN	ORBIFLOXACIN
Gram Negative				
Escherichia coli	0.25—16	0.06—2.0	0.06—2.0	0.5—4.0
Klebsiella pneumoniae	0.5	0.12—0.25	0.01—0.06	0.25
Proteus spp.	1.0	0.25—0.5	0.125	1.0
Pasteurella multocida	ND	0.016—0.03	<0.008—0.5	ND
Salmonella spp.	0.125	0.03—0.25	0.03	0.25
Bordetella bronchiseptica	4.0	0.5	0.5	2.0
Pseudomonas aeruginosa	4.0—8.0	1.0—8.0	0.06—4.0	4.0—16
Gram Positive				
Staphylococcus intermedius	1.0	0.12—0.5	0.25	0.5
S. aureus	1.0	0.12	0.25—0.5	0.5
Enterococcus spp.	ND	1.0—2.0	1.0—4.0	16—32
β-hemolytic *Streptococcus*	ND	ND	2.0	1.0—2.0
Anaerobes				
Clostridium	ND	0.5	ND	ND
Bacteroides	ND	0.5	ND	ND
Porphyromonas gingivalis	ND	1.5	ND	ND
Bifidobacterium	ND	2.0	ND	ND
Prevotella oralis group	ND	1.0	ND	ND

ND, Not determined.
Data from Walker RD. 2000. The use of fluoroquinolones for companion animal antimicrobial therapy, *Aust Vet J* 78:84–90; Pirro F, Edinglh M, Schmeer N. 1999. Bactericidal and inhibitory activity of enrofloxacin and other flurorquinolones in small animal pathogens, *In* Proc Third Int Vet Symp Fluoroquinolones. *Compend Contin Educ Pract Vet 21*(suppl):19–25; Boeckh A et al. 2001. Time course of enrofloxacin and its active metabolite in peripheral leukocytes of dogs, *Vet Ther* 2:334–344; Nielsen D. 1999. Clinical experience with an enrofloxacin-metronidazole combination in the treatment of periodontal disease in dogs and cats, *In* Proc Third Int Vet Symp Fluoroquinolones, *Compend Cont Educ Pract Vet* 21:88–94.
[a]Lower concentration indicates greater susceptibility. This table should be used as a guide to efficacy. Isolates of the same bacterial species can differ in their antimicrobial resistance depending on differences in time, geography, laboratory methodology, and prior exposure to antimicrobial drugs.

compounds; therefore extremely high concentrations of fluoroquinolones can cause systemic toxicity. Rapid IV administration of 10 to 30 mg/kg of certain quinolones to anesthetized dogs or cats produces systemic hypotension, presumably related to histamine release. Hypotension and tachycardia have also been seen after oral administration. In people, the newer quinolones, sparfloxacin and grepafloxacin have caused prolongation of the QT interval and rare arrhythmias and have been withdrawn from human use for this reason. All quinolones have the potential to cause this effect because of presumed gene inhibition involving the potassium channel. Moxifloxacin, gatifloxacin, and levofloxacin carry precautionary statements about this effect.

Central Nervous System

Abnormal electroencephalographic activity has been observed in dogs and cats after IV administration of 25 mg/kg or greater.[69] Quinolones directly inhibit gamma-aminobutyric acid and stimulate N-methyl D-aspartate receptors. Tremors and ataxia have been reported. Seizures developed in some animals, presumably those with low seizure threshold. Seizures have been precipitated by administration of quinolones parenterally with concurrent nonsteroidal antiinflammatory drugs, such as fenbufen and ibuprofen. The authors (CEG and ADJW) have also observed drug-induced seizures in a dog

receiving quinolones and antiemetic phenothiazines concurrently. An accidental administration of a fourfold overdose of enrofloxacin caused a dog with CNS lymphoma to seizure.

Ocular

Quinolones have limited solubility at alkaline pH and may crystallize in various tissues. Dogs given high doses had subcapsular lenticular cataract formation and associated inflammation after treatment for 8 to 12 months. Cats given high or IV doses of enrofloxacin have developed acute blindness from retinotoxicity and photoreceptor damage.* They develop acute blindness and mydriasis. Experimentally, administration of oral dosages greater than 30 mg/kg/day for 21 days resulted in retinal degeneration, abnormal electroretinograms, and microscopic changes in the retina.[1,409] In case studies, cats receiving oral dosages ranging from 4.6 to 54 mg/kg/day developed retinal toxicity within 2 days to 12 weeks.[124] A majority of the cats received dosages much higher than 5 mg/kg/day given twice daily or were given IV infusions of the drug. Label recommendations indicate that cats should not receive a dose greater than 5 mg/kg/day, and IV injections of enrofloxacin should be avoided. Similar toxicity has been observed with orbifloxacin at higher than recommended

*References: 1, 84, 124, 420, 423.

Table • 34-13

Peak Serum Concentrations of Quinolones in Dogs and Cats Given Various Dosages

DRUG	SPECIES	ROUTE	DOSE (mg/kg)	PEAK SERUM CONCENTRATION (µg/ml)
Difloxacin	Dogs	PO	5.0	1.1—1.8
			10.0	3.6
Enrofloxacin	Dogs	PO	2.75	0.7
			5.0	1.2—1.41
			5.5	1.4
			7.5	1.9
			11.0	2.1
		SC	20.0	4.4—5.2
			5.0	1.3
Marbofloxacin	Dogs	PO	1.0	0.8
			2.0	1.4—1.47
			2.5	2.0
			2.75	2.0
			4.0	2.9
			5.0	4.2
			5.5	4.2
Orbifloxacin	Dogs (cats)[a]	PO	2.5	1.37—2.3 (1.6—2.1)[a]
			7.5	6.0—6.9 (5.0)[a]
Ibafloxacin	Dogs	PO	7.5	3.72
			15	6.04
			30	12.15

PO, By mouth; SC, subcutaneous.

Data Adapted from: Walker RD. 2000. The use of fluoroquinolones for companion animal antimicrobial therapy, *Aust Vet J* 78:84-90; Boothe DM et al. 2002. Plasma concentrations of enrofloxacin and its active metabolite ciprofloxacin in dogs following single oral administration of enrofloxacin at 7.5, 10, or 20mg/kg, *Vet Ther* 3:409-419; Heinen E. 1999. Comparative pharmacokinetics of enrofloxacin as well as their main metabolites in dogs. *In* Proc Third Int Vet Symp on Fluoroquinolones, *Compend Cont Educ Pract Vet* 21:12-18. Drug Insert, Orbax Tablets, Schering Pharmaceuticals. Drug Insert, Zeniquin, Pfizer Animal Health; and Boeckh A, Boothe DM, Wilkie S. 1999. Time course of enrofloxacin and its active metabolite in peripheral leukocytes of dogs. *In* Proc Third Int Vet Symp on Fluoroquinolones, *Compend Cont Educ Pract Vet* 21:40-43; Coulet M et al. 2002. Pharmacokinetics of ibafloxacin following intravenous and oral administration to healthy beagle dogs. *J Vet Pharmacol Ther* 25:89-97; Heinen E. 2002. Comparative serum pharmacokinetics of the fluoroquinolones enrofloxacin, difloxacin, marbofloxacin, and orbifloxacin in dogs after single oral administration, *J Vet Pharmacol Ther* 25:1-5.

[a]Data for cats.

Table • 34-14

Fluoroquinolone Toxicity in Dogs and Cats

SYSTEM INVOLVED	ADVERSE REACTIONS OBSERVED
Central nervous system	Seizures, retinal blindness (cats)
Cardiovascular	Cardiac arrhythmias (people)
Musculoskeletal	Arthropathy in juveniles
Hepatic	Increased hepatic transaminases and alkaline phosphatase concentrations
Renal	Crystalluria-induced renal dysfunction
Gastrointestinal	Anorexia, vomiting, diarrhea
Dermatologic	Urticaria, photosensitization, pruritus

dosages.[190,420] Quinolone-associated retinal degeneration is a dose-related toxicity and not an idiosyncratic reaction. Use of co-administered drugs that increase quinolone plasma concentrations should be avoided. The blindness may be transient if it is recognized early and medication is discontinued.

Hepatic

Therapeutic doses may cause increased blood hepatic enzyme activities, especially in combination with other hepatotoxic drugs. Quinolones inhibit cytochrome P450–mediated drug metabolism.[168] As a result, they may increase the concentrations and potential toxicity of co-administered drugs that are metabolized by this system. Increased hepatotoxicity or delayed metabolism causing anorexia and increased blood hepatic transaminase concentrations have occurred when these drugs were co-administered with others, such as itraconazole, that are also metabolized by the liver and potentially hepatotoxic.[140] Trovafloxacin, a fourth-generation quinolone, was withdrawn from the market because of hepatotoxicity.

Renal

At high or supratherapeutic dosages in dogs, renal toxicity developed from crystalluria and crystal deposition in tubular lumens, especially at alkaline urine pH. Nephrotoxicity has also occurred uncommonly in people and dogs treated with usual therapeutic dosages. Temafloxacin, a fourth-generation quinolone, was withdrawn from the market because it caused hemolytic uremic syndrome and hypoglycemia.

Glucose Homeostasis

Some quinolones such as ciprofloxacin, levofloxacin, and moxifloxacin have caused minor alterations in blood glucose and insulin production in people. Gatifloxacin has been associated with more severe disruptions, especially in persons with diabetes and older adults.

Skeletal

Quinolones inhibit mitochondrial dehydrogenase activity and proteoglycan synthesis, resulting in cartilaginous damage.[163] Quinolones also chelate magnesium, altering chondrocyte-surface integrin receptors and cartilage-matrix integrity.[56] These findings are accentuated by magnesium deficiency. Cartilaginous defects in growing cartilage of young dogs[54,55] were accentuated by exercise and prevented by exercise restriction. Dose levels may be important in the production of joint damage, given that juvenile dogs did not develop arthropathy if they were treated with ofloxacin at lower doses.[431,434] Nevertheless, quinolones are contraindicated in dogs during the rapid-growth phase, between 2 to 8 months in small and medium breeds, up to 1 year in large breeds, and up to 18 months in giant breeds. Tendonitis and tendon ruptures have occurred in people.

Systemic

Allergic reactions are characterized by erythema and edema of the face and ears with shivering or shaking. Cats given high doses of ciprofloxacin developed pinnae erythema, vomiting, and clonic muscle spasms.

Reproductive

Because of effects on DNA synthesis and known fetal toxicity in other species, these drugs should not be given to young (under 6 months of age) or pregnant dogs or cats. High doses have been fetotoxic in animals. Because these drugs are excreted in milk, they should be avoided in lactating animals. High doses (100 mg/kg) for longer than 3 months have been associated with impaired spermatogenesis and testicular atrophy in dogs.

Cutaneous

Allergic and photosensitive dermal reactions have developed in people being treated with quinolones. Suspected photosensitization, exhibited by inflammation of the planum nasale, was observed each time a dog was treated with enrofloxacin.[140] Quinolones have a high affinity for melanin pigments and are taken up by the iris, choroids, and dermal melanocytes. Thus the ocular and cutaneous toxicities may have a similar mechanism. The absorption of UV light results in the formation of cytotoxic photodegradation products that may lead to the cutaneous inflammation observed.

STREPTOGRAMINS AND OXAZOLIDINONES

Quinupristin-dalforpristin are two streptogramin antibacterials marketed in combination, as a 30:70 ratio mixture, for treating *resistant* gram-positive bacterial infections in people.[110] They act synergistically on bacterial ribosomal protein synthesis for a bactericidal effect. This combination has been licensed to treat methicillin- and vancomycin-resistant staphylococci and *Enterococcus faecium* infections in people. Quinupristin-dalforpristin are inactive against *Enterococcus faecalis*. These drugs are effective also against

Mycoplasma spp. and *Clostridium perfringens*. Worldwide, gram-positive bacteria from people have been highly susceptible; however, genes mediating dalfopristin inactivation have been found in resistant strains of *E. faecium* recovered from some animals such as chickens where antibacterials have been used as food additives.[159,246] Linezolid is a synthetic oxazolidinone antimicrobial that also inhibits ribosomal protein synthesis. It is well absorbed when given orally. As with streptogramins, linezolid is effective against gram-positive bacteria, including both *E. faecium* and *E. faecalis*, and has been licensed for similar resistant strains of bacteria.[110] Because of their important role in drug-resistant human bacterial infections and the risk of inducing resistant bacterial strains in food or companion animals, the use of these two groups of drugs should be restricted or avoided in veterinary patients.

PLEUROMUTILINS

Tiamulin and valnemulin are members of a novel antibiotic class that is marketed for use only in food-producing animals. These drugs act by interfering with ribosomal protein synthesis. This group of drugs is highly active against *Mycoplasma* and spirochetes. They have been used to treat drug-resistant spirochetal infections in swine such as swine dysentery, porcine proliferative enteropathy and porcine colonic spirochetosis, and porcine respiratory disease caused by mycoplasmas. Tiamulin and valnemulin are formulated as feed additives and have not been studied in dogs or cats. Valnemulin was used to treat drug-resistant *Mycoplasma* infections in two immunocompromised people.[160] Toxicity occurs when these drugs are given in combination with ionophore antimicrobials.

KETOLIDES

Telithromycin is the first drug licensed in this new class of antibiotics. It has a spectrum of activity against gram-positive organisms. Indications for people are treatment of upper and lower respiratory tract infections. Because of their important role in drug-resistant human bacterial infections and the risk of inducing resistant bacterial strains in food or companion animals, the use of these drugs should be restricted or avoided in veterinary patients.

URINARY ANTISEPTICS

Methenamine (hexamethylenetetramine), a highly water-soluble organic compound, is rapidly absorbed after oral administration and excreted primarily in urine. It decomposes in acidic urine to form formaldehyde and is used only for long-term treatment and prophylaxis of UTIs. The tablets are enteric-coated to prevent degradation by gastric acid and often contain organic acids (mandelic, hippuric, sulfosalicylic salts) to lower urine pH and facilitate formaldehyde production. Antibacterial activity is largely confined to the bladder because transit through the upper urinary tract is rapid, allowing insufficient time to generate formaldehyde.

ANTITUBERCULOUS DRUGS

Isoniazid

This hydrazide derivative of isonicotinic acid is one of the most active compounds against *M. tuberculosis*. Isoniazid interferes with synthesis of mycolic acids in mycobacterial cell walls and acts only against replicating bacteria, leaving slow-growing or inactive organisms unaffected. Absorption of isoniazid from the intestine is rapid but inhibited by antacids, and much of the dose is excreted unchanged in the urine within 24 hours. Isoniazid penetrates most tissues well. CSF concentration is 20% of that of plasma but increases to 100% in the presence of CNS inflammation. Most strains of *M. tuberculosis* are sensitive to isoniazid, but resistance usually develops during therapy. Therefore drug susceptibility testing is recommended.

The principal side effects of isoniazid, hepatotoxicity and increased blood hepatic enzyme concentrations, are reversed if therapy is discontinued immediately. Peripheral neuropathy and CNS excitability may be caused by monoamine oxidase antagonism. Seizures, tremors, and hyperexcitability were seen in dogs that were overdosed.[100] Immune-mediated thrombocytopenia occurred in one dog treated with isoniazid.[88] GI irritation, allergic skin reaction, and vasculitis have also been reported in people.

Rifampin (Rifampicin)

This semisynthetic hydrazone derivative of rifampin B interferes with RNA synthesis. It is well absorbed from the GI tract. Rifampin is lipid-soluble and 75% to 90% of the drug is bound to serum protein. It penetrates all body tissues and reaches higher concentrations than those in blood in lung, liver, bile, cholecystic wall, and urine. Therapeutic concentrations of rifampin are attained in pleural exudate, ascites, milk, urinary bladder wall, soft tissue, and CSF. Much of the drug is metabolized by the liver and excreted in the bile. Only 6% to 30% appears in the urine.

Rifampin has antibacterial, antichlamydial, and some antiviral activity. It is primarily used to treat infections caused by *M. tuberculosis* and other mycobacteria. Rifampin is also one of the most active antibiotics against *Staphylococcus* and is effective against some gram-negative pathogens. This antibiotic is frequently helpful in combination with β-lactam drugs to treat resistant staphylococcal endocarditis or osteomyelitis. The drug has been combined with vancomycin or with cephalosporins to enhance efficacy against *Staphylococcus*. Rifampin was superior to tetracycline for treatment of experimental *Brucella* infection in laboratory animals but was inferior to minocycline in treating naturally occurring canine brucellosis. Rifampin also has effectiveness in treatment of feline bartonellosis (see Chapter 54). Although ineffective against fungi when administered alone, rifampin has been shown to enhance the effect of amphotericin B and miconazole against *Candida*.

Resistance to rifampin may develop rapidly when it is used alone, but it can be hindered by combining it with other drugs. Side effects include orange-colored urine, tears, saliva, and sweat. Rash, GI signs, and increased liver enzyme concentrations may be associated with long-term daily administration. Many other side effects have been noted at higher doses; therefore it should always be reformulated to the calculated dose when given to dogs and cats. Rifampin accelerates hepatic metabolism of other drugs and reduces the activity of concurrently administered glucocorticoids, digoxin, quinidine, barbiturates, isoniazid, dapsone, and theophylline.

Rifabutin

This drug is structurally similar to rifampin but is more lipid-soluble. Rifabutin has better tissue distribution but lower oral bioavailability. Rifabutin is extensively metabolized to active intermediates, and it can be used as a substitute for rifampin and has less effect on hepatic metabolism of other drugs.

Ethambutol

This tuberculostatic drug interferes with RNA synthesis and is active only against dividing organisms. It is well absorbed from the GI tract and is widely distributed in body tissues, including CSF. Most of the drug is excreted unmetabolized in urine, and the dose should be reduced in patients with renal failure. The main toxic effect is optic and peripheral neuritis.

Miscellaneous Drugs

Para-aminosalicylic acid is an analog of PABA that is mycobacteriostatic, interfering with folic acid synthesis. It potentiates the effect of isoniazid by delaying its metabolism. Pyrazinamide, a tuberculostatic drug with an unknown mode of action, is relatively hepatotoxic. Cycloserine inhibits bacterial cell wall synthesis and is excreted primarily by the kidneys. Ethionamide inhibits protein synthesis and has widespread tissue distribution. PABA is combined in therapy when resistance is found to other drugs. Viomycin, capreomycin, kanamycin, and amikacin have all been shown to be effective against mycobacteria when combined with other drugs. See Chapter 50 for a discussion of tuberculosis in dogs and cats.

DRUGS AGAINST RAPIDLY GROWING OPPORTUNISTIC MYCOBACTERIA

Some antituberculous drugs, such as isoniazid, rifampin, and AGs, are effective in treating other mycobacteria. Other antimicrobials have also been successful in some cases, including erythromycin, clarithromycin, doxycycline, minocycline, enrofloxacin, clofazimine, T-S, and drugs used to treat human leprosy (see Therapy sections, Chapter 50).

Dapsone is a sulfone derivative that is bacteriostatic to bactericidal against *Mycobacterium leprae*. It is absorbed completely from the bowel, metabolized in the liver, and eliminated mainly by renal excretion. Toxic effects in dogs have consisted of hemolytic anemia, leukopenia, thrombocytopenia, and increased liver enzyme activities. Acedapsone is a derivative with longer duration of action. Clofazimine, a dye with antiprotozoal and antifungal activity, is active against *M. leprae*, *M. avium*-complex organisms, and opportunistic mycobacteria. This drug should always be given in combination with other drugs. For additional information on dapsone and clofazimine, see Chapter 50 and the Drug Formulary (Appendix 8).

TOPICAL ANTIBACTERIAL DRUGS

Bacitracin

This mixture of cyclic peptides has bactericidal activity against many gram-positive aerobic pathogens, including *Staphylococcus*, *Streptococcus*, *Corynebacterium*, *Clostridium*, and *Actinomyces*. Bacitracin is not absorbed to any extent after topical or oral administration and is nephrotoxic when given parenterally. Accordingly, its use is limited to surface application for treating infections of skin, ear, and eye. Bacitracin is often given in conjunction with an AG (usually neomycin) and polymyxin. The principal toxic effect of bacitracin is hypersensitivity associated with topical application.

Mupirocin

This novel antibiotic, unrelated in structure and action to other known antimicrobials, inhibits bacterial protein synthesis. It is bactericidal against *Staphylococcus*, *Streptococcus*, and some gram-negative aerobic pathogens. The drug is available commercially as a topical ointment. The only side effect observed has been local dermal hypersensitivity reaction at the site of application in some animals.

Fusidic Acid

The principal interest in fusidic acid lies in its excellent activity against *Staphylococcus* spp., including β-lactamase–producing and methicillin-resistant strains. Fusidic acid is available in some countries in enteral, parenteral, and topical preparations.

Topical Buffered EDTA Solution

Many gram-negative bacteria are susceptible to chelating agents such as ethylenediaminetetraacetic acid (EDTA). The bactericidal effect appears to occur by removal of cations from the bacterial cell wall, resulting in leakage of cell solutes. Alkaline pH appears to facilitate bactericidal activity. Research has proved EDTA to be safe when applied topically to animal tissues. Appropriate pH is maintained by combining it with stable amino buffers, such as tromethamine (TRIS) hydrochloride at pH 8. Administration of this combination is restricted to topical application or irrigation because toxicity can result from removal of blood cations such as calcium and production of nephrocalcinosis. The buffered EDTA solution can be made with easily obtainable ingredients or it is available commercially (Table 34-15). Incorporation of sodium dodecyl sulfate, an ionic detergent, improves efficacy. Buffered EDTA solutions have been administered alone and in combination with several antimicrobial agents to treat various resistant bacterial infections in dogs and cats. A primary use has been against *Pseudomonas* organisms, which are resistant to many antibacterial drugs. Use with lysozyme, gentamicin, or oxytetracycline has been attempted to increase the potency of these drugs and to decrease the incidence of antimicrobial resistance.[112,113,349] The increased permeability of gram-negative bacterial cell walls may facilitate drug penetration and

antimicrobial activity. Overgrowth of fungi may occur during such treatment unless an antifungal drug is used simultaneously. Such overgrowth may be more likely when treating infections in body regions lacking a normal competitive microflora, such as the urinary bladder. Repeated catheteriza-

Table • 34-15

Improved Formula for Buffered EDTA Solution[a]

1. Dissolve 1.2 g of EDTA in 1 L of 0.05 M (6.05 g) tromethamine (hydroxymethyl) aminomethane (TRIS) and 1.9 g/L sodium dodecyl sulfate[b]
2. Adjust pH to 8.0 (usually requires concentrated NaOH)
3. Sterilize in autoclave (121°C for 20 min) or filter with 0.22-μm filter.
4. Store in sterile bottles at room temperature. Stable for 1 year.
5. Can add gentamicin (3 mg/ml) or amikacin (9 mg/ml).

EDTA, Ethylenediaminetetraaceticacid; *NaOH,* sodium hydroxide.
[a]Also available commercially: Tricide® and Tricide (Neo), Molecular Therapeutics LLC, Athens, GA.
[b]Sodium dodecyl sulfate improves efficacy.

Table • 34-16

Safety of Antimicrobial Drugs in Various Clinical Situations

	RENAL DYSFUNCTION	HEPATIC DYSFUNCTION	PREGNANCY	NEONATE
Probably safe	Chloramphenicol, doxycycline, griseofulvin, macrolides, penicillins (including clavulanate)	Aminoglycosides, cephalosporins, penicillins (including clavulanate)	Cephalosporins, erythromycin, lincomycin, penicillins (including clavulanate)	Cephalosporins, macrolides, penicillins (including clavulanate)
Consider dosage adjustment	Fluoroquinolones, lincomycin, trimethoprim-sulfonamide (dog)	Clindamycin, metronidazole	Nitrofurantoin, sulfonamides, trimethoprim-sulfonamide, tylosin	Lincomycin
Use caution, can accumulate[a]	Chloramphenicol (cat), flucytosine, nitrofurantoin, tetracyclines (not doxycycline)	Chloramphenicol, lincomycin, macrolides, metronidazole, sulfonamides, tetracyclines	Aminoglycosides, amphotericin B, chloramphenicol, fluconazole, flucytosine, ketoconazole, metronidazole	Aminoglycosides, polymyxins
Potentially toxic; avoid use	Aminoglycosides,[b] amphotericin B, polymyxins, trimethoprim-sulfonamide (cat)	Chlortetracycline, erythromycin estolate, griseofulvin, ketoconazole, trimethoprim-sulfonamide (dog)	Fluoroquinolones, griseofulvin, nalidixic acid, tetracyclines	Fluoroquinolones, nitrofurans, chloramphenicol, sulfonamides, tetracyclines, trimethoprim-sulfonamide

[a]Or, potentially damaging in pregnancy.
[b]If an aminoglycoside must be used in renal failure, maintain the dose but lengthen the interval by multiplying the usual interval in hours by patient's creatinine divided by the higher reference value for creatinine.

Table • 34-17

Some General Guidelines for Antibacterial Drug Selection[a]

ORGANISMS	CLINICAL CONDITIONS	FIRST CHOICES	ALTERNATIVES	GENERALLY INEFFECTIVE
Staphylococcus	Canine pyoderma, osteomyelitis	First-generation cephalosporins, isoxazolyl penicillins, macrolides, clindamycin	Chloramphenicol, trimethoprim-sulfonamide, amoxicillin-clavulanate, quinolones	Penicillin G, aminopenicillins
Pseudomonas	Soft-tissue infections	Gentamicin, ticarcillin, ceftazidime	Cefoperazone, carbenicillin, quinolones	Aminopenicillins, first- and second-generation cephalosporins
	Urinary tract infections	Tetracyclines, quinolones	Carbenicillin	
Helicobacter	Gastric inflammation and ulceration	Combination of bismuth, doxycycline, metronidazole	Azithromycin, clarithromycin	
Leptospira, Borrelia	Leptospirosis, Lyme borreliosis	Aminopenicillins, tetracyclines, aminoglycosides	Macrolides	Third-generation cephalosporins, azithromycin
Intracellular persistent organisms[b]	Pyogranulomatous inflammation, granulomas	Combinations of tetracyclines and aminoglycosides	Clarithromycin, azithromycin, quinolones, clofazamine, rifampin	β-Lactams
Other gram-positive aerobes and facultatives, plus Pasteurella	Oral infections, bite wounds, upper respiratory infections	Penicillin G, isoxazolyl penicillins, macrolides, lincosamides	Aminopenicillins, trimethoprim-sulfonamide, chloramphenicol	Third-generation quinolones
Other gram-negative aerobes and facultatives	Urinary tract infections, small and large intestinal infections	Amoxicillin-clavulanate, first-generation cephalosporins, trimethoprim-sulfonamide	Aminoglycosides, second- and third-generation cephalosporins, quinolones, tetracyclines	Penicillin G, isoxazolyl penicillins, aminopenicillins
Obligate anaerobes[c]	Stomatitis, gingivitis, bite wounds, abscesses, pleuritis, colitis, peritonitis	Clindamycin, metronidazole, penicillin G	Amoxicillin-clavulanate chloramphenicol cefoxitin, cefotetan	Fourth-generation quinolones

[a]For specific guidelines, see chapters listed under clinical conditions. For *Mycoplasma* and chlamydiae, see therapy tables in Chapters 30, 31 and 32.
[b]*Brucella, Mycobacteria,* and *Bartonella.*
[c]*Clostridium, Prevotella, Bacteroides, Fusobacterium,* etc.

tion and flushing with these solutions may also favor introduction and persistence of resistant bacterial strains.

SAFETY OF ANTIBACTERIAL DRUGS AND GUIDELINES FOR SELECTION

A listing of the safety factors of various antimicrobial drugs in various medical conditions is provided in Table 34-16.

Table 34-17 lists general guidelines for antibacterial drug selection.

SUGGESTED READINGS*

4. Albarellos G, Montoya L, Ambros L, et al. 2004. Multiple once-daily dose pharmacokinetics and renal safety of gentamicin in dogs, *J Vet Pharmacol Ther* 27:21-25.

8. Anadon A, Reeves-Johnson L. 1999. Macrolide antibiotics, drug interactions and microsomal enzymes: implications for veterinary medicine, *Res Vet Sci* 66:197-203.

29. Bloom PB, Rosser EJ. 2001. Efficacy of once-daily clindamycin hydrochloride in the treatment of superficial bacterial pyoderma in dogs, *J Am Anim Hosp Assoc* 37:537-542.

37. Boothe DM, Boeckh A, Boothe HW, et al. 2002. Plasma concentrations of enrofloxacin and its active metabolite ciprofloxacin in dogs following single oral administration of enrofloxacin at 7.5, 10, or 20 mg/kg, *Vet Ther* 3:409-419.

73. Cohn LA, Gary AT, Fales WH, et al. 2003. Trends in fluoroquinolone resistance of bacteria isolated from canine urinary tracts, *J Vet Diagn Invest* 15:338-343.

95. Dimitrova DJ, Pashov DA, Dimitrov DS. 1998. Dicloxacillin pharmacokinetics in dogs after intravenous, intramuscular, and oral administration, *J Vet Pharmacol Ther* 21:414-417.

105. Dowers KL, Oliver C, Radecki SV, et al. 2002. Use of enrofloxacin for treatment of large-form Haemobartonella felis in experimentally infected cats, *J Am Vet Med Assoc* 221:250-253.

108a. Eddlestone SM, Neer MT, Gaunt SD, et al. 2005. Failure of imidocarb dipropionate to clear experimentally induced *Ehrlichia canis* infection in dogs, Abstract # 134, 23rd Meeting ACVIM, Baltimore, Md., *J Vet Intern Med* 19:436-437.

119. Frazier DL, Thompson L, Trettlen A, et al. 2000. Comparison of fluoroquinolone pharmacokinetic parameters after treatment with marbofloxacin, enrofloxacin, and difloxacin in dogs, *J Vet Pharmacol Ther* 23:293-302.

134. Gookin JL, Trepanier LA, Bunch SE. 1999. Clinical hypothyroidism associated with trimethoprim-sulfadiazine administration in a dog, *J Am Vet Med Assoc* 214:1028-1031.

162. Heinen E. 2002. Comparative serum pharmacokinetics of the fluoroquinolones enrofloxacin, difloxacin, marbofloxacin, and orbifloxacin in dogs after single oral administration, *J Vet Pharmacol Ther* 25:1-5.

184. Jauernig S, Schweighauser A, Reist M, et al. 2001. The effects of doxycycline on nitric oxide and stromelysin production in dogs with cranial cruciate ligament rupture, *Vet Surg* 30:132-139.

191. Kay-Mugford PA, Weingarten AJ, Ngoh M, et al. 2002. Determination of plasma and skin concentrations of orbifloxacin in dogs with clinically normal skin and dogs with pyoderma, *Vet Ther* 3:402-408.

210. Lacy MK, Nicolau D, Nightingale CH, et al. 1998. The pharmacodynamics of aminoglycosides, *Clin Infect Dis* 27:23-27.

216. Lavy E et al. 1999. Pharmacokinetics of clindamycin HCl administered intravenously, intramuscularly, and subcutaneously to dogs, *J Vet Pharmacol Ther* 22:261-265.

237. Marier JF, Beaudry F, Ducharme MP, et al. 2001. A pharmacokinetic study of amoxicillin in febrile beagle dogs following repeated administrations of endotoxin, *J Vet Pharmacol Ther* 24:379-383.

249. McGrotty YL, Knottenbelt CM. 2002. Oesophageal stricture in a cat due to oral administration of tetracyclines, *J Small Anim Pract* 43:221-223.

263. Montesissa C, Villa R, Anfossi P, et al. 2003. Pharmacodynamics and pharmacokinetics of cefoperazone and cefamandole in dogs following single dose intravenous and intramuscular administration, *Vet J* 166:170-176.

307. Regnier A, Concordet D, Scheider M, et al. 2003. Population pharmacokinetics of marbofloxacin in aqueous humor after intravenous administration in dogs, *Am J Vet Res* 64:889-893.

327. Sanchez S, McCrackin Stevenson MA, Hudson CR, et al. 2002. Characterization of multidrug-resistant *Escherichia coli* isolates associated with nosocomial infections in dogs, *J Clin Microbiol* 40:3586-3595.

379. Trepanier LA, Danhof R, Toll J, et al. 2003. Clinical findings in 40 dogs with hypersensitivity associated with administration of potentiated sulfonamides, *J Vet Intern Med* 17:647-652.

400. Walker RD. 2000. The use of fluoroquinolones for companion animal antimicrobial therapy, *Aust Vet J* 78:84-90.

409. Watson PM. 2002. Idiosyncratic reaction to enrofloxacin in cats, *Vet Rec* 150:556.

415. Westfall DS, Jensen WA, Reagan WJ, et al 2001. Inoculation of two genotypes of *Hemobartonella felis* (California and Ohio variants) to induce infection in cats and the response to treatment with azithromycin, *Am J Vet Res* 62:687-691.

420. Wiebe V, Hamilton P. 2002. Fluoroquinolone-induced retinal degeneration in cats, *J Am Vet Med Assoc* 221:1568-1571.

427a. Woods JE, Brewer M, Radecki SV, et al. 2004. Treatment of *Mycoplasma haemofelis* infected cats with imidocarb dipropionate, Abstract # 192, 22nd Meeting ACVIM, Minneapolis, Minn.

428. Wright K, Tyler J. 2003. Recognizing metronidazole toxicosis in dogs, *Vet Med* 98:410-418.

438. Zetner K, Schmidt H, Pfeiffer S. 2003. Concentrations of clindamycin in the mandibular bone of companion animals, *Vet Ther* 4:166-171.

*See the CD-ROM for a complete list of references.

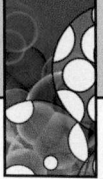

CHAPTER • 35

Streptococcal and Other Gram-Positive Bacterial Infections

STREPTOCOCCAL INFECTIONS

Craig E. Greene and John F. Prescott

Streptococci are gram-positive, nonmotile, facultatively anaerobic cocci that cause localized to widespread pyogenic infections in animals and people. Although numerous are pathogenic, many species are commensal microflora of the oral cavity, nasopharynx, skin, and genital and gastrointestinal (GI) tracts. Species differences among streptococci are responsible for the varying host ranges and virulence. Several classification systems exist for streptococci based on cultural characteristics, antigenic composition, and biochemical features. Because it tends to correlate with pathogenicity, Lancefield classification[82] based on antigenic differences in cell wall carbohydrates is used to distinguish the groups. The action on erythrocytes in culture medium has also been used to distinguish different groups of streptococci. β-Hemolysis is characterized by complete lysis of erythrocytes and clearing around the bacterial colonies. α-Hemolysis is characterized by a greenish-colored zone and intact erythrocytes in the discolored region. Some are nonhemolytic. β-Hemolytic strains tend to be most pathogenic. Lancefield groups A, B, C, E, G, L, and M are usually β-hemolytic. Group D is usually α-hemolytic but can be nonhemolytic and contains numerous species that have been reclassified as *Enterococcus* (see Enterococcal Infections section in this chapter). Organisms in the α-hemolytic and nonhemolytic categories are found on mucous membranes and skin of clinically healthy animals. If present in an infectious process, they are usually regarded as contaminants or unimportant invaders. When they do cause illness, it may take the form of valvular endocarditis or embolic abscess. The precise species classification of streptococci in numerous disease processes described next is in doubt, especially in the older literature. Increasingly, Lancefield grouping combined with detailed phenotypic characterization by commercial identification systems classifies streptococci correctly and defines more clearly the strains responsible for significant infections in dogs and cats.

Group A Streptococcal Infections of Dogs and Cats

People are the principal natural reservoir hosts of group A streptococci, and most human infections are caused by this group, which includes *Streptococcus pyogenes* and *Streptococcus pneumoniae*. Dermatitis, pharyngitis, and scarlet and rheumatic fevers are the main syndromes caused by *S. pyogenes* (Table 35-1). Rarely, these organisms produce perianal cellulitis, vaginitis, and localized abscesses. Certain strains produce pyrogenic exotoxins, which may cause toxic shocklike syndrome. *S. pneumoniae* produces lower respiratory infection with occasional dissemination. Of all the streptococcal groups, group A

organisms have the greatest virulence for human adults, whereas organisms of the other groups, such as B, C, D, F, and G, cause the most severe manifestations in neonates.

S. pyogenes

S. pyogenes is the predominant cause of group A infections of people and is the type species for this group. The sites of greatest carriage of group A streptococci in people are the caudal aspects of the pharynx and tonsillar region. Group A streptococci can survive extremes in environmental temperature and humidity; however, most infections are associated with direct or close contact among susceptible individuals (Fig. 35-1). As is true with many streptococcal infections, some individuals can harbor the infection for extended periods in the absence of clinical illness. Prevalence rates for group A streptococci are higher in young children, especially those in day-care or classroom situations. The prevalence of positive throat culture findings in such circumstances may approach 50%, even in the absence of an obvious epidemic.[59] Symptomatic rather than carrier children are most likely to bring infection into the home. Under such circumstances the isolation rate in other people in the household approaches 25% to 50%. If the child is asymptomatic, the rate is only 9%.[72] Dogs and cats have been suggested as possible sources of reinfection of treated household members, but no convincing evidence shows that dogs and cats are significant reservoirs of infection for people. However, veterinarians may need to be consulted on this topic.

Whenever streptococcal typing has been performed on the oropharyngeal region of dogs and cats, groups G, C, L, and M have been present (in order of decreasing frequency). However, screening for group A streptococcal colonization of the tonsils of dogs and cats from random households in urban environments has shown the apparent prevalence to range between 1% and 10%. In one study in which recurrent group A streptococcal pharyngitis occurred in people, the prevalence for households was said to be 42% for dogs and 36% for cats. However, because only bacitracin susceptibility was used to distinguish group A from non–group A strains in many of these studies, the findings of high prevalence must be regarded as unproven at best and fictitious at worst. When Lancefield typing has been done, the prevalence of true group A streptococcal carriage has varied from 0% to 3% of dogs and has not correlated with the presence of infection in the owner.[28,169] Biochemical testing of isolates from dogs and cats cannot accurately distinguish between those from groups A and G.[115]

Domestic pets that come into close contact with infected individuals can sometimes apparently develop pharyngeal colonization with group A streptococci. Infected pets show no clinical illness or tonsillar enlargement. Because clinical symptomatology is absent in these animals, the main consideration

Table • 35-1

Summary of Streptococcal and Enterococcal Infections of People, Dogs, and Cats

SPECIES (SEROGROUP)	HOST SPECIES[a]	MICROFLORAL DISTRIBUTION[b]	DISEASE SYNDROMES[b]
Streptococcus			
S. pyogenes (A)	P	Tonsils	Tonsillitis, pharyngitis, otitis, impetigo, bacteremia, toxemia,[12,13] toxic shock, necrotizing fasciitis
	B	None (human reservoir)	Asymptomatic
S. pneumoniae (A)	P	Tonsils	Pneumonia, otitis, bacteremia, polyarthritis, meningitis
	C	None (human reservoir)	Polyarthritis, bacteremia[14]
S. agalactiae (A)	P	Anorectum, vagina	*Neonatal:* sepsis[16,18] *Immunosuppressed:* bacteremia, meningitis, endocarditis[23,27,28] *Postparturient:* metritis; septic arthritis; pharyngitis; respiratory, skin, and wound infection
	D	Urogenital region	Fatal septicemia in pups, necrotizing pneumonia, bacteremia, endocarditis, pyelonephritis[100]
	C	Urogenital region	Peritonitis, septicemia, placentitis[36]
S. equi ssp. zooepidemicus (C)	D	Skin, genitourinary tract	Endocarditis, septicemia,[114] acute fibrinopurulent bronchopneumonia death,[37,47] UTIs
S dysgalactiae ssp. quisimilis (C)	P	None (animal reservoir)	Pharyngitis, glomerulonephritis,[55,58] pericarditis
S. suis (D or none)	C	Oropharynx	Dermatitis, fibrinonecrotic pleuropneumonia[37]
S. milleri S. intermedius (F)	P, D	Skin, mucosae	Opportunistic infections, abscesses in many tissues[45]
S. dysgalactiae (G)	P	Tonsils, vagina	Pharyngitis, tonsillitis, wound infections, neonatal and puerperal sepsis, endocarditis
S. canis (G)	C	Nasopharynx, genitalia, skin	Abscesses, neonatal sepsis, umbilical infections,[67,71,74,80] pyelonephritis[91]
	D	Tonsils, anorectum,[92] genitalia	Otitis media, neonatal sepsis (fading puppy?), umbilical infections, polyarthritis, abscesses, dermatitis, meningoencephalitis,[21] mastitis,[33,96,98,99,100] genital infections: infertility, anestrus, abortion, failure to conceive,[111] UTI; pericarditis,[130] streptococcal toxic shock syndrome/necrotizing fasciitis
Streptococcus sp. (L)	D	Genitalia	Abortion, fading puppy syndrome, sterility in bitch, endometritis[12,101,102]
Streptococcus sp. (M)	D	Tonsils[101]	Asymptomatic colonization
Streptococcus sp. (E)	D	Skin, upper respiratory tract[96]	Asymptomatic colonization found as mixed flora in mucosal inflammation[111]
Enterococcus[c]			
E. faecalis, E. avium, E. faecium (all D)	D, P, C	Intestine, feces,[96] tonsils	Asymptomatic colonization, urinary tract infection, nosocomial surgical infections
E. hirae (D)	D	Intestine, feces	Diarrhea, symptomatic upper intestinal colonization[37,83]

[a]P, Human; B, dog and cat; C, cat; D, dog; UTI, urinary tract infection.
[b]Numbers footnote symbols in this *column* refer to the reference list on the CD-ROM.
[c]Also includes E. cecorum, E. durans, and E. zymogenes.

is their potential public health risk. If pets are overlooked during treatment of their infected owners, they might serve as possible reservoirs for reinfection of family members. However, pets usually lose their infection within 2 to 3 weeks after they are removed from the household. Infected people are carriers of group A streptococci for much longer periods.[117] It is not acceptable to consider culturing and treating a dog and or cat in a household in which reinfection occurs without doing so for the human contacts.

The recovery of group A streptococci is affected by the method used when swabbing the throat, because overgrowth by indigenous microflora can result in the death of group A streptococci. Sedation may be needed, because sterile swabs should be rubbed over the surface of the exposed tonsils in their crypts. Swabs that are unrefrigerated during transport should be kept dry, otherwise overgrowth by contaminating microflora occurs. Latex agglutination and enzyme-linked immunosorbent assay (ELISA) tests are available for rapid detection of group A streptococci in children. Their value in detection of asymptomatic group A infections in dogs and cats is likely to be low.

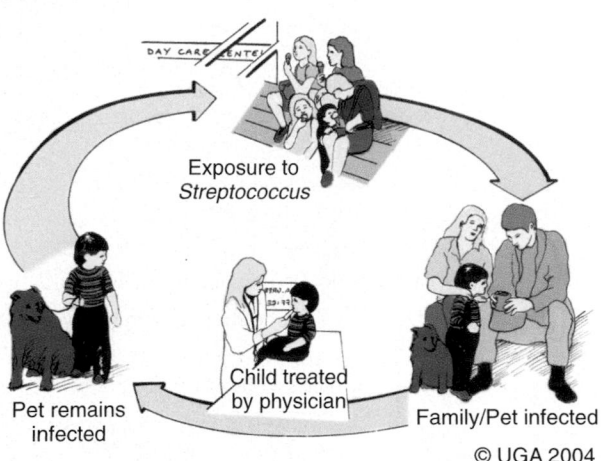

Fig 35-1 Zoonotic aspects of group A streptococcal infection in pets. Children usually acquire the infection at school. When they are treated, reinfection may result if a household pet has acquired infection and is not simultaneously treated. Treatment of additional family contacts is equally important in breaking the cycle. (Courtesy University of Georgia, Athens, Ga.)

The spectrum of effective antimicrobials for treatment of group A streptococcal infection in pets is the same as that for human strains. It is judicious to treat pets when they may be a source of recurrent infection of household members. Isolates of group A streptococci from dogs have shown the greatest susceptibility to penicillin, erythromycin, and chloramphenicol. Recommended total daily dosages are listed in Table 35-2. Resistant strains can be treated with cephalosporins.

S. pneumoniae

S. pneumoniae (formerly Diplococcus pneumoniae) can produce pneumonia, bacteremia, otitis media, endocarditis, and meningitis in people but is of no significance in dogs and cats. A single report of bacteremia and septic arthritis in a cat attributed the infection to transmission of S. pneumoniae from a human infant in the same household.[132] A French bulldog developed hyperesthesia and central vestibular disease from meningoencephalitis caused by S. pneumoniae.[70]

Group B Streptococcal Infections of Dogs and Cats

Group B streptococci (Streptococcus agalactiae) have been associated mainly with neonatal septicemia and postpartum metritis in people and mastitis in cows. Skin, pharyngeal, and wound infections can occur. Immunosuppressed individuals can develop disease in many tissues (see Table 35-1). Group B streptococci are more frequently isolated than group G from people with these syndromes. Factors at the time of delivery, such as low birth weight or difficult delivery, precipitate the development of clinical illness.

Group B streptococcal infections are rare in dogs and cats. They have been reported to cause septicemia in a dog, endometritis, and "fading puppy syndrome," symptoms of which include bacteremia, pyelonephritis, and necrotizing pneumonia. Group G streptococci have been far more commonly isolated than group B as causes of neonatal sepsis. Similarly, peritonitis with septicemia and parturient endometritis and placentitis have been described in cats. Whether canine and feline strains are indigenous or of human or other animal origin is uncertain. In one dog the organism was isolated from the skin and may have been a transient resident from a human source.[50] Treatment is similar to that for group A streptococcal infections (see Table 35-2).

Group C Streptococcal Infections of Dogs and Cats

Disease associated with group C streptococci has been described only in dogs (although dogs and cats may carry these organisms as commensal flora) in lower frequency than group G. Identification of group C streptococci in the lower respi-

Table • 35-2

Drug Therapy for Streptococcal Infections in Dogs and Cats[a]

DRUG[b]	SPECIES	DOSE[c] (mg/kg)	ROUTE	INTERVAL (HOURS)	DURATION (DAYS)
Penicillin G	Dog and cat	10,000–20,000 U/kg	IM, SC	12–24	5–7
Penicillin V	Dog and cat	8–30	PO	8	5–7
Erythromycin	Dog	3–20	PO	12–24	5–7
Chloramphenicol	Dog	15–25	PO, IV, SC	8	5–7
	Cat	10–15	PO, IV, SC	12	5–7
Cephalexin	Dog and cat	10–40	PO	12	5–7

IM, Intramuscular; SC, subcutaneous; PO, by mouth; IV, intravascular.
[a]For specific dosages for perinatal group G infections in cats, see Table 35-4.
[b]For additional information, see Appendix 8.
[c]Dose per administration at specified interval, expressed as mg/kg unless otherwise stated.

ratory tract washings of clinically healthy dogs and dogs with chronic infectious respiratory infections in kennels was associated with more severe respiratory disease in infected populations.[20] Histologic analysis revealed that dogs with group C streptococci were more likely to have intraalveolar neutrophils than those without this infection.

Acute hemorrhagic and purulent pneumonia has been described as a cause of acute respiratory infection with group C organisms, primarily in racing greyhounds or research dogs.[137,171] Weakness, coughing, dyspnea, fever, hematemesis, and red urine have been the predominant clinical signs. Many of the dogs developed septicemia, and some died suddenly without signs of clinical illness. Gross lesions at necropsy of diseased animals consisted of widespread petechial and ecchymotic hemorrhages and pulmonary congestion with mediastinal and free pleural hemorrhage. Microscopically, streptococci were found in clusters intracellularly throughout the lung parenchyma and in the spleen. The circumstances leading to group C streptococcal septicemia or pneumonia in adult dogs kept in kennels or groups are unclear, and these infections appear to be rare. The isolates have been identified as *Streptococcus equi* subsp. *zooepidemicus*, although more details of the bacterial characterization are needed to determine whether this finding is correct (see streptococcal toxic shock syndrome discussion in this chapter). Other group C streptococci isolated from less severe infections (urinary tract infections [UTIs] or abscesses) in dogs have been identified as *Streptococcus dysgalactiae* subsp. *equisimilis*, although this subspecies also has caused serious losses through septicemia and pneumonia in captive coyotes.[55] Drugs and dosages recommended for treatment are similar to those for group A infections (see Table 35-2).

Group G Streptococcal Infections
Cats
β-Hemolytic streptococci are commensal microflora of the skin, pharynx, and upper respiratory and genital tracts of cats. The majority of β-hemolytic streptococcal infections in cats are caused by Lancefield group G streptococci and are apparently *Streptococcus canis*. Whether more virulent disease-producing strains of this organism exist is uncertain, but these organisms can cause severe infections in kittens. Neonatal kittens are infected with the streptococci from the vagina of the queen. Streptococci can gain entrance via the umbilical vein and can spread by direct extension into the peritoneal cavity or through the ductus venosus and portal circulation of the liver, resulting in bacteremia. In juvenile kittens (3 to 7 months old), cervical lymphadenitis may follow a subclinical episode of pharyngitis and tonsillitis. Group G infections of older cats are often opportunistic and result from wounds, trauma, surgical procedures, viral infections, and immunosuppressive conditions. These suppurative infections can result in septicemia and embolic lesions, most often in the lung and heart.

Although infections in juveniles and older cats are generally sporadic, several kittens in a litter can be affected at one time, most frequently in the first litter of queens younger than 2 years. Young queens that become infected carry higher numbers of organisms in the vagina, and the carrier state persists throughout pregnancy, whereas older, multiparous queens can eliminate the carrier state by midgestation.

The prevalence of infection is low in kittens born to older or multiparous queens. A higher prevalence of infection occurs in cats housed in groups. Occasional outbreaks of neonatal infections with high mortality can occur in breeding catteries, especially after the introduction of group G streptococci into a naïve population. Approximately 50% of female household cats younger than 2 years and 70% to 100% of similarly aged queens in breeding catteries may carry group G streptococci in the vagina. Queens in endemically affected cat-

teries can develop protective levels of antibodies by 8 months of age. Kittens receive levels of antibodies equivalent to those of the dam via the colostrum.

Group G streptococci also can be found in the tonsils and pharynx or in the prepuce of the tom. Age, exposure, and immune responses are all important in determining whether this commensal organism causes illness.

The clinical signs vary with the site of infection and host immunocompetence. Sites of streptococcal infections in cats are listed in Table 35-3. Although cats of any age may be affected, most cases involve neonatal kittens (younger than 2 weeks of age). Most infected kittens gain less weight than littermates, and occasionally an affected kitten has a swollen, infected umbilicus. Death usually occurs by 7 to 11 days of age, but kittens born to queens with minimal prior exposure may die suddenly at younger than 3 days of age with overwhelming sepsis. In kittens with septicemia the febrile response is transient, occurs within 24 hours before death, and frequently remains undetected. Older kittens are febrile and anorexic with swelling and purulent exudate at the site of infection. Cervical lymphadenitis is a unilateral or bilateral swelling in the ventral cervical lymph nodes (Fig. 35-2). Abscess, pharyngitis, pneumonia, diskospondylitis, osteomyelitis, and arthritis are other localizations of the infectious process in this age group.[66] Animals with respiratory localization with pneumonia have fever, anorexia, coughing, and dyspnea. Those with diskospondylitis have fever, paraspinal hyperesthesia, and progressive paresis. Fever, joint swelling, and lameness are characteristic of arthritis and may involve one or more joints or extremities.

The leukogram shows a typical neutrophilic inflammatory response with a left shift. Neonatal kittens (younger than 2 weeks of age) usually have a degenerative left shift in the leukogram because of the limited bone marrow storage pool. With overwhelming sepsis, cocci may be found in the cytoplasm of circulating neutrophils.

Gram staining of exudates from affected tissues reveals single and chains of gram-positive cocci. Confirmation is based on bacteriologic culture of the affected tissues. Aerobic culture of exudates or needle aspirates of enlarged lymph nodes yield β-hemolytic, gram-positive cocci on sheep and

Table • 35-3

Anatomic Distribution of ß-Hemolytic Streptococcal Isolates[a] from Lesions in Cats

SOURCE	NUMBER OF ISOLATES	NUMBER OF PURE ISOLATES[b]
Integumentary system	57	23
Respiratory system	38	11
Genital (female) tract	28	12
Urinary tract	17	4
Serous cavities	22	9
Neonatal sepsis	12	6
Other[c]	34	13
TOTAL	208	78

Data compiled from cases during a 17-year period at the Veterinary Medical Teaching Hospital, University of California, Davis, Davis, Calif.
[a]Of 38 isolates tested, 34 were Lancefield group G positive.
[b]Number of times isolated in pure culture (only organism isolated).
[c]Other sites include oral cavity, lymph node, central nervous system, eye, ear, joint, or mammary gland.

Table • 35-4

Therapy for Group G Streptococcal Infections in Cattery Cats Based on Age

DRUG[a]	AGE	DOSE[b]	ROUTE	INTERVAL (HOURS)	DURATION (DAYS)
Prevention at Parturition					
Ampicillin (amoxicillin)	N	25 mg/kg	PO, SC	8	5—7
Procaine and benzathine	N	6,250 IU[c]	SC	48—72	3—5[d]
penicillin	Q	150,000 IU[c]	SC	48—72	3—5[d]
Infection (Lymphadenitis or Arthritis)					
Procaine and benzathine	J,A	75,000—	SC	48—72	3—5[d]
penicillin		150,000 IU[c]			
Procaine penicillin	J,A	50,000 IU[c]	SC	24	5
Penicillin V	J,A	20 mg/kg	PO	8	5

N, Neonates; *Q*, queens; *J*, juveniles; *A*, adults; *IU*, international units;
[a] For additional information, see Appendix 8.
[b] Dose per administration at specified interval.
[c] Total dose needed for each drug in a fixed combination, based on 2- to 3-kg cat. This drug has been associated with injection-site sarcomas.
[d] Only one or two doses are usually given during this treatment regimen.

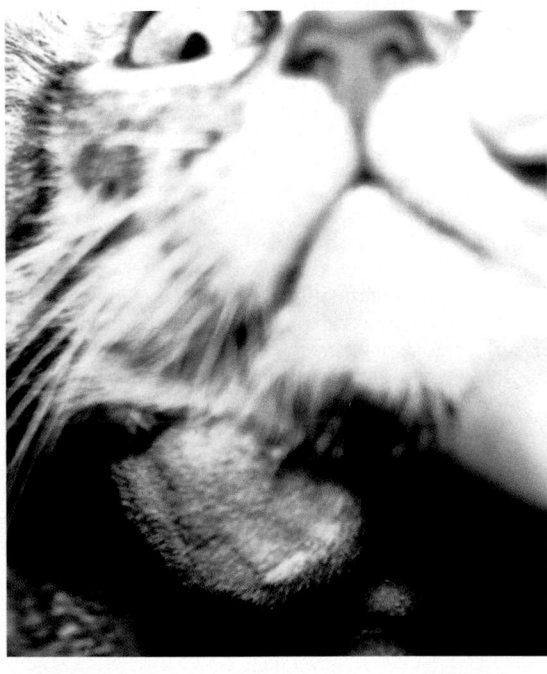

Fig 35-2 Unilateral *S. canis* cervical lymphadenitis in a 4-month-old kitten. (From Timoney JF, et al [eds]. 1998. *Hagan and Bruner's microbiology and infectious diseases of domestic animals*, ed 8. Cornell University Press, Ithaca, N.Y.)

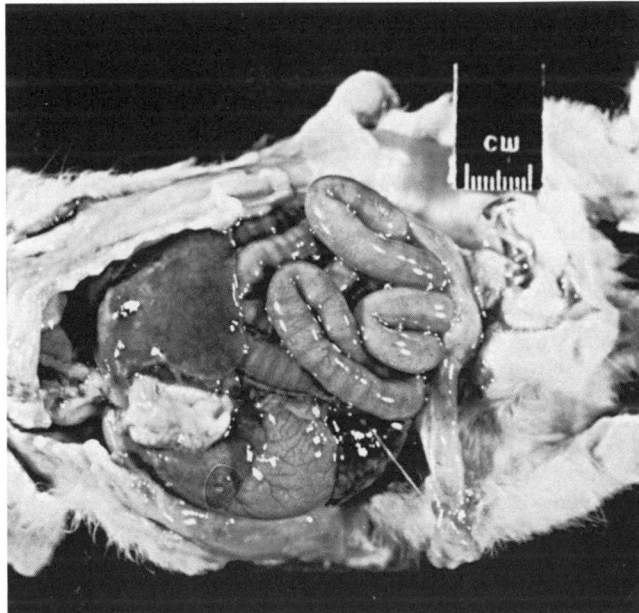

Fig 35-3 Peritonitis and umbilical vein abscess with extension into the liver in a 7-day-old kitten.

bovine blood agar plates. In fatally affected neonates the organism is found most consistently in the liver, lung, umbilicus, and peritoneal cavity (Fig. 35-3).

Necropsy findings in affected neonatal kittens with septicemia include omphalophlebitis, peritonitis, and less frequently, embolic hepatitis, pneumonia, diskospondylitis, and myocarditis. Untreated cases of cervical lymphadenitis in juvenile cats can progress to embolic myocarditis and embolic pneumonia with secondary pulmonary infarction and pleuritis and pyothorax.[170] Valvular endocarditis has also been described.[94] Older cats are less susceptible to systemic spread of streptococci.

Group G streptococci are very sensitive to penicillin and its derivatives. Juvenile and older cats with lymphadenitis should be treated immediately with oral or parenteral therapy (Table 35-4). Draining and flushing the abscesses hasten recovery. These cats should be examined for predisposing conditions such as feline leukemia, feline infectious peritonitis, feline immunodeficiency virus or viral respiratory infections, feline urologic syndrome, and wounds.

For prevention of infection in newborn kittens, dipping the navel and umbilical cord in 2% tincture of iodine and treating of all kittens at birth with ampicillin, amoxicillin, or procaine combined with benzathine penicillin have been successful. A much higher dose of combined procaine and benzathine penicillin should be given immediately to the queen of an infected litter or as a single preventive dose at parturition. Although the population of group G streptococci can be temporarily suppressed by antimicrobial therapy, the carrier state cannot be eliminated.

Treatment of infected juvenile or adult cats with lymphadenitis or arthritis can be accomplished with parenteral or oral therapy (see Table 35-4). Doses are higher than normally recommended because the organism can be harbored in the tonsillar crypts, and a considerable amount of pus forms in the abscess. Cats with diskospondylitis have required up to 6 months of therapy. Parenteral therapy can be instituted in the veterinarian's office, and medication can be dispensed for subsequent oral administration.

Group G streptococci have received increasing attention as a cause of pharyngitis, tonsillitis, wound infection, cellulitis, neonatal and puerperal septicemia, and endocarditis in people. Group G streptococci in cats appear to be *S. canis* and to be distinct from human group G streptococci.[115] In a review of all reported human group G infections in Great Britain, a majority of the patients had underlying immunosuppressive illness.[66]

Dogs

Group G streptococci are the major streptococcal type isolated as commensal flora from the skin and mucosa of dogs.[13,14] The majority of group G isolates from dogs are *S. canis*. Nevertheless, some group G isolates have the biochemical characteristics of human group G streptococci. More work is needed to define the biotypic variation within *S. canis* and the identity of unusual group G streptococci isolated from dogs. Historically, the veterinary literature has contained numerous reports of diseases in dogs caused by these organisms, including abortion, infertility, sterility, and neonatal death. In addition, cellulitis, mastitis, pharyngitis, pericarditis, tonsillitis, polysynovitis, and genital infection have been described (see Table 35-1). Metaphyseal osteomyelitis may occur in growing pups.[52] Some of the historical descriptions of disease, especially pharyngitis, tonsillitis, infertility, and sterility, caused by group G streptococci should be carefully considered because of the frequency with which these organisms are isolated from clinically healthy animals and the lack of clear description of the microbiology of the infections. However, it is also likely that streptococcal infections have declined in importance in the last 50 years with the widespread use of penicillin and its derivatives in dogs.

S. canis is generally an opportunistic pathogen of dogs and is isolated from an array of nonspecific infections, including genitourinary tract, wound, mammary gland, and skin (especially otitis externa). In addition, it may cause bacteremia or septicemia and polyarthritis in neonatal puppies, forming part of the fading puppy syndrome, in which the pup is predisposed because of lack of warmth, improper navel disinfection, and lack of nursing. Infection in these pups may come from microflora or the environment; no correlation was found between the organisms found in the milk of bitches with those isolated from dead septicemic pups.[122] Group G streptococci have also been associated with a rapidly progressive systemic infection in older dogs (see streptococcal toxic shock syndrome discussion in this chapter) *S. canis* is a common commensal of the genital tract. It may be an opportunistic organism associated with vaginitis, but its historical role in infertility in bitches is not supported by current findings. Historical but no current accounts exist of the association of this organism with acute tonsillitis and suppurative cervical lymphadenitis in dogs in kennels and other settings. Group G streptococci have also been isolated from the cerebrospinal fluid (CSF) of dogs with

meningoencephalomyelitis as a result of hematogenous spread or penetrating injuries.[21] Space-occupying abscess formation may occur within the confines of the central nervous system (CNS) in some cases. Results of CSF analysis are marked pleocytosis (usually greater than 100 cells/μl) with a predominance of neutrophils and in some cases, intracellular bacterial cocci. Antimicrobial choices for group G infections are similar to that for group A streptococcal infections (see Table 35-2). For CNS infections, therapeutic options include high-dose intravenous (IV) penicillins, trimethoprim-sulfonamide, or IV third-generation cephalosporins.

Streptococcal Toxic Shock Syndrome and Necrotizing Fasciitis

The last decade has had a resurgence of severe group A human streptococcal infections characterized by septic shock associated with multiple organ failure and with or without necrotizing fasciitis (NF) (Table 35-5). It usually originates from bacterial seeding of internal or soft tissues. One report has been made of this syndrome in a person; the source was group G streptococcus.[156] Group G dog (*S. canis*) isolates that resisted phagocytosis were examined for virulence genes comparable to those found in group A (*S. pyogenes*) human isolates. Only M-protein genes associated with surface fibrillar material and streptolysin O genes were identified in most of the canine isolates.[39] Increased invasiveness of streptococci correlates with a change in the M-protein, which inhibits phagocytosis by neutrophils and macrophages. Once the streptococci develop this new protein, they can enter the body and avoid host defenses.

Multiple organ involvement in streptococcal toxic shock syndrome (STSS) suggests a toxin produced by the pathogenic bacteria might also be involved in the pathogenesis.[113] Bacterial superantigens, a family of highly mitogenic proteins secreted by the organisms, are suspected. Superantigens simultaneously bind to major histocompatibility complex class II molecules and T-cell receptors simultaneously, resulting in sudden high cytokine levels. In vitro, the fluoroquinolone enrofloxacin caused bacteriophage-induced lysis of an *S. canis* strain that had been isolated from a dog with STSS.[69] Bacteriophage induction was associated with an enhancement of expression of a superantigen gene relative to the same organism in noninduced cultures. The presence of this gene on enrofloxacin-induced bacteriophages may explain the association between this drug treatment and the occurrence of STSS in dogs. Most of the dogs reported with this type of infection had received enrofloxacin in the early stages of disease; however, the drug was not effective in halting the progression of the disease, despite in vitro susceptibility in some cases. In fact, enrofloxacin may have been responsible for triggering the pathologic events caused by these virulent streptococci.

The dramatic and severe multisystemic (STSS) and locally invasive (NF) group A streptococcal infections in people have been dubbed *toxic shock infections* and *flesh-eating bacterial infections*, respectively, in the popular media. A similar clinical picture caused by various isolates of *S. canis* or other group G streptococci has been identified in dogs[96,101,102,111,112] and cats.[146a,163] In most cases, affected animals were previously healthy adult dogs or cats younger than 1 year. The dogs had a history of mild trauma, bite wound, or respiratory or urinary tract disease. Affected kittens had suppurative lymphadenomegaly typical of group G infection. In addition, they had multifocal purulent ulcerative skin lesions. They were generally depressed but afebrile.[163] All the dogs were febrile (40° C to 41° C [104° F to 105.8° F]) at admission. Dogs with NF had severe, rapidly developing cellulitis, usually of a limb but in one case of the ventral thorax. The most consistent clinical sign in the history and on physical examination was intense,

Table • 35-5

Clinical Features of Systemic Streptococcal Infections

Case Definition of Streptococcal Toxic Shock
I. Isolation of streptococci from normally sterile site
II. Hypotension
III. Previous two factors in addition to two or more of the following:
    A. Renal impairment (elevated creatinine)
    B. Coagulopathy (thrombocytopenia or disseminated intravascular coagulation)
    C. Liver abnormalities (elevated aminotransferase activities or bilirubin levels)
    D. Acute respiratory distress (pulmonary capillary leakage, edema)
    E. Extensive soft-tissue necrosis (fasciitis, myositis, gangrene)
    F. Erythematous rash

Case Definition of Necrotizing Fasciitis
I. Necrosis of soft tissue with fascial involvement
II. Previous factor in addition to one or more of the following
    A. Death
    B. Shock (hypotension <90 mmHg)
    C. Disseminated intravascular coagulation
    D. Organ system failure
        1. Respiratory
        2. Hepatic
        3. Renal
    E. Isolation of hemolytic streptococci from normally sterile site

Clinical Findings
I. Hyperesthesia, vomiting, diarrhea, dyspnea, tachycardia, fever
II. Hypotension, localized erythema, localized swelling and edema

Laboratory Findings
I. Hypoalbuminemia, hypocalcemia, elevated liver transaminases and creatinine activities
II. Prolonged coagulation times, high creatine kinase with fasciitis

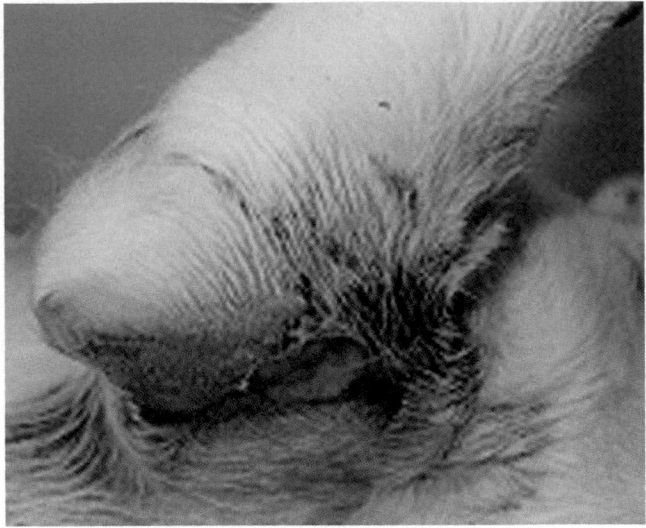

Fig 35-4 Necrotic skin lesion with underlying discoloration at elbow of dog with streptococcal necrotizing fasciitis. (Courtesy University of Georgia, Athens, Ga.)

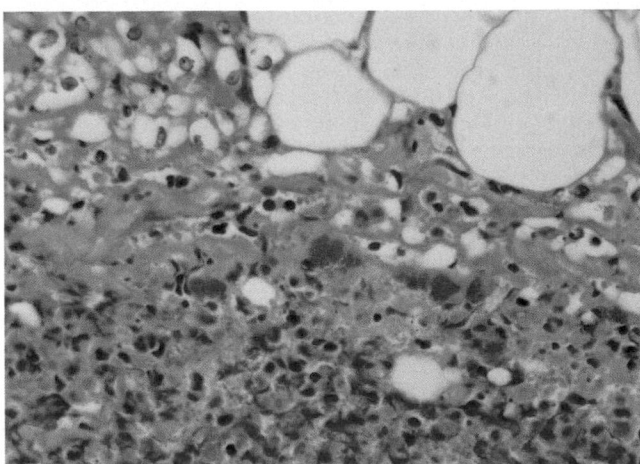

Fig 35-5 Histopathologic appearance of necrotizing fasciitis with large number of colonies of streptococci in chains in the fascial layers overlying the muscle (H and E stain, ×400). (Courtesy University of Georgia, Athens, Ga.)

excruciating pain localized around the affected area but sometimes involving the whole body. Localized heat and swelling were identified at presentation or within 2 days of hospitalization. Once evident, the cellulitis developed rapidly (Fig. 35-4). Colonies of streptococci in chains can be readily demonstrated in fluid aspirated from the cellulitis or in underlying tissues by histopathologic examination (Fig. 35-5). Dogs with NF were extremely depressed when examined and eventually went into shock. They had extensive exudate accumulation along fascial planes. The fascia required surgical debridement. In two dogs, acute onset of posterior paresis with lower motor neuron deficits developed because of the presence of septic emboli in blood vessels of the gray matter of the spinal cord and because of extension of infec-tion into the surrounding connective tissue and peripheral nerves.

Other dogs with severe invasive *S. canis* infection developed STSS without clinically apparent NF. The dogs with STSS had severe depression, fever, and rapidly developing hypotension and shock. In most the lungs were considered the primary site of infection, and acute infection appeared to be superimposed on chronic preexisting pulmonary infection. In one dog a urinary infection was the presumed source.[101]

Some kittens with NF responded favorably to treatment with amoxicillin-clavulanate, supportive care, and wound management with topical antibiotic application, while in other cases, the kittens were moribund or dead.[196a,163] The dogs with STSS died or were euthanized within 48 hours of hospitalization, but those with NF survived. All dogs had full-thickness skin sloughs and required debridement of necrotic tissue, appropriate antibiotic treatment, and intensive supportive medical care (crystalloids, colloids, plasma, low-dose heparin) aimed at treating shock with disseminated intravascular coagulation. IV plasma has been used in people to control hypotension and neutralize bacterial toxins.[78] IV IgG therapy has also shown some benefit in clinical improvement and reduction of mortality in treated versus control human patients.[29,135] Less commonly, glucocorticoid treatment was used. More appropriate antibiotics for treatment of this condition are penicillin G, aminopenicillins (ampicillin, amoxicillin), erythromycin, and clindamycin. In human STSS or NF, clindamycin is regarded as the drug of choice. In addition to its antibacterial activity, clindamycin is a potent suppressor of bacterial toxin synthesis, inhibits M-protein synthesis (which facilitates phagocytosis), and suppresses lipopolysaccharide-induced monocyte synthesis of tumor necrosis factor (TNF).[134] The authors (CEG and JFP) have found this drug to be valuable in the treatment of affected pets.

Public Health Considerations

In general, public health risks from *S. canis* colonization of infection in dogs or cats are low. Only rarely have people been infected with this organism.[162] Nevertheless, when veterinarians drain and debride NF lesions, they should recognize the extreme risk of inadvertent infection of cuts on their hands. This risk can probably be contained by wearing latex gloves and protective clothing when handling dogs with STSS or NF. Group G streptococci are normal inhabitants of the skin, oropharynx, GI tract, and female genital tract of people. Human strains generally belong to the species *S. dysgalactiae* rather than *S. canis*. Asymptomatic pharyngeal carriage of group G streptococci is found in up to 23% of people. The organisms commonly colonize human skin, and approximately 5% of asymptomatic puerperal women harbor them on the genital mucosa. Group G streptococcal infections in people are not common and involve primarily dermatitis and pharyngitis; however, bacteremia and septicemia, endocarditis, peritonitis, peripheral sepsis, soft-tissue infection, and septic arthritis are unusual.

Little evidence shows that dogs are a significant source of human infection.[16] In one report,[16] dogs were mentioned as a possible source of group G streptococcal arthritis in people, but the association was speculative. The source of infection was more likely autogenous. In one report of meningitis,[71] the isolate was not completely characterized. In another report, *S. canis* was isolated from the blood of a person with septicemia.[9] The organism was specifically typed on the basis of biochemical and genetic analysis. It was presumably transmitted from the family dog and colonized the varicose ulcers of the person's legs. The occurrence of such infections probably involves close contact between the animal and open skin wounds. Routine hand washing after animal contact and not allowing dogs to lick people, especially their wounds, are always advisable.

Other Streptococcal Infections of Cats and Dogs

Group L streptococci have been similarly associated with syndromes that parallel some of those reported historically for group G streptococci (abortion, infertility, and septicemia in puppies), although their isolation frequency from normal and diseased dogs has been low (see Table 35-1). Groups M and E have been found as normal microflora of dogs, although they are isolated with very low frequency from the oral, urogenital, and respiratory mucosae. Group D streptococci are considered normal GI flora of dogs, and many of these species have been classified as enterococci. These enteric cocci are often found in urinary tract or nosocomial tissue infections of dogs. *Streptococcus suis* has been isolated rarely from pleuropneumonic conditions in cats but appears to be of little significance.

ENTEROCOCCAL INFECTIONS

Craig E. Greene and John F. Prescott

Enterococci are gram-positive cocci that grow into short chains and are impossible to distinguish morphologically from streptococci. They were initially classified as group D streptococci but now have their own genus, which contains species such as *Enterococcus faecalis*, *Enterococcus faecium*, and *Enterococcus hirae*. These organisms can survive under more adverse environmental conditions than the less robust streptococci. In addition to being saprophytes, their major habitat in the host is the GI tract, where they are normal microflora (Table 35-6).[34] In fact, they have been used in probiotic preparations and fed to dogs in an attempt to suppress more enteropathogenic bacteria.[153] Under certain circumstances, enterococci may proliferate and colonize the entire surfaces via fimbriae that adhere to the brush border of enterocytes. Although inflammation is minimal and toxin production is absent, they may cause a decrease in activity of brush border digestive enzymes. Enterococci are not as virulent as other streptococci, but their resistance to many antimicrobials allows them to persist in host tissues after antimicrobial therapy. In people and pets, they have predominantly caused infections in hospitalized patients as nosocomial complications. Systemic infections such as bacteremia and endocarditis and localized infections of the abdominal cavity, genitourinary tract, soft tissue, or respiratory tract have been most frequent.[122] The multiple antibiotic resistance of some isolates, including notable resistance to vancomycin in rare cases, has led to the increasing prominence of these poorly virulent bacteria.

Vancomycin-resistant enterococci (VRE) are becoming a major threat to human health. People often become infected in hospital settings or their home environments. In Europe, community-acquired infections are presumably more

Table • 35-6

Enterococcal and Streptococcal Species Isolated from the Anal and Tonsillar Mucosae of Dogs and Cats[34]

	DOGS		CATS	
	ANUS	TONSILS	ANUS	TONSILS
Enterococcus				
E. faecalis	45	48	60	40
E. hirae	37	8	15	4
E. faecium	12	20	15	19
E. avium	12	0	0	0
E. avium-like	13	12	0	0
E. raffinosis	2	0	0	27
E. durans	2	0	0	0
E. cecorum	2	8	14	12
Streptococcus (Lancefield Group)				
S. canis (G)	12	32	30	19
S. bovis (D)	10	8	32	12
S. suis (S, R)	0	20	5	12
S. alactolyticus (D)	2	8	5	0
S. dysgalactiae (G)	0	8	0	0

common because a vancomycin-related glycopeptide, avoparcin, has been used extensively as a growth promoter for food-producing animals.[97] VRE have been recovered from dogs with urinary tract infections[126] and dog food sold in the United States.[43] VRE with the same genotype as those found in people have been recovered from the feces of pet dogs and cats.[38,118,154]

Enterococci are generally resistant to several antimicrobials used to treat gram-positive organisms[95,121] Nevertheless, penicillin, ampicillin, and rarely vancomycin combined with aminoglycosides are the treatments of choice. Trimethoprim-sulfonamide is not effective, despite in vitro susceptibility, because these organisms can circumvent the folate synthesis block in vivo.

Dogs

Although resistant nosocomial enterococcal infections have primarily been observed in the veterinary hospital, published reports have implicated *E. hirae* as a cause of diarrhea in dogs. *E. hirae* was isolated from the small intestine of an 11-day-old pup.[23,36] The pup was one of three that died in a litter affected with acute diarrhea. Microscopically, bacterial colonization of the apical surfaces of the enterocytes in the jejunum was diffuse with mild inflammatory infiltrates. A mixed growth of *Escherichia coli* and *E. hirae* was cultured. Although bacterial attachment has been seen in the ileum and colon of healthy pups, it is not usually found in the upper small intestine. Although enterococci have been associated with malabsorption and diarrhea in other animals, their exact role in the diarrhea or death of these three puppies is uncertain. Concurrent infection with an undetected organism may have been possible. Bacterial adhesion has also been reported in two other mature dogs with diarrhea.[74] *E. faecium* was one of many floral organisms isolated from feces of one of these affected dogs. Replication and adherence of bacteria in the upper small intestine must be distinguished from bacterial overgrowth because it can develop as a result of other small intestinal disorders.

Cats

E. hirae was identified as a cause of anorexia and diarrhea with fatal outcome in a 2-month-old Persian kitten.[83] The kitten was from a commercial breeding colony in which kittens had a history of anorexia and diarrhea at weaning and queens had a history of weight loss by the end of gestation. The kitten had intermittent anorexia for 4 weeks postweaning followed by diarrhea for 4 days and eventual shock. Fluid and antimicrobial therapy was only temporarily beneficial. Continuous mats of enterococci were adherent to the brush border epithelium of the small intestine of this kitten at necropsy. Similar bacteria were located in the hepatobiliary and pancreatic duct systems associated with suppurative inflammation in the periductal regions of the liver and pancreas. A 10.5-year-old Himalayan queen had intermittent vomiting and diarrhea for 7 days.[64] Continuous mats of bacterial cocci were adherent to the brush border epithelium; the bacterium was identified as *E. faecium*.

RHODOCOCCUS EQUI INFECTION

Craig E. Greene

Rhodococcus equi (previously *Corynebacterium equi*) is a soil-borne, pleomorphic, gram-positive bacillus that has been primarily associated with suppurative infections in domestic livestock, especially foals. It is acquired by inhalation from soil, inoculation into a wound or mucous membrane, or ingestion. Reports of infections in cats are rare but increasing and probably associated with immunosuppressive illness such as that caused by retrovirus infection. Cats with *R. equi* infection should be examined for predisposing immunocompromising viral infections. Although isolates of the organism have been made from dogs, they have generally been clinically healthy, and the prevalence of infection is rare. Disseminated infection and death was reported in one dog.[19]

R. equi commonly produces purulent pneumonia in foals, suppurative lymphadenitis in pigs, and granulomatous lymphadenitis in cows. *R. equi* has also been isolated from lesions in dogs, but isolation from abscesses in cats have been most commonly reported. It is increasing in prominence in human beings because immunocompromised people, particularly those infected with the human immunodeficiency virus (HIV), have been affected. Pulmonary lobar infiltration with cavitation, similar to that observed with tuberculosis, has been the most frequently observed syndrome in patients with the acquired immunodeficiency syndrome (AIDS).[146,155] *R. equi*, a saprophyte, is commonly recovered from soil that has herbivore manure and from feces of herbivores. The organism may enter the body through a penetrating wound contaminated by the environment and subsequently spread via lymphatics to regional lymph nodes and via the blood to the liver, spleen, and visceral lymph nodes. It is also commonly inhaled in dust. *R. equi* is a facultative intracellular parasite that invades lymphatic tissues and macrophages, resulting in granulomatous inflammation. Underlying immunosuppression is usually thought to be responsible for this hematogenous dissemination. The organism has virulent properties, which interfere with phagolysosomal fusion. In horses, *R. equi* virulence has been related to a plasmid that encodes a virulence protein, VapA, which allows its persistence in macrophages. This protein has not been consistently identified in human or other animal infections.[19,144,145] In nonequine species, immunodeficiency in the host likely allows less virulent strains to persist intracellularly.

Pyogranulomatous lesions are the characteristic finding, and most cats have had primary involvement of an extremity.[46] Localized swelling with ulcerations or fistulas and purulent drainage have been found. Unlike typical bite wound abscesses, the lesions are generally not painful, and systemic signs of fever and anorexia are usually absent. Pyothorax from mediastinal lymphadenitis is manifest by anorexia, weight loss, and dyspnea. Abdominal distention with a palpable fluid wave, hepatomegaly, and mesenteric lymphadenomegaly may be found with dissemination.

In the one infected dog, generalized hyperesthesia was present.[19] Dissemination to many organs caused necrotizing pyogranulomatous hepatitis, osteomyelitis, and polymyositis. Osteolytic and osteoproliferative changes were seen in the bones via radiography. Gross findings included intramuscular swelling.

Hematologic abnormalities may consist of leukocytosis with a left shift. Gram staining of the purulent discharge shows large, pleomorphic, gram-positive bacilli, which may be found inside macrophages. Thoracic or abdominal effusions are typically exudates with high protein (>3.5 g/dl) and nucleated cell counts (>10,000 cells/μl); the majority of cells are lymphocytes or nondegenerate neutrophils. Organisms may not be apparent.

Peripheral abscesses often have many sinus tracts with purulent drainage. Lymph nodes may be enlarged and necrotic with a similar discharge on sectioning. Histologic examination reveals that the lesions have been pyogranulomatous or granulomatous with necrotic foci. Macrophages contain phagocytized gram-positive bacteria. Pyogranulomatous lesions containing bacteria may be observed in parenchymal organs such as the liver and lung in animals with disseminated disease. In the laboratory the organism grows readily in an aerobic environment and has distinctive colonial characteristics, but laboratories not familiar with horse isolates may fail

Table • 35-7

Drug Therapy for Rhodococcus equi Infection in Cats

DRUG[a]	DOSE[b] (mg/kg)	ROUTE	INTERVAL (HOURS)	DURATIO...
Gentamicin	2	SC	12	5[c]
Lincomycin	20	PO	12	7–10[c]
Erythromycin	10	PO	8	14
Erythromycin	15	PO	12	14
Rifampin[d]	5	PO	12	14
Amoxicillin-clavulanate	12.5	PO	12	14–16

PO, By mouth; SC, subcutaneous.
[a]For additional information, see Appendix 8.
[b]Dose per administration at specified interval.
[c]A second course of therapy may be used with a 1-week interval between courses.
[d]Rifampin should be used only in combination with another drug such as erythromycin.

to identify it correctly. Clinicians should communicate their suspicion to the laboratory to ensure that proper microbiologic techniques are used to enhance colony growth. Culture of tissue specimens following maceration appears to be superior to taking swabs of exudates or infected tissues for isolation of this intracellular bacterium.[109] Growth of the organism in culture is optimal at 30° C.

Surgical removal of extremity lesions is only temporarily effective, and new lesions commonly develop even after limb amputation. Surgical drainage of abscesses is an essential adjunctive procedure. Antimicrobial susceptibility testing should always be performed because resistant strains have been identified. In general, in vitro susceptibility is greatest to erythromycin, rifampin, aminoglycosides, glycopeptides, and imipenem.[160] Premafloxacin, an extended spectrum quinolone, has the greatest in vitro activity against R. equi compared with numerous other antimicrobials, including other quinolones.[15] In cats, treatment with lincomycin and gentamicin has been most effective, and results with erythromycin have varied (Table 35-7). Cats treated with penicillin and streptomycin have responded poorly because the organism is not very susceptible to these drugs. Cats with disseminated lesions also respond poorly. Amoxicillin-clavulanate therapy has been effective in reducing the size of the lesions when it was used for a minimum of 14 to 16 days.[46] In people with pneumonia, only long-term treatment with erythromycin, combined with either rifampin or vancomycin, has been the effective chemotherapy.[155] As with treatment of other persistently intracellular organisms, combination treatment is superior. The standard, highly effective treatment in foals is prolonged oral administration of erythromycin and rifampin. This combination can be recommended for cats, although greater toxicity may occur. Infected cats have not been considered a source of infection for people, who usually acquire the infection from environmental exposure. Nevertheless, infected cats with discharge could pose a theoretical risk to immunocompromised owners.

CORYNEBACTERIUM INFECTIONS

Craig E. Greene

Numerous seemingly nonpathogenic corynebacteria have been isolated as microflora of dogs and cats. Some have been reported as causing otic infections or UTIs.[24] Corynebacterium ulcerans has been isolated from nasal swabs from two cats with nasal discharge.[147] These isolates were found to contain the

diphtheria toxin and may have been responsible for the clinical illness in these cats. Human infection with this organism is rare; however, it may result in similar respiratory signs. Consumption of raw milk or its unpasteurized products or close association with horses or cows is often a source of infection for people.

LISTERIOSIS

Craig E. Greene

Listeria monocytogenes is a pathogenic, β-hemolytic, gram-positive, rod-shape facultative anaerobe that is morphologically indistinguishable from diphtheroids and may be mistaken for a contaminant in tissues. It is capable of growing in a wide range of temperatures, including refrigerator temperatures (4° C to 10° C). Although at least 16 serotypes of the organism exist, most infections are caused by only a few serotypes. As a ubiquitous saprophyte, L. monocytogenes can be isolated from soil, water, sewage, dust, and decaying vegetation. Commonly, it can be found in farm animal feed and silage and in food products made from these animals. A study of fecal specimens from animals in Japan found a prevalence of 0.9% in dogs, but no bacteria were isolated from cats.[67]

L. monocytogenes differs from nonpathogenic species in that it possesses a hemolytic toxin, a factor that has been implicated in its virulence. This species is also able to persist as a facultative intracellular organism indefinitely in macrophages and to escape humoral immune responses. A cell surface protein, internalin, interacts with epithelial cells inducing phagocytosis. Once in the cell, listeriolysin O, along with phospholipases, enables the bacterium to escape host cell killing via phagosomes. In the cytoplasm the organism pushes pseudopod-like projections outward, which are ingested by adjacent macrophages, enterocytes, or hepatocytes. Thus the organism can move among cells in a new way without being exposed to antibodies. Host immunity is extremely important in the development of illness. Exposure via ingestion is common, but the disease is rare. Cell-mediated immunity (CMI) appears to be an important factor in preventing the intracellular persistence of the organism and in the development of clinical listeriosis. Coinfection with canine distemper virus has been reported as an immunosuppressive factor in disseminated listeriosis in a raccoon dog (Nyctereutes procyonoides).[4]

Natural infection usually results from ingestion of contaminated food; damage to the intestinal mucosal integrity is

...ion organisms are needed to ...inization of the stomach by ...tion. Foodborne epidemics are ...f contaminated feed or silage by ...contaminated meat and dairy prod- ...infection in dogs and cats is uncom- ...t is usually associated with ingestion of ...or meat by-products. Exposure in itself ...roduce disease. The incubation period in ...m 11 to 70 days. Reports of septicemic lis- ...and cats after oral ingestion of contaminated ...n rare. Pathogenic strains of *L. monocytogenes* can ...d from the GI tracts of asymptomatic animals. ...etration of the intestinal mucosa, *L. monocytogenes* ...s a bloodborne bacteremia, localization in mononu- ...phagocyte tissues, and septic embolization of many ...ans, including the CNS. The organism has a predilection for localizing in the CNS and placenta.

Clinical signs are caused by the degree of intestinal inflammation and the sites of embolic microabscess formation. Fever, diarrhea, and vomiting have been most frequent. Neurologic signs have been apparent in some cases. Abortion was suspected in one bitch.[136] Localized infections have also been infrequently reported.[80a] Peritonitis was reported in one cat as a result of a plant awn migrating through the bowel into the peritoneal cavity.[152] Another cat developed an abscess of the front paw 2 weeks after an insect bite at the same location.[77]

Cytologic evaluation of bone marrow from one dog with septicemia had coccobacilli within macrophages and neutrophils.[123] In the case of CNS infection the organism may be recognized premortem with gram-stained sediment of CSF. Organisms appear as short, intracellular and extracellular gram-positive bacilli to coccobacilli. Diagnosis of infection is usually made at necropsy, because infected animals often succumb to the septicemia. Microabscess formations and focal necrotic lesions may be grossly or microscopically visible in many organs, especially the liver and spleen. Immunohistochemical staining of formalin-fixed, paraffin-embedded brain sections has been used to confirm infection.[159] In the absence of contaminating organisms, *L. monocytogenes* can grow and be identified within 36 hours on routine media at suitable incubation temperature. Laboratory cultivation of the organism from a nonsterile site is difficult unless special precautions are taken. Selective media and cold cultivation (4° C) have been used to isolate the organism, but weeks of cold enrichment are needed because of the slow growth at this temperature. Because the organism can be commonly isolated from the GI tract of asymptomatic animals, rectal cultures may not be meaningful. (See Appendix 5 for a list of laboratories that perform the test for *Listeria* organisms.)

Antimicrobial agents effective against *Listeria* bacteria in vitro are penicillin and ampicillin, erythromycin, chloramphenicol, rifampin, tetracycline, trimethoprim-sulfonamide, and aminoglycosides. Trimethoprim-sulfonamide and aminoglycosides are bactericidal and recommended as the first choices for clinical use. Gentamicin and tobramycin have more activity than the other aminoglycosides. The combination of gentamicin and ampicillin is considered the most desirable therapy, although high doses or alternative, widely distributed drugs such as trimethoprim-sulfonamide and rifampin may be needed to reach the CNS or treat resistant infection. Chloramphenicol therapy has been associated with failure and relapse in treated people. Quinolones are ineffective.

Listeria infection in animals has not always been considered a public health risk because animals and people are exposed to the same source of environmental contamination. Nevertheless, an association has been made between human outbreaks and contact with food-producing animals or their products. Direct transmission from animals has occurred in veterinarians and farm workers through contact of unprotected skin or mucous membranes with infected animal tissues.[99] Most outbreaks occur in urban areas, where foodborne contamination is suspected. Infants, older adults, and pregnant women are most commonly affected. In a case of reverse zoonosis, listerial gastroenteritis was suspected in a litter of puppies and a newborn infant that received *Listeria*-infected milk discarded from the human mother's mammary gland.[138]

ANTHRAX

George E. Moore and Craig E. Greene

Etiology

Anthrax, a disease found in mammals worldwide, is caused by *Bacillus anthracis*, a large (1 to 1.2 μm × 3 to 6 μm), gram-positive, aerobic, spore-forming bacillus. The disease and species name is derived from the black, charcoal-appearing cutaneous lesion it causes in people. Microscopically the organisms may appear as long chains of gram-positive, square-ended bacteria, similar to a string of boxcars; shorter chains of two to three cells may be seen. Vegetative *B. anthracis* cells produce a polypeptide capsule visible when the organism is stained with methylene blue or Giemsa stains. Encapsulated anthrax organisms are refractory to phagocytosis, enhancing their ability to produce disease. Toxin production and capsule synthesis by the bacteria are mediated by plasmids designated pX01 and pX02, respectively.

B. anthracis begins to sporulate at the end of the growth phase in its life cycle, an adaptation crucial to the perpetuation of the organism in nature. Spores are not seen on direct staining of specimens; however, they appear in culture when nutrients are depleted. Atmospheric oxygen is considered necessary for sporulation because sporulation does not occur in the unopened carcass of an animal succumbing to anthrax. Anthrax spores are very resistant to heat, radiation, disinfectants, and desiccation, resulting in their persistence for more than 40 years in certain soils and environments.

Epidemiology

As mentioned, anthrax has a worldwide distribution. It has been sporadically reported in the United States, most commonly in the central and the Mississippi Delta regions. Warm temperatures (>18 ° C, or 60° F), moisture, and alkaline soils with high nitrogen content allow vegetative growth and proliferation of spores that have been released into the soil from carcasses of animals that died of anthrax.[57] Epizootics tend to occur in summer or fall after heavy rainfall or flooding preceded by drought conditions. Livestock usually become infected by ingesting spores while grazing or by eating contaminated feed. Isolated infections in dogs have been recorded during major anthrax outbreaks in farm animals. Infections in captive canids and felids have also been recorded after feeding raw meat from contaminated carcasses; however, they are relatively resistant to inhalation anthrax.

Recent events in the United States have involved documented terrorist dissemination of anthrax spores to induce inhalation anthrax in humans.[75] Companion animals in urban environments, although at reduced risk from infection through contact with infected livestock, are presumed to be at greater risk for infection from terrorist acts.

Pathogenesis

Infection occurs after inert *B. anthracis* spores enter the host body by ingestion, by inhalation, or through a break in the skin. The incubation period is usually 3 to 7 days. Based on evidence from natural and experimental infections, dogs and cats are considered relatively resistant,[27] people have intermediate resistance, and ruminants and horses are most susceptible to infection. In experimentally infected dogs, lesions have been restricted to local foci in the lungs because the organisms are generally contained by fibrin and cellular infiltrations.[56]

After spores contact the pulmonary alveoli, they are phagocytized by macrophages that migrate through the alveolar membrane and enter pulmonary lymphatics, eventually reaching hilar lymph nodes. At the point of entry in the GI mucosa, a primary focal hemorrhagic lesion is produced. Bacteria migrate to regional lymph nodes and the spleen. Within host cells the spores quickly germinate into fully encapsulated vegetative cells that release toxins. Vegetative cells respond to the host factors of high body temperature and carbon dioxide levels, resulting in transcriptional activation of capsule and toxin genes. The capsule is thought to be an antiphagocytic factor, and the toxin induces large-scale generation of cytokines such as interleukin (IL)-1 that result in septic shock.[93] Multiplication of the bacteria results in intoxication and death of the phagocytes, resulting in a continuous bacterial release into the blood. Additional replication of bacilli in high numbers in the bloodstream intensifies the systemic manifestations.

Although most *Bacillus* species are nonpathogenic to animals and people, *B. anthracis*, through its pXO1 plasmid, produces three toxin proteins: protective antigen (PA), edema factor (EF), and lethal factor (LF). The three components are serologically distinct and cause no lesions when injected separately, but in binary combinations they produce edema toxin (PA and EF) and lethal toxin (PA and LF). Protective antigen mediates the entry of either EF or LF into the cytosol of host cells. EF is an adenylyl cyclase that inhibits TNF-α synthesis and impairs host defenses. LF, a metalloprotease, inhibits mitogen-activated protein kinases and induces macrophage lysis.

If not superceded by septicemia and death, the host response involves specific IgG antibodies against PA, with antibodies functioning to inhibit spore germination and stimulate phagocytosis by macrophages. Antibiotic therapy started after initial infection does not interfere with the immune response to *B. anthracis*.

Clinical Findings

Anthrax infections can be characterized by either the rate of disease progression (peracute, acute, or subacute/chronic) or the primary route of inoculation (inhalational, GI, or cutaneous). The two characterizations are somewhat parallel, but clinical signs are influenced by species susceptibility to anthrax. Various reports of anthrax in dogs and cats suggest that some animals may be exposed to but not develop infection or are asymptomatic during infection. Thus morbidity and mortality caused by anthrax in companion animal species are reduced but not necessarily eliminated.

Cutaneous anthrax, the most common manifestation in people worldwide, is rarely the primary clinical form in canids or felids. After entering a cut or abrasion in the skin, the organisms multiply and produce toxin. The cutaneous lesion appears first as a papule, progresses to a vesicle, ruptures, and develops into a black eschar secondary to focal necrosis. Although cutaneous infection usually resolves without medical treatment, antibiotics are recommended because cases may progress to systemic involvement and fatal septicemia.

Naturally occurring anthrax in free-roaming, captive, or domestic canids or felids is most commonly GI in origin and caused by ingestion of meat or hides from infected carcasses.

After oral exposure, the infection in dogs and cats is usually manifest as fever (39.4° C to 40.5° C, or 103° F to 105° F); anorexia; and local inflammation, necrosis, and edema of tissues of the upper GI tract—the first tissues to contact the swallowed organism. Swelling of the head and neck tissues is usually apparent. Subsequent spread to the local and mesenteric lymph nodes, spleen, and liver typically occurs, causing enlargement. Acute gastroenteritis, which is often hemorrhagic, can occur, as may sudden death, particularly in younger animals. Signs in younger or immunocompromised dogs and cats may resemble systemic anthrax in more susceptible species, described as fulminating septicemia in which the principal lesions are edema, hemorrhage, and necrosis.

Experimental exposure of dogs to aerosolized anthrax spores did not reliably produce clinical disease other than short-term fever and anorexia in some dogs.[56] In more susceptible species with suspected natural inhalational exposures, clinical signs include fever, lethargy, cough, dyspnea, and septicemia.

Diagnosis

Pus or tissue specimens from animals suspected of infection should be stained with Gram's stain to show gram-positive bacilli (which have the "boxcar" appearance) and methylene blue to show the polypeptide capsule (which has the "string of pearls" appearance).

Serologic testing, using an ELISA to detect IgG to *B. anthracis* PA and capsular antigen in people, is highly sensitive; however, positive results are not completely specific for this type of anthrax.[63] A fourfold changing titer is needed to confirm active infection or recent exposure. Some people with prior exposure to herbivorous animals or their by-products have seropositive test results. Few other premortem tests are recommended. A skin test for diagnosis of anthrax in people was used in the former Soviet Union. This anthrax skin test, which detects heightened CMI against the organism, was usually positive after 3 days of illness in 97% of those affected.[125]

Necropsy of affected carcasses is not advisable because sporulation occurs, releasing the resistant spores into the environment. Examination of the stained smears of blood from a peripheral vein or of fine-needle aspirates is the most effective and safest means of making a diagnosis.

Bacterial culture is used for confirmation of anthrax in specimens. The organisms can be isolated from samples on routine culture media if the materials are fresh. Colonies are gray-white to white and nonhemolytic. The isolates are nonmotile and have a capsule; they show catalase positivity, lysis by γ-bacteriophage, penicillin susceptibility, and endospore production. Prior treatment with antibiotics may reduce the ability to isolate the organism. Vegetative cells may be isolated from blood, sputum, CSF, eschar, and feces (if the animal had GI anthrax). In cases of suspected inhalation exposure, *B. anthracis* spores may be collected for culture using sterile-water moistened swabs taken from the nares and haired muzzle or face within 24 to 48 hours of exposure to aerosolized spores.[61]

Immunocytochemical direct fluorescent antibody examination of nasal swab smears, pleural fluid smears, or pulmonary biopsy specimens using antibodies to *B. anthracis* cell wall and capsule has been used to diagnose inhalation anthrax in people.[31] If available, polymerase chain reaction (PCR) of sterile body fluids (blood or pleural effusion) can be helpful in rapidly confirming a diagnosis. Another means of specific identification is laboratory animal inoculation. Commercially available test strips (API Products, Plainview, N.Y.) can be used to aid identification.

Diagnostic pathology laboratories and shippers should always be alerted before receiving shipments of materials suspected of containing *B. anthracis*. Specimens or intact carcasses should be shipped using a biosecure procedure; they should be wrapped in plastic and kept refrigerated during transit. Public health authorities should also be notified when a diagnosis is suspected or confirmed in an animal.

Pathologic Findings

Carcasses of animals that have died of anthrax generally show little or no rigor mortis, and dark, nonclotting blood is usually seen oozing from the oral and nasal cavities and anus. The carcass often is bloated and decomposes rapidly. It is not advisable to necropsy or cut into such carcasses because exposure to air causes the vegetative organisms to form resistant spores that contaminate the environment. Blood or tissue samples for cytologic examination or culture can be obtained by taking blood from a large vein or through percutaneous aspiration. Should necropsy be inadvertently performed on an infected animal, characteristic lesions will be observed. GI anthrax has significant pathologic symptoms associated with the alimentary tract region where the ingested organisms penetrated the mucosal surface. Extensive gelatinous edema with focal areas of hemorrhage and necrosis are commonly seen and may be present around lymph nodes and in any area of the tract, from oral cavity to rectum. Diphtheritic membranes and ulcers may be present on the tonsillar surfaces. Gram-positive bacterial colonies may be present in the fibrinous exudates in the surface ulcerations of the GI mucosae. Extensive areas of necrosis in submucosal tissues are accompanied by neutrophilic infiltrates. Splenomegaly and a friable liver are often observed. Petechial hemorrhage secondary to septicemia may be noted on serosal surfaces. GI anthrax is typically also associated with extensive edema around and hemorrhage within pharyngeal and mesenteric lymph nodes.

Studies of inhalation anthrax symptoms in dogs describe discrete, dark, firm pulmonary lesions, consisting of a hemorrhagic core surrounded by dense masses of fibrin and a highly cellular periphery formed from dense accumulation of neutrophils, plasma cells, monocytes, and large macrophages.[56] This intense fibrinous and cellular local response has been interpreted as a restrictive reaction by the resistant canine host to contain the *B. anthracis* invasion (Fig. 35-6). Intrathoracic

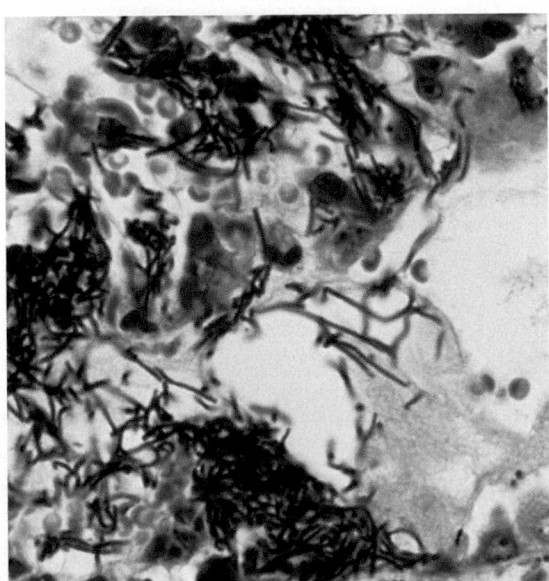

Fig 35-6 Vegetative *B. anthracis* with edema and hemorrhage in lung of inhalation anthrax laboratory model (Brown and Hopps, ×400). (Courtesy Armed Forces Institute of Pathology, Washington, D.C.)

lymph nodes were commonly enlarged because of reactive hyperplasia, but bacilli were not observed during histologic examination. In people, lymph node enlargement causes mediastinal widening, a pathognomonic radiographic sign in the diagnosis of inhalation anthrax. Mild pulmonary infiltrates and pleural effusion may also be detected radiographically.

Diagnosis of anthrax can be confirmed in pathologic specimens by specific immunohistochemical staining with an antibody conjugate that specifically identifies the galactose-N-acetyl-D-glucosamine polysaccharide unique to *B. anthracis*.[98] Electron microscopy with specific immunogold labeling of the vegetative organisms can also be used. Cultivation of the organism (as described previously) can be performed on tissue specimens

Therapy

Information regarding the recommended treatment of dogs or cats with suspected or confirmed clinical anthrax is extrapolated from literature reports of other species. *B. anthracis* is susceptible to a wide range of antimicrobials, including penicillin (which is historically the treatment of choice), ciprofloxacin/enrofloxacin, and tetracyclines (Table 35-8; see also Appendix 8, Drug Formulary). Other antimicrobials showing in vitro efficacy but that have not been clinically evaluated are chloramphenicol, erythromycin, aminoglycosides, and sulfonamides. Because of bacterial production of a cephalosporinase, *B. anthracis* isolates are typically resistant to cephalosporin antibiotics; potentiated sulfonamides are also ineffective. Initial doses of antimicrobials should be administered IV because of the potential rapid development of bacteremia and septicemia in infections. IV penicillin G is the drug of choice for people with bacteremia and should be used in dogs and cats. Although tissue cultures become negative within 24 hours after treatment is started, antibiotics are usually administered for 7 to 14 days. Postexposure prophylaxis protocols for people recommend at least 60 days of antibiotic administration because of concerns about environmental and pulmonary spore persistence.[17] Amoxicillin or ampicillin may be substituted when the treatment course is prolonged or pregnancy or lactation are contraindications for the preferred drugs.

Additional supportive care as needed is also indicated. Animals with respiratory compromise from cervical edema may need treatment with glucocorticoids or tracheostomy. Pleural effusion may require drainage. Skin or superficial lesions should never be surgically removed. Dressings with drainage from lesions should be incinerated, autoclaved, or disposed of as biohazardous waste. A dog or cat with suspected coat or skin exposure to anthrax aerosol should be immediately decontaminated by a soap and water rinse. A 0.5% sodium hypoclorite solution inactivates or kills the anthrax spores but is too caustic for prolonged use on skin. This solution should be reserved for gross decontamination only and rinsed after a few minutes.

Prevention

In endemic areas or during an outbreak, all meat fed to dogs and cats should be thoroughly cooked to eliminate the risk of exposure. Livestock at risk should receive annual vaccinations. Livestock or human anthrax vaccines currently marketed have not been tested in companion animals nor are they licensed or recommended for use. Animal vaccines approved for large animals commonly use an avirulent nonencapsulated (pXO2-deficient) spore strain, which was discovered by Sterne in 1939.[164] Two subcutaneously (SC) administered doses 2 to 3 weeks apart are recommended, as are annual boosters for animals in anthrax-endemic areas. Localized vaccine reactions, presumably caused by the adjuvant, are occasionally reported. In contrast, a U.S.-licensed anthrax vaccine for people is a cell-

Table • 35-8

Antibiotic Treatment for Anthrax Exposure or Clinical Anthrax in Dogs and Cats

DRUG[a]	SPECIES	DOSE[b]	ROUTE	INTERVAL (HOURS)	DURATION[c] (DAYS)
Penicillin	B	$20-40 \times 10^3$ U/kg	IV	8	prn
Doxycycline	D	5 mg/kg	PO	12	60
	C	50 or 100 mg per cat	PO	12	60
Amoxicillin	B	11—22 mg/kg	PO	8	60
Ciprofloxacin	D	10—15 mg/kg	PO	12	60
Enrofloxacin	D	2.5—10 mg/kg	IV, PO	24	60
	C	2.5—5 mg/kg	PO	24	60

B, Both dog and cat; *D*, dog; *C*, cat; *IV*, intravenous, *PO*, by mouth; *prn*, as needed.
[a]For additional information on each drug, see Appendix 8.
[b]Dose per administration at specified interval.
[c]Because of the persistence of the organism in the environment, a long treatment interval is recommended to prevent exposure or reinfection during an outbreak. IV treatment is used only initially in the course of treating acutely ill animals to control manifestations of bacteremia.

free filtrate containing protective antigen and alum. Six SC injections (at 0, 2, and 4 weeks and 6, 12, and 18 months) are required for immunity, and annual booster injections are recommended for maintenance. Local and systemic reactions have been reported with this vaccine.[149] Inflammatory reactions to the vaccine have been more common in women. An attenuated live vaccine for people, which was developed in the former Soviet Union, has been effective; however, it is not available in other countries.

Public Health Considerations

Anthrax is a natural disease of herbivores, and people, dogs, and cats are incidentally infected. Anthrax is a notifiable disease and should be reported to state and federal agencies. Care must be taken when handling infected tissues or carcasses, because the organism can penetrate cuts in the skin, resulting in localized infection with subsequent dissemination. In developed countries, most of the naturally occurring cases in people are cutaneous in origin. Lesions are painless, pruritic papules, sometimes surrounded by vesicles, with an ulcerated, circular, black necrotic scab. Although less common, inhalation or ingestion can result in either a highly fatal septicemia caused by hemorrhagic pneumonitis or an oropharyngitis and gastroenteritis, respectively. Anthrax has been developed as a biologic warfare agent by Japan, the United Kingdom, the United States, Iraq, and the former Soviet Union. One millionth of a gram of inhaled anthrax spores is a lethal dose to a person. Apart from terrorist events, infection in people is almost always transmitted from infected animals or their by-products. To minimize environmental contamination by anthrax spores, carcasses of animals dying from anthrax should be destroyed by incineration or buried deep with a covering of quicklime (anhydrous calcium oxide). Personnel who are cleaning up after an outbreak or terrorist attack that kills livestock and contaminates or injures more resistant dogs and cats should wear protective clothing and respirators. Decontamination involves a sporocidal solution of lye because ordinary disinfectants are ineffective (5% NaOH for 1.5 hours at 27.8° C or 3.6 hours at 21.1° C kills 99% of spores).[165] In the laboratory, surfaces can be decontaminated with either 5% hypochlorite or 5% phenol (carbolic acid). Instruments used should be autoclaved or boiled at 100° C for 10 minutes.[165] All areas, equipment, and buildings that may have contacted infected animals should be cleaned and disinfected. Control

of flying insects and scavenging insects and animals should be implemented. (For additional information on decontaminating the environment for *B. anthracis*, see Chapter 94.)

ERYSIPELOTHRIX INFECTIONS

Craig E. Greene

Erysipelothrix rhusiopathiae (insidiosa) and *Erysipelothrix tonsillarum* are small gram-positive nonmotile, nonsporulating pleomorphic facultatively anaerobic rods. These organisms, which are found worldwide, are associated with swine production. *E. rhusiopathiae* is the causative agent of swine erysipelas and other diseases in animals such as joint-ill in sheep and cattle and septicemia in turkeys, ducks, and laboratory mice. The anaerobes can be cultured from the tonsils of clinically healthy swine, the skin of freshwater and saltwater fish, and the decomposing plant and animal matter in their environments. Occupational exposure to these sources of bacteria may cause localized cutaneous or systemic infections in people.

Initially, the genus *Erysipelothrix* was thought to have a single species—*rhusiopathiae*—but biochemical and genetic analyses have identified *E. tonsillarum*, a nonpathogenic commensal of the tonsils of swine.[141] In dogs, endocarditis and septicemia were initially thought to be caused by *E. rhusiopathiae* after natural[65] and experimental[58] inoculation. However, all available isolates from endocarditis reported in dogs have been now reclassified as serovar 7 of *E. tonsillarum* and have been nonpathogenic for swine.[80,141] DNA hybridization studies have confirmed this relationship.[142] Clinical signs of fever, shifting-leg lameness, and recent onset heart murmur are characteristic of infected dogs.

The isolated strains have been susceptible to penicillin and ampicillin in vitro but resistant to aminoglycosides and sulfonamides.[141] Most cases of *Erysipelothrix* bacteremia are associated with endocarditis, therefore high doses of antimicrobials are recommended for at least 6 to 8 weeks. Relapses and reinfection are common in infected animals and people. Most human infections are acquired through occupational exposure; infections are found in slaughterhouse workers, food handlers, and animal trappers.[99] Infected dogs do not seem to pose a public health hazard.

SUGGESTED READINGS*

8. Bell DM, Kozarsky PE, Stephens DS. 2002. Clinical issues in the prophylaxis, diagnosis, and treatment of anthrax, *Emerg Infect Dis* 8:222-225.

19. Cantor GH, Byrne BA, Hines SA, et al. 1998. VapA-negative *Rhodococcus equi* in a dog with necrotizing pyogranulomatous hepatitis, osteomyelitis, and myositis, *J Vet Diagn Invest* 10:297-300.

20. Chalker VJ, Brooks HW, Brownlie J. 2003. The association of *Streptococcus equi* subsp. zooepidemicus with canine infectious respiratory disease, *Vet Microbiol* 95:149-156.

21. Cizinauskas S, Tipold A, Fatzer R, et al. 2001. Streptococcal meningoencephalomyelitis in 3 dogs, *J Vet Intern Med* 15:157-161.

24. Collins MD, Hoyles L, Lawson PA, et al. Phenotypic and phylogenetic characterization of a new *Corynebacterium* species from dogs: description of *Corynebacterium auriscanis* sp. Nov, *J Clin Microbiol* 37:3443-3447, 1999.

39. DeWinter LM, Low DE, Prescott JF. Virulence of *Streptococcus canis* from canine streptococcal toxic shock syndrome and necrotizing fasciitis, *Vet Microbiol* 70:95-110, 1999.

40. DeWinter LM, Prescott JF. 1999. Relatedness of *Streptococcus canis* from canine streptococcal toxic shock syndrome and necrotizing fasciitis, *Can J Vet Res* 63:90-95.

46. Fairley RA, Fairley NM. 1999. *Rhodococcus equi* infections of cats, *Vet Dermatol* 10:43-46.

113. Proft T, Sriskandan S, Yang L, et al. 2003. Superantigens and streptococcal toxic shock syndrome, *Emerg Infect Dis* 9:1211-1218.

122. Schäfer-Somi S, Spergser J, Breitenfellner J, et al. 2003. Bacteriological status of canine milk and septicaemia in neonatal puppies-a retrospective study, *J Vet Med B Infect Dis Vet Public Health* 50:343-346.

146a. Taillefer M, Dunn M. 2004. Group G streptococcal toxic shock–like syndrome in three cats, *J Am Anim Hosp Assoc* 40:418-422.

148. Tessier-Vetzel D, Carlos C, Dandrieux J, et al. 2003. Spontaneous vegetative endocarditis due to *Enterococcus faecalis* in a Rottweiler puppy, *Schweiz Arch Tierheilkd* 145:432-436.

162. Whatmore AM, Engler KH, Gudmundsdottir G, et al. 2001. Identification of isolates of *Streptococcus canis* infecting humans, *J Clin Microbiol* 39:4196-4199.

170. Wu CC, Kiupel M, Taymond JT, et al. Group G streptococcal infection in a cat colony, *J Vet Diagn Invest* 11:174-177.

*See the CD-ROM for a complete list of references.

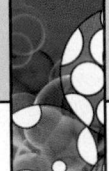

CHAPTER • 36

Staphylococcal Infections

Hollis Utah Cox

ETIOLOGY

Staphylococci are facultatively anaerobic, gram-positive cocci. Their principal habitats are the skin and mucous membranes of mammals and birds.[70] Staphylococci are classified into over 36 species (nine of which contain subspecies) based on genotypic differences and consideration of habitat or pathogenic processes.[55,70] Co-evolution of animal hosts and their species of *Staphylococcus* has occurred.[1,12,70,120] Although geographic differences between the distribution of *Staphylococcus* species in apparently similar human populations have been demonstrated, studies comparing dog and cat populations have not been reported.[70] All species of staphylococci isolated from normal animals are potentially pathogenic. However, individual species display a wide spectrum of virulence, host preference, and site specificity; and relatively few species are commonly isolated from infections of dogs and cats.* Host-adapted species may transiently colonize another host species when contact between hosts is frequent or infections are present. Staphylococci are readily acquired from environments (e.g., fomites, soil, air, water) associated with animals and from a variety of animal products. Of the nonsporulating bacteria, staphylococci survive well in the environment because they are among the more resistant bacteria to drying and disinfection.

Staphylococci are not inherently invasive and can colonize the intact epithelium of healthy animals without causing disease. In this sense, normal animals are subclinical carriers of both transient and resident colonizing staphylococci. Rather, as opportunistic pathogens, staphylococci invade epithelium damaged by traumatic insult (e.g., incisions, wounds), other infections (e.g., demodicosis, dermatophytosis), or clinical conditions (e.g., seborrhea, thyroid dysfunction, immunosuppression).[8] Disease therefore results from a disturbance in the natural host-parasite balance. The typical feature of staphylococcal disease is abscess formation because leukocytes are the primary host defense mechanism against these bacteria.

Knowledge of the pathogenesis of staphylococcal infections remains limited. In general, the obvious associations between disease and the genetic profile of individual strains have not been shown.[8] Although many underlying causes are known to predispose animals to canine pyoderma, the specific host defect that allows staphylococci to proliferate and the bacterial factors that contribute to lesion development and tissue damage are not known. Virulence is often equated with the presence of specific cell envelope components and extra-

*References: 25, 54, 83, 106, 124.

cellular toxins and enzymes that potentially produce a wide variety of biologic effects on the host after tissue invasion. None of these virulence factors alone has been consistently implicated in clinical infections, although intradermal injections of staphylococcal extracts and protein A produce epidermal lesions and histologic changes similar to those observed in clinical cases of canine superficial pyoderma and pustular dermatitis.[64] However, little genetic diversity is found between isolates of *S. intermedius* from diseased and healthy dogs.[8] Attempts to determine whether subpopulations of virulent and nonvirulent staphylococci reside on dogs are inconclusive. Staphylococci can produce various exotoxins that modulate the host immune systems.[45,59a] In people, exotoxins produced by certain strains of *S. aureus* and group A streptococci act as superantigens by bypassing phagocytes with direct activation of V5B receptors on large numbers of T cells, causing massive cytokine release, which can result in necrotic lesions and systemic toxicity (toxic shock). Because superantigens work directly on cytokine release, this reaction can occur even in severely immunosuppressed animals.[29] The exotoxin production, which exists for *S. intermedius* isolated from dogs, does not contribute to pruritus or recurrence of pyoderma[19,25,45] but may contribute to cellulitis and toxic shock syndrome. Based on analysis of digests of DNA after restriction endonuclease treatment, *S. intermedius* isolates from canine pyoderma differ from *S. intermedius* isolates from normal dogs but do not differ in recognized virulence factors or exoproteins.[3] If dogs are colonized by more than one strain of *S. intermedius*, apparently the recognized toxins are not important virulence markers, and an as yet unrecognized factor may be involved.[3] Genetic constructs encoding staphylococcal enterotoxins have been used as immunogene therapy for neoplasia in dogs.[116] Staphylococcal extracts have also been used for a variety of immunotherapeutic purposes in dogs and cats (see Immunomodulators, Chapter 2).

Coagulase, an enzyme present in most clinically significant staphylococci, polymerizes fibrinogen and clots plasma. Although coagulase is not toxic itself, its presence in a strain correlates with the presence of the other recognized virulence factors or extracellular products. *S. aureus, S. intermedius,* and three other species often produce coagulase and are generally more pathogenic relative to species that do not. Coagulase-negative staphylococci are also constituents of the normal microflora and capable of producing infections in hosts that are immunosuppressed or following invasive procedures. Protein A, an extracellular or a cell-bound protein produced by some canine and feline strains of *S. intermedius,* may enhance virulence by activating complement and by nonspecifically binding to immunoglobulins. These and other biologic effects may provoke various inflammatory and allergic responses, particularly delayed hypersensitivity, which intensify the pyogenic process and heighten the damage produced by staphylococcal infections. Some of these responses may be related to the high concentrations of circulating immune complexes that are found in dogs with recurrent pyoderma and pyoderma secondary to generalized demodicosis.[27,67] Complex polysaccharide capsules and slime layers (glycocalyx) produced by many strains of staphylococci may also enhance virulence by promoting bacterial adherence, inhibiting host phagocytosis, and resisting antibacterial drugs. Increased bacterial adherence may explain why certain breeds (German shepherd, English bulldog, and bull terrier) are predisposed to developing severe, often deep and recurrent, pyoderma.[33,66] Staphylococci are able to adhere to biomaterials used as surgical implants resulting in common infections.[7] Survival of *S. epidermidis* inside macrophages has been an important factor involved in infections associated with surgical implants. Administration of interferon (IFN)-γ to mice protected them against biomaterial-associated infection.[15] In endocarditis,

causative staphylococci have been shown to produce bacterial factors such as adhesins and toxins that allow their cellular invasion and attachment to the endocardial surfaces.[46] Acetylsalicylic acid has been used in vitro and in experimental models to reduce vegetative growth and attenuate the progression of *S. aureus*–induced valvular lesions.[58,69] *S. intermedius* isolates from dogs, cats, people, and other animals, in contrast to coagulase-negative staphylococci from these same hosts, contain some enterotoxin genes and produce enterotoxins in vitro.[9]

Transmissible plasmids are common in human strains of *S. aureus*. They may carry genes for virulence factors and for antimicrobial resistance to penicillin, ampicillin, amoxicillin, lincomycin, erythromycin, tetracycline, chloramphenicol, cephalosporin, kanamycin, and gentamicin. Other staphylococcal species infrequently carry similar plasmids, and most antibiotic resistance resides in chromosomal genes.[41,71,101] However, the potential exists for transfer of virulence and antimicrobial resistance genes from human strains of *S. aureus* to animal strains of staphylococci. The antimicrobial susceptibility patterns of clinically important isolates of staphylococci from dogs and cats have not changed considerably.* Although not common, multiresistant staphylococci are sometimes isolated from dogs with deep pyoderma or a history of antibiotic therapy.[53] Nosocomial transfer is known to modify the staphylococcal flora because nasal carrier rates for coagulase-positive staphylococci increase considerably with prolonged hospitalization of humans and dogs.

The predominant staphylococcal species of the resident bacterial microflora of dogs is *S. intermedius*. Specific biotypes have been persistently isolated in temporal studies from the hair coat and mucous membranes of individual dogs. However, the subpopulations at these two sites cannot be differentiated on the basis of antibiotic or phage susceptibility profiles, ribotyping, or other techniques.† Random amplified polymeric DNA–polymerase chain reaction (PCR) analysis has been the best method used to identify different genotypes in dogs and other host species.[96,120] Although agreement as to the natural anatomic habitat for *S. intermedius* is still debated, cultural studies have clarified the situation. Puppies acquire *S. intermedius* from the dam within 8 hours after birth.[4,95] The oral and nasal mucosae are the most frequently colonized sites, followed by abdominal skin. The level of colonization of the dam influences the level of colonization of pups.[95] Although many different genotypes are transferred to the pups, only one or two predominate and persist.[96] In adult dogs, large populations of several species of staphylococci reside at moist sites such as the nasal, anal, and oral mucosae and in rather occluded areas of the interdigital spaces and the ear canal.[4,21,43] The staphylococcus of the genital mucosae of breeding bitches following parturition is almost exclusively *S. intermedius*.[4,13] Lesser populations found at the skin surface and the distal hair coat probably indicate contamination or transient colonization rather than true resident status.[4,92] Because staphylococci can survive in inhospitable areas that are drier, more salty, and less humid, they are able to displace less tolerant species.[21] Other studies have suggested the possibility of a resident population within the pilosebaceous units from which secondary surface colonization can occur. The staphylococci on the distal hair shaft are contaminants whose origin is the resident population on the mucosae.[43] A temporal study compared the carriage of *S. intermedius* on normal dogs with that of atopic dogs in clinical remission and concluded that atopic lesions had become secondarily colonized from mucous membrane sites (nares, oral cavity, and anus).[92] When secondary staphylococcal infections were resolved, significant differences in isolation of *S.*

*References: 10, 35, 39, 51, 61, 80, 84, 85, 87, 118, 123.
†References: 3, 40, 43, 44, 48, 49, 74.

intermedius at any single site of the two groups of dogs was not evident. Dogs with pyoderma had significantly denser populations of *S. intermedius* at mucosal sites than did healthy household pets, a further indication that mucosal sites are the source for skin contamination. Results from one study indicated that nasal carriage was dependent on skin colonization.[44] However, when mucosal populations of *S. intermedius* were decreased by application of fusidic acid to mucosal surfaces, *S. intermedius* at nontreated skin sites was significantly reduced, further illustrating that mucosal carriage serves as the significant reservoir of infection in the dog.[91]

The coagulase-negative species *S. scirui* is widespread in nature and has been isolated from mucous membranes (anterior nares and mouth) and from the haired skin of dogs.[110] *S. epidermidis*, a coagulase-negative commensal of the skin and mucous membranes, was isolated from a dog with diskospondylitis.[2] This disease is most commonly caused by *S. intermedius* (see Chapter 86). Coagulase-negative *S. schleiferi* subsp. *schleiferi* and coagulase-positive *S. schleiferi* subsp. *coagulans* have been isolated from the skin of dogs with recurrent pyoderma.[34]

The predominant resident staphylococcal species of cats are *S. felis* and *S. xylosus*.[54] *S. intermedius* and *S. aureus* are isolated primarily from the hair coat of household cats and rarely from mucous membranes or from cats confined in a cattery. Apparently, they are transient residents acquired from contact with people or other animals. Coagulase-negative species are generally considered nonpathogenic commensals, and only a few isolations from pathologic lesions have been made. *S. felis* was isolated from cutaneous lesions of cats with otitis externa, paronychia, and excoriated skin lesions.[79] *S. auricularis* was isolated in combination with anaerobic bacteria in an inner ear infection in a cat.[23] In general, a less heterogeneous population of staphylococci is associated with cattery cats when compared with household cats or dogs.

CLINICAL FINDINGS

Coagulase-positive staphylococci are most frequently isolated from pyogenic infections of dogs and, less commonly, cats. As significant pathogens, they can affect every organ system independently or concurrently but are most common in abscesses and infections of the skin, eyes, ears, respiratory and genitourinary tracts, skeleton, and joints. In dogs, *S. intermedius* is the most common staphylococcal species isolated from pyoderma, otitis externa, diskospondylitis, bacteremia, conjunctivitis, and urolithiasis. Staphylococci are also found in valvular endocarditis and pericarditis.[86,109]

Other syndromes have been associated with staphylococcal infections in dogs. Botryomycosis, a poorly understood lesion caused by staphylococci and resembling mycetoma or actinomycosis, was found as an intraabdominal mass in a dog.[104] As with toxigenic streptococci (see Chapter 35), staphylococci have also been associated with skin scald, toxic shock, and necrotizing fasciitis.[37] Staphylococci were associated with an unusual cutaneous reaction, similar to psoriasiform-lichenoid dermatitis in people, that developed after topical treatment with cyclosporine A.[122] Staphylococci, unlike other potentially pathogenic microflora, are not usually associated with septicemia in neonatal pups.[97]

The infection sites are similar for cats; however, *S. felis* is the most frequent (45%) species, whereas *S. aureus* (13%) and *S. intermedius* (10%) are less common.[54] Abscesses or inflammatory granulation tissue with eosinophilic infiltration has been attributed to infection of cats with methicillin-resistant staphylococci.[75] The most frequently associated location of the lesions were subcutaneous or lymph nodes of the neck, or in the abdominal cavity, with or without mesenteric lymph node involvement.

DIAGNOSIS

Staphylococcal infections can be diagnosed presumptively by direct microscopy. Staining of a clinical specimen with Gram's stain or rapid cytologic stain will reveal neutrophils and cocci arranged singly or in pairs, short chains, or, rarely, irregular clusters. For culture, collection methods other than swabbing should be used whenever possible and should be designed to avoid superficial contamination. Surfaces of intact pustules, furuncles, or abscesses should be gently cleansed with alcohol, and the exudate directly aspirated or expressed onto a sterile swab without touching the skin (see Specimen Collection, Chapter 33). Punch biopsy procedures are suitable for both superficial and deep skin infections. Otic specimens are best obtained with a swab protected by a sterile otoscope cone inserted to the level of the horizontal ear canal. Before obtaining blood by venipuncture or urine by cystocentesis for culture, hair around the area should be shaved and the skin scrubbed as if for surgery. Respiratory tract specimens should be taken by transtracheal aspiration technique, bronchoscopic wash, or percutaneous transthoracic aspiration to bypass the oral flora. Specimens from deep-seated infections are often taken by direct biopsy or during surgery, such as aspirates or bone fragments curetted in cases of diskospondylitis.

Staphylococci in clinical specimens survive for up to 48 hours when kept cool (4° C [39.2° F]), particularly on commercial swabs containing a holding medium. Clinically significant staphylococci and normal flora contaminants grow best aerobically and may overgrow other pathogens when specimens are cultured on general-purpose, nonselective media.

Serologic assays, especially for antibodies reactive with teichoic acid or nucleases, are used as clinical aids in the diagnosis and management of bacteremia, endocarditis, and other deep-seated staphylococcal infections in people. However, the use and interpretation of results of these assays are controversial. Dogs with deep recurrent staphylococcal skin infections have high serum antistaphylococcal IgG levels compared with clinically unaffected dogs.[67,105] Dogs with superficial pyoderma secondary to atopy had high IgE levels. Despite these findings, serotesting will not likely be adapted for clinical use in animal infections.[52] High titers are more a reflection of bacterial hypersensitivity that perpetuates the inflammatory response.

THERAPY

Dosages for antimicrobials used to treat staphylococcal infections are listed in Table 36-1 and the Drug Formulary (see Appendix 8) and also under skin infections, Table 85-3. Staphylococci are rarely resistant (less than 5% of isolates) to first-generation cephalosporins (cephalexin, cefadroxil), β-lactamase-resistant synthetic penicillins (oxacillin, dicloxacillin, amoxicillin-clavulanate), gentamicin, tobramycin, enrofloxacin, mupirocin, bacitracin, and polymyxin B.[78] These drugs should be the drugs of first choice when culture and susceptibility results are unavailable and staphylococcal infection is suspected. Resistance to trimethoprim-sulfonamide combinations, chloramphenicol, and tylosin is relatively infrequent (6% to 19% of isolates).[102] Resistance to lincomycin, clindamycin, and erythromycin is relatively frequent (20% to 37% of isolates). Clinical isolates of staphylococci from dogs and cats are most frequently resistant (40% to 83%) to penicillin, ampicillin, amoxicillin, neomycin, and tetracycline.[57,60,72] Antimicrobials for which resistance is common should not be given for staphylococcal infections unless an isolate is shown to be susceptible by antimicrobial testing or by lack of β-lactamase production. Deep pyoderma or a history of antimicrobial therapy for staphylococcal infection indicates a need to culture regardless of the antimicrobial

Table • 36-1

Drug Therapy for Staphylococcal Infections in Dogs and Cats

DRUG[a]	SPECIES	DOSE[b] (mg/kg)	ROUTE	INTERVAL (HOURS)	DURATION (DAYS)
Amoxicillin-clavulanate	B	12.5–20	PO	8–12	prn
Oxacillin	B	22	PO	8	prn
Cephalexin or cefadroxil	B	22	PO	12	prn
Clindamycin	B	11	PO	24	14–42
Quinolones[c]	B	5	PO	24	prn
Erythromycin	D	10–15	PO	8	prn
Chloramphenicol	D	15–25	PO, IV, SC	8	prn
	C	10–15	PO, IV, SC	12	prn
Trimethoprim-sulfonamide	D	22	PO	12	prn

B, Dog and cat; *D*, dog; *C*, cat; *PO*, by mouth; *prn*, as needed; *IV*, intravenous; *SC*, subcutaneous.
[a]For additional information on these drugs, see Appendix 8.
[b]Dose per administration at specified interval.
[c]Includes marbofloxacin, danofloxacin, orbifloxacin, and enrofloxacin.

agent being considered for therapy.[71] Increased resistance of *S. intermedius* to chloramphenicol, clindamycin, and erythromycin has been associated with previous unspecified antimicrobial therapy of canine pyoderma. *S. intermedius* has been observed to acquire its macrolide-aminoglycoside resistance genes by horizontal transfer.[16] However, during a 1-year study in which dogs with recurrent folliculitis were treated with repeated courses of cephalexin, antimicrobial susceptibility patterns of *S. intermedius* from lesions and noninfected body sites were unchanged.[24] Canine isolates of *S. aureus* are more resistant to antibiotics than are *S. intermedius* isolates.[51] Clindamycin has been shown to be efficacious in the treatment of canine pyoderma[14,260] and experimentally induced *S. aureus* osteomyelitis in dogs.[18] Increasing resistance has been observed with the quinolone antibiotics.[59]

PUBLIC HEALTH CONSIDERATIONS

S. aureus Infections in Animals

People are the natural hosts for *S. aureus*, which colonizes the nasal passages of up to 40% of healthy adults and rarely other body sites in the absence of dermatoses. Although variants adapted to other hosts (ruminants, horses, and pigs) occur, *S. aureus* comprises less than 10% of clinical isolates from normal dogs and cats and apparently is not indigenous or site-specific in these hosts. Methicillin-resistant *S. aureus* (MRSA) is problematic as a cause of nosocomial infections and increasingly as a community-acquired, human pathogen. Staphylococcal resistance to methicillin has been attributed to multiple genetically controlled mechanisms. Most notable is their possession of a low-affinity penicillin-binding protein, PBP2a, which is encoded by an extra 30- to 50-kilobase chromosomal gene mecA. Nosocomial MRSA are considered resistant to all commonly used antibiotics, regardless of in vitro test results. This finding is justified based on the poor clinical response of MRSA to these antimicrobials. MRSA have been isolated from wound infections of a dog and cat in Japan,[31] from three dogs and a horse in Ontario,[73] from dogs in Korea,[76] a postsurgical wound of a dog in the Netherlands,[119] and from 11 canine infections associated with surgical treatment, especially orthopedic surgery, and recurrent pyoderma in Wisconsin, North Carolina, and London.[117] In another report, identical strains of MRSA were isolated from two dog owners, one concurrently colonized and one infected the previous year following surgery.[73] Two other owners had been hospitalized or had frequent out-

patient visits. The MRSA isolated from these four animals were indistinguishable from the major human clones found in Ontario. Human mupirocin- and MRSA-strains have been identified in the nasal passage of clinically healthy pet dogs and their human contacts in a household.[29a,63,104a,108,119a] Clinical infection in the people was eliminated only after successful treatment of the organism in the dog.

These cases suggest an antroponotic source for MRSA isolated from animals. However, unlike nosocomial MRSA, canine infections caused by community-acquired MRSA respond favorably to oral antibiotics to which the isolates are susceptible in vitro and are usually resistant only to β-lactam antibiotics.[117] In people, infections with MRSA have become a critical health complication. The emergence of community-acquired MRSA and the possible colonization of pets may become an increasing problem to monitor in the future. In multiresistant strain infections, newer peptides such as vancomycin and teicoplanin, and oxazolidones such as linezolid, are the only effective antimicrobials. For this reason, use of these drugs, which might induce resistant strains, should be restricted or avoided in pets (see also Chapters 85 and 99).

S. intermedius Infections in People

Staphylococci of dogs and cats are true zoonotic opportunistic pathogens. However, for many years, other than bite wound infections, zoonotic transmission of staphylococci of dogs and cats was thought to be uncommon. In early studies, only 1 of 144 veterinary hospital personnel had nasal colonization with *S. intermedius*.[112] In later reports, nosocomial transmission of *S. intermedius* in veterinary hospitals was considered to be rare.[17] For additional on transmission of staphylococci between people and dogs and cats, see Chapters 85 and 99.

Among the general pet-owning public, the transfer of *S. intermedius* from pets to people has become of concern. In past surveys, *S. intermedius* was rarely found in people, even among individuals with frequent animal exposure.[111] A study of hospitalized people identified only two *S. intermedius*-positive isolates among 3397 consecutive isolates of coagulase-positive staphylococci.[62] A human case of pneumonia in a surgical patient was described as the first case of invasive methicillin-resistant *S. intermedius* (MRSI).[36] In another human case involving otitis externa, identical strains of *S. intermedius* were isolated from the patient and her dog.[113] Mastoid cavity infection caused by *S. intermedius* developed in a person who had a dog that licked the owner's ears following mastoidectomy.[56] Bacterial strains from the dog's saliva and the otic discharge in the patient were genetically identical.

In a study of 13 individuals with dogs affected by deep pyoderma and 13 without daily contact with dogs, seven of the dog owners and only one of the nonowners carried multiple antimicrobial-resistant *S. intermedius*.[42] In six of the dog owners, genetic analysis found identical strains in the dogs and their owner. Strains detected were resistant to up to five different antimicrobial groups, including penicillins, fusidic acid, macrolides and lincosamides, tetracyclines, and chloramphenicol. MRSI are infrequently isolated from animal infections; however, they have resistance patterns similar to community-acquired MRSA.* These data are alarming with regard to spread of animal staphylococci, or potential spread of transferable antimicrobial resistance genes to human pathogenic staphylococci. In multiresistant strain infections, newer peptides such as vancomycin and teicoplanin, and oxazolidones such as linezolid are the only antimicrobials that are effective. For this reason, use of these drugs, which might induce resistant strains, should be restricted or avoided in pets.

SUGGESTED READINGS†

42. Guardabassi L, Loeber ME, Jacobson A. 2004. Transmission of multiple antimicrobial-resistant *Staphylococcus*

*References: 10, 22, 38, 39, 51, 68, 80, 84, 85, 87, 107, 118, 123.
†See the CD-ROM for a complete list of references.

cus intermedius between dogs affected by deep pyoderma and their owners, *Vet Microbiol* 98:23-27.
45. Hendricks A, Schuberth HJ, Schueler K, et al. 2002. Frequency of superantigen-producing *Staphylococcus intermedius* isolates from canine pyoderma and proliferation-inducing potential of superantigens in dogs, *Res Vet Sci* 73:273-277.
51. Hoekstra KA, Paulton RJL. 2002. Clinical prevalence and antimicrobial susceptibility of *Staphylococcus aureus* and *Staphylococcus intermedius* in dogs, *J Appl Microbiol* 93:406-413.
63. Manian FA. 2003. Asymptomatic nasal carriage of mupirocin-resistant, methicillin-resistant *Staphylococcus aureus* (MRSA) in a pet dog associated with MRSA infection in household contacts, *Clin Infect Dis* 36:26-28.
75. Ozaki K, Yamagami T, Nomura K, 2003. Abscess-forming inflammatory granulation tissue with gram-positive cocci and prominent eosinophil infiltration in cats: possible infection of methicillin-resistant *Staphylococcus*, *Vet Pathol* 40:283-287.
95. Saijonmaa-Koulumies LE, Lloyd DH. 2002b. Colonization of neonatal puppies by *Staphylococcus intermedius*, *Vet Dermatol* 13:123-130.
119. van Duijkeren E, Box AT, Mulder J, et al. 2003. Methicillin-resistant *Staphylococcus aureus* (MRSA) infection in a dog in the Netherlands, *Tijdschr Diergeneeskd* 128:314-315.

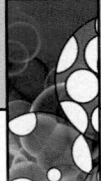

CHAPTER 37

Gram-Negative Bacterial Infections

Stephen A. Kruth

ETIOLOGY

Each gram-negative bacterial species has evolved a relatively complex outer membrane in addition to its cytoplasmic membrane and peptidoglycan layer. This outer membrane distinguishes the group from gram-positive bacteria and spirochetes. The outer surface of this membrane consists predominantly of a lipopolysaccharide (LPS, or endotoxin), which has a lipid portion embedded in the membrane (lipid A—the active component of endotoxin) and a polysaccharide portion extending from the bacterial surface (the O antigen; Fig. 37-1). In addition to conferring a gram-negative staining characteristic, these structures are important virulence factors and partially determine antibiotic susceptibility.

Gram-negative bacteria fall into numerous heterogeneous phylogenetic groups, and many can be pathogenic in dogs and cats. Some of these bacteria are discussed in other chapters: *Pasteurella* spp. (see Chapters 52 and 53), *Bordetella bronchiseptica* (see Chapters 6 and 16), and *Salmonella* spp. (see

Chapter 39). This chapter focuses on the general characteristics of *Escherichia coli*, *Proteus* spp., *Klebsiella* spp., and *Pseudomonas* spp. infections. Information and references to other chapters are also provided for *Citrobacter* spp., *Acinetobacter baumannii*, *Providencia alcalifaciens*, *Serratia* spp., and *Enterobacter cloacae* infections.

Classification

E. coli, *Proteus* spp., and *Klebsiella* spp. are members of the family Enterobacteriaceae. They are non–spore-forming, non–acid-fast, facultative, anaerobic gram-negative rods that are natural inhabitants of the intestinal tract of mammals. The Enterobacteriaceae family has 28 genera, with more than 100 well-defined species. Important species include *E. coli*, *Proteus mirabilis*, *Proteus vulgaris*, and *Klebsiella pneumoniae*.

Pseudomonas spp. are ubiquitous, non-Enterobacteriaceae, gram-negative bacteria that are found in soil, water, decaying vegetation, and animals. The most important and ubiquitous pathogenic pseudomonad is *Pseudomonas aeruginosa*. In Asia,

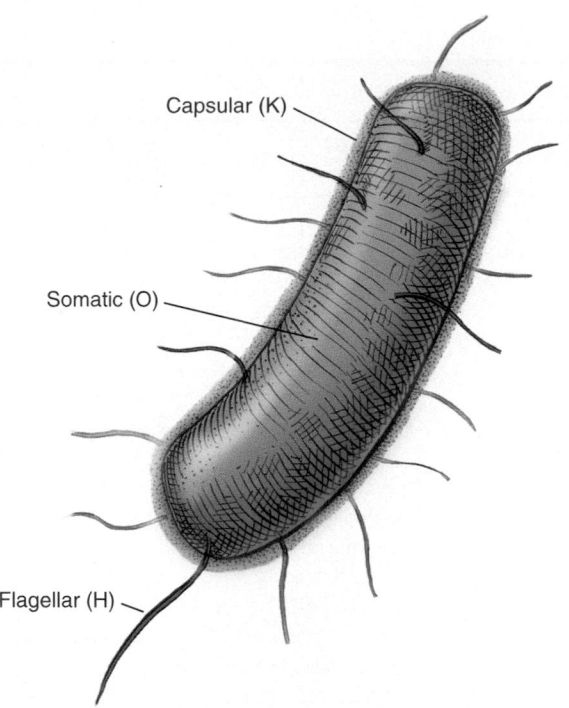

Fig 37-1 Structure of cell surface of gram-negative bacterium. (Courtesy University of Georgia, Athens, Ga.)

Eastern Europe, and Africa, *Pseudomonas mallei* is the cause of equine glanders; dogs and cats can become infected from the horse reservoir (see Chapter 46). *Burkholderia* (formerly *Pseudomonas*) *pseudomallei* is a soil organism found in Asia, central Africa, and Australia. In dogs and cats, it can cause syndromes ranging from a benign pulmonary infection to a lethal systemic disease (see Chapter 46).

Antigenic Structure

An internationally recognized serologic classification scheme has been developed for the Enterobacteriaceae based on antigenic differences in highly variable bacterial surface molecules. The *serogroup* is determined by the O *antigens*—sugars on the most external part of LPS (Fig. 37-2). The *serotype* is determined by flagellar H *antigens*. Additionally, K *antigens* can be identified in strains with a capsule. The antigenic formula of the strain indicates the presence of specific antigens (e.g., O55:K5:H21). However, for most strains, only O and H antigens are determined. At least 170 different serogroups have been identified for *E. coli*, and some correlation has been found between serogroup and virulence (e.g., O157:H7 and hemolytic uremia syndrome in humans).

EPIDEMIOLOGY AND PATHOGENESIS

The bacteria are commonly isolated from normal epithelia and spontaneously arising clinical infections of several different organ systems of dogs and cats (Table 37-1). They can

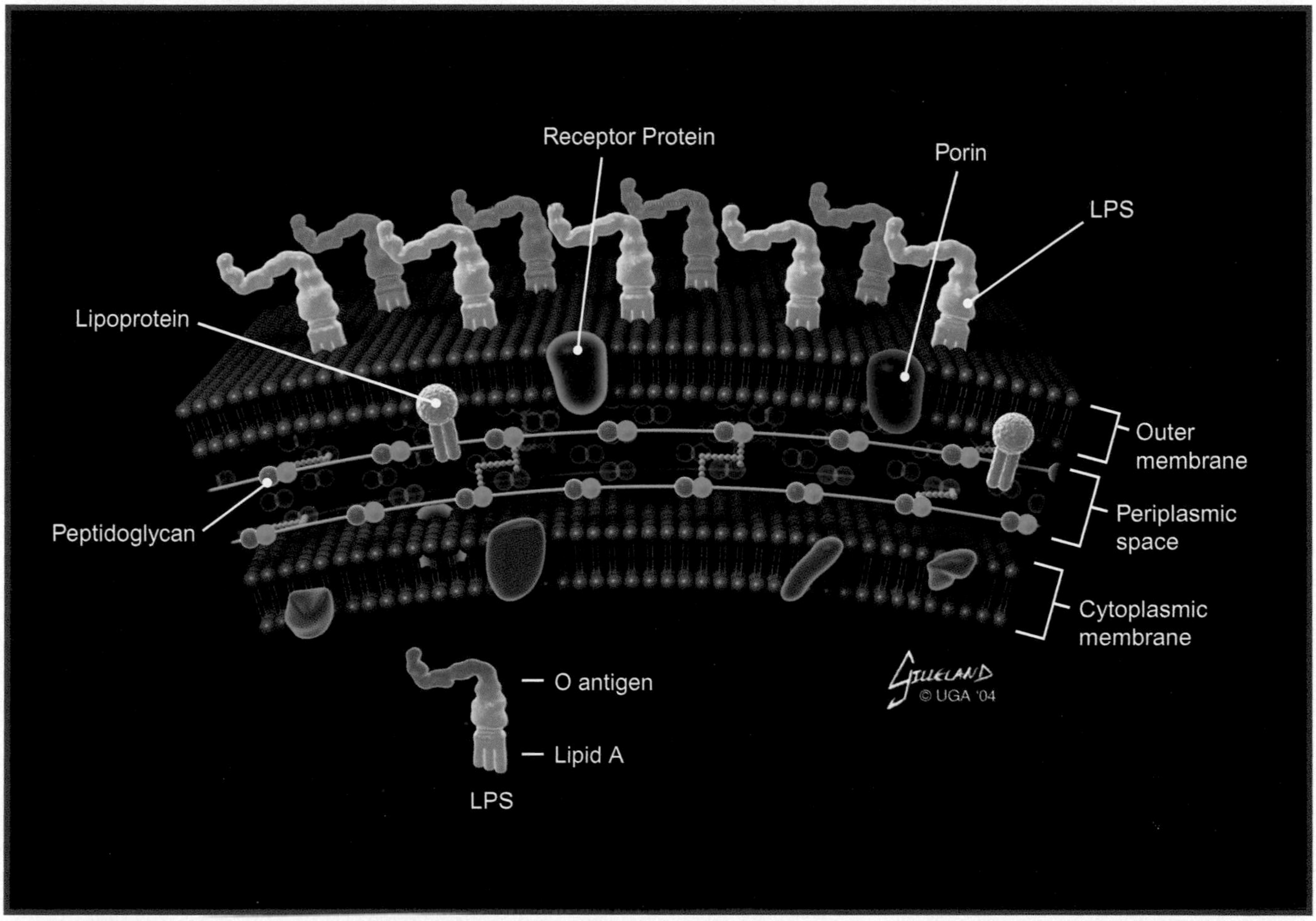

Fig 37-2 Structures of gram-negative bacteria that comprise various antigens. (Courtesy University of Georgia, Athens, Ga.)

Table • 37-1

Examples of Isolation and Infection Sites of Enterobacteriaceae and Pseudomonas Bacteria

NORMAL TISSUE SITES[a]	ESCHERICHIA COLI INFECTIONS	KLEBSIELLA INFECTIONS	PROTEUS INFECTIONS	PSEUDOMONAS INFECTIONS
Gut	Enterocolitis	Lower urinary tract infections, prostatitis	Deep pyoderma otitis externa, media, and interna	Corneal ulcers
Nasal cavity	"Small intestine bacterial overgrowth"	Pneumonia, pyothorax	Conjunctivitis, keratitis	Deep pyoderma
Mouth, tonsils, oral pharynx	Cholecystitis, cholangitis, cholelithiasis, hepatic abscess	Cholelithiasis, cholangiohepatitis	Lower urinary tract infections, pyelonephritis, prostatitis	Otitis externa, media, interna
Trachea, bronchi (Klebsiella and Pseudomonas organisms)	Peritonitis	Enteritis	Osteomyelitis	Lower urinary tract infections, prostatitis
Distal urethra, prepuce, semen, vagina	Metritis, pyometra, vaginitis	Sepsis, including neonatal septicemia	Pneumonia, pyothorax	Osteomyelitis
Conjunctiva	Mastitis	Meningitis	Cholelithiasis	Chronic rhinitis (cats)
E. coli can translocate from gut lumen to mesenteric lymph nodes	Deep pyoderma, anal sacculitis	Infection from IV catheters	Sepsis	Pneumonia, pyothorax
	Otitis externa		Infection from IV catheters	Sepsis
	Osteomyelitis			Bacterial endocarditis
	Conjunctivitis, keratitis			
	Tonsillitis, pharyngitis			
	Lower urinary tract infections, prostatitis, pyelonephritis			
	Endocarditis			
	Bronchitis, pneumonia, pyothorax			
	Sepsis, including neonatal septicemia			
	Meningitis			
	Infection from IV catheters			

[a]Tissue from which E. coli, Klebsiella, Proteus, or Pseudomonas or all of these bacteria can be cultured.

cause sepsis, nosocomial infections, and opportunistic infections in immunocompromised animals. Isolates can be endogenous or exogenous to the individual. These types of infections may be increasing in frequency because of the overuse of new antibiotics, invasive procedures, and immunosuppressive therapies.

Virulence Factors

Some strains of E. coli are true pathogens; however, most E. coli, Klebsiella, Proteus, and Pseudomonas organisms are opportunistic pathogens. The pathogenicity of gram-negative bacteria depends on the presence of various virulence factors (e.g., adhesins, toxins, iron-acquisition systems, capsules) expressed by the organism. It is the set of virulence genes carried and expressed by the organism that confers pathogenicity rather than the genus or species designation. Examples of virulence factors follow.

The establishment of infection first depends on bacteria adhering to an epithelium. Adhesins are located on bacterial pili (or fimbriae), the slender external structures that facilitate attachment to host cells. Colonization factor antigen I (CFA-I) and colonization factor antigen II (CFA-II) are specific pilus adhesins-hemagglutins that promote colonization by some enteropathogens. Another fimbrial antigen is the vir antigen, which is associated with sepsis in some species. Bacterial capsules are polysaccharides, which protect the outer membrane from the membrane attack complex of complement and also inhibit the attachment of phagocytic cells. Colonization with Pseudomonas spp. occurs when the fibronectin

coat covering host cells is disrupted by infection or mechanical trauma. The pili and exozyme S of Pseudomonas spp. promote attachment to epithelial cells, and the extracellular slime is antiphagocytic. Siderophores, such as aerobactin, aid the bacterium in competing with the host for iron in low-iron environments.

The production of various toxins is important in the pathogenesis of gram-negative infections. Secreted α-hemolysin damages host cell membranes. Endotoxin (LPS) stimulates various cytokine cascades, as well as the complement cascade. Excessive activation of these systems leads to sepsis and septic shock (see Chapter 38). Pseudomonas spp. variably produce collagenase, lecithinase, lipase, proteases, hemolysins, fibrinolysin, leukocidin (also called cytotoxin), and enterotoxin. Many strains also secrete exotoxin A, a cytotoxin that causes tissue necrosis, allowing the organism to colonize deep tissues in burn and trauma cases. As with the Enterobacteriaceae, Pseudomonas LPS can act as an endotoxin.

Virulence Factors Associated with E. coli Intestinal Infections

The documentation of pathogenic E. coli infections is confusing because many of these organisms exist as normal enteric constituents and can be found in the microflora of clinically healthy animals. Analysis for specific toxin genes or molecular typing can be done to differentiate among the different isolates. Toxin analysis is important in addition to genetic studies because many of the genes identified may not be expressed by the organisms isolated. Pathogenic E. coli have been classified on the basis of their virulence properties into virotypes (Table 37-2). Virotypes usually contain more than one serotype. Virotypes are not clear-cut distinctions; some enteropathogens isolated from dogs have predominantly "uropathogenic" traits, but they cause diarrhea. Groups that have been described in dogs and cats based on phenotypic and genotypic factors are discussed in the following sections.

Systemic Infections

E. coli with particular pathogenic features are a frequent cause of extraintestinal and extraurinary tract infections. Such isolations include a report of *E. coli* endocarditis in a cat.[20] An outbreak of fatal hemorrhagic pneumonia and bacteremia in kenneled dogs was attributed to a pathogenic *E. coli* that was positive for virulence factors α-hemolysin and cytotoxic necrotizing factor 1 and for the adhesin factor class-III papG allele.[45] These organisms have the phenotypic and genotypic characteristics of extraintestinal virulent bacteria that are a risk for people and other animals.

Enteropathogenic E. coli

Enteropathogenic *E. coli* (EPEC) adhere to mucosal cells of the small intestine and colon, causing loss of microvilli (effacement, or attaching and effacing lesions) and the formation of filamentous actin pedestals or cuplike structures under the organisms. These changes in microvillous morphology are associated with an inflammatory response. EPEC also occasionally invade mucosal cells. Clinically, EPEC cause watery diarrhea as a result of host cell invasion and alteration of signal transduction systems rather than as a result of production of toxin.[9,111]

Enterotoxigenic E. coli

Enterotoxigenic *E. coli* (ETEC) adhere to small intestinal mucosal cells and produce diarrhea by elaborating toxins. Little inflammation and usually no histologic changes develop in mucosal tissues to which the bacteria are attached. Heat-labile toxins (LTs) and heat-stable toxins (STs) are well characterized. LTs (LT-I, LT-II) alter adenyl cyclase activity in epithelial cells of the small intestine. This results in inhibition of sodium and chloride absorption in villous epithelial cells and in active secretion of chloride by crypt cells, causing extensive loss of water and chloride. Data conflict about whether LT-producing *E. coli* have been isolated from dogs.[9,25,43,78,111]

STs (STa, STb) are a family of small toxins, some forms of which deregulate guanylyl cyclase, with resultant fluid secretion similar to that induced by LTs. Other forms stimulate cyclic nucleotide-independent secretion. ST-secreting *E. coli* have been isolated from dogs and cats with enteritis, supporting a causal association.[9,43]

Table • 37-2

Characteristics of Pathogenic Escherichia coli *Strains*

CLASSIFICATION	GENES	PATHOGENIC FACTORS	CLINICAL FEATURES
Enteropathogenic *E. coli* (EPEC)			
Class I	Locus for enterocyte effacement (LEE) coding for adhesion, intimin, and Tir proteins	Attaching and effacing; adhere to Hep-2 cells	Loss of microvilli; watery and chronic diarrhea
Class II	Unknown	No adherence to Hep-2 cells	Unknown
Enterotoxigenic *E. coli* (ETEC)	Heat labile (LT) and heat stable (ST) toxin genes and Type 1 fimbria	Attachment factors; LTs and STs	No histologic mucosal changes with diarrhea; no fever; hypersecretion of water and electrolytes
Enterohemorrhagic *E. coli* (EHEC) and *E.coli* O157:H7	Two types of Shiga toxin or vero toxin (VT) genes; LEE; plasmid with hemolysin gene	LTs and STs; Shiga-like (VT) toxins; vascular damage to endothelium	Hemorrhagic colitis, diarrhea; hemolytic uremic syndrome
Necrotoxigenic *E. coli* (NTEC)	Cytotoxic necrotizing factor (CNF) genes: CNF-1 chromosomal and CNF-2 plasmid	CNFs	Diarrhea, bacteremia, and urinary tract infections in people
Uropathogenic *E. coli* (UPEC) or extraintestinal *E. coli* (ExPEC)	papG gene, CNF1 gene, adhesin hemolysin and aerobactin genes	Adhere to uroepithelium via pili	Dysuria, hematuria, urinary tract inflammation; pneumonia, sepsis, meningitis
Enteroaggregative *E. coli* (EAEC or EaggEC)	Adhesins (plasmid encoded fimbria); hemagglutinins	Adhere to intestinal epithelium via pili	Nonbloody, watery diarrhea with some inflammation
Enteroinvasive *E. coli* (EIEC)	Outer membrane proteins (plasmid encoded)	Invade epithelium	Hemorrhagic diarrhea with mucus and leukocytes (dysentery)

Enterohemorrhagic E. coli and E. coli O157:H7

Enterohemorrhagic *E. coli* (EHEC) and *E.coli* O157:H7 bind tightly to epithelial cells and produce the same type of attachment-effacement lesions as EPEC. EHEC are minimally invasive but do incite an inflammatory response. They preferentially localize in the colon. EHEC produce verotoxins (VTs), which have two major antigenic forms (VT-I and VT-II). These toxins are sometimes called *Shiga toxins* (Stx 1 and Stx 2) or *Shiga-like toxins* (SLT). VTs inhibit protein synthesis by interfering with 28S rRNA, leading to damage of the vascular endothelium in target organs such as the kidney, gastrointestinal (GI) tract, and central nervous system (CNS). Within these bacteria, gammalike phages harbor the Stx genes. Chemical agents or drugs that damage DNA may activate dormant viral particles, allowing it to infect susceptible *E. coli* within the host and create new toxin-possessing bacteria.[94] Therefore although their use is widespread, antimicrobials such as quinolones might induce more virulent bacteria when they are used to treat virulent *E. coli* infections.

In people, EHEC infections have been associated with diarrhea, hemorrhagic colitis, and hemolytic-uremic syndrome (HUS). In almost all humans the toxin-producing organism has originated from the GI tract; however, one report includes a urinary source of infection.[104] EHEC have been isolated from stools of normal dogs and cats and those with diarrhea. A case-control study suggested that VT-II-positive isolates may be causally associated with diarrhea in dogs, whereas VT-I-positive isolates are carried but do not appear to cause diarrhea.[9]

In kenneled greyhounds, enterotoxin genes were identified in *E. coli* from dogs with and without diarrhea; however, only the presence of Shiga toxin Stx1 correlated with diarrhea (Staats et al, 2003). The presence of toxigenic *E. coli* in clinically healthy and diseased dogs indicated a potential zoonotic risk.

E. coli O157:H7 is an EHEC serotype responsible for foodborne and waterborne infection in people. It is harbored by cattle but does not cause them to develop any clinical illness. Undercooked beef and water contaminated by feces from infected animals or people are the most common source for spread. Large numbers of cattle tested at slaughterhouses harbor this bacterium; however, not all strains carry the virulence factors incriminated in severe disease. Dogs living on farms and feed lots have been documented as harboring *E. coli* O157:H7.[44,58,94,109] The dogs were not clinically ill, and the organism was isolated from their feces. Infected cattle were considered the source of infection. Infection was also documented in a pet dog that was fed food scraps[87] and in dogs frequenting beaches.[29] In all these reports the dogs were asymptomatic for infection, and the public health risk was of most concern.

Cats in Ontario, Canada were examined to determine the prevalence of verotoxigenic *E. coli* (VTEC) in feces related to the presence or absence of clinical disease.[98] Organisms were screened for VT genes by the polymerase chain reaction (PCR); the overall prevalence of enteric VTEC in 179 cats was 12.3%. However, no statistical association was found between the presence of the bacteria and clinical illness. Cats were positive for generic VT but not for VT-I or VT-II genes, suggesting that the VT may have been a new, nonpathogenic variety. Some of the isolated serotypes were similar to those found in people and cattle, suggesting that cats might be capable reservoirs for human infection.

Correlation of Pathogenic E. coli and Diarrhea

Samples of feces from clinically healthy dogs in kennels or households and in dogs with acute or chronic diarrhea were analyzed for various pathogenic *E. coli* including EPEC, ETEC, VTEC, EHEC, enteroinvasive (EIEC), and enteroaggregative (EAggEC) strains.[93] More of the dogs with diarrhea were excreting EPEC and VTEC than the kenneled or household control dogs. The EPEC attaching and effacing A (*eaeA*) gene and the verocytotoxin 1 (*VR1*) gene encoding for VTEC were often found together. Isolates from dogs with diarrhea had more aggregate and cytotoxic effects on cultured cells in vitro.

Hemolytic-Uremic Syndrome and Cutaneous and Renal Glomerular Vasculopathy of Greyhounds ("Alabama Rot" or "Greenetrack Disease")

HUS in people is characterized by acute renal failure, microangiopathic hemolytic anemia, fever, and thrombocytopenia and is often associated with diarrhea or upper respiratory infection. One cause of HUS is infection with the VT-producing O157:H7 serotype of *E. coli*, usually acquired through contaminated water or meat. VTs bind to vascular endothelial cells and induce necrosis, microthrombosis, and consumptive thrombocytopenia. A syndrome similar to HUS, characterized by hemorrhagic gastroenteritis, acute renal failure, and microangiopathic hemolytic anemia has been described in a small number of dogs; however, evidence of *E. coli* infection was not shown in these cases.[51]

Cutaneous and renal glomerular vasculopathy (CRGV) of greyhounds is an acute, potentially lethal syndrome of unproven etiology that was recognized in 1985.[47] CRGV typically occurs in young racing greyhounds but has also been described in a Great Dane.[92] It is characterized by distinctive, slowly healing, sharply demarcated cutaneous ulcers involving the limbs but sparing the head and dorsum. Some affected dogs have no other signs and appear otherwise healthy. However, in addition to cutaneous lesions, some dogs develop fever, distal limb edema, and acute renal failure (with some dogs developing renal failure without fever or other systemic signs), whereas other dogs develop renal failure before the cutaneous lesions. Normocytic, normochromic anemia with evidence of microangiopathic hemolysis, thrombocytopenia, elevated alanine transferase and creatine kinase activities, hypoalbuminemia, azotemia, hematuria, proteinuria, and isosthenuria are variably present. Partial thromboplastin and one-stage thrombin times are usually normal, activated partial thromboplastin time can be prolonged, and fibrinogen degradation products are usually low. Treatment is supportive, and the mortality of dogs developing renal failure is high.

Histologically, the glomerular lesions are similar to those seen in the childhood form of HUS. It was common practice for racing and training greyhounds to be fed beef of *4D quality* (i.e., diseased, debilitated, dying, or dead) from rendering plants. O157:H7 has been isolated from this type of meat and recovered from the stools of dogs with CRVG. Based on some clinical similarities (although children do not develop the cutaneous lesions), the histologic and ultrastructural glomerular abnormalities, and the association with O157:H7, it was hypothesized that CRGV is caused by VT-producing *E. coli*. The role of O157:H7 is not completely clear, because the oral or intravenous (IV) inoculation of adult greyhounds with high doses of the VT-producing O157:H7 does not cause CRGV. Age, genetics, concurrent infection, or other factors may be involved. Anecdotally, it appears that the prevalence of CRGV has diminished dramatically, possibly because of better feeding practices.[26,88,92]

Necrotoxigenic E. coli

Cytotoxic necrotizing factors (CNFs) are protein toxins that were originally called "vir toxin." CNF1 and CNF2 have been associated with diarrhea, bacteremia, and urinary tract infections (UTIs) in people. *E. coli* producing CNF1 have been isolated from stools of normal dogs and cats, as well as dogs (but not cats) with enteritis.[9,103] Serogroups of necrotoxigenic *E. coli*-1 (NTEC)-1 strains have been the same as those that infect people.[22] NTEC may have been responsible for rhabdomyolysis in a cat with chronic renal failure and an episode of acute enteritis.[69]

Uropathogenic *E. coli*

Some strains of *E. coli* can cause extraintestinal infections, including UTIs, pneumonia, sepsis, and meningitis; these strains are designated *extraintestinal pathogenic E. coli (ExPEC)*, in keeping with the terminology used for strains causing enteritis. This classification has some overlap, and some *E. coli* isolated from dogs with diarrhea have characteristics of uropathogenic and necrotoxigenic strains.[103] (See the previous Systemic Infections section for an additional discussion of *E. coli* causing infections outside the urinary and GI systems.)

E. coli is the most common isolate from dogs with first-time and recurrent UTIs and the second most common isolate from dogs with uroliths.[63,77] Some strains of *E. coli* express virulence factors that facilitate the colonization of the urinary system; uropathogenic *E. coli* strains are designated *UPEC*. The major determinant of their pathogenicity is the ability to adhere to the uroepithelium via adhesins such as type 1 pili or P fimbriae, the gene of which *(papG)* has been identified in canine isolates.[54,56] After attachment, pili and endotoxin incite neutrophil migration and induce the release of cytokines, leading to an inflammatory response and characteristic signs of urgency, discomfort, and hematuria.

Exotoxins, especially hemolysins, may also be important in the development of clinical signs of lower UTIs. Iron acquisition is also an important virulence factor, as are bacterial capsules and antiphagocytic systems. Numerous virulence factors have been identified in canine and feline UPEC strains, including CNF1 and genes encoding adhesins, hemolysin, and aerobactin.[28,127] The ability of some UPEC to actually invade uroepithelial cells has been reported in strains isolated from people, and it is possible that this characteristic may explain some relapsing UTIs in dogs and cats. UPEC are carried in the colon of many dogs; comparing phylogenetic background, O antigens, and extended virulence genotype, 54% of urinary isolates were also found in the gut. This is consistent with the idea that UPEC have a special type of pathogenicity, and UTIs are not the result of exposure to high numbers of "normal" *E. coli*.[53] Hemolytic *E. coli* have also been found in UTIs in cats.[108]

Studies based on the identification of genes encoding adhesins, hemolysins, CNF1, and aerobactin suggest that canine uropathic strains may be similar if not identical to some human uropathic strains.[56] Similarly, *P. mirabilis* strains isolated from the urine of dogs have been characterized and found to be similar to human uropathogenic *P. mirabilis* strains. The significance of these findings for people and dogs is not known.[34] ExPEC can also infect almost any anatomic site. Pneumonia, sepsis, and meningitis are some of the infections that have been observed. Multidrug-resistant strains have been isolated from animals with recurrent infections that have been treated with several types of drugs.[107]

Klebsiella Infections

Klebsiella organisms, which are found in the nasopharyngeal and intestinal flora, can be associated with clinically significant infections of the GI and genitourinary tracts and systemic bacteremia. *Klebsiella* organisms have also been implicated in nosocomial infections in veterinary hospitals.[38]

Pseudomonas aeruginosa Infections

P. aeruginosa is an environmentally stable organism that causes infection in animals whose immune systems or host defenses are impaired. Although it can be isolated from the upper respiratory, genital and GI tracts, and intertriginous areas of the skin, numbers of organisms are usually controlled by competition from normal bacterial flora. Inflammation or injury to these mucosal areas or chronic antibacterial therapy can lead to a proliferation of *P. aeruginosa*. In addition, open wounds or surgical incisions can become contaminated and subsequently infected with antimicrobial-resistant strains from the hospital environment. Defective flexible endoscopes that became contaminated were incriminated as a source of an outbreak in people.[100] *Pseudomonas* bacteria also have the ability to invade a healthy cornea in its warm, moist state. Through small scratches, the organism can enter the cell cytoplasm, where it rapidly replicates. However, some strains produce an exoenzyme toxin that kills epithelial cells and macrophages. In dogs with otitis externa, *P. aeruginosa* and *Proteus* organisms could be cultured from the ears but were not found in the ears of clinically healthy dogs.[126] *Pseudomonas* bacteria are also isolated from mixed infections in dogs.[102] *P. aeruginosa*, which has few nutritional requirements, thrives in moist environments outside the host and creates microcolonies that allow it to grow on moist surfaces such as those in bath tubs and plumbing and drainage systems. Animals that are immunosuppressed or have implanted catheters or open wounds are particularly susceptible to contamination from these moist environments or surfaces. In hospital environments, many of the *P. aeruginosa* strains have acquired multidrug–antimicrobial resistance. Exposure to quinolones in vitro or in vivo causes *P. aeruginosa* from dogs to develop resistance more rapidly than other bacteria.[15,106]

Pasteurella Infections

Pasteurella organisms are usually associated with the oral cavities of dogs and cats and are frequently found in wound infections caused by their bites (see Bite Infections, Chapter 53). Many *Pasteurella* spp. are covered with a layer of capsular polysaccharide, which gives rise to their specific serotypes. As with most gram-negative bacteria, they have cell-surface LPSs with endotoxic activities. Several outer membrane proteins are also involved in virulence. *Pasteurella canis* was isolated from newborn puppies with systemic infection.[21] These organisms are susceptible to various commonly used antimicrobial drugs. Quinolones have been shown to exert a postantibiotic effect on isolates of *Pasteurella multocida* from cats.[27]

Citrobacter Infections

Citrobacter freundii, a member of the bacterial family Enterobacteriaceae, is a ubiquitous bacterium in the environment. The GI tract is the likely source of systemic infection in dogs and cats. Neonatal or immunosuppressed animals develop enteritis with bacteremia, and the systemic infections often involve additional organs. Systemic spread can result in hepatitis, peritonitis, meningitis, interstitial pneumonia, and sepsis.[35]

Acinetobacter baumannii Infections

The *Acinetobacter baumannii* bacteria, which is a pleomorphic rod, is a gram-negative, aerobic, oxidase-negative, catalase-positive, and nonfermentative bacterium. It is short and nonmotile during rapid growth and becomes more coccoid during static growth periods. It is a low-grade pathogen, producing endotoxin in vivo, adhesins, and some enzymes. Of most concern is its ability to develop and transfer antimicrobial resistance in a short time. Nosocomial infections with this organism have been recognized for many years in people; however, infections in hospitalized dogs and cats have been reported.[12,32]

This ubiquitous organism can be isolated from food, water, and soil in the environment. In the hospital environment, it can contaminate surfaces; animals undergoing invasive procedures, such as placement of chest tubes, central venous lines, or indwelling urinary catheters, are most likely to be affected. Outbreaks can occur as the infection is transmitted to susceptible patients through the hospital environment, the hands of hospital staff members, or medical devices. Outbreaks in human hospitals suggest that airborne dissemination has a role in nosocomial infections, and air handling systems may become contaminated. Once animals become infected, they may shed the organism into the environment. Antimicrobial therapy selects for resistant isolates and increases the risk of developing resistant nosocomial infection. Use of cephalosporins has been a risk factor for these infections in people and animals.[32] (See Chapter 94 for additional information on control of nosocomial infections.)

Providencia alcalifaciens Infection

Providencia alcalifaciens, a gram-negative member of the family Enterobacteriaceae, has been identified as a human enteric pathogen and is associated with being one cause of travelers' diarrhea. It is not a typical enteric resident of animals; however, environmental contamination through feces of infected people and from flies may spread the infection. In experimental oral infections of rabbits, the organism proliferated and colonized the intestinal tract, displacing the resident flora.[2] *P. alcalifaciens* was associated with diarrhea in pups raised in a low socioeconomic area with exposure to raw human sewage.[74] The litter of 2-week-old pups stopped nursing over a 2-day period, began vocalizing, and had yellow-green, blood-tinged diarrhea. Wright-stained fecal smears contained a homogeneous population of short bacilli, degenerate neutrophils, and desquamated epithelial cells containing the same bacteria. Dead pups had yellow pseudomembranous exudates throughout the small intestine. Microscopy revealed this symptom was associated with severe, diffuse superficial necrosis of epithelium. Large numbers of short, gram-negative bacilli were adhered to enterocytes.

Serratia Infections

Serratia organisms are gram-negative bacteria. Like *Pseudomonas* bacteria, they thrive in the environment and can grow in moist environments, even in the presence of antiseptic agents such as benzalkonium chloride. They have been linked to nosocomial infections associated with medical procedures in hospitalized dogs and cats[31] (see Chapter 94).

Enterobacter cloacae Infections

As with *Serratia* bacteria, *Enterobacter cloacae* have been associated with nosocomial infections in dogs and cats[7] (see Chapter 94).

CLINICAL FINDINGS

All of the bacteria discussed colonize normal tissues and maintain a commensal relationship in dogs and cats. Most of the bacteria are opportunists, requiring alterations in local or systemic defenses and immune function for disease to develop. However, disease cannot develop unless the colonizing strain carries at least some virulence factors. Examples of clinically significant infections with these organisms are listed in Table 37-2.

Some important clinical associations have been reported. *E. coli* sepsis and lesions consistent with acute respiratory distress syndrome can develop in puppies with parvoviral enteritis.[112] *E. coli* and *Klebsiella* spp. neonatal septicemia have been identified in puppies with either signs of failure to gain weight, dyspnea, cyanosis, hematuria, and sloughing of extremities or acute death.[82] *K. pneumoniae* has also been reported to cause severe enteritis and sepsis in adult dogs.[90] *Klebsiella* spp. produce urease, which splits urea into ammonia; this can damage the uroepithelium and alter urine pH, favoring the development of struvite uroliths. *Klebsiella*

spp. are also associated with extensive, necrotizing, consolidating pneumonias. *Pseudomonas* spp. are pathogenic only when they colonize areas devoid of normal defenses. Debilitated patients are at risk for infection, as are those with malignancies, immunodeficiencies, urinary or IV catheters, traumatized tissues, or altered normal flora secondary to the administration of antibiotics. *Pseudomonas* spp. are also associated with rapidly progressive corneal ulcers caused by proteolytic enzymes secreted by the bacteria.

Cholestasis associated with nonhepatic bacterial infections—including *E. coli* UTIs and *E. coli*, *Klebsiella* spp., and *Proteus* spp. soft tissue infections—has been described in people. In dogs, it has been reported infrequently and associated with *E. coli* and gram-positive bacterial infections.[104] Characteristic findings include hyperbilirubinemia; slight increases in liver enzyme activities; bile retention within hepatocytes, Kupffer's cells, and canaliculi; and minimal hepatocellular inflammation or necrosis. The condition is considered a "functional" cholestasis (because no obstruction is present), resulting primarily from decreased excretion of conjugated bilirubin from hepatocytes to canaliculi; the prevalence and prognostic significance of this finding is not known for dogs or cats.[60]

A. baumannii infections produce localized or systemic signs depending on the organ system of localization. Genitourinary, cutaneous, and respiratory signs are the most common, whereas systemic inflammatory responses are characteristic of dogs with sepsis.

Signs associated with *C. freundii* infections vary, as do those caused by *A. baumannii*. Mucohemorrhagic diarrhea has been observed in animals affected with extraintestinal signs, likely indicating the source of spread. Sepsis is more consistent in *C. freundii*–infected animals that are immunosuppressed.

DIAGNOSIS

Specimens such as urine, blood, exudates, spinal fluid, airway samples, and feces and equipment such as catheter tips should be submitted for culture in the routine manner. Special transport media are not necessary.

By direct microscopy the Enterobacteriaceae are seen as gram-negative, medium-size short rods that can be motile. Stained morphologic findings vary significantly in clinical specimens. *Klebsiella* spp. capsules are large and regular. The *Pseudomonas* bacterium is a motile rod and can be found as a single bacterium, in pairs, or in short chains. Capsules may be produced.

Enterobacteriaceae grow well on ordinary unenriched media. On blood agar, the bacteria look similar, typically appearing as circular, smooth colonies with distinct edges. *Klebsiella* spp. colonies are large and mucoid and tend to coalesce with prolonged incubation. *Proteus* spp. are actively motile, resulting in "swarming" on solid media. Some strains of *E. coli* produce hemolysis on blood agar. Selective media such as MacConkey's or triple-sugar iron agar contain specific dyes and carbohydrates, and may be used for rapid preliminary identification. The IMViC reactions (indole, methyl red, Voges-Proskauer, citrate) can be used to further differentiate among *E. coli*, *Klebsiella* spp., and *Proteus* spp.

Pseudomonas spp. are obligate aerobes that also grow on ordinary nutrient media. Some strains are hemolytic, and some produce a sweet or grapelike odor caused by the production of aminoacetophenone. *P. aeruginosa* forms smooth, round colonies that are fluorescent green, and various pigments can be produced. A single strain can form multiple colony types on the same plate, giving the impression that several species are present. *Pseudomonas* spp. can grow at 42° C, a characteristic that is used to differentiate it from other bacteria.

The metabolic characteristics of Enterobacteriaceae are commonly used in their identification. In general, they ferment glucose with the production of acid or acid and gas, are catalase positive and oxidase negative, and reduce nitrate to nitrite. Many biochemical tests can help to characterize carbohydrate fermentation patterns and the activity of amino acid decarboxylases and other enzymes. Several test kits are commercially available.

Several schemes have been developed to differentiate *E. coli* strains, including serotyping, biotyping, phage-susceptibility typing, electrophoretic typing of enzymes, colicin typing, and pulsed-field gel electrophoresis. Genetic methods have been used to determine sources of fecal pollution in the environment.[72] These tests may not be available in general veterinary reference laboratories.

The routine culture and identification of *E. coli* from blood or deep tissue samples are all that is required to diagnose *E. coli* sepsis (see Chapter 38 for the diagnosis of endotoxemia) and soft tissue infection. Quantitative urine culture is necessary to diagnose UTIs. Dogs and cats with diabetes mellitus, with hyperadrenocorticism, or those receiving glucocorticoids may have occult UTIs (i.e., no identification of bacteriuria and pyuria on sediment examination) and should have a urine culture to identify UTIs.[30,71] Dogs with urolithiasis may also have occult UTIs. In one study, 18.5% of negative results of urine cultures from dogs with urolithiasis had positive culture results from either the urolith or those bladder mucosal biopsies. Swabs of bladder mucosa were no more sensitive than a routine urine culture.[42]

Enteric pathogens can be differentiated from enteric commensals by evaluating cultured isolates for O, H, and K antigens and testing for production of enterotoxins. Several bioassays based on cell cultures have been described, as well as the enzyme-linked immunosorbent assay and other binding techniques. Cytotoxin (VT) assays can be performed on fecal specimens when EPEC and EHEC strains are suspected. Infected animals develop rising levels of VT-neutralizing antibodies, which can be identified serologically. Isolates can also be tested for toxin- or other virulence-encoding genes by DNA hybridization or PCR; the suggested PCR screening tests for *E. coli* isolates from dogs and cats include the *LT, STa, STb, SLT1, SLT2, CNF1, CNF2,* and *EAE* (attaching and effacing) genes.[19,101] Normal dogs and cats may carry *E. coli* with these genes, but the bacteria do not always produce the gene product and may not be pathogenic; toxin must be identified in feces to ensure a correct diagnosis.[50] Histologic examination is necessary to describe attaching and effacing lesions.

Pseudomonas spp. are typically catalase and oxidase positive and split sugars by oxidation, not fermentation. They are citrate and indole negative and reduce nitrate. Strains can be identified by serotyping, immunotyping with cross-protection studies in mice, pyocin typing, or phage typing.

Additional descriptions of the isolation and identification of these bacteria can be found in veterinary microbiology texts, and the reader is encouraged to consult with their specific laboratory on questions regarding methodology and interpretation of test results.

PATHOLOGIC FINDINGS

ETEC typically attach to the brush border of enterocytes of the distal jejunum and proximal ileum but cause minimal histologic changes. EPEC colonize the small intestine and adhere to villi of epithelial cells, where they induce attaching and effacing lesions, destroying the brush border and forming microscopic pedestal-like structures on the surface of enterocytes. EHEC colonize the colon, also cause attaching and effacing lesions, and induce necrosis of the tips of villi. The lamina propria can be edematous and infiltrated with neutrophils, lymphocytes, plasma cells, and macrophages. Submucosal blood vessels may be occluded by thrombi. Fibrinonecrotic debris can form a pseudomembrane. The lesions of CRGV (putatively caused by EHEC O157:H7) involve the skin and kidneys and are primarily vascular. Cutaneous lesions include fibrinoid necrosis of small to medium arterioles and full-thickness necrosis of the epidermis. Renal changes are predominantly glomerular, with thrombotic microangiopathy and necrosis.

In soft tissue, gram-negative bacteria elicit an acute neutrophilic response, and the histopathologic findings of acute cystitis reflect this reaction. Granulomatous inflammation (nodular infiltrates of lymphoid cells and macrophages) can develop with chronic lower UTI. Polypoid changes can also complicate chronic lower UTIs and can only be differentiated from neoplasia by biopsy. Bacterial fermentation of glucose within a chronically inflamed and devitalized bladder wall can lead to emphysematous cystitis in dogs and cats with poorly controlled diabetes mellitus. Histologic findings associated with pyelonephritis include papillitis, pyelitis, and interstitial nephritis. Chronic pyelonephritis can lead to infarction, fibrosis, and the development of end-stage kidneys.

THERAPY

Therapy is based on the administration of appropriate antibacterial drugs, as well as debridement and surgical drainage where appropriate. The gram-negative cell wall confers some inherent resistance to antibacterial drugs, and appropriate dosages are important. Acquired resistance to antibacterial drugs is common and under the control of resistance (R) plasmids, which are transferred between bacteria by conjugation. Acquired resistance can also develop through other mechanisms, such as mutations in genes encoding the A subunit of DNA gyrase or genes determining bacterial permeability, leading to resistance to fluoroquinolone antibiotics.[117] Increased fluorquinolone resistance over time has been observed in *E. coli* isolates from dogs with UTIs.[16] Acquired antibiotic resistance varies greatly, and laboratory testing of isolates for specific susceptibility is always indicated.

Empiric recommendations for suspected soft tissue infections with the Enterobacteriaceae vary, and most are not substantiated by susceptibility data. However, the antibiotic susceptibilities of numerous isolates obtained from dogs in a teaching hospital are presented in Table 37-3. In general the Enterobacteriaceae are not susceptible to chloramphenicol, tetracycline, ampicillin, or trimethoprim-sulfonamide. Based on antibacterial susceptibility trends, it is rational to treat clinically stable animals that have non–life-threatening infections suspected to be caused by gram-negative rods with either amoxicillin-clavulanate or first- or second-generation cephalosporins until susceptibility results are known. Pending culture and susceptibility results, animals with life-threatening bacteremia should be treated with either amikacin, a third-generation cephalosporin, or enrofloxacin.

Renal excretion results in a high urine concentration of some antibiotics, which facilitates the management of lower UTIs caused by gram-negative rods. Lower UTIs caused by *E. coli* can usually be treated effectively with trimethoprim-sulfadiazine. *Klebsiella* infections can be treated effectively with cephalexin, and *Proteus* spp. infections can be treated with ampicillin. (See Chapter 91 for an additional discussion of UTI management.)

Data regarding changes in *E. coli* resistance patterns are conflicting. The patterns may depend on geographic location

Table • 37-3

Guidelines for Initial Antibiotic Therapy for Infections with Gram-Negative Bacteria[a]

DRUG[c]	SPECIES	DOSE[d] (mg/kg)	ROUTE[e]	INTERVAL (HOURS)	ORGANISM (PERCENTAGE SUSCEPTIBILITY)[b]			
					ESCHERICHIA COLI	KLEBSIELLA	PROTEUS	PSEUDOMONAS
Amikacin	B	5—10	IV, IM, SC	8—12	99	95	96	97
Amoxicillin-clavulanate	B	11—22	PO	8	NR	NR	95	NR
Carbenicillin	B	20—30	PO	8	—	—	—	High[f]
		30—100	IV, IM	6—8				
Cefotaxime	B	20—80	IV, IM, SC	8 (D) 6 (C)	99	100	98	NR
Ceftazidime	B	25	IM, SC	8—12	—	—	—	High
Ciprofloxacin	B	10—15	PO	12	—	—	—	High
Enrofloxacin[g]	D C	2.5—1 2.5—5	IV, PO	24	95	90	91	NR
Gentamicin	B	2—4	IV, IM, SC	8	92	NR	NR	NR
Imipenem-cilastatin	B	2—5	IV	8	—	—	—	High
Ticarcillin	B	40—75	IV, IM	6—8	—	—	—	High
Ticarcillin-clavulanate	B	30—50	IV	6—8	NR	NR	96	92
Tobramycin	B	1	IV, IM, SC	8 (D)	—	—	—	High
		2	SC	8 (C)				

B, Both dog and cat; *D*, dog; *C*, cat; *NR*, not reported; *IV*, intravenous; *IM*, intramuscular; *SC*, subcutaneous; *PO*, by mouth.
[a]Specific therapy should be based on sensitivity testing results.
[b]Data from Hirsh D, Jang SS. 1994. Antimicrobial susceptibility of selected infections bacterial. *J Am Anim Hosp Assoc* 30:487–494.
[c]See Appendix 8 for additional information on each drug.
[d]Dose per administration at specified interval.
[e]Oral route not recommended for initial therapy of serious infections.
[f]*High* is generally greater than 80% to 90% unless it is a very resistant hospital strain.
[g]Little independent information exists regarding the clinical efficacy of marbofloxacin, difloxacin, or orbifloxacin for treating these bacteria in dogs or cats.

and antibiotic usage. In vitro, enrofloxacin and ciprofloxacin had additive effects against *E. coli* isolated from dogs.[61] An increase in enrofloxacin-resistant *E. coli* in teaching hospital and community uropathogenic isolates has been reported in California.[16] Isolates were resistant to enrofloxacin and multiple antibiotics, including ampicillin, amoxicillin-clavulanate, chloramphenicol, cephalexin, tetracycline, and trimethoprim-sulfonamide. Several strains were identified, suggesting a collective increase in *E. coli* resistance in the population.[16] Another large study in Illinois found that ExPEC susceptibility remained "fairly stable" from 1990 to 1998, with amikacin, gentamicin, norfloxacin, and enrofloxacin having the highest efficacy. Orbifloxacin and sulfamethoxazole-trimethoprim were less effective, whereas susceptibility to tetracycline fell from 80% to less than 50% during the study period.[79] Similarly, a large retrospective study in Scotland from 1989 to 1997 documented increasing *E. coli* resistance to amoxicillin, amoxicillin-clavulanate, and streptomycin but not to ampicillin, chloramphenicol, enrofloxacin, gentamicin, oxytetracycline or trimethoprim-sulfonamide. No increase in the proportion of isolates showing multiple drug resistance was found.[76]

Therapy for *Pseudomonas* spp. infections can be difficult because natural and acquired resistance is common. The bacteria also have the ability to up-regulate impermeability to or active efflux of many antimicrobial drugs.[64] Furthermore, some hospital-acquired *P. aeruginosa* strains can be highly virulent. Gentamicin, amikacin, tobramycin, carbenicillin, ticarcillin, ceftazidime, or ciprofloxacin (isolates may be resistant to enrofloxacin) can be used for initial empirical therapy (Table 37-4); however, it is essential that antimicrobial susceptibility testing be performed for all suspected *P. aeruginosa* infections. Most *P. aeruginosa* bacteria can produce chromosomally mediated β-lactamases, which hydrolyze all penicillins except ticarcillin, and many isolates have plasmid-mediated resistance to other β-lactamases. Ticarcillin is much more active against *P. aeruginosa* than carbenicillin; however, cross-resistance occurs. Antipseudomonal cephalosporins are ceftazidime, cefoperazone, and cefsulodin, which are all third-generation drugs. Some of the fourth-generation drugs such as cefepime are also antipseudomonals. Aztreonam is the only monobactam available to treat the bacteria; however, ceftazidime is more effective. Carbapenems such as imipenem and meropenem are very effective, and cross-resistance with

Table • 37-4

Antimicrobial Drugs Effective Against Pseudomonas Infections

β-Lactams
Ticarcillin
Carbenicillin
Piperacillin
Azlocillin
Aztreonam
Imipenem
Meropenem

Cephalosporins
Ceftazidime
Cefoperazone
Cefsulodin

Quinolones
Ciprofloxacin
Clinafloxacin
Trovafloxacin

Aminoglycosides
Gentamicin
Tobramycin
Netilmicin
Amikacin
Isepamicin

other β-lactams does not usually occur. Of the quinolones, ciprofloxacin has the highest efficacy for treating *P. aeruginosa;* only a few of the newer quinolones have this activity. Many of the aminoglycosides are effective against this organism. In life-threatening situations in which susceptibility testing results are not yet available, *P. aeruginosa* infections should be treated with imipenem-cilastatin as a single agent or with either ticarcillin or carbenicillin in combination with an aminoglycoside. *Pseudomonas* spp. are usually resistant to penicillin, ampicillin, tetracycline, first- and second-generation cephalosporins, chloramphenicol, and trimethoprim-sulfadiazine. Most lower UTIs can be treated effectively with tetracycline. (The management of *Pseudomonas* otitis externa is discussed in Chapter 85.)

PREVENTION

The Enterobacteriaceae are killed readily by sunlight and desiccation but not by freezing. *E. coli* can survive in feces, dust, and water at ambient temperature for months. Contaminated drinking water has been an important source of infection for people or pets. An improperly chlorinated swimming pool has also been a vehicle for transmission to people[33]; the outbreak was suspected to have been caused by a person whose feet were contaminated with animal feces when the individual entered the pool. Fomite transmission may be important, and hand washing and disinfection of fomites are essential for prevention. Rabbits have been shown to be a reservoir for enterohemorrhagic *E. coli*,[36] so people who handle rabbits might be at risk for acquiring infection, as may dogs and cats that prey

on rabbits. *Pseudomonas* spp. are important nosocomial pathogens that survive well in hospital environments in locations such as water faucets, utensils, floors, instruments, humidifiers, baths, and respiratory care equipment. *Pseudomonas* spp. can also survive in disinfectant solutions, antiseptics, and liquid fluorescein drops. Appropriate management of IV and urinary catheters is extremely important in the prevention of nosocomial infection.[65]

Orally administered autogenous vaccines have been reported to prevent and treat kennel-acquired enteric *E. coli* infections in dogs and cats, with significant decreases in morbidity and mortality; however, these are not available for general use.[6,119,120]

PUBLIC HEALTH CONSIDERATIONS

Most *E. coli*, *Klebsiella* spp., and *Proteus* spp. are opportunistic pathogens; however, some pathogenic strains could be carried by dogs or cats and transmitted to people (or vice versa). In one study, seventeen uropathogenic *E. coli* isolates from dogs were characterized by phylogenetic background and virulence genotype and compared with human clinical isolates with similar serotypes. The genotypes of canine origin *E. coli* were similar to (and in some cases indistinguishable from) human ExPEC strains, suggesting that canine isolates, rather than being dog-specific pathogens, may pose an infectious threat to people.[54,56] Furthermore, 30% of canine fecal samples collected from a residential neighborhood in St. Paul, Minn., contained ExPEC strains known to be virulent to humans.[55]

R plasmids are transmitted between gram-negative organisms, and multiple drug resistance could be a human health problem. Twenty-one *E. coli* isolates from wounds, urine, and a veterinary teaching hospital intensive care unit environment had multiple drug resistance (to most cephalosporins, β-lactams and clavulanic acid, tetracycline, spectinomycin, sulfonamides, chloramphenicol, and gentamicin).[94] Thus it has been suggested that the use of fluoroquinolone and third-generation cephalosporins in veterinary settings be considered carefully and possibly even be restricted. The theoretical potential for animal owners (especially those who are immunocompromised), veterinarians, and technicians to be infected by resistant pathogens needs to be recognized.[86,117]

SUGGESTED READINGS*

12. Boerlin P, Eugster S, Gaschen F, et al. 2001. Transmission of opportunistic pathogens in a veterinary teaching hospital, *Vet Microbiol* 82:347-359.
16. Cooke CL, Singer RS, Jang SS, et al. 2002. Enrofloxacin resistance in *Escherichia coli* isolated from dogs with urinary tract infections, *J Am Vet Med Assoc* 220:190-192.
32. Francey T, Gaschen F, Nicolet J, et al. 2000. The role of *Acinetobacter baumannii* as a nosocomial pathogen for dogs and cats in an intensive care unit, *J Vet Intern Med* 14:177-183.
35. Galarneau J-R, Fortin M, Lapointe J-M, et al. 2003. *Citrobacter freundii* septicemia in two dogs, *J Vet Diagn Invest* 15:297-299.
45. Handt LK, Stoffregen DA Prescott JS, et al. 2003. Clinical and microbiologic characterization of hemorrhagic pneumonia due to extraintestinal pathogenic *Escherichia coli* in four young dogs, *Comp Med* 53:663-670.

68. Martin Barrasa JL, Lupiola Gomez P, Gonzalez Lama Z, et al. 2000. Antibacterial susceptibility patterns of *Pseudomonas* strains isolated from chronic canine otitis externa, *J Vet Med B Infect Dis Vet Public Health* 47:191-196.

90. Roberts DE, McClain HM, Hansen DS, et al. 2000. An outbreak of *Klebsiella pneumoniae* infection in dogs with severe enteritis and septicemia, *J Vet Diagn Invest* 12:168-173.

101. Staats JJ, Chengappa MM, DeBey MC, et al. 2003. Detection of *Escherichia coli* Shiga toxin *(stx)* and enterotoxin *(estA* and *elt)* genes in fecal samples from non-diarrheic and diarrheic greyhounds, *Vet Microbiol* 94:303-312.

104. Taboada J, Meyer DJ. 1989. Cholestasis associated with extrahepatic bacterial infection in five dogs. *J Vet Intern Med* 3:216-221.

*See the CD-ROM for a complete list of references.

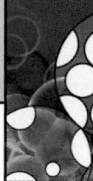

CHAPTER • 38

Endotoxemia

Stephen A. Kruth

ETIOLOGY

Clinically significant bacteremia in dogs and cats is expected to occur in a variety of infections (e.g., peritonitis, mastitis, prostatitis, pneumonia, pulmonary abscess, pyothorax, pyometra, pyelonephritis, intraabdominal abscess, biliary tract infections), as well as during dentistry. It probably also occurs during rectal palpation, intestinal endoscopy and surgery, and when indwelling venous or arterial catheters have been placed. Normally, circulating bacteria are cleared by the mononuclear-phagocyte system. Bacterial molecules are recognized by macrophages and other cells, which initiate a complex local inflammatory response, as well as up-regulating systemic host defenses, thus preparing the animal for the potential spread of infection. Typical clinical signs of bacteremia include altered body temperature, tachycardia, tachypnea, and neutrophilia or neutropenia; these signs are part of the systemic inflammatory response syndrome (SIRS). SIRS can be initiated by trauma, pancreatitis, and other insults in addition to infection and is characterized by a complex cytokine-mediated response. The host benefits if SIRS is controlled and balanced by antiinflammatory pathways. However, in some cases, bacterial virulence factors, inoculum size, coexisting disease, host genetic determinants, or any combination of these leads to the inappropriate, dysregulated generalized systemic response of severe sepsis, septic shock, and ultimately multiple organ dysfunction syndrome (MODS). The terminology referring to SIRS and sepsis was clarified in the 1990s in human medicine; relevant terms are defined Table 38-1.

Endotoxemia is the best-studied cause of SIRS and its complications in people and horses. Endotoxin (lipopolysaccharide [LPS]) consists of a lipid A moiety (the toxic component) and polysaccharides (O antigens). LPS is released from the outer membrane of gram-negative bacteria when they lyse and is normally confined within the gut and portal circulation. Animals have evolved mechanisms that recognize and respond to LPS in tissues and fluids early in gram-negative infections, and *endotoxemia* occurs when SIRS develops in response to the presence of LPS. The source of endotoxin is usually a member of the Enterobacteriaceae family (*Escherichia* spp., *Klebsiella* spp., *Enterobacter* spp., *Proteus* spp.), as well as *Pseudomonas* spp. The term *endotoxemia* implies only that toxin is present in the blood; in some cases, bacteria are also present. In other cases, the bacteria remain compartmentalized in the gut or tissues, with only toxin being absorbed (i.e., it is common to have negative blood cultures in endotoxemia).

EPIDEMIOLOGY

The prevalence of naturally occurring endotoxemia in dogs and cats is unknown, even though the dog has been used for many years as a biomedical model of endotoxemia and SIRS for people, and the acute syndromes are well described. Risk factors for dogs include canine parvoviral (CPV) enteritis, gastric dilation or volvulus, pyometra, mastitis, other gram-negative infections, and heat stroke. Endotoxemia can develop when hepatic clearance of LPS is reduced, as in hepatic insufficiency and portosystemic shunts. Obstructive biliary disease may be a risk factor because bile salts bind endotoxin in the gut. Endotoxin may also play a significant role in the pathogenesis of severe acute pancreatitis in dogs.[34]

Endotoxemia is recognized less commonly in cats. Risk factors for severe sepsis in cats include pyothorax, septic peritonitis, bacteremia secondary to gastrointestinal (GI) disease, pneumonia, endocarditis, pyelonephritis, osteomyelitis, pyometra, and bite wounds.[7] Endotoxemia is likely a component of some of these infections. Endotoxemia is also recognized as a cause of neonatal death in puppies and kittens.

Approximately 25% of individuals with gram-negative aerobic bacteremia develop endotoxic shock, with a 50% to 80% mortality rate. Predisposing conditions for endotoxic shock in those include diabetes mellitus, hepatic cirrhosis, burns, cancer, surgery, irradiation, cytotoxic drug therapy, administration of glucocorticoids, indwelling devices, and blood transfusions.

Uncomplicated SIRS-sepsis is not a negative prognostic finding if managed appropriately; however, the prognosis worsens as an animal develops severe sepsis, septic shock, and MODS.

Table • 38-1

Definitions Associated with Systemic Inflammatory Response Syndrome (SIRS)

Septicemia	Systemic signs caused by the spread of microbes or their toxins via the blood stream
Sepsis	SIRS that has a proven or suspected microbial etiology; may be caused by circulating toxins; microbial invasion of the blood is not necessary
Severe sepsis	Sepsis with signs of organ dysfunction, hypoperfusion, or hypotension, including metabolic acidosis
Septic shock	Sepsis with hypotension that is not responsive to appropriate fluid therapy
Endotoxemia	SIRS associated with increased blood endotoxin levels
Multiple organ dysfunction syndrome (MODS)	Dysfunction of more than one organ, requiring intervention to maintain homeostasis

PATHOGENESIS

Endotoxin is released into the intestinal lumen or tissues when gram-negative bacteria lyse, as occurs with rapid bacterial replication or with bactericidal action of effective antibiotics. Within the intestinal lumen, most endotoxin is bound by bile salts and contained by the mucosal barrier; the small amounts absorbed into the portal circulation are cleared by hepatic macrophages. Endotoxin absorbed through the lymphatic system is cleared in regional lymph nodes. Thus endotoxin levels in the systemic circulation are usually extremely low to immeasurable. Clinical signs of endotoxemia occur only when binding and clearance mechanisms are overwhelmed.

Within hepatocytes, endotoxin interferes with transport mechanisms, causing functional cholestasis. Endotoxin can also directly activate complement via the alternative pathway. In terms of clinical signs, these effects are relatively minor; the more significant effect of endotoxin is its ability to stimulate macrophages and other cells to release a variety of proinflammatory and antiinflammatory cytokines.

In blood, endotoxin is bound by a specific carrier lipoprotein called lipopolysaccharide binding (LPB) protein (the canine molecule has been described and cloned[38]); this complex binds to monocytes and macrophages via the receptor CD14, which amplifies the effect of endotoxin on the cell. The endotoxin-CD14 complex interacts with other cell surface receptors, called toll-like receptors, which trigger a signal transduction pathway, protein synthesis, and subsequent cytokine secretion. Soluble (free) CD14-endotoxin complexes bind to endothelial cells and induce a similar cytokine response. The endotoxin-triggered cytokine response is what leads to the clinical signs of SIRS.

The early macrophage response to endotoxin is characterized by release of multifunctional proinflammatory cytokines, especially interleukin-1β (IL-1) and tumor necrosis factor-α (TNF-α). In dogs, TNF-α levels increase within 15 minutes of exposure to LPS, peak at 2 hours, and return to baseline levels in 4 hours. TNF-α mediates many immune and inflammatory functions, as well as further stimulating macrophages to secrete IL-1, IL-6, macrophage colony-stimulating factor, and granulocyte-macrophage colony-stimulating factor. IL-1 is released in similar burst fashion; it is a major co-stimulator of type 2 helper T (Th2) cells, stimulates the acute-phase response, induces fever, and has a multitude of other proinflammatory effects. Other cytokines, such as IL-6, IL-8 and interferon (IFN)-α, are becoming recognized as additional early mediators in SIRS-sepsis (see Tizard[36] for further discussion of the various cytokines involved in SIRS-sepsis). IL-1, TNF-α, and so forth are released early and transiently in response to endotoxin, before the animal is presented with clinical signs. Novel therapeutics directed toward these mediators have not demonstrated significant benefit in most human clinical trials. However, late mediators of SIRS, such as *high-mobility group 1 protein*, are now being described and may be more appropriate therapeutic targets.[1]

The cytokine cascades increase the levels or activity (or both) of inflammatory phospholipid-derived mediators (prostacyclin, thromboxane, and platelet-activating factor),[37] coagulation factors, complement, reactive oxygen species, and nitric oxide (which is emerging as an important molecule associated with hypotension),[11,22,24,33] endothilin-1 (a vasoconstrictor),[23] β-endorphin, histamine, serotonin, vasopressin, angiotensin II, and catecholamines. The biologic effects of these mediators include neutrophil activation, aggregation, and chemotaxis; platelet activation and aggregation; a procoagulable state; increased activity of plasma proteases; and vasodilation and potentially systemic hypotension, generalized endothelial inflammation, increased vascular permeability, and GI ulceration.[21,25] Lysosomal enzymes such as elastase and chymotrypsin deplete fibronectin and activate blood clotting, triggering disseminated intravascular coagulation (DIC).

If the systemic inflammatory state progresses, structural and metabolic changes develop in vascular endothelial cells. Endothelial adhesion molecules are up-regulated, and neutrophils and platelets are sequestered in various organs. The endothelium also becomes more permeable, and plasma proteins move from the intravascular space to the interstitium, resulting in edema.

Concurrent with inflammatory mediator up-regulation, antiinflammatory mediators are secreted to balance and limit the inflammatory response. An insufficient or inappropriate antiinflammatory response can allow sepsis to progress.[21]

Until recently, the prevailing theory has been that sepsis is a result of a *cytokine storm*, leading to uncontrolled systemic inflammation. Studies now indicate that, for at least some patients, the hyperinflammatory state is followed by severe acute immunosuppression, caused by the apoptosis of B cells, CD4 T cells, and follicular dendritic cells. The mechanism of immunosuppression is not known; however, release of endogenous glucocorticoids may be an important contributor.[16] Thyroid hormone production and secretion have been impaired in endotoxin-treated dogs.[31]

In summary, endotoxin acts as a signal to the immune system that gram-negative bacterial infection has occurred. A localized response along with a primed or controlled systemic response is beneficial, while an uncontrolled response leads to systemic inflammation, immunosuppression, severe sepsis, septic shock, and ultimately organ failure (Fig. 38-1).

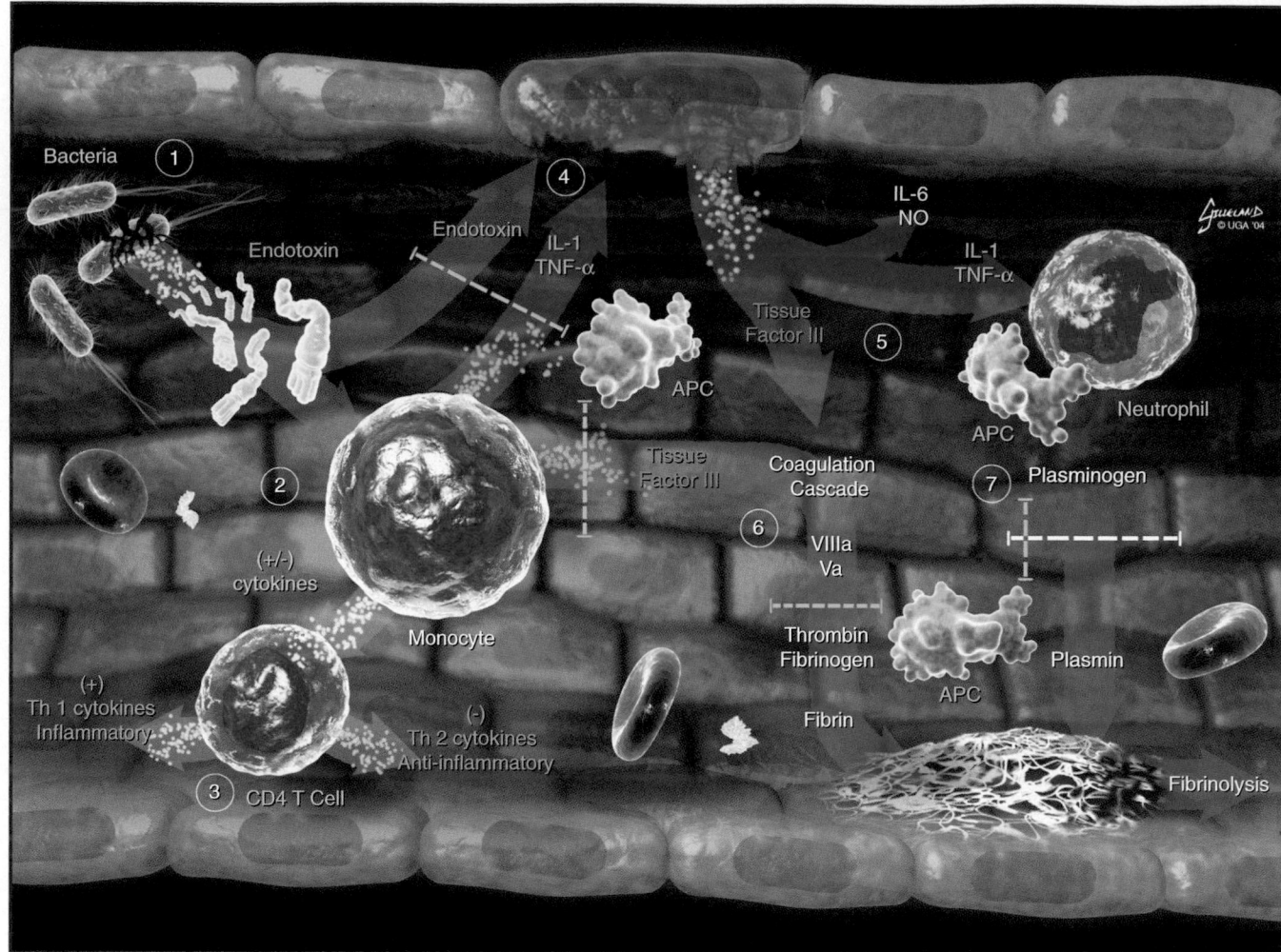

Fig 38-1 Pathophysiology of endotoxemia. 1, Intracellular or extracellular gram-negative bacterial death leads to the release of endotoxin. 2, Endotoxin stimulates monocytes to release inflammatory cytokines, including TNF-α and IL-1 and a procoagulant (tissue factor, Factor III). 3, Monocytes are activated to release cytokines, which, in turn, stimulate CD4 T cells to release inflammatory or antiinflammatory mediators. The type of pathogen, size of the bacterial exposure, and the site of infection are factors that influence which pathway is stimulated. Monocytes, previously ingesting necrotic cells, release interleukins, which induce Th1 cells to secrete inflammatory cytokines (TNF-α, IFN-γ, and IL-2). Monocytes, previously ingesting apoptotic cells, release interleukins, which induce antiinflammatory Th2 cell activation with the release antiinflammatory cytokines, IL-10, and IL4, which suppresses monophage activation. 4, Endotoxin, IL-1, and TNF-α cause endothelial injury and the further release of inflammatory mediators (IL-1, TNF-α, IL-6, and nitric oxide [NO]) and procoagulatory tissue factor. 5, Tissue factor from damaged endothelium and activated monocytes initiates the coagulation cascade. Inflammatory cytokines IL-1 and TNF-α stimulate neutrophil chemotaxis. 6, The coagulation cascade, once activated, triggers the development of a fibrin clot. 7, Fibrinolysis is activated, converting plasminogen to plasmin, which leads to the breakdown of formed clots. Activated protein C (APC) has direct antiinflammatory and antiendotoxic properties at several sites in the pathway as designated by blue dashed lines. It blocks the production of cytokines by monocytes and the effects of endotoxin on cells. APC also blocks neutrophil adhesion. It inactivates factors Va and VIIIa, thereby preventing the generation of thrombin. In addition to inhibiting the coagulation pathway, APC blocks inhibitors of fibrinolysis thus accelerating the fibrinolytic pathway and clot dissolution. *PAI,* Plasminogen activator inhibitor; *TAFI,* thrombin activating factor inhibitor. (Courtesy University of Georgia, Athens, Ga.)

CLINICAL FINDINGS

Dogs

No clinical signs have been found that are pathognomonic for endotoxemia. Animals show either signs associated with infection (e.g., purulent vaginal discharge with pyometra, coughing with pneumonia, mastitis) or localizing signs such as inactivity and inappetence. Tachycardia, tachypnea, and fever are the clinical hallmarks of SIRS (Table 38-2). If a dog is progressing towards severe sepsis or septic shock,

signs associated with the GI tract (the canine *shock organ system*) can develop, including vomiting or diarrhea, or both (with melena if GI bleeding secondary to ulceration or DIC occurs). In addition, portal hypertension, hepatosplanchnic pooling of blood, ileus, decreased jejunal absorption of water, electrolytes and glucose, increased colonic motility, and increased bacterial translocation have been described in experimental canine models. Cholestatic jaundice can develop and is not necessarily associated with a poor prognosis.

Table • 38-2

Clinical Criteria for Diagnosis of Systemic Inflammatory Response Syndrome (SIRS)

CLINICAL PARAMETERS	DOGS	CATS
Heart rate	>120 bpm	<140 bpm or >225 bpm
Respiratory rate	>40 brpm or $PaCO_2$ <30 mm Hg	>40 brpm
Temperature	<100.4° F or >104.0° F	<100.0° F or >104.0° F
Leukogram	>18,000 or <5000 WBC/μl	>19,000 or <5000 WBC/μl

bpm, Beats per minute; *PaCO₂*, arterial carbon dioxide pressure; *brpm*, breaths per minute; *WBC*, white blood cells.
Data from Brady CA, Otto CM. 2001. Systemic inflammatory response syndrome, sepsis, and multiple organ dysfunction, *Vet Clin North Am Small Anim Pract* 31:1147-1162.

The initial cardiovascular signs are associated with a hyperdynamic response, including brick-red mucous membranes, tachycardia, and bounding arterial pulses. Myocardial contractility is usually normal, and cardiac output is increased.[32] Hours later, a hypodynamic phase can develop, with decreased central venous pressure, low systemic vascular resistance, decreased arterial blood pressures, pooling of blood in the viscera, and eventual myocardial failure. Cold extremities, pale mucous membranes, weak pulse, and prolonged capillary refill times can be seen. In model systems, dogs that survive endotoxic shock can have cardiovascular abnormalities that peak at 2 to 3 days and return to normal 7 to 10 days later. In some dogs, myocardial damage is progressive, and death from heart failure can occur up to 7 days following infusion of endotoxin.

Signs associated with an infected focus may be obvious or the focus may be occult, necessitating an aggressive diagnostic workup. Dogs may be presented for signs associated with either damage to intestinal barriers (gastric dilation or volvulus, CPV enteritis) or portal-systemic shunts.

Signs associated with MODS can be related to intestinal, hepatic, cardiovascular, renal, or respiratory insufficiency. Edema is associated with increased vascular permeability and hypoalbuminemia, and bleeding can occur if DIC is present.

Hematologic findings can include hemoconcentration, leukocytosis with left shift or leukopenia, toxic changes in neutrophils, and thrombocytopenia. Prolonged coagulation times, low antithrombin III levels, and elevated fibrin degradation products are consistent with DIC. Lactic acidosis caused by poor perfusion is an early finding. Serum biochemical abnormalities can include hypo- or hyperglycemia, hypoalbuminemia, and increased serum alkaline phosphatase (ALP) and alanine aminotransferase activities. Azotemia, casts, and proteinuria are consistent with acute renal failure. Organ failure can cause other clinical pathologic abnormalities, depending upon the organ system.

Cats

Endotoxemia is rarely reported and poorly described in cats. In a retrospective case series of cats with confirmed severe sepsis (9 of 29 cats had confirmed *Escherichia coli* or *Pseudomonas* spp. infections; endotoxin was not assayed), clinical signs included lethargy, pale mucous membranes, weak femoral pulses, tachypnea, hypothermia or fever, diffuse pain on abdominal palpation, bradycardia, and icterus (Table 38-3). Anemia, thrombocytopenia, neutrophilia with increased bands, hypoalbuminemia, and hyperbilirubinemia were the most frequent hematologic abnormalities (Table 38-4). Functional cholestasis was not identified histologically; thus icterus may have been caused by hemolysis.[7] The lung is the feline shock organ, and pulmonary edema and respiratory failure may be the predominant signs in cats developing MODS.

Table • 38-3

Clinical Findings of 29 Septic Cats[a,b]

PERCENTAGE AFFECTED	MEDICAL PROBLEMS
100%	Lethargy
100%	Pale mucosae
79%	Poor pulse
66%	Bradycardia <140 beats per minute
35%	Hyperthermia 38.9° C (102° F)
59%	Hypothermia <37.8° C (100° F)
72%	Tachypnea (>40 breaths per minute)
76%	Diffuse abdominal pain
72%	Icterus

[a]Uncommon pyrexia, tachycardia, moist gums.
[b]Brady CA, Otto CM, Van Winkle TJ, et al. 2000. Severe sepsis in cats: 29 cases (1986-1998), *J Am Vet Med Assoc* 217:531-535, with permission.

DIAGNOSIS

A variety of assays have been described for the quantification of endotoxin in body fluids, with variations on the classical Limulus amebocyte lysate assay most commonly used in clinical research settings. These are specialized assays, notoriously difficult to standardize and not available for general veterinary clinical use. The interpretation of results is confounded by poor concordance with blood culture results.[17,27,30] Improved assays are becoming available for clinical use, but these need to be validated and their utility determined.[18] The diagnosis of endotoxemia remains presumptive in the majority of canine and feline clinical cases.

Assays for TNF-α, IL-1, and other cytokines are useful research tools but are also not generally available. Elevated cytokine levels are consistent with SIRS, for which endotoxin is only one stimulus. The diagnosis of sepsis is based on the identification of an infected focus in a patient with SIRS; clinical suspicion of sepsis depends on recognition of risk factors, along with the clinical signs outlined previously.

The diagnosis of severe sepsis or septic shock is dependent on hemodynamic and perfusion indices; these include rectal and toe web temperature, heart rate, mucous membrane color, pulse character, arterial blood pressure, and arterial blood gases, which should be determined at initial physical examination and then monitored. Serum electrolyte, glucose, urea nitrogen and creatinine levels, and liver enzyme activities should be determined, along with a complete blood count (CBC), platelet count, and coagulation testing. Culture spec-

Table • 38-4

Laboratory Parameters from Septic Cats[a]

PARAMETER	RANGE	NUMBER TESTED	% LOW	% HIGH
HCT	27%—45%	27	45	7
WBC	$5.5–19 \times 10^3/\mu l$	15	0	33
Bands	0	15	40	60
Glucose	75—119 mg/dl	27	44	0
Sodium	148—157 mEq/L	26	54	0
Potassium	3.5—5.0 mEq/L	26	23	14
Albumin	2.7—3.9 mg/dl	12	100	0
Bilirubin	<1.0 mg/dl	16	0	63
ALP	23—107 U/L	14	0	0
ALT	20—107 U/L	11	0	18

HCT, Hematocrit; *WBC*, white blood cells; *ALP*, alkaline phosphatase; *ALT*, alanine aminotransferase.
[a]Brady CA, Otto CM, Van Winkle TJ, et al. 2000. Severe sepsis in cats: 29 cases (1986-1998), *J Am Vet Med Assoc* 217:531-535, with permission.

imens of wounds, urine, and blood should be taken before antibiotic therapy is initiated. For a review of specimen collection, see Chapter 33.

The infected site should be identified as soon as the animal is stable. Radiography of the thorax and abdomen, abdominal ultrasonography, echocardiography, or any combination of these tools may be helpful in locating sources of sepsis. Diagnostic peritoneal lavage, tracheal or bronchoalveolar lavage, arthrocentesis, cerebrospinal fluid collection, or any combination of these should be performed if indicated.

PATHOLOGIC FINDINGS

No specific gross or histopathologic findings that are diagnostic for endotoxemia have been found. Histologic findings associated with SIRS include widespread vascular endothelial injury, neutrophil margination, edema, and microthrombosis. The most important pathologic findings will be associated with the infected focus (CPV enteritis, pyometra, bacterial endocarditis).

Autopsy studies have not revealed why human patients with sepsis die, and discordance often occurs between histologic findings and the degree of organ dysfunction. The concept of *cell stunning* has been suggested in which sepsis activates defense mechanisms that cause cellular processes to be reduced to basic housekeeping roles. As discussed previously, some patients have widespread B-cell, CD4 T-cell, and follicular dendritic cell apoptosis, consistent with a state of severe immunosuppression.[16] The exact cause of death in people with sepsis receiving supportive care remains elusive.

THERAPY

Current therapy of endotoxemia consists of aggressively managing SIRS and its complications while treating the infection with appropriate antimicrobials, drainage, and so forth, as outlined in Table 38-5. Treatment must be aggressive and instituted based on clinical signs and suspicion of sepsis because definitive diagnostic tests are not available. Because early treatment can be critical for survival, empiric therapy should be initiated as soon as clinical signs of SIRS are observed. Specific treatment for endotoxemia is more controversial because studies in people and animals have given variable outcomes. The discussion to follow is divided into routinely accepted

Table • 38-5

Therapeutic Recommendations for Endotoxemia in Dogs and Cats

1. Establish central venous catheter.
2. Obtain laboratory specimens for CBC, biochemical profile, urinalysis.
3. Replace fluid volume within the first hour.
4. If blood pressure remains reduced, begin plasma or colloid.
5. Administer heparin as indicated to control hypercoagulability.
   Low prophylactic doses in low grade DIC
   Higher doses with acute or severe organ thrombosis
   Low prophylactic doses plus plasma or whole blood in end-stage DIC
6. Administer parenteral antimicrobial therapy depending on source of infection.[a]
   Skin: β-lactamase—resistant penicillin, first-generation cephalosporin
   Soft tissue: β-lactamase—resistant penicillin plus clindamycin or metronidazole
   Urinary tract: ampicillin plus aminoglycoside, third-generation cephalosporin
   Pneumonia: macrolide plus second- or third-generation cephalosporin
   Meningitis: third-generation cephalosporin
   Intraabdominal: third-generation cephalosporin plus metronidazole or clindamycin
   Uncertain site: ticarcillin-clavulanate, clindamycin and quinolone (possibly combined)
7. Consider oxygen delivery, increasing inspired concentration and reducing consumption.
8. Consider glucocorticoids at modest physiologic dosages.

CBC, Complete blood count; *DIC*, disseminated intravascular coagulation.
[a]See Chapter 34 and Appendix 8 for information on drugs listed.

therapy followed by a review of treatments specifically directed against endotoxemia. None of the measures aimed at endotoxin can be universally accepted for treatment of dogs and cats.

Routine Management

SIRS is managed supportively with an emphasis on maintaining tissue perfusion. Aggressive volume resuscitation is probably the most important intervention to minimize the time period of reduced organ perfusion. Intravenous access should be established, a urinary catheter placed, and a shock (volume replacement) dose of an isotonic crystalloid solution administered. If the animal does not respond adequately within the first hour, fresh or fresh-frozen plasma should be given along with a synthetic colloid such as hydroxyethyl starch. Colloids are more likely to stay in the vascular space longer than crystalloids and are more likely to prevent pulmonary edema, the most serious complication of fluid resuscitation. Fluid support should be aggressive and adjusted as dictated by the animal's response. Whole blood or erythrocytes should not be used in septic shock unless the hemoglobin level is reduced below 10 g/dl. If blood pressure cannot be maintained, vasoactive agents such as dopamine or dobutamine should be infused. See Brady and Otto[6] and Hardie[14] for a more detailed review of hemodynamic resuscitation of septic dogs and cats. For drug dosages for this therapy, see Table 38-6.

Once fluid therapy has been initiated, infected sites should be cultured, drained, and débrided. Antibacterial therapy is

Table • 38-6

Drug Dosages for Sepsis[a]

DRUG[b]	SPECIES	DOSAGE[c]	ROUTE	INTERVAL (HOURS)
Volume Expanders				
Isotonic crystalloid solutions (Plasma-Lyte® 148,	D	≥90 ml/kg	IV	1[d]
lactated Ringer's, normal saline)	C	≥60 ml/kg	IV	1[d]
Colloids (fresh or fresh-frozen plasma, pentastarch,	D	20 ml/kg	IV	24
hetastarch 120, dextran 70)	C	10 mg/kg		
Sympathomimetic Drugs				
Dopamine	B	1—10 µg/kg	IV	1 min
Dobutamine	B	5—20 µg/kg	IV	1 min
Antibacterial Drugs[e]				
Ampicillin	B	22 mg/kg	IV	8
Gentamicin	B	6 mg/kg	IV	24
Amikacin	B	20 mg/kg	IV	24
Cefazolin	B	5—15 mg/kg	IV	6—8
Cefoxitin	B	30 mg/kg once, then 15 mg/kg	IV	4
Ceftazidime	B	22 mg/kg	IV	6—8
Enrofloxacin	D	10 mg/kg	IV	24
	C	5 mg/kg	IV	24
Clindamycin	B	10 mg/kg	IV	8
Imipenem-cilastatin	B	5 mg/kg	IV	8
Ticarcillin-clavulanate	B	50 mg/kg	IV	6
Antiulcer Drugs				
Ranitidine	B	2 mg/kg	IV	8—12
Sucralfate	C	250 mg total	PO	8—12
	D (<20 kg)	500 mg total	PO	8—12
	D (>20 kg)	1 g total	PO	8—12
Misoprostol	B	2—5 µg/kg	PO	8—12
Portosystemic Shunt Therapy				
Lactulose	B	0.5 ml/kg	PO	8
Neomycin	B	2.5—20 mg/kg	PO	8—12

D, Dog; *B*, dog and cat; *C*, cat; *IV*, intravenous; *PO*, by mouth.
[a]From Brady CA, Otto CM. 2001. Systemic inflammatory response syndrome, sepsis, and multiple organ dysfunction, *Vet Clin North Am Small Anim Pract* 31:1147-1162.
[b]For additional information on each antibacterial drug, see Appendix 8.
[c]Dose per administration at specified interval.
[d]Reassess perfusion and hemodilution after first hour before continuing.
[e]Combination therapy is usually indicated until culture results are available. Choices include: ampicillin + amikacin or gentamicin, cefazolin + amikacin or gentamicin, ampicillin + ceftazidime, ampicillin + enrofloxacin, clindamycin + enrofloxacin. Single-agent therapy choices include cefoxitin, imipenim-cilastatin, or ticarcillin-clavulanate. Criteria include likely organism or organisms based on infection site, knowledge of resistance patterns, severity of illness, signalment, renal or hepatic dysfunction, and cost.

one of the most important aspects of treatment. Antibiotic therapy should be directed toward the primary site of infection; however, with endotoxemia from any source, translocation of bacteria from the GI lumen to the portal circulation is increased, and antibiotic therapy should include drugs effective against anaerobes and Enterobacteriaceae. Chronic low-level endotoxemia can complicate portosystemic shunts and other forms of hepatic insufficiency. Lactulose and nonabsorbable antimicrobials such as neomycin potentially lower portal endotoxin levels by suppressing numbers of enteric bacteria.

Antimicrobic regimens are listed in Table 38-6. Effective antimicrobial therapy, especially with bactericidal drugs such as cephalosporins and quinolones, theoretically might increase the release of endotoxin[14]; this was demonstrated in some experiments in vitro and in animals following intravenous or intraperitoneal administration of bacteria. Data are insufficient in veterinary medicine to make management recommendations concerning the avoidance of specific drugs in septic dogs and cats. In people treated with severe, naturally occurring gram-negative bacteremia, bactericidal antibiotics did not increase circulating levels of endotoxin, TNF-α, IL-6, or IL-8.[19]

Anticoagulant therapy has been used to modulate complications of sepsis because hypercoagulability and DIC are inevitable manifestations.[8,43] DIC is treated with fluids and with plasma to replace the anticoagulants antithrombin 3, protein C, and thromboplastin, as well as depleted clotting factors.[6] The use of heparin to treat DIC in sepsis remains controversial[6,14]; however, it is the most practical means of anticoagulation therapy for veterinary patients. Depletion of antithrombin 3 with DIC has been of greatest concern given that it is important as a co-factor for heparin activity. Recombinant human antithrombin therapy has been implemented in the treatment of septic people; however, the effects were only demonstrable when the patients were also receiving heparin.[42] Protein C, a potent anticoagulant, inhibits coagulation through Factors Va and VIIa and limits thrombin production in addition to activating fibrinolysis. Activated protein C has been shown to reduce mortality in people with sepsis.[4]

Patients receiving parenteral nutrition may develop bacterial infections associated with their catheter or as a result of their underlying disease. Thrombosis of large veins has been a frequent complication in human patients receiving parenteral nutrition that were concurrently injected with endotoxin.[39] Prolonged bowel rest and inclusion of lipids may enhance the coagulatory response to endotoxin. Prophylactic anticoagulation may be indicated in dogs and cats with predisposing hypercoagulation. For a summary of therapy in the various stages of DIC, see Table 38-7.

Glucocorticoids have been recommended to treat sepsis because they have effects against inflammatory cytokines and mediators. People with septic shock have shown a relative adrenal insufficiency as exhibited by marginally low levels of serum cortisol. At higher doses, benefits of glucocorticoids are unproven and potentially contraindicated; however, improved survival has been observed in people with septic shock when slightly supraphysiologic doses of 0.5 to 1 mg/kg were used.[3,5]

Lazaroids are steroid compounds with free-radical scavenging and antioxidant properties. They decrease neutrophil migration and TNF-α production. These drugs have increased survival in animal studies with minimal toxicity in treated people. Pentoxifylline is a phosphodiesterase inhibitor and, among other influences, inhibits the release of TNF-α. Data on its beneficial effects in people are conflicting.

GI ulceration is a common complication of SIRS, and management should include an H₂ blocker, sucralfate, and misoprostol as necessary. Other complications such as noncardiogenic pulmonary edema, acute renal insufficiency, and cardiac failure should be managed as discussed in other sources. Nutritional support is important in animals with SIRS, and enteral alimentation is preferable to partial or total parenteral nutrition to maintain mucosal integrity and minimize bacterial translocation.[14]

Treatment of Endotoxemia

Specific therapy for endotoxemia has been investigated for many years in people and animals; however, the results of experimental and clinical studies are often contradictory. The utility of these interventions is not well established in septic dogs and cats, and the majority of substances are not currently available for use in veterinary practice; therefore they cannot be universally recommended. Table 38-8 summarizes the mechanisms of these investigational modalities and their established efficacy.

Table • 38-7

Treatment of Various Stages of Disseminated Intravascular Coagulation in Dogs and Cats

STAGE	PLATELET COUNTS	COAGULATION TIMES	DOG	CAT
Early or low grade	L	Within reference interval	Prophylaxis Aspirin: 10–15 mg/kg/day Heparin: 100 U/kg SC every 8 hrs	Prophylaxis Aspirin: 25 mg/kg/day Heparin: 50 U/kg SC every 8 hrs
Acute or fulminant	LL	Slight prolonged	Heparin: 200–300 U/kg SC every 8 hrs	Heparin 100–150 U/kg SC every 8 hrs
End stage	L	Very prolonged or incoagulable	Heparin: 100 U/kg SC every 8 hrs or added to blood products consisting of whole blood or plasma transfusion	Heparin: 50 U/kg SC every 8 hrs or added to blood products (5 U/kg) consisting of whole blood or plasma transfusion

L, Low (<200,000 and >50,000); LL, very low (<50,000); SC, subcutaneous.

Table • 38-8

Therapeutic Modalities Used in Treatment of Endotoxemia

DRUG	MECHANISM	CLINICAL AVAILABILITY	COMMENTS
Inhibitors of Inflammatory Cytokines			
TNF-α receptor fusion protein	Lowers TNF-α activity	Lenercept, Entanercept	Protects rats from shock and improves outcome in people
Antibody to TNF-α or TNF-α receptors	Interferes with TNF-α activity		
IL-1 or IL-1 receptor antagonist	Blocks IL-1 activity	Investigational	
Glucocorticoids	Antiinflammatory, inhibit TNF-α, IL1, nitric oxide synthesis, decrease release PAF	Many	Controversial results of benefits in sepsis. Low doses most benefit
Pentoxifylline	Phosphodiesterase inhibitor. Elevates intracellular cAMP, inhibits TNF release	Available	Conflicting benefits
PAF antagonists	Recruits neutrophils and platelets inducing endothelial cell and organ injury	Investigational	Reduce thrombocytopenia in dogs given endotoxin
PAF-AH	Inactivates PAF	Recombinant Investigational	Beneficial in preliminary studies in people
Antiinflammatory Cytokines			
IL-10	Reduced proinflammatory cytokines	Investigational	Effective in treated mice
Proinflammatory Mediators, Immunostimulants			
IFN-γ	Reverses monocyte inactivation caused by sepsis	Available for people	No effect on infectious complications in people in controlled studies
G-CSF	Maintain neutrophil numbers and responses	Filgrastim	Conflicting results in people
Immunoglobulins	Increase resistance to bacterial toxins by unknown mechanisms	Human and equine lyophilized	Investigational for this problem
Anticoagulants			
Antithrombin	Natural inhibitor of thrombin and other procoagulant serine proteases	Investigational	No advantage over heparin
Heparin	Inhibits coagulation	Widely available	Helpful in reducing mortality
Activated protein C	Inhibits coagulation via factors IIa, Va and VIIa, and stimulates fibrinolysis	Drotrecogin-α	Increases survival in people but can cause hemorrhage
Lazaroids	Free radical scavengers, membrane stabilization	Available, expensive	Increase survival in experimental animals
NSAIDs and Arachadonic Acid Antagonists			
Prostaglandin E1 and PGI2 (prostacyclin)	Antagonize arachadonic acid and metabolites	Investigational	Not effective
Ibuprofen, etc.	Cyclooxygenase inhibitors	Widely available	No effect on shock or survival
Ketoconazole	Thromboxane synthetase inhibitor	Available clinically	Not effective in controlled studies
Methylxanthines	Improved hemodynamics, inhibit platelet aggregation, decreased mediators	Pentoxifylline	Conflicting data on efficacy

Continued

Table • 38-8

Continued

DRUG	MECHANISM	CLINICAL AVAILABILITY	COMMENTS
Antitoxins			
LPS elimination	Polymyxin B on blood filter absorbs endotoxin	Investigational use in people	Some favorable results
Bactericidal permeability–increasing (BPI) protein	Binds to lipid-A of gram-negative bacterial endotoxin	Available for people	Used in meningococcal sepsis people. Not effective in canine parvoviral infection
Salmonella endotoxin antisera	Binds gram-negative endotoxins	Septi-serum®	Some benefit in parvoviral enteritis in pups
LPS analogues and antibodies	Interfere with LPS action	Investigational in animals	Analogues effective in mice, antibodies effective in horses
Antioxidants			
Nitric oxide inhibition	Restores blood pressure but also increases pulmonary and systemic vascular resistance	Investigational and methylene blue	Some favorable response in small studies in people
N-acetylcysteine	Replenishes intracellular glutathione; scavenges oxygen radicals	Available	Variable efficacy
Selenium	Scavenger of oxygen free radicals via dependent glutathione peroxidase	Available	Improved outcome and less renal failure in people

TNF, Tumor necrosis factor; *IL*, interleukin; *PAF*, platelet activating factor; *cAMP*, cyclic adenosine monophosphate; *PAF-AH*, PAF-acetylhydrolase; *IFN*, interferon; *NSAIDs*, nonsteroidal antiinflammatory drugs; *LPS*, lipopolysaccharide; *G-CSF*, granulocyte colony-stimulating factor.

Physical methods of decreasing LPS concentration in peripheral blood through hemofiltration have been described, including plasma exchange, extracorporeal activated charcoal hemoperfusion, and hemoperfusion or plasmapheresis over polymyxin B; these therapies are not generally available in veterinary medicine. Antibodies designed to bind LPS, lipid A analogues designed to competitively bind LBP and LPS receptors, and use of polymyxin B, which avidly binds lipid A, have been described, but their clinical utility appears to be low in people, likely because SIRS has already been initiated.[26]

Bactericidal permeability–increasing (BPI) protein, a protein of neutrophil granule origin, binds lipid A, and the human recombinant amino-terminal fragment of BPI (rBPI$_{21}$) was investigated in a randomized, blinded, placebo-controlled trial in dogs with CPV enteritis. When examined, affected dogs had elevated endotoxin levels; rBPI$_{21}$ did not have a significant effect on outcome, duration of hospitalization, or plasma endotoxin levels.[28]

Therapies designed to antagonize the cytokine and other mediators of SIRS have also been described and include IL-1 and TNF-α receptor antagonists, anti-TNF-α monoclonal antibodies, soluble TNF-α receptors, glucocorticoids, lazaroids, various nonsteroidal antiinflammatory drugs (NSAIDs), platelet-activating factor (PAF) blockers, inducible nitric oxide synthase inhibitors, and activated protein C, among others.

TNF-α has been identified as an important mediator in sepsis. It produces many of the acute pathophysiologic manifestations; however, administration of monoclonal anti-TNF-α antibody has not been beneficial in protecting people from complications of septic shock.

IL-1 acts synergistically with TNF-α and a receptor antagonist (IL-1RA), which is a naturally produced cytokine produced by macrophages, has shown variable efficacy on survival of septic people.[29]

Trials in people using PAF-antagonists have not shown improved survival rates[41]; however, use of enzymes that degrade endogenous PAF have been more favorable.[20] Dogs given endotoxin had less thrombocytopenia and neutropenia when they were pretreated with a PAF antagonist.[37]

Proinflammatory mediators, such as IL-10, and immunostimulants such as IFN-γ and granulocyte colony-stimulating factor have also been investigated in people.[26,41,16] Some data suggest that some people respond to pretreatment or early treatment with IFN-γ.[10] Because animals are evaluated clinically after inflammatory mediators have been released, the benefits of these drugs in clinical settings have been less than anticipated.

Prostaglandins and leukotrines are increased in sepsis from activation of cyclooxygenase and lipooxygenase pathways. Natural inhibitors prostaglandin E1 (PGE1) and PGI2 (prostacyclin) have not been effective in therapeutic studies. Inhibitors of cyclooxygenase and thromboxane synthetase, such as ibuprofen or ketoconazole, have had variable effects in treating human sepsis depending on the study.[41]

Antitoxins can be used to neutralize cytotoxic intermediates released in endotoxemia. A salmonella endotoxin antiserum has been developed to treat endotoxic shock in horses and dogs. BPI protein is an endotoxin-binding protein that can damage the cell membrane of gram-positive and gram-negative bacteria. Recombinant BPI inhibits inflammation caused by bacterial Group B protective surface protein. Endotoxin was also removed from sera by extracorporeal perfusion through polymyxin B filters.

Antioxidants, such as N-acetylcysteine, have been variably effective in septic patients while selenium produced a beneficial response.[2,13] Nitric oxide is increased in sepsis, and although inhibition increases blood pressure, vascular resistance and use of methylene blue have been favorable in small studies.

PREVENTION

Immunization against CPV and proper management of large- and giant-breed dogs to lessen the occurrence of gastric dilation or volvulus will help prevent endotoxemia of intestinal origin. Appropriate surgical technique and postsurgical management, avoidance of indiscriminant use of antimicrobials and glucocorticoids, and careful management of IV and urinary catheters will minimize iatrogenic and nosocomial infections. Aggressive infection control measures should be developed and implemented in intensive care facilities. Finally, animals at risk for endotoxemia, especially those with established infections, should be managed promptly and appropriately for the primary disorder and monitored for signs of SIRS.

SUGGESTED READINGS*

6. Brady CA, Otto CM. 2001. Systemic inflammatory response syndrome, sepsis, and multiple organ dysfunction, *Vet Clin North Am Small Anim Pract* 31:1147-1162.
8. Dellinger RP. 2003. Inflammation and coagulation: implications for the septic patient, *Clin Infect Dis* 36:1259-1265.
14. Hardie EM. 2000. Therapeutic management of sepsis, pp 272-275. *In* Bonagura JD (ed), Kirk's current veterinary therapy XIII Small animal practice, WB Saunders, Philadelphia.
16. Hotchkiss RS, Karl IE. 2003. The pathophysiology and treatment of sepsis, *N Engl J Med* 348:138-150.

*See the CD-ROM for a complete list of references.

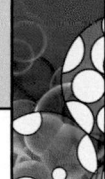

CHAPTER • 39

Enteric Bacterial Infections

CAMPYLOBACTER INFECTIONS

James G. Fox

Etiology

Campylobacter is a genus of gram-negative, slender, curved, motile rods (1.5 to 5 μm × 0.2 to 0.5 μm) that are found singularly, in pairs, or in chains with three to five spirals (Fig. 39-1). The cells can also be curved, S shape, or gull shape. *Campylobacter* species have a single, nonsheathed polar flagellum and microaerobic growth requirements. *Campylobacter jejuni* is the organism routinely associated with diarrheal disease in dogs, cats, and people as well as other domestic, wild, and laboratory animals. *Campylobacter coli*, distinguished from *C. jejuni* on the basis of hippurate hydrolysis, is also isolated from diarrheic animals and people. Other intestinal catalase-negative campylobacters, *Campylobacter upsaliensis* and *Campylobacter helveticus*, have been being isolated more frequently from asymptomatic and diarrheic dogs and cats.* Table 39-1 summarizes the features of these *Campylobacter* species.

Epidemiology

Privately owned adult dogs and cats generally have a lower isolation rate of *C. jejuni* than strays or those maintained in kennels or catteries, laboratories, and animal shelters.[147] It has been isolated from 21% and 29% of diarrheic cats and dogs, respectively, compared with 4% of clinically healthy cats and dogs.[82] In other studies the isolation rate from feces of mature dogs and cats with and without diarrhea has varied from 0% to 50%.[427] Prevalence of *C. jejuni* in clinically normal dogs in one report was significantly greater (p < 0.05) in dogs younger than 6 months old, dogs living in high-density and cohabitation housing conditions for long periods, and the autumn months.[454] Cats less than 1 year old had a higher (30%) isolation rate of *Campylobacter* spp. compared with cats older than 1 year (3%).[31a]

In a 6-year study, 64 of 227 commercially reared cats without clinical signs of diarrhea had microaerobic bacteria isolated from their feces.[400] All the isolates were initially identified as *Campylobacter*-like organisms (CLOs) based on biochemical and phenotypic characteristics. DNA extractions from 51 of these isolates were subjected to the polymerase chain reaction (PCR) using primers specific for *Helicobacter* spp. and *Campylobacter* spp. Of the isolates, 92% (47 isolates) were positive for *Campylobacter* spp., 41% (21 isolates) were positive for *Helicobacter* spp., 33% (17 isolates) were positive for both genera, 59% (30 isolates) were positive only for *Campylobacter* spp., and 8%[4] were positive only for *Helicobacter* spp. Sixteen of the 47 *Campylobacter*-positive cultures were positive for more than one species of *Campylobacter*. Based on a species-specific PCR assay, 83% of the isolates were identified as *C. helveticus*, 47% of the isolates were identified as *C. upsaliensis*, and 6% of the isolates were classified as *C. jejuni*. This study demonstrated that biochemical and

*References 99, 117, 145, 184, 383, 381, 400.

phenotypic characteristics of microaerobic organisms in cat feces were insufficient to characterize mixed *Helicobacter* and *Campylobacter* infections. The finding of C. *helveticus* in a high percentage of the cats confirms the findings of a previous study in England in which the organism was cultured from the feces of healthy cats.[423] Others have observed a high prevalence of C. *upsaliensis* and C. *helveticus* in rectal swab specimens from dogs and cats and the lack of correlation between serotypes and genotypic analysis.[311]

Investigators in the Netherlands have documented a 26% prevalence of multiple *Campylobacter* species in *Campylobacter*-containing feces of dogs.[243] Using multiple isolation methods (different antibiotic-supplemented media plus filtration), selecting 12 suspicious colonies per plate, and rapidly processing the samples, the authors were able to identify C. *jejuni*, C. *upsaliensis*, and *Campylobacter lari*. In two samples, all three species were isolated, whereas in the other four fecal samples, two species of *Campylobacter* were identified. Interestingly, none of the dogs infected with multiple species of *Campylobacter* had diarrhea.[243] This asymptomatic characteristic was also true for cats harboring multiple species of *Campylobacter* and *Helicobacter*.[400]

Alterations in *Campylobacter* may occur with changes in intestinal microflora. In dogs, fecal *Campylobacter* species counts increased in a majority of dogs fed a probiotic containing *Enterococcus faecium*, whereas counts of *Salmonella* were higher and those of *Clostridium* species were lower.[462] Feeding of probiotics containing *E. faecium* favors the adhesion and colonization of C. *jejuni* and the dissociation from and reduction of *Clostridium perfringens* in the canine intestine.[370]

Puppies and kittens appear more likely to acquire C. *jejuni* and show clinical disease, probably because of a lack of previous exposure and development of protective antibody. Studies of pups show that shedding of *Campylobacter* species ranges from less than 5% to as high as 90%.

As with most enteric microbial pathogens, fecal-oral spread with foodborne and waterborne transmission appears to be the principal avenue for infection. Suspected sources of *Campylobacter* infection include contaminated meat products, particularly poultry and unpasteurized milk. Asymptomatic carriers can shed campylobacters in their feces for prolonged periods and directly infect other animals or contaminate food products or water. Nosocomial infection of hospitalized animals occurs, as does exposure through other pets in a household (e.g., ferrets, hamsters, birds, rabbits) and rural farm animals that may shed the organism.

Pathogenesis

The severity of the disease depends on the number of organisms ingested by the host as well as previous exposure and development of protective antibody. Other enteric pathogens, such as parvovirus and coronavirus, *Giardia* organisms, or *Salmonella* organisms, may play a synergistic role.[45,384] Environmental, physiologic, and surgical stresses may also exacerbate the severity of the disease. Various virulence factors, such as enterotoxins, cytotoxins, or adherence or invasion properties, are expressed by different C. *jejuni-coli* isolates. A cytotoxin referred to as *cytolethal distending toxin* has been identified in C. *jejuni*, but its role in production of intestinal disease is not known. However, in vitro the cytotoxin causes distension of cell lines and cell cycle arrest in the G_2M1 phase in the cell cycle. Blood and leukocytes in the feces, congestion,

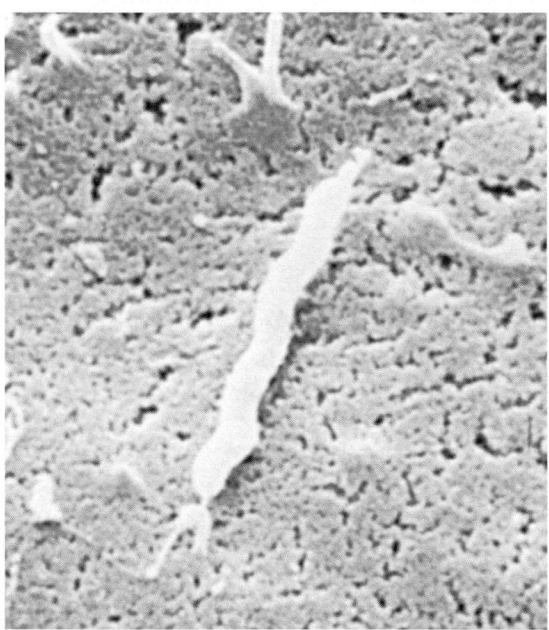

Fig 39-1 Scanning electron microscopy view of *Campylobacter jejuni* adhered to chick embryo cell (×15,900).

Table • 39-1

Comparative Features of Campylobacter *Species That Infect Dogs or Cats*

CAMPYLOBACTER ORGANISM	MORPHOLOGIC AND DISTINGUISHING FEATURES	HOSTS	CLINICAL FEATURES
C. *jejuni*; C. *coli*	Slender, curved, motile rods; found singularly, in pairs, or in chains with three to five spirals; curved S or gull shape; single, polar, nonsheathed flagellum; *C. coli:* hippurate negative	Dogs, cats, ferrets, cattle People	Neonates—diarrhea, adults—asymptomatic Diarrhea, systemic manifestations
C. *upsaliensis*	Catalase negative	Dogs, cats People	Asymptomatic Diarrhea, abscess, placental damage
C. *lari*	Grows at 42°C	Dogs People	Asymptomatic Bacteremia, urinary tract infections
C. *helveticus*	Catalase negative	Cats	Asymptomatic

edema, mucosal ulcers, and occasional sepsis in people suggest that the organism can be invasive. Experimental challenge in laboratory animals also indicates that the organism can be isolated from blood several days after challenge inoculation. Experimental infections of puppies and kittens with strains isolated from people with diarrhea are less severe than those observed in the people from which the organisms were isolated. Animals appear to be more resistant or better adapted to the pathogenic effects of various different *C. jejuni* isolates and usually only develop watery mucoid diarrhea.[278,360,362]

Clinical Findings

Dog

In many cases, dogs are asymptomatic carriers of *Campylobacter* species. The clinical syndrome occurs most frequently in dogs younger than 6 months. Animals may be more susceptible to clinical disease when stressed by hospitalization, concurrent disease, pregnancy, shipment, or surgery. *Campylobacter*-associated diarrhea has a wide clinical spectrum in dogs as well as people, ranging from mild, loose feces to watery diarrhea to bloody mucoid diarrhea. Acute campylobacteriosis that develops in puppies and some adult dogs is manifest by mucus-laden, watery, or bile-streaked diarrhea (with or without blood and leukocytes) for 5 to 15 days, partial anorexia, and occasional vomiting.[142,144,146] Elevated temperature and leukocytosis may also be present. In certain cases, diarrhea can be chronic and last 2 or more weeks, can be intermittent, or in some cases can be present for several months.[114] In people, *C. jejuni* can cause extraintestinal complications such as arthritis, meningitis, myocarditis, cholecystis, and abortions. *C. jejuni* has been isolated from two dogs with bacteremia and cholecystitis.[335] Clinical signs included anorexia, fever, and icterus. Ultrasonography showed a fluid-filled, abnormally thickened gallbladder wall in both dogs. *C. jejuni* and *Campylobacter fetus* are also recovered from the bile of people with cholecystitis, although infrequently.[165,471] Insofar as *Helicobacter* species are present in liver and bile of various hosts (see Intestinal and Hepatic Helicobacters section in this chapter), detailed biochemical and phenotypic descriptions are necessary to fully characterize and validate whether microaerophilic organisms isolated from the hepatobiliary tract of dogs are *Campylobacter* or *Helicobacter* species. *Campylobacter*-associated abortion has also been noted in dogs, although it is infrequent.

Cat

In cats, clinical signs of campylobacteriosis are poorly documented in the absence of other pathogens. As with dogs, campylobacteriosis is usually asymptomatic. If clinical signs are evident, the animal generally is younger than 6 months. In a prevalence survey of 159 cats from pounds, 17 shed *C. jejuni* in the feces, but of these only 2 had bloody, mucus-laden diarrhea. *Giardia* species were present in both, combined with *Isospora* species in one cat and *Toxocara* species in the other. Another cat concurrently infected with *Salmonella* species and *C. jejuni* was depressed and anorectic but not diarrheic. Culture results from the two cats' feces after antibiotic therapy and clinical improvement were negative for *C. jejuni*.[129] Chronic diarrhea in another cat that had serum antibodies to *C. jejuni* plus positive culture results for the organism abated when treated with chloramphenicol. *C. jejuni* could not be recultured from the stool after therapy.[132]

Diagnosis

Microscopic Examination

Rapid presumptive diagnosis is possible using either dark-field or phase-contrast microscopy. Fresh fecal samples are examined for curved bacteria with the characteristic darting motility of *C. jejuni*. This method is especially sensitive in people (and perhaps dogs and cats) during the acute stage of clinical diarrhea. With Gram stain, faintly staining, gram-negative, gull-wing-shape slender rods are apparent. Maintaining the safranin counterstaining improves their visualization.[296] However, based on morphology alone, these organisms could also be enteric helicobacters. Presence of fecal leukocytes should be ascertained, because leukocytes may be found in enteritis caused by natural or experimental infections with *C. jejuni*.

Cultural Identification

Rectal swab specimens can be obtained, or fresh feces can be collected. For diagnosis of *C. jejuni* cholecystitis and bacteremia, appropriate diagnostic testing, including abdominal ultrasonography, gallbladder aspiration with bile culture, and blood culture, should be performed.[335] Transport of fecal specimens usually does not present isolation difficulties because *C. jejuni-coli* remain viable in feces at room temperature for at least 3 days and at refrigeration temperatures for at least 1 week. However, higher rates of isolation can be achieved with shorter time delays.

Swabs obtained from fresh feces are streaked onto *Campylobacter* blood agar plates (Campy-BAP, Scott Laboratories, Fiskeville, R.I.), which are then placed in an oxygen-reduced atmosphere. The standard method for culture uses commercially available selective medium that inhibits fecal flora; however, it may not be necessary for isolating thermophilic *Campylobacter* strains from acute cases of enteritis. Similarly, broth enrichment procedures have not been more effective than direct plating on Campy-BAP for isolation of *C. jejuni* from canine feces.

Plates are incubated at 37° C to 42° C and examined at 72 to 96 hours. Colonies composed of curved gram-negative rods are round, raised, translucent, and sometimes mucoid. Isolates are identified as *C. jejuni* on the basis of positive oxidase and catalase reactions, susceptibility to nalidixic acid, resistance to cephalothin, and inability to grow at 42° C under aerobic conditions. *C. upsaliensis* and *C. helveticus* are catalase negative, and isolation is enhanced by selective filtration of feces to be cultured through a 0.45-μ filter.[171] Investigators in South Africa have published results for a protocol that has been in use in their diagnostic laboratory since 1990 and allows primary isolation of multiple species of *Campylobacter* and *Helicobacter* from the diarrheic specimens of individual children.[258,259] Filtrates are plated onto antibiotic-free blood agar plates and incubated in an H$_2$-enriched atmosphere. These authors not only documented an increase in the number of CLOs isolated but also were able to culture *C. upsaliensis* for the first time. They have reported a 16.2% prevalence of multiple species of CLOs based on primary isolation, biochemical characterization, and serologic confirmation. They frequently recovered between two and five species of CLOs from one stool sample, with *C. jejuni* (different serotypes), *C. coli*, *C. upsaliensis*, *Helicobacter fennelliae*, and *Helicobacter cinaedi* being commonly isolated.[258] Additional analysis using the filtration isolation technique with cat and dog feces may yield prevalence rates for mixed *Helicobacter* and *Campylobacter* infections even higher than those reported recently in cats.[400]

Various procedures have been used, especially during outbreaks, to identify different serotypes of *C. jejuni-coli* by using thermostabile and thermolabile surface antigens.[302] Isolates from people and various animal species have shown that extensive serologic heterogeneity exists within *C. jejuni-coli*. Many of the isolates frequently found in diarrheic and normal dogs and cats have had serotypes frequently encountered in human patients.[133] For example, serotype 4 (commonly associated with outbreaks of *C. jejuni*-associated diarrhea in people) was also a common serotype isolated from commercially reared beagles.[133,443] Plasmid characterization, restriction enzyme analysis, and ribotyping can also be used for strain identity, but these techniques require specialized methodologies. The technique of restriction enzyme analysis of whole genomic DNA allowed verification of *C. jejuni* zoonotic transmission to personnel in vivaria caring for wild-caught coyotes.[152]

Serologic Testing

Various techniques can detect serum antibodies to various antigens of *Campylobacter*. A specific bactericidal assay has been used to demonstrate a rising antibody titer in people and animals. Other serologic assays, such as the enzyme-linked immunosorbent assay (ELISA), have been developed to survey human populations during outbreaks of campylobacteriosis and ascertain previous exposures to the organism. Unfortunately, no systematic studies have been performed in dogs and cats to ascertain the importance of antibody titers as an indicator of infection in animals with or without diarrhea.

Pathologic Findings

Gross visible findings in naturally and experimentally infected canine neonates are abnormally fluid colonic contents as well as thickening, congestion, and edema of the colonic mucosa.[68] Microscopically, the colon and cecum show decreases in epithelial cell height, brush borders, and numbers of goblet cells. Hyperplasia of epithelial glands results in a thickened mucosa. Subepithelial congestion, hemorrhage, and inflammatory infiltrates have also been seen. Findings in adult animals inoculated with *C. jejuni* were similar to those in some dogs with natural campylobacteriosis: stunting of intestinal villi, infiltration of lamina propria with inflammatory cells, and hyperplastic Peyer's patches.[278] Naturally occurring intestinal lesions in adult dogs have consisted of mucosal hyperplasia in the colon characterized by immature hyperchromatic, hyperplastic epithelial cells with a high mitotic index, and deep and irregular crypts.[142] With Warthin-Starry stain, CLOs have been demonstrated attached to but not within colonic epithelium. However, in experimentally produced *C. jejuni* colitis in macaques, intraepithelial invasion of *C. jejuni* was demonstrated by electron microscopy (EM).[378] A relative increase had been noted in the number of lymphocytes infiltrating the lamina propria. Ileal lesions consisted of focal, shallow crypts and blunt, irregular villi, which occasionally fused. Mild congestion and dilatation of lacteals has been found. Stunting and fusing of intestinal villi and mononuclear cell infiltrates in lamina propria have also been noted in subacute stages of parvovirus infection and in a dog with protracted *Campylobacter*-associated diarrhea.[75] Experimentally, selected strains of *C. jejuni* produce hepatitis in mice, and the organism has been isolated from inflamed livers of dogs.

Therapy

The efficacy of antibiotic therapy and treatment of *Campylobacter*-associated diarrhea in the dog and cat is not known—nor is it known whether antibiotics effectively alter the course of enteric disease. However, in some dogs and cats with severe diarrhea, antibiotic therapy may be warranted. Antibiotic treatment of infected animals may be instituted to minimize exposure to people and other pets in the household. Fortunately, strains of *Campylobacter* isolated from animals and people are susceptible to several antimicrobial agents (Table 39-2). Erythromycin, the drug of choice for *Campylobacter*-induced diarrhea in people, may also be effective in the treatment of the disease in animals. Treatment of clinically affected cats and dogs has resulted in resolution of the illness and elimination of the organism as determined by *Campylobacter*-negative fecal culture results. However, failure to eliminate *C. jejuni* with oral erythromycin from ferrets housed in a research

environment has also been noted.[128] Erythromycin can also cause gastric irritation and vomiting in some animals.

Chloramphenicol has been given with mixed results to treat *Campylobacter*-associated diarrhea in dogs and cats. Treatment in dogs has resulted in abatement of clinical signs. However, the same organism has been reisolated after therapy has been completed. It is possible that these dogs developed an antibiotic-induced carrier state (as occurs in enteric *Salmonella* infections), experienced a protracted period of *Campylobacter* shedding, or became reinfected. Clinical improvement was noted in a diarrheic cat treated with chloramphenicol, and fecal culture results after completion of the treatment were negative for *C. jejuni*. *C. jejuni*-associated bacteremia and cholecystitis have been successfully treated with IV cefoxitin, a second-generation cephalosporin, or oral erythromycin (see Table 39-2) for 21 days, which resulted in complete resolution of all clinical and laboratory abnormalities.[335]

Several other antibiotics are active against *Campylobacter* strains isolated from dogs and cats. These strains show in vitro susceptibility to furazolidone as well as gentamicin, neomycin, clindamycin, and tetracycline. However, resistance in many strains to various tetracyclines and kanamycin is caused by plasmids that confer resistance and are transmissible within *C. jejuni* serotypes. Antimicrobial agents that are usually ineffective include penicillin, ampicillin, polymyxin B, trimethoprim, and vancomycin. In vitro resistance also develops to metronidazole and sulfadimethoxine.[139] Many *Campylobacter* strains produce β-lactamase, which accounts for the resistance to penicillin and ampicillin. Before therapy is instituted, isolation and sensitivity tests should be done. Some animals continue to shed the organism despite antibiotic therapy. Quinolone antibiotics may be useful in eliminating *C. jejuni* and *C. coli* in asymptomatic carriers, but drug resistance can develop to this class of antibiotics.

Public Health Considerations

Although *C. jejuni-coli* exist as commensal gastrointestinal (GI) microflora of domestic animals, they are a leading cause of enteric disease in people. The infectious dose of *C. jejuni* for humans is as low as a few hundred organisms. The disease is often severe in people and in addition to diarrhea may be characterized by vomiting, fever, and abdominal discomfort. When dogs or cats are the incriminated reservoirs for human infection, they usually have been recently acquired from pet stores or kennels and have had diarrhea. However, asymptomatic dogs and cats can also be a source of infection to people. A survey conducted in Seattle, Washington, indicated that 6% of sporadic *C. jejuni* infections were linked to exposure to diarrheic kittens.[13] Another study reported that 30% of the cases in university students were associated with healthy cats.[122] Risks from pet exposure have been very high among infants and children.[446,497] Other nonpet sources of exposure risk include contact with cattle or chickens, eating salad vegetables, swimming in natural water sources, and drinking natural bottled mineral water.[11,104,393a] These are all risks associated with fecal contamination in the environment. In all studies a consistent risk factor for acquiring *C. jejuni* enteritis has been the consumption of unpasteurized milk or raw or undercooked meat, particularly chicken or foods that have contacted this meat during preparation.[11,122] Nevertheless, veterinary practitioners should alert owners of the zoonotic implication of *Campylobacter* infection for other household members and stress the importance of exercising appropriate hygienic measures, especially when pets have diarrhea. An alarming concern is that *Campylobacter* strains worldwide from human and animal patients are developing increased antibacterial resistance to drugs such as the quinolones.[276,409,440,319a] Presumably, this has been linked to the use of these drugs in animal husbandry situations. An addi-

Table • 39-2

Drug Therapy for Nonenteric Salmonellosis and Other Enteric Bacterial Infections in Dogs and Cats

DRUG[a]	SPECIES	DOSE[b] (mg/kg)	ROUTE	INTERVAL (HOURS)	DURATION (DAYS)	INDICATED INFECTIONS
Erythromycin	D	20	PO	12	5–21	Campylobacteriosis, nongastric helicobacteriosis
	C	10	PO	8	5	
Trimethoprim-sulfonamide	B	12–15	PO, IV	12	7–10	Salmonellosis, shigellosis, yersiniosis
Amoxicillin/ampicillin	B	10–20	PO, IV	8	7–10	Salmonellosis, shigellosis
Chloramphenicol	D	15–25	PO, SC, IV	8	5–7	Salmonellosis, shigellosis, campylobacteriosis, nongastric helicobacteriosis
	C	10–15	PO, SC	12	8	
Metronidazole	B	8–10	PO	8	5–10	Bacterial overgrowth, nongastric and gastric helicobacteriosis
Tetracycline	B	10–20	PO	8	42	Shigellosis, yersiniosis, bacterial overgrowth
Gentamicin[c]	D	2	IM, SC	12	5	Yersiniosis, salmonellosis, nongastric helicobacteriosis
Tylosin	B	11	PO	8	42	Bacterial overgrowth
Cephalosporins (first generation)	B	20	PO	8	7	Yersiniosis
Cephalosporins (second generation)	B	22	IV	8	21	Campylobacteriosis, nongastric helicobacteriosis
Enrofloxacin[d]	B	5	PO, SC	12	5–7	Campylobacteriosis, salmonellosis

B, Dog and cat; *C*, cat; *D*, dog; *PO*, by mouth; *IV*, intravascular; *SC*, subcutaneous; *IM*, intramuscular.
[a]See Appendix 8 for additional information on each drug.
[b]Dose per administration at specified interval.
[c]Monitor for renal failure.
[d]Other quinolones such as ciprofloxacin, difloxacin, or marbofloxacin, are alternatives, although dosages vary.

tional zoonotic risk is the development of Guillain-Barré syndrome, a polyradiculoneuritis in people, which may occur after infection with *C. jejuni*. The GM, gangliosides of peripheral nerves, share epitopes with lipopolysaccharides of these bacteria.[309,332,]

C. jejuni has been linked to immunoproliferative small bowel disease, also known as α-*chain disease* in people.[265] This disease is a form of lymphoma that arises in small intestinal tissue. Interestingly, early forms of the disease respond to antibiotics, similar to *Helicobacter pylori*-associated mucosa-associated lymphoid tumor (MALT) lymphoma, which has tumors that regress in responsive to antibiotic therapy.

C. upsaliensis has been isolated from a person with bloody diarrhea as well as his pet dog, which also had diarrhea. The plasmid profile of the two strains were identical, suggesting that *C. upsaliensis* infection may also be a zoonosis.[171] *C. upsaliensis* was isolated from the blood and fetoplacental tissue of a woman with diarrhea who was 18 weeks pregnant and had been in contact with a cat that had a similar strain of *C. upsaliensis* isolated from its feces, also suggesting zoonotic transmission.[181] Others have also reported *C. upsaliensis* gastroenteritis in people who have had contact with pets.[345]

Human and canine isolates of *C. upsaliensis* have distinct ribotypes and plasmid profiles, suggesting that host-specific genotype differences may exist among strains of *C. upsaliensis*.[424] However, these analyses or other molecular fingerprinting techniques must be used on suspected pet-associated *C. upsaliensis* zoonoses before the definitive transmission can be defined.

GASTRIC *HELICOBACTER* INFECTIONS

James G. Fox

Etiology

Gram-negative, microaerophilic, curved to spiral-shape bacteria isolated from gastric mucosa of people and animals have created a great deal of interest because of their causal role in gastric disease.[267] The genus *Helicobacter* includes 24 formally named species as well as other unnamed closely related organisms.* Once considered a predominantly sterile organ pro-

*References 80, 131, 137, 153, 165, 268, 331, 426, 425.

Table • 39-3

Comparative Features of Gastric Helicobacter Species That Infect Dogs and Cats

GASTRIC HELICOBACTER ORGANISM[a]	MORPHOLOGIC AND DISTINGUISHING FEATURES	HOSTS	CLINICAL FEATURES
H. pylori	Small (2—4 μ); curved to spiral shape	People, nonhuman primates Cats	Gastritis, peptic ulcer; gastric neoplasia, also asymptomatic Gastritis in catteries
H. (Flexispira) rappini (Lockard type 1)	Fusiform shape; entwined with multiple periplasmic fibers; multiple bipolar sheathed flagella	Sheep People and animals Dogs	Abortion, hepatic necrosis Intestinal disease Asymptomatic, gastric and fecal isolate
H. felis (Lockard type 2)	7—10 μ long; superficial periplasmic fibers; sparse; exist singly or in groups; multiple bipolar flagella with sheaths	Cat, dogs, people	Cultured from stomach, subclinical (histologic) gastritis
H. bizzozeronii (Lockard type 3, Gastrospirillum hominis, H. heilmannii)	7—10 μ long; tightly spiraled; no periplasmic fibers and difficult to culture deep in gastric glands and parietal cell canaliculi	Dogs, cats, people, swine, nonhuman primates	Common gastric colonizer Inflamed gastric tissue of people mucosa-associated lymphoid tumor (MALT) in people
H. salomonis	5—7 μ long by 0.8—1.2 μ wide; tufts of sheathed flagella at each end; not as tightly spiraled as in H. bizzozeronii; isolated from glands of corpus of stomach	Dogs	Subclinical

[a]Previously used terms for organisms are in parentheses.

tected from microbial colonization by low gastric pH, the euchlorhydric stomach is now known to be colonized with gastric bacteria belonging to the newly named genus *Helicobacter* (Table 39-3 and Fig. 39-2), whereas the hypochlorhydric stomach is resistant to their replication. These organisms possess a high level of urease activity that allows them to survive in an acidic environment. The type species *H. pylori* colonizes the stomach of 20% to 95% of human adult populations worldwide (see Fig. 39-2, *A*).[172] *H. pylori* causes persistent, active, chronic gastritis and peptic ulcer disease in people and has been linked to the development of gastric adenocarcinoma and gastric mucosa-associated lymphoma.[341] *H. pylori* has also been isolated from inflamed gastric tissue of cats in a commercial cattery and can experimentally infect cats.[188,349]

Other gastric helicobacters have been linked to gastritis in various mammalian hosts.* Many of these infected animals have asymptomatic gastric inflammation. Additional species of gastric *Helicobacter* have been isolated from stomachs of various mammalian hosts, including dogs (*Helicobacter rappini, Helicobacter felis, Helicobacter bizzozeronii, Helicobacter heilmannii*-like, *Helicobacter salomonis, Helicobacter bilis*), cats (*H. felis, H. heilmannii*-like, *Helicobacter pametensis*), ferrets (*Helicobacter mustelae*), cheetahs (*Helicobacter acinonychis*), dolphins, whales, harp seals (*Helicobacter cetorum*), and nonhuman primates (*H. heilmannii*-like). (See Table 39-3 and Fig. 39-2 for a summary of the gastric helicobacters infecting dogs and cats.)

Historically, these *Helicobacter* organisms in dogs and cats have been described histologically as gastric *spirilla*.[123] Three

morphologically distinct forms have been described in dogs and cats.[274,480,481] More than one of these morphologic types of bacteria can be seen in the stomach of one animal. Lockard type 1 is a bacterium with multiple bipolar, sheathed flagella entwined with periplasmic fibers, which appear to cover the entire surface of the organism (see Fig. 39-2, *B*). A similar organism was isolated from aborted ovine fetuses and was classified as *Flexispira rappini*.[242,331] This bacterium, classified as a *Helicobacter* species based on 16S RNA sequencing, has been isolated from the feces of asymptomatic mice, dogs, and cats as well as from the stomach of dogs.[274,391] *Helicobacter bilis*, a member of the *Flexispira* taxa associated with hepatitis and inflammatory bowel disease (IBD) in mice, has also been cultured from the stomachs of dogs. Lockard type 2 also has periplasmic fibers, but they are most sparsely distributed on the organism and can appear singly or in groups of two, three, or four. This organism has been cultured from the feline stomach and has been named *H. felis* (see Fig. 39-2, *C*).[344] The third type of organisms, called *gastrospirilla*, are the bacteria most commonly found in mammalian stomachs. These are also very tightly spiraled, but they have no periplasmic fibrils. On the basis of morphologic characteristics, it appears that the Lockard type 2 organism primarily is restricted to cats and dogs, whereas type 3 has been seen in cats, dogs, nonhuman primates, cheetahs, swine, and people. The type 3 bacterium has been given various names in different hosts, including *Gastrospirillum hominis*, and *H. heilmannii*.[191,412] *H. heilmannii* is a provisional name given to closely related or perhaps identical organisms that have not yet been cultured on artificial media. These organisms (see Fig. 39-2, *D*) are morphologically similar to *H. bizzozeronii* (see Fig. 39-2, *E*) found in the gastric mucosae of nonhuman primates, dogs, cats and pigs. *H. biz-*

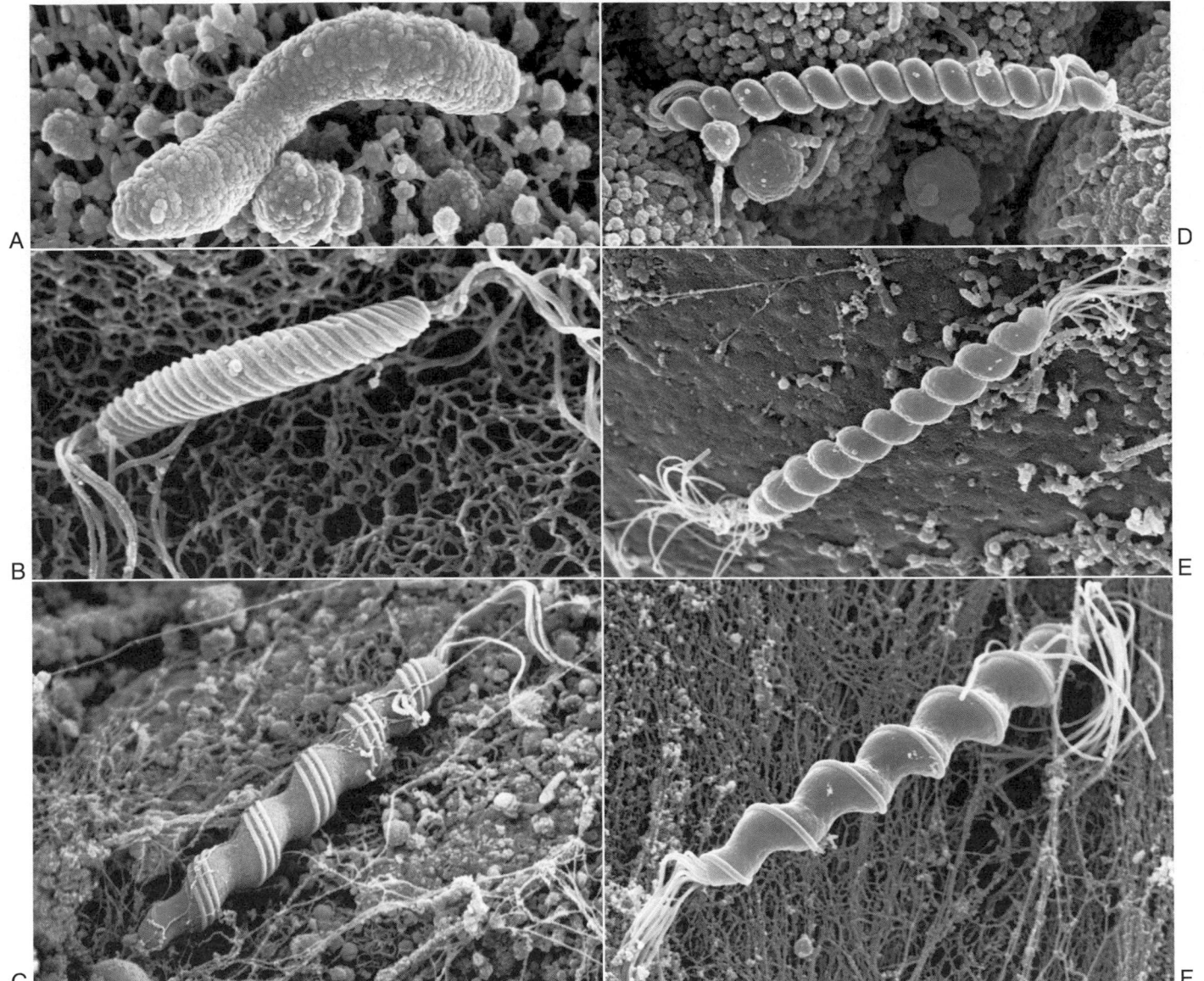

Fig 39-2 Scanning electron microphotographs of **(A)** *H. pylori*, **(B)** *H. rappini*, **(C)** *H. felis*, **(D)** *H. heilmannii*, **(E)** *H. bizzozeronii*, and **(F)** *H. salomonis*. (Courtesy M.H. Stoffel, University of Bern, Bern, Switzerland.)

zozeronii has also been cultured from the inflamed gastric tissue of people.[12] EM shows that this organism lacks periplasmic fibers, unlike *H. felis*. This morphologic distinction is confounded with the observation of two gastric *Helicobacter*-like organisms (GHLOs). These GHLOs from canine stomachs lacking periplasmic fibers had genetic analysis compatible with *H. felis*.[93] *H. salomonis* (see Fig. 39-2, *F*) is a gastric helicobacter with unique molecular characteristics that has been isolated from dogs.[191,219] Because of the difficulty in cultivating these organisms to determine their phenotypic properties, *H. bizzozeronii* and *H. salomonis* from dogs are the only formally named *gastric helicobacters* based on defined biochemical and genetic analyses.[190]

In cats, *H. felis*, *H. pylori*, *H. pametensis* (first isolated and characterized in birds), and *H. heilmannii* have been isolated or identified in gastric tissues.

Epidemiology

Although infected animals and people mount a significant systemic IgG response to gastric organisms, the antibodies are not protective and the organisms persist in the mucous layer or closely adhere to the gastric epithelium, protected from the gastric acidic milieu. The mechanisms of transmission are poorly understood. Gastric helicobacters have specific enteric tissue tropism and colonize only gastric and not intestinal epithelium. Fecal-oral transmission has been suggested, and gastric helicobacters have been isolated from feces of animals and people.[342] *H. mustelae* was isolated from feces of ferrets, particularly when ferrets had drug-induced hypochlorhydria.[148] *H. pylori* has been isolated from feces of children from a third-world country as well as from infected adults from a more developed country.[236,450] In pups, experimentally inoculated gastric helicobacters have been acquired during the lactation period, and puppies have infected each other.[190] Gastric helicobacters have been isolated from the environment in surface waters,[195] likely a result of fecal contamination. Indirect transmission in this manner might result in more widespread dissemination. One concern is that helicobacters are more resistant than coliforms to chlorination.

Oral-oral transmission is more likely and is supported by clinical observations of people being infected by exposure to gastric secretions,[342] isolation of *H. pylori* from dental plaque and tissue, and nosocomial infection from improper disinfection of gastric pH probes and endoscopic equipment. Similar transmission routes are also probable for gastric *Helicobacter* in animals. Vomitus containing gastric *Helicobacter* is another likely source for transmission.[111] Cats naturally infected with *H. pylori* were screened by culture and PCR for the organism in salivary secretions, gastric juices, gastric tissues, and feces.[149] *H. pylori* was cultured from salivary secretions (50%) and gastric fluid samples (91%) from cats. A PCR product specific for an *H. pylori* surface protein was amplified in 42% of feline dental plaque specimens and 80% of feline fecal specimens. Isolation of *H. pylori* from feline mucosal secretions suggests a zoonotic risk exists from personnel handling of *H. pylori*-infected cats in vivaria.[188] In comparison, *H. pylori* infection was not detected in stray cats,[96] which may reflect an anthroponosis in the closed commercial cattery where *H. pylori* was present in 100% of the animals. Additional studies using molecular, cultural, and histologic techniques are needed to ascertain whether *H. pylori* naturally colonizes dogs and cats.

The prevalence of gastric *Helicobacter* spp. infections in clinically healthy colony-raised dogs and cats in high population densities routinely approaches 100%, indicating the organisms' unique ability to colonize the stomach of numerous hosts selectively and efficiently.[404] In laboratory-reared beagles, *H. felis* and other spiral helicobacters were observed in high numbers in the gastric glands of the fundic-pyloric junction and the cardia. These organisms were associated with lymphoid hyperplasia and parietal cell degeneration.[197,274] In pet dogs and cats a series of gastric biopsy samples were examined for the presence of GHLOs.[200] GHLOs were observed in 82% of dogs and 76% of cats; the bacteria were present in the mucus of foveolar epithelia, gastric pits, and parietal cells. More lymphoid follicles are found in the stomachs of older random-source cats with high numbers of GHLOs in their gastric mucosae than in younger cats with lower numbers of GHLOs.[336]

Pathogenesis

Because gastric helicobacteriosis is widespread but the clinical disease is less common, host factors are likely responsible for adverse outcomes caused by infection. Chronic or chronic active gastritis resulting from oral inoculation of *Helicobacter* species has been experimentally produced in people, germ-free pigs and dogs, specific-pathogen–free (SPF) cats, mice, and nonhuman primates with *H. pylori*; in ferrets with *H. mustelae*; in kittens with *H. acinonychis* and *H. heilmannii*; and in germ-free dogs, SPF dogs, mice, and rats with *H. felis*.[123] The *H. pylori*-associated gastritis in people consists of polymorphonuclear cells as well as mononuclear cell infiltrates and is classified as active chronic gastritis. Persistent *H. pylori* infections in people (particularly children) and the domestic cat also are often characterized by lymphoid aggregates and gastric lymphoid follicles.[130,189] Inflammation and associated lymphoid follicles were primarily located in the antrum, which corresponded to the heaviest concentration of *H. pylori*.[188] Ultrastructurally the organisms were numerous in the gastric mucus, were less frequently adhered tightly to gastric epithelia, and formed pedestals between bacterial membranes and the epithelial microvilli.[188]

In the past, gastric lymphoid elements were considered a normal histologic finding in dogs and cats. However, experimental and clinical evidence suggests that they are the result of host responses to *Helicobacter* antigens.[407] The presence of GHLOs is often associated with a reduction in mucous content of surface epithelia, occasional intraepithelial leukocytes, and some degenerating glands. The gastritis observed in dogs and cats with non–*H. pylori* helicobacters is generally mild. Eosinophils in gastric mucosae of animals can also be a major component of the inflammation, particularly in the acute phase of the infection.[130,268,365] Neutrophils and eosinophilic infiltrates, interepithelial globule leukocytes, epithelial dysplasia, and up-regulation of certain mucosal proinflammatory interleukins (IL-1β and IL-8), and interferon-γ (IFN-γ) are noted in *H. pylori*–infected cats but not in uninfected control cats.[103,406,432] Despite the inflammatory and infiltrative changes, mild gastritis caused by *H. felis* in cats did not alter gastric secretion.[407] In dogs with naturally acquired gastritis, mucosal pathology was related to cytokine mRNA expression with neutrophils to IL-8 and IFN-γ, macrophages and lymphocytes to IFN-γ, and fibrosis to INF-1β.[492a]

The degree of GHLO colonization and lymphoid follicles correlated well in cats but not in dogs. If the number of GHLOs in dogs was classified as high, then lymphoid follicles were more likely to be present. In high-grade GHLO infections, glandular degeneration was more pronounced in cats than dogs.[200] The majority (91%) of naturally infected pet cats had gastric helicobacters.[316] All cats had mild to moderate gastritis in the antrum or body, regardless of the presence or density of bacteria. In other naturally infected cats, infected sick cats had a higher degree of pyloric but not fundic inflammation than healthy infected cats and uninfected cats.[433] In dogs[261] the severity of gastritis correlated with infection but not with the clinical sign of vomiting. In other studies,[92] 100% of laboratory and shelter dogs and 67% of pet dogs were colonized with GHLOs that were morphologically consistent with *H. heilmannii* or *H. felis*. Regardless of the colonization intensity, all dogs had mild to moderate gastritis, and *H. pylori* was not isolated.

Experimentally, *H. felis* infection in dogs for 26 weeks did not correlate with number of *H. felis* observed and degree of inflammation or number of affected lymphoid follicles.[403] Furthermore the gastric secretory axis was not perturbed in *H. felis*–infected dogs or dogs naturally infected with GHLOs.[405]

Competitive inhibition may occur in gastric helicobacteriosis; the colonization by one organism suppresses proliferation of other helicobacters. *H. pylori*-infected cats did not have large gastric spiral organisms colonizing the gastric mucosa. When 6-week-old pups with gastric *H. salomonis* were experimentally infected with *H. bizzozeronii*, infection by *H. salomonis* was suppressed.[190] This phenomenon has also been suggested to account for the rare occurrence of concurrent infection in people and nonhuman primates with large gastric spiral organisms and *H. pylori*.[86,87,196,267,429] Experimental inoculation of the feline *H. pylori* strain into naive cats without gastric infection caused by GHLOs confirmed that *H. pylori* produces a persistent gastritis identical to that noted in cats naturally infected with *H. pylori*.[130] *H. pylori* was isolated on serial biopsies and at necropsy 7 months after inoculation from all cats.[130] Additional studies are required to ascertain whether duodenal and gastric ulcers have an infectious component in dogs and cats.[134]

Clinical Findings

Although gastric helicobacters produce gastritis in people and animals, they usually cause asymptomatic infection in their hosts. The reason most infected individuals remain asymptomatic but some have more serious disease is unclear.[92,188] However, clinical signs in pet animals attributable to *Helicobacter*-associated gastritis do occur.[492a] Signs include chronic vomiting, weight loss, and in some cases, severe emaciation or diarrhea.[93,200] Vomiting in dogs with chronic superficial gastritis attributed to gastric spiral organisms has been characterized as intermittent, consisting of mucus or gastric secretions, sometimes containing bile. Pica, belching, anorexia, and weight loss also are occasionally noted. Signs attributed to gastric helicobacteriosis have been based on finding these

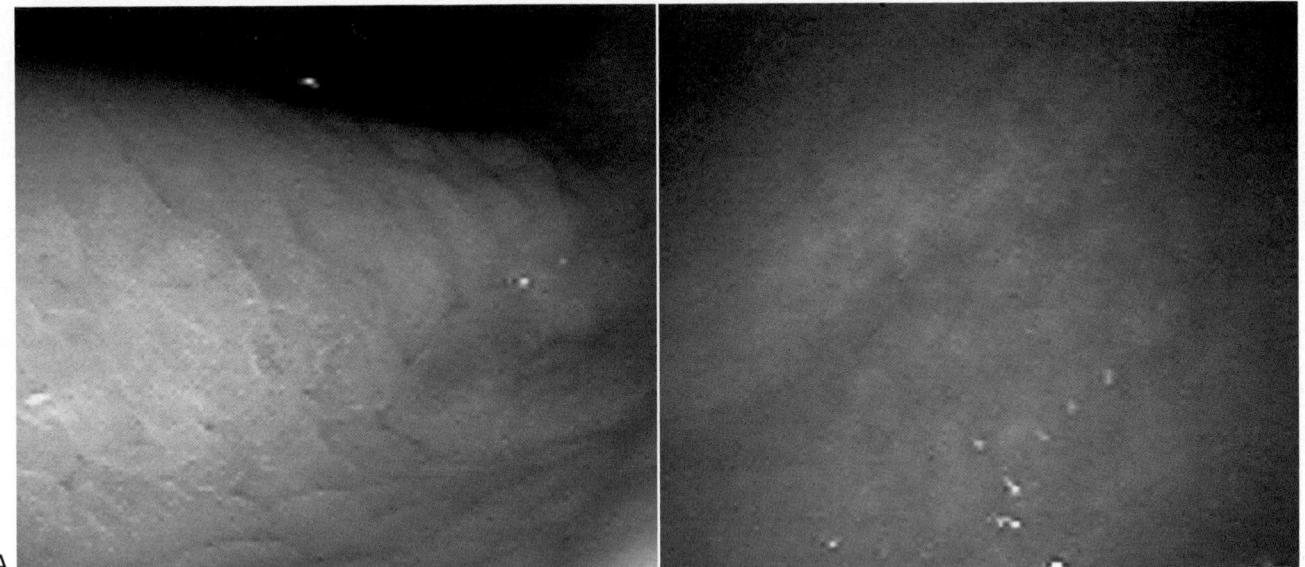

Fig 39-3 **A,** Swollen gastric mucosa with excessive folds and secretions from a dog with *Helicobacter* gastritis. **B,** Congested region of mucosa is evident. (Courtesy University of Georgia, Athens, Ga.)

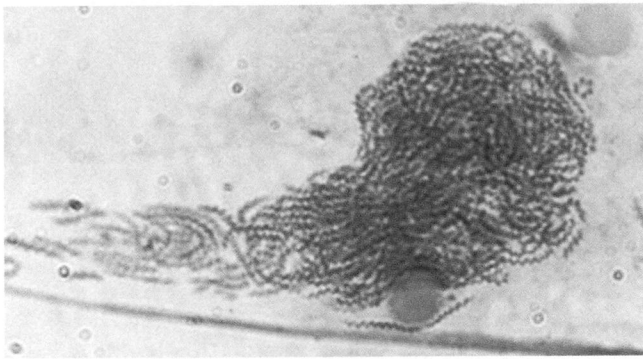

Fig 39-4 *Helicobacter* organisms visible on Giemsa stain of smear made from gastric biopsy forceps (×1000). (Courtesy University of Georgia, Athens, Ga.)

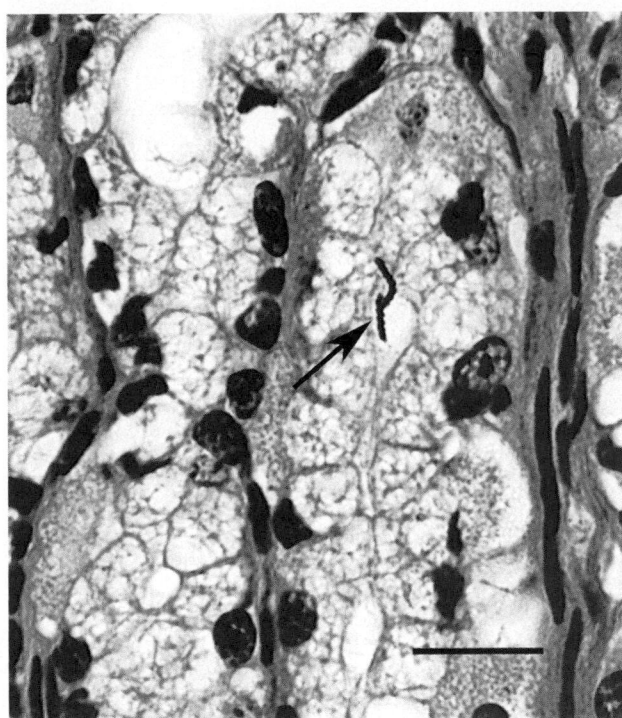

Fig 39-5 *H. pylori* in crypt of cat stomach (Warthin-Starry stain, ×1000). (Courtesy Elizabeth Howerth, University of Georgia, Athens, Ga.)

organisms in gastric biopsy samples from animals with GI illness. Because these organisms can be present in clinically healthy animals, the direct cause-and-effect relationship to clinical illness cannot always be ascertained.[319]

Diagnosis

As in people a diagnosis of chronic gastritis in animals cannot be made by gross visual endoscopic examination of the gastric mucosa (Fig. 39-3). Cytologic examination of impression smears made from gastric biopsies can reveal the presence of spiral bacteria (Fig. 39-4); however, their role if any in the inflammatory process cannot be determined. Histologic evaluation of gastric biopsy samples using a special silver stain or modified Giemsa stain to reveal the presence of GHLOs is required (Fig. 39-5). A definitive diagnosis requires culture and isolation of the specific species of *Helicobacter*. Unfortunately, *H. bizzozeronii* is the most common spiral organism in dogs and cats, and it has been extremely difficult to culture on artificial media.[191] *H. felis* is also difficult to isolate. In practice, histologic findings of inflammatory changes accompanied by gastric spiral organisms on the gastric mucosa or in the gastric mucous layer have been used for diagnosis. *H. felis* cannot be distinguished from *H. heilmannii* by histologic examination; EM and molec-

ular evaluation are necessary. Cytologic examination of gastric biopsy specimens in dogs has proven equal to or better for detecting infection than histologic examination or the rapid urease test.[192] For cytologic information, mucus covering the gastric mucosa is collected with a cytology brush during endoscopic examination and before lavage. It is smeared on a slide, dried, and preferably stained with May-Grünwald and Giemsa. The numbers of organisms can be evaluated. However, no information regarding inflammatory changes in the stomach can be obtained.

Helicobacter organisms are difficult to recognize histologically with hematoxylin-eosin stains. Silver (Warthin-Starry, Genta, or Steiner methods) and immunohistochemical stains are needed to identify these organisms. In infected cats, reactive inflammation varies in intensity and location within the stomach. *H. heilmannii*–like infected cats have had moderate lymphoid follicular hyperplasia and mild inflammatory infiltrates composed of lymphocytes, plasma cells, and macrophages in the mucosae.[390] *H. pylori*–infected cats have more severe inflammatory lesions in the pyloric mucosae with additional inflammatory cells such as neutrophils and eosinophils. In addition, diffuse fibrosis and atrophy of the pyloric mucosae were observed.[390]

Because oral bacteria and bacteria refluxed from the duodenum (e.g., Enterobacteriaceae, diphtheroids, streptococci, and anaerobes) may overgrow the fastidious *Helicobacter* species, selective media are available for isolation. Media consist of *Brucella* agar with 10% horse blood containing vancomycin (10 mg/L), polymyxin B (2500 U/L), and trimethoprim (5 mg/L). Fresh media are recommended for optimal growth. Various *Helicobacter* spp. have different antibiotic susceptibilities, and selection of the type and quantity of antibiotics in culture media may determine success of isolation. Helicobacters, like campylobacters, require special environmental and cultural conditions for their growth. The organisms are thermophilic and grow at 37° C, with some species growing at 42° C. Growth on chocolate or blood agar takes 3 to 5 days. For *H. bizzozeronii* isolation, incubation requires 5 to 10 days.[191] Helicobacters do not grow under aerobic or anaerobic conditions but achieve optimum growth in high humidity with microaerobic conditions.

A comparison of the advantages and disadvantages of diagnostic modalities for gastric helicobacteriosis is summarized in Table 39-4. Isolation of helicobacters is enhanced by proper processing of gastric tissue. Mincing the gastric tissue with sterile scalpel blades or using a tissue homogenizer enhances isolation. If immediate processing of the biopsy sample is not possible, the tissue can be placed in sterile 30% glycerol in

Table • 39-4

Comparison of Techniques to Diagnose Gastric Helicobacter Infection

TECHNIQUE	ADVANTAGES	DISADVANTAGES
Invasive		
Endoscopy	Provides biopsies for histopathologic confirmation	Requires anesthesia
	Allows detection of ulcers and neoplasia	Is invasive and expensive
	Permits culture and susceptibility testing	Has prolonged culture (~2 wk) with low sensitivity
	Allows for biopsies and rapid urease-based tests	Yields false positives with bacterial overgrowth
		Yields false negatives with antacids
Rapid urease test	Analyzes biopsy specimen quickly (<3 hr)	May indicate false-positive strains with other urease-producing organisms
		Occasionally indicates false-negative strains
Touch cytology	Allows identification of organism's morphology and numbers	Provides no information regarding inflammation in gastric mucosae
Histopathology	Allows observation of gastric pathologic changes	Inflammation not always correlated with clinical signs
Culture	Provides specific identification about infecting strain	Is difficult and prolonged and may be impossible for many helicobacters
Polymerase chain reaction (PCR)	Allows rapid detection and classification of organism	Positive indicates live or dead organisms, not clinical disease
Electron microscopy	Allows for morphologic differentiation of species	Is an expensive research tool
Noninvasive		
Serologic testing	Is minimally invasive with low exposure	Does not allow visualization of lesions or identification of organisms
	Allows retrospective evaluation	Is not reliable in animals
	Is useful for monitoring	
Urea breath test	Is minimally invasive and provides rapid results	Does not allow visualization of lesions or identification of organisms
		Gives false negatives during therapy
Urea blood test	Is minimally invasive and allows evaluation of therapy	Does not allow visualization of lesions or identification of organisms
		Requires fecal specimen
Stool antigen testing	Is noninvasive and convenient	Requires fecal specimen
Salivary IgA testing	Is noninvasive and convenient	Has low accuracy and specificity
PCR of tissue or secretions	Allows rapid detection and classification	Is a research tool that is expensive and has limited availability
		Does not distinguish between live and dead organisms
		Close similarity of currently used genes

Brucella broth at 4° C for at least 5 hours. Specimens in this media can also be frozen at −80° C for longer periods for subsequent culture of the biopsy sample or transport of previously characterized organisms.

A provisional diagnosis of gastric helicobacters takes advantage of a biochemical feature of these organisms: the ability to produce large quantities of urease. Gastric biopsy samples can be placed in a urea broth containing a pH indicator (phenol red) and a preservative (sodium azide). Rapid urease test kits are available commercially (CLOtest, Kimberly-Clark Healthcare, Roswell, Ga.) and can be used very effectively and economically in dogs.[500] A positive result correlates with the presence of gastric spiral organisms but does not definitively determine their pathogenic potential. Another urease test for people (that has been perfected only in research animals), is the urea breath test, which measures expired radiolabeled carbon dioxide, a by-product of a carbon-labeled urea test meal that is ingested by the patient.[476]

Serologic assays are being used to diagnose *H. pylori* infection in people and *H. mustelae* infection in ferrets, and *Heliobacter* spp. infection in dogs,[134,421,434] and cats.[433] However, they do not provide a routine, reliable, noninvasive diagnostic test for gastric *Helicobacter* infection in dogs and cats. ELISA analyses of serum and mucosal secretions from cats naturally infected with *H. pylori* revealed an *H. pylori*–specific IgG response and elevated anti-*H. pylori* IgA levels in salivary and local gastric secretions.[149] This assay probably cannot be used clinically in cats because of the high prevalence of the large spiral GHLOs in pet cats and the cross-reactive antigens shared by these bacteria and *H. pylori*.

In a survey of 101 dogs a combination of ELISA and immunoblotting using ureA, ureB, and heat shock protein antigens appeared to be a highly specific and moderately sensitive indicator of GHLO infection.[434] However, the degree of seropositivity assessed by ELISA was not related to degree of gastric helicobacter-colonization density, degree of mucosal inflammation, or presence of lymphoid follicles.

In a study of 17 of 45 cats naturally infected with *H. heilmannii* (9 of 17), *H. felis* (4 of 17), both infections (3 of 17), and unclassified *Helicobacter* species (7 of 17), antibody titers to high molecular cell-associated protein fraction of *H. felis* were higher for infected cats regardless of the infecting species.[433] Neither age nor clinical signs affected the results of the assay. A weak correlation was observed between the level of the titer and degree of inflammatory and lymphoid changes in the stomach.

Stool antigen tests have been used as a noninvasive method to detect and monitor *H. pylori* infection in people; however, as with antibody measurements, cross-reactivity in animal infections is anticipated. Similarly PCR, using 16S ribosomal RNA (16S rRNA) primers, has been used to detect and specifically identify corresponding helicobacter in gastric biopsies and the feces of dogs.[401]

Therapy

Therapy for gastric *Helicobacter* spp. infections has become somewhat controversial as newer information has been discovered. These organisms may cause subclinical infections in the majority of people and animals. Very few controlled studies in dogs and cats document the benefits of therapy. For people, treatment to eradicate *H. pylori* is beneficial for those with peptic ulcers or gastric lymphoma or requiring long-term treatment with nonsteroidal antiinflammatory drugs.[343] Unfortunately for people, limited studies indicate that treatment may increase the risk of esophageal cancer or worsen gastroesophageal reflux. However, this data requires confirmation in large controlled clinical trials. Antimicrobial resistance is another concern because it rapidly develops against drugs such as clarithromycin.[355]

Table • 39-5

Therapeutic Options for Gastric Helicobacteriosis

DRUG TYPES	THERAPEUTIC CHOICES
Antisecretory agents	1. Bismuth 2. H_2 antagonist 3. Proton pump inhibitor
Antimicrobials	1. Metronidazole and amoxicillin 2. Metronidazole and tetracycline 3. Metronidazole and clarithromycin 4. Amoxicillin and clarithromycin 5. Clarithromycin 6. Amoxicillin or clarithromycin and metronidazole and tetracycline

Various clinical trials using different antisecretory and antimicrobial drug combinations have been used in people to treat *H. pylori* infections (Table 39-5). Most regimens combine two to three antibacterial agents (including bismuth-containing drugs) with antisecretory drugs such as proton pump inhibitors (PPIs). Increased pH inhibits helicobacters and improves the efficacy of the antimicrobial agents. A triple-therapy regimen consisting of amoxicillin and an imidazole (either [1] metronidazole or tinidazole or [2] a tetracycline and metronidazole) and a macroclide (clarithromycin) in combination with bismuth subsalicylate given for 2 to 3 weeks has proved to be the most efficient in eradication of *H. pylori*. Indeed, this antimicrobial regimen, plus antisecretories such as ranitidine, has proved successful in treating patients with *Helicobacter*-induced gastric and duodenal ulcers. In studies comparing this treatment with ranitidine alone, ulcers not only healed faster, but the recurrence was also significantly less than in those receiving only antibiotics. Therapy regimens using PPIs (e.g., omeprazole) in combination with antibiotics (e.g., amoxicillin) also have shown considerable efficacy in eradicating *H. pylori*. Antisecretories likely improve the effect of antimicrobials by increasing gastric pH, which inhibits helicobacters and improves antibiotic activity. Whether antimicrobial therapy should be instituted in domestic dogs and cats with gastritis or ulcer disease has not been consistently evaluated. Many protocols have been adapted from treatment of *H. pylori* in people. Suggested combination drug regimens based on those that are effective for *H. pylori*–infected people[476] with dosages for dogs and cats are listed in Table 39-6. Studies in ferrets indicate that the triple therapy consisting of amoxicillin, metronidazole, and bismuth subsalicylate three times a day for 3 to 4 weeks has successfully eradicated *H. mustelae* from ferrets.[336] Omeprazole given to ferrets once daily effectively induces hypochlorhydria and can be given in conjunction with antibiotics to treat *H. mustelae*–associated duodenal or gastric ulcers. Clarithromycin and ranitidine bismuth citrate combinations have also been effective in treating these infections when the appropriate dosages were used.[285] Cases of acute bleeding ulcers must be treated as emergencies, and fluid and blood transfusions are essential.

Because GHLO infections are so common in clinically healthy dogs and cats, the decision to treat should be based on evidence of gastric lesions with compatible clinical illness. The duration of treatment of dogs and cats with helicobacteriosis has not been extensively substantiated. Cats naturally infected with *H. pylori* have received a 21-day course of oral amoxicillin, metronidazole, and omeprazole.[350] All six treated cats were culture negative at several sites (saliva, gastric juice, and gastric mucosa) for *H. pylori*. However, as determined by

Table • 39-6

Therapy for Gastric Helicobacteriosis in Dogs and Cats

DRUG[a]	SPECIES	DOSE[b]	ROUTE	INTERVAL (HOURS)	DURATION (DAYS)[c]
Coating Agents					
Bismuth subsalicylate[d]	D	0.5–2 ml/kg	PO	4–6	14–28
	C	0.5–1 ml/kg	PO	4–6	14–28
Bismuth subcitrate	B	6 mg/kg	PO	12	14–29
Antibacterials					
Metronidazole[e]	C	62.5 mg total	PO	24	14–28
	B	15 mg/kg	PO	12	14–28
Amoxicillin	B	20 mg/kg	PO	12	14–28
Tetracycline	B	22 mg/kg	PO	8	14–28
Clarithromycin[f]	B	7.5–10 mg/kg	PO	12	14–28
Antisecretories					
H₂ Antagonists					
Cimetidine[g]	B	5–10 mg/kg	PO, IV	8	14–28
	B	5–6 mg/kg	IM, IV	8[h]	14–28
Famotidine	B	0.5	PO	12	14–28
Ranitidine	D	1–2 mg/kg	PO, IV	12	14–28
	C	2.5 mg/kg	IV	12	14–28
		3.5 mg/kg	PO	8–12	14–28
Ranitidine bismuth citrate[f]	C	24 mg/kg	PO	8	14–28
Proton Pump Inhibitors					
Omeprazole	B	0.5–1 mg/kg[i]	PO	24	14–28
	D (>20 kg)	20 mg total	PO	24	14–28
Prostaglandin Analogue					
Misoprostol	D	1–5 µg/kg	PO	8	14–28
Gastric Protectant for Ulcers					
Sucralfate[j]	B	0.5–1 g	PO	4	7

B, Dog and cat; *C*, cat; *D*, dog; *PO*, by mouth; *IV*, intravenous; *IM*, intramuscular.
[a]See Appendix 8 for additional information.
[b]Dose administration at specified interval.
[c]Treatment duration in people has taken up to 8 weeks for suecessful resolution.
[d]Bismuth subsalicylate, original formula (Procter Cincinnatic OH). Dose is 17.5 mg/kg when using other products. Salicylate compounds must be used judiciously in cats, and other substitutes such as bismuth subcitrate should be considered.
[e]Metronidazole resistance has been noted with increasing frequency in people with *H. pylori* infections.[144a] A combination regimen of metronidazole (30 mg/kg/day), spiramycin (15,000 IU/5 kg/day), and omeprazole (1 mg/kg) for 7 days has been used in dogs.[264]
[f]Ranitidine bismuth citrate (*Tritec*, Glaxo, SmithKline, Research Triangle Park NC) and clarithromycin have been used as a combined bimodal therapy with high efficacy in experimentally infected ferrets.[285]
[g]Cimetidine inhibits absorption of ketoconazole; metoclopramide inhibits cimetidine absorption. Other than ranitidine, similar drugs include nizatidine and roxatidine.
[h]Not as a bolus but by slow infusion.
[i]Available as 20-mg capsule; maximum dose for dog is 20 mg. Granules must be fractionated and placed in gelatin capsules for lower doses. Alternative drugs include lansoprazole, pantoprazole, esomeprazomole, and rabeprazole.
[j]Must avoid using within 2 hr of administering many of the oral drugs because it interferes with their absorption.

PCR, 2 and 4 weeks after treatment the majority of cats at had gastric biopsy samples positive for *H. pylori*. Six weeks after treatment, all six cats had *H. pylori*–negative cultures for samples from several gastric sites taken at necropsy, and only one cat had *H. pylori* cultured from gastric juice. PCR analysis revealed that five of six cats still had *Helicobacter* DNA present in plaque, saliva, and gastric biopsy samples using *Helicobacter*-specific 26 kDa primers. However, it is known that these primers amplify DNA of other *Helicobacter* species. It is likely though not proven that the PCR helicobacter primers were amplifying DNA from enteric helicobacters present in the cats. In pet dogs with histologic GHLO gastritis, treatment in combination for 10 days with amoxicillin, tetracycline, metronidazole, and omeprazole, most dogs tested helicobacter-negative and had resolving gastrointestinal signs.[193] However, no change in the histologic lesions was found, and all dogs checked months later had a reoccurrence of infection. GI signs did not return. Reoccurrence is most likely in dogs that have intimate contact with other dogs.[500]

Treatment with amoxicillin, metronidazole, and famotidine resulted in clinical improvement in over 90% of 63 dogs and cats colonized with GHLOs and when reexamined by endoscopy, they were reportedly negative.[78] Unfortunately the diagnostic test used to assess the presence of GHLOs was not stated, nor was the time interval of the endoscopy after treatment specified. Another study, using amoxicillin, metronidazole, and famotidine for 2 weeks, indicated that at 28 days after treatment the urea breath test was still positive in most dogs.[69] Similar poor results have been documented in cats with azithromycin, tindazole, bismuth, and raniditine or with clarithromycin, metronidazole, bismuth, and raniditine for 4 to 7 days.[318] The less-than-favorable results of all these studies makes uniform recommendations of treating infected cats and dogs unlikely.

In people with severe GHLO infection (i.e., *H. heilmannii* or *H. felis*), bismuth subsalicylate, amoxicillin, tetracycline, and metronidazole in various combinations successfully eradicated GHLOs from the gastric mucosa with resolution of gastritis.[196,451] Antimicrobial therapy has also been used successfully to treat GHLO-inducedd MALT lymphoma in humans.[33a] In two separate reports, prolonged treatment with bismuth subsalicylate (4 weeks) or bismuth subcitrate (8 weeks) also successfully eradicated the GHLOs from patients.[196,310] No systematic antibiotic trials have been conducted in dogs and cats to test for efficacy in eradicating either *H. heilmannii* or *H. felis* from gastric mucosa.

Public Health Considerations

Because *H. heilmannii* (which is currently classified as *H. bizzozeronii* in dogs) and to a lesser extent *H. felis* colonize a small percentage of people with gastritis and no environmental source for these bacteria has been recognized, pets have been implicated in zoonotic transmission. In one report of *H. heilmannii* infection in a child, the child's household had two cats. A gastric biopsy from one cat indicated it was infected with gastric spiral organisms that had morphologic characteristics similar to those detected in the child's stomach.[266] In another report, a girl who moved to a rural environment developed an 18-month history of epigastric pain, nausea, vomiting, and anorexia. Antral active chronic gastritis associated with *H. heilmannii* was confirmed.[451] Institution of various anti-*Helicobacter* antimicrobial treatments was only temporarily successful. The girl had two dogs—one that frequently licked the girl's face and had chronic intermittent vomiting and another that was asymptomatic. The symptomatic dog had active chronic gastritis associated with large numbers of *H. heilmannii*, whereas the asymptomatic dog had mild gastritis associated with fewer *H. heilmannii*. The girl and the dogs were simultaneously placed on a 6-week course of amoxicillin and bismuth. The symptoms in the dog resolved, but the girl required additional therapy with omeprazole. Although DNA analysis of the *H. heilmannii* strains was not performed to confirm the organim's identity, the zoonotic association is highly suggestive. Multiple *H. heilmannii* strains were found in a person with gastric ulcers, and one genetic strain was identical to one derived from his cat.[81] Another child who acquired an *H. heilmannii* infection had a strain that matched the isolate from a cat.[469]

In Germany a survey of 125 individuals infected with GHLOs provided information in a questionnaire regarding animal contact. Of these patients, 70.3% had been in contact with one or more animals, compared with 37% of the clinically healthy control population.[429] More than three times as many male patients had GHLOs than female patients. Because *H. bizzozeronii* and *H. felis* can be cultured on artificial media, a comparison is needed among the various species infecting animals and their genetic markers. A researcher performing physiologic studies with cat stomachs developed an acute gastritis presumably resulting from *H. felis* on the basis of EM.[260] Similar gastric spiral bacteria were demonstrated in gastric mucosa of cats being used by this scientist.

If *H. pylori*, as demonstrated in commercially reared cats,[149,188] is isolated from pet cats, the zoonotic potential of helicobacteriosis from cats would obviously increase substantially. *H. pylori* infection is an important cause of human gastritis, peptic ulcer disease, MALT lymphoma, and gastric adenocarcinoma. Most epidemiologic studies do not incriminate pet contact with *H. pylori* human infection. Cats can be experimentally infected with certain strains of *H. pylori*, and they develop persistent gastritis.[349] However, cats tested generally have rare evidence of infection.[92]

In serologic studies of people with *H. pylori* infection, owning pets was inversely related to *H. pylori* IgG antibody titers; however, pet ownership in these studies was associated with a higher socioeconomic status.[111,172] Furthermore, pet ownership was not segregated by whether the pets were dogs or cats, the number and age of pets, or the length of pet ownership. In another study, even though the number of patients with pets was small, exposure to cats or dogs in the preceding year was not statistically associated with *H. pylori* infection.[470] An epidemiologic survey conducted in Germany did not show an increased risk of *H. pylori* because of cat ownership.[19] In a serologic survey measuring antibodies to *H. pylori*, lower socioeconomic status—not pet ownership or day care attendance—was associated with seropositivity.[421] In a survey of male employees in England, pet ownership as a child was marginally associated with current *H. pylori* infection; however, overcrowding plus person-to-person contact was found to be the major risk factor.[479] In veterinarians, no serologic evidence for increased risk of exposure was found.[317] Only one study suggested an epidemiologic risk. IgG anti–*H. pylori*-seropositive farm workers were more likely to report more contact with cats than dogs.[449]

INTESTINAL AND HEPATIC *HELICOBACTER* INFECTIONS

James G. Fox

Etiology

In addition to their association with the gastric mucosae, an increasing number of other *Helicobacter* species have been isolated from the lower intestinal tract of mammals and birds (Table 39-7). Some of these (e.g., *H. cinaedi*, *H. fennelliae*, and *H. rappini*) have been linked to proctitis, colitis, and septicemia in immunocompromised people.[239,455] In addition, *H. hepaticus* and *H. bilis* have been isolated from livers of mice with hepatitis and hepatocellular carcinoma as well as from intestines of asymptomatic mice sampled from United States and international sources.[137,153] *H. bilis* also has been isolated from a gastric sample of a dog and *H. canis* from the liver of a dog with hepatitis.[92,138]

One of these gram-negative spiral organisms with sheathed bipolar flagella was given the name *H. canis* group because it has a weak DNA homology to *H. cinaedi* and *H. fennelliae* but is phenotypically distinguishable from these organisms by its morphologic characteristics (Fig. 39-6); it is also resistant to polymyxin B and unable to reduce nitrate. Like *H. hepaticus*, *H. bilis*, and *Helicobacter pullorum*, the marked resistance of *H. canis* to bile probably enables the organism to colonize the liver.[137,153,425,426]

Also of interest is the isolation (on the basis of cellular fatty acid analysis) of *H. cinaedi* from the feces of dogs and a cat.[239] *H. cinaedi* was isolated from a rhesus monkey with colitis and hepatitis as well from rhesus monkeys without diarrhea.[110,140] *H. fennelliae* has also been identified in the feces of a dog and macaque monkey. Like *H. cinaedi*, *H. fennelliae* (previously

*References 127, 137, 153, 397, 426, 425.

Table • 39-7

Comparative Features of Intestinal and Hepatic Helicobacter Species That Infect Dogs and Cats

HELICOBACTER ORGANISM	MORPHOLOGIC AND DISTINGUISHING FEATURES	HOSTS	CLINICAL FEATURES
H. cinaedi and H. fennelliae	Single bipolar, sheathed flagella; catalase positive	Dogs and cats Nonhuman primates and people Hamsters	Fecal isolate Experimental and natural infection (H. cinaedi) Often asymptomatic, colitis and proctitis if immunosuppressed, diarrhea and septicemia in immunocompetent hosts
H. canis	Sheathed, bipolar flagella; resists bile; resists polymyxin B; cannot reduce nitrate	Dogs, cats People	Liver with multifocal hepatitis Diarrhea or asymptomatic
H. marmotae	Single bipolar flagella; catalase positive	Cats, woodchucks	Asymptomatic in cats, hepatitis in woodchucks
H. rappini	Fusiform—slightly spiral periplasmic fibers	Cats, dogs, people	Asymptomatic, hemorrhagic enteritis

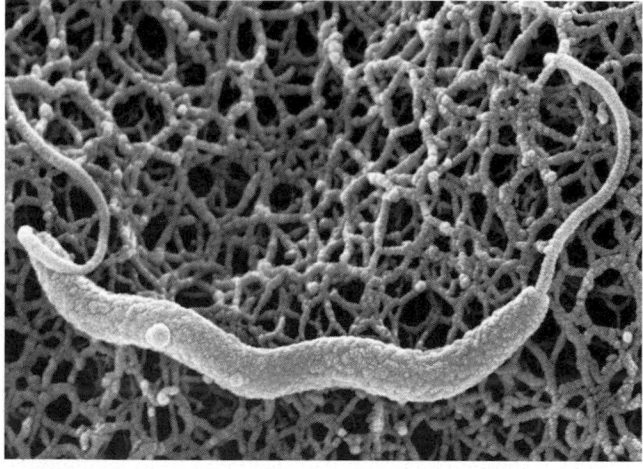

Fig 39-6 Scanning electron microphotograph of *H. canis*. (Courtesy M.H. Stoffel, University of Bern, Bern, Switzerland.)

known as *Campylobacter fennelliae*, or CLO-2) was first isolated from gay individuals who were infected with human immunodeficiency virus (HIV) and had colitis and proctitis.[455] However, unlike *H. cinaedi*, this enteric *Helicobacter* species does not often cause bacteremia in adult humans.[237,321]

Epidemiology

On the basis of biochemical, phenotypic, and 16S rRNA analyses, *H. canis* was isolated from Bengal cats with and without chronic diarrhea.[117] Because the cats were coinfected with other potential pathogens, including *C. helveticus*, and because *H. canis* was isolated from nondiarrheic cats, the causal role of *H. canis* in producing the diarrhea could not be proved. Isolation of *H. canis* in cats raises the possibility that *H. canis*, like *H. hepaticus* and *H. bilis* in mice, can cause inflammation of the colon, particularly in hosts with immune dysregulation. Additional studies are needed to determine the importance of *H. canis* as a primary enteric pathogen in cats and the role of cats in the possible zoonotic spread of *H. canis* to people.

In epidemiologic studies regarding incidence of CLOs in 1000 dogs, 4% of the animals had an organism, which was later identified as *H. canis*, isolated from their feces.[49,425] The organism was also isolated from the feces of a child with gastroenteritis during a similar survey of children to determine prevalence of CLOs.[51]

On the basis of 16S rRNA data, *H. canis* has also been identified from the liver of a puppy diagnosed as having an active, multifocal hepatitis.[138] Determining whether this organism is capable of experimentally inducing hepatitis in dogs or occurs as a natural liver infection in people requires additional study. The pathogenic potential is strengthened by isolation of *H. canis* from a bacteremic person[331] and by studies that demonstrate that *H. hepaticus*, an intestinal *Helicobacter* of mice, can experimentally induce hepatitis in both inbred and germ-free mice.[143,154,477] *H. hepaticus* can also cause liver tumors in susceptible strains of mice.

The entire genome of *H. hepaticus* has been sequenced recently.[437] It is anticipated that by analyzing this sequence data, a great deal will be learned about how this organism (as well as other enterohepatic helicobacters) exerts its pathogenic potential on its hosts.

In the 6-year study of 64 of 227 commercially reared cats, microaerobic bacteria were isolated from their feces. All the isolates were initially identified as CLOs based on biochemical and phenotypic characteristics. DNA extractions from 51 of these isolates were subjected to PCR using primers specific for *Helicobacter* species and *Campylobacter* species. Of the isolates, 92% (47 of 51 isolates) were positive for *Campylobacter* spp., 41% (21 of 51 isolates) were positive for *Helicobacter* spp., 33% (17 of 51 isolates) were positive for both genera, 59% (30 of 51 isolates) were positive only for *Campylobacter* spp., and 8% (4 of 51) were positive only for *Helicobacter* spp.

The 1.2-kb PCR products of the 16S rRNA genes of 19 *Helicobacter* species isolates were subjected to restriction fragment length polymorphism (RFLP) analysis. Of the five different RFLP patterns obtained, two clustered with *Helicobacter (Flexispira)* taxon 8, one clustered with *H. bilis*, one clustered with *H. canis*, and the remaining pattern was closely related to a novel *Helicobacter* strain isolated from a woodchuck. The sequence data for the 16S rRNA genes of 10

Helicobacter species validated the RFLP-based identification of these isolates.

Woodchucks *(Marmota monax)* have a high incidence of hepatocellular carcinoma (HCC) associated with chronic infection with woodchuck hepatitis virus and serve as a model of hepatitis B virus–associated HCC in people. To determine whether woodchucks harbor a *Helicobacter* species that might play a role in potentiating hepatic inflammation or neoplasia, a study was undertaken to determine whether the woodchucks' livers were infected with a *Helicobacter* species.[151] A 1200-base pair *Helicobacter* species-specific sequence was amplified from 14 liver samples. Southern hybridization confirmed the specific identity of the PCR products. A urease-, catalase-, and oxidase-positive bacterium was isolated from one liver sample from a woodchuck with a positive liver tumor. By 16S rRNA analysis and biochemical and phenotypic characteristics, the organism was classified as a new *Helicobacter* species. Subsequently, four additional bacterial strains isolated from feces of cats and characterized by biochemical, phenotypic, and 16S rRNA analysis were determined to be identical to the woodchuck isolate. The new helicobacter was named *Helicobacter marmotae*.[151]

Given that cats are often diagnosed with chronic cholangiohepatitis of unknown etiology, it will be interesting to ascertain whether this new *Helicobacter* species causes liver disease in cats and other mammals.[161,39a]

Pathogenesis

The normal ecologic niche of certain helicobacter species is the lower intestine; the mechanism by which they colonize the liver is unknown. Like another intestinal enteropathogen, *Salmonella typhi*, the organisms may gain access to the liver by initial enterocyte or M cell uptake in the intestine and spread to the liver via the portal circulation. The bacteria may then be discharged from the liver into the biliary tract.[208] Alternatively, helicobacters may migrate retrograde from the lumen of the gut into the bile duct. Whether the presence of intestinal parasites facilitates the ability of *H. canis* (and other helicobacters) to colonize the liver and cause hepatitis is unknown. Organisms with *H. bilis* morphologic characteristics have been noted previously in bile canaliculi of rats experimentally infected with *Fasciola hepatica*.[121] In addition, *Flexispira (H.) rappini* has been associated with abortion in sheep, necrotic hepatitis in the aborted fetuses, and intestinal disease in animals and people. Experimentally, *H. rappini* causes similar abortions and necrotic hepatitis in guinea pigs.[21,242,374] It is conceivable but certainly has not been proven that puppies can be infected in utero; however, its importance as a pathogen in pet animals has not been determined.

Pigtail macaques *(Macaca nemistrina)* were experimentally challenged orally with *H. cinaedi* and *H. fennelliae*.[115] Although infection occurred in these monkeys and caused abnormal feces and focal large-bowel lesions, only one of five monkeys infected with *H. fennelliae* had acute proctitis, and *H. cinaedi* induced only lymphoid hyperplasia.[115]

Clinical Findings

It is not known whether intestinal *Helicobacter* can cause primary diarrheal disease in immunocompetent companion pet animals or only those that are immunocompromised. *H. hepaticus* and *H. bilis* are increasingly linked to severe IBD and colon cancer in immunocompromised mice,[101,135] and select germ-free mice inoculated with the organism develop segmental enteritis.[137,143,154] A 4-month-old British Blue cat developed hemorrhagic enteritis and died. The animal was heavily colonized with spiral to fusiform bacteria in the stomach, small intestine, and cecum. A robust inflammatory response in lamina propria of stomach and intestine was noted. Immunohistochemistry using antihelicobacter antibody indicated that these spiral organisms were strongly positive. EM showed that these organisms had a morphology similar to *H. rappini*.[241] If helicobacters are determined to be a common cause of hepatitis and enteritis in dogs and cats, appropriate liver function tests as well as microaerobic culture of liver and intestinal biopsies should provide insight.

Diagnosis

Many hospital laboratories have difficulty isolating helicobacters. For example, because of the slow growth of *H. cinaedi*, laboratory diagnosis is unlikely if blood culture procedures that rely on visual detection of the culture media are used.[239,240] In a retrospective study of people with *H. cinaedi*–associated illness, most of the patients had the organism isolated from blood using automated blood culture system.[240] Dark-field microscopy or use of acridine orange staining of blood culture media rather than Gram stain increases the likelihood of seeing the organism. Likewise, fecal isolation is difficult; selective antibiotic media are required, and recovery is facilitated by passing fecal homogenates through a 0.45-μ filter.[164,398] In addition, some strains of *H. cinaedi* and *H. fennelliae* are inhibited by concentrations of cephalothin and cefazolin used frequently in selective media for isolation of enteric microaerophilic bacteria.[239] These organisms also require an environment rich in hydrogen for optimum in vitro growth. *H. canis* can be distinguished from *H. fennelliae* by its ability to grow at 42° C, its failure to produce catalase, and its marked tolerance to bile.

For the best recovery of *Helicobacter*-like organisms (HLOs), fecal samples should be placed in glycerol medium for transportation. Higher hydrogen levels (5% to 10%) are required for optimal *Helicobacter* species isolation. Unfortunately, this atmosphere is not available in the commercially available diagnostic kits used for *Campylobacter* isolation.

Microaerobic conditions were maintained in vented GasPak jars (Becton Dickinson, Franklin Lakes, N.J.) without a catalyst by evacuation to –20 mm Hg and then repressurization with a gas mixture consisting of 80% nitrogen, 10% hydrogen, and 10% carbon dioxide to yield a final oxygen concentration of 5%.[145]

Identification of multiple species of microaerobic bacteria in the feces of an animal poses a diagnostic challenge, particularly when these microaerobes grow on similar media in comparable atmospheric conditions. Primary isolation of these microaerophilic bacteria may be misleading because *Helicobacter* species may be present in smaller numbers and grow at a slower rate than *Campylobacter* species. The similar phenotypic traits and biochemical profiles of these genera also complicate the diagnosis. Using *Campylobacter* and *Helicobacter* genus-specific PCR assays allow distinction between the two genera. The PCR-RFLP assay was also useful for *Helicobacter* species identification.

Pathologic Findings

Although the normal ecologic niche of *H. canis*, *H. hepaticus*, and *H. marmotae* is the crypts of the intestine, these organisms can also colonize the liver. The best characterized liver lesion caused by a *Helicobacter* is *H. hepaticus*–associated hepatitis in A/JCr mice. In infected mice the organism causes a multifocal hepatic lesion with cholangitis and vasculitis, which progresses in severity to include bile duct hyperplasia, hepatomegaly, oval cell hyperplasia, hepatocellular proliferation and—in aged male A/JCr, B6C3F1, AXB mice—hepatoma or hepatocellular carcinoma.[137,143,477] The *H. canis*–associated liver lesion noted in a young dog consisted of an acute multifocal necrotizing hepatitis.[138] Interestingly, HLOs were present at the periphery of the hepatic lesion and appeared to be located in bile canaliculi. This pattern of colonization is also noted in *H. hepaticus*– and *H. bilis*–infected livers.[137,143,153,472]

Isolation of "*H. rappini*" from the blood of experimentally infected guinea pigs 1.5 weeks after inoculation indicates the ability of these organisms to cause bacteremia.[46] For example, *H. rappini*–like organisms were recently isolated from a 9-year-old child with bacteremia and pneumonia.[445] In addition the observation of translocation of *H. rappini*–like organisms in enterocytes of cotton-top tamarins *(Saquinus oedipus)* with ulcerative colitis or mice coinfected with *Serpulena hyodysentereae* supports this viewpoint.[59,210]

Several recent studies have been undertaken to determine whether *Helicobacter* species are associated with cholecystitis and other hepatobiliary diseases in people. In these studies the presence of *Helicobacter* species detected specific DNA by PCR and sequencing.[23,136,150,324-326] The difficulty in obtaining gallbladder and liver tissues from selected populations highlights the need for noninvasive serologic assays to determine the prevalence of hepatic *Helicobacter* organisms in various biliary and hepatic diseases of people and animals.

To date, none of these studies have reported that they have been able to culture *Helicobacter* from bile or liver. Additional studies using specific and sensitive detection methods are needed to ascertain the association of *Helicobacter* infection with hepatobiliary diseases in different human populations as well as dogs and cats.

Enterohepatic helicobacters cause IBD and lower bowel cancer in immunodysregulated mice. In addition, multiple new *Helicobacter* species have been isolated from rhesus monkeys and cotton-top tamarins with chronic debilitating colitis.[100,141,389] It will be interesting to ascertain whether chronic colitis and lower bowel cancer in dogs and cats is related to *Helicobacter* infection.[117]

Therapy

Antimicrobial susceptibility testing of *H. cinaedi* indicates that tetracycline, chloramphenicol, and various aminoglycosides should be effective in treating infections with *H. cinaedi*.[240] (See Table 39-2 for appropriate dosage information.) Apparent relapses of *H. cinaedi* bacteremia have occurred in people treated with ciprofloxacin despite its previous use to successfully treat *H. cinaedi* infection. The development of in vitro resistance of *H. cinaedi* isolates to ciprofloxacin suggests that fluoroquinolones should be used with caution.[239,240]

H. rappini–like organisms isolated from a child with bacteremia and pneumonia was successfully treated with erythromycin.[444] Recurrent *H. rappini*–associated bacteremia over a period of several months, despite several courses of antibiotics, has also been noted in two patients with prolonged cellulitis and X-linked agammaglobulinemia (XLA).

One patient was first diagnosed as having *H. rappini* at age 4. In vitro antibiotic testing using E-test strips indicated the bacteria were resistant to ampicillin, azithromycin, ceftriaxone, chloramphenicol, ciprofloxacin, and clindamycin.[487] The organism was sensitive to imipenem, metronidazole, minocycline, and rifampin and showed intermediate sensitivity to doxycycline. Based on these findings the patient was initially treated with doxycycline and metronidazole with noted clinical improvement of the cellulitis. However, blood cultures remained positive, and treatment was changed to oral amoxicillin-clavulanate, minocycline, and rifampin.[487] Initial improvement was again noted, but symptoms recurred. IV gentamicin and imipenem were then initiated and continued for 5 months. This regimen resolved the systemic infection, and follow-up blood cultures were normal.[487]

In the second case of XLA, the patient's symptoms began when he was 6 months old. He had been diagnosed as having pyoderma granulosum with nonhealing skin ulcers and swelling of the leg at age 17. One year later, he developed pyrexia and was treated with IV gentamicin, metronidazole, and vancomycin. The fever resolved and the skin ulcers healed but after treatment was terminated, the lesions recurred. Three years later, his clinical signs had not improved. Blood samples were taken, and *H. rappini*–like organisms were cultured on several occasions. Magnetic resonance imaging also indicated that the patient had osteomyelitis. Surgical bone debridement of the affected bone was performed, and *H. rappini*–like organisms were cultured from these sites. Treatment with IV imipenem and gentamicin successfully resolved the fever and macular rash; gradual improvement of the ulcers was also noted. Gentamicin was discontinued (because of hearing loss) and replaced by IV meropenum. After 9 months of IV antibiotics the ulcers regressed and therapy was discontinued. These two cases of XLA highlight the apparent susceptibility of a B-cell (humoral) immunodeficiency in people to *H. rappini*-like infections. The resultant intravascular and intralymphatic infections in people are difficult to treat with antibiotics. If these clinical signs are present in dogs and cats, clinicians should attempt to ascertain whether helicobacters are associated with the disease syndrome.

Public Health Considerations

Because *H. cinaedi* has been isolated from normal intestine flora of hamsters, it was suggested that pet hamsters could serve as a reservoir for transmission to people.[164] *H. cinaedi* was isolated from the blood and feces of a neonate with septicemia and meningitis.[333] The mother of the neonate had worked with hamsters during her first two trimesters of pregnancy and had a diarrheal illness during the third trimester. The newborn was likely infected during the birthing process, although this was not proven. Additional studies are needed to confirm the zoonotic risk of handling *H. cinaedi*–infected hamsters and possibly other animals as well.[164]

H. rappini was first reported in two people with chronic diarrhea and their pet dogs.[21] *H. rappini*–associated cellulitis ensued after a cat scratch; perhaps the patient had *H. rappini* colonization his bowel, and the organism gained access to the blood via translocation. Nevertheless, zoonotic transmission of this organism is possible.[21,374,416]

Even though *H. canis, H. cinaedi, H. fennelliae,* and *H. rappini* have been isolated from dogs, cats, and people, additional investigations are needed to ascertain whether these helicobacters in dogs and cats constitute a potential reservoir for zoonotic transmission to people. Although *H. canis* and *H. pullorum* have been isolated from children and adults with gastroenteritis and diarrhea, evidence that either organism can cause hepatitis in people is indirect. *H. canis* has been isolated from the blood of people, which increases the likelihood that liver infection with *H. canis* in people also occurs.[83,331] In addition a patient with *H. pullorum*–associated diarrhea had persistent increases in liver enzymes as well as hepatomegaly on abdominal ultrasonography.[50] With the use of appropriate diagnostic media and microaerobic culture conditions, various other *Helicobacter* species will also be isolated from people with hepatitis and companion animals.

ANAEROBIOSPIRILLUM INFECTION

Craig E. Greene

Similar to *H. rappini* and *H. cinadei*, the motile, spiral-shaped anaerobic bacteria *Anaerobiospirillum thomasii, Anaerobiospirillum succiniciproducens* and other *Anaerobiospirillum* spp. have been implicated as a cause of diarrhea with or without bacteremia in people. They are not isolated from feces of clinically healthy people but are commonly found in feces of clinically healthy dogs and cats.[284] In fact the organisms were first isolated from the pharynx and fecal contents of beagle dogs.[77] In one puppy with bloody diarrhea, spiral bacteria consisting of *C. upsaliensis, H. cinaedi, H. rappini,* and two *Anaerobiospirillum* species were isolated.[303] Organisms closely related to *A. succiniciproducens* were identified in intestinal lesions of 6 cats with ileocolitis.[77a] Vomiting, diarrhea, or signs not related to the GI tract were observed. As with *Campylobacter* infections, the risk of people developing *Anaerobiospirillum* infection from their diarrheic dogs or cats is great, and some instances have been reported.[168,282-284,445] These organisms can be distinguished from other spiral bacteria by genetic and ultrastructural methods.

SALMONELLOSIS

Craig E. Greene

Etiology

Salmonella are primarily motile, non–spore-forming, gram-negative bacilli of the family Enterobacteriaceae. Members of the genus *Salmonella* are ubiquitous pathogens that infect a wide variety of mammals, birds, reptiles, and even insects. Although they are primarily intestinal parasites, they can cause systemic disease and be isolated from other organs and blood. Salmonellae from animals have important public health implications because they are capable of causing mild to severe gastroenteritis in people.

The taxonomy of salmonellae has undergone many changes, with classification schemes being based on biochemical or serologic differences. Because the salmonellae are related, they are thought to belong to a single species: *Salmonella enterica*. The practice of substituting serotype names as species is commonly accepted. The more than 2400 serotypes of *S. enterica* are identified by agglutination reactions of their somatic (O) and flagellar (H) antigens. The species (serotypes) recognized to be of major pathogenic significance in veterinary and human microbiology include *S.* ser *choleraesuis, S.* ser *arizonae, S.* ser *enteritidis,* and *S.* ser *typhimurium. S.* ser *typhi,* which is extremely important as the cause of typhoid fever in people, is not normally pathogenic for animals; it is of little if any zoonotic importance. *S.* ser *enteritidis* has been further divided into more than 1700 bioserotypes, each with a distinguishing name such as *S. enteritidis dublin.* Although taxonomically incorrect, the species name is often omitted in favor of using the bioserotype alone (e.g., *S. dublin*).

Some species of salmonellae show a preference for certain animal hosts, and each domesticated farm animal species appears to have an adapted *Salmonella* species: horse—*Salmonella abortus equi,* cow—*S. dublin,* sheep—*Salmonella abortus ovis,* pig—*Salmonella choleraesuis,* and fowl—*Salmonella pullorum* and *Salmonella gallinarum.* Rarely, *S. choleraesuis* and *S. dublin* produce disease in people or other animals.

The remaining serotypes of *Salmonella* show little or no specific host adaptation and are equally pathogenic for people and other animals. Many have been isolated from vertebrates and invertebrates and the environment. These *Salmonella* serotypes or individual isolates of certain serotypes vary widely in their ability to infect and produce disease within a given animal host, and more virulent serotypes appear to be able to multiply intracellularly. Mucoid and encapsulated strains are more pathogenic than other strains; *S. typhi,* which produces prolonged and systemic infections in its human hosts, is noted for these features. The species most commonly isolated from diseased animals and people is *S. typhimurium.*

Epidemiology
Source of Infection

In nature, most serotypes of *S. typhimurium* are ubiquitous and readily transmitted among animals and people and the environment (Fig. 39-7). The most common source of infection, which occurs through the GI route, is contact with contaminated food, water, or fomites. Airborne transmission, which produces respiratory infection, may occur occasionally because the organism is able to survive on dried airborne particles in the absence of organic material.

Salmonellae can survive for relatively long periods outside the host. Finding *Salmonella* in the environment usually indicates direct or indirect fecal contamination. A large portion of the aquatic biosphere is now contaminated with *Salmonella* organisms, probably as a result of pollution of streams and lakes with untreated sewage, garbage, and other refuse. Fish and shellfish living in previously infected waters are microbiologic monitors, because they can harbor the organisms in their digestive tracts for extended periods after direct isolation from the water is no longer possible. Dogs and cats may acquire an infection by drinking contaminated water, although this is less of a problem in areas where pets drink from chlorinated municipal water supplies. Environmental contamination from carrier dogs was suggested in one dog that may have acquired its infection while on exercise walks.[387]

Another source of infection for dogs and cats as well as for their human owners is contamination of food. This was a major problem in the past because pets were fed uncooked or unprocessed foods. Meat and meat by-products, especially those from contaminated horse meat, were the foods most commonly incriminated. Isolation of *Salmonella* from infected animals has been most common from swine, cattle, turkeys, and horses (in that order). *S. typhimurium* was by far the most common isolate. Meat from clinically healthy animals intended for human consumption is not sterile and can contain enteropathogens. Bacterial microflora are deposited on the meat during processing. Racing greyhounds and working sled dogs are frequently fed diets containing raw meat because it is believed they need it to increase their endurance; some people want to provide uncooked meat diets for their pet animals as well.[53] Racing sled dogs are fed diets that are extremely palatable and have a high caloric content. These diets generally comprise high-fat commercial food supplemented with raw or partially cooked beef, horse, lamb, fish, or fat.[53] Carnivores in zoos being fed raw, meat-based diets are commonly exposed to and shed salmonellae in their feces.[66] Pet dogs fed pieces of whole, raw chicken meat and vegetables (a current trend involving a "natural" diet) had a 30% prevalence of salmonellae in their feces; no salmonellae were isolated from control animals fed commercially prepared food diets.[223] Salmonellae were isolated from 80% of the purchased raw chicken being fed to the animals. In other surveys, salmonellae have been found in 20% to 35% of poultry carcasses intended for human consumption.[25,54] Raw, dehydrated, or improperly cooked cat or dog food products prepared from contaminated sources have a higher prevalence of contamination than pelleted and heat-processed foods, which are less likely to be infected because they are adequately sterilized during preparation. Imported commercial dog chews made from animal hides have been found to contain *Salmonella* organisms.[495] Animal-derived dog treats sold in the United States were found to contain various *Salmonella* isolates, some of which were multidrug-resistant strains.[490] Even commercially processed foods can become contaminated if they are exposed to infected mammals, birds, reptiles, amphibians, or insects or to unsanitary conditions. Salmonellae can multiply quickly in moistened food left at room temperature. Supplementation of processed foods with uncooked food scraps or meat by-products is another common source of infection. In the United States, raw meat *(4-D meat)* used to feed racing greyhounds is highly contaminated with *Salmonella.*[63,430,494]

Contaminated fomites such as food dishes, hospital cages, endoscopic equipment, and bathtubs can spread the disease

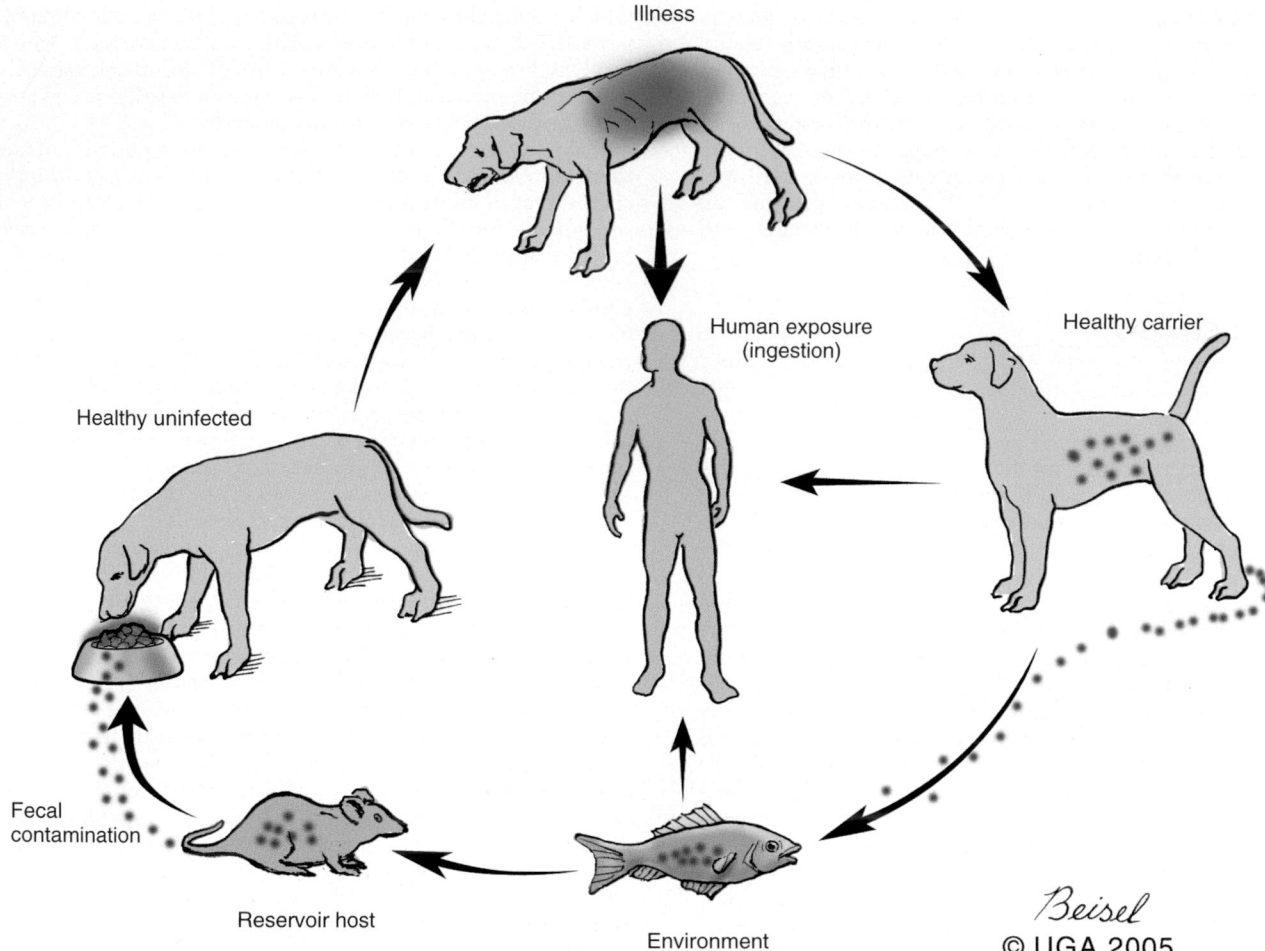

Illness

Human exposure (ingestion)

Healthy carrier

Healthy uninfected

Fecal contamination

Reservoir host

Environment

Beisel
© UGA 2005

Fig 39-7 Epidemiology of salmonellosis. (University of Georgia, Athens, Ga.)

throughout a veterinary hospital. Salmonellae can occasionally be transmitted through contaminated pharmacologic or diagnostic preparations of animal origin, such as pancreatic extracts, liver extracts, bile salts, gelatin, vitamins, and hormonal extracts. Free-roaming dogs and cats have ample opportunity for exposure to *Salmonella* because they are carnivorous and occasionally coprophagous. Such animals may be infected with and shed numerous strains simultaneously.[48,438,481,501] Cats may have greater resistance to infection than dogs, as suggested by the less frequent isolation of *Salmonella* from cats.

Infected animal handlers may also be a source of *Salmonella* infection in a hospital, kennel, or cattery. Human infections with nontyphoid salmonellae are usually self-limiting, and shedding of the organism is usually not a persistent problem. Animal infections are more important in maintaining the organism in animal-holding facilities. Human carriers chronically infected with salmonellae that cause typhoid fever pose no health hazard for animals.

Prevalence

Salmonellosis in dogs and cats is more common than the prevalence of clinical disease suggests, with numerous serotypes being isolated from each species. The frequency of fecal isolation from clinically healthy or hospitalized dogs is reported to be 1% to 36% and from healthy cats is 1% to 18%. The actual prevalence of infection is probably higher than that estimated from fecal swab culture results and routine isolation procedures, because culture of intestinal lymph node specimens taken at necropsy yields a much higher prevalence of *Salmonella* organisms. The prevalence is probably decreas-

ing because more pets are now fed commercially processed foods. *Salmonella* infection is still a problem in zoologic gardens where exotic carnivores are fed raw-meat diets.

Host Resistance

The ability to experimentally infect animals with *Salmonella* and establish clinical illness depends on many factors. Age is an important variable. Puppies and kittens younger than 1 year are more susceptible to infection and clinical illness than adult animals. Neonates may acquire infections from contaminated secretions of their dams. In utero transmission may result in death and abortion of the fetuses or birth of weak or ill puppies and kittens.

Nutritional considerations are also important in the establishment of salmonellosis. Obesity and overfeeding decreased the resistance to salmonellosis of experimentally infected dogs. Dietary deficiencies of methionine or choline in pregnant animals increase the susceptibility of their offspring to salmonellosis.[320a]

Stress caused by hospitalization, anesthesia, surgical and medical therapy, and overcrowding has been correlated with an increased risk of salmonellosis in dogs and cats. Thiamylal anesthesia enhanced the virulence of *Salmonella* endotoxin for experimentally infected animals.

The impairment of host immune defenses that occurs with malnutrition, malignancy, and glucocorticoid therapy may increase the prevalence of clinically severe salmonellosis. Immunosuppression associated with diabetes mellitus and feline leukemia virus infection may have contributed to the development of salmonellosis in two cats.[84] Intranasal modified live virus feline panleukopenia virus vaccination was suspected to cause immunosuppression and an outbreak of salmonellosis in kittens.[118] An increased postoperative prevalence of clinical salmonellosis in dogs given high-dose glucocorticoid therapy for intervertebral disc and intraocular surgery has been noted. Salmonellosis has also been reported as a complication of anticancer chemotherapy in dogs and one cat with multicentric lymphosarcomas[204] and in a dog with cyclic hematopoiesis.[307] The severity of salmonellosis is increased in people with chronic or severe hemolytic anemia, when the mononuclear-phagocyte system is overwhelmed by erythrophagocytosis.

The intestinal tract normally is protected against colonization by enteric pathogens, which explains why the clinical prevalence of gastroenteritis is lower than the frequency of *Salmonella* isolation from the pet population. Normal intestinal motility propels ingested *Salmonella* to the cecum and colon. There the resident bacterial population produces volatile fatty acids, including acetic and butyric acids, which limit further replication of the pathogens. Thus any factor that suppresses the animal's indigenous microbial population increases its susceptibility to infection by *Salmonella*. Dogs fed probiotic diets containing large numbers of *E. faecium* had a minor reduction in concentration of *Salmonella* and *Campylobacter* organisms in their stools but a significant reduction in *Clostridia* organisms.[462] Intestinal mucus itself is not bactericidal; however, it contains humoral and cellular immune factors that are important in protection against salmonellosis.

Antibiotic therapy reduces resistance to salmonellosis and prolongs the course of the illness in experimental animals. A single dose of penicillin or streptomycin greatly increases the susceptibility of mice to salmonellosis by altering the normal intestinal microflora that protects the bowel against colonization by enteric pathogens. In hospitals where outbreaks of salmonellosis had occured, dogs receiving antimicrobials that alter GI flora, such as ampicillin, were at greater risk of developing salmonellosis.

Pathogenesis

Experimentally, numerous organisms[106-109] must be ingested to produce GI colonization by *Salmonella* with or without clinical illness. Because a large proportion of ingested organisms are destroyed by the low pH of the stomach, reducing the amount of gastric acidity by administration of buffered compounds or performing vagotomy or partial gastrectomy induces a greater risk of salmonellosis in experimental animals. The organisms that survive passage through the stomach are able to colonize the middle portions of the ileum on the day of ingestion. Here they attach preferentially to the tips of villi, which they invade and in which they multiply. *Salmonella* strains of a given species vary in their virulence, which is partially determined by their ability to invade nonphagocytic host epithelial cells. Salmonellae have pili-like projections that facilitate insertion of bacterial proteins into epithelial cells following contact. This triggers a cascade that results in uptake of the bacteria by enterocytes or M cells.[162] Localization and persistence of the organisms in the intestinal epithelium and lymph nodes account for shedding, which occurs for 3 to 6 weeks in most cases. The shedding is continual for the first week but then becomes intermittent. Phagocytic cells in the intestinal lymph nodes, liver, or spleen may harbor the organism persistently, even in the absence of shedding. Reactivation of shedding or clinical illness may occur after stress, immunosuppression, concurrent systemic viral infections, and crowding.

Mucosal invasion, host inflammatory response, and resultant GI epithelial injury and sloughing are more common with salmonellosis than with bacterial diarrhea resulting from other kinds of infections. *Salmonella* strains differ in their pathogenicity, which correlates with their ability to attach to and invade mucosa, a property associated with their cell adherence and invasion. However, the extent of injury is not sufficient to explain the amount of fluid loss associated with diarrhea.[57] Adequate evidence suggests that some salmonellae produce heat-labile enterotoxins, which increase adenyl cyclase. This increase stimulates secretion of fluid by the intestinal mucosa, a process that occurs in other diarrheas associated with noninvasive enterotoxigenic bacteria (see Fig. 89-8, A).

Endotoxemia or bacteremia may occur during overt enteric infection or in the absence of signs of intestinal illness. Fever, leukopenia, endotoxic shock, and death may result. In surviving animals, focal suppuration with localization of organisms can occur in the biliary tract, kidneys, heart, spleen, meninges, joints, and lungs. A decrease in bacteremia and clearance of organisms from the blood are associated with a rising antibody titer to cell wall O antigen; the flagellar H antigen has no role in protection. Prolonged bacteremia or overwhelming sepsis is usually indicative of compromised host defense mechanisms. Prolonged intermittent bacteremia after salmonellosis is not as common a problem in animals as it is in people with *S. typhi* infection. The K, or capsular, antigen (called Vi for *S. typhi*) of this organism allows it to persist intracellularly for long periods despite adequate host defenses. Virulence plasmids found in some *Salmonella* serotypes enhance their extraintestinal growth and production of bacteremia.[112,247] For salmonellae to cause bacteremia, they must possess virulence factors allowing them to resist killing by phagolysosomes within leukocytes.

Endotoxemia from overwhelming salmonellosis is associated with various effects on the host and is related to the lipopolysaccharide composition of their cell wall (see Endotoxemia, Chapter 38). Pooling of leukocytes, erythrocytes, and platelets in the peripheral vasculature; hypoglycemia; complement activation; release of vasoactive amines; and development of disseminated intravascular coagulation (DIC) may occur.

Clinical Findings

Clinical findings in salmonellosis vary according to the number of infecting organisms, the immune status of the host, and the complicating factors or concomitant diseases. The syndromes can be artificially divided into gastroenteritis, bacteremia and endotoxemia, organ localization, and persistence of an asymptomatic carrier state.

Gastroenteritis

The clinical signs associated with *Salmonella* gastroenteritis vary. Most acute episodes begin within 3 to 5 days of exposure to the organism or after stress in carriers. Very young or old animals show the most severe clinical signs. Fever of 40° C to 41.1° C (104° F to 106° F), malaise, and anorexia are noted initially and are followed by vomiting, abdominal pain, and diarrhea. Cats frequently hypersalivate as a result of persistent vomiting. The diarrhea varies in consistency from watery to mucoid, and fresh blood is present in severe cases. Weight loss and dehydration become evident within several days after the onset of illness. Severely affected animals have pale mucous membranes, weakness, marked dehydration, cardiovascular collapse, shock, and icterus just before death. Central nervous system signs in some animals include hyperexcitability, incoordination, posterior paresis, blindness, and convulsions. Pneumonia can be associated with acute *Salmonella* gastroenteritis. Coughing, dyspnea, and epistaxis are seen in affected animals.

Bacteremia and Endotoxemia

Bacteremia and endotoxemia are usually transient subclinical features of *Salmonella* gastroenteritis and become clinically significant in either very young or immunosuppressed dogs and cats. Cats fed a raw-meat diet heavily contaminated with

Salmonella have developed severe gastroenteritis, septicemia, and death.[428] Other dogs and cats may have bacteremia and persistent fever in the absence of GI signs. Affected kittens and puppies younger than 7 weeks may not show a febrile response despite bacteremia or endotoxemia. In severe cases, mental depression, pale mucosae, weakness, tachycardia, hypothermia, and cardiovascular collapse may be seen with or without GI signs. Organ dysfunction from thrombosis or hemorrhagic tendencies can occur from DIC.

Organ Localization

Metastatic infection may occur after clinical or subclinical bacteremia. Organisms may localize in particular organ systems for a period before producing overt clinical signs. Localization is most likely to occur in tissues previously damaged or devitalized but may spread to healthy structures. The clinical signs are referable to the organ system of localization. For example, a cat developed pneumonia caused by *S. choleraesuis* without enteric manifestations or positive fecal culture results.[372] Abscesses, pyothorax, meningitis, osteomyelitis, and cellulitis are other examples of focal disease.

Other Syndromes

Abortion, stillbirth, and birth of weak puppies or kittens may result from in utero infection. Vaginal discharges, placentas, and meconia usually contain *Salmonella*. The bitch or queen generally has prolonged vaginal discharges and delayed postpartum involution. Puppies that survive are weak, unthrifty, and emaciated, and *Salmonella* can be isolated from various organs. Conjunctivitis has been a major manifestation in some infected cats that also have regional lymphadenomegaly and persistent fecal shedding of salmonellae. (See Chapter 93 for an additional discussion of ocular lesions.)

Songbird Fever

Seasonal bird migrations have been associated with *S. typhimurium* and an acute febrile illness in cats that usually lasts 2 to 7 days. Reports have been documented from wild birds migrating in the northeastern United States and Sweden.[442] Affected cats have primarily been outdoors and preyed on birds or frequented bird feeders. Clinical signs include acute depression, anorexia, fever (40° C to 40.6° C [104° F to 105° F]), diarrhea, which is often hemorrhagic, and variable vomiting. Recovery usually is rapid, but in some cases normal feeding behavior does not return for several weeks. Mortality may be as high as 10%, and other diseases causing immunosuppression may increase this number. Therapy for and prevention of this syndrome are the same as for other *Salmonella* infections.

Subclinical Infections and Clinical Recovery

Only a small proportion (less than 10%) of infected animals die during the acute stages of salmonellosis. Dogs and cats infected with few organisms and those that have otherwise normal defense mechanisms have transient or no clinical illness. Some cats may have a persistent chronic febrile illness characterized by anorexia and lethargy without diarrhea. Animals affected by acute diarrhea usually recover after 3 to 4 weeks. Rarely, chronic or intermittent diarrhea that lasts for up to 8 weeks is reported.[84] Recovered and clinically normal animals usually shed the organisms for up to 6 weeks.

Diagnosis

Salmonellosis should be suspected in animals with any acute or chronic GI illness. It has frequently been overlooked in favor of the more notorious viral enteritis caused by canine parvovirus or coronavirus and feline panleukopenia virus. The clinical and pathologic features of these diseases may be indistinguishable from those of salmonellosis (see Clinical Findings, Chapters 8 and 10).

Clinical Laboratory Findings

Hematologic abnormalities vary depending on the stage of illness. Nonregenerative hypochromic anemia, lymphopenia, thrombocytopenia, neutropenia with a left shift, and toxic leukocytes are found in animals with systemic disease and endotoxemia. Bacterial rods may be found in the leukocytes of dogs or cats with overwhelming sepsis. A mature neutrophilic leukocytosis is more characteristic of chronically infected animals or animals with localization of infection in a particular organ system. Prolonged coagulation test times are apparent in animals with severe DIC.

Biochemical abnormalities are usually present only in animals with severe clinical illness. These abnormalities include hypoproteinemia, especially hypoalbuminemia, hypoglycemia, and moderate prerenal azotemia. Dogs with salmonellosis have had electrolyte abnormalities, hyponatremia, and hyperkalemia typical of primary hypoadrenocorticism.

Bacterial Isolation

Isolation of *Salmonella* organisms is the most definitive means of confirming infection. However, mere isolation from the oral cavity, vomitus, or feces does not indicate that the organisms are causing clinical disease, because the prevalence of subclinical carriers in dog and cat populations is high. Animals recovering from clinical salmonellosis shed organisms for at least 4 to 6 weeks, and shedding can be reactivated by stress or recurrent illness.

Finding organisms in samples of normally sterile secretions or body fluids, such as blood, urine, synovial fluid, transtracheal washings, cerebrospinal fluid (CSF), and bone marrow, may allow a definitive diagnosis of systemic salmonellosis to be made from chronically febrile animals or during the acute phases of illness. Samples for culture should be taken from the liver, spleen, bone marrow, lung, mesenteric lymph nodes, and intestinal tract at necropsy. The gallbladder and bile do not appear to be consistent sites of localization of infection in animals, although they are in people infected with *S. typhi*.

Normal culture results do not necessarily eliminate the possibility of infection, because it is difficult to isolate salmonellae in the presence of other organisms. Specimens from normally sterile tissues, such as blood, bone marrow, joint fluid, and CSF, can be cultured on ordinary media. Samples taken from the oral cavity or bowel, both of which have a high concentration of commensal organisms, must be cultured on special media. Treated animals should not be considered free of infection during monitoring until at least three successive attempts at culture have been made over 2- to 3-week intervals. To avoid losing organisms during shipment to a laboratory, fresh fecal specimens should be placed in Amies transport medium with charcoal.

Enrichment broths (e.g., selenite and tetrathionate) are used to increase the yield and inhibit growth of competing organisms. Numerous improved plating media have been developed.[90,376] Atmospheric oxygen can be damaging to *Salmonella*. Commercial media (SPRINT, Oxoid Ltd, Basingstoke, England) is available that contains oxygen scavengers to facilitate cultivation.[207] After 24 hours, subculturing is performed on an inhibitory medium, such as deoxycholate, that favors the growth of *Salmonella*. After isolation, salmonellae are identified by Gram staining, motility, and biochemical reactions. They ferment certain sugars, including glucose (but not lactose) and react positively with substances such as urea, indole, and methyl red.

Immunologic and Genetic Identification

Other nonculture methods can help identify infected hosts. The real-time PCR method has been used to detect salmonellae in canine fecal specimens.[251] In addition an ELISA with monoclonal antibody *(mab)* has been used to detect *Salmonella* antigens in urine of bacteremic people.

Serologic Testing

Demonstration of a rise in serum antibody titer to O and H antigens has been used in human medicine as a less specific means of detecting clinical illness. Not all subclinically infected dogs and cats have positive serologic titers, thus serologic testing is not an accurate means of detecting carriers. Cats respond consistently with increased titers only when they are clinically ill. For these reasons, culture of body fluids or secretions is a simpler and more definitive means of making a diagnosis.

Cytologic Examination

Cytologic examination is helpful in detecting invasive GI pathogens in diarrheal illnesses. The presence of leukocytes in feces can identify diseases that cause disruption of the intestinal mucosa. A wet mount is prepared by mixing small flecks of mucus with a drop of new methylene blue on a microscope slide and placing a coverslip on the mixture. The absence of fecal leukocytes indicates a viral, mild bacterial, or nonspecific diarrhea that does not require extensive therapy. The presence of large numbers of leukocytes is typical of acute salmonellosis and other forms of diarrhea that cause extensive mucosal disruption. These cases usually require intensive parenteral fluid and antibiotic therapy.

Pathologic Findings

Gross lesions are found at necropsy in only a small percentage of infected animals that develop severe clinical illness. Pale mucous membranes and dehydration accompany a diffuse mucoid to hemorrhagic enteritis. Lesions in the intestinal mucosa vary from catarrhal inflammation to mucosal sloughing with extensive denudation of the gut. GI lesions may be extensive but are usually confined to the distal small bowel, cecum, and colon. Diffusely scattered petechial to ecchymotic hemorrhages present throughout most organ systems are associated with focal thrombosis and necrosis. A serohemorrhagic effusion may be present in the abdominal cavity, with fibrin adhered to inflamed viscera. The lungs are frequently edematous or consolidated, and mesenteric and peripheral lymph nodes are enlarged and hemorrhagic.

Histologically, variable lesions are a fibrinous to fibropurulent pneumonia, multifocal necrotizing hepatitis and splenitis, and suppurative meningitis, all of which are associated with necrotic intestinal lymphadenitis and hemorrhagic ulcerative gastroenteritis. Histologic or cytologic examination may reveal that bacteria have disseminated to many organs, including the bone marrow, spleen, and lymph nodes.

Therapy

Appropriate therapy for canine and feline salmonellosis varies according to the type and severity of clinical illness. Acute *Salmonella* gastroenteritis without systemic signs is best treated with parenteral polyionic isotonic fluids to replace losses from vomitus and diarrhea. Fluids can be administered orally when vomiting is not a problem. Hypertonic glucose-containing solutions have been effective in reversing fluid loss in infectious diarrhea (see Chapter 89). Transfusion of plasma may be more beneficial than fluid therapy when mucosal disruption and increased GI permeability lower serum albumin concentration to less than 2 g/dl.

Prostaglandin inhibitors such as indomethacin have been effective in reducing fluid losses in animals with experimentally induced *Salmonella* gastroenteritis. Increased net water loss in the lower bowel results from increased intestinal secretion induced by bacterial endotoxin and mediated through prostaglandin synthesis. Prostaglandin inhibitors must be used early in the disease to be effective and must be used cautiously if GI hemorrhage is severe. Flunixin meglumine has been more commonly administered in dogs and cats, but GI bleeding and renal failure have been associated factors.

Paradoxically, osmotically active laxatives such as lactulose have been recommended for treating acute *Salmonella* gastroenteritis. As a nonabsorbable sugar, lactulose produces osmotic diarrhea through the formation of acid metabolites in the distal small bowel and colon. Shortened transit time and an acidic environment shorten the survival time of *Salmonella* organisms. Such therapy should be used only in unresponsive cases in which fluid deficits have already been corrected.

Routine antibiotics reported to be effective against *Salmonella* include chloramphenicol, trimethoprim-sulfonamide, and amoxicillin. Aminoglycosides such as gentamicin and amikacin may be considered when bacterial resistance is anticipated, but the risk of renal toxicity precludes their routine use. Isolates are generally sensitive to the quinolones and imipenem; however, high cost and the desire to reduce the development of antimicrobial resistance make these second choices unless overwhelming sepsis is apparent. Variable resistance to erythromycin, clindamycin, ampicillin, cephapirin, sulfonamides, or nitrofurans is reported. Resistance is greatest to streptomycin, tetracycline, and sulfonamides alone. Unfortunately, the in vivo response of *Salmonella* to antibiotics does not always correlate with the results of in vitro testing. For example, a cat with salmonellosis that did not respond to amoxicillin or cephapirin was effectively treated with cephalexin.[84]

Antibiotic therapy has not been advocated for treating animals with uncomplicated *Salmonella* gastroenteritis but has been recommended for animals with concurrent signs of nonenteric (systemic) infection or histories of immunosuppression (see Table 39-2). Studies in human patients have indicated that routine antimicrobial use in treating salmonellosis induces drug-resistant strains and prolongs the convalescent excretion period. However, this widely held view has been questioned in studies that demonstrate effective eradication of *Salmonella* from people and animals by combined antibiotic therapy. One hypothesis is that antimicrobial therapy may suppress endogenous flora that normally inhibits intestinal colonization by *Salmonella* species. Competitive exclusion is a procedure that has been used on farms to reduce the carriage of enteric salmonellae by livestock. Animals are treated with antimicrobials to eliminate the *Salmonella* followed by oral administration of a probiotic. Probiotics (feed supplements containing live organisms that help reestablish the intestinal flora) have not been used in dogs, but in a controlled study in *Salmonella*-infected horses, no benefits were found.[339]

Another inherent problem with routine antibiotic administration for *Salmonella* gastroenteritis is that infecting organisms may acquire transferable (plasmid-mediated) resistance. An increased prevalence of transferable resistance has been demonstrated among *Salmonella* isolates from dogs, cats, and people. The fluoroquinolones have a reduced tendency to produce plasmid-mediated resistance in bacteria compared with other antibacterials; however, fluoroquinolone-resistant salmonellae have been found in human outbreaks associated with frequent use of the drug in hospitals.[330] Similar concerns have been addressed for veterinary isolates.[354] Other disadvantages of routine antibiotic therapy for salmonellosis are that it may enhance susceptibility to infection or activate clinical illness in a latent carrier.

Animals with more severe signs of endotoxemia or bacteremia should be treated differently from those with simple gastroenteritis. Plasma transfusions of at least 250 ml for dogs larger than 15 kg have reduced mortality in those dogs that had been given *Salmonella* endotoxin. Equal volumes of isotonic fluid or smaller volumes of plasma were not helpful. Like untreated dogs, plasma-treated dogs developed leukopenia, thrombocytopenia, and extensive tissue injury, but they had better survival rates. Dogs with experimentally induced endotoxic shock were protected by infusion of *mabs* directed against the endotoxic lipid A cell wall component of *Salmonella*.[377] A commercially available polyclonal antiserum is available for this purpose (see discussion of antiendotoxin serum in Therapy, Chapters 8 and 38).

Prevention

Prevention of salmonellosis in dogs and cats can be frustrating because of the tendency of some animals to develop a chronic subclinical carrier state or latent infection. Nontyphoid salmonellae that infect pets are also harbored by many other animals and persist in the environment, making eradication difficult.

Hygiene and isolation of individual pets should be enforced during hospitalization because of the highly infectious and contagious nature of salmonellosis. To prevent development and spread of infections in a veterinary teaching hospital, newly admitted horses were only placed in stalls where *Salmonella* had been previously isolated, after two cycles of cleaning and disinfection.[6] Infection from food sources can be minimized by using commercially available heat-processed products. Proper sanitation during handling and storing of processed foods is also important, because they frequently become contaminated by contact with utensils, rodents, or insects. Meat, eggs, and dairy products given as food should be stored or thawed at temperatures lower than 4.4° C (40° F) and should be cooked to internal temperatures of at least 74° C (165° F). Imported commercial dog chews made from animal hides have been found to contain *Salmonella* organisms.[495]

Cages in hospitals, kennels, or catteries should be routinely cleaned and disinfected between uses by different animals (see Chapter 94). Phenolic compounds or household bleach (diluted 1:32, or 4 oz per gallon of water) can be applied as surface disinfectants, but their contact with cats should be avoided. Animals brought into a group confinement situation should be segregated if they have or develop diarrhea or vomiting. Food dishes and utensils should be cold disinfected, or preferably autoclaved, between uses. Disposable dishes can simply be thrown away. Endoscopic equipment, which is shown to be a source of infection in human hospitals, should also be properly disinfected (i.e., subjected to ethylene oxide gas or immersed in glutaraldehyde [2%] or formalin [20% for a minimum of 1 hour). The equipment must be thoroughly aerated or rinsed before use (see Chapter 94).

Human carriers of nontyphoid *Salmonella* may transmit the infection as a reverse zoonosis, a possibility that should not be overlooked in an animal-holding facility that has a recurrent problem with salmonellosis. Long-term boarders or blood donors should not be housed with the transient hospital population because they may be exposed and become future sources of *Salmonella* infection.

Public Health Considerations

Clinical signs of animal-acquired salmonellosis in people include abdominal tenderness, nausea, vomiting, and diarrhea accompanied by fever, myalgia, headache, and dehydration. Like animals, people may develop localized or septicemic forms of illness, depending on their immunocompetence.

Salmonellosis is a disease of major zoonotic importance. All *Salmonella* organisms, except those causing human typhoid fever (*S. typhi* and *S. paratyphi*), infect people and animals. Considerable emphasis has been placed on foodborne outbreaks of nontyphoid salmonellosis in people through contaminated products of animal origin. Foods such as meat, eggs, or milk products that have been improperly stored, prepared, or handled before consumption are most often incriminated. Sporadic pet-associated infections have not received as

much attention. Dogs have been recognized as important vectors for non-foodborne infections in people because of the canine habits of coprophagy and ingesting carrion coupled with long-term shedding of organisms and close proximity to people. Infants and older adults are especially prone to infections from pets.[338] Dogs and horses have the greatest zoonotic potential for those with occupational exposure. Reptiles and amphibians are most frequently incriminated in pet-associated cases.[97,216] Outbreaks in people caused by exposure to infected horses have been commonly reported.[453] Contact with feces from infected pets has been an important source of exposure for young children. Cats, proved to be important but less frequently infected reservoirs, shed organisms orally, conjunctively, and focally. Thus they may contaminate their food, fur, or water source, any of which may serve as a source of infection for people. Salmonellosis caused by multidrug-resistant organisms occurred in three small animal practices where inadvertent contamination of the environment by cats with diarrhea caused outbreaks of infection in people and cats in the facilities.[17] Inadvertent ingestion of animal feces or food contaminated by feces likely occurred as a result of suboptimal hygiene in and sanitation of the veterinary facilities. The use of antimicrobial agents in the animals likely contributed to the drug-resistant strains. People who handle raw-meat diets or who are exposed to the feces of domestic or wild dogs or cats being fed such diets are also at increased risk of exposure. *S. ser enteritidis* infections are largely associated with egg products. Multidrug-resistant *S. ser typhimurium* strain DT 104, which has been a prevalent foodborne animal strain that infects people in the United Kingdom and the United States, has also been found in cats, dogs, and other nonfood animals.[14,366] Most isolates possess chromosomally encoded resistance to ampicillin, chloramphenicol, streptomycin, sulfonamides, and tetracycline, and some isolates are resistant to quinolones and trimethoprim.[382]

To reduce the risk of infection from pets, hands should be thoroughly washed with soap and water after handling animals or fomites such as animal bedding, footwear, or clothing contaminated with feces. Detergents and household bleach added to the laundry eliminate the organisms in these fomites.

Of increasing concern is the frequency with which antibiotic-resistant *Salmonella* strains have been isolated from dogs and cats. Most of the resistance is plasmid mediated and intensified by indiscriminate or frequent administration of antibiotics by veterinarians.[76,167] Antibiotic resistance has made recently acquired salmonellosis more difficult to treat in people. Quinolone resistance has been feared and reported in salmonellae in the United States, necessitating the restricted use of these drugs in food animals.[199] In the United Kingdom, antimicrobial resistance has been documented in salmonellae from food animals and their environment.[229] *Salmonella* infections have been more frequent and severe in people infected with HIV.

SHIGELLOSIS

Craig E. Greene

Etiology

Shigella is a genus of nonmotile gram-negative bacteria that are morphologically indistinguishable from other enterobacteria and cause a diarrheal condition known as *bacillary dysentery* in apes and people. On the basis of biochemical and serologic properties, they are divided into four serogroups: *Shigella dysenteriae*, *Shigella flexneri*, *Shigella boydii*, and *Shigella sonnei*. Each group is further divided into numerous subserotypes that vary in pathogenicity. Shigellae are not as environmentally resistant as salmonellae; they cannot survive a temperature of 55° C for longer than 1 hour, and they are destroyed by dilute (1%) phenol within 30 minutes. They are susceptible to inactivation by sunlight and acid pH but can remain viable for a few days in nonacidic stools maintained in the dark. Shigellae survive best in dried fecal matter on cloth that is kept in a dark, moist place. Because of their short survival time, the carrier host is most important in maintaining these organisms in nature.

Epidemiology

Shigellae are principally primate pathogens, causing severe hemorrhagic enteritis (dysentery). The disease, which spreads primarily via fecal-oral contact, is most commonly a problem in nonhuman primate colonies with substandard sanitation or hygiene practices. Although rare, waterborne outbreaks in people may occur with sewage contamination of domestic water supplies.

Dogs may become infected after contamination of their food or water supplies with infected human feces. Because of their coprophagous habits, pets may become exposed in areas with improper sewage disposal. Once they contract an infection, dogs are probably not carriers and only transiently excrete the organisms. Cats have not been reported to be naturally infected.

Pathogenesis

Shigellae may damage the body because of a gram-negative endotoxin that is produced. Shiga toxin is one of the most toxic biologic agents when given systemically. Certain organisms (e.g., *S. dysenteriae* type 1) produce enterotoxins that increase intestinal fluid secretions and can cause ulceration. Shigellae probably produce diarrhea by intestinal epithelial cell invasion with resultant necrosis and hemorrhage and by effects of the Shiga toxin. Shiga toxin is also synthesized by and may be an important virulence factor of other pathogenic bacterial species. Systemic manifestations of the toxin in infected people include DIC with renal failure, thrombocytopenia, and microangiopathic hemolytic anemia.

Clinical Findings

In primates the organism causes severe hemorrhagic, mucoid, large-bowel diarrhea. Lesions are usually ulcerative, and they spread from the distal to the proximal colon with time. In children and, although rarely, in adults, septicemia may develop with or without diarrhea. Unlike primates, dogs are relatively resistant and cats are highly resistant to infection with *Shigella*. Organisms have been isolated from a small number of clinically normal dogs, but they have not been directly implicated as a cause of diarrhea in this species.

Diagnosis

Demonstration of organisms in culture is essential to differentiate *Shigella* enterocolitis from diarrhea caused by other bacteria. Because of the fastidious nature of the organism, samples collected on swabs should be transported to the laboratory immediately and not be exposed to sunlight. Cytologic examination of the stool reveals large numbers of inflammatory cellular exudates associated with invasion of the bowel wall by *Shigella*.

Therapy

Symptomatic treatment with parenteral fluids and antimicrobial therapy are similar to those in salmonellosis and enteropathogenic diarrhea (see Table 39-2). Unlike *Salmonella* organisms, many shigellae are still sensitive to ampicillin, sulfonamide, tetracycline, and streptomycin. Antimotility therapy was detrimental to people with experimentally induced shigellosis.[89]

Prevention

Control measures for shigellae are very similar to those outlined for salmonellae. Shigellosis is easier to prevent in dogs and cats than salmonellosis because the reservoir of *Shigella* organisms is restricted to the primate host.

YERSINIOSIS

Craig E. Greene

Etiology and Epidemiology

Three major pathogenic members of the genus *Yersinia* infect dogs and cats: *Yersinia enterocolitica*, *Yersinia pseudotuberculosis*, and *Yersinia pestis*. (*Y. enterocolitica* and *Y. pseudotuberculosis* are discussed in this section, and *Y. pestis*, the cause of plague, is discussed in Chapter 47.) *Y. enterocolitica*, which is 0.5 to 1 μm × 1 to 3 μm, is a motile, gram-negative, facultative coccobacillus that causes an enterocolitis in people. An unusual feature of this bacterium is that it replicates in culture at refrigeration temperatures, which allows its selective growth in the laboratory and refrigerated food. Heating food to 60° C for a few minutes kills the organism. The bacterium, which has been isolated from the feces of various domestic and wild animal reservoirs and the environment, has a worldwide distribution. The prevalence of isolation of this organism from animals increases in colder months, perhaps because of its affinity for colder temperatures. The organism causes illness by invading many body tissues and elaborating a heat-stable enterotoxin. Virulence-related factors of the organism appear primarily at lower temperatures, making human acquisition of infection more likely through contamination of the environment or food rather than directly from the carrier host. People appear to be unnatural hosts for this organism because they develop fever, diarrhea, abdominal pain, septicemia, or skin rashes, all signs that closely mimic those of acute appendicitis. Nonsuppurative arthritis may develop as a sequela after recovery from GI illness. Conditions associated with iron overload appear to predispose the host to systemic spread of the organism.

Y. pseudotuberculosis is a cause of enteritis in many animals, especially during the wet, cold winter and spring months. Various animals, including birds, rodents, cats, and pigs, have been incriminated as reservoir hosts. People are more severely affected and develop mesenteric lymphadenitis and septicemia.

Clinical Findings

Because *Y. enterocolitica* has been isolated from feces of clinically normal dogs and cats, it is thought to be a commensal organism. It has also been isolated from people with clinical illness who presumably contracted the infection through contact with the excreta of infected household pets. Experimental infections in adult dogs have produced no clinical illness, despite periodic fecal shedding for 52 days and recovery of the organism from mesenteric lymph nodes and other tissues.[422] Feeding of contaminated raw pork produced subclinical transfer of infection to dogs.[155] Infected dogs have developed resistance to reinfection. *Y. enterocolitica* has also been cultured from the feces of young dogs with symptomatic GI illness.[105,337] The syndrome has been characterized by a several-week history of diarrhea associated with increased frequency of stools, tenesmus, blood, and mucus. In contrast to infected people, infected dogs were not systemically ill. Dogs and cats may be asymptomatic carriers of *Y. pseudotuberculosis*. A Persian cat infected with *Y. pseudotuberculosis* developed anorexia, abdominal discomfort and weight loss, and dehydration.[212] In a 4-month-old Rottweiler pup infected with *Y. enterocolitica*, sudden death was caused by transmural myocarditis. Multifocal granulomatous hepatitis was apparent. Bacteremic spread from the bowel to the liver and the systemic circulation was suspected.[491]

Diagnosis

Diagnosis of yersiniosis has been based on culture of the organism from the feces or deeper tissues of affected animals. As with other enteropathogenic bacterial infections, mere isolation from the intestinal tract may not be diagnostic of pathogenicity because the organism can be found in clinically healthy animals. Isolation of the organism from deeper tissues such as blood, urine, lymph nodes, wounds, or abscesses is more meaningful. *Yersinia* are not usually cultivated on conventional media because they produce small colonies that are later overgrown by normal floral organisms. A selective medium containing cefsulodin, irgasan, and novobiocin greatly improves the ability to isolate *Yersinia* from enteric specimens. Serotyping of *Yersinia* strains is similar to that of *Salmonella*. In systemically affected individuals, small, pale-yellow abscesses are scattered on the surface and throughout the parenchyma of the liver and spleen. Histologic examination in one clinically affected dog with *Y. enterocolitica* infection revealed a chronic enteritis with mononuclear and plasma cell infiltrates in the intestinal mucosa and mesenteric lymph nodes.[105] A cat with *Y. pseudotuberculosis* infection had focal microabscesses with microthrombosis in the liver and spleen.[212]

Therapy

Yersiniosis therapy should be attempted in younger dogs or cats from whose feces the organism has been isolated and that have diarrhea or are in contact with people with confirmed infections. The organism is usually sensitive to routine dosages of chloramphenicol, tetracycline, gentamicin, cephalosporins, and trimethoprim-sulfonamides (see Table 39-2). Penicillin and its derivatives are not usually effective in routine dosages. As with other enteropathogenic bacteria, consumption of raw dairy or meat products or of wildlife carcasses predisposes the animals to infection and should be avoided. Raw meat should not be fed to pets.

Public Health Considerations

Outbreaks of gastroenteritis have been reported in people exposed to infected pet dogs.[182] Young children who drank water from puddles and played in a sandbox frequented by a stray cat became infected with *Y. pseudotuberculosis*.[159] The organism could be isolated from the water, sand, and soil. Precautions should be taken to avoid exposing young children to these types of situations. As mentioned, raw meat should not be fed to pets.

PLESIOMONAS SHIGELLOIDES INFECTION

Craig E. Greene

A motile, gram-negative facultatively anaerobic bacterium in the family Vibrionaceae, *Plesiomonas shigelloides* is a zoonotic cause of acute diarrhea in people. (Rarely, infection spreads systemically in immunocompromised people.) This water- and soil-associated organism is found in temperate and tropical freshwater environments and is prevalent in the intestinal tract of aquatic animals. The usual means by which people acquire infection is through ingestion of water or foods contaminated by feces from infected animals such as shellfish, poultry, livestock, and dogs or cats.[3] Feeding of fish, shellfish, or aquatic foodstuffs to dogs or cats may be a source for infection.[217]

Diarrheic illness has sometimes been attributed to *P. shigelloides* in dogs and cats[120,217]; however, it is found in the feces of clinically healthy research cats[418] and was isolated from fecal swabs and postmortem material from cats.[28] In contrast, most infected people develop diarrhea that can vary from mildly self-limiting to diarrhea that is severe and has a bloody mucoid consistency. Bacteremia, which can result in embolic spread to many organs, generally occurs in immunocompromised people. Similar serotypes have been isolated from people and associated cats, suggesting zoonotic transmission.[168a] The organism is often susceptible to trimethoprim-sulfonamides, quinolones, cephalosporins, and penicillin-clavulanate combinations. Should the organisms be found in the feces of a diarrheic dog or cat, another cause should be investigated.

TYZZER'S DISEASE

Boyd R. Jones and Craig E. Greene

Etiology

Tyzzer's disease is caused by *Clostridium piliforme* (formerly "*Bacillus piliformis*"), a spore-forming, gram-negative obligate intracellular parasite measuring 0.5 μm × 10 to 40 μm that moves by means of peritrichous flagella. RNA sequences of this organism are closely related to those of the clostridia, so the new name—*C. piliforme*—has been adopted. Originally described as a disease of rodents, it is now known to affect a wide range of animals. Reports of spontaneous disease in dogs and cats have been described.*

Epidemiology

C. piliforme, which appears to be a commensal organism of the intestinal tracts of laboratory rodents, is found on fecal cultures of normal and diseased animals. Clinical illness in rodents seems to be precipitated by stress, such as crowding, unsanitary conditions, weaning, or transportation and irradiation, glucocorticoid therapy, or other forms of immunosuppression.

Dogs and cats may acquire infection by contact with or ingestion of rodent feces containing bacterial spores, although such interspecies transmission has never been reported. Experimental disease has been difficult to produce in healthy dogs and cats. Most feline cases have occurred in laboratory-reared cats, some with known contact with rodents. It is possible that dogs and cats harbor the organism.

A majority of infected animals have had naturally or experimentally induced immunosuppressive diseases such as feline leukemia, feline panleukopenia, feline infectious peritonitis, and canine distemper.[214,215,224] One group of affected kittens had familial lipoprotein lipase deficiency and were persistently lipidemic.[226]

In experimental studies the severity of the disease has been enhanced by overcrowding, administration of glucocorticoids or cyclophosphamide, splenectomy, irradiation, partial hepatectomy, and mononuclear-phagocyte blockade.

Pathogenesis

The pathogenesis of Tyzzer's disease is uncertain. The mechanisms by which *C. piliforme* attaches to and enters host cells are unknown. Endogenous or exogenous infection is followed by local proliferation of organisms in the intestinal epithelial cells. After stress or immunosuppression of the host, organisms spread by portal circulation to the liver. Colonization in the hepatic parenchyma results in multifocal periportal hepatic necrosis, presumably as the result of an unidentified toxin.

Clinical Findings

Clinical signs have been relatively consistent among dogs and cats in which the disease has been reported. The onset of

*References 32, 40, 226, 246, 249, 298, 314, 357, 358, 364, 392, 393, 493.

lethargy, depression, anorexia, and abdominal discomfort is very rapid. Hepatomegaly and abdominal distention are followed by hypothermia, with the animal becoming moribund, resulting in death within 24 to 48 hours. Diarrhea has been infrequent; scant amounts of pasty feces are more characteristic. Icterus has been apparent in some animals, especially cats.

Diagnosis

Because of the rapidly fatal course of Tyzzer's disease, diagnosis usually has been made by gross examination of specimens collected at necropsy. Just before death, marked elevations of alanine transaminase activity have been found. Characteristic findings are multiple whitish-gray to hemorrhagic foci, 1 to 2 mm in diameter, on the capsule and cut surface of the liver (Fig. 39-8). Similar lesions may be apparent on other viscera. The intestinal mucosa may be thickened and congested in the region of the terminal ileum and proximal colon. Foamy, dark-brown feces are usually present in the lumen, and mesenteric lymph nodes are generally enlarged.

Histologic findings usually include multifocal periportal hepatic necrosis and necrotic ileitis or colitis; other tissues, such as the myocardium, may be affected in some animals. Infiltrates of neutrophils and mononuclear cells are usually present at the margins of necrotic lesions. Numerous intracellular filamentous organisms are only faintly visible by hematoxylin and eosin stain in the hepatocytes at the margins of necrotic lesions and in the intestinal epithelial cells. Special stains such as Giemsa stain or Warthin-Starry or Gomori silver stain must be used to confirm the morphology of the organisms, which have a characteristic beaded appearance (Fig. 39-9). The organisms also can be demonstrated in methylene-blue–stained impression smears made from lesions in fresh tissues. Filamentous and spore forms of *C. piliforme* have been found. *C. piliforme* cannot be isolated on artificial medium that lacks living cells and so far has been cultured only in eggs or cell cultures.[419]

Serologic methods have become a common tool for diagnosing latent infections in rodent colonies. *Mab*-based tests have aided investigation of the disease. Flagellar antigens have been purified from *C. piliforme* from different species, and significant antigenic differences exist. Nevertheless, such serologic tests could be applied to investigations of the dog and cat.

Therapy and Prevention

Thus far, treatment of Tyzzer's disease has not been successful, because affected animals die before it can have an effect.

Antibiotic efficacy is undetermined. Success has been achieved with formalin-inactivated vaccines, which produce immunity to infection in mice. When possible, predisposing factors that have been associated with infection in dogs and cats should be identified and avoided.

CLOSTRIDIUM PERFRINGENS— AND CLOSTRIDIUM DIFFICILE—ASSOCIATED DIARRHEA

Stanley L. Marks and Elizabeth J. Kather

Diarrhea in dogs is a common problem facing the small animal practitioner, and bacterial enteropathogens play an important role in many cases.[178] *Clostridium perfringens* and *Clostridium difficile* are two of the most commonly incriminated bacteria in canine diarrhea[56,248,361,459,178]; however, it is important to appreciate that these bacterial species are but a small representation of putative pathogenic enteric bacteria.

Clinical signs associated with *C. perfringens* and *C. difficile* infections can range in severity from a mild, self-limiting diarrhea to a potentially fatal acute hemorrhagic diarrheal syndrome.[56] Clinical documentation of clostridial-associated diarrhea in dogs is clouded by the presence of these organisms existing as normal constituents of the indigenous intestinal microflora. In addition, isolation rates for *C. perfringens* and *C. difficile* are often similar in diarrheic and nondiarrheic dogs. Canine fecal enteric panels, which involve fecal cultures and toxin assays, are expensive ($70 to $100), are time consuming, and require technical expertise. Most small animal veterinarians do not have the facilities or expertise to perform these tests, which involves mailing fecal specimens to commercial veterinary diagnostic laboratories for evaluation (see Appendix 5, Laboratory Testing of Infectious Diseases of Dogs and Cats). No universal consensus exists among veterinary diagnostic laboratories as to which diagnostic assays should be used. This problem is compounded by the lack of validations for sensitivity and specificity of commercial toxin assays commonly used in the dog. The indications for performing fecal enteric panels on diarrheic dogs are poorly defined, resulting in indiscrimi-

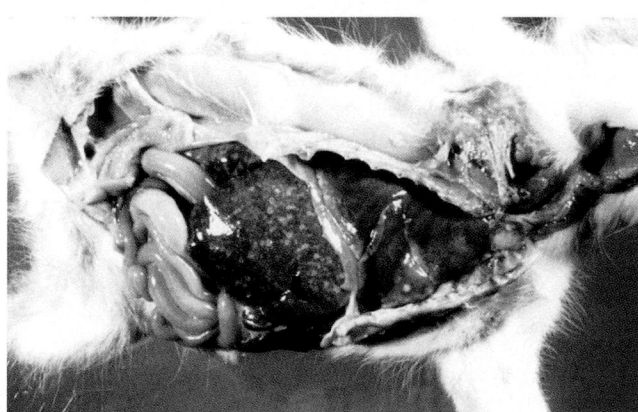

Fig 39-8 Tyzzer's disease in kitten. Multifocal white spots on liver are hepatocellular necrosis. Similar-appearing lesions visible through pericardial sac are caused by focal myocarditis. (From Jones BR, Johnstone AC, Hancock WS. 1985. Tyzzer's disease in kittens with familial primary hyperlipoproteinaemia, *J Small Anim Pract* 26:411-419.)

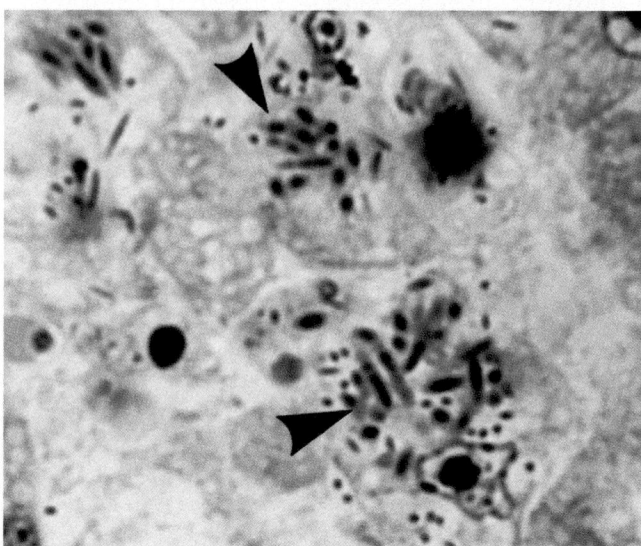

Fig 39-9 Hepatocytes at margins of necrotic focus in Tyzzer's disease. Bacteria resembling *C. piliforme* (*arrows*) are present within viable cells and extracellularly on necrotic tissue (toluidine blue, ×1500). (From Jones BR, Johnstone AC, Hancock WS. 1985. Tyzzer's disease in kittens with familial primary hyperlipoproteinaemia, *J Small Anim Pract* 26:411-419.)

nate testing and misinterpretation of results. The results of fecal cultures may take up to 72 hours to complete, and many dogs are treated with antibiotics indiscriminately before results of fecal cultures or toxin assays are available. In addition the resolution of clinical signs of diarrhea is often wrongly equated with eradication of the "incriminating" pathogen.

Clostridium perfringens—Associated Diarrhea
Etiology
The anaerobic, gram-positive, spore-forming bacillus *C. perfringens* may be one of the most widespread pathogenic bacteria, inhabiting the GI tract of people and animals as well as terrestrial and marine environments.[410] The organism is divided into five biotypes, A to E, based on the possession of one or more of four major toxin genes (Table 39-8): alpha (α), beta (β), iota (ι), and epsilon (ε).

Each biotype may also express a subset of at least 10 other established toxins, including *C. perfringens* enterotoxin (CPE). Although all five types can harbor the enterotoxin gene *(cpe)*, the global distribution of enterotoxigenic strains is relatively low (approximately 5%), with the majority of strains belonging to type A.[245,414,463] Virtually all strains isolated from dogs are type A, with only one published report documenting a type C infection in five cases of canine peracute lethal hemorrhagic enteritis.[22,299] A published study evaluating 843 *C. perfringens* isolates collected from 103 dogs revealed that all isolates tested were type A, with 15% harboring the *cpe* gene.[288] Enterotoxigenic *C. perfringens* type A has been associated with human food poisoning and sporadic diarrhea, canine acute and chronic, large and small bowel diarrhea, and an acute hemorrhagic diarrheal syndrome.[56,288,300,386] Although several studies have shown an association between the immunodetection of CPE in fecal specimens and canine diarrhea, the pathogenesis of *C. perfringens*–associated diarrhea (CPAD) in dogs is not fully understood; CPE is also detected in up to 14% of nondiarrheic dogs.[288,456,485] In addition, numerous other virulence factors such as the ß2 toxin may also play a role in diarrhea. These virulence factors may explain why the isolation of nonenterotoxigenic type A strains from a diarrheic specimen does not preclude involvement in disease. *C. perfringens* ß2 toxin has been associated with necrotic enteritis in piglets and typhlocolitis in horses.[163,166,198] The role of ß2-toxigenic *C. perfringens* in dogs is less well understood; only a single study evaluating 24 isolates collected from diarrheic dogs has been published to date.[448] In the study, isolates were positive for the *cpe* gene (33%), the ß2-toxin gene (33%), or both (17%); however, interpretation of the results of that study was difficult because of the small number of dogs and lack of a nondiarrheic control population.[448] The presence of the ß2-toxin gene was evaluated in 269 *C. perfringens* isolates obtained from 24 diarrheic and 44 nondiarrheic dogs. ß2-toxigenic *C. perfringens* was isolated from 22% and 15% of diarrheic and nondiarrheic dogs, respectively, providing no support for the role of ß2-toxigenic *C. perfringens* in canine diarrhea to date.

CPAD in the dog appears to be a complex disease with a poorly understood pathogenesis. It is still uncertain whether *C. perfringens* is a primary cause of canine diarrhea or a secondary phenomenon. In addition, much of the historical and anecdotal information regarding canine *C. perfringens* needs to be revised. Research has shed light on the several aspects of CPAD in dogs, and Table 39-9 summarizes what is known about the condition.

Pathogenesis
Knowledge about the pathogenesis of canine CPAD is limited and largely anecdotal. This phenomenon is further complicated by the fact that *C. perfringens* is a part of the normal canine intestinal microflora and readily cultured from more than 80% of diarrheic and nondiarrheic dogs.[289,485] Canine CPAD has been attributed to CPE, which has been shown to induce fluid accumulation and diarrhea in a dog model when administered orally or directly into the intestinal lumen.[30] The role of CPE in the development of diarrhea is unclear because CPE is detected in up to 34% of diarrheic dogs and in 5% to 14% of nondiarrheic dogs.[289,485] In addition, sporulated enterotoxigenic isolates are detected in up to 14% of nondiarrheic dogs.[289] In contrast to people, in whom CPAD is usually a result of ingestion of enterotoxigenic isolates, CPAD in dogs appears more likely to be secondary to disruption of the intestinal microenvironment, enabling proliferation or sporulation of commensal enterotoxigenic *C. perfringens*.

CPE is a 35-kDa protein encoded by the *cpe* gene, whose expression is coregulated with sporulation of the organism.[72,73] Several studies have shown that the *cpe* gene can be localized on either a conjugative plasmid or on the chromosome.[67,70,306] *C. perfringens* strains that carry a chromosomal *cpe* gene have primarily been associated with human foodborne disease, whereas strains with a plasmid *cpe* gene have been associated with human non–foodborne diseases and animal diseases, including canine diarrhea.[306] The reason for this distinct difference is not yet fully understood. The current model of the mechanism of CPE, which has evolved primarily from the studies of McClane[292] and Kokai-Kun et al,[245] is very complex and involves several steps. CPE is first produced in large quantities

Table • 39-9

Summary of Clostridium perfringens—Associated Diarrhea in Dogs

- Clinical signs of CPAD are not limited to colitis.
- Fecal endospore counting is not a reliable test for establishing CPAD in the dog.
- Results of *C. perfringens* enterotoxin (CPE) immunodetection assays should be cautiously interpreted, particularly the reverse passive latex agglutination assay (RPLA), which has been shown to produce more discordant results than other immunodetection methods.
- Isolation of nonenterotoxigenic strains from a diarrheic specimen does not preclude involvement in disease because other virulence factors may be involved.
- The use of tetracyclines for management of CPAD in the dogs is discouraged.
- The optimum diagnostic approach for canine CPAD is the use of an ELISA for CPE in conjunction with PCR for detection of enterotoxigenic strains procured after a heat or alcohol shock treatment.

Table • 39-8

Typing Scheme for Clostridium perfringens

TYPE	MAJOR TOXIN				ENTEROTOXIN
	α	β	ι	ε	
A	+	−	−	−	+/−
B	+	+	−	+	+/−
C	+	+	−	−	+/−
D	+	−	−	+	+/−
E	+	−	+	−	+/−

+, Positive; −, negative; +/−, positive or negative.

(15% of total protein present) by enterotoxigenic strains during sporulation and is then released during lysis of the mother cell.[73,292] In the foodborne model, food contaminated with large numbers of enterotoxigenic C. perfringens is ingested. Isolates that survive passage through the acid milieu of the stomach then undergo sporulation in the small intestine, releasing large amounts of enterotoxin.[293] Non–foodborne diseases associated with CPE are thought to involve commensal enterotoxigenic strains that are somehow triggered to undergo massive sporulation. The trigger may be one of several different factors including changes in diet, antibiotic administration, or coinfection with another intestinal pathogen. Once released into the intestinal lumen, CPE interacts with specific epithelial tight junction proteins forming a small protein complex of approximately 90 kDa, where it then becomes trapped on the membrane surface.[244,293,492] The small CPE complex then interacts with additional host proteins, forming several larger complexes, including an approximately 155-kDa complex and an approximately 200-kDa complex that contains the tight junction protein occluding.[293] Studies have suggested the 155-kDa complex is responsible for the cytotoxic and histopathologic damage that provides CPE access to occludin, causing alterations in tight junction structure and function, leading to paracellular permeability changes that contribute to diarrhea.[293] In the rabbit model, CPE binds to small and large intestinal epithelia, with the greatest histopathologic effect occurring in the ileum, and little or no cytotoxic effect is observed in colonic loops.[294,295] It is unknown whether this phenomenon occurs in the canine intestine, but investigation is warranted in the face of reports of colitis being the primary clinical manifestation in canine CPAD.

Clinical Findings

Canine C. perfringens has been characterized as a pathogen of the large intestine, causing clinical signs of increased pathogen of the fecal mucus, increased defecation frequency, tenesmus, and hematochezia.[459] However, several studies have provided evidence that C. perfringens may be associated with signs of small bowel diarrhea and diffuse disease (of the small and large intestine).[56,485] Severity of disease ranges from a mild, self-limiting diarrhea to a potentially fatal acute hemorrhagic diarrhea with severe inflammation of the intestinal mucosa.[56,386]

Diagnosis

No gold standard exists for confirmation of canine CPAD. Historically, the diagnosis has been contingent on the simultaneous occurrence of "typical" clinical signs, the detection of large numbers of C. perfringens endospores in fecal smears (=3 per high-power field), and the immunodetection of CPE in fecal specimens. The authors discourage the implementation of cytologic methods and emphasize that the optimal diagnostic approach uses a combination of fecal CPE immunodetection and molecular techniques.

Clinical Signs No pathognomonic clinical signs are indicative of CPAD in the dog, and the spectrum of disease attributed to the responsible organism varies greatly. As previously mentioned, CPAD can manifest with small intestinal, large intestinal, or diffuse clinical signs. CPAD should also be considered as a potential cause of acute hemorrhagic diarrhea in dogs. The authors discourage the oversimplistic characterization of CPAD by anatomic localization of clinical signs.

Culture Because C. perfringens is a normal commensal organism of the intestinal microflora, the mere culture of an isolate from the stool is of little diagnostic significance.[289,290,485] In addition, isolation rates for C. perfringens are similar in diarrheic and nondiarrheic dogs. Culture may be useful in procuring isolates for the application of molecular techniques such as

PCR for detection of specific toxin genes or molecular typing of isolated strains to establish clonality in suspected outbreaks.

Fecal Endospores Because sporulation is coregulated with enterotoxin production, fecal endospore counting of Wright- or Gram-stained fecal smears (=3 spores per high-power field) has been suggested as a tool for diagnosing enterotoxigenic CPAD.[178,458] Several studies have reported no association between fecal endospore counts and the presence of diarrhea or between spore counts and the detection of CPE in fecal specimens.[289,290,485] Furthermore, it has been demonstrated that sporulation of enterotoxigenic strains continually occurs in nondiarrheic and diarrheic dogs.[289]

Fecal Enterotoxin Immunodetection Detection of CPE in fecal specimens is the most widely used diagnostic tool for C. perfringens in humans and animals. Two commercially available immunoassays are currently used in veterinary diagnostic laboratories: a reverse passive latex agglutination assay (RPLA PET-RPLA, OXOID, Ogdensburg, N.Y.) and an ELISA (C. perfringens Enterotoxin Test, TECHLAB Inc., Blacksburg, Va.). Commercial veterinary diagnostic laboratories and veterinary institutions have used both assays; however, the performance characteristics for these assays have not been analyzed in the dog, and some concerns have been raised about their sensitivities and specificities. Use of the RPLA has been associated with false-positive results when compared with several different ELISA methods, thus adversely influencing the specificity of the RPLA.[34,308] Sensitivities of immunodetection methods are extremely important considering that disease associated with CPE may depend on the concentration of CPE present within the intestinal lumen. This phenomenon is underscored by the finding that up to 14% of healthy dogs have detectable concentrations of CPE using the qualitative TECHLAB ELISA.[289] In addition, time delays in sample processing can result in false-positive or false-negative results.[286]

Molecular Techniques Analysis of fecal CPE and fecal endospore counts and isolation and PCR detection of enterotoxigenic C. perfringens after a heat shock treatment were performed in 32 diarrheic and 100 nondiarrheic dogs (Fig. 39-10)[289] CPE was detected in fecal specimens via ELISA in 14% of nondiarrheic and 34% of diarrheic dogs. Although this association was significant, the fact that more than half of the ELISA-positive specimens were from nondiarrheic dogs obscures the association. However, fecal specimens from nondiarrheic dogs were far less likely to be positive for both CPE and the cpe gene (4%) than diarrheic dogs (28%).

Therapy

Animals with acute disease (hemorrhagic gastroenteritis) should have appropriate antimicrobial therapy, although antibiotics are commonly administered even in cases of mild or chronic diarrhea. Antibiotics that have been recommended for the treatment of canine CPAD include ampicillin, erythromycin, metronidazole, tylosin, and tetracycline (Table 39-10).[174,458] However, evidence has shown an alarmingly high rate (21%) of in vitro resistance to tetracycline.[287] Most isolates were susceptible to ampicillin, metronidazole, and macrolide antibiotics, although resistant strains were identified. In two dogs, recurrent diarrhea associated with metronidazole-resistant C. perfringens was treated with a prolonged course of oral cephalexin and dietary modification.[483]

Public Health Considerations

Injudicious antibiotic administration to diarrheic animals has likely contributed to the increased prevalence of resistance, which underscores the importance of routine susceptibility screening of bacterial pathogens. Preliminary studies have documented a high prevalence (96%) of isolates that carry a gene encoding an efflux pump for tetracyclines—the *tetA*(P) gene.[233] Tetracycline minimum inhibitory concentrations (MICs) for these isolates ranged from 1 μg/ml to 64 μg/ml. These findings are extremely important in light of the fact that tetracycline has been touted as a drug of choice for the treatment of dogs with suspected CPAD or small intestinal bacterial overgrowth, and subinhibitory concentrations have actually been recommended as a long-term therapeutic approach.[178,458,459] Furthermore, these results raise speculation of the potential for canine commensal *C. perfringens* to serve as a reservoir capable of interspecies and intraspecies transfer of antibiotic resistance genes.[375,402]

Clostridium difficile—Associated Diarrhea
Etiology

The anaerobic, gram-positive, spore-forming bacillus *C. difficile* was first discovered in 1935 and named *"Bacillus difficilis"* because of it was so difficult to culture.[185] The organism was not considered a significant pathogen because it was isolated from the feces of healthy newborns. However, the organism has become recognized as one of the most common causes of human nosocomial infections since the association between *C. difficile* and antibiotic-associated colitis was made in the 1970s.[29,235,256] The role of *C. difficile* has been extensively characterized in people and horses, in which infections vary in severity from asymptomatic (in carriers) to a potentially fatal pseudomembraneous colitis in people and a reported acute necrotizing hemorrhagic enterocolitis in foals.[227,234,235] Three toxins produced by *C. difficile* have been described: toxin A (an enterotoxin), toxin B (a cytotoxin), and *C. difficile* toxin (CDT, an ADP-ribosyltransferase). Diseases associated with *C. difficile* have primarily been attributed to the activity of toxins A and B, and strains have historically been thought to produce both toxins (toxigenic isolates) or neither toxin (nontoxigenic). More reports are being made from human clinical cases of *C. difficile*–associated diarrhea (CDAD) of variant strains isolated that produce only toxin A or toxin B.[2,27,250] The role that *C. difficile* plays in disease in the dog is not as well documented as it is in people and horses, and most of the literature focusing on *C. difficile* in dogs is based on isolation of the organism, which ranges from 0% to 40% in apparently healthy and diarrheic dogs.[289,369,435,485] Despite the lack of difference in isolation rates between healthy and diarrheic dogs, an association has been documented between detection of toxin A or toxin B and canine diarrhea. An outbreak of diarrhea in dogs and cats that was attributed to *C. difficile* occurred in a small animal veterinary teaching hospital.[482] Toxin A or B or both were identified in one or more fecal samples from 52% of the dogs involved.

Fecal carriage of *C. difficile* was found in 9.4% of 245 cats in a teaching hospital, and 8 (38.4%) of these cats harbored toxigenic strains.[280] Toxigenic isolates were identified by toxin A and B gene sequences, and infected cats had risk factors of immunosuppression, concurrent disease, or antibiotic therapy. Four of the cats harboring *C. difficile* had clinical signs of GI disease. No clinically healthy outpatient cats or cats from an SPF colony were found to harbor *C. difficile*. *C difficile* was associated with diarrhea in two cats described in another report.[486]

C. difficile is a significant enteropathogen in human beings and horses, in which infection is most commonly associated

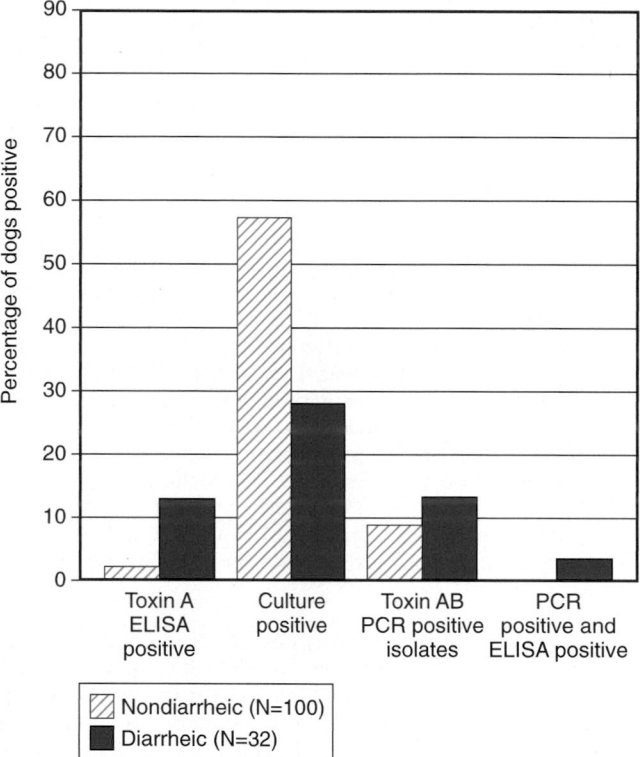

Fig 39-10 Percentage of nondiarrheic and diarrheic dogs positive for *C. perfringens* enterotoxin (CPE) by ELISA, *C. perfringens* culture, and enterotoxigenic *C. perfringens* by PCR. (From Marks SL, Kather EJ, Kass PH, et al. 2002. Genotypic and phenotypic characterization of *Clostridium perfringens* and *Clostridium difficile* in diarrheic and healthy dogs, *J Vet Intern Med* 16:533-540.)

Table • 39-10

Antimicrobial Therapy for Clostridium perfringens—Associated Diarrhea

DRUG[a]	SPECIES	DOSE[b]	ROUTE	INTERVAL (HOURS)[c]	DURATION (DAYS)
Metronidazole	D	10 mg/kg	PO	8—12	5—7
	C	62.5 mg total	PO	12	5—7
Tylosin	B	10—20 mg/kg	PO	12—24	5—7
Ampicillin	B	22 mg/kg	PO	8—12	5—7
Amoxicillin-clavulanate	B	22 mg/kg	PO	12	5—7
Clindamycin	B	10 mg/kg	PO	12	5—7
Tetracycline	D	22 mg/kg	PO	8	5—7

B, Dog and cat; *C,* cat; *D,* dog; *PO,* by mouth.
[a]See Appendix 8 for additional information on selected drugs.
[b]Dose per administration at specified interval.
[c]For chronic recurring signs, animals may be treated at the indicated dose every 12 to 24 hours.

with a disruption of the normal microflora followed by colonization with toxigenic strains. The role that *C. difficile* plays in dogs and cats is not well defined. Table 39-11 summarizes the current available information about CDAD in dogs.

Pathogenesis

In one hypothesis of the pathogenesis of *C. difficile* infection, hospitalized human patients are intermittently exposed to *C. difficile* but do not become susceptible to infection until after receiving antimicrobial therapy.[222] At that point, infection occurs, resulting in a clinically evident or subclinical colonization. If asymptomatic colonization occurs, the patient is at decreased risk of developing CDAD. Antibiotic administration, especially in hospital environments, is the most commonly reported predisposing factor for the development of CDAD in people and horses,[31,44,235] although some reports have been made of CDAD developing in the absence of antibiotic administration.[203,228] Although any antimicrobial can predispose an individual to CDAD, cephalosporins, penicillins, and clindamycin are most commonly incriminated. In contrast, administration of antibiotics does not appear to predispose dogs to CDAD.[56,289,485]

Toxins A and B Toxins A and B are the principal virulence factors thought to be involved in the pathogenesis of CDAD. The genes encoding these two toxins have been sequenced; together with three accessory genes, they form an approximately 19.6-kb pathogenicity locus, which is found only in toxigenic strains.[186] The mechanism of action for both toxins involves inactivation of Rho proteins by glucosylation, thereby causing the depolymerization of actin filaments, disruption of the cytoskeleton, cell rounding, and cell death.[203,231] Toxin A has been shown to induce histologic damage with hemorrhagic necrosis of the mucosa as well as hemorrhagic secretion in small intestinal loops of rabbits, hamsters, and mice.[277,304] Administration of toxin A to rabbit colonic loops produces similar histologic damage as that seen in toxin A–treated ileum but with less hemorrhage and cellular infiltration.[304] In contrast, no tissue damage or fluid secretion is seen in toxin B–treated intestinal loops, although it is cytotoxic for in vitro cell lines.[272,277] However, several studies suggest that toxins A and B may have a synergistic effect, with mucosal damage caused by toxin A enabling cytotoxic activity of toxin B.[277,304] The effects of both toxins have been shown to be dose and species dependent, with certain animal species appearing to be more sensitive to the cytopathic effects of the toxins. No studies have evaluated the sensitivity of canine intestinal epithelia to either toxin A or B. In addition the effects of toxins A and B appear to be age dependent in people; high levels of toxins are detected in the feces of neonates in the absence of clinical signs of disease.[271,472] This phenomenon may also occur in dogs. Toxigenic *C. difficile* can be isolated from up to 94% of neonatal dogs in the absence of clinical signs of disease.[351] The traditional view that pathogenic strains of *C. difficile* always produce toxins A and B is now being questioned because of additional reports of toxin A-negative, toxin B-positive strains that have been isolated from clinical *C. difficile* cases.[2,4,250,356] No toxin variant strains have been reported in canine isolates.

ADP-Ribosyltransferase CDT The *C. difficile* ADP-ribosyltransferase is a binary toxin consisting of two independently coded protein components: a binding component (CDTb) and an enzymatic component (CDTa), which catalyzes the ADP-ribosylation of monomeric actin, inducing alterations in the cytoskeleton.[179,359] All *C. difficile* strains that harbor the CDTa and CDTb genes also contain some part of the pathogenicity locus containing the toxin A and B genes.[436] As a result the role that CDT-producing (binary) strains play in human and equine CDADs is still unclear. The prevalence of binary-positive strains isolated from clinically affected patients has been reported to be between 6% and 13% for human strains and 24% for equine strains.[41,348,346] CDT-positive *C. difficile* strains have not been found in any canine isolates.[41]

Clinical Findings

Dogs Clinical signs that have been associated with canine CDAD range from asymptomatic carriage to a potentially fatal acute hemorrhagic diarrheal syndrome.[56,289] As with *C. perfringens*, no specific anatomic localization of clinical signs seems to exist, and studies have shown that dogs with suspected CDAD commonly have signs of small and large intestinal diarrhea as well as diffuse disease characterized by concurrent involvement of the small and large intestine.[56,289,485]

Cats An acute onset of anorexia and watery diarrhea was the predominant clinical feature in six reported clinically ill infected cats.[280,486] One cat had vomiting, fever (40.5° C [104.9° F]), and abdominal discomfort.

Diagnosis

Culture As with *C. perfringens*, isolation of *C. difficile* from diarrheic specimens is of little diagnostic value, because isolation rates in nondiarrheic and diarrheic dogs are similar (0% to 40%).[289,435,485] Culture may be useful for procuring strains for detection of toxin genes and typing.

Fecal Toxin Detection Only a few studies evaluate the presence of toxins in diarrheic and nondiarrheic animals. In addition, no consensus has been formed among veterinary diagnostic laboratories regarding diagnosis of CDAD in the dog. The current gold standard assay is the cell culture cytotoxicity assay, which detects toxin B activity; however, this assay is expensive and requires up to 48 hours for confirmation of a negative result.[255] Routine diagnosis of CDAD has been made based on positive fecal assays for toxins A or B.[107,235] Currently, several commercially immunoassays are available for detection of *C. difficile* toxin A or toxins A and B in fecal specimens. Because of increasing numbers of reports of toxin A-negative, toxin B-positive strains isolated from clinical cases, the use of ELISA kits that detect both toxins is gaining preference. However, none of the commercial ELISA kits have been validated in the dog, and no standard assay is used by veterinary diagnostic labs. This is concerning given the wide range of specificities (66% to 100%) and sensitivities (33% to 95%) that have been reported for many of the kits when analyzed for human fecal toxin detection.[5,255,329] In addition, serious concerns have been raised about the specificities

---

Table • 39-11

Summary of Clostridium difficile–Associated Diarrhea in Dogs

- CDAD is not limited to clinical signs of colitis.
- The lack of a standardized diagnostic assay makes interpretation of positive fecal toxin assays difficult. Although toxin A-negative, toxin B-positive strains have not been isolated from dogs, the potential role of these toxin-variant strains cannot be dismissed.
- The implementation of PCR for detection of toxin A or B genes in diarrheic fecal specimens combined with fecal ELISA tests for detection of toxins A and B should be used for diagnosing canine CDAD.
- Information concerning CDAD in cats is limited, although the responsible bacterium has been isolated from a higher percentage of cats with diarrhea.

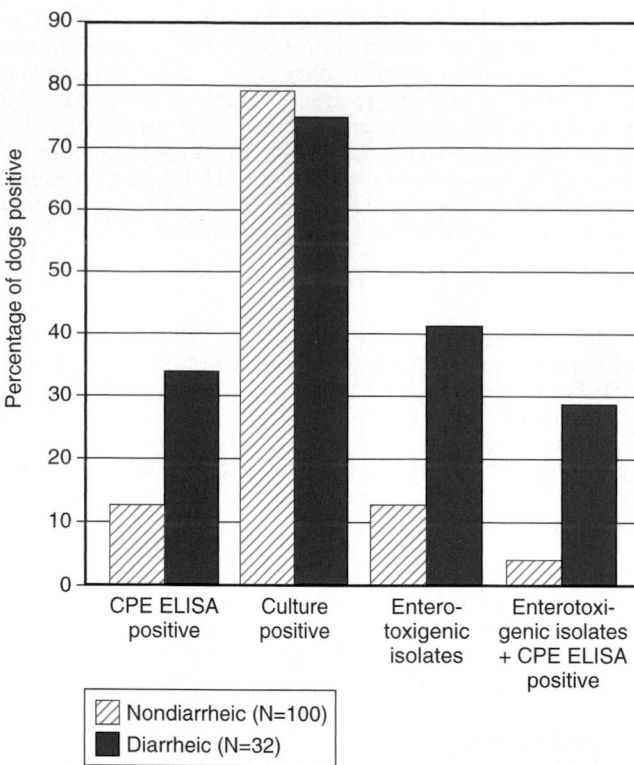

Fig 39-11 Percentage of nondiarrheic and diarrheic dogs positive for *C. difficile* toxin A by ELISA, *C. difficile* culture, and toxigenic *C. difficile*. (From Marks SL, Kather EJ, Kass PH, et al. 2002. Genotypic and phenotypic characterization of *Clostridium perfringens* and *Clostridium difficile* in diarrheic and healthy dogs, *J Vet Intern Med* 16:533-540.)

of a relatively new assay (*C. DIFFICILE* TOX A/B II, TECHLAB, Blacksburg, Va.) because of a high number of toxin-positive, culture-negative results from fresh canine fecal specimens, despite cultures being processed in an anaerobic chamber.[485] The TOX A/B ELISA kit used for dogs was also used in the diagnosis of *C. difficile* infection in two cats.[486] This kit has not been validated for use in testing feline feces. It must be evaluated to ensure that no species-specific differences could affect the test results.[486]

Molecular Techniques The detection rates of toxigenic *C. difficile* strains after culture is similar in diarrheic and nondiarrheic dogs (Fig. 39-11), decreasing the diagnostic value of more isolation from dogs. In addition, isolation of the organism is difficult, costly, and time consuming. Nevertheless, studies in human beings have begun bypassing culture of the organism and directly determining the presence of specific toxin genes in DNA obtained from fecal specimens. Sensitivities of PCR detection methods used in people have been reported to be between 96% and 100%, compared with the less effective cytotoxicity assay.[180,496] Although most commercial veterinary diagnostic laboratories do not currently offer PCR as a diagnostic test for CDAD, these techniques may be beneficial, especially considering the potential false-positive ELISA results for detection of toxins A or B. In cats with *C. difficile* infections, PCR was used to detect gene sequences for toxin A and B. In addition, DNA analysis has been used to classify individual isolates.

Therapy

Metronidazole is the drug of choice for treatment of dogs suspected to have CDAD. Although metronidazole-resistant *C.*

difficile isolates obtained from foals and adult horses have been reported, a study evaluating the in vitro susceptibilities of 70 canine *C. difficile* isolates did not demonstrate any evidence of resistance to metronidazole.[287] The second drug of choice for humans and occasionally horses is vancomycin; however, it is used only in cases of unresponsive CDAD or when metronidazole-resistant strains have been found. In a study of 70 fecal isolates from dogs, all isolates had MICs of 1 μg/ml for metronidazole and vancomycin.[287] Diarrheic cats harboring toxigenic strains of *C. difficile* have responded to metronidazole treatment.[280,486]

Prevention

Should CDAD be identified, infection control measures should be implemented to restrict contamination through the environment. Affected animals must be quarantined and barrier precautions must be taken (e.g., wearing gowns, gloves, and overboots) by personnel when handling these animals. Housing areas should be decontaminated with dilute (10%) bleach, and disinfectant footbaths should be placed at the entrance to these areas. Common exercise areas are considered a potential source of contamination.

Public Health Considerations

Although animal reservoirs of *C. difficile* infection exist for humans, the incidence of community-acquired CDAD in people is low. In contrast, nosocomial infection in hospitalized humans receiving antimicrobial therapy is high.[222] Pseudomembranous colitis, now known to be caused by *C. difficile*, is a toxin-mediated infection that is predisposed by immunosuppression or an imbalance in the intestinal microflora.

SUGGESTED READINGS*

118. Foley JE, Orgad U, Hirsh DC, et al. 1999b. Outbreak of fatal salmonellosis in cats following use of a high-titer modified-live panleukopenia virus vaccine, *J Am Vet Med Assoc* 214:67-70.

127. Fox JG. 2002. The non-*H. pylori* helicobacters: their expanding role in gastrointestinal and systemic diseases, *Gut* 50:273-283.

193. Happonen I, Linden J, Westermarck E. 2000. Effect of triple therapy on eradication of canine gastric helicobacters and gastric disease, *J Small Anim Pract* 41:1-6.

287. Marks SL, Kather EJ. 2003a. Antimicrobial susceptibilities of canine *Clostridium difficile* and *Clostridium perfringens* isolates to commonly utilized antimicrobial drugs, *Vet Microbiol* 94:39-45.

366. Randall LP, Cooles SW, Osborn MK, et al. 2004. Antibiotic resistance genes, integrons and multiple antibiotic resistance in thirty-five serotypes of *Salmonella enterica* isolated from humans and animals in the UK, *J Antimicrob Chemother* 53:208-216.

404. Simpson K, Neiger R, DeNovo R, et al. 2000a. The relationship of *Helicobacter* spp. infection to gastric disease in dogs and cats, *J Vet Intern Med* 14:223-227.

428. Stiver SL, Frazier KS, Mauel MJ, et al. 2003. Septicemic salmonellosis in two cats fed a raw-meat diet, *J Am Anim Hosp Assoc* 39:538-542.

442. Tauni MA, Österlund A. 2000. Outbreak of *Salmonella typhimurium* in cats and humans associated with infection in wild birds, *J Small Anim Pract* 41:339-341.

485. Weese JS, Staempfli HR, Prescott JF, et al. 2001b. The roles of *Clostridium difficile* and enterotoxigenic *Clostridium perfringens* in diarrhea in dogs, *J Vet Intern Med* 15:374-378.

*See the CD-ROM for a complete list of references.

486. Weese JS, Weese HE, Bourdeau TL, et al. 2001c. Suspected *Clostridium difficile*-associated diarrhea in two cats, *J Am Vet Med Assoc* 218:1436-1439.

491. Wibbelt G, Kelly DF. 2001. Sudden death in a Rottweiler puppy with myocardial yersiniosis, *Eur J Vet Pathol* 7:135-137.

497. Wolfs TFW, Duim B, Geelen SPM, et al. 2001. Neonatal sepsis in *Campylobacter jejuni*: genetically proven transmission from a household puppy, *Clin Infect Dis* 32:849, 97-99.

503. Young JK, Baher DC, Burney DP. 1995. Naturally occurring Tyzzer's disease in a puppy, *Vet Pathol* 32:63-65.

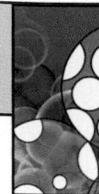

CHAPTER • 40

Canine Brucellosis

Craig E. Greene and Leland E. Carmichael

ETIOLOGY AND EPIDEMIOLOGY

Brucella canis is a small (1.0 to 1.5 μm), gram-negative, aerobic, coccobacillary organism. Its rough colonial morphology and differences in biochemical and antigenic reactions distinguish it from other members of the genus *Brucella*. Unlike the smooth Brucella organisms that infect several domestic animal species, *B. canis* has a limited host range; only dogs and wild *Canidae* have been found to be susceptible. Cats can be infected experimentally, having a transient bacteremia, but are relatively resistant. Rabbits and nonhuman primates also have been found to be susceptible to experimental infections. No other animal species has developed significant agglutination titers. Human cases have been reported as a result of laboratory accidents and contact with infected dogs, but people appear to be relatively resistant (see Public Health Considerations).

The *Brucella* genus is composed of six classical species based primarily on host preference: *Brucella abortus* (cattle), *Brucella canis* (dogs), *Brucella melitensis* (goats, sheep), *Brucella neotomae* (rodents), *Brucella ovis* (sheep), and *Brucella suis* and its biovars (pigs, cattle, hares, rodents, and wild ungulates). Novel *Brucella* (*Brucella maris*) have been isolated from cetaceans and pinnipeds[14]; however, the isolates appear to uniquely infect marine mammals. Dogs also are susceptible to infection with *B. abortus*[7,29,67] and *B. suis*.[11] Even attenuated vaccine strains of *B. abortus* can infect dogs.[61] Natural infection is thought to occur after ingestion of contaminated placentas and aborted fetuses from livestock. Dogs usually harbor the organisms in the lymph nodes of the gastrointestinal tract for extended periods. Dogs are not believed to be important in the spread and maintenance of these infections. Testing and removal of affected dogs from infected farms are the optimal preventive measures for eradication.

B. canis infects a susceptible host by penetrating the mucous membranes, especially those of the oral cavity, vagina, and conjunctiva. The minimum oral infectious dose for dogs is approximately 10^6 bacteria, and the conjunctival dose is 10^4 to 10^5 organisms. Because they contain the highest concentration of organisms, vaginal discharges and semen are the most likely sources for infection by mucosal contamination.

Natural transmission of canine brucellosis occurs by several routes. Infected female dogs transmit *B. canis* during estrus, at breeding, or after abortion through oronasal contact with vaginal discharges. Transmission is most common by oronasal contact with aborted materials because they contain up to 10^{10} organisms/ml. Shedding of *B. canis* may occur for periods up to 6 weeks after an abortion. Milk of infected bitches contains lower concentrations of organisms and appears to be less important in transmitting infection to surviving pups; most have already been infected in utero or congenitally.

Seminal fluid and urine have been incriminated as sources of infection from male dogs that harbor the organisms in their prostates and epididymides. The rate of isolation of *B. canis* from the semen of infected dogs is usually high for the first 6 to 8 weeks postinoculation (PI). Intermittent shedding of the organism in low numbers has been noted for up to 60 weeks PI and may continue for at least 2 years. Urinary excretion begins a few weeks after the onset of bacteremia and continues for at least 3 months. Concentrations of 10^3 to 10^6 organisms/ml of urine have been found in male dogs, with lesser numbers of bacteria in the urine of females. At one time, urine of infected males was thought to contain too few organisms to be infectious by the oronasal route; however, studies have demonstrated that *B. canis* can be transmitted from infected to uninfected mature male dogs after several weeks or months of close contact.[18,69] The propensity of males to shed the organism in the urine is probably related to its localization in the prostate and epididymis, which are in close association with the urinary bladder. Neutering helps reduce this risk to a large extent.

Alternative means of transmission occur less frequently under natural circumstances. Transmission via fomites has been reported after vaginoscopy, blood transfusion, artificial insemination, and use of contaminated syringes. *B. canis* is relatively short lived outside the dog and is readily inactivated by common disinfectants.

The prevalence of infection varies according to the animal's age, housing conditions, breed, and geographic location. Pet dogs in suburban environments have a lower prevalence compared with stray dogs in economically depressed areas, which may reflect increased population density and uncontrolled breeding of dogs. A relatively low prevalence has been reported in the United States and Japan (range, 1% to 18%) compared with rates as high as 28% in Mexico and Peru.[15] The southern United States appears to have a relatively higher (approximately 8%) prevalence of infection. Among breeds in this region, beagles and Labrador retrievers have a higher prevalence of infection as do feral dogs. Determination of seroprevalence is strongly influenced by the means of testing and interpretation. Cases have also been identified in other countries in Central and South America and in Germany, Spain, Czechoslovakia, and Tunisia.[20] The disease also appears to be prevalent in regions of the People's Republic of China.[36]

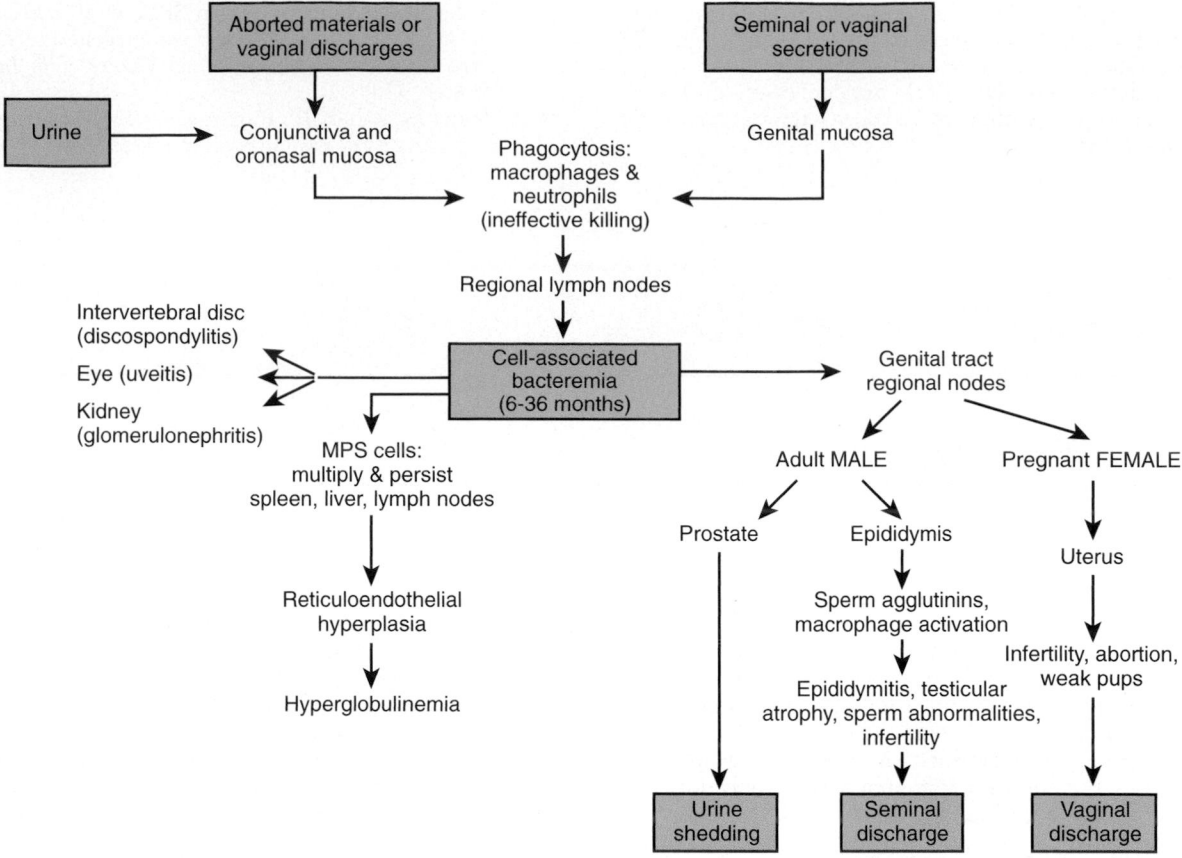

Fig   40-1   Sequential pathogenesis of canine brucellosis.

Given the insidious nature of *B. canis* in dogs, isolated infections have been found in imported dogs, even in countries such as the United Kingdom, where quarantine standards are very stringent.[26]

PATHOGENESIS

The general sequence of events after infection by *Brucella* is summarized in Fig. 40-1. The bacteria are probably phagocytized at contaminated mucosal sites by tissue macrophages and other phagocytic cells and transported to lymphatic and genital tract tissues where they multiply. They persist intracellularly within mononuclear phagocytes.[64] Brucellae evade phago-lysosome fusion and replicate in a compartment within the cell's endoplasmic reticulum.[25] A leukocyte-associated bacteremia occurs beginning 1 to 4 weeks PI and can last 6 to 64 months. Generalized lymphoreticular hyperplasia (Fig. 40-2) and development of hyperglobulinemia occur during the course of infection. As with other intracellular parasites, cell-mediated immunity is probably the most important defense mechanism against *B. canis*. Studies in people have indicated decreased T-lymphocyte responsiveness to *Brucella* cytoplasmic proteins in more chronic infections.[32] Persistent nonprotective antibody titers are characteristic of such infections and appear to have little influence on the level of bacteremia or number of organisms in tissues. The greatest numbers of *B. canis* organisms are found in the lymph nodes, spleen, and tissues of gonadal steroid dependency. Although usually confined to mononuclear phagocytes, they may enter other cells such as placental epithelium. In fact, the uterus is not a favored site of growth in the nongravid or diestrual female. Inflammation of the epididymides and testes in males causes sperm leakage, which provokes the immune system to

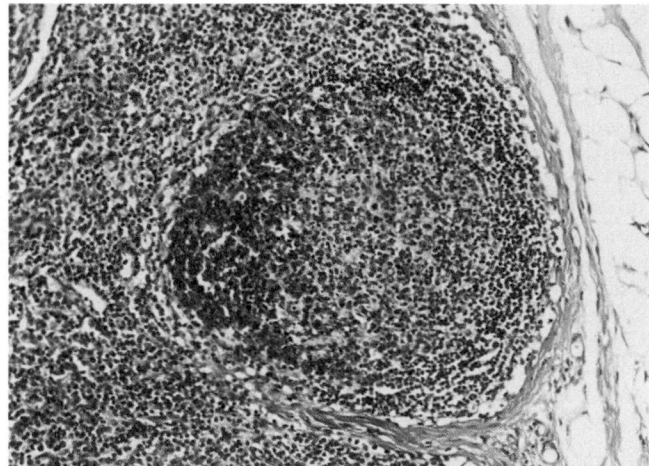

Fig   40-2   Follicular hyperplasia in the lymph node from a dog with chronic *B. canis* infection (H and E stain, × 40).

produce a complex of antisperm agglutinating antibodies and delayed-type hypersensitivity reactions against sperm that are unrelated to the antibodies against *B. canis*. The immune responses produced against spermatozoa contribute to the epididymitis, infertility, and eventual spermatogenic arrest seen in most infected male dogs.

B. canis, similar to other blood-borne bacteria, may localize in nonreproductive tissues such as the endarterial circulation of the intervertebral disk, causing diskospondylitis. Other tissues that filter blood-borne organisms or immune complexes may become involved, including the eye (anterior uveitis), kidney (glomerulopathy), and meninges (meningoencephalitis).

Spontaneous recovery from infection may occur within 1 to more than 5 years PI. Therapy accelerates the recovery process. Some dogs may have persistent bacteremia throughout this time, whereas others can harbor bacteria in tissues for several months after the bacteremia ceases. The prostate gland may be a site of this persistence in male dogs. Despite tissue persistence, when *B. canis* is no longer detected in the blood, serum agglutination titers decrease.

Dogs that recover naturally have low or negative agglutination titers and yet are immune to reinfection, suggesting that protective immunity is cell mediated. Recovered dogs that were challenged orally or intravenously as long as 4 years after spontaneous recovery from experimental infection were completely immune.[55] However, chronically infected dogs that were successfully treated with antibiotics were found to be fully susceptible to oronasal challenge 12 weeks after treatment had been halted. Natural recovery from *B. canis* infection appears to be a requirement to sustain protective immunity. Immunosuppression with glucocorticoids and antilymphocyte serum appears to increase the susceptibility of dogs to initial infection, but it does not augment the severity of the disease or alter the course of infection in experimentally infected dogs.

CLINICAL FINDINGS

Despite generalized systemic infection with *B. canis*, adult dogs rarely are seriously ill. Fever is uncommon and, with the exception of males who commonly have epididymitis, most infections will not be diagnosed by routine history or physical examination. Owners of working dogs have occasionally reported dry, lusterless coats, loss of vigor, and decreased exercise tolerance. Nongravid females show no signs of illness other than lymphadenomegaly, which occurs in both sexes.

Overt clinical signs usually involve reproductive disturbances in sexually mature animals. Bitches usually abort dead pups between 45 and 60 days of gestation but show no other clinical signs. Pups are usually partially autolyzed, with subcutaneous edema and congestion and hemorrhage of the abdominal subcutaneous region (Fig. 40-3). Moderate quantities of serosanguineous peritoneal effusions are found. Their appearance suggests fetal death in utero some time before abortion. Decomposed fetuses are not usually found because the bitch ingests them. Abortion is characterized by a brown or greenish-gray vaginal discharge that lasts for 1 to 6 weeks. Brucellosis should be suspected under any circumstance when apparently healthy bitches abort 2 weeks before term.

Although abortion of dead puppies is the primary clinical sign reported with brucellosis, conception failures could occur at any time after breeding. In utero death with fetal resorption or abortion and ingestion of fetuses may be suspected if a bitch fails to conceive after an apparently successful mating. Embryonic death may occur as early as 20 days after mating, although most conception failures are actually undetected abortions. Less commonly, bitches may carry infected puppies to term and whelp both live and dead puppies within a single litter. Most pups that are born alive will die within a few hours or days, but those that survive or that are infected as neonates usually have generalized peripheral lymphadenomegaly as the primary clinical manifestation of disease until they reach sexual maturity. Such puppies usually have persistent hyperglobulinemia (Fig. 40-4), and some may have transient fever, leukocytosis, or seizures as the systemic manifestations of their infections.

As with brucellosis in other species, infections with *B. canis* do not interfere with normal estrous cycles. A high proportion of bitches that abort may have normal litters subsequently. However, even after having normal litters, some infected bitches experience intermittent reproductive failures.

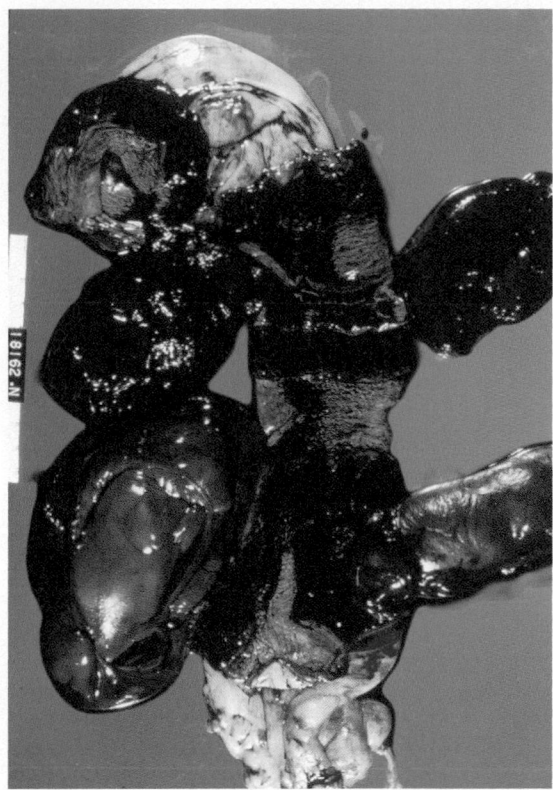

Fig 40-3 Partially autolyzed fetuses with placenta and uterus from a dog infected with *B. canis* that was neutered at 45 days gestation. (Courtesy University of Georgia, Athens, Ga.)

Because of the prominent testicular abnormalities, male dogs are presented for examination more often than are females, even though impairment of male reproductive performance often is less noticed. Nevertheless, infertility occurs. Males appear to be in good health but may have an enlarged scrotum because of accumulation of serosanguineous fluid in the tunica. Scrotal dermatitis is the result of constant licking and secondary infection with nonhemolytic staphylococci (Fig. 40-5). A major cause of testicular swelling is enlargement of the tail of the epididymis (Fig. 40-6); orchitis and primary testicular enlargement are rarely apparent. In fact, chronically infected males usually develop unilateral or bilateral testicular atrophy. A decreased volume of ejaculate without loss of libido is usually present. Acute pain is not usually evident on scrotal or testicular palpation, but discomfort may be seen at the time of ejaculation.

Nonreproductive abnormalities can also occur. Splenomegaly may accompany the diffuse lymphadenomegaly in some dogs. Dogs with diskospondylitis initially experience spinal pain and later paresis and ataxia if spinal cord compression develops (Fig. 40-7). Osteomyelitis or polyarthritis of the appendicular skeleton causes lameness of the affected limb. Meningoencephalitis has been reported after experimental and natural infections; however, neurobrucellosis in dogs, as in people, is uncommon.[53] The author has observed that a male dog with confirmed *B. canis* infection had behavioral changes, anisocoria, ataxia, hyperesthesia, head tilt, and circling. Neurologic signs began within 3 weeks after the dog's first breeding. Chronic multifocal pyogranulomatous dermatitis that resembled lick granuloma lesions has also been reported in an infected dog, but a direct causal relationship was not established. Ocular lesions include anterior uveitis, secondary glaucoma, hyphema, retinal detachment, chorioretinitis, optic neuritis vitreal haze, enophthalmitis with sec-

Fig 40-4 Electrophoretic pattern of serum proteins in a dog with a wide-based hyperglobulinemia from chronic *B. canis* infection. (Courtesy University of Georgia, Athens, Ga.)

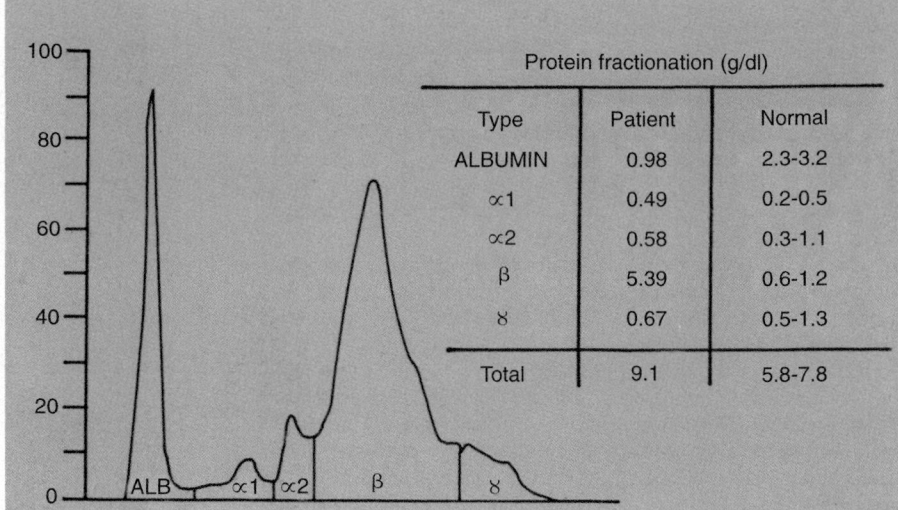

Protein fractionation (g/dl)

Type	Patient	Normal
ALBUMIN	0.98	2.3-3.2
α1	0.49	0.2-0.5
α2	0.58	0.3-1.1
β	5.39	0.6-1.2
ɣ	0.67	0.5-1.3
Total	9.1	5.8-7.8

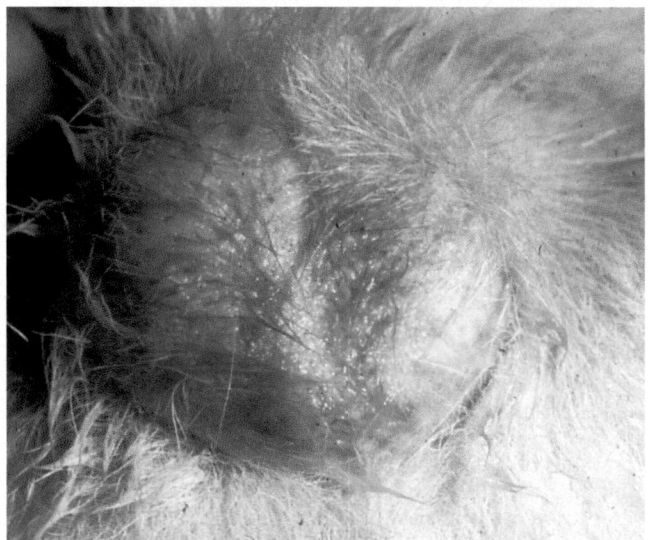

Fig 40-5 Testicular enlargement and scrotal dermatitis in an experimentally infected dog 35 weeks PI. (Courtesy Leland Carmichael, Cornell University, Ithaca, N.Y.)

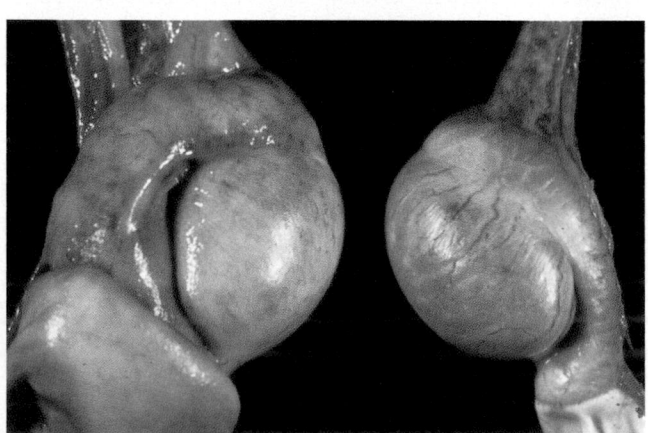

Fig 40-6 Enlargement of the tail of the epididymis on the testicle from an experimentally infected dog 60 weeks PI as compared to that of a noninfected dog. (Courtesy Leland Carmichael, Cornell University, Ithaca, N.Y.)

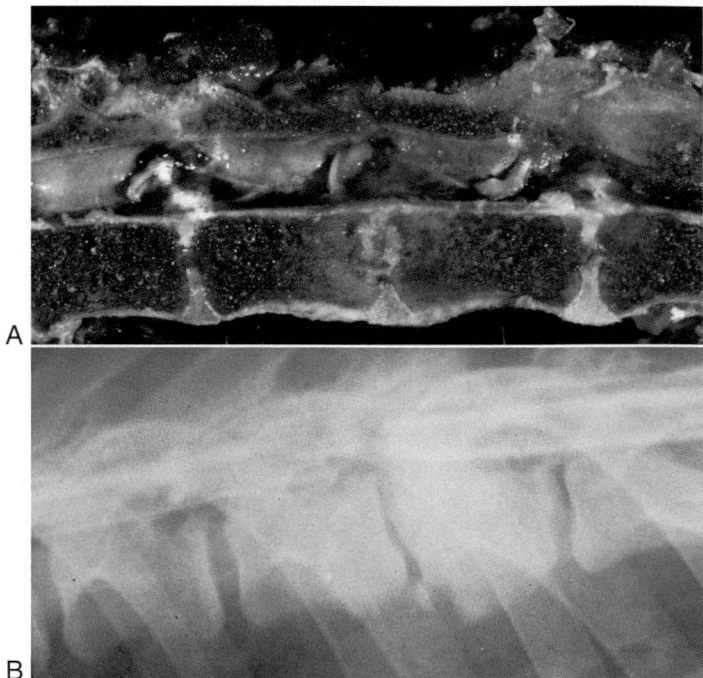

Fig 40-7 **A,** Sagittal section of the spinal canal of a dog with diskospondylitis. Lytic bone is evident at the vertebral interspace. **B,** Myelogram of a dog with diskospondylitis showing thoracic and abdominal hyperesthesia and pelvic limb paralysis. Note obstruction of the flow of radiographic contrast medium over the affected disc space. (Courtesy University of Georgia, Athens, Ga.)

ondary glaucoma or phthisis bulbi, and corneal edema with opacification (Fig. 40-8).[76] The author has observed residual chorioretinal lesions following treatment of dogs with uveitis. See Chapter 93 for a review of ocular brucellosis.

DIAGNOSIS

Clinical Laboratory Findings

Hematologic and biochemical values are either unaltered or nonspecific in canine brucellosis. Hyperglobulinemia (β and γ) with concomitant hypoalbuminemia has been the most consis-

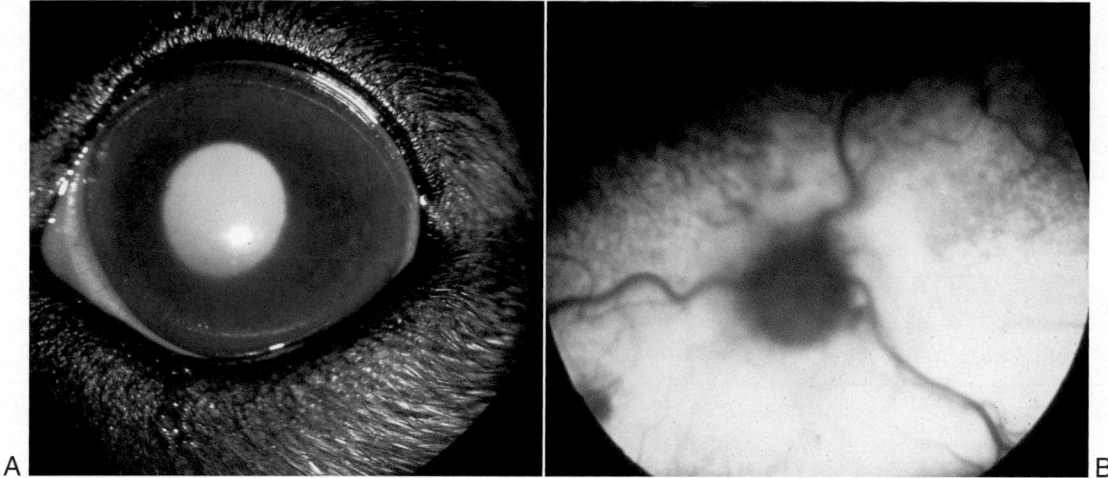

Fig 40-8 A, Uveitis and healed (B) chorioretinal lesions *(arrows)* from a dog with brucellosis. (Courtesy Leland Carmichael, Cornell University, Ithaca, N.Y. [A] and University of Georgia, Athens Ga [B].)

tent finding in chronically infected dogs. An increased incidence of positive Coombs' test findings in the absence of anemia has been reported. Examination of aspirates or biopsy samples from enlarged lymph nodes usually reveals lymphoid hyperplasia with large numbers of plasma cells. Cerebrospinal fluid analysis results are pleocytosis, primarily consisting of neutrophils, and increased protein concentration with meningoencephalitis, but they are unremarkable when diskospondylitis alone is present. Urinalysis is usually normal despite the variable presence of bacteriuria. Radiographic demonstration of intervertebral disk infection should always be followed by serologic testing and, when possible, bacteriologic confirmation of *B. canis*. Radiographic changes of diskospondylitis may be difficult to visualize in the first weeks of infection because brucellar spondylitis is a slow process. Brucellar diskospondylitis can be unifocal or multifocal. The infection centers on the disk space; vertebral architecture is usually preserved, and minimal adjacent spinal soft-tissue involvement is typical. Radionuclide scintigraphy is a sensitive way of detecting inflammatory alterations in the bone, and additional imaging modalities such as computed tomography or magnetic resonance imaging may also be helpful.

Semen Examination
Semen abnormalities, evident by 5 weeks PI, become pronounced by 8 weeks PI. Abnormalities include immature sperm, deformed acrosomes, swollen midpieces, and retained protoplasmic droplets. By week 15 PI, bent tails, detached heads, and head-to-head agglutination is seen. Large aggregates of inflammatory cells, usually consisting of neutrophils, surround adherent macrophages containing phagocytized sperm (Fig. 40-9). More than 90% of the sperm are abnormal by 20 weeks PI. Aspermia without inflammatory cells corresponds with the development of bilateral testicular atrophy. Semen morphology should always be evaluated in dogs with infertility because of the obvious abnormalities that occur with brucellosis.

Serologic Testing
Serologic testing is the most frequently used diagnostic method for detecting canine brucellosis. These tests are subject to considerable interpretive error because lipopolysaccharide (LPS) antigens of several bacterial species cross-react with *B. canis*.[49,51] The problem of false-positive cross-reactions therefore is more common than that of

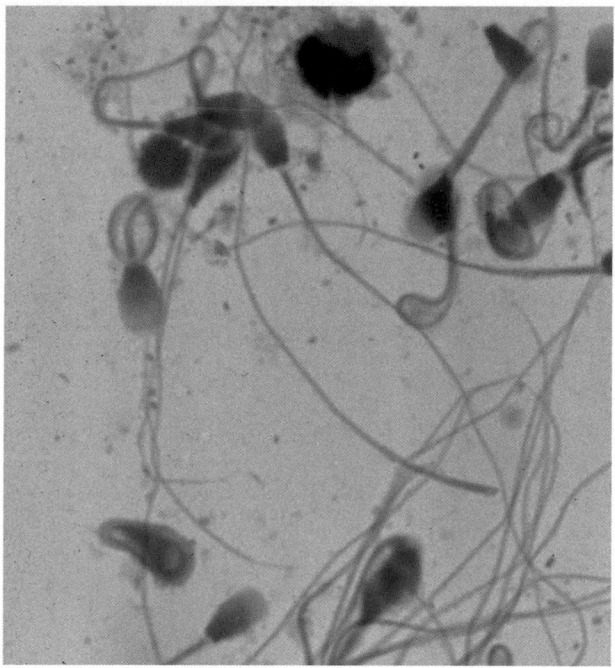

Fig 40-9 Stained smear of semen sample from a dog 35 weeks PI. Sperm abnormalities are present. (Courtesy Leland Carmichael, Cornell University, Ithaca, N.Y.)

false-negative reactions. All sera should be free of hemolysis because hemoglobin causes false-positive agglutination of the tube test antigen.

Serologic test results often are negative during the first 3 to 4 weeks PI despite the presence of bacteremia by 2 weeks PI. For this reason, newly acquired animals should be tested sequentially at least twice at 30-day intervals before introduction into a breeding kennel. Titers by any method are usually positive by 8 to 12 weeks after infection. Low or intermediate titers may mean previous disease or very recent infection, and testing should be repeated or attempts made to isolate the organism by hemoculture. Male dogs may harbor the organism in the prostate glands and epididymides for extended periods after bacteremia ceases and agglutination titers have declined. Serologic titers may remain positive for up to 36 months in some dogs after they become abacteremic.

Chronically infected female dogs may have diagnostically equivocal antibody titers and negative blood cultures. In females, recrudescence of bacteremia and increased antibody titers develop during proestrus, estrus, pregnancy, or abortion. These times are the most reliable to screen female dogs for infection.

Antibiotic therapy may suppress bacteremia and the associated serologic response, possibly contributing to false-negative serology and failure to isolate the organism from infected dogs. Antibacterials should not be given until diagnostic tests have been completed. Tetracycline drugs cause a bacteremia and a corresponding decrease in antibody titer that may rebound after treatment is discontinued because tetracyclines are not bacteriocidal.

Table • 40-1

Comparison of Serologic Procedures for Canine Brucellosis

SEROLOGIC TEST	ANTIGEN USED	EARLIEST TITER[a] (WEEKS PI)	ADVANTAGES	DISADVANTAGES
Antibody Detection Methods				
Mercaptoethanol (ME) rapid slide agglutination test (ME-RSAT)	Cell wall	3—4	Quick, high sensitivity, few (1%) false-negative results	False-positive results common; must confirm by other tests
Tube agglutination test (TAT)	Cell wall	3—6	Semiquantitative determination	False-positive results similar to RSAT
ME-TAT	Cell wall	5—8	Same at TAT, somewhat increased specificity	Longer to get positive titer compared with TAT
Agar-gel immunodiffusion (AGID) cell wall (somatic) antigen	Cell wall (LPS)	5—10	Very sensitive, positive earlier than with CPAg	Procedure and interpretation complex, nonspecific reactions
Internal cytoplasmic protein antigen (CPAg)-AGID	CPAg	8—12	Most specific (confirmatory) test, detects chronic cases when other tests have negative results; detects infections by other *Brucella* species	Complex procedure, least sensitive for initial screening, variable duration of time with positive result; may stay positive for up to 1 year after recovery from infection
Indirect FA	Cell wall (LPS)	Unknown	Available and convenient for diagnostic laboratories	May be less sensitive than ME-TAT as screening test; not extensively evaluated
ELISA	Cell wall (LPS) or CPAg	Unknown	Good results with mutant (M-) *B. canis* for cell wall extracts, or *B. abortus* for CPAg	Antigen purity and preparation critical
Organism Detection Methods				
Blood culture	Not applicable	2—4	A positive result is confirmed infection	False-negative results possible
PCR	Not applicable	2—4	Rapid results, a positive results indicates infection if specific primers are used and contamination is excluded	False-positive results possible with contamination and false-negative results with inadequate extraction methods

FA, Fluorescent antibody; *ELISA*, enzyme-linked immunosorbent assay; *PCR*, polymerase chain reaction.
[a]First significant titer to appear. Data based on adult dog.

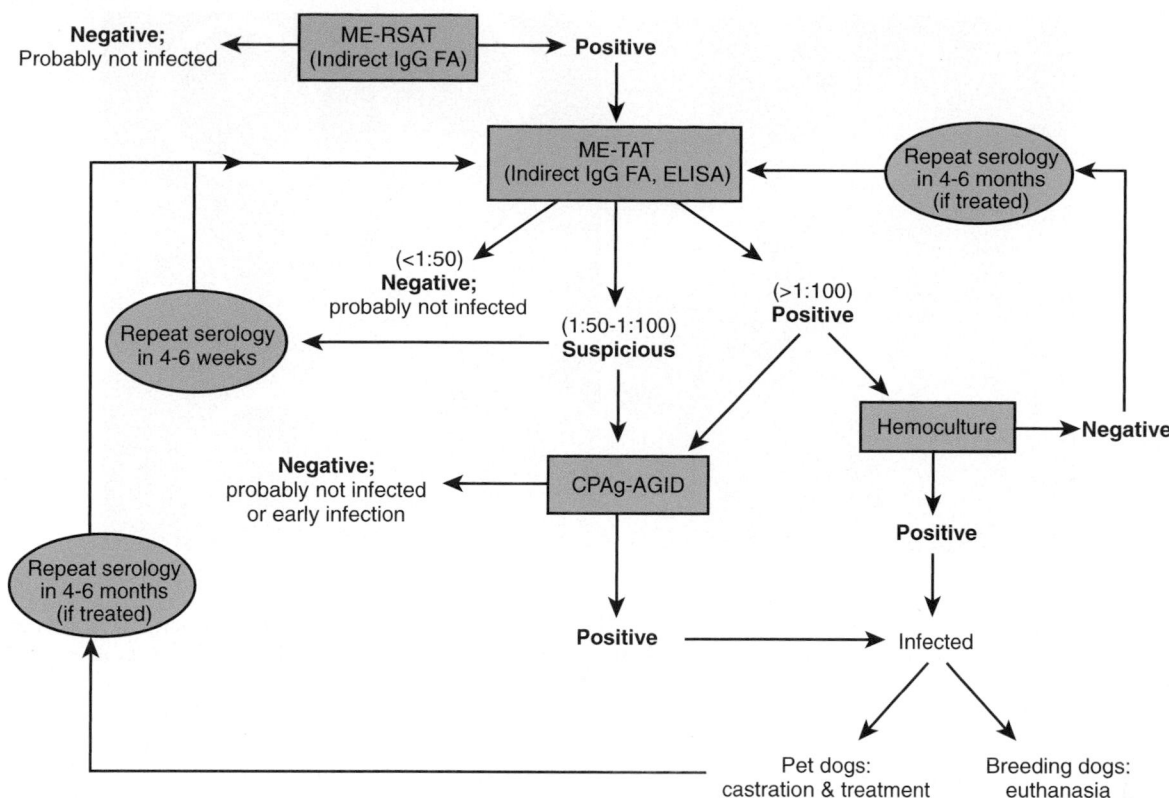

Fig 40-10 Diagnostic algorithm for canine brucellosis. The indirect FA and ELISA tests are being used more as screening tests because of unavailability of ME-RSAT and ME-TAT test antigens (see text). Titer is equal to numeral of the dilution ratio following the colon.

Table 40-1 compares the serologic tests described next. Consult Appendices 5 and 6 for information concerning commercially available testing. Serologic tests should be evaluated in light of clinical findings in the dog being evaluated (Fig. 40-10). A single high agglutination titer to *B. canis* usually indicates active infection, but this should be substantiated by additional tests. Dogs that are asymptomatic but have positive results on agglutination procedures should never be condemned as infected until blood culture results or the more specific cytoplasmic protein antigen (CPAg)–agar gel immunodiffusion (AGID) test results confirm the positive findings. All tests, with the exception of the CPAg-AGID method, measure antibodies to LPS antigens and may give nonspecific test results.

Rapid Slide Agglutination Test
The 2-mercaptoethanol rapid slide agglutination test (ME-RSAT) is preferred as an in-office screening procedure because it is inexpensive, rapid, and sensitive; it also detects antibodies early (D-Tec CB, Synbiotics, San Diego, Calif.). A 99% correlation exits between a negative test and lack of infection. The test kit used rose Bengal–stained *B. ovis* because its growth is less mucoid than *B. canis*. *B. canis* cross-reacts with all rough Brucella and with certain other bacterial species, such as mucoid strains of *Pseudomonas*, *Bordetella bronchiseptica*, and *Actinobacillus equuli*, to which serum antibodies may be present. Most causes of cross-reactions, however, have not been identified. Some breeds (e.g., Irish wolfhounds and Old English sheepdogs) have an exceptionally high false-positive test result rate for unknown reasons.[20] The ME-RSAT substantially reduces false-positive reactions by eliminating less specifically reacting IgM antibodies. 2-mercaptoethanol (ME) is labile and must be kept in a dark, tightly stoppered bottle at 4° C; use of inactivated ME gives false-positive results. A modification of the RSAT, using a less mucoid variant of *B. canis*, further reduces the rate of false-positive

results.[49,51] The ME-RSAT with the *B. canis* M-antigen therefore can be employed for confirmation of positive results of screening tests.

Tube Agglutination Test
The tube agglutination test (TAT) has been the most widely used serodiagnostic procedure for confirmation of infection in ME-RSAT–positive dogs. However, availability of antigen formerly provided by the U.S. Department of Agriculture is erratic. As with the RSAT, the TAT is also troubled by heterospecific reactions with other infectious agents and by equivocal titers in chronically infected animals; therefore the ME modification is used. Unfortunately, the ME-TAT also shows a lack of specificity, and the increase in ME-TAT antibody titers usually lags 1 to 2 weeks behind those of the TAT and 2 to 4 weeks behind those of the ME-RSAT. Nevertheless, results of the ME-RSAT correlate well with the ME-TAT, both of which should be considered as screening tests.

Lack of standardized reagents or methods makes absolute ME-TAT titer comparisons difficult. Nevertheless, a titer of 1:50 may indicate either very early (less than 3 weeks) or recovering infections. Titers of 1:50 to 1:100 should be considered suspect for infection; and titers of 1:200 or greater are highly presumptive of active infection because they often correlate with positive hemocultures. However, sera from noninfected dogs have been found to have titers from 1:50 to 1:100 and occasionally higher. As a semiquantitative test, the ME-TAT is best in control programs to quantitate serologic responses of dogs over months to determine whether infection has been eliminated with chemotherapy (see Therapy).

Agar Gel Immunodiffusion Test
This test, using selected antigens, has been developed as both a sensitive and specific procedure for the serodiagnosis of canine brucellosis. With regard to sensitivity, AGID tests reveal precipitins in the sera of infected dogs only after 5 to

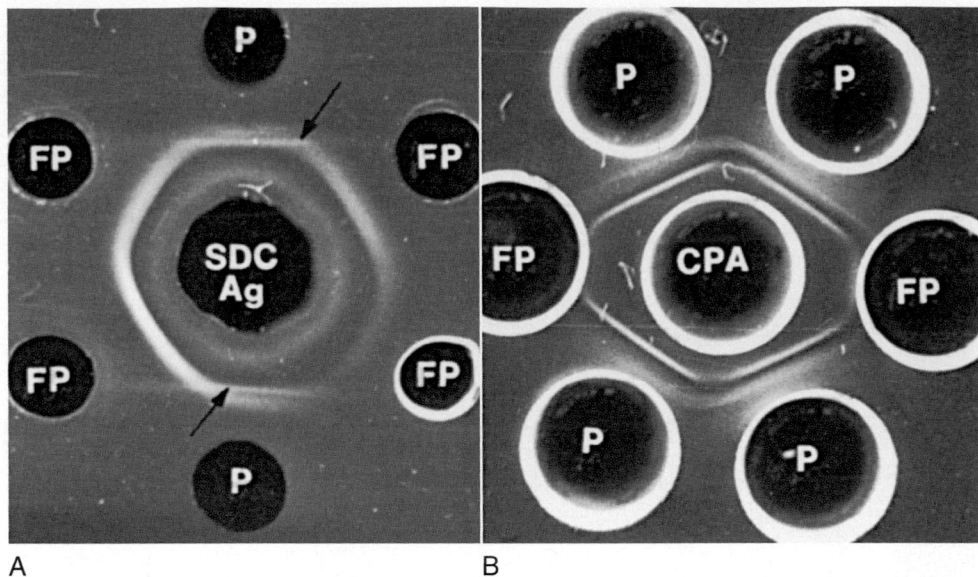

Fig 40-11 A, AGID patterns using sodium desoxycholate (SDC)-extracted somatic (LPS) antigens reacted with positive (P) and false-positive (FP) sera. Cross-reactions are evident. Arrows indicate *B. canis*–specific precipitin line. **B,** Cytoplasmic protein antigen (CPA). Precipitin lines occur only with sera from *Brucella*-infected dogs using CPA.

10 weeks PI; however, antibodies persist for several weeks or months after the bacteremia has ceased. The AGID test, using cell wall (somatic) LPS antigen, has the same problems of cross-reactions as do agglutination tests, but positive sera may be distinguished from false-positive sera by a distinct precipitin band for *B. canis* (Fig. 40-11, *A*). The somatic LPS antigen is seldom employed in the diagnostic regimen because of the lack of standardization and difficulty of interpreting test results.

The CPAg-AGID test, which is highly specific for *Brucella*, uses internal cytoplasmic antigens liberated by sonication of *B. canis* (see Fig. 40-11, *B*) or *B. abortus*.[9] Cytoplasmic antigens are shared only among Brucella organisms and will not react with antibodies to other genera of bacteria as seen with agglutination testing. The CPAg test has been able specifically to detect precipitins in the sera from dogs after other tests have become equivocal or even negative. It should be used as a confirmatory test following other serologic methods. A high proportion of sera sent to a reference laboratory for CPAg-AGID testing that are positive or suspect in the commercial ME-RSAT or the ME-TAT are found to be false-positive reactions.[20]

A disadvantage of tests with CPAg is the longer period between infection and the presence of detectable precipitins[19] (see Table 40-1). Furthermore, one or more precipitin lines may persist up to 12 months after bacteremia has ceased. In contrast to LPS antigens, both rough and smooth *Brucella* share the internal protein antigens. Thus the possibility of infection with other *Brucella* (e.g., *B. suis* or *B. abortus*) must be considered when CPAg is used. False-positive reactions have not been observed with non-Brucella species. False-negative results can occur in some dogs, presumably with early infections, whose sera are RSAT positive and AGID negative. Hemoculture is the only definitive way to resolve these differences.

Indirect Fluorescent Antibody Testing

As a result of a production shortage in the RSAT test kit and the unavailability of TAT reagents, many diagnostic laboratories have switched to the indirect fluorescent antibody (FA) test or enzyme-linked immunosorbent assay (ELISA) for sero-logic screening. Although these tests are being widely performed, they have not been as consistently evaluated as have the ME-RSAT, ME-TAT, and AGID methods. The indirect FA allows for visualization of the organism in the test procedure, and potential use of IgG-specific conjugates; however, nonspecific reactions still occur. With any test the purity and specificity of the antigen and homogeneity of the antibody conjugate are critical. The sensitivity of the indirect FA method is uncertain but may be lower than that of the ME-TAT and ELISA, meaning that some infected dogs may be missed during screening.

Enzyme-Linked Immunosorbent Assay

Newer methods for detection of *Brucella* infection have involved the use of ELISA.[46] As with other assays, the antigen source is critical in establishing test specificity. An antigen-specific, sandwich ELISA using highly purified *B. canis* cell wall antigen has been developed as a serologic test for *B. canis* infection.[70] Though very specific, ELISA may be less sensitive than the TAT in screening for infected dogs. Cytoplasmic Brucella protein (CP) extracts or lumazine synthase (LS) treatment of *B. abortus* proteins have also been used[9,10] in an attempt to improve ELISA test accuracy.[10] Recombinant ribosome recycling factor from *Brucella melitensis* has also been used to test human and canine sera.[22] The sensitivity of the ELISA has also been improved by a hot saline (HS) extract of the M-variant strain of *B. canis*.[52] HS, CP, or LS protein–based ELISAs were 97%, 94%, and 88% sensitive and 94.3%, 96.7%, and 96.7%, specific, respectively, in detecting dogs with confirmed or suspected brucellosis.[78] ELISA results usually were positive within 30 days after infection.[78] ELISAs have also been developed using recombinant produced proteins of *Brucella*.[5] Because of their convenience, ELISA methods may be further evaluated as screening tests and for quantitating serologic responses in naturally and experimentally infected dogs.[9,48]

Bacterial Isolation

Isolation of *B. canis* is time consuming but not difficult because the organism grows well aerobically on conventional media used for other *Brucella*. Of the *Brucella* infecting dogs or people, *B. canis* is the only one with a consistent *mucoid* (rough) colonial morphology because its cell wall contains truncated LPS moieties. However, less common rough strains of the other species develop, especially after culture on artificial media.

Blood is the most practical tissue or fluid for isolating the organism. Isolation of the organism from blood is the most definitive diagnostic procedure. Hemoculture should not be the sole criterion for infection because the bacteremia, although generally sustained, may be absent or intermittent in more chronically infected animals. Antibiotic administration may interfere with successful isolation of the organism. Blood culture can be helpful if serologic tests are ambiguous. Whole blood must be taken for culture because the organisms are associated with the leukocyte fraction. Bacteremia is detected 2 to 4 weeks after oronasal infection and, if untreated, persists for long (1 to 2 years or more) periods. Experimentally infected dogs have remained blood-culture positive for as long as 5.5 years. Bacterial numbers in the blood exceed 10^3/ml after 4 to 5 weeks PI and remain high for many (generally at least 6) months.[21]

Urine culture is positive in some dogs, especially males, when blood cultures are negative; however, unless cystocentesis is performed, urinary isolation of *B. canis* may be difficult because of overgrowth by urethral contaminants. However, urine collected via the urethra may have greater levels of semen, which is a predominant source of *B. canis* organisms. Collection of semen by ejaculation is valuable for culture during the first 3 months of infection, when the concentration of organisms is greatest. With diskospondylitis, culture of disk or bone specimens removed at surgery, or material from needle aspiration of the disk space, may also be cultured.

B. canis can be isolated at necropsy from several tissues of hemoculture-positive dogs. The lymph nodes, spleen, liver, bone marrow, and male reproductive organs are the most common sources, even though gross lesions are seldom present. In females, the gravid or estrual uterus, the placenta, and vaginal or uterine fluids are most consistent tissues for isolation.

Laboratory Cultivation

Contamination of specimens for culture of *B. canis* should be avoided because of overgrowth by faster-growing bacteria. Antibiotics such as bacitracin, polymyxin, and cycloheximide are usually added to the media before cultivation. Whole blood or fluid samples are usually cultured for 4 to 5 days at 37° C in Albimi, Trypticase soy, or Tryptose broth (Difco Labs, Detroit, Mich.), with citrate added as an anticoagulant. After 4 to 7 days of growth, cultures are streaked on solid media such as *Brucella* broth (BBL, Cockeysville, Md.), Tryptose agar, horse or cow blood agar, Trypticase soy agar (BBL, Cockeysville, Md.), or Thayer-Martin media (Difco Labs, Detroit, Mich.). Automated culture systems (Bact/Alert System, Organon Teknica, Durham, N.H.) have been helpful in giving consistent isolation times between 48 to 72 hours from the time of whole blood sample submission.[65] Tissue swabs or specimens may be streaked directly onto solid media and incubated aerobically at 37° C. Growth is not usually seen before 48 hours. Initially, colonies appear small and translucent but become mucoid after several days of incubation. Biochemical and immunologic methods and phage typing help identify isolates of *B. canis*.

Genetic Detection

Polymerase chain reaction (PCR) has also been used to detect *Brucella* species in tissues and fluids.[13] A genus-specific PCR, based on the gene encoding BCSP31, an antigenic periplasmic protein, is conserved in all species.[8,24,13] PCR has been more sensitive than blood culture and serology in detecting infec-

tion in human patients.[56] Using this method, at least two biovars of *B. canis* have been identified.[43] Molecular characterization of isolates has been helpful for differentiating among Brucella in the clinical laboratory.[30] That the conserved 16S rRNA sequences of *Brucella* species of domestic animals are over 98% similar indicates these organisms are closely related to *Bartonella* and *Agrobacterium*. The interspace region of this gene is unique for *Brucella* and is useful in differentiating them from other isolated bacteria.

PATHOLOGIC FINDINGS

Macroscopic changes in adults or surviving pups are usually confined to lymphadenomegaly and splenomegaly. Histologic changes are relatively uniform. Lymph node enlargement is the result of diffuse lymphoreticular hyperplasia (Fig. 40-12). In dogs with chronic bacteremia, lymph node sinusoids and the spleen are filled with plasma cells and macrophages containing phagocytized bacteria. Special stains (e.g., Brown-Brenn stain) must be used to detect intracellular organisms.

Diffuse submucosal lymphocytic infiltration occurs in all genitourinary organs. A necrotizing vasculitis occurs in the target tissues of gonadal steroids, including the prostate, scrotum, sheath, or vulva. Lesions are most prominent in the prostate, epididymis, and uterus, whereas milder changes are observed in the renal pelvis, testes, ductus deferens, urinary bladder, and ureters. Extensive necrosis of the prostatic parenchyma and seminiferous tubules is caused by inflammatory cell infiltration, which eventually results in atrophy or fibrosis (Fig. 40-13). A chronic to subacute endometritis can be seen in the uterus, with glandular hyperplasia and reticular cell nodules (Fig. 40-14). Focal hepatic necrosis, myocarditis, and meningoencephalitis also have been described. Renal abnormalities occur in some dogs and consist of hyaline thickening of the basement membrane of glomeruli with minimal cellular infiltration or proliferation. A mild interstitial nephritis has been noted. Ocular disease includes granulomatous iridocyclitis and exudative retinitis, consisting of diffuse infiltration of lymphocytes, plasmacytes, and neutrophils. Corneal endothelium has vacuolated cytoplasm with variable plasma cell infiltration; exudates with leukocytes are present in the anterior chamber (see Systemic Disease, Chapter 93).

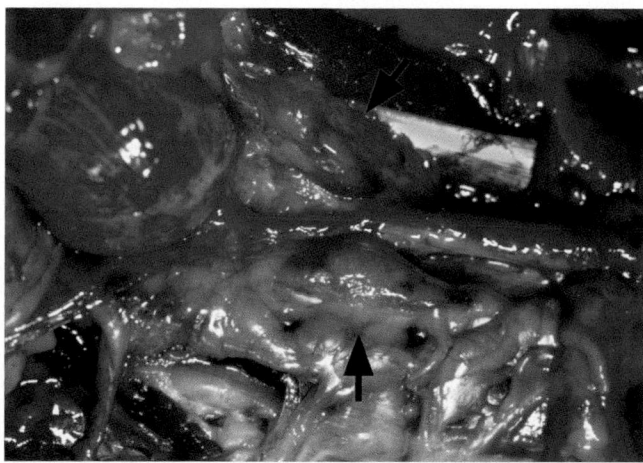

Fig 40-12 Enlarged sublumbar lymph nodes *(arrows)* at necropsy from a dog with chronic brucellosis. (Courtesy University of Georgia, Athens, Ga.)

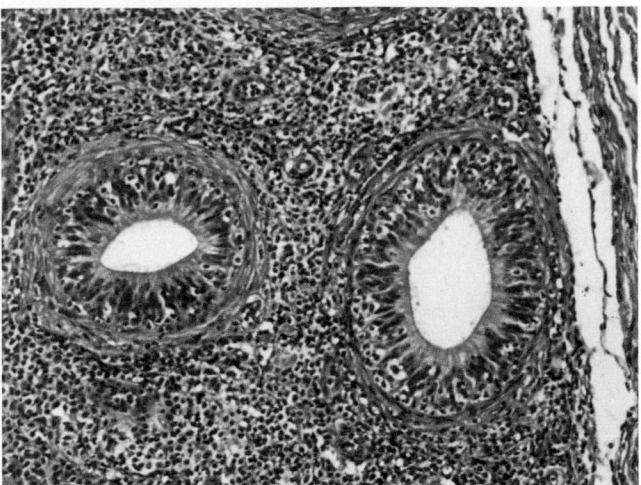

Fig 40-13 Early focal inflammatory cell cluster *(arrow)* in the head of the epididymis from a dog infected with *B. canis* (H and E stain, ×40). (Courtesy Leland Carmichael, Cornell University, Ithaca, N.Y.)

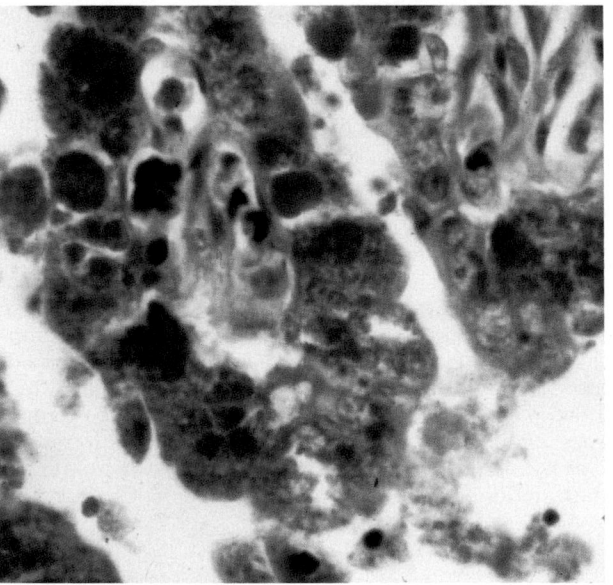

Fig 40-14 Endometritis with glandular hyperplasia and multifocal inflammation from a dog with *B. canis* infection. (Courtesy Leland Carmichael, Cornell University, Ithaca, N.Y.)

THERAPY

Because of the persistent intracellular location of *B. canis*, the outcome of antibiotic therapy of canine brucellosis is uncertain. The organism is susceptible to several antibiotics, but the ineffectiveness of in vivo therapy commonly leads to failures or relapses. None of the treatment regimens is 100% successful. Dogs with brucellosis should *never* be treated with a *single* antibiotic regimen; in all cases, combination therapy should be used. Unfortunately, the most studied regimen (tetracycline plus dihydrostreptomycin) is unobtainable because of the restricted availability of dihydrostreptomycin. Bacteremia often recurs days to months after treatment is discontinued, making follow-up evaluation essential because animals can still harbor infection in certain tissues. The reproductive tissues of the ovary and uterus and testes and epididymis should be surgically removed. In addition, ocular infections may require enucleation of severely affected eyes.

Breeding Animals

It is strongly recommended that infected dogs be isolated and eliminated from breeding programs as soon as a diagnosis is confirmed. Treatment should be considered only under exceptional circumstances, because therapy is expensive and often unsuccessful, especially in chronically infected animals. Aborting females may subsequently produce normal litters, but even in those cases the success of therapy is uncertain. Clinically normal, infected bitches may transmit infection to their surviving offspring. Despite treatment, intact males frequently develop irreversible sterility, making their prognoses as breeding animals poor. Limited studies suggest inability to clear infection in the prostate gland in most instances. Infected female dogs have been reinstated in breeding programs but only after prolonged isolation and therapy and with great risk of failure. The risk of infecting males when breeding with previously infected females has been minimized by judicious artificial insemination. Breeding of such animals should be done only under exceptional circumstances when it is considered essential (e.g., the loss of a valuable blood line) and after the risk is explained to an owner.

Pet Animals

Infected pets should, minimally, be neutered and given a regimen of antibiotic therapy to reduce the chance of infecting family members via genital secretions. The organism can persist in tissues of neutered animals, but shedding is believed less likely. Repeated courses of antibiotic therapy are recommended on the basis of follow-up serologic testing and blood cultures.

Cures of brucellosis must not be assumed because bacteremia may recur weeks or months after antibiotics are discontinued. Attempted culture of bacteria or serologic testing immediately after treatment is halted is deceiving. Reports of successful cures should be viewed with caution unless subsequent cultures and serology have been performed for at least 6 months.

Use of quantitative ME-TAT titers is the best means of monitoring successful elimination of the organism. Testing should be performed at 6- to 9- month intervals after a treatment regimen. Titer values should decrease if therapy is effective. Titers below 1:100 should be reached or else additional courses of treatment are indicated. Corresponding AGID titers results should also become negative. Persistence of increased (more than 1:100) titers should make evoke suspicion that the infection still exists.

Antibiotic Therapy

Several drugs have been used to treat canine brucellosis, but the organism is rarely eliminated if the appropriate antibiotic combination and regimen are not used.[57] Single-antibiotic therapy is not efficacious to eradicate *Brucella* species. By mean inhibitory concentration, in vitro susceptibility has been demonstrated for tetracycline, chloramphenicol, aminoglycosides, spectinomycin, rifampin, third-generation cephalosporins, ampicillin, and fluoroquinolones. Synergy has been noted in vitro among tetracycline and fluoroquinolones and aminoglycosides and sulfonamides.[50] Infected dogs respond poorly or not at all to those drugs when they are given alone or for a single course of therapy. Relapse occurs within a short time period after therapy is discontinued. Partial in vitro susceptibility occurs with erythromycin, penicillin, novobiocin, and lincomycin. Decreased susceptibility to cephalosporins, nalidixic acid, and cycloserine exists. None of the antibiotics in these last two groups should be given to treat canine brucellosis. Quinolones such as ciprofloxacin, norfloxacin, and enrofloxacin have been shown to be effective in vitro against *Brucella* species,[39] but limited in vivo studies have not. Fluoroquinolone monotherapy has been associated with treatment failures and relapses, especially in cases of uveitis or diskospondylitis. Azithromycin has combined with gentamicin to treat brucellosis in people with less efficacy than doxycycline and gentamicin.[71]

High-dose oral minocycline or doxycycline therapy combined with intramuscular streptomycin (Table 40-2) has given the highest rate of success in experimentally infected dogs. Lower doses of this combination or other antibiotics alone or in combination were not as effective. Because of the unavailability of streptomycin and its derivatives, gentamicin has been substituted for streptomycin, but efficacy was less than that with dihydrostreptomycin.[58] Gentamicin is currently used as the most available aminoglycoside for combination regimens. Treatment regimens that are less expensive but generally less effective have been described (see Table 40-2). A longer treatment regimen of tetracycline for 28 days combined with streptomycin for 14 days has had success, especially in treating dogs infected for less than 1 to 2 months.[57]

Diskospondylitis

Localized infections in hard-to-reach areas such as in the intervertebral disk should be treated with at least two or more sequential or intermittent 4-week courses of antimicrobial therapy after neutering. Doxycycline and aminoglycoside combination is recommended for this treatment. Recurrence of hyperesthetic episodes is common in dogs with canine brucellosis diskospondylitis. Owners of infected animals should be cautioned about the potential need for repeated treatment. Surgical intervention is rarely needed unless the diagnostic workup requires obtaining intervertebral tissues for culture. Decompressive surgery should be avoided in paraparetic dogs when possible by first evaluating the clinical response to antimicrobial therapy. Sequential radiography and titers at 3- to 6-month intervals are used to monitor progress. Serologic monitoring should be done with quantitative methods so that relative changes can be detected.

Ocular Infection

Uveal infections with *B. canis* have been exceedingly difficult to treat. No reports have been issued of successful elimination of ocular infection in dogs, as based on an animal becoming seronegative. The organism can be cultured from the aqueous humor in such cases,[34] and the ocular tissues are difficult to penetrate, especially with aminoglycosides. Enucleation is required if the eye has been severely damaged because vision will never return and the eye acts as a persistent nidus for the organism. Even use of two antimicrobials is associated with

Table • 40-2

Recommended Tetracycline and Aminoglycoside Combination Therapy for Canine Brucellosis[a]

DRUG[b]	DOSE[c] (mg/kg)	ROUTE	INTERVAL (HOURS)	DURATION (WEEKS)
Tetracyclines				
Minocycline or doxycycline[d,28]	25	PO	24	4
	12.5	PO	12	4
Tetracycline[57]	30	PO	12	4
Aminoglycosides				
Dihydrostreptomycine[e,28]	10	IM, SC	12	2 (treatment weeks 1 and 4)
	20	IM, SC	24	2 (treatment weeks 1 and 4)
Gentamicin	2.5	IM, SC	12	2 (treatment weeks 1 and 4)
	5.0	IM, SC	24	2 (treatment weeks 1 and 4)
Streptomycin[d,e,57]	20	IM, SC	24	2 (treatment weeks 1 and 4)
Fluroquinolones				
Enrofloxacin	5	PO	24	4
Ocular Involvement				
Rifampin	5	PO	24	4
Prednisone acetate (1%)	1 drop	Topical in eye	8	prn
Gentamicin (0.3%)	1 drop	Topical in eye	8	prn
Flurbiprofen (0.03%)	1 drop	Topical in eye	8	prn
Cyclosporin (0.2%)	1 drop	Topical in eye	8	prn

PO, By mouth; *IM*, intramuscular; *SC*, subcutaneous.
[a]Combination therapy is *always* indicated. One tetracycline and one aminoglycoside should be chosen and administered over a 4-week interval as indicated with the aminoglycoside being given for 2 of the weeks. Dogs should be tested at the end of treatment, and, again 1 and 3 months later. If treatment unsuccessful, improved therapeutic efficacy has been reported by repeating the regimen. Rifampin has been given as a fourth possibility, in combination with either tetracyclines and/or fluoroquinolones in the successful treatment of human and canine brucellosis.[76]
[b]See Appendix 8, Drug Formulary, for more information on these drugs.
[c]Dose per administration at specified interval.
[d]Generic doxycycline may be substituted at the same dose at a lower cost.
[e]Dihydrostreptomycin and streptomycin are not currently available to veterinarians in the U.S. Gentamicin may be substituted at the dose indicated, but its efficacy is uncertain.

relapse rates of ocular inflammation of 6% to 21%. Multiple-drug combination therapy with doxycycline, gentamicin, enrofloxacin, and subsequent addition of rifampin was successful in eliminating the ocular inflammation in an infected dog.[76] This finding was the first reported instance of clinical resolution of the ocular inflammation over 3 years of monitoring. Lesions of inactive chorioretinitis were evident. The AGID titer results were negative; however, the dog still maintained an indirect FA titer of a reduced level suggesting persistence of the organism. Topical or subconjunctival glucocorticoid therapy or topical ocular medications may be needed on a temporary or continual basis to control the intraocular inflammation to prevent irreversible panophthalmitis. Adjunctive topical therapy includes other antiinflammatory drugs such as flurbiprofen or cyclosporine and gentamicin.

Meningoencephalitis

As with other central nervous systems (CNS) infections, therapy with antimicrobials must be at maximal levels to obtain reasonable drug concentrations at the site of infection. Furthermore, as the blood-CNS barrier heals, concentrations will be much more difficult to achieve. Aminoglycosides are of little use in clearing infections from the CNS.

CONTROL IN INFECTED KENNELS

Control of canine brucellosis in a kennel with cases confirmed by serologic tests and isolation of the organism is a difficult, time-consuming, and agonizing experience for both dog owners and their veterinarians. Difficulties are compounded if antibiotic therapy is instituted when brucellosis is suspected but not confirmed because isolation of *B. canis* becomes uncertain and serologic tests results are questionable. A kennel should be quarantined as soon as the diagnosis of *B. canis* is ascertained, and infected animals should be promptly eliminated. Appropriate disinfection procedures should be implemented to arrest spread of infection via fomites. Persons working with infected dogs and their discharges or secretions in an infected kennel should wear gloves until serotesting can be done to determine the extent of the infection. Animals should not be admitted to or released from the kennel until the disease is eradicated. Movement of dogs within a colony also should be restricted to removal of proven and suspect cases to isolation quarters. New additions are at high risk for infection, especially if dogs are not individually penned, which also increases the number of animals requiring repeated testing during the eradication process. Animals must not be released for sale or any other purpose because they may spread the disease. All dogs in an infected kennel should be serotested for at least 3 months after seronegative status is achieved, especially before each breeding, even if artificial insemination is used. If animals are retained as pets or working dogs, or if treatment is contemplated, they should be neutered and moved to separate housing. Although determining the origin of infections is important, this has proved difficult because of the reluctance of owners to reveal actual or suspected sources.

Carrier dogs are important in maintaining *B. canis* in the dog population because its survival outside the host is short lived, and disinfection with quaternary ammonium compounds or iodophors has been effective in killing the bacterium.

PREVENTION

In brucellosis-free areas where importation regulations exist, vigilance should be maintained by serotesting incoming animals similar to what has been implemented in evaluating rabies protection and ehrlichial infections. A dog entering the United Kingdom was later found to be infected.[26] Neutered animals pose less of a risk of transmitting infection should they inadvertently enter such areas.

Preventive measures are particularly important in large breeding kennels or wherever a large number of dogs are kept, but no legally mandated control measures exist, and in the United States, canine brucellosis is not a reportable disease in most states. Prevention is accomplished by quarantine of all new acquisitions until two serotest results at a 1-month interval are negative. Animals from kennels known to have had breeding problems should be rejected unless test results are negative.[37] Animals with any clinical sign of canine brucellosis should be rejected. Animals used for breeding should be tested 3 to 4 weeks before each mating to allow time for test results to be reported. Brood bitches should not be mated to stud dogs unless they have been tested and certified negative. If dogs leave a colony, they should be tested before readmission. All canine blood donors should be screened for brucellosis because infections have been documented in people by transfusion of contaminated blood products.[1]

No vaccine is available, and results of experimental studies have been unsatisfactory. The desirability of a vaccine is questionable, especially when diagnostic testing is available, because an effective vaccine would be required to provide serviceable immunity but not confound the serodiagnosis.

PUBLIC HEALTH CONSIDERATIONS

Brucella spp. vary in their virulence for people, but exposure to animals or their tissues or secretions is a common denominator. Brucellosis is the most commonly reported laboratory-acquired infection.[68] Veterinarians can also be infected by accidental inoculation or ocular absorption of the live attenuated vaccines for *B. abortus* or *B. melitensis*. The highest virulence is seen with infections caused by *B. melitensis* and biovars of *B. suis*, while *B. abortus* has a modest virulence. In such infections, spondylitis, polyarthritis, conjunctivitis, and uveitis are among the more common manifestations of infection. Rare complications include thrombocytopenia, valvular endocarditis, meningitis, pneumonia, neuroretinitis, glomerulonephritis, hepatitis, and visceral abscesses.* Laboratory infection with the *B. maris* group of isolates from marine mammals has been reported.[23]

Natural and laboratory-acquired infections with *B. canis* have been reported in several countries; however, the actual number of cases is unknown because human infections are often misdiagnosed.[15,62,73] Contact with aborting bitches was the source of infection for the majority of infected pet owners, whereas male dogs and undetermined sources were present in other cases. People are relatively resistant to infection with *B. canis*, and the disease is relatively mild compared with infections caused by other *Brucella*. However, infection has even been reported with the so-called *less virulent* laboratory M strain of *B. canis* that is used for serologic diagnosis.[77] A proportion of human *B. canis* infections are asymptomatic, as determined by serotesting, but the overall rate of infection relative to exposure is low. Fever, chills, fatigue, malaise, lymphadenomegaly, and weight loss have been present in symptomatic patients. In people, *B. canis* infections produce bacteremia, and in some cases endocarditis.[79] Spondylitis has not been described in people infected with *B. canis*.[72] Diagnosis of human infections should include bacteriologic examination by blood culture and serologic evaluation. Antibodies to *B. canis* in human sera will react in serologic tests used in

*References: 2, 35, 54, 80, 81.

dogs and, as in dogs, they do not cross-react with *B. abortus* antigen used in routine testing for human brucellosis. Titers of 1:200 or more, using the ME-TAT, are seen in most active cases. Human infections can be readily and effectively treated with tetracycline therapy. As with infected dogs, people have suffered relapse with ampicillin.

Clients should always be informed of the potential health hazard in keeping *B. canis*–infected pets. Veterinarians should practice good hygiene when examining suspected dogs, especially aborting bitches.

Laboratory workers should always use personal protection including goggles, masks, gloves and protective clothing and only work with the organism in a biologic safety cabinet. Biohazard precautions should be taken in the laboratory when handling or pipetting samples submitted for diagnostic testing. All waste materials should be autoclaved.

SUGGESTED READINGS*

13. Bricker BJ. 2002. PCR as a diagnostic tool for brucellosis, *Vet Microbiol* 90:435-446.

18. Carmichael LE, Joubert JC. 1998. Transmission of *Brucella canis* by contact exposure, *Cornell Vet* 78:63-73.
44. Kustritz MV. 2000. Theriogenology question of the month. Agarose gel immunodiffusion (AGID) serologic testing for brucellosis, *J Am Vet Med Assoc* 216:181-182.
47. Lucero NE, Escobar GI, Ayala SM, et al. 2002. Sensitivity and specificity of an indirect enzyme-linked immunoassay for the diagnosis of *Brucella canis* infection in dogs, *J Med Microbiol* 51:656-660.
68. Scheftel J. 2003. *Brucella canis*: potential for zoonotic transmission, *Compend Cont Educ Pract Vet* 25:846-853.
76. Vinayak A, Greene CE, Moore PA, et al. 2004. Clinical resolution of *Brucella canis*–induced ocular inflammation in a dog and a review of ocular brucellosis in dogs at North American veterinary schools 1964-2003, *J Am Vet Med Assoc*, 1804-1807.
79. Ying W, Nguyen MQ, Jahre JA. 1999. *Brucella canis* endocarditis: case report, *Clin Infect Dis* 29:1593-1594.

*See the CD-ROM for a complete list of references.

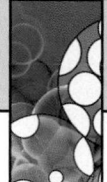

CHAPTER • 41

Anaerobic Infections

Craig E. Greene and Spencer S. Jang

ETIOLOGY

Obligate anaerobes are either gram-positive or gram-negative rods or cocci (Table 41-1). They cannot grow in the presence of molecular oxygen because they do not make superoxide dismutase, and most do not produce catalase. These enzymes are necessary for the breakdown of reactive oxygen intermediates (e.g., superoxide anion, hydrogen peroxide) that are normally generated when bacteria grow in the presence of oxygen. Only species of the genus *Clostridium* form endospores anaerobically, distinguishing them from the genus *Bacillus*, which forms spores under aerobic conditions. The most commonly encountered anaerobes are listed in Table 41-2.

Anaerobes make up a significant portion of the normal bacterial flora of dogs and cats.[11,49] The predominant microorganisms living on most mucosal surfaces are anaerobes, and metabolic by-products produced by this group of microorganisms are important in the regulation of the numbers of aerobic species (facultative and obligate) that also comprise the normal flora. Thus anaerobic bacteria play an important role in protection of mucosal surfaces from interactions involving other microorganisms with pathogenic potential. For example, approximately 1 million salmonellae are needed to produce disease in animals with intact anaerobic flora, whereas fewer than 10 salmonellae are needed to produce disease in animals with few anaerobes. The importance of this observation is seen clinically; dogs are more prone to develop salmonellosis when they are medicated with antibi-

otics, especially those effective in reducing the anaerobic component of the normal flora (e.g., ampicillin).[80]

Aside from being responsible for a significant portion of innate immunity (the normal flora), anaerobes may be important participants in clinical disease.[29,34,39,46,47] Compromise of a mucosal surface by perforation or of a surface or an area contiguous to a mucosal surface may lead to inoculation of members of the normal flora into a normally sterile site. At this point, introduced anaerobes become clinically relevant in addition to other members of the normal flora. These are important facts because antibiotic therapy is almost always started before results of microbiologic analysis of exudative material are received. Therefore an educated guess about the microorganisms present must be made. If anaerobic bacteria are involved in an infectious process, an average of two different species are almost always admixed with aerobic bacteria. The most commonly associated aerobic bacteria are enterics (mainly *Escherichia coli*), members of the genus *Pasteurella*, and coagulase-positive staphylococci (Table 41-3; see Bite Wound Infections, Chapter 53).

If they contain the appropriate virulence factors, anaerobic bacteria may also produce disease on a mucosal surface. In addition to periodontal disease, anaerobes are associated with disease in other regions of the gastrointestinal tract (see Chapter 89); the most important of these anaerobes within the intestine are *Clostridium difficile* and *Clostridium perfringens* (see Chapter 39).[74,78] Both of these species may be a part of the normal flora of dogs and cats, although evidence suggests that both may be passed to previously uncolonized animals.[45,60,66]

Table • 41-1

Characteristics of Obligate Anaerobic Bacteria Most Commonly Isolated from Dogs and Cats

MICROORGANISM	GRAM REACTION	SHAPE
Bacteroides spp.	Negative (pale)	Rod
Prevotella spp.	Negative (pale)	Rod (coccobacillus)
Porphyromonas spp.	Negative (pale)	Rod (coccobacillus)
Fusobacterium spp.	Negative (pale)	Rod (usually thin)
Peptostreptococcus anaerobius, anaerobic gram-positive cocci	Positive	Coccus
Clostridium spp.	Positive	Rod (spores)
Eubacterium spp.	Positive	Coccus
Actinomyces spp.	Positive	Rod (spores)

Table • 41-2

Species of Obligate Anaerobic Bacteria Isolated from Dogs and Cats

ORGANISM	NUMBER	PERCENTAGE OF ISOLATES (n-316)
Bacteroides spp.	74	23
• B. fragilis group[a]	38	12
• Other Bacteroides	36	11
Peptostreptococcus anaerobius, anaerobic gram-positive cocci	57	18
Fusobacterium spp.[b]	43	14
Porphyromonas spp.[c]	34	11
Clostridium spp.[d]	28	9
Prevotella spp.[e]	16	5
Miscellaneous spp.	39	12

Data compiled from cases from Veterinary Medical Teaching Hospital, University of California, Davis, Calif., 1991–1995.
[a]B. fragilis was most commonly isolated.
[b]F. nucleatum was most commonly isolated.
[c]P. asaccharolyticus was most commonly isolated.
[d]C. perfringens was most commonly isolated.
[e]P. heparinolyticus was most commonly isolated.

EPIDEMIOLOGY

Infectious processes involving a normally sterile site are usually a consequence of "contamination" by members of the normal flora. The composition of the normal flora of the contiguous surface usually mirrors what is found in the infectious process. In human patients, infectious processes involving structures above the diaphragm are more likely to contain

Table • 41-3

Most Commonly Isolated Aerobic Microorganisms Associated with Anaerobic Infections in Dogs and Cats

MICROORGANISM	PERCENTAGE OF ISOLATES	
	DOGS (505 ISOLATES)	CATS (85 ISOLATES)
Enterics[a]	29	18
Pasteurella spp.[b]	12	28
Coagulase-positive Staphylococcus spp.	11	7

Data compiled from cases from Veterinary Medical Teaching Hospital, University of California, Davis, Calif., 1991–1995.
[a]Most common isolate was E. coli, accounting for 70% of the enteric isolates from dogs and 53% of the enteric isolates from cats.
[b]Most common isolate was P. canis, accounting for 48% of the isolates from dogs, and P. multocida, accounting for 75% of the isolates from cats.

anaerobes originating in the mouth, whereas disease below the diaphragm usually involves anaerobes from the intestinal tract.[75] In animal patients the various species of anaerobes do not seem to have different predilections for a particular site or location.[41]

Although disease produced by C. difficile is the result of its proliferation in the enteric tract of the host after a trigger event (e.g., certain antibiotics and chemotherapeutic agents), epidemiologic evidence from human hospitals suggests that the agent can be spread from patient to patient, resulting in outbreaks of C. difficile–associated disease (see Chapter 39).[70] Such observations imply that the organism either is or has the potential to be contagious. However, determining whether C. difficile is truly a contagious pathogen is difficult because it is also found in the enteric tract of clinically healthy animals.[66,74]

It is unclear whether toxigenic C. perfringens is contagious. It likely causes disease by proliferating in the intestinal tract and producing enterotoxin. The trigger that stimulates the proliferation is unknown. What also remains to be determined is whether the source of the agent is endogenous, acquired from another infected animal, or acquired from the environment. The report of outbreaks of C. perfringens–associated diarrhea in small animal hospital settings suggests it is contagious, although it is important to remember that some C. perfringens are present in the enteric tract of clinically healthy dogs.[45,78] Detectable levels of C. perfringens enterotoxin are not often found in the feces of asymptomatic animals (see Chapter 39).[78]

The genus Fusobacterium includes numerous species, one of which—Fusobacterium nucleatum—has five subspecies.[8] One of the new subspecies, Candidatus Fusobacterium canifelium, is common in the oral cavity of dogs and cats and has been isolated from dog and cat bite wounds in people. Unfortunately, this organism is often more resistant to quinolones than are human isolates.

PATHOGENESIS

Anaerobic bacteria cannot live in healthy tissue. On mucosal surfaces (e.g., intestinal tract, gingival crevices, genital tract), they live with other microorganisms that scavenge molecular

Table • 41-4

Factors Contributing to Development of Anaerobic Infections

PHYSIOLOGIC INJURY	CAUSES
Immunosuppression	Cytotoxic chemotherapy
	Glucocorticoid therapy
	Malignancies
	Neutropenia
	Hypogammaglobulinemia
	Narrow-spectrum aerobic antibacterial therapy
	Diabetes mellitus
Altered tissue oxygenation	Vascular compromise
	Hypotension
	Tissue anoxia
	GI obstruction or stasis
	Tissue trauma
Tissue contamination	GI or urogenital perforation
	Bite or puncture wounds of soft tissues
	Foreign body migration

oxygen, resulting in a local environment with very low pH (a measure of oxygen tension). Likewise, in compromised tissue, inflammatory cells and coinoculated aerobic microorganisms lower the pH sufficiently for anaerobes to grow. Numerous factors that predispose the body to anaerobic infections are listed in Table 41-4.

Components of anaerobic bacteria have been shown to elicit potent inflammatory responses. Gram-negative anaerobes possess lipopolysaccharides with endotoxic activity, as do their aerobic counterparts. The peptidoglycan of gram-positive anaerobes incites the same inflammatory response as gram-positive aerobic microorganisms. Some anaerobic bacteria produce capsules (e.g., *Bacteroides fragilis*, pigmented *Prevotella* organisms, and *Porphyromonas* organisms), which incite inflammatory responses that result in abscess formation; in other words, capsules without viable bacteria induce abscess formation.[79] Some evidence suggests that coinoculated aerobic microorganisms induce anaerobe capsule formation. Capsules also play a more traditional role by discouraging association with phagocytic cells.[7,32]

Aerobic and anaerobic microorganisms can have a synergistic relationship.[7] Anaerobes act with facultative aerobes such as *E. coli* to induce abscess formation more rapidly than either bacterial group alone. *Actinomyces*, a genus of facultative anaerobes, is commonly found in association with anaerobic infections from foreign body migrations and in association with pyothorax or peritonitis (see Chapter 49). The facultative bacteria lower the oxidation-reduction potential of the tissue environment, facilitating anaerobic proliferation. The necrotic and abscessed tissue may protect the facultative organisms from antimicrobials and body defenses such as phagocytosis. In addition to helping trigger capsule formation, aerobic organisms scavenge oxygen and curtail phagocytosis of the anaerobic component of the sample (and vice versa).[81] Enzymes such as β-lactamase produced by one member of the aerobic-anaerobic partnership protect susceptible microorganisms in the vicinity from being killed by β-lactam antibiotics. These synergistic interactions are important to keep in mind when designing therapeutic regimens, because antibiotic

therapy should be directed at both populations for optimal resolution of the infection.

Some anaerobic bacteria produce toxins. *Fusobacterium necrophorum* produces a toxin that forms pores in leukocyte membranes.[32] *C. difficile* produces toxins (A and B) that disrupt the cytoskeletal elements of the intestinal epithelial cell, resulting in cell death.[1,69] *C. perfringens* produces an enterotoxin that interacts with the target cell membrane, resulting in the formation of pores that are made partly by the enterotoxin and partly by the target cell.[69] Electrolytes are lost through these pores, resulting in reversal of ion and water flow (diarrhea) and finally, death of the cell.

Some species of anaerobes produce adhesin molecules (pili or fimbriae).[32] These proteins are usually associated with more virulent anaerobes. However, adhesins probably do not play a role other than association with specific sites or locations on mucosal surfaces. Adhesin molecules probably are not expressed and do not have an important role when exposed to phagocytic cells to which they might adhere—an event that leads to phagocytosis and the demise of the anaerobe. In keeping with this model, it has been shown that blood or abscess isolates of *B. fragilis* are rarely piliated, whereas those found on the mucosal surface almost always have pili.[7]

CLINICAL FINDINGS

Conditions involving anaerobic bacteria infecting a normally sterile site vary according to location, but all involve the formation of a pyonecrotic process. This process stems primarily from the inflammatory response triggered by anaerobe capsule material, cell wall constituents of the anaerobic and aerobic microorganisms that may be present, and thwarted attempts of phagocytosis, leading to deposition of lysosomal contents into surrounding tissue. The most commonly encountered sites of anaerobic isolation are listed in Table 41-5. The clinical findings of such infections are listed in Tables 41-6 and 41-7. Exudate from infectious processes that contain anaerobes is often malodorous.

Bacteremia is often associated with seemingly localized anaerobic infections, although it is not often recognized. Animals with intraperitoneal or intrapleural infections experience a systemic spread of organisms into the blood stream. Fever, leukocytosis, hypoglycemia, increased serum alkaline phosphatase activity, and hypoalbuminemia reflect the systemic manifestations of an acute-phase reaction to the anaerobic infection. The hypoalbuminemia may be compounded by loss of serum proteins into effusions or from draining wounds.

DIAGNOSIS

In addition to clinical features, the cytologic analysis is often helpful in determining whether an anaerobic infection is present. Abundant degenerative neutrophils are usually found with multiple and often morphologically diverse forms of intracellular and extracellular bacteria. Large and filamentous morphology is often typical of anaerobes. Extracellular bacteria may be a result of bacterial contamination of a specimen or contamination of the staining solution. Microscopic evaluation for morphologic shape and Gram staining should be performed when the specimen is collected so that the results can be compared with culture results or the type of organism can be predicted by its shape and staining properties (see Table 41-1). The standard for determining the presence of anaerobic bacteria in an infectious process is their isolation from clinical samples. They are difficult to isolate in clinical practice unless precautions are taken. Errors in specimen handling and submission are the primary reasons anaerobes are not routinely

Table • 41-5

Relative Frequency of Obligate Anaerobic Bacteria with Respect to Disease Process or Site in Dogs and Cats

DISEASE PROCESS OR ANATOMIC SITE	SPECIES	RANKING	PERCENTAGE CULTURE POSITIVE	PERCENTAGE WITH ANAEROBES
Draining tract	Dog	1	79	39
Pleural fluid	Dog	2	43	31
	Cat	1	44	40
Abscess	Dog	3	81	30
	Cat	2	82	40
Bone	Dog	6	22	6
	Cat	3	46	36
Abdominal fluid	Dog	4	52	19
	Cat	4	50	27
Respiratory tract	Dog	5	50	9
	Cat	5	70	17

Data compiled from Veterinary Medical Teaching Hospital, University of California, Davis, Davis, Calif., 1991–1995; data also reported in Jang SS, Breher JE, Dabaco LA, et al. 1997. Organisms isolated from dogs and cats with anaerobic infections and susceptibility to selected antimicrobial agents, *J Am Vet Med Assoc* 210:1610-1614.

Table • 41-6

Clinical Findings Suggestive of Anaerobic Infection

Fever, pain, and swelling
Bite or puncture wound
Foul-smelling wounds or discharges
Gas in tissues or body cavities
Abscess formation
Contiguous infection to mucosal surface with anaerobic microflora
Necrotic or devitalized tissue
Gangrenous tissue
Dark, discolored exudates
Presence of sulfur granules in exudate
Mixed population of organisms or filamentous forms shown by microscopy
Failure to culture organisms with routine methods

isolated. Their growth is enhanced by use of an anaerobe chamber, improved transport media, and collection practices.[4] When attempting to isolate anaerobic bacteria, the samples should be handled with extreme care before they are given to laboratory personnel (Table 41-8). As mentioned, anaerobes are sensitive to oxygen and because of their slow growth are also easily overgrown in samples containing aerobic microorganisms; greater than 70% are mixed. Therefore transport media, transport time, and temperature are important issues (see Chapter 33). Refrigeration has been shown to be detrimental to the isolation of anaerobic bacteria, thus samples should not be placed at temperatures lower than 4° C. In comparison, aerobic microorganisms in samples maintained at 25° C multiply and in some cases overgrow the anaerobic component. However, at 15° C, aerobes do not multiply to any extent, nor do the anaerobes die. Because swabs tend to dry out and become oxygenated, their use is discouraged. If swabs are used, the tip should be moistened with a prereduced media such as brain-heart infusion broth. The amount of time between sample collection and culture depends on the type of sample, whether transport medium is used, and the volume of the sample. Anaerobic microorganisms in large pieces of tissue or quantities of fluid (greater than 2 ml) are relatively protected from toxic interaction with oxygen and can survive for up to 24 hours before culture, whereas anaerobes in smaller samples or swabs usually cannot. Anaerobic transport media greatly increase the survival of anaerobes and discourage the growth of aerobes. Anaerobic media are available for transport of aspirated material, tissue or biopsy material, and material collected on swabs.[50]

At the laboratory, media must be inoculated with specimens as soon as they are received. Use of prereduced, anaerobically sterilized media improves the success of isolation. After inoculation, media is placed in oxygen-free carbon dioxide until it can be put in an anaerobic chamber with an atmosphere of 5% carbon dioxide, 5% hydrogen, and 90% nitrogen. Anaerobic cultivation is time consuming and expensive. The plates must always be handled in an anaerobic hood or a chamber that has been flushed with anaerobic gas. For example, the isolation and demonstration of an anaerobe in a sample containing only one species of anaerobe takes at least 4 days. The cost is approximately $10 (in American dollars) for media alone. Because most infectious processes contain an average of two different species of anaerobes and at least one aerobe, significantly more effort is required, as is money.

A diagnosis can be made using other methods. Depending on the site, condition, characteristics of the exudate (e.g., odor), and contents observed in stained smears, a presumptive diagnosis of anaerobic bacterial involvement can be made (see Tables 41-6 and 41-7 and Fig. 41-1). When viewed microscopically, some gram-negative anaerobic rods are pale staining and have shapes suggestive of anaerobes—they are often thin, can be sometimes misshapen, and occasionally have pointed ends.

Disease produced by anaerobes while they are on a mucosal surface is somewhat more difficult to diagnose. Isolation from sites where obligate anaerobes are part of the normal flora, such as the oral or pharyngeal cavity, vagina, external auditory meatus, conjunctiva, or skin, can be difficult to associate with pathogenicity. Isolating *C. difficile* and *C. perfringens* harbored in the intestinal tract involves using specialized agar for isolation, immunologic tests to determine the presence of microorganism or toxin in feces or in broth culture, or the polymerase chain reaction for toxin genes in

Table • 41-7

Comparative Clinical Features of Anaerobic Infections

SITE	PARTICULAR CLINICAL FEATURES	SOURCES
Head and neck	Cranial or cervical abscesses, exophthalmos, pain when opening mouth, subauricular swelling, anorexia, difficulty swallowing, gingivitis and stomatitis, para-aural abscesses, tonsillar abscesses, brain abscesses, inner ear infections, panophthalmitis, meningoencephalitis	Traumatic ear canal separations,[51] pharyngeal foreign body penetration (stick injuries),[62] dental infections, chronic sinusitis,[82] tonsillar abscesses, chronic otitis media,[10] bite wounds, meninges[65]
Intrathoracic		
Pulmonary	Coughing, fever, dyspnea, lobar or multifocal consolidation (abscesses), hypertrophic osteopathy	Pneumonia, endocarditis,[18] aspiration pneumonia[27]
Intrapleural or mediastinal	Fever, dyspnea, muffled heart sounds, leukocytosis, pyothorax	Penetrating chest injuries, inhaled foreign bodies, esophageal foreign body perforation[68,64]
Intraabdominal		
Peritoneal	Fever, abdominal distention, anorexia, intraabdominal abscesses, adhesions	Postoperative foreign suture materials (e.g., silk, multifilament nylon, braided material), ovariohysterectomy, bowel leakage, genital tract infections, actinomycosis
Hepatic	Anorexia, lethargy, vomiting, diarrhea, fever, dehydration, hepatomegaly, mucosal bleeding	Bacteremia, hepatic neoplasia, ascending biliary infection, immunosuppression in diabetes mellitus[16]
Enteric	Chronic diarrhea, blood, mucus	Intestinal stasis, blind loop syndrome, colitis, colonic ulceration
Retroperitoneal	Swelling in lumbar flank, sinus tracts or drainage, pain, fever, anorexia, reluctance to walk	Osteomyelitis of lumbar vertebrae from plant awns, ovarian or uterine ligatures,[43] actinomycosis, ruptured urethra and perirenal abscess
Paraspinal	Pain, reluctance to walk, fever, paresis or paralysis	Usually epidural from local penetration or extension of paraspinal infection, bite wounds, *meningitis:* less likely anaerobic and often from hematogenous sources
Subcutaneous	Fever, swelling, discharge, leukocytosis	Bite wounds, penetrating injuries (see Chapters 52 and 53)

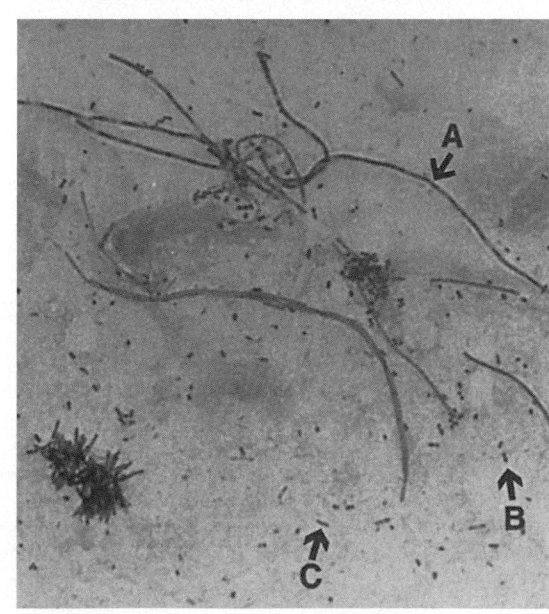

Fig 41-1 Gram-stained smear of exudate obtained from a cat with pyothorax. The filamentous microorganism *(A)* is probably *Filifactor (Clostridium) villosus*[9,47,76]; the cocci are probably *Peptostreptococcus (B)*; and the rods are either an enteric microorganism (e.g., *E. coli*), a nonenteric microorganism (e.g., *Pasteurella*), an anaerobe (*Bacteroides, Prevotella, Porphyromonas, Fusobacterium*), or a combination. Filamentous microorganisms *(C)* in the chest of a dog would most likely be microaerophilic members of the genus *Actinomyces*.

Table • 41-8

Specimen Collection for Anaerobic Isolation

Proper Collection Methods

Percutaneous needle aspiration into deeper tissues

Surgical curettage or scraping of mucosal surfaces

Tissue biopsy of deeper specimens (soft or bony)

Bone sequestrae—deep aspirates of drainage

Female genital tract—(1) laparoscopic or surgical specimens or (2) aspirates

Body fluid aspiration (synovia, peritoneal fluid, plueral fluid, bile, urine)

Lung specimens—always by aspiration or biopsy

Dental or respiratory sinus tissue—should be biopsied or aspirated after decontamination

Specimen Handling

Fluids—injected via syringe directly into anaerobic transport media

Infected tissue pieces—preferably stored in sterile, capped containers in anaerobic bags

Kept at room temperature, not refrigerated

Transported to the laboratory as soon as possible

Items and Specimens That Should Not Be Submitted

Tissue specimens with abundant microflora (mucosal surfaces)

Contents in plastic syringes

Surface swabs

Nasopharyngeal, gingival, or bronchial washings

Voided urine

feces or isolates.[59] (See Chapter 39 for an additional discussion of diagnosis for these enteric clostridial disorders.)

THERAPY

Successful treatment of infectious processes containing an anaerobic microorganism involves medical and surgical interventions (e.g., correction of fluid and electrolyte imbalances, drainage) combined with appropriate antimicrobial therapy. Antimicrobial therapy without surgical drainage is usually unsuccessful. Because anaerobic infections are often polymicrobic, antimicrobial therapy of infectious processes with an anaerobic component should focus on the anaerobic *and* the presumed aerobic components. The most commonly isolated aerobes have been enterics *(E. coli)*, members of genus *Pasteurella*, and *Staphylococcus intermedius*.[39] The susceptibility of these microorganisms to aerobic antimicrobial agents is shown in Table 41-9. (See Chapter 49 for treatment of infections associated with *Actinomyces* organisms.)

It is difficult and expensive to determine the susceptibility of anaerobes to antimicrobial agents. Guidelines for such testing have been established; however, the assay results have not always been repeatable or consistent for all anaerobic species.[26] For these reasons, few laboratories perform such assays (although the disk test is used for therapeutic predictions to determine whether an isolate produces a β-lactamase; Nitrocefin Disc, Difco Laboratories, Detroit, Mich.). In this test a portion of an isolated colony is smeared onto a disk containing a substrate that changes color if a β-lactamase is present. The most common anaerobic β-lactamases are cephalosporinases (which act on first-generation cephalosporins such as cephalexin and cefazolin), penicillin G, ampicillin, and amoxicillin. Clavulanate irreversibly binds to these enzymes. Table 41-10 summarizes the prevalence of β-lactamases found in various anaerobes isolated from dogs and cats.

Table • 41-9

Percentage Susceptibility of Selected Infectious Bacterial Agents from Dogs[a]

DRUG	BORDETELLA BRONCHISEPTICA	ESCHERICHIA COLI	KLEBSIELLA PNEUMONIAE	PASTEURELLA SPP.	PSEUDOMONAS AERUGINOSA	COAGULASE-POSITIVE STAPHYLOCOCCUS SPP.
Amikacin	90	99	95	100	97	100
Ampicillin	45	57	7	100	8	54
Amoxicillin-clavulanate	95	67	52	100	8	99
Ceftizoxime	5	99	100	100	8	100
Ceftiofur	5	91	80	100	1	96
Cephalothin	35	32	48	100	8	99
Chloramphenicol	90	67	54	100	0	92
Enrofloxacin	—	95	90	100	2	94
Erythromycin	0	0	0	38	0	85
Gentamicin	90	92	71	100	70	99
Tetracycline	95	64	59	100	0	71
Ticarcillin-clavulanate	—	65	42	100	92	—
Trimethoprim-sulfamethoxazole	75	74	72	97	6	94

—, No data reported.

[a]Data excluding that from *Enterococcus* spp., *Enterobacter* spp., and *Proteus mirabilis*.

Data from Hirsh DC, Jang SS. 1994. Antimicrobial susceptibility of selected infectious bacterial agents obtained from dogs. *J Am Anim Hosp Assoc* 30:487–494.

Table • 41-10

Prevalence of β-Lactamase–Producing Strains of Anaerobic Gram-Negative Bacteria Isolated from Dogs and Cats

ORGANISM	SPECIES	NUMBER	β-LACTAMASE POSITIVE	PERCENTAGE β-LACTAMASE POSITIVE
Bacteroides spp., B. fragilis	Dog	34	27	79
	Cat	10	8	80
B. fragilis group[a]	Dog	51	38	75
	Cat	21	13	62
Other Bacteroides	Dog	24	3	13
	Cat	10	5	50
Porphyromonas spp.	Dog	49	7	14
	Cat	13	5	38
Prevotella spp.	Dog	22	4	18
	Cat	10	1	10
Miscellaneous spp.	Dog	11	4	36
	Cat	13	3	23

Data compiled from Veterinary Medical Teaching Hospital, University of California, Davis, Calif., 1994–2000.
[a]Includes B. fragilis.

Table • 41-11

Susceptibility to Antimicrobial Agents of Selected Obligate Anaerobic Isolates from Dogs and Cats

| MICROORGANISM | NUMBER | METRONIDAZOLE | PERCENTAGE SUSCEPTIBLE | | | |
			CHLORAMPHENICOL	AMOXICILLIN-CLAVULANATE	AMPICILLIN	CLINDAMYCIN
Bacteroides spp.	41	100	100	100	68	81
• B. fragilis group	26	100	100	100	65	77
• Other Bacteroides	15	100	100	100	73	87
Peptostreptococcus spp.	9	100	100	100	100	100
Fusobacterium spp.	25	100	100	100	100	100
Porphyromonas spp.	4	100	100	100	100	100
Clostridium spp.	5	100	100	100	100	80
Prevotella spp.	13	100	100	100	100	100

Data compiled from Veterinary Medical Teaching Hospital, University of California, Davis, Calif., 1994–1995. Determined by use of the E-test (Epsilometer, AB Biodisk, Solna, Sweden). Results interpreted using interpretive categories and correlative minimum inhibitory concentrations as described by the National Committee for Clinical Laboratory Standards.

Because of the difficulty of antimicrobial susceptibility testing, antimicrobial treatment aimed at the anaerobic component is usually empiric and based on retrospectively acquired data. Anaerobic bacteria are inherently resistant to certain antibiotics (e.g., the aminoglycosides and the quinolones), although extended-spectrum quinolones (e.g., temafloxacin, grepafloxacin, trovafloxacin, cinafloxacin, sparfloxacin, gemifloxacin, and moxifloxacin) and desfluoroquinolones such as garenoxacin act on anaerobic bacteria (see Quinolones, Chapter 34).[6,20,21] The most active antimicrobials for anaerobic bacteria are metronidazole, amoxicillin-clavulanate, chloramphenicol, and clindamycin (Tables 41-11 and 41-12).[26a] Numerous newer β-lactamase inhibitor combinations such as ampicillin-sulbactam, ticarcillin-clavulanate,

Table • 41-12

Drug Dosages for Anaerobic Infections

DRUG[a]	SPECIES	DOSE[b]	ROUTE	INTERVAL (HOURS)
Penicillin G	Dog and cat	20,000 U/kg	IM, IV	6—8
Amoxicillin-clavulanate[c]	Dog and cat	20 mg/kg	PO	8—12
Cephalexin	Dog and cat	10—20 mg/kg	PO	8
Cefoxitin	Dog and cat	10—20 mg/kg	IV, IM	8
Clindamycin	Dog and cat	5—10 mg/kg	PO, IV	12
Chloramphenicol	Dog	15—25 mg/kg	PO, SC, IV	8
Metronidazole	Dog and cat	10 mg/kg	PO, IV	8

IM, Intramuscular; *IV*, intravascular; *PO*, by mouth; *SC*, subcutaneous.
[a]See Drug Formulary, Appendix 8 for specific information on each drug.
[b]Dose per administration at specified interval.
[c]Recommended to use amoxicillin with clavulanate for anaerobic infections. Other combinations, such as ampicillin-sulbactam, ticarcillin-clavulanate, and piperacillin-tazobactam, are also effective.

and piperacillin-tazobactam have been shown to be very active against human anaerobic isolates but have not been tested on veterinary isolates.[3,26a] Drugs in the broad-spectrum carbapenem group such as imipenem, meropenem, and ertapenem have been very effective in anaerobic infections associated with mixed aerobic populations. Although anaerobes may be susceptible to trimethoprim-sulfonamides in vitro, inhibitors (mainly thymidine) are found in vivo that make this drug combination an unpredictable treatment for anaerobic microorganism infections.[37] The tetracyclines are unpredictable as well.[29] Isolates of C. *difficile* are susceptible to metronidazole and vancomycin in vitro, and disease produced by this microorganism responds to either drug. Isolates of C. *perfringens* are susceptible to and respond to treatment with the macrolides (tylosin, erythromycin), metronidazole, and ampicillin.[78] Among the quinolones, only extended-spectrum drugs, such as moxifloxacin and gemifloxacin, and the newer desfluoroquinolones, have reasonable activity against anaerobes at generally used therapeutic dosages.[22]

PUBLIC HEALTH CONSIDERATIONS

It is estimated that several million people are bitten by dogs and cats every year (see Chapter 53).[19] Although most of the wounds resulting from animals bites contain aerobic microorganisms, approximately one third contain anaerobes. All are thought to be members of the normal flora of the mouth of dogs and cats. The most common anaerobes belong to the same genera as the anaerobes found in disease processes in dogs and cats.[19,55] Some members of the oral flora of dogs and cats produce serious disease in immunocompromised individuals and those that are asplenic or have liver disease (see Chapter 53).

C. *difficile* is an important cause of disease in human beings. Data indicate that strains of C. *difficile* found in animals are not the same ones found in human patients.[28,60] No data exist

concerning the communicability of C. *perfringens* from dogs and cats to people. However, because it appears that this microorganism can be acquired from contaminated environments, it seems likely but has not been proved that C. *perfringens* from any source can infect dogs, cats, or people. Whether disease results depends on a trigger event, which remains undetermined.

SUGGESTED READINGS*

8. Citron DM. 2002. Update on the taxonomy and clinical aspects of the genus *Fusobacterium*. *Clin Infect Dis* 35(Suppl 1):S22-S27.
14. Edmiston CE, Krepel CJ, Seabrook GR, et al. 2002. Anaerobic infections in the surgical patient: microbial etiology and therapy. *Clin Infect Dis* 35(Suppl 1):S112-S118.
15. Even H, Rohde J, Verspohl J, et al. 1998. Investigations into the occurrence and the antibiotic susceptibility of gram-negative anaerobes of the genera *Bacteroides*, *Prevotella*, *Porphyromonas*, and *Fusobacterium* in specimens obtained from diseased animals. *Berl Munchen Tierarztl Wochenschr* 111:379-386.
22. Goldstein EJC. 2002. Intra-abdominal anaerobic infections: bacteriology and therapeutic potential of newer antimicrobial carbapenem, fluoroquinolone, and desfluoroquinolone therapeutic agents. *Clin Infect Dis* 35(Suppl 1):S106-S111.
40. Jang SS, Hirsh DC. 2000. Prevalence of beta-lactamase producing strains of anaerobic bacteria isolated from domestic animals. *Anaerobe* 8:155.
44. Jousimies-Somer H, Summanen P. 2002. Recent taxonomic changes and terminology update of clinically significant anaerobic gram-negative bacteria (excluding spirochetes). *Clin Infect Dis* 35(Suppl 1)S17-S21.

*See the CD-ROM for a complete list of references.

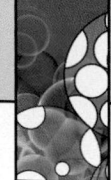

CHAPTER • 42

Botulism

Jeanne A. Barsanti

ETIOLOGY

Botulism is a neuroparalytic illness resulting from intoxication with a neurotoxin produced most commonly by the organism *Clostridium botulinum*. *C. botulinum* is a group of culturally distinct organisms that are alike only in that they are clostridia that produce toxin with the same pharmacologic properties, even though the toxins themselves are antigenically distinct.[7,26,39] *C. botulinum* organisms are gram-positive, straight to slightly curved, motile, spore-forming, saprophytic, anaerobic rods that are distributed in soil worldwide.[7,8] They are 0.5 to 2.0 μm in width, 1.6 to 22 μm in length, with oval subterminal spores.[7] The spores are resistant to heat, light, drying, chemicals, and radiation. Anaerobic conditions and the appropriate nutrient environment (high quantities of organic material) are necessary for spore germination and cell division. The organism grows best under anaerobic conditions and with warmth (15° to 45° C), although some strains can grow at temperatures as low as 6° C. The organism produces toxin under anaerobic, low acid (pH over 4.6), and low solute conditions.[39]

Seven types of *C. botulinum* have been identified, distinguished by the antigenically distinct types (A, B, C1, D, E, F, and G) of botulinum neurotoxin that they produce.[7,17] All of these types have similar structure and the same neurotoxic effect. The nucleotide sequences for all types have been determined,[2,39] but the three-dimensional structure of only type A is known.[26] Types A, B, E, and F are associated with human disease.[6,18] Types C and D cause disease in birds and other mammals.[7,39] Type G has not been confirmed as a cause of disease in any species.[7] All canine cases to date have been caused by type C toxin, with the exception of two cases of type D reported from Senegal.[18] Although the disease has been experimentally produced in cats,[3] no natural cases have been reported. A cat that ate contaminated yogurt did not become ill even though two people eating the same yogurt did.[12] Type C botulism has been reported in lions (*Panthera leo*), but jaguars (*P. onca*) and coatis (*Nasua nasua*), eating the same food as did the lions, were not affected.[3,11] Most cases of feline dysautonomia have been reported in the United Kingdom, while most canine cases have been seen in the United States. The cause of this syndrome has been elusive. In an outbreak of dysautonomia in a closed colony of cats, immunoglobulin A (IgA) antibody titers to *C. botulinum* surface antigens and toxoid were increased in the ileum and feces of affected compared with control cats.[31] Toxin was detected in the feces of affected and some subclinical cats but not control cats, even without enrichment culture. In addition, toxin was found in dry cat food. The results support the role of botulinum intoxication in this syndrome.

Usually a single organism expresses a single toxin type.[8] Types C and D toxins are produced by a *C. botulinum* group that is partially proteolytic and does not ferment glucose.[8] Although mildly alkaline pH stimulates growth of most types of *C. botulinum*, pH 5.7 may be optimal for type C producing strains.

Botulinal toxins are the most potent, naturally occurring, acutely toxic substances known.[2] In people, botulinal toxin is 10,000 times more toxic than cyanide[8] and 15,000 times more potent than sarin gas, used in the terrorist attack in Tokyo.[39] Significant differences exist in species susceptibility to botulinal toxin of different types as noted previously. Botulinal toxin is released from vegetative cells only by lysis of the cell or spore. The toxin is not secreted from the cell or spore.[8] The amount of toxin in spores is only approximately 1% of that found in vegetative cells, but the intrasporal toxin is resistant to heat denaturation. Type C toxin is stable at a pH range from 2.7 to 10.2.[21] Vegetative cells produced by germinating spores begin to produce toxin within several days after germination. All the different serotypes of botulinal toxin are a single polypeptide of 150 kDa that is inactive when initially released.[2] All the botulinal neurotoxins are composed of a heavy (H) chain of 100 kDa and a light (L) chain of 50 kDa. The H chain consists of an amino-terminal domain of 50 kDa and a carboxy-terminal end of 50 kDa.[7] The H and L chain are bridged by a single interchain disulfide bond (Fig. 42-1).[2,22] Activation is achieved by a specific proteolytic cleavage of a single peptide bond within a surface exposed loop.[2,36] Bacterial or host proteases can accomplish this cleavage. After cleavage the toxin remains as an associated H and L chain via the disulfide bridge and via noncovalent protein-protein interactions as described in the next paragraph.[32] The interchain disulfide bond is essential for toxicity.[36]

After release from the bacterial cell, the toxin is bound noncovalently with nontoxic proteins to form complexes known as progenitor toxins. The progenitor toxin is very stable at low pH, protecting the neurotoxin from proteolytic attack in the gastric environment. This stability allows the complex to reach the small intestine, where the alkaline pH is conducive to dissociation of the complex, releasing the neurotoxin,[8,26] which explains why the progenitor toxin is more toxic than neurotoxin alone when administered orally.[22] The number and size of the associated nontoxic proteins differ between toxin types. Type C toxin may be associated with up to five additional proteins, resulting in a released complex of molecular size of 500 or 900 kDa.[8]

PATHOGENESIS

The basis of the production of lower motor neuron (LMN) paralysis in botulism is that the toxin prevents the presynaptic release of acetylcholine at the neuromuscular junction. Both the spontaneous release of acetylcholine and its release caused by a nerve action potential are inhibited.[26] Signs of autonomic dysfunction (parasympathetic and sympathetic) co-exist with skeletal neuromuscular dysfunction.[26]

Botulism is usually caused by ingestion of the preformed toxin, although two variants of the disease in people, infant botulism and infantlike botulism, are caused by in vivo production

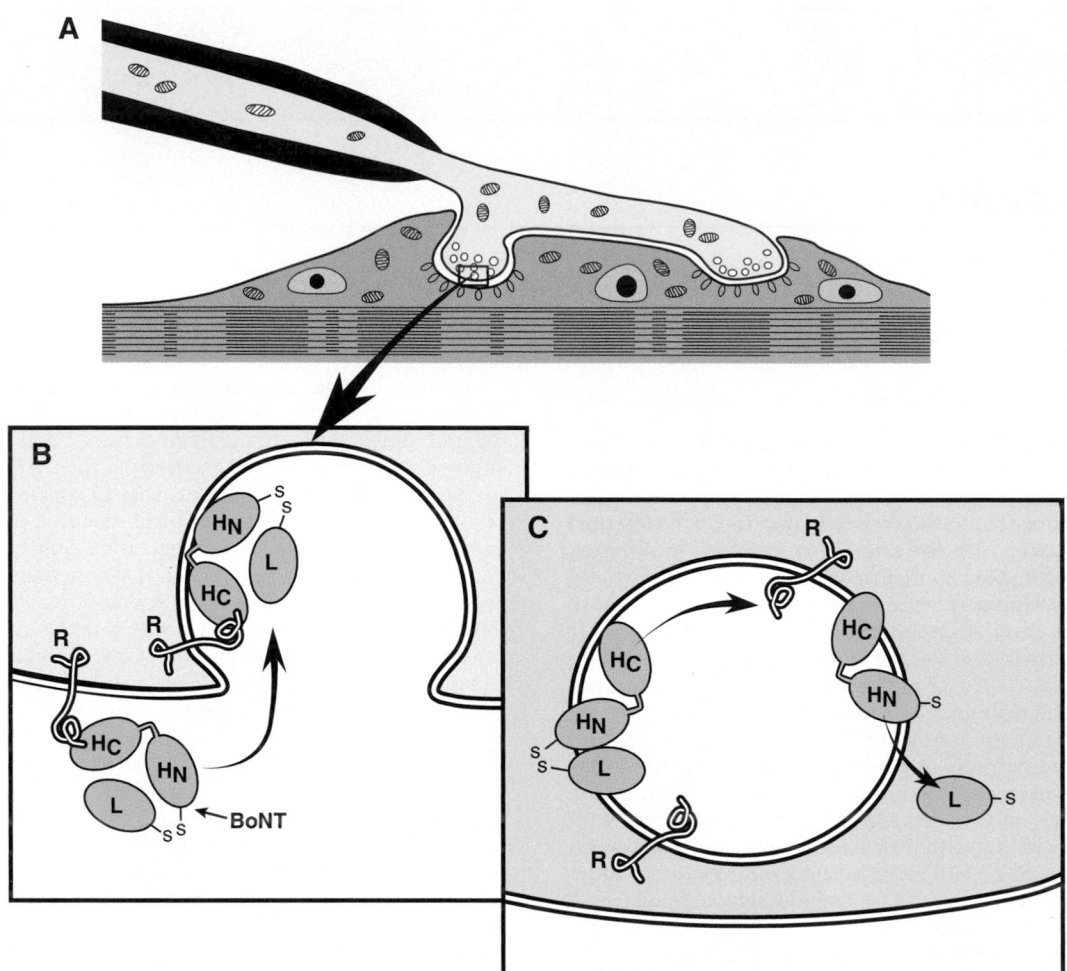

Fig 42-1 Schematic drawing of the binding of botulinal toxin by a membrane receptor (R) at the neuromuscular junction (**A**). The toxin is composed of a heavy chain with carboxyl (HC) and amino (HN) terminal ends and a light (L) chain containing zinc. The carboxyl end of the heavy chain binds to the receptor at the nerve ending (**B**). The HN terminal end is thought to be involved in the membrane translocation of the L chain into the nerve cell by inserting itself into the membrane lipid bilayer (**C**). The L chain, free in the cytosol and by its zinc-endopeptidase activity, selectively cleaves SNARE proteins involved in the exocytosis of acetylcholine (**C**).[13,18,22] (Courtesy University of Georgia, Athens, Ga.)

of toxin in the intestine after germination of spores and intestinal colonization with neurotoxigenic clostridia, not necessarily *C. botulinum*.[7,16] Normal human adults are resistant to intestinal colonization with *C. botulinum*, largely because of intestinal microflora. Colonization can be induced in adult animals or people only if they are germ free or are being treated with antibiotics.[3] Persistent intestinal colonization in adults with *C. botulinum* rarely causes clinical illness.[3] Intestinal colonization was established experimentally in 8- to 11-day-old puppies, but no intoxication occurred.[3] Intestinal colonization has been found in a natural case of botulism in a 6-month-old dog.[3] However, the dog recovered without antibiotic therapy, even though intestinal colonization continued for several months. Wound botulism, in which the organisms infect a wound and produce toxin, is another rare form of botulism in people, usually associated with illicit, injectable drug use.[7] A concern associated with bioterrorism is that aerosolized botulinum toxin type A can be absorbed through the lungs.[39]

The source of botulinal toxin is rarely found in reported canine cases. Type C toxin has been isolated from fly larvae (maggots) and from carrion, and most canine cases are thought to be associated with ingestion of carrion.[15,18,25] An outbreak in cats was associated with ingestion of carrion.[14a] Other intoxications are associated with wetlands during

warm weather, the areas associated with avian botulism epizootics.[34]

Once ingested, types C and D toxins are absorbed primarily from upper small bowel into the lymphatic system via endocytosis similar to nutrient proteins. Toxin can continue to be absorbed from the lower small bowel and colon, but this process proceeds more slowly. From the lymphatic system, the toxin enters the bloodstream. The absorbed toxin is in its disulphide-bonded di-chain form.[8] Neural intoxication occurs in four steps: binding to cell surface receptors by the carboxy-terminal of the H chain, internalization of the toxin into endosomal-like compartments, membrane translocation facilitated by the amino-terminal of the H chain, and enzymatic cleavage of target proteins by the L chain (see Fig. 42-1).

The carboxy-terminal end of the H chain is responsible for binding to the presynaptic membrane (see Fig. 42-1).[22,31] This end of the H chain is composed of two sub-domains, an N-terminal and a C-terminal.[8,24] The C-terminal end is the most critical to binding and is the most variable between toxin types, perhaps explaining part of the difference in species susceptibility to different toxins.[24,36] Binding occurs very quickly and is irreversible, unaffected by temperature and independent of neural activity. The cell membrane receptors for the toxin must have very high affinity for it because only minute quantities (fewer than 10^{-12} mol) of botulinal toxin are sufficient to cause death.[18,22] The receptor sites on the neuron are not well understood, but it is postulated that binding requires both polysialoganglioside and other protein components.[7,8,24] The toxin binds to the presynaptic nerve endings of the peripheral nervous system and cranial nerves.[39] Variations in receptor affinity for different types of toxin also help explain the different sensitivities of animal species to the different botulinal toxins.[18,22,31] During this stage, the toxin is susceptible to inactivation by antitoxin. After binding, the toxin passes through the cell membrane by receptor-mediated endocytosis.[6] Once inside the cell, the toxin is more resistant to inactivation by antitoxin. However, some experiments show that some types of antibody can enter cholinergic neurons and inactivate internalized neurotoxin.[2]

The amino-terminal end of the H chain governs toxin translocation (see Fig. 42-1).[25] This process is temperature and energy dependent.[31] The translocation is pH dependent and requires a low pH step. Low pH triggers a change in the toxin to a state of greater hydrophobicity, leading to ability to penetrate the membrane lipid bilayer.[8]

The L chain is a metallo-protease containing zinc. The blockage of acetylcholine release is caused by zinc-dependent cleavage of protein components of the neuroexocytosis apparatus (the SNARE proteins).[8,26] The SNARE proteins are essential to the docking and fusion of synaptic vesicles with the presynaptic membrane, events that lead to the release of acetylcholine into the neuromuscular junction.[7,8] A remarkable finding is that proteolysis of a small amount of the total SNARE present is sufficient to block acetylcholine release.[36] Different types of botulinal toxin cleave different bonds within this membrane protein system. Type C toxin targets syntaxin and SNAP-25 proteins, with syntaxin cleavage being most significant.[26,36] Syntaxin cleavage by type C toxin prevents G-protein regulation of calcium channels associated with presynaptic neurotransmitter release sites. Normally calcium influx through these ion channels stimulates fusion of the vesicles and release of neurotransmitter into the synapse. Thus, with type C toxin, the formation of synaptic vesicles, their number, and their distribution along the presynaptic membrane are all normal, but neurotransmitter cannot be released because the vesicles cannot fuse with the presynaptic membrane.[2] The life time of intracellular toxin can be quite long; and until the last molecule of the L chain is degraded, toxin-mediated SNARE proteolysis will occur.[36]

Mutations in the amino acid sequence of the toxin targets make them resistant to proteolysis.[26] Differences in the targets for the toxins between species are also thought to account for species insensitivity to certain toxin types.

Botulinal neurotoxins do not cause death of the affected neuron. They cause only paralysis and degeneration of the intoxicated synapse. Under light microscopy, no lesions are apparent at the neuromuscular junction. However, changes in terminal axons, synaptic clefts, and adjacent muscle fibers have been noted in neuromuscular junctions by electron microscopy (EM) from human cases. If the animal survives, recovery occurs by reformation of functional neuromuscular junctions. Thus animals with botulism have the potential for a complete recovery of neurologic function with no sequelae.

CLINICAL FINDINGS

In all species, botulism is characterized by generalized LMN dysfunction, leading to weakness and flaccid paralysis.[8] Autonomic dysfunction also occurs. In the most severe cases, failure of respiratory muscles leads to death. Botulism should be considered in all dogs with diffuse LMN disease.

The clinical signs in type C canine botulism have been the same whether experimentally or naturally induced.[3,34,41] The severity of signs varies with the amount of toxin ingested and individual susceptibility. The first sign is a progressive, symmetric, ascending weakness from the rear to the forelimbs that can result in quadriplegia (Fig. 42-2). Tail wag is maintained. A complete neurologic examination will show hyporeflexia and hypotonia, indicating generalized LMN dysfunction. Cranial nerves are often affected: mydriasis with sluggish pupillary responses, decreased jaw tone, decreased gag reflex with excess salivation, diminished palpebral reflexes, and weak vocalization have been found in affected dogs. Pain perception and alert mental attitude are maintained (Fig. 42-3). Unlike inflammatory LMN diseases such as polyradiculoneuritis and polymyositis, dogs with botulism do not show hyperesthesia to muscle flexing, stretching, or palpation. In severely affected dogs, decreased abdominal muscle tone and primarily diaphragmatic respiration may occur.

The heart rate is variable (increased or decreased), and constipation and urinary retention may develop. Megaesophagus has been noted in some affected dogs. Muscle atrophy is variable. No hyperesthesia is present. Conjunctivitis and ulcerative keratitis may develop because of the weak palpebral reflex. Bilateral keratoconjunctivitis sicca has been noted because tear production may be reduced with neurochemical paralysis. Death may result from respiratory paralysis or from secondary respiratory or urinary infections. On necropsy, no

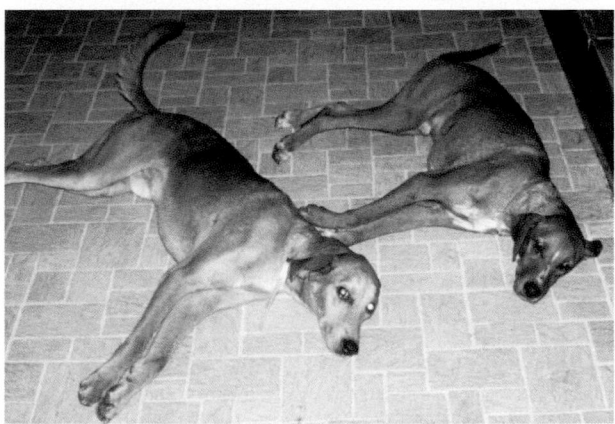

Fig 42-2 Dogs with quadriplegia resulting from botulism. (Courtesy University of Georgia, Athens, Ga.)

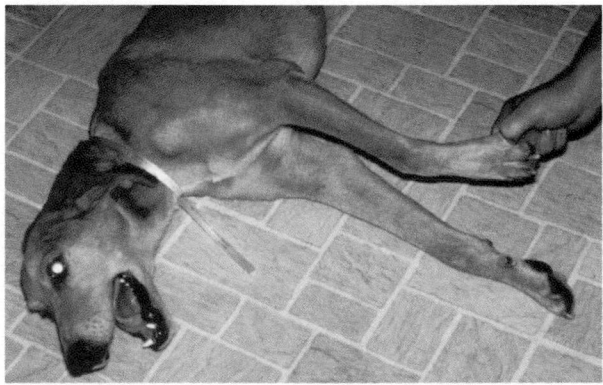

Fig 42-3 Dog with botulism showing normal pain perception but lack of a withdrawal reflex. Note the dilated pupil as evidenced by the reflective tapetum. (Courtesy University of Georgia, Athens, Ga.)

gross or light microscopic abnormalities can be seen in the nervous system.

The progression of signs is explained by differences in affected muscles, the diaphragm being much more resistant than skeletal muscle to paralysis with progressive neuromuscular blockade.

The incubation period after ingestion of contaminated food in dogs has been from hours to 6 days. The earlier the signs appear, the more serious is the disease. The duration of illness in dogs that recovered has ranged from 14 to 24 days. Cranial nerve, neck, and forelimb functions tend to return first in affected dogs. If recovery occurs, it is complete (Fig. 42-4). Recovery is expected unless secondary infections or respiratory failure occur.

In the reported cases of type D botulism, the dogs died suddenly with signs of generalized hemorrhage and without observed neurologic deficits.[3] The signs may have been caused by a different toxin, C2 toxin, which increases vascular permeability and induces hemorrhage and edema.[33]

The possible causes of LMN disease in dogs include polyradiculoneuritis, myasthenia gravis, organophosphate toxicity, and tick paralysis. Coral snake venom toxicity and the dumb form of rabies have also been considered in the differential diagnosis.[9] Although signs in these diseases can overlap, cranial nerve abnormalities and cholinergic signs are more common in botulism than in polyradiculoneuritis or tick paralysis.

Affected cats have shown a similar diffuse ascending LMN paralysis.[14a] Some cats died with severe signs, whereas cats with less severe illness had marked recovery by 56 hours.

In the dysautonomia associated with Key-Gaskell syndrome in dogs and cats, clinical signs include regurgitation or vomiting, variable anorexia, dysphagia, constipation, urinary retention, and pupillary dilation. In addition to autonomic dysfunction, dogs with this syndrome can also show lower motor neuron paralysis of the skeletal muscle.[31] Further studies will be needed to substantiate this syndrome is associated with botulism.

DIAGNOSIS

All results of routine laboratory work (complete blood count [CBC], blood chemistry profile, urinalysis) are within reference limits unless secondary complications, such as cutaneous (decubital ulcer) or respiratory (aspiration pneumonia) infec-

tions, develop.[3,34] Cerebral spinal fluid is normal in affected dogs and people. Thoracic radiographs may show megaesophagus in dogs (Fig. 42-5).

Electromyography (EMG) shows that LMN dysfunction in clinically affected dogs is caused by a problem at the neuromuscular junction and perhaps to peripheral nerve conduction.[3,43] When a motor nerve is stimulated, motor unit potentials are subnormal in amplitude but not polyphasic (Fig. 42-6). Decrements in motor unit potentials are variable after repetitive stimulation. Fibrillation potentials were noted in one study but not in another,[3] which may be related to the difference in the time of performance of EMGs (mean of 16 and 12 days, respectively). Nerve conduction velocity was mildly decreased in one report, even with correction for hypothermia. As the dogs recovered, increased electrode insertional activity and positive sharp waves were found. The main EMG findings in affected people are decreased compound muscle action potentials with normal nerve conduction.[34] The most specific EMG test for people is rapid repetitive stimulation: a 50% greater increase in the evoked train of compound muscle action potentials with rapid repetitive stimulation at 50 Hz indicates botulism.[1] Positive results may be found in only one muscle, although many muscles may be weak.[7] As in dogs, EMG findings in people vary and sometimes lead to incorrect initial diagnoses because findings are relatively nonspecific and experienced electromyographers are essential.[39]

Confirmatory diagnosis of botulism is based on the finding of the toxin in serum, feces, vomitus, or in samples of the food

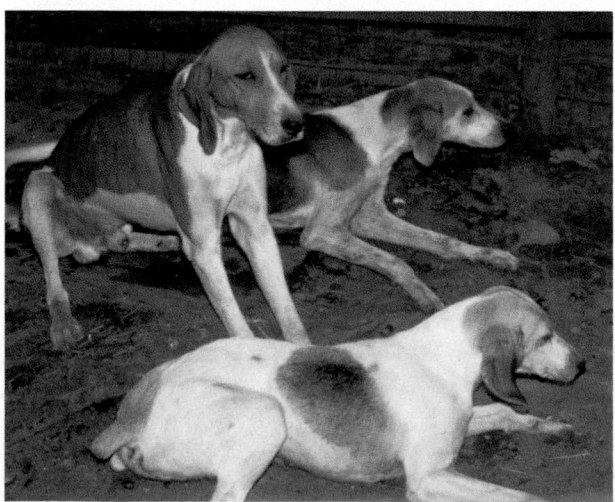

Fig 42-4 Dogs recovering from botulism, having regained the ability to resume sternal recumbency and move the head and neck. (Courtesy University of Georgia, Athens, Ga.)

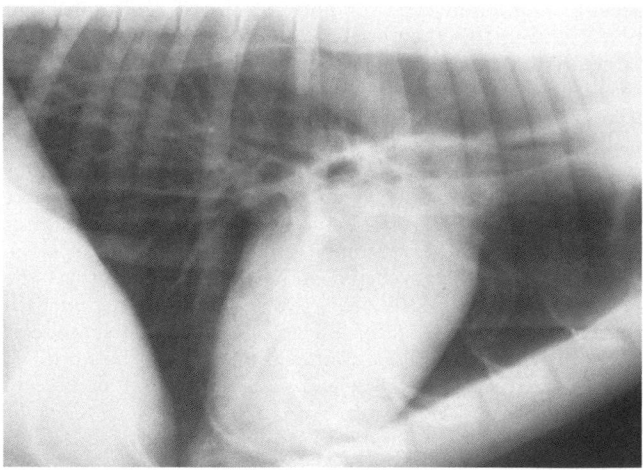

Fig 42-5 Lateral thoracic radiograph of a dog with botulism showing megaesophagus. (Courtesy University of Georgia, Athens, Ga.)

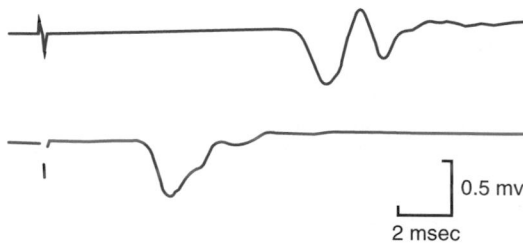

0.5 mv

2 msec

Fig 42-6 EMG tracing after stimulation of the right tibial nerve of a dog with botulism. The upper tracing is the response to stimulation at the level of the femoral trochanter, and the lower tracing is the response to stimulation at the popliteal fossa. The amplitudes of the evoked potentials are markedly subnormal.

that was ingested. Serum should be collected as early in the disease course as possible and when clinical signs are maximal. Approximately 10 ml of serum or 50 g of feces, vomitus, or food are needed to conduct diagnostic tests. Specimens should be refrigerated, but not frozen unless delay of analysis of several days is likely, and examined as soon as possible. Freezing does not affect the toxin but does affect the ability to detect the organism. Specimens sent to a distant laboratory should be placed in sterile, leak-proof containers and then in insulated shipping containers with coolant. The container should be labeled that it contains a potential biologic hazard, refrigerated on arrival, and should be shipped by the most rapid means available.[7] Refer to Appendix 5 for a list of laboratories that perform these tests.

The standard and most reliable method of identifying the toxin remains the mouse inoculation test.* In this test, serum or an extract of feces, vomitus, or food is injected alone and in combination with type-specific antitoxin into the peritoneal cavity of mice. The mice are then observed for signs of botulism. Survival of one group protected with one type of antitoxin and death of the other groups with signs consistent with botulism confirm the presence of botulinal toxin. This test is highly sensitive but is expensive and involves the death of research animals. Safety is also an issue, especially with strains that affect people. Notably, type C toxin has been shown to be as effective as type A in human therapeutic uses[35]; thus type C toxin may also affect people contaminated via laboratory exposure. Minute quantities of botulinum toxin acquired by ingestion, inhalation, or absorption through the eye or a break in the skin might cause intoxication. Therefore experienced personnel, preferably immunized with botulinal toxoid, must handle all test materials.[7]

With increasing concern about such bioassays, a need has developed for in vitro tests. A variety of enzyme-linked immunosorbent assays (ELISAs) have been developed to measure the endopeptidase activity of botulinal toxin by the cleavage of artificial substrates.[8,17] These assays have been used to detect botulinal toxin in food in human outbreaks. Some of these assays appear to match the sensitivity and specificity of the mouse bioassay and measure functional toxin.[8,17] They are more rapid compared with the mouse test. These tests will be important in replacing the mouse bioassay as the diagnostic test of choice when they are validated further and more readily accessible.[8] Polymerase chain reaction (PCR) assays for toxin are also being developed.[17]

An attempt to isolate *C. botulinum* from feces or gastric contents is recommended in people.[1,7,39] The organism can be isolated from feces of approximately 60% of people with botulism. Isolation of the organism in association with clinical signs provides evidence for the diagnosis, but it is not as conclusive as is toxin identification. Isolation for the organism from food or the environment is usually considered of little significance given that spores are ubiquitous in the environment.[39] The type C organism is one of the most difficult to culture because it is a strict anaerobe. The presence of toxin in an extract of cultured feces is often used as evidence of the organism's presence.[3,12] Because isolation of the organism is time consuming and requires specialized facilities and specifically trained personnel, other ways to identify the organism are being sought. The molecular characterization of the genes for the organisms has led to the possibility that DNA analysis might be useful. PCR-based detection tests have been developed for toxin types A, B, E, and F. However, the potential for false-positive results caused by normally unexpressed genes for toxin production has rendered these tests inadequate for establishing the neurotoxicity of a bacterium. At this point in time, these tests are not being used as routine diagnostic

tools in people.[8] A PCR test for *C. botulinum* type C was used on avian and environmental samples in an outbreak of avian botulism.[19] The results of the PCR test for the organism correlated well with the mouse bioassay conducted after sample enrichment. However, the problem is that the presence of part of the gene from the organism does not confirm that the organism produces neurotoxin.[19]

In human beings, at least one laboratory test for botulism was positive in 65% of patients suspected to have the disease. Large outbreaks have occurred in people in which none or only a low percentage of specimens yielded a positive result. Thus, in people, the diagnosis is often made on history and clinical findings.[7]

THERAPY

Supportive Care

Supportive treatment is most important because spontaneous recovery will occur if the amount of toxin ingested is not too large and if respiratory and urinary tract infections can be avoided. If ingestion is recent, removal of material from the intestinal tract via gastric lavage, cathartics, or enemas may be useful. Cathartic agents containing magnesium should be avoided because of the theoretical concern that magnesium may enhance the action of botulinum toxin.[39] Affected animals should be assisted to eat, drink, and move about. Waterbeds or cage padding will reduce the incidence of decubital sores. Ability to urinate should be monitored and the bladder expressed as needed. Enemas and stool softeners should be given for constipation. Parenteral fluids should be used as necessary to avoid dehydration, especially if swallowing is impaired. Antibiotics should be provided if infection develops, but aminoglycosides should be avoided because they also have the potential to block neuromuscular transmission. To avoid altering the intestinal microflora, which might allow *C. botulinum* to grow, antibiotics should be given only when necessary.[3] Topical nonmedicated or antibiotic ophthalmic ointments should be provided to prevent exposure keratitis in dogs with poor palpebral function. In the most severe cases, mechanical ventilatory support may be needed. Aggressive ventilatory support and meticulous intensive care has lead to markedly improved survival in affected people.[7]

Antitoxin

Antitoxin therapy is most effective if given early in the disease course because equine antitoxin, the only one currently available, is not effective after the toxin has bound to the nerve endings, which occurs rapidly after the toxin is absorbed.[7] Antitoxin may prevent further toxin binding if intestinal absorption and circulation are still occurring. Because cases in dogs in the United States to date have been type C, that specific antitoxin is needed. Unfortunately, the available antitoxin in the United States is an equine product with antibodies to toxin types A, B, and E[39] and thus is not useful in dogs.

Antibiotics

Penicillin or metronidazole has been administered in dogs and people in an attempt to reduce any potential intestinal population of *C. botulinum*.[3] The efficacy of these drugs is doubted because disease is usually caused by ingestion of preformed toxin and because neither drug is certain to eradicate *C. botulinum* from the intestine.[3] The possibility that these drugs might make the disease worse by releasing more toxin through bacterial lysis or by promoting intestinal infection has also been raised.[3] Even in infant botulism, which may involve intestinal colonization with *C. botulinum*, penicillin has no effect on recovery.[3] Therefore antibiotic administration is not indicated in the treatment of this disease.

*References: 1, 7, 16, 17, 39.

Neuromuscular Potentiators

Two drugs, guanidine hydrochloride and 3,4 diaminopyridine, were used in clinical cases in animals, based on literature in people.[3,12,13] Administration of guanidine hydrochloride to an affected lion resulted in seizures and pyrexia with death 2 days after drug administration.[3] Diaminopyridine was given to two lions, with improvement in signs for only 30 minutes. That neither of these drugs, or related drugs, will work with type C toxin is now known because they cannot block the specific effect of this toxin. No drug is available for people or animals that counter the effects of botulinal neurotoxins.[2]

Antibody Therapy

Because of the threat of bioterrorism using botulism toxin, a sustained research effort has led to the first compound that can be mass-produced to prevent or treat adult human botulism.[10] Scientists have isolated and identified three antibodies against botulism toxin and combined them. Each antibody is capable of binding to a different part of the toxin, neutralizing the toxin more effectively than a single antibody. A single dose protects people for 6 months, and only small doses are required.

Intravenous administration of human botulism immune globulin is in clinical trials for use in human infant botulism. Infants treated with this product within 3 days of onset of signs recover more rapidly.[8]

Neither of these therapies may be useful in dogs and cats. The antibodies being produced are of human origin and are directed primarily against the toxin types common in people, rather than the type C toxin common in animals. An investigational equine heptavalent botulism immune globulin fragment has been under study.[27]

PREVENTION

Heating food to 80° C for 30 minutes or to 100° C for 10 minutes destroys the botulinal toxin. Preventing access to carrion and thorough cooking of any food fed to dogs will prevent the disease. Foxhounds appear predisposed to the disease because they may be fed raw meat. Recovered animals do not develop immunity because the amount of toxin necessary to produce clinical signs is so low.[9]

Vaccination with a toxoid against toxin types A, B, C, D, and E has been successful in cattle, abattoir personnel, exposed laboratory workers, and some military personnel.[8] This vaccine has a significant number of disadvantages. It does not result in equal protection against all serotypes (mainly protects against types A and E), and it requires the production of the active toxin. It is unlicensed, protection requires several months, and immunity is not lifelong.[39] Efforts have been directed toward producing recombinant vaccines that can be prepared without isolating toxin from clostridia, and early reports are encouraging.[8] For example, a recombinant type C variant in which three amino acids were replaced in the L chain was nontoxic to mice and did not cleave syntaxin in vitro.[2] This product stimulated high antibody levels and protective immunity in mice when given orally or subcuta-

neously. These studies suggest that new vaccine strategies are possible. Vaccination will probably not be recommended for the general human population because it would block current use of botulism toxin for overactive muscular disorders such as dystonias.

Antibody administration, as described under Therapy, is also being developed for prevention of disease in people.

The recent increased research on prevention is caused by the potential for intentional poisoning. As many as 17 countries are suspected to be developing biologic weapons.[39] Botulinum toxin is often one of these agents because it is relatively easy to produce and is highly lethal in small quantities. Whether dogs and cats would be affected in such an attack would depend on the type of toxin and the method of administration.

THERAPEUTIC USE OF BOTULINAL TOXIN

As previously noted, botulinal toxin is used therapeutically in people for dystonias and wrinkling. One canine case of probable essential blepharospasm responded well to botulinum toxin A therapy.[28] A total dose of 200 mouse units was used per eye. This total dose was divided and injected with a 25-gauge needle in six subcutaneous sites per eye in the area of the orbicularis oculi muscle. The dog was retreated with 100 mouse units per eye as needed thereafter. The first retreatment was at 1 month, the next at 3 months, and then every 4 months. After more than 3 years of therapy, no adverse effects were noted. Botulinum toxin was evaluated as a potential long-term treatment for excessive mucosal secretions such as in vasomotor rhinitis.[38] Type A botulinum toxin (50 units) was packed in a nasal passage of dogs for a 1-hour period. Saline-soaked gauze was a control in the other nostril. When tested by electrostimulation 6 days later, the toxin side had reduced rhinorrhea. Local injection of botulinum toxin have also been evaluated for reducing tone in the sphincter of Oddi controlling biliary retention in dogs.[42]

SUGGESTED READINGS*

2. Atassi MZ, Oshima M. 1999. Structure, activity, and immune (T and B cell) recognition of botulinum neurotoxins, *Critical Rev Immunol* 19:219-260.
5. Barsanti JA, Walser M, Hatheway CL, et al. 1978. Type C botulism in American foxhounds, *J Am Vet Med Assoc* 172:809-813.
15. Fain Binda JC, Fernandez RA, Blotta RE, et al. 1998. Natural botulism in dogs due to ingestion of botulinum toxin, *Vet Argentina* 15:216-221.
31. Nunn F, Cave TA, Knottenbelt C, et al. 2004. Association between Key-Gaskell syndrome and infection by *Clostridium botulinum* type C/D, *Vet Rec* 153: 111-115.
41. Tjalsma EJ. 1990. Three cases of *Clostridium botulinum* type C intoxication in the dog, *Tijdschr Diergeneeskd* 115:518-521.

*See the CD-ROM for a complete list of references.

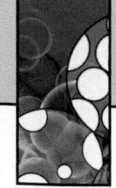
Tetanus

Craig E. Greene

ETIOLOGY

Tetanus is caused by the action of a potent neurotoxin formed in the body during the vegetative growth of *Clostridium tetani*. *C. tetani* is a motile, gram-positive, nonencapsulated, anaerobic, spore-forming bacillus. Although strain differences of *C. tetani* exist throughout the world, an antigenically homogeneous toxin is produced by all strains. Resistant spores of the organism can be found in the environment, especially in the soil, where increased moisture, cultivation, and fertilization favor their survival. Organisms are routinely isolated from the feces of many domestic animals, including the dog and cat.[9] Isolation from human feces occurs with greater frequency in those occupationally exposed to farm animals. Spores can survive adverse weather conditions in the absence of direct sunlight for months or years and can be found readily in dust and debris in indoor environments. Spores are resistant to boiling water, phenol, cresol, and mercury bichloride, and they resist an autoclave temperature of 120° C for 15 to 20 minutes. However, the vegetative phase of *C. tetani* is no more resistant to chemical and physical inactivation than other microorganisms.

EPIDEMIOLOGY

Tetanus develops when spores are introduced into wounds or penetrating injuries. The spores vegetate in response to anaerobic conditions at the site of injury. The presence of a foreign body, tissue necrosis, other microorganisms, or abscess formation contributes to germination. Two toxins from *C. tetani* have been identified. *Tetanolepsin* causes hemolysis of erythrocytes during rapid in vitro growth of the bacteria; however, it is not considered clinically significant. In contrast, *tetanospasmin* (molecular weight = 176,000) enters the body from the wound site and produces marked effects on neurologic function. It is not absorbed from the gastrointestinal (GI) tract because digestive juices usually destroy it. Its high molecular weight precludes its entry into the placenta.

The prevalence of the disease in dogs and cats is relatively low compared with that in other domestic animals, which may be related to the natural resistance of dogs and cats to this toxin (Table 43-1). The resistance is related to the inability of the toxin to penetrate and bind to nervous tissue; direct central nervous system (CNS) injections of toxin produce the same signs in different species.

PATHOGENESIS

Many experimental studies have been performed with dogs, cats, and other laboratory animals to elucidate the mechanism by which tetanospasmin enters and affects the CNS. The site and route of administration of toxin are important in determining the type of disease that develops. Localized tetanus can be produced by intramuscular (IM) or subcutaneous (SC) injection of toxin at a specific site. Tetanospasmin is a dimer composed of (1) a heavy chain (100 kDa) that binds to neuronal cells and transport proteins and (2) a light chain (50 kDa) that blocks the release of neurotransmitters.[24] Toxin enters the axons of the nearest motor nerves at the neuromuscular end-plate and migrates by retrograde transport within motor axons at a rate of 75 to 250 mm per day to the neuronal cell body within the spinal cord (Fig. 43-1). Within the spinal cord, toxin ascends bilaterally until it reaches the brain (Fig. 43-2).

Systemic intravenous (IV) administration of large amounts of toxin usually results in intracranial signs, such as convulsions, facial muscle spasms, or respiratory arrest, before development of generalized limb rigidity. Small amounts of bloodborne toxin are thought to enter the CNS through the intact blood-brain barrier. Alternatively, hematogenously disseminated toxin may localize preferentially in the neuromuscular endings of many motor nerves throughout the body, from which it may ascend by retrograde axonal transport simultaneously into many areas of the nervous system. The initial involvement of facial musculature after hematogenous spread of toxin is explained by the fact that cranial nerve motor axons (e.g., facial nerves) are shorter than those of the limbs. Although all muscles are affected in generalized tetanus, characteristic postures such as outstretched limbs or a closed jaw are observed. The stronger of the opposing muscle groups predominates, such as the extensors rather than the flexors for antigravity support or the muscles used for closing rather than opening the jaw.

The clinical signs of tetanus infection can be explained by the known pathophysiologic effects of tetanus toxin on the nervous system. It inhibits release of glycine and γ-aminobutyric acid (GABA)—neurotransmitters of inhibitory interneurons of the brain and spinal cord. Presynaptic blockade of synapses of Renshaw cells and 1a fibers of alpha motor neurons occurs. Most experimental evidence has confirmed the effect of toxin at the spinal cord; however, the brain, neuromuscular junctions, and the autonomic nervous system can also be affected. Tetanus toxin has an affinity for gangliosides within the gray matter of the CNS, which may explain the cerebral signs that appear in some animals without obvious spinal cord involvement. The effects of tetanus toxin have also been ascribed to its affinity for binding at the neuromuscular junction, which may induce direct neuromuscular facilitation before the migration of toxin to the CNS. Tetanus toxin may affect sympathetic preganglionic neurons in the same way it affects lower motor neurons within the spinal cord, causing signs of autonomic dysfunction. Bradycardia associated with tetanus probably results from vagal-parasympathetic hyperactivity. Tetanus toxin also blocks neurotransmitters in the parasympathetic cardiac inhibitory center of the nucleus ambiguous, resulting in increased vagal tone and pronounced

Table • 43-1

Relative Susceptibility of Animals to Tetanus Toxin

ANIMAL	SUSCEPTIBILITY[a]
Horse	1 (most susceptible)
Guinea pig	2
Human	3
Mouse	12
Rabbit	24
Dog	600
Cat	7200
Chicken	360,000 (least susceptible)

[a]The horse has been assigned an arbitrary value of 1, with 1 indicating *most susceptible*. Susceptibility values relate to the comparative amount of toxin required to produce clinical illness, with increasing values indicating decreasing susceptibility.

bradyarrhythmias. Increased catecholamine release associated with adrenergic stimulation can also cause episodes of hypertension or tachycardia in tetanus.

The binding of tetanus toxin to presynaptic sites of inhibitory neurons is irreversible; recovery depends on sprouting of new axon terminals.[24]

CLINICAL FINDINGS

Clinical signs of tetanus usually occur within 5 to 10 days after receiving a wound, although ranges of 3 to 18 days have been reported.[16] This time varies and is shorter when the wound is closer to the CNS, has numerous organisms, and has a more anaerobic environment, which favors toxin production. Because of the increased resistance of cats and dogs to tetanus, disease onset may be delayed for up to 3 weeks. This delay may account for the absence of a detectable wound at the time of examination. However, because of greater innate

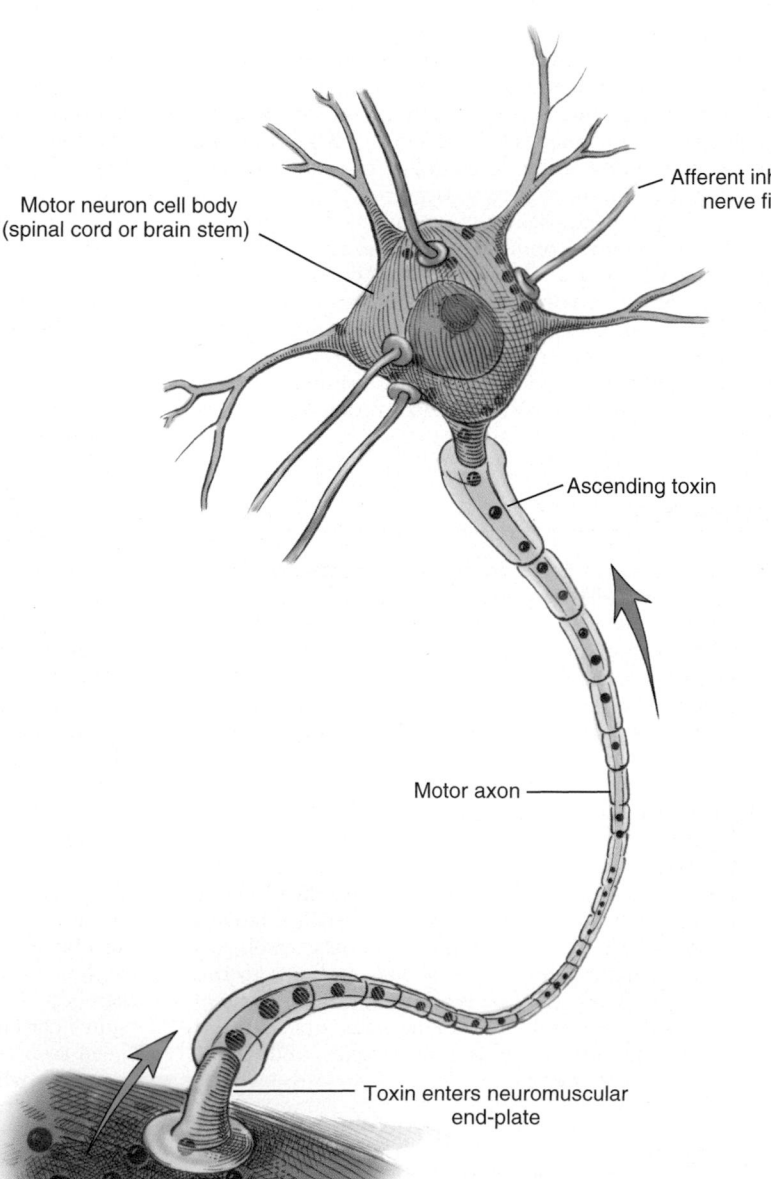

Fig   43-1   Retrograde intraaxonal transport of tetanus toxin into the CNS. (Courtesy University of Georgia, Athens, Ga.)

Afferent inhibitory nerve fiber

Motor neuron cell body (spinal cord or brain stem)

Ascending toxin

Motor axon

Toxin enters neuromuscular end-plate

Beisel
© UGA 2004

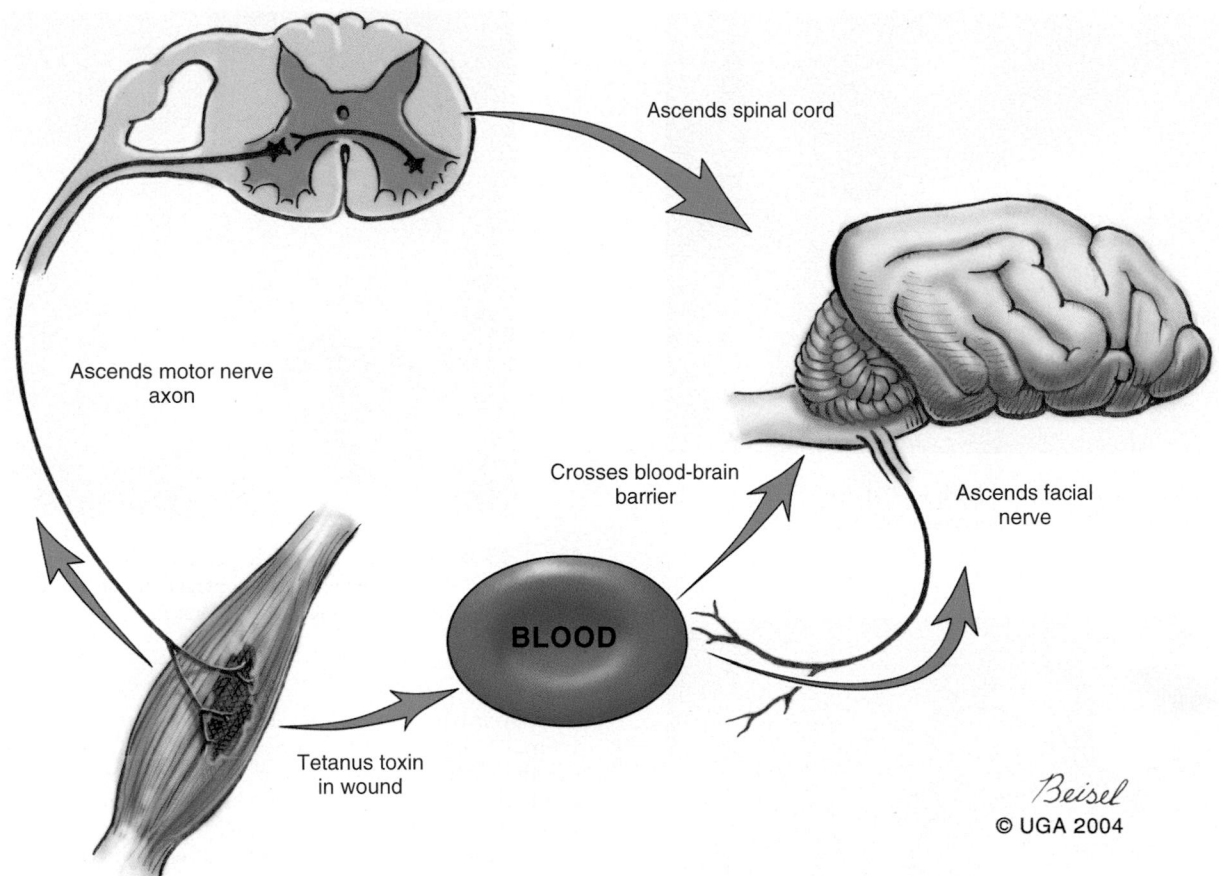

Ascends spinal cord

Ascends motor nerve
axon

Crosses blood-brain
barrier

Ascends facial
nerve

BLOOD

Tetanus toxin
in wound

Beisel
© UGA 2004

Fig 43-2 Potential routes of tetanus toxin spread into the CNS. (University of Georgia, Athens, Ga.)

resistance of cats, the wound required to produce disease is so extensive that it is usually obvious. Wounds closer to the head (i.e., brain) are associated with more rapid onset and generalized CNS signs than injuries to distant extremities. Tetanus has also been frequently observed as a complication of ovariohysterectomy, pregnancy, or parturition associated with fetal death.[2,14,16]

Localized tetanus is more common than *generalized tetanus* in dogs and cats than it is in people and other domestic animals because of the relative resistance of carnivores to the toxin. Increased stiffness of a muscle or an entire limb is first noted in close proximity to the wound site (Fig. 43-3). In the thoracic limb the elbow is usually extended, and the carpus may be held flexed or extended. The stiffness usually spreads, gradually involving the opposite extremity. This process usually progresses over a variable length of time and eventually involves the entire CNS.[18] Localized tetanus in the pelvic limbs has been commonly associated with the female reproductive tract of dogs and cats. In animals in which a single extremity is affected, the diagnosis may be unclear.

Animals affected with *generalized* tetanus walk with a stiff gait and generally have an outstretched or a dorsally curved tail. They are not in pain but have difficulty in standing or lying down in comfortable positions because of the extreme muscle rigidity (Figs. 43-4 and 43-5). The rectal temperature is usually increased because of the excessive muscular activity. Postural reaction testing, such as a proprioceptive positioning evaluation, usually reveals normal initiation but stiff performance of the motor response. If the animal is extremely rigid, attempts to correct the knuckled limb may fail. When

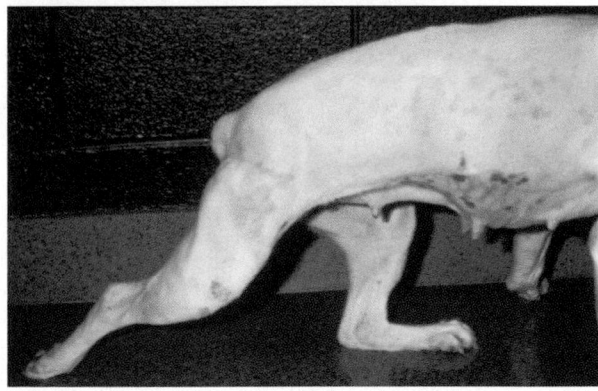

Fig 43-3 Localized tetanus in rear right limb of dog with postpartum metritis. Stiffness progressed to involve all four limbs as well as facial muscles. (Courtesy University of Georgia, Athens, Ga.)

performing this type of testing, providing weight support is important for obtaining a more accurate evaluation. Myotactic reflexes are generally accentuated and flexor reflexes are depressed, but both may be difficult to elicit because of muscle stiffness.

Intracranial signs develop in the late stages of localized tetanus. They begin earlier in animals with generalized tetanus and usually generalized muscular stiffness. Cranial nerve motor nuclei are affected, resulting in hypertonicity of respec-

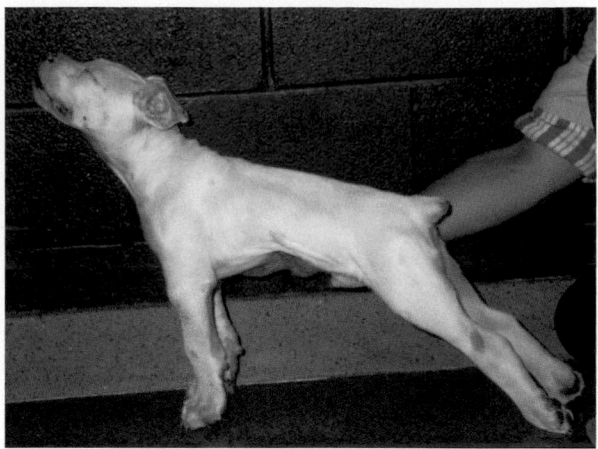

Fig 43-4 Characteristic "sawhorse" stance of dog with generalized tetanus. (Courtesy University of Georgia, Athens, Ga.)

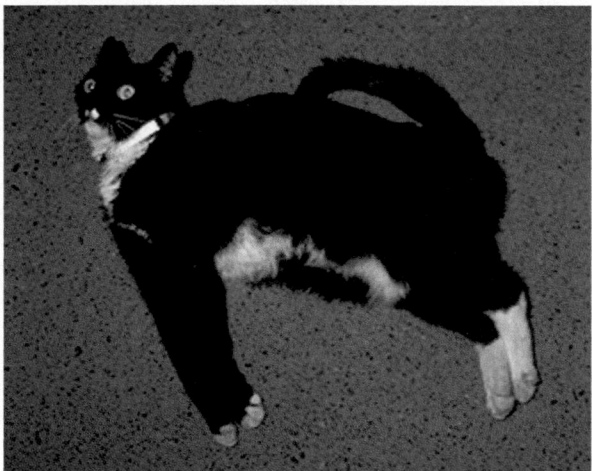

Fig 43-5 Characteristic posture of cat with generalized tetanus, showing stiff limbs and outstretched tail. (Courtesy University of Georgia, Athens, Ga.)

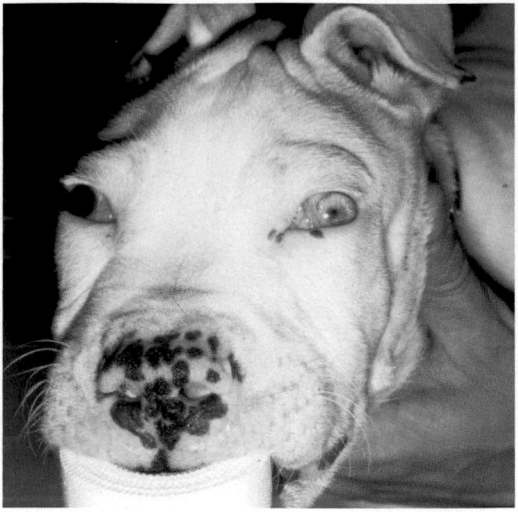

Fig 43-6 Pit bull dog with generalized tetanus, showing protrusion of third eyelid and contracture of facial muscles. (Courtesy University of Georgia, Athens, Ga.)

tive musculature. Protrusion of the third eyelid and enophthalmos result from retraction of the globe, which is caused by extraocular muscle hypertonicity (Fig. 43-6). In addition, miosis is frequently present. The ears are held erect, the lips are drawn back (risus sardonicus), and the forehead is wrinkled as a result of facial muscle spasms. Trismus ("lockjaw") is caused by contraction of masticatory muscles. Increased salivation, increased heart and respiratory rates, laryngeal spasms, and dysphagia can result from involvement of parasympathetic and somatic cranial nerve nuclei.

Reflex muscle spasms occur in animals with generalized tetanus or intracranial involvement. Animals become apprehensive and react strongly to tactile or auditory stimulation. Mild stimulation may precipitate periodic generalized tonic contraction of all muscles with opisthotonus or cause grand mal convulsions. When tonic contractions begin to occur, the interval between spasms decreases until the animal reaches a convulsive state. Dogs and cats usually remain conscious until they develop convulsions. Reflex muscle spasms are painful, so animals may vocalize during such episodes. Animals with tetanus usually have a desire to eat but because of jaw stiffness, they may have trouble prehending or swallowing solid

food. Animals with complicating hiatal hernia begin regurgitating.[7,28] Dysuria and urine retention, constipation, and gaseous distention are common results of persistent anal and urethral sphincter contractions. Hyperthermia is a consistent complication from constant muscle contractions or seizures. Nosocomial pneumonia is a common complication of tetanus and is caused by factors such as recumbency, reintubation or tracheostomy, aspiration, use of paralytic agents, or autonomic disturbances.[4] The progression of clinical signs culminates in death, which is usually caused by respiratory compromise resulting from rigidity of the respiratory musculature, reflex spasms of the larynx, increased airway secretions, and central respiratory arrest from medullary intoxication or anoxia.

DIAGNOSIS

History of a recent wound and clinical signs are the primary means of diagnosing tetanus. Wounds that may be present cause hematologic abnormalities, including leukocytosis with neutrophilia and left shift. Serum biochemistry and cerebrospinal fluid (CSF) values are unaffected, although moderate to marked elevations of muscle enzyme (creatine kinase, aspartate aminotransferase) activities may be present. Presumably this elevation results from the muscle injury caused by sustained hypertonicity and recumbency.

Tachyarrhythmias and bradyarrhythmias may be noted in individuals with tetanus. Rapid heart rates are usually associated with sinus tachycardia. Bradycardia (less than 70 beats/min) is characterized by atrioventricular heart block, sinus arrest, and ventricular escape complexes.

In dogs that develop hiatal hernia and megaesophagus, thoracic radiographic changes occur in the caudal region and include increased density and esophageal dilation.

The muscle spasms that develop in animals with tetanus are usually reduced but not always abolished by general anesthesia. Deep anesthesia in mildly affected animals may resolve all evidence of muscle hypertonicity. Even when clinically evident relaxation occurs, characteristic electromyographic changes can usually be detected. Insertion of the needle or tapping of the muscles or tendons is followed by persistent electrical motor unit discharges rather than the expected period of electrical silence. Muscle biopsy results are usually normal in acute cases of tetanus, and any observed abnormalities may be attributed to muscle trauma caused by constant hypertonicity or prolonged recumbency.

Measurement of serum antibody titers to tetanus toxin has been used to substantiate the diagnosis of tetanus. Values must be compared with those from control animals. Such measurements might be helpful in a clinical setting to confirm the cause of undiagnosed muscle stiffness.

Isolation of *C. tetani* from wounds can be a difficult procedure and is unrewarding in a majority of cases. The organisms are usually present in very low concentrations, and although gram-stained smears may demonstrate gram-positive rods and dark-staining spherical endospores, the morphology of *C. tetani* is not unlike that of many other anaerobic bacteria. If culture is attempted, it should be performed under strict anaerobic conditions at 37° C for 12 days. Biochemical reactions or bioassays can be evaluated in an attempt to classify the organism. Mouse inoculation with isolates is not a readily available procedure.

THERAPY

Therapy for tetanus in severely affected animals is costly and time consuming, and owners must be advised of the possibility of complications and a lengthy hospitalization. Fortunately the disease is often localized or mild in dogs and cats because of their innate resistance. However, untreated cases can prove fatal. Because of their natural resistance, dogs and cats are not vaccinated with toxoid as a means of prophylaxis or treatment. Recommended dosages for the drugs used in the following treatment are summarized in Table 43-2.

Antitoxin

The antitoxin for tetanus consists of antitetanus equine serum (ATS) or human tetanus immune globulin (TIG). In the United States, TIG is approved for IM use, whereas ATS is licensed for IM or IV use. The TIG contains thimerosal and immunoglobulin aggregates and may be more likely to produce reactions when given by other than the IM route.[1]

The immediate concern when treating tetanus is administration of antitoxin to neutralize any toxin that has not bound to the CNS or has not yet been formed. The timing and route of antitoxin administration are important in determining the effectiveness of detoxification. Use of antitoxin should be routine; however, the elimination of bound toxin by the affected animal is gradual, and the administration of antitoxin does little to hasten the process. Thus recovery is usually slow and progressive. The dose for prophylaxis is much less than that for treatment. In mildly affected dogs or cats or in those with localized tetanus, antitoxin therapy may not be necessary because of their innate resistance to the toxin.

IV administration of antitoxin is superior to IM or SC administration in producing a rapid and marked increase of circulating antitoxin. It takes 48 to 72 hours for SC-administered antitoxin to reach therapeutic concentrations. The equine antitoxin dose is given slowly over 5 to 10 minutes. Larger animals should receive a proportionally lower dose on the basis of body weight. Total doses greater than 20,000 U do not appear to be more effective because they increase the antigenic mass; they are also more costly.

Unfortunately, IV antitoxin is associated with a high prevalence of anaphylaxis, therefore appropriate precautions should be taken during administration. An initial test dose (0.1 to 0.2 ml) of antitoxin should be given SC or intradermally (ID) 15 to 30 minutes before the administration of the IV dose. A wheal at the site of injection may indicate that an anaphylactic reaction is going to develop. Epinephrine, glucocorticoid, and antihistamine should be readily available in case of an adverse reaction, or glucocorticoid and antihistamine may be given before an antitoxin IV injection if a reaction is anticipated. IV administration of 0.1 ml/kg of epinephrine (diluted 1:10,000) is the drug dose of choice to treat an anaphylactic reaction. It is not advisable to repeat the dose at any time during the course of therapy. A therapeutic blood level of antitoxin persists in dogs for 14 days after the injection, and repeated doses increase the chance of an anaphylactic reaction.

Local IM injection of a small dose of antitoxin (1000 U) around and proximal to the wound site has been shown to be beneficial in experimental studies of localized tetanus.

Intrathecal injection of antitoxin in laboratory animals has been shown to be beneficial in treating tetanus under experimental conditions. Use in affected people has not been proven to be effective.[1,29] Intrathecal injection of as little as 1% of the recommended IV dose reduced the mortality and morbidity in dogs with mild or moderate tetanus compared with similarly affected animals given IV or lumbar intrathecal injections. The advantage of antitoxin being injected into the CNS and CSF rather than providing a similar systemic dose is that it does not need to penetrate the blood-brain barrier and may partially neutralize bound toxin. Because it is a foreign protein, antitoxin may be toxic in the subarachnoid space. For these reasons, intracisternal therapy should be reserved for severely affected animals.

Antimicrobial Therapy

Local and parenteral antibiotic therapy should be instituted in an attempt to kill any vegetative *C. tetani* organisms present in the wound (see Table 43-2). Although antibiotics by themselves may not neutralize circulating toxin, they reduce the amount of antitoxin required to treat experimental tetanus once clinical signs are apparent. Penicillin G, the drug of choice, can be given IV in the form of an aqueous potassium or a sodium salt or IM as the procaine salt. A portion of the dose, in the form of procaine penicillin, can be injected IM close to an identified wound site. Because the effectiveness of penicillin on the vegetative organisms may vary, tetracycline has been recommended as an alternative. Penicillin derivatives, such as ampicillin, are not as effective against the organism, and their use may cause little or no response. Metronidazole has been shown to be superior to penicillin G and tetracycline in treating clinical and experimental tetanus, although it has a higher risk for causing toxicity. Metronidazole may be more active and preferred for treatment of tetanus because it is bactericidal, affecting most anaerobes, and builds effective therapeutic concentrations, even in anaerobic tissues. Penicillin is also a known antagonist of GABA, as is tetanus toxin. Clindamycin and tetracyclines are also effective against *C. tetani*, although they are not generally used. The efficacy of fluoroquinolones against *C. tetani* is questionable, so they should not be used. Tetanus in a cat progressed from a localized form to a generalized form despite treatment with enrofloxacin.[19]

Sedatives

Various drugs alone and in combination have been given to control the reflex spasms and convulsions associated with tetanus. These drugs also help control the hyperthermia that results from the excessive muscle contractions. An ideal agent is one that controls excitability and spasticity without interfering with voluntary motor function or consciousness. Unfortunately, no such drug is available; however, a combination of phenothiazine and barbiturate comes closest to the ideal.

When provided alone or in combination with barbiturates, phenothiazines appear to be highly effective in controlling the

Table • 43-2

Recommended Drug Dosages for Tetanus

DRUG[a]	SPECIES	DOSE[b]	ROUTE	INTERVAL (HOURS)	DURATION (DAYS)
Antimicrobials					
Penicillin G	B	20,000–100,000 U/kg	IV, IM, SC	8–12	10
	B	20,000 U/kg	IV	4–6	10
Amoxicillin-clavulanate	B	12 mg/kg	PO, SC	12	10
Metronidazole	D	10 mg/kg	PO, IV	8	10
	C	250 mg total	PO	12–24	10
	B	15 mg/kg	PO,IV	12	10
Tetracycline	B	22 mg/kg	PO, IV	8	10
Clindamycin	B	3–10 mg/kg	PO, IV, IM	8–12	10
Immunotherapeutic agents					
Equine antitoxin[c]	B	100–1000 U/kg	IV, IM, SC		Once
		1000 U per site	Intralesional		Once
		1–10 U/kg	Intrathecal		Once
Sedatives and Relaxants					
Acetylpromazine	B	0.02–0.06 mg/kg[e]	IV	2	prn
	B	0.1–0.25 mg/kg[e]	IM	4	prn
	B	1.0 mg/kg	PO	6–8	prn
Chlorpromazine	B	0.5–2 mg/kg	IM, IV, PO	8–12	prn
Midazolam	B	0.1–0.2 mg/kg	IM, IV	2–4	prn
Diazepam	D	5.0–10 mg total	IV, PO, IM	2–4	prn
	B	0.2–10 mg/kg	IV	prn	prn
Methocarbamol	B	15–50 mg/kg	PO	6–12	prn
Pentobarbital	B	3–15 mg/kg	IV, IM	2–3	prn
Phenobarbital	B	1–4 mg/kg	PO, IM	6–12	prn
Autonomic Agents					
Atropine[d]	B	0.05 mg/kg	SC	prn	prn
Glycopyrrolate[d]	B	0.005 mg/kg	SC, IV	prn	prn
		1 mg total	PO	8	prn
Metoclopramide	B	0.28 mg/kg	PO[f]	8	prn

B, Dog and cat; *D*, dog; *C*, cat; *IV*, intravenous; *IM*, intramuscular; *SC*, subcutaneous; *PO*, by mouth; *prn*, as needed.

[a]See Appendix 8, Drug Formulary, for additional information on these drugs.

[b]Dose per administration at specified interval. Always infuse IV drugs slowly via diluted drip solution or infusion pump. Lowest range value applies to animals with greatest body weight.

[c]IV route is most preferred and efficacious. Administration of an intradermal or a subcutaneous test dose (0.1–0.2 ml) before IV infusion is recommended to detect hypersensitivity.

[d]Use as necessary to control bradyarrhythmias.

[e]Maximum dose IV of 3 mg in any dog.

[f]May have to be given IV as a continuous infusion during the early course of treatment.

hyperexcitable state. Chlorpromazine is the drug of choice, although acetylpromazine and methotrimeprazine can be given as substitutes. Phenothiazines are ineffective in treating similar-appearing signs caused by strychnine or other causes of convulsions. Tetanus is one exception of a condition for which phenothiazines are used in seizure-prone animals. They are thought to work centrally on the brainstem to depress descending excitatory input on the lower motor neurons within the spinal cord.

Barbiturates can be administered for successful control of grand mal convulsions, generalized body stiffness, and opisthotonus, all of which may occur. Pentobarbital may have to be given every 2 to 3 hours, but the actual dose should be adjusted according to the severity of the clinical signs of the patient, because an overdose may unnecessarily suppress the

respiration rate and consciousness. Oral or injectable phenobarbital can be given when a longer-acting drug is needed. When a combination of phenothiazine and pentobarbital is used, less barbiturate is needed to control the tetany, although bradycardia can result from this combination. When the heart rate decreases to less than 60 beats/min, glycopyrrolate can be administered as needed to reverse the bradycardia.

Benzodiazepine derivatives such as diazepam or midazolam are alternatives to barbiturates in the control of seizures and nervous hyperexcitability. They block polysynaptic reflexes within the medulla and spinal cord. Methocarbamol is frequently recommended but less commonly used as a central-acting muscle relaxant. It has a relatively short duration of action, as does diazepam. Baclofen, a depressant and antispasmolytic that acts as a GABA agonist in the CNS, has been beneficial when given intrathecally to treat severe tetanus in people.[23,29] Dantrolene, a direct-acting muscle relaxant, has been used to control spasticity in human tetanus.[22,25] It must not be used when underlying hepatic disease is present. Respiratory depression has been a complicating factor in some cases. Curare has only been used in human patients.

Narcotics should never be included in tetanus therapy because they depress the respiratory centers and may stimulate other areas of the CNS. Parasympatholytic drugs such as atropine should also be avoided in routine cases; however, bronchospasm, bronchial hypersecretion, and cardiovascular instability have been controlled by continuous atropine infusions in people with severe tetanus.[8]

Severely affected animals with respiratory compromise from uncontrollable tetanic spasms may be sedated or anesthetized, intubated, and placed on positive-pressure ventilation. These measures often become too costly for owners of veterinary patients and often result in cardiorespiratory complications.

Surgery and Wound Management

Surgery may be required if tissue necrosis or abscess formation is extensive. Antitoxin should be administered before surgery because toxin is released into the circulation during tissue manipulation. General anesthesia is usually required to debride wounds and remove necrotic tissue. Devitalized tissue and visible foreign material should be removed and the wound irrigated. Hydrogen peroxide may be beneficial in flushing the wound because it increases oxygen tension, which inhibits obligate anaerobes. The prognosis for recovery is always greater if the wound site is located and can be debrided.

Autonomic Agents

Autonomic agents are occasionally required to control the cardiac rhythm. Sympatholytic agents generally are not provided in the management of tachyarrhythmias, because other sedatives usually control this complication. Bradyarrhythmia (a heart rate of less than 60 beats/min) that persists can be controlled by short-term administration of a parasympatholytic agent such as atropine or glycopyrrolate as needed. This type of arrhythmia often resolves after a few days in animals that begin to show resolution of their muscle stiffness. Continuous atropine infusion has been used in the management of severe tetanus in people.[8] In addition to assisting with cardiovascular arrhythmias, bronchospasm, bronchial hypersecretion, and hypersalivation are reduced. Clonidine, a central-acting sympathoplegic, reduces autonomic dysfunction in tetanus and might benefit severely affected animals.[27]

Glucocorticoid therapy has never been proven to be beneficial in tetanus and generally should be avoided. In a controlled study of human patients with severe tetanus, betamethasone reduced the need for tracheostomy and ventilation from laryngeal spasm. Hyperbaric oxygenation has been provided for people and dogs with tetanus in an attempt to inactivate *C. tetani*; however, insufficient proof of its benefits exists to justify the time and cost of such a procedure. Neuromuscular blocking agents have been used in humans with tetanus in an attempt to control convulsions or paralyze the patients, who are then placed on artificial respirators. However, this type of therapy is impractical in veterinary medicine because of the intensive monitoring required.

Nursing Care

Supportive measures are imperative in the successful management of an animal with tetanus. Constant nursing may be required for severely affected animals. The animals should be placed in a dark, quiet environment with minimal stimulation. Cages should be shrouded to reduce light, and pledgets of cotton or gauze should be placed in their ears to reduce sound transmission. All therapeutic measures should be coordinated and take place at the same time each day so the least amount of handling and stimulation occurs. Soft, comfortable bedding should be provided because tetanus causes incapacitation, frequently leading to decubital ulcers. Animals should be encouraged to eat and drink on their own. Rinsing the mouth with a solution of 0.1% chlorhexidine acetate helps to cleanse and lubricate the mucosal surfaces. Tetanic animals frequently have difficulty prehending and swallowing solid foods, but they can usually eat blended foods or fluids by sucking through clenched teeth. A stomach tube may be placed if the animal is reluctant to eat, but this is frequently stressful for conscious animals, and esophageal spasm or hiatal hernia may restrict passage of the tube or cause subsequent regurgitation. Only frequently offered, small amounts of food should be given through a stomach tube because of the high risk of gastroesophageal reflux or vomiting and resultant aspiration pneumonia. Animals with tetanus frequently have gastroesophageal reflux, and their laterally rigid posture prevents gravity from assisting their swallowing efforts. A gastrostomy tube may be required for feeding severely affected animals. The hematocrit (HCT) level, plasma protein level, and body weight should be evaluated daily to determine whether adequate fluid balance is being maintained. Balanced polyionic isotonic fluids should be given parenterally to correct any deficits. Parenteral alimentation may be helpful to meet the caloric needs of some animals; however, it requires continual IV administration of special fluids through a central venous catheter and is expensive.

Complications in dogs and cats with tetanus are numerous. Decubital ulcers may develop over bony prominences of recumbent dogs, but they can be prevented by adequately padding the cage and rotating the animal every few hours. Fractures of the long bones, spine, or skull may result from trauma incurred during sudden muscular spasms or convulsions. Other problems include sepsis from IV catheterization and aspiration pneumonia caused by difficulties swallowing. Esophageal hiatal hernia and megaesophagus may result in gastroesophageal reflex and regurgitation. A tracheostomy may be required if breathing is obstructed from laryngeal spasms. Urinary and fecal retention occurs as a result of hypertonic anal and urethral sphincters. Repeated urinary catheterizations may be needed if dysuria or reflex dyssynergia occurs. Intermittent clean catheterization as needed is preferred to maintaining an indwelling catheter because the patient is less likely to establish a bacterial infection. Orally administered simethicone, gastric intubation, and enemas may help relieve GI gas or obstipation. A glutamine solution (10 g per 500 ml of water) can be given orally at a dose of 0.5 g/kg/day on a divided basis by gavage or indwelling tube as a supplement to help maintain GI mucosal integrity. Hyperthermia from generalized muscle contractions may be controlled by parenteral fluids, fans, and application of alcohol to the footpads and pinnae. Nosocomial pneumonia is a serious complication of patients with severe tetanus.[4] Reasons for its occurrence in animals with tetanus include diaphragmatic immobility, recumbency with atelectasis or aspiration of ingesta, prolonged mechanical ventilation, having tracheostomy, and use of paralytic agents or sedatives.

Prognosis

The prognosis for recovery from tetanus varies depending on the severity of the rigidity at the time therapy is instituted. Most dogs and cats have a self-limiting course of tetanus when rapid and appropriate therapy is instituted. Those with localized tetanus have a better prognosis and more rapid recovery than those with generalized forms. Individuals with rapidly progressing disease have a poorer prognosis.

Animals with stiffness that prevents them from maintaining a standing position or walking rigidly without assistance have the most guarded prognosis. Animals with opisthotonus or continual convulsive episodes that cannot move from a rigid lateral recumbent position often are at risk of respiratory arrest. Those with secondary complications are also at risk. The duration, intensity, and cost of treatment are all greater for animals with generalized tetanus. Mortality from complications also is high in those with generalized disease. Improvement after institution of treatment is usually noticeable within 1 week, and gradual but complete recovery is generally noted by 3 to 4 weeks. Occasionally, stiffness persists for longer periods of up to 16 weeks.

PREVENTION

Active immunoprophylaxis with tetanus toxoid is not recommended for dogs and cats; it is used for more susceptible species such as people and horses. Routine tetanus boosters or postexposure prophylaxis is not required. Appropriate care of infected wounds and rational antibiotic therapy should minimize the occurrence of tetanus. Epizootics have occurred in veterinary hospitals that inadequately sterilize their surgical instruments. Cold sterilization of instruments used for surgical procedures should not be used.

SUGGESTED READINGS*

3. Baral RM, Catt MJ, Malik R. 2002. What is your diagnosis? Localized tetanus in a cat, *J Feline Med Surg* 4:221-224.
17. Loose NL, Carey S. 2004. A dog with generalized muscle stiffness, *Vet Med* 99:26-32.
19. Malik R, Simpson DJ, Church DB. 1998. What is your diagnosis? Tetanus, *J Small Anim Pract* 39:217-252.

*See the CD-ROM for a complete list of references.

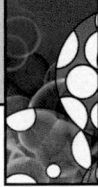

CHAPTER • 44

Leptospirosis

Craig E. Greene, Jane E. Sykes, Cathy A. Brown, and Katrin Hartmann

ETIOLOGY

Leptospirosis, a zoonotic disease of worldwide significance that affects many animal species, is caused by infection with antigenically distinct serovars of the species *Leptospira interrogans sensu lato*, of which at least 10 are of most importance for dogs and cats. Leptospiral nomenclature and taxonomy is complicated. Before 1989, the genus was divided into two species, *L. interrogans*, containing all pathogenic strains, and *Leptospira biflexa*, with all saprophytic strains from the environment. Since that time, the genus has been classified into at least 16 new species on the basis of genetic relatedness (Table 44-1).[39,113] Both pathogenic and nonpathogenic serovars occur within the same species in this new genetic classification. Over 200 serovars of *L. interrogans* have been described and further classified into antigenically related serogroups. Serogroups currently have no taxonomic basis; however, they have been useful for an epidemiologic tracking and understanding of the disease. Serovars are maintained in nature by numerous subclinically infected wild and domestic animal reservoir hosts that serve as a potential source of infection and illness for people and other incidental animal hosts (Table 44-2). When infected, incidental hosts develop more severe clinical illness and shed organisms for shorter periods. Epidemiologic studies have shown that host preferences can change with time and geographic region of the world.

Leptospires are thin, flexible, filamentous (0.1 to 0.2 μm wide and 6 to 12 μm long) bacteria made up of fine spirals with hook-shaped ends (Fig. 44-1). They are composed of a protoplasmic cylinder that is wound around a straight central axial filament. The outer envelope is composed of lipopolysaccharide (LPS) and antigenic mucopeptide. Leptospires are motile, making writhing and flexing movements while rotating along their long axis.

The most commonly incriminated serovars in canine leptospirosis have been canicola, icterohaemorrhagiae, grippotyphosa, pomona, and bratislava, which belong to serogroups Canicola, Icterohemorrhagiae, Grippotyphosa, Pomona, and Australis, respectively. Theories suggest that since the introduction of vaccines containing serovars canicola and icterohaemorrhagiae over 30 years ago, an apparent epidemiologic change in canine leptospirosis has taken place in which dogs are routinely vaccinated, with decreasing reports of disease caused by serogroups Canicola and Icterohaemorrhagiae and increasing reports of disease caused by serogroups such as Australis, Grippotyphosa, and Pomona. Serovars canicola and icterohaemorrhagiae were the predominant serovars associated with canine disease at the time vaccination was first instituted, and thus early vaccines contained only these serovars.[197] Emergence of disease associated with other serogroups may stem from several factors, including the use of vaccination and the greater exposure of unnatural hosts such as dogs to wildlife reservoir hosts in rural or suburban environments. Raccoons have been implicated as a source of the serogroup Grippotyphosa infections in the northeastern regions of the United States and Eastern Canada.[118,159,165] Increased testing for these serogroups may also contribute to their increased recognition because before 1970 most assays for dogs only detected serogroups Canicola and Icterohaemorrhagiae. The duration of shedding and potential spread of these serogroups from infected dogs to other dogs or people is uncertain. In serologic surveys, the prevalence of seroreactivity is greater than that of clinical disease, suggesting that subclinical infections occur. In other areas, the prevalence of seroreactivity is

Table • 44-1

Genomospecies Identified with Selected Serovars of Leptospira *Isolated Worldwide*[a]

SEROVAR	GENOMOSPECIES[b]
australis	*interrogans*
autumnalis	*interrogans*
bratislava	*interrogans*
canicola	*interrogans*
grippotyphosa	*interrogans, kirschneri*
hardjo	*interrogans, borgpetersenii, meyeri*
icterohaemorrhagica	*interrogans, inadai*
pomona	*interrogans, noguchii*
saxkoebing	*interrogans*
sejroe	*borgpetersenii*

[a]Most common serovars reported in canine infections. Data adapted from Brenner DJ, Kaufmann AF, Sulzer KR, et al. 1999. Further determination of DNA relatedness between serogroups and serovars in the family Leptospiraceae with a proposal for *Leptospira alexanderi* sp. nov. and four new *Leptospira* genomospecies. *Int J Syst Bacteriol* 49:839-858.
[b]Other genospecies not listed here are *biflexa, wolbachii, parva, illii,* genomospecies 1, genomospecies 2, genomospecies 3, genomospecies 4, genomospecies 5.

low.[141] Despite the presence of leptospiral antibody titers in the feline population, clinical reports of leptospirosis in cats are infrequent. Although cats seroconvert after exposure to leptospires, they appear to be less susceptible than dogs to both spontaneous and experimental infections.[5,55,208]

EPIDEMIOLOGY

Leptospires are transmitted between animals by direct or indirect contact. Direct transmission occurs through contact with infected urine, venereal and placental transfer, bite wounds, or ingestion of infected tissues. Crowding of animals, as may occur in a kennel situation, enhances the direct spread of infection. Recovered dogs excrete organisms in urine intermittently for months after infection. Once outside the host, leptospires do not replicate. Indirect transmission occurs through exposure of susceptible animals to contaminated water sources, soil, food, or bedding. The spirochete may remain viable for several months in moist soil that has been saturated with urine. Although evidence exists that spirochetes survive in insects and other invertebrate hosts, the significance of this finding with regard to disease transmission is unknown. The indirect transmission of leptospires may increase when environmental factors favoring the survival of leptospires are optimal.

Table • 44-2

Range for *Common Serovars of* Leptospira interrogans sensu lato *Infecting Animals*[a]

SPECIES SELECTED SEROVARS[b]	KNOWN PRIMARY RESERVOIR HOSTS	INCIDENTAL HOSTS			OTHER DOMESTICATED ANIMALS	REPRESENTATIVE WILD ANIMALS
		DOG	CAT	PEOPLE		
L. interrogans sensu stricto						
bratislava	Rat, pig, horse?	+	–	+	Cow, horse	Mouse, raccoon, opossum, hedgehog, vole, fox, skunk, bandicoot, weasel, nutria
autumnalis	Mouse	+	–	+	Cow	Rat, raccoon, opossum, bandicoot
icterohaemor-rhagiae	Rat	+	+	+	Cow, horse, pig, cavy[c]	Mouse, raccoon, opossum, hedgehog, fox, woodchuck, nutria, ape, skunk, civet, muskrat, mongoose
pomona	Cow, pig, skunk, opossum	+	+	+	Horse, sheep, goat, rabbit, cavy	Mouse, raccoon, hedgehog, wolf, fox, woodchuck, vole, sea lion, deer, civet
canicola	Dog	+	+	+	Cow, horse, pig	Rat, raccoon, hedgehog, armadillo, mongoose, bandicoot, nutria, vole, jackal, skunk
bataviae	Dog, rat, mouse	+	+	+	Cow	Hedgehog, vole, armadillo, bandicoot, shrew, leopard cat
hardjo	Cow	+	–	+	Pig, horse, sheep	Wild bovidae
L. kirschneri						
grippotyphosa	Vole, raccoon, skunk, opossum	+	+	+	Cow, pig, sheep, goat, rabbit, gerbil, cavy	Mouse, rat, fox, bandicoot, squirrel, bobcat, shrew, hedgehog, muskrat, weasel, mole, leopard cat

[a]Classification based on Ramadass P, Jarvis BDW, Corner RJ, et al. 1992. Genetic characterization of pathogenic *Leptospira* species by DNA hybridization. *Int J Syst Bacteriol* 42:215-219.
[b]Less common serovars for dogs include hebdomadis, javanica, panama, pyrogenes, and tarassovi; for cats include javanica and ballum.
[c]Guinea pig.

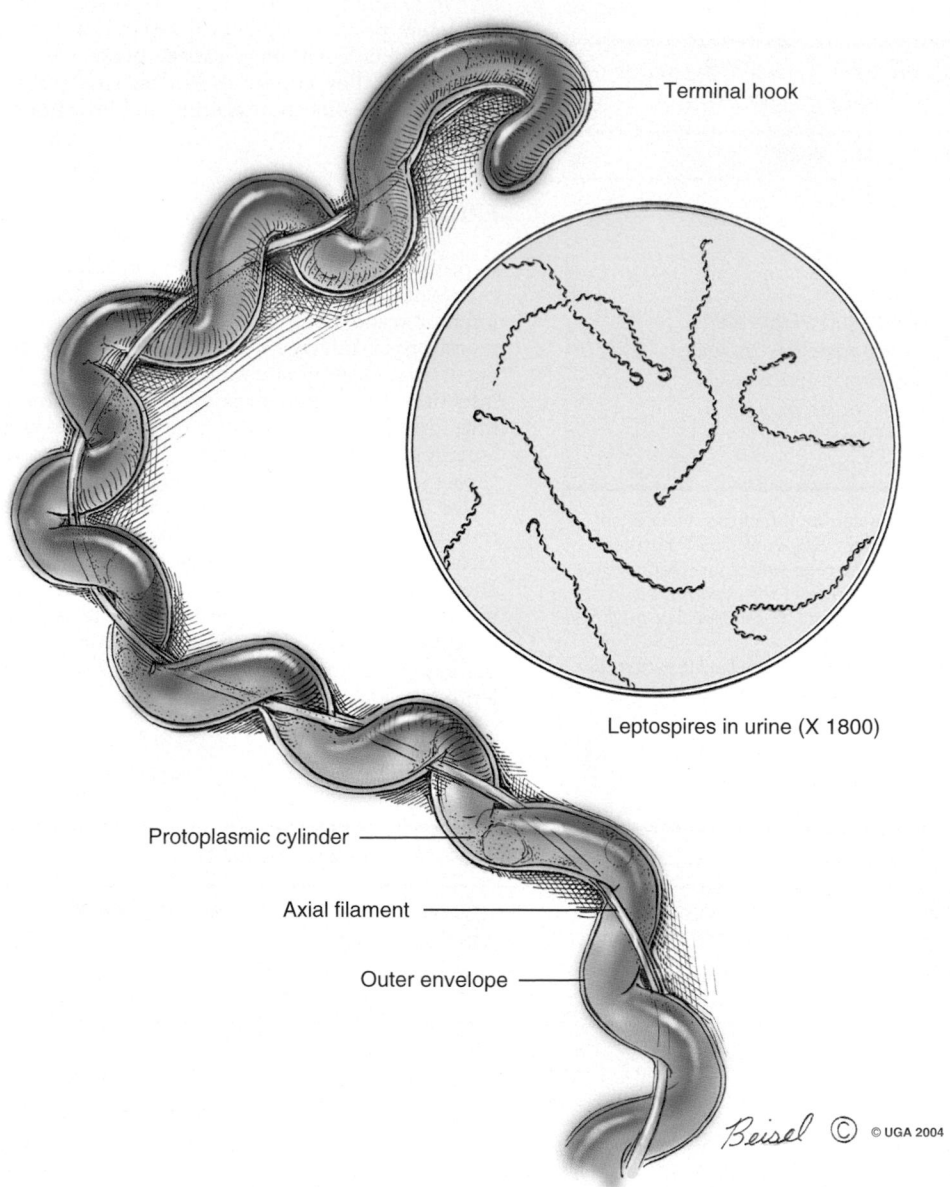

Terminal hook

Leptospires in urine (X 1800)

Protoplasmic cylinder

Axial filament

Outer envelope

Beisel © © UGA 2004

Fig 44-1 Ultrastructure of pathogenic leptospires. (Courtesy University of Georgia, Athens, Ga.)

Stagnant or slow-moving warm water, although not essential, provides a suitable habitat for spirochetes. Optimal survival in soil is favored by a neutral or slightly alkaline pH. Spirochetes survive only transiently in undiluted acidic urine (pH 5.0 to 5.5), whereas the opposite conditions provide more suitable habitats. Ambient temperatures between 0° C and 25° C favor the survival and replication of leptospires, whereas freezing markedly decreases survival. The temperature and pH requirements for maximal leptospiral survival may explain the apparent increased seasonal incidence of canine leptospirosis in the late summer and early fall[41,136] and in the southern semitropical belt of the United States and similar climatic regions worldwide. Outbreaks have occurred in association with high rainfall, especially in tropical regions. In the United States and Canada, a correlation was found between a greater number of cases of leptospirosis in dogs at veterinary teaching hospitals and higher average rainfall.[206]

Several scenarios exist for the occurrence of leptospirosis in dogs and similar observations have been made for the disease in people. Where seasonality exists throughout the world, most cases are observed during warmer months of the year. Because of the water requirement, disease incidence or outbreaks often increase during periods of higher rainfall or flooding, respectively. In arid areas or during drought conditions, infections of accidental hosts are more common around water sources. Infections are observed in rural or suburban dogs that through activities or utility are exposed to standing water, lakes, or streams. Herding dogs, hounds, working dogs, and mixed-breed dogs have been at greatest risk in the United States.[207] The number reports of disease in urban-dwelling dogs or dogs used to track scents in urban areas has increased, presumably through their contact with infected rodents or their urine.[72] Polymerase chain reaction (PCR) has detected infection in rodents from such inner-city areas.[4] Leptospirosis also appears to be of higher prevalence dogs kept in crowded kennels with unsanitary conditions.[177]

Although the prevalence of clinical leptospirosis in cats is very low, they are probably exposed to leptospires excreted by wildlife. Serosurveys generally show exposure rates of 10%

or less. Outdoor cats have the highest seroprevalence. Serovars canicola, grippotyphosa, and pomona have been isolated from cats. Cats may also be exposed to urine of cohabitating dogs, and transmission from rodents carrying serovars ballum or icterohaemorrhagiae is suspected.

PATHOGENESIS

Leptospires penetrate intact mucous membranes of the mouth, nose, or eyes or abraded, scratched, or water-softened skin. They multiply rapidly after entering the blood vascular space (Fig. 44-2). They then spread and further replicate in many tissues, including the kidney, liver, spleen, central nervous system, eyes, and genital tract. The incubation period until clinical signs appear is approximately 7 days but can vary according to the infecting strain and host immunity. Increases in serum antibodies thereafter clear the spirochetes from most organs, but organisms may persist in the kidney and be shed in urine for weeks to months. The extent of damage to internal organs is variable depending on the virulence of the organism and host susceptibility.[134] Certain serovars have the propensity to produce acute hemorrhagic, hepatic, or most commonly renal involvement. Many animals develop more than one of these clinical manifestations, and disease expression can vary among outbreaks and geographic areas with a given serovar. Tissue edema and vasculitis may occur in rapid and severe infections that result in acute endothelial injury and hemorrhagic manifestations. *Leptospira* LPS stimulates neutrophil adherence and platelet activation,[94] which may contribute to the inflammatory and coagulatory abnormalities that occur.

Generally, infections of dogs with serovars canicola, bratislava, and grippotyphosa have been associated with predominantly renal dysfunction and with minimal liver involvement, whereas serovars icterohaemorrhagiae and pomona produce more hepatic disease. Younger dogs (under 6 months) seem to develop more signs of hepatic dysfunction in any disease outbreak.

Renal colonization occurs in most infected animals because the organism replicates and persists in renal tubular epithelial cells, even in the presence of serum neutralizing antibodies (see Fig. 44-2). The organism penetrates the renal capillaries and enters the interstitium; and by 2 weeks after infection, leptospires may be seen within the proximal tubular cells and tubular lumen, which coincides with the onset of shedding. The invasive capacity of leptospires may be related to their pathogenicity because nonpathogenic leptospires do not penetrate cells as readily as pathogenic leptospires.[21] Acute impairment of renal function may result from decreased glomerular filtration caused by kidney swelling that impairs renal blood perfusion. Damage to the endothelium of small blood vessels may result in ischemic damage to the renal parenchyma. In addition, several leptospiral factors have a toxic effect on cells located within the renal parenchyma. Significant renal damage probably results from the leptospiral LPS and other outer membrane components. Leptospiral LPS is a potent activator of macrophages, and stimulates secretion of interleukin (IL)-1 and interferon by these cells, in addition to augmenting their killing capacity.[95] Incubation of peripheral blood mononuclear cells with leptospiral LPS results in the dose-dependent release of tissue necrosis factor-α and IL-10. These cytokines may play a role in the inflammatory response to leptospires.

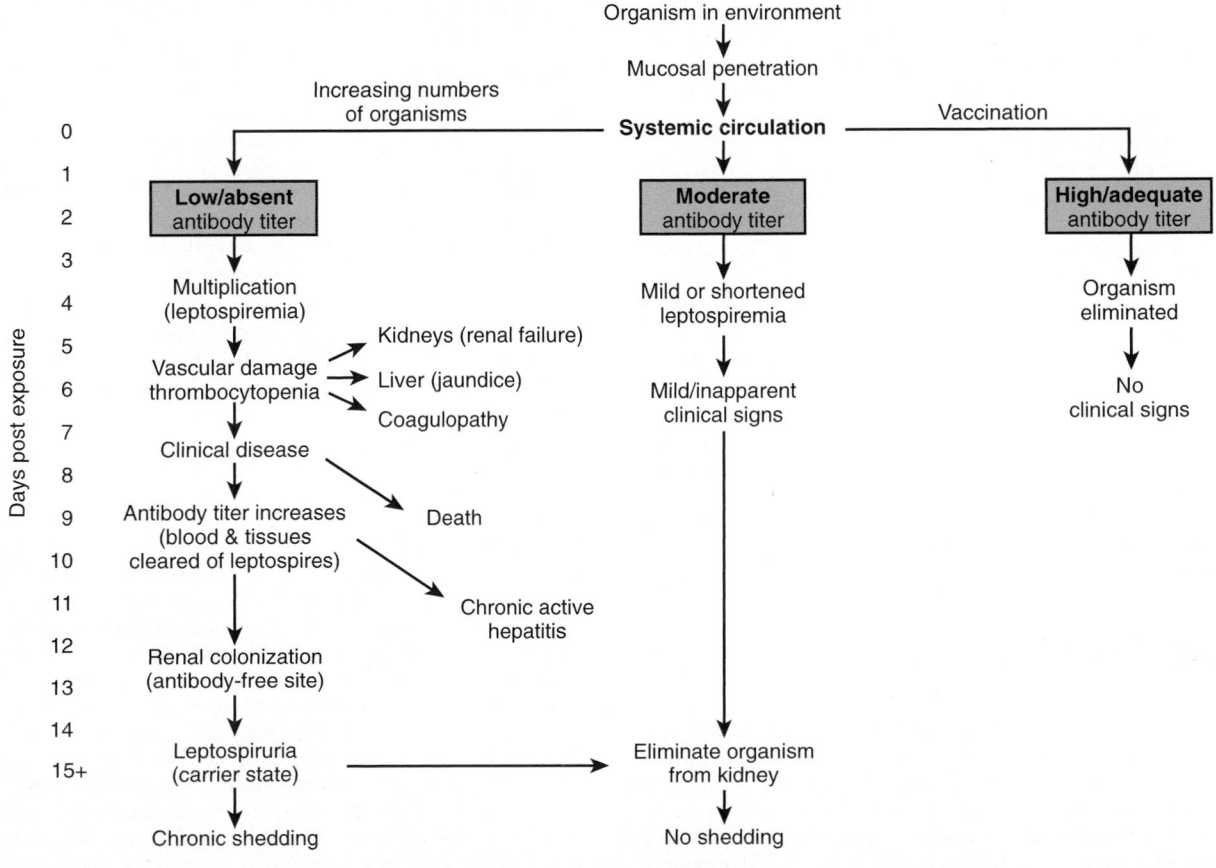

Fig 44-2 Pathogenesis of leptospirosis.

Unsaturated fatty acids in a glycolipid fraction from leptospires specifically inhibit sodium-potassium adenosine triphosphatase (Na^+-K^+ ATPase), which might account for the urinary potassium wasting observed in many patients with leptospirosis.[120,142,214] Endotoxin fractions from *L. interrogans* have been shown to interfere with renal concentrating mechanisms.[43]

Two hemolysins have been identified in pathogenic leptospires. The first (sphingomyelinase C) was purified from *Leptospira borgpetersenii hardjo*.[26] Sphingomyelinase H causes pore formation in target cell membranes, and is highly conserved only in pathogenic leptospires.[109] The extent to which these factors cause tissue damage in leptospirosis remains to be investigated.

Eventual recovery depends on increased specific antibody in the circulation within 7 to 8 days after infection. Animals with adequate functional kidney tissue will recover. Pathologic changes will persist in the severely affected kidney tissue despite clinical improvement. In surviving reservoir hosts, renal colonization will be long term, with shedding in urine for months to years. Although dogs are known to be persistent renal carriers of serovar canicola, the duration of shedding of other serovars has not been determined.

The liver is the second major parenchymatous organ damaged during leptospiremia. Profound hepatic dysfunction may occur without major histologic changes because of subcellular damage produced by leptospiral toxins. The degree of icterus in both canine and human leptospirosis usually corresponds to the severity of hepatic necrosis. In contrast, icterus, hemoglobinemia, and hemoglobinuria that develop in cattle with leptospirosis result from a serovar-specific hemolytic toxin produced by serovar pomona. Decreased osmotic fragility has been detected in canine leptospirosis,[172] making hemolysis less likely.

Chronic active hepatitis has been a sequela to serovar grippotyphosa and infection in dogs.[29] Dogs in a breeding colony of beagles in France had similar disease from serogroup Australis.[2] Presumably, initial hepatocellular injury and persistence of the organism in the liver result in altered hepatic circulation, fibrosis, and immunologic disturbances that perpetuate the chronic inflammatory response. Extensive hepatic fibrosis and failure may result from this process. Dogs with hepatic inflammation or fibrosis should be serotested for leptospirosis.

Acute lung injury occurs as a result of the effects of the toxins of the organism on pulmonary tissue. Fluid exudation within the lung may result from vasculitis, and rarely, acute severe pulmonary hemorrhage may occur.[28] The degree of pulmonary impairment is often reflective in the prognosis for recovery.[66,124]

Other body systems are damaged during the acute phase of infection. A benign meningitis is produced when leptospires invade the nervous system. Uveitis occasionally is present in naturally and experimentally occurring leptospirosis. Abortion or infertility resulting from transplacental transmission of leptospires associated with serovar bataviae infection has occurred in a dog.[58]

CLINICAL FINDINGS

Dog

Table 44-3 summarizes all the clinical features of leptospirosis. Clinical signs in canine leptospirosis depend on age and immunity of the host, environmental factors affecting the organisms, and virulence of the infecting serovar. The clinical severity cannot always be correlated with the serotype of the infecting pathogen. One factor is that the serotypes are genetically heterogeneous throughout the world. Nevertheless, certain gener-

---

Table • 44-3

Medical Problems Associated with Leptospirosis

HISTORY

Young animals more severely affected than adults; large breed, outdoor dogs commonly affected

CLINICAL FINDINGS

Acute: fever 39.5° C to 40° C (103° F to 104° F), shivering, muscle tenderness, vomiting, dehydration, peripheral vascular collapse, tachypnea, rapid irregular pulse, poor capillary perfusion, hematemesis, hematochezia, melena, epistaxis, widespread petechiae, icterus, intestinal intussusception

Subacute: fever, anorexia, vomiting, dehydration, polydipsia and polyuria, reluctance to move, paraspinal hyperesthesia caused by muscular, meningeal or renal inflammation, congested mucous membranes, petechial or ecchymotic hemorrhages, conjunctivitis, uveitis, rhinitis, tonsillitis, oliguria or anuria, coughing or dyspnea, icterus

CLINICAL LABORATORY FINDINGS

Hematology: leukocytosis, thrombocytopenia

Biochemistry: hyponatremia, hypochloremia, hypokalemia or hyperkalemia, hyperphosphatemia, hyperglycemia, ↑ ALT activities, ↑ AST activities, ↑ LDH activities, ↑ ALP activities, ↑ bilirubin, ↑ sulfobromophthalein retention, ↑ serum amylase activities (intussusceptions), ↑ serum lipase activities, azotemia

Urinalysis: glucosuria, tubular or glomerular proteinuria, bilirubinuria, ↑ numbers of granular casts, pyuria, hematuria

IMAGING FINDINGS

Interstitial to nodular alveolar densities

Ultrasound of urinary system: renomegaly, pyelectasia, ↑ cortical echogenicity

---

ALT, Alanine aminotransferase; *AST,* aspartate aminotransferase; *LDH,* lactic (acid) dehydrogenase; *ALP,* alkaline phosphatase.

---

alizations can be made. A comparison of the historical and physical findings is in Table 44-4. Young animals are more severely affected than are adults. Large breed (over 15 kg), outdoor, adult dogs are the most commonly affected.[136] In a survey of reported cases from veterinary teaching hospitals in the United States, herding dogs, hounds, and working dogs had a higher risk of infection compared with other breeds.[207] Peracute leptospiral infections can be exhibited by massive leptospiremia and death with few premonitory signs. In acute infections, pyrexia (39.5° C to 40° C [103° F to 104° F]), shivering, and generalized muscle tenderness are the first clinical signs. Subsequently, vomiting, rapid dehydration, and peripheral vascular collapse occur. Tachypnea, rapid and irregular pulse, and poor capillary perfusion have been noted. Coagulation defects and vascular injury are apparent with hematemesis, hematochezia, melena, epistaxis, and widespread petechiae. Terminally ill dogs become depressed and hypothermic, and renal and hepatic failure does not have time to develop.

Subacute infections are characterized by fever, anorexia, vomiting, dehydration, and increased thirst. Reluctance to move and paraspinal hyperesthesia in dogs may result from muscular, meningeal, or renal inflammation. Mucous membranes appear congested, and petechial and ecchymotic hemorrhages are widespread. Coughing and dyspnea usually accompany conjunctivitis, rhinitis, and tonsillitis. Progressive deterioration in renal function is exhibited by oliguria or anuria. Renal function in some dogs surviving subacute infections may return to normal within 2 to 3 weeks, or chronic compensated polyuric renal failure may develop.

Icterus is more common in dogs affected with the acute form of the disease (Fig. 44-3). Intrahepatic cholestasis from hepatic inflammation may be so complete that fecal color changes from brown to gray. Dogs with chronic active hepatitis or chronic hepatic fibrosis as a sequela to leptospirosis may eventually demonstrate overt signs of liver failure, including chronic inappetence, weight loss, ascites, icterus, or hepatoencephalopathy. Chronic progressive hepatic disease can occur in the clinical absence of other organ system involvement.[2]

Intestinal intussusceptions occur with some frequency in dogs with acute infections presumably associated with gastrointestinal (GI) inflammation. Careful abdominal palpation should be performed in dogs that develop persistent vomiting and diarrhea. Feces become scanty in such cases, and hematochezia or melena will be apparent.

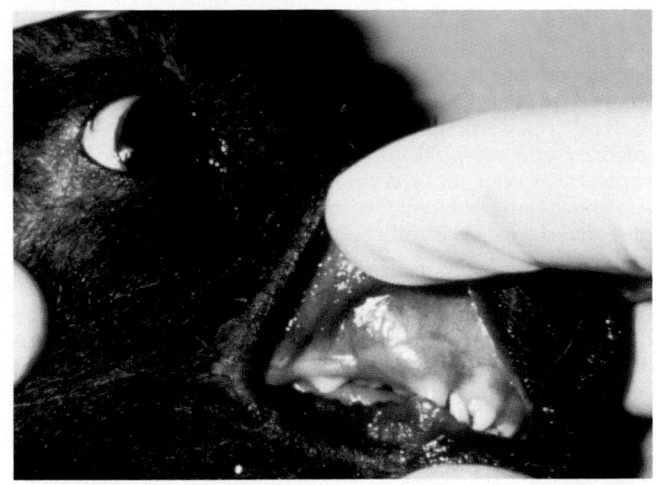

Fig 44-3 Icterus of mucous membranes of a young pup with acute leptospirosis. (Courtesy University of Georgia, Athens, Ga.)

Table • 44-4

Clinical Signs of Leptospirosis in Dogs[a]

CLINICAL FINDINGS	PREDOMINANT SEROGROUP								
	GRIPPOTYPHOSA				AUTUMNALIS n=11[f] (%)	POMONA			POMONA & AUSTRALIS n=11[j] (%)
	n=15[b] (%)	n=35[c] (%)	n=49[d] (%)	n=17[e] (%)		n=36[g] (%)	n=36[h] (%)	n=17[i] (%)	
Lethargy/Depression	13	83	67	88	90	65	58	88	NR
Anorexia	66	80	57	88	81	68	67	65	73
Vomiting	53	57	61	88	81	88	50	71	82
Fever	13	40	10	6	13	15	11	6	18
Hypothermia	NR	20	4	18	NR	22	NR	12	36
Dehydration	NR	31	NR	NR	53	NR	36	NR	27
Weight loss	7	20	37	29	NR	NR	44	NR	9
Polyuria/polydipsia	33	NR	31	35	42	NR	50	18	27
Abdominal or lumbar pain	NR	20	20	29	65	42	33	35	45
Stiffness, arthralgia, myalgia	NR	NR	10	41	35	23	25	24	NR
Renomegaly[k]	NR	NR	30	31	10	NR	56	20	NR
Diarrhea	NR	40	14	24	NR	29	33	6	36
Icterus	NR	46	10	NR	29	NR	33	24	36
Oculonasal discharge	NR	NR	8	18	3	NR	42	NR	9
Posterior paresis, weakness	NR	54	NR	24	NR	NR	39	NR	18
Respiratory signs[l]	NR	NR	NR	18	35	NR	3	NR	NR

As, Australis; *At,* Autumnalis; *B,* Bratislava; *C,* Canicola; *G,* Grippotyphosa; *H,* Hardjo; *I,* Icterohemorrhagica; *P,* Pomona; *Sa,* Saxkoebing; *Se,* Sejroe

[a]See Table 44–5 for data related to serum biochemical alterations from dogs in these studies.
[b]From Ill., USA, 1996-2001: G = 80%, G and B = 20%.[36]
[c]From Southern Germany, 1999-2000: B = 34%, Sa = 23%, I = 14%, C = 14%, B = 9%, Se = 3%, B = 3%[83]
[d]From Ga., USA, 1990-2000: G = 47%, B = 12%, C = 12%, P = 8%, I = 6%, G, P = 6%, H = 2%, B, G = 2%, C, I = 2%, C, G, I = 2%[41,56]
[e]From Mass., Conn., N.H., and Maine, 1986-1989: G = 41%, P = 29%, P, G = 29%, C = 0%, C = 0%, H = 0%, I = 0%[164]
[f]From Ontario, Canada, 1998-2000: At = 75%; remaining serovars not specified.[160]
[g]From Calif., USA, 1900-1998: P = 44%, B = 25%, P, B = 22%, G, C = 3%, G, P, B, C = 3%, H = 3%[3]
[h]From N.Y., USA, 1980-2001: P = 59%, G = 26%, P, G = 6%, H = 3%, I = 3%, At = 3%[28]
[i]From N.J. and Mich., USA, 1990-1995: P = 20%, P, G, At = 20%, P, G = 13%, At = 7%, H = 7%, G, At = 7%, P, H, At = 7%, G, H, I, At = 7%, P, G, I, At = 7%, P, G, I, At, B = 7%[80]
[j]From Bern, Switzerland, 1991-1996: P, As = 36%, P, As, G = 18%, P, As, I = 18%, P = 9%, P, G = 9%, P, I, G = 9%[192]
[k]Greatest percentage from either physical examination, radiography, or ultrasound.
[l]Includes coughing, dyspnea; or includes tachypnea.

Pulmonary manifestations include labored respiration and coughing.[164] Both interstitial pneumonia and pulmonary hemorrhage have been documented as the cause in people,[25,92] and in dogs (Fig. 44-4, *A* and *B*).[23,28]

Based on serologic surveys of clinically healthy dogs, a majority of leptospiral infections in dogs are chronic or subclinical.[177] Other medical disorders that subsequently follow subclinical infections such as meningitis and uveitis have been observed in people or other animals.[48,61] Serologic and microbiologic evaluation for leptospirosis might be performed on dogs with fever of unknown origin, unexplained renal or hepatic disease, anterior uveitis, or meningitis and on healthy dogs in kennels, multidog households, neighborhoods, or other environs where infection in other members has been documented.

Cat

Clinical signs are usually mild or unapparent in feline leptospirosis despite the presence of leptospiremia and leptospiruria and histologic evidence of renal and hepatic inflammation. More widespread testing of cats with acute hepatic or renal disease for leptospirosis may lead to increased recognition of clinical disease in this species.

DIAGNOSIS

Clinical Laboratory Findings

Hematologic findings in typical cases of canine leptospirosis include leukocytosis and thrombocytopenia. Leukocyte counts fluctuate depending on the stage and severity of infection. Leukopenia, common in the leptospiremic phase, develops into leukocytosis with a left shift. In later stages, white blood cell counts usually range from 16,500 to 45,000 cells/µl. A majority of dogs with leptospirosis have renal failure on initial examination.

Serum urea nitrogen and creatinine increases are found in dogs with varying severity of renal failure (Table 44-5). Electrolyte alterations usually parallel the degree of renal and GI dysfunction. Hyponatremia, hypochloremia, hypokalemia, and hyperphosphatemia are present in most cases, whereas hyperkalemia develops in dogs with terminal oliguric renal failure. In people, hypokalemia in the presence of acute renal failure has been thought to be likely associated with leptospirosis.[142] Similar associations have not been made for the infection in dogs. Mild hypocalcemia is related to hypoalbuminemia and decreased concentration of the protein-bound calcium fraction. Blood pH and serum bicarbonate concentration are reduced in severely affected animals, reflecting metabolic acidosis. Hypoglycemia is occasionally present with severe hepatic failure. Hepatic dysfunction may be apparent in some dogs, but it usually is less dramatic than renal failure or is associated with concurrent renal failure. Liver damage is demonstrated by increased serum alanine aminotransferase (ALT), aspartate aminotransferase, lactate dehydrogenase, and alkaline phosphatase (ALP) activities and bilirubin concentration. The increase in serum ALP activity is often proportionally greater than that of ALT activity. Bilirubin levels may be increased in serum and urine, and the magnitude is usually proportional to the degree of liver impairment. Marked bilirubinuria usually precedes hyperbilirubinemia. Serum bilirubin peaks by days 6 to 8 after onset of disease. Increased sulfobromophthalein retention (more than 5%) can be found in acute leptospirosis before the onset of icterus and in dogs that later develop chronic active hepatitis. Increased serum amylase and lipase activities may result from their release from inflamed hepatic and small intestinal tissues and from decreased renal excretion. Dogs with intussusception have the highest serum amylase concentrations. Serum creatine kinase activity is increased when skeletal muscle inflammation occurs. Urinalysis can be characterized by glucosuria, tubular or glomerular proteinuria, and bilirubinuria and by increased numbers of granular casts, leukocytes, and erythrocytes in the sediment. Some dogs have an increased protein to creatinine ratio in their urine in the presence of an acellular urinary sediment, which indicates the kidney as the source of the urine protein. Leptospires will not be observed in the urine without special staining or darkfield microscopy.

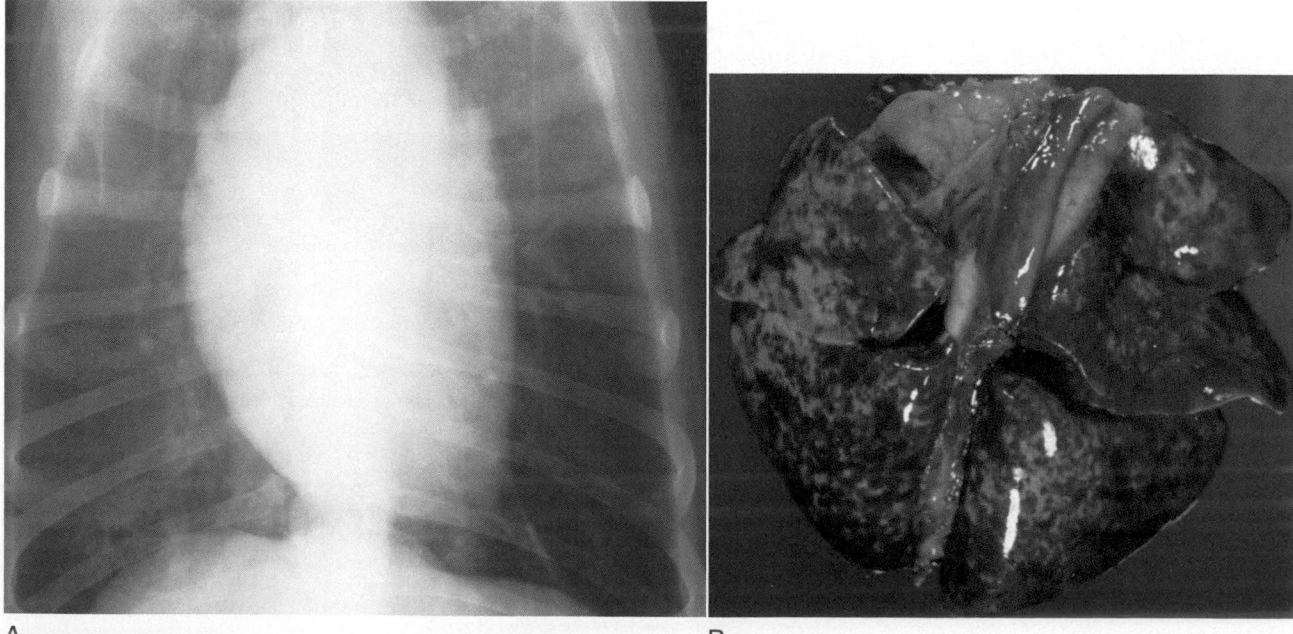

A

B

Fig 44-4 **A,** Thoracic radiograph from a dog with acute leptospirosis showing interstitial pulmonary infiltrates. **B,** Petechial and ecchymotic hemorrhages on the serosal surfaces of the lungs from a fatally infected dog. (Courtesy University of Georgia, Athens, Ga.)

Table • 44-5

Serum Biochemical Alterations in Dogs with Leptospirosis

SERUM BIOCHEMICAL ALTERATIONS	IL, USA[36]	SOUTHERN GERMANY[83]	GA, USA[56,41]	MA, CT, NH, ME, USA[164]	ONTARIO, CAN[160]	CA, USA[3]	NY, USA[28]	NJ, MI, USA[80]	BERN, SWITZERLAND[192]
	n = 15 (%)	n = 35 (%)	n = 49 (%)	n = 17 (%)	n = 31 (%)	n = 36 (%)	n = 36 (%)	n = 17 (%)	n = 11 (%)
Increased serum urea	73	60	91	100	94	100	81	82	55
Increased creatinine	80	NR	91	100	87	100	83	82	55
Hypoalbuminemia	NR	NR	37	18	NR	NR	NR	NR	55
Hypocalcemia	NR	NR	20	29	NR	NR	NR	NR	NR
Hypercalcemia	NR	NR	26	0	NR	NR	NR	NR	NR
Hyperphosphatemia	NR	46	74	59	NR	NR	50	47	55
High ALP	33	74	41	59	58	19	56	65	55
High ALT	33	77	27	35	26	NR	33	35	55
Hyperbilirubinemia	33	86	17	24	68 (total)	22	17	41	NR
Hyperkalemia	NR	14	20	18	NR	NR	NR	12	NR
Anemia	NR	48	29	24	45	NR	33	18	NR
Leukocytosis	NR	89	54	47	58	55 (n = 31)	31	53	73
Glucosuria	NR	NR	10	53	NR	26	9	NR	NR
Granular casts	NR	NR	17	18	NR	26	24	0	18
Hematuria (microscopic)	NR	79	13	NR	NR	17	27	42	NR
Proteinuria	NR	79	77	NR	NR	83	28	33	82
Dilated renal pelvis	NR	NR	27	27	NR	NR	17	13	NR
Hyperechoic renal cortices	NR	24	62	NR	NR	22	33	25	NR

ALP, Alkaline phosphatase; *ALT*, alanine aminotransferase; *NR*, not reported.
See Table 44-4 for data related to clinical signs from dogs in these studies.

Thrombocytopenia and increased fibrinogen degradation products have been found in dogs experimentally infected with serovar icterohaemorrhagiae. In a majority of dogs, other clotting parameters are normal, suggesting compensated hemostatic mechanisms. Severely affected dogs frequently have vascular endothelial damage with hypofibrinogenemia and thrombocytopenia resulting from disseminated intravascular coagulation (DIC). With meningitis, increased protein concentration with a predominance of neutrophils can be detected by cerebral spinal fluid (CSF) analysis.

In people, assessment of clinical laboratory findings has allowed prediction of severity and mortality in affected patients.[57,124] Dyspnea and severe alveolar infiltrates on thoracic radiography, elevated blood leukocyte counts, oliguria, and repolarization abnormalities on electrocardiograms are all poorer prognostic findings. Similar associations have not been made for affected dogs.

Radiographic and Ultrasonographic Findings

Although coughing and dyspnea are not consistent features of canine leptospirosis, interstitial to nodular alveolar densities, likely associated with pulmonary hemorrhage from endothelial damage and vasculitis, are found in thoracic radiographs of some dogs.[23] Lesions are most consistently detected in the caudodorsal lung fields. A complete clearance of the lesions occurs in recovered dogs. In decreasing order of prevalence, ultrasonographic abnormalities of the urinary system have included renomegaly, pyelectasia, increased cortical echogenicity, mild perirenal fluid accumulation, and a medullary band of increased echogenicity (Fig. 44-5).[63] The

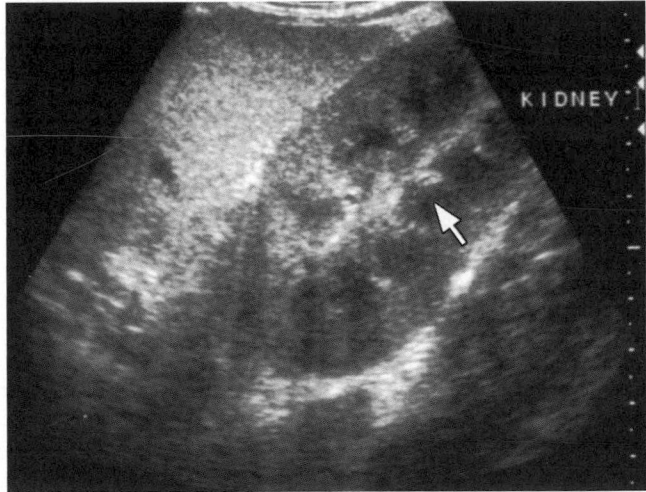

Fig 44-5 Ultrasonographic appearance of the kidney with a band of medullary hyperechogenicity. (Courtesy University of Georgia, Athens, Ga.)

medullary echogenic banding is not specific for leptospirosis in dogs and corresponds to a region of renal necrosis and hemorrhage seen grossly and histologically.

Serologic Testing

Microscopic Agglutination

This standard serologic means to diagnose leptospirosis requires darkfield microscopy, and samples must be sent to commercial laboratories. Organisms grown in liquid media are exposed to serial dilutions of the patient's sera. The end point is the highest serum dilution that causes 50% of the organisms to agglutinate. Contrary to popular belief, the microscopic agglutination (MA) test is a serogroup-specific assay; it does not discriminate organisms at the serovar level.[113] Screening with multiple antigens helps identify the suspected serogroup causing disease in a given patient or population; sera are usually screened at an initial dilution of 1:100. Further twofold dilutions are done against positive-reacting antigens to determine which antibody is present in highest concentration. Many laboratories stop at dilutions of 1:3200; however, others will report the results to end point.

The report to the veterinarian lists the various serovars used as antigens and the respective titers. Dogs with positive titers generally have sera that cross-react to a variety of serovars and that with the highest titer is interpreted as belonging to the infecting serogroup, and lower titers represent antibody cross-reactivity between serovars. Therefore interpreting titers as serogroup specific rather than serovar specific is appropriate. For example, in dogs naturally and experimentally infected with serovar grippotyphosa, the highest titer is against this serovar with lower titers to serovars pomona and bratislava. When titers are equal or greater than 1:3200 for more than one serovar, the causative serogroup is classified as mixed and occurs from shared epitopes among organisms of the same group. Unfortunately, if the infecting serogroup is not included as a test antigen, false negative results will occur, or titers may be low because of less affinity to any cross-reacting antigens used. Furthermore, even if the infecting serogroup is included, the MA test does not always correctly identify the infecting serogroup (paradoxical reactions).[113] Cross-reactions tend to be worse during the acute phase of the disease; the infecting serogroup is more likely to be identifiable in convalescent sera.

The magnitude expected for a single titer to be positive is always dependent on the background exposure in a population. In any geographic region, measured titers in dogs that are clinically healthy or suffering from other disease syndromes can help with determination and interpretation of background seroreactivity. In some circumstances, background titers may be found from certain serovars that are not associated with clinical disease.[192]

Demonstration of a fourfold increase or decrease in MA titer is classically required for serologic confirmation of an acute, potentially self-limiting disease such as leptospirosis. Many naturally infected dogs will have titers of 1:800 or greater, which on a single specimen is presumptive of leptospirosis with compatible clinical illness and knowledge of no recent vaccinations. Because titers can be negative in the first week to 10 days of acute illness, a second and sometimes a third serum sample should be obtained within 2- to 4-week intervals. Other affected dogs will have high (at least from 1:1600 to 1:12,800) titers when they are hospitalized, with no further increases noted. The magnitude of rise in titer does not always parallel the severity of clinical illness. In some dogs, very high titers or hyperglobulinemia suggests persistence and replication of the organism. Previous infection or vaccination is usually associated with an MA titer of less than 1:400, although higher titers are occasionally observed.[10] If higher vaccination titers (at or above 1:800) develop, they generally do not persist for longer than 3 months, although occasionally titers as high as 1:800 have been observed to persist for 9 months after vaccination.[195] Generally, titers at or above 1:800 indicated active infection or a subclinical renal carrier state. However, some dogs infected with serovar canicola to which they are well adapted may have titers less than 1:400 while being actively infected and excreting organisms.

Antimicrobial therapy very early in the course of disease may decrease the magnitude of the titer rise. Antibody titers will often reduce fourfold over weeks to months after successful antimicrobial therapy of established infections.[80] Therefore a fourfold increase or decrease in titer is considered indicating active or recent infection. When the renal carrier state has been successfully eliminated, serologic titers will decrease to at the most 1:200 within a 6- to 9-month period, or sooner. Testing of treated animals after this interval is important to determine if the animal is a safe public health risk. Lower levels of antibodies to leptospiral antigens used in the MA test may also indicate some exposure to infection with nonleptospiral spirochetes. Dogs exposed to ticks harboring Borrelia burgdorferi that developed high titers to that organism did not show significant increases in titers on the MA test.[185] In contrast, leptospiral infections can affect serotest results for borreliosis when whole-cell assays are used (see Diagnosis, Chapter 45). A summary of criteria for diagnosis using the MA titer and other testing is in Table 44-6.

Enzyme-Linked Immunosorbent Assay

Assay methods such as enzyme-linked immunosorbent assay (ELISA) have been used in dogs to detect IgG or IgM antibodies to leptospires.[166,209] In comparison, increases in the MA titer parallel the ELISA IgM titer more closely than the IgG titer, although both classes of antibody can cause agglutination. The IgM ELISA increases within 1 week after initial infection, and the maximum titer develops within 2 weeks, with a subsequent decrease thereafter. The IgM ELISA appears to be more sensitive in detecting antibody and is more serogroup specific than the MA test for determining very early infection in dogs. Dogs that died within the first week of illness have had high IgM titers, despite having negative MA titers.

In dogs, increased IgG ELISA titers develop 2 to 3 weeks after infection, with a maximum titer in approximately 1 month. IgG ELISA titers better parallel protection against

---

Table • 44-6

Criteria for Diagnosis of Leptospirosis

Serologic Testing by Microscopic Agglutination
Vaccination more than 3 months prior
Fourfold rise in paired titers at 3-week interval or 1:800 or greater single titer
Other compatible clinical findings

Microscopy
Lesions compatible by gross or microscopic examination in specimens taken by biopsy or necropsy
Silver or immunostaining of tissues

Organism Identification
Darkfield microscopy of urine
Immunostaining of urine sediment
Polymerase chain reaction positive results on tissues or body fluids
Culture

infection than do MA titers. In contrast to MA and IgM titers, IgG titers increase dramatically after vaccination and persist for many months. By using combined IgG and IgM measurements, the ELISA is better suited to distinguish between natural infection and vaccine-induced immunity than is the MA test. ELISA testing in dogs that have received more than one vaccination demonstrates a high IgG titer accompanied by a low or negative IgM titer, even within the first few weeks after vaccination. The ELISA is not widely available for clinical application. A recombinant antigen-based ELISA method has also been developed that can detect antibodies to a whole variety of pathogenic serovars.[54a]

Other Immunoassays

A macroscopic slide agglutination test, developed for the diagnosis of human leptospirosis, detects antibodies as early in the course of infection as does the IgM ELISA.[38] The advantage of this assay is that it can be used as a field test because it can be done without microscopy. Slide agglutination and indirect hemagglutination assays, available as a commercial kits, have also been used to detect recent or active infections in people and dogs.[116] (See Appendix 6.) The slide agglutination and hemagglutination assays may be used on a variety of animals without modification. A commercial screening testing using a broadly reactive leptospiral antigen is incorporated into an ELISA test strip (LEPTO Dipstick assay, Dutch Royal Tropical Institute).[180,187] This human-specific test strip is a screen for IgM antibodies in serum and has been used in people to determine recent or active infection.

Organism Identification

Bacterial Culture

Proper timing and technique are essential for the recovery of leptospires because of their fastidious growth requirements and susceptibility to adverse environmental conditions. Samples should be taken before initiation of antibiotic therapy. Dogs are leptospiremic during the first week of infection, but the numbers of circulating organisms subsequently decrease as serum antibody titers increase. However, urinary shedding develops thereafter.[173] Occurrence of leptospires in CSF parallels that in blood.[167] Urine is the ideal fluid to be cultured; however, multiple sampling is required because of intermittent shedding of organisms. If animals are adequately hydrated, administration of a low dose of a diuretic such as furosemide (0.5 mg/kg) just before urine collection may facilitate recovery of organisms.

Premortem isolation is preferred because postmortem tissue contaminants will overgrow fastidious leptospires unless selective media are employed. A small volume of tissue (preferably liver or kidney) or body fluid for culture should be collected aseptically in a clean, sterile glass container. Catheterized or voided urine is frequently contaminated by normal flora that interferes with the growth of leptospires; therefore cystocentesis is preferred. Inhibiting substances such as antibody in host tissues and fluids require dilution of the sample by at least 1:10 (vol/vol) with buffered saline, 1% bovine serum albumin, or culture medium. As an alternative, 0.25 to 0.5 ml of blood, urine, or CSF taken at the appropriate stage of infection can be directly inoculated into 7 to 10 ml of transport media. Blood should be anticoagulated with preservative-free heparin or sodium polyethylene sulfonate (as in blood culture bottles) for transport to the laboratory if it cannot be diluted immediately. Citrate anticoagulants should be avoided because they inhibit leptospires. Urine should be alkalinized to pH 8 or greater during transport because leptospires cannot survive acidic conditions for more than a few hours. Tissue or fluid samples, if shipped, should be kept in transport medium or on ice but not frozen. For research purposes, organisms can be frozen in semisolid or transport media and stored at temperatures of −60° C to −70° C for up to 6 years before culture.

Media for isolation of leptospires are liquid, semisolid, or solid in nature. Ellinghausen, McCullough, Johnson, Harris (EMJH) is a liquid or semisolid medium containing polysorbate 80 and fetal calf serum or bovine serum albumin. Modification of standard medium by adding antibiotics or 5-fluorouracil has produced improved results in isolation of certain leptospiral serovars. Leptospires commonly lose their virulence on culture in artificial media, but this loss can be reversed by passage in susceptible animals. Culture of spirochetes from tissues or body fluids is not by itself diagnostic of clinical illness because leptospires can be recovered from both fluids and tissues of healthy dogs.

Identification of the infecting serovar requires application of serologic or genetic typing techniques following isolation. MA test with polyclonal or monoclonal antibodies is the best means of serologic classification. Pulsed-field gel electrophoresis following restriction digestion of full-length chromosomal DNA accurately types serovars, and is more rapid than serologic methods.[49,90]

Microscopic Evaluation

Darkfield examination is necessary for rapid identification of viable leptospires because they cannot be stained by simple methods with aniline dyes. Wet-mount preparations are also necessary to help characterize their writhing and flexing movements. A variety of bacteria that can be confused with leptospires produce more random movement in wet mount preparations. Cellular fibrils or extrusions and fibrin strands can be mistaken for organisms. Darkfield microscopy can also fail to detect active infections because approximately 10^5 organisms/ml are required.[32] Centrifugation can be used to concentrate specimens. Because of the inaccuracies of darkfield examination, it should always be followed by cultural or serologic procedures. Because of these inaccuracies, darkfield examination is no longer recommended.

Leptospires can be seen by light microscopy in tissue sections or on air-dried smears with Giemsa stain or silver impregnation.

Direct fluorescent antibody (FA) techniques have been adapted to identify leptospiral serovars in tissues imprints of liver and kidney and in body fluids such as blood or urine (Fig. 44-6). Direct FA testing can be used as a screening method to identify animals shedding organisms in urine when culture is impossible or too time consuming. Organisms may not be shed in urine until 4 to 10 days after the onset of clinical signs. Generally, available conjugates do not discriminate among serovars, and the method cannot differentiate viable and nonviable organisms.

Immunodetection

Agglutination-adsorption techniques using monoclonal antibodies have been employed in specialized laboratories to serotype isolates. Antigen capture using similar antibodies in dot ELISA has been developed to detect *Leptospira* antigen in urine of infected people.[170] Although not widely available, this method is highly sensitive and specific and can be used at low cost without specialized equipment.

Genetic Detection

Leptospires have been detected in biologic fluids by the very sensitive PCR. PCR can be used to rapidly differentiate pathogenic from nonpathogenic isolates.[149] Genetic methods allow for more specific determination of the infecting strains, which is not possible with measurement of serum antibody titers. Genetic probes have been used to detect leptospires in blood, CSF, aqueous humor, and urine.[18,131,167] PCR has been used to detect leptospires in the aqueous humor of people and horses

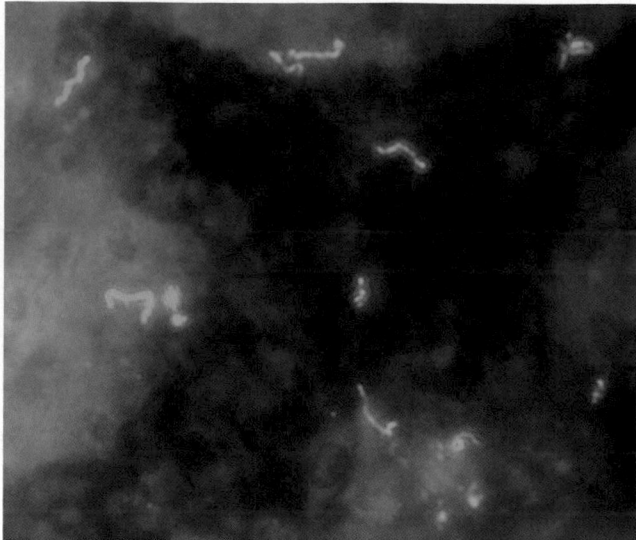

Fig 44-6 Direct FA stain of leptospires in the kidney (×60). (Courtesy Wayne Roberts, University of Georgia, Athens, Ga.)

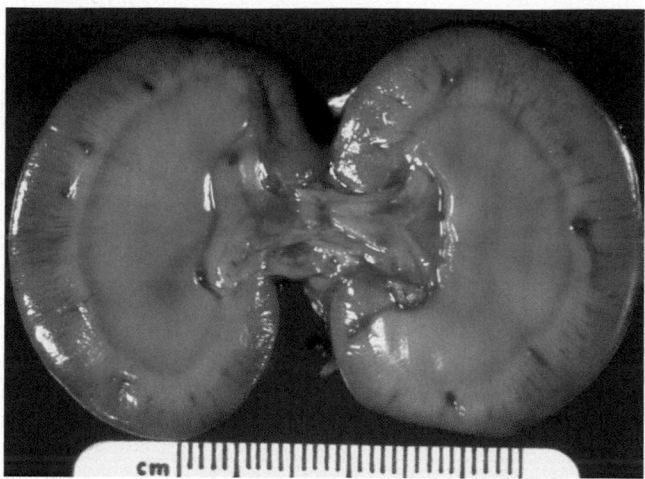

Fig 44-7 Swollen kidney from a dog that died of acute leptospirosis. (Courtesy University of Georgia, Athens, Ga.)

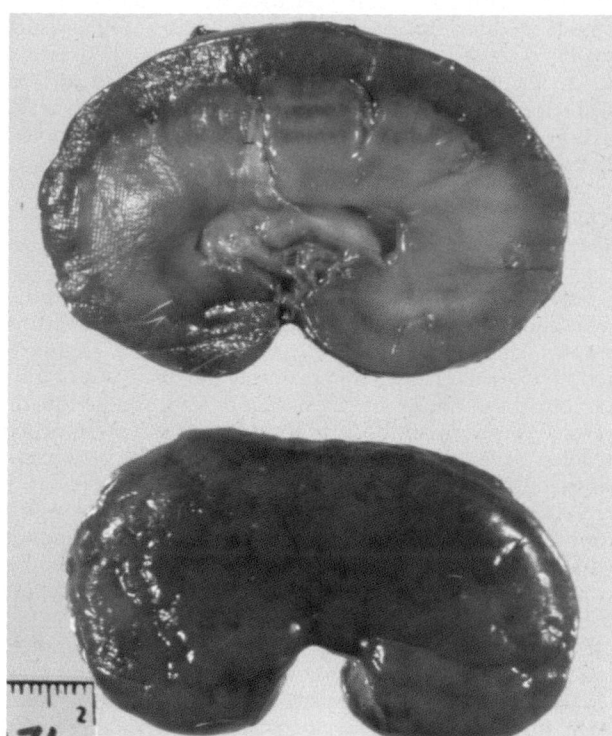

Fig 44-8 Shrunken and fibrotic kidneys from an 8-month-old puppy that had acute icterus and renal failure; the illness had been diagnosed as leptospirosis by serologic testing 5 months previously. The dog had been treated and was clinically normal until the time of death from an automobile accident. (Courtesy University of Georgia, Athens, Ga.)

with uveitis.[48,61] Because of higher concentration of leptospires in urine, testing that fluid is essential to ensure the accuracy of genetic detection methods. In people, PCR is more reliable than serologic testing or culture of urine for very early diagnosis.[42] Multiplex or arbitrarily primed PCR methods have been sensitive and specific for detection of leptospires in canine urine.[44,81,82,111] Although some of these assays offer the advantage of rapid speciation of the infecting organism, discrimination at the serovar level has not been possible. Magnetic immunocapture has been used to increase the sensitivity of PCR detection.[196] Restriction endonuclease analysis of DNA amplified using PCR has allowed differentiation between many serovars and has the potential to be used on DNA obtained directly from clinical samples. Unfortunately, some of these methods have failed to detect certain serovars, and others did not permit differentiation of all-important serovars infecting dogs. PCR methods such as arbitrarily primed PCR have allowed epidemiologic tracking of the source and commonality of particular strains involved in disease outbreaks in people.[151] PCR results in urine have been more sensitive in giving positive results than those of MA testing of sera in evaluating dogs with suspected leptospiral infection.[81,82] As with culture, PCR results may have false positive results and may detect organisms in subclinical carriers. Therefore positive results must always be interpreted in light of the clinical signs. Furthermore, genomic sequences of nonviable Leptospira can be detected in recovered or treated dogs. Further studies are needed to determine the sensitivity and reliability of this method for diagnosis.

PATHOLOGIC FINDINGS

External gross lesions vary greatly depending on the severity of the disease and may include congested and icteric mucous membranes with diffuse petechiae. Focal ulcerations may be seen on the tongue and in the buccal cavity and are likely secondary to uremia. Tonsillar or lymphoid tissue enlargement may be present. Kidneys are enlarged in animals that die of acute infection. They are pale and yellow-gray in color and bulge on the cut surface (Fig. 44-7). The renal capsule may be adherent to the surface of the kidneys, and subcapsular hemorrhages are common. In less acute cases, focal, white spotting may be seen in the renal cortex on cut sections and is most prominent along the corticomedullary junction. In chronically infected or treated and recovered dogs, the kidneys may be scarred and shrunken (Fig. 44-8). Leptospires can be cultured from macerated kidney tissue. More commonly, with serovar icterohaemorrhagiae infection, the respiratory tract may be edematous with pulmonary congestion, and spotty, diffuse, pneumonic infiltrates may be present. Petechial and ecchymotic hemorrhages are commonly found on the pleural surface (see Fig. 44-4, B). With hepatic involvement, the liver is enlarged and friable, with pronounced interlobar markings

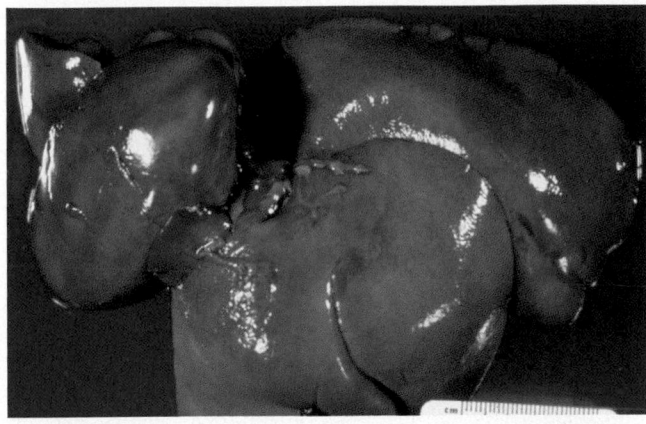

Fig 44-9 Swollen necrotic liver from a dog with acute leptospirosis. (Courtesy University of Georgia, Athens Ga.)

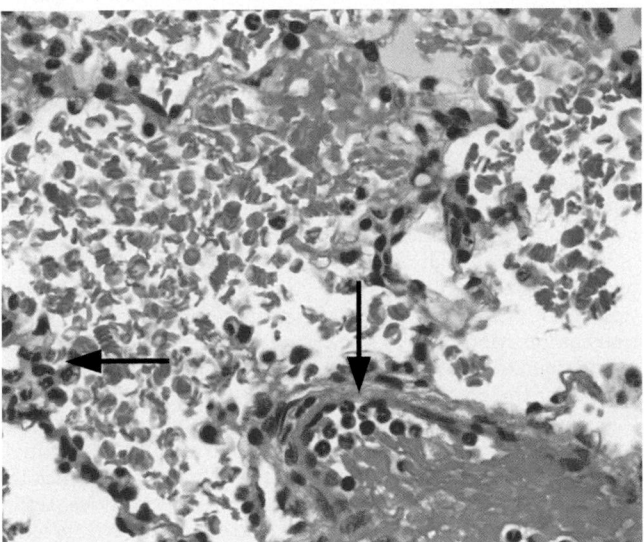

Fig 44-10 Acute pulmonary hemorrhage in a dog with acute leptospirosis. Alveoli contain large numbers of extravasated erythrocytes. Note margination of neutrophils within blood vessels *(arrows)* (H and E stain, ×400). (Courtesy Cathy Brown, University of Georgia, Athens, Ga.)

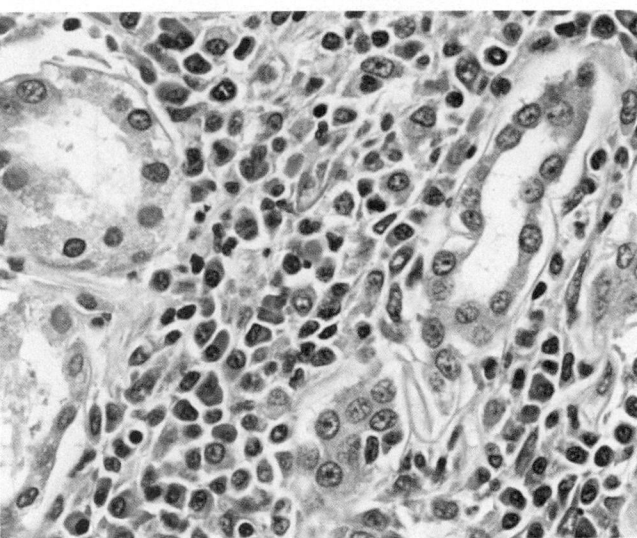

Fig 44-11 Renal lesions of subacute leptospirosis. Renal tubules in the deep cortex are separated by a large number of plasma cells, small numbers of macrophages, and scattered neutrophils (H and E stain, ×400). (Courtesy Cathy Brown, University of Georgia, Athens, Ga.)

and yellow-brown discoloration (Fig. 44-9). Petechiae and ecchymoses are found throughout the leptomeninges. Ulcerative and hemorrhagic gastritis is often present in uremic animals.

Necrosis and hemorrhage are occasionally present in the bowel with intestinal intussusceptions. Free blood or acholic feces may be found in the colon and rectum of some animals. The spleen may be pale and shrunken.

Some variability exists in the histologic appearance of the kidney; this variability is attributed to the virulence of the infecting serovar and the duration of the infection. Dogs with acute leptospirosis, which occurs before a significant serologic response (i.e., titers are frequently negative), have severe renal dysfunction. Histologically, however, the renal lesions are subtle, consisting of mild renal tubular necrosis and interstitial edema. Interstitial inflammation is absent or minimal. Secondary lesions of uremia, such as pulmonary mineralization, gastric mucosal mineralization, and vascular fibrinoid necrosis, are common. Severe multifocal pulmonary hemorrhage is apparent (Fig. 44-10). The subacute form of leptospirosis is characterized by diffuse interstitial renal inflammation, which is most severe at the corticomedullary junction (Fig. 44-11). The infiltrate is composed primarily of plasma cells, with lesser numbers of lymphocytes and macrophages. Scattered neutrophils and necrotic epithelial cells are often present within tubular lumina. Kidneys of chronically affected dogs are characterized primarily by diffuse renal interstitial fibrosis, with only mild to moderate multifocal lymphoplasmacytic inflammation, and scattered macrophages. These histologic lesions of more chronic leptospirosis are nonspecific and are found in most end-stage kidneys.

Special stains are needed to visualize leptospires in tissues. With silver staining, which is relatively nonspecific, globular debris and intact spirochetes can be found adhered to the luminal surface of renal tubular epithelial cells. Intact organisms are most often detected in subacute cases; silver stains often fail to detect organisms in acute or chronic cases. Although no more sensitive than silver stains, immunohistochemical stains are highly specific for detecting leptospires.[210] Immunohistochemical staining is uniformly positive in subacute cases, appearing primarily as globular material within tubular lumina, tubular epithelial cells, and interstitial macrophages. Widely scattered intact organisms may be detected in clumps or individually within tubules in some but not all subacute cases (Fig. 44-12). Positive staining material is also seen in the inflammatory foci in chronic leptospiral renal disease. Leptospiral antigen is detected immunohistochemically in some, but not all, of the acute cases. FA examination of unfixed kidney is a more sensitive, widely available, method for detecting leptospiral antigen and will detect both intact organisms and leptospiral debris.

Histologic changes in the lung consist of fibrinoid necrosis of blood vessels and perivascular, intraalveolar, and subpleural hemorrhages. Mononuclear cell infiltrates surround thrombosed pulmonary vessels. Focal necrosis of hepatic parenchyma may be present. Hepatocytes are rounded, with pyknotic nuclei, and contain an eosinophilic granular cytoplasm. Intrahepatic bile stasis and severe hepatocellular injury are usually evident in icteric animals. The clinical severity of hepatic disease parallels the severity of histologic changes in the liver. Subclinical cases usually have mild fatty changes in

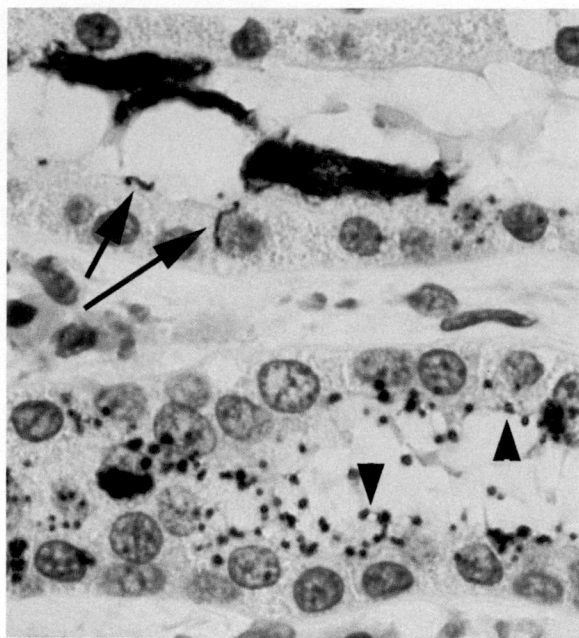

Fig 44-12 *Leptospira* immunohistochemistry; subacute leptospirosis. Large clumps of positive staining debris and occasional intact spirochetes *(arrows)* are present within tubules, in addition to prominent globular intraepithelial staining *(arrowheads)* (peroxidase, ×60). (Courtesy Cathy Brown, University of Georgia, Athens, Ga.)

hepatocytes, whereas moderately ill dogs have fragmented hepatic cords, with lymphocytic infiltrates in areas of necrosis, and severely affected dogs have widespread necrosis of hepatic parenchyma and disintegration of nuclei. Chronically infected dogs develop chronic active hepatitis and hepatic fibrosis. Organisms may be demonstrated in intercellular locations within hepatic cords.

Neurologic damage includes perivascular hemorrhage (uncommon in the cat), mononuclear cell infiltrate, and occasionally, vascular thrombosis. When a silver stain is applied, leptospires can be found in pericapillary areas. Although gross lesions are absent in the heart, focal lymphocytic myocarditis may be evident on histologic examination.

Immunohistochemical procedures that have been developed to detect leptospires in canine tissues[210] have been effective on formalin-fixed specimens, and the monoclonal antibodies provide a high degree of specificity.

THERAPY

Supportive therapy for animals with leptospirosis depends on the severity of infection and the presence of renal or hepatic dysfunction and other complicating factors. Dehydration and shock occur in severely affected animals. Placement of a jugular or central venous catheter is usually recommended to assist with repeated sampling, high-volume fluid administration, and measurement of central venous pressure. Indwelling urinary catheters may be needed in oliguric animals to obtain precise measurements of urine output; however, they often result in complicating nosocomial bacterial infections. Fluid loss results from vomiting and diarrhea, and balanced polyionic intravenous (IV) fluids should be used to correct the deficits. Oral alimentation must be discontinued in vomiting animals. Uremia and uremic gastritis are chemical and visceral causes for vomiting in these animals. Centrally acting antiemetics and parenterally administered gastric protectants (e.g., H2-receptor blockers, proton-pump inhibitors) may be needed; however, oral administration of gastric protectants may be impossible if vomiting persists. Petechial and ecchymotic hemorrhages indicate thrombocytopenia from vasculitis or DIC in severely affected animals. Plasma or fresh whole blood transfusions should be given with caution and only with concurrent low-dose heparin for ongoing DIC or severe hypoalbuminemia.

Oliguria (under 2 ml/kg/hr) and anuria are treated initially with rehydration. Osmotic diuretics, such as 10% to 20% glucose (5 ml/kg) or 20% mannitol (0.5 g/kg), should be given IV over 30 to 60 minutes when impaired renal function persists after rehydration. If treatment with these diuretics fails, dopamine (5 μg/kg/min) or dopaminergic agents may be administered by IV infusion. Tubular diuretics such as furosemide (2 to 4 mg/kg) should be administered parenterally in conjunction with dopamine to increase urine flow; however, the effect on improving glomerular filtration is debated. An essential element is that fluid therapy be adjusted to the individual patient's urine output. Peritoneal dialysis or preferably hemodialysis (when available) should be considered if oliguria persists because acute renal dysfunction is potentially reversible.[3] Predicting which dogs will respond to fluid diuresis is not always possible based on laboratory values.

In people, massive pulmonary hemorrhage is often associated with high mortality. Adjunctive therapy has consisted of hemofiltration to remove cytokines and use of nitric oxide inhalation to help open up blood-filled alveoli.[66]

Antibiotics usually reduce fever and bacteremia within a few hours after administration. They immediately inhibit multiplication of the organism and rapidly reduce fatal complications of infection such as hepatic and renal failure. The sooner in the course of infection that antimicrobial agents are used, the better the chance is for reversal of tissue injury caused by the spirochetes. Therefore this therapy should be instituted immediately on suspicion and before return of definitive testing results. In vitro and experimental in vivo susceptibilities exist to the penicillins, cephems, aminoglycosides, tetracyclines, and macrolides. Penicillin and its derivatives are the antibiotics of choice for terminating leptospiremia (Table 44-7), but they do not eliminate the carrier state. Initially, penicillin or ampicillin can be given parenterally to the vomiting, uremic, or hepatically compromised animal. Once oral alimentation is begun, oral therapy with amoxicillin is recommended because of its superior absorption. Other drugs such as the tetracyclines, aminoglycosides, or macrolides should be provided after therapy with the penicillins and after oral alimentation is possible to eliminate the carrier state. Doxycycline can be used for initial therapy or for elimination of the carrier state. It can be given IV or by mouth, depending on the animal's state of alimentation. The dose does not need to be adjusted in animals with renal failure because doxycycline is predominantly excreted in the feces. Aminoglycosides, although highly effective in clearing the renal carrier state, should never be given to clear the carrier state unless results of renal function tests have returned to reference ranges. Streptomycin is less available and it has been replaced, in treatment of people, by gentamicin, tobramycin, and isepamicin.[104] In experimental studies in animals, ampicillin and first-generation cephalosporins have not been effective in eliminating the organisms from tissues and body fluids, whereas tetracyclines and macrolides such as erythromycin and its derivatives (clarithromycin, azithromycin) were effective.[7] Third-generation cephalosporins, such as ceftiofur, have cleared the renal carrier state in cattle.[8] Ceftriaxone, which is often used to treat human borreliosis, was as efficacious in

Table • 44-7

Recommended Therapy for Leptospirosis

DRUG[a]	SPECIES	DOSE[b]	ROUTE	INTERVAL (HOURS)	DURATION (WEEKS)
Penicillin G	B	25,000—40,000 units/kg	IM, SC, IV	12	2
Ampicillin	B	22 mg/kg	PO, SC, IV	6—8	2
Amoxicillin	D	22 mg/kg	PO	8—12	2
Doxycycline[c]	D	5 mg/kg	PO, IV	12	2
Tetracycline[d]	B	22 mg/kg	PO	8	2
Azithromycin[e]	D	20 mg/kg	PO	24	1

B, Dog and cat; D, dog; IM, Intramuscular; SC, subcutaneous; IV, intravenous; PO, by mouth.

[a]Refer to Appendix 8 for additional information on these drugs.

[b]Dose per administration at specified interval.

[c]Can be used as primary therapy or to clear renal carriers since excretion not affected by azotemia.

[d]Used to clear the renal carrier once azotemia has resolved. Repositol oxytetracycline (LA-200) has been used to treat large numbers of affected foxhounds at an IM dose of 20 mg/kg once weekly for 4 weeks.

[e]Efficacy of macrolides has not been well studied although they have an appropriate in vitro spectrum. Other alternatives are erythromycin or clarithromycin.

treating severe leptospirosis in people.[148] Ineffective drugs include chloramphenicol and sulfonamides. Ciprofloxacin is effective in vitro and in vivo against virulent strains of leptospires, but its clinical application has been limited.[184] Orbifloxacin at recommended dosages was not effective compared with oral amoxicillin in treating one dog,[71] and quinolones have not been effective in clearing experimentally infected animals.[199]

PREVENTION

Prevention of leptospirosis involves elimination of the carrier state. Unfortunately, wild animal reservoirs and subclinically affected domestic animals continue to harbor and shed organisms. Control of rodents in kennels, maintenance of environmental conditions to discourage bacterial survival, and isolation of infected animals therefore are important to prevent spread of the disease. Doxycycline has been given at a low dose (200 mg once weekly) to people in endemic areas for prophylaxis when vaccination with appropriate serovars is unavailable. Use at this lower level does not prevent infection but helps reduce morbidity and mortality in people who become infected.[179] Such therapy may result in development of bacterial resistance and is not generally recommended for people or their pets.

Bacterins that contain four main serovars—canicola, icterohaemorrhagiae, grippotyphosa, and pomona—are available for dogs. Some preparations contain only grippotyphosa and pomona; others contain only canicola and icterohaemorrhagiae. Current vaccines are not completely cross-protective against other significant disease-causing serogroups such as *Sejroe* and *Autumnalis*. Experimental studies have documented that the LPS antigens are responsible for homologous protection, whereas protein antigens give both homologous and some heterologous protection.[190] Many currently marketed vaccines are chemically inactivated whole cultures, which makes them relatively allergenic in comparison with the tissue culture lines of virus vaccines (see Postvaccinal Complications, Chapter 100). Immunization has been effective in reducing the prevalence and severity of canine leptospirosis. Previously, inactivated bacterins did not prevent the carrier state, which is associated with potential zoonotic risk. Newer vaccines marketed for dogs and other species have pre-

vented renal colonization and shedding.[34] Protection against postinfection shedding, which varied among tested vaccines, was observed when dogs were challenged up to 7 weeks after the second of two doses of three commercial vaccines.[10]

Adequate initial immunization, employing many of the available products, takes up to two to three injections 2 to 3 weeks apart to produce immunity to challenge infection that will last at least 6 to 8 months. Challenge studies in dogs have shown some leptospiral vaccines provide some protection against challenge at 3, 27, and 56 weeks (see Table 100-12A).[102] Protection was complete at 3 weeks, but some organisms may be isolated from the blood of some animals at 27 and 56 weeks, indicating some decline in sterile immune protection with time.

Vaccines have been produced from the outer envelope fraction of leptospires, which is the site of leptospiricidal activity of antibody and complement.[127] Antigenic material has been reduced by culture in a protein-free media; adjuvants have been removed, and up to five Leptospira serovars have been included in such vaccines. Maximal antibody titers have been produced in dogs within 2 weeks after a single vaccination, and dogs have been protected against infection and urinary shedding after challenge. Recombinant-produced outer surface immunogenic lipoproteins (LigA-m and LigB-m) have shown promising results in challenge studies in mice.[105a]

Agglutination titers, which are predominantly IgM, do not increase to very high levels following vaccination. IgG titers, which are primarily responsible for protection, are produced for at least 1 year after the third vaccination in dogs. Because immunity wanes with time, and because highest titers are produced by multiple injections, yearly (and sometimes biannual) vaccinations should be given to dogs in endemic areas, and all dogs in highly endemic regions should receive at least three injections in their primary vaccination series. For further guidelines concerning leptospirosis vaccination, see Chapter 100.

PUBLIC HEALTH CONSIDERATIONS

People acquire infection through occupational, recreational, or avocational activities. Leptospira require humid conditions for their survival, and infected dogs, as with other animals,

Table • 44-8

Outbreaks of Leptospirosis in People Associated with Exposure to Dogs

LOCATION AND DATE	NUMBER AFFECTED	EXPOSURE SOURCE	PRESUMPTIVE SEROGROUP	INFECTING SEROVAR ISOLATED	REFERENCE
North Dakota, 1950	9	Infected family dog	Canicola	NI	85
Georgia, 1952	26	Swimming in creek; dogs suspected	Canicola	NI	211
Japan, 1953	114	Swimming in river; dogs suspected	Canicola	canicola	138
Texas, 1971	7	Pet dogs	Canicola	canicola	19
Portland, Oregon, 1972	9	Infected family dog	Autumnalis	fort bragg	64
St. Louis, Missouri, 1972	5	Infected pet dogs	Icterohaemorrhagiae	icterohaemorrhagiae	62
Morón, Cuba, 1986	6	Swimming in creek; dogs suspected	Canicola	NI	89
Barbados, 1988	1	Kennel dogs	Autumnalis	bim	60
Nicaragua, 1995	100	Flooding, walking in creek; dogs suspected	Canicola	portlandvere	198, 216

NI, Not isolated.

may disseminate the organism through urination in drinking, bathing, or recreational water sources. Seasonal flooding has been a major risk factor in some outbreaks in developing countries. Flooding elevates the water table, saturates the soil with leptospires, prevents evaporation of contaminating animal urine, and prolongs the survival of the spirochetes in surface water. The majority of infections in people are among those who experience occupational exposure to infected wildlife or domestic animal hosts, or engage in water sports activities, or contact animal urine or contaminated fomites in their daily lives.* Veterinary students have been documented to become infected during their course of training during the clinical years in the areas of food inspection, farm work, and contact with pet carnivores and animal traders.[186] A few outbreaks have been associated with eating food contaminated with rodent urine.[104] Exposure to outdoor water-related activities have been a concerned risk for infection; however, a high rate of infection of leptospirosis has been identified in inner cities.[27] Exposure of people living in unsanitary environments to rodent urine has been suspected. The chance that dogs might be involved has not been eliminated.

In some outbreaks, simultaneous exposure of people and dogs can occur (Table 44-8).[202] Contaminated urine is highly infectious for people and for susceptible animal species; therefore contact on mucous membranes or skin abrasions should be avoided. Spirochetes do not penetrate intact skin; however, open skin wounds, or softening or maceration of the skin from prolonged immersion in water, or exposure to mucous membranes, or swallowing water, greatly increases the risk of infection.[77,153]

During treatment of animals suspected to be infected, precautions should be taken. The animals should be physically separated to prevent inadvertent contact with other animals or people. Latex gloves should be worn when handling urine or urine-contaminated items from animals. Facemasks and goggles should be worn when hosing contaminated kennel areas. Canine infection and leptospiruria have been found in healthy vaccinated dogs with resultant development of the disease in people. All known or suspected shedders should be treated with antibiotics. Once appropriate antimicrobial therapy has been instituted to affected animals, the public health risk is minimized because viable organisms will not be actively shed. Reshedding can occur when antimicrobial therapy is discontinued if drugs used to clear the renal carrier state are not used. Areas contaminated by infected urine should be washed with detergent and then treated with iodophor disinfectants (see Chapter 94) to which the organism is very susceptible. People with human immunodeficiency virus (HIV) are at particular risk for severe infection[97]; therefore if they live in an endemic area, their dogs should be screened serologically for exposure and possible infection, and thereafter these animals should receive multivalent vaccination on a periodic basis. Chemoprophylaxis with tetracyclines has been used to prevent infection in people temporarily exposed to high-risk environments.

SUGGESTED READINGS*

3. Adin CA, Cowgill LD. 2000. Treatment and outcome of dogs with leptospirosis: 36 cases (1990-1998), *J Am Vet Med Assoc* 216:371-375.
10. Andre-Fontaine G, Branger C, Gray AW, et al. 2003. Comparison of the efficacy of three commercial bacterins in preventing canine leptospirosis, *Vet Rec* 153:165-169.

*References: 6, 13, 14, 24, 96, 140, 178, 182, 198.

*See the CD-ROM for a complete list of references.

36. Boutilier P, Carr A, Schulman RL. 2003. Leptospirosis in dogs: a serologic survey and case series 1996-2001, *Vet Ther* 4:178-187.
44. Cai HY, Hornby G, Key DW, et al. 2002. Preliminary study on differentiation of *Leptospira grippotyphosa* and *Leptospira sejroe* from other common pathogenic leptospiral serovars in canine urine by polymerase chain reaction assay, *J Vet Diagn Invest* 14:164-168.
82. Harkin KR, Roshto YM, Sullivan TJ, et al. 2003b. Comparison of polymerase chain reaction assay, bacteriologic culture, and serologic testing in assessment of prevalence of urinary shedding of leptospires of dogs, *J Am Vet Med Assoc* 222:1230-1233.
114. Levett PN. 2003. Usefulness of serologic analysis as a predictor of the infecting serovar in patients with severe leptospirosis, *Clin Infect Dis* 36:447-452.
160. Prescott JF, McEwen B, Taylor J, et al. 2002. Resurgence of leptospirosis in dogs in Ontario: recent findings, *Can Vet J* 43:955-961.

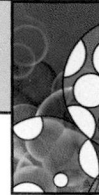

CHAPTER • 45

Borreliosis

Craig E. Greene and Reinhard K. Straubinger

Members of the genus *Borrelia*, which contains at least 37 species, are usually categorized into one of two groups: the relapsing-fever borreliae or the Lyme borreliosis borreliae. Both groups contain pathogenic species and other borreliae that have been isolated only from ticks or asymptomatic animals. Lyme borreliosis is the most commonly diagnosed vectorborne disease in people. It has been reported in North America, Europe, and Asia. Unconfirmed accounts of the disease have come from Australia, South America, and Africa. This disease is one of a larger group of vectorborne borrelioses that affect mammalian and avian hosts (Table 45-1). Experimentally and spontaneously induced Lyme borreliosis has been described in dogs, cats, and other animals. Because of the difficulty in confirming a diagnosis and the diversity of borrelial species being isolated from ticks, controversy still exists regarding the exact prevalence and geographic distribution of infection. The relapsing-fever borreliae affect people and domestic animals. Only one confirmed case in which these organisms were isolated from clinically ill dogs has been reported.[25] The discussion that follows focuses on Lyme borreliosis (about which more information is available) unless otherwise indicated.

ETIOLOGY

Lyme Borreliosis

Like most spirochetes, borreliae are small (0.2 × 30 µm), and dark-field or phase microscopy is needed for proper visualization of live organisms (Fig. 45-1). The genospecies of *Borrelia burgdorferi* sensu lato, the causative agent of Lyme borreliosis, has been divided into at least four genomic species groups (see Table 45-1).[35,66] Analysis of outer surface proteins (Osps) such as the lipoproteins OspA and OspB and of genetic and amino acid sequences have been used to subgroup the *Borrelia* species. Group 1 (*B. burgdorferi* sensu stricto) is the primary isolate seen in the United States. In people, it is associated with annular skin lesions, polyarthritis, and meningitis. In the United States, *Borrelia andersonii* and *Borrelia bissettii* have been isolated from *Ixodes* ticks on rabbits or rodents and birds, respectively; their pathogenic significance is uncertain. In Europe, groups 1, 2, and 3 have been isolated from people, with groups 2 (*Borrelia garinii*) and 3 (*Borrelia afzelii*) predominating. In most European countries, *B. garinii* is the most abundant species being isolated from *Ixodes ricinus* ticks.[212] The three main *Borrelia* genospecies in Europe appear to have common rodent hosts, and many of these hosts harbor multiple infectious agents.[207] The greater diversity among species in Europe suggests that this complex of organisms originated in Eurasia.[262] However, other evidence suggests that *B. burgdorferi* sensu stricto may have been reintroduced into Europe from transported mammalian hosts. *Borrelia valaisiana* has been isolated from *I. ricinus* ticks on vegetation and birds; however, its pathogenic significance if any is uncertain. Meningopolyneuritis (Bannwarth's syndrome) is the primary clinical sign in people with group 2 infection, whereas in Europe, group 3 seropositivity has been associated with chronic arthritis and dermatitis (erythema chronica migrans [ECM]).[57] *B. afzelii* has been isolated from a naturally infected dog,[238] and mixed infections with this and other European species has been described.[238] A new species, *Borrelia japonica* (group 4), has been isolated from ticks found on dogs and people in Japan.[9] In the same region two additional species, *Borrelia takunii* and *Borrelia turdi*, have been isolated from ticks from small mammals; however, their pathogenic significance is uncertain. In the northeastern United States, *B. andersonii* has been found in ticks from rabbits. In the southeastern United States, more than 200 *Borrelia* strains have been isolated that can be classified molecularly into *B. burgdorferi* sensu stricto.[188] They feed on principal small mammal reservoirs such as the cotton mouse, the cotton rat, the eastern wood rat, and the cottontail rabbit. Other yet unidentified pathogenic and nonpathogenic strains of *Borrelia* exist.[169] A variant *Borrelia* species has been associated with ECM skin lesions in people in Missouri.[164] Southern tick-associated rash illness (STARI) is a Lyme borreliosis-like illness that occurs in people in the southeastern and south central United States, and the organism *Borrelia lonestari* has been cultured from these individuals.[257] The differences in strains or species may account for the regional differences in clinical findings that have been reported.

On the basis of in vitro borreliacidal assays, North American and European isolates of *B. burgdorferi* are divided into at least five seroprotective groups that differ from the species groups previously described.[149] Although North

Table • 45-1

Borrelial Species of Medical and Veterinary Importance

SPECIES	DISEASE	GEOGRAPHIC LOCATION	VECTOR	WILD ANIMAL RESERVOIR	DOMESTIC HOSTS
Lyme Borreliae					
B. burgdorferi sensu lato B. burgdorferi sensu stricto (group 1)	Lyme borreliosis, erythema migrans (annular skin lesions), polyarthritis, meningitis, carditis	North America	Ixodes scapularis, Ixodes pacificus and Ixodes neotomae	*Larvae and nymphs:* Rodents, small mammals, birds *Adults:* Deer, larger mammals, birds	People, dog, cat
	Lyme borreliosis	Europe	Ixodes ricinus	Same as above, except birds more prevalent for all stages	People, dog
B. garinii (group 2)	Erythema chronica migrans (ECM), meningopolyneuritis, arthritis	Europe, Asia	I. ricinus, Ixodes persulcatus	Small mammals, birds	People dog?, cat?
B. afzelii (group 3)	ECM, meningopolyneuritis, arthritis, acrodermatitis chronica atrophicans (ACA)	Europe, Asia	I. ricinus, I. persulcatus	Small mammals	Humans, dog?, cat?
B. japonica (group 4)	Unknown	Japan	Ixodes ovatus, I. persulcatus	Rodents, birds	Unknown
B. bissettii sp. Nov.	ECM, lymphocytoma	Slovenia	I. ricinus	Rodents, birds	People
Relapsing-Fever Borreliae					
Borrelia spp.	Visible spirochetemia, lymphadenomegaly, lameness, anterior uveitis, fever	Florida, United States	Unknown	Unknown	Dog
B. lonestari	Southern tick-associated rash illness (STARI)	Southeastern & south central United States	Amblyomma americanum	Deer	People
B miyamotoi sensu lato		Japan Connecticut, Europe	Ixodes spp.	Rodents?	Unknown
B. recurrentis	Epidemic louse-borne relapsing fever	Central and East Africa, South America, Europe, Asia	Pediculus humanus (body louse)	None	People
B. anserina	Avian spirochetosis	Worldwide	Argas persicus	Birds	Poultry
B. hermsii, B. turicatae, B. parkeri	Endemic tick-borne relapsing fevers, visible spirochetemia	North America	Ornithodoros spp.	Rodents, small mammals	People
B. persica	As above	Asia	As above	As above	As above
B. hispanica	As above	Spain	As above	As above	As above
B. duttonii	As above	East Africa	As above	As above	As above
B. coriaceae	Enzootic abortion	Western United States	Ornithodoros coriaceus	Deer	Cow

?, Uncertain involvement

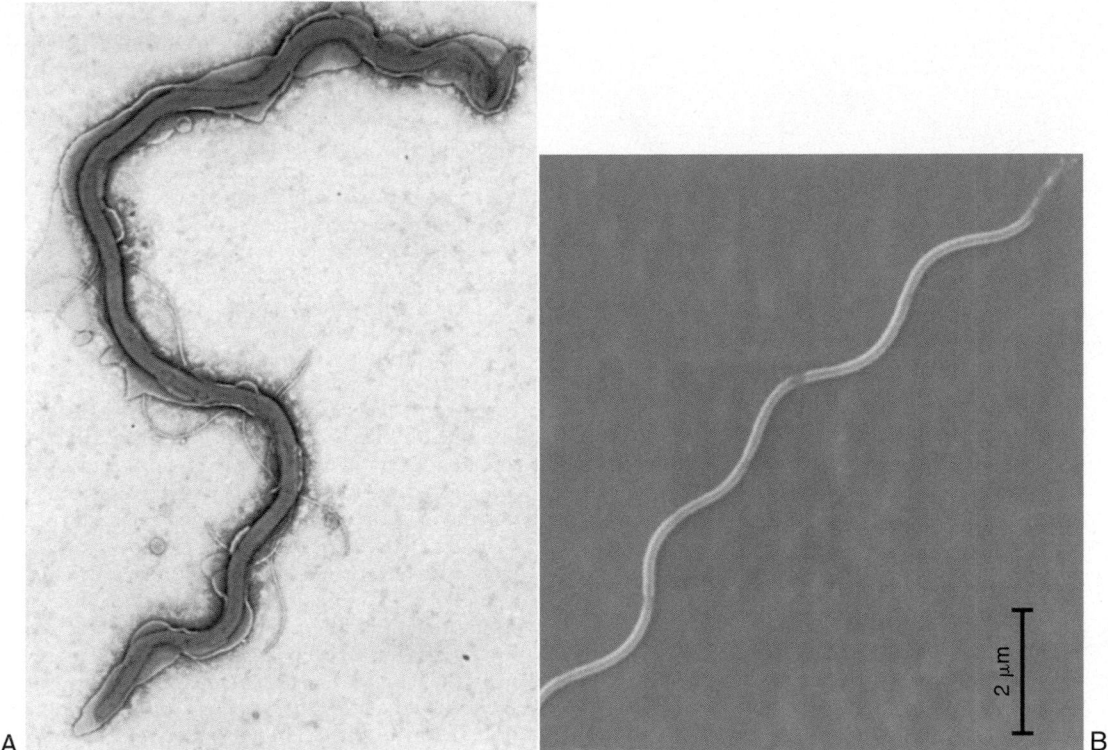

Fig 45-1 **A,** Transmission electron micrograph of *B. burgdorferi* showing periplasmic flagella that have been released from the confines of the outer membrane secondary to specimen preparation (phosphotungstic acid, ×7100). **B,** Scanning microscopic view of *B. burgdorferi* (×15,000). (Courtesy R. Straubinger, University of Leipzig, Leipzig, Germany.))

American isolates have been thought to be more homogeneous than European strains, isolates from the United States have substantial genetic heterogeneity with regional differences.[166]

Relapsing-Fever Borreliosis

Numerous borreliae species comprise the relapsing-fever group of vectorborne agents that cause disease in domestic animals and people (see Table 45-1). Except for *Borrelia recurrentis*, which causes louseborne relapsing fever, all are transmitted by ticks. The occurrence of most of these infections in dogs and cats have not been substantiated. A previously unrecognized borrelial species was described in dogs from Florida; spirochetemia was visible.[25]

EPIDEMIOLOGY

Lyme Borreliosis

Unlike *Leptospira* organisms, borreliae cannot survive as free-living organisms in the environment. They are host associated, being transmitted between vertebrate reservoir hosts and hematophagous arthropod vectors. *B. burgdorferi* sensu lato infections are geographically dispersed (see Table 45-1). In general, Lyme borreliosis occurs in temperate latitudes with cooler climatic conditions. In the United States, it has been reported in people in 50 states; however, approximately 85% of the cases were from eastern coastal states from Massachusetts to Virginia, 10% were from the upper Midwest (Wisconsin and Minnesota), and 4% were from northern California (Fig. 45-2, *A*). Although 1% of the reports were from other states, the organism has never been cultured from people or dogs outside the mentioned endemic areas. In Canada, Lyme borreliosis is endemic in southeastern Ontario. Less is known about the national seroprevalence of canine infection or exposure.

The principal vectors of *B. burgdorferi* sensu lato are various species of slow-feeding hard ticks of the *Ixodes* complex, whose distribution is associated with the prevalence of disease (Table 45-2). In the United States, closely related black-legged ticks, *Ixodes scapularis* (in the northeastern, midwestern, and southeastern states) and *Ixodes pacificus* together with *Ixodes neotomae* (in the western states)[27] appear to be involved (Fig. 45-2, *B*). Differences in the northern and southern populations of *I. scapularis* influence the prevalence of disease in these respective areas. *I. scapularis* in the northeastern states was previously designated "*Ixodes dammini.*" Debate continues over whether it is distinct from *I. scapularis*. Ticks in the north central United States prefer deciduous, dry to mesic forests and sandy or loamy soils overlying sedimentary rock.[95] Ticks were not associated with grasslands, conifer forests, or acidic soils with low fertility or a claylike consistency.

These small (less than 3 mm) ixodid ticks generally feed on more than one host during their life cycle (Fig. 45-3). The number of hosts varies depending on the tick species. In North America, where approximately 50 to 80 vertebrate species are hosts, larvae and nymphs of *I. scapularis* (the northern variety) generally feed on small mammals, whereas *I. scapularis* (the southern variety) and *I. pacificus* feed on reptiles. Adults of these ticks feed on deer or larger mammals. Because reptiles are not competent reservoir hosts, the infection rate of southern *I. scapularis* ticks (less than 1%) is much lower than that of northern *I. scapularis* ticks in the northeastern United States (10% to 50%). Lizards possess a borreliacidal substance similar to complement in their blood that reduces or prevents infection with *B. burgdorferi*.[129] Furthermore, because the southern *I. scapularis* ticks do not always feed on mammals, the prevalence of Lyme borreliosis in people and domestic animals is low in the southern regions.[269] Infected *Ixodes* ticks may be dispersed to new areas by feeding on migratory birds.[111,127,225,234]

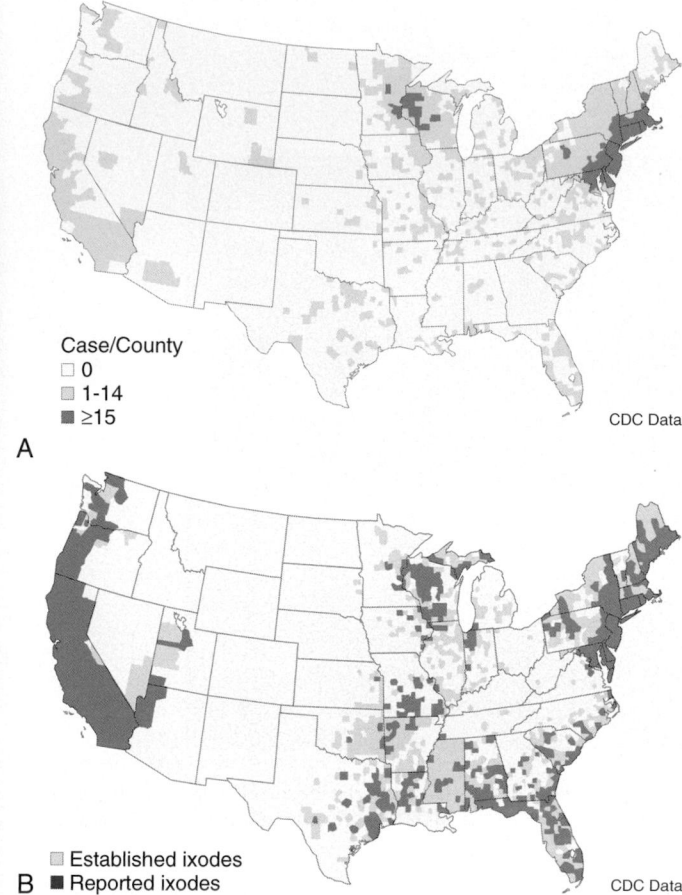

Case/County
- ☐ 0
- ▨ 1-14
- ■ ≥15

CDC Data

A

☐ Established ixodes
■ Reported ixodes

B   CDC Data

Fig 45-2 **A,** Annual incidence in 2000 of Lyme borreliosis in the United States by county. Darker color indicates higher concentration of cases as indicated in the legend. **B,** Distribution of *Ixodes* species ticks in the United States by county. (Data from Centers for Disease Control and Prevention, Atlanta, Ga. Maps courtesy University of Georgia, Athens, Ga.)

I. ricinus and *Ixodes persulcatus* are the primary vectors in Europe and Eurasia, respectively. In Europe, most cases have been documented in the Scandinavian countries and in central Europe, especially in the Alpine countries of Germany, Austria, and Switzerland in association with *I. ricinus* (Fig. 45-4). *B. burgdorferi*, *B. garinii*, and *B. afzelii* are responsible for the infection. The distribution of infection stretches eastward across Eurasia, corresponding to the habitat of the tick *I. persulcatus*, which transmits only *B. garinii* and *B. afzelii*. Infection with *B. burgdorferi* sensu lato, *B. burgdorferi* sensu stricto, and *B. garinii* has also been found in *I. ricinus* ticks in northern Africa.[214] Other isolated enzootic cycles exist in nature between *Ixodes* ticks and rodents infected with new *Borrelia* species.[182] For example, *I. ricinus*-complex ticks have also been infected with the other genospecies, including *B. valaisiana*, *B. bissettii*, and *Borrelia lusitaniae*.[209] In these cases, the infection is being maintained in nature; however, the clinical significance of such infections in people or domestic animals is unknown.

In Europe and Asia, *I. ricinus* and *I. persulcatus*, respectively, parasitize more than 200 vertebrate species. Several species of mice, voles, and rats are important reservoir hosts. Squirrels, hedgehogs, shrews, and birds are also involved in the maintenance of the infection cycle. On both continents, larger ungulates such as deer and moose are important in the life cycle because adult *Ixodes* species feed on them. However,

the level of infection in these large mammals is insufficient to transmit to feeding ticks, making them unsuitable reservoir hosts.[114,178,254]

The *Ixodes* species ticks that transmit Lyme borreliosis have a 2-year life cycle and maintain infection in nature by over-wintering as infected nymphs (see Fig. 45-3). In the northeastern and upper midwestern United States, *I. scapularis* primarily becomes infected when immature stages feed on infected white-footed mice *(Peromyscus leucopus)*. Direct transmission of borreliae between reservoir hosts is unlikely, and transovarial transmission in ticks is relatively nonexistent.[196] When infected nymphs that have over-wintered feed in the spring, they transmit organisms to competent reservoir hosts. Nymphs are thought to be primarily responsible for the transmission of infection to domestic animals and people. The larvae from the current year's generation feed in late summer and fall off the host and become infected by feeding on an infected reservoir host.[30a] Larvae and other stages of ticks can also become infected from previously uninfected hosts by cofeeding with infected ticks that have attached in close temporal and spatial proximity.[185,205] However, in other studies, cofeeding of *I. ricinus* ticks was not as efficient in transmitting *B. afzelii* infection as horizontal transmission of the organism from previously infected mice to uninfected larvae.[207,208] After molting, nymphs become infected and over-winter for the next tick season (see Fig. 45-3). Adult female ticks feed on white-tailed deer *(Odocoileus virginianus)* to maintain the tick population, but deer are not effective reservoir hosts for infection.[114] Despite the zoonotic risk from nymphal ticks, adult ticks appear to have the highest rate of infectivity among stages, presumably because of their longevity and repeated exposure to infected mammals and birds.

In the western United States, transmission of infection by *I. pacificus* involves two sylvan cycles. The maintenance cycle involves *Ixodes spinipalpus* feeding on dusky-footed wood rats *(Neotoma fuscipes)* and kangaroo rats *(Dipodomys californicus)*. Immature *I. pacificus* become infected by feeding on these rodent reservoirs, and the adult ticks transmit the infection to larger mammals during subsequent feedings. As in Europe, birds may be more important in the sylvatic cyle of infection in the western United States.[270]

Ixodes ticks can be simultaneously infected with additional animal and human pathogens, including *Rickettsia helvetica*, *Anaplasma phagocytophilum* (formerly classified as *Ehrlichia* species; see Chapter 28 and Table 28-1), *Babesia* species *(Babesia microti, Babesia odocoilei,* and *Babesia gibsoni)*, and multiple *Borrelia* species.[107,175] *Amblyomma americanum* (the Lone Star tick) can be coinfected with *B. lonestari, Ehrlichia ewingii,* and *Ehrlichia chaffeensis*. Diagnosis and interpretation of serologic tests is problematic when a coinfection exists.

Numerous hematophagous arthropods, including other tick species, fleas, flies, and mosquitoes, have been found to be infected in nature. Whether these infections indicate vector competency is uncertain, but their role relative to ticks is insignificant. Contamination from feeding on infected vertebrates is suspected; however, these other arthropods have not been documented to transfer infection to new hosts.[201] Only *I. scapularis*—not *A. americanum* or *Dermacentor variabilis*—has effectively transmitted a diverse collection of *B. burgdorferi* strains from North America.[201] Nevertheless, *A. americanum* has been found to harbor *B. lonestari*, a presumptive species that causes an ECM-like rash in people and may be associated with seropositivity in people and animals in areas where *Ixodes* species ticks are not found.[226] Experimentally, deer but not mice were infected with *B. lonestari*, and organisms were observed in Giemsa-stained blood smears.[146] Deer may be reservoir species for this organism.

Contrary to media reports, Lyme borreliosis is not spreading in epidemic proportions; it is likely being overdiagnosed

Table • 45-2

Selected Vectors of Borrelia burgdorferi[a]

SPECIES	GEOGRAPHIC LOCATION	FEEDING PREFERENCE		INFECTION PREVALENCE
		LARVAE, NYMPH	ADULTS	
Northern				
Ixodes scapularis (previously Ixodes dammini)	United States (New England, northern Midwest)	White-footed mouse (Peromyscus leucopus), small mammals, birds	Deer, larger mammals	<1% larvae 10%–25% nymphs 10%–50% adults
Southern				
I. scapularis	United States (southeastern)	Lizards	Lizards (occasionally mammals)	<1% larvae <1% nymphs <1% adults
Ixodes pacificus, Ixodes neotomae	United States (western)	Lizards	Lizards (occasionally mammals)	1%–5%
Ixodes ricinus	Europe (western and central)	Small mammals, birds, mice (Apodemus flavicollis, Apodemus sylvaticus, Clethrionomys glareolus)	Deer, larger mammals	10%–25%
Ixodes persulcatus	Eurasia, Soviet Republics	Small mammals, birds	Deer, larger mammals	10%–25%

[a]B. burgdorferi or related organisms have been recovered from numerous other ticks and arthropods in nature, but the significance is uncertain. Many sylvan cycles exist in nature in which tick vectors do not feed on large mammals. Only the established vectors for people or domestic animals are listed here.

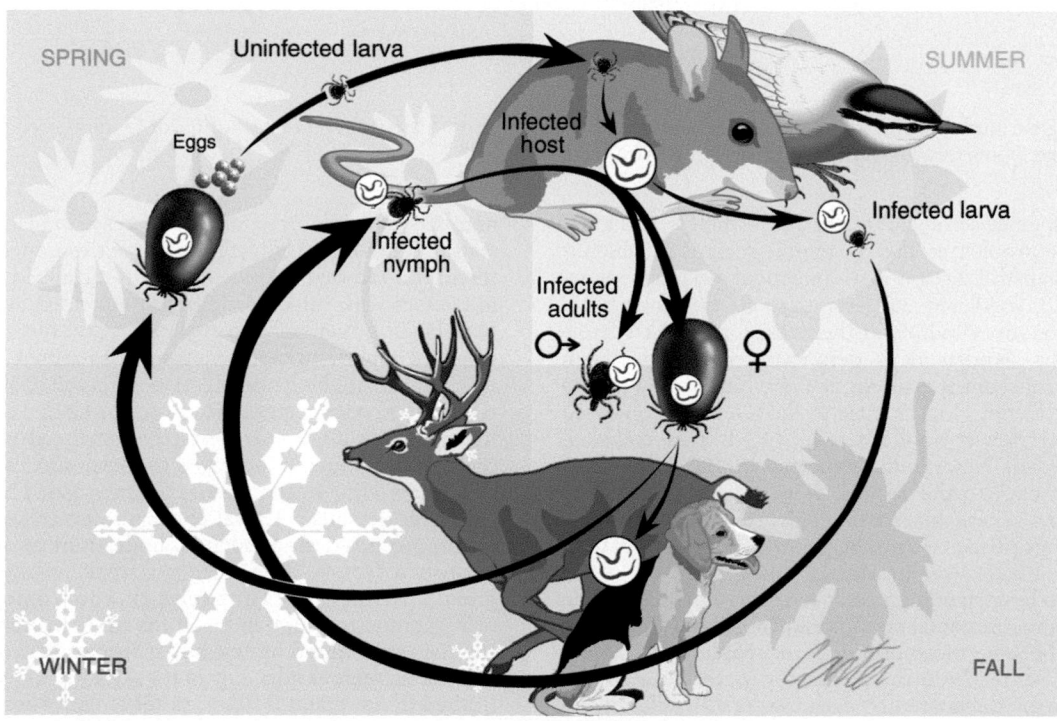

Fig 45-3 The life cycle of northern *I. scapularis* ("*dammini*") lasts 2 years. Eggs are oviposited in the spring, and the larvae emerge approximately 1 month later. They feed once in the summer, usually on birds and small mammals, and then over-winter. The following spring, the larvae molt into nymphs, which then feed in late spring or early summer. The nymphs feed on mice or larger mammals such as dogs, deer, or humans and are considered the most likely source of infection for dogs and people. Nymphs then molt into adults in the fall. The adults usually feed on larger mammals (often the white-tailed deer), where they mate. The females die after laying their eggs, and the 2-year cycle is repeated. (Courtesy University of Georgia, Athens, Ga.)

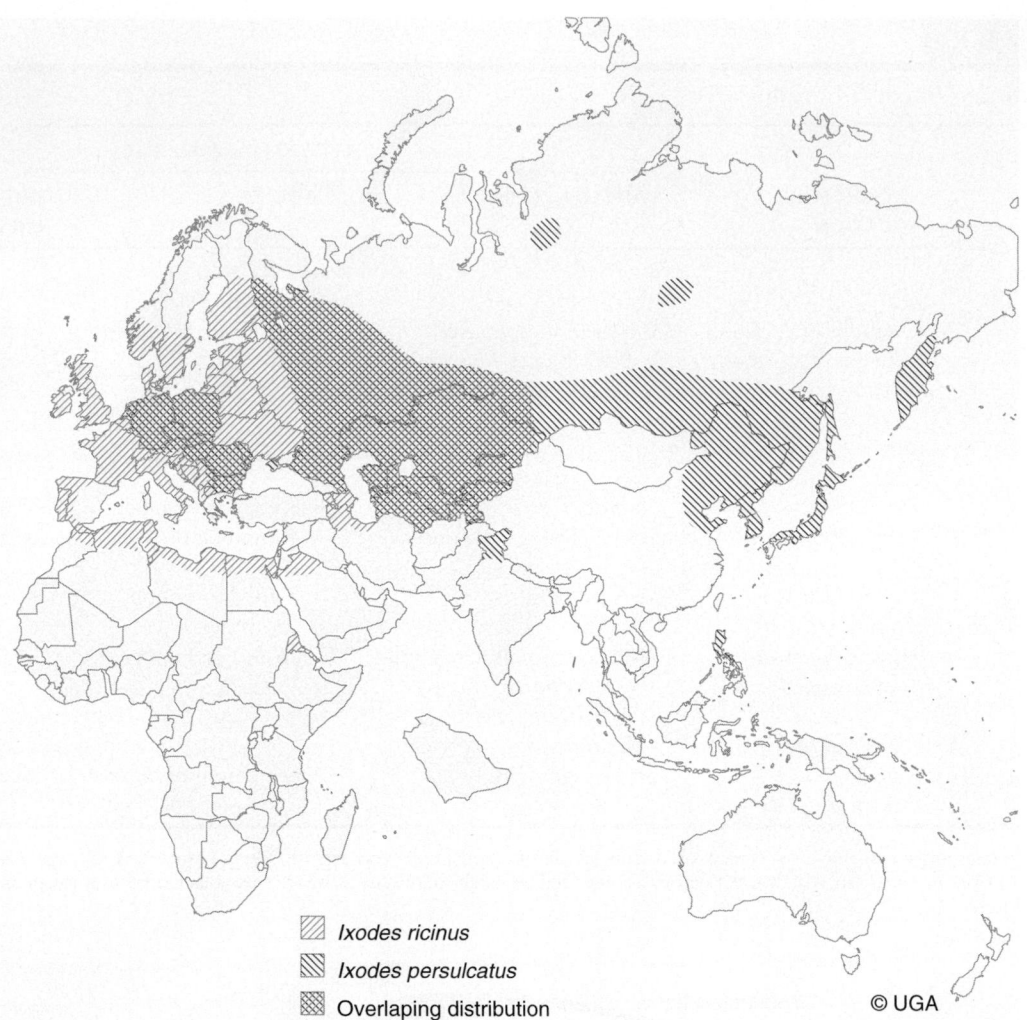

Ixodes ricinus
Ixodes persulcatus
Overlaping distribution
© UGA

Fig   45-4   Distribution of *I. ricinus* and *I. persulcatus* ticks in the Eastern Hemisphere. Distribution of Lyme borreliosis follows this geographic range. (Courtesy University of Georgia, Athens, Ga.)

by use of nonspecific serologic testing. Nevertheless, it is a significant disease problem in the geographic regions in which it occurs. Although the disease in Connecticut was first recognized in 1975, evidence suggests that *B. burgdorferi* has infected indigenous wildlife and their respective tick vectors for many years. Studies have demonstrated that ear skin samples from museum specimens of the white-footed mouse collected near Dennis, Massachusetts, during 1894 contained *B. burgdorferi* DNA.[162] Similarly, embalmed ticks collected from Long Island, New York, from the 1940s[199] and from Europe dating back to the 1880s[168] have also been found to contain borrelial genetic material.[110] The disease has been recognized in Europe since the beginning of the twentieth century.

Despite the long-standing presence of the borrelial sylvan cycle, certain environmental conditions probably caused Lyme borreliosis to become more prevalent in people in the twentieth century. Before 1900 the habitat of the eastern United States was heavily deforested by early settlers. Populations of deer and their associated ticks, such as *I. scapularis*, were reduced. During this time, a sylvan cycle maintaining *B. burgdorferi* most likely existed between *Ixodes muris*, a one-host tick, and rodent species, which were most prevalent in forest-free areas. After the turn of the century, farms were abandoned and reforestation occurred, as did a continual increase in the deer population. With an increase in deer

numbers came a corresponding increase in black-legged ticks. As the numbers of infected ticks of these species increased, the likelihood that people and domestic animals would come in contact with infected ticks also increased. Although Lyme borreliosis is generally associated with forests, it may be acquired in parks in major metropolitan centers. In these areas, rats appear to be the effective reservoir host for feeding ticks.[167,235] In the northern midwestern United States, seropositivity among dogs was positively associated with numerous risk factors including increased tick exposure, time spent outdoors, and living in forested or urban wooded habitats and on sandy, fertile soils.[97] Larval and nymphal *Ixodes* are found in moist, protected areas such as under humus on the floor of hardwood forests. They feed on small rodents, lizards, and ground-feeding birds. The adult ticks climb onto tips of grasses or vegetation to quest and wait for larger mammals to contact them. In the United States, *Ixodes* species ticks are distributed in wooded regions adjacent to the Atlantic Coast, lake regions of the Midwest, and Pacific coastal ranges. These regions have high humidity and more temperate climates moderated by the abundant adjacent bodies of water.

No evidence proves that infected pet dogs or cats pose a direct risk to people other than that they introduce unfed ticks in various life cycle stages into a household. The ticks do not survive long indoors and if fed, they do not reattach without molting. However, partially fed ticks can pose a greater risk of

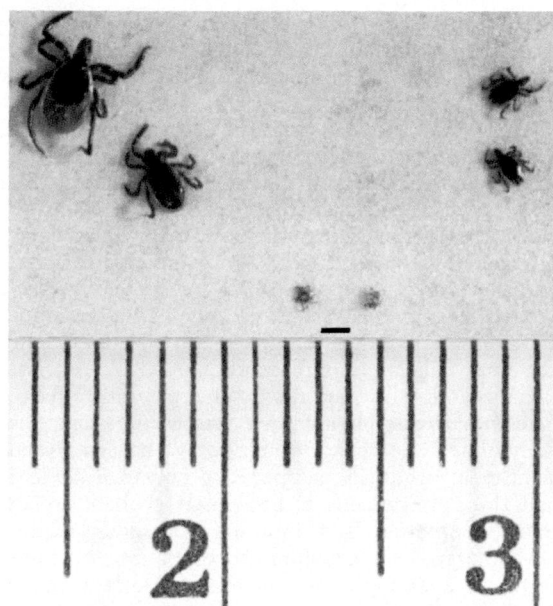

Fig 45-5 Northern *I. scapularis* ("*dammini*") is smaller than other ticks commonly found on dogs. From largest to smallest, two adults (male, female), two nymphs, two larvae (bar = 1 mm). (Courtesy Mike DeRosa, West Somerville, Mass.)

infection to the second mammalian host because a shorter period of attachment is required to transmit infection to the second host. *Ixodes* ticks are extremely small and detected in only a low percentage of cases of Lyme borreliosis (Fig. 45-5). Unfortunately, pets may be blamed for a human infection when ticks are actually the source of the infection. Experimentally, dogs that became infected with *B. burgdorferi* after exposure to infected adult ticks were able to transmit infection to feeding immature ticks.[165] Therefore dogs could increase the human risk of exposure by serving as competent reservoirs of infection for ticks, although dogs are not the preferred hosts for these ticks.

Direct horizontal spread from dogs and cats to people is unlikely; pets merely serve as sentinels for human infection. Most contact studies in which horizontal transmission occurred in dogs have been performed by exposure coincident to the time of parenteral inoculation.[40] Pregnant bitches were inoculated parenterally every 2 weeks during pregnancy induced by artificial insemination (AI) of semen from infected male dogs.[98] Infection in the offspring was determined by polymerase chain reaction (PCR) detection of DNA sequences. A majority of the females had at least one infected neonate when the pups were tested up to 6 weeks of age. The presence of IgM antibodies in a pup that did not nurse suggested that the infection occurred in utero. However, infection by parenteral inoculation may have superseded the uterine-placental barrier.

In a more natural infection model study with ticks, control dogs that were in direct contact with infected dogs for up to 1 year did not undergo seroconversion, and organisms could not be isolated from the urine or urinary bladder of infected dogs.[6] Canine urine is an unlikely source of infection. These investigations also could not document any evidence of in utero spread despite seroconversion of the dam. *B. burgdorferi* can survive freezing and storage, making semen intended for AI a potential source of infection.[126] Blood transfusions could be another source of infection for dogs and cats. *B. burgdorferi* organisms can survive in blood processed for transfusion and stored under blood-bank conditions.[116,177] However, not a single case of *B. burgdorferi* infection caused by blood trans-

fusion has been documented in people[74,21] or animals, and no animal model exist in which Lyme borreliosis can be induced by intravenous (IV) injection of *B. burgdorferi* organisms.

Relapsing-Fever Borreliosis

Relapsing fever is a typical zoonotic disease in which the pathogen is maintained in nature between susceptible reservoir hosts and competent soft ticks. Because of the susceptibility of soft ticks to the environment, their reservoir hosts are a variety of burrow-inhabiting mammals. In contrast to Lyme borreliosis, a wide variety of vertebrates such as rodents, lagomorphs, and ungulates can serve as hosts for the ticks. Despite this fact the borreliae causing relapsing fevers have more restricted geographic ranges and niche vectors than those causing Lyme borreliosis (see Table 45-1). In the western United States and Mexico, *Ornithodoros turicata* infests burrows of rodents, terrapins, and snakes, as well as domestic habitats of people and animals. In the western United States, *Ornithodoros hermsi* and *Ornithodoros parkeri* feed on rodents and squirrels and live in dead trees, fallen logs, and cabins and homes. Tickborne relapsing fever in the United States has not been reported in states east of Texas and Oklahoma; however, sporadic isolations have been made from ticks and people outside this area. Relapsing-fever—like borreliae have been isolated from *Ornithodoros erraticus*, an important vector in northern Africa that feeds on rats, mice, gerbils, and other small mammals. *Ornithodoros tholozani* inhabits the Middle East, the Balkans, and the southern former Soviet Republic, where it inhabits man-made shelters and caves while feeding on various wild and domestic animal hosts and people. A relapsing-fever—like spirochete, *Borrelia miyamotoi*, has been isolated from *I. persulcatus* ticks in Japan.[70] New relapsing-fever borreliae have been identified in North American *I. scapularis* ticks[224] and European *I. ricinus* ticks.[209] The clinical significance of these infections in people and animals is unknown.

PATHOGENESIS

Lyme Borreliosis

Spirochete transmission requires at least 50 hours[51] of tick attachment, during which time organisms multiply and cross the gut epithelium into the hemolymph, disseminate to the salivary glands, and infect the host through tick saliva.[195] OspA, the predominant surface protein, is expressed on the outer surface of borreliae in the midgut of infected nymphal ticks. In unfed ticks, virtually all spirochetes reside in the midgut. OspA has been shown to help the spirochetes adhere to midgut epithelial cells. During feeding and because of the warmth and ingested blood meal, spirochetes down-regulate their expression of OspA protein and express OspC. The up-regulation of OspC correlates with the migration of the spirochetes from the midgut into the hemolymph and finally to the salivary glands of the feeding tick.[195] OspC facilitates the adherence of spirochetes to the tick salivary gland cells and likely to host tissues as well. Levels of the immunodominant lipoprotein component VlsE, which is important in serodiagnosis, increase during the last 2 days of tick engorgement.[202] Sufficient numbers of virulent spirochetes are not present in the salivary glands until approximately 53 hours have elapsed.[187]

Despite the numerous people and animals that are bitten, only a few develop clinical disease. Host immune reactions are likely involved in preventing many of these infections. From the vector perspective, up to 50% (see Table 45-2) of *Ixodes* ticks may be infected in endemic regions, whereas less than 2% of people bitten by these ticks become infected. The implication is that most ticks are removed before this patent period.

As the number of attached ticks and correspondingly the number of inoculated spirochetes increase, the likelihood increases that clinical illness will result; host immunity is important in this regard. It is likely that borreliae proliferate locally in skin at the site of tick attachment and spirochete inoculation for the duration of infection. From there, they replicate and migrate through tissues, beginning close to the tick bite. Later, they can spread through and infect many tissues, including the joints. Active migration in tissues is more common than passive dissemination via the blood. Not all animals infected after tick bites develop clinical illness. In fact, evidence suggests that the percentage of dogs developing clinical disease is very low (5% to 10%) compared with the frequency of exposure based on seropositivity (75% in endemic areas) and the rate of infection demonstrated in ticks.[140] Part of this seropositivity may represent an exposure to infectious but nonpathogenic isolates of *Borrelia* in addition to indicating infection with low numbers of *B. burgdorferi* organisms in a host with an efficient immune system.[2] Even among genetically similar *B. burgdorferi* sensu stricto strains, pathogenicity may vary. Development of disease in genetically identical susceptible mice was determined by the pathogenic properties of the infecting *B. burgdorferi* isolate.[261]

Once in the body, *B. burgdorferi* acts as a persistent pathogen. Experimental evidence suggests the spirochetes exist extracellularly and in an undetermined way can evade immune clearance for extended periods in the skin, connective tissues, joints, and nervous system. Data suggest that these spirochetes undergo major changes in surface protein expression as they enter the host.[49] Other studies have shown that *Borrelia* organisms are capable of modifying not only their outer surface profile but also their entire shape. Spiral, motile borreliae can change into spherical life forms within minutes after they have encountered unfavorable environmental conditions (Fig. 45-6).[1,26] In this form they survive for days without nutrition and revert back into the well-known spiral form when conditions improve. Furthermore, these spherical borreliae were able to infect mice.[94] This may explain the reason *B. burgdorferi* can still persist and be detected in tissue samples by PCR or occasionally by culture even after months of antibiotic treatment. After a few weeks of infection, *B. burgdorferi* is difficult to detect or isolate from body fluids or internal organs of incidental hosts such as dogs, and exceedingly few are detected in other tissues.[6,45,82] Clinical illness results from the host's own inflammatory response. Some of the immunopathologic events may be related to immune responses generated against specific borrelial antigens. Flagellin, one of the most immunogenic proteins, can elicit an antibody that binds to host neuroaxonal proteins.[230] This sequence may in turn stimulate the inflammatory response in nervous tissue.[231] Clonal accumulation of activated CD8+ T cells has been observed in the cerebrospinal fluid (CSF) of people during the early phase of neuroborreliosis.[112] The cytokine release may help the inflammatory response clear the organism but also results in damage to nervous tissue. Results of PCR on synovial fluid are often positive in human patients, because genetic sequences for plasmid-encoded genes such as OspA, OspB, and OspC are readily detected[198]; results of culture studies are usually negative.[198] The inflammatory response to a small number of spirochetes may be explained by autonomous replications of plasmid DNA.[266] Up-regulation of interleukin-8 (IL-8), which recruits neutrophils to inflammatory sites, has been found in the synovial membranes of experimentally infected dogs.[248] This may be an important mechanism in producing suppurative polyarthritis. In a few animals the development of arthritis is probably related to pathologic perpetual host immune reactions. People with certain haplotypes of the major histocompatibility complex are prone to more severe, treatment-resistant clinical manifestations of the disease in which *B. burgdorferi* cannot be detected.[240]

The tissues of preferential localization may vary by *Borrelia* species, affect pathogenicity, and therefore determine the difference in clinical manifestations seen in different geographic regions. *B. garinii* was found in the liver of dogs having elevated liver enzyme activities, a finding not associated with *B. burgdorferi* sensu stricto.[109]

The Jarisch-Herxheimer reaction (JHR) is a severe systemic reaction that is observed after receiving antimicrobial therapy for spirochetal or other bacterial infections. It is associated with the systemic release of cytokines (e.g., tumor necrosis factor-α [TNF-α], IL-6, and IL-8). The JHR has many similarities to severe sepsis. Clinical signs include fever, rapid pulse and respiration rates, an increasing blood pressure, and leukopenia. Pretreatment with antibodies against TNF-α keeps the JHR from developing in people.[65]

Relapsing-Fever Borreliosis

Tickborne relapsing fever, caused by *Borrelia hermsii* and transmitted by *O. hermsi*, is the model spirochetal disease of the relapsing-fever group. The principal mammalian reservoirs for this infection are diurnal rodents; people and other animals become infected as incidental hosts. Unlike the *Ixodes* species,

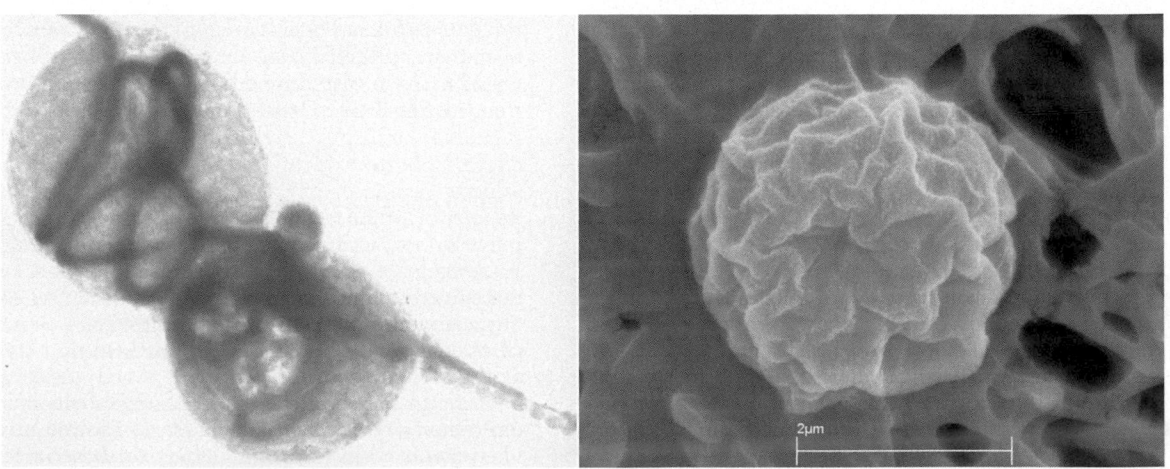

Fig 45-6 **A,** Transmission electron microscopic (×12,000) and **B,** scanning electron microscopic (×12,000) appearance of cystic form of *B. burgdorferi*, a defense mechanism of organism for survival under adverse conditions such as antimicrobial therapy or host immune defenses. (Courtesy R. Straubinger, University of Leipzig, Leipzig, Germany.)

Ornithodoros ticks harbor spirochetes for extended periods because their life cycle takes years to complete. Mammalian hosts are only intermittently spirochetemic for 14 to 30 days, thus the ticks are most responsible for maintaining the infection in nature. Unlike other *Ornithodoros* species, *O. hermsii* does not excrete coxal fluid while feeding; it must transmit the organism while biting the host. Whereas the organisms in *B. burgdorferi*–infected *Ixodes* ticks migrate from the midgut to the saliva, the salivary gland, midgut, and other tissues of *O. hermsii* are permanently contaminated with *B. hermsi* organisms, which allows for rapid transfer of the spirochetes. Furthermore, orgasid ticks feed and transfer infection more rapidly than ixodid ticks and can immediately infect the host during the short tick-feeding interval.

In the mammalian host, *B. hermsii* has been shown to be highly adapted and has developed mechanisms to evade the immune system. Each inoculated spirochete may produce 30 unique antigenic variants, each expressing a major immunodominant protein that defines a specific serotype. In the mammalian host, episodes of cyclic spirochetemia are caused by waves of replicating spirochetes with relatively homogenous serotypes. As each new wave of replication becomes recognized by the host defenses, a new one is expressed, allowing the subsequent generation to proliferate—hence the relapsing nature of infection. Analyses of the surface proteins of *B. hermsii* have shown that the organism expresses a variable major protein, Vsp 33; however, after ingestion by the tick, a new major protein is up-regulated on the cell surface and confers the unique specific serotype. The Vsp 33 protein is homologous to the OspC protein of *B. burgdorferi* and as a result allows the organism to maintain its infectivity within the nonfeeding tick.

CLINICAL SIGNS

Lyme Borreliosis

The clinical features of Lyme borreliosis in people include dermatitis, arthritis, meningoencephalitis, and myocarditis.

Dogs

Initial attempts to recreate experimental Lyme borreliosis in dogs using laboratory-derived strains were unsuccessful, as they were in cats.[31,89] However, fever and polyarthritis have been experimentally produced after inoculation or natural exposure to tick-derived *B. burgdorferi*.[6,40,82,263] The use of spirochetes directly inoculated during feeding of field-collected ticks has been most successful.[6] Clinical illness in experimentally infected dogs occurs 2 to 6 months after tick exposure, and the severity and propensity to develop signs of illness seem to vary inversely with the animal's age and immune status. The onset of clinical illness usually correlates with the initial increase in serum antibody titer.

Systemic Signs Acute signs of fever (39.5° C to 40.5° C [103.1° F to 104.9° F]), shifting leg lameness, articular swelling, lymphadenomegaly, anorexia, and general malaise, all of which are responsive to antimicrobials, most commonly develop in naturally exposed seropositive dogs.[136,140,145,170] The accuracy of the diagnosis in many spontaneously diseased dogs is difficult to determine because limb and joint signs (swelling, lameness, and pain) with fever and inappetence have been observed with equal frequency in dogs with and without *B. burgdorferi*–specific antibodies.[44,156,155]

Arthritis Polyarthritis is the best experimentally documented syndrome caused by acute *B. burgdorferi* infection in dogs (Fig. 45-7). Spread of the organism in skin, connective, joint, and muscle tissues is most likely responsible for some of the observed lameness. The first limbs affected are usually closest to the site of tick attachment. The onset of lameness can correspond to an increased body temperature. Lameness in a particular limb often lasts for a few days and then may shift to another limb or disappear. Despite the transient nature of the arthritis, pathologic changes in the joints are progressive. Chronic nonerosive polyarthritis, the primary condition found in more animals with prolonged infections than in untreated patients, may persist despite antimicrobial therapy at a lower frequency. Lesions have been most consistently found in skin, lymphatic tissues, and joints, even though the organism can be isolated from other tissues and body fluids.

Renal Disease Protein-losing glomerulopathy has been described in a few naturally infected dogs.[81,172] An acute progressive renal failure associated with azotemia, uremia, proteinuria, peripheral edema, and body cavity effusions has been characterized in 49 dogs from *Borrelia*-endemic areas.[46] A preponderance of Labrador and golden retrievers was affected. The duration of clinical illness was 24 hours to 8 weeks, with a sudden onset of anorexia, vomiting, lethargy, and weight loss. Some dogs had recent or concurrent lameness. All dogs died or were euthanized as a result of renal failure. The dogs had antibodies to *B. burgdorferi*. Natural exposure to *B. burgdorferi* was likely involved but has not yet been proven. In rapidly progressing glomerular disease, the role if any of vaccination in the development of the lesion is undetermined.

Meningitis Often a later manifestation of lyme borreliosis infection in people is neurologic signs. Experimental infections of nonhuman primates have produced similar features.[210]

Fig 45-7 Experimentally induced borrelial arthritis in **(A)** thoracic limb of beagle dog and **(B)** pelvic limb of hound. Fever and shifting leg lameness develop 60 to 90 days after inoculation. Lameness occurs earliest and is most severe in limb closest to inoculation site. **A,** Courtesy R. Straubinger, University of Leipzig, Leipzig, Germany; **B,** Courtesy University of Georgia, Athens, Ga.)

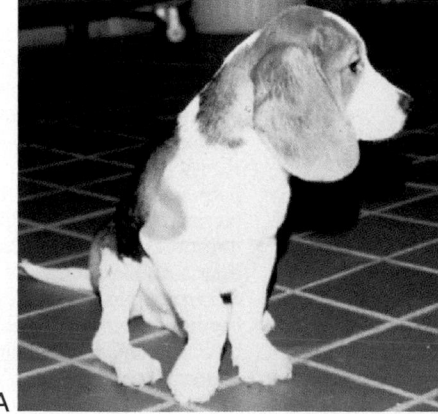
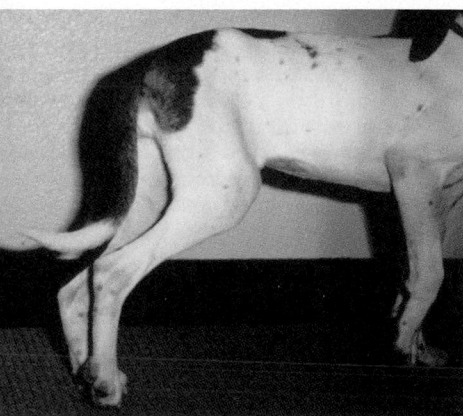

A

B

The rhesus monkey is the only animal model to exhibit this predominant form of Lyme borreliosis. Experimentally infected dogs developed mild focal meningitis, encephalitis, and perineuritis; however, neurologic signs were not observed.[42]

Other Manifestations A small, reddish lesion develops in the skin at the site of tick attachment but disappears within the first week (Fig. 45-8). However, the organism can be isolated from the skin for extended periods. This lesion is not like the dramatic lesion associated with ECM in people. Erythematous rashes, suggestive of early Lyme borreliosis, may not be specific for this disease. In the southern United States, focal rashes (Fig. 45-9) and transient fever and malaise associated with the bite of *A. americanum* ticks were attributed to infection with *B. lonestari*, an organism more closely related to *Borrelia miyamotoi*, a relapsing-fever spirochete in Japan, and the unnamed species isolated from dogs in Florida.[34,115]

Other syndromes reported in a few spontaneously diseased dogs include rheumatoid arthritis[211] and myocarditis-induced cardiac arrhythmia.[138] These other signs are similar to those that have been reported in people. Unfortunately, the diagnoses in these naturally diseased dogs were often circumstantial—based on serologic data or microscopic evidence but no organism isolation. In people, conjunctivitis, vitreitis, choroidi-

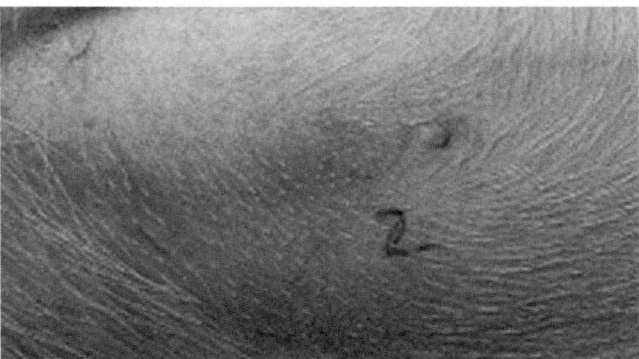

Fig 45-8 Small reddened lesion *(arrow)* in skin at site of inoculation of an experimentally inoculated dog. (Courtesy University of Georgia, Athens, Ga.)

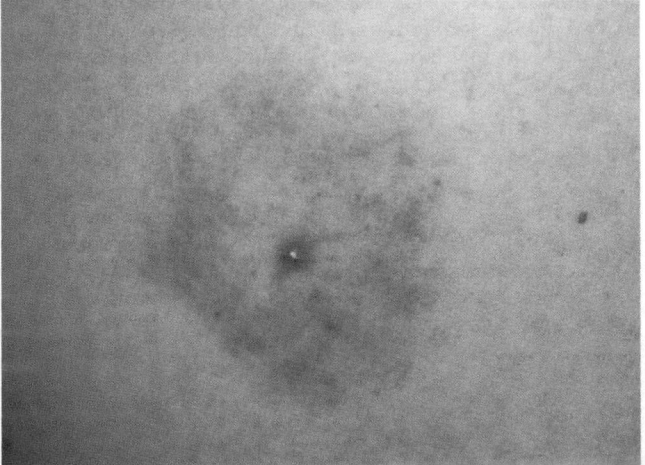

Fig 45-9 Erythematous lesion at attachment site of *A. americanum* associated with human infection by *B. lonestari* in Georgia. (Courtesy University of Georgia, Athens, Ga.)

tis, hepatitis, and myositis or fasciitis have been reported as rare syndromes and have not been reported in dogs. The strain used or the relatively short observation period in experimental studies may be the reason that the nonarthritic syndromes have not been reproduced in experimentally inoculated animals.

Cats

Despite evidence for seropositivity for *B. burgdorferi* in cats, natural disease has not been described as a distinct clinical entity. Cats examined in endemic areas of the northeastern United States had infestations with *Ixodes* ticks.[154] Approximately 13% of cats were seropositive according to indirect fluorescent antibody (FA) testing or an enzyme-linked immunosorbent assay (ELISA); however, no difference in positive results was found between cats with or without lameness. Similarly, cats that were screened as clinical patients in the United Kingdom had a low rate (4.2%) of seroreactivity.[171] The seropositive cats in the United Kingdom study had no symptoms of lameness.

Cats may be more resistant than dogs to the development of clinical signs of Lyme borreliosis. As in dogs, inoculation of cultivated borreliae is associated with reduced virulence or immune recognition. Cats inoculated by various routes (i.e., parenteral, oral, conjunctival) with cultivated spirochetes developed IgG seropositivity; however, organisms were found only in the blood of the IV-infected and ocularly infected cats.[32] The spirochetemia was transient, clearing by day 24, and only one cat had organisms in its tissues at necropsy. In contrast, when cats were inoculated with organisms directly from arthropods, they developed multiple-limb lameness and had joint, pulmonary, lymphoid, and central nervous system (CNS) inflammation at necropsy.[75,76] Arthritis or meningitis seems to be the predominant manifestation that would warrant investigation of Lyme borreliosis in cats.

Relapsing-Fever Borreliosis

Borreliosis caused by a new borrelial spirochete was reported in two dogs from Florida.[25] Clinical signs included elevated rectal temperature, shifting leg lameness, hepatosplenomegaly, visible spirochetemia, and anterior uveitis, all similar to the signs of endemic tickborne relapsing fever. Many of the relapsing-fever spirochetes may infect dogs and cats as incidental hosts in the same way they are known to infect people (see Table 45-1). Additional studies are needed to determine the clinical significance of these infections.

DIAGNOSIS

Reports of Lyme borreliosis in people often exceed the geographic boundaries of known endemic foci.[36] Although travel accounts for a minor number of disparities, the overestimation of numbers of cases results from cross-reactivity to other infectious agents and from the inaccuracies of serologic procedures. Better studies to define the distribution of the disease in nature must be based on examination of ticks and wildlife, because isolation of the organism from ticks or reservoir hosts is more successful than from people and domestic animals.

Clinical Laboratory Findings

No specific hematologic or biochemical changes are pathognomonic of borreliosis, although CSF, joint fluid, and urine may show evidence of inflammatory changes. If a dog in an endemic area for borreliosis has leukopenia or thrombocytopenia, these hematologic abnormalities are likely caused by infection or coinfection with a rickettsial pathogen (e.g., *A. phagocytophilum*, see Chapter 28). The synovial fluid changes in dogs with borreliosis have been best substantiated by increased cell counts of 5000 to 100,000 cells/µl with neutrophils predominating (up to 95%). Protein concentration and turbidity are increased. CSF from human patients with neuroborreliosis demonstrates lymphocytic pleocytosis and a mild protein increase. Consistent CSF values have not been found in dogs with suspected neurologic dysfunction.

Serologic Testing
Lyme borreliosis is probably overdiagnosed in human and veterinary medicine because it has become a "trendy" illness.[243] The presence of an elevated antibody titer to *B. burgdorferi* signifies exposure to the spirochete but does not prove that a current clinical illness is caused by the organism. In endemic areas, asymptomatic animals are often seropositive, possibly a result of adequate host immune responses or exposure to nonpathogenic forms of *B. burgdorferi* or other closely related spirochetes.[7] In addition to seropositive results with a validated assay, the animal should have a history of tick exposure with compatible clinical signs and a rapid response to antimicrobial therapy. Unfortunately, the diagnosis of Lyme borreliosis has become more of a laboratory diagnosis than a clinical diagnosis. Clinicians depend on serologic testing because culture and microscopic detection of the organism from specimens of tissues or body fluids are uncommon. Rather than being thought of as a "test for Lyme borreliosis," serologic studies should be viewed as determining "seroreactivity to *B. burgdorferi*."[230] Commercially available ELISA tests can be used to screen for potential exposure to *B. burdgorferi*; however, these should be followed by quantitative serial measurement of antibody titers or by immunoblotting to help determine the specificity of the infection.

Antibody Measurements Using Whole Spirochetes
Various problems have been noted with serologic testing. First, antigen preparations, techniques, and interpretations of different laboratories are not standardized. Matched sera sent to 10 commercial laboratories for antiborrelial serologic testing resulted in only 53% agreement among all sera tested.[87] Furthermore, nonspecificity of whole-cell borrelial assays is apparent in that other inflammatory conditions in people, such as autoimmune diseases, rheumatoid arthritis, syphilis, and periodontal disease, are known to produce cross-reactive antibodies, and similar reactivities probably occur in the dog and cat.

Serologic *screening procedures* clinically available for animals are the ELISA and indirect FA techniques. These assays use whole cells with many proteins that are present in other bacteria and therefore induce production of cross-reactive antibodies.[33,68,144,170,229] The ELISA and indirect FA results have shown that *Leptospira*-positive sera can have low levels of reactivity to *B. burgdorferi*. Seroreactivity caused by infection with *B. burgdorferi* likely gives the highest titers, although cross-reactions should always be considered with any positive result. False-negative antibody tests results are rare.

Antibodies to the relapsing-fever–like organism described in dogs in Florida[25] cross-reacted with *B. burgdorferi*-derived antigens. They caused lower titers in the assay than the antigen from the new organism. Some of the reports of human and animal Lyme borreliosis in the western United States, where relapsing fever occurs, may be related to the nonspecificity of whole-cell ELISA or indirect FA. An immunoreactive protein, GlpQ, may be able to help distinguish these infections when used in immunoassays.[223]

The time course of serologic testing is also important in determining whether active or past infection is responsible for seropositivity. Early serodiagnostic results are usually negative because the immune response to *B. burgdorferi* develops gradually. Experimentally infected dogs developed IgG-ELISA-positive (whole bacterial cell) titers by 4 to 6 weeks after exposure.[6] Titers were at their highest levels by 3 months after exposure and lasted for at least 2 years.[250] Persistence of antibody responses have been found in people 10 to 20 years after they were diagnosed with active Lyme borreliosis.[118] Antibody titers may decline after treatment and patients may become clinically healthy, but antibodies remain detectable for many years. Titer increases almost always precede clinical lameness and fever in experimentally infected dogs.[6,82] High or persistent IgG titers could indicate infection and as such are difficult to interpret on single specimens. Absolute values of titers can vary widely, therefore paired-sample titers should be submitted simultaneously to the same laboratory. Simultaneous measurements of IgG and IgM in a single specimen would theoretically provide more meaningful information than either titer alone. After experimental inoculation, IgM titers have been the first to increase and remain elevated for 2 months, after which they decline. However, in naturally infected dogs and people, IgM persists for many months so that a positive titer does not help to confirm recent exposure or infection.[104,113]

In general, data from many laboratories obtained from indirect FA or ELISA methods suggest that titer results greater than 1:64 to 1:128 indicate the least significant level of reactivity. Titer results can be much higher in recently exposed, actively infected animals. High serum antibody levels seem to decline or disappear with antibiotic treatment, but increases that occur 6 months or later after termination of therapy are interpreted as proliferation of surviving spirochetes.[246,248] Vaccinated dogs show seroreactivity for months to years after vaccination, making a diagnosis of *B. burgdorferi* infection difficult with whole-cell antigen preparations, although protective antibody titers after vaccination may decrease with time.

Immunoblotting
In most cases a two-step testing procedure should be used to confirm positive results from ELISA or indirect FA and substantiate the presence of Lyme borreliosis. Evaluating reactivity to selected antigens of *B. burgdorferi* organisms in a supplemental immunoblot (Western blot) helps identify sera that produce false-positive results in whole-spirochete assays because of cross-reactive antibodies; in addition, it is a powerful tool to differentiate infected from vaccinated animals (Fig. 45-10). The pattern of antibody reactivity after natural tick infection differs from that produced by vaccination. Sera from some dogs in endemic areas that are vaccinated with any product (lysate or recombinant antigens derived from *B. burgdorferi* organisms) exhibit reactivity to specific antigens that are expressed only on the surface of *B. burgdorferi* organisms in ticks or on borreliae raised in culture.[71,83,106,158,228] The actual measured size of the bands (in kilodaltons) described in the following section varies in different investigations because of varied techniques and strain differences and should only be used as a guideline. After natural exposure to *B. burgdorferi*, antibodies develop to proteins in the range of 58, 41, 39, and 22 kDa, which represent p58, flagellin, periplasmic protein, and OspC, respectively.

Reactivity, particularly to OspA, OspB, and possibly OspF (31-, 34-, and 28-kDa bands, respectively), and 93-kDa bands occurs in vaccinated or parenterally inoculated dogs but is normally absent or occurs (rarely) very late in naturally infected dogs.[6,90,92,139]

Newer ELISA tests using OspC proteins or using preparations derived from OspA- and OspB-deficient mutant *B. burgdorferi* strains, or using new recombinant *B. burgdorferi*–relevant antigens may help to improve the accuracy of serodiagnosis.

Antibody to Specific Outer Surface Proteins
ELISA testing for antibodies against specific recombinant proteins allows for discriminating between an active infection and

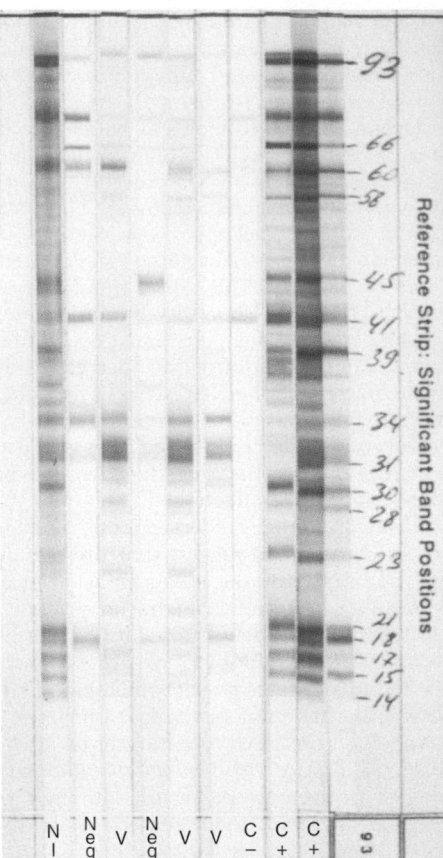

Fig 45-10 Immunoblot of sera from control-positive (C+) and control-negative (C−), vaccinated (V), and naturally infected (NI) dogs. (Courtesy R. Straubinger, University of Leipzig, Leipzig, Germany.)

past exposure and vaccination. The outer surface proteins of *B. burgdorferi* change from OspA and OspB to OspC after the tick ingests warm blood. Genetic expression of OspC proteins allows the organism to leave the midgut and enter the salivary glands and penetrate the host. The surface proteins revert to OspA and OspB again when *B. burgdorferi* organisms reside within the arthropod host after it drops off, molts, and begins questing or when organisms are grown in culture for vaccine or diagnostic purposes. Whole-spirochete ELISAs using both OspA- and OspB-containing strains and deficient mutant strains are able to discriminate between natural and vaccine exposure,[272] especially when recombinant vaccine containing OspA was used. Using these ELISAs as an alternative to immunoblots, vaccinated animals can be differentiated from infected animals. Antibodies to OspA and OspB proteins rarely if ever appear later in the course of infection of the mammalian host because the organism alters its surface proteins in an attempt to avoid the host's immune system.

Although antibodies to OspA and OspB can indicate exposure to vaccines, detection of antibodies to OspC may be used to screen for active host infection. Proteins to OspC, which are only expressed by the organism during infection, are produced by recombinant technology. In ELISA testing of human sera for IgM, use of recombinant-produced OspC antigen had a higher degree of sensitivity in detecting recent infection than ELISA of whole cells or immunoblotting.[73,192] Antibodies to recombinant OspC have also been most specific in determining infection in people with the varied borreliae that exist in Europe.[101] Detection of borreliacidal antibodies against OspC was helpful in detecting experimentally infected dogs, and the magnitude of the titer paralleled the severity of infection and

wider dissemination of the organism.[37] Borreliacidal antibodies to an OspC-containing strain did not increase after vaccination, which helped differentiate vaccinated from naturally infected dogs.

Variation in the genes that encode for the immunodominant VlsE surface lipoprotein of *B. burgdorferi* allows the spirochete to escape the host immune response when it enters the host. One immunodominant region of VlsE known as IR_6, originally isolated from a European species of *B. garinii*, is genetically, structurally, and antigenically conserved among *B. garinii*, *B. afzelii*, and different *B. burgdorferi* strains and genospecies. The genes for IR_6 are only expressed during infection of and replication in the mammalian host, and the protein is not found on organisms in unfed ticks or those grown at ambient temperatures for vaccine or diagnostic antigen. A recombinant-produced peptide known as C_6 reproduces the IR_6 sequence. Host antibody response to C_6 has been used in serodiagnostic testing of people and animals as a marker for host invasion and active infection. Testing for C_6 has been substituted for conventional whole-cell ELISA and subsequent immunoblotting in diagnosis of human borreliosis.[11,161]

A commercial test—SNAP 3DX(TM) (IDEXX Laboratories, Westbook, Me.)—is available that tests for antibody to the C_6 peptide. The C_6 commercial test can be used to more accurately differentiate between vaccinated and infected dogs compared to the whole-spirochete and immunoblot test methods (Table 45-3). In studies of dogs, C_6 protein has been used in ELISA testing of experimentally[143,200] and naturally[134] infected animals. The anti-C_6 antibody response increased and waned more quickly after treatment than the antibody response measured by ELISA using whole-spirochete antigen extracts of *B. burgdorferi*.[200] C_6 did not react with sera from healthy dogs, those with other infections (e.g., dirofilariasis, babesiosis, ehrlichiosis, Rocky Mountain spotted fever, leptospirosis), or those vaccinated with either OspA, whole-spirochete vaccines, or commonly used vaccines for other diseases.[143,184] Use of this protein in serotesting may help determine the presence of active infection and if treatment has been successful may help eliminate the infection. Because not all dogs infected with virulent spirochetes become ill—and *B. burgdorferi* sensu lato and other closely-related strains and genospecies vary in pathogenicity—the C_6 antibody response may not always correlate with clinical illness in dogs. Clinical illness in seropositive animals may also relate to disease caused by other organisms that were present in the feeding tick.

The C_6 ELISA test has also been evaluated in cats on a limited basis.[141] Of 24 cats tested in an endemic area, 17 had seropositive test results that matched those obtained by a whole-spirochete FA method. Five cats had negative antibody test results for both assays, and two negative test result samples had positive results at low dilutions with the FA method; one of these specimens had positive test results using immunoblotting. Cats were selected for their likeliness of exposure, and no correlation was made with clinical illness. As with dogs, if a cat is evaluated with clinical signs such as fever and joint swelling, the C_6 assay may be helpful as an adjunctive test for diagnosis of Lyme borreliosis; however, coinfections with *A. phagocytophilum* (see Chapter 28) or other coincidental diseases must also be considered.

Cerebrospinal Fluid Antibody

Other approaches have been proposed to assist in the diagnosis of borreliosis. CSF antibody titers have been compared with those of serum in an attempt to diagnose neuroborreliosis in human patients.[103,265] Intrathecal production of specific antibodies to *B. burgdorferi* can be demonstrated if the ratio of CSF or serum *B. burgdorferi* antibody is greater than the CSF or serum albumin, total IgG, or specific IgG to another infec-

Table • 45-3

Comparative Serologic Test Results for Borreliosis in Dogs

SEROLOGIC TEST	NATURALLY INFECTED VIA TICK	RECOVERED FROM NATURAL INFECTION	VACCINATED WHOLE CELL	VACCINATED OSPA OR OSPB
IgM whole-cell ELISA or indirect FA[a]	Positive within first 60—90 days	Negative	Transient increase after vaccination	Transient increase after vaccination
IgG whole-cell ELISA or indirect FA[b]	After 60—90 days, positive for months or years	Positive for months to years	Positive for months to years	Positive for months to years
Immunoblot[c]	Numerous bands but *not* OspA or OspB[e]	Numerous bands but *not* Osp A or B[e]	Numerous bands *including* Osp A or B[e]	*Only* Osp A or B protein bands[e]
C_6 ELISA assay[d]	Positive	Negative	Negative	Negative

ELISA, Enzyme-linked immunosorbant assay; *FA,* Fluorescent antibody.

[a]IgM whole-cell assays are the most nonspecific. Low to moderate titer increases occur with reaction to many spirochetes and some other bacteria. Only very high titers should be considered caused by spirochetes. Indirect FA may be more specific in this regard.

[b]IgG whole-cell false-positive results caused by previous infections in recovered animals, vaccine, and reactions to many other closely related spirochetes. Indirect FA is more specific in this regard.

[c]Immunoblot false-positive results include reactions with pathogenic and nonpathogenic isolates. Positive titer results persist even after infection has been eliminated.

[d]C_6 false-positive results are caused by infection with *B. burgdorferi* sensu lato strains; some may be nonpathogenic. Subclinical infection occurs with *B. burgdorferi* strains when host immunity is adequately controlling infection.

[e]P31 and P34 proteins.

tious agent (see Chapter 3, Diagnosis of Distemper, and Chapter 80, Toxoplasmosis). When the same assay method is used for specific IgG, the specific method has the most reliability.[99,240] Increased CSF IgM antibody directed against OspA, OspB, and OspC that did not have a corresponding increased in serum has been documented in people with neuroborreliosis.[216]

An increased intrathecal antibody concentration was demonstrated in dogs with neurologic dysfunction.[64,160] These results are difficult to assess because the dogs were from endemic areas, and no supporting histopathologic or culture findings were supplied.

Detection of Organism

Microscopic Detection

B. burgdorferi can be visualized in body fluids such as synovial fluid using dark-field microscopy or in tissues after nonspecific silver or specific immunologic staining methods. However, the spirochete density in clinical specimens is low.[260] Microscopy is best used to detect organisms in the tissues of ticks. Table 45-4 compares various features of organism detection methods.

In Vitro Cultivation

Culture of spirochetes from specimens of a diseased patient is the most definitive means of diagnosis but in most cases is difficult because of the low numbers of organisms present. The probability of isolating borreliae from blood is low because spirochetes migrate through connective tissues and only incidentally enter the circulatory system.[249] Large quantities (20 ml) of ethylenediaminetetraacetic acid (EDTA) noncoagulated blood have improved isolation rates in people.[267] A special medium called *Barbour-Stoenner-Kelley (BSK) medium* is required for borreliae isolation. Skin and collagen-rich connective tissues (fascia, pericardium, peritoneum, meninges, synovium) are the most consistent tissues for premortem or postmortem culture from dogs when specimens are taken at or near the site of tick attachment.[37,249] The skin is clipped to remove the hair, a local anesthetic is instilled, and the area is carefully disinfected. Biopsy is performed using a 6-mm punch, and the specimen is placed in sterile tubes. Samples are processed with sterile pestles in medium, sequentially transferred to larger volumes of media, cultured at 33° C, and microscopically examined at 2-week intervals. Culture may be more sensitive than PCR before antimicrobial therapy[246]; however, culture is more time consuming than PCR (see Table 45-4).

Nucleic Acid Detection

Heralded as the supreme test for organism detection, PCR does have restrictions that have limited its use. Although most investigators claim its high specificity and sensitivity, PCR results can vary according to the designs of the selected primers (which are short stretches of artificially produced DNA used to induce specific DNA amplification). In contrast to culture, samples submitted for PCR require extensive handling. After enzymatic digestion of the sample matrix, DNA is recovered either by phenol/chloroform extraction (which is more efficient for DNA recovery but is considered more laborious) or by column purification. Subsequently, only a fraction of the pure eluted DNA (approximately 1% of the total amount, depending on the technique applied) is used for PCR analysis. With a low prevalence of organisms in the tissue sample, this statistically reduces the sensitivity of this assay tremendously, whereas the entire sample is submerged in medium during culture. Primers that target conserved DNA sequences can be used to detect various strains. Primers targeting plasmidial DNA are thought to be much more sensitive because of the multiple copies of plasmids present in the bacterium.[198,245] PCR should be performed on synovial tissue biopsy rather than on joint fluid because it is more likely to contain the organism in infected patients. PCR cannot distinguish live from dead organisms. PCR has been used to detect *Borrelia* in the CSF of people with acute or chronic neuroborreliosis; however, the sensitivity is limited, and false-negative results[180] may occur. Instead, PCR performed on skin specimens was more sensitive than PCR on CSF or urine samples in these patients.[132] PCR has been a valuable experimental tool and will likely become a more important clinical method for diagnosis in dogs. PCR of skin is superior to culture in dogs that have been treated with antimicrobials or in untreated animals with long-term infections.[246]

Table • 45-4

Comparison of Detection Methods of Borrelia burgdorferi in Clinical Specimens

DIAGNOSTIC METHOD	SPECIFICITY	SENSITIVITY	ACCURACY	QUANTIFICATION	USES
Microscopic detection, silver staining	Poor	Poor	Fair	Yes	Detection in tick and animal tissues
Microscopic detection, immunochemical staining	Good	Poor	Good	Yes	Detection in tissues
Antigen-capture ELISA	Poor	Fair	Poor	Yes	Screening method (substantiate with other tests)
Cultural isolation	Excellent	Good	Good	No	Definitive for laboratory use (takes 2—3 wk)
PCR probe	Good	Good	Good	Yes	Detection of infection in clinical specimens
Real-time PCR	Good	Excellent	Good	Yes	Detection and quantification for experimental studies

Modified from Wang G. 2002. Direct detection methods for Lyme Borrelia, including the use of quantitative assays. *Vector Borne Zoonotic Dis* 2:223-231.

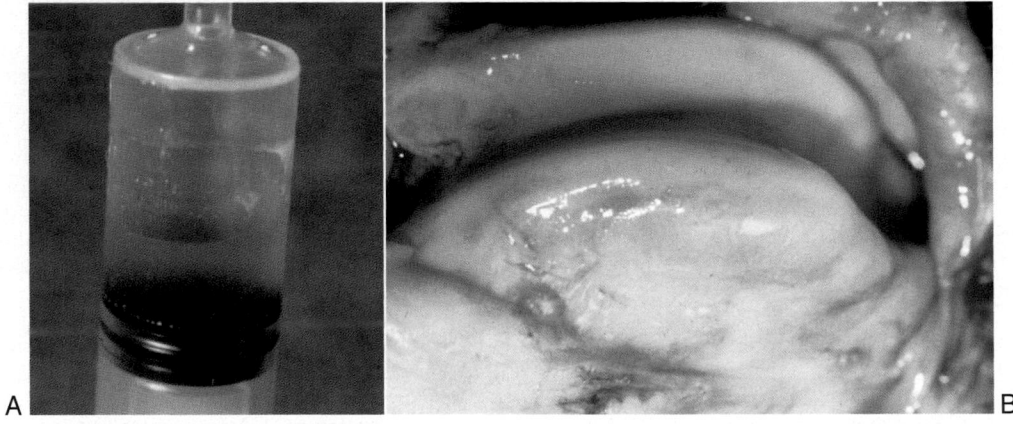

Fig   45-11   **A,** Cloudy synovial fluid containing large numbers of neutrophils from dog experimentally infected with *B. burgdorferi*. **B,** Gross appearance of chronic arthritic change in joint of experimentally infected dog. (Courtesy University of Georgia, Athens, Ga.)

Detection of Borreliae by Other Techniques

Tissue specimens can be examined microscopically for pathogenic spirochetes by using specific antibodies labeled with fluorescent dyes or enzymes that produce a signal in a subsequent color reaction or with gold particles that are visible on transmission electron microscopy (EM). Xenodiagnosis, in which naïve ticks become infected after feeding on suspect infected hosts, has proved very reliable in the research laboratory setting but is expensive and time consuming.

PATHOLOGIC FINDINGS

Severely affected animals have grossly swollen joints with synovial effusion (Fig. 45-11). Inflammation within the synovial membrane is mild, and the effusion consists of fibrin and neutrophils in acute cases. In more chronic infections, dogs that have undergone seroconversion develop nonsuppurative inflammation within the synovial membrane and joint capsule. Peripheral lymphadenomegaly is present, especially in nodes draining the affected limbs.

In experimentally infected dogs, histologic lesions have developed in the lymph nodes, joints, pericardium, and skin.[6] In addition, blood vessels (vasculitis, arteritis), peripheral nerves (perineuritis), and meninges (meningitis) have associated inflammation (Fig. 45-12).[251] Histologically, follicular enlargement and increased size of parafollicular areas in lymph nodes are evident. Skin biopsy samples have superficial perivascular lymphoplasmacytic infiltrates with mast cell accumulations. Renal lesions have not been found in experimentally infected dogs but were evident in naturally diseased dogs.[46] Glomerulitis, diffuse tubular necrosis with regeneration, and interstitial inflammation were found. These symptoms are more commonly found in certain breeds such

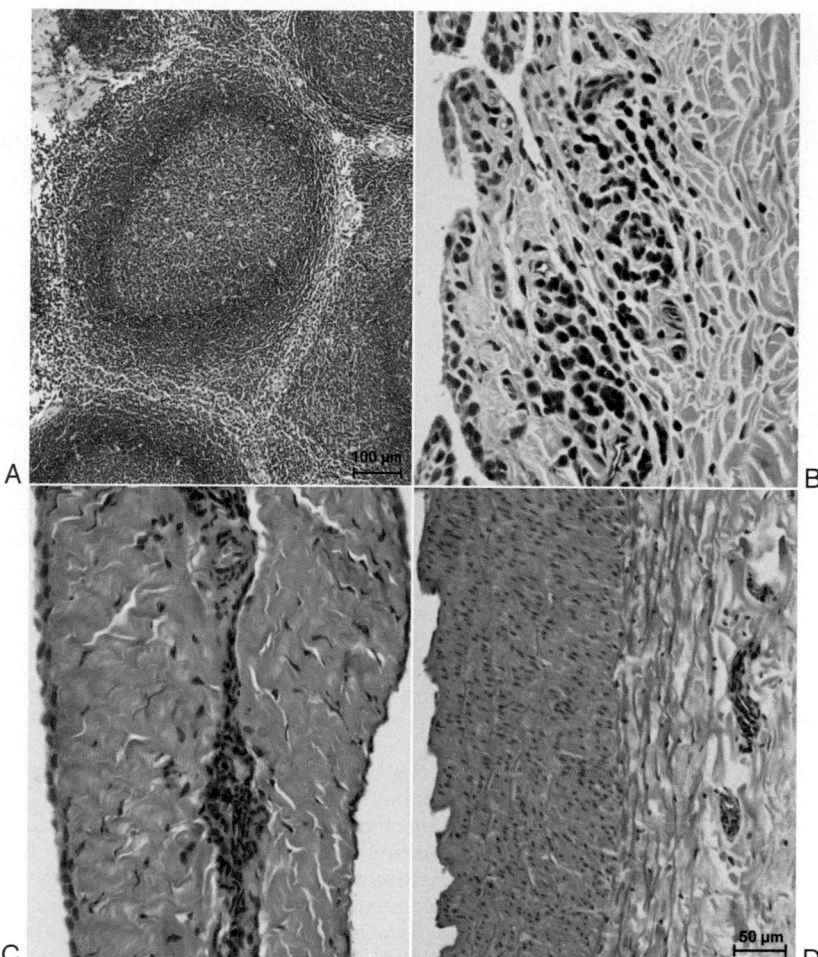

Fig 45-12 Histopathologic lesions in dog infected with *B. burgdorferi*. Representative tissue sections of inflammatory lesions (hematoxylin-eosin stain). **A,** Severe follicular hyperplasia of left axillary lymph node. **B,** Synovial membrane of left elbow with moderate nonsuppurative arthritis. Note accumulation of plasma cells in subsynovial tissue. **C,** Mild nonsuppurative pericarditis with several cellular aggregates—mostly mononuclear cells in tissue. **D,** Tunica media and tunica adventia of artery with small cuffs of mononuclear cells around branch of vasa vasorum *(arrows)*. (Courtesy R. Straubinger, University of Leipzig, Leipzig, Germany.)

as Labrador and golden retrievers. Borreliae can be demonstrated in tissues using silver impregnation methods or cytologic specimens with Giemsa stain. Silver stain of the kidneys of these dogs revealed rare spirochetes unrelated to lesion development.[46] In addition to hepatic degeneration, splenic hyperplasia, regional lymph node plasmacytosis, nonsuppurative meningoencephalitis, and pneumonitis, similar renal lesions have been noted in experimentally infected cats.[75,76]

THERAPY

Because of the difficulty in obtaining an accurate diagnosis, antibiotics are often given empirically in an attempt to make a therapeutic diagnosis. Many reports exist of successful recovery after administration of antimicrobial drugs in dogs diagnosed with Lyme arthritis. Improvement often occurs within 24 to 48 hours after antimicrobial therapy is initiated. The greatest success is achieved with treatment in the initial phases of clinical illness. Clinical improvement after any therapeutic intervention should be viewed with caution because the acute limb and joint dysfunction is intermittent and often resolves after several days to weeks regardless of whether antimicrobials are given.[156] In addition, doxycycline can cause nonspecific antiinflammatory changes in injured joints and has been shown to be chondroprotective in noninfectious arthritis in dogs.[271]

Early treatment is associated with a reduction in antibody titers and organisms in tissues and prevention or cure of clinical lameness and joint lesions.[249,251] Most treatment is instituted for a minimum of 30 days, and amoxicillin, azithromycin, ceftriaxone, and doxycycline have all been used. However, on the basis of research studies, clearance of the organism after 30 days of treatment in dogs and rodents is questionable, and relapse and recrudescence of infection can occur after the antimicrobial therapy is discontinued.* Similar treatment outcomes have been reported for human patients.[53] In addition to an inability to clear the organism, chronic inflammatory changes that occur in various tissues such as the joints may become self-perpetuating. Intraarticular persistence of *B. burgdorferi* nucleic acids occurs even though they cannot be cultured.[23,251] The persistence may stimulate chronic immune and inflammatory processes. Those with more chronic borreliosis are less likely to improve or more likely to have relapses, even if treatment continues for weeks or months. Using clinical improvement after treatment as the basis for diagnosing borreliosis or other causes of bacterial or rickettsial polyarthritis is difficult because fever, joint distention, and lameness may appear and then disappear spontaneously. Furthermore, some antimicrobial drugs such as the tetracyclines have antiinflammatory effects.

Nevertheless, antimicrobial therapy is still the mainstay for treatment of borreliosis (Table 45-5). In vitro antimicrobial susceptibility testing has shown ceftriaxone, erythromycin, amoxicillin, cefuroxime, doxycycline, tetracycline, and penicillin G to range from most to least effective.[116] Tetracycline,

---

*References 20, 159, 193, 246, 249-251.

Table • 45-5

Suggested Antibiotic Regimens for Lyme Borreliosis

DRUG[a]	DOSE[b]	ROUTE	INTERVAL (HOURS)	DURATION (DAYS)	PREFERRED USES
Doxycycline	10 mg/kg	PO	12	30	Early disease, arthritis or neurologic manifestations, not for pups or kittens
Amoxicillin	20 mg/kg	PO	8	30	Early, arthritis or neurologic manifestations, young patients
Azithromycin	25 mg/kg	PO	24	10—20	Early disease
Penicillin G	22,000 U/kg	IV	8	14—30	Persistent arthritis, neurologic manifestations, or carditis
Ceftriaxone	25 mg/kg	IV, SC	24	14—30	Late neurologic or cardiac manifestations, persistent arthritis
Cefotaxime	20 mg/kg	IV	8	14—30	Neurologic manifestations
Chloramphenicol	15—25 mg/kg	PO, SC	8	14—30	Neurologic manifestations

PO, By mouth; IV, intravenous; SC, subcutaneous.
[a]See Appendix 8 for additional information. Information on many drugs is based on extrapolation from literature on humans.
[b]Dose per administration at specified interval.

ampicillin, and erythromycin classically have been used to treat human and animal patients. Newer erythromycin derivatives, such as azithromycin, or third-generation cephalosporins, such as ceftriaxone, have been administered for more refractory human cases.[47] They are most effective for treatment of chronic infections. High-dose IV penicillin G has been advocated in an attempt to treat unresponsive animals. Borreliae are resistant to aminoglycosides and quinolones.

Doxycycline is generally the drug of choice because it is a lipid-soluble tetracycline and is relatively inexpensive. The theoretical advantages of lipid solubility are that a lower dosage is needed, tissue distribution is greater, and intracellular penetration is better than that achieved with conventional tetracycline. For growing animals, amoxicillin is recommended because doxycycline may stain the nails, skin, and enamel teeth. Doxycycline is less likely to cause this staining than other tetracyclines.[56] Ceftriaxone is reserved as parenteral therapy for meningitis in people. Treatment of people with ceftriaxone (2 g given IV once daily for 30 days) was effective in treating chronic Lyme encephalopathy.[148] Oral doxycycline (for 3 weeks to 2 months) may also be effective because it has been used to treat spirochetal meningitis in people.[48,55]

Treatment of clinically healthy seropositive dogs with antimicrobial therapy is controversial. Many infected hosts have a natural immunity that prevents the organism from causing clinical disease. Furthermore, treatment of many dogs in endemic areas that might have antibody titers could lead to the development of additional resistant strains of spirochetes and other resident bacterial microflora. In contrast the incubation period can be prolonged; as immunopathologic consequences of infection develop, treatment may help to prevent the progression of these events during a subclinical period. Some veterinarians with this view advocate vaccination of animals in conjunction with treatment to prevent additional reinfection should the organism be eliminated.[135]

Nonsteroidal compounds offer relief for many of the painful arthritic complications, but judicious use is warranted because of their tendency to produce GI irritation. Glucocorticoids have also been hesitantly provided at very low antiinflammatory dosages in the management of persistent pain and swelling from chronic arthritis that cannot be completely controlled with one or more courses of antibiotics. An unfortunate consequence of persistence is that immunosuppression, such as that associated with administration of prednisolone in a dosage of 2 mg/kg daily for 2 weeks, reactivates latent disease.[250] Dogs show no clinical signs of lameness while being treated but after therapy is discontinued, they develop signs of arthritis within 1 week.[250] Immunosuppressive doses of glucocorticoids should definitely be avoided in chronically infected dogs because of infection exacerbation, or they should be given in combination with antibiotics.

Treatment and prognosis of renal dysfunction associated with Lyme borreliosis varies according to the stage and severity of the illness at the time diagnosis is made. With progression, marked proteinuria can lead to the nephrotic syndrome and systemic hypertension. In the early stages, ACE inhibitors and antiinflammatory drugs may be considered. As the disease progresses, animals may develop severe hypoproteinemia and decreased renal perfusion, which necessitates volume expanders, vasoactive agents, and osmotic diuresis. Unfortunately, like the polyarthritis, renal manifestations are usually progressive despite therapy.

PREVENTION

Antimicrobial Therapy

In people a single dose of doxycycline given at the time of identified tick attachment was 87% effective in preventing Lyme borreliosis.[176] Implementing this practice in dogs would be possible; however, the high exposure rate compared with the lower incidence of clinical illness in endemic geographic regions suggests a low degree of transmission and generally effective host immune responses. Early removal of ticks makes prophylactic treatment expensive and impractical.

Vaccination

Vaccines are marketed to prevent borreliosis in dogs.[122] In Europe, the multiplicity of infecting species may make protection by vaccination more difficult. Recombinant protein OspA vaccines and whole-cell bacterins are commercially available for dogs (Table 45-6 and Appendix 3). Adjuvanted recombinant vaccine with expressed OspA and OspB proteins has protected dogs against tick-induced infection.[45] Unadjuvanted OspA, a lipoprotein, appears to offer equal protec-

Table • 45-6

Comparison of Vaccines Licensed for Lyme Borreliosis in the United States[a]

COMPANY	PRODUCT NAME	TYPE OF VACCINE	ADJUVANTED	ROUTE	MINIMUM AGE (WEEKS)	RECOMMENDED BOOSTER INTERVAL (YEARS)	CHALLENGE INTERVAL (DAYS)
Fort Dodge	LymeVax	Whole-cell bacterin	+	SC, IM	*First dose:* 6 *Second dose (interval):* 2–3	1	150
Schering Plough	Galaxy Lyme[b]	Whole-cell bacterin	+	IM	*First dose:* 12 *Second dose (interval):* 3–4	1	230
Intervet	ProLyme	Recombinant-bacterin OspA protein	+	SC	*First dose:* 4 *Second dose (interval):* 3–4	1	366
Merial	Recombitek Lyme	Recombinant-produced lipidated OspA protein	–	SC	*First dose:* 9 *Second dose (interval):* 3–4	1	366

SC, Subcutaneous; *IM,* intramuscular.
[a]See Appendix 3 for availability and combinations of antigens available.
[b]Contains two strains of *B. burgdorferi* sensu stricto.

tion.[122] The vaccines are recommended for use beginning at 4 and 12 weeks of age, depending on the product. Primary vaccination schedules consist of two inoculations 3 weeks apart. Vaccines given early in life before exposure offer the best means of protection. Vaccination should not be universally recommended or provided as a replacement for adequate tick control measures. Dogs should be selected for vaccination based on the geographic area in which they reside or travel and by their geographic location, activities, and habits. That is, outdoor, hunting, or field-trial dogs that frequent known tick-infested areas should receive priority for vaccination. Dogs that are vaccinated with adjuvanted whole-cell vaccines or recombinant Osp vaccines before infection develop enhanced resistance to infection as demonstrated by an increased level of protective antibodies mainly directed against OspA (recombinant OspA vaccine) and minor antigens such as OspB and other currently unidentified antigens (bacterin vaccine).[6,89,149,206,247,252] This type of protection does not appear to develop in the naturally infected animals. Reinfection is possible in animals that are treated or recover from natural infections. Although OspA is an abundant protein on culture-derived *B. burgdorferi*, vertebrate hosts infected by tick bites rarely seroconvert to OspA.[17,51] The OspA is expressed by borreliae in the midgut of unfed ticks, and the organism down-regulates this protein in response to a blood meal during transmission from the vector to the vertebrate host (see Pathogenesis in this chapter).[219] OspA allows the organism to adhere to and colonize the vector, and it is not present on spirochetes in engorged ticks.[194] Therefore to be effective, the vaccine-induced antibodies *must* be present in the host *before* the tick feeds. During tick feeding, OspC is expressed on the surface of the spirochete and appears on organisms that infect the feeding host.[51,221,244]

In the presence of complement, the antibodies to OspA from the host cause an arrest of growth and prevention of salivary gland invasion in the ticks that feed on previously vaccinated animals.[50,51] The borreliae are not eliminated in these ticks—their numbers are only diminished. In this manner, vaccine-induced immune protection begins in the tick before spirochetes enter the host. If experimentally infected animals are given passively administered OspA antibodies after tick engorgement, the animals stay infected. Vaccination of an already infected animal does not clear the infection or prevent clinical illness.[18] In a study of naturally infected dogs in a highly endemic area, the C_6 ELISA revealed that dogs vaccinated annually with a whole-spirochete bacterin had a much lower rate of infection (5%) than unvaccinated dogs (64%).[135]

Because commercial OspA vaccines do not sustain protective titers, annual revaccination is recommended for high-risk dogs to maintain adequate titers. Furthermore, an anamnestic response against OspA does not occur because borreliae entering the host's skin no longer express this surface protein. In parenteral challenge studies, it was shown that protection is not afforded by prior immunization vaccines based on OspC.[203] Although OspC is highly immunogenic, considerable variation in OspC among strains of *B. burgdorferi* and other species such as *B. afzelii* makes heterologous protection with this antigen difficult.[105] Existing *B. burgdorferi* infection in mice was cleared with passively administered sera from mice previously vaccinated with OspC. However, when actively vaccinated with OspC, mice had no beneficial protection against infection.[273] Culture-confirmed reinfection of a person with different strains of *B. burgdorferi* sensu stricto has been reported, therefore cross-protection may be limited or does not exist among closely related strains and *Borrelia* species within the same genus.[78] In addition, cross-protection between *B. burgdorferi* sensu lato species inoculated into mice was not found.[15]

The disadvantage of vaccination is that the induced antibodies cause positive serologic test results for months or years and hamper the identification of infected animals. This problem may be resolved with use of the more specific immunodiagnostic tests, such as the previously described immunoblotting and C_6 assays. More important, whole-cell vaccines could theoretically lead to immunologic reactions that produce cross-reactive antibodies to host antigens. An additional theoretical but not yet documented disadvantage of the vaccine is the possibility that a hypersensitivity reaction may occur if it is given to a dog harboring large quantities of the organism.[113] This has been more of a potential concern for whole-cell than recombinant Osp products, because the OspA targeted by the recombinant vaccines is missing on tissue-adapted *Borrelia* spirochetes. Therefore screening of older dogs for past infection is recommended, and those that have been previously exposed should not be vaccinated. Other concerns have been expressed about the exclusive use of recombinant OspA vaccines. Successful vaccination using these products requires high titers of OspA antibodies to be present at the time of natural infection because borrelicidal antibody titers are not maintained at high levels for extended periods. Regular revaccination may be very important. OspA is antigenically distinct among different *B. burgdorferi* species and other species such as those in Europe, so cross-reactive antibodies may not be protective. The additional antigens in a whole organism can assist in adjuvanting and broadening the immune response. Using one experimental whole-cell sonicated unadjuvanted vaccine produced more sustained borreliacidal antibody titers and a superior response to challenge infection in dogs compared with an OspA vaccine.[247]

Local and systemic allergic reactions have been noted with whole-cell vaccines, but their prevalence rate is relatively low.[139] Borreliae are known to change their genotypic and phenotypic make-up to survive in the presence of organism-specific antibodies, so vaccine protection could lapse in the future or in particular geographic areas. Protection afforded by canine *Borrelia* vaccines is not absolute. Recommendations are to give two initial doses of the vaccine at a 2-week interval (see Table 45-6). Annual vaccination is recommended. In people, immunity was often much stronger after the third vaccine in the series.[232,241]

Vector Control in the Dog and Cat

Supportive measures are needed to reduce the prevalence of infection in people and pets. Personal protection methods have received the most attention for tick control on pets. Individually applied products have included collars, topical powders, shampoos, dips or foams, sprays, spot applications, and oral products. Collars are impregnated with permethrin or amitraz. Amitraz-impregnated flea collars have prevented transmission of *Borrelia* infection to vector-exposed dogs.[60] Topical solutions contain selamectin, fipronil, and permethrin. Topical selamectin is effective in control of *Rhipicephalus* and *Dermacentor* species; however, it is not as effective in treating dogs as permethrin.[61] As a noninsecticidal method, daily combing to remove attached ticks may also be effective, as are the tick checks that are used on people. (For personal protection for people, see Public Health Considerations in this chapter. See Chapter 94 for an additional discussion of vector control.)

Vector Control in the Environment

Application of acaricides to relatively large environmental areas is expensive and difficult. *Ixodes* species have a 2-year life cycle and become redistributed by various hosts after feeding, making it difficult to treat all stages with one application. Residual environmentally destructive compounds, such as the chlorinated hydrocarbons, have been the most successful method of controlling ticks, but their disadvantages are obvious.

A unique approach in tick control on wild mice has been adopted. The Maxforce Tick Management System (http://www.maxforcetms.com/maxforce_tms.html) is a small plastic box containing fipronil, as an acaricide, and a bait that is attractive to mice. Mice enter the box through a small hole. As a mouse moves through the box, it passes under a small applicator wick containing the fipronil.

Another method is to target infested rodents by placing cotton impregnated with permethrin insecticides near entrances to their burrows. To be effective, such acaricides have to target all reservoir hosts in a limited area. Treatment of all deer in a region with acaricides would inhibit the survival and reproduction of adult *I. scapularis*; however, the logistics of such an approach are overwhelming. Even if effective, vaccination of reservoir species would be impossible. Reduction of the deer population might help to decrease the number of ixodid ticks, but other mammalian hosts could still propagate the vectors.

PUBLIC HEALTH CONSIDERATIONS

The case definition of human Lyme borreliosis is (1) an erythematous rash or one objective sign of musculoskeletal, neurologic, or cardiovascular disease and (2) laboratory confirmation of infection.[4] In 2000, 17,730 cases were reported from 44 states and the District of Columbia; the northeastern United States accounted for approximately 85% of the total cases. Since surveillance for human Lyme borreliosis was established in 1982, more than 140,000 cases have been reported from 50 states (www.cdc.gov). The sylvan cycle in nature has been found in only 19 states. Errors in reporting are probably due to underreporting, misclassification, and overdiagnosis. For example, tickborne relapsing fever caused by *B. hermsii* causes false seropositivity in Lyme borreliosis testing, resulting in unrecognized and underreported cases of relapsing fevers and overreported cases of Lyme borreliosis.[58] Serodiagnosis with older whole-spirochete antigen tests likely overestimated the prevalence of disease because of cross-reactivity.

The highest annual incidence of Lyme borreliosis is among children younger than 14 years and adults older than 30 years. Clinical signs usually begin from several days to 1 month after a tick bite. An expanding nonpruritic ringlike erythematous lesion of at least 5 cm—an *erythema migrans*—may develop in the vicinity of the bite. Fever, myalgia, arthralgia, and headache (flulike symptoms) may accompany the lesion. Tick-bite–associated ECM lesions can be found on individuals in nonendemic regions and may be associated with organisms inoculated by bites of ticks that are not competent vectors of *B. burgdorferi*. These people have mild constitutional symptoms but test seronegative for *B. burgdorferi*. In contrast, people who become ill from *B. burgdorferi* infection develop recurrent joint swelling and musculoskeletal soreness. Meningeal signs include pain, sensory loss, behavioral changes, and recurrent headaches. Myocarditis is characterized by development of symptoms characteristic of atrioventricular conduction disturbances. Subclinical infections are also thought to occur; however, these are less frequent than previously realized because of cross-reactivity with older immunoassay methods.[242] Treatment of Lyme borreliosis in people is most rewarding during the early phases of illness. In chronically infected people with musculoskeletal or neurocognitive impairments, antimicrobial therapy is no more effective than placebo.[123]

Personal protection measures for human tick control are not difficult to institute.*[102] The most effective precautions include avoiding tick habitats, wearing long pants and long-sleeved shirts, taping socks over cuffs, tucking pants into socks, wearing light-colored clothing (to help identify ticks for early removal), and treating clothing and exposed skin with repellents. Agents containing diethyltoluamide (DEET) repel ticks and can be applied to clothing or exposed skin. Those containing permethrin kill ticks on contact but can only be applied to clothing. Additional measures include avoiding areas with tall grass and dense brush. Daily tick removal helps prevent transmission of infection. A delay exists between the beginning of tick feeding and the appearance of infectious spirochetes in tick saliva. Studies in animals show that little risk of infection exists within the first 24 hours of attachment and a maximum rate of infection between 48 to 72 hours of attachment or if the infected tick feeds until engorgement.[52] The incidence of disease is also greater in people when ticks are attached for 72 hours or more.[236] A single dose of doxycycline administered within 72 hours of a recognized *I. scapularis* bite efficiently prevented ECM in people living in endemic areas.[176]

Although Lyme borreliosis is classified as a zoonosis, dogs, cats, and people are incidental hosts for a sylvan cycle that exists in nature. Lyme borreliosis is associated with outdoor activities that result in exposure to tick vectors. Dogs and cats do not appear to be a source for infection in people because they do not excrete infectious organisms in their body fluids (including urine) to any appreciable extent.[6] Uninfected control dogs kept in direct contact with infected dogs for up to 1 year did not become infected or underwent seroconversion.[6]

Dogs and cats appear to be sentinel hosts but not reservoir hosts for human infection. In the same environment, dogs and cats have a greater risk of exposure than their human counterparts because of their greater likelihood of contacting the tick vector. Pets may bring infected ticks into the household, but ticks generally do not refeed after detachment. As with other tickborne illnesses, improper handling of ticks resulting in release of midgut contents onto abraded skin or mucous membranes might allow percutaneous penetration of infectious material. Even in areas where borreliosis is endemic, the risk of infection from a recognized ixodid tick bite is so low that prophylactic antimicrobial therapy of exposed people is not routinely recommended.[227]

*Additional information on Lyme borreliosis in people is available from (1) state and local health departments, (2) the Centers for Disease Control and Prevention (CDC) voice information system (404-332-4555) and Bacterial Zoonoses Branch (970-221-6453) and the Office of Communications at the National Institutes of Health (301-496-5717).

The human vaccine that had been marketed in the United States was based on recombinant OspA because of the concern about whole-cell vaccine safety.[130] Although recombinant vaccines have been shown to be efficacious when used before exposure,[232,241] their use has been limited because of concerns about potential but unproven side effects, and the product was withdrawn from the market in 2000.

SUGGESTED READINGS*

37. Callister SM, Jobe DA, Schell RF, et al. 2000. Detection of borreliacidal antibodies in dogs after challenge with *Borrelia burgdorferi*-infected *Ixodes scapularis* ticks. *J Clin Microbiol* 38:3670-3674.
42. Chang YF, Novosel V, Chang CF, et al. 2001. Experimental induction of chronic borreliosis in adult dogs exposed to *Borrelia burgdorferi*-infected ticks and treated with dexamethasone. *Am J Vet Res* 62:1104-1112.
124. Korshus JB, Munderloh UG, Bey RF, et al. 2004. Experimental infection of dogs with *Borrelia burgdorferi* sensu stricto using *Ixodes scapularis* ticks artificially infected by capillary feeding. *Med Microbiol Immunol (Berl)*. 193:27-34.
134. Levy S, O'Connor TP, Hanscom JL, et al. 2002. Utility of an in-office C₆ ELISA test kit for determination of infection status of dogs naturally exposed to *Borrelia burgdorferi*. *Vet Ther* 3:308-315.
135. Levy SA. 2002. Use of a C₆ ELISA test to evaluate the efficacy of a whole-cell bacterin for the prevention of naturally transmitted canine *Borrelia burgdorferi* infection. *Vet Ther* 3:420-424.
141. Levy SA, O'Connor TP, Hanscom JL, et al. 2003. Evaluation of a canine C₆ ELISA lyme disease test for the determination of the infection status of cats naturally exposed to *Borrelia burgdorferi*. *Vet Ther* 4:172-177.
220. Schwan TG, Piesman J. 2002. Vector interactions and molecular adaptations of Lyme disease and relapsing fever spirochetes associated with transmission by ticks. *Emerg Infect Dis* 8:115-121.
246. Straubinger RK. 2000. PCR-based quantification of *Borrelia burgdorferi* organisms in canine tissues over a 500-day postinfection period. *J Clin Microbiol* 38:2191-2199.
247. Straubinger RK, Rao TD, Davidson E, et al. 2002. Protection against tick-transmitted Lyme disease in dogs vaccinated with a multiantigenic vaccine. *Vaccine* 20:181-193.
250. Straubinger RK, Straubinger AF, Summers BA, et al. 2000. Status of *Borrelia burgdorferi* infection after antibiotic treatment and the effects of corticosteroids: an experimental study. *J Infect Dis* 181:1069-1081.

*See the CD-ROM for a complete list of references.

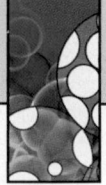

CHAPTER • 46

Miscellaneous Bacterial Infections

Carolyn R. O'Brien, Craig E. Greene, and Russell T. Greene

MELIOIDOSIS

Melioidosis is an infection caused by *Burkholderia pseudomallei* (formerly *Pseudomonas pseudomallei*), an aerobic, gram-negative, motile bacillus with a single polar flagellum. The organism, which is restricted to latitudes within 20 degrees north or south of the equator, is a ubiquitous saprophyte, endemic to Southeast Asia, northern Australia, and the South Pacific where it is primarily isolated from moist soil and water-holes. Heavy monsoonal rains and winds may increase the risk of inhaling *B. pseudomallei*.[8] Infection is thought to occur via cutaneous inoculation through wounds contaminated with soil or from bites of arthropod vectors, inhalation of dust, and ingestion of soil or contaminated carcasses. Infection can spread into the environment from an infected animal via caseous nodules that rupture.

The organism is a facultative intracellular organism, and the spectrum of clinical syndromes it causes in people and animals range from acute, fulminant septicemia and pneumonia, and chronic abscess formation and granuloma formation to mild or unapparent infections. Disease may appear many years after presumed exposure.[24] Cell-mediated immunity is important for successful elimination of infection in a host.[13]

Cases of canine and feline melioidosis appear infrequently in the literature, although anecdotal evidence suggests that infection in these species is more common in endemic areas than the literature would suggest.[17] Seven military dogs stationed in Vietnam developed fever, myalgia, and abscess formation of multiple organs, including the dermis, lung, liver, kidneys, spleen, epididymis and testis,[21] and an Australian dog developed disseminated cutaneous melioidosis after ingesting part of a goat carcass that had died of the disease.[15] Of the four cases of feline melioidosis reported,[7,17,22] three were presumed to have acquired the infection in Malaysia, with the remaining case having domicile in Northern Australia. Multifocal abscesses, lymphadenomegaly, hepatomegaly, and splenomegaly were most common in the affected cats (Figs. 46-1 and 46-2).

The diagnostic technique of choice is isolation of the organism from blood or lesions. Generally, *B. pseudomallei* is easily and inexpensively grown on routine media, although selective media such as Ashdown's agar may be needed to isolate the organism from sites where contaminating microorganisms are present. Thorough examination of Gram-stained smears of pus from lesions can sometimes identify small numbers of bipolar-staining gram-negative rods that may raise suspicion of the infection in endemic areas (Figs. 46-3 and 46-4). Immunologic assays for the detection of *Burkholderia* antigen and antibodies are available; however, none have been developed specifically for use in the dog or cat. In people, antibody detection may reflect exposure rather than active disease. Polymerase chain reaction can detect the organism in buffy coat and pus samples,[2,9,20] and immunohistochemical methods can detect the organism in affected tissues.[23] Pathologic findings are abscesses in affected organs and draining lymph nodes (Figs. 46-5 and 46-6).

Treatment of melioidosis may be prolonged and is often unsuccessful, and relapses may occur. Surgical drainage of large abscesses may be required in conjunction with antimicrobial therapy. Antibacterial treatment is recommended for small or disseminated lesions. The organism tends to be susceptible in vitro to trimethoprim-sulfonamide, fluoroquinolones, amoxicillin-clavulanate, some third-generation cephalosporins, tetracyclines, and carbapenems. Combinations of penicillins and aminoglycosides are ineffective. The most effective treatment of acute melioidosis in human patients appears to be high doses of parenteral ceftazidime given for at least 10 days, followed by a maintenance drug regimen of orally administered doxycycline, trimethoprim-sulfonamide, chloramphenicol, or any combination for 8 to 10 weeks.[6] Adjunctive treatment with granulocyte colony–stimulating factor has helped reduce the mortality in people with septic shock due to melioidosis.[6a] These drug regimens would likely also be effective in veterinary patients. However, amoxicillin-clavulanate has also shown to be adequate for maintenance treatment.[19] It might be combined with an initial short concurrent course of parenteral imipenem.[17] For appropriate therapeutic dosages, see Appendix 8. Following a response to treatment, affected animals should be closely monitored for any signs of relapse.

Nosocomial transmission of infection has been suspected. The organism has survived in a parenteral anesthetic solution and an antiseptic cleaning agent containing cetrimide 3% and chlorhexidine 0.3%.[16] Zoonotic transmission is thought to be extremely rare, although anecdotal reports of animal to human transfer have been documented.[12,16] Generally, people in endemic areas become infected from the environment, as do animals.

GLANDERS

Pseudomonas mallei is a coccoid to filamentous, non–spore-forming, unencapsulated, nonmotile, gram-negative organisms that is a soil saprophyte of worldwide distribution. It affects primarily solipeds that ingest contaminated food or water, or the organism spreads between infected horses via aerosols. Cloven-hoofed animals are relatively resistant. Other animals, such as dogs and cats, and people have intermediate susceptibility. Glanders are infected by inadvertent contact with diseased horses, by consumption of contaminated horsemeat, or occasionally by wound contamination.

After intestinal or local wound infection, the organism produces bacteremia and spreads to the lymph nodes, nasal passages, and lungs where it produces nodular lesions resembling those of tuberculosis.

The organism grows on laboratory media, a process that can be facilitated by the addition of antimicrobials and growth factors. Serologic testing is used to confirm a diagnosis in solipeds, but accuracy in detecting canine and feline infection is uncertain.

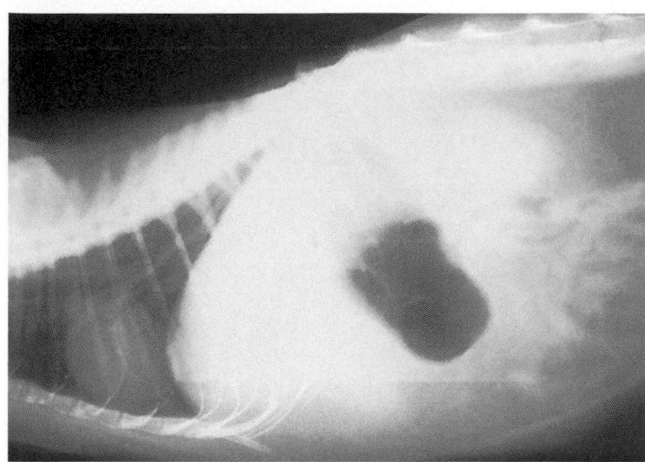

Fig 46-1 Lateral thoracoabdominal radiograph of a cat with disseminated melioidosis. Sternal lymph node is enlarged and the liver is enlarged extending beyond the costal arch. (Reprinted from O'Brien CR et al. 2003. Disseminated meliodosis in two cats, *J Feline Med Surg* 5:83-89; with permission from European Association of Feline Medicine.)

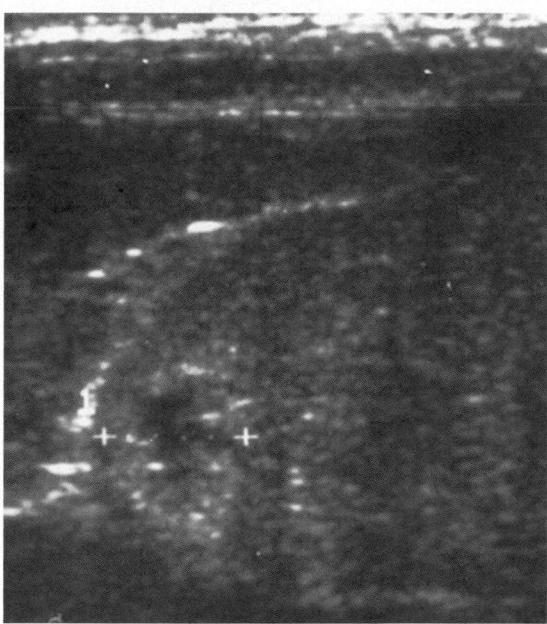

Fig 46-2 Ultrasonogram of the liver of a cat with disseminated meloidosis showing cavitary anechoic lesion within the liver. At necropsy, this was an abscess. (Reprinted from O'Brien CR et al. 2003. Disseminated meliodosis in two cats, *J Feline Med Surg* 5:83-89; with permission from European Association of Feline Medicine.)

Burkholderia mallei are sensitive to sulfonamides and tetracyclines. Dosages are listed in Appendix 8.

CHRYSEOMONAS INFECTIONS

Chryseomonas luteola (formerly Ve-1) has been recognized as a cause of infection in people with bacteremia and of peritonitis from peritoneal dialysis.[11,14,18] In people, *C. luteola* is usually associated with infections involving foreign materials, such as central venous catheters or joint prostheses. The 16S rRNA sequence of *C. luteola* supports the close relationship of this genus to *Pseudomonas*[1] and *Flavimonas*.

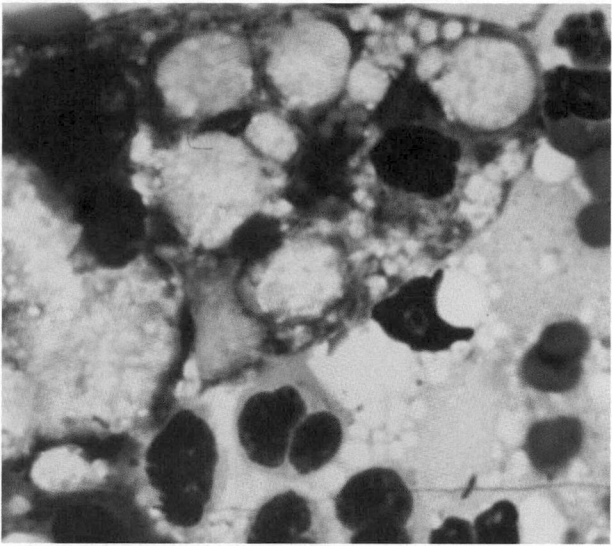

Fig 46-3 Squash preparation of liver lesion from cat with disseminated melioidosis obtained at necropsy. Note the suppurative inflammation (Diff Quik; original magnification ×330). (Reprinted from O'Brien CR et al. 2003. Disseminated meliodosis in two cats, *J Feline Med Surg* 5:83-89; with permission from European Association of Feline Medicine.)

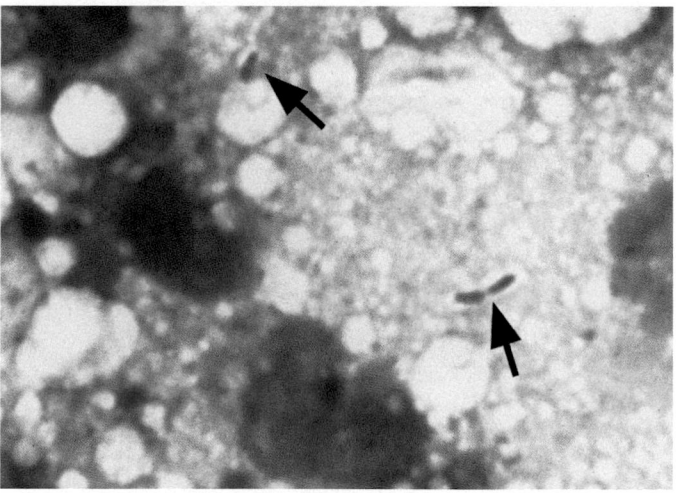

Fig 46-4 Squash preparation of liver lesion from cat with disseminated melioidosis obtained at necropsy. Note the extracellular gram-negative bacilli (Burke's modification of the Gram stain; original magnification ×330). (Reprinted from O'Brien CR et al. 2003. Disseminated meliodosis in two cats, *J Feline Med Surg* 5:83-89; with permission from European Association of Feline Medicine.)

In a dog with pyogranulomaltous dermatitis and lymphadenitis, *C. luteola* and *Aeromonas caviae* were isolated as presumptive opportunistic bacteria from inguinal lymph node aspirates.[16a] Infection with *C. luteola* was documented in a cat. Approximately 1 year after being diagnosed with diabetes mellitus, a 4.8-kg, 8- to 10-year-old domestic shorthaired cat was presented with a 4 × 8 cm swelling with purulent drainage from the right hip (Fig. 46-7). The animal was receiving subcutaneous insulin once daily. Pus from the mass was surgically drained, and amoxicillin, 20 mg/kg, was prescribed for 2 weeks. Four days later, the mass was still present; thus it was

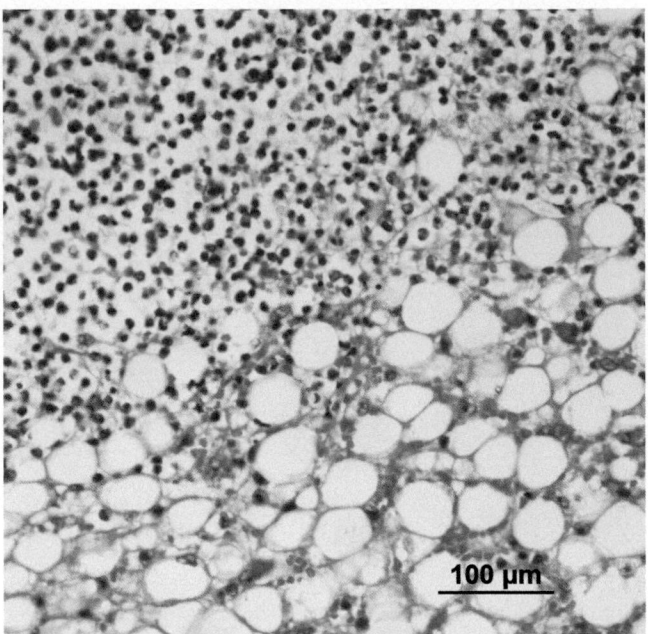

100 μm

Fig   46-5 Histopathology of liver microabscesses from a 5-year-old domestic shorthair cat with melioidosis. Note the relatively well-circumscribed aggregation of the neutrophilic aggregation and the surrounding fatty degeneration of hepatocytes (H and E stain, bar = 100 μm). (Courtesy Mark Krockenberger, University of Sydney, Sydney, Australia.)

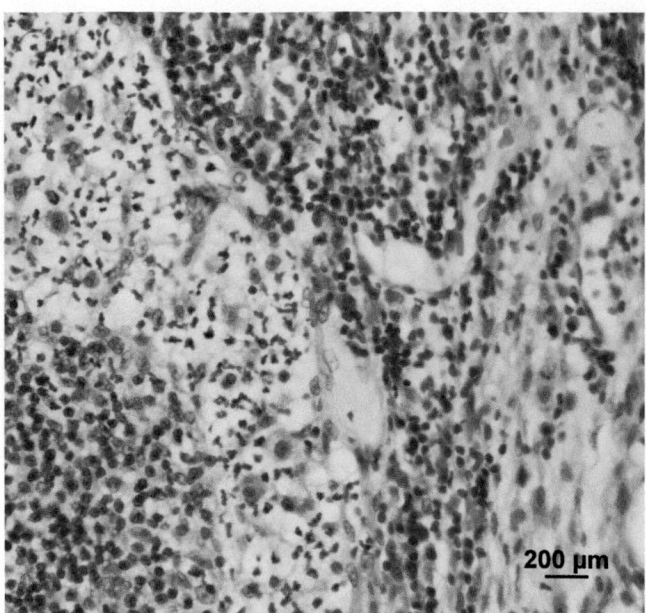

200 μm

Fig   46-6 Histopathology of sternal lymph node from the same case. Note the neutrophilic exudate present in the cortical sinus. Involvement of the sternal lymph node was presumed secondary to the hepatitis observed in this case (H and E stain, bar = 200 μm). (Courtesy Mark Krockenberger, University of Sydney, Sydney, Australia.)

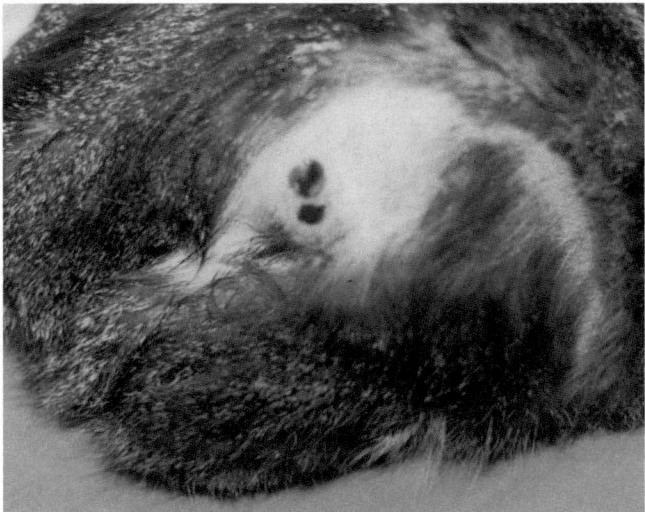

Fig   46-7 Draining abscess on the hip of a cat containing C. luteola. (Courtesy Russell Greene, Phoenix Veterinary Internal Medicine Service, Phoenix, Ariz.)

surgically removed and a drain was placed. The mass was submitted for histopathology. Six months later, a smaller mass developed at the lesion site. Cytologic examination of the exudate revealed large gram-negative rods. Biopsy findings were marked suppuration with primarily polymorphonuclear cell infiltration. Very large rod-shaped organisms were found within the inflammation.

Specimens for bacterial culture yielded a convex, circular, yellow-pigmented colony within 24 hours on sheep blood agar. Lysis of the red blood cells was noted under the colony. Gram stain revealed it to be a very large, gram-negative rod. The isolate was identified as C. luteola. Kirby-Bauer testing revealed sensitivity to tetracycline, aminoglycosides, trimethoprim-sulfonamide, and enrofloxacin. The isolate was resistant to ampicillin, cephalothin, and oxacillin. The cat was treated with oral enrofloxacin, 22.7 mg (total dose), twice daily for 3 weeks and the lesion resolved.

SUGGESTED READINGS*

3. Brett PJ, Woods DE. 2000. Pathogenesis of and immunity to melioidosis, *Acta Trop* 74:201-210.
15. Lloyd JM, Suijdendorp P, Soutar WR. 1988. Melioidosis in a dog, *Aust Vet J* 65:191-192.
16. Low Choy J et al. 2000. Animal melioidosis in Australia, *Acta Trop* 74:153-158.
17. O'Brien CR et al. 2003. Disseminated melioidosis in two cats, *J Feline Med Surg* 5:83-89.
18. Rahav G, Simhon A, Mattan Y, et al. 1995. Infections with *Chryseomonas luteola* (CDC group Ve-1) and *Flavimonas oryzihabitans* (CDC group Ve-2), *Medicine* 74:83-88.
24. Woods DE, DcSharzer D, Moore RA, et al. 1999. Current studies on the pathogenesis of melioidosis, *Microbes Infect* 1:157-162.

*See the CD-ROM for a complete list of references.

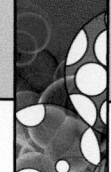

CHAPTER • 47

Plague

Dennis Macy

ETIOLOGY

Plague is caused by *Yersinia pestis*, a coccobacillus of the family Enterobacteriaceae, is a nonmotile, non–spore-forming, facultative anaerobic, gram-negative, bipolar-staining bacteria. The organism is nonsaprophytic and sensitive to desiccation and temperatures higher than 40° C, which make fomite transmission unlikely. This coccobacillus can survive for several weeks to months in organic material such as infected carcasses. Cold temperatures or freezing may prolong the viability of this organism for years. The organism grows slowly in culture even at its optimum temperature (28° C on blood agar or MacConkey agar), so cultures should be held for at least 48 hours before discarding. Colonies are much smaller than other Enterobacteriaceae and may be overlooked. *Y. pestis* produces a lipolysaccharide endotoxin and a capsular envelope containing the antiphagocytic principal fraction I antigen. Three geographic variants of *Y. pestis (orientalis, antiqua,* and *mediaevalis)* can be distinguished biochemically but have identical virulence. Environmental and temperature fluctuations moderate the bacteria's expression of transmission and virulence factors. In this way the bacillus can survive in arthropods, transmit easily to mammalian hosts, and replicate readily in its new host, thus the infection has spread to most continents.

EPIDEMIOLOGY

Plague is a zoonotic infection transmitted among natural animal reservoirs. Infection is maintained by an obligatory flea-rodent-flea cycle involving chronically bacteremic rodent hosts and their resident fleas (Fig. 47-1). People and domestic animals are alternate hosts for *Y. pestis.* More than 230 species of rodents and 1500 species of fleas infected with the plague organism have been found. Despite this wide host range, only 30 to 40 rodent species serve as permanent natural reservoirs for plague; other rodent species are considered only temporary or amplifying hosts for the organism. Natural reservoir hosts are relatively resistant to plague infections, but susceptibility varies tremendously within a species and is based on geographic location, flea species, and environmental factors. Dog and cat fleas (*Ctenocephalides* species) are considered poor vectors for plague. In the United States, prairie dogs (*Cynomys* species), rock squirrels *(Spermophilus variegatus),* and ground squirrels such as *Spermophilus richardsoni* are commonly infected wild hosts. Mortality approaches 100% in these species.

Plague exists in various discontinuous regions on every continent except Australia (Fig. 47-2). These foci of plague are most frequently associated with semiarid, cooler climates that are usually adjacent to deserts. Each focus is unique in terms of its rodent reservoirs, flea vectors, and environmental factors. Common characteristics of endemic areas include the availability of rodent hosts with a short life expectancy and high reproductive potential and year-round flea activity. In the United States, plague foci are located throughout an area bounded on the east by the Rocky Mountains and on the west by the Pacific Ocean as well as in Hawaii (Fig. 47-3). In reservoir animals the disease may have explosive and often devastating sporadic or periodic epizootics among susceptible rodents. During epizootic outbreaks, the geographic area has spread into the high plains of Colorado, western Kansas, Oklahoma, and Texas. These temporary geographic expansions are caused by spread of the disease into highly susceptible ground squirrel populations but are usually not maintained for more than several years because of high mortality in these species. High mountain parks in Colorado and grasslands in California are also susceptible to rapid expansion of plague because of the presence of amplifying rodent species. People and pets exposed to infected rodents during these epizootics may develop plague pneumonia.

Rodent-burrowing systems maintain plague ecosystems by providing a moist environment for flea reproduction and housing very large numbers of animals such as prairie dogs. Burrows allow the exchange of infected fleas and allow interspecies spread when abandoned burrows are used by another species, such as rabbits, seeking refuge from a predator.

Cats and dogs acquire plague by ingestion of infected rodents or lagomorphs or possibly by bites from their prey's plague-infected fleas. Of 60 cats diagnosed with plague, 75% had hunted rodents.[11] Ten days after ingestion of rodents infected with *Y. pestis,* plague organisms can be isolated from the oropharynx and blood stream in approximately 50% and 20% of dogs, respectively. Dogs develop only mild clinical symptomatology, including fever and lymphadenomegaly, and undergo seroconversion. Wild and domestic cats are more susceptible to plague than dogs or other carnivores.

Domestic and wild cats have a susceptibility to *Y. pestis* that is similar to that of people and can be a source of infection for people. Disease in cats has been more common in the summer months; fewer cases are reported in the spring and winter. However, the time of year should not be used to exclude plague from the differential diagnosis. Raptors and other birds; wild carnivores, including black bears, coyotes, badgers, skunks, and raccoons; and domestic dogs are remarkably resistant to *Y. pestis* infection but may transport infected fleas or rodent carcasses. Rabbits, although not considered reservoir hosts, may become infected during enzootic outbreaks and serve as sources of infection in hunters.

PATHOGENESIS

The proventriculus of the flea is a valve-like organ with rough inner lining covered by cuticle that is interposed between the esophagus and the stomach (midgut). It mechanically lyses ingested erythrocytes, allowing smoother passage into the stomach while acting as a valve to prevent regurgitation of stomach contents.

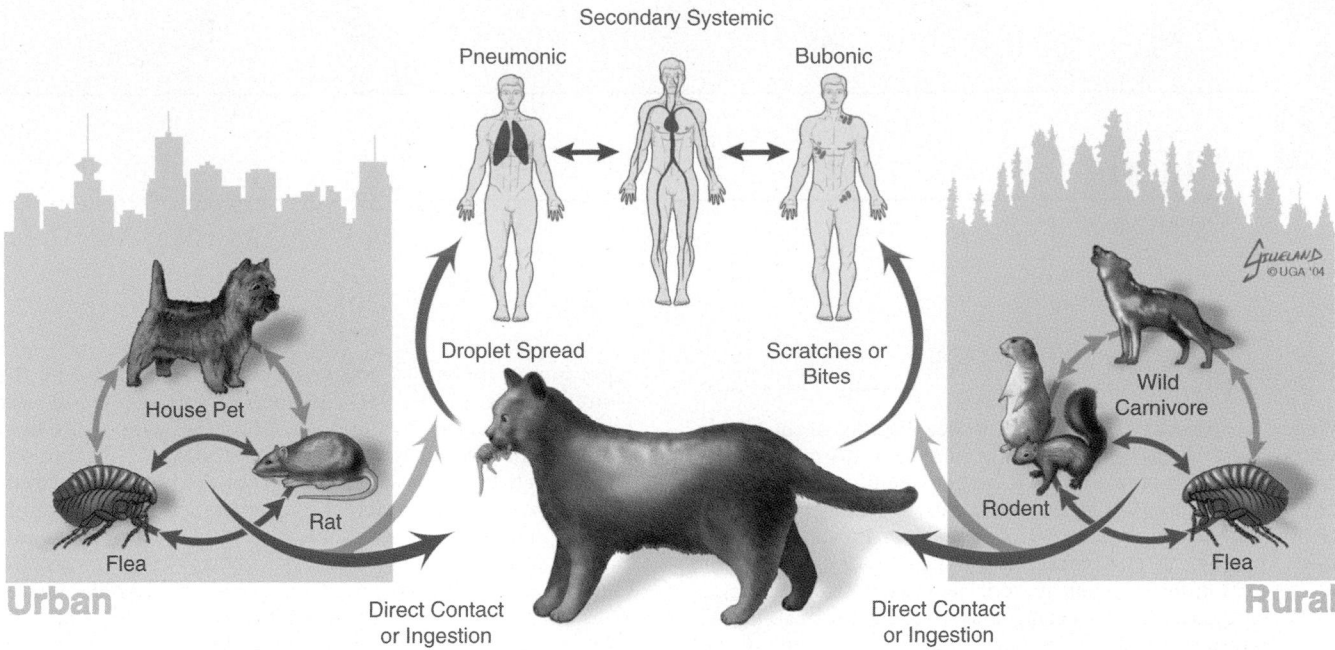

Fig 47-1 Epidemiologic features of plague. (Courtesy University of Georgia, Athens, Ga.)

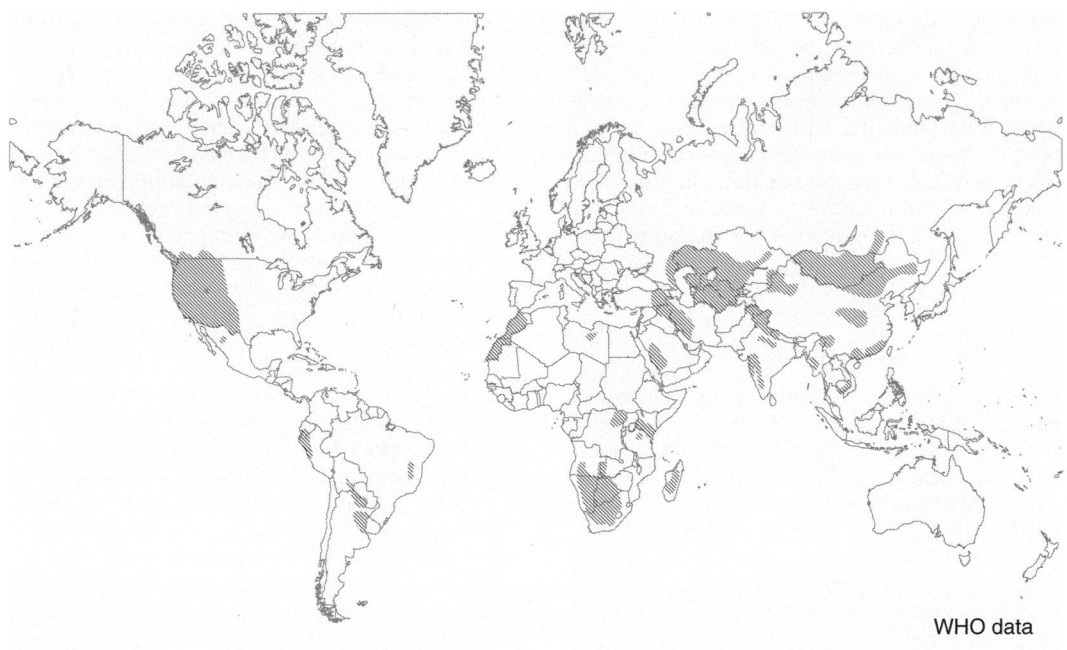

Fig 47-2 Known foci and areas of plague. (Data from the World Health Organization, Geneva, Switzerland. Map courtesy University of Georgia, Athens, Ga.)

Following ingestion of blood from an infected reservoir host, *Y. pestis* may be cleared by some fleas. In others, it replicates in high numbers in the flea stomach. A genetically encoded cytokine factor, *Yersinia* murine toxin (Ymt, a plasmid-encoded phospholipase D), is produced by virulent *Y. pestis* strains and allows the organisms to survive and replicate in the flea midgut by either antagonizing or down-regulating their antibacterial defenses.[15] Ymt activity arises within *Y. pestis* after exposure to plasma ingested with the blood meal. After several days of successful replication, bacterial cells aggregate and attach themselves to the lining of the proventriculus. A second pathogenic factor, hemin storage phenotype (Hms), found in virulent strains of *Y. pestis* is required for the bacteria to colonize and block the proventriculus, resulting in a blocked flea. Hms genes facilitate the production of an extracellular matrix and biofilm that attach to the acellular surface of spines lining the interior of the proventriculus and cause the blockage.[17a] Blocked fleas become starved for blood and attempt to feed more often. During these attempts, they regurgitate plague organisms into the bite wound of an uninfected host. Only blocked fleas transmit infection; they may die of starvation and dehydration. Fleas may remain infected for more than a year, allowing transmission of the disease long after the death of the host.

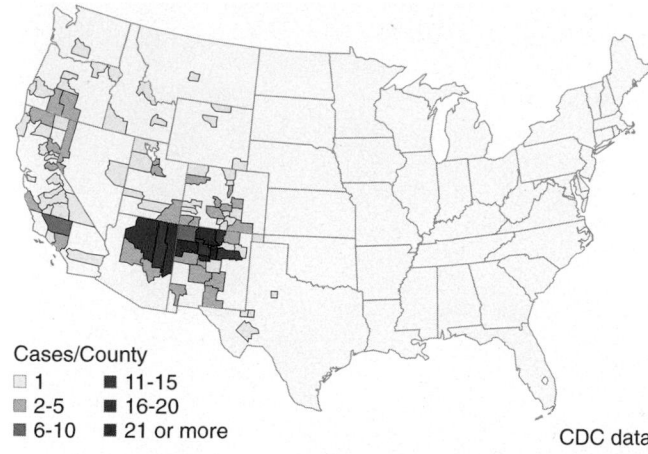

Fig 47-3 Distribution of human plague in United States from 1970 to 1997 by county. (Data from the Centers for Disease Control and Prevention, Atlanta, Ga. Map courtesy University of Georgia, Athens, Ga.)

Cases/County
1 ☐   11-15 ■
2-5 ■   16-20 ■
6-10 ■   21 or more ■

CDC data

Transmission of *Y. pestis* between most hosts occurs by flea bite. Although less common, transmission can also occur through contact of the organism with mucous membranes or broken skin or by inhalation of droplets from animals with pneumonic plague (see Fig. 47-1). Depending on whether the organism enters from a flea bite or through mucous membranes or broken skin, two distinct pathogeneses are possible. After a flea bite the organism is phagocytized by polymorphonuclear cells, in which *Y. pestis* cells are destroyed, and by mononuclear cells, in which *Y. pestis* not only survives but also multiplies. Infected mononuclear cells are carried to regional lymph nodes. As *Y. pestis* replicates, the lymph nodes become inflamed and swell, forming the bubo. Bubo most frequently develop in the submandibular and sublingual lymph nodes in the cat. Bubo eventually undergo necrosis and abscess formation, with eventual dissemination of the organism after 2 to 6 days via either the lymphatic channels or the blood stream to other organs, including the lungs. Replication in the mononuclear cells results in the production of a capsular envelope, which renders the organism resistant to further phagocytosis. When the organism is ingested or inhaled from contaminated tissues or fluids (rather than being transmitted through a flea bite), which is common in cats and other carnivores, the organism has already acquired this phagocytosis-resistant capsule from the previous host's mononuclear cells. Infection spreads more quickly, resulting in a shorter incubation period of 1 to 3 days.

Lesions at the site of inoculation are usually minimal. The most common visible lesions are in the lymph nodes that drain the site of inoculation. Marked lymphadenomegaly (bubo formation) develops, and nodes may abscess and drain a thick, creamy pus through fistulous tracts. Both deep and superficial lymph nodes in other parts of the body may become similarly infected after hematogenous or lymphogenous spread of the organism. In the bacteremic state, other tissues, such as the eye, liver, kidney, heart, spleen, brain, and lung, may become infected. Coalescing areas of infection and necrosis may result in parenchymal abscesses. *Y. pestis* contains endotoxins that may result in edema, septic shock, and disseminated intravascular coagulopathy. The clinical course may last 6 to 20 days.

Sixteen healthy cats that were experimentally infected with *Y. pestis* exhibited one of three responses. Thirty-eight percent died within 4 to 9 days after ingestion of a plague-infected mouse. The clinical course included fever (40.7° C to 41.2° C [105° F to 106° F]), depression, and submandibular lymphadenomegaly. Forty-four percent developed transient infections characterized by fever, depression, and lymphade-

nomegaly. In contrast to cats that maintained an elevated body temperature and eventually died of plague, the cats that survived demonstrated a sharp drop in body temperature by day 4 and had clinically recovered by day 14. Nineteen percent of the cats exposed to a plague-infected mouse showed no signs of clinical illness and had no hematologic changes.[14] Most cats fed infected mice had *Y. pestis* cultured from their oropharynx and could have transmitted plague. In the natural environment the mortality in cats approaches 50%.[20] Cats with previous antibody titers to plague by either vaccination or natural infection generally have a more protracted illness but are not protected from bacteremia or death.

CLINICAL FINDINGS

Cats

In people and cats, three clinical forms of the disease have been recognized: bubonic, septicemic, and pneumonic plague. The most common and probably the least fatal form is bubonic plague. In cats, bubonic plague is associated with high temperature (40.6° C to 41.2° C [105° F to 106° F]), dehydration, lymphadenomegaly, and hyperesthesia. It is usually acquired by ingesting infected rodents, and the submandibular, retropharyngeal, and cervical lymph nodes in the area of inoculation become enlarged, form abscesses, and may drain. Drainage is not always apparent; however, cats with abscesses that spontaneously drain are more likely to survive. If allowed to progress, the bubonic form of plague may spread hematogenously or through the lymphatics to become the septic form.

Septicemic plague may develop with or without bubo formation. Hematogenous spread may result in involvement of virtually every organ in the body, although the most frequently involved organs are the spleen in people and lungs in cats. Features of septic shock, such as fever, anorexia, vomiting, diarrhea, tachycardia, weak pulse, hypotension, cold extremities, DIC, and marked leukocytosis are characteristic of the septic form of the disease in the cat. The septic form is usually fatal within 1 to 2 days after the presence of bacteremia.

Pneumonic plague in cats can develop *secondary* to hematogenous or lymphogenous spread of the organism and may be considered a sequel to bubonic or septic forms of the disease, whereas *primary* pneumonic plague is contracted through droplet transmission. Although cats normally do not contract primary pneumonic plague, they have been responsible for primary pneumonic plague in people who have contact with them. Pneumonic plague, whether primary or secondary, has the worst prognosis. In addition, persistent fevers of greater than 40° C (104° F) in cats are associated with poor prognoses. In people, untreated pneumonic plague is 100% fatal. In summary, plague should be considered when examining any febrile cat in endemic areas. Other atypical clinical signs have included ocular discharge, vomiting, diarrhea, dehydration, weight loss, a poor hair coat, a swollen tongue, tonsillar enlargement, necrotic stomatitis, facial ulceration, cellulitis, and abdominal distention.[5,11]

Dogs

Clinical illness is less likely in dogs because of their apparent resistance to infection. Fever, anorexia, cervical and mandibular lymphadenomegaly and abscessation, and coughing have been observed in naturally infected dogs.[23]

DIAGNOSIS

Although a clinician may be highly suspicious of plague in an animal on the basis of clinical and epidemiologic information, the diagnosis must be confirmed. Pneumonic plague may be indicated by pneumonic lesions visualized with thoracic radi-

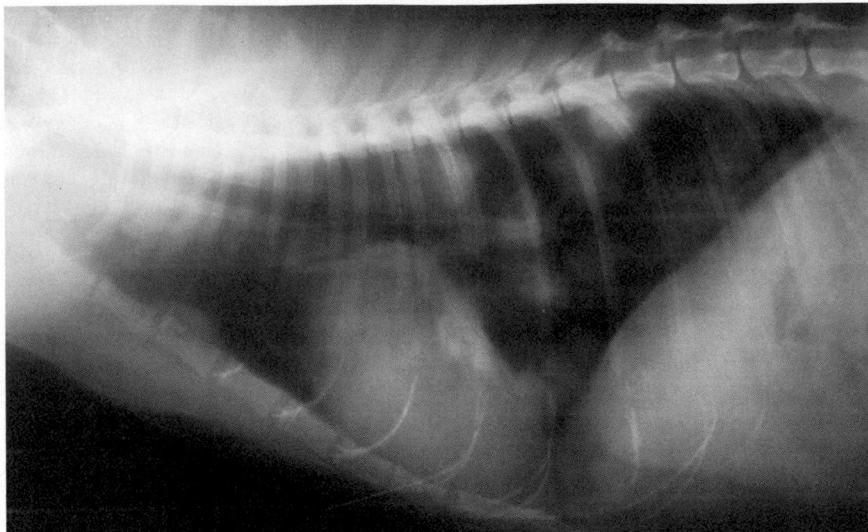

Fig 47-4 Thoracic radiograph of a cat with pneumonic plague. (Courtesy Dennis Macy, Colorado State University, Fort Collins, Colo.)

ographs (Fig. 47-4). *Y. pestis* is usually found in large numbers in infected tissues. In the clinical setting, it is important to collect samples and start antimicrobial therapy before the disease is confirmed. Needle aspirates from lymph nodes, blood, or infected tissue may be selected based on the clinical form of the disease in the patient. A quick Gram stain of these tissues usually reveals a monomorphic population of gram-negative organisms (Fig. 47-5), whereas common cat bite abscesses usually contain a mixture of organisms found in the feline oral cavity. Aseptically collected samples of fluids, tissues, lymph node aspirates, or blood should be submitted. Cultures of tonsils from experimentally infected cats have given consistently positive results, and the tonsils may serve as a source of infection of the saliva. Four or more slides for bacterial stains should be prepared by making impression smears or cytologic smears, allowing them to air dry, and then lightly heat fixing them over a flame. Care should be taken to avoid contact with purulent material while obtaining and preparing these samples. Individuals with the expertise to conduct plague tests are generally only found in public health laboratories in endemic areas and in the United States at the plague laboratory of the Centers for Disease Control and Prevention (CDC).

To make smears for direct fluorescent antibody testing, fluid specimens are applied to clean, thin, glass slides. One or two drops of sample fluid are placed on the slide into two circles made with a wax pencil. The drops are spread with a loop. With tissue specimens, impression smears are made within each circle. Slides are allowed to air dry and should be frozen if they cannot be shipped or examined immediately. This test provides the most rapid, presumptive diagnosis with good reliability.

For serologic confirmation, two serum samples should be collected 10 to 14 days apart for antibody titers against *Y. pestis*. Because dogs and cats in endemic areas frequently have high titers to *Y. pestis* that persist for a year or longer after exposure, a fourfold rise in titer is needed to distinguish active disease from previous exposure. Early in the course of disease, results of serologic testing are often negative.

Alternatively, specimens for culture may be collected using a sterile syringe by aspiration (before antimicrobial therapy is instituted) and placed in blood tubes or inoculated into transport media (Stuarts [Difco, Detroit, Mich.] or Cary-Blair [BBL, Cockeysville, Md.]). Refrigerated but not frozen, they are sent to a reference laboratory for confirmation. No fixa-

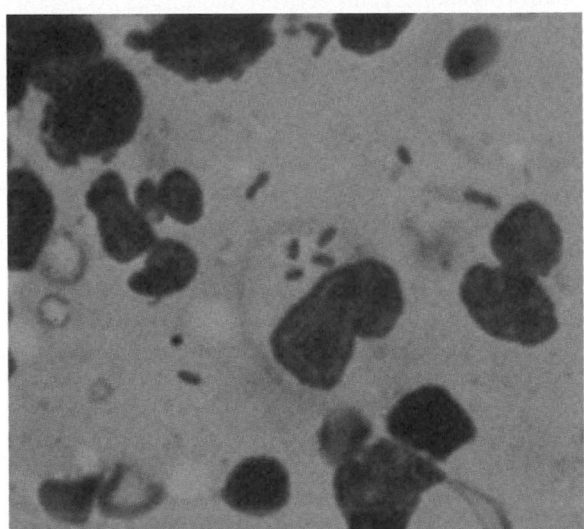

Fig 47-5 Fine-needle aspirate of bubo from cat with plague. Note monomorphic population of bipolar staining coccobacillus organisms. (Courtesy Dennis Macy, Colorado State University, Fort Collins, Colo.)

tives or preservatives should be used. Veterinarians should not attempt to culture specimens, because class II precautions must be taken when isolating and identifying cultures from animals with possible plague. Samples should be wrapped in a double-thickness of plastic and padded to prevent breakage and leakage, which complies with federal requirements for transporting hazardous agents. It is recommended that the state veterinarian or health department be contacted before shipping samples to the Division of Vectorborne Infectious Disease.[970]* Local public health officials may recommend that regional or state laboratories conduct the specialized serologic or cultural testing for plague (see Appendix 5).

At the laboratory, Gram stains are performed to determine staining characteristics, and Giemsa or Wayson stains are per-

*Division of Vectorborne Infectious Disease, Centers for Disease Control and Prevention, P.O. Box 2087, Fort Collins, CO 80522, 970-221-6400.

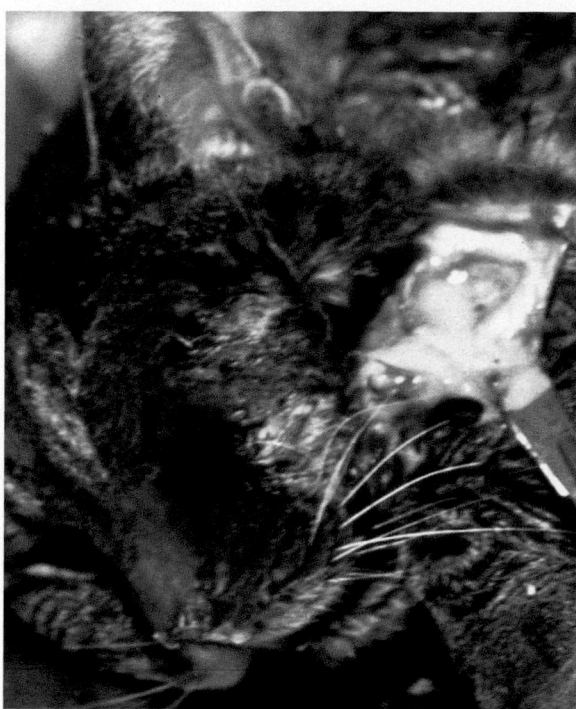

Fig 47-6 Necropsy of cat infected with plague. Note marked swelling (bubo) and purulent exudate from abscess visible on incision of the superficial cervical lymph node. (Courtesy P.W. Gasper, University of Maryland, College Park, Md.)

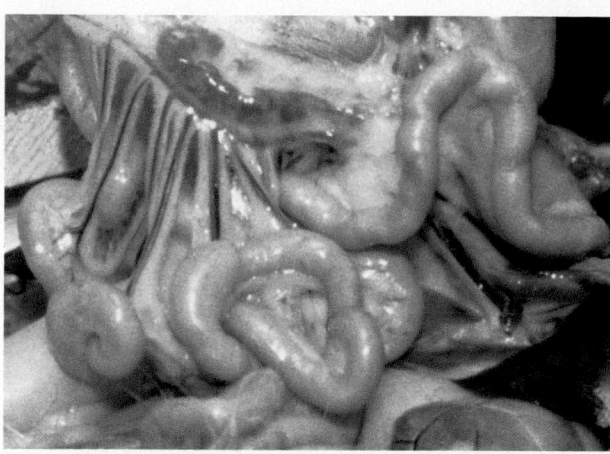

Fig 47-7 Mesenteric lymph node from cat infected with plague. Node is markedly enlarged and hemorrhagic. (Courtesy P.W. Gasper, University of Maryland, College Park, Md.)

formed to determine whether the bipolar "safety-pin" appearance suggestive of *Y. pestis* is present. *Y. pestis* can be cultured on enriched blood agar but grows slowly, requiring 48 hours of incubation at an optimum temperature of 28° C to produce nonmucoid 1- to 2-mm gray colonies. If growth is observed, suspect isolates can be shipped to a reference laboratory. A polymerase chain reaction procedure has been developed to identify the presence of the organism in tissues, blood, and fleas.[16]

PATHOLOGIC FINDINGS

Cats, of which 50% die acutely, may have focal necrotic lesions of the adrenal glands, spleen, and liver, with evidence of secondary pneumonic spread of the disease. Those surviving for longer periods develop cervical or submandibular abscesses or bubos (Fig. 47-6). Consistent involvement of the cranial and cervical lymph nodes was apparent when cats were experimentally infected by the oral route.[29] In fatal cases, tonsils and submandibular, cranial thoracic, and mesenteric lymph nodes were also affected (Fig. 47-7). The normal nodal architecture is totally replaced by hemorrhage, suppuration, and necrosis (Fig. 47-8). Lymph nodes from cats that were euthanized after clinical recovery showed only lymphoid hyperplasia. Bacterial infiltration of the lung parenchyma, resulting in diffuse interstitial pneumonia, is characterized by focal areas of hemorrhage with clusters of bacteria. Coalescing areas of necrosis and abscess formation can occur. Because experimentally infected dogs develop only transient fever and lymphadenomegaly, no pathologic features have been described.

THERAPY

The decision to treat an animal for plague is seldom based on a definitive diagnosis. When plague is suspected on the basis of clinical or epidemiologic information, clinicians should not wait for laboratory confirmation before beginning specific antimicrobial therapy. All plague suspects should be handled by persons wearing gloves, gowns, eye protection, and high-density surgical masks. Animals with respiratory signs should have thoracic radiographs taken to determine whether they have pneumonic plague. Animals should be examined for fleas; if any are found, patients in surrounding cages and examination rooms should be treated with carbamates or pyrethrins. Bubos should be lanced and flushed with chlorhexidine diacetate (Nolvasan, Fort Dodge, Fort Dodge, Ia). Organic material, including tissues or pus-containing gauze pads, should be double bagged and incinerated. Routine disinfectants are effective in killing the plague organism and should be applied as a precautionary measure on cages and examination tables used in the care of infected animals.

Y. pestis is susceptible to a wide variety of antimicrobial agents (Table 47-1). Unfortunately, multiple drug-resistant strains are being isolated with increasing frequency.[9] Although *Y. pestis* appears to be sensitive in vitro to penicillin, it is resistant to β-lactam antibiotics in vivo. Aminoglycosides such as streptomycin and gentamicin are considered the most effective antibiotics against *Y. pestis*.[2a] Treatment efficacy with penicillins or aminoglycosides has been increased in experimentally infected mice by using successive therapy with rifampin.[21] Chloramphenicol is used in the treatment of patients with central nervous system spread of plague organism. Administration of tetracyclines has been associated with relapse, presumably caused by the development of bacterial resistance or poor absorption from the gastrointestinal tract. Tetracyclines (with doxycycline being preferred) are given primarily for the bubonic form of the disease and for prophylaxis. The fluoroquinolones and doxycycline have been shown to be effective in the treatment of plague in mice.[4,27] No clinical data exist on the effectiveness of fluoroquinolones, so their use in treating cats or dogs is not recommended. Infected cats should be treated for a minimum of 21 days. Treatment should continue far beyond the resolution of bubos and pneumonic changes. Patients should be isolated during the first 48 to 72 hours of antibiotic therapy. Animals with plague pneumonia should remain hospitalized for slightly longer periods to avoid inadvertent exposure to caregivers in their home environment.

Prophylactic therapy with a tetracycline is indicated in asymptomatic animals exposed to plague and should be continued for 7 days. People exposed to plague while caring for plague-infected animals are usually treated with a similar

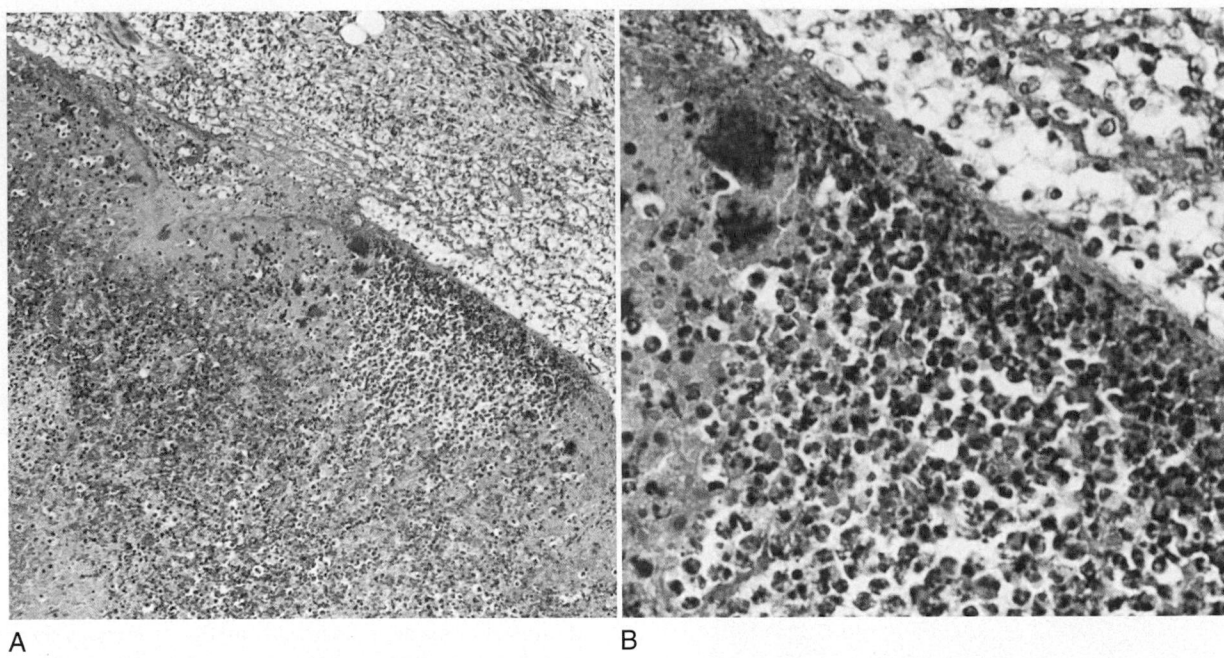

A   B

Fig   47-8   Low power **(A)** and high power **(B)** view of lymph node suppuration and necrosis from cat infected with plague. Note massive necrosis of lymphocytes, hemorrhage, and colonies of bacteria (H and E stain, ×10 **[A]** and ×40 **[B]**). (Courtesy Armed Forces Institute of Pathology, Washington, D.C.)

Table • 47-1

Antimicrobial Therapy for Plague

DRUG[a]	DOSE[b] (MG/KG)	ROUTE	INTERVAL (HOURS)	DURATION (DAYS)
Streptomycin[c]	5	IM	12	21
Kanamycin[c]	5–7.5	IM	12	21
Gentamicin[c]	2–4	IM	12–24	21
Trimethoprim-sulfonamide	15	PO, IV, IM	12	21
Tetracycline	20	PO	8	21
Doxycycline	5–10	PO	12	21
Chloramphenicol	15	PO, SC	12	21

IM, Intramuscular; *PO*, by mouth; *IV*, intravenous.
[a]See Appendix 8 for more information about these drugs.
[b]Dose per administration at specified interval (see Appendix 8).
[c]Renal function must be closely monitored because of potential nephrotoxicity.

therapy by a physician. The prognosis depends on the clinical form of the disease and the species infected.

PREVENTION

People and domestic animals have intruded into the natural ecosystem in which plague circulates. Elimination of plague in wild rodent populations is generally impossible. Risk factors for cats include living in or visiting rural areas in endemic regions, flea infestation, and hunting or eating rodents and rabbits. Veterinarians should be especially alert when evaluating sick cats during plague outbreaks and take appropriate precautions to protect themselves, their employees, and their clients. Examination of fleas taken from patients may quickly reveal whether they are of rodent source. Flea control in dogs and cats should be stressed in enzootic areas, because pets have ample opportunity to spread fleas to their owners.

Fipronil has been effective in control of vector fleas from ground squirrels.[22] Dogs and cats should not be allowed to come in contact with burrows or have access to carcasses of dead rodents or lagomorphs. Residents in endemic areas should be encouraged to decrease the availability of food and habitats (such as trash or garbage piles) for peridomestic host species, which may become infected during enzootic outbreaks. Climate dynamics such as increased rainfall that augment flea and small mammal populations enhance the risk of plague. Local and state health officials may institute rodent control measures but not before flea control has been instituted in the area.

In the veterinary hospital, inadvertent nosocomical spread to the veterinary hospital staff is a serious problem that can occur before a diagnosis has been confirmed. Therefore veterinarians in endemic regions should be extremely aware of possible plague. Risk of droplet or airborne spread to caregivers can be decreased with protective well-fitted surgical masks and eyewear. Droplets, which can travel up to 2 m, can be generated by coughing, by sneezing, or during lavage or aspiration of abscesses. Infected or possibly infected animals should be isolated from other animals and have their movement restricted. Contaminated droplets do not remain suspended, so special measures for ventilation and air handling are not required. After pneumonia has been discounted or the animal has been treated for at least 72 hours, standard precautions for handling contagious diseases can be implemented. Standard precautions include washing hands before and after contact with animals, wearing gloves when contacting body fluids or tissues, and wearing gowns to minimize transfer of the organism to clothing, other animals, and the surrounding environment.*

Killed and modified live vaccines for *Y. pestis* have been produced for human use. The killed formalin-fixed virulent whole-organism preparation was used in the United States until 1999. No plague vaccine is approved for use in the United States. Even in areas where vaccine is available, vaccination of veterinary staff is not recommended.[12] Immunization of cats with the killed vaccine did not protect them against bacteremia or death and prolonged the clinical course of the disease. In the past, vaccination has been recommended for all laboratory and field personnel who are working with *Y. pestis* and for persons engaged in field operations in areas of enzootic plague. Experimental subunit vaccines have been evaluated and appear to protect against bubonic and pneumonic plague.[28]

PUBLIC HEALTH CONSIDERATIONS

Human plague is seasonal, with most cases in the Northern Hemisphere occurring between March and October. A total of 377 cases in people were reported from 1970 to 2001.[23] The incidence of human plague in the United States is increasing. The 105 cases that occurred in 8 western states during the 1970s represented the largest number in the continental United States in any decade since 1900 to 1909. In decreasing order of number of cases, 90% of the human cases of plague reported were from New Mexico, Arizona, Colorado, and California. Since 1949, New Mexico has reported annually more than 50% of plague cases. In one survey, 82% of human plague cases were transmitted by flea bites, 15% by direct contact with infected wild animals, and 3% by contact with infected domestic cats. A review of 297 cases of plague in the western United States found that 7.7% of the cases in people were associated with handling infected cats.[7]

From 1977 to 1998 the CDC confirmed 23 human plague infections acquired through inhalation of *Y. pestis*–infected droplets expelled from cats with secondary plague pneumonia.[12] Approximately one fifth of those infected died, and one fourth of those infected were veterinarians or their technicians. The remaining three fourths of those infected were owners of or people caring for sick cats. Approximately three fourths of the people developed bubonic plague, one person developed septicemic plague, and the remainder developed a pneumonic infection.[23] The overall death rate in the United States for humans treated for plague is 15% to 22%. The two primary reasons people die from this treatable disease are that (1) they delay seeking medical attention, and (2) a clinician does not recognize the disease as plague. These factors are even more likely to play a role when people acquire the infection in enzootic areas and travel to areas of the United States where clinicians have never seen patients with plague. The death rates in such instances has been 80%. Enhanced awareness is needed for early diagnosis and successful treatment.[7]

All free-roaming cats in an endemic area must be considered at risk for exposure to plague. Veterinarians and their assistants are more likely to be exposed to plague because of their occupations. People may become infected by inhaling respiratory droplets from animals infected with secondary pneumonic plague, through broken skin or mucous membranes while handling infected tissues and body fluids, or through bites of plague-infected fleas. Patients suspected of having plague should be hospitalized and isolated immediately, and attempts should be made to limit the number of individuals caring for infected animals. They should be educated about plague transmission and advised to wear protective clothing and gloves while treating and caring for infected pets. Routine disinfectants should be applied to cages and examination tables, and flea control should be instituted in the area housing affected infected animals. Veterinarians who diagnose plague in cats should advise the cat owners to contact their physicians immediately. Local and state health authorities should be notified early in the management of plague-infected animals.

PLAGUE AS A BIOLOGIC WEAPON

Plague has caused more human deaths than most other diseases and wars combined. It is estimated to have killed one fourth to one third of Europe's population in the Middle Ages. Antibiotic therapy and public health advances make a natural global pandemic unlikely. However, because *Y. pestis* is extremely virulent, can be transmitted from human to human, and has antibiotic-resistant strains that have emerged naturally or been developed in the laboratory, plague is considered a high-priority bioterrorism agent. The plague bacillus has been classified as a Category A, Critical Biologic Agent, by the CDC.[1] Plague was first used as a weapon in the 14th century when the Tatar army catapulted diseased corpses over enemy walls in the Crimea. In World War II the Japanese army secret unit 731 reportedly sprayed grain laced with plague-infected fleas over Chinese cities, causing plague outbreaks. In the 1950s and 1960s the American and the Soviet biological weapons programs developed techniques to aerosolize plague particles. The intentional release of a plague cloud could result in an outbreak of fatal pneumonic plague. In 1970 the World Health Organization reported that, in a worst-case scenario, 50 kg of aerosolized *Y. pestis* released over a city of 5 million people would cause 150,000 people to develop pneumonic plague, 36,000 of whom would die. Plague bacilli would remain viable as an aerosol for 1 hour for a distance of up to 10 km. Inhabitants attempting to leave the area would spread the disease even more. The most likely first indication of an attack would be a sudden outbreak of severe pneumonia and sepsis. The presence of hemoptysis in previously healthy people and symptoms of fever, cough, shortness of breath, cheat pain, and rapid death suggest plague. The secondary spread of plague from person to person, animal to person, and person to animal would be likely.

SUGGESTED READINGS*

12. Gage KL, Dennis DT, Orloski KA, et al. 2000. Cases of cat-associated human plague in the Western US, 1977-1998. *Clin Infect Dis* 30:893-900.

14. Gasper PW, Barnes AM, Ovan TJ. 1993. Plague *(Yersinia pestis)* in cats: description of experimentally-induced disease. 1993. *J Med Entomol* 30:20-26.

17a. Jarrett CO, Deak E, Isherwood KE, et al. 2004. Transmission of *Yersinia pestis* from an infectious biofilm in the flea vector, *J Infect Dis* 190:783-792.

*See www.cdc.gov/ncidod/hip/ISOLAT/Isolat.htm for additional information on biocontainment of plague-infected animals.

23. Orloski KA, Lathrop SL. 2003. Plague, a veterinary perspective. *J Am Vet Med Assoc* 222:444-448.
27. Russell P, Eley SM, Green M, et al. 1998. Efficacy of doxycycline and ciprofloxacin against experimental *Yersinia pestis* infection. 1998. *J Antimocrob Chemother* 41:301-305.
29. Watson RP, Blanchard TW, Mense MG, et al. 2001. Histopathology of experimental plague in cats. *Vet Pathol* 38:165-172.

*See the CD-ROM for a complete list of references.

CHAPTER 48

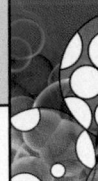

Tularemia

Craig E. Greene and Brad M. DeBey

ETIOLOGY

Tularemia is an acute bacterial infection of many avian and mammalian species, including dogs and cats and occasionally people. Terrestrial and aquatic mammals serve as reservoirs for the disease. It occurs throughout the temperate region of the Northern Hemisphere, predominantly between 20 and 70 degrees latitude.[17] The etiologic agent, *Francisella tularensis*, is a small (0.2 × 0.2 to 0.7 μm), pleomorphic, gram-negative, non–spore-forming bacillus. The tularemia bacillus has two main biovars: type A (subsp. *tularensis*; previously *nearctica*) and type B (subsp. *holarctica*; previously *palearctica*). Type A strains ferment glycerol and are highly virulent for laboratory rabbits *(Oryctolagus cuniculus)*, and type B strains do not ferment glycerol and are avirulent for rabbits. Type A strains are associated with a tick-rabbit cycle of infection and occur only in North America. Type B strains have a more complex epidemiology—involving rodents, ticks, mosquitoes, mud, muskrats, beavers, and water—and occur throughout the Northern Hemisphere. Both type A and B strains have been isolated from cats in the United States.[3] Human illness is generally more severe with type A strain infections.[28] Two less frequently isolated biotypes include subspecies *mediasiatica*, found in Kazakhstan and Uzbekistan, and *novicida*, primarily from North America. Subspecies *novicida* is of low virulence.

EPIDEMIOLOGY

Tularemia is endemic in the Northern Hemisphere between the latitudes of 30 degrees N and 71 degrees N (Fig. 48-1). This area includes much of Eurasia to countries on the Mediterranean coast of Africa. In North America, this region ranges from the Arctic Circle as far south as Guadalajara, Mexico. Tularemia is a rural disease in people and in their pets as a result of contact with wildlife reservoirs, their vectors, or the contaminated environment.

In Eurasia, cricetine rodents (e.g., meadow voles, lemmings, muskrats), hares, and bites of infected mosquitoes are important sources of infection. In North America, the principal animal sources are the cottontail rabbit (*Sylvilagus* spp.) and wild hares and rodents, as well as the ticks that infest them. Biting flies mechanically transfer the infection.

In the United States, four tick species constitute the primary vectors for dogs and cats: the wood tick *(Dermacentor andersoni)* found in the Rocky Mountain region; the American dog tick *(D. variabilis)* found in the eastern two-thirds of the country, as well as in the Pacific coastal states; the Pacific Coast tick *(D. occidentalis)* found in California and Oregon; and the Lone Star tick *(Amblyomma americanum)* found in the southern central and southeastern states. The incidence of infection for people in the United States is presented in Fig. 48-2.

Because the epidemiology of tularemia is complex, and its host species so diverse,[17] only the aspects that are important in its transmission to dogs and cats are discussed here (Fig. 48-3). Various tick species, which are true biologic vectors for the disease, serve as both reservoirs and vectors of tularemia. Infection can pass transovarially in ticks, and infection persists for life. Amplification of the infection rate in a tick population occurs when uninfected ticks feed on bacteremic animals. Although ticks are capable of transmitting tularemia at all three stages of their development, the adult and, less commonly, nymphal stages are most important in transmission to dogs, cats, and people.

Cats and dogs may also be infected when they hunt or eat infected rabbits or rodents. Transmission can also occur through bites or scratches from other predators with contaminated teeth or claws. Infection in people has developed following inhalation of aerosols or dusts or ingestion of food or water contaminated with the organism. Numerous blood-feeding insects (such as mosquitoes or biting flies) can serve as mechanical vectors for the disease when their mouthparts become contaminated when they bite infected hosts.

PATHOGENESIS

In the laboratory, *F. tularensis* requires enriched growth media and replicates in a variety of cells. In vivo, it is a facultative intracellular pathogen. Macrophages are the major host cell, and the organism's capsule is thought to be important in its intracellular survival. The infectious dose is extremely low, and inhaling 10 to 50 colony-forming units is enough to induce disease.

The clinical presentation of human tularemia varies by route of infection and initial sites of localization. Typically, a localized infection occurs at the primary inoculation site and is associated with prominent regional lymphadenomegaly. In a highly susceptible host, only less than 50 organisms can cause

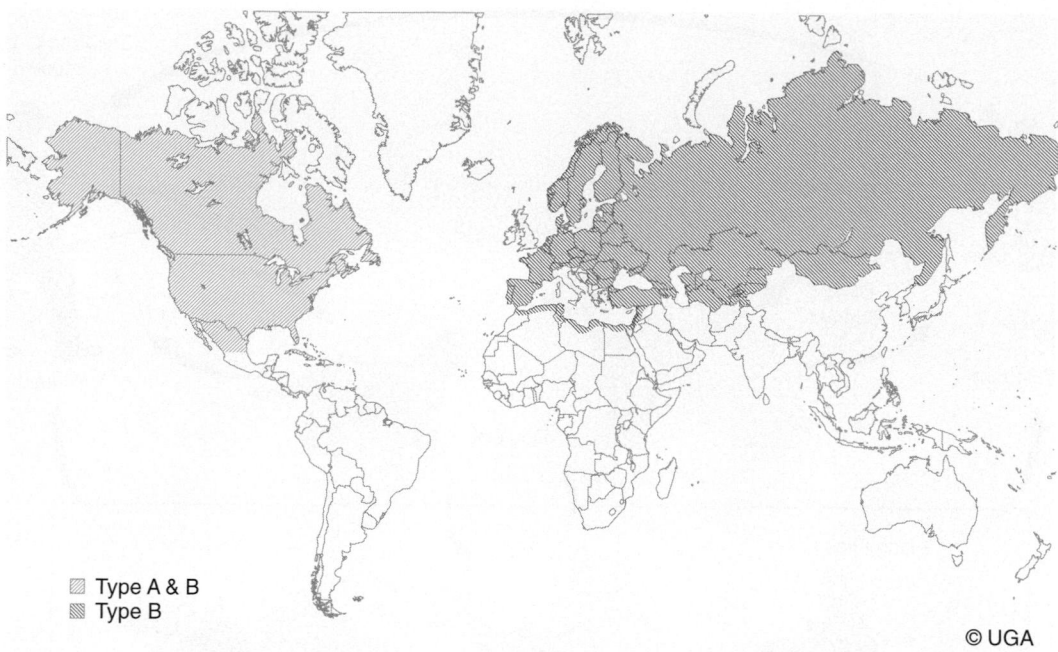

☐ Type A & B
☒ Type B

© UGA

Fig 48-1 Worldwide distribution map of tularemia. (Map courtesy University of Georgia, Athens, Ga.)

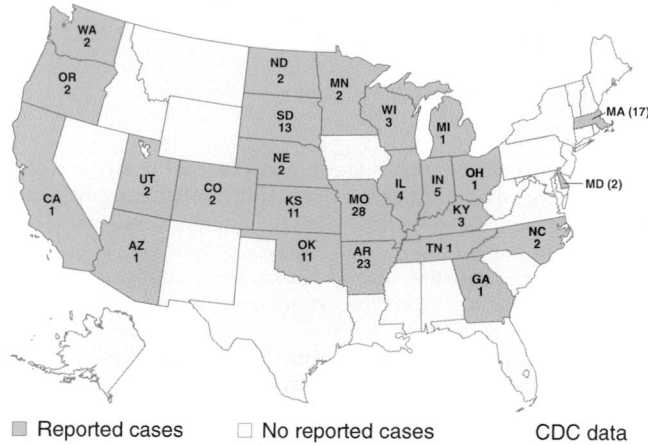

■ Reported cases   ☐ No reported cases   CDC data

Fig 48-2 Yearly incidence data of tularemia in the United States for 2002. (Data from the Centers for Disease Control and Prevention, Atlanta, Ga. Map courtesy University of Georgia, Athens, Ga.)

infection by parenteral inoculation, while at least 10^8 are needed for oral infection. Subsequent bacteremia and multiorgan involvement are common. The lungs, spleen, liver, lymph nodes, and skin are the sites of embolic spread (Fig. 48-4). Early embolic lesions, which begin as microabscesses, progress to granulomatous inflammation as the body attempts to wall off the infection. Bacteremic disease without antecedent localized infection is referred to as typhoidal tularemia. Cell-mediated immunity plays an important role in recovery.

A similar disease pattern appears to occur in dogs and cats. The severity of illness in experimentally infected dogs varies with age; puppies are more susceptible than are young adults. Ingestion of infected tissues or intradermal (ID) challenge produced milder disease than intranasal (IN) challenge.[13,19] When dogs were fed infected tissues, an acute 5-day illness began after a 48-hour incubation period.[19] Fever (40.2° C [104.4° F]) and a mucopurulent discharge from the nose and eyes

were present. Transient ulceroglandular tularemia follows ID challenge with concomitant development of fever, pustules at the inoculation site, and regional lymphadenomegaly.

More serious illness characterized by septicemia and high mortality follows subcutaneous (SC) or intramuscular (IM) inoculation. Draining abscesses develop at the inoculation sites and are associated with regional lymphadenomegaly and high temperature and with systemic dissemination of the disease after 1 week. At this time, the dogs appear obviously ill, have mucopurulent ocular and nasal discharges, and develop a vesiculopapular skin rash.

Cats have become ill after eating experimentally infected guinea pigs.[30] Although some cats appear unaffected, younger cats succumb primarily to systemic (typhoidal) infection characterized by generalized lymphadenomegaly and miliary abscess formation involving the liver and spleen.

After SC inoculation, similar findings have been apparent, and young kittens appear most susceptible.[30] Some SC- and IN-inoculated cats have had areas of bronchopneumonia from which *F. tularensis* was isolated, as well as splenomegaly and multifocal hepatic necrosis.

Respiratory disease resulting from inhaling *F. tularensis* has a more virulent course. This form has been observed more in people than animals. Coughing, fever, hilar lymphadenomegaly, and pulmonary infiltration occur. Mortality is more common with this form of illness.

CLINICAL FINDINGS

Dogs

Despite the ability to produce experimental infections and high seroprevalence, indicating exposure in endemic areas, naturally acquired infections in dogs have been rare.* Dogs are considered relatively resistant to tularemia. Typically, a dog develops a brief episode of anorexia, listlessness, and low-grade fever. Sudden death of uncertain cause has occurred in a dog a few days after sniffing a dead infected rabbit.

*References: 5, 8, 13, 17, 24, 24a.

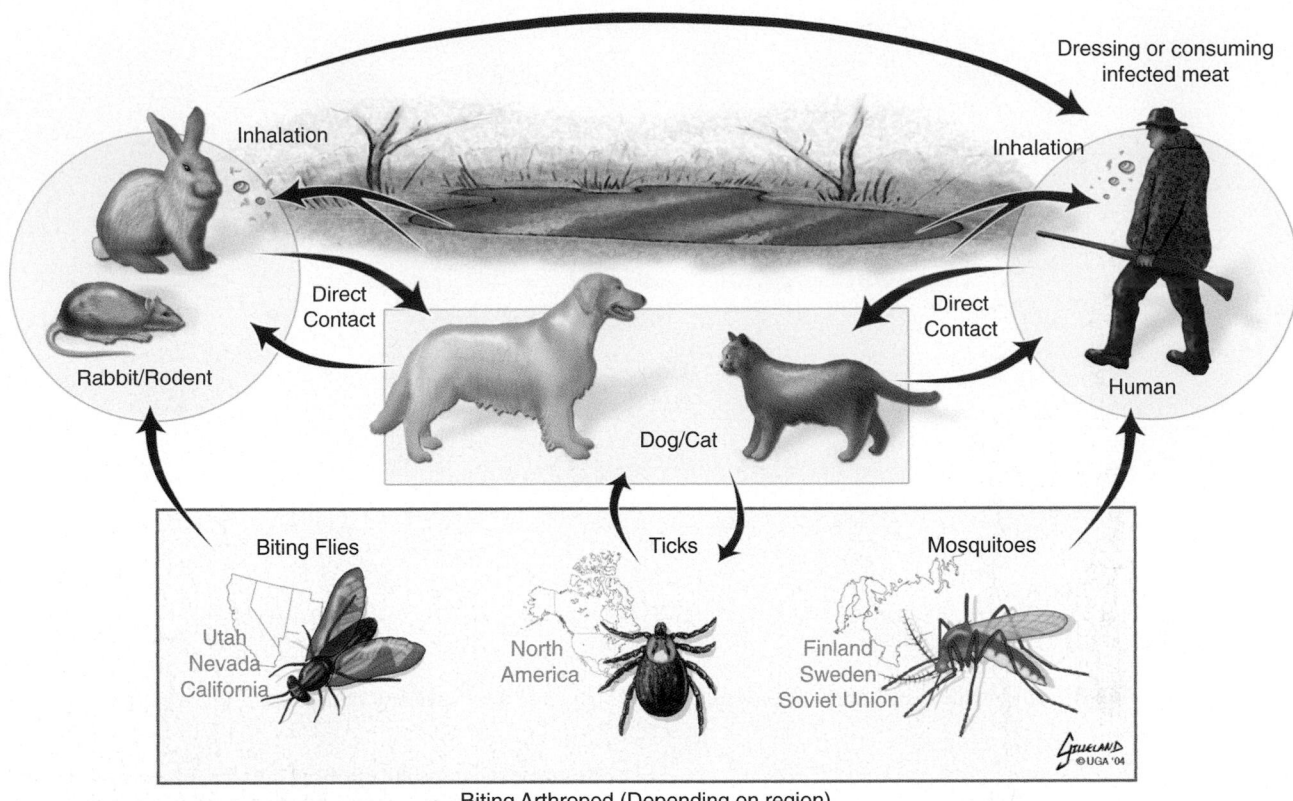

Fig 48-3 Sylvatic cycle of *F. tularensis* in the environment. (Courtesy University of Georgia, Athens, Ga.)

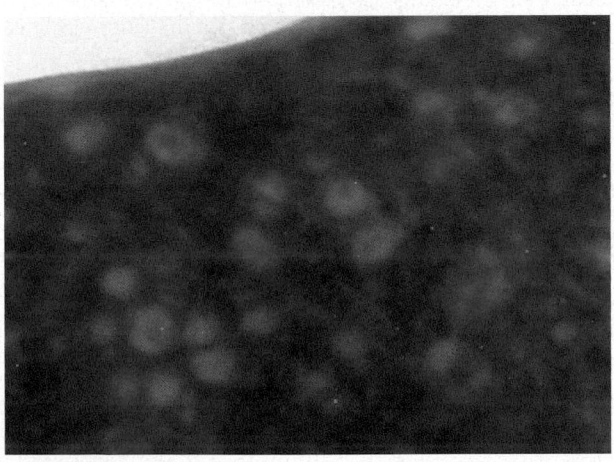

Fig 48-4 Multifocal necrosis with fibrinosuppurative and granulomatous inflammation in the spleen of a cat infected with *F. tularensis*. (Courtesy Dept. of Veterinary Pathology, Kansas State University, Manhattan, Kans.)

Another dog developed multifocal draining abscesses in the SC tissue and superficial lymph nodes in addition to fever, anorexia, myalgia, and shivering. Uveitis and conjunctivitis developed in the left eye, with subsequent transient conjunctivitis and corneal clouding in the right eye.

Cats

Based on the large number of reports, cats are more susceptible to tularemia compared with dogs. The spectrum of illness associated with spontaneous feline tularemia has not been well described. In a series of three typhoidal cases, pertinent clinical signs included fever; marked depression; pharyngeal, cervical, mesenteric, regional, or generalized (or any combination) lymphadenomegaly; palpable splenomegaly and hepatomegaly; acute shallow oral or lingual ulcers (or both); icterus; and panleukopenia with severe toxic changes of neutrophils.[3] The oral and lingual ulcers were compatible with infection resulting from ingestion of infected rodents or rabbits.

Other cases in cats have been briefly described in epidemiologic reports of human cases.* Implicated cats had frequently eaten or mouthed wild rabbits before the onset of clinical signs. Variable signs of fever, anorexia, listlessness, lymphadenomegaly, draining abscesses, and, occasionally, icterus and death were reported. Some cats had no signs of illness.

DIAGNOSIS

Laboratory abnormalities in tularemia have been leukocytosis with a left shift, thrombocytopenia, increased serum hepatic transaminases, and hyperbilirubinemia.

Testing for serologic evidence of microscopic agglutinating (MA) antibody is the most commonly used diagnostic procedure. Both dogs and cats develop antibodies, but titers tend to be lower than those observed in people. Titers from 1:140 to 1:160 are typical of recent infections in dogs.[19,28] Using an MA method in cats, serum antibody titers to *F. tularensis* have been above 1:20.[37]

Enzyme-linked immunosorbent assay techniques have been developed to detect antibodies to specific *F. tularensis* antigens in infected people,[4] but their usefulness for testing canine and feline sera is uncertain. Indirect fluorescent antibody methods have also been used for serotesting. A fourfold increase in antibody titer is required to confirm active disease;

*References: 6, 15, 17, 22, 26, 30.

however, a single titer of at least 1:160 suggests active disease.[38] Direct FA methods can be used to detect the coccobacillary organisms in exudates and tissues, even with paraffin-embedded tissues. Polymerase chain reaction (PCR) has also been used to confirm infection. Lymph node aspirates have been of a mixed lymphoid cell population characteristic for hyperplasia.

The isolation of *F. tularensis* from exudates or tissue specimens is the definitive method of diagnosis. The organism is fastidious and must be isolated on special media, such as supplemented chocolate agar, or by initial inoculation of a susceptible laboratory animal with subsequent culture of the liver and spleen. Blood-glucose-cysteine agar or brain-heart infusion agar supplemented with blood is needed for isolation at 37° C. Characteristic dewdrop colonies are isolated. Biosafety level 3 measures must be used to handle infected tissue. Refer to Appendix 5 for a listing of laboratories that perform this isolation.

The infectious dose for humans is less than 100 organisms, inhaled as an aerosol, accidentally inoculated, or splashed in the conjunctival sac. Cultures of *F. tularensis* and necropsies of animals with suspected tularemia should be performed therefore only in laboratories with adequate biosafety equipment. Testing of aspirated pus with PCR has been used for definitive diagnosis of this infection in people.[10]

PATHOLOGIC FINDINGS

Gross necropsy findings in affected dogs and cats are similar. Most of this information has been obtained in experimentally infected animals. Lymph nodes are often markedly enlarged in a regional or more generalized pattern and they often contain multiple foci of necrosis. Draining sinus tracts may arise from the nodes. Hepatomegaly or splenomegaly, or both, may be present. Multiple small, grayish foci representing necrosis are commonly found in the spleen, liver, lung, and, occasionally, heart (Figs. 48-4 and 48-5). Segmental to diffuse hemorrhage of the small and large intestines has been reported in cats.[3] These same cats had prominent ulceration in Peyer's patches and colonic lymphoid follicles. Fibrinosuppurative to granulomatous inflammation is observed in many parenchymal organs (Figs. 48-6, *A* and *B*, 48-7, and 48-8). The causative bacteria are not easily demonstrated in the lesions except by specific FA or other immunohistochemical stains (Fig. 48-9).[9] Where small numbers of organisms are present in lesions,

culture may be more sensitive than immunohistochemistry for diagnosis.[35]

THERAPY

No substantial reports have been made on antimicrobial therapy of canine or feline tularemia. In one cat, surgical removal of a localized subcutaneous mass followed by treatment with amoxicillin-clavulanate was curative.[35] In people, the aminoglycosides (streptomycin and gentamicin) are currently considered the drugs of first choice, but streptomycin is available only on a limited case-by-case basis.[12,25] Therefore parenteral gentamicin treatment is the drug of choice

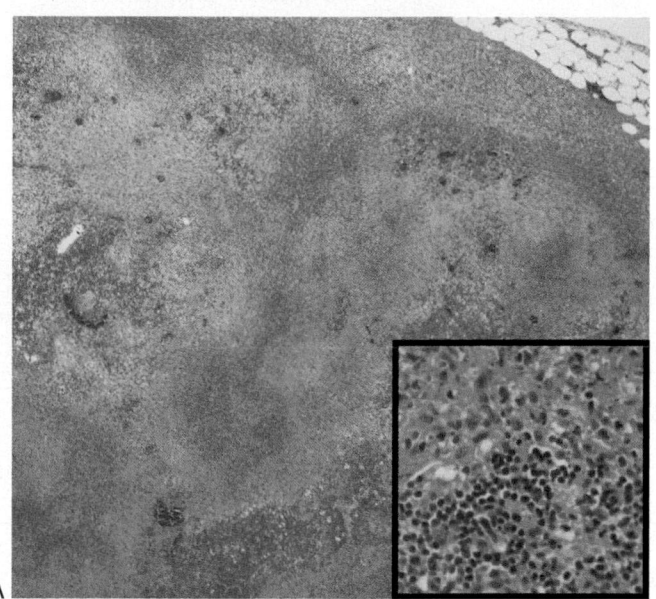

Fig 48-6 **A,** Photomicrograph demonstrating necrosis, fibrinosuppurative and granulomatous inflammation in a mesenteric lymph node of a cat infected with *F. tularensis.* **B,** Inset with higher magnification (H and E stain). (Courtesy Brad DeBey, Kansas State University, Manhattan, Kans.)

Fig 48-5 Multifocal necrosis and granulomatous inflammation in the liver of a cat infected with *F. tularensis.* (Courtesy Brad DeBey, Dept. of Veterinary Pathology, Kansas State University, Manhattan, Kans.)

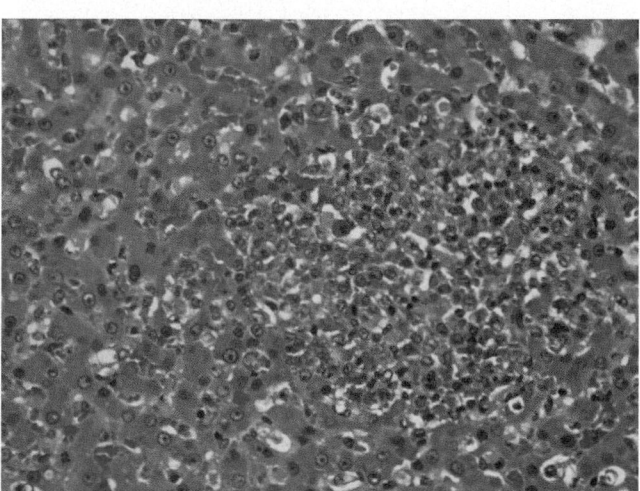

Fig 48-7 Photomicrograph demonstrating focal hepatic necrosis and granulomatous inflammation in a cat infected with *F. tularensis* (H and E stain). (Courtesy Dept. of Veterinary Pathology, Kansas State University, Manhattan, Kans.)

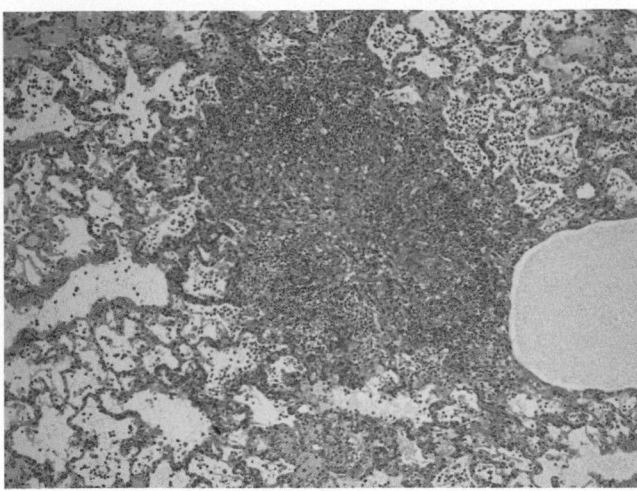

Fig 48-8 Photomicrograph revealing granulomatous and suppurative inflammation in the lung of a cat infected with *F. tularensis* (H and E stain). (Courtesy Dept. of Veterinary Pathology, Kansas State University, Manhattan, Kans.)

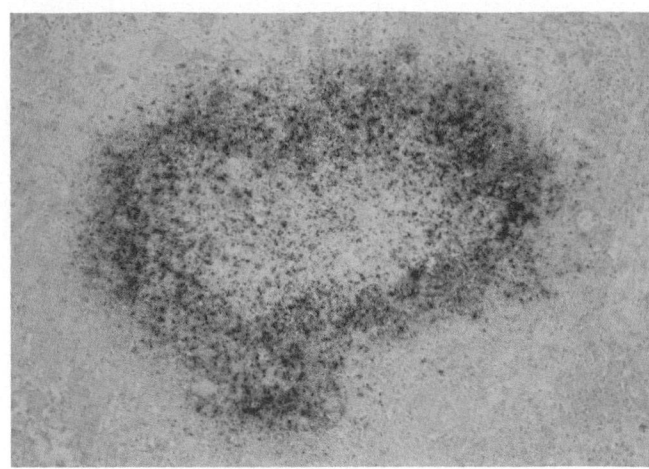

Fig 48-9 Immunohistochemical stain of the spleen of a cat infected with *F. tularensis*. Red areas indicate the location of specific bacterial antigen (peroxidase with hematoxylin counterstain). (Courtesy Dept. of Veterinary Pathology, Kansas State University, Manhattan, Kans.)

Table • 48-1

Drug Therapy for Tularemia

DRUG[a]	SPECIES	DOSE[b]	ROUTE	INTERVAL (HOURS)	DURATION (DAYS)
Gentamicin	B	5 mg/kg	SC, IV, IM	24	7—14
Doxycycline	D	5 mg/kg	PO	12	14
	C	50–100 mg[c]	PO	12	14
Chloramphenicol	C	50 mg/kg	PO, SC, IM	12	14
Enrofloxacin[d]	D	5 mg/kg	PO, SC	12	10
	C	5 mg/kg	PO	24	10

B, Dog and cat; *D*, dog; *C*, cat; *SC*, subcutaneous; *IV*, intravenous; *IM*, intramuscular; *PO*, by mouth.
[a]For additional information on selected drugs, see Drug Formulary, Appendix 8.
[b]Dose per administration at specified interval.
[c]Do not break or crush tablets because they are irritating to the esophagus. Relapses can occur with bacteriostatic drugs such as doxycycline or chloramphenicol.
[d]Other veterinary quinolones such as orbifloxacin, danofloxacin, or marbofloxacin may be substituted at an appropriate dose.

(Table 48-1). Precautions should always be taken to monitor renal function during the treatment interval. Tetracycline and chloramphenicol are potential alternative drugs, but relapses occur frequently with their use. Doxycycline would be the preferred tetracycline because of its superior penetration. Historically, both streptomycin and tetracycline have been given successfully in controlled trials of antibiotic prophylaxis in human tularemia.[27] Quinolones, such as ciprofloxacin and norfloxacin, may be effective[29,31]; however, treatment failures have been described.[7] A significant number of these drugs, such as enrofloxacin, are marketed for animal use. Consult the Drug Formulary, Appendix 8, for dosages and further information on each drug. Because of the potential risk of handling an infected dog or cat, maximal precautions should be used for handling contaminated secretions with gloves and wearing face and eye protection during wound care of hospitalized animals.

PUBLIC HEALTH CONSIDERATIONS

In people, tularemia occurs in two main syndromes: ulceroglandular and typhoidal.[25] Both syndromes have an incubation period of 2 to 10 days followed by acute onset of high temperature, chills, myalgia, and other nonspecific constitutional symptoms. Ulceroglandular tularemia is characterized by a skin ulcer developing at the portal of infection with associated regional lymphadenomegaly. In typhoidal tularemia, few localizing signs of bacteremia occur, pneumonia is more common, and the case-fatality ratio can exceed 30% if the illness is untreated. Other less common syndromes that occur localized to the site of exposure include oculoglandular (Parinaud's syndrome) from conjunctival exposure, glandular with localized lymphadenomegaly, oropharyngeal (characterized by pharyngitis and tonsillitis), and primary pneumonia from inhalation.

In the United States, the incidence of human tularemia is low: fewer than 225 cases annually in the last 10 years.[1] Most cases have resulted from tick-borne infection and to a lesser extent contact with tissues of wild animals such as rabbits. Of the 1041 human cases reported in the southwestern central United States from 1981 to 1987, 17 (1.6%) cases were associated with cat bites and scratches.[32] At least 53 additional cat-associated cases and 8 dog-associated cases have been reported in North America, but some of these have not been well substantiated.* Although cat bites have been associated with these human infections, no cases have emerged of human tularemia from nonbite exposure to cats with systemic infection.[35]

Exposure to airborne organisms is a particular hazard. Before the availability of live vaccines and protective biosafety hoods, accidental infection of laboratory workers was frequent. Occasional outbreaks, in the general population from incidental aerosol exposure to organisms in the environment, are a reminder of its virulence. Nonlaboratory occupations or avocations that have been associated with an increased risk of infection are farmer, veterinarian, sheep worker, hunter or trapper, and cook or meat handler. Landscapers that whack weeds, mow lawns, and blow leaves have become infected in outbreaks.[14]

Cat-associated cases usually involved people being bitten or scratched, with the initial lesion typically developing at the trauma site.[2,6,22,36] Although the cats often have no obvious illness, a common feature has been a history of hunting or eating wild animals, particularly rabbits.

None of the eight dog-associated cases involved bites or scratches. In one case, a young girl developed typhoidal tularemia 3 days after the onset of a vague illness in her pet puppy, which presumably had contact with rabbits.[17] The dog frequently licked the young girl, and its saliva was considered her probable source of infection. In another instance, a family of seven persons staying at a cottage with their dogs during a 1-week period developed pulmonary tularemia.[33] After the dogs finished hunting for rabbits, they would shake the water from their hair when they entered the cottage. The resultant aerosol was considered the most likely source of infection. The dogs never appeared ill but subsequently were found to have antibodies to *F. tularensis*.

Although no cases have been associated with removing ticks from pets, the finding of infected ticks on dogs does indicate a potential hazard.[28] See Therapy section earlier in this text for recommendations on handling infected dogs or cats.

*References: 6, 17, 22, 33, 36.

Owners should be advised concerning risk factors for exposure from their pets.

In Scandinavia, type B infections in people have been more common and have been associated with contaminated water and infected animals that inhabit aquatic environments. Infections with type B in people are less severe and have lower mortality than with type A infections. Most outbreaks have occurred in farmers who processed hay contaminated by dead animals or their secretions, or by contact with mosquitoes. However, epidemiologic assessment of an outbreak showed farming and owning a cat as inherent risk factors.[11] Use of protective clothing and facemasks may be needed when working outdoors in endemic areas.

Bioterrorism Risk and Vaccination

Tularemia has been classified as a potential bioterrorism agent, and outbreaks of infection in people or animals must be reported to public health officials. A live attenuated vaccine is available on an investigational basis for people working in high-risk environments such as research laboratories. The vaccine provides partial protection against severe infection in some people and complete protection in others.

SUGGESTED READINGS*

9. DeBey BM, Andrews GA, Cnard-Bergstrom C, et al. 2002. Immunohistochemical demonstration of *Francisella tularensis* in lesions of cats with tularemia, *J Vet Diagn Invest* 14:162-164.
16. Gustafson BW, DeBowes LJ. 1996. Tularemia in a dog, *J Am Anim Hosp Assoc* 32:339-341.
35. Valentine BA, DeBey BM, Sonn RJ, et al. 2004. Localized cutaneous infection with *Francisella tularensis* resembling ulceroglandular tularemia in a cat, *J Vet Diagn Invest* 16:83-85.
37. Woods JP, Crystal MA, Morton RJ, et al. 1998a. Tularemia in two cats, *J Am Vet Med Assoc* 212:81-83.

*See the CD-ROM for a complete list of references.

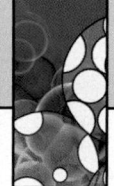

CHAPTER • 49

Actinomycosis and Nocardiosis

David F. Edwards

ACTINOMYCOSIS

Etiology and Epidemiology

Actinomycosis is a chronic, pyogranulomatous disease characterized by pleural and peritoneal exudates, dense fibrous masses, frank abscesses, and fistulous tracts with draining sinuses. The disease is caused by anaerobic actinomycetes that are endogenous saprophytes of mucous membranes and members of the family Actinomycetaceae. *Actinomyces bowdenii, Actinomyces canis, Actinomyces catuli, Actinomyces hordeovulneris, Actinomyces odontolyticus, Actinomyces turicensis,*[67a] *Actinomyces viscosus,* and *Arcanobacterium pyogenes* (formerly *Actinomyces pyogenes*) have been recovered from

infected dogs.* *A. bowdenii, A. viscosus, Actinomyces meyeri,* and *A. pyogenes* have been recovered from infected cats.[12,13,90,91,108] Anaerobic actinomycetes are part of the normal bacterial flora of the mucous membranes. In addition to streptococci, actinomycetes colonize the peridontal mucosal surfaces and adhere to the tooth surface to form plaque.[145] *A. viscosus, A. odontolyticus, Actinomyces israelii, Actinomyces bovis,* and *Actinomyces naeslundii* have been cultured from the dental plaque of dogs, and *Actinomyces colecocanis* has been cultured from the canine vagina.[64] *A. viscosus, A. hordeovulneris,* and *Actinomyces denticolens* have

*References 13, 24, 37, 43, 49, 63, 65, 67a, 108, 123.

been cultured from normal feline gingiva.[92] These endogenous saprophytes are not normally pathogenic, but if *Actinomyces* species are inoculated into tissues with associated bacteria, an insidious pyogranulomatous disease can develop. (Use of the term "*Actinomyces* species" refers to [1] species currently classified in the genus *Actinomyces* and [2] related *Actinomyces*-like bacteria classified in other genera but that cause the clinical disease recognized as actinomycosis.)

Actinomycosis occurs most commonly in young adult to middle-age large-breed male dogs that are used or kept in an outdoor environment.[58,74] Hunting dogs have the highest prevalence of disease, and males and females seem to be affected equally. Actinomycosis in outdoor dogs is related in large part to their chronic exposure to grasses.[19,46,47,67,106] Inhaled or ingested florets or awns contaminated in the oropharynx migrate to various sites and act as the nidus of infection. Although infrequently reported in cats, actinomycosis is often attributed to bite wounds.[90] Because of the difficulty in culturing *Actinomyces* species and their susceptibility to many antibiotics, the true prevalence of actinomycosis in dogs and cats is greater than that suggested by the literature.

Pathogenesis

Actinomyces species are opportunistic pathogens that depend on mechanical disruption of normal mucosal barriers. Because of the organism's normal habitat, infections must somehow be linked to the mucous membranes, usually the oropharyngeal area. The disease characteristically spreads by direct extension and is unimpeded by normal tissue planes; however, rare instances of hematogenous dissemination occur.[67a] The most common clinical forms of actinomycosis in cats and dogs involve the cervicofacial region, thorax, abdomen, retroperitoneal space, and subcutaneous tissue.* Infection of the cervicofacial region can develop from bite wounds, perforation of the oropharynx by a foreign body, or chronic gingivitis-periodontitis. Pulmonary infections can develop by aspiration of oropharyngeal material, which may include inhalation of a contaminated grass awn. Preexisting lung disease (e.g., neoplasia) can act as a nidus for infection.[42] Alternative routes of thoracic infection include involvement of the mediastinum from esophageal perforation and direct extension of cervicofacial or abdominal disease. Intraabdominal actinomycosis develops from swallowed organisms or plant material penetrating the gastrointestinal (GI) mucosa. In people, GI disease, abdominal trauma, or surgery often precedes infection. Penetration of the GI tract by a bullet or other foreign bodies, including plant material, also increase the risk of infection for animals. Like thoracic infections, abdominal involvement can occur by direct extension. Infection of the retroperitoneal space in dogs is often associated with grass foreign bodies. Theoretically, contaminated grass florets or awns migrate to the space by migrating through the lung and up the crus of the diaphragm to its dorsal attachment, or by perforating the intestinal wall and migrating via the mesentery to its dorsal attachment. Actinomycosis of the limbs is caused by bite wounds, foreign bodies, and lacerations contaminated by licking. Infection of the subcutaneous tissue in dogs usually represents an extension of cervicofacial, thoracic, or retroperitoneal disease, whereas in cats it is caused by bite wounds. Central nervous system (CNS) infections develop from hematogenous or lymphatic dissemination from a primary site or direct extension from a contiguous infection.

Actinomycosis is characteristically a polymicrobial infection, and the pathogenicity of *Actinomyces* species is dramatically increased in mixed infections. The associated bacteria are commensal organisms from the oral cavity or intestinal tract that produce and maintain an anaerobic tissue environment. Inoculation of pure cultures of *Actinomyces* species or

*References 12, 37, 47, 58, 67, 74, 90, 91, 106.

the associated bacteria alone often do not produce infection. *Actinomyces* species with fimbriae bind to specific cell surface receptors on other bacteria. This coaggregation markedly inhibits neutrophil phagocytosis of and bactericidal activity on the bacterial complex.[107] If not bound to other bacteria, actinomycetes bind to specific receptors on neutrophils, initiating phagocytosis and degranulation. Additionally, *Actinomyces* species induce neutrophil chemotaxis, activate macrophages, and stimulate B-lymphocyte hyperplasia. These bacterial-cellular interactions produce the characteristic actinomycosis lesion—a dense mat of *Actinomyces* species and associated organisms surrounded by neutrophils, macrophages, and plasma cells. Proteolytic enzymes from the associated bacteria, macrophages, and degranulated neutrophils destroy connective tissue, facilitating extension of the disease through normal tissue planes.[145]

Clinical Findings

Dog

Cervicofacial actinomycosis produces acute to chronic subcutaneous soft tissue swelling in the head or neck region.[37,42,106,128] The lesion can be fluctuant or firm, may be indurated, and can be ulcerated or have draining sinuses. The mandible, submandibular region, and ventral or lateral cervical area are most frequently affected, but infections involving the face, retrobulbar space, and temporal area have been reported. Radiographically, adjacent bone can have periosteal new bone formation, and a chronic infection may be characterized by osteomyelitis. Ultrasonography and magnetic resonance imaging can be used to identify linear grass awn foreign bodies.[46a,124a] Material aspirated from fluctuant masses or discharged from sinuses appears serosanguineous to purulent and may contain macroscopic, yellow-tan granules (i.e., *sulfur granules*), which are small, soft macroscopic colonies of actinomycetes that are often present in exudates or infected tissue. The term *sulfur granule* was derived from the frequently seen yellow pigmentation of the granule; however, granule color can vary from white to tan to gray (Fig. 49-1). Aspiration of firm lesions may yield only a few drops of blood.

Actinomycosis involving the thoracic or abdominal cavity is characteristically chronic and progressive; weight loss, often severe, and fever are the most common clinical signs. *Thoracic actinomycosis* may be limited to the lung parenchyma but can involve multiple structures within the thorax, including the

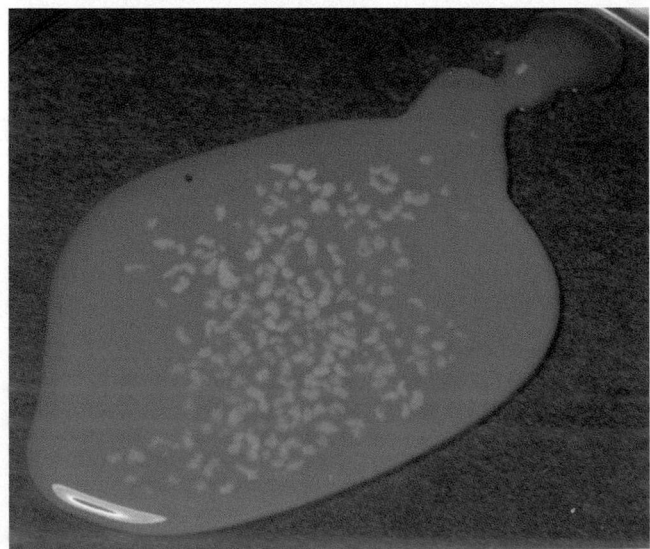

Fig 49-1 Thoracic exudate in Petri dish containing numerous macroscopic sulfur granules. (Courtesy David F. Edwards, University of Tennessee, Knoxville, Tenn.)

mediastinum, pleura, heart, and chest wall.* Other clinical features include cough, tachypnea, dyspnea, decreased lung sounds (from empyema or a mass lesion), and subcutaneous soft tissue masses on the lateral thorax. Thoracic wall masses often develop a draining sinus. Radiographically, lung disease appears as alveolar and interstitial infiltrates with consolidation. Variable findings include pleural thickening, pleural effusion (often loculated to one side), pericardial effusion, widening of the mediastinum, mass lesions, and periosteal new bone formation or osteomyelitis involving adjacent ribs, vertebral bodies, or sternebrae. Clinical features of *abdominal actinomycosis* include palpable masses and abdominal distention (effusion).[29,43,49,58] Subcutaneous masses, which may have draining sinuses, are rarely present unless the abdominal disease develops from an extension of thoracic or retroperitoneal infections. Radiographic manifestations include variable amounts of peritoneal effusion and mass lesions that incorporate or displace adjacent structures. Pleural, pericardial, and peritoneal effusions resemble the exudate from cervicofacial abscesses.

Retroperitoneal actinomycosis is characterized by back pain and rear leg paresis or paralysis.[37,47,67,77] A subcutaneous mass with a draining sinus involving the caudal thorax or flank area is often present. Radiographic findings include periosteal new bone formation involving the ventral aspects of two or three adjacent vertebral bodies (usually T-13 through L-3); involvement of disk spaces is uncommon (Fig. 49-2). Chronic disease may cause the vertebral bodies to develop osteomyelitis and compression fractures. This finding contrasts with diskospondylitis caused by embolic spread of bloodborne bacteria or fungi to the disk space (see Chapters 40, 64, and 86).

Cutaneous-subcutaneous actinomycosis is characterized by a soft to firm mass, which may have a draining sinus.[37,47,74,106,128] These infections are typically located in the head and neck area, lateral thoracic wall, and flank region and are usually extensions of cervicofacial, thoracic, or retroperitoneal actinomycosis.

Rare cases of actinomycosis involving the extremities and CNS have been reported. Lameness, mass lesions with draining sinuses, and periosteal new bone formation are characteristic of limb involvement.[20,58] Actinomycosis of the brain is rare,[128,5,34] whereas involvement of the spinal cord is a common sequela to subvertebral infections.[43,67,77] Clinical findings associated with brain infections are nonlocalizing and

include altered behavior, decreased consciousness, neck pain, ataxia, abnormal reflexes, and seizures. With spinal cord involvement, pain, paresis, paralysis, and abnormal reflexes are noted, and radiographic evidence of a bony change in adjacent vertebral bodies is present. Cystitis in dogs has been associated with *Arcanobacterium pyogenes* and a *Nocardia*-like organism, which most likely represents *A. turicensis*, a common isolate from wogenital tract infections.[13,66,68,117]

Cat

Pyothorax and subcutaneous bite wound abscesses are the most common disorders in cats from which *Actinomyces* species are isolated.[90,91] The abscesses have a malodorous, yellow to sanguineous exudate without a granulomatous mass, and the *Actinomyces* species is always mixed with two to five other pathogens. Actinomycosis as described in the dog has been reported infrequently in cats. The feline cases have involved the cervicofacial region,[30,84,147] thoracic cavity,[60] and subcutaneous tissue with extension to the spinal canal.[12,127] Otitis external secondary to *A. pyogenes* has been reported in a cat.[13]

Diagnosis

Clinical Laboratory Findings

Hematologic test results in animals with actinomycosis vary according to the location and duration of disease. Animals with focal lesions (e.g., cervicofacial and limb infections) may have few abnormal results, whereas animals with more extensive, chronic disease have mild to moderate nonregenerative anemia, leukocytosis with a left shift and monocytosis, hypoalbuminemia, and hyperglobulinemia (sometimes marked). Dogs with body cavity effusions may be hypoglycemic. Aspirates of abscesses or effusions, tracheal lavages, and sinus discharges are suppurative to pyogranulomatous, whereas aspirates of firm masses may reveal only blood. In some specimens, especially those from effusions, sulfur granules are visible macroscopically (see Fig. 49-1). Microscopically, mixed bacterial populations containing rods and cocci are common. The actinomycetes appear individually or in dense aggregates (sulfur granules) as gram-positive, non–acid-fast filamentous organisms that are occasionally branched (Fig. 49-3). *Nocardia* species and *Filifactor villosus*–gram-positive filamentous rods can be confused with *Actinomyces* species.[91,135]

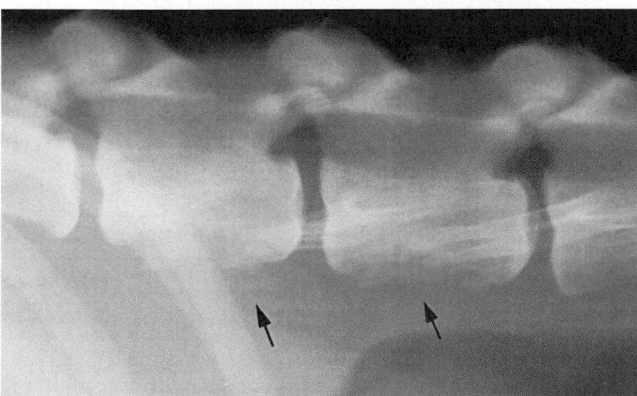

Fig 49-2 Spinal radiograph of an 8-year-old pointer with retroperitoneal actinomycosis. Periosteal new bone growth *(arrows)* is present on ventral aspect of vertebral bodies of L-2 and L-3. (Courtesy David F. Edwards, University of Tennessee, Knoxville, Tenn.)

*References 18, 28, 37, 43, 46, 47, 58, 89, 115, 124, 128.

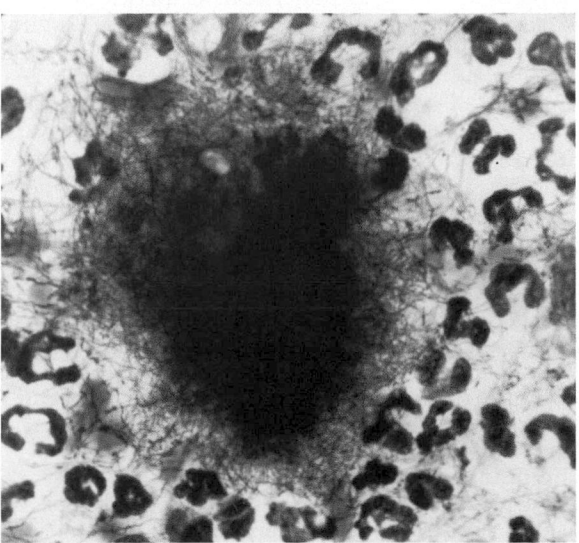

Fig 49-3 Smear of thoracic fluid. Dense mat of infrequently branched, filamentous rods (i.e., sulfur granule). Note presence of other bacterial species (×198). (Courtesy David F. Edwards, University of Tennessee, Knoxville, Tenn.)

Bacterial Isolation and Identification

The disease is confirmed by culture of the organism, but frequently culture results are negative or contain only associated bacteria. *Actinomyces* species either are facultative *(A. canis, A. catuli, A. coleocanis, A. bowdenii, A. denticolens, A. hordeovulneris, A. naeslundii, A. odontolyticus, A. viscosus, A. pyogenes)* or obligate *(A. bovis, A. israelii, A. meyeri)* anaerobes.[16,63-65,108] Specimens should be collected and processed anaerobically and cultured on blood agar or enriched thioglycolate media in the presence of 5% to 10% carbon dioxide. Species that are facultatively anaerobic are variably aerotolerant and can grow aerobically. *A. viscosus* actually grows best in aerobic conditions. All species cultured aerobically require carbon dioxide, except *A. bowdenii, A. naeslundii,* and *A. odontolyticus.*[61]

Growth of *Actinomyces* species can be observed within 48 hours but usually requires 5 to 7 days. It may be necessary to hold plates 2 to 4 weeks. Colonies on blood agar are flat to convex, circular with entire or irregular margins, and translucent to opaque and white; surfaces are smooth and moist or rough (*bread crumb* or *molar tooth* surface). Some strains of *A. israelii* produce aerial filaments, resulting in a powdery, or cotton ball, appearance. Microscopically *Actinomyces* species are gram-positive, non–acid-fast short rods and filaments. The filaments are less than 1 μm wide, vary considerably in length, may branch, and can stain irregularly, producing a beaded appearance.[18,29,43,58,74] *Actinomyces* species are heterogeneous, and species identification using traditional biochemical tests is difficult.[120] Results of 16S rRNA gene sequence analysis of previously identified species indicates that several genera in addition to *Arcanobacterium* and *Actinobaculum* will emerge from the species now classified in the genus *Actinomyces.*[31,56,112] Variants of *A. hordeovulneris* that are cell wall deficient have been produced in culture, suggesting that L forms of *Actinomyces* species may be associated with clinical disease; however, because of special culture requirements, these variants would be isolated infrequently.[23]

Actinomycosis is characteristically a mixed bacterial infection.* Three to five associated bacteria are typically recovered from properly handled specimens. The most commonly isolated organisms are resident flora of the oral cavity or intestinal tract and include *Bacteroides* species, *Corynebacterium* species, *Escherichia coli*, *Eubacterium* species, *Fusobacterium* species, *Pasteurella multocida*, *Peptostreptococcus* species, *Staphylococcus aureus*, and *Streptococcus* species. Most of the associated bacteria are facultative or obligate anaerobes, therefore isolation requires appropriate specimen handling. Unfortunately, the growth of a mixed microflora can impair the isolation of *Actinomyces.*[61]

Because *Actinomyces* species are sensitive to many antibiotics, the treatment of animals before obtaining specimens for culture can prevent recovery of the organisms. This fact, compounded by improperly handled specimens and polymicrobial growth, accounts for the frequent failure of *Actinomyces* isolation from infected animals. The diagnosis is often based on the cytologic or histologic identification of the organism in specimens from animals with appropriate clinical signs. Because *Actinomyces* is a commensal oral bacteria, it is commonly swallowed, inhaled, and transferred by licking, therefore culture of the organism from the airways, GI tract, or skin does not necessarily constitute infection.

Pathologic Findings

Actinomycosis is characterized by a poorly defined, often indurated mass that incorporates adjacent structures.† The mass may contain one or more pockets of a reddish-brown exudate. Fistulas and sulfur granules may be found. Thoracic and abdominal infections produce a diffuse, red, velvety to granular thickening of the parietal pleura and peritoneum and omentum. The visceral pleura and peritoneum may be less affected. A variable amount of a reddish-brown exudate that may contain sulfur granules is present. Lung involvement is usually localized and may appear as a consolidation or mass; infrequently, multiple pulmonary nodules are present. Masses can affect multiple internal structures (e.g., heart, mediastinum, lung, diaphragm, and chest wall) and produce an external subcutaneous swelling that may have a draining sinus. With abdominal disease, only one organ may be affected (e.g., liver), but typically a mass or masses involve multiple adjacent structures.[29,43,49] Subcutaneous masses may be ulcerated and in dogs are usually an extension of cervicofacial, thoracic, or retroperitoneal disease.[37,47,67]

The histologic reaction to *Actinomyces* species infection is characterized by a core of neutrophils encapsulated by fibrosing granulation tissue. The granulation tissue contains macrophages, plasma cells, and lymphocytes in a dense, fibrous tissue matrix. The centrally located actinomycotic (sulfur) granule or grain can be very difficult to find, so multiple tissue sections may be needed to confirm the diagnosis. When associated with appropriate clinical signs, identification of true actinomycotic granules is diagnostic of actinomycosis. In tissue sections stained with hematoxylin and eosin (H and E), the granules appear as round, oval, or scalloped amphophilic solid masses with an outer basophilic band (Fig. 49-4, *A*). The granules vary in size (from 30 to 3000 μm in diameter) and often are rimmed by partially confluent radiate, eosinophilic serrate, or club-shaped structures (i.e., the Splendore-Hoeppli phenomenon). Neutrophils frequently contact or appear enmeshed in this material. Individual actinomycete filaments are not delineated by H and E stain or Gridley's fungal or periodic acid-Schiff reactions, whereas Gram staining of tissues (i.e., the Brown-Brenn procedure) reveals clumps of tangled, intermittently branched, thin (less than 1 μm in diameter) filaments that are gram-positive and slightly beaded (Fig. 49-4, *B*). Gram-positive or gram-negative nonfilamentous bacteria can be mixed with the *Actinomyces* species. *Actinomyces* species are non–acid-fast when stained by the Fite-Faraco modification of the Ziehl-Neelsen technique, which uses a weaker decolorizing agent of 1% sulfuric or 1% hydrochloric acid. With the rare exception of some *Nocardia* species, other fungi and bacteria that produce tissue granules can be reliably distinguished from *Actinomyces* by tinctorial and morphologic properties.[27] Features of nocardiosis that distinguish it from actinomycosis are listed in Table 49-1.

Therapy

Successful treatment of actinomycosis involves prolonged administration of antibiotics; the role of surgery varies with the form of the disease. Large doses of penicillin given for prolonged periods (weeks to months) is the treatment of choice (Table 49-2).[81] No strains of *Actinomyces* species have shown in vitro resistance to easily attainable serum concentrations of penicillin, and acquired resistance in vivo has not been confirmed. Poor drug penetration of the dense granulomatous tissue reaction necessitates the prolonged, high-dose therapy. A minimal dose of penicillin G (benzyl penicillin) or penicillin V (phenoxymethyl penicillin) of 40 mg/kg every 8 hours is recommended.[43] Units of penicillin equivalency per milligram depend on the formulation (see Appendix 8). The therapeutic advantage of initial parenteral administration is questionable, therefore if the animal is stable clinically, oral therapy can be started from the outset.[43,105] Because food reduces the absorption of most penicillins, medication should be given 1 hour before or 2 hours after feeding. Therapy must be extended significantly (weeks to months) beyond resolu-

---

*References 19, 47, 58, 74, 90, 91, 134.
†References 28, 29, 43, 60, 89, 128, 134.

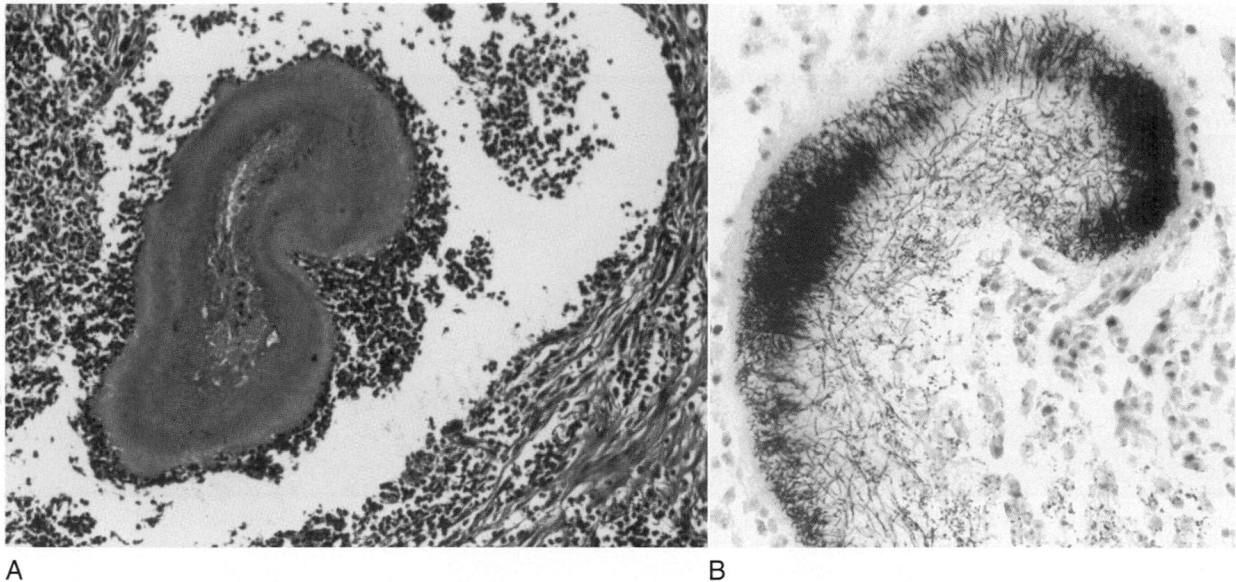

A   B

Fig 49-4 **A,** H and E stained section of abdominal mass from 5-year-old neutered female boxer dog. Actinomycotic tissue granule is surrounded by neutrophils. Encapsulating fibrous tissue has mononuclear cell infiltrate. (The long dimension of the granule measures 695 μm; ×13.2). **B,** Tissue section (Gram stain, Brown-Brenn procedure) of intrathoracic mass from 4-year-old German shorthaired pointer. Actinomycotic tissue granule showing infrequently branched, filamentous rods characteristic of *Actinomyces* organisms (×132). (**A,** Courtesy David F. Edwards, University of Tennessee, Knoxville, Tenn.)

Table • 49-1

Comparison of Actinomycosis Versus Nocardiosis

ACTINOMYCES SPECIES	*NOCARDIA* SPECIES
Culture	
1. Facultative or obligate anaerobe	1. Aerobe
2. Fastidious growth requirements; often not cultured	2. Usually cultured
3. Two to five associated microbes usually recovered	3. Sole isolate unless from contaminated sample (e.g., tracheal wash, ulcerated skin)
Staining Characteristics	
1. Irregular staining that can produce slight beading	1. Irregular staining that can produce marked beading
2. Gram-positive and non—acid-fast using Fite-Faraco modification of Ziehl-Neelsen technique	2. Gram-positive and partially acid-fast using Fite-Faraco modification of Ziehl-Neelsen technique
Cytopathologic Characteristics	
1. Suppurative to pyogranulomatous inflammation with a mixed bacterial population; macroscopic and microscopic dense mats of long filamentous bacteria often present (see Fig. 49-3)	1. Suppurative to pyogranulomatous inflammation; long filamentous bacteria typically present singly or in loose aggregates (see Fig. 49-6); infrequently macroscopic and microscopic dense mats of long filamentous bacteria present
Histopathologic Characteristics	
1. Pyogranulomatous inflammation with marked encapsulating fibrosis (see Fig. 49-4)	1. Pyogranulomatous inflammation; significant fibrosis present only in chronic skin infections (see Fig. 49-7)
2. Variable presence of tissue granules (30—3000 μm diameter)	2. Granules present only in skin infections (15—200 μm diameter)
Clinical Disease	
1. In adult outdoor dogs (especially hunting breeds); with bite wounds and pyothorax in cats	1. In dogs younger than 2 years old; from fight wounds in cats
2. Direct spread to adjacent structures	2. Hematogenous spread; can see lesions at noncontiguous sites
3. Sensitive to high doses of penicillin	3. Variable sensitivity to sulfonamides
4. Low mortality	4. Moderate to high mortality

Table • 49-2

Drugs Used to Treat Actinomycosis in Dogs and Cats

DRUG[a]	SPECIES	DOSE[b]	ROUTE	INTERVAL (HOURS)
Penicillin G	B	100,000 U/kg	IV, IM, SC	6–8
Penicillin G[c]	B	40 mg/kg[d]	PO	8
Penicillin V	B	40 mg/kg[d]	PO	8
Clindamycin	B	5 mg/kg	SC	12
Erythromycin	B	10 mg/kg	PO	8
Chloramphenicol	D	50 mg/kg	PO, IV, IM, SC	8
	C	50 mg/kg	PO, IV, IM, SC	12
Rifampin	D	10 mg/kg	PO	12
Minocycline	B	5–25 mg/kg	IV, PO	12
Ampicillin (amoxicillin)[c]	B	20–40 mg/kg	IM, SC, PO	6

B, Dog and cat; *D*, dog; *C*, cat; *IV*, intravenous; *IM*, intramuscular; *SC*, subcutaneous; *PO*, by mouth.
[a]See Appendix 8 for more information on these drugs.
[b]Dose per administration at specified interval. For duration, see text.
[c]Give at least 1 hr before or 2 hr after feeding to facilitate GI absorption.
[d]Minimum recommended dose (see text); 1 mg = 1600 U (see Appendix 8).

tion of measurable disease to prevent relapse; in some cases, treatment can exceed 1 year.[43,58] Drugs other than penicillin that are effective against most *Actinomyces* species include erythromycin, clindamycin, ampicillin, tetracycline, minocycline, doxycycline, chloramphenicol, imipenem, and first-generation cephalosporins and ceftriaxone.[81,123,146] Anecdotal success with ciprofloxacin was reported in a human patient with recalcitrant actinomycosis of 20 years' duration;[94] however, recently described *Arcanobacterium bernardiae* and *Actinomyces neuii* are resistant to ciprofloxacin, and in vitro resistance to fluorinated quinolones was reported for an *Actinomyces* species isolate from a dog with thoracic disease.[16,41] Oxacillin, dicloxacillin, cephalexin, metronidazole, and aminoglycosides have poor in vitro activity against most *Actinomyces* species; however, *A. pyogenes* is sensitive to aminoglycosides (other than streptomycin) but resistant to tetracycline, minocycline, and doxycycline.[55] Poor response to appropriate doses of penicillin may be attributable to poor surgical drainage and failure to eliminate associated bacteria.[81] Infections by these organisms usually resolve with penicillin, but on occasion they require broader spectrum antibiotics during the initial treatment period followed by long-term administration of penicillin. Cats with pyothorax or subcutaneous abscess that have not developed a granulomatous tissue reaction often can be cured with drainage and a shorter duration of antibiotic treatment.

Surgery has a controversial role in the treatment of actinomycosis. Draining of abscesses and effusions (thoracic, abdominal, and pericardial) should always be used as an adjunct to antibiotic treatments.[58,60,115] Continuous suction and intermittent drainage techniques have been used for thoracic effusions in dogs.[46,134] Drain tubes are removed when the purulent exudate changes to a serosanguineous transudate, usually within 4 to 10 days. Daily lavage with fluids containing crystalline penicillin G may be beneficial. Using sodium penicillin rather than potassium penicillin in the lavage fluid prevents the development of cardiotoxicity from hyperkalemia. (Crystalline potassium penicillin G contains 1.7 mEq potassium per 10^6 U.) Complications of drainage include pneumothorax and subcutaneous abscess formation at the drain tube insertion site. Animals not responding to drainage

and appropriate antibiotic therapy warrant exploratory surgery.[46,115,134] In animals with pulmonary abscesses, diseased lung lobes often require removal. The characteristic invasive fibrotic lesions obliterate tissue planes, preventing conservative dissection, and the tissue is well vascularized, therefore moderate to severe bleeding is common. With diffuse disease involving body cavities, tissue resection should be restricted to decrease the chance of death. In dogs with solitary masses involving the thoracic and abdominal walls, radical surgical excision has a high cure rate, although repeat surgeries may be needed.[46] The masses often can be reduced and better defined by an initial period of antibiotic therapy. Frequently, grass florets or awns are found in these lesions and during surgical exploration of diseased retroperitoneal regions.[46,46a,67,124a] Surgery should never be performed in lieu of and should always be followed by appropriate antibiotic therapy.

Appropriate treatment of dogs with actinomycosis, which can involve extremely prolonged use of antibiotics and surgery, results in a cure rate of greater than 90%.[43,46,58] Because of the infrequent documentation of actinomycosis in cats, a meaningful cure rate is not available, but it is likely similar to the cure rate in dogs.

Public Health Considerations

No reports exist of actinomycosis being transmitted from clinically infected animals to humans or to other animals; however, humans bitten by dogs, cats, or other people can develop actinomycosis.[113] Nevertheless, animal care workers handling infected tissues or discharge should wear protective gloves to avoid inadvertent contact by inoculation or through damaged skin.

NOCARDIOSIS

Etiology and Epidemiology

Nocardiosis is a suppurative to granulomatous, localized or disseminated bacterial infection caused by aerobic actinomycetes that are members of the family Nocardiaceae.[10,11] *Nocardia asteroides* is the most commonly isolated species in dogs and cats, but infections by *Nocardia brasiliensis* (in the dog and cat), *Nocardia otitidiscaviarum* (in the dog and cat), *Nocardia nova* (in the cat), and *N. africana* (in the cat) have been reported.* As historically defined, *N. asteroides*,[126,116] *N. brasiliensis*,[136] *N. nova*,[33] *N. otitidiscaviarum*[108a] and *Nocardia transvalensis*[142] consist of several subtypes and species. Recent publications cite approximately 34 valid species of *Nocardia*; to date, at least 20 species have been implicated in human infections. It is certain previous reports of nocardiosis in dogs and cats understate the number of species producing disease. These aerobic actinomycetes are ubiquitous soil saprophytes that degrade organic matter and are found in soil, in water, and on plants.[10,99] Infections are considered opportunistic, occurring by either inhalation of organisms or inoculation through puncture wounds.

In a survey of 53 dogs with nocardiosis, males were infected three times more frequently than females; 65.4% of the dogs were younger than 1 year, 82.7% were younger than 2 years, and only 7.8% were older than 6 years; 26.9% had an underlying condition, most often canine distemper.[11] Apparently in dogs, like in people, predisposing factors (i.e., diseases) increase susceptibility to nocardiosis. Approximately 40% of people with nocardiosis have primary disorders that involve immunosuppressive drug therapy, obstructive pulmonary disease, metabolic disorders (e.g., hyperadrenocorticism, diabetes mellitus), neoplasia (lymphosarcoma, leukemia), immunologic disease (systemic lupus erythematosus, dysgammaglobulinemia), or infectious diseases (e.g., acquired immunodeficiency syndrome).[10,99] In 20 reported cases of feline nocardiosis, 15 involved males and 4 involved females.† Ages ranged from 2 to 15 years (with a median age of 7 years). Fourteen of the cats had draining wounds or abscesses that were associated with scratches or bite wounds.

Pathogenesis

Similar to the systemic mycoses, pulmonary nocardiosis probably results from inhalation of soil organisms. Nocardial lesions develop in alveolar spaces and frequently erode into blood vessels, resulting in systemic spread of the disease. Secondary lesions from systemic spread can develop in any tissue. Involvement of contiguous structures within the thorax (e.g., pleura, mediastinum, pericardium) is also common. Localized cutaneous, subcutaneous, and regional lymph node infections result from inoculation through a puncture wound (e.g., bite, scratch, foreign body). Other solitary extrapulmonary sites of infection are likely caused by localization from a transient bacteremia. The primary source may be an inapparent pulmonary infection.[10,99]

Pathogenicity of *Nocardia* species is influenced by the strain and growth phase of the organism and host susceptibility. Normal host response to infection is characterized by an initial neutrophil mobilization that may inhibit growth but not kill the organism. Subsequent cell-mediated immunity consisting of activated macrophages and T lymphocytes is normally bactericidal. Diminished host resistance is a primary factor in nocardiosis, but not all diseased animals have identifiable predisposing conditions. Virulent strains of *Nocardia* are facultative intracellular pathogens that inhibit phagosome-lysosome fusion, neutralize phagosomal acidification, resist oxidative burst, and alter lysosomal enzymes within neutrophils and macrophages. These effects are partly related to the content and structure of mycolic acids within the bacterial cell wall, which vary among strains and during the growth phase. Some strains exhibit organ-specific trophism (e.g., brain), and the filamentous, logarithmically growing organisms

are 10 times more virulent than the coccoid stationary-phase cells.[10,99]

Clinical Findings
Dog
Pulmonary nocardiosis can have a peracute onset characterized by inspiratory dyspnea, hemoptysis, hypothermia, collapse, and death[85]; however, subacute to chronic clinical symptoms are more characteristic.[1,26,36,76,96] The signs are often similar to those of distemper and include mucopurulent oculonasal discharge, anorexia, weight loss (often emaciation), cough, dyspnea, diarrhea, and hyperthermia. Lung sounds may be increased (from bronchopneumonia) or decreased (from a mass lesion or empyema). Coinfection by the canine distemper virus is commonly reported.[11] The radiographic appearance of lesions varies and includes multiple, diffuse pulmonary nodules, intrapulmonary or extrapulmonary solitary masses, focal or diffuse bronchointerstitial to alveolar infiltrates, lobar consolidations, pleural effusions, and often, dramatic hilar lymphadenopathy (Fig. 49-5).

Systemic, or *disseminated*, *nocardiosis*, defined by lesions at two or more noncontagious sites within the body, is typically associated with pulmonary disease and rarely develops without obvious associated pulmonary disease.* The most frequently involved extrathoracic organs are skin and subcutaneous tissue, the kidney, the liver, the spleen, lymph nodes, the CNS, bone, and joints. The cutaneous-subcutaneous lesions are characterized by firm to fluctuant swellings that may ulcerate or develop fistulous tracts through which a reddish-brown exudate is discharged. Involvement of the liver, the spleen, and lymph nodes is detected because of organomegaly. CNS lesions may cause seizures. Bone or joint infection results in swelling and lameness; radiographic findings include soft tissue swelling, bone lysis, and periosteal new bone growth.

Solitary extrapulmonary nocardiosis develops infrequently and usually occurs as a cutaneous-subcutaneous abscess[8] or an actinomycotic mycetoma.[20,119] A case of humeral osteomyelitis has been reported.[40] Mycetoma is a localized, subcutaneous granulomatous tumor that contains organized aggregates (grains or granules) of free-living or exogenous, geophilic actinomycetes (actinomycotic mycetoma) or fungi (eumycotic mycetoma). Mycetomas usually develop on extremities, may involve underlying bone, and typically form abscesses that result in fistulas to the skin. Because *Actinomyces* is endogenous, tumorous infections of subcutaneous tissues are not classified as mycetomas. *Nocardia* infections have been reported in 10 dogs with thoracolumbar vertebral osteomyelitis and in one dog with cystitis[66]; however, many of these dogs were probably infected with *Actinomyces* species (see Actinomycosis, Clinical Findings, in this chapter).[17,103,122,125]

Cat
The clinical forms of feline nocardiosis (pulmonary, systemic, and solitary extrapulmonary) are similar to those described in the dog; however, in cats, cutaneous-subcutaneous† disease (abscesses and actinomycotic mycetomas) is the most common clinical form. Of 20 reported cases of nocardiosis, 14 cats had cutaneous-subcutaneous lesions involving the extremities,† inguinal area,[5,59,62,102] and neck.[23,62] Five cats had pulmonary disease (nodules or empyema),[3,6,78,95,109] one had peritonitis,[131] and five had systemic nocardiosis.[2,3,59,95,141] All those with systemic disease had a primary cutaneous-subcutaneous lesion. Macroscopic sulfur granules were noted in the

---

*References 2, 11, 59, 62, 93.
†References 2, 3, 6, 9, 26, 38, 59, 62, 78, 93, 95, 102, 109, 131, 141.

*References 1, 8, 72, 73, 76, 96, 114, 121, 129.
†References 72, 38, 62, 93, 95, 141.

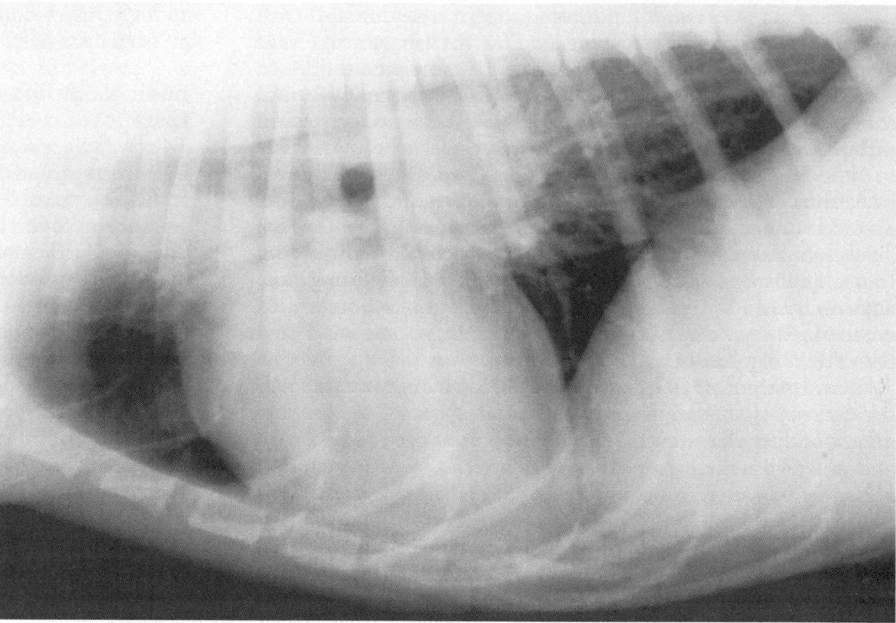

Fig 49-5 Right lateral thoracic radiograph of 8-month-old male Labrador retriever with pulmonary nocardiosis. Radiographic abnormalities include bronchointerstitial pattern and marked hilar lymphadenopathy. (Courtesy Royce Roberts, University of Georgia Veterinary Teaching Hospital, Athens, Ga.)

exudate of five cats (representing all three forms of clinical disease).[26,38,62,131]

Diagnosis
Clinical Laboratory Findings
Animals with nocardiosis have nonregenerative anemia, neutrophilic leukocytosis with a left shift, monocytosis, and hyperproteinemia. Hypercalcemia associated with granulomatous disease has been reported.[102] Pleural effusions, bronchial lavages, and aspirates of abscesses are suppurative to pyogranulomatous. Gram-positive, partially or weakly acid-fast, beaded, branching filamentous organisms are often observed individually or in loose aggregates (Fig. 49-6). Macroaggregates (i.e., sulfur granules) have been noted infrequently in effusions. Unlike actinomycosis, mixed bacterial populations from deep tissue sites are rare and probably caused by contamination of the sample (e.g., bronchial lavage, ulcerated skin abscess).[1,8,76,96]

Bacterial Isolation and Identification
The presence in clinical specimens of a gram-positive, partially acid-fast, beaded, branched filamentous organism 0.5 to 1 μm in diameter warrants specific therapy for nocardiosis, but the diagnosis is confirmed by culture of the organism. *Nocardia* species grow aerobically at a wide temperature range on simple media (e.g., Sabouraud's glucose agar, blood agar). Growth is enhanced by 10% carbon dioxide, modified Thayer-Martin medium and buffered charcoal-yeast extract agar but is retarded by inhibitory medium used for fungal isolation. Organisms are usually recovered in pure cultures, and colonies are often visible after 2 days. However, 2 to 4 weeks of incubation may be necessary, especially if samples contain multiple bacterial species (e.g., bronchial lavage) or are from animals receiving antibiotics. Colonies can be smooth and moist or rugose with a powdery surface from aerial filaments. Because most *Nocardia* species produce carotenoid-like pigments, colony color varies (cream, yellow, orange, pink, or red).[10,82,99] Microscopically, *Nocardia* species grown on solid media appear as branched filaments that fragment into pleomorphic, rod-shape, or coccoid elements. *Nocardia* species are gram-positive and variably acid-fast. In clinical specimens or primary isolates, *Nocardia* species are often partially acid-fast, but a Fite-Faraco modification of the Ziehl-Neelsen technique decolorized with 1% sulfuric or 1%

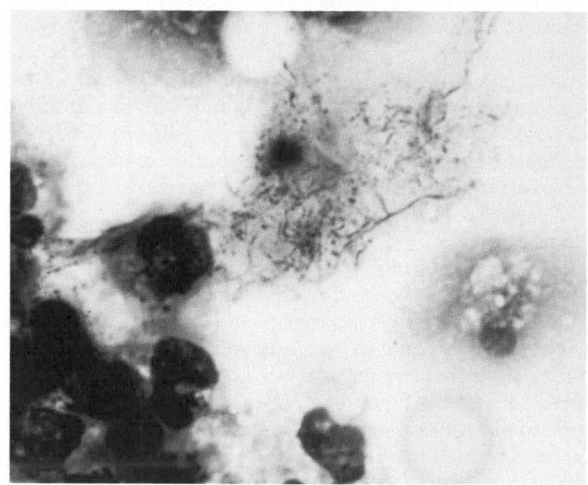

Fig 49-6 Impression smear of chronic (15 months duration), ulcerated cutaneous lesion on lateral thorax of 3-year-old female domestic shorthaired cat. Loose aggregate of infrequently branched, filamentous rods with beading from irregular staining is typical of *Nocardia* organisms (×330). (Courtesy David F. Edwards, University of Tennessee, Knoxville, Tenn.)

hydrochloric acid must be used. Not all pathogenic strains of *Nocardia* species are acid-fast—a characteristic that may disappear after subculture.[10,82,99]

Identification of the species of *Nocardia* isolates is important for prediction of antimicrobial susceptibility. Traditionally, species have been distinguished by phenotypic features, including growth characteristics and antibiotic susceptibility patterns; however, modern molecular methods have provided a more reliable and rapid means of speciation.[32,75,138] Restriction fragment length polymorphism (RFLP) analysis of polymerase chain reaction (PCR) products from the 16S rRNA gene identifies most pathogenic *Nocardia* organisms at a level of therapeutic relevance, but ultimate differentiation of closely related *Nocardia* species may require RFLP analysis of *hsp* gene products, 16S rRNA and *hsp* gene sequencing, or DNA-DNA hybridization.[33,116,142] L-form *Nocardia* spp., cell wall–deficient variants, have been associated with clinical disease in people and a dog.[22] These bacteria require special media for isolation and culture (see Chapter 33).

Pathogenic *Nocardia* species are not common laboratory contaminants, therefore the isolation of a single colony from a closed lesion is significant. Because *Nocardia* organisms are ubiquitous in soil and in certain circumstances may act as respiratory saprophytes, the isolation of small numbers of organisms from ulcerated skin lesions or the respiratory tract must be interpreted in conjunction with clinical signs.[10,82,99]

Pathologic Findings

Nocardiosis is characterized by suppurative necrosis and abscess formation and infrequently produces granulomas. The gross lesions on internal organs typically are numerous small (1 mm) to large (1 cm), discrete to coalescing, raised white or gray-white nodules.[72,114,121,129] The nodules are usually subserosal and when cut appear caseous to purulent. Affected lung tissue may appear congested. Lymph nodes are enlarged, often massively, and are firm to fluctuant with a caseous to purulent core.[36,76,114] A reddish-brown exudate may be present in the pleural or peritoneal space or within abscesses.[1,8,128] Yellow granules in the exudate have been noted.[76,131]

The histologic reaction to nocardial infection is characterized by a central region of necrosis and suppuration surrounded by macrophages, lymphocytes, and plasma cells.[114,121,129] Clusters of epithelioid macrophages and multinucleated giant cells may be observed. Except with some skin infections, fibrous tissue is usually poorly structured, producing thin or incomplete encapsulation of the lesion. In chronic cutaneous-subcutaneous infections, pyogranulomatous foci may be interspersed within a dense fibrous tissue matrix.[20,36]

Nocardial organisms are usually present and often abundant in the necrotic and suppurative tissue reactions. Gram staining of tissue (e.g., the Brown-Brenn procedure) is best for seeing the filaments, but tissues can also be stained by methenamine silver preparations, especially with prolonged silver nitrate exposure (i.e., 80 to 100 minutes). *Nocardia* filaments are not visible in tissue sections stained with H and E or with Gridley's fungal or periodic acid-Schiff reactions. The organisms are characteristically but not invariably partially acid-fast when a weak decolorizing solution is used (i.e., 1% sulfuric or 1% hydrochloric acid). *Nocardia* species appear as beaded, branching filaments that are 10 to 30 μm or more long and 0.5 to 1.0 μm wide. The filaments usually appear individually or in tangled, loose aggregates. In chronic skin infections, tissue granules characterized by colonies arranged in large, rosette-like arrays have been reported (Fig. 49-7). In human nocardiosis, tissue granules are uncommon; when present, the granules are small (15 to 200 μm), usually not associated with the Splendore-Hoeppli phenomenon, and usually produced in chronic skin infections by *N. brasiliensis*.

Therapy

Sulfonamides, including trimethoprim-sulfonamide combinations, are the primary drugs for treating nocardiosis (Table 49-3). Most *Nocardia* species, with the possible exception of *N. otitidiscaviarum*, are susceptible to sulfonamide therapy, but treatment must be continued for a prolonged period. From 1 to 3 months is recommended in people with cutaneous infections, up to 6 months for uncomplicated pulmonary infections, and 12 months or longer for systemic infections or infections in those who are immunocompromised. Clinical improvement should be observed within 7 to 10 days of starting treatment. Abscesses or empyema usually must be surgically drained to cure the patient.[82,99]

Antibiotics in addition to or other than sulfonamides may be needed because not all *Nocardia* isolates are sensitive to

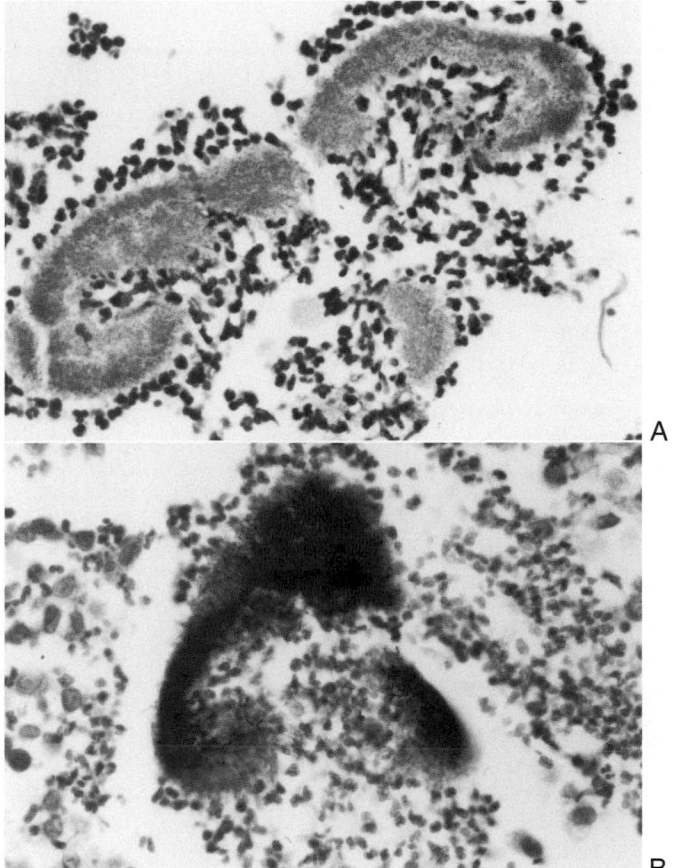

Fig 49-7 A, H and E–stained section of chronic, ulcerated cutaneous lesion on flank of 3-year-old male domestic longhaired cat. *Nocardia* tissue granules are surrounded by pyogranulomatous inflammatory reaction. (Long dimension of largest granule is 110 μm; ×66.) **B**, Acid-fast stain (Fite-Faraco modification of Ziehl-Neelsen technique) of same tissue section (×132). (Courtesy David F. Edwards, University of Tennessee, Knoxville, Tenn.)

Table • 49-3

Drugs Used to Treat Nocardiosis in Dogs and Cats[a]

DRUG[a]	DOSE[b]	ROUTE	INTERVAL (HOURS)
Triple sulfa no. 4	60 mg/kg[c]	IV	12
Sulfadiazine	80 mg/kg	PO	8
Sulfasoxazole[d]	50 mg/kg	PO	8
Amikacin	8–12 mg/kg	IV, IM, SC	8
Imipenem-cilastatin	2–5 mg/kg	IV	8
Cefotaxime	20–80 mg/kg	IV, IM	6
Minocycline	5–25 mg/kg	IV, PO	12
Erythromycin	10 mg/kg	PO	8
Ampicillin	20–40 mg/kg	IV, IM, SC, PO	6
Linezolid	8–20 mg/kg	PO	24

IV, Intravenous; *PO*, by mouth; *IM*, intramuscular; *SC*, subcutaneous.
[a]See Appendix 8 for more information on these drugs.
[b]Dose per administration at specified interval. For duration, see text; usually a minimum of 6 weeks is required with all the drugs.
[c]120 mg/kg IV initially.
[d]Also sulfamethizole.

Table • 49-4

Percentage of Pathogenic Nocardia Species Isolates with Sensitivity or Intermediate Sensitivity to Various Drugs In Vitro[a]

ISOLATE	AMK	A-C	AMP	CTX	CTA	CIPRO	ERY	IMP	GENT	LNZ	MINO	T-S	SULFA
N. asteroides complex													
Type I: N. abscessus[140] (1)	S	S	S	S	—	R	I	S	—	—	—	S	S
Type II: N. brevicatena[b]													
N. paucivorans[c,44,140] (3)	S	S	S	S	S	S	S	—	S/I	—	—	S	—
Type III: N. nova type strain[21,101,137,140]	100	6	84	96	96	0	100	100	—	100	98	88	—
N. africana[144]	—	—	100	—	—	—	100	—	0	—	—	—	0
N. veterana (5)[33,52,110,14]	S	I/S	S	I/R	R/I	R	S	S	S/R	S	I	S	—
Type V: N. farcinia[21,101,132,139,140]	99	79	7	6	17	80	9	83	3	100	96	76	95
Type IV: N. asteroides sensu stricto (3)[21,104]	S	R/S	—	I/S	I/S	R	—	I/R	—	100	I	S	S
N. cyriacigeorgici (1)[132]	S	—	—	—	S	—	S	—	—	—	—	—	S
N. brasiliensis COMPLEX													
N. brasiliensis[21,54,137]	100	100	<10	94/<50[d]	92/<50[d]	<17	0	<10	100	100	98	97	83
N. pseudobrasiliensis[21,14]	100	29	10	78	9	95	—	<10	—	100	26	94	—
N. otitidiscaviarum COMPLEX[e,14,21,45,51,140]	100	15	10	9	29	78	55[f]	57	86	100	100[f]	31	31
N. transvalensis COMPLEX[e,21,100]	—	—	10	50	50	60	50	90	—	100	54	82	90
N. transvalensis sensu stricto[142]	0	0	—	—	—	—	—	—	20	—	—	—	—
New taxon 1[142]	12	87	—	—	—	—	—	—	12	—	—	—	—
New taxon 2 (1)[87,142]	33	100	R	S	S	S	—	—	0	—	S	—	S
Type IV: N. asteroides COMPLEX[126,142]	3	87	—	—	—	—	100	—	4	—	—	—	—

AMK, Amikacin; A–C, amoxicillin-clavulanate;; AMP, ampicillin; CTX, cefotaxime; CTA, ceftriaxone; CIPRO, ciprofloxacin; ERY, erythromycin; IMP, imipenem; GENT, gentamicin; LNZ, linezolid; MINO, minocycline; T-S, trimethoprim-sulfamethoxazole; SULFA, sulfonamides; S, sensitive; I, intermediate sensitivity; R, resistant.

[a]If data from only a small number of clinical isolates were available, the number of isolates is indicated in parentheses following the species name and susceptibility patterns are designated by S (sensitive), I (intermediate sensitivity) and R (resistant). When 2 letters (e.g., S/I) are present the first letter represents the susceptibility pattern of the majority of isolates.

[b]To date, no clinical isolates have been tested.

[c]N. paucivorans has tentatively been categorized as a type II N. asteroides complex based on a 99.7% 16S rRNA gene sequence similarity to N. brevicatena. (Yassin AF, et al. 2000. Int J Sys Evol Microbiol 50:803-809.)

[d]Cited references report significantly different susceptibility patterns to third-generation cephalosporins.

[e]Susceptibility data for N. otitidiscaviarum and N. transvalensis complex isolates are confounded by lack of separation of more recently identified species.

[f]Approximately 50% of isolates were of only intermediate sensitivity.

sulfonamides, in vitro susceptibility may not be associated with clinical response, and resistance can develop during treatment.[82,99,111] Adverse drug reactions may prevent prolonged sulfonamide administration.[133] High doses of trimethoprim-sulfadiazine given for long periods to dogs and cats produces reversible myelosuppression (anemia and leukopenia).[35,88] Drug susceptibility testing of Nocardia isolates is technically difficult and should be done at experienced laboratories. The National Committee for Clinical Laboratory Standards has approved a standard for susceptibility testing by broth microdilution,[143] and a comparative study of several conventional susceptibility testing methods has been published.[4] PCR identification and drug susceptibility testing of Nocardia species can be done at the University of Texas Health Center at Tyler.*

*Mycobacteria/Nocardia Research Laboratory, Department of Microbiology, University of Texas Health Center at Tyler, 11937 US Highway 271, Tyler, TX 75708. Phone: 903-877-7685; Fax: 903-877-7652.

Susceptibility studies have identified relatively characteristic species-associated resistance patterns (Table 49-4) and led to the use of various antibiotics other than or in conjunction with sulfonamides to treat nocardiosis in people. In vitro, combinations of imipenem with cefotaxime or trimethoprim-sulfamethoxazole and amikacin with trimethoprim-sulfamethoxazole were synergistic, increasing minimum inhibitory concentrations four times or more for the majority of 26 isolates of *N. asteroides* complex. Combinations of amikacin with imipenem or cefotaxime were predominantly additive.[53] Linezolid, an oxazolidinone, had in vitro activity against all *Nocardia* species tested.[21,33,54] Based on in vitro data, topical imidazoles and ketaconazole may be effective against some *Nocardia* species.[41] Treatment success has been reported with amikacin, ampicillin, broad-spectrum cephalosporin, clarithromycin, doxycycline, erythromycin, imipenem, minocycline, ofloxacin, and linezolid alone or in combination.[82,99,83,104,130] Nocardiosis in animals that are severely ill, have systemic diseases, or have predisposing conditions may warrant initial combination drug therapy. If CNS disease is present, use of drugs with excellent CNS penetration, which include third-generation cephalosporins, imipenem, and linezolid, may be more effective than sulfonamides alone. Longer term use of linezolid in humans produces a reversible myelosuppression (anemia and thrombocytopenia)[50] and rarely has been associated with optic and peripheral neuropathies.[79,80] Ideally, drug selection should be based on susceptibility studies of the isolate but if the information is not available, logical choices can be made using the in vitro data in Table 49-4. Substitution of antibiotics within a class of drugs may not provide effective treatment; for example, although sensitive to amikacin, *Nocardia farcinia* isolates are resistant to gentamicin (see Table 49-4), and although sensitive to minocycline, *N. brasiliensis* isolates are mostly resistant to doxycycline.[54] Drug susceptibility patterns of *Nocardia* species more recently isolated from human patients (*Nocardia abscessus, Nocardia asiatica, Nocardia cyriacigeorgici, Nocardia inohanensis, Nocardia yamanashiensis, Nocardia niigatensis,* and *Nocardia beijingensis*) have not yet been fully characterized.[48,68-71]

In a review of 53 dogs with nocardiosis, 50% of the dogs died and 38.5% were euthanized.[11] Nine of 19 cats with nocardiosis either were euthanized or died.* The high mortality rate is partly attributable to predisposing conditions (distemper in dogs), delayed diagnosis, and inappropriate therapy. With earlier diagnosis and multidrug therapy, mortality of nocardiosis in animals may decrease to the rate reported in people. Only 19.8% of people with primary infections died, whereas 42.4%

of patients with predisposing conditions and more than 50% of patients with either systemic or CNS nocardiosis died.[10]

Public Health Considerations

No cases of human nocardiosis acquired from direct contact with an infected dog or cat have been reported; however, several cases of cutaneous nocardiosis transmitted to people by a scratch or bite from clinically healthy cats and dogs have been documented.[7,15,45,86,118] *Nocardia* species, which are ubiquitous in the soil, can contaminate the claws and teeth of dogs and cats, although the risk of a person contracting nocardiosis by an animal bite or scratch wound is no greater than the risk associated with getting a puncture wound while gardening. Special precautions are warranted when a person with suppressed immunity (e.g., who is receiving immunosuppressive drug therapy, who has human immunodeficiency virus infection) is caring for a dog or cat with nocardiosis.

ACKNOWLEDGMENT

The author would like to thank Barbara Brown-Elliott, Mycobacteria/Nocardia Research Laboratory, Department of Microbiology, University of Texas Health Center at Tyler, for her comments regarding the methods used for speciation of Nocardia isolates.

SUGGESTED READINGS*

31. Clarridge III JE, Zhang Q. Genotypic diversity of clinical *Actinomyces* species: phenotype, source, and disease correlation among genospecies. 2002. *J Clin Microbiol* 40:3442-3448.
108. Pascual C, Foster G, Falsen E, et al. *Actinomyces bowdenii* sp. nov., isolated from canine and feline clinical specimens. 1999. *Int J Syst Bacteriol* 49:1873-1877.
116. Roth A, Andrees S, Kroppenstedt RM, et al. Phylogeny of the genus *Nocardia* based on reassessed 16S rRNA gene sequences reveals underspeciation and division of strains classified as *Nocardia asteroides* into three established species and two unnamed taxons. 2003. *J Clin Microbiol* 41:851-856.
124. Sivacolundhu RK, O'Hara AJ, Read RA. Thoracic actinomycosis (arcanobacteriosis) or nocardiosis causing thoracic pyogranuloma formation in three dogs. 2001. *Aust Vet J* 79:398-402.
135. Walker AL, Jang SS, Hirsch DC. Bacteria associated with pyothorax of dogs and cats: 98 cases,1989-1998. 2000. *J Am Vet Med Assoc* 216:359-363.

*References 2, 3, 6, 9, 26, 38, 59, 62, 78, 93, 95, 102, 109, 131, 141.

*See the CD-ROM for a complete list of references.

CHAPTER 50

Mycobacterial Infections

Mycobacterial infections are caused by bacteria that belong to the family Mycobacteriaceae, order Actinomycetales. *Mycobacterium* is a genus comprising morphologically similar, aerobic, non–spore-forming, non-motile bacteria with wide variations in host affinity and pathogenic potential. Historically, these bacteria have been subdivided into several groups and individual species, according to characteristic biochemical and cultural reactions (Table 50-1). Genetic sequencing studies have corroborated and extended this taxonomic classification. Molecular diagnostics have become more useful than phenotypic traits by classifying isolated mycobacteria according to their genetic relationships. Although cultural characteristics are less useful, growth rates and pigment formation continue to be a practical means of classifying these bacteria in the laboratory. This trait is because growth and biochemical characteristics often correlate with the virulence and form of disease produced in the mammalian host.

Mycobacteria have the distinctive property of retaining hot carbolfuchsin and other stains after subsequent treatment with acid or alcohol, or both. The high lipid content of mycolic acid in the cell wall causes this acid-alcohol fastness. Cord factor and wax D, other surface constituents of mycobacterial cells, are partly responsible for the host's granulomatous response to the organism.

Mycobacteria are more resistant to heat, pH changes, and routine disinfection than are other pathogenic, non–spore-forming bacteria. Common disinfectants are often added to samples collected from nonsterile sites (e.g., sputum) for culture of mycobacteria to kill extraneous contaminating organisms. The minimum criteria established for pasteurization and heat disinfection were developed to kill mycobacteria. Mycobacteria are highly susceptible to dilute (5%) phenol or direct sunlight. Although they are relatively more stable in the presence of organic material, mycobacteria are killed by dilute (5%) household bleach within 15 minutes at room temperature.

On a clinical basis, mycobacteria are classified by their growth in culture—as being slow, difficult to cultivate, or rapid—whether they produce tubercles or granulomatous disease with or without dissemination. These features generally relate to the properties of the organisms that depend on their genetic relatedness. In this chapter, the organisms and diseases they cause will be divided into (1) slow-growing organisms that do or do not produce tubercles, (2) leproid granuloma–producing organisms, which cannot be cultured using standard methods, and (3) rapidly growing mycobacteria that are easy to cultivate. These organisms and the syndromes they cause will be discussed under the respective headings that follow.

INFECTIONS CAUSED BY SLOW-GROWING MYCOBACTERIA

Craig E. Greene and Danielle A. Gunn-Moore

Etiology

Tuberculous Mycobacteria

Mycobacterium tuberculosis and Mycobacterium bovis These highly pathogenic tubercle-producing mycobacteria are facultative or obligate intracellular parasites. *M. tuberculosis* is the type species, and evidence of human disease dates back to the dawn of civilization. *Tuberculous bacilli* (TB) are closely related species of mycobacteria that have been difficult to distinguish, except by using a few biochemical tests and nucleic acid probes. They possess mycolate-containing molecules in their cell walls, including the original cord factor trehalose 6,6'-dimycolate. These substances are associated with virulence and the production of characteristic tubercles (i.e., grossly small round translucent granulomatous lesions that histologically have central caseation surrounded by granulomatous inflammation). *M. bovis* is genetically and evolutionarily considered a subtype of *M. tuberculosis*. To be maintained in nature, they require infection of reservoir mammalian hosts because environmental survival is limited to a maximum of 1 to 2 weeks on infected fomites. The other members of the *M. tuberculosis* complex are *M. canettii*, a human pathogen; *M. microti*, a rodent pathogen that historically was reported to infect cats and has been found to infect people; *M. pinnipedii*, a seal bacillus; and *M. africanum*, a rare cause of human TB infections in Africa.

Mycobacterium microti–like An unclassified variant with properties intermediate to *M. tuberculosis* and *M. bovis* (previously termed *M. tuberculosis–M. bovis* variant) has been identified as a common cause of TB infection in cats in Great Britain.[20,70,71]

Mycobacterium microti This organism of voles has been found in cats and was identified as a cause of infection in people using genetic analysis of mycobacterial isolates.[148,186]

Nontuberculous Mycobacteria

Mycobacterium avium Complex Other opportunistic, saprophytic mycobacteria that occur as granuloma-producing pathogens, which sometimes disseminate, are organisms related to and include *M. avium*. Considerable overlap occurs between the properties of *M. avium* and a closely related pathogen *M. intracellulare*. Because of this indistinct separation, *M. avium–M. intracellulare* or *M. avium* complex (MAC) has been used to refer to these organisms. In classification systems, they are labeled nontuberculous mycobacteria (NTM) or mycobacteria other than tuberculosis-complex organisms and produce granulomas but not true tubercles. Their slow growth during cultivation makes them similar to tuberculous bacteria. In adult humans, MAC organisms

Table • 50-1

Characteristics of Selected Species of Mycobacterium of Veterinary Interest

GROUP SPECIES	AFFECTED NATURAL HOSTS (EXPERIMENTAL HOSTS)	MEANS OF EXISTENCE	PECULIAR CULTURAL AND BIOCHEMICAL FEATURES
Tuberculous			
M. tuberculosis	People, dog, cat, pig (guinea pig, mouse, hamster)	FI	Niacin positive, glycerol enhances
M. bovis	People, cat, dog, cow, pig, buffalo, and other captive zoo species (guinea pig, rabbit, mouse)	FI	Niacin negative, glycerol inhibits
M. microti—like	Cats, seals, other captive zoo species, rodents?	FI	Niacin variable, pyruvate enhances
M. microti	People, cat, mice, voles, llamas, ferrets	FI	
Lepromatous			
M. leprae	People (armadillo, mouse)	OI	Unable to cultivate
M. lepraemurium	Mouse, cat	OI	Difficult to cultivate, requires complex media
M. visibilis (provisional)	Cat	?	?
Other			
M. avium subsp. paratuberculosis	Cattle	FI	Requires mycobactin
Opportunistic, Nontuberculous			Runyon's Classification[a]
Slow Growing			
M. kansasii	People, dog (hamster; variable in mouse)	S, FI	I
M. avium—intracellulare complex[b]	Birds, people, dog, cat (variable in rabbit and mouse)	S, FI	III
M. genavense	Birds, people, dog, cat, ferret	S, FI	Requires mycobactin
M. terrae complex	People, cat	S, FI	III
M. simiae	Monkey, cat (mouse)	S, FI	I
Rapid Growing			
M. thermoresistible	Cat	S	II
M. xenopi	Cat	S	III
M. chelonae— abscessus[c] group	Dog, cat, ferret	S	IV
M. fortuitum group	Dog, cat (mouse)	S	IV
M. phlei	Cat	S	IV
M. smegmatis group	Cat	S	IV

FI, Facultative intracellular; *OI*, obligate intracellular; *S*, saprophyte; *?*, uncertain.
[a]Older (Runyon's) classification system for atypical mycobacteria bases on cultural properties:
I photochromogens: produce yellow pigment on exposure to light, buff color on growth in dark.
II scotochromogens: produce orange pigment, independent of light.
III nonchromogens: filamentous forms, buff or yellow regardless of amount of light; slow growth (nonphotochromogens).
IV nonchromogens: rapid growth, mature colonies in 4 to 6 days at 37° C, most others require 1 to 2 weeks.
[b]Included in tuberculous group in this chapter because produces clinically similar disease. Growth enhanced by glycerol and 42° C.
[c]Because of taxonomic uncertainties, organisms of *M. chelonae* and *M. abscessus* are hyphenated.

produce pulmonary infiltrates and disseminated disease, generally in immunocompromised hosts. In cats and children, localized lymphadenitis can occur. When newer methods of genetic analysis have been performed, some cases clinically classified as feline leprosy syndrome (see next section) have been attributed to MAC infection. Although in cats, MAC disease often becomes disseminated, in dogs, granuloma formation often occurs in visceral organs with only occasional

dissemination to other tissues. As an opportunistic disease, MAC infection is more likely in immunocompromised hosts.[66] Among opportunistic mycobacteria in people and animals, MAC organisms are the most likely to produce bacteremia and multiple-organ disseminated disease.

Serotyping by agglutination reactions has been classically used to differentiate MAC isolates. However, now, nucleic acid probes are used for their rapid identification. Using serologic methods, MAC organisms consist of 28 serovars; 1 through 6 and 8 through 11 are assigned to *M. avium*, and 7, 12 through 17, 19, 20, and 25 are assigned to *M. intracellulare*.[89,181] Serotypes 1 and 4 have been isolated from cats, and serotypes 1, 2, and 4 have been isolated from dogs.[96] Currently, MAC organisms are distinguished by nucleic acid profiles (see Organism Detection later in this chapter).

Other Slow-Growing Saprophytic Mycobacteria *M. kansasii*, *M. genavense*, *M. simiae*, and the *M. terrae* group (including *M. terrae*, *M. nonchromogenicum*, and *M. triviale*) are all slow-growing saprobes that have cultural characteristics in common with the MAC organisms. In dogs and cats, they generally produce disease similar to MAC organisms, characterized by localized pyogranulomatous lesions, usually in the lungs with complicating pyothorax or as a cause of widely disseminated disease. Although classified in this group, the *M. terrae*–group organisms often cause cutaneous lesions similar to the rapid-growing organisms (see later discussion).

Epidemiology
Tuberculous Mycobacteria

M. tuberculosis Human beings are the only reservoir hosts for *M. tuberculosis*. Dogs and cats are susceptible to infections by *M. tuberculosis* and *M. bovis*. Cats are naturally much more resistant to *M. tuberculosis* than they are to *M. bovis*, while both dogs and cats are more resistant than

people are to infection by MAC organisms. Despite this inherent resistance, exposure to MAC organisms is much greater because they are ubiquitous in the environment. Canine and feline infections with *M. tuberculosis* are considered an anthropozoonosis; the direction of transmission is from people to animal (Fig. 50-1). Although pets acquire the infection from people, the spread back from dogs or cats to people has not been reported. Dogs have had a higher prevalence of infection with *M. tuberculosis* than have cats. Dogs with tuberculous pneumonitis discharge organisms in the sputum as do infected people. Aerosolized droplets are the primary means of transmission of this disease. Airborne droplet nuclei from respiratory secretions fall to the ground where they temporarily remain viable but stationary and thus relatively noninfectious for other people and pets. Only small (3 to 5 μm) diameter particles can successfully bypass upper respiratory clearance mechanisms and deposit in alveoli. Discharges that are not airborne may potentially be infectious to dogs and cats exposed through close contact. In general, tubercle bacilli are not as transmittable as other bacterial pathogens because prolonged, frequent exposure or large inocula are usually required. Because of measures imposed to control infection in people, the overall prevalence of human and animal *M. tuberculosis* infections had been decreasing in developed countries. Relative increases have occurred in densely populated urban areas and in economically depressed areas. The interrelated factors of homelessness, illicit drug use, and human immun-

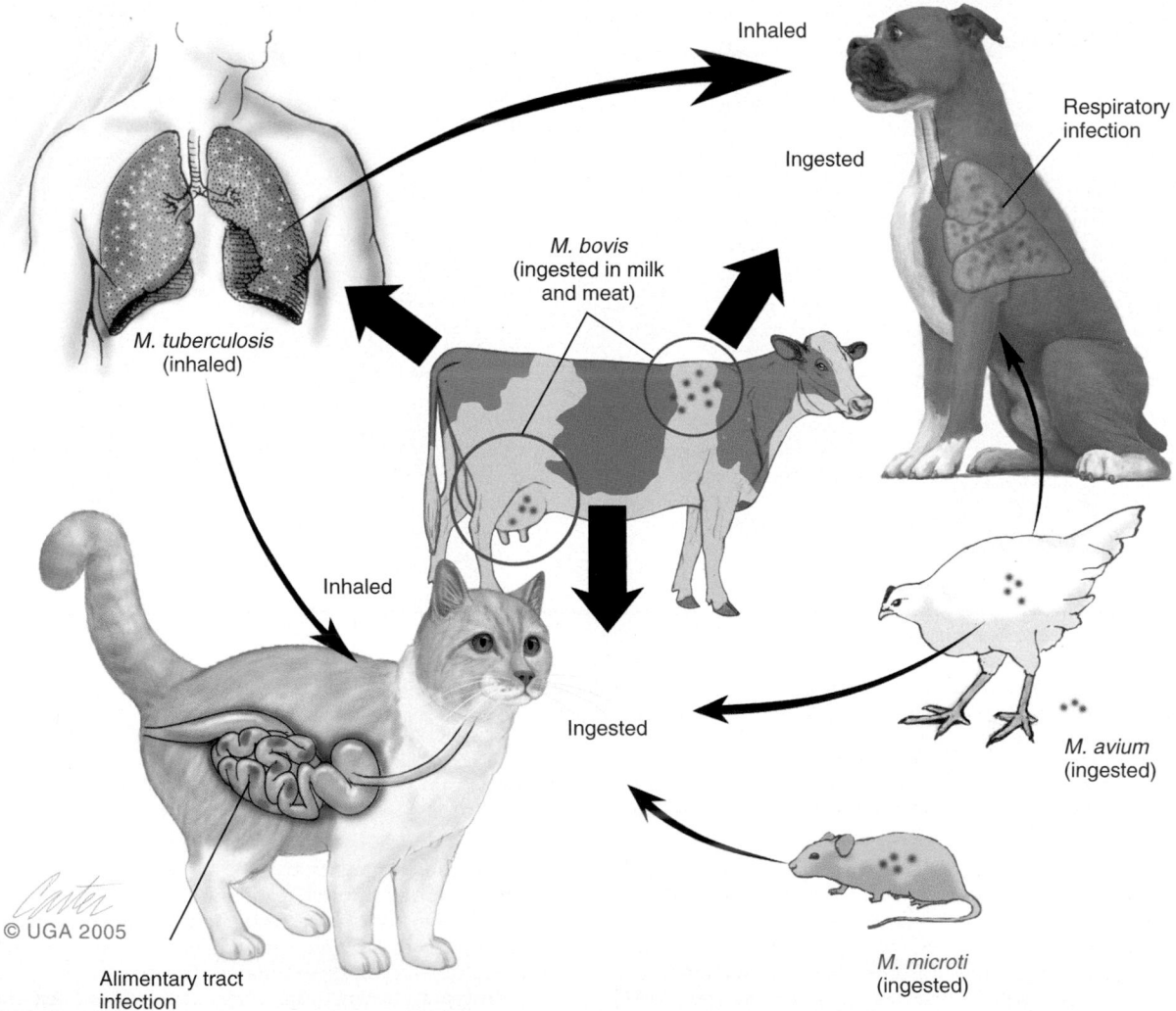

Inhaled

Respiratory infection

Ingested

M. bovis (ingested in milk and meat)

M. tuberculosis (inhaled)

Inhaled

Ingested

Ingested

M. avium (ingested)

© UGA 2005

Alimentary tract infection

M. microti (ingested)

Fig 50-1 Epidemiology of tuberculosis in the dog and cat. Width and direction of arrows indicate the relative frequency and usual sources of infection. (Courtesy University of Georgia, Athens, Ga.)

odeficiency virus (HIV) infection have caused unanticipated increases in its prevalence. Multiple-drug–resistant tuberculosis has emerged in these so-affected populations because of irregular compliance with drug therapy. Pets in such environments will have an increased risk of becoming infected. The incidence of *M. tuberculosis* infections in the United States is highest in Atlantic coast metropolitan regions and in the southeastern regions.

M. tuberculosis infection has become an important emerging anthropozoonosis in free-ranging wildlife. Until recently, the infection was identified only in wildlife or captive zoo animals such as elephants that had close and prolonged contact with people.[135,143] Infections caused by *M. tuberculosis* have been increasing in recent years, especially in underdeveloped countries, as a result of the acquired immunodeficiency syndrome (AIDS) epidemic. In Africa, expansion of ecotourism and changing land use have increased contact between infected people and free-living animals. Wild animals living in close proximity to human habitations and refuse sites have become infected. Certain wildlife populations have become endemically infected, such as the banded mongoose *(Mungos mungo)* in Botswana and suricates *(Suricata suricatta)* in South Africa.[3]

Mycobacterium bovis This organism has a wide host range, including many animals and people, and a worldwide geographic distribution.[72] In most industrialized countries, bovine tuberculosis has been controlled with surveillance, testing and slaughter, and pasteurization of dairy products. In developing countries, tuberculosis caused by *M. bovis* has become widespread and a potential risk for exposed people and animals.[41] With respect to *M. bovis* infections, the gastrointestinal (GI) tract is the most common portal of entry. Cats and dogs can be potential disseminators of disease when the organism preferentially localizes in the intestinal or respiratory tracts. Because of localization of infection, cats usually excrete the organism via feces and dogs via sputum. *M. bovis* does not endure long in the environment, and reservoir hosts are essential for survival of the organism. Outside its hosts, the organism survives for a period varying from 4 days in summer to less than 28 days in winter.[92] Organisms may persist for several months in organic material such as feces or carcasses.[166,178] Dogs and cats acquire infection when they consume contaminated milk or scavenge contaminated carcasses. Dogs and cats may be involved in the maintenance of bovine tuberculosis on farms, where it is enzootic, and may be rarely responsible for transmission of the bovine bacillus to people (see Fig. 50-1). Subclinically, infected dogs and cats sometimes remain on farms after reactor cattle have been identified and removed from the herd, and farms or families with recurrent TB infections should have their pet animal contacts checked periodically. Rarely, spread of *M. bovis* between people has been reported.

Cats are more commonly infected with the bovine bacillus than dogs are; and on an experimental basis, cats appear to be more susceptible to bovine than to human TB. Part of this affinity is related to the frequent ingestion of contaminated, unpasteurized milk or uncooked meat or offal from infected cattle. Milk is an ideal medium for the organism because it buffers the gastric acid that normally prevents colonization of the lower GI tract with TB. Dogs and cats may also acquire TB from uncooked, infected meat used as cat and dog foods. As a result of eradication measures, the prevalence of bovine tuberculosis is low in the United States. Increased use of commercial foods and trends to urban living have reduced the prevalence of bovine tuberculosis in dogs and cats.

Despite the reduction of infection in domestic animals, bovine TB remains a problem worldwide, except in Australia, because it has become established in wildlife hosts that have acquired infection from cattle and that act as continued reservoirs for infection. As a result, domestic animals such as cattle, cats, and dogs continue to become infected.[46,47,159,185] For example, in Great Britain and Ireland, badgers *(Meles meles)* and foxes *(Vulpes vulpes)* have become a major wildlife reservoir.[44] Although transmission between badgers is predominantly by aerosols, *M. bovis* has also been found in their bite wounds suggesting cutaneous inoculation. Following a cattle outbreak in Cornwall, infection in domestic cats on the farm and local badgers all shared the same spoligotype.[141] Interestingly, no cattle had been recently kept on the premises suggesting that local badgers had somehow infected the resident cat population. In New Zealand, feral brushtail possums *(Trichosurus vulpecula)* and deer act as reservoir hosts; wild ferrets, pigs, cats, and goats are amplifier hosts whose carcasses infect carrion-eating animals. Amplifier hosts can become infected from carnivorous ingestion. Sheep, horses, and hedgehogs are spillover hosts that are incidentally infected.[40] Stoats, dogs, hares, rabbits, and many small rodents, are occasional dead-end hosts.

Captive and free-living exotic wildlife carnivores, including nondomestic canids and felids, and domestic and feral dogs and cats have been most commonly infected with *M. bovis*. Ingestion of infected carrion is the most common source of infection. The infection is maintained in gregarious herbivores, while carnivorous predators such as lions *(Panthera leo)*, cheetahs *(Acinonyx jubatus)*, leopards *(P. pardus)*, spotted hyaenas *(Crocuta crocuta)*, Iberian lynx *(Lynx pardina)*, Siberian tiger *(P. tigris longipilis)*, snow leopard *(Uncia uncia)*, and feral domestic cats have become secondarily infected.* Additional subsequent transmission of infection via aerosol or biting between gregarious carnivores, such as lions, has been suspected.[103]

M. microti—like Identified in Great Britain, the variant species was found predominantly in rural cats with avid hunting behavior. The source of infection is believed to be a prey species. Some previous reports of this infection from the United Kingdom may have been mistaken for *M. bovis* infections.[20] Currently, the relationship of this variant to *M. microti* is uncertain, but it is likely that they are very closely related.

M. microti Infection with *M. microti* has been described in cats.[85] Infection from rodents is considered the source of infection for cats and people. Pulmonary infection was found in the people who had no underlying evidence of immunodeficiency.

Nontuberculous Mycobacteria

M. avium Complex These organisms are ubiquitous worldwide in soil and water under certain conditions. MAC organisms have been shown to be present in acidic (pH 5.0 to 5.5) conditions and soils high in organic matter.[107] These conditions are met in acidic swamp areas, coastal plains, and brackish coastal waters. Feces of infected birds contain large numbers of bacilli, and infection of dogs and cats occurs from ingestion of infected meat or contact with infected soil or with fomites contaminated by poultry carcasses or feces (see Fig. 50-1). Unlike *M. tuberculosis* and *M. bovis*, MAC organisms remain viable for at least 2 years in the environment, including municipal water supplies, soil, dairy products, and tissues of birds and mammals. Natural, potable, and even treated water supplies in temperate and tropical regions can harbor nontuberculous mycobacteria. These organisms can exist within biofilms that coat the internal surfaces of water pipes, fixtures, and storage tanks. MAC organisms are likely to be found in recirculating water systems commonly used in human hospitals.[154] Hot water has a higher degree of colonization and chlorine does not inactivate these organisms, especially at higher temperatures. In hospital environments,

*References: 14, 25, 103, 112, 121, 180.

bathing, rinse, lavage, and disinfectant solutions made with potable water can become contaminated with MAC and NTM organisms. Endoscopy equipment can be similarly infected during cleaning.

Despite the widespread nature of MAC organisms, infections in dogs and cats have been rare owing to their innate resistance. Poultry and swine are primarily susceptible to MAC infection after contact with infected food or water.

The importance of infection with MAC organisms is that they produce granulomas of deeper tissue and parenchymal organs that are grossly indistinguishable from those caused by mammalian tubercle bacilli. No evidence has been found for spread of MAC organisms between or within animals and people.

Other Slow-Growing Saprophytic Mycobacteria The natural habitat of organisms such as *M. kansasii*, *M. simiae*, *M. terrae*, and *M. genavense* is likely the environment. They can be isolated from the sputum and stool of clinically healthy people and animals indicating exposure and contamination or colonization without establishment of clinical infection. The pathogenicity of these organisms is thought to be low, and they cause disease mainly in immunocompromised hosts.

Pathogenesis

Tubercle bacilli enter the body through either the respiratory or alimentary tract or skin penetration, depending on the initial route of exposure. Local multiplication of the bacillus may develop at the initial site of deposition—termed a primary complex—as well as in the regional draining lymph node. Granuloma formation occurs at both sites. Incomplete primary complex refers to infection and localization in the lymph node without lesion formation at the site of deposition. Cats more commonly form incomplete primary complexes whether tonsils, mandibular lymph nodes, or ileocecal lymph nodes are infected; the last are the most common sites for localization and shedding of *M. bovis* organisms. Dogs, which more commonly acquire *M. tuberculosis*, tend to develop respiratory infections with complete primary complex formation and lesions both in the lungs and hilar lymph nodes. *M. tuberculosis* more readily infects the respiratory tract because of its high oxygen requirements. Infections involving MAC organisms in dogs and cats have often been disseminated throughout lymphoid and many other tissues, without indications of a primary granuloma at the site of entry.

The cytokine staining pattern of feline mucocutaneous mycobacteriosis is similar to that described for human leprosy in which T cell–mediated response leads to epithelioid granulomas with abundant CD4+ type 1 helper T (Th1) cells and upregulation of the cytokines interleukin (IL)-1b, tumor necrosis factor (TNF)-α, IL-6, and granulocyte-macrophage colony-stimulating factor.[106]

Not all initial exposures to mycobacteria result in the formation of persistent granulomas because in most individuals, immune responses usually limit further multiplication and spread of the agent. The initial inflammatory response may then subside and resolve, with healing and fibrosis if the remaining tubercle bacilli can be eliminated. The production of persistent focal or disseminated disease is suggestive of defective cell-mediated immunity (CMI). With decreased immunologic resistance, the mycobacteria merely become confined within phagocytic cells where they continue to multiply because of the body's inefficiency in eliminating these intracellular pathogens. Granuloma formation is therefore a reflection of the body's attempt to contain remaining organisms. These viable organisms may remain dormant only to break out later and spread as a result of immunosuppression.

In a certain percentage of animals, the mycobacteria appear to outpace the host defense mechanism, resulting in progressive disease. This increased virulence may result from alterations in the route of exposure, size of inoculum, strain pathogenicity, and CMI defense mechanisms. Having produced primary lesions, the tuberculous mycobacteria may disseminate throughout the body, spreading the infection into adjacent tissue by direct extension or by mechanical means. Aspiration and gravitation of infectious exudates may spread the disease through other areas of lung tissue. Intracellular multiplication of the bacteria is unimpeded as the infection spreads to other tissues by lymphatic or hematogenous means.

A higher prevalence of *M. tuberculosis* infection has been observed in people with AIDS. In contrast, no clear association has been made between feline retroviral infection and mycobacteriosis. Certain breeds, such as the basset hound, the miniature schnauzer, Siamese cat, and Abyssinian cat, are over-represented in reports of MAC infection. Siamese cats are similarly predisposed to infections with other persistent intracellular organisms. Although likely, the precise defects in the immune system of these breeds have not been determined.

The factors that contribute to mycobacterial resistance by the host are unclear.[91] CMI is typically associated with protection against facultative intracellular pathogens such as mycobacteria. Increased resistance seems to be associated with the enhanced capacity of activated macrophages to kill tubercle bacilli or to inhibit their intracellular multiplication. In people with refractory pulmonary mycobacteriosis caused by non–*M. tuberculosis* organisms, a defect in interferon (IFN)-γ secretion has been documented.[165]

Infection with MAC organisms usually begins with ingestion of the organism from the environment or contaminated food or infected uncooked viscera. These organisms are closely related to *M. avium* subspecies paratuberculosis, the cause of Johne's disease, which is chronic granulomatous enteritis of ruminants and other herbivores. With Johne's disease, animals may acquire infection as neonates, through eating contaminated food or exposure to a contaminated environment. The mycobacteria may be phagocytized by intestinal macrophages at which time the infection becomes quiescent. Eventually, with stress or acquired or inborn immunosuppression, the organisms replicate and the disease occurs. Similar events are suspected to occur in MAC infections of dog breeds, such as the basset and miniature schnauzer, which develop illness within the first few years of life, likely as the result of unrecognized defects in CMI. In some animals with severe immunosuppression, bacteremia may result and multiple organ dissemination ensues.

Clinical Findings

Table 50-2 reviews the clinical features of disease caused by the various mycobacterial species.

Tuberculous Mycobacteria

M. tuberculosis* and *M. bovis Canine and feline tuberculosis is frequently a subclinical disease. Many pets become inadvertently infected with *M. tuberculosis* while living in the same household with tuberculous owners. Farm pets also may serve as subclinical reservoirs of *M. bovis* for susceptible cattle.

When clinical signs occur in dogs and cats, they reflect the site of granuloma formation. *M. tuberculosis* is more likely to cause pulmonary infections than is *M. bovis*, which often affects the GI tract. With respiratory involvement, bronchopneumonia, pulmonary nodule formation, and hilar lymphadenomegaly are most common in dogs, causing fever, weight loss, anorexia, and harsh nonproductive coughing.[61] Dogs and cats may develop dysphagia, retching, hypersalivation, and tonsillar enlargement, all the result of ulcerated and chronically draining oropharyngeal lesions. Cats develop primary intestinal localization more commonly than dogs, and they exhibit weight loss,

Table • 50-2

Comparison of Species of Mycobacterium Infecting Dogs and Cats

ORGANISM	ENVIRONMENTAL FACTORS	CLINICAL FEATURES	DRUG SUSCEPTIBILITY OR REPORTED SUCCESSFUL THERAPY[a]
Slow-Growing Tuberculous: Tubercles and Lymphadenitis, Occasional Dissemination			
M. tuberculosis	Urban, close contact affected person	Usually respiratory, pulmonary localization, can disseminate systemically	Isoniazid, rifampin, ethambutol, pyrazinamide
M. bovis	Rural cats, ingest raw beef or dairy products	Usually alimentary disorders, may get respiratory, cutaneous or lymphatic involvement, sometimes systemic dissemination	Rifampin, clarithromycin, fluoroquinolones, ethambutol, isoniazid, surgical excision of skin lesions
M. microti—like	Rural, suburban, hunter, bite wounds, prey exposure	Nodular cutaneous lesions draining, ulceration, peripheral lymphadenomegaly, local myositis, arthritis, osteomyelitis, sometimes systemic dissemination	Clarithromycin, fluoroquinolones, rifampin
Lepromatous: Cutaneous Nodular Dermatosis			
M. lepraemurium	Cooler wet climates, winter months, cats under 3 yrs of age exposed to infected rodent prey	Single to multiple cutaneous and subcutaneous dermal nodules on head and extremities, ulcers, fistulas, abscesses regional spread only	Clofazamine, clarithromycin, doxycycline or minocycline, rifampin, surgical removal
Feline leprosy, novel species	Central coast New South Wales, Australia, New Zealand, older cats over 10 yrs of age, feline immunodeficiency virus predisposes	Multiple subcutaneous dermal nodules, no ulceration, sometimes dissemination	Clarithromycin, rifampin, clofazimine
Candidatus *M. visibilis*	Environmental exposure	Cutaneous and disseminated	Clofazamine
Nontuberculous: Pyogranulomatous			
Saprophytic Slow Growing: Cutaneous Lesions, Lymphadenitis, Dissemination in Immunocompromised Hosts			
M. avium—complex	Exposure to infected soil, water or dust; acidic soils contaminated with bird feces or carcasses, Bassett hounds and Siamese cats most prevalence	Dermal and regional lymph node granulomas, alimentary infiltration, corneal granulomas, systemic dissemination	Clarithromycin, clofazimine, doxycycline or minocycline, rifabutin, ethambutol; rifampin preferred if central nervous system involvement for better penetration
M. genavense	Environmental exposure in immunocompromised host	Disseminated lymphadenitis	Clarithromycin, ethambutol, fluoroquinolones, clofazimine
M. terrae complex	Environmental exposure	Cutaneous lesions	Clarithromycin, fluoroquinolones, rifampin
M. simiae	Environmental exposure	Cutaneous and disseminated	Clarithromycin, fluoroquinolones, rifampin?
Canine leproid granuloma, novel species	Probably worldwide, biting flies	Subcutaneous nodules especially on the head and ears	Surgical removal, rifampin, clarithromycin

Continued

Table • 50-2

Continued

ORGANISM	ENVIRONMENTAL FACTORS	CLINICAL FEATURES	DRUG SUSCEPTIBILITY OR REPORTED SUCCESSFUL THERAPY[a]
Saprophytic Fast Growing: Cutaneous and Subcutaneous Pyogranulomatous Infections			
M. thermoresistibile	Soil and house dust, inhaled water, wound contaminant	Pyogranulomatous pneumonia, pyothorax, cutaneous and subcutaneous pyogranulomas	Doxycycline, clarithromycin
Other fast-growing opportunistic species	Soil and water exposure; bite and puncture wounds; immunocompromised host	Cutaneous and subcutaneous granulomas, especially inguinal region, ulcers, drainage, with regional spread only Secondary wound infections	Surgical removal, wide excision, variable susceptibility to fluoroquinolones, doxycycline, aminoglycosides, clofazimine, clarithromycin, trimethoprim-sulfonamide

[a]For dosages and detailed information on each, see Tables 50-4 to 50-7 and 50-9 and Drug Formulary, Appendix 8. A minimum of two and often three drugs should always be used in combination.

anemia, vomiting, and diarrhea as signs of intestinal malabsorption. Mesenteric lymph nodes are palpably enlarged. Abdominal effusion is present in some cases.

A continuum of clinical signs develops with disseminated disease. Direct extension of lung disease can result in pleural or pericardial effusion with signs of dyspnea, cyanosis, and right-sided heart failure. Dissemination from the GI tract to other tissues including the lungs has been commonly reported with longstanding infections in lions and cheetahs.[102,103] Dissemination from cutaneous lesions to the lungs has been observed in cats with *M. bovis* infections and can cause respiratory dysfunction. Disseminated disease may be the first sign of illness in many dogs and cats, and clinical signs are correlated with the organ localization in each case. Generalized lymphadenomegaly, anorexia, weight loss, fever, and sudden death may be observed. Masses or enlargement may be detected in many abdominal organs, especially the liver and spleen. Dermal nodules and nonhealing, draining ulcers have been noted commonly in cats and sometimes in dogs. Cats with *M. bovis* infections have developed tuberculous choroiditis and retinal detachments.[56] Granulomatous uveitis and central nervous system (CNS) signs have occurred in some cases. Lameness and spontaneous fractures have been observed with bone localization. Additional clinical signs have included hemoptysis, hematuria, and icterus.

***M. microti*—like** Cats with these infections usually develop cutaneous granulomas at the site of a bite or scratch wound or other penetrating injury (Figs. 50-2, *A* and *B*). Lesions often develop drainage and associated regional lymphadenomegaly. Organisms may disseminate subsequently causing infection of multiple organs.

Nontuberculous Mycobacteria

Mycobacterium avium Complex The ubiquitous distribution of MAC organisms in the environment compared with the low prevalence of the disease also suggests that subclinical infections are common. Dogs with MAC-induced disease have usually had extensive granulomatous disease of the bowel, spleen, liver, and mesenteric lymph nodes. Most dogs have been less than 4 years of age, and it is evident from lesions that the disease has been subclinical and progressive. Weight loss and lethargy are predominating clinical signs. Vomiting, anorexia, fever, diarrhea, and hematochezia have been

observed, but these may be intermittent. Other signs in some dogs have been paraspinal hyperesthesia, paresis, lameness, subcutaneous swellings, anterior uveitis, and respiratory difficulty.[78]

Cats with MAC infections often have developed enlargement of regional lymph nodes and subcutaneous swellings, especially around the head and face, and in some cases keratitis (Fig. 50-3).* These infections often follow bite or scratch wounds to the face. Weight loss, anorexia, and fever have been observed. Dissemination can occur to many tissues in some cats, and the clinical signs reflect the area involved.[12] Cats can develop visceral disease similar to dogs where thickened intestinal loops, hepatomegaly, splenomegaly, and intestinal lymph node enlargement can be palpated or observed (Fig. 50-4). Dissemination from GI viscera can produce respiratory dysfunction from pulmonary nodular interstitial infiltration.

Being environmentally resistant and an opportunist, *M. avium* infection has been implicated in outbreaks of hypersensitivity or granulomatous pneumonitis in people.[53] Aerosolized droplets of disinfected (e.g., chlorinated) water has been responsible for inflammatory reactions in the lungs of people and might also occur in their animals.

Other Slow-Growing Saprophytic Mycobacteria *M. genavense*, a fastidious MAC-like organism, is the cause of muscle wasting, small-bowel wall thickening, and hepatic granulomatous infiltration in birds and in humans with AIDS.[23] Pulmonary and disseminated infection with *M. genavense* has been found in dogs and an immunodeficiency virus (FIV)–infected cat.[82,104] *M. kansasii* caused pneumonia with pulmonary abscess formation and pyothorax in a dog.[158] *M. terrae* complex caused nodular dermal thickening of a digit of a cat.[74] Disseminated disease associated with multiple cutaneous nodules and ocular (chorioretinitis) and pulmonary involvement was found in a cat with *M. simiae* infection.[49]

Diagnosis

Clinical Laboratory Findings

Clinical laboratory findings in mycobacterial infections are frequently nonspecific and include moderate leukocytosis and anemia. The anemia is usually nonregenerative, but in some cats with intestinal infections, is reportedly macrocytic.[96]

*References: 48, 101, 123, 139, 174.

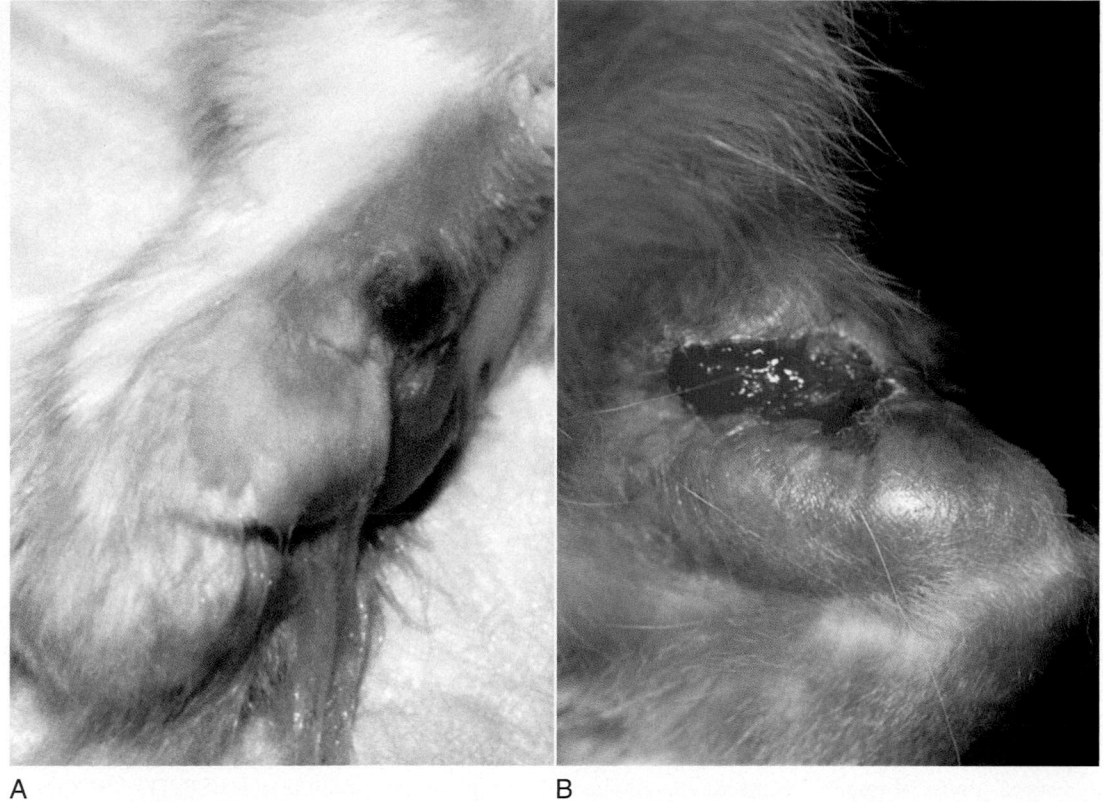

A   B

Fig 50-2 Nodular **(A)** and ulcerative **(B)** lesions of the extremities of cats with *M. microti*–like infection. (Courtesy D. Gunn-Moore, University of Edinburgh, Edinburgh, Scotland.)

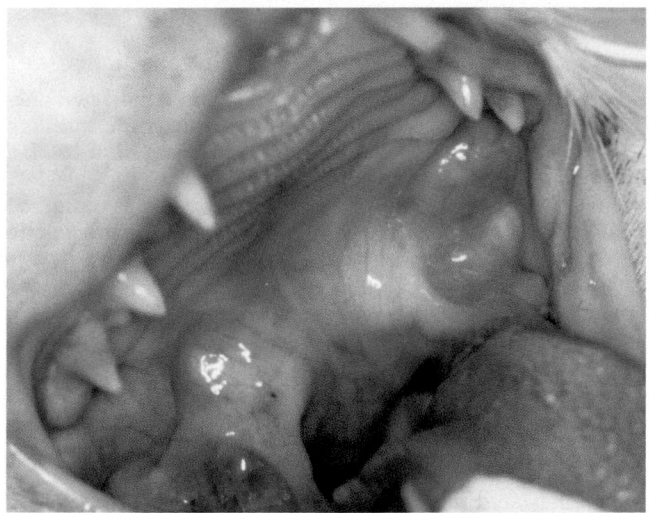

Fig 50-3 Mass lesion in the upper palate and maxillary region of a cat from localized *M. avium*–intracellulare infection. (Courtesy University of Georgia, Athens, Ga.)

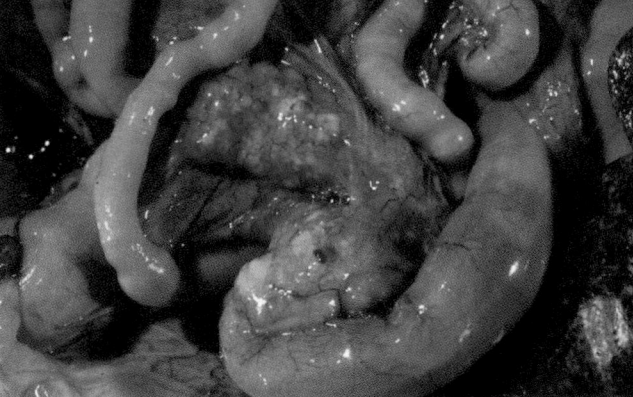

Fig 50-4 Intestinal mesenteric granulomas examined by exploratory laparotomy of a cat with disseminated *M. avium*–intracellulare infection. (Courtesy B. Flatland, University of Georgia, Athens, Ga.)

Normal to reduced serum albumin levels and hyperglobulinemia are frequently apparent. Hypercalcemia may be present as a result of the granulomatous inflammation as observed in other mycobacterial infections.[1,133] Organisms may be visualized in leukocytes of blood and bone marrow smears or buffy coat preparations or urine.[38,183] The lipid-containing cell wall does not stain with Romanovsky's stains so that bacilli appear as unstained bars within leukocytes.

With MAC infection, dogs have had anemia, leukocytosis, lymphopenia, hypoalbuminemia, and increased liver enzyme activities. Hilar lymphadenomegaly is often visible with thoracic radiography. In one dog, organisms were observed with acid-fast stained fecal smears.[78] Cats typically have anemia, neutrophilic leukocytosis, and hyperglobulinemia.

Radiographically and ultrasonographically visible masses may be apparent in various organ systems. Abnormalities on thoracic radiography can include tracheobronchial lymphadenomegaly and interstitial pulmonary infiltrates; calcified pulmonary lesions may be observed (Fig. 50-5). Lung consolidation and granuloma formation have been associated with diffuse radiopaque densities in lung lobes. Metastatic lesions from dissemination are seen as diffuse miliary densities (Figs.

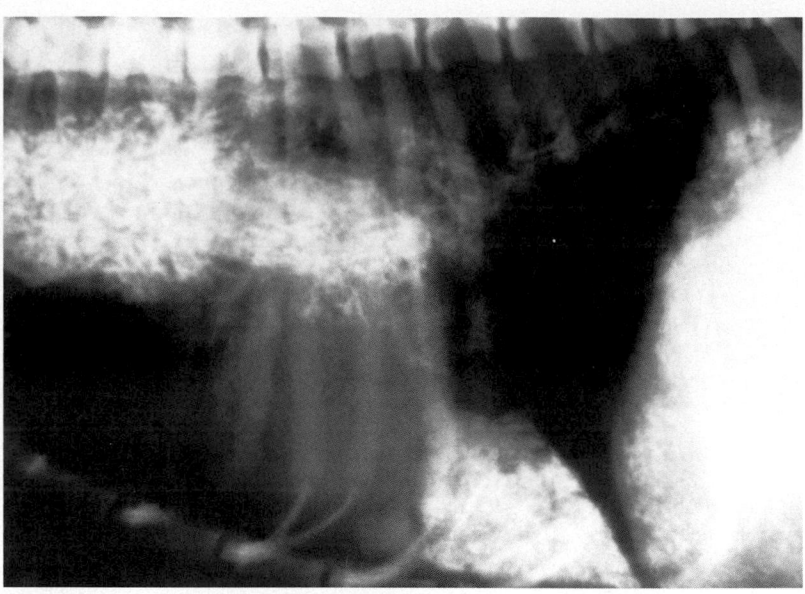

Fig 50-5 Lateral thoracic radiograph of a 3-year-old male Yorkshire terrier with tuberculosis. Note the multiple irregular mineralization of soft tissue in the craniodorsal thorax and cranial abdomen. (From Lui S, Weitzman L, Johnson GG. 1980. Canine tuberculosis, *J Am Vet Med Assoc* 177:164–167. Reprinted with permission.)

50-6, *A* and *B*). Fluid may be present in the pleural or pericardial cavities. Abdominal radiography may reveal enlargement of parenchymal organs such as the liver and spleen or solitary abdominal masses. Fluid may be present in the abdominal cavity, and calcified mesenteric lymph nodes may be evident. Bony lesions consist of small, circumscribed, radiolucent areas. Thoracic involvement may be associated with hypertrophic pulmonary osteopathy. Diskospondylitis or vertebral osteomyelitis may be apparent.

Cytology

Specimens should be obtained from tissue aspirates or impression smears taken by biopsy or at necropsy. The acid-fast stain is the most widely available method for making a rapid presumptive diagnosis of mycobacterial infection. Acid-fast stains will be positive for specimens from many but not all animals with mycobacterial infections. It is more consistent for organisms recovered in culture. Mycobacteria can be stained for acid fastness with carbolfuchsin or fluorescent dyes (i.e., auramine-rhodamine). The fluorochrome stains are more sensitive and technically less difficult to examine than conventional carbolfuchsin stains. For enteric infections with organisms such as *M. avium* or *M. bovis*, acid-fast staining of rectal scrapings or fecal mucus may detect organisms.

Tuberculin Testing

Tuberculin is a purified protein derivative (PPD) from *M. tuberculosis*. People or animals infected with tubercle-producing mycobacteria develop a delayed hypersensitivity reaction when this antigen is injected intradermally (ID). Nontuberculosis mycobacteria contain proteins analogous to *M. tuberculosis*, and considerable cross-reactivity exists. ID skin testing has been used as an aid in the detection and diagnosis of human tuberculosis and to evaluate delayed-type hypersensitivity in animals. The two types of tuberculin used for ID testing are summarized in Table 50-3. Depending on whether a history of infection or disease exists, various strengths (1, 5, or 250 tuberculin units/0.1 ml) of PPD are usually selected in human skin testing. However, the highest concentration is needed to test dogs. ID tuberculin testing in dogs is reportedly inconsistent and unreliable. In contrast, use of the pinna showed reliability in detecting dogs previously sensitized with bacille Calmette-Guérin (BCG) vaccine, an attenuated mutant strain of *M. bovis* that has been used in people as a vaccine to induce resistance to tuberculosis and as a nonspecific immunostimulant. In addition, infected dogs have been shown to respond well to ID skin testing with BCG. A disadvantage of BCG is that it can induce later false-positive reactions in skin testing with PPD. Although not studied in animals, false-positive results have been more common in people using certain brands of PPD.[164] BCG must be handled cautiously to avoid inadvertent inoculation because immunosuppressed people, especially those with AIDS, or immunocompromised animals being tested may develop disseminated disease.[177,188,189] Both tuberculous and nontuberculous mycobacterial infections give positive results with ID tuberculin or BCG testing.

Tests are performed by injecting BCG or PPD ID on the medial side of the proximal hind limb or, preferably, on the inner surface of the pinna. A positive reaction is indicated only if a raised, indurated, and subsequently necrotic swelling appears at the site of injection between 48 and 72 hours later. Necrosis and ulceration may take up to 2 weeks to develop. Mild erythema after ID BCG injection in dogs is considered nonspecific. False-positive results caused by cross-reactivity with other bacterial species have been observed.

Another method of tuberculin testing for dogs, recommended by the U.S. Department of Agriculture (USDA), requires that a baseline rectal temperature be taken. If it is in the reference range, inject Subcutaneous (SC) 0.75 ml PPD bovis (as supplied by USDA, see Table 50-3). The rectal temperature is monitored every 2 hours for 12 hours. A 1.1° C (2° F) rise in temperature is interpreted as a positive test result.

Unlike many species, cats do not react strongly to ID-administered tuberculin. Despite their lack of response to PPD, cats still have adequate immunity to tuberculosis. SC or intravenous (IV) challenge with tuberculin is no more reliable, and cats do not respond well to ID BCG. Cats sensitized to BCG have responded to PPD injected ID in the pinna; unfortunately, the response has usually been inconsistent, infrequent, or transient. The SC method has not been evaluated in cats, and biopsy, culture, and necropsy are more definitive tests. Tuberculin testing has been effectively used in lions by inoculating ID in the cervical region.[103]

Serologic Testing

Although unreliable compared with skin testing, serologic testing for antimycobacterial antibodies includes hemagglutination and complement fixation. Serologic testing has been employed to detect infected dogs and cats when skin testing

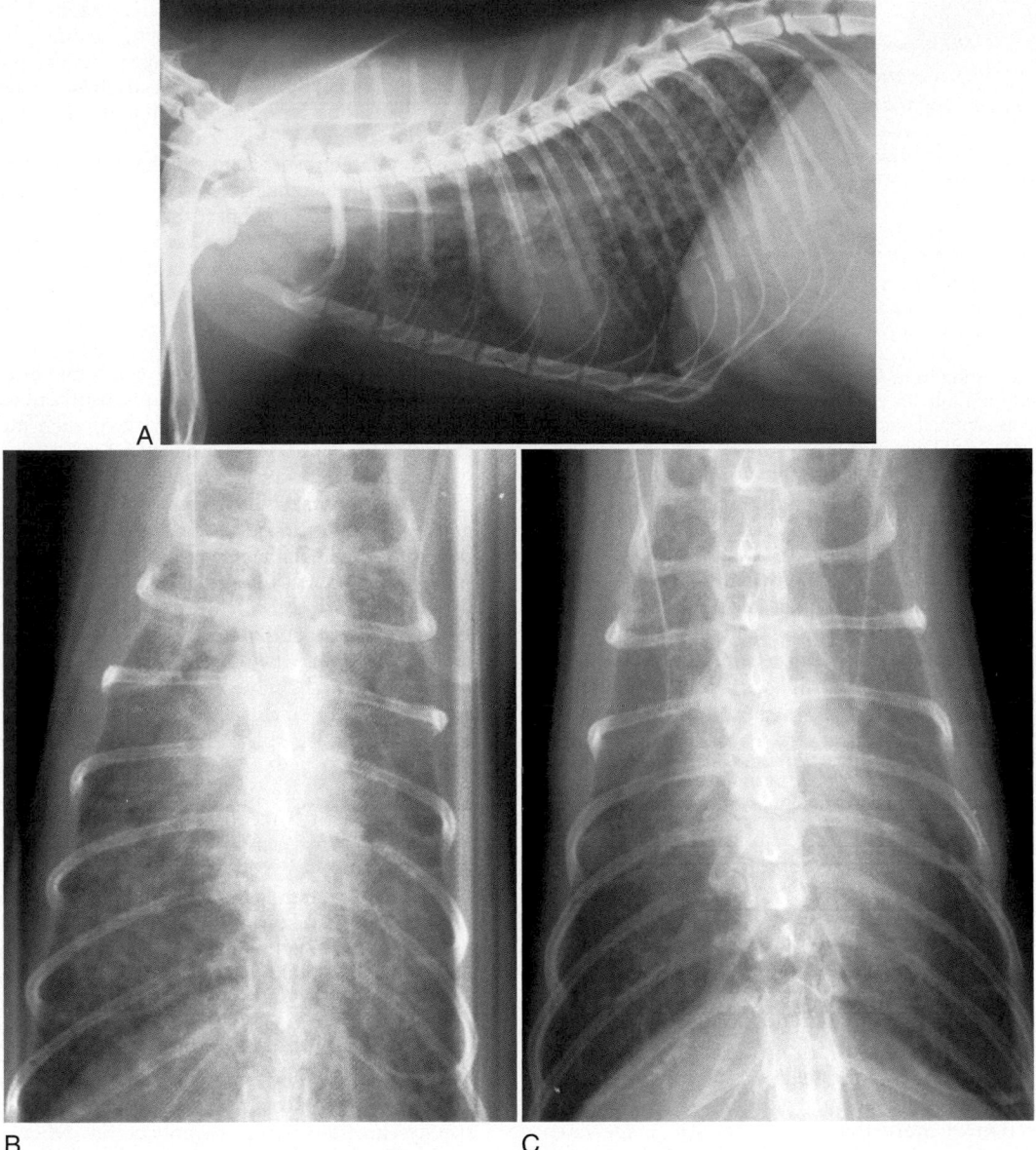

Fig 50-6 **A,** Lateral thoracic radiograph of a cat with disseminated *M. bovis* infection and dorsoventral thoracic radiograph of a cat with disseminated *M. avium*–intracellulare infection before **(B)** and after **(C)** therapy. (Part **A** courtesy D. Gunn-Moore, University of Edinburgh, Edinburgh, Scotland. Parts **B** and **C** courtesy University of Georgia, Athens, Ga.)

was inconclusive. The serologic response to *M. bovis* BCG vaccination in cats and dogs has been evaluated with immunoblotting against specific protein antigens.[21] Antibody increases were detected 3 to 5 weeks after vaccination and remained increased for 23 weeks and longer than 1 year in dogs and cats, respectively. Serologic testing may potentially detect exposure to mycobacteria similar to ID skin testing. Unfortunately, antibodies to mycobacteria such as BCG react with a wide variety of bacteria, fungi, and protozoa. This feature has been employed as a histochemical procedure to detect microorganisms in tissues.[22]

Bacterial Isolation

Mycobacterial culture is the reference standard for diagnosis. In collection of specimens for *M. tuberculosis*, direct inoculation of pleural exudates into media gives a greater yield than that following transport of the specimen to the laboratory.[35] Addition of heparin to the specimen gave similar results to direct inoculation, presumably because the organisms trapped in coagulated material could not be cultured. For culture, tissue- or mucosa-derived samples are usually treated with 4% sodium hydroxide and another disinfectant such as N-acetyl-L-cysteine to eliminate any contaminating micro-

Table • 50-3

Summary of Intradermal Skin Testing for Tuberculosis in Dogs and Cats[a]

SUBSTANCE	PREFERRED SITE	DOSE
PPD	Inner surface pinna	250 TU[b] (0.1 ml)
BCG	Inner surface pinna	0.1–0.2 ml[c]

BCG, Bacilli Calmette-Guérin; PPD, purified protein derivative of tuberculin; TU, tuberculin units.

[a]See text for information on performance and interpretation of the test.

[b]PPD for bovine testing from U.S. Department of Agriculture is 30,000 TU/ml (1 mg/ml). To prepare at least 250 TU/0.1 ml, remove 0.1 ml as supplied; add to 1.1 ml sterile water for injection; mix in sterile glass vial. Diluted solutions of PPD should be made fresh and used soon after preparation. Human (M. tuberculosis) or bovine (M. bovis) strains can be used for tuberculin source because cross-reactions exist to cell wall components. The human strain might give a stronger reaction to M. tuberculosis but bovine is available in higher concentration. Higher concentrations are used to test animals than people when sensitivity rather than specificity is more important when public health risk exists. NOTE: in people, 5 TU units in 0.1 ml of solution (50 TU/ml) are used on volar aspect forearm and read in 48–72 hours. If human tuberculin is supplied in milligrams, the conversion factor is 50,000 U of PPD equals 1 mg of PPD.

[c]BCG vaccine USP contains 8–26 million colony-forming units/ml of living bacillus. Reconstitute freeze-dried preparation into 1-ml aliquots according to manufacturer's recommendation. BCG may sensitize the animal to false-positive results to further tuberculin testing.

organisms. Specimens that are usually sterile (internal tissues, cerebral spinal fluid, urine, blood) should not be decontaminated because the viability of low numbers of mycobacteria present can be lost. When specimens are small and contain acid-fast organisms, the entire sample should be placed in a broth-based culture medium. Broth or liquid media facilitate more rapid growth and higher yields of mycobacteria. Solid media are still required for optimal isolation of mycobacteria and for detection of more than one species in a specimen. Pathogenic tuberculous mycobacteria are slow-growing, often requiring 4 to 6 weeks to establish visible colonies on solid media, and their growth is inhibited unless enrichment media are used. Egg-enrichment media such as Lowenstein-Jensen (LJ) and agar-based media such as Middlebrook (both from Difco Labs, Detroit, Mich.) are preferred as solid media for isolating tubercle bacilli. Glycerol, which is added to media such as LJ to enhance the growth of M. tuberculosis, actually inhibits the growth of M. bovis. Stonebrink's or B83 media are used when M. bovis is suspected.[42] Growth is more rapid in 5% to 10% carbon dioxide. Some saprophytic species such as M. genavense grow better under microaerophilic conditions of reduced (2.5%) oxygen tension.[161] Pathogenic and saprophytic mycobacteria have been identified and differentiated by colony growth and biochemical characteristics (see Table 50-1).

Commercial methods have been developed that facilitate rapid detection and classification of the mycobacteria. The lysis-centrifugation method (Isolator system, Wampole Labs, Cranbury, N.J.) has also been used to facilitate culture of intracellular pathogens such as mycobacteria from blood. Radiometric automated methods for broth culture such as the BACTEC system (Becton Dickinson Microbiology Systems, Sparks, Md.), ESP-AFB (Difco Labs, Detroit, Mich.), and MB/Bact (BioMerieux, Durham, N.C.) have reduced time for initial detection of mycobacterial growth to an average of

10 to 13 days. Using the BACTEC system, LJ media could be eliminated without compromising accuracy.[171] Final identification can be 4 to 6 weeks longer, but the polymerase chain reaction (PCR) followed by restriction analysis and nucleic acid hybridization has shortened this time to a few days.[34,155,181,187]

Mycobacterial isolates can have been identified and specialized laboratories determine their susceptibility to antimicrobial drugs. In the United States, some of these laboratories are the National Animal Disease Laboratory in Ames, Iowa, and the National Jewish Medical and Research Center in Denver, Colo. (see Appendix 5).

Organism Detection

Mycobacterial components are detectable in body fluids such as CSF using enzyme-linked immunosorbent assay (ELISA) or radioimmunoassay. The sensitivity of such methods is much greater than acid-fast staining is to detect organisms in leukocytes. Detection of mycobacterial antigens in sputum by ELISA is more difficult because they are often lost in the processing of such fluids for analysis. MAC organisms have been detected within phagocytes in acid-fast stained fecal smears from animals with GI infections.[78]

Animal inoculation has been performed historically to identify mycobacterial species and those, such as M. leprae and M. lepraemurium, that are difficult to culture. Laboratory animals such as guinea pigs, rabbits, mice, and hamsters have been inoculated intraperitoneally with suspensions of lymph node, spleen, and granulomas from suspected cases.

PCR can be used on tissue specimens or body fluids to detect or identify mycobacteria that grow slowly or cannot be cultured in the microbiology laboratory. The Direct Test (Gen-Probe, San Diego, Calif.) targets ribosomal RNA, and the AMPLICOR Test (Roche Molecular Systems, Branchburg, N.J.) targets DNA. Such nucleic acid hybridization methods are best used for specific identification of the organisms found in culture. These methods have been helpful investigating outbreaks because genotyping strains may help determine their pathogenic significance or facilitate epidemiologic tracking of their source. Nucleic acid methods should complement but not replace conventional methods of mycobacterial isolation for detection of infection. These methods have a high sensitivity in identifying mycobacteria when organisms are prevalent in cytologic specimens, but a low sensitivity when organisms are few or unapparent.

Genotyping M. tuberculosis isolates is usually done via restriction-fragment-length polymorphism analysis of the distribution of an insertion sequence (IS6110) in different strains.[10] The genome of M. tuberculosis also contains many mycobacterial interspersed repeat units which can be distinguished. The detection of these spacers can be used in a process called spacer oligonucleotide typing (spoligotyping). Genotyping offers the advantage of evaluating different isolates for drug susceptibility, epidemiologic tracking, and environmental control purposes.

Tissue Biopsy

Definitive diagnoses can be made by demonstrating acid-fast organisms within a lesion via biopsy and histologic examination of lesions or by direct smears of exudates or fluids. Although often present in low numbers, intracellular tubercle bacilli are recognized by their clubbed-shape and beaded appearance. M. tuberculosis bacilli may be prominent in extracellular locations.[106] In comparison to tubercle bacilli, MAC organisms are generally smaller and present in high numbers within infected cells. The acid-fast staining method is ideal for aspirates of tissue and granulomas and for identifying organisms in bacterial cultures. A modified Dieterle stain was more sensitive in detection of low numbers of mycobacteria in lesions than acid-fast methods.[24] Unfortunately, this silver impregnation stains *Nocardia* and *Bartonella* in a similar fashion so that other stains such as acid-fast, which also stains *Nocardia*, must be used. Mycobacteria can also be more specifically identified by direct fluorescent antibody methods or PCR. A high percentage of human patients have positive results based on culture and PCR yet have negative staining results by acid-fast methods. Such acid-fast false negative results may relate to a dormant state shown by *M. tuberculosis* in which an alteration in cell-wall composition develops with persistence of infection.[168]

Pathologic Findings

In dogs and cats, generalized emaciation is a frequent finding on gross necropsy. Multifocal granulomas are grayish-white to yellow, circumscribed, nodular lesions and appear in many organs. Lung and bronchial lymph nodes are usually the primary lesion sites in dogs, and ileocecal and mesenteric lymph nodes are similarly involved in cats. Generalized spread is more common in dogs than in cats; pleura, pericardium, liver, kidney, heart, intestine, and CNS lesions are the most frequent (Fig. 50-7). The mesenteric lymph nodes, spleen, and skin are more commonly involved in cats. Rarely, bone, joint, and genital lesions may be observed in dogs and cats, and conjunctival lesions have been observed in cats and ferrets. Unlike larger solitary primary granulomas, metastatic lesions are frequently small (1 to 3 mm) and multifocal or appear as large clusters of coalescing tubercles in many organs.

Histologically, granulomatous lesions consist of areas of focal necrosis surrounded by infiltrations of plasma cells and macrophages. Evidence of encapsulation is apparent by peripheral layers of densely packed fibroblasts in a thin, fibrous, connective tissue capsule. Calcification of the granuloma is sometimes present; however, liquefaction of the necrotic central caseous portion is rarely, if ever, observed in carnivores (Fig. 50-8). Epithelioid or histiocytic cells usually border the necrotic zone; giant cell formation, which occurs in other species, is uncommon. Short-chained, beaded, slightly pleomorphic, acid-alcohol–fast bacilli may be detected intracellularly in the periphery of necrotic lesions (see Fig. 50-8). Organisms within macrophages and epithelioid cells are usually more numerous in MAC and *M. genavense* infections than they are in infections caused by *M. bovis* and *M. tuber-*

culosis (compare Figs. 50-9, *A* and *B* with Fig. 50-8). Infection with *M. microti*–like variant can result in variable numbers of intracellular bacilli. In contrast, *M. tuberculosis* infections are characterized by extracellular bacilli.[106]

Therapy

Because of the delay in definitive isolation of mycobacteria, treatment should be instituted based on cytologic or histologic diagnosis. Single-drug treatment of any mycobacterial infection of animals is not advised; rather, for best efficacy, combination therapy is always needed (Table 50-4). Antimicrobial resistance may develop when single-agent therapy is used.[2] At least two, if not three, drugs should be given simultaneously. For additional information on antimycobacterial drugs, see Antibacterial Chemotherapy, Chapter 34, and respective agents in the Drug Formulary, Appendix 8.

M. tuberculosis *Infection*

Treatment of human tuberculosis involves several drug regimens, depending on whether the patient has been exposed and whether the subclinical or active disease has been demonstrated. Long-term (6 to 12 months), single-drug (isoniazid) regimens are given prophylactically when exposure with concurrent immunosuppression increases the likelihood of producing active disease. Treatment of active *M. tuberculosis* infection involves the combination of at least two agents for a minimum of 6 to 9 months. In people, the isoniazid-ethambutol-rifampin combination is the most effective course of therapy, although pyrazinamide is being substituted for ethambutol more frequently. Drugs such as these have made human tuberculosis a curable disease, and surgical removal of

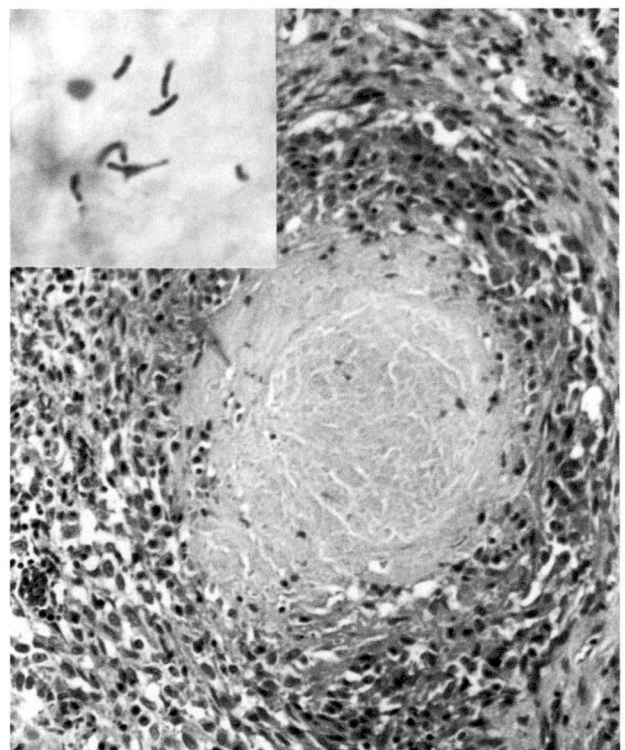

Fig 50-8 Photomicrograph of a liver from a 2-year-old female German shepherd showing a caseous tubercle with central necrosis, proliferation of histiocytes and fibroblasts in the middle zone, and encapsulation in the periphery (H and E, ×100). Inset: beaded bacilli (acid-fast, ×1000). (From Lui S, Weitzman I, Johnson GG. 1980. Canine tuberculosis, *J Am Vet Med Assoc* 177:164–167. Reprinted with permission.)

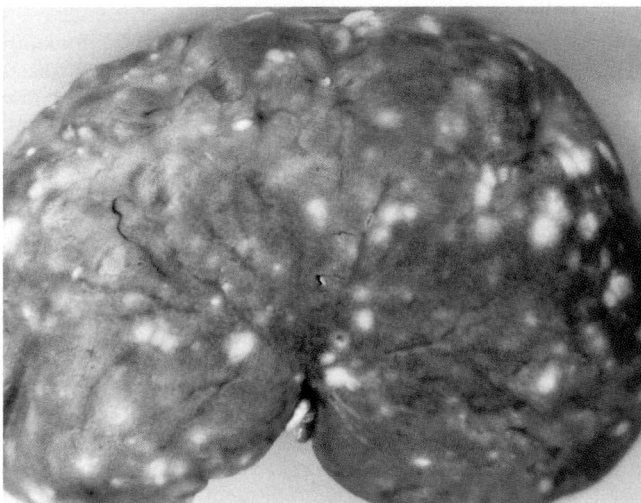

Fig 50-7 Multifocal granulomas in the kidney of a 3.5-year-old male boxer with systemic spread of *M. tuberculosis* infection. (From Lui S, Weitzman I, Johnson GG. 1980. Canine tuberculosis, *J Am Vet Med Assoc* 177:164–167. Reprinted with permission.)

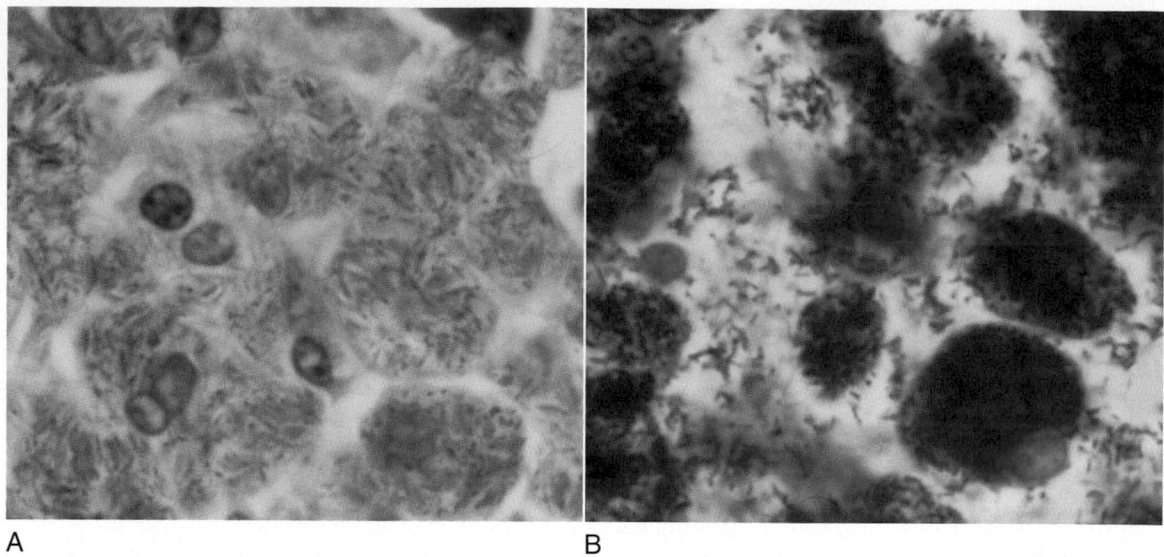

Fig 50-9 A, Multinucleated macrophages in the tissues of a cat with disseminated *M. genavense* infection (H and E, ×1000). **B,** Same sections with aggregates of macrophages and multinucleated cells packed with acid-fast, beaded Gram-variable, short (1.5 to 4.0 μm) straight bacilli (acid-fast, ×1000). (Courtesy Paul Canfield, University of Sydney, Sydney, Australia.)

tuberculous granulomas is no longer required. However, increasing antimicrobial resistance to these drugs is cause for concern and routine treatment of animal infections might contribute to the development of this resistance.

Similar guidelines might apply when considering treatment of pets (see Table 50-4). Chemotherapy of spontaneous canine tuberculosis has been successful in certain cases in which it has been provided. Rapid regression of experimentally produced lesions in dogs has been achieved by combined IV administration of rifampin and isoniazid and intramuscular administration of streptomycin for 23 months. Increases in coagulation times and liver enzyme activities were side effects of this extended therapy. Other drugs that have been shown to have activity against tuberculous mycobacteria are fluoroquinolones, metronidazole, oxazolidinones, azithromycin, and clarithromycin.

The decision to treat infected dogs and cats must be taken seriously because of the obvious human health hazard that exists, particularly when *M. tuberculosis* or *M. bovis* is responsible. It is not recommended for confirmed infections. Diagnosis by skin or serologic testing is not as reliable in detecting exposed or latently infected animals, and placing dogs or cats exposed to human or bovine tuberculosis on prophylactic chemotherapy may be desirable.

M. bovis *Infection*

M. bovis is resistant to pyrazinamide. Cats with *M. bovis* infection have been treated effectively by surgical excision of localized skin lesions and oral rifampin at 4 mg/kg/day for 2 to 5 months and by using long-term protocols including rifampin, a fluoroquinolone, and either clarithromycin or azithromycin.[47,69] Unfortunately, use of rifampin alone has the potential to induce bacterial resistance.

M. microti–*like Infection*

Cats with *M. microti*–like infections have been treated successfully in some cases with a combination of rifampin, enrofloxacin or marbofloxacin, and clarithromycin or azithromycin (see Table 50-4).[69] Given that single cutaneous lesions have the most favorable prognosis, assessing the cat for evidence of disseminated infection before starting treatment is important. Thoracic radiography is a valuable diagnostic aid

for this purpose. Cats with disseminated infection may still respond to treatment but usually require more prolonged courses (longer than 6 months).

M. avium *Complex Infection*

Unlike opportunistic rapid-growing mycobacteria, MAC strains are often resistant in vitro to the quinolones and a large number of other antimicrobials. Treatment of dogs with MAC infection has not been very rewarding; however, in most cases, advanced, disseminated visceral infection occurred before diagnosis. One dog was treated with a combination of clofazimine, ciprofloxacin, and rifampin with limited success.[140] Anemia and hepatotoxicity were side effects of rifampin therapy. A basset hound with disseminated infection that was on continuous combination therapy of enrofloxacin, clarithromycin, and clofazimine (dosages as outlined in Table 50-4) was in remission for 2 years before experiencing relapse.[19] In another basset hound, this same regimen was successful in halting progression of the disease and no relapse had occurred in 2.5 years.[63] A third basset hound developed a CNS granuloma during posttreatment remission with enrofloxacin, clarithromycin, and clofazimine, and the progression of the intracerebral lesion was halted by substitution of rifampin with clarithromycin as a better CNS-penetrating drug.[63] In human patients with AIDS, the three-drug regimen of rifabutin, ethambutol, and clofazimine is more effective compared with rifampin, ethambutol, clofazimine, and ciprofloxacin.[170]

In cats, localized or cutaneous infections have been treated with more success. One cat with a localized MAC granuloma had surgical removal alone, but the mass subsequently returned.[175] A cat with localized MAC infection was successfully treated with surgical removal of a portion of the mass followed by combination therapy with clofazimine and doxycycline.[101] Another cat treated with clofazimine alone following surgical debulking had complete remission.[123] In another cat with cutaneous infection, treatment with enrofloxacin alone was unsuccessful.[139] An Abyssinian cat with disseminated infection involving the mesentery and lungs was successfully treated with a combination of clofazimine, clarithromycin, and doxycycline at dosages in Table 50-4.[63] Clinical resolution of the problem occurred within 2 months, and

Table • 50-4

Dosages of Some Antimicrobial Drugs for Treatment of Slow-Growing Mycobacterial Infections

DRUG	SPECIES	DOSE (MG/KG)[a]	ROUTE	INTERVAL (HOURS)	TOXICITIES
M. tuberculosis infection					
Chemoprophylaxis[b]					
Isoniazid	D	10[c]	PO	24	Hepatotoxic
Treatment (minimum of two of the following drugs in combination)[d]					
Isoniazid	D	10–20[e]	PO	24	Hepatotoxic
Rifampi(ci)n	D	5–10[f]	PO	12–24	Hepatotoxic; discolors mucosae, tears, and urine
Ethambutol	D	10–25	PO	24	Optic neuritis
Dihydrostreptomycin	D	15	IM	24	Ototoxic
Pyrazinamide[g]	D	15–40	PO	24	Hepatoxic, GI signs, arthralgia
M. microti—like, M. terrae Group, and M. simiae Infections[h]					
Rifampi(ci)n	C	10–20	PO	24	Hepatotoxic, cutaneous erythema
Enrofloxacin	C	5	PO	24	Vomiting, retinal toxicity
Marbofloxacin	C	2	PO	24	Retinal toxicity
Clarithromycin	D	7.5–12.5	PO	12	Cutaneous erythema
	C	62.5 mg total[i]	PO	12	Cutaneous erythema
Azithromycin	C	7–15	PO	24	
M. avium—Complex Infection					
Clarithromycin	D	7.5–12.5	PO	12	Cutaneous erythema, hepatotoxicity
	C	62.5 mg total[i]	PO	12–24	Cutaneous erythema, hepatotoxicity
Clofazimine[j]	D	4–12	PO	24	Orange staining
	C	8–10	PO	24	Orange staining
	C	25 mg total	PO	24	Orange staining
Rifampi(ci)n	B	10–15	PO	24	Hepatotoxic, cutaneous erythema
Doxycycline	B	5–10[k]	PO	12	Vomiting, esophagitis

D, Dog; *C*, cat, *B*, both, *PO*, by mouth, *IM*, intramuscular.
[a]Dose per administration at specified interval. After daily dosing for weeks to months, switch to twice weekly administration for 6–9 months. See also Appendix 8. See Table 50–2 for general susceptibility guidelines and recommended combination therapy for each organism.
[b]For 6–12 months.
[c]Dosages are extrapolated from human child and adult recommendations. Treatment of *M. tuberculosis* or *M. bovis* infections is not recommended for dogs and cats.
[d]*Localized*: isoniazid and rifampin daily for 6 months with pyrazinamide added during the first 2 months or isoniazid and rifampin alone for 9 months. *Disseminated*: isoniazid and rifampin, with ethambutol or pyrazinamide, or both, initially and treat daily beyond 9 months.
[e]Maximum 300 mg daily.
[f]Maximum 600 mg daily.
[g]Ineffective for *M. bovis* strains.
[h]Treatment for 2 months minimum with three drugs in combination (e.g., rifampin with a fluoroquinolone [either enrofloxacin or marbofloxacin] and with either clarithromycin or azithromycin). Maintenance therapy for 4 months thereafter consists of the same dosages of any two of the three drugs.[69]
[i]Some large cats require higher doses.
[j]Because of difficulty of fractionating liquid in capsules, for convenience cats are usually given one 50-mg capsule per dose. The contents of capsule may be cut into halves with a scalpel blade while wearing disposable gloves and dividing it into two gelatin capsules. Alternatively a compounding pharmacist can provide the optimal dosage size. Currently not available in the United States.
[k]Can increase dosage up to 10 mg/kg for improved efficacy but only if this level is tolerated; give with food or administer water to avoid esophageal injury; if possible use monohydrate salt to minimize gastrointestinal irritation.

treatment was continued for 7 months until hepatotoxicity was heralded by anorexia and marked increase in serum alanine aminotransferase activity. Substituting enrofloxacin for clarithromycin solved this problem, and treatment was continued for an additional 3 months at which time it was discontinued. No relapse occurred during an additional 12 months of monitoring. Several Abyssinian cats with disseminated MAC infections were successfully treated using clofazimine and clarithromycin in combination.[8,122] Appropriate therapy for potentially resectable granulomatous masses should involve excision of the majority, if not all, of the lesions, when possible, followed by multiple drug therapy. With pulmonary dissemination, effectiveness of therapy can be monitored by repeating thoracic radiography for a clearing of the lung fields (see Fig. 50-6, C). Abdominal ultrasonography is best for monitoring resolution of mesenteric lesions.

Other Slow-Growing Mycobacteria

Enrofloxacin, rifampin, and clarithromycin, in combination, were effective in treating a cat with localized *M. terrae* complex infection[74] and another with disseminated *M. simiae* infection.[49]

Adjunctive Therapy

In vitro and in vivo, phenothiazine drugs inhibit mycobacterial growth.[4] Levels that were effective were greater than what could be achieved therapeutically. However, these drugs concentrate in macrophages and may potentiate antimycobacterial agents. Use of low daily levels of a drug such as acepromazine may be considered as adjunctive therapy to help facilitate antimicrobial efficacy. Immunotherapy with avirulent mycobacteria, such as *M. vaccae*, has been advocated to treat people with tuberculosis; however, results in controlled trials have not been effective.[43] Low antiinflammatory dosages of glucocorticoids have been given to immunocompromised people with *M. avium* infection when antimicrobial treatment has failed.[50] Fever and malaise were reversed, and new opportunistic infections were not noticeably increased.

Prevention

Tuberculosis is a major human public health problem. People are susceptible to *M. bovis*, *M. tuberculosis*, *M. microti*, and MAC organisms. This susceptibility is important with respect to control in animals. Identification of *M. tuberculosis* infection in people should be followed by serologic testing or clinical evaluation of pet contacts as possible reservoirs. Outbreaks of *M. bovis* infection in cattle should also be followed by evaluation of dogs and cats on the farm. Feeding of unpasteurized milk or raw offal to pets must be discontinued. Live BCG vaccine has been administered to protect people against infection with *M. tuberculosis*. Live recombinant DNA vaccines have been produced using nonvirulent mycobacteria.

The effectiveness of such products is being evaluated on an experimental basis. The attempt to control tuberculosis in dogs with modified live vaccines has had moderate success in that some dogs have shown increased resistance to infection, but immunity is partial, and vaccination has not been generally recommended. This approach also can produce false-positive skin test results as it does in other species.

Handling of saprophytic mycobacteria-infected dogs or cats is not a major health risk for immunocompetent people because these bacteria are normally found in the environment in large numbers. However, they do pose a risk for immunodeficient people and animals. As compared with other pathogenic bacteria, mycobacteria are among the most resistant organisms to disinfection, elevated temperature, or ultraviolet light. Disinfection efficacy depends on the chemical used, its time of application, concentration, and duration of contact. Instruments that contact mucous membranes should be treated with the utmost care to avoid inadvertent transfer of organisms to uninfected patients. Instruments that will contact tissue surfaces must have a high level of disinfection yet be nonirritating. Table 50-5 summarizes appropriate disinfectants and their properties. Glutaraldehyde at 2% should be used for 10 minutes at 20° C. Ethyl and isopropyl alcohols are mycobactericidal agents that can be used as the terminal rinse in disinfection. Regardless of the disinfectant used, manual precleaning with neutral detergents has the greatest effect in decontaminating equipment that has been in contact with mycobacteria. Tap water should never be used as a final rinse to remove disinfecting agents.

Public Health Considerations

Tuberculous Mycobacteria

Although *M. tuberculosis* and *M. bovis* infections are not maintained in canine and feline reservoirs, infected dogs and cats may serve as temporary sources for dissemination of bacteria into the environment. Because respiratory or intestinal secretions may be contaminated, it is recommended that *M. tuberculosis*–infected animals be either treated or euthanized. *M. tuberculosis* infections have developed in animals in zoologic

Table • 50-5

Comparison of Available Environmental Disinfectants for Mycobacteria[a]

DISINFECTANT	CONCENTRATION	ADVANTAGES	DISADVANTAGES	COMMENTS[b]
Glutaraldehyde	2%	Noncorrosive; active in presence of organic matter	Expense, harmful vapors, contact irritation	20 min at 20 °C Manual precleaning Final alcohol rinse
Iodophors	50—100 ppm	Minimal irritation	Stains contacted materials; organic matter decreases activity	Moderate activity, increased with dilutions
Alcohols	70%—90%	Inexpensive	Weakens glues, damages rubber and plastics	Rapid evaporation, limits contact time
Chlorine	1000 ppm	Inexpensive	Weakens certain materials, toxic with acids; ineffective in hard water in presence of organic matter	Common for water system disinfection; less active at hot water temperatures
Hydrogen peroxide	6%	For nebulizers, inhalation equipment	Expensive, may damage certain materials	Mucosal irritation after use for endoscopy

ppm, Parts per million.

[a]Nontuberculous mycobacteria such as *M. avium*–complex organisms may be more resistant to environmental inactivation compared with *M. tuberculosis* and *M. bovis*.

[b]Contact times for disinfection as outlined by U.S. Food and Drug Administration are 45 minutes at 25° C. Final rinses with alcohol and drying are recommended for most equipment in contact with tissue or mucosae to remove the irritating chemicals.

gardens.[135,137,143,150] Zoos are a major public health concern because of the unique value of the exhibited animals and their close contact with zoo personnel and visitors. Animals in these exhibits acquire their infection from people they contact. However, spread from the animals back to human personnel has not been documented.[135,150] Although *M. bovis* infections have been frequent in New Zealand, infected cats did not appear to be a major risk to their owners.[46,47] Nevertheless, owners should be advised that this organism is a known transmitted pathogen. *M. microti*–like infections in cats are probably acquired from hunting infected prey species; therefore restriction of this activity is the only known preventive measure. This species is not known to infect people. However, occasional cases of human infection with closely related *M. microti* have been reported.[148]

Nontuberculous Mycobacteria

Because they are soil saprophytes, MAC organisms are just as likely to be acquired from environmental sources by people as by pets. Infections with saprophytic mycobacteria, MAC and *M. microti*–like, are the appropriate ones to treat in companion animal practice.[71,96,101,140] However, to avoid any potential concern, families with members who are immunocompromised should generally be advised not to keep *Mycobacterium*-infected pets.

FELINE LEPROSY SYNDROMES

Richard Malik, M. Siobhan Hughes, Patricia Martin, Denise Wigney

The term *feline leprosy* is used to refer to a mycobacterial disease in which single or multiple granulomas form in the skin or subcutis in association with large numbers of acid-fast bacilli (AFB), which microbiologists are unable to culture using standard methods. The condition was first recorded in the literature by Australian and New Zealand researchers in the early 1960s.[115,194] Since then, the disease has been reported in Western Canada, the Netherlands, France, the United Kingdom, and United States.[195]

Etiology

Historical Perspective

Historically, the causative agent of feline leprosy was purported to be *M. lepraemurium*. This bacterium causes murine leprosy, a systemic mycobacterial infection of rats. Cats are thought to contract *M. lepraemurium* following bite injuries from infected rodents.[163]

M. lepraemurium is a fastidious, slow-growing mycobacterial species that can be cultured with difficulty from large inocula on Ogawa's egg yolk medium under strictly controlled conditions or in enriched liquid medium at a critical pH (6.0 to 6.2).* Although a few investigators have successfully grown *M. lepraemurium* from infected cats, the basis of ascribing this bacterium as the etiologic agent of feline leprosy was dependent on transmission studies and the results of delayed hypersensitivity reactions to ID-injected tissue extracts. Several groups were able to show that material obtained from feline lesions can be used to transmit disease to rats, and subsequently back to cats.[115,117] In such studies, the incubation period varied from 2 months to 1 year or more. Interestingly, among cats, some had a higher degree of susceptibility than others.

Current Perspective

Molecular methodologies have been used to investigate presumptive feline leprosy. Data from such studies have revealed

---

*References: 7, 100, 147, 149, 151.

that a large number of different organisms are responsible for what is called the *feline leprosy syndrome*. Of eight cases of invasive or disseminated cutaneous mycobacterial disease investigated by Hughes and colleagues[83] using material collected largely from New Zealand cats, four were shown to have *M. lepraemurium* infections. Of the remaining cats, one had a disseminated *M. avium* infection, the cause in one cat was undetermined, and in two cats, infection was attributable to a novel mycobacterial species. In a reappraisal of Australian feline leprosy cases, cats could be divided into two groups on the basis of the patient's age, lesion histology, clinical course, and sequence of 16S rRNA PCR amplicons obtained from lesions.[84,124] One syndrome in young cats was caused by *M. lepraemurium* and another in immunosuppressed elderly cats was caused by a single novel mycobacterial species. Other investigators found a third novel organism responsible for a lepromatous infection in cats from western North America.[5,131]

Epidemiology

Feline leprosy is more common in certain geographic locations such as the North Island of New Zealand, the Netherlands, and British Columbia. Furthermore, feline leprosy appears to be more prevalent in temperate coastal areas and port cities, as opposed to inland or tropical habitats.

Clinical Findings

According to the literature, cats with feline leprosy have typically been young adults (younger than 5 years of age), with a preponderance of males. Presumably these patient characteristics reflect the need for the cat to interact with a rat to become infected. The initial lesion is a focal granuloma of the subcutis. Owners become aware of solitary, or more commonly multiple, painless, raised, fleshy, tumorlike lesions, from a few millimeters up to 4 cm in diameter. These granulomas are freely movable over underlying tissues. Lesions can develop rapidly and, when large, may ulcerate. Infection spreads to adjacent areas and may invade underlying tissues and drain to regional lymph nodes. Lesions can occur anywhere but tend to be concentrated on the head and limbs. Small lesions are occasionally found on the tongue, lips, and nasal plane. Lesions, even if multiple, tend to be initially concentrated in one region and have the propensity to recur following excision. In some cases, widespread cutaneous lesions develop.

M. lepraemurium *Infection*

This disease generally occurs in young cats (typically younger than 4 years of age), which initially develop localized nodular disease affecting the limbs. Lesions progress rapidly and sometimes ulcerate (Fig. 50-10). Sparse to moderate numbers of AFB can be identified using cytology or histology, typically in

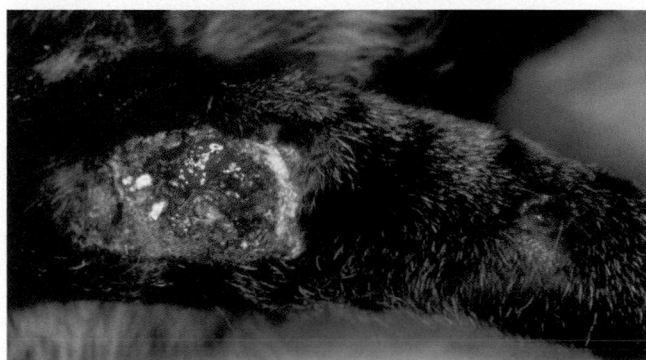

Fig 50-10 Ulcerated *M. lepraemurium* lesions on the forelimb of a young cat. (Courtesy of Peter Ihkre, University of California, Davis, Calif.)

areas of caseous necrosis and surrounded by pyogranulomatous tuberculoid inflammation. Organisms do not stain with hematoxylin and range from 2 to 6 μm (usually 2 to 4 μm). *M. lepraemurium* can be diagnosed based on the sequence of a 446 bp fragment encompassing the V2 and V3 hypervariable regions amplified from lesions using PCR and mycobacterial primers. Based on gene sequence data, *M. lepraemurium* shows greatest nucleotide identity with *M. avium* subsp. *paratuberculosis* and *M. avium*. The clinical course of *M. lepraemurium* infections is aggressive, with a tendency towards local spread, ulceration, recurrence following surgery, and development of widespread lesions over several weeks. Cats tend to reside in suburban or rural areas where contact with other cats is likely.

Novel Mycobacterial Infection

A second group of *feline leprosy* cases occurs in old cats (older than 9 years) with generalized nodular skin lesions (Fig. 50-11) associated with multibacillary lepromatous histology.[124] Some cats initially have localized disease that subsequently becomes widespread, while others have generalized disease from the outset. Disease progression is protracted, typically taking months to years, and skin nodules do not ulcerate. Microscopically, lesions consist of sheets of epithelioid macrophages containing large to enormous numbers of AFB, 2 to 8 μm (mostly 4 to 6 μm), which stain also with hematoxylin (Figs. 50-12 and 50-13). A single unique sequence spanning a 557 bp fragment of the 16S rRNA gene can be identified in lesions from these patients. The sequence was characterized by a long helix 18 in the V3 region, suggesting the new species is likely to be a fastidious, slow grower. The 16S rRNA sequence has greatest nucleotide identity with *M. leprae*, *M. haemophilum*, and *M. malmoense* and contained an additional "A" nucleotide at position 105 (the only other mycobacterial database sequence with the same extra nucleotide being *M. leprae*). A very slow, pure growth of a mycobacterial species was observed on LJ medium (supplemented with iron) and semisolid agar in 1 of 3 cases in which culture was attempted at a reference laboratory.[124] The environmental niche of this new mycobacterial species has yet to be determined, although the preponderance of cats from rural or semirural areas suggests it is a saprophyte found more commonly in these locations than in metropolitan environments. The organism may normally reside in soil or stagnant watery environments that favor the proliferation of saprophytic mycobacteria and subsequently become inoculated into the

subcutis through contamination of traumatic injuries (from cats or native wildlife) or via a biting arthropod.

The establishment or spread of infection with the novel mycobacterial species suggests a requirement for decreased immunologic surveillance to permit the development of disease with an organism of limited virulence. Furthermore, the etiopathogenesis needs to account for the absence of young cats among this cohort of patients. The presence of a foamy histiocytic infiltrate of the dermis and subcutis in human patients with mycobacteriosis is observed almost exclusively in association with profound immunodeficiency such as that seen with terminal HIV infection. Feline leprosy caused by the novel mycobacterial species may similarly represent a manifestation of deteriorating immune competence in elderly cats with longstanding FIV infection, and indeed one half of the cats so far tested in Australia have been FIV positive. Decreased cellular immunity associated with renal

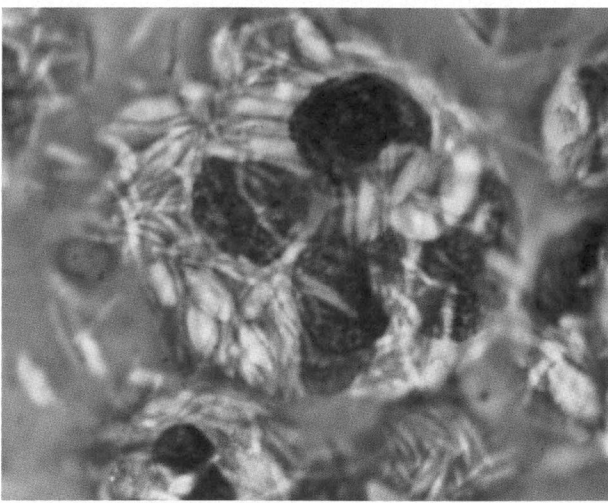

Fig 50-12 Biopsy material from a cat with novel mycobacterial species. Negatively stained bacilli are evident individually and in bundles, predominantly within macrophages (DiffQuik®, ×1000). (Courtesy Patricia Martin, University of Sydney, Sydney, Australia.)

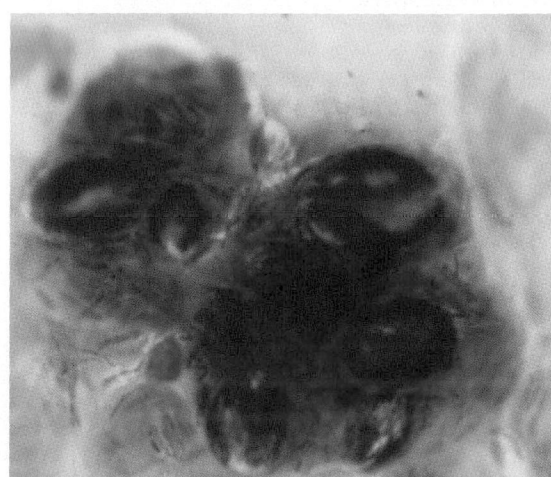

Fig 50-13 Biopsy material from a cat infected with the novel mycobacterial species. Macrophages laden with abundant intracellular AFB appear pink as a result of taking up the carbol fuchsin stain. The AFB are often grouped in ovoid bundles (acid-fast, ×1000). (Courtesy Patricia Martin, University of Sydney, Sydney, Australia.)

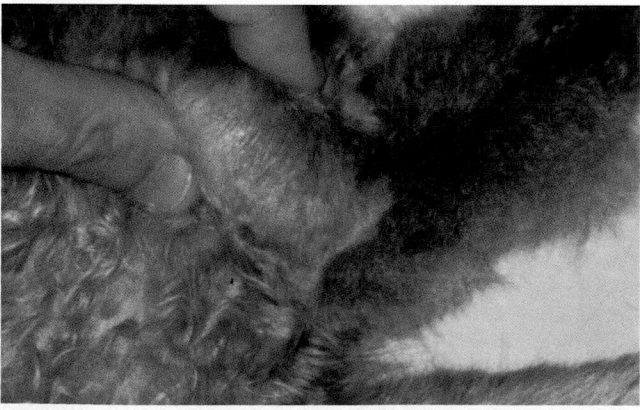

Fig 50-11 Granuloma on the hock of an 11-year-old, FIV-negative Persian cat infected with the novel mycobacterial species. Although this was the largest lesion evident, numerous similar lesions were present elsewhere over the integument. (Courtesy Richard Malik, University of Sydney, Sydney, Australia.)

disease may also predispose cats to infection, as renal disease is common among infected cats. Alternately, renal disease may occur as a consequence of the mycobacterial infection, as it does in rats with disseminated *M. lepraemurium* infection, presumably as a result of immune complex deposition in glomeruli. Thankfully, these infections seem quite sensitive to antimycobacterial therapy.[81,124]

Feline Multisystemic Granulomatous Mycobacteriosis

To make matters even more complex, work by Appleyard and Clark[5] and Matthews and Liggitt[131] has demonstrated a third mycobacterial syndrome in cats from western Canada and the United States (Idaho and Oregon) called *feline multisystemic granulomatous mycobacteriosis*. This disease is caused by slow-growing taxa provisionally called *M. visibilis* that gives rise to diffuse (rather than nodular) cutaneous disease and widespread dissemination to multiple internal organs. Sequence analyses demonstrate a large number of nucleotide differences between *M. visibilis* and both *M. lepraemurium* and the novel species reported by Hughes and colleagues.[84]

Diagnosis

Microscopic Appearance

Diagnosis of the *feline leprosy* syndromes is usually straightforward, provided that the clinician has a high index of suspicion for the condition. Needle aspirates, crush preparations of biopsy material and histologic sections stained with Ziehl-Neelsen (ZN) or similar methods contain easily demonstrable AFB surrounded by variable granulomatous to pyogranulomatous inflammation. In DiffQuick® (Baxter Diagnostics, Bellevue, Wash.) or Geimsa-stained smears mycobacteria can be recognized by their characteristic negative-staining appearance of slender rods located within macrophages and giant cells (see Fig. 50-12). In smears or sections stained with modified acid-fast stains such as ZN or Fite's stain, organisms take up the pink carbol fuchsin and are acid-alcohol fast (see Fig. 50-13).

Bacterial Isolation

Material should also be submitted also for culture, because occasionally slowly-growing species such as MAC and *M. geneavense*[82] and the tubercle bacilli (*M. bovis* or *M. microti*[32]) can produce an identical clinical presentation. In such animals, optimal antimycobacterial therapy can be selected more readily on the basis of in vitro susceptibility results and information available in the literature. *M. lepraemurium* cannot be cultured easily or quickly and is best detected using PCR, and the same is true for the novel mycobacterial species.

Nucleic Acid Detection

In the majority of cases, conventional mycobacterial culture gives a negative result caused by the fastidious nature of the causal organisms. Thus a mycobacterial etiology can only be proven using molecular techniques such as PCR amplification and nucleotide sequence determination of gene fragments, as described previously. PCR has the additional advantage of providing a rapid diagnosis. Fresh (frozen) tissue delivered to a diagnostic laboratory with mycobacterial expertise and PCR facilities provides the optimal sample, although freeze-dried specimens may be more conveniently sent when tissues need to travel long distances. Sometimes PCR can be performed successfully on formalin-fixed paraffin-embedded material, although fixation conditions invariably cause some DNA degradation that may limit the success of the procedure. Recently, Hughes and colleagues[84] have developed specific PCR assays to diagnose infections caused by *M. lepraemurium* and the novel species.[84] Furthermore, use of a simple restriction enzyme digest allows these assays to distinguish *M. visibilis* strains also.

Pathologic Findings

Pathologically, feline leprosy has been subdivided into two forms based on the number of visible AFB present (multibacillary versus paucibacillary), which corresponds with the host immunologic response (lepromatous versus tuberculoid, respectively). Because the causal mycobacteria are slow-growing organisms capable of intracellular survival, the histologic picture depends on the host's immune response. When this response is poor, lepromatous (multibacillary) disease develops with infiltration of the dermis with large sheets of *incompetent* foamy macrophages containing an enormous number of organisms. AFB are usually arranged in the cytoplasm of macrophages as dense parallel accumulations, which displace the nucleus to an eccentric position. Lymphoid cells and plasma cells are virtually absent from the lesions. If the host's immune response is more effective, histiocytic cells are accompanied by a moderate number of lymphoid cells and plasma cells and multiplication of the organism is limited—the so-called tuberculoid response. The tuberculoid form accounts for perhaps two thirds of the cases in western Canada, a large proportion of cases in New Zealand and the Netherlands, but a minority of the cases encountered in Australia.[124] Invasion of local nerves, a prominent feature of human leprosy, is rarely observed in patients with feline leprosy, although a report described a cat without skin lesions which had mycobacterial infiltration of one sciatic nerve.[152]

Therapy

The existence of multiple diseases, rather than one, clearly has important implications for prevention, diagnosis, and therapy of feline leprosy. For example, most authors recommend wide surgical excision as the treatment of choice for focal lesions.[195] This option is practical in *M. lepraemurium* infections, at least when cats are treated in a timely manner when lesions are localized. On the other hand, although surgery may have a place in reducing the bulk of particularly large lesions in infections caused by the novel mycobacterial species, medical therapy with a combination of drugs generally represents a better first line of treatment.

Only a few cases have been treated, with a documented organism established by PCR, to provide definitive treatment guidelines. Although *M. lepraemurium* and the novel species can be cultured in vitro, isolating these organisms is currently not routine or reliable because of their slow growth and fastidious requirements. Determination of in vitro susceptibility data for individual isolates is therefore not possible.

Only limited experimental studies have been undertaken to determine effective drug therapy for *M. lepraemurium* in vitro or in vivo, and, as yet, data only for the novel mycobacterial species are limited. In one report,[157] the minimum inhibitory concentration (MIC) for rifampin of two strains of *M. lepraemurium* was 4 and 8 μg/ml, levels that should be just obtainable in vivo based on extrapolation from pharmacokinetic studies in people and dogs. Other drugs shown to have activity against *M. lepraemurium* in vitro include ansamycin compounds (rifabutin) and sulpha drugs. Substantial evidence exists that clofazimine has efficacy in vivo, although it is likely that clarithromycin would also be effective based on its wide spectrum of activity against slow-growing mycobacterial species.[153]

The literature suggests that when *M. lepraemurium* infection is diagnosed early, while disease is localized, wide surgical excision of infected tissues provides the best chance to simply and rapidly effect a cure.[195] Aggressive resection techniques should be adopted, with en bloc resection of all lesions, and reconstruction of resulting tissue deficits using appropriate surgical techniques. An approach such as this one should be combined with adjunct antimicrobial therapy beginning a few days before surgery so that effective levels of drugs are

Table • 50-6

Drug Dosages for Treatment of Lepromatous Mycobacterial Infections[a]

DRUG[b]	SPECIES	DOSE[c]	ROUTE	INTERVAL (HOURS)	DURATION (WEEKS)
Clofazimine[d]	C	25—50 mg/cat	PO	24—48	≥8
	C	8—10 mg/kg	PO	24	≥8
Clarithromycin	C	62.5 mg /cat	PO	12	≥12
Rifamp(ic)in	C	10—15 mg/kg	PO	24	≥12

PO, By mouth; C, cat.

[a]Surgical removal is the most effective therapy. For medical therapy use at least two drugs to include clarithromycin, rifampin or clofazimine.
[b]For specific information about each drug consult Drug Formulary, Appendix 8.
[c]Dose per administration at specified interval.
[d]Because of difficulty of fractionating liquid in capsules, cats are usually given one 50-mg capsule per dose. Alternately, the contents of capsule may be cut into halves with a scalpel blade while wearing disposable gloves and dividing it into two gelatin capsules. Alternatively a compounding pharmacist can provide the optimal dosage size.

present in blood and tissues intra- and postoperatively to ensure primary intention healing.

Clofazimine, at a dose listed in Table 50-6 given every 24 to 48 hours, has the best reported success rate, although combination therapy using two or more drugs likely will prove superior. Drugs that can be combined with clofazimine include rifampin and clarithromycin, although sulfonamides, doxycycline, new fluoroquinolones such as gatifloxacin, linezolid, or amikacin may in time also prove to be useful. In some patients with advanced disease, the response to treatment is poor.

In feline leprosy cases caused by the novel mycobacterial species, we believe that combination therapy using two or three drug choices of clofazimine, clarithromycin, or rifampin represents optimal therapy. However, we are currently unsure of which drug will prove to be the best combination, and side effects in individual cats may affect which two drugs are used in a given patient. Currently, we recommend a combination of rifampin and clarithromycin as initial therapy. For appropriate dosages and formulating the drugs, see Table 50-6 and Drug Formulary, Appendix 8. Given that clofazimine and rifampin both can produce reversible hepatotoxicity, biochemical monitoring of cats regularly during therapy is mandatory, while vomiting or inappetence (or both) suggests the need for dose reduction or temporary discontinuation of therapy. We have encountered photosensitivity and pitting corneal lesions in some cats during clofazimine therapy. Of these different agents, clarithromycin is the least likely to cause worrisome side effects; however, monotherapy with this agent is not recommended because of the possibility of resistance developing during treatment.

Guidelines for duration of therapy are hard to define, although mycobacterial infections should be generally treated for several months and continued for at least 2 months (the life of a macrophage in the tissues) after disappearance of lesions.

Treatment has been attempted only in one cat with *M. visibilis* infection, which was cured using clofazimine and clindamycin.[5]

CANINE LEPROID GRANULOMA SYNDROME (CANINE LEPROSY)

Richard Malik, M. Siobhan Hughes, Patricia Martin, and Denise Wigney

Etiology

Canine leproid granuloma syndrome (CLGS) or canine leprosy is the most common mycobacterial disease of dogs in

Australia. A gene sequence was identified representing a novel mycobacterial agent.[83] Although the causal organism (see Nucleic Acid Detection later) has a worldwide distribution, its prevalence in other countries has not been documented. Patients with this infection have one or more nodules in their subcutis or skin but are otherwise well.* The condition was first described in a boxer and a bullmastiff from Zimbabwe in 1973,[172,173] with similar reports from Australia appearing soon afterwards.[54,130,193]

Epidemiology

CLGS has a wide geographic distribution, with cases recorded from coastal and inland regions of all states of Australia. The causal organism is likely to have a worldwide distribution because the condition has also been reported in New Zealand, Zimbabwe, Brazil, California, and Florida.[55,63,113] The authors are also aware of unreported cases of affected boxers in New York and foxhounds and other dogs in Georgia in the United States. The condition appears to be especially common in Australia and Brazil.

Interestingly, a strong propensity exists for short-coated breeds to be affected, with boxer and boxer-cross dogs accounting for nearly one half of the cases reported. Despite the fact that CLGS was first reported nearly 30 years ago, its etiopathogenesis has not been fully elucidated. The initial report of the disease by Richard Smith observed that, "lesions appear suddenly and are usually seen on dogs bothered by biting flies.[172,173] This finding might suggest that flies or some other biting arthropod, such as midges or mosquitoes, inoculate mycobacteria from an environmental niche into susceptible hosts. The predilection for lesions to develop in regions of the body favored by biting insect vectors, such as the head and particularly the ears, is consistent with this hypothesis, as is the overrepresentation of short-coated, large breed dogs, which are generally housed outdoors.

Clinical Findings

Primary skin lesions consist of single or multiple, well-circumscribed nodule or nodules. These lesions can appear anywhere on the dog, although they are usually located on the head and typically on the dorsal fold of the ears. The nodules are hard, painless, and vary in size from 2 mm up to 5 cm in diameter (Fig. 50-14, *A* and *B*). Small nodules are detected as hard subcutaneous lumps, while larger nodules may show superficial hair loss. Very large lesions may ulcerate.

Leproid granulomas are confined to the subcutis and skin and do not involve regional lymph nodes, nerves, or internal organs. Consequently, affected dogs suffer no apparent sys-

*References: 33, 55, 83, 126, 127, 130, 160.

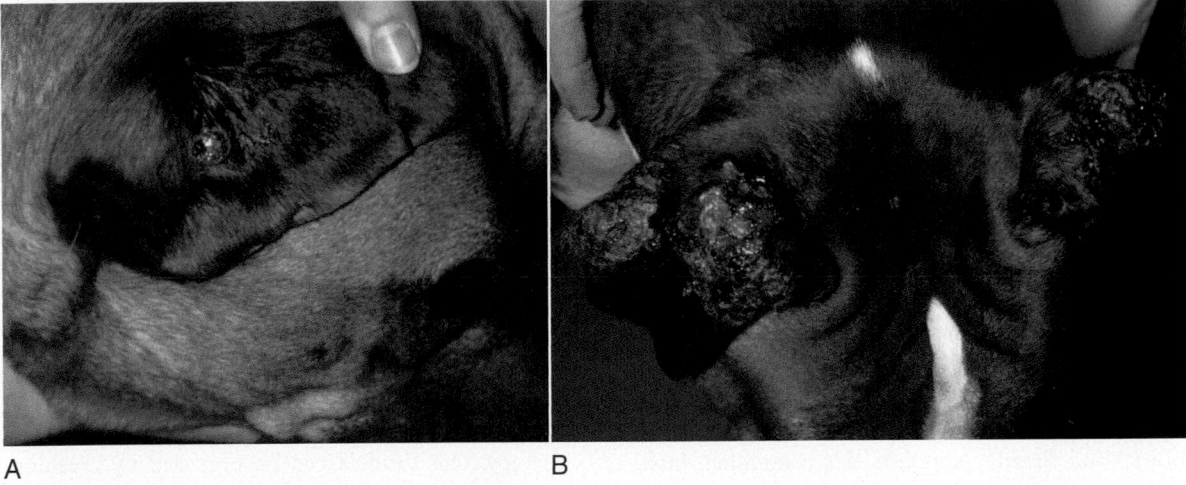

Fig 50-14 Appearance of CLGS lesions in dogs. **A,** Solitary lesion on the dorsal ear fold of a mastiff dog. **B,** Multiple, ulcerated lesion on both ear folds of a boxer dog. (Courtesy Richard Malik, University of Sydney, Sydney, Australia.)

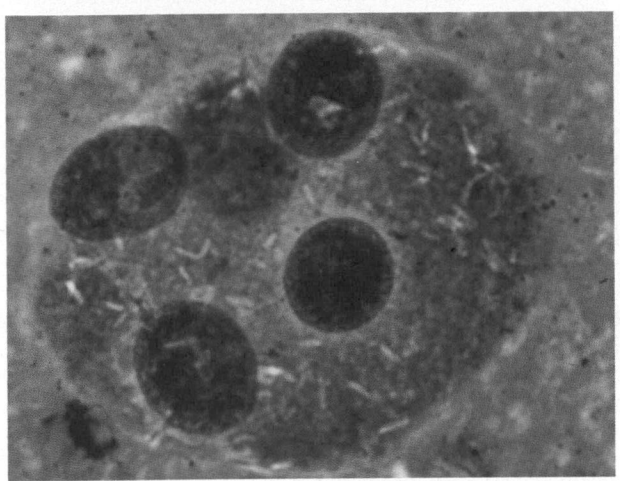

Fig 50-15 Cytology of an aspirate from a CLGS lesion. Note the negatively stained bacilli within the Langerhans-type giant cell (DiffQuik®, ×750). (Courtesy Patricia Martin, The University of Sydney, Sydney, Australia.)

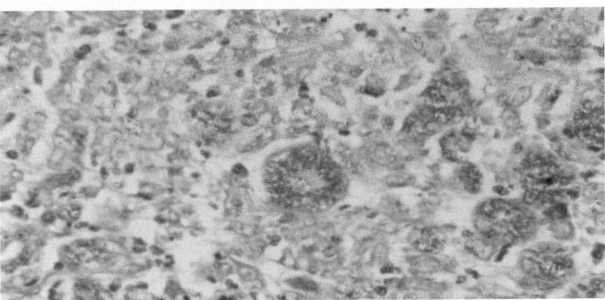

Fig 50-16 Microphotograph of CLGS. Mycobacteria stain positively (i.e., acid-fast) with the carbol fuchsin (pink stain) (ZN, ×300). (Courtesy Patricia Martin, University of Sydney, Sydney, Australia)

temic ill effects. This finding suggests that the causal organism has low pathogenicity or special prerequisites, such as a requirement for low temperature, which permits them to survive and multiply in superficial tissues only. Lesions can be disfiguring and cause irritation, especially when lesions are multiple and secondarily infected with *Staphylococcus intermedius*.

Diagnosis
Clinical and Pathologic Findings
Diagnosis is usually straightforward, given the distribution of lesions (especially the propensity for the dorsal ear fold to be affected), coupled with the tendency for lesions to be multiple, particularly in an at-risk breed, is strongly suggestive of CLGS. Diagnosis can be confirmed by obtaining specimens of representative lesions for cytologic or histologic examination.[33] DiffQuik®-stained smears from needle aspirates typically demonstrate numerous macrophages with a variable number of lymphocytes and plasma cells and lower numbers of neutrophils. Usually a few-to-moderate number of negatively stained, medium-length bacilli can be detected within macrophages or extracellularly (Fig. 50-15). Histologically,

lesions within the subcutis and dermis consist of pyogranulomas composed chiefly of epithelioid macrophages, Langerhans-type giant cells with scattered neutrophils, plasma cells, and small lymphocytes (Fig. 50-16). The number and morphology of AFB in ZN-stained sections are highly variable from case to case. Confirming the diagnosis by culture is impossible because the in vitro growth requirements for this fastidious organism have not been determined. A negative culture result, however, can exclude other mycobacteria as the etiologic agent. The skin surface must be thoroughly disinfected before obtaining specimens for culture because saprophytic mycobacteria can easily be cultured erroneously from dirt present on canine skin.

Nucleic Acid Detection
PCR methods using universal and purpose-designed primers designed to amplify regions of the bacterial 16S rRNA gene have been performed on leproid granuloma specimens from dogs.[83] Using sequence capture PCR for paraffin-embedded specimens and nested PCR on DNA from fresh tissue specimens, a novel PCR product has been identified with identical sequence over a 350 bp region. Analysis of the partial 16S rRNA sequence supports the notion that the novel species is a fastidious, slow-growing mycobacterium. In total, molecular methodologies identified this proposed novel mycobacterial sequence in material from more than 16 Australian cases of CLGS, indicating that the species represented by this sequence is probably the principal causative agent of CLGS.[83] Our continuing experience and those of colleagues

Table • 50-7

Drug Dosages for Treatment of Canine Leproid Granuloma Infection[a]

DRUG[b]	SPECIES	DOSE[c]	ROUTE	INTERVAL (HOURS)	DURATION (WEEKS)
Rifamp(ic)in	D	10—15 mg/kg	PO	24	4—8
Clarithromycin	D	7.5—12.5 mg/kg	PO	12	4—8
Doxycycline[d]	D	5—7.5 mg/kg	PO	12	4—8

PO, By mouth; D, dog.
[a]Surgical removal is the most effective therapy. For medical therapy use at least two of the drugs in this table in combination. Topical therapy may also be considered. See text for further information on using topical formulations.
[b]For specific information about each drug consult Drug Formulary, Appendix 8.
[c]Dose per administration at specified interval.
[d]Use monohydrate salt, if available, and administer with food or follow with water.

in California[55] and Brazil[113] supports this contention. Interestingly, the species represented by this sequence has never been recorded from mycobacterial granulomas affecting the skin or subcutis of cats, horses, people, or other noncanine mammalian species. Hence no public health risk is believed to exist to the owners of affected dogs.

Therapy

Very little has been written concerning the treatment of CLGS. Many cases are self-limiting, with the nodular skin lesions regressing spontaneously with time, typically within 1 to 3 months of initial appearance. The stated time frame is based on our experiences consulting with veterinarians in relation to cases diagnosed histologically; by the time the sections are submitted, processed, reported on, and a dialogue established with the clinician, lesions have often already started to regress, either spontaneously or in response to antimicrobials (useful for secondary *S. intermedius* but with unlikely efficacy for mycobacteria). This *self-cure* occurs presumably as a result of an effective CMI response mounted by the patient.

In cases with a limited number of lesions, surgical excision can be curative and provides material with which to confirm the diagnosis histologically and using PCR. In other cases, however, the infection progresses to produce chronic, disfiguring lesions that may persist indefinitely. Limited information suggests that treatment with conventional antimicrobial regimens using β-lactam drugs, doxycycline, or a quinolone (as monotherapy) fails to have a significant impact on the course of infection,[126] although these drugs may be of some benefit by effectively treating secondary pyogenic infections. One report concerning two dogs from Brazil suggested topical antibacterial treatment and orally administered rifampin may be effective.[113] Our experience treating *canine leprosy* suggests that this infection responds to therapy with combinations of antimicrobial agents known to be effective against nontuberculous mycobacteria, including rifampin, clarithromycin, clofazimine, and doxycycline. Based on our evolving experience, a combination of rifampin and clarithromycin given orally at the dosages listed in Table 50-7 is recommended for treating severe or refractory CLGS cases.[130] Unfortunately, the clarithromycin component of therapy is extremely expensive in large dogs. A far more affordable combination consists of rifampin and doxycycline at the dosages listed in Table 50-7, and further studies may prove this to have similar efficacy to the former regimen. Treatment should be continued until lesions are substantially reduced in size (typically for 4 to 8 weeks) and ideally until lesions have resolved completely. Monitoring hepatic function periodically during treatment is prudent because rifampin may cause hepatotoxicity in some patients. A topical formulation containing clofazimine in petroleum jelly may be used as an adjunct to systemic drug therapy. This formula can be prepared by crushing (with a hammer) 40 50-mg clofazimine *capsules* in a plastic bag; the extracted liquid dye is mixed into an ointment with 100 g of petroleum jelly.[130] Further work is required to determine the most cost-effective treatment regimen for this condition, and to this end, a topical treatment using multiple chemotherapeutic agents in a permeant vehicle is under development in Australia.[122]

INFECTIONS CAUSED BY RAPIDLY GROWING MYCOBACTERIA

Richard Malik, Patricia Martin, Denise Wigney, and Sue Foster

Etiology

Rapidly growing mycobacteria (RGM, previously termed opportunistic or atypical mycobacteria) are a heterogeneous group of organisms that produce colonies on synthetic media within 7 days when cultured at 24° to 45° C (see Tables 50-1 and 50-2). They are distributed ubiquitously in nature and can be isolated from soil, dirt, and bodies of water (including tap water).[26] RGM include the *M. fortuitum* group (including *M. fortuitum*, *M. peregrinum*, and the third biovariant complex), the *M. chelonae* and *M. abscessus* group, the *M. smegmatis* group (including *M. smegmatis sensu stricto*, *M. goodii*, and *M. wolinskyi*), and a variety of other species including *M. phlei* and *M. thermoresistibile*. The taxonomy of the RGM has been revised and because of this, the word *group* is used when referring to isolates recorded in early publications.[26]

In both people and animals, RGM are strongly linked with localized infections of immunocompetent hosts* because the organisms are well adapted to a saprophytic existence and have inherently low virulence for mammals. Thus they do not produce disease unless a breakdown in normal defense barriers provides them with a portal of entry to a favorable tissue environment. RGM are not generally transmitted between hosts. Once introduced, RGM are generally constrained by a vigorous immunologic response that may or may not eradicate them from the tissues but which is effective enough to prevent hematogenous or lymphatic spread. RGM can produce widely disseminated disease but only in severely immunocompromised individuals. They are, however, much less common pathogens in this group of patients than other mycobacterial species, such as the *M. avium* complex.[26] RGM produce three different syndromes in cats and dogs: (1) mycobacterial panniculitis, (2) pyogranulomatous pneumonia, and (3) disseminated systemic disease.[67] In certain dairy herds, RGM are a significant cause of mastitis.[179]

*References: 26, 87, 111, 129, 195.

Mycobacterial panniculitis refers to a syndrome characterized by chronic infection of the subcutis and skin with RGM.[195] This condition is quite common in cats, especially in Australia, and series of up to 49 cases have been reported.[111,125,129] The condition is less common in dogs.[68,94,111,128,142] RGM replicate in mammalian tissues when introduced through some breach in the skin, which typically follows penetrating injury, especially when the wound is contaminated by debris or soil. Preference of RGM for fat is a key factor in the pathogenesis of these infections and results in a tendency for disease to occur in obese individuals and in tissues rich in lipid, such as the subcutaneous panniculus and especially the inguinal fat pad of cats. Experimental infections cannot be induced in cats that do not have appreciable subcutaneous fat depots.[119] Similarly, experimental infections of the ovine mammary gland require instillation of oil in addition to organisms to induce mastitis. The same phenomenon accounts for situations in which RGM give rise to human infections, for example, athletes that inject anabolic steroids in oily vehicles from contaminated multiuse vials, as a complication of lipoid pneumonia, and following augmentation mammoplasty, liposuction, and median sternotomy.[26] Adipose tissue offers a favorable environment for survival and proliferation of RGM by providing triglycerides for growth of organisms or protecting them from the phagocytic or immune responses of the host.

Initial reports suggested mycobacterial panniculitis was more common in warm humid climates[111]; however, cats from temperate regions, including parts of Australia, Canada, Finland, and Germany, have subsequently been reported to develop these infections, and RGM can be cultivated from soil samples from Japan and throughout the United States.[26] In Australia, the *M. smegmatis* group accounts for the majority of feline cases, whereas it is a much less common cause of equivalent infections in human patients. The *M. fortuitum* group are the predominant pathogens in people.[129] Interestingly, the swimming pool or fish tank bacillus *M. marinum*, a common cause of subcutaneous mycobacterial disease in people, has not been isolated from feline or canine patients.

Mycobacterial pneumonia has been reported in several dogs[90,94,182,197] and a few cats.[195] *M. thermoresistibile* caused pulmonary abscessation and pleurisy in a cat.[57] Insufficient cases have been recorded to identify predisposing factors, apart from a cat examined by Wilkinson in which the infection was thought to be secondary to aspiration of liquid paraffin administered as a fur-ball treatment.[195] In people, as in animals, disseminated infection caused by rapidly growing mycobacteria is uncommon; however, it has been observed in patients with CMI defects or co-infections (or both) with other opportunistic pathogens.[36]

Clinical Findings

In cats, infections tend to start in the inguinal region, usually following environmental contamination of catfight injuries (e.g., raking wounds inflicted with the hind claws). The infection may spread to contiguous subcutaneous tissues of the ventral and lateral abdominal wall and perineum. Penetrating injury by sticks, metallic objects, and vehicular trauma may also give rise to these infections, as can cat and dog bite injuries contaminated with soil or dirt. Sometimes infections start in the axillae, flanks, or dorsum and spread into adjacent tissues.[195]

Early in the clinical course, infections can resemble catfight abscesses but without the characteristic fetid odor and turbid pus. Instead, a circumscribed plaque or nodule is apparent at the site of injury. Later, the nearby subcutis, to which overlying skin becomes adherent, progressively thickens. Affected areas become denuded of hair and numerous punctate fistu-lae appear, discharging a watery exudate. Fistulae are intermingled with focal purple depressions, which correspond to thinning of the epidermis over accumulations of pus (Fig. 50-17, *A*, *B*, and *C*). The *lesion* gradually increases in area and depth and may eventually involve the entire ventral abdomen, adjacent flanks, or limbs. If cats promptly receive veterinary attention, and the lesion is confused with an anaerobic cat bite abscess, surgical drainage and administration of a synthetic penicillin are typically followed by wound breakdown and development of a nonhealing suppurating tract surrounded by indurated granulation tissue (see Fig. 50-17, *D*). Most cats, even those with extensive cutaneous lesions, have few signs of systemic illness. Some affected cats with severe infections develop constitutional signs; they become depressed, pyrexic, inappetent, lose weight, and are reluctant to move. Occasionally, cats develop the hypercalcemia of granulomatous disease, although this is rarely if ever symptomatic. Surprisingly, other cats remain comparatively well despite extensive disease. The problem usually remains localized to the skin and subcutis. Although adjacent structures such as the abdominal wall can be affected eventually, spread to internal organs or lymph nodes is very unusual.[195]

In dogs, RGM infections should be suspected when the clinician is confronted with patients with chronic nonhealing wounds unresponsive to drainage and *conventional* antimicrobial therapy. Lesions typically consist of firm to fluctuant subcutaneous swellings or nodules that ulcerate, drain, and spread centrifugally (with the development of new lesions at the edges of older lesions). Some infections behave differently and instead spread widely to produce multifocal lesions through the entire subcutaneous panniculus. Lesions tend to be neither painful nor pruritic and are generally located in regions subjected to bite wounds or injections, such as the neck, shoulders, flank, or dorsum. A prior history of penetrating injury is common, for example, a bite wound or veterinary intervention (injections, previous surgery). A minority of animals may demonstrate pyrexia, pain, or lameness.[68,94,111,142]

Dogs and cats with pyogranulomatous pneumonia show coughing, dyspnea, fever, malaise, and often have lost weight because of poor appetite. Young dogs appear to be overrepresented. One patient developed hypertrophic osteopathy secondary to the pulmonary pathology.[197]

Diagnosis
Sample Collection, Cytology, and Histology
A tentative diagnosis of mycobacteriosis can be confirmed by collection of pus or deep tissue specimens. This material is used to confirm the diagnosis using appropriately stained cytology preparations, histologic sections, and mycobacterial culture. A histologic diagnosis is generally unnecessary if appropriate samples for cytology and culture have been procured.[125,129] Apprising the laboratory that a mycobacterial origin is suspected is vital so special procedures for processing the specimens can be adopted.

Specimen Collection and Submission
In our experience, samples of pus obtained from needle aspirates of affected tissues through intact skin provide the best laboratory specimens in panniculitis cases. This material can be obtained from a palpably abnormal portion of the subcutis. Pockets of fluid can also be visualized using high-resolution ultrasonography, facilitating aspiration. The overlying skin should be carefully disinfected with 70% ethanol before obtaining the specimen to preclude the isolation of saprophytic mycobacteria residing on the skin surface. It may be necessary to carefully move the needle in the subcutaneous space, while applying constant negative pressure, until a pocket of purulent material is encountered. High-resolution

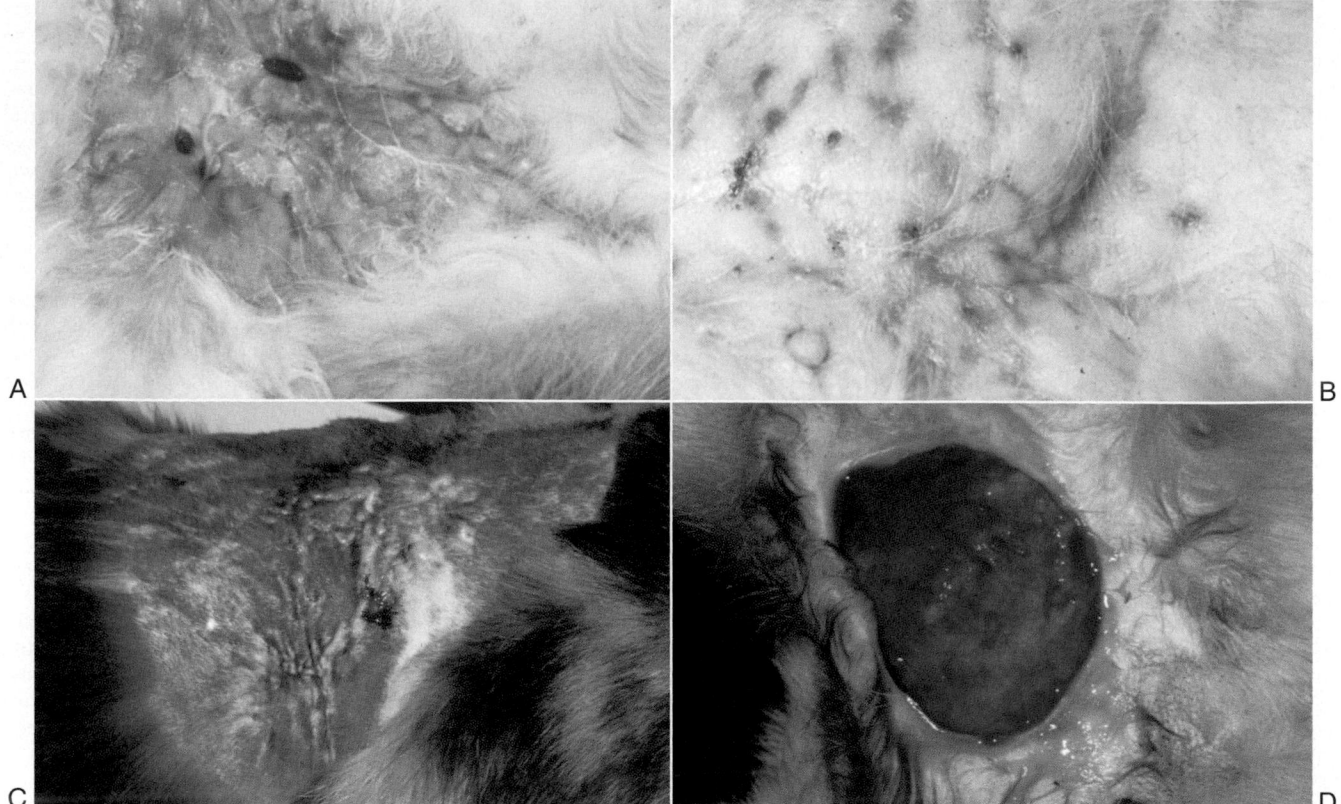

Fig 50-17 Inguinal panniculitis. **A,** Inguinal panniculitis caused by *M. smegmatis* in a cat before any therapy. Suppuration from draining sinus tracts is obvious. **B,** Inguinal panniculitis caused by *M. smegmatis* in a cat. Note the "pepper pot" appearance of the skin, caused by draining sinus tracts, some of which are covered by a thin layer of epidermis. The draining tracts are drying out in response to doxycycline therapy. **C,** Panniculitis caused by *M. smegmatis* on the dorsum of a cat. Infection at this site is unusual. **D,** Inappropriate treatment with a penicillin and surgical drainage results in a nonhealing fistulous granuloma. (Courtesy Richard Malik, University of Sydney, Sydney, Australia.)

ultrasound can be useful in canine patients to identify anechoic foci suitable for aspiration. Aspirated purulent fluid should be submitted to the laboratory for cytology and mycobacterial culture or inoculated immediately into a commercially prepared mycobacteria culture bottle, which is subsequently submitted to the laboratory. Only a small amount of liquid material needs to be aspirated into the hub of the syringe. Submitting the entire syringe to the laboratory after replacing the needle with a sterile cover is easiest. Exudate from draining sinus tracts is heavily contaminated with secondary invaders and represents an inferior sample. If deep biopsies are obtained, they should be titrated in brain heart infusion broth using a sterile mortar and pestle to produce a tissue homogenate suitable for cytology and culture. In animals suspected of having mycobacterial pneumonia, deep bronchial washings, bronchoalveolar lavage specimens, or ultrasound-guided transthoracic fine needle aspirates provide optimal specimens.

Cytologic Examination

Multiple smears prepared from aspirates of purulent exudate, bronchial washings, or tissue homogenates should be stained using Diff Quik®, Burke's modification of the Gram stain, and a modified acid-fast procedure (decolorizing with 5% sulfuric acid for only 3 to 5 minutes because RGM are not as acid-fast as other mycobacteria). Cytology invariably demonstrates pyogranulomatous inflammation, visualizing gram-positive or acid-fast bacteria, or both, is generally possible (Fig. 50-18), although an exhaustive search of several smears is sometimes required.[125,129] Organisms often demonstrate beading. Speck-

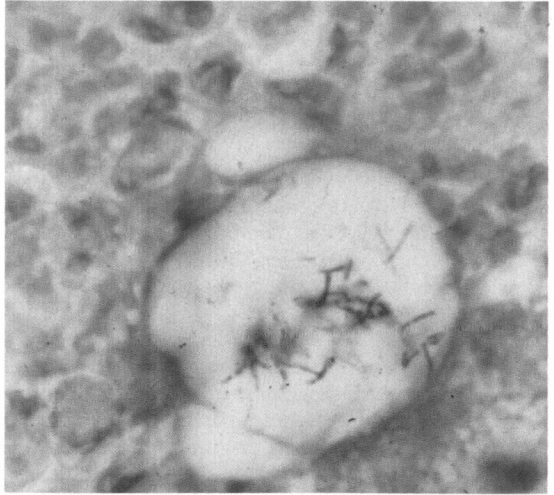

Fig 50-18 Modified acid-fast stain of purulent fluid of a cat with inguinal panniculitis. Note the acid-fast bacilli in the extracellular lipid vacuole. (Courtesy Patricia Martin, University of Sydney, Sydney, Australia.)

led structures or nonstaining *ghosts*, corresponding to poorly staining or nonstaining bacilli, may be observed in smears stained with Romanowsky-type stains[94] but are much harder to appreciate than in *M. avium* infections, feline leprosy, or canine leproid granuloma cases.

Organism Cultivation and Antimicrobial Susceptibility Testing

Tissue homogenates and pus should be streaked onto duplicate 5% sheep blood agar plates and a mycobacterial medium such as LJ medium or 1% Ogawa egg yolk medium and incubated aerobically at 37° C and 25° C, respectively. If available, the BACTEC system (Becton Dickenson Systems, Sparks, Md.) can also be used. Moderate to heavy growth of pinpoint, nonhemolytic colonies is usually detected after 2 to 3 days (occasionally longer) on sheep blood agar at 37° C. When only contaminated specimens are available, tissue homogenates can be treated with 4% sodium hydroxide followed by neutralization with dilute hydrochloric acid before inoculation onto media. Another method that can be used to selectively differentiate RGM from contaminant flora is primary isolation around antibiotic sensitivity disks (first-generation cephalosporins or isoxazolyl penicillins) applied to the plate after inoculation. We prefer this method to alkali-pretreatment when dealing with specimens contaminated with staphylococci.

Determining species identification and susceptibility data is of great value in every case because this has a big impact on antimicrobial drug strategies. Species identification can be carried out in a well-equipped veterinary bacteriology laboratory, although sending the strain to a mycobacteria reference laboratory following primary isolation is often more convenient. See Appendix 5 for a listing of specialized mycobacterial laboratories. Table 50-8 contains a summary of information concerning phenotypic features used to identify mycobacteria in the laboratory.

MICs for ciprofloxacin, gentamicin, trimethoprim, clarithromycin, and doxycycline can be determined easily using the Etest (AB Biodisk, Solna, Sweden) method.[75] This methodology is less demanding than is the *gold standard* of broth microdilution. Antimicrobial susceptibility of clinical isolates can also be determined using disk diffusion methodology. Typically, isolates are tested against disks containing representative antimicrobials including doxycycline (30 µg), gentamicin (10 µg), ciprofloxacin (5 µg), trimethoprim (5 µg), tobramycin (10 µg), polymyxin B (300 µg), enrofloxacin (5 µg), and clarithromycin (30 µg). Some antibiotics are included to determine a suitable agent for long-term oral therapy, while others (trimethoprim, polymyxin B, tobramycin) are used to provide phenotypic information concerning strains. Suspensions of each organism in saline or nutrient broth are sown onto sensitivity agar and incubated at 37° C. Results are recorded after incubation for 48 and 72 hours.[129]

Pathologic Findings

Histologically, pyogranulomatous inflammation of subcutaneous adipose tissue, overlying dermis, and underlying abdominal fascia and musculature is noted. AFB may be difficult or impossible to find in ZN-stained tissue sections and are typically located in lipid vacuoles.

Therapy

The management of mycobacterial panniculitis continues to evolve over time according to ongoing clinical experience, availability of new antimicrobial agents, and development of new surgical techniques.[125,129] Variation in the severity and extent of lesions from patient to patient is great. Difficulty in making a prompt diagnosis is partly responsible for the chronicity, severity, and refractoriness of these infections.[94] Briefly, treatment should commence with one or more oral antimicrobials (doxycycline, a fluoroquinolone, or clarithromycin) initially chosen empirically but subsequently based on in vitro susceptibility data. Dosages for these drugs are listed in Table 50-9. Long-term administration of such an agent or agents is sometimes sufficient to effect a cure, but in more severe cases, surgical resection of recalcitrant tissues is eventually necessary so that oral antimicrobial therapy will be able to cure the infection permanently. Given the extent and severity of the pathology in many of these cases, understandably, adequate levels of antimicrobials may not be achieved throughout all affected tissues. In these cases, the best chance for a successful outcome is to remove as much infected tissue as possible following preliminary antimicrobial therapy.[156] Residual foci of infection can then be targeted by the high concentrations of antibiotics achieved during and after surgery. Peri- and postoperative antimicrobial therapy is vital to ensure primary intention healing of the surgical incision.

Once a tentative diagnosis of mycobacterial panniculitis is made, immediately starting treatment is desirable. Because positive primary culture takes 3 to 4 days, with an additional similar period required for susceptibility testing, the initial choice of one or more antimicrobials must be guided by retrospectively acquired microbiology data. This data is different in different regions. In Australia, *M. smegmatis* and *M. fortuitum* infections are encountered with similar frequency in companion animals; whereas in the southern United States, *M. fortuitum* and *M. chelonae* infections predominate.[68,94,111] *M. smegmatis* strains are susceptible to a wide range of antimicrobial agents suitable for treating chronic infections, except for clarithromycin to which a majority of strains show inherent resistance. In contrast, *M. fortuitum* strains generally demonstrate resistance to one or several agents and often have higher MICs for agents to which strains are susceptible, while *M. chelonae* strains tend to be resistant to all common agents available for oral dosing apart from clarithromycin, gatifloxacin, and linezolid.[26] In Australia, doxycycline or a fluoroquinolone are thus sensible choices for first-line therapy; whereas in the United States, clarithromycin is the drug of

Table • 50-8

Phenotypic Features That Aid in the Identification of Mycobacterial Species[a]

Organism morphology in Ziehl-Neelsen—stained smears of growth taken from Lowenstein-Jensen medium

Colonial morphology (rough or smooth)

Pigmentation when cultivated in the dark or lighted environment

Degree of acid-fastness

Rate of growth at room temperature and at 37° C

Ability to grow at 42° C to 52° C

Arylsulphatase activity at 3 days

Iron uptake

p-amino salicylic acid degradation

Nitrate reduction

β-galactosidase activity

Acid production from carbohydrates (glucose, inositol, mannitol)

Utilization of compounds (glucose, fructose, inositol, mannitol, citrate) as the sole carbon source

Tolerance to 5% sodium hydroxide in Lowenstein-Jensen medium

Susceptibility to polymyxin B, trimethoprim, tobramycin, and other agents

[a]In specialized laboratories, a variety of molecular techniques are also used.[26,129]

Table • 50-9

Drug Dosages for Treatment of Rapidly Growing Mycobacterial Infections

DRUG[a]	SPECIES	DOSE[b] (MG/KG)	ROUTE	INTERVAL (HOURS)	DURATION (WEEKS)
Gentamicin	B	2 mg/kg	SC, IM	8—12	2—4[c]
Amikacin	B	5—10 mg/kg	SC, IM	8—12	2—4[c]
Doxycycline	B	5—10 mg/kg	PO	12	12—52[d]
Trimethoprim-sulfonamide	D	15—30 mg/kg	PO	12	4—6[e]
	C	10 mg/kg	PO	12	4[e]
Ciprofloxacin	B	10—20 mg/kg	PO	12	12—52[f,g]
Enrofloxacin	D	5—15 mg/kg	PO	24	12—52[f,g]
	C	5 mg/kg	PO	24	12—52[f,g,h]
Clofazimine[i]	B	8—12 mg/kg[i]	PO	24	12—5g[g]
Clarithromycin	B	10—15 mg/kg	PO	12	12—52
	C	62.5 mg total	PO	12—24	12—52

B, Both dog and cat; C, cat; D, dog; SC, subcutaneous; IM, intramuscular; PO, by mouth.

[a]For specific information about each drug consult Drug Formulary, Appendix 8.

[b]Dose per administration at specified interval.

[c]Monitor blood-urea-nitrogen weekly for evidence of nephrotoxicity; often combined with other drugs. Cannot use long term.

[d]Use monohydrate salt, if available; to minimize esophageal irritation give before or with food, or followed by a small amount of water.

[e]Must check hemogram weekly for evidence of myelosuppression. Cannot use long term.

[f]For the dosage of other quinolones, see Drug Formulary.

[g]Avoid in young animals.

[h]Avoid higher doses or parenteral use in cats because of risk of retinal toxicity.

[i]Because of difficulty of fractionating liquid in capsules, cats are usually given one 50-mg capsule per dose. The contents of capsule may be cut into halves with a scalpel blade while wearing disposable gloves and dividing it into two gelatin capsules. Alternatively a compounding pharmacist can provide the optimal dosage size.

choice for empiric therapy. Recommendations from human infectious disease experts emphasize the possibility of RGM developing resistance to quinolones during a course of therapy.[26] Thus using quinolones strategically after surgical debulking or using them initially in concert with another effective antimicrobial may be prudent to reduce the likelihood of resistance developing. Such considerations are said not to be applicable to doxycycline or clarithromycin.[26] For this reason, many veterinary dermatologists in Australia routinely use combination therapy with doxycycline and a fluoroquinolone from the outset. Emphasis should be made that, although some RGM strains show in vitro susceptibility to amoxicillin-clavulanate, this drug combination has no efficacy in vivo.

Once susceptibility data becomes available, the optimal drug or drugs are selected. The in vivo response to a drug (or drugs) known to be effective in vitro can then be assessed. It general, using doses as high as possible is necessary because affected subcutaneous tissues are not well perfused, and considerable diffusion barriers prevent blood levels of antibiotics from reaching organisms in fat. Treatment should commence using standard dose rates. Subsequently, the dose is increased slowly (over several weeks) until adverse side effects (inappetence, vomiting) suggest the need for slight dose reduction or until a convincing clinical improvement is observed.

Some animals treated in a preliminary fashion using orally administered agents respond progressively to such an extent that surgery becomes unnecessary. These animals can be cured using medical therapy alone, although treatment with oral antimicrobials for 3 to 12 months may be required. As a generalization, lesions that resolve without the need for further surgical intervention involve a lesser depth of tissues than those that require surgery. Some lesions are so severe, however, that only a limited improvement can be achieved with antimicrobial therapy alone, and surgical intervention is required to affect a cure. Because predicting which cases will require operative débridement is impossible, our recommendation is to start empiric therapy, determine the in vitro sus-

ceptibility pattern, then reassess the patient every 3 to 4 weeks to decide if continued improvement is occurring or whether therapy has plateaued and surgery is required.

Preliminary medical therapy is of great benefit because, first, it reduces the amount of tissue requiring resection, and second, it minimizes the possibility of wound dehiscence.

Surgical resection, drainage, or debulking of large pyogranulomatous masses has traditionally been more beneficial in treatment of dogs than it has been in cats. However, recurrence may occur at the wound margins, especially in cats. Obtaining more radical surgical margins has been of benefit in our hands. If surgery is required, a drug with known efficacy against the causal strain that can be administered by injection. For example, gentamicin should be administered intraoperatively (2 mg/kg every 8 hours or 6 mg/kg every 24 hours; IV or SC) and in the early postoperative period (ideally for several days if economically possible). Gentamicin is a good choice because it is bactericidal, available in a parenteral form, inexpensive, and displays good in vitro activity against all RGM. Amikacin is superior to gentamicin, although it is substantially more expensive in Australia.

The critical surgical consideration is to remove as much abnormal subcutaneous tissue as possible (Fig. 50-19), which in some animals may necessitate the removal of very large portions of infected tissue. Severe cases benefit from the radical excision technique developed by Hunt (Fig. 50-20) in which infected tissues are resected en bloc followed by rearrangement of nearby skin to fill the often substantial tissue deficits created.[87,88] In some cases, however, panniculitis is so extensive that this technique is not feasible. Advanced cases with extensive lesions optimally require the skill of an experienced soft-tissue surgeon to reconstruct the resulting wound without undue tension, particularly in feline cases. The large amount of dead space created by the débridement requires judicious use of latex or closed suction drains for several days postoperatively.

Following surgery, drugs thought to be of greatest theoretical efficacy against the causal organism are used in the postop-

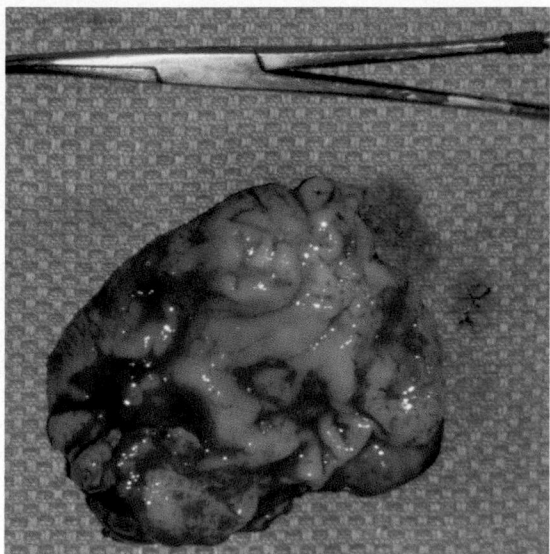

Fig 50-19 Subcutaneous fat and skin removed from a cat with panniculitis. The large portion of tissue was removed by en bloc resection. (Courtesy Richard Malik, University of Sydney, Sydney, Australia.)

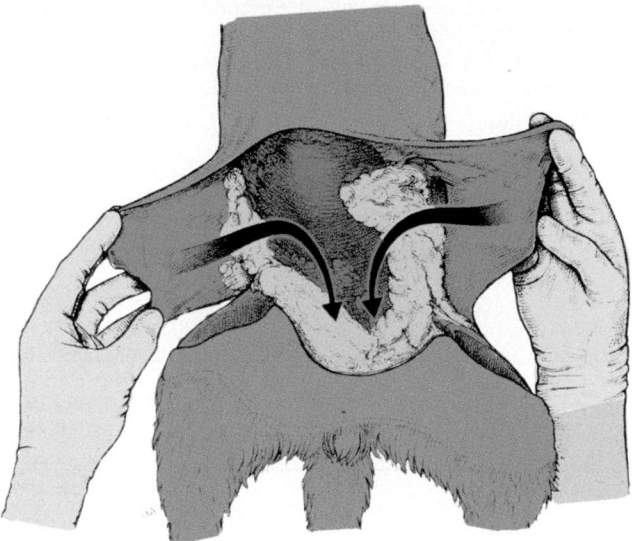

Fig 50-20 Diagrammatic representation of mobilizing both flank folds to reconstruct the tissue deficit resulting from surgical resection of an infected inguinal fat pad. (From Hunt GB. 1995. Skin-fold advancement flaps for closing large sternal and inguinal wounds in cats and dogs. *Vet Surg* 24:172–175; and Hunt GB, Tisdall PLC, Liptak JM, et al. 2001. Skin-fold advancement flaps for closing large proximal limb and trunk defects in dogs and cats. *Vet Surg* 30:440–448.)

erative period to ensure that primary intention healing occurs. Residual bacteria at the wound margins are thus targeted by high levels of the effective agent or agents. Because of cost considerations and other practicalities, the choice is generally reduced to one or a combination of a fluoroquinolone, doxycycline, or clarithromycin based on in vitro susceptibility. Dosages for these drugs are listed in Table 50-9.

Of the agents suitable for postoperative therapy, the fluoroquinolones (enrofloxacin, marbofloxacin, orbifloxacin, gatifloxacin) and doxycycline are generally the agents of choice for treating RGM infections in Australia, where *M. smegmatis* and *M. fortuitum* strains predominate. In the United States,

clarithromycin or fluoroquinolones, or both, represent the cornerstones of therapy for RGM, although doxycycline still has a place in the treatment of susceptible strains.

Fluoroquinolones are bactericidal, penetrate well into tissues (including fat), and are concentrated in polymorphs and macrophages. Current concerns about the retinotoxic potential of enrofloxacin when given to cats in daily doses exceeding 5 mg/kg probably preclude its use in this species, whereas ciprofloxacin, gatifloxacin, or other *veterinary quinolones* may be safer choices at the high doses likely to be required for these infections. However, retinal toxicity may be a potential problem with higher doses of any fluoroquinolones in cats (see Drug Formulary, Appendix 8). The authors have had no experience using marbofloxacin or orbifloxacin in the treatment of mycobacterial infections, and unfortunately no published data on their use is available. Doxycycline has a cost advantage over the quinolones and, based on our experience, has similar efficacy and is equally suited to long-term oral therapy. Doxycycline monohydrate is the tetracycline of choice for use in small animal patients because it is well tolerated, is present in a readily available form (VibraVet tablets; Pfizer Animal Health, Sydney, NSW, Australia), and has good lipid solubility. This drug is not readily available in many other countries, which is problematic because other doxycycline salts are more irritating, causing vomiting or, worse, esophageal ulceration.[134] For this reason, doxycycline should be either given immediately before meals with butter or margarine, or it should be followed by a small amount of liquid (see Appendix 8). Clarithromycin, a macrolide with an extended spectrum of activity and prolonged pharmacokinetics, has proved extremely useful in treating RGM infections in human and veterinary patients. Its major disadvantages is its high cost, which becomes an issue in the treatment of large dogs. Information is insufficient to recommend routine combination therapy in these animals, but the possibility of resistance emerging during therapy should be considered in animals in which a favorable response (especially to fluoroquinolones) is not sustained during a course of therapy or if relapse occurs.

In human infections caused by RGM, single-drug therapy is recommended for localized or minor disease. In contrast, severe or disseminated disease and pulmonary infections usually require multiple antimicrobials, including both IV (e.g., amikacin) and oral medications (e.g., clarithromycin, ciprofloxacin) at least for the first 2 weeks of therapy.

The total duration of therapy should be at least 3 to 12 months. Agents should be administered for at least 1 to 2 months after affected tissues look and feel completely normal. In occasional refractory cases, clofazimine,[136] cefoxitin, or amikacin may be used for monotherapy or in conjunction with other agents shown to be effective in vitro. Cefoxitin and amikacin can be given only by injection. Several new oral agents for treating refractory RGM infections have become available, including gatifloxacin and linezolid.[26] Although these agents hold great promise for some previously untreatable mycobacterial infections, high cost precludes their routine use. We have had limited experience with gatifloxacin in feline patients in which it has proven to be well tolerated and helpful in two refractory cases. This drug has greater activity against *M. fortuitum* and *M. chelonae* strains than older quinolones such as ciprofloxacin.[27]

In summary, mycobacterial panniculitis is an eminently treatable disease. Diagnosis is straightforward, especially for practitioners familiar with the syndrome. The prognosis is excellent, even in cases with severe, extensive, and longstanding disease. Treatment involves long courses of antimicrobials chosen on the basis of laboratory testing, sometimes combined with extensive surgical débridement and wound reconstruction. Finally, the routine prophylactic use of doxycycline following treatment of penetrating injuries in obese dogs and cats may prevent the development of these deep-seated infections.

Similar considerations apply to the treatment of pyogranulomatous pneumonia caused by RGM. Empiric treatment should be started immediately after obtaining diagnostic specimens for cytology and culture. Therapy may need to be altered in the light of susceptibility data. Treatment should initially consist of high levels of two agents known to be effective in vitro, including IV gentamicin and amikacin. Nebulization using gentamicin or amikacin is likely to be a useful adjunct to systemic therapy. Pulmonary lesions that respond incompletely to appropriate medical therapy may need to be surgically resected to affect a cure.*

Public Health Considerations

Rapid-growing mycobacteria are free-living saprophytes; the risk of transmission of these infections between animals or from animal to people is small. However, wound disinfection and contact precautions are usually advised, especially if immunosuppressed people are present in the same environment. Sodium hypochlorite (100 ppm available chlorine) rapidly kills these organisms on contaminated surfaces or inanimate objects.

SC inoculation of *M. chelonae* organisms reportedly occurred through penetration of dog hair into the owner's Achilles tendon by prolonged and vigorous rubbing of the person's ankle on that person's pet terrier.[132] Tendonitis caused by *M. chelonae* resulted. Cultures of the dog's hair and of tap water from the patient's home were negative for mycobacteria. Human hospital–acquired infections have also occurred. Contamination of multiple dose–injection syringes, peritoneal

*References: 57, 90, 94, 182, 197.

dialysis and hemodialysis machines, bronchoscopes, and some surgical equipment has led to severe nosocomial infections. Similar problems have not been reported in veterinary hospitals, but the potential exists.

SUGGESTED READINGS*

6. Aranaz A, Liebana E, Pickering X, et al. 1996. Use of polymerase chain reaction in the diagnosis of tuberculosis in cats and dogs, *Vet Rec* 138:276-280.
33. Charles J, Martin P, Wigney D, et al. 1999. Pathology of canine leproid granuloma syndrome, *Aust Vet J* 77:799-803.
55. Foley JE, Borjesson D, Gross TL, et al. 2002. Clinical, microscopic and molecular aspects of canine leproid granuloma in the United States, *Vet Pathol* 9:234-239.
94. Jang SS, Hirsh DC. 2002. Rapidly growing members of the genus *Mycobacterium* affecting dogs and cats, *J Am Anim Hosp Assoc* 38:217-220.
98. Kaneene JB, Bruning-Fann CS, Dunn J, et al. 2002. Epidemiologic investigation of *Mycobacterium bovis* in a population of cats, *Am J Vet Res* 63:1507-1511.
99. Kaneene JB, Thoen Co. 2004. Tuberculosis. *J Am Vet Med Assoc* 224:685-691.
129. Malik R, Hughes MS, James G, et al. 2000. Infection of the subcutis and skin of cats with rapidly growing mycobacteria: a review of microbiological and clinical findings, *J Feline Med Surg* 2:35-48.
141. Monies RJ, Cranwell MP, Palmer N, et al. 2000. Bovine tuberculosis in domestic cats, *Vet Rec* 146:407-408.

*See the CD-ROM for a complete list of references.

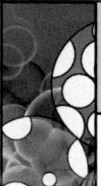

CHAPTER • 51

Dermatophilosis

Craig E. Greene

ETIOLOGY AND EPIDEMIOLOGY

Dermatophilosis (cutaneous streptothrichosis) is an exudative skin disease caused by the actinomycete *Dermatophilus congolensis*. Chronic exposure of the skin to trauma or moisture and immunosuppressive therapy or concurrent debilitating diseases may predispose the patient's skin to overgrowth and colonization by *D. congolensis*. This aerobe or facultative anaerobe is a normal dermal inhabitant of numerous mammalian species, including horses, sheep, goats, and cattle. Although not primary hosts, cats[5,9,12,13] and dogs[2,6] can be naturally infected. Acquisition from the soil, contact with another carrier animal, or latent infection in an affected animal cannot be excluded in reported cases.

Dermatophilosis has been produced experimentally in dogs after inoculation of the organism onto previously damaged skin[14] and in cats by subcutaneous inoculation.[9] Trauma associated with insect bites may predispose an animal to or transfer infection. Contamination of puncture wounds is presumed to occur in infected cats.

CLINICAL FINDINGS

Dogs

Spontaneous dermatophilosis in dogs is confined to the skin. As a primary dermatologic disease, dermatophilosis produces minimal signs of systemic illness, although emaciation and debilitation may be associated with an underlying immunosuppressive disease process. Lesions in dogs are frequently found on haired portions of the skin and consist of dry, adherent scabs that become entrapped in surrounding hair (Fig. 51-1). Removal of the crusts reveals underlying erythematous and ulcerated skin.

Cats

In affected cats, deeper abscesses in muscle, lymph nodes, and subcutaneous tissues have been more characteristic. The lesions are submucosal or subcutaneous pyogranulomas that can produce chronic draining fistulas. Fever, anorexia, and regional lymphadenomegaly or abscess formation

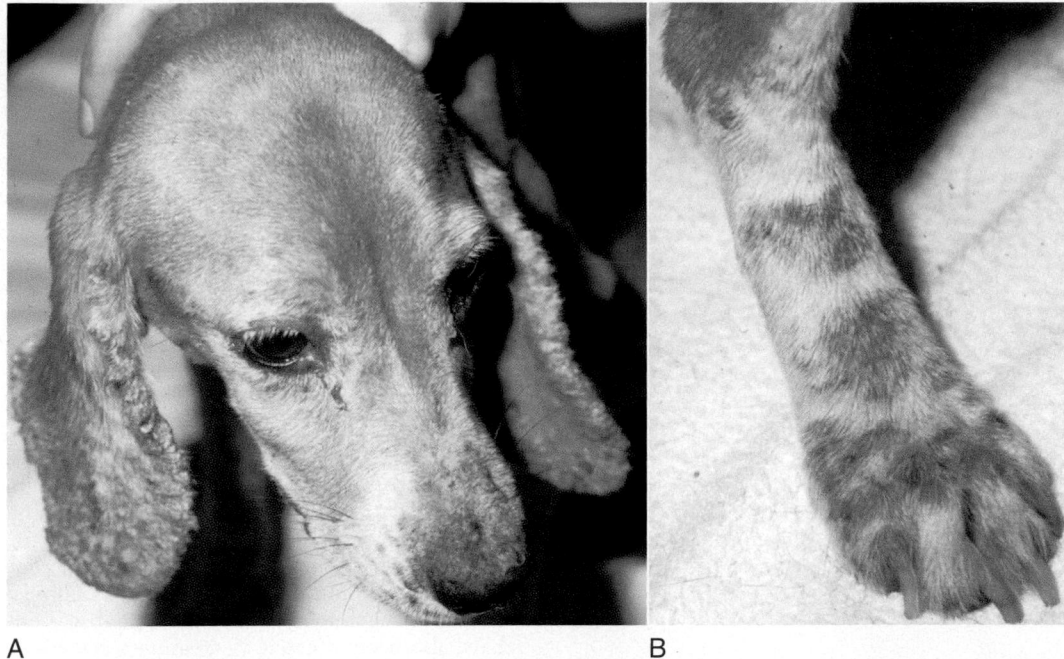

A   B

Fig 51-1 Skin lesions of dermatophilosis in a beagle. Crusty lesions surround tufts of hair on **(A)** ear margins and **(B)** extremities. (Courtesy University of Georgia, Athens, Ga.)

are common. Ulcerative granulomas in cats that involve the tongue or urinary bladder have also been described.[1,13]

DIAGNOSIS

The simplest and most rapid means of establishing a diagnosis involves removing the dried scabs from epidermal lesions or taking biopsy samples of deeper tissues where abscesses are found. Samples are minced in small amounts of sterile saline or nutrient broth. Some of the material is also used to prepare wet mounts or air-dried smears for microscopic examination, and the remainder is submitted for culture. Wet mounts can be stained with new methylene blue; dried specimens are heat-fixed and best stained by Giemsa methods, although Wright and Gram stains are suitable. Exudates or minced preparations usually contain large numbers of neutrophils in clusters around gram-positive branching filamentous organisms. The filaments are recognized by characteristic transverse and longitudinal divisions that result in three to eight paired rows of coccoid spores arranged linearly (Fig. 51-2). Monoclonal antibodies to *D. congolensis* have been used with indirect fluorescent antibody staining to specifically identify the organism in clinical samples.[8]

Sterile specimens from scabs or biopsy samples may be cultured aerobically at 25° C and aerobically or anaerobically at 37° C on solid nutrient agar such as blood or brain-heart infusion media. Small, grayish, raised colonies surrounded by a zone of hemolysis are typically produced. The organism can be more specifically identified by its biochemical properties or after experimental inoculation in laboratory animals. The cocci are vigorously motile when taken from fresh cultures.

PATHOLOGIC FINDINGS

Histologically, the organism produces an exudative, suppurative dermatitis characterized by epidermal hyperkeratosis and

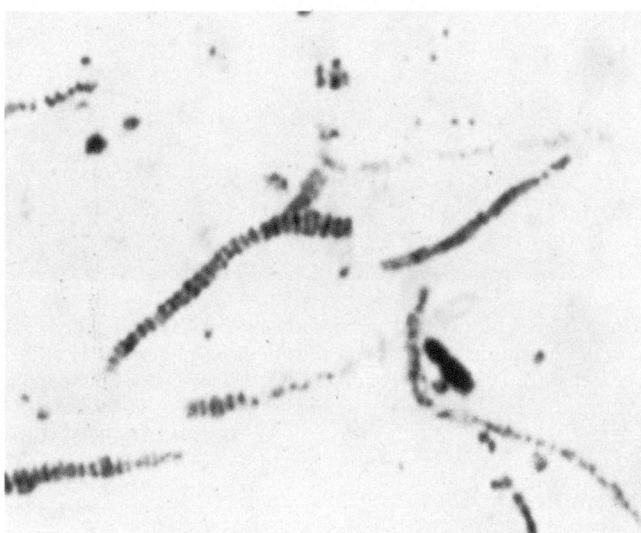

Fig 51-2 Cytologic characteristics of *D. congolensis*. Note filaments of paired rows of cocci, which have a "stacked coins" appearance (Gram stain, ×4300). (Courtesy Emmett Shotts, University of Georgia, Athens, Ga.)

subcorneal abscesses with underlying dermal edema and hemorrhage. Branching hyphae and clusters of coccoid bodies are usually in the parakeratotic layer (Fig. 51-3). Hair follicles are minimally affected. In cats the lesions consist of pyogranulomas in subcutaneous tissues or lymph nodes. The organism may be identified by hematoxylin-eosin–stained preparations in the periphery of necrotic lesions. The banded filamentous nature is best demonstrated by Twart's modified Gram stain. Immunostaining with polyclonal bacille Calmette-Guérin antibody has also been used[3]; however, the procedure is not specific for particular bacteria.

Table • 51-1

Drug Therapy for Dermatophilosis

DRUG[a]	SPECIES	DOSE[b] (mg/kg)	ROUTE	INTERVAL (HOURS)	DURATION (DAYS)
Penicillin V[c]	Dog, cat	10	PO	12	7—10
Gentamicin	Dog, cat	2	IM	12	7
Ampicillin or amoxicillin	Dog, cat	20	PO	8—12	7—10
Doxycycline	Dog, cat	5—10	PO	12	7—10

PO, Oral; IM, intramuscular.
[a]See Appendix 8 for additional information on these drugs.
[b]Dose per administration at specified interval.
[c]Penicillin may be given alone or in combination with gentamicin.

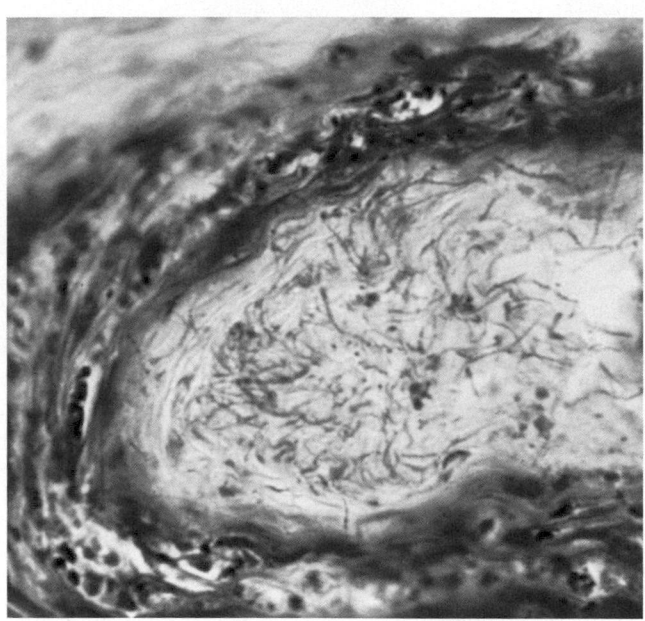

Fig 51-3 Biopsy specimen showing hyphae and individual coccoid organisms within parakeratotic layer of dermis (H and E stain, ×400). (Courtesy Emmett Shotts, University of Georgia, Athens, Ga.)

THERAPY

Treatment involves keeping the animal's skin dry and hair clipped around the periphery of the lesions or over the entire body if lesions are widespread. Clipping the hair and subsequently bathing with 2% lime sulfur or organic iodine preparations facilitate the softening and removal of the impervious, dry, adherent crusts. Bathing and crust removal should continue for a minimum of 2 weeks.

The infecting organism is susceptible to numerous antimicrobial agents in vitro; however, on the basis of cost and efficacy, penicillin derivatives are the most practical choice (Table 51-1). Penicillin may be given alone or in combination with an aminoglycoside. Ampicillin or amoxicillin has been administered successfully to treat cats with abscesses.[5] Tetracyclines have also been effective in treating a cat with an isolate that was not sensitive to penicillins.[10] For dermatophilosis treatment to be successful and permanent, its causes must be found and eliminated.

PUBLIC HEALTH CONSIDERATIONS

People are accidental secondary hosts of *D. congolensis*. People handling infected carcasses or tissues can develop exudative pustular dermatitis.[4] The disease in people is extremely rare, and approximately 10 cases have been reported in the literature.[4] Lesions usually consist of multiple white pustules 2 to 5 mm in diameter at the site of contact. These lesions neither spread nor coalesce but resolve within 2 weeks or more rapidly if the lesions are opened to drain.

SUGGESTED READINGS*

6. Chastain CB, Carithers RW, Hogle RM, et al. 1976. Dermatophilosis in two dogs. *J Am Vet Med Assoc* 169:1079-1080.
10. Kaya O, Kirkan S, Unal B. 2000. Isolation of *Dermatophilus congolensis* from a cat. *J Vet Med* 47:155-157.
11. Larrasa J, Garcia A, Ambrose NC, et al. 2002. A simple random amplified polymorphic DNA genotyping method for field isolates of *Dermatophilus congolensis*. *J Vet Med B Infect Dis Vet Public Health* 49:135-141.

*See the CD-ROM for a complete list of references.

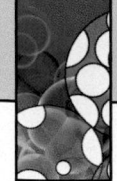

CHAPTER • 52

Abscesses and Pyogranulomatous Inflammation Caused by Bacteria

Craig E. Greene

ABSCESSES

Etiology and Pathogensis

Abscesses, which are characterized by an accumulation of pus, can occur in almost any tissue (Table 52-1). Percutaneous abscesses are the most common bacterial infections of feline skin and probably the most common site of abscess formation in dogs and cats. The following discussion will focus on feline abscesses, although the principles of diagnosis and treatment are similar in any location. See infections in the various system chapters for a discussion of abscesses in these locations. Abscesses develop more frequently in cats than they do in dogs, owing to the tough, elastic nature of feline skin, which readily seals over contaminated puncture wounds, causing the accumulation of subcutaneous exudates. Sharp teeth and fighting behavior, especially of adult males, are important predisposing factors to abscess formation. The size and degree of abscess formation depend on many factors, including the overlying skin tension, amount of dead space, and gravitation of exudate below the point of penetration. Pus-filled cavities that form above the puncture site drain easily. Cavities that gravitate below the puncture site become overdistended and may repeatedly drain through the puncture site without complete resolution.

Because feline abscesses usually result from bites and scratches, the most common organisms found within them are resident oral microflora (Table 52-2).* Although more difficult to cultivate, anaerobes are more frequently isolated than are aerobes. The supposition that *Pasteurella multocida* is the most common organism involved in cat abscesses is incorrect. Anaerobes can often be isolated in greater frequency. *P. multocida* is likely the most common facultative aerobic organism contaminating cat bite wounds (see Table 52-2). Cats that sustain bite injuries are more likely to become infected with feline immunodeficiency virus (FIV) (see Chapter 13).

Clinical Findings

The clinical signs of abscess formation in cats reflect the site and severity of the infection. Abscesses are usually located around the cat's legs, face, back, and base of the tail (Fig. 52-1). Some cats have a noticeable swelling with few other signs of illness, whereas more extensive infection is associated with fever (39.7° to 40.6° C [103.6° to 105.2° F]), anorexia, depression, and regional lymphadenomegaly. Pain is usually present at the site of infection, and obvious swelling or warmth may or may not occur. Mature abscesses that are ready to discharge are usually tender with a soft, fluctuant central area. Feline skin easily stretches over distended abscesses. Redness or discoloration is rarely apparent unless

*References: 7, 8, 14, 15, 23, 25, 32, 34.

the blood vascular supply has been compromised. Drainage of white, creamy, purulent material occurs spontaneously or after surgical lancing. Foul-smelling, red-brown discharges occur, especially with tissue necrosis and virulent anaerobic bacterial infection. Systemic signs often abate once the abscess ruptures, and the only evidence of infection may be matted hair at the site of drainage. Careful examination in the area of swelling usually reveals a small puncture wound covered by a crust. Recurrent abscesses at the same site suggest underlying osteomyelitis or neoplasia, poor surgical drainage, immunodeficiency (e.g., FeLV or FIV infection), antimicrobial resistance, or the presence of a foreign body. Abscesses associated with foreign bodies, underlying osteomyelitis, or certain organisms such as *Nocardia* or *Mycobacterium* also tend to recur, persist, or spread in tissues (Fig. 52-2). Abscesses in dogs and cats are often associated with noticeable regional lymphadenomegaly. Sometimes the overlying skin may become necrotic, and exudate drains externally (Fig. 52-3).

Additional clinical manifestations reflect various sequelae that can occur. Lameness or paralysis will be apparent with myositis, osteomyelitis, septic arthritis, or discospondylitis. Depression, stiffness, lethargy, nuchal rigidity, or seizures can be seen with meningitis. Osteomyelitis also causes chronic or recurrent draining fistulas that only temporarily respond to antibiotics. Respiratory distress, dyspnea, and stridor are noted with pyothorax, sinusitis, and rhinitis. Vestibular signs can be noted if otitis media or interna develops. Signs of bacteremia and systemic infection include malaise and fever or reflect those of another organ system of hematogenous localization.

Retrobulbar abscess or cellulitis is associated with proptosis, decreased globe mobility, oculonasal discharge, chemosis, conjunctival congestion, protrusion of the third eyelid, pain while opening the mouth, periocular swelling or discomfort, lethargy, weight loss, and fever. Corneal ulcers may develop from exposure keratitis or physical trauma caused by the discomfort. Swelling may be present behind the last upper molar.

Diagnosis

Determining the presence of an abscess is usually based on clinical history and examination. Abscesses should be expected in cats that develop an acute onset of unexplained fever, anorexia, or lameness, even in the absence of an obvious swelling, given than abscess formation may be delayed or hidden. The differential leukocyte count can help in determining the extent of infection and the animal's ability to control it. A low count with an inappropriate shift is associated with diffuse infection or cellulitis. A mature neutrophilia is more characteristic of a walled-off or mature abscess. Severe leukopenia (a cell count of under 4000/mm^3), with or without an associated anemia, may be present in cats infected with feline leukemia virus (FeLV) or FIV that develop chronic or recurrent abscesses as a result of immunosuppression.

Table • 52-1

Various Anatomic Locations of Canine and Feline Abscesses

DOG	PHYSICAL CAUSES	CHAPTER
Retrobulbar[20,37]	Suppurative myositis, cellulitis, or abscess	93
Retropharyngeal[38]	Penetrating foreign bodies	89
Pyothorax[44,49]	Inhaled foreign bodies, pneumonia, pulmonary abscess	88
Mediastinal[27,47]	Penetrating or inhaled foreign bodies	88
Paravertebral, epidural[5,11,40]	Foreign bodies, penetrating wounds, diskospondylitis	86, 92
Fascial[43]	Necrotizing fasciitis, gram-positive infections	35
Prostatic[9,22,45,51]	Urinary infection, intact males, urolithiasis, neoplasia	91
Hepatic or splenic[16]	Bacterial translocation	89, 90
Perirenal[19,35]	Pyelonephritis	91
Pericardial[42]	Bacterial translocation, penetrating foreign bodies	87
Intraabdominal[48,53]	Gut perforations, penetrating injuries, pancreatitis	89
Para-aural[12,28]	Pinna trauma or lacerations	85
Subcutaneous[14,39]	Fight wounds	52,53
Intracranial[26,47]	Bacteremia, otitis interna	92

Table • 52-2

Bacteria Isolated from Feline Abscesses[a]

GENUS	SPECIES	PERCENTAGE[b]
Anaerobes		
Porphyromonas[c]	gingivalis, tectum, heparinolyticus, salivosa, melaninogenicus, corrodens, fragilis, circumdentaria, others	26—76
Fusobacterium	nucleatum, necrophorum, russii, others	17—64
Peptostreptococcus	anaerobius	11—45
Clostridium	perfringens, novyi, sordellii, septicum, chauvoei, tetani, villosum	6.5
Propionibacterium	acnes, freudenreichii	4.2
Bifidobacterium	spp.	1.2
Lactobacillus	spp.	1.2
Eubacterium	lentum	0.6
Aerobes/Facultative		
Pasteurella	multocida[d]	13—27
Actinomyces	viscosus, odontolyticus	7—18
Nocardia	spp.	
Staphylococcus	spp.	14
Rhodococcus	equi	27
Enterobacteriaceae	other than E. coli listed below	13
Streptococcus	spp.	4.8—13
Enterococcus	spp.	12
Lactobacillus	spp.	1.8
Escherichia	coli	0.6

[a]Summarized from data in references 7, 8, 14, 15, 17, 21, 23, 25, 32–34, 39.
[b]Percentage of the class of isolates (anaerobes or aerobes) cultured from feline abscesses.
[c]Previously *Bacteroides*.
[d]Has been reclassified, see Etiology, Chapter 53.

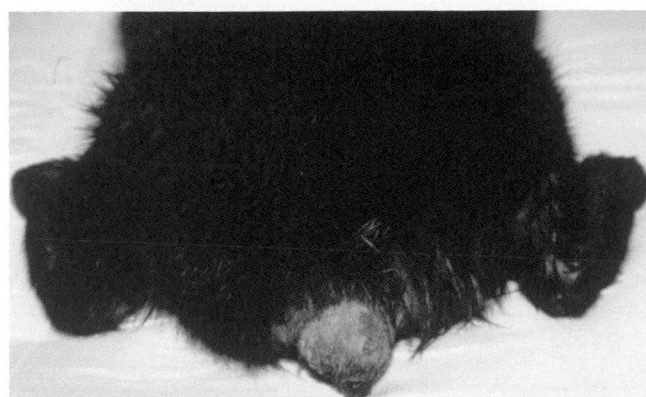

Fig 52-1 Abscess of tailhead from bite wounds in a cat with fever, leukocytosis, and caudal hyperesthesia. The tail was amputated because of severe infection and tissue necrosis. (Courtesy University of Georgia, Athens, Ga.)

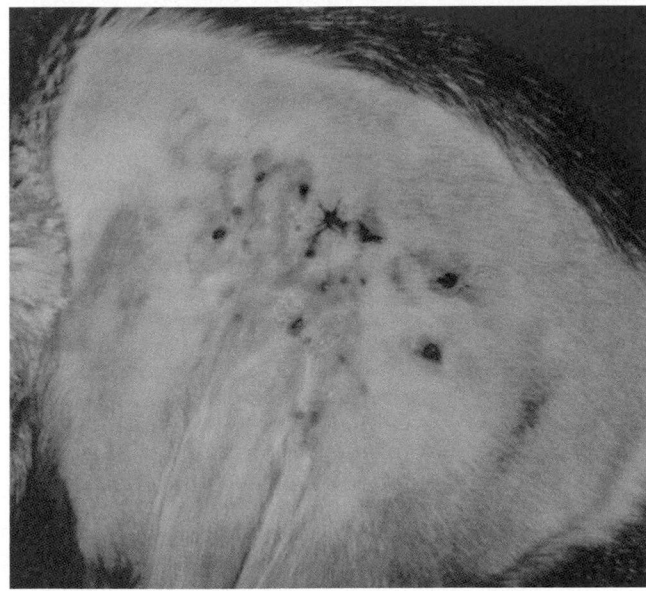

Fig 52-2 Recurrent draining tracts over the thoracic region in a cat with a bite wound infection caused by *Nocardia* sp. (Courtesy University of Georgia, Athens, Ga.)

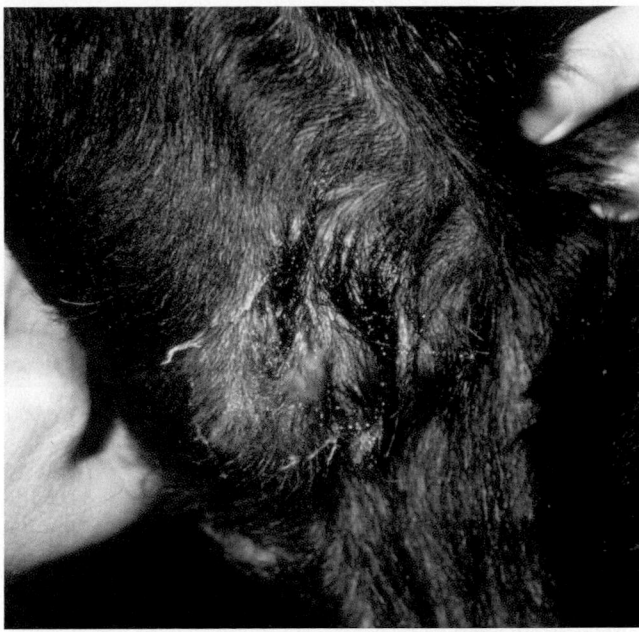

Fig 52-3 Abscess of cervical lymph node with drainage in a dog caused by a stick puncture wound injury of the oropharynx. *Actinomyces* sp. was isolated. (Courtesy University of Georgia, Athens, Ga.)

Unlike those in FeLV- or FIV-infected cats, the leukograms usually improve in immunocompetent cats after the abscesses drain.

Ultrasonography can be used to view the extent of a swelling and accumulation of fluid or pus in soft-tissue planes.[3,1a] Radiographic contrast procedures may be helpful in determining the extent or depth of a draining fistulous tract. Injection of contrast via an indwelling Foley catheter can be followed by radiography, computerized tomography (CT) scans, or magnetic resonance imaging (MRI). Cerebrospinal fluid evaluation and radiographic imaging is needed to detect central nervous system abscesses within the cranial vault or spinal canal.[38a]

Causes of recurrent or nonhealing abscesses in cats include retroviral infections, as previously discussed, underlying osteomyelitis, neoplasia or foreign body, or infection with organisms such as *Nocardia, Mycobacterium,* fungi, or parasites such as *Cuterebra*. Chronic or recurrent draining abscesses should be evaluated by radiography for underlying osteomyelitis, by cytology and culture for possible fungal or unusual bacterial infection, or by surgical exploration for the presence of a foreign body or parasite. Culture of abscess wounds for bacteria is not generally indicated because surgical débridement and empiric antimicrobial therapy are often effective. Anaerobic bacteria are difficult to culture.

Therapy

Abscesses vary in severity and in the extent of therapeutic intervention required. Small, localized abscesses that drain spontaneously by the time animals are presented for examination require that the hair around the wound be clipped, and the margins of the wound should be cleaned. Should abscesses not be open, surgical drainage and débridement may be needed. Whether opened naturally or by surgery, the cavity should be flushed with hydrogen peroxide, dilute chlorhexidine, or dilute iodophor solutions. More extensive infections that cause signs of systemic illness may require antibiotic administration, surgical drainage, or supportive care.

Antibiotic Therapy

Antibiotic therapy has a decided but not absolute role in the management of abscesses in cats. Although mortality and complications resulting from abscesses have been reduced with the use of antibacterials, these agents should not be given indiscriminately or in the absence of other adjunctive measures. Antibiotics alone are ineffective in penetrating walled-off abscesses that require drainage. Empiric antibiotic therapy should be discontinued and extensive diagnostic investigation initiated if abscesses or fever persist longer than 1 to 2 weeks or reform after repeated surgical drainage.

Penicillin derivatives are antibiotics of choice for treating abscesses because they are bactericidal and have marked activity against the more frequently encountered organisms (Table 52-3). Penicillin V, amoxicillin, or ampicillin may be dispensed in oral formulations to be administered by the client. How-

Table • 52-3

Drug Therapy for Feline Abscesses[a]

DRUG[b]	DOSE[c]	ROUTE	INTERVAL (HOURS)	DURATION (DAYS)[d]
Penicillin G	30,000—50,000 U/kg	SC, IM, IV	12	5—7
Penicillin V	20 mg/kg	PO	12	5—7
Ampicillin (amoxicillin)	20 mg/kg	PO, SC, IV	8—12	5—7
Chloramphenicol	15 mg/kg	PO, SC, IV	8	5—7
Clindamycin	10 mg/kg	PO, IM	12	5—7
Metronidazole	10 mg/kg	PO, IV	8—12	5—7
Doxycycline	5—10 mg/kg	PO, IV	12	5—7

SC, Subcutaneous; *IM*, intramuscular; *IV*, intravenous; *PO*, by mouth.
[a]See also Drug Therapy for Anaerobic Infections, Table 41–10, and Rhodococcal Infections, Table 35–6.
[b]See Appendix 8, Drug Formulary, for additional information on these drugs.
[c]Dose per administration at specified interval.
[d]Treatment is required for at least 14 to 28 days if surgical drainage is not performed.

ever, amoxicillin or ampicillin may not always be as effective as penicillin is in treating anaerobic infections. Because of a similar antibacterial spectrum, chloramphenicol can be substituted for penicillin, but it is bacteriostatic and frequently causes anorexia; it can also be hazardous to people. If anaerobes are suspected, penicillin, second- or third-generation cephalosporins, chloramphenicol, clindamycin, and metronidazole have the greatest efficacy. Certain *Fusobacterium* spp. have also been susceptible to erythromycin and doxycycline (see also Therapy, Chapter 41).[33] *Rhodococcus* has been primarily susceptible to aminoglycosides, chloramphenicol, and erythromycin (see also Rhodococcal Infections, Chapter 35).[15] Topical application or direct instillation of antibiotics into the abscess cavity is ineffective because, with the exception of nitrofurans, none work in the presence of pus. Hydrogen peroxide or chlorhexidine solutions and nitrofurazone powder or solution are empirically placed in surgically opened abscess cavities without documented efficacy. Systemic antibiotic therapy may be beneficial in minimizing abscess formation when given immediately after bite wound contamination or with diffuse cellulitis (see also Bite Wound Infections, Chapter 53). Within 24 hours of injury, a single injection of procaine penicillin G can thwart the development of an abscess.[24] Although therapeutic drainage has been advocated for most abscesses, medical therapy alone has proved efficacious in treating affected people.[4] Antimicrobial treatment of abscesses in cats may be considered when surgical intervention will alter delicate anatomic structures or will involve considerable anesthetic risk. Less favorable outcomes are associated with large (over 5 cm) lesions or with mixed bacterial populations.[4] Without surgical drainage, medical therapy must be continued for longer periods of at least 14 to 28 days.

Surgery

Surgical intervention is reserved for mature or ruptured abscesses. Diffuse cellulitis or early abscesses should be allowed to mature before surgical drainage is performed. Applying warm compresses daily or soaking affected extremities in warm, saturated Epsom salt solutions may hasten the maturation process. Both measures have been beneficial in keeping already established drainage sites open until proper healing can occur. Surgical therapy usually involves creating drainage openings at the most ventral portion of an abscess cavity. Controversy exists as to the degree and type of surgical closure indicated. Most veterinarians débride the abscess cavity and remove a small portion of overlying skin to prevent premature closure. Placement of soft rubber tubing that exits at the lowest point of incision with partial closure is fre-

quently used to maintain a drainage opening. A few veterinarians, advocating complete primary closure of the abscess cavity after extensive débridement, argue that more rapid healing and less postoperative drainage are achieved.[2] Systemic antibiotic therapy is probably essential whenever partial or complete surgical closure is performed because the likelihood of organisms remaining in the wound is high, and the risk of systemic spread increases.

Surgical drainage must be established whenever abscess formation occurs within closed cavities. Retrobulbar abscesses must be drained by passing a probe from immediately behind the last upper molar upward into the retrobulbar space. Infraorbital abscesses are usually associated with infection of the upper carnassial tooth, which must be extracted. Sinusal, nasal, and chronic middle-ear abscesses also require surgical drainage with débridement of bone because of the loculation of pus within cavities surrounded by bone. Abscesses associated with underlying osteomyelitis must be treated by surgical débridement of infected bone. Foreign bodies or material must be removed from abscess cavities before they will heal.

Castration is recommended as a preventive measure to abscess formation because it reduces the fighting and roaming behavior of male cats. Progestogens can be given similarly to modify behavior, but the necessity of their continued use induces many undesirable side effects.

FELINE PSEUDOMYCETOMA, BOTRYOMYCOSIS, PYOGRANULOMATOUS INFLAMMATION

A chronic pyogranulomatous inflammatory reaction caused by bacteria and resembling a fungal growth is known as botryomycosis. Literally, the gross appearance of these proliferative growths resembles a bunch of grapes. Eosinophilic infiltration is commonly found. Grossly, the lesions have microabscesses surrounded by fibrous granulation tissue. This funguslike condition is often caused by *Staphylococcus* spp. (presumably, *intermedius*); however, other unidentified rod-shaped bacteria have been observed.[41] Lesions are usually localized masses with embedded yellow-white grains that resemble bacterial colonies (similar to *Actinomyces* or *Nocardia*). These lesions are composed of infiltrating eosinophils and macrophages surrounding necrotic tissue. A large number of saprophytic bacteria and fungi, in addition to staphylococci, can produce similar lesions and must be considered (Table 52-4).

These lesions are thought to be caused by chronic unresolved abscesses. The reason for development of these lesions

Table • 52-4

Organisms Causing Pyogranulomatous Infections

Bacteria:
Bartonella[a] (Chapter 54)
Staphylococcus[b] (Chapter 36)
Mycobacterium (Chapter 50)
Nocardia (Chapter 49)
Actinomyces (Chapter 49)

Fungi:
Blastomyces (Chapter 59)
Histoplasma (Chapter 60)
Cryptococcus (Chapter 61)
Coccidioides (Chapter 62)
Aspergillus (Chapter 64)
Miscellaneous fungi (Chapter 67)

Oomycetes:
Pythium (Chapter 67)

Protozoa:
Toxoplasma (Chapter 80)
Neospora (Chapter 80)

[a]Especially in nonreservoir hosts.
[b]Especially antimicrobial resistant strains; see text.

has not been determined; however, neutrophils surrounding bacterial colonies are replaced by fibrosing granulation tissue later in the encapsulation of the abscess. Only a few cats had positive antibody test results for FIV; none had positive results for FeLV.

Lesions are commonly found in the cervical and extremity regions in addition to the abdominal mesentery of cats. Lesions usually develop as localized masses.

Diagnosis of this condition is first made by cytologic examination of exudates. Degenerate neutrophils, macrophages, lymphocytes, plasma cells, and intracellular bacteria (often cocci) will be observed. The grains when squashed on a slide consist of masses of bacteria. Should staphylococci not be isolated, further diagnostic testing should include histopathologic examination and aerobic and anaerobic bacterial culture. Special staining should include methenamine silver and acid-fast methods.

Treatment involves surgical removal and drainage of infected tissues. Antibacterial therapy by itself is usually futile; however, it can be helpful as an adjunctive measure. Long-term antimicrobial therapy for up to 4 months is often needed. Methicillin-resistant staphylococci have been cultured or suspected as the cause of this condition; thus antimicrobial therapy may require prior culture and susceptibility testing.

SUGGESTED READINGS*

3. Armbrust LJ, Biller DS, Radlinsky MG, et al. 2003. Ultrasonographic diagnosis of foreign bodies associated with chronic draining tracts and abscesses in dogs, *Vet Radiol Ultrasound* 44:66-70.
9. Boland LE, Hardie RJ, Gregory SP, et al. 2003. Ultrasound-guided percutaneous drainage as the primary treatment for prostatic abscesses and cysts in dogs, *J Am Anim Hosp Assoc* 39:151-159.
11. Cherrone KL, Eich CS, Bonzynski JJ. 2002. Suspected paraspinal abscess and spinal epidural empyema in a dog, *J Am Anim Hosp Assoc* 38:149-151.
13. Daigle JC, Kerwin S, Foil CS, et al. 2001. Draining tracts and nodules in dogs and cats, *Clin Tech Small Anim Pract* 16:214-218.
16. Ginel PJ, Lucera R, Arola J, et al. 2001. Diffuse splenomegaly caused by splenic abscessation in a dog, *Vet Rec* 149:327-329.
27. Koutinas CK, Papazoglu LG, Saridomichelakis MN, et al. 2003. Caudal mediastinal abscess due to a grass awn (*Hordeum* spp.) in a cat, *J Feline Med Surg* 5:43-46.
41. Ozaki K, Yamagami T, Nomura K, et al. 2003. Abscess-forming inflammatory granulation tissue with gram-positive cocci and prominent eosinophil infiltration in cats: possible infection of methicillin-resistant *Staphylococcus*, *Vet Pathol* 40:283-287.
47. Seiler G, Rytz U, Gaschen L. 2001. Radiographic diagnosis—cavitary mediastinal abscess, *Vet Radiol Ultrasound* 42:431-433.

*See the CD-ROM for a complete list of references.

CHAPTER • 53

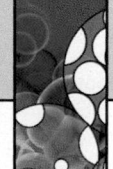

Bite Wound Infections

Craig E. Greene and Ellie J. C. Goldstein

DOG AND CAT BITE INFECTIONS

Veterinarians can be an important source of information for the public concerning animal bites. Approximately 50% of Americans will be bitten by an animal at some point in their lifetime. In addition to the zoonotic concern, dogs and cats frequently bite each other, resulting in injuries that must be treated as emergencies.

Epidemiology of People Bitten by Animals

Animal bite wounds are fourth among the most commonly reported human illnesses each year in the United States.

Although it is reported that 4.7 million people are bitten by animals in the United States annually,[10,34,128,140] less than half of the bites are ever reported and only 18% of the people seek medical attention.[123] Bites from animals that are pets are even more drastically underreported. Approximately 90% of animal bites of people are from dogs and cats.[151] Approximately 1% (with a range of 0.3% to 1.1%) of emergency hospital visits by people involve bite injuries.[164] Data from Switzerland suggest that similar statistics are found in Europe. Dogs accounted for more than 60% and cats for 25% of all bites inflicted by vertebrate animals.[106]

Veterinarians and animal health personnel are at greater risk for injury by dogs and cats than the general population.[93] Results of a survey of a group of veterinarians in the United States indicated that approximately 65% had sustained a major animal-related injury.[93] Animal bites and scratches accounted for 34% and 3.8%, respectively, of the traumas. Dogs were involved in 24% and cats in 10% of the injuries. In their careers, 92% of the veterinarians surveyed had sustained dog bites, 81% cat bites, and 72% cat scratches. The following epidemiologic discussion focuses on bite injuries that are not related to veterinary practice and for which a veterinarian may be consulted to determine the disposition of the dog or cat responsible for the bite. (However, the information can be applied to injuries that occur within a veterinary practice setting.) The procedures for injured people can also be applied to treating wounds of dogs and cats that are bitten during a fight. The characteristics of dog- and cat-related injuries are summarized in Table 53-1.

Dog Bites

An estimated 34 million American households own dogs, with a total canine population of 68 million. Dog prevalence varies worldwide, and developing countries have a greater percentage of feral domestic dogs. Risk factors for dog bites include the dog's age, breed, size, medical health, sex, and reproductive status.[57,97,122,134,167] Bites are more likely to be delivered by reproductively intact male, large-size (greater than 22.7 kg [50 lb]), 6-month-old to 4-year-old dogs that are mixed breeds, German shepherds, or chow chows. However, breed-specific statements can be inaccurate because of breed popularity and misidentification, inaccurate estimates of a breed's prevalence, and differences in aggressive behavior.

Of the 800,000 annual dog bites in the United States that require medical attention, approximately 20 are fatal.[8,49,141,164] Approximately 350,000 emergency room visits related to dog bites occur each year[10,164]; the number of admissions is second only to baseball and softball injuries as admissions for recreational injuries. Reports citing large dogs as the most frequent biters may underestimate the number of bites from smaller dogs.[167] However, serious bites to children are commonly inflicted by large dogs.[24,57,97] Regardless of size, dogs can exert a jaw force of 450 psi, enough to do extensive damage to tissues. Additional pulling and tearing can cause shearing injuries. Dogs cited for causing a high percentage of the severe or fatal bites have included pit bulls, Rottweilers, German shepherds, chow chows, cocker spaniels, and huskies.[112,141,142] However, a study in one Florida county found that golden retrievers and cocker spaniels have bitten more people than German shepherds. In one observation, Labrador retrievers and golden retrievers commonly bit their owners or someone petting them, whereas German shepherds, Bernese mountain dogs, and collies tended to be aggressive to strangers.[107] Dominance aggression has been linked to unprovoked attacks of people by dogs. In one behavior clinic, the most prevalent breeds for which dominance aggression was treated were the English springer spaniel, cocker spaniel, Labrador retriever, golden retriever, Dalmatian, Rottweiler, and German shep-

herd.[123] In addition to breed behavior, another important contributory factor to biting is the degree of responsibility exercised by the animal's owner.

A survey of fatal dog-bite attacks in the United States from 1979 to 1998 listed the pit-bull–type, Rottweiler, German shepherd, husky-type, malamute, Doberman, chow chow, Great Dane, and Saint Bernard as the most prevalent breeds.[142] These data were acquired by searching news accounts and the Humane Society of the United States registry databank. Dog bite statistics from media reports in North America show that up to 77% of 931 dog attack fatalities and maimings resulted from dogs that were pit-bull types, Rottweilers, wolf hybrids, or a mix of these breeds.[33] These data, which may be biased by media interest, show that pit-bull types are the only breed that attack adults as frequently as children; these dogs may lack normal canine inhibition. In contrast, Rottweilers and other breeds attack children 3 times more often than they attack adults, indicating that the children's size may play a role. Wolf hybrids predominantly attack young children (younger than 7 years), suggesting that predation rather than territoriality or reactivity is the reason for their attacks.[33] Some are concerned that data from news services may sensationalize and bias reported incidents.[123] Furthermore, the data on fatal attacks should not overshadow the medical importance of nonfatal bite injuries, which likely do not have the same breed bias. Lastly, dog owners can play a significant role in increasing or decreasing aggressive pet behaviors by the socialization of their dogs and the way they handle aggressive behaviors. No dog is born aggressive, but it can become aggressive through improper discipline and training. Therefore veterinarians should emphasize and support educating their clients about aggressiveness and legislation directed at controlling undesirable animal behaviors or negligent owners.[110] Legislation on breed-specific prohibitions is unlikely to be legally enforceable.[162] Veterinarians should always report aggressive incidents that happen during a pet's hospitalization to the pet's owners and others handling the involved pets (Table 53-2).

Less than one half of dog bites are provoked; males and children are more likely to be involved in provoked attacks.[124] Most dog bites involve a dog owned by the family or a neighbor, and they are often unprovoked. For example, fatal dog bites of newborns often occur when infants are sleeping. The majority of cat bites are provoked, and females and adults are more likely to be bitten.

Other factors involved with dog bites include the person bitten, the dog-person relationship, and the setting.[168] Approximately 75% of bite injuries are in people younger than 21 years, with peak incidence at 5 to 9 years. Children are more likely to provoke dogs and often do not understand the dog's body language. Reports of the high prevalence of bites among children may be related to the additional attention given to dog bites of children compared with those of adults. Although males comprise approximately 65% of all those bitten, boys and girls younger than 6 years account for almost 60% of all fatal bite injuries. More than 50% of injuries among children occur on the head, face, or neck. *Any* movements in the presence of *certain* dogs can cause the dogs to become aggressive, especially when children are involved.[104,134] Bending over, reaching toward, hugging, or grabbing the collar of a dog are typical human behaviors that may increase the risk of being bitten, especially if a dog is afraid, possessive, or dominant. Other kinds of dog aggression and their eliciting behaviors are discussed elsewhere.[168,170]

In general, people are more likely to be bitten by a dog if they own a dog, they are in the presence of a dog owned by someone else, or the dog lives in a household with at least one child.[57,104,167] Recipients of reported bites are more likely to be neighbors of families who own dogs, with the next likely

Table • 53-1

Epidemiologic Characteristics Associated with Dog- and Cat-Related Bites or Scratches

CHARACTERISTICS OF CATS AND DOGS EXHIBITING AGGRESSION

	CATS	DOGS
Age	Insufficient data	Less than 5 years (49%)
Sex	Female (67%)	Male (70%—79%)
Ownership Status	Stray (57%)	Owned (a significant number of these owned aggressive dogs live in a household with at least one child)
Reproductive Status	Insufficient data	Intact (not neutered)
Size	Insufficient data	Large dogs (> 50 lbs)
Breed	Insufficient data	Total annual # bites: mixed breed and German shepherds Bite rates: German shepherds and Chow-Chows. Highest rate of severe/fatal bites: pit bulls, German shepherds, Chow-Chows

CHARACTERISTICS OF PEOPLE INJURED BY CATS AND DOGS

	VICTIMS OF AGGRESSION BY CATS	VICTIMS OF AGGRESSION BY DOGS
Age	25—34 years	< 20 years old, with significant occurrence in 5—9 years old
Sex	Females (59%)	Males (62%)
Relationship to animal	Victim does not own cat	Victim is family member or acquaintance to the owners Dog's owners are most frequently bitten by dogs — not necessarily by their own dogs (family's dog-30%; neighbor's dog-50%)

CHARACTERISTICS OF THE INJURY EVENT

	COMMON CAT-BITE SCENARIO	COMMON DOG-BITE SCENARIO
Kinds of aggression	Fear-related aggression, play aggression, redirected aggression, "biting and petting syndrome"	Dominance aggression, possessive aggression, fear-related aggression, protective/Territorial aggression, punishment-induced aggression, pain-elicited aggression
Time of Year	May through August (warm weather)	May through August (warm weather)
Time of Day	9:00 am to noon	Late afternoon
Other Factors	If the cat is owned, 50% of the victims are the owners	Unusually high incidence of bites by chained dogs who are restrained on their own property
Typical wound characteristics	80% of all bites require medical attention	20%—60% of all bites require medical attention
	50% of all wounds become infected	Insufficient data on number of wounds that become infected
	29% of all cat-bite victims return to doctor after initial visit due to complications	5% of all dog-bite victims return to doctor after initial visit due to complications
	Wounds consist of scratches (70%); punctures (27%) and tears (3%) to finger (21%), arm (18%), foot or leg (8%), face or neck (7%); and multiple body locations (3%).	Wounds consist primarily of puncture and tears to the extremities (76%) and to face (15%), 70% fatal injuries to children < 9 yrs old. Highest death rate to neonates (< 1 month old). Death rates of neonates 295/100 million; for children 1—11 months old 47/100 million

Table • 53-1

Continued

	LOCATION OF BITE WOUNDS[a]	
	CAT BITES (%)	DOG BITES (%)
Face, scalp, or neck	2	16
Trunk	0	2
Shoulder, arm, or forearm	23	12
Hand	63	50
Thigh or leg	9	16
Feet	3	4

[a]Adapted from Talan DA, Citron DM, Abrahamian FM, et al. 1999. Bacteriologic analysis of infected dog and cat bites, *N Engl J Med* 340:85–92.

Table • 53-2

Recommendations for Limiting Dog Bites

Animal Health Professionals
1. Use extra caution when handling pit bulls, Rottweilers, wolf hybrids, and chow chows.
2. Separate aggressive dogs from one another, and protect handling personnel. Provide leashes and carriers.
3. Always muzzle dogs with known or suspected aggressive tendencies.
4. Use a metal choke collar and chain leashes on aggressive dogs.
5. Snap bolt cages or runs containing aggressive dogs. Place signs on cages and runs to identify aggressive dogs.
6. Always have two people in a room when handling or working around aggressive dogs.
7. Educate clients on pet selection, conditioning, and handling.

Dog Owners
1. Avoid selecting dog breeds with known aggressive tendencies.
2. Do not bother ill animals or those who are eating, sleeping, or nursing pups.
3. Socialize dogs at an early age.
4. Take dogs to obedience classes when they are pups.
5. Have pets neutered, especially males.
6. Always supervise children when pets are present.
7. Never leave any dog alone with an infant or a child.
8. Select dog breeds based on known bite tendencies.
9. Never take a pet with a history of aggression into a household with children.
10. Be sensitive to children's fears of pets, and delay or avoid acquiring one until they are comfortable.
11. Spend time with a pet before taking it home.
12. Teach dogs submissive behavior when they are being reprimanded or fed.
13. Immediately notify your veterinarian if your dog shows aggressive tendencies.
14. Never pet a dog until it has had time to see and sniff you.
15. Do not play aggressively with dogs or stare at them directly.
16. Teach children not to approach unfamiliar dogs without allowing the pets to smell them first. When reaching out to a dog, the child should present a balled fist to keep fingers protected.
17. Children should not disturb sleeping dogs or run and scream around them.
18. If a dog becomes aggressive, children and adults should remain motionless, avoid direct eye contact, and if knocked over, lie curled up and motionless.
19. Report all bite incidents to adults or proper authorities.

Community Efforts
1. Disseminate information to children and parents.
2. Provide bite prevention courses in schools and for parent organizations.
3. Institute animal control laws and enforcement.
4. Target chronically irresponsible dog owners rather than specific breeds.

recipients being the owners, although bites to owners are probably underreported.[24,170]

Other factors that can affect a dog's likelihood of biting include whether the dog is chained for long periods,[57] geographic location, time of year, time of day, and weather. A majority of dog bite injuries occur between April and September, when warm weather is conducive to outdoor activity (see Table 53-1).[167] A booklet on bite prevention is available at www.statefarm.com/consumer/dogbite.htm or www.avma.org. Additional information on dog bite prevention can be found at www.hsus.org. Information concerning variations in dog bite statutes in the United States has been reviewed.[68] An excellent review on the community approach to dog bite prevention was published in a report by an American Veterinary Medical Association task force.[9]

In a study of dog bites involving caregivers in a veterinary teaching hospital, caregivers interacting with older dogs were more likely to be bitten than those interacting with younger ones.[43] Dogs with a propensity to bite already had warning signs posted on their cages.

Cat Bites
Compared with dog bites, much less has been reported about feline aggression (biting and scratching) toward people. Approximately 400,000 cat bites are reported each year in the United States, and cat-induced wounds have a greater propensity for becoming infected than dog-induced wounds. Cat bites constitute 5% to 25% of animal-related injuries in people, whereas other domestic and wild animals account for less than 1% of reported bites.

The most commonly reported cat bites and scratches involve unowned female cats that have injured adult women (see Table 53-1). Scratches and bites are more common in warm weather (the summer season) and the late afternoon. Cat-induced wounds have been described as being scratches, punctures, or tears.[166] Owned cats have bitten people on the neck, face, and multiple sites, whereas strays are more likely to injure the hand. Older people are more likely to be bitten on the hand.

Bite Wounds
Of the injuries for which medical attention is sought, it is estimated that between 4% to 20% of dog bite wounds and 20% to 50% of cat bite wounds become clinically infected.[151] Clinical infections usually occur within 8 to 24 hours after injury. Dog bite injuries may result in significantly more functional impairments, although cat bite wounds have a greater risk of developing a progressive infection.[96] The small incisors of cats cause deep punctures that can penetrate underlying bones, connective and muscle tissues, and joints. Most bite infections are minor; however, at least 10% require suturing, and between 1% and 5% result in hospitalization.[163]

The infecting organism in bite or scratch injuries usually corresponds to the normal oral microflora of dogs and cats (Table 53-3; compare with Table 89-1), although organisms from the environment or skin around the injury may also contaminate the wound. Bite wounds are usually polymicrobial, with a median of five isolates per wound comprising three aerobes and two anaerobes.[42,151,152] Although greater than 80% of cultures produce pathogens, only 15% to 20% of bite wounds become clinically infected.[61] The risk of infection is highest (approximately 40%) for crush injuries, puncture wounds, wounds in areas of preexisting edema, and hand wounds.[60] Despite the numerous aerobic and anaerobic organisms that contaminate bite wounds, only a few such as *Pasteurella multocida*, Eugonic fermenter-4a (EF-4a), and *Capnocytophaga canimorsus* consistently cause systemic manifestations. In the past the role of strictly anaerobic bacteria in bite wounds has been overshadowed by such notorious genera

as *Pasteurella*. However, with modern methods of anaerobic cultivation, the role of these bacteria in bite wounds has been realized. When present, anaerobic bacteria are usually isolated in mixed cultures. *Fusobacterium* species, *Bacteroides* species, *Porphyromonas* species, *Prevotella* species, and other anaerobic gram-negative bacilli are often involved.[4,91] *Erysipelothrix rhusiopathiae* has been isolated from dog and cat bites.[1,151] An unusual form of motor neuron disease suspected to be caused by a virus occurred after a cat bite.[80]

The public health aspects of rabies, tetanus, and bartonellosis are discussed in Chapters 22, 43, and 54, respectively. People who have been bitten may have to be hospitalized if they develop significant local or systemic infections; are unresponsive to oral antibiotics; have penetrating wounds of tendons, joints, or the central nervous system (CNS); have open fractures; have significant blood loss or airway injuries; require reconstructive surgeries; require wound elevation; have head or hand injuries; or are immunocompromised.[163]

Bacteria Relatively Unique to Dog and Cat Bites
Bite wounds caused by dogs and cats may contain some unique bacteria that have not been previously identified in people. Although some such as *Pasteurella* organisms are commonly found in animal bite wounds, others such as *Riemerella anatipetifer* in the cat mouth and *Bacteroides tectum*, which is found in cat and dog bites, are unique to these animals. *Eikenella corrodens*, a pathogen often found in wounds caused by human bites, has been reported once each as a result of a dog bite and a cat bite.[151] Unfortunately, some of the unusual isolates may not be responsive to conventionally used antibacterials.

Pasteurella *Pasteurella* organisms are small, nonmotile, gram-negative, bipolar-staining bacilli that are clinically significant in many dog- and cat-bite wounds. These organisms normally inhabit the nasal, gingival, and tonsillar regions of approximately 12% to 92% of dogs and 52% to 99% of cats, as well as many other animals. *Pasteurella* species have been reclassified based on their DNA homology. *P. multocida* ssp. *multocida* and ssp. *septica* have been the most common isolates from clinically healthy cats, whereas *Pasteurella canis* has not been frequently isolated from healthy dogs.[20,108] This same distribution is found with bite-associated infections. Strains isolated from cats were more commonly pathogenic (71%) than those from dogs (8%). *P. multocida* ssp. *multocida* and ssp. *septica* have been isolated in more serious or systemic infections caused by biting or licking of wounds by dogs or cats.[76,121] The frequency of isolation is as follows: in cat wounds, *P. multocida* is 50% and *P. septica* is 30%; in dog bite wounds, *P. canis* is 27%, *P. multocida* is 13%, and *Pasteurella septica* is 13% (see Table 53-3).[62] Isolation of *Pasteurella dagmatis* is rare.[38] Although many cats and dogs harbor *Pasteurella* organisms in their saliva, the risk of infection in people is low if they have not been bitten.[138]

Although dog bites account for more than 80% of emergency room visits related to animal bites, cats are responsible for approximately 75% of bites or scratches contaminated with *Pasteurella*. More than 50% of all cat-bite wounds and 20% to 30% of all dog-bite wounds are contaminated with *Pasteurella*.[96] *Pasteurella* infections also have been reported after bite injuries caused by large exotic Felidae. Scratch injuries from dogs are less likely to cause *Pasteurella* infections than cat scratches, unless the scratch is also associated with a bite injury.[105] Cats frequently lick their paws and usually hiss when they scratch, thereby producing aerosolized secretions that contaminate the wounds, which is probably related to the higher incidence of *Pasteurella*-infected scratches. A person who was licked daily on her hands by her dog devel-

Table • 53-3

Organisms Isolated from Infected Human Wounds Caused by Dog or Cat Bites or Scratches

ORGANISM	REPORTED% OF ISOLATES[a]		ORGANISM (CONTINUED)	REPORTED% OF ISOLATES[b]	
	DOG	CAT		DOG	CAT
VIRUSES			Gram-Negative Aerobes (Chapter 37)		
Rabies virus (Chapter 22)	NA	NA	*Brevibacterium*	6	4
Motor paralysis agent	NR	R	*Gemella morbillorus*	6	4
BACTERIA			*Lactobacillus*	4	2
Gram-Negative Aerobes			*Stenotrophomonas maltophila*	4	NR
Yersina pestis (Chapter 47)	NR	NA	*Riemerella anatipestifer*	5	4
Francisella tularensis (Chapter 48)	R	R	*Aeromonas hydrophila*	NR	2
Bartonella henselae (Chapter 56)	NR	NA	**Gram-Positive Aerobes** (Chapter 35)		
Pasteurella spp.[b]	25—54	50—78	*Enterococcus*[f]	4—9	NR
Eugonic Fermenter 4b (EF 4b)	10	16	*Streptococcus* spp.[g]	40—46	46—52
Pseudomonas spp.[c]	6—8	5	*Staphylococcus* (coagulase-positive)	23—36	33
Actinobacillus actinomycetemcomitans	6	NR	*Staphylococcus epidermidis*	19	7—70
Capnocytophaga canimorsus (DF-2)	NA	NA	*Corynebacterium* spp.[i]	8—20	11—28
Capnocytophaga cynodegmi (DF-2-like)	NA	NA	*Micrococcus* spp.	6	NR
Flavimonas oryzihabitans (VE-2)	2—4	2	Diphtheroids	4	25
Bergeyella (Weeksella) zoohelcum (CDC IIj)	4	7	*Bacillus* spp.[j]	4	NR
Neisseria weaveri (formerly CDC M-5)	5	11	*Nocardia* (Chapter 49)	R	R
Neisseria spp.[d]	2	11—25	*Rhodococcus* (Chapter 35)	NR	2
Brucella suis	NA	NR	*Erysipelothrix rhusiopathiae*	R	R
Acinetobacter lwoffi and *Acinetobacter baumannii*	NR	7—1	**Anaerobes**		
Moraxella spp.[e]	NA	22	*Porphyromonas*[k]	32	22
Hemophilus aphrophilus	4	NR	*Prevotella*[l]	23—28	22
Streptobacillus moniliformis	R	NR	*Propionibacterium* spp.[m]	18—21	NR
Chromobacterium	2	NR	*Bacteroides* spp.[n]	11—32	22
Flavobacterium spp.	4	NR	*Eubacterium* spp.	4—11	2
Eikenella corrodens	2	2	*Fusobacterium* spp.[o]	5—36	30—33
Escherichia coli	2—6	NR	*Peptostreptococcus* spp.[p]	5—18	5—16
Spirillum minor	NR	R	*Clostridium* spp.	5	11
Proteus mirabilis	2—4	NR	*Clostridium tetani* (Chapter 43)	R	R
Enterobacter cloacae	R	11	*Leptotrichia buccalis*	5	NR
Klebsiella	2—4	2	*Veillonella*	5	2
Nonoxidizer-1 (NO-1)	2	R	*Actinomyces* (Chapter 49)[q]	R	NR
Eugonic Fermenter 4a (EF-4a)	6	R	*Filifactor villosus*	NR	5
M-5 (*Moraxella*-like)	R	R	**FUNGI**		
Citrobacter spp.	4	NR	*Blastomyces dermatitidis* (Chapter 59)	R	NR
Mycobacterium fortuitum (Chapter 50)	R	R			

Table notes on following page

Notes to Table 53-3

D, Dog; *C*, cat; *NA*, not available and may vary based on geographic location; *R*, rare or isolated reports; *NR*, not reported.
Data from Talan DA, Citron DM, Abrahamian FM, et al. 1999. Bacteriologic analysis of infected dog and cat bites. *N Eng J Med* 340:85–92; Talan D, Goldstein EJC. 1996. Emergency Medicine Animal Bite Infection Study Group. *Bacteriology of infected dog and cat bite wounds.* Society for Academic Emergency Medicine, Denver; Greene CE, Lockwood R, Goldstein EJC. 1990. Bite infections, pp 330–337. In *Infectious diseases of the dog and cat.* WB Saunders, Philadelphia, Pa; Citron DM, et al. 1996. *Clin Infect Dis* 23(Suppl)S78–S82.

[a]Percentages are based on isolates of wounds for which patients sought medical attention and are listed in order of relative frequency of isolation. For breakdown of specific genera, see respective footnotes, in which percentage is listed for individual dog or cat isolates.

[b]*P. multocida* subsp. *multocida* C: 52%, D: 14%; *P. multocida* subsp. *septica* C: 30%, D: 14%; *P. dagmatis* C: 4%, D: 5%; *P. stomatis* C: 4%; *P. canis* D: 27%; *P. multocida* subsp. *gallicida* D: 5%; *P. pneumotropica* D: 5%; *P. stomatis* D: 5%.

[c]*P. aeruginosa* D: 2%; *P. vesicularis* C: 2%, D: 2%; *P. diminuta* D: 2%; *P. putida* C: 2%; *P. stutzeri* C: 2%.

[d]*N. subflava* C: 2%, D: 2%; *N. cinera-flavescens* C: 2%; *N. mucosa* C: 2%.

[e]*M. catarrhalis* C: 11%; *M. osloensis* C: 11%; *M. atlantae* C: 7%; *M. nonliquefaciens* C: 4%.

[f]*E. faecalis* C: 4%, D: 6%; *E. avium* D: 2%; *E. malodoratus* D: 2%; *E. durans* C: 9%.

[g]*S. mitis* C: 23%-33%, D: 22%-36%; *S. sanguis II* C: 19%, D: 18%; *S. equinus* C: 11%, D: 5%; *S. pyogenes* C: 6%-9%; *S. constellatus* C: 4%, D: 4%; *S. mutans* C: 4%-11%, D: 4%-12%; *S. agalactiae* C: 4%, D: 2%; *S. sanguis* C: 4%, D: 2%, D: –5%; *S. sanguis I* C: 4%, D: 2%; *S. sanguis II* C: 12%, D: 8%; *S. intermedius* C: 4%, D: 6%; *S. dysgalactiae* D: 1%.

[h]*S. epidermidis* C: 7%, D: 23%; *S. wameri* C: 7%, D: 5%; *S. aureus* C: 4%, D: 14%; *S. cohnii* D: 5%; *S. intermedius* C: 4%, D: 9%; *S. coagulase* neg D: 5%; *S. xylosus* D: 4.5%; *S. haemolyticus* C: 4%; *S. hominis* C: 4%, D: 1%; *S. hyicus* C: 4%; *S. sciuri/lentus* C: 4%; *S. simulans* C: 4%; *S. auricularis* D: 1%; *S. capitis* C: 2%; *S. saprophyticus* C: 2%.

[i]*Corynebacterium* Group G C: 5%, D: 6%; *C. minutissimum* C: 7%, D: 4%; *C. aquaticum* C: 14%, D: 2%; *C. jeikeium* C: 2%, D: 1%; *C. afermentans,* Group E, and *C. pseudodiphtheriticum,* all D: 2%; Group B, Group F-1, *C. kutscheri, C. propinquum,* and *C. striatum,* all C: 2%.

[j]*B. firmus* C: 4%, D: 4%; *B. circulans* C: 2%, D: 2%; *B. subtilis* D: 2%.

[k]*P. macacae* C: 7%, D: 6%; *P. gingivalis* C: 7%, D: 9%; *P. cangingivalis* C: 4%, D: 5%; *P. canoris* C: 9%, D: 4%; *P. salivosa* C: 4%, D: 4%; *P. circumdentaria* C: 5%, D: 2%; *Porphyromonas* spp. D: 5%; *P. cansulci* C: rare, D: 6%; *P. levii*-like D: 2%; *P. cangingivalis* C: 4%, D: 4%.

[l]*P. bivia* C: 11%; *P. heparinolytica* C: 9%, D: 14%; *P. intermedia/nigrescens* D: 5%; *P. melaninogenica* C: 2%, D: 5%; *Prevotella* spp. C: 8%; *P. zoogleoformans* C: 2%, D: 4%; *P. denticola* D: 2%.

[m]*P. acnes* C: 16%, D: 14%; *P. acidi/propionicus* D: 2%; *P. avidum* C: 2%; *P. lymphophilium* C: 2%.

[n]*B. tectum* C: 28%, D: 14%; *B. forsythus* D: 4%; *B. ureolyticus* D: 9%; *B. gracilis* D: 5%; *B. fragilis* C: 2%, D: 5%; *B. ovatus* D: 2%.

[o]*F. nucleatum* C: 26%, D: 18%; *F. russii* C: 15%, D: 5%; *F. gonidiaformans* C: 4%, D: 5%; *F. alocis* D: 2%.

[p] *Peptostreptococcus* spp. C: 5%, D: 8%; *P. asaccharolyticus* D: 2%.

[q]*A. viscosus* C: 2%, D: 4%; *A. neuii* subsp. *anitratus* D: 2%.

oped a *Pasteurella* throat abscess after tonsillectomy.[76] *Pasteurella* meningitis developed in a person with extensive dental caries who regularly kissed the family dog. *Pasteurella* has been isolated from the oral cavity of some people who have kissed their dogs and cats but not from those who have not.[11,12] *Pasteurella* acquired from pets may also cause various upper respiratory tract infections, including tonsillitis,[171] sinusitis,[13,116] and epiglottiditis.[139] Submandibular cellulitis (Ludwig's angina) developed in a previously healthy person 10 days after playing with a dog.[44] *Pasteurella* peritonitis developed in dialysis patients after a cat scratch or bite that penetrated the tubing of their home dialysis machines.[98] Nontraumatic domestic cat exposure has also been associated with *Pasteurella* peritonitis in people with hepatic cirrhosis.[89] Joint arthroplasties have become infected with *P. multocida* when people have been bitten by cats.[23,52]

Most *Pasteurella* infections occur in people who have frequent contact with farm or pet animals. Presumably, bites in people in urban environments are related to dog, cat, or other small animal or rodent exposure.

Although a majority of human *P. multocida* infections are related to animal bites, people also may develop pasteurellosis from general animal exposure. In most of these cases, licking of the human's intact or injured skin by the pet and inhalation or ingestion of animal secretions are the most likely sources of entry. Infections associated with inhaled or disseminated microorganisms frequently localize in the gastrointestinal or respiratory tracts or CNS. Patients who are immunosuppressed or have a predisposing underlying illness such as diabetes mellitus and hepatic dysfunction are more likely to develop bacteremia and die. Meningitis has been reported in infants and children who have been licked in the face by family dogs.[156] Even neonatal puppies may be susceptible to certain virulent strains of *Pasteurella,* presumably acquired from the oral cavity of their dam. A virulent strain of *P. canis* biotype 1 was determined to be the cause of mortality in neonatal puppies with multisystemic infection.[41]

Bergeyella (Weeksella) zoohelcum *Bergeyella (Weeksella) zoohelcum,* a gram-negative bacillus previously classified as CDC IIj, is a component of the normal oral flora of dogs, cats, and other animals. Few instances have been reported of infection in people caused by a bite wound from dogs or cats.[109,151] Abscesses, tenosynovitis, meningitis, and pneumonia have occurred. The organism is susceptible to β-lactam antibiotics, quinolones, and chloramphenicol.

Eugonic Fermenter-4 EF-4 are unclassified bacteria that are resident oropharyngeal and nasal microflora of dogs and cats. Isolation rates vary, with 30% to 90% of clinically healthy animals having these bacteria.[54] EF-4 bacteria are more prevalent than *Pasteurella* in the oropharynx of dogs. They can cause severe illness in immunocompromised people or when inoculated into deep bite puncture wounds. EF-4 bacteria have been divided by biochemical features into two biovars, EF-4a and EF-4b, which have different pathogenic potentials.[6] EF-4a has been isolated from infected dog bite wounds in people and has been associated with deeper or systemic infections in people. In contrast, EF-4b has been found in wounds caused by bites from dogs and cats.[151] EF-4b has also been the predominant isolate associated with virulent pneumonia in dogs and cats (see Respiratory Infections, Chapter 88).

Capnocytophaga *Capnocytophaga* species are capnophilic (carbon dioxide-flourishing), gram-negative, gliding bacteria that are closely related to *Fusobacterium* and *Bacteroides* species. They are commonly isolated from the oral cavity of people and animals. The organisms are divided into two main groups: (1) species from the human oral cavity (*Capnocytophaga ochracea, Capnocytophaga gingivalis,* and *Capnocytophaga sputigena*—previously Centers for Disease Control (CDC) biogroup dysgonic fermenter-1 [DF-1]) and (2) species found in the oral cavity of dogs, cats, and other animals (*C. canimorsus* and *Capnocytophaga cynodegmi*—previously CDC biogroup DF-2). In immunocompetent hosts, *Capnocytophaga* can produce various infections including in the respiratory tract, wounds, bone, and abdomen. In immunocompromised hosts, fatal bacterial sepsis can result. *C. canimorsus* is a slow-growing (3 to 11 days in culture), thin, filamentous, non–spore-forming, nonmotile, pleomorphic, facultative aerobic, gram-negative bacillus. It has been associated with fatal septicemia in people, predominantly after dog bites and less commonly after cat bites or scratches.[102,160] It has been isolated from the oral cavity of 16% and 18% of clinically healthy dogs and cats, respectively.[163] Many cases with a 30% mortality rate have been reported in the literature. *C. canimorsus* has an unusual propensity to cause systemic bacteremia, presumably because of its tropism for endothelial surfaces and its inherent resistance to serum complement. The majority of *C. canimorsus* infections have occurred in immunocompromised individuals older than 40 years. A veterinarian who had undergone a splenectomy died from an illness after a dog bite. Most people who develop fatal complications of *C. canimorsus* infection have underlying contributing factors, such as cytotoxic chemotherapy–induced or surgical splenectomy, glucocorticoid therapy, Hodgkin's disease, macroglobulinemia, alcoholism, peptic ulcer, arteriosclerotic heart disease, hemoglobinopathy, immune-mediated thrombocytopenia, granulomatous or other chronic lung disease, chronic arthritis, macroglobulinemia, neutropenia, intestinal malabsorption, or old age (older than 65 years). Presumably, the factors caused defects in the phagocytic immune defenses, and the individuals could not eliminate the organism from the blood. As with pasteurellosis, some patients with *C. canimorsus* sepsis have been exposed to dogs, cats, or other carnivores or to outdoor environments but had no known bites.

Ocular keratitis and blepharitis have developed in people who were closely associated with their pet dogs or cats but have also developed in other people with no known animal exposure. Corneal scratch injuries from cats have also produced keratitis in people. Results from DNA hybridization and biochemical studies have shown that the more virulent species isolated from people with septicemia were *C. canimorsus*, and those from localized (noninvasive) wound infections or keratitis were *C. cynodegmi* (DF-2-like). Other *Capnocytophaga* species are part of the normal gingival flora of people and cause problems such as conjunctivitis, periodontitis, gingivitis, abscesses, and body cavity infections.[46] In addition, they can cause bacteremia in immunocompromised individuals.[63] Infections with these other *Capnocytophaga* are not associated with animal exposure.

Nonoxidizer-1 The nonoxidizer-1 group of bacteria (CDC NO-1) comprises isolates of an unusual bacterium that has been only recovered from people bitten by dogs (77%), cats (18%), and other animals (5%).[84] The bites were on various parts of the body. Isolates have been described as fastidious, gram-negative pleomorphic rods. The organisms are similar to asaccharolytic strains of *Acinetobacter*. Numerous other bacteria can be isolated from infected wounds; however, isolation of these bacteria appears to be unique to animal bites. Dogs and cats should be considered reservoirs for these bacteria.

Epidemiology of Bitten Dogs and Cats

The incidence of bite wounds in dogs and cats has not been well established; however, estimates are that they comprise approximately 10% and 15% of trauma-related emergencies for dogs and cats, respectively.[90] As with humans who are bitten, many incidents likely go unreported, and owners do not seek immediate veterinary attention. Dogs can cause puncture wounds, but their strong jaws also tear, lacerate, crush, and avulse bones and soft tissues. Cats with small, thin teeth often produce piercing injuries of deeper tissues. Although open wounds have more immediate tissue injuries,

those from deep punctures are more likely to result in deep infections and abscesses with secondary damage.

In one study a majority of dogs bitten were intact males.[146] Bitten dogs often weigh less than the overall population of dogs and have a median weight of 20 kg. Dog bites peak in the warmer months of the year, a similar finding with cat bites (Table 53-4). Small dogs are more likely than large dogs to have thoracic and back lesions (Fig. 53-1). In medium-weight dogs the most common bite sites are the neck, back, and extremities. They have a higher prevalence of back and perineal injuries than small dogs. In large dogs the head and extremities are the most commonly involved sites. Penetrating wounds have been seen in 31% of thoracic bites and 79% of abdominal wounds.[146]

Clinical Findings
People
The types of injuries caused by dogs biting humans vary and include abrasions, punctures, avulsions, and lacerations. Dog bites cause severe crushing injuries and lacerations with ligamentous tearing and tissue necrosis. A majority of lesions in adults are primarily on the upper extremities and trunk (Figs. 53-2 and 53-3). Young children generally have facial injuries because of their small stature and lack of experience with dogs and because dogs tend to bite the face and mouth when being aggressive. In comparison, dogs biting other dogs most commonly injure the extremities followed by the head, neck, thorax, and abdomen (Fig. 53-4; see Table 53-1).[35]

Cat bites are deep, and the sharp teeth are more likely than dog teeth to produce wounds that become foci for abscess formation and resultant complications such as sepsis, meningitis, endocarditis, septic arthritis, or osteomyelitis. Cat scratches frequently occur on the handler's arms and hands and usually are associated with attempts to restrain the animal (see Table 53-1). Scratches can become colonized by the same organisms as bites. (See Bartonellosis, Chapter 54, for a discussion of cat scratch disease.)

Signs indicating wound infection include localized swelling or reddening and pain with or without a purulent drainage. The type of organism causing infection and the bite site are the most important factors in determining the clinical course of the injury. The two most clinically significant organisms are *C. canimorsus* and *Pasteurella* species.

Pasteurella *Infections* Almost two thirds of infections with *Pasteurella* in people are cutaneous and often caused by bites or licking of wounds or damaged mucous membranes by animals.[45] Systemic spread or penetration of deeper tissues has caused respiratory infections, septicemia, and urogenital and intraabdominal infections. Bite infections caused by *Pasteurella* organisms are more progressive than those produced by many other bacteria. The time from bite until onset of infection has been 12.3 hours, 15 hours, and 24 hours for streptococci, *Pasteurella* species, and staphylococci, respectively.[152] Usually within 8 to 48 hours, cellulitis develops at the site of injury with *Pasteurella* species infections. Erythema, tenderness, and swelling occur in association with a serosanguineous to purulent, malodorous, dark yellow discharge. Lymphadenomegaly and low-grade fever (less than 38° C [100.5° F]) develop in some patients. Cellulitis can lead to extensive infection of deeper tissues or potentially fatal septicemia. Septicemia is characterized by persistent chills, fever, and collapse. Chronic osteomyelitis, septic or posttraumatic arthritis, tenosynovitis, meningitis, and smoldering abscesses also can develop.[94]

Eugonic Fermenter-4 Infections As with *Pasteurella* species, EF-4 organisms have been associated with cutaneous, systemic, respiratory, and intraabdominal infections in people.

Table • 53-4

Characteristics of Bitten Dogs and Cats

PARAMETER	DOGS[a] (n = 004 185)	CATS[a] (n = 11)
Median age (range)	4 yr (2–7)	1 yr (0.2–9)
Weight	61% small[b] 16% medium 24% large[c]	NR
Sex	71% male; 99% intact[b] 29% female; 58% intact[b]	55% male; 67% intact 45% female; 100% intact
Peak times	April (14%), March (11%), and September (11%)	April (14%), March (11%), and September (11%)
Most prevalent breeds	37% mixed breeds 27% pinschers[b] 5% terriers[b] 5% Pekingese[b] 4% German shepherds	82% domestic 9% Persians 9% Siamese
Peak time of hospital arrival	6–10 PM (43%)	6–10 PM (43%)
Time interval until arrival	Mean <3 hr (55%); median 2 hr (0.3–96 hr)	Mean <3 hr (55%); median 2 hr (0.3–96 hr)
Number of injured sites	Small: one, 42%; multiple, 58% Medium: one, 25%; multiple, 75% Large: one, 62%; multiple, 38%	NR
Location of injuries (totals for all breeds)	35% thorax 35% extremities 31% head 31% back 28% neck 24% abdomen 19% pelvic limbs 12% thoracic limbs 8% perineum 3% tail	46% back 36% thorax 27% abdomen 27% extremities 18% neck 18% perineum 18% pelvic limbs 9% head 9% thoracic limbs 0% tail

Data from Shamir MH, Leisner S, Klement E, et al. 2002. Dog bite wounds in dogs and cats: a retrospective study of 196 cases, *J Vet Med A Physiol Clin Med* 49:107–112.
[a]NR, Not reported. For dogs: small, ≤10 kg; medium, 11–20 kg; large, >20 kg.
[b]Significantly higher than hospital population.
[c]Significantly lower than hospital population.

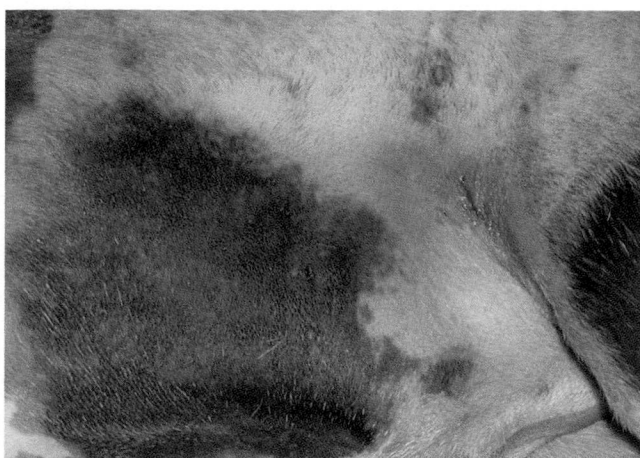

Fig 53-1 Bite wound to abdominal wall with puncture entering underlying abdominal cavity. (Courtesy University of Georgia, Athens, Ga.)

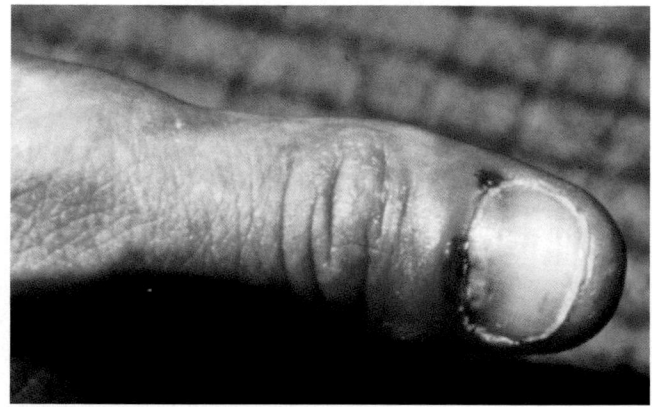

Fig 53-2 Bite wound to thumb showing discoloration. (Courtesy University of Georgia, Athens, Ga.)

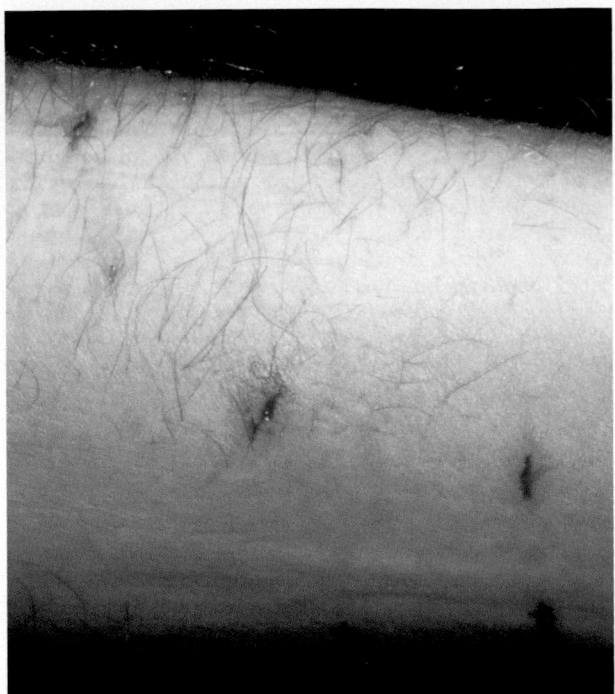

Fig 53-3 Bite wound to forearm. (Courtesy University of Georgia, Athens, Ga.)

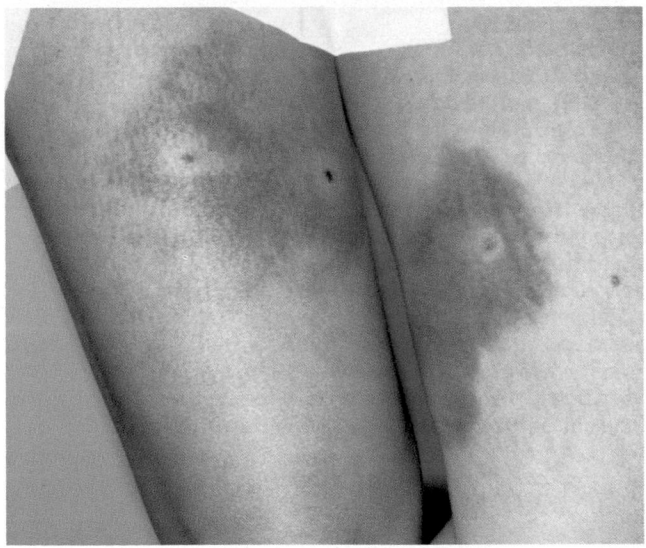

Fig 53-4 Bite wound to thighs. (Courtesy University of Georgia, Athens, Ga.)

Their presence in a human infection is generally correlated with close aerosol, salivary, or bite contact with dogs or cats. Otitis externa and media developed in a man whose dogs frequently licked his ears.[137]

Capnocytophaga Infections Although inconsistent, cellulitis is the most common finding associated with bite wounds contaminated by *C. canimorsus* and *C. cynodegmi*. Bite infections caused by *Eubacterium plautii* can appear to be similar to those of *C. canimorsus*.[56] In some cases, eschariform lesions, characterized by formation of purplish-black necrotic tissue around the bite site, are seen. Patients who have undergone splenectomy or are immunosuppressed, including those with older age or cirrhosis, develop the most severe illness from septicemia, which is characterized by fever, malaise,

myalgia, vomiting, diarrhea, abdominal pain, dyspnea, hypotension, thrombocytopenia with purpura, symmetric peripheral gangrene, oliguria, disseminated intravascular coagulopathy, and death.[126] The fatality rate has been higher than 25%, and acute myocardial infarction has been reported in some people. Regardless of the clinical spectrum, most patients have continuous bacteremia. Localization of the septic process without death can occur, and some people develop endocarditis, purulent meningitis, and polyarthritis. The organisms may not be demonstrated on microscopic examination of tissues, although they may be found in blood films of some patients with severe bacteremia and in blood culture.

Capnocytophaga isolates may be detected within 72 hours in culture, but 7 to 10 days is typical. Growth is enhanced in the presence of carbon dioxide and with serum-enriched media. The laboratory should be advised when *Capnocytophaga* is suspected so that specific tests can be performed to detect these unusual gram-negative organisms. Because identification of the organisms takes a relatively long time, antimicrobial therapy must be instituted immediately without definitive identification.

Nonoxidizer-1 Infections Infections caused by NO-1 appear to be local and result in abscesses or cellulitis. Purulent drainage, hyperesthesia, erythema, and swelling are characteristic. In rare situations, sepsis can develop with fever and chills; however, patients from which this organism has been isolated did not have identified preexisting immunodeficiencies.

Dogs and Cats
In the mobile, elastic skin of dogs and cats, bite injuries may be less noticeable or may migrate through deeper tissues and go undetected, whereas animal bite wounds in people are more apparent. As in dog or cat bite injuries of people, the organisms inoculated into dog and cat tissues after bites are the inhabitants of the oral flora. Bacteria come from the local environment, skin surfaces, and the oral cavity. Infections are often mixed and include a combination of aerobic and anaerobic bacteria. Infections may dissect along tissue planes and into deeper body cavities or visceral organs. Many of these subsequent infections may be delayed and go unrecognized until signs of systemic infection are observed. (See Chapter 52 for a discussion of feline abscesses.)

Bite wounds are considered contaminated as soon as they occur. Organisms inoculated into damaged tissue are likely to proliferate and produce considerable infection. Aerobic bacterial flora are the predominant isolates from canine and feline bite wounds (Table 53-5); however, this is likely a result of inferior techniques in collection and processing of specimens and the additional cost associated with anaerobic culture in clinical practice. Studies that have used fastidious collection and processing of anaerobic specimens have resulted in higher yields.

Management and Therapy
Animal Bites in Dogs and Cats
Transport and Evaluation When possible, owners should be advised on transportation procedures for bitten animals. Hemorrhage from wounds should be controlled with gentle pressure applied to affected wounds using a clean, lint-free, dry compress (Table 53-6). The animal should be strapped to a large, flat board or wrapped in bedding. Internal injuries are impossible to assess immediately, so it is much better for an initial physical examination to be performed as a baseline evaluation. Bitten animals are often in severe pain, so they should be muzzled during transport. The owner should be advised to bring vaccination documents to the clinic. At that time,

Table • 53-5

Organisms Isolated from Dog and Cat Bite Wounds

ORGANISMS	FREQUENCY OF ISOLATION	
	Dog[a]	Cat[b]
VIRUSES		
Rabies	U	U
Feline Foamy (Syncytium forming) Virus	ND	U
Feline Immunodeficiency Virus	ND	U
MYCOPLASMA		
Mycoplasma spp.	U	C
BACTERIA		
Gram-negative Aerobes		
Pasteurella multocida	5	13–27
Escherichia coli	13–18	0.6
Pseudomonas aeruginosa	5	ND
Serratia marscens	3	ND
Proteus spp	3	ND
Enterobacter	3	ND
Acinetobacter spp	3	ND
Gram-positive Aerobes		
Staphylococcus intermedius (see Chapter 36)	20–23	14
Enterococcus spp. (see Chapter 35)	15	12
Staphylococcus (coagulase negative)(see Chapter 36)	13	ND
Streptococcus (alpha) (see Chapter 35)	7	4–13
Actinomyces spp (see Chapter 49)		7–18
Corynebacterium	3	ND
Anaerobes (See Chapter 41)		
Porphyromonas		26–76
Bacillus	7	ND
Clostridium	7	6.5
Bacteroides	ND	ND
Peptostreptococcus	ND	11–45
Fusobacterium	ND	17–64
Proprionibacterium	ND	ND
FUNGI	ND	ND
PROTOZOA		
Babesia gibsoni? (see Chapter 77)	ND	ND

U, = Uncommon or less common; N, no data; C, common or frequent.
[a]Data compiled from references 67, 39, 152, 32, 86. (These wounds were caused by dogs biting dogs.)
[b]Data from references cited in Table 52–3. (These wounds were caused by cats biting cats.)

obtaining a more complete history of the bite incident will help determine whether the animal needs rabies prophylaxis or special precautions should be taken while handling and observing the bitten patient (see Rabies, Chapter 22, and Compendium, Appendix 4). Refer to these sources for specific guidelines as published by the American Association of State Public Health Veterinarians and the Centers for Disease Control and Prevention.

Diagnostic Procedures Assessing the animal's vital signs, such as body temperature, pulse, and respiration rate, and performing a general systems evaluation are paramount for stabilizing the traumatized patient. Hypotension from shock, infection, or hypovolemia should be managed with IV fluids; antibiotics and short-term glucocorticoids may be necessary. Physical examination of the site determines the extent of injury to nerves, tendons, or bones. The need for cosmetic repair must be gauged immediately to reduce the amount of

scar tissue in the final healing. Chemical restraint or local lidocaine infusion may been needed to better assess and probe the wound. Injuries can include punctures, lacerations, and crush or avulsion injuries. Injuries to nerves, tendons, ligaments, or bones should be evaluated by checking for sensation, mobility, and palpable swellings. A diagram or photograph of the injury may be valuable. A radiograph may detect underlying bony injuries or the presence of a foreign body such as a tooth and can serve as a baseline for evaluation of potential osteomyelitis in the future.

Cultures and Gram stains are helpful if signs of local drainage or regional lymphadenomegaly are present. Signs of infection are usually apparent beginning 12 to 24 hours after the injury. For cultures, areas around the wounds should be clipped with a number 40 clipper blade followed by cleansing with chlorhexidine and the procedure outlined in Table 53-6. Culture swabs are satisfactory for open wounds, whereas tissue aspiration is best for deep puncture wounds.

Table • 53-6

Evaluation and Care of Bite Wounds: Tips for Veterinarians

Dog or Cat Bitten by Animal
Obtain animal information
  History of injury
    1. Identify species of biting animal. If wildlife species, obtain biting animal or its body or head if possible.[a]
    2. Note time bite occurred.
    3. Note behavior of biting animal or provocation causing bite.

  Physical examination of injuries
    1. Measure and classify depth, tissue damage, and risk for cosmetic damage and infection.
    2. Determine range of motion and extent of muscle and tendon swelling.
    3. Perform neural exam for sensory function and motor response.
    4. Evaluate circulation by assessing warmth and color.

Diagnostic measures
1. Obtain baseline radiographs if injury is over bone.
2. Obtain cultures of wounds (optional).
    a. Aerobic: culturettes with transport media[b]
    b. Anaerobic: culturettes with reducing media[c]
3. Cytologic or Gram stain evaluation of exudates is essential.
4. Perform complete blood count or chemistry panel if anesthesia is warranted.
5. Provide rabies booster (see Chapter 22 and Appendix 4).

Treatment
1. Clip the hair away with a #40 clipper blade.
2. Cleanse with antiseptic scrub to skin edges surrounding wound.
    a. Chlorhexidine[d]
    b. Povidone-iodine[e]
3. Flush wound with copious amounts of soap and water, saline, or both.
    a. 18-gauge needle or tubing on 35–50 cc syringe or fluid bag
    b. Lavage: 8 psi to facilitate bacterial cleansing
    c. Isotonic warm Ringer's or saline solution
    d. Disinfectant solution of chlorhexidine[d] or povidone-iodine[e]
4. Prepare wound with surgical debridement of devitalized structures.
5. Close wound only under special circumstances (see text).
6. Cover wound with bandage or sterile water-based ointment.
7. Give antimicrobial therapy (prophylactic if indicated by depth or severity).
8. Immobilize and elevate wound.
9. Provide staged debridement with periodic application and removal of adherent bandages.

Human Bitten by Dog or Cat
Obtain animal information
  History of injury
    1. Note whether the attack was provoked.
    2. Identify precipitating events.
    3. Note time bite occurred.

  Information about biting animal's health
    1. Evaluate immunization status of animal, especially for rabies (see Chapter 22 and Appendix 4).
    2. Note recent or present illnesses.
Confinement and observation of animal
Notification of public health officials

Immediate first-aid measures for bitten person
1. Cleanse wound with copious amounts of soap and water.
2. Immobilize and elevate wound.
3. Insist person seek immediate medical attention.

[a]Be cautious; wild animals or stray dogs may be rabid (see Chapter 22).
[b]Culturette: Becton Dickinson Co, Sparks, Md.
[c]BBL Port-A-Cul Envelope: Becton Dickinson Co, Sparks, Md.
[d]Chlorhexidine 2% stock solution: 1 part diluted with 39 parts sterile water or 0.9% sodium chloride solution to final 0.05% concentration. May precipitate within 4 hours but is still effective.
[e]Povidone-iodine 10% stock solution: 1 part diluted with 9 or 19 parts sterile water or isotonic electrolyte solution to final 1% or 0.5% concentration, respectively.

General Management Wounds to the head and neck, including injuries to the esophagus, spinal cord, or cervical and cranial nerves, may damage vital respiratory or vascular structures. Subcutaneous emphysema, pneumomediastinum, esophagitis, esophageal strictures, and pneumothorax may develop. Pneumothorax is unlikely unless the parietal pleura are damaged. Damage to the thoracic cavity may cause a flail chest from broken ribs or intrathoracic hemorrhage or pneumothorax from vessel or airway damage. Continuous pleural suction may be needed to evacuate fluid or air in the chest cavity. Abdominal injuries can result in damaged or necrotic viscera. Exploratory celiotomy may be required after the animal has become stable enough for anesthesia. Complications of celiotomy include peritonitis, diaphragmatic hernia, or abdominal wall hernias. Neurologic injury may result if the axial skeleton or the peripheral nerves are damaged. Fractures and luxations require immediate consideration for decompressive and stabilization surgery, whereas nondisplaced structures should be managed conservatively. As with other compressive spinal cord injuries, pain sensation is the last to disappear and can be used as a prognostic indicator. Meningitis can be caused by penetrating injuries of the subarachnoid space and is more difficult to treat once it becomes established.

Wound Management Wounds must be irrigated with copious quantities of isotonic saline, cleansing agents mixed with isotonic saline, or both. Soap and detergents have antiviral properties and have been shown to provide some local rabies virus prophylaxis. Antibiotic-containing solutions are not physiologic, are frequently irritating, and do not work well on direct contact for short periods (see Table 53-4). For lavage, diluted povidone-iodine solutions can serve as antimicrobials, but in the organic milieu of the wound they are less effective. Chlorhexidine has much better antibacterial activity in this regard and does not interfere with healing.

Any scabs, foreign bodies, or necrotic tissue should be removed during the initial debridement period. Necrotic muscle or fat should be removed cautiously to prevent damage to the remaining blood or nerve supply. Care should be taken to minimize the amount of tissue removed from viable tissue. Conservative removal allows for later evaluation (within 72 hours) to better determine demarcation of viable tissue.

Wounds that are already infected or have been present for longer than 24 hours should be treated as open wounds. Suturing bite wounds is generally not advocated unless the opening is approximated and drains are placed. Facial wounds with a rich blood supply are often closed to prevent scarring, as are extremity wounds that have less underlying tissue in which deep infections can hide. Such closures require close monitoring, and the animal should remain hospitalized or be checked daily.

Whether open or closed, wounds should be bandaged, elevated, and immobilized to prevent swelling and dehiscence. Collars or other restrictive devices are often needed to prevent animals from removing bandages and interfering with wound healing. For extremities, splinting and bandaging is the primary method of immobilization. Bandages protect tissue and absorb drainage from the open wound. Wet dressings may be applied if exudates are thick; however, moist bandages have the propensity to macerate tissue and allow for bacterial overgrowth. Antibiotic- or petrolatum-impregnated gauze prevents bacterial overgrowth or maceration of wounds; however, they may interfere with granulation tissue or epithelial growth within the wound. Contact layers of dressing should be nonadherent if the wound has minimal drainage and active granulation. Adherent and moistened contact layers are indicated if the wound has necrotic areas with viscous drainage. Adsorbent layers in moist dressings are soaked in antiseptic or saline solutions and placed in the wound cavity before dressing with dry layers. For example, calcium alginate, a hydrophilic fiber, has been incorporated into wound dressings. Bandage material on the outer surface of open wounds should always be porous to allow ventilation of the lower layers. Moist bandages are changed several times daily; necrotic tissue is removed, and the wound is dressed and flushed with solutions before rewrapping. In later stages of wound healing, occlusive bandages are used to create a moist environment for granulation and epithelial growth. Hydrogels, hydrocolloids, or polyurethane foams are incorporated into bandages as nonadherent dressings in this phase.

Chemical restraint is often indicated for wound dressings and bandaging. Systemic narcotic analgesics may be used alone or in combination with sedatives or local anesthesia. Local anesthetics may interfere with epithelial growth and should be avoided in later stages of healing.

Drainage is an important component of wound management. Punctures or lacerations that caused injuries below the surface may have to be soaked daily with warm compresses and opened for drainage after seroma or abscess formation occurs. Healing may be by second intention. When dead space remains below the wound surface or drainage is excessive, a passive or an active drainage system must be instituted. Passive drainage relies on capillary action or gravity, whereas active drains rely on constant external suction. Drains should be removed when drainage becomes tenacious and exudative or septic.

Surgical closure of bite wounds is a controversial and complex subject beyond the scope of this chapter. Surgical texts and other reviews should be consulted for a more extensive discussion.[40,77] Primary closure is indicated early if tissues appear vital, infection or contamination is minimal, and dead space can be eliminated. Delayed primary or secondary closure may be indicated within 5 days after the wound occurs, when the wound is actively healing and has minimal exudation. The delay helps prevent scarring that develops from unapposed wound margins. Second-intention healing involves granulation, contraction, and epithelialization to close the entire wound and results in the most scarring; however, it must be used when excessive drainage, tissue loss, or infection within the wound exists.

Antimicrobial Therapy Topical antimicrobial therapy is reserved for wound dressings on the outer skin surfaces. Empirical systemic antimicrobial therapy may be instituted to treat a broad spectrum of organisms, although antimicrobials alone have not been shown to prevent bite wound infections. Bite wounds are always contaminated with various environmental and commensal microflora. Antibiotics should be considered for wounds involving deep punctures or extensive surgical debridement. Animals that are immunocompromised because of various conditions, such as cats with retroviral infections or dogs with ehrlichiosis or infection with another persistent intracellular organism, may require more aggressive antimicrobial therapy. In general, intravenous therapy may be more effective than oral antibiotics in preventing infections associated with bite wounds. More rapid delivery of antibiotic in higher concentrations occurs with parenteral use.

Antibiotic selection should be broad so that it can be effective against most of the anticipated oral microflora of the dog and cat (Table 53-7). The most effective therapy is instituted within the first 3 hours of wounding. Few single agents can effectively treat the broad spectrum of organisms in the oral cavity. Amoxicillin-clavulanate has been the drug of choice during the contamination period, because it has a broad spectrum of efficacy and low toxicity. It acts against most of the organisms in the oral cavity of dogs and cats that can also be cultured from bite wounds.[67] Oral therapy is often used in

Table • 53-7

Recommended Therapy for Bite Infections

DRUG[a]	SPECIES	DOSE[b] (mg/kg)	ROUTE	INTERVAL[c] (HOURS)	ANTIBACTERIAL SPECTRUM
Amoxicillin-clavulanate	D	10–20	PO	8	Most gram-positive and gram-negative aerobes and anaerobes; first-choice drug for most bite wounds
	D	13.75	PO	12	
	C	10–20	PO	12	
Ampicillin (amoxicillin)	B	22	PO	8	Some gram-positive and gram-negative aerobes
	B	11–22	SC, IV	6–8	
Ticarcillin	D	20–50	IV	6–8	Gram-positive and gram-negative aerobes and anaerobes
Cefotaxime	B	15–30	IV, IM, SC	6–8	Sepsis from bite wounds caused by gram-negative aerobes or anaerobes
Doxycycline	D	5	PO, IV	12	Some aerobes and anaerobes; mycoplasmas
Clindamycin	B	5–11	PO	8–12	Gram-positive aerobes and anaerobes
Enrofloxacin[d]	D	5	PO, SC	12–24	Gram-negative aerobes
Difloxacin[d]	D	5–10	PO	24	Gram-negative aerobes
Orbifloxacin[d]	D	2.5–7.5	PO	24	Gram-negative aerobes
Marbofloxacin[d]	D	2–4	PO	24	Gram-negative aerobes
Azithromycin	D	20	PO	24	Gram-positive aerobes; mycoplasmas and mycobacteria
Chloramphenicol	D	25–50	PO, IV, IM, SC	8	Some anaerobes; variable with gram-positive and gram-negative aerobes
Metronidazole	B	10	PO, IV	8	Anaerobes

D, Dog; *C*, cat; *B*, dog and cat; *PO*, by mouth; *SC*, subcutaneous; *IV*, intravenous; *IM*, intramuscular.
[a]See Appendix 8 for additional information on these drugs.
[b]Dose per administration at specified interval.
[c]Treatment should continue for 3–4 days after evidence of infection is no longer apparent.
[d]See text for a list of appropriate combinations to achieve a broader spectrum. Use of only quinolones may predispose wound to necrotizing fasciitis from overgrowth of anaerobes and gram-positive bacteria.

conscious patients or for home treatment, although parenteral therapy often accompanies sedation or anesthesia for wound management and is used to achieve more effective blood levels. Bacteria are often resistant to many penicillins without ß-lactamase inhibitors and first-generation cephalosporins. Second-generation cephalosporins are not as effective as third-generation cephalosporins against anaerobes, although they are often preferred by veterinary surgeons. *Pasteurella* strains are commonly resistant to erythromycin, clindamycin, penicillin, and first-generation cephalosporins. Therefore when treating cat bite infections, these drugs should only be used in combination with other agents. For example, in severe and established wound infections, clindamycin can be combined with a fluoroquinolone or aminoglycoside to counteract a wide array of aerobic and anaerobic bacteria. Similarly, a first- and third-generation cephalosporin combination could be combined to create a similar broad-spectrum treatment. Drugs with an anaerobic spectrum of activity, such as metronidazole, must be given with other drugs that are effective against aerobic bacteria. Prophylactic therapy should continue for 3 to 5 days after infection is no longer apparent unless significant cellulitis is present; this may require longer treatment periods for management. If osteomyelitis is present, therapy often continues for a minimum of 6 weeks. Should the infection already be established at the time of first examination, therapy should also involve surgical drainage. A swab can be taken for culture, and additional material should be examined using a Gram stain to help the clinician choose more effective antibiotics. Therapy is often instituted before getting the results, and then the drug selection is modified based on the report.

Dog and Cat Bites in People

Judging from the discrepancy between the numbers of reported versus estimated bites, not all people who are bitten seek medical attention. In areas where it is required, bites should be reported to public health officials, whose job it is to investigate the incidents and make recommendations concerning the treatment of the person who was bitten and the disposition of the animal. Only a few states have developed formal guidelines for handling animal bites. Individuals who are immunocompromised and have been bitten or scratched should *always* be instructed to seek medical attention immediately. The need for prophylaxis for tetanus, rabies, or potential bacterial complications should be emphasized by medical professionals.

Although not primarily responsible for the treatment of bitten humans, veterinarians should be aware of the proper protocols for medical care (see Table 53-6). As in treating animal bites in dogs and cats, thorough washing of all bite wounds and scratches with soap and water is essential. Soaking in an aqueous organic iodine solution (1% povidone-iodine) may also be beneficial, but it may also irritate tissue and lead to secondary infection caused by contamination with bacteria such as *Pseudomonas* and may delay healing. Surgical scrubbing should not be performed because it is toxic to tissue. It is important that wounds be irrigated with physiologic solutions such as normal saline or lactated Ringer's solution. Intermittent, pulsating, high-pressure irrigation, which streams isotonic fluids directly into the wound, is most effective in dislodging contaminating bacteria. Irrigation is usually performed with an 18- to 20-gauge blunted needle or catheter, a 20- to 50-ml syringe, and approximately 150 ml of solution.[96]

The degree of surgical intervention frequently depends on the site and type of bite. Facial injuries bleed profusely and produce highly visible scarring, so they are routinely sutured. Extremity wounds are less visible and often more contaminated and prone to infection, so they are often treated as open wounds. Puncture wounds with minimal hemorrhage should be irrigated, although some physicians cautiously excise the margins of the wound, leaving it open to drain. Unfortunately, this may create a larger, nonhealing wound. Any wound that becomes infected should be cultured. The affected extremity should be elevated to prevent swelling.

Whether antibiotics prevent infection after bite wounds is controversial. Antimicrobial therapy with penicillin or ampicillin-amoxicillin for 3 to 5 days has been recommended for all penetrating bite injuries, even though studies have questioned routine prophylaxis. This recommendation is based on the fact that most animal bite wound isolates, with the exception of staphylococci, are susceptible to penicillin G. Amoxicillin-clavulanate has also been recommended because of its broader and anaerobic spectrum.[49]

Early initiation of antimicrobial prophylaxis can reduce the severity of infection, but the difference in overall numbers of infections that develop is not statistically significant when empirical prophylaxis is used. Therefore some question the need for routine treatment. When therapy is empirical, drugs with a gram-positive and anaerobic spectrum such as β-lactams are usually effective for this purpose. Therapy is generally used for 3 to 7 days for penetrating wounds. Amoxicillin-clavulanate has been a first-choice therapy; penicillin V is an alternative for less severe injuries. Increasing numbers of reports of β-lactamase–producing strains of organisms such as *Capnocytophaga* species have warranted the use of the penicillins combined with inhibitors such as clavulanate. Doxycycline has been an alternative for patients who are allergic to penicillin. Generally, little need exists for culture of clinically uninfected bite wounds. Because of their polymicrobic nature, clinically infected bite wounds should be cultured. Resistant bacteria must be treated with cephalosporins or penicillinase-resistant antibiotics. Tetracycline is an alternative for patients who are allergic to β-lactam drugs. Use of erythromycin, clindamycin, first-generation cephalosporins, or dicloxacillin is often associated with microbial resistance, especially to *Pasteurella* spp. (For a discussion of therapy of wounds infected with rabies virus, anaerobic bacteria, or *Clostridium tetani*, see Chapters 22, 41, and 43, respectively.)

***Pasteurella* Infections** Penicillin and its analogs such as ampicillin are the single most effective antibiotics for controlling *Pasteurella* infection in adults. Tetracyclines, chloramphenicol, trimethoprim-sulfonamides, quinolones, and second- and third-generation cephalosporins are similarly effective. Bacterial resistance to β-lactamase–resistant penicillins and to cephalosporins has been reported in 18% to 50% of animal isolates. Erythromycin does not control infection, and relapses can occur after its use is discontinued.

***Capnocytophaga* Infections** Many cases of *C. canimorsus* sepsis are fatal in people who are immunocompromised, although some people may completely recover even without antimicrobial therapy. Physicians and veterinarians should realize the potential risk that dog ownership creates for people who are immunocompromised and advise them to seek immediate medical care and antimicrobial treatment after bite injuries. Response to therapy in individuals treated early enough in the course of septicemia has generally been dramatic but not always curative. The organism shows in vitro susceptibility to many antimicrobials, including penicillin, ampicillin, amoxicillin-clavulanate, cephalosporins, tetracycline, carbenicillin, clindamycin, chloramphenicol, erythromycin, imipenem, and quinolone. *C. canimorsus* isolates have been resistant to the typical drugs, such as colistin, gentamicin, and kanamycin, selected to treat gram-negative infections. Susceptibility to trimethoprim-sulfamethoxazole has varied. Penicillin should be used as a first choice. In severely ill people a third-generation cephalosporin has been recommended to be given concurrently with penicillin because penicillin-resistant strains of *Capnocytophaga* and *Pasteurella* have been isolated on occasion.

Nonoxidizer-1 Infection NO-1 bacteria are susceptible to various antibiotics. All strains have been susceptible to aminoglycosides, β-lactams, tetracyclines, quinolones, and sulfonamides.[84] At least 50% of the strains have been resistant to trimethoprim. β-Lactams should be the first choice for treating these infections.

Prevention

Avoiding actions that precipitate aggression in dogs and cats is key in preventing bite injuries (see Table 53-2). Pet owners can avoid selecting breeds or breed mixes with known aggressive tendencies. Male, unneutered, free-roaming dogs of German shepherd, pit bull, or chow chow breeding seem to present the greatest risk. Neutering aggressive male dogs is advised. Early experiences and socialization, including proper handling and attention during the neonatal period, are essential for puppies and kittens. Veterinarians should advise clients with children to obtain a young dog so that it can be more easily socialized in the new environment. They can educate families who want to acquire new animals about the known relative risks associated with particular dog breeds. During initial training, dogs should be taught not to sleep on furniture or eat or beg at meals and that the people in the household are in charge. Children should be educated about proper behavior around dogs. They should avoid running or screaming in the presence of dogs. They should not reach outward with their hand to greet unknown dogs or hug them as they would another person. Children should always allow a dog to sniff them before they pet the animal. People with a higher risk for bites because of their occupations, such as animal control officers, postal employees, meter readers, and animal health workers, should be provided education programs to help them interpret canine and feline communicative behaviors. Crown reduction, an endodontic method for disarming the canine teeth, has been used to reduce the injury caused by biting dogs and cats[147] but is probably not very effective in preventing injuries from dog bites.[133,169]

RAT BITE INFECTIONS

Two commensal organisms of rodents are responsible for a bacterial disease that develops in dogs, cats, and people who have direct or indirect contact with rodent tissues or their secretions. *Streptobacillus moniliformis* is a small (0.25 to 0.5 μm × 1 to 3 μm), motile, aerobic, pleomorphic gram-negative bacillus with unipolar flagella. *Spirillum minus* is a motile, gram-negative spiral organism (3 to 5 μm) that has polar flagellar bundles.

These species of bacteria are resident nasopharyngeal flora in up to 50% of wild or laboratory rodents. Subclinical infections of rats with *S. moniliformis* are prevalent worldwide, although some rats have abscess formation and develop a purulent infection. Other rodents such as mice and guinea pigs more commonly develop clinical illness when infected. The prevalence of infection with *S. minus* in rats is more variable and depends on the geographic location, although most are inapparently infected.

Dogs and cats contaminate their oral cavities with these bacteria while catching rodents. They can also harbor the agents subclinically and act as mechanical vectors because they can transmit their recently acquired infection to people by biting.[125] Occasionally, abscesses develop in dogs or cats, presumably as a result of a rat bite.

Infected people have fever, myalgia, arthralgia, lymphadenitis, and generalized exanthematous eruptions that may develop weeks or months after bites.[16] Epidemic infections have rarely been reported after laboratory or foodborne contamination. Endocarditis and polyarthritis are chronic sequelae. With infections caused by *S. moniliformis*, the site of the original bite usually heals by the time clinical signs are seen. With infections caused by *S. minus*, the healed wound may become reinflamed and later ulcerate during the course of febrile illness. Regional lymphadenitis and lymphangitis are common in the region of the bite.

S. moniliformis can be isolated in culture on serum-enriched media, and a diagnosis requires notifying the laboratory that the organism may be involved. Isolation from blood must not be made in blood culture media because the typical anticoagulant—polyanethol sulfonate—inhibits the organism's growth. *S. moniliformis* has the propensity to convert to pleomorphic, cell-wall–deficient, L forms in vivo or in vitro, during unfavorable growth conditions, or during β-lactam therapy (see L-Form Infections, Chapter 32). *S. minus* does not grow on laboratory media, so dark-field examination of exudates or inoculation of mice with blood from affected patients is necessary to confirm the infection.

Penicillin is the drug of choice for infection caused by either organism. Tetracyclines are indicated for animals with resistant or L-form infections (see Table 32-2 and Appendix 8 for dosages). Oral infections of dogs and cats are usually inapparent, so treatment is unnecessary. In animals with abscess formation, surgical drainage should accompany antimicrobial therapy.

SUGGESTED READINGS*

9. Anonymous. 2001. A community approach to dog bite prevention. *J Am Vet Med Assoc* 218:1732-1749.
10. Anonymous. 2003. Nonfatal dog bite-related injuries treated in hospital emergency departments-United States, 2001. *MMWR* 52:605-610.
67. Griffin GM, Holt DE. 2001. Dog-bite wounds: bacteriology and treatment outcome in 37 cases. *J Am Anim Hosp Assoc* 37:453-460.
87. Kelly PJ, Mason PR, Els J, et al. 1992. Pathogens in dog bite wounds in dogs in Harare, Zimbabwe. *Vet Rec* 131:464-466.
99. Love DN, Malik R, Norris JM. 2000. Bacteriological warfare amongst cats: what have we learned about cat bite infections? *Vet Microbiol* 74:179-193.
123. Overall KL, Love M. 2001. Dog bites to humans—demography, epidemiology, injury, and risk. *J Am Vet Med Assoc* 218:1923-1934.
142. Sacks JJ, Sinclair L, Gichrist J, et al. 2000. Breeds of dogs involved in fatal human attacks in the United States between 1979 and 1998. *J Am Vet Med Assoc* 217:836-840.

*See the CD-ROM for a complete list of references.

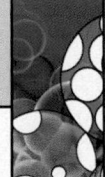

CHAPTER • 54

Bartonellosis

Bartonella is a fastidious genus of hemotropic bacteria, the members of which have each become highly adapted to preferential mammalian reservoir hosts and within which the adapted bacterial species usually causes a long-lasting intraerythrocytic bacteremia.[115,131] *Bartonella* spp. are vector transmitted, and the vector preference for particular host species has resulted in the evolution of individual sylvatic transmission cycles. In the natural reservoir host, chronic bacteremia with a *Bartonella* spp. can frequently be detected by culture or polymerase chain reaction (PCR) testing in seemingly clinically healthy individuals. Until recently, mechanisms that facilitate persistent *Bartonella* bacteremia in mammals were not well understood. However, the intraerythrocytic localization for these bacteria is a unique strategy for bacterial persistence.* Nonhemolytic intracellular colonization of erythrocytes would preserve the organisms for efficient vector transmission, protect *Bartonella* from the host immune response, and potentially contribute to decreased antimicrobial efficacy.[195]

Species of *Bartonella* are small, curved, gram-negative bacteria and include organisms that once comprised the genera of *Bartonella, Rochalimaea,* and *Grahamella* (Fig. 54-1 and Table 54-1).[17,30,212] *B. bacilliformis,* the original type species, causes a focally occurring vasculoproliferative and hemolytic disease of people in the Andes Mountains of Peru. *B.* (formerly *Rochalimaea*) *quintana,* the cause of trench fever in World War I, also causes bacillary angiomatosis, endocarditis, and chronic lymphadenomegaly, predominantly in immunocompromised people.[58,70,127,130] *B. quintana* is transmitted by the body louse and has also been detected in cat fleas in France[197]; however, this potentially incidental finding may relate to recent feeding on an infected host. *B. (Rochalimaea) henselae,* a feline-adapted *Bartonella* species, has usually been isolated from clinically healthy cats, although some strains of the organism have been associated with relatively mild illnesses and histopathologic lesions. In contrast, people with *B. henselae* infections have developed bacillary angiomatosis, visceral bacillary peliosis (extravasation of blood), relapsing fever with bacteremia, meningitis, encephalitis, neuroretinitis, endocarditis, and pyogranulomatous lymphadenitis (cat-scratch disease [CSD]).[128,187,193,215] *B. henselae* was detected using PCR testing in the liver of a dog with peliosis hepatis,[126] the liver of a dog with granulomatous hepatis,[85] and blood of three dogs with other serious illness or immunosuppression.[†] Closely related to *B. henselae, B. clarridgeiae* comprises approximately 10% to 30% of *Bartonella* isolates from clinically healthy cats[‡] and was found in endocarditis lesions in one dog[52] and in another dog with hepatopathy using PCR testing[85] (see Canine Bartonellosis later). *B. clarridgeiae* has been serologically associated with CSD-like illness in people.[135,147,20,105] *B. koehlerae*[71] was isolated from two healthy cats and a human with endocarditis[4a]; and *B. bovis* (formerly *B. weissii'*)[15,188] was isolated from four cats; the pathogenic significance of these two species in cats has not been determined. *B. (Rochalimaea) elizabethae* was isolated from a human immunodeficiency virus infected person with endocarditis.[62] PCR testing in blood of a moribund dog with renal failure and anemia.[166] *B. (Rochalimaea) vinsonii* subsp. *vinsonii* has only been isolated from voles. *B. vinsonii* subsp. *berkhoffii* has been isolated from the blood of healthy and diseased dogs, healthy coyotes, and from one human being with endocarditis.[39,137,202] *B. vinsonii* subsp. *arupensis* was isolated from a cattle rancher with fever and bacteremia.[230] Species from the former genus *Grahamella, B. talpae,* and *B. peromysci,* and three new species, *B. grahamii, B. taylorii,* and *B. doshiae* isolated from small feral mammals, were unified in the genus *Bartonella.*[17] *B. grahamii* was associated with neuroretinitis in one person.[123] Additional species or subspecies, isolated from woodland mammals and for which the pathogenic potential in cats, dogs, or people has yet to be defined, include *B. alsatica, B. birtlesii, B. capreoli, B. schoenbuchii, B. tribocorum,* and *B. chomeli.*[§] The possibility exists that new *Bartonella* pathogens and disease manifestations will be observed in the future. With respect to feline and canine infections, the following discussion of *Bartonella* in animals focuses on *B. henselae, B. clarridgeiae,* and *B. vinsonii* subsp. *berkhoffii.* These and other species of *Bartonella* infecting people and their zoonotic implications are discussed under Public Health Considerations.

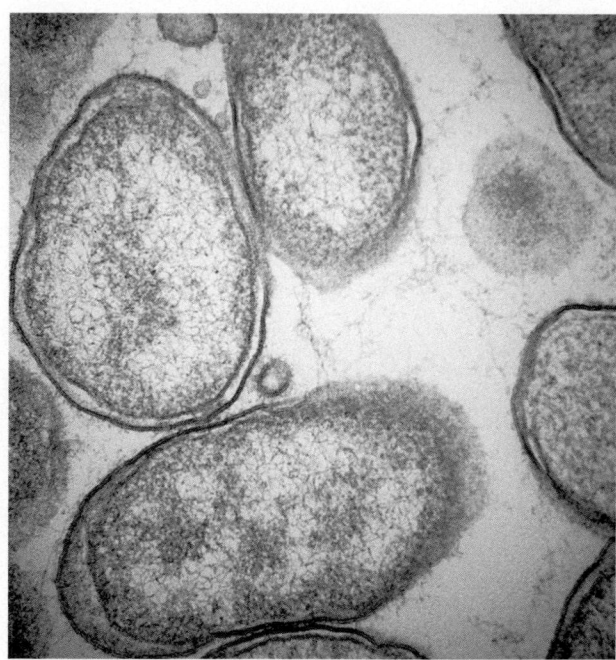

Fig 54-1 Transmission electron photomicrograph of *B. henselae* organisms in culture media (methanol uranyl acetate and then lead citrate, ×120,000). (Courtesy Stanley Hayes, Rocky Mountain Laboratories, Hamilton, Mont.)

FELINE BARTONELLOSIS

Lynn Guptill-Yoran

Epidemiology

Since the first recognition of feline *B. henselae* infection in 1992,[190] it has been established that cats may be naturally infected with four *Bartonella* species: *B. henselae, B. clarridgeiae, B. koehlerae,* and *B. bovis.*[*] Serologic and blood culture data indicate that exposure to *Bartonella* spp., most frequently *B. henselae,* is prevalent among cats in the United States and throughout most temperate regions of the world. Domestic and wild cats throughout North America, Eastern and Western Europe, Africa, Australia, and Southeast Asia have been found to be infected with *Bartonella* species.[169] Prevalence in domestic cats is lowest in Northern Europe and the Rocky Mountain regions of the United States and Canada, and greatest in warmer, more humid regions (Fig. 54-2). There are two main genotypes of *B. henselae.* The Houston 1 genotype is more prevalent in the Far East, and the genotype Marseille is predominant in western Europe, Australia, and the western United States. Both genotypes are equally prevalent in the eastern United States.[49a] A third genotype, designated Berlin, was indentified in a cat from Germany.[4] Seroepidemiologic studies in cats generally show a higher prevalence of seroreactivity with age, warmer temperature, and higher humidity, and in feral cats and those infested with fleas.[†] *B. henselae* bacteremia affects approximately 5% to 40% of cats in the United States, depending on geographic location and is most common in temperate areas.[‡] Prevalence rates of *B. clarridgeiae* infections were reported to be approximately 10% in cats with *Bartonella* bacteremia evaluated in the United States, 16% to 31% of cats with *Bartonella* bacteremia in France,

---

*References: 16, 64, 65, 115, 131, 195, 211, 210.
†References: 63, 80, 166, 215, 236.
‡References: 20, 48, 100, 101, 136.
§References: 15, 16, 66, 106, 107, 152.

*References: 15, 71, 128, 147, 188.
†References: 12, 19, 20, 45, 48, 60, 105, 116, 128, 137, 156, 241, 225.
‡ References: 26, 45, 99, 156, 158.

Table • 54-1

Comparison of Recognized Disease-Producing Members of the Genus Bartonella[a]

ORGANISM (CLASSIC DISEASE)	GEOGRAPHIC OCCURRENCE	VECTOR[b]	RESERVOIR HOST	INCIDENTAL HOST	CLINICAL FEATURES
B. bacilliformis (Oroya fever)	Andes Mountains	Sandfly (Lutzomyias)	Human[b]	Human	Hemolytic anemia, fever, nonsymptomatic bacteremia, indolent angiomatous skin lesions (verruga peruana)
B.[c] quintana (trench fever)	Focal WWI worldwide	Body louse (Pediculus humanis) and cat flea (Ctenocephalides felis)	Human[b]	Human	Bacteremia, localized tissue infection; angiomatosis, peliosis, granulomatous and pyogenic inflammation, lymphadenitis, endocarditis
B.[c] henselae (cat-scratch disease)	Worldwide	Cat flea, tick (Ixodes ricinus)[d]	Cat	Dog, human	Dog: peliosis hepatis Human: similar to B. quintana, plus neuroretinitis, focal retinochoroiditis
B. clarridgeiae	Worldwide	Cat flea[d]	Cat	Dog, human	Dog: endocarditis Human: similar to B. quintana
B.[c] vinsonii subsp. berkhoffii or berkhoffii	Worldwide?	Brown dog tick (Rhipicephalus sanguineus)[d]	Coyote	Dog, human	Dog: endocarditis, bacteremia, granulomatous and pyogenic inflammation Human: endocarditis, fever, lymphadenopathy
B.[c] elizabethae	?	Rat flea (Xenopsylla cheopis)[d]	Urban rat	Dog, human	Dog: possible opportunist, bacteremia Human: endocarditis, bacteremia
B. koehlerae	?	Cat flea[d]	Cat[e]	Human	Human: endocarditis
B. bovis (B. weissii), B. chomeli	?	?	Ruminants	Cow	?
B. grahamii	Europe, United States	?	Rodents	Human	Neuroretinitis
B. vinsonii subsp. arupensis	?	Deer tick (Ixodes scapularis)[d]	Rodents, Peromyscus	Human	Bacteremia, fever, neurologic signs
B. washoensis	?	Tick[d]	Rodent, ground squirrels[e]	Human, dog	Cardiac disease, endocarditis

WWI, World War I; ?, unknown.

[a]Also includes other organisms of uncertain pathogenicity—B. alsatica (rabbit), B. birtlesii, B. bovis, B. capreoli, B. doshiae (rodent), B. koehlerae (cat), B. peromysci (rodent), B. schoenbuchii, B. talpae (rodent), B. taylorii (rodent), B. tribocorum (rodent), B. vinsonii subsp. vinsonii (Canadian vole agent)—that infect small woodland mammals and herbivores, and domesticated animals (fish and birds?).

[b]Nonhuman primates have been experimentally infected.

[c]Formerly Rochalimaea.

[d]Suspected, but not proven, vector.

[e]Suspected involvement as reservoir host.

and 31% of cats in the Philippines that had Bartonella bacteremia.[48,105,136] B. koehlerae was isolated from two cats (from the same household in California), and B. bovis was isolated from two cats in Utah and two in Illinois.[71,188] Domestic cats are considered the major reservoir and vector for human infections with B. henselae and for B. clarridgeiae. Cattle are the reservoir for B. bovis. The reservoir for B. koehlerae is unknown. In France, molecular methods detected B. quintana, B. koehlerae, B. henselae, and B. clarridgeiae in cat fleas, along with rickettsial pathogens.[197] This finding suggests that fleas may be involved in

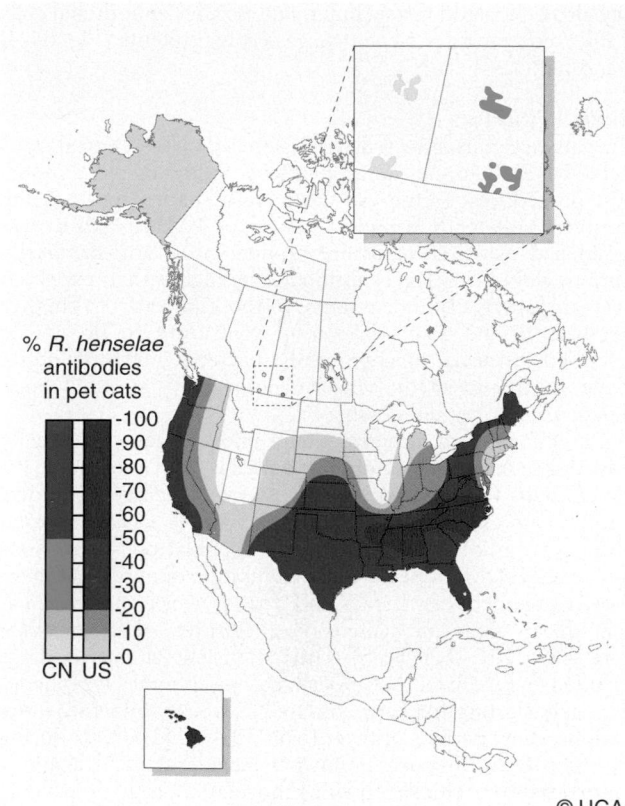

% R. henselae
antibodies
in pet cats

-100
-90
-80
-70
-60
-50
-40
-30
-20
-10
-0
CN US

© UGA

Fig 54-2 Percentage of pet cats with *B. henselae* antibodies throughout the United States and selected areas in Canada based on samples received from 29 geographic regions of the United States and from four parks in Canada. (Map data from references 116 and 149; inset courtesy University of Georgia, Athens, Ga.)

the transmission of many of these bartonellae for people and animals; however, the fleas had just fed on their host. Additional evidence that arthropods serve both as reservoirs and vectors of some *Bartonella* species comes from finding these organisms in questing ticks.[36,169b] Biting flies have also been infected with *Bartonella*.[55a]

Wild felids are also exposed to *Bartonella* spp.; 18% of panthers in Florida and 28% of mountain lions in Texas had serum antibodies to *B. henselae*, and the prevalence of serum antibodies to *B. henselae* in free-ranging and captive wild felids in California was 30% to 53%.[201,240] Prevalence of serum antibodies to *B. henselae* in pumas (*Felis puma concolor*) and bobcats (*Lynx rufus*) in Mexico, Central America, and South America ranged from 0% to 33%.[51] *Bartonella* infection has also been documented in free-ranging wild and captive African lions (*Panthera leo*) and cheetahs (*Acinonyx jubatus*), using serology, PCR testing, and blood culture.[169,49a]

B. henselae contains multiple genetically diverse strains. Two recognized 16S rRNA types of *B. henselae* (Houston 1 [type 1] and Marseille [type II]) and at least two subgroups are within each type.[157,242] Cats can be co-infected with *B. henselae* 16S rRNA types I and II and co-infected with *B. henselae* and *B. clarridgeiae*.[100] In cats, co-infection also exists with hemotrophic *Mycoplasma* spp. that cause erythrocytic mycoplasmosis (haemobartonellosis), given that they are also transmitted by cat fleas (see Chapter 31).[145] Regional differences in prevalence of infection of cats exist with different rRNA types of *B. henselae*.[13,93,101,105] Some evidence is suggestive of genomic variation in *B. henselae* during the course of infection in cats.[119]

Such variation may enhance the ability of *B. henselae* to persist in an infected cat for prolonged periods. Whether the 16S rRNA type is the most accurate means of describing genetic differences among *B. henselae* isolates has not yet been determined. Multiple other methods are under investigation, and the full extent of genetic diversity within *B. henselae*, is yet to be defined.[68,113,114,141] Genetic variation makes vaccine development difficult (see Pathogenesis) but is useful in epidemiologic studies and may also be useful in furthering the understanding of the pathogenicity of various *Bartonella* isolates.

Pathogenesis

B. henselae is believed to be naturally transmitted among cats by cat fleas *(Ctenocephalides felis felis)*. The exact role of the flea in transmission has not been determined. *B. henselae* was transmitted among cats by transferring fleas fed on infected cats to specific specific-pathogen–free (SPF) cats, and by intradermal (ID) inoculation of flea excrement.[49,78] Cats exposed to *Bartonella*-infected fleas that were confined to capsules that permitted fleas to feed, but prevented contamination of cats' skin and hair coat with flea excrement, did not become infected with *B. henselae*.[78] This finding suggests that transmission does not occur via flea saliva. Ticks may have a role in transmission; *B. henselae* and other *Bartonella* spp. were detected by PCR test in questing ticks in California,[36,38] and from *Ixodes ricinus* ticks in Italy.[208] Ticks have been proposed as the vectors for transmission of some *Bartonella* infections in people, dogs, and other mammalian hosts.[11,183,215,230]

Cats were experimentally infected with *B. henselae* through intravenous (IV) or intramuscular (IM) inoculation with infected cat blood,[134] and by IV, subcutaneous, ID, or oral (PO) routes of inoculation with plate-grown bacteria.[1,91,92,177] *B. henselae* transmission has not occurred when infected cats cohabit with uninfected cats in a flea-free environment,[1,92] indicating that transmission among cats does not occur through cat bites, scratches, grooming, or sharing of food dishes and litter boxes. Transmission did not occur when cats were inoculated IM with urine of bacteremic cats.[132] Transmission also did not occur between bacteremic female cats and males during mating, or to the kittens of infected females either during gestation or in the neonatal period,[1,96] again in flea-free environments.

Bacteremia with *B. henselae* and *B. clarridgeiae* is commonly chronic and waxes and wanes; periods occur when bacteremia cannot be detected either by culture or by PCR testing. Measured increases in IL-4 and serum antibody titers in response to the peak of bacteremia subsequently decrease the bacteremia to low or undetectable levels.[119a] Experimentally infected cats maintained *B. henselae* or *B. clarridgeiae* bacteremia for as long as 454 days.[134] Naturally infected cats maintained recurrent bacteremia for periods of as long as 3 years; however, reinfection via fleas of cats living in private homes may occur.[138]

Immune mechanisms are important in the suppression or elimination of infection in cats. Complete protection against reinfection is highly specific, even with strains of a given species of *Bartonella* and likely in reactivity to the outer membranes of the organism.[41] A lack of protection against reinfection has been demonstrated in cats previously infected with *Bartonella*. Cats previously infected with *B. henselae* 16S rRNA type II were susceptible to infection with *B. henselae* 16S rRNA type I.[237] Cats infected with *B. henselae* type I or II were susceptible to challenge infection with *B. clarridgeiae*, and cats infected with *B. koehlerae* or *B. clarridgeiae* were susceptible to challenge infection with *B. henselae* type I or type II.[239] In contrast, cats infected with *B. henselae* type I were partially or completely protected against challenge infection with *B. henselae* type II.[239] The level of bacteremia and degree of susceptibility to reinfection following challenge inoculation is likely to vary with strains, as well as with species, of *Bartonella*.[237]

Despite the lack of protection against heterologous challenge, cats can become immune to ID challenge with homologous strains of the organism.[89,237] Cats can still be reinfected with the same strain through blood transfusions.[89,132] These findings suggest that the intracellular localization of the organism provides protection from immune clearance mechanisms.

The extent of localization of *Bartonella* in cats has not been completely determined. *Bartonella* are intracellular bacteria. *B. henselae* have been detected within erythrocytes of naturally infected cats[198,210,211] and in vitro (Fig. 54-3).[164] *Bartonella*

may also be located intracellularly in vascular endothelial cells of infected cats as has been suggested for rodents (Fig. 54-4, *A* and *B*).[65]

Clinical Findings

Few cats naturally infected with *Bartonella* have clinical signs (Table 54-2). Four cats developed fever following elective surgical procedures.[21] One cat with uveitis had a serologically positive result for *B. henselae*[144] and 7 of 49 cats with uveitis (14%) had evidence of ocular production of anti-*Bartonella* immunoglobulin G (IgG) antibodies by higher than expected levels in aqueous humor relative to those in sera.[146] Whether members of the genus *Bartonella* contribute to previously described instances of argyrophilic bacteria in lymph nodes of cats with persistent lymphadenomegaly[125] or to peliosis hepatis in cats[32] is unknown.

Clinical signs in experimentally infected cats are usually mild and transient; therefore naturally infected cats may have clinical signs that owners do not observe. Severity of clinical signs in cats experimentally infected with *B. henselae* varied with the strain of *B. henselae* used for inoculation.[95,134,177] Cats inoculated ID developed areas of induration or abscess at inoculation sites between 2 days and 3 to 4 weeks after inoculation* from some of which pure cultures of *B. henselae* were obtained[95] (Fig. 54-5). Other transient clinical findings included generalized or localized peripheral lymphadenomegaly (lasting for approximately 6 weeks following inoculation), short periods of fever (over 39.4° C [103° F]) during the first 48 to 96 hours following inoculation and again at approximately 2 weeks following inoculation, mild neurologic signs (nystagmus, whole body tremors, focal motor seizures, either decreased or exaggerated responses to external stimuli, behavior changes), and epaxial muscle pain. Some cats are lethargic and anorexic during febrile periods.† Reproductive failure occurred in some cats experimentally infected with *B. henselae*.[96] Cats experimentally infected with *B. koehlerae* exhibited no clinical signs.[238]

B. henselae type I was associated with fatal blood culture–negative vegetative aortic valve endocarditis in two cats.[53,49a]

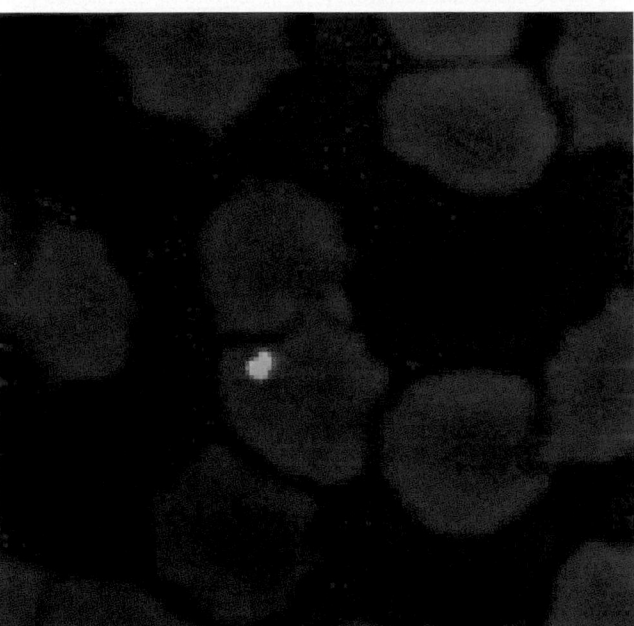

Fig 54-3 Intraerythrocytic *B. henselae* viewed by confocal microscopy. (Courtesy J.-M. Rolain, Unité des Rickettsies, Marseille, France.)

*References: 90, 95, 134, 168, 177.
†References: 95, 132, 134, 168, 177.

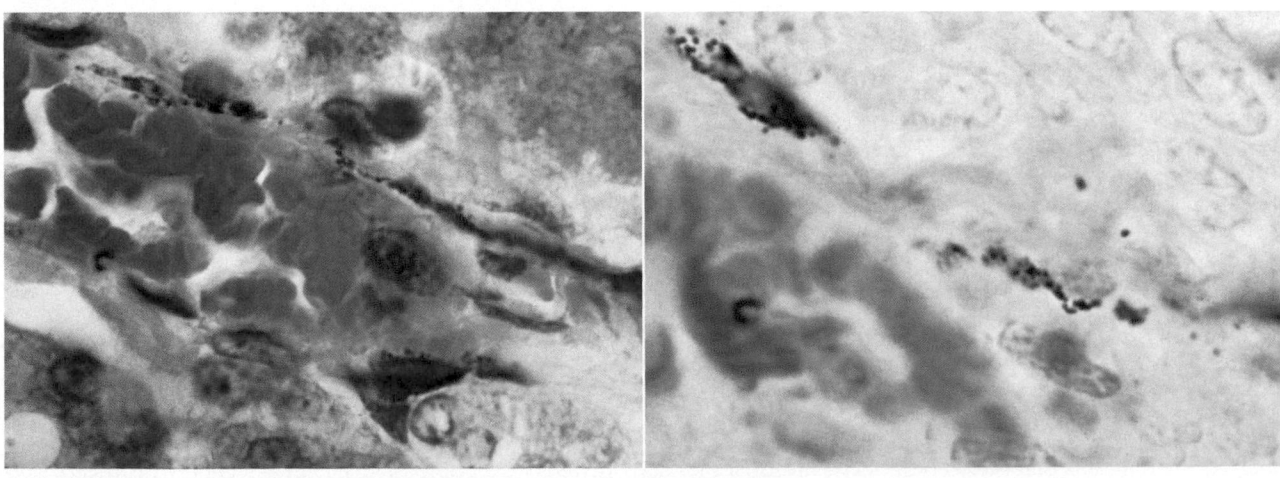

A   B

Fig 54-4 Liver from a cat with experimentally induced chronic *B. henselae* infection. In both specimens, organisms are visible in the periendothelial region with (**A**) Warthin–Starry silver stain and (**B**) Giemsa stain (×1000). (Courtesy Edward Breitschwerdt, North Carolina State University, Raleigh, N.C.)

Table • 54-2

Medical Problems of Cats Associated with Bartonella Infections[a]

Experimental Infection

B. henselae
Subclinical[90,192]
Papules or small abscesses at site of inoculation[95,177]
Transient fever, lethargy, anorexia[95,132,177]
Lymphadenomegaly[95,132,177]
Lymph node and splenic hyperplasia, splenic microabscesses, focal pyogranulomatous nephritis, interstitial myocarditis[95]
CNS signs: nystagmus, tremors, focal motor seizures[95,132,168,177]
Myalgia[168,177]
Reproductive failure[96]

B. henselae or *B. clarridgeiae*
Lymph node and splenic hyperplasia[134]
Lymphocytic infiltrates in liver, heart, and kidney[134]

B. koehlerae
Subclinical[238]

Natural Infection as Determined by Bacterial Isolation or PCR Identification

B. henselae
Fever[21]
Valvular endocarditis[3]

B bovis (formerly *B. weissii*)
Subclinical (suspected)[188]

Natural Infection as *Suspected* by Serum Antibody Measurement

B. henselae
Stomatitis and urologic disease?[69a,86,c]
Gingivitis with FIV coinfection?[224,c]
Uveitis? [144,146,d]
Keratitis, Uveitis?[124,e]

CNS, central nervous system; *PCR*, polymerase chain reaction; *FIV*, feline immunodeficiency virus.
[a]Most consistently seen with experimental infections and signs vary according to the tested strain. *B. koehlerae* has not been tested.
[b]Sample obtained from to a commercial diagnostic laboratory where health status of the cat was unknown.
[c]*Bartonella* infection in these retrospective studies was diagnosed by serologic fluorescent antibody testing.
[d]*Bartonella* infection in these studies was diagnosed by serologic enzyme-linked immunosorbent assay.
[e]Serologic testing was performed with an immunoblotting procedure.

B. henselae DNA was detected in the aortic valve. Occasional silver-stained coccoid structures were seen in endothelial cells of the myocardium, but no bacteria were seen on transmission electron microscopy of the aortic valve.

A potential causative role of *Bartonella* spp. in chronic diseases of cats has been proposed because *Bartonella* bacteremia is prolonged. A Japanese study suggests that co-infection of cats with *B. henselae* and feline immunodeficiency virus was more likely to cause gingivitis or lymphadenomegaly than was either infection alone.[224] Results of a Swiss study suggest

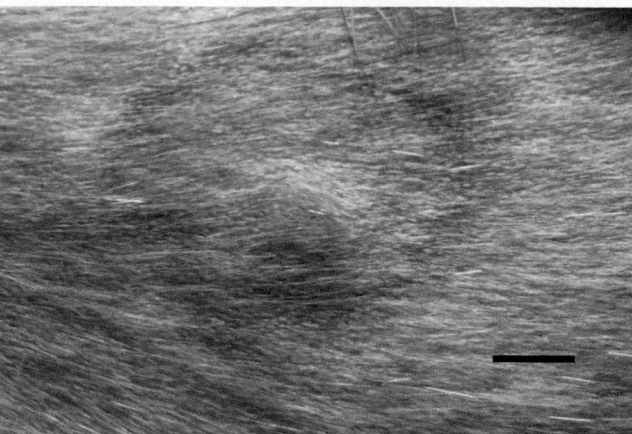

Fig 54-5 Postinoculation papule 20 days after ID inoculation of *B. henselae* in a cat. The size of the papule increased from the time of inoculation and only *B. henselae* was isolated from bacterial culture of an aspirate. Bar = 1 cm. (Courtesy Lynn Guptill, Purdue University, West Lafayette, Ind.)

possible associations between *B. henselae* seropositivity and stomatitis and various urinary tract disorders.[86] Both studies obtained serum and historical information about cat health from practicing veterinarians. Plexiform vascularization of the lymph nodes, which has been described as a clinical entity in cats,[232] resembles visceral peliosis of people that is associated with *B. henselae* infections. Further studies are needed on this and other conditions (see Table 54-2) to determine whether they are associated with *B. henselae* infections in cats.

A contribution of *Bartonella* infections to development of chronic illnesses in domestic cats has not been verified. For example, suggestions indicate that infected cats have a greater prevalence of chronic gingivitis, stomatitis, or ocular lesions, but this is not proven.[103a-b] No significant differences were found in the prevalence rate for PCR or serum antibody-positive results between cats with stomatitis and age-matched control cats.[69a] Because of the high prevalence of *Bartonella* infection in the domestic cat population, proof of a causative association between any disease or syndrome and *Bartonella* infection will require extensive, carefully controlled epidemiologic investigations.

Diagnosis

As a result of the transient and protean nature of clinical signs, determining which cats are likely to have *Bartonella* infection is difficult. In addition to the need to test for *Bartonella* infections in sick cats, veterinarians will be asked to test healthy pet cats belonging to clients with *Bartonella*-related illnesses or to screen healthy cats that are being considered as pets for people considered most susceptible to *Bartonella* infections (see Public Health Considerations).

Clinical Laboratory Findings

Most experimentally infected cats had no abnormalities on complete blood counts, serum biochemical tests, or urinalysis. Some cats had transient anemia early in the course of infection, and some had persistent eosinophilia.[134] Mature neutrophilia occurred in some cats during periods of skin inflammation.[95]

Cytologic Detection

Finding *B. henselae* in erythrocytes of infected cats has not been an effective means of detection using conventional staining methods. Special confocal microscopy (see Fig. 54.3) and staining has been used.[210] Intraerythrocytic location of *B. clarridgeiae* and *B. koehlerae* have also been documented in cats using fluorescent antibody (FA) detection methods.[197,199] In addition, extracellular *B. henselae* have been documented in peripheral blood and other tissues of infected cats using immunocytochemical and immunohistochemical methods.[98]

Bacterial Isolation

A positive blood culture result or culture of other tissue is the *most reliable test for definitive diagnosis* of active *Bartonella* infection. However, because of the relapsing nature of feline *Bartonella* bacteremia, culture is not always a sensitive diagnostic tool. Blood culture is indicated for sick cats whose history and clinical presentation suggest possible *Bartonella* infection or when a client's physician requires such testing of pet cats. Blood for culture should be obtained using sterile technique, and the blood placed in ethylenediaminetetra-acetic acid (EDTA)-containing tubes or lysis centrifugation blood culture tubes (Isolator tubes, Wampole, Cranbury, N.J.). If blood is collected into EDTA tubes, the blood should be chilled or frozen during shipment; ideally, plastic EDTA tubes should be used. Blood should be sent to laboratories familiar with the culture of these fastidious organisms (see Appendix 5). Laboratories should be contacted for specific instructions for sample collection and submission. Blood culture is not recommended for absolute screening of cats because of potential false-negative results during lapses in bacteremia. Initial screening to eliminate any potential for infection is probably best done using serology, which overestimates the number of infected cats.

Serologic Testing

Measuring serum antibodies has limited value for determining whether an ill cat has an active *Bartonella* infection but is useful for epidemiologic surveys and can be useful for screening. Serum IgG antibodies persist in experimentally infected cats for prolonged periods. How long antibodies persist following clearance of infection is not known. Indirect FA, enzyme immunoassay (EIA), and Western blot tests are available. Because of the genetic diversity of *Bartonella* organisms, infections with some strains or species of *Bartonella* may be missed using any method, depending on the antigen preparations used.[84] The positive predictive value of indirect FA or EIA (IgG) serologic tests for bacteremia is only 39% to 46%. The utility of a negative serologic result is greater because the negative predictive value for these tests for bacteremia is high at 89% to 97%.[12,45,93,101] Nevertheless, some seronegative bacteremic cats exist.[55,93,185] A positive correlation may exist between indirect FA titer and level of bacteremia[239]; however, cut-off values allowing use of serologic testing to determine whether a cat is currently infected with *Bartonella* have not been established.

Immunoblotting

The use of Western blot tests has been advocated for serodiagnosis of feline *B. henselae* infections, but the diagnostic accuracy of Western blot tests awaits further investigation. In human medicine, variability in Western blot testing remains problematic. Serologic responses of people as evaluated by immunoblot vary from patient to patient.[205] Results of studies of Western blot analyses of cats infected with *B. henselae* have differing results. Results of one study indicated no differences in Western blot patterns of cats evaluated over the course of infection when sera from multiple time points were incubated with polyacrylamide gel-separated proteins of bacterial isolates from multiple time points in infection.[134] Results of another study indicated that antibodies in sera of infected cats reacted with an increasing number of bands of polyacrylamide gel-separated proteins over the course of infection.[81,93]

Nucleic Acid Detection

Standard PCR testing for the presence of *Bartonella* DNA is often no more sensitive than blood culture is for detecting active *Bartonella* infection, and detecting DNA does not always equate to detection of living organisms. Using PCR, *B. henselae* DNA has been detected in the dental pulp of 1-year-old and 800-year-old cat cadavers.[1a,141a] Extraction methods from blood are extremely critical in determining the sensitivity of PCR test and can be responsible for false-negative results when compared with blood culture.[89,176] Nested PCR testing may increase sensitivity for detection of *Bartonella* DNA in cat blood[204] and may be available through some research laboratories (see Appendix 5). A benefit of PCR testing is that the product obtained in the reaction may be sequenced and the species or strain (or both) of *Bartonella* therefore identified. In addition, the results of PCR testing are often available more quickly than are those of blood culture. PCR methods have been described that allow for rapid differentiation of pathogenic *Bartonella* spp.[117,221] Blood samples for PCR testing should be obtained using the same sterile technique recommended for blood culture. Care must be taken in collection and sample processing to avoid sample contamination and DNA degradation. Contact individual laboratories for submission guidelines (see Appendix 5).

Pathologic Findings

Acutely and chronically infected cats had hyperplasia of lymphoid organs, small foci of lymphocytic, pyogranulomatous, or neutrophilic inflammation in multiple tissues (lung, liver, spleen, kidney, heart) (Figs. 54-6 and 54-7)—or necrotic foci associated with pyogranulomatous inflammation—usually in liver or lymphoid tissues (Fig. 54-8).[95,134]

Therapy

Documentation of clearance of *Bartonella* infections through antibiotic treatment is difficult because of the prolonged relapsing bacteremia of infected cats. No regimen of antibiotic treatment has been proven effective, in controlled studies

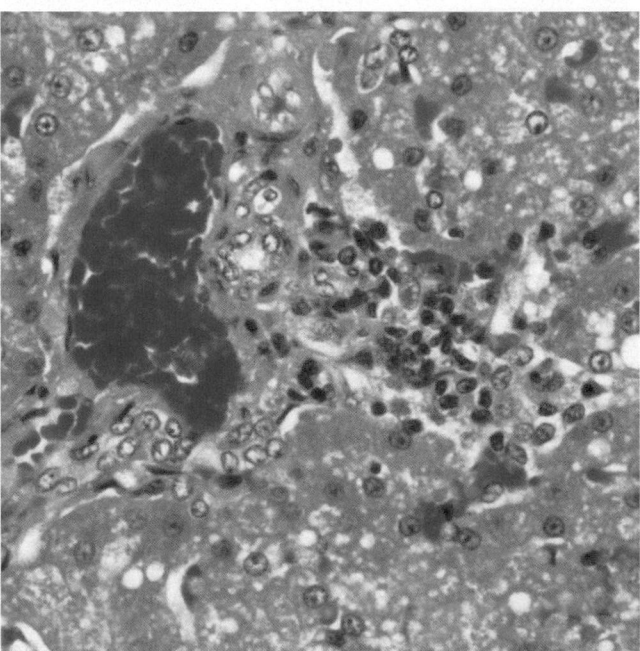

Fig 54-6 Perivascular microscopic focus of inflammation in the liver from an experimentally infected cat with chronic *B. henselae* infection (H and E stain, ×400). (Courtesy T. Brown and E. Breitschwerdt, North Carolina State University, Raleigh, N.C.)

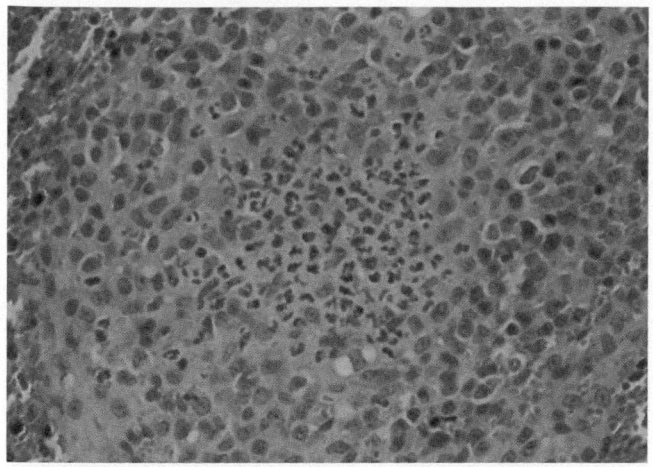

Fig 54-7 Histologic section of feline spleen showing a microabscess 14 days following inoculation with *B. henselae*. (H and E stain, ×400). (Courtesy Lynn Guptill, Purdue University, West Lafayette, Ind.)

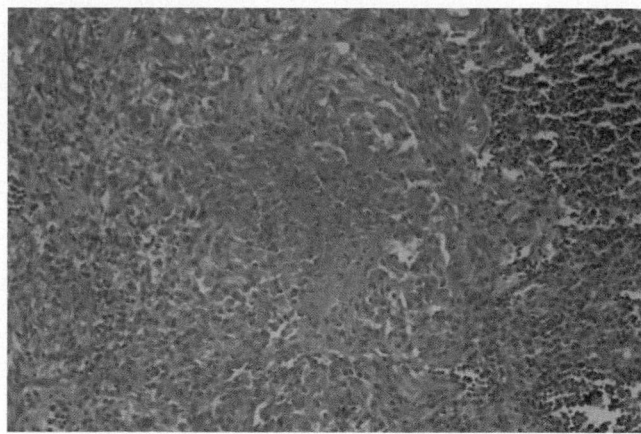

Fig 54-8 Necrotizing granuloma in the lymph node of a cat infected with *B. henselae*, 56 days following inoculation (H and E stain, ×200). (Reprinted from Guptill et al. 1997. Experimental infection of young specific pathogen–free cats with *Bartonella henselae*, J Infect Dis 176:206–216. Used with permission.)

Table • 54-3

Suggested Antibiotic Dosage for Bartonellosis Infections of Cats[a]

Drug[b]	DOSE[c] (mg/kg)	ROUTE	INTERVAL (HOURS)	DURATION[d] (WEEKS)
Enrofloxacin[e]	5 mg/kg	PO	24	2—4
Doxycycline	10—22 mg/kg[f]	PO	12	2—4
Rifampin[g]	10 mg/kg	PO	24	2
Azithromycin	10 mg/kg	PO	24	1[h]

[a]Data from references 136, 89, 90, and 124. Efficacy of these drugs in clearing bacteremic cats is controversial.
[b]For further information on these drugs, see Drug Formulary, Appendix 8.
[c]Dose per administration at specified interval.
[d]Giving these drugs for 4 weeks appears to be more efficacious than for 2 weeks.
[e]Doses greater than 5 mg/kg/day have been associated with retinal degeneration in cats, but 5 mg/kg may be ineffective.
[f]The dose should be rounded up to give whole tablets or capsules to avoid esophageal irritation.
[g]Rifampin is effective alone or in combination with doxycycline but has to be reformulated so that the dose given here can be administered. Rifampin should ideally be given in combination with another drug in treatment-resistant cases to reduce the possibility of inducing antibacterial resistance in *Bartonella* that might eventually pose a public health risk.
[h]After the first week, the same dose is given every other day for 5 weeks.

with long-term follow-up, for definitively eliminating *Bartonella* infections in cats.[11,90,136,192] Enrofloxacin (5.4 to 7.6 mg/kg, given PO, every 12 hours) for 14 or 28 days appeared to clear *B. henselae* or *B. clarridgeiae* infection in 4 of 6 or 5 of 7 treated cats, respectively, that were followed for 12 weeks after treatment.[136] However, studies show that enrofloxacin causes retinal degeneration in cats, and use of doses of greater than 2.5 mg/kg, given every 12 hours, is contraindicated.[234] Doxycycline (4 to 12 mg/kg, given PO, every 12 hours) cleared bacteremia in only one of six cats treated for 14 days and one of two cats treated for 28 days.[136] Antibiotics tested in other studies, including erythromycin, amoxicillin, amoxicillin-clavulanate, and tetracycline, rapidly decreased the level of bacteremia in infected cats. However, in one study, treated and untreated cats became blood-culture negative after the same period, making proof of efficacy of antibiotics difficult. In another study, cats were not followed for more than 8 weeks after treatment, thereby making it difficult to assess drug efficacy resulting from the possibility of chronic relapsing bacteremia in these cats.[90,192] In experimental infections, the effective doxycycline dose in cats has been a minimum of 10 mg/kg twice daily,[88] which is similar to that recommended in treating infections with other related persistent intracellular organisms such as *Brucella canis* and *Ehrlichia canis* in dogs.

In experimental studies in cats, rifampin alone and in combination with doxycycline has been effective in clearing *B. henselae* bacteremia.[88] Azithromycin has been recommended for treatment of infected cats, but data from controlled efficacy studies with long-term follow-up are lacking. Azithromycin was used to treat seropositive cats with uveitis[103b,124]; however, documentation of infection by detection of organisms was lacking. Similarly, azithromycin has been used to treat seropositive cats with gingivitis and stomatitis and other inflammatory conditions.[103a] Despite clinical improvement in some cats, no proof has been found that the serologic titer results indicate exposure to this or oral microorganisms responsible for the inflammation. Azithromycin appears to have important immunomodulatory and antiinflammatory properties in addition to the broad antimicrobial spectrum of this antibiotic.[61,142,143,178] These properties may make it difficult to determine whether beneficial effects reported following azithromycin treatment of cats are solely a result of anti-*Bartonella* activity or instead are a result of azithromycin's other properties, of the antimicrobial action of azithromycin on other bacteria, or of a combination of all of these.

Recommended dosages are listed in Table 54-3. However, because of the uncertainty of antibiotic efficacy, several followup blood cultures should be performed at 4- to 8-week intervals *after* discontinuation of antibiotic treatment.[90,136,192] Because routine treatment with antibiotics may induce resistant strains, recommendations are to treat only cats showing clinical signs or when euthanasia is the only alternative to treatment.[136] Although treatment decreases the level of bacteremia in cats, no concrete evidence has been found that treatment of the cat will decrease the probability of transmission of *Bartonella* infection to an owner. Client education regarding the uncertainty of treatment efficacy and the need for prolonged followup is important. The importance of flea control and other means of preventing transmission (see Prevention) should be emphasized.

People with *Bartonella* infections causing bacillary angiomatosis or peliosis or endocarditis are treated with a variety of antibiotics, including doxycycline, erythro-mycin, ciprofloxacin, rifampin, gentamicin, trimethoprim-sulfamethoxazole, clarithromycin, and azithromycin.[9,155] Azithromycin was shown in a controlled clinical trial to have some efficacy for decreasing lymph node size in people with CSD.[9]

Prevention

Prevention of *Bartonella* infections in cats is best accomplished by avoiding exposure to infected animals and their fleas. Because *B. henselae* and *B. clarridgeiae* have been transmitted through inoculation of infected cat blood,[132] cats should not receive blood transfusions from cats of unknown *Bartonella* status or cats that are seropositive for *Bartonella*. A vaccine to prevent *Bartonella* infection in cats is not available. If a vaccine were developed, it would by necessity have to protect against a wide variety of strains.

Public Health Considerations

People are susceptible to infection with at least nine *Bartonella* species or subspecies, including *B. quintana*, *B. bacilliformis*, *B. henselae*, *B. clarridgeiae*, *B. vinsonii* subsp. *berkhoffii*, *B. vinsonii* subsp. *arupensis*, *B. grahamii*, *B. elizabethae*, and *B. washoensis*, the latter seven of which are considered zoonotic. Cats are the reservoir and vector for transmission of *B. henselae* and possibly (but uncommonly) *B. clarridgeiae* to people. Coyotes are probably a reservoir for *B. vinsonii* subsp. *berkhoffii*. Rodents are likely reservoirs for other zoonotic *Bartonella* spp. The role of fleas, ticks, and other arthropods in direct transmission of any of these species of *Bartonella* to people is not certain. Transmission of *B. henselae* from cats to people is believed to occur through contamination of cat scratches with flea excrement.[49] Transmission may also occur through cat bites if cat blood or flea excrement contaminates the bite site.[232a]

Bartonella spp. cause a wide variety of clinical syndromes in people, including CSD (typical and atypical forms, including encephalopathies in children); bacillary angiomatosis and peliosis; parenchymal bacillary peliosis; relapsing fever with bacteremia; endocarditis; optic neuritis; pulmonary, hepatic, and splenic granulomas; and osteomyelitis.* Immunocompetent individuals usually have more localized infections (Fig. 54-9), whereas infections in immunocompromised individuals are more often systemic and can be fatal. Diagnosis in people is usually made by serologic testing or PCR testing because of the low level or absence of bacteremia in immunocompetent hosts. In one study, a high prevalence of antibodies to *B. henselae* was found among children in Italy, without evidence of obvious illness.[161] This finding suggests that exposure and nonsymptomatic infection occurred during exposure early in life with spontaneous resolution. Evidence suggests that certain genotypes of *Bartonella* may induce different pathologic features in infected people.[35,235] For example, only rRNA type I isolates were associated with hepatosplenic peliosis. Close typing of isolates from people and their cats'

*References: 80, 127, 155, 173, 202, 215, 230, 233.

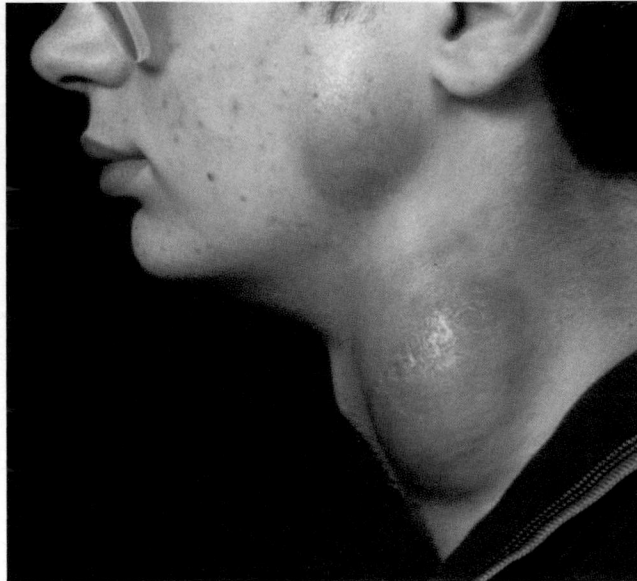

Fig 54-9 Enlarged lymph nodes in a person with CSD. (Courtesy University of Georgia, Athens, Ga.)

contacts show them to be related, thus incriminating the cats as the source of human infection. Clients should be informed of the current understanding of how dogs and cats acquire *Bartonella* infections and how these infections may be transmitted to people, including the possibility of transmission by ticks or fleas.

Common sense precautions for avoiding transmission of *Bartonella* spp. from pets to people include ongoing flea and tick control, avoiding interactions with cats and dogs that result in scratches or bites, thoroughly washing bite or scratch wounds, and acquiring new pets of known good health status that are and have been ectoparasite free. Stray or impounded cats less than 1 year are most likely to be infected. No evidence has been found that declawing cats decreases the probability of transmission of *B. henselae* between cats and human beings. The United States Public Health Service/Infectious Diseases Society of America (USPHS/IDSA) *Guidelines for Preventing Opportunistic Infections Among HIV-Infected Persons*[226] recommends the following when acquiring a new cat: adopt a cat older than 1 year of age that is in good health, avoid rough play with cats, maintain flea control, wash any cat-associated wounds promptly, and do not allow a cat to lick wounds or cuts. The USPHS/IDSA Guidelines note that no evidence has been found to indicate any benefit to cats or their owners from routine culture or serologic testing of cats for *Bartonella* infections.

CANINE BARTONELLOSIS

Edward B. Breitschwerdt and Bruno B. Chomel

Epidemiology

B. vinsonii subsp. *berkhoffii* was isolated from a dog with endocarditis in our laboratory in 1993.[27,137] Retrospectively, long-term administration of immunosuppressive doses of glucocorticoids for a presumptive diagnosis of systemic lupus erythematosus may have facilitated the isolation of the original type strain of *B. vinsonii* subsp. *berkhoffii* from this dog with endocarditis. Because of the relatively recent recognition that dogs can be infected with *B. vinsonii* subsp. *berkhoffii* and potentially other *Bartonella* spp., seroprevalence data is limited.[6,109,111,183] Seroprevalence was determined in 1920 sick dogs from North Carolina or surrounding states that were evaluated at a veterinary teaching hospital.[183] Using a titer of over 1:32, only 3.6% of sick dogs had antibodies to *B. vinsonii* subsp. *berkhoffii*. Risk factors, expressed as odds ratio (OR), that may be associated with seroreactivity included heavy tick exposure (OR 14.2), cattle exposure (OR 9.3), rural versus urban environment (OR 7.1), and heavy flea exposure (OR 5.6). These data were interpreted to support the possibility that exposure to *B. vinsonii* subsp. *berkhoffii* was more likely in dogs in rural environments that were allowed to roam. In addition, these dogs were likely to have a history of heavy tick infestation. Using sera from dogs experimentally infected with *Rickettsia rickettsii* or *Ehrlichia canis*, cross-reactivity to *Bartonella* antigens was not detected. However, 36% of serum samples derived from dogs naturally infected with *E. canis* were reactive to *B. vinsonii* antigens. Because *E. canis* is transmitted by *Rhipicephalus sanguineous*, this tick may be involved in the transmission of *B. vinsonii*. The possibility of tick transmission was further supported by two additional studies involving dogs infected with one or more *Ehrlichia* spp. from the same geographic region, in which seroreactivity to *B. vinsonii* subsp. *berkhoffii* antigens was 30% and 89%, respectively.[25,139] Seroprevalence, using *B. vinsonii* subsp. *berkhoffii* antigens, was 10% (4 out of 40 dogs) in those with suspected tick-borne illness from Israel and 36% in dogs with fever and thrombocytopenia from Thailand.[6,220] Using an enzyme-linked immunosorbent assay, 35% of 869 samples, derived from coyotes (*Canis latrans*) in California, contained antibodies to *B. vinsonii* subsp. *berkhoffii* antigens.[40] The organism has been isolated from wild coyotes incriminating them as a likely wildlife reservoir in the western United States.[39] Dogs with *Bartonella*-induced endocarditis in California also had positive antibody titers to *Anaplasma phagocytophilum*, suggesting common tick vector exposure.[151] In the southeastern United States, epidemiologic evidence suggests that *Amblyomma americanum* or *Dermacentor* may be involved in transmission because co-infections with other tick-borne organisms carried by these ticks have been documented.[25,139,183] Current data indicates that exposure to *B. vinsonii* subsp. *berkhoffii* can be found throughout much of the United States and most tropical and subtropical regions of the world. The organism has been identified in *Ixodes* with PCR methods.[119a]

Other Bartonellae

Based on cultural and molecular evidence, *B. vinsonii* subsp. *berkhoffii* is considered the most frequent *Bartonella* species that causes disease in dogs. However, this conclusion may not be accurate because sera from dogs have not been screened systematically against a large panel of *Bartonella* spp. antigens, and minimal PCR testing has been performed. Studies from Hawaii, the United Kingdom, and Japan identified *B. henselae* seroprevalence of 6.5% (2 of 31 dogs), 3.0% (3 of 100 dogs) and 7.7% (4 of 52 dogs), respectively.[8,67,222] Although the pathogenicity of all *Bartonella* spp. in dogs is poorly characterized, it is becoming increasingly clear that species other than *B. vinsonii* subsp. *berkhoffii* can infect dogs.[122,140,222] For example, *B. henselae* was amplified and sequenced on two independent occasions from the liver of a dog with peliosis hepatis.[126] This is a unique pathologic lesion that is induced only by *B. henselae* infection in people.[115] Recently, *B. henselae* DNA was amplified from a dog with granulomatous hepatis, a histopathologic lesion that is reported with some frequency in children infected with *B. henselae*.[85] Similarly, *B. clarridgeae* DNA has been amplified and sequenced from the liver of a Doberman pincher with copper storage disease and from the aortic valve of a dog with vegetative valvular endocarditis.[52,85] *B. elizabethae*, a species for which rodents are the

reservoir, was PCR amplified and sequenced from an EDTA blood sample obtained from a dog that had experienced chronic weight loss culminating in sudden unexplained death.[166] *B. henselae*–specific antibodies were detected in the sera of healthy (10.8 %) and sick (28.5%) dogs from North Carolina[217] and in 14% of clinically healthy dogs that were tested.[119a] Many of the dogs showed seroreactivity to other vector-borne diseases, indicating the potential for combined infections. Cross-reactivity to infection with other closely related *Bartonella* cannot be eliminated in some animals. These observations indicate that, although presumably infrequent, the *Bartonella* spp. that frequently infect cats or rodents and are transmitted by fleas among reservoir hosts may cause disease manifestations in dogs. Genetic methods have been used to substantiate many of the *Bartonella* infections in dogs, inasmuch as they are presumably unnatural hosts and levels of organisms are low and difficult to cultivate. *Bartonella* is closely related to members of the α-*Proteobacteria*, and bacteria in this group or other as yet unclassified members of the genus *Bartonella* may also be important as causes of infection in dogs.[22]

Pathogenesis

Although as yet unproven, *B. vinsonii* subsp. *berkhoffii* is presumably transmitted to dogs by the bite of an infected tick. If similar to other *Bartonella* spp., the organism causes chronic intraerythrocytic and endothelial cell infections and is presumably well tolerated by the dog for extended periods. Similar to other highly adapted intracellular vector-transmitted pathogens, the factors that ultimately result in these organisms causing disease manifestations are yet to be determined. If similar to babesiosis, another intraerythrocytic pathogen, stress, hard work, parturition, or concurrent infection with other organisms may contribute to the development of pathology. Following experimental inoculation of SPF dogs with culture grown *B. vinsonii* subsp. *berkhoffii*, sustained suppression of peripheral blood CD8+ lymphocytes was noted accompanied by an altered cell surface phenotype and an increase in CD4+ lymphocytes in the peripheral lymph nodes.[179,181] Therefore infection with *B. vinsonii* subsp. *berkhoffii* might induce a degree of chronic immunosuppression that may predispose dogs to secondary infections, resulting in a wide array of clinical manifestations in naturally infected dogs.

The extent to which infection with *Bartonella* influences the pathophysiology of ehrlichiosis, a disease of much longer historical venue, deserves critical reappraisal. For example, infection with *Bartonella* in dogs concurrently infected with *E. canis* may contribute to the tendency to develop epistaxis (see Chapter 28). Of similar potential concern in both canine and human medicine is the finding of co-segregation of *Borrelia burgdorferi* (Chapter 45), *Anaplasma phagocytophilia* (previously *Ehrlichia equi* or human granulocytic ehrlichiosis, Chapter 28), *Babesia microti* (Chapter 77), and *Bartonella vinsonii* (*arupensis*) in *I. scapularis* ticks in the northeastern and north-central United States. Regional differences in tick species, accompanied by differences in the bacterial, viral, and protozoal organisms that ticks transmit, create substantial challenges for the clinician in regard to diagnosis and medical management. From an evolutionary perspective, it is obvious that vectors, vector-borne organisms, and animal and human hosts have developed a highly adapted form of mutual interaction. In general, vectors need blood for nutrition; the bacterial, rickettsial, and protozoal organisms need an intracellular environment to survive; and immunologically, most hosts appear able to support chronic infection with many vector-borne organisms for months to years without obvious deleterious effects. These factors serve to illustrate the potential difficulty in establishing causation in dogs or people co-infected with individual or multiple tick-transmitted pathogens.

Clinical Findings

B. vinsonii *subsp.* berkhoffii

The spectrum of disease associated with *Bartonella* infection in dogs and most other animal species is continuing to expand (Table 54-4). Endocarditis associated with *B. vinsonii* subsp. *berkhoffii* occurs in large breed dogs with a potential predisposition for aortic valve involvement.[22,27,52] Boxer dogs have been especially prevalent in this syndrome. In some dogs, intermittent lameness, bone pain, or fever of unknown origin can precede the diagnosis of endocarditis for several months, whereas other dogs will show an acute history of cardiopulmonary decompensation (Fig. 54-10). Cardiac arrhythmias secondary to myocarditis can be detected in dogs without echocardiographic evidence of endocarditis. Leukocytosis, thrombocytopenia, hypoalbuminemia, azotemia, and proteinuria with a clean sediment are found in a majority of affected dogs.[23,151]

Bartonella-induced granulomatous lymphadenitis, involving the left submandibular lymph node, was diagnosed in a dog based on seroreactivity to *B. vinsonii* subsp. *berkhoffii* antigens, visualization of Warthin-Starry silver-staining bacteria within the lymph node (Fig. 54-11), and PCR amplification followed by Southern blot hybridization.[180] Seven days before enlargement of the lymph node, the owners removed an engorged tick from the left ear. This case provides the best evidence to date that ticks can transmit *Bartonella* spp. to dogs and potentially to people. The granulomatous lymphadenitis in this dog is analogous to acute bartonellosis CSD in people, in which a scratch or bite injects the inoculum (usually *B. henselae*), rather than inoculation by the bite, of a tick.[115] Based on serologic evidence in dogs, *B. vinsonii* subsp. *berkhoffii* or closely related *Bartonella* spp. appear to contribute to the development of dermatologic lesions indicative of a cutaneous vasculitis, anterior uveitis, polyarthritis, rhinitis, meningoencephalitis, or immune-mediated hemolytic anemia.[23] Anterior uveitis and choroiditis were observed in one dog.[167]

Co-Infections

As with other tickborne illnesses, infections from multiple agents can occur simultaneously. This finding may cause confusion because of additional unexplained clinical signs that do not resolve with therapy. *Babesia canis* and *B. vinsonii* subsp.

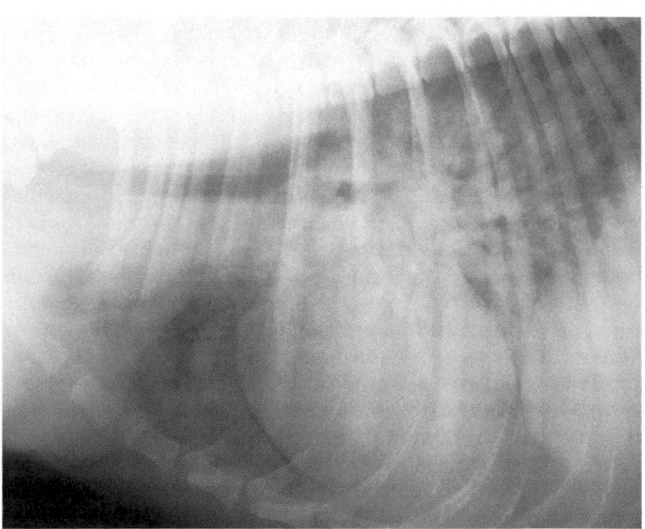

Fig 54-10 Perihilar pulmonary edema and cardiomegaly from aortic insufficiency–induced heart failure in a dog with *B. vinsonii* subsp. *berkhoffii* endocarditis. (Courtesy University of Georgia, Athens, Ga.)

Table • 54-4

Medical Problems of Dogs Associated with Bartonella *Infections*

B. vinsonii subsp *berkhoffii*
Granulomatous rhinitis[180]
Granulomatous to pyogranulomatous lymphadenomegaly[180]
Myocarditis[22,27]
Endocarditis[22,27]
Cardiac arrhythmias, lethargy, anorexia, vomiting, weakness, collapse, sudden death[22,27,151]
Cutaneous vasculitis[23]
Anterior uveitis[23,29]
Anterior uveitis and choroiditis[167]
Polyarthritis[23]
Meningoencephalitis[23]
Leukocytosis[22,23]
Thrombocytopenia[23]
Eosinophilia[23]
Hemolytic anemia[23]

B. henselae
Peliosis hepatis[126]
Granulomatous hepatitis[85]
Systemic illness receiving glucocorticoids[166]
Penetrating abdominal injury[166]

B. clarridgeiae
Lymphocytic hepatitis[85]
Endocarditis[52,151]

B. elizabethae
Moribund dog with chronic renal failure[166]

B. washoensis
Mitral valve endocarditis[54]

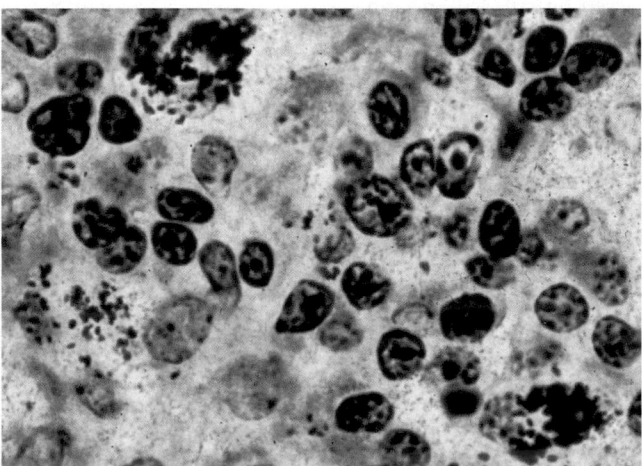

Fig 54-11 Granulomatous lymphadenitis in a dog with *B. vinsonii (berkhoffii)*. Coccobacilli are in clusters among lymphoid elements (Warthin-Starry silver, ×200). (Courtesy T. Brown and E. Breitschwerdt, North Carolina State University, Raleigh, N.C.)

berkhoffii infection occurred in a dog and resolution of signs only occurred after both infections were treated.[223]

Other Bartonellae

A dog with peliosis hepatis caused by *B. henselae* developed generalized weakness and abdominal distention. Biochemical abnormalities were high serum alkaline phosphatase (ALP) activity, hyponatremia, and hypochloremia. A serosanguineous abdominal effusion was found as were multiple fluid-filled cysts in the liver.[126] Another dog with chronic hepatis, where *B. henselae* DNA was detected, had fever, anorexia, weight loss, icterus, and increased serum ALP and alanine aminotransferase activities.[85]

B. elizabethae DNA was amplified and sequenced from the blood of a dog with chronic weight loss and sudden unexplained death presumably from cardiac dysfunction.[166] *B. clarridgeiae* DNA was amplified and sequenced from the aortic valve of a dog with vegetative valvular endocarditis and manifestations of third-degree heart block, causing heart failure.[52] *B. clarridgeiae* DNA was found in the liver of a Doberman pinscher with hepatic copper storage disease that had high hepatic enzyme activities on a routine preanesthetic blood testing.[85]

B. washoensis was isolated from a dog with a heart murmur and congestive heart failure caused by vegetative endocarditis.

Diagnosis

Clinical Laboratory Findings

Thrombocytopenia, anemia, which frequently can be immune mediated, and neutrophilic leukocytosis are the most commonly detected hematologic abnormalities in dogs that are seroreactive to *B. vinsonii* subsp. *berkhoffii* antigens. Thrombocytopenia is found in approximately one half of the dogs with disease manifestations. Eosinophilia is also found in approximately one third of infected dogs. Monocytosis can also occur in *B. vinsonii*–infected dogs, particularly those with endocarditis. Hemoglobinuria, generally unaccompanied by hematuria, is a frequent finding, particularly in dogs with immune-mediated hemolytic anemia. Serum biochemical abnormalities are usually very mild or nonexistent. Antinuclear antibodies have been detected in dog sera that were reactive to *B. vinsonii* subsp. *berkhoffii*, *E. canis*, and *Leishmania infantum* antigens.[216] These titers may represent cross-reactive antinuclear antibodies that are induced by exposure to bacterial DNA which has analogous sequences of the mammalian host.

Radiographic Imaging

Dogs infected with *B. henselae* may have hypoechoic cystic lesions in parenchymal organs (Fig. 54-12). In *B. vinsonii* subsp. *berkhoffii* infections, valvular endocarditis leads to cardiac failure, with the left side most commonly involved. Pulmonary edema will develop in cases of advanced insufficiency (see Fig 54-10). Echocardiographic changes are valvular vegetations and regurgitant flow can be observed with color-flow Doppler studies (Fig. 54-13, *A* and *B*).

Bacterial Isolation or Detection

Attempts to isolate *B. vinsonii* or other *Bartonella* from immunocompetent dogs with serologic or molecular evidence of *Bartonella* infection have not been successful in most instances. When using the currently recommended microbiologic techniques, considerable variation appears to exist in the degree of difficulty associated with the isolation of different *Bartonella* spp. from the blood of different animal species. Because blood culture is insensitive, serology and PCR amplification of *Bartonella* DNA are the mainstays of diagnosis. Because seroprevalence to *B. vinsonii* subsp. *berkhoffii* antigens

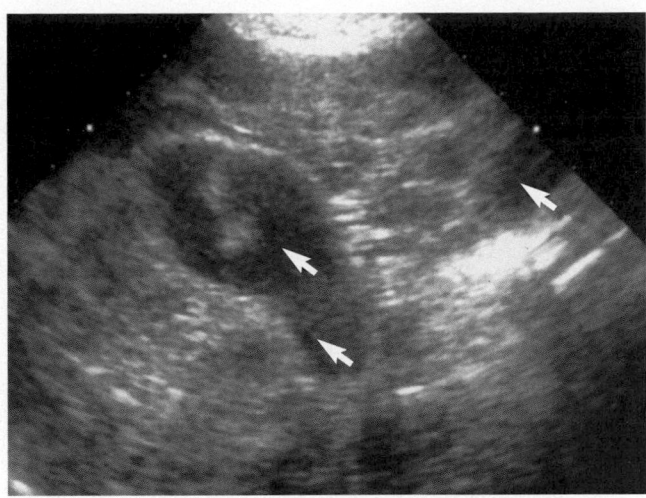

Fig 54-12 Ultrasonographic appearance of the liver of a dog with peliosis hepatis, associated with *B. henselae* infection showing hypoechoic areas (*arrows*) representing vascular peliosis. (Courtesy Barbara Kitchell, University of Illinois, Urbana, Ill.)

is infrequently detected (under 4%) in sick dog populations in endemic regions, detection of antibodies in a sick dog provides strong clinical evidence for prior exposure and potentially active infection. For this reason, treatment of seroreactive dogs or dogs from which *Bartonella* spp. DNA is detected in blood or tissue samples would be recommended. A titer of 1:64 or greater is considered indicative of prior exposure to or active infection with *B. vinsonii* subsp. *berkhoffii*. Given that isolation of *Bartonella* from dogs is usually unsuccessful, PCR testing on blood or tissues is the best method of detecting species other than *B. vinsonii* subsp. *berkhoffii*. Because more recent evidence indicates that *B. henselae* may contribute to the development of disease manifestations, such as polyarthritis and hepatitis, serologic testing for *B. henselae* antibodies has been validated using canine sera. In the southeastern United States, *B. henselae* seroprevalence is approximately 10% in healthy dogs and 26% in sick dogs.[217,218] This finding indicates that exposure to *B. henselae* is much more frequent than exposure to *B. vinsonii* subsp. *berkhoffii* is in dogs in the southeastern United States. Therefore, until additional research is completed, canine seroreactivity to *B. henselae* antigens should be interpreted with caution.

Serologic and molecular evidence indicates that coinfection in dogs with *Ehrlichia*, *Babesia*, *Rickettsia*, and *Bartonella* spp. may be more frequent than previously realized.* Because certain *Borrelia*, *Ehrlichia*, *Babesia*, and *Bartonella* spp. can cause chronic, insidious infection in dogs, the relative role of each organism to the pathogenesis of specific disease manifestations in a sick, naturally infected dog will remain difficult to establish in the clinical setting. When dealing with sick dogs with a history of tick exposure, clinicians should screen by serologic or molecular testing modalities for a panel of tick-transmitted pathogens.

Pathologic Findings

In dogs, pathologic findings associated with *Bartonella* spp. infections include endocarditis (Fig. 54-14), myocarditis, granulomatous lymphadenitis or hepatitis, and peliosis hepatis (Fig. 54-15). Multifocal areas of severe myocardial inflammation can be found in dogs with *B. vinsonii* endocarditis.

*References: 22, 25, 27, 139, 183, 220.

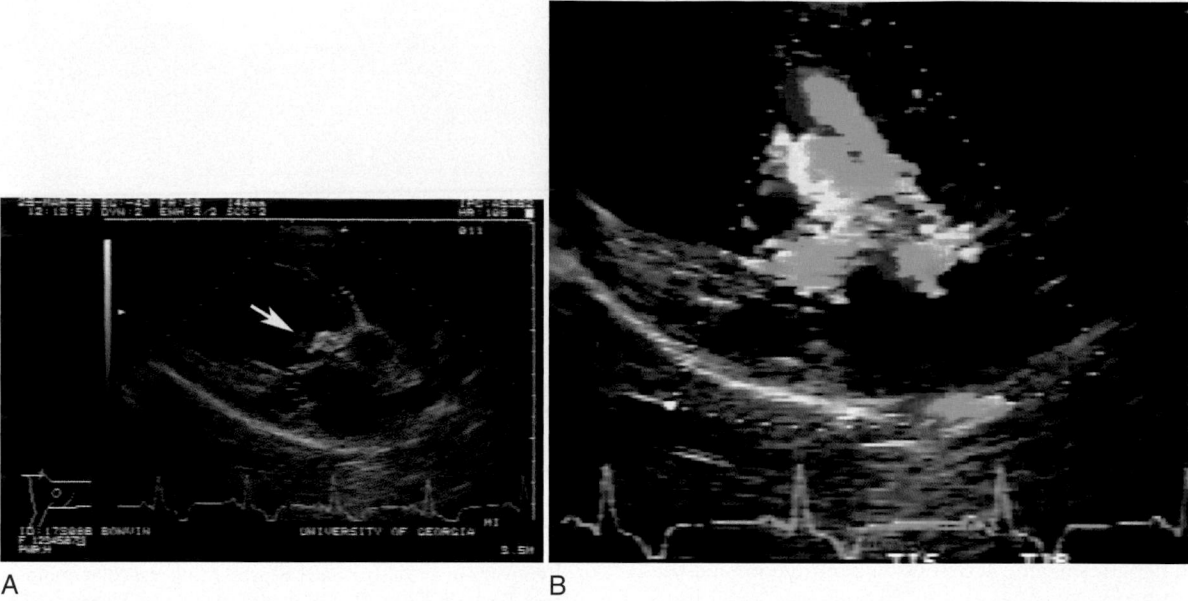

Fig 54-13 **A,** Echocardiogram showing vegetative lesion (*arrow*) on the aortic valve of a dog with *B. vinsonii* subsp. *berkhoffii* aortic endocarditis. **B,** Color flow Doppler study of the same dog showing regurgitant blood flow from aortic valvular leakage. (Courtesy University of Georgia, Athens, Ga.)

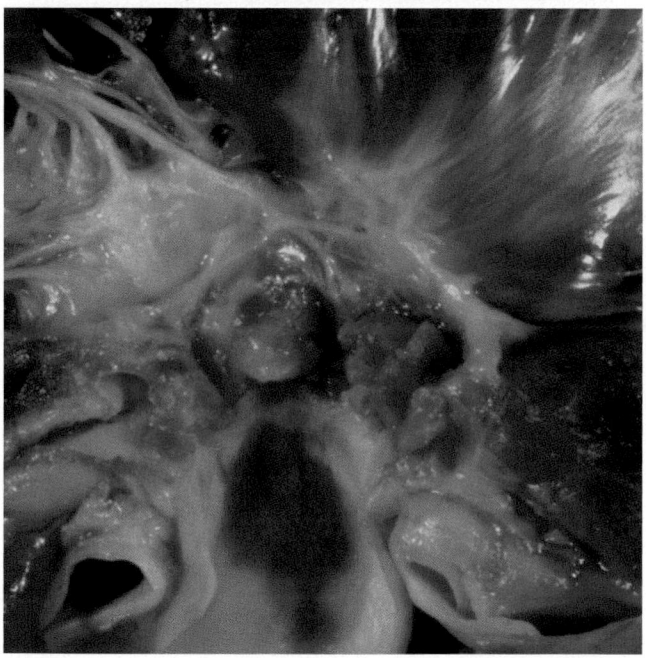

Fig 54-14 Heart valve with vegetative lesions caused by infection with *B. clarridgeae*. (Courtesy B. Chomel, University of California, Davis, Cal.)

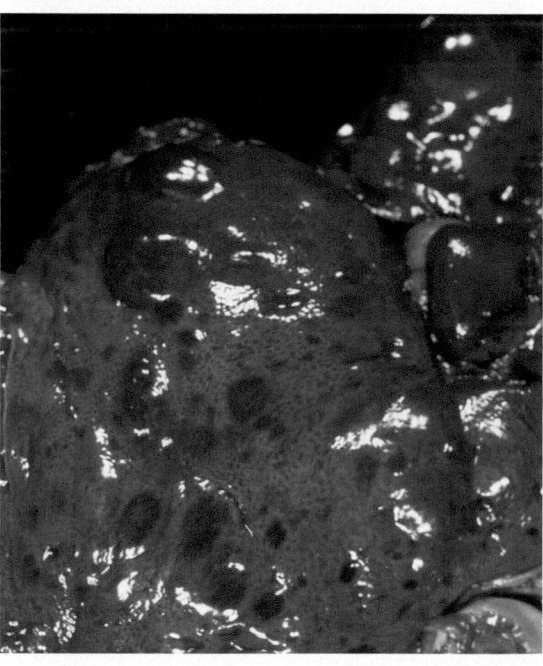

Fig 54-15 Liver from a dog with peliosis hepatis associated with *B. henselae* infection. (Courtesy Tim Fan, University of Illinois, Urbana, Ill.)

Although not specific for *Bartonella* infections, organisms can be detected in acutely diseased tissues, such as acute regional lymphadenitis, using silver stains (see Fig. 54-11). During chronic infections, organisms are presumably too few in number to be detected in tissues by silver staining, unless localized to heart valves.

Therapy

To date, an optimal protocol has not been established for the treatment of *Bartonella* infections in cats, dogs, or people.[162,200] Regardless of the antibiotic that is used for treatment, a long duration of antibiotic administration (4 to 6 weeks) may be necessary to eliminate the infection (Table 54-5). Macrolides (erythromycin, azithromycin) most probably represent the oral antibiotic class of choice for treating *Bartonella* infec-

Table • 54-5

Suggested Antibiotic Dosage for Bartonellosis Infections of Dogs[a]

DRUG[b]	DOSE[c] (mg/kg)	ROUTE	INTERVAL (HOURS)	DURATION (WEEKS)
Doxycycline	10–15	PO	12	4–6
Enrofloxacin	5	PO	12	4–6
Azithromycin[d]	5–10	PO	24	6

PO, By mouth.
[a]Efficacy of these drugs to treat dogs with these infections is poor, especially with endocardial lesions.
[b]See Drug Formulary, Appendix 8, for additional information on these drugs listed below.
[c]Dose per administration at specified interval.
[d]Azithromycin is given every 24 hours for the first week then every 48 hours for the next 5 weeks.

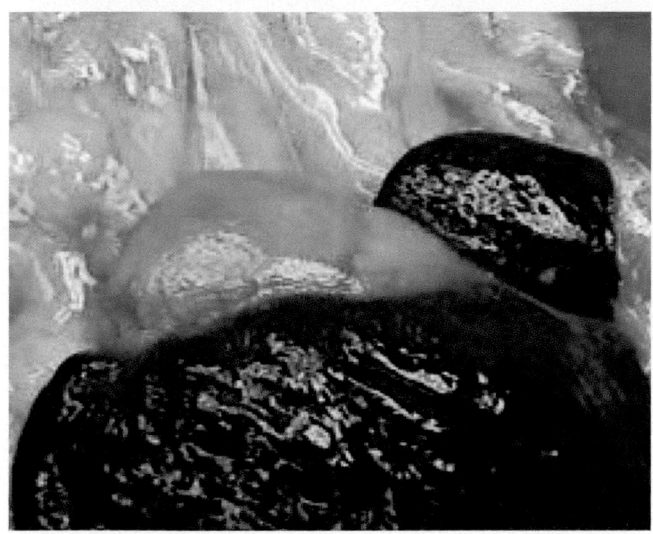

Fig 54-16 Abscess in the spleen from a dog (Fig. 54-13, *A* and *B*) with endocarditis from *B. vinsonii* subsp. *berkhoffii*. (Courtesy University of Georgia, Athens, Ga.)

tions.[162,200] Fluoroquinolones alone or in combination with amoxicillin have also elicited a positive therapeutic response in dogs, which is accompanied by a progressive decrease in *B. vinsonii* antibody titers.[23] Doxycycline may be effective for treatment of *B. vinsonii* subsp. *berkhoffii*, but data from cats experimentally or naturally infected with *B. henselae* or *B. clarridgeae* indicates that a high dose (10 mg/kg every 12 hours) for 4 to 6 weeks may be necessary to eliminate *Bartonella* infection in dogs, cats, or other animal species. *B. vinsonii* subsp. *berkhoffii* has been cultured from the blood of dogs that were treated with doxicycline for weeks to months for ehrlichiosis.[20] Following effective antimicrobial therapy, apparently, *Bartonella* serum antibody titers decrease rapidly (3 to 6 months) and are generally no longer detectable in dogs that recover completely following antimicrobial therapy. Persistence of *Bartonella* antibodies may be indicative of treatment failure. Therefore posttreatment serology may be a useful adjunct to determine therapeutic elimination of *Bartonella* infections. Dogs with *B. vinsonii* subsp. *berkhoffii* infection often have large valvular vegetative lesions by the time a diagnosis is made. Antibiotic penetration is difficult in these lesions, and signs of heart failure eventually occur. Surgical valve replacement is often used to treat people with this condition; however, it is not being done in animals.

Prevention

Increasingly, veterinarians play an important role in advising the public as to the epidemiologic and zoonotic implications associated with vector-borne pathogens. Nondomestic animals frequently serve as the primary reservoir for *Bartonella* spp. For example, the coyote appears to be an important reservoir host for *B. vinsonii* subsp. *berkhoffii*.[39] Although somewhat circumstantial, increasing evidence suggests that *Bartonella* spp. can be transmitted by fleas and ticks to cats, dogs, and people.[22,36,183] Based on scientific evidence generated during the last several decades, vector-transmitted pathogens can induce clinical manifestations ranging from acute fatal illness (e.g., Rocky Mountain spotted fever, ehrlichiosis, babesiosis, bartonellosis) to chronic debilitating disease states (ehrlichiosis, babesiosis, borreliosis, and bartonellosis). Therefore minimizing or eliminating flea and tick exposure is perhaps of greater veterinary and public health importance today than during any previous time in history. When rigorous flea and tick control measures are instituted, it is highly probable that transmission of *Bartonella* spp. will be greatly reduced or eliminated.[133]

Public Health Considerations

B. vinsonii subsp. *berkhoffii* was isolated from a human endocarditis patient.[202] The extent to which dogs can serve as a reservoir host for *B. vinsonii* subsp. *berkhoffii* or other *Bartonella* spp., such as *B. henselae*, *B. clarridgeae*, or *B. elizabethae*, is poorly characterized. Although dogs have been implicated in the direct transmission of *B. henselae* to people by a scratch or bite, this mode of transmission is as yet poorly established.

SUGGESTED READINGS*

25. Breitschwerdt EB, Hegarty BC, Hancock SI. 1998. Sequential evaluation of dogs naturally infected with *Ehrlichia canis*, *Ehrlichia chaffeensis*, *Ehrlichia equi*, *Ehrlichia ewingii*, or *Bartonella vinsonii*, *J Clin Microbiol* 36:2645-2651.

29. Breitschwerdt EB, Suksawat J, Chomel B, et al. 2003. The immunologic response of dogs to *Bartonella vinsonii* subspecies *berkhoffii* antigens as assessed by Western immunoblot analysis, *J Vet Diagn Invest* 15:349-354.

52. Chomel BB, MacDonald KA, Karsten RW, et al. 2001. Aortic valve endocarditis in a dog due to *Bartonella clarridgeiae*, *J Clin Microbiol* 39:3548-3554.

85. Gillespie TN, Washabau RJ, Goldschmidt MH, et al. 2003. Detection of *Bartonella henselae* and *Bartonella clarridgeae* DNA in hepatic specimens from two dogs with hepatic disease, *J Am Vet Med Assoc* 222:47-51.

*See the CD-ROM for a complete list of references.

97. Guptill L, Slater L, Wu C-C, et al. 1999. Immune response of neonatal specific pathogen-free cats to experimental infection with *Bartonella henselae*, *Vet Immunol Immunopathol* 71:233-243.
126. Kitchell BE, Fan TM, Kordick D, et al. 2000. Peliosis hepatis in a dog infected with *Bartonella henselae*, *J Am Vet Med Assoc* 216:519-523.
139. Kordick SK, Breitschwerdt EB, Hegarty BC, et al. 1999. Co-infection with multiple tick-borne pathogens in a Walker hound kennel in North Carolina, *J Clin Microbiol* 37:2631-2638.

151. MacDonald KA, Chomel BB, Kittleson MD, et al. 2004. A prospective study of canine infective endocarditis in Northern California (1999-2001): emergence of *Bartonella* as a prevalent etiologic agent, *J Vet Intern Med* 18:56-64.
180. Pappalardo BL, Brown T, Gookin JL, et al. 2000b. Granulomatous disease associated with *Bartonella* infection in 2 dogs, *J Vet Intern Med* 14:37-42.

*See the CD-ROM for a complete list of references.

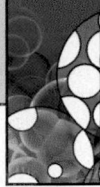

CHAPTER 55

Surgical and Traumatic Wound Infections

Craig E. Greene and Michael G. Dearmin

Virtually every surgical wound becomes contaminated, but only a few become infected. Bacterial infections have hindered successful healing of operative wounds throughout the history of surgery. The use of aseptic methods and minimization of tissue trauma were major breakthroughs in reducing postoperative infections. Subsequent development and use of antibiotics in surgery further reduced numbers of surgical infections. The prevalence of nosocomial infections is increasing again because of the more invasive and prolonged surgical procedures, synthetic implants being used today, and drug-resistant bacteria.

ETIOLOGY

The skin serves as a barrier to contamination but is compromised by surgical incisions, so the resulting wound must progress through the predictable stages of wound healing. As mentioned, contamination of the wound bed occurs with every surgical procedure, but most surgical wounds do not develop an infection. The success of wound healing is influenced by the overall health of the patient, the surgical procedure and type of wound created, and the type and number of contaminating organisms introduced into the wound.

The major source of bacteria contaminating surgical wounds is the patient's endogenous microflora. Skin-associated bacteria can be reduced but not eliminated by disinfection. Bacteria residing in the deeper parts of the skin such as the hair follicles and sebaceous glands are not removed or killed by preparative scrubbing, and they may enter deeper tissues during the initial incision. Nosocomial infections can also arise from inadequate sterilization of surgical equipment, operating room air flow, or the veterinary staff or hospital environment. Microbes indigenous to the hospital environment are most problematic because they are often antimicrobial resistant. A National Research Council (NRC) wound classification system of human surgical wound contamination can be applied to veterinary practice and is summarized in Table 55-1. In a study of 1574 dogs and cats with clean, clean contaminated, contaminated, or dirty surgical wounds, infection rates were 4.7%, 5%, 12%, and 10%, respectively.[6]

Anaerobic bacteria should always be assumed to be a component of mixed surgical infections,[13] or numerous therapeutic failures could result.

Clean surgical wounds involve surgical incision sites with no prior trauma or inflammation, no breaks in sterile technique during surgery, and mucosal surfaces such as the respiratory, genitourinary, or alimentary tracts that are not compromised. Infection rates in animals with clean surgical wounds are very low when experienced surgeons perform the procedures and in some reports have been as low as 0.9%.[32] *Clean contaminated surgical wounds* involve minor breaks in surgical technique (such as a torn glove), contact with normal mucosae of the gastrointestinal (GI) tract without spillage of visceral contents, or contact with uninfected genitourinary, biliary, or respiratory tracts. They also include otherwise clean procedures involving drain placement. Infection rates in people for these surgical procedures are less than 10% when aseptic techniques are used.[31] Oral antimicrobial prophylaxis may be needed for upper alimentary surgery when antacids have been used preoperatively to decrease gastric acidity, possibly causing gastric bacterial flora to proliferate. *Contaminated surgical wounds* have accidental GI tract spillage from penetration of an infected viscus or tissue, foreign bodies, devitalized tissue, or pus or involve a break in sterile technique. Bacterial contamination is suspected, but purulent discharge is absent. Clean lacerations of the skin or subcutaneous tissues that are not already infected are often categorized as contaminated. Contaminated surgical wounds have a high risk for developing postoperative infections and are two times more likely to become infected than clean contaminated wounds.[31] For example, after colonic spillage, isolated pathogens are often mixed, and up to five species may be present. Aerobic species usually include *Escherichia coli* and enterococci, and anaerobes include *Bacteroides* species, anaerobic cocci, and clostridia (see Chapter 89, Intraabdominal Infections).[29] *Infected (dirty) surgical or traumatic wound infections* are surgical wounds or nonsurgical defects that are already infected or have breaks in the skin associated with blunt trauma. Devitalized tissues, foreign bodies, or purulent discharges are often observed. Examples of dirty wounds include previously perforated viscera, devitalized wounds, compound fractures,

Table • 55-1

Classification of Surgical Wounds and Indications for Prophylaxis[a]

CLEAN	CONTAMINATED
1. Wound from elective surgery 2. Nontraumatic 3. No entry into mucosal surface 4. No break in asepsis 5. No inflammation or drainage encountered 6. 2.5%[c]–4.7%[d] infection rate	1. Fresh traumatic wound 2. Break in sterile technique 3. Spillage from GI surface 4. Acute inflammation 5. Dental prophylaxis[b] 6. Mucosal surgery 7. 5.8%[c]–12%[d] infection rate

CLEAN CONTAMINATED	INFECTED (DIRTY)
1. Bacterial entry into GI, genitourinary, or respiratory tract mucosae with minimal spillage or simple laceration 2. No unusual contamination, no suppurative inflammation 3. Minor break in asepsis 4. 4.5%[c]–5%[d] infection rate	1. Abscessed material present 2. Viscus perforated or fecal contamination 3. Older (>4-hr) traumatic wound 4. Suppuration 5. Major break in asepsis 6. 18.1%[c]–10%[d] infection rate

GI, Gastrointestinal.
[a]Modified from National Academy of Sciences/National Research Council, 1964. Postoperative wound infections: the influence of ultraviolet irradiation of the operating room and of various other factors, *Ann Surg* 160(Suppl): 1-132.
[b]For dental prophylaxis information, see Gingivitis and Periodontitis, Chapter 89.
[c]Prevalence of wound infections in dogs and cats from a veterinary teaching hospital.[42]
[d]Prevalence of wound infections in dogs and cats from a veterinary teaching hospital.[6]

foreign bodies, pus pockets, and acute cellulitis. Traumatic wounds are assumed to be contaminated and have a high risk of infection because microbes bypass the anatomic and immunologic barriers of the host. Necrotizing soft tissue infections are almost always colonized by numerous anaerobic and aerobic bacteria.[14] Bacteria from these wounds have often already spread systemically. Establishment of tissue infection depends on the type and depth of the injury, extent of damage to the vascular supply, extent of tissue devitalization, and length of delay in seeking treatment. With orthopedic injuries, posttraumatic osteomyelitis occurs when a broken bone has a contaminated open wound, an avascular fragment, and a milieu of damaged necrotic tissue or hemorrhage[5] (see Musculoskeletal Infections, Chapter 86). Subsequent to trauma and hospitalization, urinary and IV catheter infections are the most common infections, followed by pneumonia, intraabdominal infections, and wound infections. Responsible organisms are often staphylococci, *E. coli*, *Enterobacter*, *Pseudomonas*, and *Klebsiella*. (See Chapter 53 and reviews by Holt and Griffin[20] and Underman[40] for a discussion of bite wound infections; see Chapter 35 for a discussion of necrotizing fasciitis; see Chapter 94 for a thorough discussion of surgical preparations needed to prevent postoperative infections.)[32]

The NRC wound classification system has been widely used since its development in 1964. However, the risk for development of infection depends on many factors other than the wound environment. In an attempt to account for such other factors in estimating the risk of wound infection, the National Nosocomial Infections Surveillance System (NNISS) developed an index to predict risk of surgical infection.[10] A risk index score of 0, 1, 2, or 3 is based on the sum of three risk factors: (1) an American Society of Anesthesiologists preoperative assessment score of 3, 4, or 5 (Table 55-2); (2) an operation with an NRC classification of *contaminated* or *dirty*, and (3) an operative time of X hours, where X represents the time in which 75% of the given surgical procedures are completed. When the index was developed, it was compared with

Table • 55-2

American Society of Anesthesiologists: Preoperative Assessment Scores

I.	Healthy, no organic disease
II.	Local disease with no systemic signs
III.	Disease causing moderate systemic signs that limit function
IV.	Disease causing severe systemic signs that threaten life
V.	Moribund; not expected to live 24 hours with or without surgery

Modified from Owens WD, 1978. Physical status classification: a study on consistency of ratings, *Anesthesiology* 49:239-243.

the NRC classification of surgical wound infections from more than 80,000 surgical procedures. Surgical wound infection rates for the NRC classification system were 2.1%, 3.3%, 6.4%, and 7.1% for each respective category. The NNISS index surgical wound infection rates were 1.5% with zero risk factors present, 2.9% with one risk factor present, 6.8% with two risk factors present, and 13% with three risk factors present. Compared with the NRC classification, risk stratification was significantly increased with the NNISS index. Such an index may not be practical in many veterinary situations; however, the results of this comparison highlight the need to consider factors other than simply the wound type when evaluating infection risk.

The process of wound healing should be viewed as a complex interaction between the patient, the local wound environment, and the contaminating pathogen. Each facet of this interaction has many associated factors, the combination of which are unique to each situation. A thorough assessment of these factors and the common sources of perioperative contamination (Table 55-3) should be considered when prepar-

Table • 55-3

Sources of Infection Associated with Surgical Manipulations

PREOPERATIVE
Preexisting infection
Abscess formation
Traumatic wounds
Foreign bodies
Viscus perforation

INTRAOPERATIVE
Airborne microbes, inadequate air filtration
Operating room personnel
Hands or torn gloves
Mucosae or skin of patient
Drain placement
Hematogenous dissemination
Opening viscus
Surgical materials or suction tip

POSTOPERATIVE
Intravenous catheters
Urinary catheters
Drains
Hematogenous to implants

Table • 55-4

Methods for Reducing Risk of Surgical Wound Infection

PREOPERATIVE
Minimize length of preoperative hospitalization.
Treat with antimicrobial or do not perform surgery on animals with concurrent infections.
Treat remote sites of infection before operating.
Widely clip hair around incision site.
Shave skin just before surgery.
Prepare skin with povidone-iodine or chlorhexidine.

INTRAOPERATIVE
Use prophylactic antimicrobials when (1) manipulating contaminated tissues or intestine, (2) for prolonged surgical procedures (>3 hr), and (3) with synthetic implants.
Keep surgical room free of dust and insects.
Keep surgical field clean, and use routine antiseptic technique.
Ensure that incision and dissection are accurate and sharp.
Avoid excessive use of electrocautery.
Prevent normal skin or mucosal flora from contacting body cavities or internal tissues.
Minimize drying and exposure of handled tissues.
Surgically debride all tissues to healthy vascular areas.
Remove all foreign bodies, avascular tissue, and dead space.
Irrigate contaminated areas with antimicrobial or disinfectant solutions.
Avoid circulatory compromise.
Use meticulous hemostasis to decrease risk of tissue hemorrhage and blood clots (hematoma formation).
Place stab wounds drains at other than incision sites.
Delay surgical closure with dead space.
Handle soft tissues and abdominal viscera gently.
Change suction tips during prolonged surgical procedures.
Reduce number of people in the operating room.

POSTOPERATIVE
Delay closure of contaminated wounds.
Change intravenous catheters routinely.
Prevent aspiration pneumonia.
Keep drainage established, and irrigate healing wounds.

ing for each surgical procedure so that the most appropriate steps can be taken to minimize the risk for the development of postoperative infection (Table 55-4).

Preoperative preparation of the surgical site is a critical factor in preventing wound infection (see Chapter 94). Skin trauma produced during surgical preparation greatly increases the local bacterial population. Preoperative clipping time is an important factor in the development of postoperative wound infections.[6] Animals with surgical sites that were clipped before anesthesia induction rather than immediately before surgery were 3 times more likely to develop surgical wound infections. Animals clipped hours or days before the surgery because ultrasonographic studies were performed had a postoperative infection rate 3 times greater.[6] Animals with endocrinopathies such as hypothyroidism or hyperadrenocorticism are much more likely to develop postoperative wound infections.[28] Intact males were also found to have a higher risk of wound infection, which parallels findings in people and rodents and is presumably a result of the inhibitory effect of testosterone on some inflammatory cytokines.[36]

Use of proper surgical technique is perhaps the single most important factor in preventing postoperative infections. The risk of tissue infection is directly proportional to the increased amount of tissue handling and trauma. Vascular compromise to tissue, excessive electrocautery, and bleeding into tissue spaces are the major contributory factors. Foreign material and blood clots allow for adherence and replication of microorganisms. Experimentally, use of fibrinolytic agents prevents infections, abscesses, and adhesions after surgery. Bacteria that invade surgical sites or implants can remain dormant for months to years and although less common, the sites can be entered during the healing and recovery phases. In some animals, occult orthopedic infections develop. The bacteria remain at the site of the healed fracture but do not cause clinical or radiographic evidence of osteomyelitis.[12] The infection may persist locally until the orthopedic implants are removed.

Surgical wounds may be colonized with *Staphyloccoccus aureus*, a human commensal flora, which may lead to infections that are resistant to treatment if methicillin-resistant staphylococci are involved.[38]

Orthopedic implants have greatly improved treatment of bone fractures and noninfectious arthritis, but they are associated with an increased risk for orthopedic-device–related infection.[47] Immediately after implantation, all synthetic materials undergo a race in colonization of their surface by tissue and bacterial cells in the local area. In addition to body fluids containing serum proteins (albumin) and platelets, bacteria such as staphylococci have adhesins that attach bacteria to the biomaterial. Adherence leads to colonization of the foreign body surface, which can result in overt infection or bacteremia. Under these conditions, bacteria become sessile and develop antimicrobial resistance in this quiescent phase. Standard antimicrobial therapy at this time may eliminate the clinical illness, but the bacteria may persist in the biofilm. Various organisms such as coagulase-negative staphylococci and *Pseudomonas aeruginosa* produce a pathogenic biofilm composed of polysaccharide glycocalix (slime). With strict anaerobic conditions or with molecular identification techniques, anaerobes such as *Propionibacterium* species are often recognized.[39] They form an additional layer on the surface of prosthetic implants that can originate during the surgical procedure.[2] The glycocalix slime promotes intercellular adhesion, captures nutrients, and protects microorganisms from antibacterial therapy.

The use and timing of prophylactic antimicrobial therapy affects infection rates in animals with clean surgical wounds. In a study at a teaching hospital, 72.5% of 1100 animals with clean surgical wounds received perioperative antibiotics, which was associated with a lower infection rate.[42] However, in another comparable study in which 41% of 1146 animals with clean surgical wound received antibiotics at varying times, the infection rate varied according to the timing of the antibiotic administration.[6] Animals with clean wounds receiving perioperative antibiotics, no antibiotics, or postoperative antibiotics had infection rates of 2.2%, 4.4%, and 8.2%, respectively. In another study at a teaching hospital, dogs undergoing elective orthopedic surgery were divided into three groups and given either no antimicrobials, penicillin G, or cefazolin 30 minutes before surgery, and again if the surgery lasted longer than 90 minutes.[46] Dogs in both antibacterial treatment groups had lower infection rates, therefore the control group was abandoned. Results in these studies emphasize the importance of having maximal antibacterial activity at the time of the surgical procedure. (See Tables 55-5 and 55-6 and the Drug Formulary, Appendix 8, for a list of dosages.)

The duration of surgery has a major influence on the overall risk of wound infection.[28] Drying of tissue and airborne contamination are also major factors. Tissue counts of less than 100,000 organisms per gram of tissue are needed to ensure proper incisional healing. Bacterial counts may double during each additional hour of operative time. Nosocomial infections develop in 1% of patients after procedures lasting less than 30 minutes and in 14% after procedures lasting more than 3.5 hours. In a study of dogs and cats the risk for postoperative infection was 2 times higher for those undergoing procedures lasting 90 minutes than for those undergoing procedures lasting 60 minutes.[6] Ultra-clean surgical rooms have been shown to reduce the prevalence of postoperative infection; however, in most operating rooms with high-volume air exchange and perioperative antimicrobial use in extended procedures, the risk of postoperative infections can be minimized. For each additional person in the operating room, the risk of surgical-site infection in dogs and cats was 1.3 times greater.[74a]

Localized infections in areas far from the surgical site can spread to operative wounds hematogenously. Bacterial translocation denotes the spread of viable bacteria from the lumen of the GI tract into the blood stream via the portal circulation. Manipulation of the intestines during surgery may lead to distant postsurgical infection or sepsis. The majority of culturable translocating bacteria in mesenteric lymph nodes and blood are *E. coli*.[34] In corresponding experiments, anesthesia without intestinal manipulation produced minimal bacteremia. Prolonged fasting (greater than 48 hours) before and after surgery caused increased bacteremia in animals with intestinal manipulation, presumably because of intestinal stasis and bacterial overgrowth. Bacterial translocation also increases with endotoxemia, abdominal irradiation, splenectomy, biliary obstruction, and hemorrhagic shock.

Host immunosuppression by a concurrent disease or an inherent immunodeficiency disorder may increase the risk of postoperative infection. In a study of dogs that were immuno-deficient because of treatment with glucocorticoid and aza-thioprine had a higher prevalence of infected vascular grafts than immunocompetent dogs.[2] Diabetes mellitus, hyper-adrenocorticism, obesity, and malnutrition are predisposing factors. An immunodeficient state may be induced in traumatized animals as a result of hemorrhage, glucocorticoid therapy, and reduced cell-mediated immunity from cytokine dysregulation. Previous urinary outflow obstruction has been shown to predispose cats to a higher risk of postoperative infection after perineal urethrostomy than cats without obstruction that are having the same surgery.[18] Although anesthesia has been associated with in vitro alterations in leukocyte chemotaxis, mobility, and lymphocyte stimulation, actual documentation of impaired host immune responses in vivo has not been confirmed. Bacterial colonization of suction tips was a source of infection during surgery in dogs and cats.[37] Staphylococci were the most common contaminating organisms, and they appeared to originate from operating room air.

Delayed wound healing caused by excessive numbers of sutures, foreign implants, or devascularized tissues can serve as a focus for infection after contamination.[2] Dead space between tissues should be avoided, and all surgical wounds should be closely approximated. Although surgically placed drains allow for removal of blood or pus from dead space areas, they may delay closure or allow entry of organisms into wounds. Intravenous (IV) catheters and intubation used in trauma patients or those that have undergone surgery also increase the risk of infection. Drains and IV catheters should be removed as soon as possible during the recovery period to minimize the direct or hematogenous colonization of the surgical site.

Prolonged hospitalization increases the risk of infection with antimicrobial-resistant bacteria. Wet dressings reduce the fibrin seal formation on a wound and may allow for the maceration of tissue and proliferation of bacteria at the incision site. Prophylactic antibiotics should not be used indiscriminately during surgical procedures and should only be used when contamination of tissues is expected (see Antimicrobial Prophylaxis in this chapter).

CLINICAL FINDINGS

The signs of infection are often masked in the traumatized patient, and complicating infection should be considered when any clinical signs worsen. Fever and leukocyte changes are not always predictive of infection. Some local inflammation or serous discharge should be expected at the incision site of any surgical procedure. A diagnosis of posttraumatic infection can be made from soft tissue swelling, hyperesthesia, fever, and leukocytosis. Additional signs that may be associated with systemic infections are increased respiratory distress, hyperglycemia or hypoglycemia, renal failure, thrombocytopenia, icterus, and severe mental depression.

DIAGNOSIS

Postsurgical infections are characterized locally by heat, swelling, pain, and erythema at the incision site. Unfortunately, the same signs may be part of the initial healing phases after surgery. Systemic manifestations of infection, such as rectal temperature elevations and leukocytoses or left shifts in the hematologic test findings, are more indicative of infection. A correlation has been made between elevation of rectal temperature 24 hours postoperatively and increased duration of surgical procedure.[42] However, an elevation of the rectal temperature the day after surgery does not always indicate the development of wound infection. A wound is considered

Table • 55-5

Indications and Drugs for Antimicrobial Prophylaxis or Treatment in Surgery

SURGICAL CLASS	EXAMPLES	ASSOCIATED BACTERIA	RECOMMENDED THERAPY[a]	
			FIRST CHOICE	ALTERNATIVES
Prophylaxis				
Clean	Routine surgery	None	None	None
Clean contaminated	Genital surgery	Aerobes: gram-negative Anaerobes	Cefazolin[b]	Fluoroquinolone
	Prolonged (> 3 hrs) surgery, orthopedic prosthesis, amputation, open fracture reduction	*Escherichia coli*, staphylococci, streptococci	Cefazolin[b]	β-lactamase-resistant penicillin
	Intra-abdominal	Aerobes: gram-negative Anaerobes	Cefoxitin[c]	Gentamicin, metronidazole
	Dentistry	Aerobes: gram-positives and anaerobes	Cefazolin[b]	Ampicillin, amoxicillin, chloramphenicol
Contaminated	Bite wounds	Aerobes and anaerobes	Ampicillin or amoxicillin-clavulanate	Clindamycin
	Enterotomy with leakage, abdominal trauma	Aerobes: streptococci, enterococci Anaerobes: bifidobacteria, clostridia, fusobacteria, *Bacteroides*	Cefoxitin[c]	Aminoglycoside, metronidazole
	Biliary infection cholecystectomy	Enterobacteriaceae (*E. coli, Klebsiella, Proteus*), *Bacteroides*, *Clostridium*	Cefoxitin[c], cefotaxime[d]	Gentamicin
	Colonic resection[e]	*E. coli, Bacteroides*	Neomycin and metronidazole preanesthesia, and enemas	Cefoxitin, gentamicin, clindamycin
Treatment				
Infected	Abscesses	Aerobes	Ampicillin or amoxicillin-clavulanate	Aminoglycoside, clindamycin
	Ruptured bowel, colonic leakage	Anaerobes	Cefotaxime[d]	Metronidazole
	Pyometra	Aerobic and anaerobes	Cefazolin[b]	Fluoroquinolone

[a]For additional information, see Drug Formulary, Appendix 8.
[b]Can substitute another first-generation drug; see also Table 34–4 and Drug Formulary, Appendix 8.
[c]Can substitute another second-generation drug; see also Table 34–4 and Drug Formulary, Appendix 8.
[d]Can substitute another third-generation drug; see also Table 34–4 and Drug Formulary, Apendix 8.
[e]Oral therapy starting 48 hours before surgery and before anesthesia includes neomycin and metronidazole, along with enemas for cleaning. Parenteral cefoxitin may also be given during the procedure. Routine prophylaxis not recommended with soft tissue (cyst removal, laparotomy not involving a viscus, inguinal hernia repair, mastectomy, tonsillectomy, simple lacerations); neurologic (laminectomy, fenestration); ophthalmic (lens extraction); orthopedic (rhinotomy or rhinoplasty).

Table • 55-6

Recommended Preoperative Therapy for Surgical Prophylaxis

DRUG[a]	SPECIES	DOSE[b]	ROUTE	TIMING (MINUTES PREOPERATIVELY)	ANTIBACTERIAL SPECTRUM AND INDICATIONS
Penicillin G	D	40,000 U/kg	IV	30	Gram-positive and anaerobic bacteria, with some antibacterial resistance noted among isolates
Amoxicillin-clavulanate	D	10–20 mg/kg	PO	30	Most gram-positive and gram-negative aerobes and anaerobes; first-choice drug for most bite wounds
	D	13.75 mg/kg	PO	30	
	C	10–20 mg/kg	PO	30	
Ampicillin, (amoxicillin)	B	22 mg/kg	PO	30	Some gram-positive and gram-negative aerobes
	B	11–22 mg/kg	SC, IV	30	
Ticarcillin	D	20–50 mg/kg	IV	30	Gram-positive and gram-negative aerobes and anaerobes
Cefazolin[c]	B	20–30 mg/kg	IV	16–60	First-generation drug: gram-positive aerobes, oral, gastroduodenal; and orthopedic surgery; clean surgery
Cefoxitin	B	30 mg/kg	IV	16–60	Second-generation drug: gram-negative aerobes
Cefotaxime	B	15–30 mg/kg	IV	16–60	Third-generation drug: gram-negative aerobes or anaerobes; ileocolic and gynecologic surgery
Clindamycin	B	5–11 mg/kg	PO	16–60	Gram-positive aerobes and anaerobes
Metronidazole	B	10 mg/kg	PO, IV	16–60	Anaerobes

B, Dog and cat; D, dog; C, cat; IV, intravenous; PO, by mouth; SC, subcutaneous.
[a]For additional information, see Drug Formulary, Appendix 8.
[b]Dose per administration at specified interval.
[c]Drug concentrations of greater than 4 μg/ml were achieved in the surgical wound by using 20 mg/kg every 6 hours.[33] A second dose is given if the surgical procedure lasts longer than 90 minutes.[46] (See Table 34-4 for a review of the cephalosporin-generation drugs.)

infected if during the postoperative period (1) discharge from the incision site is found, or (2) dehiscence develops in one or more wound layers and is accompanied by drainage, warmth, or swelling (Fig. 55-1). Wounds involving intestinal perforation and burns are always contaminated and therefore require immediate attention. With deeper wounds, radiographs of the skeleton or ultrasonograms of the soft tissues may reveal deeper tissue damage, soft tissue swelling, or gas formation. With chronic orthopedic infections, bony lysis, bone proliferation, or sequestra develop. Cytology of exudates and biopsy or culture of tissues is most definitive. Deep-sample culturing of infected wounds must be performed with surgical entry or needle penetration because surface contaminants are common. Material obtained in this way should be sealed in an airtight container and submitted to a laboratory as soon as possible so that the anaerobic agents that often are present can be cultured.

THERAPY

Tables 55-4 and 55-5 describe drug indications and recommendations for surgical prophylaxis. Extensive debridement or surgical drainage of wounds may be required to prevent wound infection and reduce extensive swelling or abscess formation. Wounds should be covered to prevent extensive drying of devitalized tissues, and drainage should be encouraged by incomplete closure or drain placement. Occlusive dressings containing adequate absorbent material should be changed whenever drainage is present. To encourage formation of sufficient granulation tissue, limbs should be immobilized or supported. Chronic nonhealing scar tissue should be resected from the wound. Prolonged hospitalization and indiscriminate use of topical or systemic antibiotics favor the overgrowth of resistant bacteria. Surgical drains, IV catheters, and intubations in trauma patients also increase the risk of infections. For intraabdominal infections and suspected or documented ruptured viscus, antimicrobial therapy should be provided to combat fecal flora, including anaerobes and gram-negatives such as Enterobacteriaceae species (see Intraabdominal Infections, Chapter 89). For orthopedic injuries with mandibular and maxillary or open fractures, penicillins or cephalosporins, respectively, are often administered. If implants are involved, stabilization, irrigation, antimicrobial carriers, implant removal, or wound debridement is often indicated.[11]

PREVENTION

Skin Disinfection and Wound Irrigation

Antiseptics are important for reducing the prevalence of postoperative infections. Tincture of chlorhexidine (0.5% in 70% ethanol), povidone-iodine (0.75% available iodine), and detergents of chlorhexidine (4%) or iodine are the most commonly used agents for skin preparation.[30,32] Alcoholic solutions of chlorhexidine are preferable to aqueous preparations because the alcohol is bactericidal and promotes drying of the exposed lesions. Various formulations of povidone-iodine have no deleterious effects on wound healing.[17] Chlorhexidine diacetate as a 0.05 % w/v nondetergent antiseptic solution has been used to lavage open wounds and prevent contamination of dog tissues with *Staphylococcus intermedius*.[25] Chlorhexidine gluconate and alcohol were equally effective as stabilized glutaraldehyde, with or without alcohol, as a presurgical skin disinfectant in dogs.[143a] Chlorhexidine solution has been more effective than povidone-iodine as an antibacterial treatment.[24,35] In some instances, povidone-iodine solutions have harbored such organisms as *Pseudomonas*. In addition, the iodophors have less residual antibacterial activity than chlorhexidine. Despite its effectiveness, chlorhexidine can be irritating to intraarticular structures.[1] Although effective, hexachlorophene is no longer used because of its potential neurotoxicity in animals and people. Traumatic wounds are commonly irrigated with sterile saline. However, in a study with children, lacerations had the same infection rate whether irrigated with sterile saline or running tap water,[41] suggesting that physical flushing is more important in contaminated traumatic injuries to reduce bacterial levels. With regard to tissue injury, Ringer's lactate has been less traumatic than normal saline or tap water to canine connective tissues in vitro,[8] so it might be the most desirable flush solution to preserve tissue healing (see Bite Wound Infections, Chapter 53).

Surgical Equipment Disinfection

The disinfection of surgical tools and facilities is an intimate part of the operative procedure. (See Chapter 94 for a review of hospital and equipment disinfection procedures.) The animal's hair should always be shaved and its skin prepared for surgery before it enters the operating room. Care should be taken not to injure the skin during the clipping procedure. Surgical equipment should be appropriately sterilized using steam autoclaves or ethylene oxide rather than cold disinfection and should be stored in dust-free, enclosed cabinets. Cold disinfection should be avoided when possible because it may be associated with an increased risk of infections from soil saprophytes such as *Clostridium tetani* (see Chapter 43). All surfaces in operating rooms that do not contact the patient should be routinely disinfected with phenolic compounds. Floors can be washed with disinfectants and wet mopped or polished. Wet mops or vacuums with filtered exhaust elements can pick up excess disinfectant and loose debris. Built-up disinfectant films can be removed with a solution of 0.12 L (one-half cup) of vinegar in 3.8 L (1 gallon) of water. Dry mops and brooms should never be used to clean hospital floors because they disseminate microorganisms in dust. Personnel should wear face masks to minimize aerosol contamination in surgery areas. Washing hands and wearing gloves are superior to hand washing alone in minimizing the spread of skin microflora to the patient during surgery. Antisepsis of the skin at the incision site is similar to the procedure used to prepare IV catheter sites, but a final application of tincture of iodine or iodophor solution is used just before the animal is draped. (See Chapter 94 for a discussion of cleanliness and sterility of anesthesia and nebulizer equipment.)

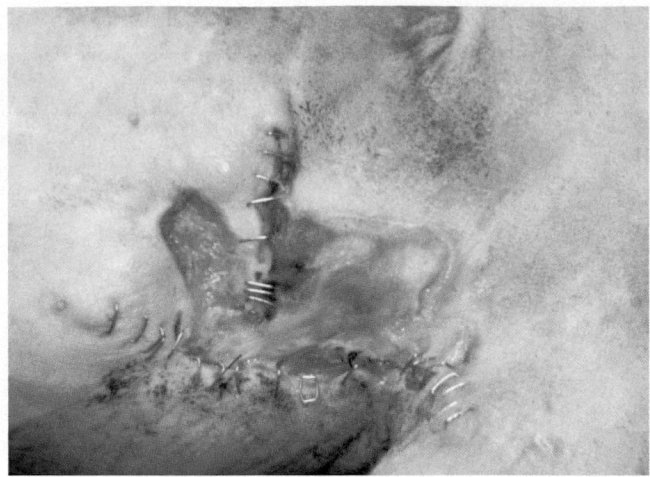

Fig 55-1 Secondary closure in a wound contaminated by bacteria. At this stage, the area must heal by secondary granulation tissue.

Lavage

Contaminated wounds should be lavaged with copious amounts of prewarmed saline solution. Pressure is delivered by a 35-ml syringe and 18-gauge needle or similar size catheter. Lavage without jet irrigation is not effective. Local antibiotic instillation may achieve higher concentrations of drugs in the desired tissue with minimal toxicity. Because antibiotics are readily absorbed, they should not be instilled in body cavities. Chlorhexidine has been used as a successful wound disinfectant.

Antimicrobial Prophylaxis

A majority of nosocomial infections occur in hospitalized animals undergoing surgery. Preoperative and intraoperative antimicrobials have been shown repeatedly to reduce the prevalence of postoperative infection when strict antisepsis cannot be maintained, such as during surgery of the bowel, respiratory, or biliary tracts or of the oropharyngeal region. (See Chapter 89 for a discussion of prophylaxis during dental procedures.) Organisms that contaminate relatively avascular subcutaneous tissues, bone fragments, or serosal surfaces are often commensals of skin and mucosal surfaces. In certain surgical situations, antimicrobial therapy administered before the procedure for an anticipated infection may be beneficial (see Table 55-5). Antimicrobial prophylaxis was not better than placebo in decreasing infection rates for short-term, clean surgical procedures in dogs and cats performed by experienced surgeons.[23,43] However, when veterinary surgical procedures required longer than 90 minutes, antimicrobial therapy was beneficial in reducing infection rates.[42] In contrast, the administration of antibiotics significantly reduced the frequency of wound infection in clean surgical procedures performed by senior veterinary students.[42] In human surgeries, procedures of more than 2 hours have been associated with a much higher prevalence of postoperative infection.[31] Prophylactic antimicrobial therapy is beneficial in conjunction with surgical drainage of abscesses.

The success of prophylaxis depends significantly on the chosen antimicrobial (see Tables 55-5 and 55-6). Because of their low toxicity and effectiveness against the commonly infecting staphylococci, cephalosporins have been the mainstay of prophylaxis for surgery. Because of its prolonged duration of activity, cefazolin has been a popular choice among surgeons.

The timing of administration of antibiotics is an important factor in the prevention of surgical wound infections. The success involves timing the administration of the drug slightly before (less than 1 hour) or during the surgery to achieve the maximum possible concentration during the operative procedure and not continuing the administration for longer than 24 hours after surgery. Parenteral infusion has been preferred for antimicrobial prophylaxis, with an optimal administration time of between 16 and 60 minutes, depending on the route of administrations before the first incision.[15] Administration more than 1 hour before surgery is associated with lower drug levels at the time of incision. If antimicrobial prophylaxis is considered as an afterthought, it will *not* be effective.

Oral therapy is given 1 hour before, intramuscular injections one-half hour before, and IV therapy immediately at the beginning of the anesthetic induction as an IV bolus (see Table 55-6). With the exception of colonic surgery, in which prophylaxis is started earlier, the initial dose of a systemically administered drug should be given parenterally at the time of anesthetic induction. For colonic surgery, systemic antimicrobial therapy combined with mechanical cleaning of the large bowel to reduce the microflora is started 48 hours before surgery. Enemas with isotonic lavage fluids and cathartics are often used.

Even with clean surgeries, the operating field is considered to be contaminated if the procedure lasts longer than 3 hours. Another dose of antimicrobial should be given at that time to maintain concentrations during the operation. Providing another dose of the drug at the time of closure may be needed if the procedure takes longer than 3 more hours. Antimicrobials penetrate formed tissue exudates and blood clots poorly but are readily incorporated into clots if they are present in the plasma during the clot formation. The risk of contamination is present until a firm fibrin seal forms between the wound edges 3 to 5 hours postoperatively. For this reason a final dose of antimicrobial is recommended during contaminated procedures when the closure is being completed. Perioperative antimicrobials should be chosen based on the procedure being performed and the contaminants most likely to enter the wound site. Specific dose and frequency guidelines are available based on the pharmacokinetic and pharmacologic variables of the chosen antimicrobial.

When contamination is suspected but infection is not documented, antimicrobial therapy should never be given for more than 12 to 24 hours after surgery. Measures should be taken to reduce the risk of infection after antimicrobial prophylaxis because infection with resistant organisms is more likely. Hospitalization, stress, and invasive procedures should be avoided in immunosuppressed patients. If perioperative antibiotics are used, they should be bactericidal drugs with effectiveness that is limited as much as possible to the suspected contaminant (see Table 55-6). Systemic antibiotics are thought to enter host tissues at the time of surgery and should be maintained at high concentrations during the entire procedure. A full course of antibiotics at the proper dosage should be provided; anything less is often ineffective in animals with an adequate immune system. If results of susceptibility testing conflict or indicate that organisms are not susceptible to a particular drug, antibiotics should not be changed if the patient appears to be responding.

Antimicrobial chemoprophylaxis has several disadvantages, some of which are so serious that the risks might outweigh the benefits. For example, bacterial resistance or drug toxicities may develop. In addition, chloramphenicol may interfere with barbiturate metabolism, some cephalosporins (cefamandole, cefoperazone, and cefotetan) may cause hypoprothrombinemia, and aminoglycosides may cause neuromuscular blockade or nephrotoxicity. Prophylaxis with antimicrobials may suppress normal microflora and increase the risk of infection with resistant microorganisms (superinfection). Multiple antibiotic-resistant bacteria such as enterococci, staphylococci, and *Klebsiella* species have been isolated that have increasing levels of resistance. (See Antimicrobial Chemotherapy, Chapter 34, and the Drug Formulary, Appendix 8, for additional information on drugs and their dosages.)

SUGGESTED READINGS*

6. Brown DC, Conzemius MG, Shofer F, et al. 1997a. Epidemiologic evaluation of postoperative wound infections in dogs and cats. *J Am Vet Med Assoc* 210:1302-1306.

19. Heldman E, Brown DC, Shofer F. 1999. The association of propofol usage with postoperative wound infection rate in clean wounds: a retrospective study. *Vet Surg* 28:256-259.

28. Nicholson M, Beal M, Shofer F, et al. 2002. Epidemiologic evaluation of postoperative wound infection in clean contaminated wounds: a retrospective study of 239 dogs and cats. *Vet Surg* 31:577-581.

37. Sturgeon C, Lamport AI, Lloyd DH, et al. 2000. Bacterial contamination of suction tips used during surgical procedures performed on dogs and cats. *Am J Vet Res* 61:779-783.

46. Whittem TL, Johnson AL, Smith CW, et al. 1999. Effect of perioperative prophylactic antimicrobial treatment in dogs undergoing elective orthopedic surgery. *J Am Vet Med Assoc* 215:212-216.

74a. Eugster S, Schawalder P, Gaschen F, et al. 2004. A prospective study of postoperative surgical site infections in dogs and cats, *Vet Surg* 33:342-550.

*See the CD-ROM for a complete list of references.

Fungal Diseases

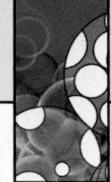

CHAPTER • 56

Laboratory Diagnosis of Fungal and Algal Infections

Spencer S. Jang and Richard L. Walker

Specific diagnosis of fungal and algal infections in animals requires laboratory procedures that include direct microscopic examination and culture, frequently supported by serologic tests. Many such direct examinations and primary cultures and some serologic tests are now well within the scope of in-office diagnostic procedures for veterinary practice. The development of improved methods for mycologic diagnosis is directed at rapid procedures using prepackaged identification kits and reagents, serologic kits, automated systems, and molecular techniques.[16] In a high proportion of such cases, confirmation by a specialty laboratory will still be necessary to establish a definitive diagnosis. Refer to Appendix 5, Laboratory Testing for Infectious Diseases of Dogs and Cats.

SPECIMENS FOR LABORATORY DIAGNOSIS

A satisfactory sample should be representative of the focus of infection and of adequate size to permit direct examination and culture. Except in systemic infections suggesting fungemia and requiring blood culture, samples should be obtained from the site of infection as indicated by lesions, signs, or symptoms. Because systemic mycoses are usually acquired via the respiratory tract, lung tissue or airway exudates are preferred samples. In certain disseminated mycotic infections, urine may also be an appropriate specimen to culture.

SAMPLE COLLECTION

When collecting skin scrapings for dermatophyte culture, clean the lesion, particularly the periphery, with 70% alcohol. Avoid using iodine, which is harmful to dermatophytes. Surface antisepsis, when feasible, aids in minimizing the collection of environmental bacterial and fungal contaminants and thereby ensures a meaningful result. Before venipuncture, the skin must be disinfected by swabbing with 70% alcohol followed by 2% iodine.

Scrapings for dermatophyte culture are best obtained with a scalpel blade or the edge of a glass microscope slide from the marginal, most active portion of the ringworm lesion. Use of a Wood's lamp may identify hairs infected with certain dermatophyte species. The hair roots are then plucked with forceps for culture. Nails are collected by clipping. The surface of heavily keratinized structures is scraped away for access to deeper portions. Claw surfaces are disinfected with alcohol. The surface of skin pustules, nodules, vesicles, and so forth is disinfected, and aspiration is done with sterile needle and syringe. A biopsy may be required if fungi fail to grow from the aspirate, scraping, or swab. Normal tissue, along with portions from all zones of the lesion, should be taken. Opened skin lesions are not disinfected or cleaned because such procedures may remove or kill the organisms of interest.

Swabs are of limited value in fungal isolation, and their use is discouraged. If no alternative collection method is available, specimens received on swabs in a suitable transport medium (see Chapter 33) should be cultured without delay. Swabs for direct smears, preferably, should not consist of cotton because recovery rates are poor, and inexperienced observers may mistake cotton fibers for hyphae.

Blood for cultures are collected directly via syringe and needle into conventional and biphasic blood culture bottles, automated blood systems, and lysis-centrifugation systems (see Isolation).[1,11] A fresh needle is used for transfer of blood, 1 ml per 9 ml of culture medium, from syringe to the culture bottle. Blood samples taken from indwelling intravenous (IV) catheters are not recommended.[1,11]

Urine is best taken by percutaneous cystocentesis, which ensures a sample uncontaminated by bacterial or fungal flora in the lower genitourinary tract (see Chapter 91).

Stool specimen cultures for diagnosis of fungal infections of the gastrointestinal tract are generally misleading. Biopsy specimens for histologic examination is best.

Fluids and contents of abscesses are collected through aspiration by needle and syringe. Large volumes, adequate for centrifugation, are best. Any granules should be included and characterized. Bone marrow is similarly sampled by needle and syringe or core needle biopsy. At least 3 ml of cerebral spinal fluid (CSF) is desirable via lumbar or cisternal puncture. For lung sampling, a transtracheal or bronchial wash or bronchial brushing is done (see Chapter 88).

Necrotic material or curettings and other surgically collected material should be handled aseptically pending examination and culture. Corneal lesions are sampled by scraping several times with a sterile Kimura spatula or nylon brush (see Fig. 93-9). Slide preparation and culture are done at the site and time of collection.

TRANSPORTATION AND PRESERVATION

For referral to a diagnostic laboratory, tissue and fluid samples should be shipped by the most expeditious route in secure, sturdy, leak-proof containers. Accompanying information on the type of sample being submitted and any clinical information and other circumstances will assist the laboratory clinician in selecting methods of processing the sample, including appropriate media, incubation conditions, and safety precautions.

Specimens that cannot be promptly processed can be held in a suitable bacterial transport medium (see Chapter 33). They are refrigerated at 4° C but not frozen for periods of up to 12 to 15 hours. Refrigeration may delay proliferation of slow-growing fungi for 1 to 2 days. *Aspergillus* and zygomycetes are sensitive to refrigeration. If a specimen suspected of harboring a zygomycete cannot be promptly cultured, overnight storage at room temperature in a bacteriologic transport medium is permissible. Some fungi have been recovered from specimens up to 2 weeks in transit, but this type of delay is not recommended.

Urine specimens may be kept under refrigeration for up to 12 hours before culture. Most bacteria and yeasts will multiply in urine kept at room temperature. The Urine C & S Transport Kit (Becton Dickinson, Franklin Lakes, N.J.) delays growth of bacteria and *Candida albicans* for up to 48 hours at room temperature. Vaginal swabs in transport medium or aspirates may be held under refrigeration before processing.

Blood culture bottles or lysis-centrifugation tubes (see Isolation), if subject to delay in processing, can be held at room temperature for up to 16 hours. CSF and fluids from serous cavities and joints should be processed as soon as possible. The presence of proteins and carbohydrates in CSF contributes to its qualities as a maintenance medium. CSF should be held at room temperature if not cultured immediately.

Nasal curettings and excised polyps may be divided between sterile containers for culturing and jars of 10% buffered formalin for histologic preparation aimed at diagnosing rhinosporidiosis (Fig. 56-1). Impression or scrape smears of nasal tissue should be made before fixation of specimens (see Fig. 83-3). Tissue and bone marrow may be moistened with a small amount of sterile saline if transport is delayed.

Skin scrapings, nails, and hairs can be collected in a clean envelope or a sterile culture dish for mailing. Skin scrapings also can be held in place between glass slides taped at both ends. Such samples should not be kept in tightly sealed containers because resulting accumulation of moisture can lead to overgrowth by saprophytes. Storage is best at room temperature; refrigeration can be harmful for some dermatophytes.

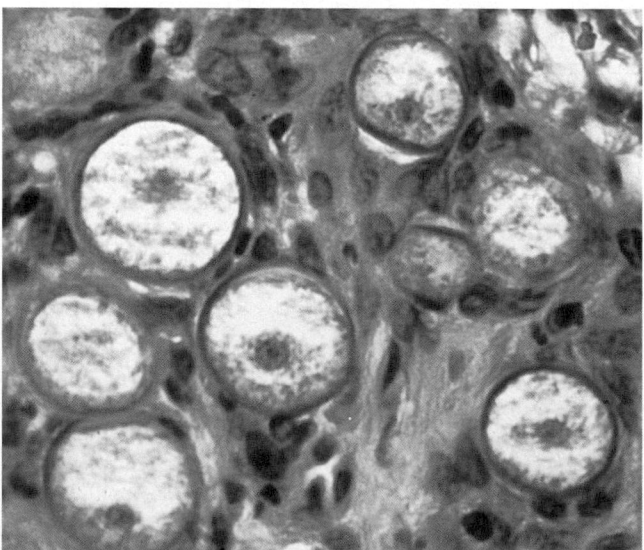

Fig 56-1 *Rhinosporidium*. Section of nasal polyp, dog. Thick-walled proliferating spherules (H and E stain, ×500). (Courtesy Spencer Jang, University of California, Davis, Calif.)

PROCESSING OF SPECIMENS

The complete processing of specimens involves direct microscopic examination, isolation, identification, and serology. In the following sections, some of the procedures are considered, with particular reference to their feasibility as in-office tests. No special equipment, beyond that required for basic clinical bacteriology, is needed for fungal diagnosis. For incubation purposes, an undisturbed area where room temperature (approximately 25° C) remains fairly constant is adequate. A hand lens (8 to 10×) or a dissecting microscope is helpful in the early recognition of fungal colonies.

Direct Examination

The search for diagnostically significant fungal structures may involve preparation of stained or unstained wet mounts, fixed stained smears, and histologic sections. Some of these techniques are simple and rapid and may provide the clinician with a presumptive or even definitive diagnosis and a time-saving guide to therapy (Table 56-1).

Wet Mounts

Specimen material may be suspended on a slide in saline, water, or, preferably, 10% potassium hydroxide (KOH), which clears the preparation of tissue admixtures, leaving fungal elements intact. Examination should begin under low power (100×) and with subdued light, with the condenser racked down to achieve maximal contrast. When structures suggestive of fungal elements are seen, higher magnification (400×) is needed for confirmation.

The KOH digestion method is employed universally in preparation of cutaneous samples suspected of harboring dermatophytes (see Chapter 58). The hair or skin scraping to be examined is placed into a drop of 10% KOH on a clean slide (Fig. 56-2, *A*). Material may require soaking in KOH for a period before further processing. The crusty material is teased apart with forceps or dissecting needles and covered with a coverslip. Gently press the coverslip down to expel any bubbles. This preparation is passed over an open flame several times, but care must be taken not to boil the mixture. This slide is examined immediately for the presence of arthroconidia or fungal chains embedded in the material (see Fig. 56-2, *B* and C). If no organisms are initially observed, the slide is reexamined in 30 minutes. A mixture of 20% KOH and 36% dimethyl sulfoxide or 25% KOH or sodium hydroxide (NaOH) with 5% glycerol increases penetration and clarity of specimens. Nails may require up to 2 hours for better clearing.

India ink (Pelikan) or nigrosin (1% aqueous), when mixed on a slide with fluids or exudates containing *Cryptococcus neoformans*, provides a dark background that outlines the large capsules surrounding the yeast cells (see Fig. 61-6,*B*). Placing a drop of test material and a drop of India ink separately on a slide and then adding a coverslip will allow for a proper mixture gradient to form. Less than 50% of culture-positive human CSF samples are proved to be infected by this method.[1]

Less generally available but useful methods of unstained wet mount study include phase microscopy, in which the visibility of fungal structures against a background of tissue debris is improved, and fluorescent microscopy, in which a specimen is prepared by mixing with an equal volume of 10% to 20% KOH and 0.5% calcofluor white (Difco, Detroit, Mich.) on a slide. The specimen is examined on a fluorescent microscope equipped with a 365-nm exciter filter and a barrier filter that will transmit light at 410 nm. The fungal wall will fluoresce brilliantly. This procedure would be available at commercial diagnostic laboratories. See Appendix 5.

Table • 56-1

Direct Examination of Fungi in Clinical Specimens

STAIN OR REAGENT	USAGE	TEXT FIGURES/DISADVANTAGES
Gram	Stains bacteria, yeasts, and other fungi	*Cryptococcus neoformans* (Fig. 56-3); *Malassezia pachydermatis* (Fig. 56-4); *Sporothrix schenckii* (Fig. 56-5); some fungi stain variably or not at all
Potassium hydroxide	Clearing tissue and cellular debris from variety of specimens to provide greater visibility of fungal elements	Dermatophytes (Fig. 56-2); artifacts develop after preparation time; experience required
India ink	Observation for presence or absence of capsules of fungal cells against a dark background	*C. neoformans* (Fig. 61-6); problems of artifacts can occur in the stain, poor sensitivity
Calcofluor white	A fluorescent brightener binding to polysaccharide such as cellulose and chitin	Detects variety of fungal elements; requires a fluorescent microscope
Wright	Stain for cytologic examination of peripheral blood, bone marrow, body fluids, and organ impressions	*Histoplasma capsulatum* (Fig. 60-8); *Aspergillus* (Fig. 64-5); *Candida* (Fig. 65-1,*A*), *Prototheca* (Fig. 69-6); limited use
Gomori's methenamine silver	Detection of fungal elements in histologic section	*Candida albicans* (Fig. 65-5); not readily available to most clinical laboratories
Periodic acid-Schiff reaction	Detection of fungal elements in histologic section	*C. albicans* (Fig. 65-6); not readily available to most clinical laboratories
Hematoxylin and eosin	Routine histologic stain used for detection of some fungal elements	*Rhinosporidium* (Fig. 83-4); *Coccidioides immitis* (Fig. 62-8); *Prototheca* (Fig. 69-1); usually requires large numbers of fungi to be detected with this stain

Fixed Smears

Gram stain is commonly done on most routine clinical specimens and will detect most fungi. It is of limited use in differentiating fungi because most specimens will stain gram positive or unpredictably, and it produces distortion in cell morphology. Yeasts can often be detected because they retain the primary crystal violet stain (Fig. 56-3). Fungal cell walls often appear as unstained halos. The usefulness of Gram stain is generally limited to smears in which *Candida*, *Malassezia* (Fig. 56-4), *Geotrichum*, *Trichosporon*, or the yeast form of *Sporothrix* spp. (Fig. 56-5) is suspected.

Romanowsky-type stains, such as Wright, Giemsa Leishman's, and Diff-Quik, will stain many fungi, especially yeasts, and are the stains of choice for the tissue phase of *Histoplasma capsulatum* (see Fig. 60-8). As with Gram stain, fungal cell walls remain unstained by these procedures.

A modified periodic acid-Schiff (PAS) reaction is applicable to direct smears and colors mycotic structures and some other extraneous and tissue components selectively red. This application is beyond the scope of most routine office laboratory work but should be obtainable as a service through any histology laboratory (see Appendix 5).

Fluorescent microscopy has had some limited application in mycologic diagnosis. Currently, no fluorescent diagnostic reagents are available commercially, and no diagnostic services use this approach.

Molecular-based methods for the direct detection of fungal pathogens have advanced substantially in recent years and are finding their way into use in the clinical laboratory. At present, use of these methods is predominately restricted to large clinical laboratories or reference laboratories because of the associated expense and technical complexity of the tests. Refer to Appendix 5 for laboratories performing these tests.

The most common molecular methods for identification of specific fungal agents employ either nucleic acid hybridization, which use genus- or species-specific nucleic acid probes or nucleic acid amplification methods such as the polymerase chain reaction (PCR).[16] PCR uses DNA primers to amplify specific segments of fungal genome from the sample. In some cases, PCR is coupled with the use of internal probes or restriction fragment length polymorphism analysis to improve sensitivity and specificity. Alternatively, DNA sequencing can be performed on fungal-specific, PCR products amplified directly from tissues or fluids using universal primers derived from conserved regions in the fungal genome. Once the DNA sequence is obtained, a database can be searched to determine what the sequence most closely matches. This method allows for identification of fastidious or noncultivable fungi.

Histology

Stained sections from biopsy and necropsy specimens often provide critical diagnostic information about mycotic infections. Routine hematoxylin and eosin stain permits detection of the tissue phase of dimorphic fungi causing systemic

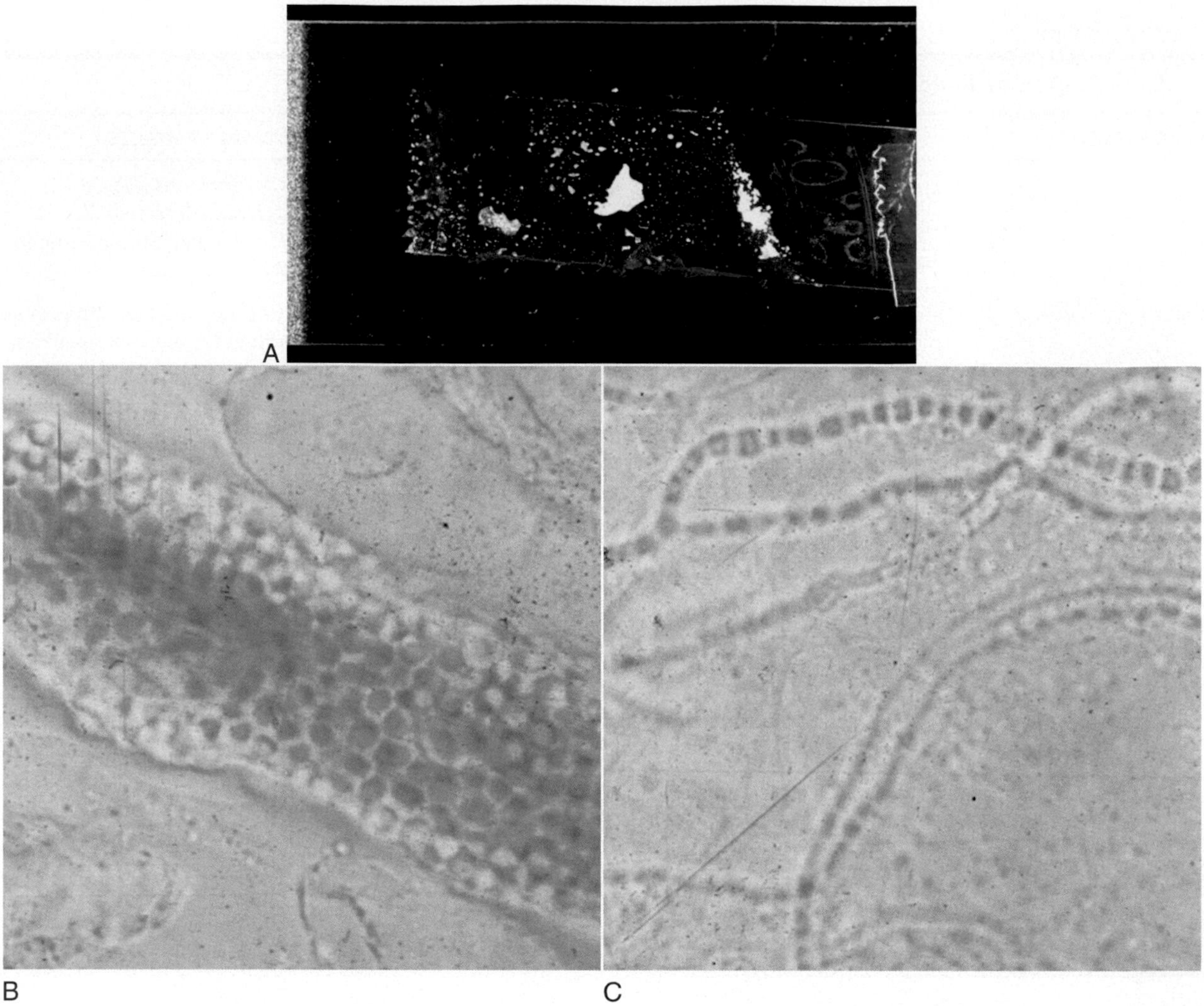

A

B   C

Fig 56-2 A, Hairs from a crusty skin lesion, in a KOH preparation under 40× magnification with **(B)** arthrocondia along or on the hair shaft or **(C)** chains of arthroconidia embedded in crusty material. (Courtesy Spencer Jang, University of California, Davis, Calif.)

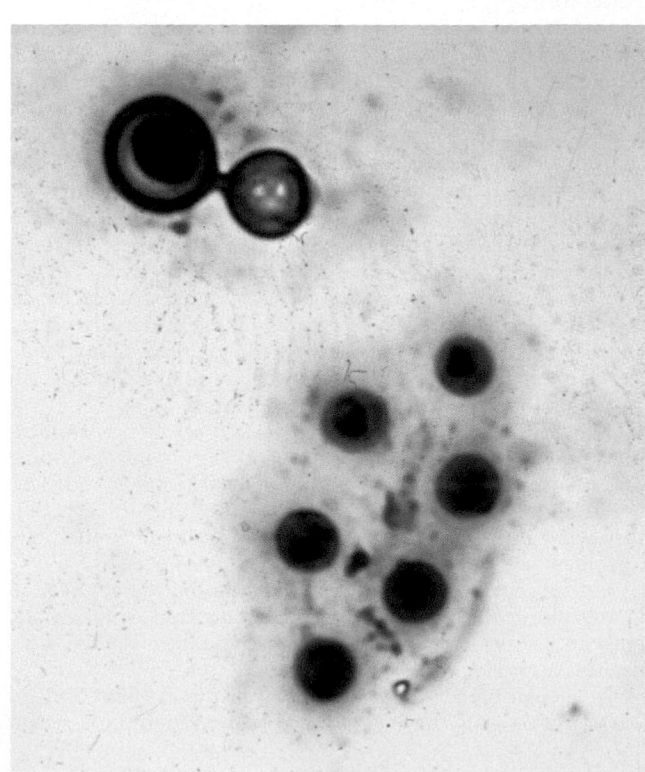

Fig 56-3 *C. neoformans.* Nasal granuloma of a cat. Budding forms, *top;* hazy zone around the six cells below represent capsules (Gram, ×5000). (Courtesy Spencer Jang, University of California, Davis, Calif.)

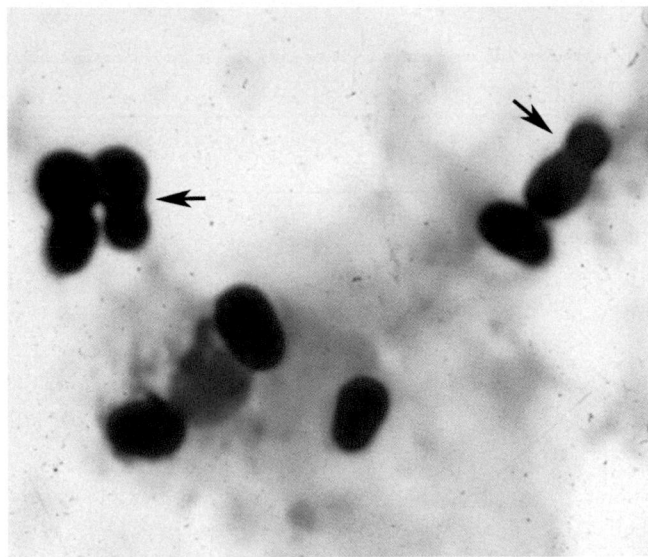

Fig 56-4 *Malassezia pachydermatis.* Ear exudate, dog. Broad-based budding yeast cells *(arrows)* have "shoe print" appearance (Gram, ×5000). (Courtesy Spencer Jang, University of California, Davis, Calif.)

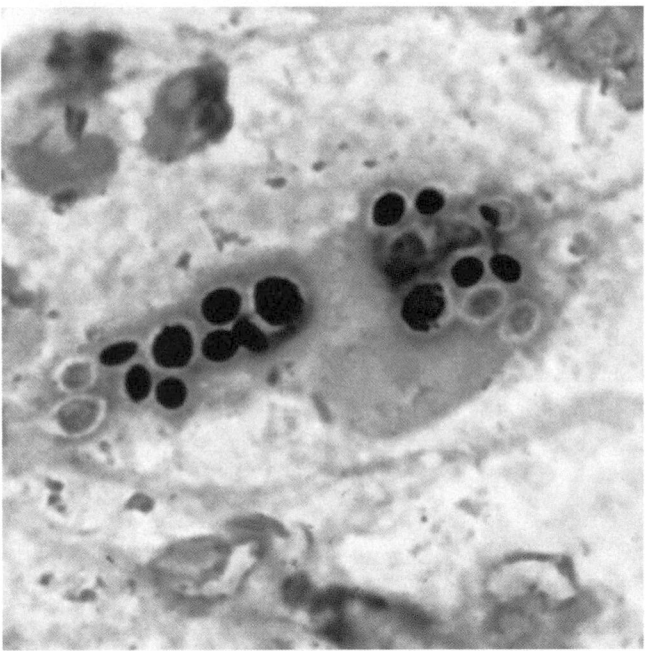

Fig 56-5 *Sporothrix schenckii.* Cutaneous exudate of a cat. Note budding yeasts, oval, rod, and cigar-shaped forms (Gram, ×2000). (Courtesy Spencer Jang, University of California, Davis, Calif.)

mycoses (coccidioidomycosis, histoplasmosis, blastomycosis, cryptococcosis). With filamentous fungi, it may demonstrate hyphae in tissues, often providing an indication as to their septate or nonseptate nature and whether they are pigmented or nonpigmented, and thereby helping with their classification. More specific for fungi is the preferred Gomori's methenamine silver stain, which stains fungal structures brownish-black against a pale green background, or a PAS reaction, which makes mycotic elements appear dark red

against a contrasting background, depending on the counterstain. Many laboratories use hematoxylin and eosin as a counterstain or hematoxylin alone, which permits better pathologic characterization of the lesion than do other procedures. Mayer's mucicarmine can be used to demonstrate capsules on *C. neoformans.*

Isolation

Inoculation of a suitably prepared specimen on any appropriate medium is required. Preparation of specimens may include centrifugation of fluid samples, grinding of biopsy and other tissues, surface sterilization of necropsy specimens by searing, repeated washing of granules from mycetomas with saline, or filtration of CSF and blood. Scrapings, swabs, and blood may be inoculated directly without further preparation.

Because many pathogenic fungi, when propagated on agar media, constitute airborne health hazards, laboratories often prefer tubes and bottles to Petri plates for isolation purposes. If plates are used, they should be secured with oxygen-permeable tape. All examinations of cultures producing aerial mycelium should be carried out in biologic safety cabinets. Most fungi grow on media used routinely in microbiologic diagnosis (Table 56-2). These media should be used when the sample is obtained from an uncontaminated site, such as the central nervous system, internal organ, or joints. These sites have no resident flora and are not exposed to the external environment. Samples originating from cutaneous sources or mucous membranes that harbor such flora are cultured on selective media that may contain broad-spectrum antibacterial and antimycotic agents (see Table 56-2) for the suppression of bacteria and nonpathogenic fungi, respectively. A low pH (no higher than 6.0) of the medium may further limit bacterial overgrowth. Yeasts can be selectively recovered from specimens heavily contaminated with bacteria by propagation on a medium of pH 3.5 to 4.0. Fungal cultures are optimally incubated at 25° C to 30° C. Incubation at 37° C allows bacterial overgrowth and causes failure of some fungal pathogens to grow. An atmosphere of 40% to 50% humidity is favorable for most fungi.

The Isolator system (Wampole Laboratories, Cranbury, N.J.) has improved the number and rate of fungal isolations from blood.[11] This system involves lysis and centrifugation of 10 ml of blood. The supernatant is removed from the upper stopper, and the concentrate is removed from the bottom stopper and plated. The isolation rates of *H. capsulatum, C. immitis,* and *C. neoformans* have improved with the Isolator.[11] Vented broth bottles used for bacterial blood cultures should not be expected to detect fungi other than certain yeasts. Biphasic bottles contain 50 ml of brain-heart infusion broth and brain-heart infusion agar. A biphasic bottle is inoculated with 10 ml of blood, vented, and incubated in an upright position. After daily examination, it is tilted so that the broth floods the agar surface. Automated blood culture systems have been used and are an efficient means for laboratories dealing with large volumes of blood cultures.

Identification

Microscopic morphology of fungal reproductive structures is the most helpful criterion for identification. Other criteria are macroscopic colonial features under different conditions of incubation, nutritional and metabolic properties, antigenic characteristics, and pathogenicity for experimental animals.

Agar cultures are examined daily during the first 2 weeks of incubation and twice weekly thereafter. Allow 4 to 6 weeks for slow-growing fungi. Some common zygomycetes (*Mucor, Rhizopus* spp.) grow rapidly and abundantly, filling a tube or Petri dish within 2 or 3 days. Fruiting bodies may be visible

Table • 56-2

Isolation Media for Fungi

MEDIUM (COMMERCIAL SOURCE)	SELECTIVE FEATURES	PRINCIPAL USE/LIMITATION IN MYCOLOGIC DIAGNOSIS
Blood agar (Remel Labs, Lenexa, Kan.)	Highly nutritious for most fungi	General purpose, converts some dimorphic fungi to yeast form; noninhibitory, nonselective, easily overgrown
Potato flake agar (Remel Labs, Lenexa, Kan.)	Low pH, highly nutritious for most fungi	To induce sporulation of fungi
Inhibitory mold agar (Remel Labs, Lenexa, Kan.)	Gentamicin and chloramphenicol for bacterial suppression	General purpose; not for dermatophytes
Sabouraud's dextrose agar (Remel Labs, Lenexa, Kan.; marketed as SAB DUET with DTM in a two-compartment plate by Bacti-lab, Mountain View, Calif.)	Low pH, modest nutritional quality; addition of chloramphenicol and cycloheximide inhibits bacteria and some fungi	General purpose; added antibiotics for isolation from contaminated environment such as recovery of dermatophytes; cycloheximide inhibits *Cryptococcus; Aspergillus, Scedosporium apiospermum, (Pseudallescheria boydii),* some *Candida* spp.; chloramphenicol inhibits some yeast
DTM (Remel Labs, Lenexa, Kan.; Bacti-lab, Mountain View, Calif.)	Gentamicin, tetracycline, and cycloheximide are inhibitors; glucose and phenol red are indicators	Isolation of dermatophytes, which turn yellow medium to red in 48 hours; not for sporulation; may produce atypical colonial growth; natural pigmentation obscured; nondermatophytes turn yellow medium to red eventually
RSM (marketed as DERM DUET with DTM in a two-compartment plate by Bacti-lab, Mountain View, Calif.)	Cycloheximide and chloramphenicol are inhibitors; glucose and bromothymol blue are indicators	For dermatophytes, which turn blue medium green early; prompt conidial and pigment development permits identification; color change of RSM not as intense as of DTM with some dermatophytes

DTM, Dermatophyte test medium; *RSM,* rapid sporulation medium.

as black specks in the colorless mycelium (Fig. 56-6). Aerial mycelium is grossly less prominent but more intensely pigmented by the presence of fruiting structures with *Aspergillus* (Fig. 56-7) and *Penicillium* spp. (Fig. 56-8). Some fungi produce soluble pigment that diffuses through the medium (e.g., *Microsporum canis*). In others, pigment is confined to parts of the organism and may be best observed either on the surface or on the reverse side of the colony. The colonial surface varies according to mycelial growth patterns from smooth ("glabrous") to powdery, velvety, and cottony. Yeasts, which form no or little pseudomycelium, produce mucoid, creamy, pasty, or waxy colonies.

Low-power (25 to 50×) microscopy helps in early detection of mycelial growth and such diagnostic features as macroconidia and microconidia of dermatophytes (Figs. 56-9, 56-10, 56-11). Once colonial growth is established, identification is based largely on microscopic examination for hyphal characteristics: septate versus nonseptate, pigmented (dematiaceous) (Fig. 56-12) versus nonpigmented (hyaline), and conidia and their supporting structures. This step obviously involves the opening of a culture vessel and should be done only by trained, experienced personnel and under conditions in which

exposure to people and animals and contamination of the environment can be avoided.

At the in-office laboratory level, it is feasible to make *teased preparations* or transparent cellophane tape lactophenol aniline blue mounts (LPAB, Remel Labs, Lenexa, Kan.) from mold cultures by using appropriate precautions. Diagnostic features are usually better preserved in their natural interrelationships in cellophane tape mounts (Figs. 56-13 and 56-14). In the absence of a laminar flow biosafety cabinet, such attempts should be restricted to macroscopically positive dermatophyte cultures.

The slide culture procedure probably exceeds the capabilities of most veterinary practices and should be left to clinical laboratories. This procedure permits study of undisturbed fungal structures by using LPAB (Figs. 56-15 and 56-16).

The germ tube test allows rapid differentiation of *C. albicans* (see Chapter 65) from most of the other, usually nonpathogenic, *Candida* spp. Serum, 0.5 to 1 ml, is inoculated lightly with suspect growth and incubated at 35° C for 2 to 3 hours. A drop of the suspension is then examined microscopically (100× and 400×) for the presence of germ tubes

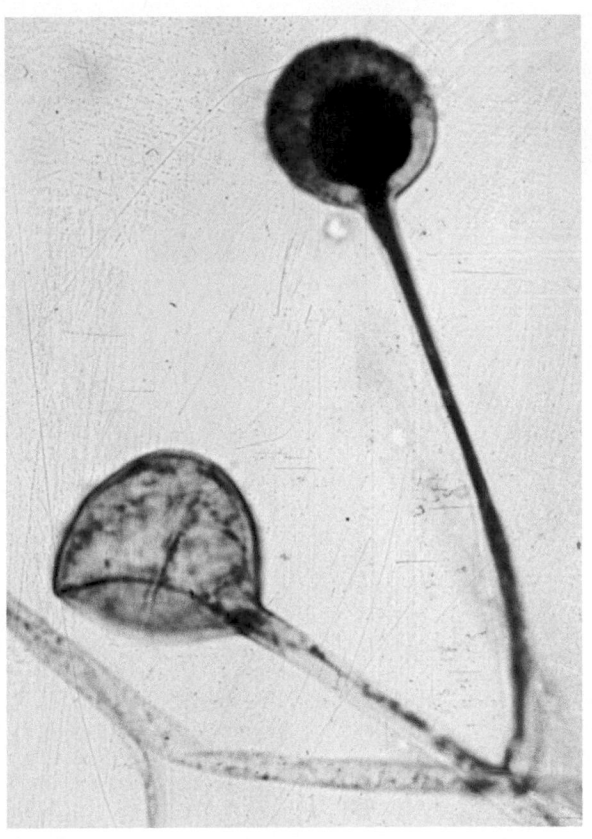

Fig 56-6 *Mucor* in culture. Sporangia form on sporangiophores; note nonseptate, broad hyphae (Lactophenol analine blue, ×2000). (Courtesy Spencer Jang, University of California, Davis, Calif.)

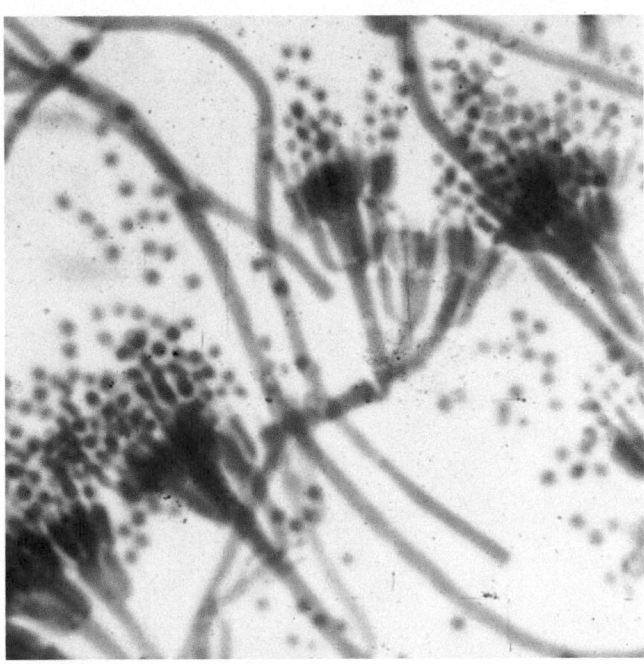

Fig 56-8 *Penicillium*. Fruiting heads give brushlike appearance (Lactophenol analine blue, ×500). (Courtesy Spencer Jang, University of California, Davis, Calif.)

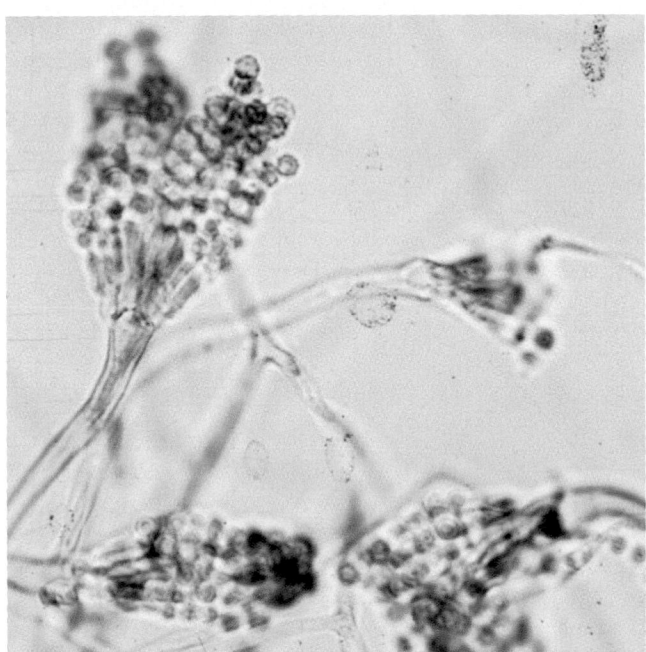

Fig 56-7 *Aspergillus deflectus*. Columnar conidial head resembling a briar pipe and biseriate arrangement of phialides (Lactophenol analine blue, ×500). (Courtesy Spencer Jang, University of California, Davis, Calif.)

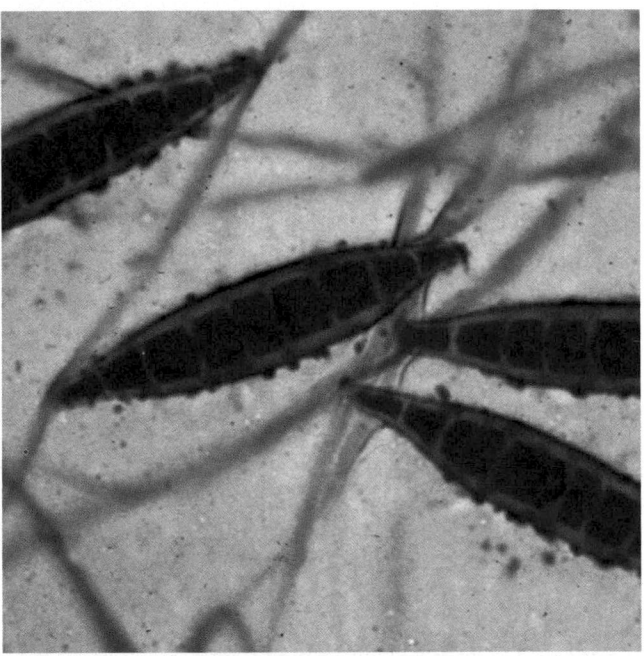

Fig 56-9 *M. canis* in culture. Rough and thick-walled multicellular spindle-shaped macroconidia. Note curved, pointed ends (Lactophenol analine blue, ×2000). (Courtesy Richard Walker, University of California, Davis, Calif.)

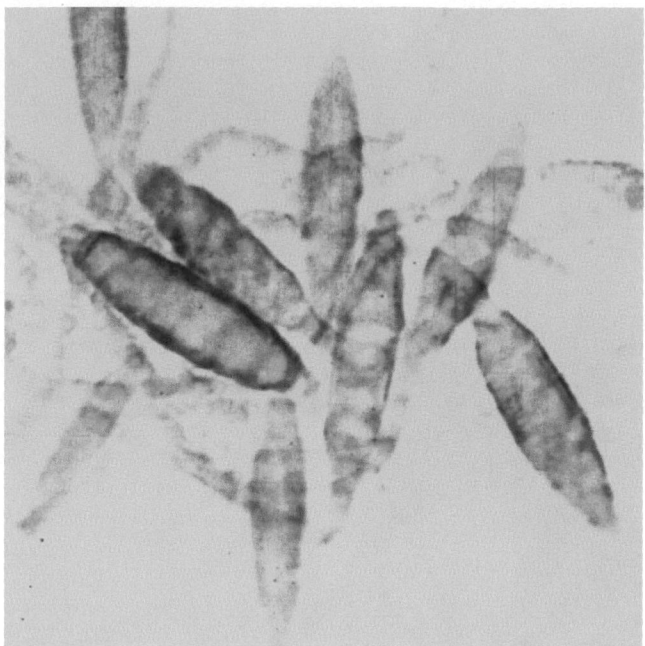

Fig 56-10 *Microsporum gypseum* in culture. Numerous multicellular, fairly thin-walled macroconidia with rounded ends (Lactophenol analine blue, ×2000). (Courtesy Spencer Jang, University of California, Davis, Calif.)

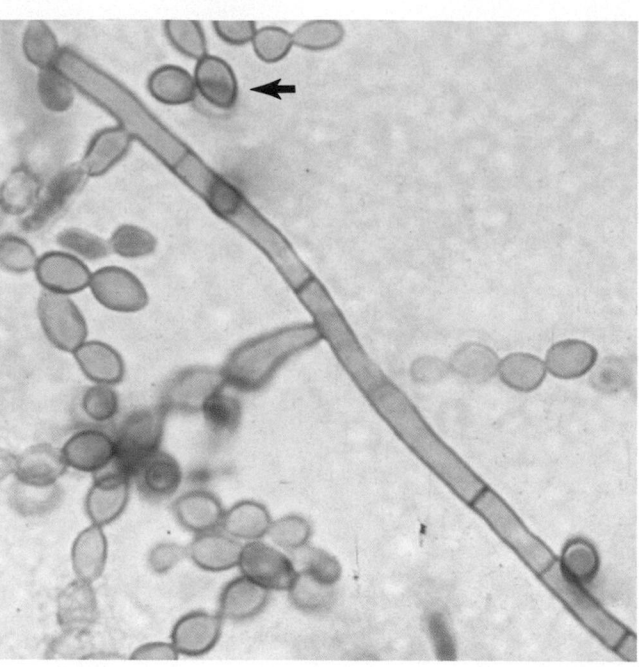

Fig 56-12 *Cladophialophora bantiana* in culture. Oval conidia occurring in chains. Note dematiaceous (dark-pigmented) appearance of some conidia and mycelium *(arrows)* (Lactophenol analine blue, ×2000). (Courtesy Spencer Jang, University of California, Davis, Calif.)

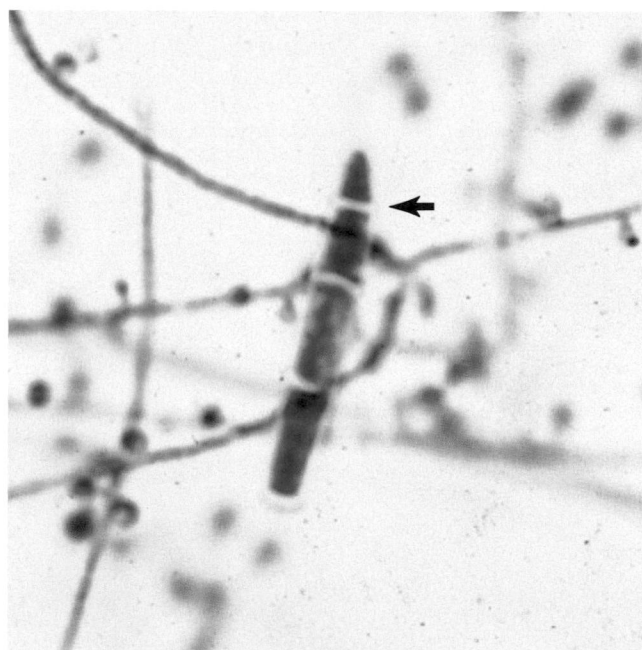

Fig 56-11 *Trichophyton mentagrophytes* in culture. Spherical microconidia and one thin-walled, multicellular, cigar-shaped macroconidium *(arrow)* (Lactophenol analine blue, ×2000). (Courtesy Spencer Jang, University of California, Davis, Calif.)

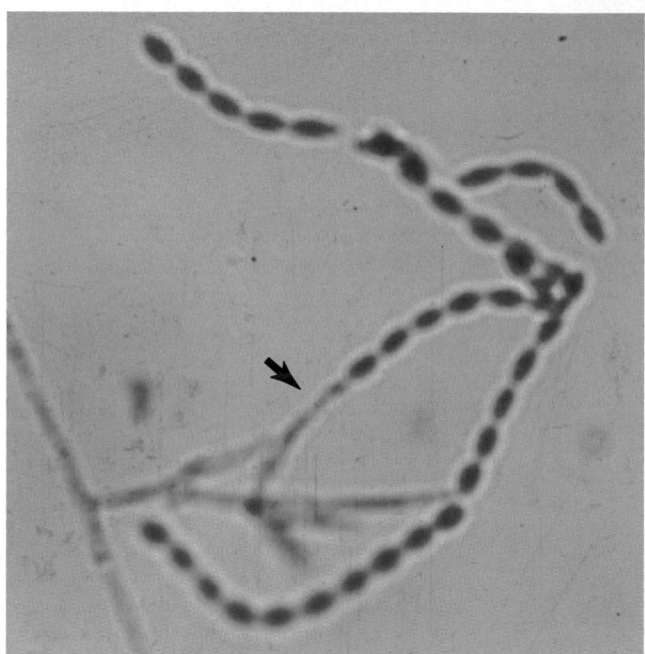

Fig 56-13 *Paecilomyces* in culture. Ovoid chains of conidia attached to a phialide *(arrow)* that is usually tapered (not visible) (Lactophenol analine blue, ×2000). (Courtesy Spencer Jang, University of California, Davis, Calif.)

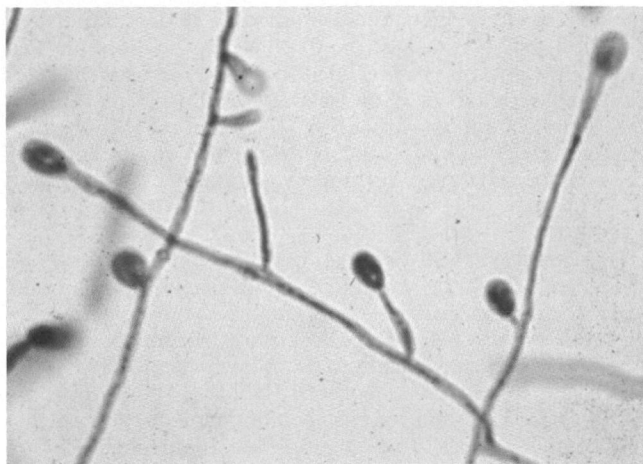

Fig 56-14 *Pseudallescheria boydii* (= asexual stage of *Scedosporium apiospermum*). Single elliptical conidia attached to tips of conidiophores arising along the hyphae (Lactophenol analine blue, ×2000). (Courtesy Spencer Jang, University of California, Davis, Calif.)

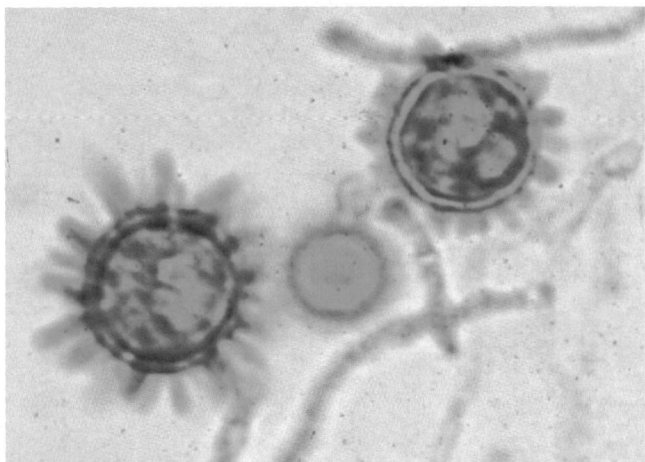

Fig 56-15 *H. capsulatum* in culture. Tuberculate macroconidia (Lactophenol analine blue, ×2000). (Courtesy Spencer Jang, University of California, Davis, Calif.)

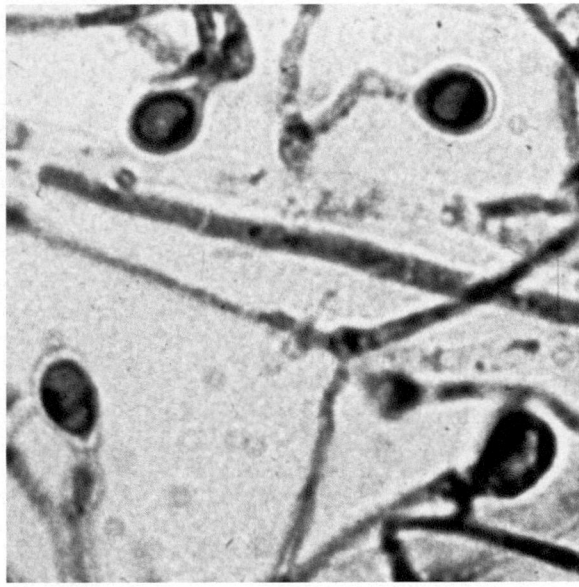

Fig 56-16 *Blastomyces dermatitidis* in culture. One-celled conidia on short conidiophores, "lollypop" appearance (Lactophenol analine blue, ×2000). (Courtesy Spencer Jang, University of California, Davis, Calif.)

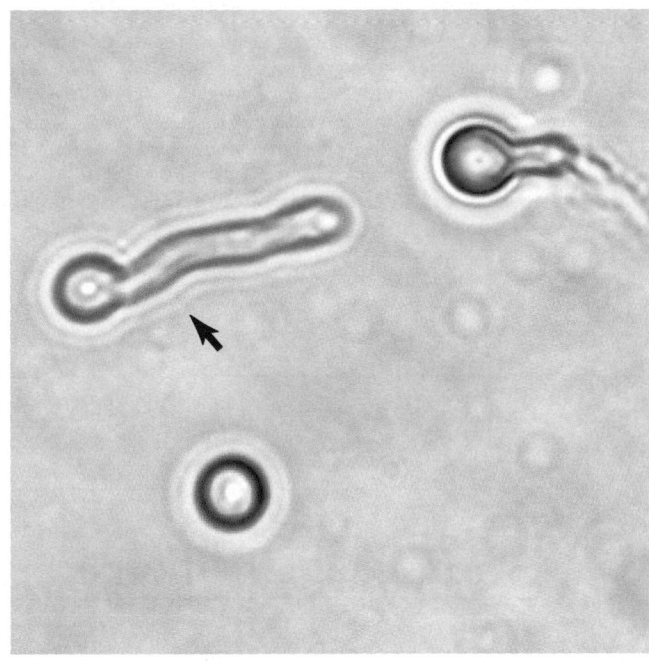

Fig 56-17 Germ tube test. Formation of germ tube *(arrow)* characteristic of *C. albicans*. Blastoconidia on left (wet mount, ×2000). (Courtesy Richard Walker, University of California, Davis, Calif.)

sprouting from yeast cells (blastoconidia) of *C. albicans* (Fig. 56-17).

Commonly used differential media include Czapek agar (Difco, Detroit, Mich.) for the differentiation of *Aspergillus* spp.; cornmeal agar for the demonstration of chlamydospores in *C. albicans* and their absence in most other *Candida* spp.; Trichophyton agars (Remel Labs, Lenexa, Kan.) for the identification of *Trichophyton* spp.[2] by their growth factor needs; Christensen's urea agar (Difco, Detroit, Mich) for production of urease by *Cryptococcus, Rhodotorula, Trichophyton,*[2] and *Trichosporon* spp. and CHROMagar *Candida* (Hardy Diagnostics, Santa Maria, Calif.) for culture and identification of *C. albicans, C. krusei, C. tropicalis,* and *Trichosporon* spp.[6]

For definitive identification of the dimorphic fungi *Coccidioides immitis, H. capsulatum,* and *Blastomyces dermatitidis* antisera are commercially available (ImmunoMycologics, Norman, Okla.) for use in agar immunodiffusion exoantigen test. The antigen is prepared from an extract of mycelial growth.[7,10]

Fungal isolates can be identified to genus or species level, or both, by many molecular-based methods. Universal primers to regions in the 28S rRNA gene have been used in PCR to amplify DNA that is then tested with specific nucleic acid probes.[12] The use of a multiplex PCR approach for identification of a battery of commonly encountered yeasts and molds has also been described.[9] Commercially available DNA probes such as the Accuprobe system (Genprobe Inc., San Diego, Calif.) are available for identification of the important fungal agents, such as *C. immitis, B. dermatitidis,* and *H. capsulatum.*

DNA sequencing of specific regions of the fungal genome can also be used for identification purposes. The ribosomal RNA genes are most commonly used because they contain conserved areas present in most fungi and therefore serve as sites for amplification of DNA from a variety of different fungi with a single pair of primers. The rRNA genes also contain variable regions that are used in sequence analysis for making the identification. At present, the most commonly used region is the D2 variable region of large subunit rRNA gene. Commercial sequencing kits are available (MicroSeq D2 rDNA Fungal Identification System, Applied Biosystems) that use this region, but the method is complex and generally relegated to use by reference laboratories that have access to DNA sequencing facilities. A few commercial laboratories provide nucleic acid sequencing services for identification of fungal isolates (Accugenix, Newark, Del. and MIDI Labs, Newark, Del.). Sequence analysis of the internal transcribed spacer (ITS) regions (ITS-5.8S rRNA-ITS2) has also been used to identify a large number of fungal species.[5] Oomycetes in the genus *Pythium* and *Lagenidium* are not true fungi but produce fungal-like granulomatous diseases (see Chapter 67). PCR has been used to determine the specific cause of these infections.[4] Real-time PCR has been used to test peripheral blood for the diagnosis of invasive aspergillosis in people.[8] A panfungal PCR has been used to detect *Candida* and *Aspergillus* in the blood of people with suspected disseminated infections.[13]

Molecular-based test results should be combined with clinical findings and morphologic features of the agent in tissues or in culture, or both, before making a final diagnosis.

Among miniaturized prepackaged identification kits for yeast and algae isolates belonging to the genus *Prototheca* spp. isolates, the API 20C (bioMerieux Vitex, Inc., Hazlewood, Mo.), the Uni-yeast-tek system (Remel Labs, Lenexa, Kan.), and RapID yeast plus panel (Remel Labs, Lenexa, Kan.) are used.[14] All rely on tests that are scored to yield a single profile code, which is listed in a code book and translates into a species name. Identification can be completed within 4 hours to several days and more conveniently and generally more rapidly than by conventional methods. Rapid multiple biochemical test systems lack the database for the more unusual yeasts. Automated systems such as Vitex Yeast biochemical card (bioMerieux Vitex, Inc., Hazlewood, Mo.)[14] and Microbial Identification System (MIS), (Microbial ID [MIDI], Inc., Newark, Del.) require continued expansion and updating of the veterinary database for improved quality.

Serologic Testing

Reagents designed to detect antigens and antibodies in body fluids are becoming commercially available in increasing numbers. An antigen detection kit, the *C. neoformans* latex agglutination test (Meridian Diagnostics, Cincinnati, Ohio), is one of several kits available that has been adapted for use in office laboratories (see Chapter 61, Table 61-3, and Appendix 6). Testing for antigens for *Histoplasma capsulatum* is available on a commercial basis (see Chapter 60 and Appendix 6).[15] The accuracy of this procedure for use in dogs and cats is not known. An enzyme-linked immunosorbent assay has been developed for the serologic diagnosis of pythiosis (see Chapter 67 and Appendix 6).[4] For a discussion of serum antibody testing of particular fungal infections, see the respective chapters.

SUGGESTED READINGS*

4. Grooters AM, Leise BS, Lopez MK, et al. 2002. Development and evaluation of an enzyme-linked immunosorbent assay for the serodiagnosis of pythiosis in dogs, *J Vet Intern Med* 16:142-146.
5. Hendolin PH, Paulin L, Koukila-Kahicola P, et al. 2002. Panfungal PCR and multiplex liquid hybridization for detection of fungi in tissue specimens, *J Clin Microbiol* 38:4186-4192.
16. Yeo SF, Wong B. 2002. Current status of nonculture methods for diagnosis of invasive fungal infections, *Clin Microbiol Rev* 15:465-484.

*See the CD-ROM for a complete list of references.

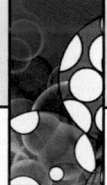

CHAPTER • 57

Antifungal Chemotherapy

Craig. E. Greene

SYSTEMIC ANTIFUNGALS

Table 57-1 lists various systemic antifungal drugs and the circumstances in which they are used. Chapters 58 to 68 provide information on their use for specific diseases, and details on dosage and usage are given in the Drug Formulary, Appendix 8.

Griseofulvin

Griseofulvin is an orally administered antifungal drug produced by *Penicillium griseofulvum*. Absorption from the gastrointestinal (GI) tract is facilitated by addition of fat to the diet. The drug has also been improved by production of micro-sized and ultramicrosized formulations. Griseofulvin is effective against infections caused by dermatophytes but not yeasts.

Griseofulvin is deposited in the epidermal layers of the skin and dermal appendages as they are formed. Several weeks of therapy are required for complete drug distribution throughout cell layers and for inhibition of fungal growth. Resistance rarely develops during therapy. Despite its teratogenic effects, griseofulvin does not have deleterious effects on semen quality in dogs.[138]

Iodides

A solution of 20% sodium iodide or 100% (supersaturated) potassium iodide has been given orally to treat cutaneous

Table • 57-1

Systemically Used Antifungal Drugs

GENERIC NAME (TRADE NAME)	ROUTE	CLINICAL FORMULATION	INDICATIONS	
			FIRST	**ALTERNATE**
Griseofulvin (Fulvicin, Grisactin)	PO	Capsules, tablets, Suspension	Dermatophytosis	None
Sodium or potassium iodide	PO	Solution (20% NaI-100% KI)	Sporotrichosis	None
Amphotericin B (Fungizone, AmBiosome, Amphocil, Abelcet)	IV, SC	See Table 57-2	Rapidly progressive or severe systemic mycosis, systemic aspergillosis, sporotrichosis, or mucormycosis	Imidazole-resistant cryptococcosis or other systemic mycoses
Flucytosine (Ancobon)	PO	Capsules (250 mg, 500 mg)	In combination with amphotericin B for cryptococcosis	Systemic candidiasis
Miconazole (Monistat IV)	IV	Ampules (10 mg/ml in 20 ml)	Systemic mycoses	None
Ketoconazole (Nizoral)	PO	Tablets (200 mg)	Systemic mycoses in dogs, systemic aspergillosis, miscellaneous fungal infections	Adjunctive with enilconazole for resistant aspergillosis, systemic mycoses in cats, dermatophytosis
Itraconazole (Sporanox)	PO	Capsules (100 mg) Oral suspension (100 mg/10 ml)	Cutaneous sporotrichosis, systemic mycoses in cats and small dogs, miscellaneous fungal infections, malasseziosis	Adjunct with nasal aspergillosis, systemic mycoses if funds available, dermatophytosis
Fluconazole (Diflucan)	PO, IV	Capsules (50, 100, 150, 200 mg) Oral suspension (10 or 40 mg/ml in 35 ml) IV solution (2 mg/ml in 50 or 100 ml)	CNS, meningeal or ocular systemic mycosis	Systemic mycoses in cats, candidiasis
Voriconazole (Vfend)	PO	Capsules (50 mg and 200 mg) Oral suspension (40 mg/ml, 75 ml) IV solution (200-mg vial)	Invasive aspergillosis, CNS mycosis	Candidiasis
Terbinafine (Lamisil)	PO	Tablets (250 mg) Topical solution (1%)	Onchomycosis, aspergillosis	Miscellaneous mold fungal infections
Caspofungin (Cancidas)	IV	IV solution (50- and 70-mg vials)	Invasive and disseminated aspergillosis	None

PO, By mouth; *IV,* intravenous; *SC,* subcutaneous; *CNS,* central nervous system.
For additional information on drugs and dosages, see Drug Formulary, Appendix 8.

sporotrichosis (see Chapter 63). The mechanism of action of the iodides is uncertain because they are not directly toxic to *Sporothrix* species in vitro. Iodides are all less toxic than amphotericin B (AMB), which should be reserved as a second-choice drug or for disseminated disease. Iodism, manifested clinically as dermal eruption with hair loss, may occur as a result of therapy.

Amphotericin B and Other Polyenes

AMB is a lipophilic polyene isolated from *Streptomyces nodosus* that binds to sterols in cell membranes of eukaryotic organisms and causes increased permeability and leakage of nutrients and electrolytes. Nystatin is another polyene and is applied topically (see Topical Antifungals in this chapter). AMB has greater binding affinity for ergosterol, the major sterol of fungal cell membranes, than for cholesterol, which is present in mammalian host cells. Because it is poorly absorbed across the GI mucosa or skin, AMB must be given parenterally (usually intravenous [IV]) for the treatment of systemic mycoses. Most of the drug is metabolized locally at tissue sites, and lesser amounts are excreted in the urine. Standard IV preparations contain lyophilized AMB combined with deoxycholate and buffer in a colloidal state (ABD). ABD has been diluted and given subcutaneously, which appears to delay its absorption and reduce its nephrotoxicity, allowing larger amounts of the drug to be given.[83] Lipid-based formulations are now available with lower toxicity (Table 57-2); however, merely giving ABD in a fat emulsion did not alter nephrotoxicity.[109,139] In contrast, commercially prepared lipid-encapsulated formulations are taken up well into organs of the mononuclear phagocyte system where the organism resides; they accumulate at relatively low levels in the kidneys.[4,73] Lipid-based formulations can be given at a higher dose and may be effective in treating resistant or ABD-unresponsive mycoses.[100] The overall dose rate for these drugs can be higher because of their lower toxicity. The cost of these lipid formulations is usually prohibitive for veterinary patients. Occasionally, the AMB formulations are used for topical therapy of mycotic disease. (See the Drug Formulary, Appendix 8, for information about the various preparations and specific information regarding AMB use.)

The fungal organisms affected by AMB are listed in Table 57-1. Zygomycetes (family Mucoraceae) are variably susceptible, and *Aspergillus* species are usually resistant. Because higher effective AMB dosage levels can be achieved, lipid-based formulations are more effective against zygomycosis and fusariosis, and they might be the first choice for treating these diseases.[54]

AMB was the first line of therapy for rapidly progressive or disseminated deep mycotic infections. Resistance rarely if ever develops during treatment, but relapses may occur when the drug is discontinued. Oral azoles such as ketoconazole (KTZ), itraconazole (ITZ), and fluconazole (FCZ) have become alternatives for treatment of uncomplicated systemic mycoses.

Hamycin is another polyene that is effective against *Candida*, *Cryptococcus*, *Histoplasma*, *Blastomyces*, and *Aspergillus* species. It has been given orally, topically, and intraperitoneally to treat various mycotic conditions, although toxicity does occur. A dog with disseminated aspergillosis was treated with some success.[66] Liposomal encapsulation of this drug has been associated with increased efficacy and reduced toxicity.[93]

Flucytosine

Flucytosine, or 5-fluorocytosine (FCY), is a fluorinated pyrimidine originally synthesized as an antineoplastic agent. It interferes with pyrimidine metabolism and resultant DNA synthesis in yeasts.

FCY is effective against *Cryptococcus* species, *Candida* species, and other yeasts but has little or no effect on other deep mycotic agents or on *Aspergillus* species. Localized candidiasis or cryptococcal infections respond best, but resistance to FCY frequently develops during therapy. For this reason, the drug is always given in combination with AMB. Skin eruptions similar to those caused by azoles have been observed in treated dogs.[85]

Azole Derivatives

Synthetic imidazole derivatives were originally produced as broad-spectrum anthelmintics with activity against some gram-positive bacteria and protozoa. Like AMB, they inhibit sterol synthesis via fungal cell cytochrome P-450 as one of their main effects, but they are generally less toxic. They also inhibit nucleic acid, triglyceride, and fatty acid synthesis and alter oxidative enzyme biochemistry. At low concentrations they are fungistatic, and at higher concentrations, which cannot be achieved systemically, they are fungicidal. When given systemically, they vary in pharmacokinetic parameters such as oral bioavailability, protein binding, plasma clearance, and volume of distribution (see Drug Formulary, Appendix 8). They all undergo hepatic metabolism by cytochrome P-450 enzymes. The metabolism can lead to drug interactions in which their level is decreased by coadministered drugs that reduce their absorption or accelerate their metabolism (Table 57-3). Unexpected toxicity of coadministered drugs may result because of their delayed metabolism (see Table 57-3). Of the imidazole group, thiabendazole was initially recognized as being effective in treating human dermatophytoses. Miconazole, clotrimazole, and enilconazole are available in creams and lotions and can be formulated into solutions for topical treatment of fungal infections of the skin, such as dermatophytosis and candidiasis (see Topical Antifungals in this chapter and Drug Formulary, Appendix 8). However, oral therapy with an azole, griseofulvin, or terbinafine, is needed for nail infections. Of the orally administered azoles, KTZ is an imidazole, whereas newer drugs are triazoles such as ITZ and FCZ. The orally administered azoles are becoming widely used in human and veterinary medicine to treat systemic and opportunistic fungal infections. Oral administration has been preferred in many situations because it is easier than IV administration of AMB. In vitro susceptibility testing of the drugs shows variable efficacy against different fungi, but it does not always parallel in vivo efficacy.

Ketoconazole

KTZ is less active than miconazole but is better absorbed from the GI tract, making it convenient for the treatment of systemic mycoses and chronic mucocutaneous candidiasis. Absorption is improved when taken with a meal or acid media, therefore antacids and H_2-receptor antihistamine antagonists should not be given concurrently. The drug is predominantly bound to plasma albumin, entering all tissues and body fluids in therapeutic concentrations with the exception of seminal, central nervous system (CNS), and ocular locations. The drug is distributed throughout the skin and subcutaneous tissues and therefore has been used in treating superficial fungal infections of the skin and hair. Metabolites of the drug, produced in the liver, lack antifungal activity.

Occasional nausea, partial anorexia, and vomiting in dogs can be overcome if the drug is given with meals and by dividing the daily dose into three or four administrations. Additional side effects of KTZ are similar to those of other azoles. Frequently, reversible subclinical increases in activities of hepatic transaminases and alkaline phosphatase in blood occur as manifestations of hepatotoxicity. Less commonly, clinical hepatitis develops, and if treatment continues or dosages are

Table • 57-2

Comparison of Clinical Formulations of Amphotericin B[a]

ABBREVIATION	FORMULATION	BRAND NAME (MANUFACTURER)	DIAMETER (nm)	COMPOSITION	RATIO	LD$_{50}$ (MURINE)
ABD	Deoxycholate	Fungizone[b]	≥300	Detergent deoxycholate/buffer/AMB	0.8:0.5:1	3
L-AMB[1]	Liposome Encapsulated	AmBiosome[c]	55–75	Hydrogenated soy phosphatidylcholine (HSPC)/cholesterol(Chol)/distearoylphosphatidylglycerol (DSPG)/AMB	2:1:0.8:0.4	175
ABCD[31,37]	Colloidal dispersion, lipid disk particle	Amphocil[d]	~115	Cholesterylsulfate/AMB	1:1	38
ABLC[61]	Lipid complex, ribbon shape	Abelcet[e]	2,000–11,000	Dimyristoylphosphatidytcholine/dimyristoylphosphatidylglycerol/AMB	7:3:10	40
PEG-AMB-LIP[f]	Liposomal complexed to PEG	Experimental	95–105	PEG-DSPE-HSPC-Chol-AMB	0.21:1.79:1:0.32 (PEG/AMB/LIP)	ND
AMB-H[f]	Cholesterol hemisuccinate vesicles	AMB hydrosomes,[g] experimental	~105	AMB in hemisuccinate vesicles	ND	ND

PEG, Polyethylene glycol; AMB, amphotericin B, ND, no data; LD$_{50}$, lethal dose killing 50% of treated mice; ABD, colloidal dispersion of amphotericin B and the bile salt, deoxycholate; L-AMB, amphotericin B with encapsulated unilamellar liposomes; ABCD, amphotericin B with cholesteryl sulfate; ABLC, amphotericin B with lipid complex; LIP, liposomal complex; H, hemisuccinate vesicles.

[a]For additional information, see Drug Formulary, Appendix 8.
[b]Squibb, Bristol Myers-Squibb, Princeton, N.J.
[c]NeXstar, San Dimas, Calif.
[d]Sequus, Menlo Park, Calif.
[e]Liposome Co, Princeton, N.J.
[f]Investigational only; not commercially available.
[g]Access Pharmaceuticals.

Table • 57-3

Drug Interactions of Commonly Used Antifungal Drugs[30,40,89]

DRUG	USE	ANTIFUNGAL DRUG INTERACTION	CLINICAL COMPLICATION
Cimetidine, ranitidine[a]	H$_2$-receptor antacids	ITZ, KTZ	Decreased azole absorption
Cyclosporine	Immunosuppressant	ITZ, KTZ, FCZ, VCZ	Nephrotoxicity of cyclosporine
Digoxin	Cardiac inotrope	ITZ	Digoxin toxicity
Phenytoin	Anticonvulsant	ITZ, KTZ, VCZ, FCZ	Increased azole metabolism; phenytoin toxicity
Felodipine, nifedipine, amlodipine	Calcium-channel blockers	ITZ	Edema, calcium-channel concentrations
Isoniazid	Antimycobacterial	KTZ	Increased azole metabolism
Lovastain	Lipid control	ITZ, VCZ	Rhabdomyolysis
Midazolam, diazepam	Sedative	ITZ, KTZ, FCZ, VCZ	Sedation
Nortryptyline	Antidepressant	FCZ	Sedation, cardiac arrhythmias
Omeprazole[b]	Antacid	ITZ, KTZ	Decreased azole absorption
Phenobarbital	Anticonvulsant	ITZ, KTZ	Increased azole metabolism
Rifampin	Antibacterial	ITZ, KTZ, FCZ, VCZ	Increased azole metabolism
Terfinidine	Antihistamine	ITZ, VCZ	Cardiac arrhythmias, death
Sucralfate	GI-coating agent	ITZ, KTZ	Decreased azole absorption
Sulfonylureas	Hypoglycemic agents	ITZ, KTZ, FCZ, VCZ	Severe hypoglycemia
Zidovudine (AZT)	Antiretroviral	FCZ	Zidovudine toxicity

FCZ, Fluconazole; *ITZ*, itraconazole; *KTZ*, ketoconazole; *VCZ*, voriconazole.
[a]Any antacid that raises gastric pH will interfere with absorption of azoles.
[b]This interaction is used to increase the drug concentration of cyclosporine to help reduce the required dosages for treating perianal fistulas in dogs.

high enough, it may be fatal. Histologic findings in affected animals include enlarged portal tracts, bile duct proliferation, and infiltration with mononuclear cells. KTZ may produce endocrine dysfunction by suppressing testosterone and cortisol synthesis.

KTZ is most effective in vitro against yeast and dimorphic fungi such as *Candida, Malassezia, Coccidioides, Histoplasma,* and *Blastomyces* species and is less effective against *Cryptococcus, Sporothrix,* and *Aspergillus* species. Evidence suggests that in rapidly progressing systemic mycoses, such as in many cases of blastomycosis, patients should first be treated with AMB and then maintained on KTZ (see Amphotericin B and Other Polyenes in this chapter). The action of KTZ alone often occurs so slowly (over 5 to 10 days) that the disease progresses before the drug has a chance to take effect. In contrast, KTZ has been given alone in dogs and cats to successfully treat coccidioidomycosis and some cases of histoplasmosis and cryptococcosis, although relapses are common when host defenses are inadequate. Preference for more active and generally less toxic ITZ or FCZ has been apparent for treatment of these infections. If underlying immunosuppression is thought to be responsible for the fungal disease, concurrent treatment with AMB is recommended. No evidence suggests that KTZ provides synergistic effects with other antifungals except AMB, and even that evidence is inconclusive. (For dosing and detailed information on administration, see Drug Formulary, Appendix 8, and Chapters 58 to 68.)

Unfortunately, as noted with many of the other antifungal drugs, eradication of systemic fungi with azole drugs is often incomplete. Relapses can occur when maintenance therapy is discontinued. Infections in areas where the drug cannot easily reach such as bone and the CNS are especially difficult to treat. Therapy should always continue at least 4 weeks after disease is no longer detectable clinically.

Itraconazole

ITZ is a broad-spectrum azole with more potent activity than KTZ against *Candida* species, *Aspergillus* species, and dermatophytes. It can be given orally or parenterally and is widely distributed in body tissues other than the CNS. The best success in treating human patients has been in those with (in decreasing order) paracoccidioidomycosis, blastomycosis, sporotrichosis, noninvasive aspergillosis, meningeal cryptococosis, and aspergilloma. Some patients with zygomycosis or other fungal infections also respond to ITZ treatment. In small animal practice, it has been most effective in treating blastomycosis (see Chapter 59), histoplasmosis (see Chapter 60), cryptococcosis (see Chapter 61), and coccidioidomycosis (see Chapter 62). ITZ seems to be less toxic than KTZ, probably because ITZ more selectively inhibits fungal rather than mammalian enzymes. Therefore unlike KTZ, ITZ has minimal effects on androgen or cortisol metabolism. Higher dosages should be expected to cause side effects similar to those of KTZ. Dosage adjustments do not appear to be necessary in the presence of renal dysfunction. Bioavailability after oral administration is erratic, but it can be maximized by giving ITZ with a food or fats. An oral solution improves absorption, especially in cats.[9] An IV formulation is also available for treatment of severe resistant infections such as aspergillosis, and high, steady-state plasma concentrations can be reached without the loading period required for oral formulations (see Drug Formulary, Appendix 8).

Fluconazole

FCZ is an orally active agent that has been used to treat systemic mycoses, including cryptococcal meningitis, blastomycosis, and histoplasmosis and to treat superficial infections, including candidiasis and dermatophytosis. FCZ crosses the blood-brain and blood-cerebrospinal fluid (CSF) barriers better than the older azole derivatives. It is effective for treating cryptococcosis because of its CNS penetration.[101] Voriconazole (VCZ), an FCZ derivative, also has excellent CNS penetration. The advantages of FCZ are that it is well absorbed orally and has a long half-life, making it valuable for treating susceptible fungal infections in various tissues. However, it generally is less active than ITZ, especially against filamentous fungi. It seems to be less toxic than KTZ. It is not very effective against *Aspergillus* species. Most FCZ is excreted unchanged in the urine, which makes it valuable for treating urinary yeast infections caused by *Candida* species.

Voriconazole

VCZ (Pfizer Ltd, Sandwich, UK) is a synthetic derivative of FCZ. VCZ is licensed for treatment of drug-resistant *Candida* and *Aspergillus* infections in people. It is the first among a second generation of triazoles, including posaconazole and ravuconazole, to be licensed. These three drugs have enhanced broad-spectrum antifungal activity against *Candida*, *Trichosporon*, *Cryptococcus*, *Histoplasma*, *Blastomyces*, *Aspergillus*, and *Fusarium* species and against some zygomycetes. The drugs have also demonstrated potent therapeutic efficacy in treatment of invasive pulmonary aspergillosis and disseminated and oropharyngeal candidiasis in experimental animals. This group of drugs is also effective against the filamentous fungi, and VCZ can penetrate the CNS barrier. VCZ has been more effective than AMB in the initial treatment of invasive aspergillosis in people,[53] but it has shown some tendency to produce hepatotoxicity in people.[108] (See Drug Formulary, Appendix 8, for additional information on VCZ.)

Posoconazol

Posoconazol (PCZ, previously SCH 56592; Schering-Plough Inc, Kenilworth, N.J.), a hydroxylated analogue of ITZ, is least active against *Candida* species that are resistant to FCZ or ITZ. However, its in vitro activity against *Aspergillus* species is greater than that of ITZ and VCZ. Bioavailability after oral administration is good. It has been formulated as an oral tablet and suspension and is in clinical trials in human medicine. Preliminary trials in rodents with experimental pulmonary invasive aspergillosis have shown it to be superior to AMB or other triazoles reducing fungal burden compared.

Ravuconazole

Ravuconazole (RVZ; Bristol-Myers Squibb Inc, Wallingford, Conn.) is structurally similar to FCZ and VCZ. It has fungicidal activity and is 47% to 74% bioavailable, with absorption enhanced by food. In rodents with invasive pulmonary aspergillosis, it has been equally or more effective than AMB and the other triazoles.

Terbinafine

Terbinafine is an antifungal allylamine derivative that has been extremely effective for treating people with chronic dermatophytosis of the skin or nails and superficial yeast infections. High concentrations are reached in these tissues. Improvement or resolution of onychomycosis usually occurs after 3 to 6 months of therapy. Side effects have been minimal. This drug has potential value for treating canine and feline onychomycosis. Terbinafine has been used alone or in combination with other antifungals for treatment of aspergillosis and other filamentous fungal infections (see Drug Formulary, Appendix 8).

Inhibitors of Chitin Synthesis and Cell Wall Synthesis

Fungal cell walls are composed of polysaccharides, predominantly chitin, chitosan, glucan, and mannan. Newer compounds that are being investigated as systemic antifungals are the polyoxins and nikkomycins, drugs that inhibit chitin synthesis in the fungal cell walls. Nikkomycins are nucleoside-peptide antibiotics that are competitive analogues for a substrate of the enzyme chitin synthase and have effects similar to those of β-lactams on gram-positive bacteria. In vitro studies have shown marked efficacy against *Coccidioides* and *Blastomyces* species and lesser activity against *Candida* and *Cryptococcus* species. Filamentous fungi seem more resistant. Nikkomycin Z was less effective in many experimental fungal infections in rodents; however, combination therapy may be more beneficial.[82] Lufenuron, a benzoylphenyl urea and chitin-synthesis inhibitor used to control fleas, has been reported to be effective in the treatment of dermatophytosis and coccidioidomycosis; however, in controlled studies the results have been equivocal (see Chapters 58 and 62, respectively, and Drug Formulary, Appendix 8).[3,7,8] The benanomicins and pradimicins damage the mannan component of the fungal cell wall by calcium chelation, but their use is limited by their poor oral bioavailability.

Echinocandins

Aculeacins, echinocandins, and papulacandins are lipopeptides that inhibit the synthesis of 1, 3-β-glucan, a polysaccharide in the cell wall of many pathogenic fungi. Together with chitin, ropelike glucan fibrils give the cell wall integrity and strength. One early echinocandin, cilofungin, was effective against systemic candidiasis and *Aspergillus* species in laboratory animals when given by continuous IV infusions. Caspofungin, micafungin, and anidulafungin have been most promising for clinical use.

Caspofungin

Caspofungin (MK-0991, L-743,872, *Cancidas*; Merck, Rahway, N.J.) has been approved for treatment of mucosal and invasive candidiasis and invasive aspergillosis in people refractory to AMB or triazoles. It is a fungicidal, water-soluble drug that must be given parenterally because of its low oral bioavailability. Metabolism is predominantly via the liver. Fungal growth is required, so the onset of action in vivo is slower than that of AMB. It has also been shown to be equal or more effective than AMB in treatment of invasive candidiasis.[94] This class of drugs has few side effects. The drugs are currently only available for IV infusion on a once daily basis. Interactions are apparent with other drugs that undergo hepatic metabolism. In vitro studies have shown an enhanced antifungal effect in the presence of sera or phagocytes, suggesting damage to hyphae is followed by enhanced fungicidal activity. Toxicity has been low in investigational studies in people. *Micafungin* (FK463; Fujisawa Healthcare, Deerfield, IL) has shown high in vitro activity against *Aspergillus* species that is greater than that of AMB or ITZ. Preliminary results in clinical trials have been favorable. *Anidulafungin* (VER-002, LY-303366; Vicuron, King of Prussia, Pa.) has the longest half-life of any of the echinocandins and has fungistatic activity that has been higher than AMB or ITZ during in vitro studies. In studies in rodents with invasive aspergillosis, anidulafungin in combination with glucocorticoids proved highly fatal.[17] This is thought to be a complication that can occur with the any drug in the echinocandin class.[126]

Combination Therapy

Simultaneous administration of antifungal agents is indicated in certain circumstances. Combined use of AMB and FCY is synergistic in treating cryptococcal infections; presumably, AMB facilitates penetration of FCY into the fungal cell. Synergism has also been subjectively assessed in the treatment of blastomycosis, coccidioidomycosis, and histoplasmosis by combining AMB and azole derivatives. Generally, AMB and azoles are started simultaneously in cases of rapidly advancing infection because of the 2- to 3-week delay of the azole derivatives to be effective. After this time the AMB may be discontinued. The therapeutic combination of ITZ and AMB as a combination for resistant infections is highly controversial. Lipophilic azoles such as KTZ and ITZ block the interaction of AMB with the fungal cell membrane.[129] Water-soluble azoles such as FCZ enter the fungal cell membrane and do not cause this interaction. Synergism between FCZ and AMB has been observed in treatment of systemic candidiasis, whereas combinations of echinocandins with azoles, AMB, or nikkomycins have not shown antagonism and deserve more study.[42] In invasive aspergillosis, combination therapy using AMB and 5-FCY or AMB and rifampin was more efficacious than either drug alone and superior to AMB and ITZ.[127] Combinations of allylamine antifungals such as terbinifine and azoles have been more effective in vitro and in vivo than either drug alone.[119] Fluoroquinolones appear to enhance the antifungal activity of AMB or FCZ.[119]

Immunotherapy

Disseminated fungal infections are often indicative of impaired host immunity. A direct relationship has been established between immunosuppressive dosages of glucocorticoids or cyclosporine and fungal dissemination. Glucocorticoids can suppress the ability of phagocytes to kill conidia through inhibition of nonoxidative processes and impairment of lysosomal activity.[126] Glucocorticoids predominantly suppress macrophages, whereas cytotoxic chemotherapy decreases neutrophil numbers and function. Recombinant hemopoietic cytokines such as G-CSF, M-CSF and GM-CSF reduce periods of neutropenia and the risk of developing invasive mycoses.[96,112] Pretreatment of neutrophils or phagocytes with their respective stimulatory cytokines may reverse or attenuate the inhibitory effect on cytotoxic antifungal activity. Granulocyte transfusions have not been very beneficial in potentiating treatment of fungal infection in people unless donors have been primed with G-CSF. Therefore the effect of the cytokine may be critical in this facilitation. Leukocyte colony-stimulating factors and additional cytokines such as interferon-γ (IFN-γ), which can enhance the activity of phagocytes against fungi, have shown some efficacy during in vitro and in vivo animal studies. Antifungal drugs combined with IFN-γ or interleukin-12 (IL-12) were synergistic in treating systemic infections in laboratory rodents.[15,42] Antifungal therapy and immunotherapy have also been combined and may have a synergistic effect. Vaccines composed of whole *Pythium insidiosum* cells or concentrated soluble antigens have been used for treatment of infection in horses and dogs.[51] The effectiveness of such immunotherapy requires additional investigation. IV immunoglobulin therapy may help reduce the prevalence of fungal infections in immunocompromised hosts; however, additional controlled studies are needed (see Immunotherapy, Chapter 2, and Drug Formulary, Appendix 8).

Antifungal Drug Use in Pregnancy

Griseofulvin, FCZ, and KTZ are all teratogenic or embryotoxic in animals and should be avoided. KTZ also interferes with steroidogenesis and may alter sexual differentiation. Iodides may cause congenital goiter in fetuses, thereby causing dystocias. AMB and its lipid preparations are not teratogenic and are probably the drugs of choice for systemic chemotherapy of pregnant animals. FCZ is safe at low dosages in pregnancy; however, higher levels produce congenital malformations. At higher than therapeutic dosages, ITZ produced maternal and embryotoxic effects and teratogenicity in rats and mice. Whenever possible, topical therapy for dermatomycoses is recommended during gestation.

Fungal Biofilms

Nosocomial fungal infections may be caused by organisms that have adapted to produce biofilms on inanimate objects, which allows them to infect or colonize patients that are hospitalized for various medical conditions requiring indwelling catheters, endoscopy, or invasive or prosthetic procedures. For example, *Candida* species biofilms have been identified on indwelling IV catheters (see Chapter 65). Once attached to the surface of the implanted device, the organisms can proliferate, forming dense colonies of yeasts, hyphae, or pseudohyphae. Subsequently, organisms detach, producing septicemia. The clinical significance of such infections is host and antimicrobial resistance.[59] The lipid formulations of AMB and the echicocandins have been shown to be most effective in penetrating these biofilm-associated infections.

Antifungal Resistance

An increased risk of invasive fungal infections such as aspergillosis has been noted in immunosuppressed people who received previous treatment with FCZ.[121] Resistance of *Aspergillus* species to ITZ in vitro has been associated with up-regulation transporter genes, and previous treatment with FCZ has made *Aspergillus* species more resistant to the effects of AMB in vitro.[70] These observations suggest that indiscriminate antifungal prophylaxis for immunocompromised hosts may lead to more resistant fungal infections and should be avoided. The total cumulative dose of FCZ administered and the use of subtherapeutic intermittent dose schedules are the factors most likely to contribute to emergence of fungal resistance.[145]

Adjunctive Surgical Therapy

Surgery is often needed to debride fungal infections in areas that are difficult for antifungal agents to penetrate. Fungal diskospondylitis may require debridement and stabilization of infected intervertebral lesions. Osteoproliferation does not often occur with such infections as with bacterial diskospondylitis. It is also difficult to eliminate infections in the testes or epididymis, so neutering is recommended when infection is detected in these tissues. Endogenous enophthalmitis often develops as a result of systemic fungal dissemination. Fungal infection localizes in the retinal vessels and choroid, with exudative lesions developing along blood vessels; later the infection spreads to the vitreous. The capillaries of the CNS and aqueous are nonfenestrated and as a result are more resistant to the entry of antifungal drugs. Early choroidal infections can be treated with systemic therapy. Even AMB cannot penetrate the inflamed eye. In such circumstances, AMB is sometimes injected directly into the vitreous. In some cases the vitreous or eye must be surgically removed. Of the azoles, FCZ is most lipid soluble and reaches intraocular concentrations between 25% and 50% serum concentrations. It is likely that higher-than-recommended dosages of FCZ may be needed for intraocular infection.

TOPICAL ANTIFUNGALS

Many formulations are used in the treatment of dermatophytosis and superficial yeast infections (Table 57-4; see Dermatophytosis, Chapter 58). Undecylenic acid is an unsaturated fatty acid given in combination with zinc to treat dermatophytosis. Its mechanism of action is unknown. Mercaptans—organic mercurial compounds—have been used as plant fungicides and can be a low-cost, dilute dip for affected animals. Tolnaftate, a synthetic lipid-soluble compound, has also been used, but hyperkeratotic plaques must be removed before its application to ensure its effectiveness. Topical cuprimyxin is a copper-containing compound that is highly

Table • 57-4

Agents Commonly Used Topically Against Fungi and Yeasts

GENERIC NAME	CLINICAL FORMULATION (% ACTIVITY)	SUSCEPTIBLE ORGANISMS (MOST TO LEAST)	COMMENTS AND RECOMMENDATIONS FOR VETERINARY USAGE
Miscellaneous			
Mercaptans	Captan Technical-grade powder (45%)	Dermatophytes	Not recommended, toxic, carcinogenic, ineffective
Chlorhexidine	Nolvasan,[a] chlorhexiderm[a,b] solution (1%), shampoo (0.5%)	Dermatophytes	Poor efficacy
Tolnaftate	Tinactin[c] Cream, powder, solution, aerosol, liquid (1%)	Dermatophytes	Spot treatment: animals can ingest, bitter taste
Undecylenic acid and salts	Powder, ointment, cream, 2%–10% soap, liquid, foam[c]	Dermatophytes	Spot treatment: animals can ingest, bitter taste
Halprogin	Halotex[d] Cream solution (1%)	Dermatophytes, *Malassezia*	Spot treatment, ear medicant
Lime sulfur	Lymdyp[b]	Dermatophytes	Has odor, stains hair, good for dermatophytosis, very safe in puppies and kittens, stains jewelry
Ciclopiroxolamine	Loprox[e] Cream, lotion (1%)	*Malassezia* dermatophytes, *Candida*	Spot treatment
Naftifine hydrochloride	Naftin[f] Cream, gel (1%)	Dermatophytes	Spot treatment
Polyenes			
Amphotericin B	Fungizone[g] Cream, lotion, ointment (3%)	*Candida*	Limited use as irrigant for affected mucosal tissues
Nystatin	Mycostatin[c] Ointment, cream, or powder (10^5 μg); suspension (10^5 U/ml); tablets 5×10^5 U	*Candida* dermatophytes, variable *Aspergillus*	Limited as irrigant for affected mucosal tissues
Imidazoles			
Thiabendazole	Solution (13%)	Dermatophytes, *Candida Aspergillus*	Third choice for nasal aspergillosis
Ketoconazole	Nizoral[h] Cream, shampoo, solution (2%)	Dermatophytes, *Malassezia*	Poor efficacy in dermatophytosis
Econazole nitrate	Spectazole,[i] Sebazol Cream, spray, powder (1%)	Dermatophytes, *Candida*	Spot treatment, may need to treat whole animal
Miconazole nitrate	Micatin[i] Powder, shampoo, cream, lotion (2%)	Dermatophytes, *Candida Malassezia Leishmania*	Spot treatment, shampoo efficacy undocumented
Clotrimazole	Lotrimin, Mycelex[c] Cream, lotion, solution (1%)	Dermatophytes, *Candida Aspergillus*	First choice for nasal aspergillosis, urinary flush for resistant candidal urinary infection
Enilconazole	Imaverol[h] Solution (10%)	Dermatophytes, *Aspergillus*	Second choice for canine nasal aspergillosis, toxic to cats

[a]Fort Dodge, Fort Dodge, Iowa.
[b]DVM Pharmaceuticals, subsidiary of IVAX Corp., Miami, Fla.
[c]Various, over the counter.
[d]Westwood Squibb, subsidiary of Bristol-Myers Squibb, Montreal, Canada.
[e]Medicis, Inamed, Scottsdale, Ariz.
[f]Allergan, Irvine, Calif.
[g]E-R Squibb, Bristol-Myers Squibb, Princeton, N.J.
[h]Janssen, Titusville, Tenn.
[i]Ortho-McNiel, Raritan, N.J.

effective against *Malassezia* species. Iodochlorhydroxyquin is a halogenated oxyquinoline that has been given orally as an antifungal, antiprotozoal, and antibacterial agent in dogs, although overdosages have caused CNS toxicity. Chlorhexidine solution (0.5%) has been recommended as a daily dip or shampoo for persistent dermatophyte infections, although its efficacy is poor.[25,147] Haloprogin is a broad-spectrum topical antifungal drug that may be more helpful against dermatophyte and *Candida* species infections.

Nystatin is a polyene antibiotic that is closely related to AMB and produced by *Streptomyces noursei*. It is poorly absorbed after oral administration or topical application to skin or mucous membranes. Because it is very toxic to internal tissues, parenteral administration must be avoided. Although nystatin is somewhat effective against dermatophytes and *Aspergillus* species, its primary use has been to treat candidiasis. Liposomal nystatin has lower toxicity than the conventional preparation; however, the in vitro and experimental in vivo efficacy has not been superior to AMB.[126]

Although azole derivatives were discussed in the systemic antifungal drugs section, several agents are only used topically. *Thiabendazole* (13%) has been used as a dip 3 times weekly for 3 weeks to treat cats with dermatophytosis. *Miconazole* was initially licensed for systemic use, but it is no longer used in this way because of its toxicity. Miconazole is now used topically in a variety of veterinary preparations for dermatophyte or yeast infections of the skin or ears. Polymyxin B, included in some of these preparations to treat bacteria, and miconazole may have a synergistic effect against bacteria and fungi. Shampoos containing miconazole and chlorhexidine are available for topical treatment of cutaneous fungal infections. Miconazole has often been used as a topical treatment for dermatophytosis in conjunction with simultaneous systemic therapy with griseofulvin. *Clotrimazole* is very effective against yeasts, dermatophytes, and *Aspergillus* species. Because of its limited absorption, severe irritation of the GI tract, and sys-

temic toxicity, it has been confined to topical application, especially for treatment of dermatophytosis (see Chapter 58) and nasal aspergillosis (see Chapter 65 and Drug Formulary, Appendix 8).[20] It was more effective than miconazole in treating dermatophytosis in dogs and cats when applied as a 1% solution twice daily for 2 weeks. Clotrimazole has also been instilled in the urinary bladder to treat *Candida* species cystitis in dogs and cats[34,134] (see Chapter 65). *Enilconazole* is a topically applied derivative that has been valuable in the treatment of nasal aspergillosis (see Chapter 64 and Drug Formulary, Appendix 8). Several other topical azole preparations from human medicine are listed in Table 57-4.

SUGGESTED READINGS*

4. Bekersky I, Boswell GW, Hiles R, et al. 1999. Safety and toxicokinetics of intravenous liposomal amphotericin B (AmBiosome) in Beagle dogs. *Pharm Res* 16:1694-1701.
8. Ben-Ziony Y, Arzi B. 2001. Updated information for treatment of fungal infections in cats and dogs. *J Am Vet Med Assoc* 218:1718.
16. Castanon-Olivares LR, Manzano-Gayosso P, Lopez-Martinez R, et al. 2001. Effectiveness of terbinafine in the eradication of *Microsporum canis* from laboratory cats. *Mycoses* 44:95-97.
23. DeBoer D, Moriello K. 2002. Efficacy of pre-treatment with lufenuron for prevention of *Microsporum canis* infection in a feline cohabitant challenge model. *Vet Dermatol* 13:215.
27. de Jaham C, Paradis M, Papich MG. 2000. Antifungal dermatologic agents: azoles and allylamines. *Compend Cont Educ Pract Vet* 22:548-566.

*See the CD-ROM for a complete list of references.

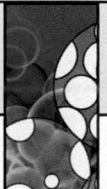

CHAPTER • 58

Cutaneous Fungal Infections

DERMATOPHYTOSIS

Douglas J. DeBoer and Karen A. Moriello

Etiology
Pathogenic Dermatophytes
Dermatophytosis is a superficial cutaneous infection with one of a group of keratinophilic fungi. The great majority of canine and feline dermatophyte infections worldwide are caused by *Microsporum canis*, *Trichophyton mentagrophytes*, or the geophilic species *Microsporum gypseum*,[38,124] although the list of species of dermatophytes that have been reported occasionally or rarely from symptomatic or asymptomatic dogs and cats is extensive (Table 58-1). The prevalence of infections caused by each of the three common etiologic agents varies geographically.

In cats, over 90% of infections are caused by *M. canis* worldwide. The prevalence of *M. gypseum* infection, which is most common in humid tropic and subtropic areas, varies seasonally, being more common in summer and autumn.[124] Simultaneous infection of dogs with more than one dermatophyte species may occur. Of combined infections, those caused by *M. gypseum* and *T. mentagrophytes* have been the most common.

Phenotypic[128] and genotypic[88,111] diversity within different strains of the same dermatophyte species is now widely recognized. Various DNA fingerprinting techniques have demonstrated strain variability within species such as *M. canis* and *T. mentagrophytes* and have also led to potential reclassification of some of the minor *Microsporum* spp.[88,111,116] The practical importance and clinical implications of this variation are as yet uncertain.

Table • 58-1

Dermatophyte Species Reported from Specimens from Dogs and Cats

SPECIES	HOSTS	GEOGRAPHIC RANGE/COMMENT
Zoophilic		
Microsporum canis[a] (includes *M. distortum*)	B	Worldwide; common
M. equinum (horses; resembles *M. canis*)	D	?; rare
M. nanum (pigs)	B	Worldwide
M. gallinae	B	Worldwide
Trichophyton equinum (horses)	B	Worldwide
T. verrucosum (cattle, sheep)	B	Worldwide
Sylvatic		
T. mentagrophytes includes *T. mentagrophytes erinacei* (hedgehogs) and *T. mentagrophytes quinckeanum* (mice)	B B	Worldwide; common
M. persicolor (voles)	B	Europe and Canada; not in hair
Geophilic		
M. cookei	B	Worldwide
M. fulvum (resembles *M. gypseum*)	B	Worldwide
M. vanbreuseghemi[a]	B	Eurasia and North America
T. simii	B	India; frequently infects monkeys and poultry
M. gypseum	B	Worldwide; especially warm climates; common
T. terrestre	B	Worldwide; not very pathogenic; not in hair
T. ajelloi	B	Worldwide; not very pathogenic; not in hair
Anthropophilic		
Epidermophyton floccosum	B	Worldwide
M. audouini[a]	B	Worldwide
T. megninii	B	Africa, Europe
T. rubrum	B	Worldwide
T. schoenleinii	B	Africa, Asia; rare in Americas
T. tonsurans	B	Worldwide; especially Latin America
T. violaceum	B	Worldwide; rare in North America

B, Both dog and cat; *D*, dog; ?, uncertain.
[a]This species fluoresces when illuminated with ultraviolet light.

Fungal Microflora on the Hair and Skin

Dogs and cats harbor many saprophytic molds and yeasts on their haircoats and probably on dermatitic skin as well. The most common fungi isolated from the haircoats of clinically healthy cats are *Alternaria, Aspergillus, Cladosporium, Penicillium, Rhizopus,* and *Trichoderma.*[162,163,171] From dogs, the same fungi are isolated with somewhat different frequencies.[189]

At one time, it was proposed that cats are reservoirs of pathogenic dermatophytes (*M. canis, M. gypseum, Microsporum vanbreuseghemii, Trichophyton verrucosum, T. mentagrophytes, Trichophyton rubrum, Epidermophyton* spp.). To investigate this possibility, many populations of cats have been surveyed by culture.[79,153,189,203] Using similar techniques, fungal isolates from the haircoats of pet, stray, or cattery cats from various geographic regions were collected. The prevalence of dermatophyte isolation, specifically *M. canis,* varied among the populations, depending on the geographic region, whether or not the cat was a stray or pet cat, and the presence or absence of skin disease at the time of sampling. *M. canis* was most commonly isolated from stray cats or those in multiple cat facilities and from warm geographic regions.

In surveys of pet cats from the United States, Belgium, and the United Kingdom, the prevalence of *M. canis* isolation in 172 cats was 0%, in 467 was 2.1% and in 181 cats was 2.2%.[153] In the last study, all four of the cats with positive culture results were from multiple-cat households and were allowed to roam freely outside. Interestingly, in the United States study, *T. rubrum* was isolated from 14 cats; this organism is the human pathogen associated with tinea pedis (athlete's foot).[79] This point highlights the importance of fomite carriage by the haircoat of dogs and cats of potentially pathogenic dermatophytes; *T. rubrum* infection is rare in cats.

In catteries, the isolation of *M. canis* depends greatly on whether the cattery has a history of dermatophytosis. In one study of catteries from temperate regions of the United States, cats had either negative culture results, or, in *M. canis*–affected catteries, virtually all cats had positive culture results.[163] These findings were identical to those of a smaller study from a warmer region of the United States that also failed to isolate *M. canis* from the haircoat of cattery cats from facilities that were free of the disease.[224]

In surveys of stray and shelter cats, the incidence of *M. canis* isolation was higher. In the United States, the isolation of *M. canis* from animal shelters in a subtropic climate was 17.5% compared with 4% from a temperate climate.[171] Both isolations were performed at the same time of the year. In a study conducted in Belgium, 134 cats were cultured and *M. canis* was isolated from 15.7%.[153] A study from Italy emphasizes the impact that climate and geography has on the prevalence of *M. canis* isolation.[203] In this study, 173 stray cats without skin disease were sampled, and 47% had positive culture results for *M. canis*. These studies on the fungal flora of dogs and cats highlight two important points. First, pathogenic dermatophytic fungi (e.g., *M. canis*) should not be considered part of the *normal* fungal flora of cats (or dogs). If they were, they would have been isolated routinely from healthy dogs and cats regardless of geographic region, lifestyle (indoor or outdoor), or status (pet or stray). Second, isolating pathogens from clinically healthy animals is possible. The isolation of a pathogenic organism indicates either infection (obvious or subclinical) or fomite carriage from exposure to a contaminated environment. However, if the animal is lesion free, distinguishing between these possibilities is often impossible. Regardless, animals with positive culture results should be treated because dermatophytosis is an important zoonotic disease.

Epidemiology

The exact prevalence of dermatophytosis is unknown because the disease is not reportable, even though it is a zoonosis. In clinical practice, dermatophytosis is overdiagnosed, most likely because of its similarities to other skin diseases. In all studies of skin disease of dogs and cats in which fungal cultures have been performed, the prevalence of dermatophyte infections seems to be approximately 2% of all dermatologic cases. The percentage of positive culture results among specimens submitted from suspected ringworm cases has ranged from less than 4% to 50%.[28,124,134,214] In the United Kingdom, a survey showed that culture results were positive from only 16% of 8349 specimens from dogs or cats suspected of having dermatophytosis, whereas in Turin, Italy, the figure was 40% of cases examined.[134,214] These figures may reflect not only geographic variation, but also differences in the types of cases chosen for dermatophyte culture. Environmental factors, such as increased warmth and high humidity, and animal background, such as existence of debilitation or concurrent disease, extremes of age, feral behavior, or congregated housing, may increase the prevalence of infection in dogs and cats.[160] Long haircoats, especially in cats, may predispose the animal to infection because the hair may become matted or protect the spores from removal by grooming and increase contact with the underlying skin.[160]

Pathogenesis

Transmission and Predisposing Factors

Dermatophytes are spread between animals or to persons from animals by direct contact, by contact with infected hair and scale in the environment, or via fomites. The typical infective portion of the organism is the arthrospores, formed from the segmentation and fragmentation of fungal hyphae. These infective spores are small and can be carried on air currents and dust particles or fomites. Fleas from infected animals can also transmit the disease. The dose or quantity of infective material needed to establish spontaneous infection is unknown; under experimental conditions, at least 100 spores typically are required. Infections have been traced to contact with contaminated brushes, collars, environments, and casual contact with subclinically infected cats. Casual contact is of particular concern for individuals working in multiple-animal facilities because not many infected hairs are needed to transmit the infection. Transmission to a child from the interior of a used car was reported.[225]

After reaching the haircoat, infective spores must compete with natural host defense mechanisms to establish infection. Under optimal conditions of temperature (25° C to 37° C), infective spores can germinate within 6 hours of adherence to keratinocytes. Arthrospores adhere very strongly to keratin. Arthrospores cannot penetrate healthy intact skin; some type of superficial trauma is needed to facilitate infection. The amount of trauma required is relatively minimal based on experimental models of infection.[55] Increased hydration and maceration of the skin (e.g., within footwear) is a common predisposing factor to infection in people. Moisture enhances the ability of dermatophytes to penetrate the skin and favors germination. In general, the normally dry condition of the skin surface and fungistatic properties of serum and sebum are natural host defense mechanisms. Normal grooming behavior of cats distributes sebum from areas of high concentration and production (chin and dorsum) to other areas of the body and may remove spores.

The incubation period is 1 to 3 weeks. With *M. canis* infections, the source is typically an infected cat or fomites contaminated by cats. In contrast, most *Trichophyton* infections are suspected of being caused by contact with rodents or their nests. *M. gypseum* is a geophilic organism that inhabits rich soil; dogs and cats are exposed by digging and rooting in contaminated areas. Infections with anthropophilic species are acquired, albeit uncommonly, as *reverse zoonoses* by direct contact with infected persons.

Dermatophytosis is more common in hot, humid environments, which may contribute to conditions favoring outbreaks of dermatophytosis in multiple-animal facilities. Excessive bathing and grooming of cats or dogs may predispose them to infection by removing normal host defense mechanisms (fungistatic sebum and serum), removal of epidermal cells that act as an intact barrier, and increasing the humidity of the skin and haircoat. In addition, routine sanitation in multiple-cat facilities may also increase humidity, favoring development of infection.

Dermatophyte infections of dogs and cats involve the hair shaft, follicle, and surrounding stratum corneum. Infected hair shafts are fragile, and dislodged hair fragments containing infective spores are the most efficient means of transmission to other hosts. Such material may remain infectious in the environment for many months. One study found that samples of hair stored for 18 months could yield positive culture results.[221]

Virulence Factors

Several different proteolytic enzymes (keratinase, elastase, and collagenase) have been isolated from dermatophyte fungi, and a role for these proteases has been proposed in the initiation and progression of infection.[1,29,30,69] The enzymes are produced under in vitro culture conditions, as well as being detectable in infected skin biopsies.[154] The number and quantity of enzymes produced varies from strain to strain and may, in part, explain variability in clinical presentation.[1]

Immunology

When infective dermatophyte arthrospores contact the hair and skin, many factors influence whether infection will ensue. Some of these factors are not dependent on development of a specific immune response to the fungus. Trauma facilitates development of infection. Normal serum inhibits growth of dermatophytes, as do fungistatic fatty acids present in sebum. Physical occlusion leads to increased hydration of the normally dry skin surface, with subsequent maceration and easier infection. The overall immunologic status of the host influences development of infections. Infections are more easily established in very young, very old, or immunocompromised animals and people. For example, an increased frequency of isolation of *M. canis* was reported in feline immunodeficiency virus–infected cats.[129] These innate factors in *resistance* are distinct from the specific immunologic responses acquired as a consequence of infection.

Dermatophyte Antigens Three different physical components of dermatophytic fungi have received the most attention for their role as antigens in the host immune response: cell wall carbohydrates, cell wall proteins, and secreted keratinases. Fungal mycelium is composed of approximately 10% protein, 20% carbohydrate (notably chitin and mannan), and 70% lipid. The immunologically active portion of the cell wall is of glycopeptide composition, with the carbohydrate portion chiefly involved in immediate-type hypersensitivity and the peptide portion important in delayed-type hypersensitivity. These glycopeptides are not fungal species specific; abundant cross-reactivity is present across different genera of keratinophilic fungi. Most infected individuals also develop humoral and cell-mediated immunity (CMI) against fungal keratinases, proteolytic enzymes secreted at the tips of the invading hyphae. Fungal keratinases, including those from *M. canis* of feline origin, have been isolated and characterized chemically and immunologically.[150-152] Antibodies developed against dermatophyte antigens cross-react with mycelial antigens from common saprophytic fungi such as *Penicillium, Hormodendrum, Aspergillus,* and so forth, and attempts to classify dermatophytes according to serologic reactivity were not successful.

Acquired Immunity During Infection Though the host immune response to dermatophyte infection has been the subject of investigation for nearly a century, only relatively recently has the immunology of this disease been closely studied in companion animal species, and most information comes from studies performed in cats. Overall, early animal studies generally concluded that CMI, rather than humoral immunity, is more important in resistance to reinfection. The majority of human patients with acquired dermatophytosis develop positive intradermal test (IDT) reactions to dermatophyte antigens. Development of a delayed (48 to 72 hours) IDT reaction represents CMI and correlates well with both a positive lymphocyte blastogenesis test result and at least partial immunity to reinfection. Development of an immediate (15 to 30 minute) IDT reaction represents development of reaginic antibody–mediated hypersensitivity. Attempts have been made to relate the type of positive skin test reaction (immediate or delayed) to clinical status of the patient. As a general rule, human patients who recover from acute dermatophyte infections develop positive delayed IDT reactions and usually are relatively immune to further infection. In contrast, some human patients develop chronic, unrelenting dermatophytosis that persists for months or years. These patients develop strong immediate IDT reactions but often fail to exhibit delayed reactions even after prolonged disease. This evidence led to early speculation that a strong cell-mediated, delayed-type hypersensitivity response is responsible for elimination of the infection, whereas an immediate-type, antibody-mediated hypersensitivity response tends to inhibit or delay recovery.[99]

Natural infection of cats with *M. canis* is accompanied by both a humoral antibody response (rising immunoglobulin G [IgG] titers, and sometimes positive immediate IDT result) and a cell-mediated response (positive lymphocyte blastogenesis and delayed IDT results) against dermatophyte components, including glycoprotein extracts.[54,56,168] Available data suggest that these responses are not completely *Microsporum*-specific; that is, cross-reaction is present with *Trichophyton.* Delayed IDT reactions are often weaker in cats with active infections and in cats whose infection was aborted with anti-fungal treatment, suggesting that the infection must run its entire natural course for development of full immunity.[168] Both IDT and in vitro data in cats supports the concept that recovery from dermatophytosis depends on development of a strong CMI response.

Genetic factors also influence the development of chronic dermatophytosis in people, as evidenced by the higher prevalence of chronic infections among related individuals versus unrelated individuals living in the same household. Genetic factors may be important in cats as well. In one cattery study, chronic dermatophytosis was found most commonly in three facilities where the cats were genetically related.[163] Cats with chronic dermatophytosis had significantly higher antidermatophyte antibody levels and different lymphocyte blastogenic responses.

Once an individual recovers from dermatophytosis, generally, at least partial immunity to reinfection is present. This resistance varies in degree and duration, depending on the individual, host species, strain of dermatophyte, and the site of the original infection. Resistance is often observed to be generalized (the whole body) but typically is greatest at or near the previously infected site. Resistance is relative: experimentally inducing a second infection in a recovered person or animal is generally possible, but it requires a much greater number of spores or more occlusive conditions, or both. Additionally, the subsequent infections are cleared sooner than the first. Maximal resistance may take two or more episodes of infection to develop.

Clinical Findings

Dermatophytosis is a pleomorphic disease and cannot be diagnosed based on clinical signs alone. Dermatophytosis is primarily a follicular disease, and the most common clinical signs include hair loss, scaling, and crusting. Pruritus is variable. Some patients may develop a classic ringlike lesion with central healing and fine follicular papules on the periphery. Generally, however, signs and symptoms are highly variable and depend on the degree of inflammation and hair shaft destruction (Table 58-2).

Table • 58-2

Diverse Clinical Features of Dermatophytosis

Cats	Alopecia, frayed hairs
	Pruritus
	Erythema
	Scaling and crusting
	Comedones (feline acne)
	Hyperpigmentation
	Paronychia
	Pruritic ear pinnae (*M. canis*)
	Miliary dermatitis (one cause)
	Granulomatous nodules or ulcers
	Facial fold pyoderma, conjunctivitis
Dogs	Alopecia
	Papules or pustules
	Crusts, scales, hyperpigmentation
	Facial furunculosis
	Nodular skin lesions (kerion reactions)
	Onychomycosis
	Urticaria and papular eruptions

Cat

Dermatophytosis can seemingly mimic almost any described feline skin disease. *M. canis* infection is not generally a localized disease, despite appearances to the contrary. Clinical lesions maybe focal or multifocal, but spores or areas of inapparent infection, or both, will be present throughout the haircoat. Pruritus varies from none to self-mutilation. Hyperpigmentation of the skin is rare in cats but is most likely seen in cats with dermatophytosis. Scaling may be limited or generalized and diffuse or multifocal. Because hair loss is a common finding, a usual owner complaint is excessive shedding. Cats with generalized dermatophytosis often ingest large amounts of hair while grooming and may have a history of vomiting, constipation, hairball problems, or any combination of these. Erythema and scaling of the inner or outer pinnae (or both) is another common presentation in adult cats. Patches of scale with minor alopecia or hair breakage is one of the most common presentations in longhaired cats. Feline skin reaction patterns where dermatophytosis should be considered as a differential diagnosis include miliary dermatitis, symmetrical alopecia, eosinophilic plaques, and indolent ulcers.

Dermatophyte lesions in kittens tend to consist of areas of hair loss and scaling; erythema is variable and is often difficult to detect in dark-haired cats. Lesions are often first seen as areas of hair loss on the muzzle, face, ears, and forelegs (Fig. 58-1). Depending on the overall health of the kitten, lesions may be focal, multifocal, or generalized. Kittens with limited dermatophyte lesions that develop upper respiratory infections or gastrointestinal (GI) diseases, or both, are at increased risk for the development of generalized lesions. *M. canis* can cause comedone-like lesions (i.e., *chin acne*) in young cats.

Uncommon presentations of feline dermatophytosis include an appearance clinically identical to pemphigus foliaceus, with scaling and crusting over the bridge of the nose and the face or crusting exudative paronychia, or both. Unilateral or bilateral pinnal pruritus is another under-recognized presentation of *M. canis*. In the cats examined by the author (KAM), infected hairs were limited to the ear margin or long hairs within the "bell" of the ear, or both. *M. canis* is uncommonly a cause of recurrent otitis externa.[89] Rarely, diffuse alopecia with hyperpigmented patches of long hair has been observed.[200]

Granulomatous dermatitis, in the form of well-circumscribed, ulcerated dermal nodules, is infrequently recognized in cats (Fig. 58-2). The lesions occur on cats afflicted with more generalized typical *M. canis* infections. Interestingly, one report described different strains of *M. canis* isolated from the granulomatous lesions and from the surface infections of the same cat.[155] These lesions have been called mycetomas, pseudomycetomas, and Majocchi's granulomas. This form of disease carries a poor prognosis for resolution.[201]

Dog

Lesions in puppies usually consist of focal or multifocal areas of hair loss and are clinically indistinguishable from other common causes of focal hair loss in a puppy, specifically demodicosis and bacterial pyoderma. As in kittens, the overall health of the puppy is an important factor in the severity of the infection.

Unlike cats, dogs are more likely to develop the *classic* foci of alopecia with follicular papules, scales and crusts, and a central area of hyperpigmentation (see Table 58-2). Dermatophytosis should be considered in any papular or pustular eruption. Facial folliculitis and furunculosis, superficially mimicking an autoimmune skin disease, can develop (Fig. 58-3). Nodular skin lesions called *kerion reactions* may occur on the face and legs (Fig. 58-4). These lesions appear as areas of deep pyoderma and are most often caused by *M. gypseum* or *Trichophyton* spp. infections. More generalized, widespread lesions should prompt a search for a potential underlying systemic cause predisposing to the infection.[39a] Onychomycosis may be exhibited by chronic ungual fold inflammation, with or without footpad involvement, or the claw alone may be infected, which causes claw deformity and fragility. Dermatophytic granulomas have been reported rarely in dogs.[7] One of the authors (DJD) has seen several shorthaired dogs

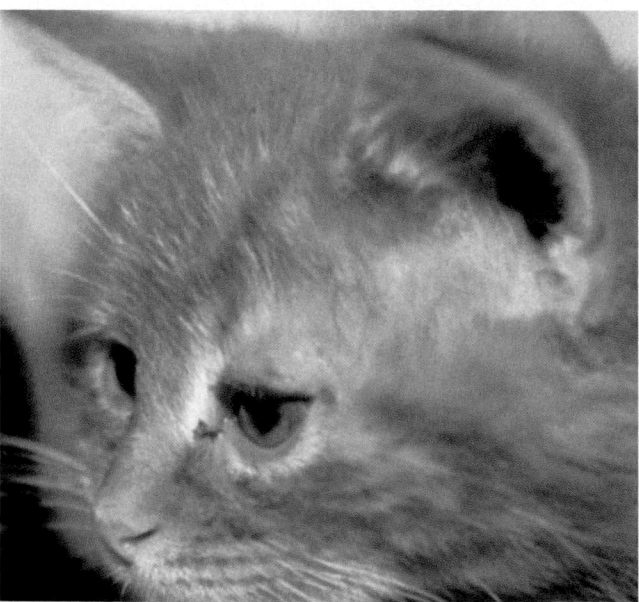

Fig 58-1 Dermatophytosis in this kitten with *M. canis* is characterized by patchy alopecia with marked scaling and hyperkeratosis. (Courtesy University of Wisconsin Teaching Materials, University of Wisconsin, Madison, Wisc.)

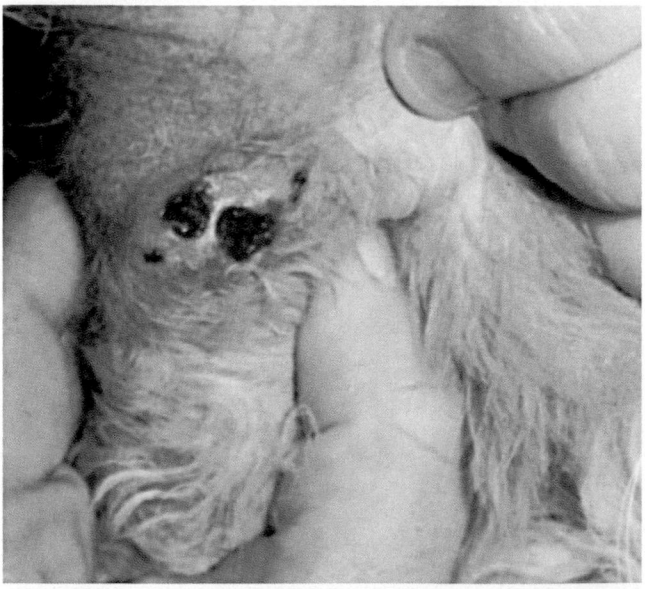

Fig 58-2 Granulomatous dermatitis has developed in this cat with generalized dermatophyte infection caused by *M. canis*. Microscopically, this lesion resembled a mycetoma. (Courtesy Gail Kunkle, University of Florida, Gainsville, Fla.)

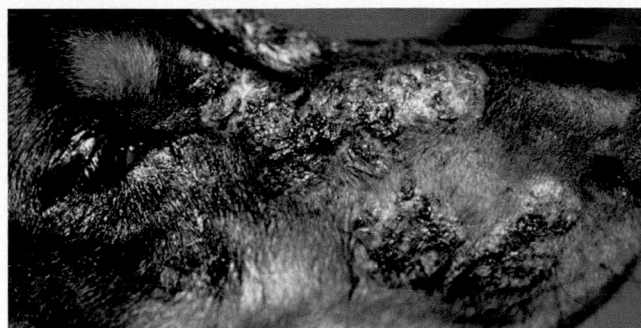

Fig 58-3 Facial folliculitis and furunculosis in this dog was caused by *T. mentagrophytes*. This dog was referred as a suspected pemphigus foliaceus case. (Courtesy University of Wisconsin Teaching Materials, University of Wisconsin, Madison, Wisc.)

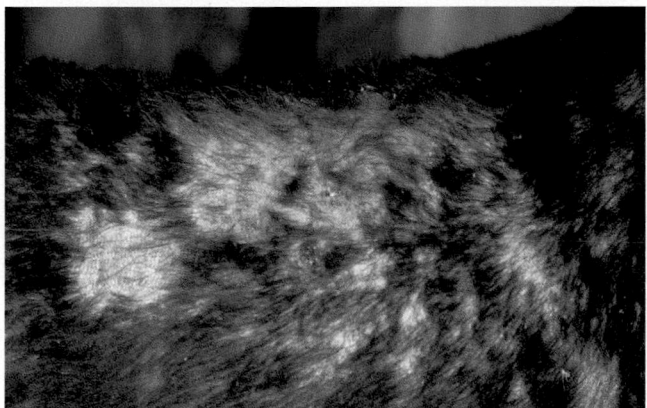

Fig 58-4 This nodular skin lesion on a dog is a kerion caused by *M. gypseum*. (Courtesy University of Wisconsin Teaching Materials, University of Wisconsin, Madison, Wisc.)

with histories of recurrent urticaria and papular eruptions caused by dermatophytosis.

Demodicosis and dermatophytosis can be clinically indistinguishable but can be reliably differentiated by a skin scraping. Superficial folliculitis, especially when accompanied by the spreading rings of erythema and exfoliation that have been characterized as *staphylococcal hypersensitivity* or *superficial spreading pyoderma*, is more often mistaken for dermatophytosis. Staphylococcal skin lesions of seborrheic spaniels are also often misdiagnosed as dermatophytosis.

Diagnosis

Although some research has focused on cellular and humoral responses to dermatophyte infections,[56,63,217,219] only preliminary work has been reported on serologic diagnosis of canine dermatophytosis.[194,81a,184a] Followup studies examining cross-reacting antibodies in experimental and naturally occurring feline dermatophytosis are needed because serology might be a useful tool for protecting cat breeders from importing infected animals to their facilities. Additionally, investigating the appropriateness of the immune response to infection in groups of persistently infected animals may soon become possible.[218] Other new developments in diagnosis include the production of polymerase chain reaction probes and immunohistochemical stains for the various species of dermatophytes.* Such techniques promise more rapid identification in clinical

*References: 9, 87, 88, 111, 125, 192, 226.

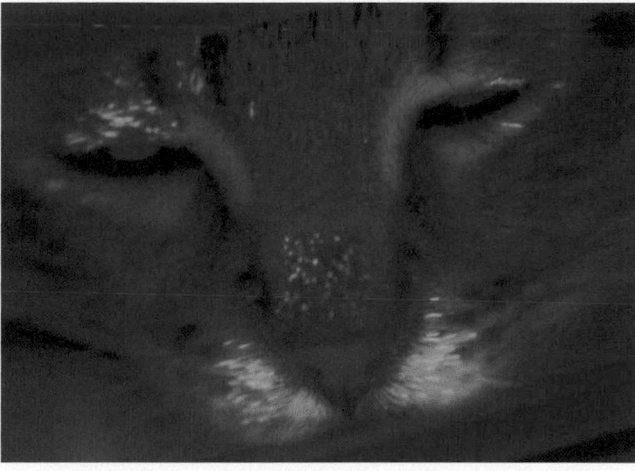

Fig 58-5 Wood's light examination of a cat with dermatophytosis showing positive fluorescence results. (Courtesy Jeanne Barsanti, University of Georgia, Athens, Ga.)

specimens but have yet to be developed for commercial use. Calcofluor white has been mentioned to improve the diagnostic accuracy of direct microscopic examination of hairs (see following discussion).[220]

Wood's Light Examination

Examination of the haircoat with a Wood's (ultraviolet, 320 to 400 nm wavelength, light) lamp is a quick and easy initial screen for presence of certain dermatophyte infections but clearly is not definitive. Perhaps only one half of all strains of *M. canis* will show fluorescence and other animal dermatophyte species will not, rendering the Wood's lamp an insensitive test. The fluorescence results from a fungal metabolite produced only when the organism is growing on hair and not on scale or claw material. Thus true fluorescence is bright "apple green" in color and occurs only along hair shafts, never in scale (Fig. 58-5). Debris, scale, lint, and topical medications commonly produce false fluorescence. Because of these pitfalls, suspected fluorescing hairs should always be cultured or examined microscopically, or both, to confirm presence of the infection. Compared with culture, the Wood's lamp examination was found to have a sensitivity of approximately 50% for *M. canis* infection.[214] Wood's lamp examination is most useful when monitoring infection status in a cattery or multiple-animal facility where endemic infection with a fluorescing strain is involved. In examining a patient with a Wood's lamp, make sure that the lamp has been allowed to warm up for a few minutes before the examination, and spend several minutes (with room lights out) examining the haircoat slowly and closely both to allow sufficient time for dark-adaptation and to avoid missing small areas of fluorescence.[166] The authors find that the larger, more powerful lamps that operate on household current are superior to smaller, battery-operated models.

Direct Microscopic Examination

Mineral oil is often used to remove and suspend hairs for microscopic evaluation. However, the hair shafts are opaque reducing visualization of the fungal elements. Hair and scale may be wet mounted in 10% to 20% potassium hydroxide (KOH) overnight or heated gently in the same solution for 10 minutes for clearing of keratin and visualization of fungal elements. Mounting in chlorphenolac (50 g chloral hydrate, 25 ml liquid phenol, and 25 ml liquid lactic acid) solution accomplishes the same task in a few minutes without heating, but the solution is not commercially available and is cumbersome to prepare. Even in experienced hands, direct examination is time consuming and may be diagnostic in only a few cases. It may lead to misinterpretation if saprophytic fungal spores are present in the specimen; debris and the complex structure of normal hair shafts can be misinterpreted as fungal elements. Dermatophytes never form macroconidia in tissue, but rather form hyphae and arthroconidia *(ectothrix spores)* on hair and scale. One investigation has recommended hair examination with a solution of 0.5 % calcofluor white stain (Beckton Dickenson, Franklin Lakes, N.J.) and Evans blue dye (1:9 solution) in equal volume of 20% KOH for superior visualization of fungal elements.[220] Direct microscopic examination is most useful when fluorescing hairs are found and can be directly plucked with a forceps under a Wood's lamp. The Wood's

lamp can be used as a light source for the microscope to aid in visualization. In this case, the finding of ectothrix spores along the hair or mycelium, or both, growing down the center of the hair shaft (Fig. 58-6, *A* and *B*) is justification for beginning treatment while awaiting more definitive culture identification of the pathogen. Compared with normal hairs, infected ones are thicker, frayed, and indistinct with a filamentous appearance.

Fungal Culture

Definitive diagnosis of dermatophytosis is made by culture, although it is neither perfectly sensitive nor always specific for the diagnosis.[214] Proper specimen collection techniques, regular examination of the growing cultures, and microscopic confirmation of the fungal species are all necessary for ideal performance of this test.

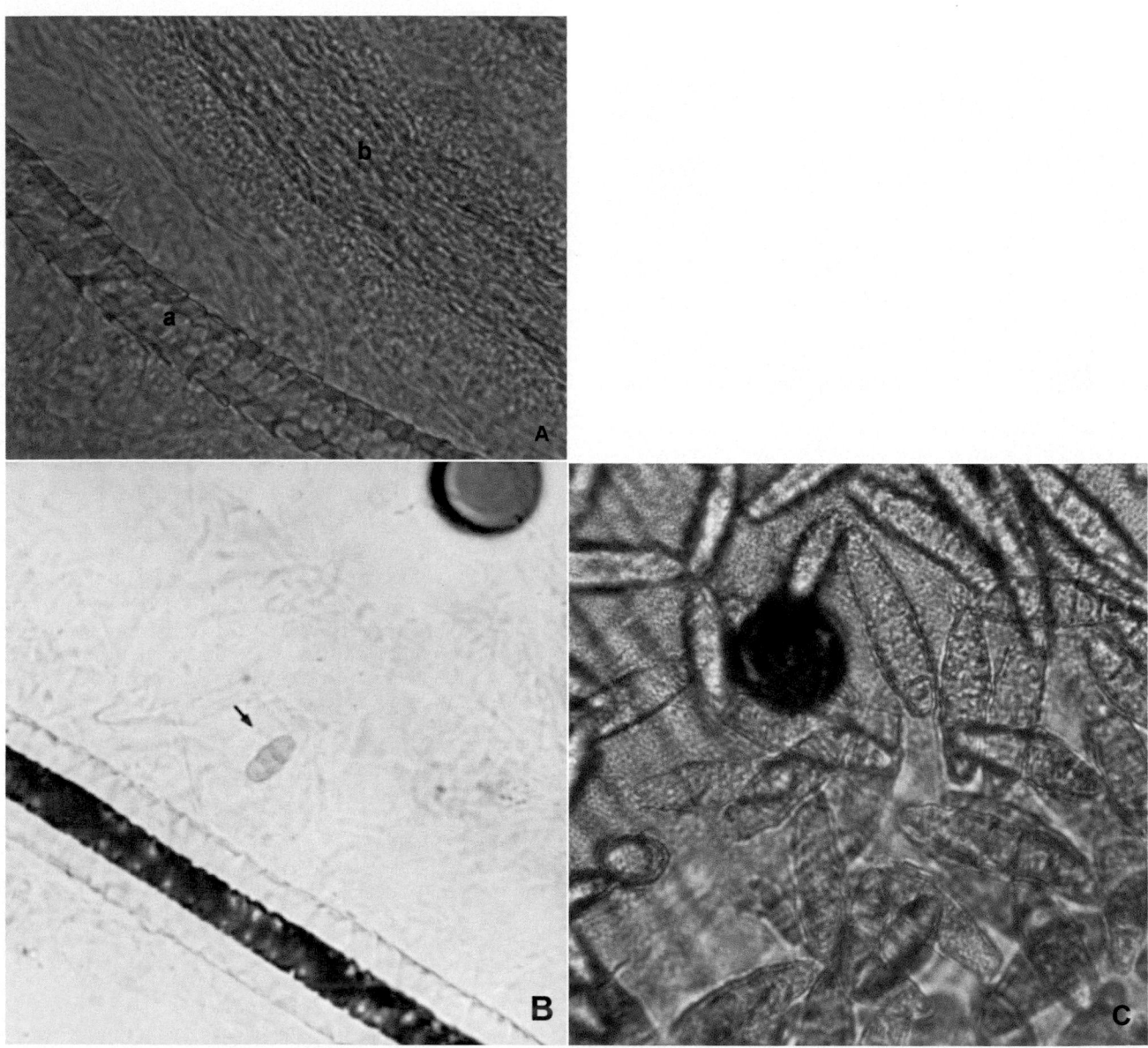

Fig 58-6 **A,** Microscopic appearance of infected hairs cleared with KOH. The lower hair (A) is normal; note the upper hair (B) is swollen, misshapen, and has tiny spherical ectothrix spores on the surface (unstained, ×100). **B,** This KOH-digested microscopic preparation of hair and scale from a dog contains a multiloculated fungal spore that may be mistaken for a dermatophyte macroconidium. It is an *Alternaria* spore. Dermatophytes never produce macroconidia in tissue. **C,** Microscopic appearance of macroconidia *(arrow)* from a positive dermatophyte test medium culture, displaying typical morphology for *M. canis* (unstained, ×100). (Courtesy University of Wisconsin Teaching Materials, University of Wisconsin, Madison, Wisc.)

Specimen Collection Specimens can be taken either by plucking hair and scale from suspected lesions or by using a brushing method; the latter method is highly recommended. If hairs are to be plucked, the area should be patted clean with an alcohol-moistened gauze and then allowed to dry. Hair shafts should be collected from several suspect sites by pulling them with a forceps or hemostat. Hairs that appear broken and near active inflammation should be selected. Scales should be included in the sample. Exudate or antiseptics should not be transferred to the medium. Brushing techniques have become favored in recent years because they allow sampling of much larger areas of the haircoat simultaneously such that the chance of missing an active area of infection is less. For this method, a new inexpensive human toothbrush is vigorously combed over regions of suspected infection (or, alternatively, all parts of the haircoat) for 2 to 3 minutes. These brushes are mycologically sterile in their original wrapping and need not be sterilized. Hairs should be visible in the bristles after brushing. The bristles and attached hairs are then pressed lightly and repeatedly (20 to 30 times) onto the surface of the culture medium, attempting to ensure contact of all sides of the sampling brush with the medium. Leaving collected hairs on top of the medium, or "planting" the hairs into the medium is unnecessary. Care must be taken not to press too firmly into the medium such that agar is removed with the brush. The toothbrush can be discarded after a single use. For followup cultures, owners can be taught to sample their pets at home, brushing the animals one at a time and depositing the brush into an individual, sealed plastic bag marked with the pet's name. This procedure avoids having to transport potentially infected animals to a clinic, with contamination of the vehicle and veterinary premises. Note that the toothbrush method requires use of culture medium in a plate format, rather than in tubes or vials, because insertion of the brush to inoculate into a narrow tube or vial is mechanically impossible.

Special Specimen Collection Situations The toothbrush method excels in identification of animals with mild, subclinical, or asymptomatic infections. In this case, every square inch of the entire animal—from nose to tail, including limbs and all trunkal surfaces—is sampled by vigorous brushing for several minutes, and the medium is inoculated as previously detailed. In kittens, brushing the face and in the hairs on the inside of the *bell* of ear is important. Early lesions of dermatophytosis often start at these sites, and, unfortunately, these sites are often undersampled or not sampled at all during coat brushes.

When dermatophytosis is suspected as a cause of claw or nailbed infection, special culture techniques may be needed.

In many cases, the hair surrounding the ungual fold may be infected and may be cultured, as is done elsewhere on the body. However, in dogs, geophilic fungi may contaminate preexisting foot lesions; thus correlating cultural findings with histologic demonstration of fungi in hair or claw may be necessary. Otherwise, repeated isolation of fungus from the lesions may be regarded as evidence of causation. If the claws alone are affected, a scalpel blade may be used to shave fine pieces from the proximal end of clipped or surgically excised specimens for culture.

If surgical biopsy is performed on nodular lesions, aseptically collected and transported tissue should be submitted for cultural and histologic examination.

Media, Incubation, and Interpretation Culture can readily be performed as an in-office procedure employing dermatophyte test medium (DTM). DTM consists of a nutrient medium plus inhibitors of bacterial and saprophytic growth and phenol red as a pH indicator. Several variants are available, some of which claim to speed growth of the culture, but all perform similarly.[71,95] DTM is sold in either vials or plates; the latter are preferable because they permit inoculation with a toothbrush. For incubation, DTM containers should be loosely covered or capped at room temperature and protected from ultraviolet light and desiccation, for example, in a covered container containing a damp paper towel. Dermatophyte colonies may appear as soon as 5 to 7 days after inoculation, but the culture plates should be retained for 3 weeks before calling the culture result negative. Plates should be inspected daily for a color change of the medium to red and growth of a white to buff colored, powdery to cottony mycelium. The color change must occur *at the same time* the colony is first visible, never later. All fungal growth, including nonpathogens, will produce a red color change after the colony has grown for several days to a week. Dermatophyte colonies are never green, gray, brown, or black.

Dysgonic varieties of *M. canis* (sometimes called *M. canis* var. *distortum*) may occasionally be isolated, particularly from cat colonies.[188,206] These varieties grow under the surface of the agar, giving a feathery or snowflakelike appearance. They do not produce conidia or a red color change on DTM[166] and can be converted to more typical forms by a diagnostic laboratory for identification.[140] Plates should be kept for 21 days, especially in monitoring treated animals, because fewer viable fungal spores will be present and their growth rate is often reduced.

Most often, large numbers of colonies of the dermatophyte will appear on the plate if the animal is truly infected. Table 58-3 describes the appearance of the most common isolates.

Table • 58-3

Comparison of Dermatophytes Isolated from Dogs or Cats

ORGANISM	COLONY CHARACTERISTICS	MICROSCOPIC APPEARANCE
Microsporum canis	White top surface, yellow-orange reverse pigment undersurface; flat with depressed center; cotton or wool consistency	Macroconidia: spindle or canoe shaped; each contains ≥6 cells with thick walls with outer spines on surface and terminal knob
Microsporum gypseum	Cinnamon brown top surface, yellow to tan reverse pigment undersurface; flat colonies; face powder consistency	Macroconidia: row-boat shaped; each contains <6 cells with thin walls Microconidia: single cell
Trichophyton spp.	White to cream top surface, tan to brown to red reverse pigment under surface	Macroconidia: rare; cigar shaped Microconidia: common; often spiral hyphae

The number of colonies decreases as the infection resolves spontaneously or from treatment. In some cases, only one or a few dermatophyte colonies appear. In addition to recovery, this finding may indicate either early or mild infection or poor sampling technique. This result can also be seen in uninfected cats that are living in the same environment as are infected cats; in this case, the cat's coat has become contaminated with spores from the environment (i.e., the cat is acting as a fomite). Such *innocent carrier* cats are impossible to distinguish from cats with a mild infection using culture alone, and if any question arises, the suspect cat should be treated.

One of the most common problems with in-house culturing is the lack of sporulation or growth, or both, of *M. canis* on DTM. Noting that growth will be slow in animals that are being treated is important. Additionally, a recent study challenges the common recommendation to *incubate at room temperature*. Increased sporulation was found when plates were incubated at higher temperatures (21° C to 23.8° C [70° F to 75° F]).[95] This finding has been confirmed in our laboratory.[161] Ambient temperature in many veterinary clinics, especially during warm weather months when the air conditioning is being used, is well below this temperature. The current recommendation by the authors is to incubate cultures at higher temperatures.

Microscopic Confirmation The principle of DTM is not perfect, and even an immediate red color change is not diagnostic. For example, colonies of the nonpathogen *Scopulariopsis* can appear grossly identical to those of dermatophyte colonies and cause an immediate red color change. Therefore suspect colonies must be examined microscopically to confirm presence of a pathogen. After 7 to 10 days of growth, most colonies will begin to produce spores, which will allow specific identification. To accomplish this task, brush a small strip of clear cellophane tape lightly over the colony surface to collect spores. Place the tape (sticky side down) onto a drop of lactophenol cotton blue stain on a microscope slide. Add another drop of stain on top of the tape, then coverslip and examine at 100× magnification. Among the many hyphal strands will be dermatophyte macroconidia (spores), which have typical shapes according to the species (see Fig. 58-6, C; Table 58-3; and Chapter 56). If spores are not visible, wait 4 to 7 days and try again; some colonies may not sporulate until they are quite old. A suspect colony that fails to produce spores or is difficult to identify, as is sometimes the case in *Trichophyton* species, should be sent to a qualified diagnostic laboratory.

Histopathologic Findings

Biopsy examination is not as sensitive as culture is in the diagnosis of dermatophytosis. When the significance of culture results is questioned, demonstration of the organism in biopsy specimens is more definitive. Histologic examination is most helpful in detecting the nodular forms of dermatophytosis (the kerion and granulomatous ringworm), especially because these lesions often have negative culture results. Shaved, clipped, or surgically excised specimens of claws may be submitted for histologic examination in cases of paronychia, onychorrhexis, or onychomadesis. If fungal organisms are present, they will be readily visible within the substance of the claw. When submitting such specimens to the pathology laboratory, indicate the suspicion of fungal disease so that special fungal stains may be performed if necessary.

Therapy

An important point to recognize is that, in an otherwise healthy animal, dermatophytosis is generally a self-curing disease, with full resolution following development of an appropriate CMI response. In dogs, localized lesions and even generalized *M. canis* or *M. gypseum* infections can resolve without treatment.[58,142,165] Cats and kittens with seemingly localized disease can also self-cure, but infection can be prolonged (from at least 60 to 100 days). Positive culture results from cats do not prove that the dermatophyte is causing the clinical illness given that they can innocently harbor the organisms as a fomite, and the signs are variable, mimicking other diseases. Treatment is recommended nevertheless because it will accelerate resolution, thus minimizing the time course of the infection and minimizing the potential that it will spread to other animals or people. Wherever possible, curing the infection in the cat and decontaminating the environment is desirable. Systemic treatment is mandatory under certain circumstances such as recurrent or recalcitrant infection or with any immunocompromised state. See Table 58-4 for treatment guidelines based on the health status and environment of affected cats. Drugs and dosage regimens are summarized in Table 58-5.

Experimental infection studies have emphasized that the ideal treatment regimen is composed of three elements (topical, systemic, and environmental treatment), each of

Table • 58-4

Treatment Recommendations for Dermatophytosis in Cats

CAT ENVIRONMENT/OWNER	THERAPEUTIC PROCEDURES

Infected cat:
  No zoonotic risks
  Only cat in household or up to four other cats
	Shorthaired with <5 lesions: clip focally with blunt metal scissors.
	If longhaired or more lesions: clip entire body.
	Administer topical and systemic antifungals until 2—3 negative culture results.
	Culture starting 4 weeks after treatment initiated.

Exposed cat:
  Housemate of infected cat
  Member of infected cattery
  Show cat in contact
	Obtain toothbrush culture (see text).
	Clip *entire* haircoat of cats with positive culture results.
	Provide whole body topical therapy (6 times).

Infected cat with public health risk:
  Children in household
  Cosmetologist
  Immunosuppressed
  Human or animal health care worker
	Administer systemic antifungals.
	Culture starting 4 weeks after treatment initiated at weekly or biweekly intervals until three successive negative culture results.

Table • 58-5

Drugs for Systemic Therapy of Dermatophytosis in Dogs and Cats

DRUG[a]	SPECIES	DOSE[b] (mg/kg)	ROUTE	INTERVAL (HOURS)	DURATION[c] (WEEKS)
Griseofulvin					
Microsize[d]	B	25—50	PO	24[e]	6—10
Ultramicrosize[f]	B	5—10	PO	24[e]	6—10
Ketoconazole[g]	D	10	PO	24	4—8
Itraconazole[g]	D	5—10	PO	24	4—8
	C: daily therapy	10	PO	24	4—8, or until cured
	C: continuous/pulse	10	PO	24	4 then every other week, until cured (~8—10 weeks)
	C: low-dose cycle	1.5—3	PO	24	Variable[i]
Terbinafine[j]	B	30—40	PO	24	3—18

B, Both dog and cat; *D*, dog; *C*, cat; *PO*, by mouth.
[a]See Drug Formulary, Appendix 8, for additional information on each drug.
[b]Dose per administration at specified interval.
[c]Followup brush culture results should be negative before discontinuing therapy. Two negative culture results are recommended.
[d]Trade names: Grifulvin V, Fulvin U/F, Grisactin. For small kittens, usually culture negative at 8 weeks and cured at 10 weeks.
[e]Dose can be divided and given every 12 hours. Dose of 50 mg/kg daily has often been effective after 41–70 days of therapy.
[f]Dose is approximately two thirds that of microsize preparation. Some preparations contain polyethylene glycol to facilitate absorption. Trade names: Fulvicin P/G, Grisactin Ultra, Gris-PEG. Effective dosages are higher than manufacturer suggests and may be toxic. Note: manufacture of this drug may be discontinued.
[g]Trade name: Nizoral; generic available; cats often receive 50 mg total dose daily; with side effects, every other day treatment is used. Not recommended for use in cats because of adverse effects: vomiting, inappetence.
[h]Trade name: Sporanox (human). Capsules may be opened and contents divided to administer recommended doses, or use oral solution.
[i]After 15 days, fungal culture is performed and cycle is repeated until negative culture result is obtained. Usually takes 1–3 cycles (15–45 days).
[j]Trade name: Lamisil. Not yet evaluated in dogs. Monitor liver enzymes in cats. Can be substituted for itraconazole in various regimens.

which has a somewhat different role. Topical therapy reduces contamination on the haircoat (and thus environmental contamination) and results in a faster mycologic cure than systemic therapy alone.[216] However, with the exception of lime-sulfur or enilconazole, topical therapy appears to do little to accelerate complete clinical resolution in the animal. Systemic therapy, in contrast, benefits the individual animal by reducing the number of weeks to complete cure. Environmental treatment also reduces the chances that the infection will spread to other animals or people in the same household.

Clipping of the Haircoat

Clipping of the haircoat will mechanically remove fragile hairs that will fracture and spill spores into the environment and onto the haircoat. It allows for thorough penetration of topical medications, reducing the amount and duration of treatment. Clipping of the entire haircoat is the optimal treatment in all cases of dermatophytosis; however, this is not always possible or practical. Clipping is time consuming and often requires sedation and can be irritating to cats. The following guidelines are offered. Shorthaired animals with less than five focal lesions do not need to be clipped. Cats or dogs with long hair, more than five focal lesions, generalized lesions, concurrent skin or systemic illnesses, or any combination of these should have their entire haircoat clipped. Clipping of the entire haircoat with a #10 electric clipper blade is usually adequate in animals with generalized lesions. Clipping of the haircoat in catteries with dermatophytosis is helpful for successful eradication. Important to note is that clipping of the haircoat may temporarily exacerbate lesions; however, this should not be used as a reason to not clip the haircoat. The use of adequate sedation and a #10 blade will minimize skin trauma.

Topical Therapy

To date, no evidence has been found to support the use of localized or *spot treatment* for dermatophytosis in dogs or cats. In fact, evidence has been found suggesting that use of spot-treatment products alone may predispose individuals to chronic subclinical infections.[27] Rather, whole-body shampooing, dipping, or rinsing with topical antifungal agents is much preferred. General topical treatment recommendations are summarized in Table 58-6.

Topical therapy, in addition to clipping of the haircoat, will help decrease contamination of the environment by hairs and spores, decrease the chance of spread of the disease to other animals and people, and help speed mycologic cure of the infection. The choice of topical antifungal treatment is important because studies have shown that many common topical agents are ineffective.* The relative efficacies of various topical antifungal drugs is summarized in Table 58-7. In vitro and in vivo studies have shown that the most consistently effective topical antifungal whole body treatments are lime-sulfur, enilconazole, and miconazole (the latter with or without chlorhexidine).† Captan, povidone-iodine, and chlorhexidine are consistently ineffective against *M. canis* and should not be used in lieu of the following products listed.

Lime-sulfur has been extensively tested in in vitro models, and when used at concentration of 8 ounces/gallon of water (1 : 16 dilution) has shown superior antifungal activity.[79,170] Lime-sulfur used at 4 ounces/gallon has been ineffective in the treatment of cats with dermatophytosis in one of the author's experience (KAM). Lime-sulfur treatment alone, twice weekly at this concentration, has been used by one of the authors (KAM) to successfully treat dermatophytosis in

*References: 34, 58, 166, 170. 230.
†References: 97, 103, 136, 182, 187, 216.

single and multiple cat households when combined with whole body clipping and appropriate environmental treatment. Lime-sulfur is virtually nontoxic if applied properly and can be used even on newborn kittens and puppies.

Enilconazole topical solution is also an effective treatment; unfortunately, it is not available in the United States and is licensed only for use in dogs and horses. Because of its superior antifungal activity, the safety and efficacy of enilconazole have been evaluated in cats.[96,103] In two studies, enilconazole was evaluated as a sole topical therapy (after whole body clipping) for the treatment of naturally occurring *M. canis* infection in Persian cats.[67,103] In one study, cats were dipped with

either water (control) or 0.2% (2 mg/ml) enilconazole twice weekly for 8 weeks.[67] In the enilconazole-treated cats, results of fungal cultures were negative as early as 5 weeks after initiation of therapy, and remained negative to the end of the 10-week monitoring period. In contrast, 75% of control cats still had culture-positive results at the end of 10 weeks of monitoring. In the second study, 22 Persian cats in a cattery were treated with 0.2% enilconazole every 3 days for a total of eight applications.[103] All cats improved clinically and had culture-negative results by day 28 of therapy. In both studies, cats were observed for adverse effects, and serum biochemistry panels were monitored. Enilconazole was well tolerated but may have been associated with hypersalivation, anorexia, weight loss, emesis, idiopathic muscle weakness, and slightly elevated serum alanine aminotransferase concentrations. Anecdotal reports have surfaced of uncommonly severe toxicity, and even death, occurring in cats after topical application of enilconazole. These cases are thought to be associated with ingestion of the solution by the cat via grooming after application. Enilconazole appears safe for use on cats if the animals are fitted with an Elizabethan collar for a few hours after each treatment, to prevent grooming, until the cat is dry. See Drug Formulary, Appendix 8, for further information.

Miconazole is also an effective topical antifungal in both in vitro and in vivo studies.[136,187] Important to note is that, in the in vivo studies, miconazole was used twice weekly as an adjunct to systemic therapy, rather than as sole therapy. As with all medicated shampoos, a skin contact time of 10 minutes is recommended for optimal therapeutic effect. This product can be irritating to the eyes and can cause skin irritation. Synergism between miconazole and chlorhexidine has been demonstrated in vitro,[187] and shampoos with this combination of ingredients are documented to hasten mycologic cure.[216]

Systemic Therapy

The role of systemic therapy in treating dermatophytosis is to accelerate resolution of the infection in the individual animal. Several effective drugs are available, and the appropriate choice must be made depending on cost considerations, fungal species, patient species, and potential toxicities. Development of standardized methods for antifungal susceptibility testing of dermatophytes[104,109] permits testing of apparently resistant strains to determine which systemic drug may be optimal, but

---

Table • 58-6

General Recommendations for Topical Antifungal Therapy

- The most consistently used antifungal topical agents are lime-sulfur, enilconazole, and miconazole.
  - Lime-sulfur: 8 ounces/gallon of water
  - Enilconazole (Imaverol™) available in the United States as Clinafarm EC™; see Drug Formulary, Appendix 8; 0.2% emulsifiable concentrate, licensed for use as an environmental disinfectant, used off-label in the treatment of dermatophytosis at a dilution of 55.6 ml/gallon of water as a topical antifungal.
  - Miconazole available as shampoo formulation, either as a sole agent or combined with chlorhexidine.
- Twice weekly application as a whole body rinse or shampoo recommended.
- Topical therapy best used in conjunction with systemic antifungal drugs.
- If topical therapy used as a sole therapy, hair coat should be clipped and either lime-sulfur or enilconazole used.
- Do not use spot treatment.
- Do not allow cats to lick or groom off the antifungal solutions.

Modified and used with permission from Moriello KA. 2003. Dermatophytosis Symposium, Parts 1–4, *Vet Med* 98:844–891.

Table • 58-7

Efficacy of Various Topical Agents Recommended for Treatment of Dermatophytosis in Dogs and Cats[a]

TOPICAL AGENT	AVAILABLE FORMULATIONS	COMMENTS ON EFFICACY
Captan	Shampoo, rinse	Poor performance in vitro
Chlorhexidine	Shampoo, rinse	No advantage over control treatment in experimental clinical infection; inferior in in vitro tests[b]
Clotrimazole	Cream, lotion	Creams and lotions not formulated to penetrate infected hair
Enilconazole	Rinse, fogger	Superior in in vitro tests
Ketoconazole	Shampoo, cream	Tested in animal models, fair efficacy; creams not formulated to penetrate infected hair
Lime-sulfur	Rinse	Superior at 1 : 16 dilution in in vitro tests
Miconazole	Shampoo, cream	Superior in in vitro tests[b]
Povidone-iodine	Shampoo, rinse, ointment	Poor performance in vitro
Sodium hypochlorite	Rinse	Inferior (1 : 10 dilution) in in vitro tests

[a]In vitro tests performed with infected hair.
[b]Combined 2% miconazole/chlorhexidine shampoo has been more effective than either agent alone.

such testing is currently limited in availability. These drugs should be used only when the diagnosis is certain. See Chapter 57 and Drug Formulary, Appendix 8, for further information on each of these drugs discussed here.

Griseofulvin Griseofulvin (GFV) is declining in use because of its still relatively high cost, potential toxicities, and availability of other drugs. GFV is poorly water soluble; thus GI absorption after oral dosing is variable and incomplete. Absorption is enhanced by administration with a fat-containing meal. The original microsize-particle formulations are mostly no longer manufactured, being replaced by ultra-microsize formulations in polyethylene glycol, which are better absorbed. Even the latter formulations are increasingly difficult to obtain because popularity of the drug has declined. Dosages recommended for dogs and cats differ and are not based on modern pharmacologic studies. Dosages that have proved to be effective in the largest number of cases are higher than manufacturer recommendations, and significant toxicities may be encountered. The most common adverse effects are vomiting, diarrhea, and anorexia. These effects can be partially avoided by dividing the daily dose into two administrations. Bone marrow suppression and neurologic signs have occurred, unrelated to dose or treatment length, as idiosyncratic reactions. Myelosuppression has particularly been reported in cats with feline leukemia virus and feline immunodeficiency virus infection, and this drug should not be used if such infection is present. Leukopenias can be severe (even life threatening) and unpredictable; thus blood counts at monthly intervals are recommended when using GFV. The drug should not be used in animals younger than 6 weeks of age. GFV is teratogenic and must never be given during the first two thirds of pregnancy.

Imidazoles and Triazoles Ketoconazole (KTZ) is a moderately effective fungistatic drug against *M. canis* and *T. mentagrophytes*. It has been used successfully to treat canine and feline[143] dermatophytosis. Less favorable results were reported in longhaired animals. Because of its potential toxicity, KTZ should be reserved for patients in which intolerance of GFV is a problem and in which itraconazole (ITZ) cannot be substituted because of greater expense. Side effects of KTZ include vomiting, hepatotoxicity, and inhibition of steroidal hormone synthesis.

ITZ is an oral triazole antifungal that is fungistatic at low tissue concentrations but fungicidal at higher concentrations. ITZ is better tolerated by cats and dogs compared with either KTZ or GFV and is comparable or superior to GFV in its efficacy against *M. canis*.[126,132,165] In human medicine, ITZ has proved helpful in chronic, recalcitrant dermatophytosis, including onychomycosis.[64,98,100,208] Signs of hepatotoxicity have been reported rarely in cats, and idiosyncratic cutaneous vasculitis is reported in dogs. Nearly all patients, however, tolerate the drug well at the dosages recommended for treatment of dermatophytosis. ITZ is not recommended in pregnancy. The drug is available in 100-mg capsules that can be opened, divided, and dispensed to small animals in butter or food in the appropriate doses or as an oral liquid (10 mg/ml) that is useful for dosing very small animals or kittens (see Drug Formulary, Appendix 8). Many clinicians have used ITZ in kittens as young as 6 weeks.

ITZ, along with the other triazoles, persists in skin and nails for weeks to months after administration to people, and intermittent or *pulse* therapy is frequently prescribed for skin infections or onychomycosis.[106] Persistence of ITZ in the skin of dogs or cats has not been studied, but intermittent administration protocols appear effective. One study reported efficacy in cats with daily administration for 28 days, then every-other-week administration until cured.[46] The authors routinely use ITZ for feline dermatophytosis on a one-week-on, one-week-off schedule, with apparent efficacy at one half the total drug cost. ITZ solution (Itrafungol, 52 mg/ml) is licensed for use in cats in some countries but not in the United States; however, a similar preparation is licensed for use in people. ITZ has become a common, and perhaps even preferred, treatment for feline dermatophytosis because of its strong efficacy, ease of administration, and low incidence of toxicity. Because of its relatively high cost, this treatment is generally not practical for dermatophytosis in medium- to large-breed dogs.

Fluconazole (FCZ) is another triazole antifungal used primarily for treating human candidiasis. It has not been evaluated for its efficacy in treatment of dermatophytosis in dogs or cats. In an experimental guinea pig model, FCZ and ITZ administered at the same dosages were equally effective in clearing *T. mentagrophytes* infections.[176] However, in vitro studies, examining minimum inhibitory concentrations (MIC) of antifungal agents for various dermatophyte species, reported that mean MICs for FCZ were approximately 10 to 100 times higher than the MICs for ITZ, KTZ, or voriconazole.[83,186] These data suggest that FCZ may be less useful for treatment of dermatophytosis than are other drugs of the same class, and limited clinical experience supports this contention. Thus no therapeutic or cost advantage can be found of FCZ over ITZ for dermatophyte infections. Triazole derivatives on the horizon include voriconazole and posaconazole; neither is primarily intended for dermatophytosis, and neither has been extensively evaluated in dogs or cats.

Terbinafine This allylamine antifungal agent is indicated primarily for dermatophytosis but also has activity against other fungi such as *Aspergillus* and *Candida*.[205] Terbinafine is fungicidal by virtue of its inhibition of the enzyme squalene epoxidase, which is necessary for fungal ergosterol biosynthesis. It is available in both topical (cream) and oral (tablet) formulations. Oral doses necessary to achieve fungicidal concentrations in hair of cats are higher by twofold to sixfold than human doses because of the differences in drug metabolism in cats.[120,131] Various dosages ranging from 8 to 40 mg/kg/day have been used for treatment of feline *M. canis* infection.[119,120,131] Doses at the higher end of this range (30 to 40 mg/kg) are demonstrably superior to lower doses, which may not produce resolution faster than spontaneous recovery.[39,120] One cat with dermatophytic pseudomycetoma was treated with terbinafine at only 15 mg/kg/day without success.[25] Reported adverse effects include occasional vomiting[131,160] and elevation in serum ALT concentrations.[42] The latter occurs in approximately one third of cats treated and is typically without clinical significance, but monitoring of liver enzymes is advised with use of terbinafine in cats. The drug reaches especially high concentrations in sebum and the stratum corneum, and fungicidal concentrations may persist in the skin for several weeks after administration in people, suggesting that intermittent dosing regimens may be possible.[131] Intermittent dosing has not been evaluated in human beings or cats to date. Terbinafine is not licensed for veterinary use, is very expensive, and its use in dogs has not been reported.

Lufenuron Lufenuron (LFN), a benzoylphenylurea drug that disrupts chitin synthesis, is used worldwide for the control of fleas on cats and dogs. Chitin is a critical structural component of the exoskeleton of arthropods, such that interference with its synthesis prevents normal development of immature fleas and leads to disruption of the flea life cycle.[53] Chitin is also a component of the outer cell wall of fungi, including dermatophytes. Possibly, some compounds that disrupt chitin synthesis might also have antifungal activity. An early, uncontrolled trial of LFN in dogs with *Coccidioides* *immitis* infection suggested possible clinical efficacy.[4] However, in further controlled studies, LFN treatment resulted in neither in vitro inhibitory activity of *C. immitis* nor in extended survival of mice with experimental coccidioidomycosis.[110] A case report described apparent success in treating equine fungal endometritis with LFN.[101] In a retrospective epidemiologic study, LFN treatment was strongly associated with recovery of a large number of dogs and cats from a variety of superficial fungal infections, including dermatophytosis.[6] This study led to widespread speculation about the potential usefulness of LFN as an antifungal treatment or preventative drug (or both) for dermatophytosis.

In a controlled experimental infection study,[168a] LFN treatment of cats at 30 or 130 mg/kg orally (PO) did not prevent establishment of *M. canis* infection, when the challenge infection was induced by application of fungal spores to the skin. However, a slight delay was noted in establishment of the infection in the LFN-treated cats, as compared with control cats. In a subsequent study, clinically healthy cats treated with four doses of LFN at 100 to 133 mg/kg PO or 40 mg/kg subcutaneously (SC) at monthly intervals were exposed to a cat with mild *M. canis* infection.[62] Treated cats received five monthly doses thereafter. All treated healthy cats became infected, although it again appeared that the onset of the infection was delayed slightly. Continued LFN treatment did not result in faster resolution of the infection than did the placebo treatment. A field study in two *M. canis*–infected catteries reported that addition of LFN to topical enilconazole treatment resulted in more rapid improvement of clinical signs in one cattery but not the other.[96] Thus inconsistent clinical results have been obtained with treating feline dermatophytosis with LFN, which may reflect fungal strain variation or variation in study methodology. Current evidence does not favor use of LFN for prevention or treatment of dermatophytosis, particularly with the availability of drugs with documented efficacy, such as ITZ.

Duration of Treatment and Followup Examinations

Cats or dogs with dermatophytosis should be treated until complete resolution of clinical signs (*clinical cure*), and then continued until the fungus cannot be cultured from the haircoat, on at least two sequential cultures a week or more apart (*mycologic cure*). The followup cultures can begin as early as 3 to 4 weeks after treatment is instituted and thereafter on a 2-week schedule. Once the culture results are negative, monitoring can be on a once-weekly basis. At least two negative culture results in single-cat households and three in multiple-cat environments are recommended. Cats can appear clinically healthy before their skin and hair are cleared of fungal organisms. Although a Wood's light can help screen for dermatophytes, it is not a good tool to monitor the progress of infection in an individual cat because positive fluorescence may occur in some hair shafts in which fungus has been inactivated.[158]

Treatment Failure

With competent immune systems, cats with dermatophytosis usually resolve their clinical illness within 100 days.[160] Clinical improvement usually begins to occur within 2 to 4 weeks of starting treatment. Early improvement is characterized by a reduction in pruritus, erythema, scaling, and hyperpigmentation. If the animal's hair has been clipped, hair growth will begin but may not be complete for several months. Incorrect diagnosis and lack of elimination of infection or reinfection are reasons that therapy can be unsuccessful. Given that dermatophytosis mimics many other skin diseases, an incorrect diagnosis is a major reason that clinical signs may not resolve following use of antifungal therapy. Relapses usually result from inadequate duration or type of therapy. Failures are caused by owner compliance, incorrect dosing, or antifungal resistance. The muzzle should be checked carefully, given that it can remain affected because of the hesitancy to put topical medications near the face or from reexposure through facial contact with the environment or carrier animals. Immunosuppression can be caused by concurrent infections, systemic illnesses, or medications. These conditions include endocrine diseases such as hyperadrenocorticism, hyperthyroidism or hypothyroidism, cytotoxic or glucocorticoid therapy, demodicosis, and retroviral infections. Reinfection is caused by inadequate decontamination of the environment or elimination of infection in inapparent carrier animals. Clipping of the haircoat may be imperative in some animals.

Environmental Control

M. canis spores can persist in the environment for long periods; spores have remained viable in the authors' laboratory for several years. The spores are microscopic and can easily be spread via air currents, contaminated dust, heating vents, and so forth. Contaminated environments are underrecognized in their importance as reservoirs of infection for people and other cats. In addition to general cleanliness, the amount of environmental contamination is directly related to the number of animals involved in the outbreak and the duration the animals have spent in the home before the infection is recognized.[160] General environmental control recommendations are summarized in Table 58-8.

Label claims of fungicidal activity for disinfectant products are determined by testing the compound against the mycelial form of a dermatophyte or macroconidia and not against the form actually found in contaminated premises (i.e., infected hair fragments, arthrospores). A disinfectant inactivates virtually all recognized pathogenic microorganisms on inanimate objects but not necessarily all physical forms (spore forms) of the microorganism. In the case of dermatophytosis, a product may be appropriately labeled as fungicidal (because it kills mycelial forms) yet be ineffective against arthrospores (i.e., the naturally infective state in the environment). Studies have shown that many previously recommended disinfectants and products commonly used in veterinary clinics are ineffective as agents for dermatophytosis.[166,169] The only solutions shown to be 100% fungicidal after a single application were agents such as 1% formalin and undiluted household chlorine bleach. Neither of these solutions can be used in the home because of the human health safety concerns and because both are too caustic. The antifungal activity of many products is limited in the presence of organic material. In addition, fungal elements within hair shafts may be protected from disinfectants. Also important to note is that these products may not be effective on contact; a minimal wetting time for the surface of 10 minutes is recommended.

Studies using isolated infected hairs or spores or field studies using dermatophyte-contaminated environments have shown that the following disinfectant products are consistently effective: lime-sulfur (1:33), enilconazole (0.2%), and 1:10 to 1:100 household chlorine bleach.[97,159,169,230] In addition, a study has also shown that strain variation of *M. canis* with respect to susceptibility to disinfectants is not present.[169] In this study, all 10 strains were susceptible to lime-sulfur, enilconazole, and 1:10 bleach. None of the strains were susceptible to any dilution of, including four times the recommended concentration of, chlorhexidine or detergent-peroxide disinfectant. Rather than variations in strain susceptibility to disinfectants, *resistant* infections are likely caused by inadequate decontamination procedures.

For treatment of routine infections with one or a few animals in the household, extensive environmental decontamination is generally impractical and unnecessary. Thorough vacuuming and mechanical cleaning will remove much

Table • 58-8

Recommendations for Mechanical Cleaning and Disinfection of Surfaces[a]

To Start
- Remove and discard or disinfect all cat rugs, blankets, collars, brushes, fabric toys, etc.
- Discard any other object that cannot be repeatedly vacuumed, scrubbed, and disinfected.
- Purchase a new vacuum cleaner with hose attachments in price range that will allow it to be ultimately discarded.
- Remove all drapes, decorative objects, and so forth from the room and clean them.
- Remove all heating duct covers and vents for washing. Install piece of disposable furnace filter behind the metal duct plates before replacing them. These can purchased at almost all home improvement stores and will help keep spores from being spread through heating ducts.
- Commercial cleaning of heating and cooling ducts may be needed in some catteries.
- If possible, put a fan in the window and set it so it draws air out of the room to the external environment.
- Thoroughly vacuum ALL surfaces of the room.
- Dust all surfaces, ledges, and so forth with disposable dusting cloth.
- Scrub all surfaces with a detergent that is safe to use around pets. Rinse all surfaces well; ideally, use a wet-dry vacuum to remove the dirty water.
- Apply a 1 : 10 to 1 : 100 dilution of household bleach to all nonporous surfaces, or use enilconazole emulsifiable concentrate (Clinafarm EC™ [Janssen Pharmaceuticals, Titusville, N.J.]; distributed by American Scientific Laboratories, Union, N.J.) or smoke generator. Note: read labels for contact and wetting time. Surfaces treated with bleach need to be wetted for at least 10 minutes for maximal fungicidal action. USE APPROPRIATE VENTILATION AND PERSONAL PROTECTIVE EQUIPMENT (gloves, eye protection).
- Use a portable dehumidifier in cat rooms to keep humidly low; humid environments favor spore viability.

Daily
- Vacuum all surfaces and use disposable dust cloths to remove dirt and spores.
- Depending on the number of cats in the room, wash floors and any surfaces contacted by cats with detergent. Use of mops with disposable detergent pads is recommended.

Weekly
- Thoroughly vacuum, dust, and scrub all surfaces in contact with cats.
- Apply disinfectant to all surfaces. Allow adequate contact time. Rinse thoroughly.

Preventing Spread in Catteries
- Use plastic sheeting on the inside of the doorway to prevent spores from escaping.
- Use disposable trash bags to cover clothes while treating cats or cleaning rooms.
- Change shoes before and after leaving cat treatment area.
- Do not run air conditioners in room if this action blows air throughout the house.

[a]Modified and used with permission from Moriello KA. 2003. Dermatophytosis Symposium, Parts 1–4, *Vet Med* 98:844–891.

infective material. All hard surfaces should be mopped with disinfectant such as a 1:100 bleach solution. During treatment, these few animals should be confined to a small easily cleaned room without carpeting until they have received systemic antifungal therapy for at least 2 weeks and have been dipped at least four times with topical preparations such as lime-sulfur. Cat beds and blankets can be washed daily in hot water and bleach.

In the instance that an infected cat has been introduced into a previously unaffected household, the extent of infection in other cats and the environment can often be limited with early intervention. Where the new animal has not been confined, infection is first noted in the most social cats and often is found on their head and ears. The degree of environmental contamination is usually low. However, if culture results reveal infection in the least social cats, the environment must be considered as contaminated, and disinfection procedures are warranted.

In an animal shelter or cattery with endemic infection, extensive environmental disinfection is critical. A thorough vacuuming of the environment is the first step; no visible hairs should be present. This step is followed by thorough cleaning with a routine household detergent; suction of the wet solution from surfaces is recommended and can be accomplished using inexpensive wet-dry vacuum cleaners. After cleaning, liberally apply 1:10 to 1:100 (i.e., 1 ounce/gallon) bleach, or appropriately diluted enilconazole. The latter is available in the United States as an emulsifiable concentrate or smoke generator. See Drug Formulary, Appendix 8, for further information. In the United States, enilconazole products are registered with the Environmental Protection Agency for use in poultry houses to control aspergillosis in the environment but are not registered for other uses. Enilconazole is safe for human exposure when guidelines are followed, but it can be corrosive. Chlorhexidine is not an effective disinfectant for dermatophytes. In an animal shelter or similar facility, environmental disinfectants may be conveniently applied (with suitable skin and respiratory protection used by personnel) using a pressurized garden-type sprayer.

Special Considerations for Infected Multiple-Animal Facilities

Endemic dermatophytosis has a profound effect on the health, community reputation, and economic status of animal breeding colonies and animal shelters. Breeding programs must be interrupted because newborn animals are rapidly and easily infected, leading to debilitation and sometimes death. Adoption of shelter pets must be temporarily halted to avoid spread of the infection to new owners. Eradication of dermatophytosis from such a facility is completely possible but very expensive and time consuming; thus every attempt must be made to do the job correctly the first time and to institute preventive measures against future outbreaks.

Important to recognize is that animals with visible, obvious lesions represent only *the tip of the iceberg* in an endemic colony, particularly in a *M. canis*–infected cattery. Many animals will also have subclinical infections, and many more will be innocently carrying dermatophyte spores on their haircoats. Therefore the eradication process must begin by toothbrush culturing (see previous discussion, Specimen Collection) every animal in the facility, regardless of clinical appearance. Beginning an eradication effort with 50% to 100% of animals with culture-positive results is not unusual, though not all of these may be actually infected. While awaiting the initial culture results, quarantine any animals with obvious or suspected infection. This precaution requires isolation in a separate *contaminated* room or building, with floor surfaces that can be disinfected easily. A Wood's lamp is very helpful here, if the outbreak is caused by a fluorescing strain. A separate *clean* room or building must also be prepared into which cured animals will be gradually moved. If new animals must be introduced into the colony during the eradication effort, as is common for an animal shelter, a separate, third *intake* room or building must be prepared, where new arrivals will be quarantined until it is certain they are not infected. Environmental decontamination procedures should begin immediately in all three rooms, as previously detailed, and repeated monthly for the duration of the entire decontamination effort.

Once the initial results are known, the animals can be divided into two groups based on culture result and clinical appearance. The first group consists of lesion-free animals with negative culture results, and is typically fairly small. These animals should be bathed with a miconazole-chlorhexidine or KTZ-chlorhexidine shampoo, followed by a dip in lime-sulfur or enilconazole. They can be immediately transferred to the *clean* room. Animals that have visible lesions or have positive culture results, or both (even if normal in appearance), are assigned to the *contaminated* room, and this will initially be the majority of animals.

All animals in the *contaminated* room are treated. If feasible, clipping the hair short on all longhaired animals is desirable. If clipping is not practical, at the very least, any visible lesional areas should be clipped. This step will eliminate a great deal of infective material that otherwise would be spread into the environment. All animals are bathed with an antifungal shampoo and dipped in lime-sulfur, and the bath and dip are repeated twice weekly for the duration of the effort. Concurrently, begin oral antifungal treatment on all animals, with daily GFV or alternate-week ITZ as previously detailed. See Table 58-5.

A key to successful eradication is careful monitoring by culture. Followup toothbrush fungal cultures are obtained from animals at intervals of approximately 2 weeks. Animals in the *clean* room should be recultured once after being transferred to that room, as a precautionary measure. Animals in the *contaminated* room are cultured every 2 weeks until each animal has a negative result on at least two successive times. Animals that initially had positive culture results but only carrying a few spores (as opposed to being actively infected) will develop negative results rapidly, and as they achieve two cultures with negative results, they can be transferred to the *clean* room. It will soon become obvious which animals are truly infected because these individuals will have multiple successive positive culture results even during treatment. Treatment is continued in the *contaminated* room until all animals are cured and moved to the *clean* room. At this point, the *contaminated* room should be thoroughly cleaned and decontaminated before further use.

During treatment, watch for animals that have persistently positive culture results, with many colonies on the culture plate and little apparent resolution despite treatment. These animals, which will typically be only one or a few, may be chronically infected by virtue of their failure to develop appropriate CMI, and they represent a potent threat to the continued health of the entire colony. Recommendations are that these chronically infected animals be removed entirely to a separate facility for treatment or euthanized.

Each animal in the *contaminated* room may require from 4 to 12 weeks of treatment before having two consecutive negative culture results. In a typical animal shelter with 50 to 100 cats, the entire eradication process will last 5 to 6 months. If, for some reason, separate *clean* and *contaminated* areas cannot be prepared, the authors have had occasional success in eradication by simply treating all animals in the entire facility as *contaminated* and continuing treatment until all animals have two consecutive negative culture results.

If new animals are entering via the *intake* room, as each animal enters, it should be immediately toothbrush cultured, followed by an antifungal bath and dip. Most animals will have negative culture results and can be transferred to the *clean* room as the culture results become known. Any animal that has a positive culture result is transferred to the *contaminated* room and treated as previously noted. After the eradication effort is concluded, this *intake* procedure should be maintained indefinitely. In the authors' experience, for 1 out of every 15 to 20 new animals entering a shelter to have positive culture results is not unusual, and this animal would be capable of starting a new endemic infection in the whole facility if not discovered. In a show cattery, this principle applies also to any cat coming back into the facility from a cat show or breeding loan.

Prevention

In an indoor-cat household, the most likely risk of infection is introduction of an infected cat or exposure of an existing cat that has been to a veterinary hospital or boarding or grooming facility where the infection exists. All new dogs or cats entering a dermatophyte-free environment should be screened for infection by culture and simultaneously treated with lime-sulfur if it originates from a multiple-cat environment. Cats that come into contact with spores from the outside on short absence should generally be able to eliminate the spores through grooming; however, at least, a preventative dip in lime-sulfur is warranted. Longhaired cats that become exposed for several days or more constitute the greatest risk and should be quarantined and cultured until the results are known. For catteries without dermatophytosis, periodic screening of the environment and animals by culture will detect reintroduction or relapses before they spread. Strict cleaning and disinfection in the environment, as previously outlined, are beneficial in preventing introduction and spread. Cats at shows should be placed in carriers with cloth coverings to help protect against spore contamination. Visitors to the cattery should wear protective clothing and should not have contact with cats if they have had been handling infected cats.

Knowledge of the immunology of dermatophytosis has led to some dramatically effective programs of vaccination and eradication of ringworm from food and fur-bearing animals in many countries, and reasonable hope exists that the same observations extended to companion animals will someday result in the possibility of prophylactic vaccination in these species.

Vaccine Development

Early investigations demonstrated that inoculation of various preparations of living or killed dermatophytes by SC, intramuscular, intraperitoneal, or even topical routes produced both positive intradermal test results and partial resistance to further infection. The resistance was often incomplete and of short duration. In species such as cattle and fur-bearing animals, further investigation of the immunologic response of the host to dermatophytic fungi led to the development of highly effective vaccines. Historically, the greatest successes came with injection of live mycelium or viable spores. The biologics industries in Eastern Europe were active early in development of vaccines for use in cattle, horses, and foxes. Vaccines that were developed included LTF-130 for cattle, SP1 for horses, and TM-135 for foxes and rabbits. Vaccination programs have essentially eradicated bovine dermatophytosis from several European countries, with a concomitant decrease in human infections. All of these vaccines were intended to prevent animals from developing *Trichophyton* infections.

Two experimental vaccine preparations have been studied in cats. A killed *M. canis*–cell wall vaccine induced both antibody titers and CMI in laboratory cats, but these responses were not as strong as those seen in natural infection and did not confer resistance to challenge infection.[56,58,62] Combined live-inactivated dermatophyte vaccine, consisting of attenuated live *Trichophyton* with killed *Microsporum* components, was tested in cats under laboratory conditions. Again, the vaccine induced a specific immune response; the response was not protective against direct challenge infection but produced a trend for reduced severity of initial infection.[61] The most recent vaccination efforts involve injection with recombinant proteases of *M. canis* origin, but initial studies in guinea pigs have been disappointing.[70] A commercial product (Fel-O-Vax MC-K) consisting of killed dermatophyte components in adjuvant had been marketed in the United States for feline use but is no longer available. The major indication for this commercial vaccine was for reduction in severity of the clinical signs of dermatophytosis in cats; it was not protective against infection induced by direct topical application of spores.[61] Apparently, the goal of a truly prophylactic vaccine against feline dermatophytosis has not been attained, but success in other species and increasing knowledge regarding the immune response of cats and experimental infections hold promise that this goal will be eventually achieved.

Public Health Considerations

Pet Owners and Animal Health Workers

Dermatophytosis is a zoonotic disease and is of particular concern in certain at-risk populations. These groups include children, transplant and cancer patients, people with debilitating or immunocompromising diseases, and older adults. Immunocompromised persons may be at increased risk for infections and for more serious infections.[117] In addition, everyone in the health care professions must take precautions to avoid contracting the disease because it can limit their ability to work with patients. One of the authors is aware of a physician who contracted *M. canis* from a kitten and was not able to return to work for 4 months. Any animal acquired from an animal shelter, rescue agency, or breeding facility poses an increased risk of being infected or mechanically carrying spores on its haircoat. These animals should have fungal cultures performed on toothbrush-collected specimens as part of their routine examination and testing. Cats used in facilitated therapy for human rehabilitation should be tested on a biannual basis. Approximately 50% of people exposed to either symptomatically or asymptomatically infected cats develop lesions (Fig. 58-7), and in 70% of all households with an infected cat, at least one person usually contracts the disease.[185] Worldwide, the reported number of cases of human

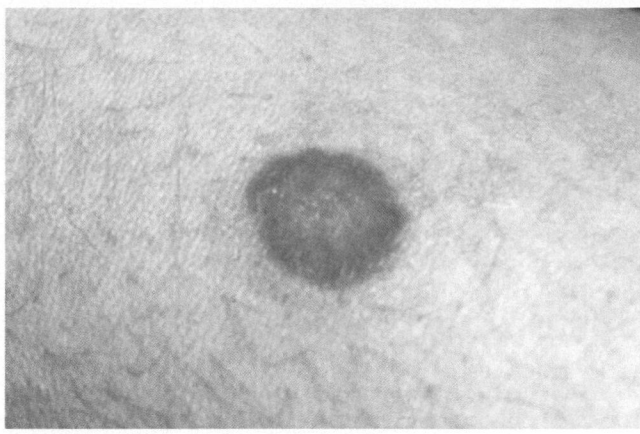

Fig 58-7 Ringworm lesion on the forearm of a cat owner. (Courtesy University of Georgia, Athens, Ga.)

infection with *M. canis* continues to increase.[201] The author's opinion holds that a fungal culture should be part of all new animal examination and testing procedures.

For handlers of small animals, the occupational risk of acquiring dermatophytosis is not as great as it is for those working with cattle, for whom ringworm is the most commonly reported zoonosis. Not surprisingly, *M. canis* is most often implicated in cases involving small animal practitioners and their employees. An investigation of veterinary clinics in Italy revealed that, in 15 of 50 clinics, *M. canis* could be isolated from the floors of waiting rooms, examination rooms, radiology rooms, and wards.[130] Veterinary practitioners must be vigilant in protecting themselves and their employees from this zoonosis.[118]

Interspecies Transmission

In one study on the fungal flora of cats, 14 isolates of *T. rubrum* were noted; this organism is an important human pathogen associated with tinea pedis (athlete's foot).[79,162] After the report of this finding one of the authors (KAM) became aware of a household in which at least one cat was diagnosed with clinical dermatophytosis caused by *T. rubrum*. When informed of the diagnosis, the owner admitted to having chronic athlete's foot fungus and that he commonly rubbed his bare feet against the cat's haircoat.[209] *M. canis* may be transmitted from people to household pets as well. *M. canis*–infected cats have been implicated as the source of infection in farm animals, including pigs, lambs, and rabbits.[85,105]

MALASSEZIA DERMATITIS

Ross Bond

Etiology

Malassezia spp. (previously *Pityrosporum* spp.) are lipophilic yeasts that reproduce asexually by monopolar or sympodial budding. They are most often isolated from the skin and mucosal sites of clinically healthy mammals and birds. The genus is divided into two groups based on their lipid dependency in culture media. *Malassezia pachydermatis* is unique within the genus in that it can be cultivated on routine mycologic media without lipid supplementation. *M. pachydermatis* has been found to be genetically heterogeneous and to be in the process of differentiation, probably linked to animal hosts. Following a taxonomic revision of the genus, six lipid-dependent *Malassezia* species are recognized, namely

M. furfur, M. sympodialis, M. globosa, M. obtusa, M. restricta, and *M. slooffiae*; these species require lipid supplementation for growth in vitro. Dogs are very frequently colonized by *M. pachydermatis* but very rarely colonized by lipid-dependent *Malassezia* spp.[50] Further information regarding the species within the genus and their identification by molecular methods has been published.[90,93] Clinically healthy cats and cheetahs (*Acinonyx jubatus*) are often colonized by *M. pachydermatis* and occasionally by lipid-dependent species, including *M. sympodialis, M. globosa,* and *M. furfur.*[16,49,51,102] A variant of *M. sympodialis* has also been isolated from a cat with otitis externa.[102] Lipid-dependent species are frequently isolated from human skin where they are associated with a number of diseases,[115] but *M. pachydermatis* is rarely isolated from human skin.

In dogs, *M. pachydermatis* is frequently isolated from the haired skin of the chin and lips, interdigital skin, and external ear canal and less often from other intertriginous areas such as the axilla and groin. Population sizes in healthy dogs are generally low but are markedly increased, often up to 10,000-fold, in many cases of *Malassezia* dermatitis, although overlap in population densities can be found between some healthy and affected dogs. The anatomic sites most often colonized in healthy animals correlate with regions most often affected in dogs with skin disease caused by the yeast. For a discussion of *M. pachydermatis* in otitis externa, see Chapter 85.

Malassezia dermatitis is commonly seen in dogs but is much less frequent in cats. A change in host immunity, altered skin microclimate, or disruption in epidermal physiology may predispose animals to develop clinical disease, although the factors that favor the transition from commensalism to parasitism are poorly understood. Further studies are required to elucidate the innate and adaptive events involved in the immunoregulation of the yeast and its interaction with the cells of the epidermis in both health and disease. *Malassezia* dermatitis may be the only disease recognized in some dogs, but in others, concurrent disorders such as allergies, especially atopic disease, keratinization defects, endocrinopathies, and the presence of skin folds may be important in favoring the yeast. Breed predilections vary between geographic regions but may include basset hounds, West Highland white terriers, cocker spaniels, toy and miniature poodles, dachshunds, boxers, Cavalier King Charles spaniels, shih tzus, Australian and silky terriers, and German shepherd dogs. Affected cats may also have underlying allergic and metabolic diseases, but immunosuppressive viruses such as feline leukemia virus and feline immunodeficiency virus, and paraneoplastic disorders (pancreatic paraneoplastic alopecia, exfoliative dermatitis with thymoma), may also favor infection. Bull terriers with lethal acrodermatitis are known to have impaired immune function, and they harbor large numbers of *Malassezia* on their skin.[141] *Candida albicans* co-infection may be partly responsible for lesions in the nails and footpads of these dogs.

Both healthy and affected dogs develop serum IgG antibodies that recognize *Malassezia*-derived proteins; titers are increased in dogs with disease.[14,178] Western immunoblotting showed that more protein bands are detected by sera from diseased dogs.[21,44] Some dogs with atopic disease show immediate reactivity to intradermal injections of *Malassezia* antigens, suggesting that hypersensitivity to yeast antigens may exacerbate the clinical signs of atopic disease in some individuals.[13,172] Elevated serum IgE titers to *M. pachydermatis* have also been demonstrated in dogs with atopic disease,[178] frequently associated with immunoreactivity to allergens of 45, 52, 56 and 65 kDa.[45] By contrast, basset hounds with *Malassezia* dermatitis usually show delayed rather than immediate skin test reactivity to *Malassezia* antigens, indicating that a spectrum of immunologic responsiveness is present in dogs with *Malassezia* dermatitis.[24]

Clinical Findings

Dogs

Clinical signs may be localized or generalized. In dogs, the disease is most often seen at anatomic sites that create a relatively warm, moist skin environment. Thus the interdigital skin, ventral neck, lip region, ear canal, axilla, groin, and folded areas are most often affected. Pruritus is normally reported and ranges in degree from mild to severe. Erythema accompanied by greasy exudation is commonly observed, especially in intertriginous areas where a brown exudate may mat the lower portion of the hair; malodor may be noted with extensive exudative lesions (Figs. 58-8 and 58-9). Traumatic alopecia, lichenification, and hyperpigmentation may develop in dogs with marked pruritus (Fig. 58-10). Paronychia (nail fold inflammation) associated with *M. pachydermatis* may lead to pedal pruritus accompanied by reddish-brown discoloration of the claw and or exudation in the nail fold. The isolation rate of *M. pachydermatis* from the eyes of dogs with corneal ulcers was greater than that from clinically healthy dogs,[196a] suggesting some role for its presence in the development of these lesions.

A seasonal increase in case numbers may be observed in geographic regions where a noticeable change to warm, humid climatic conditions is present. Typically, the response to glucocorticoid therapy is poor.

Cats

M. pachydermatis appears to be a relatively infrequent pathogen in cats, at least when compared with dogs. This finding may reflect the lower carriage rates of the yeast in healthy cats[15,16,52] The isolation rate from the ear canal is lower in clinically healthy cats compared with those with otitis.[176b] Ceruminous otitis externa responsive to antifungal eardrops is the most common clinical presentation of *M. pachydermatis*–associated skin disease in cats but occasional cases of localized or generalized *M. pachydermatis*–associated dermatitis have been described. Exfoliative erythroderma, greasy exudation, and varying degrees of pruritus may be seen. Cats with exfoliative dermatitis associated with thymoma[80] and paraneoplastic alopecia may have concurrent proliferations of *Malassezia.*[84]

The pathogenicity of lipid-dependent *Malassezia* spp. in cats has not yet been fully determined[51,52]; *M. sympodialis* has been isolated from the external ear canals of cats with otitis externa. The author is aware of sporadic unpublished cases in which *M. sympodialis* has been implicated in more generalized dermatitis in cats.

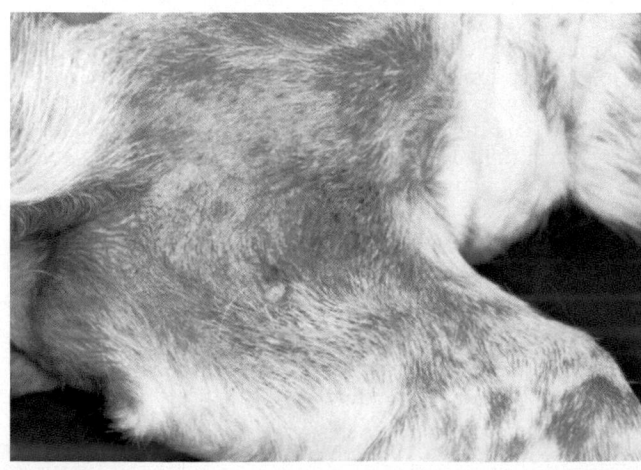

Fig 58-8 Marked erythema with greasy exudation in the axilla of a basset hound with *Malassezia* dermatitis. (Courtesy Ross Bond, Royal Veterinary College, Herts, United Kingdom.)

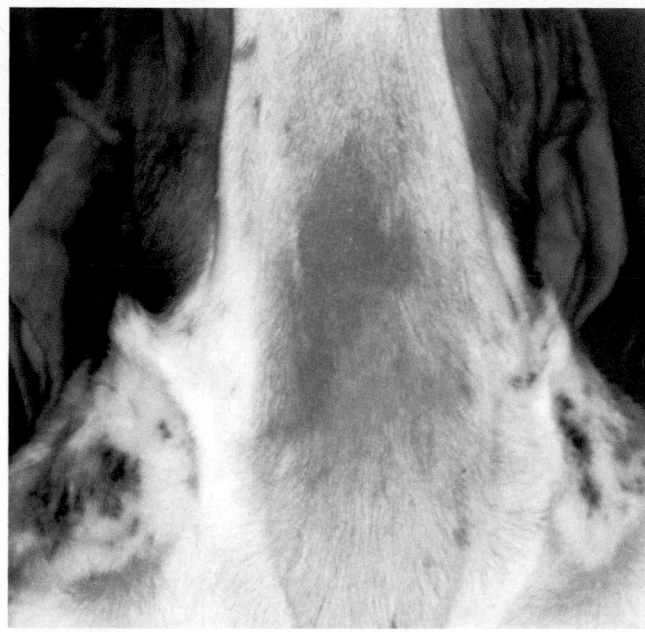

Fig 58-9 Intense erythema and brown discoloration of the hair in the neck fold of a basset hound with *Malassezia* dermatitis. (Courtesy Ross Bond, Royal Veterinary College, Herts, United Kingdom.)

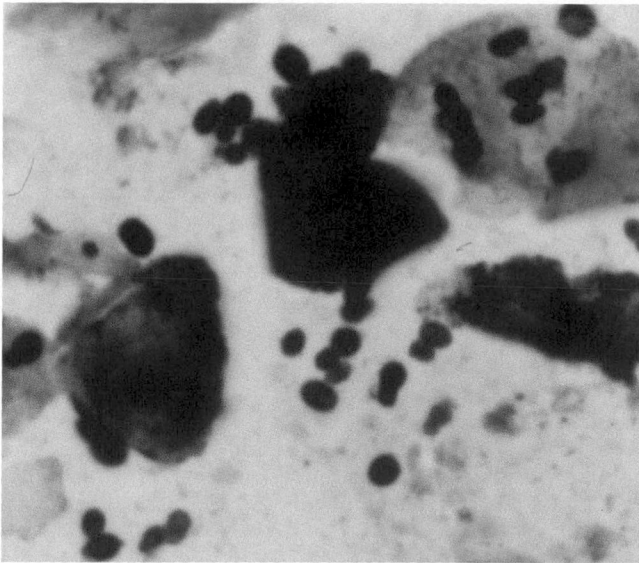

Fig 58-11 Tape-strip preparations stained with Diff-Quik and examined using the ×100 objective are useful in the assessment of *Malassezia* populations on skin. Numerous *Malassezia* yeast cells with their characteristic morphology associated with monopolar budding can be seen amongst stratum corneum cells, indicating an elevated population. (Courtesy Ross Bond, Royal Veterinary College, Herts, United Kingdom.)

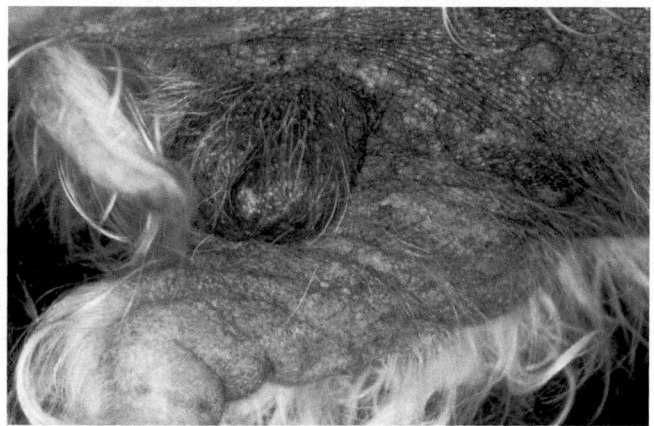

Fig 58-10 Marked erythema, skin thickening, hyperpigmentation and alopecia of the medial aspect of the hind limb of a West Highland white terrier with *Malassezia* dermatitis. (Courtesy Ross Bond, Royal Veterinary College, Herts, United Kingdom.)

Diagnosis

The clinical signs of *Malassezia* dermatitis are not pathognomic, and the disease should be routinely suspected in dogs with inflammatory skin diseases, especially those with erythema or greasy exudation as a dominant presenting sign. *Malassezia* dermatitis may mimic or complicate atopic disease and dietary sensitivity. Seborrheic presentations and fold-associated diseases should also prompt an evaluation of the presence and numbers of the yeast.

The diagnosis is based on clinical signs, presence of elevated numbers of the yeast in lesional skin, and a clinical and mycologic response to antifungal therapy. In clinical practice, yeast numbers are most usefully assessed by cytologic examination. Impression smears can be made directly onto glass slides, or

exudate can be transferred to the slide using swabs. However, the author prefers the tape-strip method; clear cellophane tape is pressed on the surface of the skin, thus collecting the stratum corneum cells and any superficial microbes. Unlike direct impressions, tape stripping can be used effectively in most anatomic sites and in dry or greasy lesions. The tape is stained, usually with a modified Wright stain, and examined using the light microscope (Fig. 58-11). Normally, the characteristic peanut-shaped *Malassezia* spp. yeast cells are rarely seen in healthy skin but are usually readily identified in specimens from affected individuals.

Although some authors have proposed guidelines on the number of yeasts needed for significance (e.g., one or more yeast per high powered field), this approach does not accommodate the overlap seen in yeast population densities in skin samples from healthy and diseased dogs. In addition, quantitative cultural investigations have demonstrated important breed and anatomic site differences in population sizes in healthy dogs. Also possible is that hypersensitivity responses to yeast-derived allergens might enable a relatively small number of organisms to generate skin disease in sensitized individuals. Thus trial therapy is an important component in the diagnostic evaluation of *Malassezia* dermatitis. Therapy should be given whenever the yeast is readily identified in cytologic specimens obtained from consistent lesions.

Quantitative cultural techniques involving contact plates and detergent scrubs are primarily used in research rather than routine clinical practice, although the contact plate method is a useful method of isolating the yeast from the skin. Cellophane tape strip sampling described for cytology above can also be used to transfer cells to the surface of culture plates,[180] although the potential for an antimicrobial effect of the adhesive tape should be considered. *M. pachydermatis* can be isolated using Sabouraud's dextrose agar, modified Dixon's agar, or Leeming's medium, with optimal growth at temperatures between 32° C and 37° C (89.6° F and 98.6° F).[92] Lipid-dependent species may be recovered using modified Dixon's agar or Leeming's medium; use of these media is preferred when samples are taken from cats in case lipid-dependent species are present. Skin biopsy specimens typically show marked irregular epidermal hyperplasia, spongiosus, and a superficial perivascular or interstitial infiltrate of mononuclear cells, with focal accumulations of neutrophils, eosinophils, and mast cells. Yeast cells may be seen in the stratum corneum, but the disruption of this layer that occurs during routine tissue processing may lead to an absence of the yeast; biopsy has a low sensitivity for yeast detection when compared with cytology (Fig. 58-12).

Therapy

Therapy is based around topical and or systemic antifungal therapy (Table 58-9).

Topical Therapy

The yeast is located in the stratum corneum, and thus topical therapy alone can be successful when potent antifungal agents are correctly applied. This approach depends on

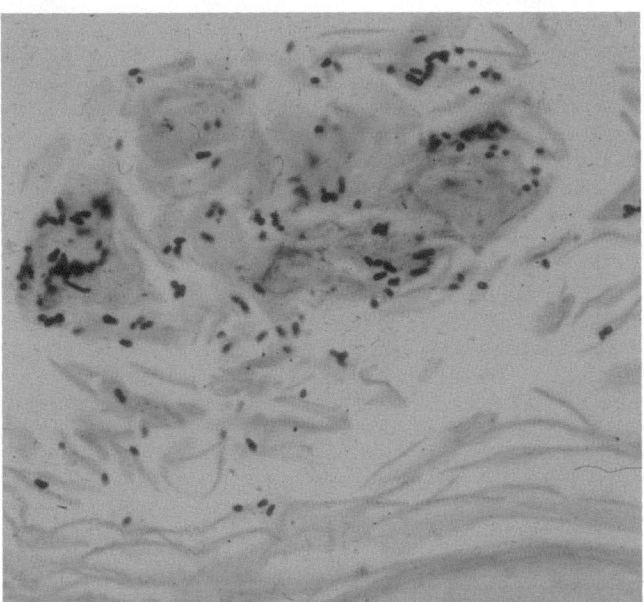

Fig 58-12 Skin biopsy specimen from a dog with *Malassezia* dermatitis. Large numbers of peanut-shaped *Malassezia* yeasts are present in the stratum corneum (methenamine silver, ×1000). (Courtesy Ross Bond, Royal Veterinary College, Herts, United Kingdom.)

good compliance and availability of effective products. Topical therapy avoids the expense and potential toxicity of systemic azole drugs but is more labor intensive for the owner. A 2% miconazole–2% chlorhexidine shampoo has been available in a significant number of countries for several years and has been shown to be highly effective when used every 3 days for 3 weeks as the sole treatment. Other topical agents include azole-containing rinses, lotions and creams, and selenium sulphide and benzoyl peroxide–containing shampoos.

Systemic Therapy

Both KTZ and ITZ are effective when given orally. KTZ may be used at doses ranging from 5 to 10 mg/kg, either once or twice daily, for 14 to 28 days. The antiinflammatory effects of this drug may also be beneficial. ITZ can be given at 5 to 10 mg/kg, PO, once daily for 2 to 4 weeks, and is less toxic and has better tissue penetration compared with KTZ. A pulse-therapy regimen of ITZ, 5 mg/kg daily, PO, for 2 successive days each week, has been described as an alternative to daily dosing.[193] For additional information on these drugs, see Drug Formulary, Appendix 8. GFV, the medication used to treat dermatophyte infections, is not effective in *Malassezia* infections.

Prevention

Failure to identify and correct concurrent diseases may result in relapsing infection. Intermittent or continuous maintenance therapy is often necessary in animals that experience relapsing disease, particularly in dogs with poorly controlled allergic disease or in dogs in which the reason for disease susceptibility cannot be identified.

Public Health Considerations

M. pachydermatis, for which dogs are natural reservoirs, is rarely associated with diseases in people. Owners of dogs with inflamed skin had a high rate of carriage of the organism.[173a] A potentially fatal fungemia has been reported in premature babies and less often in immunocompromised adults.[3] Most of the affected neonates were premature, had concurrent serious underlying disease, had central or peripheral catheters placed, and in some cases were receiving lipid emulsions as a component of parenteral nutrition. In one outbreak, *M. pachydermatis* was thought to have been transmitted from neonate to neonate on the hands of health care workers; the original source of the yeast was not identified, but transfer from pet dogs was suspected.[40]

Table • 58-9

Drugs for Systemic Therapy of Malassezia Infection in Dogs and Cats

DRUG[a]	SPECIES	DOSE[b] (mg/kg)	ROUTE	INTERVAL (HOURS)	DURATION[c] (WEEKS)
Ketoconazole[d]	D	5—10	PO	12—24	2—4
Itraconazole[e]	D	5—10	PO	24	2—4
	C: daily therapy	10	PO	24	2—4
	B: pulse treatment	10	PO	24	First 2 days of each week
Terbinafine[f]	D	30	PO	24	3—4

D, Dog; *C,* cat; *B,* both dog and cat; *PO,* by mouth.
[a]See Drug Formulary, Appendix 8, for additional information on each drug.
[b]Dose per administration at specified interval.
[c]Followup brush culture results should be negative before discontinuing therapy.
[d]Trade name: Nizoral; generic available; cats often receive 50 mg total dose daily; with side effects, every other day treatment is used.
[e]Trade name: Sporanox; capsules may be opened and contents divided to administer recommended doses, or use oral solution.
[f]Effective in reducing *Malassezia* concentration in basset hound skin.[90a]

SUGGESTED READINGS*

13. Bond R, Curtis CF, Hendricks A, et al. 2002. Intradermal test reactivity to *Malassezia pachydermatis* in atopic dogs, *Vet Rec* 150:448-449.
62. DeBoer DJ, Moriello KA, Blum JL, et al. 2003. Effects of lufenuron treatment in cats on the establishment and course of *Microsporum canis* infection following exposure to infected cats, *J Am Vet Med Assoc* 222:1216-1220.
96. Guillot J, Malandain E, Jankowsk, F, et al. 2002. Evaluation of the efficacy of oral lufenuron combined with

topical enilconazole for the management of dermatophytosis in catteries, *Vet Rec* 150:714-718.
160a. Moriello K. 2004. Treatment of dermatophytosis in dogs and cats: reviews of published studies, *Vet Dermatol* 15:99-107.
193. Pinchbeck LR, Hillier A, Kowalski JJ, et al. 2002. Comparison of pulse administration versus once daily administration of itraconazole for the treatment of *Malassezia pachydermatis* dermatitis and otitis in dogs, *J Am Vet Med Assoc* 220:1807-1812.

*See the CD-ROM for a complete list of references.

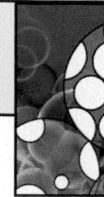

CHAPTER • 59

Blastomycosis

Alfred M. Legendre

ETIOLOGY

Blastomycosis is a systemic mycotic infection caused by the dimorphic fungus *Blastomyces dermatitidis*. In nature, *Blastomyces* grows in a saprophytic mycelial form *(Ajellomyces dermatitidis)* that reproduces sexually, producing infective spores (aleurioconidia). At body temperature in tissues the organism transforms into the yeast form and replicates asexually. The gene *bys-1* controls the change of the fungus from a mycelial to a yeast phase.[21] Budding yeasts are 5 to 20 μm in diameter and have a thick, refractile, double-contoured cell wall. Dogs and people are the most commonly infected with *Blastomyces*, but cats, horses,[78] sea lions,[86] wolves, ferrets, and polar bears as well as lions and other captive nondomestic felines such as tigers, cheetahs, and snow leopards[77] have developed systemic blastomycosis.[49,52] Blastomycosis was recently identified in a rhesus monkey.[80]

EPIDEMIOLOGY

Natural Reservoir

The reservoir for *Blastomyces* is thought to be the soil; however, recovery of the organism from sites of suspected exposure is uncommon. Growth of the organism in the environment appears to require sandy, acid soil and proximity to water. Decaying wood by-products and animal waste substrates support growth of organisms.[11] Environmental survival of *Blastomyces* is also restricted because normal soil organisms in most areas destroy *Blastomyces* inoculated into the soil. A special set of environmental conditions—an *ecologic niche*—is required for proliferation of the organism. Organisms were recovered from a beaver dam where numerous schoolchildren were exposed to the organism.[46] Living near a waterway is a risk factor for blastomycosis infection. In Wisconsin studies, 95% of dogs with blastomycosis lived within 400 m of a body of water at altitudes less than 500 m above sea level.[14,14a] The importance of proximity to water also was recognized in a Louisiana study in which dogs with blastomycosis were 10 times more likely to live within 400 m of water than control dogs.[2] Although proximity to water is a risk factor, exposure to the outside environment is not necessary because blastomycosis develops in strictly indoor dogs and cats.[2,13,64] Rain or heavy dew appears to facilitate the release of infectious spores. Access to sites that have been excavated also increases the risk for infection because of exposure to organisms deep in the soil.[14] In people, involvement in dirt-moving activities significantly increased the risk of developing blastomycosis.[64] Even within endemic regions, *Blastomyces* species are not widely distributed. Most people and dogs living in such areas show no serologic or skin test evidence of exposure. A point source of exposure within an enzootic area is more likely. For example, it is not unusual to find neighborhoods in which numerous dogs with blastomycosis are identified in a short time. In 14% of households in which blastomycosis has been diagnosed in the people or dogs, another case is diagnosed in the same household in the next several years.[13] Dogs and people being exposed to a common source of infection while duck and raccoon hunting has been reported.[4,72]

In other systemic fungal infections such as histoplasmosis (see Chapter 60), coccidioidomycosis (see Chapter 62), and aspergillosis (see Chapter 64), many animals are exposed, but few develop significant disease. However, in canine blastomycosis, subclinical infection is uncommon. When tissues from pound dogs in endemic areas were cultured for fungal organisms, *Blastomyces* organisms were found in 2%, and *Histoplasma* organisms were found in 50% of the dogs.[79]

Two of 48 healthy dogs from an enzootic area for blastomycosis had antibodies to *Blastomyces* according to a radioimmunoassay (RIA), but an agar-gel immunodiffusion assay (AGID) for both dogs was negative.[45] The dogs had no history of respiratory disease, which suggested they had a subclinical, self-resolving infection.[45]

Geographic Distribution

Blastomycosis, caused by *B. dermatitidis*, is principally a disease of North America, but it has been identified in Africa, India, Europe, and Central America. In North America, blastomyco-

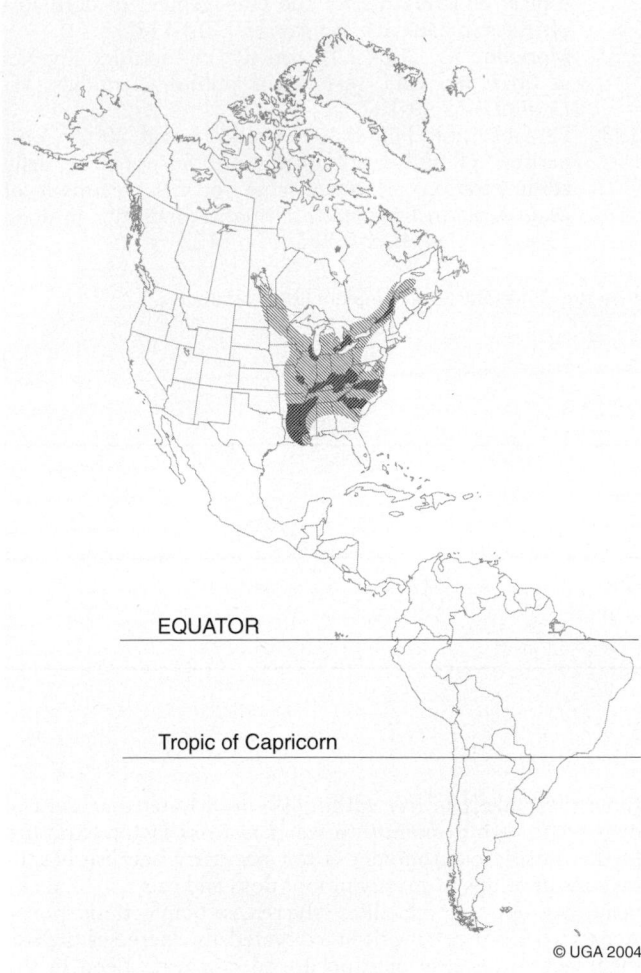

EQUATOR

Tropic of Capricorn

© UGA 2004

Fig 59-1 Dotted lines indicate area of endemic blastomycosis. Areas of highest incidence are cross-hatched. (Courtesy University of Georgia, Athens, Ga.)

sis has a well-defined endemic distribution that includes the Mississippi, Missouri, and Ohio River valleys, the mid-Atlantic states, and the Canadian provinces of Quebec, Manitoba, and Ontario (Fig. 59-1)[66]; however, the distribution may be greater than previously recognized or may be enlarging with sporadic cases in New York.[24,26] Occupationally acquired blastomycosis was identified outside the recognized endemic area in two people from Boulder, Colo., who became infected by digging to relocate prairie dogs.[1,26] Seven dogs with blastomycosis were reported from Colorado State University Veterinary Hospital from 1980 to 1990,[68] although the complete travel history on the animals was not available. Pets visiting or hunting in enzootic areas may become infected. Therefore the areas of risk might be greater than previously recognized. A history of travel to an endemic area should increase suspicion for blastomycosis.

Genetic analysis of isolates from soil and human patients has resulted in three isolates—A, B, and C—and each has numerous subtypes.[58] All type A isolates were from North America in the upper Midwestern states or Canada. B and C isolates were also found in this region, the rest of the United States, and other endemic regions in the world. Genetic identification could discriminate isolated strains for epidemiologic investigations of outbreak sources and the geographic area of infection. Serologic differences in serum antibody responses were found in dogs and rabbits infected with Tennessee and

Wisconsin *Blastomyces* isolates, supporting regional differences in the organisms.[5]

Mode of Infection

Most cases of blastomycosis are acquired by inhalation of the spores from mycelial growth in the environment. The spores enter the terminal airway and establish a primary infection in the lungs. When the yeast grows at body temperature, it is too large to enter the terminal airway in an aerosol, therefore transmission by coughing is very unlikely. Inoculation of *Blastomyces* into a wound from soil appears to be uncommon in the dog, but in dogs with solitary skin infections without systemic disease the possibility of direct inoculation cannot be excluded.[36,56] Because of the rarity of disease restricted to a focal skin area, cutaneous blastomycosis in the dog should be considered a manifestation of disseminated disease.

PATHOGENESIS

Host Signalment

No breed, age, or sex predisposition for blastomycosis has been recognized in the cat.[51] In dogs, males are more frequently infected than females, although in a Louisiana study the male/female ratio simply reflected the clinic population.[2] In dogs with equally severe blastomycosis, a greater percentage of females survived treatment in one study,[55] but in another study no differences in survival were found.[2] An epidemiologic study using the Veterinary Medical Data Base (Purdue University, West Lafayette, Ind.) identified sporting dogs and hounds to be at greater risk for blastomycosis.[68] This finding was attributed to outdoor activity as a risk factor for developing blastomycosis, but as mentioned previously, blastomycosis also develops in strictly indoor dogs and cats.[13,64] Many of the sporting breeds are brought to high-risk areas to hunt. Certain nonsporting breeds such as Doberman pinschers were also at increased risk.[2,50,68] In general, large-breed dogs are more commonly infected than small-breed dogs. This finding also may reflect increased exposure from outdoor activities and roaming in larger dogs. The highest prevalence is in 2-year-old dogs; most infections develop in dogs 1 to 5 years of age. No seasonal differences in disease are found in Tennessee, but more cases occur from late spring through late fall in Wisconsin.[3] In Louisiana, more cases were reported in August, September, October, and January than in the rest of the year.[2]

Dissemination of Organisms

After a *Blastomyces* infection becomes established in the lungs, it disseminates throughout the body. The preferred sites in the dog are the skin, eyes, bones, lymph nodes, subcutaneous tissues, external nares, brain, and testes. Less commonly affected sites are the mouth, nasal passages, prostate, liver, mammary gland, vulva, and heart. Intestinal lesions have rarely been found in dogs with systemic disease.[7,62] Dissemination is thought to occur via vascular and lymphatic routes. Although organisms enter the lung in almost all cases, lung lesions may resolve by the time the sites of disseminated infection become apparent. Occasionally, a focal lesion develops from a puncture wound,[36,56] but generally a solitary lesion should be considered part of a systemic process.

Host Response

Distinct species differences in susceptibility to *Blastomyces* seem apparent. The dog appears to be more susceptible to infection than people, and in enzootic areas of Arkansas and Wisconsin, the incidence of blastomycosis is 10 times higher in dogs than in people.[9,14] The incidence in dogs was 1420 per 100,000 dogs per year.[14] Young age and close proximity to a shoreline were risk factors.[15]

Dogs appear to have a shorter prepatent period and tend to develop the disease more quickly than people when exposed at the same time.[72] Dogs may inhale a larger inoculum of organisms than people because they are closer to the ground. Larger doses of inoculum cause the disease to progress faster and death to occur sooner.[81] The pathogenicity of isolated strains varies considerably.[61] Cats rarely are infected with *Blastomyces*. A 5-year survey of the Veterinary Medical Data Program identified three infected cats, whereas 324 dogs with blastomycosis were found.[50]

An effective immune response to *Blastomyces* requires a T-lymphocyte, cell-mediated immune (CMI) response directed partly to a surface adhesion virulence factor Wisconsin 1 (WI-1) now called *Blastomyces adhesion 1 (BAD-1) antigen*.[43] The BAD-1 antigen is an important virulence factor that depresses the production of tumor necrosis factor-alpha (TNF-α). TNF-α is important for phagocyte killing of the *Blastomyces* organisms and recovery from blastomycosis.[19,28,44] Antibodies against the WI-1 antigen produced no protection against infection in a mouse model,[85] a finding that is consistent with high antibody concentrations specific for *Blastomyces* organisms in dogs with life-threatening, progressive blastomycosis. A majority of dogs *experimentally* infected by exposure to contaminated soil recover from blastomycosis without treatment.[76] It is likely that when *naturally* exposed, some dogs develop mild respiratory signs and recover spontaneously. Antibodies in 2 of 48 healthy dogs from an endemic area with no history of illness suggest that occasionally dogs do develop a subclinical, self-resolving disease.[45] However, almost all dogs with clinical signs that have warranted veterinary attention have disseminated disease and should be aggressively treated. Dogs[2] and people[71] occasionally recover from symptomatic blastomycosis without treatment.

CLINICAL FINDINGS

Dogs

Dogs with blastomycosis usually have clinical signs that include anorexia, weight loss, cough, dyspnea, ocular disease, lameness, or skin lesions. Signs of disease usually have been present for a few days to a week but may have been apparent for up to a year. In some dogs the disease process seems to plateau; animals show few signs for weeks to months, but then the disease suddenly progresses and symptoms worsen. Many of the dogs have a history of antibiotic therapy with minimal or temporary improvement.

The physical findings in blastomycosis vary greatly. Mental depression is frequent but inconsistently noted. About 40% to 60% of dogs have a fever of 39.4° C (103° F) or greater. Dogs with chronic lung disease are often severely emaciated. Lymphadenomegaly of one or more lymph nodes is a common finding.

A majority (85%) of dogs with blastomycosis have lung lesions with characteristic dry, harsh lung sounds. Dogs with mild lung disease show exercise intolerance, and severely affected dogs have dyspnea at rest. Coughing is a variable finding. Thoracic radiographs are indicated for dogs suspected of having blastomycosis because some dogs have lung changes without respiratory signs. On radiographs, diffuse, nodular interstitial and bronchointerstitial lung changes are the most common findings (Fig. 59-2). Other less common manifestations include well-marginated solitary to multiple cystic or solid nodules or masses. Tracheobronchial lymphadenomegaly develops in some dogs. Pleural effusion, pneumomediastinum, and cavitary lung lesions are also observed. Chylothorax and solid fibrous masses are uncommon manifestations of thoracic blastomycosis. Solid fibrous masses may partially occlude the great vessels. An obstructive anterior vena caval syndrome and *Blastomyces*-induced granulomas causing chylothorax was

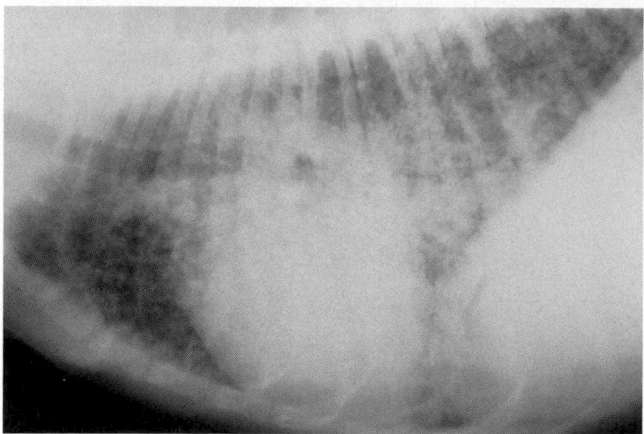

Fig 59-2 Severe, diffuse miliary to nodular interstitial pulmonary infiltrate.

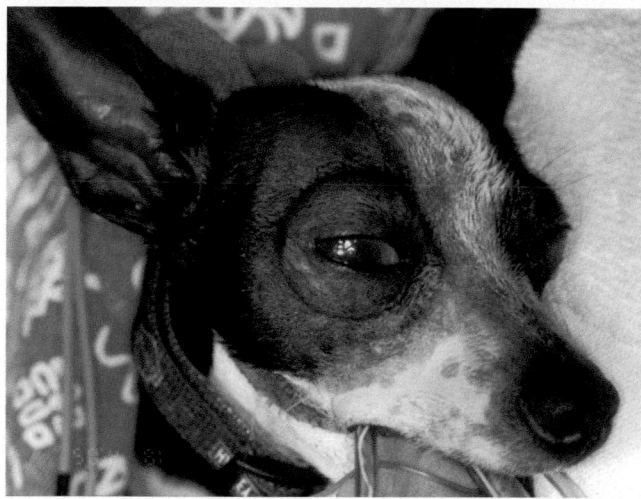

Fig 59-3 Panophthalmitis with associated orbital inflammation in a dog with blastomycosis. (Courtesy Diane Hendrix, University of Tennessee, Knoxville, Tenn.)

diagnosed in a young dachshund.[38] Pulmonary thromboembolism secondary to blastomycosis can increase the degree of dyspnea that develops with the fungal pneumonia.[59]

Up to 40% of dogs with blastomycosis have ocular lesions, the most common of which is uveitis. Early signs of uveitis are conjunctival hyperemia, iridial hyperemia, aqueous flare, and miosis (Figs. 59-3 and 59-4). Chorioretinitis (Fig. 59-5), optic neuritis, retinal detachment, retinal granulomas, vitritis, and vitreal hemorrhage are also caused by blastomycosis. Severe corneal edema may prevent good visualization of the internal ocular structures. Glaucoma secondary to angle closure also develops.[17] Lens rupture occurred in 40% of eyes with endophthalmitis requiring enucleation. The lens material probably contributed to cataract formation and ocular inflammation.[37] Panophthalmitis with associated orbital inflammation is common in severe ocular disease. Keratitis, conjunctivitis, and inflammation of periorbital tissues are frequently observed. A review by Krohne discusses the spectrum of lesions and specific therapy for blastomycosis in the eye.[48] Uveitis in conjunction with signs of respiratory or skin disease should alert the clinician that an animal may have blastomycosis. Early diagnosis and appropriate treatment are essential to preservation of vision in blastomycosis (see Ocular Infections, Chapter 93).

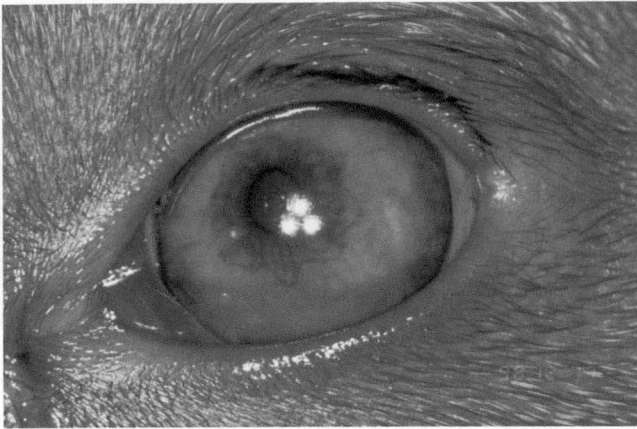

Fig 59-4 Anterior uveitis with iridial hyperemia, aqueous flare, and miosis in a dog with blastomycosis. (Courtesy Diane Hendrix, University of Tennessee, Knoxville, Tenn.)

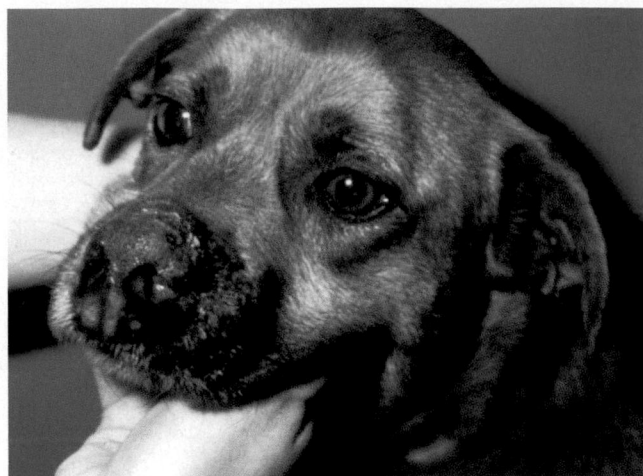

Fig 59-6 Ulcerative lesion on nasal planum associated with blastomycosis in a dog.

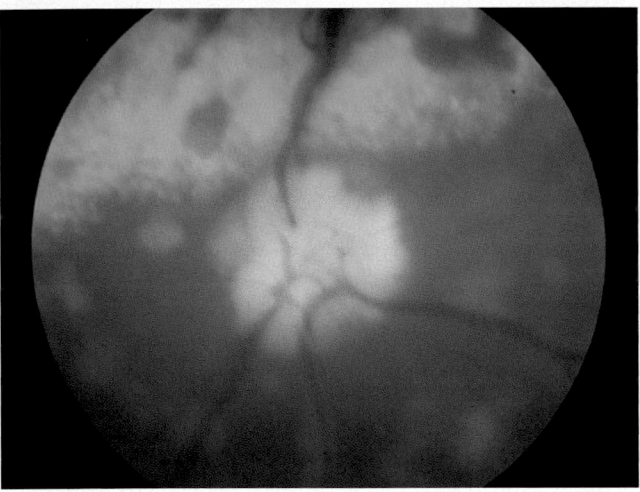

Fig 59-5 Chorioretinitis and retinal detachment associated with blastomycosis in a dog. (Courtesy Diane Hendrix, University of Tennessee, Knoxville, Tenn.)

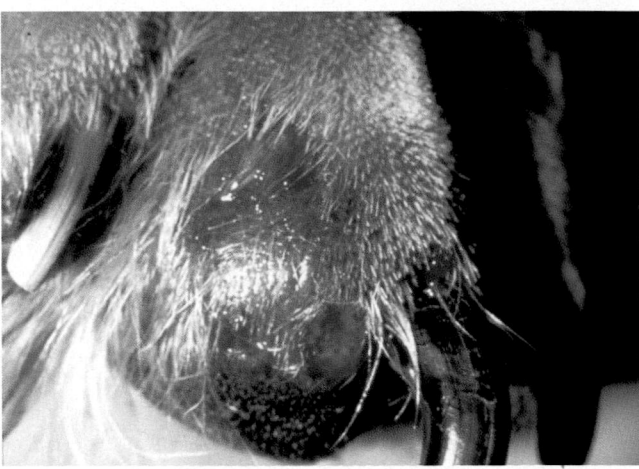

Fig 59-7 Granulomatous lesion of nail bed associated with blastomycosis in a dog. (Courtesy Linda Frank, University of Tennessee, Knoxville, Tenn.)

Skin lesions, found in 20% to 50% of dogs with blastomycosis,[2,49,52] may be ulcerated with drainage of a serosanguineous or purulent fluid. Other lesions may be granulomatous, proliferative, and meaty. Well-defined subcutaneous abscesses may develop. Calcinosis cutis developed in three dogs during amphotericin B (AMB) treatment.[34] The lesions resolved completely after the completion of treatment. Although the skin lesions may be found anywhere, the planum nasale (Fig. 59-6), the face, and the nail beds (Fig. 59-7) appear to be preferred sites.

Bone involvement occurs in up to 30% of infected dogs. Lameness is the primary sign in affected animals and may be the only sign of disease. Special procedures, such as bone scans, may identify a greater percentage of dogs with bone involvement. Lesions usually involve the appendicular skeleton and are typically osteolytic with periosteal proliferation and soft tissue swelling (Fig. 59-8). A majority of the bone lesions are solitary and develop distal to the stifle and elbow. Fungal osteomyelitis must be differentiated from primary and metastatic bone tumors and bacterial osteomyelitis.

Various other tissues may be less commonly infected, including testes, prostate, kidney, bladder, brain, mammary gland, joints, and nasal passages.[2,49,52] The testes and epididymis may be greatly enlarged and painful. Involvement of the prostate gland produces swelling and pain. Dogs with involvement of the kidneys, bladder, or prostate may have organisms in the urine. Meningeal and secondary brain involvement usually develops with widely disseminated disease but may develop without multisystemic manifestations. Depression, seizures, and neurologic deficits are noted with central nervous system (CNS) infections. Changes in the periventricular and third ventricle area were found on contrast enhanced computed tomography (CT) imaging of the brain in a dog with CNS blastomycosis.[69] Nasal discharge and obstruction of airflow through the nose develop when blastomycosis involves the nasal passages. Lesions have been found in most organs of infected dogs. Blastomycosis of the gastrointestinal (GI) tract is rare but was identified in two dogs with generalized blastomycosis.[7,62] Sites of *Blastomyces* infection in dogs can be identified using positron emission tomography (PET) imaging.[57] This is a very sensitive technique but unfortunately is not widely available.

Cats

Cats with blastomycosis have lesions similar to those of dogs, but too few cats have been evaluated to derive a reliable

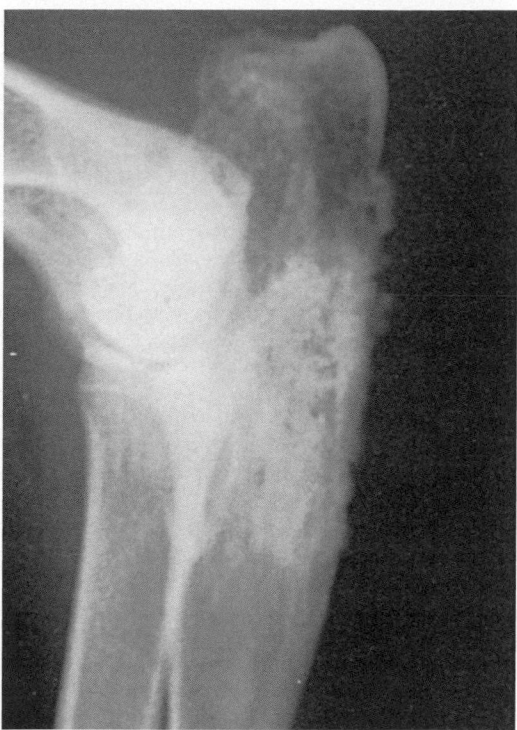

Fig 59-8 Semiaggressive bone lesion characterized by osteolysis and amorphous bone production of proximal tibia of a dog.

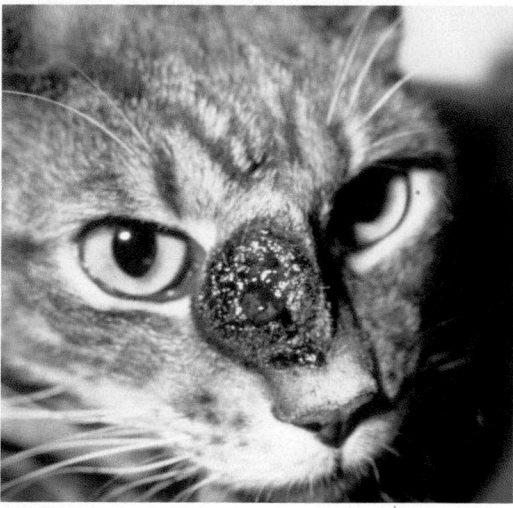

Fig 59-9 Ulcerative lesion of nasal planum of a cat. (Courtesy University of Georgia, Athens, Ga.)

characterization of predominant signs. Dyspnea, visual impairment, draining skin lesions (Fig. 59-9), and weight loss have been the most frequent findings. Eye involvement generally produces a pyogranulomatous uveitis.[31] Intracranial CNS disease and posterior paralysis also have been reported.[60] Clinical signs reflect the involved tissues: lung, lymph node, kidney, eye, CNS, skin, GI tract, pleura, and peritoneum.[60]

DIAGNOSIS

Clinical Laboratory Testing
On preliminary laboratory evaluation, a mild normocytic, normochromic anemia develops that can be attributed to chronic

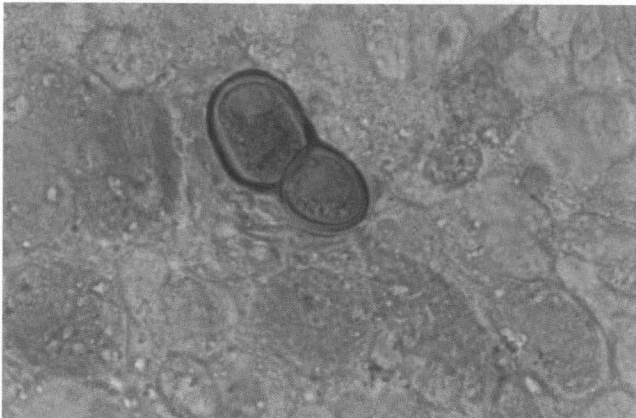

Fig 59-10 Budding yeast form of *Blastomyces* (new methylene blue stain, ×1260). (Courtesy University of Georgia, Athens, Ga.)

inflammation. Most dogs have a moderate leukocytosis (17,000-30,000 white blood cell count [WBC]/µl) with a mild left shift, and lymphopenia is common. They usually have hyperglobulinemia and hypoalbuminemia. The increased globulin concentrations are caused by an increase in α_2-globulin and a polyclonal increase in other immunoglobulins. The only other biochemical change that may be seen is hypercalcemia of granulomatous disease (12.5 to 17.5 mg/dl), which may occur without bone lesions.[27] Twelve of 87 dogs with blastomycosis had hypercalcemia, but the increase was less than 13.4 mg/dl in all but one dog, which had a 16.8 mg/dl increase in serum calcium.[2] Increased serum calcium concentrations return to normal after treatment. Hypercalcemia may be associated with renal failure.

Organism Identification
Diagnosis should be made by identifying the organism through cytologic or histologic evaluation. Any of the common cytologic stains can be used. Because of the cost of therapy, a definitive cytologic rather than a serologic diagnosis is preferred. The combination of aspirates of enlarged lymph nodes and impression smears of skin lesions or cytology of draining exudates reveal *Blastomyces* organisms in more than half the cases (Fig. 59-10). The cytologic reaction is characteristically pyogranulomatous and include nondegenerate neutrophils and macrophages (which have an epithelioid appearance), with occasional multinucleated giant cells. Plasma cells, lymphocytes, and fibroblasts are also seen. Occasionally, a suppurative reaction predominates.[30] Organisms are usually plentiful in fulminating disease. When the disease is primarily ocular and less invasive diagnostic procedures have failed, vitreous aspirates or histologic examination of enucleated blind eyes can be used to diagnose the disease as blastomycosis. In dogs with productive coughs, a tracheal wash may be used to identify the organism, but this test is less reliable than other procedures, probably because of the primarily interstitial site of infection. Lung aspirates can be used when the lung is the only affected site and the results of the tracheal wash are negative. Ultrasound-guided fine needle aspirates of focal lung lesions identified organisms in five of six dogs with blastomycosis without complications.[82] Pneumothorax is a potential complication of lung aspiration, although severe complications are uncommon. Premedication with atropine is recommended before lung aspiration to prevent excessive vagal stimulation. In dogs with urinary tract or prostatic blastomycosis, the organism may be found on urinalysis. In a dog with *Blastomyces*-induced peritonitis, peritoneal

lavage recovered the organism.[62] *Blastomyces* organisms may be found in stool samples if the organism has been coughed up and swallowed.[12] Although rare, in dogs with brain involvement, organisms may be found on examination of the cerebrospinal fluid (CSF). Culture of cytologic specimens is not recommended for in-clinic laboratories because personnel may become infected with the mycelial form of the organism (see Fig. 56-16).[25] The polymerase chain reaction (PCR) can be used to confirm the identity of *Blastomyces* organisms. PCR was positive only in infected tissues in which organisms were seen on histopathologic examination.[16]

Atypical pulmonary fibrous masses containing organisms in small inflammatory foci may develop in lieu of the usual granulomatous reaction. These fibrous masses have few organisms, and cytology of aspirates is usually unsuccessful. Surgical biopsies are required, and multiple histologic sections with fungal staining are needed to find the organisms.

Serologic Testing

Only after searching for organisms should serologic testing be done to help establish a diagnosis. Although serologic testing alone is not definitive, a combination of compatible history, clinical signs, and suggestive radiographs in conjunction with positive serology tests may be substituted for identification of the organism.

The AGID test has replaced the complement fixation test and is the most commonly used serologic test for blastomycosis. It has a sensitivity of 41% to 90% and specificity of 90% to 100%.[45,53,63] AGID test results in dogs may be negative early in the development of infections. A positive AGID result is strongly supportive of *but not* definitive for blastomycosis. The AGID test has been used in only a few infected cats, and results were positive in only one of three cats tested.[60] Although the intensity and the number of bands seen on the AGID tend to decrease after successful treatment, the persistence of antibodies in cured animals precludes AGID for evaluating response to therapy or recurrence of disease. An RIA for detecting antibodies against *Blastomyces* was more sensitive than the AGID, detecting 92% of infected dogs, whereas the AGID detected 41%.[45] Enzyme-linked immunosorbent assay (ELISA) methods using *B. dermatitidis* have also been developed[6,23]; however, their accuracy and sensitivity have not been as extensively evaluated. (See Appendix 5 for a listing of laboratories that offer this test.)

PATHOLOGIC FINDINGS

Blastomyces produces purulent to pyogranulomatous lesions in infected tissues of dogs and cats. The yeasts are admixed with neutrophils, macrophages, and multinucleated giant cells. Lymph nodes are hyperplastic and have increased numbers of plasma cells and macrophages. In tissue, the broad-based, budding yeasts are best seen with special stains, such as periodic acid–Schiff, Gridley's fungal, or Gomori's methenamine silver stain. Filamentous forms rather than the yeast form have been found in the tissue of people and dogs,[42] and giant forms of the organism measuring 30 to 35 μm in diameter rather than the usual 20 μm have been seen.[40] *Blastomyces* organisms in the eyes are primarily found in the choroid and rarely in the retina or anterior segment.[22]

THERAPY

For a summary of the dosage regimens, see Table 59-1 (and the Drug Formulary, Appendix 8, for additional information).

Amphotericin B

AMB is an effective, rapidly acting, fungicidal drug for the treatment of various systemic fungal infections, including blastomycosis. Because AMB is nephrotoxic and has to be given intravenously (IV), it has been replaced as the drug of choice for blastomycosis by itraconazole (ITZ), which is equally effective and safer.[54] (See Drug Formulary, Appendix 8, for additional information on AMB and its precautions.)

In dogs that cannot absorb oral medications or have not responded to ITZ treatment, AMB can be a life-saving drug. AMB deoxycholate should be given at a dose of 0.5 mg/kg every other day. The serum urea concentration should be

Table • 59-1

Drug Therapy for Blastomycosis

DRUG[a]	SPECIES	DOSE[b] (mg/kg)	ROUTE	INTERVAL (HOURS)	DURATION[c] (DAYS)
Itraconazole (ITZ)	Dog[d]	5	PO	24	60
	Cat	5	PO	12	60
Fluconazole (FCZ)	Dog	5	PO	12	60
Amphotericin B (AMB) lipid complex[e]	Dog	1	IV	3 times weekly	Varies[f]
AMB	Dog	0.5	IV	3 times weekly	Varies[g]
	Cat	0.25	IV	3 times weekly	Varies[h]

PO, By mouth; *IV*, intravenous.
[a]See text and Drug Formulary, Appendix 8, for additional information concerning administration of each drug.
[b]Dose per administration at specified interval.
[c]Minimum duration of therapy. Ideally, therapy should continue for at least 1 month beyond the last detection of clinical illness or infection.
[d]ITZ is preferred drug and dosage therapy. ITZ should be given every 12 hours for the first 5 days (see text). A 12-hour interval (10 mg/kg/day total dose) is recommended when intraocular involvement is present.[32] When expense is a factor, other regimens may be considered. FCZ may also better penetrate the eye when treating intraocular infections; however, it is not as active. Enucleation may be needed.
[e]Three lipid formulations are available (see Drug Formulary, Appendix 8). Efficacy at this dose has been established for ABLC (Abelcet, Liposome Co., Princeton, N.J.).
[f]Stop when cumulative dose reaches 12 mg/kg.
[g]Stop when azotemic or cumulative dose reaches 4–6 mg/kg, then start azole, or when cumulative dose is 8–10 mg/kg when given alone.
[h]Stop when azotemic or cumulative dose reaches 4 mg/kg, then use ITZ.

monitored closely and the AMB discontinued when the urea level approaches 50 mg/dl. A cumulative dose of 8 to 10 mg/kg is required to cure blastomycosis. Cats should be given no more than 0.25 mg/kg every other day.

AMB lipid complex (see Drug Formulary, Appendix 8) has been less toxic when given to treat dogs with systemic blastomycosis.[47] The effective dose is somewhat higher than that of AMB deoxycholate and it is considerably more expensive, but the drug is much less nephrotoxic. Unless the dog has preexisting renal disease, it is difficult to justify the high cost of the lipid complex AMB as the initial treatment with AMB.

Itraconazole

Dogs

ITZ is an azole drug of the triazole group (see Drug Formulary, Appendix 8). Dogs with blastomycosis respond to treatment with ITZ as rapidly as they do with AMB and more rapidly than they do with ketoconazole (KTZ). Compared with AMB, ITZ is easier to administer and has fewer side effects. Because ITZ is given orally, dogs can be treated at home. Although ITZ is more costly than AMB, the cost of treatment with ITZ is similar if the expense of IV administration and frequent monitoring of renal function with AMB is considered. Dogs that cannot take oral medications can receive an IV form of ITZ; however, it is expensive.

Seventy-four percent of dogs treated with 5 mg/kg/day of ITZ responded to treatment; a 77% response rate was found in a historic control group treated with AMB.[54] Of the dogs that responded initially, 20% of the AMB-treated dogs and 20% of the ITZ-treated dogs had a recurrence of disease after completing the ITZ treatment.[54] Likewise, in another study, 21 of 31 dogs (68%) responded to a 60- to 90-day course of ITZ. In responding dogs, 5 of 21 dogs (24%) had a recurrence, and 4 of those dogs were successfully retreated with a second course of ITZ.[2] The mortality rates of ITZ-treated and AMB-treated dogs are very similar. The 5 mg/kg/day dose of ITZ is better than the 10 mg/kg/day dose. The cure and relapse rates are similar, but the lower dose group had fewer adverse effects. ITZ appears to penetrate the eye in dogs with active disease, because the dogs with ocular blastomycosis of the posterior chamber often respond to ITZ treatment.[20] Twice-daily dosing with 5 mg/kg has been recommended for intraocular infections.[32] Voriconazole, a related azole, has been effective in treating CNS blastomycosis in a person.[6a] ITZ is not excreted in the urine. so it cannot be used in urinary tract disease. Fluconazole (FCZ) is excreted in the urine and should be considered in these cases. The ease of administration, the decreased likelihood of toxicity, and the efficacy of ITZ make it the drug of choice for the treatment of blastomycosis. The only disadvantage of ITZ treatment is the relatively high cost of the drug.

For dogs, ITZ should be started at a dosage of 5 mg/kg every 12 hours for 5 days to maximize blood concentrations rapidly. The dosage is then reduced to 5 mg/kg/day for the remainder of the treatment. ITZ treatment should be continued for at least 60 days and for at least 1 month after all signs of disease have resolved. Most dogs with mild to moderate lung involvement can be cured with a 60-day course of treatment. Dogs with severe lung involvement should be treated for at least 90 days. Recurrence occurs in about 20% of responding dogs—usually within 1 year of treatment completion. FCZ can be used for the treatment of blastomycosis but it is not as effective as ITZ. (See Drug Formulary, Appendix 8, for additional information on ITZ.)

Cats

Cats with blastomycosis have been successfully treated with ITZ at 5 mg/kg given every 12 hours. This is an effective, safe treatment for most cats. No studies have been done on the efficacy of lower drug dosages.

Adverse Effects

The most common adverse effect of ITZ treatment is anorexia associated with hepatotoxicity. Ninety-two percent of dogs receiving 5 mg/kg/day had no clinical signs of toxicity.[54] Only 1 of 24 dogs studied had serum ALT activities above 200 U/L. Increases in liver enzymes correlate with serum concentrations of ITZ. Serum concentrations of ITZ can vary tremendously in dogs receiving the same dose of drug. If toxicity occurs, medication should be stopped until the appetite returns and the serum liver enzyme activities return to less than 100 U/L. The medication should be reinstituted at half the former dose and serum liver enzymes monitored every 2 weeks.

Ulcerative dermatitis developed in 7.5% of dogs receiving 10 mg/kg/day of ITZ, but it did not develop in any dog receiving 5 mg/kg/day (Fig. 59-11).[54] Ulcers were usually focal, 1 to 2.5 cm in diameter, and circular, with ischemic dermis from an underlying vasculitis. The lesions healed quickly after ITZ was stopped. Lesions did not recur when ITZ was restarted at a decreased dose. This reaction must not be interpreted as a recurrence of blastomycosis.

Serum concentration of ITZ can be measured to ensure that the dog is receiving enough drug.[54] Serum ITZ concentrations of 2 µg/ml or greater appear to be adequate. Serum samples can be sent to the Fungus Testing Lab, University of Texas Health Science Center, 7703 Floyd Curl Drive, San Antonio, TX 78284.

Prognosis

The prognosis for dogs and cats with blastomycosis is good. One way to monitor response to therapy is to perform follow-up thoracic radiography of treated animals after clinical remission (Fig. 59-12). The two prognostic factors for survival are brain involvement and severity of lung disease. Dogs with brain involvement usually die but occasionally can be treated successfully. Dogs with CNS signs should be treated initially with AMB. The severity of lung infiltrates may worsen in the first 2 to 3 days of treatment, and the worsening of signs has been attributed to an inflammatory response to dying organisms in the lungs. Death usually results from respiratory failure and occurs in 50% of the dogs with severe lung disease during the first 7 days of treatment. Dexamethasone at a dose of 0.25 to 0.5 mg/kg IV for 2 to 3 days can be given to dogs that

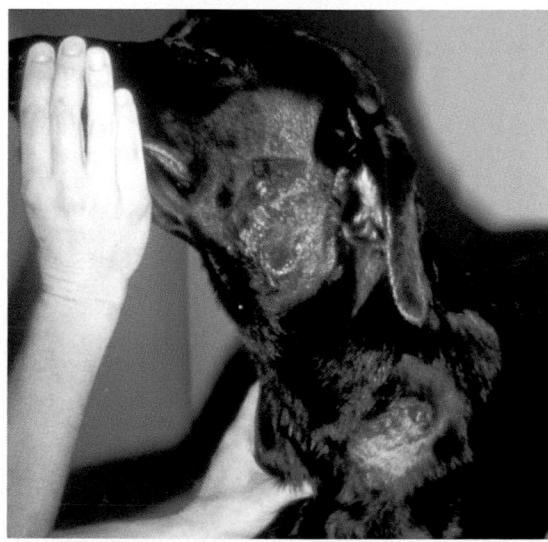

Fig 59-11 Ulcerative dermatitis may occur in some dogs treated with 10 mg/kg/day of itraconazole. (From Legendre AM, Rohrbach BW, Toal RL. Treatment of blastomycosis with itraconazole in 112 dogs. *J Vet Intern Med* 10:365-371, 1996.)

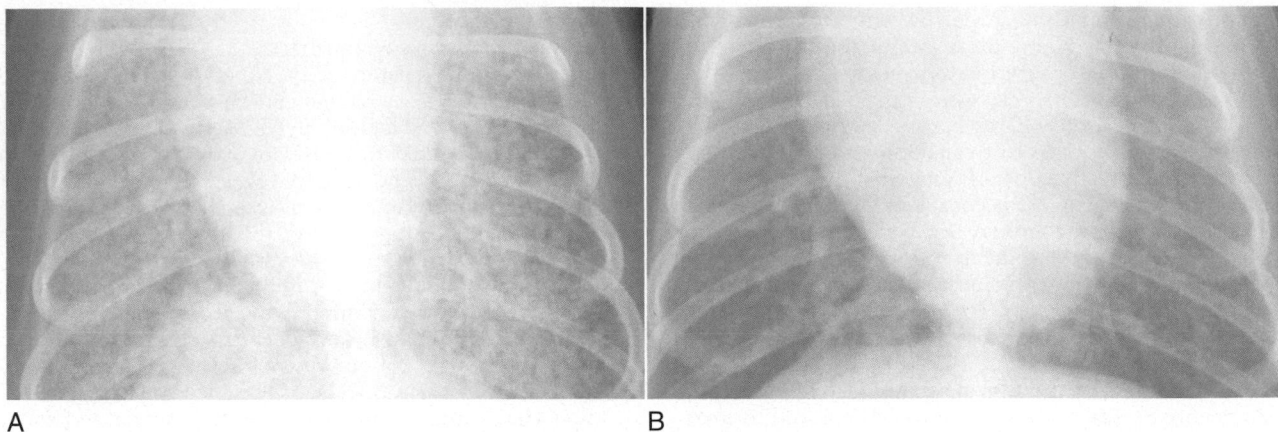

A   B

Fig   59-12   Thoracic radiographs from dog with blastomycosis. **A,** Before treatment. **B,** After therapy, showing reduced pulmonary alveolar-interstitial density. (Courtesy University of Georgia, Athens, Ga.)

develop life-threatening respiratory disease after starting anti-fungal treatment. The glucocorticoids must only be given in conjunction with antifungal treatment. This should reduce the inflammatory response in the lung enough to avoid respira-tory failure. Dogs that receive glucocorticoids should be treated for at least 90 days with antifungal drugs. Improved survival rates can be achieved only with earlier diagnosis of the condition before severe lung disease occurs. For ocular lesions, dogs with mild posterior segment disease, without complete retinal separation, have good prognoses for retain-ing vision.[17] Dogs with severely affected eyes with endoph-thalmitis, glaucoma, or both have poor prognoses for improvement in vision.[48,49,52]

Budding, apparently viable, *Blastomyces* organisms were found in 85% of enucleated, blind eyes despite ITZ treat-ment.[37] Blind eyes should be enucleated after the animal can safely tolerate anesthesia to eliminate a persistent focus of infection.

Treatment of Relapse

Approximately 20% to 25% of the dogs relapse after treat-ment with ITZ, AMB alone, or AMB plus KTZ treatment.[2,54,55] Recurrence after apparently successful treatment usually occurs in the first 6 months after completion of therapy, but recurrences can occur up to 3 years after completion of therapy.[2,54,55] Likelihood of relapse is related to severity of the initial lung disease. Reinfection after successful treatment does not appear to occur, and the recurrence of infection is prob-ably a result of reactivation of a residual site of infection. Recurrence of disease can be effectively treated with another 60- to 90-day course of ITZ. The *Blastomyces* organisms do not appear to develop resistance to the ITZ. Retreatment has an 80% or greater chance of producing a cure.

PREVENTION

The ecologic niche for growth of *Blastomyces* has not been identified, therefore preventive measures are impossible. Even if the site were identified, sterilization of the soil is impossi-ble. Restricting animals from lakes and creeks in areas where other dogs have become infected may be helpful. Dogs should be kept away from construction sites where people have been digging. Dogs kenneled in a heavily shaded area where the soil remains moist may be at increased risk. Removal of some tree branches to allow sunshine into the kennel area may be helpful in reducing the risk of infection. A potential modified

live vaccine for prevention of blastomycosis has been devel-oped by deletion of the WI-1 or BAD-1 virulence factor gene. This modified organism protects mice against challenge with *Blastomyces* organisms.[83,84] This potential vaccine needs to be evaluated in dogs.

PUBLIC HEALTH CONSIDERATIONS

The yeast phase of the organism cannot be transmitted from animals to people or from people to people through aerosols. Penetrating wounds by objects contaminated by the organism have produced infections in people.[36] Care should be taken to avoid bites when handling a dog with blastomycosis.[33] Contaminated knives or needles can accidentally inoculate clinicians during necropsy or fine-needle aspiration.[35,65] The organism should be cultured only in laboratories with proper facilities. Primary pulmonary blastomycosis has readily devel-oped in laboratory workers exposed to cultures of the mycelial form of *B. dermatitidis*.[8,25]

SUGGESTED READINGS*

  2. Arceneaux KA, Taboada J, Hosgood G. 1998. Blastomy-cosis in dogs: 115 cases, 1980-1995. *J Am Vet Med Assoc* 213:658-664.

 16. Bialek R, Cirera AC, Herrman T, et al. 2003. Nested PCR assays for detection of *Blastomyces dermatitidis* DNA in paraffin-embedded canine tissues. *J Clin Microbiol* 41:205-208.

 34. Gortel K, McKiernan BC, Johnson JK, et al. 1999. Calci-nosis cutis associated with systemic blastomycosis in three dogs. *J Am Anim Hosp Assoc* 35:368-374.

 37. Hendrix DVH, Rohrbach BW, Bochsler PN, et al. 2004. Comparison of histologic lesions of endophthalmitis induced by *Blastomyces dermatitidis* in untreated and treated dogs: 36 cases,1986-2001. *J Am Vet Med Assoc* 15:1317-1320.

 62. Nielsen C, Olver CS, Schutten MM, et al. 2003. Diag-nostic peritoneal lavage for identification of blastomyco-sis in a dog with peritoneal involvement. *J Am Vet Med Assoc* 223:1623-1627.

 77. Storms TN, Clyde VL, Munson L, et al. 2003. Blastomy-cosis in nondomestic felids, *J Zoo Wildl Med* 34:231-238.

*See the CD-ROM for a complete list of references.

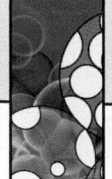

CHAPTER • 60

Histoplasmosis

Craig E. Greene

ETIOLOGY

The etiologic agent of American histoplasmosis is the soil-borne, dimorphic fungus *Histoplasma capsulatum*. This organism can survive wide fluctuations in environmental temperature and prefers areas with warm (mean ambient temperatures of 22° C to 29° C [71° F to 84.2° F]) moist (annual precipitation 35 to 50 inches), and humid (67% to 87%) conditions. These conditions are generally between latitudes 45 degrees north and 30 degrees south. *H. capsulatum* grows best and accelerates its sporulation in soil containing nitrogen-rich organic matter such as bird and bat excrement. Although most affected animals have exposure to the outdoor environment, some affected cats have been housed exclusively indoors. This finding suggests that even accumulations of household dust or soil-containing houseplants may be potential sources of infection.

EPIDEMIOLOGY

H. capsulatum is endemic throughout large areas of the temperate and subtropical regions of the world (Fig. 60-1). Although infections have been documented from every continent except Antarctica, they are most prevalent in the Americas, India, and southeastern Asia. Infection has been documented in dogs in Japan.[26,43] The organism in these infections may be *H. capsulatum* var. *farciminosum*. The organism *H. capsulatum* var. *duboisii*, the cause of African histoplasmosis, is confined to that continent, while *H. capsulatum* var. *capsulatum* (*H. capsulatum*) has been isolated from soil in 31 of the continental United States. Most clinical cases occur in the central United States in the region of the Ohio, Missouri, and Mississippi Rivers. Histoplasmosis can appear in traditionally nonendemic regions if local environmental conditions are altered to favor fungal growth. Soil rich in bird or bat feces, such as where poultry is raised or in caves, respectively, is most likely to harbor the fungus. Obtaining a detailed travel history is important to identify patients that may have acquired infection while in endemic regions.[19,25a]

Determining true rates for histoplasmosis in companion animals is difficult because most infections are subclinical. The prevalence of infection probably parallels that in the human population in endemic regions.

PATHOGENESIS

The life cycle of *H. capsulatum* is similar to that of other dimorphic fungi. The free-living, environmentally resistant mycelial stage in soil at 25° C (77° F) produces macroconidia (5 to 18 μm) (see Fig. 56-15) and microconidia (2 to 5 μm) that are the source of infection for mammals. Histoplasmosis is probably acquired by inhalation of microconidia that are small enough to reach the lower respiratory tract. The incubation period after exposure in susceptible hosts is approximately 12 to 16 days.[15] In the body at 37° C, the microconidia convert to the yeast phase in the lung and reproduce by budding. The yeast organisms are phagocytized by cells of the host's mononuclear phagocyte system and undergo further intracellular replication. Infection may be grossly limited to the pulmonary tree; however, lymphatic and hematogenous dissemination of *H. capsulatum* can occur early in the course of the disease because of the intracellular location of the fungus. Severe clinical disease can result if the dose of infective spores is large or if the immune system of the host is compromised. The cellular immune system, predominantly involving cytokine-mediated macrophage killing, will rapidly bring the infection under control in most patients. T-cell immunity is critical for clearance of the organism. In immunocompetent hosts, *H. capsulatum* may establish a dormant phase and may not be totally eliminated from the mononuclear phagocyte system.[16] With subsequent immunosuppression, reactivation of infection can occur. Dissemination involves primarily organs that are rich in mononuclear phagocytes.

The yeast form of *H. capsulatum* may be more resistant to host defense mechanisms because it is more invasive. Only in endocarditis does the mycelial form sometimes appear on the valve leaflets. When conidia are incubated at 34° to 37° C, genes producing heat shock proteins 70 and 83, M-phase cell cycle enzymes, and tubulin proteins are activated. The walls of yeasts contain more chitin and less mannose and amino acids than do mycelial-phase cells. These transformed yeasts readily enter the cytoplasm of phagocytes where they are engulfed by phagolysosomes. The yeasts raise the intracellular pH slightly by releasing urease, ammonia, and bicarbonate, thus facilitating their absorption of intracellular iron.

In addition to phagocyte impairment, the fungus induces nonspecific anergy, as demonstrated in people and mice with disseminated infections. The yeast cells overproduce interleukin (IL)-4, which at high levels can interfere with the cellular immune response. The yeast also synthesizes melanin or melanin-like compounds, as do other pathogenic yeasts, and this may be an important virulence factor.[37]

The occurrence of gastrointestinal (GI) histoplasmosis without respiratory tract involvement suggests that the GI tract may also be a primary site of infection. However, experimental studies have failed to produce GI disease reliably after oral administration of *H. capsulatum* spores.

CLINICAL FINDINGS

Cats

Cats are very susceptible hosts and are at least as likely as dogs are to develop clinical histoplasmosis. The age range of cats affected with histoplasmosis is 4 months to 14 years; the majority of cases occur in young cats (under 4 years).[24] No

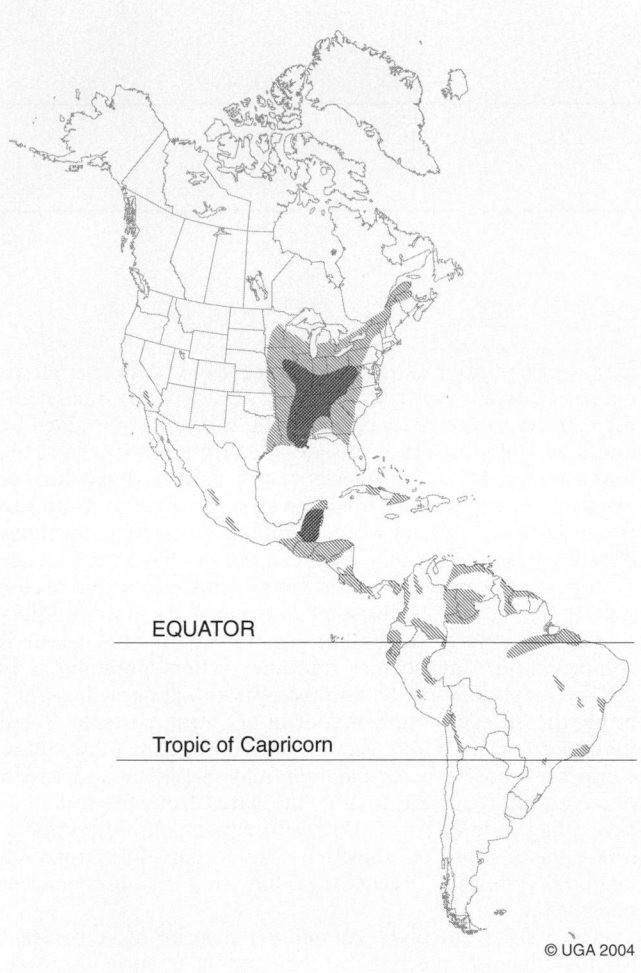

Fig 60-1 The prevalence of histoplasmosis in North and South America based on seropositivity in people. The darker-shaded areas indicate zones of very high endemicity. (Courtesy University of Georgia, Athens, Ga.)

apparent breed predilection is present; females appear to be more commonly affected than are males.[24]

Most infected cats have disseminated disease and exhibit a wide range of nonspecific clinical signs, including depression, weight loss, fever, anorexia, and pale mucous membranes.[10] Coughing is uncommon, but dyspnea, tachypnea, and abnormal lung sounds are found in more than one half of affected cats. Other frequent findings include peripheral or visceral lymphadenomegaly, splenomegaly, and hepatomegaly. Occasionally, *Histoplasma* infects the eye, causing conjunctivitis, granulomatous blepharitis, granulomatous chorioretinitis, retinal detachment, and optic neuritis.[24,25,34] Some cats have had osseous lesions, causing soft-tissue swelling and lameness. The skin is infrequently affected with nodular or ulcerated lesions.[38] Rare clinical findings include oral ulcers, nasal polyps, vomiting, and diarrhea.

Dogs

Histoplasmosis has been reported in dogs ranging in age from 2 months to 14 years. Most affected dogs are young (under 4 years), and no apparent sex predilection is present. Pointers, Weimaraners, and Brittany spaniels are overrepresented in some published reports.[2,51,52]

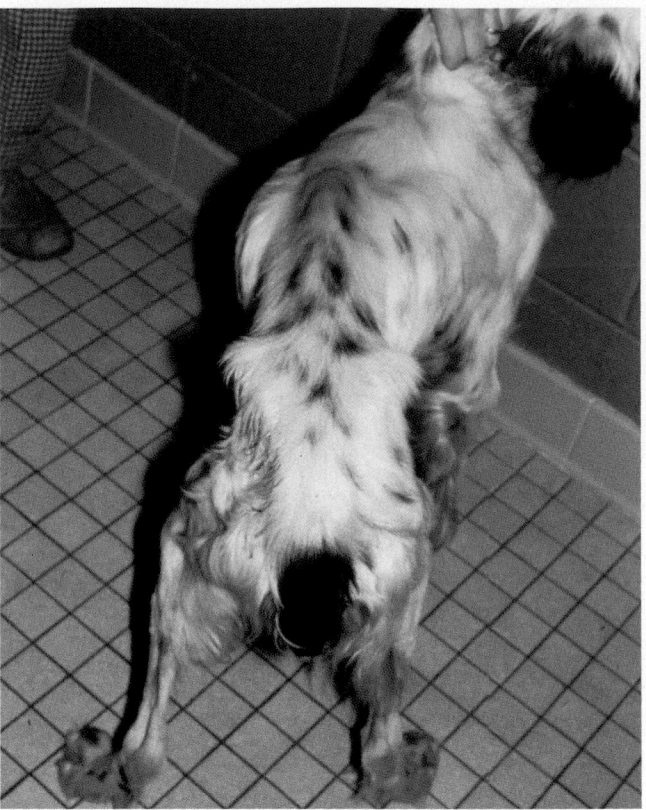

Fig 60-2 Dog with severe weight loss caused by malabsorption from *Histoplasma* enteritis. (Courtesy University of Georgia, Athens, Ga.)

Inappetence, weight loss, and fever unresponsive to antibiotic therapy occur in most cases of canine histoplasmosis (Fig. 60-2). In some dogs, the clinical signs may be limited to the respiratory tree and include dyspnea, coughing, and abnormal lung sounds. However, in most dogs, clinical signs result from disseminated histoplasmosis with GI involvement.[11,30] Signs of large-bowel diarrhea with tenesmus, mucus, and fresh blood in the stool are the most common clinical findings. Pale mucous membranes often are found in patients with bone marrow involvement or GI blood loss. Extensive *Histoplasma* infiltration of the small bowel can cause a voluminous, watery stool with an accompanying protein-losing enteropathy (Fig. 60-3). Hepatomegaly, visceral lymphadenomegaly, splenomegaly, icterus, and ascites are frequent associated findings. Unusual signs include vomiting, peripheral lymphadenomegaly, and lameness as a result of osseous infection. Ocular lesions and skin lesions as described for cats have also been reported in the dog. Neurologic involvement, recognized with dissemination of infection in dogs, is rare.[36] Lesions in infected dogs from Japan have been confined to the skin or gingival, and pulmonary or GI lesions have not been grossly apparent.[26]

DIAGNOSIS

Clinical Laboratory Findings

The most common hematologic abnormality in both dogs and cats with disseminated histoplasmosis is normocytic, normochromic, nonregenerative anemia. The anemia probably results from chronic inflammatory disease, *Histoplasma* infection of the bone marrow, and intestinal blood loss in GI disease. Leukocyte counts are variable. Neutrophilic leukocy-

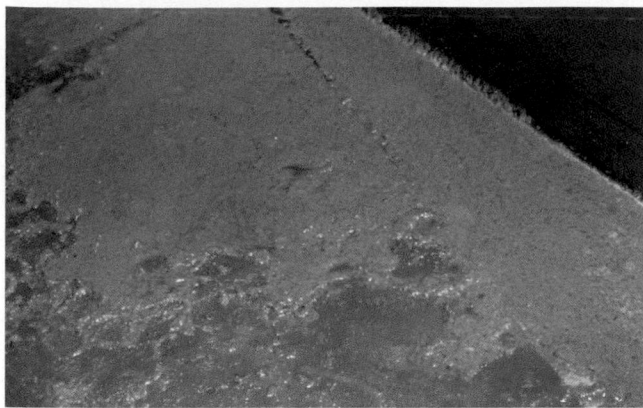

Fig 60-3 Severe watery diarrhea from malabsorption found in the dog in Figure 60-2. (Courtesy University of Georgia, Athens, Ga.)

tosis with monocytosis and eosinopenia is found most frequently. Leukopenia and thrombocytopenia have also been reported. In a survey of neutropenic dogs, histoplasmosis was associated as a risk factor.[6] Severe pancytopenia has been observed in some cats. *Histoplasma* organisms may be found during routine blood film examination in circulating monocytes, neutrophils, and, rarely, eosinophils. Performing 1000-cell differential counts or examining buffy coat smears will enhance detection of infected cells.

Abnormal coagulation function tests have been found in some thrombocytopenic dogs with disseminated histoplasmosis, suggesting the presence of microangiopathic hemolysis. Disseminated intravascular coagulation (DIC) in these dogs may occur as a result of extensive *Histoplasma* infiltration of the liver. Hemolysis and an increased bleeding tendency associated with DIC may enhance the severity of the anemia in these patients.

Biochemical profiles are usually unremarkable in dogs with pulmonary histoplasmosis. Hypoalbuminemia is a fairly consistent finding in cats with disseminated histoplasmosis. Some cats have had hyperproteinemia, hyperglobulinemia, and mild elevations of serum glucose and alanine aminotransferase (ALT) activities. Dogs with disseminated disease may have hypoproteinemia and severe hypoalbuminemia as a result of intestinal blood loss or protein-losing enteropathy. Liver dysfunction in affected dogs may cause hypoalbuminemia, hyperbilirubinemia, elevated serum alkaline phosphatase and ALT values, and abnormal results on liver function tests.[7] Hypercalcemia (probably associated with granulomatous disease) has been reported in several cats.[24]

Urinalyses are usually normal in dogs and cats with histoplasmosis. Most cats have tested negative for feline leukemia virus and feline immunodeficiency virus infections.

Radiography and Ultrasonography
Thoracic radiographs of dogs and cats with active pulmonary histoplasmosis usually exhibit a linear or diffuse pulmonary interstitial pattern associated with granulomatous fungal pneumonia (Fig. 60-4, *A*). The infiltrates often are coalescing and may appear miliary or grossly nodular. True alveolar involvement in pulmonary histoplasmosis is rare. Hilar lymphadenomegaly is common in dogs but rare in cats (see Fig. 60-4, *B*). Pleural effusion occurs infrequently in the dog. Pulmonary calcification, indicative of inactive pulmonary histoplasmosis, is occasionally seen in dogs.

The interpretation of abdominal radiographs in dogs with GI histoplasmosis may be difficult because of the emaciated

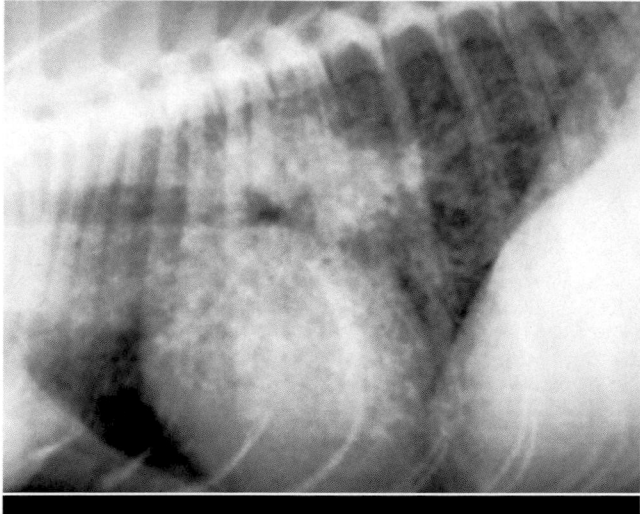

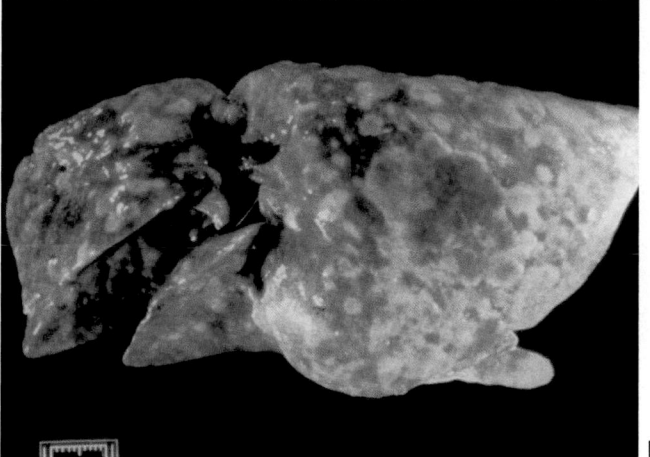

Fig 60-4 **A,** Lateral radiograph of a *Histoplasma*-infected dog with tracheobronchial lymphadenomegaly and linear nodular diffuse interstitial infiltrates. **B,** Lungs from a 2-year-old domestic shorthaired cat that died from widespread, fulminating, granulomatous pneumonia caused by *H. capsulatum.* (Part A courtesy Department of Radiology, University of Georgia, Athens, Ga.; Part B courtesy Alice Wolf, Texas A&M University, College Station, Tex.)

condition of the patient or the presence of abdominal fluid. Noncontrast studies may demonstrate hepatomegaly, splenomegaly, or ascites (Fig. 60-5). Barium contrast examination may reveal irregularities of the intestinal mucosa and thickening of the intestinal walls.

Ultrasound examination of dogs with liver involvement reveals hyperechoic liver parenchyma (Fig. 60-6).[7] Nodular and infarctive lesions have also been observed.

Osseous involvement with histoplasmosis is rare in the cat and even less common in the dog. The typical radiographic appearance of bony lesions is a mixed pattern of osteolysis, subperiosteal bone proliferation, and periosteal new bone formation (Fig. 60-7). Intraarticular infection has been observed in both dogs and cats but is rare.[25] In the cat, *Histoplasma* most frequently infects the metaphyses of long bones with a predilection for the bones of and adjacent to the carpal and tarsal joints.

Endoscopy
Endoscopic examination of dogs with colonic histoplasmosis reveals mucosal thickening, granularity, friability, and ulceration.[30] Cytologic or histologic examination of rectal scrapings

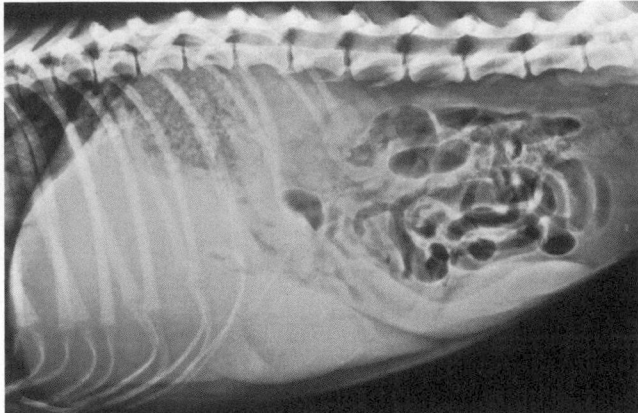

Fig 60-5 Lateral radiograph of the abdomen of a 5-year-old male English setter with disseminated histoplasmosis and resultant severe hepatomegaly and splenomegaly. (From Clinkenbeard KD et al. 1989. Canine disseminated histoplasmosis, *Compend Cont Educ Pract Vet* 11:1355. Reprinted with permission.)

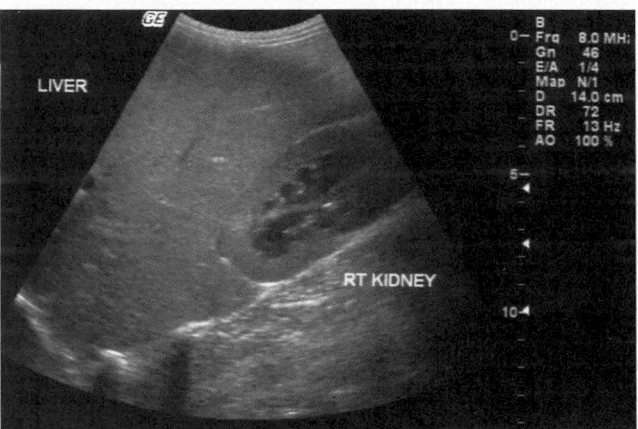

Fig 60-6 Ultrasonographic appearance of hepatomegaly in a dog with visceral histoplasmosis. (Courtesy Department of Radiology, University of Georgia, Athens, Ga.)

and biopsy samples usually reveals large numbers of *Histoplasma* organisms.

Transtracheal Wash and Bronchoalveolar Lavage

Transtracheal wash (TTW) and bronchoalveolar lavage (BAL) have been suggested as methods to evaluate patients with suspected pulmonary mycotic infections in which organisms were not recovered by other noninvasive methods.[22] Generally, BAL is superior to TTW because the collected cells are more representative of the interstitial and distal portions of the airway. BAL requires anesthesia and causes more respiratory compromise than does TTW; therefore patients must be evaluated carefully before undergoing this procedure. Fungal organisms may not be numerous in specimens recovered with either procedure, and the sensitivity of these tests has not been thoroughly evaluated.

Cytologic and Histologic Findings

Histoplasma organisms are usually numerous in infected tissues. A definitive diagnosis can often be made by fine-needle aspiration and exfoliative cytology.[38] The organisms are usually contained within cells of the mononuclear phagocyte system; single or multiple yeast cells may be present within

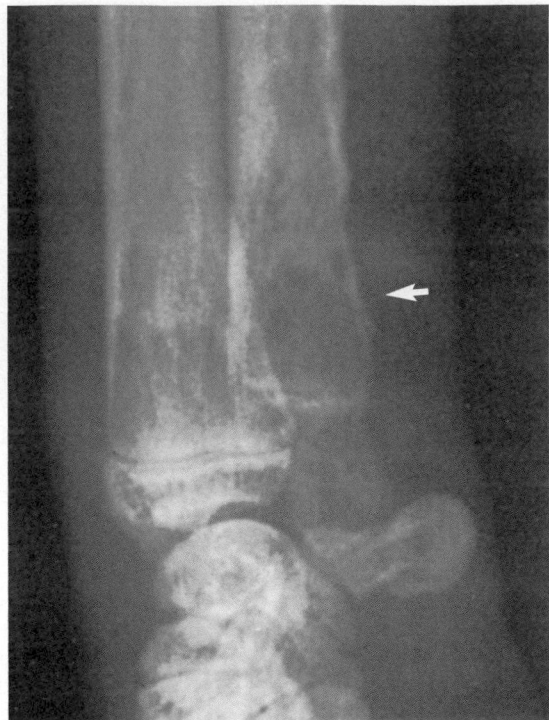

Fig 60-7 Lateral radiograph of the distal radius and ulna of a 5-year-old cat showing diffuse osteolysis and new reactive bone formation (*arrow*) characteristic of osseous histoplasmosis. (Courtesy Alice Wolf, Texas A&M University, College Station, Tex.)

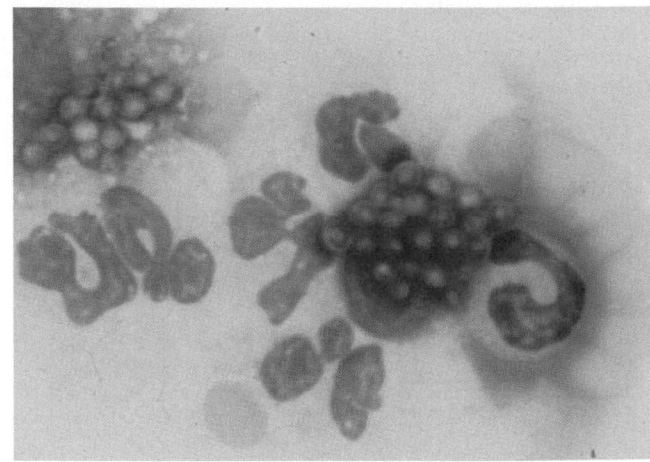

Fig 60-8 *H. capsulatum* in circulating blood monocytes. This organism can also be found in neutrophils and, rarely, in eosinophils (Wright, ×1000). (Courtesy Ken Latimer, University of Georgia, Athens, Ga.)

each phagocytic cell. Routine Wright or Giemsa's hematologic stains demonstrate the organism as a small (2 to 4 μm) round body with a basophilic center and lighter halo caused by shrinkage of the yeast during staining (Fig. 60-8). In the cat, *Histoplasma* organisms are most easily recovered from bone marrow, lung, and lymph node aspirates. Rectal scrapings, imprints of colonic biopsy specimens, and aspirates of liver, lung, spleen, and bone marrow are most productive in the dog. *Histoplasma* organisms have been found in macrophages in peritoneal and pleural effusions, and these and other tissues should be examined as warranted by the clinical signs in each case.[28]

Tissue biopsy may be required if exfoliative cytology is not diagnostic. Affected tissues demonstrate granulomatous inflammation, but *Histoplasma* organisms are difficult to detect with routine hematoxylin and eosin stain. Special fungal stains (periodic acid-Schiff, Gomori's methenamine silver, Gridley's fungal stain) should be used to enhance detection of the organisms if histoplasmosis is suspected. Immunostaining with polyclonal anti-*Mycobacterium bovis* (Bacille Calmette-Guérin) was used to identify *Histoplasma* and other infectious agents in skin biopsy specimens in animals.[4]

Cerebrospinal Fluid

Central nervous system (CNS) involvement is rare in dogs or cats with histoplasmosis. Cerebrospinal fluid (CSF) specimens from affected dogs demonstrate increased protein and cellularity.[36] The granulomatous cellular response consists of nondegenerate neutrophils, macrophages, monocytes, and occasional lymphocytes. *Histoplasma* organisms have been identified in CSF macrophages in some patients.

Fungal Isolation

Attempts to culture *H. capsulatum* in a routine practice setting are *not* recommended because of the pathogenic potential of this organism. *H. capsulatum* can be cultured from tissue specimens, fine-needle aspirates, and body fluids. The yeast phase produces white, moist colonies when inoculated on blood agar and incubated at 30° or 37° C (see Chapter 56 and Fig. 56-15). The mycelial phase will develop within 7 to 10 days on routine fungal culture media incubated at room temperature. Microconidia produced by the mycelial phase are infectious, and cultures exhibiting fluffy white or buff-brown mycelial growth should be handled with caution.

Immunodiagnosis

Intradermal skin tests for reactivity to histoplasmin are unreliable in companion animals and cannot be used to confirm the diagnosis of histoplasmosis. Serologic tests (agar-gel immunodiffusion, complement fixation) for antibodies directed against *Histoplasma* antigens are often falsely negative in animals with active naturally occurring disease.[24,28] Test results may be false positive in an animal with prior exposure that has recovered from infection. Sera from dogs with histoplasmosis cross-react with *Blastomyces dermatitidis* antigens used in enzyme-linked immunosorbent assay (ELISA) for detection of antibodies.[45] Currently, no consistently reliable antibody detection test is available for identification of histoplasmosis in companion animals.

An antigen detection assay, which identifies a polysaccharide antigen of *H. capsulatum* in serum, CSF, or urine, has been used in the diagnosis of human infections[46a] (MiraVista Diagnostics, Indianapolis, Ind.; http://www.miravistalabs.com; see Appendix 6). This assay has become important in the monitoring of immunosuppressed people because it gives generally 90% positive results in patients with progressive disseminated histoplasmosis. Positive rates are much lower with confined pulmonary lesions. Antigen concentrations decrease during therapy, and increases have been correlated with relapses.[47] Even in human infections, cross-reactivity of the urine test for *Histoplasma* antigens occurs in people with blastomycosis, coccidioidomycosis, and penicilliosis.[48] The test might be of value as a provisional diagnostic aid for animals with serious infections caused by one of these organisms; however, further studies are needed.

Polymerase chain reaction (PCR) has been used on a limited basis in diagnosis of human infections. Infection was confirmed in one dog by nested PCR on paraffin-embedded biopsy specimens.[43] PCR has also been used to examine different strains in soil and those from corresponding human and canine infections in the same geographic region.[17]

PATHOLOGIC FINDINGS

The organs affected in histoplasmosis will depend on whether the disease is pulmonary or disseminated. In the pulmonary form, the lesion can be active, with miliary or larger gray foci, or chronic and calcified. With dissemination, many visceral organs are generally involved. The surface of the intestinal tract is thickened and the mucosa often hemorrhagic (Fig. 60-9). The liver is enlarged and has a variegated pale pattern resulting from inflammatory infiltration (Fig. 60-10). With disseminated disease, many parenchymal organs are affected. The hilar and mediastinal lymph nodes may be grossly enlarged

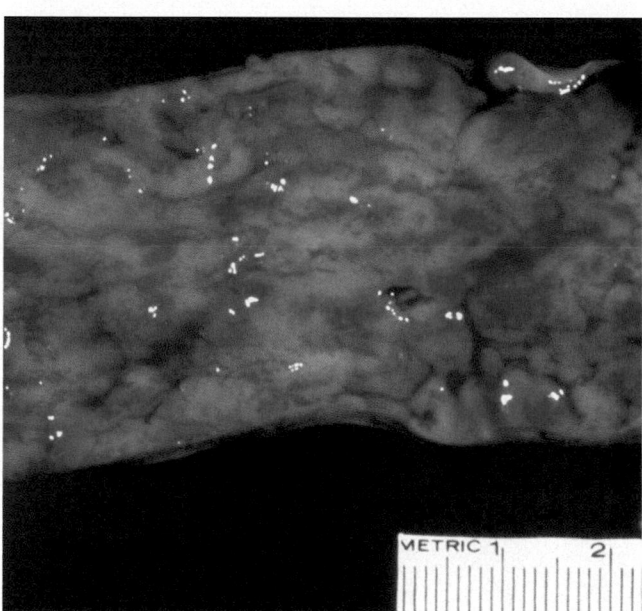

Fig 60-9 Mucosal surface of the colon showing thickening and ulceration caused by disseminated histoplasmosis. (Courtesy University of Georgia, Athens, Ga.)

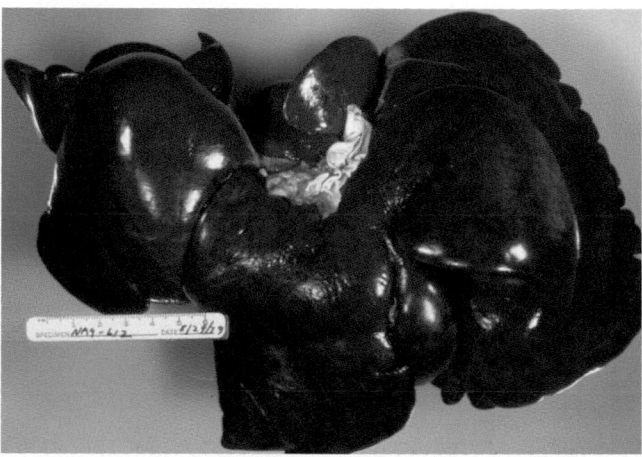

Fig 60-10 Enlarged liver with variegated appearance from a dog with disseminated histoplasmosis. (Courtesy University of Georgia, Athens, Ga.)

and firm (Fig. 60-11). This enlargement may be sufficient enough to cause tracheal or vascular compression. Histologically, granulomatous nodules are infiltrated by macrophages containing *Histoplasma* organisms. *Histoplasma* organisms may be difficult to visualize (Fig. 60-12). Neutrophils are often seen in close association, and occasional infiltration with lymphocytes and plasma cells can be observed. Within the lungs, interstitial and peribronchial thickening can encroach on and fill alveoli.

THERAPY

Antifungal Drugs

Pulmonary histoplasmosis in the dog may be self-limiting and can resolve without treatment.[15] However, antifungal chemotherapy is recommended because dissemination can occur early in the course of infection (Table 60-1). Itraconazole (ITZ) is currently the drug of choice for the treatment of histoplasmosis in animals. Treatment is usually initiated once daily; however, pharmacokinetic studies in cats indicate significant variability in the oral absorption of ITZ, and twice daily dosing (at 10 mg/kg) may be required in some cats to achieve the desired therapeutic effect.[5] The oral solution is more consistently absorbed, when compared with capsules, allowing for 10 mg/kg once daily dosing. See Drug Formulary, Appendix 8, for detailed information on the use of ITZ.

Despite the reportedly poor penetration of ITZ into the CNS and eye, several cats with *Histoplasma*-induced ocular lesions had complete resolution of disease with a standard course of ITZ therapy.[24,53] Liposomal amphotericin B (AMB) has been used to treat people with CNS histoplasmosis.[46a]

In dogs or cats with severe or fulminating pulmonary or GI histoplasmosis with dissemination, AMB or combination therapy with AMB and ITZ or high loading doses of ITZ may provide more rapid control of the fungal infection (see Table 60-1). See the Drug Formulary, Appendix 8, for further information on AMB. ITZ treatment is initiated simultaneously with AMB administration and is continued after termination of the AMB regimen.

The duration of antifungal treatment required for each patient is variable and is determined by the severity of infection and the patient's clinical response. The response to therapy should be evaluated by monitoring for the resolution of clinical signs, hematologic and biochemical abnormalities,

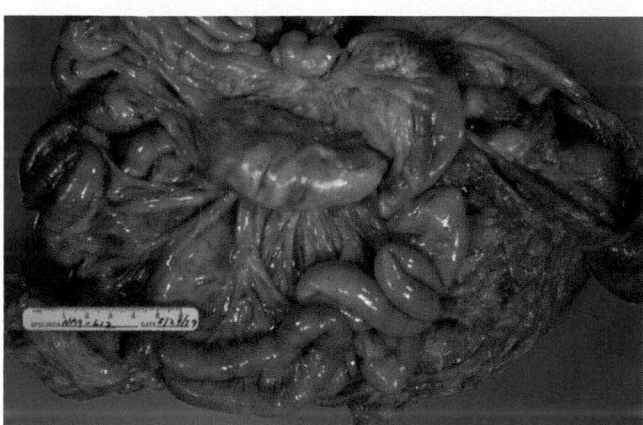

Fig   60-11   Enlarged mesenteric lymph node and inflamed intestines from the dog in Figure 60-9. (Courtesy University of Georgia, Athens, Ga.)

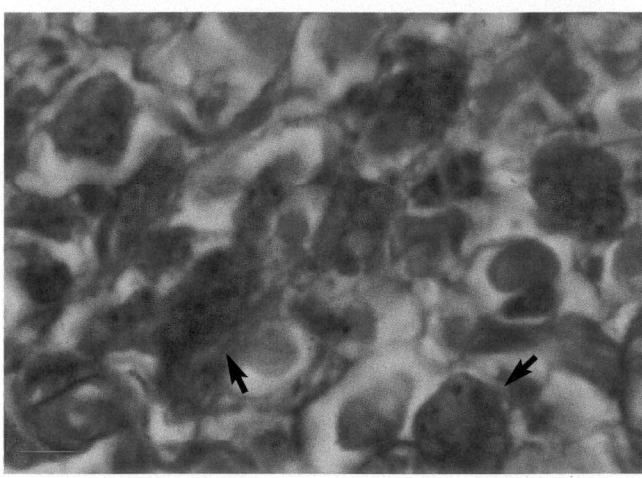

Fig   60-12   Many intracellular *Histoplasma* organisms in a tissue biopsy specimen from a dog with disseminated histoplasmosis (PAS, ×400). (Courtesy University of Georgia, Athens, Ga.)

Table • 60-1

Therapy for Histoplasmosis

DRUG[a]	SPECIES	DOSE[b] (mg/kg)	ROUTE	INTERVAL (HOURS)	DURATION (MONTHS)
Itraconazole	B	10	PO	12–24	4–6[c]
Ketoconazole	D	10–20	PO	12	4–6
AMB[d]	B	0.25–0.5	IV	48[e]	[f]

B, Both dog and cat; *D*, dog; *AMB*, amphotericin B; *PO*, by mouth; *IV*, intravenous.
[a]See Drug Formulary (Appendix 8) for further information.
[b]Dose per administration at specified interval.
[c]Minimum time; each case must be evaluated independently; see text. Treat for at least 2 months after resolution of clinical signs.
[d]Given in conjunction with a concurrently administered oral azole. See Table 57-2 and Drug Formulary, Appendix 8, for alternate formulations and dosages of AMB.
[e]Monday-Wednesday-Friday schedule usually used.
[f]Continue until cumulative dose of 5 to 10 mg/kg is reached in dogs, 4 to 8 mg/kg in cats.

and radiographic lesions. Generally, most patients are treated with oral antifungal drugs for at least 4 to 6 months.

Another orally administered triazole, fluconazole (FCZ), has better penetration into the CNS and eye than does ITZ (see Drug Formulary, Appendix 8). FCZ is theoretically preferred for patients with neurologic involvement or ocular lesions that are refractory to AMB or ITZ treatment. FCZ may also be used for animals that do not tolerate ITZ therapy; however, it is not as effective as ITZ is in treating people with histoplasmosis.[35] Similar studies in animals outlined later indicate that FCZ is not very effective in the treatment of histoplasmosis. FCZ but not ITZ antagonized the effectiveness of AMB when these combinations were used to treat mice with disseminated histoplasmosis.[31] In mice with experimental *Histoplasma* meningitis, FCZ monotherapy and AMB and FCZ combined therapy was less effective compared with AMB monotherapy.[23] Therefore FCZ is not recommended over AMB or ITZ for treatment of histoplasmosis. ITZ has been effective in treating CNS histoplasmosis in people in which AMB and FCZ treatment have failed.[1] ITZ is more active than FCZ is against *H. capsulatum* in vitro, which parallels its superior in vivo effectiveness. Although concentrations of ITZ in CSF are negligible, those in CNS tissue exceed that in plasma and may explain the benefits of this drug in treating CNS mycoses.

Ketoconazole (KTZ), the first licensed oral azole antifungal agent, has lower potency against *Histoplasma* and increased relative toxicity compared with ITZ and FCZ. For these reasons, it is not recommended as a first-choice treatment unless expense becomes a limiting factor. See Drug Formulary (Appendix 8) for further information.

Voriconazole is active against *Histoplasma* and penetrates the CSF, making it a consideration for treating CNS infection. Posaconazole (PCZ, SCH 56592) is a newer triazole structurally related to ITZ. It was shown to be highly effective when compared to AMB or ITZ in treating immunosuppressed mice with disseminated histoplamosis.[12]

The ability to treat animals with histoplasmosis effectively has improved significantly because of the availability of safe and efficacious oral azole antifungal drugs. Dogs and cats with pulmonary histoplasmosis have a fair to excellent prognosis. The prognosis for animals with disseminated histoplasmosis is fair to good, depending on the severity of fungal involvement. *Histoplasma*-infected areas most difficult to treat with histoplasmosis are CNS, ocular, boney, and epididymal infections. For the epididymal infections, orchiectomy is advised. For the others, prolonged antifungal therapy is needed, although the prognosis for complete recovery is guarded. The prognosis for return of vision depends on the severity of retinal damage before the control of infection.[20,29]

Antiinflammatory Drugs

Life-threatening infection with histoplasmosis is caused by rapid proliferation of the organism in many tissues, including the lung, and from chronic airway obstruction from hilar lymphadenomegaly. Glucocorticoids have been used to treat people with active inflammatory disease and chronic airway obstruction. Clinical signs and airway obstruction associated with hilar lymphadenomegaly resolved more rapidly in dogs treated with glucocorticoids with or without antifungal chemotherapy.[42] Coughing decreased more rapidly, and the glucocorticoid-treated animals had improvement in their overall well being. Clinical improvement was noted in a mean of less than 1 week, 2.6 weeks, and 8.8 weeks, in dogs with suspected chronic pulmonary histoplasmosis treated respectively, with glucocorticoids, glucocorticoids and antifungals, and antifungals alone. Dogs were included in the study if they had serum antibodies against *H. capsulatum* and thoracic radiographic and bronchoscopic indications of airway obstruction.

They were excluded from the study if evidence of active histoplasmosis (organisms recovered on cytologic or biopsy specimens) or other current disease was detected. None of the dogs treated with glucocorticoids had a worsening or dissemination of their disease as a result of glucocorticoid treatment. Prednisone was used at a dosage range of 2 mg/kg orally, given every 24 hours, to 2 mg/kg orally, given every 12 hours. Treatment was continued for a mean of 6.5 weeks, with a gradually tapering dosage. Glucocorticoids are not generally recommended in the treatment of active histoplasmosis in people or animals because they may induce immunosuppression and dissemination of infection.

Immunostimulants

Interferon (IFN)-γ has been administered alone and in combination with a suboptimal regimen of AMB in the treatment of experimental disseminated histoplasmosis in mice.[8] IFN-γ alone given subcutaneously postinfection prolonged survival over untreated controls, and combined regimens of AMB and IFN-γ reduced the fungal burden in organs as compared with either drug alone. For further information on IFN-γ see Drug Formulary, Appendix 8.

PREVENTION

Effective immunoprophylaxis is not clinically available for histoplasmosis. In laboratory experiments, several constituents extracted from the cell wall and cell membrane of *H. capsulatum* protect mice against infection.[16] A genetic recombinant-produced version of one of these extracts, heat shock protein 60, protects mice against challenge with yeast cells.[19] Prevention consists of avoiding exposure to *Histoplasma*-infected soil in endemic areas. Soil containing bird or bat excrement enhances the growth of *Histoplasma* and is particularly dangerous. People or animals disturbing the soil, or in areas of poor ventilation such as caves, are at greatest risk. Formalin (3%) or formaldehyde solution may be used for soil decontamination if small, focal sources of infection can be identified.

PUBLIC HEALTH CONSIDERATIONS

Both companion animals and people residing in or traveling through endemic regions of the country are at risk of exposure to *H. capsulatum*. Concurrent common-source infection of people and animals has been observed; however, as with the other systemic mycoses, direct transmission of histoplasmosis from animal to animal or animal to people has not been reported.[15,49] Fungal cultures containing mycelial growth of *H. capsulatum* are highly infectious and should be handled with extreme caution. Infections in people have occurred after kidneys, taken from donors in endemic regions, have been transplanted into patients outside endemic areas.[32] Such risks might also occur in animals if such procedures become more widely used.

SUGGESTED READINGS*

17. de Medeiros Muniz M, Pizzini CV, Peraita JM, et al. 2001. Genetic diversity of *Histoplasma capsulatum* strains isolated from soil, animals, and clinical specimens in Rio de Janeiro State, Brazil, by a PCR-based random amplified polymorphic DNA assay, *J Clin Microbiol* 39:4487-4494.

*Please see the CD-ROM for a complete list of references.

31. LeMonte AM, Washum KE, Smedema ML, et al. 2000. Amphotericin B combined with itraconazole or fluconazole for treatment of histoplasmosis, *J Infect Dis* 182:545-550.
43. Ueda Y, Sano a, Tamura M, et al. 2003. Diagnosis of histoplasmosis by detection of the internal transcribed spacer region of fungal rRNA gene from a paraffin-embedded skin sample from a dog in Japan, *Vet Microbiol* 94:219-224.
46. Wheat LJ, Garringer T, Brizendine E, et al. 2002. Diagnosis of histoplasmosis by antigen detection based upon experience at the histoplasmosis reference laboratory, *Diagn Microbiol Infect Dis* 43:29-37.
46a. Wheat LJ, Musial CE, Jenny-Avital E. 2005. Diagnosis and management of central nervous system.

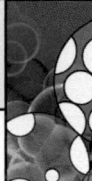

CHAPTER • 61

Cryptococcosis

Richard Malik, Mark Krockenberger, Carolyn R. O'Brien, Patricia Martin, Denise Wigney, and Linda Medleau

ETIOLOGY

Cryptococcosis is an important disease in people and animals and the most common systemic mycosis of cats.[41] The infection is thought to be acquired from the environment, and no cases of disease transmission from one affected animal to another have been reported.[19,40] Thus cryptococcosis is not a contagious or anthropozoonotic disease. Occasional outbreaks of infection in people and animals, such as in British Columbia, Canada, may be the result of a common environmental source.[57,92]

Cryptococcosis is most commonly caused by two encapsulated yeast species of the genus Cryptococcus—*Cryptococcus neoformans* and *Cryptococcus gattii* (formerly *C. neoformans* var. *gattii*, also *Cryptococcus bacillisporus*), although other species (such as *Cryptococcus laurenti* and *Cryptococcus albidus*) very rarely cause disease in people and animals.[51] *Cryptococcus magnus* was isolated from the external ear canal of a cat with otitis externa.[43a] The ability of *C. neoformans* and *C. gattii* to grow at 37° C may be a factor in their pathogenicity, because other members of the genus grow poorly at this temperature. Elaboration of a polysaccharide capsule and the enzymes laccase and phospholipase by *C. neoformans* and *C. gattii* are additional virulence factors that contribute to pathogenicity of these species.[15]

C. neoformans and *C. gattii* are dimorphic, basidiomycetous fungi.[50] They exist in animal tissues as the yeast form (*Cryptococcus* species) but are capable of transforming under special laboratory conditions into a filamentous form (*Filobasidiella* species). Unlike other dimorphic fungi, the yeast phase of *Cryptococcus* is found under routine laboratory conditions and in infected tissues. Thus far, the filamentous phase has been demonstrated only under strictly controlled laboratory conditions, but this perfect state is likely to exist in certain natural environments. The importance of the *perfect state* is that spores resulting from sexual or asexual filamentous reproduction could well represent the infectious propagules that give rise to mammalian disease.[21,93] An unusual temperature-sensitive isolate of *C. neoformans*, which would not grow at 37° C, produced hyphal elements in a granuloma within the nasal passage of a cat and in culture at 35° C.[6]

In animal tissues, *C. neoformans* and *C. gattii* exist as a round to oval yeast with a variably sized polysaccharide capsule as its distinguishing feature. The capsule provides protection from environmental insults (e.g., desiccation) and the phagocytic response of the host. In tissues, *Cryptococcus* reproduces by forming one or two daughter cells (buds) that are connected to the parent cell by a narrow isthmus. Buds may break off when small, and thus the cell population varies in size.[41]

Cryptococcus has a worldwide distribution and in addition to people infects various domestic and native mammals, including cats,[69] dogs,[62] ferrets,[60] horses, goats, sheep, cattle, dolphins, birds,[64] and koalas[47] and other marsupials. In contrast to the other systemic mycoses, the prevalence of cryptococcosis in cats exceeds that in dogs. Historically, five serotypes (A, B, C, D, AD) were recognized on the basis of antigenic differences in capsular polysaccharide. Recent advances in the taxonomy of the genus *Cryptococcus* have led to a new nomenclature that was proposed at the Fifth International Conference on *Cryptococcus* and Cryptococcosis and is now generally accepted with the modification to elevate C. *neoformans* var *gattii* to species status (Table 61-1).[51]

C. neoformans and *C. gattii* differ biochemically, genetically, ecologically, and epidemiologically. *C. neoformans* has a worldwide distribution, whereas *C. gattii* is largely restricted to tropical and subtropical climates.[22] *C. neoformans* can be divided into two varieties based on serotyping, *C. neoformans* var. *grubii* and *C. neoformans* var. *neoformans*. Both varieties are strongly associated with disease in human patients who are immunocompromised, although the same may not be true for companion animals. *C. neoformans* var. *grubii* is by far the most common isolate worldwide from people and animals with cryptococcosis, although *C. gattii* is important in certain geographic regions such as Australia, Papua New Guinea, Southeast Asia, and Central Africa. Strong evidence suggests that several species of Australian eucalyptus trees provide a natural environmental niche for *C. gattii*.[22,49] Interestingly, koalas (*Phascolarctos cinereus*) serve as a sentinel host for infection and at the same time, they seem capable of amplifying the number of cryptococci in certain environments.[49] The definitive environmental niche for *C. neoformans* has not been determined, although a strong historical association exists between weathered bird (especially pigeon) guano[41] and growth in decaying plant matter in hollows of certain trees.[56] *C. gattii* (serotype B) in Australia exists in highest concentra-

Table • 61-1

Major Causative Agents of Cryptococcosis

YEAST FORM (*CRYPTOCOCCUS* SPP.)		FILAMENTOUS FORM (*FILOBASIDIELLA* SPP.)	ENVIRONMENTAL NICHE	GEOGRAPHIC DISTRIBUTION
CURRENT NOMENCLATURE	PREVIOUS NOMENCLATURE			
C. neoformans var. *grubii*	*C. neoformans* var. *neoformans* (serotype A)	*F. neoformans*	Avian guanos	Worldwide
C. neoformans var. *neoformans*	*C. neoformans* var. *neoformans* (serotype D)	*F. neoformans*	Avian guanos	Europe
C. gattii	*C. neoformans* var. *gattii, C. bacillisporus, C. hondurianus* (serotypes B and C)	*F. bacillispora*	Hollows of eucalyptus trees and some other trees	Tropical and semitropical climates—many countries; Temperate climates— Vancouver and Vancouver Island, British Columbia

tion within the dead plant material in eucalyptus tree hollows (e.g., *Eucalyptus camaldulensis* and *Eucalyptus teriticornis*). In British Columbia, Canada, the organism is consistently found on living tree bark (Garry oak, maple, cedar, and pine) and air.[4,57] *C. neoformans* passes through the gut of pigeons, but systemic infection of pigeons is extremely rare. Perhaps the pigeon's high body temperature protects it from infection.[64] Pigeon guano provide an alkaline, hyperosmolar environment that is rich in many nitrogen-containing compounds including creatinine that favor cryptococcal growth. Cryptococci may remain viable for at least 2 years in environments such as pigeon lofts, where accumulations of pigeon guano are protected from drying or sunlight.

Most basidiomycetes reproduce sexually in their natural environment, and the teleomorphs of *C. neoformans (Filobasidiella neoformans)* and *C. gattii (Filobasidiella bacillisporus)* can be induced to undergo sexual reproduction in the laboratory and produce dikaryotic hyphae, blastoconidia, basidia, and basidiospores. The recent documentation of α- and a-mating types of *C. gattii* in *E. camaldulensis* trees suggests that this may occur in nature.[32] However, recent work has suggested that *C. neoformans* may be evolving into an asexual fungus,[26] and basidiospores may result from haploid (monokaryotic) fruiting as well as by sexual recombination.[102] In either case, the notion that the basidiospore is the infectious propagule for *Cryptococcus* is attractive, as this stage is suited to dispersal by air currents and has physical properties that favor penetration into the respiratory system, thereby facilitating primary infection of mammalian hosts.[21,93]

Cryptococcus has various virulence factors, including its capsule, melanin, mannitol, laccase, and other enzymes. After it infects a host, the capsule thickens considerably. The capsule is a key virulence factor and is composed of glucuronoxylomannan (GXM). Two capsular genes—CAP59 and CAP64—have been associated with virulence. Capsule is continuously shed into the host's cerebrospinal fluid (CSF) and blood, where it circulates for an extended period. Capsules of the A and D serotypes are chemotactic for neutrophils. Comple-

ment fixation also results in attraction of leukocytes. The capsule may help protect the organism because it blocks the Fc portion of bound antibodies from interacting with the receptors on host phagocytes. Furthermore, encapsulated organisms do not stimulate proinflammatory cytokines and are not phagocytyized or killed by phagocytes to the same degree as unencapsulated mutants. Phenotypic switching, characterized by stable alterations in cell membrane sterol composition and GXM structure, has been identified in *C. neoformans* and allows them to persist in the host by minimizing the inflammatory response.

PATHOGENESIS

The exact mode of infection is unproven, but the most likely route is via inhalation of air-borne organisms, such as basidiospores or yeast cells desiccated by environmental exposure. Shrunken, poorly capsulated cryptococci that are small enough for alveolar deposition have been isolated from pigeon guano and soil. Although human patients with cryptococcosis usually show neurologic signs referable to meningoencephalitis, strong circumstantial evidence suggests that the disease starts in the lungs and subsequently spreads hematogenously via macrophages to the nervous system. People have been shown to be colonized with *C. neoformans* var. *grubii* long before they are clinically ill.[27] Respiratory involvement usually does not result in human illness, although lesions can be detected in thoracic radiographs, thoracic computed tomography scans, or at necropsy. The small particle size of infectious propagules is said to be the reason the lung is primary site of infection, because only very small particles are capable of penetrating deep into the lower respiratory tract.[40] Primary cutaneous cryptococcosis is a rarely described phenomenon that occurs in people; a solitary skin lesion in unclothed areas is most common.[82] *C. neoformans* can be found on the skin of healthy people without infection. Participation in outdoor activities or exposure to bird droppings are risk factors. Clinically healthy people are susceptible to this form of infection and a feline case was reported presumably as a result of a contaminated cat scratch injury.[68a]

Unlike in people, in cats, dogs, koalas, and psittacine birds, the nasal cavity is usually the primary site of infection.[47,62,64,69] The reasons for this difference are a matter of conjecture, but the more developed nasal passages in animals, which more efficiently filter small particles, may provide part of the explanation. It appears that most cases of canine and feline cryptococcosis begin as mycotic rhinitis after asymptomatic colonization of the nasal cavity. *C. neoformans* var. *grubii* has been shown to be a transient colonizer of the nasal mucus of cats, dogs, and koalas in Australia,[47,70] whereas *C. gattii* can be isolated in sufficient numbers and with sufficient frequency to be actually considered part of sinonasal normal flora of koalas in certain environments.[47] Studies in koalas have shown that self-limiting, subclinical infection is common, with limited invasion, granuloma formation, and successful eradication or containment of organisms.[47]

When disease ensues, clinical signs of rostral nasal cavity disease such as sneezing, epistaxis, and nasal discharge are conspicuous, and granulomatous protuberances occasionally can be seen at the nares. In some cases, destruction of adjacent facial bones facilitates spread of infection to contiguous regions, such as the bridge and side of the nose, the planum nasale, or hard palate.[69] When facial distortion develops, the clinical symptoms strongly suggest either fungal rhinosinusitis or nasal neoplasia. In contrast, when infection begins in the caudal portion of the nasal cavity, signs of mycotic rhinitis may be subtle or absent. In other cases, caudal nasal cavity involvement gives rise to a mass lesion, which occludes one or both choanae, resulting in nasopharyngeal signs (e.g., stertor, snoring, dyspnea, open-mouth breathing).[39,65] Occasionally the infection spreads to the middle ear via the auditory tube.[5] It is possible to confirm the sinonasal region as the primary site of infection using cytology, culture, endoscopy, or cross-sectional imaging.

Cryptococcal infection tends to localize in the cooler areas of the body such as the respiratory passages and the subcutaneous tissue. Further spread, when evident, typically involves the central nervous system (CNS). Although the exact means of the organisms' spread into the CNS is uncertain, infection in some cases appears to extend through the cribriform plate into the olfactory bulbs and olfactory tract, giving rise to meningoencephalitis. In these cases the anatomic proximity of the optic nerves frequently results in concurrent cryptococcal optic neuritis and secondary retinitis. Clinically, symptoms include widely dilated pupils that respond poorly to light, swelling of the optic disc, and focal retinal hemorrhage. The infection typically spreads caudally within the meninges along the floor of the cranial vault. As a result, multiple cranial nerve abnormalities can develop subsequently, especially in dogs. Infection may also spread via the CSF pathways to other surfaces of the CNS, such as the dorsal aspects of the brain, and out the foramen magnum along the spinal cord. Hematogenous spread of organisms to the CNS is also possible. Cryptococcal antigen has been persistently identified in the CSF within days following experimental parenteral (subcutaneous [SC] or intravenous [IV]) inoculation of cats with *C. neoformans*.[74] Whether this represents viable organisms remains to be determined.

Multifocal cutaneous involvement in cats and dogs reflects hematogenous dissemination from the primary site of infection, as do lesions in bone (e.g., digits) or periarticular soft tissues. In ferrets[60] and the occasional cat, localized cutaneous cryptococcosis can develop after a penetrating skin injury. In some cats, infection spreads to the mandibular lymph nodes, presumably via the lymphatics from the nasal cavity. Rarely, mandibular lymphadenomegaly can be massive and require surgical debridement. Occasionally salivary gland infection

has been documented, although the way the organisms reach this site is a mystery. In cattle, cryptococci from the environment enter the mammary gland via the teat canal and cause granulomatous mastitis. Primary gastrointestinal (GI) cryptococcosis can occur in very rare circumstances, with involvement of segments of bowel, mesenteric lymph nodes, stomach, and other intraabdominal structures.[60,63]

Cryptococcosis can occur in healthy or immunodeficient individuals, although those with T-cell deficiencies are most commonly infected. In Australia, about half of infected human patients have no detectable T-cell defects. In the remaining 50%, some deficit in cellular immunity exists caused by conditions or treatments such as malignancy, chemotherapy, human immunodeficiency virus/acquired immunodeficiency syndrome (HIV/AIDS), immunosuppressive drug therapy, diabetes, or sarcoidosis.[91] In metropolitan communities, about 10% of patients with HIV/AIDS are likely to develop cryptococcosis in the absence of highly effective antiretroviral therapy.[17] Interestingly, whereas cryptococcosis patients with HIV/AIDS invariably become infected by *C. neoformans*, *C. gattii* infections tend to develop almost exclusively in healthy hosts (i.e., who do not have HIV/AIDS).[80,91] In people with cell-mediated immunodeficiencies, severe meningitis and disseminated infections are common. After experimental inoculation of mice, the magnitude of fungemia has been correlated with the degree of brain infection.[16]

In eastern Australia, about 20% to 30% of human cryptococcosis cases are caused by *C. gattii*,[80,91] with similar percentages in cats and dogs.[62,69] Animals in rural environments tend to be infected with *C. gattii*, presumably because of increased exposure to eucalyptus material, and all cases recorded in koalas have been attributable to *C. gattii*. The development of granulomatous intracranial or pulmonary mass lesions (cryptococcomas) is strongly associated with immunocompetence. Thus in human patients, cryptococcomas are more typical of *C. gattii* infections,[80,91] whereas *C. neoformans* infections in patients who are immunodeficient typically result in meningitis with little involvement of the brain parenchyma.

Infections with feline leukemia virus (FeLV) and feline immunodeficiency virus (FIV) have been thought to predispose cats to cryptococcosis. In North America, evidence suggests that some FeLV-positive cats develop cryptococcosis as a result of immune dysfunction because they respond more slowly or fail to respond to treatment and are much more likely to have relapses.[41] In Australia, FeLV-positive cats with cryptococcosis are exceedingly rare, probably because of the very low prevalence of persistent FeLV infection in the cat population.[69] Although several reports have been made of one or two cats with cryptococcosis allegedly caused by FIV infection, studies in Australia involving large numbers of cats have failed to produce convincing evidence that cryptococcosis is a feline, AIDS-defining disease.[69,100] Rather, it is thought that coinfection usually reflects the high prevalence of FIV infection in Australia. Leukocyte and lymphocyte subset numbers in FIV-positive and FIV-negative cats with cryptococcosis were the same, and a positive FIV status did not mean the cat had an unfavorable prognosis.[100] Indeed, many FIV-positive cats with cryptococcosis are cured of the fungal infection and do not relapse, despite cessation of therapy. Cryptococcosis is rarely reported in cats receiving immunosupressive therapy or chemotherapy for malignancy.[43] Thus underlying diseases are typically not detected in cats with cryptococcosis, and factors predisposing to disease remain elusive. Two FIV-negative cats with cryptococcosis were treated and subsequently developed malignant lymphoma. Although no relationship was established between the two conditions, a similar association has been the subject of previous reports.[38,59,103] In addition, two FIV-positive cats with cryptococcosis developed lymphoma

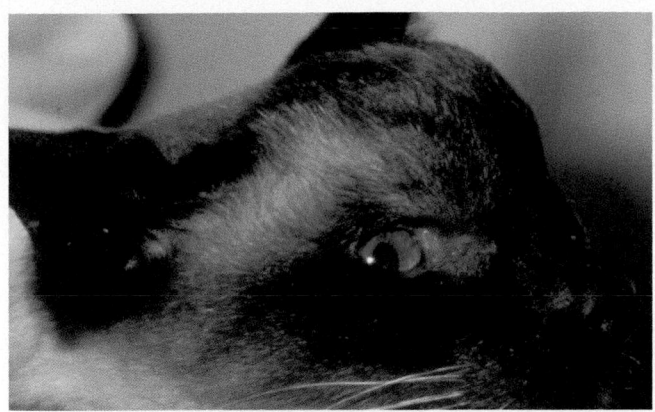

Fig 61-1 Siamese cat with long-standing, invasive *C. neoformans* infection of nasal cavity. Infection has penetrated bones overlying nasal cavity, and cat's nasal bridge and forehead are swollen markedly. At surgery, this subcutaneous swelling was shown to consist almost exclusively of cryptococcal organisms rather than host tissue. (Courtesy R. Malik, University of Sydney, Sydney, Australia.)

and mast cell neoplasia, respectively, subsequent to developing other opportunistic infections.[3] Long-standing FIV infection may have predisposed the animals to cryptococcosis and the terminal malignancies. Genetic factors may be involved in the predisposition toward development of cryptococcosis; Siamese (Fig. 61-1), Birman, and ragdoll cats and German shepherd and American cocker spaniel dogs are affected significantly more than other breeds in reported cases.[41,69] In dogs, immunosuppressive diseases such as ehrlichiosis have been associated with cryptococcosis, but in one study, immunosuppressive factors were identified in fewer than 6% of affected dogs.[7]

CLINICAL FINDINGS

Cats

Cryptococcosis is the most common of the systemic mycoses of cats.[23,28,40,42] No gender predisposition exists, and the age range of affected cats is broad,[69] although young adult cats (2 to 3 years old) appear to be at increased risk. It is likely that exposure and self-limiting infection occur in the first few years of life, with disease in older cats reflecting reactivation of viable cryptococci in residual granulomatous foci. Upper respiratory tract signs are most common and include sneezing; snuffling; and mucopurulent, serous, or hemorrhagic nasal discharge that is unilateral or bilateral. Signs are usually chronic and in some cases, a polyplike mass is evident in the nostril (Fig. 61-2). In others, a firm to fluctuant subcutaneous swelling over the bridge of the nose is present (see Figs. 61-1 and 61-2). Cats with nasopharyngeal cryptococcosis develop stertor, inspiratory dyspnea, a tendency to use open-mouth breathing, and occasionally, secondary otitis media.[46,65] Often, mandibular lymphadenomegaly is evident, and ulcerated or proliferative lesions in the oral cavity occasionally develop. Lower respiratory tract signs are rare in cats. Thoracic radiographs are usually normal, although small nodular lesions may be present. Rarely, large pulmonary nodules, a mediastinal granuloma, or cryptococcal pleurisy are found.[41]

Neurologic signs associated with cryptococcal infection in cats vary depending on the location of lesions in and around the CNS. Common signs include depression, changes in temperament and bizarre behavior, seizures, circling, head pressing, ataxia, paresis, head tilt and other vestibular signs,

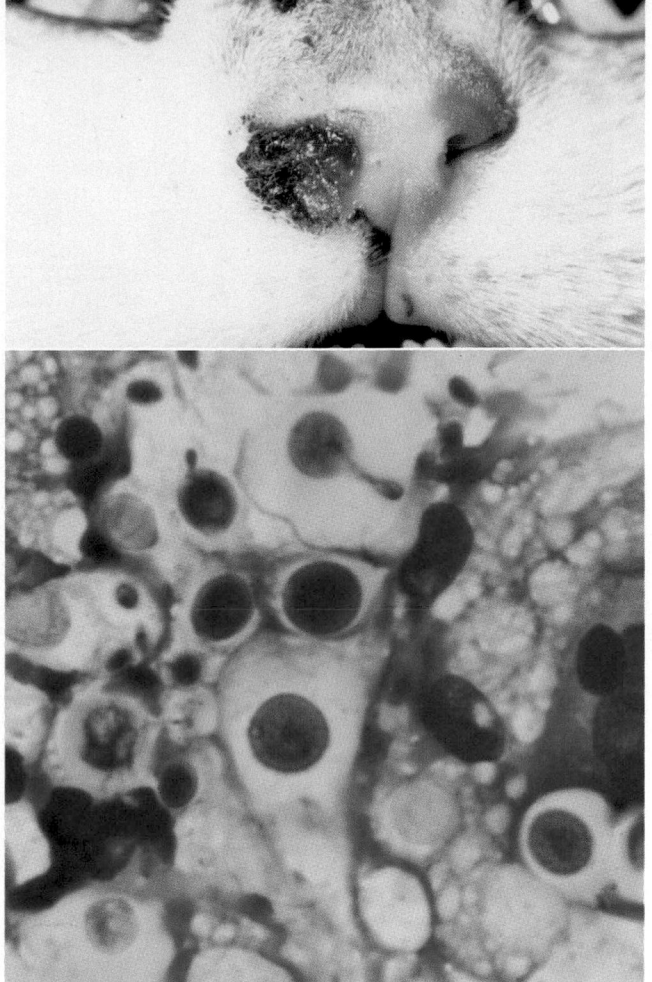

Fig 61-2 **A,** Domestic shorthaired cat with invasive cryptococcal rhinitis that has extended to involve subcutaneous tissues on side of cat's nose. The cat was treated successfully using surgical debridement of lesion and a long course of fluconazole. **B,** Cytology shows capsulate yeasts, with narrow-neck budding in a DiffQuik-stained smear. (Courtesy R. Malik, University of Sydney, Sydney, Australia.)

anosmia, and blindness. These signs may develop individually or in association with other physical findings and may result from the presence of masslike cryptococcomas or meningoencephomyelitis. In people, cerebral cryptococcosis is often associated with increased intracranial pressure,[80] and the same is likely in cats and dogs.

Ocular abnormalities develop in some affected cats and almost always are a marker for CNS involvement. The most common sign is peripheral blindness with dilated, unresponsive pupils (Figs. 61-3, *A* and *C*) because of optic neuritis, exudative retinal detachment, and granulomatous chorioretinitis (see Figs. 61-3, *B* and *D*; see cryptococcosis section in Chapter 93).

Cutaneous lesions are common in cats with cryptococcosis, principally from secondary involvement of the planum nasale (see Fig. 61-2, *A*). Although very rare, localized cutaneous cryptococcosis can develop after inoculation of propagules

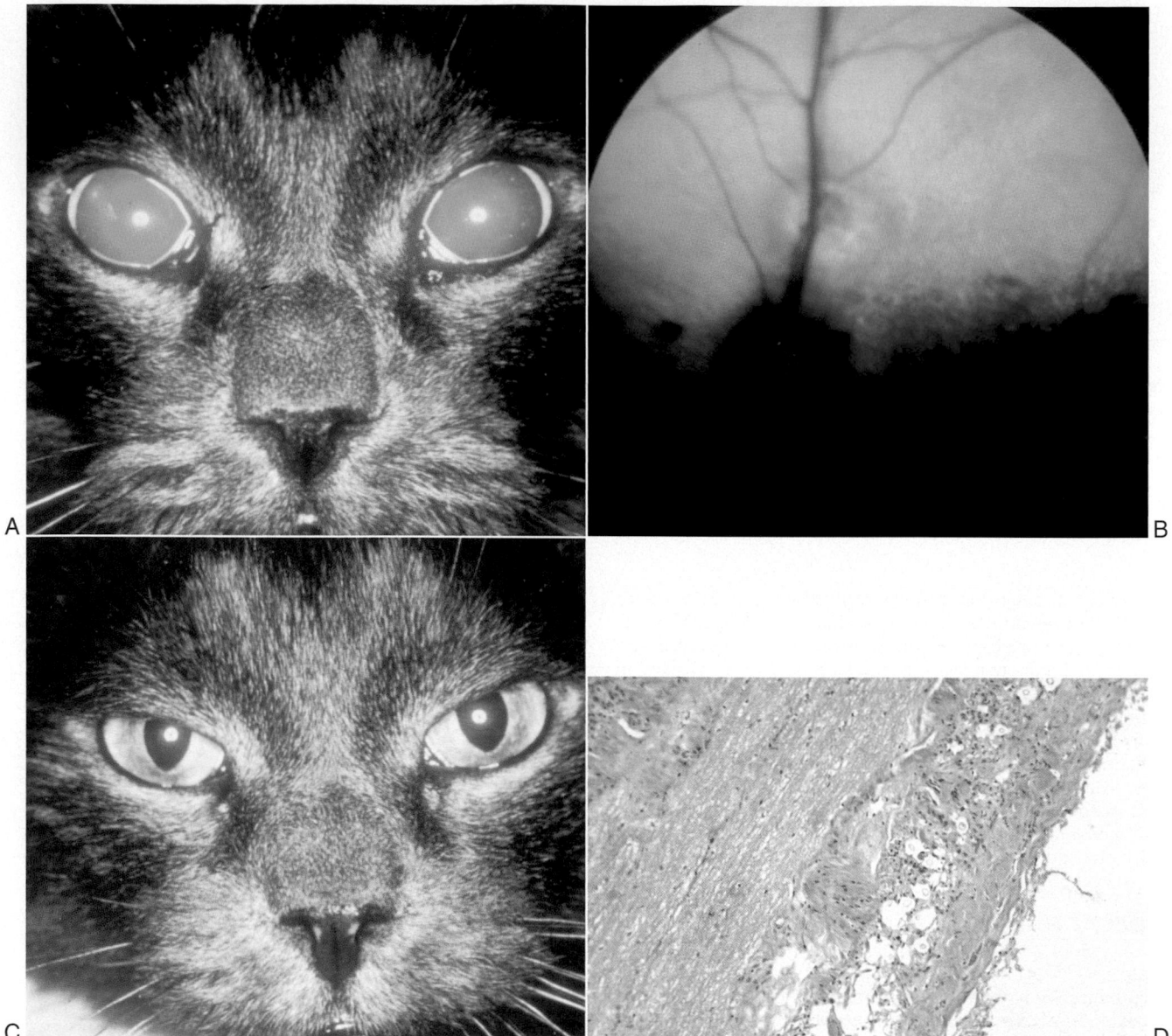

Fig   61-3   Photographs of widely dilated pupils (**A**) and fundus (**B**) of cat with cryptococcal optic neuritis and retinitis. Nasal cavity was shown by culture to be primary site of infection. **C,** Patient was successfully treated using subcutaneous amphotericin B, oral flucytosine, and fluconazole. **D,** Cryptococcal optic neuritis in cat that died of CNS cryptococcosis. (**A, B,** and **C,** Courtesy Nancy Bombaderi and Tony Reid, Adelaide, Australia; **D,** courtesy R. Malik, University of Sydney, Sydney, Australia.)

(e.g., after a cat scratch; Fig. 61-4). Multifocal skin lesions are the result of hematogenous dissemination and consist of papules and nodules that are fluctuant to firm and range from 1 to 25 mm in diameter. Larger lesions tend to ulcerate, leaving a raw surface with a serous exudate (Fig. 61-5).

Cats with disseminated disease also may have enlargement of one or more lymph nodes, with cryptococci evident in aspirates from affected nodes. Fever is uncommon in affected cats. Cryptococcosis is typically a chronic infection, causing listlessness and weight loss due to poor appetite. Other reported signs include change in personality or behavior, peripheral lymphadenomegaly (unassociated with skin lesions), bone lysis, swollen digits, chronic cough, and renal failure due to kidney involvement.[41]

Dogs

Cryptococcosis is a disease that develops predominantly in young adult dogs, and most dogs are younger than 4 years old at diagnosis.[62] No gender predisposition exists. Doberman pinschers, German shepherd dogs, and American cocker spaniels are affected more than other breeds.[41,62] German shepherd dogs susceptible to cryptococcosis presumably have the same genetic predisposition that is responsible for their susceptibility to other systemic fungal infections such as disseminated aspergillosis.

Weight loss and lethargy are common nonspecific findings. Major organ systems affected by canine cryptococcosis include the nasal cavity, CNS, and the eyes. CNS signs are typically multifocal, caused by meningitis and progressive meningoencephalomyelitis, and include head tilt; nystagmus; facial paralysis; paresis, paraplegia, or tetraplegia (usually the upper motor neuron type); ataxia; circling; seizures; and cervical hyperesthesia.[7,8] The most common ocular abnormalities consist of optic neuritis, exudative granulomatous chorioretinitis, and retinal hemorrhage associated with dilated pupils and blindness. Occasionally, anterior uveitis develops, as does

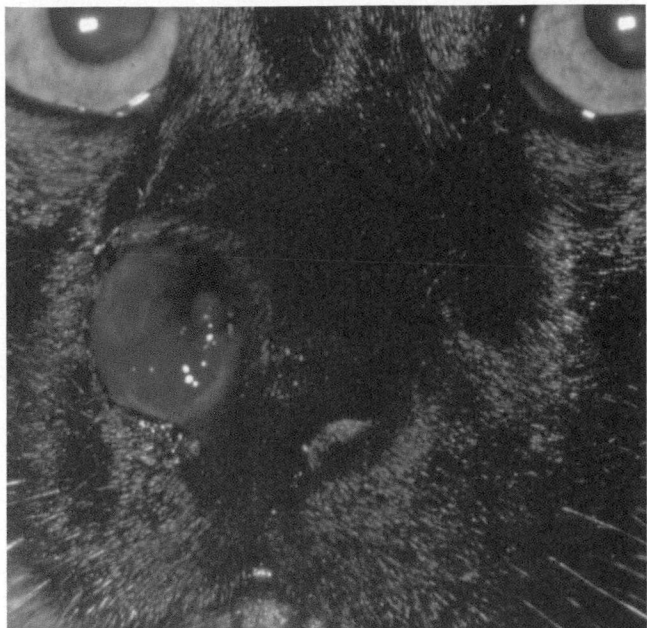

Fig 61-4 Localized cutaneous cryptococcosis in Siamese cat. It was suspected that this lesion resulted from inoculation with numerous infectious propagules of *C. neoformans* after a cat-scratch injury. The cat had no concurrent nasal signs and responded rapidly to short course of fluconazole. (Courtesy R. Malik, University of Sydney, Sydney, Australia.)

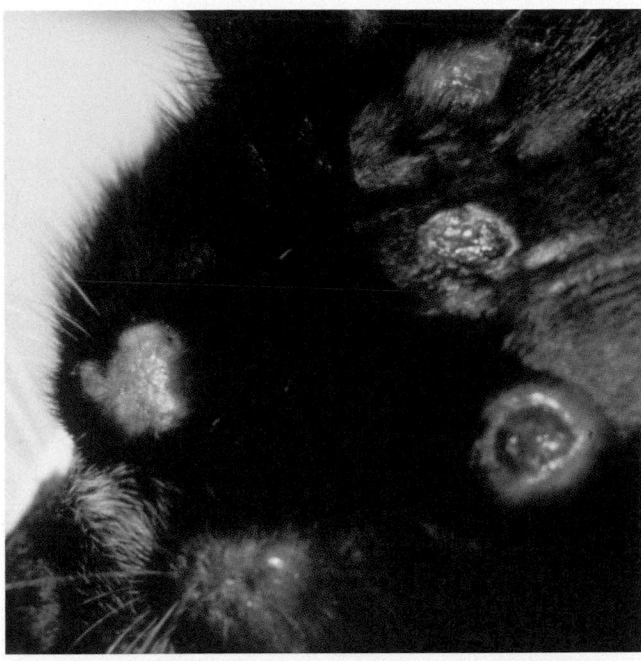

Fig 61-5 Disseminated *C. neoformans* infection in FIV-positive cat. Multiple cutaneous nodules, some of which have ulcerated, are evident on head and trunk. The nasal cavity was demonstrated to be primary site of infection. This cat was successfully treated using a long course of fluconazole. (Courtesy R. Malik, University of Sydney, Sydney, Australia.)

periorbital swelling. Rhinosinusitis from cryptococcosis may be subclinical, thus its incidence may be underestimated because respiratory signs are frequently not reported in dogs that show florid neurologic signs.[22,62]

Cutaneous involvement, as in the cat, is a marker for disseminated disease. Skin lesions consist of papules, nodules, or ulcers that may involve any portion of the integument, the nose, tongue, gums, hard palate, lips, or nail beds. Some dogs develop fever. Less common clinical signs include lameness caused by lytic bone lesions and peripheral lymphadenomegaly. Table 61-2 summarizes medical problems associated with cryptococcosis in dogs and cats.

DIAGNOSIS

Specimen Collection

In most of the previously mentioned conditions, definitive diagnosis is straightforward and based on obtaining representative tissue specimens for cytology, culture, and occasionally histology.[19] Suitable specimens may include deep nasal swabs, nasal washings, needle aspirates from cutaneous nodules or enlarged lymph nodes, bronchoalveolar lavage specimens, pleural fluid, and CSF. A definitive diagnosis of cryptococcosis can be made by culture and identification of the organism by a reputable laboratory. However, it is possible to obtain a high index of suspicion of cryptococcosis by identifying characteristic capsulate, narrow-necked budding yeasts in cytologic smears or histology sections.

Cytologic Examination

Romanowsky-type stains (DiffQuik, Giemsa, and Wright), new methylene blue, and Gram stain are all satisfactory for making a cytologic diagnosis. DiffQuik is simple and reliable (Fig. 61-6, *A*). With Gram stain the organism retains the

Table • 61-2

Medical Problems Associated with Cryptococcosis in Cats and Dogs

Nasal discharge
Deforming sinonasal disease
Nasal plane disease
Nasopharyngeal disease
Multiple cutaneous nodules (including digital swellings)
Regional or generalized peripheral lymphadenomegaly
Peripheral blindness, optic neuritis, retinitis
Intracranial disease, especially vestibular syndromes
Spinal cord disease
Nodular lung disease
Pleural effusion
Middle ear disease

crystal violet, whereas the capsule stains lightly pink with safranin. The organism is often most easily visualized at low power (×10). India ink has been used historically to examine CSF for cryptococci, which appear unstained and silhouetted against a black background (see Fig. 61-6, *B*). In the authors' experience, India ink is not as helpful as other stains because lymphocytes and fat droplets are easily confused with the organism. More success demonstrating yeasts in CSF has been achieved using cytocentrifuged preparations stained with DiffQuik and then culture, than with India ink preparations. Cytologic examination can also be performed on crush preparations of biopsy samples.

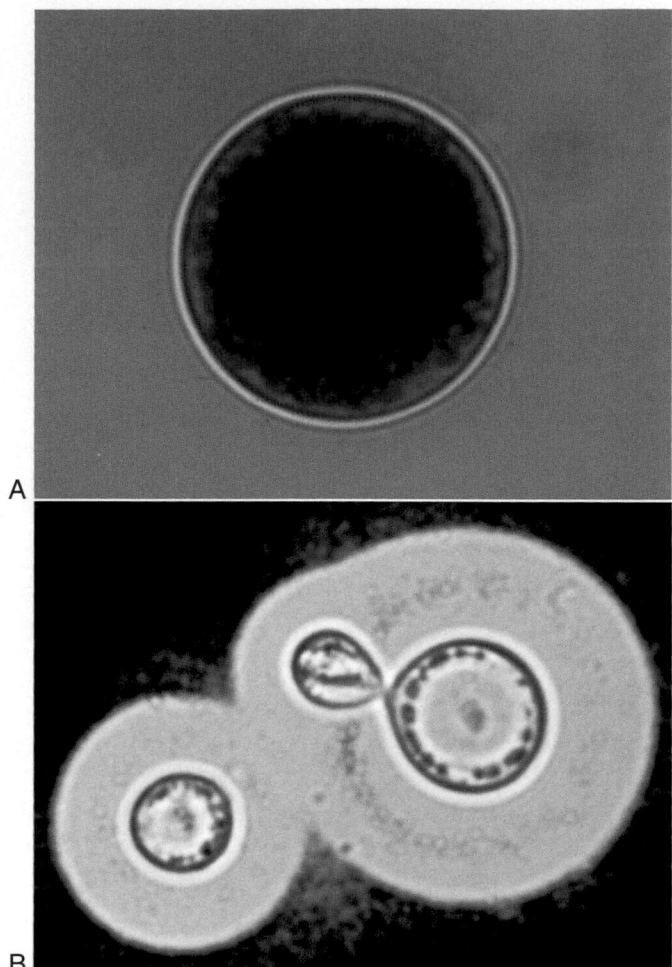

Fig 61-6 **A,** New methylene blue stain of CSF showing internal structure of *C. neoformans* (×1000). **B,** Corresponding India ink preparation of the same CSF with two organisms. One shows characteristic budding (×1000). (Courtesy University of Georgia, Athens, Ga.)

Cytologic examination of nasal or cutaneous exudates, masses, CSF, or ocular fluid demonstrate organisms in a majority of cases, although culture can be a more sensitive test. Urine sediment should be evaluated because many dogs and some cats have subclinical renal infection.[41] In human patients, blood culture is often useful; however, it has not been well evaluated in dogs or cats. Although cytologic examination is a rapid test, negative test results do not eliminate the possibility of cryptococcosis. Poorly capsulated organisms may be overlooked unless large numbers are present; if a sufficient index of suspicion exists, additional diagnostic tests are indicated. Generally, cryptococcal organisms are only found by cytologic examination of CSF in only 40% to 70% of humans and 60% of veterinary patients.[24]

Serologic Testing

The detection of cryptococcal capsular antigen by the latex agglutination procedure is the most widely used serologic test and is very useful in a veterinary setting.[66,76] Various detection methodologies exist.[19] The test used in the authors' laboratory detects polysaccharide antigen using latex particles coated with anticryptococcal antibodies. Tests detect all known serotypes and can be used for serum or CSF. They provide a rapid diagnosis when organisms have not been visualized or cultured (Table 61-3). In human studies, commercial kits typically demonstrate 90% to 100% sensitivity and 97% to 100% specificity.[81,95] Results have been similar for animals.[47,60,64,66] The sensitivity and specificity of polysaccharide antigen test has been improved by pretreatment of test specimens with pronase (a proteinase).[31] This digestion step is included with some test kits but should be performed routinely, even when the enzyme is not supplied by the manufacturer.[19,66]

Testing for cryptococcal antigen in serum may prove advantageous when CSF collection is unacceptably risky or a diagnosis of cryptococcosis is unlikely but should be excluded. For example, all cats and dogs with intracranial signs should be tested for cryptococcal antigen before CSF collection or brain imaging. Numerous canine and feline patients have experienced a marked deterioration in neurologic status after CSF collection, despite the use of appropriate anesthetic regimens. This is hardly surprising, considering that many animals have intracranial mass lesions or increased CSF pressure—with the additional risk of brain herniation following a cister-

Table • 61-3

Immunodiagnostic Kits for Detection of Cryptococcal Antigen in Clinical Specimens

NAME	MANUFACTURER	WEB SITE
Latex Agglutination Tests		
Crypto-LA	Wampole Laboratories, Princeton, N.J.; International Biological Laboratories, Cranbury, N.J.	www.wampolelabs.com; www.doctorfungus.org
CALAS	Meridian Diagnostics, Cincinnati, Ohio	www.cimascientific.com
Immy Latex-Crypto Antigen	Immunomycologics Inc., Norman, Okla.	www.immy.com
MYCO-Immune	American Micro Scan, Mahwah, N.J.	www.doctorfungus.org
ELISA Test Kits		
Premier EIA	Meridian Diagnostics, Cincinnati, Ohio	www.cimascientific.com
Premier Crypto	Meridian Diagnostics, Cincinnati, Ohio	www.cimascientific.com
Omega Crypto Enzyme Immunoassay	Immunomycologics Inc., Norman, Okla.	www.immy.com

nal tap. If cryptococcal meningitis is suspected, only limited amounts of CSF should be removed to reduce the risk of brain shifts during the procedure.

Antigen titers can be extremely high (>1:65,536) in cats and dogs with disseminated disease, but even a titer of 1:2 is considered a positive result.[66] Titer results from different kits can vary considerably, thus the methodology should not be altered when monitoring the response to treatment. When monitored consistently, titers have proven useful in evaluating patients' progress during therapy. A good prognosis is indicated by a decrease in antigen titer, whereas a persistent titer after treatment suggests continued infection. Reductions in the titer typically lag behind clinical improvement. No correlation has been found between pretreatment antigen titer and outcome.

In human patients, measurement of the antigen titer in CSF is often more sensitive than cytology or culture and therefore is theoretically preferable to serum in animals with neurologic signs. However, the authors' experience is that most patients with CNS cryptococcosis have positive antigen titers in serum, presumably because sufficient antigen is released from the primary site of infection. Cryptococcal antigen can also be detected in other body fluids such as pleural fluid or bronchoalveolar lavage fluid.

Although cats, dogs, and koalas all make anticapsular antibodies in response to infection, subclinical disease with seroconversion is common. Because titer cutoffs have not been determined with certainty, antibody determinations are currently a research tool rather than a clinical tool.[23,68]

Tissue Biopsy

Because of the rapidity of cytologic evaluation, impression smears or potassium hydroxide (KOH) preparations should always be made from suspect biopsy samples. If no organisms are seen, part of the sample can be used for culture, and the rest can be processed for routine histology. In sections stained with hematoxylin-eosin (H and E) stain, the organism appears as a faint, eosinophilic, round to oval body surrounded by a clear halo (the unstained capsule). The organism is more easily visualized with periodic acid–Schiff, methenamine silver, or Fontana-Masson stain, although the capsule still does not stain well with these methods. Mayer's mucicarmine is the definitive stain; the cryptococcal capsule takes on a rose-red color, and the organism appears pink against a blue background. Other fungi with similar morphologic features do not stain with this method. The large capsule and the thin cell wall of *Cryptococcus* species differentiate them from *Blastomyces* organisms. The budding and lack of endospores of cryptococcal organisms distinguish them from *Coccidioides* species. However, some *C. neoformans* strains have poorly developed capsules. When unsure about the presence of cryptococci and only formalin-fixed tissues are available, immunohistology can be used to differentiate the organisms from other fungi and identify their species and serotype.[48] This technique is also very useful for examination of archived material.

Genetic Identification

The polymerase chain reaction (PCR) could be used as a highly sensitive and specific means of identifying cryptococcal infection if other means fail. However, it is not regarded as a routinely useful clinical tool. Detection of the CAP59 gene was used to detect *C. neoformans* in a cat,[43] and a nested PCR was developed to detect *C. neoformans* in CSF.[88] The CAP59 gene was also detected in urine, serum, and biopsy samples of two cats with cryptococcosis.[85]

Mycology

The organism can be easily cultured from aspirates, exudate, CSF, urine, and tissue specimens. Although *C. neoformans* and

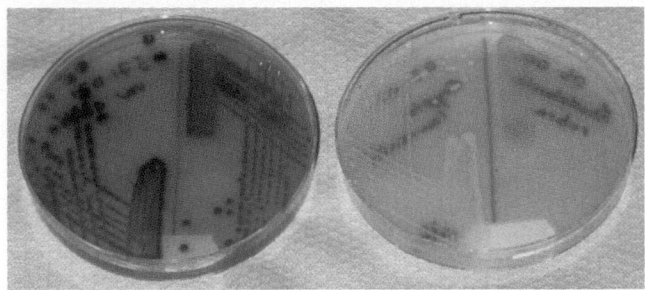

Fig 61-7 *C. neoformans (left)* and *C. albicans (right)* plated onto Staib's birdseed agar. Note prominent brown-color effect of *C. neoformans* colonies. (Courtesy R. Malik, University of Sydney, Sydney, Australia.)

C. gattii grow on almost all laboratory media, Sabouraud's dextrose agar is preferred when fungi are being considered in the differential diagnosis. Standard Sabouraud's agar, without antibacterial additives, is optimal when culturing a normally sterile site such as CSF, because antibiotics included in the media may inhibit the growth of some cryptococcal strains.[19] During sampling of a site normally contaminated by bacteria (e.g., the nasal cavity), inclusion of antibiotics in the medium improves the chances for isolating cryptococci. Growth of *Cryptococcus* species is inhibited by media containing cycloheximide. Culture should be performed at 25° C and 37° C. Colonies become visible within 2 to 10 days, but typically in 2 to 3 days. The organisms form white, creamy colonies that yellow with age, are mucoid if the strains are heavily capsulated, and are dry of the capsules are poorly developed. *C. gattii* colonies are typically much more mucoid than *C. neoformans* colonies. Characteristics used to identify the organism include its morphology (presence of a capsule, narrow-necked budding), growth at 37° C, hydrolysis of urea, brown-color effect on bird seed agar, growth and color change on canavanine glycine bromothymol blue agar,[52] and response to the various assimilation tests that are available as commercial kits. Culture results of CSF are usually positive in patients with CNS cryptococcosis. Thus fungal culture is recommended when CSF is collected from patients with inflammatory CNS disease, even if the organism cannot be demonstrated cytologically or serologically.

Birdseed agar that contains antibiotics can be useful in the diagnosis of cryptococcosis, especially with sampling sites expected to be heavily contaminated with bacteria, such as nasal exudate.[49] It is also an ideal media for environmental studies. Normally, bacteria and other fungi outgrow *C. neoformans* and *C. gattii* on plates; birdseed agar containing antibiotics suppresses growth of contaminants while distinguishing colonies of *Cryptococcus* species from other yeasts and filamentous fungi by the brown-color effect produced in the agar (Fig. 61-7).

Fungal susceptibility testing using disk diffusion, Etest strips (e.g., AB Biodisk, Solna, Sweden), or broth microdilution provides useful information concerning therapy. Although not as accurate as bacterial in vitro susceptibility testing, the strains that have a low minimum inhibitory concentration for a given drug in vitro tend to be susceptible to the drug in vivo, although the converse is not always true.

PATHOLOGIC FINDINGS

A lesion associated with cryptococcosis can vary from being a gelatinous mass consisting almost exclusively of organisms to

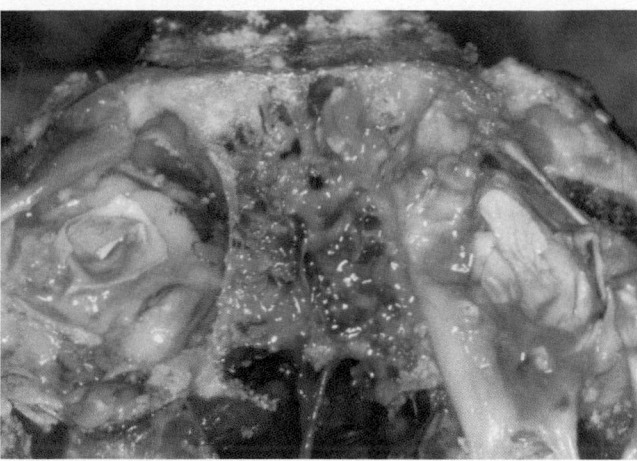

Fig 61-8 Necropsy photograph of cross-section of nasal cavity of Burmese cat with granulomatous cryptococcal rhinitis. The cat developed FIP during therapy and was euthanized. Note diffuse thickening of turbinates. (Courtesy R. Malik, University of Sydney, Sydney, Australia.)

being a well-ordered, cell-mediated immune (CMI) response resulting in granuloma formation. The gelatinous appearance is a reflection of the large amount of capsular polysaccharide present in lesions. The primary cellular response comprises neutrophils, macrophages and giant cells, with a few plasma cells and lymphocytes. Generally, the presence of a granulomatous response is indicative of an immunocompetent host. A weak or absent response suggests either overwhelming disease or immunodeficiency (although the center of large lesions, even in immunocompetent hosts, often has a limited response to organisms).

Cats

In cats that die or are euthanized, granulomatous rhinitis is usually evident (Fig. 61-8), and in rare instances the lungs are affected also. Cerebral cryptococcosis consists of either primary meningoencephalitis[41] or a cerebral granuloma (Fig. 61-9).[25,29] Optic neuritis (see Fig. 61-3, *D*) is common in cats that die of cerebral cryptococcosis, and in some cats the olfactory bulbs are replaced by a gelatinous mass of yeast cells. Other affected organs include skin and subcutaneous tissues, kidneys, and lymph nodes that drain infected areas. Renal granulomas have been found in some cats with disseminated disease, as have lesions in the spleen, adrenal glands, thyroid glands, and liver.

Dogs

Dogs that die or are euthanized because of cryptococcosis infection usually have CNS infection, ocular involvement, or widely disseminated disease. The lesions consist of meningoencephalitis; neuritis of the optic, facial, or vestibular nerves; and granulomatous chorioretinitis. At least 50% of dogs in reported cases have lesions in the respiratory tract—usually the nasal cavity (Fig. 61-10), lungs, or mediastinum.

PROGNOSIS

The prognosis for many cats and dogs with cryptococcosis is good or excellent if they have diligent, cooperative owners who are prepared to medicate their pets for many months and pay for the costs of drugs and monitoring.

Animals with longstanding, extensive disease have a less favorable prognosis than patients diagnosed early with mild signs of disease, although even longstanding, severe cases can

be cured. Patients with neurologic signs always have a guarded prognosis, although many (perhaps two out of three) can be treated successfully using combination therapy including amphotericin B (AMB). Two additional considerations apply to patients with cryptococcal meningoencephalitis. First, neurologic status often deteriorates soon after starting therapy, presumably because death of cryptococci and the resulting inflammation give rise to a dangerous increase in intracranial pressure.[63] Second, neurologic deficits such as blindness and gait abnormalities may persist, even after successful therapy.[62]

Cats in which a persistent positive FeLV status is confirmed by testing on at least two consecutive occasions have a poor long-term outlook, so drug therapy for cryptococcosis in these animals should be considered palliative.[75] In contrast, many FIV-positive cats can be cured, although some need a prolonged course of treatment, and recurrence or the development of other clinical problems remain possible.

THERAPY

One of the reasons for renewed veterinary interest in cryptococcosis was the availability of a new generation of triazole antifungal drugs (fluconazole [FCZ], itraconazole [ITZ], and voriconazole [VCZ]) suitable for long-term oral administration and the development of new ways to use AMB more easily and safely. The main problems in treating cryptococcosis is the high cost of therapy, the multiple hospital visits, and the regular medication of pets for a protracted period.

Treatment of immunocompetent animals may be curative; immunocompromised hosts may have recurrences or persistent infection. Table 61-4 lists factors that play a role in the therapeutic approach to dogs and cats with cryptococcosis.

Surgical Intervention

When it is feasible, surgical excision of large aggregations of fungus-infected tissue before or shortly after starting medical therapy is a prerequisite for successful treatment. For example, cats with extensive involvement of the nasal bridge, large nasopharyngeal masses (Fig. 61-11), or massively enlarged lymph nodes benefit enormously if abnormal tissue is removed surgically early in the course of treatment.[39] This prevents problems with diffusion of antifungal agents into poorly perfused tissues, because they may consist almost exclusively of cryptococcal elements. In some cases the nasal masses can be dislodged by "traumatic" flushing or by simultaneous massaging through the soft plate. Endoscopic visualization can be helpful during these procedures. In other animals, surgical incisions must be made through the soft palate to remove granulomas. Nasopharyngeal lymphoma can appear very similar to cryptococcal caudal nasal granulomas.

Therapeutic Agents

Five drugs are available for treating cryptococcosis in cats and dogs (Table 61-5). Each has a role in therapy, which varies depending on the individual animal being treated.

Amphotericin B

AMB is the most effective anticryptococcal agent. It is the only drug that is fungicidal and whose ability to permanently eradicate CNS infections has been proven. It must be given parenterally, therefore its administration requires a hospital visit. It is nephrotoxic, although the condition is at least partially reversible. The combination of AMB and flucytosine (FCY) is considered the optimal therapy for cats and dogs with severe or widely disseminated disease, especially when the CNS is involved. Newer forms of AMB such as liposomal and lipid complex preparations[46] are not necessarily more

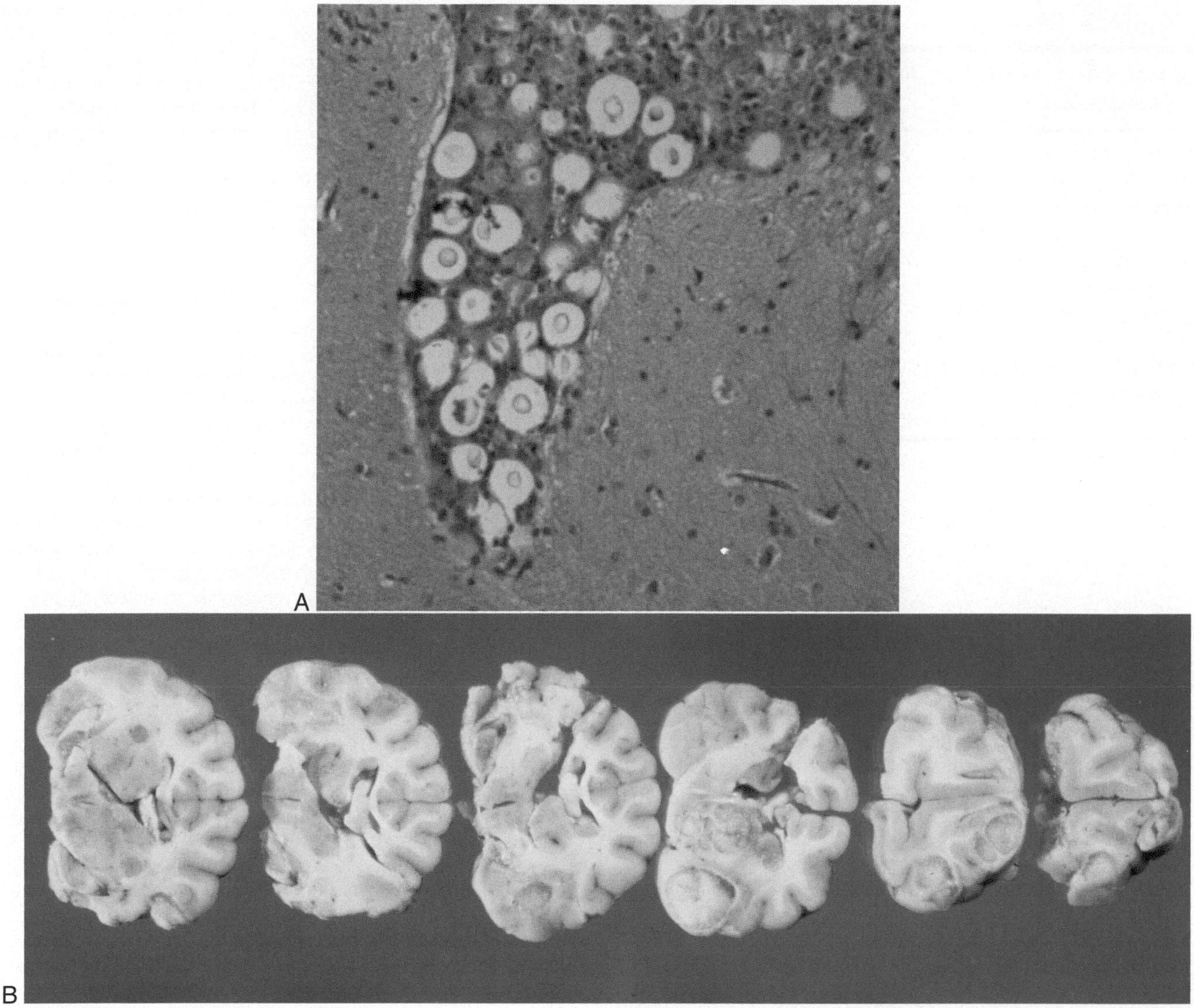

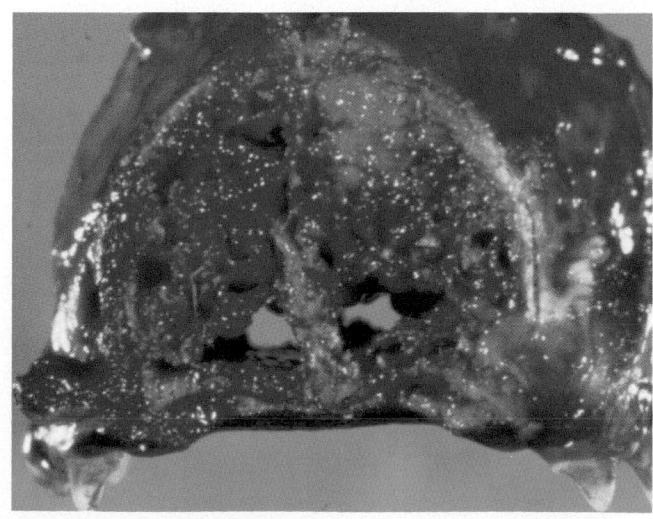

Fig 61-9 **A,** Meningoencephalitis in cat with cryptococcosis with superficial granulomatous inflammation in sulcus of brain (H and E stain, ×100.) (Courtesy University of Georgia, Athens, Ga.) **B,** Multiple cerebral cryptococcal granulomas in brain of cat that died as result of *C. gattii* infection. The cat was initially presented with signs of nasal cavity disease. Note cryptococcomas at many levels of sectioned brain. (Courtesy R. Malik, University of Sydney, Sydney, Australia.)

Fig 61-10 Necropsy cross-section of nasal cavities of greyhound with granulomatous cryptococcal rhinitis. Treatment was not attempted. Note diffuse thickening of turbinates rather than the turbinate atrophy that is seen characteristically with canine nasal aspergillosis. (Courtesy R. Malik, University of Sydney, Sydney, Australia.)

Table • 61-4

Factors Affecting Therapy for Dogs and Cats with Cryptococcosis

Duration of infection
Extent of local invasion and dissemination
Tissue involvement, especially the presence or absence of
  central nervous system and ocular involvement
Feline immunodeficiency virus and feline leukemia virus
  status
Age and physical condition
Renal and hepatic function
Temperament and appetite
Owner's financial resources
Owner's emotional commitment

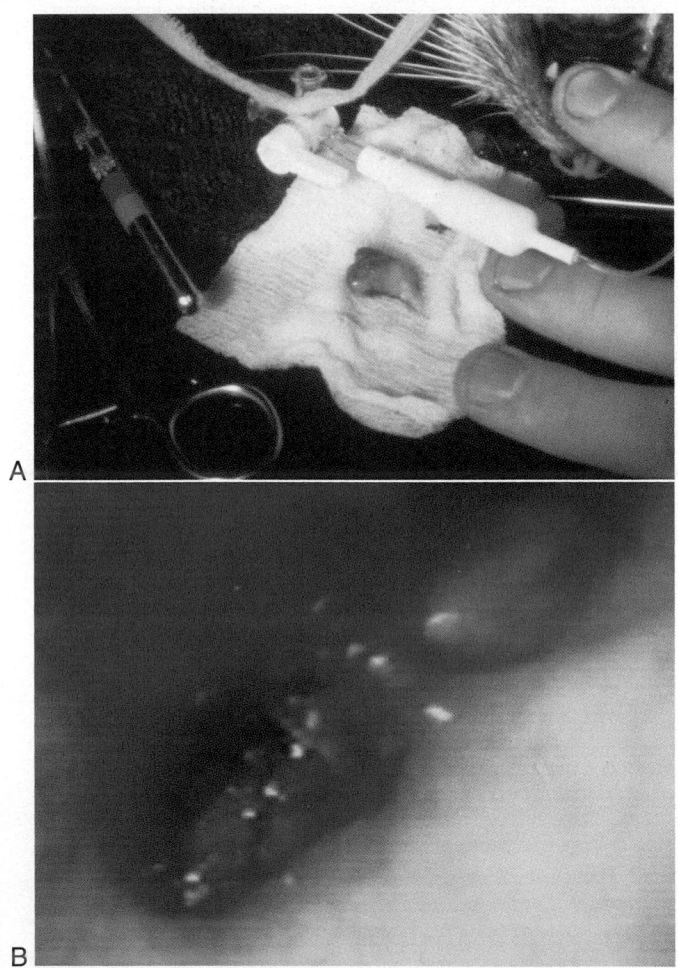

Fig 61-11 **A,** Nasopharyngeal cryptococcal granuloma removed from cat presented for stertor and inspiratory dyspnea. Traumatic flush with saline dislodged the caudal nasal cavity mass. **B,** Retroflexed-endoscopic appearance of cryptococcal granulomas in choanae of boxer dog showing neurologic signs and stertor. (Courtesy R. Malik, University of Sydney, Sydney, Australia.)

effective but are less nephrotoxic, which in a veterinary setting may translate into greater efficacy, although at a substantially increased cost. Heat-pretreatment (60° C to 70° C for 10 minutes) of standard formulations of AMB immediately before administration (see Drug Formulary, Appendix 8) substantially reduces nephrotoxicity, thereby increasing the dose that can be given safely.[54,55,87] Because AMB is an established drug that has been used for quite some time, it is relatively inexpensive, apart from the costs associated with the administration IV or as an SC infusion.[61]

Flucytosine

FCY is a useful, effective, and moderately expensive drug. Because of the rapid resistance that can develop when it is used alone, it is used chiefly to improve the efficacy of other antifungal drugs.[37] It shows true synergy when combined with AMB and is particularly good at penetrating the CSF and blood-brain barriers.[61] Thus combination therapy using AMB and FCY is the ideal initial treatment for cryptococcosis in human patients, and the authors believe the same is true for canine and feline patients. Relapses in people are lower when FCY is combined with another drug during the first 2 weeks of therapy.[89] Unfortunately, dogs receiving FCY almost invariably develop a severe drug reaction, typically 10 to 14 days after starting therapy.[67] This reaction is so severe that it precludes additional FCY therapy and causes a temporary setback in the patient's clinical course. FCY has also been given together with azoles to improve their efficacy.[61,78]

Fluconazole

Undoubtedly, FCZ may be the most desirable and effective drug for treating cryptococcosis and is certainly more effective than ketoconazole (KTZ) for the majority of isolates, with its good penetration of the brain, eye, and urinary tract and its minimal side effects. It is water soluble and excreted by the kidney, reaching high concentrations in urine. Cryptococcus is not usually a urinary pathogen, so this is not a deciding factor for FCZ's use. It has been recommended for treating CNS infections because of its penetration of the CNS[44,89]; however, its efficacy in this treatment has not yet been substantiated (see Management of CNS Infections in this chapter). However, FCZ is so expensive that only very wealthy or dedicated owners can afford it, particularly for long courses of therapy. In situations involving no financial limitations, FCZ may be a drug to consider for initial therapy.[69] Cost considerations are directly proportional to the size of the patient. When the drug is out of patent, the availability of generic preparations should reduce the current high cost of therapy.

Itraconazole

ITZ is currently the drug of choice for treatment of most cases of cryptococcosis in cats.[42,74,75] It is more effective than KTZ, with generally fewer side effects and a higher therapeutic index, and it is given only once daily. An oral suspension containing cyclodextrin has greater bioavailability than oral capsules (see Drug Formulary, Appendix 8). Importantly, it is significantly less expensive than FCZ, with which it has comparable to slightly inferior efficacy for infections that are not in the CNS, eye, or urinary tract. Adverse effects include anorexia, vomiting, and hepatic disease associated with elevated alanine aminotransferase (ALT) activity. Rarely, vasculitis with severe cutaneous ulceration can develop. It is metabolized by the liver and extensively distributed to lipophilic tissues. Its concentration in kidney, liver, and skin is 2 to 20 times greater than in plasma. Although it is not well distributed into the CNS, ITZ still has been used to successfully treat humans, cats, and dogs with cryptococcal meningitis.[18,40,75] Like KTZ, ITZ should be given with food to maximize its bioavailability.

Table • 61-5

Therapy for Cryptococcosis

DRUG[a]	SPECIES	DOSE[b] (mg/kg)	ROUTE	INTERVAL	DURATION (MONTHS)
Flucytosine	C	30	PO	6 hr	1–9
		50	PO	8 hr	1–9
		75	PO	12 hr	1–9
	C (≥3.5 kg)	250 mg total	PO	6–8 hr	1–9
	D	50–75	PO	8 hr	1–12
and/or					
Amphotericin B (deoxycholate)	B	0.5	IV	3 times/week	Varies[c]
	B	0.5–0.8	SC	2–3 times week	Varies[d]
Amphotericin B (lipid complex)	D	1.0	IV	3 times/week	Varies[e]
Ketoconazole	C	5–10[f]	PO	12 hr	6–18[g]
		10–20[f,h]	PO	24 hr	6–18[g]
		50 mg total	PO	24 hr	6–18[g]
	D	5–15	PO	12 hr	6–18[g]
		30	PO	24 hr	6–18[g]
Itraconazole	D	10	PO	24 hr	6–18[g]
	C	10–20	PO	24 hr	6–18[g]
	C (≤3.5 kg)	50 mg total	PO	24 hr	6–18[g]
	C (>3.5 kg)	100 mg total	PO	24 hr	6–18[g]
	C (≤3.5 kg)	100 mg total	PO	48 hr	6–18[g]
Fluconazole	B	5–15	PO	12–24 hr	6–18[g]
	C	30–50 mg total	PO	12 hr	6–18[g]

C, Cat; D, dog; B, both dog and cat; PO, by mouth; IV, intravenously; SC, subcutaneously; ITZ, itraconazole; FCZ, fluconazole AMB, amphotericin B.

[a]See Appendix 8, Drug Formulary, for additional information on these drugs.
[b]Dose per administration at specified interval.
[c]Until a minimum cumulative dosage of 10 mg/kg is reached. For some dogs, cumulative dosages as high as 40 mg/kg have been given over prolonged periods of several months. For cats receiving 2 infusions per week, 0.5 to 0.8 mg/kg is given per infusion.
[d]Add each dose to 400 ml of 0.45% saline, 2.5% dextrose; for dogs over 20 kg, add AMB to 900 ml of 0.45% saline and 2.5% dextrose.[61] See text of this chapter, and the Drug Formulary, Appendix 8 for special precautions using this method.
[e]With lipid-complex drug, dose per administration and cumulative dosage may be slightly increased; has been effective for blastomycosis (see Chapter 59); until a cumulative dosage of 8 to 12 mg/kg has been reached; for various formulations of AMB see Table 57–2 and Drug Formulary, Appendix 8.
[f]If toxicity develops, the dose should be changed to 50 mg/kg cat every other day.
[g]Range may vary from 6 to 10 months depending on remission of clinical signs and antigen titers.
[h]If lack of response to therapy or toxicity is noted at these dosages, then ITZ, FCZ, or AMB lipid preparations should be used.

Ketoconazole

KTZ is the least expensive of the available drugs, although doses that have good efficacy in vivo often result in inappetence and vomiting, especially in cats with capricious appetites. However, in some patients, it is effective even when given as monotherapy. It also seems useful against *C. gattii* isolates from the Vancouver Island region.[57]

Management Regimens

Based on these considerations, an optimal plan has been developed for dealing with cryptococcosis in small animals. First, procure material to culture the organism, determine the species and variety, and ideally, obtain in vitro susceptibility data. Second, obtain a serum sample to determine baseline biochemical measurements, FeLV and FIV status, and permit future measurement of the pretreatment cryptococcal antigen titer. A portion of the serum sample should be stored frozen, because sequential antigen titers used to monitor therapy should ideally be processed in the same assay run. Third, surgically debulk easily accessible, localized accumulations of fungus-infected tissues. This may be done at the outset or after

a short period of drug therapy, depending on convenience, the physical status of the patient, and the initial response to therapy. The subsequent management of the case depends on the severity of disease and whether the CNS is involved.

Cats with Mild to Moderate Disease without CNS Involvement

Commence therapy with ITZ, 50 to 100 mg per cat once daily with food. Medium- to large-size cats should receive 100 mg once daily, whereas cats weighing 3.5 kg or less should receive 50 mg daily or 100 mg every other day.[74,75] ITZ capsules can be opened and split into two 50-mg portions using empty gelatin capsules or with the help of a compounding pharmacist. Alternately, the content of the capsules can be mixed with small portion of a tasty food treat or butter and given at the start of the meal; the ITZ formulation has no discernable effect on texture or palatability of food. The oral suspension should also be considered to achieve appropriate dosing and better systemic absorption. Many cats eventually develop liver toxicity during therapy with ITZ, especially when given high doses. The toxicity can take several weeks to months to develop, and its clinical symptoms include reduced appetite and possibly vomiting. Invariably a concurrent elevation in serum ALT activity occurs. ITZ-induced hepatoxicity is reversible on discontinuation of the drug, although it can take as long as 7 days for cats to regain their appetite and demeanor. Once this occurs, it is generally possible to safely administer the drug again, albeit at a reduced dose—typically 50% of the dose given originally. In a minority of animals, it is necessary to change therapy to FCZ.

Therapy should be continued until the cat appears completely healthy, with resolution of all clinical signs and eradication of viable organisms from accessible tissues (as assessed by cytology and culture). Typically, this takes 3 to 12 months, although some cats require even longer. When this stage has been reached, a second serum sample should be obtained from the cat to determine the extent of the antigen titer decrease caused by therapy. A fourfold to fivefold reduction suggests successful therapy, so when this level has been obtained, it is recommended to continue ITZ (possibly at a reduced dose) or alter therapy to KTZ (50 mg once daily with food) until the antigen titer decreases to zero. If the antigen titer has decreased but is still substantial, then ITZ therapy should be continued as before, because it is likely that a substantial amount of viable fungus remains in the cat's tissues. If the antigen titer has not decreased, then more aggressive therapy should be implemented as described in the following section.

Generally speaking, the antigen titer should drop by at least 1 dilution (twofold) per month during effective therapy; failure to observe a decrease of this order strongly suggests the need for more aggressive therapy. However, in the interests of economy, the antigen titer does not need to be determined for several months if the cat is doing well and visible lesions have been regressing.

FCZ can be used in the same way as ITZ, although in some locations, it is substantially more expensive. It is a very effective agent for treating cryptococcosis,[69] well tolerated even at high doses, and largely devoid of serious side effects. The authors generally use an oral dose of 30 to 50 mg per cat every 12 hours, for small and large cats, respectively. Some pharmacokinetic studies suggest lower doses achieve therapeutic blood levels,[99] but experience shows that higher doses are required in vivo to successfully treat many cats with cryptococcosis. One advantage of FCZ over ITZ is that it reaches effective concentrations in the CNS and CSF (even in the absence of inflammation) and is less likely to cause hepatic or other toxicities. Largely for financial reasons, the use of FCZ is often reserved for cats with CNS involvement or in cats that develop exaggerated toxicity during ITZ therapy. The latter subgroup of cats generally responds favorably to FCZ.

Cats with Severe Disease, with CNS Infections, or Failing to Respond Adequately to Azoles

Cats with advanced, disseminated, or severe disease and patients with CNS involvement may improve with oral azole therapy; however, these cats respond more quickly and have better outcomes if treated with AMB and FCY.[61] If the animals are sufficiently debilitated to require IV fluid therapy, give the AMB as a continuous IV infusion (0.5 mg/kg/day) in 0.45% saline and 2.5% dextrose supplemented with 20 mmol of potassium chloride per liter at 4 ml/kg/hour (twice the maintenance requirements).

Otherwise, use a protocol in which AMB is administered 2 or 3 times weekly as a SC infusion.[61] AMB is prepare by adding 10 ml of sterile distilled water to a 50-mg vial of Fungizone® (Bristol-Myers Squibb, Princeton, N.J.) to produce a 5 mg/ml colloidal suspension. Once prepared, the AMB suspension can be stored frozen for up to 4 weeks without a loss of efficacy. When required the stock solution is thawed, and the calculated dose is aseptically aspirated from the vial,

which is subsequently refrozen. Thawing the frozen AMB in very hot tap water may reduce its nephrotoxicty, which was discussed in a previous section. To prepare an SC infusion of AMB, a 500-ml bag of 0.45% saline in 2.5% dextrose is heated to 40° C in a microwave oven and then connected to a fluid-administration set; 100 to 150 ml is discarded. The calculated dose (0.5 to 0.8 mg/kg; typically 0.4 to 0.8 ml) of the stock AMB suspension is injected into the fluid bag through its injection port. Fluid is then aspirated and injected back and forth into the syringe repeatedly to ensure effective transfer of AMB to the bag.

A 19-gauge needle is then attached to the fluid administration set and inserted into the SC space between the scapulae roughly on the midline. The fluid is allowed to flow as fast as gravity allows. Raising the bag of fluid as high as possible facilitates rapid delivery of the infusion, which usually takes approximately 10 minutes. It is preferable to deliver the entire volume (350 to 400 ml) in one site, although the needle occasionally may be repositioned caudally if the cat becomes very uncomfortable after half or more of the fluid has been administered. In general, the SC infusion is well tolerated by cats that do not resent restraint per se. In fractious cats, sedation using midazolam/ketamine or light anesthesia using sevoflurane (Abbott Laboratories, Abbott Park, Ill.) is necessary. The fluid moves extensively through the SC space, tending to pool ventrally for several hours before being absorbed.

The infusions are continued 2 to 3 times per week until obvious clinical improvement and a corresponding decrease in the antigen titer are noted. Typically the cumulative dose of AMB required is 10 to 20 mg/kg. Interestingly, it is the cumulative dose that appears to be important rather than the period over which the drug is administered. Using AMB SC as a dilute suspension delays its absorption into the systemic circulation. This type of administration prevents the high peak blood levels that cause renal damage. Administering AMB together with a large volume of fluid (and sodium) also reduces the likelihood of developing nephrotoxicity, because of the protective effect of the ensuing diuresis. Therefore it is possible to administer larger and thus more effective quantities of AMB using this protocol than have been administered traditionally. It is prudent to monitor serum urea and creatinine concentrations regularly during therapy and temporarily discontinue therapy if azotemia develops. Owners are also advised to add a small amount of salt to the cat's diet, because it should also help minimize renal toxicity.

FCY is administered orally in concert with AMB at a dose of 250 mg (1/2 tablet) every 8 hours for average-sized cats and every 6 hours for large cats. This drug is generally well tolerated by cats, although the authors know of one cat that became thrombocytopenic during therapy. In some cats with neurologic signs, FCZ is administered also, although the use of azoles is often reserved for a later stage in therapy.

AMB is continued on a schedule of 2 or 3 times per week. If animals are hospitalized, treatment is given on a Monday-Wednesday-Friday schedule (0.5 mg/kg per infusion), whereas cats treated as outpatients receive two infusions per week (0.5 to 0.8 mg/kg per infusion) for the owner's convenience. After this therapy is started, it is usually continued for at least 6 to 12 weeks, at which time the patient is usually well enough to be given follow-up oral azole therapy until the antigen titer decreases to zero. In some cats, an additional course of AMB infusions is required later (e.g., if the decrease in the antigen titer is not sustained during azole therapy). If mild azotemia develops, it is necessary to discontinue combination therapy for a few weeks. This is usually more of a problem in older cats that have lost some renal reserve. Cats are given ITZ or FCZ while AMB/FCY therapy is temporarily discontinued.

Based on the authors' experience of managing numerous cases of cryptococcosis in cats, dogs, and koalas, it is certain that therapy incorporating AMB is more effective than oral therapy using either ITZ or FCZ, thus this regimen is recommended for severe or intractable cases and all cats with CNS disease. However, treatment using this combination requires much more effort and dedication from the owner and the veterinary team. Because many patients with CNS involvement deteriorate during initial treatment with AMB and FCY, short-acting glucocorticoids such as prednisolone may be necessary to support patients during a critical 1- to 2-day period of increased intracranial pressure.[63] Occasionally, cats develop sterile abscesses at sites of fluid administration, but they usually resolve spontaneously; in some cats, it may be more expedient to aspirate an obvious accumulation of pus. These infusion reactions appear in some cats and not others and are more likely to occur when the infusion remains localized rather than spreading extensively through the SC space. Tonicity of the solution should also be reduced to help alleviate the occurrence of this reaction (see Dogs section that follows).

Finally, it is vital to support these cats during the initial phase of therapy. This may involve IV fluid therapy, force feeding, or tube feeding. Generally, cats improve significantly within 1 to 2 weeks of starting therapy, and it is unusual for them to be hospitalized for longer than this at the outset.

Dogs

The majority of dogs with cryptococcosis have severe disease, and it is typically disseminated, has CNS involvement, or both. Furthermore, dogs affected are often the large breeds, which makes dosing with azoles (especially FCZ) too expensive for most owners. No reports have been published of CNS cryptococcosis in dogs that have been cured with FCZ alone. In one dog, surgical debridement of an extradural spinal cord granuloma combined with fluconazole treatment (an oral dose of 5.5 mg/kg daily) controlled spinal cord infection.[44] In a dog with disseminated CNS cryptococcosis, FCZ therapy (ranging from 4.2 to 9.1 mg/kg/day over 47 weeks) resulted in prolonged substantial clinical improvement for 1 year with eventual progression of neurologic signs.[96] In another dog with disseminated cryptococcosis that included the CNS, continual therapy with FCZ (5 mg/kg every 12 hours) caused clinical improvement in neurologic signs during 60 weeks of monitoring; however, the recovery was incomplete, and active chorioretinitis persisted despite therapy.[86]

In people, initial AMB and FCY combination therapy is preferred to FCZ for CNS infections; however, FCZ is used as a follow-up therapy on a long-term basis after remission has been achieved. The vast majority of dogs with cryptococcosis are young adults, and they are much more tolerant of AMB than cats, therefore higher individual and cumulative doses can be safely administered. In most canine patients, especially large dogs or those with meningoencephalitis, AMB therapy is the most effective and inexpensive treatment. ITZ is an important drug for treating less severe cases or maintaining treatment after an initial 2-month induction period of AMB therapy. In people and in some dogs, a dramatic worsening of signs may be seen during institution of combination therapy, presumably because of the release of organisms or fungal antigens into the CSF and resultant osmotic or inflammatory changes. Repeated removal of CSF or temporary antiinflammatory therapy may be needed to keep animals from developing complications of severe increases in intracranial pressure.

SC infusions are given to dogs in a similar way that they are given to cats—either 2 or 3 times per week—and it is even possible to train exceptional owners to give the infusions at home, because dogs are much more tolerant of the procedure than cats. When making up AMB infusions, it is important to remember that the drug is irritating, so a concentration of 20 mg/L should not be exceeded. Thus when treating dogs that weigh more than 20 kg, it is necessary to suspend the AMB in 1000 ml of 0.45% saline and 2.5% dextrose, whereas dogs weighing less than 20 kg usually require a 500-ml infusion. Despite this precaution, some dogs develop sterile abscesses at the site of fluid administration, although they usually resolve spontaneously. Occasionally, the abscesses are severe; in these individuals, AMB can be given as an IV infusion over several hours preceded by 30 to 50 ml/kg of crystalloid solution IV (over 1 hour) on a twice-weekly basis.

It is difficult to recommend routine adjuvant FCY therapy in dogs. Like many human infectious disease physicians, the authors believe that FCY enhances the efficacy of AMB. However, the drug eruption that invariably ensues is a real setback to patients.[67] Currently, we therefore recommend that if FCY is given, therapy should be closely monitored and discontinued at the first sign of malaise, fever, facial pruritus, or mucocutaneous ulceration. Almost certainly, FCY should not be continued for longer than 14 days in any patient unless a very strong clinical justification exists. Many veterinarians may feel more comfortable using combination therapy consisting of AMB and ITZ (10 mg/kg orally with food once daily) from the outset to avoid this potential complication.

Most young dogs are very tolerant of AMB, and cumulative doses as high as 40 mg/kg can be given safely over a prolonged period, although it is sometimes necessary to temporarily discontinue therapy for several weeks in the middle of a course of therapy to permit azotemia to resolve. ITZ is given during this period. The ability to safely administer a large dose of AMB results in less need of follow-up azole therapy in canine patients. Although ITZ (5 to 10 mg/kg orally once daily) should be continued until the antigen titer is zero, the authors have had many patients in which this was not possible but whose antigen titers continued to decline to zero after 2 to 3 months of AMB infusions. The antigen titer does not distinguish between the polysaccharide material elaborated by viable yeast cells and the dead organisms being phagocytized by the host.

Long-Term Follow-Up

One of the greatest challenges in treating animals is to ensure that the infection is eliminated from the patient permanently. Serial antigen titer determinations are most useful in this regard because patients typically improve clinically long before viable fungus is eliminated from the body. This is especially true during monotherapy with azoles, which are fungistatic and rely on a CMI response and phagocytosis to actually remove cryptococci from the host. For example, most cats treated with ITZ alone require a median of 8 months of therapy.[42] Having observed disease recurrences as long as 10 years after apparently successful therapy, the authors now recommend continuing antifungal therapy until the cryptococcal antigen titer is zero. In some cases, this may take quite a considerable time, possibly up to 2 years or more. In these circumstances, usually only one drug is prescribed, and in some situations KTZ may be used instead of ITZ or FCZ because it is less expensive. Patients that have received a large cumulative dose of AMB in concert with FCY typically require a shorter duration of therapy, presumably because this combination is fungicidal, and residual antigen titers reflect dead fungus undergoing phagocytosis. In cats that are FeLV or FIV positive, it may be prudent to continue maintenance therapy with ITZ or KTZ indefinitely, even if the titer decreases to 0, and the same may be true for German shepherd dogs. Alternatively, the titer can be monitored regularly, perhaps every 6 months, so that any recurrence is diagnosed early. In studies in HIV-infected people with cryptococcosis, persistent infection has been attributed to relapse rather than reinfection or antifungal drug resistance.[11]

Therapeutic Perspective

The diagnosis and treatment of cats and dogs with cryptococcosis remains a challenge. A high index of suspicion for this disease is required, especially in cases with nasal cavity or neurologic disease, because early diagnosis markedly improves outcomes. The cost of therapy is likely to decline over time as the new azoles come out of patent, while new formulations of AMB using delivery systems such as liposomes or lipid emulsions will further improve the prognosis. Although well documented trials have yet to be conducted, many infectious disease physicians consider liposomal AMB to be a useful advance over the deoxycholate formulation, owing to comparable efficacy, reduced toxicity, and thus a greater therapeutic index. Unfortunately the very high cost of this formulation makes it difficult to use in a veterinary setting, even in cats, because cost-efficient strategies to use the contents of a reconstituted vial have not been developed.

PUBLIC HEALTH CONSIDERATIONS

Cryptococcosis is the most important opportunistic fungal infection of people infected with HIV. Cryptococcosis is not considered to be a zoonotic disease, so infected cats and dogs pose no public health threat to owners or veterinarians.[40] The organism does not aerosolize from sites of tissue infection, so the disease cannot spread among people or animals. The major public health significance of infected pets is that they may act as a sentinel species for human beings. In the diagnostic laboratory, culture of *Cryptococcus* is not a health hazard, because only the yeast form is grown routinely, and this form does not aerosolize from media. During handling of the yeast or infected tissues, precautions should be taken to prevent inadvertent inoculation of the organism directly into the body, which has produced infection in experimental animals.

SUGGESTED READINGS*

16. Chrétien F, Lortholary O, Kansau I, et al. 2002. Pathogenesis of cerebral *Cryptococcus neoformans* infection after fungemia. *J Infect Dis* 186:522-530.
57. Lester SJ, Kowalewich NJ, Bartlett KH, et al. 2004. Clinicopathologic features of an unusual outbreak of cryptococcosis in dogs, cats, ferrets, and a bird: 38 cases (January to July 2003), *J Am Vet Med Assoc* 225:1716-1722.
61. Malik R, Craig AJ, Wigney D, et al. 1996a. Combination chemotherapy of canine and feline cryptococcosis using subcutaneously administered amphotericin B. *Aust Vet J* 73:124-128.
84. O'Brien CR, Krockenberger MB, Wigney DI, et al. 2004. Retrospective study of feline and canine cryptococcosis in Australia from 1981 to 2001: 195 cases. *Med Mycol* 42:449-460.
86. O'Toole TE, Sato AF, Rozanski EA. 2003. Cryptococcosis of the central nervous system in a dog. *J Am Vet Med Assoc* 222:1722-1725.
92. Stephen C, Lester S, Black W, et al. 2002. Multispecies outbreak of cryptococcosis on southern Vancouver Island, British Columbia. *Can Vet J* 43:792-794.

*See the CD-ROM for a complete list of references.

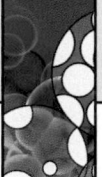

CHAPTER • 62

Coccidioidomycosis and Paracoccidioidomycosis

Russell T. Greene

COCCIDIOIDOMYCOSIS

Etiology

Coccidioides is a soil-borne fungus restricted to certain geographic regions. It grows in soil and culture medium as a mycelium. Unlike other fungal pathogens, *Coccidioides* is a haploid organism with no known sexual state.[16] The vegetative mycelia germinates to form thick-walled, barrel-shaped, rectangular, multinucleate arthroconidia, 2 to 4 μm wide and 3 to 10 μm long (Fig. 62-1). Within the mycelium, viable arthroconidia alternate with smaller, thin-walled, nonviable cells and can persist within the soil indefinitely. Activities that disturb the soil cause the intervening nonviable cells to degenerate, releasing the environmentally resistant arthroconidia, which are dispersed by wind. The arthroconidia can germinate to yield new hyphae or serve as the infecting form for animals and people (Fig. 62-2). When inhaled, arthroconidia, at higher temperature (37° C [98.6° F]) and in the presence of increased carbon dioxide, convert into a different morphologic form. They shed all but one nucleus, round up, and enlarge to produce an immature spherule. The nucleus undergoes division, which is followed by inward partitioning of the cytoplasm, resulting in a mature spherule with endospores in the center. The spherule gradually enlarges to 20 to 200 μm in diameter and eventually breaks open to release 200 to 300 endospores (3 to 5 μm). These endospores form new spherules at 37° C or mycelia at room temperature. Transformation from arthroconidia to immature spherules can be completed within 2 to 3 days. Intact spherules are poorly chemotactic for neutrophils. The neutrophils that do attach cannot penetrate the wall of the spherule (Fig. 62-3). However, the endospores are the most vulnerable stage of *Coccidioides* in the body. They attract a large number of neutrophils and are small enough to be phagocytized.

Epidemiology

The mycelial phase of *Coccidioides* has been found in nature only in a specific ecologic region, the Lower Sonoran life zone. Geographically, the Lower Sonoran life zone is within the southwestern United States, Mexico, and Central and South America (Guatemala, Honduras, Colombia, Venezuela, Paraguay, and Argentina) (Fig. 62-4). This zone is character-

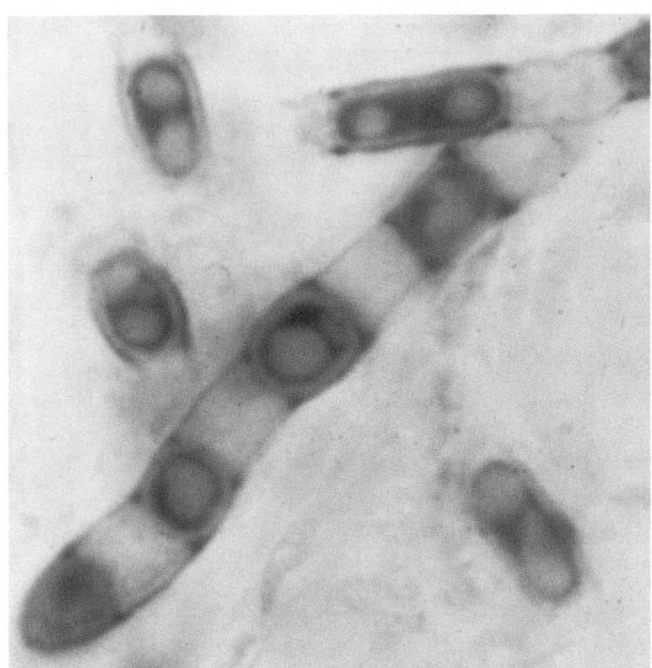

Fig 62-1 Lactophenol cotton blue preparation from a *Coccidioides immitis* colony. The arrangement of the barrel-shaped arthroconidia of *C. immitis* is a characteristic alternating pattern of live and dead arthroconidia. These arthroconidia are extremely dangerous, and mycelial cultures should only be handled within a biosafety hood (×100). (Courtesy University of Georgia, Athens, Ga.)

ized by sandy, alkaline soils, high environmental temperatures (summer mean above 26.6° C [79.9° F]; winter mean 4° to 12° C [39.2° to 53.6° F]), low annual rainfall (3 to 20 inches), and low elevation (sea level to a few hundred feet). During prolonged periods of high temperature and low soil moisture, *Coccidioides* survives below the soil surface at depths as great as 20 cm where competitive organisms are few. After a period of rainfall, *Coccidioides* replicates in the upper soil surface, sporulates, and releases a large number of arthroconidia to be disseminated by the wind. Epidemics in people have occurred after dust storms, following the rainy season, or after earthquakes.[52] People and animals residing in or visiting endemic areas are at high risk of exposure during these periods. Endemically, the incidence of disease is highest in the early fall and winter, when the soil is dry and crops are being harvested. Occupational and recreational exposure of people and animals in the outdoors leads to a greater risk of infection. In the United States, the disease is often referred to as *valley fever* after the occurrence of an epidemic in the San Joaquin Valley of California, but it is also prevalent in Arizona and southwestern Texas. The disease is less common in New Mexico, Nevada, and Utah. A few endemic areas are found in Central and South America, particularly Venezuela. From a taxonomic perspective, *Coccidioides immitis* is the species of organism distributed in the San Joaquin Valley, while *Coccidioides posadasii*, formerly the non-California isolate, is found in all other endemic areas.[20]

Although the majority of infections in animals and people are diagnosed within the southwestern United States, an occasional case may be identified outside this area. Usually, individuals involved in these "stray" cases have a history of residence or travel within an endemic area. The patient may have been in an endemic area several years earlier, and the organism had remained dormant for some time period.[10] Sero-

logic surveys indicate that most human and canine inhabitants in endemic areas become infected; however, most infections are subclinical or cause only mild, transient respiratory signs. Estimates are that only 40% of infected people develop respiratory symptoms, and very few develop systemic manifestations. In the remaining 60%, the only evidence of infection is seroconversion. Although not proven, the theory suggests that the same statistics concerning infections and clinical signs are similar in domestic animals. In contrast to other species, dogs appear more susceptible to developing disseminated disease.

Pathogenesis

The disease is highly infectious, but not typically contagious. The major route of infection is by inhalation. Very few (fewer than 10) arthroconidia must be inhaled to produce disease. The incubation period from inhalation to onset of abnormal respiratory signs is 1 to 3 weeks. Primary localized infection of skin lesions from penetrating wounds has rarely been reported. Experimentally, intradermal inoculation or skin scarification produces only localized infection in a small percentage of animals. After inhalation, the arthroconidia first enter the bronchioles and alveoli and then extend into the peribronchiolar tissue, eventually causing subpleural lesions. The first cellular response is neutrophilic, followed by monocytes, lymphocytes, and plasma cells. As with all fungal infections, cell-mediated immunity (CMI) is more important than humoral immunity is in eliminating infection. Mononuclear phagocytes are responsible for removing the organism from tissues and body fluids. Endospores are most susceptible to host CMI. The wall of spherules provides a means of immune evasion by the organism. Although not protective, antibody response to two different antigens of the fungus has been used to detect infection (see Diagnosis).

Recovery from initial infection in people results in lifelong immunity, but resistance to reinfection in animals is uncertain. With massive exposure, pregnancy, or depressed cellular immunity, pulmonary infection can become more extensive, and the organism can invade the hilar lymph nodes and distant tissues. Interleukin levels may play a role in resistance to infection, as has been demonstrated in mice.[19] In people, race is a known risk factor,[46] but no definite breed predilection has been defined in dogs. In one report,[50] the authors stated greyhounds may be more susceptible.

If disease progresses beyond the hilar lymph nodes, which it can do within 10 days of exposure, it is considered to have disseminated. Dissemination involves the reproductive cycle from spherules to endospores to new spherules. If the disease disseminates, the organs that are usually affected are, in decreasing order of frequency, bones, eyes, heart and pericardium, testicles, brain, spinal cord, and visceral organs (primarily spleen, liver, and kidney). Ocular lesions begin as a chorioretinitis and extend into the anterior chamber. The intestinal mucosa and endocardium are rarely affected. Virtually all other tissues can be affected. Signs referable to dissemination usually occur approximately 4 months after pulmonary signs develop, but this period is variable, and the respiratory infection may have never been noticed. Disseminated cases usually follow a chronic course of months to years. However, the author has seen disseminated disease in a puppy only 10 weeks of age. Widespread dissemination was also observed in a dog with concurrent multicentric lymphosarcoma.[30]

Intrauterine transmission has typically been thought not to occur because of the large size of the spherules. Neonatal disease transmission has generally been thought to occur from contact of the neonate with the female genital tract or vaginal secretions as the neonate is being born. However, in a case report in a human infant delivered by cesarean section, transplacental transmission from mother to baby was well

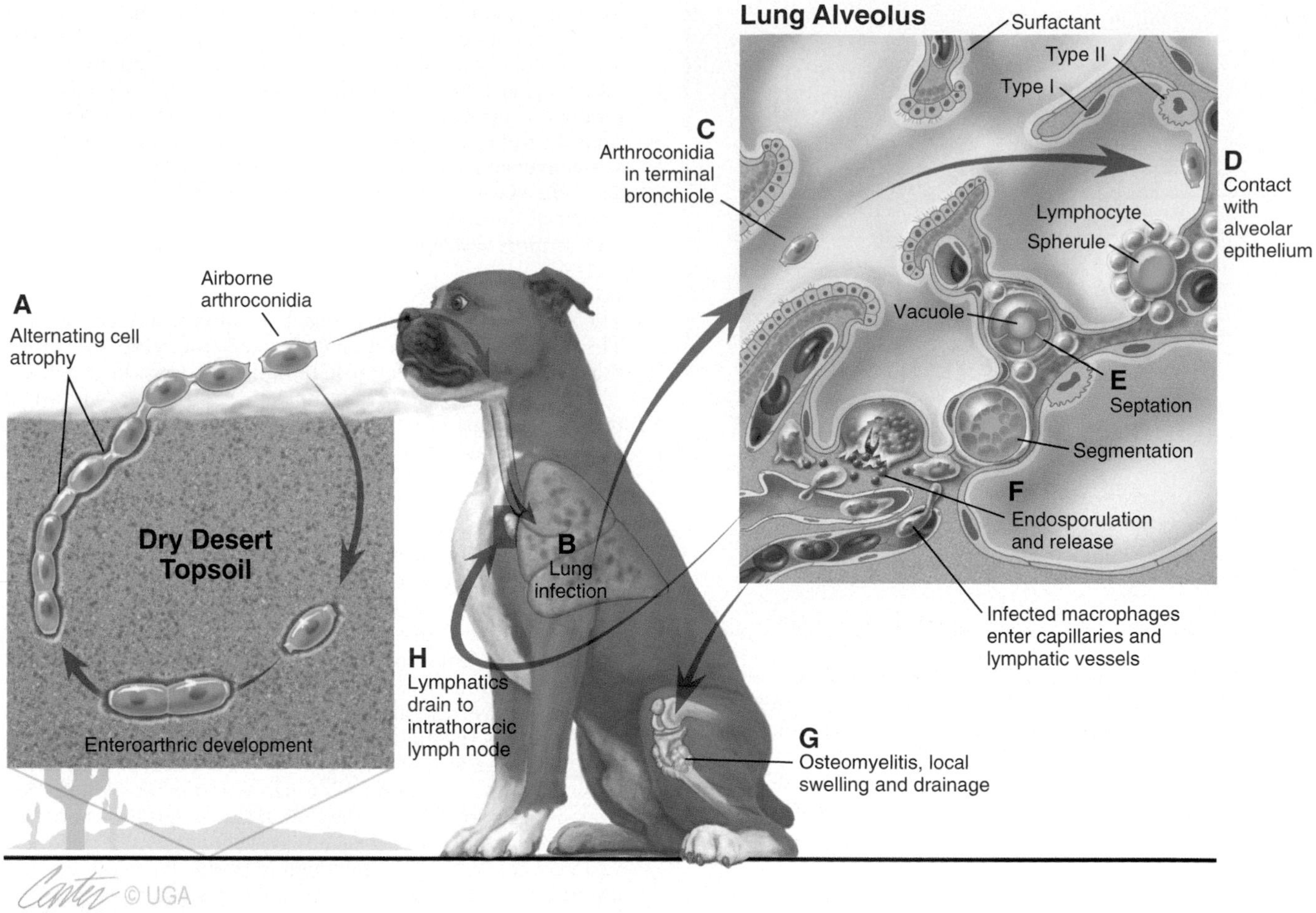

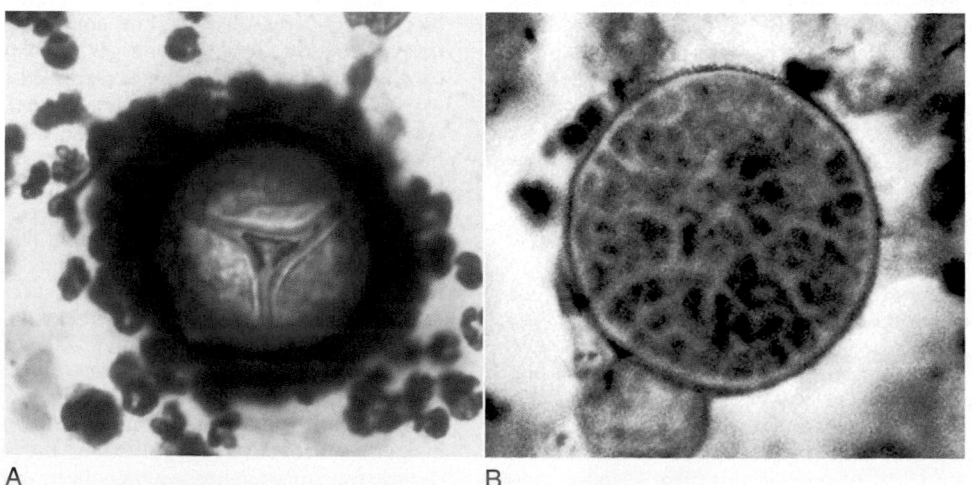

Fig 62-2 Life cycle of C. *immitis*. **A,** In the soil (an arthroconidium) or in culture of infected tissues (an endospore), the single cell germinates to become hyphae, which eventually form arthroconidia that alternate into becoming live and dead cells. The hyphae can break off at the nonviable segments, releasing arthroconidia that can disseminate in the air or enter the soil to form new hyphae. **B to E,** Once airborne arthroconidia are inhaled, they enter the lung and change morphologically to a round spherule that undergoes repeated internal divisions until it is filled with thousands of endospores. Each endospore has the capacity to become a new spherule. **F,** They also disseminate via phagocytes to infect distant tissues, causing granuloma formation. **G,** Swelling and drainage occur at lesion sites close to skin surfaces and underlying infected bone. **H,** Regional lymph nodes draining sites of infection become enlarged. (Courtesy University of Georgia, Athens, Ga.)

Fig 62-3 Spherule of C. *immitis* containing visible endospores as observed on cytologic examination. **A,** Note the pyogranulomatous inflammation consisting of neutrophils and macrophages surrounding the spherule (Wright, ×20). **B,** Similar magnification of a free spherule in an inflammatory exudate (Wright, ×1000). (Courtesy University of Georgia, Athens, Ga.)

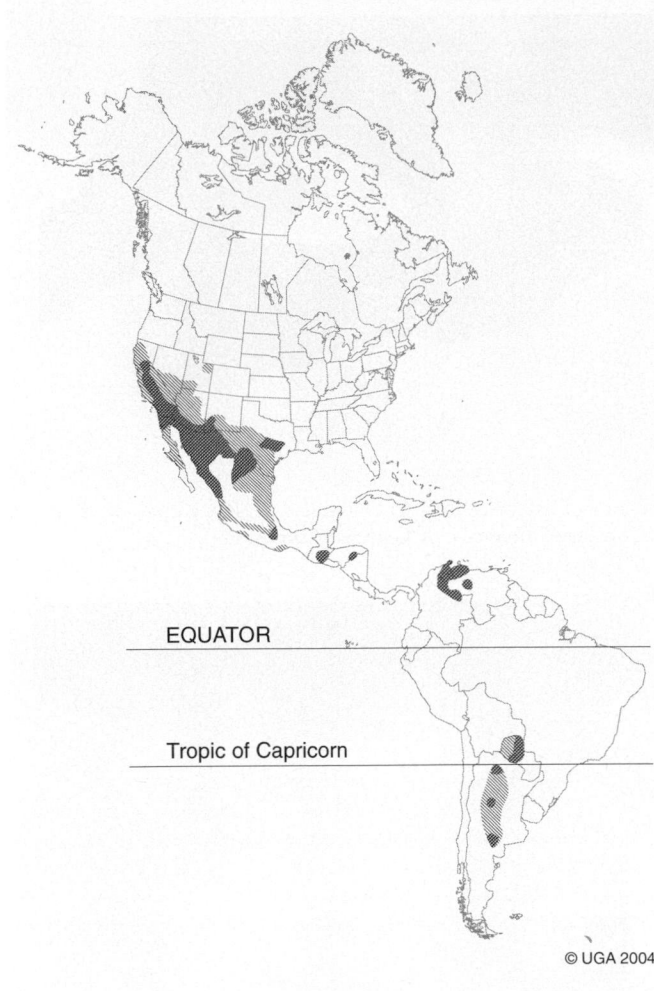

Fig 62-4 Worldwide distribution of incidence and prevalence of coccidioidomycosis. The areas marked by horizontal lines indicate incidence; the cross-hatched areas indicate regions of high endemicity. (Courtesy University of Georgia, Athens, Ga.)

documented.[11] This baby girl developed disease at 15 days of age.

Although very rare, reports have surfaced of C. *immitis* fungal hyphae, rather than endospores or spherules, being recovered from disseminated infections involving the central nervous system (CNS) in people.[42,61] In many instances, but not always, this type of infection has been found in association with a surgically placed CNS shunt for hydrocephalus.[29] This unusual form of infection has not been reported in animals.

Clinical Findings
Dogs
The high prevalence of positive skin test reactions in epidemiologic surveys of healthy dogs indicates that the most common form of coccidioidomycosis is an asymptomatic or mild, undiagnosed, lower respiratory tract infection. When clinical respiratory disease develops, it can be characterized by either a dry, harsh cough similar to that associated with tracheobronchitis or a wet, moist, productive cough. A dry cough is usually the result of hilar lymphadenomegaly or diffuse pulmonary interstitial disease. A productive cough is usually the result of alveolar involvement. Fever, partial anorexia, and

weight loss are commonly present in both situations. The pulmonary disease can resolve or worsen. The latter course leads to severe generalized pneumonia with a worsening of respiratory signs.

Clinical signs most commonly associated with disseminated disease include, in decreasing order of frequency, persistent or fluctuating fever, anorexia, weight loss, depression and weakness, lameness, localized peripheral lymphadenomegaly, draining skin lesions, seizures, bone or paraspinal hyperesthesia, keratitis, uveitis, and acute blindness. Gastrointestinal (GI) signs, as well as generalized peripheral lymphadenomegaly, are extremely uncommon. Other systemic lesions are common in dogs in endemic areas. The occurrence of clinical signs relative to each organ system depends on the specific localization of infection and is reviewed here.

Signs of right- or left-sided congestive heart failure can also occur. Cardiac dysfunction arises from disturbances in blood flow, conduction, and myocardial contractility resulting from granulomatous lesions in the pericardium.[55] The lesion often spreads within the pericardial sac, resulting in constrictive pericarditis.

Cranial or paraspinal hyperesthesia is typical for dogs with early CNS localization as a result of meningeal localization and inflammation.[32] Seizures, ataxia, behavioral changes, and coma have been associated with subsequent encroachment on the CNS by granulomatous meningoencephalomyelitis.[7]

Lameness is usually accompanied by painful bone swellings (Fig. 62-5). Bone lesions usually are initially localized to one bone but may progress to involve multiple sites. The lesions generally occur in the long bones in the distal diaphysis, metaphysis, and epiphysis, and a combination of bony lysis and production is usually noted. Lesions occur in the axial skeleton but only at a 10% prevalence compared with the appendicular skeleton. Joint infection is not typical, although secondary immune-mediated polyarthritis can develop in infected dogs.

Most cutaneous involvement results from systemic hematogenous spread of the organism. Skin lesions that begin as small bumps and progress to abscesses, ulcers, or draining tracts are almost always found over sites of infected bone (see Fig. 62-5). Naturally occurring primary cutaneous infection from penetrating injury is extremely rare in dogs.[48]

Cats
Signs associated with C. *immitis* infection in cats are similar to those described in dogs.[28] However, skin lesions are the most frequent type of infection found in cats. Skin infections without underlying bone involvement is common. Fever, inappetence, and weight loss are commonly found concurrently with skin lesions. Coughing, wheezing, and respiratory difficulties are only occasionally recognized with feline C. *immitis* infections, possibly because cats limit their physical activity. Appendicular bone lesions, similar to lung lesions, are rarely recognized in feline infections compared with canine infections. When bone lesions are present in cats, the radiographic changes are similar to those observed in dogs. Ocular lesions of chorioretinitis and anterior uveitis occur with about the same frequency in cats as they do in dogs.

Diagnosis
Clinical Laboratory Findings
Hematologic changes may include mild nonregenerative anemia and moderate neutrophilic leukocytosis, often with a left shift and monocytosis. Eosinophilia of blood and cerebrospinal fluid (CSF), common in human coccidioidomycosis, is quite variable in animals. Hyperglobulinemia and hypoalbuminemia are common, reflecting a chronic persistent inflammatory disease. Hypercalcemia unassociated with bone lesions has not yet been described in affected dogs or cats but has

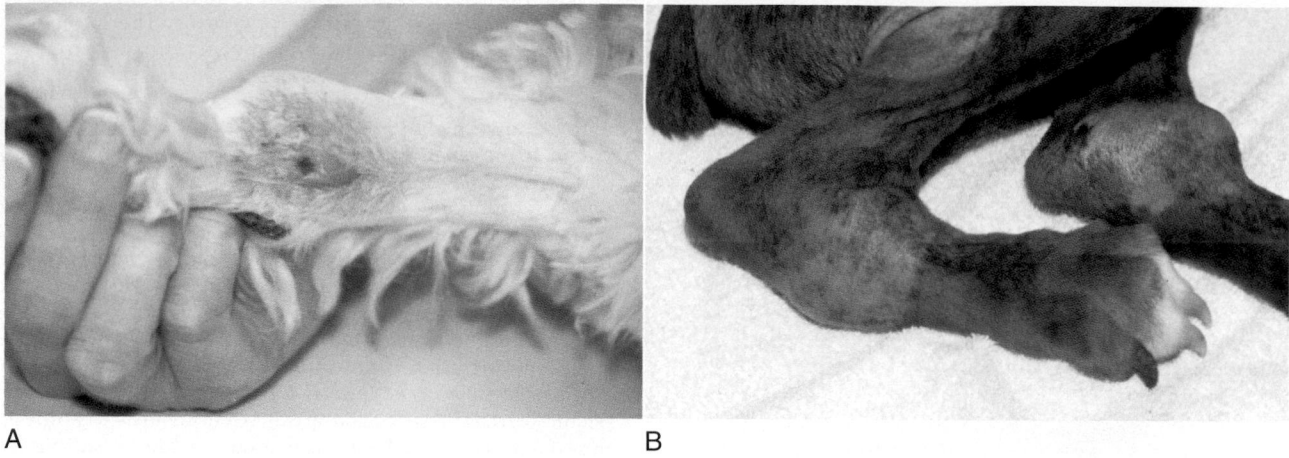

A   B

Fig 62-5 Two dogs with disseminated coccidioidomycosis with evidence of osteomyelitis. **A,** One dog with left carpal swelling had a draining fistula, and **(B)** the second dog had bilateral tarsal swelling. (Courtesy University of Georgia, Athens, Ga.)

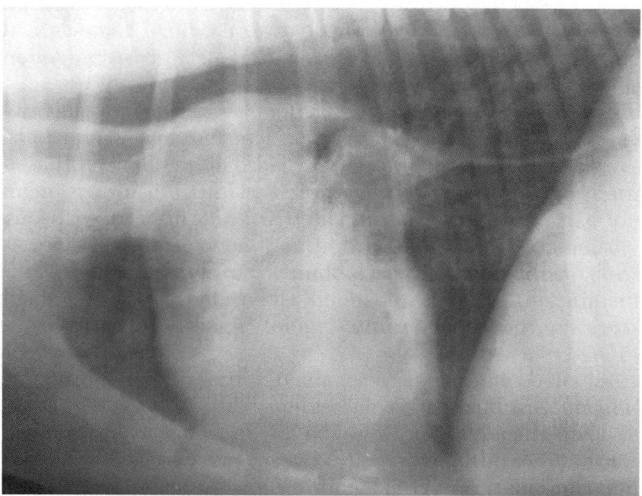

Fig 62-6 Lateral thoracic radiograph of a dog with pulmonary coccidioidomycosis, showing a hilar lymphadenomegaly and diffuse interstitial lung pattern. (Courtesy Russell T. Greene, Phoenix Veterinary IM Services, Phoenix, AZ.)

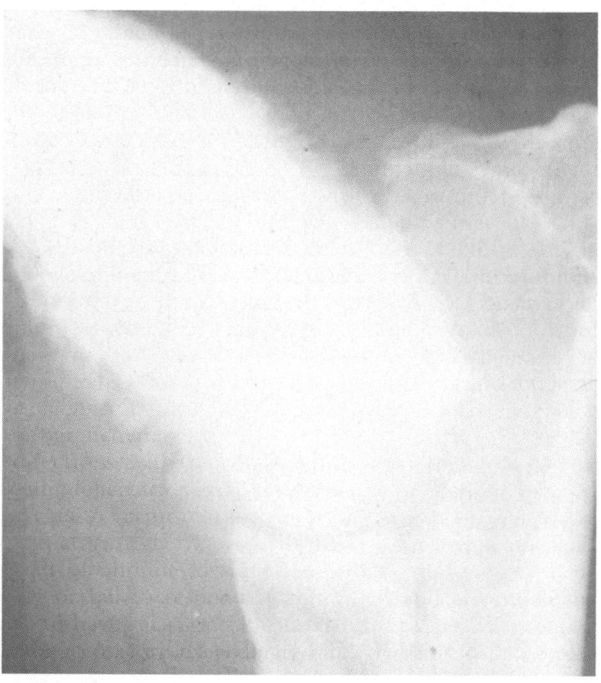

Fig 62-7 Radiograph of the distal humerus of a dog with disseminated coccidioidomycosis. Lesions are classically a mixture of lysis and production of bone. (Courtesy University of Georgia, Athens, Ga.)

been found with other systemic mycoses and in some human patients. An osteotrophic factor similar to that causing humoral hypercalcemia of malignancy has been postulated.

Radiography

Thoracic radiographic findings vary with the severity of the disease. A diffuse interstitial pattern is most common but is often mixed with a localized alveolar pattern (Fig. 62-6). Miliary to nodular interstitial densities may be found. If solitary nodules are found, they are often found in the periphery. If computed tomographic scans are used for evaluation of these nodules, central necrosis or cavitation may be found in up to 30% of the lesions.[35] A halo of homogeneous attenuation around the nodule is often found. Pulmonary abscess formation, fibrosis, and bronchiectasis (rarely calcification) may be sequelae to severe pulmonary infection. Hilar lymphadenomegaly is quite common, affecting most dogs with chronic illness, but calcification of the hilar lymph nodes or sternal lymphadenomegaly is rare. Pericardial and pleural effusion may occur secondary to right-sided myocardial failure or, more frequently, to pericarditis.[55] Radiographic findings

of osteomyelitis are typically a mixture of both lysis and production (Fig. 62-7).

Reports of magnetic resonance imaging (MRI) changes in animals are lacking. In people with acute meningitis, if MRI is performed, focal or diffuse enhancement may be found along with ventricular enlargement and deep infarcts.[18]

Cytology

Coccidioidomycosis is conclusively diagnosed by cytologic or histologic visualization of the organism. However, because of lesion localization or costs associated with invasive procedures, demonstration of the organism is often not possible. In such cases, a diagnosis is based on history, clinical findings, and serologic test results.

As with other nodular interstitial diseases, false-negative results are common with transtracheal or bronchial washings.

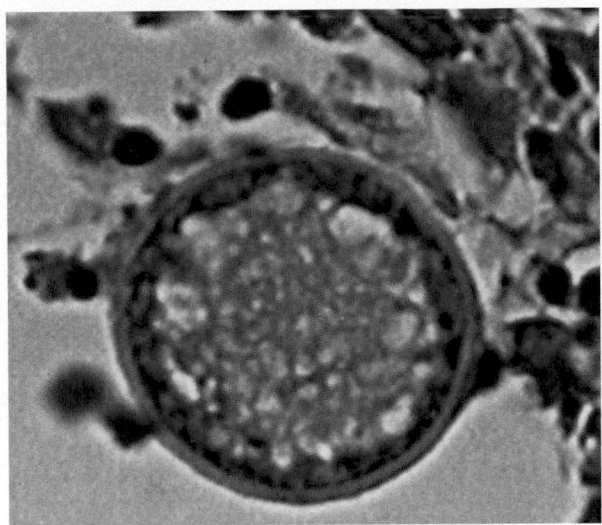

Fig 62-8 Histopathology of *C. immitis*–induced lesion with a large *C. immitis* spherule surrounded by pyogranulomatous inflammation (H and E stain, ×100).

The chance of a positive yield increases if alveolar disease is present. In human patients with diffuse lung disease, Papanicolaou's (Pap) stain was found to be superior in detecting organisms compared with 10% potassium hydroxide or calcofluor white.[51] Spherules are frequently found in aspirates of enlarged nodes or in impression smears of draining lesions (Fig. 62-8). CSF abnormalities include pleocytosis with a predominance of neutrophils and a lesser number of mononuclear cells and are consistent with granulomatous inflammation. Organisms may not always be observed.

The organism can be seen in unstained preparations under reduced light as a large (10 to 80 μm), round, double-walled structure containing endospores. Ten percent potassium hydroxide can clear an unstained specimen, although stained preparations are more typical. The organism is readily recognized with standard Wright's stain, but to specifically stain the fungal structures, the best stains are Pap and periodic acid-Schiff (PAS). With Pap stain, the capsular wall is refractile and purple-black, the cytoplasm yellow, and the endospores red-brown. Not all spherules contain recognizable endospores. Smaller spherules may have a crumpled, transparent wall. With PAS stain, the wall is deep red to purple and the endospores are bright red. A large number of neutrophils may surround the spherules, making visualization difficult.

Biopsy
In histopathology specimens, the organism usually can best be found in microabscesses. Spherules are detected employing routine hematoxylin and eosin stains, but for optimal visualization, special stains such as PAS or Grocott-Gomori's methenamine silver should be used. Spherules may be difficult to find in bone biopsy samples because of the reactive bone that forms within lesions. Repeated biopsies may be necessary to find the organism. Pathologists recommend that several biopsy samples be taken from the same lesion. Redirecting the biopsy needle through the same insertion site to obtain several core samples is often most successful. Immunofluorescence techniques can also be used to identify *C. immitis* spherules in tissues or cytologic preparations, but false-negative results can occur, and these techniques are rarely needed.

Fungal Isolation
C. immitis grows on a wide range of common fungal culture media and blood agar. *No* attempts should be made to culture

and identify this organism within veterinary practices. Instead, samples should be sent to laboratories familiar with biosafety precautions (see Appendix 5, Laboratory Testing for Infectious Diseases in Dogs and Cats). The mycelial phase grows best at 25° to 30° C. It usually grows within 3 days but may require more time if the number of organisms in the sample is low. The characteristic pattern of alternating live and dead arthroconidia associated with the appearance of the fungal colony allows for presumptive identification, but additional in vitro and in vivo methods can further definitively identify the organism. Veterinarians, technicians, and laboratory personnel must recognize that arthroconidia from mycelial growth are highly infectious.

Serologic Testing

Dogs When the organism cannot be demonstrated by cytology or biopsy, detection of antibodies to the organism is commonly used as a presumptive test. The two classic antigens for serotesting are the tube precipitin (TP) and complement fixation (CF) antigens. The names for these differently prepared antigens were based on the types of tests that were initially used to detect antibodies. The antibody response to the TP antigen is primarily immunoglobulin (IgM), whereas the antibody response to the CF antigen is associated more with IgG. For interpretation of TP and CF antibody titers in naturally infected dogs, refer to Table 62-1. Refer to Appendix 5 for laboratories that perform these tests.

Advances in molecular diagnostics have brought new methods of antibody detection. For example, use of a purified recombinant proline-rich antigen of *Coccidiodes* was used to detect infection and monitor progress of disease in people.[45] Clinicians should always check with the laboratory performing the serologic tests to determine which method is being used. Instead of the TP and CF methods, some laboratories employ the latex agglutination, agar gel immunodiffusion (AGID), or enzyme-linked immunosorbent assay (ELISA) methods for detection of these same antibodies. See Table 62-2 for a comparison of these methods. TP and CF antigens are still used in performing the AGID tests. Because the antigens and the antibody responses were named well before these newer techniques, the serologic terminology becomes confusing. Even more confusing is the fact that many of these new assays have not been fully evaluated using animal sera. Assumptions have often been made concerning their accuracy based on limited research in testing human sera. Because of the nature of the disease and the studies that have been completed to date, determining which of the tests are correct versus incorrect is usually difficult when discrepancies are noted. Further serologic studies with corresponding histologic, cytologic, or mycologic confirmation are needed. Advantages of the AGID and the ELISA methods over the classic CF test are that these newer methods are less complicated to perform, and interference by anticomplementary factors, which can be found in 15% to 25% of normal dog sera, does not occur.

Negative serologic test results, despite microbiologically confirmed coccidioidomycosis, occur on occasion. A published series of cases in people have suggested a prevalence of up to 15% to 20%. The author's opinion is that a 5% to 10% prevalence rate is more typical for dogs. In many cases, dermatologic cases and primary hilar lymphadenopathy cases are the ones that tend to have seronegative results.[27]

Tests to detect antigenemia in people have been developed and used on an investigational basis in rodents. Antigen detection would be helpful in early cases before seroconversion or in patients with immunodeficiencies in which seroreactivity does not develop. Interference by various components in serum has been a major problem with antigen tests. However, newer techniques are being evaluated. Appendix 5 should be

Table • 62-1

Interpretation of Serologic Testing for Coccidioidomycosis in Dogs and Cats

	TP ANTIBODY: NEGATIVE	TP ANTIBODY: POSITIVE (PREDOMINANTLY IgM)
CF ANTIBODY: NEGATIVE	1. No infection 2. Early infection; if disease suspected, repeat test in 4 to 6 wks to detect positive TP or CF test results 3. Rapidly fatal, fulminating infection in severely immunocompromised animal	1. Early or mild infection: TP test results become positive 2 wks postexposure and may become negative after 4 to 6 wks
CF ANTIBODY: POSITIVE (PREDOMINANTLY IGG)	1. Past exposure or disease, healing or localized lesions, or long-standing residual titer (especially if weak CF titer, 1 : 4 or less) 2. Chronic infection: TP antibody frequently disappears after 4 to 6 wks; the higher the CF titer, the more likelihood of severe or disseminated disease 3. Higher CF titers ≥ 1 : 64 are most frequently seen with severe pulmonary or disseminated lesions	1. Early or active infection: the greater the CF titer, the more likely disease is severe or disseminated 2. Chronic infection: positive TP tests occur later in infections or at the time of dissemination or recrudescence

TP, Tube precipitin; *CF*, complement fixation.

Table • 62-2

Comparison of Serologic Tests for Coccidioidomycosis[a]

TEST (ABBREVIATION)	MEASURED IMMUNOGLOBULIN	COMMENTS
TP	IgM	Positive results early in disease. Titer may increase with reactivation or dissemination.
CF	IgG	Good test for quantitative titers. Considered reference test for IgG. Positive results occur later in infection and rise with dissemination. Titer remains elevated months after successful treatment or if arrested. Titer gradually decreases with successful treatment. False-negative results occur in some immunosuppressed or anergic animals.
Latex agglutination	IgM	Some false-positives occur in canine sera. Detects acute (<1 mo) infections.
Immunodiffusion (AGID)		
TP antigen (IDTP)	IgM	More sensitive than TP in detecting recent (<1 mo) infections.
CF antigen (IDCF)	IgG	Good correlation with ELISA IgG with quantitative immunodiffusion. Most sensitive screening test for IgG.
ELISA		
IgM	IgM	Some (~15%) false-positives when compared with IDTP; also cross-reacts with some blastomycosis sera.
IgG	IgG	Good correlation with CF and IDCF: OD readings do not always correlate directly with CF titers. Cross-reacts with some blastomycosis sera.

TP, Tube precipitin; *CF*, complement fixation; *AGID*, agar gel immunodiffusion; *IDTP*, immunodiffusion tube precipitin; *IDCF*, immunodiffusion complement fixation; *ELISA*, enzyme-linked immunosorbent assay; *OD*, optical density.
[a]Based on data from Greene RT, unpublished observations, 1996; Pappagianis D, Zimmer BL. 1990. *Clin Microb Rev* 3:247–268.

consulted for a list of laboratories that perform these serologic tests for coccidioidomycosis.

Cats Early publications suggest that serologic tests were not useful diagnostic aids. However, a review of 48 feline cases indicated that both TP and CF antibodies were routinely detected in feline infections.[28] Both antibodies appear to persist for long periods in cats, even when therapy is initiated and maintained.

Skin Testing

Skin testing is used for epidemiologic surveys and evaluation of immunocompetence to *C. immitis* rather than as a diagnostic tool. The accuracy of intradermal testing with coccidioidin is subject to antigen variability. A positive reaction is defined as an area of induration of 5 mm or greater at 24 to 36 hours after injection. A positive test result indicates past or present infection. In people, the test result becomes positive within 1 week, after development of respiratory signs, whereas in dogs, a positive test result has been found within 3 to 8 weeks of natural exposure. In healthy people, positive skin test result indicates past exposure and resistance to infection and remains positive for years. Approximately 5% of people and 10% of dogs with disseminated disease have a negative skin test results, owing to severe immunosuppression. Skin testing is not especially specific because cross-reactions with histoplasmin and blastomycin can occur. Use of an antigen from the spherule phase, spherulin, has not proven diagnostically superior to coccidioidin in people.

Pathologic Findings

The lesions induced by *C. immitis* in dogs and cats are usually pyogranulomatous and are most often seen in the lungs. On gross inspection, lesions may vary from miliary to massive, from red to gray to white, from nodular to diffuse, and from firm to caseous or liquefactive (Fig. 62-9). Tracheobronchial lymph nodes are often increased in size and firm. Bone enlargement is found in dogs with coccidioidal osteomyelitis. At the time bone lesions are observed, lung lesions may have resolved. With CNS involvement, granulomas have been found in the cerebrum, midbrain, and cord. A granulomatous uveitis, retinitis, and keratitis may be present. In dogs with granulomatous pericarditis, the organism can be found in pericardial fluid. In dogs, right-sided heart failure is more commonly caused by coccidioidal pericarditis than by myocarditis. Fungal spherules can be found within granulomatous lesions.

Therapy

Because of the lack of controlled studies and the wide range of disease manifestations, ranging from spontaneously clearing uncomplicated illness to aggressive disseminated illness, the standard of care for treatment of coccidioidomycosis has not been fully defined.[34] Therapy in dogs and cats typically involves long-term antifungal drug treatment (Table 62-3). However, success is unpredictable. Controversy exists as to whether animals with primary pulmonary disease should be treated because these cases may resolve spontaneously. In people with initial mild primary pulmonary involvement, therapy is avoided unless chronic (6 weeks' duration) debilitation is present.[22] In dogs and cats, therapy has generally been instituted earlier for fear of dissemination. Animals with severe pulmonary infections, those with increasing titers of CF antibody (especially at or above 1:16), and those with fever, weakness, lameness, or worsening clinical signs are candidates for therapy. All animals with disseminated disease should be treated.

Because of the cost and potential toxicity of treatment, caution should be exercised when a diagnosis is based on serologic data alone. Positive CF titers of 1:8 or less are suspect for infection in animals. Patients with clinical illness may be treated, and serotesting should be repeated in 3 to 4 weeks to determine whether the titer is rising. Many dogs in enzootic areas have titers of 1:4 or less from prior exposure. Symptomatic animals with these low titers should have additional diagnostic procedures performed rather than be treated. Although relatively infrequent, animals can be infected yet be seronegative.

Deciding whether to terminate therapy is based on resolution of the clinical disease, radiographic appearance of bone and lung lesions, and serologic titers. Serologic titers alone may not be helpful in determining whether the disease is in remission because CF titers may stabilize or decrease only slightly. However, long-term monitoring of serologic response is beneficial to determine whether the titer is rising. Rising titers suggest poor absorption of drug or poor therapeutic response. If blood levels of the drug suggest adequate absorption, an alternate therapy should be considered.

If uveitis is the only sign of active infection, and it is not improving with antifungal therapy, enucleation should be performed. Uveitis has been curative, without further treatment, in at least one cat.[28]

The three azole drugs, ketoconazole (KTZ), itraconazole (ITZ), and fluconazole (FCZ), are most commonly prescribed. Because of the marked drop in cost of the newer azoles (ITZ

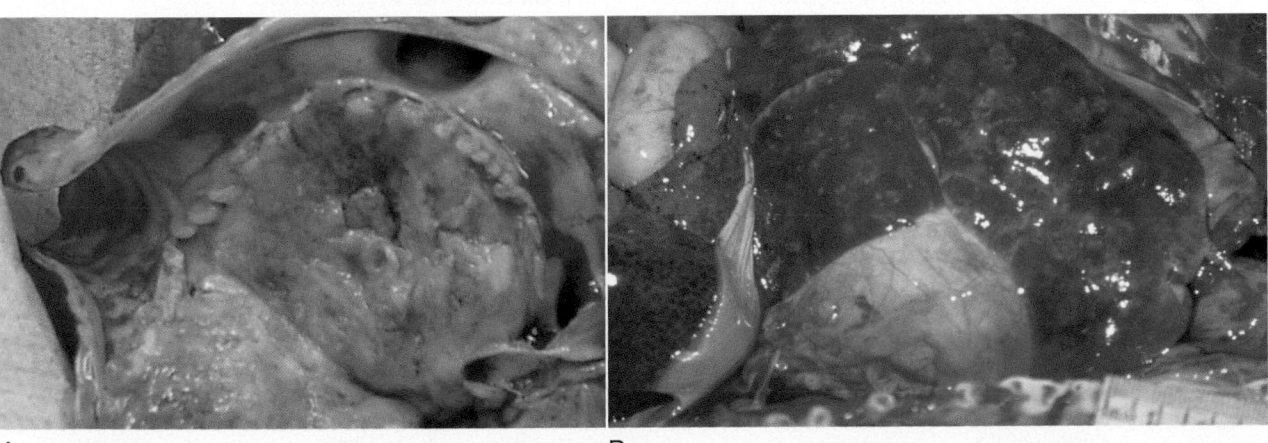

A   B

Fig 62-9 Lungs from dogs with severe pulmonary coccidioidomycosis showing (**A**) markedly enlarged hilar lymph node and (**B**) multiple light-colored granulomas throughout the lung lobes. (**A**, courtesy Russell T. Greene, Phoenix Veterinary IM Services, Phoenix, AZ; **B**, courtesy University of Georgia, Athens, Ga.)

Table • 62-3

Antifungal Therapy of Coccidioidomycosis

DRUG[a]	SPECIES	DOSE[b]	ROUTE	INTERVAL (HOURS)	DURATION (MONTHS)
Ketoconazole	D	5–10 mg/kg	PO	12	8–12[c]
	C	50 mg (total)	PO	12–24	[c]
Itraconazole	D	5 mg/kg	PO	12	[c]
	C	25–50 mg (total)	PO	12–24	[c]
Fluconazole	D	5 mg/kg	PO	12	[c]
	C	25–50 mg (total)	PO	12–24	[c]
Amphotericin B[d]	D	0.4–0.5 mg/kg	IV	48–72[e]	[f]
Lufenuron	D	5 mg/kg	PO	24	4[g]

D, Dog; C, cat; PO, by mouth; IV, intravenous.

[a]For additional information, see Drug Formulary, Appendix 8.

[b]Dose per administration at specified interval.

[c]Not based on controlled studies, but typical duration with dissemination is generally 12 months. Primary respiratory diseases often require shorter therapy. Ketoconazole or itraconazole have been the drugs of choice for treating dogs, and itraconazole has been preferred in treating cats.

[d]Amphotericin is rarely used because of its nephrotoxicity. It can be used alone or in combination with an azole. If used in combination, the recommended cumulative dose is often one half. The newer lipid encapsulated amphotericin B preparations are less toxic, but ideal dosages and intervals have not been determined.

[e]Given Monday and Thursday or Monday, Wednesday, and Friday (i.e., two to three times weekly).

[f]Until cumulative dose is 8 to 11 mg/kg.

[g]Efficacy of therapy and minimum dosage regimen has not been established. Maintenance therapy may be needed for longer periods. This treatment is still experimental and not generally recommended by the author.

and FCZ) when prepared by compounding pharmacies, these drugs are increasingly being used as the first drugs of choice in small animals. Although, no small-animal studies have been done that demonstrate a superiority of outcome in patients treated with these drugs, side effects with them tend to be fewer. FCZ is thought to have the best tissue penetration and the fewest side effects and is recommended for meningeal coccidioidomycosis. Interestingly, a recent randomized, double-blind comparison study between ITZ and FCZ in people with nonmeningeal coccidioidomycosis was completed.[23] It compared response rates in people with pulmonary, soft-tissue and skeletal lesions, when treated with either drug for 8 months. This excellent study showed no statistical difference between the efficacy of ITZ or FCZ. However, patients treated with ITZ tended to do better. This tendency for better success was most pronounced in people with skeletal lesions. Of interest was the relapse rate of approximately 15% of patients after these drugs were discontinued. Possibly, these patients needed to receive more than 6 months of therapy to prevent a relapse.

Using these drugs for 3 to 6 months beyond resolution of clinical signs and normalization of serologic titers is standard. As in people, how low the titer should go and how long the course of therapy should be to prevent relapses is controversial and undetermined.[44,58]

Ketoconazole

The drug of choice for initial treatment of coccidioidomycosis in dogs has been KTZ. See the Drug Formulary, Appendix 8, for detailed information about this drug. The recommended dosages for KTZ are listed in Table 62-3. The duration of therapy has been variable, depending on the site and extent of disease. Relapses are common if the drug is not administered on a daily basis for an adequate period. Treatment of animals with bone or disseminated coccidioidomycosis typically requires a minimum of 1 year of therapy. Because GI absorption of the drug is variable, measuring a 2- to 4-hour postpill KTZ blood level after 2 to 3 weeks of treatment is helpful. An acidic gastric environment increases the absorption of KTZ; therefore a dose of vitamin C is often concurrently administered.

Poor response and relapses sometimes occur with KTZ. Serologic tests should be repeated after 4 to 6 weeks of therapy. If the CF titer has continued to rise or clinical signs are deteriorating, an alternative azole or, rarely, amphotericin B (AMB) should be considered (see Table 62-3).

In people with nonmeningeal coccidioidomycosis, KTZ appears to be fungistatic; most patients improve, but relapses are common even at higher-than-recommended doses, and cures occur in only approximately 30% of patients. For meningeal disease, KTZ has been considered a poor choice for treatment because of its decreased penetration into the CSF and CNS. In the past, intrathecal AMB was given for CNS coccidioidomycosis, but the drug is irritating by this route. Because of its excellent pharmacokinetics and CNS penetration, FCZ is recommended for these cases (see Fluconazole, Chapter 57, and Drug Formulary, Appendix 8).

Itraconazole and Fluconazole

The newer azoles, ITZ and FCZ, are thought to have fewer side effects and to be more efficacious for treating coccidioidomycosis in people as compared with KTZ; however, no controlled studies in dogs or cats demonstrating similar efficacy have been conducted. Cats generally tolerate ITZ better than they do KTZ, with fewer side effects. A multiinstitutional, randomized, double-blind study evaluating the efficacy of FCZ and ITZ in nonmeningeal Coccidioides infections revealed a trend towards greater efficacy with ITZ as compared with FCZ, especially if skeletal lesions were involved.[23] Concern has surfaced that a high relapse rate (40%) may occur in human patients following discontinuation of FCZ therapy, which was higher than that noted for ITZ therapy. In some patients, the newer azoles have failed when they were tried first only to have the infection subsequently controlled with KTZ. As with KTZ, some of the animals treated with ITZ or FCZ develop relapses. These drugs may be an alternative to KTZ but not a panacea. Side effects such as hepatic dysfunction, GI upsets, and skin reactions[48] can also occur, as they do with KTZ. Hypertriglyceridemia has been seen with itraconazole.[60] An acidic gastric environment is not needed for FCZ absorption.

Although expense is a major concern for the use of azoles, compounding pharmacies in the United States currently formulate capsules at a reasonable cost. Newer formulations of ITZ, as an oral solution with the carrier cyclodextrin, appear to confer increased bioavailability.

Other Triazoles

Novel triazole compounds, such as voriconazole have become available for treating resistant infections, and posaconazole (SCH 56592), UR-9746, and UR-9751 are being developed. These have been evaluated in vitro and in experimental models of coccidioidomycosis.*

Amphotericin B

For many years, AMB was the only antifungal drug available; however, because of its potential renal toxicities and need for intravenous administration, it is currently less commonly used. The newer route of subcutaneous administration has not been evaluated in this disease (see Drug Formulary, Appendix 8). Now, new lipid-encapsulated formulations of AMB are on the market, with reportedly fewer renal complications, that have been used in treating human patients,[3] but their exact efficacy and optimal dosages have not been determined for dogs and cats. In a dog with concurrent multicentric lymphoma, simultaneous treatment with lipid formulation of AMB and cytotoxic chemotherapy was successful in producing initial remission of both diseases.[30] Other case reports have been issued of the efficacy of lipid-encapsulated formulations of AMB in people with coccidioidomycosis and of dogs and cats with other fungal infections. These lipid-encapsulated formulations of AMB are often cost prohibitive for general use.

Lipid formulations of AMB are available and have less toxicity but have not been clinically tested in dogs or cats (see Drug Formulary, Appendix 8). In people, case reports with successful outcomes have been issued.[37] The drug is indicated as the first choice in treating people with clinically severe pulmonary infections.[22] In a rabbit model of meningeal coccidioidomycosis, systemically administered lipid encapsulated AMB led to fungal eradication from brain and spinal cord in 3 out of 8 animals, a result not previously seen with any other systemic therapy studied.[14] Several lipid-encapsulated AMB formulations are commercially available. No study has determined the efficacy of one over the other, but a single case report has been done of a potential anaphylactic reaction in a human patient that started out receiving one compound and then was switched to another one.[33]

AMB, previously the drug of choice for treating canine coccidioidomycosis, may be indicated in animals that are unable to tolerate an azole compound. The toxicities and difficulties of administering AMB make it less desirable than are the azoles for dogs (see Chapter 57).

The dose of AMB to induce remission, when used alone or in combination, is listed in Table 62-3. In people, using intrathecal AMB in combination with an oral azole for coccidioidal meningitis is common.[59] A subcutaneous route of administration has been reported for the treatment of cryptococcosis, but this method of delivery has not been adequately tested on a series of dogs. The author has tried it on a few dogs with bone lesions and the clinical signs remained unchanged.

Chitin Synthesis Inhibitors

Chitin synthesis inhibitors are newer antifungal agents that also interfere with formation of the cell wall of fungi. One drug, Nikkomycin-Z (Shaman Pharmaceuticals, Inc., San Francisco, Calif.), is nearing clinical trials. This compound is fungicidal, rather than fungistatic, as are the azoles. By com-

*References: 8, 15, 25, 40, 43.

parison, Nikkomycin-Z requires relatively low doses for shorter time periods; it is orally administered. Lufenuron, another chitin synthesis inhibitor, is licensed for control of flea infestation in dogs and cats. In one pilot canine study, instead of once-monthly treatment, the drug was given daily for 16 weeks.[5] Clinical improvement began after 1 week, and resolution of radiographic lesions in the lungs was minimal. Dogs that showed some improvement did not start showing any changes until after 10 weeks. The drug did not appear to affect titers, and it has never been shown to be effective for successful treatment of this disease.

Caspofungin, which has received United States Food and Drug Administration approval for salvage therapy of invasive *Aspergillus* infections, is the first of the echinocandins (these inhibit 1,3 β D-glucan synthetase) to become available. Caspofungin was therapeutically effective in a murine model of *C. immitis* infection, despite its lack of in vitro activity against the fungus when minimum inhibitory concentrations were determined, using National Committee of Clinical Laboratory standards.[24,25] For further information, see Drug Formulary, Appendix 8.

Terbinafine

Terbinafine is a naftifine analog with a mechanism of action distinct among antimycotics. It inhibits fungal growth by inhibiting the fungal enzyme squalene epoxidase, a key enzyme in the synthesis of the fungal sterol ergosterol. Terbinafine has a broad range of in vitro activity and distributes widely into adipose and keratin-rich tissues. However, in a rabbit model of coccidioidal meningitis, it did not do as well as did FCZ alone, although some attenuation of the lesions was noted. Terbinafine was not detectable in the CSF, suggesting that it did not pass through the blood-brain barrier well. However, this finding was not considered the cause of the poor response because other drugs, such as ITZ, have efficacy in this model but cannot be measured in the CSF. The possibility exists that, in combination with another drug, terbinafine may provide synergistic activity. Further studies will be needed to define the role of this drug in coccidioidal infections.

Cytokines

Interferon-γ has been used as an adjunct in the treatment of a person with *C. immitis* infection and respiratory failure that failed to respond to conventional therapy alone.[39] For a further discussion of use of cytokines in treating disseminated fungal infections, see Antifungal Chemotherapy, Chapter 57.

Prognosis

The prognosis for localized respiratory coccidioidomycosis without treatment is good. However, many dogs are routinely treated to decrease the chance of dissemination. Without treatment, dogs with disseminated disease will usually die, or they have to be euthanized shortly after the disease is discovered. In more than 90% of these dogs, signs resolve with KTZ therapy. However, complete recovery rates in animals that require no further maintenance therapy are much lower. Complete recovery rates vary with the severity of the disease and degree of dissemination, ranging from 90% with only pulmonary involvement to 0% with multiple bone involvement. An overall recovery rate of approximately 60% has been noted. CNS involvement has a guarded to poor prognosis because of difficulty of drug penetration. Many infected cats show clinical improvement with KTZ therapy, although relapses have been common, especially when medication was discontinued.[14,28] Some cats experience a relapse each time that treatment is stopped (i.e., multiple relapses).

Prevention

The most beneficial strategy to prevent infection in people or animals would be through vaccination; however, a commercial vaccine is not available. A killed spherule vaccine was found to be highly protective against coccidioidal infection in mice. A similar vaccine in people failed to demonstrate protection. Current studies are examining the use of purified or recombinant antigens as vaccines.[1,31,54,62]

Evidence suggests that a patient's immune reaction to the organism may protect against dissemination.[6] Immunotherapy has been tried with little to variable success in people using a variety of drugs and cytokine inducers. Similarly, levamisole and acemannan have been empirically given to infected dogs with little success. All immunosuppressive drugs, including glucocorticoids, should be avoided or withdrawn before and during therapy. Synthetic immunomodulators or those produced by recombinant DNA techniques may offer an approach in the future.

Public Health Considerations

Coccidioidomycosis is generally accepted as being noncontagious because the infectious arthroconidial form of the agent is typically not produced in tissues. Except for one unusual case in which disseminated meningeal coccidioidomycosis developed in a veterinarian who performed a necropsy on a horse with disseminated disease,[38] no known direct spread from animal to people occurred. This veterinarian may have been exposed to arthroconidia growing in improperly preserved infected tissue or, less likely, to aerosolized or inoculated spherules from fresh tissues or discharges. In general, infected animals are not considered public health hazards. However, veterinarians should be cognizant of the potential problem of placing bandages over draining lesions. The tissue drainage may contaminate the bandage material and provide a suitable environment for arthroconidia development.

In contrast, handling mycelial cultures of the organism in the laboratory is extremely dangerous, and precautions must be taken to prevent arthroconidia release into the air. Laboratory technicians have also developed primary cutaneous lesions while working with the mycelial phase or while injecting suspected cultures into laboratory rodents. *C. immitis* has been considered a potential bioweapon.[17] Considering this

organism, the implementation of such use has many limitations, and the efficacy would likely be highly variable.

PARACOCCIDIOIDOMYCOSIS

Paracoccidioidomycosis, a systemic fungal disease of people and rarely of animals in Central and South America, is caused by the dimorphic fungus *Paracoccidioides brasiliensis*. It is characterized by granulomatous pulmonary and disseminated lesions. The organism was isolated from a dog with cervical lymphadenomegaly. Budding yeasts were surrounded by granulomatous inflammation. The organism was identified by immunochemistry and genetic analysis. This was the first report of the disease in a dog.[48a]

SUGGESTED READINGS*

20. Fisher MC, Koenig GL, White TJ, et al. 2002. Molecular and phenotypic description of *Coccidioides posadasii* sp. *nov.*, previously recognized as the non-California population of *Coccidioides immitis*, *Mycologica* 94:73-84.
28. Greene RT, Troy GC. 1995. Coccidioidomycosis in 48 cats: a retrospective study (1984-1993), *J Vet Intern Med* 9:86-91.
30. Jeroski A. 2003. Multicentric lymphoma and disseminated coccidioidomycosis in a dog, *Can Vet J* 44:62-64.
32. Johnson LR, Herrgesell EJ, Davidson AP, et al. 2003. Clinical, clinicopathologic, and radiographic findings in dogs with coccidioidomycosis: 24 cases (1995-2000), *J Am Vet Med Assoc* 222:461-466.
39. Kuberski TT, Servi RJ, Rubin PJ. 2004. Successful treatment of a critically ill patient with disseminated coccidioidomycosis, using adjunctive interferon-gamma, *Clin Infect Dis* 38:910-912.
48a. Ricci G, Mota FT, Wakamatsu A, et al. 2004. Canine paracoccidioidomycosis, *Med Mycol* 42:379-383.
50. Rubensohn M, Stack S. 2003. Coccidiomycosis in a dog, *Can Vet J* 44:159-160.

*See the CD-ROM for a complete list of references.

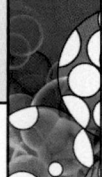

CHAPTER • 63

Sporotrichosis

Edmund J. Rosser, Jr. and Robert W. Dunstan

ETIOLOGY AND EPIDEMIOLOGY

Sporotrichosis is a mycotic disease of animals and people caused by the dimorphic fungus *Sporothrix schenckii*. The fungus exists in a mycelial form at environmental temperatures (25° to 30° C [77° to 86° F]) and in a yeast form at body tissue temperature (37° C [98.6° F]). In the environment the organism changes phases into an ascomycete telemorph that can survive on living or decaying plant material.[54] The organism is found worldwide and prefers soils that are rich in decaying organic matter. It has also been isolated from barberry and rose bush thorns, sphagnum moss, tree bark, and mine

timbers.[34,39,48] Sphagnum moss has been associated with sporadic outbreaks of sporotrichosis,[16] including a multistate outbreak among forestry workers and seedling handlers.[11] The sphagnum moss was harvested in Wisconsin and used as a packing for conifer seedlings.[9] *S. schenckii* does not grow on the living sphagnum moss in bogs but does grow and sporulate well on moist, dead sphagnum moss after harvest.[57] The handling of stored hay bales and moldy hay have also been associated with outbreaks.[7,10] In addition, some case reports have described sporotrichosis associated with puncture wounds from fish spines, squirrel bites, and the stings of fire ants.[15,28,42] Many cases in people have related to scratches acquired during armadillo hunting. Infected cats develop many draining lesions and have also been responsible for many infections in people.[3]

Infection is usually caused by traumatic inoculation into tissues of soil, plant material, or organic matter contaminated with the fungus.[39,48] The disease in dogs is often associated with a puncture wound caused by a thorn or wood splinter and therefore is most frequently observed in hunting dogs. In cats, sporotrichosis is most commonly identified in intact male cats that are allowed to roam outdoors. Infection presumably occurs when the organism is inoculated into a puncture wound caused by the contaminated claw or oral cavity of another cat.[12,39,47] Similar to other systemic mycosis, widespread cutaneous lesions in cats likely arise from primary respiratory infection followed by hematogenous dissemination to involve skin sites.[45]

Although contamination of a puncture wound by organisms in the environment is considered an important mechanism in human acquisition of the disease, human contact with cats infected with *S. schenckii* or clinically healthy cats that are exposed while living with infected cats with *S. schenckii* are now considered significant methods of zoonotic infection.[24,36,43,56] The organism can be isolated from nail clippings of cats in households where an infection has been reported.[47] *S. schenckii* can be isolated from 100% of skin lesions, 66.2% of nasal cavities, 41.8% of oral cavities, and 39.5% of nails of cats with sporotrichosis.[43] In addition, 3.57% of clinically healthy cats with domiciliary contact with diseased cats had positive results from oral cultures. (See Public Health Considerations in this chapter for an additional discussion of these implications.)

After the organism enters the tissues, it converts into a yeastlike form. It can propagate locally and produce lesions at the inoculation site, it can spread up regional lymphatics and produce lymphangitis and lymphadenitis, or it can disseminate systemically in immunocompromised hosts. Many mammalian species, including dogs and cats, can become infected and develop clinical illness.

CLINICAL FINDINGS

Sporotrichosis has three clinical forms: cutaneous, cutaneolymphatic, and disseminated. In many instances, an animal may have more than one form simultaneously. In addition to the cutaneous manifestations, dogs and cats may have a history of lethargy and anorexia, with the physical examination revealing depression and fever, which suggests *disseminated* disease. This finding should indicate to the clinician that the animal may be immunocompromised. In general the clinical symptoms of this disease are different in dogs and cats.

Dogs
Sporotrichosis in dogs usually develops in the cutaneous or cutaneolymphatic form; the disseminated form of the disease is extremely rare.[39,41] The *cutaneous* form is a multinodular condition, typically occurring on the trunk or head, with nodules in the dermal and subcutaneous layers. Nasal masses protruding from the nostrils have been observed.[49] The nodules may be ulcerated. Ulcerated nodules are associated with purulent exudate and crust formation. Dogs with the *cutaneolymphatic* form usually develop nodules on the distal aspect of one limb (Fig. 63-1). The infection then ascends proximally, following lymphatic vessels. Secondary nodules develop (referred to as *cording* of the lymphatics), which may also ulcerate and drain a purulent exudate. The cutaneolymphatic form is usually associated with regional lymphadenomegaly. Coinfection with *Cryptococcus neoformans* was reported in one dog.[49]

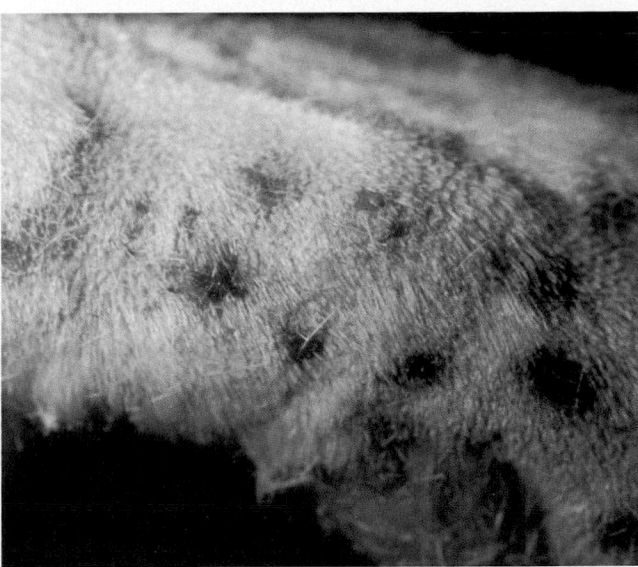

Fig 63-1 Canine sporotrichosis with multiple nodules on the lateral aspect of paw. (Courtesy University of Georgia, Athens, Ga.)

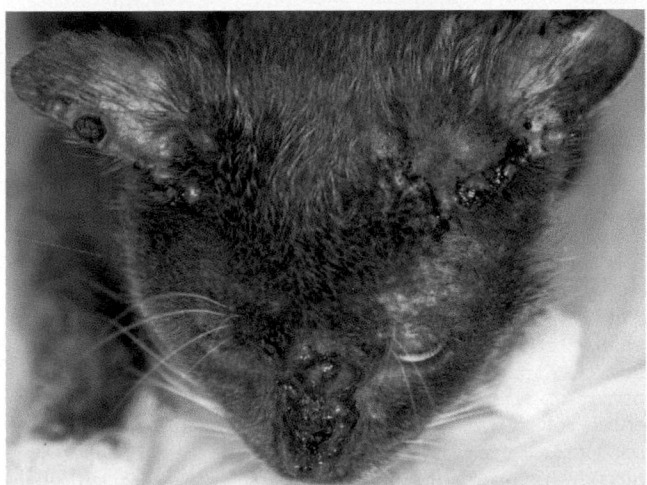

Fig 63-2 Feline sporotrichosis with multiple nodules, ulceration, and draining tracts on head. (Courtesy University of Georgia, Athens, Ga.)

Cats
Lesions usually occur on the distal aspects of the limbs, head, or tail-base region, sites that are commonly exposed or inoculated during cat fights. Draining puncture wounds that first appear are similar to fight-wound abscesses or cellulitis. Previous treatment with soaks and systemic antibiotics for bacterial infection results in poor or partial improvement. Subsequently, the affected areas become ulcerated, drain a purulent exudate, and form large, crusted lesions (Fig. 63-2). Extensive areas of necrosis may develop, exposing muscle and bone. The disease process may be further complicated by autoinoculation, occurring when the cat licks and scratches the lesions and then continues with normal grooming behavior, which results in multiple lesions on the extremities, face, and ears (Fig. 63-3). The involvement of the lymphatic system may not be apparent during the physical examination of affected cats. However, with necropsy or biopsy of internal

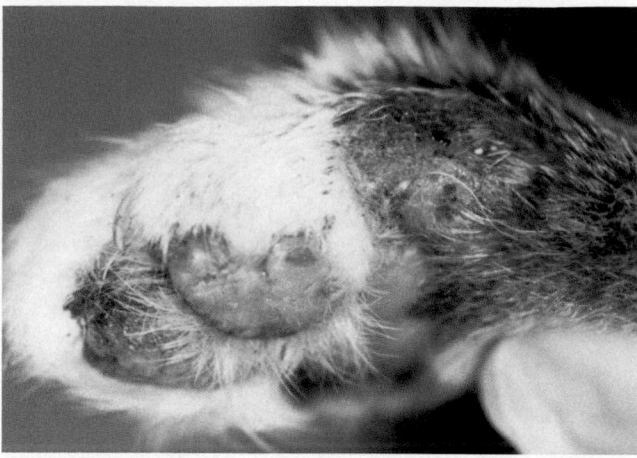

Fig 63-3 Feline sporotrichosis lesions on paws of cat in Fig. 63-2. These lesions were likely caused by autoinoculation during grooming. (Courtesy University of Georgia, Athens, Ga.)

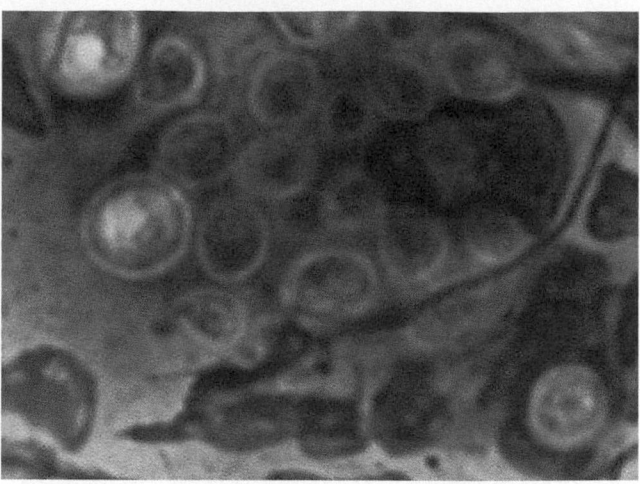

Fig 63-4 Photomicrograph of impression smear from ulcerated nodule in cat with sporotrichosis. Notice numerous fungal organisms within a macrophage. (Courtesy Patrick Hensel, University of Georgia, Athens, Ga.)

organs, most cats have evidence of disseminated disease with lymph node and lymphatic vessel involvement. The lung and liver are predominant sites for gross dissemination[44,54]; however, many other organs can be microscopically or culturally affected. *Sporothrix* organisms are commonly present and may be cultured from the blood of cats with disseminated cutaneous disease.[43,44] Coinfection with feline immunodeficiency virus (FIV) has been documented in some of the cats with disseminated disease,[44] although a direct association has not been documented.

DIAGNOSIS

The initial symptoms of dogs or cats with sporotrichosis are similar to that of an animal with a deep cutaneous bacterial infection and other deep cutaneous fungal infections. The clinician should become suspicious of the possibility of sporotrichosis or other deep cutaneous fungal infections if the appropriate use of systemic antibiotics for a deep pyoderma or cellulitis results in minimal or partial improvement. Diagnosis is often suspected after cytologic or histopathologic visualization of the organism and is confirmed by cultural isolation. When bacterial cultures have been performed, the ulcerative and exudative lesions of sporotrichosis are often secondarily infected with bacterial organisms, especially *Staphylococcus intermedius*.

Cytology

Exudates from draining lesions should first be examined cytologically and stained for the presence of yeastlike organisms, which can be visualized by Wright (Romanowsky-type) stain and confirmed as the fungus using either culture or periodic acid–Schiff (PAS) or Gomori's methenamine silver (GMS) stains. The organism is often difficult to find in the exudates from dogs, and sporotrichosis should not be ruled out on the basis of negative cytologic findings. In contrast, *S. schenckii* is often easily identified in the exudates from cats. However, one case report[20] and our own experience have indicated that the organism can be difficult to find on cytologic examination of exudates from cats and dogs. When present, *S. schenckii* appears as a pleomorphic yeast, 3 to 5 μm wide and 5 to 9 μm long, that is round, oval, or cigar-shape and may be found within macrophages and inflammatory cells or extracellularly (Fig. 63-4; see Fig. 56-5).

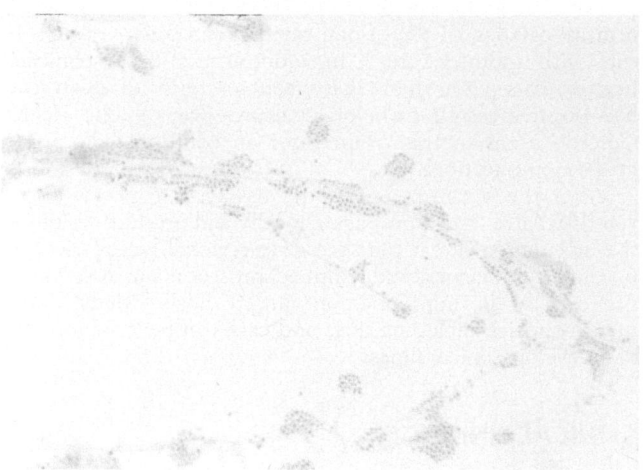

Fig 63-5 Cytologic appearance of *Sporothrix* organisms in culture showing chains of organisms on hyphal elements (Lactol Phenol Cotton Blue stain, ×100). (Courtesy University of Georgia, Athens, Ga.)

Fungal Isolation

When culturing for the presence of *S. schenckii*, samples of the exudate from deep within a draining tract and a piece of tissue surgically removed for a macerated tissue culture should be submitted. This approach is especially important in the dog, because usually very few organisms are present in the lesion. It is also advisable to alert the laboratory to which samples have been submitted that a diagnosis of sporotrichosis is being considered. Organisms in culture at 25° C are characterized by formation of septate hyaline hyphae, conidiophores, and conidia (Fig. 63-5). Hematogenous dissemination can be documented by blood culture of infected cats.[45]

Histopathologic Findings

Whenever possible, the best specimens to submit for histologic examination are biopsy samples of early-forming, intact nodules. The histologic pattern observed in sporotrichosis of the dog and cat is a nodular to diffuse pyogranulomatous inflammatory reaction. It is primarily located in the dermal and subcutaneous tissues and may extend to involve the underlying skeletal muscle. As with cytologic examination, it is easier to find the organism in lesions from cats than from dogs. In the feline lesions, organisms are frequently so numerous that they are readily demonstrated within the pyogranulomatous reaction, even on sections stained with hematoxylin-eosin stain. However, experience has indicated that in cases of feline sporotrichosis the organism can occasionally be difficult to demonstrate on histopathologic examination of tissues. Because usually only a few organisms exist in canine tissues, slides should be counterstained with a fungal stain such as PAS or GMS and even then, each section of tissue should be carefully examined.

Immunofluorescence Testing

Specific fluorescent antibody (FA) detection of the organism (*Sporothrix* antigen-specific direct FA test) is most useful in establishing the diagnosis in dogs when the results of the just-mentioned procedures have been negative or when attempts at culturing the organism have failed.[39] This diagnostic procedure can be performed by the Centers for Disease Control and Prevention in Atlanta, Ga., on a sample of exudate or preferably on affected tissue from a patient suspected of having the disease (see Appendix 5). Serologic testing for antibodies to the organism is available, but a positive result indicates exposure and not necessarily active infection.

Genetic Detection

Molecular detection was used to identify *S. schenckii* directly in biopsy specimens from an infected cat.[17a]

THERAPY

In the management of sporotrichosis in dogs and cats, the use of glucocorticoids or any immunosuppressive drug is contraindicated both during and after the treatment of the disease. Immunosuppressive doses of glucocorticoids have been shown to cause a recurrence of the clinical disease after it has apparently resolved.[39] Any concurrent bacterial infection should be simultaneously treated for 4 to 8 weeks with an appropriate antibiotic on the basis of the results of culture and susceptibility testing.[37]

Dogs

The treatment of choice for dogs is the oral administration of a supersaturated solution of potassium iodide (SSKI) with food for 30 days beyond apparent clinical cure (Table 63-1). When sporotrichosis is not treated for an adequate time, it often recurs. Care should be taken to observe the dog for any signs of iodism (e.g., ocular and nasal discharge, dry hair coat with excessive scaling, vomiting, depression, and collapse). If iodism is observed, the medication should be discontinued for 1 week. If the side effects were mild, they may not recur, and therapy should then be reinstituted. If the side effects recur or the initial reactions were severe, an alternative treatment should be considered. Ketoconazole (KTZ) can be given to dogs that do not tolerate SSKI and to those that are refractory to iodide therapy (see Table 63-1). The authors have successfully treated a dog with sporotrichosis using KTZ at 15 mg/kg, given orally every 12 hours for 1 month beyond the apparent clinical cure (which required 3.5 months of treatment). KTZ is usually well tolerated by dogs, but potential hepatotoxicity should be monitored during therapy (see Appendix 8, Drug Formulary).[37,50] Itraconazole (ITZ) has also been shown to be a relatively safe and effective drug in the treatment of sporotrichosis in people,[26,53,55] and was used successfully in the treatment of a case of canine sporotrichosis at 7.3 mg/kg, given orally every 12 hours with food for 5 days, then every 24 hours for 1 month beyond the apparent clinical cure (which required 3 months of treatment).[51] However, hepatotoxicity was reported to occur in about 10% of dogs when ITZ was given at a dosage of 5 mg/kg twice daily and about 5% of dogs when ITZ was given at a dosage of 5 mg/kg once daily.[22,23] This study involved the use of ITZ for the treatment of 112 dogs with blastomycosis. The subsequent recommended dosage for the use of ITZ in the treatment of blastomycosis was 5 mg/kg once daily, because this dosage minimized the adverse and toxic reactions without compromising the effectiveness of the drug[23] (see Appendix 8, Drug Formulary). In addition, the twice-daily dosing of ITZ has been associated with adverse cutaneous drug reactions (espe-

Table • 63-1

Drug Therapy for Sporotrichosis[a]

DRUG[b]	SPECIES	DOSE (mg/kg)[c]	ROUTE	INTERVAL (HOURS)	DURATION (MONTHS)
SSKI[d]	Dog	40	PO	8	≥2
	Cat	10–20	PO	12	
Ketoconazole[e]	Dog	5–15	PO	12	≥2
	Cat	5–10	PO	12–24	
Itraconazole capsules[f]	Dog and cat	5–10	PO	12–24	≥2
	Cat	15	PO	24	≥2
Itraconazole solution[f]	Cat	1.25–1.5	PO	24	≥2
Terbinafine[g]	Cat	30	PO	24	≥2

PO, By mouth; *SSKI*, supersaturated solution of potassium iodide.
[a]Continue treatment at least 30 days beyond resolution of all clinical signs—usually 2 or more months of treatment.
[b]See Drug Formulary, Appendix 8, for additional information.
[c]Dose per administration at the specified interval.
[d]Supersaturated solution of potassium iodide (see Iodide, Drug Formulary, Appendix 8); treatment of choice for dogs.
[e]Preferred therapy for dogs; toxicity more likely in cats on higher dosages.
[f]Preferred therapy for cats; toxicity more likely in dogs on higher dosages.
[g]Recommended for use in combination and only in resistant cases.[46]

Cats

Treatment of sporotrichosis in the cat is more difficult than in the dog because of the cat is more likely to develop toxic side effects from iodides (e.g., vomiting, anorexia, depression, twitching, hypothermia, cardiovascular failure) and KTZ (e.g., anorexia, depression, vomiting, diarrhea, fever, neurologic signs, jaundice).[22,39] ITZ is recommended as the treatment of choice for sporotrichosis in cats (see Table 63-1). ITZ solution is preferred to the capsules because of its improved absorption and bioavailability at the recommended dosage of 1.25 to 1.5 mg/kg once daily.[4] Because of lower bioavailability, dosage of the capsular form of the drug is 5 to 10 mg/kg once to twice daily.[44] The treatment should be continued for at least 1 month beyond the apparent clinical cure. ITZ has been shown to be effective in the treatment of systemic or disseminated sporotrichosis in people and is becoming the recommended treatment of choice.[18,26,30,53,55] Because disseminated sporotrichosis commonly occurs in cats, the use of ITZ seems most rational. ITZ appears to be an effective alternative for the treatment of feline sporotrichosis and is better tolerated by cats than either iodides or KTZ.[4,6,22,27,50] The potential for hepatotoxicity exists, and it is recommended that serum liver enzymes be monitored monthly during therapy. The most common side effect of ITZ in cats is anorexia; other reported side effects include vomiting, weight loss, and depression.[27] With concern over the development of imidazole and triazole derivative drug resistance in some deep fungal infections, terbinafine (a fungicidal allylamine) may be a useful alternative when toxicities, side effects, or a poor response to treatment develop with the use of ITZ. Terbinafine has been used as an effective treatment for feline dermatophytosis infections caused by *Microsporum canis*, with the only reported side effect being vomiting, which was alleviated by giving the medication with food.[5,21,25] Most recently, terbinafine has been shown to be effective in the treatment of cutaneous sporotrichosis in people.[8,17,52] Amphotericin B has only been used to treat people with life-threatening or extensive pulmonary infection.[19] In a retrospective study involving 68 of 347 cats that were cured (as measured by repeated culture) with various regimens of antifungal therapy, initial treatment with ITZ and sodium iodide were most commonly used, but some of the "cured" cats were initially treated with combinations of ITZ plus fluconazole or ITZ plus terbinafine or KTZ alone.[46] Eight cats that had positive test results for FIV antibody were clinically cured. Many of the cats that were "not cured" had improved clinical conditions; however, positive fungal culture results were subsequently documented. The length of treatment for clinical resolution ranged from 16 to 80 weeks, with a mean of 36 weeks, when 41 of the cats were given two treatment regimens.

PUBLIC HEALTH CONSIDERATIONS

Traditionally, sporotrichosis has been considered to have minimal zoonotic potential. However, several reports have documented the transmission of sporotrichosis to people through contact with an infected wound or exudate from an infected cat.[36,39,56] In recent years, hundreds of cases in people associated with cats have been reported from Brazil.[3,44] The ready transmission of sporotrichosis from animals to people,

even (although rare) in the absence of a skin-penetrating injury, appears to be a feature limited to feline sporotrichosis, presumably because of the copious numbers of organisms found in tissues, exudates, and feces of infected cats. However, inoculation of the organism may occur through the puncture wound caused by the contaminated claw or oral cavity of the cat[12,39,47] or contact with clinically healthy cats that share living space with cats infected with *S. schenckii*.[43] Theoretically, transmission from infected dogs seems less likely because it is often difficult to demonstrate the presence of the organism. Similarly, this infection does not spread from person to person.[19]

The population at greatest risk for acquiring sporotrichosis from an infected cat includes veterinarians, veterinarian assistants, and anyone exposed during treatment. An outbreak of sporotrichosis occurred in a metropolitan area among people of lower socioeconomic status who had contact with domiciled cats that roamed the neighborhood.[3] In some instances, infection has occurred after nontraumatic exposure to an infected cat; one person had no known preexisting injury or penetrating wound before contracting the disease. However, inadvertent exposure to the organism may have been caused by the cat rubbing its faces against the person.

The appearance of lesions in people can be nodular, pustular, cystic, ulcerated, ulcerovegetative, or plaquelike, with or without lymphangitis. The lesions in people are frequently lymphocutaneous, localized cutaneous, mucosal (including nasopharyngeal or ocular), or widespread cutaneous lesions. Disseminated sporotrichosis is uncommon and has been observed in immunocompromised people with the acquired immunodeficiency syndrome, alcoholism, or diabetes mellitus or who are being treated with immunosuppressive therapy.[14] These individuals may acquire their infection from the air or percutaneously and should not directly handle or closely associate with infected cats. Pulmonary sporotrichosis in people is difficult to treat effectively. SSKI solution has been effective in the treatment of cutaneous sporotrichosis in people. However, gastrointestinal side effects have been problematic. ITZ has been the most effective drug for treating in all forms of the disease and has had few adverse effects. In a few cases, ITZ resistance has necessitated treatment with SSKI.[40]

People handling cats suspected of having sporotrichosis should wear disposable gloves. Afterward, they should remove the gloves carefully and wash their forearms, wrists, and hands with either a chlorhexidine or povidone-iodine scrub.

SUGGESTED READINGS*

3. Barros MBL, Schubach AO, Valle ACF, et al. 2004. Cat-transmitted sporotrichosis epidemic in Rio de Janeiro, Brazil: description of a series of cases. *Clin Infect Dis* 38:529-535.
43. Schubach TM, de-Oliveira-Schubach A, dos-Reis RS, et al. 2002. *Sporothrix schenckii* isolated from domestic cats with and without sporotrichosis in Rio de Janeiro, Brazil. *Mycopathologia* 153:83-86.
46. Schubach TMP, Schubach AO, Okamoto T, et al. 2004. Evaluation of an epidemic of sporotrichosis in cats: 347 cases,1998-2001. *J Am Vet Med Assoc* 224:1623-1629.
54. Welsh RD. 2003. Sporotrichosis. *J Am Vet Med Assoc* 223:1123-1126.

*See the CD-ROM for a complete list of references.

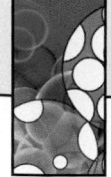

CHAPTER • 64

Aspergillosis and Penicilliosis

*A*spergillus and *Penicillium* are saprophytic fungi, ubiquitous in the environment, that generally cause either nasal or pulmonary and disseminated infections in dogs and cats. Everything in the environment, even pet foods, have high levels of contamination.[12] *Penicillium* spp. are often confused with *Aspergillus* spp. on gross or histologic appearance, and culture is required to distinguish the two. Cats may have gastrointestinal (GI) mucosal localization. Rarely do solitary lesions occur outside the nasal passages; nasal infections have not been suspected to disseminate to distant locations.[61]

Nasal infection has been associated most commonly with *Aspergillus fumigatus*. *Aspergillus* and *Penicillium* are common contaminants of body or mucosal surfaces and of the respiratory tract; therefore culture without either histologic or cytologic evidence of associated inflammation can be misleading. These organisms are generally opportunistic pathogens. Host immunocompetence is an important determinant in the development of these opportunistic fungal infections. Cell-mediated immunity (CMI) is probably the major factor in limiting systemic spread of infection.

Immunosuppressive conditions such as diabetes mellitus, persistent granulocytopenia, cytotoxic chemotherapy, glucocorticoid therapy, concurrent infection, and hereditary cell-mediated immunodeficiency are often associated with disseminated disease. German shepherd dogs are as predisposed to opportunistic infections, especially aspergillosis and hyalohyphomycosis, as they are to rickettsial diseases (see Chapters 28 and 29). For a discussion of infection with other opportunistic saprophytic fungi, see Chapter 67.

CANINE NASAL ASPERGILLOSIS-PENICILLIOSIS

Kyle G. Mathews and Nick J. H. Sharp

Etiology

Nasal aspergillosis is encountered much more frequently than is nasal penicilliosis. The two conditions are indistinguishable other than by the microscopic appearance of their conidiophores (Fig. 64-1). *A. fumigatus* is the most common species encountered, although *Aspergillus niger*, *Aspergillus nidulans*, and *Aspergillus flavus* are occasionally involved. The species of *Penicillium* causing nasal penicilliosis have not been defined. These organisms all branch dichotomously (branches are approximately equal in diameter to the stem) at 45-degree angles and form septate, nonpigmented hyphae of approximately 3 to 8 μm diameter in culture and in tissue specimens.[79] Both groups of fungi are ubiquitous saprophytes and are regarded as opportunistic pathogens.

Pathogenesis

Aspergillus is found in the environment living and growing on organic debris. Its airborne conidia of 2 to 3 μm are released in such large numbers that they land on most inanimate and animate objects. Their small size keeps them airborne indoors and out, with most hosts inhaling hundreds of conidia daily.[60]

In immunocompetent individuals, these organisms are eliminated by innate immune mechanisms. To invade the host, *Aspergillus* must adhere to and penetrate the respiratory epithelia and kill surrounding cells and resist phagocytosis.[81] Conidia bind to various surface proteins; however, only a few of the existing adhesion systems, such as hydrophobins, have been identified. *A. fumigatus* also produces a toxic metabolite known as gliotoxin, which inhibits macrophage phagocytosis and has a broad range of immunosuppressive actions. Other metabolites can impair mucociliary action and prolong the organism's epithelial residence. Enzymes such as proteases allow for tissue invasion.

Nasal aspergillosis is a common disease in dogs that affects primarily young to middle-aged mesaticephalic and dolichocephalic breeds. In one report of 60 dogs with nasal aspergillosis, the age of affected animals ranged from 3 months to 11 years (mean 3.3 years).[85] In contrast, nasal neoplasia tends to occur in older animals.[57] A history of nasal trauma is uncommon but has been reported in some dogs.[55] Nasal aspergillosis can occur concomitantly with, and probably secondary to, nasal tumors and nasal foreign bodies such as grass awns. Other differential diagnoses should include extension of dental disease and cleft palate, as well as lymphoplasmacytic, bacterial, and allergic rhinitis. Nasal infection with *Cryptococcus neoformans* is less common but has also been reported in dogs and should be considered as a potential differential diagnosis (see Chapter 61).[84] Dogs with disseminated aspergillosis do not generally have any clinically overt nasal involvement (see the following section).

Some dogs with nasal aspergillosis may have an underlying immunodeficiency that predisposes them to infection, and impaired lymphocyte blastogenesis responses have been reported.[3,127] However, whether impaired CMI is a cause or a result of infection is unclear because *A. fumigatus* products have been shown to inhibit lymphocyte transformation in vitro.[23] Impaired CMI can also persist long after the organism has been eliminated.[127] In immunocompromised people receiving low-dose itraconazole (ITZ) for prevention of aspergillosis, infection developed with non-*Aspergillus* fungi that were less susceptible to the drug.[96]

Invasion of bone is usually restricted to nasal turbinates; however, infection from the nasal passages can spread through the cribriform plate, palatine bone, or through the orbit, causing osteolysis. In people, invasive sinonasal aspergillosis occurs primarily in immunocompromised hosts. Mucosal invasion is followed by infarction and necrosis and spread of infection in a centrifugal fashion to adjacent mucosae and bone.[138]

Pulmonary aspergillosis is the primary form of localized disease observed in people. The long nasal passages of dogs may more effectively trap *Aspergillus* spores before they reach the lower airways. Pulmonary aspergillosis caused by *A. niger* was documented in a dog.[74]

Clinical Findings

Clinical and historical signs consistent with nasal aspergillosis in dogs include mucopurulent nasal discharge, sneezing, signs

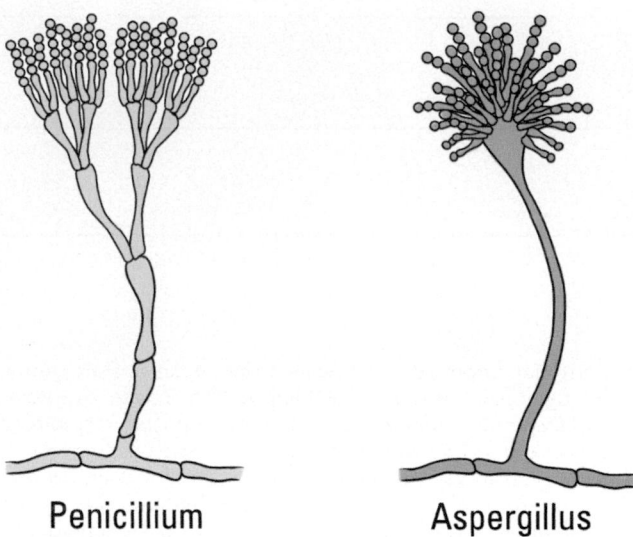

Penicillium **Aspergillus**

Fig 64-1 *Aspergillus* spp. *(right)* Septate hyphae (2 to 8 μm) give rise to unbranched conidiophores. Each conidiophore has a rounded tip (vesicle) covered with flask shaped phialides, which support chains of round conidia. *Penicillium* spp. *(left)* Septate hyphae (2 to 5 μm) give rise to branched or unbranched conidiophores with secondary branches. Secondary branching gives *Penicillium* its brushlike appearance. Flask-shaped phialides support chains of round conidia.

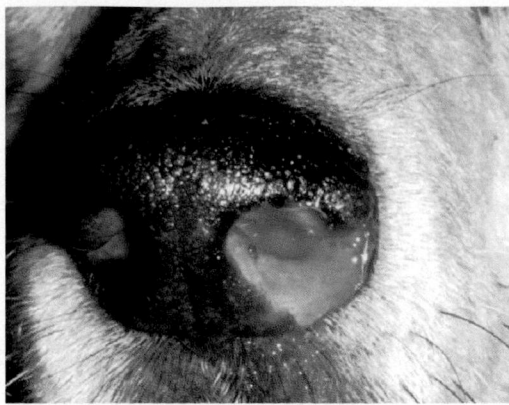

Fig 64-2 Ulceration of the external nares in association with *A. fumigatus* infection. (Courtesy Kyle Mathews, North Carolina State University, Raleigh, N.C.)

of nasal discomfort (pawing at the face or pain on palpation), epistaxis, decreased appetite, lethargy, and nasal planum depigmentation or ulceration (Fig. 64-2). Stertor, stridor, openmouth breathing, or any combination may also be noted. Nasal discharge is initially unilateral in most cases but often progresses to bilateral involvement caused by destruction of the midline nasal septum. *A. fumigatus* has been shown to produce an endotoxin that is both hemolytic and dermonecrotic.[143] This toxin presumably causes the turbinate necrosis and erosion of the rhinarium, which occur in infected animals. With time, paranasal extension may result in facial swelling; nasolacrimal duct obstruction or destruction may result in epiphora. Orbital invasion can result in oculonasal discharge, exophthalmos, discomfort on opening the mouth, corneal injury, or strabismus. Enophthalmos and phthisis bulbi may be found in the healing stages.[160] Erosion of the cribriform plate, if it occurs, usually does not result in clinical signs but may preclude topical therapy. On rare occasions, with fulminant invasive fungal rhinitis or sinusitis, an animal will show signs of intracranial disease that are caused by extension of nasal or frontal sinus infection.[100] In other animals, with more long-standing and less virulent nasal fungal infections, arthrolithiasis or pastelike exudates may develop within the nasal passages or sinuses as a result of caseous sinusitis caused by the organism.[94] With this mycetoma formation, radiographic studies may show sinus opacification often with flocculent calcification. Mucopurulent, cheesy or claylike material is often found by surgical or endoscopic examination. Histopathologic changes are a dense conglomeration of hyphae separate from but adjacent to mucosa of the sinus. The mucosa itself has chronic suppurative inflammation without fungal invasion.

Signs of pulmonary aspergillosis include fever, cough, and mucopurulent nasal discharge. See disseminated infection later in this chapter for other signs should systemic spread develop.

Diagnosis

Physical examination should include facial palpation for evidence of pain or asymmetry, evaluation of airflow through

each nostril, and an oral examination. Established guidelines used to make a definitive diagnosis, include positive results on biopsy, a positive titer with positive culture results, or a positive titer with radiographic or computed tomography (CT) scan changes suggestive of fungal rhinitis (turbinate loss).

Organism Cultivation

Aspergillus spp. can be isolated from cultures of the nasal passages as a result of colonization of the immunocompetent host. Unfortunately, confirmation of the diagnosis usually requires multiple independent tests because *Aspergillus* spp. are often part of the endogenous flora in the nasal cavity of many animals, and culture alone is unreliable and misleading (Fig. 64-3).[56] Culture should be performed from biopsy specimens of healthy and diseased nasal and sinus mucosae and bone adjacent to areas of necrosis. Paired specimens should also be evaluated for histopathology. Laboratory culture is also needed to differentiate *Aspergillus* or *Penicillium* infections from other saprophytic infections, such as those caused by *Mucorales* or *Alternaria* spp. In addition, fungal culture results may also be negatively affected by secondary bacterial overgrowth. *Pseudomonas* spp. and Enterobacteriaceae cause common secondary infections of necrotic tissue within the nasal chamber.

Serologic Testing

Numerous techniques for determination of *Aspergillus* serum fungal-specific antibody titers have been evaluated, including agar gel double diffusion (AGDD), counter-immunoelectrophoresis (CIE), and enzyme-linked immunosorbent assay (ELISA) techniques. AGDD and CIE tests have been reported to be highly sensitive and specific, while ELISA appears to be less reliable.[73,77,110] However, negative AGDD results should be viewed with some skepticism if the clinical, radiographic, and rhinoscopic picture is consistent with fungal rhinitis. Earlier studies using this method had low false-negative results, but multiple *Aspergillus* antigens preparations were used. Current AGDD tests typically use only one antigen, and their accuracy has not been well documented. We (KGM and NJHS) have obtained several false negative results using AGDD (Meridian Diagnostics, Inc., Fungal immunodiffusion system, Cincinnati, Ohio) early in the disease process from histologically confirmed cases of nasal aspergillosis. Many of these cases had positive titer results when retested at a later date. Furthermore, nasal *Penicillium* infection, which is clinically indistinguishable from aspergillosis, can result in a negative AGDD test result if only *Aspergillus* antigens are used.[56]

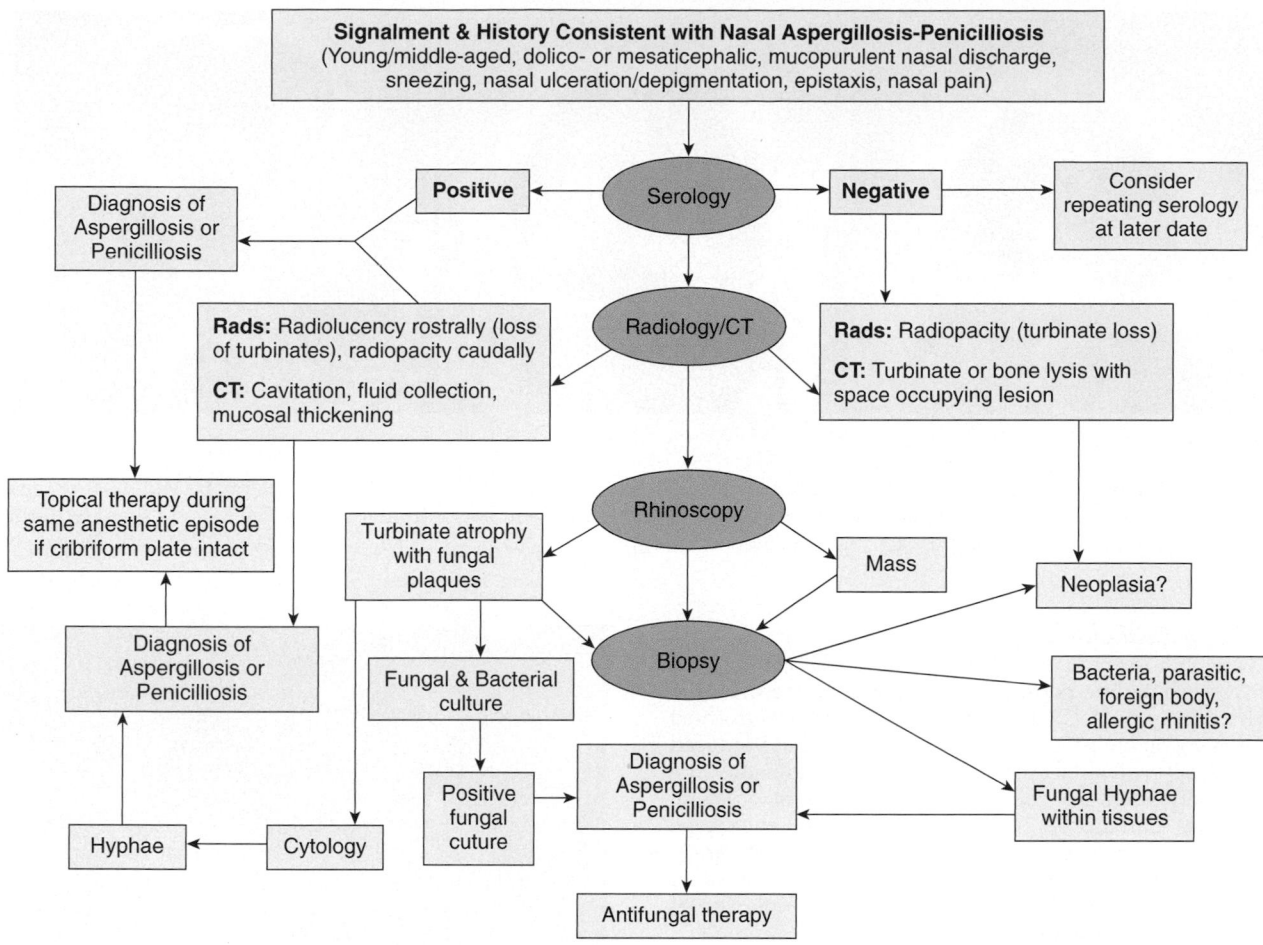

Fig 64-3 Decision-making algorithm for the diagnostic evaluation of dogs with clinical signs consistent with nasal aspergillosis-penicilliosis.

In addition, a positive result does not eliminate the possibility of a concurrent disease process such as neoplasia. Request for an *Aspergillus* titer, followed by general anesthesia, a radiographic evaluation, and rhinoscopy with the intent to perform biopsy and culture, is a logical diagnostic approach (see Fig. 64-3).

Antigen or Genetic Detection
See these topics later in this chapter under Disseminated Aspergillosis in Dogs.

Radiographic Imaging
Nasal and frontal sinus radiographs can be used as a screening tool to evaluate dogs with suspected fungal rhinitis. Rostral radiolucency (cavitary destruction) caused by turbinate lysis or a mixed pattern of caudal lucency and opacity (or both) are usually seen on dorsoventral views, while increased radio opacity and frontal bone thickening on rostrocaudal "skyline" views are typical.[139] Nonspecific thickening of the mucosa of the inner surface of bones of the frontal sinus, maxillary recess, and nasal cavity is often noted.[119] Changes may be asymmetrical because the disease may affect one nasal cavity initially and then spread to the opposite side. The CT and magnetic resonance imaging (MRI) anatomy of the mesaticephalic canine nasal cavity has been well described.[36,48] Studies have shown that CT is superior to radiography for defining the extent of nasal disease, detection of cortical bone lesions, and in differentiating infectious from neoplastic rhinitis.[25,99] MRI was helpful in differentiating between a thickened mucosa and secretions or fungal colonies.[116a] Nasal neoplasia results in loss of turbinates and bone, but these structures are replaced by a soft-tissue density (mass). Fungal rhinitis is typified by loss of turbinates with resultant air-filled cavities and mucosal thickening resulting from edema and inflammation (Fig. 64-4).[118,119] In some cases of nasal aspergillosis, even CT images may be difficult to interpret because significant accumulations of fluid may occur and obscure fungal granulomas, concomitant masses, or turbinate and frontal sinus detail. CT or MRI is required to evaluate the integrity of the cribriform plate.

Response to Empirical Therapy
Topical treatment may be performed without advanced imaging techniques if nasal radiographs and other diagnostic tests are suggestive of fungal infection. However, if evidence of caudal nasal involvement exists, referral for CT is recommended. This course of action is recommended because erosion of the cribriform plate may contraindicate the use of topical infusions. Although complications arising from leakage of antifungal medications into the central nervous system (CNS) of dogs with fungal rhinitis have not been well described, neurologic complications resulting in euthanasia following topical therapy have been reported in two animals with suspected cribriform damage.[85] Owners of affected dogs should be informed of this concern before attempting topical therapy with large volumes of antifungal medication infused under pressure. If cribriform involvement is detected on CT, dogs may be treated with oral ITZ.

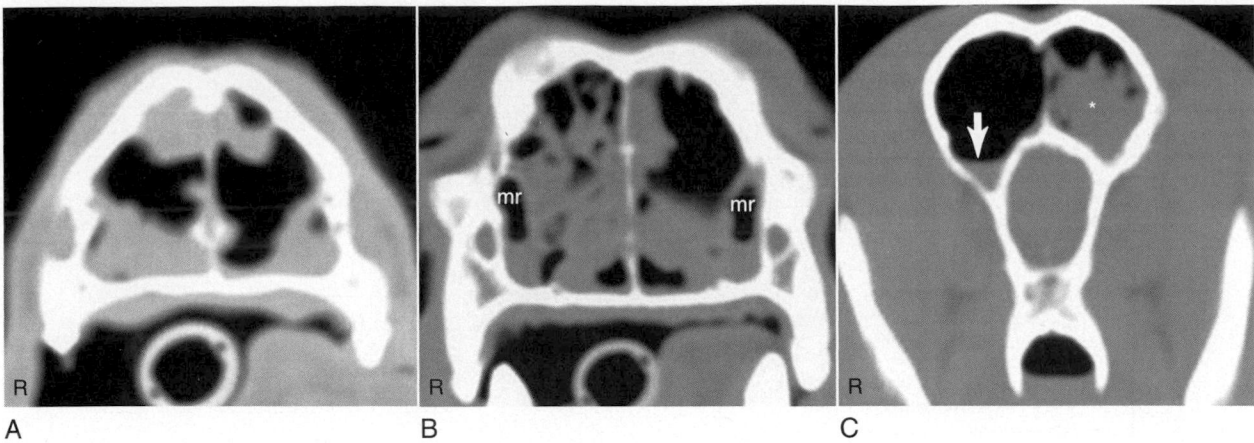

Fig 64-4 CT transverse images of a dog with nasal aspergillosis (same dog as in Figure 64-8). **A,** Rostral; **B,** Mid-nasal at the level of the maxillary recesses *(mr)*; **C,** Caudal at the level of the cribriform plate and lateral frontal sinuses. Cavitation caused by turbinate destruction *(*)*, fluid accumulation *(arrow)*, fungal granuloma. (Courtesy Kyle Mathews, North Carolina State University, Raleigh, N.C.)

Endoscopic Evaluation

Following radiographic or CT evaluation of the nasal cavity, rhinoscopy should be performed, preferably during the same anesthetic episode.[88] Nasal examination is never performed before radiographic procedures because hemorrhage induced by rhinoscopy will alter the results. A sterile rigid endoscope is commonly used for rhinoscopy. Evaluation of a lateral frontal sinus can also be performed with a rigid endoscope after penetrating the dorsal wall of the sinus with a Steinman pin. A flexible bronchoscope has the added advantage of allowing visualization of the nasopharynx by retroflexion of the bronchoscope around the soft palate.

After inserting the endoscope through the rostral nares, it is first directed into the ventral nasal meatus toward the nasopharynx. It is then directed into the dorsal nasal meatus toward the olfactory epithelium, the openings (ostia) of the frontal sinuses, and the cribriform plate. If dorsal examination were performed first, hemorrhage may potentially result in an inability to explore the ventral nasal cavity thoroughly. The advantages of direct visualization of the nasal cavity include a more thorough understanding of the nature of the disease process and the potential to place a biopsy instrument at the area of interest. Many endoscopes are equipped with biopsy ports or sleeves that simplify tissue sampling. In addition, a biopsy instrument may be inserted alongside the endoscope if space permits. Additionally, a cuffed endotracheal tube is required, as is packing the pharynx with laparotomy sponges to prevent aspiration of blood, flush, and nasal secretions.

Biopsy specimens are placed in 10% buffered formalin for histologic examination, in appropriate media for bacterial and fungal cultures, and are also rolled onto glass slides for immediate cytologic examination (Fig. 64-5). Following resolution of hemorrhage and before recovery from anesthesia, pharyngeal sponges are removed, and the pharynx is suctioned.

Rhinoscopic evaluation of dogs with aspergillosis typically reveals areas of turbinate atrophy, mucopurulent discharge, and fungal plaques. Fungal plaques may be white, off-white, or have a greenish tint. The surface of a plaque may be fuzzy in appearance resulting from the presence of conidiophores (fruiting bodies) (Fig. 64-6, *A* and *B*). Collections of exudate should not be mistaken for plaques.

If a diagnosis of nasal aspergillosis is rendered following nasal examination based on consistent radiographic or CT findings and the presence of fungal plaques or hyphae, or both, on cytologic examination, topical treatment may be performed during the same anesthetic episode.

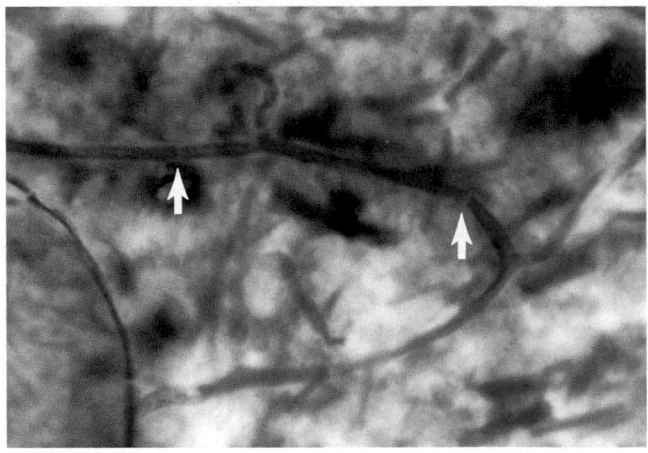

Fig 64-5 Nasal cytologic specimen collected during rhinoscopic evaluation of a dog nasal aspergillosis. Note septate hyphae *(arrows).* (Courtesy Eleanor Hawkins, North Carolina State University, Raleigh, N.C.)

Pathologic Findings

Biopsy of suspicious lesions is required to demonstrate mucosal invasion. Histopathologic abnormalities of tissue biopsy specimens are erosions and ulcerations of respiratory epithelium, submucosal infiltrates with lymphocytes, plasma cells and neutrophils, and a neutrophilic exudate surrounding large mats of branching septate fungal hyphae. The hyphae have terminal bulbs with swellings consistent with *Aspergillus* spp.

Therapy
Systemic Therapy

Treatment of nasal aspergillosis with systemic antifungal medications such as thiabendazole, ketoconazole (KTZ), and fluconazole has been disappointing in that the reported successful response rate is only 43% to 60%.* Response to oral administration of ITZ has been approximated at 60% to 70%,[83] but currently, no large studies evaluating systemic treatment with ITZ have been done, and cost of the drug is often prohibitive. Hepatic toxicosis may mandate temporary or permanent discontinuation of ITZ in 5% to 10% of dogs,

*References: 54, 55, 56, 123, 125, 127, 129, 130.

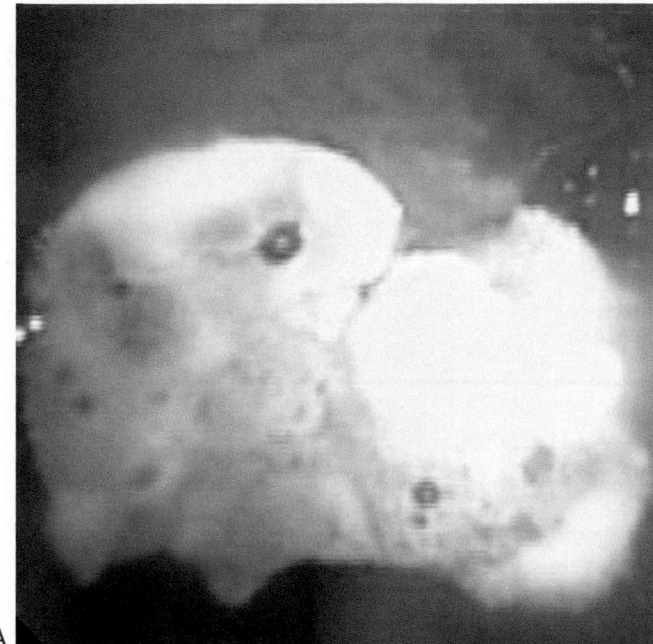

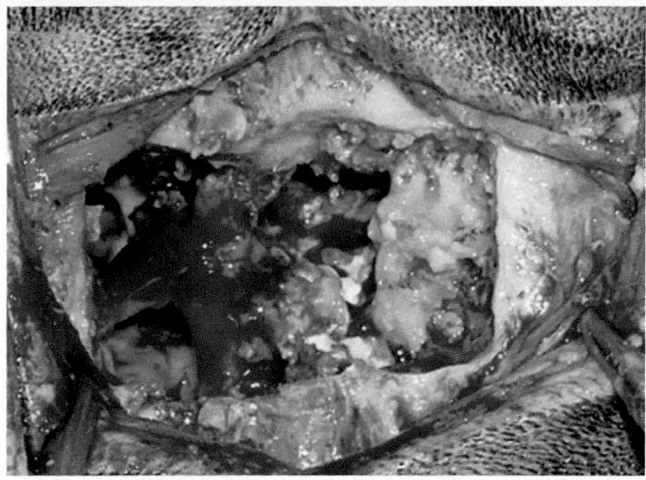

Fig 64-6 **A,** Endoscopic appearance of a fungal granuloma from within the nasal passage near the connection with the frontal sinus. Loss of turbinate bone is apparent, and the mass is golden-brown in color. Some of the surface is white and fuzzy in appearance caused by the presence of *Aspergillus* conidiophores. **B,** Similar fungal granuloma within the lateral frontal sinus of Rottweiler with nasal aspergillosis, as viewed by surgical sinusotomy and rhinostomy. (**A** courtesy Christiane Stengel, University of Georgia, Athens, Ga.; **B** courtesy Kyle Mathews, North Carolina State University, Raleigh, N.C.)

and serial monitoring of serum alanine aminotransferase (ALT) concentration is recommended.[83] Fluconazole at oral doses of 2.5 to 5.0 mg/kg was effective for treatment of canine nasal aspergillosis; however, the success was lower than that using topical enilconazole.[125]

Systemic therapy is indicated as part of the treatment regimen if the fungus has invaded extranasal structures. For dosages of recommended antifungal drugs, see Table 64-1. The results obtained for systemic therapy are not as good as those obtained for topical agents. Systemic antifungal therapy can be associated with side effects of hepatotoxicity or cutaneous eruptions.

Amphotericin B (AMB) has been used in the past to treat nasal aspergillosis in dogs.[5,134] The results were generally

unsuccessful, and it is not recommended. Given that AMB has some efficacy against pulmonary disseminated infections in people and disseminated infections in dogs (see later discussion), the problem likely relates to insufficient concentrations in the nasal passages by systemic administration. Terbinafine, an antifungal drug used to treat disseminated aspergillosis in people, has been tried on an empirical basis, alone and in combination with azole drugs, to treat refractory cases of nasal aspergillosis. Further studies are needed to determine the efficacy of this drug in nasal aspergillosis.

Topical Therapy

Topical administration of enilconazole and clotrimazole is more effective compared with orally administered antifungal medications.* Intranasal administration of enilconazole requires a sinusotomy to place indwelling catheters into the nasal cavity or frontal sinuses, or both.[127,131] However, intrasinusal administration of enilconazole was described using endoscopically placed catheters passed into the frontal sinuses and nasal passages.[163] After catheter placement, 5 to 10 ml (50 mg/ml = 10 mg/kg) of enilconazole are administered twice daily for 1 to 2 weeks. Larger volumes are avoided because of risk of aspiration. Nasal discharge resolved in 19 (80%) of 24 dogs treated solely with topical administration of enilconazole.[131] Common complications include premature removal of catheters, transient postoperative subcutaneous emphysema, inappetence, and ptyalism.[127,130,131] As previously noted, erosion of the cribriform plate may be a contraindication to infusion of large volumes of topical medications under pressure. However, one of the authors (NS) has treated two dogs with small volumes of enilconazole, as noted here, without adverse effect.

A 1-hour infusion of clotrimazole, administered to anesthetized dogs, resulted in the resolution of clinical signs in many cases.[13,29,85] Topical administration of clotrimazole causes direct damage to fungal membranes and inhibits fungal ergosterol synthesis.[63] Although a surgical procedure (sinusotomy) was used for catheter placement into the frontal sinuses, many cases resolved after a single treatment.[27] In addition, the complications associated with indwelling catheters were eliminated, and hospitalization times were substantially reduced.

In a study evaluating the distribution of dye injected into cadaver skulls of normal dogs, a noninvasive technique for intranasal infusion resulted in better distribution of infusate within the nasal cavity and paranasal sinuses than did techniques that used catheters placed via sinusotomy (Fig. 64-7.).[109] Large volumes of infusate may be administered and leakage minimal because the nares and nasopharynx were occluded during intranasal infusion. With cadaver skulls placed in dorsal recumbency, bilateral administration of 50 ml (100 ml total) through the nares resulted in excellent distribution of infusate to the entire nasal cavity and frontal sinuses with minimal leakage into the pharynx.[109] This noninvasive intranasal technique resulted in good distribution of infusate to the nasal cavity and frontal sinuses, as determined by evaluation of pre- and postinfusion images on CT scans, in 12 dogs with confirmed fungal rhinitis.[86] The percentage of the lateral sinus filled with infusate varied from 10% (enough to cover the roof of the lateral sinus) to 100% (mean, 42%). The infusate that mixed with present exudates, as outlined previously, obscured fungal granulomas.[86]

One study evaluated 60 dogs with nasal aspergillosis treated with 1-hour infusions of clotrimazole.[85] The goals of the study were to examine the clinical response to topical administration of clotrimazole in dogs with nasal aspergillosis and to compare the efficacy of surgical versus nonsurgical placement of

*References: 13, 29, 83, 85, 119a, 127, 130, 131, 133, 160, 163.

Table • 64-1

Therapy for Nasal Aspergillosis

DRUG[a]	SPECIES	DOSE[b] (mg/kg)	ROUTE	INTERVAL (HOURS)	DURATION
Amphotericin B (deoxycholate)	D	0.25	IV	48	[c]
Itraconazole	B	5	PO	12	prn[d]
Fluconazole	D	2.5—5.0	PO	24	prn[d]
Amphotericin B lipid complex	D	2—3	IV	3 days per week	[e]
	C	1	IV	3 days per week	[f]
Terbinafine	D	5	PO	12	prn[g]

D, Dog; B, dog and cat; C, cat; PO, by mouth; IV, intravenous; prn, as needed.

[a]For additional information, see Drug Formulary, Appendix 8.

[b]Dose per administration at specified interval.

[c]Until a cumulative dose of 4 to 8 mg/kg is reached for cats and 8 to 12 mg/kg for dogs.

[d]Therapy to control infection may require months to years, although clinical remissions may be achieved; the infection may reactivate in a variable time period after discontinuing treatment. Topical therapy with azole drugs is generally superior to systemic administration for nasal aspergillosis; see text and reference 119a.

[e]For a total of 9 to 12 treatments until a cumulative dose of 24 to 27 mg/kg is reached.

[f]For a total of 12 treatments until a cumulative dose of 12 mg/kg is reached.

[g]This dose is extrapolated from human studies. No efficacy studies have been conducted on this drug for treatment of aspergillosis in dogs or cats; however, it has been used empirically in nonresponsive cases.

catheters. Topical 1% clotrimazole solution was infused during a 1-hour period via surgically placed frontal sinus and nasal catheters (27 dogs) and via nonsurgically placed intranasal catheters (18 dogs). An additional 15 dogs required and received two to four infusions by either route. Topical administration of clotrimazole resulted in resolution of clinical disease in 65% of dogs after one treatment and in 87% of dogs after one or more treatments. No difference in outcome was noted between surgically and nonsurgically placed catheters.

Topical administration of clotrimazole, using either technique, is therefore an effective treatment for nasal aspergillosis in dogs. The use of noninvasive intranasal infusion of clotrimazole eliminates the need for surgical trephination of the frontal sinuses in many dogs and is associated with fewer complications.[13,85,133] The most common posttreatment complication in dogs treated by trephination of the frontal sinuses was subcutaneous emphysema. Subcutaneous and retrobulbar leakage and nasolacrimal duct filling of clotrimazole have also occurred with no apparent adverse effects. Nasal discharge ceases in most dogs by 2 weeks after topical clotrimazole therapy.[85] A repeat treatment is recommended if nasal discharge continues without improvement 2 weeks after the initial treatment. Sequential evaluation of Aspergillus titers does not aid in the decision to re-treat because titers may remain elevated for years despite resolution of disease.[126,127]

The volume of the nasal cavity and frontal sinuses varies depending on the size of the dog, the extent of turbinate destruction, and the volume of accumulated exudate. Based on a study in cadavers, the average volume of the frontal sinuses in breeds predisposed to fungal rhinitis was 25 ml per side.[109] The nasal cavity and sinuses can be flooded with a larger volume of infusate (50 to 60 ml per side), resulting in distribution of the infusate to all areas of the nasal cavity and frontal sinuses. A 1% formulation of clotrimazole in a polyethylene glycol base (Lotrimin® solution, Schering Corporation, Kenilworth, N.J.) is readily available in a 30-ml vial, which makes treatment with two vials per side convenient. Sixty ml per side is used in mid-sized to large breed dogs, regardless of head size. Thirty ml per side should be adequate for smaller breeds. Formulations that contain polyethylene glycol, isopropyl alcohol, and propylene glycol (Canesten® solution, Miles Canada, Etobicoke, Ontario, Canada) should be used with caution because they may result in pharyngeal irritation and edema.[19,28]

Preliminary information on the use of enilconazole (Imaverol, Janssen-Cilag SA, Beerse, Belgium) administered in a similar fashion was not favorable. Of four dogs treated in this manner, one resolved after two treatments, one died from sepsis after the second treatment, and two developed profuse fungal growth in the face of therapy.[10] In a group of 10 dogs treated with a 1-hour Imaverol infusion, five were cured and five failed treatment.[59] In both cases, fairly high concentrations of enilconazole were given (5% to 10%). These concentrations are probably much higher than necessary to kill the fungus, and the carrier detergent may result in irritation of the nasal mucosa if left in place for 1 hour.[10] Subsequent studies using 1% Imaverol as a 1-hour soak have reported more favorable results.[117,163] Twenty of 36 dogs (56%) were cured after a single treatment, and 34 of 35 (94%) were cured after one to three treatments.[117] Enilconazole is available for poultry in the United States as Clinafarm-EC (Sterwin Labs, Inc., Millsboro, Del.). Clinafarm-EC contains alcohol and therefore should be used with some caution until more information is available. Clinifarm-EC (5%) has been used as a 1-hour infusion.[89] In this study, the drug was administered to six anesthetized dogs after endoscopic placement of catheters in the caudal portion of the nasal cavity and frontal sinuses.[89] The dogs received two to three treatments, with 50 to 200 ml infused during each treatment. All six dogs showed favorable clinical response soon after treatment. Two dogs were treated with ITZ concurrently. Three dogs that were followed for a mean of 16.5 months had marked clinical improvement. Using similar endoscopic placement of infusion catheters, 2% enilconazole (Imaverol) infused over 1 hour resulted in cure in all six dogs in one report.[163] Three of the six dogs were treated simultaneously with oral KTZ.

A 1-hour infusion with 1% clotrimazole or enilconazole (Imaverol) should now be considered the treatment of choice for nasal aspergillosis-penicilliosis when the cribriform plate is intact. If the cribriform plate is damaged, then systemically active drugs should be given. Re-treatment with infusions should be performed if nasal discharge does not cease within 2 weeks. In one study, clotrimazole was infused directly in the frontal sinuses via trephine holes.[44] Whether an advantage to using enilconazole exists for the second treatment if the first was with clotrimazole, and vice versa, is unclear. The decision to treat via intranasal infusion with the patient in dorsal recumbency versus sinusotomy with the patient in sternal

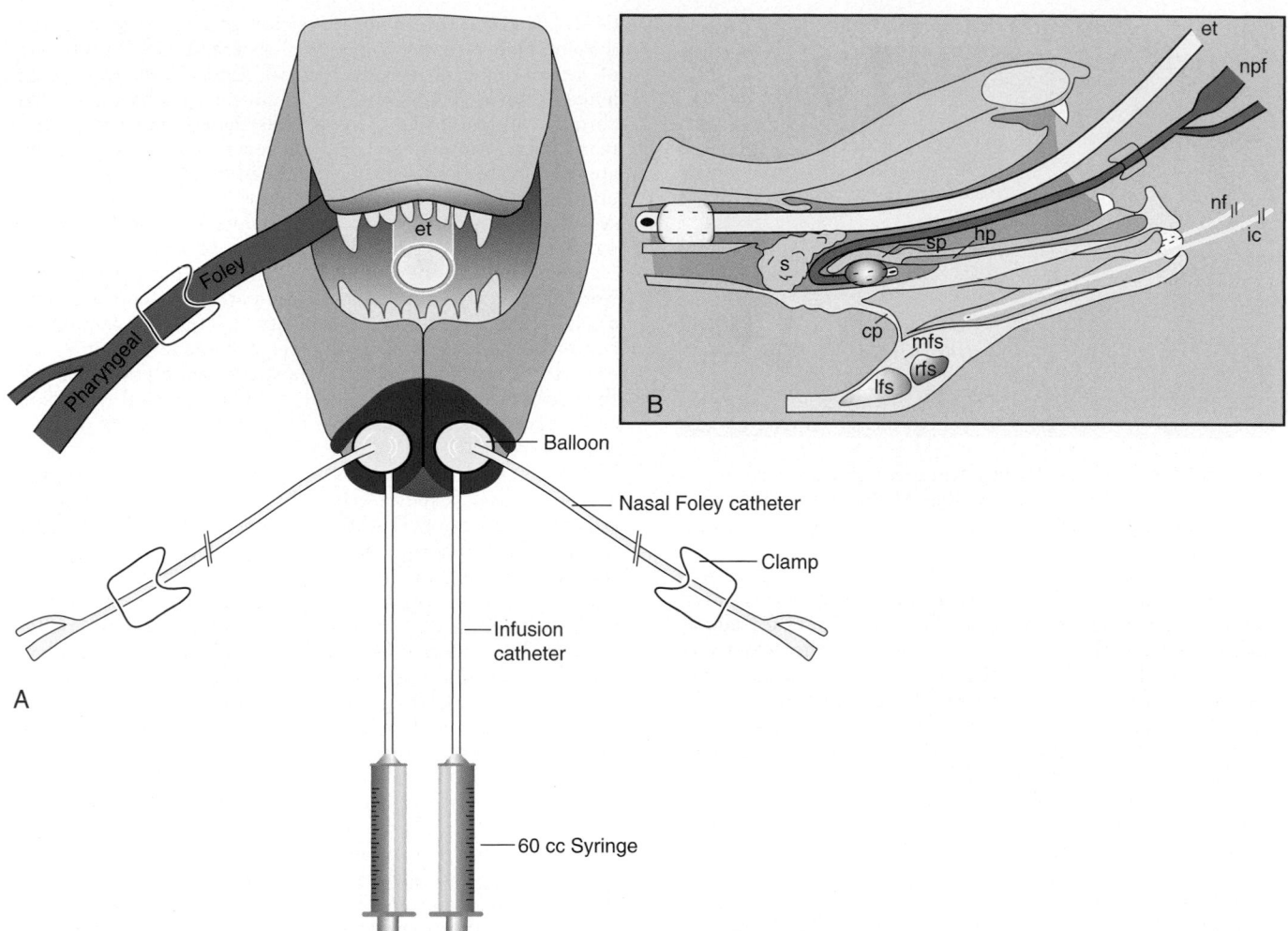

Fig 64-7 **A,** Catheter position with the dog in dorsal recumbency. A Foley catheter with the balloon inflated in the nasopharynx and pharyngeal gauze sponges (not shown) minimize leakage of infusate caudally. A cuffed endotracheal tube *(et)* further diminishes the risk of aspiration. Sixty-milliliter syringes are used to inject infusate into the dorsal nasal meatus via polypropylene infusion catheters. Inflated Foley catheter balloons obstruct the nares to diminish leakage of infusate rostrally. Tubing clamps on Foley catheters are closed when fluid is observed within the catheter lumen. **B,** Sagittal section showing the position of the endotracheal tube *(et)*, nasopharyngeal Foley catheter *(npf)*, pharyngeal sponges *(s)*, infusion catheter *(ic)*, and rostral nasal Foley catheter *(nf)* in relation to the hard palate *(hp)*, soft palate *(sp)*, cribriform plate *(cp)*, rostral frontal sinus *(rfs)*, medial frontal sinus *(mfs)*, and lateral frontal sinus *(lfs)*. (From Mathews KG et al. 1996. Computed tomographic assessment of noninvasive intranasal infusions in dogs with fungal rhinitis, *Vet Surg* 25:309–319, 1996. Reprinted with permission.)

recumbency should be based on the presence or absence of fungal granulomas within the frontal sinuses. We (KGM and NJHS) have seen several cases fail with topical clotrimazole therapy when a large granuloma was evident within a frontal sinus. Clinical signs typically improve but do not completely resolve. Our assumption is that penetration of the drug into the center of the granuloma is inadequate and results in regrowth. Following sinusotomy, curettage, lavage, and suction to remove large fungal balls, topical treatment via the sinusotomy is usually effective.

In the few cases in which 1-hour topical infusions of 1% clotrimazole or enilconazole (Imaverol) fail, the placement of indwelling tubes for instillation of enilconazole over 1 to 2 weeks (as previously noted) might be considered as a salvage treatment.

Topical therapy will often fail when the organism invades soft-tissue structures outside of the nasal cavity. These cases require a combination of topical therapy (assuming the cribriform plate is intact) with a systemically active agent such as ITZ.[85,113,131]

Open nasal cavity treatment of nasal aspergillosis with povidone-iodine solution has been reported but is used only for cases that fail less aggressive treatment options.[93,104]

We have had to resort to this method in one animal which failed to resolve following sinusotomy and multiple treatments with both enilconazole and clotrimazole. Resolution of nasal aspergillosis (mixed infection with *A. fumigatus* and *A. niger*) in this case required a combination of open nasal cavity treatment with simultaneous oral administration of ITZ (Fig. 64-8).

Surgery
Rhinotomy or sinusotomy and turbinectomy have no roles in the treatment of fungal rhinitis other than to remove fungal granulomas, fungus balls, or mycetomas. The tendency to continue with a turbinectomy should be strongly resisted. Turbinectomy is of no benefit in controlling the nasal discharges and is often detrimental.* Care must be taken to cause as little damage as possible to nasal and turbinate mucosa and to the nasofrontal ostia.[86,149]

Prognosis
The best indication of successful therapy is the rapid resolution of nasal discharge or epistaxis, pain, and ulcerated nares. In some dogs, a mild serous to mucopurulent, crusty discharge

*References: 54, 78, 131, 152, 153.

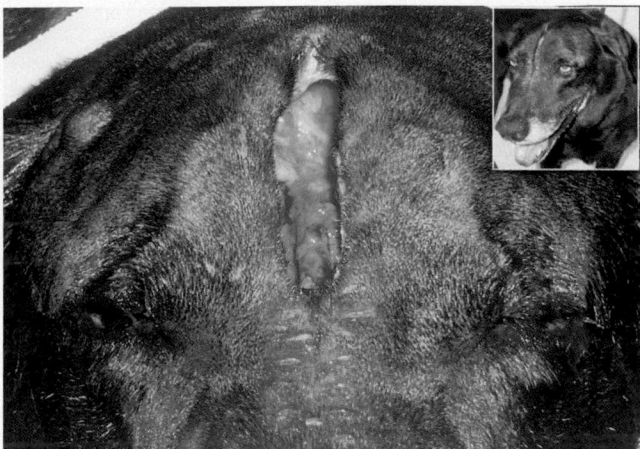

Fig 64-8 Open nasal cavity treatment of a dog with recurrent nasal aspergillosis. (Courtesy Kyle Mathews, North Carolina State University, Raleigh, N.C.)

may persist at one or both nostrils, presumably as a result of the reorganized nasal architecture. In evaluation of CT abnormalities, no correlation was found between the severity of changes on CT with the response to intranasal infusion of enilconazole; however, dogs with the least abnormalities had the best clinical response to one infusion.[117] Serology is of only limited value in assessing the response to treatment. Although titers tend to decline within 1 to 2 years of successful therapy, this occurrence is not a reliable indicator. Positive titer results may persist for more than 2 years using ELISA methodology or for 5 years using agar gel immunodiffusion (AGID) in dogs that remain free of disease.[127]

Relapse of fungal disease does not appear to be a common problem with canine nasal aspergillosis-penicilliosis once the clinical signs of infection have been eliminated. Of 43 dogs that had shown complete resolution of clinical signs after treatment with a variety of systemic and topical antifungal drugs, only one suffered a relapse of fungal rhinitis during followup periods, ranging from 6 months to 5.5 years.[127] Similarly, recurrent fungal rhinitis was documented in only 1 of 60 dogs following clotrimazole treatment.[85] A bacterial rhinitis may develop in up to 12% to 25% of dogs after successful resolution of the primary fungal disease, possibly because of previous destruction of the nasal anatomy by the fungus. Bacterial rhinitis is characterized by a return of the profuse mucopurulent nasal discharge but usually without epistaxis or facial pain. Fungal plaques are absent in these dogs, and the discharge responds to antibiotic therapy based on culture and antimicrobial susceptibility results.[78,85,131,152]

Public Health Considerations
No instances of infection in people arising from dogs or cats have been documented. Infection in all species occurs from common environmental sources. A prudent course of action, however, for the clinician is to inform an owner that immunosuppressed individuals should not be exposed to affected animals that may be discharging large quantities of fungal hyphae and spores.

FELINE NASAL ASPERGILLOSIS-PENICILLIOSIS

Kyle G. Mathews and Kamil Tomsa

Although rarely reported, both *Aspergillus* and *Penicillium* spp. have been incriminated in sinonasal infections in cats (Table

64-2). Systemic immunosuppression is not critical to the development of nasal or paranasal aspergillosis.[2,123] Only one of seven reported cats with nasal aspergillosis was feline leukemia virus (FeLV) positive.[49] Clinical signs have included chronic mucopurulent nasal discharge, epistaxis, and mandibular lymphadenomegaly. In several cases, the infection appeared to begin in, or then extended into, the extranasal or orbital tissues, causing exophthalmos.[51,52,105,157] The clinical symptoms are usually localized to one side of the nasal-paranasal-orbital cavities, but the disease can be bilateral. Nasal aspergillosis-penicilliosis is clinically indistinguishable from chronic viral rhinitis and nasal-paranasal neoplasia, and, as in these conditions, secondary bacterial infection is common. Bone erosion and focal soft-tissue opacities are typical but are nonspecific diagnostic imaging findings in all the previously listed clinical entities. Chronic viral rhinitis in cats is usually bilateral and does not cause loss of teeth, as does nasal neoplasia.[97]

Identification of irregular mineralized densities in the nasal-paranasal cavities should raise the suspicion of *Aspergillus* infection (Fig. 64-9, *A* and *B*).[94,144] Rhinoscopic findings were reported in three affected cats and included diffuse reddening of nasal mucosa, copious white-grey discharge, profound loss of turbinates, and the presence of a white-yellow mass.[144] The diagnosis of feline nasal aspergillosis-penicilliosis should be based on typical clinical and diagnostic imaging findings accompanied by histologic evidence of pyogranulomatous fungal rhinitis, with variable degrees of tissue invasion and necrosis. Fungal culture should be best attempted on samples taken directly from fungal colonies within the respiratory passages. However, culture was successful in only two of seven reported cases.[52,105] Presence of serum anti-*Aspergillus* antibodies in affected cats has been documented by AGID test[49] and serum immunoelectrophoresis[144] and may be considered useful noninvasive diagnostic information. Further studies may be needed to determine the prevalence of these antibodies in clinically healthy cats and those with other non-*Aspergillus* nasal disorders.

Currently, only limited information is available regarding the best therapeutic approach. Systemic therapy with ITZ was attempted in two animals. One cat with extranasal involvement had progressive worsening of clinical signs and was euthanized despite treatment with ITZ, topical clotrimazole, and surgery.[52] Another animal with disease confined to the nasal-paranasal cavity had to have ITZ therapy stopped after 6 weeks because of hepatotoxicity.[144] Clinical signs recurred in this cat, but they abated following a single treatment with intranasal clotrimazole. Treatment with noninvasive 1-hour infusion of topical clotrimazole, combined with systemic therapy, if extranasal involvement is present, is a reasonable approach until more information is available. ITZ is preferable to KTZ for systemic therapy in cats and should be given at a dosage of 10 mg/kg once daily.[83,91] Sinusotomy may be a final resort to remove fungal balls or mycetomas and provide drainage.[49,162] The prognosis for a resolution of clinical illness and fungal infection in feline sinonasal aspergillosis is generally poor.

CANINE DISSEMINATED ASPERGILLOSIS

Michael J. Day

Etiology and Pathogenesis
Most cases of canine disseminated aspergillosis have occurred in German shepherd dogs (age range, 2 to 8 years) and have been reported from Australia[31,72,154] and California.[31,66] The disease has also been documented in Spain,[101,106] Belgium,[24]

Table • 64-2

Summary of Cases of Feline Nasal Aspergillosis-Penicilliosis

SIGNALMENT HISTORY[a]	DIAGNOSIS	IMMUNOLOGY (I) CULTURE (C)	HISTOPATHOLOGY	RADIOGRAPHY	TREATMENT (T) OUTCOME (O)
6.5 yr, F, DSH, exophthalmos[105]	Bilateral sinonasal penicilliosis with orbital extension and fungal pneumonitis	I: None C: *Penicillium* spp.	Inflammation with necrosis and fungal hyphae	Increased opacity of sinuses, zygomatic lysis	T: None O: Euthanized
4 yr, M, DLH, exophthalmos[157]	Bilateral orbital aspergillosis with extension into frontal sinuses	I: None C: *Apsergillus* spp., *Pasteurella*	Inflammation with necrosis and fungal hyphae		T: None O: Euthanized
4 yr, M, DSH with previous viral URI, unilateral nasal discharge[49]	Right sided sinonasal aspergillosis	I: AGID positive for *A. fumigatus*; FeLV-positive C: Negative for fungus; heavy growth of hemolytic streptococci		Turbinate loss / nasal radiolucency, increased frontal sinus opacity	T: Rhinotomy O: Slow improvement, resolved 3 mos postoperatively
8 yr, M, Persian with epiphora, nasal discharge, exophthalmos[52]	Unilateral orbital, bilateral sinonasal, and nasopharyngeal aspergillosis	I: None C: *Aspergillus* spp., *Staphylococcus* spp.	Inflammation with fungal hyphae — morphology consistent with *Aspergillus* spp.	CT: soft-tissue mass effect in left orbit, and dorsal to soft palate; increased nasal and frontal sinus opacity	T: ITZ, sinusotomy, orbitotomy, topical clotrimazole O: Orbital involvement progressed requiring exenteration; euthanized 4 mos later for difficulty swallowing
2 yr, FS, Siamese with unilateral nasal discharge[144]	Unilateral nasal aspergillosis	I: IEP positive for *A. fumigatus*; C: Negative for fungus; *Pasteurella dagmatis*, α-hemolytic *Streptococcus* spp.	Inflammation with fungal hyphae		T: None O: Resolved spontaneously
12 yr, MN, Persian with bilateral nasal discharge, epiphora, epistaxis, sneezing[144]	*Aspergillus* or *Penicillium* fungal rhinitis with anterior uveitis	I: FeLV, FIV, coronavirus negative; IEP negative for *A. fumigatus* C: Negative for fungus; *Escherichia coli*	Inflammation with necrosis, calcification, and fungal hyphae	CT: unilateral turbinate loss with nasal object of similar density to teeth	T: None O: Euthanized
8 yr, MN, Persian with chronic unilateral nasal discharge[144]	Unilateral sinonasal aspergillosis	I: IEP positive for *A. fumigatus* C: Negative for fungus and bacteria	Frontal sinus inflammation with fungal hyphae, nasal inflammation	CT: unilateral turbinate loss, fluid in sinuses, vomer deviation, orbital bone thinning	T: 6 wks ITZ, followed by topical clotrimazole O: ITZ hepatotoxicity developed, stopped treatment; clinical signs recurred; treated with topical clotrimazole and oral enrofloxacin; clinically normal within 10 days.

Table • 64-2

Continued

SIGNALMENT HISTORY[a]	DIAGNOSIS	IMMUNOLOGY (I) CULTURE (C)	HISTOPATHOLOGY	RADIOGRAPHY	TREATMENT (T) OUTCOME (O)
8 yr, MN, DSH with sneezing, epistasis[153a]	Unilateral nasal, sinonasal *Aspergillus* or *Penicillium* infection	I: None C: None for fungus	Multifocal inflammation with fungal hyphae	CT: left nasal cavity	T: 4 mos ITZ O: Resolved for 8 mos after therapy stopped
9 yr, MN, Persian with purulent nasal discharge, periorbital swelling[153a]	Unilateral nasal mass and inflammation	I: AGID negative for *A. fumigatus* C: None	Chronic active inflammation with bone loss and hyphae	CT: fluid and mass unilateral in nasal passage, punctate bone lysis	T: 10 wks ITZ then fluconazole at relapse O: Resolved but then recurred 8 mos later
4 yr, MN, Himalayan with chronic purulent nasal discharge[153a]	Bilateral fungal rhinitis	I: None C: *A. niger*	Inflammation and disseminated fungal hyphae	CT: bilateral fluid and soft tissue accumulation, areas of bony lysis	T: 2 mos itratconazole, developed toxicity O: Recovered, one episode 9 mos later
8 yr, Sex not reported, sneezing and unilateral epstaxis[153a]		I: None C: None	Inflammation with fungal hyphae	CT: masses in both nasal cavities	T: ITZ just started O: No long-term follow-up available yet

MN, Male neutered; *FS,* female spayed; *URI,* upper respiratory infection; *CT,* computed tomography; *AGID,* agar gel immunodiffusion; *IEP,* serum immunoelectrophoresis; *FeLV,* feline leukemia virus; *FIV,* feline immunodeficiency virus; *ITZ,* itraconazole
[a]Numbers in this column indicate references cited at the end of this chapter or on the CD.

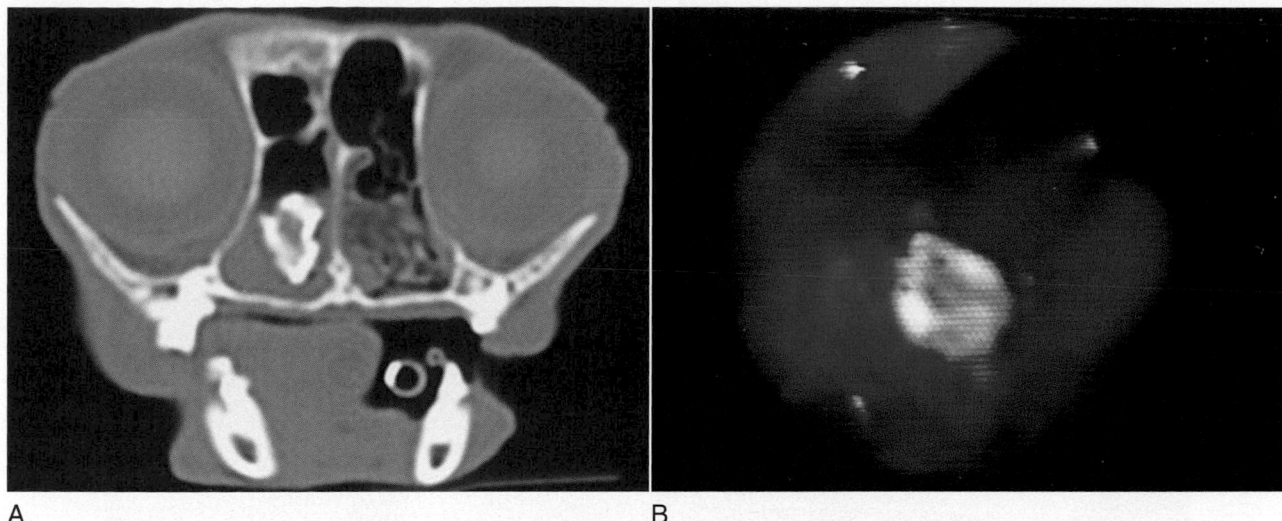

Fig 64-9 **A,** CT scan from a cat with nasal aspergillosis showing loss of turbinates and exudate bilaterally with a calcified density in the ventral aspect of the nasal passage. **B,** Endoscopic view of the same cat. (Courtesy Tomsa K, Glaus TM, Zimmer C, et al. 2003. Fungal rhinitis and sinusitis in three cats, *J Am Vet Med Assoc* 222: 1380–1384.)

the United Kingdom,[15] South Africa,[8] and the eastern United States.[15,26,47,70] Canine disseminated aspergillosis is probably more ubiquitous than the reports suggest. In cases in which the species has been identified, infection has involved, in decreasing frequency, *Aspergillus terreus*, *Aspergillus deflectus*, *Aspergillus flavipes*, and *A. fumigatus*. This finding contrasts with nasal aspergillosis (see previous discussion on Nasal Aspergillosis) in which *A. fumigatus* is most common. The portal of entry of *Aspergillus* is thought to be via the respiratory tract with subsequent hematogenous spread. Rare cases of infection restricted to the lungs are recorded.[45] As with any blood-borne pathogen, common sites of embolic dissemination of fungal organisms are the intervertebral disks, renal glomeruli, and uveal tracts. Other parenchymatous organs or muscles and long bones may be affected.

Disseminated aspergillosis in people is usually secondary to immunodeficiency or immune suppression, although invasive *Aspergillus* has been described in immunocompetent individuals.[69] The most common underlying predisposing factors are leukemia, neutrophil or macrophage dysfunction, neutropenia, acquired immunodeficiencies, and prior chronic antibacterial therapy.[1] The protective immune response to *Aspergillus* has been well characterized in murine models of infection and includes a variety of innate mechanisms (e.g., expression of Toll-like receptor-2 by pulmonary dendritic cells) in addition to T-helper cell (Th)1-regulated adaptive immunity characterized by the production of cytokines such as interleukin (IL)-18, IL-12, tumor necrotizing factor (TNF)-α, and interferon-γ (IFN-γ). Individuals that have dominant Th2 immunity develop progressive disease, and glucocorticoid therapy is known to stimulate Th2-driven immune responses.[7,22,82] In an experimental system, mice vaccinated with *Aspergillus* antigens developed a protective Th1 immune response; however, vaccination for aspergillosis is unlikely to have a role in a clinical setting.[21] In experimental infections, a sonicate vaccine given before the administration of glucocorticoids protected mice against lethal pulmonary aspergillosis.[62]

Predisposing factors for canine aspergillosis may include a combination of optimal climatic conditions, an access to particular strains of *Aspergillus*, and a subtle defect in mucosal immunity that may have a genetic basis.[33] German shepherd dogs are also susceptible to disseminated infection, with a range of other opportunistic fungi.[153] Glucocorticoids should

never be administered to dogs with aspergillosis, and their inadvertent use has precipitated dissemination of the infection in some cases.

Clinical Findings

Disease involves multiple organ systems and develops over several months, but most dogs are terminally ill when first examined. The most consistent clinical features are vertebral pain progressing to paraparesis, paraplegia, or limb lameness with pronounced swelling and discharging sinus tracts. A sudden onset of paraplegia may result from rupture of an infected intervertebral disk or vertebral subluxation from instability.

Other nonspecific clinical signs include anorexia, weight loss, muscle wasting, pyrexia, weakness, lethargy, and vomiting. Occasionally, dogs have clinical evidence of CNS involvement, lymphadenomegaly with cutaneous edema, and pyometra. Uveitis or endophthalmitis may be clinically apparent some months before generalized illness develops and thus may be important in early diagnosis.

Although uncommon, aspergillosis can also infect body cavities, either from hematogenous spread, or from local extension from a penetrating wound or foreign body. Further systemic spread can occur from these sites. Pericarditis and associated effusion can result in signs of right-sided heart failure such as abdominal distention from a modified transudate.[17] It can arise from rupture of a myocardial abscess, contiguous spread from the lung or hematogenous source. Intraabdominal infections can result from a perforating bowel or transabdominal catheter placement or penetrating wounds. Fever, GI signs, abdominal distention, and anorexia are the most common findings with abdominal infections.

Diagnosis

Clinical Laboratory Findings

The most consistent hematologic abnormality is the presence of mature neutrophilia. Eosinophilia or monocytosis may be apparent. Biochemical analysis may reveal elevations in total protein concentration, serum urea, and serum alkaline phosphatase (ALP), ALT, and amylase activities. Radiography of affected long bones reveals areas of lysis and cortical destruction, with similar changes in sternebrae and vertebral bodies associated with diskospondylitis (Fig. 64-10, *A* and *B*). In the few cases with bronchopulmonary involvement, inter-

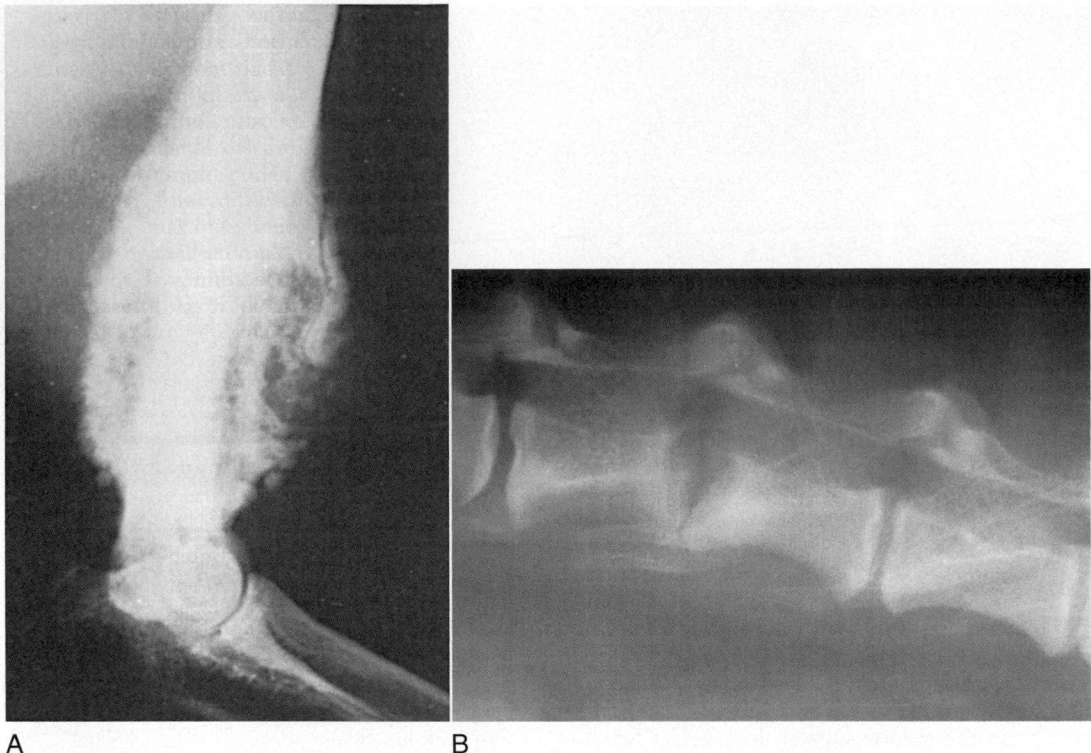

A   B

Fig   64-10   Canine disseminated aspergillosis. **A,** Radiograph of humeral lesion. Note extensive cortical destruction and new bone formation. **B,** Diskospondylitis in a dog with disseminated aspergillosis. (Courtesy Michael Day, University of Bristol, North Somerset, United Kingdom.)

stitial alveolar or consolidated alveolar patterns have been observed.[24]

Organism Identification

Methods to detect *Aspergillus* include cytology, culture, and histopathology. An effective and simple diagnostic test involves examination of an aseptically collected urine sample for the presence of hyphal elements (Fig. 64-11). Urinary tract *Aspergillus* infections are generally a consequence of hematogenous spread and are usually observed in immunocompromised hosts. Fungal elements may also be observed on cytologic examination of blood, synovial fluid, lymph node, bone, or intervertebral disk material. Confirmation of fungal involvement by culture on Sabouraud's dextrose agar requires at least 5 to 7 days.

Antibody Testing

Because *Aspergillus* is ubiquitous, establishing a definitive diagnosis by measuring serum antibodies can be confusing if other results of diagnostic modalities are not considered during the evaluation. Several methodologies are available to measure *Aspergillus*-specific antibodies in serum. The AGID, CIE, ELISA, and fluorescent antibody (FA) test may provide rapid serologic confirmation, but not all dogs with disseminated infection have detectable *Aspergillus* antibodies. For example, kits using *A. fumigatus* as an antigen may not detect antibodies in dogs with disseminated infection caused by *A. terreus*.[136] Serologic responses can have positive results in animals that are exposed to the fungus but not persistently infected. Titers may be relatively lower in these animals.[45] For further information on laboratories and test kits for antibody assays, see Appendices 5 and 6, respectively.

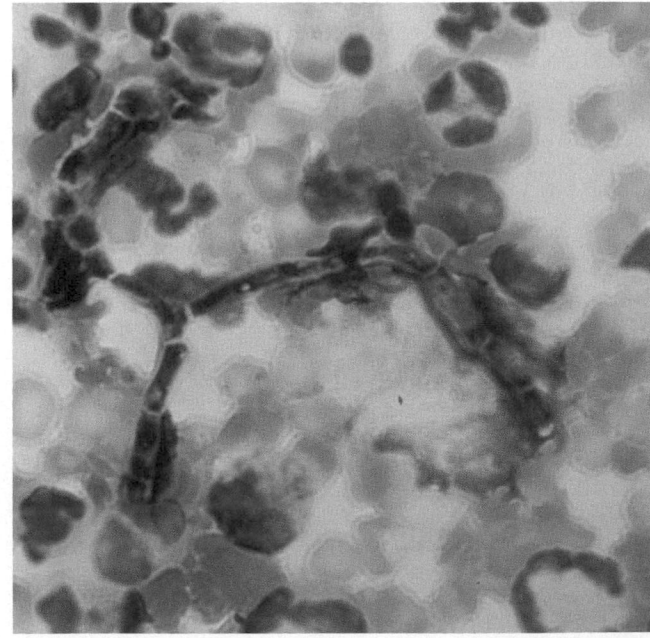

Fig   64-11   Microscopic appearance of stained urine sediment from a dog with disseminated aspergillosis. Branching hyphal elements amid leukocytes and erythrocytes (Wright, ×1000). (Courtesy Edward Mahaffey and Abby Kaufman, University of Georgia, Athens, Ga.)

Antigen Detection

In people with invasive aspergillosis, efforts to detect *Aspergillus* antigens in body fluids have focused on detection of *Aspergillus* galactomannan (GM) or other carbohydrates in serum, cerebrospinal fluid (CSF), respiratory washings or urine by latex agglutination (Pastorex *Aspergillus* latex agglutination test; Sandofi Diagnostics Pasteur, Marnes-La-Coquette, France) or ELISA (Platelia™ *Aspergillus* EIA; Sandofi Diagnostics Pasteur, Marnes-La-Coquette, France and Bio-Rad Laboratories, Redmond, Wash.) or immunoblot methods.[61a,120,147] This component of the polysaccharide cell wall of the organism is released in viable quantities in body fluids during fungal growth in tissues. False-negative results in serum correspond to low test sensitivity, whereas false-positive results in urine correspond to reaction to other fungi and organisms causing urinary tract infections.[68,140,155] In people, ELISA tests are more sensitive and reproducible than are latex methods. Furthermore, the presence of serum *Aspergillus* antibody may interfere with the ELISA test.[58] Rising GM levels have been associated with treatment failures in patients with invasive aspergillosis.[9] Application of tests for GM for the diagnosis of canine aspergillosis has been limited.[45] Detection of GM levels was inconsistent in dogs with disseminated disease.

Genetic Detection

The application of polymerase chain reaction (PCR) to diagnosis is now becoming more widespread in human medicine, and it has been applied to samples of whole blood, serum, urine, CSF, and bronchoalveolar lavage fluid. A range of target genes are used, including those within the 18S, 5.8S and 28S rDNA gene complex that are relatively conserved among fungal species, mitochondrial genes, and the variable sequences of the intervening internal transcribed spacer regions.[64,107] In one case of canine disseminated aspergillosis, the identity of the organism was confirmed by partial sequencing of 18S rDNA.[111] In people, positive PCR results were comparable to those of serum GM levels.[11] Quantitative (real-time) PCR has been used to monitor infectious load in human patients with invasive aspergillosis, and the increased sensitivity of this assay permits an earlier diagnosis (by days to weeks) compared with serologic methods.[67,159] PCR results may be positive in patients that are culture negative,[108] and PCR-positive people with invasive aspergillosis become PCR negative after successful treatment.[80] Additional studies will be needed to determine if PCR is a sensitive and reproducible predictor of disseminated illness.

Pathologic Findings

Gross changes include focal osteomyelitis and multiple, pale granulomas in kidneys and spleen that may also be seen in lymph nodes, myocardium, pancreas, and liver. Occasionally, pulmonary congestion or GI mucosal reddening or erosions may be found. Microscopic granulomas may be associated with areas of slow vascular flow in liver, lungs, eyes, and pancreas and occasionally in prostate, thyroid, uterine submucosa, and brain. Infarcted areas secondary to thrombi containing fungal elements have been found in spleen, kidneys (Fig. 64-12), and liver. Lesions are granulomatous and contain varying numbers of septate, branching hyphae that may have characteristic lateral branching aleuriospores (Fig. 64-13, *A*). Intralesional hyphae are best visualized by periodic acid-Schiff or Gomori's methenamine silver stain, and they have been identified by immunostaining with specific antisera (see Fig. 64-13, *B*).[15,106] The cellular infiltrates may be predominantly neutrophilic or may also include macrophages, giant cells, lymphocytes, and plasma cells.[34,106]

Therapy and Prognosis

Severely ill dogs have poor prognoses. Treatments, including supportive therapy of fluids and antibiotics, together with thi-

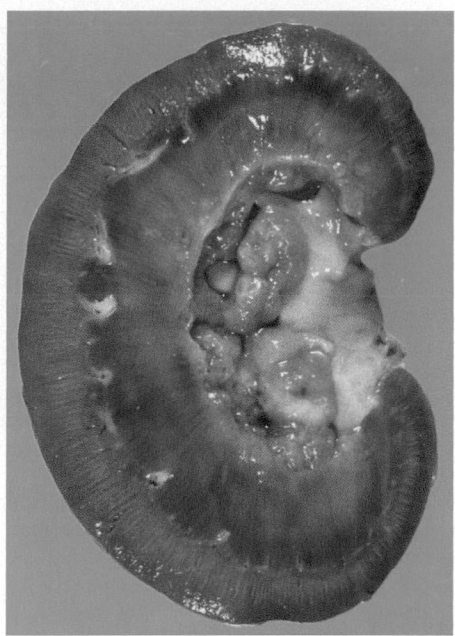

Fig 64-12 Canine disseminated aspergillosis. Sagittal section of kidney with fungal mass in renal pelvis and scattered fungal granulomata *(A. terreus)*. (Courtesy Michael Day, University of Bristol, North Somerset, United Kingdom.)

abendazole or KTZ with and without concurrent 5-fluorocytosine, have been unsuccessful. Hamycin, an experimental polyene related to AMB, showed partial effectiveness in treating one dog.[70] Only two systemic antifungals have shown evidence of efficacy to date: AMB and ITZ (Table 64-3). The potential fungicidal and immunomodulatory effects of AMB are counterbalanced by its nephrotoxicity, which limits its use in patients with renal dysfunction. This problem has been addressed by the use of novel delivery systems that enhance uptake of the drug by reticuloendothelial cells at sites of inflammation and reduce accumulation in the kidneys. These formulations are AMB-lipid complex (Abelcet, Liposome Co., Princeton, N.J.), AMB-colloidal dispersion (Amphocil/Amphotec, Sequus Pharmaceuticals, Menlo Park, Calif.), and liposome-encapsulated AMB (AmBisome, Fujisawa Healthcare, Deerfield, Ill. and Nexstar, San Dimus, Calif.).[41] AMB-lipid complex has been used to treat disseminated aspergillosis in people[22a] and has been evaluated in companion animals, but use is limited by expense. An alternative intravenous lipid formulation has proven efficacious in the treatment of canine leishmaniasis but has not been evaluated for aspergillosis.[76] New lipid delivery systems are currently under development, for example, cochleate lipid cylinders that are a lipid bilayer sheet rolled into a spiral without internal aqueous space.[151]

The induction of long-term clinical remission has been achieved in four dogs with oral ITZ (5 to 10 mg/kg daily for up to 1095 days).[72,153] In one dog, the infection was eliminated; others had resolution of clinical illness but eventually died from disseminated aspergillosis after therapy was discontinued. One dog was euthanized while improving clinically during treatment because of radiographic evidence of additional spondylitic lesions. The surviving dog was not a German shepherd. In people with disseminated aspergillosis, ITZ is also a useful drug in treatment, but similar failures or relapses are common in the most immunocompromised patients.[39]

Because azole-resistant strains of *Aspergillus* and other fungi are now recognized, a new generation of triazole drugs has now been developed for human medicine. Voriconazole,

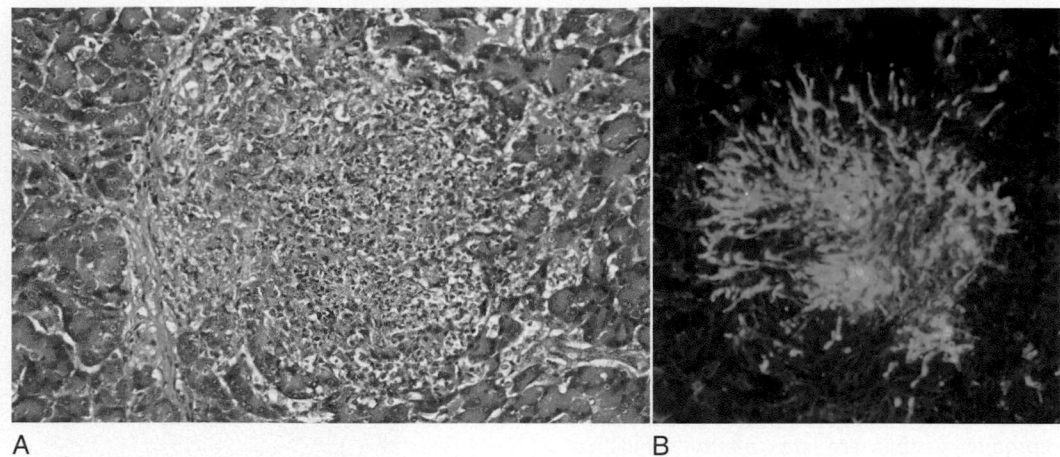

Fig 64-13 Canine disseminated aspergillosis. **A,** Fungal granuloma in pancreas (H and E stain, ×140). **B,** Fungal hyphae within a granuloma marked with antiserum to *A. terreus* (Fluorescent antibody, ×320). (Courtesy Michael Day, University of Bristol, North Somerset, United Kingdom.)

Table • 64-3

Therapy for Disseminated Aspergillosis

DRUG[a]	SPECIES	DOSE[b] (mg/kg)	ROUTE	INTERVAL (HOURS)	DURATION
Amphotericin B (deoxycholate)	D	0.25	IV	48	[c]
Itraconazole	D	2.5–5.0	PO	12	prn[d]
	C	10	PO	24	prn[d]
Amphotericin B lipid complex	D	2–3	IV	3 days per wk	[e]
	C	1	IV	3 days per wk	[f]
Terbinafine	D	5	PO	12	prn[g]

D, Dog; *B,* dog and cat; *C,* cat; *IV,* intravenous; *PO,* by mouth; *prn,* as needed.
[a]For additional information, see Drug Formulary, Appendix 8.
[b]Dose per administration at specified interval.
[c]Until a cumulative dose of 4 to 8 mg/kg is reached for cats and 8 to 12 mg/kg for dogs.
[d]Therapy to control infection may require months to years, although clinical remissions may be achieved; the infection may reactivate in a variable time period after discontinuing treatment.
[e]For a total of 9 to 12 treatments until a cumulative dose of 24 to 27 mg/kg is reached.
[f]For a total of 12 treatments until a cumulative dose of 12 mg/kg is reached.
[g]Extrapolated human dose. Tablets may have to be reformulated to achieve this dose level. No dog studies on pharmacokinetics or studies of efficacy with aspergillosis have been conducted.

posaconazole, and ravuconazole all have activity against *Aspergillus* spp.[150] These agents have not yet been tested in companion animal patients. Terbinafine, an allylamine drug that inhibits fungal sterol synthesis, has been used to treat resistant disseminated aspergillosis in people, alone and in combination with other antifungal drugs. Use of this drug in treating fungal infections in dogs and cats has been empirical and requires further studies on efficacy. A new class of antifungal drug, the β-glucan synthase inhibitors (e.g., caspofungin), acts by blocking synthesis of 1,3-β-D-glucan, a component of fungal cell walls that is not found in mammalian cells. Caspofungin is efficacious in invasive aspergillosis of people but has not been evaluated in veterinary species.[71] Combination therapy that uses AMB with azoles, flucytosine, or rifampin has been beneficial in in vitro and in some animal experiments, but further use in invasive disease of people is needed to confirm efficacy. Caspofungin has been used in combination with ITZ in effectively treating invasive aspergillosis in people.[114] See Chapter 57 and the Drug Formulary, Appendix 8, for more information on these drugs.

Immunomodulatory therapy (e.g., recombinant cytokine therapy) is sometimes used as an adjunct treatment in human invasive mycotic disease, and although such agents are available for use in the dog (e.g., recombinant granulocyte colony-stimulating factor [G-CSF], granulocyte-macrophage colony-stimulating factor [GM-CSF]) they have not been applied to cases of canine disseminated aspergillosis.[18,43]

FELINE DISSEMINATED ASPERGILLOSIS

Michael J. Day

Feline aspergillosis largely occurs in cats up to 2 years of age, although, in one study, the majority of affected cats were middle aged or older. No clear breed predispositions have been discovered. Unlike dogs with aspergillosis, most affected cats have concurrent immunosuppressive diseases, such as panleukopenia, feline infectious peritonitis, FeLV infection, or multiple diseases, or they have had dystocia or have been receiving glucocorticoid or antibiotic therapy.[98] Aspergillosis has not been reported in cats with feline immunodeficiency virus (FIV) infection, although such cats may have other opportunistic mycoses.[16] Cats infected with FeLV or FIV had a greater diversity of fungal genera cultured from their skin or mucous membranes compared with noninfected control cats. Clinical signs are referable to GI or pulmonary involvement, with nonspecific findings similar to those in dogs. Hematologic findings are variable and may reflect other underlying diseases. Feline aspergillosis is so uncommon that treatment options have not been extensively reviewed. Rare cases of localized *Aspergillus* infection have recovered following complete surgical débridement of affected tissue.

Diagnosis is often made at necropsy, and findings may include pulmonary granulomata, GI ulcers, or pseudomembranes and involvement of urinary system or CNS. The lesions are characterized by hemorrhage and necrosis, with variable numbers of inflammatory cells and fungal hyphae that may invade blood vessels, leading to thrombosis.

SUGGESTED READINGS*

45. Garcia ME, Caballero J, Cruzado M, et al. 2001a. The value of the determination of anti-*Aspergillus* IgG in the serodiagnosis of canine aspergillosis: comparison with galactomannan detection, *J Vet Med* 48:743-750.
93. Moore AH. 2003. Use of topical povidone-iodine dressings in the management of mycotic rhinitis in three dogs, *J Small Anim Pract* 44:326-329.
117. Saunders JH, Duchateau L, Stork C, et al. 2003a. Use of computed tomography to predict the outcome of a noninvasive intranasal infusion in dogs with nasal aspergillosis, *Can Vet J* 44:305-311.
153a. Whitney BL, Broussard J, Stefanacci JD. 2005. Four cats with fungal rhinitis, *J Feline Med Surg* 7:53-58.
163. Zonderland JL, Stork CK, Saunders JH, et al. 2002. Intranasal infusion of enilconazole for treatment of sinonasal aspergillosis in dogs, *J Am Vet Med Assoc* 221:1421-1425.

*See the CD-ROM for a complete list of references.

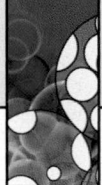

CHAPTER • 65

Candidiasis and Rhodotorulosis

Craig E. Greene and Francis W. Chandler

CANDIDIASIS

Etiology

Members of the genus *Candida* are dimorphic fungi in the family Cryptococcaceae. In the yeast phase, *Candida* species normally inhabit the alimentary, upper respiratory, and genital mucosae of mammals. A sexual stage has not been identified, and the small (2- to 6-μm), thin-walled, ovoid, yeastlike cells (blastoconidia) reproduce by budding. Not all *Candida* species are adapted to colonize normal mucosae. *Candida* species, especially *Candida albicans* and *Candida parapsilosis*, have been the most commonly cultured fungi from the ears, nose, oral cavity, and anus of clinically healthy dogs. In contrast, in cats with or without retrovirus infections, *Candida* species were less commonly isolated from the oropharyngeal mucosa (5.9%) or haircoat (9.4%) than other fungi.[39] Occasionally, *Candida tropicalis*, *Candida pseudotropicalis*, *Candida guilliermondii*, and *Candida krusei* have been found on human and animal body surfaces. These four species require an immunocompromised host to effectively colonize the mucosae and produce disease. In one study of *Candida* urinary infections, *C. albicans* was the most common isolate from dogs and cats, whereas *Candida rugosa* and *C. krusei* were only isolated from dogs, and *Candida* (previously *Torulopsis*) *glabrata* and *C. parapsilosis* were only isolated from cats.[35] *Candida* species become more prevalent in environments where people or animals live. Only rarely are *Candida* species isolated from soil or as laboratory contaminants.

C. glabrata is part of the normal microbial flora of the skin and mucosal surfaces of people and animals and is an environmental saprophyte. It is considered to be a nonpathogenic inhabitant of mucosal surfaces, but in immunosuppressed animals, clinical illness can occur. *C. glabrata* is different from other *Candida* species because of its nondimorphic blastoconidial morphology and haploid genome.

Epidemiology

Candida species, first acquired by neonates as they pass through the birth canal, colonize the oral, gastrointestinal (GI), upper respiratory, and genital mucosae for the life of the animals, but their presence normally evokes no reaction. The intact skin is an abnormal site for *C. albicans* except at mucocutaneous junctions of body orifices. Opportunistic infections may result if the skin becomes chronically traumatized or moistened. Under certain circumstances, *Candida* species also can invade deeper host tissues and proliferate as blastoconidia, pseudohyphae, and branched, septate hyphae. In other instances, they may disseminate via the blood stream to many tissues.

C. glabrata has been implicated more frequently as the cause of nosocomial infections in immunocompromised and neutropenic human patients.[43] As with other *Candida* species, it can be cultured from surfaces in the hospital environment. Hospitalized human or animal patients may become colonized with *Candida* organisms during their hospital stay from contact with contaminated surfaces or during medical diagnostic or therapeutic procedures. Urinary tract infections (UTIs) have been observed in immunocompromised dogs and cats. The yeast gains access to the genitourinary tract from local contamination and ascending infection or from embolic spread to the kidneys in disseminated infection. Disseminated infections are not as common but are associated with similar immunosuppressive conditions. Immunosuppression or chronic antibacterial therapy contributes to colonization and subsequent overgrowth of the fungus.

Pathogenesis

Pathogenic factors of *Candida* species are important in determining their relative virulence in the host. *C. albicans* can colonize and invade stratified squamous epithelia with varying degrees of keratinization and columnar epithelia in the intestines. *C. albicans* is also the most polymorphic species of the genus; whereas yeast cells can colonize epithelia, hyphae are thought of as the more invasive forms and are found with deeper tissue invasion. Hyphae of this organism consistently adhere more readily than yeast cells to host epithelial tissues. When cells of *C. albicans* enter the blood stream, they become rapidly coated with host platelets as a result of fibrinogen-binding ligand. This coating likely reduces the immune-visibility of the fungus to the host, thereby allowing dissemination.

Local proliferation of *Candida* species in wounds or on mucosal surfaces is the first step in the spread of infection. Overgrowth of *Candida* is probably inhibited under most circumstances by various factors, including intestinal, genital, and cutaneous microflora. Factors that upset the balance of normal endogenous microflora, such as prolonged broad-spectrum antibiotic therapy, may allow *Candida* organisms to proliferate, especially in the external auditory meatus, oropharynx, and GI tract.[26,41] Similarly, disruption of cutaneous or mucosal barriers by burns, surgery, cytotoxic agents, trauma, or indwelling vascular or urinary catheters provides a pathway for *Candida* organisms to enter the body from the body surfaces or the environment. Intestinal candidiasis may be a sequela to parvoviral infections[31,38] or alterations in microflora caused by antibacterial chemotherapy.[44] Dogs and cats may be more likely to contract urinary tract candidiasis from (1) increased intestinal colonization, such as after antimicrobial use or viral enteritis; (2) decreased cellular immunity from glucocorticoids or cytotoxic agents, irradiation, or granulocytopenia; or (3) alterations in the urinary environment, such as those caused by glucosuria, an altered pH, dilute urine, a bacterial infection, urolithiasis, neoplasia, urethrostomy, cystostomy, indwelling catheters, or urinary stasis.[17,35]

Bull terriers with lethal acrodermatitis are known to have impaired T-cell function and have been shown to harbor higher numbers of *Malassezia* and *Candida* organisms on their skin, especially at lesion sites.[25] *C. albicans* was frequently isolated from lesional skin and haircoat, mucous membranes, nails, and foot pads from affected dogs but not from control healthy dogs or those with atopic dermatitis. Fungal hyphae or pseudohyphae were demonstrated in lesions of hyperkeratosis of the foot pads and nail dystrophy.

Cell-mediated immunity (CMI) and circulating neutrophils appear to be major defenses against disseminated candidiasis. Multinucleated giant cells containing fungal organisms can be observed within lymph nodes and lymphatic vessels draining the mucosal lesions and may provide a mechanism for dissemination. Once in the body, CMI appears to be an important determinant of additional spread of infection. Evidence also shows that mannan, a *Candida* cell wall glycoprotein, has immunosuppressive properties that facilitate persistent intracellular infection. As with surface infections, prolonged immunosuppression, cytotoxic chemotherapy causing persistent neutropenia, diabetes mellitus, long-term glucocorticoid therapy, and prolonged antibiotic therapy have resulted in an increased incidence of disseminated candidiasis in people. Candidiasis has developed in dogs with experimentally induced and spontaneous neutropenia.[2] Similar predispositions have not been substantiated for the occurrence of disseminated candidiasis in cats. However, a cat with disseminated infection had concurrent toxoplasmosis, diabetes mellitus, and suspected hyperadrenocorticism.[12,42]

In disseminated candidiasis, the microcirculation in tissues, such as lungs, skin, kidneys, liver, brain, myocardium, eyes, intervertebral discs, and skeletal muscle, filters and clears the blood of yeasts. This activity results in embolic colonization and microabscess formation at these sites.

Clinical Findings

Localized candidiasis is found in chronically immunosuppressed dogs and cats and in those with nonhealing ulcers of the oral, upper respiratory, GI, or genitourinary mucosae. Clinical signs reflect the anatomic location and extent of the mucosal damage (Table 65-1). Lesions are characterized by nonhealing ulcers covered by whitish-gray plaques with hyperemic margins. A white vaginal or preputial discharge may be seen in candidiasis of the genital mucosa. Dysuria and hematuria are features of *Candida* urocystitis (Fig. 65-1).[11] Some urinary infections are subclinical. Chronic lesions of the skin or nail beds may appear as nonhealing, erythematous, moist, greasy exudations, and crusting (Fig. 65-2).[29] Pruritus varies. Crusts may be superficial and may be peeled off to reveal eroded skin. Superficial ocular infections appear as conjunctival congestion and corneal ulceration.[12] Chronic otitis externa characterized by erythema, exudation, and pruritus, may be apparent.[26,32]

Disseminated candidiasis has been recognized in dogs and cats. Although clinical signs frequently reflect involvement of particular organ systems, lesions in dogs and cats with multisystemic infections are often widespread.[17] Fever and the sudden appearance of multiple raised erythematous to hemorrhagic skin lesions have been described in canine systemic candidiasis. The lesions begin as small wheals or macules that eventually ulcerate (Fig. 65-3). Pain and reluctance to move are common manifestations of myositis. Dogs with systemic candidiasis also have peripheral lymphadenomegaly and fistulous drainage resulting from underlying osteomyelitis. Cats with systemic infections have developed uveitis, chorioretinitis, neurologic deficits, and pleural effusions.[12] Enophthalmitis has also been observed in a dog,[22] and intraocular infections are considered sequellae to disseminated infections.

Diagnosis

Hematologic findings usually are normal in localized infections; however, leukopenia and thrombocytopenia may be associated with disseminated disease. Muscle and liver enzyme concentrations may be increased, depending on the tissues affected. Cytologic examination of impression smears, aspirates of the lesions, or urine sediment, may reveal the yeast cells (see Fig. 65-1).

Isolation methods, which first involve lysis centrifugation, release fungi from leukocytes, increasing the ability to grow *Candida* species and decreasing the time between inoculation and growth of the organism. *Candida* species grow well on blood agar, therefore they are often isolated from specimens submitted for bacterial culture. *Candida* grow rapidly at room temperature or 37° C (98.6° F), producing smooth or wrinkled, creamy white, yeast colonies. Colonies are composed of spherical to oval yeast cells that are 5 to 7 µm in diameter (Fig. 65-4), pseudohyphae, and septate hyphae that are 3 to 5 µm wide. Pseudohyphae are composed of elongated yeast cells that remain attached end to end in chains. They can be distinguished from true hyphae by their prominent constrictions at points of attachment between adjacent cells. Septate hyphae are tubular with parallel contours. The thick-walled chlamydoconidia, 8 to 12 µm in diameter, are spherical. *C. albicans* is also identified by a positive germ tube test (see Fig. 56-17 and associated text) and patterns of carbohydrate metabolism.

Table • 65-1

Clinical Features of Candidiasis in Various Body Systems

LOCALIZATION[a]	CLINICAL SIGNS	PREDISPOSING FACTORS	ORGANISMS[a]
Integument	Erythema, pruritus, oily and watery exudation	Chronic antibacterial therapy, lethal acrodermatitis	*C. guilliermondii*[29]; *Candida* spp.[34]; candidal acrodermatitis[25]
Ears	Erythema, pruritus, oily and watery exudation	Chronic antibacterial therapy	*C. albicans*[32]
Gastrointestinal	Diarrhea	Chronic antibacterial therapy	*Candida* spp.[31, 2, 44, 21]; *C. famata*[27]
Urinary	Dysuria	Diabetes mellitus, hyperadrenocorticism, urinary catheters	*C. parapsilosis*[20]; *C. albicans*[10]; *C. glabrata*[42]; *Candida* spp.[35]
Ocular	Uveitis, chorioretinitis	Lymphocytic enteritis, disseminated candidiasis	*C. albicans*[22]
Disseminated	Fever, leukocytosis, tachycardia, weak pulse, disseminated intravascular coagulation	Urinary or vascular catheters, parvoviral infection, d iabetes mellitus, hyperadrenocorticism	*Candida* spp.[7, 18, 14, 38]; *C. albicans*[17]

[a]Number indicates reference cited at the end of this chapter or on the CD-ROM.

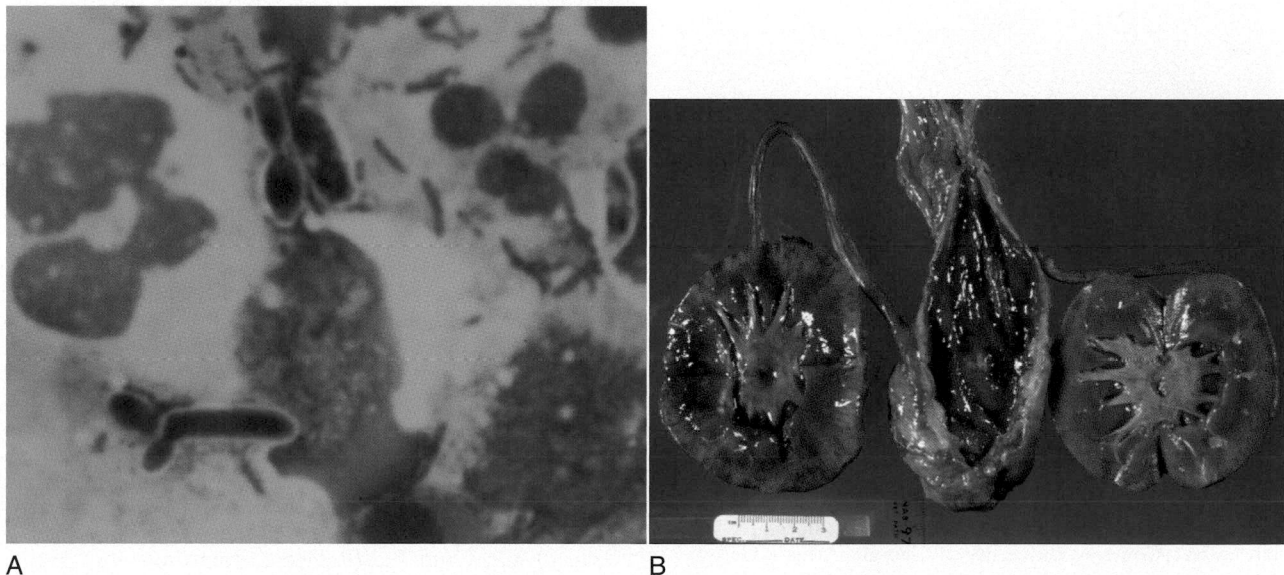

A   B

Fig   65-1   A, Stained urinary sediment contains blastoconidia with leukocytes from a dog with secondary *Candida* cystitis as a result of long-term cyclophosphamide therapy. **B,** Bladder and kidneys from same dog. (Courtesy University of Georgia, Athens, Ga.)

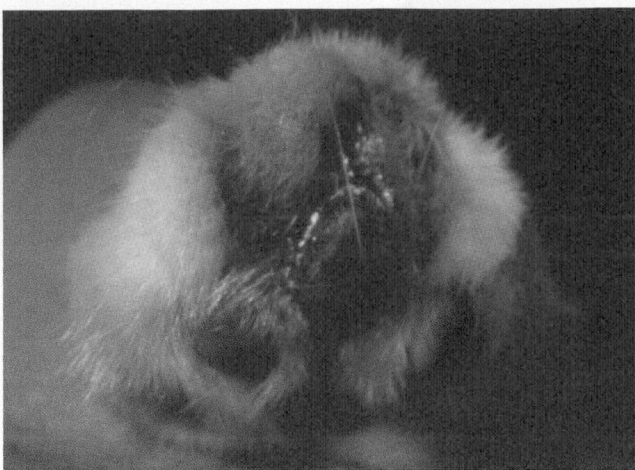

Fig 65-2 Cat with localized ulcerated proliferative *Candida* infection of the nail bed with underlying osteomyelitis. (Courtesy University of Georgia, Athens, Ga.)

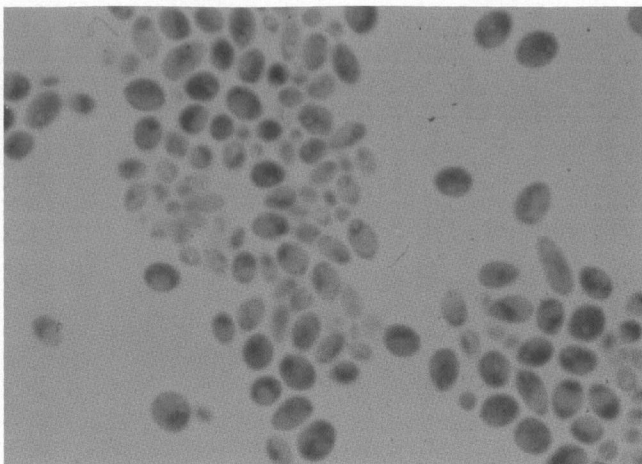

Fig 65-4 Culture of *Candida* species from urinary infection showing variable-size budding yeasts (Lactol Phenol Cotton Blue stain, ×100). (Courtesy University of Georgia, Athens, Ga.)

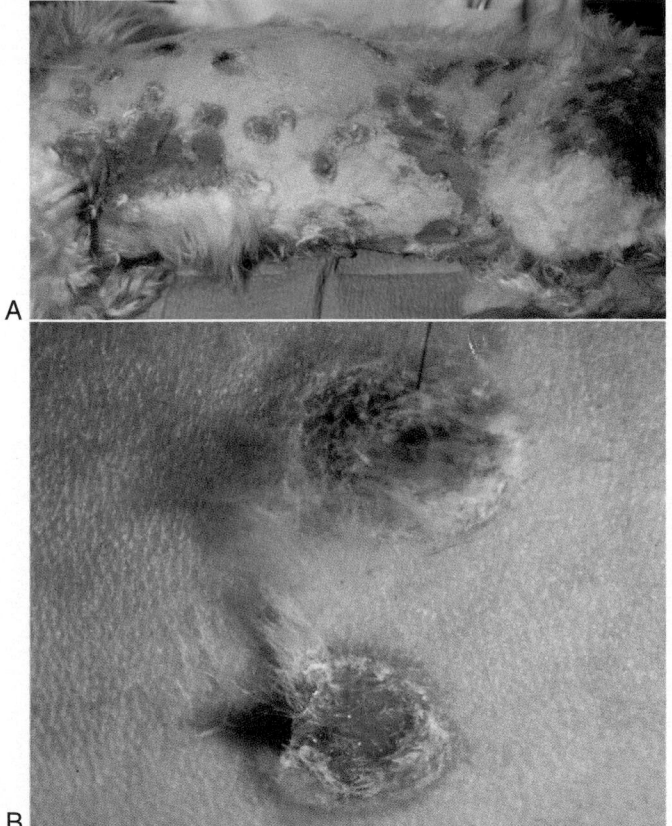

Fig 65-3 **A,** Ulcerative dermatitis in dog with concurrent polymyositis. *Candida* organisms were cultured from lesions, and disease responded to therapy with ketoconazole. **B,** Closer view of skin lesion. (Courtesy University of Georgia, Athens, Ga.)

Antemortem blood samples for culture are best obtained from peripheral arteries, because most of the organisms, effectively filtered out by tissues, never reach the systemic venous circulation. Because consistent renal embolization occurs with disseminated infection, *Candida* species are more easily isolated from urine than from the blood. Candiduria in patients without lower urinary tract signs or indwelling urinary catheters usually reflects hematogenous spread to the kidneys. Recovery of *Candida* species from a normally sterile fluid such as cerebrospinal fluid or joint fluid is indicative of invasive candidiasis. Organisms may sometimes be cultured from many tissues at surgery or necropsy, but such results should be interpreted cautiously. Culture of *Candida* species from cutaneous or mucosal surfaces or exudates alone should not be considered an absolute indicator of infection. Histologic confirmation of invasion and host reaction are essential. Cutaneous or mucosal biopsy specimens should be submitted for histologic and cultural examinations simultaneously. Biopsies of liver, spleen, lung, and kidney may be needed to document hematogenous spread. A definitive histologic diagnosis can sometimes be made in the presence of negative culture results.

Numerous nonculture methods have been developed for the diagnosis of disseminated candidiasis in serum, whole blood, or urine specimens.[36] D-arabinitol, a low molecular weight metabolite, is occasionally increased in serum of humans with disseminated candidiasis. Artifactual increases of D-arabinitol that develop during renal failure are identified by comparing its concentration with that of serum creatinine.

As a more rapid alternative to culture methods, the polymerase chain reaction (PCR) has been used to detect *Candida* species in blood and urine.[28,28a] PCR of urine from dogs allowed for direct detection of *Candida* within 2 days.[20] Numerous tests also have been developed on an experimental basis to detect soluble antigens of *Candida* species such as mannan in blood and urine using the enzyme-linked immunosorbent assay (ELISA) and latex agglutination (LA) immunoassay.[16] Two LA tests are commercially available for clinical detection of *Candida* antigens in body fluids: Pastorex *Candida* (Sanofi Diagnostics Pasteur, Marres-la Coquette, France) and Cand-Tec (Ramco Laboratories, Inc., Houston, Tex.).

Pathologic Findings

Animals that die of disseminated candidiasis have gross lesions consisting of multiple white foci in the heart, liver, spleen, lymph nodes, central nervous system, kidneys, or other organs. Microscopic evaluation reveals multifocal abscesses or areas of necrosis that contain abundant blastoconidia (budding, yeast-like cells), pseudohyphae, and true hyphae surrounded by

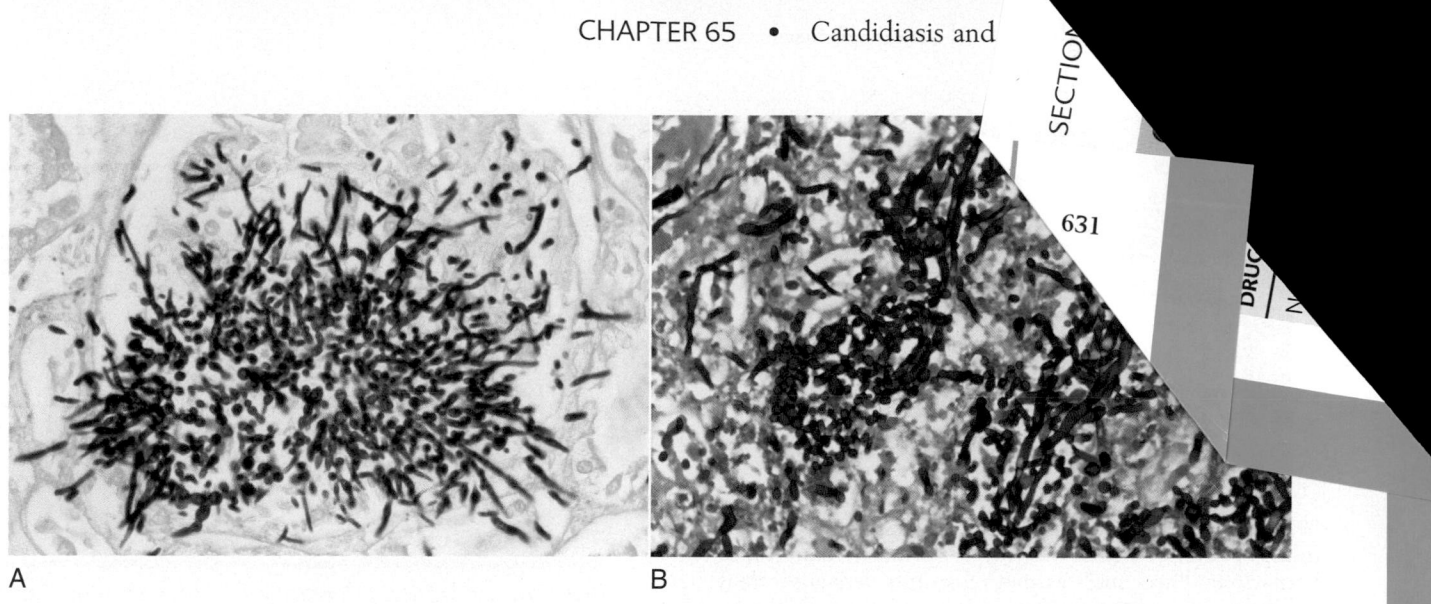

A   B

Fig   65-5   Hematogenous renal candidiasis caused by *C. albicans*. **A,** Glomerulus contains spherical to oval blastoconidia and periph- eral, radially oriented pseudohyphae (GMS stain, ×300). **B,** Blastoconidia and branched, septate hyphae with parallel contours prolifer- ate within a necrotic renal papilla (GMS stain with H and E counterstain, ×300). (Courtesy Francis Chandler, Medical College of Georgia, Augusta, Ga.)

mixed inflammatory cells (Fig. 65-5). Infiltrates are usually minimal in profoundly immunosuppressed or leukopenic animals. Occasionally, hyphal angioinvasion or occlusion of small and medium-size arteries by systemic candidal emboli results in nodular, hemorrhagic infarcts.

Caution must be exercised in diagnosing localized, super- ficial candidal infections on the basis of cytologic or histologic study of mucocutaneous lesions unless invasive hyphal ele- ments and numerous inflammatory cells are present (Fig. 65- 6). The different *Candida* species are morphologically and tinctorially indistinguishable in clinical specimens. Culture is needed for definitive species identification. Test kits are avail- able to confirm genus identity in clinical or culture specimens (see Appendix 6).

In smears and sections of infected tissue, *C. glabrata* closely resembles *Histoplasma capsulatum*, but they do have some distinguishing characteristics. In tissues stained with hema- toxylin-eosin (H and E) stain, *C. glabrata* does not show the pseudocapsule, or "halo," effect shown by *H. capsulatum*. With Gomori's methenamine silver (GMS) stain, *C. glabrata* are larger, bud more frequently, are more often extracellular, and are not in clusters. Unlike other *Candida* species, *C. glabrata* reproduces only by budding and is always a yeast form in tissue or culture.

Therapy

Treatment of superficial candidiasis involves drying of non- mucosal lesions. Antifungal susceptibility testing is unreliable. Skin lesions can be treated by systemic azoles and shampoos containing chlorhexidine, azoles, and selenium sulfide. Topical therapy may need to continue for up to 8 weeks.

Mucosal lesions can be treated with topical nystatin, gentian violet (1:10,000), or topical amphotericin B (AMB) lotions (Table 65-2). However, treatment of mucocutaneous candidiasis is generally dominated by the azole antifungal drugs, and they can be used topically or systemically. Intrav- esicular administration of clotrimazole was used to treat a *Candida* UTI in a cat.[42] Lufenuron also has been used to treat cutaneous infections.[4] In a diabetic hypothyroid dog with a UTI caused by systemic drug-resistant *C. albicans*, local intravesicular infusion of clotrimazole was successfully used.[10] Previous treatment with fluconazole (FCZ), terbinafine, and flucytosine (FCY) was unsuccessful. AMB, which is usually effective against *C. albicans*,[37] was contraindicated in this dog.

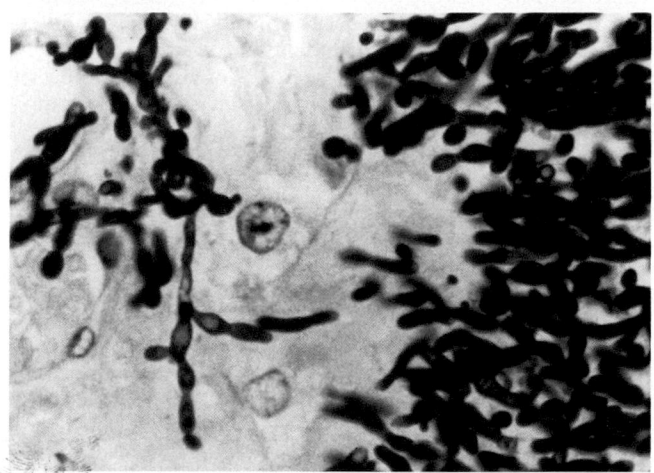

Fig   65-6   Invasive candidiasis. Budding yeastlike cells (blas- toconidia) and segmentally constricted pseudohyphae of *C. albicans* invade esophageal mucosa (PAS stain, ×700). (Courtesy Francis Chandler, Medical College of Georgia, Augusta, Ga.)

Similarly, intravesicular administration of clotrimazole was successful in controlling UTI in a cat with diabetes mellitus and iatrogenic hyperadrenocorticism and *C. glabrata* infection.[42] Unfortunately, with intravesicular infusions, infec- tion above the bladder cannot be controlled unless systemic therapy is used. Systemic antifungal therapy is generally reserved for renal parenchymal disease and is not often effec- tive against lower urinary tract fungal infections because of the low concentrations of polyene and azole drugs in the urine. Use of FCY may be beneficial in these cases because it reaches a high concentration in the urine. Voriconazole (VCZ), a newer antifungal in this class, is equally as effective against *Candida* but is not widely available (see Drug Formulary, Appendix 8). Clotrimazole infusions may be effective in treating *Candida* lower UTIs; however, if the infection is deeper in the kidney than the renal pelvis or within the wall of the bladder or ureters, infection may not

65-2

...ended Drugs for Topical Treatment of Dermal Candidiasis and Trichosporonosis

GENERIC (BRAND)	FORMULATION	INTERVAL (HOURS)	DURATION (WEEKS)
...ystatin (Nilstat)	100,000 U/g	8–12	1–2
Miconazole (Conofite)	2%	12–24	2–4
Clotrimazole (Lotrimin)[a]	1%	6–8	1
Amphotericin B (Fungizone)	3%	6–8	1

[a]For intravesicular infusion in the treatment of cystitis, see text and Drug Formulary, Appendix 8.

be effectively controlled without simultaneous topical infusion along with systemic antifungal administration. Urinary acidifiers such as methenamine derivatives may be helpful because they produce a low pH that inhibits fungal growth. For additional information on the bladder infusion method, see Table 65-3 and clotrimazole in Drug Formulary, Appendix 8.

Treatment of lower UTIs caused by *C. glabrata* would involve local infusion of antifungal solutions, although systemic antifungal therapy, as outlined for candidiasis, would be more convenient and appropriate should disseminated infections be diagnosed. Unfortunately, *C. glabrata* is innately resistant to azole antimycotic agents. AMB or FCY must be used at higher levels.[9,37] FCY should only be used in combination with another antifungal cell-wall active drug such as AMB. Lipid formulations of AMB might be considered; however, the urinary excretion of these drugs is lower than with unmodified AMB. Higher levels of FCZ would be needed for treating UTIs caused by *C. glabrata* than by the other *Candida* species (Table 65-4).

Systemic candidiasis is the most refractory form of infection. Animals with systemic candidiasis should always be evaluated for uveitis or chorioretinitis, because intraocular localization is difficult to resolve. Systemic candidiasis can be treated with intravenous (IV) AMB, but the drug's nephrotoxicity in otherwise compromised hosts can be fatal. Lipid formulations of AMB are relatively effective and recommended for conditions in people for whom expense is less of a concern. Ketoconazole (KTZ) and other related benzimidazoles are currently the drugs of choice for treating infected dogs (see Table 65-4). Supplemental oral administration of vitamin A might be recommended in any form of candidiasis because it has been shown to increase resistance to infection by *Candida* species.

Caspofungin, the first echinocandin antifungal agent, has activity against *Candida* and *Aspergillus* species. It is only available as a parenteral preparation, and dosages for dogs and cats are not available. VCZ, the previously mentioned newer azole, is effective against FCZ-resistant strains of *Candida*.[33]

RHODOTORULOSIS

Yeasts of the genus *Rhodotorula* are saprophytes, found in domestic environments on shower curtains, in bathtub grout, and as commensals of moist skin. They can be isolated as environmental or dermal contaminants and are rarely isolated from clinical specimens of the urinary tract or surgical wounds. Granulomatous epididymitis was associated with this infection in a dog,[19] and disseminated infections have developed in immunocompromised people.[1]

This yeast may gain access to the genitourinary tract through local contamination. The yeast has caused septicemia

Table • 65-3

Protocol for Infusing Urinary Bladder of Dogs and Cats with Clotrimazole[a]

1. Put animal under general anesthesia and in dorsal recumbency.
2. Cleanse genitalia with physiologic saline.
3. Insert balloon-tipped (Foley) catheter, where possible, and inflate cuff.
4. Attach three-way stopcock and remove urine from the bladder through this port.
5. Attach syringe containing 1% clotrimazole.[b]
6. Infuse 5 to 10 ml/kg while palpating bladder to avoid overdistention.
7. Keep solution inside urinary system for 15 to 25 minutes.
8. Rotate animal for several minutes on each side to ensure contact with all urinary bladder surfaces.
9. Recover animal from anesthesia.
10. Keep catheter in place until animal voids spontaneously.
11. Deflate cuff and remove catheter at the appropriate time.
12. Provide at least three to four treatments, 1 week apart.
13. Check urinalysis each week and monthly thereafter to ensure yeasts are not found in sediment. Repeat clotrimazole-infusion if infection is still present.
14. Repeat fungal culture after third treatment.
15. Repeat fungal culture 1 to 2 months after last treatment.
16. Recommend at least one treatment after yeasts are no longer visible.
17. Recommend concurrent fluconazole therapy because infection may ascend to the kidneys.

[a]Modified from Pressler BM, Vaden SL, Lane IF, et al. 2003. Candida spp. urinary tract infections in 13 dogs and seven cats: predisposing factors, treatment, and outcome. *J Am Anim Hosp Assoc* 39:263–270.
[b]Commercially available solution with polyethylene glycol 400.

and meningitis in people on long-term IV therapy. Contamination of IV catheter sites is the presumed route of these infections.[23] As with candidiasis, immunocompromised states are associated with disseminated infections.

Rhodotorula species can be isolated on routine mycologic media at room temperature after 3 to 4 days incubation. Colonies are smooth, are salmon pink, and contain 10 μm-diameter encapsulated yeasts. Biochemical characteristics have been described.[19]

Table • 65-4

Recommended Drugs for Systemic Treatment of Candidiasis

SYSTEMIC DRUG[a] (INDICATIONS)	SPECIES	DOSE[b]	ROUTE	INTERVAL (HOURS)	DURATION[c] (WEEKS)
Ketoconazole	D	5—11 mg/kg	PO	12	5
	C	50 mg total	PO	12—24	4
Itraconazole	B	2.5—10 mg/kg[d]	PO	12	4
Fluconazole (urinary infection)	B	3.5—7 mg/kg[d]	PO	12	4
	B	7—10 mg/kg[d]	PO	24	4
(C. glabrata infection)	B	8 mg/kg[d]	PO	12	4
(C. glabrata infection)	B	12 mg/kg[d]	PO	24	4
Amphotericin B[e]	D	0.25—0.5 mg/kg	IV	48	4—6
(disseminated or urinary	C	0.1—0.2 5 mg/kg	IV	48	4—6
C. glabrata infection)	D	35 mg/kg	PO	8	4
Flucytosine[f]	B	28 mg/kg	PO	12	4
Methenamine (urinary infection)	D	46—68 mg/kg[g]	PO	24	4—8
Lufenuron (cutaneous infection)	C	50—200 mg/kg[g]	PO	24	4—8
Caspofungin	H	50 mg total	IV	24	4

D, Dog; C, cat; B, both; H, human; PO, by mouth; IV, intravenous.
[a]For additional information on these drugs, see Drug Formulary, Appendix 8.
[b]Dose per administration at specified interval.
[c]May have to extend therapy based on response.
[d]Higher dosage within given range may be needed for systemic and urinary C. glabrata infections; however, increased risk of toxicity is more likely. Monitor animals by noting decreased appetite and increased serum ALT activity.
[e]For additional information on amphotericin B dosing regimens, see Drug Formulary, Appendix 8.
[f]Always use in combination with a cell-wall–acting drug such as amphotericin B or an azole.
[g]Dose per kilogram varies inversely with body weight (see Drug Formulary, Appendix 8, for complete breakdown by weight).

In a dog with granulomatous epididymitis, severe swelling of the scrotum was observed.[19] Treatment with antibiotics was ineffective, and the scrotum became firm. The testes and epididymides were surgically removed. The epididymides were swollen and when sectioned, were found to contain fibrous connective tissue, multifocal hemorrhages, and abscesses. On histopathologic examination, marked infiltration of neutrophils and macrophages with fibrosis was found in the dilated and partially ruptured ductus deferens. In surrounding stroma, focal collections of macrophages contained eosinophilic, spherical, 5- to 8-μm diameter, yeastlike structures. The intracellular yeasts stained positive by periodic acid–Schiff and GMS procedures. Removal of the affected testes and epididymides was curative. In disseminated infections, systemic antifungal therapy, as for candidiasis, is indicated.

SUGGESTED READINGS*

10. Forward ZA, Legendre AM, Khalsa HDS. 2002. Use of intermittent bladder infusion with clotrimazole for treatment of candiduria in a dog. J Am Vet Med Assoc 220: 1496-1498.

22. Linek J. 2004. Mycotic edophthalmitis in a dog caused by Candida albicans. Vet Ophthalmol 7:159-162.

29. Mueller RS, Bettenay SV, Shipstone M. 2002. Cutaneous candidiasis in a dog caused by Candida guilliermondii. Vet Rec 150:728-730.

35. Pressler BM, Vaden SL, Lane IF, et al. 2003. Candida spp urinary tract infections in 13 dogs and seven cats: predisposing factors, treatment, and outcome. J Am Anim Hosp Assoc 39:263-270.

42. Toll J, Ashe CM, Trepanier LA. 2003. Intravesicular administration of clotrimazole for treatment of candiduria in a cat with diabetes mellitus. J Am Vet Med Assoc 223:1156-1158.

*See the CD-ROM for a complete list of references.

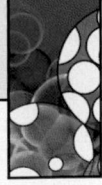

CHAPTER • 66

Trichosporonosis

Craig E. Greene and Francis W. Chandler

ETIOLOGY

Trichosporon spp., yeastlike fungi that exist in nature as soil saprophytes, are members of the family Cryptococcaceae. In culture, they form hyaline yeastlike cells, mycelia, and characteristic arthroconidia. *Trichosporon* spp. are not considered to be primary pathogens because they are distributed in the environment worldwide and form a minor component of normal cutaneous and mucosal flora of people and animals. They cause superficial, cutaneous, and deep-seated mucosa-associated infections in immunocompetent hosts and disseminated, life-threatening infections in immunocompromised or postoperative patients.

The causative agent of disease was previously classified as *T. cutaneum*; however, taxonomic genomic analysis has indicated that six species (*T. asahii, T. asteroides, T. cutaneum, T. inkin, T. mucoides,* and *T. ovoides*) are important for human infections. The genus is also classified serologically into four types (I: *T. cutaneum, T. mucoides;* II: *T. asahii, T. asteroides, T. ovoides;* III: *T. brassicae, T. domesticum;* and also in I-III, *T. dulcitum* and *T. gracile*).

T. beigelii (= T. cutaneum), a transient skin commensal, is recognized as the agent of white piedra, a nodular mycosis of hair shafts affecting people, monkeys, and horses in temperate to tropical climates. A synergistic coryneform bacterial infection is often present in this condition, suggesting a pathogenic co-infection.[37] *T. beigelii*, along with *T. asahii* and *T. mucoides*, have been linked to the syndrome of human summer-type hypersensitivity pneumonitis in Japan[22,25] and catheter-associated infections. *T. beigelii* has been found in the urine of human patients with indwelling urinary catheters and may be an opportunist in causing urinary tract infections (UTIs).[16] *T. mucoides* was incriminated as a cause of nosocomial infection in children associated with a faulty bronchoscope.[28] *T. beigelii* was associated with outbreaks of mastitis in dairy herds.[7] *T. capitatum (= Blastoschizomyces capitatus, Geotrichum capitatum)* has been incriminated as causing abortion in a cow and horse. Both *T. beigelii* and *T. capitatum* have caused systemic infections in people, especially in patients being treated for hematologic malignancies, in those with hereditary phagocyte deficiencies, and in recipients of renal and bone marrow transplants. *T. pullulans* and *T. beigelii* have caused infections in three cats. Biochemical and genetic studies indicate that cutaneous, mucosal, and environmental isolates differ from those that cause disseminated illness.[14,17,29]

PATHOGENESIS

Most cases of trichosporonosis in people have been disseminated and fatal, and they have occurred in patients with severe immunosuppression who were also neutropenic. Many patients had received multiple or broad-spectrum antibiotics for documented or presumed bacterial infections, whereas others had neoplastic diseases or organ transplants. Presumably, the fungus invades mucosal surfaces of the respiratory, gastrointestinal, or urogenital tracts of immunosuppressed hosts, with subsequent dissemination. A few cases of valvular endocarditis caused by *Trichosporon* spp. have been reported.[1,13] Phenotypic switching, a process by which pathogenic species of these yeasts vary their surface characteristics and enzyme production, may be a way they avoid host defense mechanisms.[11]

Feline infections have been characterized by mixed suppurative and granulomatous inflammation of the mucosal and submucosal or subcutaneous tissues. Evidence for immunosuppression has not been apparent in all affected cats, but one had multicentric lymphosarcoma.

CLINICAL FINDINGS

One cat was reported to have a fever, an inspiratory stertor, and a protruding unilateral nasal mass (Fig. 66-1) similar to that caused by *Cryptococcus neoformans*.[10] Later spread to regional lymph nodes and pulmonary tissues was suspected. Another cat had a chronic ulcerative subcutaneous lesion at the site of a bite wound.[4] A third cat suffered from chronic hematuria and dysuria as a result of chronic cystitis complicated by the yeast infection.[4] Another cat in which *T. domesticum* was isolated also had persistent lower urinary tract signs of hematuria and dysuria.[27] In people, clinical findings are usually those of fungal sepsis, with fever that is unresponsive to antibiotic therapy. Cutaneous lesions, chorioretinitis, and signs referable to renal glomerular and pulmonary vascular localization are most frequent.

DIAGNOSIS

Mere culture of *Trichosporon* spp. from cutaneous or mucosal surfaces can be misleading because the organism is a normal constituent of the endogenous microflora in these areas. Biopsy with histopathologic confirmation of host reaction and invasion of the deeper tissues by characteristic fungal elements is more specific for documentation of pathogenicity. In the animals with UTIs, yeasts may be observed microscopically in the urine sediment.

Trichosporon spp. can be grown on Sabouraud's or Mycosel agar (Becton Dickinson Microbiology Systems, Cockeysville, Md.) at 25° C, and after several days, spreading cream-colored yeastlike colonies are formed. Wet-mount lactophenol blue-stained preparations show hyaline, septate hyphae, arthroconidia (10.4 × 2.5 μm), and pleomorphic blastoconidia (2.5 to 8.0 μm in diameter). The characteristic arthroconidia are produced by segmentation and fragmentation of hyphae. Unlike those of *C. neoformans*, blastoconidia of the *Trichosporon* spp. do not show a capsule when stained with mucin stains or India ink. The species are distinguished from

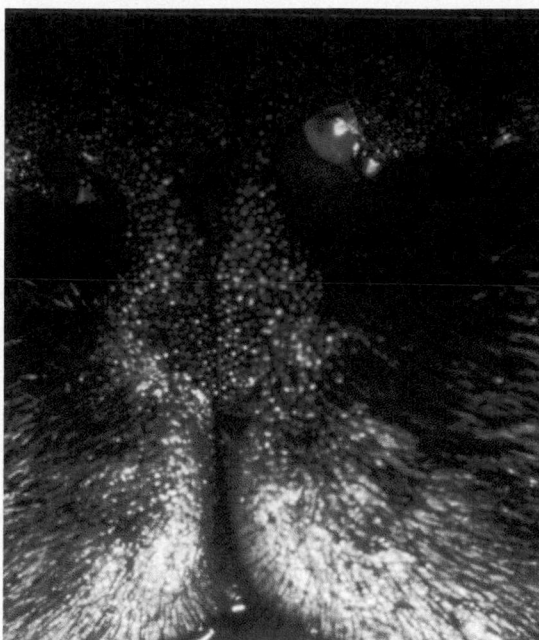

Fig 66-1 Mass *(arrow)* protruding from the nostril of the cat with nasal trichosporonosis. (Courtesy University of Georgia, Athens, Ga.)

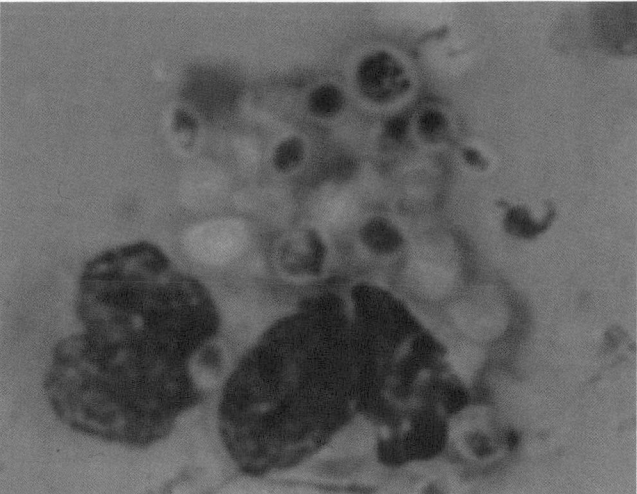

Fig 66-2 Macrophage with multiple intracytoplasmic yeasts *(arrows)* in an impression smear made of the excised mass shown in Fig. 66-1 (Wright, ×800). (Courtesy University of Georgia, Athens, Ga.)

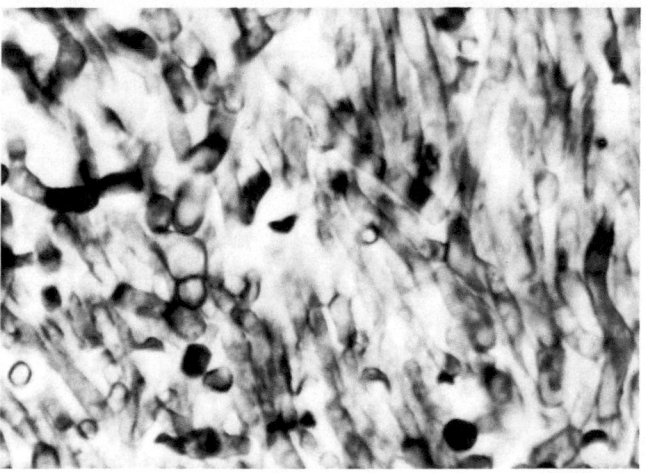

Fig 66-3 Disseminated trichosporonosis. Pleomorphic blastoconidia and branched, septate hyphae of *T. beigelii* occupy a nodular splenic infarct (GMS stain, ×850). (Courtesy Francis Chandler, Medical College of Georgia, Augusta, Ga.)

each other by differences in various carbon and nitrogen sources for growth.

T. beigelii produces a heat-stable, cell-wall antigen that is similar to the capsular polysaccharide of *C. neoformans*. The latex agglutination test, used to detect cryptococcal capsular polysaccharide antigen (see Chapter 61), has been used to diagnose disseminated *T. beigelii* infection in people and in experimentally infected rabbits.[21,32] Pretreatment of sera with pronase, which presumably disrupts immune complexes and nonspecific protein binding to the fungal capsule, increased the sensitivity of the antigen detection test. In a cat with nasal infection caused by *T. pullulans*, cryptococcal antigen test findings of serum were negative before clinical evidence of dissemination.[10]

Polymerase chain reaction has been used to develop genus-specific primers for detection of *Trichosporon* spp. in clinical specimens and culture.[27,30] Pathogenic *Trichosporon* sp. can be detected with this method, while DNA sequences of other similar pathogenic yeasts such as *Malassezia* spp., *Candida* spp., and *C. neoformans* are not amplified.

PATHOLOGIC FINDINGS

Histologic findings in trichosporonosis are similar to those of disseminated aspergillosis and consist of abscesses and nodular infarcts, with mycotic vascular invasion, thrombosis, and infiltration of neutrophils and macrophages.[3] Spherical to oval yeastlike organisms (blastoconidia), 3 to 8 μm in diameter, arthroconidia, and septate hyphae can be seen in tissue sections and impression smears (Figs. 66-2 and 66-3). In disseminated lesions, fungal elements often proliferate from a central nidus to produce a radial or sunburst pattern of growth (Figs. 66-4 and 66-5). All fungal elements are readily stained with periodic acid-Schiff and Gomori's methenamine silver stains as a result of abundant polysaccharides in the fungal cell walls. The arthroconidia, formed by hyperseptation and disarticulation of hyphal segments, are frequently difficult to demonstrate in tissue sections. When this problem occurs,

Trichosporon spp. and *Candida* spp. can be mistaken for each other and must be distinguished by immunohistologic or cultural studies.[15]

THERAPY

In general, *Trichosporon* spp. are more susceptible in vitro to benzimidazole compounds than they are to amphotericin B (AMB) or flucytosine. Resistance can vary among particular pathogenic species. Multifocal cutaneous *T. asahii* infection in a person was treated successfully with liposomal AMB and fluconazole in combination.[35] AMB has been effective in treating disseminated infection in an infant.[36] Resistance to AMB often has been demonstrated when treating infected people,[34] but itraconazole (ITZ) has been effective.[1] Multiple drug–resistant *Trichosporon* spp. from people have been susceptible to voriconazole.[5,6] Caspofungin has also been used to

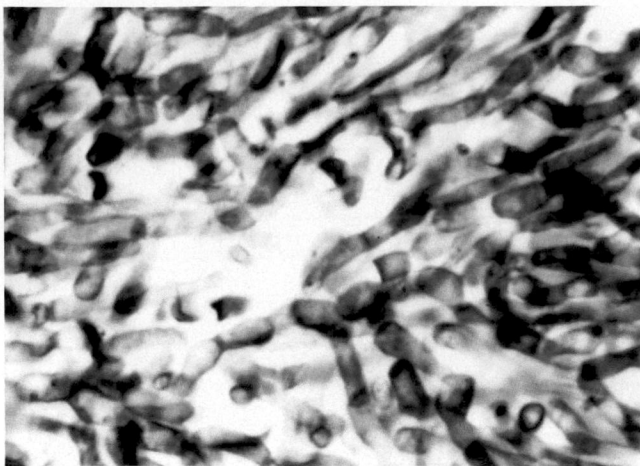

Fig 66-4 Disseminated trichosporonosis. A microcolony of *T. beigelii* consists of yeast-like cells, true hyphae, and arthroconidia formed by septal disarticulation of hyphae (GMS stain, ×850). (Courtesy Francis Chandler, Medical College of Georgia, Augusta, Ga.)

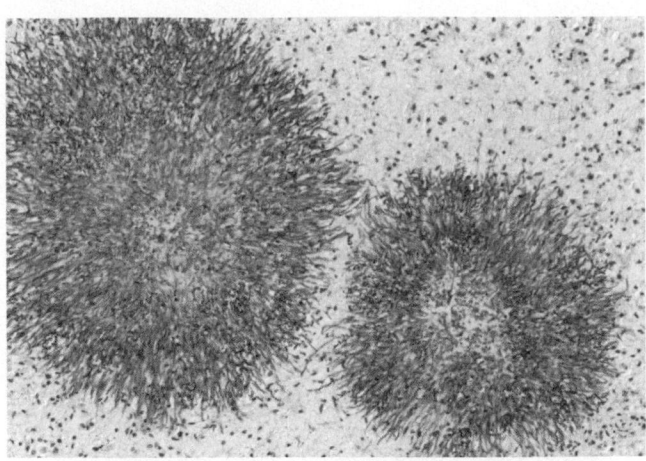

Fig 66-5 Disseminated trichosporonosis involving the spleen. Fungal elements proliferate in a radial or sunburst pattern to form two microcolonies of *T. beigelii* (PAS reaction, ×120). (Courtesy Francis Chandler, Medical College of Georgia, Augusta, Ga.)

Table • 66-1

Recommended Drugs for Topical Treatment of Trichosporonosis

SYSTEMIC DRUG[a]	SPECIES	DOSE[b]	ROUTE	INTERVAL (HOURS)	DURATION (WEEKS)[c]
Ketoconazole	D	5—11 mg/kg	PO	12	5
	C	50 mg total	PO	12—24	4
Itraconazole	B	5—10 mg/kg	PO	12	4
Fluconazole	B	5 mg/kg	PO	12	4

D, Dog; *C*, cat; *B*, dog and cat; *PO*, by mouth.
[a]For additional information on these drugs, see Drug Formulary, Appendix 8.
[b]Dose per administration at specified interval.
[c]May have to extend therapy based on response.

treat drug-resistant *Trichosporon* infections in people.[18] See Drug Formulary, Appendix 8, for further information on these novel antifungal drugs. Cats should initially be treated orally with ITZ when antifungal susceptibility data is not available (Table 66-1). Cats that develop anorexia, vomiting, or diarrhea may need to have the dosage reduced to 50 mg total on alternate days. ITZ is not as hepatotoxic in cats as is ketoconazole (KTZ). Reduction of ITZ dosage has been associated with relapse of disease. Surgical removal of a nasal granuloma in one cat with *T. pullulans* infection was incomplete, and later dissemination occurred despite treatment with KTZ or AMB and flucytosine.[10]

PUBLIC HEALTH CONSIDERATIONS

No documented zoonotic risk of *Trichosporon* infections exists in animals. These yeasts are ubiquitous in the environment and on the mucosa of clinically healthy animals and people; however, they can proliferate to large numbers in the lesions of affected animals. Contamination of human skin and mucosal surfaces is possible when handling infected animals. Transmission of infection in a dairy between cows was suspected via the handlers and the milking equipment or other fomites. Therefore wearing of gloves and hand washing is important to prevent colonization of people working in a contaminated environment.

SUGGESTED READINGS*

5. Falk R, Wolf DG, Shapiro M, et al. 2003. Multidrug-resistant *Trichosporon asahii* isolates are susceptible to voriconazole, *J Clin Microbiol* 41:911.
23. Moylett EH, Chinen J, Shearer WT. 2003. *Trichosporon pullulans* in 2 patients with chronic granulomatous disease: an emerging pathogen and review of the literature, *J Allergy Clin Immunol* 111:1370-1374.
27. Sakamoto Y, Kano R, Nakamwa Y, et al. 2001. Case report. First isolation of *Trichosporon domesticum* from a cat, *Mycoses* 44:518-520.
30. Sugita T, Nishikawa A, Shinoda T. 1998. Rapid detection of species of the opportunistic yeast *Trichosporon* by PCR, *J Clin Microbiol* 36:1458-1460.
37. Youker SR, Andreozzi RS, Appelbaum PC, et al. 2003. White piedra: further evidence of a synergistic infection, *J Am Acad Dermatol* 49:746-749.

*See the CD-ROM for a complete list of references.

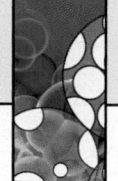
Miscellaneous Fungal Infections

Amy M. Grooters and Carol S. Foil

Infections caused by miscellaneous fungal and pseudofungal pathogens include pythiosis and lagenidiosis, which are caused by aquatic pathogens in the class Oomycetes and several opportunistic fungal infections that affect dogs and cats sporadically. Although identification of specific fungal pathogens is usually impossible without culture, these infections can often be categorized to some degree on the basis of their morphologic features, such as pigmentation, hyphal diameter, and septation in tissue. Infections caused by opportunistic fungi are generally classified by the form of the fungal elements in tissue and whether they are pigmented; for example, phaeohyphomycosis is caused by pigmented hyphal forms, hyalohyphomycosis by unpigmented hyphal forms, and eumycotic mycetoma by fibrosing granuloma with sulfur grains containing pigmented or unpigmented fungal elements. The diseases and agents are summarized in Table 67-1.

Clinically, distinguishing these infections is important because of differences in epidemiology, treatment, and prognosis. Therefore uncultured lesions should not be classified by pathologic features without the aid of serology, the polymerase chain reaction (PCR), or immunohistochemistry. In addition, diagnosis of any infection caused by a saprophytic fungus must be made on the basis of isolation of the organism from tissue (not exudate) and histologic evidence of tissue invasion by a morphologically compatible organism.

Pythiosis, lagenidiosis, and zygomycosis are caused by a taxonomically diverse group of pathogens but share similar clinical and histologic characteristics; all cause lesions characterized by pyogranulomatous and eosinophilic inflammation associated with broad, sparsely septate hyphae. Because of these similarities, they were previously grouped together in the category of *phycomycosis*. Although phycomycosis is a convenient label for cases in which a definitive culture-based diagnosis has not been made, the term is no longer an appropriate taxonomic designation and should be replaced in current literature with the more specific terms *pythiosis*, *lagenidiosis*, and *zygomycosis*. The obsolete term "chromomycosis" occasionally still appears in the veterinary literature as a synonym for either phaeohyphomycosis or chromoblastomycosis, the latter of which has not yet been described in animals.[15] Another difficulty for clinicians is the confusion that arises from taxonomic revisions in medical mycology, which results in confusing synonymy in fungal nomenclature. Excellent resources for updated fungal nomenclature can be found in the literature[24] and online at www.doctorfungus.org.

PYTHIOSIS

Pythiosis is best known as a cause of gastrointetinal (GI) or cutaneous disease in dogs[29,89] and of cutaneous granulomas in horses.[18] It has also been described as an uncommon cause of cutaneous or subcutaneous lesions in cats[9,25,40,121] and calves[91] and of arteritis, keratitis, or periorbital cellulitis in people.[4,61,113,122]

Etiology

Pythium insidiosum[22] is an aquatic pathogen belonging to the class Oomycetes in the kingdom Stramenopila (Chromista). *Pythium* species and other oomycetes differ from true fungi in producing motile, flagellate zoospores and having cell walls that contain cellulose and β-glucan but not chitin. In addition, ergosterol is not an important component of the oomycete cell membrane. Furthermore, members of the genera *Pythium* and *Lagenidium* are sterol auxotrophs—they incorporate sterols from their environment rather than producing them. Other members of the genus *Pythium* are plant pathogens of some economic importance. Based on molecular studies, the pathogens most closely related to oomycetes are the *Prototheca* species.[67] The infective stage of *P. insidiosum* is thought to be the biflagellate aquatic zoospore, which is released into warm water environments and likely causes infection by encysting in damaged skin or GI mucosa.[40] Although the specific factors that favor sporulation of *P. insidiosum* in the environment are unknown, some evidence suggests that certain types of plant material may be involved in the life cycle as a natural host.[88]

Epidemiology

In the United States, pythiosis is encountered most often in the Gulf Coast states but has been recognized with some frequency in animals living as far north as New Jersey, Virginia, Kentucky,[81] southern Illinois, and southern Indiana and as far west as Oklahoma, Missouri, and Kansas. Surprisingly, during the past 2 years, GI pythiosis was confirmed in several dogs that lived in Arizona but had not traveled outside the Southwest.[41] In addition, in fall 2003, GI pythiosis was confirmed in two dogs living in northern California.[51] Globally, pythiosis is most often encountered in Southeast Asia (especially Thailand and Indonesia), eastern coastal Australia, New Zealand, and South America but has also been recognized in Korea, Japan, and the Caribbean.

Pythiosis is most often identified in young, large-breed male dogs and is especially common in outdoor working breeds such as Labrador retrievers.[28] Affected dogs are taken to the veterinarian more often in the fall, winter, and early spring than in the late spring and summer months.[89] In cats, specific breed and sex predilections have not been apparent in the few cases that have been reported. However, of 11 cats with cutaneous pythiosis diagnosed through the authors' laboratory since 1999, six were younger than 10 months old, with an age range of 4 months to 9 years.[42]

Infected dogs often have a history of recurrent exposure to warm, freshwater habitats. However, some infections develop in suburban house dogs with no known access to a standing body of water. Because *P. insidiosum* zoospores have been shown to have an affinity for damaged skin,[83] it would make sense to assume that animals with cutaneous wounds or parasite-induced injury to GI mucosa are more likely to become infected. However, solid epidemiologic evidence to support this assumption is lacking. Other risk factors for the devel-

Table • 67-1

Miscellaneous Fungal Infections of Dogs and Cats

DISEASE	AGENT[a]	FUNGAL CHARACTERISTICS	SPECIES	LESION DISTRIBUTION AND ASSOCIATED CONDITIONS
Pythiosis	Pythium insidiosum[b]	Broad, poorly septate hyphae	Dog, cat	GI, subcutaneous, rarely disseminated
Lagenidiosis	Lagenidium sp	Broad, poorly septate hyphae	Dog	Cutaneous, subcutaneous, disseminated
Zygomycosis				
Mucormycosis	Mucor, Rhizopus, Rhizomucor, Absidia	Broad, poorly septate hyphae	Dog, cat	CNS, GI, disseminated
Entomophthoromy-cosis	Conidiobolus, Basidiobolus	Broad, poorly septate hyphae with eosinophilic sleeves	Dog	Conidiobolus: Nasal, pharyngeal, subcutaneous, pulmonary Basidiobolus: Subcutaneous, pulmonary
Adiaspiromycosis	Emmonsia[c] parva	Adiaspores	Dog	Lung
Hyalohyphomycosis	Acremonium[d]	Branching septate hyphae with chlamydospores	Dog	Cutaneous nodules, disseminated, keratomycosis
	Chrysosporium	Swollen hyphae and yeastlike bodies	Dog	Diskospondylitis
	Fusarium	Branching, septate hyphae with ballooning ends	Dog, cat	Pyelonephritis, cutaneous, disseminated, keratomycosis, meningitis
	Geotrichum	Short, septate hyphae and yeastlike bodies	Dog	Cutaneous, disseminated
	Paecilomyces	Branching septate hyphae, dilated hyphae, and yeastlike bodies	Dog, cat	Nasal granuloma, CNS, disseminated, diskospodylitis, prostatitis, cystitis
	Pseudallescheria[e]	Septate, branching hyphae and racket hyphae	Dog	Cutaneous, osteomyelitis, nasal granuloma, keratomycosis, abdominal cavity, disseminated
	Metarhizium	Long adherent chains of olive-green cylindrical conidia	Cat	Rhinitis
	Monocillium indicum	Septate hyphae with large chlamydospores and small yeastlike bodies	Dog	Disseminated granulomatous lymphadenitis and splenitis[72a]
Phaeohyphomycosis	Alternaria	Darkly pigmented septate hyphae with swollen bodies	Dog, cat	Nasal, subcutaneous, keratomycosis
	Bipolaris[f]	Branching, septate, lightly pigmented hyphae with globose elements	Dog, cat	Subcutaneous, paranasal sinusitis, rarely disseminated
	Cladophialophora[g]	Lightly pigmented septate hyphae, bizarre forms, yeastlike cells	Cat, dog	CNS, keratomycosis, cutaneous, disseminated
	Curvularia	Moderately pigmented hyphae with swollen forms and yeastlike bodies	Dog, cat	Subcutaneous, keratomycosis
	Exophiala	Pigmented hyphae and yeastlike bodies	Cat	Subcutaneous, on face and feet; rhinitis; disseminated including CNS
	Fonsecaea	Moderately pigmented hyphae and yeastlike bodies	Cat	Dermal on nose

Table • 67-1

Continued

DISEASE	AGENT[a]	FUNGAL CHARACTERISTICS	SPECIES	LESION DISTRIBUTION AND ASSOCIATED CONDITIONS
	Macrophomina	Septate hyaline or pigmented hyphae	Cat	Subcutnaeous mass from pyogranulomatous inflammation[51b]
	Microsphaerosis arundinis	Yeastlike bodies and septate pigmented mycelia	Cat	Draining sinuses on extremity[65a]
	Moniliella	Darkly pigmented pseudohyphae and yeastlike cell	Cat	Subcutaneous
	Ochroconis	Pigmented hyphae?	Cat	Disseminated
	Phialemonium	Pleomorphic with darkly pigmented hyphae and swollen yeastlike elements	Dog	Osteomyelitis, cutaneous nodules, tracts
	Phialophora	Pigmented pseudohyphae with globose yeastlike bodies	Cat	Subcutaneous
	Phoma	Lightly pigmented thick-walled hyphae	Cat	Cerebral
	Pseudomicrodochium	Pigmented hyphae with bizarre forms	Dog	Cutaneous
	Scolecobasidium	Septate pigmented hyphae with globose swellings	Cat	Subcutaneous
	Stemphyllium	Pigmented hyphae	Cat	Subcutaneous
Eumycotic mycetoma (white grain)	Acremonium	Unpigmented tissue grains with hyphae and chlamydospores	Dog (possibly)	Intraabdominal and disseminated
	Pseudallescheria	Unpigmented tissue grains with phphae and chiamydospores	Dog	Intraabdominal
Eumycotic mycetoma (black grain)	*Cladophialophora bantiana*	Pigmented tissues grains	Dog	Subcutaneous on thorax[51a]
	Curvularia	Pigmented tissue grains with hyphae and chlamydospores	Dog, cat	Subcutaneous on extremities
	Madurella	Pigmented tissue grains with hyphae and chlamydospores	Dog	Intraabdominal
	Phaeococcomyces[h]	Possibly: pigmented tissue grains with hyphae and chlamydospores	Cat	Subcutaneous, tailhead
	Staphylotrichum coccosporum	Possibly: pigmented tissue grains with hyphae and chlamydospores	Cat	Subcutaneous

GI, Gastrointestinal; *CNS*, central nervous system
[a]An excellent resource for taxonomic synonyms is www.doctorfungus.org
[b]Synonyms: *Hyphomyces destruens, P. destrans, P. gracile.* An oomycete in the kingdom Stramenopila
[c]Synonym: *Chrysosporium*
[d]Synonym: Cephalosporium
[e]Synonyms: *Petriellidum; Allescheria*; sprophytic stage = *Scedosporium apiospermum*
[f]Synonyms: *Cladosporium, Drechslera*
[g]Synonyms: *Cladosponum bantianum, Xylohypha bantiana, Torula bantiana, Cladosporium trichoides*
[h]Synonym: *Phaeococcus*

opment of pythiosis have not been identified. Affected animals are typically immunocompetent and otherwise healthy.

Clinical Findings

Clinical signs caused by *P. insidiosum* infection are the result of cutaneous or GI lesions or of disease extension into adjacent tissues or regional lymph nodes. Cutaneous and GI lesions are rarely found together in the same patient. Systemic dissemination of pythiosis has only been described once.[29]

Cutaneous pythiosis in small animals typically causes nonhealing wounds and invasive masses that contain ulcerated nodules and draining tracts (Figs. 67-1 and 67-2).[29,121] Affected dogs are usually taken to the veterinarian because of solitary or multiple cutaneous or subcutaneous lesions involving the extremities, tailhead, ventral neck, perineum, or medial thigh. When present, regional lymphadenomegaly often reflects extension of infection rather than just reactive inflammation. Lesions in 11 cats with cutaneous pythiosis recently evaluated through the authors' laboratory have included subcutaneous masses (some of which were highly invasive) in the inguinal, tailhead, or periorbital regions, and draining nodular lesions or ulcerated plaquelike lesions on the extremities (see Fig. 67-1), occasionally centered on the digits or footpad. Two cats with pythiosis had large subcutaneous masses affecting the extremities and cranioventral thorax but no cutaneous involvement.[121] In a third case, *P. insidiosum* infection resulted in nasal cavity and nasopharyngeal lesions and bilateral retrobulbar masses.[9]

GI pythiosis in dogs is characterized by severe segmental transmural thickening of the stomach, small intestine, colon, rectum, or (although rarely) the esophagus or pharyngeal region (Fig. 67-3).[28,54,89,99] Mesenteric lymphadenomegaly is common and occasionally observed without accompanying GI tract lesions. The gastric outflow area, duodenum, and ileocolic junction are the most frequently affected portions of the GI tract, and it is not uncommon to find two or more segmental lesions in the same patient. Inflammation in affected regions is typically centered on the submucosa, with variable mucosal ulceration and occasional extension of disease through serosal surfaces, resulting in adhesion formation and peritonitis. Involvement of the mesenteric root may cause severe enlargement of mesenteric lymph nodes, which are often embedded in a single, large, firm granulomatous mass that is palpable in the midabdomen. Extension of disease into mesenteric vessels may result in bowel ischemia, infarction, perforation, or acute hemoabdomen.[100] In addition, infection may extend from the GI tract into contiguous tissues such as the pancreas and uterus.[28,89] In one report, a prostatic abscess caused by *P. insidiosum* was observed in a dog with an adjacent colonic lesion.[62] Clinical signs associated with GI pythiosis include weight loss, vomiting, diarrhea, hematochezia, or all of these symptoms. Physical examination often reveals a very thin body and a palpable abdominal mass. Signs of systemic illness such as lethargy or depression are not typically present unless intestinal obstruction, infarction, or perforation occurs. Similar to clinical signs observed in dogs, those of GI pythiosis in cats have been attributed to partial intestinal obstruction, palpable abdominal masses, and mesenteric lymphadenomegaly.[101a]

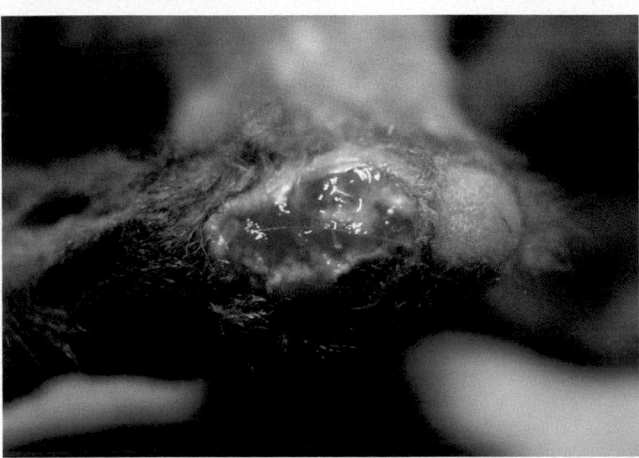

Fig 67-1 Ulcerative lesion caused by pythiosis on tarsus of cat. (Courtesy Carol Foil, Louisiana State University, Baton Rouge, La.)

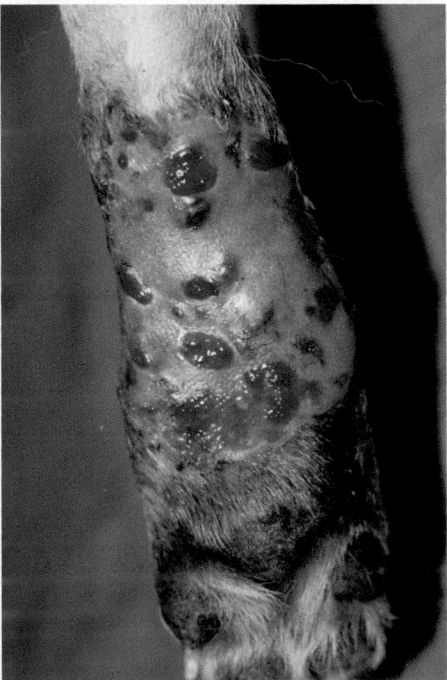

Fig 67-2 Cutaneous pythiosis in dog. Split-thickness graft was performed after resection of subcutaneous pythiosis lesion and became infiltrated with new granulomatous nodules. Leg was amputated, curing the disease. (Courtesy Carol Foil, Louisiana State University, Baton Rouge, La.)

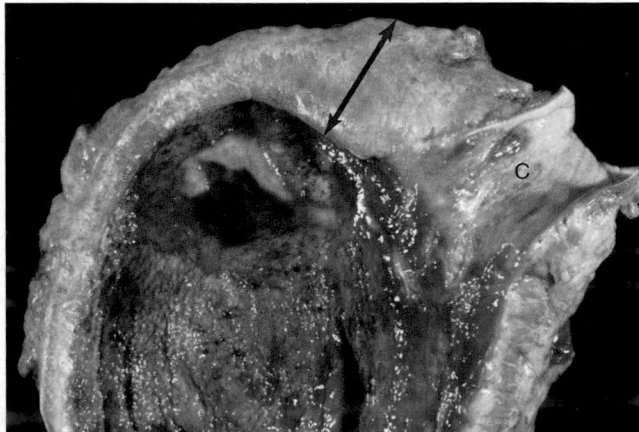

Fig 67-3 Gastric pythiosis in dog. C, Cardia. Note extreme thickening of gastric wall (*arrow*). (Courtesy Amy Grooters, Louisiana State University, Baton Rouge, La.)

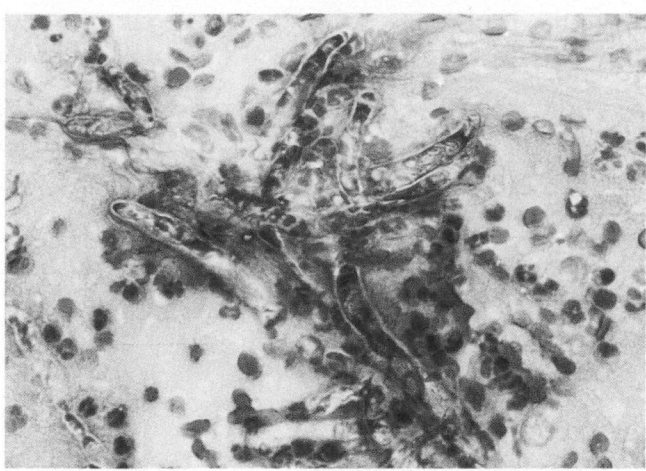

Fig 67-4 Cytologic specimen obtained by fine needle aspiration of enlarged inguinal lymph node in 1-year-old female spayed Labrador retriever with a large tailhead lesion caused by pythiosis. Note presence of multiple broad, poorly septate hyphal structures (modified Wright stain). (Courtesy Casey LeBlanc, Louisiana State University, Baton Rouge, La.)

Diagnosis

The definitive diagnosis of pythiosis has traditionally been challenging because histologic features are not specific and culture is often not performed successfully. However, numerous highly specific serologic, immunohistochemical, and molecular-based tools for the diagnosis of pythiosis have been developed. These assays are likely to make the definitive diagnosis of pythiosis possible in the majority of affected animals, even when culture is unsuccessful. In addition, they may provide clinicians with an opportunity to make a diagnosis earlier in the course of disease, when lesions may be more amenable to surgical or medical therapy.

Culture

Isolation of *P. insidiosum* from infected tissues is not difficult when appropriate sample handling and culture techniques are used. For best results, unrefrigerated tissue samples should be wrapped in a sterile saline-moistened gauze sponge, shipped at ambient temperature, and arrive at the laboratory within 24 hours of collection. However, when samples cannot be processed for more than 2 to 3 days after collection, they should be shipped with ice packs, stored in the refrigerator, or stored at ambient temperature in an antibiotic solution to decrease proliferation of bacterial contaminants.[50] The use of selective media significantly increases the likelihood of isolating pathogenic oomycetes. The authors routinely use vegetable extract agar[50] amended with streptomycin (200 µg/ml) and ampicillin (100 µg/ml) for the isolation of *P. insidiosum*. As a commercially available alternative, Campy blood agar (Remel, Inc., Lenexa, Kan.), which contains trimethoprim, vancomycin, polymyxin B, cephalothin, and amphotericin B (AMB), is also effective. Small pieces of fresh, nonmacerated tissue should be placed directly on the surface of the agar and incubated at 37° C (98.6° F); growth is typically observed within 12 to 24 hours.

Although the identification of oomycetes is generally based on morphologic features of sexual reproductive structures such as oogonia and antheridia, isolates of *P. insidiosum* rarely produce these structures in vitro. Therefore identification of *P. insidiosum* should be based on colonial and hyphal characteristics; growth at 37° C; production of motile, reniform,

biflagellate zoospores; and if possible, specific PCR amplification or ribosomal RNA (rRNA) gene sequencing. Colonies on vegetable extract, Sabouraud's dextrose, or cornmeal agar are typically submerged, are white to colorless, and have an irregular radiate pattern.[7,23] Microscopically, hyphae are broad (4 to 10 µm in diameter), hyaline, sparsely septate, and tend to branch at right angles. Zoospores can be readily produced by placing boiled grass blades on the surface of a 1- to 2-day-old colony growing on 2% water agar, incubating at 37° C for 18 to 24 hours, and then placing the infected grass blades in a dilute salt solution.[19,35,86] After 2 to 4 hours of incubation at 37° C, terminal vesicles from which zoospores are released can be seen extending from the cut edges of the infected grass blades. Although the production of zoospores is an important supporting feature for the identification of pathogenic oomycetes, it is not specific for *P. insidiosum*.

Serology

Immunoblot analysis has been used successfully to demonstrate the ability of sera from *Pythium*-infected horses,[85] dogs,[66] and cats[101a] to recognize antigens of *P. insidiosum* and has the added advantage of high specificity and sensitivity. Because of these advantages, immunoblot analysis is currently the authors' serologic test of choice for evaluation of dogs and cats suspected of having pythiosis, lagenidiosis, or zygomycosis. In addition, a soluble mycelial antigen-based enzyme-linked immunosorbent assay (ELISA) for the detection of anti-*P. insidiosum* antibodies in dogs and cats has been found to be highly sensitive and specific for the diagnosis of pythiosis.[47] In addition to providing a means for early, noninvasive diagnosis, the ELISA also appears to be useful for monitoring response to therapy in affected patients. In 11 dogs and 2 cats assessed through the authors' laboratory, a dramatic decrease in antibody levels approaching the range of healthy animals was detected 2 to 3 months after successful surgical resection of infected tissues. In contrast, antibody levels remain high in animals that have a clinical recurrence after surgical treatment. Therefore the ELISA appears to be a promising tool for the early detection of postoperative recurrence and may also be used to guide the duration of postoperative medical therapy.

Molecular Assays

To circumvent the difficulties associated with obtaining a culture-based diagnosis of pythiosis, a *P. insidiosum*-specific PCR assay was recently developed.[43] This assay can be applied to DNA extracted either from cultured isolates or appropriately preserved infected tissue samples.[126] In addition, this technique has been successfully used with DNA extracted from paraffin-embedded tissues sections.[62] The major advantage of this assay is its high specificity.

Immunohistochemistry

Immunohistochemical techniques based on polyclonal antibodies developed first by Brown et al[13] and later by Newton[99] have been used regularly during the past 10 years as confirmatory tests for pythiosis. An advantage of these techniques is that they can be used with paraffin-embedded tissues, permitting the evaluation of archival samples. However, at least one of these antibodies has demonstrated cross-reactive staining when used to evaluate tissues from dogs with conidiobolomycosis[58] and lagenidiosis.[46] Therefore the specificity of this antibody for the immunohistochemical diagnosis of pythiosis may be questionable. A new polyclonal anti-*P. insidiosum* antibody raised in chickens and adsorbed with sonicated *Lagenidium* and *Conidiobolus* hyphae appears to be highly specific for the immunohistochemical detection of *P. insidiosum* hyphae in tissues.[49]

Pathologic Findings

A presumptive diagnosis of pythiosis, lagenidiosis, or zygomycosis can occasionally be established cytologically if lesions are accessible (Fig. 67-4). Cytologic examination of exudate from draining tracts, impression smears made from ulcerated skin lesions, and fine needle aspirates of enlarged lymph nodes often reveal pyogranulomatous, suppurative, or eosinophilic inflammation (or all of these). In addition, macerated tissue fixed in 10% potassium hydroxide (KOH) may be examined microscopically for the presence of typical wide, poorly septate, branching hyphal elements.

Histologic findings associated with pythiosis are characterized by eosinophilic granulomatous to pyogranulomatous inflammation with fibrosis. Affected tissues typically contain multiple foci of necrosis surrounded and infiltrated by neutrophils, eosinophils, and macrophages. In addition, discrete granulomas composed of epithelioid macrophages, plasma cells, multinucleate giant cells, and fewer neutrophils and eosinophils may be observed.[28,29,59] Vasculitis is occasionally present. Organisms are usually found within areas of necrosis or at the center of discrete granulomas.[89] Although *P. insidiosum* hyphae are difficult to visualize on sections stained with hematoxylin-eosin (H and E) stain, they may be identified as clear spaces (*hyphal ghosts*) surrounded by a narrow band of eosinophilic material.[89] Hyphae are easily visualized in sections stained with Gomori's methenamine silver (GMS) but not with periodic acid–Schiff (PAS). They are broad (mean, 4 μm; range, 2 to 7 μm), rarely septate, and occasionally branching.[29,89]

Cutaneous pythiosis typically causes severe nodular to diffuse ulcerative dermatitis and panniculitis. Because areas of inflammation are most often found in the deep dermis and subcutis, wedge biopsies are preferred to punch biopsies when pythiosis is suspected. Similarly, because inflammation in GI pythiosis centers on the submucosal and muscular layers rather than mucosa and lamina propria,[89] the diagnosis of pythiosis may be missed on endoscopic biopsies that fail to reach deeper tissues. Therefore pythiosis should be considered as a differential diagnosis when endoscopic biopsies reveal eosinophilic or pyogranulomatous inflammation without identification of an etiologic agent.

Therapy

Aggressive surgical resection is the treatment of choice for pythiosis. Because it provides the best opportunity for a long-term cure, complete excision of infected tissue should be pursued whenever possible. When cutaneous lesions are limited to a single distal extremity, amputation is recommended. In animals with GI pythiosis, segmental lesions should be resected with 3- to 4-cm margins whenever possible. Despite the fact that mesenteric lymphadenomegaly is almost always present, *P. insidiosum* hyphae are often absent in enlarged mesenteric nodes. Therefore the presence of nonresectable mesenteric lymphadenomegaly should not dissuade the surgeon from pursuing complete resection of a segmental bowel lesion. In this situation, enlarged lymph nodes should be biopsied and cultured for prognostic information. Unfortunately, most dogs with GI pythiosis are not taken to the veterinarian until late in the course of disease, when complete excision is not possible. In addition, the anatomic location of the lesion may prevent complete surgical excision when the esophagus, gastric outflow tract, rectum, or mesenteric root is involved.

Local postoperative recurrence of pythiosis is common and can occur either at the site of resection or in regional lymph nodes. For this reason, combination medical therapy with itraconazole (ITZ) and terbinafine is recommended for at least 2 to 3 months after surgery (Table 67-2). To monitor for recurrence, ELISA serology should be performed before and 2 to 3 months after surgery. In animals that have had a complete surgical resection and do not have a recurrence of disease, serum antibody levels drop significantly within 3 months of surgery.[47] If this occurs, medical therapy can be discontinued, with subsequent reevaluation of serum antibody levels in 3 months. If antibody levels remain elevated 2 to 3 months after surgery, medical therapy should be continued, with periodic reevaluation of ELISA serology.

Medical therapy for pythiosis has traditionally been unrewarding, likely because ergosterol (the target for most currently available antifungal drugs) is generally lacking in the oomycete cell membrane. Despite this fact, clinical and serologic cures have been obtained using medical therapy with ergosterol-targeting drugs in a small number of *P. insidiosum*-

Table • 67-2

Drug Therapy for Miscellaneous Fungal Infections[a]

DRUG[b]	SPECIES	DOSE (MG/KG)[c]	ROUTE	INTERVAL	DURATION (MONTHS)
Itraconazole[d]	B	10[e]	PO	24 hr	3–9
	B	5–15[f]	PO	24 hr	3–9
Terbinafine[d]	D	5–10[e]	PO	24 hr	3–9
Amphotericin B lipid complex (ABLC)	D	2–3[g]	IV	3 times weekly	
Amphotericin B lipid complex (ABLC)	C	1[h]	IV	3 times weekly	

B, Dog and cat; *D*, dog; *C*, cat; *PO*, by mouth; *IV*, intravenous.
[a]Including pythiosis, lagenidiosis, zygomycosis, hyalohphomycosis, and phaeohyphomycosis.
[b]See Appendix 8, Drug Formulary, for more information on these drugs.
[c]Dose per administration at specified interval.
[d]Combination of itraconazole and terbinafine recommended for treatment of pythiosis and lagenidiosis.
[e]Recommended dose for pythiosis and lagenidiosis.
[f]Recommended dose for zygomycosis, phaeohyphomycosis, and hyalohyphomycosis.
[g]For a cumulative dose of 24 to 27 mg/kg.
[h]For a cumulative dose of 12 mg/kg.

infected dogs, as well as with an infection in a 2-year-old child.[113] In the authors' experience during the past 5 years at Louisiana State University, a small number of dogs with GI pythiosis have responded to either ITZ or amphotericin B (AMB) lipid complex (see Table 67-2). More recently, the authors have observed clinical and serologic improvement or resolution in several cases of canine and feline cutaneous pythiosis treated with the combination of ITZ and terbinafine. Although the percentage of animals responding is still low (less than 20%), based on our subjective observations, the combination protocol seems superior to ITZ or AMB alone.

Caspofungin, the first antifungal in the newly developed echinocandin class of β-glucan synthase inhibitors to gain United Sates Food and Drug Administration approval, has the potential to be a much more effective drug for the treatment of oomycosis because of the large amount of β-glucan present in the oomycete cell wall. However, it is extremely costly and likely to be used only on rare occasions.

A vaccine derived from soluble mycelial antigens and secreted exoantigens of *P. insidiosum* has been used successfully to treat cutaneous granulomas in horses and vasculitis in people.[60,120] Unfortunately, although controlled trials have not been completed, the efficacy of *Pythium* vaccines in dogs appears to be poor, and clinical improvement has not been observed in any of the authors' patients.

The limited published information currently available regarding the efficacy of *Pythium* vaccines in dogs is anecdotal.[84] In one canine case report that suggested a vaccine-related therapeutic effect,[56] tissues were submitted to Louisiana State University that were obtained after the initial diagnostic wedge biopsies but before vaccine administration. The tissue culture was negative for oomycetes and failed to show any hyphae in multiple GMS-stained sections, suggesting that the disease may have been resolving before the vaccine administration.[39] Interestingly, the authors of this chapter are aware of one additional dog in which lesions associated with cutaneous pythiosis resolved completely without additional therapy after incomplete surgical resection.

Public Health Considerations
Infections caused by *P. insidiosum* are acquired from the environment. No evidence suggests transmission between hosts; however, routine precautions should be taken when handling infected tissues or exudates.

LAGENIDIOSIS

Until recently, *P. insidiosum* was considered to be the only mammalian pathogen in the class Oomycetes. However, in 1999 a second pathogenic oomycete was isolated from tissue taken from a dog with severe multifocal cutaneous lesions and regional lymphadenomegaly. The dog died acutely after rupture of a caudal vena caval aneurysm, and necropsy revealed severe sublumbar lymphadenitis and pyogranulomatous vasculitis. Sequencing of a portion of the rRNA gene of the isolate recovered from this dog identified it as member of the genus *Lagenidium*.[45] More than 40 dogs with serologic, histologic, or culture evidence (or all of these) of *Lagenidium* species infection have been identified.

Etiology
The majority of species in the genus *Lagenidium* are parasites that infect algae, fungi, rotifers, nematodes, crustaceans, *Daphne*, and insect larvae. The best studied species, *Lagenidium giganteum*, is a larval mosquito pathogen approved by the United States Environmental Protection Agency for use as a biocontrol agent for mosquitos.[64] Although antigenic and molecular similarities suggest that the canine pathogenic

Lagenidium species is closely related to *L. giganteum*, differences in their in vitro growth characteristics and the failure of *L. giganteum* to infect rodents in mammalian safety studies[63] suggest that they are likely distinct species. Little is known about the life cycle of the canine pathogenic *Lagenidium* species, although it is likely similar to that of *P. insidiosum* and *L. giganteum*.

Epidemiology
The epidemiologic and clinicopathologic features of lagenidiosis that have thus far been identified are similar in many respects to those that have previously been associated with cutaneous pythiosis. Affected animals are typically young to middle-age dogs living in the southeastern United States. Although most of these dogs have been from Florida or Louisiana, dogs in Texas, Tennessee, Virginia, and Indiana have been identified as well. Numerous infected dogs frequented lakes or ponds. Two of the dogs were unrelated housemates,[46] suggesting that environmental exposure to the pathogen may play an important role in infection.

Clinical Findings
Dogs with lagenidiosis are typically taken to the veterinarian with progressive cutaneous or subcutaneous lesions (often multifocal) involving the extremities, mammary region, perineum, or trunk.[46] Grossly, these lesions appear as firm dermal or subcutaneous nodules or as ulcerated, thickened, edematous areas with regions of necrosis and numerous draining tracts (Fig. 67-5). Regional lymphadenomegaly is often noted and may develop in the absence of cutaneous lesions. Animals

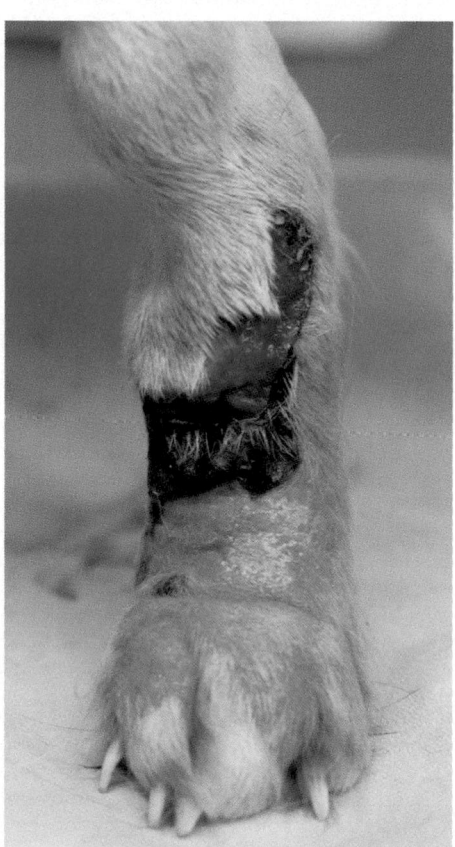

Fig 67-5 Ulcerative dermatitis caused by *Lagenidium* species infection in young dog with progressive multifocal skin lesions and generalized lymphadenopathy. (Courtesy Amy Grooters, Louisiana State University, Baton Rouge, La.)

with great vessel or sublumbar lymph node involvement often develop hind limb edema. Similar to the clinical course associated with cutaneous pythiosis, skin lesions in dogs with lagenidiosis tend to be progressive, locally invasive, and poorly responsive to therapy. However, in contrast to pythiosis the majority of dogs with lagenidiosis have been found to have lesions in distant sites, including great vessels, sublumbar and inguinal lymph nodes, lung, pulmonary hilus, and cranial mediastinum. Lagenidiosis has not been identified in cats.

Diagnosis

Immunoblot serology for the detection of anti-*Lagenidium* antibodies in canine serum can provide a presumptive diagnosis of lagenidiosis, but must be interpreted in conjunction with results of serologic testing for *P. insidiosum* infection because of the potential for cross-reactivity in serum from dogs with pythiosis.[46] A definitive diagnosis of lagenidiosis is best made by culture. Isolation techniques for *Lagenidium* species are similar to those described for *P. insidiosum* but involve peptone-yeast-glucose (PYG) agar amended with ampicillin (100 μg/ml) and streptomycin (200 μg/ml).

Identifying *Lagenidium* isolates based on morphologic characteristics is more difficult than identifying *P. insidiosum* because zoospores are only occasionally produced with the techniques used for sporulation of *P. insidiosum* and because sexual reproductive structures have not been identified. Colonies of *Lagenidium* species on PYG agar are submerged and white to colorless. Microscopically, mature hyphae are broad (25 to 40 μm in diameter), are occasionally to frequently branching or budding, and often appear as segmented chains of rectangular to oval structures in mature colonies. Because of the current limitations associated with morphologic characterization of this pathogen, definitive identification of *Lagenidium* species should be based on rRNA gene sequencing or specific PCR amplification.[39] The same PCR assay can also be used to detect *Lagenidium* DNA in infected tissue samples.[126]

Pathologic Findings

The histologic features of lagenidiosis, which are similar to those associated with pythiosis and zygomycosis, are characterized by pyogranulomatous and eosinophilic inflammation associated with broad, irregularly branching, sparsely septate hyphae. In contrast to *P. insidiosum*, *Lagenidium* species hyphae are usually visible on sections stained with H and E. On GMS-stained sections, numerous broad, thick-walled, irregularly septate hyphae are easily recognized (Fig. 67-6). *Lagenidium* hyphae typically vary significantly in size but in general are much larger than *P. insidiosum* hyphae, ranging from 7 to 25 μm in diameter, with an average of 12 μm.[46] Cytologic examination of lymph node aspirates or exudate from draining tracts may reveal pyogranulomatous to eosinophilic inflammation with or without broad, poorly septate hyphal elements.[40]

Therapy

Aggressive surgical resection of infected tissues is the treatment of choice for lagenidiosis. In animals with lesions limited to a single distal extremity, amputation is recommended. In those with cutaneous or subcutaneous lesions in other areas of the body, the surgeon should pursue aggressive resection with wide margins. Because dogs with lagenidiosis often have occult systemic lesions, radiographic imaging of the chest and abdomen and sonographic imaging of the abdomen are recommended to determine the extent of disease before attempting surgical resection of cutaneous lesions. Unfortunately, the majority of *Lagenidium*-infected dogs have nonresectable disease in regional lymph nodes or distant sites by the time the initial diagnosis is made. Medical therapy for lagenidiosis

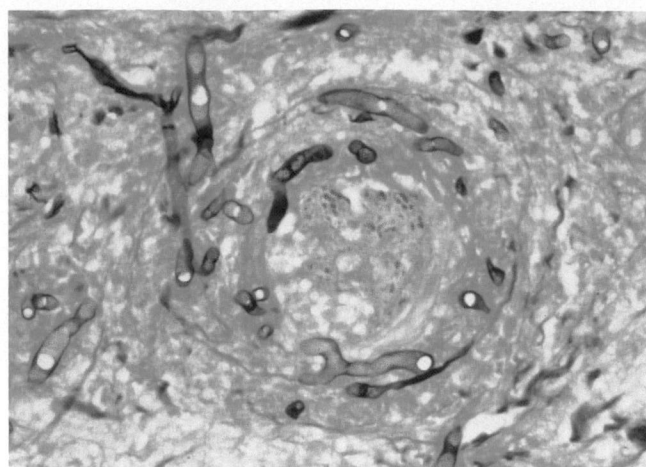

Fig 67-6 Broad, thick-walled, irregularly septate hyphae associated with granulomatous vasculitis in lymph node from 2-year-old dog with *Lagenidium* species infection (GMS stain). (Courtesy Amy Grooters, Louisiana State University, Baton Rouge, La.)

is typically ineffective. However, a combination of ITZ with terbinafine combined with aggressive surgical resection was effective in resolving a *Lagenidium* species infection in two dogs with multifocal cutaneous lesions but no systemic lesions (see Table 67-2). In general, the prognosis for dogs with lagenidiosis is grave.

Public Health Considerations

Infections caused by *Lagenidium* species are acquired from the environment. No evidence suggests transmission between hosts; however, routine precautions should be taken when handling infected tissues or exudates.

ZYGOMYCOSIS

The term *zygomycosis* refers to infections caused by fungi in the class Zygomycetes, including the genera *Basidiobolus* and *Conidiobolus* in the order Entomophthorales, and the genera *Rhizopus, Absidia, Mucor, Saksenaea,* and others in the order Mucorales. In humans and veterinary patients, the Mucorales organisms tend to cause an acute, rapidly progressive disease in debilitated or immunocompromised individuals, whereas the Entomophthorales organisms typically cause chronic localized infections in subcutaneous tissue or nasal submucosa of immunocompetent patients.[108] Culture-confirmed infections caused by pathogens in the order Mucorales have not been well documented in small animals. However, in dogs, *Basidiobolus* and *Conidiobolus* species have been reported to cause cutaneous pyogranulomatous lesions that are grossly and histologically similar to those caused by *P. insidiosum* and *Lagenidium* species.

Etiology and Epidemiology

Basidiobolus ranarum (previously *Basidiobolus haptosporus*), *Conidiobolus coronatus, Conidiobolus incongruus,* and *Conidiobolus lamprauges* are saprophytes that are widely distributed in nature. *Conidiobolus* and *Basidiobolus* species are found in soil and decaying plant matter, and *Basidiobolus* species are also commonly isolated from insects and the feces of amphibians and reptiles.[108] Cutaneous infection with *Basidiobolus* or *Conidiobolus* species likely occurs by percutaneous inoculation of spores through a minor trauma or insect bites. Dogs with hard palate lesions caused by *Conidiobolus* species may become infected by direct implantation of spores when chewing on decaying pieces of wood. Infection may also result from inhalation or ingestion of spores. Affected animals are typically immunocompetent.

Clinical Findings

In humans, horses, sheep, and other mammalian species, conidiobolomycosis is usually a nasopharyngeal infection with possible local dissemination into tissues of the face, retropharyngeal region, and retrobulbar space. In two dogs evaluated by the authors, a presumptive diagnosis of nasopharyngeal conidiobolomycosis was made on the basis of histologic and serologic findings. One of the dogs showed signs of chronic nasal cavity disease, and the other had a severe chronic ulcerative dermatitis of the nasal planum. In two other dogs evaluated in the authors' hospital, culture-confirmed conidiobolomycosis was associated with ulcerative lesions of the hard palate (Fig. 67-7). Both dogs had radiographically apparent involvement of the nasal cavity or nasopharynx. In a fifth dog described in the literature, *Conidiobolus* infection was associated with multifocal nodular draining subcutaneous lesions and regional lymphadenomegaly. In addition, a *Conidiobolus* species was recently confirmed as the cause of pneumonia in a dog that was receiving chemotherapy for treatment of lymphoma.[44] Culture-confirmed cases of zygomycosis in cats have not been well described. However, the authors have made a presumptive diagnosis of conidiobolomycosis based on histopathology and serology in a 3-year-old cat with an ulcerative lesion of the hard palate.

Basidiobolomycosis is a rare cause of ulcerative draining skin lesions in dogs (Fig. 67-8) and in one case was reported as a cause of tracheobronchitis.[38] Disseminated *Basidiobolus* species infection involving the GI tract and other abdominal organs have been described in two dogs.[88,92] In addition, the authors have evaluated samples from two dogs (one with a focal preputial lesion and another with a focal vulvar lesion) in which a presumptive diagnosis of basidiobolomycosis was made on the basis of histologic and serologic findings. Complete surgical resection of the infected tissue cured both animals.

Diagnosis

Because serologic and immunohistochemical techniques are not currently available for the diagnosis of conidiobolomycosis and basidiobolomycosis in small animals, a definitive diagnosis must be based on isolation and identification of the pathogen. Entomophthorales organisms typically grow well on media routinely used for the isolation of pathogenic fungi, such as Sabouraud's dextrose agar, potato flakes agar,[109] potato dextrose agar, or cornmeal agar. The authors routinely use potato flakes agar amended with ampicillin (100 μg/ml) and streptomycin (200 μg/ml) for initial isolation of *Conidiobolus* and *Basidiobolus* species.

Identification of zygomycetes in the laboratory is generally based on morphologic characteristics of asexual reproductive structures (conidia) and sexual reproductive structures (zygospores).[24] *Conidiobolus* isolates on potato flakes agar or half-strength cornmeal agar readily produce primary conidia that are forcibly discharged and can be visualized on the underside of the petri dish lid. Primary conidia of *C. coronatus* are spherical, 40 μm in diameter and have a prominent basal papilla. Because *C. coronatus* is a heterothallic species, zygospores are not observed in clinical isolates. However, *C. incongruus* is a homothallic species that produces large (15- to 25-μm), round, smooth, thick-walled zygospores without beaks. Reproductive structures of *B. ranarum* are readily produced after 3 to 5 days of incubation on half-strength cornmeal agar. Zygospores are easily identified as large (20- to 50-μm), thick-walled, round intercalary structures with beaklike protuberances that represent the remains of copulatory tubes. Primary conidia (often with a hyphal tag still attached), secondary conidia (morphologically similar to primary conidia but often smaller), and capilliconidia (oval to elongate spores with a terminal adhesive knob that develop at the end of a thin supporting hypha) may all be seen on the inside of the petri dish lid.

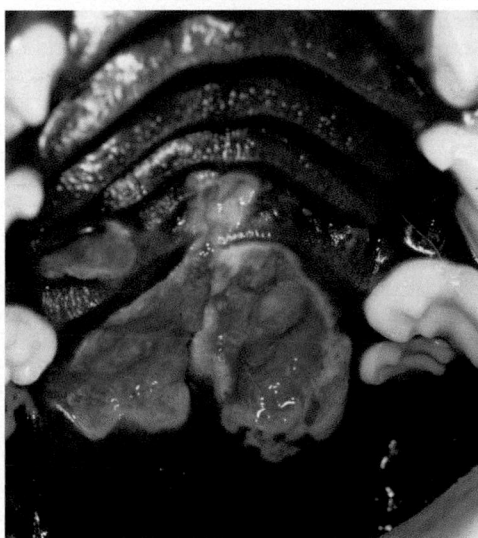

Fig 67-7 Irregular and deep palatal ulcer in dog with conidiobolomycosis. Lesion resolved after treatment with itraconazole, and dog had no recurrence. (Courtesy Carol Foil and Steve LeMarie, Louisiana State University, Baton Rouge, La.)

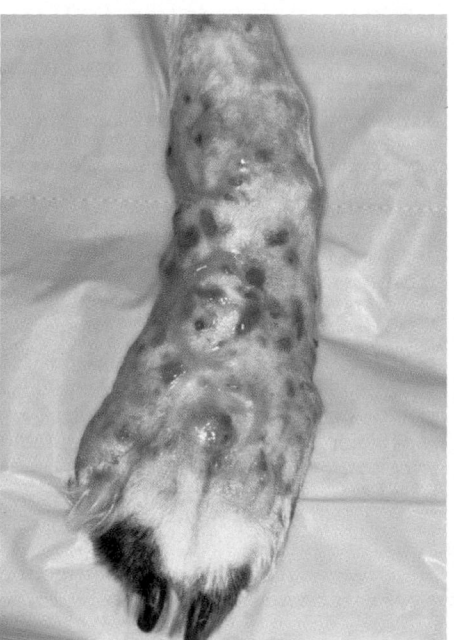

Fig 67-8 Dog with multifocal cutaneous and subcutaneous draining lesions caused by *B. ranarum* infection. Notice resemblance of this lesion to lesion caused by *P. insidiosum* (see Fig. 67-2). (Courtesy University of Georgia, Athens, Ga.)

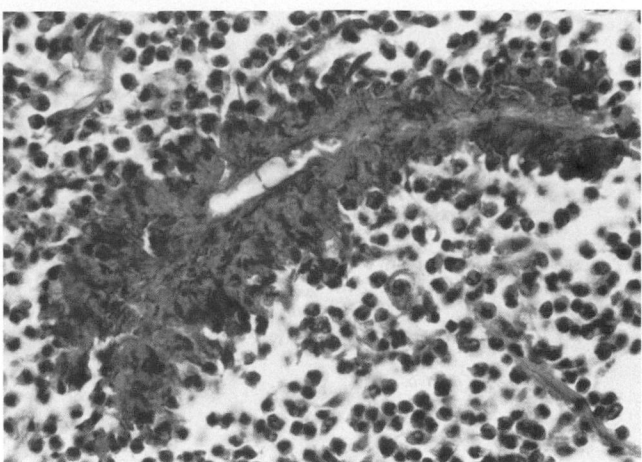

Fig 67-9 *Conidiobolus* species hyphae in tissue biopsy from ulcerative hard palate lesion in 3-year-old female boxer. Note large amount of amorphous eosinophilic material (sleeve) surrounding the hyphal segment (H and E stain). (Courtesy Amy Grooters, Louisiana State University, Baton Rouge, La.)

Pathologic Findings

The histologic features of zygomycosis are similar to those associated with pythiosis and lagenidiosis. On GMS-stained sections, hyphae appear broad, thin-walled, and occasionally septate. The histologic hallmark of zygomycosis is the presence of a wide (2.5- to 25-µm) eosinophilic sleeve surrounding the hyphae and making them easily located on sections stained with H and E (Fig. 67-9). This finding helps to differentiate zygomycosis from pythiosis and lagenidiosis, in which eosinophilic sleeves tend to be thin or absent. In addition, the hyphal diameter tends to be significantly larger for *Basidiobolus* species (mean, 9 µm; range, 5 to 20 µm) and *Conidiobolus* species (mean, 8 µm; range, 5 to 13 µm) than for *P. insidiosum* (mean, 4 µm; range, 2 to 7 µm).[90]

Therapy

Recommendations for the treatment of zygomycosis are not straightforward because attempted therapy has only been described in a few patients with culture-confirmed diagnoses. Although anecdotal information and a small number of cases in the literature suggest that cutaneous zygomycosis may be less aggressive than cutaneous pythiosis or lagenidiosis, progression of lesions and occasionally even dissemination despite treatment have also been described in zygomycete-infected dogs. This may reflect variability in the susceptibility of *Conidiobolus* and *Basidiobolus* isolates, as suggested by results of in vitro susceptibility testing performed in a limited number of isolates.[125] The most appropriate recommendation for the treatment of zygomycosis in small animal patients is aggressive surgical resection of infected tissues when possible, followed by ITZ therapy for 2 to 3 months (see Table 67-2). If resection is not possible, therapy with either ITZ or AMB lipid complex should be recommended.

Public Health Considerations

Zygomycetes are saprophytic and acquired from the environment. They are not transmitted directly between hosts.

HYALOHYPHOMYCOSIS

Hyalohyphomycoses are opportunistic infections caused by nondematiaceous fungi that form hyphal elements in tissue.

By convention, aspergillosis and penicilliosis are not included (see Chapter 64). Cases of hyalohyphomycosis described in dogs or cats are summarized in Table 67-1.

Etiology

In animals and humans, at least 50 species of fungus classified in more than 20 genera in 3 phyla (Deuteromycota, Ascomycota, and Basidiomycota) have been implicated as agents in hyalohyphomycosis.[77] An unidentified species of *Acremonium* has been associated with disseminated disease[116] and multifocal subcutaneous disease.[37] *Acremonium hyalinulum* has been associated with osteomyelitis and nephritis,[52] and *Acremonium kiliense* has been associated with keratoconjunctivitis in dogs.[82] A *Fusarium* species was the cause of an unilateral pyelonephritis[22] and an undocumented case of disseminated disease in Australian dogs. *Fusarium solani* was isolated from an ear lesion of a cat.[21] *Geotrichum candidum* infection has been reported in disseminated diseases[107] and in infections after bite wounds; it has also been reported as a cause of cutaneous nodules[103] and superficial dermatitis[114] in dogs and as a cause of disease in cats.

Paecilomyces fumosoroseus, *Paecilomyces variotii*, *Paecilomyces lilacinus*, and other *Paecilomyces* species[96] have been associated with cutaneous and disseminated lesions in dogs and cats.[30,98,123] Hypercalcemia, as with other granulomatous diseases, has been associated with disseminated infection.[73] *Pseudallescheria* (which is also called *Allescheria*, *Petriellidium*, and *Scedosporium apiospermum*) *boydii* has been isolated from dogs with pneumonia and from dogs with osteomyelitis and disseminated disease.[5,110,123]

The fungi that cause hyalohyphomycosis are generally ubiquitous soil saprophytic molds and are common contaminants of laboratory cultures. *P. lilacinus* is found in tap water and contaminates "sterile" solutions. *Fusarium* species have been found in water systems in human hospitals, a source of infection that has been responsible for many nosocomial infections in immunocompromised people.[2] *Geotrichum* species may also be considered a normal part of the oral and GI flora.[68] Unfortunately, in some reported cases the identification of invasive infection in animals and humans as being caused by *Geotrichum* is questionable.[68] *P. boydii*, which is a much more common cause of hyalohyphomycosis in people than the other causative agents, causes disparate syndromes, especially in those who are immunocompromised, including sinusitis, keratitis, brain abscess, arthritis, fungal ball, endocarditis, cutaneous disease, and disseminated disease. Similar clinical localizations have been observed in infected dogs.[14] *Metarhizium anisopliae* was the cause of rhinitis in a cat.[95] *Trichoderma* species have been recognized as an emerging cause of infection in people[20]; however, they have not yet been documented in dogs and cats.

Although saprophytic fungi are considered opportunistic infectious agents in local or disseminated disease in dogs and cats, rarely is an associated predisposing condition identified. In particular, *Fusarium* infections are associated with neutropenia in humans, and *P. boydii* is associated with neutropenia and human immunodficiency virus (HIV) infection[77]; these types of associations have not yet been made for companion animals. However, a tendency for saprophytic fungi to infect German shepherd dogs[123] and dissemination after treatment with glucocorticoids[107] have been noted.

Clinical Findings

Clinical features that characterize the individual infections are difficult to generalize because so few cases have been reported. *Geotrichum* species in particular and *Paecilomyces* species may colonize epithelial surfaces and thus be more likely to begin as local disease after wounding or to remain confined to skin or mucosae. However, for each species, reports of disseminated disease have been made and can result from immunosuppression caused by terminal illness, immunosuppressive drugs, or long-term antibiotic usage. Dissemination is apparently hematogenous. Signs vary with the organ system affected, which can be the nasal passages, sinuses, lungs, central nervous system (CNS), myocardium, bone and bone marrow, lymph nodes, spleen, kidneys, liver, peritoneum, and pleura. Pneumonia has been prominent in dogs with disseminated geotrichosis.[107] One case of unilateral pyelonephritis with local extension into the retroperitoneal space was associated with a *Fusarium* species.[22] Some cases of cutaneous and subcutaneous nodules have been reported, both of which may be localized or widespread. *Acremonium*, *Fusarium*, and *Pseudallescheria* organisms have been reported as causes of canine keratomycosis.[75,117]

Diagnosis and Pathologic Findings

Many potentially pathogenic fungi that cause hyalohyphomycosis are common laboratory contaminants. Furthermore, most can frequently be isolated from the skin and hair coats of clinically healthy animals. Mycology laboratories frequently have problems identifying members of this group of fungi, which is unfortunate because species-specific treatment guidelines have been developed in human medicine for the fungal agents.[119] PCR-based identification is available for *Pseudallescheria* species, the fungi most often implicated in human disease.[124] Documentation of invasive disease involves cultural and histologic correlation. Evidence of tissue invasion and morphologic characteristics compatible with a fungus isolated from cultures properly obtained from clinical specimens renders the most definitive diagnosis (see Figs. 56-13 and 56-14). Specimens should not be contaminated with epithelial flora or obtained from open wounds. When appropriate specimens are not obtained for fungal culture or when histologic specimens are the only material available, many pathogenic fungal species can be tentatively identified with immunohistochemical techniques. However, in the United States, this type of testing is generally obtainable only by referring the specimens to the Centers for Disease Control and Prevention (CDC) in Atlanta, Ga.

Therapy

Animals with disseminated or CNS disease have a grave prognosis. In many reported cases, treatment has been attempted with AMB or imidazoles (see Table 67-2). Many reports have described treatment with ITZ in particular. In a report of disseminated paecilomycosis in a dog, the initial positive response to combined flucytosine (FCY) and fluconazole therapy was followed by recurrence and death.[96] Temporary remission was also observed after treatment with ketoconazole (KTZ) in a dog with disseminated *Paecilomyces* infection.[10] In some cases, treatment seems to prolong the survival of dogs with disseminated disease,[73,116,123] but few dogs have been reported to survive disseminated hyalohyphomycosis. If treatment is attempted, the isolate should be identified and subjected to in vitro susceptibility testing to formulate a rational therapeutic plan.[78,119] In humans with keratitis or a deep infection with *Pseudallescheria boydii*, combination therapy with AMB and antifungal azoles is recommended.[77] When disease is localized, surgical removal is the treatment of choice, although dissemination might be expected. Keratitis is often treated with topical natamycin or miconazole. When treating *Paecilomyces* infections, it is important to note that its various species have apparently widely differing drug susceptibilities. *P. varioti* is reportedly sensitive to AMB and FCY, whereas *P. lilacinus* is resistant to them but sensitive to imidazoles and even griseofulvin.[17] A cat with invasive *M. anisopliae* rhinitis improved after treatment with ITZ; however, the animal had a relapse after therapy was discontinued.[95]

Public Health Considerations

The fungi that cause hyalohyphomycosis are mostly saprophytic and acquired from the environment. They are not transmitted directly between hosts.

PHAEOHYPHOMYCOSIS

Etiology and Epidemiology

Phaeohyphomycoses are uncommon opportunistic infections caused by numerous ubiquitous saprophytic and plant pathogenic molds. They form characteristic pigmented (dematiaceous) hyphal elements in tissue. The pigment is melanin, and the fungus may be very pale to very dark, generally staining with Masson-Fontana melanin in histologic sections. The presence of melanin in their cell walls may be their virulence factor. Taxonomy of the commonly implicated agents is confusing, and the generic names change frequently. Fungi classified as Deuteromycetes, which belong to more than 100 species and 60 genera, have been described as agents of phaeohyphomycosis in animals or humans.[77] The number of reports about these types of infections in humans and animals is increasing.[105,106,115] These fungi are thought to be one of the major emerging groups of pathogenic fungi in laboratory diagnoses.[33]

Hyphae in phaeohyphomycosis differ from those associated with most hyalohyphomycoses by their thick walls, varying diameters, and yeastlike swellings. Phaeohyphomycosis differs from the human disease chromoblastomycosis in that the spherical yeastlike bodies do not have septa in two perpendicular planes like the sclerotic bodies of the chromoblastomycosis infection. Phaeohyphomycosis is also different from dark-grain mycetomas, which are discussed in the following section. All of the infections caused by pigmented fungi are often called *chromomycoses*.

The organisms that have been isolated from canine and feline phaeohyphomycotic infections are listed in Table 67-1.

Alternaria, *Bipolaris*, *Exophiala*, *Phialemonium*, *Phialophora*, and *Stemphyllium* species are ubiquitous wood and soil saprophytes. Interestingly, *Exophiala* organisms and other dematiaceous fungi may be easily isolated from oligotrophic water sources such as hospital water supplies, sauna facilities, and bathroom drain pipes.[76,97] *Moniliella* organisms have been recovered from cheese, butter, and margarine. *Ochroconis* species are usually a cause of phaeohyphomycosis in cold-blooded vertebrates. Several of the potentially pathogenic species have been cultured from the skin of clinically healthy people, cats, and dogs.[16,36,93,94] Animals and people presumably are exposed to infection with dematiaceous fungi by wound contamination, especially through wood slivers, although initial respiratory tract colonization cannot be ruled out in systemic cases. The route of exposure in cerebral phaeohyphomycosis is not understood, although extension from sinus infections, orbital injuries, and middle ear infections has been postulated as a route in humans. *Bipolaris* species are usually associated with paranasal sinus infections in humans,[77] and rhinitis has been described in a cat.[87] Some species of *Cladophialophora* demonstrate neurotropism.[3,74]

Only rarely are cases of localized phaeohyphomycosis in animals associated with other systemic disorders or obvious immunosuppression. These infections are not associated with HIV-induced immunosuppression in humans; however, central venous catheters have been implicated in some cases.[71] Intact granulocyte function is an important defense mechanism against these infectious agents.[77] Persistent lymphopenia has been either a cause or an effect of infection in dogs with systemic infections.[72] Hyperglobulinemia can occur as a result of a persistent but an ineffective humoral response. Of the reported cases, one dog was treated with long courses of glucocorticoids, one dog had ehrlichiosis, one cat had leukemia, and another cat was treated with glucocorticoids. All of these immunosuppressed patients had disseminated phaeohyphomycosis.

Clinical Findings

Subcutaneous and Dermal Phaeohyphomycosis

Singular or multifocal, poorly circumscribed, and ulcerating or fistulating nodules and plaques characterize subcutaneous and dermal phaeohyphomycosis (Figs. 67-10 and 67-11). The fungal pigmentation is often apparent in the tissue (Fig. 67-12). In cats the lesions may resemble chronic bacterial abscesses or thick-walled cysts, which may evolve over weeks

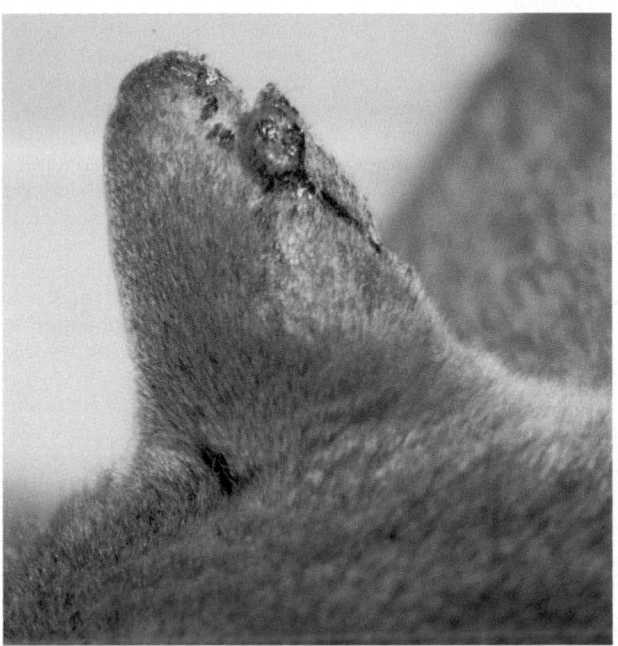

Fig 67-10 Cutaneous phaeohyphomycosis on pinna of cat with ulcerated and crusted nodule. Lesion was pigmented clinically and on cut surface. Disease was resolved by routine excisional biopsy. (Courtesy Carol Foil, Louisiana State University, Baton Rouge, La.)

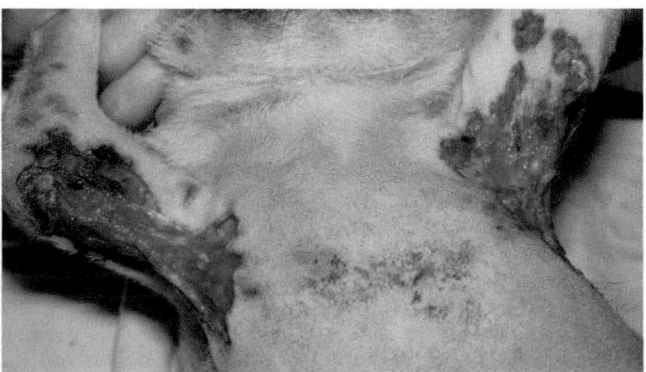

Fig 67-11 Extensive cutaneous ulceration caused by subcutaneous phaeohyphomycosis caused by *Bipolaris spicifera*. (Courtesy Kenneth Kwochka, The Ohio State University, Columbus, Ohio.)

to months. In dogs, cutaneous lesions have been associated with osteomyelitis. In a report of a dog with phaeohyphomycosis caused by *Curvularia geniculatum*, the lesions had a sporotrichoid appearance involving lymphatics and lymph nodes on the affected limb.[6] In one report of disseminated cutaneous infection with *Curvularia* species in a dog that had been treated with glucocorticoids, organisms were seen histopathologically within hair follicles and furunculosis lesions.[57] The authors speculated that the hair follicle could be a route of infection in a dog without a penetrating skin wound.

Most cases of subcutaneous and dermal phaeohyphomycosis have been described in cats, and lesions in this species most often occur on the face or distal extremities. *Bipolaris spicifera*, *Exophiala jeanselmei*, and *Phialophora verrucosa* are the most common isolates. *Alternaria alternata*, *Cladophialophora bantiana*—which usually causes cerebral phaeohyphomycosis—and *Fonsecaea pedrosoi*—the agent most often implicated in human chromoblastomycosis—have been associated with nasal dermal nodules in cats.[1,31,79]

Cerebral (Encephalitic or Brain Abscess) Phaeohyphomycosis

The agents involved in cerebral phaeohypohomycosis are almost always *Cladophialophora* (formerly *Cladosporium*, *Xylohypha*) species (Fig. 67-13). Authors of a recent case report of a cat tentatively identified a new agent, *Phoma eupyrena*.[70] Dogs and cats are both affected.[11,32,74] CNS disease can also develop as a manifestation of disseminated phaeohyphomycosis. Neurologic dysfunction varies with the site of disease, because most cases involve localized brain abscesses.

Keratomycosis in a cat has been associated with *Cladophialophora* species and in dogs with *Alternaria* and *Curvularia* species. A recent report of intraocular granulomatous uveitis in a cat is the first published instance of intraocular phaeohyphomycosis.[8]

Disseminated Phaeohyphomycosis

Systemic phaeohyphomycosis usually has an acute to subacute course, with symptoms varying according to the organ system involved. As noted, CNS disease is prominent and invariably fatal, and some patients have potentially immunosuppressive conditions. A report of disseminated *C. bantiana* in a Maltese dog with ehrlichiosis is an example.[111] In addition a report of disseminated *Phialemonium obovatum* in a German shepherd dog was associated with depressed

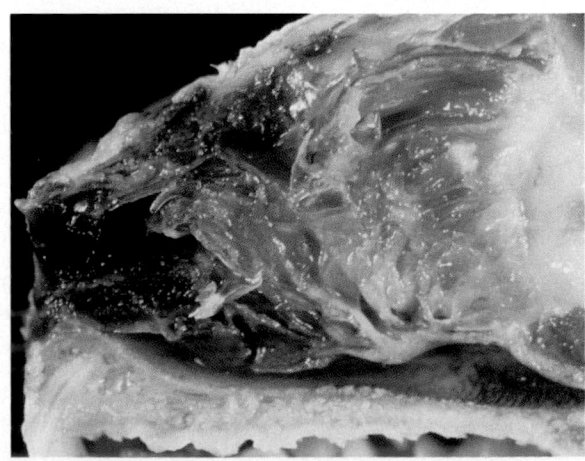

Fig 67-12 Necropsy specimen of cat with nasal phaeohyphomycosis illustrating darkly pigmented nature of infiltrate. Pigment is imparted by fungal melanin. (Courtesy Richard I. Miller, Idexx Laboratories, Brisbane, Australia.)

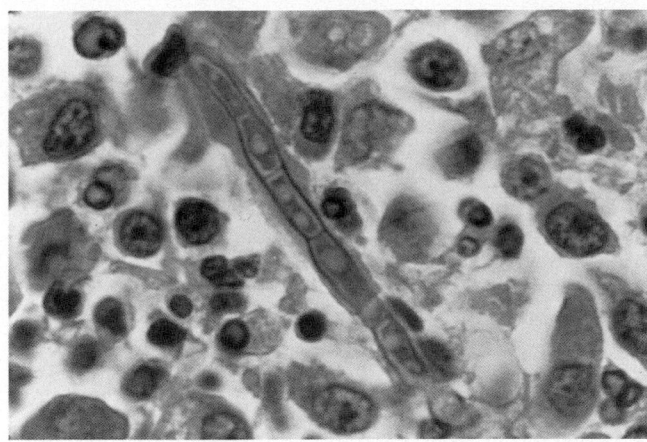

Fig 67-13 Pigmented hyphae in brain of cat with abscess caused by *Cladophialophora* species (H and E stain, ×500). (Courtesy Joe Kornegay, University of Missouri, Columbia, Mo.)

lymphocyte blastogenesis.[118] In contrast, there is a report of multifocal disease caused by *E. jeanselmei* in a 14-year-old spayed domestic short-haired cat had no known immunosuppressive condition.[55] Multifocal lesions in this cat were detected ultrasonographically in the liver and kidneys. On necropsy, multifocal granuloma-like masses were seen on the liver, kidneys, abdominal wall, mesentery, thoracic wall, pericardium, and epicardium. Similar lesions were found on the cervical portion of the spinal cord, cerebrum, and cerebellum.

Diagnosis

Direct examination of exudate or macerated tissue mounted in KOH may reveal the pigmented fungal elements. As with other opportunistic mycoses, confirmation of the diagnosis is based on the concomitant demonstration of hyphae in tissue and culture of a morphologically compatible organism from properly obtained tissue specimens. Histopathologically, dematiaceous fungi may appear darkly pigmented or need to be visualized using special lighting, processing techniques, or stains to demonstrate the presence of melanin in the fungal elements.[102] These organisms grow readily on Sabouraud's dextrose agar, although specialized agar may be required to encourage production of the identifying fruiting bodies (see Fig. 56-12). Regardless, some expertise is required for specific mycologic identification,[33] and a referral to a specialized laboratory such as the Fungus Testing Laboratory at the University of Texas Health Science Center in San Antonio, Tex., may be required (see Appendix 5, Laboratory Testing for Infectious Disease). When culture cannot be obtained, specific identification of the most commonly pathogenic species may be performed with experimental immunohistochemical techniques available at the CDC.

CNS lesions may be investigated with magnetic resonance imaging, computerized tomographic (CT) imaging, and cerebrospinal fluid analysis. In one report of sterotactic CT-guided biopsy of a brain lesion in a dog caused by *C. bantiana*, a tentative diagnosis was obtained cytologically from a smear preparation of the material, a histologic diagnosis was made, and the organism was obtained in culture for specific diagnosis.[3]

Therapy

An animal with disseminated CNS disease or widespread cutaneous disease has a grave prognosis. Successful treatment of the localized cutaneous forms often seen in cats has been

described (see Table 67-2). When the lesions are excisable, surgery may be curative,[79] but recurrence at the same or new sites is common.

In animals with unexcisable lesions or recurrent disease, antifungal chemotherapy may be helpful, but the response is unpredictable. Drugs should be chosen on the basis of in vitro sensitivity and susceptibility testing if possible; the imidazoles have variable in vitro activity against saprophytic organisms. A cat apparently was cured after multiple excisions and treatment with KTZ,[87] and yet another was treated successfully with AMB and FCY.[80] In other feline cases, treatment with both KTZ and FCY was unsuccessful.[65] In a published report a dog with disseminated cutaneous infection with *Phialemonium curvatum* was cured long term with KTZ at 5 mg/kg/day (2.3 mg/lb/day).[12] ITZ treatment of human subcutaneous and musculoskeletal phaeohyphomycosis has been reviewed[112]; of 17 patients assessed, only 3 were cured, although another 6 improved. In all cases the fungal isolates were reported to be susceptible to ITZ on in vitro testing. A cat with granulomatous rhinitis caused by *E. jeanselmei* was successfully treated with oral ITZ given for 30 days. Another cat with *Fonsecaea* nasal granuloma responded to 4- to 6-month courses of ITZ at 5 mg/kg (2.3 mg/lb) every 12 hours but relapsed 6 to 9 months after cessation of treatment each time.[31] Terbinafine, an allylamine, has been shown to be useful in some people with phaeohyphomycosis.[27,101]

Public Health Considerations

The fungi that cause phaeohyphomycosis are mostly saprophytic and acquired from the environment. They are not transmitted directly between hosts.

EUMYCOTIC MYCETOMAS

Mycetomas are pyogranulomatous nodules that contain tissue grains or granules. The grains contain dense colonies of organisms and host-derived matter—usually necrotic debris.

Etiology

When mycetomas are caused by fungi, they are classified as *eumycotic mycetomas* to distinguish them from *actinomycotic* lesions (see Chapter 49) and *botryomycosis*, a bacterial pseudomycosis caused by organisms such as staphylococci. Eumycotic mycetomas must also be differentiated from the pseudomycetomas seen in long-haired cats with generalized dermatophytosis (see Chapter 58).

Eumycotic mycetomas may be caused by fungi that impart their pigmented appearance to the grains in tissue; they are called *black-grain*, or *dark-grain*, *mycetomas*. Black-grain mycetomas have been associated with infections by *Curvularia* species, *Madurella* species, and *Staphylotrichum coccosporum*. Unpigmented organisms cause white-grain mycetomas. White-grain mycetomas have been caused by *Acremonium* and *Pseudallescheria* species. Most eumycotic mycetomas are confined to the subcutaneous tissues, but white-grain mycetomas on the body wall may be extensions of abdominal cavity disease. Fungal isolation from affected dogs and cats has not been done in all cases. Of the black-grain mycetomas, *Curvularia geniculata* is the most common isolate, and infections caused by *Curvularia spicifera*, *Curvularia lunata*,[26] and *Curvularia senegalensis*[21] have been reported. In abdominal and body wall white-grain mycetomas of the dog, *P. boydii* and *A. hyalinum* have been isolated. Disseminated infection was caused by *Acremonium* species in a dog.[116] *Madurella grisea* has been isolated from a cat with mycetoma, and *Madurella mycetomatis* has been isolated from a dog.[69] A cat positive for feline leukemia virus was reported to have simultaneous dermatophytic pseudomycetoma and subcutaneous black-grain mycetomas caused by an agent not previously reported to be pathogenic—*Staphylotrichum coccosporum*.[34]

Clinical Findings

In white-grain mycetomas, most infections have involved abdominal cavity organs. Dogs have developed peritonitis or abdominal masses after contamination from unrelated surgical wound dehiscence. As with aspergillosis, German shepherd dogs have the greatest prevalence rate of infection. Peritonitis and intraabdominal granulomas accompanied by symptoms typical of septic peritonitis are noted. Lesions within the abdomen have tissue grains and are usually caused by *P. boydii*. Systemic infection caused by *Acremonium* was characterized by signs of neurologic dysfunction, uveitis, and visceral granulomas.[116] A black-grain mycetoma caused by *M. mycetomatis* developed at the site of a uterine stump subsequent to wound dehiscence after ovariohysterectomy.[69]

Cutaneous mycetoma has been the typical finding of black-grain infection. Infection probably develops at the site of a superficial wound, possibly contaminated by a plant foreign body. Such cases are more often reported in dogs than in cats and are most often caused by *Curvularia* species. In one cat, a black mycetoma developed after a bite wound. Lesions are cutaneous nodules, relatively poorly circumscribed, and usually on the extremities or the face. They do not often ulcerate widely, but fistulas may form within the nodule. Most become surmounted by alopecic and hyperkeratotic epidermis. Cycles of healing and ulceration may lead to firm swelling and scarring. Black tissue grains may be visible within the exudate, or the exudate or the tissue itself may appear black. Some nodules are so heavily pigmented that they are mistaken for cutaneous melanomas. On the limbs and feet, the infectious process may involve underlying bone.

Diagnosis and Pathologic Findings

A presumptive diagnosis of mycetoma can be made if grains are found within exudate from any draining tract. Cytologic investigation must be directed at the tissue grains, because organisms are often scant or absent elsewhere within exudates or tissues. Grains may be crushed and smeared on a slide for staining in some cases. Black grains are often gritty and may require digestion in 10% KOH before they can be mounted for microscopic study. The fungal elements are usually quite evident in thinly smeared or flattened grains. Serum may be tested for specific antibodies by agar gel immunodiffusion. In histologic specimens, common fungi may be identified by immunohistochemical techniques.

Investigation by culture technique is otherwise necessary to confirm cytologic findings and identify the causative organism. Tissue grains may be collected from exudate and washed in sterile saline for culturing. Alternatively, if surgically excised tissue contains grains, it can be cultured. Fungal isolates should be retained for possible in vitro sensitivity and susceptibility testing. The agents associated with mycetomas in dogs and cats are readily cultured on standard media.

Therapy

The prognosis in abdominal mycetoma is guarded, because patients described to date have had extensive involvement of abdominal organs, have not responded to debridement, chemotherapy, or both. Cutaneous mycetoma is not a life-threatening disease but is difficult to resolve. Radical surgical excision is the treatment most often used for humans. Amputation of affected limbs may be necessary; spontaneous resolution does not occur. Any attempt at antifungal chemotherapy should be based on in vitro susceptibility testing of the isolate. Even if an antifungal chemotherapeutic agent that may be helpful is identified, it is apparently difficult to attain effective levels within the tissue grains where the organism resides. Successful outcomes have been reported in humans with local hyperthermia treatments and improvement with high-dose ITZ.[104] Scattered reports have been made of successful treatment of mycetomas in people with terbinafine with or without other agents.[53]

Public Health Considerations

The fungi that cause eumycotic mycetomas are saprophytic and acquired from the environment. They are not transmitted directly between hosts.

SUGGESTED READINGS*

30. Foley JE, Norris CR, Jang SS. 2002. Paecilomycosis in dogs and horses and a review of the literature. *J Vet Intern Med* 16:238-243.

43. Grooters AM, Gee MK. 2002. Development of a nested PCR assay for the detection and identification of *Pythium insidiosum*. *J Vet Intern Med* 16:147-152.

46. Grooters AM, Hodgin EC, Bauer RW, et al. 2003. Clinicopathologic findings associated with *Lagenidium* sp infection in six dogs: initial description of an emerging oomycosis. *J Vet Intern Med* 17:637-646.

47. Grooters AM, Leise BS, Lopez MK, et al. 2002. Development and evaluation of an enzyme-linked immunosorbent assay for the serodiagnosis of pythiosis in dogs. *J Vet Intern Med* 16:142-146.

126. Znajda NR, Grooters AM, Marsella R. 2002. PCR-based detection of *Pythium* and *Lagenidium* DNA in frozen and ethanol-fixed animal tissues. *Vet Dermatol* 13:187-194.

*See the CD-ROM for a complete list of references.

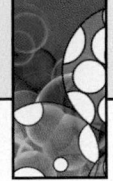

CHAPTER 68

Pneumocystosis

Craig E. Greene, Francis M. Chandler, and Remo Lobetti

ETIOLOGY

Pneumocystis carinii, the etiologic agent of pneumocystosis, occurs worldwide and infects virtually all mammalian species, including people. A saprophyte of low virulence, *Pneumocystis* spp. exist in temperate and tropical climates at altitudes up to 5000 feet. Its primary habitat is the mammalian lung where it causes opportunistic infection. Estimates of latent human infections range from 1% to 10% of the population. Subclinical or latent infections are common in rats, mice, guinea pigs, rabbits, cats, sheep, and various wild animals. Clinical pneumonia has been reported to occur spontaneously in dogs, pigs, horses, goats, nonhuman primates, and people. Airborne transmission is suspected because healthy animals become infected when they are housed with infected animals.[6] The presumption is that the organism may have a yet undiscovered dormant life stage in the environment. Most reports of clinical *P. carinii* pneumonia are linked with documented or suspected cell-mediated immunodeficiency in the host. Rarely, *P. carinii* disseminates to extrapulmonary sites.

The taxonomy of *P. carinii* is uncertain. It has been classified using freeze-fracture techniques as a unicellular protozoan belonging to the phylum Sarcomastigophora, subphylum Sarcodina. Ultrastructurally, the reproductive behavior of *P. carinii* is similar to the ascospore formation of yeast cells, and its organelles and staining properties by light microscopy resemble those of most pathogenic fungi. Phylogenetic classification based on 16S-like rRNA sequences indicates that *P. carinii* is most closely related to the fungi of the class Ascomycetes, especially *Saccharomyces cerevisiae*. Biologically, however, it behaves similar to a protozoan and is sensitive to drugs used to treat sporozoan infections but resistant to most antifungal drugs. The morphology of the organisms and the histopathology of the lesions produced by both human and animal isolates throughout the world are similar. Only a single species name had been assigned to the genus *Pneumocystis*, but antigenic differences suggest that several strains may exist. Biologic differences between isolates from different hosts are suggested by the relative difficulty of experimental interspecies transmission. Although controversial, the designated species infecting people, known previously as *P. carinii* f. sp. *hominis*, is now named *Pneumocystis jiroveci*.[30,51] The species found in the rat continues to be called *P. carinii*. Species designations for the organisms isolated from dogs and other animals will require further genetic and biologic study. For purposes of this chapter, and with few exceptions listed later in this text, the organism infecting dogs and people will continue to be labeled *P. carinii*.

EPIDEMIOLOGY

P. carinii appears to be maintained in nature by transmission from infected to susceptible animals within a species. Although spore collections suggest an environmental source, none has been determined. The primary mode of spread is thought to be airborne droplet transmission between hosts. The contagious nature of pneumocystosis is suggested by the epidemic spread that has occurred in institutionalized people. Sporadic case reports may represent an activation of latent infection by stress, crowding, and immunosuppressive therapy during hospitalization of latent carriers. Clinical disease has also been experimentally activated after glucocorticoid therapy, cytotoxic chemotherapy, and irradiation of laboratory rodents. A higher prevalence of infection has been found in dogs with canine distemper compared with a corresponding control population.[52] However, genetic analysis of isolates in people indicate that most infections are not acquired early in life but rather result from an infected source that is likely of the same species within a given geographic region.[7] Therefore recent acquisition of infection, rather than reactivation of infection, may be responsible for clinical illness.[35] The greater prevalence of pneumocystosis is probably caused not only by an increased awareness of it, but also by the increased use of immunosuppressive therapy.

The entire life cycle of *P. carinii* is completed within the alveolar spaces where organisms adhere in clusters to the lining cells. Ultrastructural studies have contributed a large body of information concerning the life cycle of *P. carinii* (Fig. 68-1). Two main forms, the trophozoite (1–4 μ) and cyst (8 μm), are found there. Although *Pneumocystis* infections are usually confined to the lungs, in human cases and an infection in one dog, organisms have been reported in extrapulmonary sites. Causes of severe cell-mediated immunodeficiency in humans, such as acquired immunodeficiency syndrome (AIDS), can be associated with lymphatic or hematogenous dissemination of organisms from the lungs to other tissues. Transmission of infection to an offspring can occur via aspiration of contaminated amniotic fluid from placental infection.

PATHOGENESIS

Pneumocystis can be inhaled from the environment and then can colonize the lower respiratory tract of clinically healthy mammals. *Pneumocystis* organisms rarely multiply to large numbers in the lungs of clinically healthy hosts. In conditions in which impaired host resistance (especially reduced CD4 T-lymphocyte counts) or preexisting pulmonary disease is present, rapid proliferation of organisms can occur. The overgrowth and clustering of *P. carinii* within alveolar spaces can then lead to alveolocapillary blockage and decreased gaseous exchange. Intraalveolar organisms are often accompanied by thickening of alveolar septa, but they seldom invade the pulmonary interstitium and are rarely phagocytosed by alveolar macrophages. With an adequate immune response, the body may eliminate the infection, but the removal of large numbers of organisms and cellular debris may take up to 8 weeks. Organisms and the minimal inflammatory response they provoke contribute to the pulmonary alveolar damage.

In infected people, when extrapulmonary pneumocystosis occurs, it is rare and occurs primarily when accompanied by

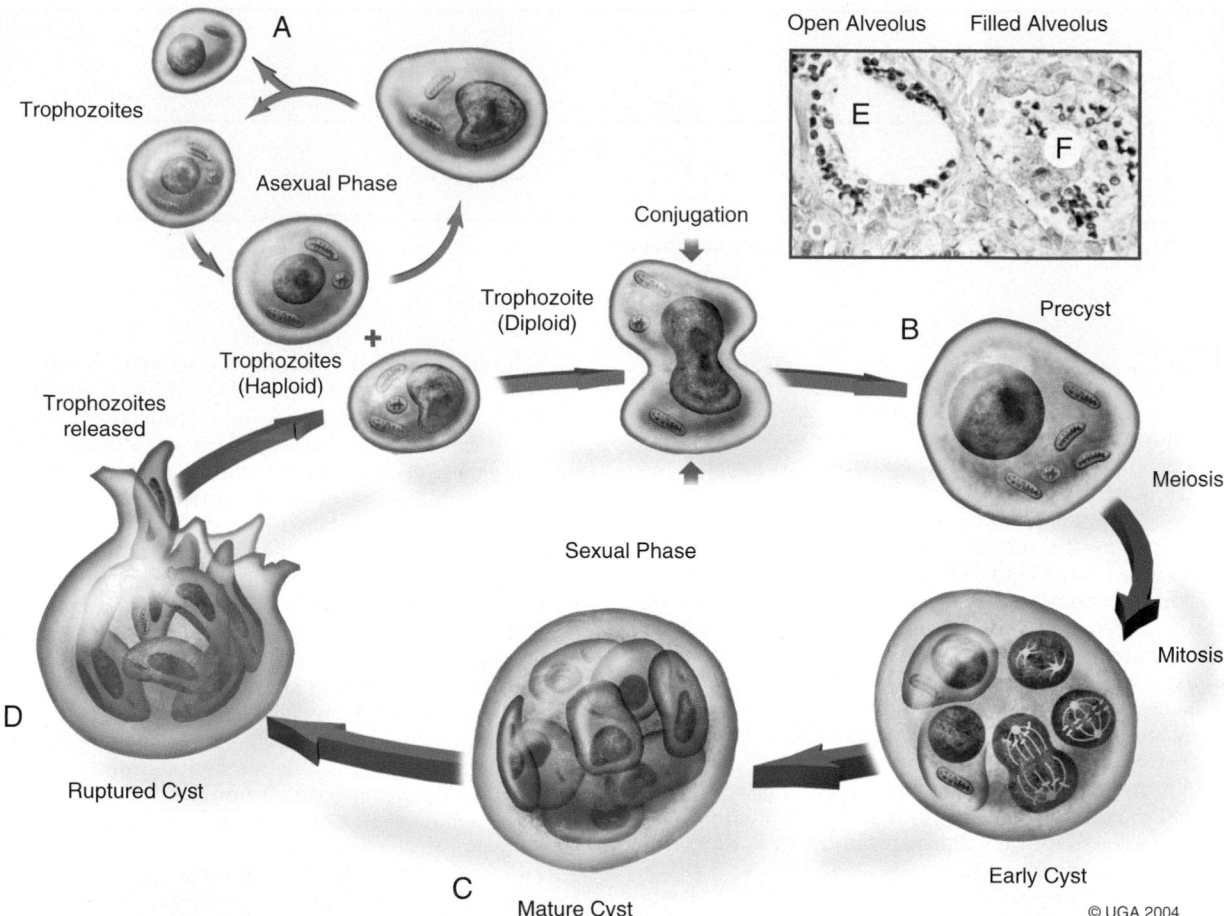

Fig 68-1 Haploid trophozoites replicate asexually by mitosis *(A)* and also conjugate to form a precyst *(B)*. The cyst undergoes meiosis and subsequent mitosis eventually producing a mature cyst containing eight haploid organisms *(C)*. The cyst matures and finally ruptures releasing the ovoid- or crescent-shaped trophozoites *(D)*. As the process continues, the once open alveolus *(E)* becomes filled obstructing ventilation *(F)*. See Figure 68-10 for more detailed view of *E* and *F*. (Courtesy University of Georgia, Athens, Ga.)

overwhelming pulmonary infection, profound underlying immunodeficiency, and long-term use of aerosolized pentamidine for prophylaxis against *P. carinii* pneumonia in human immunodeficiency virus (HIV)-infected individuals.[57] Sites of extrapulmonary infection include lymph nodes, spleen, liver, bone marrow, gastrointestinal tract, eyes, thyroid gland, adrenal glands, kidneys, heart, pancreas, and external auditory canal.

CLINICAL FINDINGS

Cats

In general, pneumocystic infections of cats are latent or subclinical, as they are in people. The organism has been found in the lungs of cats, but clinical disease has not been reported. Lung specimens examined from cats suffering from feline leukemia virus infection, interstitial pneumonia, or both have not shown evidence of pneumocystosis. Cats that were experimentally infected with *P. carinii* isolated from mice developed a cough, tachypnea, and pneumonia if they were immunosuppressed with concurrent glucocorticoid administration.[58] In contrast, subclinical infections occurred in cats that did not receive immunosuppressive therapy.

Dogs

Most canine cases have been in miniature dachshunds younger than 1 year with a suspected congenital immunode-

ficiency,[36,38] although cases of pneumocystosis have been reported in a Shetland sheepdog and Yorkshire terrier,[11] as well as in adult Cavalier King Charles spaniels.[10,13,45,53] The syndrome of common variable immunodeficiency (CVID) in which B cells produce little or no antibody in association with normal or reduced B-cell numbers has been suspected to occur in affected miniature dachshunds.[36] Immunologic studies on these dogs showed hypogammaglobulinemia; deficiency of serum IgA, IgG, and IgM; decreased lymphocyte transformation response to phytohemagglutinin and pokeweed mitogens; and absence of B lymphocytes with presence of T lymphocytes in the lymphoid tissue stained with CD3 and CD79a lymphocyte markers. Immunoglobulin deficiencies have also been observed in affected Cavalier King Charles spaniels.[56]

The clinical features of pneumocystic pneumonia in dogs are similar to those caused by other pulmonary pathogens except for dry lung sounds, nonproductive cough, and low-grade or absent fever. The typical clinical history is that of gradual weight loss and respiratory difficulty progressing over 1 to 4 weeks (Fig. 68-2). The weight loss, which occurs in spite of a good appetite in most dogs, may be associated with diarrhea and occasional vomiting. Coughing is not always reported, but reduced exercise tolerance is uniform. Infected animals have responded minimally or temporarily to antibiotic and glucocorticoid therapy.

Abnormalities on physical examination include dyspnea, tachycardia, and increased dry respiratory sounds on thoracic

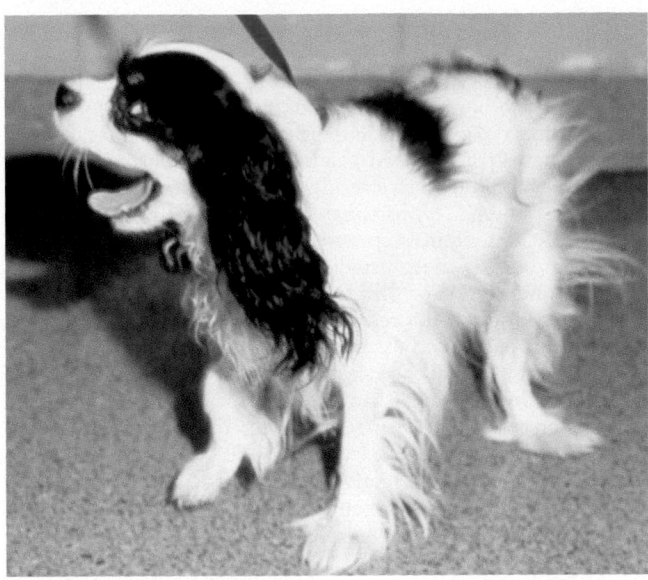

Fig 68-2 A 3-year-old Cavalier King Charles spaniel with severe dyspnea and weight loss as a result of pulmonary pneumocystosis. (Courtesy University of Georgia, Athens, Ga.)

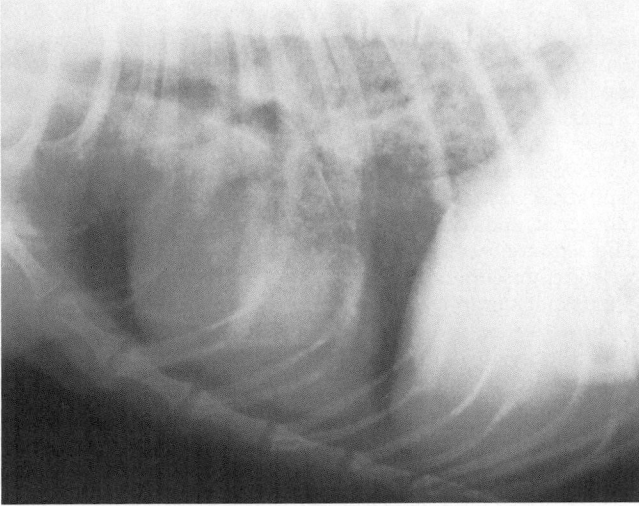

Fig 68-3 Lateral survey thoracic radiograph from a dog with pneumocystosis showing a diffuse miliary interstitial density. (Courtesy University of Georgia, Athens, Ga.)

auscultation. Animals are usually in poor condition, cachectic, and may show dermatologic changes, such as superficial bacterial pyoderma and demodicosis. Although the mucous membranes are generally of normal color, they may be cyanotic in severely affected animals. Affected dogs remain relatively alert and afebrile, although slight (1° to 2° C [1.8° to 3.6° F]) elevations of rectal temperature have been reported. Fluid may be present in the thoracic and peritoneal cavities of some dogs. Ocular fundic lesions known as "cotton wool spots" rarely occur in people with pneumocystosis, and they represent infarction of the nerve fiber layer. They have not been reported in animal infections.

DIAGNOSIS

Hematologic abnormalities are usually nonspecific, and a neutrophilic leukocytosis with a shift suggesting inflammation is seen most consistently. Less frequently, eosinophilia and monocytosis are found. Polycythemia may occur secondarily to arterial hypoxemia from impaired gaseous exchange. Thrombocytopenia, which can be significant enough to cause bleeding, has been a complication in people. In contrast, thrombocytosis may be present in miniature dachshunds. Artifactual thrombocytopenia and megathrombocytosis has been observed in Cavalier King Charles spaniels[3]; however, this finding has a hereditary basis likely unrelated to the suspected immunodeficiency. Biochemical alterations are usually nonspecific. Total serum proteins are usually within reference limits with a low to borderline-low globulin level, which correlates with low γ-globulin levels on serum protein electrophoresis.[38] Low globulin levels and decreased lymphocyte function have been reported in a Cavalier King Charles spaniel.[26] Low levels of IgA, IgG, and IgM have been apparent. Arterial hypoxemia (oxygen tension [PO_2] at or below 80), hypocapnia (carbon dioxide tension [PCO_2] at or below 35), and increased arterial blood pH indicate an uncompensated respiratory alkalosis. The PO_2 is often lower than would be expected from the clinical signs and thoracic radiographs.

Findings on thoracic radiography include diffuse, bilaterally symmetric, miliary-interstitial to alveolar lung disease (Fig. 68-3), with compensatory emphysema in severely infected animals. Solitary lesions, unilateral involvement, cavitary lesions, spontaneous pneumothorax, and lobar infiltrates are occasionally present. Tracheal elevation, right-sided heart enlargement, and pulmonary arterial enlargement reflect cor pulmonale secondary to diffuse pulmonary disease.

For detecting human infections, serologic tests have been developed, but their diagnostic value is uncertain. Unfortunately, many immunodeficient patients who develop pneumocystosis fail to produce antibody titers, and healthy contacts of these patients frequently have higher titers than the patients themselves. Increased antibody titers to *P. carinii* persist for long periods, offering a valuable index of infection in epidemiologic studies. However, they are of limited use for an immediate diagnosis. An increase in titer over 2 to 3 weeks is needed to confirm active infection. Circulating *Pneumocystis* antigen has been detected in human serum by counterimmunoelectrophoresis and enzyme-linked immunosorbent assay (ELISA) methods. However, antigenemia also is found in up to 15% of clinically normal people who have been tested.

P. carinii has been successfully propagated in cell cultures but not on a continual basis. Immunosuppressed rodents have been used to propagate organisms for serologic and experimental testing. Because of the difficulty of isolation of organisms, diagnosis requires direct demonstration of *P. carinii* in biopsy specimens, respiratory fluids, or occasional extrapulmonary sites. Sputum, transtracheal or endotracheal washings, gastric contents, and oropharyngeal secretions may contain organisms. Transtracheal aspirates have been effective for identifying organisms in dogs.[38] Samples for cytology may be obtained by endobronchial brushing and transbronchoscopic biopsy, but these procedures require special endoscopic equipment and involve the risks of general anesthesia. Transtracheal or endotracheal lavage and percutaneous transthoracic needle aspiration are more available to practitioners and have been shown to have good correlation with transbronchoscopic biopsy findings in confirming a diagnosis. None of the cytologic techniques are as reliable or as definitive as is histopathologic examination of lung biopsy specimens for documenting active pneumocystosis. Lung biopsy is unfortunately more invasive, has potential complications of hemorrhage or pneumothorax, and is associated with additional costs and hospitalization.

Of 24 reported cases in dogs reported in the literature, diagnosis was made antemortem in 15 dogs. When premortem diagnosis was attempted, multiple procedures were often used. Tracheal washing was performed in nine dogs, and the organism was found in seven dogs by one group of investigators.[32,38] Bronchoalveolar lavage results were positive in one of the two cases in which it was used.[45,53] Transthoracic needle aspiration was performed in three dogs; two developed pneumothorax, and one died as a direct result of the procedure.[21,45] The aspirate was diagnostic in only one of the dogs. Unfortunately, endoscopic or percutaneous lung biopsy has the greatest risk of complications. Hemorrhage, secondary infection, pneumothorax, and death from anesthesia have been reported after biopsy in dogs. Open surgical biopsy is the preferred method and gives a definitive diagnosis.[3,21] The least traumatic and invasive method involves a laparotomy with a transdiaphragmatic approach.[3] Antimicrobial therapy can begin 24 to 48 hours before specimen collection in a patient suspected of having pneumocystosis, without the drug masking the presence of organisms in the sample.

To facilitate early diagnosis and treatment, impression smears for cytologic study should be made from all tissues before fixation for histologic evaluation. The cytologic material obtained is placed on a glass microscope slide to dry, after which it is selectively stained with methenamine silver for cysts or with Giemsa for nuclei of intracystic sporozoites and trophozoites (Figs. 68-4 and 68-5). Diff-Quik (a modified Giemsa stain) can be used as a fast and inexpensive screening stain after which negative results can be confirmed with more sensitive staining.[17] Unfortunately, *Pneumocystis* organisms are difficult to detect in respiratory secretions or washing, and success in finding them usually depends on the experience of the examiner and the collection and processing of specimens. Direct or indirect fluorescent antibody (FA) test has been effective in specifically detecting organisms in sputum, tracheal aspirates, or pulmonary tissue (Fig. 68-6).[43] Immunoperoxidase techniques also can be used to identify *P. carinii* in impression smears and in formalin-fixed, paraffin-embedded lung sections (Fig. 68-7, *A* and *B*).[34] Polymerase chain reaction (PCR) has been effective in the detection of *P. carinii* in bronchoalveolar lavage specimens from people[33,35,39,46] and in lung tissue from dogs.[26,53] Sensitivity of PCR on bronchoalveolar lavage fluids from infected people has been greater than that of conventional staining without loss of specificity.[22] DNA analysis of *Pneumocystis* isolates has been used for epidemiologic monitoring of isolates from people and animals.[20]

PATHOLOGIC FINDINGS

Pathologic findings in pneumocystosis are primarily confined to the lungs, although dissemination to regional lymph nodes, spleen, liver, bone marrow, and other organs has been reported. On gross examination, the lungs are firm, consolidated, and pale brown or gray (Fig. 68-8). They do not collapse when the chest cavity is opened. Unlike in many pneumonic processes, fluid is not expressed from cut surfaces of the lung. The pulmonary and mediastinal lymph nodes are often enlarged. Despite the apparent lack of pleural inflammation, small amounts of fluid may be found in the pleural cavity. Cardiac enlargement, when present, has been right sided in all cases.

Appropriate histologic staining is essential to ensure detection of *P. carinii* organisms (Table 68-1). The routine hema-

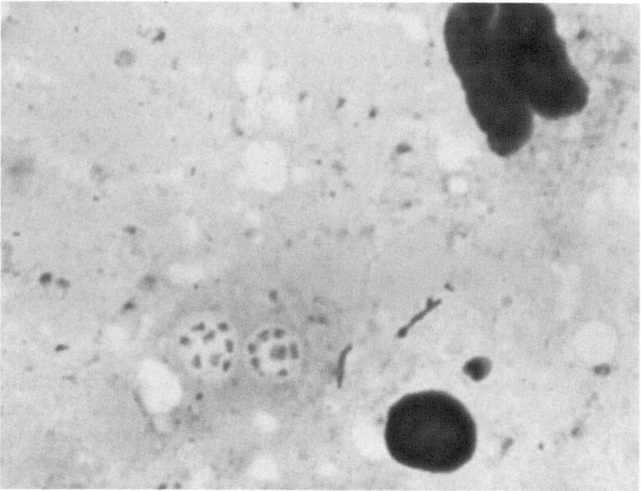

Fig 68-4 Lung smear of rat containing two *Pneumocystis* cysts with intracystic organisms (Giemsa, ×1500). (Courtesy J. P. Dubey, Beltsville, Md.)

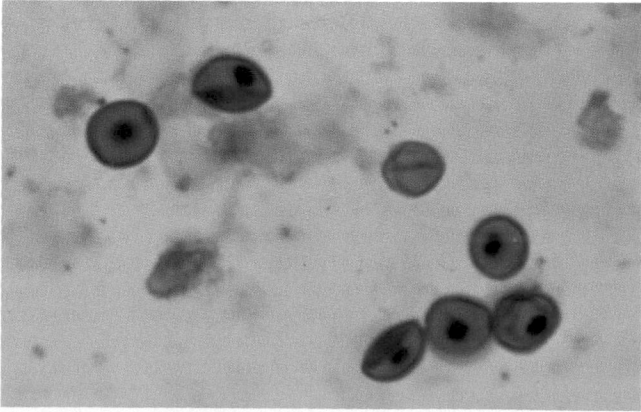

Fig 68-5 *P. carinii* cysts in touch imprint contain spherical to oval foci of enhanced staining that in profile are contiguous with cyst wall (GMS stain, ×400).

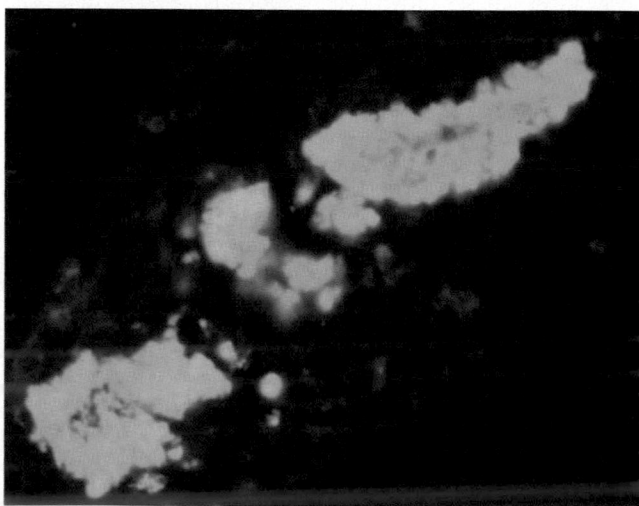

Fig 68-6 Brightly decorated intraalveolar aggregates of *P. carinii* cysts and trophozoites demonstrated with monoclonal antibody 2G2 in a routinely processed histologic section of lung (Immunofluorescence, ×160).

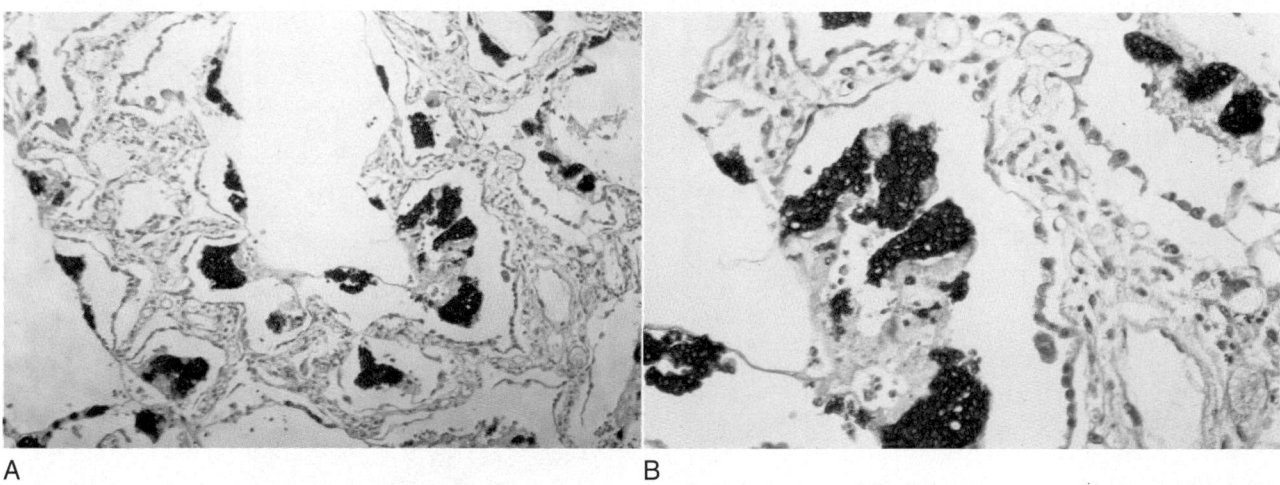

Fig 68-7 Immunoperoxidase staining of intraalveolar cysts and trophozoites of *P. carinii* in a human patient with AIDS using monoclonal antibody 2G2 in a routinely prepared biopsy specimen **(A)** (×25). **B,** Higher magnification of **A** showing detail of organisms (×100).

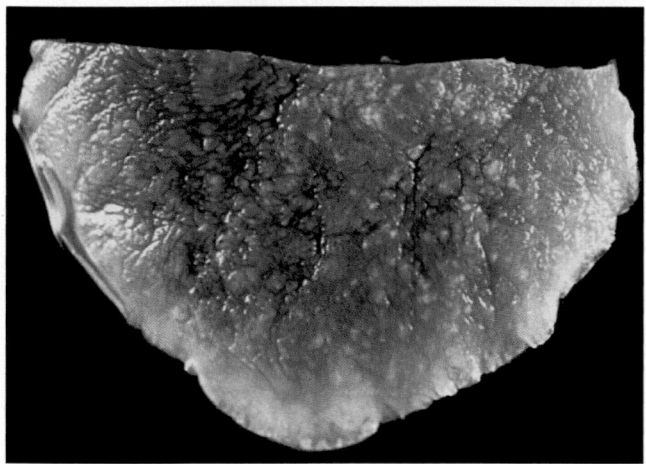

Fig 68-8 Lung of a rhesus monkey with *Pneumocystis* pneumonia in an early stage. The surface of the lung is covered with scattered, pinpoint, grayish-white lesions which are filled alveolar spaces. These lesions were found throughout the lung when it was sectioned (×3).

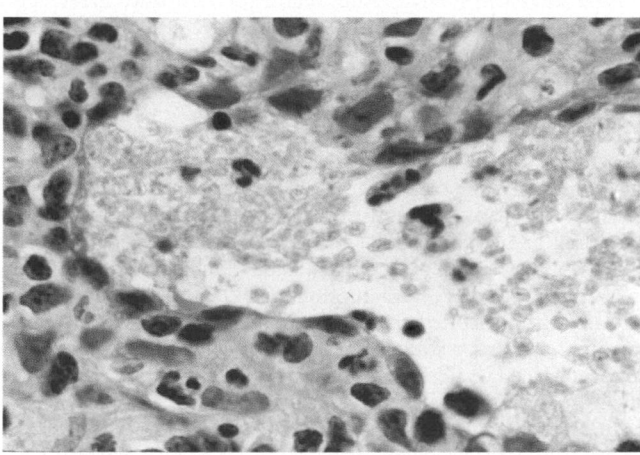

Fig 68-9 *P. carinii* within alveolar spaces in a dog with *Pneumocystis* pneumonia. Only the nuclei of the organisms are visible making it difficult to identify. (Courtesy University of Georgia, Athens, Ga.)

Table • 68-1

Comparison of Staining Methods for Demonstrating Pneumocystis *in Clinical Specimens*

	REACTION OF		
STAIN	**TROPHOZOITE**	**CYST WALL**	**INTERNAL STRUCTURES**
Hematoxylin and eosin	Unstained	Unstained	Weakly basophilic
Methenamine silver	Unstained	Brownish-black	Unstained
Toluidine blue	Unstained	Purplish-violet	Unstained
Periodic acid-Schiff	Unstained	Red	Unstained
Giemsa	Unstained	Unstained	Magenta
Gram	Unstained	Positive	Positive

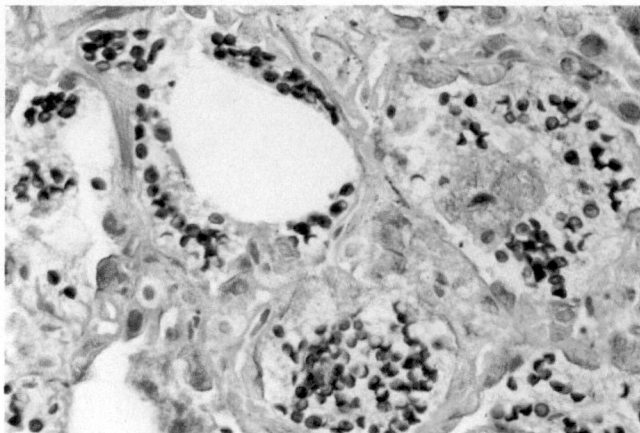

Fig 68-10 *P. carinii* within alveolar spaces in a person with AIDS and *Pneumocystis* pneumonia. Light, honeycombed matrix contains trophozoites and cellular debris. Darker ovoid, irregular, and crescent-shaped structures are cysts (GMS, ×400). See Figure 68-1 for further orientation.

toxylin and eosin stain does not readily demonstrate the developmental forms of *P. carinii*, which may explain why the disease is not recognized more frequently (Fig. 68-9). With this stain, only the hematoxylinophilic nuclei of intracystic sporozoites and trophozoites are demonstrated. Various modifications of methenamine silver staining can be employed to stain the cyst walls brownish-black, but trophozoites will not be detected (Fig. 68-10). Overstaining with Gomori's methenamine silver (GMS) may cause blackened and crenated erythrocytes in alveolar spaces to be mistaken for cyst forms of *Pneumocystis*. Polychrome stains, such as Wright's, Giemsa, and methylene blue, will demonstrate nuclei of trophozoites and intracystic sporozoites in cytologic specimens, but the walls of cyst and trophozoites will not be apparent (see Fig. 68-5, *A*). The cysts of *P. carinii* do not reproduce by budding and should not be confused for small yeast-form fungi in GMS-stained tissue sections. Polarization microscopy has also been used to demonstrate *P. carinii* in tissues.[1]

On histologic examination, alveolar spaces are filled with cohesive aggregates of amorphous, foamy, eosinophilic material that has a honeycomb-like pattern (see Fig. 68-9). A few macrophages and detached alveolar lining cells also may be present, but polymorphonuclear leukocytes are absent. Special staining methods are needed to identify cyst forms (see Fig. 68-10). Little or no phagocytosis of intact *Pneumocystis* organisms is present. However, nonviable organisms, such as those seen after treatment, are often phagocytosed, and macrophages may contain GMS-positive granular material that represents the residuum of cyst wall degradation. In some instances, alveolar septa are markedly thickened by dense accumulations of plasma cells, lymphocytes, and macrophages. The septa may be widened by fibrosis in chronic infections, especially after treatment. With GMS stain, cyst forms appear as spherical, ovoid, or crescent-shaped structures that range from 4 to 7 μm in diameter and have dotlike, argyrophilic, focal, cyst wall thickenings (Fig. 68-11). Cyst walls also can be demonstrated with other stains (see Table 68-1), and they will fluoresce when stained with orange G of a Papanicolaou stain. Trophozoites in tissue sections and smears are best demonstrated with Giemsa stain, especially Wolbach's procedure. On ultrastructural examination, intact alveoli are filled with compact aggregates of trophozoite and cyst forms. Trophozoites commonly line alveoli.

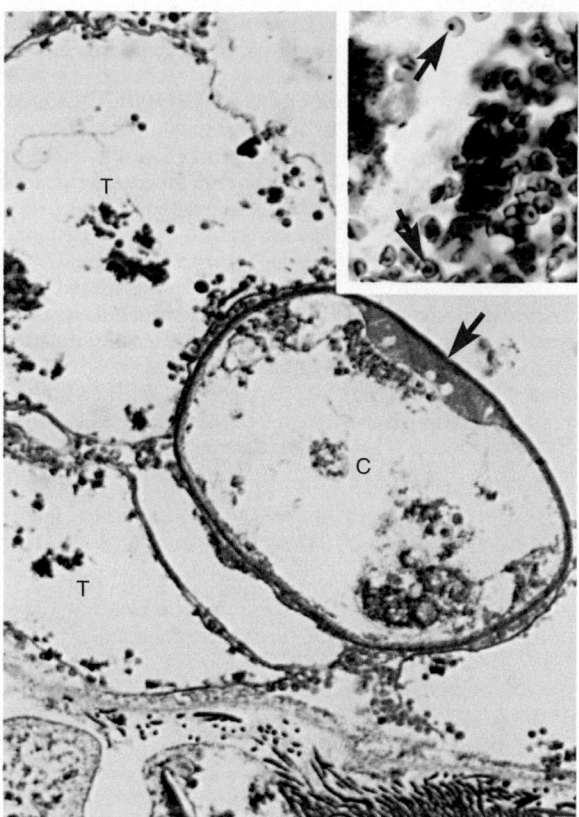

Fig 68-11 Pulmonary pneumocystosis. Alveolar space contains thin-walled trophozoites *(T)* and a cyst form *(C)* of *P. carinii*. Segmental, lamellated thickening of cyst wall *(arrow)* corresponds to darkly stained "intracystic" foci seen by light microscopy (transmission electron microscopy uranyl acetate and lead citrate, ×22,000). *Inset, P. carinii* cysts in touch imprint contain spherical to oval foci of enhanced staining *(arrows)* that in profile are contiguous with cyst wall (GMS, ×560).

THERAPY

Supportive care is essential for any patient with pneumocystic pneumonia because of disturbed alveolar gaseous exchange. Oxygen therapy administered by cage, mask, or intubation is needed, and ventilatory assistance may also be required. Bronchodilators may help reduce airway resistance. If a patient is receiving immunosuppressive agents, they should be temporarily discontinued; however, antiinflammatory drugs may be indicated. Antimicrobial chemotherapy of pulmonary pneumocystosis results in a decline in arterial oxygen related to the inflammatory reaction to dying organisms. Administration of antiinflammatory doses of glucocorticoids has been shown to improve pulmonary function and survival in people,[2,9,40] although subsequent studies have not been as supportive.[19] Immunosuppressive levels of glucocorticoids should *never* be given because they are known to facilitate the unchecked replication of the organism and fatal dissemination in people and experimental animals.

Specific chemotherapy is most beneficial in cases in which the disease is suspected or diagnosed during its early stages (Table 68-2). Despite their close genetic resemblance to fungi, *Pneumocystis* organisms are most sensitive to drugs used to treat protozoal infections. The two major chemotherapeutic agents that have successfully been used to treat pneumocystosis are pentamidine isethionate and the combination of trimethoprim and sulfonamide (TMS).

Table • 68-2

Therapy for Pneumocystosis

DROUG[a]	DOSE[b]	ROUTE	INTERVAL (HOURS)	DURATION (WEEKS)
Specific Agents				
Trimethoprim-sulfonamide	15—20 mg/kg	PO	8	3—16[c]
	30 mg/kg	PO	12	3
Pentamidine isethionate	4 mg/kg	IV, IM	24	3
Trimetrexate	45 mg/m^2	IV	24	3
Clindamycin and primaquine	3—13 mg/kg	PO	8	3
Atovaquone	15 mg/kg	PO	24	3
Adjunctive Agents				
Aminophylline	10—20 mg/kg	PO	8	3
Prednisone	1 mg/kg	PO	12—24	1
Cimetidine	5 mg/kg	PO	12	3
Levamisole	5 mg/kg	PO	48	3

PO, By mouth; *IV,* intravenous; *IM,* intramuscular.
[a]See Drug Formulary, Appendix 8, for additional information on each drug.
[b]Dose per administration at specified interval.
[c]Trimethoprim-sulfonamide is generally used alone or following remission with one of the other drugs. Treatment duration depends on the response to therapy. With use beyond 4 weeks, periodic monitoring for myelosuppression from folate synthesis antagonism is essential. Clinical response is monitored by repeated thoracic radiography.

Pentamidine isethionate is an aromatic diamidine that has been provided to reduce fatalities from the disease in people. Its major side effects include impaired renal function, hepatic dysfunction, hypoglycemia, hypotension, hypocalcemia, urticaria, and hematologic disorders (see Chapter 71). Serum urea nitrogen and glucose are monitored daily during treatment, and the drug is discontinued or dosage is reduced if complications or azotemia occur. Intramuscular (IM) and intravenous (IV) administration of pentamidine is associated with local inflammation and systemic hypotension, respectively, in people such that aerosolized delivery has been the preferred route of administration. IM administration of this drug has been successful in treating a dog with pneumocystosis with the only side effect being localized pain at the injection site. To lower its toxic side effects, pentamidine also has been successful, at a reduced dosage, in combination with sulfonamides. Levcovorin (folic acid) has been used as a supplement to avoid myelosuppression during long-term treatment.[54]

The combination of TMS has been found more effective and less toxic than pentamidine is in treating and preventing *Pneumocystis* pneumonia in immunodeficient people. A relatively high oral dosage of 30 mg/kg given every 6 hours for 2 weeks has been recommended in people so that the drug reaches therapeutically effective serum concentrations. Long-term (up to 2 years) prophylactic therapy for pneumocystosis at this dosage has not caused bone marrow toxicity in children, although changes in oral and fecal microflora have been noted as has increased prevalence of mucocutaneous candidiasis.

In dogs, treatment has been reported in eight dogs,[32,38,53] and four were dachshunds that recovered with treatment.[32] A TMS dose of 15 mg/kg, every 8 hours, or 30 mg/kg, every 12 hours, for 3 weeks was used in treating these dogs; the longest reported followup in these studies was for 4 months. Only one King Charles spaniel has been successfully treated, and the followup has been for a 3-year period (Fig. 68-12,*A* and *B*).[3] TMS was initially administered at a dose of 15 mg/kg, every 8 hours, daily for 4.3 months. After this time, medication was discontinued because of clinical resolution of signs of dyspnea, exercise intolerance, and pulmonary infiltrates, and the development of nonregenerative anemia suspected from folate antagonism. During the subsequent 3 years of monitoring, maintaining remission has required two re-treatment periods of 45 and 208 days in length. For dosage recommendations in treating dogs or cats, see Table 68-2.

In human infections, IV TMS therapy has been shown to be as or more effective than is oral therapy and has the advantage of ease of administration in severely depressed or comatose patients. Unfortunately, genotypic resistance to sulfonamides has been noted among some strains of *P. jiroveci* isolated from people.[12] Folic acid supplementation should be given if side effects such as leukopenia and anemia are observed or if long-term therapy is required.

Atovaquone, a hydroxynaphthoquinone, is licensed for the treatment of people with pneumocystosis.[28,50] This drug is not as effective as is pentamidine or TMS but has lower toxicity. Bioavailability is increased when the drug is given with food with a high fat content. It also has been used, as has pentamidine, in aerosol administration.[15]

Combination therapy using clindamycin and primaquine has been effective in vivo and in vitro, but neither drug is effective alone. Further investigation on the naturally occurring disease is needed. Aromatic diamidines, such as diminazene, imidocarb, and amicarbalide, have been more effective than pentamidine in treating experimental *P. carinii* pneumonia (see Chapter 71). Dapsone and trimethoprim or pyrimethamine, in combination, has been effective in experimental animals and clinical trials in immunosuppressed people with pneumocystosis.[29] Trimetrexate, a lipid-soluble antifolate, has been given concomitantly with leucovorin in people with *Pneumocystis* pneumonia and AIDS. As with most of the other drugs, neutropenia with or without thrombocytopenia has been the main side effect. In experimentally infected animals, *P. carinii* is resistant to imidazole antifungal drugs,[5] but the anthelmintics benzimidazole and albendazole have been effective.[4] Dapsone, alone or in combination with trimethoprim or pyrimethamine, has potent anti-*Pneumocys-*

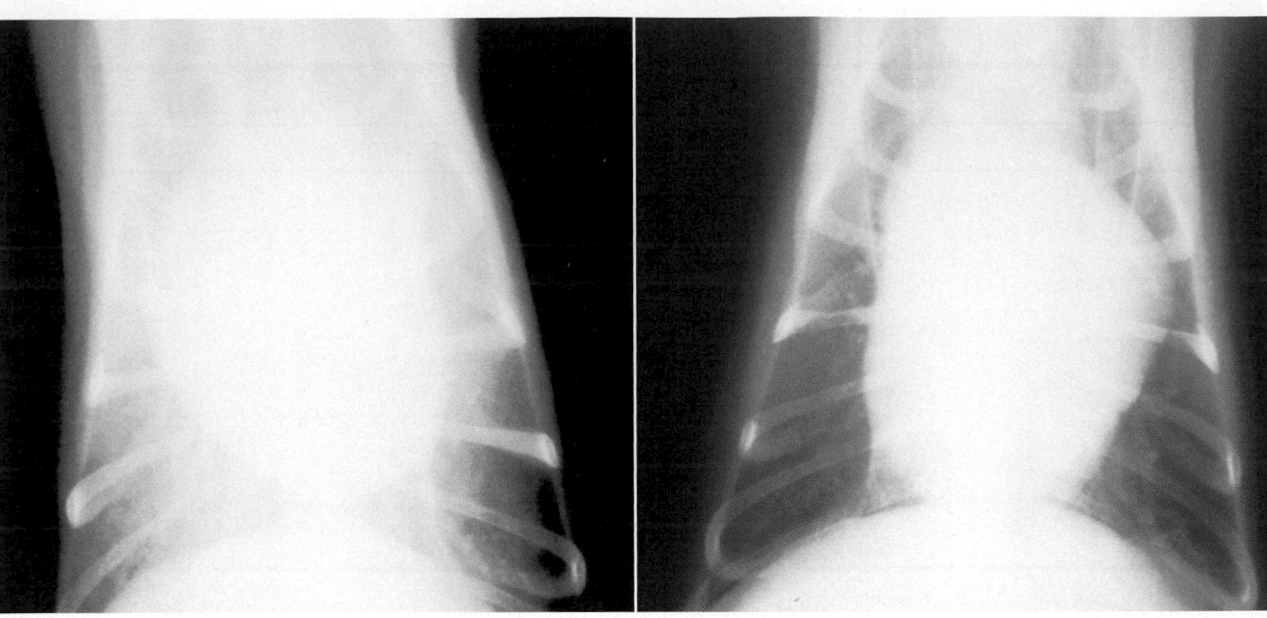

A   B

Fig   68-12   Ventrodorsal radiographs from a dog with *Pneumocystis* infection **(A)** before and **(B)** after therapy for 2 months. (Courtesy University of Georgia, Athens, Ga.)

tis activity in vitro and in animal studies.[29] When given at weekly, biweekly, or monthly intervals dapsone appeared effective in clearing organisms in the lung and might serve as a prophylactic measure to prevent infection in people.

Pneumocystosis in people and animals is *prima facie* evidence of immunodeficiency. For this reason, prophylactic treatment with TMS has been used in hospitalized people who are receiving irradiation or immunosuppressive agents or who have immunodeficiencies and debilitating diseases. Nonspecific immunostimulants such as cimetidine and levamisole (see Immunotherapy, Chapter 2) have been given adjunctively to treat affected miniature dachshunds.[21] Similar precautions are not warranted in pets because pneumocystosis has not been recognized with similar frequency in such instances.

PUBLIC HEALTH CONSIDERATIONS

Pneumocystis organisms are ubiquitous in the environment. The primary health risk is immunodeficiency syndromes. People and animals are exposed to the same environmental sources of *Pneumocystis*. Molecular and epidemiologic evi-

dence does suggest that spread occurs between people because of localized outbreaks. Clinically affected people and animals have the greatest concentrations of organisms in their airway secretions. Host immunocompetence is the most critical factor in determining whether illness develops. Therefore the most potential risk for a person acquiring infection from a pet would be if the animal was clinically ill from *Pneumocystis* pneumonia and the person in close contact was immunocompromised.

SUGGESTED READINGS*

3. Ayoob AL, Singer MJ, Brockus C, et al. 2004. Treatment of *Pneumocystis carinii* pneumonia in a dog, *J Small Anim Pract*, in press.
7. Beard CB, Carter JL, Keely SP, et al. 2000. Genetic variation in *Pneumocystis carinii* isolates from different geographic regions: implications for transmission, E*merg Infect Dis* 6:265-272.

*See the CD-ROM for a complete list of references.

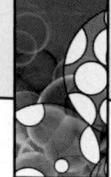

CHAPTER • 69

Protothecosis

Craig E. Greene, Pauline M. Rakich, and Kenneth S. Latimer

ETIOLOGY

Protothecosis is caused by *Prototheca*, a saprophytic achlorophyllous alga that is closely related to the green algae of the genus *Chlorella*. In culture or tissue, the cells are spherical to oval and range from 1.3 to 13.4 μm in diameter and 1.3 to 16.1 μm in length. The size varies with the stage of development, the species, and the medium used for culture. Organisms have a hyaline cell wall approximately 0.5 μm thick; a granular, basophilic cytoplasm; and a small, centrally located nucleus. In smaller, immature forms, a nucleus may not be evident. Reproduction is by endosporulation, with irregular nuclear and cytoplasmic cleavage resulting in 2 to 20 or more endospores. The mother cell ruptures, discharging tiny replicas that enlarge, mature, and repeat the life cycle. Empty cell casings scattered among intact algal cells may be seen in lesions. Figure 69-1 shows typical *Prototheca* in tissue.

Of the three recognized species of *Prototheca*—*Prototheca stagnora*, *Prototheca zopfii*, and *Prototheca wickerhamii*—the last two have been incriminated as pathogens. The species can be differentiated by sugar and alcohol assimilation tests or by fluorescent antibody (FA) methods.

EPIDEMIOLOGY AND PATHOGENESIS

The disease has been identified in people and animals in Europe, Asia, Africa, Australia, islands of the Pacific Ocean, and North America; a preponderance of the cases in North America are restricted to the southeastern United States.[18] Ecologically, *Prototheca* species are primarily found in raw and treated sewage, slime flux of trees, and animal wastes.[31] From these sources, *Prototheca* organisms secondarily contaminate water systems, soil, and food, from which they may be ingested by or come into contact with injured skin or mucosa of people and animals. Although *Prototheca* organisms can be isolated from freshly voided human and animal feces, the algae are regarded as transient contaminants and only rarely cause disease. Protothecosis is a sporadic illness that primarily develops when the host's immune resistance is suppressed or altered, often by a preexisting or concurrent disease. People with hematologic malignancies and who are receiving chemotherapy have been highly susceptible.[41] Lack of cell-mediated immunity seems to be a more important factor than decreased humoral responses in allowing entrance of *Prototheca* organisms into tissues and establishment of infection. An association has been made between the development of protothecosis and the acquired immune deficiency syndrome (AIDS) in people.[22,46] Infections have also occurred in people at sites of prolonged endotracheal intubation or peritoneal catheterization.[14,19] Another pathogenetic mechanism noted in some infected people is a deficiency in the ability of the host's neutrophils to destroy *Prototheca* organisms after phagocytosis. No other evidence has been found of failure of either humoral immunity or cell-mediated immunity in such

patients. Evaluation of immune function in one dog with disseminated protothecosis revealed depressed T-lymphocyte function and neutrophil inhibition.[32] A serum inhibitory factor may have been responsible for both findings. Inflammatory infiltrates are minimal in active lesions with large numbers of organisms; however, mononuclear infiltrates increase once therapy is instituted and numbers of organisms decrease in the tissues.[29] In people with mild immunosuppression that become colonized by *Prototheca* organisms, progression of the infection is accompanied by a reduction in measures of host immunosurveillance.[39]

In people, infection is usually cutaneous, subcutaneous, or bursal, although mucosal, catheter-related, and disseminated infections also occur. Cutaneous and localized infections are frequently seen in cats. In contrast, in nearly all infected dogs, evidence of protracted colitis with multisystemic dissemination has been reported. This finding suggests that after ingestion by dogs, the colon may be the common site of replication, with the infection subsequently spreading to other organs by blood and lymph.

Virulence of the various *Prototheca* species may differ. Only *P. wickerhamii* has been isolated from dogs and cats with cutaneous infections. In contrast, *P. zopfii* is almost always isolated from dogs with disseminated infections. Breed susceptibility may also be a factor in dogs because a disproportionate number of cases have been reported in collies.[40] No age predilection is known, but a majority of the infected dogs are females.

CLINICAL FINDINGS

Dogs

The most frequently reported clinical observation in dogs is bloody diarrhea, which is usually intermittent and protracted. Melena or hematochezia may be observed. However, dogs generally develop widely disseminated disease; types and severity of clinical signs vary depending on the tissues involved. The kidney, liver, heart, intestine, brain, and eye are the most common sites of systemic dissemination. Weight loss and debility become more pronounced over the course of the disease. Clinical signs attributed directly to involvement of the central nervous system (CNS) have been reported in about 40% of the dogs and have included marked depression, ataxia, circling, incoordination, and paresis. Deafness has developed, as have signs of renal failure. Only a few cases of cutaneous infection have been reported in dogs. Skin lesions usually last for several months and are characterized by nodules, draining ulcers, and crusty exudates on the trunk, extremities, and mucosal surfaces (Fig. 69-2). Even in those with cutaneous infections, lesions may become disseminated, involving other organs such as the joints, lymph nodes, heart, and lungs.

The eyes are involved in two thirds of the cases, and in some dogs blindness may be the primary symptom. Leukokoria resulting from vitreous clouding is common when dogs are

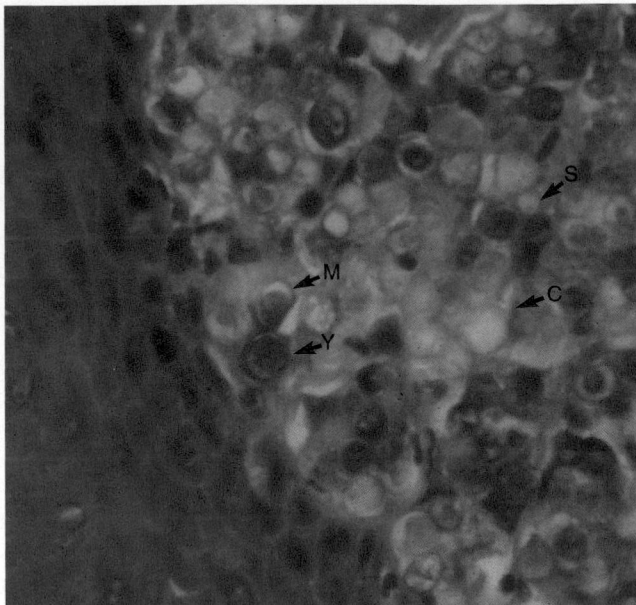

Fig 69-1 *Prototheca* organisms in various stages of development; lesion in skin of dog with disseminated protothecosis. Dermis is replaced by numerous *P. zopfii* organisms, including young spherical cells *(Y)* , more mature oval cells *(M)*, sporulating cells *(S)*, and scattered empty casings *(C)* of organisms (H and E stain, ×400). (Courtesy Pauline Rakich, University of Georgia, Athens, Ga.)

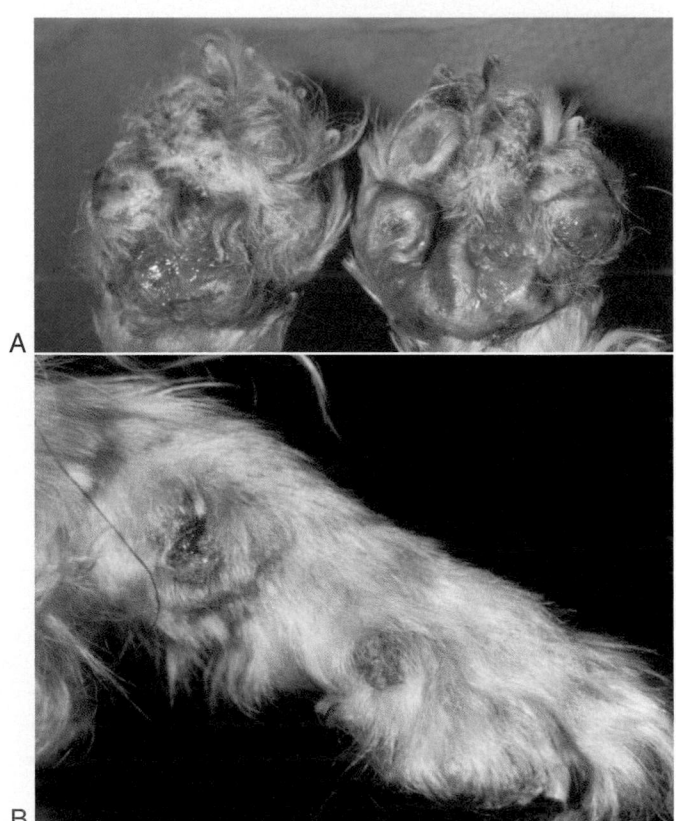

Fig 69-2 A, Heavy crusts on footpads of dog with rare cutaneous form of protothecosis. All four footpads were involved, as were **(B)** other areas of the skin. (Courtesy University of Georgia, Athens, Ga.)

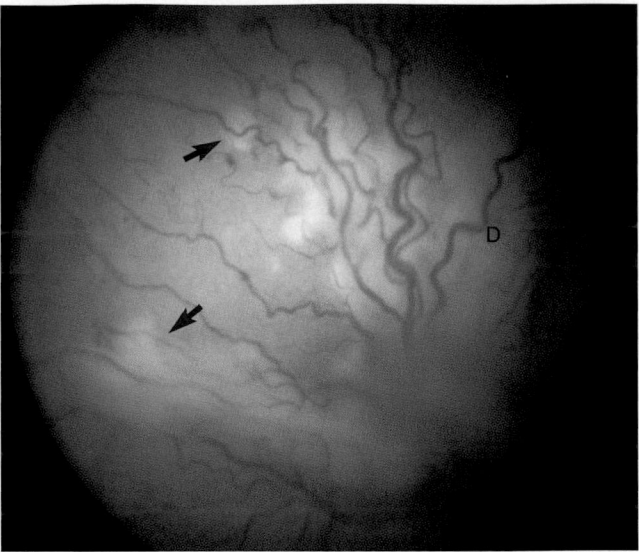

Fig 69-3 Ophthalmoscopic appearance of ocular fundus from dog with protothecosis. Posterior granulomatous uveitis is characterized by multifocal, round, and elongated, white subretinal infiltrates *(arrows)* with serous retinal detachment *(D)*. (Courtesy Charles Martin, University of Georgia, Athens, Ga.)

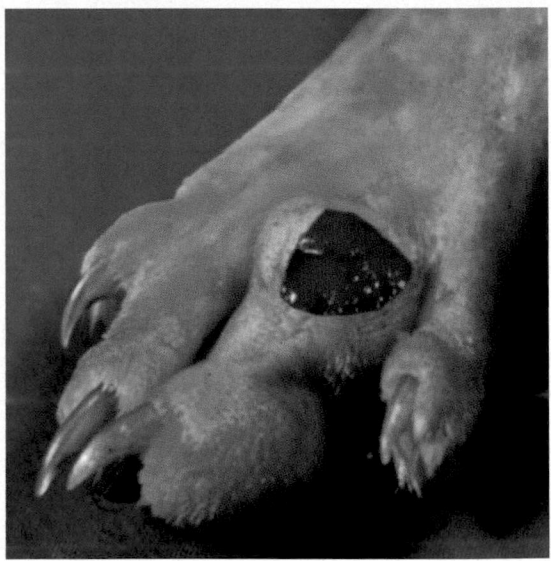

Fig 69-4 Cat's paw containing ulcerated cutaneous nodule *(arrow)* caused by localized infection with *P. wickerhamii*. (Courtesy Pauline Rakich and Ken Latimer, University of Georgia, Athens, Ga.)

first brought to the veterinarian for an examination.[24] Generally, ophthalmoscopic examination reveals exudative clouding of the fluid in one or both chambers and multiple white, raised foci or streaks in the retina (Fig. 69-3), often accompanied by small hemorrhages. Retinal detachment is usually evident.

Cats

Only the cutaneous form of protothecosis has been reported in cats.[8,11,12,20] Lesions usually consist of large, firm cutaneous nodules on the limbs or feet (Fig. 69-4). They have also been reported on the nose, forehead, pinna, and base of the tail. All cats were in good health otherwise. No published reports included results for feline leukemia virus (FeLV) and feline immunodeficiency virus (FIV) status, making any association uncertain.

DIAGNOSIS

Clinical Laboratory Findings

Laboratory data have not been well characterized in cats and dogs with prototothecosis. Generally, the results of the complete blood count (CBC) are within reference ranges. Rarely, serum hepatic enzyme activities are slightly elevated. Acute renal failure may develop in some dogs, resulting in azotemia and increase serum creatinine concentrations.[31a] Abnormalities in the cerebrospinal fluid (CSF) may include marked pleocytosis (greater than 100 cells/μl), with granulocytes and lymphocytes being the predominant nucleated cell types, and an increased protein concentration (greater than 100 mg/dl).[32,43]

Cytologic Examination

Whenever a dog that has ocular lesions and a history of protracted bloody diarrhea, protothecosis should be suspected. Diagnosis is often made by cytologic or histologic evaluation of affected tissues. For lower alimentary tract infections diagnosis can be made by cytologic examination of rectal and colonic scrapings (Fig. 69-5). Cytologic examination of scrapings is the most cost effective direct means of diagnosis. If necessary, full-thickness biopsy of the intestinal tract also can be performed. Fine-needle aspiration of other lesions also may be diagnostically useful. Cats that develop nodular and ulcerative skin lesions should also be checked for protothecosis. Because Prototheca organisms commonly invade Bowman's space and renal tubules after embolization, the presence of the organism in urinary sediment is an accurate indication that dissemination of infection has occurred (Fig. 69-6).[31a,32]

Algal Identification and Isolation

For all lesions, microbiological isolation and identification is the most accurate way to confirm a diagnosis. Clinically, organisms have been found by culture of CSF or fluid obtained by vitreous centesis or fine-needle aspirates and from histologic evaluation of lesion biopsy specimens or enlarged lymph nodes.

Prototheca species grow readily on various laboratory media, such as Sabouraud's cycloheximide-free dextrose agar at 25° C to 37° C, forming white to light tan colonies within 2 to 7 days. Characteristic organisms in all stages of development can be recognized by staining a smear from the colony with Gram iodine stain (Fig. 69-7). Ribostamycin-impregnated disks have been used to differentiate *Candida* and *Prototheca* colonies grossly on Sabouraud's glucose agar.[5] *Prototheca* colonies develop a halo of inhibition around the disks, whereas *Candida* colonies do not. *Prototheca* species can be differentiated by the use of clotrimazole-impregnated discs, because *P. wickerhamii* is susceptible to clotrimazole, whereas *P. zopfii* is resistant.[4] For specific differentiation, the slower but more routine method of culturing followed by sugar and alcohol assimilation testing can be done in most diagnostic laboratories.

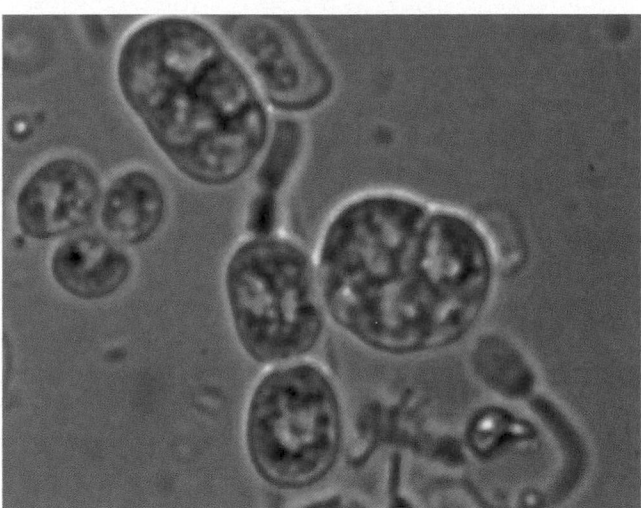

Fig 69-6 Urine sediment from dog with disseminated protothecosis. *P. zopfii* organisms are numerous and exhibit anisocytosis and occasional sporulation. Scattered spermatozoa also are present (unstained urine sediment, ×1000). (Courtesy Robert Duncan, University of Georgia, Athens, Ga.)

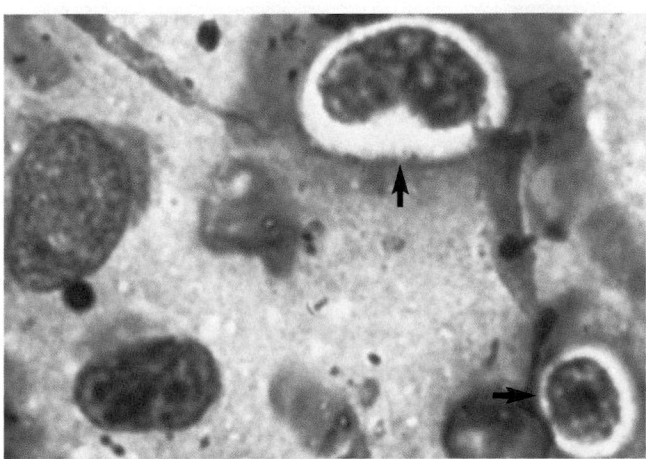

Fig 69-5 Prototothecal cells *(arrows)* in smear of rectal scraping from dog with disseminated protothecosis. *P. zopfii* organisms vary in size and have granular basophilic to magenta cytoplasm surrounded by a clear capsule. Scattered columnar epithelial cells, erythrocytes, two neutrophils, and small lymphocyte are present also (Wright stain, ×1008). (Courtesy Ken Latimer, University of Georgia, Athens, Ga.)

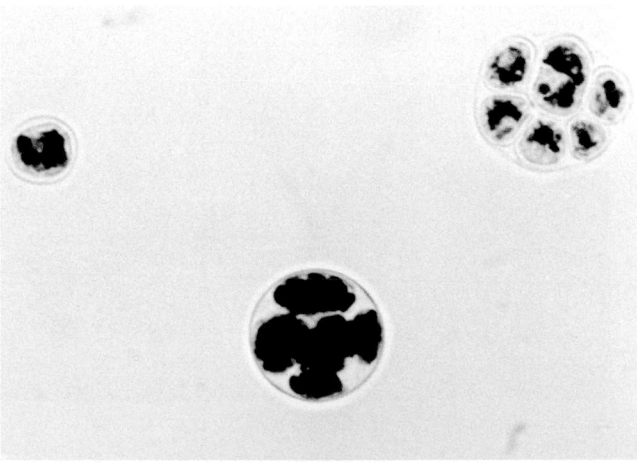

Fig 69-7 Sporulating and nonsporulating forms of *P. zopfii* isolated from canine CSF (Gram iodine stain, ×1000). (Courtesy David Tyler, University of Georgia, Athens, Ga.)

PATHOLOGIC FINDINGS

Dogs

Protothecosis is predominantly a disseminated disease, producing lesions in a wide variety of tissues. Lesions in parenchymatous organs and on serosal surfaces are diffusely scattered throughout the tissues as white to tan granular foci measuring 0.5 to 2 mm in diameter or as streaks measuring 0.5 × 2 to 3 mm wide. This pattern is particularly common in the myocardium, skeletal muscle, intestinal muscularis, lymph nodes, thyroid, liver, and loose connective tissue (Fig. 69-8).[9] In the kidney, lesions tend to be larger, often measuring up to several centimeters, and are surrounded by a peripheral ring of hemorrhage. They also have a radiating linear pattern and may appear in either the cortex or medulla. Gross lesions may develop throughout the intestinal tract, but the colon is most commonly affected. The lesions in the mucosa may vary from diffuse reddening to marked nodular thickening and scattered,

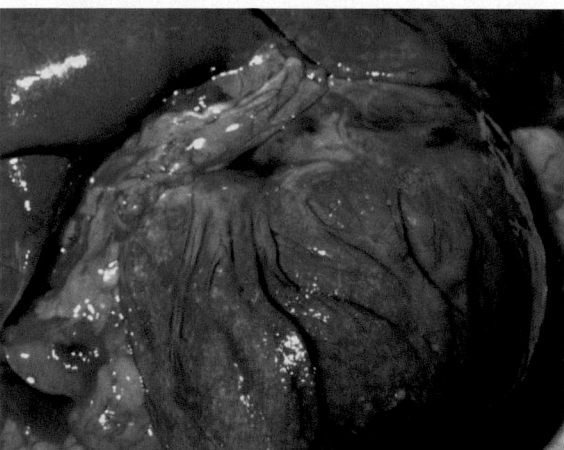

Fig 69-8 Heart and lungs of dog that died from disseminated infection with *P. zopfii*. Small, granular, white to tan foci are visible on surface of myocardium. (Courtesy Ken Latimer, University of Georgia, Athens, Ga.)

often hemorrhagic, ulcers. Tiny white foci are frequently seen in the muscularis and serosa. Sections of affected eyes contain gray-white cloudy exudates, often with red streaks, in one or both chambers and beneath the retina, which is often detached.

Microscopically, various host reactions may be seen. Inflammation is usually mild and composed of mixed inflammatory cells at the periphery of clusters of numerous *Prototheca* organisms (Figs. 69-9). The infiltrate consists of macrophages, lymphocytes, neutrophils, and plasma cells, which may be particularly numerous. Although less common, inflammation is pronounced and granulomatous or pyogranulomatous. In such lesions, macrophages and multinucleate giant cells contain many phagocytosed *Prototheca* cells. Hemorrhage and necrosis occur more commonly in the kidneys, heart, and intestines.

In the colon the mucosal surface is multifocally ulcerated and hemorrhagic. Masses of organisms, often arranged in cords or nodules, replace much of the mucosa and extend into and replace the submucosa. Small focal colonies of organisms are scattered throughout the muscularis and serosa. As in other tissues, inflammation is usually mild and composed of mixed cells. When infection is prolonged, granulation tissue may be intermingled with organisms in the mucosa and submucosa. In the kidney, multiple aggregates of *Prototheca* cells are distributed in the interstitium of the cortex, medulla, and occasionally the papillae. Inflammation and necrosis may vary from minimal to marked. Lesions in the brain and spinal cord usually develop as widely scattered, small foci of necrosis containing mixed inflammatory cells and rare to multiple aggregates of *Prototheca* cells. Similar lesions may be present in the inner ear. Focal to diffuse granulomatous chorioretinitis, retinal detachment, and severe retinal degeneration are the most common ocular lesions seen microscopically. Masses of organisms are in the vitreous and between the retina and choroid. Fewer develop focally in the choroid. The inflammatory infiltrate is mixed and may be pyogranulomatous.

In cutaneous lesions, masses of *Prototheca* cells are distributed in the dermis, subcutis, and subjacent skeletal muscle. The epidermis is variably hyperkeratotic, ulcerated, and inflamed. Ulcerated surfaces are commonly secondarily infected with bacteria. Cutaneous lesions may extend into the

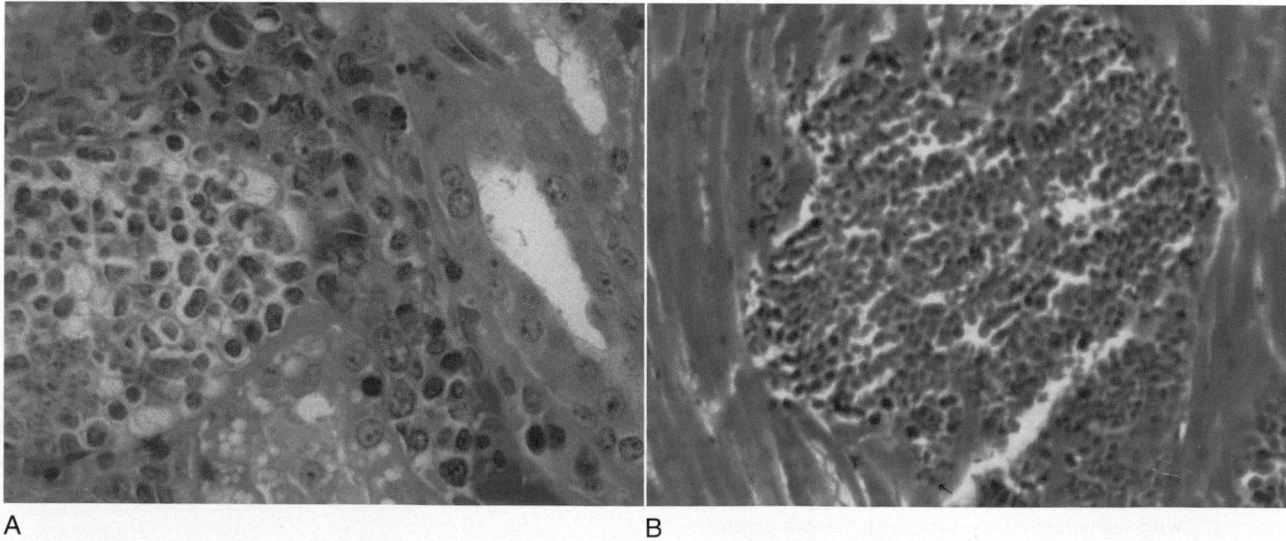

A   B

Fig 69-9 Sections of kidney (**A**) and heart (**B**) from dog with disseminated *P. zopfii* infection. **A,** Renal interstitium is infiltrated by *Prototheca* organisms. Inflammation is minimal and consists of a few lymphocytes and plasma cells (H and E stain, ×400). **B,** Myocardium contains large infiltrates of *Prototheca* organisms in absence of inflammation (H and E stain, ×400). (Courtesy Ken Latimer, University of Georgia, Athens, Ga.)

nasal mucosa and produce necrosis, ulceration, hemorrhage, and infiltration of neutrophils and plasma cells mixed with large masses of proliferating *Prototheca*.[38] Typically the regional lymph nodes are invaded secondarily. In one dog with cutaneous protothecosis, inflammation before treatment was mild but increased during treatment even though the number of organisms decreased.[29] These findings suggested that viable organisms inhibited the immune response or were less immunoreactive in tissues than dead organisms.

P. zopfii and *P. wickerhamii* may have sufficient morphologic differences to be identified histologically[7]; however, the differences are too subtle for pathologists who see these organisms infrequently to make the distinction. When species identification is required, preserved biopsy and necropsy tissues and unstained histologic sections can be examined at specialized laboratories by the indirect FA technique.

Cats

Localized cutaneous lesions in cats consist of gray-white subcutaneous or dermal masses that extend deeply into the underlying tissue and infiltrate tendons, nerves, and blood vessels. Histologically, they are granulomas characterized by numerous epithelioid macrophages and scattered multinucleated giant cells. Neutrophils and plasma cells may be prominent in some lesions. Masses of *Prototheca* in all stages of reproduction constitute the bulk of the lesion.

Special Staining

Prototheca and *Chlorella* species are morphologically indistinguishable in tissues stained with hematoxylin-eosin (H and E)

but can be differentiated using Gomori's methenamine silver (GMS) or periodic acid–Schiff (PAS) stain (Fig. 69-10). With these stains, large starch granules are seen in *Chlorella* species but not in *Prototheca* species. The presence of chloroplasts is characteristic of *Chlorella* species, but they are not visible in light microscopy of fixed tissues. No reports have been made of *Chlorella* organisms infecting dogs or cats; however, they have infected several other animal species and frequently are identified improperly as *Prototheca* species.

THERAPY

Cutaneous

Because protothecosis usually occurs as a single focal cutaneous lesion in people and cats, wide excision has been successful; and the preferred therapeutic approach for solitary lesions is resection in conjunction with systemic antimicrobial chemotherapy. Human cutaneous infections are usually caused by *P. wickerhamii*, which appears to be more susceptible to antifungal chemotherapy. In vitro studies on *P. wickerhamii* have shown a synergistic effect between amphotericin B (AMB) and other drugs such as tetracycline. Treatment of human cutaneous *P. wickerhamii* infection with AMB alone, in combination with oral tetracycline, or with ketoconazole (KTZ) or fluconazole (FCZ) has been successful.[21,44]

One human with a *P. wickerhamii*-infected wrist wound was successfully treated with orally administered KTZ.[28] Hepatotoxicity, which developed in response to the treatment, resolved spontaneously after cessation of treatment.

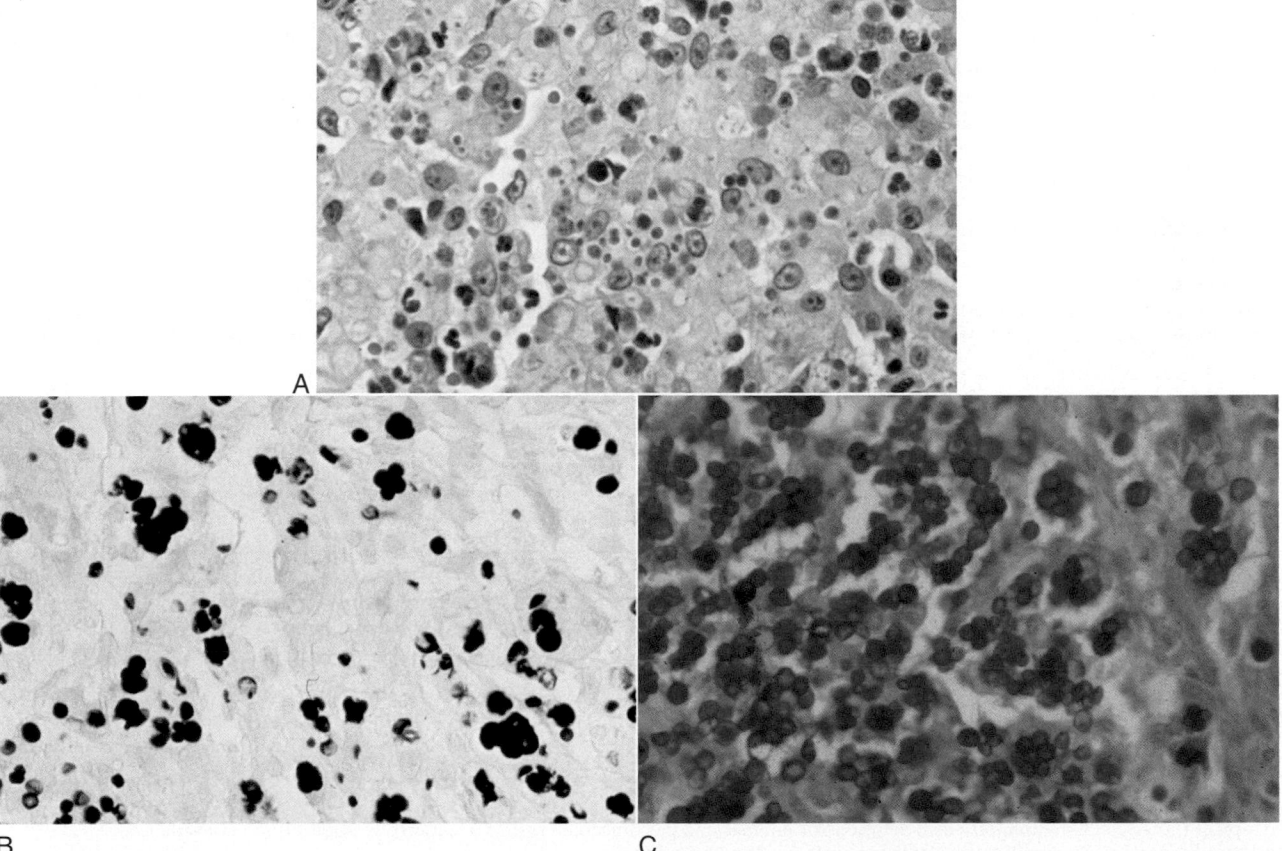

Fig 69-10 *Prototheca* organisms are readily identified in tissue section using special stains. Organisms stain **(A)** magenta with H and E stain, **(B)** black with GMS, or **(C)** magenta with the PAS technique (**A, B,** and **C,** ×400). (Courtesy Ken Latimer, University of Georgia, Athens, Ga.)

Chemotherapy with itraconazole (ITZ) resolved a dermal infection with *P. wickerhamii* in one person.[26] An immunocompetent person who developed a localized granuloma was also successfully treated with ITZ.[30] In a more unusual reported case of localized dermal *P. zopfii* infection, successful treatment involved local infiltration of FCZ solution into the lesion.[36] In another case of localized *P. zopfii* infection in a person, amikacin and tetracyclines were combined for successful therapy.[47] Cutaneous *P. wickerhamii* infection in a human with AIDS did not respond to ITZ but did resolve with AMB therapy.[2] Susceptibility testing was predictive in this case and may be indicated in other cases of protothecosis because of the variable clinical responses achieved from various isolates from human and animal infections.

KTZ was effective in causing regression of multifocal cutaneous abscesses caused by infection with *Prototheca* species in a dog.[23] Treatment continued for 4 months, although long-term follow-up information was not available. The organism showed marked in vitro susceptibility to KTZ. In another dog with cutaneous manifestations of *P. wickerhamii* infection, oral KTZ therapy for 6 months resolved all the lesions except for a scrotal granuloma, which was surgically removed.[15] However, a clinical relapse occurred 5 months later.

In vitro, clotrimazole (CTZ) is not effective for treating *P. zopfii* but is highly efficacious against *P. wickerhamii*.[4] It is only available in topical preparations. Because cutaneous protothecosis in dogs and cats is caused by *P. wickerhamii*, topically applied CTZ might be the drug of choice for this form of protothecosis. Topical CTZ did not appear to alter the course of successful therapy with systemic KTZ in one dog.[15]

Disseminated

Various antimicrobial agents have been used to treat people and animals with disseminated infection. However, in most instances, treatment was unsuccessful. Therapies have included systemic administration of various antibacterial drugs, AMB, griseofulvin, potassium iodide, and pentamidine isethionate and topical application of antibiotics, copper sulfate, AMB lotion, gentian violet, brilliant green, and chlorinated lime.

A few human beings with disseminated protothecosis have been treated successfully with AMB and transfer factor.[10] An immunocompetent person with disseminated *P. wickerhamii* infection was successfully treated with AMB for several weeks in conjunction with 3 months of KTZ treatment.[6]

Dogs often develop the disseminated disease, and consequently the prognosis is guarded to poor. Unfortunately the disease is insidious, often widespread, and often involves many organs by the time clinical signs are evident. Ocular involvement causes endophthalmitis, which results in visual loss. Diarrhea may wax and wane initially, but it progresses inevitably. Treatment may prolong the course of infection, but the outcome is invariably fatal. Of almost 30 cases of disseminated *P. zopfii* infection reported in dogs since 1969, treatment has been uniformly unsuccessful in eliminating infection or preventing dissemination.

Aminoglycosides such as gentamicin have in vitro activity against *Prototheca*, but their clinical usefulness has not been well substantiated.[17a] Ribostamycin, an aminoglycoside antibiotic closely related to kanamycin, is an effective agent in vitro against all species of *Prototheca*, especially *P. zopfii*.[3] Although not commercially available, ribostamycin was used experimentally to treat a dog with chorioretinitis as the primary manifestation of infection with *P. zopfii*.[34] The drug was administered at a dose of 12.5 mg/kg given intramuscularly twice daily. Ocular manifestations improved, but the dog later died with disseminated lesions.

AMB was not effective in the treatment of ocular protothecosis *(P. zopfii)* in a dog.[25] The initial treatment reduced the size of the lesion in the eye, and blood culture results became negative, but therapy was discontinued because renal toxicity developed. Subsequently, lower doses failed to stop the progression of the lesions. Simazine (an algicidal drug used to clean fish tanks), gentamicin, and KTZ also were tried in the same dog without success. In another dog with ophthalmic lesions, ITZ therapy did not eliminate the lesions; however, the progression of infection was slowed, and the dog survived for 11 months.[35]

In one dog with prothecal colitis, treatment with KTZ for 30 days may have slowed the progression of illness; the dog had a 4-month period of clinical remission after treatment.[33] In another dog with *Prototheca* enterocolitis, systemic AMB therapy was followed by an enema with 3% AMB cream.[37] Some of the clinical signs resolved, and the number of organisms in colonic cytologic specimens decreased. The dog was discharged from the hospital receiving a maintenance treatment of ITZ for 4 weeks; however, it died 6 weeks after treatment was instituted.

Treatment with AMB alone was successful in slowing the progression of clinical signs for 1 year in a dog with cutaneous and systemic infection with *P. wickerhamii*.[45] The more favor-

Table • 69-1

Proposed Systemic Drug Therapy for Protothecosis[a]

DRUG[b]	SPECIES	DOSE (MG/KG)[c]	ROUTE	INTERVAL (HOURS)	DURATION (DAYS)
Amphotericin B	Dog	0.5–1	IV	3 times weekly	Varies[d]
	Cat	0.25	IV	3 times weekly	Varies[e]
plus					
Itraconazole[f]	Dog and cat	5–10	PO	12	28–42

IV, Intravenous; *PO*, orally.
[a]For topical therapy a 3% amphotericin B solution for enemas and clotrimazole cream for cutaneous application are available.
[b]See Drug Formulary, Appendix 8, for additional information on each drug.
[c]Dose per administration at specified interval.
[d]Until cumulative dose is 8–12 mg/kg. Higher doses of lipid formulations are used; see Drug Formulary, Appendix 8.
[e]Until cumulative dose is 4 mg/kg. Higher doses of lipid formulations are used; see Drug Formulary, Appendix 8.
[f]Continue while receiving amphotericin B. More effective against *Prototheca wickerhamii* than *Prototheca zopfii*.

able outcome in this case may be because *P. wickerhamii* is more susceptible to antifungal drugs than *P. zopfii*.

Based on previous reports and in the absence of susceptibility data, disseminated disease in dogs caused by *P. zopfii* should be treated with AMB alone or in combination with ITZ. Aminoglycosides or tetracyclines could be alternative additional drugs. See Table 69-1 for appropriate drugs dosages for treating protothecosis.

PUBLIC HEALTH CONSIDERATIONS

Protothecosis is considered to be acquired from environmental exposure and is not transmissible between hosts. People, dogs, and cats are continually exposed to this ubiquitous organism but infrequently develop disease. Immunocompetent people and animals have less risk of developing clinical disease or dissemination than individuals with compromised immunity. Handling wastes or exudates from infected pets carries no greater risk of infection than environmental exposure. However, in general, immunocompromised people should be advised to avoid close contact with infected animals. People who are hospitalized and receiving immunosuppressive or surgical therapy or those with intravenous, endotracheal, or peritoneal catheters are at greatest risk for infection.

SUGGESTED READINGS*

31a. Pressler BM, Gookin JL, Sykes JE, et al. 2005. Urinary tract manifestations of protothecosis in dogs, *J Vet Intern Med* 19:115-119.

33. Rallis TS, Tontis D, Adamama-Moraitou KK, et al. 2002. Protothecal colitis in a German Shepherd dog. *Aust Vet J* 80:406-408.

41. Torres HA, Bodey GP, Tarrand JJ, et al. 2003. Protothecosis in patients with cancer: case series and literature review. *Clin Microbiol Infect* 9:786-792.

47. Zhao J, Liu W, LV G, et al. 2004. Protothecosis successfully treated with amikacin combined with tetracyclines. *Mycoses* 47:156-158.

*See the CD-ROM for a complete list of references.

SECTION • IV
Protozoal Diseases

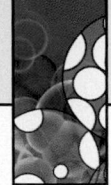

CHAPTER • 70

Laboratory Diagnosis of Protozoal Infections

Susan E. Little

Protozoa are responsible for some of the easiest and some of the most difficult infections to diagnose in clinical practice. When organisms are readily apparent and present in large numbers, diagnosis can be quickly achieved by direct microscopic examination of appropriate samples. However, in many cases, the protozoal organisms responsible for an infection are not present in high numbers, are not being shed or circulating at the time of sample collection, or they are difficult to identify because of their small size, subtle diagnostic features, or because of damage associated with mishandling of the sample before submission for diagnosis. Detection of organisms can also be hindered by prior treatment with antimicrobials. Although immunologic and molecular assays are becoming increasingly available to aid in the diagnosis of protozoal infections in dogs and cats, direct microscopic examination of feces, blood, or other clinical samples remains the mainstay of reaching a diagnosis for most of these organisms.

Many of the assays described in this chapter can be readily performed in clinic by trained personnel. However, because confirmation and consultation are often desired when reaching a diagnosis of an unusual parasite, collection and preservation of samples for submission to veterinary diagnostic laboratories are also discussed. Detailed descriptions of diagnosis of specific protozoal infections also are available in the appropriate chapters of this text.

MICROSCOPIC EXAMINATION

Feces
Protozoa are commonly found in fecal samples. Although samples should ideally be examined as quickly as possible following collection, some stages of some protozoans will still be evident in refrigerated or fixed samples.

Collection and Storage of Feces
To maximize the likelihood of identifying a parasite, at least 5 g of feces should be collected and placed in a clean, dry, airtight container. The amount of material retrieved by use of a fecal wand is insufficient for reaching a diagnosis of most intestinal parasites. Although interpretation of a positive result on direct smear from a fecal wand sample is possible, a negative result is all but meaningless because of the small sample size examined. If possible, the fecal sample should be held at room temperature and examined immediately (within 30 minutes) after collection. Protozoal trophozoites may lyse during refrigeration or long-term storage and thus fail to be detected. If samples cannot be examined immediately, however, then feces should be refrigerated. Tightly sealed, refrigerated samples may be examined for the presence of cysts or oocysts, which

are hardier and persist in the environment for up to 1 week after collection.[7]

Examination of Feces
Table 70-1 lists the recommended microscopic procedures for the diagnosis of intestinal protozoal infections.

Direct Saline Smear The direct smear technique, which can be performed on diarrheic or formed fecal samples, is most important when used with diarrheic specimens. To enhance detection, the substage condenser of the microscope should be adjusted to maximize contrast; unstained organisms may otherwise be overlooked. When available, the phase-contrast or dark-field microscope may aid in the demonstration of motile trophozoites but is not a necessary piece of equipment for reliable diagnosis of protozoal infection.

A direct smear is made by placing a drop of saline on a clean microscope slide and then mixing in a minute amount of fecal material; the amount that adheres to the tip of a wooden applicator stick is sufficient. A coverslip is then applied and the slide systematically scanned using the 10× objective but alternating with the 40× objective whenever structures morphologically resembling protozoal trophozoites or cysts are encountered. The fecal-saline mixture should be transparent enough that newsprint can be easily read through the material. Motility and structural features of protozoa are best examined using the high-dry objective (40× to 43×). The oil immersion objective (100×) is not recommended for examining fresh wet mounts because pressure on the coverslip from the oil objective displaces the fluid medium between the coverslip and the slide, making viewing difficult. If necessary, once motility has been observed, stain may be added to the smear to aid in specific identification of the organisms.[9]

Stained Smear Although not required, adding stain to the wet mount through the edge of the coverslip may aid in visualizing internal structures of some protozoa. Because staining the preparation kills the organism, examination for motility must be performed first. Table 70-2 describes the trophozoites found on direct smears from fecal samples of dogs and cats.

Iodine is the most common stain used to reveal the internal structure of protozoans and is especially useful for confirming the identity of *Giardia* cysts and trophozoites. The iodine stains the cytoplasm of cysts dark gold, while the nuclei remain pale and refractile. Other stains used to identify protozoa in feces include methylene blue, acid methyl green, aqueous eosin, and crystal violet. Methylene blue is useful for identifying trophozoites, especially those of *Entamoeba histolytica*, while acid methyl green stains the macronucleus of *Balantidium coli*. Aqueous eosin and crystal violet are both

Table • 70-1

Recommended Procedures for the Diagnosis of Gastrointestinal Protozoans of the Dog and Cat

ORGANISM	STAGE	PROCEDURE
Balantidium coli	Trophozoites	Direct smear
	Cysts	Zinc sulfate centrifugation flotation technique
Coccidia (Toxoplasma, Isospora, Sarcocystis, Hammondia, Besnoitia, and Cryptosporidium)	Oocysts	Sheather's sugar centrifugation flotation technique
Entamoeba histolytica	Trophozoites	Direct smear
	Cysts	Direct smear
Giardia	Trophozoites	Direct smear, occasionally seen on flotation
	Cysts	Direct smear, zinc sulfate centrifugation flotation technique
Pentatrichomonas	Trophozoites	Direct smear

Table • 70-2

Protozoal Trophozoite Identification by Direct Fecal Smear

ORGANISM	SIZE (μm)	DISTINGUISHING MORPHOLOGY	
		FRESH SMEAR	STAINED SMEAR
Balantidium coli	50—150	Oval shape; revolving movement by means of cilia; macronucleus may be visible	Large kidney bean—shaped macronucleus is prominent; occasionally micronucleus may be seen
Entamoeba histolytica	12—50	Constantly changes shape when active; moves by means of finger-like projections of cytoplasm; one nucleus that is difficult to see; may contain erythrocytes	Nucleus usually has evenly distributed peripheral chromatin and centrally located, compact karyosome
Giardia	9—21 × 5—15 × 2—4	Bilaterally symmetric; pear shaped on dorsoventral view; crescentic on lateral view; rolling movement by means of flagella; contains two nuclei	Two large nuclei, each with prominent karyosomes and axonemes and median bodies give monkey-faced appearance
Pentatrichomonas	5—20 × 3—14	Oval to pear shaped; wobbly, jerky, rapid movement by means of flagella; undulating membrane visible	Oval nucleus in anterior half of body; axostyle protruding from posterior end

negative stains, which stain fecal debris but leave parasitic cysts and trophozoites, which exclude the dye, highlighted by their colorless appearance against the stained background.[2]

Fecal Flotation Fecal concentration methods are often necessary to reveal the presence of protozoal cysts or oocysts. With this technique, sugar or salt solutions are used with centrifugation to concentrate the cysts or oocysts present in several grams of feces into a small volume of fluid that can be examined on a single slide. Standard sodium nitrate tabletop flotation alone is not adequate for detecting most protozoa, although coccidia oocysts are often revealed by this method. Although killed by the hypertonic solution and almost always lysed, trophozoites, especially those of Giardia, may also occasionally be seen on fecal flotation.

Solutions used in centrifugal fecal flotation methods include zinc sulfate and Sheather's sugar. Five to 10 g of feces are mixed with water to a liquid consistency, and the mixture is strained with gauze. Two parts Sheather's sugar solution (500 g sugar, 300 ml water, and 6.5 g melted phenol crystals) are added to one part fecal suspension and centrifuged in a capped centrifuge tube. Care should be taken not to fill the tube to the top to prevent spills or aerosols. After centrifugation at 1000× G for 10 minutes, remove 1 to 2 drops from the meniscus by a dropper, place on a microscope slide, cover with a coverslip, and examine at low-power (×100) magnification. To assist in the examination of very mucoid or fatty fecal samples, 2 to 3 g of feces should first be combined with 5 to 10 ml of water, strained through a double layer of cheesecloth, the mixture centrifuged for 5 to 10 minutes at approximately 650 × G, and the supernatant discarded. The sediment should then be mixed with 5 to 10 ml 33% zinc sulfate with a specific gravity of 1.18 or Sheather's sugar solution, strained through cheesecloth, and centrifuged for 5 to 10 minutes at approximately 650 × G.[9]

When available, a centrifuge with a swinging bucket rotor is ideal for the flotation step. With this protocol, the strained feces–flotation solution mixture is poured into a 15-ml conical centrifuge tube and enough flotation solution added to form a reverse meniscus at the top of the tube. A coverslip is then placed on top of the meniscus and the tube spun with the coverslip in place; a second tube is needed to balance the centrifuge. Once completed, the coverslip is removed, transferred along with the adherent fluid to a slide, and the slide is examined. If only a fixed angle bucket rotor is available, fecal flotation with centrifugation can still be performed. In this case, the feces–flotation solution mixture should be poured into a 15-ml centrifuge tube to the point at which it is almost full but does not spill when placed into the centrifuge bucket (approximately 13 ml). The tube is then spun without a coverslip. After centrifugation is complete, the top layer of the centrifuged material can be collected by carefully touching the base of a small test tube or a microbiological loop to the surface and then transferring the adherent fluid to a slide. A coverslip is then applied and the preparation examined. Prepared slides should be completely examined using the 10× and, when necessary to confirm the identification of an organism, the 40× objectives. Scanning a slide at 4× is not sufficient to allow detection of most protozoa.[9]

Preservation of Feces

If examining a fecal sample for protozoa is delayed, or if the sample is to be sent to a diagnostic laboratory for microscopic examination, the feces should be thoroughly mixed with a preservative before shipment. Enough fixative solution should be added to the feces to ensure adequate fixation. Some commonly used solutions include potassium dichromate, polyvinyl alcohol (PVA), and 10% formalin.[2]

Potassium dichromate is the solution of choice for storing samples containing oocysts of coccidia because it allows the oocysts to sporulate, permitting the precise measurements of sporocysts and sporozoites and complete evaluation of oocyst structure that are needed for identification. Historically, PVA has been considered the best choice for fixing trophozoites because permanently stained slides can be prepared from PVA-fixed fecal material. However, both PVA, which contains mercuric chloride, and potassium dichromate are potent toxicants and should be handled with great care. In recent years, less toxic, more environmentally safe substitutes for PVA have become available, including Proto-Fix (AlphaTec Systems, Inc., Vancouver, Wash.) and ECOFIX (Meridian Diagnostics, Inc., Cincinnati, Ohio).[6]

Whole Blood

Protozoa may be detected in both fresh blood samples and in samples collected into anticoagulants. The most common method used to detect protozoa in blood is by preparing and staining a blood smear and examining the preparation microscopically. Blood-borne and systemic protozoa that can be detected in blood smears are listed in Table 70-3.

Collection

Appropriate collection procedures for blood samples are dictated, in part, by the protozoa suspected to be the cause of disease. For samples from which blood smears will be performed, care should be taken in collection and handling the blood to avoid hemolysis that may destroy parasites and thus preclude detection. Smears from fresh whole blood should be made immediately following collection; samples of blood collected into ethylenediaminetetraacetic acid (EDTA) anticoagulant can be submitted for smears to be made at a later time. Some protozoa, especially *Babesia* spp., are more easily found in the peripheral circulation of microcapillary beds; detection of these parasites may be enhanced by collecting from an ear margin or clipped toenail.

Preparation of Blood Films

Preparing blood films that will be useful in diagnosis of parasitic protozoa requires care and skill. Thick films allow examination of a larger volume of blood, increasing the likelihood of detecting any parasitic protozoa present, but thin films are necessary to allow morphologic identification of the organisms. If possible, both thick and thin films should be prepared. When submitting slides to a diagnostic laboratory, multiple slides (at least two thick and two thin) should be prepared and submitted unstained.[7]

Thin Films

Thin films are prepared by placing a small drop of blood at one end of a clean microscope slide and then using a second slide to spread the blood. The short edge of the spreader slide is placed in the middle of the slide at a 30-degree angle and pulled back toward the blood. The blood is allowed to spread

Table • 70-3

Practical Techniques for the Diagnosis of Blood-Borne and Systemic Protozoal Infections

ORGANISM	BLOOD FILMS	ASPIRATE IMPRESSIONS	TISSUE IMPRESSIONS
Babesia	+	−	−
Cytauxzoon	+	−	+
Encephalitozoon	−	+[a]	−
Entamoeba histolytica	−	+	+
Hepatozoon	+	−	+
Leishmania	−	+	+
Neospora	−	+	+
Toxoplasma	−	+	+
Trypanosoma	+	+	+

+, Useful or indicated; −, not used or recommended.
[a]May give negative results in seropositive animals.

along the width of the spreader slide; then, in a fairly rapid and even motion, the spreader slide is pushed across the length of the slide, dragging the blood along behind it. The blood should not be pushed across the slide because this will rupture many cells and parasites.

Thick Films

To prepare thick films, 2 to 3 drops of blood are placed on a clean microscope slide and spread with the corner of another slide in a circular motion over a 2-cm area. Fresh blood should be stirred on the slide for an additional 30 seconds to prevent formation of fibrin strands. EDTA-anticoagulated blood does not need to be stirred after spreading.[7]

Both thick and thin films should be air dried at room temperature on a flat surface. The choice of stain will determine the need for additional preparation and fixation before staining. Some stains require thick films to be laked (i.e., immersed in distilled water to rupture and remove erythrocytes) before staining. Thin films that are not stained within 48 hours should be fixed in 100% methanol. Both thick and thin films should be stored in a cool, dry, clean place in a sealed box.[7]

Staining Blood Films

Although personal preferences vary, Giemsa, Wright, and Wright-Giemsa are the most commonly used stains for detecting and identifying hemoprotozoa on blood smears. Stains such as Diff-Quik can be used, but both detection of the presence of protozoa and subsequent morphologic identification to species are more difficult.[5] Giemsa-stained blood smears have the added advantage of permanency; Wright-stained blood smears will fade over time.

Examination of Blood Films

Stained blood films may be examined with or without a coverslip. When a coverslip is not used, a drop of immersion oil can be placed on the stained smear to reduce diffraction and facilitate microscopic examination at low (10×) power and with the high-dry (43×) objectives. Additional oil should then be added and the feathered edge of the stained smear examined closely using the oil immersion (100×) objective. If preferred, a thin (#1) coverslip can be applied with neutral mounting medium before examination. The mounting medium prevents the coverslip from moving around on the stained smear and also reduces diffraction in a manner similar to immersion oil applied directly to the smear.[7] One advantage of using a coverslip is that it allows the slide to be thoroughly cleaned with lens cleaner and reexamined at a later date by another diagnostician; the surface of stained smears that do not have a coverslip cannot be cleaned.

Other Samples

Protozoa may also be visualized directly by histologic examination of biopsy samples or tissues collected at necropsy or by direct microscopic examination of body fluids (other than blood), fine needle aspirates, and impression smears from biopsy samples. Blood-borne and systemic protozoa that can be detected in aspirates and impression smears are listed in Table 70-3.

Histopathology

Parasitic protozoa are often readily seen on histologic examination of tissues with routine hematoxylin and eosin staining. Special stains may be used to improve detection or enhance morphologic characteristics of the stage of parasite seen, allowing more confident identification. Tissue samples to be examined by histology should be collected and submitted quickly for frozen section when an immediate diagnosis is desired and resources to complete frozen section evaluation are available, or they should be placed in 10% formalin if pro-

cessing will be delayed. Tissues on which electron microscopy will be performed should be placed in a glutaraldehyde-based fixative.[7]

Other Body Fluids

Protozoa are rarely found on direct microscopic examination of aqueous humor, cerebrospinal fluid, synovial fluid, urine, or transtracheal wash or bronchoalveolar lavage. *Giardia* trophozoites may occasionally be seen in duodenal aspirates collected at endoscopy. To determine if motile protozoa are present, all body fluids should be examined by direct smear immediately following collection; storage of samples for even a short period may result in lysis of organisms and subsequent failure to detect infection. Specimens are processed for examination by centrifuging collected fluid at $2000 \times G$ for 5 minutes and then making smears with the sediment and adding a small amount of associated fluid. After drying, smears should be stained as described for blood smears and examined for protozoa.

Fine Needle Aspirates

Protozoa are occasionally found in fine needle aspirates of lymph node, spleen, liver, and bone marrow. Aspirated material should be placed on a slide and then the material teased apart and thoroughly spread across the slide with a small-gauge needle to distribute it in a thin layer without disrupting cells. Alternatively, the material can be compressed between two slides and the slides pulled apart to distribute the material. Dried smears of fine needle aspirates are stained with Giemsa, Wright, or Wright-Giemsa and examined for protozoa as described for blood smears.

Impression Smears

Examination of stained impression smears of superficial lesions or of tissue collected at biopsy or necropsy may also reveal the presence of protozoa. For this reason, impression smears should be made of all biopsy material for which a protozoal diagnosis is suspected. Impression smears are made by blotting the cut edge of the tissue on an absorbent surface before touching the tissue to the surface of a glass slide. The small amount (ideally, a single cell layer) of material transferred to the glass slide is allowed to air dry and then stained and examined microscopically as described for blood smears.

CULTURE AND ANIMAL INOCULATION

Feces

Fecal protozoal culture is rarely performed in small animal practice. Specialized diagnostic laboratories that perform fecal culture must be identified before sample submission. See Appendix 5 for a listing of these laboratories. The sample should be fresh and sent by the most rapid means available; preservative should not be added to feces to be cultured. Although fecal culture for diagnosis of protozoal infections is rarely employed, specific media have been developed that will support the growth of *E. histolytica*, *B. coli*, and trichomonads. However, identifying enteric protozoa present in feces as specifically as possible is essential, based on morphologic appearance of the organisms before submitting samples for fecal culture.

Confirming the identity of some coccidia present in feces can be facilitated by inoculation of animals. This approach is most often reserved for pursuing research questions and is rarely undertaken in clinical veterinary medicine. The diagnostic laboratory or research facility that will perform the animal inoculation trials should be contacted before shipment of specimens for specific instructions on collection, handling, and transport of material. In general, feces containing oocysts suspected to be *Toxoplasma gondii, Neospora caninum,* or another coccidian of interest are shipped fresh to the research facility where the oocysts are collected from the feces and then fed to mice or another suitable intermediate host model. After allowing time for asexual stages to develop in the intermediate host, tissues are collected and examined to identify the species of parasite present.

Whole Blood

Although usually reserved for research projects, blood culture and animal inoculation with whole blood are occasionally performed to detect and document the presence of parasitic protozoa. However, because it is rarely performed for clinical diagnosis, protozoal blood culture or animal inoculation should be arranged with the laboratory before submission of samples and specific instructions obtained on sample collection and handling. In general, samples are collected aseptically into EDTA and then submitted to the participating laboratory as soon as possible.

Xenodiagnosis

Xenodiagnosis is another rarely performed procedure for clinical diagnosis in which laboratory-reared, parasite-free arthropods are allowed to feed on suspected infected hosts, and then, after appropriate time for development has elapsed, the arthropods are examined for the presence of parasites. Xenodiagnosis has historically been used for the diagnosis of trypanosomiasis but may also be useful in detecting other protozoal parasites.

Other Samples

In some cases, culture of tissue aspirates, biopsy samples, or body fluids other than blood may be desired. When indicated, an aliquot of the sample collected for cytologic evaluation is placed in a sterile tube at the time of collection. Culture or animal inoculation can then be performed with this sample as indicated. Rapid submission to an appropriate diagnostic laboratory will increase the likelihood of successfully culturing any protozoa present. To facilitate the process and receive exact instructions on sample handling and submission, the diagnostic laboratory to be used should be contacted before collection of samples. See Appendix 5 for laboratories performing these tests.

ANTIGEN DETECTION

Protozoal antigen present in clinical samples may be detected by enzyme-linked immunosorbent assay (ELISA) or by staining via direct fluorescent antibody (FA) or immunohistochemistry. In these assays, specific antibodies bind to surface proteins of the protozoa of interest, and the bound antibody is detected through subsequent steps. Although not a substitute for direct microscopic examination, these assays can augment diagnosis greatly by enhancing the detection of protozoa that are present in low numbers in clinical samples.

Commercial immunodiagnostic assays are available for detecting and identifying cysts of *Giardia* and *E. histolytica* and oocysts of *Cryptosporidium* spp. in feces. See Appendix 6 for information on these test kits. Some of these assays, which were originally developed for use in diagnosis of human infections, have been successfully used in veterinary species, including dogs and cats. Comparison of zinc sulfate centrifugation flotation with an ELISA developed for use in human samples found that the flotation method was slightly more sensitive.[3] Because false-negative results can occur, these tests should always be performed along with microscopic examination of feces following centrifugal concentration using an appropriate flotation solution.

Fine needle aspirates and biopsy samples can also be evaluated for the presence of parasite antigen. Aliquots of samples should be placed in a separate sterile tube at the time of collection and submitted to appropriate laboratories for direct FA or immunohistochemistry specific for the parasite in question. Paired samples should always be submitted for cytologic or histologic examination whenever direct FA or immunohistochemical detection is pursued.

NUCLEIC ACID DETECTION

Detection of nucleic acid sequences characteristic of a given protozoa also provides direct evidence of current or very recent infection. The most commonly used techniques for detecting protozoa in clinical research projects are polymerase chain reaction (PCR) and in situ hybridization. PCR amplification of specific gene sequences has been used extensively in research projects to evaluate fecal samples for the presence of *Giardia* spp. and *Cryptosporidium* spp. Although promising, this technique is not yet available for routine testing of clinical samples. PCR is also becoming increasingly important in evaluating blood samples for the presence of hemoprotozoa. Whole blood samples to be submitted for PCR assay should be collected into new blood tubes containing the anticoagulant specified by the testing laboratory; EDTA is the most common anticoagulant used in samples to be tested by PCR. PCR can also be performed on samples of other body fluids, fine needle aspirates, and biopsy samples. If they will not be assayed immediately, samples on which PCR will be performed should be frozen at the time of collection and held frozen until submission to the diagnostic laboratory. In situ hybridization involves detection of nucleic acid in tissue sections using labeled specific probes. At present, in situ hybridization is only performed at specialized research laboratories for a few protozoal parasites. Refer to Appendix 5 for a listing of laboratories performing nucleic acid tests.

SEROLOGY

Serologic assays to detect antibodies reactive to parasitic protozoa of dogs and cats are widely available and provide indirect evidence of past or current infection. Although indirect FA tests are the most common type of serologic assay employed, ELISA and parasite agglutination tests are also available and are occasionally used to detect antibodies reactive to a given protozoa (see Appendix 5). Serology is not available for all parasitic protozoa of dogs and cats, and not all veterinary diagnostic laboratories are equipped to run the assays that are available. Individual laboratories should be consulted before submitting samples. Blood collected for serologic testing should be placed in a tube free of anticoagulant; care should be taken to prevent hemolysis during sample collection or handling. Serum separated from the clot may be frozen before testing. Details on the tests available and information on interpreting results can be found in the individual chapters for each protozoan.

Serologic testing for protozoal infections has several advantages, including ease of sample collection, low cost of most procedures, and wide availability of assays. However, most of these assays are based on detection of IgG, which develops later in infection, often after clinical disease has begun, and remains elevated for months to years after initial infection, complicating interpretation of a single titer in a clinically ill animal. Diagnosis of active infection with an IgG-based test requires demonstrating a fourfold change in titer in two paired serum samples. In general, IgM is produced early in the course of an infection, and some IgM-based tests are available.

However, the presence of antibodies in the serum does not correlate directly with clinical illness in all animals. Many healthy animals have detectable antibodies to protozoan parasites, and immunosuppressed animals may not develop antibodies despite infection and clinical disease. Different assays also vary in sensitivity and specificity. The diagnostic laboratory performing the assay should be consulted for assistance in interpreting results (see Appendix 5).

SUGGESTED READINGS*

2. Ash LR, Orihel TC. 1987. Parasites: a guide to laboratory procedures and identification, ASC Press, Chicago.

5. Hahn N. 1994. Parasites of the blood, pp 101-120. *In* Sloss MW, Kemp RL, Zajac AM (eds), Veterinary clinical parasitology, ed 6, Iowa State University Press, Ames, Iowa.
9. Zajac AM. 1994. Fecal examination in the diagnosis of parasitism, pp 3–93. *In* Sloss MW, Kemp RL, Zajac AM (eds), Veterinary clinical parasitology, ed 6, Iowa State University Press, Ames, Iowa.

*See the CD-ROM for a complete list of references.

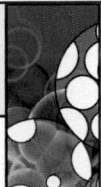

CHAPTER • 71

Antiprotozoal Chemotherapy

Craig E. Greene and Sidney A. Ewing

Table 71-1 summarizes the indications for current antiprotozoal drugs. See Chapters 72 to 82 for details about chemotherapy for specific diseases. Dosages of various drugs are available in the Drug Formulary, Appendix 8.

AZO-NAPHTHALENE DRUGS

Trypan blue was one of the first compounds used to treat babesiosis. Because local irritation and abscesses develop after subcutaneous (SC) injection, it is administered intravenously (IV). Trypan blue does not completely eliminate *Babesia* organisms, but infected animals recover from illness and remain in a state of premunition. They must be treated with aromatic diamidines (see Aromatic Diamindines) within 1 month to be cured. A disadvantage of trypan blue is that it stains all body tissues and secretions for several weeks.

ACRIDINE DYES

Quinacrine, developed as a human antimalarial drug, has been administered to dogs as an alternative treatment to nitroimidazoles for giardiasis. It becomes incorporated into the DNA of the organism and inhibits nucleic acid synthesis. Evidence of toxicity includes vomiting, fever, pruritus, neurologic signs, yellow discoloration of urine and tissues, and hepatic dysfunction. It is no longer available in the United States.

QUINOLINE AND QUINOLONE DERIVATIVES

Diiodohydroxyquin and iodochlorhydroxyquin are halogenated oxyquinolines that have been provided as topical antifungal drugs. They are also amebicidal when administered orally. They are not absorbed systemically and have relatively low toxicity. Signs of toxicity are abdominal pain, diarrhea, and neurologic signs, all of which have been reported in dogs.

Atovaquone is a closely related hydroxynaphthoquinone derivative licensed to treat *Pneumocystis* species infections. It has been used in combination with azithromycin to treat babesiosis in people and dogs (see Chapter 77).[44] Buparvaquone, which has been used to treat theileriosis in herbivores, has not effectively treated leishmaniasis or cytauxzoonosis in dogs or cats, respectively.[96] Decoquinate, an hydroxyquinolone licensed for treating coccidiosis in poultry, is effective in ameliorating the signs of hepatozoonosis (see Chapter 74 and Drug Formulary, Appendix 8).[54]

AROMATIC DIAMIDINES

Phenamidine, pentamidine, diminazene, amicarbalide, and imidocarb, which are diamidine derivatives, are the drugs of choice for treating *Babesia*, *Cytauxzoon*, and African *Trypanosoma* species infections in dogs and cats. They also effectively treat some other protozoa (see Table 71-1) by interfering with nucleic acid metabolism. These drugs are formulated as salts to reduce irritation after parenteral (intramuscular or SC) injection. Pentamidine has also been used to treat leishmaniasis.[77]

Diamidines are rapidly effective and usually resolve clinical signs and parasitemia within 24 hours. They do not completely eradicate the organisms but have residual activity after a single injection. The drugs become highly concentrated in parenchymal organs such as the liver and brain and are slowly metabolized or excreted unchanged. The slow metabolism and elimination of diamidines contribute to their prophylactic effects for many weeks after a single injection. Subtherapeutic dosages may allow organisms to develop resistance to these drugs.

NITROIMIDAZOLES

Nitroimidazoles are effective against anaerobic enteric protozoa that cause trichomoniasis, amebiasis, giardiasis, and

Table • 71-1

Properties of Antiprotozoal Drugs

GENERIC NAME (TRADE NAME)[a]	INFECTIONS INDICATED	
	FIRST CHOICE	ALTERNATE CHOICE
Azo-Naphthalene Dyes		
Trypan blue	None	*Babesia*
Acridine Dyes		
Quinacrine hydrochloride (Atabrine, Keybrin)	None	*Giardia*
Quinoline and Quinolone Derivatives		
Diiodohydroxyquin (iodoquinol; Diodoquin, Yodoxin)	*Balantidium*	*Entamoeba*
Iodochlorhydroxyquin (clioquinol; Vioform)	*Balantidium*	*Entamoeba*
Decoquinate (Deccox)	*Hepatozoon*	Coccidiosis
Hydroxynaphthoquinones		
Atovaquone (Mepron)	None	*Babesia, Pneumocystis, Toxoplasma*
Aromatic Diamidines		
Pentamidine isethionate (Lomidine, Pentam, NebuPent); also phenamidine	*Babesia, Acanthamoeba*	*Leishmania, Pneumocystis*
Diminazene aceturate (Berenil, Ganaseg)	*Cytauxzoon, Babesia,* African *Trypansoma*	*Hepatozoon canis*
Imidocarb dipropionate (Imizol)	*Babesia, Hepatozoon canis, Cytauxzoon*	*Ehrlichia*
Amicarbalide (Diampiron)	*Ehrlichia*	None
Nitroimidazoles		
Metronidazole (Flagyl, Stomorgyl[b])	*Giardia, Pentatrichomonas*	*Entamoeba* (invasive), *Balantidium*
Dimetridazole (Emtryl)	*Entamoeba, Balantidium*	None
Tinidazole (Fasigyn)	*Pentatrichomonas*	*Babesia, Giardia*
Benzimidazoles		
Fenbendazole (Panacur)	Helminths, *Giardia*	None
Albendazole (Valbazan)	*Giardia, Encephalitozoon*	None
Febantel-Praziquantel-Pyrantel pamoate (Drontal-plus)	Helminths	*Giardia*
Ionophores		
Monensin (Rumensin, Coban)	Coccidia	*Toxoplasma*
Lasalocid (Bovatec)	Coccidia	None
Salinomycin (Bio-cox)	Coccidia	None
Antimonials		
Sodium stibogluconate (Pentostam)	*Leishmania*	None
Meglumine antimoniate (Glucantime)	*Leishmania*	None
Antibacterials		
Paromomycin (Humatin, Aminosidine)	*Cryptosporidium, Pentatrichomonas*	*Entamoeba, Giardia, Leishmania*
Furazolidone (Furoxone)	Coccidia	*Giardia*
Nifurtimox (Lampit)	*Trypanosoma cruzi*	*Leishmania*
Tetracycline, doxycycline (many formulations)	*Balantidium*	*Hepatozoon canis*
Trimethoprim-sulfonamide (Tribrissen, Ditrim, Bactrim, Septra)	*Pneumocystis,* Coccidia, *Cyclospora, Neospora*	*Acanthamoeba*
Pyrimethamine (Daraprim)	*Toxoplasma, Neospora*	*Pneumocystis*
Spiramycin (Rovamycin, Stomorgyl[b])	*Cryptosporidium*	*Toxoplasma*

Continued

Table • 71-1

Continued

GENERIC NAME (TRADE NAME)[a]	INFECTIONS INDICATED	
	FIRST CHOICE	ALTERNATE CHOICE
Clindamycin (Antirobe, Cleocin)	*Toxoplasma, Neospora*	*Babesia*
Azithromycin (Zithromax)	*Toxoplasma*	*Babesia, Cryptosporidium*
Miscellaneous		
Bismuth-*N*-glycolylarsanilate (Milibis-V)	None	*Entamoeba, Giardia*
Amprolium (Amprol, Corid)	None	Coccidia
Amphotericin B (Fungizone, Albecet[c])	*Acanthamoeba*	*Leishmania*
Phosphocholine (Oleyl-Pc, Miltefosine)	*Leishmania*	*Trypanosoma*
Toltrazuril (Baycox)	Coccidia	*Toxoplasma, Hepatozoon*
Ponazuril (Marquis)	*Neospora*	*Sarcocystis*
Ketoconazole (Nizoral)	*Leishmania*	None
Allopurinol (Zyloprim[d])	*Leishmania*	*Trypanosoma cruzi*
Fumagillin	*Encephalitozoon*	*Entamoeba*
Suramin (Metaret)	African *Trypanosoma*	Feline leukemia virus
Interferon-γ[d]	*Leishmania*	None

[a]See Drug Formulary, Appendix 8, for additional information on these drugs.
[b]Combination of metronidazole (25, 125, 250 mg) with spiramycin (46.9, 234, 469 mg) in tablets.
[c]Lipid formulations preferred.
[d]Used in combination with antimonials for leishmaniasis.

balantidiasis. They can be used to treat intraintestinal and invasive parasites. The nitrogroup within anaerobic protozoa and bacteria undergoes a reduction to produce various unstable metabolites, some of which have antimicrobial activity. The drugs are generally much less effective against microaerophilic or aerobic microorganisms. Metronidazole, tinidazole, nimorazole, dimetridazole, secnidazole, and ornidazole are close structural analogs marketed in various regions of the world. Metronidazole is the most widely used of these compounds. In addition to protozoa, it is active against obligate spore-forming anaerobes such as *Clostridium*, some non–spore-forming anaerobes such as *Campylobacter*, and microaerophilic organisms such as species belonging to the Enterobacteriaceae. Metronidazole is generally preferred for treating giardiasis.[83] *Giardia* infections that are resistant to metronidazole have been effectively treated by combining treatment with quinacrine.[66] Metronidazole is the drug of choice for treating invasive amebiasis in people.

Metronidazole is almost completely absorbed after oral administration. Food does not reduce the extent of absorption but may delay the rate. IV administration of metronidazole may be preferable in severely ill patients but is expensive and potentially more neurotoxic. The drug distributes widely and penetrates body tissues, extracellular fluids, and even pus-filled cavities. Metronidazole achieves good concentrations in the central nervous system (CNS) even in the absence of inflammation. It is extensively metabolized in the liver, but renal excretion of active drug also occurs.

Metronidazole has been administered alone and with spiramycin to treat periodontal disease and stomatitis and in combination with aminoglycosides to treat mixed infections associated with bowel perforation and intraabdominal sepsis (see Chapter 89). In people the drug effectively treats intraabdominal, pelvic, pleuropulmonary, CNS, and bone and joint infections.

Side effects of metronidazole include gastrointestinal irritation with signs of vomiting and anorexia, glossitis, and stomatitis. Neurologic signs may be seen in dogs and cats after 7 to 10 days of treatment with high dosages (greater than 66 mg/kg/day) and may be resolved when therapy is discontinued.[12] Some dogs have developed fatal encephalopathy, persistent seizures, or cerebellar and central vestibular ataxia after therapy; diazepam helped the dogs recover (see Drug Formulary, Appendix 8).[20]

BENZIMIDAZOLES

Fenbendazole and albendazole are broad-spectrum benzimidazoles that are used to treat a wide range of infections with helminths and selected protozoa. They affect microtubule synthesis in the protozoal cytoskeleton. Both drugs have been effective in the treatment of intestinal giardiasis and are often more potent than metronidazole.[30] Fenbendazole is relatively safe, and dosages used for treating helminths (50 mg/kg for 3 days) are effective in treating giardiasis.[30,82,100] The drug was not as effective in cats that were coinfected with *Cryptosporidium*.[41] Fenbendazole use was associated with development of granulocytopenia as an idiosyncratic reaction in one dog.[23a] Myelotoxicity has been caused by albendazole use in dogs and cats[89] but can be reversed after treatment is discontinued. Febantel, which is metabolized to fenbendazole, is one component of an antihelmentic combination that is effective against *Giardia*.[6,70]

AZOLES

The antifungal drugs ketoconazole, fluconazole, and terbinafine have some antileishmanial activity, because the infecting organism has ergosterol in its cell wall. In experimental animal models, these drugs have been less effective than other antiprotozoal drugs. Another antifungal, amphotericin B (AMB), has been more effective (see below, Miscellaneous drugs).

IONOPHORES

Ionophores are compounds that form lipid-soluble complexes with cations, which facilitate transport of the ions across biologic membranes. They are antibiotics isolated from *Streptomyces* spp. and are provided primarily as coccidiostats. Monensin, lasalocid, and salinomycin, the compounds used in veterinary medicine, cause accumulation of intracellular ions within the parasite, interfering with its metabolism. They have been used primarily as growth promoters in food animal practice, although monensin has been effective in reducing shedding of *Toxoplasma* oocysts by cats. The ionophores also have antibacterial activity and have been used experimentally to treat endotoxic shock in dogs. Because of their stimulatory effects on cardiac contractility and myocardial perfusion, their toxicity may be increased by concurrent administration of cardiac glycosides.

ANTIMONIALS

Sodium stibogluconate and meglumine antimoniate are pentavalent antimony compounds and two of the main agents used in the treatment of leishmaniasis.[27,84,91-93] The dosage is based on the amount of antimony compound administered. Treatment with these drugs is not curative, and two or three courses may be necessary. Side effects include anorexia, vomiting, nausea, myalgia, and lethargy. Electrocardiogram abnormalities and nephrotoxicity can develop at higher dosages. Although these antimonials are often given parenterally, a cyclodextrin formulation was found to have good bioavailability in mice.[16]

ANTIBACTERIALS

Paromomycin (aminosidine) and furazolidone are nonabsorbable antibacterials (previously discussed; see Chapter 34). They are effective in treating some intestinal protozoal infections. Because of potential intestinal absorption and nephrotoxicity, paromomycin—an aminoglycoside—must be administered with caution when treating amebiasis or trichomoniasis when bowel lesions are extensive. Paromomycin has also been used to treat leishmaniasis. Furazolidone and sulfonamides are effective in treating intestinal coccidial infections. Nifurtimox, a nitrofuran derivative, can suppress but not cure *Trypanosoma cruzi* infections. Nausea, vomiting, and convulsions may be side effects.

Trimethoprim, an antibacterial diaminopyrimidine compound that inhibits folic acid synthesis, has broad-spectrum antimicrobial activity (see Chapter 34). Combined with sulfonamides, it has been used to treat *Pneumocystis* and coccidial infections. Pyrimethamine is closely related to trimethoprim but is more effective against protozoa. It has been used in combination with sulfonamides to treat infections with *Neospora* and *Toxoplasma* organisms.

Several newer antifolate drugs (see Chapter 80) under development may also be active against these two protozoa. Clindamycin, a lincosamide antimicrobial drug, and certain macrolides (azithromycin, clarithromycin) are also active against these two protozoa.

Spiramycin, a macrolide antibiotic, has an antibacterial spectrum similar to that of erythromycin but is less effective. Absorption after oral administration is adequate for therapeutic purposes. It is widely distributed and reaches high concentrations in tissues, from which it is slowly eliminated in the bile and urine. Its usefulness has been limited for treating bacterial infections in veterinary medicine, but it is now marketed in combination with metronidazole, primarily to treat periodontal and oral infections. Spiramycin has been found to be somewhat effective for treating intestinal cryptosporidiosis and has been given to people to treat acute toxoplasmosis.

MISCELLANEOUS DRUGS

Bismuth-*N*-glycoloylarsanilate is an antihelmintic drug that is a second choice for treating giardiasis. Amprolium is a thiamine inhibitor that is commonly chosen to treat coccidiosis in dogs, although it is not approved by the Food and Drug Administration for this purpose (see Chapter 81). Overdoses may produce neurologic signs. As mentioned previously, the antifungal drug AMB is effective in treating leishmaniasis because the infecting protozoa have ergosterol in their cell walls. It is much more efficient than other drugs in treating human patients.[61] Lipid emulsions may improve this efficacy and lower toxicity.[15] Toltrazuril is an anticoccidial agent that is unrelated to the others. It appears to be very effective in eliminating coccidia in most animals without interfering with a persistent host immune response.[25,26] Toltrazuril has been used to control oocyst shedding by cats acutely infected with *Toxoplasma* organisms.[52] The drug can be given by mouth in water or food, systemically by SC injection, or by topical application. A sulfone derivative of the drug (ponazuril) is effective in treating *Sarcocystis neurona* infection in horses,[22] and it has been used to treat *Neospora caninum* infection in calves and dogs[45] (see Drug Formulary, Appendix 8). Nitazoxanide is a thiazolide compound that has been approved for use in people with drug-resistant *Giardia* and *Cryptosporidium* infections. Allopurinol is a pyrazolopyrimidine that interferes with nucleic acid synthesis in *Leishmania* and *T. cruzi* organisms. It has been licensed to treat hyperuricemia and gout in people but is now being used to treat American trypanosomiasis and leishmaniasis in endemic areas (see Chapters 72 and 73).* Miltefosine (hexadecylphosphocholine) is a membrane active drug that accumulates in macrophages and is active against *Leishmania* while simultaneously stimulating T-cell activation and production of toxic intracellular intermediates. Although the orally administered drug has been effective in treating *Leishmania*-infected people,[75,90] side effects are more severe in dogs, so other derivatives of phosphocholine are recommended (see Drug Formulary, Appendix 8). Antihelmintics containing febantel have been used to treat dogs with giardiasis.[70]

SUGGESTED READINGS†

1. Abboud P, Lemee V, Gargala G, et al. 2001. Successful treatment of metronidazole- and albendazole-resistant giardiasis with nitazoxanide in a patient with acquired immunodeficiency syndrome. *Clin Infect Dis* 32:1792-1794.
5. Baneth G, Shaw S. 2002. Chemotherapy of canine leishmaniasis. *Vet Parasitol* 106:315-324.
6. Barr SC, Bowman DD, Frongillo MF, et al. 1998. Efficacy of a drug combination of praziquantel, pyrantel pamoate, and febantel against giardiasis in dogs. *Am J Vet Res* 59:1134-1136.
11. Cavaliero T, Arnold P, Mathis A, et al. 1999. Clinical serologic and parasitologic follow-up after long-term allopurinol therapy of dogs naturally infected with *Leishmania infantum*. *J Vet Intern Med* 13:330-334.

*References 17, 24, 35, 43, 48, 51, 55, 95.
†See the CD-ROM for a complete list of references.

17. Denerolle P, Bourdoiseau G. 1999. Combination allopurinol and antimony treatment versus antimony alone and allopurinol alone in the treatment of canine leishmaniasis (96 cases). *J Vet Intern Med* 13:413-415.

29. Greene CE, Latimer K, Hopper E, et al. 1999. Administration of diminazene aceturate or imidocarb dipropionate for treatment of cytauxzoonosis in cats. *J Am Vet Med Assoc* 215:497-500.

41. Keith CL, Radecki SV, Lappin MR. 2003. Evaluation of fenbendazole for treatment of *Giardia* infection in cats concurrently infected with *Cryptosporidium parvum. Am J Vet Res* 64:1027-1029.

45. Kritzner S, Sager H, Blum J, et al. 2002. An explorative study to assess the efficacy of toltrazuril-sulfone (Ponazuril) in calves experimentally infected with *Neospora caninum. Ann Clin Microbiol Antimicrob* 1:4.

70. Payne PA, Ridley RK, Dryden MW, et al. 2002. Efficacy of a combination febantel-praziquantel-pyrantel product, with or without vaccination with a commercial *Giardia* vaccine, for treatment of dogs with naturally occurring giardiasis. *J Am Vet Med Assoc* 220:330-333.

78. Riera C, Valladares JE, Gallego M, et al. 1999. Serological and parasitological follow-up in dogs experimentally infected with *Leishmania infantum* and treated with meglumine antimoniate. *Vet Parasitol* 84:33-47.

79. Sánchez S, Sallovitz J, Savio E, et al. 2000. Comparative availability of two oral dosage forms of albendazole in dogs. *Vet J* 160:153-156.

95. Vercammen F, Fernandez-Perez FJ, del Amo C, et al. 2002. Follow-up of *Leishmania infantum* naturally infected dogs treated with allopurinol: immunofluorescence antibody test, ELISA and Western blot. *Acta Trop* 84:175-181.

CHAPTER • 72

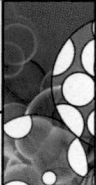

Trypanosomiasis

AMERICAN TRYPANOSOMIASIS

Stephen C. Barr

Etiology and Life Cycle

Trypanosoma cruzi, the etiologic agent of American trypanosomiasis or Chagas' disease, is a hemoflagellate protozoan of the class Zoomastigophorea and family Trypanosomatidae. The organism exists in three morphologic forms. The trypomastigote or blood form is 15 to 20 μm long, with a flattened spindle-shaped body and a centrally placed vesicular nucleus. A single, free flagellum originates from a basal body near the large subterminal kinetoplast (situated posterior to the nucleus) and passes along the body to project anteriorly (Fig. 72-1). The intracellular or amastigote form is approximately 1.5 to 4.0 μm in diameter and ovoid, and it contains a large, round nucleus and rodlike kinetoplast. The flagellum is small and not always obvious under light microscopy. Epimastigotes, the third morphologic form, are found in the reduviid vector (subfamily Triatomae), commonly known as the kissing bug. This flagellated and spindle-shaped form has a kinetoplast situated anterior to the nucleus.

Infection usually occurs when trypomastigotes are deposited in the insect vector's feces at the bite site (Fig. 72-2). Oral ingestion of infected insects will cause infection in opossums and might be a possible route of infection in dogs.[79] Other less common sources of infection include blood transfusions, congenital factors, or ingestion of meat or milk from infected lactating animals.[24] Trypomastigotes usually enter macrophages and myocytes, either locally or systemically, after hematogenous spread. Once they are intracellular, trypomastigotes transform into amastigotes, which multiply by binary fission. These amastigotes transform into trypomastigotes before rupture of and release from the cell. Rapid intracellular multiplication cycles ensure a rapid rise in parasitemia before effective immunity develops. The vector becomes infected by ingesting circulating trypomastigotes, which transform to epimastigotes and multiply by binary fission. Transformation of the epimastigotes back into trypomastigotes occurs in the vector's hindgut before the trypomastigotes are passed in the feces (Fig. 72-2).

Trypanosoma evansi, or a closely related trypanosome, has been isolated from animals in the Pantanal region of Brazil.[6,95] *T. evansi* has previously been isolated from animals in the Eastern hemisphere.

Epidemiology
T. cruzi *Infection*
T. cruzi infects people and a wide range of domestic and wild animal species in the Americas (Fig. 72-3, *A*). It is a major human health problem in South America (especially Brazil, Venezuela, Argentina) and Central America and is gaining importance in Mexico. Few human cases involving transmission by vectors have been reported in the United States. However, a large number of people have emigrated from endemic regions to the United States, where an estimated 50,000 to 100,000 *T. cruzi*–infected people now reside. Consequently, the number of cases associated with blood transfusion transmission have steadily risen.[61,104] Screening of canine blood donors for this infection has also been controversial.[118] Most canine cases in the United States, the number of which in fact may be rising, occur in Texas, especially in areas close to the Mexican border.[10,78] Isolated canine cases occur in other southern states,* although the infection was found to be endemic in a group of Walker hounds in Virginia.[24] A bitch and a majority of her pups were found to be infected, suggesting transplacental or transmammary infection. Other kennels of dogs have been studied throughout the United States for evidence of serum

*References: 10, 23, 30, 106, 110.

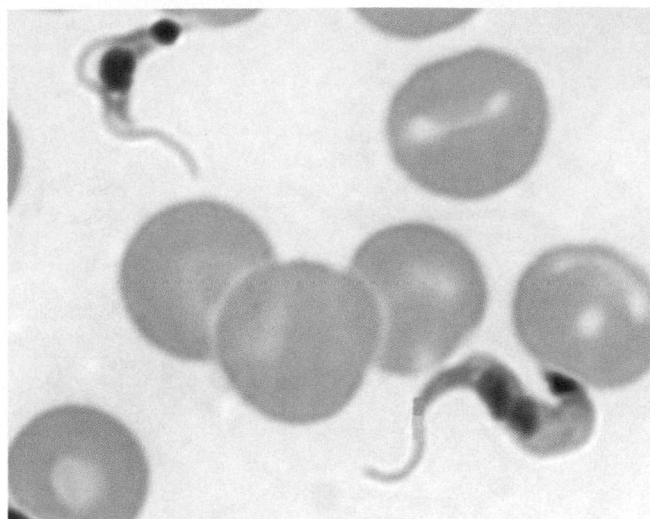

Fig 72-1 Trypomastigote form of *T. cruzi* in a blood film (Wright, ×1000).

antibody titers to *T. cruzi* (see Fig. 72-3, *B*). Presumably, vector and other means of transmission maintain infection within these populations. Transplacental transmission has been experimentally documented in rodents suffering acute parasitemia following inoculation before conception with a dog strain of *T. cruzi*.[80]

Usual transmission of *T. cruzi* in endemic countries depends on the confluence of reservoirs, vectors, parasites, and hosts (people or animals) in a single habitat. Two extremes of vector behavior have been noted: those that are habitually domiciliated and those that are habitually sylvan; many species are intermediate in behavior. Because of this variation, vectors tend to have either domestic or sylvan cycles, with crossover between the two occasionally. Of the many triatomid species that can feed on people in South America, only three, *Triatoma* spp., *Triatoma dimidiata*, and *Rhodnius prolixus*, are related to the epidemiology of human infections. They are efficient vectors for human infection because they feed on blood from both people and domestic reservoir mammals (dogs, cats, guinea pigs), reproduce prolifically while co-habiting close to people, and defecate soon after taking a blood meal. Infection rates in these vectors can be as high as 100% south of the Equator. Twelve species of triatomines are found in the United States. The most important are *Triatoma sanguisuga* in the eastern United States, *Triatoma gerstaeckeri* in Texas and New Mexico, and *Triatoma rubida* and *Triatoma protracta* in Arizona and California.[25,65] In comparison, infection rates of the two principal vectors in the United States, *T. protracta* and *T. sanguisuga*, are 20%. These two vectors are peridomestic, and their inability to adapt to living in human dwellings, their different feeding and defecation habits, and their lack of access to people with a higher standard of housing are some reasons for low infection rates in the United States. As a comparison, in Oklahoma, impounded or owned dogs had 3.6% rate for positive antibody titer results, while those in rural areas of Argentina have had seropositive result rates as 65%.[35]

The principal sylvan reservoir hosts of *T. cruzi* in the southern United States are opossums, raccoons, and armadillos.* Similarly, in Maryland,[116] Oklahoma,[56] North Carolina,[60] South Carlina,[123] and Georgia,[93,94,123] raccoons and opossums are the main reservoir hosts. In California and New Mexico, the main sylvan hosts are various mouse, squirrel, and rat species.[10] Although *T. cruzi* isolates from infected vectors,

*References: 15, 16, 32, 60, 77, 84, 124.

animal reservoirs, and people in North America show similar in vitro characteristics to those from South America,[17] these isolates tend to be less pathogenic in mice than do South American isolates.[15] Because inoculation of *T. cruzi* isolates from opossums and armadillos into dogs experimentally produces a similar disease described in naturally acquired cases of acute and chronic canine trypanosomiasis, dogs in nature are likely infected with the same isolates as are these sylvan hosts.[20-22]

T. evansi *Infection*

T. evansi, a previously recognized African trypanosome, was isolated from coati *(Nasua nasua)*, horses, and dogs in the Pantanal region of Brazil.[95] *T. evansi* has one of the widest geographic distributions and mammalian host ranges of any trypanosome and is thought to have evolved from *Trypanosoma brucei*. When inoculated into rats, the isolates had a varied virulence and fluctuating parasitemia typical of the African trypanosomes. The data suggest that the organism is transmitted between domestic and sylvatic hosts in the region via as yet undetermined vectors. For a further discussion of *T. evansi* infection, see African Trypanosomiasis later in this chapter.

Pathogenesis

T. cruzi trypomastigotes enter host cells soon after infection, multiply unhindered, avoid the immune response, and are transported throughout the body primarily within macrophages. Parasitemia develops within a few days and peaks 2 to 3 weeks postinoculation (PI), coinciding with acute clinical disease.[20] The pathogenesis of the acute phase is thought to result from cell damage as trypomastigotes rupture from host cells, especially cardiac myocytes and in some cases neurologic tissue. Most clinical signs during the acute stage are referable to this cell destruction. The period from infection to development of acute disease is variable, with puppies showing severe disease 2 weeks PI. Dogs infected after age 6 months may show no signs of acute disease other than slight depression and low-rising parasitemia. In contrast to these events, some *T. cruzi* isolates that infect dogs in the United States are not pathogenic but can produce a marked serologic response and a low parasitemia during times of stress or immunosuppression.

Generally, by 4 weeks PI, parasitemias in infected dogs have dropped to undetectable levels probably the result of a rising specific immune response to the parasite, and signs of acute disease diminish. Dogs tend to remain asymptomatic for months or years. During this time, a progressive development of myocardial degeneration occurs, leading eventually to biventricular dilative cardiomyopathy of unknown pathogenesis.[3] Many theories have been offered concerning the cause of the cardiomyopathy, including damage by toxic parasite products and immune-mediated mechanisms leading to autonomic nervous system disruption within the myocardium.[53,69] Further studies suggest that local spasm of the coronary microvasculature will lead eventually to myocardial ischemia and possibly to progressive cardiac myocyte destruction.[12] Infected human patients with progressive myocardial disease develop alterations in the conduction system and gradual cardiac insufficiency caused by mononuclear cell infiltration, microvascular alterations, ventricular remodeling, and fibrosis. Cardiac dilatation occurs when fibrosis no longer permits efficient compensatory hypertrophy.[1,108] As a possible explanation, people with myocardiopathy have had high levels of transforming growth factor (TGF)-β1 in association with myocardiopathy, intracellular activation of the TGF-β1 pathway, and tissue fibrosis.[8]

Benzimidazole (BZ) compounds, used to treat *T. cruzi* infections, have their greatest efficacy during the acute rather than the chronic stage of infection. Furthermore, the efficacy of

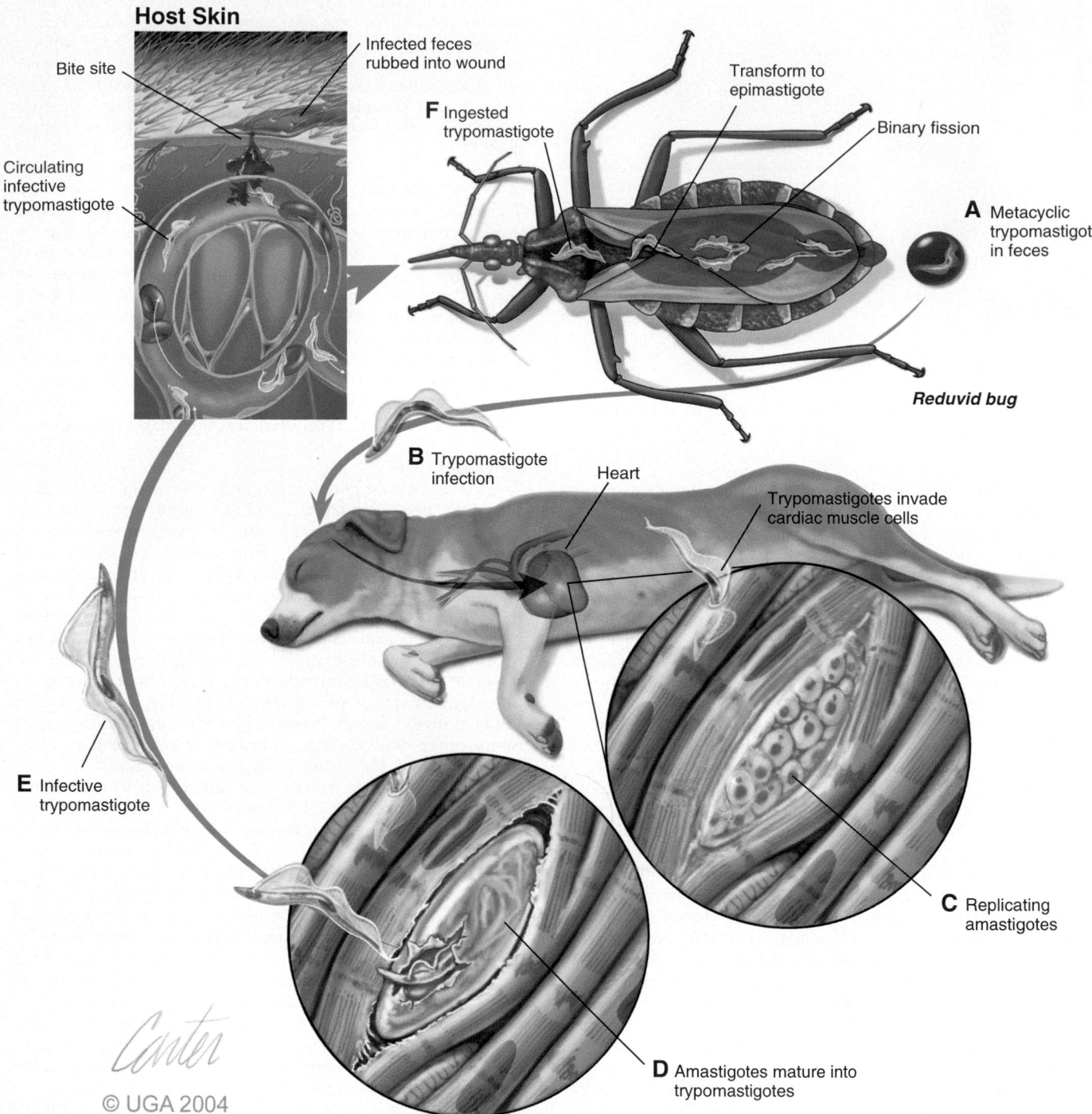

Host Skin

Bite site

Infected feces rubbed into wound

F Ingested trypomastigote

Transform to epimastigote

Binary fission

Circulating infective trypomastigote

A Metacyclic trypomastigote in feces

Reduvid bug

B Trypomastigote infection

Heart

Trypomastigotes invade cardiac muscle cells

E Infective trypomastigote

C Replicating amastigotes

D Amastigotes mature into trypomastigotes

© UGA 2004

Fig   72-2   Life cycle of *T. cruzi*. **A,** Metacyclic trypomastigote in feces is deposited in close proximity to the bug bite and can enter the site following abrading fecal material in the site. **B,** Within the body, the trypomastigotes enter the blood and **(C)** spread to many organs including the cardiac and skeletal muscle which are preferred replication sites and become amastigotes. **D,** Within host tissues, replicating amastigotes mature into motile trypomastigotes that re-enter the circulation. Rupture of host cells during the replication process causes clinical illness. **E,** The circulating trypomastigote is ingested in blood obtained by the vector during feeding. **F,** The trypomastigote converts to an epimastigote which replicates in the vector's gut. (Courtesy University of Georgia, Athens, Ga.)

chemotherapy in clearing *T. cruzi* infection appears dependent on an adequately functioning immune system. In experimental infections in knockout mice with various cytokine deficiencies, the presence of interferon-γ and other cytokines was critical in determining the efficacy of BZ treatment.[99]

Clinical Findings

Dogs

Clinically affected dogs develop either acute or chronic disease. Acute disease occurs mainly in dogs younger than 1 year of age and is sudden in onset, with signs referable to

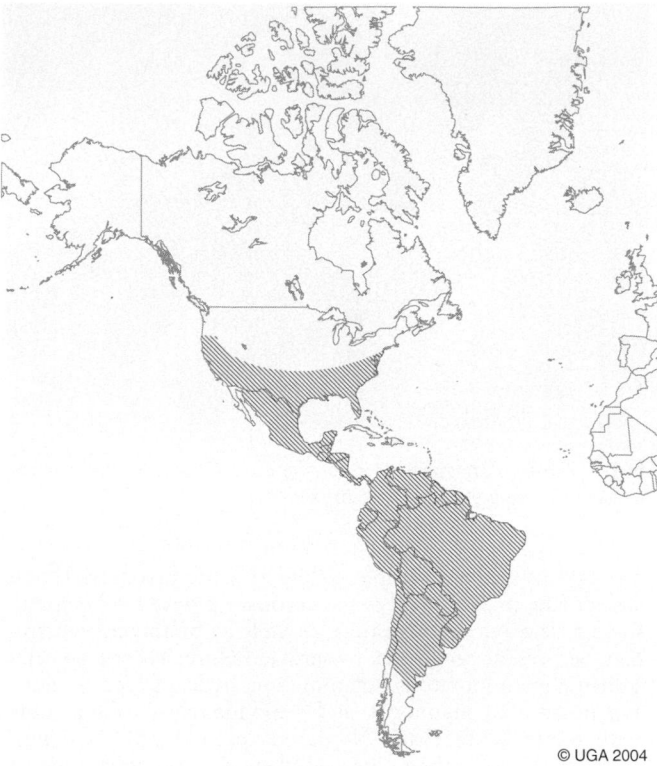

A

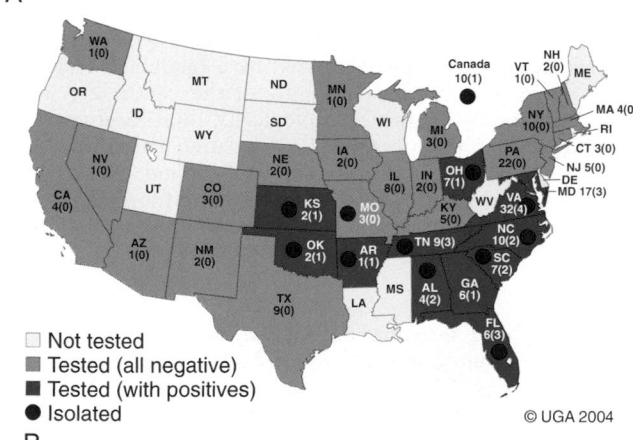

□ Not tested
▨ Tested (all negative)
■ Tested (with positives)
● Isolated

© UGA 2004

B

Fig 72-3 **A,** Geographic distribution of endemic American trypanosomiasis in animals and vectors. **B,** Distribution of antibodies to *T. cruzi* in kenneled foxhound dogs in the United States. (Number of dogs tested and number positive in parentheses.) Dots represent states where organisms have been isolated from dogs. (Data courtesy Zandra Duprey, Atlanta, Ga. Maps courtesy University of Georgia, Athens, Ga.)

right-sided heart failure and cardiac arrhythmias. Generalized lymphadenomegaly may precede and is invariably present during acute illness. Signs referable to acute myocarditis, such as sudden collapse and death of a previously normal young dog, have been reported most frequently. Pale mucous membranes, slowed capillary refill time, weak pulse with deficits, tachyarrhythmia, and terminal hypothermia and respiratory distress are common. Most infected dogs that do not die suddenly develop ascites, hepatomegaly, and splenomegaly caused by right-sided heart failure. Anorexia and diarrhea are also common during acute disease. Neurologic signs referable to meningoencephalitis, including pelvic limb ataxia, profound

weakness, and hyperreflexive spinal reflexes suggestive of distemper, have been found in naturally and experimentally infected dogs.[10,20,26] During acute disease, dogs, similar to experimentally infected mice, probably suffer a profound immunosuppression because of altered interleukin-2 activity.[108] Such immunosuppression has been proposed as the cause of the development of distemper in pups with acute canine trypanosomiasis after they received modified live distemper vaccine.[24] Electrocardiographic (ECG) changes during acute disease are highly variable and include alteration in ST-T segments, T-wave inversion, low-amplitude QRS complexes, positive polyphasic ventricular premature contractions, and first- and second-degree heart block.[21]

Survivors of acute myocarditis will become aparasitemic and asymptomatic, and they develop chronic myocarditis with cardiac dilatation over the next 8 to 36 months.[20,21] During the long asymptomatic period between acute and chronic disease in the dog, ECG readings may be normal except for the intermittent occurrence of ventricular arrhythmias, which can be exacerbated by exercise or excitement.[11] Sudden death during this stage can occur and is thought to be caused by fatal cardiac arrhythmias. As cardiac dilatation occurs, ECG abnormalities become more prevalent, and clinical signs referable to right-sided and eventually, in some cases, left-sided chamber failure occur. Dogs diagnosed at an older age (mean of 9 years) survived between 30 to 60 months, whereas dogs diagnosed at a younger age (mean of 4.5 years) survived only up to 5 months postdiagnosis.[78] These cases are indistinguishable from chronic dilative cardiomyopathy seen in large breeds of dogs and are often diagnosed as such until histology or immunohistochemical findings are available.[22-24] Trypanosomiasis should be considered in any dog with signs of myocarditis or cardiomyopathy.

Megaesophagus and other megaviscus syndromes described in people with chronic Chagas' disease have not been described in dogs spontaneously or experimentally infected with *T. cruzi*. Morphometry of the myenteric esophagus was not altered in dogs with experimentally induced chronic *T. cruzi* infection.[70]

Cats

Cats are reported to be susceptible to South American isolates of *T. cruzi*, but little information is available regarding clinical disease. No reports of domestic feline trypanosomiasis from North America have been submitted.

Diagnosis
Radiographic and Clinical Laboratory Findings

Thoracic radiography is of value in the diagnosis of pleural effusion, pulmonary edema, and chamber dilation in both acute and chronic myocarditis. ECG information is valuable in the diagnosis of the dilative cardiomyopathy of chronic disease. Thinning of ventricular walls, large end-diastolic volumes, and low shortening fractions (usually under 20%) are often present.[21]

Hematology is of little specific diagnostic value. Lymphocytosis may occur in the acute phase in a small number of cases. Alanine aminotransferase activity may be elevated as a result of hepatic hypoxia. Creatine kinase (CK) and lactate dehydrogenase activities are rarely elevated during acute disease. Elevations of serum CK (isoenzyme MB) do occur but are too variable and transient to be of any diagnostic value in the dog.[20] The abdominal effusion is typically a modified transudate from cardiac causes.

Cytology

Trypomastigotes can be identified in the blood just before and during acute disease (see Fig. 72-1). Although organisms are identified in most cases of acute trypanosomiasis, rarely are they found in chronic cases. Parasitemias are often so low, however, that organisms can be missed during routine examination of Wright-stained blood films. Trypomastigotes may be pelleted for examination from plasma (obtained by centrifugation of 50 ml of heparinized blood at $800 \times G$ for 10 minutes) by further centrifugation ($8000 \times G$ for 15 minutes). High-power (400×) examination of the buffy coat-plasma interface of a centrifuged microhematocrit tube may reveal characteristically motile parasites. A thick-film buffy coat smear, stained with Wright's or Giemsa stain or examined as a wet preparation for trypomastigote movement, is also an effective means of concentrating trypomastigotes. Lymph node aspirates or impression smears may be positive even when parasitemias are very low. Abdominal effusions may contain organisms that can be identified cytologically. Polymerase chain reaction (PCR) has been shown to have higher sensitivity than microscopic methods in detecting parasitemia.[63]

Isolation

Isolation of organisms into germ-free hosts or cell culture systems is a sensitive but time-consuming practice. Blood agar slants overlaid with liver infusion tryptose (LIT) medium or LIT alone are effective for isolating trypomastigotes from blood of an infected animal, but from 2 to 20 weeks may be needed for the results to become positive for epimastigotes.[66] Direct inoculation of blood into a Vero cell monolayer will usually result in the development of intracellular amastigote forms and trypomastigotes in media after 2 to 4 weeks.

Weanling laboratory inbred mice (C3H) inoculated intraperitoneally or subcutaneously with the patient's blood will usually develop detectable parasitemias 10 to 30 days later. Treating mice with glucocorticoids before and after inoculation increases the sensitivity.

Serologic and Polymerase Chain Reaction Testing

The indirect fluorescent antibody (FA) test, enzyme-linked immunosorbent assay (ELISA), and radioimmunoprecipitation assays are most commonly used.[30,114] These tests confirm the presence of antibodies to *T. cruzi* but most cross-react with antibodies to *Leishmania*.[48] Positive titer results should be confirmed by additional testing for *Leishmania* to determine which has more seroreactivity. In an experimental infection in dogs, PCR, antibody testing, and xenodiagnostic methods were evaluated. The serologic testing results were positive in all dogs for parasite-specific antibody. A PCR assay with high specificity for *T. cruzi* had sensitivity ranging from 67% to 100% with more accuracy if multiple (2 to 9) serially collected samples were examined.[7] However, xenodiagnostic methods only yielded positive results ranging between 11% to 22%. In a subset of people with myocardiopathic signs consistent with *T. cruzi* infection, serologic test results have been negative, despite positive results using PCR.[102] This finding is a major concern with regard to diagnosis, therapeutic monitoring, and blood donor screening. Similar information is not available for dogs. Serologic testing for *T. cruzi*–specific antibodies in association with clinical signs is considered the gold standard for the diagnosis of Chagas' disease in dogs. Central laboratories in North America perform serologic assays for *T. cruzi* (see Appendix 5). Titer results usually become positive by 3 weeks PI at the time when parasitemias are declining and persist for the life of the animal.[18] Because of the cross-reactivity with *Leishmania* spp., all positive sera results should be confirmed by also testing the sera for reactivity to *L. donovani*. The cross-reactive titer should be 1 to 2 dilutions less than the reactivity to *T. cruzi*.[25]

Pathologic Findings

In acute disease, lesions usually are confined to the heart, especially the right side. Subendocardial and subepicardial hem-

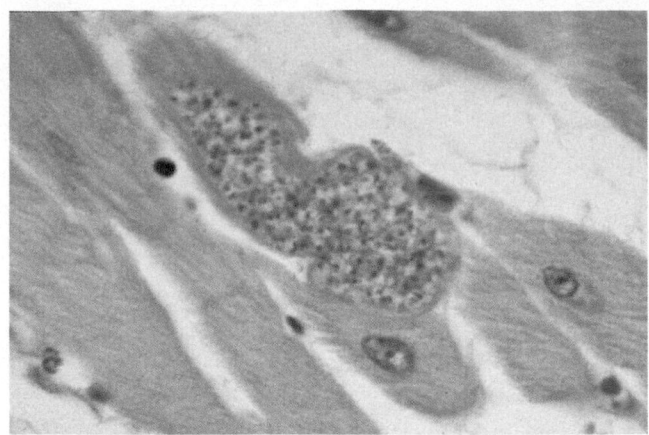

Fig 72-4 Amastigotes in a pseudocyst within the cardiac muscle of a dog (H and E stain, ×1000).

orrhages, as well as multiple yellow to white myocardial spots and streaks, mainly involve the coronary groove.[22,120] Hepatic, splenic, and renal congestion, as well as pulmonary edema, may be present secondary to cardiac failure. Microscopically, a diffuse granulomatous inflammation, hydropic degeneration and necrosis of myofibrils, and a mononuclear cellular infiltrate typify acute cases. Numerous pseudocysts containing amastigotes are often associated with the inflammatory response (Fig. 72-4). Mild granulomatous myositis and organisms can be found in other organs, including the smooth muscle of the stomach, small intestine, bladder, and skeletal muscle. Nonsuppurative encephalitis has also been found.

Chronic disease is characterized by a bilaterally enlarged flaccid heart with areas of thinning of the ventricular walls caused by fibrous plaques. Histologically, multifocal coalescing areas of lymphoplasmacytic inflammation and mild necrosis with extensive loss of myocardial fibers and replacement by fibrous tissue occur. Organisms are seldom found in tissues. The apex of the heart is one of the more likely areas to find them.[22]

Therapy

Two drugs have shown some efficacy in the treatment of American trypanosomiasis (Table 72-1). The investigational drug nifurtimox (Bayer 2502 or Lampit, Bayer Ag, Leverkusen-Bayerwerk, Germany) has been reported to be successful in treating experimental and natural cases of canine trypanosomiasis, but severe side effects often preclude its use.[51] Improved survival has been shown to occur in dogs treated concurrently with antiinflammatory doses of glucocorticoids.[2] Benznidazole (Ragonil®, Roche SA, Buenos Aires, Argentina) has been shown to produce cures in acute Chagas' disease in people and dogs and has less side effects compared with nifurtimox. Although neither drug shows any efficacy during the chronic stage of disease, benznidazole and nifurtimox are considered the recommended therapies for Chagas' disease.[113] Both drugs are available in the United States from the Centers for Disease Control and Prevention, Atlanta, Georgia. Ketoconazole, gossypol, and allopurinol have been investigated, but the results of these studies are less than convincing.[45,74,100] Albaconazole, an experimental triazole, was effective in suppressing parasite proliferation and death in infected dogs; however, a cure was not achieved.[41a] The calcium channel blocker, verapamil, decreases mortality in acutely infected mice[81] and decreases the severity of cardiac pathology in chronically infected mice[109] but does not have the same efficacy in dogs with Chagas' disease.[13] For further information on nifurtimox, see Drug Formulary, Appendix 8.

Table • 72-1

Therapy for American and African Trypanosomiasis

DISEASE/DRUG[a]	DOSE (MG/KG)[b]	ROUTE	INTERVAL (HOURS)	DURATION (MONTHS)
American Trypanosomiasis				
Nifurtimox[c]	2–7	PO	6	3–5
Benznidazole	5–7	PO	24	2
African Trypanosomiasis				
Diminazene aceturate[d]	3.6–7	IM	2 wks[38]	[e]
Melarsoprol	2.2	IV	24	10

[a]See Drug Formulary, Appendix 8, for additional information on each drug.
[b]Dose per administration at specified interval.
[c]Lampit (Bayer) is an investigational drug in the United States. Available only from the Centers for Disease Control and Prevention, Atlanta, Georgia, for treatment of human infections.
[d]Available for use in endemic areas.
[e]Repeat therapy as needed to control relapse or reinfection.

Supportive therapy, including furosemide and theophylline, is indicated in cases of dilatational myocarditis. Cardiac arrhythmias may require specific therapy, depending on the source and severity of the disturbance. If the disease is diagnosed and treated early enough, the mortality rate of acute disease can be decreased. However, dogs surviving acute disease invariably develop chronic cardiac disease in 1 to 5 years. The prognoses of these animals must be guarded because the outcome is usually fatal.

Prevention

Preventing contact between dogs and infected vectors by upgrading housing of the dogs will do much to limit infection. Residual insecticides should be sprayed monthly in peridomiciliary structures (woodpiles, chicken houses) and dog kennels. Oral cythioate (Proban, Bayer, Shawnee, Kan.), 3 mg/kg every other day, given to dogs housed outdoors will reduce vector numbers. Once vector numbers are reduced, the dose can be given twice a week. Limiting contact between dogs and infected reservoir hosts (opossums, raccoons, armadillos) and their vectors is virtually impossible but would limit infection. Most cases in the United States have been reported in hunting dogs, which do have an increased risk of exposure.[19] Dogs should not be fed raw meat of reservoir hosts. Blood donors in endemic areas should be screened serologically to determine previous exposure to *T. cruzi*.

Persistent immunity does not develop in dogs infected with *T. cruzi*. Experimentally, dogs have been reinfected five times over a 3-year period.[71] Levels of parasitemia decreased and antibody titers increased with each successive reinfection. Neither amastigotes nor *T. cruzi* DNA was detected in tissues of infected dogs after the fifth infection; however, progressive myocarditis was observed.

Public Health Considerations

An estimated 20 million Latin Americans are infected with Chagas' disease, but only three naturally acquired cases have been reported in the United States.[84] Several factors are probably responsible for this low prevalence of Chagas' disease. First, the North American species of *Triatoma* usually leave the host before defecating, unlike the South American insect, which defecates while still on the host. Because contact with infected insect feces is the usual mode of transmission in people, this behavior limits the chance of contact. Second, the density of infected *Triatoma* in human dwellings is much less in the United States than it is in endemic areas of South America. Third, more cases of human Chagas' disease may

have occurred in the United States but have gone unrecognized because of a low index of suspicion. Because estimates are that 50,000 to 100,000 infected people now reside in the United States, the risk of catching *T. cruzi* from blood transfusion is greater than it is from infected vectors. Blood transfusion has been a major risk of infection for people in many Latin American countries.

Chagas' disease in dogs and wild hosts is of considerable public health significance because of the severity of and difficulty in treating the disease in people. Dogs cohabitating premises with people in endemic areas may serve as reservoir hosts for an insect species that is considered a zoonotic vector. Dogs diagnosed with this disease serve as sentinels for potential human infection and likelihood of infected bug infestation of a domicile.[25] Veterinarians should take particular care in treating animals with *T. cruzi* infection and make owners aware of the potential zoonotic risk. Blood samples taken from infected dogs are potentially infective, and laboratory staff should be appropriately instructed in handling suspected body fluids and tissues.

AFRICAN TRYPANOSOMIASIS

Craig E. Greene and George Matete

Etiology and Epidemiology

Trypanosomiasis is an important hemoparasitic disease of animals and people in Africa (i.e., sleeping sickness). Human infections occur in 36 African countries between 14 degrees North and 29 degrees South latitude (Fig. 72-5).[75] *T. brucei* comprises a group of indistinguishable flagellated hemoparasites in the subgenus *Trypanozoon*. Some of the subspecies cause human sleeping sickness. *T. brucei brucei* and *Trypanosoma congolense*, a species in the subgenus *Nannomonas*, are parasites of wild and domestic animals but do not infect people. Host species differ in their susceptibility to infection, and dogs are particularly susceptible to *T. congolense* and *T. brucei brucei*.[90] *T. evansi* is thought to have evolved from *T. brucei*.

Dogs are susceptible to various trypanosomes, including *T. brucei brucei*, *T. brucei rhodesiense*, *T. brucei gambiense*, *T. congolense*, and *T. evansi*.[75] In Nigeria, canine trypanosomiasis occurs in the *T. brucei gambiense* region causing ocular, lymphatic, and meningeal forms.[89] In Kenya, outbreaks of infection with *T. brucei rhodesiense* are associated with development of corresponding outbreaks of blindness in dogs and

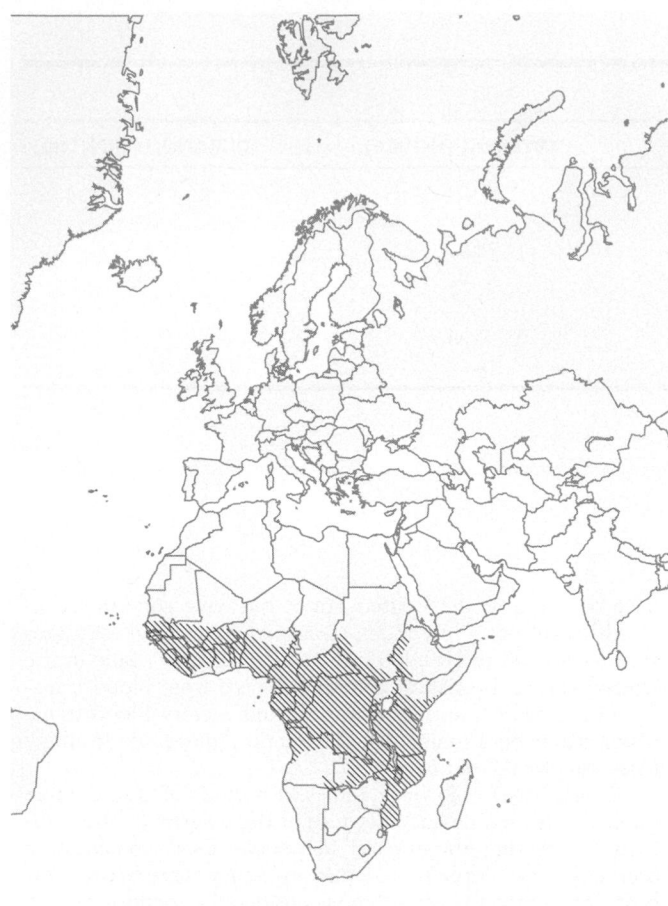

© UGA 2004

Fig   72-5   Geographic distribution of African trypanosomiasis. (Courtesy University of Georgia, Athens, Ga.)

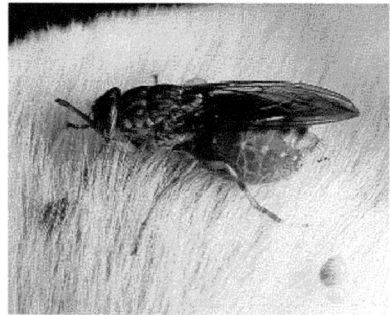

Fig   72-6   Tsetse fly, the vector of African trypanosomiasis.

sleeping sickness in people.[75] Dogs may be more important as sentinels for infection rather than reservoir hosts. Dogs, which have a course of disease of 2 to 4 weeks until death, are unlikely to maintain the infection in nature.

These parasites are transmitted by tsetse flies of the genus *Glossina*, which are widespread in Africa (Fig. 72-6). Transmission of infection in nature occurs primarily around water sources frequented by hosts and the vector flies. Mechanical transmission by other vectors and congenital transmission does not occur in nature. Rare laboratory inoculations have developed into disease.

In the cycle of infection, flies become infected after ingesting blood containing trypomastigotes (Fig. 72-7). The organism has a developmental cycle in the insect vector and transforms into slender trypomastigotes, which enter the salivary glands and become infective epimastigotes. Transmission occurs when these forms are inoculated by the fly during feeding on a new host.

Pathogenesis

Once they enter the mammalian host, African trypanosomes also replicate unimpeded by immune defenses. Unlike *T. cruzi*, African trypanosomes undergo continual antigenic variation of their outer glycoprotein coat as a means of immune evasion. Replication in the host results in widespread hemolymphatic dissemination. From the site of inoculation, inflammation spreads to the lymph nodes and spleen. Pericarditis and myocarditis, anemia, thrombocytopenia, leukocytosis, and disseminated intravascular coagulation can occur. Ocular involvement is thought to occur via the localization of organisms or associated immune complexes in the uveal tract with deposition along the inner surface of the cornea. Damage to the corneal endothelium, with resultant corneal edema, or granular deposits along the inner corneal surface may cause clouding of the cornea, similar to the "blue eye" observed in infectious canine hepatitis (see Chapter 4). Invasion of the central nervous system occurs in final stages of the disease with a diffuse meningoencephalitis.

The spleen is important in the production of antibodies and immune response to these hemoprotozoa. Splenectomy delays the onset of anemia and increases parasitemia and febrile responses.[42]

Clinical Findings

Clinical signs in acutely infected dogs consist of anorexia and fever (mean, 39.8° C [102.2° F]); edema of the face, genitalia, and subcutaneous tissues; purulent ocular and nasal discharges; orchitis in male dogs; and pale mucosae and weakness. Petechial hemorrhage and mucosal bleeding, lymphadenomegaly, and splenomegaly also occur. Weight loss is typical of chronically infected animals. As in people, sleepiness is an apparent feature, and it may relate to meningoencephalitis. In Nigeria, *T. brucei gambiense* infections are associated with ocular inflammation and lymphadenomegaly. In Kenya, ocular manifestations with *T. brucei brucei* and *T. brucei rhodesiense* predominate. Other clinical features, not previously described, include pale mucosae, dyspnea, rough haircoat, and subcutaneous edema of the head and neck.[75] The swelling of the thoracic limbs and neck has been associated with the development of decubital ulcers and limb edema caused by prolonged recumbency. Neurologic abnormalities include mental dullness and postural reaction deficits with intact reflexes, indicating upper motor neuron dysfunction. Neurologic signs are progressive and result in mental deterioration and behavioral changes similar to those of rabies. Ocular lesions include corneal opacity, conjunctivitis with a mucopurulent oculonasal discharge, uveitis with hemorrhage and turbidity in the anterior chamber, and visual loss (Fig. 72-8).[75]

Diagnosis and Pathologic Findings

Hematologic changes during the course of infection include a decline in hematocrit with reticulocytosis and elevated mean corpuscular volume. The white blood cell count often decreases with neutropenia, lymphopenia, and eosinopenia and thrombocytopenia. In other cases, leukocytosis with neutrophilia has been noted. Trypanosomes may be demonstrated in the blood of infected dogs and in the cerebrospinal fluid (CSF) of those with neurologic signs (Fig. 72-9). CSF analysis changes are pleocytosis with a predominance of lymphocytes.

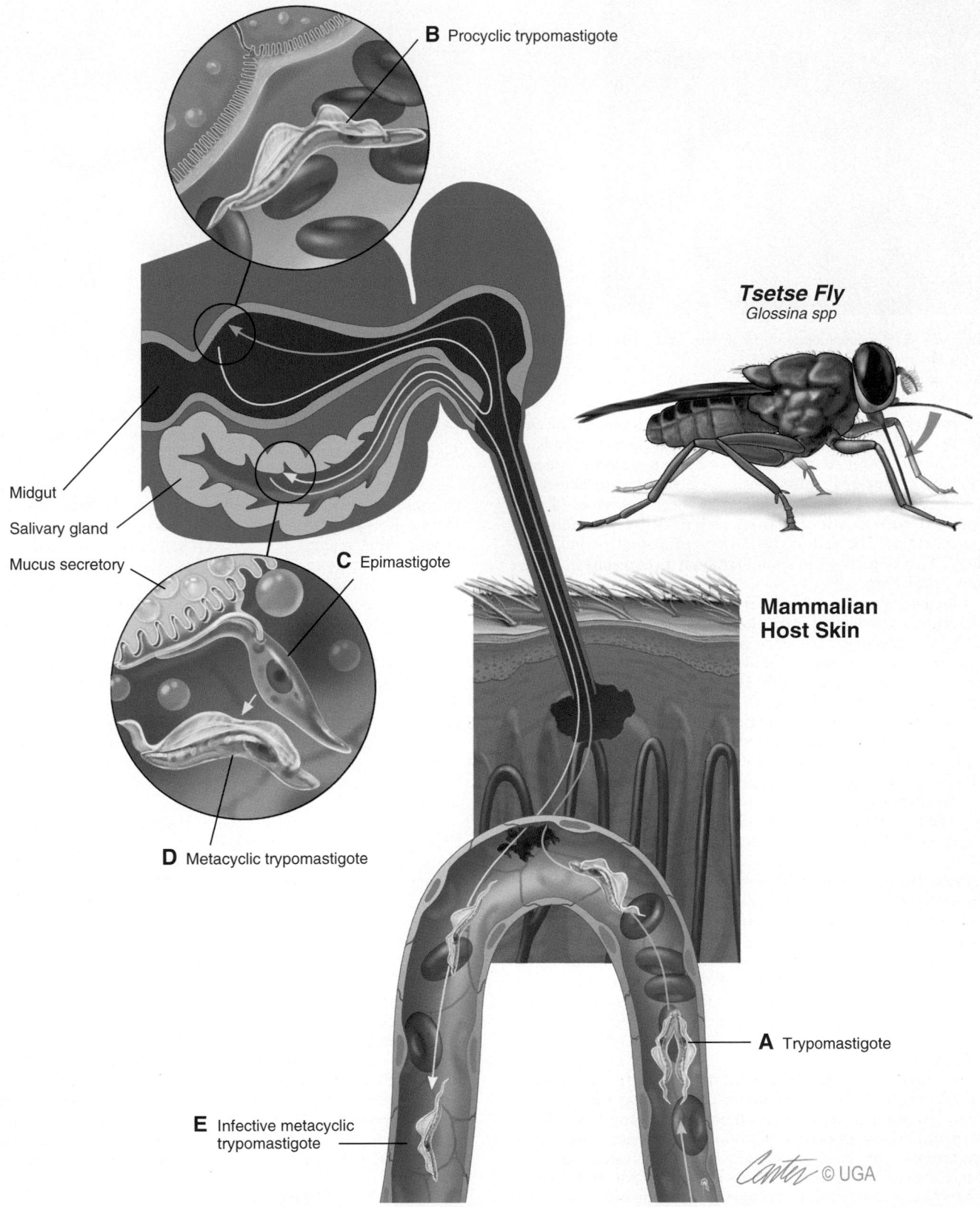

B Procyclic trypomastigote

Tsetse Fly
Glossina spp

Midgut

Salivary gland

Mucus secretory

C Epimastigote

Mammalian Host Skin

D Metacyclic trypomastigote

A Trypomastigote

E Infective metacyclic trypomastigote

Carter © UGA

Fig 72-7 Life cycle of African trypanosomiasis. **A,** The organism is ingested by the insect vector as a trypomastigote in the blood. **B,** Within the vector midgut, the organism transforms into slender procyclic trypomastigotes that enter salivary glands. **C,** There, transformation takes place into epimastigotes, and **D,** subsequently to metacyclic trypomastigotes which are **(E)** inoculated into an uninfected susceptible host during feeding. (Courtesy University of Georgia, Athens, Ga.)

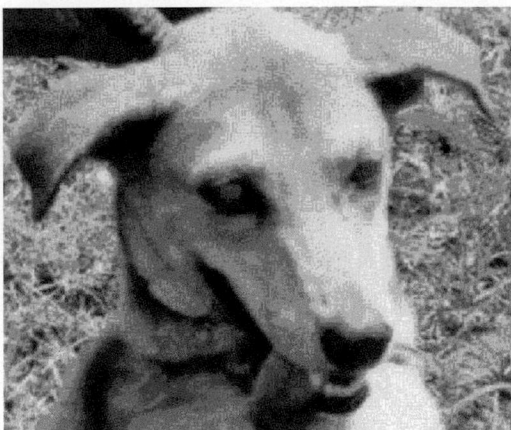

Fig 72-8 Corneal opacity in a dog with naturally acquired African trypanosomiasis.

Immunodiagnostic methods include detection of an antibody response using indirect FA and ELISA methods, of which the latter is more sensitive. Trypanosome species–specific monoclonal antibodies have been used to detect circulating antigen in infected dogs.[43] The parasitemia of dogs infected with *T. evansi* was characterized by an undulating parasitemia.[6] The end of the 2-week prepatent period correlated with an increase in serum antibody titer results that were not protective.

Genetic detection methods are being studied as a way to determine carriers of infection. The organism expresses a 743 bp molecular mass gene product that allows the organism to survive within the blood of human hosts.[117] A unique serum resistance–associated (SRA) gene is found in *T. brucei rhodesiense* isolates, allowing the detection of this pathogen in the mammalian host and in tsetse vectors without the need for strain characterization of this species.[86] This SRA gene has been found in trypanosomes infecting a dog, which suggests that dogs may carry trypanosomes that infect people.[75]

At necropsy, edema and subcutaneous hemorrhages may be visible in many organs. Hepatosplenomegaly and lymphadenomegaly may be apparent. The carcass is often emaciated, with edema of the face, ventral thorax, abdomen, and extremities. The mucopurulent exudate mats the hairs surrounding the eyes. Skeletal muscles show various degree of atrophy. The pericardial sac may be filled with turbid fluid, which may contain flakes of fibrin. Lymphoplasmacytic infiltrates are found in many organs. Throughout various regions in the central nervous system, cellular infiltration of the leptomeninges with macrophages, neutrophils, plasma cells, and lymphocytes is apparent.

Therapy

Few drugs exist in the treatment of African trypanosomiasis (see Table 72-1). Isometamidium chloride was the first drug used. Suramin is the drug of choice for treating East African trypanosomiasis in people who do not have neurologic manifestations. For meningoencephalitis, the trivalent arsenical Melarsoprol® (Melarsen, France) is used. Melarsoprol® is effective in penetrating the nervous system but is available only on an experimental basis. Treatment of one dog with Melarsoprol® caused clearing of organisms in the blood within 24 hours and progressive clearing of the uveal inflammation.[75] However, the neurologic signs eventually progressed and the organism was found in impression smears of brain tissue at necropsy. Eflornithine is used to treat West African disease involving the central nervous system. Other arsenicals such as cymelarsan (RM 110, Merial, Iselin, N.J.) and an

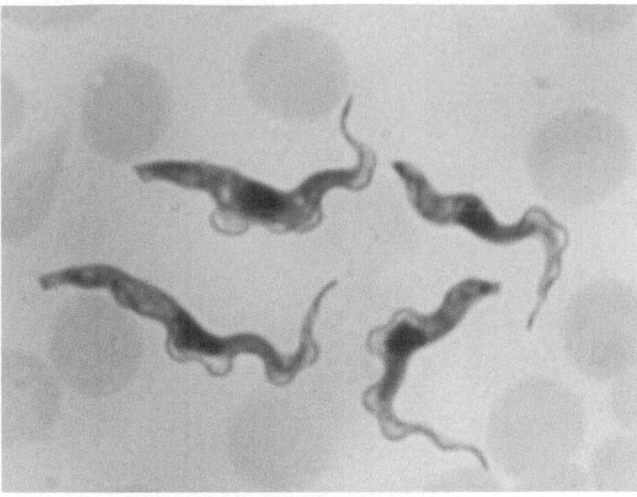

Fig 72-9 Trypomastigotes in the blood of a dog with African trypanosomiasis. (From Gardiner CH, Fayer R, Dubey JP, et al. 1988. An atlas of protozoan parasites in animal tissues, USDA Agricultural Handbook No 651, Beltsville, Md.)

enzyme inhibitor, difluoromethylornithine (DFMO; Hoechst Marion-Roussel, Somerville, N.J.), have shown efficacy in experimental studies.[90,107] DFMO has been combined with diminazene in treating infected dogs. Although relapses have occurred with this combination, they were lower than those that developed with either drug alone. Trypanosomes may cross the blood-brain barrier, evading the effective drugs, which are molecularly too large to cross.[38] Diminazene appears to be the most effective drug against relapses and is available for treatment of affected cattle. Concentrations of diminazene are higher in brain tissue of infected dogs compared with healthy dogs,[90,91] presumably as a result of inflammation of the blood-brain barrier. Appropriate dosages for some of the previously listed drugs are listed in Table 72-1. Further information on their use appears in the Drug Formulary, Appendix 8.

Public Health Considerations

Sleeping sickness is an endemic disease of sub-Saharan Africa caused by *T. brucei rhodesiense* in East Africa and *T. brucei gambiense* in West Africa. Following the bite of a tsetse fly, people develop fever, lethargy, rash, headache, gastrointestinal signs, neurologic signs, and myalgia. A local chancre at the site of the bite, lymphadenomegaly, splenomegaly, and signs of renal or cardiovascular dysfunction may also be observed. Laboratory abnormalities include leukopenia, anemia, thrombocytopenia, elevated hepatic transaminases, coagulation abnormalities, azotemia, and hyponatremia.[105] Definitive diagnosis relies on demonstrating the organism in peripheral blood, CSF, or the inoculating wound site. Examination of lymph node aspirates is not as helpful. Early treatment with suramin prevents the more resistant meningoencephalitic form of the disease. Animals pose minimal risk for human infection. Rather, they act as sentinels for the same infection.

SUGGESTED READINGS*

7. Araujo FM, Bahia MT, Magalhaes NM, et al. 2002. Follow-up of experimental chronic Chagas' disease in dogs: use of polymerase chain reaction (PCR) compared with parasitological and serological methods, *Acta Trop* 81:21-31.

*See the CD-ROM for a complete list of references.

25. Beard CB, Pye G, Steurer FJ, et al. 2003. Chagas disease in a domestic transmission cycle in Southern Texas, USA, *Emerg Infect Dis* 9:103-105.
30. Bradley KK, Bergman DK, Woods JP, et al. 2000. Prevalence of American trypanosomiasis (Chagas' disease) among dogs in Oklahoma, *J Am Vet Med Assoc* 217:1853-1857.
75. Matete GO. 2003. Occurrence, clinical manifestation and the epidemiological implications of naturally occurring canine trypanosomosis in western Kenya, *Onderstepoort J Vet Res* 70:317-323.

78. Meurs KM, Anthony MA, Slater M, et al. 1998. Chronic *Trypanosoma cruzi* infection in dogs: 11 cases (1987-1996), *J Am Vet Med Assoc* 213:497-500.
80. Moreno EA, Rivera IM, Moreno SC, et al. 2003. Vertical transmission of *Trypanosoma cruzi* in Wistar rats during the acute phase of infection, *Invest Clin* 44:241-254.
99. Romanha AJ, Alves RO, Murta SMF, et al. 2002. Experimental chemotherapy against *Trypanosoma cruzi* infection: essential role of endogenous interferon-γ in mediating parasitologic cure, *J Infect Dis* 186:823-828.

CHAPTER • 73

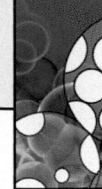

Leishmaniases

The leishmaniases are a group of infectious diseases that affect people and domestic and wild animals worldwide and are caused by members of the genus *Leishmania*. The infection is transmitted by sandflies of the genus *Phlebotomus* in the Old World and *Lutzomyia* in the New World. Visceral leishmaniasis, the most severe disease form, is a frequent cause of clinical illness in dogs in some regions but is less common in cats. Reservoir hosts vary within different geographic areas and can include domestic or wild animals. Infected domestic dogs serve as reservoirs of the disease for people in several areas where leishmaniasis is endemic. Dogs are reservoirs for *Leishmania infantum* infection in an area that stretches from Portugal to China. They are also reservoirs of infection for foxes and opossums in an area of *Leishmania chagasi (infantum)* that extends from southern Mexico to South America. Canine leishmaniasis is also sometimes found in nonendemic countries because of international tourists and immigrants who bring infected pets or because of dog importation. Dogs can be asymptomatic carriers of leishmaniases that are infectious to sandflies, and infection may go unnoticed for a long time. In this chapter, a global coverage of leishmaniasis will be presented, followed by two recognized geographic forms of emerging disease in animals in the New World.

LEISHMANIASIS

Gad Baneth

Etiology

Leishmaniasis is caused by diphasic protozoans of the genus *Leishmania* in the class Kinetoplasta and family Trypanosomatidae. About 30 different leishmanial species are found in various parts of the Old World and New World (Fig. 73-1). Of these, about 20 are responsible for a wide spectrum of clinical illnesses in people.[15] Most *Leishmania* spp. that infect people are zoonotic, and only a few are strictly *anthroponotic* (i.e., transmitted directly from person to person via sandflies). Leishmaniasis is endemic in 88 countries—66 in the Old World and 22 in the New World. Approximately 12 million people are infected with leishmaniasis, and some 350 million people are at risk of acquiring the disease, with a yearly incidence of 1 to 1.5 million new cases of cutaneous disease and

500,000 new cases of the potentially fatal visceral form.[55,56] Dogs are frequently involved in sylvan and urban cycles of zoonotic *Leishmania* spp. that cause disease in people in many parts of the world.[217] Based on seroprevalence studies from Spain, France, Italy, and Portugal, it has been estimated that 2.5 million dogs in these countries are infected with visceral leishmaniasis.[142] The number of infected dogs in South America is also estimated to be in the millions, with high infection rates being reported in some areas of Brazil.

The genus *Leishmania* is divided into the subgenera *Leishmania* and *Viannia* based on the differences in sandfly development. Many species are recognized within these subgenera. Classification is primarily based on DNA sequence comparisons, electrophoresis migration patterns of isoenzymes (zymodemes), and reactivity to monoclonal antibodies and to membrane-shed antigens.

The diseases caused by the various *Leishmania* spp. in people are divided into three forms according to their clinical manifestations (Table 73-1): cutaneous leishmaniasis (CL), mucocutaneous leishmaniasis (MCL), and visceral leishmaniasis (VL). Some species cause more than one form of the disease.

Canine leishmaniasis is often classified as VL because it is associated with some of the *Leishmania* spp. that cause VL in people; however, dogs usually have visceral and cutaneous involvement. *L. chagasi*, the VL agent in South America, is considered to be synonymous with *L. infantum* based on various genetic analyses.[135] The low genetic variability of *L. chagasi* is consistent with recent importation to the New World, and it is thought that it was introduced by infected dogs from Europe that arrived with settlers.

Epidemiology

The natural cycle of *Leishmania* infection involves a sandfly vector and a vertebrate host in which different forms of the parasite are found. Hematophagous female sandflies harbor *Leishmania* promastigotes in their guts and transmit the parasite during a blood meal to wild or domestic animals and people, where the amastigote form develops. Phlebotomine sandflies of the genus *Phlebotomus* in the Old World and *Lutzomyia* in the New World are the natural vectors of leishmaniasis. Sandflies are small insects with a body length seldom exceeding 3 mm.[105] The biting activity of sandflies is crepuscular and nocturnal. In the Mediterranean region and Asia,

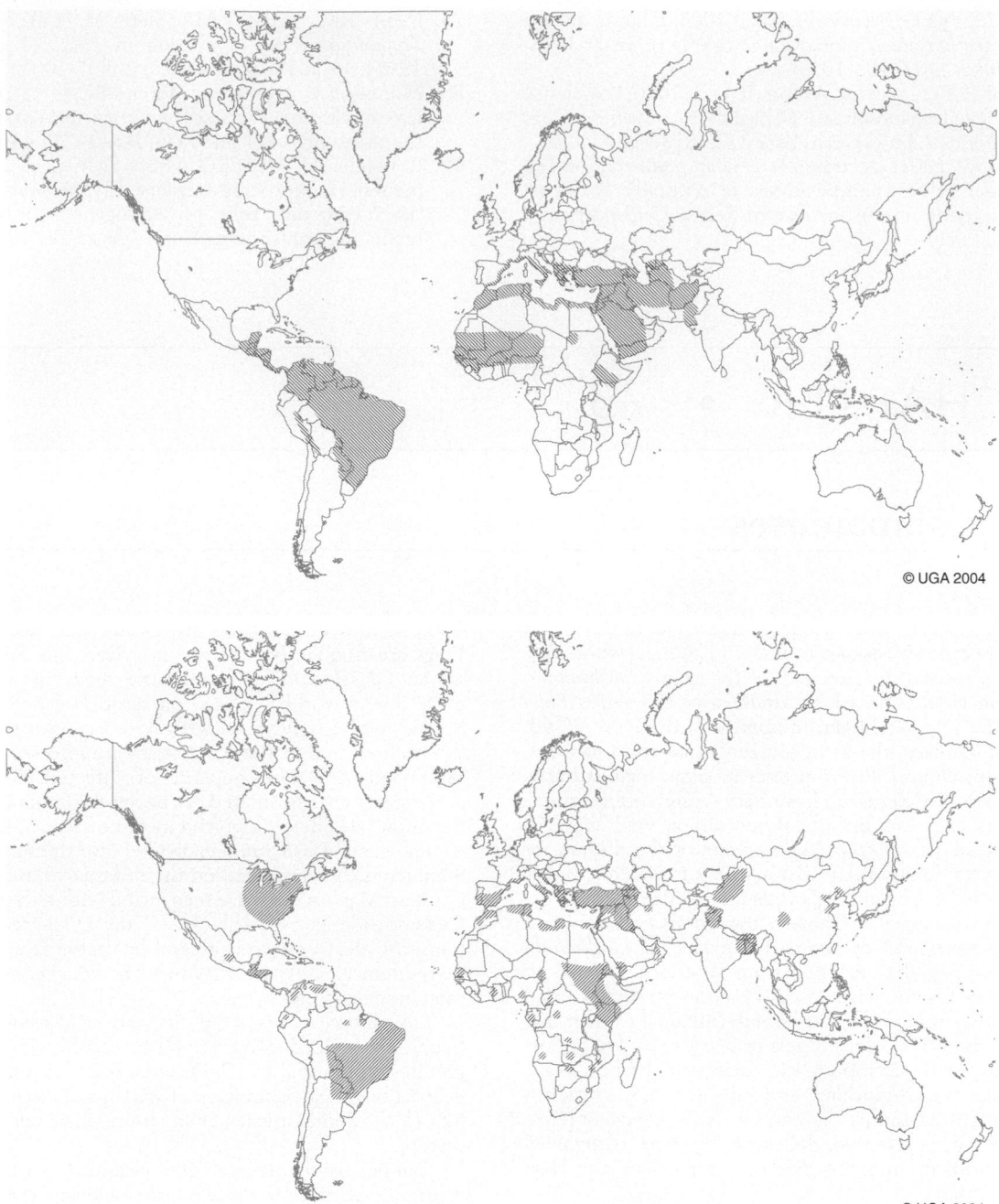

Fig   73-1 Distribution of cutaneous and mucocutaneous (**A**) and visceral (**B**) leishmaniasis. (Data modified from World Health Organization. 1984. *The leishmaniases*. The WHO Expert Committee. WHO Technical Report Series No. 701. Geneva, WHO; map courtesy University of Georgia, Athens, Ga.)

sandflies are primarily active in the warm months—from spring to late fall. In Latin America, some sandflies are active throughout the year. They do not move long distances, and studies have shown that they are seldom dispersed more than 1 km from their breeding sites. Many species of sandfly exist, but only some of them act as disease vectors. Different vector species may be found in distinct geographic regions and ecologic niches. Some sandfly species exclusively transmit only one *Leishmania* species, whereas others are vectors for more than one species. The vectorial capacity of different sandfly species appears to be related to the ability of promastigotes to specifically bind to receptors in the sandfly gut. When they do not bind to the sandfly gut, the parasites that initially replicated in the gut lumen are excreted with the sandfly feces and

presumably do not reach the critical mass needed to infect a host during a second blood meal. Organisms of the *Viannia* subgenus of *Leishmania braziliensis* replicate in the hindgut, in contrast to the midgut replication characteristic of all other *Leishmania* species.

In vertebrate hosts, *Leishmania* is found in macrophages in its nonflagellate form, the amastigote. Amastigotes are ovoid or round, 2.5 to 5 μm long and 1.5 to 2 μm wide. In addition to a basophilic-staining nucleus, a rod-shape, darker staining kinetoplast is visible with Wright's or Giemsa stain (Fig. 73-2). Amastigotes multiply by binary fission, rupture out of the macrophage, and infect new cells. Sandflies can ingest the amastigotes when they become engorged with blood from an infected host. In the sandfly, amastigotes are freed from their

Table • 73-1

Leishmanial Species and Types of Diseases

CLINICAL DISEASE	OLD WORLD	NEW WORLD
Visceral	*L. donovani*	*L. chagasi*[a]
	L. infantum[a,b]	(*L. infantum*)[a]
	L. tropica[c]	
Cutaneous	*L. aethiopica*	*L. mexicana*[b]
	L. major	*L. amazonensis*
	L. infantum	*L. venezuelensis*[b]
	L. tropica	*L. (Viannia) braziliensis*[b,d]
		L. panamensis[d]
		L. peruviana[d]
		L. guyanensis
		L. lainsoni
		L. naiffi
		L. shawi
Mucocutaneous		*L. braziliensis*
		L. guyanensis
		L. panamensis

[a]Main causative agents of canine visceral leishmaniasis.
[b]Reported to infect domestic cats.
[c]Rare cause of canine leishmaniasis.
[d]Causative agents of American tegumentary leishmaniasis in dogs in South or Central America.

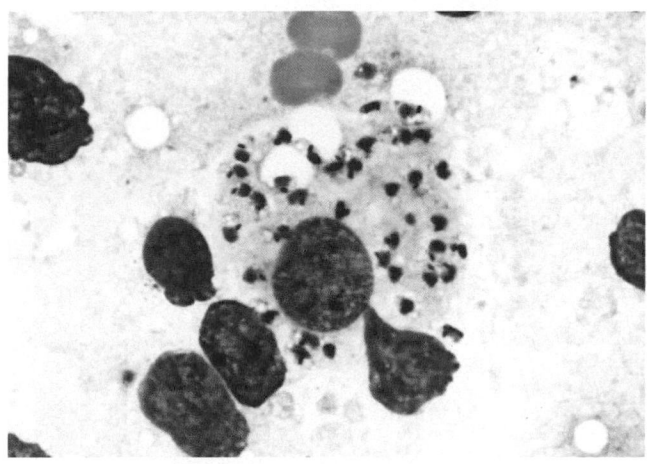

Fig 73-2 *L. infantum* amastigotes in canine macrophage from popliteal lymph node aspirate (May-Grunwald-Giemsa stain, ×500).

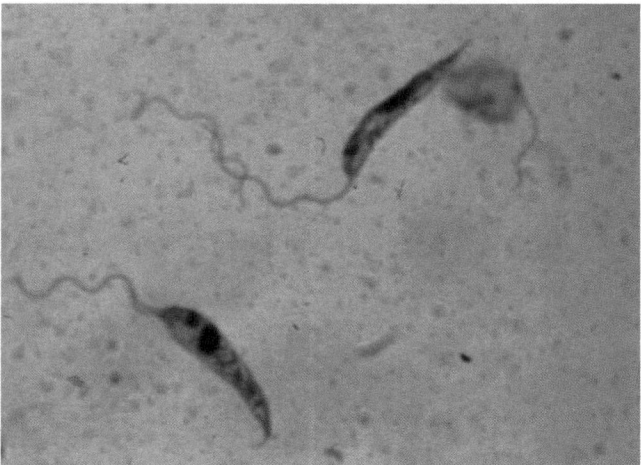

Fig 73-3 *Leishmania* promastigotes grown in culture. Note round nuclei and rod-shape kinetoplast (May-Grunwald-Giemsa stain, ×1000).

host cells, undergo a series of morphologic alterations, transform into the extracellular flagellated promastigote form, and replicate in the sandfly gut (Fig. 73-3). Promastigotes are injected with saliva into the skin of a vertebrate host when the female feeds again. After inoculation into the host, the promastigotes lose their flagella and transform back into amastigotes (Fig. 73-4).

Domestic dogs (*Canis familiaris*) are considered the main VL reservoirs for people in the Mediterranean basin, Middle East, and South America, where *L. infantum (L. chagasi)* is the causative agent of infection. In regions with a high infection rate among dogs, the incidence of clinical VL in the general human population is generally low[217]; however, human exposure rates (as determined by the prevalence of specific antibodies or positive leishmanin skin test results), which indicate past exposure to *Leishmania* organisms, may be high.[2,4,141,216]

In the Indian subcontinent and East Africa, where *Leishmania donovani* is the agent of VL, people are the reservoir hosts, and animals do not appear to play a significant role in the anthroponotic epidemiology of infection. The main reservoir hosts for *Leishmania* spp. causing CL and MCL in people are rodents and other wild animal species. Domestic cats are rarely hosts.

Canine VL caused by *L. infantum* is an important cause of zoonotic disease in many endemic countries and areas, including Spain, Portugal, southern France, Italy, Malta, Greece, Turkey, Israel, Egypt, Tunisia, Algeria, Morocco, Iraq, Iran, the former Asian republics of the Union of the Soviet Socialist Republics, Pakistan, and some parts of China.[18,131,137,170,208] Recent information indicates that VL may occur also in a part of southern Germany.[112] Reports have been made of sporadic cases of canine leishmaniasis caused by importation or trans-

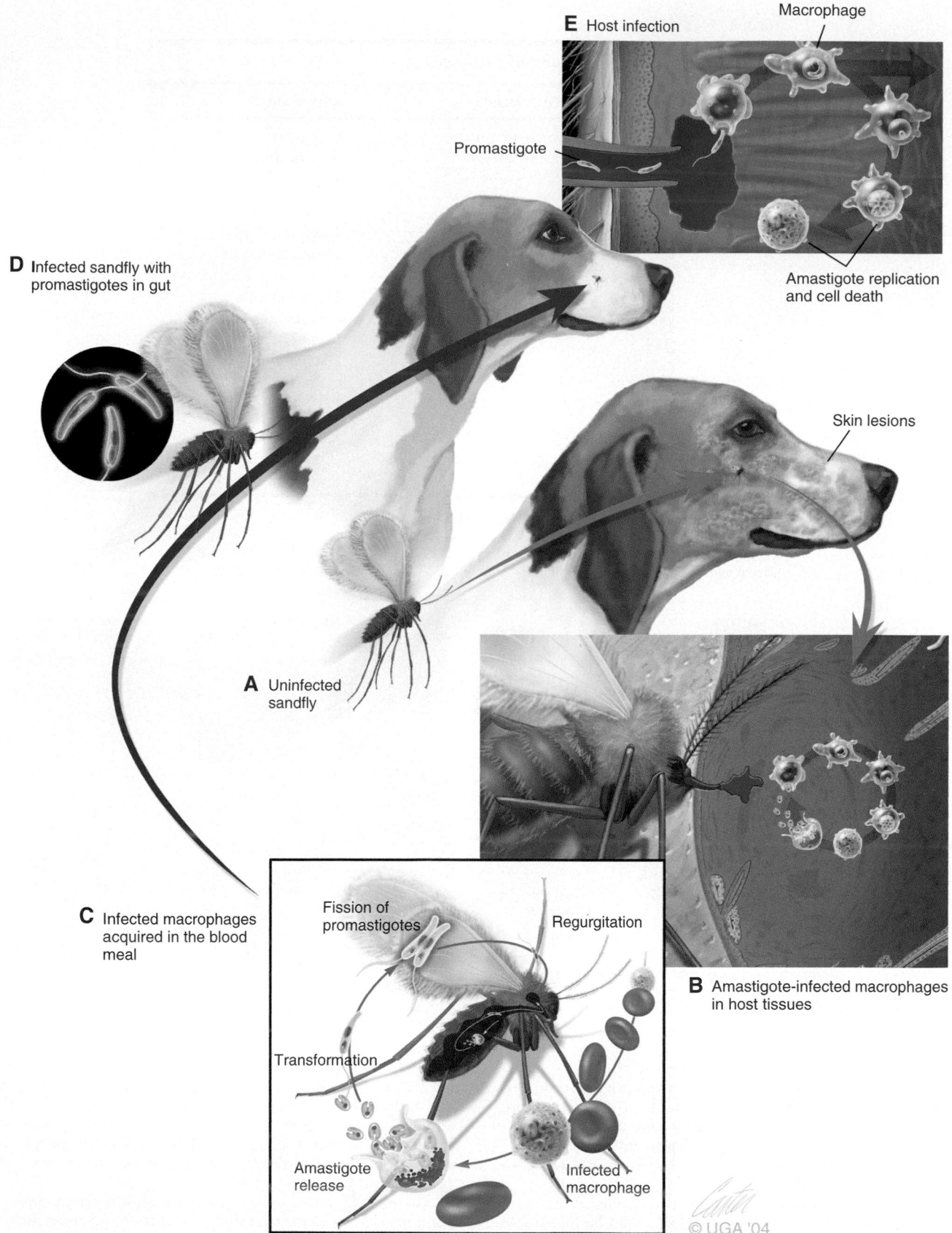

Fig 73-4 The life cycle of *L. infantum*. **A,** Uninfected sandfly feeds on an infected host and **(B)** ingests infected macrophages in host tissues. **C,** The organisms are released from the infected macrophages into the sandfly gut and **(D)** transform into motile promastigotes which replicate in the sandfly gut. **E,** The promastigotes are regurgitated during feeding of the infected sandfly. The infected sandfly transmits the infection to the new host during feeding. (Courtesy University of Georgia, Athens, Ga.)

port of infected dogs to countries where sandfly transmission of VL does not occur, such as Holland, England, and Sweden.[206] Similarly, dogs are a reservoir of *L. infantum (L. chagasi)* infection for people in South America.[41] Because many dogs in endemic areas harbor asymptomatic infections, infection rates are often estimated not only by the presence of clinical signs compatible with the disease, but also by serologic methods, the presence of parasite DNA in the tissues or blood, or both as determined by the polymerase chain reaction (PCR). Canine infection rates as shown by PCR and serology in highly endemic foci such as the Balearic Islands of Spain,[199] the Marseille area in France,[26] and Greece[118] approach 70% to 80%. This is a much higher prevalence of infection than that associated with symptomatic disease or determined by serology alone. It is thought that most or all dogs in these areas are infected during their lives. Some dogs succumb to the infection, others harbor the pathogen and are resistant to the development of clinical disease, and some dogs are able to eliminate the pathogen before developing clinical disease. In other areas, infection is not as highly prevalent, possibly because of less favorable environmental conditions for transmission and vectors.[142,221]

Canine infection occurs mostly in rural areas or the outskirts of towns; however, urbanization of canine and human infection has been reported and poses a threat to the well-being of large dogs and humans.[49,142] *L. infantum* infection has been reported in wild canids such as foxes *(Vulpes vulpes)* and jackals *(Canis aureus)* in Europe and the Middle East and in crab-eating foxes *(Cerdocyon thous)* in South America.* These wild canine species may demonstrate signs of disease or be asymptomatic. Infected crab-eating foxes were found to have low rates of transmission to the sandfly *Lutzomyia longipalpis* and were therefore not considered important as reservoirs of VL in Brazil.[45] The particular role of wild canids in the epidemiology and spread of sylvatic *L. infantum* infection to domestic dogs *(Canis familiaris)* and people is not well understood and should be separately investigated in every ecosystem where this disease is found. Although *L. infantum* is naturally transmitted through the bites of sandflies, vertical in utero transmission from a dam to its offspring has been documented in a few reports.[58] *Rhipicephalus sanguineus* has been shown to acquire *Leishmania* organism in their guts after feeding on infected dogs[40a]; however, its competence as a vector has not been confirmed.

Leishmania tropica occurs in the Old World and is a rare cause of infection in dogs. *L. tropica* is an important agent of CL in people in some parts of the Middle East and Africa. It also caused VL in American soldiers returning from the Persian Gulf after the 1991 Operation Desert Storm[124] and in patients from India.[179] It has been sporadically found in dogs with CL from Tunisia and Morocco[54] and from another dog from Morocco with VL and no dermal abnormalities.[92] However, *L. tropica* infection is rare compared with the common canine *L. infantum* infection.

Pathogenesis

As the sandfly bites, *Leishmania* promastigotes are transferred with the sandfly saliva into the vertebrate host's skin. The promastigotes are then phagocytized by macrophages and multiply as amastigotes within phagolysosomes that separate them from the host cell defense mechanisms. When the macrophage ruptures, freed amastigotes penetrate additional host cells and disseminate from the local bite site. They travel throughout the host's body but primarily to the hemolymphatic system organs and remote dermal areas to create a generalized infection.

As mentioned previously, not every dog naturally or experimentally infected with *Leishmania* develops disease.[107,162] The

immune responses mounted by dogs at the time of infection and thereafter appear to be the most important factor in determining whether they develop a generalized infection and whether and when the infection will progress from a asymptomatic state into symptomatic disease. Infection initially has no apparent symptoms but later might progress into a symptomatic disease unless the replication of amastigotes is halted by immune mechanisms. Dogs that are able to resist an infection by either resolving it and eliminating the parasite or restricting the infection and remaining consistently asymptomatic are *clinically resistant*. Animals that are predisposed to developing an infection and symptomatic disease are considered *susceptible*. The innate, or nonspecific, immune response is the first line of defense encountered by *Leishmania* parasites when entering the susceptible host. One of several suggested mechanisms by which *Leishmania* parasites depress the innate host immune defenses involves the ability of amastigotes to survive and replicate within macrophage phagolysosomes by producing compounds such as lypophosphoglycans that inhibit phagosome maturation.[180]

Specific immune responses play a major role in susceptibility to infection. An experimental model of cutaneous leishmaniasis in mice infected with *Leishmania major* has shown that a susceptible mouse strain, which typically develops a T-helper (Th) type 2 (Th2) cellular response, succumbed to infection. This Th2 response resulted in secretion of specific cytokines such as interleukin-4 (IL)-4 and interleukin-10 (IL)-10 and production of a significant antibody response. Other mouse strains that respond with a different set of cytokines, including interferon-γ (IFN-γ) and interleukin-12 (IL)-12, typical of a Th1 response are resistant to infection.[93,187] IFN-γ secreted from T cells activates macrophages for the elimination of parasites. This general concept derived from the experimental CL model of a Th-cell dichotomy—in which one type of Th-cell response produces resistance or cure and a second type produces susceptibility and disease exacerbation—has been applied to infections with other pathogens in many hosts. However, whether this concept applies to VL is unclear. In experimental murine VL, both types of responses develop,[103,140] and it is the balance of the Th1/Th2 responses that is considered to be important in controlling parasite replication, disease progression, or a cure. The balance between the two types of cellular immune responses also appears to be important in natural canine and human VL.

Protective immunity to leishmaniasis in dogs is mediated by T cells.[162] Resistance to experimental infection with *L. infantum* in dogs is associated with proliferation of peripheral blood lymphocytes, which produce IL-2, tumor necrosis factor, and IFN-α with parasite antigen-specific stimulation. In addition, *L. infantum*–infected macrophages are lysed in a histocompatibility complex-restricted manner by CD8+ cytotoxic T cells, CD4+ cytotoxic T cells, or both. These processes are suppressed in symptomatic dogs, in which T-cell proliferation with leishmanial antigen and antigen-specific IFN-γ production are depressed and a marked IgG response to the parasite ensues.[51,133,162,163] A strong delayed-type hypersensitivity response with the leishmanin intradermal skin test indicative of a cell-mediated response to *Leishmania* infection is found in infection-resistant dogs that have been exposed to the parasite and is absent in highly symptomatic dogs.[162,197,198] In addition, intracellular killing of the parasite by neutrophils and monocytes is impaired.[34] During the infection, dogs become increasingly immunosuppressed and develop lower CD4+ lymphocyte counts and experience a decrease in the CD4+/CD8+ ratio.[32,143] This finding is commonly associated with retroviral diseases, such as the human immunodeficiency virus (HIV) in people and feline immunodeficiency virus (FIV) in cats, and is proportional to the degree of susceptibility to opportunistic pathogens. Moreover, it has been demon-

*References 1, 18, 43, 47, 97, 125, 190.

strated that the infectiousness of dogs with leishmaniasis to sandflies increases proportionally with the decrease in CD4+ counts.[91]

Susceptibility and resistance to canine VL appear to have a genetic basis. The prevalence of overt VL among Ibizan hounds in the Balearic Islands is lower than among other breeds, and it has been shown that this breed mounts a predominantly cellular immune response against *L. infantum.*[198] A study on the polymorphism of the canine NRAMP1 gene, which encodes an iron transporter protein involved in the control of intraphagosomal replication of parasites and macrophage activation, has implied that susceptible dogs have mutations in this gene.[7] A DLA class II DLA-DRB1 genotype, which is a dog major histocompatibility complex class II allele, has been linked to the risk of being infected in an endemic area in Brazil.[169]

Canine VL is usually a chronic disease, and clinical signs of disease may develop 3 months to 7 years after infection. T-lymphocyte regions in the lymphoid organs become depleted, and antibody-producing B-cell regions proliferate. The proliferation of B lymphocytes, plasma cells, histiocytes, and macrophages results in generalized lymphadenomegaly, splenomegaly, and consistent hyperglobulinemia. The immunoglobulin response is usually massive; however, it is not a protective response and can eventually be detrimental. Autoantibodies that may be associated with the development of pathologic phenomena such as immune-mediated thrombocytopenia and anemia are also frequently produced. Another potential hazard of impaired T-cell regulation with exuberant B-cell activity is the generation of large amounts of circulating immune complexes (CICs).[121] CIC deposition in the walls of blood vessels may cause vasculitis, polyarthritis, uveitis, and glomerulonephritis. In dogs, CIC deposition in the kidneys eventually results in renal failure, which is the main cause of death of dogs with leishmaniasis. Systemic vasculitis may lead to local ischemia that causes visceral and cutaneous necrosis and, although rare, to nervous system involvement.[77,168] CICs may also include cryoglobulins. These proteins may precipitate in the blood vessels of the extremities when exposed to cold and cause ischemic necrosis.[192]

Canine leishmaniasis is most often associated with various skin lesions, which are generalized rather than local because *L. infantum* disseminates all over the body.[167] It may also be detected in healthy-looking skin and not necessarily in dermal lesions.[196] The more rare form of generalized nodular lesions (the nodular form of leishmaniasis) probably indicates that a dog mounted a less effective immune response than that associated with generalized alopecia.[72] Although rare, skin lesions could be restricted to a few ulcerations or nodules.

Dogs with leishmaniasis may show signs of a hemorrhagic diathesis—primarily epistaxis. Histopathology of the nasal mucosa of 10 dogs with CL, three of which had a history of epistaxis, revealed that all 10 dogs had ulcerative and inflammatory lesions that could be involved with bleeding.[102] Other than nasal ulcers, possible causes include paraglobulinemia, which may interfere with fibrin polymerization and which in association with uremia may inhibit thrombocyte function. In addition, thrombocytopenia may develop as a result of CIC, autoantibodies, splenic pooling, or bone marrow suppression. Anemia usually develops as a sequel to the decreased erythropoiesis of chronic disease or to chronic renal failure but may be aggravated by blood loss, an immune-based destruction of erythrocytes, or both.

Clinical Findings

Dogs

Canine VL is a chronic systemic disease. The signs of disease are highly variable and often begin with slight but progressive

Table • 73-2	
Clinical Findings in 80 Dogs with Leishmaniasis[191]	
FINDINGS	**PERCENTAGE OF DOGS**
CLINICAL AND HISTORICAL FINDINGS	
Decreased endurance	67.5
Weight loss	64
Somnolence	60
Increased fluid intake	40
Anorexia	32.5
Diarrhea	30
Vomiting	26
Polyphagia	15
Epistaxis	15
Melena	12.5
Sneezing	10
Coughing	6
Fainting	6
PHYSICAL EXAMINATION ABNORMALITIES	
Lymphadenomegaly	90
Skin involvement	89
Cachexia	47.5
Abnormal locomotion	37.5
Hyperthermia	36
Conjunctivitis	32.5
Palpable spleen	32.5
Abnormal nails	20
Rhinitis	10
Keratitis	7.5
Pneumonia	2.5
Icterus	2.5
Uveitis	1.3
Panophthalmitis	1.3

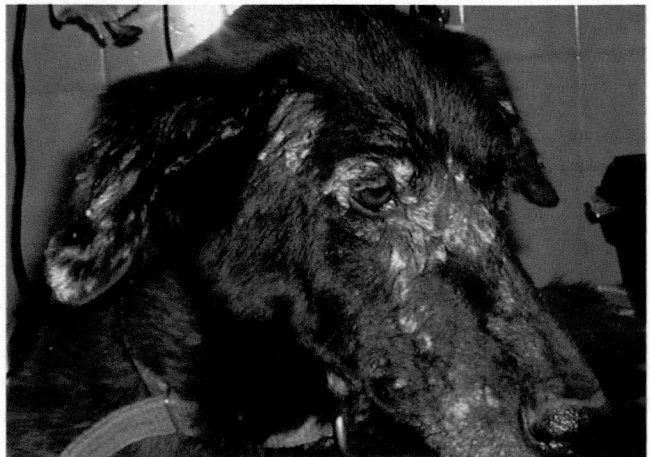

Fig 73-5 Canine leishmaniasis showing exfoliative dermatitis and scaling on face.

dullness and insidious exercise intolerance. The clinical findings in canine leishmaniasis are presented in Table 73-2.

The prevalence of cutaneous lesions in dogs with symptomatic leishmaniasis ranges between 56% to 90%.[40,109,191] Dermatologic abnormalities may occur in the apparent absence of

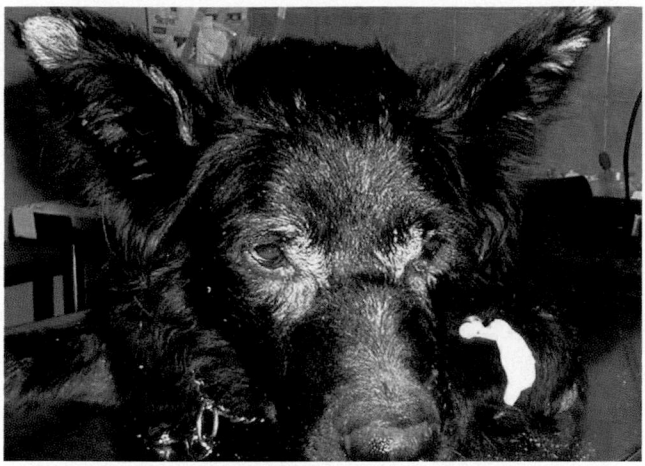

Fig 73-6 Canine leishmaniasis showing scaling on pinna and face.

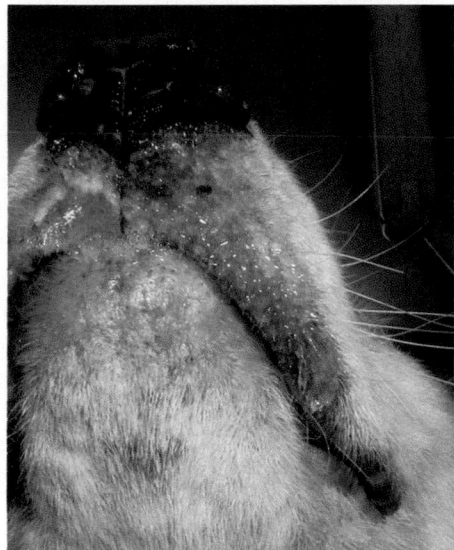

Fig 73-7 Mucocutaneous ulceration in a dog with leishmaniasis.

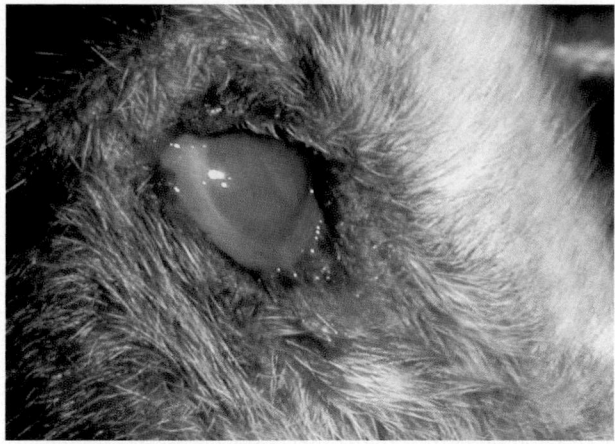

Fig 73-8 Ocular lesions in leishmaniasis showing junctivitis in a dog with uveitis.

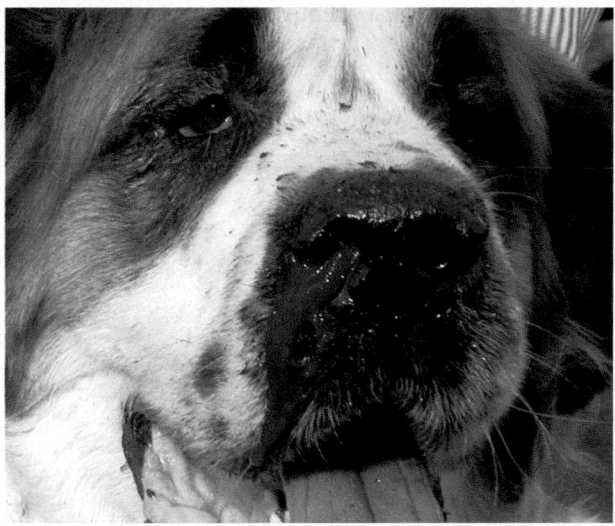

Fig 73-9 Epistaxis in St. Bernard with leishmaniasis and no dermal lesions.

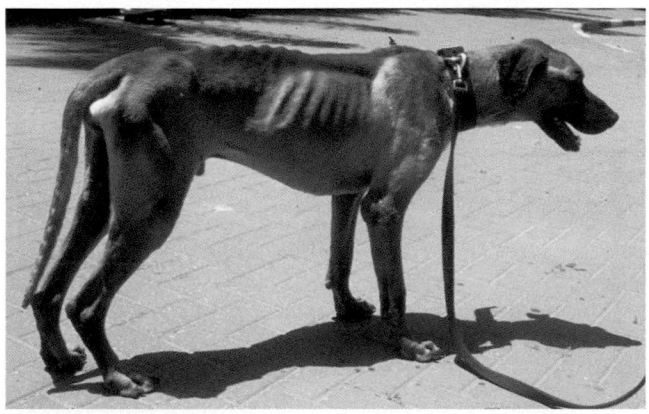

Fig 73-10 Dog with characteristic features of leishmaniasis. Note cachexia, muscle atrophy, and excessive scaling.

other obvious signs of disease, but any animal with dermal manifestations of leishmaniasis should be presumed to have visceral involvement, because the parasites disseminate throughout the body before generalized skin lesions develop. Dermatologic abnormalities vary in character and extent but are rarely pruritic. Most dogs develop a progressive and symmetric alopecia with exfoliative dermatitis and desquamation, usually commencing on the head and extending to the rest of the body (Fig. 73-5). In addition, some animals develop ulcerations on the nose and the pinna (Fig. 73-6) or chapping of the muzzle or the footpads. Less frequently, mucocutaneous ulcers (Fig. 73-7), cutaneous nodules, mucosal nodules, or pustular eruptions develop.[78,109,111,71a] Lymphadenomegaly of multiple superficial lymph nodes frequently develops in canine VL[119b] with lymph nodes enlarging 2 to 6 times their normal size and occasionally mimicking clinical findings of lymphosarcoma. Splenomegaly is also frequently detected by abdominal palpation.

Approximately 20% to 40% of the dogs diagnosed with VL have ocular lesions, including keratoconjunctivitis and lymphoplasmacytic or granulomatous uveitis (Fig. 73-8).[40,80,160,191] In some cases, ocular abnormalities are the only clinical signs.[160] Abnormally long or brittle nails (onychogryphosis), a rather specific finding, develop in a small proportion of the

patients. Epistaxis is another clinical sign that may be develop in conjunction with other typical abnormalities or as the only presenting sign in canine VL (Fig. 73-9).[102]

Weight loss and muscle atrophy are the most common signs of visceral involvement (Fig. 73-10). Some dogs lose weight despite having a ravenous appetite. A serious worsening of condition is often associated with ensuing renal failure. Progressive renal failure may be accompanied by anorexia, mental depression, polyuria, polydipsia, and vomiting. Transient diarrhea may occur. Renal failure may be the sole apparent abnormality in dogs with VL; dogs with this condition in endemic areas should be tested for leishmaniasis.

In cases of overt disease, decreased physical activity is obvious and related to somnolence, decreased endurance, and locomotion disturbances. Locomotion disturbances may be caused by neuralgia, polyarthritis, polymyositis, footpad clefts, interdigital ulcers, osteoarticular and osteolytic lesions, or proliferative periostitis.[5,28,200b] Body rectal temperature may fluctuate but is usually normal or subfebrile. Immunosuppression may promote the occurrence of concomitant infections, hence the clinical picture may be complicated by conditions such as demodicosis, pyoderma, gastrointestinal disease, and pneumonia. Combined infections with *Ehrlichia, Babesia, Hepatozoon, Trypanosoma,* and *Dirofilaria* are quite common when *Leishmania* infection occurs in regions where these organisms are also endemic. Other less common manifestations may include pericardial tamponade,[75] masticatory myositis,[210] pancreatitis,[36] meningitis,[215] chronic colitis,[67] pemphigus,[83] and polyarthritis.[201] Thrombosis has also occurred as a result of the nephrotic syndrome caused by glomerulonephritis.[72,74] Signs caused by disseminated intravascular coagulation or its complications may occur.[76]

Cats

Feline leishmaniasis is rare. Symptomatic leishmaniasis in domestic cats have included infection with *L. infantum,*[154,165,180a] *Leishmania mexicana,*[20,46] *Leishmania venezuelensis,*[29,30] *L. (Viannia) braziliensis,*[186] and unspecified species.[96]

Sporadic cases of feline leishmaniasis in southern Europe caused by *L. infantum* have been described. The cats had cutaneous ulcerative or nodular lesions essentially similar to those found in dogs (Fig. 73-11).[96,165,178a,160a] One cat had visceral involvement that included hepatosplenomegaly, icterus, lymphoplasmocytic gastroenteritis with abundant *Leishmania* parasites, and membranous glomerulonephritis.[96] A second cat from which *L. infantum* MON-1 zymodeme was cultured had disseminated crusty cutaneous lesions and amastigotes in the bone marrow.[154] Another cat with disseminated disease had uveitis as a predominant finding.[119a] Infected cats were seropositive for *Leishmania* antigen by various serologic methods.[96,154,165] Infection was reported in cats with feline leukemia virus and FIV[165] and also from cats with no retroviral disease.[154] Serologic or PCR surveys of cat populations in canine leishmaniasis-endemic regions in southern Europe indicate that feline infection might be more widespread than indicated by clinical manifestations.

Reports of feline leishmaniasis in the New World have primarily discussed cutaneous infections with species that cause CL in people. Pinnal nodules caused by *L. mexicana* were diagnosed in a cat from southern Texas.[46] Thirty months after radical pinnectomy was performed, the cat developed similar pinnal lesions that progressed to more diffuse lesions on the muzzle and in the nasal mucosa. No visceral organ involvement was found on necropsy.[20] Nodular lesions on the nose and ears have been observed in cats with CL in a *L. venezuelensis*–endemic region of Venezuela.[29] Infection with a dermatotrophic *Leishmania (Viannia)* species in a cat from Brazil was detected in a proliferative interdigital lesion on the cat's posterior paw.[159] In other instances, *L. (V.) braziliensis* was isolated from cutaneous lesions from two cats in Brazil.[186,200a] Experimental studies showed that cats were susceptible to a generally self-limiting infection with a human isolate of this organism.[190a] *L. chagasi* DNA sequences were amplified from a lesion on a cat's nose; the cat was from a previously nonendemic area in Brazil.[181]

Diagnosis
Clinical Laboratory Findings
A summary of the clinicopathologic findings from three large case series studies on canine leishmaniasis[40,110,191] is shown in Table 73-3. The most consistent serum biochemistry findings in dogs with clinical VL are serum hyperproteinemia with hyperglobulinemia and hypoalbuminemia resulting in a decreased albumin/globulin ratio. Marked hyperglobulinemia in dogs from *Leishmania*-endemic regions with no apparent cause or in dogs that have traveled to such areas should be investigated for VL. Mild increases of liver enzyme activities are frequent; however, grossly elevated liver enzyme activities, severe azotemia, or both are found in only a minority of dogs with VL. Proteinuria and some pathologic renal symptoms develop in most dogs with this disease, and subsequent renal failure caused by immune-complex glomerulonephritis eventually develops in dogs with progressive pathologic renal

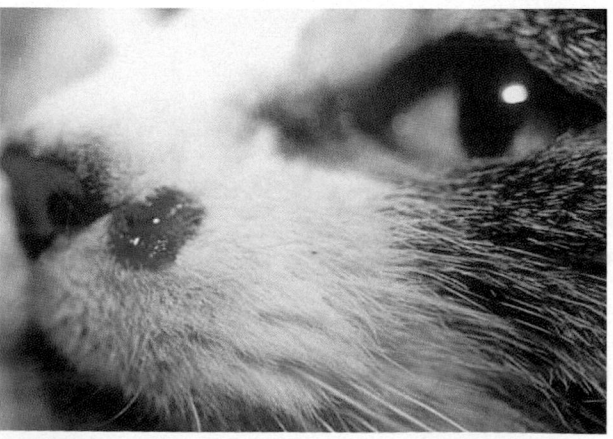

Fig   73-11   Cutaneous ulcer in cat with leishmaniasis. (Courtesy Maria Grazia Pennisi, University of Messina, Messina, Italy.)

Table • 73-3

Clinicopathologic Abnormalities in Dogs with Visceral Leishmaniasis[40,110,191]

ABNORMALITY	PERCENTAGE OF DOGS
Hyperproteinemia	63.3–72.8[40,110]
Hyperglobulinemia	76–100[40,191]
Hypoalbuminemia	68–94[40,191]
Decreased albumin/globulin ratio	76[40]
Azotemia	16–45[40,191]
Increased serum alkaline phosphatase activity	16–51[40,191]
Increased alanine aminotrasferase activity	16–61[40,191]
Proteinuria	71.5–85[110,191]
Anemia	60–73.4[110,191]
Leukocytosis	24[40]
Leukopenia	22[191]
Thrombocytopenia	29.3–50[40,191]
Positive for antinuclear antibody	31–53[40,191]
Positive Coombs' test	21–84[40,191]

symptoms. The urinary protein/creatinine ratio and enzymuria have been proposed as tests for assessing renal damage in affected animals.[156,157]

Mild to moderate nonregenerative anemia is frequently found. More rarely, regenerative hemolytic anemia caused by immune-mediated mechanisms is detected. Thrombocytopenia, mild leukocytosis, or leukopenia are inconsistent findings. However, lymphopenia is frequently reported in dogs with VL. Test results for antinuclear antibodies can be positive in dogs with *L. infantum* infections, especially if co-pathogenic infections are present.[195] Parasites are rarely detected in peripheral blood.[71b]

Definitive diagnosis of leishmaniasis can be confirmed by microscopic demonstration of parasites in cytologic preparations or histopathologic specimens, serology, culture of the organism in appropriate medium, or detection of parasite DNA using molecular methods.

Serologic Testing
Various serologic methods have been used to detect serum anti-*Leishmania* antibodies. Methods have included indirect fluorescent antibody testing, the enzyme-linked immunosorbent assay (ELISA), direct agglutination assays, and Western blotting.* A purified recombinant antigen for ELISA, rK39, has been used for detection of VL in people and dogs.[176,182,152a] In general, these methods have good sensitivities and specificities for the diagnosis of clinical VL. In naturally infected dogs, antibodies are present usually long before clinical signs of disease appear. Asymptomatically infected dogs that are slowly developing overt disease are often seropositive. However, a low positive titer result may be detected in animals that have been exposed but have not developed disease or in dogs that are persistent asymptomatic carriers. In an animal with compatible disease signs, a positive titer result strongly supports the preliminary diagnosis. Antibodies are very rarely undetectable in dogs with clinical signs of leishmaniasis. However, serology is thought to underestimate the true prevalence of asymptomatic infection in canine populations in endemic regions.[118,199] In cases with inconclusive serologic results, additional detection methods are advised.[100]

Decreasing titer results have been used to monitor therapy,[13,66,213] but titer results may decrease with the reduction in parasitic burden and not necessarily with total parasite elimination. Therefore results are often not consistent with parasitic cure, and relapses can occur frequently despite an initial lowering in antibody titer results. Serologic cross-reactivity with other pathogens is a problem in regions where *Trypanosoma* spp. are found, particularly in South and North America, where *Trypanosoma cruzi* is a pathogen of domestic canines and wild carnivores.[90]

Organism Identification by Microscopy and Culture
Definitive diagnosis is usually based on cytologic or histologic identification of amastigotes—either contained in macrophages or free—in routinely stained smears from lymph nodes, splenic aspirates, skin touch impressions, or bone marrow. The specificity of these methods is virtually 100%, but depending on the time spent searching for parasites, the maximum sensitivity is ±80% in dogs with clinical signs of the disease and lower in asymptomatic seropositive dogs. Cytologic studies may reveal few or no demonstrable parasites in dogs with overt clinical signs of disease. Identification of amastigotes in formalin-fixed, paraffin-embedded sections of canine skin or visceral tissues may be facilitated by immunohistochemical methods such as immunoperoxidase staining.[33,68] The diagnosis may also be established by the culture of parasites from tissues in Novy-MacNeal-Nicolle medium or Schneider's *Drosophila* medium or by the inoculation of hamsters.

*References 71, 94, 126, 152, 184, 211, 214.

Polymerase Chain Reaction
PCR demonstration of leishmanial DNA in tissues of infected animals is sensitive. It is routinely used for diagnostic purposes, epidemiologic studies, and screening for human and canine blood donors.[13,134] Several protocols with different target gene sequences have been used in laboratories. The small-subunit rRNA gene, the internal transcribed spacer of the ribosomal operon, and high-copy sequences of kinetoplast DNA (kDNA) are frequently used as PCR targets.[113] PCR can be performed on DNA extracted from tissues, blood, or even histopathologic specimens.[99,178] Noninvasive conjunctival PCR has recently been shown to be accurate in the direct diagnosis of canine infection.[202]

Pathologic Findings
Severely affected patients with chronic symptomatic disease are usually cachectic. The organs primarily affected are the skin and hemolymphatic organs. Generalized enlargement of lymph nodes and splenomegaly are usually present. Hepatomegaly may be present but is less common. Small, light-colored focal nodular granulomas may develop in various organs, including the skin and the kidneys. Mucosal ulcerations in the stomach, intestine, and colon are occasionally observed. Petechiae and ecchymotic bleeding in mucosal and serosal membranes develop in some cases. Osteolytic or proliferative periosteal lesions may be found in various parts of the skeleton.[5]

Histopathology reveals granulomatous perifolliculitis and perivascular dermatitis. Multifocal or diffuse plasmacytic infiltration of the skin, spleen, lymph nodes, liver, kidneys, bone marrow, intestine, and conjunctiva may be observed, with an occasional or large numbers of amastigotes in macrophages. Renal lesions include glomerulonephritis, interstitial nephritis, and occasionally amyloidosis.[147,222] Amyloidosis may also be present in the liver and other organs. Nervous system involvement with *Leishmania* organisms in choroid plexus inflammatory cells has been reported.[149]

Therapy
Dogs
Canine leishmaniasis in dogs is more resistant to therapy than human leishmaniasis, and only rarely are *Leishmania* organisms completely eliminated with available drugs.[19] Relapses necessitating retreatment are the rule rather than the exception, although some dogs may eventually become cured of the clinical disease (Table 73-4).

For decades, pentavalent antimonials (Sb^{5+}) have been the primary drug for treatment of canine and human VL. They selectively inhibit the protozoal enzymes required for glycolytic and fatty acid oxidation. Two Sb^{5+}-containing agents have been administered to dogs: meglumine antimoniate (trade name Glucantime; Merial, Lyon, France) and sodium stibogluconate (trade name Pentostam; Wellcome Foundation Ltd, United Kingdom; see Drug Formulary, Appendix 8). Both agents must be injected daily and may cause serious adverse effects. Meglumine antimoniate appears to cause milder side effects, but it is not licensed for use in some countries, including the United States. Sodium stibogluconate is currently involved in an investigational new drug protocol for human physicians through the Centers for Disease Control and Prevention (CDC) in the United States. The development of *L. infantum* strains that are resistant to Sb^{5+} has been reported in France, Spain, and Italy and is a major veterinary and public health concern.[37,38,86,116]

Dosage regimens for Sb^{5+} vary widely. Sb^{5+} is quickly excreted in the urine. Only a small part is reduced to the toxic Sb^{3+}, which may accumulate in the body. However, normal doses of the drug rarely cause signs of toxicity unless administered daily for longer than 2 months or administered to a patient with renal, cardiac, or hepatic failure. Antimonials may

Table • 73-4

Antimicrobial Therapy for Canine Leishmaniasis

DRUG[a]	DOSE (MG/KG)[b]	ROUTE	INTERVAL (HOURS)	DURATION[c] (WEEKS)
Meglumine antimoniate (Glucuantime)	100	IV, SC	24	3—4
Sodium stibogluconate[d] (Pentostam)	30—50	IV, SC	24	3—4
Allopurinol[e]	20	PO	12—24	Indefinitely

IV, Intravenous; *SC*, subcutaneous; *PO*, by mouth.
[a]For additional information on use of these drugs, see Drug Formulary, Appendix 8.
[b]Dose per administration at specified interval.
[c]All long-term survivors must be treated on multiple occasions because of relapses.
[d]Available in the United States for treatment of human infections by special request from the Centers for Disease Control and Prevention, Atlanta, Ga.
[e]Some studies suggest that combined therapy with allopurinol and antimony compounds is the most effective for treating *L. infantum* infections.

be injected intramuscularly (IM), subcutaneously (SC), or intravenously (IV). IM injections in the thigh have resulted in severe lameness as a result of muscle fibrosis. Possible local complications of SC administration are less serious but include local inflammation. IV injections may cause thrombophlebitis and hence thrombosis. Results of pharmacokinetic studies of Sb^{5+} compounds in dogs are controversial,[205,209] but the clinical effect and parasitologic clearance is the same when 100 mg/kg of meglumine antimoniate is given IV once daily or SC divided into two daily doses.[193]

An alternative to Sb^{5+} injection in dogs is therapy with allopurinol[39,110] (see Drug Formulary, Appendix 8). Allopurinol is a hypoxanthine compound that is metabolized by *Leishmania* spp. to produce an analogue of inosine. The analogue is incorporated into leishmanial RNA, causing faulty protein translation and inhibition of parasite multiplication. This drug is less expensive than Sb^{5+} compounds, can be administered orally, has few adverse effects, and is readily available, even in the United States and other countries. Use of allopurinol causes hyperxanthinuria, which may incidentally produce urolithiasis. It is used with increasing frequency by veterinarians, often in combination with Sb^{5+}.[8,52,66,82,207] Dosage schedules vary widely, and the optimal dose has not been defined. Clinical remission is frequently obtained by treating with allopurinol alone. A dose of 20 mg/kg once daily often results in remarkable clinical improvement within 4 weeks and reduction of parasites to undetectable numbers. However, relapses consistently occur once therapy has been discontinued. Even after conscientious administration of the drug for 6 months, complete recovery is rare.[119] Relapses develop more insidiously and are often less serious than with meglumine; however, deterioration of kidney function may commence during allopurinol therapy despite resolution of dermal lesions and general improvement in the clinical condition. This progression is likely caused by continuation of immune complex deposition. When Sb^{5+} is used as the initial drug for treatment, allopurinol may be used in combination.[158b] At the end of combined treatment, allopurinol is commonly recommended for long-term maintenance therapy or even indefinitely for dogs diagnosed with symptomatic leishmaniasis. In a study from Holland, dogs treated with 20 mg/kg per day of allopurinol had a 78% chance of survival for more than 4 years (if they did not have severe renal failure when therapy was started).[194]

Amphotericin B (AMB), a polyene macrolide primarily used as an antifungal drug, also has activity against some protozoa. It acts by binding to ergosterol and altering the cell membrane permeability. AMB has a profound toxic effect on the canine kidney by causing renal vasoconstriction and reduction of the glomerular filtration rate and possibly by acting directly on renal epithelial cells. It can be administered to dogs with leishmaniasis in a highly nephrotoxic free form, lipid emulsion, or liposomal formulation that reduces its toxic effects and directs the drug to being taken up by macrophages and accumulating in visceral organs. Liposomal AMB is effective in the treatment of people and has largely replaced therapy of human patients with antimonials in Italy and other European countries.[86] However, a study on the use of liposomal AMB in dogs failed to show that treated dogs had long-term clinical improvements with elimination of the infection.[150] The use of AMB in a lipid emulsion of soybean oil administered IV to dogs pretreated with saline and mannitol has had higher clinical cure success rates and more negative posttreatment parasitologic tests in some animals. This therapy is associated primarily with transient side effects of anorexia and vomiting and requires careful monitoring of renal parameters.[42,115]

Additional drugs that are not recommended as first-line therapy for canine VL because of the adverse effects associated with treatment include pentamidine and aminosidine.[166,175] Pentamidine, an aromatic diamidine used also for pneumocystosis, babesiosis, and trypanomiasis, is injected IM in dogs and can cause severe irritation at the site of injection, hypotension, tachycardia, and vomiting. Aminosidine sulphate is an aminoglycoside antibiotic that is toxic at doses that are clinically effective against *Leishmania*. Other drugs that are being investigated for the treatment of canine leishmaniasis include alkylphosphocholine derivatives related to the drug miltefosine, which is used for treating some forms of human VL,[199a] and metronidazole.

In a trial comparing the efficacy of conventional treatment with meglumine antimoniate and allopurinol against use of metronidazole and spiramycin, treated dogs showed some clinical improvement without a parasitologic cure, similar to control dogs.[160a]

If dogs are seriously ill, and especially if they are in severe renal failure, it may be necessary to restore fluid and acid-base balances before antileishmanial drugs are administered. Because of its lower toxicity, allopurinol is preferred to a Sb^{5+} compound in these cases. The prognosis of canine leishmaniasis depends on the severity of injury to the dog's systems at the time of diagnosis and the dog's individual response and rate of deterioration. In dogs that have not reached a progressive state of renal failure, treatment frequently significantly improves dermal and visceral signs of the disease. Immune responses were monitored in dogs before and after treatment and have indicated that in some cases, parasite-specific cell mediated immunity that is absent before therapy is regained after drug administration but may deteriorate again during a clinical relapse.[53,143,175]

Cats

Almost no published information is available on drug therapy for feline leishmaniasis. One cat in Spain with primarily cutaneous lesions was treated with 5 mg/kg of meglumine antimoniate SC combined with 10 mg/kg ketoconazole orally. A 4-week course of combined therapy was repeated three times, with 10 days without therapy between each course, and resulted in the resolution of the cutaneous lesions.[96] Topical treatment of cutaneous *L. mexicana* infection in a cat with clotrimazole and subsequently with paromomycin did not improve the dermal lesions.[20]

Control and Prevention

Efforts to control leishmaniasis in the canine populations in endemic countries are controversial and generally have not been considered to be successful.[14,44,59,158] Killing symptomatic and seropositive dogs is obviously unacceptable to the owners, but it is also ineffective because nonsymptomatic dogs, occasionally seronegative dogs, and possibly wild canids are sources of parasite transmission. Furthermore, available methods for testing do not identify all infected dogs, and a population of young susceptible puppies can replace the culled animals.[145] Spraying for sandfly vectors and eradicating their presumptive breeding places has limited effectiveness in preventing spread of the disease. No prophylactic drug has yet been shown to be effective against infection, and medical treatment of infected dogs with antileishmanial drugs is ineffective in eliminating the parasite.

Sandfly vectors of VL are primarily active outside houses, therefore selective spraying inside houses is ineffective. However, spraying inside and around kennels could reduce the risk of infection. Measures to protect the individual dog include keeping the animal indoors as much as possible from 1 hour before sunset to 1 hour after dawn during the vector season and installation of fine-mesh screens to keep sandflies out of kennels. Topical insecticides for protecting dogs against sandfly bites include solutions, spot-on tubes, sprays, and collars. A spray containing permethrin and pyroproxyfene (trade name Duowin; Virbac, Fort Worth, Tex., www.virbacorp.com) is recommended every 3 weeks for adult dogs and every 2 weeks for puppies.[139] A spot-on containing imidacloprid and permethrin (K9 Advantix,® Bayer, Leverkusen, Germany) is recommended for dogs every 4 weeks for repelling sandflies. Deltamethrin-impregnated collars (trade name Scalibor; Intervet, Boxmeer, Netherlands; *www.intervet.com*) have been shown to protect dogs for about 8 months from more than 90% of bites from *Phlebotomus perniciosus*, the primary vector of *L. infantum* in France, and *Lutzomyia longipalpis*, a major South American vector.[50,106] A controlled study on the effect of using collars on dogs in a focus of VL in Iran indicated that the seroconversion rate after 1 year in dogs and children in intervention villages was significantly lower than in control villages.[136] Topical insecticide protection appears to be valuable for dogs in endemic regions during transmission seasons and for dogs traveling to these areas. Use of collars on client-owned infected dogs treated medically and living in infected areas is warranted.

Vaccination of dogs against VL could be a major preventative measure. Trials with several types of candidate vaccines for *Leishmania* in animal models have been carried out during the past 4 decades. These included the assessment of attenuated or killed whole parasites, purified parasite fractions, recombinant antigens, live bacteria expressing *Leishmania* antigens, DNA vaccines, and the use of numerous adjuvants.[31,31a,85] A canine vaccine is now commercially available in Brazil, and another vaccine brand is likely to be marketed in Europe in the near future.

Public Health Considerations

VL is a serious human disease that may be fatal if untreated. Malnutrition appears to be a predisposing factor for the progression of infection.[11,17] Traditionally, VL primarily affected young children and infants, but now it is also often a complication in adults infected with HIV or those receiving cytostatic or immunosuppressive drugs.[88,101,177,218]

Transmission of *L. infantum* from dogs or wild canids to people via sandflies is considered to be the primary route of infection involved in zoonotic VL. Asymptomatically infected dogs have been shown to be infectious to sandflies, and symptomatic dogs may be infectious shortly after treatment with antileishmanial drugs.[8] Ownership of an infected dog does not appear to be a major risk factor for human infections in Europe, where the ratio of clinically affected people to dogs is usually low. However, a study from Iran indicated that dog ownership is a significant risk factor for childhood seropositivity.[137] The link between dog and human infections probably differs from one region and life style to another and could depend on multiple factors including human nutrition, time spent outdoors, the density of dogs, and the behavior of sandfly vectors. Transmission by direct contact between dogs and people is speculated to be rare, if it occurs at all, and although it has not been well documented, it cannot be ruled out. Transmission of *L. infantum* through blood products has been reported in dogs that received blood transfusions from infected canine donors and in people.[153] Studies in Spain of humans who use IV drugs and share needles have indicated that the infection was transmitted through the needles.[48] Therefore direct contact with contaminated hypodermic needles or with open wounds or exudates from dogs with leishmaniasis should be avoided.

Infected pets may remain disease carriers despite treatment. In areas where sandfly vectors are found, this poses a problem to owners, veterinarians, and local public health and environmental agencies who are concerned with the risk to people and animals. Before deciding on the fate of an infected pet, owners should be consulted and educated about the disease, its zoonotic nature, the prognosis for their dog, what should be expected from therapy, and safety precautions that should be taken. A clear, official policy based on relevant research and a calculated estimation of the risk to the community is desirable.

CANINE AND FELINE AMERICAN TEGUMENTARY LEISHMANIASIS

Gad Baneth

Cutaneous (tegumentary) leishmaniasis is caused by *L. (V.) braziliensis*, *L. (V.) peruviana*, or related species and affects dogs and people in South America. Infection in dogs has been reported from Brazil, Argentina, Bolivia, Peru, Ecuador, Colombia, Venezuela, and Panama.[123,173] Sporadic infection of cats has also been reported.[159,186,59a,200a] Outbreaks of American tegumentary leishmaniasis have been associated with deforestation of jungle areas.[155]

The clinical signs of disease in dogs include chronic ulcerative lesions on the ears or other areas of the skin, mucocutanous erosive lesions, and lymphadenomegaly.[129,155,164] Ulceration sometimes involves the nasal or auricular cartilage.[129] Hematogenous dissemination of parasites in dogs is likely, and the presence of parasite DNA has been demonstrated by PCR of the blood and bone marrow from symptomatically and asymptomatically infected dogs.[174] Cats have developed cutaneous nodular lesions on their skin. Diagnosis can be confirmed by microscopic detection of parasites in lesions, in culture, by specific serologic tests, or by PCR. The number of parasites found in canine dermal lesions is usually low. Infected dogs respond to antimonial therapy; however, they remain infected after therapy and commonly have clinical relapses.[164] Numerous wild animals including opossums and rodents have been reported to be infected with the agents of tegumentary leishmanaisis. Although it is involved in this disease, the dog does not appear to be a significant reservoir host of infection for people.[173]

CANINE VISCERAL LEISHMANIASIS IN NORTH AMERICA

Edward B. Breitschwerdt and Peter Schantz

Endemic VL is an emerging disease in dogs in North America. Although human and canine VL are well established in parts of Asia, Africa, southern Europe, Central America, and South America, VL has been infrequently reported in people and domestic animals in the United States and Canada.

Etiology

Before 2000, most cases of canine VL in the United States and Canada were associated with a history of international travel.[98,119,183,219] However, between 1980 and 2001, four reports of canine VL were made in which the dogs had no history of foreign travel. These reports included an American foxhound from a kennel in Oklahoma, an English foxhound maintained in a closed research colony at The Ohio State University, a pet basenji from Texas, and a pet toy poodle from Maryland.[9,62,189,204] The infected dogs in these reports had not traveled outside of the United States, and neither a source of infection nor an insect vector was ever identified. Two additional outbreaks of VL in foxhounds were recognized by one of the authors in kennels in Michigan in 1989 and Alabama in 1994. Since that time, several laboratories have identified serologic, molecular, or culture-based evidence of *L. infantum* infection in numerous foxhounds that are indigenous to the United States (Fig. 73-12).[60] Retrospectively, it now appears that canine VL was established as an autochthonous disease in American foxhounds in North America, at least after 1979.[9] Investigation of a disease outbreak among foxhounds in an index kennel located in Duchess County, New York, ultimately led to the discovery that infection with *L. infantum* was well established in foxhounds throughout much of North America. The initial outbreak investigation involved a cooperative effort among the College of Veterinary Medicine at North Carolina State University, the Division of Parasitic Diseases in the National Center for Infectious Diseases of the CDC (Atlanta, Ga.), the Walter Reed Army Institute of Research (Washington, DC), the New York State Department of Agriculture and Markets and Department of Health, local veterinarians, and the kennel owners and staff.[81] At the time VL was diagnosed in the four index cases, 46 (41%) of 112 dogs in the New York foxhound kennel were infected. Infection was diagnosed by a positive *Leishmania* culture result, PCR amplification of *Leishmania* DNA, identification of amastigotes by cytology or histopathology, or seroreactivity (all titers equal to or greater than 1:64) to *Leishmania* antigens. This suggested a high rate of exposure or infection with *Leishmania* species within the kennel population, particularly because serologic testing tends to underestimate the prevalence and incidence of *Leishmania* infections in endemic regions. After infection, dogs or people can remain subclinically infected for months to years before the onset of disease manifestations.

Subsequent to the New York kennel investigation, the CDC screened more than 10,000 foxhounds and found seropositive foxhounds in 69 kennels in 21 states and 2 Canadian provinces.[185] Now that this disease has become endemic in the United States, it is possible that leishmaniasis will be recognized more often in dog breeds other than American foxhounds. In addition, autochthonous human cases may be diagnosed in the United States in the future.

Epidemiology

In endemic regions, Phlebotomine sandflies (genus *Lutzomyia* in the New World) are the primary insect vectors for transmission of *Leishmania* spp.[70,173] In addition to dogs and humans, cats, horses, coyotes, foxes, and rodents can be infected with *Leishmania* spp. However, dogs are considered the primary *L. infantum* reservoir in endemic countries in southern Europe (France, Italy, Spain, and Malta). Based on isoenzyme electrophoresis, many of the North American isolates obtained from 40 foxhounds, including the isolate obtained from a foxhound in Oklahoma in 1980, are *L. infantum* MON-1, which is the predominant *Leishmania* zymodeme found in southern Europe.[9,81,89] In endemic regions the protozoal life cycle begins when the infective form—the promastigote—is injected into the skin of the vertebrate host by the sandfly (see Fig. 73-4).[104] After entering the host, the promastigote is transformed into the nonflagellated form—the amastigote. Amastigote multiplication in macrophages occurs by binary fission either locally in the cutaneous or mucocutaneous forms or systemically throughout the reticuloendothelial system in the visceral form. Vectors ingest amastigotes while obtaining a blood meal from the infected host. If ingested by an unsuitable vector, the amastigotes are either destroyed or passed out in the feces. If the vector is suitable, ingested amastigotes transform into promastigotes and attach to the midgut epithelium of the sandfly. Promastigotes then detach and move cranially to the foregut, where some attach and others remain free for subsequent transmission through a bite, which completes the transmission cycle. In certain regions, additional epidemiologic complexity is created by the ability of certain sandflies to serve as hosts to multiple *Leishmania* spp.

Fourteen species of *Lutzomyia* sandflies have been recorded in North America, and only three (*Lutzomyia shannoni*, *Lutzomyia diabolica*, and *Lutzomyia vexator*) have been suspected as vectors for *Leishmania* spp.[104,117,220] Because of the lack of human leishmaniasis in the United States, protozoal research laboratories have only recently evaluated indigenous sandfly species for their ability to transmit *L. donovani*. The most prevalent sandfly in the southeastern United States (all Atlantic coastal states south of Pennsylvania and west to Louisiana) is *L. shannoni*. Previous studies have demonstrated that *L. shannoni* develop a very heavy parasitemia when feeding on dogs infected with *L. infantum*; however, the vector

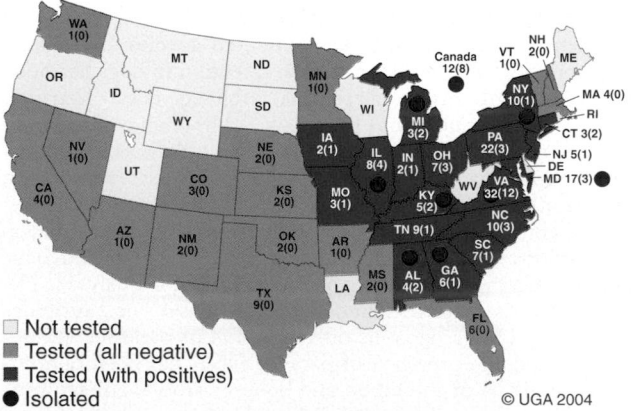

Fig 73-12 Seroprevalence of leishmaniasis in dog kennels. Numbers tested are shown, and number with positive results are in parentheses. Solid dots indicate states where organism has been isolated from affected dogs. (Data courtesy Zandra Duprey, Centers for Disease Control and Prevention, Atlanta, Ga.; map courtesy, University of Georgia, Athens, Ga.)

competence of *L. shannoni* for transmission of *L. infantum* has not been established. In the previously mentioned New York kennel, a significant correlation was found between a positive *Leishmania* status and *Ehrlichia canis* seroreactivity ($p = 0.03$).[81] Although not thought to occur in nature, *L. infantum* has been experimentally transmitted by *Rhipicephalus sanguineus*, a known vector for *E. canis*.[138] Foxhounds with a positive *Leishmania* status were 5 times more likely to have traveled to the southeastern United States or to have been older than 18 months of age. These factors tend to support the presence of a competent insect vector, potentially in the southeastern United States. No evidence supports vector transmission in the northeastern United States; adjacent foxhound kennels and beagles and basset hounds housed on the same premises during the summer months had no serologic evidence of exposure to *L. infantum*.[81] Serologic screening of pet dogs, coyotes, and foxes from the United States has not resulted in the detection of *L. infantum* antibodies.[81] The mode of *L. infantum* transmission among foxhounds in North America has not yet been determined.

Foxhound kennels are geographically distributed throughout much of the United States. Because of the substantial number of foxhounds with serologic evidence of exposure to *Leishmania* species, dog-to-dog transmission via direct contact, exposure to blood products from an infected dog, or possibly during parturition or breeding may explain the high prevalence of leishmaniasis in this breed. Historic evidence from nonendemic countries supports dog-to-dog transmission by direct contact (referred to as *mechanical transfer*) and perinatal transmission.[127,194] Leishmaniasis can also be transmitted from dog to dog by blood transfusions.[153] In these instances, macrophages containing amastigotes serve as the source of infection. The Penn Animal Blood Bank at the Veterinary Hospital of the University of Pennsylvania has documented transmission of *L. infantum* from foxhound donors to canine patients.[153] Because of the high *L. infantum* seroprevalence, the use of foxhounds as blood donors in North America may not be advisable, particularly because serologic testing may not detect chronically infected dogs.

Clinical Findings

Clinical manifestations in foxhounds included chronic wasting, conjunctivitis, anterior uveitis, retinitis, facial alopecia, severe muscle atrophy, lymphadenopathy, polyarthritis, and protein-losing nephropathy, which may be accompanied by renal failure.[81,153] These are the same abnormalities associated with canine VL in endemic regions. Despite chronic infection, hematologic and biochemical abnormalities may be mild or absent. When present, anemia, thrombocytopenia, lymphocytosis, hypoalbuminemia, hyperglobulinemia, hyperamylasemia, and azotemia are the most frequently detected laboratory abnormalities. In addition to foxhounds, other breeds of dogs with unexplained wasting disease, especially if accompanied by hypergammaglobulinemia, bilateral facial alopecia similar to the pattern observed for demodectic mange, or unexplained glomerulonephritis and protein-losing glomerulonephropathy, should be tested for exposure to *L. infantum*. In pet dogs, owners have reported behavioral changes, including an increase in aggressive tendencies, as the first indication of leishmaniasis.

Diagnosis

VL can be diagnosed by cytologic or histopathologic identification of organisms, isolation of amastigotes, detection of serum antibodies, or PCR amplification of leishmanial DNA. Antibody titers of greater than 1:16 are considered indicative of *Leishmania* exposure.[185] However, serologic cross-reactivity between *Leishmania* spp. and *T. cruzi* can occur, a factor that should be considered, particularly in kennel or hunting dogs.

Although *T. cruzi* is enzootic among wild animals throughout much of North America, reports of infections in domestic dogs have generally been limited to Texas, Louisiana Oklahoma, and Virginia (see Chapter 72).[21,22,79] The extent to which infection with *T. cruzi* contributes to the high level of seroreactivity to *Leishmania* species antigens in North American foxhounds remains unclear. Western immunoblotting or the use of a *T. cruzi*–specific ELISA test (developed for humans) may help differentiate between exposure to *L. infantum* and to *T. cruzi*. Although presumably infrequent, dogs can be infected with *Leishmania* species without developing a detectable antibody response. In foxhounds, this is particularly true when a dog is chronically infected but has not developed clinical disease manifestations. As an alternative to serologic testing, PCR can be used to confirm the diagnosis. Of the seroreactive foxhounds from the New York kennel, infection in 65% (26 out of 40) was confirmed by PCR detection of *Leishmania* species DNA in peripheral blood anticoagulated by ethylenediaminetetraacetic acid (EDTA).[81] Peripheral blood was selected as the diagnostic sample for PCR because of convenience; however, the sensitivity of PCR to confirm *Leishmania* infection in seropositive dogs or to detect subclinical infection can be enhanced by examination of lymph node or bone marrow aspirates rather than blood.[13,171] For diagnostic assistance with leishmaniasis, serum (for antibody determination) or EDTA blood (for PCR) samples can be submitted to the Vector-Borne Diseases Diagnostic Laboratory, North Carolina State University, Raleigh, N.C. (Contact the laboratory for appropriate submission forms before submitting specimens; see Appendix 5 for specific contact information for this laboratory.)

Therapy

For details regarding treatment of sick dogs, refer to the previous general *Leishmaniasis* section in this chapter. No treatment protocol has been proved to cure VL in dogs.[65] Despite clinical improvement or a clinical cure (i.e., a healthy appearance after treatment), relapses are common, and chemotherapeutic elimination of *L. infantum* has not been achieved with any drug tested. However, continuous chemotherapy with allopurinol most likely decreases the parasitemia to a level that has little risk of direct or sandfly transmission (see Table 73-4).[39,52] Therefore this approach could be used for the medical management of pet or kennel dogs in the United States; however, periodic (every 6 months to 1 year) serologic screening of uninfected dogs in the kennel or household is recommended. In nonendemic regions, euthanasia has been promoted to prevent leishmaniasis from becoming established. Some foxhound kennels have adopted a test-and-elimination approach in an effort to remove infected dogs from the environment.

Public Health Considerations

Because of sandfly exposure in endemic regions, the incidence of leishmaniasis in people is about 2 million cases per year (1.5 million cases of the cutaneous form and 500,000 cases of the visceral form).[217] If untreated, leishmaniasis is generally fatal. Disease manifestations in people can be quite nonspecific in immunocompetent individuals; however, children and severely immunocompromised people are most likely to develop serious disease manifestations. *L. infantum* was detected by PCR and culture in asymptomatic carriers who were blood donors in France.[67]

Numerous pet dogs belonging to military personnel and other individuals from *Leishmania*-endemic regions are being transported to the United States.[151] Although potentially chronically infected, these dogs can remain healthy for months to years after being introduced or reintroduced to United States. If sandflies in North America are able to transmit VL from infected to susceptible dogs, then vector transmission of this serious human pathogen from infected dogs to humans is possible. An autochthonous human case of VL from the United States has not been reported, and no data supports vector transmission among dogs in North America.

SUGGESTED READINGS*

7. Altet L, Francino O, Solano-Gallego L, et al. 2002. Mapping and sequencing of the canine NRAMP1 gene and identification of mutations in leishmaniasis-susceptible dogs. *Infect Immun* 70:2763-2771.

19. Baneth G, Shaw SE. 2002. Chemotherapy of canine leishmaniosis. *Vet Parasitol* 106:315-324.

40. Ciaramella P, Oliva G, De Luna R, et al. 1997. A retrospective clinical study of canine leishmaniasis in 150 dogs naturally infected with *L. infantum*. *Vet Rec* 141: 539-543.

44. Courtenay O, Quinell RJ, Garcez LM, et al. 2002a. Infectiousness in a cohort of Brazilian dogs: why culling fails to control visceral leishmaniasis in areas of high transmission. *J Infect Dis* 186:1314-1320.

85. Gradoni L. 2001. An update on antileishmanial vaccine candidates and prospects for a canine *Leishmania* vaccine. *Vet Parasitol* 100:87-103.

91. Guarga JL, Moreno J, Lucientes J, et al. 2000. Canine leishmaniasis transmission: higher infectivity amongst naturally infected dogs to sand flies is associated with lower proportions of T helper cells. *Res Vet Sci* 69: 249-253.

103. Kaye PM, Curry AJ, Blackwell JM. 1991. Differential production of Th1- and Th2-derived cytokines does not determine the genetically controlled or vaccine-induced rate of cure in murine visceral leishmaniasis. *J Immunol* 146:2763-2770.

118. Leontidas LS, Saridomichelakis MN, Billinis C, et al. 2002. A cross-sectional study of *Leishmania* spp. infection in clinically healthy dogs with polymerase chain reaction and serology in Greece. *Vet Parasitol* 109:19-27.

136. Mazloumi Gavgani AS, Hodjati MH, Mohite H, et al. 2002a. Effect of insecticide-impregnated dog collars on incidence of zoonotic visceral leishmaniasis in Iranian children: a matched-cluster randomized trial. *Lancet* 360:374-379.

140. Miralles GD, Stoeckle MY, McDermott DF, et al. 1994. Th1 and Th2 cell-associated cytokines in experimental visceral leishmaniasis. *Infect Immun* 62:1058-1063.

143. Moreno J, Nieto J, Chamizo C, et al. 1999. The immune response and PMBC subsets in canine visceral leishmaniasis before, and after, chemotherapy. *Vet Immunol Immunopathol* 71:181-195.

173. Reithinger R, Davies CR. 1999. Is the domestic dog (*Canis familiaris*) a reservoir host of American cutaneous leishmaniasis? A critical review of the current evidence. *Am J Trop Med Hyg* 61:530-541.

184a. Schantz P, Steurer FJ, Duprey ZH, et al. 2005. Autochthonous visceral leishmaniasis in dogs in North America, *J Am Vet Med Assoc* 226:1316-1322.

199. Solano-Gallego L, Morel P, Arboix M, et al. 2001b. Prevalence of *Leishmania infantum* infection in dogs living in an area of canine leishmaniasis endemicity using PCR on several tissues and serology. *J Clin Microbiol* 39:560-563.

*See the CD-ROM for a complete list of references.

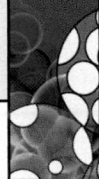

CHAPTER • 74

Hepatozoonosis

Hepatozoonosis is an arthropod-borne infection caused by apicomplexan protozoa from the family Hepatozoidae in the suborder Adeleorina.[16] Based on analysis of 18S ribosomal DNA sequences and morphologic features, parasites in the genus *Hepatozoon* are believed to be most closely related to other apicomplexan parasites such as *Plasmodium* spp. and piroplasms.[17] More than 300 different species of *Hepatozoon* have been described in amphibians, reptiles, birds, marsupials, and mammals.[94] Of these, more than 120 species infect snakes, and approximately 50 have been reported in mammals. The genus was named *Hepatozoon* because merogonic development of the type strain *Hepatozoon muris* was observed in the liver of rats.[68] However, the liver is not necessarily a major target tissue for other *Hepatozoon* spp. *Hepatozoon* spp. that infect amphibians, reptiles, and avian hosts parasitize mainly erythrocytes, whereas gamonts of *Hepatozoon* spp. infecting mammals are found primarily in leukocytes. *Hepatozoon* spp. have a basic life cycle that includes asexual development with merogony followed by gamontogony in a vertebrate intermediate host such as the dog and sexual development leading to sporogony in a hematophagous invertebrate definitive host such as a tick. A variety of blood-sucking arthropod vectors serves as definitive hosts for different *Hepatozoon* spp. These hosts include ticks, mites, mosquitoes, sand flies, tsetse flies, fleas, lice, and reduviid bugs.[94] Unlike many vector-borne protozoal and bacterial pathogens that are transmitted via the salivary glands, *Hepatozoon* transmission takes place by ingestion of the definitive host, an invertebrate that contains mature oocysts, by the intermediate vertebrate host. Two species that use domestic dogs as the intermediate host, *Hepatozoon canis* and *Hepatozoon americanum*, have been identified. Infections caused by *H. canis* and *H. americanum* will be discussed in two separate sections in this chapter.

HEPATOZOON CANIS INFECTION

Gad Baneth

Etiology
Dogs
H. canis infection (HCI) in dogs was first described from India in 1905,[48] and until 1997, the presumption was that canine hepatozoonosis was caused by a single species. However,

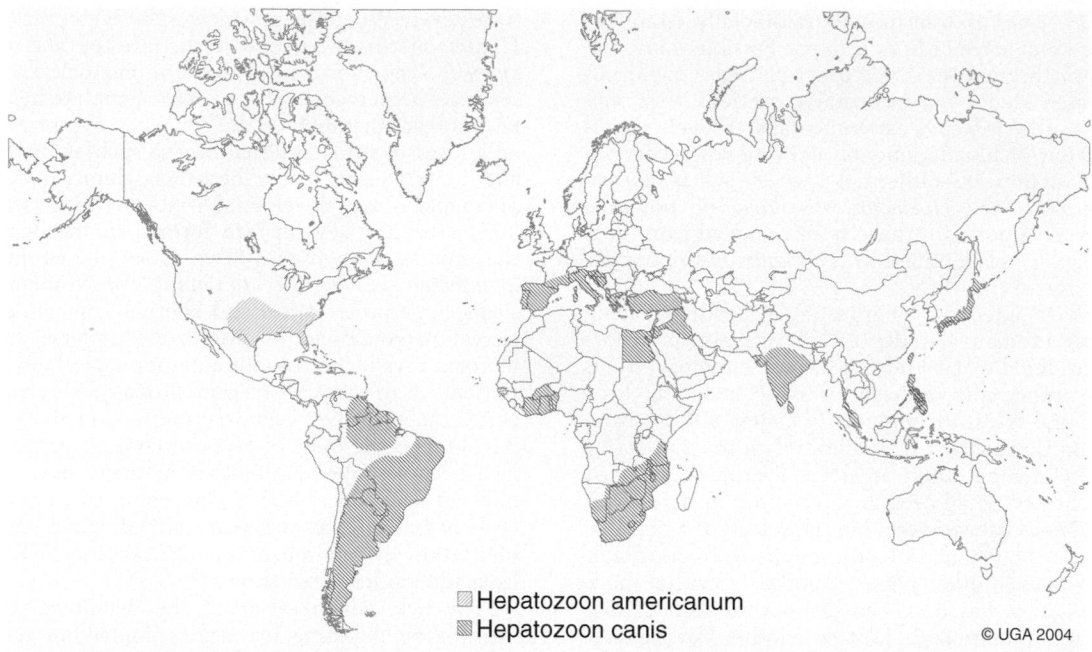

Fig 74-1 A map of the reported geographic distributions of *H. canis* and *H. americanum*. (Map courtesy University of Georgia, Athens, Ga.)

research elucidating the pathologic and clinical syndromes associated with hepatozoonosis,* its transmission by tick species, the parasite life cycle,[9,63,64] and genetic and antigenic characterization of *Hepatozoon* isolates,[4,66] has led to the recognition that two distinct *Hepatozoon* spp. infect dogs. This finding resulted in naming the parasite that infects dogs in the southern United States *H. americanum*[100] and separating it from the previously described *H. canis.*[8] The discussion in this first section will focus on *H. canis* infection.

Cats and Wild Carnivores

The host range of *H. canis* in mammalian carnivores other than the domestic dog has not been clarified. *H. canis* or *Hepatozoon* spp. morphologically resembling *H. canis* have been reported from several wild canine species, from domestic and wild felines, and from other carnivore species, including the red fox *(Vulpes vulpes),*[21,24,62] crab-eating fox *(Cerocyon thous),*[1] black-backed jackal *(Canis mesomelas),*[67] golden jackal *(Canis aureus),*[92] African wild dog *(Lycaon pictus),*[96] hyena *(Crocuta crocuta),*[67] palm civet *(Paradoxurus hermaphroditus),*[55] cheetah *(Acinonyx jubatus),*[67] leopard *(Panthera pardus),*[67] lion *(Panthera leo),*[28] and Pallas cat *(Felis manul).*[15] Although the probability that *H. canis* may infect other animals species is high, particularly those that are closely related to the domestic dog, this has not been demonstrated by experimental transmission or genetic characterization and comparison of isolates. Reports before 1997 of *H. canis*–like organisms in North American wild carnivores are possibly related to the species known today as *H. americanum* or to a species other than *H. canis.* For a further discussion on feline hepatozoonosis, see the following section.

Epidemiology

Geographic Distribution and Prevalence

HCI is prevalent in regions of tropical, subtropical, and temperate climate. HCI has been reported from the domestic dog *(Canis familiaris)* from most continents and numerous countries, including Greece,[54] Italy,[39] France,[89] Spain[49] and Portu-

*References: 14, 34, 61, 80, 100.

gal in southern Europe; Israel[50] and Egypt[36] in the Middle East; South Africa[67] and Nigeria[35] in Africa; India,[48] Sri Lanka, Singapore,[55] Malaysia,[88] The Philippines,[77] Thailand,[90] and Japan[75] in Asia; and Brazil,[40] Argentina, and Venezuela in South America (Fig. 74-1). In addition, imported cases of HCI in dogs brought into nonendemic areas have been detected in several countries, including Germany and Holland.[25,37] The homogeneity of different *H. canis* isolates using comparison of conserved DNA sequences has not been studied thoroughly. However, a phylogenetic analysis of a partial sequence of the 18S ribosomal RNA gene from *Hepatozoon* isolates from dogs in Japan indicated that these isolates had a 99% identity with *H. canis* sequenced from Israel and were more distant to *H. americanum.*[47]

The prevalence of HCI in different regions ranges considerably. Circulating *H. canis* gamonts were detected in 39% of the dogs surveyed in rural areas of Rio de Janeiro state in Brazil,[78] in 22% of dogs surveyed in Zaria in Nigeria,[35] and in 1.2% in Malaysia.[88] Serologic studies of HCI revealed that 33% of the dogs surveyed in Israel[12] and 4.2% in the Yamaguchi region in Japan[46] had been exposed to the parasite, as indicated by the presence of anti-*H. canis* antibodies demonstrated by indirect fluorescent antibody (FA) testing. As found also for other tick-borne diseases, including canine ehrlichiosis, babesiosis, and Lyme disease, the exposure rate for HCI in endemic areas is often much greater than the prevalence of clinical disease. Most dogs that are infected with *H. canis* probably undergo a subclinical infection. Among the dogs surveyed for *H. canis* antibodies in Israel, of 33% seropositive dogs, 3% had detectable blood gamonts, and only 1% had severe clinical signs associated with the infection.[12]

Transmission

The distribution of canine hepatozoonosis is tied closely to its acarine definitive hosts. The primary vector of *H. canis* is the brown dog tick, *Rhipicephalus sanguineus.*[9,20,103] It is a three-host tick that is considered to be the most widely distributed tick species in the world.[101] *R. sanguineus* is adaptable to different environmental conditions and is found in warm and temperate regions, making the potential distribution of HCI widespread. *H. canis* is transmitted transtadially from the nymph to the adult stage in *R. sanguineus*. Possible transovarial transmission through the tick's ovary and eggs could not be demonstrated under experimental conditions.[12] *R. sanguineus* ticks can be infected experimentally through percutaneous injection of blood gamonts, allowing researchers to study the disease in ticks.[9] Other tick species such as *Haemophysalis longicornus* and *Haemophysalis flava* are potential vectors and were reported to have been removed from dogs with HCI in Japan and identified with *Hepatozoon*-like oocysts in their hemocoel.[73]

In addition to infection by ingesting ticks that contain mature oocysts, alternative modes of HCI transmission to dogs should be considered when studying the epidemiology of this disease. As for other apicomplexan parasites, including *Toxoplasma gondii* and *Neospora caninum* (Chapter 80), horizontal transmission through the uterus from dam to its offspring has also been demonstrated in HCI. Naturally infected pregnant bitches were allowed to give birth in a tick-free environment. Meronts were found in the spleen of a pup that died 16 days after birth, and blood gamonts were detectable as early as 21 days in other pups.[72] Another potential mode of transmission that has not been demonstrated in HCI is predation of one intermediate host on another intermediate or transport host. Experimentally, infection did not result from parenteral inoculation of tissues or blood from infected dogs but from inoculation of emulsified tick tissues.[104] Some species of *Hepatozoon* that infect snakes, lizards, and frogs are transmitted through predation and ingestion of tissue cysts found in intermediate host tissues.[94]

Epidemiologic Characteristics

No gender or breed predilection for HCI has been noted. HCI was reported in all age groups, from pups younger than 3 months of age to old dogs.[2,12,14] In a case series of dogs from Greece, the female-to-male ratio was 1.2:1, and the mean age was 4.2 years.[54] Dogs with HCI are more likely to be from a rural community as compared with an urban setting, which is probably the result of a higher exposure rate to ticks.[14]

Most HCI cases are detected during the warmer months of the year, when tick vectors are more abundant. In a case-control study of 100 dogs with HCI from Israel, 77% were admitted during the warm period of May through November.[14] A follow-up study on the periodic appearance of *H. canis* gamonts in the blood of dogs in Japan indicated that the peak parasitemia was from spring to autumn.[74] However, HCI is also diagnosed during the colder months, when transmission by vector ticks is less likely, caused by chronic persistence of the infection.[14]

Pathogenesis

The presumption is that most dogs become infected with *H. canis* through grooming ticks from their haircoat or feeding on prey infested with parasitized ticks. *R. sanguineus* is a three-host tick that drops off its host when engorged with blood and, following molt, seeks another animal on which to feed. An adult tick stage might therefore acquire the HCI, as a nymph feeding on a parasitemic dog, and then after molting, attach and feed on a new host, not necessarily a dog. Experimental evidence has shown that both male and female adult *R. sanguineus* can harbor *Hepatozoon* oocysts and are potentially infective to dogs.[9]

The life cycle of *H. canis* involves the sequential formation of several distinct life forms in each of its two hosts, the dog serving as intermediate host and the tick as definitive host (Fig. 74-2). Some confusion has been caused by synonymous use of terms relating to life cycle stages of *H. canis*. Older literature often relates to schizonts and gametocytes, whereas current texts commonly use the terms meronts and gamonts, respectively. When the dog ingests the vector tick or tick parts, *H. canis* sporozoites release in the intestine and penetrate the gut wall. The sporozoites invade mononuclear cells and disseminate hematogenously or via the lymph to hemolymphatic target organs that include the bone marrow, spleen, and lymph nodes and to other internal organs such as the liver, kidney, and lungs. Respectively, hepatitis, glomerulonephritis, and pneumonitis may develop. Meronts in which asexually dividing merozoites develop are formed in the dog's tissues in the process of merogony. Two types of meronts are found in infected tissues, one containing approximately 20 to 30 slender micromerozoites and another containing up to four larger macromerozoites. Merozoites release from mature meronts, invade neutrophils and monocytes, and develop into gamonts in the process of gamontogony. Alternatively, merozoites can produce secondary meronts in the target tissues. Small monozoic cysts of *H. canis* containing a single parasite have been described in tissues of naturally and experimentally infected dogs (Fig. 74-3).[10] The role of these cysts in the life cycle of *H. canis* has not been clarified. However, they resemble cysts described in lizards and snakes in which transmission by predation has been shown.[94]

The tick, which serves as the definitive host, becomes infected by ingesting leukocytes containing gamonts when feeding on a parasitemic dog. Morphologically indistinguishable male and female *H. canis* gamonts release from the dog leukocytes within the tick gut, associate in syzygy, and differentiate in the process of gametogenesis to distinct gametes. After fertilization, the zygote divides and sporogony takes place with the formation of oocysts that release into the tick's hemocoel. The oocysts are large, spherical forms consisting of a membrane that envelops hundreds of sporocysts in which the infective sporozoites are found.[64] Sporozoites do not migrate to the feeding parts or salivary gland of the tick; therefore it must be ingested to infect the dog.

The life cycle of *H. canis* can be completed within 81 days. In an experimental transmission study, adult-stage *R. sanguineus* ticks were infective by ingestion to dogs 53 days after the ticks fed as nymphs on a naturally infected dog. Meronts were first detected in the experimentally infected dog's bone marrow 13 days postinoculation, and gamonts appeared in the blood, thereby completing the life cycle in 28 days.[9]

The pathogenesis of HCI is influenced by immunodeficient conditions, an immature immune system in young pups, a congenital defect, or concurrent infectious agents. Conditions that weaken the immune responses increase the susceptibility to new infection with *H. canis* or allow existing infections to reactivate. Co-infections with *Toxoplasma*, *Leishmania*, *Babesia*, or *Ehrlichia* predispose to clinical illness. In a litter of Dalmatians that were diagnosed with *H. canis* parasitemia, pups that contracted parvoviral enteritis demonstrated a significantly higher parasitemia than did their littermates.[2] In addition, treatment of experimentally infected dogs with an immunosuppressive dose of prednisolone was followed by the appearance of parasitaemia.[9]

Infection with *H. canis* elicits a distinct humoral immune response during the early stages of the disease.[9,11] No information is currently available on the cellular response to HCI; however, because *H. canis* is an intracellular parasite, cell-mediated immunity probably constitutes a major role in the immune mechanism mounted by the host against HCI.

Clinical Findings

Dogs

A variety of clinical presentations is associated with HCI, ranging in severity from an incidental hematologic finding in an apparently healthy dog to a debilitating and life-threatening illness. A low level of *H. canis* parasitemia with gamonts found in less than 5% of neutrophils is the most common pres-

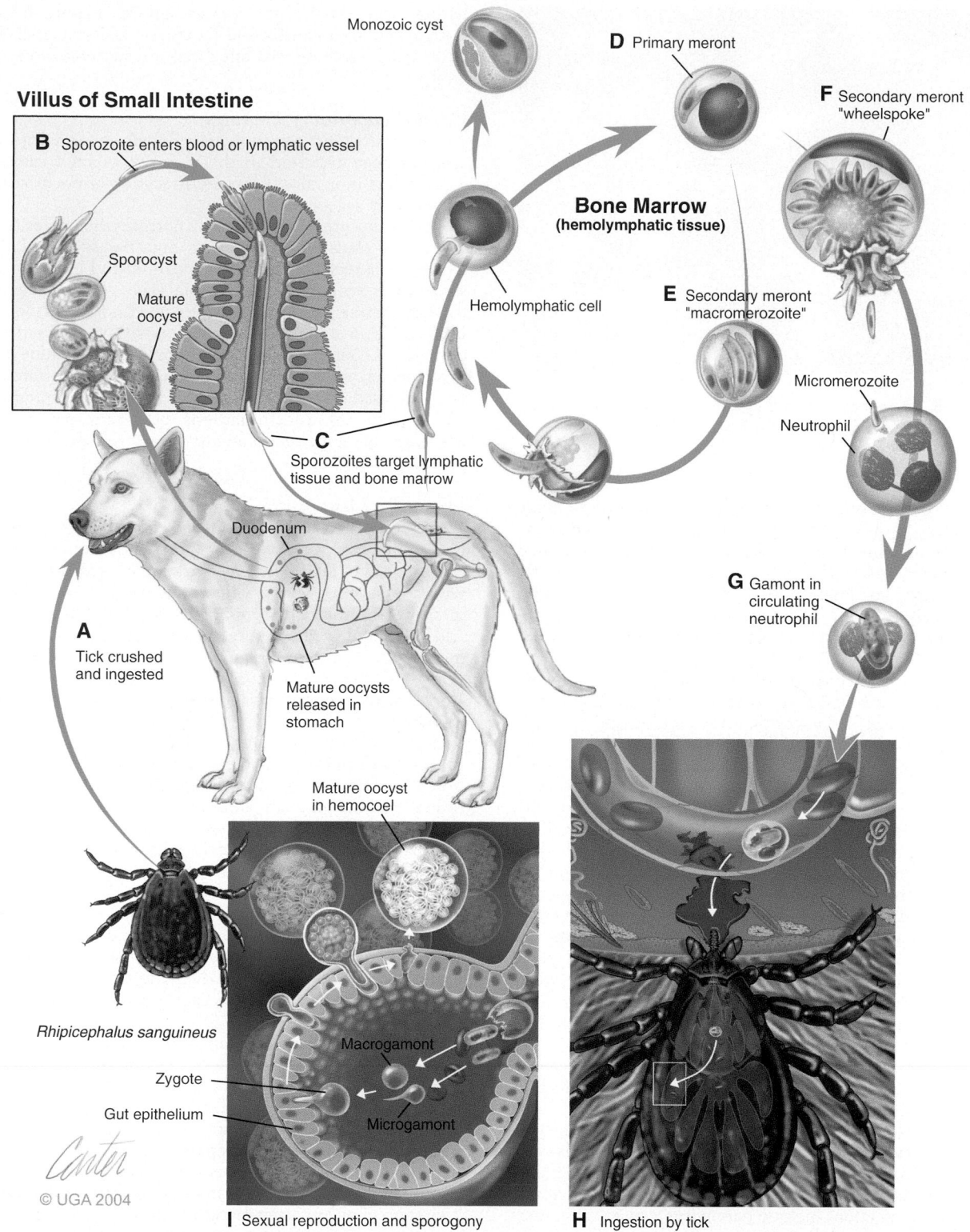

Fig 74-2 Stages in the life cycle of *H. canis*. **A,** Infected tick is ingested by the dog. **B,** Sporozoites are freed from the sporocyst in the dog's intestine, **(C)** penetrate the gut wall and reach the hemolymphatic target tissues (e.g., bone marrow) hematogenously or via the lymph. **D,** Merogony occurs in the target tissues, producing meronts containing **(E)** macromerozoites which can be released from the meront to invade new host cells to form secondary meronts containing macro- or micromerozoites. **F,** The secondary 'wheel-spoke' shaped meront releases micromerozoites which invade myeloid cells to form gamonts, or alternatively produce further generations of meronts. **G,** Gamontogony occurs with a developing gamont in a neutrophil. Neutrophils with mature gamonts circulate in the blood. **H,** Gamonts are taken up by a tick during a blood meal. **I,** Morphologically indistinguishable male and female gamonts are released in the tick's gut, and associate in syzygy. Male and female gametes transform during gametogenesis prior to fertilization and produce a zygote. Sporogonic development in the gut leads to the formation of large oocysts found enveloping numerous sporocysts. Oocysts release into the hemocoel, and each sporocyst within them contains the infective sporozoites. (Courtesy University of Georgia, Athens, Ga.)

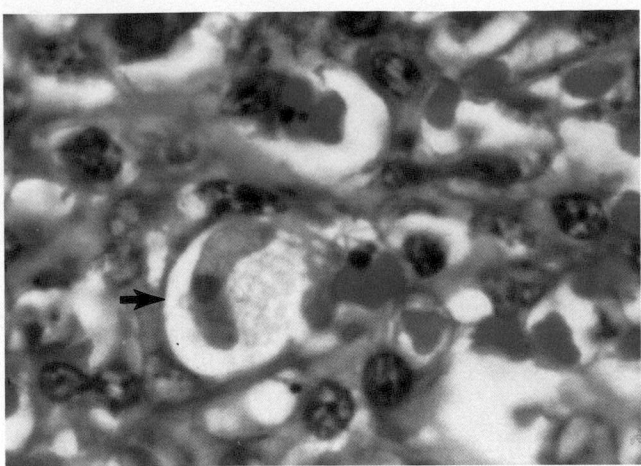

Fig 74-3 A monozoic tissue cyst of *H. canis* in splenic tissue of a naturally infected dog (H and E stain, ×500).

entation of HCI. It is usually associated with an asymptomatic to mild disease. A high parasitemia sometimes approaching 100% of neutrophils with a leukocytosis is usually associated with a severe disease. High parasitemia rates are frequently found with extreme leukocytosis, reaching as high as 150,000 leukocytes/μl of blood.[6,14] The mechanism causing this elevation in leukocytes, most commonly in neutrophils, has not been elucidated.

In a case-control study of 100 dogs with HCI, dogs were categorized into low and high parasitemia groups. Eighty-five percent of the dogs had a low parasitemia level and 15% had a high number of circulating parasites.[14] Dogs with low parasitemia were more anemic and had lower platelet counts than did the control dogs with other disease conditions. However, dogs with high circulating parasite numbers suffered mainly from fever, lethargy, weight loss, anemia, and hyperglobulinemia. The high numbers of circulating gamonts, in some cases ranging between 50,000 and 100,000 gamonts/μl of blood, are indicative of the large extent of tissue parasitism present in highly infected dogs. Tissue meronts produce the numerous merozoites that eventually invade leukocytes. The load of blood and tissue parasites present in dogs with high parasitemia levels takes its toll by demanding nutrients and exerting tissue injury. This finding explains the weight loss leading to cachexia and the profound lethargy observed in this subgroup of infected dogs.

Concurrent infections involving *H. canis* and other canine pathogens are common. Some of the reported co-infecting organisms, including *Ehrlichia canis* (Chapter 28)[86] and *Babesia canis* (Chapter 77),[54] are transmitted by the same tick vector, *R. sanguineus*, and are likely to be found in dogs with tick infestations in areas where these diseases are endemic in the dog population. Other pathogens reported to be involved in concurrent infections include parvovirus, canine distemper, *Anaplasma phagocytophilum*, *Anaplasma platys*,[54] *Toxoplasma gondii*,[42] and *Leishmania infantum*.[54,89] Co-infections may influence the susceptibility to establishing a new infection or the progression of an existing one.[2,39,42] In the case of concurrent infection, clinical signs attributed to HCI must be interpreted cautiously and separated from manifestations of the concomitant pathogen.

Diagnosis

The pathogenesis, vectorial capacity, tissue tropism, and clinical signs associated with HCI differ from *H. americanum* infection. *H. canis* is found primarily in hemolymphatic

tissues, whereas *H. americanum* infects mainly muscular tissues, causing myositis and lameness. The principal differences between these two infections are summarized in Table 74-1.

Clinical Laboratory Findings

Anemia is the most common hematologic abnormality in HCI and has been reported in the majority of HCI cases.[14,40,54] The anemia is, in most cases, normocytic normochromic and occasionally regenerative.

The leukocyte count is usually normal when parasitemia is low and is elevated in dogs with high parasitemia. Extreme neutrophilia reaching 100,000 neutrophils/μl blood occurs in some cases with high parasitemia (Fig. 74-4). Thrombocytopenia is present in approximately one third of the dogs with HCI and is, in some cases, associated with concurrent canine ehrlichiosis. Serum chemistry abnormalities include hyperproteinemia with hyperglobulinemia and hypoalbuminemia and increased creatine kinase (CK) and alkaline phosphatase (ALP) activities. Electrophoresis of serum proteins from the sera of hyperglobulinemic dogs revealed polyclonal gammopathy.[14,39]

Organism Identification

Microscopic detection of *H. canis* gamonts in Giemsa- or Diff-Quik–stained blood smears is the most common method for diagnosis of HCI. The concentration of organisms increases with the severity of the illness. The gamonts are ellipsoidal in shape and measure approximately 11 × 4 μm (Fig. 74-5) and are found in the cytoplasm of neutrophils and rarely in monocytes. Gamonts are enveloped in a thick membrane (Fig. 74-6) and are often situated in the center of the neutrophil and compress its lobulated nucleus toward the cell membrane.[102]

H. canis meronts can be detected in histopathologic specimens or in cytologic preparations made from aspirates or touch impressions of hemolymphatic tissues. Meronts are round to oval and are approximately 30 μm in diameter. Immature meronts appear as round opacities filled with globular foamlike material. As the meront matures, basophilic-staining chromatin material forms as either 2 to 4 larger macromerozoites or more than 20 micromerozoites. The shaping micromerozoites align in a circle close to the meront wall around a central opaque core. The mature meront visualized in histopathologic specimens creates a typical "wheel spoke" form when the circle of micromerozoites is incised in cross-section through their mid-shaft (Fig. 74-7).

H. canis can also be identified in vector ticks. Mature oocysts can be seen even without magnification as small white globular forms in wet preparations of the hemocoel. The observation of oocysts is verified and differentiated from the tick's organs and salivary glands by microscopy of hemocoel smears as unstained wet preparations or as Giemsa-stained specimens (Fig. 74-8). Oocysts are enveloped in an easily torn membrane and contain hundreds of smaller oval sporocysts. Free sporocysts are often present scattered outside the oocyst, and infective sporozoites are packed as elongated slender forms within the sporocysts.

Serologic Testing

The indirect FA test and the enzyme-linked immunosorbent assay (ELISA) for the serodiagnosis of HCI using gamont antigen have been developed and are used mainly for epidemiologic studies.* Antibodies of the IgM and IgG classes were detectable in the sera of experimentally infected dogs as

*References: 5, 12, 13, 38, 41, 46, 93.

Table • 74-1

Comparative Characteristics of Hepatozoon canis *and* Hepatozoon americanum *Infections*

VARIABLE	*HEPATOZOON CANIS*	*HEPATOZOON AMERICANUM*
Geographic distribution	Asia, Southern Europe, Africa, South America	Southern United States
Principal vector tick	Brown dog tick, *Rhipicephalus sanguineus*	Gulf Coast tick, *Amblyomma maculatum*
Major target organs	Spleen, bone marrow, lymph nodes	Skeletal muscles, myocardium
Common clinical examination findings	Fever, lethargy, weight loss	Gait abnormalities, fever, muscle hyperesthesia, mucopurulent ocular discharge, lethargy
Severity of clinical disease	Usually mild when parasitemia is low; a severe disease with large numbers of circulating gamonts	Severe
Hematologic findings	Anemia; extreme neutrophilia is infrequent and found in dogs with large numbers of circulating gamonts; circulating blood gamonts are common and found mainly in neutrophils and rarely in monocytes; parasitemia ranges from 1% to 100% of the neutrophils	Anemia; neutrophilia is common and often extreme; circulating blood gamonts are infrequent and usually found in less than 0.1% of the leukocytes
Radiographic findings	Nonspecific	Periosteal proliferation
Histologic findings	Hepatitis, splenitis, nephritis, and pneumonia associated with presence of *H. canis* meronts	Pyogranulomatous myositis
Unique morphologic features	"Wheel spoke" meront; small monozoic splenic tissue cysts	Large muscle "onion skin cysts"
Main diagnostic procedure	Demonstrating gamonts in blood smear	Muscle biopsy demonstrating tissue cysts and pyogranulomas associated with developing parasitic stages
Serologic tests	Indirect FA test, ELISA (gamont antigens)	ELISA (sporozoite antigens)

FA, Fluorescent antibody; *ELISA*, enzyme-linked immunosorbent assay.

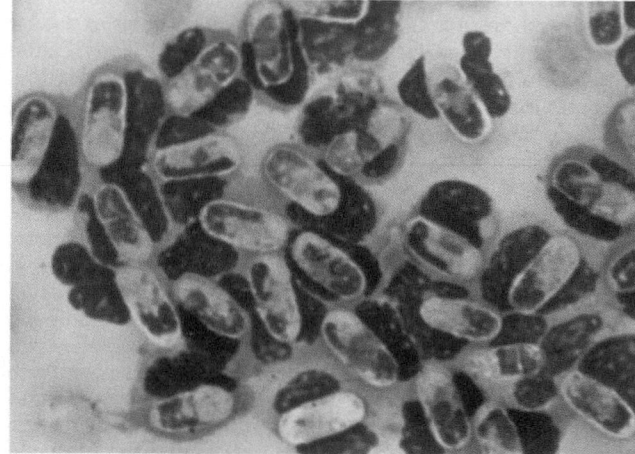

Fig 74-4 Feathered edge of a Giemsa-stained blood smear from a dog with leukocytosis and a high *H. canis* parasitemia. Note that close to 100% of the neutrophils are parasitized with gamonts (×1000).

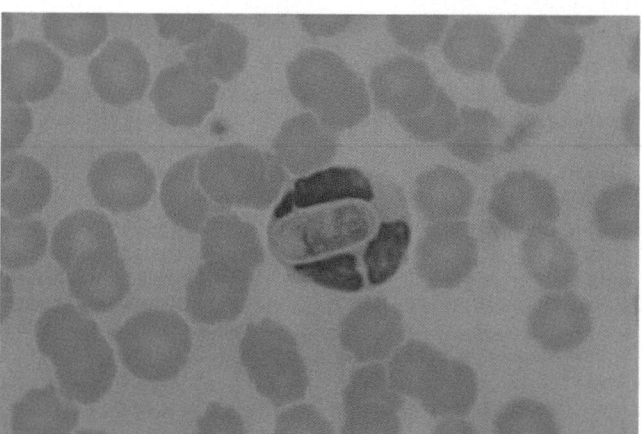

Fig 74-5 *H. canis* gamont in a Giemsa-stained blood smear. Note the location of the gamont in the cytoplasm of a neutrophil compressing the lobulated nucleus to the margins of the cell (×1000).

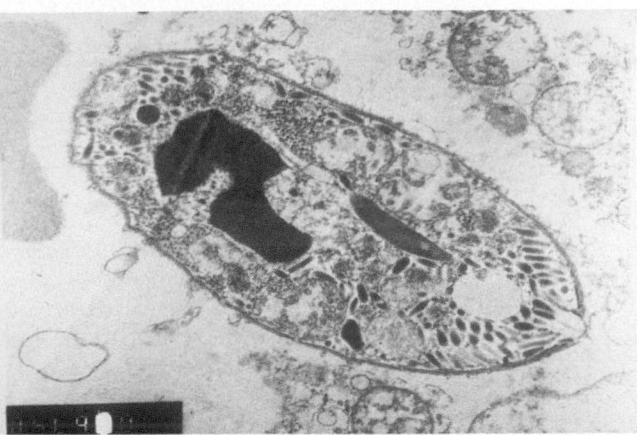

Fig 74-6 A transmission electron microscopic image of *H. canis* gamont from the blood of a naturally infected dog. Note the conoid at the anterior end of the parasite. A three-layer membrane envelopes the gamont.

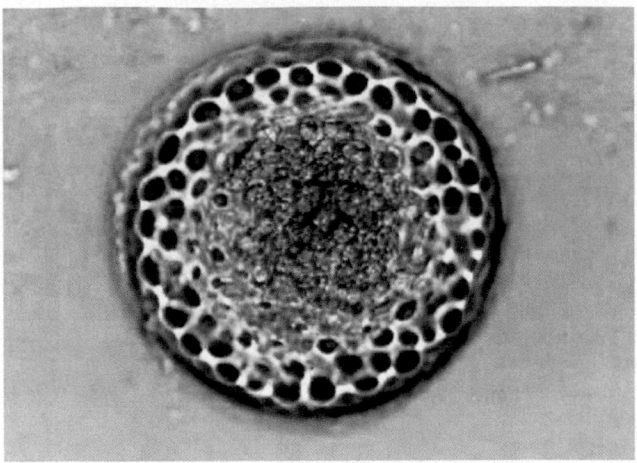

Fig 74-8 Unstained *H. canis* oocyst containing numerous sporocysts from the hemocoel of an adult stage *R. sanguineus* tick (×200).

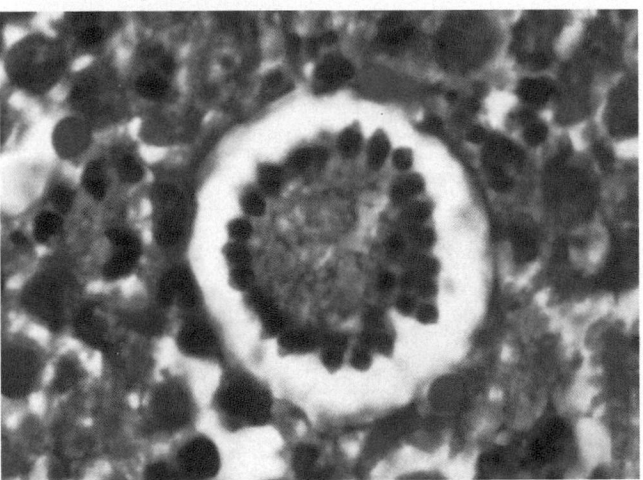

Fig 74-7 *H. canis* meront containing micromerozoites forming a "wheel-spoke" shape in splenic tissue (H and E stain, ×400).

early as 16 and 22 days postinfection, respectively, peaked at 7 to 9 weeks, and persisted for more than 7 months.[5,11,41]

Pathologic Findings

Pathologic descriptions of infected dogs range from reports on infrequent tissue meronts termed as incidental findings[50] to severe and occasionally fatal multiple-organ involvement.* A considerable variation is found in the spectrum of lesions and the number of parasitic life forms. The major macroscopic lesions found in dogs with heavy infections include splenomegaly and hepatomegaly, with a diffuse pattern of small white necrotic foci 1 to 2 mm in diameter.[6,43] Necrotic foci may be larger and nodular in appearance and are also found in other tissues, including the pancreas and on the pleura.[6,14,42] Pneumonia may be evident, and lymph nodes are typically enlarged.

Histopathology reveals a varying number of developing or mature meronts with their "wheel spoke" pattern in the affected tissues. These meronts are associated with a mild

*References: 6, 14, 42, 43, 67.

inflammatory response in some cases, ranging to severe responses in others.[67] Focal splenic necrosis is associated with *H. canis* merogony in red and white pulp regions, with white pulp necrosis located primarily in lymphoid follicles.[43] Hepatitis with Kupffer cell hyperplasia and mononuclear and neutrophil infiltration is associated with developing meronts in the liver.[14,67] The presence of *H. canis* in the lung is associated with interstitial pneumonia and the thickening of alveolar septa with inflammatory cell infiltrates. Renal lesions include glomerulonephritis and interstitial nephritis with multifocal necrosis. Mild to extensive parasitism with meronts and developing gamonts is described in the lymph nodes and bone marrow.[14,67]

Therapy

The current treatment protocol for HCI is imidocarb dipropionate at 5 to 6 mg/kg (2.5 to 3.0 mg/lb), subcutaneously or intramuscularly, every 14 days, until gamonts are no longer present in the blood smears. One or two injections may suffice; however, the elimination of gamonts in heavy infections using imidocarb dipropionate may require treatment for 8 weeks or longer.[14] Oral doxycycline at 10 mg/kg/day (5 mg/lb/day) for 21 days is also frequently used in combination with imidocarb dipropionate to treat potential or identified tickborne co-infections. No controlled studies on the therapy of HCI have been published.

The rate of survival of treated dogs with a low *H. canis* parasitemia is generally good and is frequently dependent on the prognosis of any concurrent disease, if present. The prognosis for dogs with a high parasitemia is guarded. Only 7 of 15 dogs (47%) with a high parasitemia survived 2 months despite specific treatment.[14]

Prevention

Prevention of HCI should consist of an effective control of vector ticks on dogs and in the environment using *external* parasiticides. Dogs must be prevented from ingesting ticks while grooming or scavenging. To prevent congenital transmission, infected dams should be treated effectively before being bred. Until the certainty that HCI may be transmitted by ingestion of infected tissues is reached, dogs in endemic areas should be prevented from eating raw or prey meat.

Public Health Considerations

The spectrum of natural hosts for HCI is not currently known. Only one report of infection with a *Hepatozoon* sp. in a person from the Philippines has been issued.[19] This patient was anemic and icteric, and gamonts were detected in the blood. However, no parasites were found in liver and bone marrow biopsies. Although the zoonotic importance of *H. canis* is not known, and it is unlikely to be a significant pathogen in immunocompetent people, caution should be used when handling infected dogs infested with ticks or when removing ticks from dogs.

FELINE HEPATOZOONOSIS

Gad Baneth

Hepatozoonosis of domestic cats has been reported from India,[85] South Africa,[95] Nigeria,[57] the United States,[29] Israel,[3,7,51] and France.[18] The species of *Hepatozoon* that infect cats has not been identified. Whether only a single species is found in cats and whether it is similar to any species described in other animals is unknown. The vector of feline hepatozoonosis (FeHPZ) is also unknown. See Cats and Wild Carnivores, under Etiology earlier in this chapter, for the host range of reported infections.

FeHPZ is associated with infection of muscle tissues. *Hepatozoon* meronts have been identified in the myocardium and skeletal muscles of cats with hepatozoonosis,[18] and elevated activities of the muscle enzyme CK were found in the majority of cats with FeHPZ in a retrospective study of this disease.[3] Retroviral diseases are frequently found in association with FeHPZ and appear to be a predisposing factor. Feline immunodeficiency virus and feline leukemia virus (FeLV) were detected in four of six cats reported with FeHPZ from Israel and in two cats from France.[3,18]

A wide variety of clinical signs has been described in cats with FeHPZ.* In a parasitemic cat from Israel, weakness, hypersalivation, lingual mucosal ulceration, and lymphadenomegaly were observed.[7] The cat was treated with doxycycline and recovered. Two parasitemic cats from France that also had positive test results for FeLV had lethargy, anorexia, anemia, and thrombocytopenia.[18] A cat from Hawaii had weight loss, ulcerative glossitis, pyrexia, progressive anemia, serous ocular discharge, and icterus.[29] The cat also had cytologic evidence of liver infection consistent with hepatozoonosis. The diagnosis of FeHPZ is usually performed by detection of gamonts in blood smears. The gamonts are located in the cytoplasm of neutrophils, have an ellipsoidal shape, and posses a round or pleomorphic nucleus (Fig. 74-9). The level of parasitemia is frequently low with less than 1% of the neutrophils containing gamonts. FeHPZ has been treated with the oral administration of doxycycline at 5 mg/kg (2.5 mg/lb)[7] or oral oxytetracycline at 50 mg/kg (25 mg/lb) twice daily with a single dose of oral primaquine at 2 mg/kg (1 mg/lb).[95]

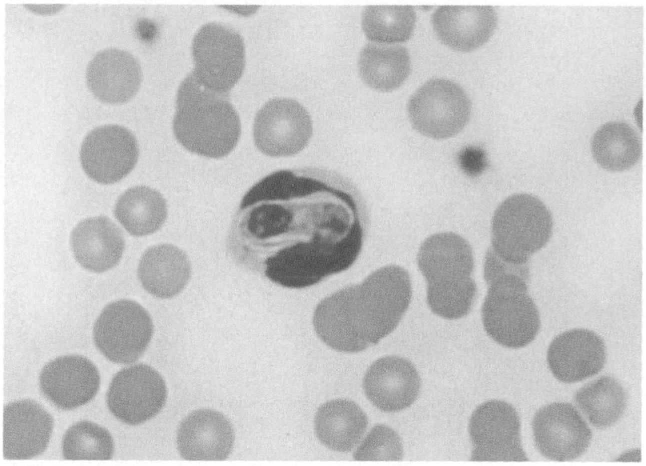

HEPATOZOON AMERICANUM INFECTION

Douglass K. Macintire, Nancy A. Vincent-Johnson, and Thomas M. Craig

Etiology and Epidemiology

All canine infections were once attributed to *H. canis* because of the similar appearance of *Hepatozoon* gamonts in canine white blood cells. In 1997, however, a new species, *H. americanum*, was identified based on differences in tissue stages, tick vector, clinical syndrome, ultrastructure, geo-

*References: 3, 7, 18, 29, 95.

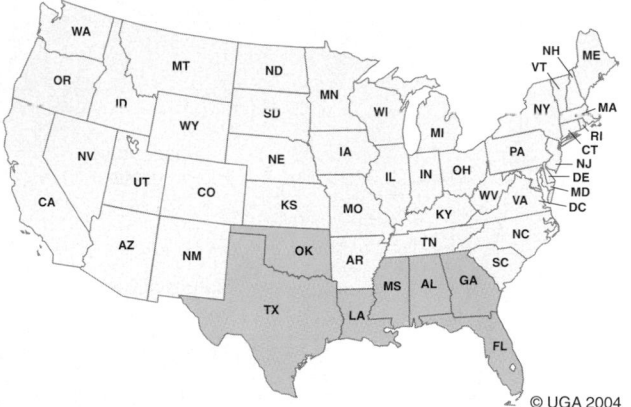

Fig 74-9 *Hepatozoon* sp. gamont in the cytoplasm of a neutrophil from a domestic cat. The blood smear was stained with Giemsa (×500).

Fig 74-10 Map showing known distribution of reported cases of *H. americanum* infection. (Courtesy University of Georgia, Athens, Ga.)

graphic distribution, and genetic and antigenic characteristics.[4,100] Table 74-1 compares the clinical features of *H. canis* with *H. americanum*.

In the United States, hepatozoonosis was first described in the Texas Gulf Coast in 1978.[23] Since that time, it has been reported also in Louisiana, Alabama, Georgia, Mississippi, Oklahoma, Tennessee, and Florida[59,61] (Fig. 74-10). The definitive host for *H. americanum* is the Gulf Coast tick, *Amblyomma maculatum*.[63,30] The geographic distribution of this tick was once confined to the warm, humid areas of the Texas gulf coast, but the range of this tick now has expanded as far north as Kansas and Kentucky.[91] *H. americanum* infection appears to be an emerging disease that is spreading north and east from the area where it was initially detected. In addition to dogs, *H. americanum* or a similar organism has been diagnosed in coyotes, bobcats, and ocelots in the southern United States by identifying cysts or meronts in muscle or gamonts in blood smears.[23,52] Whether the hepatozoonosis reported in dogs from Brazil[40,78,79] was caused by *H. canis* or *H. americanum* is uncertain.

In contrast to *H. canis*–infected dogs, most dogs with *H. americanum* exhibit severe clinical signs even in the absence of concurrent disease or immunosuppression.[59] Because the parasite appears to be poorly adapted to dogs as a natural host,

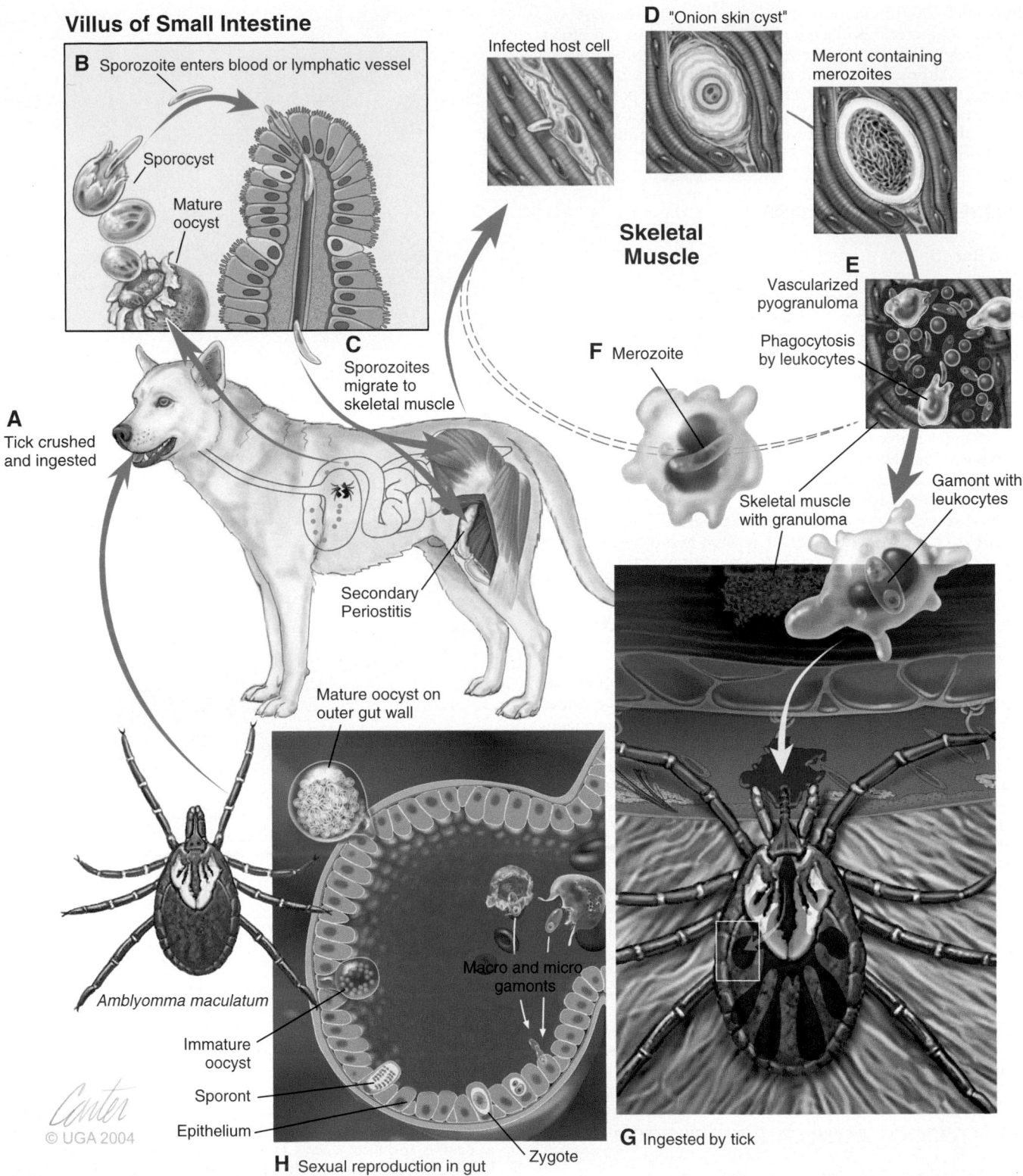

Villus of Small Intestine

B Sporozoite enters blood or lymphatic vessel

Sporocyst

Mature oocyst

D "Onion skin cyst"

Infected host cell

Meront containing merozoites

Skeletal Muscle

E Vascularized pyogranuloma

Phagocytosis by leukocytes

F Merozoite

C Sporozoites migrate to skeletal muscle

A Tick crushed and ingested

Secondary Periostitis

Skeletal muscle with granuloma

Gamont within leukocytes

Mature oocyst on outer gut wall

Amblyomma maculatum

Immature oocyst

Sporont

Epithelium

Macro and micro gamonts

Zygote

G Ingested by tick

H Sexual reproduction in gut

© UGA 2004

Fig   74-11 Stages in the life cycle of *H. americanum*. **A,** Infected tick is ingested by the dog. **B,** Sporozoites are freed from the sporocyst in the dog's intestine and penetrate the gut wall. **C,** They migrate to the skeletal and cardiac muscle target tissues hematogenously or via the lymph where they lodge in a presumed phagocytic cell between myocytes. **D,** Concentric layers of mucopolysaccharide material (onion skin) are deposited around the cyst. Some remain dormant while others undergo merogony forming meronts containing many merozoites. **E,** Upon maturation the meront ruptures releasing merozoites and induce a pyogranulomatous inflammatory reaction. Migrating phagocytes ingest the organisms. **F,** The ingested organism can circulate to other sites and continue asexual cycle. Others enter circulating phagocytes (monocytes or neutrophils) and transform into gamonts. **G,** Infected leukocytes are ingested by *Amblyomma* tick. **H,** Syngamy (sexual cycle) occurs in the tick gut epithelium producing macro- and microgamonts which fuse to form a zygote that matures to an oocyst. See text. (Courtesy University of Georgia, Athens, Ga.)

H. americanum is likely a natural parasite of some other species in the wildlife reservoir. Dogs become an accidental host after ingesting infected ticks. In the United States, the wildlife reservoir for domestic dogs infected with *H. americanum* has yet to be elucidated.

The life cycle is similar to that of HCI; however, notable differences exist (Fig. 74-11). In contrast to *H. canis*, the primary tissue sites for development of meronts in dogs with *H. americanum* infection are skeletal and cardiac muscle.[80] Infective sporozoites ingested by the dog are transported to striated muscle and other target organs where they develop within an unidentified host cell, which is most likely a phagocytic cell that initially lodges between myocytes.[81,83] Concentric layers of a mucopolysaccharide material are deposited around the host cell to form a large cystic structure of 250 to 500 μm diameter. This structure has been referred to as an "onion skin cyst" and is the most common tissue stage of *H. americanum* found in infected dogs. Some cysts appear to go into a dormant state, while others undergo merogony. On maturation, numerous merozoites are released from the ruptured cyst, inducing a severe inflammatory response. Migration of neutrophils and monocytes into the area results in the formation of a pyogranuloma where the meront once existed. The pyogranuloma becomes highly vascularized, and inflammatory cells that have phagocytized single zoites return to circulation where they may travel to distant sites to continue the asexual cycle or may become circulating gamonts that can complete the life cycle when ingested by *A. maculatum* ticks feeding on the dog. In experimental infections, completion of the life cycle from ingestion of infected ticks to development of circulating gamonts can occur in as few as 35 days.[81] In the tick, 42 days are needed for the organism to develop into mature oocysts that are present in the hemocoel of newly molted adults.[64] Experimental infections have been produced in both dogs and coyotes fed infected *A. maculatum* ticks.[53]

The primary mode of transmission of *H. americanum* is through ingestion of the *A. maculatum* tick.[31] Recent studies have shown that experimentally infected larval ticks are infectious to dogs after molting to nymphs.[30] Adult-stage ticks that have acquired infection at the nymph stage are also infectious to dogs. Gulf Coast tick larvae and nymphs feed primarily on ground-inhabiting birds and small mammals, while adults feed on larger wild and domestic mammals. This wide range of potential intermediate hosts can allow the organism to maintain an endemic life cycle in the geographic distribution area of the *A. maculatum* tick. The number of different species of animals that are susceptible to infection with *H. americanum* is not known, nor is the number of species that serve as the natural reservoir of disease.

In utero or congenital transmission of *H. americanum* from dam to puppies has not been documented but is probable given that it has been shown to occur with *H. canis*.[23] Also suggested is that dogs may potentially become infected by eating animals that have tissue stages of the organism. Although this type of transmission has not been proven, it does occur with other species of *Hepatozoon* and would seem plausible for *H. americanum* as well.

The geographic distribution of *H. americanum* parallels that of the definitive host, *A. maculatum*. Researchers at Auburn University, Auburn, Alabama, and Oklahoma State University, Stillwater, Oklahoma, were unable to transmit the disease with *R. sanguineus* or *Dermacentor* spp. ticks but were able to transmit the disease readily with *A. maculatum* ticks.[31,97]

The occurrence of hepatozoonosis appears to be seasonal in the warmer months or in early fall when dogs are most likely to be exposed to ticks. Dogs with *H. americanum* usually exhibit waxing and waning clinical signs that occur throughout the year as repeated cycles of asexual reproduction and pyogranulomatous inflammation take place.

Pathogenesis

The progression of *H. americanum* infection in dogs from ingestion of sporozoites in ticks until the onset of clinical signs has been investigated in experimentally infected dogs[81] and coyotes.[53] The earliest lesions are seen at 3 weeks postinfection, when the organism can be observed within a host cell located between myocytes. As the zoite matures, the host cell produces the layers of mucopolysaccharides that surround the host cell and protect it from the dog's immune system. No inflammatory response is associated with the organism when it appears as the onion skin cyst. Clinical signs occur when the cyst ruptures inducing severe pyogranulomatous myositis. Although some cysts rapidly undergo merogony, others can apparently remain dormant for years after the initial infection. Activation of these cysts and continued reproduction of the organism through repeated cycles of merogony result in the waxing and waning course of the disease and the occurrence of relapses following treatment. A prolonged infection may result from a single infecting episode perpetuated by repeated asexual cycles. Cysts have been found in muscle biopsies taken from dogs for up to 5 years after the initial infection.[34] Pyogranulomatous myositis in muscles adjacent to bones may stimulate a marked periosteal reaction along bone surfaces, especially in younger animals. Chronic infection causes persistent antigenic stimulation and may result in vasculitis, immunoproliferative glomerulonephritis, and amyloid deposition in various organs. Prolonged infection usually results in chronic cachexia and progressive weight loss and muscle wasting with death generally occurring within 12 months postinfection.

Clinical Findings
Dogs

In contrast to the usually mild disease seen with HCI, *H. americanum* causes a debilitating and usually fatal disease. Antibiotic unresponsive fever (39.3° to 40.9° C [102.7° to 105.6° F]), cachexia, depression, generalized muscle atrophy, and hyperesthesia (especially noticeable over the paraspinal regions), purulent ocular discharge, and mild anemia are seen in most dogs.[23] The clinical signs may wax and wane with the degree of pyogranulomatous inflammation. Many dogs have been treated for fever of unknown origin with several courses of antibiotic therapy before it became evident that the waxing and waning course is not a positive response to treatment. Chronic weight loss most likely results from muscle atrophy and the increased caloric demands associated with the prolonged inflammatory state. Mucopurulent ocular discharge is a fairly consistent finding and may be secondary to pyogranulomatous inflammation of extraocular muscles or destruction of the lacrimal gland. Approximately one third of the dogs with matted eyes have decreased tear production on a Shirmer tear test.[59] Other occasionally reported ocular abnormalities have included focal retinal scarring, hyperpigmentation and hyperreflectivity, mild papilledema, and uveitis with active inflammatory fundic lesions.[23]

The pain that accompanies the myositis may show as cervical, back, joint, or generalized pain. Hyperesthesia, stiffness, neck guarding, and fever can easily be mistaken for meningitis or diskospondylitis, but analysis of cerebrospinal fluid is usually unremarkable. Gait abnormalities can include stiffness, generalized weakness, rear-limb paresis and ataxia, and an inability or unwillingness to rise.

The stiffness and reluctance to move cause many dogs to assume a "master's voice" stance (Fig. 74-12). Pain, particularly in the lumbar region, may resemble traumatic or degenerative disease of the spine. Because of fever, lumbar pain, and

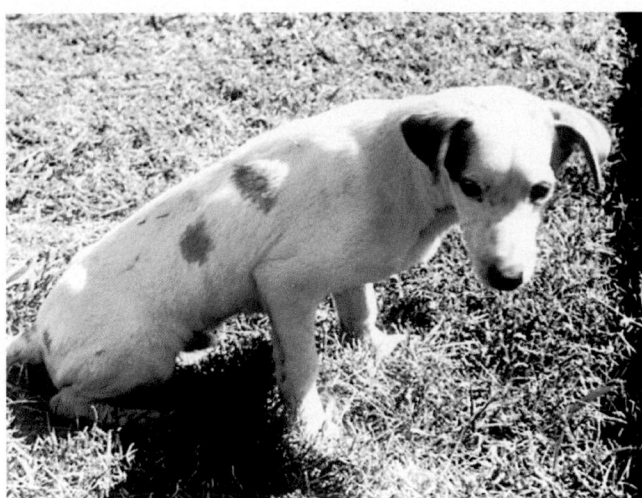

Fig 74-12 Six-month-old terrier mix with hepatozoonosis. Notice the extreme emaciation and "master's voice" posture.

leukocytosis, a few cases were initially suspected of having pyelonephritis or closed pyometra.[23] Dogs may have a history of polyuria and polydipsia, especially if secondary glomerulonephritis or amyloidosis is present. Less common clinical signs include transient bloody diarrhea, abnormal lung sounds, cough, pale mucous membranes, and lymphadenomegaly.[23] Despite progressive weight loss and muscle wasting, many dogs continue to maintain a fairly normal appetite.

Diagnosis
Clinical Laboratory Findings
The most consistent laboratory abnormality for dogs with *H. americanum* is an elevated leukocyte count that commonly ranges from 20,000 to 200,000 cells/µl.[59] Infection with *H. americanum* is usually associated with a mature neutrophilia, but occasionally a mild to moderate left shift may be present. A mild normocytic, normochromic, nonregenerative anemia has been a consistent finding, with reported cases of hepatozoonosis. The platelet count is typically normal to elevated, and marked thrombocytosis (up to 916,000 platelets/µl) has been evident in some dogs.[61] The finding of thrombocytopenia should prompt the clinician to suspect concurrent infection with other tick-borne diseases such as ehrlichiosis (Chapter 28), Rocky Mountain spotted fever (Chapter 29), or babesiosis (Chapter 77).

The most common abnormalities detected on serum chemistry panels in dogs with *H. americanum* include mildly increased serum ALP activity, hypoglycemia, and hypoalbuminemia.[59] The increase in serum ALP activity may be associated with the periosteal inflammation that occurs secondary to myositis. Hypoglycemia, generally in the range of 40 to 60 mg/dl, is thought to be the result of in vitro metabolism of glucose by white blood cells. When sodium fluoride is used as the anticoagulant to block glucose metabolism by the cells, the blood glucose value is usually in the normal reference range. Hypoalbuminemia is a consistent finding and may be associated with decreased protein intake, chronic inflammation, or renal loss. Serum urea values are usually low unless significant renal damage has occurred from chronic disease. Decreased serum urea values may represent reduced protein intake or disordered protein metabolism secondary to negative nitrogen balance and production of inflammatory proteins. Low serum urea values may contribute to the polyuria seen in some dogs because of a reduced renal medullary concentration gradient. With chronic disease, dogs may develop protein-losing nephropathy with high urine protein-creatinine

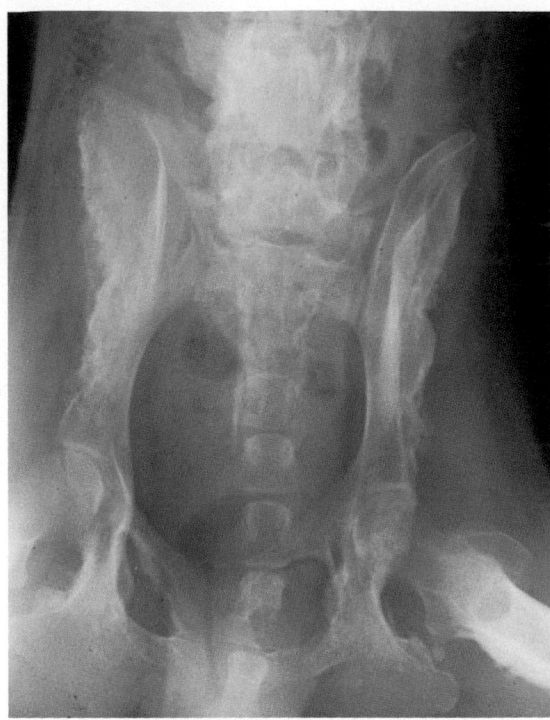

Fig 74-13 Radiograph of the pelvis and lumbar vertebrae of a dog with periosteal new bone proliferation associated with *H. americanum* infection.

ratios secondary to glomerulonephritis or renal amyloidosis. Although hypoglycemia, hypoalbuminemia, and low serum urea levels are often associated with liver disease, serum bile acids are usually normal or only slightly elevated in dogs with *H. americanum* infection. Despite the muscle inflammation, CK activity is almost always within reference limits. Hyperglobulinemia is relatively uncommon. Generalized polymyopathy may be found with electromyography. Lymph node aspirates are characterized microscopically by hyperplasia. Results of synoviocentesis analysis reveal nonseptic inflammation.[61] Bone marrow cytologic findings are granulocytic hyperplasia and erythroid hypoplasia with a high myeloid-erythroid ratio.

Radiography
Periosteal bony lesions have not been described in dogs infected with *H. canis* and have only been reported in dogs from North America, with the exception of one dog in Japan.[23] For dogs infected with *H. americanum*, radiographic findings may range from spectacular to nonexistent. Periosteal bone proliferation has been associated with the attachment of muscle on most bones of the body except the skull (Figs. 74-13 and 74-14). Bony changes have been noted in the vertebrae, pelvis, radius, ulna, humerus, femur, fibula, and tibia.[27,59] Not all infected dogs develop this unique lesion. Radiographic lesions are more common in younger dogs (younger than age 1 year) than they are in older dogs. Whether the radiographic changes are associated with rapid skeletal growth or are indicative of a more severe infection in the young is unknown. Morphologically, the lesions resemble hypertrophic osteopathy.[83]

Radiographs can be used as a screening test to provide supportive data for a diagnosis of hepatozoonosis. Pelvic radiographs or radiographs of the long bones may show subtle irregular periosteal exostoses or smooth lamellar thickening of the periosteum. Nuclear bone scintigraphy can detect changes in the bone beginning between 35 and 67 days after infection.[27]

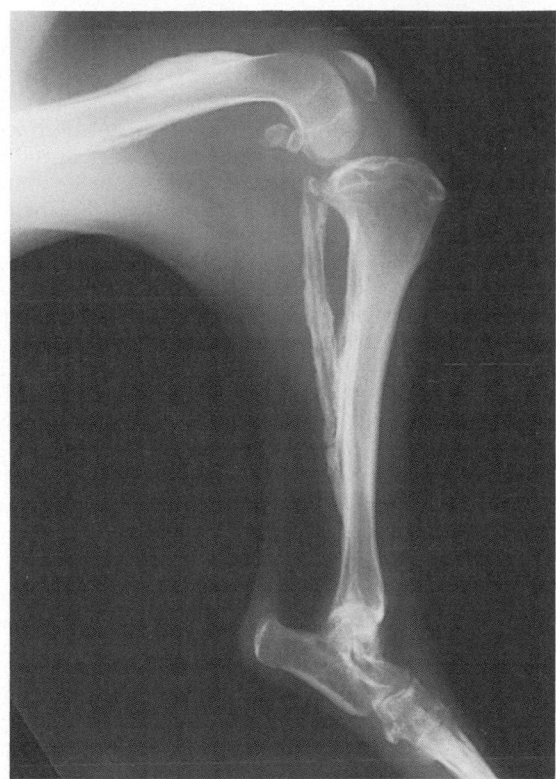

Fig 74-14 Radiograph of femur, tibia, and fibula of a dog infected with *H. americanum*.

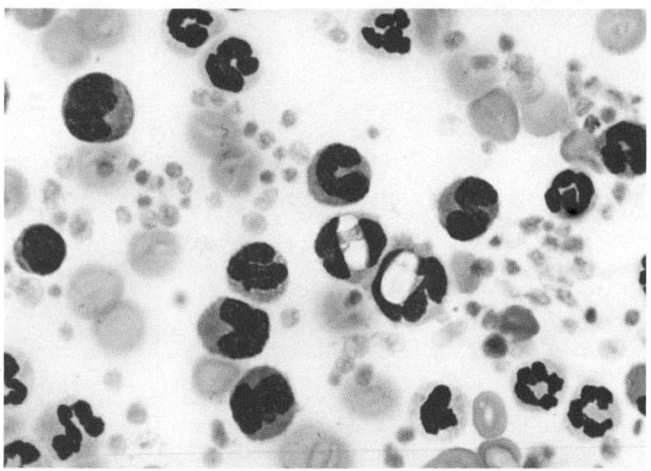

Fig 74-15 Gamonts of *H. americanum* in circulating neutrophils appear identical to *H. canis* gamonts (Giemsa, ×1200).

Organism Identification

In contrast to HCI, the gamonts of *H. americanum* are difficult to find because usually less than 0.1% of neutrophils or monocytes are infected. When seen, the gamonts of *H. americanum* appear as a light blue to clear oblong capsule measuring approximately 8.8 × 3.9 μm with a faintly staining nucleus (Fig. 74-15). Special staining techniques have been advocated, but they are laborious and often unrewarding because of the low degree of parasitemia. Examination of buffy coat smears may increase the chance of finding a gamont-infected cell.

Muscle biopsy is a convenient and more consistent means of establishing a diagnosis of *H. americanum* in infected dogs

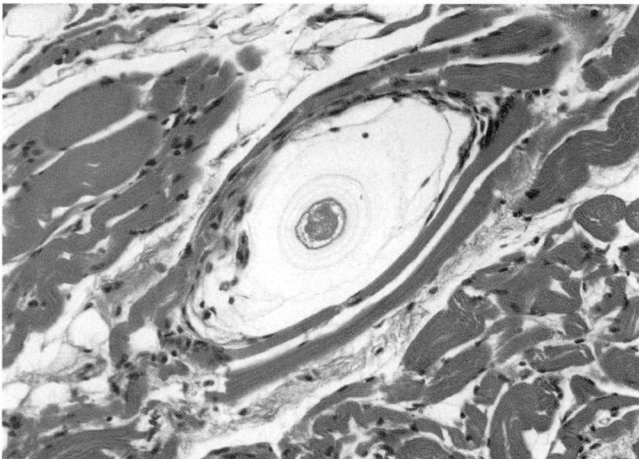

Fig 74-16 "Onion skin cyst" of *H. americanum*. Concentric layers of a mucopolysaccharide material surround a host cell to form a large cystic structure in the skeletal muscle (H and E stain, ×400).

(see Pathologic Findings). Two or three small pieces of muscle (2 × 2 cm) are taken from the biceps femoris or semitendinosus muscle with the dog under general anesthesia. Cysts, meronts, and pyogranulomas with zoite-containing neutrophils and monocytes are diagnostic of *H. americanum* infection. Myositis is a less specific but common finding. False-negative results sometimes occur when a sample does not contain any lesions, but this rarely happens because of the extremely high number of organisms in infected dogs. Taking several samples or repeating the procedure sequentially may reduce the probability of obtaining a false-negative result. Xenodiagnosis, whereby adult ticks are examined for infection after feeding at the nymph stage on a suspected dog, is the most sensitive means of detection; however, it is practical only in an experimental setting.[34]

Serologic Testing

Researchers at Oklahoma State University have developed an ELISA method for *H. americanum* using sporozoites as the antigen. This test showed a 93% sensitivity and 96% specificity when compared with muscle biopsy results.[65]

Pathologic Findings

Consistent gross findings in dogs with *H. americanum* are cachexia and muscle atrophy. Roughened, thickened bone surfaces may be seen. Grossly, pyogranulomas may appear as multiple, 1 to 2 mm, white to tan foci scattered diffusely throughout muscle and other tissues. Microscopically, the cysts (Fig. 74-16), meronts (Fig. 74-17), and pyogranulomas (Fig. 74-18) are found primarily in skeletal and cardiac muscle but may also be found sporadically in other tissues, including adipose tissue, lymph node, intestinal smooth muscle, spleen, skin, kidney, salivary gland, liver, pancreas, and lung. An immunohistochemical staining procedure has been developed to identify specifically muscle cysts.[84] Vascular changes in various organs include fibrinoid degeneration of vessel walls, mineralization and proliferation of vascular intima, and pyogranulomatous vasculitis. Renal lesions are common and include focal pyogranulomatous inflammation with mild glomerulonephritis, lymphoplasmacytic interstitial nephritis, mesangioproliferative glomerulonephritis, and occasionally amyloidosis. Amyloid deposits can also be found in the spleen, lymph nodes, small intestines, and liver. Less common findings include pulmonary congestion, splenic coagulative necrosis, lymphadenomegaly, and congestion of the gastric mucosa.

Therapy

Table 74-2 describes treatment regimens for hepatozoonosis.

Treatment of *H. americanum* has been frustrating because no therapy is effective in eliminating the tissue stages of the organism. Palliative therapy with nonsteroidal antiinflammatory drugs at standard dosages can provide immediate relief from fever and muscle pain while definitive antiprotozoal therapy is initiated. Remission of clinical signs can usually be obtained quickly by administering a combination of trimethoprim-sulfadiazine, clindamycin, and pyrimethamine (TCP combination) for 14 days. (See Table 74-2 for dosages.) Although the clinical response is dramatic, it is often short-lived. Most dogs relapse within 2 to 6 months following treatment because of continued release of merozoites into muscle and other tissues as the meronts undergo replication and development. No treatment is available that is able to penetrate the host cell and arrest development of the meronts when they are in the cystic stage. Although response to treatment is generally good with subsequent relapses, they may recur more frequently over time. Persistent recurrent infections can lead to glomerulonephropathy, amyloidosis, vasculitis, and chronic cachexia.

A relatively new treatment to assist in preventing clinical relapses is decoquinate (Deccox), an anticoccidial drug for food animals. This drug is given daily for 2 years once clinical signs have resolved (see Table 74-2). In some cases, mild relapses can occur even when dogs are receiving decoquinate. If fever and leukocytosis are present, another course of antiprotozoal therapy is warranted. Decoquinate is available as a livestock feed additive at a concentration of 27.2 grams of decoquinate per pound of premix. The powder can be mixed into moist dog food at a rate of 0.5 to 1.0 teaspoons per 10 kg body weight and fed twice daily.

In the past, the prognosis for dogs with *H. americanum* infection was guarded to poor.[23] With the advent of the TCP combination therapy followed by daily decoquinate administration, the prognosis has markedly improved. Relapses are less frequent and severe, and glomerulonephritis and amyloidosis are less common. In a comparison of treatment protocols, the 2-year survival rate for dogs receiving only antiprotozoal therapy was 12.5% but increased to greater than 84% survival for dogs receiving antiprotozoal treatment followed by long-term decoquinate.[60] Dogs treated with TCP combination therapy followed by decoquinate for 2 years have been disease free for over 5 years.

Prevention

Control of ticks with an effective acaricide is important to limit the spread of disease. The transmission of *H. canis* occurs only transtadially; transovarial transmission is unknown. Environmental control of the vector by preventing it from feeding on infected dogs therefore will help prevent spread. Home or kennel environments should be sprayed on a routine basis. Regular dipping of dogs from infested premises will kill any ticks feeding at that time.

Although transmission by ingestion of infected tissues has not been proven, it does occur with other species of *Hepato-*

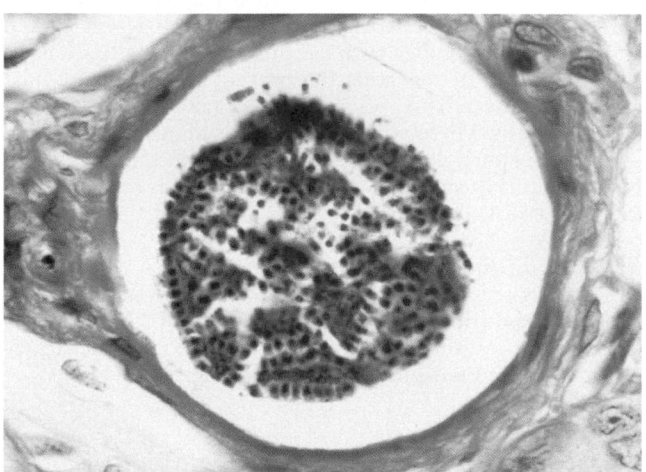

Fig 74-17 A mature *H. americanum* meront just before release of merozoites. Note the lack of inflammation surrounding the cystic structure (H and E stain, ×1200).

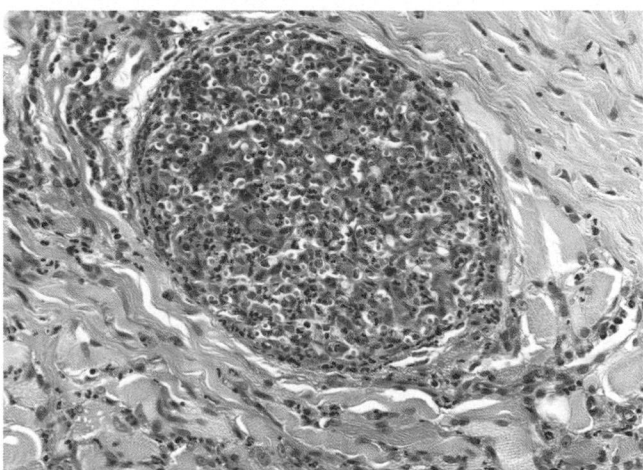

Fig 74-18 Pyogranuloma associated with the invasion of merozoites released from a cyst in a dog with *H. americanum*. Phagocytized merozoites can either reenter circulation to become gamonts or form a new "onion skin cyst."

Table • 74-2

Therapy for Hepatozoon americanum *Infection in Dogs*

DRUG[a]	DOSE[b] (MG/KG)	ROUTE	INTERVAL (HOURS)	DURATION (DAYS)
TCP combination: trimethoprim-sulfonamide *and*	15	PO	12	14
clindamycin *and*	10	PO	8	14
pyrimethamine	0.25	PO	24	14
and decoquinate	10–20	PO	12	730

TCP, Trimethoprim-sulfadiazine, clindamycin, and pyrimethamine; *PO,* by mouth.
[a]See Drug Formulary, Appendix 8, for additional information on each drug.
[b]Dose per administration at specified interval.

zoon. For this reason, dogs should not be fed raw meat or organs from wildlife in endemic areas.

Public Health Considerations

Only one report of human infection with a *Hepatozoon* spp. has been issued[23] (see previous discussion on *H. canis* infection). Transmission of *H. americanum* to people is unlikely because the disease is transmitted by ingestion of a tick rather than by a tick bite. The danger of direct transmission from dogs to people is apparently low.

SUGGESTED READINGS*

3. Baneth G, Aroch I, Tai N, et al. 1998a. *Hepatozoon* sp. infection in domestic cats: a retrospective study, *Vet Parasitol* 79:123-133.

4. Baneth G, Barta JR, Shkap V, et al. 2000a. Genetic and antigenic evidence supports the separation of *Hepatozoon canis* and *Hepatozoon americanum* at the species level, *J Clin Microbiol* 38:1298-1301.

27. Drost WT, Cummings CA, Mathew JS, et al. 2003. Determination of time of onset and location of early skeletal lesions in young dogs experimentally infected with *Hepatozoon americanum* using bone scintigraphy, *Vet Radiol Ultrasound* 44: 86-91.

34. Ewing SA, Panciera RJ, Mathew JS. 2003. Persistence of *Hepatozoon americanum* (Apicomplexa: Adeleorina) in a naturally infected dog, *J Parasitol* 89: 611-613.

60. Macintire DK, Vincent-Johnson NA. 2001. Treatment of dogs infected with *Hepatozoon americanum*: 53 cases (1989-1998), *J Am Vet Med Assoc* 218:77-82.

63. Mathew JS, Ewing SA, Panciera RJ, et al. 1998. Experimental transmission of *Hepatozoon americanum* (Vincent-Johnson et al, 1997) to dogs by the Gulf Coast tick, *Amblyomma maculatum*, Koch, *Vet Parasitol* 80:1-14.

65. Mathew JS, Saliki JT, Ewing SA, et al. 2001. An indirect enzyme-linked immunosorbent assay for diagnosis of American canine hepatozoonosis, *J Diagn Inves* 13: 17-21.

81. Panciera RJ, Ewing SA, Mathew JS, et al. 1999. Canine hepatozoonosis: comparison of lesions and parasites in skeletal muscle of dogs experimentally or naturally infected with *Hepatozoon americanum*, *Vet Parasitol* 82:261-72.

*See the CD-ROM for a complete list of references.

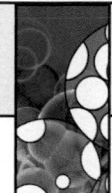

CHAPTER • 75

Microsporidiosis

Peter J. Didier, Karen Snowden, Xavier Alvarez, and Elizabeth S. Didier

ETIOLOGY

Microsporidiosis in dogs and cats is primarily caused by the obligate, intracellular parasite *Encephalitozoon cuniculi*, which is a member of the phylum Microsporidia. More than 1000 species of microsporidia—classified into approximately 100 genera—infect insects and members of all classes of vertebrates.[6,23] Medically important species of the genus *Encephalitozoon* (*Encephalitozoon hellem*, *Encephalitozoon intestinalis* [previously named *Septata intestinalis*], and three strains of *E. cuniculi*)[5,22,29,33] that have been described may infect dogs, cats, and birds.[23] Another microsporidian species, *Enterocytozoon bieneusi*, a common intestinal opportunistic parasite in patients with the acquired immunodeficiency syndrome (AIDS), has been identified in stool samples from cats, farm dogs, nonhuman primates, and numerous asymptomatic pigs.[12,17,20,38] Although no disease from *E. bieneusi* or *E. intestinalis* has been described in dogs and cats, the zoonotic potential of these subclinical infections needs additional investigation by analysis of diagnostic materials.[66]

Because *E. cuniculi* is the most commonly described microsporidian in pet animals, this chapter will focus primarily on this species. Mature spores of *E. cuniculi* are small and oval, measuring approximately 1.5 μm wide and 2.5 μm long. They contain the distinctive coiled polar tubule or filament-and-extrusion apparatus that distinguish microsporidia from all other organisms (Fig. 75-1). The polar tubule is used to propel the sporoplasm (containing the microsporidian nucleus) into the host cell. Spores also contain a posterior vacuole, ribosomes, endoplasmic reticulum, and Golgi-like membranes, but they lack mitochondria and peroxisomes. The spore coat contains an outer glycoprotein coat, a middle layer containing chitin, and an internal plasma membrane.[20]

Infection of most mammalian hosts with *E. cuniculi* occurs by ingestion or inhalation of spores from contaminated urine or feces that are shed by infected hosts.[6,23] Infection by transplacental transmission and traumatic inoculation have been reported as well.[50] Once internalized, infectious spores invade host cells by propelling the sporoplasm through the everting polar tubule by a process called *germination*. The sporoplasm of *E. cuniculi* develops within a host-cell–derived membrane-bound parasitophorous vacuole (Fig. 75-2). The organisms undergo schizogony (also called *merogony*), which is an asexual process of cell division or binary fission. During sporogony and maturation, organisms develop the spore coat and organelles (the polar tubule, endoplasmic reticulum, and polar cap). The host cells eventually rupture and release organisms that infect new cells or environmentally resistant spore forms, which are shed in the urine or feces.[6] Typical organs of localized infection in dogs and cats include the kidney, liver, and brain.[50]

EPIDEMIOLOGY

Natural infections with *E. cuniculi* have been described in a wide range of hosts, including rabbits, mice, cats, dogs, foxes,

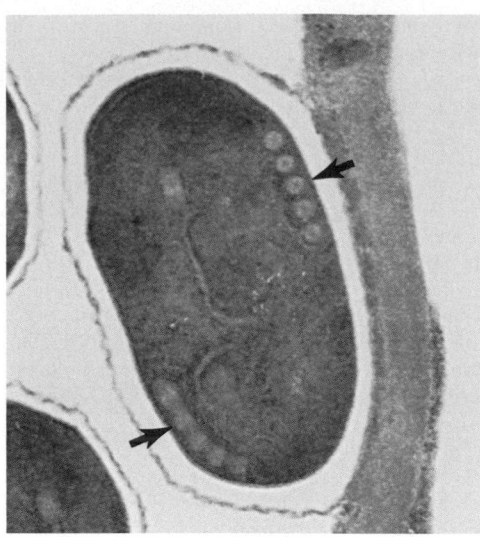

Fig 75-1 Electron microscopy of a mature *E. cuniculi* spore. Anterior polaroplast *(P)*, loops of the polar filament *(F)* in longitudinal and cross-section views, nucleus *(N)*, posterior vacuole *(V)* and electron-lucent spore wall are shown (bar = 200 nm). (From Shadduck JA, Bendele R, Robinson GA. 1978. Isolation of the causative organism of canine encephalitozoonosis, *Vet Pathol* 15:449–460. Used with permission.)

and people.[6,23,50,52] Of the three strains (genotypes) of *E. cuniculi*, strain I has been identified in rabbits and people. Strain II has been identified in mice, rats, and blue foxes, and strain III has been found in dogs and people.[11,21-23,41,66] Strain III has also caused fatal infections in nonhuman primates.[43] Differences in these isolates have been confirmed by protein electrophoresis, Western blot immunodetection, and small subunit ribosomal RNA (SSU rRNA) gene sequence analysis. Although epidemiologic information is sparse, one report suggests that *E. cuniculi* was transmitted to a dog groomer with AIDS.[66] However, strain I (primarily from rabbits) can infect mice, cats, and sheep in experimental situations.[23,44,50] A comparison of isolates from people and rabbits suggests the infecting strain is zoonotic.[13,14,23] A strain of *E. cuniculi* from a dog produced a subclinical infection in immunocompetent monkeys.[23,54] Relatively few isolates of *E. cuniculi* are available for comparison, so the host specificity of the *E. cuniculi* strains is still unclear.

A few studies have been published on the prevalence rates of naturally acquired *E. cuniculi* infections.[23] In a group of stray dogs that were housed three per cage in a London kennel, 13.3% of the dogs were found to express specific antibodies to *E. cuniculi*.[30] In South Africa a serologic study of 220 serum samples submitted for clinical evaluation suggested a prevalence of 18% in domestic dogs.[49] Among 52 dogs with renal failure, 12 (23%) expressed specific antibodies for *E. cuniculi*, compared with 2 of 42 (5%) control dogs.[48] Based on the presence of specific antibodies, a prevalence of 70% was also reported in 50 dogs housed in kennels. This high prevalence may have been a result of confinement and closer contact to contaminated urine or feces.[23,49] In an urban animal shelter, 6 of 20 dogs were found to be excreting

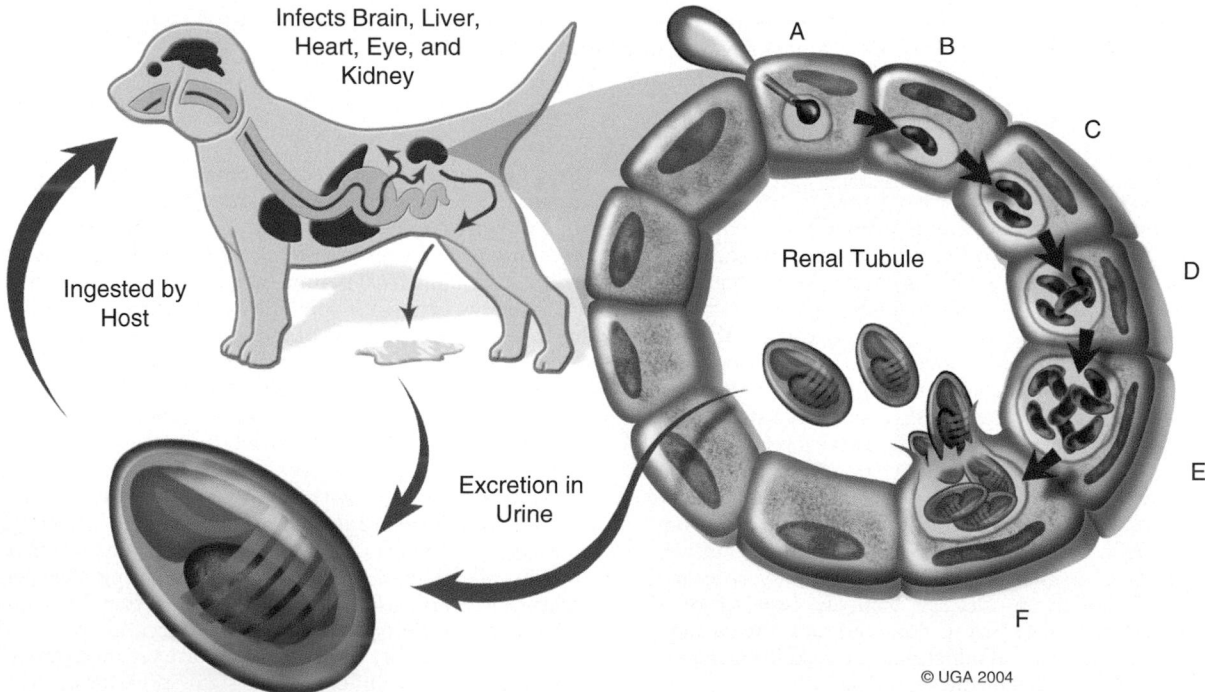

Fig 75-2 Intracellular life cycle of *E. cuniculi* in the renal tubular epithelium. Diagram is based on light and electron microscopic examination of parasites. Spore is ingested or inhaled and penetrates the gut wall, entering the systemic circulation. Spore can spread to many organs, such as the kidney shown here. **A,** Mature spore uses polar tubule to propel its sporoplasm into host cell. **B-F,** Proliferative forms of parasite *(schizonts)* replicate within parasitophorous vacuole. Binary fission occurs during contact with membrane of intracellular vacuole. As maturation progresses, spores collect in center of vacuole. **D** and **E,** Parasitophorous vacuole containing spores and proliferative forms. These stages are visible under light microscope. **F,** Vacuole ruptures, releases its spores into renal tubule lumen, and is excreted in urine. (Courtesy University of Georgia, Athens, Ga.)

microsporidial spores in the stools.[32] In Norway, biochemical testing did not identify antibody titers to *E. cuniculi* in sera from dogs of unknown health status.[1] Natural *E. cuniculi* infections of cats are rare, and no prevalence data have been published.[50]

Clinically significant infections of *E. cuniculi* generally develop in neonatal and young puppies and are acquired by transplacental transmission and ingestion or inhalation of spores shed from the mother.[23,50] Older dogs may become infected with microsporidia by inhalation or ingestion of spores from contaminated urine or feces or by ingestion of tissues from rabbits or mice infected with *E. cuniculi*.[40,50] Experimental canine infections also may be transmitted by intraperitoneal (IP) inoculation, whereas kittens may be infected experimentally by intracerebral, IP, or oral inoculation. Cats and older dogs generally show few or no clinical signs of disease but do sporadically shed organisms in the urine. Younger dogs infected with microsporidia have clinical signs associated with renal disease.[48,50] In experimental studies of other mammals, microsporidiosis has been chronic and asymptomatic in healthy immunocompetent animals but severe and lethal in T-cell–depleted animals.

CLINICAL FINDINGS

Dogs

Clinical signs in neonatal dogs appear within a few weeks postpartum, and several pups in a litter may have stunted growth and general unthriftiness.[23] As infection progresses, animals show signs of renal failure and neurologic abnormalities such as depression, ataxia, convulsions, and blindness.[8,39,40,50] Animals may develop aggressive behavior consisting of viciousness, biting, and abnormal vocalizations. The high frequency of anti-*E. cuniculi* antibodies in dogs with azotemia suggests that *E. cuniculi* may contribute to chronic renal disease in dogs.[48,50]

Clinical laboratory findings are available only for experimentally infected dogs.[23,50,51] A normochromic, normocytic anemia is a consistent finding and may result from severe renal lesions with depression of erythropoietin production. In contrast, leukocyte numbers, especially those of lymphocytes and monocytes, are higher. Bone marrow is hypercellular, with a preponderance of large mononuclear cells. Serum biochemical findings include increased alanine aminotransferase and alkaline phosphatase concentrations (in the high normal to slightly elevated range), variable serum urea nitrogen and creatinine levels, and increased total serum protein levels. Cerebrospinal fluid (CSF) may have more protein and cells in animals with behavioral and neurologic signs and higher anti-*E. cuniculi* IgG levels in the CSF than in serum. Urinalysis may demonstrate hematuria and pyuria.

Cats

Clinical signs in feline encephalitozoonosis vary. Severe muscle spasms, superficial corneal infection with blepharospasm, depression, paralysis, and death have occurred in those with natural infections, but the results could not be duplicated in experimental trials.[23,50] Clinical laboratory findings specifically for cats have not been reported.

DIAGNOSIS

Immunologically competent hosts produce specific antibodies to *E. cuniculi*, which can be detected by methods such as indirect fluorescent antibody (FA) staining and an enzyme-linked immunosorbent assay (ELISA).[23,50] An indirect FA titer greater than 1:20 or an ELISA titer of 1:800 or greater is considered to be positive for the presence of antibodies to *E. cuniculi*.[23,30,49,50] However, serologic tests are not commercially available, and some are concerned about the diagnostic reliability of serologic tests in immunologically immature puppies or casually exposed hosts. Therefore, diagnostic methods have focused on detecting the microsporidian spores in urine, stool, and tissue specimens.

The small size and poor staining qualities of *Encephalitozoon* organisms have made them difficult to visualize with routine parasitologic and histologic techniques. They are easily missed with hematoxylin-eosin (H and E) staining, especially when few organisms are present.

Transmission electron microscopy (EM) has been considered the standard for the specific diagnosis of microsporidiosis. Presence of the polar tubule distinguishes microsporidia from other organisms (see Fig. 75-1).[6,23,50] However, transmission EM is relatively insensitive, costly, and time consuming and requires technical expertise.[18,23]

Cytologic examination of body fluids is extremely important when making a clinical diagnosis in animals with disseminated infections. Spores shed into the urine from parasitized renal tubular epithelial cells are readily identifiable in the sediment with Gram or Ziehl-Neelsen staining.[23,26,28,50] Stained spores are gram-positive, whereas spores in the proliferative stages are gram-negative. Microsporidia in stool specimens are also difficult to distinguish from other gram-positive bacteria; however, indirect FA methods using monoclonal antibodies or hyperimmune polyclonal antisera can specifically identify microsporidia[23,56] (Fig. 75-3, *A*), but reagents are not commercially available. When viewed with cross-polarizing filters, *Encephalitozoon* species and other microsporidia

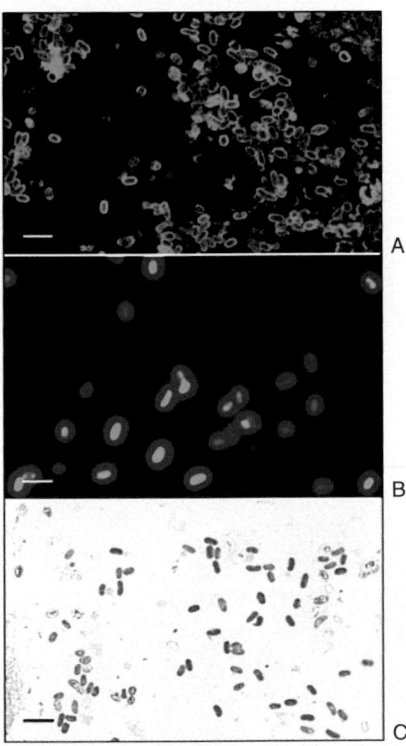

Fig 75-3 Diagnostics for urine and feces. **A,** *E. cuniculi* stained with rabbit polyclonal antiserum, secondary antibody linked to Alexa 468 fluorochrome, and visualized with fluorescence confocal microscopy. **B,** *E. cuniculi* stained with calcofluor white. White organisms with blue halo viewed with ultraviolet microscopy. **C,** *E. cuniculi* stained with trichrome and viewed by light microscopy. Of the three techniques, this provides the best demonstration of size and polar vacuole (bar = 5 μ).

have a birefringent appearance, unlike the coccidians *Toxoplasma gondii* and *Isospora* species. Chitin-staining fluorochromes (e.g., Calcofluor White 2MR, American Cyanamid, Princeton, N.J.) are useful for detecting the microsporidia, which stain as white to turquoise oval halos when viewed with ultraviolet (UV) microscopy (see Fig. 75-3, *B*).* Microsporidia are easily stained with the modified trichrome stains (using tenfold higher concentrations of chromotrope 2R) and appear bright pink with a diagonal pink band and a clear posterior vacuole. Bacteria stain with the counterstain (see Fig. 75-3, *C*).† Yeasts also stain bright pink but lack a posterior vacuole, and they are usually larger and more round than the oval-shape microsporidia. However, these staining methods cannot be used to discriminate between species of microsporidia. Molecular identification by the polymerase chain reaction (PCR) may soon replace EM as the method of choice for confirmation of microsporidiosis because experimental studies suggest PCR is significantly more sensitive and specific.‡

PATHOLOGIC FINDINGS

Based on experimental infections, gross lesions of canine encephalitozoonosis include hepatomegaly, petechiae on multiple organs, patchy consolidation and edema of the lungs, fibrinous pericarditis, regional enteritis, focal myocardial degeneration, swollen kidneys, hemorrhagic cystitis, and splenomegaly.[23,50] The kidney may contain mild petechiae or severe cortical cysts and infarcts (Fig. 75-4). The brain may

*References 10, 18, 23, 26, 37, 55, 57.
†References 10, 18, 23, 26, 27, 35, 62.
‡References 11, 21-23, 26, 29, 41, 59, 60, 64, 66, 67.

contain thrombosed meningeal blood vessels, focal encephalomalacia, and cystic spaces within the parenchyma. In naturally infected blue foxes, nodular thickening of the extramural coronary arteries and lymphadenomegaly have been seen.[50]

Histologically, dogs and blue foxes with encephalitozoonosis consistently have nonsuppurative meningoencephalitis (Fig. 75-5).[23,39,50] Fibrinoid necrosis of small and medium-size arteries of the brain can result in thrombosis and encephalomalacia. Parasitophorous vacuoles develop in endothelial and glial cells. Kidneys of dogs, cats, and foxes have multifocal nonsuppurative interstitial nephritis. Para-

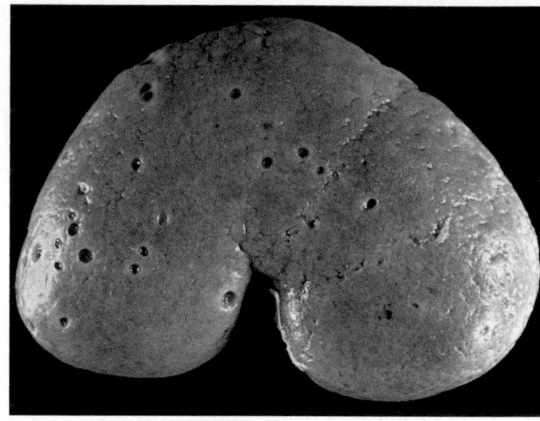

Fig 75-4 Kidney with pale, firm cortex that has irregular-subcapsular surface and numerous projecting cysts filled with clear fluid. (From Shadduck JA, Bendele R, Robinson GT. 1978. Isolation of the causative organism of canine encephalitozoonosis, *Vet Pathol* 15:449-460.)

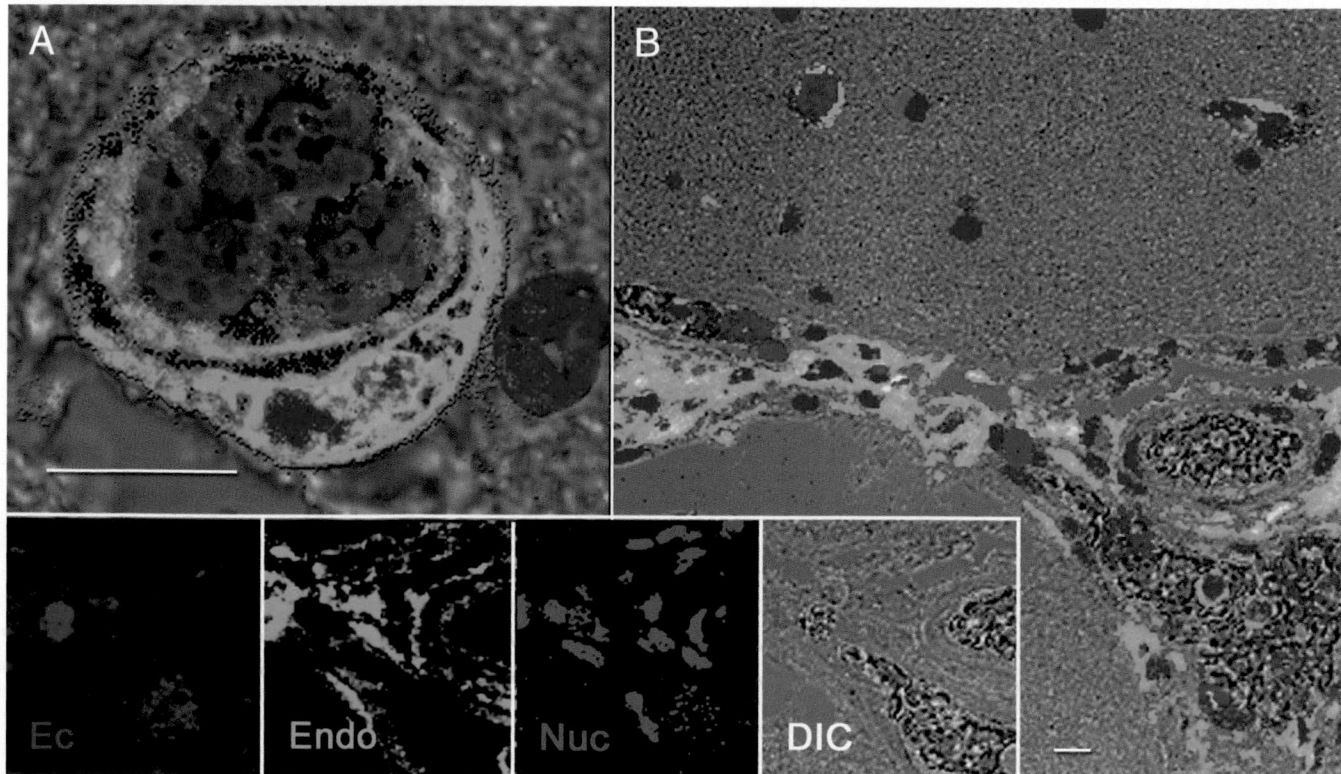

Fig 75-5 **A,** Parasitophorus vacuole packed with *E. cuniculi (red)* in endothelial cell *(green)* of nearly occluded cerebral capillary from fetal dog with transplacental infection. **B,** Lower power confocal image demonstrates *E. cuniculi* in and near cerebral vasculature. Small numbers of inflammatory cell and resident nuclei are blue (TO-PRO-3 dye). Background *(gray)* is differential interference phase contrast. *E. cuniculi* is stained with rabbit antiserum and secondary antibody linked to Alexa 468; endothelium is marked with isolectin B4 and Alexa 568 (bar = 5 μm).

sitophorous vacuoles with organisms are present in the renal tubular epithelia. In the heart, focal myocardial necrosis, vasculitis, and fibrinoid necrosis of small and medium-size arteries are associated with *E. cuniculi* in endothelial cells and smooth muscle cells. In experimental infections, livers of dogs and cats developed vascular fibrinoid necrosis, focal hepatic necrosis, and lymphoplasmacytic infiltration associated with *E. cuniculi* in hepatocytes, Kupffer's cells, and endothelial cells. In blue foxes, ocular lesions are attributable to arterial lesions of the short and long ciliary arteries and retinal vessels. Other nonspecific lesions include pulmonary edema, nonsuppurative interstitial pneumonia and enteritis, lymphadenomegaly, reticuloendothelial hyperplasia of the spleen, and hyperplasia of the bone marrow.[50]

THERAPY

No treatment has been reported for either canine or feline encephalitozoonosis. In vitro experiments demonstrate that the antibiotic fumagillin inhibits the replicative ability of the organism without damaging the host cell, but the drug is toxic when used systemically in mammals.[23,50] Topical fumagillin has successfully treated microsporidial keratitis in people infected with the human immunodeficiency virus (HIV). No information regarding its use in dogs and cats with microsporidiosis has been reported.[19,23,24] An analogue of fumagillin, known as *TNP-470*, was effective in vitro and in vivo in mice with experimental intraperitoneal infections.[9] Resveratrol, a natural compound in grapes, has sporicidal activity in vitro and was not toxic to cultured cells, suggesting a potential use for treatment.[35a] The benzimidazole albendazole has successfully treated *Encephalitozoon* infections in patients with AIDS.[3,11,19,23,42,55] No information regarding its use for treating dogs and cats with microsporidiosis has been published. *E. intestinalis* and only some *E. bieneusi* strains, both of which can infect dogs, are susceptible to albendazole. In adult humans, the dosage is 400 mg every 12 hours for 4 weeks or longer. In vitro and in vivo studies suggest that the parasite is inhibited by antifolate drugs. Trimethoprim or pyrimethamine and sulfonamides alone or in combination with albendazole have effectively treated people with disseminated infections.[23,25] Clindamycin effectively treated a disseminated *Encephalitozoon*-like species infection in an immunocompromised person.[34] (See the Drug Formulary, Appendix 8, for canine dosages and precautions.)

PREVENTION AND PUBLIC HEALTH CONSIDERATIONS

Identification of several species of microsporidia in people and animals (Table 75-1) suggests the possibility of zoonotic transmission.[12,14] In people with AIDS, *E. bieneusi*, *E. intestinalis*, and *E. hellem* are the most frequent causes of disease and probably result from opportunistic spread of endogenous microflora. In people infected with HIV, intestinal microsporidiosis is associated with male homosexuality and swimming pools, suggesting fecal-oral transmission by sexual and waterborne routes.[31] However, one report describes a 10-year-old girl who underwent seroconversion to *E. cuniculi* after close contact with an infected puppy[23,40]; transmission of *E. cuniculi* and *E. bieneusi* to a dog handler was suspected in another case.[66] No direct evidence proves that dogs infect people with microsporidia, people infect dogs, or both. Isolates of *E. cuniculi* strain III have been identified in dogs and immunocompromised individuals, suggesting that this species has a zoonotic potential, a common source of exposure, or both.[46]

Table • 75-1

Species of Microsporidia Infecting People and Animals

MICROSPORIDIA	HUMAN CONDITION	NATURALLY INFECTED ANIMALS
Brachiola algerae	Keratitis	Mosquitoes
Brachiola connori	Disseminated infection	Invertebrates
Enterocytozoon bieneusi[a]	Diarrhea, malabsorption, weight loss, rhinitis, bronchitis	Monkeys, swine, farm dogs, cats
Encephalitozoon cuniculi	Peritonitis, hepatitis, rhinosinusitis, seizures, nephritis, disseminated infection	*Strain I:* rabbits, humans; *strain II:* mice, blue foxes, rats; *strain III:* dogs, cats, humans, tamarins Foxes, rodents, monkeys, birds, cattle
Encephalitozoon hellem	Conjunctivitis, keratoconjunctivitis, rhinosinusitis, bronchiolitis pneumonia, disseminated infection	Budgerigars
Encephalitozoon intestinalis[a]	Diarrhea, disseminated infection pneumonia, cholecystitis, cholangitis	Dogs, goats, cattle, swine
Pleistophora species[a]	Myositis	Australian terrestrial mammals, insects, neon tetra fish
Trachipleistophora hominis	Myositis, keratitis, rhinosinusitis	Unknown
Trachipleistophora antheiopopthera	Disseminated infection	Unknown
Microsporidium species[b]	Keratitis	Unknown
Nosema ocularum[a]	Keratitis	Invertebrates
Vittaforma corneae[a]	Keratitis, disseminated infection	Unknown

[a]Water and/or food contamination also reported in addition to known animal sources.
[b]Collective term for unclassified microsporidia.

Maintaining sanitary conditions is important when handling suspected cases of encephalitozoonosis because environmentally resistant spores may be shed in urine or feces. Spores can readily be rendered uninfective by various disinfectants; the most commonly available are 2% phenol, 10% formalin, and 70% ethyl alcohol. Infectivity is unaffected by sonication, freezing and thawing, and pH levels ranging from 4 to 9. Infectivity of spores stored in neutral buffer at 4° C and 20° C persists for more than 24 days, indicating that spore survival is possible in a humid environment at ambient temperatures.[23,50]

ACKNOWLEDGMENT

We would like to thank John A. Shadduck, mentor, scientist, and author of this chapter in previous editions, for his continued support and inspiration in the field of microsporidiosis.

SUGGESTED READINGS*

20a. Didier ES, Didier PJ, Stovall ME, et al. 2004. Epidemiology of microsporidiosis: sources and modes of transmission, *Vet Parasitol* 126:145-166.

26. Garcia LS. 2002. Laboratory identification of the microsporidia. *J Clin Microbiol* 40:1892-1901.

46. Snowden K, Logan K, Didier ES. 1999. *Encephalitozoon cuniculi* strain III is a cause of encephalitozoonosis in both humans and dogs. *J Infect Dis* 180:2086-2088.

52. Tosoni A, Nebuloni M, Ferri A, et al. 2002. Disseminated microsporidiosis caused by *Encephalitozoon cuniculi III* (dog type) in an Italian AIDS patient: a retrospective study. *Mod Pathol* 15:577-583.

*See the CD-ROM for a complete list of references.

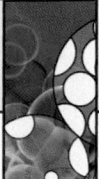

CHAPTER • 76

Cytauxzoonosis

Craig E. Greene, James Meinkoth, and A. Alan Kocan†

ETIOLOGY AND EPIDEMIOLOGY

Cytauxzoon felis causes a tick-borne blood protozoal disease of domestic cats *(Felis domesticus)* and exotic Felidae from several central, south central, and southeastern states in the United States (Fig. 76-1). This distribution corresponds somewhat with the only known tick vector, *Dermacentor variabilis*. Infection of domestic cats results in a rapidly progressive, usually fatal, disease. The natural reservoir host appears to be the North American bobcat *(Lynx rufus)*, in which infection is usually exhibited as a persistent, but asymptomatic, erythroparasitemia. Other wild cats may also harbor the organism. In a study of naturally exposed exotic cats in Florida, the prevalence of asymptomatic infection for transplanted Texas cougars was 39% and for Florida panthers was 35%.[30] Fatal cytauxzoonosis was reported in a captive-reared white tiger *(Panthera tigris)* at a private breeding facility in northern Florida.[10] Florida panthers *(Puma concolor coryi)* and a Texas cougar *(P. concolor stanleyana)* at this facility were also suspected of being infected. In Germany, a captive Bengal tiger *(Panthera tigris)* developed fatal cytauxzoonosis, presumably after contact with bobcats imported from North America.[16] The organism has previously been recognized in the erythrocytes of cheetahs *(Acinonyx jubatus)*.[33] Iatrogenic transmission from a Florida panther to a domestic cat has been reported.[4] Cytauxzoonosis, caused by similar organisms as evaluated by light microscopy, was first described in African ungulates. Electron microscopic examination of a natural, fatal case of African cytauxzoonosis in a tsessebe calf *(Damaliscus lunatus)* showed the size and appearance similar to those described for *C. felis*.[17] Organisms genetically similar to *C. felis* have been identified in cats in Spain,[6] South Africa,[1] and in a Pallas' cat *(Otocolobus manul)* from Mongolia.[18] Therefore this disease may be more widespread than was previously recognized. Reservoir hosts and vectors will need to be determined for these newly recognized foci of infection.

Cytauxzoon has been classified in the order Piroplasmida and family Theileriidae. This family has both an erythrocytic and a leukocytic, or tissue, phase. In the case of *C. felis*, the tissue phase consists of large schizonts that develop within macrophages, whereas *Theileria*, a more familiar genus of this family, has its exoerythrocytic phase primarily within lymphocytes. The Babesiidae, a related family, is characterized by having only or primarily an erythrocytic (piriform) phase in the mammalian host that is indistinguishable from the erythrocytic form in *Cytauxzoon*. Although no serologic cross-reactivity has been reported between *C. felis* and the South African parasites *Theileria taurotragi* and *Babesia felis*, RNA gene sequence analysis links *C. felis*, *Babesia equi*, and *Babesia rodhaini* to both the theilerias and babesias, with some suggestion that these three organisms be reclassified within a separate family.[1,7]

In the life cycle of *C. felis*, schizonts develop primarily within mononuclear phagocytes, first as indistinct vesicular structures within the cytoplasm of infected cells and later as large, distinct, nucleated schizonts that actively undergo division by schizogony and binary fission (Fig. 76-2).[22] The phagocytes line the lumens of vessels within almost every organ and become huge and numerous, often occluding the vessel similar to a thrombus. Multiplication of schizonts within host cells is observed ultrastructurally to be true schizogony, without host cell division. Later in the course of the disease, schizonts develop buds (merozoites) that separate and eventually fill the entire host cell. The host cell probably ruptures, releasing the merozoites into the blood or tissue fluid. Merozoites appear in macrophages 1 to 3 days before they are observed in erythrocytes. These organisms then invade uninfected erythrocytes and produce late-stage para-

†*Deceased.*

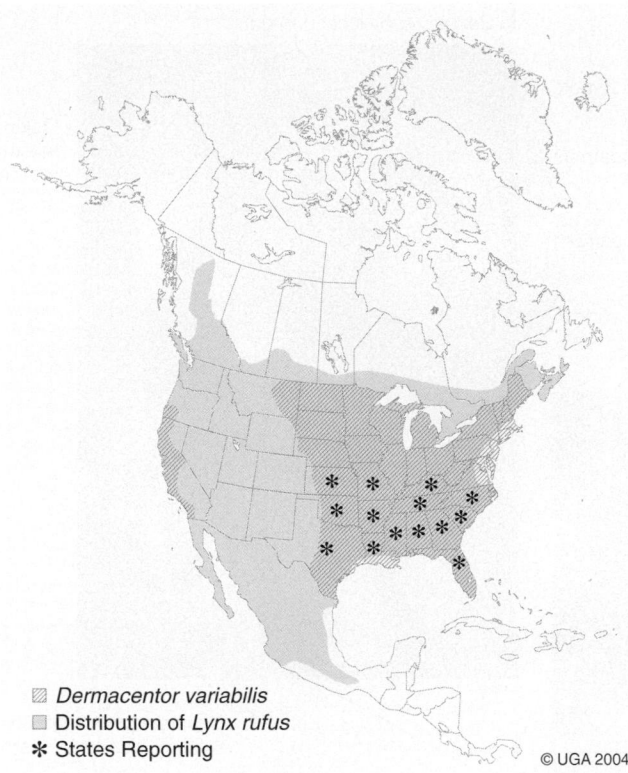

Fig 76-1 Map of distribution by state of reported cytauxzoonosis in the United States, along with overlapping distribution of the tick and reservoir host. (Courtesy University of Georgia, Athens, Ga.)

- ▨ *Dermacentor variabilis*
- ☐ Distribution of *Lynx rufus*
- ✳ States Reporting

© UGA 2004

sitemias that are detected on examination of blood films, usually 1 to 3 days before death.[20]

The apparently sporadic occurrence, short course of illness, and usually fatal nature of the disease indicate that the domestic cat is likely an incidental dead-end host. However, at least two cats with naturally occurring infections and two experimentally inoculated, untreated cats have survived.[13,28,32] In contrast, the schizogenous phase is limited and transient in infected bobcats that usually develop a nonfatal erythroparasitemia and serve as potential carriers.[3] Infection rates as high as 60% in clinically healthy, wild-trapped bobcats has been reported.[12] However, fatal disease has been reported sporadically in some bobcats.[3,21,29]

Ticks likely are the natural vector for *Cytauxzoon* because most cases have been associated with the presence of ticks on the hosts. Tick *(Dermacentor variabilis)* transmission from wild-caught, splenectomized bobcats with parasitemia to two splenectomized domestic cats resulted in the fatal form of the disease. Conversely, subinoculation of blood from bobcats to cats appeared to transmit only the erythrocytic piroplasm stage resulting in asymptomatic parasitemia.[2] The fatal form of the disease with extraerythrocytic stages develops only, or primarily, after tick transmission of the organism or inoculation of schizont-containing tissues from fatally infected cats. In the white tiger that developed naturally occurring fatal disease in Florida, two female Lone Star ticks *(Amblyomma americanum)* were present on the inguinal skin.[10]

PATHOGENESIS

The prepatent period of natural infection is between 2 to 3 weeks. Rapid, intravascular multiplication of the tissue phase of the parasite is responsible for the severe clinical illness seen in domestic cats, most likely the result of mechanical obstruction of blood flow, especially through the lungs. By-products of tissue parasites may be toxic, pyrogenic, and vasoactive. The blood phase may induce destruction and phagocytosis of erythrocytes, although erythroparasitemia in the absence of schizogenous development is of little clinical significance. Disseminated intravascular coagulation (DIC) has been a complication based on laboratory findings in naturally infected cats.[10,13] Infected cats appear to die from a shocklike state.

CLINICAL FINDINGS

In the naturally occurring disease, affected cats develop nonspecific clinical signs that lead to a rapid course of illness and death, usually in fewer than 5 days. Most cats are presented from March through September, and geographic clusters of infection may be observed. Access to an outdoor, wooded environment or tick exposure is typically noted. Anorexia, dyspnea, lethargy, dark urine, dehydration, depression, icterus and pallor, anemic heart murmur, capillary refill time greater than 2 seconds, and fever (39.4° to 41.6° C [103° to 107° F]) have been observed (Fig. 76-3). Some cats vocalize as if in pain. Hypothermia, recumbency, and coma are clinical findings in terminally ill cats.

Clinical signs in experimentally induced cytauxzoonosis have been similar to those in naturally occurring cases. Incubation periods have varied from 5 to 20 days, probably attributable to type and dose of inoculum, method of cryopreservation, and individual cat response. After a febrile period (39.9° to 40.1° C [103.8° to 104.2° F]), the temperature may become subnormal, and the cat may have difficulty breathing. Parasitized erythrocytes are observed late in the disease, during the febrile episode. Cats usually die 2 or 3 days after the temperature peak, and the entire course of clinical illness usually takes less than a week.

DIAGNOSIS

Cytauxzoonosis should be considered in the differential diagnosis when a cat that is allowed access to tick-infested, wooded areas becomes depressed and develops high temperature and possibly anemia and jaundice. Confusion with hemotrophic mycoplasmosis (formerly haemobartonellosis) is most frequent (see Chapter 31). Generally, cytauxzoonosis can be suspected when anemia is mild relative to the degree of icterus. Instead of the strongly regenerative anemia typical of hemolysis, the anemia of cytauxzoonosis is normocytic, normochromic, and nonregenerative. The leukocyte count may be variable, but a profound leukopenia or thrombocytopenia, or both, are present, particularly late in the course of disease. High serum concentrations of total bilirubin and bilirubinuria are common findings. Other clinical chemistry changes are variable and less specific but include low serum concentrations of albumin, cholesterol, and potassium and high serum glucose and alanine aminotransferase activity.[15] Although serum urea nitrogen and ammonia concentrations and hepatic enzyme activities may be elevated in febrile or comatose animals, they may not be elevated earlier in the course of disease. Along with thrombocytopenia, prolonged activated coagulation, activated partial thromboplastin time (APTT), and prothrombin time tests and increased fibrin split products will be present in cats with DIC.[10,13,14] Cats with cytauxzoonosis do not always have prolongation of all coagulation values; the APTT, in conjunction with thrombocytopenia, is usually most consistently elevated.

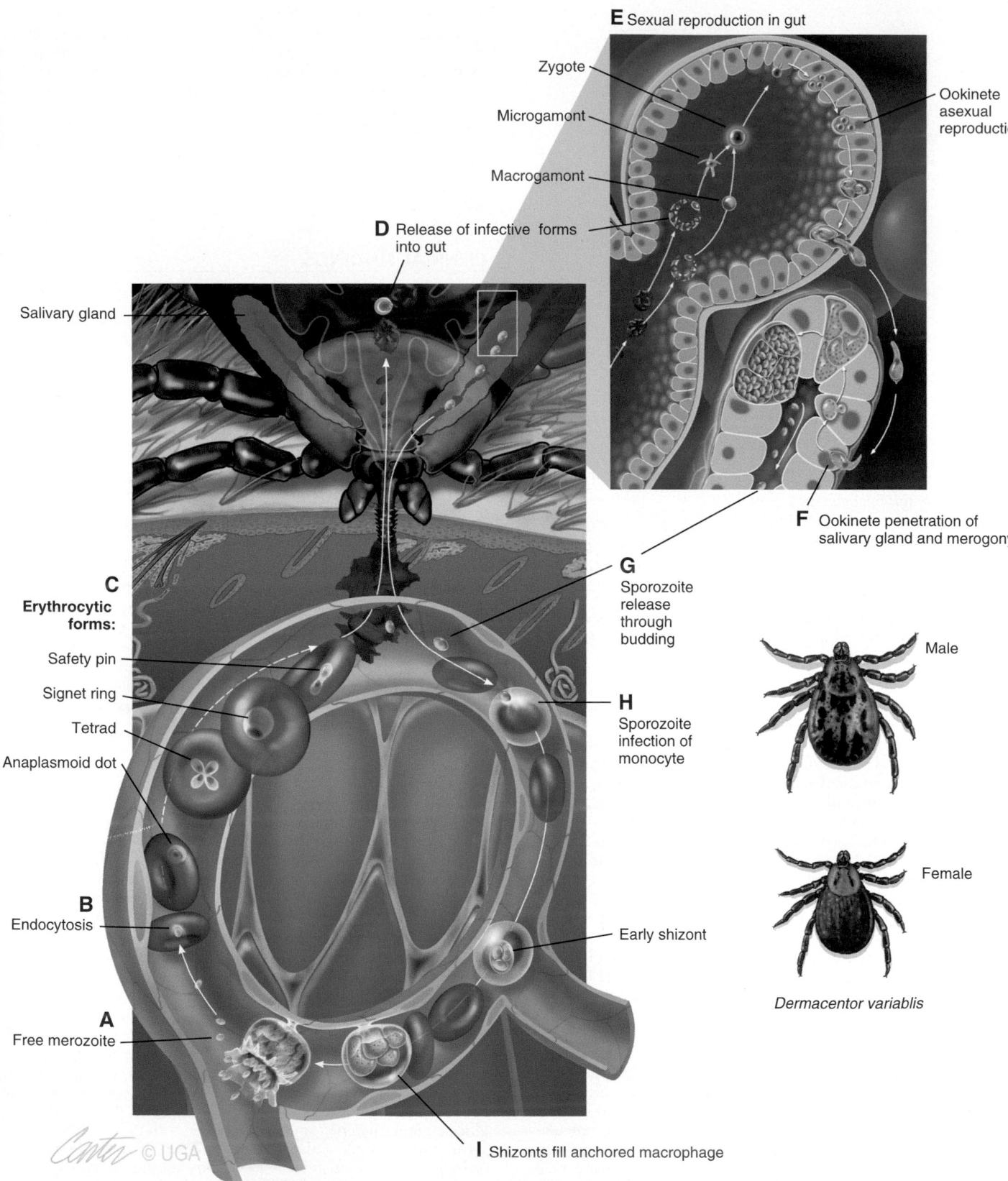

E Sexual reproduction in gut

Zygote

Microgamont

Macrogamont

Ookinete asexual reproduction

D Release of infective forms into gut

F Ookinete penetration of salivary gland and merogony

Salivary gland

G Sporozoite release through budding

C Erythrocytic forms:

Safety pin

Signet ring

Tetrad

Anaplasmoid dot

H Sporozoite infection of monocyte

B Endocytosis

Early shizont

A Free merozoite

Male

Female

Dermacentor variablis

I Shizonts fill anchored macrophage

Fig 76-2 Life cycle of C. *felis*. **A,** Free merozoites, released from schizonts, **(B)** enter circulating erythrocytes by endocytosis and **(C)** undergo replication in a variety of forms. The circulating parasitized erythrocytes are ingested by the tick and **(D)** are released into the gut. **E,** These differentiate into macro- and micro-gamonts which unite to form a zygote. This differentiates into an ookinete which replicates by asexual reproduction and finally penetrates the gut wall and migrates to the salivary gland. **F,** Once there, asexual reproduction by merogony results in salivary infection, **(G)** via budding of organisms from the cell surface. **H,** During feeding, the organism is inoculated by the tick and enters mononuclear phagocytes. **I,** Within the phagocytes, replication by schizogony and binary fission leads to large parasitized cells that often occlude the blood vessel lumen. Merozoites engorge the cell until it ruptures releasing the merozoites into the blood and the cycle continues (Courtesy University of Georgia, Athens, Ga.)

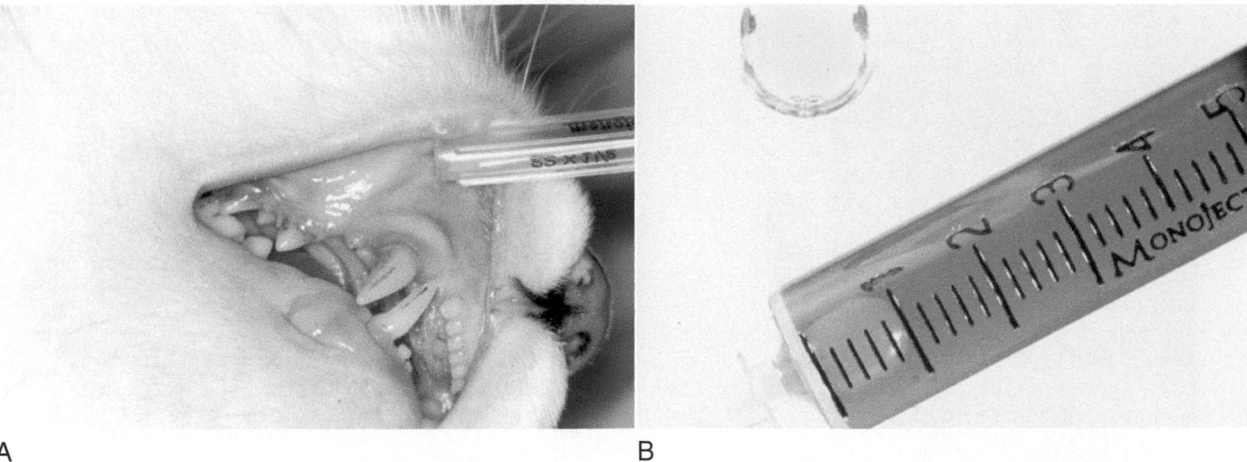

A B

Fig 76-3 **A,** Cat showing paleness from *Cytauxzoon* infection. **B,** Serum *(glass tube, top left)* and urine *(syringe, bottom right)* show high bilirubin content. (Courtesy University of Georgia, Athens, Ga.)

Definitive diagnosis is most commonly made by demonstrating the erythrocyte phase (piroplasms) in Wright's- or Giemsa-stained thin blood films. The piroplasms within erythrocytes appear as round "signet ring"–shaped bodies, 1 to 1.5 μm in diameter; bipolar oval "safety pin" forms, 1 × 2 μm; tetrad forms; or anaplasmoid round "dots," less than 0.5 μm in diameter (Fig. 76-4). All forms may occur in a single blood film, the signet ring–shaped organisms being most characteristic. A single cell usually contains only one parasite, but pairs and tetrads (Maltese crosses) are observed occasionally. The nucleus of the piroplasm is round to elongated and stains purple to dark red. The cytoplasm stains light blue or may appear as an indistinct clearing of the erythrocyte adjacent to the nucleus. The erythrocytic stage of *Cytauxzoon* may appear similar to other hemoparasites. The prominent, well-defined nuclear area of *C. felis* piroplasms allows differentiation from the ring form of hemotrophic mycoplasmas. Piroplasms of some small *Babesia* spp., such as *B. felis,* and *Theileria* spp. are morphologically indistinguishable from those of *C. felis.* However, these organisms have not yet been reported to infect domestic cats in the United States.

The number of parasitized cells varies from cat to cat and with the stage of the disease, increasing as the disease progresses. The development of schizogenous tissue phases, which is responsible for clinical signs of disease, precedes the appearance of piroplasms in the peripheral blood by a few days. Therefore some cats examined early in the course of disease may not be parasitemic on initial evaluation. The number of parasites in peripheral blood smears may increase dramatically in a 24-hour period; therefore reevaluation may be helpful when cytauxzoonosis is suspected despite a negative blood smear. When quantitated, the percentage of parasitized erythrocytes during illness ranges from 0.5% to 4%. In terminally ill, moribund cats, parasitemia has been higher. The number of nucleated erythrocytes and erythrocytes with Howell-Jolly bodies may increase slightly.

If the parasitemia is absent or low, the schizogenous tissue phase may be found in Wright's- or Giemsa-stained aspirates or impression smears of spleen, lung, liver, bone marrow, or lymph node.[9] Phagocytes containing tissue-phase schizonts are sometimes found on the feathered edge of a peripheral blood smear. Schizonts are first recognized as basophilic areas within the cytoplasm of macrophages (Fig. 76-5). As the developing schizont enlarges to fill the cytoplasm of the macrophage completely, the parasitized host cell enlarges greatly and develops a large, prominent nucleolus (Fig. 76-6). As the schizont matures, the purple nuclei of developing merozoites can be seen within the basophilic schizont (Fig. 76-7).

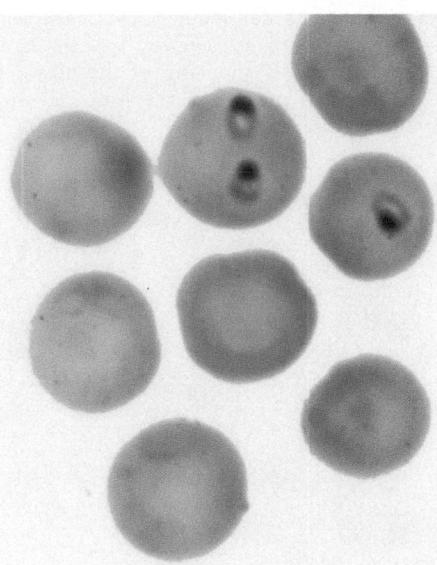

Fig 76-4 Feline erythrocytes infected with characteristic, signet ring–shaped *Cytauxzoon* piroplasms. The large, clearly evident nuclear area allows the organisms to be differentiated from hemotrophic *Mycoplasma* organisms (Wright-Giemsa, ×330).

Thoracic radiographs may show a bronchointerstitial pulmonary pattern, presumably related to the schizogony occurring in the pulmonary tissues.[25] Endotracheal washings from one cat had a mixed cell pattern of macrophages, eosinophils, neutrophils, and lymphocytes, in decreasing order. Intracellular schizonts were observed in pulmonary macrophages.

In cats that die, histologic confirmation should be made from standard formalin-fixed tissues (lung, lymph node, spleen, liver, heart, brain) sent to a veterinary pathology laboratory for parasite evaluation because hemotrophic mycoplasmosis and babesiosis do not have a tissue stage. A direct fluorescent antibody test for the detection of the tissue phase[31] and a microfluorometric immunoassay system for the detection of the serum antibody to *C. felis*[5] have been developed; however, neither test is commercially available. Polymerase chain reaction (PCR) has been used to document and follow infection in cats that survived infection, and it may become commercially available.[27,1a] In one treated cat, the PCR results were positive 18 months after treatment,

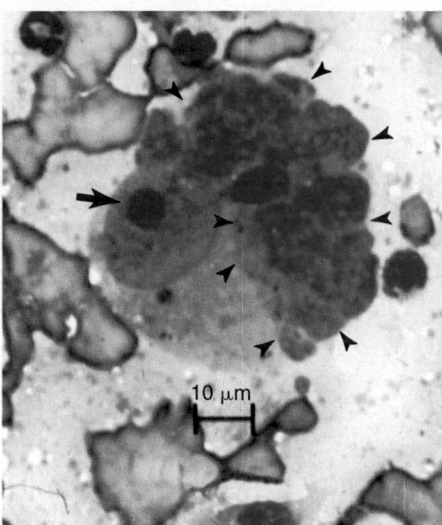

Fig 76-5 Impression smear from a feline liver showing a macrophage contains a developing *Cytauxzoon* schizont. The early schizont *(outlined by arrowheads)* appears as a lobulated basophilic area within the cytoplasm of the host cell. A large, prominent nucleolus is present in the host cell nucleus *(long arrow)* (Wright-Giemsa, ×165).

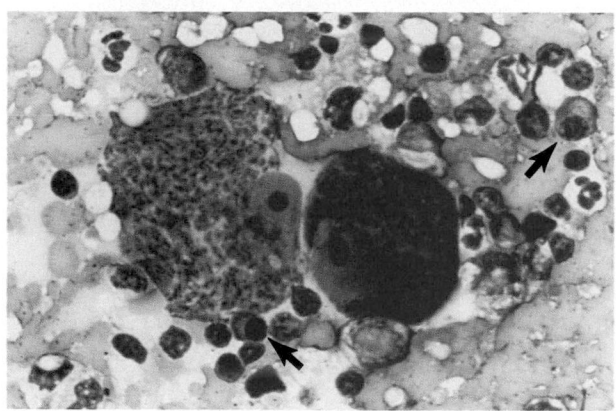

Fig 76-6 Two schizont-containing macrophages in an impression smear of feline spleen. The host cells are greatly enlarged as can be seen by comparison with the numerous small lymphocytes and plasma cells *(arrows)* in the background (Wright-Giemsa, ×66.)

although no organisms were detected on blood smear examination.[27] Because of the usually rapidly progressive nature of the disease, such tests are not needed in most routine cases.

PATHOLOGIC FINDINGS

Gross findings in domestic cats include dehydration; pallor; icterus; hydropericardium; hydrothorax; enlarged, edematous, and hemorrhagic lymph nodes; accentuated hepatic lobular pattern; intraabdominal venous distention; splenomegaly; and petechial and ecchymotic hemorrhages on the serosal surfaces of abdominal organs and lungs (Fig. 76-8). The lungs are frequently congested and edematous, often with petechiae throughout (Fig. 76-9).

The characteristic lesion on histologic examination of feline cytauxzoonosis is the accumulation of a large number

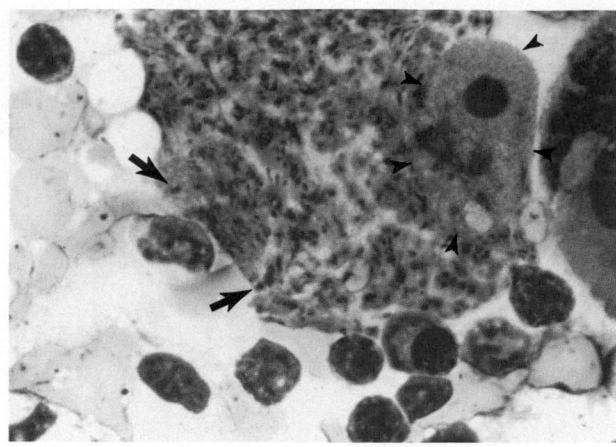

Fig 76-7 Higher magnification of cell in Fig. 76-6. The host nucleus *(outlined by arrowheads)* with an enlarged nucleolus is visible. The developed schizont completely fills the cytoplasm and the nuclear material of the developing merozoites is evident *(small arrows)* (Wright-Giemsa, ×330).

of parasitized mononuclear phagocytes containing schizonts in various stages of development. These cells are particularly prevalent within the lumens of veins of the lungs, liver, lymph nodes, and spleen, making these vessels appear partially or completely occluded (Fig. 76-10). Minimal inflammatory reaction is present in affected tissues. Spleen and lymph node should be used for tissue impression films, which should be stained with Wright's or Giemsa stain.

THERAPY

Preliminary attempts to treat cats that have either naturally or experimentally induced disease have had very limited success. The domestic cat as an unnatural host appears highly susceptible to this organism. Some evidence for more recent adaptation exists in that cats are being presented for clinical illness rather than at postmortem.[13,27] Strains from different geographic areas may also vary in virulence. Since 1997, an increasing number of cats from a limited geographic area in northwestern Arkansas and northeastern Oklahoma have survived natural infection, most without receiving any specific, potentially effective antiprotozoal treatment.[27] These cats appear to be immune to subsequent challenge with virulent *C. felis*.[26] In most other reports, even with the most effective drugs, the mortality is extremely high. Of the recovered cats, supportive care is essential. Supportive diuresis with isotonic intravenous fluids and adjunctive heparin is necessary to control concomitant DIC.[14]

Parvaquone, sodium thiacetarsemide, buparvaquone, and tetracycline appear to be ineffective. One cat treated with fluids, enrofloxacin, and tetracycline survived, although therapy was likely not related to survival in this animal.[32] This cat came from the area in northeastern Oklahoma in which survivors have subsequently been commonly reported and may in fact represent an early infection with a less virulent strain. Most success in treatment has been with the carbanilide compounds, diminazene, or imidocarb. Imidocarb is commercially available in the United States (see Drug Formulary, Appendix 8).[14] The drug is given as two injections within a 1- to 2-week interval. Parasympatholytic drugs such as atropine or glycopyrrolate should be given before treatment to counteract potential parasympathetic side effects. Morphologic examination of the organisms in blood smears showed a degenerating appearance within 48 hours after drug therapy was

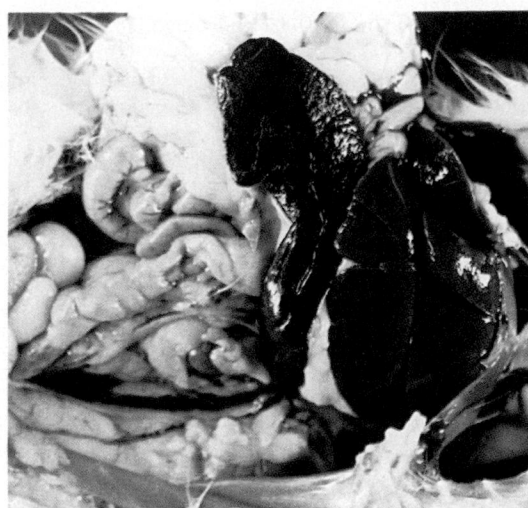

Fig 76-8 Gross lesions in a cat experimentally infected with *C. felis* include a greatly enlarged spleen and a slightly enlarged liver with rounded edges and distended veins.

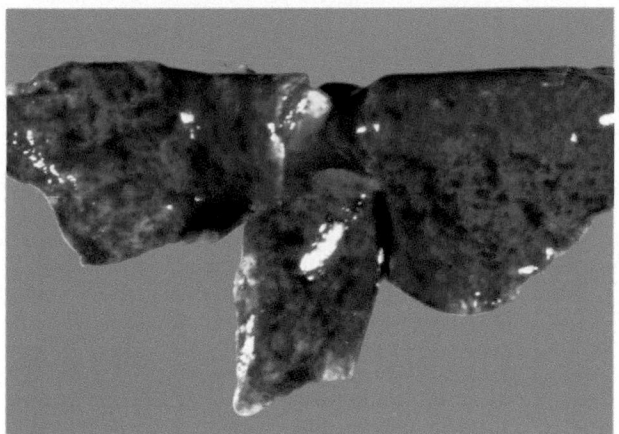

Fig 76-9 Petechial and ecchymotic hemorrhages throughout the lungs of a cat that died from cytauxzoonosis. (Courtesy Oklahoma State University Veterinary Pathobiology Teaching Set, Stillwater, Okla.)

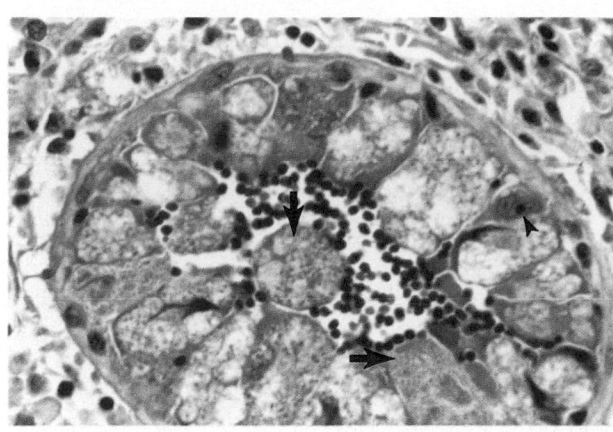

Fig 76-10 Section of lung from a cat with cytauxzoonosis. Schizont-containing macrophages completely line the endothelial surface and nearly occlude the lumen of a large vessel. The enlarged nucleoli of host cell nuclei are visible in some cells *(arrowheads)*. Developing organisms can be seen as a faint granular appearance to the cytoplasm of some of the cells *(arrow)* (H and E stain, ×66).

instituted. Enrofloxacin has also been used in a limited number of cats, in combination with the carbanilides; however, its efficacy has not been substantiated. Recommended dosages for these drugs are listed in Table 76-1. Within the first week following treatment, the cat develops a hemolytic anemia, presumably as a result of destruction of dying organisms in infected erythrocytes. Cats that recover subsequently have an increase in their erythrocyte neutrophil and platelet counts. Blood transfusions may be required in cats that have the most severe hemolytic anemia following treatment.

PREVENTION

A conscientiously applied ectoparasite control program and confinement indoors during tick season may be beneficial in preventing cytauxzoonosis because all naturally occurring cases have involved cats that were free to roam in wooded, tick-infested areas. See Chapter 94 for more extensive information on tick control.

Table • 76-1

Therapy for Cytauxzoonosis

DRUG[a]	DOSE[b]	ROUTE	INTERVAL	DURATION (DAYS)
Heparin	100–150 U/kg	SC	8 hours	As needed
Atropine	0.04 mg/kg	IV, IM, SC	24 hours	1[c]
Glycopyrrolate	0.005–0.01 mg/kg	IV, IM, SC	24 hours	1[c]
Enrofloxacin[d]	5.0 mg/kg	PO, SC	12 hours	7–10
Imidocarb dipropionate	5.0 mg/kg	IM	14 days	14
Diminazene aceturate	2.0 mg/kg	IM	7 days	7

SC, Subcutaneous; *IV*, intravenous; *IM*, intramuscular; *PO*, by mouth.
[a]See Drug Formulary, Appendix 8, for specific information on each drug. Adjunctive isotonic fluid therapy is extremely important for this disease. See text.
[b]Dose per administration at specified interval.
[c]Given once, 15 minutes before injection of imidocarb or diminazene.
[d]The efficacy of this drug alone for cytauxzoonosis is uncertain. Use of imidocarb or diminazene is recommended instead or in combination. Higher dosages of enrofloxacin previously used have been associated with retino toxicity.

SUGGESTED READINGS*

6. Criado-Fornelio A, Gonzalez-del-Rio, Buling-Sarana A, et al. 2004. The "expanding universe" of piroplasms, *Vet Parasitol* 119:337-345.
14. Greene CE, Latimer K, Hopper E, et al. 1999. Administration of diminazene aceturate or imidocarb dipropionate for treatment of cytauxzoonosis in cats, *J Am Vet Med Assoc* 215:497-500.
18. Ketz-Riley CJ, Jazson MV, Van den Bussche R, et al. 2003. An intraerythrocytic small piroplasm in wild caught Pallas cat *(Otocolobus manul)* from Mongolia, *J Wild Dis* 39: 42-430.
25. Meier HT, Moore LE. 2000. Feline cytauxzoonosis: a case report and literature review, *J Am Anim Hosp Assoc* 36:493-496.
27. Meinkoth J, Kocan AA, Whitworth L, et al. 2000. Cats surviving natural infection with *Cytauxzoon felis:* 18 cases (1997-1998), *J Vet Intern Med* 14:521-525.

*See the CD-ROM for a complete list of references.

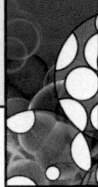

CHAPTER • 77

Babesiosis

Joseph Taboada and Remo Lobetti

Canine babesiosis (piroplasmosis) is an important worldwide, tickborne disease caused by hemoprotozoan parasites of the genus *Babesia*.[82,138,141] *Babesia* organisms primarily cause erythrocyte destruction, and the severity of illness can range from a relatively mild to a fatal disease. Although hemolytic anemia is the hallmark of infection, numerous variations exist and complications involving multiple organs may develop.

ETIOLOGY

Babesia canis and *Babesia gibsoni* have been the two predominant species capable of naturally infecting a dog. Strains of these organisms are found worldwide (Table 77-1). A small *Babesia* organism resembling *B. gibsoni* has been described and may be a third species affecting dogs in California.[32,75] In Spain an organism resembling *Babesia microti* and tentatively being described as *Theileria annae* has been described in dogs.[172,173] *Babesia equi* has been isolated from dogs in Spain.[33] In cats, *Babesia felis, Babesia cati, Babesia herpailuri, Babesia leo,* and *Babesia pantherae* have been reported (see Table 77-1).[82,141]

Dogs
B. canis is a large (2.4 μm × 5 μm), piriform-shape organism that exists singly or paired within erythrocytes (Fig. 77-1, *A*). Its expansive geographic range includes most of southern Europe, Africa, Asia, North America, Central America, and South America. Based on genetic, serologic, and cross-immunity studies, as well as differences in pathogenicity and vectors, a trinomial nomenclature system for *B. canis* has been proposed.[26,149,174] *B. canis vogeli* is the proposed name for the strain that is found in tropical and subtropical regions of most continents and transmitted by the brown dog tick *Rhipicephalus sanguineus*. It is the least pathogenic of the three strains and is the one found in the United States. *B. canis canis* is the name proposed for the strain in Europe and parts of Asia. It intermediately pathogenic and transmitted by ticks of the *Dermacentor* genus. *B. canis rossi* is the proposed name for the highly pathogenic strain that is found in South Africa and transmitted by *Heamaphysalis leachi*. A large strain, a yet unclassified *Babesia*, was isolated from a dog with hemolytic anemia, leukopenia, and thrombocytopenia.[14a]

B. gibsoni is a small, pleomorphic (1 μm × 3.2 μm) organism usually observed singly within erythrocytes (see Fig. 77-1, *B*). Initially, it was found primarily in northern Africa and the southern parts of Asia but has now been found in Australia, Europe, and the United States.

Other small *Babesia* species have been isolated from clinically ill dogs. The organisms were likely acquired from ticks that fed on infected wildlife reservoirs. In the western United States an unnamed species similar to the CA1 strain that infects people in the region causes hemolytic anemia in dogs.[75] Another unnamed species closely related to *B. microti* or *Theileria*, tentatively named *Theileria annae*, was found in the Pyrenean region of Spain.[172] A Spanish isolate of *B. equi* was identified in a dog.[33]

Cats
Feline babesiosis has not been studied as extensively as the canine form. *B. felis* is a small, highly pathogenic strain that infects domestic cats in southern Africa and the Sudan. Infection of domestic cats primarily has been identified in the strip along the coast of South Africa.[68,119] The other small strain, *B. cati*, is less pathogenic and found primarily in India. Genetic sequences of *B. canis canis* have been amplified from the blood of three cats from Spain and Portugal[34]; however, no organisms were visualized. *B. canis* ssp. *presentii* was identified in two cats in Israel.[9] The ill cat was coinfected with feline immunodeficiency virus (FIV) and *Mycoplasma haemominitum*. No cases of feline babesiosis have been reported in the United States. *B. herpailuri* and *B. pantherae* are large *Babesia* organisms of wild Felidae in Africa and have been transmitted experimentally to the domestic cat.[82] A small piroplasm *(B. leo)* similar to but serologically distinct from *B. felis* was isolated from lions *(Panthera leo)* in Kruger National Park.[92]

EPIDEMIOLOGY

B. canis and *B. gibsoni* are the two species that cause canine babesiosis worldwide (see Table 77-1). *B. canis canis* is transmitted by *Dermacentor reticulatus* in Europe, and *B. canis vogeli*

Table • 77-1

Common Babesia *Species, Vectors, and Distribution*

SPECIES	GEOGRAPHIC DISTRIBUTION	TYPICAL MORPHOLOGIC CHARACTERISTICS	RECOGNIZED TICK VECTORS	CLINICAL FINDINGS
Canine				
Babesia canis vogeli	Africa, Asia, Central America, South America, North America, northern and central Europe, Australia,	Large (2.4—3 × 4—5 μm), single or paired piriform bodies	Rhipicephalus sanguineus, Hyalomma plumbeum (?)	Mild disease with inapparent clinical signs; more severe in young animals
B. canis canis	Europe, foci in Asia	Large (2.4—3 × 4—5 μm), single or paired piriform bodies	Dermacentor reticulates	Transient parasitemia and organ congestion
B. canis rossi	South Africa	Large (2.4—3 × 4—5 μm), single or paired piriform bodies	Haemaphysalis leachi	Highly virulent hemolytic or immune disease
Babesia (large strain)[14a]	North Carolina	Large (2.5—5 μm)	Unknown	Hemolytic anemia, thrombocytopenia, leukopenia
B. gibsoni (many strain variants)	Asia, including Japan, Sri Lanka, Malaysia, and India; northern and eastern Africa; Australia; midwestern and eastern United States; southern Europe	Small (1—2 × 3—4 μm), usually single annular bodies (signet rings)[b]	Haemaphysalis bispinosa?[a] R. sanguineus?[a]	Hemolytic anemia or chronic subclinical infection with weight loss and debilitation
Small Babesia organisms	California	Small (1 × 2.5 μm), usually single; occasional maltese crosses	Unknown (suspect wildlife reservoir)	Hemolytic anemia
B. microti-like (Theileria annae)[c]	Northwestern Spain	Small (1 × 2.5 μm), usually single	Ixodes hexagonus? (suspect wildlife reservoir)	Severe hemolytic anemia, some animals develop renal failure
B. equi (Spain isolate 1)	Spain	Small (1 × 2.5 μm) usually single	Unknown	Hemolytic anemia
Feline[d]				
B. felis	Africa, southern Asia, Europe	Small (0.9 × 0.7 μm), single or paired annular bodies	Unknown	Hemolytic anemia with chronic course; seen in domestic cats in South Africa
B. herpailuri	Africa, South America?	Large (1 × 2.5 μm), single or paired annular bodies	Unknown	Isolated from jaguarundi (Herpailurus yagurundi) in South America
B. cati	Indian subcontinent	Small (1 × 1.5 μm), single or paired annular bodies	Unknown	Isolated from Indian wildcat (Felis catus)
B. canis ssp. presentii	Israel	Large (2.7 × 1.7 μm) round to oval or ring-shape	Unknown	Profound anemia and icterus or nonsymptomatic
Human[e]				
B. microti	North America: northeastern United States and Great Lakes region; Europe	Small, pleomorphic bodies	North America: I. scapularis; Europe: I. trianguliceps, I. ricinus	Hemolytic anemia, fever, chills, mild or subclinical anemia

Continued

Table • 77-1

Continued

SPECIES	GEOGRAPHIC DISTRIBUTION	TYPICAL MORPHOLOGIC CHARACTERISTICS	RECOGNIZED TICK VECTORS	CLINICAL FINDINGS
B. divergens	Europe	Small, pleomorphic bodies	*I. ricinus*	Hemolytic anemia, more severe than *B. microti*, often in those that have had a splenectomy
B. divergens—like	North America: Washington state, Missouri (MO1), Kentucky	Small, pleomorphic bodies, high-level parasitemia	Unknown	Hemolytic anemia, more severe than *B microti*, often in those that have had a splenectomy
B. odocoilei—like (EU1)	Austria, Italy	Small, pleomorphic bodies, occasional *maltese crosses*	Unknown	Fever, hemolytic anemia in those that have had a splenectomysplenectomy
B. gibsoni—like (CA1—CA4)	North America: California	Ring forms and tetrads	*Dermacentor?* (identical isolates from deer and bighorn sheep)	Hemolytic anemia—severe if immunosuppressed or have had a splenectomy
B. gibsoni—like, WA-1, CA5—CA6	North America: Washington state, California	Ring forms and tetrads	*Dermacentor?* (only infects hamsters, not dogs)[145]	Hemolytic anemia

?, Association as a tick vector has not been proved but is suspected.

[a]Definitive studies identifying vectors for *B. gibsoni* have not been published; most evidence is circumstantial.

[b]Some *B. gibsoni* isolates are larger and have a heterogenous appearance resembling *B. canis*, so PCR testing gives the most reliable differentiation.

[c]*Theileria annae* has been proposed as a new name for this organism.[23,172]

[d]Also includes *B. pantherae*, which has been isolated from a leopard cat *(Panthera pardus)* in Kenya, and a small piroplasm that has been isolated from lions *(Panthera leo)* in the Kruger National Park, South Africa.[92]

[e]People are thought to be accidental hosts for babesias of reservoir animal hosts (e.g., *B. microti* [rodents], *B. divergens* [cattle]).

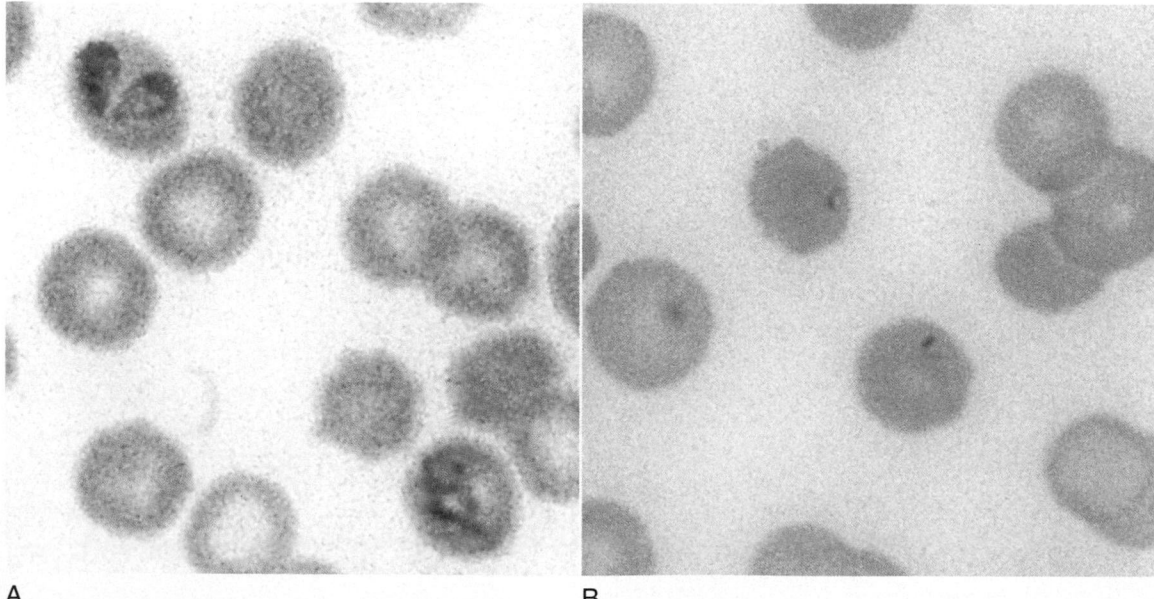

A   B

Fig   77-1   Blood smears from dog with babesiosis. **A,** Pair of large, piriform-shape merozoites of *B. canis* within erythrocytes. **B,** Individual merozoites of *B. gibsoni* in erythrocytes (Wright stain, ×1000). (Courtesy Ken Latimer, University of Georgia, Athens, Ga.)

is transmitted by *R. sanguineus* in many temperate and tropical countries. *B. canis rossi* is transmitted by *H. leachi* in South Africa. Experimentally, *B. canis* isolates have been transmitted by *Dermacentor andersoni* and *Hyalomma marginatum*.[40,82] In the United States, canine babesiosis caused by *B. canis vogeli* is most common along the Gulf Coast and in the southern, central, and southwestern states. Reported prevalence has ranged from 3.8% to 59%.[140] The seroprevalence is higher in adult dogs than in dogs younger than 1 year.[15] In a serosurvey of dogs in Florida, 46% of 393 greyhounds were seropositive. The prevalence within kennels ranged from 17% to 100%; the lower prevalence was noted in kennels with more intensive tick control. None of 50 adult pet dogs that were not greyhounds surveyed were seropositive, implicating both environment and breed susceptibility as factors in determining seroprevalence in endemic areas.[140] Outbreaks may occur and are often localized to a relatively small area or to a kennel. Veterinarians in one practice may see affected dogs often, whereas neighboring practices in the same area may not see any at all.[138] Transplacental transmission of *B. canis* infections is suspected but unproven.[47]

Infections with *B. gibsoni* occur throughout the world, and the insidious nature of this infection has allowed the inadvertent transport of the organism from Asia to other areas. Definitive proof identifying the vectors in this infection is lacking. In its original endemic area of Asia, the geographic range of *B. gibsoni* correlated with that of the suspected vector ticks, *Haemaphysalis bispinosa*, and *R. sanguineus*.[82] *Haemaphysalis longicornis* and *H. leachi* were also incriminated in some areas. Most of the isolations have been from dogs in the eastern and midwestern regions of the United States. Transmission studies proving vector competence for both *R. sanguineus* and *Dermacentor variabilis*, both of which are found in the United States, have been unsuccessful or inconclusive.[167] Various stages of the parasite were found in the salivary glands of engorged *R. sanguineus*; however, infection could not be transovarially or transstadially transmitted to other dogs.[167]

Infections with *B. gibsoni* occur sporadically in the United States, most often in American Staffordshire and American pit bull terriers or dogs that have been in fights with them.[10,13,60,93] The identified strains are those likely imported from Asian countries. American pit bull terriers in Australia have also been found to have the imported infections,[70,108] and isolated infections have been reported in Europe.[157] Although seroprevalence shows exposure to *B. gibsoni* to be highest in adult dogs, those younger than 1 year are most susceptible to clinical illness.[63] Because pups and many dogs within the same breed are infected, transmission from dam to offspring is suspected, although an exact mode of transmission is uncertain. Dogs younger than 2 months may be protected by maternal antibodies. Younger age is not a significant factor in the severity of clinical disease caused by *B. gibsoni*. In kennels where *B. gibsoni* infections have been problematic, nonvector transmission is suspected. The high prevalence of babesiosis among American pit bull terriers in many countries is likely a result of breed susceptibility and environmental factors that lead to extensive exposure to vector ticks.[10,93] In addition, fighting may play a role in transmission—through bite wounds and intermingling of blood, through saliva, or through ingested blood.[10,98] Dogs who became infected after fighting with infected dogs developed clinical signs of illness within 2 weeks. Sharing instruments for surgery, such as those used for tail docking, and reusing needles for vaccinations can result in transmission of all *Babesia* species. However, transmission via fomites has not been documented in the previously mentioned kennels, so fighting is still considered the most likely mechanism of infection.

Small-strain (CA1) organisms reported in California infect various dog breeds in different housing situations, and older dogs have a greater prevalence of seropositivity.[166] The parasite most closely resembles *Babesia* isolated from mule deer (*Odocoileus hemionus*) and bighorn sheep (*Ovis canadensis nelsoni*) in the western United States.[75] It was also similar to the WA1-type strains, which have been isolated from people in the western United States.[75,120,121] Babesial developmental stages have been detected in *R. sanguineus*; however, transmission has not been shown.[167]

The previously mentioned Spanish isolate of *Babesia* (tentatively classified as *T. annae*) is closely related to *B. felis*, *B. microti*, and isolates from wild felids in Africa.[75,92,172] Based on ticks collected from infected dogs, *Ixodes hexagonus* is the suspected principal vector.[25]

The characteristic geographic ranges established for the various *Babesia* species is based on close vector relationships. Because of the international transport of dogs and cats, new infections may be reported any time they are identified in new areas. In addition, exposure of these infected animals to vectors in new regions may allow the infection to become established in new vectors and hosts. Furthermore, people and animals are becoming exposed to new pathogens as they settle and reproduce in new environments in which sylvatic cycles between vectors and their reservoir hosts exist. This has been apparent with the increasing number of new isolates of *Babesia* in people and animals.

Babesias are transmitted through the bite of infected ixodid ticks (Fig. 77-2). The adult female tick is most important in transmission, but with *B. canis*, all stages of the tick are likely to be infected.[40] Of the *Babesia* organisms that are not transmitted transovarially, larvae are not infected. Once in the host, *Babesia* species attach to the erythrocyte membrane and are engulfed by endocytosis.[58] Once in the erythrocyte, the red blood cell membrane that surrounds the parasite disintegrates, and all subsequent stages are in direct contact with the host cell cytoplasm. *B. canis* multiplies within the erythrocytes by repeated binary fission, creating merozoites. As many as 16 merozoites of *B. canis* may be seen in a single erythrocyte, but they most commonly exist singly or in pairs. Ticks are infected by ingesting merozoites during feeding. A complex life cycle involving transtadial and transovarial transmission results in sporozoite formation in cells of the tick's salivary glands.[40,58] When infected ticks feed, the sporozoites are passed with saliva into the circulation of the host. The tick must feed a minimum of 2 to 3 days for transmission of *B. canis* to occur.[96]

Several differences in life cycles have been identified in non-*B. canis* infections. Transovarial transmission in ticks is not a feature of *B. gibsoni* infections. Furthermore, the California strain of *Babesia* replicates into tetrads or Maltese crosses and does not undergo binary fission.

PATHOGENESIS

The pathogenic sequence of events in babesiosis is summarized in Fig. 77-3. After infection, a significant host immune response usually is generated. The immune system does not appear able to completely eliminate the infection, and animals that recover are usually chronic carriers of the parasite. Poor humoral immune response is common in pups younger than 8 months. Transplacental transmission of *B. canis* is likely and may result in weak or fading puppies.[20,47,139] In one instance, *B. canis* infection was diagnosed in a 36-hour-old greyhound pup that was born to a seropositive bitch. The pup's hematocrit (HCT) was lower than the levels of its four littermates.[139]

The pathogenicity of *Babesia* organisms is determined primarily by the species and strain involved.[125,149,163] Host factors, such as the age of the host and the immunologic response generated against the parasite or vector tick, are also important.[151] Infected erythrocytes incorporate parasite antigens into their

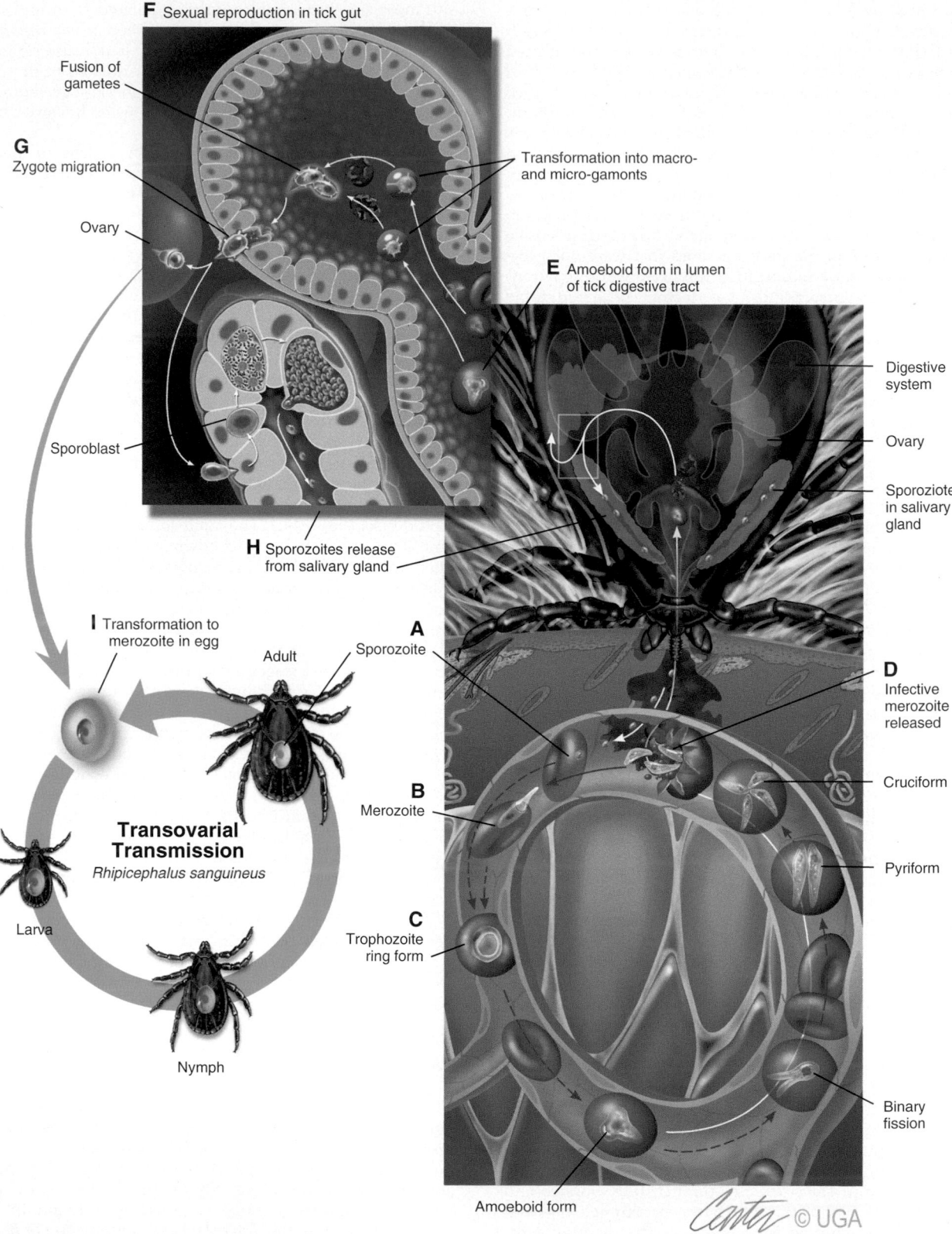

F Sexual reproduction in tick gut

Fusion of gametes

G
Zygote migration

Ovary

Transformation into macro- and micro-gamonts

Sporoblast

E Amoeboid form in lumen of tick digestive tract

Digestive system

Ovary

Sporoziote in salivary gland

H Sporozoites release from salivary gland

I Transformation to merozoite in egg

Adult

A Sporozoite

D Infective merozoite released

B Merozoite

Cruciform

Pyriform

Transovarial Transmission
Rhipicephalus sanguineus

Larva

C Trophozoite ring form

Nymph

Binary fission

Amoeboid form

Carter © UGA

Fig 77-2 Life cycle of *B. canis*. **A,** Sporozoites of the organism enter the blood following tick feeding, and infect erythrocytes by focal host erythrocyte membrane invagination and dissolution. **B,** The organisms differentiate into merozoites, and then **(C)** pleomorphic trophozoites (forms). These divide within erythrocytes by binary fission causing eventual cell lysis. The asexual reproduction (merogony) also produces more merozoites **(D)** which infect new erythrocytes. If infected erythrocytes are ingested by ticks **(E),** organisms appear in the tick gut about 10 hours after feeding. **F,** They differentiate into gametes which penetrate the tick gut epithelium fuse to form a zygote. **G,** The zygote penetrates the gut, enters the hemolymph, and migrates to the salivary gland tissue. **H,** Sporozoite replication occurs within the salivary gland and cells become filled and they eventually bud from the surface epithelium into the tick's saliva. (Courtesy University of Georgia, Athens, Ga.)

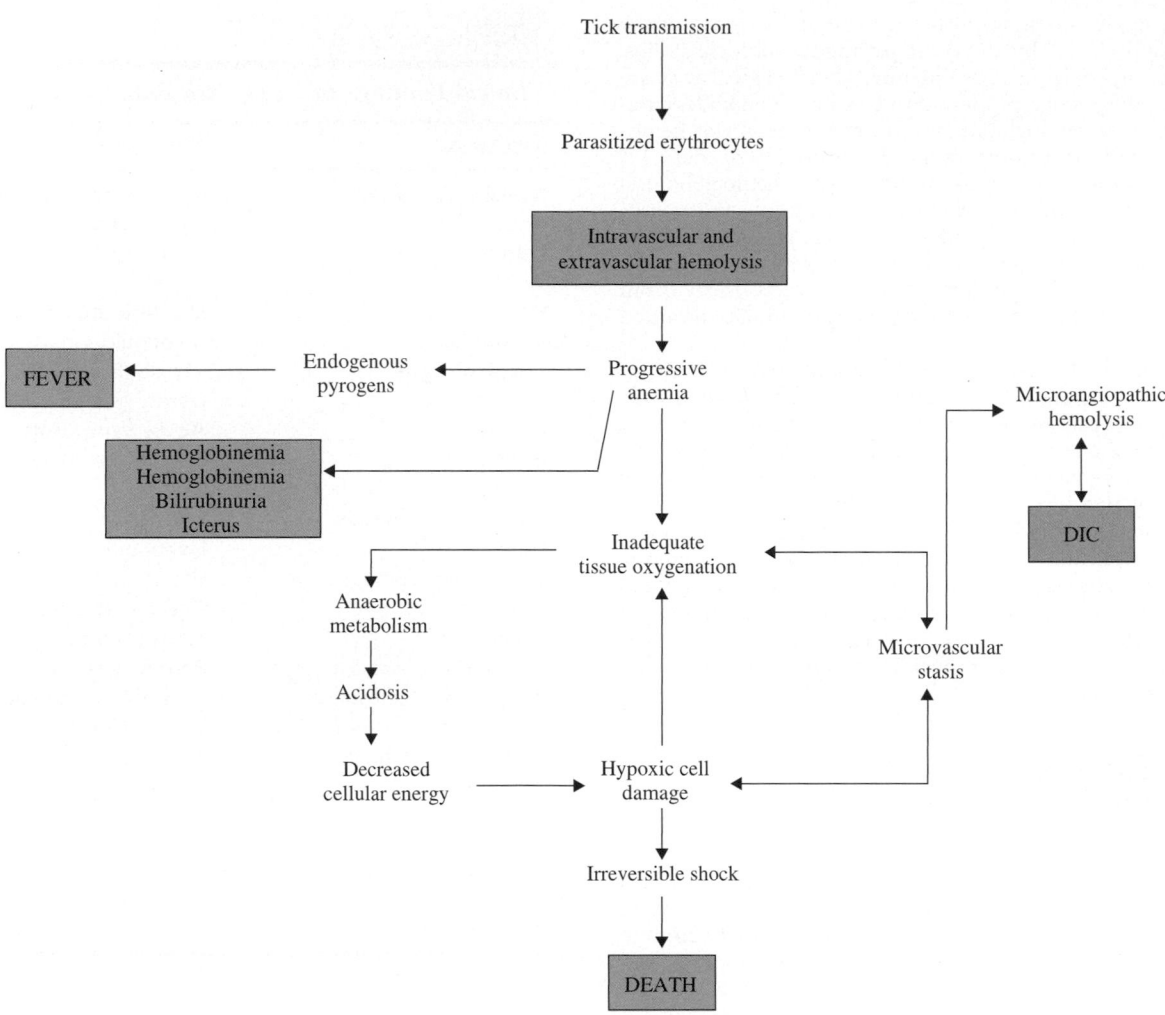

Fig 77-3 Proposed pathogenesis of canine babesiosis.

surface and induce antibodies in the host that opsonize the erythrocytes, which leads to removal of infected erythrocytes by the mononuclear-phagocyte system. Splenectomy makes the anemia and parasitemia more severe.[24]

Two syndromes, one characterized by hemolytic anemia and the other by multiple-organ dysfunction syndrome (MODS), account for most of the clinical signs observed in animals with babesiosis (see Fig. 77-2).[62,63] MODS has primarily been associated with the most pathogenic *B. canis rossi* infections found in South Africa and often causes intravascular hemolysis. Parasitemia results in osmotically fragile erythrocytes, hemolysis, and subsequent anemia.[94] However, the severity of anemia is not proportional to the low degree of parasitemia usually observed. Direct parasitic damage contributes to the anemia. However, induction of serum hemolytic factors, increased erythrophagocytic activity of macrophages, and damage induced by the secondary immune system after formation of antierythrocyte membrane antibodies are also important to the pathogenesis.[3-5,107,109,111,112] Serum from infected dogs inhibits erythrocyte 5'-nucleosidase, which can lead to the accumulation of cyclic nucleotides and may contribute to erythrocyte damage.[56] Oxidative stress is another possible cause of damage to erythrocytes that also results in increased susceptibility to phagocytosis.[110] Increased production of superoxide has been demonstrated in erythrocytes infected with *B. gibsoni*, which may relate to oxidative damage from lipid peroxidation.[114] Increased urinary methemoglobinemia levels have been found in dogs with naturally

occurring *B. canis* infections.[90] Lipid peroxidation occurring during *Babesia* infection increases rigidity of parasitized and nonparasitized erythrocytes and slows their passage through capillary beds. Soluble parasite proteases activate the kallikrein system and induce fibrinogen-like protein (FLP) formation. The FLPs make erythrocytes more "sticky," leading to additional erythrocytes sludging in the capillaries. Vascular stasis from sludging of parasitized cells and erythrocyte stroma within capillary beds is thought to contribute to the acute anemia and many of the other potential clinical signs. The most severe sludging appears to occur in the central nervous system (CNS) and muscles.[163] Rhabdomyolysis and acute renal failure have been complications of babesiosis.[64,91]

Thrombocytopenia alone is observed in many cases of babesiosis and may relate to immune or coagulatory consumption of platelets from hemolytic or vascular injury. Abnormal coagulation results are not found in many dogs.[45] However, overt disseminated intravascular coagulation (DIC) can be a devastating complication of the severe forms of canine babesiosis caused by *B. canis rossi*. *Babesia* proteases may induce increases in plasma kallikrein levels, which can activate the intrinsic cascade at factor XII. Thrombocytopenia is common, especially in dogs infected with *B. gibsoni*. This condition can be a result of DIC but is also likely a result of immune-mediated platelet destruction. Membranoproliferative glomerulonephritis is seen in some infected dogs and may have an immune-mediated pathogenesis.

Tissue hypoxia is an important contributor to many of the clinical signs caused by the most pathogenic *Babesia* strains. Causes of hypoxia include anemia, shock, vascular stasis, excessive endogenous production of carbon monoxide, parasitic damage to hemoglobin, and decreased ability of hemoglobin to offload oxygen from *Babesia*-infected dogs.[63,90] Hypoxia appears to be more important than hemoglobinuria in damaging the kidneys of experimentally infected dogs.[91] Lactic acid generation from tissue hypoxia is considered the main reason for metabolic acidosis that develops in animals with babesiosis.[84] Respiratory alkalosis results partly from compensation but more directly from hyperventilation caused by hypoxemia.

Many atypical signs or complications can develop in animals with babesiosis, especially if caused by *B. canis rossi* infection; they cannot be directly explained by hemolysis but appear to be the result of the host inflammatory response. The resultant tissue damage probably causes the release of cytokines, which would be expected to support widespread inflammation and additional damage to multiple organs.[63] MODS complications resulting from the so-called *systemic inflammatory response syndrome (SIRS)* have been acute renal failure, hepatopathy, immune-mediated hemolysis, pulmonary edema, rhabdomyolysis, and cerebral dysfunction.[160] Pulmonary, CNS, and renal complications were associated with a higher rate of mortality.

CLINICAL FINDINGS

Dogs

General Features

Babesiosis may have a hyperacute, an acute, a chronic, or a subclinical course (Table 77-2). Acute disease characterized by fever and lethargy, and acute anemia is the most common clinical syndrome, whereas the hyperacute presentation characterized by extensive tissue damage is rare.[32,38] *B. canis rossi*, prevalent in South Africa, is highly virulent and causes a hemolytic anemia or an acute overwhelming inflammatory response.[124] *B. canis canis* results in a low-level parasitemia (less than 1%), and clinical disease is associated with congestion of organs of the mononuclear phagocyte system.[127] *B. canis vogeli* results in mild clinical disease, generally without overt signs.

Acute clinical signs are typical of initial infections with *B. gibsoni* and the more virulent strains of *B. canis*.[19,32] Acute disease is characterized by anorexia, hemolytic anemia, thrombocytopenia, lymphadenomegaly, and splenomegaly.[2,61,63] Anorexia, lethargy, fever, and vomiting are also common. Fatalities may occur, especially in puppies and occasionally in *B. gibsoni*–infected adults, but most animals with this acute disease recover with treatment. Hematuria and icterus may be noted, especially in *B. canis*–infected dogs. The acute presentation is most typical of *B. gibsoni* infections encountered in Asia and the United States and *B. canis* infections encountered in Africa, Australia, and southern Europe. Immune-mediated hemolytic anemia (IMHA) and systemic lupus erythematosus are the primary diseases that must be differentiated from this form of babesiosis.

Chronic manifestations of *B. canis* infection are poorly characterized.[63] Most infected dogs with *B. canis vogeli* in the United States are subclinical carriers.[140] Low-grade or subclinical manifestations can also be seen with certain strains and more commonly with *B. gibsoni* infections.

Specific Clinical Features

B. canis rossi in South Africa *B. canis rossi* is the most virulent form of canine babesiosis. Two general and severe manifestations have been described.[124] Clinical disease is often

Table • 77-2

Clinical Findings in Dogs with Babesiosis[138]

SPECTRUM	DURATION
Nonspecific Signs	**Hyperacute Symptoms**
Anorexia	Hypothermia
Lethargy	Shock
Weakness	Coma
Pyrexia	Disseminated intravascular
Weight loss	coagulation
Atypical Signs	Metabolic acidosis
Ascites	Death
Edema	**Acute Symptoms**
Constipation	Hemolytic anemia
Diarrhea	Icterus
Ulcerative stomatitis	Splenomegaly
Hemorrhage	Lymphadenopathy
Congested mucous	Vomiting
membranes	**Chronic Symptoms**
Polycythemia	Intermittent pyrexia
Ocular and nasal discharge	Partial anorexia
Respiratory distress	Loss of body condition
Masticatory myositis	Lymphadenopathy
Temporomandibular	
joint pain	
Back pain	
CNS signs	
Seizures	
Ataxia	
Paresis	

correlated with the degree of parasitemia.[127] Thrombocytopenia is a consistent finding in babesiosis and may be considered a screening test.[73] Severely anemic dogs had hypoxic hepatic disease and increased concentrations of serum urea without creatinine. Nonanemic dogs had severe azotemia and electrolyte disturbances. Hypoglycemia was a common finding in virulent canine babesiosis and was common in dogs with mental depression or other neurologic signs.[72] As with *B. gibsoni* infections, fighting breeds such as bull terriers, American pit bull terriers, and Staffordshire bull terriers had a higher prevalence of *B. canis rossi* infections, with high mortality indicating increased susceptibility to or greater exposure risk of babesiosis.

B. canis vogeli in greyhounds in the United States The prevalence of babesiosis among greyhounds in the United States is high.[140] The likely organism affecting greyhounds is the Gulf Coast strain of *B. canis vogeli*, which rarely causes clinical disease in adults. No evidence suggests that these dogs are more susceptible than other breeds after experimental inoculation.[31]

B. gibsoni in Asia, Africa, Europe, the United States, and Australia Typical clinical signs of *B. gibsoni* infection are intermittent fever, pale mucous membranes (Fig. 77-4), decreased appetite, and marked loss of body condition.[27] A low-grade or compensated hemolytic anemia and variable thrombocytopenia may be observed with laboratory testing. The chronic form of the disease has been frequently observed, especially in the United States. Dogs develop mild fever, pale mucous membranes, splenomegaly (Fig. 77-5), hepatomegaly,

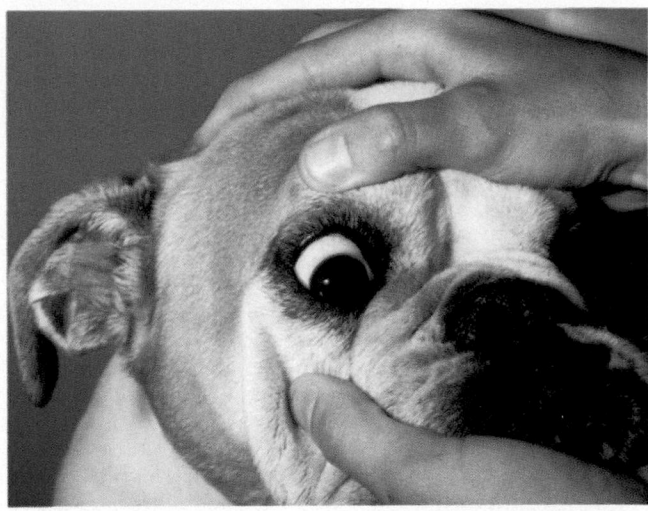

Fig 77-4 Pale mucous membranes of pit bull dog with *B. gibsoni* infection. (Courtesy University of Georgia, Athens, Ga.)

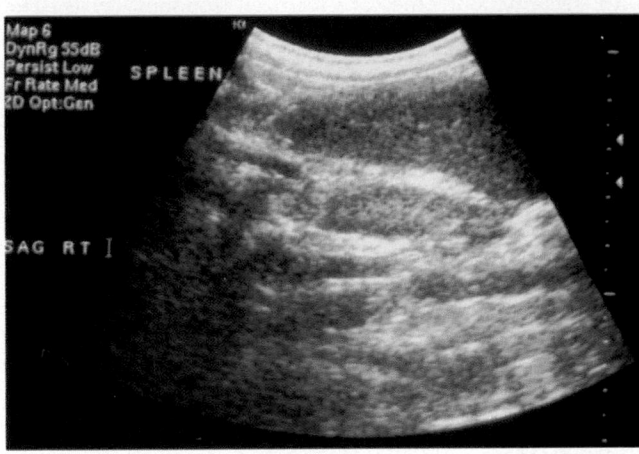

Fig 77-5 Ultrasonographic appearance of spleen from dog with *B. gibsoni* infection. (Courtesy University of Georgia, Athens, Ga.)

lymphadenomegaly, and lethargy without many of the complicating factors associated with other *Babesia* infections.[101]

California isolate Clinical signs of dogs affected by the California *Babesia* isolate have included lethargy, vomiting, elevated rectal temperature, and pale mucous membranes caused by anemia.[32] Most infected animals have developed acute severe hemolytic anemia and accompanying thrombocytopenia.

Spanish isolate In Spain, disease caused by the *B. microti*-like agent (and being called *T. annae*) is associated with pale mucosae, weakness, hemoglobinuria, tachycardia, tachypnea, and elevated rectal temperature caused by regenerative hemolytic anemia and thrombocytopenia that in some cases was accompanied by renal failure.[23,24,46,172] In animals with renal failure, nonregenerative anemia, azotemia, and proteinuria with high urine protein/creatinine ratios was found.[22]

Uncomplicated Babesiosis
Canine babesiosis can be classified clinically as uncomplicated or complicated. The course and severity of the disease

depends on the virulence of the infecting organism and the host's immunocompetency. Coinfections with other organisms can create a confusing clinical illness and cause immunosuppression.[147]

Animals with uncomplicated babesiosis typically have clinical signs relating to acute hemolysis, including fever, anorexia, depression, pale mucous membranes, splenomegaly, and water-hammer pulse. This form can be further classified as mild, moderate, or severe according to the severity of the anemia. Mild, uncomplicated babesiosis case can progress to become severe complicated babesiosis with life-threatening anemia.

Complicated Babesiosis
The clinical manifestations of complicated babesiosis are not easily explained by the hemolytic disease process. The development of many clinical or laboratory abnormalities often correlates with a greater degree of parasitemia. Rare complications include gastrointestinal (GI) disturbances, myalgia, ocular involvement, upper respiratory signs, cardiac involvement, necrosis of the extremities, fluid accumulation, and the chronic form of the disease. Overlap among the different categories of the complications can also occur. Complications are most frequently reported in *B. canis rossi* infections in dogs from South Africa.

Acute renal failure Acute renal failure (ARF) associated with babesiosis typically includes symptoms of anuria or oliguria despite adequate rehydration but is an uncommon complication. Evidence of renal damage, reflected on urinalysis by the presence of proteinuria, casts, and renal tubular epithelial cells, is common in complicated and uncomplicated cases but does not necessarily predict renal failure. An elevated serum urea alone is an unreliable indicator of renal insufficiency in animals with babesiosis, as a disproportionate rise in urea (compared with creatinine) has been related to catabolism of lysed erythrocytes.[35a] Renal failure is diagnosed on the basis of ongoing evaluation of urine volume, urinalysis, and degree of azotemia.

Acute intrinsic renal impairment without overt ARF occurs in humans with malaria—a clinical picture very similar to canine babesiosis. Renal tubular epithelial and other cells in the urine sediment, enzymuria, proteinuria, and variable azotemia have been observed in dogs with *B. canis rossi* infections.[91] ARF was also documented in numerous dogs in the same study.

Cerebral babesiosis Cerebral babesiosis is defined as the concurrent presence of neurologic signs in an animal with babesiosis. The signs, typical of peracute onset, include a combination of incoordination, hind-quarter paresis, muscle tremors, nystagmus, anisocoria, intermittent loss of consciousness, seizures, stupor, coma, aggression, paddling, or vocalization.[63] Pathologic changes in the brain are congestion, macroscopic and microscopic hemorrhages, sequestration of parasitized erythrocytes in capillary beds, and pavementing of parasitized cells against the endothelium.

Coagulopathy The most consistent hemostatic abnormality in babesiosis is profound thrombocytopenia, which is a routine finding in complicated and uncomplicated cases, but clinically apparent hemorrhages are relatively rare. DIC has been reported in animals with babesiosis; however, confirmation of DIC in animals with babesiosis is difficult because of the nature of the underlying disease process and the reported unreliability of the human fibrin degradation product test.[63] Clinical signs of DIC are difficult to recognize until hemorrhages develop in the hypocoagulable phase. In the hypercoagulable phase, signs are related to microthrombi-induced organ dysfunction.

Icterus and hepatopathy In some cases of babesiosis, icterus, elevated liver enzyme levels, and elevated bile acid levels develop, which indicate a liver insult.[102] Whether the insult is caused by inflammatory cytokines, hypoxic damage, or a combination of these is not known. Icterus does not solely appear to be caused by hemolysis or hepatic obstruction. Therefore liver dysfunction appears to be at least contributory. Histologic changes usually associated with icterus include diffuse and periportal lesions, whereas icteric dogs with babesiosis have a centrilobular lesion. However, it is possible that the liver has a diffuse, mild or moderate lesion that does not cause histologic changes but is severe enough to cause a functional change. Hypoxic insults are known to cause diffuse hepatocellular swelling, thus the hypoxia in severe babesiosis may be severe enough to cause a transient hepatopathy.

Immune-mediated hemolytic anemia Immune-mediated hemolysis is an increased destruction of erythrocytes caused by erythrocyte-membrane–associated antibodies. This destruction can either be primary, in which the membrane is normal, or secondary, in which the membrane is altered and recognized as foreign. Secondary destruction is assumed to occur in babesiosis.[146] The cardinal feature of babesiosis-associated IMHA is continuing hemolysis despite successful antibabesial treatment. Diagnosis is confirmed by finding autoagglutination with saline dilution of blood, detection of spherocytosis, or both. The Coombs' test cannot be used to confirm a diagnosis because uncomplicated cases and cases complicated with IMHA have a positive test result.

Acute respiratory distress syndrome Acute respiratory distress syndrome (ARDS) is a severe and frequent catastrophic complication of babesiosis. Typical clinical signs are a sudden increase in respiratory rate (which may be caused by other factors, such as pyrexia and acidosis), dyspnea, moist cough, and blood-tinged frothy nasal discharge. The diagnosis of ARDS is based on the presence of diffuse pulmonary infiltrates on thoracic radiography, hypoxemia from ventilation-perfusion mismatch, normal pulmonary capillary wedge pressure, and reduced pulmonary compliance.[39] In most clinical situations, pulmonary wedge pressure, blood-gas analysis, and compliance cannot be measured. Thus diagnosis depends on the recognition of risk factors for ARDS, thoracic radiographs, and exclusion of other causes of pulmonary edema, particularly cardiogenic causes and fluid overload. Excluding fluid overload is particularly important in animals with oliguric renal failure. Fluid loads that can be tolerated by normal dogs may fatally exacerbate pulmonary edema in ARDS.

Hemoconcentration The paradoxical phenomenon of severe intravascular hemolysis combined with hemoconcentration constitutes the syndrome "red biliary." The clinical features are congested mucous membranes, visible hemoglobinemia, hemoglobinuria, or all of these and high-normal or elevated hematocrit levels.[63] Hemoconcentration has been associated with other complications, such as cerebral babesiosis, DIC, ARF, and ARDS. Hemoconcentration in babesiosis is thought to be a result of reduction in blood volume as a result of fluid shifts from the vascular to the extravascular compartment. Because plasma protein concentrations are normal, plasma—rather than a filtrate of plasma—shifts from the vasculature. The widespread increase in capillary permeability, which occurs in SIRS, may play an important role in the pathogenesis. Concurrent hypoalbuminemia may relate to a loss of albumin into the interstitium because of lost endothelial integrity associated with SIRS.

Hypotension Dogs with severe and complicated babesiosis are frequently in a state of collapse and clinical shock. Shock can resemble the hyperdynamic phase of septic shock. In a study, it was shown that hypotension occurs frequently in dogs with babesiosis, and the presence and severity of hypotension increases with increased disease severity.[66] The presence of hypotension in a large proportion of dogs with complicated babesiosis is consistent with the hypothesis that inflammatory mechanisms play a major role in this disease and can result in a sepsislike state. It is likely that hypotension in animals with babesiosis is a combination of vasodilation, reduced vascular volume caused by increased vascular permeability, dehydration, or all of these and myocardial depression. Hypotension can play a role in the pathophysiologic symptoms of the disease because it has been hypothesized to facilitate parasite sequestration.

Cardiac changes In one study, dogs with complicated and concurrent IMHA-babesiosis had significantly higher cardiac troponin I and T concentrations.[87] In this study, dogs with babesiosis developed important electrocardiogram (ECG) changes such as heart blocks, ventricular premature complexes (VPCs), and prolonged QRS changes and ST segment changes. However, most of the changes were not associated with severity, outcome, and cardiac troponin levels. The exception was the presence of VPCs because a correlation was found between troponin concentrations and VPCs. Cardiac histologic changes reported in the study were hemorrhage, necrosis, inflammatory infiltrate, and fibrosis.

Acute pancreatitis A retrospective study reported acute pancreatitis as a complication of canine babesiosis.[103] In this study, four dogs had histologic evidence of pancreatitis, and another 16 dogs had serum amylase elevations, lipase activity elevations, or both of a magnitude that supported a diagnosis of acute pancreatitis. The median time of pancreatitis diagnosis was 2.5 days postadmission, with primarily young (a median age 3 years), sexually intact dogs being affected. The development of pancreatitis was unrelated to the degree of anemia at time of admission. In addition to pancreatitis, 80% of dogs had other babesial complications, namely icterus, ARDS, IMHA, renal failure, hemoconcentration, and cerebral syndrome. Acute pancreatitis may represent the previously reported gut form of babesiosis.

Acid-base disturbances Dogs with severe *B. canis rossi* infection have an arterial pH that varies from acidemia to alkalemia.[84] A high anion gap metabolic acidosis is present in many dogs, whereas almost all have concurrent metabolic acidosis and respiratory alkalosis. The severity of these abnormalities could not be linked to clinical outcome.

Subclinical Infections

Subclinically infected dogs are common in certain populations.[98c] Greyhounds in the United States have a very high seroprevalence of disease, but adult dogs rarely show clinical signs. Likewise, American pit bull terriers appear to have a high prevalence of infection based on polymerase chain reaction (PCR) studies.[93] *B. canis* parasites are rarely found on blood smears from asymptomatic carriers, making identification of this group of dogs difficult without performing serologic screening tests or PCR. A slightly higher likelihood of finding *B. gibsoni* on blood smears from asymptomatic American pit bull terriers exists if the clinician examines the smears very thoroughly. However, serology and PCR are also more sensitive screening tools in this population of dogs. The primary importance of this group of dogs may be in their role as a potential source of infection to susceptible puppies in breeding colonies or as a source of infection through blood transfusion or fighting.[38,140] Babesiosis can be a significant and underdiagnosed cause of morbidity and mortality of puppies from breeding colonies located in endemic areas. The seroprevalence among adults in affected kennels often is higher than 75% and can serve as a serologic marker for the disease. In comparison, the seroprevalences are typically less than 20% in well-managed kennels from endemic areas where anemic puppies are less likely to be encountered.[140] Most subclinical carriers never show clinical signs of babesiosis; however, although rare, they may have symptoms when subjected to stress or treated with glucocorticoids.[19,97]

Cats

The reports of clinical infection in domestic cats have been predominantly from South Africa. Cats with naturally occurring babesiosis usually are younger than 3 years and have no breed or sex predilection. Affected cats generally have lethargy, anorexia, weakness, a rough hair coat, or diarrhea.[68] Fever and icterus are less common. Anemia can be severe and is the underlying reason for the clinical signs. The disease is chronic, and signs may not be apparent until a later stage of illness. Cats usually adapt to the anemia and may have only mild clinical signs until they experience the stress of a physical examination or diagnostic evaluation.[104] Complications of the hemolytic anemia included hepatopathy, pulmonary edema, renal failure, CNS signs, and concurrent infections.

DIAGNOSIS

Clinical Laboratory Findings

Dogs

The primary differential diagnoses for acute uncomplicated babesiosis are hemolytic states such as parasitic, immune-mediated, oxidative, and traumatic insults to erythrocytes and GI hemorrhage mimicking a hemolytic anemia. The clinical pathologic changes are nonspecific; the primary hematologic abnormalities are anemia and thrombocytopenia.[2,61,99,113] The prevalence of thrombocytopenia is higher than that in dogs with ehrlichiosis. A mild, normocytic, normochromic anemia is generally noted in the first few days after infection, and the anemia then becomes macrocytic, hypochromic, and regenerative as the disease progresses. The reticulocytosis is proportional to the severity of the anemia. Uncommonly, a relative polycythemia with normal plasma protein concentration may be noted.[63] Leukocyte abnormalities are inconsistently observed but may include leukocytosis, neutrophilia, neutropenia, lymphocytosis, and eosinophilia.[61,113] A leukemoid response similar to that in cases of IMHA is occasionally seen.[86] Autoagglutination of erythrocytes in saline was noted in 21% of 134 dogs with babesiosis in one study, and almost 85% of infected dogs were positive on direct antiglobulin (Coombs') test in another, making it difficult to differentiate the disease from IMHA if organisms are not apparent.[63] Thrombocytopenia is generally a feature of canine babesiosis, regardless of whether concurrent anemia is present.[147]

Serum chemistry values are usually normal. Hypokalemia may be found in severely affected animals but is probably nonspecific because of decreased potassium intake. Hyperkalemia and hypoglycemia were noted in severely affected animals in one study.[61] Dogs with mild and severe babesiosis have low total serum protein and albumin levels, albumin/globulin ratios, and α-globulin levels. They also have an acute-phase response characterized by elevated α_1-acid glycoproteins.[89] A study of dual infections with B. canis and Ehrlichia canis showed that the prevalence of hyperglobulinemia was higher in dogs with dual infections than in dogs infected with a single infection caused by either organism.[99] Azotemia and metabolic acidosis are common in animals with severe intravascular hemolysis and appear to contribute to morbidity and mortality. More severely affected animals have high serum transaminase and alkaline phosphatase activity and increased serum bilirubin levels. Hyperbilirubinemia is a consistent finding during acute disease caused by B. canis strains but not by B. gibsoni.[61,156] Liver enzyme activity may be increased during severe disease. Urinalysis may reveal bilirubinuria, hemoglobinuria, proteinuria, and granular casts. In B. canis rossi infections in anemic South African dogs, animals can develop hypoxic hepatic disease with an increased serum urea and profound leukocytosis with a left shift.[124] Nonanemic dogs may have severe azotemia, marked electrolyte changes, and in some cases, leukopenia.

Cats

In feline babesiosis, which is caused by B. felis, the anemia is typically macrocytic, hypochromic, and regenerative.[130] No characteristic change in total or differential leukocyte counts occurs, and thrombocytopenia is an inconsistent finding. The in-saline agglutination test may also be positive.[130]

Cats infected with B. felis typically have elevated hepatic cytosol enzyme activity and total bilirubin concentrations. Serum protein values are primarily normal, but polyclonal hyperglobulinemia can occur. Renal parameters are unaffected. Although various electrolyte abnormalities were reported, no consistent pattern was found.[130]

Microscopic Identification

The definitive diagnosis of babesiosis depends on demonstration of organisms within infected erythrocytes, amplification of babesial DNA extracted from infected blood or tissue, or positive serology results. B. canis are large, piriform-shape organisms and usually exist singly or in pairs (see Fig. 77-1, A), whereas smaller single intracellular organisms are likely to be B. gibsoni (see Fig. 77-1, B). Parasitemia is often low, especially in B. canis–infected dogs, making thorough examination of thin blood smears necessary. With B. canis infections, blood collected from the peripheral capillary beds of the ear tip or nail bed may yield higher numbers of parasitized cells.[61] Erythrocytes adjacent to the buffy coat of centrifuged specimens are also more likely to be infected because the organism favors reticulocytes that have higher levels of nucleic acids, amino acids, and adenosine triphosphate (ATP) and lower levels of glutathione.[169,170] Occasionally, phagocytized organisms and erythrocyte fragments are seen in neutrophils. Although the organisms within erythrocytes may be numerous in some acutely infected animals, they are rarely evident in chronically infected or asymptomatic carriers. Evaluation of stained slides can be tedious and requires a significant time commitment on the part of the laboratory technician. Flow cytometric techniques correlate closely with conventional light microscopic techniques for identification of Babesia-parasitized erythrocytes and degree of reticulocytosis.[9b,41,148] In addition, the methods of concentrating and staining of buffy coat improve the sensitivity of parasite detection.[100] Electron microscopy can also be used by research laboratories to better characterize the parasite.[122]

Serologic Testing

Because of the difficulties in detecting Babesia parasites, especially in chronic carriers, immunodiagnostics may be used to screen for infected hosts. Serodiagnostics have proved reliable as a method of indirect parasite detection in either patent or occult infections that have been present long enough for an immune response to be generated.[123,158] For canine babesiosis, the indirect fluorescent antibody (FA) test is probably the most specific and most commonly used test for detection of babesial antibody.[123] Although laboratory methods differ, generally titers to B. canis that are greater than or equal to 1:80

on a single sample are sufficient for diagnosis. A cut-off titer of 1:320 or greater has been established for incriminating *B. gibsoni* infection.[168] A titer level of 1:1280 or greater has been considered as the cut-off to increase certainty for incrimination of infection in some serologic studies.[168] Titers to multiple species must be measured if serology is performed in geographic areas where more than one type of *Babesia* infection exist. Cross-reactivity between *B. canis* and *B. gibsoni* make parasite identification or PCR necessary to differentiate between the two species. However, very young dogs or dogs tested early in the disease course may be serologically negative, making it necessary to evaluate convalescing serum in some cases.[15] Antibodies were not detected in 36% of dogs with *B. canis* parasitemia in one study.[15] Enzyme-linked immunosorbent assay (ELISA) and dot-ELISA techniques for antibody detection have been developed. ELISA results are much more sensitive and less specific than those from indirect FA. ELISA testing is used more for seroepidemiologic studies than clinical diagnosis.[15,123,156a] Using some tests based on whole-cell antigens, dogs infected with *B. gibsoni* may have false-positive serologic test results for *Toxoplasma gondii* and *Neospora caninum* as well as for *B. canis*, especially at lower serum titers.[168] Recombinant-produced P50 protein ELISA testing has been more specific for *B. gibsoni* infection than immunoblotting and indirect FA testing.[42,156a]

Nucleic Acid Detection

Because organisms vary or are infrequent in blood smears, genetic methods are the most sensitive and specific means of detecting infection. Genus-specific screening for *Babesia* can be performed by PCR of DNA extracted from blood samples.[7,44] Species identification can then be accomplished by comparing small subunit (SSU) ribosomal RNA (rRNA) gene sequences found with known sequences of *B. gibsoni* and *B. canis*.[37a,58b,115a,76,135] Use of a seminested PCR allows for detection and differentiation of *B. gibsoni* and *B. canis* DNA in blood.[11] PCR has been used to identify a third *Babesia* species endemic to the western portion of the United States,[76,93] a new strain from a dog in North Carolina,[14a] and another species from northwestern Spain.[172] PCR also detected an organism similar to *Babesia odocoilei* and *Babesia divergens* in ticks from dogs in Japan.[59]

PATHOLOGIC FINDINGS

Pathologic findings include staining of tissues with hemoglobin or bilirubin, hepatosplenomegaly, lymphadenopathy, and kidneys that are a dark-reddish color.[150] Edema and hemorrhage, which may indicate vascular injury and poor tissue oxygenation in severely affected dogs, are often most severe in the lungs. Large numbers of parasitized erythrocytes may be noted in capillary beds, especially in the brain (Fig. 77-6). Nonparasitized cells often line the endothelial surface with parasitized cells sludged in the lumen. Microthrombi of many tissues may be evident in animals exhibiting signs of DIC. Large numbers of parasitized cells are often evident in the spleen. Impression smears of the spleen may substantiate the diagnosis of babesiosis at necropsy. Organisms can be found in erythrocytes within the microvasculature (Fig. 77-7). Nonspecific findings include erythroid hyperplasia in the bone marrow, extramedullary hematopoiesis of the liver and spleen, mononuclear phagocyte system hyperplasia, and centrolobular necrosis of the liver. Vasculitis has been observed in *B. gibsoni* infections and is associated with hepatitis and lymphadenitis with multifocal deposits of IgM in inflamed arteries and renal glomeruli.[162] In chronic cases of canine babesiosis and cases of feline babesiosis, the only gross finding may be splenomegaly.

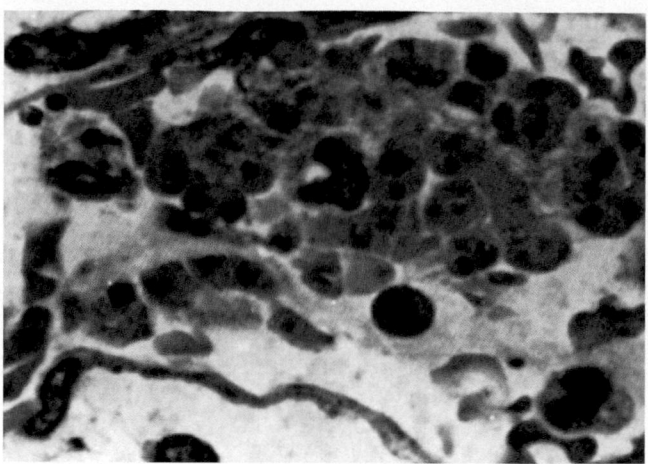

Fig 77-6 Cerebral vessel filled with numerous erythrocytes parasitized by *B. canis* (H and E stain, ×1200). (Courtesy Charles W. Qualls, Jr., Stillwater, Okla.)

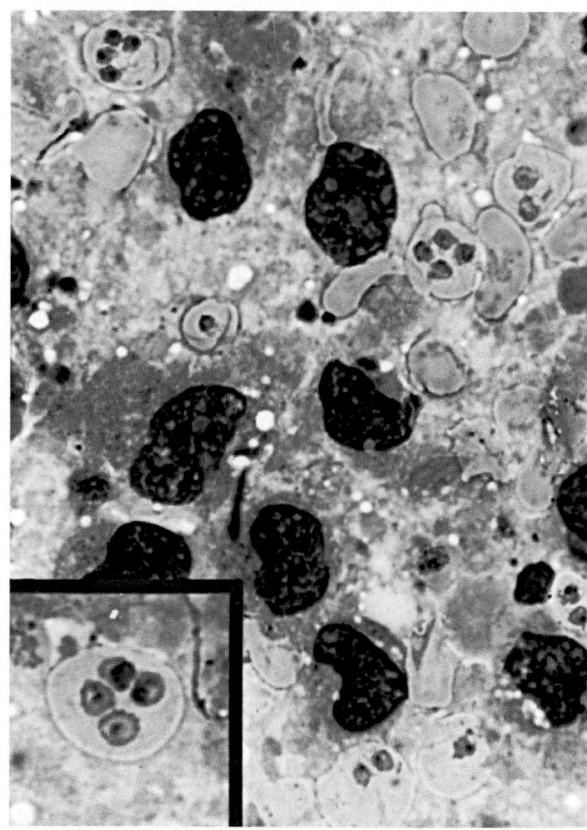

Fig 77-7 Impression smear of spleen obtained at necropsy from naturally infected dog. Numerous erythrocytes contain one or more *B. canis* organisms (Wright-Giemsa stain, ×1100). (Courtesy Peter MacWilliams and Charles W. Qualls, Jr., Stillwater, Okla.)

THERAPY

Dogs

Dogs generally show clinical improvement within 24 hours of treatment with antibabesial drugs (Table 77-3[81]; see the Drug Formulary, Appendix 8, for additional information). Few drugs have been shown to eliminate the parasites, and most dogs sur-

Table • 77-3

Selected Babesiacidal Compounds Used in the Treatment of Canine and Feline Babesiosis

GENERIC (BRAND)[a]	DOSE (mg/kg)[b]	ROUTE	INTERVAL (HOURS)	DURATION (DAYS)	ORGANISM BABESIA CANIS	BABESIA GIBSONI	BABESIA FELIS
Imidocarb dipropionate (Imizol)	5—6.6	IM	Once	Repeat in 14	+++	+	—
	7.5	IM	Once	NA			
Diminazene aceturate (Berenil, Ganaseg)[c]	3.5—5	IM	Once[d]	NA	+++	++	+
Phenamidine isethionate (Lomadine, Phenamidine)[c]	15—20	SC	24	2	+++	++	—
Pentamidine isethionate (Pentam 300)[e]	16.5	IM	24	2	++	++	?
Quinuronium sulfate (Acaprin)	0.25	SC	48	2	++	—	—
Trypan blue	10	IV	Once	NA	++	—	—
Primaquine phosphate (Primaquine)	0.5	PO	24	1–3	?	—	+++
	1 mg per cat	IM	36	6	—	—	+++
Clindamycin (Antirobe, Cleocin)[f]	12.5—25	PO	12	7—10	?	?	?
Doxycycline (Vibramycin)[g]	10	PO	12	7—10	+	?	?
Azithromycin (Zithromax)[h]	10	PO	24	10	?	+++	?
Atovaquone (Mepron)[h]	13.3	PO	8	10	?	+++	?
Quinuronium sulfate (Acaprin)	0.25	SC	48	2	++	?	?

IM, Intramuscular; *SC*, subcutaneous; *IV*, intravenous; *PO*, by mouth; +++, very good; ++, good; +, fair to poor; —, not effective; ?, unknown; *NA*, not applicable.

[a]For specific information on each drug, see Drug Formulary, Appendix 8.
[b]Dose per administration at specified interval.
[c]Drugs not approved for use in the United States. Available in other countries as oxopirvedine (trade name Merial, Lyon, France), where it is combined with antihistamine, oxomemazine.
[d]For *B. canis*, this dose is sufficient; for *B. gibsoni*, repeat dose in 24 hours. These total dosages of 7 mg/kg or higher are associated with an increased risk of neurotoxicity.
[e]Orphan drugs.
[f]Anecdotal evidence for effectiveness against *B. canis*.
[g]Only shown to reduce or prevent parasitemia in dogs that were infected during treatment.
[h]Effective against *B. microti* in people and hamsters. Also effective against *B. gibsoni* in dogs when both azithromycin and atovaquone are used in combination.[14]

viving the acute hemolytic crisis develop premunition in which a delicate balance exists between their immune response and the persistent parasite. Unfortunately, two of the most effective of the babesiacidal drugs for *B. canis* infection, diminazene aceturate and phenamidine isethionate, are not approved for use in the United States. Diminazene aceturate is the most commonly used drug worldwide.[80] It is an aromatic diamidine derivative in the same class of drugs as phenamidine isethionate and pentamidine isethionate. Diminazene aceturate is effective when given intramuscularly (IM), although clearance of infection is inconsistent even at higher doses. *B. gibsoni* infections are less responsive to diminazene than *B. canis* infections. Dogs are more susceptible to the toxic effects of the drug than other species. Side effects include pain and swelling at the injection site, GI irritation, and neurologic manifestations.

Phenamidine isethionate is available in many countries as a licensed drug for treatment of canine babesiosis. Pentami-dine isethionate (trade name Pentam 300; Abbott Labs, Abbott Park, Ill.) has been approved for use in the United States by the Food and Drug Administration as an orphan drug for treatment of *Pneumocystis* pneumonia in people. The drug has been effective against *B. canis* and *B. gibsoni*.[81] The drug has not been as extensively studied as the other diaminidines. Side effects include injection site pain, hypotension, tachycardia, and vomiting.

A carbanilide member of the diaminidine family, imidocarb dipropionate, is an effective drug against *B. canis*.[6,81] It is available in the United States (see Drug Formulary, Appendix 8). It is less effective against *B. gibsoni*. At the suggested dose (see Table 77-3), imidocarb eliminates the *Babesia* infection and eliminates the infectivity of ticks engorging on treated animals for up to 4 weeks after treatment. A single dose of 7.5 mg/kg or a single dose of 6 mg/kg the day following a dose of diminazene at 3.5 mg/kg has also been shown to clear infections.[117] A dose of 7 mg/kg imidocarb given on days 15 and 27 following experimental *B. canis* infection cleared infection but inhibited the protective response associated with gradual recovery, making the animals more susceptible to reinfection parasitemia than untreated control dogs.[18] Because PCR was not performed and antibody titers persisted, immune stimulation caused by premunition caused by subclinical persistence of the parasite is possible. Imidocarb is also effective against *E. canis* and is therefore the drug of choice in dual infections.[6] It has protective prophylactic activity up to 6 weeks after a single injection.[155] Side effects are uncommon and thought to be related to an anticholinesterase effect of the drug. They include transient salivation, lacrimation, vomiting, diarrhea, muscle tremor, restlessness, tachycardia, and dyspnea.[1] An overdose of 10 times the proper amount resulted in hepatic necrosis and death in one dog.[77]

Atovaquone is an antiprotozoal drug approved for the treatment of *Pneumocystis carinii* pneumonia in human patients with the human immunodeficiency virus (HIV). The mechanism of action is not completely understood, but the site of action appears to be inhibition of electron transport at the cytochrome bc 1 complex (Complex III) in *Plasmodium* species. Atovaquone and azithromycin are effective against *B. microti* in hamster models[57,159] and *B. gibsoni* in vitro and in vivo in dogs.[98b] The combination has proved effective in treating *B. gibsoni* in a pilot study involving a small number of dogs with naturally acquired infection.[14a] Atovaquone (13.3 mg/kg given orally every 8 hours) and azithromycin (10 mg/kg given orally once daily) were given for 10 days. The treatment appeared to sterilize *B. gibsoni* infections or reduce the parasitemia below detectable limits. Although additional studies on more strains are needed, this may be the treatment of choice for *B. gibsoni* infections in dogs. Atovaquone is difficult to obtain in some countries, and the expense can be much greater than that of other treatments. Recrudescence of infection was observed greater than 30 days following atovaquone monotherapy for *B. gibsoni* infection in dogs.[98a] Increased resistance to the drug was found by in vitro testing. For this reason, it should always be used in combination with other drugs.

Quinuronium sulfate has been effective in treating dogs with *B. canis* infection.[78] Dogs showed clinical improvements within 24 to 48 hours of treatment.

Trypan blue (1% solution) is effective in treating dogs with mild to moderate signs of infection with *B. canis* (see Table 77-3).[67,133] It has also been recommended for patients with severe infections because it lacks the anticholinergic properties of imidocarb and the CNS toxicity of the other diamidines.[81] Trypan blue does not clear infections and results in bluish discoloration of tissues and plasma.

Aggressive supportive care and clindamycin (25 mg/kg given orally every 12 hours for 7 to 21 days) has been recommended if the specific antibabesial drugs are not available. Clindamycin is the treatment of choice for *B. microti* in people, and numerous anecdotal reports describe success in treating canine babesiosis at 25 to 50 mg/kg/day. However, many infected dogs recover completely without specific babesiacidal therapy if adequate supportive measures are taken, making interpretation of uncontrolled treatment observations difficult. Clindamycin proved effective in managing the acute complications of *B. gibsoni* infections in experimentally infected dogs but did not clear the organisms.[164] Clindamycin at 25 mg/kg given orally every 12 hours for 7 to 21 days after infection resolved anemia and other clinical findings. However, no significant differences were found between treated and untreated dogs in parasitemia levels or antibabesial IgG titers. Nevertheless, morphologic changes in circulating parasites showed degenerative changes. Levels of

parasitemia fluctuated in subsequent monitoring in both groups; however, treated dogs had stronger humoral and cell-mediated immune responses against the parasite. Clindamycin was also ineffective compared with oxytetracycline or diminazene for treating experimental *B. canis* infection in mice.[8]

Doxycycline has been effective in preventing or reducing parasitemia in dogs that were being treated at the time of infection.[155]

Cats

Treatment of feline babesiosis has not been as critically evaluated as its canine counterpart.[81] Most babesiacidal drugs appear to be ineffective. Primaquine phosphate, an antimalarial compound, administered orally or as an IM injection, is effective and currently the drug of choice (see Table 77-3). However, the effective dose, 0.5 mg/kg, is very close to the lethal dose of 1 mg/kg. In experimental studies, rifampicin and trimethoprim-sulfadiazine were not as effective as primaquine.[118] Danofloxacin, enrofloxacin, and buparvaquone had no anti-*B. felis* activity.

Blood Transfusions

Blood transfusions are usually indicated in severe, uncomplicated cases and complicated cases involving a life-threatening anemia. The decision to transfuse is based on clinical signs, history, and hematologic test results. Clinical signs that would indicate the need for transfusion are tachycardia, tachypnea, water-hammer pulse, weakness, and collapse. The acuteness of onset and the degree of red cell regeneration should also be taken into consideration. The hematocrit is the most commonly used indicator of anemia, but red cell count and hemoglobin can also be used. No HCT has been established at which a transfusion should be given, because it must be evaluated in conjunction with the clinical signs and history. Generally a transfusion is considered when the HCT is 15% or lower and is always indicated when the HCT is 10% or lower. The degree of parasitemia is not an important deciding factor because it often bears little relation to the degree of anemia. Packed red cells are the component of choice for babesiosis. The administration of the plasma component of whole blood is unnecessary in the majority of dogs with babesiosis and can place the patient at risk of volume overload. If rehydration is required, crystalloid replacement solutions are preferable. Fresh whole blood improves oxygen status and acid-base balance in *B. canis*–infected dogs, as well as replaces subfunctional hemoglobin with functional hemoglobin.

Supportive Care

Ongoing supportive therapy should be based on a thorough patient assessment and ongoing monitoring, appropriate laboratory testing, and accepted therapeutic principles for the complications that may be present.

Whether glucocorticoids are indicated is controversial. The immune system is implicated in many of the clinical manifestations of canine babesiosis, especially the hemolytic anemia. In one study, 20% of dogs with *B. canis* infection had hemolytic anemias that were not responsive to antibabesial therapy alone.[63] Treatment with immunosuppressive doses of glucocorticoids is sometimes necessary. However, long-term use is probably not indicated, and in most dogs the glucocorticoid dosage can be tapered over 2 to 3 weeks. This therapy may predispose the animals to other infections and has the potential to induce babesial relapse.[97] The monocyte-macrophage system is important in controlling *Babesia* parasitemia. Reduction in this system's function often results in more severe parasitemia shortly after glucocorticoids are initiated.

PREVENTION

General Guidelines

The difficulty in obtaining specific therapeutic compounds for treatment of *Babesia* makes prevention of paramount importance. Preventive measures alone may be sufficient to control *B. canis* outbreaks in kennels in the southeastern United States. The primary means of prevention is control of the vector tick.[134] Frequent inspection of the skin and hair coat for ticks is important because it takes a minimum of 2 to 3 days of feeding for transmission of the parasite to occur. New animals should be serologically tested, treated, and quarantined before being introduced into a colony. Flea and tick collars, although not very effective for flea control, are reasonably effective for tick control when used with inspection, topical ascaricide application, and environmental control. Fipronil (trade names TopSpot, Frontline; Merial, Iselin, N.J.) appears to be effective as a topical product for tick control.

Premunition (subclinical infection) is important in controlling clinical signs of disease in areas where more virulent strains of *Babesia* are endemic.[117] In these areas, completely clearing infections may not be desirable. The role premunition plays in immunity in areas where less virulent strains are endemic is not known.

Duration of protective immunity against *B. canis* babesiosis is limited. Antibody titers gradually decline between 3 and 5 months after infection.[149,154] Dogs are protected against homologous infection within 5 to 8 months after infection.[156] Cross-protection between strains does not occur, and seropositivity is no guarantee of protection against heterologous challenge.

A vaccine produced from cell-culture–derived exoantigens of *B. canis* is available in Europe.[106] An efficacy of 70% to 100% has been reported, with the disease occasionally seen in the vaccinates generally being mild.[105] Other field studies have been less impressive. Vaccination does not prevent infection but appears to block initiation of many of the pathologic processes involved in disease pathogenesis (see Fig. 77-3).[125,126] Vaccines may limit the parasitemia, reduction in HCT, and development of splenomegaly.[125] Differences in strain antigenicity substantially limit the usefulness of the commercial vaccine in other areas. However, heterologous protection was achieved using soluble parasite antigens from the European *B. canis vogeli* isolate and South African *B. canis rossi* isolate.[129]

Babesia organisms can be transmitted by transfusion, making control in a blood donor colony especially important.[38,136] All prospective canine blood donors should be serologically tested for babesiosis. Positive animals should be identified and culled from the program because seropositivity overestimates the infection rate but provides a safer zone for eliminating potential carriers. PCR also offers a fairly sensitive way to detect carriers. When PCR is not available, splenectomy has been used to increase the likelihood of finding parasites in animals with occult infection and therefore is indicated. Blood smears should be examined for *Babesia* daily for 2 weeks after splenectomy and then periodically thereafter.

Babesiosis in Greyhounds and American Pit Bull Terriers

Of the 16,000 greyhounds that were adopted through rescue leagues in 1995, 20% to 60% were likely to have positive serotest results for *B. canis*. Much of this screening was done before the availability of PCR, and serologic testing results likely overestimate the true prevalence of infection. This concern about babesiosis developing in adopted greyhounds is common among adopting owners, greyhound rescue organizations, and veterinarians. The question of what to do with these animals is not an easy one to answer. The likelihood of the adopted greyhound developing clinical babesiosis is low, as is the likelihood of the dog serving as an epidemiologic significant source of spread of the disease. However, the risk to other dogs is great if the infected animal is placed in a breeding kennel in which dogs are housed together and tick control is not adequate or if the animal is used as a canine blood donor. A single IM dose of imidocarb dipropionate at 7.5 mg/kg apparently eliminates the *B. canis* carrier status. This approach should be considered in situations in which risk of spread is likely. In other situations, the owner should be made aware of the seropositive status so that should clinical signs consistent with babesiosis arise, the attending veterinarian can be alerted to the possibility of the disease.

The organism affecting American pit bull terriers is *B. gibsoni*. Most reported cases of *B. gibsoni* in the southeastern United States have been associated with American pit bull terriers. It is common for dogs that are not pit bull dogs and are infected with *B. gibsoni* to have recently been in fights with pit bull dogs.[10,93] It is therefore important to include questions about recent fights in the history when evaluating a dog for hemolytic anemia.

PUBLIC HEALTH CONSIDERATIONS

Babesiosis is a significant tickborne zoonosis of people found throughout Europe and in the northeast and upper Midwest of the United States, and isolated cases of uncharacterized *Babesia* have been reported in Africa and Mexico.[74] The majority of infections are mild or asymptomatic; however, some result in severe illness and death. People who have had a splenectomy or are older (older than 55 years) are especially at risk.[36,120] No *Babesia* organism has been identified that is host specific for people. Sylvan cycles with wild animal reservoirs occur in nature. As for other tickborne zoonoses, people serve as accidental hosts for *Babesia* of animals when they are bitten by infected ticks. *B. microti* is the primary parasite affecting people in the northeast and upper Midwest of the United States (see Table 77-1). The vector tick is *Ixodes scapularis (dammini)*, the vector tick of Lyme borreliosis (see Chapter 45). The hemolytic disease with flulike symptoms is usually mild and self-limiting or easily managed with clindamycin and quinine. As in dogs, complications of the disease occur in people that have had a splenectomy or have other immunosuppressive illnesses.[48,52,53]

A severe form of human babesiosis is caused by *B. divergens* in Europe and *B. equi* in the United States. This form of the disease usually occurs in people who have had a splenectomy and is often fatal. An organism closely related to *B. divergens*—MO1—was isolated from a person in Missouri who had had a splenectomy and had a fatal illness.[52] Babesiosis was also identified in Italy and Austria with a new strain (EU1) that was more closely related to *B. odocoilei* than *B. divergens*.[49] In both instances the people had previously had splenectomies and developed characteristic signs of hemolytic anemia. Identical isolates of *Babesia* have been found in *Ixodes ricinus* ticks from Slovenia, indicating a more widespread distribution of this organism in Europe.

A syndrome of severe anemia that has been reported in people who have had a splenectomy occurs in the western United States.[121,120] Genetic analysis has shown that this northern California and Washington strain (WA1) is more closely related to (but distinct from) the ilerial species and the California strain of piroplasm in dogs than to other *Babesia*.[74,120] Historic case reports of human babesiosis caused by domestic animal piroplasms such as *Babesia bovis* or *B. canis* have not been well documented.[54] However, domestic animals are a source of exposure to the ticks, which may harbor other organisms more likely to infect humans.

SUGGESTED READINGS*

9. Baneth G, Kenny MJ, Tasker S, et al. 2004. Infection with a proposed new subspecies of *Babesia canis, Babesia canis* subsp. *presentii*, in domestic cats. *J Clin Microbiol* 42:99-105.
11. Birkenheuer AJ, Levy MG, Breitschwerdt EB. 2003b. Development and evaluation of a seminested PCR for detection and differentiation of *Babesia gibsoni* (Asian genotype) and *B. canis* DNA in canine blood samples. *J Clin Microbiol* 1:4172-4177.
18. Brandão LP, Hagiwara MK, Myiashiro SI. 2003. Humoral immunity and reinfection resistance in dogs experimentally inoculated with *Babesia canis* and either treated or untreated with imidocarb dipropionate. *Vet Parasitol* 114:453-265.
22. Camacho AT, Guitián FJ, Pallas E, et al. 2004. Azotemia and mortality among *Babesia microti*-like infected dogs. *J Vet Intern Med* 18:141-146.
32. Conrad P, Thomford J, Yamane I, et al. 1991. Hemolytic anemia caused by *Babesia gibsoni* infection in dogs. *J Am Vet Med Assoc* 199:601-605.
73. Kettner F, Reyers F, Miller D. 2003. Thrombocytopenia in canine babesiosis and its clinical usefulness. *J S Afr Vet Assoc* 74:63-68.
93. Macintire DK, Boudreaux MK, West GD, et al. 2002. *Babesia gibsoni* infection among dogs in the southeastern United States. *J Am Vet Med Assoc* 220:325-329.
108. Muhlnickel CJ, Jefferies R, Morgan-Ryan UM, et al. 2002. *Babesia gibsoni* infection in three dogs in Victoria. *Aust Vet J* 80:606-610.
118a. Penzhorn BL, Schoeman T, Jacobson LS. 2004. Feline babesiosis in South Africa, a review. *Ann NY Acad Sci* 1026:183-186.
160. Welzl C, Leisewitz AL, Jacobson LS, et al. 2001. Systemic inflammatory response syndrome and multiple-organ damage/dysfunction in complicated canine babesiosis. *J S Afr Vet Assoc* 72:158-162.

*See the CD-ROM for a complete list of references.

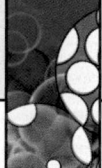

CHAPTER • 78

Enteric Protozoal Infections

The enteric protozoa covered in this chapter are limited to four protozoan genera: *Giardia, and Trichomonas,* and *Entamoeba* in the phylum Sarcomastigophora and *Balantidium* in the phylum Ciliophora. Salient characteristics of these organisms and the diseases they may cause are presented in Table 78-1. Enteric protozoa of the phylum Apicomplexa are discussed in Chapters 80 (Toxoplasmosis and Neosporidiosis), 81 (Enteric Coccidiosis), and 82 (Cryptosporidiosis and Cyclosporiasis). Detailed coverage of laboratory methods for diagnosis of enteric protozoan infections is presented in Chapter 70.

GIARDIASIS

Stephen C. Barr

Etiology and Epidemiology

Giardia duodenalis (syn. *G. intestinalis, G. lamblia*), a protozoan parasite found in the intestinal tracts of human beings and most domestic animals throughout the world, has two morphologic forms.[128] The intestinal lumen-dwelling motile form, the trophozoite, is approximately 15 µm long and 8 µm wide. Under light microscopy, the trophozoite is easily identified by its "smiling face" appearance formed by the two nuclei in the anterior third (forming the eyes), the axonemes passing longitudinally between the nuclei (forming the nose), and the median bodies (forming the mouth) situated transversely in the posterior third (Fig. 78-1). Four pairs of flagella complete the rather comical appearance of this form. The second form, the cyst, is responsible for transmission and environmental survival. It is approximately 12 µm long and 7 µm wide. Because the cyst contains two incompletely separated but formed trophozoites, the axonemes, fragments of the ventral disks, and up to four nuclei can be seen within (Fig. 78-2). The cyst is susceptible to desiccation under dry, hot conditions but can survive for several months outside the host in wet, cold conditions. Transmission is fecal-oral route by ingestion of feces or fecal-contaminated water, food, or fomites. The life cycle is direct (Fig. 78-3). After ingestion, cysts (trophozoites are noninfective) excyst in the duodenum on exposure to gastric acids and pancreatic enzymes. The two released trophozoites separate, mature, and attach to the brush border of the villous epithelium (Fig. 78-4). The distribution of trophozoites within the intestinal tract varies with host and diet. In dogs, the organism seems to prefer the duodenum and jejunum[132] but has been found from the ileum to the duodenum.[34] Circumstantial evidence indicates that trophozoites occupy the upper intestinal tract (duodenum) in infected symptomatic dogs[76] and the lower tract (jejunum) in infected asymptomatic dogs.[9,140] In cats, trophozoites have been found throughout the intestinal tract.[63,76] In dogs, a high-carbohydrate diet rather than a high-protein diet[132] may favor trophozoite habitation of the upper tract. In people, *Giardia* is often found in chronic atrophic gastritis (often associated with *Helicobacter pylori* infection or gastric adenocarcinoma) when a decrease in gastric acidity occurs.[33,110] Trophozoites adhere (using a ventral adhesive disk) to the brush border of the intestinal mucosa and move from one attachment site to another using flagella. Encystation of trophozoites is stimulated by bile salts and fatty acids at slightly alkaline pH[46]; however, the site and mechanism are unknown. Trophozoites may be passed in diarrheic stools, but cysts are more routinely shed. Whereas cysts may survive for

Table • 78-1

Comparison of Some Enteric Protozoa in Dogs and Cats

ORGANISM	STAGE	AVERAGE SIZE (μm)	NATURAL HOSTS	ORGAN PARASITIZED	PATHOGENIC MECHANISMS	CLINICAL SIGNS
Giardia[a]	Tr Cy	15 × 10 × 3 10 × 8	D, C, H, other mammals	Small intestine	Damage to glycocalyx and microvilli on intestinal epithelium; inhibition of some digestive enzymes; host elicits inflammatory response	None to chronic diarrhea, continuous or intermittent, malabsorption
Entamoeba histolytica	Tr Cy	25 (diam.) 12 (diam.)	D, C, H, NHP	Large intestine	Invades colonic wall, producing ulcers; may metastasize to extraintestinal sites	None to diarrhea; dysentery
Balantidium coli	Tr Cy	60 × 35 50 (diam.)	D, P, H, NHP	Large intestine	Invades colonic wall, producing ulcers metastases (rare)	None to diarrhea; dysentery
Pentatrichomonas hominis	Tr	8 × 5, five flagella	D, C, H, other mammals	Large intestine	Probably none; considered harmless commensal but may be opportunistic pathogen	None to diarrhea
Tritrichomonas foetus	Tr	8 × 5, three flagella	D, C, Ca, P	Genitalia (cattle) Intestine, nasal (swine) Large intestine (cat)	Epithelial adherent, elaboration of cytotoxins and enzymes; host elicits inflammatory response	Large bowel diarrhea in feline; infertility and fetal loss in cattle; diarrhea in co-infected pups

Tr, Trophozoite; *Cy*, cyst; *D*, dog; *C*, cat; *H*, human being; *NHP*, nonhuman primate; *P*, pig; *Ca*, cattle.
[a]Some *Giardia* species may be identical.

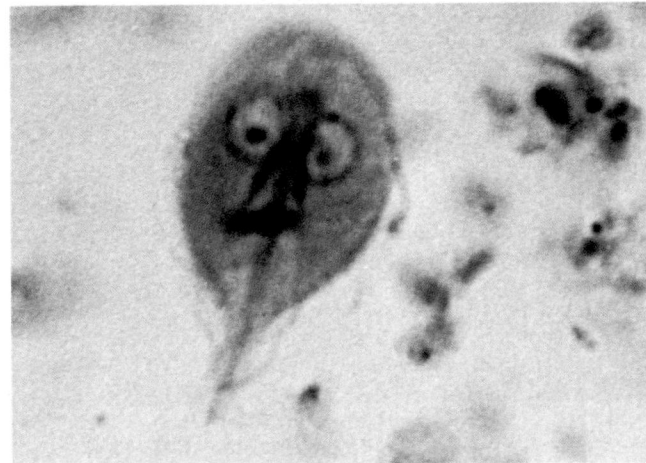

Fig 78-1 *Giardia* trophozoite in a fecal smear stained to enhance the characteristic organelles (iron hematoxylin, ×2000).

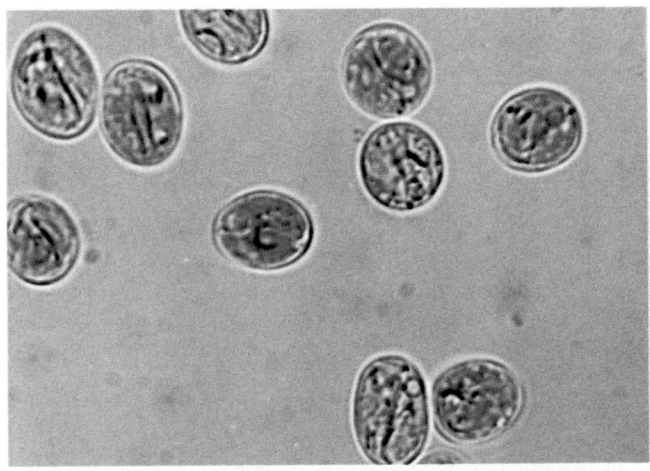

Fig 78-2 *Giardia* cysts concentrated from the feces of a cat by the zinc sulfate centrifugal flotation technique. Cyst wall, nuclei, axonemes, and median bodies are apparent in several of the cysts (iodine, ×1100).

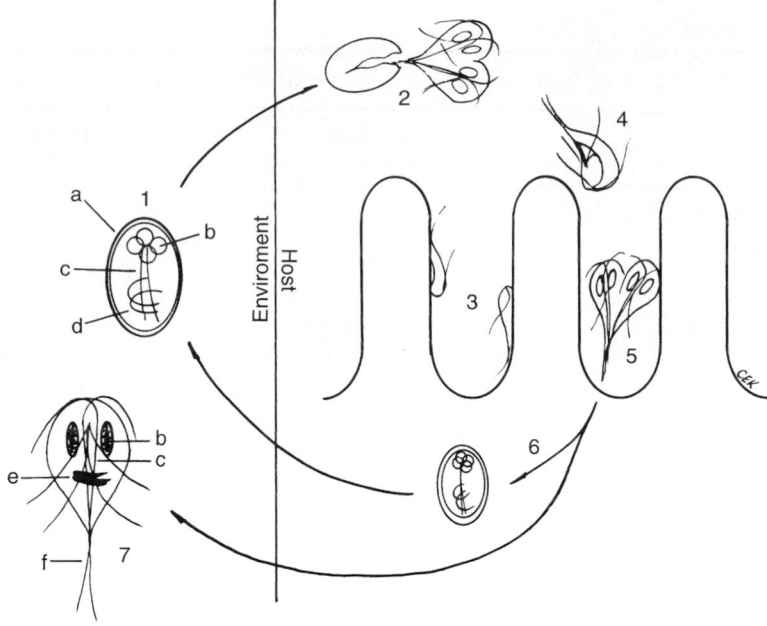

Fig 78-3 Diagram of *Giardia* life cycle, indicating organelles of cyst and trophozoite visible by light microscopy. After the cyst *(1)* is ingested by the host, excystation *(2)* occurs in the small intestine. Trophozoites *(3 through 5)* attach to the mucosa or swim freely in the lumen where they divide asexually. Following encystment, cysts are excreted *(6)* in the feces, completing the cycle. Excreted trophozoites *(7)* do not survive. Key to structural features: *a,* cyst wall; *b,* nuclei; *c,* axonemes (recurrent flagella); *d,* adhesive disk fragments; *e,* median bodies; *f,* flagella. (From Kirkpatrick CE. 1987. Giardiasis, *Vet Clin North Am* [*Small Anim Pract*] 17:1377–1387. Reprinted with permission.)

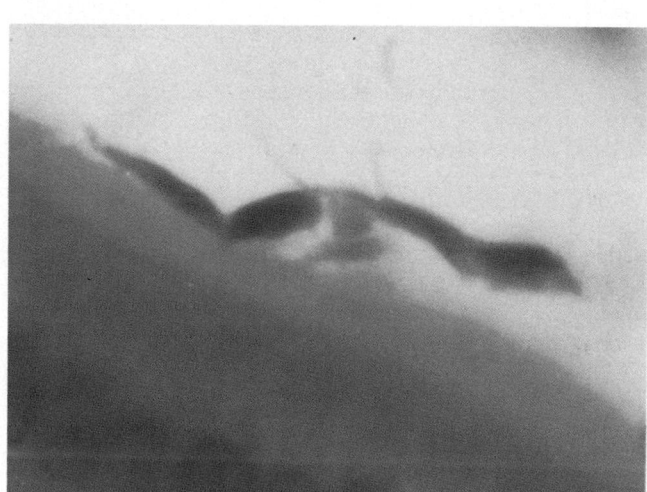

Fig 78-4 High magnification of trophozoites of *Giardia* sp. attached to intestinal villus of canary (H and E stain, ×1500). (From Gardiner CH et al. 1988. An atlas of protozoan parasites in animal tissues, USDA Agricultural Handbook No. 651, Beltsville, Md.)

days to weeks in cool, moist conditions, trophozoites do not survive long outside the host. On excretion, the relatively resistant, ellipsoidal cysts are immediately infective to another host.

The prepatent period of *Giardia* infection ranges from 5 to 12 days (mean, approximately 8 days) in dogs and from 5 to 16 days (mean, approximately 10 days) in cats. The onset of disease, when it occurs, may precede cyst shedding by 1 to 2 days.

The prevalence of *Giardia* is approximately 10% in well-attended dogs, 36% to 50% in puppies, and up to 100% in breeding kennels.[76,107a] The prevalence in cats ranges from 1.4% to 11%.[62,76] In the general population of both species, the overall prevalence averages approximately 2.5%.[89,99,129] Although the prevalence of giardiasis is high in cats and dogs, obvious clinical disease is rare. Immunodeficient adults, the young, and group-housed animals (breeding kennels, catteries, and laboratory animal colonies) have a high prevalence of clinically apparent *Giardia* infection. Glucocorticoid therapy at antiinflammatory dosages (1 mg/kg/day of prednisolone) for 10 days, allowed replication and reshedding of *Giardia*.[140]

Pathogenesis

Because virtually no studies of how *Giardia* causes clinical disease in dogs and cats have been submitted, most of the following information is extrapolated from human studies. In people, infection can cause malabsorption of vitamin B$_{12}$, folate, iron (leading to anemia),[59] triglycerides, lactose, and, less commonly, sucrose.[57] Specific histologic changes have not been identified in the small-bowel mucosa[100]; however, parasite-related pathogenic factors have been implicated in abnormally rapid sloughing of intestinal epithelial cells, leading to failure of new epithelial cells arising in the crypts to differentiate fully into columnar cells with microvilli. Blunting of intestinal villi and microvilli results in decreased absorptive surface area.[5]

Putative differences in virulence of *Giardia* strains, as well as host genetics and immune status, probably determine the outcome of an infection. Not only do morphologically identical human *Giardia* isolates vary in respect to their surface antigens,[95] susceptibility to proteases,[96] and genetic profiles,[22] they also vary in their virulence.[23,24] An intact cellular and humoral[71] immune system is important for overcoming infection and developing protective immunity.[40] Absence of an Secretory IgA (S-IgA) response to one of *Giardia* heat shock proteins is associated with persistent infection despite an IgG response to this protein and IgA responses to other *Giardia* polypeptides.[26] Few studies involve dogs or cats; the prevalence of *Giardia* infection in a colony of IgA-deficient beagles was higher than that of normal animals.[76] Administration of immunosuppressive amounts of glucocorticoids will lead to recrudescence of *Giardia* infections in dogs.[140]

Clinical Findings

Most infections in which cysts are passed in the feces are asymptomatic. Acute diarrhea tends to occur in very young puppies and kittens shortly after infection. In older cats and dogs, diarrhea may be acute and short lived, intermittent, or chronic. Despite the high prevalence of *Giardia* in cats, clinical disease is uncommon. In addition to young animals, those that are stressed, immunosuppressed, or housed in groups have the greatest prevalence of clinical disease. In clinically affected animals, feces are often malodorous, pale, and steatorrheic. Affected animals may experience weight loss secondary to diarrhea, but rarely will they become inappetent.[76] Although *Giardia* cysts and trophozoites can be seen in the stool of dogs with small- or large-bowel diarrhea with weight loss,[37] the organism is unlikely to be the sole cause of the diarrhea. Giardiasis does not in itself produce fever or emesis.

Diagnosis
Fecal Microscopy
Finding cysts or trophozoites in the feces or samples taken from the intestinal tract is the most definitive means of diagnosing giardiasis because clinical signs and laboratory test results (hemogram, serum biochemistry, radiology) are not pathognomonic. The prevalence of *Giardia* is high, even when giardiasis often goes undetected.[7] Reasons for this occurrence may include failure to consider the organism in the differential diagnosis, failure to recognize the organisms, use of inappropriate methods for fecal analysis, and intermittent excretion of organisms in feces of infected individuals. Most infected animals passing cysts are asymptomatic, while those with diarrhea shed trophozoites.

A fecal smear, especially in symptomatic patients, may reveal trophozoites that are distinctive by their erratic tumbling motion and concave ventral disk. *Giardia* trophozoites can be distinguished from those of *Trichomonas foetus* or *Pentatrichomonas hominis* (see Trichomoniasis later in this chapter). A drop of feces is mixed with a drop of normal saline on a glass slide, a coverslip is applied, and the specimen is examined immediately with 40 × with the condenser in its lowest position. Morphology of the organisms can be better appreciated by adding a drop of Lugol's iodine, which kills the parasite, thereby rendering it immobile, to a drop of feces. Finding organisms in a fecal smear provides a definitive diagnosis of *Giardia* infection, but a negative result does not rule it out.

If a direct smear provides a negative result, the zinc sulfate concentration technique (ZSCT) should be performed.[76,140] This method is also effective in demonstrating nematode eggs in the feces of cats and dogs and is superior to sucrose (of equal density) flotation because it is less likely to distort the organisms. Commercial ZSCT that do not include centrifugation have a markedly reduced specificity than do techniques that include concentration by centrifugation.[139] Because cats and dogs shed *Giardia* organisms intermittently,[61,76] and the presence of organisms in feces does not necessarily parallel the severity of clinical signs, at least three fresh fecal samples should be examined over a period of 3 to 5 days to maximize the chance of ruling out infection. Approximately 70% and 93% of *Giardia*-positive dogs can be identified with one and two ZSCTs, respectively.[76,140] For shipping, fecal samples should be refrigerated at 4° C (39° F) to ensure survival for at least 2 days; cysts will not survive in 10% formalin. Slides prepared by the ZSCT should be examined within 10 minutes of preparation because the cysts shrink with time and lose the internal morphologic characteristic appearance that differentiates them from other organisms. Cysts may be distinguished from coccidian oocysts and sporocysts by internal structure and by observing that *Giardia* cysts will take up iodine, whereas coccidia will not. Yeasts also will stain with iodine; however, yeasts are oval, not ellipsoidal, and are approximately one half the size of *Giardia* cysts. Furthermore, close observation of yeast cells may reveal budding. If steatorrhea frustrates attempts at flotation, the formalin-ethyl acetate sedimentation method to concentrate *Giardia* cysts from a fecal specimen is usually successful.

Fecal Immunoassays
Commercial enzyme-linked immunosorbent assay (ELISA) kits to detect fecal *Giardia* antigens (see Appendix 6) have over 97% sensitivity and over 96% specificity in humans.[114,145] In dogs, the ProSpecT/Giardia ELISA kit (Alexon Inc., Mountain View, Calif.) was found to be slightly less sensitive and have a slightly lower relative specificity than did the ZSCT.[9] The test may be slightly more effective compared with a single ZSCT in diagnosing *Giardia* infections in dogs.[141] In another study, the false negative rate was 31.6% compared with ZSCT, but the specificity was high at 95.7%.[108] Frozen fecal samples or samples preserved in formalin fixative can be used. Given that the ELISA kits are technically more difficult to use and more expensive compared with the ZSCT, they do not seem to offer any advantages over performing three ZSCTs for the diagnosis of giardiasis in dogs. The ELISA has not been adequately evaluated in the cat, although it will detect infected fecal samples.

Similar to the ELISA kits, the direct fluorescent antibody (FA) test (using fluorescent-labeled monoclonal antibodies to detect *Giardia* cysts in feces) is highly sensitive (100%) and specific (99.8%) in people.[145] One such test (Merifluor Cryptosporidium/Giardia Direct Immunofluorescence Assay, Meridian Diagnostics, Cincinnati, Ohio) is more sensitive than the sucrose gradient flotation and ZSCT are at identifying infected feces from cattle and sheep, especially when the cyst concentration in the feces is low.[137] In cats, the sensitivities and specificities of the fecal antigen and ZSCT were 95% and 100%, and 87.5% and 75%, respectively. One would expect a similar finding for feces from dogs. Furthermore, direct FA and fecal antigen tests are superior to the ZSCT assay for stored samples because cysts become distorted (creating false-negative readings) and yeast grows in stored samples (creating false-positive readings).[79] Because direct FA requires a fluorescent microscope, it is more likely to be used in diagnostic laboratories. Feces should be collected fresh and preserved as soon as possible in 10% formalin or sodium acetate–acetic acid formalin.

Duodenal Sampling
Two techniques used to collect a sample from the duodenum for the microscopic examination of trophozoites have reportedly had disparate findings. In one study, examination for trophozoites of duodenal aspirates collected during gastroduodenoscopy or exploratory laparotomy has been shown to be more efficacious than a ZSCT is on a single fecal sample from the same dogs suffering from clinical giardiasis.[109] However, in another study performed in asymptomatic dogs, a single sample was found to be as effective as a duodenal aspirate was for the diagnosis of giardiasis.[140] The disparity between these findings may be explained by the fact that, in subclinically infected dogs, the organism colonizes various levels (not always including the duodenum) anywhere along the small intestine.[34] However, even in animals with diarrhea, intestinal aspiration rarely identifies *Giardia* over and above ZSCT.[103] Duodenal aspiration to specifically rule out *Giardia* infection is clinically impractical but may be performed if the dog was undergoing gastroduodenoscopy for other reasons and had not previously been treated for *Giardia* or had a ZSCT performed.[103]

The second technique used to sample duodenal contents, a commercially available peroral nylon string test (Entero-test, HDC Corp., San Jose, Calif.), has been found to be both safe and accurate for the diagnosis of giardiasis in people.[113] The test is not safe or effective in diagnosing infection in asymptomatic dogs,[9] although it has been effective in detecting trophozoites in two symptomatic dogs. The test has not been evaluated in cats. See Appendix 6 for information on this product.

Nucleic Acid Detection

G. intestinalis isolates from people and animals are morphologically similar. Nucleic acid sequence analysis indicates genetic diversity among the isolates. They have been grouped into seven genetic lineages, known as assemblages, A through G (Table 78-2). Two major zoonotic genotypes (A and B) and animal-specific genotypes (assemblages C through G), such as for dogs or cats, have been found. Within the A genogroup, A-I subtypes are closely related animal and human isolates, while A-II contains only human isolates.[128] Assemblage B consists of genetically diverse groups of genotypes isolated from people and various animals. These two groups contain the isolates of zoonotic concern. Animals also have their own host-specific strains. The dog-specific types, which are more divergent, have been further divided into types C and D. Cat- and livestock-specific isolates are more closely related to the A and B genotypes, suggesting a more recent genetic divergence.[3,65,127a] This polymerase chain reaction (PCR) can be used to distinguish between strains of zoonotic risk and those specific to pets. In a study of *Giardia* isolates from domestic, farm and wild animals worldwide, genotypes A and B were widespread in nature and found among diverse types of animals.[134] Whether this finding represents a cause or effect of human infections is uncertain. In addition, one dog was infected with a mouse-type isolate. PCR has also been used to link human and animal infections (see Public Health Considerations later in this chapter). PCR appears to be sensitive in detecting low levels of infection. Microscopy, ELISA, and PCR methods were used on fecal specimens to determine the prevalence of *Giardia* infection in domestic cats, and rates of 5%, 60%, and 80%, respectively, were found.[87]

Therapy

In the United States, no drug used to treat giardiasis in small animals is officially approved for that purpose. However, a significant number of licensed drugs that have been employed commonly in human patients to treat giardiasis have been used in small animals. Drug resistance can develop in *Giardia* to any of the available regimens with repeated use, and therefore additional measures for control should be employed. Even if chemotherapy is highly effective, control measures must also be used to prevent reinfection. Some of the reportedly effective treatment regimens in dogs and cats are shown in Table 78-3.* Fenbendazole (Panacur granules 22.2%, Hoechst-Roussel Agri-Vet Co., Somerville, N.J.), at the dose approved in dogs for the control and removal of roundworms, hookworms, and whipworms, and the tapeworm *(Taenia pisiformis)*, was effective in removing *Giardia* cysts from feces in 100% of dogs (six of six dogs treated) in a controlled trial[13] and in 9 of 10 dogs in another study.[139] No side effects were seen at this dose regimen, nor is fenbendazole (similar to some other benzimidazoles) thought to be teratogenic. It is safe to treat puppies as young as 6 weeks at these doses. Mild diarrhea has been the only side effect noted. These results suggest that fenbendazole alone may be used to treat giardiasis or to rule out (by therapeutic trial) *Giardia* and whipworm infections as a cause of chronic diarrhea in the dog. Fenbendazole has been evaluated in a group of cats concurrently infected with *Giardia* and *Cryptosporidium*. Of eight cats treated with fenbendazole (50 mg/kg, orally, once daily for 5 days), four remained clear of *Giardia* for the study period (23 days). Three other cats transiently stopped shedding cysts for approximately 1 week after stopping treatment but then resumed. One cat showed only a transient reduction in cyst excretion.[73,74] A combination product, febantel-praziquantel-pyrantel (Drontal Plus, Bayer Co., Shawnee Mission, Kan.), has similar efficacy to fenbendazole in dogs when used at recommended doses for 3 consecutive days.[10] Similar but slightly lower efficacy was demonstrated when the combination was used once at double the dose or when used at the recommended dose for 2 days.[45] In six cats treated for 5 days, significant decreases in cyst shedding occurred, and the percentage of positive fecal results was reduced compared with untreated control cats.[118] Shedding was not reactivated in four of the cats after immunosuppression with glucocorticoids. The active ingredient against *Giardia* in the combination is thought to be febantel, which is converted to fenbendazole and oxfendazole by the liver. In another study, febantel-praziquantel-pyrantel combination was used in association with strict hygiene procedures to excellent effect, underlining the need to use chemotherapy in association with methods to prevent or limit reinfection.[108] Oxfendazole (11.3 mg/kg, orally, every 24 hours for 3 days; Dolthene, Merial Laboratories, Lyon, France), a benzimidazole used in Europe as a common canine anthelmintic, was also 100% effective against *Giardia* in kenneled dogs when used in combination with control methods.[135] Albendazole given to dogs for 2 days was 90% efficacious in clearing *Giardia* cysts from feces[12]; however, a longer regimen (5 days) is needed in cats.[11] No side effects were seen in cats at doses provided or in beagles treated at 30-mg/kg body weight orally once a day for 13 weeks.[126] However, albendazole is potentially toxic, causing myelosuppression in both dogs and cats. In dogs, toxicity appears to be dose dependent, while in cats, the reaction appears to be idiosyncratic.[123] Therefore its use in cats is not recommended. Albendazole, but not fenbendazole, is suspected of being teratogenic[29] and therefore should not be given to pregnant animals.

Metronidazole (a nitroimidazole) has been administered extensively in dogs and cats for the treatment of giardiasis. It has often been less effective than albendazole or fenbendazole is against *Giardia* in vitro and in vivo. The drug is only 67% effective in eliminating *Giardia* from infected dogs and has been associated with the development anorexia, vomiting, and acute neurologic signs, including progression of pronounced generalized ataxia and vertical positional nystagmus. This situation has resulted in euthanasia in some animals.[35,42] However, metronidazole benzoate was more effective than fenbendazole was in treating *Giardia* when cats were co-infected with *Cryptosporidium*.[117] Cats often resent the admin-

*References: 11-13, 16, 75, 77, 143, 144.

Table • 78-2

Genetic Groupings of Giardia duodenalis Morphologic Group[6,127]

ASSEMBLAGE (GENETIC GROUP)	HOST RANGE
A (Polish strains, Group A1, A2)	A1: People, livestock, cats, dogs, beavers, guinea pigs, slow loris A2: People
B (Belgian strains, Group 3)	People, slow loris, chinchillas, dogs, beavers, rats, siamang
C (Dogs)	Australian dog strains
D (Dogs)	Dogs
E (Livestock)	Cattle, goats, pig, sheep, alpacas
F (Cat)	Cats
G (Rat)	Rats
(Muskrat)	Muskrats, voles

Table • 78-3

Drug Therapy for Enteric Protozoal Infections[a]

DRUG	SPECIES	DOSE[b]	ROUTE	INTERVAL (HOURS)	DURATION (DAYS)	INFECTION
Fenbendazole	D	50 mg/kg	PO	24	3	G
Albendazole	D	25 mg/kg	PO	12	2	G
	C	25 mg/kg	PO	12	5	G
Metronidazole	D	15–30 mg/kg[c]	PO	12–24	5–7	G, T, A ,Ba
	C	10–25 mg/kg	PO	12–24	5–7	G, T, A, Ba
Tinidazole	D	44 mg/kg	PO	24	6	G, T?, A?, Ba?
Ronidazole	C	30–50 mg/kg	PO	12	14	T
Ipronidazole	D	126 mg/L[d]	PO	Ad libitum	7	G
Quinacrine	D	9 mg/kg	PO	24	6	G
	D	6.6 mg/kg	PO	12	5	G
Furazolidone	C	4 mg/kg[e]	PO	12	7–10	G
Tetracycline	D	22 mg/kg	PO	8	7–10	Ba
Paromomycin	C	125–160 mg/kg	PO	12	5	T, A
Combination (10:1 ratio) of Febantel *plus* praziquantel	B	Febantel: 15 mg/kg *plus* Praziquantel: 1.5 mg/kg	PO	24	5	G

D, Dog; *C*, cat; *B*, both dog and cat; *G*, giardiasis; *T*, trichomoniasis; *A*, amebiasis; *Ba* balantidiasis; *?*, uncertain efficacy.

[a]For additional information on each drug, see Drug Formulary, Appendix 8. For coccidial infections, see Chapter 81; for Cryptosporidiosis, Chapter 82.

[b]Dose per administration at specified interval.

[c]Neurotoxicity has been noted with higher doses previously recommended; see Nitroimidazoles, Chapter 77. To facilitate the dosage to smaller animals, the 250- or 500-mg tablets may be ground, or smaller tablet size (50 or 100 mg) may be used. This may be placed in a palatable base. For cats, metronidazole benzoate formulations are better tolerated than USP formulations. See Drug Formulary, Appendix 8.

[d]In drinking water.

[e]In suspension, 200 mg/day maximum.

istration of metronidazole because of the bitter taste of the tablets; however, this is less of a problem with the benzoate formulation[117] (see Drug Formulary, Appendix 8). Drug resistance to metronidazole by various isolates of *Giardia* is a serious concern in people and in some areas; it is not recommended for the treatment of giardiasis.[39,133] At high doses (see Table 78-3), quinacrine is 100% effective but is associated with a 50% rate of side effects (lethargy and fevers) toward the end of the therapeutic regimen.[76] These side effects regress spontaneously within 2 to 3 days after stopping drug administration. Similar to albendazole and metronidazole, quinacrine should not be given to pregnant animals. Quinacrine has not been demonstrated to be effective in cats.

Ipronidazole, a feed-water additive for the treatment of blackhead in turkeys caused by *Histomonas meleagridis* and *Trichomonas foetus* in cattle, has been provided effectively in drinking water to treat giardiasis in two greyhounds. Unfortunately, the drug has not been more extensively tested. Tinidazole, another nitroimidazole, has an efficacy against giardiasis similar to metronidazole,[76] but it is unavailable in the United States. Furazolidone is effective in treating giardiasis in cats, but side effects of diarrhea and vomiting can occur.[76] Furazolidone has not been well evaluated in dogs. As is the case with many of the other anti-*Giardia* compounds, furazolidone is suspected of being teratogenic and should not be used in pregnant queens.[76] See the Drug Formulary, Appendix 8, for more information on these drugs.

Vaccination

Giardia vaccine (GiardiaVax, Fort Dodge Animal Health, Overland Park, Kan.) for cats and dogs composed of chemically inactivated trophozoites became commercially available early in 2000. Pups and kittens (age 7 weeks and naïve to *Giardia* exposure) that received one vaccine and a booster 3 weeks later were immune to a *Giardia* challenge 6 and 12 months later.[103,106] In other studies using older dogs, vaccination reduced the duration of cyst shedding and the number of cysts shed.[104] Of 817 dogs receiving the vaccine, 97% showed no local or systemic vaccine-associated reactions, and those that did react developed only mild, transient, injection site reactions.[102] The vaccine has been used as an immunotherapeutic agent in dogs. Thirteen dogs that failed to be cured of giardiasis using chemotherapeutic measures showed clinical cures and cessation of fecal cyst shedding between 3 to 10 weeks postvaccination (some dogs required up to three vaccines).[104] However, in other studies, vaccination failed to prevent reinfection.[108] *Giardia* vaccination has not been an effective treatment for asymptomatic canine *Giardia* infections.[5a] Furthermore, the present author (SBC) has seen numerous asymptomatically infected dogs develop clinical symptoms of diarrhea after receiving the vaccine. *Giardia* vaccination at 4, 6, and 10 weeks after cats were experimentally infected failed to clear the infection, suggesting that the vaccine may not be efficacious in cats that already infected.[122] Although the vaccine might have a place in the treatment of some chronically infected dogs in which chemotherapy and hygiene control methods have failed, its utility appears small for use is as a general vaccine for the control of giardiasis in the general population of dogs or cats that are invariably exposed to the organism before vaccination.

Prevention

To date, no drug has been convincingly proven to be 100% effective against *Giardia*. Trials testing the efficacy of drugs against *Giardia* are based on clearing cysts from feces, not removing organisms from the intestinal tract. Thus, because the possibility exits that these compounds do not clear organisms but only inhibit cyst production for a time, whether treated animals may be a source of infection in the future is unknown. Certainly, autoinfection occurs by virtue of viable cysts present in fecal material adherent to the external haircoat or present in a cold, moist environment. Because the prepatent period can be extremely short for *Giardia*, an animal may become reinfected and start excreting cysts again within 5 days after the last treatment. Because of these factors, preventing reinfection of household pets or animals held in uncontrolled environments is virtually impossible. Preliminary trials in kittens, using a killed trophozoite vaccine (Langford/Cyanamid, Guelph, Ontario, Canada) has shown protection against diarrhea, weight loss, and cyst shedding.[105] Lesser numbers or no cysts and reduced cyst viability were found in vaccinates compared with unvaccinated kittens.

In controlled environments (cattery or kennel situation), four main approaches should be employed to control *Giardia*: (1) decontaminating the environment, (2) using drugs to treat animals, (3) cleaning cysts from coats, and (4) preventing reintroduction of infection.[8]

In a cattery or kennel, first, establishing a "clean area" is necessary. In a small facility, all the animals should be moved out of the facility while it is being cleaned. In a large facility, clean areas can be created over time by setting up a few cages or runs on a rotation basis once animals are moved out to a holding facility. Before moving animals to the holding facility, they should be treated (preferably with fenbendazole or febantel-praziquantel-pyrantel combination) and moved to the holding facility on the last day of treatment. Once moved, the cages or runs should be steam or chemically cleaned after all fecal material has been picked up. Quaternary ammonium (QUAT)-containing disinfectants (Roccal, Winthrop Labs, New York, N.Y.; Totil, Calgon Corp., St. Louis, Mo.), when used at the manufacturers' recommended concentrations, are effective in inactivating *Giardia* cysts (1 minute at room temperature).[76] QUATs lose considerable activity when used in the presence of organic matter. The kennel should be allowed to dry thoroughly after cleaning (cysts are extremely susceptible to drying) and preferably left dry and empty for several days before being repopulated. Before repopulating the clean area, the animals should be bathed to remove all fecal material from their coats with a general pet shampoo and thoroughly rinsed. The animals should be bathed again (especially the perianal area) with a QUAT compound. QUAT compounds can irritate skin and mucous membranes with repeated or prolonged exposure but appear to produce no ill effects when applied for 3 to 5 minutes followed by thorough rinsing. The coat is allowed to dry thoroughly before returning the animal to the clean area. Animals should then be treated again, preferably with a different compound than the one initially used, once back in the clean facility. Theoretically, the only way *Giardia* can be reintroduced into a clean area is by an infected animal or by fomite transmission. New animals introduced into the kennel or cattery should be treated and their coats cleansed as discussed, regardless of whether they are *Giardia* negative on fecal examination. Fomite transmission can be avoided by donning shoe covers before entering the facility or cleaning boots with a QUAT footbath. Fecal samples should be periodically checked using the ZSCT, which should detect whether the process has been effective.

Public Health Considerations

Giardia is the most common intestinal parasite, affecting people worldwide. Many infections are acquired by drinking unfiltered municipal water originating from *Giardia*-contaminated streams, rivers, or lakes.[66] Infants and children in day care facilities appear to have a particularly high risk for infection. Furthermore, giardiasis has been regarded as an emerging disease in developed countries. Approximately 200 million people in Asia, Africa, and Latin America have symptomatic giardiasis.[136] Contaminated water is an important vehicle for transmission of this infection. Although scant direct evidence links zoonotic infections from dogs and cats, molecular and immunologic analyses of assemblage A group I (A-I) and B *Giardia* isolates from animals, including dogs and cats, and people suggest that they are not highly host specific.[14,38,58] The A-I and B isolates that parasitize people have been found in cysts from fecal samples of dogs, cats, some farm animals, and wild animals, suggesting that these genotypes are widespread and possibly zoonotic.[134] Of the human genotypes, only those of the A-I type have been found in cats. Genetic studies of host infections over time suggest that mixed populations of genotypes do not persist, and the better host-adapted strain eventually predominates.[127] For example, the higher infection rate in Aboriginal dogs in Australia allows the better-adapted dog strain to dominate.[127] In these communities, both people and dogs are commonly infected. However, almost all the dogs harbor the canine-specific strain.[64,65] Similarly, in metropolitan Perth, Australia, all but one genotype isolated from cats was a dog strain.[87] This situation contrasts with some urban areas where the prevalence of infection has been lower, but the infecting strain in dogs is usually a zoonotic one from assemblages A-I or B. In kennels in central Italy, 23% of the isolates from dogs were assemblage A-I with potential zoonotic implications and the remainder was the dog genotype.[17] In genetic studies on a focus of infection in a remote Indian subcontinent community, canine isolates were in the human assemblages A-I and B.[130,131] An epidemiologic association was made between the prevalence of *Giardia* infection in people and dogs within the same households.

Chlorine disinfection of public drinking water is not completely effective in controlling *Giardia* contamination, and filtration should also be used.[110a] Organic chlorine compounds such as *N*-halamines are stable in water and have shown marked efficacy in inactivating *Giardia* cysts within 2 minutes at 22° C (72° F).

AMEBIASIS

Stephen C. Barr

Etiology and Epidemiology

Entamoeba histolytica is a facultatively parasitic ameba that predominantly infects people and nonhuman primates. Genetic analysis has shown that, within a given geographic region, families of closely associated people harbor unique strains.[142] This finding suggests that household members, including pets, are at risk for exposure. Although the prevalence of amebiasis in the United States has declined considerably over the last several decades, *E. histolytica* remains an important parasite in many tropical areas around the world.

Trophozoites either inhabit the colonic lumen as commensals or invade the colonic wall. Rarely do they disseminate to other organs such as the liver, lungs, brain, perianal skin, and genitalia (Figs. 78-5 and 78-6). Various strains of *E. histolytica* differ in virulence. Cysts, passed in human feces, are the infective stages. Because encystment of trophozoites rarely occurs in dogs and cats, amebiasis is among the unusual diseases that are transmissible from people to pets but seldom vice versa.

Willaertia is a genus of free-living saprophytic amebas that are closely related to *Naegleria*. The latter species has been identified in human infections in which trophozoites are

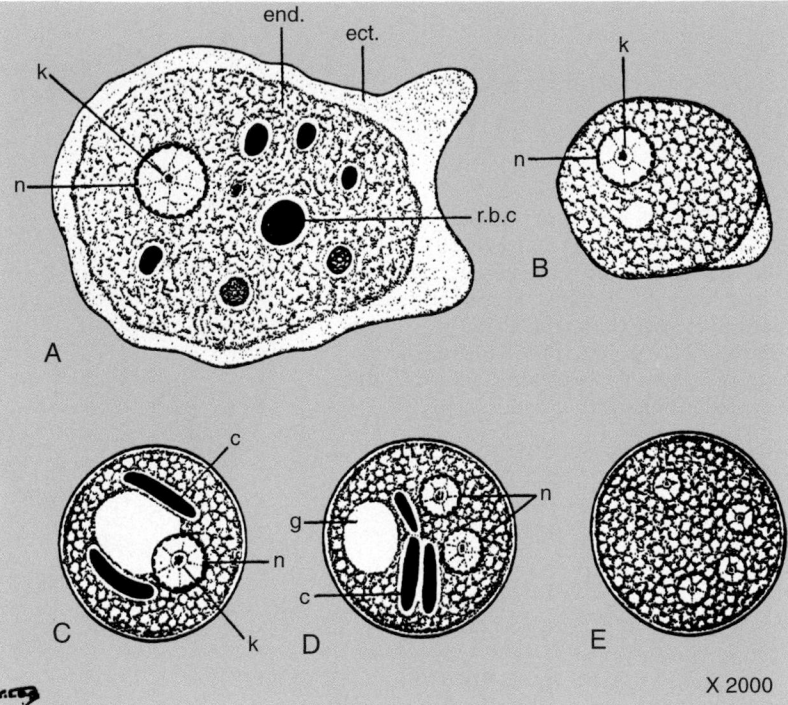

Fig 78-5 Schematic depiction of *E. histolytica* trophozoite **(A)** and various stages of cyst development **(B through E)**. Key: *c*, chromatoid bodies; *g*, glycogen vacuole; *k*, karyosome; *n*, nucleus; *r.b.c.*, red blood cell; *end.*, endoplasm; *ect.*, ectoplasm. (From Brown HW, Neva FA. 1983. Basic clinical parasitology, ed 5, Appleton-Century-Crofts, Norwalk, Conn., with permission.)

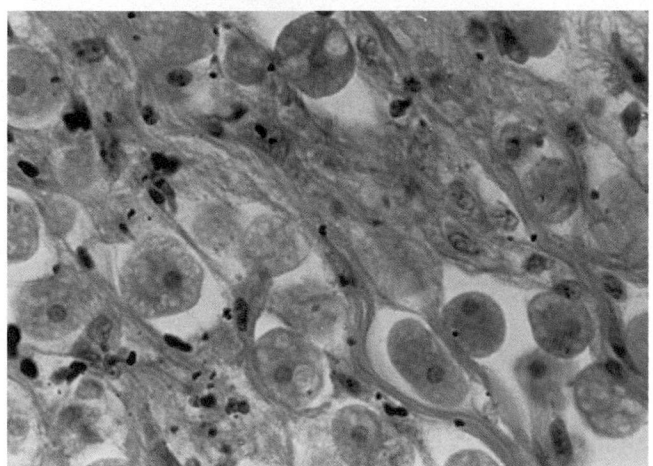

Fig 78-6 Numerous *E. histolytica* trophozoites in a section from the wall of a human colon. Each organism contains a single, darkly stained nucleus; in some of the trophozoites, pale vacuoles are apparent (H and E stain, ×540).

found in tissues. In contrast to these locally invasive infections, *Acanthamoeba* disseminates to other tissues and encysts (see Chapter 79).

Pathogenesis and Pathologic Findings

E. histolytica trophozoites damage the intestine by attaching to and lysing host cells and secreting enzymes that disrupt intercellular connections. The presence of certain bacteria and a host with deficient protein intake contribute to parasite virulence. The host's own cellular immune response to tissue-invading amebas can exacerbate the damage. Secretory diarrhea may be induced by serotonin and other factors secreted by the trophozoites.

Mucosal IgA antibodies to the amebic adherence lectin have been shown to provide resistance to enteric infection in people.[120] However, immunity is transient and reinfections are common. Secretory immunity is also important in preventing dissemination and subsequent development of hepatic abscesses.

Invasive amebiasis results in erosion or ulceration of the colonic mucosa. Microscopic examination of infected colonic tissue may reveal the classic flask-shaped ulcer of amebiasis, which is the result of mucosal undermining by trophozoites in the submucosa. Trophozoites may be seen in sections stained with hematoxylin and eosin, iron hematoxylin, or periodic acid-Schiff reaction.

Clinical Findings

E. histolytica infections are usually asymptomatic but can lead to signs of severe ulcerative colitis, including dysentery. Fulminant, untreated amebiasis may prove fatal. Extraintestinal amebiasis, a serious complication, is rare in dogs and unknown in cats. In such cases, signs would be referable to the parasitized tissue (e.g., lung). Vulval swelling and bloody vaginal discharge have been reported in a dog with uterine, cervical, and vaginal invasion with trophozoites.

A gastric infection with *Willaertia* was described in a dog with gastric ulceration and adenocarcinoma.[121] The dog had been receiving glucocorticoids for paraparesis and was vomiting and had melena.

Diagnosis and Therapy

Definitive diagnosis of amebiasis in dogs and cats requires finding *E. histolytica* trophozoites in feces or tissues (see Table 78-1). Trophozoites are difficult to detect in fecal specimens. Direct smears of fresh feces reveal the sluggish, ameboid motility of the trophozoites. In invasive amebiasis, trophozoites may contain erythrocytes. Macrophages in feces may be confused with trophozoites. Methylene blue staining of a wet mount may be helpful in revealing amebas. Trichrome- or iron-hematoxylin–stained fecal smears are ideal for diagnosis, but these techniques are best left to a reference laboratory (see Appendix 5). Fecal concentration methods (e.g., flotation, sedimentation) are unsuitable for *E. histolytica*

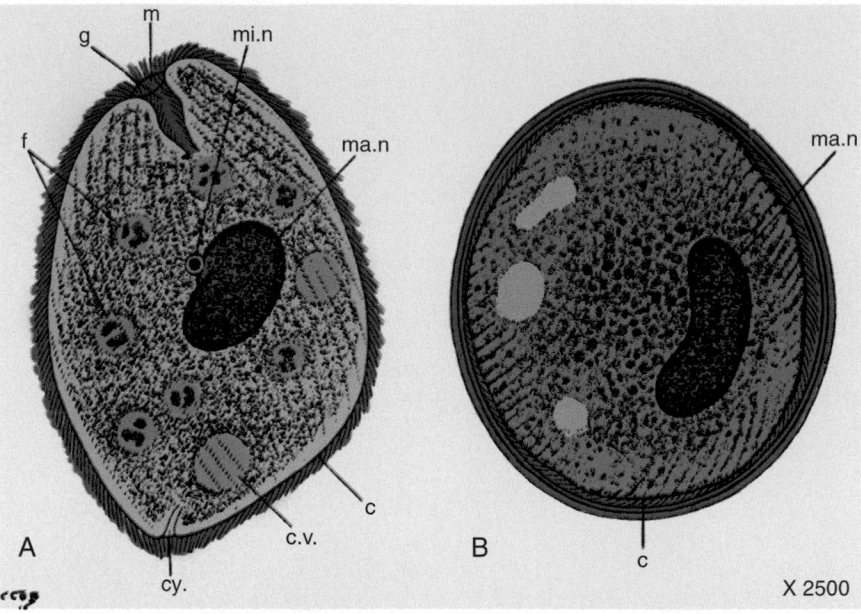

Fig 78-7 Schematic diagram of a *B. coli* trophozoite (**A**) and cyst (**B**). Key: *c*, cilia; *cv.*, contractile vacuole; *cy.*, cytopyge; *f*, food vacuole; *g*, gullet; *m*, mouth; *ma.n*, macronucleus; *mi.n*, micronucleus. (From Brown HW, Neva FA. 1983. Basic clinical parasitology, ed 5, Appleton-Century-Crofts, Norwalk, Conn., with permission.)

trophozoites. In clinically affected animals, a more reliable means of detecting the trophozoites is the microscopic examination of a sectioned biopsy specimen of colonic mucosa (see Fig. 78-6). An ELISA-based antigen test has been shown to be parasite specific in dogs,[98] but its clinical application has not been evaluated. For available test kits, see Appendix 6.

Colitis caused by *E. histolytica* rapidly responds to metronidazole at doses recommended for treatment of giardiasis (see Table 78-3), but dogs can continue to shed organisms.[5,70] Paromomycin has been used to treat people; however, precautions should be used because of potential nephrotoxicity (see Therapy under Trichomoniasis).

Diagnosis of free-living amebiasis is best achieved by tissue biopsy. Trophozoites, rather than cysts, are identified in tissue margins of the ulcer and in the serosal exudate. Immunostaining can be used to determine the species of ameba present.[114] For further information on Acanthamebiasis, see Chapter 79.

Public Health Considerations

Although amebiasis is a potentially serious human disease, dogs and cats are not likely significant reservoirs of these parasites for people. Dogs and cats more likely acquire their infections from human feces or from food or water contaminated by human feces. Although amebiasis is not a zoonosis, the finding of *E. histolytica* in a pet should prompt the veterinarian to suggest that the owners seek medical advice. The owners may have infected the pet or been exposed to a common source of *E. histolytica* cysts. With free-living amebiasis, people and animals are at risk for exposure to the same environmental sources. Immunocompetency is important in determining whether infection becomes established.

BALANTIDIASIS

Stephen C. Barr

Etiology and Epidemiology

Balantidium coli is a relatively large (see Table 78-1), ciliated protozoan (Figs. 78-7 and 78-8) found throughout the world. Although the pig is the most frequently infected animal, dogs

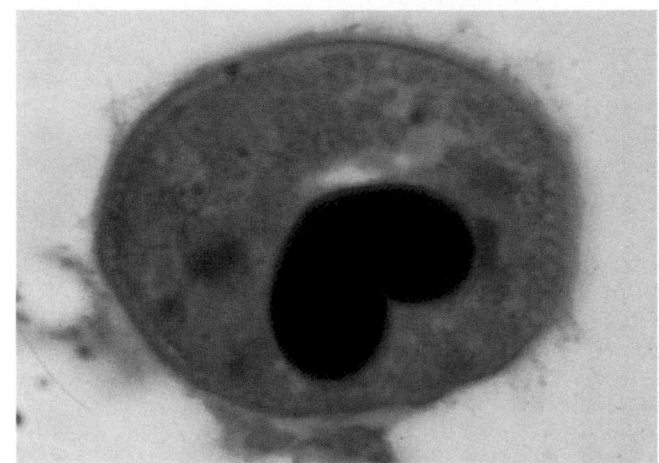

Fig 78-8 Large intestine of gorilla containing *Balantidium* sp. with large macronucleus and distinct cilia (×1500). (From Gardiner CH et al. 1988. An atlas of protozoan parasites in animal tissues, USDA Agricultural Handbook No. 651, Beltsville, Md.)

and people sometimes become infected with *B. coli*. Infection in the cat has not been reported. In a large survey of 56 mammalian species in Japan, nonhuman primates and artiodactyls were infected, and no rodents or carnivores, including dogs or cats, were infected.[94] Similar to *E. histolytica*, *B. coli* trophozoites inhabit the colon, either as commensals or invasive parasites, and cysts are passed in the feces. Cysts are infective when ingested by a susceptible host.

Pathogenesis and Pathologic Findings

The question as to why normally commensal *B. coli* trophozoites may become virulent in some instances remains unanswered. Certain colonic bacteria and concurrent whipworm (*Trichuris vulpis*) infections may contribute to *B. coli* invasiveness.

The gross and microscopic features of balantidiasis closely resemble those of amebiasis in the colon. Unlike amebiasis, extraintestinal metastasis of *B. coli* trophozoites is rare.

Routinely processed sections of affected colonic tissue will reveal the trophozoites with their characteristic cilia and bean-shaped macronucleus (Fig. 78-9).

Clinical Findings

Balantidiasis is clinically indistinguishable from some other causes of hemorrhagic colitis, including amebiasis and trichuriasis. A history of contact with swine may be present, although pigs are usually asymptomatic.

Diagnosis and Therapy

B. coli cysts and, occasionally, trophozoites may be detected on fecal flotation using the ZSCT. Fresh fecal smears in an isotonic solution are preferred to demonstrate the motile trophozoites. The distinctive macronucleus of both cyst and trophozoite (see Figs. 78-8 and 78-9) is invisible unless stained. A drop of acidic methyl green solution (1 g methyl green, 1 ml glacial acetic acid, 100 ml water) added to the preparation will reveal the macronucleus in most of the organisms after a few minutes of contact.

Reports of therapy of canine balantidiasis are few.[28] Tetracyclines and phenethylamines have been used. Based on human clinical studies, oral metronidazole should also prove effective in the dog. See Table 78-3 for dosages.

Public Health Considerations

Because *B. coli*–infected dogs may excrete cysts in feces, the potential for transmission from dog to people exists. Compared with swine, because dogs are rarely infected, they cannot be considered significant reservoirs of *B. coli* for people.

BLASTOCYSTOSIS

Craig E. Greene

Etiology and Epidemiology

Blastocystis hominis, a waterborne commensal, is now a protozoan that inhabits human and animal intestinal tracts. Its pathogenicity in causing gastrointestinal illness in people is controversial. *Blastocystis* organisms isolated from various animals are similar to *B. hominis*.[4,36] Genetic analysis has separated the isolated strains into seven groups.[1] Using this phylogenetic data, animal isolates have been given unique species

names, and others can be found in people, indicating zoonotic potential. The organisms found in dogs and cats were slightly smaller and had few vacuoles compared with *B. hominis* by light and by transmission electron microscopy.[36] In Brisbane, Australia, prevalence rates of organisms in the stools from domestic dogs and cats predominantly in animal shelters were over 0.8% and 67.3%, respectively. In the presumed life cycle, resistant fecal cysts are ingested and develop into vacuolar forms that replicate by binary fission.[125a] Some of these forms mature into cysts that are shed in the feces. Prevalence of infection is highest in areas of poor sanitation.

Clinical Findings

The organism has been found in a high percentage of clinically healthy animals; its pathogenic role in dogs or cats is uncertain.

Diagnosis

Blastocystis in canine feces ranged from 3 to 10 μm and irregular in shape. In unstained wet mounts, organisms had a thin outer rim of cytoplasm, containing barely discernable organelles, surrounded by a variably shaped central vacuole (Fig. 78-10, *A* and *B*).[36] In feline feces, the organisms were between 2 to 10 μm and had a similar vacuolar appearance. *Blastocystis* spp. have been cultured from canine feces in prereduced inspissated egg stunt medium covered with Forcke's solution.[36] Internal structures of the organism can be visualized by electron microscopy (Fig. 78-11, *A* and *B*). They possess a nucleus, mitochondria, Golgi complex, and endoplasmic reticulum. As is the case with light microscopy, a thin rim of cytoplasm surrounds a large central vacuole.

Therapy

Although the pathogenicity of *B. hominis* in people is controversial, people are often treated when it is the only apparent cause of diarrhea. Metronidazole for 10 days has been used to treat affected people.[97] Clinical improvement and a reduction in the number of organisms in the stool were observed. Relapses were observed after 6 months in some of the treated patients, presumably as a result of reinfection. Nitazoxanide has also been used to treat people with *Blastocystis* infection, as well as a significant number of other protozoal infections.[27,32]

Public Health Considerations

Though *Blastocystis* may be a commensal, it is associated with signs of diarrhea and cutaneous rashes in immunocompromised people. Although morphologic features suggest similarities among human and animal *Blastocystis* organisms, insufficient evidence exists to support or refute this possibility.

TRICHOMONIASIS

Jody L. Gookin

Etiology and Epidemiology

Trichomonads are spindle to pear-shaped, highly motile flagellates similar in size to *Giardia*. They exist only as trophozoites (no cyst stage), divide by binary fission, and are transmitted directly via the fecal-oral route. Trophozoites bear characteristic numbers of anteriorly directed flagella and a single, posteriorly directed flagellum that arises at the anterior end and courses along the body attached to the undulating membrane, a characteristic feature of trichomonads. A rigid, rod-shaped organelle, the axostyle, runs through the trophozoite and protrudes from the posterior end (Fig. 78-12).

Pentatrichomonas hominis has five anterior flagella, is considered to be nonpathogenic, and inhabits the large intestine

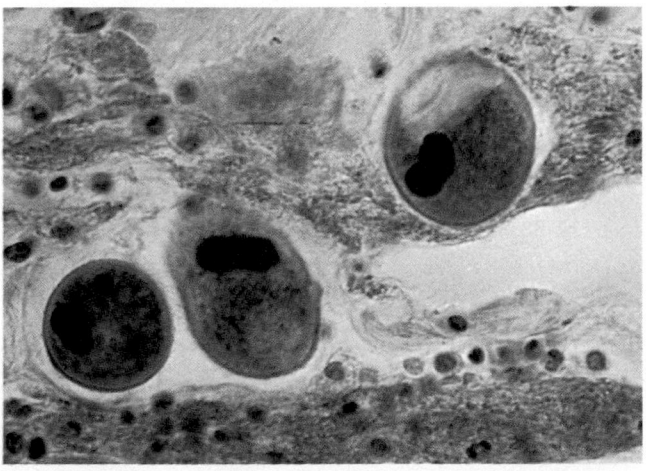

Fig 78-9 *B. coli* trophozoites in a section from the wall of a human colon. Note the prominent parasite macronuclei and the surrounding inflammatory response (H and E stain, ×250).

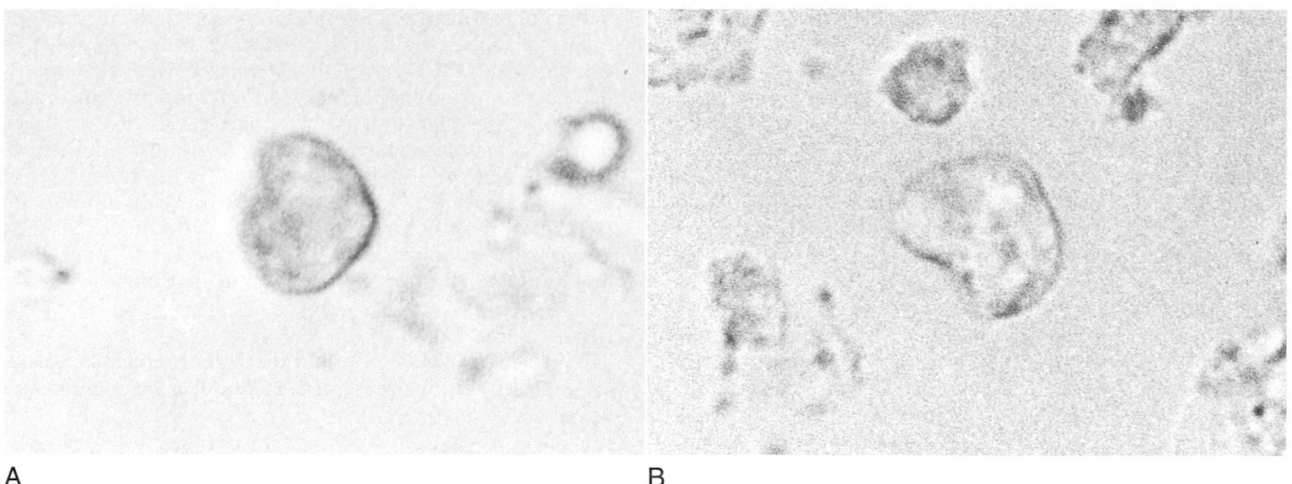

A   B

Fig   78-10 Light micrographs of *Blastocystis* sp. in canine **(A)** and feline **(B)** fecal material (unstained wet mounts, ×1000). (Courtesy Deborah Stenzel, Queensland University of Technology, Brisbane, Australia.)

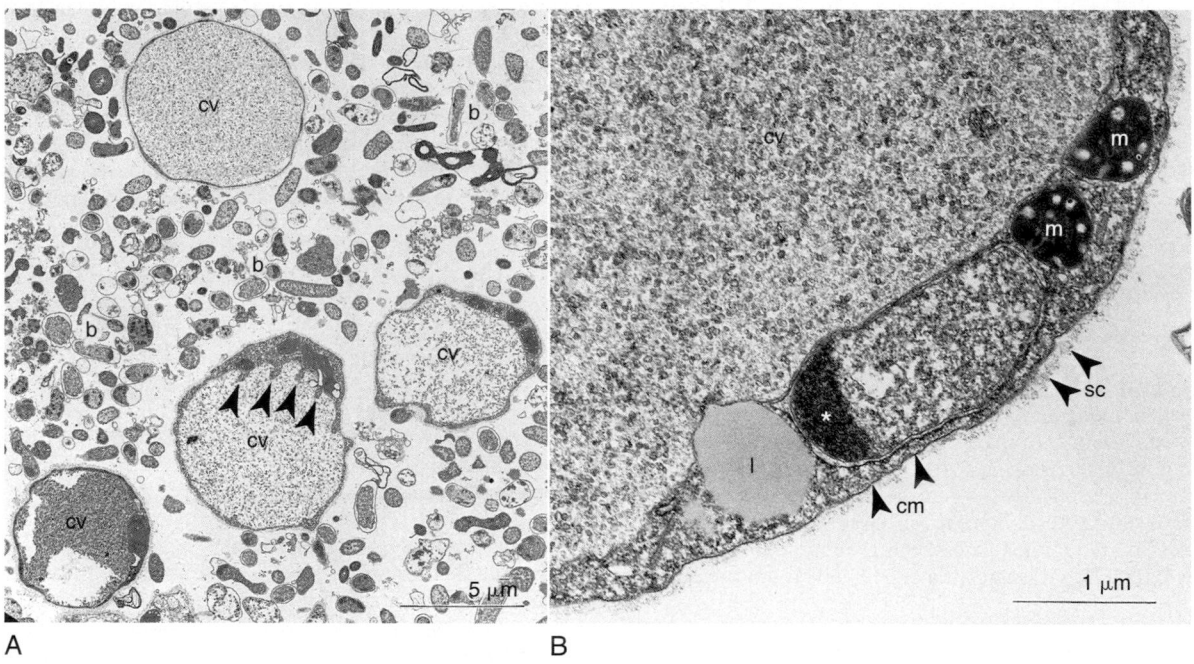

A   B

Fig   78-11 Transmission electron microscopy of *Blastocystis* sp. in culture from canine fecal material. **A,** Low magnification showing general cell morphology. Variability is noted in the central vacuolar *(cv)* contents. One cell shows projections of the cytoplasm *(as indicated by arrowheads)* into the central vacuole. Numerous bacteria *(b)* are present in the culture. **B,** High magnification showing details of the nuclear region. A crescentic band of electron opaque material *(indicated by asterisk)* is present in the nucleus. Mitochondria *(m)* and a lipid inclusion *(l)* are seen in the cytoplasm. A surface coat *(sc)* surrounds the cell. Small granules are present in the central vacuole *(cv)*. (Courtesy Deborah Stenzel, Queensland University of Technology, Brisbane, Australia.)

of a large number of mammalian hosts, including cats, dogs, and people. Natural and experimental infections with *P. hominis* in dogs and cats were described in the early 1900s; however, clinical signs were either absent or largely attributable to coexisting intestinal infection.[19] DNA of *P. hominis* was isolated from the feces of a litter of pups with diarrhea containing trichomonads and *Isospora canis* oocyst.[48a] Only one published report of feline diarrhea associated with intestinal trichomoniasis has been submitted over the 60-year period before 1996,[72] perhaps because *P. hominis* was presumed to be opportunistic. Since 1996, however, numerous reports of diarrhea associated with trichomoniasis in cats have been pub-

lished.* Detailed morphologic and genetic analyses of isolates obtained from affected cats have identified the trichomonads as *Tritrichomonas foetus*,[48,54,84] which had not been previously described in the cat.

T. foetus is recognized as an important venereal pathogen of naturally bred cattle in which the organism is transmitted from the prepuce of the bull to the vagina and uterus where infection leads to infertility and abortion.[18] The organism has also been described as an inhabitant of the porcine gastrointestinal and nasal mucosa where its pathogenicity is uncer-

*References: 49, 51, 54, 111, 112.

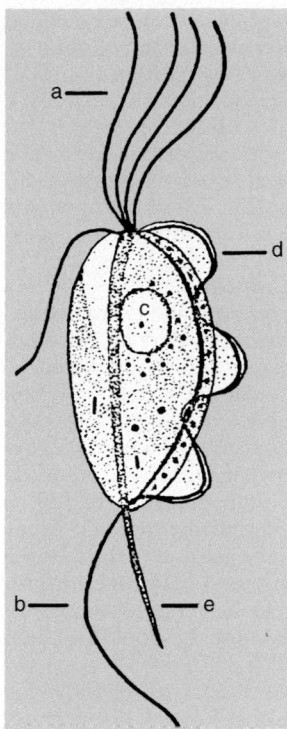

Fig 78-12 Drawing of *P. hominis* trophozoite indicating some of the characteristic organelles. Key: *a*, anterior flagella; *b*, posterior flagellum; *c*, nucleus; *d*, undulating membrane; *e*, axostyle. (Modified from Wenrich SH. 1947, The species of *Trichomanas* in man, *J Parasitol* 33:177–188, with permission.)

tain.[43,124] *T. foetus* and *T. suis* are considered to be strains of the same species based on morphology, ultrastructural analysis, random amplified polymorphic DNA analysis, enzyme homogeneity, and rRNA gene sequence identity.[125] Cross-transmission studies between cattle and swine with *T. foetus* or *T. suis* have revealed little host specificity.[43] The natural history of *T. foetus* in the feline host and any relationship to bovine or swine trichomoniasis needs further evaluation.

The prevalence of *T. foetus* infection was 31% among 117 cats from 89 cattery owners attending an international cat show.[54] Evidence of the organism was found in feces from 18 cat breeds from 17 states and Germany based on direct microscopic examination, protozoal culture, or PCR of feces. Catteries in which *T. foetus* was identified had larger numbers of cats with diarrhea and lower numbers of square feet of facility per cat, suggesting that crowding may be a significant risk factor for infection. Proximity of a cattery to agricultural species (pigs, cattle, horses), feeding of raw meat, type of water source, outdoor contact, or history of travel were not identified as significant risk factors for *T. foetus* infection. Co-infection by *T. foetus* and *Giardia* was common. *T. foetus* was not demonstrated by either direct microscopic examination or protozoal culture of feces from 100 feral cats or 20 healthy indoor cats from geographic regions comparable to those of naturally infected cats.[49] Thus *T. foetus* does not appear to be a component of the normal feline intestinal flora. DNA of *T. foetus* was identified in the diarrheic feces of pups having profuse watery diarrhea and co-existing *Giardia* infection.[48a]

Pathogenesis
Multiple organism, host, and environmental factors are likely involved in the pathogenesis of diarrhea in cats with *T. foetus* infection. Pathogenic factors associated with trichomonads include interaction with endogenous bacterial flora, adherence

to host epithelium, and elaboration of cytotoxins and enzymes.[41] Infection of specific-pathogen–free cats with axenically cultured *T. foetus* results in chronic colonization of the terminal ileum, cecum and colon, and large bowel diarrhea akin to that observed in naturally infected cats.[52] In naturally infected cats, *T. foetus* antigen can be demonstrated within the superficial mucus and in contact with the surface epithelium of the cecum and colon. Antigen uptake by surface epithelial cells is also evident. Whether long-term infection of cats with *T. foetus* is a predisposing factor for development of inflammatory bowel disease is unknown. The predominance of young cats from dense housing conditions may reflect an increased opportunity for exposure or enhanced susceptibility to infection because of environmental stress or immunologic immaturity.

Clinical Findings
The widely accepted view is that *P. hominis* does not cause disease in dogs and cats, although the possibility exits that it is an opportunistic pathogen. Though a large number of trophozoites have been described in diarrheic feces from dogs, an unambiguous, causal relationship remains to be established.

Cats with diarrhea and *T. foetus* infection are generally young but have ranged in age from 3 months to 13 years. In one study, approximately 75% of cats were younger than age 1 year at the time of diagnosis.[49] Infections are seen in both nonpurebred (sheltered) and purebred (cattery) cats.

Feline *T. foetus* infection is characterized by a waxing and waning large bowel diarrhea that occasionally contains fresh blood and mucus. Diarrhea is semiformed to cow-pie in consistency and malodorous. In very young cats and with poor housing conditions, the anus may appear edematous, erythematous, and painful; involuntary dribbling of feces or rectal prolapse may be seen. In general, cats otherwise maintain good health and body condition. A consistent feature of *T. foetus* diarrhea is improved fecal consistency and disappearance of trichomonads during administration of antimicrobial drugs with return of diarrhea containing trichomonads shortly after drugs are discontinued.[49] Misdiagnosis of *Giardia* is common in cats having *T. foetus* infection. Cats diagnosed with *Giardia* based on direct fecal smear examination and that fail to respond to appropriate antimicrobial therapy should be closely reevaluated for the possibility that the observed trophozoites were *T. foetus*.

Diagnosis
Direct Fecal Smear Examination
Diagnosis is made by observation of trophozoites in feces diluted with saline solution and examined under a coverslip using a light microscope equipped with a 20× or 40× objective (Fig. 78-13).[49] Lowering the microscope condenser to increase contrast may enhance visualization. Trichomonad trophozoites must be distinguished from those of *Giardia*. *Giardia* trophozoites have a concave ventral disk and motility reminiscent of a "falling leaf." In contrast, trichomonads are spindle shaped, possess a single nucleus with no concave disk, have an undulating membrane that courses the entire length of the body, and have a jerky, rolling forward motility (Fig. 78-14). *T. foetus* can be difficult to distinguish with any reliability from nonpathogenic intestinal trichomonads such as *P. hominis* based on light microscopic appearance because the two organisms differ in appearance only by the number of anterior flagella.

Freshly voided and diarrheic fecal samples should be examined. Detection of trophozoites can be improved by collecting samples using a fecal loop[52] and by examining multiple fecal smears. Trichomonads will not survive refrigeration and are not observed after fecal flotation or sedimentation. Sur-

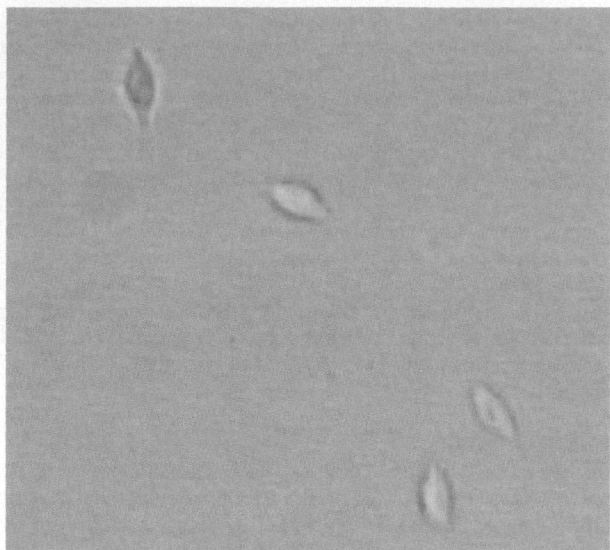

Fig 78-13 Light microscopic appearance of *T. foetus* in feces of a cat (unstained, ×200). (Courtesy Jody Gookin, Raleigh, N.C.)

vival of trophozoites in feces can be extended from 0 to 4 days by removal of adherent litter and dilution of the sample with normal saline to avoid desiccation (3 ml 0.9% saline per 2 g of feces).[44] Concurrent antibiotic therapy will diminish the number trophozoites present in feces, a fact that should be considered in cats with negative fecal smear results.[49] The sensitivity of direct fecal smear examination for diagnosis of trichomoniasis is low (2% in cats with experimentally induced infection and 14% in cats with spontaneous disease).[52,54]

Fecal Protozoal Culture

If repeated direct microscopic examination results are negative for trophozoites, feces may be cultured in-house using a commercially available system marketed for diagnosis of *T. foetus* infection in cattle (In Pouch™ TF, Biomed Diagnostics, San Jose, Calif.)[50] (Fig. 78-15). For diagnosis of feline *T. foetus*, pouches should be inoculated with 0.05 g (approximately the size of a peppercorn) of freshly voided or loop-collected feces and incubated at room temperature (25° C [77° F]) in an upright position. Before microscopic examination, pouches are tapped against a bench-top to dislodge adherent organisms and then placed within a manufacturer-provided clamp that allows the pouch to be mounted onto the stage of a light microscope. Pouch contents should be examined every other

Fig 78-14 Animated motility. **A,** *Giardia* has a ventral flattening and motility reminiscent of a "falling leaf." **B,** Trichomonads have a jerky axial rolling motion. (Courtesy University of Georgia, Athens, Ga.)

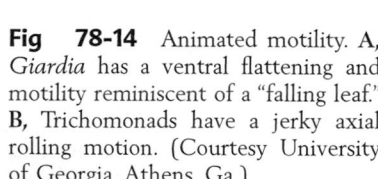

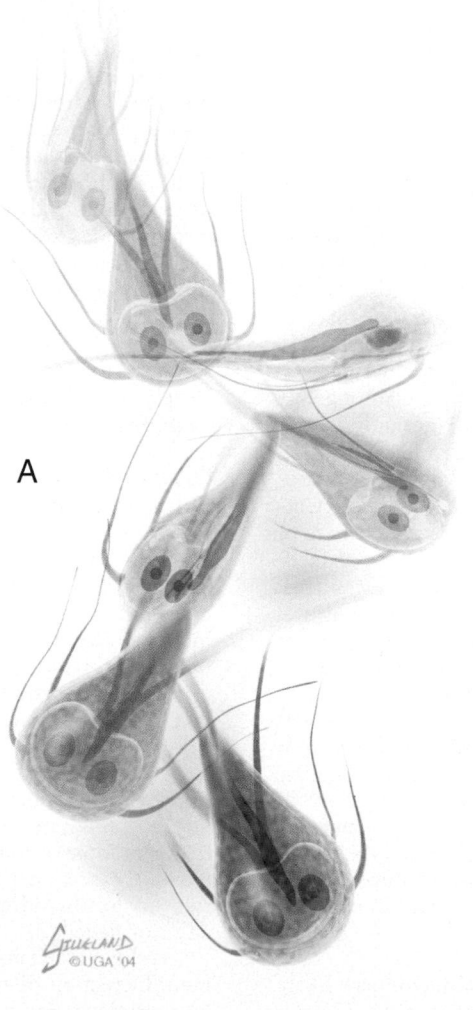

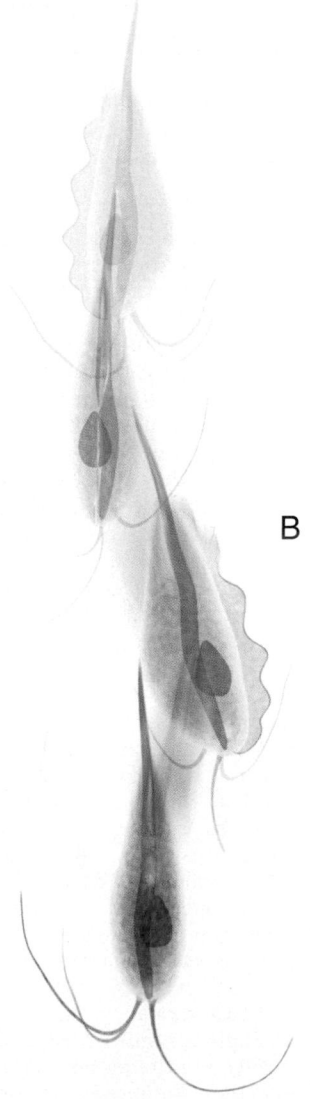

A

B

Giardia

Tritrichomonas

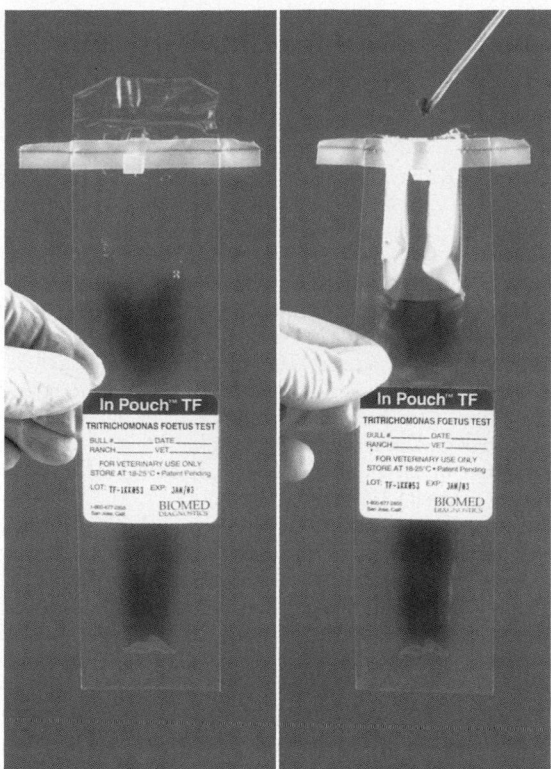

Fig 78-15 The In Pouch™ TF system consists of two chambers of culture medium connected by a channel. To inoculate the In Pouch™ TF, the upper chamber is opened by tearing off a plastic strip along the top of the pouch. Approximately 0.05 g of feces is inoculated into the upper chamber and mixed with the culture contents. The top edge is then rolled down to seal the opening and forces the contents into the lower chamber for cultivation (Courtesy Jody Gookin, Raleigh, N.C.)

day for motile trophozoites using a light microscope with 20 × or 40 × objective and discarded if still negative after 12 days. Fecal culture using In Pouch™ TF has a detection limit of greater than 1000 *T. foetus* organisms per 0.05 g feces and is superior to direct fecal smear examination for diagnosis of *T. foetus* infection.[50,54] Neither *Giardia* nor *P. hominis* organisms can survive in In Pouch™ TF for longer than 24 hours; thus positive cultures results are strongly suggestive of *T. foetus* infection.[50] Strictly speaking, however, the types of trichomonads potentially hosted by cats and the specificity of In Pouch™ TF with regard to these other types of trichomonads is unknown. Positive In Pouch™ TF culture results do not preclude the possibility of co-infection with *P. hominis* or *Giardia*.

Fecal samples can also be cultured in antibiotic-fortified, modified Diamond's medium.[48] Such cultivation requires shipment of feces to a research laboratory, preparation and maintenance of sterile medium, and 37° C (99° F) incubation. Minimal evidence exists to suggest that modified Diamond's medium culture provides any greater diagnostic sensitivity than does in-house fecal culture using In Pouch™ TF.

Polymerase Chain Reaction
A sensitive and specific single-tube nested PCR based on amplification of a conserved portion of the *T. foetus* internal transcribed spacer region (ITS1 and ITS2) and 5.8S rRNA gene from feline feces has been described.[48] The PCR test is superior to fecal culture for diagnosis of naturally infected

cats[54] and is commercially available. Refer to Appendix 6 for more information on this test.

Exclusion of Coexisting Disease
Coexisting systemic or enteric disease should be excluded in cats with trichomonas infection. Studies of experimental feline infection suggest that coexisting intestinal infection (e.g., cryptosporidiosis) worsens clinical signs of diarrhea and increases the shedding of *T. foetus* organisms.[52] Further diagnostic evaluation of infected cats may include complete blood count; serum biochemical analysis; urinalysis; tests for feline leukemia virus (FeLV), feline immunodeficiency virus (FIV), and feline enteric coronavirus; fecal flotation; *Giardia*-specific antigen testing; fecal direct FA for *Cryptosporidium*; fecal gram stain for clostridia; and colonic mucosal biopsies. Commercial ELISA kits to detect fecal *Giardia*-specific antigen do not cross-react with *T. foetus*.

Pathologic Findings
Hematologic and serum biochemical analysis results from cats with *T. foetus* infection are invariably normal. Coexisting enteric infection by recognized feline pathogens (e.g. *Giardia*, *Cryptosporidium*, internal parasites) is not a consistent feature. Infected cats usually test negative for FeLV antigen and FIV antibody.[49] Histopathologic changes in colonic mucosal biopsies from infected cats have been consistent with mild to severe lymphoplasmacytic colitis. Because trichomonads are noninvasive and extremely fragile, they are unreliably preserved in intestinal biopsy specimens (Fig. 78-16), although immunohistochemistry may be used to enhance their detection.[52]

Therapy
P. hominis is reportedly exquisitely responsive to treatment with metronidazole at the dosages that are effective for *Giardia*. An effective antimicrobial treatment for feline *T. foetus* infection has not been identified. Attempts to identify an effective treatment for economically important bovine trichomoniasis have failed; therefore specific therapy for feline infection in the near future seems unlikely.

Cats infected with *T. foetus* have failed treatment with recommended (and in many cases higher) dosages of numerous antimicrobial drugs, including metronidazole, fenbendazole, albendazole, sulfadimethoxine, trimethoprim-sulfadiazine, furazolidone, tylosin, enrofloxacin, amoxicillin, clindamycin, paromomycin, and erythromycin.[49] Furthermore, in vitro studies of feline *T. foetus* in culture have revealed multiple drug resistance (e.g., to paromomycin, furazolidone, metronidazole, anisomycin, azithromycin, ciprofloxacin, chloroquine, doxycycline, tinidazole, and clotrimazole).[82] Although nitazoxanide inhibited growth of *T. foetus* in culture, rapid resistance to the drug was acquired in vivo.[52] In contrast to prior reports, paromomycin is not an effective treatment for *T. foetus* infection and has precipitated acute renal failure in infected cats.[53]

Despite antibiotic failure to eradicate the infection, some cats have improved fecal consistency while receiving antimicrobial drugs.[49] This improvement may be related to a dependence of trichomonads on endogenous bacterial flora and host secretions for acquisition of essential nutrients. Prolonged use of antibacterial drugs has not been uniformly useful for long-term control of diarrhea and may delay the onset of clinical remission. Ronidazole, a nitroimidazole, was effective in curing infected cats with monitoring of up to 13 weeks post-treatment.[49a]

In a study of long-term outcome in 26 cats with diarrhea and *T. foetus* infection, clinical signs resolved a median of 9 months after the onset of diarrhea (range, 4 months to 2 years).[44] Relapses of diarrhea were common and associated with dietary change, medical treatments unassociated with *T. foetus* infection, and travel. Based on fecal PCR, *T. foetus*

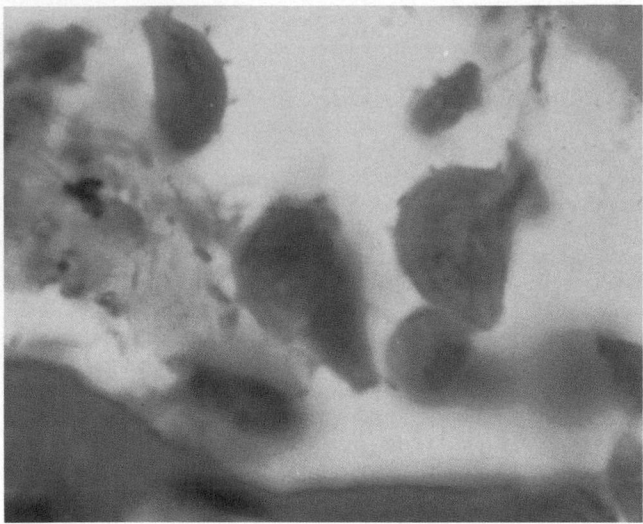

Fig   78-16 Lumen of small intestine of hamster containing trophozoites of *Pentatrichomonas* sp. With large nucleus and undulating flagellum (H and E stain, ×1500). (From Gardiner CH et al. 1988. An atlas of protozoan parasites in animal tissues, USDA Agricultural Handbook No. 651, Beltsville, Md.)

was undetectable in more than 50% of cats when tested 2 to 5 years after diagnosis. Thus cats with *T. foetus* may have a good long-term prognosis for spontaneous resolution of disease.[44]

Public Health Considerations

In light of the poor host specificity of *T. foetus* and the intimate association between infected cats and their human companions, the potential for zoonotic transmission should be considered. Only a single case of human infection with *T. foetus* appears in the literature. The infected individual had

epididymitis and meningoencephalitis following immunosuppression and peripheral blood stem cell transplantation.[101]

SUGGESTED READINGS*

2. Abe N, Kimata I, Iseki M. 2002. Identification of genotypes of *Cryptosporidium parvum* isolates from a patient and dog in Japan, *J Vet Med Sci* 64:165-168.
17. Berrilli F, DiCave D, Liberato CD, et al. 2004. Genotype characterization of *Giardia duodenalis* isolates from domestic and farm animals by *SSU-rRNA* gene sequencing, *Vet Parasitol* 122:193-199.
27. Cimerman S, Ladeira MC, Juliano WA, et al. 2003. Blastocytosis: nitazoxanide, as a new therapeutic agent, *Rev Soc Bras Med Trop* 36:415-417.
30. Decock C, Cadiergues MC, Larcher M, et al. 2003. Comparison of two techniques for diagnosis of giardiasis in dogs, *Parasite* 10:69-72.
55. Gookin JL, Stebbins ME, Hunt E, et al. 2004. Prevalence of and risk factors for feline *Tritrichomonas foetus* and *Giardia* infection, *J Clin Microbiol* 42:2707-2710.
84. Levy MG, Gookin JL, Poore MF, et al. 2003. *Tritrichomonas foetus* and not *Pentatrichomonas hominis* is the etiologic agent of feline trichomonal diarrhea, *J Parasitol* 89:99-104.
117. Scorza AV, Lappin MR. 2004. Metronidazole for the treatment of feline giardiasis, *J Feline Med Surg* 6:157-160.
122. Stein JE, Radecki SV, Lappin MR. 2003. Efficacy of *Giardia* vaccination in the treatment of giardiasis in cats, *J Am Vet Med* Assoc 222:1548-1551.
142. Zaki M, Reddy SG, Jackson TFHG, et al. 2003. Genotyping of *Entamoeba* species in South Africa: diversity, stability, and transmission patterns within families, *J Infect Dis* 187:1860-1869.

*See the CD-ROM for a complete list of references.

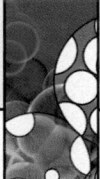

CHAPTER • 79

Nonenteric Amebiasis: Acanthamebiasis, Hartmannelliasis, and Balamuthiasis

Craig E. Greene and Elizabeth W. Howerth

ETIOLOGY

Acanthamoeba is a genus of ubiquitous free-living amoebas found in fresh and salt water, soil, dust, and sewage.[1,14,18] The classification of the genus *Acanthamoeba* and separation from the closely-related genus *Hartmannella* has had a confusing history that is becoming resolved only with the use of molecular techniques.[31,37] *Hartmannella* and *Acanthamoeba* are classified as distinct genera based on morphologic differences in the trophozoite shape and cyst wall structure, nutritional requirements, and serologic responses by infected hosts. *Acanthamoeba* has been further divided into three morphologic groups (I, II, and III) based on trophozoite and cyst size and

structure. Although this morphologic classification is used, genetic comparisons have suggested the need for additional taxonomic reevaluation.[31] *Balamuthia mandrillaris* is another free-living amoeba that can cause fatal granulomatous amebic encephalitis.

Acanthamoeba has a relatively simple life cycle with two stages, one as a dormant free-living cyst in the environment and the other as a vegetative feeding form in host tissues. The vegetative replicating trophozoite has two distinct phagotrophic niches: (1) feeding on bacteria in aquatic habitats and (2) acting as opportunists of host cells in the body. The cyst phase is often able to resist adverse environmental conditions, including desiccation[14] and possibly host immune responses. The cyst can also survive exposure to temperatures between −20° C and +42° C and a pH of 3.9 to 9.75.[1]

In the environment, *Acanthamoeba* species are omnipresent and abundant. They have been isolated from all water sources. In the atmosphere, they are carried on pollutants, and their concentrations have been used as potential monitors of air quality.

Several *Acanthamoeba* species are pathogenic for animals and people. They can subclinically colonize superficial epithelial surfaces but can also produce ocular surface infections and may disseminate in immunocompromised individuals. Disseminated infections usually involve the central nervous system (CNS). *Acanthamoeba castellanii*, *Acanthamoeba culbertsoni*, and *Acanthamoeba* sp. genotype T1 have been causes of canine infections.[3,26]

In addition to *Acanthamoeba* species, *Hartmannella vermiformis*, another free-living but potentially pathogenic amoeba, can be isolated from the ocular surfaces of people. As with *Acanthamoeba* species, *Hartmannella* have been found in corneal biopsies of people with keratitis. Clinically healthy cats have been shown to harbor *Hartmannella* on their ocular surfaces; however, compared with clinically healthy cats, those with ocular disease were more likely to harbor amoebic DNA of *Hartmannella* and its endosymbiont rickettsiae *Neochlamydia hartmannellae*.[35,36] The significance of *Hartmannella* infection as a cause of ocular surface infections in cats or dogs needs additional study. Finding a greater prevalence of *N. hartmannellae* and its amoebic host in cats with ocular disease suggests a causal association (see Chlamydial Infections, Chapter 30).

Several other forms of amoebic meningoencephalitis exist, which can be a source of confusion. Two related amoebae, *Naegleria fowleri* and *Balamuthia mandrillaris* (previously, *Leptomyxida amoebae*), also cause meningoencephalitis in people and nonhuman primates; *B. mandrillaris* caused disseminated infection with granulomatous nephritis and meningoencephalitis in a dog.[14] Systemic infections with *Acanthamoeba* species develop in immunocompromised people; however, those caused by *Naegleria* and *Balamuthia* species can affect immunocompetent people. Infection with *Naegleria* and *Balamuthia* organisms is acquired through swimming in contaminated waters, with the infection spreading through the olfactory neuroepithelium to the CNS. *Acanthamoeba* and *Hartmannella* species have spikelike (acanth) projections, which help differentiate them from the genus *Naegleria*, *Balamuthia*, or other amoebae.

EPIDEMIOLOGY

Acanthamoeba organisms cause pneumonia and encephalitis in people[14,18,34] and animals[2,11,14,15,26] and disseminated dermatitis and chronic keratitis in people.[20,22] Although rare, rhinosinusitis, osteomyelitis, and disseminated infection have been developed in human infections.

Primarily solitary cases of acanthamebiasis in dogs have been reported, although in greyhound kennels, multiple dogs have been infected.[14,15] Acanthamebiasis has not been described in cats.

In dogs, epizootics of acanthamebiasis have been observed in greyhounds,[14,15] whereas single cases were described in a German shepherd dog[2] and an immunosuppressed Akita.[26] Young dogs appear to be most susceptible. Affected greyhounds ranged from 4 to 13 months of age. During outbreaks, organisms are thought to be acquired from a common environmental source rather than from other animals. The source of infection and the incubation period in dogs are unknown.

Immunosuppressed persons, such as those who have had organ transplants, have the acquired immunodeficiency syndrome, abuse alcohol, have diabetes, or have other debilitating conditions, are at high risk for infection and particularly susceptible to acanthamebiasis.[18,38] In people who are critically ill or debilitated, *Acanthamoeba* species typically cause a chronic granulomatous meningoencephalitis that may last for weeks or months before causing death.[18] Disseminated *B. mandrillaris* infection developed in a dog given immunosuppressive doses of glucocorticoids.[14] Amebic keratitis has been seen in otherwise healthy people who wear contact lenses or have minor corneal trauma.[20,22] Using tap water to make saline solutions for contact lenses has been suggested as a source of infection.[16]

PATHOGENESIS

The pathogenesis in dogs is unknown; however, in people, routes of infection may include inhaling organisms from water while swimming or from contaminated air. The organisms can replicate in the upper or lower respiratory tract after inhalation or in skin or other tissues after penetrating injuries. They then spread to the CNS by hematogenous means. Alternatively, infection of the cornea and nasal passage might lead to a retrograde spread to the nervous system via optic and olfactory nerves, respectively.

CLINICAL FINDINGS

Clinical manifestations of canine acanthamebiasis and canine distemper are remarkably similar.[15,26] Initial signs include mild oculonasal discharge, anorexia, and lethargy. Rectal temperature varies from normal to as high as 40.5° C (105° F). Respiratory distress and neurologic signs then develop. Most dogs eventually develop neurologic dysfunction. Neurologic signs include incoordination, head tilt, stumbling, dysmetria, and seizures. Coughing and dyspnea may be observed after a few days. Severely affected dogs are tetraplegic and in lateral recumbency without the ability to right themselves. Less severely affected greyhounds have permanent disabilities that preclude performance racing. In one dog, progressive neurologic disease was caused by the meningoencephalitis; however, the brain damage also induced a syndrome of inappropriate antidiuretic hormone secretion (SIADH).[7] SIADH was associated with impaired water excretion and normal sodium excretion leading to peripheral edema, serum hypoosmolality, and an inappropriately high serum sodium concentration.

The dog with disseminated balamuthiasis developed lethargy and hematuria followed by neurologic dysfunction, including intermittent seizures, rotary nystagmus, recumbency and coma.[14]

Cats with *Hartmannella* species infection may be more likely to have clinical manifestations of keratitis or conjunctivitis such as photophobia, lacrimation, conjunctival hyperemia, and ocular discharge. However, a direct causal association between this amoeba and ocular surface inflammation has not been proven.

DIAGNOSIS

The clinical laboratory abnormalities in animals with systemic acanthamebiasis are nonspecific. Leukopenia in greyhounds is a result of marked lymphopenia[15] and in other breeds is caused by a reduction in all types of blood leukocytes.[2,26] The cause of the leukopenia is unknown but may be concurrent infectious disease, stress, or specific factors produced by the *Acanthamoeba* organisms. No laboratory findings are available for the dog that developed *B. mandrillaris* infection.

Identification of amoebae in animals with keratitis is best accomplished using corneal scrapings or biopsy. Swabs are not suitable. The specimen should be inoculated as soon as possible onto specialized media (Page's agar). Specimens can be transported to the laboratory in a sterile vial containing a few drops of sterile saline. The organisms can be visualized in the specimen by microscopy, although trophozoites do not always stain predictably.

Premortem diagnosis of *Acanthamoeba* encephalitis in dogs or people has been rare. Culture or biopsy of affected tissues would be the most specific means of confirmation. Although lung and CNS tissues are not readily accessible, the possibility of finding organisms in cerebrospinal fluid (CSF) and tracheal washings has not been evaluated.

Amoebas can be cultured from lesions by special methods that are not done in most laboratories[34] because biocontainment facilities are needed.[4] Organisms grow sparingly on potato dextrose agar, where amoebas grow as individual colonies with many cysts, or on non-nutrient agar seeded with bacteria, where they grow more rapidly as a confluent expanding ringlike mass of trophozoites with cysts at the central portion. Organisms can also be isolated in cell culture, where they cause cytopathic effects. Mouse inoculation can be used to test the pathogenicity of isolated strains. Polymerase chain reaction analysis of corneal epithelial and tear samples has been used in the diagnosis of *Acanthamoeba* keratitis.[17] Similar genetic evaluation of CSF or blood samples for diagnosis of systemic infections has not been done in human or animal infections.

PATHOLOGIC FINDINGS

In dogs with acanthamebiasis, lung and brain lesions have been observed grossly in all cases. Lung lesions vary from light-tan to deep-red, raised, semisolid nodules distributed uniformly throughout all lobes.[2,3,26] The nodules have a tendency to coalesce, and intralesional cavitations have been noted. Brain lesions may be large, multifocal, and visible on the meningeal surfaces of the cerebrum and cerebellum and vary from red to tannish brown as a result of recent hemorrhage or necrosis.

Microscopically, multifocal necrotizing and often hemorrhagic meningoencephalitis and pneumonia with purulent, pyogranulomatous or granulomatous inflammation are seen. Trophozoites and occasional cyst forms of *Acanthamoeba* are seen within alveolar spaces and terminal bronchioles (Figs. 79-1 and 79-2). In brain lesions the amoebas are best visualized in perivascular and subarachnoid spaces, because in the neural parenchyma they are often masked by the presence of infiltrating inflammatory cells. Similar necrotizing and purulent to granulomatous foci containing amoeba may be seen in other tissues, including kidney, heart, liver, adrenal, and pancreas.[2,3,26]

Histologic and direct fluorescent antibody (FA) methods are used to demonstrate and identify the organism in tissues.[34] Free-living pathogenic amoebas are difficult to differentiate microscopically from certain mammalian cells, especially macrophages.[10] The diagnostic feature of *Acanthamoeba* in histologic sections is the centrally located nucleolus[14,34] (*targetoid karyosome*) and vacuolated cytoplasm. Periodic acid–Schiff and Gomori's methenamine silver methods stain only the cyst wall. Trophozoites are 15 to 45 μm in diameter, and cysts are 15 to 20 μm. Direct FA staining is specific and reliable on deparaffinized sections of formalin-fixed tissue and with specific conjugates can be used to distinguish among the various species of *Acanthamoeba*.

In the dog with *B. mandrillaris* infection, grossly visible granulomas were found in the kidneys and brain (Figs. 79-3

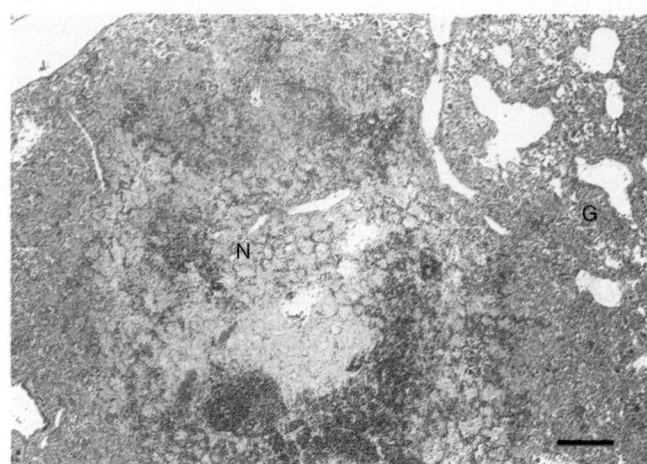

Fig 79-1 Lung from greyhound with acanthamebic pneumonia characterized by necrosis and hemorrhage *(N)* surrounded by pyogranulomatous inflammation (*G;* H and E stain, bar = 0.3 mm).

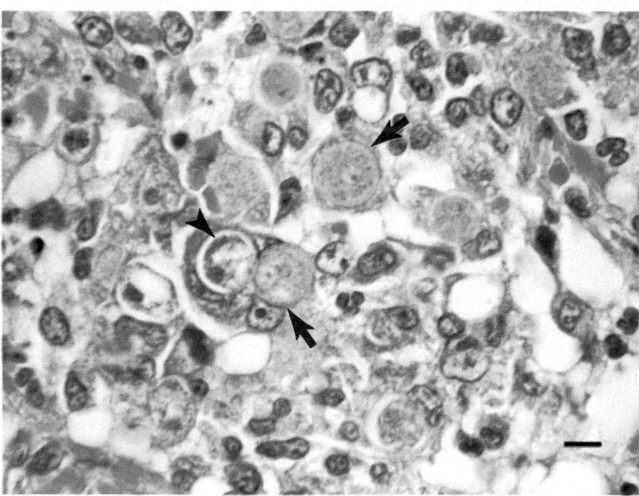

Fig 79-2 Lung from greyhound with acanthamebic pneumonia. *Acanthamoeba* trophozoites *(arrows)* and developing cysts (*arrowhead* shows mature cyst) are present in pyogranulomatous inflammation in an alveolus (H and E stain, bar = 30 μm).

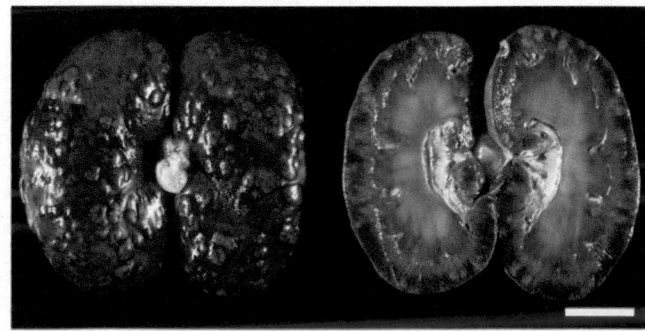

Fig 79-3 Kidney from dog with numerous granulomatous lesions throughout cortex as result of disseminated *B. mandrillaris* infection (bar = 2 cm). (From Foreman O, Sykes J, Ball L, et al. 2004. Disseminated infection with *Balamuthia mandrillaris* in a dog, *Vet Pathol* 41:506-510.)

and 79-4). In the kidneys, marked interstitial edema and necrosis with perivascular granulomatous inflammation was found (Fig. 79-5). Cyst and troph forms of amoebae were admixed with these infiltrates. Trophs were 15 to 45 µm in diameter and round to oval, with short cytoplasmic pseudopodia (Fig. 79-6). The cysts were 15 to 20 µm in diameter and surrounded by a double wall (Fig. 79-7).

THERAPY

Information on treating topical and systemic amoebic infections in animals is lacking. No therapeutic regimen for systemic acanthamebiasis in people has been well established, and drug susceptibility has been inconsistent. Drugs active against *Acanthamoeba* in vitro include polyene antifungals (amphotericin B), imidazoles (ketoconazole [KTZ]), and the antitubercular drug rifampicin, among others.[12] Rifampicin was effective in treating mice with meningitis.[12] In one immunocompromised person with disseminated skin lesions from *Acanthamoeba rhysodes* infection, successful treatment involved topical chlorhexidine gluconate and KTZ cream and systemic treatment with pentamidine followed by itracona-

zole (ITZ).[30] Treatment was likely successful in this case because it was instituted before spread to the CNS. Combination therapy with intravenous pentamidine, oral fluconazole, flucytosine (FCY), and sulfadiazine is recommended in people with disseminated and CNS infections.[21] Sulfadiazine has been beneficial in treating experimental infection in mice,[10] and trimethoprim-sulfonamide cured a child with meningoencephalitis after 8 weeks of therapy.[28] When used in combination with ITZ, 5-FCY transiently halted progression of disseminated *Acanthamoeba* infection in a person infected with human immunodeficiency virus.[9] A dog diagnosed with *Acanthamoeba* infection should be treated with one or more of these drugs. As a first choice, and because of its CNS penetration, trimethoprim-sulfonamide could be instituted at a dosage of 30 mg/kg given every 12 hours. (See Drug Formulary, Appendix 8, for additional information and dosages on the relevant drugs.)

For ocular surface or dermal infections in people, topical treatment with propamidine isethionate has been used; however, acquired drug resistance has developed. Chlorhexidine is the most available amebicidal compound for topical therapy and can be combined with propamidine. A standard treatment schedule has been 0.02% weight per volume (w/v) chlorhexidine digluconate in sterile isotonic saline and 0.1% w/v propamidine isethionate. The solution is applied at a decreasing frequency for a total of 6 months.[27] Concurrent topical antiinflammatory therapy may be needed for a brief

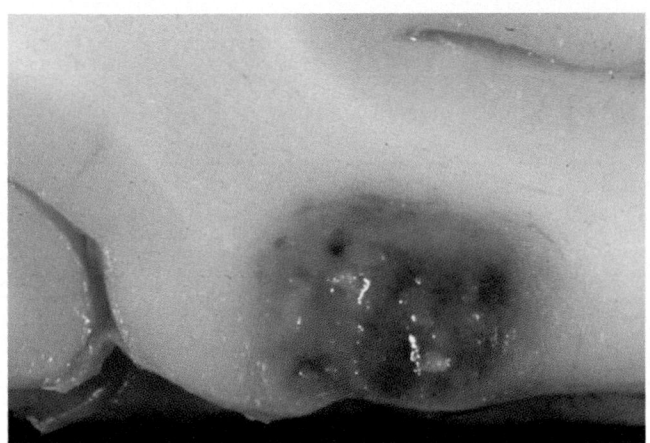

Fig 79-4 Focal necrotizing lesion in right occipital lobe of cerebral cortex of dog with *B. mandrillaris* infection. (From Foreman O, Sykes J, Ball L, et al. 2004. Disseminated infection with *Balamuthia mandrillaris* in a dog, *Vet Pathol* 41: 506-510.)

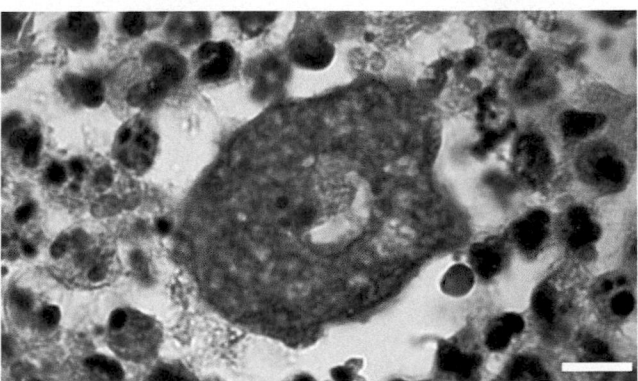

Fig 79-6 Trophozoite of *B. mandrillaris* in canine brain showing vacuolated cytoplasm (bar = 10 µm). (Courtesy Oded Foreman, Davis, Calif.)

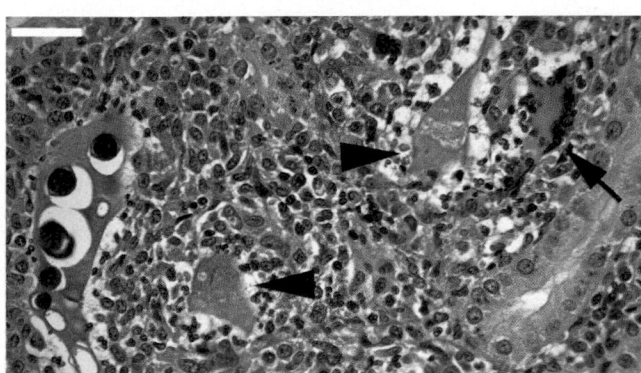

Fig 79-5 Kidney from dog with *B. mandrillaris* infection. Small cluster of organism cysts on right and trophozoite stages (*arrowheads*) are accompanied by mononuclear infiltration and multinucleated giant cell (*arrow*; H and E stain, bar = 33 µm). (From Foreman O, Sykes J, Ball L, et al. 2004. Disseminated infection with *Balamuthia mandrillaris* in a dog, *Vet Pathol* 41:506-510.)

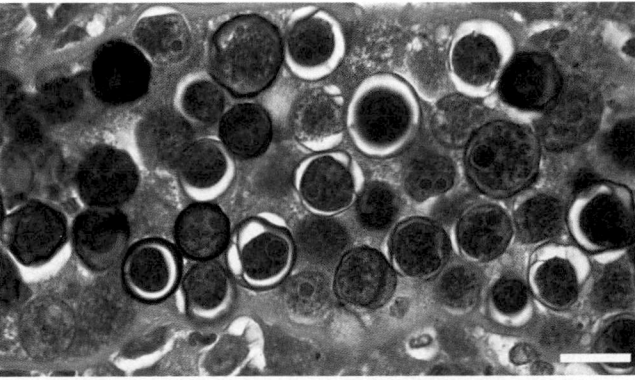

Fig 79-7 Dog kidney containing cystic stages of *B. mandrillaris* infection. Note outer undulating membrane and prominent karyosomes (Giemsa stain, bar = 15 µm). (From Foreman O, Sykes J, Ball L, et al. 2004. Disseminated infection with *Balamuthia mandrillaris* in a dog, *Vet Pathol* 41:506-510.)

period to control the surface inflammation caused by dying amoebae. Topical treatment with polyhexamethylene biguanide (a swimming pool amebicidal disinfectant) has also been effective, especially combined with propamidine, in treating human amoebal keratitis.[19,32]

PREVENTION

Dogs may be exposed to low numbers of *Acanthamoeba* organisms throughout their lifetimes. Because they are free-living amoebae, infection prevention involves avoiding access to contaminated water. Pathogenic, free-living amoebas are found more frequently in thermally enriched and polluted discharge water from industrial plants, lakes, and swimming pools.[18] Nonthermally enriched water contains fewer amoebas. A 0.5% solution of sodium hypochlorite is a satisfactory aqueous disinfectant. Because *Acanthamoeba* species feed on bacteria, water sources can be screened for amoebae initially by testing for coliforms.

PUBLIC HEALTH CONSIDERATIONS

No transmission of infection between hosts is known, and infections are thought to originate solely from environmental sources.[33] However, the dog is sentinel for human infection because of common environmental exposure.

SUGGESTED READINGS*

7. Brofman PJ, Knostman KAB, DiBartola SP. 2003. Granulomatous amebic meningoencephalitis causing the syndrome of inappropriate secretion of antidiuretic hormone in a dog. *J Vet Intern Med* 17:230-234.

12a. Dubey JP, Benson JE, Blakeley KT, et al. 2005. Disseminated *Acanthamoeba* sp. infection in a dog. *Vet Parasitol* 128:183-187.

13. Foreman O, Sykes J, Ball L, et al. 2004. Disseminated infection with *Balamuthia mandrillaris* in a dog. *Vet Pathol* 41:506-510

30. Slater CA, Sickel JZ, Visvesvara GS, et al. 1994. Brief report: successful treatment of disseminated *Acanthamoeba* infection in an immunocompromised patient. *N Engl J Med* 331:85-87.

36. Von Bomhard W, Pospischil A, Richter M, et al. 2002. Amoebic infections in cats with ocular disease. *Vet Rec* 146:556.

*See the CD-ROM for a complete list of references.

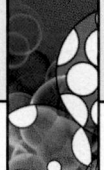

CHAPTER • 80

Toxoplasmosis and Neosporosis

J. P. Dubey and Michael R. Lappin

TOXOPLASMOSIS

Etiology

Toxoplasma gondii is an obligate intracellular coccidian parasite that infects virtually all species of warm-blooded animals, including people.[93,319] Domestic cats and other Felidae are the definitive hosts that excrete oocysts. All nonfeline hosts are intermediate hosts that harbor tissue cysts. Three infectious stages have been noted: sporozoites in oocysts, tachyzoites (actively multiplying stage), and bradyzoites (slowly multiplying stage) enclosed in tissue cysts. Oocysts are excreted in feces, whereas tachyzoites and bradyzoites are found in tissues. Most isolates of *T. gondii* can be grouped into three genetic lineages that can be used in epidemiologic monitoring. The three predominant genotypes likely resulted from a single cross between two parenteral strains approximately 10,000 years ago.[119a,319]

Epidemiology

The three major modes of transmission are congenital infection, ingestion of infected tissues, and ingestion of oocyst-contaminated food or water (Fig. 80-1). Other minor modes of transmission include lactational,[278] transfusion of body fluids, or transplantation of tissues or organs.[26,93]

Toxoplasmosis and seroreactivity to *T. gondii* are more prevalent in older animals as a factor of increasing exposure with aging and in animals from a rural or feral environment that are more apt to hunt small mammals.[251] A higher frequency of disease and exposure is found in dogs or cats that are fed raw meat instead of commercial diets.[130,131,245a] Seroprevalence is highest in older cats, and in those that are kept outdoors, are homeless, or found in shelters.[69,140,235,294a,339a] Outdoor cats in the Bangkok metropolitan area had a relatively low infection rate, presumably because they were predominantly fed well-cooked fish and rice.[321] Exotic cats in zoologic gardens have a high prevalence of infection, presumably from eating raw meat diets.[229,307,307a] *T. gondii* has also been identified as a cause of morbidity and mortality in marine mammals.[127] Presumably, these animals become infected from contaminated runoff water that enters the ocean.[91a,244b] Mollusks or marine invertebrates may act as transfer hosts. *T. gondii* can survive in and sporulate in seawater and remain viable for at least 6 months at a temperature range of 4° to 24° C.[214] Contaminated oocysts may enter the marine environment by entering storm water drainage or sewage systems by being flushed from toilets and in open public drainage.[119a]

Enteroepithelial Life Cycle

This cycle is found only in the definitive feline host (see Fig. 80-1). Most cats are thought to become infected by ingesting intermediate hosts infected with *T. gondii*. Bradyzoites are released in the stomach and intestine from the tissue cysts

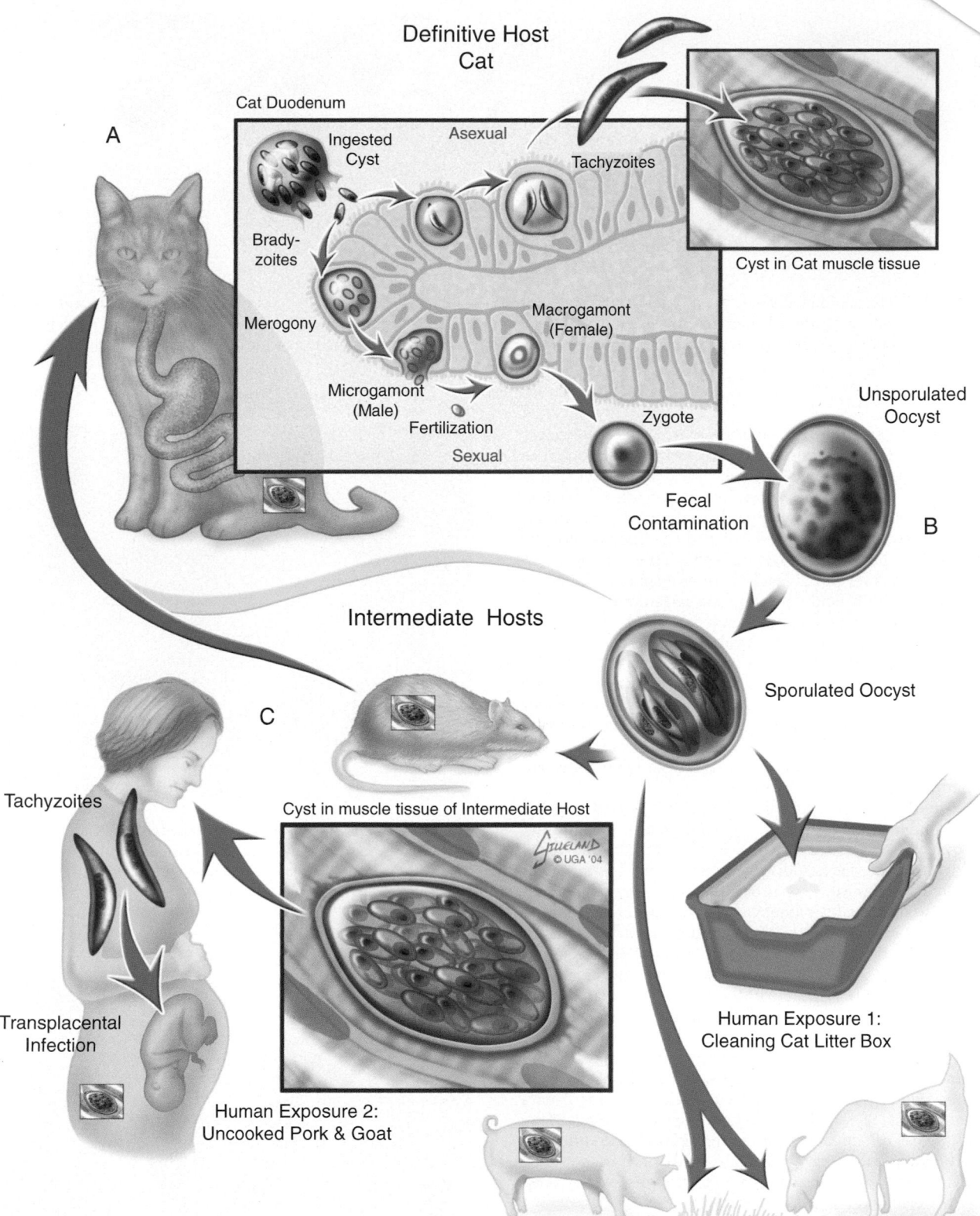

Fig 80-1 Life cycle of *T. gondii*. **A,** Enteroepithelial replication occurs in the cat intestine after ingestion of oocysts from fecal contamination or bradyzoites within tissue cysts. Following tachyzoite formation, some systemic spread to other tissues may occur with encystment. Ingested bradyzoites can also undergo merogony to form micro- and macrogamonts. An unsporulated oocyst is eventually formed following union of gamonts. **B,** The oocyst is excreted unsporulated in the feces and is noninfectious. It sporulates in the environment, becomes infectious, and then can be ingested by a variety of intermediate hosts. **C,** Muscle and tissue encystment occur in the intermediate host. In females infected for the first time during pregnancy, congenital infection of the fetus occurs. (Courtesy University of Georgia, Athens, Ga.)

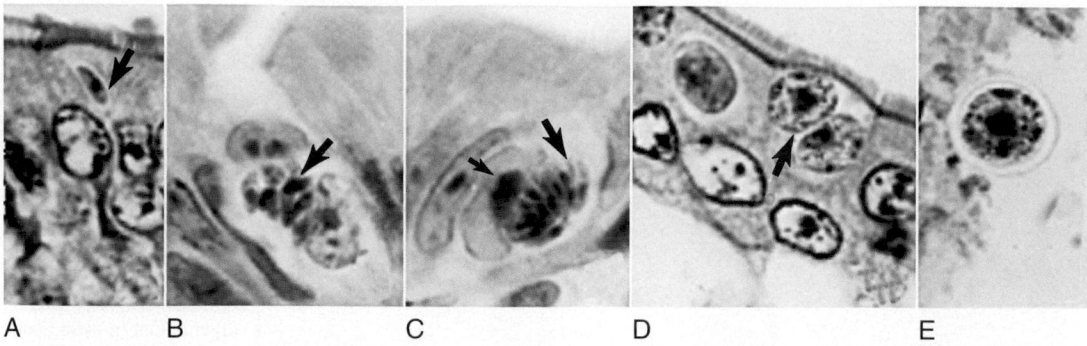

A   B   C   D   E

Fig 80-2 Enteroepithelial stages of *T. gondii* in the small intestine of cats (H and E stain, ×1000). **A,** Merozoite *(arrow)* above the epithelial cell nucleus. **B,** Type B meront *(arrow)*. **C,** Type C *(arrow)* in banana-shaped merozoites. The epithelial cell nucleus *(arrowhead)* is hypertrophied. **D,** Two gamonts on right *(arrow)*, each with one nucleus, and a male gamont on the left. **E,** Unsporulated oocyst in intestinal lumen.

when digestive enzymes dissolve the cyst wall. Bradyzoites penetrate the epithelial cells of small intestine and initiate the five types of predetermined asexual stages (Fig. 80-2). These types, A to E, are equivalent to schizonts of other intestinal coccidia.[314a] After an undetermined number of generations, merozoites released from type D or E form male (micro) or female (macro) gamonts, respectively. The microgamont divides and forms several biflagellate microgametes, which are released and swim to and penetrate macrogamonts.[314a] A wall is formed around the fertilized macrogamont to form an oocyst. Oocysts are round to oval, 10 × 12 μm, and are unsporulated (uninfective) when passed in feces (Fig. 80-3). After exposure to air and moisture for 1 to 5 days, oocysts sporulate and contain two sporocysts, each with four sporozoites. Sporozoites are banana shaped, approximately 8 × 2 μm, and can survive in the oocyst for many months, even under harsh environmental conditions. These sporozoites are the infectious form of the oocyst.

The entire enteroepithelial (coccidian) cycle of *T. gondii* can be completed within 3 to 10 days after ingestion of tissue cysts and occurs in up to 97% of naïve cats. However, after ingestion of oocysts or tachyzoites, the formation of oocysts is delayed until 18 or more days, and only 20% of cats fed oocysts will develop patency.[81,83,89] The differences in the life cycle that account for this delay and resistance are uncertain, but bradyzoites are probably precursors of enteroepithelial replication, allowing for more rapid development. Bradyzoites are more infective to cats as compared with oocysts because much fewer of the former are needed to establish patent infections.[88]

Dogs have been infected by feeding on tissue cysts.[217] Experimentally, dogs have been fed sporulated oocysts from cat feces, which passed through into their feces for 2 days postinoculation (PI).[218] Although these dogs seroconverted, no clinical signs of infection or enteroepithelial replication occurred. Dogs ingesting cat litter would serve as potential mechanical vectors for transmission to people as they shed ingested sporulated oocysts in their stool.[218]

Extraintestinal Life Cycle

The extraintestinal development of *T. gondii* is the same as it is for all hosts, including rodents, dogs, cats, and people, and is not dependent on whether tissue cysts or oocysts are ingested. After the ingestion of oocysts, sporozoites excyst in the lumen of the small intestine and penetrate intestinal cells, including the cells in the lamina propria. Sporozoites divide into two by an asexual process known as endodyogeny and thus become tachyzoites. Tachyzoites are lunate in shape, approximately 6 × 2 μm (Figs. 80-4 and 80-5), and multiply

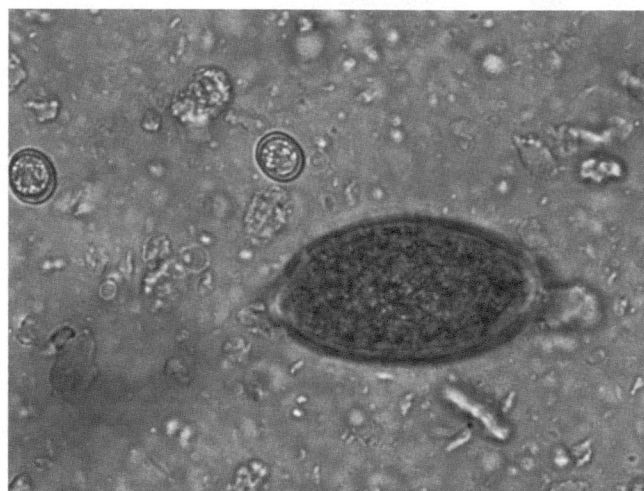

Fig 80-3 *Toxoplasma* oocysts compared with *Capillaria* eggs in feces of a naturally infected cat (unstained).

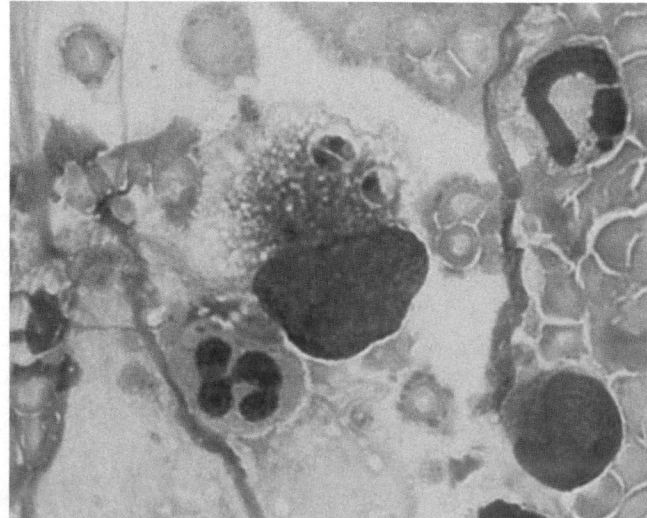

Fig 80-4 Tachyzoites of *T. gondii* in bronchial lavage from a cat. Several tachyzoites are within a macrophage (Giemsa, ×1250).

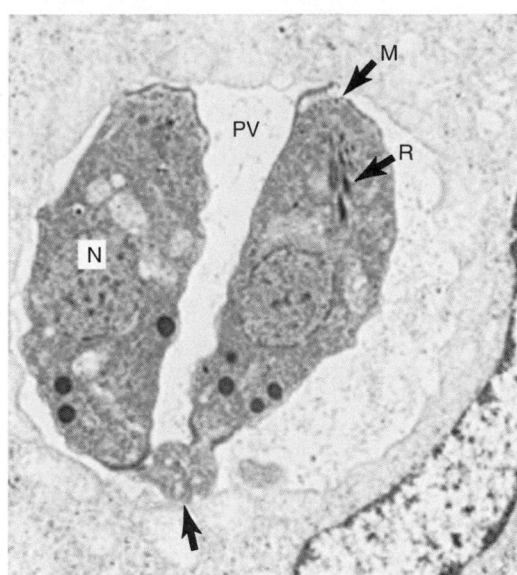

Fig 80-5 Transmission electron micrograph of tachyzoites of *T. gondii*. Tachyzoites are separated from the host cell cytoplasm by a parasitophorous vacuole *(PV)*. One tachyzoite has divided into two progeny that are still attached at the posterior end. Note central nucleus *(N)*, rhoptries *(R)*, and micronemes *(M)* anterior to the nucleus (×10,000). (Courtesy C.A. Speer, Montana State University, Bozman, Mont.)

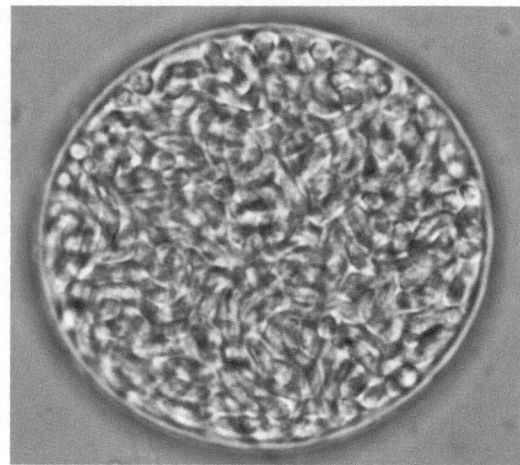

Fig 80-6 *T. gondii* tissue cyst from brain emulsion of experimentally infected mice showing a thin cyst wall and banana-shaped bradyzoites (unstained smear, ×1000).

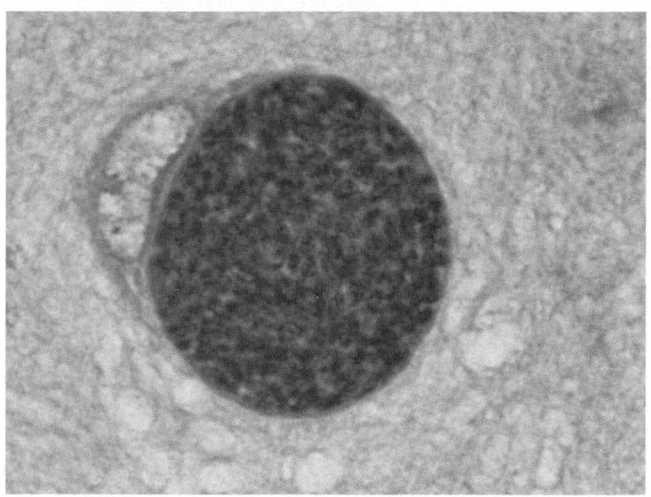

Fig 80-7 Tissue cyst in the brain of a cat (PAS stain).

in almost any cell of the body. If the cell ruptures, they infect new cells. Otherwise, tachyzoites multiply intracellularly for an undetermined period and eventually encyst. Tissue cysts grow intracellularly and contain numerous bradyzoites (Figs. 80-6, 80-7, and 80-8). Bradyzoites resemble tachyzoites in structure except that they are thinner and the nucleus is located at the posterior (nonconoidal) end of the parasite. Biologically, bradyzoites differ from tachyzoites in that they can survive the digestive process in the stomach, whereas tachyzoites are usually killed. Tissue cysts vary in size from 15 to 60 μm and usually conform to the shape of the parasitized cell. Tissue cysts are separated from the host cell by a thin (less than 0.5 μm) elastic wall (see Fig. 80-8). Tissue cysts are formed in the central nervous system (CNS), muscles, and visceral organs and probably persist for the life of the host. Some variation in tissue tropism for cyst formation has been observed.[83]

Toxoplasma-encysted organisms can injure the CNS of infected mice and rats, resulting in impaired learning and memory and behavioral abnormalities. *T. gondii*–infected rodents become less neophobic, leading to decreased aversion to the odor of cats.[24] This behavior might help ensure that rodents would be eaten by cats and the life cycle would be preserved; however, the neurologic signs were transient and corresponded with peak development of tissue cysts in the brain.[167] Wild mice (*Mus domesticus*) have been shown to transmit the infection congenitally at a rate of 75% or greater.[234] This may serve as a mechanism, other than involving cats, of maintaining the infection in nature.

Congenital Transmission

Parasitemia during pregnancy can cause placentitis followed by spread of tachyzoites to the fetus. In people or sheep, congenital transmission usually occurs when the woman or ewe becomes initially infected during pregnancy. High levels of congenital transmission have also been observed in natural urban populations of mice,[234] which may help maintain infec-

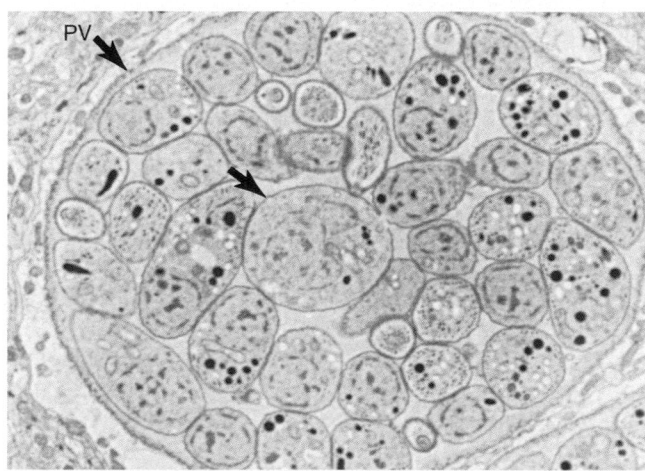

Fig 80-8 Transmission electron micrograph of a young tissue cyst of *T. gondii* in the brain of a mouse (21 days PI). The tissue cyst is separated from the cytoplasm of the neuron by a parasitophorous vacuole *(PV)*. One bradyzoite *(shorter arrow)* is dividing (×6500). (Courtesy D. J. P. Ferguson, Oxford University, England.)

tion in these rodents in the absence of cats. Bitches fed sporulated oocysts at 56, 40, and 32 days of gestation showed evidence of congenital infection and aborted.[35] The prevalence of congenital toxoplasmosis in dogs is thought to be less common than that in sheep and goats. Many kittens born to queens infected with *T. gondii* during gestation became infected transplacentally or via suckling as tachyzoites are shed in milk.* Clinical illness was common, varying with the stage of gestation at the time of infection, and some newborn kittens shed oocysts.[108] Lactational or transplacental transmission may predispose kittens to the development of ocular toxoplasmosis.[280]

Pathogenesis

The type and severity of clinical illness with *T. gondii* infections depend on the degree and localization of tissue injury. Tachyzoites are the invasive asexual forms of the parasite that require intracellular existence for replication and survival. All cell types appear susceptible. Cell necrosis is caused by the intracellular growth of *Toxoplasma*. *T. gondii* does not produce a toxin. In infections acquired after the ingestion of tissue cysts or oocysts, initial clinical signs are caused by the necrosis of intestine and associated lymphoid organs caused by tachyzoites. Enteroepithelial stages in the cat appear to have unique antigens.[325] Antibodies of the IgA class, specific for *T. gondii* enteroepithelial stages, increase in the intestinal secretions as part of the immune response to terminate the phase of intestinal replication.[259,294] *T. gondii* also spreads to extraintestinal organs via blood or lymph, and focal necrosis may develop in many organs (Fig. 80-9). The brain, liver, lungs, skeletal muscle, and eyes are common sites of initial replication and chronic persistence of infection. The clinical outcome is determined by the extent of injury to these organs, especially vital organs such as the heart, lung, liver, and adrenal glands. Although acute disseminated infections can be fatal, the host often recovers. Interferon (IFN)-γ–dependent cell-mediated immunity and humoral factors are important in resistance to *Toxoplasma* encephalitis as studied in experimentally infected rodents.[323] Resistance is caused by interplay among T and B lymphocytes, IFN-γ–producing non-T cells, microglia, astrocytes, and dendritic cells. The classical complement pathway of cats is not activated after exposure to *T. gondii*,[178] a feature that appears unique to the definitive host.

*References: 44, 96, 106, 108, 278, 297.

By approximately the third week after infection, tachyzoites begin to disappear from visceral tissues and may localize as tissue cysts (as bradyzoites). This phase is associated with a systemic immune response, which inhibits the parasitemia. These tissue cysts may persist in the host for life. Tissue cysts may rupture, and released bradyzoites may initiate a clinical relapse during immunosuppression, such as with antitumor or glucocorticoid therapy (Fig. 80-10). The mechanism of reactivation is not known.

The reason why some infected dogs or cats develop clinical toxoplasmosis while others remain well is not fully understood. Age, sex, host species, strain of *T. gondii*, number of organisms, and stage of the parasite ingested may account for some of the differences. Postnatally acquired toxoplasmosis is generally less serious than is prenatally acquired infection. Stress may also aggravate *T. gondii* infection. Concomitant illness or immunosuppression may make a host more susceptible because *T. gondii* proliferates as an opportunistic pathogen. Clinical toxoplasmosis in dogs is often associated with canine distemper or other infections, such as ehrlichiosis, or with glucocorticoid therapy or vaccination with live attenuated vaccines.[122a] In some cases, however, predisposing disorders cannot be found. Historically, the prevalence of canine toxoplasmosis has decreased with the routine use of canine distemper vaccines.[98] Some cases of clinical feline toxoplasmosis have been observed concomitantly with glucocorticoid or cyclosporin therapy, hematotropic mycoplasmal infection (haemobartonellosis), feline leukemia virus (FeLV) and immunodeficiency virus (FIV) infections, and feline infectious peritonitis.* In one serosurvey of urban stray cats, cats infected with FIV were more likely to have seropositive test results for *T. gondii*, whereas no association with concurrent FeLV infection was found.[75]

Preexisting FIV infection can produce more severe *Toxoplasma* infection in cats that are subsequently challenged with FIV.[65,197] FIV-infected cats that were subsequently co-infected with *T. gondii* had suppressed CD4+ and CD8+ lymphocyte expression of interleukin (IL)-2, IL-6, IFN-γ and IL-12 when compared with cats infected with *T. gondii* alone.[207] IL-10 levels were increased in FIV-infected cats before and after infection with *T. gondii* and may have suppressed the T1 helper cytokine response to *T. gondii* infection. In contrast to these experiments, experimental FIV and FeLV infections in

*References: 21, 65, 95, 96, 157, 210, 260, 330.

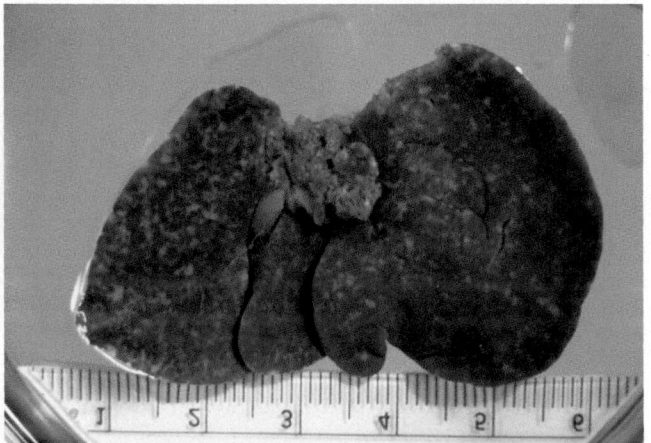

Fig 80-9 Liver of a kitten congenitally infected with *T. gondii*. Numerous white-yellowish areas of discoloration are caused by necrosis produced by tachyzoites.

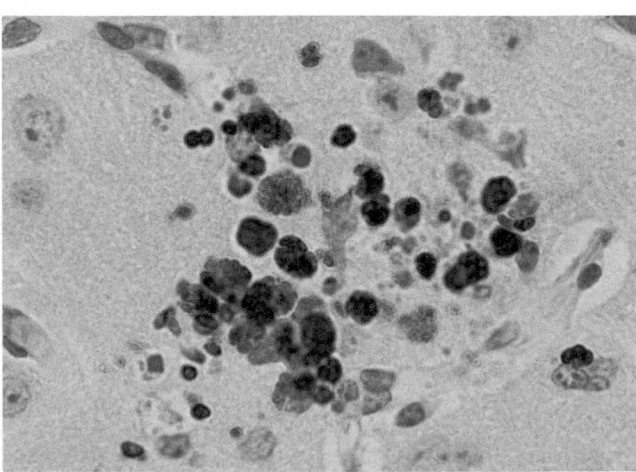

Fig 80-10 Tachyzoites and tissue cysts in section of brain (immunohistochemical stain).

cats did not produce reactivated or more severe acute infections in cats already or simultaneously inoculated with *T. gondii*.[194,199,268] Regardless of the difference in these experimental studies or which infection precedes the other, clinically, cats with FIV and *T. gondii* co-infections are more difficult to treat effectively (see sections to follow).

IL-6 activity is greatly elevated in cats with uveitis suspected to be a result of their *Toxoplasma* infection,[196] and cats with toxoplasmosis have circulating *T. gondii*–containing immune complexes[200] that may play a role in development of ocular toxoplasmosis. Feline herpesvirus 1 and *Bartonella henselae* co-infections failed to activate ocular toxoplasmosis in congenitally infected kittens.[279] Toxoplasmosis has been associated with dissemination and mortality in cats and dogs receiving immunosuppression with cyclosporine.[1,26,341b] Therefore animals to receive such therapy should be prescreened by serologic testing for the risk of reactivating a chronic infection.

Clinical Findings
Cats

Naïve cats ingesting bradyzoites from tissues can develop self-limiting, small-bowel diarrhea as a manifestation of enteroepithelial replication. Otherwise, this phase of the illness, which lasts up to 10 days, can be clinically silent and unimportant. Immunosuppressed cats can have simultaneous systemic manifestations with extraintestinal spread of tachyzoites. However, clinical toxoplasmosis from systemic spread is most severe in transplacentally or lactationally infected kittens because tachyzoite replication can be overwhelming.[96,108,117] Affected kittens may be stillborn or may die before weaning. Kittens may continue to suckle until death. Clinical signs reflect inflammation of the liver, lungs, and CNS (Fig. 80-11). Lethargy, depression, hypothermia, and sudden death can occur. Affected kittens may have an enlarged abdomen because of enlarged liver and ascites. Encephalitic kittens may sleep most of the time or cry continuously. Kittens born to infected queens develop chorioretinitis, sometimes in the absence of other signs of clinical illness.[280] Some kittens develop transient concurrent anterior uveitis.

Clinical signs in older cats can be the result of spread of tachyzoites following initial acute exposure or reactivation of a chronic encysted infection by release of bradyzoites following immunosuppression. Anorexia, lethargy, and dyspnea caused by pneumonia have been commonly recognized features of postnatal toxoplasmosis (Table 80-1). Other clinical

signs include persistent or intermittent fever, anorexia, weight loss, icterus caused by hepatitis or cholangiohepatitis, vomiting, diarrhea, abdominal effusion, hyperesthesia on muscle palpation, stiffness of gait, shifting leg lameness, neurologic deficits, dermatitis, and death.[95,159,202,4a,225a] In 100 cats with histologically confirmed toxoplasmosis, clinical syndromes were diverse, but infection of pulmonary (97.7%), CNS (96.4%), hepatic (93.3%), pancreatic (84.4%), cardiac (86.4%), and ocular (81.5%) tissues were most common.[95] Clinical signs may be sudden or have a slow onset. The disease may be rapidly fatal in some cats with severe respiratory or CNS signs. Anterior or posterior uveitis involving one or both eyes is common.* Iritis, iridocyclitis, or chorioretinitis can occur alone or concomitantly. Aqueous flare, keratic precipi-

*References: 49, 62, 95, 196, 202, 205.

Table • 80-1

Clinical Findings in Feline Toxoplasmosis

Fever
Anorexia, lethargy
Weight loss
Muscle pain, hyperesthesia
Respiratory tract disease
    Conjunctivitis
    Rhinitis
    Coughing
    Dyspnea, tachypnea
    Diffuse harsh bronchovesicular sounds
Vomiting, diarrhea
Abdominal discomfort
Icterus
Abdominal effusion
Arthritis, joint pain, shifting lameness
Cardiac arrhythmias, sudden death
Splenomegaly
Lymphadenomegaly
Pyogranulomatous dermatitis
Neurologic signs
    Ataxia
    Circling
    Behavioral changes
    Seizures
    Twitching
    Tremors
Ocular signs
    Retinochoroiditis, retinal hemorrhages
    Optic neuritis
    Optic nerve atrophy
    Anisocoria
    Blindness
    Anterior uveitis, aqueous flare, hyphema, velvety iris
    Glaucoma
    Lens luxation
    Retinal detachment
Neonatal (transplacental infection)
    Stillbirth
    Fading kittens
    Organ dysfunction (liver: hepatomegaly, icterus, ascites; lung: dyspnea; central nervous system: sleep, crying)

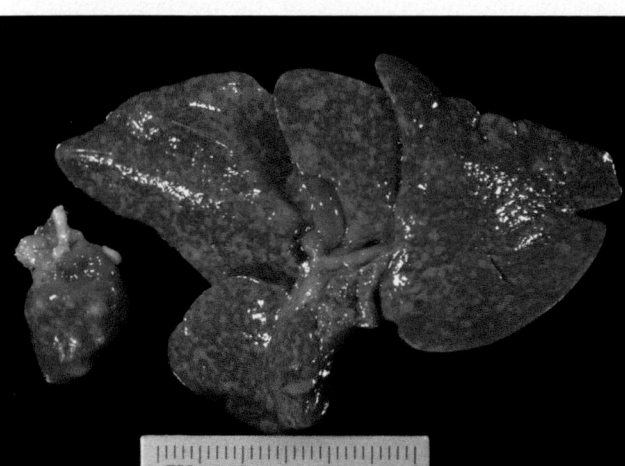

Fig 80-11 Pneumonia and necrosis in heart of a congenitally infected kitten.

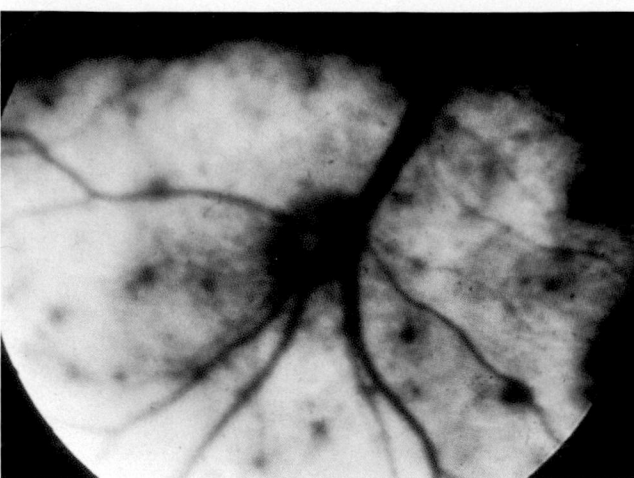

Fig 80-12 Chorioretinitis in a cat with toxoplasmosis. (Courtesy University of Georgia, Athens, Ga.)

tate, lens luxation, glaucoma, and retinal detachment are common manifestations of uveitis. Chorioretinitis, which can be unifocal or multifocal, may occur in both tapetal and nontapetal areas (Fig. 80-12) (see Toxoplasmosis, Chapter 93). Ocular toxoplasmosis occurs in some cats without polysystemic clinical signs of disease. In experimental *T. gondii* in cats, those infected concurrently with FIV developed severe pneumonitis and hepatitis, whereas those not infected with FIV developed multifocal chorioretinitis and anterior uveitis.[63,65] Neurologic and ocular manifestations that occur in the absence of other systemic signs are more common with reactivated infection rather than acute infection. Nodular pyogranulomatous dermatitis has developed in dogs and cats with disseminated infection resulting from immunosuppressive drug therapy.[4a,205a]

Dogs

Clinical signs may be localized in respiratory, neuromuscular, or gastrointestinal (GI) systems, or they may be caused by generalized infection.[93,98] The neurologic form of toxoplasmosis may last for several weeks without involvement of other systems, whereas severe disease involving the lungs and liver may kill dogs within a week.[93] Generalized toxoplasmosis is seen mostly in dogs younger than 1 year and is characterized by fever, tonsillitis, dyspnea, diarrhea, and vomiting. Icterus usually results from extensive hepatic necrosis.[286] Myocardial involvement is usually subclinical, although arrhythmias and heart failure may develop as predominant findings in some dogs. Occasionally, there is dermatitis.[341b]

The most dramatic clinical signs in older dogs have been associated with neural and muscular systems.[153] Neurologic signs depend on the site of lesion in the cerebrum, cerebellum, or spinal cord. Seizures, cranial nerve deficits, tremors, ataxia, and paresis or paralysis may be seen. Dogs with myositis may initially show abnormal gait, muscle wasting, or stiffness. Paraparesis and tetraparesis may rapidly progress to lower motor neuron paralysis. Canine toxoplasmosis is clinically similar to *Neospora caninum* infection, which was previously confused with toxoplasmosis (see Neosporosis later in this chapter).[266] Canine CNS toxoplasmosis may occur concurrently or be predisposed by canine distemper virus infection.[68,98] Although these diseases are similar, toxoplasmosis appears to be more prevalent in cats and neosporosis more prevalent in dogs.

Only a few reports have been submitted of ocular lesions associated with toxoplasmosis in dogs. Retinitis, ante-

rior uveitis, iridocyclitis, ciliary epithelium hyperplasia, and optic nerve neuritis have been noted (see Toxoplasmosis, Chapter 93).

Diagnosis

Clinical Laboratory Findings

Routine hematologic and biochemical parameters may be abnormal in cats and dogs with acute systemic toxoplasmosis. Nonregenerative anemia, neutrophilic leukocytosis, lymphocytosis, monocytosis, and eosinophilia are most commonly observed. Leukopenia of severely affected cats may persist until death and is usually characterized by an absolute lymphopenia and neutropenia with an inappropriate left shift, eosinopenia, and monocytopenia. In experimentally infected cats, neutropenia and lymphopenia persist for 5 to 12 days. Leukocytosis was seen in the recovery phase of illness.[199] Lymphocyte counts greater than 7000 cells/µl were common from 28 to 154 days after primary inoculation.[199] Secondary exposure of cats to *T. gondii* did not result in significant changes in leukocyte numbers.[199]

Biochemical abnormalities during the acute phase of illness include hypoproteinemia and hypoalbuminemia. Hyperglobulinemia has been detected in some cats with chronic toxoplasmosis.[202] Marked increases in serum alanine aminotransferase (ALT) and aspartate aminotransferase (AST) activities have been noted in animals with acute hepatic and muscle necrosis. Dogs generally have increased serum ALT and alkaline phosphatase (ALP) activities with hepatic necrosis, but this occurs less frequently in cats. Serum creatine kinase activity is also increased in cases of muscle necrosis. Serum bilirubin levels have been increased in animals with acute hepatic necrosis, especially cats that develop cholangiohepatitis or hepatic lipidosis. Cats or dogs that develop pancreatitis may show increased serum amylase and lipase activities, although these are inconsistent. Cats often show proteinuria and bilirubinuria. Cats with pancreatitis may have reduced serum total calcium with normal serum albumin concentrations.[95]

Cytology

Tachyzoites may be detected in various tissues and body fluids by cytology during acute illness (see Fig. 80-4). They are rarely found in blood, cerebrospinal fluid (CSF), fine-needle aspirates, and transtracheal or bronchoalveolar washings[36,128,155] but are more common in the peritoneal and thoracic fluids of animals developing thoracic effusions or ascites.

Inflammatory changes are usually noted in body fluids. In suspected feline toxoplasmosis of the nervous system, CSF protein levels were within reference ranges to a maximum of 149 mg/dl, and nucleated cells were a maximum of 28 cells/ml.[202] Lymphocytes predominate, but a mixture of inflammatory cells may be found.

Radiology

Thoracic radiographic findings, especially in cats with acute disease, consist of a diffuse interstitial to alveolar pattern with a mottled lobar distribution (Fig. 80-13).[296] Diffuse symmetric homogeneous increased density caused by alveolar coalescence has been noted in severely affected animals. Mild pleural effusion can be present. Abdominal radiographic findings may consist of masses in the intestines or mesenteric lymph nodes or homogeneous increased density as a result of effusion. Loss of contrast in the right abdominal quadrant can indicate pancreatitis. Abdominal ultrasonographic changes can indicate organ or tissue enlargement as a result of inflammation or granuloma formation. Lesions within the CNS may be detected by myelography, computed tomography, or magnetic resonance imaging.

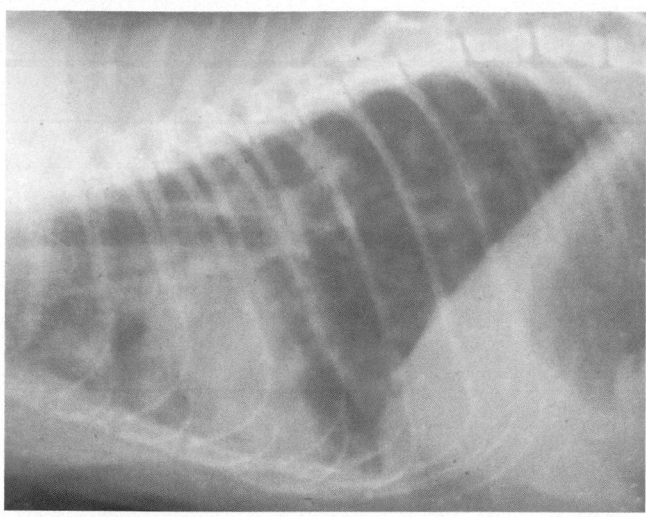

Fig 80-13 Lateral thoracic radiograph of a cat with *Toxoplasma* pneumonia. (Courtesy University of Georgia, Athens, Ga.)

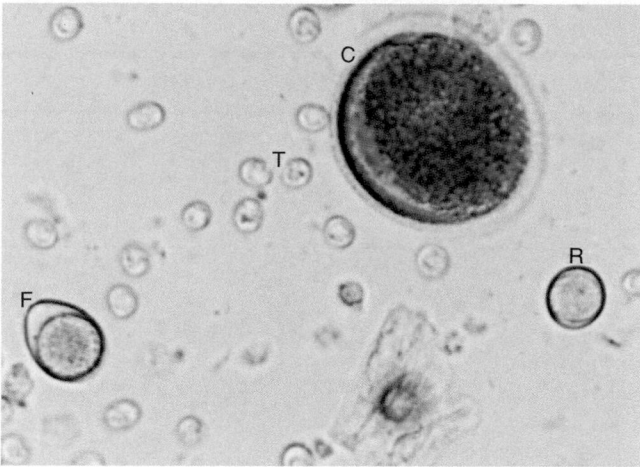

Fig 80-14 Unsporulated oocysts of *T. gondii (T)*, *I. felis (F)*, and *I. rivolta (R)*, and an egg of the roundworm *T. cati (C)* in a flotation of feline feces (unstained, ×410). (From Dubey JP. 1976. A review of *Sarcocystis* of domestic animals and of other coccidia of cats and dogs, *J Am Vet Med Assoc* 169:1061–1078. Reprinted with permission.)

Fecal Examination

Despite the high prevalence of serum antibodies in cats worldwide, the prevalence of *T. gondii* oocysts in feces is low. In the United States, approximately 1% of cats shed oocysts on any given day.[93,160,314] Because cats usually shed *T. gondii* oocysts for only 1 to 2 weeks after their first exposure, oocysts are rarely found in routine fecal examination. Moreover, cats are usually not clinically ill and do not have diarrhea during the period of oocyst shedding. Although cats are considered immune to reshedding of oocysts, they may shed a few oocysts after rechallenge with different strains more than 6 years later.[80] Cats that are immune have partial asexual development of *T. gondii* in their intestines compared with complete development cycle in naïve cats.[66] Immunosuppression with high dose (10 to 80 mg/kg, daily by mouth or intramuscularly (IM) once a week) of prednisolone will cause chronically infected cats to reexcrete oocysts, whereas a lower dose (5 mg/kg IM for 4 weeks) will not.[195]

T. gondii oocysts in feline feces are morphometrically indistinguishable from oocysts of *Hammondia hammondi*, *Besnoitia orcytofelisi* and *Besnoitia darlingi*, which also occur in cats (see Chapter 81). Oocysts of these coccidians can be differentiated only by ultrastructural and molecular examination, sporulation, and subsequent animal inoculation.[124,316] If 10 μm–sized oocysts are found, they should be considered to be *T. gondii* until proved otherwise. Because of the infectious nature of this organism, further inoculations should be attempted only in a diagnostic laboratory with competence in this procedure.

Because of their small size, oocysts of *T. gondii* are best demonstrated by centrifugation using Sheather's sugar solution. See Chapter 70 for a discussion of this technique. Examine 1 to 2 drops removed from the meniscus at low-power (×100) magnification. *T. gondii* oocysts are approximately one fourth the size of *Isospora felis* and one eighth the size of *Toxocara cati* (Fig. 80-14).

Serologic Testing

Once infected, animals harbor toxoplasmic tissue cysts for life, which stimulates a long-term humoral immune response in infected adults. Serologic surveys indicate that *T. gondii* infections are prevalent worldwide. Approximately 30% of cats and dogs in the United States have *T. gondii* antibodies (Fig. 80-

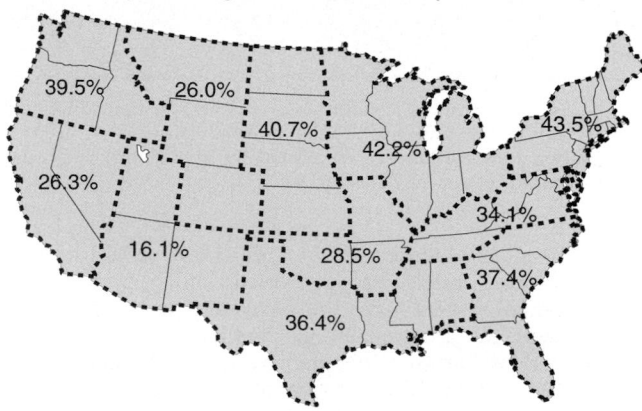

Toxoplasma gondii Feline Seroprevalence

Fig 80-15 Seroprevalence of *T. gondii* in cats in the continental United States. (Modified from Vollaire MR, Radecki SV, Lappin MR. 2005. Seroprevalence of *Toxoplasma gondii* antibodies in clinically ill cats in the United States, *Am J Vet Res* 66:874–877.

15).[69,93,339] The prevalence of seropositivity increases with age of the cat or dog because of the chance of exposure rather than susceptibility.

Multiple serologic tests for the detection of antibodies have been used in the diagnosis of toxoplasmosis (Table 80-2). The use of these tests in cats has been reviewed.[188] No single serologic assay exists that can definitively confirm a diagnosis of toxoplasmosis. The Sabin-Feldman dye test is highly sensitive and specific for human toxoplasmosis but not necessarily for cats. Moreover, the test is too technical to perform in diagnostic laboratories, and it uses live *T. gondii*.

The indirect fluorescent antibody (FA) technique is comparable to the dye test but does not require live antigen. Some false-positive polar staining that can occur with the indirect FA test has been attributed to Fc receptors on the surface of *T. gondii* tachyzoites that nonspecifically bind Ig. The indirect

Table • 80-2

Serologic Tests for Feline Toxoplasmosis

TEST	EARLIEST DETECTION (WEEKS)	ANTIBODY CLASS	TITER (LEAST SIGNIFICANT LEVEL OF REACTIVITY[a])	GUIDELINES FOR ACTIVE INFECTION
Sabin-Feldman	1–2	IgG, IgM	16	Fourfold rise over 2—3 wk
Indirect FA				
IgM	1–2	IgM	64	Titer > 1:64 with or without concurrent IgG
IgG	2	IgG	64	Fourfold rise over 2—5 wk
Indirect hemagglutination	2	IgG	64	Fourfold rise over 2—3 wk; insensitive
Latex agglutination	2	IgG	64	Fourfold rise over 2—3 wk
Modified Agglutination Test				
Acetone-fixed antigen	1–2	IgG	100	Fourfold rise over 2—3 wk or high titer with low formalin-fixed; titers remain high for 3 mo
Formalin-fixed	2	IgG	—	Fourfold rise over 2—3 wk; titers remain high for years
ELISA				
IgM	1–2	IgM	64	Titer > 1 : 64 with or without concurrent IgG
IgG	2	IgG	64	Fourfold rise over 2—3 wk

[a]Titers may vary between laboratories on the basis of individual methodologies. Whenever comparisons are being made, both samples should be processed at the same time by the same laboratory.
For additional information on test availability, see Laboratory Listings, Appendix 5.
Modified from references 211 and 188.

FA can be adapted to detect IgM, IgG, or IgA using whole or immunoblotted antigen (see later discussion).[324]

Agglutination tests have the advantage of being species independent and are available in commercial kits that have been developed for use in people. The indirect hemagglutination (IHA) test (TMP-test, Wampole Labs, Carter Wallace Inc., Cranbury, N.J.) does not require live antigen but is less sensitive compared with the dye test, indirect FA test, and enzyme-linked immunosorbent assay (ELISA).[204] The main drawback is that it primarily measures IgG and is usually not positive during acute infection.

The latex agglutination test (LAT) (Toxo-test, Eiken Chemical Co., Tokyo, Japan; Synkit Inc., Chatsworth, Calif.) is somewhat more sensitive for serologic screening; however, it cannot be used to distinguish immunoglobulin classes. The modified agglutination test (MAT) (Toxo-Screen DA, Biomerieux, Marcy-l'Etoile, France) detects only IgG but is extremely sensitive compared with the other available assays.[226] The MAT has been improved in its sensitivity and specificity in distinguishing acute and chronic Toxoplasma infections in people and cats by using acetone- or methanol-fixed and formalin-fixed trophozoites, respectively.[109] Antibodies to acetone-fixed antigen are elevated only during acute (under 3 months) infection, whereas antibodies to formalin-fixed antigen may remain high for several years.[126] For additional information on commercial laboratory testing and test kits, see Appendices 5 and 6, respectively.

ELISA, with and without immunoblotting, has been adapted for the detection of IgM, IgG, and IgA class antibodies against T. gondii in feline sera.* ELISA methods are as sensitive as is indirect FA[31] and more sensitive compared with LAT or IHA. As a result, ELISA may be less specific at lower dilutions of sera. Immunoblots of separated antigens, reacted with an animal's sera and ELISA, can be used to identify specific target antigens and improve specificity. Comparison of antigen recognition patterns by serum from infected queens and their kittens by immunoblot aids in the diagnosis of neonatal toxoplasmosis.[44] ELISA has also been compared with indirect FA and IHA tests in the kinetics of the humoral immune response in dogs experimentally infected with T. gondii.[305] Specific IgM was detected from day 7 PI and began decreasing by day 27 PI, with the ELISA showing slightly earlier and longer detection of IgM. Specific IgG was detected from day 7 PI throughout the 62 days of the study. IgM may constitute an indicator of recent or active infection in dogs.

Investigational Assays   An ELISA incorporating a recombinant-produced immunodominant surface antigen (SAG)1 and P30 was developed to measure antibodies in experimentally infected cats and in experimentally and naturally infected dogs.[181,305,306] The antigen is stage specific, being secreted by tachyzoites, and might be of consideration in the diagnosis of active clinical infections.[181] Use of recombinant SAG2 in ELISA allowed for discrete detection of experimentally infected cats with the same specificity as that for the LAT.[168,169] The test has also been adapted to an immunochromatographic method.[168] The SAG2 ELISA appears to be specific because no cross-reaction occurred between sera of Neospora- and Toxoplasma-infected mice.[181] In studies in people, IgG binding avidity for Toxoplasma antigens is low soon after primary antigenic challenge.[208] The IgG avidity increases during subsequent months of infection from chronic

*References: 39, 44, 169, 181, 188, 192, 199, 308, 328.

humoral immune stimulation. Assays that quantitate the degree of antibody avidity might be used as a single assay to discriminate between recently acquired and chronic encysted infections.

Antibody Kinetics Soon after inoculation, approximately 80% of experimentally inoculated cats develop detectable IgM titers; 100% develop detectable IgA and IgG titers. Chronic persistence of high IgG titers thereafter merely reflects continued presence of *Toxoplasma* antigen. Documentation of a positive IgM titer or an increasing IgG or IgA titer (fourfold) can verify recent infection but not necessarily oocyst shedding.[255] Some cats do not develop detectable IgM titers, and positive IgM titers can persist in some cats for months to years after infection. Persistent IgM titers have been observed in experimentally infected cats that were co-infected with FIV, after repeat exposure to *T. gondii*, or from exposure to glucocorticoids. Thus this antibody class does not accurately predict the oocyst-shedding period. Some cats may not develop IgG titers to *T. gondii* for 4 to 6 weeks, well after the completion of the oocyst-shedding period. Following the initial detection of IgG or IgA antibodies in serum, maximal titers are often reached in 2 to 3 weeks, leaving a narrow window for the documentation of an increasing titer.[189] Thus failure to document a changing IgG titer does not exclude a diagnosis of recent infection. Optimally, sequential serum samples should be assessed at the same time in the assay to avoid interassay variation. After experimental inoculation of cats, IgG titers greater than 1:30,000 are commonly detected by MAT for 6 years after inoculation; thus high IgG titers do not prove recent or active infection.[109] Some seropositive cats will shed lower numbers of oocysts after oral inoculation with *T. gondii*, and therefore the presence of serum antibodies does not prove intestinal immunity.[80] Because of these findings, the measurement of serum antibodies in healthy cats cannot accurately predict the oocyst-shedding period. IgG in kittens born to chronically infected queens is transferred in colostrum and persists for 8 to 12 weeks after birth.[257]

Public Health Risk Assessment In general, for *assessing human health risk*, serologic test results from healthy cats can be interpreted as follows:
1. A seronegative cat is not likely currently shedding oocysts but will likely shed oocysts if exposed to the organism for the first time. This cat poses the greatest public health risk.
2. An IgG test seropositive cat is probably not currently shedding oocysts and is less likely to shed oocysts if reexposed or immunosuppressed. Recommendations are that potential exposure to oocysts be minimized.

Following initial exposure, IgM levels increase followed by increases in IgG levels. An increased IgM titer by itself may indicate very recent exposure and infection correlating with a period of oocyst shedding. Any concurrent increase in IgG would indicate that the shedding period had already passed and would also be expected in a chronic reactivated infection.

Disease Assessment A *tentative antemortem diagnosis* of clinical toxoplasmosis in dogs or cats can be based on the following combination of serology and clinical parameters:
1. Serologic evidence of recent or active infection consisting of high IgM titers, or fourfold or greater, increasing or decreasing, IgG or other antibody titers (after treatment or recovery, or both)
2. Exclusion of other causes of the clinical syndrome
3. Beneficial clinical response to an anti-*Toxoplasma* drug

Because antibodies occur in the serum of both healthy and diseased cats, results of these serologic tests do not independently prove clinical toxoplasmosis. Antibodies of the IgM class are commonly detected in the serum or aqueous humor of clinically ill or FIV-infected cats but not healthy cats, and they may be a better marker of clinical disease than IgG or IgA.[197,199,202,203] *T. gondii*–specific IgM is occasionally detected in the serum of cats with chronic or reactivated infection and does not always correlate with recent exposure.

Cats with uveitis or meningoencephalitis often have seropositive test results for other ocular pathogens such as FeLV, FIV, and feline infectious peritonitis virus. These co-infections may be responsible for immunosuppressing cats and allowing *Toxoplasma* infections to reactivate. Given that these infections have been associated with uveitis, positive serologic tests may also confuse exact determination of the underlying cause. For this reason, determination of *Toxoplasma*-specific antibodies in aqueous and CSF has been recommended.

Aqueous Humor and Cerebrospinal Fluid Assessment

In dogs and cats with toxoplasmic encephalitis or uveitis, both protein and leukocytes may be increased in CSF or aqueous humor.[205] Cells are usually a mixed population of large and small mononuclear cells and neutrophils; the organism is rarely seen.

When assessing specific antibodies in aqueous humor or CSF, those produced locally must be differentiated from those passively diffusing across a damaged vascular barrier. As with serologic testing for other CNS or ocular infections, a comparison of antibody in CSF or aqueous humor can be made with that of serum for *Toxoplasma* and another nonocular infectious agent such as calicivirus.[161,205] (See also Immunologic Testing, Canine Distemper, Chapter 3.) This coefficient is calculated by the following:

$$\text{Antibody coefficient} = \frac{\substack{\textit{Toxoplasma}\text{-specific antibody} \\ \text{aqueous (or CSF)}}}{\substack{\textit{Toxoplasma}\text{-specific} \\ \text{antibody serum}}} \times \frac{\substack{\text{Other agent-specific} \\ \text{antibody serum}}}{\substack{\text{Other agent-specific} \\ \text{antibody aqueous (or CSF)}}}$$

Titers or equivalent numerical values from ELISA or other assays are substituted in the formula.

Antibody coefficient values greater than 1, and especially greater than 8, are considered stronger evidence for local production of *Toxoplasma* antibody and associated infection compared with nonselective leakage from inflammation.[205] Ideally, to avoid variables inherent in test sensitivity, the same methodologies (e.g., ELISA, indirect FA, agglutination) should be employed in the assays for both infectious agents. For examination of CSF and CNS infection, the other agent should be a pathogen that is likely to have a serum titer such as a vaccine antigen but does not cause CNS infection. Calicivirus is also suitable for this purpose in cats. In some experimentally infected cats, high *T. gondii*–specific IgG antibody coefficients can be detected for 3 to 4 months after inoculation.[50] Caution must be exercised in assuming that this increased value always correlates with CNS or ocular replication of organisms. In some cats previously exposed to *T. gondii*, nonspecific immune stimulation resulted in an increased antibody coefficient (greater than 1) on CSF or aqueous humor.[217] Analysis of IgM in aqueous humor shows better discrimination in cats with uveitis.[205]

Transient local production of *T. gondii*–specific antibodies in the eyes (IgG and IgA) and CNS (IgG) of cats has been documented after primary and secondary experimental inoculation.[50,191,210,247] Local production of *T. gondii*–specific IgM has been detected only in client-owned, naturally exposed cats with uveitis or clinical signs of encephalitis, suggesting that this antibody class in CSF or aqueous humor may be a marker of clinical disease.[188,205] *T. gondii*–specific antigens can be detected in the aqueous humor of some cats with uveitis.[205,217]

Organism Detection

Identification of *T. gondii* in body tissues or fluids is definitive for infection. The presence of *T. gondii* can be confirmed by bioassays in animals or cell culture inoculation. Laboratory mice are the most susceptible animals. Homogenized suspensions of tissues or body fluids obtained at necropsy or biopsy may be used to infect laboratory mice or tissue culture. Cleaned, sporulated oocysts obtained from feces similarly may be used to infect mice. Generally, mice are inoculated subcutaneously or intraperitoneally (IP). Beginning 4 to 6 days PI, peritoneal exudates of mice are examined for tachyzoites of *T. gondii* in IP inoculated mice. Tissue cysts are present 4 to 6 weeks PI mostly in neural tissue. *Toxoplasma* antibodies in mice have developed by 6 weeks PI and can be demonstrated by any one of the serologic tests mentioned. Lack of parasite demonstration does not mean that the mice are not infected with *T. gondii*, and serologic verification is necessary.

ELISAs that detect *T. gondii* antigen, both free and bound in immune complexes, have been studied in naturally and experimentally infected cats.[200,201] Clinically ill cats and those with ocular involvement were more likely to have immune complexes in serum. Although this finding may have a role in disease development, the detection of circulating antigen does not confirm that *T. gondii* is responsible for clinical illness in a given animal. Research is being conducted in cats with acute *Toxoplasma* infections to clinically evaluate detection in blood of two antigens (H4 and P18) known to be only secreted by tachyzoites.[47,162]

Polymerase chain reaction (PCR) can be used to verify the presence of *T. gondii* in biologic specimens.* PCR was more sensitive than the mouse inoculation bioassay was in detecting infection in the blood of experimentally infected cats.[41] The PCR results were positive for the entire time period after primary challenge up to 140 days and after rechallenge. Therefore, being so sensitive, it can detect infected cats but cannot distinguish whether they have acute or chronic subclinical encysted infection. PCR has been performed to detect *T. gondii* in the blood of people with acute toxoplasmosis.[150] False-negative results occur, and chronically infected people may not be identified. PCR followed by restriction analysis can also be used to determine genotypes of infecting strains.[166] PCR has detected *T. gondii* in the intestine[132] and aqueous humor[38] of experimentally infected cats. In the aqueous humor, *T. gondii* was detected transiently by PCR after primary and secondary inoculation of cats.[40,190] The organism was commonly identified before the detection of specific antibody in the aqueous humor of cats with and without uveitis. In client-owned, naturally exposed cats, the organism was detected in the aqueous humor from 8 of 43 cats with uveitis and 2 of 23 healthy cats.[40,190] Because *T. gondii* can be detected without the clinical signs of uveitis, positive PCR results in aqueous humor do not prove that the ocular signs are from toxoplasmosis. A multiplex PCR was developed that can detect and distinguish between *Neospora* or *Toxoplasma* DNA in CSF, skeletal muscle, or neural tissue of cats and dogs.[301]

Pathologic Findings

Cats

The gross and microscopic findings may be similar to those seen in dogs; however, in feline toxoplasmosis, necrosis is predominantly in the liver (see Fig. 80-9), mesenteric lymph nodes, pancreas, and lungs.[95,117] CNS lesions are similar to those found in dogs. Granulomas may be present in intestines

*References: 41, 170, 190, 231, 318.

and mesenteric lymph nodes. Tissue cysts in naturally infected cats have always been identified as *Toxoplasma* and not *Neospora*. Cholangiohepatitis, found in cats infected with *Toxoplasma*, has not been reported in any other host. The bile ducts are hyperplastic and plugged with desquamated bile duct epithelium and exudate. *T. gondii* schizonts (not tachyzoites) were seen in the biliary epithelium in both naturally occurring and experimentally induced disease.

Dogs

Grossly, necrosis is the predominant lesion, particularly in the brain, lung, liver, and mesenteric lymph nodes.[98] Pulmonic lesions consist of gray-white nodular foci up to 5 mm in diameter and are found in the subpleura and in the parenchyma. The bronchial lymph nodes are often enlarged and necrotic. Grossly visible necrotic foci are also seen in pancreas, liver, kidneys, and spleen. Multiple ulcers up to 10 mm in diameter are observed in the stomach and small intestines. In the CNS, areas of discoloration and necroses up to 12 mm in diameter and cerebellar atrophy have been observed.

Myositis involving the muscles of the limbs has been observed in dogs with *T. gondii* infections. The affected muscles are pale and reduced in mass and, in severe, chronic cases, are grossly replaced by connective tissue. Fibrosis and scarring are usually not as prominent as those occurring with neosporosis (see later discussion).

Microscopically, pulmonic lesions consist of fibrinous exudation and necrosis involving alveolar walls, blood vessels, and bronchioles. The alveolar lumina are filled with fibrin and occasionally with lymphocytes, neutrophils, and eosinophils. The alveolar lining and terminal epithelial cells are hypoplastic and infiltrated with lymphocytes, plasma cells, and multinucleated giant cells. Necrosis, the predominant muscular lesion, involves myofibers, small blood vessels, and surrounding connective tissues. Necrotic myofibers are replaced by fibrosis. Neural lesions consist of necrosis, gliosis, and vasculitis and are characteristic of multifocal nonsuppurative meningoencephalomyelitis. Lesions seen early in blood vessels consist of endothelial cell proliferation, necrosis, and perivascular cuffing. Neuronal necrosis, mild malacia, and some astrocytosis may be seen. Multifocal leptomeningeal infiltrates of macrophages, plasma cells, and some lymphocytes and neutrophils are found. In dogs with *T. gondii* polymyositis, noninflammatory degenerative changes are observed in peripheral nerves and nerve roots. Immunoperoxidase staining can be used to demonstrate *T. gondii* definitively in tissues to distinguish it from *N. caninum*. Electron microscopy can also be used for this purpose.[315]

Therapy

Available drugs usually suppress replication of *T. gondii* and are not completely effective in killing the parasite. Dosages for these drugs are summarized in Table 80-3.

Clindamycin is the drug of choice for treating clinical toxoplasmosis in dogs and cats.[147,202] Because of clindamycin's good intestinal absorption, oral and parenteral dosages are similar. Clindamycin dosages for treating toxoplasmosis are greater than those for treating anaerobic infections for which the drug is marketed.

Clinical signs of systemic illness usually begin to resolve within 24 to 48 hours after institution of therapy. Appetite improves, hyperesthesia disappears, and fever usually subsides. Lower motor neuron deficits and muscle atrophy may take weeks to resolve in animals with polymyositis. Clindamycin has been effective in crossing the blood-brain and bloodvascular barriers in *Toxoplasma*-infected animals and people. Neurologic deficits improve, but signs may not totally resolve because of permanent damage caused by CNS inflammation. Active chorioretinitis generally subsides within 1 week. Some

Table • 80-3

Therapy for Toxoplasmosis

DRUG[a]	SPECIES	DOSAGE (mg/kg)[b]	ROUTE	INTERVAL (HOURS)	DURATION (WEEKS)
Extraintestinal Cycle (Systemic Infection)					
Clindamycin	D	3—13[c]	PO, IM	8	4
	D	10—20	PO, IM	12	4
	C	8—17	PO, IM	8	4
	C	10—12.5	PO, IM	12	4
Sulfonamides[d]	B	30	PO	12	4
and					
Pyrimethamine[e]		0.25—0.5	PO	12	4
Trimethoprim-sulfonamide	C	15	PO	12	4
Enteroepithelial Cycle (Oocyst Shedding by Cats)					
Clindamycin	C	50	PO, IM	24	1—12
	C	12.5—25	PO, IM	12	1—2
Sulfonamides[d]	C	100	PO	24	1—2
and					
Pyrimethamine[e]		2.0	PO	24	1—2
Monensin	C	[f]	PO	24	1—2
Toltrazuril	C	5—10	PO	24	2

D, Dog; *C*, cat; *B*, dog and cat; *PO*, by mouth; *IM*, intramuscular

[a]See Appendix 8, Drug Formulary, for more information on these drugs.
[b]Dose per administration at specified interval. See Therapy, in text, for other drugs being investigated to treat systemic infections.
[c]Use proportionally higher doses per kilogram in small (<5 kg) dogs.
[d]Twice this dosage is used if sulfonamides are used alone.
[e]Available only in 25-mg tablets. For proper dosing of cats, must be divided. More effective than trimethoprim.
[f]Mixed as 0.02% (w/w) concentration in dry weight of food.

cases of anterior segment inflammation thought to be from toxoplasmosis have resolved with the administration of clindamycin alone.[49,202] However, because intraocular inflammation commonly leads to lens luxation and glaucoma, cats with anterior segment inflammation should be treated with topical, oral, or injectable glucocorticoids (see Toxoplasmosis, Chapter 93). Antiinflammatory doses of glucocorticoids are not likely to exacerbate systemic disease, although treating first with topical antiinflammatory therapy in conjunction with systemic clindamycin is better.[62,195] Clindamycin, given by itself early in the course of acute experimental infection of cats, caused increased inflammatory reaction and tumor necrosis factor-α levels.[64] These effects have not been substantiated in naturally infected cats and may be related to the increased killing of actively replicating parasites, decreased IgM titer development, or decreased phagocytic activity caused by the drug. Cats with concurrent FIV infections do not respond as well as FIV-naïve cats to therapy.

Oral clindamycin can cause anorexia, vomiting, and diarrhea in dogs and cats, especially at higher doses.[148] These side effects appear to be related to local GI irritation because parenteral therapy at similar doses does not cause them in the same animals. The side effects stop soon after the dose is reduced or therapy is discontinued. *Clostridium difficile* overgrowth has not been documented in dogs and cats as it has been in people treated with clindamycin (see Drug Formulary, Appendix 8, and Macrolides and Lincosamides, Chapter 34).

Although less suitable compared with clindamycin, the combination of pyrimethamine and rapid-acting sulfonamides, such as sulfadiazine, sulfamethazine, sulfamerazine, and triple sulfas, is synergistic in the therapy of systemic toxoplasmosis. Pyrimethamine has greater efficacy than trimethoprim has when used in combination. Because mental depression, anemia, leukopenia, and thrombocytopenia from bone marrow suppression develop rapidly in antifolate-treated cats compared with dogs, frequent hematologic monitoring is required, especially if therapy lasts longer than 2 weeks. Although trimethoprim-sulfonamide crosses the blood-brain barrier well, it has been reported to be ineffective in treating a dog with severe uveitis and optic neuritis.[103]

Bone marrow suppression can often be corrected with the addition of folinic acid (5.0 mg/day) or brewer's yeast (100 mg/kg/day) to the animal's diet. Baker's yeast, which contains folic acid, is inexpensive and as effective as is folinic acid. The parasite uses preformed folic acid better than does folinic acid. Nevertheless, pyrimethamine and sulfonamides inhibit folic–folinic acid metabolism in *T. gondii* to a greater extent than it does in the mammalian cell; therefore supplementation with folic acid does not completely reverse therapeutic efficacy when used in combination with pyrimethamine and sulfonamides.

Doxycycline and minocycline have been shown to be effective in vitro and in vivo in experimental infections in mice and on cerebral toxoplasmosis in people,[246] and they have been used to treat related intestinal coccidiosis. Doxycycline and minocycline might be considered when side effects are noted with clindamycin or antifolates or with co-infections of other pathogens that are susceptible to the tetracyclines.

Several new drugs, such as trimetrexate and piritrexim (antifolates), roxithromycin (a macrolide), atovaquone (a hydroxynaphthoquinone), and arprinocid (a purine analog and an anticoccidial drug), have been effective in treating experimental toxoplasmosis in mice,[302] but they have limited availability for clinical use in cats or dogs. Azithromycin and clarithromycin are newer macrolides that are licensed for human use and show in vitro and in vivo activity against *T. gondii*[70] (see Drug Formulary, Appendix 8). The combination of pyrimethamine and azithromycin was as effective as pyrimethamine and sulfadiazine was in treating ocular toxoplasmosis in people with the advantage of fewer side effects.[33] Trioxane derivatives have been shown to be effective against *T. gondii* in vitro. Spiramycin, used in Europe for prevention of transplacental transmission of *Toxoplasma*, has not been as effective in treating postnatally infected people.

In addition to pyrimethamine-sulfonamide combinations, pyrimethamine has been administered in combination with clindamycin or dapsone. Limited clinical and experimental studies have shown synergy with azithromycin-pyrimethamine, clarithromycin-minocycline, clarithromycin or azithromycin and sulfonamides, and atovaquone with pyrimethamine or sulfonamides.[8,346] Biologic response modifiers such as INF-γ have been given synergistically in combination therapy with antimicrobials.[9]

Oocyst Shedding in Cats

Oocyst shedding has been partially controlled only when high doses of pyrimethamine and sulfonamide have been provided (see Table 80-3). Oocyst excretion also has been reduced by the doses of clindamycin recommended for systemic chemotherapy.

Monensin, an anticoccidial drug used in poultry and cattle feeds, is effective in suppressing oocyst shedding when placed in dry cat food within 1 to 2 days PI. It did not prevent infected cats from developing immunity against shedding of oocysts in subsequent exposure to *Toxoplasma*. Toxicity in cats was not noted when the drug was fed for extended periods, despite its known tendency to produce a myopathy in dogs and horses. Toltrazuril has been highly effective when given on a daily basis in preventing oocyst shedding after infection or reshedding after glucocorticoid-induced immunosuppression. These drugs may be beneficial in treating cats owned by pregnant women to reduce the risk of potential exposure of the fetuses to oocysts.

Prevention

Preventing toxoplasmosis in dogs and cats involves measures intended to reduce the incidence of feline infections and subsequent shedding of oocysts into the environment (see also Chapter 99). Kittens raised outdoors usually become infected shortly after they are weaned and begin to hunt. Cats should preferably be fed only dry or canned, commercially processed cat food. The prevalence of canine and feline toxoplasmosis has been higher in countries where raw meat products are fed to pets. Freezing or γ-ray irradiation can kill tissue cysts without affecting meat quality.[79,125] Household pets should be restricted from hunting and eating potential intermediate hosts or mechanical vectors, such as cockroaches, earthworms, and rodents. If meat is provided, it should always be thoroughly cooked, even if frozen before feeding.[311,348] Cats should be prevented from entering buildings where food-producing animals are housed or where feed storage areas are located. Toxoplasmosis has developed in people and experimental animals after transfusion of contaminated blood products, making donor screening an important consideration.

The development of protective immunity in toxoplasmosis appears to be strain or stage specific, or both.[253] An oral vaccine containing live bradyzoites of a mutant strain (T-263) was reported for reducing oocyst shedding by cats.[82,136,137] The vaccine strain itself does not produce oocyst shedding.[136] Although not commercially available, the value of a vaccine for cats would be to reduce the environmental contamination in areas of human habitation and food production. In actual and experimental modelings, vaccination of cats living on commercial swine farms reduced oocyst shedding of the resident cats and significantly reduced the *T. gondii* seroprevalence of finishing pigs.[236,237]

Public Health Considerations

Worldwide, nearly 500 million people have *T. gondii* antibodies. The seroprevalence of *T. gondii* is highest (approaching 100%) in warm, moist, or tropical climates and lowest in the arid and the frigid regions of the world.[93,327] In the United States, prevalence is highest in the East and in the Appalachian Mountain regions and is lowest in the southwestern arid regions and northwestern mountain regions. Approximately 25% to 50% of people tested in the United States have antibodies to *Toxoplasma*.

People become infected with *T. gondii* by ingesting viable cysts in raw or undercooked meat or by ingesting oocysts shed in the feces of a recently infected cat. In the United States, estimates are that at least 50% of acquired infections are associated with ingestion of meat.[43,291] Oocyst-induced infections in people may be more severe than those acquired from ingestion of tissue cysts.[91a] Water-borne outbreaks can occur sporadically related to contamination of water supplies by domestic or wild cat feces.[7] Transplacental infection of the fetus occurs via tachyzoite spread when a pregnant woman is infected for the first time. The rate of congenital infection varies among countries, being higher in continental Europe and South America than in North America.[93] The fetus can become infected from an immunocompromised or human immunodeficiency virus–infected woman who is also chronically infected with *Toxoplasma*. The fetus is affected most severely when infection takes place during the first half of gestation. Retinochoroiditis is the primary clinical disease in congenitally infected children. Prenatal detection of fetal infection and treatment of the pregnant mother have greatly reduced the morbidity of disease in newborn infants.

Clinical disease in postnatally infected people is similar to that in other infected intermediate hosts, such as dogs.[134] Postnatally acquired infections are generally asymptomatic and self-limiting, usually persisting 1 to 12 weeks. Such infections with persistent or recurrent lymphadenomegaly may resemble infectious mononucleosis or Hodgkin's disease and are usually not fatal unless the host is severely immunosuppressed and the infection becomes disseminated. Reactivation of chronic latent (encysted) infection also is possible. Reactivated disease has been seen in patients with acquired immunodeficiency syndrome (AIDS) when *Toxoplasma* encephalitis is the predominant illness.[22] *Toxoplasma* encephalitis also occurs in non-AIDS immunosuppressed people. High-dose trimethoprim-sulfonamide has been used to reduce the risk for development of CNS inflammation.[288] Many studies have linked *T. gondii* infections in people to neuropsychiatric disorders and decreased psychomotor performance.[154] In particular, a link has been made with a high prevalence of *T. gondii*–specific serum antibodies or strong correlation of obtaining a cat during childhood in people with schizophrenia.[331] However, these studies have been serologic; one examining the presence of *T. gondii* by PCR of cortical brain tissue from psychiatric patients was not incriminating.[56]

Ingestion of undercooked meat, or contamination of uncooked foods by cutting boards used to prepare raw meat, is a common source of *Toxoplasma* infection for people. On farms housing food-producing animals, cat populations should be controlled, and pigs should be reared on concrete or indoors when feasible.[342] In France, where eating undercooked meat and toxoplasmosis is prevalent, exposure to undercooked beef, cat ownership, consumption of raw vegetables, and eating undercooked lamb were found to be risk factors, in decreasing order, for infection in pregnant women.[17] Although people generally become infected by ingesting bradyzoite-infected meat,[52,230,348] ingestion of raw goat's milk may be an additional source of human toxoplasmosis. Laboratory accidents, blood transfusions, and organ transplants are additional sources of infection.

Oocyst survival is an important determinant of the distribution and maintenance of the disease in nature.[122,211] Oocysts, which are shed by cats, contaminate the environment and are ingested by herbivorous animals, which subsequently infect carnivorous animals higher in the food chain, such as people. Sporulated oocysts can survive up to 18 months during unfavorable environmental conditions and are resistant to most disinfectants. Even unsporulated oocysts can survive for at least 11 weeks at refrigerated temperatures.[212] Dogs that eat cat feces may also act as transport vectors for sporulated oocysts as they will shed these sporulated oocysts in their feces for 2 days after ingesting them.[218]

Although oocysts are key in the epidemiology of toxoplasmosis, in most studies, no direct correlation has been found between toxoplasmosis in adults and cat ownership (see Chapter 99).* Studies showing seroconversion during pregnancy have independently linked the consumption of under cooked meat and soil contact through gardening or eating unwashed vegetables with primary infection.[185a] In one study, veterinary staff in Canada, which regularly handled cats, did not have a high prevalence of serum IgG reactive to *T. gondii*.[304] In another serologic survey, prevalence of serum antibodies to *T. gondii* were 5.2% for children living in rural environments and 1.1% among those in urban areas.[269] Seroprevalence increased with age in both groups, and cat ownership was associated with seropositivity in rural but not urban children. Rural children in a household with more cats had a much greater risk of exposure. These differences may relate to the health habits of children and the contrasting defecation habits of rural versus urban cats.

Given that individual cats provide human emotional health benefits and are not a direct risk factor for acquiring toxoplasmosis where good hygiene is practiced, relinquishing them is unnecessary.[5,340] Most cats become infected from carnivorous behavior soon after weaning and shed oocysts for only short periods (under 3 weeks) thereafter. Cats found to be shedding *T. gondii* oocysts should be hospitalized for this period and treated to eliminate shedding, particularly when a pregnant woman is present in the household. To prevent inadvertent environmental contamination, cat owners, and especially childbearing-aged women, should practice proper hygienic measures on a routine basis. Because infected cats rarely have diarrhea, and they groom themselves regularly, direct fecal exposure from handling infected cats is unlikely. Oocysts were not detected in fur of cats that had shed large numbers of *T. gondii* oocysts.[80]

Litter boxes should be changed daily because at least 24 hours are usually necessary for oocysts to reach the infective stage. Oocyst sporulation depends on environmental temperature (Table 80-4). Unsporulated oocysts are more susceptible to disinfection and environmental destruction; therefore control efforts should be directed at this stage. Litter pans should be disinfected with scalding water. Cat feces should be discarded in the septic system, incinerated, or sealed tightly in a plastic bag before placing in a sanitary landfill. Only organic litters that are biodegradable should be placed in the septic system. High-temperature composting to kill oocysts remains to be proved. Under no circumstances should litter boxes be dumped into the environment.

Oocysts survive best in warm, moist soil, a factor that helps explain the high prevalence of disease in temperate and tropical climates. Nonsporulated oocysts kept at 0° to 4° C survive and are viable for sporulation and infecting cats for at least 11

*References: 17, 57, 176, 250, 274, 320.

Table • 80-4

Effects of Temperature on Toxoplasma Oocyst Sporulation

TEMPERATURE	DAYS
23.8° C (75.8° F)	1–3
15° C (59° F)	5–8
11° C (51.8° F)	21

weeks.[212] They also withstand exposure to constant freezing temperature, drying, and high environmental temperature up to 18 months or more, especially if they are covered and out of direct sunlight. A cat's natural instinct to bury or hide its feces provides the protected environment for oocyst survival. Children's sandboxes should be covered to prevent cats from defecating in them. Mechanical vectors, such as sowbugs, earthworms, and houseflies, have been shown to contain oocysts, and cockroaches and snails are additional mechanical vectors. Control of these invertebrates will help reduce the spread of infection.

Dogs that commonly roll in foreign feces were examined for their potential to act as mechanical vectors for oocysts. Oocyst sporulation did not occur when cat feces were placed on the skin and fur of dogs kept at 19° C to 22° C (66° F to 71.6° F) and 40% to 100% relative humidity.[218]

Sporulated oocysts resist most disinfectants, and only 10% ammonia is effective when it is in contact with contaminated surfaces for 10 minutes. Because of the time required for chemical disinfection and the fumes produced by ammonia, immersing litter pans in boiling or scalding water is usually the easiest means of disinfection. Steam cleaning can decontaminate hard, impervious surfaces.

Outbreaks of human infections have been reported when oocyst-contaminated dust particles were inhaled or ingested.[7,23,329] Dispersion of oocysts can also occur by earth-moving or cultivating equipment, shoes, animal feet, wind, rain, and fomites. Streams can become contaminated via water runoff. Stray and wild cats have been known to contaminate streams. Water from streams or ponds should always be boiled before drinking. Heating utensils to 70° C (158° F) for at least 10 minutes will kill oocysts.

Prevention of human toxoplasmosis involves avoiding exposure of susceptible hosts, which includes the unborn fetus and immunosuppressed adult. Risk of exposure by contact with infected meat can be avoided by cooking all meat to an internal temperature greater than 67° C (152.6°F) (Table 80-5). Microwaving does not kill all *T. gondii* because of uneven heating.[230] Gamma-ray irradiation at doses of 5 centigray has been effective.[125] Freezing of meat in home freezers (−12° C) (152° F) for at least 24 hours is an effective method for killing organisms. Good personal hygiene dictates that hands be thoroughly washed after handling raw meat. Animal care technicians who clean cat cages should wear masks and protective clothing.

T. GONDII—LIKE INFECTION OF CATS

T. gondii is thought to be a single species despite its widespread host range. An unidentified, structurally different, *Toxoplasma*-like parasite has been found in five cats with systemic or neurologic manifestations, or both, that might be confused with toxoplasmosis.[97,100,120] Fever and multisystemic signs had been present in some cats, and some had predominant signs

Table • 80-5

Survival of Toxoplasma

CONDITIONS	MAXIMAL SURVIVAL TIME
Bradyzoites	
–3° C (26.6° F)	3 weeks
–6° C (21.2° F)	11 days
50° C (122° F)	20 min
58° C (136° F)	10 min
61° C (142° F)	4 min
64° C (147.2° F)	1 min
Oocysts	
Unsporulated	
–21° C (–5.8° F)	1 day
4° C (39° F)	30 days
37° C (98.6° F)	1 day
50° C (122° F)	10 min
Sporulated	
–20° C (–4° F)	28 days
50° C (122° F)	30 min
5% Ammonia	60 min

of cervical spinal cord injury, which are unusual for toxoplasmosis. In one cat with disseminated infection, hyperemic skin nodules were observed.[225a] Some reactivity was noted to *T. gondii* in serologic testing. In one cat in which CSF was examined, an elevated white blood cell count (117 cells/μl) and protein level (186 mg/μl) were present, and the cells were predominantly lymphocytes. Histologically, nonsuppurative inflammation was observed in many organs, including the CNS. Unlike lesions caused by *T. gondii*, many tissue cysts and free bradyzoites were present; tachyzoites in inflammatory lesions were lacking. The tissue cysts were larger than those of *T. gondii*, they had thinner walls, and, ultrastructurally, they had micronemes arranged in rows. Although not evaluated, treatment would likely be similar to that of toxoplasmosis. The significance of this parasite awaits elucidation of its life cycle and host range.

T. GONDII–LIKE CUTANEOUS INFECTION OF DOGS

A 6-year-old female Great Dane dog from Rio de Janeiro, Brazil, died from chronic illness caused by an *Ehrlichia*–like organism.[121] As a co-infection in this dog, numerous apicomplexan parasites were found in dermal lesions. The protozoan reacted with polyclonal anti-*T. gondii* sera but not with *Neospora caninum* or *Sarcocystis neurona* antibodies. Ultrastructurally, the protozoa had schizont-like structures, with merozoites arranged around a prominent residual body, and the merozoites had several rhoptries with electron-dense contents. In contrast, *T. gondii* tachyzoites are electron lucent, and a residual body is not found in groups of tachyzoites.

NEOSPOROSIS (*NEOSPORA CANINUM* INFECTION)

Etiology

N. caninum is a protozoan of the phylum Apicomplexa; before 1988, it had been confused with *T. gondii*.[92,97a,99] Its tachyzoites

and tissue cysts resemble those of *T. gondii* under light microscope. The domestic dog or the coyote (*Canis latrans*) is the definitive host and sheds oocysts following ingestion *N. caninum*–infected tissues (Fig. 80-16).[19,143b,219,241,242] The shedding period appears to be short and oocysts few. However, shedding in some instances has been documented up to 4 months by both visual inspection and PCR methods.[242] Detecting oocysts in naturally and experimentally infected wild canids has been unsuccessful.[3,221] Cats are not definitive hosts because they do not shed oocysts after consuming bradyzoites.[241] Antibodies to *N. caninum* have been detected in the sera of domestic cats from São Paulo, Brazil,[113] but the significance of this natural exposure is unknown. As with other coccidia, herbivores likely become infected by ingesting oocysts shed by the definitive host or by subclinical congenital infection from transplacental transmission or through ingestion of milk by neonates.[4] Canids can be experimentally infected by ingesting parasitized tissues from the intermediate herbivore hosts. Deer and cattle, whose carcasses may be preyed upon by dogs and coyotes, appear to be the intermediate hosts for *N. canium* infection. Larger numbers of oocysts are detected after feeding dogs infected tissues from cattle, the natural intermediate host, as compared with tissues from rodents.[124a,143] In naturally infected dogs, the predominant route of transmission is considered to be transplacental, and a clinical sign is often an exacerbation of congenitally acquired infection. Tachyzoites are 5 to 7 μm × 1 to 5 μm, depending on the stage of division (Fig. 80-17). They divide into two zoites by endodyogeny. In infected carnivores, tachyzoites are found within macrophages, polymorphonuclear cells, spinal fluid, and neural and other cells of the body. Individual organisms are ovoid, lunate, or globular. They contain one or two nuclei and are arranged singly, in pairs, or in groups of four or more. Cell necrosis occurs after rapid intracellular replication of tachyzoites. Widespread dissemination of tachyzoites to many organs may occur in the acute phases, with subsequent restriction by the host's immune response, to neural and muscular tissues in more chronically affected dogs.[13]

Nonseptate tissue cysts (up to 100 μm in diameter) are found mainly in neural cells (brain, spinal cord, peripheral nerves, and retina) and occasionally in muscles.[92,124a,270a] (Fig. 80-18). They may be round or elongated. The cyst wall is up to 4 μm thick and encloses slender, periodic acid-Schiff–positive bradyzoites.[92] Rupture of tissue cysts is associated with a granulomatous inflammatory reaction in the involved tissue.

Unsporulated oocysts (10 to 14 μm in diameter) are shed in dog feces 5 days or later after ingesting tissue cysts. Sporulation occurs after 24 to 72 hours outside the body. Sporulated oocysts contain two sporocysts each with four sporozoites.[219,241] Unlike the transient shedding associated with *T. gondii* infection in cats, *Neospora*-infected dogs may shed oocysts over an extended period of several months.[242] Susceptible hosts can become infected after ingesting food or water contaminated with *N. caninum* oocysts.

Epidemiology

Naturally occurring infections in dogs have been found throughout the world.[99,101,215,271] Seroprevalence of clinically healthy dogs is usually much less than 20% but much greater than the prevalence of clinical illness, suggesting subclinical infections.[220,334] Purebred dogs, especially German shorthaired pointers, Labrador retrievers, boxers, golden retrievers, basset hounds, and greyhounds, have been noticeably prevalent in published case reports.[215,293] Seroprevalence in canids also varies according to geographic location and whether domestic or wild populations are examined.[11,58] In the same geographic area, feral dogs have a higher prevalence rate of *N. caninum* serum antibody reactivity than do owned dogs.[9a,141] Dogs being fed raw meat have a much higher prevalence of

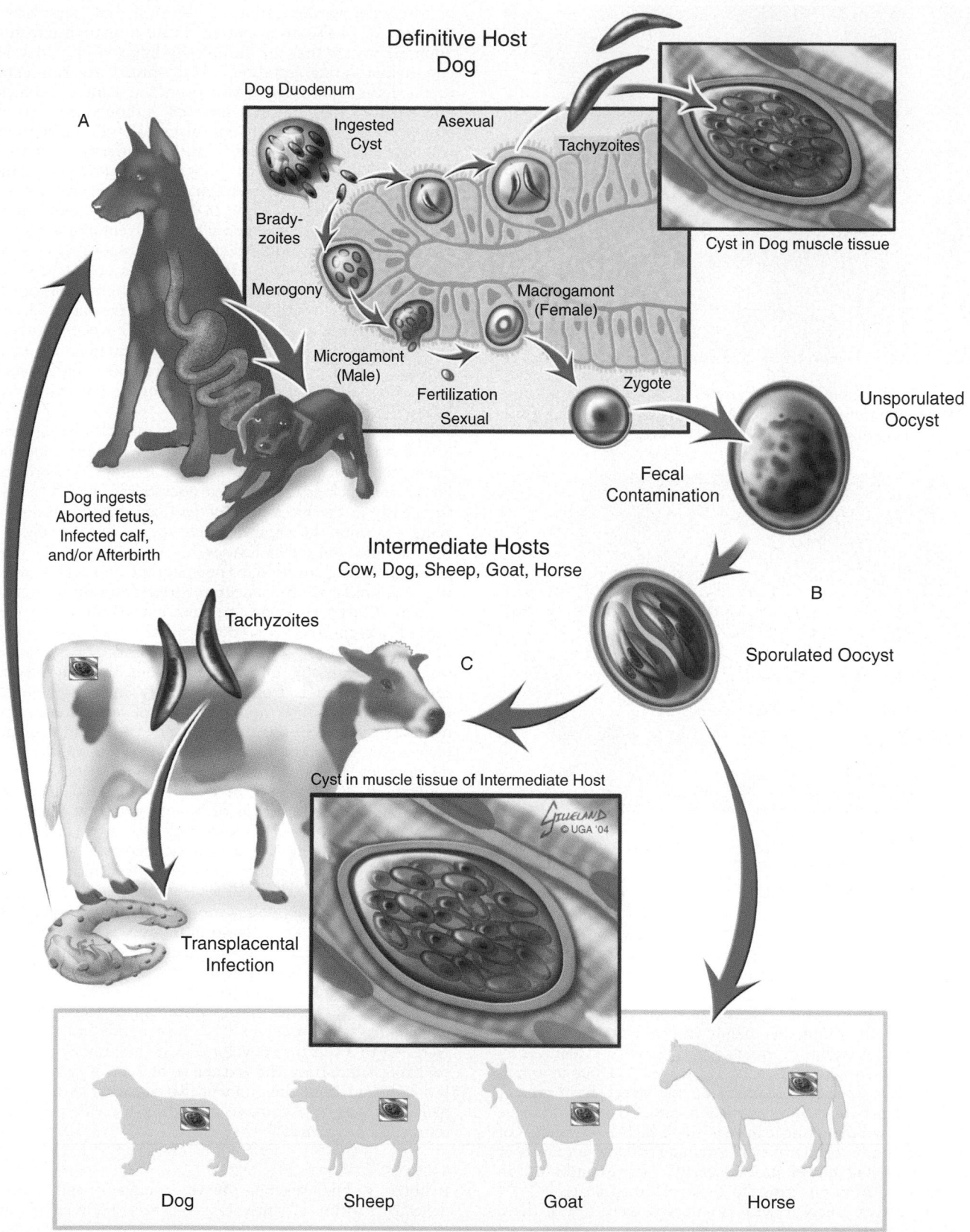

Fig 80-16 Life cycle of *N. caninum*. **A,** Following ingestion of tissue cysts, some bradyzoites transform to tachyzoites with systemic spread resulting in encystment in neural and muscle tissues. In the intestine, enteroepithelial replication also occurs with merogony leading to the development of gamonts and a zygote. **B,** Oocysts are shed unsporulated in the stool. **C,** Once mature and infectious, sporulated oocysts are ingested by a variety of herbivores. Organisms spread from the intestine as tachyzoites and encyst in muscle and nervous tissues. Spread to reproductive tissues often results in abortion. The tissues of the fetus or the infected intermediate host are ingested by a new definitive host and the cycle continues. (Courtesy University of Georgia, Athens, Ga.)

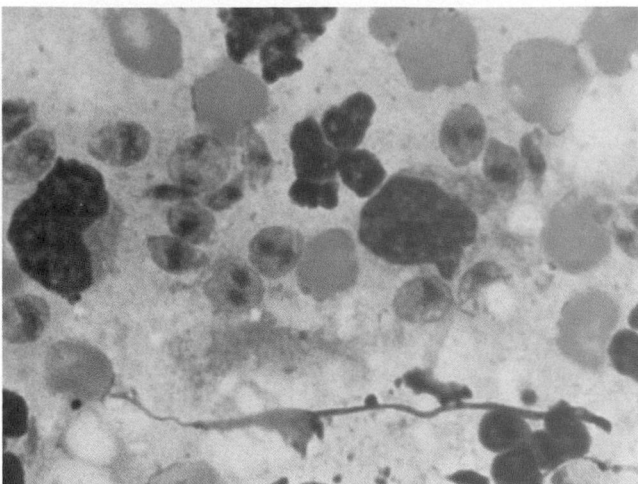

Fig 80-17 Numerous tachyzoites of *N. caninum* in a smear of an ulcer in the skin of a dog. Dividing tachyzoites *(arrows)* are thicker than nondividing tachyzoites (Giemsa, ×750).

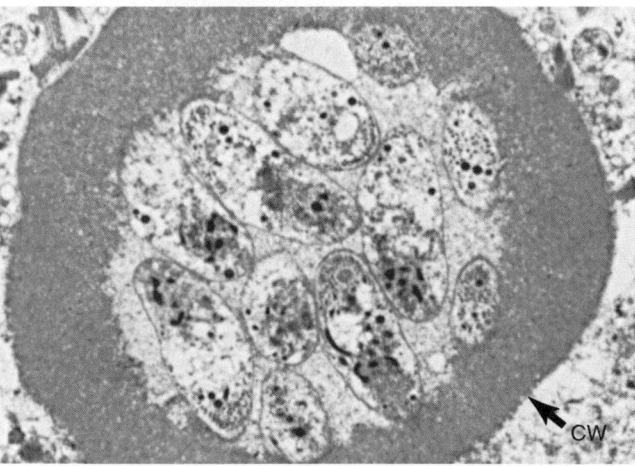

Fig 80-18 Transmission electron micrograph of a tissue cyst of *N. caninum* in the brain of a dog. Note the thick cyst wall *(CW)* and bradyzoites (×9939).

reactive antibody than do dogs on commercial diets.[185,242] Serologic prevalence is also greater in farm dogs as compared with urban dogs.[6,295,298] A strong statistical association has been found between infections in dairy herds and the presence and density of dogs on farms.[264a] Serologic studies suggest that dogs may acquire their infection mainly via horizontal transmission from ingesting tissues of infected herbivores as evidenced by the increase in seroprevalence with age.[11,45] Dogs in urban areas, which were free roaming on the street, have greater seroprevalence than do companion pets.[45] Dogs that have been fed raw bovine meat have a much higher prevalence of serum antibody reactivity to *N. caninum*.[185] Dogs on farms or dairy farms had higher prevalence of reactive antibodies in serum to *N. caninum* than did those in urban areas.[179,347,341a] In comparative analysis with uninfected dairy farms, those with established infection in cows had dogs consuming vaginal discharges, aborted materials, or milk from cows, and where dogs defecated in the food or feeding alleys.[72,73] Introduction of a previously infected dog onto a farm may also precipitate infection in a herd.[73] Ingestion of infected calf tissues appears to increase the numbers of oocysts shed compared with numbers produced following ingestion of infected mice.[143] Experimental transmission in dogs has been produced by oral or parenteral administration of *Neospora*, but transplacental transmission is also an important route in natural infections. Suppositions are that the chronically infected bitch develops parasitemia during gestation, which spreads transplacentally to the fetus. Successive litters from the same subclinically infected dam may be born infected, although perhaps at a reduced rate.[106a] However, transplacental transmission alone will not be able to propagate *N. caninum* infection in nature.[15] The majority of, but not all, puppies in a litter have clinical manifestations.[107] Other pups may carry the infection subclinically with reactivation. In contrast to toxoplasmosis, underlying immunodeficiencies or concurrent illnesses are not always apparent in adult dogs with neosporosis. However, reactivation of infection causing cutaneous, neural, or muscular disease has occurred following immunosuppressive illnesses or administration of modified live virus vaccines, cytotoxic agents, or glucocorticoids.[261] Glucocorticoids can also increase the shedding period and number of oocysts excreted by dogs.[219] With new awareness and available serotesting, postnatal infections are being recognized with increasing frequency.[242]

Infection in the intermediate hosts may also be important in maintenance of the disease in nature. This infection has a major economic impact for the cattle industry worldwide. Herbivores such as cattle ingest oocysts that have been shed transiently in the feces of infected dogs. After ingestion and acute exposure, the organism may spread systemically, cross the placenta, and infect fetuses, resulting in sporadic or epidemic infertility, abortion, or neonatal infection. This circumstance is similar to the concern of toxoplasmosis in pregnant women with oocyst exposure from cats. Point source exposure of neosporosis in a cattle herd has been linked to introduction of a dog.[73] Once cattle are infected, *N. caninum* spreads endemically in the herd from the transplacental spread of infection from congenitally infected heifers to their offspring. Calves up to 1 week of age can be experimentally infected by ingesting milk or colostrum containing tachyzoites, but lactogenic transmission is not considered epidemiologically important.[67,190] By these routes, successive generations of cows in a herd remain infected. Dogs shed oocysts following ingestion of bovine placental tissue from *N. caninum* seropositive cows but not after ingestion of colostrum containing *N. caninum* tachyzoites.[74]

Naturally occurring infections have been reported worldwide in domesticated animals such as dogs, cattle, sheep, goats, horses, water buffalo, and camels. *N. caninum* antibodies or infection have also been found in numerous wild canids (red and grey foxes, dingoes, coyotes) and their prey (deer, rhinoceros). A sylvatic transmission cycle likely exists that has evolved over time and maintains the infection in nature.[143a,337a] Dogs fed CNS tissues from white tailed deer (*Odocoileus virginianus*) shed oocysts.[143a] Subsequently, these oocysts were fed to a calf that developed a high antibody titer to *N. caninum*, supporting the existence of such a sylvatic cycle. Isolated dogs from the Amazon River region in Brazil have had antibodies to *Neospora*, indicating its widespread environmental prevalence.[45]

Clinical Findings

Rabbits, gerbils, pigeons, foxes, monkeys, and raccoons develop subclinical infections with experimental infection.[86,244] Mice, rats, pigs, and domestic cats are also susceptible experimentally and show illness.[91,110,111] A predominant manifestation in herbivores is abortion. Neonatal death and in utero mortality may result, depending on when infection occurs during pregnancy. Infection has been transmitted from mother to fetus in cattle, sheep, goats, mice, dogs, cats, monkeys, and pigs.[87] Lactogenic transmission has been experimentally proven in cattle.[335] *N. caninum* or another species of *Neospora*,

N. hughesi, has also been identified as a less common cause of equine protozoal myelitis than is *Sarcocystis neurona*.[115,232,233]

Dogs

Likely, many dogs diagnosed with toxoplasmosis before 1988 actually had neosporosis. In general, clinical findings in dogs are similar to those of toxoplasmosis, but neurologic deficits and muscular abnormalities predominate (Table 80-6). Clinical signs may also include those of hepatic, pulmonary, and myocardial involvement, but any tissue can become involved. Both pups and older dogs are clinically affected, and the infections can be transmitted congenitally. Experimental studies suggest that *N. caninum* can cause early fetal death, mummification, resorption, and birth of weak pups.[111] Although abortion is a major feature of the disease in cattle, no reports of abortion in dogs have been produced.

Puppies Younger Than 6 Months The most severe (disseminated) and frequent infections have been in young (under 6 months) dogs that showed ascending paralysis of the limbs. In the youngest pups, signs are often noticed beginning at 3 to 9 weeks of age. Features that distinguish neosporosis from other forms of paralysis are gradual muscle atrophy and stiffness, usually as an ascending paralysis; the pelvic limbs are more severely affected than are the thoracic limbs. Paralysis progresses to rigid contracture of muscles of affected limbs (Fig. 80-19). This arthrogryposis is a result of the scar formation in the muscles from lower motor neuron damage and myositis. In some pups, joint deformation and genu recurvatum may develop. Cervical weakness, dysphagia, megaesophagus, and ultimately death occur. In some dogs, the progression may become static. Dogs do not develop severe intracranial manifestations and maintain alert attitudes. They can survive for months with hand feeding and care but remain paralyzed with associated complications.

Dogs Older Than 6 Months Older dogs most likely become ill from reactivation of a chronic subclinical infection. They often have signs of multifocal CNS involvement with or without polymyositis; less common manifestations result from myocarditis, dermatitis, pneumonia, or multifocal dissemination. These latter syndromes usually result from more widespread dissemination with spread of tachyzoites. Cutaneous neosporosis has been most common in dogs that become immunosuppressed from concurrent illnesses or drug therapy.[261,326] Should a dog be examined with concurrent signs of multifocal CNS disease and myositis such as hyperesthesia, muscle swelling or atrophy, and increased creatine kinase activity, then neosporosis should be highly considered. Death from diffuse CNS or muscle inflammation can occur in dogs of any age.

Cats

N. caninum can induce a fatal infection in experimentally inoculated cats.[114] The infection is most severe in prenatally and neonatally infected kittens. Subclinical disease was found in adult cats. These cases were more severe and acute when the cats were immunosuppressed with glucocorticoids. As in dogs, encephalomyelitis, polymyositis, and hepatitis are the predominant lesions. Natural clinical infections have not been documented, although antibodies to *N. caninum* have been reported in domestic and wild felids.

Diagnosis

Hematologic and biochemical findings have been variable, depending on the organ system of involvement. With muscle disease, creatine kinase and AST activities have been increased. Serum ALT and ALP activities are increased in dogs that develop hepatic inflammation. CSF abnormalities have

---

Table • 80-6

Clinical Features of Canine Neosporosis

PUPS (<6 MONTHS)

Ascending LMN Rigid Paralysis to Tetraparesis (polymyositis, radiculitis, encephalomyelitis)[10,14,53,60,103a,106a,124a,133,156,173,175,271,281,284,336,337,343]

 Disseminated infection in many tissues
 Variable CNS signs
  Monoparesis or paraparesis to tetraparesis
  Can progress to paralysis
 Signs of myositis
  Muscle atrophy
  Rigid hyperextension
  Hyperesthesia
  Incontinence
  Respiratory muscle paralysis
  Cranial muscle paralysis (cranial myositis)
  Dysphagia
  Trismus
  Glossal paralysis

DOGS (>6 MONTHS)

LMN Flaccid Paralysis (regional or generalized myositis in older dogs)[147,227,337]

 Lameness and focal hyperesthesia
 Acute flaccid LMN signs
 Paraparesis to tetraparesis
 Diffuse hyperesthesia
 Muscle hypotonia

Central Nervous System Manifestations (meningitis, encephalomyelitis, cerebellitis)[14,46,97a,104,227,337]

 Paraparesis, tetraparesis, ataxia
 Tremors and ataxia (cerebellitis)[19a,46,97a,172,227]
 Head tilt
 Seizures
 Behavior changes
 Altered thirst
 Blindness, anisocoria (retinitis, choroiditis, optic neuritis)
 Horner's syndrome[34]
 Trigeminal neuropathy[239]

Systemic Signs

 Fever, dyspnea, cough (pneumonia)[149]
 Cardiac arrhythmias, sudden death
  (myocarditis)[14,175,252,243]
 Ulcerative, pruritic skin lesions (pyogranulomatous
  dermatitis)[33a,118,138,87,16,176,326]
 Regurgitation, megaesophagus (esophagitis,
  esophagomyositis)[14,106a]
 Fever, vomiting, icterus (pancreatitis, hepatitis)

LMN = lower motor neuron.

---

included mild increases in protein (over 20 but under 150 mg/dl) and nucleated cell (over 10 but under 100 cells/dl) concentrations. Differential leukocyte counts, in decreasing numbers, included lymphocytes, monocytes and macrophages, neutrophils, and eosinophils.[61,106a,266] CSF results can be within reference limits in some dogs.[156] Electromyographic abnormalities have consisted of spontaneous activity of fibrillation

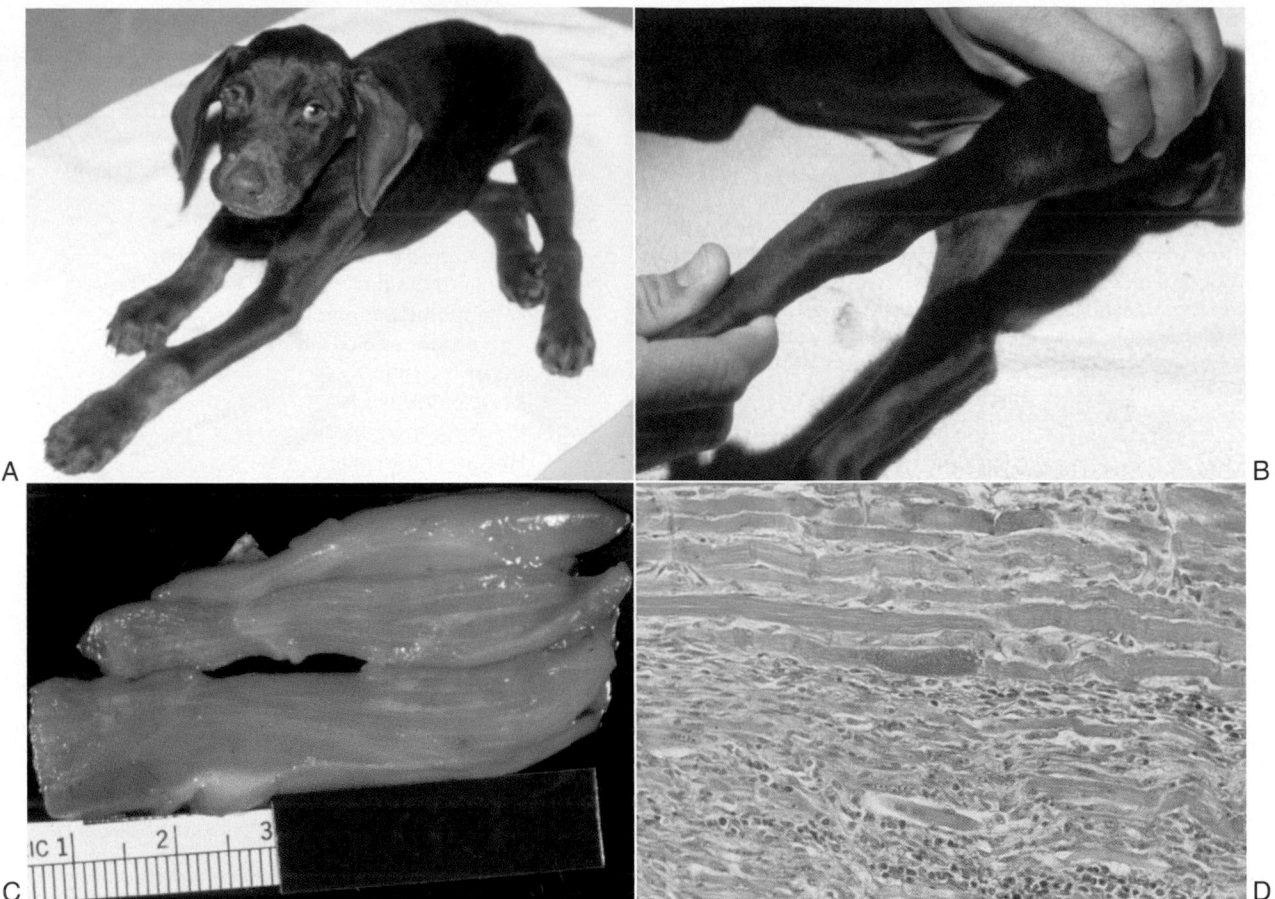

Fig 80-19 **A,** Three-month-old Doberman pinscher with tetraplegia. **B,** Atrophy and rigid contracture of the puppy's limbs are apparent. **C,** Gross and **(D)** microscopic appearances of muscle fibers in chronic myositis. A group of organisms *(arrow)* is shown in **D** (H and E stain, ×40). (Courtesy University of Georgia, Athens, Ga.)

potentials, positive sharp waves, and occasional repetitive discharges. Nerve conduction velocities may be reduced in the most severely affected limbs, especially proximally, but they are often within reference range. Low evoked action potentials may be found with myositis.

Serologic Testing

Demonstrating serum antibodies to *N. caninum* can help confirm the diagnosis of neosporosis. Assays have included indirect FA, ELISA, and immunoprecipitation.[106a,245,249,295] For indirect FA assays, serum is reacted with cell-cultured *N. caninum.* Serum indirect FA titer results can vary between laboratories; however, in one reference laboratory, values of 1:50 or greater are considered positive, and values are often greater than 1:800.[216] CSF can be tested, but titers are of lesser magnitude (1:50 to 1:800).[14] Positive titers can exist in previously exposed dogs that may be infected, but they remain nonsymptomatic, with values of 1:800 or greater for years. Indirect FA IgG titers in most species increase 1 to 2 weeks after infection.[112] Higher indirect FA results have been found in clinically versus subclinically affected dogs and in those with the longest duration of illness.[14] However, no correlation has been found between the magnitude of titer and clinical signs. Indirect FA titers appear to have high specificity at greater dilutions of sera; occasionally animals with histologically verified infections have low titer results.[99,103a,106a] Maternal antibodies may be passed from dam to offspring, making false-positive titers; however, these levels were gone in uninfected pups by day 32 of life.[106a]

Several ELISA methods are available to detect *N. caninum* antibodies. A direct agglutination test measuring IgG was as sensitive and specific as was an indirect FA test, with the advantage of being useful in a variety of host species.[289] Antibodies to *T. gondii* do not cross-react with *N. caninum* at dilutions of 1:50 or less; therefore serum or CSF antibody titers to *T. gondii* in *Neospora*-infected dogs are negative. Slight cross-reactivity with sera from dogs infected with *Babesia gibsoni* but not *B. canis* has been observed.[349] Some cross-reactivity has been observed with ELISA testing when crude extracts are used as antigens.[111] Some cross-reaction exists among cellular antigens of *T. gondii, H. heydorni,* and *N. caninum.*[213a,249] Western blots show four major antigens (17, 29, 30, and 37 kD) that appear to be specific for *Neospora.*[31]

Organism Detection

In canine feces, *N. caninum* oocysts are very similar in morphology to those of *Hammondia heydorni.*[300] Critical analysis has indicated that these are different species.[105] Immunologic cross-reactions may exist between other parasites and *N. caninum.* Tachyzoites can be found in aspirates or smears from any parasitized tissue or body fluid. With immunostaining, cross-reactions with *T. gondii* may be found in CSF or tissue aspirates and biopsies of some dogs and may be detected with any material used to stain blood films. Monoclonal antibodies have been developed for immunohistochemical staining that can distinguish between different organisms. Biopsy of affected muscle may yield a definitive diagnosis when organisms are detected.[249] Tachyzoites may be visualized in tissues, fluids, or cytopathologic samples. Muscle biopsy should be considered when serologic testing for neosporosis yields negative or inconclusive results but muscle disease is still suspected. *N. caninum* tachyzoites are similar to *T. gondii* tachyzoites by light microscopy (see Fig. 80-17) but can be differentiated by electron microscopy (Fig. 80-20). Tissue cysts of *N. caninum* have thicker walls than those of *T. gondii* (Fig. 80-21). *N. caninum* can be grown in cell culture and in mice. *N. caninum* must be distinguished from *T. gondii* in sections by immunochemical stains.[55] Structural differences can also be detected with transmission electron microscopy. *T. gondii* has a thinner cyst wall and fewer micronemes and rhoptries. PCR can be used to specifically detect *N. caninum* in biologic specimens and differentiate infection with other protozoa; however, the sensitivity has been lower relative to other diagnostic methods.[227a,310] PCR has also been used to differentiate *N. caninum* and *H. heydorni* oocysts in canine feces.[309,310,316,316a]

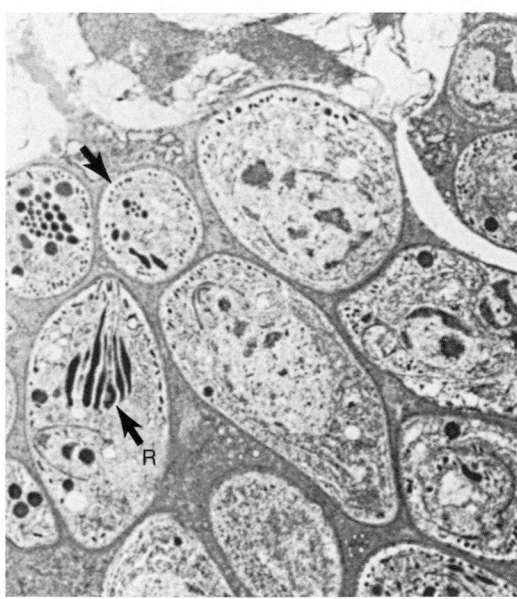

Fig 80-20 Several tachyzoites of *N. caninum* directly in the cytoplasm of a myelinated cell *(arrow)* in the spinal cord of a dog. Several tachyzoites are dividing into two by endodyogeny. Numerous electron-dense rhoptries *(R)* in tachyzoites distinguish *N. caninum* from *T. gondii* (×10,425).

The use of molecular genetics and PCR to distinguish *Neospora* from other related parasites has been reviewed.[111,316a]

Pathologic Findings

Gross lesions include multifocal streaks of necrosis, fibrosis, and mineralization of striated muscles, especially the diaphragm. Hepatomegaly, pneumonia, and discoloration of brain or spinal cord tissues may be apparent on cut section.

Pups with disseminated infection can have parasitic stages in the thymus, liver, kidney, stomach, adrenal, and skin, among other tissues. With respect to neural and muscular tissues, parasite-containing lesions are found in the muscles, heart, brain, spinal cord, nerve roots, and retina. Nonsuppurative encephalomyelitis, polyradiculoneuritis, ganglionitis, myositis (of all striated muscles), and myofibrosis are the predominant histologic findings (see Fig. 80-13). The radiculoneuritis is a more typical feature of infection in pups. The encephalomyelitis is characterized by inflammation, axonal degeneration, and formation of glial nodules in gray and white matter. Parasites are most consistently found in the cerebrum, regardless of the clinical presentation.[13] Cerebellar cortical necrosis and inflammation has been a predominant feature in some dogs.[29,146,172,227] Tissue cysts are present mainly in central or peripheral neural tissues, whereas tachyzoites are present in many tissues. Tissue cysts are often present, even in treated animals.[99,106a] Muscle lesions can range from focal necrosis to generalized inflammation of all skeletal muscles and esophageal and cardiac muscles. Inflammation and necrosis of other tissues also occur. Finding tachyzoites in lesions is diagnostic of infection. *N. caninum* appears to induce more inflammation compared with *T. gondii* and causes severe phlebitis and dermatitis. Nonsuppurative myocarditis, pneumonia, and hepatitis are commonly present as subclinical lesions. Lesions caused by *N. caninum* are similar to those caused by *T. gondii* or to granulomatous meningoencephalitis. Confirmation therefore requires serologic or immunohistochemical methods. Antibodies to *N. caninum* tachyzoites may offer more specific staining as antisera to bradyzoites may have some cross-reactivity with some antigens, such as BAG1, of *T. gondii*.

Therapy

Information on effective therapy for this disease is limited. However, drugs used in therapy for toxoplasmosis should be tried early in the course of illness. In vitro assays have shown activity of dihydrofolate reductase inhibitors (trimethoprim), ionophore antibiotics (monensin and salinomycin), macrolides

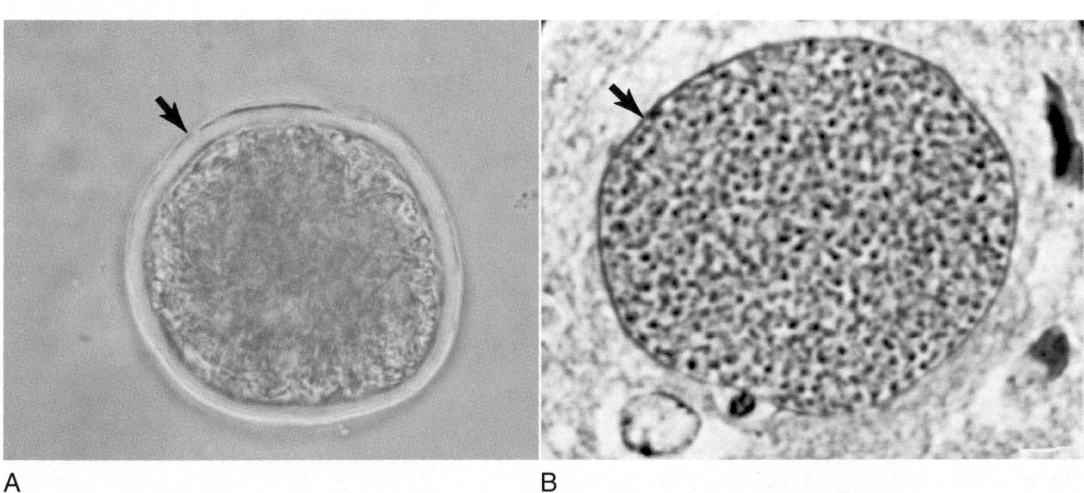

A   B

Fig 80-21 Comparison of tissue cysts of *N. caninum* from an unstained brain homogenate of a dog **(A)** and *T. gondii* **(B)** section of a brain of a mouse (H and E stain, ×750). The cyst wall *(arrows)* of *N. caninum* is thicker than that of *T. gondii*.

Table • 80-7

Drug Therapy for Neosporosis[a]

DRUG	SPECIES[a]	DOSE (mg/kg)[b]	ROUTE	FREQUENCY (HOURS)	DURATION (WEEKS)
Trimethoprim-sulfonamide	D	15—20	PO	12	4—8
		10—15	PO	8	4—8
Clindamycin[c]	D	7.5—15	PO, SC	8	4—8
		15—22	PO, SC	12	4—8
Pyrimethamine *and* sulfonamide[d]	D	1	PO	24	2—4
	D	15—30	PO	12	

D, Dog; *PO*, by mouth; *SC*, subcutaneous.
[a]For additional information on listed drugs, see Drug Formulary, Appendix 8.
[b]Dose per administration at specified interval.
[c]Also been used in combination with trimethoprim-sulfonamide or pyrimethamine.
[d]Can be substituted with trimethoprim-sulfonamide.

(azithromycin, clarithromycin, and erythromycin), tetracyclines (doxycycline and minocycline), and lincosamides (clindamycin).[213] Clindamycin, sulfadiazine, and pyrimethamine alone or in combination have been administered to treat canine neosporosis (Table 80-7).[14,106a,111] In neonates, clinical improvement is not likely in the presence of muscle contracture or rapidly advancing paralysis.[14,106a,111] To reduce the chance of illness, all dogs in an affected litter should be treated as soon as the diagnosis is made in one littermate. Older (over 16 weeks) puppies and adult dogs respond better to treatment.[14] In adult dogs with acute lower motor neuron paralysis from myositis, dysfunction is often more amenable to early treatment because scar contracture is less common.[147] Dermatitis and myositis have responded to therapy with clindamycin. With neurologic involvement, trimethoprim-sulfonamide or pyrimethamine and sulfonamide should be used because of better penetration of the CNS. No known therapy to prevent a bitch from transmitting infection to her pups is available. Clindamycin is effective in suppressing the replication and dissemination of tachyzoites but does not appear to be effective against encysted bradyzoites.[106a]

Prevention

In dogs, *N. caninum* can be transmitted repeatedly through successive litters and litters of their progeny. This tendency should be considered when planning the breeding of *Neospora*-infected bitches.[107] Dogs should not be fed uncooked meat, especially beef. On farms, dogs should not be allowed to feed on offal or aborted materials. They should be prevented, when possible, from defecating in feed troughs, watering sources, pastures, or livestock holding pens where cattle are housed. No vaccine has been developed to combat neosporosis. No drugs are known to prevent transplacental transmission.

Public Health Considerations

The zoonotic potential of *N. caninum* is unknown. Nonhuman primates can be experimentally infected.[163] There is no direct evidence that the organism can infect people, although serologic evidence suggests that people are exposed to the organism.[249,332] In examining sera from 76 women with a history of abortions, none had detectable serum antibodies to the parasite.[272] Serum samples from human agricultural workers and blood donors in Ireland had no measurable antibody reactivity to *N. caninum*.[145] Additional refinements and antigen purification may be needed in human serologic testing to clarify whether cross-reactivity or actual infection exists.

NEOSPOROSIS (*NEOSPORA HUGHESI* INFECTION)

Equine protozoal myeloencephalitis is caused predominantly by *Sarcocystis neurona* (see Chapter 80). *N. hughesi* has also been described as a cause of this disease.[232,233] *N. hughesi* is morphologically similar to, but ultrastructurally, antigenically, and genetically distinct from, *N. caninum*. Tissue cysts of *N. hughesi* are smaller compared with *N. caninum*, with thinner cyst walls. *N. caninum* has been described from infections in horses and antibodies to *N. caninum* have been found in horses.[87,151] Further molecular studies will be needed in future cases to determine which species is infecting the horse. Glucocorticoid-immunosuppressed dogs fed brains from experimentally infected mice that contained *N. hughesi* stages did not shed oocysts.[341] Dogs are likely not involved in the role of transmission of this infection, and another carnivore definitive host is likely.

SUGGESTED READINGS*

19. Basso W, Venturini L, Venturini MC, et al. 2001. First isolation of *Neospora caninum* from the feces of a naturally infected dog, *J Parasitol* 87:612-618.
22. Belanger F, Derouin F, Grangeot Keros L, et al. 1999. Incidence and risk factors of toxoplasmosis in a cohort of human immunodeficiency virus–infected patients: 1988-1995, *Clin Infect Dis* 28:575-581.
36. Brownlee L, Sellon RK. 2001. Diagnosis of naturally occurring toxoplasmosis by bronchoalveolar lavage in a cat, *J Am Anim Hosp Assoc* 37:251-255.
48. Cat Group. 2004. The Cat Group policy statement 6. Cats and toxoplasmosis: what are the risks? *J Feline Med Surg* 6:iii-vi.
69. DeFeo ML, Dubey JP, Mather TN, et al. 2002. Epidemiologic investigation of seroprevalence of antibodies to *Toxoplasma gondii* in cats and rodents, *Am J Vet Res* 63:1714-1717.
72. Dijkstra T, Barkema HW, Eysker M, et al. 2002. Natural transmission routes of *Neospora caninum* between farm dogs and cattle, *Vet Parasitol* 105:99-104.
91. Dubey JP. 2003. Review of *Neospora caninum* and neosporosis in animals, *Korean J Parasitol* 41:1-16.

*See the CD-ROM for a complete list of references.

185. Kramer L, DeRiso L, Tranquillo VM, et al. 2004. Analysis of risk factors associated with seropositivity to *Neospora caninum* in dogs, *Vet Rec* 154:692-693.
219. Lindsay DS, Dubey JP, Duncan RB. 1999. Confirmation that the dog is a definitive host for *Neospora caninum*, *Vet Parasitol* 82:327-333.
278. Powell CC, Brewer M, Lappin MR. 2001. Detection of *Toxoplasma gondii* in the milk of experimentally infected lactating cats, *J Vet Parasitol* 102:29-33.
301. Schatzberg SJ, Haley NJ, Barr SC, et al. 2003. Use of a multiplex polymerase chain reaction assay in the ante-

mortem diagnosis of toxoplasmosis and neosporosis in the central nervous system of cats and dogs, *Am J Vet Res* 64:1507-1513.
310. Šlapeta JR, Modrý D, Kyselová I, et al. 2002. Dog shedding oocysts of *Neospora caninum*: PCR diagnosis and molecular phylogenetic approach, *Vet Parasitol* 109:157-167.
319. Su C, Evans D, Cole RH, et al. 2003. Recent expansion of *Toxoplasma* through enhanced oral transmission, *Science* 299:414-416.

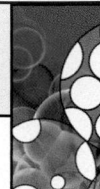

CHAPTER • 81

Enteric Coccidiosis

J. P. Dubey and Craig E. Greene

Coccidia are obligate intracellular parasites normally found in the intestinal tract. They belong to the phylum Apicomplexa, class Sporozoasida, order Eucoccidiorida, and depending on the species, family *Eimeriidae*, *Cryptosporidiidae*, or *Sarcocystidae*. Coccidian genera that infect cats and dogs are *Isospora* (also called *Cystoisospora*), *Hammondia*, *Besnoitia*, *Sarcocystis*, *Toxoplasma*, and *Neospora* species (see Chapter 80), as well as *Cryptosporidium* and *Cyclospora* species (see Chapter 82).[5] *Caryospora* infections are also discussed in this chapter. Another coccidian genus, *Eimeria*, found commonly in herbivores, birds, lagomorphs, and rodents, is found only in feces of dogs and cats after they ingest intestinal contents or feces from these animals. The oocysts pass unchanged through the feline or canine intestine. Some coccidians of dogs remain unclassified.

Intestinal coccidia discussed in this chapter are host specific. Infections of definitive or intermediate hosts generally only occur in cycles established by evolution. Some aberrant cycles exist, such as with *Sarcocystis neurona* infections in horses. Human health risks from these parasites are considered minimal to nonexistent, even in immunosuppressed humans.

INTESTINAL COCCIDIOSIS

All coccidians have an asexual and a sexual cycle. In some genera, such as *Sarcocystis*, the asexual and sexual cycles occur in different hosts, whereas in *Isospora* both cycles may occur in the same host (Table 81-1 and Fig. 81-1). The oocyst is the environmentally resistant stage in the life cycle of all coccidia and is excreted in feces of the definitive host.

A representative coccidian life cycle is best described as follows. Oocysts are passed unsporulated in feces and contain a single nucleated mass called a *sporont*, which almost fills the oocyst (Fig. 81-2). After exposure to warm (20° C to 37° C [68° F to 98.6° F]) environmental temperatures and moisture, oocysts sporulate, forming two sporocysts. Within each sporocyst are four sporozoites (Fig. 81-3). The sporozoites have a banana shape and are the infective stage (Fig. 81-4). They can

survive environmental exposure, protected inside the oocysts for many months. After the ingestion of sporulated oocysts by cats or dogs, sporozoites excyst in the intestinal lumen, and the sporozoites initiate the formation of schizonts or meronts. During schizogony or merogony, the sporozoite nucleus divides into two, three, or more nuclei, depending on the parasite and the stage of the cycle. After nuclear division, each nucleus is surrounded by cytoplasm, forming a merozoite. The number of merozoites within a schizont varies from two to several hundred, depending on the stage of the cycle and the species of coccidia. Merozoites are released from the schizont when the host cell ruptures. The number of schizogonic cycles varies with the parasitic species. First-generation merozoites repeat the asexual cycle and form second-generation schizonts or transform into microgamonts (males) and macrogamonts (females). The microgamont divides into many tiny microgametes. A microgamete fertilizes a macrogamete, and an oocyst wall is formed around the zygote. The life cycle is completed when unsporulated oocysts are excreted in feces.

Isospora Species

Members of the genus *Isospora*, the most commonly recognized coccidians infecting dogs or cats, are species specific for the definitive host. At least four species—*Isospora canis*, *Isospora ohioensis*, *Isospora burrowsi*, and *Isospora neorivolta*—infect dogs, and two species—*Isospora felis* and *Isospora rivolta*—infect cats.

Epidemiology

The life cycle of *Isospora* infecting dogs and cats is similar to the basic coccidian intestinal cycle, except an asexual cycle can also occur in the definitive or intermediate host. On ingestion by definitive or suitable paratenic (intermediate) hosts, oocysts excyst in the presence of bile, and free sporozoites invade the intestine. Some sporozoites penetrate the intestinal wall and enter mesenteric lymph nodes or other extraintestinal tissues, where they form enlarging unicellular cysts (Fig. 81-5). If no replication occurs, the host is called a *paratenic host* rather than an *intermediate host*. Monozoic cysts of *Isospora* may remain in extraintestinal tissues of definitive and paratenic hosts for the life of the host. In dogs and cats,

Villus of Small Intestine

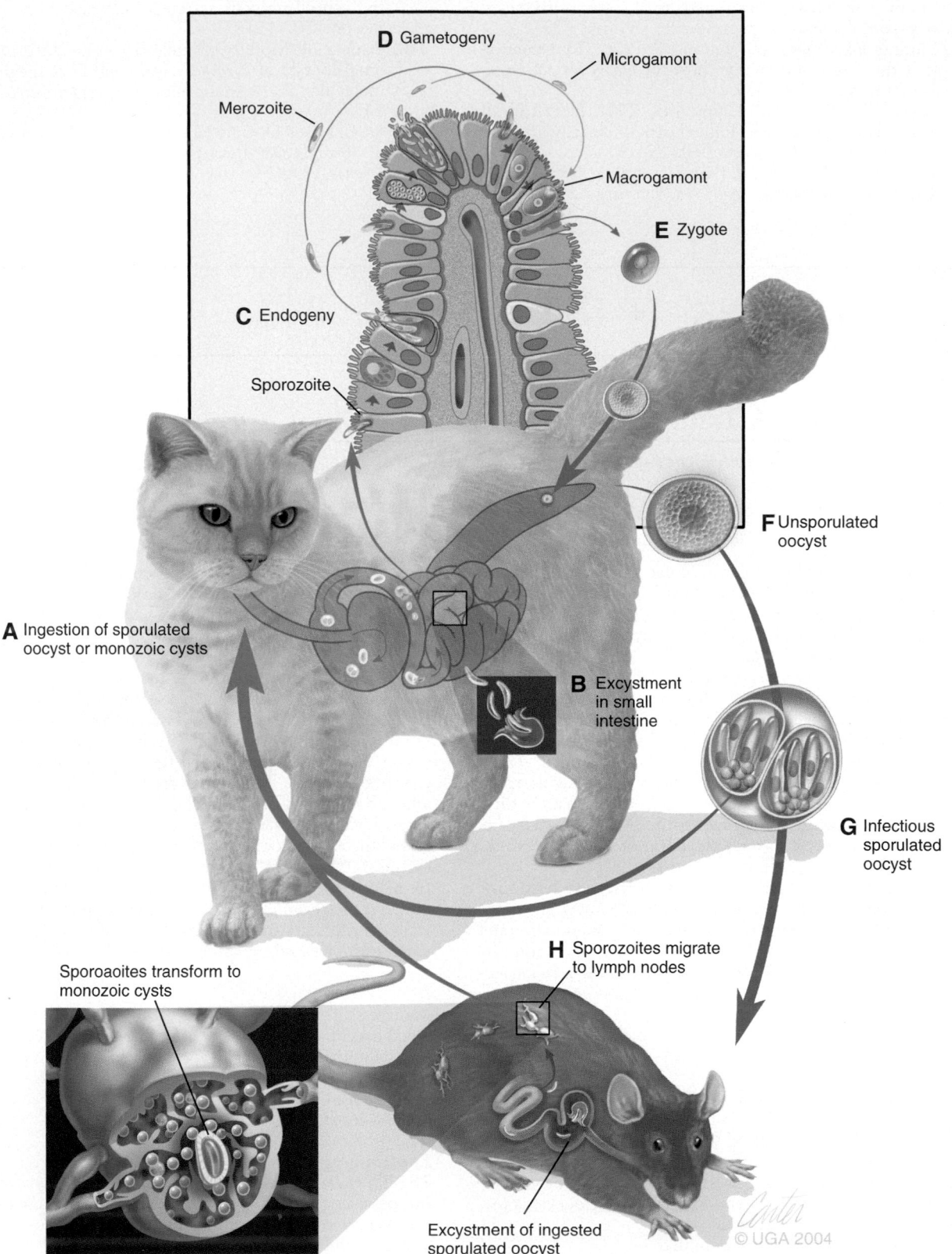

Fig 81-1 Life cycle of *I. felis*, which is typical of the *Isospora* spp. The mode of transmission may be direct, via ingestion of sporulated oocysts from the environment, or indirect via ingestion of cysts in prey animals. **A,** Either sporulated oocysts or monozoic tissue cysts are ingested. **B,** These excyst in the intestine. **C,** They undergo asexual (endodyogeny) and **(D)** sexual (merogony and gametogony) reproduction with the formation of a zygote. **E,** The zygote becomes an **(F)** unsporulated oocyst that is shed in the stool **(G).** This matures into the infectious sporulated oocyst which can be ingested by the definitive or intermediate host. **H,** In the intermediate host, the excysted sporozoites migrate to tissues and form cysts (Courtesy University of Georgia, Athens, Ga.)

Table • 81-1

Comparison of Selected Coccidial Genera That Infect Dogs and Cats

GENUS	DIRECT TRANSMISSION POSSIBLE?	SEXUAL CYCLE: INTESTINAL REPLICATION		ASEXUAL CYCLE: EXTRAINTESTINAL REPLICATION	
		DEFINITIVE HOST	FORM OF OOCYST PASSED	INTERMEDIATE OR PARATENIC HOSTS	LOCATION OF TISSUE CYSTS
Isospora	Yes	Dog and cat	U	Dog, cat, many other mammals	Extraintestinal or lymphoid tissues (monozoic)
Besnoitia	No	Cat	U	Many vertebrates	Fibroblasts
Hammondia	No	Dog and cat	U	Herbivores, rodents	Skeletal muscle
Sarcocystis	No	Dog and cat	S[a]	Many vertebrates	Cardiac and skeletal muscle
Cryptosporidium	Yes	Dog and cat	S[b]	None	None
Toxoplasma	Yes	Cat	U	Many vertebrates	Many tissues

U, Unsporulated; *S*, sporulated.
[a]Free sporocysts.
[b]Naked sporozoites.

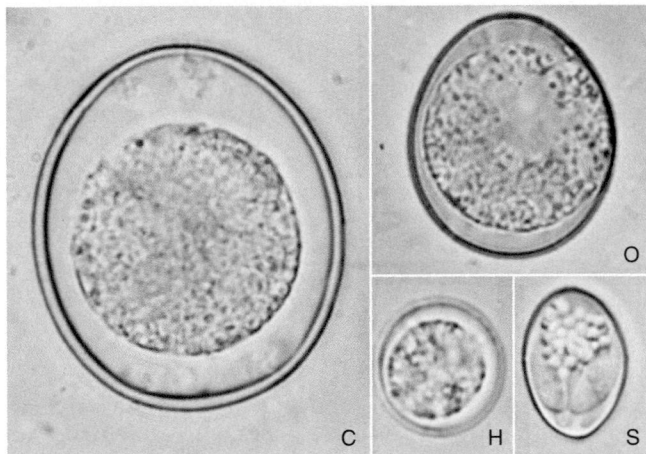

Fig 81-2 Unsporulated oocysts of *Isospora canis (C)*, *Isospora ohioensis (O)*, and *Hammondia heydorni (H)* and sporulated sporocyst of *Sarcocystis* species *(S)* from canine feces (unstained, ×1700). (From Dubey JP. 1976. A review of *Sarcocystis* of domestic animals and of other coccidia of cats and dogs, *J Am Vet Med Assoc* 169:1061-1078.)

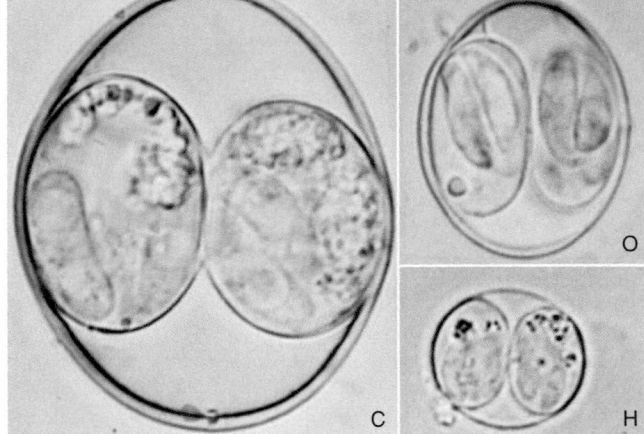

Fig 81-3 Sporulated oocysts of *I. canis (C)*, *I. ohioensis (O)*, and *H. heydorni (H)* (unstained, ×1700). Compare with Fig. 81-2. (From Dubey JP. 1976. A review of *Sarcocystis* of domestic animals and of other coccidia of cats and dogs, *J Am Vet Med Assoc* 169:1061-1078.)

these cysts may serve as a source of intestinal reinfection and relapse of enteric coccidiosis. Ingestion of monozoic cysts in paratenic hosts leads to intestinal infection in the definitive dog and cat host. The life cycle after the ingestion of paratenic host is the same as after the ingestion of sporulated oocysts from feces.

Clinical Findings

Diarrhea with coccidiosis in immunocompetent animals probably represents incidental or concurrent infections with coccidia and other infectious agents because coccidial infection can be present in the absence of clinical illness. Enzootic infections are frequently found in catteries or kennels where animals congregate. Clinical signs are most apparent in neonates. Experimental studies have shown that clinical signs of intestinal disease are uncommon unless large numbers of oocysts are fed to very young (younger than 1

month) or immunosuppressed animals. Clinically, severe diarrhea has been associated with naturally occurring coccidiosis in immunosuppressed dogs and cats. German shepherd dogs may have an increased susceptibility to clinical infection.[27,41] Diarrhea with weight loss and dehydration and, although rare, hemorrhage is the primary sign attributed to coccidiosis in dogs and cats. Anorexia, vomiting, mental depression, and ultimately death may be seen in severely affected animals. Severely immunosuppressed dogs and cats may have extraintestinal stages in macrophages of the lymphocyte-depleted mesenteric lymph nodes or extraintestinal tissues.

Intestinal coccidiosis may be manifest clinically when dogs or cats are shipped or weaned or experience a change in ownership. Diarrhea might result from the extraintestinal stages of *Isospora* returning to the intestines. Monozoic cysts do not cause clinical disease in paratenic hosts.

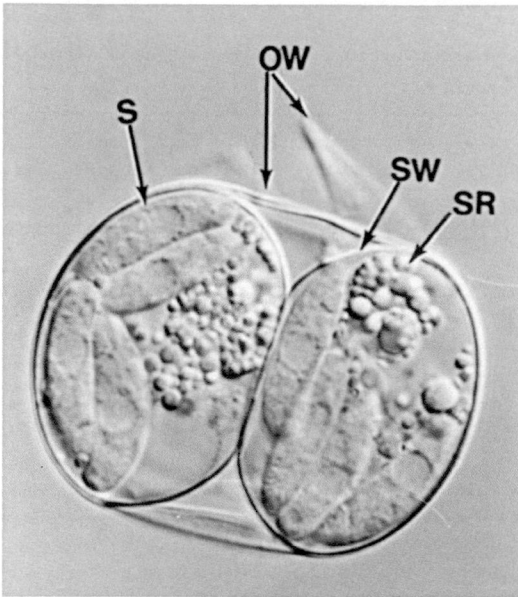

Fig 81-4 *I. canis* sporulated oocyst treated with 5.25% sodium hypochlorite solution to dissolve part of oocyst wall *(OW)*. Two sporocysts occupy most of oocyst. Each sporocyst has a thin sporocyst wall *(SW)*, four banana-shape sporozoites *(S)*, and a sporocystic residual body *(SR)*. SR may be compact or dispersed (unstained, ×1600). (From Kirkpatrick CE, Dubey JP. 1987. Enteric coccidial infections. *Isapora, Sarcocystis, Cryptosporidium, Besnoitia, and Hammondia, Vet Clin North Am Small Anim Pract* 17:1405-1420.)

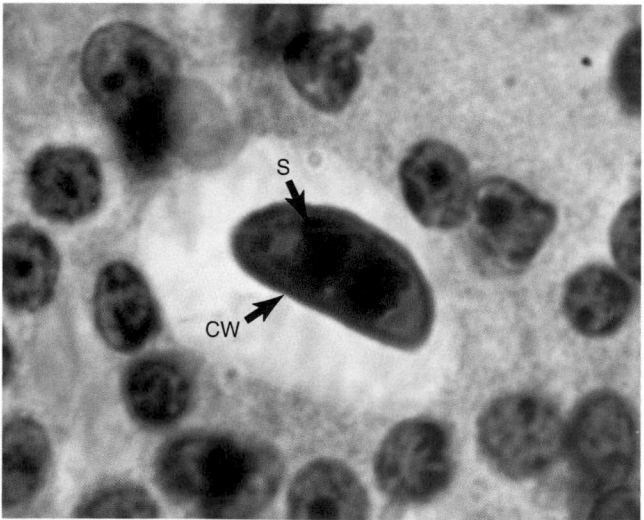

Fig 81-5 Tissue cyst of *I. ohioensis* in smear of mesenteric lymph node of an experimentally infected mouse. The sporozoite *(S)* is surrounded by a thick cyst wall *(CW)*. Vacuole around cyst wall is fixation artifact (PAS stain, ×1250).

Diagnosis

Intestinal coccidial infection in dogs and cats is diagnosed by identification of the oocysts with any of the fecal flotation methods commonly used to diagnose parasitic infections (see Fecal Examination, Chapter 70). Shedding of oocysts by some animals may be erratic, therefore repeated examinations are recommended. In dogs, only *I. canis* can be identified with certainty by oocyst size and shape (see Fig. 81-2). The two species of *Isospora* found in cats can be readily distin-

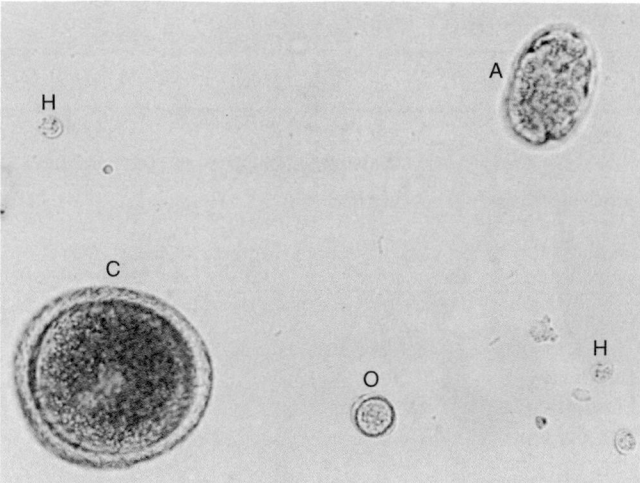

Fig 81-6 Unsporulated oocysts of *I. ohioensis (O)* and *H. heydorni (H)* compared with eggs of nematodes *Toxocara canis (C)* and *Ancylostoma caninum (A)* in flotation of canine feces (unstained, ×385). (From Dubey JP. 1976. A review of *Sarcocystis* of domestic animals and of other coccidia of cats and dogs, *J Am Vet Med Assoc* 169:1061-1078.)

guished by oocyst size (see Fig. 80-9). Oocysts of *I. felis* in cats and *I. canis* in dogs are large and easily distinguished from small oocysts, whereas it is almost impossible to distinguish *I. rivolta, I. burrowsi,* and *I. ohioensis* morphologically (Fig. 81-6; see also Fig. 80-9). Although *I. felis-, I. rivolta-, I. canis-,* and *I. ohioensis*-like oocysts are passed unsporulated in freshly excreted feces, they sporulate partially by the time a fecal examination is made. Partially sporulated oocysts contain two sporocysts without sporozoites. *Isospora* spp. may sporulate within 8 hours of excretion, and these *Isospora* are highly infectious.

Therapy

The presence of underlying disease or host immunosuppression should be suspected when coccidial infections persist for extended periods in older animals or when associated with chronic diarrhea. Treatment is often indicated in bitches and their newborn puppies because of the severity of clinical signs at this age. If diarrhea or dehydration is severe, parenteral fluid therapy must be considered as a supportive measure. Blood transfusion may be required when severe intestinal hemorrhage results in anemia.

Specific therapy involves the use of drugs that are coccidiostatic rather than curative (Table 81-2). However, as with many protozoal diseases, the presence of low-level infection may lead to premunition. The drugs shorten the prepatent period and may shorten the course of the disease.

Sulfonamides have long been the drugs of choice for the treatment of coccidiosis. Rapid-acting sulfonamides, such as sulfadimethoxine or sulfaguanidine, can be given alone or in combination with other antifolate drugs such as trimethoprim. Trimethoprim-sulfonamide offers the advantages of being readily available and being less toxic than other drugs. It should be considered a drug of first choice. Nitrofurazone can be administered alone or in combination with sulfonamides. Nitrofurazone is also available as a 4.59% soluble powder that can be added to drinking water (up to 1 g/2 L) for 7 days.

Amprolium is considered an effective preventive and treatment for coccidiosis in kenneled puppies. Although it is not currently approved for use in dogs, it can be administered as an undiluted liquid and a paste, but it is unpalatable in these forms (see Drug Formulary, Appendix 8).

Table • 81-2

Anticoccidial Drugs for Dogs and Cats

DRUG[a]	SPECIES	DOSE (mg/kg)[b]	ROUTE	INTERVAL (HOURS)	DURATION (DAYS)
Sulfamethoxine[c]	B	50—60	PO	24	5—20
Sulfaguanidine	B	100—200	PO	8	5
Trimethoprim-	D	30—60[d]	PO, SC	24	5
sulfonamide	B	15—30[e]	PO, SC	12—24	5
Ormetoprim-sulfadimethoxine	D	66[f]	PO	24	7—23
Furazolidone[g]	B	8—20	PO	12—24	5
Amprolium	D	300—400 (total)[h]	PO	24	5
	D	110—200 (total)[i]	PO	24	7—12
	C	60—100 (total)	PO	24	7
Quinacrine	B	10	PO	24	5
Spiramycin	H	50—100 (total)[j]	PO	24	5
Toltrazuril	D	15	PO	24	3—6[k]
Ponazuril	B	7.5—15[l]	PO	24	28
Roxithromycin	H	2.5	PO	12	15

B, Dog and cat; D, dog; C, cat; H, human; PO, by mouth; SC, subcutaneous.

[a]See Appendix 8, Drug Formulary, for additional information.
[b]Dose per administration at specified interval.
[c]Other sulfonamides, such as sulfadimidine and sulfaguanadine, can be used, but sulfaquinoxaline should not be used because it interferes with ditamin K synthesis and may result in hemorrhagic complications.
[d]Greater than 4 kg body weight.
[e]Less than 4 kg body weight.
[f]11 mg ormetoprim and 55 mg of sulfadimethoxine.
[g]When furazolidone is combined with sulfonamides, 50% of this dose is used.
[h]Total dose per day. Lower dose recommended for puppies, with a maximum of 300 mg total per day (see Drug Formulary, Appendix 8).
[i]Total dose per day. Combine 150 mg amprolium and 25 mg sulfadimethoxine per kilogram per day for 14 days (see Drug Formulary, Appendix 8).
[j]Total dose per day. Dose on a mg/kg basis is listed in Drug Formulary, Appendix 8.
[k]Doses of 30 mg/kg have been used for 1 day; however treatment at half that dose for at least 3 days with repeating if needed, has been more effective in treatment of pups and kittens with coccidiosis without relapses.[35]
[l]Dose extrapolated from use in horses and mice for treatment of Sarcocystis neurona infections.

Quinacrine, spiramycin, toltrazuril, tetracycline, and roxithromycin have been used on a limited basis to treat canine and feline coccidiosis.[4] Their use might be considered if more established treatment regimens fail or protozoal resistance develops.

Prevention

Coccidiosis tends to be a problem in unsanitary environments. The fecal shedding of large numbers of environmentally resistant oocysts makes infection likely under such conditions. Animals should be housed in a way that does not allow contamination of food and water bowls by oocyst-laden soil or infected feces. Feces should be removed daily and incinerated. Oocysts survive freezing temperatures. Runs, cages, food utensils, and other implements should be disinfected by steam cleaning or immersion in boiling water or by a 10% ammonia solution. Animals should have limited access to intermediate hosts and should not be fed uncooked meat. Insect control is essential in animal quarters and food storage areas because cockroaches and flies may serve as mechanical vectors of oocysts. Coccidiostatic drugs can be given to infected bitches before or soon after whelping to control the spread of infection to puppies.

Hammondia Species

Two species of Hammondia exist in domestic animals: Hammondia hammondi, with cats as definitive hosts, and Hammondia heydorni, with dogs and other canids as definitive hosts.[5,25] Unlike Isospora species, H. hammondi and H. heydorni have obligatory two-host life cycles (see Chapter 80 and Table 81-1). Goats and rodents are natural intermediate hosts for H. hammondi, and the domestic cat (Felis catus) and the European wild cat (Felis sylvestris) are the definitive hosts. H. hammondi does not invade extraintestinal tissues of the cat, and cats are infected only by eating tissue cysts. Experimentally, many warm-blooded animals, including monkeys, sheep, goats, pigs, rabbits, guinea pigs, and mice, can serve as intermediate hosts. Intermediate hosts become infected by ingesting sporulated oocysts, which resemble those of T. gondii. Sporozoites excyst in the intestinal lumen, invade the intestinal wall, and multiply as tachyzoites in the intestines, mesenteric lymph nodes, and other tissues. The parasite eventually encysts principally in muscles (Fig. 81-7).

H. heydorni's life cycle is not fully known but seems to be similar to that of H. hammondi. Dogs and other canids are definitive hosts, and cattle, sheep, goats, buffaloes, camels, moose, and deer serve as intermediate hosts.[14,26a] The structure of the parasite in the intermediate hosts is not known. H. hammondi and H. heydorni are nonpathogenic, therefore no treatment is necessary.

Besnoitia Species

Cats, not dogs, are definitive hosts for three species of Besnoitia: Besnoitia wallacei of rats and mice, Besnoitia darlingi of opossums and possibly lizards, and Besnoitia oryctofelisi of rabbits.[18,26]

The life cycle of Besnoitia is similar to that of T. gondii (see Table 81-1). Cats become infected by ingesting tissue cysts, and schizonts (Fig. 81-8) and gamonts are formed in intestinal goblet cells or lamina propria. Schizonts may be

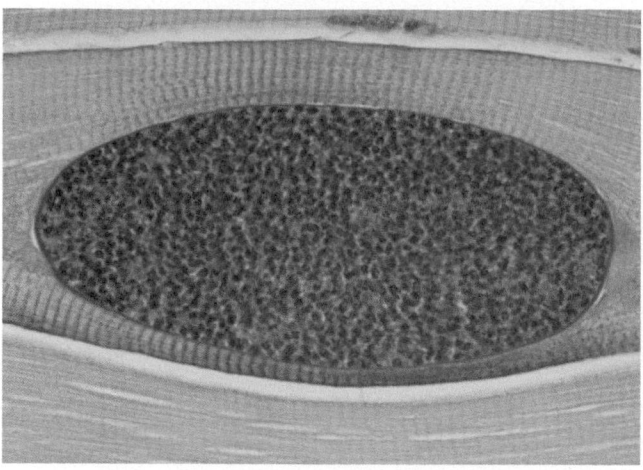

Fig 81-7 *H. hammondi* tissue cyst in skeletal muscle of mouse. Note thin cyst wall enclosing hundreds of periodic acid–Schiff-positive bradyzoites (PAS stain, ×750).

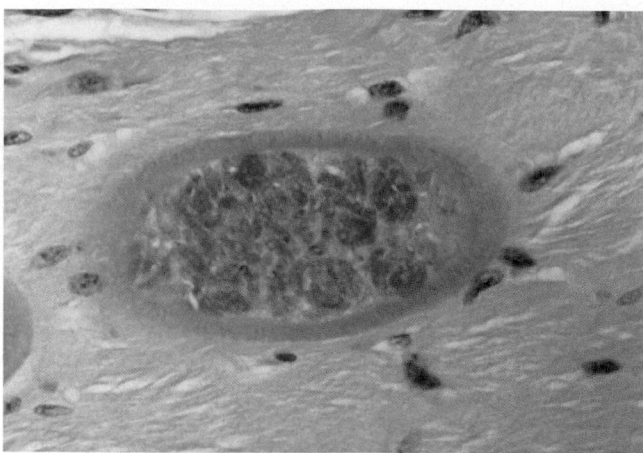

Fig 81-9 Esophageal muscle with thick-walled sarcocyst of *Sarcocystis hirsute* (H and E stain, ×630). (From Gardiner CH, Fayer R, Dubey JP. 1988. *An atlas of protozoan parasites in animal tissues*, Beltsville, Md, USDA Agricultural Handbook No 651.)

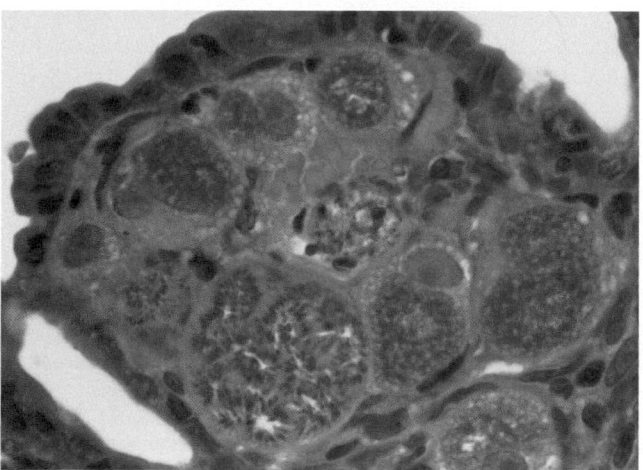

Fig 81-8 *B. oryctofelisi* schizonts in the lamina propria of jejunum of an experimentally infected cat (H and E stain, ×750).

found in extraintestinal organs.[26] Unsporulated oocysts are shed in feces, and they are difficult to distinguish from those of *T. gondii*. Intermediate hosts become infected by ingesting sporulated oocysts. The parasite develops in connective tissue, and cysts may become macroscopic. *Besnoitia* is considered nonpathogenic in cats, and no treatment is necessary.

Intestinal *Sarcocystis* Species

Infections resulting from *Sarcocystis* spp. are ubiquitous in reptiles, birds, and warm-blooded animals.[5] Virtually all cattle and sheep are infected with this parasite. More than 90 species of *Sarcocystis* have been identified, and they have an obligatory two-host life cycle (see Table 81-1). Carnivores (predators) are definitive hosts, and herbivores (prey) are intermediate hosts. As the name implies, the parasite forms tissue cysts (sarcocysts) in muscles and neural tissues of these intermediate hosts (Fig. 81-9). Sarcocysts are thin or thick walled, and the zoites are usually separated from each other by septa. Cats and dogs become infected by ingesting sarcocysts. The life cycle of *Sarcocystis* is distinct from other coccidians of domestic animals in that oocysts sporulate within the definitive host and are excreted in the feces in an infective form (Fig. 81-10).

The intermediate hosts become infected by ingesting sporocysts or oocysts. One to three generations of schizogony occur in blood vessels or hepatocytes (depending on the species of intermediate hosts). Merozoites then invade skeletal muscles and nerve cells, where they form sarcocysts (see Figs. 81-10 and 81-11). Certain species of *Sarcocystis*, transmissible via dogs, are pathogenic in cattle, sheep, goats, pigs, and mule deer, whereas species transmissible via cats are generally nonpathogenic.

More than 20 species of *Sarcocystis* infect cats and dogs. It is not possible to differentiate species on the basis of measurement of sporocysts. *Sarcocystis* is excreted in feces fully sporulated, often as free sporocysts when examined microscopically (Fig. 81-12). They are small and not very dense, so they lie at a different plane of focus than other parasites.

Sarcocystis species are not pathogenic for the intestinal tract of dogs or cats, so no treatment is necessary. Infections can be prevented by cooking all meat fed to animals. Occasionally, sarcocysts are found in skeletal muscles of immunosuppressed or wild cats and dogs, but their life cycle is unknown.[8,12]

Extraintestinal *Sarcocystis* spp.

Sarcocystis canis *Infection*

One of the extraintestinal *Sarcocystis*-like parasites *(S. canis)* has been found in Rottweiler dogs in the United States.[0a,21-23,48a] Only asexual stages (schizonts) were seen in various cells, including neurons, hepatocytes, and dermal cells (Figs. 81-13 and 81-14). Affected dogs ranged from 2 days old to adult dogs and had neurologic and hepatic signs and dermatitis. Schizonts were 5 to 25 × 4 to 20 μm and contained 6 to 40 merozoites. Occasionally, merozoites were arranged around a residual body. The parasite was named *S. canis* because it differed from other species of *Sarcocystis*. Its life cycle is unknown. An unidentified *Sarcocystis* sp. caused granulomatous myositis in a dog.[2a]

Feline Sarcocystis *Infection*

Sarcocysts have been identified in the skeletal and cardiac muscles of 11 free-ranging Florida panthers and cougars,[30] 3 domestic cats[32] and in hind-limb muscle biopsy specimens of 2 domestic cats.[28] The sarcocysts found in these studies were not specifically identified, and the immune status of the host may have been compromised. Some of these infections might

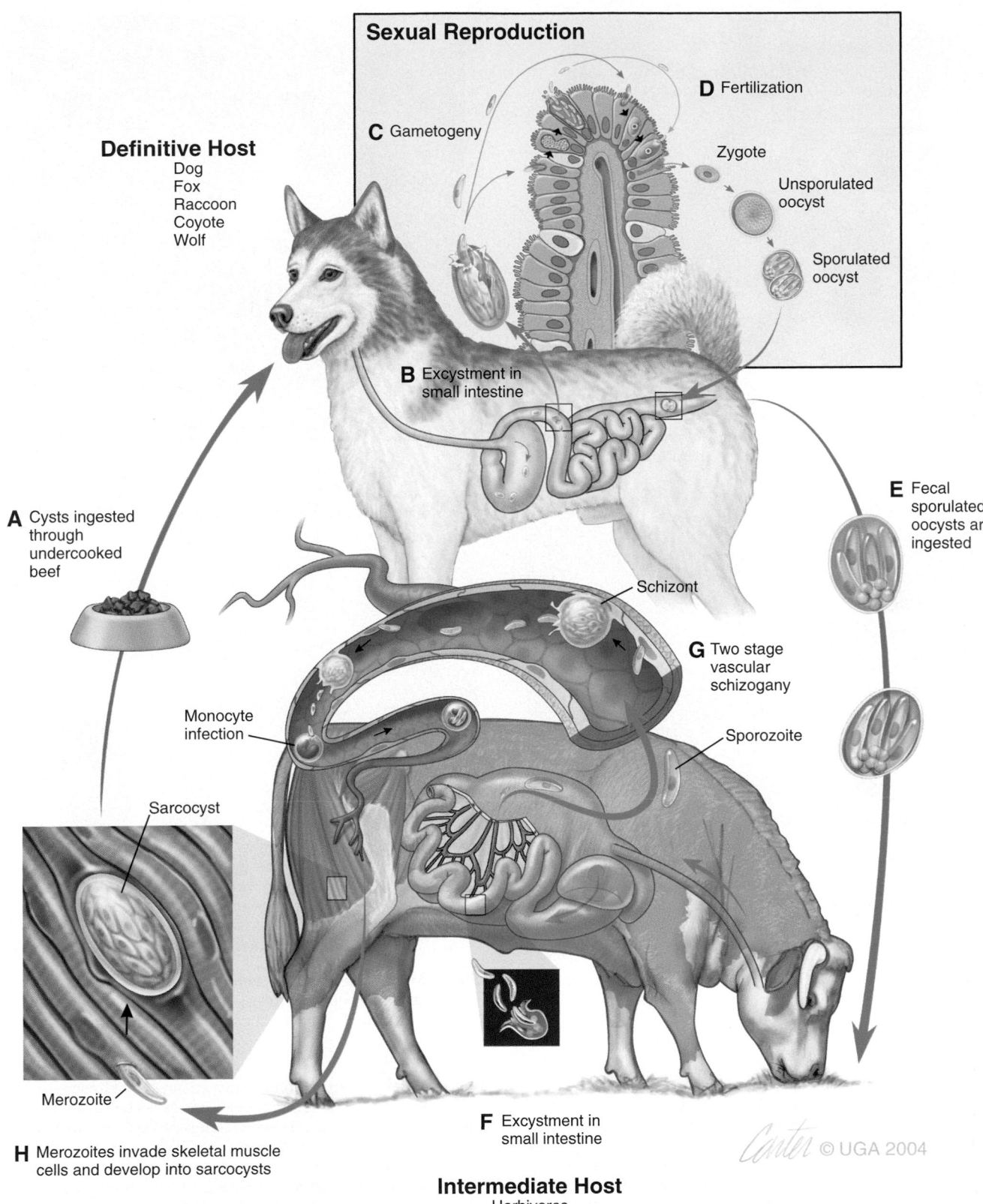

Sexual Reproduction

C Gametogeny

D Fertilization

Zygote

Unsporulated oocyst

Sporulated oocyst

Definitive Host
Dog
Fox
Raccoon
Coyote
Wolf

B Excystment in small intestine

A Cysts ingested through undercooked beef

E Fecal sporulated oocysts are ingested

Schizont

G Two stage vascular schizogany

Monocyte infection

Sporozoite

Sarcocyst

Merozoite

H Merozoites invade skeletal muscle cells and develop into sarcocysts

F Excystment in small intestine

Carter © UGA 2004

Intermediate Host
Herbivores

Fig 81-10 Life cycle of *S. cruzi*, which is typical of *Sarcocystis* spp. **A,** Muscle cyst is ingested by definitive carnivore host. **B,** These excyst in the small intestine and penetrate epithelial cells. **C,** Gametes develop in the intestinal epithelium and these (**D**) fuse to form a zygote which matures into an unsporulated and then a sporulated oocyst. **E,** Sporulated oocysts are shed in the feces. **F,** Oocysts, ingested by herbivores, excyst in the small intestine to release sporozoites. **G,** These penetrate the epithelium and migrate in the blood vasculature where they replicate in two phases of schizogony. **H,** In the final stages, mature schizonts rupture releasing merozoites which enter the muscles to form sarcocysts which contain many organisms. (Courtesy University of Georgia, Athens, Ga.)

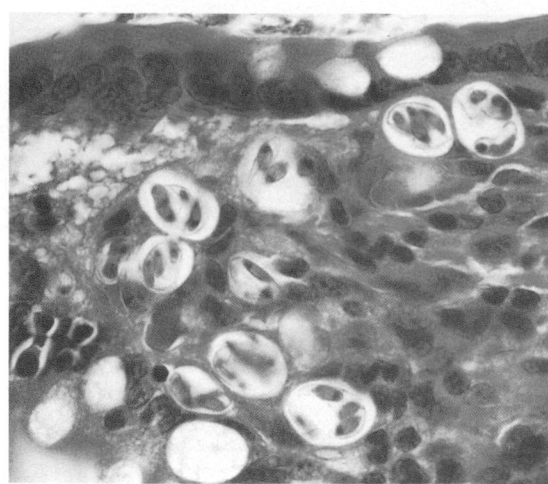

Fig 81-11 Canine small intestine with numerous sporulated oocysts in subepithelium (H and E stain, ×630). (From Gardiner CH, Fayer R, Dubey JP, 1988. *An atlas of protozoan parasites in animal tissues*, Beltsville, Md, USDA Agricultural Handbook No 651.)

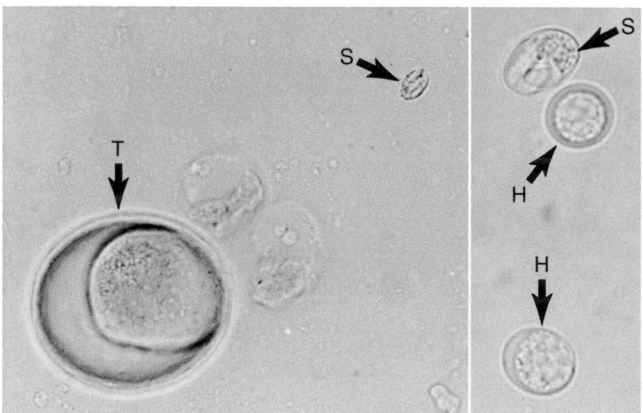

Fig 81-12 Sporulated *S. cruzi* sporocysts *(S)*, unsporulated *H. hammondi (H)*, and *Toxascaris leonina* egg *(T)* in fecal flotation of canine feces (**A,** unstained, ×430; **B,** unstained, ×1250). (From Dubey JP. 1976. A review of *Sarcocystis* of domestic animals and of other coccidia of cats and dogs, *J Am Vet Med Assoc* 169:1061-1078.)

have been caused by *Sarcocystis neurona*, which is discussed in the following section.

Sarcocystis neurona *Infection*

S. neurona is the principal parasite associated with equine protozoal encephalomyelitis, although a species of *Neospora* has also been incriminated (see Chapter 80). Opossums *(Didelphis virginiana)* are the definitive hosts for *S. neurona* (Fig. 81-15). Animals that ingest oocysts from opossums and serve as intermediate hosts by developing muscle sarcocysts are the nine-banded armadillo *(Dasypus novemcinctus)*, striped skunk *(Mephitis mephitis)*, raccoon *(Procyon lotor)*, sea otter *(Enhydra lutris)*, and brown-headed cowbird *(Molothrus ater)*.[19,36] Experimentally and naturally, cats have been shown to be intermediate hosts of *S. neurona*, although results have varied with individual isolates.[1,19,49] Cats experimentally fed sporocysts shed by opossums develop schizonts in their tissues and sarcocysts in their muscles, and infected cats develop high antibody titers (1:4000) as measured by a serum agglutination test.[17] Opossums were shown to shed *S. neurona* sporocysts after

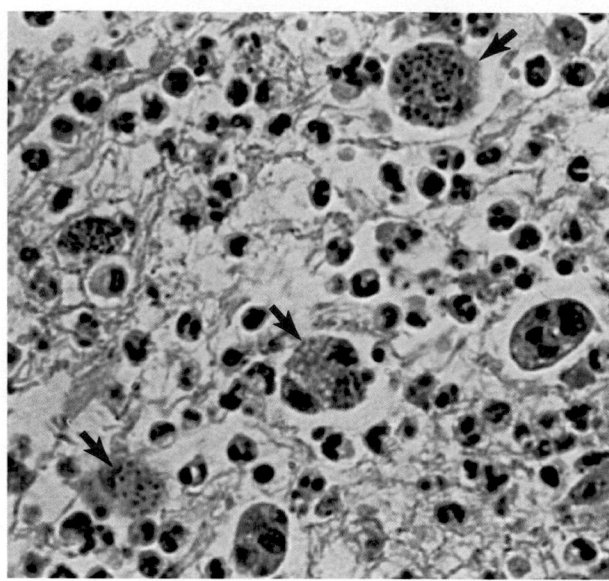

Fig 81-13 *S. canis* schizonts in section of dermal ulcer from dog. Note distended macrophages *(arrows)* with parasites in inflammatory exudate, mainly neutrophils (H and E stain, ×750).

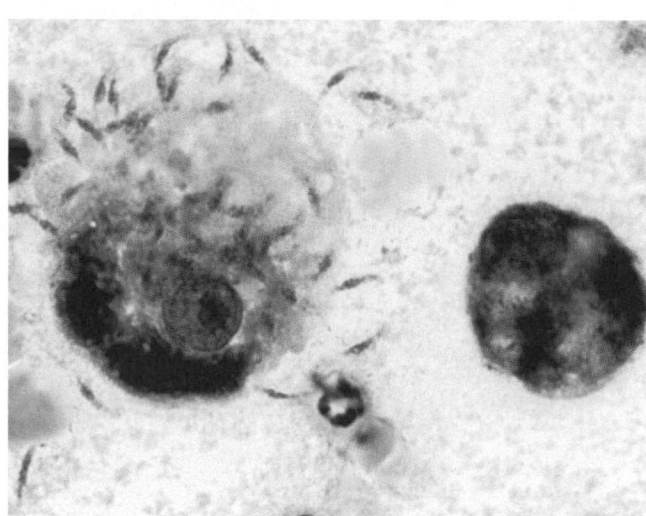

Fig 81-14 An intact *S. canis* schizont *(arrow)* and several merozoites *(arrowheads)* released from ruptured schizont in smear of exudate from dermal ulcer of dog (Giemsa stain, ×750).

ingesting feline tissues containing sarcocysts.[16] Horses are considered incidental or aberrant dead-end hosts because they only develop lesions within the central nervous system, and muscle sarcocysts have not been documented. This organism can cause fatal encephalomyelitis in dogs, raccoons, mink, and cats.

Sarcocystis-associated meningoencephalomyelitis was described in a 13-week-old Burmese kitten with lethargy, depression and crying, and progressive upper motor neuron hemiparesis.[13] Another 12-week-old kitten developed progressive neurologic dysfunction 3 days after a routine castration.[6] Encephalomyelitis was associated with numerous *S. neurona* schizonts and merozoites in the brain and spinal cord. *S. neurona* infection was also documented in a 13-year-old captive Canadian lynx *(Felis lynx Canadensis)*.[29] Serum antibodies to *S. neurona* were detected in 13% of 310 farm cats from Ohio[48] and in 5% of 196 domestic cats from Michigan whose sera were submitted for *T. gondii* antibody testing.[43]

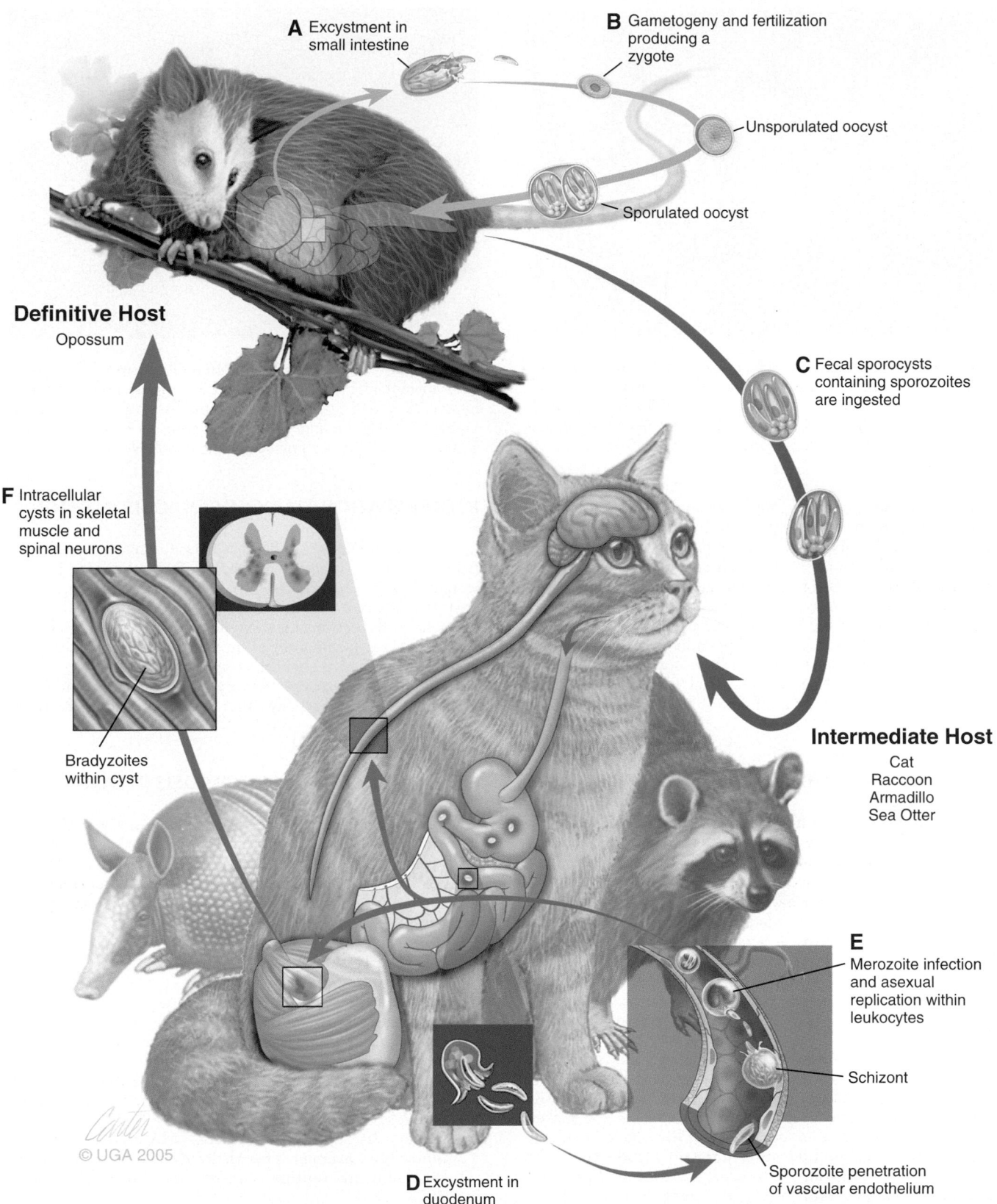

A Excystment in small intestine

B Gametogeny and fertilization producing a zygote

Unsporulated oocyst

Sporulated oocyst

Definitive Host
Opossum

C Fecal sporocysts containing sporozoites are ingested

F Intracellular cysts in skeletal muscle and spinal neurons

Bradyzoites within cyst

Intermediate Host
Cat
Raccoon
Armadillo
Sea Otter

E Merozoite infection and asexual replication within leukocytes

Schizont

D Excystment in duodenum

Sporozoite penetration of vascular endothelium

© UGA 2005

Fig 81-15 Life cycle of *S. neurona*. Opossums (*Didelphis virginiana, D. albiventris*) are its definitive hosts. They ingest organisms from the tissues of intermediate hosts. **A,** These excyst in the small intestine and enter the gut epithelium. **B,** Gametogony occurs followed by fertilization producing a zygote which eventual forms an oocyst. **C,** Sporulated oocysts shed in the feces are ingested by natural intermediate hosts such as cats, armadillos, raccoons, sea otters, skunks and possibly other mammals. **D,** Ingested sporocysts excyst in the small intestine and **(E)** replicate to a limited extent within the vascular endothelium and leukocytes within viscera and then spread, probably by leukocytes, to other tissues. **F,** There, sarcocysts, composed of bradyzoites, develop in the muscle and neural tissues. Equids are considered aberrant intermediate hosts as development does not occur beyond schizont and merozoite stages. (Courtesy University of Georgia, Athens, Ga.)

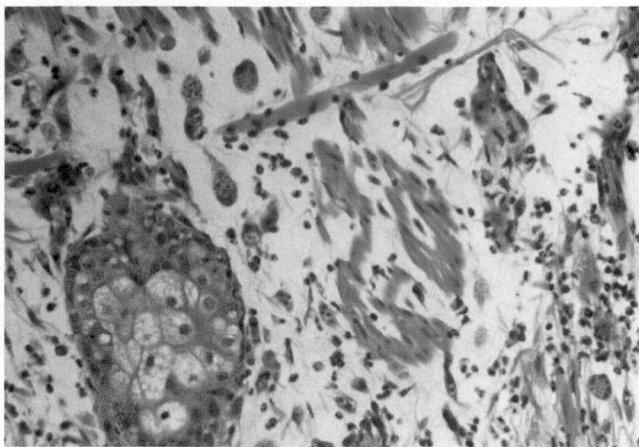

Fig 81-16 Section from skin of dog with *Caryospora* dermatitis. Note numerous *Caryospora* stages in dermal cells, including gamonts and schizonts (H and E stain, ×750; bar = 10 μm). (From Dubey JP, Black SS, Sangster LT, et al. 1990a. Caryospora-associated dermatitis in dogs, *Parasitol* 76:552-556.)

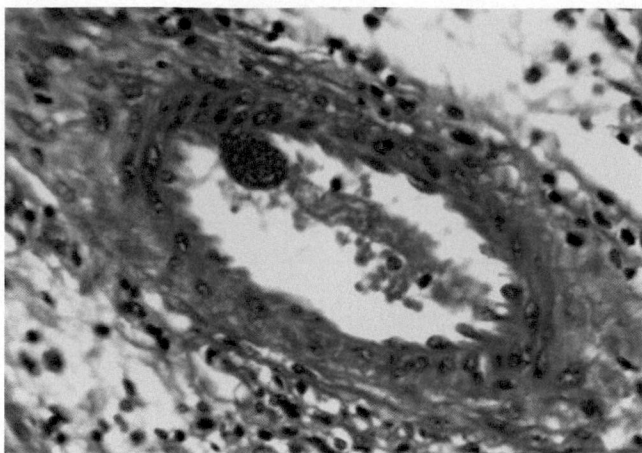

Fig 81-17 Mesenteric artery with multinucleated first-generation meront of *S. hirsute* (synonym *S. bovifelis*) protruding into lumen (H and E stain, ×630). (From Gardiner CH, Fayer R, Dubey JP. 1988. *An atlas of protozoan parasites in animal tissues*, Beltsville, Md, USDA Agricultural Handbook No 651.)

Diagnosis in horses has involved immunoblot testing for specific antibodies to *S. neurona* in cerebrospinal fluid not contaminated with blood. Use of feline antibody conjugates would be needed to apply this method for use in cats. Treatment of affected cats has not been attempted because diagnosis of clinically affected cats was made after death. Effective treatment of horses has involved the use of ponazuril. (See Table 81-2 and Drug Formulary, Appendix 8, for dosage information that has been extrapolated from dosages used to treat horses and mice.) Other anticoccidial drugs such as clindamycin, tetracyclines, or antifolate inhibitors might also be considered.

VISCERAL AND CUTANEOUS CARYOSPOROSIS

A *Caryospora bigenetica*–like organism was isolated from cutaneous nodules in five dogs ranging in age from 2 to 6 months. The dogs were thought to be concurrently affected with a distemper virus-like infection.[7] The skin nodules were up to 2 cm in diameter, and some had a central ulcerated area through which serohemorrhagic exudate could be expressed. Microscopically, the dermatitis was characterized by edema and infiltrations by polymorphonuclear cells, eosinophils, and macrophages (Fig. 81-16). Schizonts, male and female gamonts, unsporulated and sporulated oocysts, and caryocysts were seen in macrophages. In one dog, infection had spread to the lymph nodes.

Members of the genus *Caryospora* have an oocyst with one sporocyst that contains eight sporozoites, and they typically parasitize reptiles and raptors. At least two species, *C. bigenetica* and *Caryospora simplex*, parasitize rodents and snakes. *Caryospora* spp. have a complicated life cycle involving asexual and sexual multiplication in the prey (rodent) and the predator (snake). In addition to usual schizonts and gamonts, sporulated oocysts and monozoic cysts (caryocysts) are formed in connective tissue cells of the prey. The caryocysts (unlike sporocysts and oocysts) have a thin cyst wall enclosing the host cell nucleus. Two unusual features of *Caryospora* stages are noted in histologic sections of dog tissue: (1) the small size (less than 15 μm) of all developmental stages and (2) the presence of gamonts, schizonts, and oocysts in a single macrophage.

INTRAHEPATIC BILIARY COCCIDIOSIS IN DOGS

Intrahepatic biliary coccidiosis is a rare condition in dogs.[34] Clinical signs associated with hepatic disease include icterus, weight loss, and vomiting. Small and large bile ducts are enlarged because of inflammation and desquamation of epithelial cells. Lesions may extend into hepatic parenchyma. Asexual stages (schizonts) of an unidentified coccidium are found in biliary epithelial cells (Fig. 81-17). These coccida are different from *Toxoplasma*, *Sarcocystis*, *Hammondia*, and *Cryptosporidium* species and any other known coccidium found in the dog.

INTRAPULMONARY COCCIDIOSIS IN DOGS

An adult dog with clinical signs of weakness, fever, diarrhea, dehydration, weight loss, and harsh lung sounds was found to have canine distemper complicated by pulmonary infection with coccidia-like organisms.[38] Asexual stages of coccidia were observed in cytoplasmic vacuoles of many bronchiolar epithelial cells.

SUGGESTED READINGS*

1. Butcher M, Lakritz J, Halaney A, et al. 2002. Experimental inoculation of domestic cats *(Felis domesticus)* with *Sarcocystis neurona* or *S. neurona*-like merozoites. *Vet Parasitol* 107:1-142.
4. Daugschies A, Mundt HC, Letkova V. 2000. Toltrazuril treatment of cystoisosporosis in dogs under experimental and field conditions. *Parasitol Res* 86:797-799.
6. Dubey JP, Benson J, Larson MA. 2003. Clinical *Sarcocystis neurona* encephalomyelitis in a domestic cat following routine surgery. *Vet Parasitol* 112:261-267.
45. Schares G, Heydorn AO, Cüppers A, et al. 2001. *Hammondia heydorni*-like oocysts shed by a naturally infected dog and *Neospora caninum* NC-1 cannot be distinguished. *Parasitol Res* 87:808-816.

*See the CD-ROM for a complete list of references.

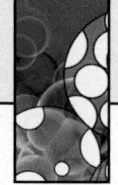

CHAPTER 82

Cryptosporidiosis and Cyclosporiasis

Stephen C. Barr

CRYPTOSPORIDIOSIS

Etiology and Epidemiology

Cryptosporidium is a ubiquitous coccidian genus in the phylum Apicomplexa, suborder Eimeria, family Cryptosporidiidae, that inhabits the epithelium of the respiratory and digestive systems of reptiles, birds, and mammals. Infections of the ileum are most common, but gastric, respiratory, and conjunctival infections have been observed in immunosuppressed hosts. Most species may be relatively host specific. *Cryptosporidium* found in reptiles and birds apparently do not infect mammals. The multiple genospecies of *Cryptosporidium* include *Cryptosporidium felis* and *Cryptosporidium canis*.* Only two morphologically distinct species are recognized mammals based on the very small oocyst size, namely *Cryptosporidium parvum* (4 to 5 μm in diameter) and *Cryptosporidium* sp. (= *Cryptosporidium muris*; 6 to 8 μm in diameter). Strains that infect cats and dogs cannot be morphologically differentiated from those that infect people. However, genetic methods can be used to differentiate different isolates of *C. parvum*. New species designations have been made for these distinct isolates (Table 82-1). Many of the newly described genospecies from animals were originally thought to be host specific. However, the host restriction may be less strict given the evidence of a complex circulation of the cryptosporidial species in the environment.[15] Oocysts are often difficult to demonstrate in the feces without special techniques. The biology of *C. muris* is not well known and its host range is limited,[5] and it will not be considered further. *C. parvum* subtype 1 is the cause of most human infections and is anthroponotic. In contrast, subtype 2 is zoonotic, with cattle being a principal reservoir host. The organism is thought to be by far the most commonly occurring species in mammals and, similar to *Toxoplasma*, has a wide mammalian host range.[97] *Cryptosporidium* has been reported in rodents, domestic livestock, cats, dogs, people, and numerous wild mammals. Ruminants, especially calves, are considered reservoir hosts for the cattle subtype. Cross-infection between various mammalian hosts occurs with this strain.[93] Despite their host specificity, experimentally, *C. parvum* from calves can induce respiratory signs in chickens[103]; however most such attempts have failed.[97] Canada geese (*Branta canadensis*) have been shown to be vectors of *C. parvum* infection and they may cause fecal contamination far from the site of its origin.[36] A high prevalence of serum antibodies to cryptosporidia in most species tested, including cats, suggests that exposure to the parasite is common.[92] Prevalence of serum antibodies to *C. parvum* in cats in various geographic regions in the United States ranges from 1.3% to 14.7%, with older animals in the southeastern states showing the highest exposure rate (15.3%).[80,81] However, young stray cats are more likely to excrete cysts in their feces. In New York, 3.8% of shelter cats between 1 and 12 months of age were excreting cysts in their feces, while in Colorado, 5.4% of cats were positive.[47] In the Colorado study, dogs and cats with diarrhea were more likely to shed cysts in their feces compared with clinically normal animals.[47] In a clinical and postmortem study in metropolitan domestic and feral cats, the prevalence of infection was 5.1% and 12.1%, respectively.[90] In rural cats from the surrounding area, the prevalence was 12.3%.[94] Fecal cyst excretion rates in dogs in California and Colorado were 2% and 3.8%, respectively, suggesting that the number of dogs excreting oocysts at any one time may be lower than that in cats.[24,47] Ranges for prevalence of fecal oocysts in various populations have been 0–38.5% in cats and 0–44.8% in dogs.[70a]

The life cycle of cryptosporidians differs from most other coccidians (Fig. 82-1). All stages of development (asexual and sexual) of cryptosporidia occur within one host.[97] After ingestion, oocysts excyst in the gastrointestinal (GI) tract, releasing infective sporozoites, which become enclosed as trophozoites within parasitophorous vacuoles of the microvillous surface of enterocytes rather than in the cytoplasm (Fig. 82-2). The trophozoites proliferate (asexually) by merogony to produce, sequentially, two types of meronts. Within 24 hours, type I meronts (containing eight merozoites) leave the parasitophorous vacuole to invade other epithelial cells where they develop into more type I meronts or type II meronts (containing four merozoites). The type II meronts do not undergo merogony but produce sexual reproductive stages (gamonts). The zygotes formed by sexual reproduction (gametogony between male microgamonts and female macrogamonts) form either thick-walled (excreted in the feces) or thin-walled (autogenous reinfection) oocysts each containing four sporozoites.

Oocysts of cryptosporidia are highly resistant and spread via the fecal-oral route. Fecal contamination of food or drinking water is a common source of infection. Large outbreaks can occur when a community water source becomes contaminated.[25a] The organism is extremely infective; as few as 100 oocysts are necessary to precipitate disease in people.[76]

Pathogenesis

Cryptosporidia are either primary pathogens or secondary invaders in a variety of immunosuppressive diseases of animals and people. Crowding and unsanitary practices increase the risk of exposure. Cryptosporidial diarrhea is common among calves in intensive raising units and among children in day care centers.

Cryptosporidiosis may cause malabsorption or secretory diarrhea, but the underlying mechanisms are complex and still not fully understood and have been reviewed elsewhere.[34] The organism remains just beneath the luminal cell membrane of the intestinal epithelial mucosa. Functional impairment (glucose-stimulated sodium and water absorption) and morphologic changes (villous atrophy, crypt hyperplasia, and inflammatory cell infiltration) have been reported in pigs experimentally infected with *C. parvum*.[4,86] Although secre-

*References: 2, 53, 88, 89, 109, 120.

Villus of Small Intestine

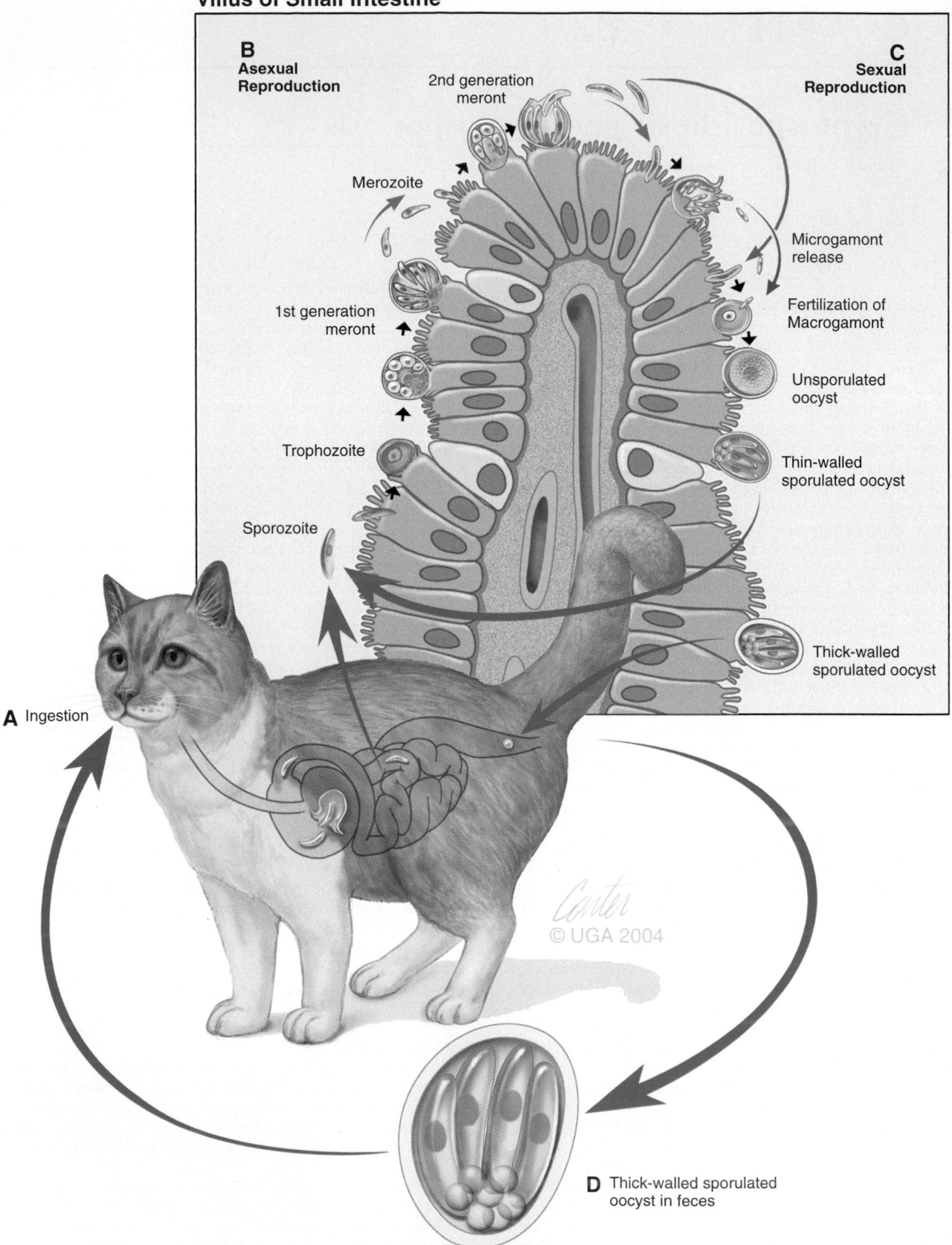

Fig 82-1 Life cycle of *Cryptosporidium*. **A,** Oocysts are ingested by the host and these excyst in the intestinal tract. **B,** They undergo replication in the intestine by two generations of merogony. **C,** Meronts then differentiate into male and female gamonts which form a zygote that matures into a sporulated oocyst within the intestine. Sporozoites from thin-walled oocysts can reinfect new cells. **D,** Thick-walled oocysts are environmentally resistant and infectious as they are passed in the stool. (Courtesy University of Georgia, Athens, Ga.)

Table • 82-1

Genospecies of Some Cryptosporidial Species Isolated from People and Animals

GENOTYPES	INFECT PEOPLE	INFECT ANIMALS	CLINICAL ILLNESS IN PEOPLE	CLINICAL ILLNESS IN DOGS OR CATS
C. hominis	+	—[a]	Yes, diarrhea	
C. parvum (bovine)	+	Cow, dog, cat, cattle, sheep, goat, horse, lab rodents	Yes, diarrhea	Diarrhea in young or immunocompromised
C. meleagridis	+	Turkey	Yes, diarrhea	
C. felis	+	Cat	Yes, diarrhea	Generally asymptomatic
C. canis	+	Dogs[b]	Generally asymptomatic	Generally asymptomatic
C. muris[c]	±	Mouse[d]	Symptomatic in immunocompromised	

−, No; +, yes; ±, uncertain.
[a]Cat experimentally infected.
[b]Isolates of this genotype from dogs and other animals are variably infective for people.
[c]Only this species has morphologically distinct oocysts.
[d]Dogs, cats, guinea pigs, rabbits, lambs, and gerbils experimentally infected, although infections not always patent.

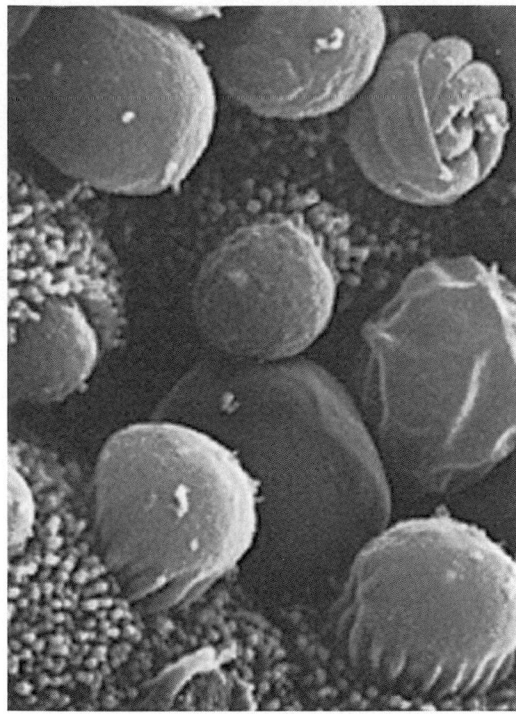

Fig 82-2 Scanning electron microscopic image of various stages of *Cryptosporidium* on the epithelial cell microvillous surface of the cloaca of a young chicken (×5000). (Courtesy of Sandy L. White, Lilly Research Labs, Greenfield, Ind. From Current WL. 1988. The biology of *Cryptosporidium, ASM News* 54:605–612, with permission.)

tory toxins have been implicated in the electrogenic chloride secretory stimulation,[39] the mechanism of action is unclear.[76] Substance P, a neuropeptide in the tachykinin family, is increased in symptomatic as compared with asymptomatic people with cryptosporidiosis related to acquired immunodeficiency syndrome (AIDS).[116] Neuropeptides such as SP are known to mediate many inflammatory processes in the intestine. Tumor necrosis factor and prostaglandins, which are released during infection, may also be involved in a disturbance of the epithelial cell function. The net effect of the cellular mediators and villous atrophy is nutrient and electrolyte malabsorption and shifts in water balance in favor of net secretion.[34] Lymphocytic duodenitis and intestinal bacterial overgrowth have been documented in a young cat with cryptosporidiosis; however, whether *Cryptosporidium* sp. caused the lesion is unknown.[46]

Both humoral and cell-mediated immunity (CMI) participate in the host response to infection with *C. parvum*.[35] CMI appears to be the major component of the protective response; the role of antibodies is unclear. In affected people, causes of immunodeficiency such as chemotherapy, IgA deficiency or interferon-γ deficiency have been associated with an increased risk infection. Although cryptosporidial cysts are excreted by asymptomatic cats or dogs, most case reports document a potential cause of systemic (feline leukemia virus [FeLV], feline immunodeficiency virus, canine distemper, parvovirus) or local (GI lymphoma, coronavirus, *Campylobacter, Isospora* spp., *Toxocara cati*) immunosuppression in infected symptomatic animals.[19,32,67,113] Concurrent infections with various organisms (*Capillaria* spp., *T. cati, Isospora felis, Pharyngostomum cordatum*) were detected in normal cats excreting cryptosporidial oocysts in the feces. Cryptosporidiosis was found to be more common among asymptomatic young and newborn kittens as compared with older (6 months or older) cats.[83]

Clinical Findings

Cats

Because experimental inoculations in healthy adult cats or 6-week-old kittens with *C. parvum* resulted in asymptomatic infections, whether cryptosporidial infections can cause diarrhea in healthy animals is questionable. Diarrhea can be self-limiting or absent in naturally infected immunocompetent cats. Pathogenicity undoubtedly is greater in immunodeficient cats. Intestinal cryptosporidiosis in other FeLV-negative or FeLV-positive cats has also been associated with chronic anorexia, marked weight loss, and persistent diarrhea.[113] The diarrhea is usually of a small-bowel nature, characterized by high-volume, low-frequency stools with significant weight loss. Tenesmus, fresh blood, swelling, and discomfort may be seen with chronicity. *C. felis* has been identified as a cause of infection in people associated with cats (see Public Health Considerations). Clinical illness, when reported, has been that of diarrhea with occasional blood.[88] Many cats are possible carriers for this species, and clinical illness may only occur following stress or immunosuppression.

Dogs

In older reports in which the infecting species was unknown, experimental infection of healthy pups resulted in oocyst shedding without accompanying disease.[113] In subsequent reports in which the infecting genospecies has been identified, a majority of dogs infected with *C. canis* have been asymptomatic. However, in two dogs, with concurrent parvovirus infection or immune-mediated thrombocytopenia, the dogs had hemorrhagic diarrhea.[19,89] In one pup, *C. canis* was found in the stomach mucosae, as a novel finding.[82] Naturally occurring cryptosporidiosis has been reported in a 1-week-old pup that died after an episode of diarrhea and dyspnea,[97] whereas other pups infected with cryptosporidia did not show clinical signs suggestive of infection.[113] As in cats, signs of diarrhea have been most severe in immunosuppressed dogs. Cryptosporidiosis has been described in immunosuppressed pups with distemper[113] and in dogs with GI lymphoma.[7] Cryptosporidial infection has been diagnosed in an adult dog with persistent diarrhea, weight loss, and malabsorption syndrome and no obvious cause for immunosuppression.[37]

Calves and Other Animals

Although cryptosporidial infection in calves without clinical signs of diarrhea is common, it is an important cause of diarrhea of varying severity (from mild intermittent to profuse watery with dehydration) among calves younger than 3 weeks.[98] The organism has also been identified in the bronchial epithelium of a calf.[77] Cryptosporidial diarrhea is also an important disease among young ruminants found in zoos. Less severe infections have been reported in young swine, lambs, and foals. The coccidian is fairly common in birds, infecting the digestive and respiratory tracts and the bursa of Fabricius, and may be a primary pathogen. In captive snakes, cryptosporidia causes gastritis and subsequent vomiting because it parasitizes the stomachs of these reptiles.[97]

People

People of all ages can become infected with cryptosporidia, and the severity of disease depends on the immunocompetence of the host. Most people develop transient clinical signs and recover. Cryptosporidiosis is an increasingly common cause of death in people with AIDS.[122] Individuals with congenital immunodeficiency disease may survive for years with cryptosporidiosis when fed parenterally. Immunocompetent persons may be infected readily with *Cryptosporidium*, as demonstrated when more than 400,000 people in Milwaukee developed diarrhea as a result of contracting the organism via the public water supply.[73] Enzootic infections by this means are very common.[11,31,74] Infection among veterinary students is common after contact with infected calves and has been documented after contact with infected lambs,[28] a dog,[37] and cats.[23,60,69] Canine and feline isolates have been found in human immunodeficiency virus (HIV)-infected people, but cat ownership by people with HIV is not associated with an increased risk to cryptosporidiosis.[30,109] Severe stress or concurrent infection by viruses or bacteria serves to exacerbate the diarrheal syndrome.

In people, a causal connection has been cited between oocysts being shed in the stool and GI signs.[56] The typical prepatent period is 5 to 7 days. Clinical signs, which may last from 2 to 26 days in immunocompetent people, may include nausea, abdominal cramps, low-grade fever, and anorexia. Occasionally, episodes last longer. Diarrhea may be profuse, and dehydration is a common sequela. Asymptomatic infections do occur, especially in recovery phases of the illness. Conversely, symptomatic patients can have intermittently negative stools.[56]

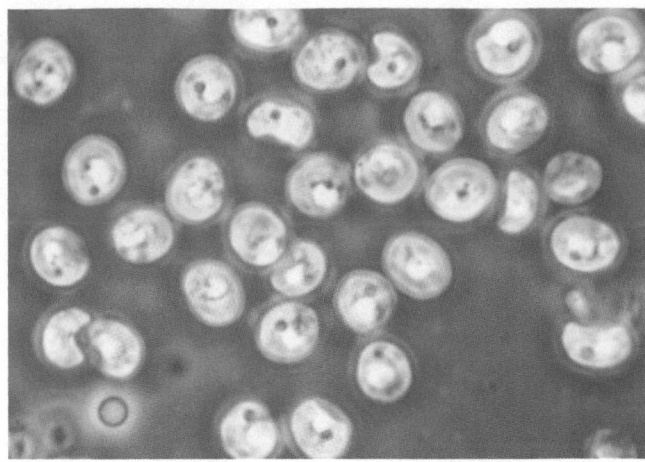

Fig 82-3 Fecal float with unstained oocysts suspended in water and viewed with bright-field microscopy (×1500). (From Gardiner CH, Fayer R, Dubey JP. 1988. An atlas of protozoan parasites in animal tissues, USDA Agricultural Handbook No. 651, USDA, Beltsville, Md.)

Diagnosis
Fecal Examination

Fecal oocyst excretion directly coincides with the onset and duration of clinical signs. Because cryptosporidial oocysts are directly infective when shed in the feces, caution must be used to avoid accidental infection. To destroy the oocyst, one part 100% formalin (38% formaldehyde) should be mixed with nine parts fluid feces before performing fecal examination procedures. Sodium acetate–acetic acid formalin is another acceptable fixative, but polyvinyl alcohol fixatives are not compatible with most staining procedures. Samples should also be formalinized before shipment to a diagnostic laboratory and should be placed in a nonbreakable container. The outside of the container should be disinfected to avoid accidental infection of laboratory personnel. The laboratory should be notified of suspicion of cryptosporidial infection. Oocysts may be seen microscopically on direct smears of feces, but concentration techniques, such as Sheather's sugar solution, can be used (see Fecal Examination, Chapter 70). Because oocysts are slightly smaller compared with erythrocytes, and because of transparency, unstained preparations using conventional light microscopy do not permit accurate identification.[113] When searching for cryptosporidial oocysts on unstained preparations, phase-contrast microscopy is often recommended; however, bright-field microscopy can be used (Fig. 82-3). A wet preparation in which crystal violet is applied to fluid stools enhances visualization of organisms. Oocysts can readily be seen because they do not stain. Because the small and refractile oocysts cling to the coverslip on Sheather's flotation, focusing immediately beneath the coverslip is imperative. Oocysts appear as circular, sometimes concave, disks that are refractile and pink with bright-field microscopy. Dark shadows of sporozoites may be seen within the oocysts.

Beagle pups experimentally infected with *C. parvum* of calf origin commenced shedding oocysts 3 to 5 days postinoculation (PI), with a peak shedding at 7 to 9 days PI. Shedding lasted for at least 80 days at a low or intermittent level.

Other procedures, used by diagnostic laboratories to demonstrate cryptosporidial oocysts in fluid stools, include formalin-ethyl acetate (FEA) sedimentation technique or examination of direct smears of feces or intestinal contents with positive stains, such as Giemsa (Fig. 82-4), or acid-fast, negative stains, such as Kinyoun's modified carbolfuchsin malachite green, and crystal violet (Fig. 82-5).* The negative stains give a clear halo around the oocysts. Using the FEA concentration method on watery stool specimens provided 100% detection with direct fluorescent antibody (FA) or acid-fast staining when 10^4 oocysts/g or more were present.[136] For formed stools, 5×10^4 oocysts/g or more was needed for direct FA and 5×10^5 oocysts/g or more for acid-fast staining. A modification of the acid-fast technique using dimethyl sulfoxide has simplified the procedure by staining the internal structure of the organism. Newer but more expensive auramine-rhodamine staining techniques are very sensitive.[75] Staining methods allow for easier detection of the oocysts and their differentiation from yeasts, which stain darker, are oval, appear in clumps, and may show budding, and are slightly smaller than cryptosporidia. Commercial kit staining methods are available.[97] A direct FA kit for staining cryptosporidial oocysts (and *Giardia* cysts) in feces is commercially available (Merifluor, Meridian Diagnostics, Cincinnati, Ohio). Although few evaluations have been reported in dogs and cats,[75b] the test is

*References: 25, 52, 71, 75, 91, 96.

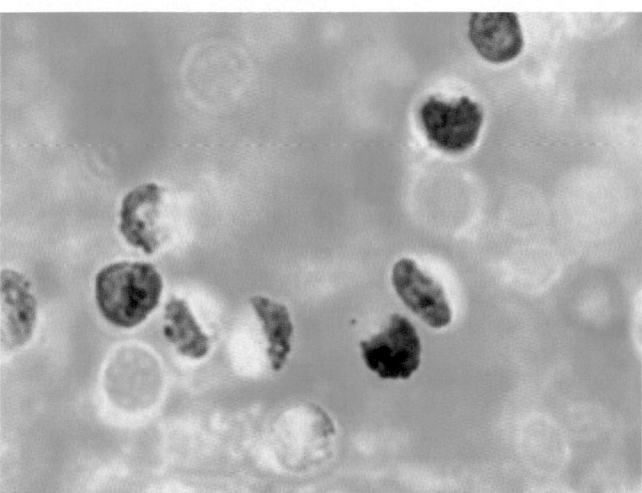

Fig 82-4 Fecal smear with cryptosporidial oocysts stained blue (Giemsa, ×750). (From Gardiner CH, Fayer R, Dubey JP. 1988. An atlas of protozoan parasites in animal tissues, USDA Agricultural Handbook No. 651, USDA, Beltsville, Md.)

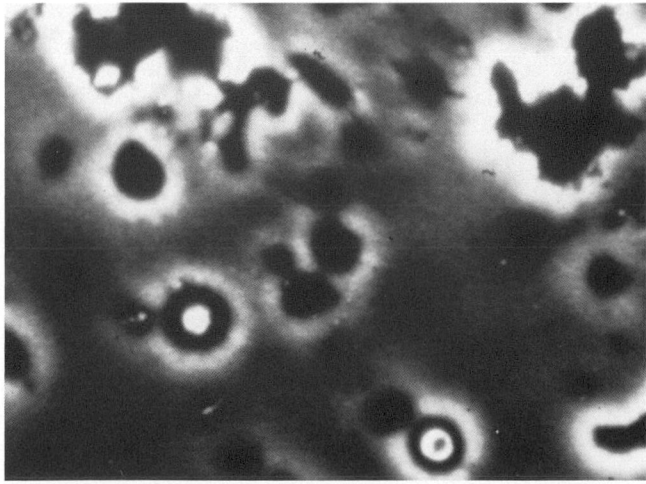

Fig 82-5 Acid-fast stained preparation of *Cryptosporidium* oocysts. Organisms are outlined well with negative staining method (×1000). (Courtesy University of Georgia, Athens, Ga.)

effective for oocyst detection in fecal samples from calves and sheep.[145] Several enzyme-linked immunosorbent assays (ELISA) (ProSpecT and ProSpecTR, *Cryptosporidium* Microtiter Assay, Alexon, Sunnyvale, Calif.; Color-Vue *Cryptosporidium*, Seradyn, Indianapolis, Ind.) for the detection of cryptosporidial antigen in feces are also available, but whether these tests will consistently reveal *C. felis* or *C. canis* is unknown. ELISA tests were more sensitive in detecting *Cryptosporidium* oocysts in a single fecal specimen of kittens compared to acid-fast staining and direct FA methods.[75b] Nested polymerase chain reaction (PCR) has been used to detect *C. parvum* DNA in feces of symptomatic people with 500 oocysts/g of feces, some of whom had negative results with acid-fast staining.[6] Similar high sensitivity has been reported for PCR detection in calf feces.[136] PCR has been used for the diagnosis and the molecular typing of isolates causing cryptosporidiosis in dogs.[3,2,121a] A nested multiplex PCR was developed that can simultaneously detect and distinguish between four zoonotic species: *C. parvum* genotypes 1 and 2, *C. canis*, and *C. felis*.[70] When compared with immunofluorescence, PCR has been shown to be 10 to 100 times more sensitive for the diagnosis of cryptosporidiosis in cats.[63,121,121a] Flow cytometry has also been used to increase the sensitivity of oocyst detection.[133] See Appendix 5 for the laboratories that perform diagnostic tests and Appendix 6 for further information on test kits available for diagnosis of this disease.

Serologic Testing

An ELISA was developed to measure *Cryptosporidium*-specific IgG in feline sera.[65] Positive antibody titers were correlated with exposure but not necessarily active infection or oocyst shedding. This test has been used as an epidemiologic surveillance tool.[80]

Animal Inoculation

Oocysts for animal inoculation may be harvested by sugar centrifugation and stored in a refrigerator in 2.5% potassium dichromate for up to 6 months without appreciable loss of viability. Neonatal mice are inoculated per os, and the intestinal tissues are examined microscopically 1 week later.

Intestinal Biopsy

Gross lesions consist of enlarged, congested mesenteric lymph nodes, and changes are most severe in the distal ileum. The mucosa is hyperemic and may contain watery, yellow contents. Giemsa and routine hematoxylin and eosin stains are effective given that most parasite stages are basophilic (Fig. 82-6). As a routine method of diagnosis, biopsy is costly, time consuming, and lacks sensitivity because only small amounts of tissue can be examined.

Specimens may be fixed in Bouin's or formalin solutions. Samples must be fixed within hours of biopsy procedure, otherwise cellular death associated with autolysis causes rapid loss of the intestinal surface that contains the organisms. Microscopic lesions vary in degree of villous atrophy, reactive lymphoid tissue, and inflammatory infiltrates in the lamina propria, consisting of neutrophils, macrophages, and lymphocytes. Blunting of the intestinal villi and crypt hyperplasia is apparent. Parasites may be found throughout the intestines but are usually most numerous in the distal small intestine. Electron microscopy (EM) readily identifies organisms by their unique ultrastructural characteristics and location within distinctive parasitiferous vacuoles.[97] EM shows that the organism is covered by the host cell microvillous membrane and therefore is intracellular but extracytoplasmic in location.

Therapy

Infections in immunocompetent animals or people are usually self-limiting, and full recovery soon ensues. To date, few drugs have been used successfully for treating cryptosporidiosis, although more than 100 have been screened.[58] Spiramycin showed early promise, but subsequent studies did not corroborate its efficacy.[108] Eflornithine,[117] oral bovine dialyzable extract,[79] and hyperimmune bovine colostrum[112] have shown clinical benefit. The aminoglycoside antibiotic, paromomycin (Humatin, Parke-Davis, Morris Plains, N.J.), is effective in treating acute intestinal cases of cryptosporidiosis in people,[18] calves,[26] mice,[42] and rats.[135] Clinical signs of disease and oocyst shedding were eliminated in cats and dogs after paromomycin was administered for 5 days (Table 82-2).[7,8] Paromomycin is not absorbed from the GI tract unless gut epithelium is injured. If injured, a resulting absorption of paromomycin, renal damage, or deafness similar to that caused by other aminoglycosides may occur. Acute renal failure has been described in four cats receiving excessive doses of paromomycin for the treatment of hemorrhagic diarrhea presumably caused by cryptosporidiosis.[35] Paromomycin was effective in preventing cryptosporidial enteritis in a controlled study in goats.[55] See the Drug Formulary, Appendix 8, for further information on this drug. Although paromomycin seems effective against ileal infections, it was ineffective against cecal and biliary tract infections in immunosuppressed rats.[115] Tylosin (11 mg/kg, orally, twice daily for 28 days) was helpful in

relieving diarrhea in a cat with cryptosporidiosis and lymphocytic duodenitis,[46,64] which may be related to its antibacterial effects. Neither prior treatment with clindamycin nor metronidazole was effective in treating this cat. Pretreatment with paromomycin was effective in prolonging the prepatent period of infection in a controlled study of calves with experimentally induced infections; however, it did not reduce the severity or occurrence of infection.[38] Paromomycin was no more effective than placebo was in treating human patients with advanced AIDS.[45] Azithromycin, a macrolide antibiotic, was more effective than paromomycin was when used at identical regimens against cryptosporidial infection involving the ileum, cecum, or biliary tract of immunosuppressed rats.[115] Azithromycin has been effective in treating an immunocompetent man with cryptosporidiosis acquired from a calf.[10] Azithromycin is being tested in human trials but has not been extensively studied for the treatment of infected dogs or cats. Azithromycin, combined with paromomycin, was highly effective in treating an immunocompromised person with AIDS.[124] Clarithromycin, a related derivative to azithromycin, was highly effective in preventing development of cryptosporidiosis in human patients with AIDS when it was combined with a rifabutin as prophylaxis for mycobacterial infections.[50] Nitazoxanide has shown some efficacy in people infected with cryptosporidiosis and has been licensed for treatment.[118,138] In one study, cats treated with nitazoxanide showed immediate cessation of cyst excretion in their feces, but administration was complicated by vomiting soon after the cats received the oral drug.[35] This drug needs further study in cats and dogs. Lasalocid, an ionophorous antibiotic, had in vitro and in vivo activity against cryptosporidia,[43] although further studies are needed. For additional information on the above drugs, see Chapter 34, and the Drug Formulary, Appendix 8.

Parenteral fluid replacement is usually indicated if dehydration is severe. Antibiotic therapy for eliminating secondary bacterial invaders may be necessary. Because absorptive-cell surface epithelium is lost and developing glutamine-dependent epithelium predominates, oral rehydration solutions containing glutamine may be helpful as supportive care.[40]

Public Health Considerations

Cryptosporidial infections in people were not recognized until 1976. Since that time, it has been diagnosed with increasing frequency. Animal handlers, medical personnel, people living or traveling in developing countries, and children in day care facilities have the highest risk of exposure. Infection is not restricted to, but is more severe in, immunocompromised hosts. Between 4% and 7% of human patients admitted to hospitals for gastroenteritis have cryptosporidiosis, and infections are more common during the warm, humid months. Aquatic transmission via drinking water, the source of infection for more than 400,000 people in Milwaukee in 1993,[73] and swimming pools[74,78] have been major sources of infection. One out-

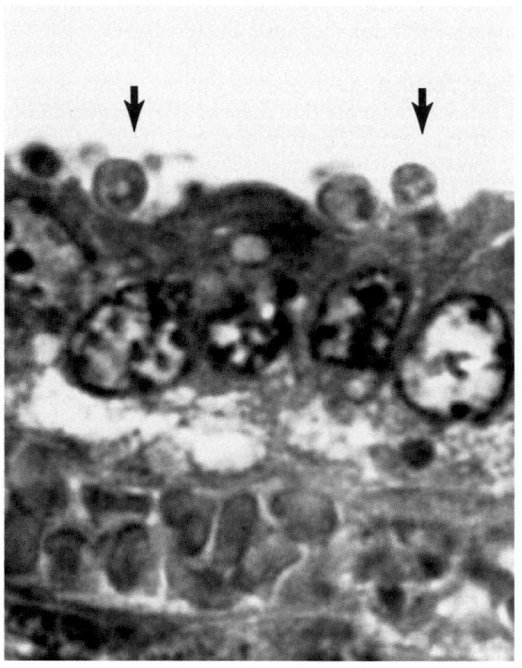

Fig 82-6 *Cryptosporidium (arrows)* in intestine from an infected calf is characteristically located at the microvillous border (H and E stain, ×250). (Courtesy University of Georgia, Athens, Ga.)

Table • 82-2

Drug Therapy for Cryptosporidiosis

DRUG[a]	SPECIES	DOSE[b] (mg/kg)	ROUTE	INTERVAL (HOURS)	DURATION (DAYS)
Paromomycin	B	125—165	PO	12	5[7,8]
Azithromycin[c]	D	5—10	PO	12	5—7
	C	7—15	PO	12	5—7

B, Dog and cat; *D,* dog; *C,* cat; *PO,* by mouth.
[a]See Drug Formulary, Appendix 8, for specific information on drugs.
[b]Dose per administration at specified interval.
[c]Dose for systemic infections; effective level for this disease has not been established.

break in the United States has also been associated with a recreational lake.[62] Although major human outbreaks of cryptosporidiosis caused by *C. hominis* and *C. parvum* have been linked to contaminated drinking water, none has incriminated *C. felis* or *C. canis*.[70a] Reports of food contamination with feces from infected people or animals are less common.[58] Owning a dog or cat does not increase the risk of humans developing cryptosporidiosis.[70a] Although epidemiologic data implicating household pets as sources of cryptosporidiosis in people is weak, several reports have been issued of human infection after contact with infected cats[60] and a dog.[37]

C. parvum of the cattle genotype has been considered as the predominant zoonotic risk for people. Dogs may also be infected with the cattle genotype, which they may conceivably pass on to people. Dogs are most commonly infected with the host-restricted species *C. canis*. Therefore dogs are not a significant reservoir for human infection. The dog isolate has been identified only in a few reports of human infection.* The people in these reports have generally been immunocompetent and nonsymptomatic. Similarly, human infection with *C. felis* has been an uncommon occurrence; however, clinical illness has been more apparent. Fourteen cases of *C. felis* infection of people have been documented with genetic methods.† Clinical illness, characterized by watery diarrhea, was observed in immunocompetent (n = 4) and immunosuppressed (n = 10) people.[12] Reports of human cryptosporidiosis acquired from cats have been published in which the infecting species was unknown.[30] A nosocomial outbreak of *C. parvum* infection in animals and people in a veterinary teaching hospital was associated with infection from a hospitalized calf.[61] Numerous reports of transmission from calves to humans have been issued.[66,68,83] Genetic analyses of human and bovine isolates have shown that two types of *C. parvum* exist.[107] One is involved with calf-to-human, human-to-human, human-to-calf, and other interspecies transmissions. The other is an exclusive anthroponotic cycle, with people being both the reservoir and affected population. Because cryptosporidiosis can be fatal in immunocompromised people, especially those with AIDS, owners of infected animals must be made aware of the zoonotic risks. *C. muris*, predominantly a rodent species that can experimentally infect dogs and cats among other animals, has been isolated from immunocompromised people.[104] Whether dogs can be reservoirs for this species is uncertain.

In immunocompetent people, GI signs, in decreasing frequency, include profuse watery diarrhea, low-grade fever, vomiting, and abdominal discomfort. Diarrhea usually lasts 3 to 12 days. Infants, children, and older adults have more chronic persistent diarrhea and dehydration. In immunodeficient individuals, especially those with AIDS, the diarrhea becomes chronic (usually 20 or more weeks), debilitating, and potentially fatal. In addition, respiratory tree, biliary, and pancreatic duct colonization has been reported in immunodeficient people with associated clinical signs.[17]

Cryptosporidia are resistant to commercial bleach (5.25% sodium hypochlorite); routine chlorination of drinking water does not affect oocyst viability.[114] Of the common disinfectants, only formol saline (10% solution) and ammonia (5% solution) were effective in destroying the viability of cryptosporidial oocysts. However, oocysts had to be in contact with the disinfectants for 18 hours. More concentrated (50%) ammonia solutions have been effective after 30 minutes. Moist heat (steam or pasteurization [over 55° C]), freezing and thawing, or thorough drying are more practical means of disinfection. Swimming pools can be disinfected by using high-chlorine concentrations for long periods (3 mg/L of water for 53 hours or 8 mg/L for 20 hours).[57] Excellent sanitation and liberal use of boiling water for scalding food and water bowls should minimize contamination in a clinical environment. Chlorination of drinking water is not effective, and because filtration of this small organism is difficult, the organism can enter treated municipal supplies. Even bottled noncarbonated mineral water has been contaminated.[95]

CYCLOSPORIASIS

Cyclospora cayetanensis is a member of subclass Coccidia in the phylum Apicomplexa that infects people and animals in warm or tropical climates worldwide. For many years, *C. cayetanensis* was considered a cyanobacterium, a blue-green alga, or a large (8 to 10 μm) strain of *Cryptosporidium*. Phylogenetically, the organism is most closely related to *Eimeria*.[110] Veterinarians should be aware that this parasite may be mistaken for *Cryptosporidium*, and parasites closely resembling *Cyclospora* have been found in animals. Both *Cyclospora* and other coccidia have similar appearing oocysts in feces and produce similar GI signs.[143] The morphology and features of *Cyclospora* that distinguish it from other coccidial oocysts are listed in Table 82-3. The life cycle of *Cyclospora* is unknown, but transmission occurs through contaminated water.[75a] Oocysts are passed in a noninfectious state and must survive long enough to sporulate and to be ingested by a susceptible host. The oocyst dies immediately when desiccated. *Cyclospora* oocysts have only been recovered in limited quantities from water sources because of technological limitations of recovery methods. At least 2 weeks at a temperature range of 25° C to 30° C (77° F to 86° F) are required outside the host for sporulation of oocysts to be infectious.[127]

Outside this range, oocyst sporulation does not occur, or the time interval is markedly prolonged. Following ingestion, sporulated oocysts excyst in the small bowel and enter epithelial cells. The upper small intestine is the site of replication in immunocompetent hosts, and more diffuse intestinal involvement occurs in the immunosuppressed hosts.[105] Asexual replication is thought to occur in the small bowel with extruded merozoites penetrating new epithelial cells. Sexual reproduction occurs in the small bowel epithelium as unsporulated oocysts are shed in the stool.[101] Malabsorption is caused by inflammation, villous atrophy, and crypt hyperplasia. Cholecystitis has also been reported in people.[148]

Outbreaks correspond to the time of the rainy season in endemic countries. Drinking contaminated water or eating unwashed berries (e.g., raspberries) or other plants (e.g., basil, salad leaves) imported from some countries in South America or Southern Europe have been implicated as risk factors in the United States,* where the prevalence in stool specimens submitted to diagnostic laboratories is generally less than 0.5%.[51,125] Carriage rates of up to 20% of people with diarrhea are found in endemic tropical countries. Animals or insects may act as reservoir hosts maintaining the organism in nature. Although other animals might be infected, this has been currently identified only as a human pathogen. *Cyclospora*-like organisms have been recovered from dogs, chickens, ducks, and primates.[127] Only in primates has the organisms been confirmed as *Cyclospora*. In other animals, inert passage through the intestinal tract cannot be eliminated. Two cases in dogs in Sao Paulo, Brazil, have been reported.[147] However, when dogs were experimentally inoculated orally with *Cyclospora* cysts, infection did not occur.[22] In Mexico, feces of cats were examined to no avail; however, a large number of oocysts morphologically and biologically resem-

---

*References: 2, 87, 106, 109, 144.
†References: 12, 14, 87, 106, 109, 144.

*References: 16, 20, 44, 48, 72.

Table • 82-3

Comparison of Coccidial Oocysts and Transmission

VARIABLE	CYCLOSPORA	CRYPTOSPORIDIUM	ISOSPORA	TOXOPLASMA
Definitive host	People, possibly animals	People, dog, cat, other animals	People, dog, cat, other animals	Cat
Intestinal biopsy				
Intracellular stages	T, S, M	T, S, M, G	T, S, M, G	T, S, M, G
Intracellular location	Deep seated	Intramembranous, extracytoplasmic	Deep seated	Deep seated
Size in tissue (µm)	4—16	2—5	3—15	3—15
Feces				
Oocyst size (µm)	8—10	4—6	10—19 × 20—30 Varies with species	12 × 10
Sporulated oocyst				
Number sporocysts	2	0	2	2
Number sporozoites per sporocyst	2	4 per oocyst (naked)	4	4
Acid-fast staining	Variable	Yes	Yes	Yes
Ultraviolet autofluorescence, 365-nm filter	Blue-green Circles	None	Yes	None
Auramine fluorescence	Weak	Bright	Variable	Variable
Infectivity in fresh feces (already sporulated)	No	Yes	No	No
Zoonotic transmission	Unknown	Many animals	None, host specific	Cat
Host-to-like-host transmission	Unknown	Yes	Yes	Yes, uncommon via oocyst

T, Trophozoite; S, schizont; M, merozoitel G, gametocyte.
Modified from Soave R. 1996. *Cyclospora*: an overview, *Clin Infect Dis* 23:429–437, with permission of the University of Chicago Press; Sun T, Ilardi CF, Asnis D, et al. 1996. Light and electron microscopic identification of *Cyclospora* species in the small intestine: evidence of the presence of asexual life cycle in human host, *Am J Clin Pathol* 105:216–220; copyright © 1996, by the American Society of Clinical Pathologists. Reprinted with permission.

bling *C. cayetanensis* was found in poultry feces.[29] Fowl feces may be involved in contamination of poultry meat, water supplies, vegetables and fruits, or any combination of these. Animal-to-human or person-to-person transmission is not yet documented.

Cyclosporiasis produces relapsing watery diarrhea, fatigue, systemic influenza-like manifestations, and weight loss in susceptible people such as those infected with HIV, those receiving organ transplants or immunosuppressants, and those traveling to different geographic areas. Clinical signs usually begin after 1 week following exposure. Clinical signs are infrequent or transient in immunocompetent hosts, who usually recover within several weeks.[101]

Diagnosis is made by microscopic detection of oocysts in fecal specimens. At present, definitive oocysts have only been identified in human feces. These oocysts can be confused with *Cryptosporidium* and *Isospora*, which also stain acid-fast in stool specimens. However, *Cyclospora* has a variable staining intensity on an individual preparation. The organisms are passed unsporulated in fresh feces and on superficial examination, they may be misidentified as a fungal spore. Although PCR has been used for specific detection of the organism in fecal specimens, cross-amplification with other coccidia has not been determined.[99,111] Organisms can also be detected on jejunal aspiration or biopsy. Unlike cryptosporidiosis, cyclosporiasis in people responds to 7 days of treatment with trimethoprim-sulfonamides with rapid cessation of diarrhea and shedding of oocysts.[49,134] Should a dog or cat be diagnosed with clinical cyclosporiasis or pose a potential risk for human infection, routine dosages of trimethoprim-sulfonamide can be used (see Drug Formulary, Appendix 8). As with other coccidia, chlorine bleach is not an effective disinfectant for *Cyclospora* spp. oocysts.

C. cayetamensis requires a period in the environment to sporulate into the infectious oocysts. Therefore direct animal-to-person or person-to-person spread would be minimal. People tend to acquire their infection from consuming contaminated water or produce. Nevertheless, cyclosporiasis in Peru has been epidemiologically associated with ownership of domestic animals, especially birds, guinea pigs, and rabbits.[9]

SUGGESTED READINGS*

2. Abe N, Kimata I, Iseki M. 2002. Identification of genotypes of *Cryptosporidium parvum* isolates from a patient and a dog in Japan, *J Vet Med Sci* 64:165-168.

34. Gookin JL, Nordone SK, Argenzio RA. 2002. Host responses to *Cryptosporidium* infection, *J Vet Intern Med* 16:12-21.

*See the CD-ROM for a complete list of references.

35. Gookin JL, Riviere JE, Gilger BC, et al. 1999. Acute renal failure in four cats treated with paromomycin, *J Am Vet Med Assoc* 215:1821-1823.
82. Miller DL, Liggett A, Radi ZA, et al. 2003. Gastrointestinal cryptosporidiosis in a puppy, *Vet Parasitol* 115:199-204.
88. Morgan UM, Sargent KD, Elliot A, et al. 1998. *Cryptosporidium* in cats—additional evidence for *C. felis*, *Vet J* 156:159-161.

89. Morgan UM, Xiao L, Monis P, et al. 2000. *Cryptosporidium* spp. in domestic dogs: the "dog" genotype, *Appl Enviro Microbiol* 66:2220-2223.
119. Saini PK, Ransom G, McNamara AM. 2000. Emerging public health concerns regarding cryptosporidiosis, *J Am Vet Med Assoc* 217:658-663.
121. Scorza AV, Brewer MM, Lappin MR. 2003. Polymerase chain reaction for the detection of *Cryptosporidium* spp. in cat feces, *J Parasitol* 89:423-426.

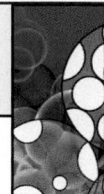

CHAPTER • 83

Rhinosporidiosis

M. Cecilia Castellano and Edward B. Breitschwerdt

ETIOLOGY

Rhinosporidiosis, a chronic granulomatous disease caused by *Rhinosporidium seeberi*, induces tumorlike growths of epithelial tissues in domestic animals, birds, and people.[6,13,15]

The taxonomy of *R. seeberi* has long been controversial. Based on its morphologic characteristics, it has been classified in the past few years as a fungus by most microbiologists. Phylogenetic analysis indicates *R. seeberi* to be a member of a newly recognized group of human and animal pathogens that form a branch in the evolutionary tree near the animal-fungal divergence.[8,10] It has been proposed that this new phylogenetic group be referred to as the class Mesomycetozoea (between fungi and animals) and *R. seeberi* be considered a monotypic genus within this class.[10,19] Genetic analysis of isolates suggests that host-specific strains of the organism may exist.[22a] Like other mesomycetozoeans, *R. seeberi* is associated with aquatic environments. Although *R. seeberi* is generally believed to be the causative agent of rhinosporidiosis, a few challenge this accepted premise. In one study, a cyanobacterium *Microcystis aeruginosa* was isolated from water in which human patients with the disease were bathing.[2,3] The organism was also identified in clinical specimens; however, additional confirmation is needed for this hypothesis. Microscopic findings of lesions indicate that *R. seeberi*, and not a bacterium, is the cause of this disease.

Although a few successful attempts to propagate *R. seeberi* in tissue culture have been described,[6,14] the results have been questioned.[18] Most microbiologists consider *R. seeberi* to be intractable to culture.[8,10,19] The infective unit is a small (7- to 15-μm), round spore that once implanted in tissues progressively develops into large (100- to 450-μm), spherical bodies known as *sporangia*. Sporangia undergo a maturation process, resulting in the production of 16,000 to 20,000 endospores that are then discharged through an apical pore, and the cycle is reinitiated.[6]

EPIDEMIOLOGY

Rhinosporidiosis is endemic in India, Sri Lanka, and Argentina and is reported sporadically from other parts of the world. In the United States, canine rhinosporidiosis has been reported only in the southern states; however, occurrence of the disease in a dog native to Ontario and in a cat from a suburb of Washington, DC, suggests the possibility of a more widespread distribution in North America. In Europe, canine rhinosporidiosis has been recognized only in northern Italy.[7]

Feline rhinosporidiosis has been reported in two outdoor cats, both in the United States.[20,23]

R. seeberi is stimulated to develop mature endospores that are released from its sporangia after exposure to water, thus the disease is associated with wet environments and the host's moist mucous membranes. Most affected animals are exposed to flowing or impounded water. Infection frequently involves the mucous membranes of the nasal cavity, but it may occasionally affect the ear, pharynx, larynx, trachea, esophagus, urogenital mucosae, and skin. Reported cases of canine and feline rhinosporidiosis have involved only the nasal cavity.

The disease is more common in large-breed dogs with a mean age of 5 years (and a range of 1.5 to 13 years) and seems to be more common in males, as it is in people and horses. Behavioral and biologic factors may be responsible for this apparent predisposition. Because of the few reported cases, it is not known whether the same tendencies are found in cats.

PATHOGENESIS

The pathogenesis of rhinosporidiosis has not been completely characterized because of the difficulties associated with in vitro propagation of the organism.

R. seeberi has not been detected in the environment, and its natural host remains unknown. Reports from endemic areas suggest that infection is acquired by mucosal contact with stagnant water. Mucous membrane trauma may be a predisposing factor. In arid countries, most human infections are ocular, and dust is postulated to be a fomite. In vitro studies suggest that endospore release from mature sporangia is stimulated by mucous secretions.[18] Once implanted in tissues, endospores elicit a severe, focal pyogranulomatous reaction.

Little is known about the immune response to *R. seeberi*. A mucoidlike layer with immunogenic properties has been recognized beneath the sporangium's cell wall.[11,18] It has been suggested that it may play a role in the immunology of the disease.

CLINICAL FINDINGS

Clinical findings include wheezing, sneezing, unilateral seropurulent nasal discharge, and epistaxis. Polypoid lesions may be visible in the nares (Fig. 83-1) and may also be visualized by rhinoscopy in the rostral nasal cavity (Fig. 83-2). Single or multiple polyps ranging in size from a few millimeters up to 3 cm are pink, red, or pale gray and covered by numerous pinpoint white-yellowish granules (sporangia). Polyps may be sessile or pedunculated, and the superficial surface is irregular, glistening, and possibly ulcerated. Duration of clinical signs in reported canine cases ranges between 2 weeks and 8 months.

DIAGNOSIS

The organism can be demonstrated by several stains: hematoxylin-eosin, Wright, Gridley's, toluidine blue, periodic acid–Schiff, and Grocott's. Cytologic examination of nasal exudate and of scrape or brush samples obtained from the surface of the polyp usually allows diagnosis through identification of single or clusters of *R. seeberi* spores. Although less common, sporangia may be observed (Fig. 83-3). Sporangia and spores should be easily recognized by histologic examination.

A polymerase chain reaction assay specific for *R. seeberi* has been developed.[8]

PATHOLOGIC FINDINGS

Microscopic examination reveals that polyps are composed of fibrovascular tissue lined by squamous or columnar epithelium that is frequently ulcerated.[6] Sporangia at different stages of maturation can be seen (Fig. 83-4) and may be releasing

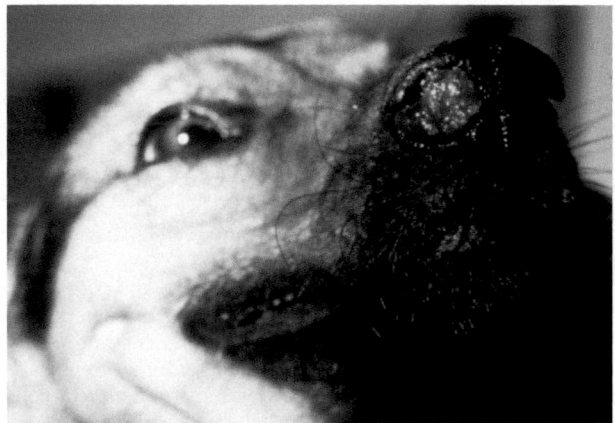

Fig 83-1 Two-year-old male dog of mixed German shepherd breeding from Argentina, with a bright red sessile growth in the right nostril. Rhinosporidiosis was diagnosed after histologic examination.

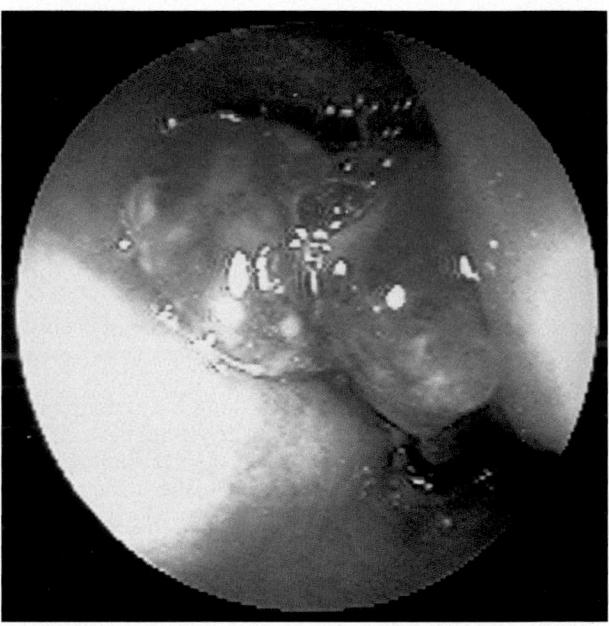

Fig 83-2 Rostral rhinoscopy in dog with rhinosporidiosis. Polyp is attached to nasal mucosa. (Courtesy University of Georgia, Athens, Ga.)

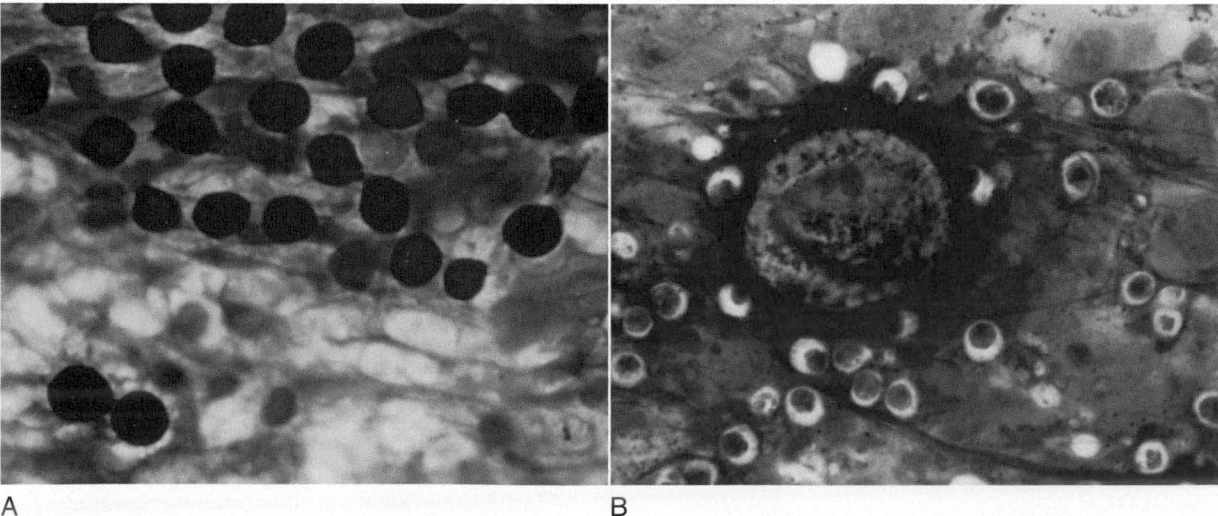

A   B

Fig 83-3 Scrape smear of nasal polyp. **A,** Numerous single endospores of *R. seeberi* dispersed in epithelial-cell background (PAS stain, ×200). **B,** Juvenile sporangium of *R. seeberi*. Note transparent capsules and numerous endospores with internal globular bodies (Wright stain, ×200).

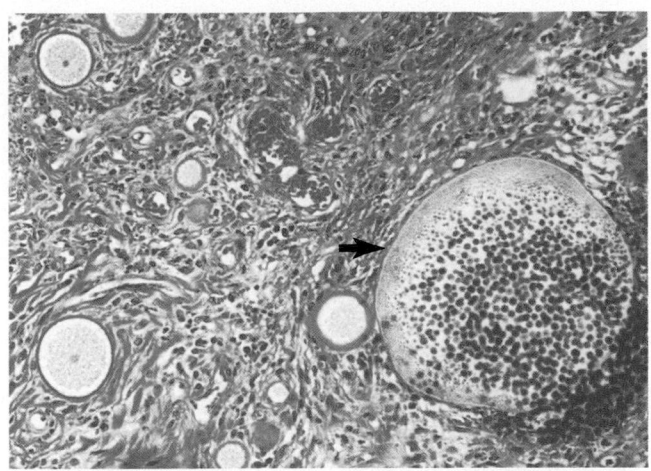

Fig 83-4 Nasal polyp. Note larger mature sporangium *(arrow)* and smaller trophic stages throughout stroma (H and E stain, ×160). (From Gardiner CH, Fayer R, Dubey JP. 1988. *An atlas of protozoan parasites in animal tissues*, Beltsville, Md, USDA, Agriculture Handbook No 651.)

spores through the epithelium to the superficial surface. A superficial exudate most prominent in areas of spore extrusion is composed of spores, neutrophils, epithelia, and erythrocytes. A mixed inflammatory response consisting predominantly of plasma cells and lymphocytes and to a lesser extent, macrophages, is scattered throughout the tissue.

THERAPY

Surgical excision remains the treatment of choice and may be curative when a single polyp is excised. Because of the frequent rostral location of the polyps, surgical excision through the nares or by anterolateral approach to the nares generally is possible, negating the necessity for the more invasive dorsonasal flap procedure. In four dogs treated with surgery alone, no recurrence was noted after 1 to 2 years.[7] Recurrence has been reported 2 to 12 months after surgery in dogs with single or multiple lesions. Dapsone has been used to treat human

rhinosporidiosis with variable success[12,6] and might be considered as an adjunct to surgical removal of lesions in dogs or cats. Light and electron microscopic studies have demonstrated that dapsone induces degenerative changes in *R. seeberi* by inhibiting division of the organism.[22] Treatment with dapsone (1 mg/kg every 8 hours for 2 weeks, followed by 1 mg/kg every 12 hours for 4 months) likely cured a dog that developed polyps after surgical extirpation.[6,17] Ketoconazole (8.7 mg/kg every 8 hours for 21 days) eliminated nasal discharge in a dog after 4 days, and visual and cytologic resolution of the polyps occurred after 21 days of therapy.[6] Although treatment continued for an additional 21 days, the disease recurred 6 months later, necessitating surgical excision of a large polyp. Medical therapy of rhinosporidiosis may be improved by screening antiparasitic drugs that have an effect on other members of the Mesomycetozoea class.

PUBLIC HEALTH CONSIDERATIONS

Although people are also affected with this disease, no evidence supports the possibility of transmission of *R. seeberi* from animals to people. Dogs and people appear to become infected from common environmental sources.

SUGGESTED READINGS*

7. Caniatti M, Roccabianca P, Scanziani E, et al. 1998. Nasal rhinosporidiosis in dogs: four cases from Europe and a review of literature. *Vet Rec* 142:334-338.
9. Fredricks DN, Jolley JA, Lepp PW, et al. 2000. *Rhinosporidium seeberi*: a human pathogen from a novel group of aquatic protistan parasites. *Emerg Infect Dis* 6:273-282.
19. Mendoza L, Taylor JW, Ajello L. 2002. The class Mesomycetozoea: a heterogeneous group of microorganisms at the animal-fungal boundary. *Annu Rev Microbiol* 56:315-344.
20. Moisan PG, Baker SV. 2001. Rhinosporidiosis in a cat. *J Vet Diagn Invest* 13:352-354.
23. Wallin LL, Coleman GD, Froeling J, et al. 2001. Rhinosporidiosis in a domestic cat. *Med Mycol* 39:139-141.

*See the CD-ROM for a complete list of references.

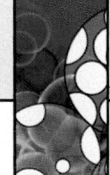

CHAPTER • 84

Neurologic Diseases of Suspected Infectious Origin and Prion Disease

GRANULOMATOUS MENINGOENCEPHALITIS

Andrea Tipold and Marc Vandevelde

Granulomatous meningoencephalitis (GME) has been reported in dogs in the United States,[16,17,31] Australia,[47] New Zealand,[4] Japan,[74] and several European countries.[137] It is a relatively common condition and is characterized by disseminated inflammatory lesions in the central nervous system (CNS) with perivascular granuloma formation.[138]

Etiology

GME is thought to be an infectious disease. However, experimental attempts to transmit the agent in dogs using GME-infected brain tissue have been unsuccessful.[85] Bacteria and fungi can cause granulomatous lesions in the CNS of small animals, but such agents would not likely have escaped detection on light microscopic examination of GME. Possibly, the periodic acid-Schiff–positive and acidophilic inclusions in macrophages in lesions in some cases may be an unidentified infectious agent.[31] Other investigators have searched unsuccessfully for an infectious organism by electron microscopic (EM) examination of the tissues.[33] Serologic tests for toxoplasmosis have been carried out in a few cases, but the results have been negative.[17] The possibility of rickettsial infection as an underlying cause should also be considered. Certain viral infections such as equine infectious anemia, feline infectious peritonitis, and visna are also associated with granulomatous lesions of the CNS. Canine distemper virus (CDV), which is responsible for a variety of CNS lesions, can be excluded as a cause of GME because systematic immunocytochemical studies in a large number of GME cases failed to find CDV antigen in the lesions.[59] The presence of anti-CDV antibody titers in the CSF of seven dogs with GME can probably be explained by unspecific invasion and amplification of B cells in the inflammatory lesions. Attempts to identify reverse transcriptase activity in the cerebrospinal fluid (CSF) failed. Results have also been negative for rabies virus antigen, fungi, bacteria, and protozoa.[72] Sophisticated culturing techniques are probably necessary to identify the agent. Some dogs with GME-compatible CSF cytologic abnormalities have had positive serologic test results to *Bartonella vinsonii* subsp. *berkhoffii* (see Chapter 54).[18] Simultaneous onset of clinical signs in two related Afghan hounds and a certain predisposition for small-breed dogs suggests that the disease may be associated with either common exposure or a genetic predisposition.[54] Lesions consist of infiltrates of major histocompatibility complex class II antigen-positive macrophages and to an equal amount of T and B cells, in contrast to virus-induced encephalitis with a predominance of T cells and bacterial and protozoal infections with a predominance of B cells in perivascular cuffs.[133] Other investigators have detected a predominance of T cells.[72] Before its recognition as a clinicopathologic entity, GME lesions were classified as reticulosis, implying some kind of proliferative disorder. The belief was that granulomatous inflammatory lesions could evolve to neoplasms of the monocytic-microglial lineage. In some instances, differentiating between GME and certain lympho-histiocytic tumors remains difficult. That GME might be a purely proliferative rather than an infectious disease cannot be dismissed.

Clinical Findings

The disease occurs most often in young to middle-aged small purebred females, but dogs of different ages, breeds, and sex can develop the disease. The prevalence for smaller breeds, especially poodles, small terrier breeds, Pekingese, and Maltese, appears to be higher.[16] The disease rarely occurs before the age of 2 years. Clinical signs usually have an acute onset, and the disease is always progressive. Two forms of the disease are described. In the acute form, clinical signs develop rapidly over the course of 1 to 10 days, and without treatment, it is rapidly progressive and fatal. In the chronic form, signs may develop more slowly over a period of 1 to 4 months. The chronic form with long-term survival for several months to years was thought to be associated with the focal form of GME when large tumorlike masses develop. However, clinical signs with slow progression can also be found with diffuse histopathologic lesions. Specific neurologic signs cannot be expected because lesions can occur anywhere in the CNS. Signs are associated with the site of most extensive damage or may reflect a multifocal lesion. Signs consist of disturbances in gait and postural reactions, with ataxia, dysmetria, paresis, and paralysis; changes in mental status, with confusion, lethargy, and coma; and cranial nerve dysfunction. In the acute stage of the disease, more than one half of

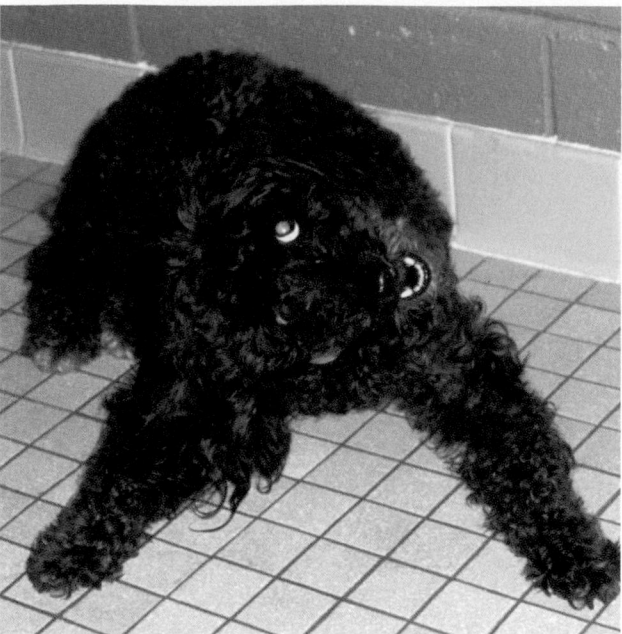

Fig 84-1 Dog showing central vestibular signs.

the animals have fever, and many exhibit paraspinal discomfort[119] or cervical pain.[31,120] In this stage of the disease, central vestibular signs are common (Fig. 84-1); seizures may also be observed. The clinical presentation can also be suggestive of a space-occupying mass referring to a single site of involvement, most frequently the posterior fossa, with brain stem and cerebellar signs. Cerebral or spinal signs sometimes predominate. A particular ocular localization of GME, previously called ocular reticulosis, occurs with acute unilateral or bilateral blindness and ophthalmoscopic evidence of optic neuritis.[16]

Diagnosis

Typical hematologic and biochemical findings are lacking. Neutrophilia may be present in the acute disease.[119,120] The CSF is abnormal, with a marked pleocytosis; cell counts of 100 to several thousand leukocytes/μl are usual. Mild pleocytosis or even a normal cell count is observed in animals pretreated with glucocorticoids. Mononuclear cells predominate, but a mixed pleocytosis can also be observed with varying numbers of neutrophils.[7] Cytologic examination of the CSF may reveal large anaplastic mononuclear cells with abundant lacy cytoplasm[16] and up to 20% are macrophages. The acute and the chronic form of the disease cannot be distinguished by differential cell count. Protein concentration is usually increased, with a range from reference values up to 1119 mg/dl and a mean of 163.2 ± 25 mg/dl.[7] Electrophoretic examination of the CSF may suggest blood-brain barrier disruption and intrathecal immunoglobulin synthesis.[119,120] Such changes are not specific for GME. Electroencephalographic (EEG) patterns studied in some dogs with GME were unspecific. In focal GME, the tumorlike lesions can be detected with computed tomography (CT)[16] after intravenous (IV) inoculation of contrast medium and magnetic resonance imaging (MRI).[95] With CT, GME lesions are contrast enhanced, however, not to the degree of meningiomas.[121] MRI features can resemble neoplasia in which lesions with T_1-weighted images appear isointense and have hypointense margins, but lesions with T_2-weighted images appear hyperintense.[82] Inflammatory lesions may have lesions on T_1- and T_2-weighted images that enhance with contrast.[82] Regardless of ancillary testing, a definitive intra vitam diagnosis still depends on histopathology of brain biopsies.

These specimens must be taken by stereotaxic equipment, surgical biopsy, or necropsy. Without these diagnostic modalities, GME can be mistaken for a neoplasm or another focal encephalitis.[125] Mixed cell patterns and increased proteins in CSF can also occur with inflammatory encephalitis produced by CDV, *Neospora caninum*, *Toxoplasma gondii*, and systemic mycoses.

Pathologic Findings

Lesions are found in the meninges, brain, and spinal cord, especially in the cervical segments. White matter is generally more severely affected compared with gray matter. Although the lesions are disseminated, the cerebral hemispheres, the midbrain, and the region around the fourth ventricle are most frequently involved. The lesions, which are strictly associated with the vasculature, consist of perivascular cuffing of monocytes, lymphocytes, plasma cells, and sometimes a few neutrophils and mast cells. The formation of eccentrically situated nodular foci of macrophages within these cuffs is a characteristic finding in GME (Fig. 84-2). The cuffs can be distinguished in three degrees of severity: small disseminated perivascular lesions, confluence of several perivascular cuffs into small granulomas, and large focal coalescing granulomas, leading to the formation of tumorlike lesions. Additionally, necrosis of the neuropil, mitosis in the perivascular cuffs, and edema may be observed in both forms of the disease. Tryptase-positive mast cells can be found in perivascular cuffs of the lesions of GME, in the meninges, and in the CNS parenchyma. Dogs with the acute form of the disease have significantly more mast cells compared with dogs with the chronic form, suggesting that this cell population may contribute to the dynamics of the lesion and to the rapid clinical deterioration of dogs with GME.[39] Antiastrocyte antibodies are increased in the CSF of dogs with GME and necrotizing meningoencephalitis (NME) but not with other inflammatory conditions of the CNS.[93] Autoantibody was also detected in some dogs with brain tumors and may represent only a secondary response to a damaged blood-CNS barrier.

Therapy

No specific therapy for GME exists, although improvement frequently has been observed following administration of glucocorticoids or diverse immunosuppressive drugs (Table 84-1). Because a final intra vitam diagnosis of GME is difficult, treatment studies have been cumbersome. However, all known patients have eventually died of the disease despite glucocorticoid or other treatments. Because glucocorticoid therapy provides only temporary improvement in many cases, other immunosuppressive drugs have been used. The use of procarbazine or cytosine arabinoside, two alternative antineoplastic drugs, may be considered.[34,99] Procarbazine is a prodrug that forms numerous active cytotoxic metabolites following metabolism. This DNA-alkylating agent is an anticancer drug that has also been used in human transplant cases. It can be used alone or in combination to treat GME.[34] Procarbazine is well absorbed orally and may cause neurotoxicity, vomiting, or hepatic dysfunction. The patient should be monitored closely for cytotoxicity, and after 1 month of daily therapy, every-other-day dosing should be used. Cytosine arabinoside, a parenteral drug, is also effective, has few side effects, and is reasonably priced.[34] Because of its parenteral route, it is used primarily for induction therapy in the hospital. Both drugs cause myelosuppression and must be monitored for signs of toxicity. Leflunomide is a pyrimidine synthesis inhibitor that suppresses activated T cells. It has been used as an alternative treatment because of the side effects or lack of responsiveness when other drugs are used. Leflunomide can affect cell replication, causing leukopenia, diarrhea, or alopecia in people. Mycophenolate mofetil (MMF) has been used to treat dogs with various immune-mediated diseases such as pemphigus foliaceus and myasthenia gravis. It inhibits an enzyme in purine synthesis, which in turn suppresses lymphocyte function. It causes minimal myelosuppression. MMF is expensive; however, it has a low degree of toxicity, which is usually associated with vomiting or diarrhea. Cyclosporine has shown to be of benefit in treating dogs with localized GME.[1] The response to cyclosporine alone or initially in combination with

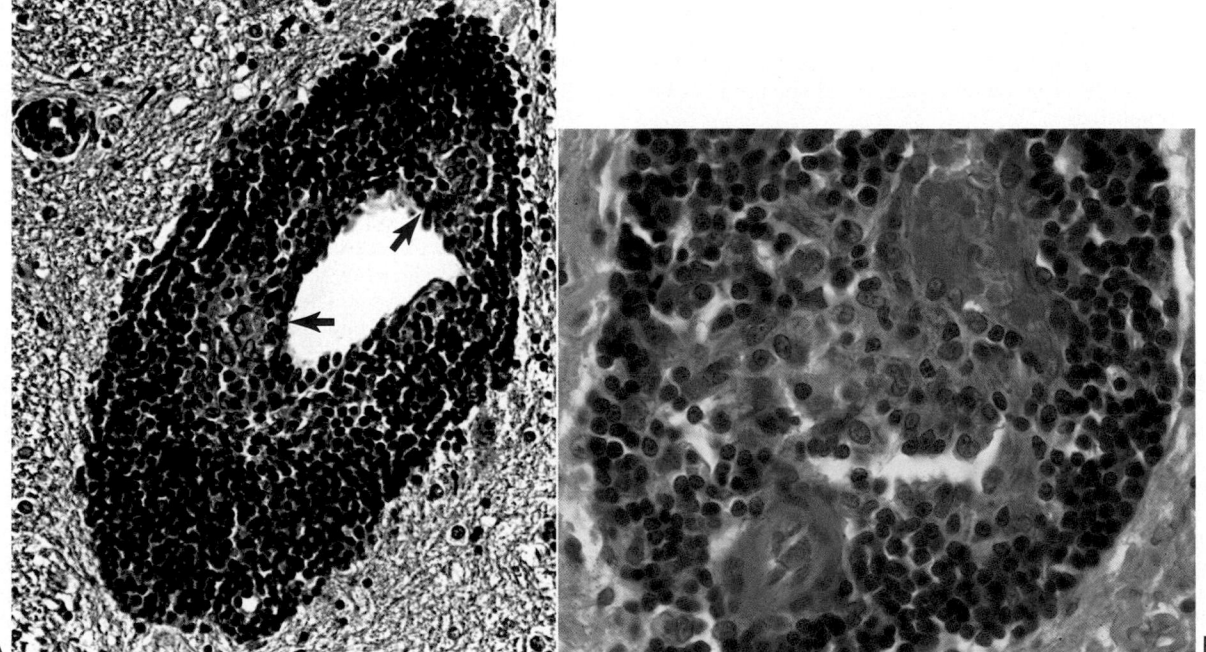

Fig 84-2 Histologic section from a dog with granulomatous meningoencephalitis. **A,** Typical perivascular mononuclear cuffing with eccentrically situated nodular foci of macrophages *(arrows)* (H and E stain, ×100). **B,** Closer view of a perivascular lesion (H and E stain, ×250).

Table • 84-1

Recommended Dosages of Immunosuppressive Drugs for Neurologic Diseases of Unknown Origin

DRUG[a]	SPECIES[b]	DOSE	ROUTE	INTERVAL (HOUR)
Prednisolone	B	2 mg/kg	IV, IM, SC	12—24[c]
Dexamethasone	B	0.2—0.4 mg/kg	PO, IM, SC	12—24[c]
Procarbazine	D	25 mg/m²	PO	30[d]
Cyclosporine	D	3—6 mg/kg	PO	12[e]
Leflunomide	D	4 mg/kg	PO	24
Cytosine arabinoside	D	100 mg/m²	IV, SC	24[f]
Mycophenolate mofetil	D	10 mg/kg	SC	12

B, Dog and cat; D, dog; IV, intravenous; IM, intramuscular; SC, subcutaneous; PO, by mouth.
[a]For more information on all drugs, see Drug Formulary, Appendix 8.
[b]Dose per administration at specified interval.
[c]Dose is gradually tapered over 4 months to the lowest that is effective in maintaining remission. Rarely can drug therapy be discontinued.
[d]After 30 days, every-other-day dosing is given. With no control, dose is increased to 50 mg/kg every other day and 25 mg/kg on alternate days.
[e]Generally, the 3-mg/kg dose is used for induction. Response to treatment and blood levels should be monitored to achieve efficacy and avoid nephrotoxic side effects. Drug levels should be checked 4 to 6 hours after last dose. Dose is usually reduced to every 24 hours for long-term maintenance.[1]
[f]Use to induce immunosuppression for 4 days in dogs.

glucocorticoids achieved remission and halted progression of neurologic signs for up to 1 year of monitoring with continued daily administration of a maintenance dosage. Use of cyclosporine without glucocorticoids avoided many of the undesirable side effects. Nephrotoxicity of cyclosporine was not observed, and blood monitoring showed safe therapeutic blood levels of the drug. Excess shedding of hair, alopecia, and potential worsening of an existing urinary tract infection were the observed side effects.

Radiation therapy with cobalt or linear accelerator has been used to slow the progression of the disease.[98] Dogs with focal lesions survive longer than do those with multifocal neurologic signs.[98] Radiation injury of cranial tissues is an adverse effect; however, this may be an alternative to systemic immunosuppression caused by chemotherapy.

Anticonvulsants may be needed to control seizures associated with inflammatory forebrain lesions in dogs with GME. Oral phenobarbital and potassium bromide are indicated for general use, and IV or rectal diazepam should be used in cases of status epilepticus.

The prognosis of GME is generally guarded given that most dogs develop progressive neurologic signs despite treatment. Dogs with multifocal GME have a rapid and virulent course of illness over several weeks that rarely respond to antiinflammatory or immunosuppressive therapy. Patients with more focal signs can have progressive illness over several months[111]; those with focal forebrain localization have the longest lifespan.[98]

ENCEPHALITIS IN PUG AND MALTESE DOGS

Andrea Tipold and Marc Vandevelde

This disease was initially described only in the Pug dog breed in the United States[32,36,49] but occurs worldwide.[11,55,79] The exact prevalence of this disease remains uncertain and seems to be a rare condition. An NME, clinically and pathologically indistinguishable from Pug dog encephalitis, has been reported in five Maltese dogs in the United States[122] and in one Maltese dog in Europe.[106] The disease may also occur in other toy breeds such as the Pekingese[25] and Papillon.[124]

Etiology

The cause of Pug and Maltese dog encephalitis is unknown. The distribution and morphologic characteristics of the lesions are unique for this disease and totally different from the histologic findings in other known CNS infections in small animals. The pathologic findings are, nevertheless, strongly suggestive of an infectious process. Bacterial, fungal, and protozoal organisms may probably be ruled out as potential causes because they would have been detected on histologic examination. The predominantly mononuclear inflammation suggests a viral cause. Viral isolation attempts in two cases, however, were unsuccessful.[36] The restriction of this disease to a few breeds is highly unusual for infections of small animals and strongly suggests predisposing genetic factors. Speculatively, these breeds may have a breed-specific tissue antigen that might act as a receptor for a hitherto unknown virus or may have a breed-specific composition of the immune-response genes, leading to an atypical immunologic reaction toward a known pathogen or perhaps an autoantigen. In this respect, the finding of an autoantibody recognizing glial fibrillary acidic protein can be explained.[136] The predilection of the cerebral hemispheres for involvement with a necrotic inflammatory process is similar to that with herpesvirus encephalitides of other species.[32,122]

Clinical Findings

The disease may occur at any age and affects both sexes. The course of the disease is usually 1 to 6 months, but occasionally dogs may die a few days after the onset of signs or survive for more than 1 year. The most consistent sign is the occurrence of focal or generalized seizures. Other signs include decreased consciousness, abnormal behavior, compulsive circling, blindness, hyperesthesia, generalized ataxia and paresis, and deficient postural reactions.[11,43a] A few animals may exhibit brain stem signs. The disease is always progressive, and many animals die as a result of severe seizures.[36]

Diagnosis

No typical hematologic and biochemical findings have been determined. CSF analysis is abnormal in most dogs, with a predominantly mononuclear pleocytosis (usually 90 to 600 cells/µl) and an increased protein concentration (usually 50 to 200 mg/dl)[32,67]; however, these are not specific because other encephalitides are associated with similar CSF changes. The massive necrotizing lesions in the cerebrum can be detected with CT or MRI.[79,122] Lesions appear as multifocal vascularization and hypodense areas with no contrast enhancement. Abnormal areas with increased signal intensity of T_2-weighted imaging can be detected with MRI. Irregular-shaped dilation and shifting of the lateral ventricles occurs with progression of the disease as a result of cerebral atrophy from loss of parenchymal tissue.

Pathologic Findings

Necrotizing lesions in the cerebrum may be visible on macroscopic examination. The histologic findings are unusual and highly typical for this disease: disseminated meningitis, choroiditis, and encephalitis, with greatest involvement in the cerebrum. The perivascular and meningeal inflammatory infiltrates consisting of lymphocytes, plasma cells, histiocytes, and macrophages have a strong tendency to invade the parenchyma. Extensive compact subpial and subventricular lesions are present and may extend deep into the underlying brain tissue, with unusually intense microglial proliferation and total destruction of the original tissue elements. In some areas, frank cerebrocortical necrosis occurs. The cerebral white matter also is severely affected, with intense perivascular cuffing and gliosis (Fig. 84-3). In some areas, leukomalacia with liquefaction and cavitation of the tissue is noted.

Therapy

No treatment for this disease has been found. Glucocorticoids do not alter the course of this necrotizing encephalitis in confirmed cases, and antiepileptic drugs are often ineffective in controlling seizures.[36,55] Animals usually develop persistent seizures and progressive neurologic signs and do not usually live longer than 7 months after the onset of clinical illness.

ENCEPHALITIS IN YORKSHIRE TERRIERS

Andrea Tipold and Marc Vandevelde

This condition appears to be restricted to Yorkshire terriers. The disease was originally reported in Switzerland[131] but

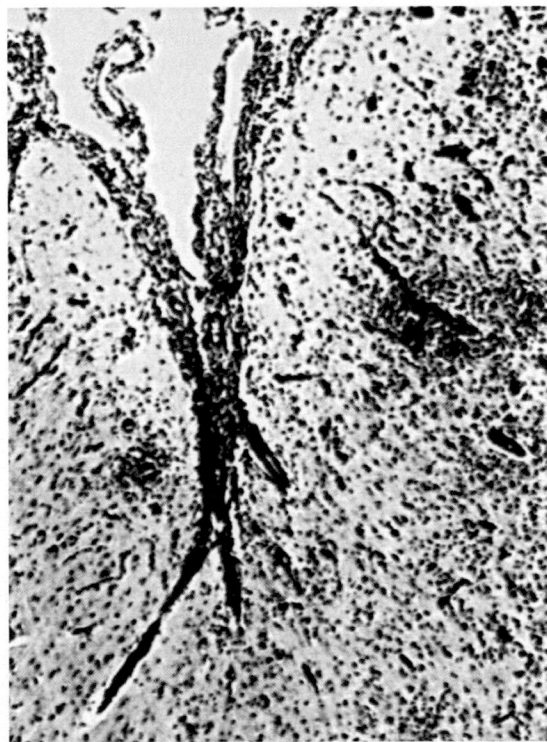

Fig   84-3   Histologic section from a case of pug dog encephalitis. Severe perivascular and meningeal inflammation, as well as necrosis of large areas of the cerebral cortex, are evident (H and E stain, ×100).

also occurs in other western European countries,[144] North America,[71,114] and Japan.[37] The disease seems to be a relatively new entity because retrospective examination of neuropathologic collections did not reveal cases before 1985. Both clinical and pathologic features of this disease differ considerably from the encephalitis in Pug and Maltese dogs.[140]

Etiology

The cause of Yorkshire terrier encephalitis remains unknown. An infectious organism is likely involved. Bacteria, fungi, and parasites can probably be excluded based on microscopic examination of the lesions using appropriate special stains. The appearance of the lesions suggests a viral cause. CDV was excluded by immunocytochemistry and in situ hybridization for CDV antigen and CDV mRNA. Rabies virus and central European tick-borne encephalitis virus were excluded using similar techniques.[140] To date, isolation studies have not been attempted.

Clinical Findings

Encephalitis in Yorkshire terriers appears to be predominantly a disease of adult dogs affecting both sexes. Although animals can show acute signs, a clear tendency exists for the disease to become protracted for months or even years.[80] No extraneural signs occur. Neurologic signs refer to a multifocal-diffuse intracranial disease involving the cerebrum (compulsive pacing, seizures, and visual deficits) and the brain stem (central vestibular signs, severe gait abnormalities with proprioceptive and multiple cranial nerve deficits).[83]

Diagnosis

No specific diagnostic test exists for this disease. Obviously, neurologic signs are not diagnostic per se. Lesions are quite large and are therefore detectable by imaging techniques.[114] In chronic cases, the lesions appear multifocal and cystic. Using CT and MRI, areas of decreased opacity and ventriculomegaly may be seen.[41,83,114] CSF changes consist of mononuclear pleocytosis, which is marked but not specific for the disease. The differential diagnosis includes chronic distemper encephalitis and GME.

Pathologic Findings

Multifocal, destructive inflammatory lesions are found in the cerebral white matter and in the brain stem. They can be visualized grossly as brownish discoloration on cut section (Fig. 84-4). These lesions have a characteristic appearance consisting of a malacic center surrounded by a rim of extremely intense perivascular infiltration. Older lesions become cystic with intense astrocytic sclerosis.[83,140]

Therapy

No treatment for this disease has been found. Glucocorticoids do not alter the course of the disease in confirmed cases, and antiepileptic drugs are often ineffective in controlling seizures.

HYDROCEPHALUS WITH PERIVENTRICULAR ENCEPHALITIS IN DOGS

Andrea Tipold and Marc Vandevelde

Hydrocephalus is probably the most common developmental abnormality of the CNS in dogs and may be the result of congenital or acquired stenosis of the mesencephalic aqueduct, resulting in internal hydrocephalus.[63] Acquired hydrocephalus is usually a result of infectious or neoplastic diseases that lead to obstruction of the CSF drainage pathways. A particular form of acquired hydrocephalus in young dogs is associated

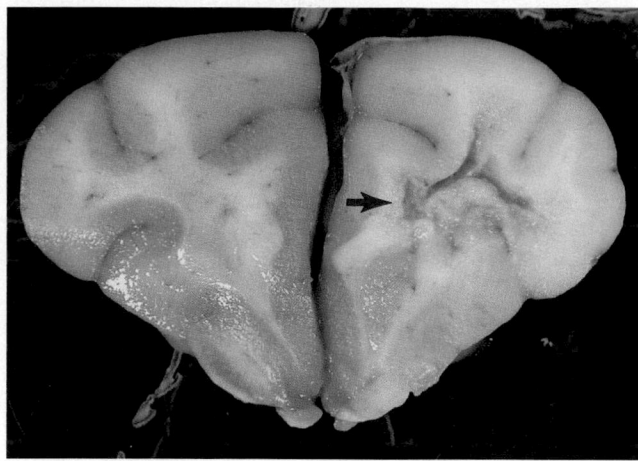

Fig 84-4 Yorkshire encephalitis. Burnt out cystic lesion in the cerebral white matter *(arrow)*.

with severe periventricular inflammation.* In one puppy, inflammation likely closed drainage from the skull, causing external hydrocephalus.[41]

Etiology

Because of the severe inflammatory changes seen with hydrocephalus, an infectious cause has been suspected. On bacteriologic examination of brain tissue and CSF in two dogs with this disease, three different bacteria were isolated; however, these were thought to be contaminants.[60,150] Staphylococci were isolated in another case.[41] Possibly, the underlying disease might be caused by a virus, although no infectious agent was found on EM study of the periventricular tissues of two dogs.[150] Canine parainfluenza virus has caused hydrocephalus in dogs after experimental inoculation (see Chapter 7).[9,10] However, the clinical and pathologic findings in experimental parainfluenza-induced hydrocephalus are totally different from those of the condition described herein. Serum-neutralizing antibodies against canine parvovirus were absent.[150]

Clinical Findings

The disease occurs in puppies between 2 and 6 months of age. No predilection for miniature breeds exists, as is the case with congenital hydrocephalus. The animals are normal at birth and exhibit normal development for the first 2 months of life. At 2 or 3 months of age, acute neurologic signs occur together with rapidly progressing skull enlargement. Neurologic signs include behavioral changes such as depression, dullness, and hyperactivity. Progressive incoordination occurs in all limbs, and most animals develop central blindness. Less consistent findings are cranial nerve deficits, which may include deafness, and abnormal eye motility, such as strabismus, head tilt, and dysphagia. The course of the disease is usually progressive over several days to a few weeks. In some animals, the clinical condition may stabilize.

Diagnosis

No consistent hematologic or biochemical findings are associated with this form of hydrocephalus. CSF abnormalities consist of xanthochromia, increased protein concentration, and pleocytosis, including erythrocytes, mononuclear cells, and macrophages containing erythrocytes. Radiographic examination of the skull reveals abnormalities such as thinning of the cranial vault and homogeneous appearance of the intracranial contents. CT and MRI confirm the enlargement

*References: 19, 24, 41, 60, 150.

of the ventricles. However, these findings are indicative of hydrocephalus, regardless of its cause.[63] The same can be said for the EEG findings indicative for hydrocephalus.[63]

Pathologic Findings

Massive enlargement of the cerebral ventricles occurs, which are filled with cloudy, hemorrhagic CSF. The internal surface of the ventricles is focally roughened, with a brownish discoloration. A typical finding is the presence of large dissecting cavities, also called false diverticula, in the cerebral mantle (Fig. 84-5, *A*). These dissecting cavities communicate with the lateral ventricles. Histologically, severe inflammation with necrosis of the ependymal and subependymal tissues can be found.[24,140] The lesions are always hemorrhagic. Hemosiderin-laden macrophages are found in old lesions. Perivascular cuffing with inflammatory cells occurs and, in acute lesions, diffuse infiltration with neutrophils and macrophages (see Fig. 84-5, *B*, and *C*). Glial mesenchymal repair tissue is formed later in the course of the disease.

Therapy

By the time the condition becomes evident to the owner, severe damage has already taken place. In most cases, the disease is rapidly progressive, leading to severe neurologic impairment. However, in cases in which the condition stabilizes, conservative therapy with glucocorticoids or surgical treatment may be considered.[63] Antibiotics and a ventriculoperitoneal shunt was successful in treating a puppy with external hydrocephalus associated with staphylococcal infection.[41] Prognosis remains cautious given that placed catheters may become obstructed by the inflammatory reaction.

NONSUPPURATIVE MENINGOENCEPHALITIS IN GREYHOUNDS

Andrea Tipold and Marc Vandevelde

A novel breed-specific meningoencephalitis has been described in young greyhounds from three different kennels in southern Ireland.[23] An infectious origin is suspected, but no inclusion bodies, fungi, or protozoal cysts were seen. Additional tests for common antigens failed to determine the cause of the disease. Neurologic signs occur with acute onset and include central vestibular signs with head tilt, ataxia, and recumbency. Additionally, circling and blindness are common findings. The animals are dull, dehydrated, and have lost weight. Hematologic and biochemical parameters reflect only dehydration. Diffuse encephalitis with perivascular, predominantly mononuclear, cuffing was described.

FELINE POLIOMYELITIS

Andrea Tipold and Marc Vandevelde

Poliomyelitis in domestic cats was first reported in North Africa and Ceylon in the 1950s. Later, additional cases were described in North America and Europe.[65,77,142] A clinically and pathologically similar condition occurs in large Felidae (lions and tigers) held in captivity.[45,94]

Etiology

Pathologic findings indicate that poliomyelitis in cats is almost certainly caused by a virus. However, ultrastructural studies to demonstrate a specific causal virus in domestic cats have not yet been performed, and the considerable efforts to identify such a virus in lions and tigers, including tissue culture studies, animal inoculation, and serologic studies for known viruses,

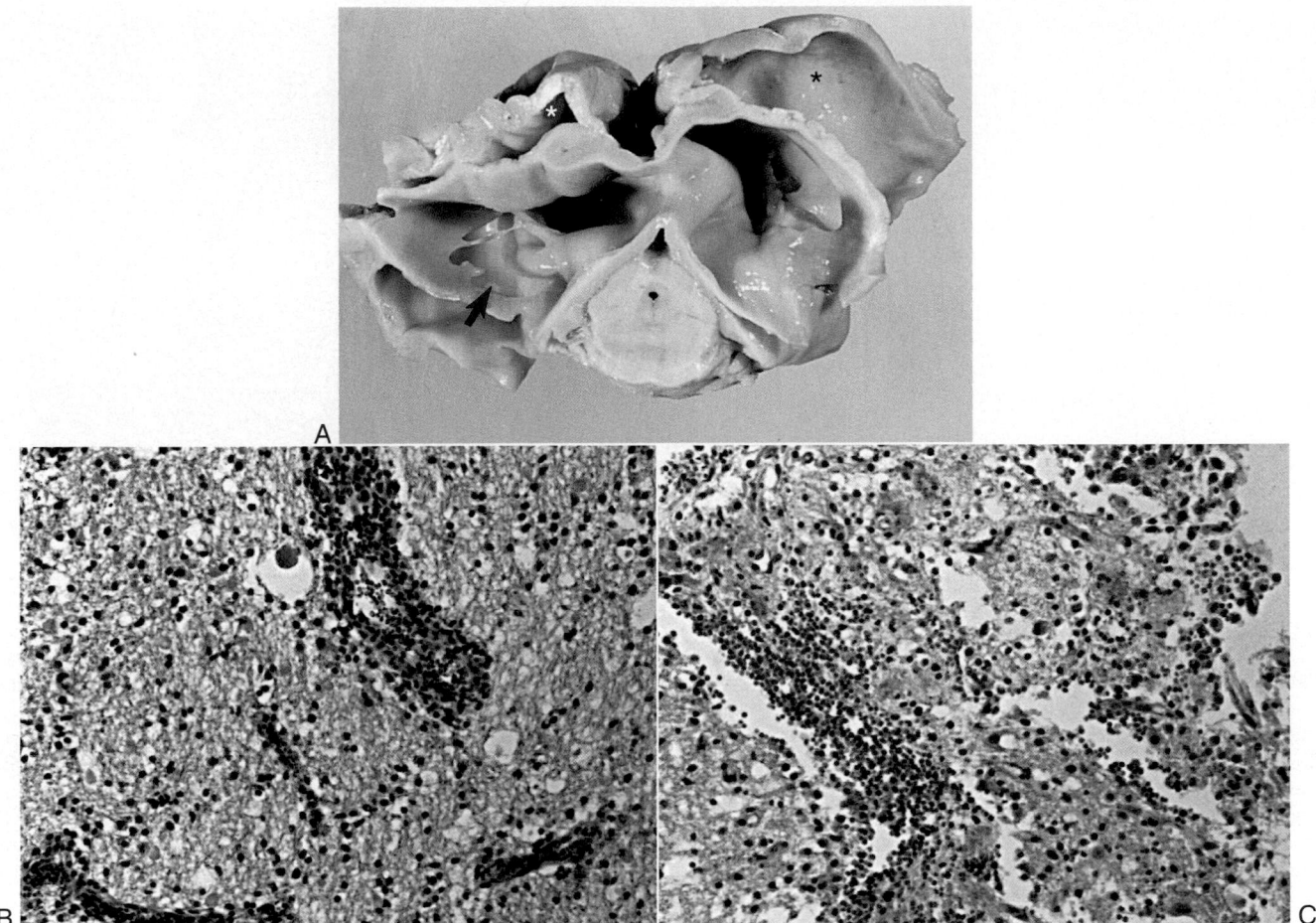

Fig 84-5 Gross and histologic specimens from a dog with periventricular encephalitis. **A,** Occipital area at the level of the midbrain showing greatly enlarged ventricles. False diverticulum *(asterisk)* communicates with the lateral ventricle through a defect *(arrow)* in the ventricular wall. **B,** Inflammatory changes (cuffing) in the periventricular tissue (H and E stain, ×100). **C,** Hemorrhage and malacia in periventricular tissue (H and E stain, ×100). (Part **A** from Wouda W, Vandevelde M, Kihm U. 1981. Internal hydrocephalus of suspected infectious origin in young dogs, *Zentralbl Veterinarmed A* 28:481-493, with permission.)

have been unsuccessful.[94] Comparative pathologic studies suggest that several known spontaneously occurring or experimentally induced viral infections of cats are unlikely to cause poliomyelitis; however, the role of togaviruses should be investigated further.[65] Nonsuppurative encephalitides in cats have been associated with *Borna* virus infection in some European countries such as Austria, Switzerland, and Sweden (see Chapter 26). Borna disease in cats has been named *staggering disease*. However, Borna disease in cats is morphologically and clinically distinct from feline poliomyelitis. In addition, poliomyelitis also occurs in countries such as the United States where Borna disease is not known.

Clinical Findings

Feline poliomyelitis is an insidious disease; its onset is slow, and it progresses over weeks to months. In many instances, the neurologic signs may stabilize, and some animals may recover. Immature and adult cats appear to be susceptible. In cats, the disease is sporadic. However, outbreaks in which several lions and tigers were simultaneously affected have occurred in zoologic gardens.[45,94] The predominant signs are problems in locomotion, including paresis, ataxia, and depressed postural reactions in the pelvic and thoracic limbs. Lower motor neuron involvement is characterized by muscle atrophy and decreased tendon reflexes. Hyperesthesia in the thoracic and lumbar areas is apparent in some cases. Additional neurologic findings, which occur rarely, include epilepsy, cerebellar signs, and pupillary abnormalities.

Pathologic Findings

Disseminated inflammatory lesions are found in the brain and spinal cord (Fig. 84-6). The spinal cord and medulla oblongata are most severely affected. The lesions consist of perivascular mononuclear cuffing, gliosis, and neuronal degeneration, the last being most obvious in the ventral horns of the spinal cord. In chronic cases, little inflammation may be seen, but neuronal loss and intense astrogliosis in the cord are striking. As a result of neuronal damage, marked diffuse wallerian degeneration of the lateral and ventral columns also occurs, resembling a primary degenerative disorder. No consistent lesions in other organ systems are found.

Therapy

No curative treatment has been found for the suspected viral infection. Contact between unaffected cats and those suspected to have the disease should be avoided. The prognosis is not always unfavorable because large Felidae suspected of having the infection have been known to recover.[45]

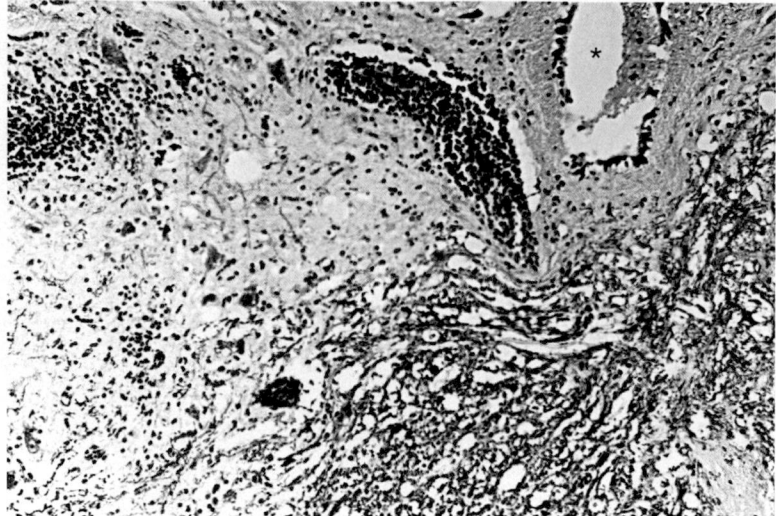

Fig 84-6 Histologic section from the spinal cord of a cat with poliomyelitis showing perivascular cuffing and nodular gliosis in the gray matter. Asterisk indicates central canal (H and E stain, ×250).

STEROID-RESPONSIVE MENINGITIS-ARTERITIS

Andrea Tipold and Marc Vandevelde

Steroid-responsive meningitis-arteritis (SRMA) has been described numerous times in veterinary literature in several areas of the world. The name may be somewhat misleading; a positive response to glucocorticoids occurs in a variety of inflammatory conditions caused by infections or their immunopathologic complications. In this chapter, a specific syndrome in dogs is covered in which immune-mediated reactions appear to involve primarily arteries and meninges of the CNS. In a certain percentage of the cases, the disease occurs in combination with polyarthritis.[146] A breed predisposition has been noted in Bernese mountain dogs,[96,107,129] boxers,[64,105,129] beagles, Toller retrievers, and basset hounds. However, other medium- to large-breed dogs, usually young adults,[64,105] may be affected.

Juvenile polyarteritis, a systemic vasculitis involving medium- to small-sized muscular arteries, predominantly associated with the coronary and meningeal vessels, has been commonly reported in purpose-bred beagles of 6 to 9 months of age. Beagles kept as companion animals and not derived from inbred colonies are equally affected. Although the *beagle pain syndrome* appears to be of a more systemic nature, it shares many characteristics with SRMA reported in other breeds and has been better characterized.[44,116]

Etiology and Pathogenesis

The epidemiology of the disease suggests an infectious origin. As in other infectious diseases, the lesions are inflammatory. SRMA, however, displays immunopathologic features especially with respect to the vascular lesions. Although resembling immune complex injury, arteritis of beagles and other breeds has not been associated with immune complex deposits in affected vessels. Nevertheless, immunoglobulin-producing plasma cells are associated with the lesions in the meninges. T cells diffusely infiltrate vessel walls.[133] In beagles, increased amounts of circulating immune complexes in one dog, increased rheumatoid factors in two dogs, and decreased C3 in one dog have been found.[56]

Further findings suggesting an immunopathologic event are markedly increased IgA levels in CSF and serum, increased B-cell/T-cell ratio in the blood, suppressed blastogenic response to mitogens, inability to generate immunoglobulin-secreting plasma cells following activation, and antineutrophil cytoplasmic antibodies in CSF and serum. However, the last finding is not specific for this disease and can be found in other CNS lesions and even in some healthy dogs.[130] A large portion of the T cells are activated, suggesting the presence of a superantigen.[44,134] Immunocytochemically, in SRMA, an overrepresentation of B cells occurred in meningeal lesions, whereas the distribution of lymphocyte subsets was similar to the one in bacterial or protozoal diseases. All attempts to find an infectious agent such as virus isolation, measurement of RT, and cultivation of bacteria failed.[130] Elevated interleukin (IL)-6 levels in serum have been found in affected beagles, and levels paralleled clinical illness. IL-6 levels decreased following glucocorticoid therapy and remission of clinical signs.[66] Elevated IL-8 levels and increased chemotactic activity in the CSF were consistent findings in SRMA. IL-8 did not decrease after glucocorticoid administration, which may explain the recurrent nature of the disease.[22] The uncontrolled IgA synthesis may be the result of immune dysregulation, perhaps induced by an infectious agent and mediated by enhanced transforming growth factor-β (TGF-β) production. Excessive IgA is likely to play a central role in the pathogenesis of the lesion.

Clinical Findings

The classic clinical presentation is episodic and recurrent and includes cervical pain of acute onset, reluctance to move, stiff gait, resistance to neck manipulation, paraspinal hyperesthesia, and high rectal temperature. Chronically affected animals develop neurologic deficits consistent with a multifocal or spinal cord lesion. In rare cases, spontaneous bleeding in the subarachnoidal space may occur and result in tetra- or paraplegia.

Diagnosis

Hematologic findings include a predominantly neutrophilic leukocytosis.[44] CSF may be turbid, blood tinged, or xanthochromic from hemorrhage occurring in the subarachnoidal space. Neutrophilic pleocytosis (up to several thousand cells/μl) and erythrophagocytosis are apparent. All dogs synthesize immunoglobulins in high concentrations in the CNS.[135]

High IgA concentrations are found in the CSF, which is synthesized intrathecally.[129] Simultaneous demonstration of high IgA levels in serum and CSF is highly diagnostic (specificity of approximately 90%). Large numbers of neutrophils are predominant in the CSF in acute cases; in chronic cases, mononuclear cells predominate. Mild-to-moderate hydro-

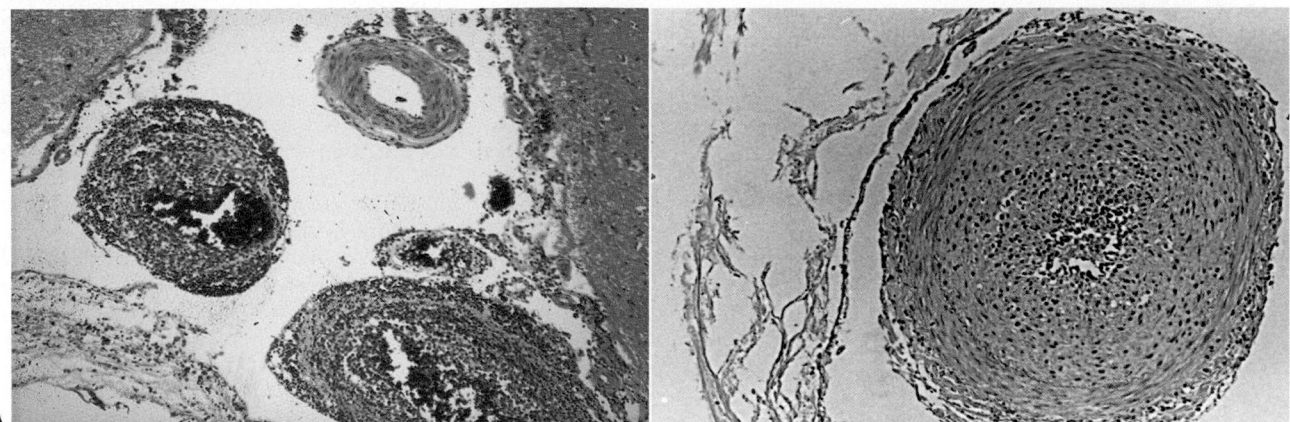

Fig 84-7   Spinal cord at ventral fissure from dog with steroid-responsive meningitis-arteritis. **A,** Marked infiltration of the vascular wall with inflammatory infiltrate in meninges (H and E stain, ×40). **B,** Closer view of a lesion from an affected dog showing stenosis of spinal meningeal artery from subintimal proliferation with associated periluminal inflammatory cell infiltrate and fibrosis of adjacent arachnoidea (H and E stain, ×100).

cephalus has been documented in some chronic cases with cisternography and neurosonographic techniques. CT reveals hyperdensities in the meningeal spaces after IV injection of contrast medium.

Pathologic Findings

At necropsy, subarachnoid hemorrhages extending over the entire length of the meninges of the spinal cord and brain stem have been found in a few cases in which the vascular lesions had led to rupture of major blood vessels. In chronic cases, fibrous thickening of the spinal meninges may be noted. Lesions outside the CNS are relatively rare in affected dogs. Extraneural arteritis is more frequently noted in affected beagles, particularly in the extramural coronary arteries and myocardium.

Histologic changes are found in the meninges of the spinal cord and to a much lesser degree in the brain stem. These changes consist of necrotizing arteritis of medium- and small-sized arteries and associated leptomeningitis (Fig. 84-7). Chronic lesions include proliferative changes of the vascular intima with stenosis and adventitial fibrosis. The intramedullary arteries and neural parenchyma can be mildly affected in chronic cases. Occasional vessels may be thrombosed. The meningeal infiltrate contains hemosiderin-laden macrophages in cases in which hemorrhage had occurred. No evidence of immune complex deposition has been found, but immunoglobulin (IgG, IgM, and IgA) deposits have been found in the vascular walls of some animals[135] with the chronic stage of the disease.

Therapy

Spontaneous remission has been observed. Response to antibiotics is therefore coincidental because relapses and intermittent episodes occur. In dogs with extremely high body temperatures, fluid therapy and ice packs are useful. In cases with the first episode of pain and mild pleocytosis in the CSF, nonsteroidal antiinflammatory drugs are administered. At the first relapse, if signs worsen, or if massive pleocytosis in the CSF occurs (several thousand cells/μl), glucocorticoids are administered. The initial response to this therapy is usually dramatic. Such an immediate and impressive therapeutic response hardly occurs in GME, which usually continues to progress despite treatment. Prednisolone is given as a long-term treatment starting with 4 mg/kg of body weight for 1 to 2 days, a dose that is tapered slowly. Response to treatment and followup examinations determine the treatment protocol.

If patients do not respond well to prednisolone or show side effects such as polydipsia or polyuria and polyphagia, immunosuppressive drugs and glucocorticoids are given on alternate days. Several studies have shown that neither glucocorticoids nor immunosuppressive drugs can influence the underlying immunopathologic condition, which appears to abate spontaneously within a certain period (usually several months). However, the described medication is necessary to prevent lasting damage to the CNS related to hemorrhage, bad perfusion, and destructive effects of inflammation. Older dogs with frequent relapses insufficiently treated with glucocorticoids and high IgA levels in the CSF seem to require a longer duration of therapy and have a less favorable prognosis. Long-term treatment studies show a good prognosis in 60% to 80% of treated dogs.[28]

PRION DISEASES AND FELINE SPONGIFORM ENCEPHALOPATHY

Marc Vandevelde and Craig E. Greene

Etiology and Pathogenesis

Feline spongiform encephalopathy (FSE) belongs to the transmissible spongiform encephalopathies (TSE), a group of neurodegenerative diseases in humans and animals (Table 84-2) characterized by a very long incubation time and degeneration of the CNS with vacuolation of the neuropil and nerve cells. The infectious agent is small and resistant to inactivation by heat, formalin, glutaraldehyde, alcohol, and radiation. Infectivity is associated with a host-encoded protein, the so-called prion protein (PrP). PrP is widely distributed in the CNS, peripheral nerve, neuroendocrine and lymphatic tissues, and many other organs.[30] They are involved in neuronal development and function and prevent cell death. The mechanism of TSE involves a misfolding of the normal prion protein (PrP^c) to a new heat-resistant protein (PrP^{Sc}; PrP^{res}). In its new conformation, the PrP^{Sc} is protease resistant and hence accumulates in the tissue. Misfolding of the PrP can also occur spontaneously and sporadically through genetic mutations in the PrP gene, leading to hereditary SE, which are exceedingly rare in people. Once formed, the modified, abnormal PrP is thought to induce additional copies of itself by interacting with normal PrP. Thus the belief holds that this misfolded protein itself becomes an infectious agent, the prion.[30] The prion theory is a revolutionary concept in biology, and many

Table • 84-2

Transmissible Spongiform Encephalopathies of People and Animals

DISEASE	HOST[a]	FIRST RECOGNIZED
Creutzfeldt-Jakob	People	1920
Kuru	People (New Guinea)	1957
Gerstmann—Straussler—Scheinker syndrome	People	1928
Fatal familial insomnia	People	1986
Variant Creutzfeldt-Jakob Disease (bovine SE in People)	People	1996
Sporadic familial insomnia	People	1999
Scrapie	Sheep	1730
	Goats	1872
Transmissible Mink Encephalopathy	Mink	1947
Chronic Wasting Disease	Mule deer	1967
	Elk	1979
Bovine SE (Mad Cow Disease)	Cattle (Europe)	1985
SE	Eland, Oryx, Greater Kudu (Africa)	1989
Feline SE	Domestic cats (Europe)	1990
	Exotic cats	1992
SE of Captive Primates	Monkeys	1996

SE, Spongiform encephalopathy
[a]Geographic location in parenthesis when restricted to a specific area.

questions remain. Prions are unique because they can be both inherited and infectious.

The PrP^c gene is highly conserved among different animals; however, knockout mice devoid of the protein develop normally with mild neuronal abnormalities. However, the presence of an abnormal PrP in the CNS is devastating. PrP^{Sc} is insoluble and aggregates as amyloid fibrils in infected brain tissue where deposits (amyloid plaques) can be observed in some TSEs. Accumulation of aberrantly folded PrP^{Sc} fibrils is central in the pathogenesis of these diseases.[30] Accumulation leads to astrocytic proliferation, microglial cell activation, loss of synapses, and finally to neuronal cell death by apoptosis.

The TSEs are transmissible to other animals, at least under experimental conditions.[35] Routes of natural transmission of TSEs involve oral ingestion, skin scarification, or congenital transmission. For example, scrapie has been consistently found in the placenta of ewes.[109] Infection has spread iatrogenically through contaminated biologics[26] and likely through other veterinary procedures or feeding practices.[118]

During the incubation period, PrP^{Sc} accumulates on membranes of follicular dendritic cells (FDC) in local lymphoid tissue.[2] A crucial phase of neuronal invasion likely occurs at the interface of FDC and nerve endings in secondary lymphoid organs. From the lymphoreticular tissues at the site of inoculation, the prion is thought to gain access to the peripheral nervous system through local nerve endings. From there the prion migrates to the CNS. Knockout mice that lack the chemokine receptor, CXCR5, have altered FDC that are closely related to nerve terminals, and they have accelerated incubation periods. When FDC are depleted from mice experimentally, infection is attenuated. Following ingestion, PrP^{Sc} may enter the gut-associated lymphoid tissue, then enter nerve endings in the intestinal tract, and migrate to the CNS via the vagus nerve. In bovine SE (BSE), the nucleus of the vagus is consistently affected following oral inoculation.[70]

Epidemiology

Scrapie, the classic TSE of small ruminants, has been recognized for approximately 275 years. Since that time, other SEs have been recognized in people and animals. TSEs became notorious in the late 1980s as a result of the BSE outbreak in Great Britain,[147] where scrapie has been endemic for centuries. BSE was spread by animal protein concentrates in cattle feed. The scrapie agent in so-called meat and bone meal is believed to be derived from abattoir offal, and fallen livestock, including scrapie-infected sheep, was no longer properly inactivated because of changes in the production procedures of the rendering industry. As a result, the scrapie agent probably became adapted to a new host and established BSE in bovines with major epidemic consequences. Animals with BSE were undoubtedly also recycled by the rendering industry until the epidemiology of the disease became understood, thus leading to a considerable enrichment of the agent in meat and bone meal before the protein-feeding ban came into effect. By 2004, the outbreak in British cattle involved approximately 180,000 cattle, and millions of animals have been slaughtered to control the outbreak.[118] BSE was not restricted to the United Kingdom. Recycling of imported live animals, processed beef, or livestock food supplements from Great Britain in the local rendering industry sparked new small-scale epidemics in many European countries. The United States banned the importation of beef from the United Kingdom since the mid-1980s, and little sheep-derived feed products enter the feed for other animals.[87] One case of BSE, imported from Canada, has occurred in the United States. Only two cases (of which one was a British import) were found in Canada. Ten cases have been detected in Japan. The incidence of BSE is declining in all European countries as a result of measures taken by the European Union.[141]

FSE was first recognized during the BSE epidemic in Great Britain.[3] Based on strain-typing experiments, FSE is undoubtedly caused by the BSE agent.[21] Cats were probably infected by ingesting BSE-contaminated feed.[152] Cats cannot be experimentally infected by the scrapie agent directly as they can by BSE and Creutzfeldt-Jakob disease (CJD) agents, which indicates an adaptation to the new hosts.[53] The first cases of FSE were diagnosed in the early 1990s,[81,152] and approximately 90 cases had been reported by the end of 2004. The outbreak was attributed to consumption of beef products contaminated by CNS tissues from infected animals.

In addition to Great Britain, one case of FSE has been described in a domestic cat in Norway that was fed commercial dry cat foods imported from Great Britain.[15] Other single cases of FSE have been reported in North Ireland, Liechtenstein, and Switzerland,[38] and more have likely occurred in domestic cats throughout Europe. Captive wild species of Felidae such as lions (Panthera leo), tigers (P. tigris), cheetahs (Acinonyx jubatus), and pumas (Felis concolor) that were fed bovine tissues have also been affected with BSE.[8,73,149] An Asiatic golden cat (Catopuma temmincki) imported into Australia from Europe was found to have prion-associated SE.[153] The number of cats being reported annually with FSE in

Great Britain has sharply decreased in the past years. The last case was reported in 2001. This decline is expected because of measures taken to prevent further spread of the bovine disease. TSE has not been documented in the dog.

Clinical Findings

Because of the long incubation time of TSE, the signs of the disease are observed only in adult cats (peak incidence at age 5 years). The neurologic signs develop progressively over several weeks to months and are characterized by behavioral changes such as aggressiveness and fear. Gait abnormalities include ataxia and inaccurate landing while jumping. Affected cats are hypersensitive to tactile stimulation. No focalization of the neurologic signs occurs. The disease is invariably progressive and fatal.

Diagnosis

No typical laboratory findings have been discovered. The suspicion of FSE is based on the age of the animal and the clinical signs. A variety of neurologic conditions have to be considered. Laboratory diagnosis of TSE is based on immunochemical detection of the protease-resistant PrP. Monoclonal and polyclonal antibodies have been generated against PrP,[115,88] and several commercial kits are on the market. Some species differences can be found in reactions to these commercially available test kits that must be recognized. A commercial test kit (BSE Test Kit®, Bio Rad, Hercules, Calif.) has been developed to detect PrP[Sc] in the brain of cattle with BSE, and it may be beneficial for testing other tissues and body fluids.[48] Western immunoblotting methods have also been effective for rapid surveillance of BSE (Prionics-Check®, University of Zuerich-Irchel, Switzerland).[115] In living individuals affected by TSE, PrP[Sc] can be detected in biopsies from lymphatic tissues. In scrapie, the abnormal prion can be demonstrated in lymphoid tissues such as the tonsils or third eyelid.[100] Given that no replication of the BSE agent occurs in lymphatic tissues, laboratory diagnosis is possible only on brain material after slaughter. In cats, extraneural PrP[Sc] accumulation appears to be inconsistent.[112] An insoluble proteinase-resistant PrP isoform is present in urine of people and animals affected with prion disease.[117] This isoform can be detected long before clinical evidence of the disease occurs. The value of these methods in testing specimens from various animals requires further study. As a potential premortem test,

pathologic PrP was detected by immunoblotting in the dorsal olfactory epithelium of people with sporadic (naturally occurring) CJD.[155] This method might serve as a means of diagnosis of disease in living animals.

Pathologic Findings

As in all other TSEs, the pathologic findings in FSE are highly characteristic. The changes consist of vacuolation in the neuropil and neurons in a bilaterally symmetric distribution, especially in the thalamus, basal ganglia, and cerebral cortex (Fig. 84-8, *A*). Immunocytochemistry for PrP[Sc] reveals accumulation of PrP in affected areas (see Fig. 84-8, *B*). Advanced cases reveal neuronal loss and gliosis. Advanced lesions are more commonly observed in human patients because affected animals are often euthanized in early stages of the neurologic disease. No inflammation is present.

Therapy

A large number of potential therapeutic agents have been used to treat TSEs. Polyene antimicrobials have been considered for use in preventing accumulation of PrP[c] and treating infection by certain scrapie strains.[76] Analogs of Congo red, quinacrine, and chlorpromazine and inhibitors of peptide syntesis might also be considered. Active and passive immunization using recombinant PrP[c] and antibodies to PrP[c] have considerable merit. TSEs are similar to Alzheimer's disease in which neurodegeneration is accompanied by massive deposition of amyloid–β-protein, and some reduction in progression occurs when immunotherapy is used.

Prevention

All TSEs are fatal diseases. Prevention of exposure is the most important control measure. Although transmitting an SE from one species to another orally is generally difficult, 13 other animal species were found to be infected with BSE in Great Britain.[21] BSE in these other species undoubtedly resulted from oral exposure. Scrapie-infected sheep were processed into meat and bone meal supplements being fed to cattle, and tissue from sick animals were recycled through the animal food supply. Because of the enormous resistance of the infectious agent to physical and chemical inactivation procedures, high titers of infectivity remain, even in extensively processed contaminated feedstuffs. To prevent exposure to other species, including people, the authorities in endemic countries confis-

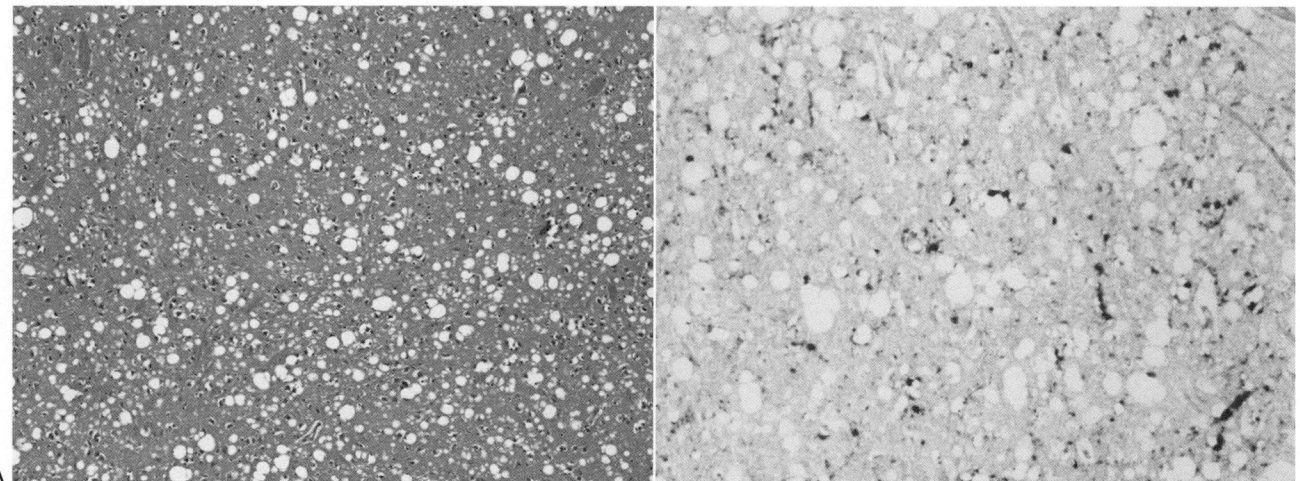

Fig 84-8 Feline spongiform encephalopathy. **A,** Area in the thalamus with many small and large vacuoles in the neuropil (H and E stain, ×100). **B,** Area with spongiform change. Punctate and plaque-like deposits *(red)* of the protease resistant PrP (immunocytochemical staining with polyclonal anti-PrP; avidin biotinylated enzyme complex [ABC] technique, ×250).

cated all tissues (CNS, lymphoid tissues, intestine) in which the infectious agent might be theoretically present from all bovines at the time of slaughter. This measure came into effect in the fourth year of the BSE epidemic and took several years to become completely effective.[118] Thus, most likely, the exposure of other species had taken place before that time. Considering an average incubation period of approximately 5 years, the peak of the epidemic in cats has certainly been passed.[14] Further spread in the bovine population in Europe was prevented by banning the feeding of animal proteins to ruminant species and finally to all farm animals. The BSE epidemic is expected to reach its end within a few years.[118] FSE should therefore soon disappear. Although BSE will be soon eradicated, scrapie remains a challenge because it is a naturally occurring disease that spreads from animal to animal. Because susceptibility to scrapie is genetically controlled, polymerase chain reaction has been used to detect alleles of scrapie-susceptible sheep to assist selection for breeding of scrapie-resistant animals.[154]

Public Health Considerations

During the outbreak of BSE in Britain, a new variant of CJD (vCJD) occurred in people.[68] The disease has also been reported in other countries. Approximately 140 cases have been detected, and the epidemic appears to be on the decline. In contrast to classical CJD, the variant disease affected primarily young adults and was suspected as being caused by ingestion of contaminated cattle products. Based on strain typing in mice, the vCJD agent is similar to the BSE agent.[52] Further evidence for the BSE etiology of vCJD is derived from electrophoretic patterns of the three PrP glycotypes (glycotyping), vCJD, and BSE showing the same type 4 pattern.[29,50] The prions of BSE, vCJD, and sporadic CJD have been inoculated into transgenic mice.[6] Although most of the mice produced type 4 prions, a few expressed type 2, which suggests the possibility that some humans with apparently sporadic CJD might be infected with BSE prions.[61] However, this finding can be explained in other ways, and such speculations that are common in the TSE field need more solid scientific evidence. Not all people are equally susceptible to the development of SE. A higher prevalence of disease is associated with homozygosity for a polymorphism at codon 129 of the PrP gene.[30]

Despite the control of the outbreak through management of livestock feeding, the number of clinically healthy people incubating the disease is still undefined. Transmission of the agent through blood transfusions or organ donation is therefore a major concern. In addition, use of medical and surgical instruments on successive patients is of theoretical concern. The danger of contaminated materials is not with contact but with ingestion or inoculation. The safest method of preventing spread of disease to a new patient is to destroy all instruments used. If this precaution is not possible, then the items should be immersed in 1 M sodium hydroxide (NaOH) and then autoclaved. Work surfaces should be flooded with 2 M NaOH and then allowed to soak for 1 hour. No effective disinfection procedure exists for delicate instruments that cannot withstand autoclave temperatures (134° C) or 1 N NaOH. For delicate equipment, repeated washing with detergent-proteinase solutions and exposing it to 6 M urea or 4 M guanidinium thiocyanate can eliminate the offending prions of TSE.[91]

CONCLUSIONS

In addition to the conditions described in this chapter, other CNS diseases of suspected infectious origin are occasionally encountered in dogs and cats during diagnostic workup. Some will remain a single sporadic observation; others will become recognized as disease entities. The ability to characterize infectious agents in these diseases is limited when formalin-fixed tissues are used. Fresh material for culture should be collected when clinical findings are compatible with one of these disorders. In addition to brain tissue taken for isolation procedures, serum and CSF should be collected and screened for antibody activity against a wide variety of known infectious agents. The advent of widely available, extremely powerful molecular biologic techniques also extends the range of etiologic studies considerably. In addition, more systematic ultrastructural studies of appropriately fixed tissues taken from lesions and sites indicated by the clinical examination may be helpful in detecting infectious agents. For a discussion of meningitis of suspected infectious or immune-mediated causes, see Bacterial Infections of the Central Nervous System, Chapter 92.

SUGGESTED READINGS*

1. Adamo FP, O'Brien RT. 2004. Use of cyclosporine to treat granulomatous meningoencephalitis in three dogs, *J Am Vet Med Assoc* 225:1211-1216.
2. Aguzzi A. 2003. Prions and the immune system: a journey through gut, spleen, and nerves, *Adv Immunol* 81:123-171.
7. Bailey CS, Higgins RJ. 1986. Characteristics of cerebrospinal fluid associated with canine granulomatous meningoencephalitis: a retrospective study, *J Am Vet Med Assoc* 188:418-421.

*See the CD-ROM for a complete list of references.

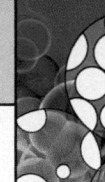

CHAPTER • 85

Integumentary Infections

BACTERIAL INFECTIONS OF THE SKIN

Peter J. Ihrke

Pyoderma is defined as a pyogenic or pus-producing bacterial infection of the skin. The diversity of clinical syndromes seen with canine pyoderma is enormous, varying from minor annoyances to disease with life-threatening potential.* Pyoderma may affect the surface, creating inflammation without the invasion of living tissue; be superficial, involving the epidermis and hair follicle units; or invade deeper, compromising structures in the dermis and subjacent fatty tissue. This tremendous diversity and pleomorphism is responsible for diagnostic and management difficulties that may be encountered. Misdiagnosis also may result from the continuum of clinical characteristics and severity of the pyoderma, among various dogs, of different anatomic sites, and between acute and chronic disease. The presence of pus cannot be used as a defining diagnostic criterion because pus may not be visible grossly. The aging and rupture of pustules leads to crusted papules that are much more difficult to use for diagnosis. In addition, accumulations of pus in the mid-dermis in deep pyoderma may not be visually obvious.

Globally, pyoderma remains one of the most common causes of canine skin disease. Pyoderma was second only to flea allergy dermatitis in frequency of diagnosis in a study from North American veterinary colleges.[67,134] An additional epidemiologic study performed in a relatively flea-free environment in Canada ranked bacterial folliculitis and furunculosis first among all canine skin diseases, comprising more than one quarter of the dermatology caseload.[133] Conversely, pyoderma is a relatively uncommon cause of skin disease in cats, other domestic animals, and humans. Bacterial skin disease in the cat is rare, with the exception of subcutaneous bite wound abscesses (see Chapter 53).

The reasons for the markedly elevated frequency of bacterial skin disease in the dog in comparison with other mammalian species are unknown. Various host factors that may result in enhanced susceptibility include the comparatively thin, compact canine stratum corneum, the relative lack of intercellular lipids in the canine stratum corneum, the lack of a lipid-squamous epithelial plug in the entrance of canine hair follicles, and the relatively high pH of canine skin.[67,86,98,132]

Etiology and Pathogenesis
Normal Microflora of the Skin and Hair
Skin microbial flora is composed of resident and transient bacteria. Resident bacteria are harmless commensals that multiply on the skin surface and in hair follicles and maintain a static, consistent population. Transient bacteria cannot compete long term with the established resident flora and may seed the skin from either mucous membranes, other animals, or the environment. The total number of resident bacteria residing on normal canine skin is not large and may comprise less than 350 organisms per square centimeter.[67] Studies examining the bacterial flora of normal dogs have documented aerobic organisms, including *Micrococcus* species, β-hemolytic streptococci, and *Acinetobacter* species, and anaerobic organisms, including *Clostridium perfringens* and *Propionibacterium acnes*.*

Published data have clarified the role of *Staphylococcus intermedius* in canine pyoderma.† This pathogen is probably not a true cutaneous resident but rather a contaminant on normal canine hair and either a contaminant or a transient, restricted, local colonist on normal canine skin. Mucous membranes such as those of the anus and nares probably play an important role as sources of this potential skin pathogen. Normal grooming in all dogs, and excessive licking in pruritic dogs, may repetitively seed the skin with *S. intermedius* from the anus and nares.‡

Staphylococcus intermedius and Other Canine Cutaneous Pathogens
S. intermedius is the primary canine cutaneous pathogen. This organism is a species separate and distinct from the human pathogen, *Staphylococcus aureus*.[50,67] Pure cultures of this bacterium are grown from most pustules or draining tracts in dogs with pyoderma. Recently, two subspecies of *Staphylococcus schleiferi* were implicated as causing some cases of recurrent canine pyoderma.[11,43] It is likely that these subspecies of *S. schleiferi* formerly were misidentified as *S. intermedius*. Limited data indicate that methicillin and fluoroquinolone resistance may be more common in strains of *S. schleiferi*.[43] Methicillin resistance also may be increasing slightly within the *S. intermedius* population.[47]

Pathogenicity of staphylococci in humans correlates with virulence factors such as various proteins and toxins. Evidence does not support virulence factors as the cause of differences in canine susceptibility or severity of infection.[19,25,59,67,68]

When potential virulence factors have been examined comparing *S. intermedius* isolates from normal dogs and dogs with pyoderma, clear differences in toxin profiles, gel electrophoresis of exoproteins, and immunoblotting of concen-

---

*References 65, 67, 68, 96, 106, 131, 132, 150.

---

*References 55, 57, 66, 67, 84, 131, 132.
†References 2, 4, 5, 41, 55, 57, 67, 84, 97, 124, 125.
‡References 2, 3, 4, 5, 67, 84.

trated extracellular proteins were not elucidated.* Production of exotoxins does not appear to play a role in the pathogenicity of *S. intermedius* for canine skin.[19] The role of various other virulence factors such as protein A, leukocidin, hemolysins, epidermolytic toxin, and other soluble products is less clear in the dog. Data suggest that host factors rather than virulence factors appear to be more important in determining susceptibility, severity, and outcome in canine staphylococcal pyoderma.†

Secondary gram-negative invaders such as *Proteus* species, *Pseudomonas* species, or *Escherichia coli* may be isolated in conjunction with *S. intermedius*, usually from deep pyoderma. However, if gram-negative bacteria are isolated from pyoderma without the concomitant isolation of *S. intermedius*, the technique used and the results obtained should be questioned, because canine pyoderma caused by gram-negative bacteria without staphylococcal coinfection is exceedingly rare. Primary infection with *S. intermedius* creates a tissue milieu that is more conducive to secondary invasion by gram-negative bacteria.[66,67]

Microbial Alterations with Skin Disease

The factors that promote the proliferation of *S. intermedius* on skin leading to pyoderma are poorly understood. However, it is well established that dogs with other skin diseases are more likely to develop secondary pyoderma. Dogs with defects in cornification exhibit a shift in the balance of bacterial species colonizing the skin such that coagulase-positive staphylococci predominate. Clinically, this correlates with an increased frequency of pyoderma in dogs with cornification abnormalities. A shift in the frequency and intensity of staphylococcal colonization has been noted in dogs with atopic dermatitis and contact dermatitis as well as seborrheic dermatitis.[67]

Zoonotic Potential of Skin Pathogens

Because *S. intermedius* is a separate and distinct species from *S. aureus*, this partially explains why humans with a normally functioning immune system are not at great risk for skin or wound infections contaminated with *S. intermedius*. Healthy owners of dogs with staphylococcal pyoderma are generally not at risk for zoonotic bacterial infection. However, subclinical transfer of the organism from dogs to people has been documented.[51,140] Many of the isolated strains have been antimicrobial resistant strains. These data indicate that a dog with suppurative pyoderma would be of medical concern if an immunocompromised household member were bitten or exposed to suppurative discharges. Dogs harbor this organism in their mouth; up to 21% of dog bite lesions in people may be infected with *S. intermedius*.[139] Nevertheless, the pathogenicity of other bite-transmitted organisms unassociated with pyoderma is greater. (For additional information on bite transmission of this organism, see Bite Wound Infections, Chapter 53.)

S. schleiferi is a recognized human pathogen, causing nosocomial infections. It has been isolated as a commensal from human skin. Antimicrobial-resistant strains of this organism have been isolated from people, dogs, and cats. In the past, many human and veterinary laboratories have likely confused this organism with *S. aureus* and *S. intermedius*, respectively. Although *S. schleiferi* has been identified in the skin of clinically healthy dogs, the prevalence of carriage has not been determined. Isolations of *S. schleiferi* in dogs have primarily been from those with otitis externa or recurrent pyoderma, and the majority of isolates have been methicillin resistant.[43] Because *S. schleiferi* has been both a commensal and pathogen in people, the concern of transferring this potentially drug-

resistant pathogen between people and pets is considerable. Additional investigations are needed.

The human pathogen, *S. aureus*, has also been isolated from animals, including dogs and cats that have close association with people.[63,90] Methicillin-resistant *S. aureus* strains have also been identified in pets, making them potential sources for infection of people. For an additional discussion of this problem, see Staphylococcal Infections, Chapter 36, and Immunocompromised People and Pets, Chapter 99.

Susceptibility and Host Response to Infection

S. intermedius does not possess the requisite virulence factors to be a potent pathogen. Consequently, most canine pyodermas probably are associated with underlying disease or other host factors. Diseases such as ectoparasitism, cornification defects (seborrhea), allergies (atopic dermatitis, food allergy, flea allergy dermatitis), hereditary skin diseases (genodermatoses)—especially those affecting hair follicles—and endocrinopathies such as hypothyroidism and Cushing's disease frequently predispose animals to pyoderma.[35,67,78,131,132] Pyoderma secondary to cornification defects and allergic diseases are best documented. More broadly, pruritus from any underlying disease, cutaneous inflammation from any cause, injudicious use of glucocorticoids (iatrogenic hyperglucocorticoidism), and poor grooming in long-coated dogs all contribute to the likelihood of secondary pyoderma.

Superficial infection of the hair follicle is the most common canine pyoderma. Follicular defects, dysplasia, obstruction, atrophy, inflammation, or degeneration predispose to folliculitis. After pyoderma is initiated, immunologic incompetence, coexisting skin disease, pruritus, inflammation, scar tissue formation, and improper initial therapy are negative prognostic factors.[67]

The initiation of staphylococcal pyoderma requires colonization and invasion of host tissues in addition to evasion of host immunity. Host defense mechanisms mobilized to prevent bacterial invasion include immunologic and nonimmunologic processes. Nonimmunologic mechanisms include the desquamation of the stratum corneum (surface and follicular), the lipid intercellular barrier, epithelial proliferation in response to injury, and the antibacterial effect of inorganic salts found in sebum and sweat. Additionally, competition among resident bacteria is a nonimmunologic, "nonhost" defense mechanism. Immunologic host defense mechanisms of the skin include proteins within the intercellular matrix; immunoglobulins within the basement membrane zone; and immunologically active cells such as Langerhans cells, dermal dendrocytes, lymphocytes, mast cells, and venular endothelial cells present in either the epidermis or dermis.[67]

Host immunologic response may be deleterious as well as beneficial. Some dogs with chronic or recurrent pyoderma exhibit depression of lymphocyte transformation testing. Exceptionally potent bacterial antigens, termed *superantigens*, may explain the troublesome nature of pyoderma secondary to canine atopic dermatitis and the marked inflammation and pruritus seen in some canine pyoderma.[67]

Bacterial hypersensitivity has long been theorized as a complicating factor in recurrent canine pyoderma. The potential importance of bacterial hypersensitivity has been underscored by work indicating that mast cell degranulation can initiate enhanced epidermal permeability to bacterial antigens in atopic dogs.[67,97] Several studies have verified an association between antistaphylococcal antibodies and various subgroups of canine pyoderma.[67,105]

Classification of Pyoderma

Classification based on depth of bacterial involvement is most useful clinically because it provides information on diagnosis, likelihood of underlying disease, prognosis, required duration

*References 1, 3, 19, 49, 50, 67.
†References 1, 3, 50, 19, 25, 67, 132.

of therapy and response to therapy. In general, the deeper the infection, the more likely that underlying triggering causes are present. Deeper infections also require that the clinician be more aggressive diagnostically and therapeutically. Using depth of bacterial infection, canine pyoderma can be described as *surface, superficial,* or *deep* (Table 85-1).[67]

Surface Pyoderma Surface pyoderma consist of inflammatory processes in the skin without strong evidence of direct bacterial invasion. Bacterial involvement probably is secondary to various factors that encourage surface bacterial overgrowth. Pyotraumatic dermatitis (acute moist dermatitis, hot spots), intertrigo (skinfold pyoderma), mucocutaneous pyoderma, and surface bacterial overgrowth are classified as surface pyoderma. Pyotraumatic dermatitis usually develops secondary to flea allergy dermatitis. Intertrigo occurs in skinfolds secondary to breed-characteristic anatomic defects and is seen in conjunction with friction, poor drainage, and maceration. In mucocutaneous pyoderma, bacterial involvement may become deeper with chronicity. Mucocutaneous pyoderma is a surface disease of unknown cause that predominantly involves the lips and perioral skin but may involve other mucocutaneous sites such as the anus.[67,70] Intertrigo and pyotraumatic dermatitis rarely are diagnostic or therapeutic challenges.

In the past, the clinical importance of surface overgrowth by staphylococci and other bacteria has not been recognized in the dog. The author feels that secondary surface bacterial overgrowth triggered by underlying, predisposing skin disease is a prime cause and perpetuator of chronic cutaneous inflammation and pruritus in dogs.

Superficial Pyoderma Superficial pyoderma is the most common type of canine bacterial skin disease. Impetigo is characterized by nonfollicular, intraepidermal pustules involving the superficial layers of the epidermis (Fig. 85-1). Superficial folliculitis affects the ostial portion of the hair follicle and is the most common subgrouping of canine pyoderma. Impetigo and superficial folliculitis may be a diagnostic challenge because pustules rupture readily, giving rise to considerably less diagnostic crusted papules. A third clinical subset of superficial pyoderma, termed *superficial spreading pyoderma,* is characterized by centrifugally expanding inflammation with characteristic peripheral epidermal collarettes. Superficial spreading pyoderma may be seen alone or in conjunction with superficial folliculitis.

Deep Pyoderma Deep pyoderma is characterized by infection that proceeds deeper in the hair follicle with or without follicular rupture. The factors that allow infection to proceed from superficial to deep folliculitis are not understood. Deep folliculitis can lead to follicular rupture (furunculosis) with a granulomatous foreign body tissue response (Fig. 85-2). Interconnecting furunculosis involving the interstitium between hair follicles, the dermis, and subcutis is termed *cellulitis.* Deep pyoderma is much less common than superficial pyoderma. Diagnosis of deep pyoderma usually is not difficult; however, therapy often is problematic.

Clinical Findings
Dermatology has a singular advantage over most other specialty medical disciplines in that skin lesions are visible for careful inspection and available for precise sampling. Excellent lighting is essential for a proper physical examination. A hand lens is beneficial. Severity, extent, and pattern of clinical findings may be clarified additionally by clipping overlying hair from an affected lesion.

Table • 85-1

Classification of Canine Pyoderma Based on Depth of Infection

SURFACE PYODERMA
Pyotraumatic dermatitis (acute moist dermatitis, hot spots)
Intertrigo (skinfold pyoderma): lip-fold, facial-fold,
    vulvar-fold, tail-fold, obesity-fold
Mucocutaneous pyoderma[a]
Surface bacterial overgrowth[a]

SUPERFICIAL PYODERMA
Impetigo (puppy pyoderma)
Superficial bacterial folliculitis[a]
Superficial spreading pyoderma[a] (exfoliative pyoderma)

DEEP PYODERMA
Deep bacterial folliculitis and furunculosis
Muzzle folliculitis and furunculosis (canine acne)
Pyotraumatic folliculitis[a]
Pedal folliculitis and furunculosis[a]
Callus pyoderma (pressure-point pyoderma)
German shepherd dog pyoderma[a]
Cellulitis (secondary to demodicosis or immunologic
    incompetence)

DISEASES FORMERLY CLASSIFIED AS PYODERMA
Juvenile sterile granulomatous dermatitis and lymphadenitis
    (juvenile cellulitis, puppy strangles, juvenile "pyoderma")
Hidradenitis suppurativa[b]

[a]Subgroups of pyoderma in which recurrence or recrudescence is more common.
[b]These diseases were most likely autoimmune subepidermal blistering diseases or were vesicular cutaneous lupus erythematosus of the Shetland sheepdog or collie.

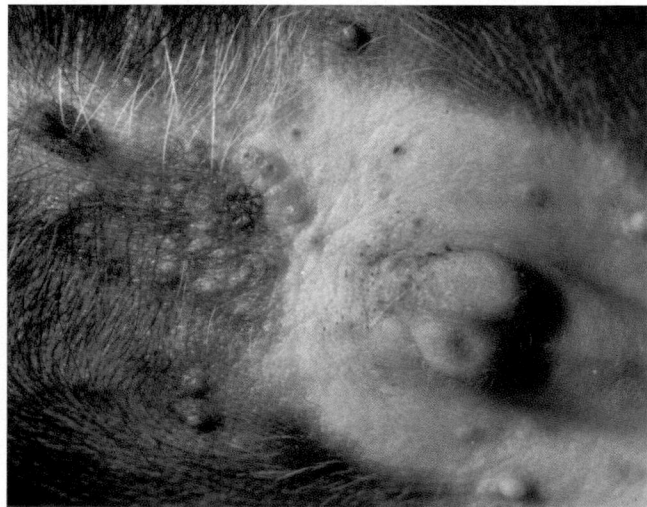

Fig 85-1 Impetigo in young pup with severe intestinal parasitism. (Courtesy University of Georgia, Athens, Ga.)

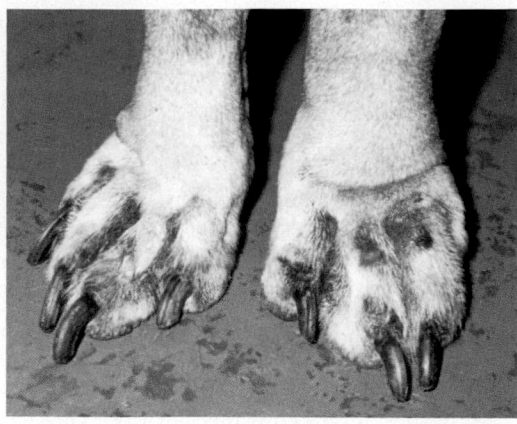

Fig 85-2 Interdigital pyoderma in dog with draining tracts and a granulomatous inflammatory reaction. (Courtesy University of Georgia, Athens, Ga.)

Primary Skin Lesions

An erythematous papule is the most common primary skin lesion seen in most superficial and milder deep pyoderma. Papules are circumscribed, solid elevations of the skin that usually form in groups. As infection proceeds, pus accumulates in intraepidermal or follicular locations, forming pustules. Small pustules may appear as papules to the unaided eye. Intact pustules often are transient in canine skin. When surface pustules rupture, crusted papules result. In deep pyoderma, more intense inflammation leads to nodule formation. Follicular rupture exacerbates inflammation in the adjacent dermis, resulting in larger nodules with fistulation. Peripheral collarettes, the "footprints" of pyoderma, are composed of detaching stratum corneum at the margins of inflammation. In deep pyoderma, host response is more intense, producing more obvious inflammation and swelling.

Secondary Skin Lesions

Pustules either rupture spontaneously or are obliterated by self-trauma, resulting in crusted papules. Clinically, crusted papules are less useful for diagnosis and may be indistinguishable from the papules seen with many other skin diseases. If crusted papules are grouped, crusts composed of dried pus, exudate, and keratin debris may mimic disorders of cornification. Self-traumatic excoriations may obliterate more diagnostic primary lesions, because pruritus is a feature of many pyodermas.

Alopecia commonly is seen secondary to pyoderma as hair fragments are shed from infected follicles. Transient, patchy (moth-eaten) alopecia probably results from premature telogenization and telogen arrest in a normally mosaic, asynchronous hair replacement pattern. Permanent, scarring alopecia secondary to deep folliculitis and furunculosis is uncommon in the dog, in contrast with pyoderma in people. Cellulitis leads to follicular obliteration.

Follicular rupture in deep pyoderma leads to nodule formation and draining fistulous tracts (see Fig. 85-2). Dermal hemorrhage resulting from follicular rupture with intense inflammation may result in hemorrhagic bullae that appear as dark bluish regions visible in the dermis.

Distribution of Lesions

Acute moist dermatitis, usually secondary to flea allergy dermatitis, is seen most commonly in the dorsal lumbosacral region. Intertrigo, or skinfold pyoderma, is observed at the spe-

cific site of the anatomic defect (lip-fold, facial-fold, vulvar-fold, tail-fold) according to breed. Mucocutaneous pyoderma occurs predominantly on and around the lips but may affect other mucocutaneous junctions. Surface bacterial overgrowth most commonly initially affects the intertriginous folds, such as those seen in the groin and axillae, but may become a generalized infection.

Uncomplicated superficial pyoderma occurs predominantly in the moist, intertriginous zones of the groin and axilla and to a lesser extent in the interdigital webs. Impetigo occurs primarily in the groin of prepubescent dogs. Superficial folliculitis and superficial spreading pyoderma are most commonly found in the groin and axilla, but lesions may generalize on the thorax. The attendant patchy, partial alopecia is more visually distinctive in short-coated breeds. Improper use of glucocorticoids may contribute to the spread of any superficial pyoderma while paradoxically decreasing visible inflammation. Bullous impetigo in the adult dog is most commonly secondary to iatrogenic hyperglucocorticoidism but can be associated with other underlying immunosuppressive diseases.

Deep pyoderma usually develop as an extension of superficial pyoderma. A characteristic distribution is seen with interdigital, pressure-point and nasal pyoderma, and canine acne. Because most canine cellulitis occurs secondary to generalized demodicosis, the distribution is similar to that of the primary disease.

Diagnosis
Differential Diagnoses

Many other skin diseases may mimic canine pyoderma. Differential diagnoses are listed in an approximate order of importance in Table 85-2. For additional information, see the Suggested Readings.[67,131]

Various diagnostic procedures may be helpful in diagnosing pyoderma and determining the presence of underlying diseases or other predisposing factors. Skin scrapings, cytologic examination, and skin biopsy usually are the most useful diagnostic procedures for the evaluation of suspected pyoderma.[67] Conversely, bacterial culture and identification and antibiotic susceptibility testing are overused procedures, because bacterial species and susceptibility to antimicrobial therapy commonly can be predicted.

Skin Scrapings Skin scrapings should be performed in all suspected cases of canine pyoderma, because demodicosis can initiate lesions that mimic uncomplicated pyoderma. It is especially important to scrape any pustular or papular lesion with a follicular orientation. In addition to mimicking pyoderma, demodicosis commonly triggers secondary pyoderma. Pyoderma secondary to demodicosis follows the distribution pattern of demodicosis, aiding diagnosis. Skin scrapings are more likely to yield demodicosis in suspected cases of lip-fold intertrigo, superficial folliculitis, deep folliculitis, furunculosis (canine acne, pedal folliculitis), and cellulitis.

Cytologic Examination Cytologic examination is a simple, cost-effective, and frequently beneficial diagnostic test for the documentation of canine pyoderma. Material from either direct smears of pustules or draining tracts often yields as much or more useful information than bacterial cultures and is more rapid and cost effective. Cytologic examinations of inflamed skin lacking primary lesions often demonstrates inappropriate surface bacterial overgrowth. Specimens should be air dried and stained with either a modified Romanovsky-type Wright's stain (Diff-Quik) or new methylene blue. Modified Wright's stain is beneficial both for documenting organisms and identifying inflammatory cells. The identification of cocci indicates the probable presence of *S. intermedius*.

Table • 85-2

Differential Diagnosis of Canine Pyoderma

SURFACE

Pyotraumatic dermatitis (acute moist dermatitis, hot spots): Pyotraumatic folliculitis, demodicosis, neoplasia (especially sweat gland adenocarcinoma), cutaneous metastasis, fixed drug eruption, early necrotizing form of idiopathic nodular panniculitis, early localized vasculitis, focal *Malassezia* dermatitis, candidiasis

Intertrigo (skin-fold pyoderma)
Lip-fold intertrigo: Localized demodicosis; fixed drug eruption; superficial necrolytic dermatitis, with or without *Malassezia* dermatitis or candidiasis; zinc-responsive dermatosis; muzzle folliculitis and furunculosis (canine acne); localized pemphigus foliaceus; early pemphigus vulgaris; early autoimmune subepidermal blistering disease

Facial-fold intertrigo: Localized demodicosis, *Malassezia* dermatitis, dermatophytosis

Vulvar-fold intertrigo: Urinary tract infection with self-trauma, vesicular cutaneous lupus erythematosus, ulcerative dermatosis of the Shetland sheepdog and collie, drug eruption, canine familial dermatomyositis, pemphigus vulgaris, early autoimmune subepidermal blistering disease

Tail-fold intertrigo: Flea allergy dermatitis

Obesity-fold intertrigo: *Malassezia* dermatitis

Mucocutaneous pyoderma: Lip-fold intertrigo, localized demodicosis, early discoid lupus erythematosus, zinc-responsive dermatosis, generic dog food dermatosis, muzzle folliculitis and furunculosis (canine acne)

Surface bacterial overgrowth: *Malassezia* dermatitis

SUPERFICIAL

Impetigo (puppy pyoderma): Early flea allergy dermatitis, superficial folliculitis

Superficial bacterial folliculitis: Superficial spreading pyoderma, flea allergy dermatitis, demodicosis, pemphigus foliaceus, sarcoptic acariasis, severe impetigo, drug eruption, erythema multiforme, seborrheic dermatitis, sterile eosinophilic pustulosis

Superficial spreading pyoderma: Superficial bacterial folliculitis, pemphigus foliaceus, erythema multiforme, seborrheic dermatitis

DEEP

Deep folliculitis and furunculosis: Demodicosis, subcutaneous and deep mycoses, opportunistic fungal infections, pythiosis, lagenidiosis, severe maladapted dermatophytosis, sterile granuloma-pyogranuloma, histiocytosis, idiopathic nodular panniculitis, juvenile sterile granulomatous dermatitis and lymphadenitis, vasculitis

Pyotraumatic folliculitis: Pyotraumatic dermatitis, demodicosis, neoplasia (especially sweat gland adenocarcinoma), cutaneous metastasis, fixed drug eruption, early necrotizing form of idiopathic nodular panniculitis, early localized vasculitis, focal *Malassezia* dermatitis, candidiasis

Muzzle folliculitis and furunculosis (canine acne): Localized demodicosis, early juvenile sterile granulomatous dermatitis and lymphadenitis

Pedal folliculitis and furunculosis: Demodicosis, dermatophytosis, subcutaneous and deep mycoses, opportunistic fungal diseases, pythiosis, lagenidiosis, pelodera dermatitis

Callus pyoderma (pressure-point pyoderma): Acral lick dermatitis, generic dog food skin disease, focal actinic comedones

German shepherd dog pyoderma: Demodicosis with secondary deep pyoderma, subcutaneous and deep mycosis, opportunistic fungal diseases, pythiosis, lagenidiosis

Cellulitis (with or without demodicosis): Juvenile sterile granulomatous dermatitis and lymphadenitis (juvenile cellulitis), subcutaneous and deep mycosis, German shepherd dog, pyoderma, sterile granuloma-pyogranuloma, idiopathic liquefying panniculitis, opportunistic fungal diseases, pythiosis, lagenidiosis

Modified from Ihrke PJ. 1996. *Bacterial skin disease in the dog: a guide to canine pyoderma.* Veterinary Learning Systems, Princeton, NJ.

The presence of degenerating neutrophils and intracellular cocci supports the diagnosis.

Skin Biopsy Skin biopsy is an often neglected valuable tool in the diagnosis of canine pyoderma. Increased reliance on skin biopsy has led to the more frequent diagnosis of pyoderma. The benefit of skin biopsy can be maximized if basic principles are followed: timing, lesion selection, method selection, technique, preparation of supportive material, and submission to a dermatopathologist are all important factors.

Bacterial Culture and Identification and Antibiotic Susceptibility Bacterial culture is overused in the evaluation and management of canine pyoderma. Bacterial culture and identification and antibiotic susceptibility tests are indicated if mixed infection is suspected (as determined by cytologic examination) or if appropriate empiric antibiotic therapy has not been effective. Cultures of intact pustules, furuncles, and nodules are more likely to yield helpful information. Bacterial cultures from open lesions are less likely to yield meaningful results. Bacterial cultures from the skin surface are not recommended.

Evaluation for Immunocompetence

Reliable diagnostic tests to determine immunocompetence in the dog are not available.[34,67] Gross information can be derived from a complete blood count (CBC) and serum electrophoresis. An absolute neutrophilia with a lymphocyte count of at least 1000 to 1500 cells per milliliter should be observed in normal dogs with ongoing or recurrent pyoderma. A broad-based elevation in the serum electrophoretic pattern in the ß and γ ranges should be present.[66,67] Assays such as in vitro lymphocyte stimulation and bactericidal tests are still primarily research tools because of their expense and lack of availability. The lack of ability to correct any defects that are documented further detracts from the clinical usefulness of these tests.[35,132] Pyoderma, especially when deep, is associated with a high prevalence of circulating immune complexes (CICs). Dogs with chronic deep pyoderma are more likely to be proteinuric, with a predominance of albuminuria, than dogs with superficial pyoderma.[10] The proteinuria is suspected to be a consequence of CICs depositing in glomerular microcapillaries.

Therapy

Systemic antibiotics usually are not needed to treat surface pyodermic infections such as pyotraumatic dermatitis and intertrigo; topical antibacterial therapy usually is sufficient. However, systemic antibiotics are necessary for the management of mucocutaneous pyoderma and surface bacterial overgrowth. Successful management of most superficial and deep pyoderma requires systemic antibiotic therapy. Topical antibacterial shampoo therapy commonly is applied as an adjunct in the management of mucocutaneous pyoderma, surface bacterial overgrowth, and most superficial and deep pyoderma to speed recovery, improve patient well-being, and potentially prevent recurrence. Immunomodulatory therapy is used less frequently, usually in an attempt to prevent or diminish the frequency of recurrent infection. Extended regimens of antibiotics should be considered a last resort in the management of recurrent pyoderma.

Antibiotic Therapy

The basic principles of systemic antibiotic therapy include the selection of an appropriate antibiotic, the establishment of an optimal dosage, and the maintenance of that dosage for enough time to ensure cure rather than transient remission. Although sequestered foci of infection may not be visible, surface lesions in deep pyoderma commonly heal before deeper lesions have resolved, leading to inappropriately early termination of therapy. Antibiotic selection can either be empiric or based on bacterial culture and susceptibility testing. An antibiotic chosen empirically should have a known spectrum of activity directed against S. intermedius and ideally should not be inactivated by β-lactamases, although most β-lactamase–resistant antibiotics are more expensive. Antibiotic therapy should be maintained for at least 1 week after the clinical cure for superficial pyoderma and a minimum of 2 weeks after the clinical cure for all types of deep pyoderma.

An ideal empiric antibiotic should have a narrow spectrum of activity, minimal side effects, and reasonable cost and have been shown to be an effective agent in the management of canine pyoderma. Little clinical evidence exists that bactericidal agents are more effective than bacteriostatic agents in the management of uncomplicated superficial pyoderma. Bactericidal antibiotics are recommended if hair follicle defects are present, in most deep pyoderma cases, and when immunosuppression is suspected or confirmed. If culture is performed, pustules or fistulous tracts should be recultured if S. intermedius was not isolated as the primary pathogen. If multiple isolates are not sensitive to a single oral antibiotic, an antibiotic effective against S. intermedius should be instituted because staphylococci create a tissue milieu favorable to the replication of secondary bacteria invaders. Results of culture and susceptibility studies and detailed information on individual antibiotics are discussed in greater detail in the Drug Formulary, Appendix 8.[67,131,132]

Antibiotics effective in the management of pyoderma are listed in Table 85-3. Penicillin, ampicillin, amoxicillin, and tetracycline are poor choices for the treatment of canine pyoderma. Previous and regional usage may alter antibiotic susceptibility.* Not surprisingly, resistant S. intermedius and gram-negative isolates are seen more commonly in referral practices than in general practice, and resistant bacterial populations are identified most frequently in deep pyoderma.[64,67,109] Many clinical trials have shown various antibiotics to be effective in managing canine pyoderma. Erythromycin, tylosin, lincomycin, clindamycin, chloramphenicol, trimethoprim and ormetoprim-potentiated sulfonamides, oxacillin, cephalexin, cefadroxil, fluoroquinolones, amoxicillin-clavulanate, and rifampin have been successful in the treatment of various canine pyoderma.†

Previously, it had been predicted that antibiotic-resistant S. intermedius would preclude the administration of many antibiotics common in dermatology. An examination of similarities and differences in antibiotic susceptibility patterns published during the past 2 decades indicates remarkably little spp.,[67] S. intermedius strains cultured from canine pyoderma in most locales apparently are no more resistant to commonly used antibiotics than they were 25 years ago. Fortunately, in comparison with S. aureus in humans and Pseudomonas spp., S. intermedius appears to lose resistance profiles rather rapidly when antibiotic pressure is removed. Consequently, many of the antibiotics just mentioned are still effective for the management of canine pyoderma. Preferred narrow-spectrum antibiotics include erythromycin, lincomycin, and oxacillin, and preferred broad-spectrum antibiotics include cephalexin, cefadroxil, ormetroprim-potentiated sulfonamides, enrofloxacin, and marbofloxacin.

Owner compliance using different dosing schedule regimens is not well studied in veterinary medicine. Perceived differences in efficacy probably correlate with differences in compliance. Compliance is easier with antibiotics given only once or twice daily than with those that need to be given 3

---

*References 44, 47, 64, 67, 68, 89.
†References 13, 67-69, 71, 129, 132.

Table • 85-3

Oral Antibiotics Useful for Treating Canine Pyoderma

DRUG NAME[a] (DOSE)	ADVANTAGES	DISADVANTAGES	ASSESSMENT
Erythromycin (10-15 mg/kg, 3 times daily)	Inexpensive, narrow spectrum	Cross-resistance with lincomycin, vomiting and diarrhea common, multiple daily dosing	Good first empiric choice
Lincomycin (22 mg/kg, 2 times daily)	Less frequent dosing narrow spectrum, few side effects	Cross-resistance with erythromycin, relatively expensive	Good first empiric choice, especially if need twice-daily drug
Clindamycin (10 mg/kg, 2 times daily, or 11 mg/kg, once daily)	Infrequent dosing	Only ~75% effective, development of resistance during therapy	Only a second-choice therapy for a once-daily drug
Ormetoprim-sulfadimethoxine (27.5 mg/kg, once daily)[b]	Less frequent dosing broad spectrum	Relatively expensive	Good first empiric choice, especially if need once-daily drug
Cephalexin or cefadroxil (22-30 mg/kg, 2 times daily)	Less frequent dosing broad spectrum, rare resistance, good tissue penetration	Cefadroxil expensive, generics moderately expensive	Excellent choice refractory-recurrent deep pyoderma, twice-daily drug
Enrofloxacin (5-15 mg/kg, once daily)	Less frequent dosing broad spectrum, rapidly absorbed, excellent tissue penetration	Expensive, cannot use in growing dogs	Excellent choice for refractory-recurrent deep pyoderma, once-daily drug
Marbofloxacin (2.5-5 mg/kg, once daily)	As above	As above	As above
Orbifloxacin (7.5 mg/kg, once daily)	As above	As above	As above
Oxacillin (22 mg/kg, 3 times daily)	Narrow spectrum, rare resistance, side effects rare	Expensive, multiple daily dosing absorption decreased by food	Good choice for refractory-recurrent deep pyoderma
Amoxicillin-clavulanate (12.5-20 mg/kg, 2 or 3 times daily)	Broad spectrum, side effects rare	Expensive, moisture sensitive, in vivo effect may not be as good as would be predicted	Efficacy low, somewhat expensive, for deep pyoderma
Trimethoprim-sulfonamide (22 mg/kg, 2 times daily)	Inexpensive, less frequent dosing broad spectrum	Side effects: keratoconjunctivitis sicca, severe cutaneous drug reactions, hepatic necrosis	Good empiric choice, concern for drug reactions

[a]For additional information on listed drugs, see Drug Formulary, Appendix 8. Treatment generally lasts for a minimum of 21 days.
[b]Give dose twice daily on the first day.
Modified from Ihrke PJ. 1996. *Bacterial skin disease in the dog: a guide to canine pyoderma*. Veterinary Learning Systems. Princeton, NJ.

times daily. Ormetoprim-potentiated sulfadimethoxine and the fluoroquinolones are the only antibiotics useful in canine pyoderma that can be administered once daily. Cephalexin, cefadroxil, and lincomycin require twice-daily dosing. Most other recommended antibiotics require three daily doses.

Various *tiered systems* for antibiotic usage have been popularized in the past.[35,67,78,131,132] The following recommendations comprise the tiered system recommended by the author. Erythromycin, lincomycin, clindamycin, and ormetoprim-potentiated sulfadimethoxine are useful for the management of uncomplicated, first-occurrence superficial pyoderma. The advantages and disadvantages of these drugs are listed in Table 85-3. Trimethoprim-potentiated sulfonamides are additional possible candidates for uncomplicated, first-occurrence pyoderma. However, the potential side effects of trimethoprim-sulfonamides are of concern.[77]

First-generation cephalosporins (cephalexin and cefadroxil), enrofloxacin, marbofloxacin, and oxacillin are rec-

ommended for pyoderma refractory to initial antibiotic therapy or recurrent pyoderma. Some veterinary dermatologists use amoxicillin-clavulanate. Chronic, deep pyoderma requires antibiotics with better penetrating ability because sequestered foci of infection and scarring prevent antibiotic access to the site of infection. Cephalexin, enrofloxacin, and marbofloxacin offer better penetrating ability. In the exceedingly rare circumstances when efficacy is not achieved with these drugs alone, rifampin (in conjunction with cephalexin or oxacillin) may be considered.

Enrofloxacin and marbofloxacin and other fluoroquinolones offer the advantages of once-daily dosing, excellent tissue penetration, activity against *S. intermedius* and gram-negative secondary invaders, and less likely development of resistance.[39,69,71] Once-daily dosing is recommended because the bactericidal effect is concentration rather than time dependent.[71,103] Uptake of enrofloxacin by macrophages leads to potent tissue-penetrating abilities.[39,71]

Oxacillin is a β-lactamase-resistant, narrow-spectrum, synthetic penicillin. Advantages include consistent efficacy in pyoderma and few side effects. Price is the primary disadvantage, even as a generic. Oxacillin must be administered 3 times daily and should be administered at least 1 hour before feeding, because food interferes with absorption.

Topical Therapy

Topical therapy is important in the management of pyoderma. Shampoos are the most commonly used delivery system. Antibacterial shampoos may be effective without concurrent antibiotics in some surface pyoderma and are frequently used as adjunctive therapy in the management of superficial and deep pyoderma. Antibacterial shampoos aid in debridement, encourage drainage, and decrease pain and pruritus. Their desired mechanisms of action are to decrease surface bacterial counts and limit recolonizing organisms, thereby diminishing the likelihood of recurrent infections. Improvement in patient attitude and owner encouragement are additional benefits.

Available antibacterial shampoos contain benzoyl peroxide with or without sulfur, chlorhexidine, ethyl lactate, or triclosan. Twice-weekly use of antibacterial shampoos with a minimum of 10 minutes contact time are recommended. Benzoyl peroxide shampoos may decrease recrudescence in susceptible dogs. This compound acts as an antiseborrheic, having antibacterial and degreasing properties.

Dogs with deep pyoderma require more aggressive topical therapy. After clipping, dogs benefit from daily antibacterial shampoos or twice-daily whirlpools or soaks. Chlorhexidine or povidone-iodine are added to warm water in whirlpools or soaks. Whirlpools remain a seldom used but very beneficial modality of topical therapy for deep pyoderma.

Antibacterial gels, creams, and ointments may be applied in the treatment of limited areas of skin. Cost, messiness, and time required for application limit their usefulness. Benzoyl peroxide is available in a gel vehicle. Mupirocin is a potent antibacterial agent with superior penetrating ability formulated for skin but not mucosal surfaces. Mupirocin should not be used when absorption of large amounts of the polyethylene glycol vehicle is likely because of the potential for nephrotoxicity.[67] Fusidic acid, a topically applied steroid antibiotic, has activity against gram-positive bacteria, such as staphylococci. It is bactericidal at higher concentrations. When applied to canine mucosal sites including the conjunctiva, nostrils, anus, and vulva, populations of *S. intermedius* were reduced on the mucosal and skin sites within 2 to 4 days after treatment was instituted and continued for up to 2 weeks after treatment was discontinued.[123]

Immunomodulatory Therapy

Immunomodulatory therapy remains controversial because of widely varying perceptions of efficacy. If immunomodulation is attempted, it should be an adjunct to antibiotic and topical therapy with the goal of diminishing the frequency or severity of recurrence of infection. Immunomodulatory therapy is most efficacious in dogs with idiopathic recurrent superficial pyoderma that respond completely to appropriate therapy, but recurrence follows within weeks after therapy has been discontinued. Most mentions in the literature referable to immunomodulatory therapy are either highly subjective or anecdotal, because it is often used in conjunction with combined systemic and topical antibacterials. Controlled trials are difficult to perform because immunomodulatory therapy rarely is the sole therapy.

Immunomodulators can be either bacterial or nonbacterial preparations. Commercial products contain either killed *Staphylococcus* or *Propionibacterium* species as the antigen.

Nonbacterial immunomodulatory drugs include levamisole and cimetidine (see Immunostimulants, Chapter 2).

Staphage Lysate (Delmont Laboratories, Swarthmore, Pa.) is the most common commercial bacterin used in North America and contains bacterial antigens of *S. aureus* isolated from humans. Staphage Lysate is the only product for which efficacy has been documented (approximately 40% of cases using 0.5 ml twice weekly[37]) by double-blinded, placebo-controlled studies. Autogenous bacterins occasionally are made from specific staphylococcal organisms isolated from a dog with pyoderma for use in that dog. Inactivation methodology is crucial because the process must kill the organism without disrupting antigenic determinants.

Nonbacterial immunomodulatory therapy is controversial; most reports are anecdotal. Levamisole, a levo-isomer of tetramisole sold as a vermifuge for large animals, may alter lymphocyte and phagocyte immune function. The recommended dosage of the sheep boluses is 2.2 mg/kg given every other day orally. Cimetidine, an H_2-histamine receptor blocker developed for treating gastric ulcers, theoretically could reduce immunosuppression by down-regulating suppressor T lymphocytes, thereby modulating cytokine production. The suggested dosage is 3 to 4 mg/kg orally given twice daily for at least 10 weeks. Controlled studies of efficacy have not been performed with either product.[67] Oral recombinant interferon-a2b has been used to treat idiopathic recurrent superficial pyoderma in dogs.[142] Only transient benefit was noted as compared with placebo.

Factors Contributing to Therapeutic Failure and Complicating Management

The most common cause of therapeutic failure in second-opinion cases noted in University of California, Davis Teaching Hospital is failure to adhere to the basic principles of systemic antibiotic therapy. The most common errors are the lack of establishment of an optimal therapeutic dosage and the failure to maintain therapy for long enough to achieve clinical cure.

Treatment failure, disease recrudescence, and disease recurrence also commonly are associated with lack of recognition of factors that can complicate management and influence prognosis. The most common complicating factors include inappropriate initial therapy, unidentified coexisting problems, sequestered foci of infection in deep pyoderma, and external environmental factors such as poor compliance that may not be known to the veterinarian.

Most antibiotic dosages for treatment of pyoderma are largely empiric, because little research has been done in this area. In deep pyoderma, sequestered foci of infection impede antibiotic penetration, and keratin debris from ruptured hair follicles encourages foreign body granulomatous response. Antibiotics that require microbial replication for activity, such as penicillins, are less effective when necrotic tissue and obstructed drainage routes create conditions that are no longer favorable for bacterial multiplication. Consequently, higher dosages usually are warranted in the management of chronic, deep pyoderma. Flexible dosage ranges approved for enrofloxacin and marbofloxacin encourage appropriate dosing.

Concomitant problems such as demodicosis, cornification disorders, hair follicle defects, hypothyroidism, and steroid abuse may hinder successful management. Pruritus, associated with either a pyoderma or an underlying pruritic disease, is an additional complicating factor.

Assessment of Therapy

All dogs receiving systemic antibiotics for pyoderma should be reevaluated within 10 to 14 days. If substantial improvement is not noted, the clinician should consider other factors that can complicate management. The clinician should consider owner compliance to the appropriate dosage regimen, drug loss through vomiting, drug inactivation by food, or malabsorption. Lack of identification of underlying triggering diseases also must be considered as should initial misdiagnosis since other diseases may closely mimic pyoderma. The alternative of referral to a veterinary dermatologist should be considered each time that clinical failure occurs.

Recurrent Pyoderma

Recurrent pyoderma can be defined as bacterial skin infections that respond completely to appropriate therapy, leaving the dog free of clinical signs of infection between episodes of pyoderma. The relatively small but unknown percentage of cases characterized by frequent recurrences is one of the most frustrating aspects of veterinary dermatology. Recurrent superficial pyoderma is the most common subgroup. Underlying skin disease or undiagnosed internal medical abnormalities are the most common causes of recurrent canine pyoderma.[35,67,78,131,132] Possible causes of recurrent pyoderma can be subdivided into persistent underlying skin disease, bacterial hypersensitivity, immunodeficiency, resistant strains of *S. intermedius*, and nonstaphylococcal pyoderma.[35] Recurrent pyoderma is considered idiopathic only if all appropriate diagnostic procedures have failed to reveal a predisposing cause.

Recurrent pyoderma triggered by continuing underlying skin disease may alter the clinical appearance of the predisposing condition, making identification of the predisposing trigger difficult. Diagnosis of the underlying disease may be facilitated by first treating with an appropriate course of antibiotics to unmask the symptomatology of the underlying disease.

Pruritus can be an important discriminating feature in evaluating recurrent pyoderma. If pruritus is totally ameliorated by antibiotic therapy, the pruritus probably was caused by the bacterial infection. If pruritus is still present after complete resolution of the pyoderma, the pruritus is most likely being caused by an as yet undiagnosed underlying disease.

Recurrent pyoderma commonly is a lifelong disease requiring extensive client communication and counseling. An informed client is more likely to make the necessary commitment to treatment. Curing underlying diseases may completely prevent recurrent pyoderma. Hypothyroidism is an example of an underlying disease in which pyoderma may be completely eliminated. In contrast, therapy for underlying flea allergy dermatitis seldom completely eliminates secondary pyoderma and requires constant flea control. Many skin diseases that act as triggers for recurrent pyoderma can be controlled but not cured, requiring continuous management. Canine atopic dermatitis and defects in cornification are examples of skin diseases that rarely respond completely to appropriate therapy and therefore continue to trigger occasional secondary pyoderma.[67]

Choices in the management of recurrent pyoderma in which successful management of an underlying disease is not possible or the pyoderma is idiopathic include long-term topical antibacterial shampoos, immunomodulatory therapy, and extended regimens of systemic antibiotics. Antibacterial shampoo therapy performed once or twice weekly should be attempted initially. If this therapy prevents recurrence, it can be maintained indefinitely. Adjunctive immunomodulatory therapy should be considered as the next option if shampoo therapy alone is unsuccessful.

Extended regimens of antibiotics using subtherapeutic dosage regimens to prevent recurrence are viewed as a last resort in the long-term management of recurrent canine pyoderma and should be used only after the current episode of the pyoderma has been brought under complete control. Antibiotics most useful for extended regimens include cephalexin, enrofloxacin, marbofloxacin, oxacillin, and amoxicillin-clavulanate.

Risks inherent in the extended administration of systemic antibiotics using subtherapeutic dosage regimens include undesirable effects in the patient, induction of antibiotic resistance, and formation and possible dissemination of resistant strains of bacteria in the environment. The relatively high cost is an additional drawback. The author currently prefers 2 or 3 consecutive days per week at the full daily dosage. Other options include every-other-week dosing at therapeutic levels followed by extending the duration of time off antibiotics in gradual increments (2 weeks, 3 weeks).[67] Long-term therapy must be monitored carefully because of inherent risks.

OTITIS EXTERNA

Craig E. Greene

Etiology

Otitis externa is inflammation of the external ear canal. The following discussion focuses on microbial factors; reviews should be consulted concerning other causes of this condition. (For a discussion of otitis media-interna, see Musculoskeletal Infections, Chapter 86.) Numerous causative agents have been associated with otitis externa (Table 85-4), and failure to identify and eliminate the underlying cause results in ineffective treatment. Most microbial infections of the external ear canal are secondary to another disease or factor that make it susceptible to colonization by normal or opportunistic microflora. Bacteria, yeasts, parasites, and viruses have all been incriminated as causing otitis externa. In many cases, an underlying disease can be found, and the role of the infectious organism as the primary cause of otitis externa cannot be substantiated. For example, cocker spaniels have ceruminous and sebaceous gland hyperplasia with chronic otitis externa, whereas other breeds develop fibrosis.[6]

The normal ear canal is colonized by various microorganisms that can proliferate with damage or inflammation from the primary factors (Table 85-5). Microfloral overgrowth can exacerbate or perpetuate inflammatory reactions. Higher concentrations of bacterial and yeast organisms have been found in the ear secretions of dogs with otitis externa than in clinically healthy dogs.[152] Coagulase-positive *S. intermedius* is the most common isolate in normal ears and in acute otitis externa, in which it is even more prevalent. β-Hemolytic streptococci are found with equal frequency in normal and diseased ears, so their pathogenic status is uncertain. Other common organisms rarely found in clinically healthy ears and isolated predominantly in cases of chronic otitis externa are *Pseudomonas* species and *Proteus mirabilis*.[152] *Pseudomonas* species have been associated with a severe, virulent form of otitis externa. These organisms are isolated from the ear canal of fewer than 1% of clinically healthy dogs and up to 20% of those with chronic otitis externa. *Pseudomonas* organisms isolated from the ear canals of dogs are often highly resistant to antibacterial drugs. In one report, *Pseudomonas aeruginosa* isolated from canine ear cultures were 32% resistant to gentamicin and 100% resistant to ampicillin, cepthalothin, trimethoprim-sulfonamide, and tetracycline.[117] Because of the multidrug resistance pattern of *Pseudomonas*, empirical therapy is not advised. Mixed infections usually are composed of *S. intermedius* in conjunction with a gram-negative rod. In cats, *Pasteurella multocida* may also be isolated.

Bacteria or the broad-based budding yeast *Malassezia pachydermatis* may proliferate in an ear canal of an animal pre-

Table • 85-4

Predisposing Factors for Otitis Externa

HOST

Anatomic

Breed	German shepherd
Conformation	Long droopy ears (cocker, bassett), stenotic canals (English bulldog, Shar pei, chow chow), hair in canals (poodle, schnauzer, bichon, Airedale, wirehaired, and fox terriers), ceruminous gland hyperplasia (cocker spaniel)
Otitis media-interna	Causing self-inflicted trauma or act as nidus
Masses	Polyps, squamous cell carcinoma, ceruminous gland tumors, papilloma, sebaceous adenoma, ceruminous adenoma, fibroma squamous cell carcinoma, basal cell carcinoma, fibrosarcoma
Hyperkeratosis	Seborrheic diseases (German and Belgian shepherds), sebaceous gland infection (standard poodles, Akitas, Samoyeds), inflammatory polyp (cats)

Immunologic Conditions

Hypersensitivities	Atopic dermatitis, juvenile cellulitis (puppy strangles, golden and Labrador retrievers, dachshunds, pointers, Lhasa apso), contact allergies (propylene glycol), food allergy, drug eruption
Immunodeficiency	Debilitation
Autoimmune	Systemic lupus erythematosus, pemphigus foliaceus

Endocrinopathic Conditions   Male-feminizing syndrome, hypothyroidism, Sertoli cell tumor, ovarian imbalance

ENVIRONMENT

Moisture	Swimming (Labrador retrievers), high environmental temperature and humidity
Foreign material	Plant material, excessive otic medicants, soil, exudates, dried wax
Medicants	Yeast infections due to chronic antibiotic and glucocorticoid therapy
Astringents	Alcohol, cleansing agents
Trauma	Iatrogenic or self-induced, lacerations of aural mucosal, excessive cleaning or medicants, cotton swabs

AGENT

Parasites	*Otodectes cynotis* (ear mite), biting flies, chiggers, ticks, *Demodex canis*, *Sarcoptes*, *Notoedres*, flea allergy
Bacteria	*Staphylococcus intermedius*, β-hemolytic streptococci, *Proteus*, *Pseudomonas*
Fungi	*Malassezia canis*, *Microsporum canis*, *Candida*

disposed to infection because of other underlying diseases or prolonged antibacterial therapy. *Microsporum canis* is considered to be a secondary invader contributing to or perpetuating and exacerbating inflammation in an already diseased ear canal. In cats the relative importance of *M. pachydermatis* in disease is less certain because it is found with equal frequency in clinically healthy cats and those with otitis externa. (For additional discussion of *M. pachydermatis* infections in dogs and cats, see Chapter 58.)

The ear mite *Otodectes cynotis* is believed to be responsible for a majority of feline cases of otitis externa; dogs have a much lower prevalence of infection. Most animals develop a hypersensitivity reaction to the mite that causes the inflammation seen clinically; however, some are nonsymptomatic carriers. In others, the inflammation may lead to a secondary bacterial or yeast infection that can eventually result in the destruction of the mites.

Clinical Findings

A complete history, with special attention to the animal's environment and exposure to vegetation and water, is helpful. Pruritus, a major problem with otitis externa, is manifest by head shaking, scratching, or rubbing the ears along the floor or other objects. On physical examination, pinnal or caudal auricular alopecia, matted hair, broken hairs, excoriations, and occasional areas of acute moist dermatitis are apparent. The external auditory meatus may be erythematous and swollen. In many uncomplicated cases of otitis externa, the clinical findings are limited to erythema and possibly a slight increase in ear wax (ceruminous otitis) (Fig. 85-3). When otitis externa is complicated by secondary bacterial or yeast infections, the character and amount of discharge may become more purulent and moist and may have a foul odor (suppurative otitis). Inflammation may be severe, the ear canals may become painful, and self-inflicted trauma may be apparent. Some animals become head shy; others show evidence of pain only when the canal is palpated. Chronic otitis is characterized by epidermal hyperplasia with thickening of the pinna and narrowing or calcification of the ear canal or both. Fibrosis is observed in most breeds with chronic otitis, although cocker spaniels have the most significant degree of ceruminous and sebaceous gland hyperplasia (Fig. 85-4).[6] A thorough examination of the ear with an otoscope is needed to determine the presence of secondary changes and the extent of the inflammation and discharge as well as the condition of the tympanic membrane. If the canal is very swollen and stenotic, treatment should proceed with a broad-spectrum topical preparation for up to 1 week before performing the otoscopic examination.

Pseudomonas ear infections are highly virulent and characterized by unilateral or bilateral aural pruritus, head shaking, scratching, and rubbing of the ears. A foul-smelling, greenish-yellow discharge is typically found.

Table • 85-5

Organisms Isolated from External and Middle Ear Canal of Dogs and Cats

ORGANISM	HOST	FREQUENCY OF ISOLATION (PERCENTAGE)[a]			PHYSICAL DESCRIPTION
		CLINICALLY HEALTHY	OTITIS EXTERNA	OTITIS MEDIA	
GRAM-POSITIVE BACTERIA					
Staphylococci (coagulase positive), includes *Staphylococcus intermedius*	Dog	9-20	22-40	18	Light brown or pale yellow exudates
Streptococci (β-hemolytic)	Dog	16	10	9	Light yellow to light brown exudates
GRAM-NEGATIVE BACTERIA					
Pseudomonas species	Dog	0.4	20	26	Painful, copious light yellow to green exudates, often ulcerated epithelium
Proteus species	Dog	0	11	6.5	Light yellow exudates, ulcerated with chronicity
Escherichia coli	Dog	0	14	2.6	Light yellow exudates
FUNGI					
Malassezia species	Dog	15-49	50-83	17	Light brown to dark (chocolate) brown exudates
	Cat	23	19		
METAZOANS					
Otodectes cynotis	Dog	0	5-10	0	Dark brown exudates
	Cat	0	50		

[a]Data on animals with otitis media are from Cole LK, Kwochka KW, Kowalski JJ, et al. 1998. Microbial flora and antimicrobial susceptibility patterns of isolated pathogens from the horizontal ear canal and middle ear in dogs with otitis extrerna, *J Am Vet Med Assoc* 212:534-538. Data on clinically healthy animals and those with otitis externa are from references cited in the text.

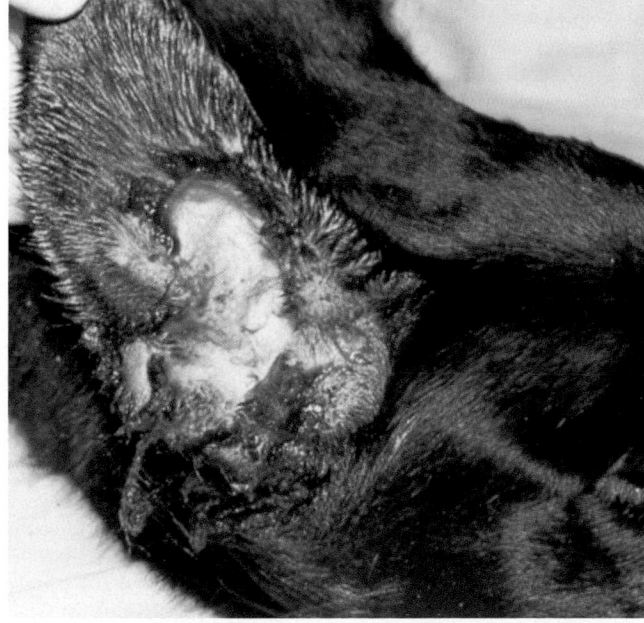

Fig 85-3 Acute otitis externa in dog with erythema and increased ocular discharge. (Courtesy University of Georgia, Athens, Ga.)

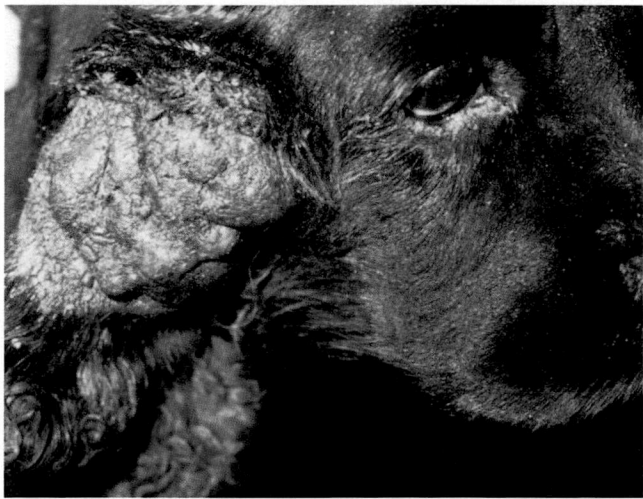

Fig 85-4 Chronic proliferative epidermal hyperplasia of ear canal of cocker spaniel dog with otitis externa. (Courtesy University of Georgia, Athens, Ga.)

Diagnosis

After a complete history and physical otoscopic examination, smears of the ear canal contents should be made. To prevent cross-contamination, a separate, clean otoscope cone must be used for each ear. Sterilized cones should be used if bacterial or fungal culture specimens are taken. The canal should be examined for its diameter, amount and type of exudate, foreign bodies, neoplasms, parasites, condition of the tympanic membrane, and integrity of the epithelium. As described by others,[28] ears can be thoroughly cleaned by placing cerumi-nolytic ear cleaners within the ear for 10 minutes to emulsify wax and debris. Ears are then flushed with warm sterile isotonic 0.9% saline using a bulb syringe to remove any loosened debris. Some ceruminolytic agents can be irritating and damage the structures of the middle and inner ear if the tympanic membrane is perforated.[92] Because the integrity of the tympanic membrane is not known before cleaning, only mild agents should be used for this purpose.

Additional examination can be done with general anesthesia or sedation. Hand-held or videoendoscopes are used to examine the horizontal canal and deeper structures. Further drying of the cleaned canal may be accomplished using swabs so that the entire canal can be visualized. Deeper irrigation of the canal is accomplished with a syringe attached to an 8 French polypropylene urinary catheter cut to approximately 9 cm, blunted using a flame, and attached to a 12-ml syringe.[28] Swabs should be inserted into the horizontal canal of each ear through a sterilized otoscope cone to recover material for microscopic examination and culture. One swab should be placed in a drop of mineral oil on a slide and examined for ear or *Demodex* mites. Another swab should be rolled onto microscope slides, and a fast stain based on Giemsa's or Wright's methods is often used. Before staining, the slide should be heat fixed by passing it over an open flame 2 or 3 times. Heat fixing melts some wax and debris, which causes them to adhere better to the glass slide. Without heat fixing, much of the wax, lipid, and associated yeasts may wash away in the staining process. More than 10 yeasts per high-power field are suggestive of their overgrowth.

Cytologic examination of exudate is needed to evaluate the type of inflammatory response and potential underlying cause. Numbers and morphology of leukocytes, neoplastic cells, and bacteria or fungi should be recorded. In one report, mean *Malassezia* counts per high-dry power (40×) field equal to or greater than 5 in the dog and equal to or greater than 12 in the cat and mean bacterial counts of ≥25 in the dog or equal to or greater than 15 in the cat were considered indicative of external ear canal infection.[45] Because commensals are cultured from normal ears, cytologic enumeration of bacteria provides a means of determining their overgrowth and a hint about their type before culture results become available. When secondary bacterial infections are contributing to the disease, leukocytes and phagocytized bacteria are usually present. When primarily wax and keratin are present, the bacteria observed are most likely incidental but can still contribute to the odor and inflammation by their lipolytic action on waxy debris.

Occasionally, *O. cynotis* or *Demodex* can be identified during examination of a smear. Failure to find mites, especially if secondary infection is present, does not rule out their existence.

Bacterial culture and susceptibility testing offer little additional information compared with good basic cytologic evaluation and are costly. Antimicrobial susceptibility can usually be determined on the basis of organism morphology (Table 85-6). Furthermore, the levels achieved by topical application are much higher than the serum levels of sensitivity disks. Bacterial isolation is of more benefit if the tympanic membrane is ruptured with otitis media or interna and the clinician is contemplating systemic antibiotic therapy. Culture and sus-ceptibility testing also are indicated in chronic otitis externa when primarily bacterial rods are found on a smear or when microorganisms persist in spite of apparent appropriate topical medication. *Malassezia* is better identified by cytology than by culture (see Fig. 56-4). Repeating cytologic examination on subsequent visits helps evaluate drug resistance or owner compliance. Persistent inflammation in the absence of abundant microorganisms suggests an allergic or ceruminous otitis.

In a prospective study of 23 dogs with chronic bilateral otitis externa, infection was identified in at least one tympanic bulla in 22 dogs.[28] Infection of the middle ear could not be determined by the presence or absence of an intact tympanic membrane. Myringotomy was used to detect infection within the tympanic bulla. Furthermore, organisms isolated from the horizontal ear canal and middle ear were only identical in 10.5% of the ears. Therefore for definitive evaluation, specimens for cultures should be taken from the horizontal ear canal and in the bulla via myringotomy during examination under general anesthesia. Myringotomy is accomplished by passing a sterile culture swab or rubber or polypropylene catheter through a sterilized otoscope cone into the cau-doventral portion of the tympanic membrane. Use of a catheter allows for lavage of the bulla should exudate be found on penetration. Duplicate specimens should be taken and submitted for cytologic and cultural examination.

Radiologic imaging should be considered with chronic or recurrent otitis when signs of vestibular dysfunction or other neurologic signs of dysfunction or cranial hyperesthesia are observed. Skull radiography allows for visualizing the tympanic bulla; however, computed tomography and magnetic resonance imaging with contrast enhancement are able to detect meningeal or intracranial involvement.

Therapy

Effective treatment and management of otitis externa are best achieved by combining several principles. If possible, predisposing causes should be identified and eliminated or prophy-lactically treated. Topical therapy is especially beneficial because drugs attain their highest concentrations with the fewest systemic effects. To obtain owner compliance, the treatment should be specific and simple. Systemic antibacterial or antifungal therapy may be needed if the external canal is occluded or otitis media is present. Systemic therapy can be selected on the basis of culture and susceptibility results. For empiric systemic bacterial therapy, drugs used to treat staphylococcal pyoderma such as erythromycin, first-generation cephalosporins, lincomycin, clindamycin, amoxicillin-clavulanate, ormetoprim- or trimethoprim-sulfonamides, or fluoroquinolones are most effective. For *Pseudomonas* species, effective drugs have included extended-spectrum penicillins (piperacillin, ticarcillin, carbenicillin), third-generation cephalosporins (ceftazidime, cefoperazone), aminoglycosides, and quinolones. *P. aeruginosa* is more likely than other organisms to develop resistance to any of these drugs during treatment. For example, isolates of *Pseudomonas* and *Enterococcus* species from dogs with otitis externa or urinary tract infection have been shown to develop resistance to enrofloxacin, whereas *Klebsiella*, *Proteus*, and *Streptococcus* species were less likely to develop resistance.[15] In one report, *Pseudomonas* organisms isolated from chronic canine otitis externa were more susceptible to tobramycin, marbofloxacin, and ceftazidime than to enrofloxacin, presumably from more extensive use of the latter drug.[94] Regardless of which antimicrobial therapy is instituted, treatment usually lasts a minimum of 3 to 4 weeks (see Table 85-6).

Cleaning

Depending on the animal's temperament, sedation or anesthesia may be needed for cleaning the ears, which should be

Table • 85-6

Antimicrobial Selection for Otitis Externa[a]

ACUTE OTITIS
Cytologic exam: gram-positive cocci; culture; staphylococci, streptococci
Topical
Neomycin (Panolog, Tritop, Quadritop, Tresaderm, Neopredef)
Povidone-iodine (Betadine) dilute 1 : 50 (intact tympanum); 1 : 100 (perforated tympanum)
Chlorhexidine (Nolvasan) dilute 1 : 40 in water
Acetic acid (white vinegar 5%) dilute 1 : 3 in water; concentrations of 2%-5% are irritating (many formulations)

Cytologic exam: gram-negative bacilli; culture; *Proteus* species, *Escherichia coli*
Topical
Neomycin (Panolog), polymyxins (Surolan), gentamicin (Gentocin otic)
Acetic acid (white vinegar 5%) dilute 1 : 3 in water (many)
Povidone-iodine (Betadine) dilute 1 : 50 (intact tympanum); 1 : 100 (perforated tympanum)

Cytologic exam: yeasts
Topical
Nystatin (Panolog), thiabendazole (Tresaderm), miconazole (Surolam, Conofite), clotrimazole (Otomax, Genotic B-C, MalOtic Ointment, Otibiotic, Otosoothe, Tri-Otic, Mometamax Otic)

CHRONIC OR RESISTANT OTITIS
Yeasts
Topical
Clotrimazole (Otomax, many formulations), miconazole (Surolam, Conofite), clotrimazole (many), Silvadene

Systemic
Ketaconazole 5 mg/kg twice daily for 2-4 weeks, itraconazole 5-10 mg/kg once daily for 2-4 weeks

Gram-negative species, usually *Pseudomonas*
Topical
Gentamicin (Gentocin otic, otomax), polymyxin B, colistin or polymyxin E (Coly-Mycin), polymyxin B (Cortisporin)
Polyhydroxidine iodine (Xenodyne, Solvay) diluted 1 : 3 to 1 : 5 in water and apply twice daily

Systemic
Ormetoprim-sulfadimethoxine, trimethoprim-sulfonamide, first-generation cephalosporin

Culture *Pseudomonas* species
Topical
Ticarcillin (Ticar suspension), add 4 g to 4-oz bottle of Oti-clens
Tobramycin (Tobrex ophthalmic)
Enrofloxacin (Baytril injectable) diluted 50% in water, 3-5 drops twice daily
Amikacin sulfate (Amiglyde-V injectable) undiluted (50 mg/ml) 5-6 drops twice daily
Silver sulfadiazine (Silvadene) diluted 1 : 1 in water, 4-12 drops twice daily
TRIS-edetic acid-gentamicin solution (Wooley's solution) (see Chapter 34, Table 34-12)

Systemic
Enrofloxacin, marbofloxacin, orbofloxacin, gentamicin

[a]Trade names appear in parentheses.

dried before initiating therapy. Initial cleaning and drying of the ear canals are essential to complete the otoscopic examination, determine the integrity of the tympanic membrane, and facilitate the penetration of topically administered drugs. Thorough cleansing of the ear canals removes small secondary foreign bodies as well as degenerated inflammatory cells, free fatty acids, bacterial toxins, wax, and debris. Ear cleaning with physical flushing of the canal may be repeated as needed, but it should not be performed more than 2 times weekly because it produces mucosal ulceration. Ear-cleaning solutions may be applied more frequently by the owner, who can instill a few drops just before an otic antimicrobial drug is given. The animal should be allowed to shake its head to disperse the solution, and the excess removed before instilling the desired medication. Cleaning and flushing solutions are generally disinfectants and are listed in Table 85-7. They are used for initial removal of debris or as ceruminolytics. Ceruminolytics are selected when excessive waxy accumulation is present. In most cases, ceruminolytic agents, such as carbamide peroxide and dioctyl sodium sulfosuccinate, are most effective in emulsifying and facilitating the cleaning procedures and are water soluble. Carbamide peroxide has a foaming action that breaks

Table • 85-7

Solutions for Management of Otitis Externa

CLASSES AND INDICATIONS	INGREDIENTS	PRODUCTS
Flushing Solutions Primary cleaning of canal, have weak antibacterial activity	Cleaning and disinfecting solutions containing dilute acids and disinfectants	Betadine, povidone-iodine 10% (dilute 1 : 10 to 1 : 50); Xenodyne, polyhyroxidine iodine 0.5% (dilute 1 : 1 to 1 : 15); Nolvasan chlorhexidine 2% (dilute 1 : 40); vinegar, acetic acid 5% (dilute 1 : 3); lactic acid 2.5%; salicylic acid 0.1%
Ceruminolytics Permeate and solubilize waxy debris	Squalenes, surfactants, carbamide peroxide, chlorhexidine, dioctyl sodium sulfosuccinate, propylene glycol	Cerumene, Clear X, Veterinary Surfactant, Sebo-o-sol, Otic Chlor-7, Otic Clear, Nolvasan Otic, Adams Pan Otic
Ceruminolytic and Drying Agent When combined, dissolve wax and dry out canal	Same as ceruminolytic ingredients, but also includes alcohols and acids such as lactic, salicylic, malic, benzoic, and acetic	Cerbin-otic, Oti-clens, Epi-otic, Chlorhexiderm Otic, Adams Ear Dessicant, Fresh Ear, VPL Otic Cleanser, Chlor-otic-L, Otic-clear
Drying Agents Have mild antibacterial activity, dry ear canal, act as astringents on exuding lesions	Organic acids, alcohols, silicone dioxide (as listed for previous combinations)	Dermal Dry, Otic Domeboro, Panodry, Otic Calm, acetic acid 5% and isopropyl alcohol in a 3 : 1 ratio

down debris. Ceruminolytic oils such as squalene, lanolin, and mineral oil are more difficult to clean up. Many combination ceruminolytic and drying products contain organic acids with a ceruminolytic agent or alcohol added. They are easier to clean up and can be used as a one-step procedure. These products must be applied with great caution if the tympanum is ruptured. In a study of several ceruminolytic agents, only a solution containing squalene and isopropyl myristate with liquid petrolatum base (Cerumene, Evsco Pharmaceutical, Buena, N.J.) was nonirritating to the middle ear in the presence of a ruptured tympanum.[92] If ceruminolytics are used before the discovery of a ruptured membrane, thorough rinsing with pure water or saline is preferred. Other rinse solutions should not contain detergents or disinfectants because they are ototoxic and contraindicated with a ruptured tympanic membrane.

Rubber bulb ear syringes are a very efficient way to flush the ear. After the initial flushing, loops can be used to remove any remaining material. Cotton swabs should be avoided because they pack exudate and debris down in the ear and may injure the tympanum or epithelial lining. In other cases, especially in animals with a ruptured tympanum, a feeding tube attached to a 12-ml syringe may be used for the final flushing as well as for cleaning out the bulla. In addition, by applying negative pressure, it is a rapid, atraumatic way of removing residual water. Head tilt, ataxia, or both may develop after cleaning as a result of otitis media or interna.

Topical Therapy

Once the ears are clean and dried, topical therapy can be effective in the treatment plan. In general, most ear products contain various combinations of glucocorticoids and antibacterial, antiyeast, and parasiticidal agents in aqueous solution or oil vehicles (Table 85-8). The most appropriate topical drug can be prescribed on the basis of clinical findings, cytology, and diagnosis. Cleaning solutions and disinfectants (antiseptics) are the first preparations that can be used to help remove debris and control overgrowth of microorganisms. Oil vehicles are best applied when the ears are dry, because they tend to moisturize the skin. In moist, exudative ears, water-soluble vehicles are preferred because they are less occlusive. Water-soluble aqueous preparations are most desirable when the tympanic membrane is ruptured. Besides selecting the most appropriate vehicle, the clinician must decide which active ingredients are most appropriate for each case. No single perfect topical ear product exists.

Topical glucocorticoids are most effective when an animal has early, acute inflammation, and high-potency fluocinolone, betamethasone, and dexamethasone are recommended. Although they are generally contraindicated in infectious processes, they do reduce the inflammation in the ear canal, which controls pruritus, swelling, exudation, wax build-up, and tissue proliferation and hyperplasia. It is difficult to find a commercial otic medication that is not formulated with glucocorticoids. Because they may predispose the patient to secondary yeast infections and hyperadrenocorticism, the lowest required potency (e.g., hydrocortisone) and frequency are recommended for long-term (greater than 3 months) treatment. Otic preparations with dexamethasone and triamcinolone have systemic effects and result in signs of hyperadrenalism with iatrogenic pituitary-adrenal suppression. With severely painful or inflamed ears or stenotic canals, systemic prednisone is recommended at a dose of 0.25 to 0.5 mg/kg twice daily for 1 to 2 weeks in dogs and twice this dose for cats.

Bacterial infections should be treated with topical antibiotics or disinfectants. In general, the aminoglycosides

Table • 85-8

Broad-Spectrum Veterinary Otic Antimicrobial Preparations

PRODUCT (MANUFACTURER)[a]	FORMULATION/ VEHICLE	ANTIBACTERIAL	ANTIINFLAMMATORY	ANTIFUNGAL
Surfacticide (Centaur)	Drops	Nitrofurazone	—	—
Terra-Cortril (Pfizer)	Suspension	Oxytetracycline	Hydrocortisone	—
Gentocin Otic (Schering)	Solution; propylene glycol, alcohol, glycerine	Gentamicin	Betamethasone	—
Betsolan (Janssen)	Drops	Neomycin	Betamethasone	—
Neo-Predef (Pfizer)	Ointment; lanolin, petrolatum, mineral oil	Neomycin	Isoflupredone	—
Betagen Otic Solution (Med-Pharmex), Garagen Otic Solution (PPC), Gentamicin Otic Solution (Butler), Genta-Otic (Vetus), Gentaved Otic Solution (Vedco)	Solution; alcohol, glycerin, propylene glycol	Gentamicin sulfate	Betamethasone valerate	—
Tritop (Pfizer)	Ointment	Neomycin sulfate	Isoflupredone acetate	—
Epi-Otic (Virbac), Epi-Otic NF (Virbac), ResiCHLOR Lotion (Virbac)	Solution; propylene glycol	Chlorhexidine	—	Chlorhexidine
Auroto (Kyron)	Solution	Neomycin	—	Thiabendazole
Baytril Otic (Bayer)	Solution; alcohol, neutral oil	Enrofloxacin	—	Silver Sulfadiazine
Fungi-Dry-Ear (Q.A. Laboratories)	Gel; alcohol, lanolin oil, acetic acid	—	—	Zinc undecylenate
Otomax Ointment (Schering), CGB Ointment (PPC), Genotic B-C (Butler), MalOitc Ointment (Vedco), Otibiotic Ointment (RXV), Otosoothe Ointment (Vetus), Tri-Otic (Med-Pharmex)	Ointment; mineral oil, hydrocarbon gel	Gentamicin sulfate	Betamethasone valerate	Clotrimazole
Mometamax Otic Suspensor (Schering-Plough)	Suspension; mineral oil hydrocarbon gel	Gentamicin Sulfate	Momethasone furoate monohydrate	Clotrimazole
Panolog (Fort Dodge), Quadritop Cream (Vetus), Oridermyl (Centaur)	Ointment; mineral oil	Neomycin	Triamcinolone	Nystatin
Otospectrine (Phenix)	Solution	Neomycin	Dexamethasone	Monosulfiram
Surolan (Janssen)	Solution	Polymixin B	Prednisolone	Miconazole
Tresaderm (Merial)	Solution; glycerine, alcohol, propylene glycol	Neomycin	Dexamethasone	Thiabendazole
Animax Ointment (Pharmaderm)	Ointment; polyethylene, mineral oil	Neomycin sulfate	Thiostrepton	Nystatin

[a]Available Internet addresses of manufacturers: Virbac (www.virbac.com), Schering (www.sp-animalhealth.com), Pfizer (www.pfizerah.com), Fort Dodge (www.wyeth.com/divisions/fort_dodge.asp), Merial (www.merial.com), Q.A. Laboratories (see Butler), Bayer (www.bayer-ah.com), Pharmaderm (www.pharaderm.com), PPC, Butler (www.accessbutler.com), Vedco (www.vedco.com), Vetus (www.burnsvet.com), RXV (www.dvmresources.com), Med-Pharmex (www.med-pharmex.com).

(neomycin, polymyxin, gentamicin) and chloramphenicol are frequently effective. Although the aminoglycosides are potentially ototoxic, especially when topically applied to an ear with a ruptured eardrum, this has not been shown to be a problem (see Aminoglycoside Toxicity, Chapter 34). Optimally, drugs that may later be needed for systemic therapy should not be used topically in acute cases because resistance may develop. Disinfectants are an effective alternative to antibiotics. Iodine and chlorhexidine are good choices for treating bacteria and yeasts, respectively, but are ototoxic when put into the middle ear. Acetic acid at 2% is generally effective against *Pseudomonas* species and at 5% is effective against most bacterial pathogens involved in otitis externa. Other acids that are effective are 2% boric acid, 2.5% lactic acid, and 0.1% salicylic acid.[29] For more resistant *Pseudomonas* infections, otic or ophthalmic medicants containing gentamicin, tobramycin, or polymyxins can be applied, and as a last resort, compounded formulations of ticarcillin or amikacin solutions can be prepared and instilled twice daily. Silver sulfadiazine, a compounded mixture of two antibacterial agents, is highly effective against *Pseudomonas* and other bacteria and yeasts in canine otitis externa.[110] Silver sulfadiazine ear solution (0.1%) is prepared by mixing 0.1 g of chemical-grade powder into 100 ml distilled water. Alternatively, 1.5 ml of cream is mixed with 13.5 ml distilled water; however, this mixture is more viscous and requires warming above ambient temperature to ease its topical application. TRIS-ethylenediaminetetraacetic acid (EDTA) preparations are also effective against *Pseudomonas* and other resistant gram-negative bacteria (see Buffered EDTA Solution, Chapter 34, and Table 34-15). *Pseudomonas* infections may be susceptible to quinolones that have been compounded into topical preparations for treatment of chronic otitis externa. (For specific information on compounding topical enrofloxacin and ticarcillin preparations for treating Pseudomonas described above, see Drug Formulary, Appendix 8.)

Secondary yeast infection may occur when systemic or topical antibacterial therapy is prolonged. Cytologic examination should be performed at repeat visits to check for this complication.

When *Malassezia* organisms are present, the topically applied antiyeast agents such as nystatin and thiabendazole contained in many ear medicants are frequently effective. Thiabendazole can be a contact irritant in some dogs. In more difficult cases, 1% miconazole or clotrimazole lotions usually work. A mixture of 2% boric acid and 2% acetic acid instilled in the ear once daily for 7 weeks was reported to be effective in treating *Malassezia* otitis.[48] If a *Malassezia* otitis media is diagnosed, then the systemic antifungal ketoconazole given 5 mg/kg every 12 hours or itraconazole given 5 mg/kg every 24 hours for 4 to 6 weeks is the preferred treatment (see Chapter 58 for further information on *Malassezia* infections).

O. cynotis is relatively sensitive to most insecticides, including pyrethrins, rotenone, and thiabendazole. In addition to treating the ears, the entire body and other in-contact animals should be treated. Ivermectin at 250 mg/kg, given orally once weekly for 3 to 4 weeks or subcutaneously once every 10 days for two treatments, is effective against *Otodectes* mites. It also eliminates mites from other areas. However, ivermectin is not approved for use in cats or dogs at this dosage. It is absolutely contraindicated in collies.

Surgical treatment of refractory otitis externa and media is total ear canal ablation and lateral bulla osteotomy. In one study, various bacteria were isolated from the subcutaneous tissues at the time of the initial skin incision, the tympanic bulla, and the tissues at the time of closure of the incision[147] (Table 85-9). In this study, susceptibility of isolates for each drug were as follows: gentamicin (50%), ampicillin (54%), amikacin (62.5%), cefazolin (70%), trimethoprim-sulfonamide (87.5%), and greater than 90% showing susceptibility to amoxicillin-clavulanate, ticarcillin, ticarcillin-clavulanate, or ciprofloxacin. Dehiscence from infection is common after this procedure and may also relate to numerous factors, including difficulty of decontaminating the recesses of the ear canal and bulla during surgical preparation and bacterial resistance to surgical preparation solutions such as chlorhexidine that are

Table • 85-9

Culture Results for Specimens Taken During Total Ear Canal Ablation and Bulla Osteotomy in 13 Dogs

BACTERIAL OR FUNGAL SPECIES	INITIAL INCISION[a] (MEAN COLONY COUNT PER GsRAM OF TISSUE)	BULLA[b] (MEAN COLONY COUNT PER GRAM OF TISSUE)	SUBCUTANEOUS TISSUE AT CLOSURE[c] (MEAN COLONY COUNT PER GRAM OF TISSUE)
Streptococcus canis	4.13	$>10^5$	$>10^5$
Streptococcus bovis	0	53	7
Staphylococci (coagulase positive)	15.4	$>10^5$	57.66
Staphylococci (coagulase negative)	10	0	18
Proteus mirabilis	0.5	$>10^5$	$>10^5$
Escherichia coli	0.14	$>10^5$	$>10^5$
Pseudomonas aeruginosa	0.67	$>10^5$	$>10^5$
Streptococci (β-hemolytic)	0	2	0
Micrococci	0	1	0
Malassezia species	1	31	1
Alcaligenes dentrificans	$>10^5$	$>10^5$	$>10^5$
Enterococci	$>10^5$	$>10^5$	$>10^5$

[a]Subcutaneous tissue immediately after skin incision.
[b]Excised epithelium from the bulla ossea.
[c]Subcutaneous tissue just before skin closure.
From Vogel et al. 1999. *J Am Vet Med Assoc* 214:1642-1643.

in many ear remedies. Therefore care should be taken to reduce bacterial contamination before and during otic surgeries, and bacterial culture with antimicrobial susceptibility testing is indicated at the incision site before closure.

Prognosis

The prognosis is generally good in acute (less than 4 weeks' duration) cases of otitis externa when the tympanic membrane is intact. Early control of the disease is important in preventing secondary changes. A guarded to good prognosis is indicated in chronic cases unless surgical intervention is advised. Whenever the tympanic membrane is ruptured, otitis media is diagnosed, and the prognosis for complete recovery becomes guarded with medical therapy alone. When secondary changes have progressed to marked fibrosis with narrowing of the ear canal or osteomyelitis of the bulla, surgical intervention may be required. In animals with calcified ear canals, surgery is also necessary to achieve good results. Lateral (horizontal) ear resection is indicated to facilitate drainage and administer medicants, but it is usually only palliative because diseased tissue often remains. Total (vertical) canal ablation is needed with tissue proliferation and calcification of the ear canal. When clinical signs of middle or inner ear disease occur and fluid density is apparent within the bulla or thickening of the bulla is seen radiographically, bulla osteotomy is the treatment of choice (see also Otitis Media/Interna, Chapter 86).[143] Total canal ablation and lateral bulla osteotomy can be done simultaneously.[76] Although these procedures may cure the otitis externa and media, postoperative complications include hearing impairment, Horner's syndrome, facial nerve paralysis, and vestibular dysfunction.

SUGGESTED READINGS*

6. Angus JC, Lichtensteiger C, Campbell KL, et al. 2002. Breed variations in histopathologic features of chronic severe otitis externa in dogs: 80 cases,1995-2001. *J Am Vet Med Assoc* 221:1000-1006.

30. Colombini S, Merchant SR, Hosgood G. 2000. Microbial flora and antimicrobial susceptibility patterns from dogs with otitis media. *Vet Dermatol* 11:235-239.

43. Frank LA, Kania SA, Hnilica KA, et al. 2003. Isolation of *Staphylococcus schleiferi* from dogs with pyoderma. *J Am Vet Med Assoc* 222:451-454.

51. Guardabassi L, Loeber ME, Jacobson A. 2004. Transmission of multiple antimicrobial-resistant *Staphylococcus intermedius* between dogs affected by deep pyoderma and their owners. *Vet Microbiol* 98:23-27.

64. Holm BR, Petersson U, Morner A, et al. 2002. Antimicrobial resistance in staphylococci from canine pyoderma: a prospective study of first-time and recurrent cases in Sweden. *Vet Rec* 151:600-605.

90. Manian FA. 2003. Asymptomatic nasal carriage of mupirocin-resistant, methicillin-resistant *Staphlococcus aureus* (MSRA) in a pet dog associated with MRSA infection in household contacts. *Clin Infect Dis* 36:e26-e28.

123. Saijonmaa-Koulumies L, Parsons E, Lloyd DH. 1998. Elimination of *Staphylococcus intermedius* in healthy dogs by topical treatment with fusidic acid. *J Small Anim Pract* 39:341-347.

141. Tejedor Junco MT, Martín Barrasa JL. 2002. Identification and antimicrobial susceptibility of coagulase positive staphylococci isolated from healthy dogs and dogs suffering from otitis externa. *J Vet Med B Infect Dis Vet Public Health* 49:419-423.

152. Yoshida N, Naito F, Fukata T. 2002. Studies of certain factors affecting the microenvironment and microflora of the external ear of the dog in health and disease. *J Vet Med Sci* 64:1145-1147.

*See the CD-ROM for a complete list of references.

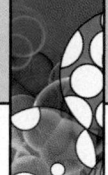

CHAPTER • 86

Musculoskeletal Infections

Craig E. Greene and Steven C. Budsberg

Musculoskeletal infections involve bones, joints, and muscles. Osteomyelitis is classically defined as inflammation of the cortical bone, medullary cavity, and periosteum.[17,46] Most cases involve infectious agents, including bacteria, fungi, and viruses. Other potential causes include irritants, such as radiation therapy, or surgical implants; however, these causes are much less common.[17,46,62] Bone infections can be divided into skeletal (including the skull and pelvis) and vertebral (including intervertebral disks and vertebral bodies). Diskospondylitis with secondary osteomyelitis developing in the opposing vertebrae is more common in dogs and cats compared with people. In humans, vertebral osteomyelitis often occurs without disk space infection. In animals, vertebral osteomyelitis usually arises from penetrating injuries (see Actinomycosis, Chapter 49) rather than from blood-borne infections that cause diskospondylitis (see Diskospondylitis and Vertebral Osteomyelitis later in this chapter).

To understand osteomyelitis, the disease process is best divided into hematogenous and posttraumatic causes. Posttraumatic osteomyelitis can be either acute or chronic.[17,46,62] Because of differences in causes, clinical findings, and treatments, skeletal osteomyelitis and diskospondylitis are discussed separately (Table 86-1). Additionally, otitis media is covered in this chapter because the bony structures of the middle and inner ear are involved. Joint and muscle infections that concern soft tissues adjacent to bone are each covered

Table • 86-1

Predisposing Causes of Musculoskeletal Infections

Diskospondylitis
    Bacteremia in mature animals[63]
    Bacterial endocarditis
    Severe stomatitis and gingivitis
    Disk fenestration—laser disk ablation[6]
    Spinal trauma, surgery, or instability
    Immunosuppression and IgG deficiency
    Lumbosacral instability; increased blood flow
    Intraabdominal or intrathoracic abscesses[109]
    Extension of paravertebral infection
    Genitourinary infections
Vertebral Osteomyelitis
    Migrating plant awns
    Paravertebral abscesses
    Penetrating paraspinal injuries
    Intraabdominal or intrathoracic abscesses
Vertebral Physitis[119]
Metaphyseal Osteomyelitis
    Bacteremia in young animals[68,47]
    Cat[14]
    Fungal dissemination[45]
    Congenital immunodeficiency[120]
Osteomyelitis
    Penetrating foreign bodies[100]
    Orthopedic implants[102]
    Bacteremia[52,15,37]
    Fungal dissemination[60]
Septic Arthritis
    Multifocal
        Hematogenous—bacteremia, endocarditis
    Solitary
        Postoperative joint surgery
        Penetrating wounds

separately. Table 86-2 lists microorganisms commonly associated with musculoskeletal infections.

OSTEOMYELITIS

Etiology

Bacterial infections cause most cases of osteomyelitis in clinical practice. In some studies, gram-positive organisms such as *Staphylococcus* accounted for 50% to 60% of cases,[46,69] and *Staphylococcus. intermedius* is the primary organism. Other gram-positive organisms found less frequently include *Streptococcus* and *Enterococcus*. In other reports, both gram-positive and gram-negative organisms have been approximately equal in their recovery rate.[29] Gram-negative organisms have included *Pasteurella, Escherichia coli, Pseudomonas, Proteus, Serratia,* and *Klebsiella*. Anaerobic bacteria include *Peptostreptococcus, Bacteroides, Fusobacterium, Actinomyces, Nocardia,* and *Clostridium*.[85] Anaerobic bacteria have been isolated with greater frequency as sample collection, transportation, and incubation techniques have improved.[69,85] Anaerobic bacteria are rarely isolated alone, and other anaerobes and microaerophilic or aerobic bacteria usually make the envi-

ronment conducive for anaerobic growth. Polymicrobial infections are becoming more common, presumably because of overuse of antimicrobial agents, which enables resistant bacterial populations to flourish, or because of better bacterial collection and detection methods. In human medicine, a poorer prognosis is found in cases of osteomyelitis when more than one organism is isolated.

A variety of fungi has been identified in osteomyelitis from regions where the organisms are endemic. In the United States, the most common isolates are *Blastomyces, Coccidioides, Histoplasma,* and *Cryptococcus*.[62,133] Other organisms reported include *Aspergillus* and *Phialoconidium*. German shepherd dogs have the highest prevalence rate for hematogenous fungal osteomyelitis, making a hereditary immune deficiency a likely contributing factor (see also Disseminated Aspergillosis, Chapter 64).

Although viral agents have been incriminated as causing inflammatory bone diseases, factual data have been limited. However, virulent and vaccine-strain canine distemper virus (CDV) has been suspected as a cause of hypertrophic osteodystrophy (HOD) and juvenile cellulitis in dogs (see Chapters 3 and 100).[71,78,130]

Pathogenesis

Hematogenous Spread

Spread of infection via the bloodstream from a distant site is rare in dogs and cats. When infection occurs, immature animals are usually affected.[53,62] The animal's predisposition of the metaphyseal region to hematogenous embolization is likely a result, in part, of the microvascular architecture of the region in growing bone. Capillaries that extend into the growth plate have both variable continuous and discontinuous epithelia.[44,53] Terminally growing capillary buds lack a basement membrane and have discontinuous endothelium.[44,53] Discontinuities allow circulating microorganisms to escape into the extravascular tissue space during a bacteremic phase. Blood flow through these capillary beds is slow, creating an ideal environment for bacterial lodgment and proliferation. Furthermore, in contrast to secondary spongiosa, leukocytes appear to be absent around primary spongiosa.[44] Bacterial invasion in the region of developing bone may be opposed by only tissue-based macrophages. Unrestricted infection in the metaphyses may spread to the epiphyses, periostea, soft tissues, and adjacent joints. In dogs and cats, unlike other species, transphyseal vessels are absent at birth; thus infection is usually restricted to the metaphyseal side of the growth plate.[33]

Posttraumatic Injuries

Normal bone is resistant to infection. Osteomyelitis is unlikely to develop in the absence of complicating factors that include tissue ischemia, bacterial contamination, bone necrosis and sequestration, fracture instability, foreign material implantation, and systemic or local alteration in immune response or tissue metabolism.[17,46,56,62] Tissue trauma and subsequent vascular compromise are important factors when discussing posttraumatic osteomyelitis. Soft tissues provide the first blood supply to the ischemic bone during the initial phases of healing. Inoculation of bacteria can occur from direct penetration of a missile or other foreign body, a bite wound, an exposure of the bone via an open fracture, or a surgical intervention. Avascular bone fragments provide an ideal ecologic niche for bacteria to colonize and proliferate. Fracture instability perpetuates the persistence of infection in the bone. Instability may occur when initial stabilization is inadequate or when initial fixation fails. In either case, disruption of the blood supply is caused by damage to proliferating capillaries, promoting tissue and bone necroses and bacterial colonization and growth.

Table • 86-2

Microorganisms Associated with Musculoskeletal Infections

INFECTION	MICROORGANISMS (CHAPTER REFERENCE)
Osteomyelitis	Viral: canine distemper virus (3, 100) Bacterial: many Fungal: *Blastomyces* (59), *Histoplasma* (60), *Cryptococcus* (61), *Coccidioides* (62), *Aspergillus* (64), *Candida* (65)
Diskospondylitis	**Dogs** Bacterial: *Staphylococcus intermedius, S. epidermidis, Enterococcus faecalis* (36), *Brucella canis* (40), *Nocardia* and *Actinomyces* (49), *Streptococcus canis, Alcaligenes, Micrococcus, Proteus* (35), *Escherichia coli, Pseudomonas aeruginosa* (37), *Mycobacterium* (50), *Corynebacterium, Pasteurella* (53), *Bacteroides* (41) Fungal: *Aspergillus terreus* (65), *Paecilomyces varioti* (67), *Fusarium, Mucor* (67) **Cats** *Streptococcus canis* (35), *Actinomyces* (49), *E. coli* (37)
Otitis Media/Interna	*Pasteurella multocida* (53)
Joint infections	Polyarthritis (hematogenous seeding or immune complex deposition) Viral: effusive feline infectious peritonitis (11), feline calicivirus (16), feline syncytium-forming virus (17) Rickettsial: granulocytic *Ehrlichia* (28), *Rickettsia rickettsii* (29), *Chlamydia* (31) Mycoplasmal: *Mycoplasma* (32), bacterial L-forms (32) Bacterial: hemolytic: *Streptococcus, Proteus, Pseudomonas, Erysipelothrix, Corynebacterium* (35), *Staphylococcus* (36), *E. coli* (37), *Salmonella, Yersinia* (39), *Brucella* (40), anaerobes (41), *Borrelia* (45), *Pasteurella* (53, 88), *Nocardia* (49), *Mycobacterium* (50) Fungal: *Blastomyces* (59), *Histoplasma* (60), *Cryptococcus* (61), *Coccidioides* (62), *Aspergillus* (64), *Candida* (65) Protozoal: *Leishmania* (73) Suspected infectious: Akita arthritis (100), shar pei fever (95)
Myositis	Polymyositis Viral: feline immunodeficiency virus (14) Bacterial: *Leptospira* (44), *Borrelia* (45), clostridia (41) Fungal: *Sporothrix* (63) Protozoal: *Trypanosoma* (72), *Leishmania* (73), *Hepatozoon* (74), *Toxoplasma gondii* (80), *Neospora caninum* (80), *Sarcocystis* (81) Local myositis: numerous bacteria, toxigenic *Streptococcus canis* (35)

Biofilm

Implantation of foreign material has been associated with increased infection rates.[39,100,112] Staphylococci are the predominant bacterial contaminants in these infections. The primary mechanism in biomaterial-centered sepsis is microbial colonization of these materials and adjacent damaged tissues.[56] Tissue necrosis and inflammation along the biomaterial's surface, associated with failure of implant integration into host tissues, serve as a glycoprotein-conditioned substratum for which bacteria have specific receptors.[56] Adherent bacteria produce a matrix of condensed exopolysaccharides known as a glycocalyx.[77] The biofilm is composed of a cluster of microorganisms and glycocalyx on an inanimate surface. Embedded in the biofilm mixture of glycocalyx, host-derived serum proteins, and cellular debris, bacteria often form into microcolonies (Fig. 86-1). Within biofilms, bacteria are protected from antibodies, phagocytes, and even antibiotics.[56,62,77] Bacteria within biofilms have been shown to intercommunicate via cytokines,[28] and this appears to assist them in adapting as a colony within their biologic environment and avoiding host defense mechanisms. The glycocalyx retards the penetration of drugs, organisms become dormant within the biofilm, and the microenvironment within adversely affects antimicrobial activity.[34] Furthermore, several different types of bacteria can both coexist and replicate in glycocalyx-enclosed microcolonies in the interstitial spaces of connective tissue associated with dead bone sequestra, causing mixed infections.

Clinical Findings

Clinical signs of osteomyelitis vary with the type and duration of disease. Acute osteomyelitis, either hematogenous or post-traumatic in origin, produces localized pain, erythema, and soft-tissue swelling. The animal is usually febrile. Elevated leukocyte counts are common. Various signs of systemic illness include lethargy and inappetence.[17,46,62] Chronic posttraumatic osteomyelitis is a localized disease with rare systemic manifestations; the most common of these is a history of trauma or surgery with a subsequent draining tract and lameness. Nonhealing wounds that continue to drain should always be evaluated by radiography for underlying osteomyelitis.

Metaphyseal Osteomyelitis

In young animals, hematogenous osteomyelitis often results in fever, lameness, and swelling of the metaphyseal region of long

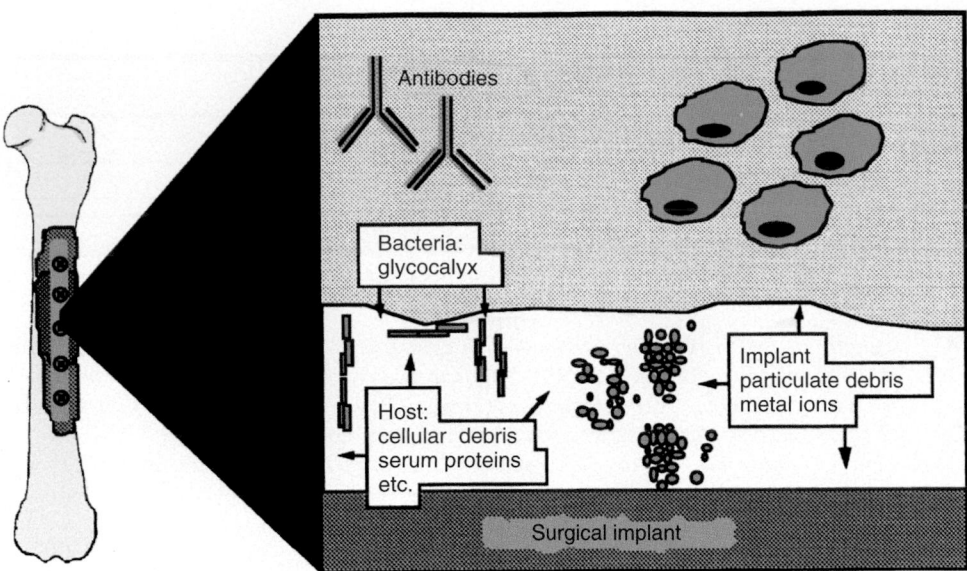

Fig 86-1 Schematic drawing showing osteomyelitis involving the femur and associated surgical implant. Bacteria produce glycocalyx, which, combined with host-derived and implant-derived materials, forms a biofilm. This biofilm protects bacteria from host defenses.

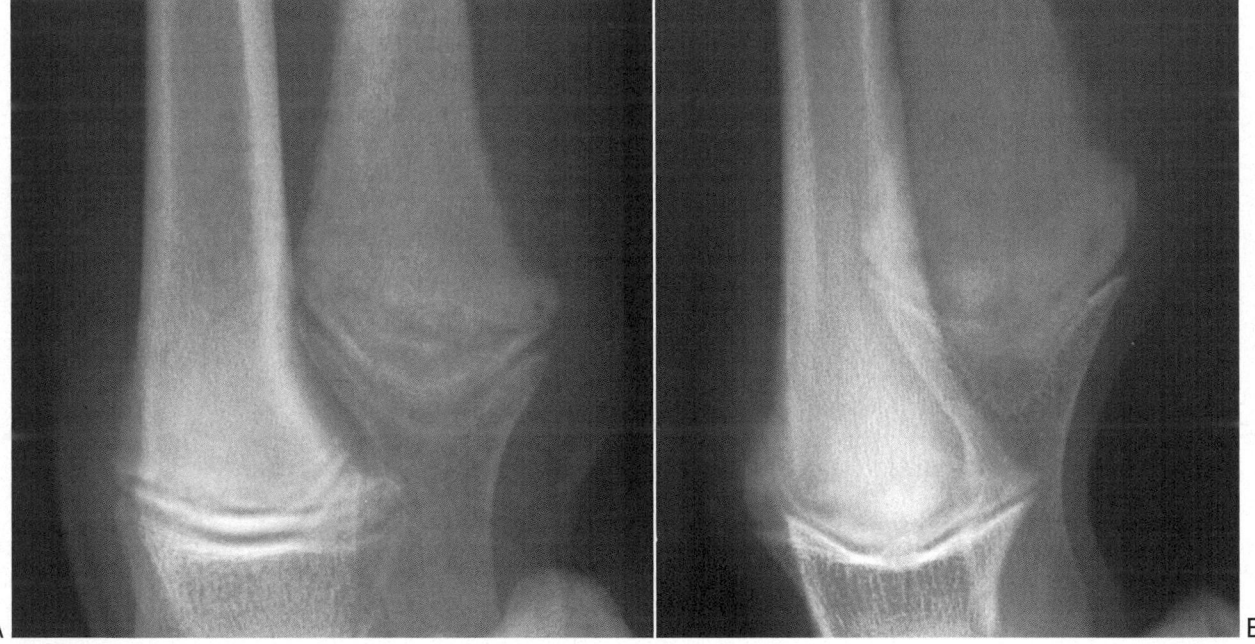

Fig 86-2 Thoracic limb radiography of dogs with (**A**) hypertrophic osteodystrophy with increased lucency and irregularity of the epiphyseal lines. **B**, Metaphyseal osteomyelitis with increased density in the metaphyseal region resulting from osteoproliferation as a result of bacterial infection. (Courtesy University of Georgia, Athens, Ga.)

bones. Dogs and cats have both been affected by this condition.[14] This area is likely predisposed to colonization in the young animal because of its high blood supply and anatomic features, as described under Pathogenesis of Hematogenous infections previously mentioned. Gram-positive bacteria such as *Staphylococcus* are often isolated. Swelling and lameness in a young animal can be confused with HOD in the dog. Radiographically, the features of the two diseases are distinct (Fig. 86-2). In HOD, epiphyseal lines show radiolucent banding with metaphyseal periostitis. In metaphyseal osteomyelitis, either increased or decreased density is observed within the metaphyseal region resulting from osteoproliferation or osteolysis, depending on the type and stage of infection. If multiple animals in a litter develop this condition, then an

underlying immunodeficiency or congenital or early neonatal infection should be considered.[120]

Diagnosis

History, physical examination, and radiography will localize the site of the lesion. Nonspecific laboratory findings may include variable leukocytosis and increased serum concentrations of calcium and phosphorus or high alkaline phosphatase activity. Radiography will localize and determine the type of lesion. In an acute case, the only finding may be soft-tissue swelling. As the infection progresses, radiographic changes include, but are not limited to, periosteal bone proliferation, bone resorption, and increased medullary density. In chronic cases, radiography can demonstrate the presence of loose or broken implants or nonviable bone (sequestra). Unfortunately, radiography reportedly has a sensitivity of 62.5% and specificity of 57% in the detection of osteomyelitis.[13] More accurate detection can be achieved with the use of nuclear scintigraphy.

Technetium-99m-methylene diphosphonate (MDP), indium-111 leukocyte, and IgG scintigraphy are radionuclide imaging techniques that can provide additional diagnostic information if radiographic findings are equivocal.[67] However, these tests are used sparingly in veterinary medicine and require the specialized equipment of referral centers.

Cytologic evaluation of exudates is informative, whereas microbiologic culture of an infectious agent is definitive. Specimens from a sterile aspirate of the lesion through intact skin or from sequestra, local necrotic tissue, or implant at the time of débridement provide the most valuable material for culture. For aspiration for cytologic or culture specimens, the site is aseptically prepared at intact, unaffected skin over the suspected lesion. A 20-gauge needle is then inserted to the level of the bone, followed by aspiration into a 12-ml syringe. Organisms isolated from discharges of draining tracts may be contaminants. Proper collection and transport of both aerobic and anaerobic samples is also imperative (see Chapter 33). In cases of hematogenous osteomyelitis, blood should be cultured, as well as the secondary site of infection.

Anaerobic infections should be suspected when affected tissue is characterized by a foul odor, sequestra, or the presence of multiple bacterial species suggested by impression smears or histologic specimens (see Chapter 41).[85] Further suspicion of an anaerobic infection should be raised if no organism is cultured from material in which cytologic findings indicate infection. Multifocal sterile pyogranulomatous osteomyelitis has been reported in dogs[22] but probably is caused by immune dysregulation rather than infection.

Therapy

The infective agent, local tissue environment, and blood supply should always be considered in any therapeutic strategy. Although treatment is customized to each patient, certain principles must be followed. Mere use of antimicrobial drugs will not eradicate the infection associated with chronic osteomyelitis. The local environment must be improved by débridement, drainage, fracture stabilization, dead-space obliteration, and antimicrobial therapy. Regardless of the situation, every effort should be made to obtain a culture and susceptibility testing for both aerobic and anaerobic bacteria. Followup evaluation involves serial clinical and radiographic evaluation and repeated culturing of the infected area.

Hematogenous Osteomyelitis

Animals with hematogenous osteomyelitis are often septic. The infections, which can occur in any skeletal site, frequently involve the metaphyseal region of the bone and do not extend into the adjacent joint (Fig. 86-3, A). However, synoviocentesis and radiography are strongly recommended to make this determination. Blood culture results may also be informative. If joints are affected, aggressive management should be undertaken as described later for monoarthropathies. If no joint involvement can be demonstrated, any fluctuant, warm, or painful area around the affected bone can be aspirated for culture and susceptibility testing. If an obvious fluctuant area is present, attempts should be made to open and copiously lavage the region with a sterile isotonic solution and to perform débridement. Systemic intravenous (IV) antibiotics should be given for a minimum of 3 to 5 days before switching to the oral route. Oral administration should continue for a minimum of 21 days. Bactericidal agents that are active against β-lactamase–producing *Staphylococcus* should be used (Tables 86-3 and 86-4). Systemic treatment for sepsis should be addressed if necessary (see Chapters 38 and 87). Radiographs taken 2 to 3 weeks after treatment can help evaluate progression and response to therapy (see Fig. 86-3, B). Sys-

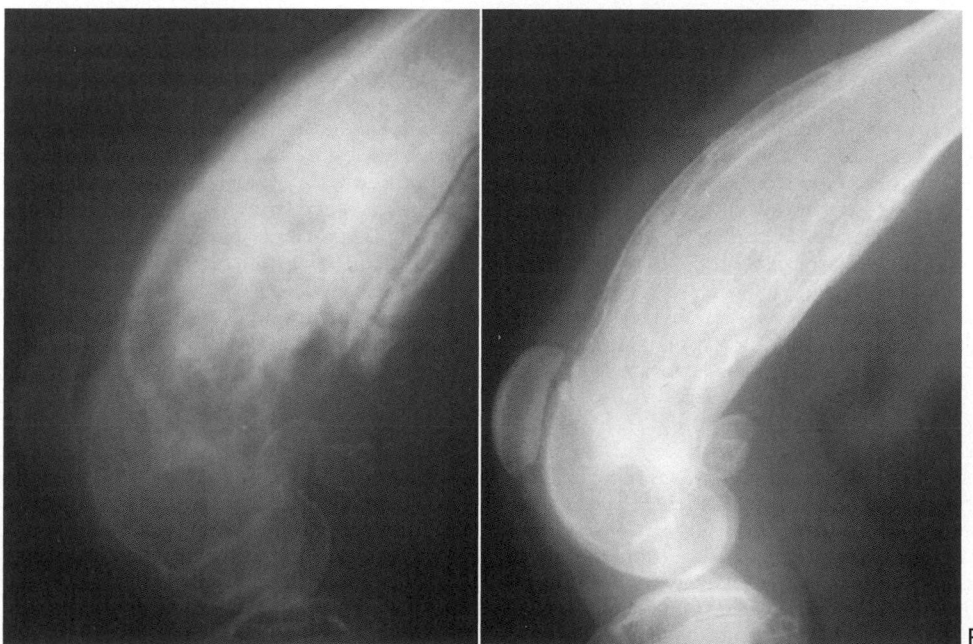

Fig 86-3 **A,** Pelvic limb radiograph of 4-month-old Doberman with lameness and painful stifle swelling of 10 days' duration. Acute hematogenous osteomyelitis with metaphyseal lysis and extensive bony production within the distal diaphysis are evident. **B,** One month after surgical biopsy and culture of *Staphylococcus intermedius* and institution of systemic antibiotic treatment. Remodeling of the femoral metaphysis with reduced sclerosis and periosteal proliferation occurs.

Table • 86-3

Recommended Therapy for Musculoskeletal Infections in Dogs and Cats

ORGANISM (CHAPTER REFERENCE)	USUAL CONDITION	SYSTEMIC ANTIBIOTICS[a]
Mycoplasma (32)	A	Tetracycline,[b] quinolones
Streptococcus sp. (β-hemolytic) (35)	D, A, I	Ampicillin, penicillin,[c] clindamycin, first-generation cephalosporin
Erysipelothrix (35)	D, A	Penicillin[d,e]
Staphylococcus coagulase negative	O	First-generation cephalosporin, nafcillin
Staphylococcus intermedius (36)	D, A, O	Amoxicillin-clavulanate, first-generation cephalosporin,[d] oxacillin[e]
Actinomyces (49)	D, O	Penicillin
Proteus, Pseudomonas, E. coli (37)	I, O	Quinolones, aminoglycoside, second- or third-generation cephalosporins, ticarcillin-clavulanate, imipenem
Brucella canis (40)	D	Lipid soluble tetracycline[b] and streptomycin,[f] quinolone
Anaerobes (41)	M, O, I	Amoxicillin-clavulanate, clindamycin, metronidazole, penicillin
Borrelia (45)	A	Ampicillin, tetracycline
Pasteurella multocida (53, 88)	I	Ampicillin, tetracycline
Blastomyces (59), Coccidioides (62)	O	Itraconazole, ketoconazole, amphotericin B
Cryptococcus (61)	A	Itraconazole, ketoconazole, fluconazole, amphotericin B
Aspergillus (64)	D	Itraconazole, amphotericin B
Toxoplasma (80)	M	Clindamycin, pyrimethamine and sulfonamides, azithromycin

A, Arthritis; D, diskospondylitis; I, otitis media/interna; O, osteomyelitis; M, myositis.
[a]Drugs are listed in order of most desirable choice first. See Chapter 34 and Appendix 8, Drug Formulary.
[b]Use minocycline or doxycycline.
[c]Substitute amoxicillin, first-generation cephalosporin, or erythromycin.
[d]Substitute any first-generation cephalosporin.
[e]Substitute any β-lactam–resistant penicillin.
[f]Substitute gentamicin or amikacin.

temic manifestations and presence of joint involvement are indicators of poorer prognoses.[53]

Acute Posttraumatic Osteomyelitis

The prevalence of osteomyelitis is increased in open fractures when bacteria have the ability to invade the wound directly from the environment. However, most cases of posttraumatic osteomyelitis are acquired in the hospital environment and involve staphylococci or enteric gram-negative organisms such as Pseudomonas. The condition is likely a result of the adherent biofilms formed by these organisms. Osteomyelitis developing within 2 to 5 days after an insult may be difficult to differentiate from a soft-tissue wound infection. However, most wound complications are restricted to soft tissues. Regardless, treatment is similar, and absolute differentiation is not always necessary. Treatment should be aggressive in an effort to prevent these infections from developing into chronic processes. Modalities include drainage and débridement, systemic antimicrobial agents, rigid stabilization, direct bone culture, and delayed wound closure (Fig. 86-4, A).[17,46,62]

Meticulous drainage and débridement of all necrotic tissues or bones, hematomas, and abscesses should be done first and is an essential component of treatment. Culture and biopsy samples are obtained at this time, followed by copious lavage of the area with lactated Ringer's solution or saline. Drainage by closed suction units and open-wound management with daily flushing are options to be considered. Initial antimicrobial therapy is similar to that of hematogenous osteomyelitis; the most common bacterium is β-lactamase–producing Staphylococcus (see Tables 86-3 and 86-4). Drugs should be given parenterally (preferably IV) for the first 3 to 5 days followed by oral therapy for a minimum of 4 weeks; many cases require 8 weeks. Therapeutic agents may be adjusted as culture results become available. Patient monitoring must be intense and regular. In all cases, radiographs should be taken 2 to 3 weeks after intervention and then sequentially as needed (see Fig. 86-4, B).

Chronic Posttraumatic Osteomyelitis

Chronic posttraumatic osteomyelitis is the most common type of osteomyelitis seen in veterinary practice. Because of devitalized tissues, therapy with antibiotics alone is usually not successful. Drugs cannot enter the tissue in which they are most needed. Without improving the ischemic, necrotic environment, success in bacterial eradication is minimal. Treatment is based on the same fundamental objectives of débridement of necrotic tissue, bony sequestra, and all foreign material, including old implants. Attempted bacterial isolation, obliteration of dead space, establishment of drainage, and rigid stabilization of bone should be done. Bone will actually heal in the presence of infection if it can be stabilized.

Débridement and sequestra removal are essential to management. During and after the surgical procedure, copious lavage is performed. Fracture stability should be evaluated intraoperatively; implants must be removed if they are loose. Rigid fixation of fractures is imperative for healing and eradication of infection. Removal of all implants, if the fracture is healed, or of implants that are not adding to the stabilization eliminates sites for biofilm formation. Eradication of dead space and removal of unnecessary foreign material, including sutures, should be performed. Establishment of drainage can be accomplished using many different techniques. Closed suction units, saucerization, and treating an open wound without suturing the skin to the soft tissues are all viable methods. Placement of vascularized muscle flaps over the defect after infection has been controlled can also be considered.

Table • 86-4

Drug Dosages for Treatment of Musculoskeletal Infections

DRUG[a]	SPECIES	DOSE[b]	ROUTE	INTERVAL (HOURS)
Amikacin	B	7.5 mg/kg	IV, IM, SC	12
Ampicillin	B	22 mg/kg	IV, IM, SC, PO	6—8
Amoxicillin	B	22—30 mg/kg	IV, IM, SC, PO	6—8
Amoxicillin-clavulanate	B	22 mg/kg	PO	8
Cefazolin	B	22 mg/kg	IV, IM, SC	6—8
Cefotetan	B	30 mg/kg	IV, IM, SC	12
Cefoxitin	B	30 mg/kg	IV, IM, SC	8
Cephalexin	B	22—30 mg/kg	PO	8
Cephradine	B	22—30 mg/kg	PO	8
Chloramphenicol	D	25—50 mg/kg	IV, PO	8
	C	25—50 mg/kg	IV, PO	12
Ciprofloxacin	B	11 mg/kg	IV, PO	12
Clindamycin	B	11 mg/kg	IV, IM, PO	8—12
Cloxacillin	B	10—15 mg/kg	IV, IM, PO	6—8
Doxycycline	B	12.5—15 mg/kg	PO	12
Enrofloxacin	D	5—15 mg/kg	SC, PO	24
Enrofloxacin	C	5 mg/kg	PO	24
Gentamicin	B	5—6 mg/kg	IV, IM, SC	24
Metronidazole	B	10 mg/kg	PO, IV	8
Minocycline	B	10 mg/kg	PO	12
Oxacillin	B	22—30 mg/kg	IV, IM, SC, PO	6—8
Penicillin G (aqueous)	B	20,000—40,000 U/kg	IV	6
Penicillin G (procaine)	B	40,000—50,000 U/kg	PO, SC	6
Penicillin-V	B	40 mg/kg	PO	6
Streptomycin	B	20 mg/kg	IM	12
Tetracycline	B	22 mg/kg	PO	8
Ketoconazole	D	10 mg/kg	PO	12
Itraconazole	D	5 mg/kg	PO	12
Itraconazole	C	50 mg total	PO	24
Fluconazole	D	5 mg/kg	PO	12—24
Amphotericin B	B	0.25 mg/kg	IV	48

B, Dog and cat; *D*, dog; *C*, cat; *IV*, intravenous; *IM*, intramuscular; *SC*, subcutaneous; *PO*, by mouth.
[a]Duration of therapy depends on the tissue, site, and duration of infection; see text for guidelines. For additional information and dosages on drugs listed below, refer to Drug Formulary, Appendix 8.
[b]Dose per administration at specified intervals.
[b]Dose until a total of 8-12 mg/kg (dog) or 4-8 mg/kg (cat) is reached.

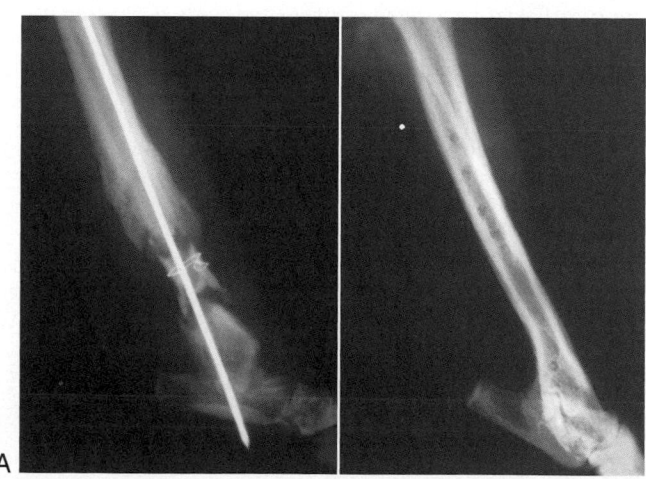

Fig 86-4 A, Radiograph of a 4-year-old dog with open segmental fracture of tibia in which an intramuscular pin was placed 3 months previously. Osteomyelitis with a nonunion and large sequestrum of bone is present in the mid tibia. **B,** Radiograph 2 years later after surgical removal of implant and bony sequestrum, obtaining tissue for culture and susceptibility, débridement, lavage, stabilization with a bone plate, cancellous bone graft, open wound management, and systemic antimicrobial therapy. (Courtesy Dennis Aron, University of Georgia, Athens, Ga.)

Antimicrobial therapy must be based on culture and susceptibility results; however, correlation of clinical response and in vitro susceptibility of some microorganisms is often lacking. These failures can be attributed in part to the inability of antibiotics to achieve sufficient concentrations in affected tissue. With this limitation, the best chance to reach and maintain levels at consistent concentrations would be IV infusions over a minimum treatment period of 4 to 6 weeks. Unfortunately, in practice, financial constraints usually limit treatment to short parenteral regimens followed by orally administered antimicrobials. Antibiotics that can be used orally for long-term treatment that are effective against β-lactamase–producing *Staphylococcus* should be considered (see Tables 86-3 and 86-4). Placement of local infusion drug delivery systems is currently receiving a great deal of research interest. Use of implants impregnated with antibiotics is common in human medicine and less frequent in veterinary medicine. Carriers are usually either a form of bone cement or a biodegradable polymer.[19,123,129] Polymethylmethacrylate (PMMA) is an implant material that has been used successfully with numerous antibacterials, including vancomycin, clindamycin, tobramycin, and gentamicin. Unfortunately, the slow release of low levels of antimicrobials, such as aminoglycosides that are often employed, may lead to colonization by antimicrobial-resistant microbial strains. After 2 to 4 weeks, elution of the antibacterials is complete, and bacterial biofilms can successfully colonize the foreign material. Treatment of severe orthopedic infections in humans and animals has used antimicrobial-impregnated beads at the site of infection. Slow release in the wound site allows for high concentrations of antimicrobials in the tissue for prolonged periods. Levels of up to 200 times that following systemic administration can be achieved for as long as 80 days after implantation.[132] Aminoglycosides have been the most commonly used antibacterials impregnated into beads. Despite the high concentrations at the wound site, serum and urine concentrations of antibiotics do not reach toxic levels. In an experimental study in dogs evaluating the effect of PMMA bead implantation on osteomyelitis, implantation had radiographic, bacteriologic, and pathologic evidence of clearing infection compared with control dogs when evaluation was performed after 6 months following implantation.[127] PMMA is less than ideal in that it is not degraded and can result in eventual inflammatory reactions. Once the antimicrobial efficacy has been lost, it may support bacterial growth, which can result in bone resorption. Use of newer biodegradable polymers has shown fewer side effects. In evaluating other polymers, polyglycolic beads containing gentamicin, staphylococcal osteomyelitis was effectively controlled in dogs.[50] Such polymers have also been used to coat metallic implants. Other polymers such as bioerodible polyanhydrides or more natural substances such as hydroxyapatite or collagen have been impregnated with antibacterials with some early success.

Management of open wounds or suction systems dictates initial postoperative management. Once this early phase is complete, weekly checks and radiographs at 3-week intervals are advised. Antibiotics must be continued for *at least* 6 to 8 weeks, regardless of any early positive response. Owners should be advised that the animal's chronic osteomyelitis can remain quiescent for weeks, months, or years with potential for relapse or reinfection.

Prevention

Prophylactic antimicrobial therapy is accepted management for dogs and cats undergoing prolonged surgical procedures or those associated with the greatest risk of postoperative infection. For orthopedic procedures, decreases in infection rates have been observed. Dogs undergoing elective orthopedic surgery had a reduced rate of infection compared with saline-treated control dogs when treatment with penicillin G or cefazolin was used.[131] The choice of antimicrobial therapy should be based on the type and location of the surgical procedure and the most likely organisms to be involved in secondary contamination. Antimicrobials are administered only 30 minutes before or during the operative period at an interval of every 90 minutes and not continued beyond the operative period. For further information, see also prophylactic antibacterial therapy in Chapter 34, Nosocomial Infections in Chapter 94, and Bacteremia and Dental Disease in Chapter 89.

DISKOSPONDYLITIS AND VERTEBRAL OSTEOMYELITIS

Diskospondylitis is defined as inflammation of an intervertebral disk and adjacent vertebral end plates and bodies. In comparison, infections located in the vertebral body usually caused by penetrating wounds, paravertebral infection, or foreign bodies are termed *vertebral osteomyelitis* and are less frequent in dogs than they are in cats. In addition to or in lieu of infection of the disk space, vertebral osteomyelitis often involves the adjacent soft tissues and vertebral bodies and meninges. The most common cause of these processes is bacterial infection; however, fungal infections have also been reported (see Table 86-2).[82] Any vertebral space can be affected; the thoracic and lumbar sites are the most commonly involved.

Etiology

Dog

S. intermedius is the most common causative bacterium identified in the dog.[63,64,82] Other frequently documented bacterial pathogens include *Streptococcus*, *Brucella canis*, and *E. coli*.[63,64,82] Less common isolates have been *Pasteurella* spp., *Proteus* spp., *Corynebacterium* spp., *Actinomyces*, *Nocardia* spp., *Bacteroides* spp., *Mycobacterium* spp., *Pseudomonas aeruginosa*, *Enterococcus faecalis*, and *Staphylococcus epidermidis*.[1,11] The wide variety of other bacterial species underscores the need to attempt to obtain bacterial isolation and susceptibility testing in each case. Fungi are involved in some infections, and most common genera have included *Aspergillus*, *Fusarium*, and *Paecilomyces*.[20,45,63,82] In addition to hematogenous exposure, migrating foreign bodies have produced spinal infections with vertebral body osteomyelitis (see Actinomycosis, Chapter 49). Plant materials have been the most widely associated foreign bodies, and geographic regional differences influence the specific causative agent.[82] Postprocedural diskospondylitis may be caused by direct inoculation during a diagnostic or operative procedure on the spinal column or by spread from other infectious foci to the intervertebral site. Injury to intervertebral endplates, operative trauma to small vessels causing tissue necrosis or hematoma formation, provides growth media for bacteria.[61] Epidural abscess and diskospondylitis can develop after epidural injections.[105] Spinal column and disk infection has also been sequelae of spinal surgery or disk fenestration.

Cat

Few reports of diskospondylitis in the veterinary literature have been published.[4,72,86,128] In all of these cases, soft-tissue injury from trauma or fighting has been the underlying cause. As spreading infections from adjacent soft tissues, most of these infections can more appropriately be termed primary vertebral osteomyelitis with secondary disk involvement. Compared with disk infection in dogs, associated meningomyelitis has also been more commonly associated with these infections in cats. *E. coli* was isolated from the cerebral spinal fluid (CSF) of one cat.[4] One author of this chapter (CEG) has also documented diskospondylitis in a 6-month-

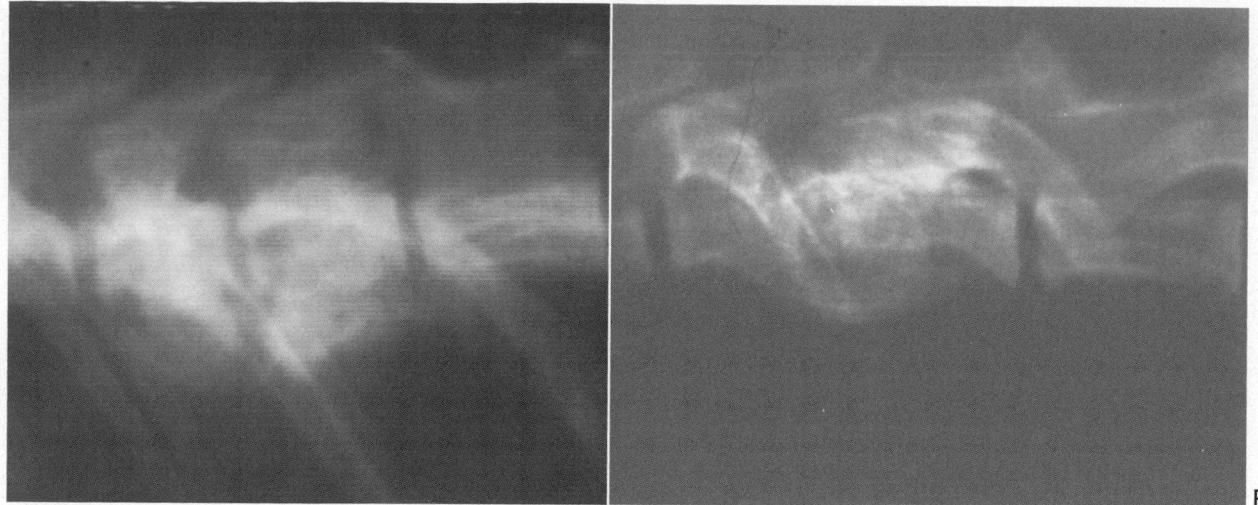

Fig 86-5 Radiograph of the thoracic spine from a cat with diskospondylitis caused by hematogenous *Streptococcus canis* infection. **A,** At the time of diagnosis. **B,** Five months later after antibacterial therapy. (Courtesy University of Georgia, Athens, Ga.)

old purebred cat caused by group G streptococcal bacteremia, presumably acquired as a neonate (see Chapter 35). In this cat, the intervertebral disk space was affected and the lesion progressed to marked involvement of the opposing vertebral bodies (Fig. 86-5).

Pathogenesis

Diskospondylitis is thought to arise from hematogenous spread of the organism into the disk space and subsequently into the adjacent vertebrae. The most commonly incriminated sources include urogenital tract and skin infections, dental disease, and valvular endocarditis. However, in many cases, no other site of infection is detected. Preferential hematogenous localization in the disk space probably occurs as a result of retrograde blood flow into vertebral sinuses or as a result of subchondral vascular loops in the vertebral epiphysis that slow blood flow.[63,64,82] Predisposing factors have included immunosuppression and previous trauma, including surgical intervention (see Table 86-1).[63,64]

Clinical Findings

Dog

Clinical presentation can vary; however, in general, signs progress slowly. Although any dog or cat is susceptible to this disease, the most common signalment is that of a young to middle-aged male large-breed dog.[63,64] Signs can vary from those of systemic infection (depression, anorexia, fever, weight loss) to musculoskeletal dysfunction. Signs of paraspinal hyperesthesia are the most characteristic of this disease and include abnormal gait and reluctance to rise or ambulate. Neurologic signs, which often develop subsequent to hyperesthesia, are those of extradural compression, resulting in paresis and ataxia, or paralysis (Fig. 86-6). The neurologic deficits depend on the site and severity of the vertebral lesion. Paraspinal hyperesthesia is often noticed earliest, although some dogs are stoic and do not show overt signs of discomfort. Neurologic dysfunction, demonstrated by paresis, can develop gradually with osteoproliferation. Sudden onset of paraplegia can occur with intervertebral disk rupture from weakened ligaments. The most commonly reported sites of infection are L7-S1, caudal cervical area, and midthoracic spine.[63,64] Monoparesis or monoparalysis can result from nerve-root involvement in patients with infection, causing chronic asymmetric osteoproliferation.

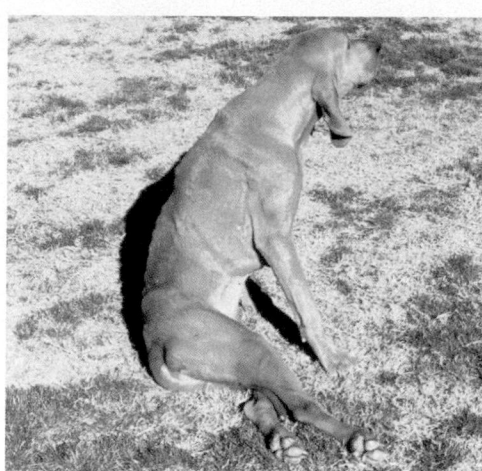

Fig 86-6 Dog with lumbar diskospondylitis showing complete paraplegia from sudden disk rupture. (Courtesy University of Georgia, Athens, Ga.)

Cat

Fever, anorexia, and paraspinal hyperesthesia have been the predominant signs in affected cats. Because of the usual association with adjacent soft-tissue infection, signs have been gradual and progressive from fever, lethargy, progressive gait dysfunction, and eventual paresis and paralysis.

Diagnosis

A tentative diagnosis is made from the patient history and the physical and neurologic examinations. Hyperglobulinemia, associated with the chronic antigenic stimulation from chronic bacterial infection, may be found with evaluation of serum proteins. Definitive diagnosis is made with spinal radiographs. Changes include concentric lysis of adjacent vertebral endplates early, with later vertebral body osteolysis or proliferative sclerosis, vertebral body shortening, narrowing of disk spaces, and ventral osseous bridging (Fig. 86-7, *A*). This situation must be differentiated from other vertebral lesions, including vertebral osteomyelitis (see Fig. 86-7, *B*), spondylosis deformans (see Fig. 86-7, *C*), and neoplasia (see Fig. 86-7, *D*). Extensive vertebral body infection may result in vertebral

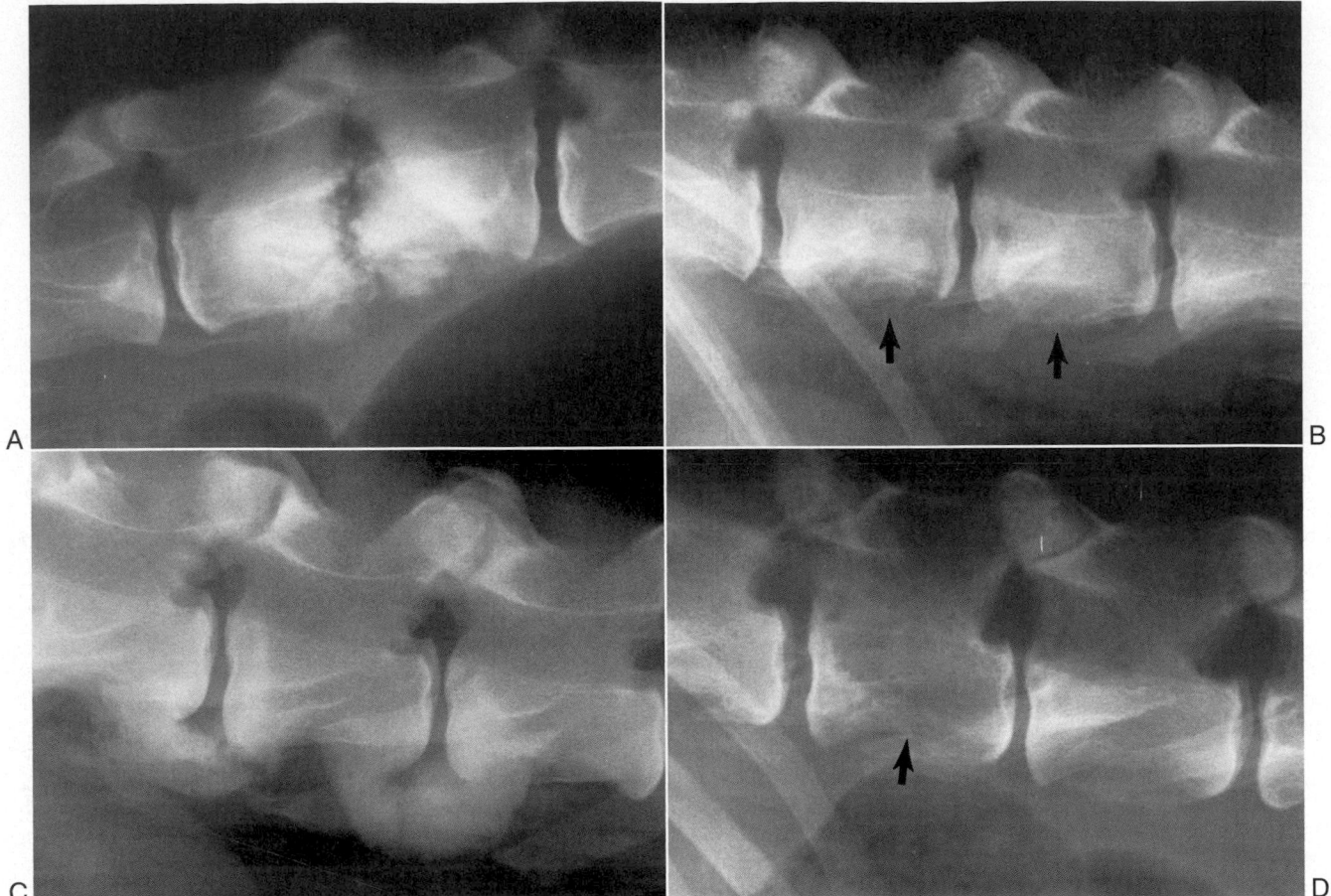

Fig 86-7 Lateral radiograph of the thoracolumbar spine from dogs with **(A)** diskospondylitis at the L2-L3 interspace from bacteremia, with indistinct endplates and new production of bone ventrally. **B,** Lumbar osteomyelitis from a migrating foreign body, involving L2-L3 *(arrows)* with ventral periosteal proliferation. **C,** Spondylosis deformans at the L3-4 and L4-5 interspaces. **D,** Vertebral neoplasia with focal lucencies in the L3 lumbar vertebrae; the process does not involve the interspace. (Courtesy University of Georgia, Athens, Ga.)

body collapse or subluxation.[16] Radiographic changes associated with diskospondylitis can take 2 to 4 weeks to develop after the initiation of the infection.[64] Thus sequential radiographs may be needed to confirm the diagnosis in an animal with initial signs of hyperesthesia. Clinical signs and radiographic severity of lesions do not always correlate. Computed tomography (CT) and magnetic resonance imaging (MRI) have added a new dimension to detection of infectious lesions of the spine. These measures are always indicated when spinal radiography is inconclusive because radiography may not detect lesions until up to 2 to 6 weeks after infection. CT can also be used to guide fine-needle aspiration and tissue-core biopsy.[125] With MRI, early changes are decreased intensity and definition on T1-weighted images and increased intensity of the disk and endplate on T2-weighted images. Later, destruction of the vertebral endplate occurs. With T1-weighted scans after gadolinium–diethylenetriamine pentetic acid, enhancement occurs between the disk and endplate. Bone scans may show increased uptake of radiopharmaceuticals at the affected disk space and endplates. Unfortunately, changes are not detected unless radiographic abnormalities are already visible. In people and dogs, tissue-core biopsy has been superior to fine-needle aspiration for obtaining positive culture results.[125] For aspiration, which is often done with fluoroscopy, 0.5 ml of sterile saline is injected in the disk space and immediately aspirated to retrieve a specimen.

When hyperesthesia and neurologic dysfunction are absent, diskospondylitis may be overlooked. Spinal radiography should be considered as an initial screening test for animals with chronic, recurrent urinary tract infection or fever of unknown origin. Dogs with confirmed diskospondylitis should always be immediately screened serologically for *B. canis* (see Chapter 40). Should serologic test results be negative, disk-space culture provides the most consistent recovery of the offending organism. However, culturing the disk is often impractical because of the inaccessibility of the lesion unless decompressive surgery is performed. If the lesion is caudal to the thoracolumbar junction and fluoroscopy is available, guided direct aspiration of the disk can be attempted.[43] Blood and urine cultures should be performed therefore in an attempt to recover the organism before instituting therapy. Positive blood culture results range from 45% to 75% and should be considered in all cases. This approach is especially warranted in dogs with increased rectal temperatures or animals with signs of sepsis in hematologic parameters.[64] Organisms may be cultured from urine approximately 40% of the time.[64] Other sources of infection from which possible dissemination has occurred may be investigated. If infection is detected in urine and blood, the entire urinary tract and the heart valves, respectively, may be evaluated by radiologic or ultrasonographic testing.

Other imaging techniques may aid in the diagnosis of early radiographically undetectable diskospondylitis. CT, MRI, and

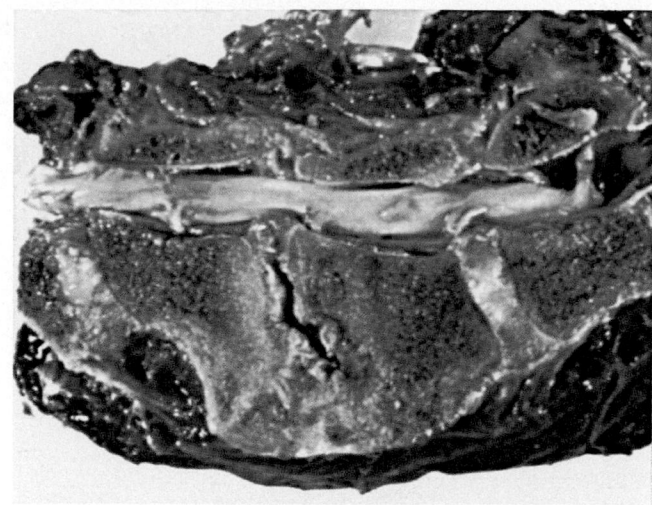

Fig 86-8 Lateral view of transected vertebral column from a 6-year-old female Great Dane with tetraparesis and depression of 6 weeks' duration. The C6-C7 interspace is at the center of the picture. The caudal aspect of the vertebral body of C6 and the cranial aspect of the vertebral body of C7 are irregular in appearance, suggesting vertebral lysis. Fibrous tissue and new bone present dorsal to the disk space compress the spinal cord ventrally. The intervertebral disk at C6-C7 is absent. Considerable new bone occurs ventral to the C6-C7 disk space and sclerosis of the caudal aspect of the vertebral body of C6 and the cranial aspect of the vertebral body of C7. A diagnosis of diskospondylitis was made. (From Kornegay JN. 1979. Canine diskospondylitis, *Compend Cont Educ Pract Vet* 1:931. Used with permission.)

radionuclide scans, including MDP, gallium-67, and indium-111–labeled leukocytes, may become more routine in veterinary referral centers to augment the diagnosis of occult diskospondylitis. Gross pathologic findings include lysis of the vertebral endplates with purulent material in the disk interspace (Fig. 86-8).

Therapy

Ideally, antimicrobial treatment should be based on culture results from blood, urine, or optimally affected bone. Initial empiric treatment is recommended while culture results are still pending. The initial assumption should be that the offending bacterium is a *Staphylococcus*-producing β-lactamase, rendering penicillin, amoxicillin, and ampicillin ineffective. Use of a bactericidal, β-lactamase–resistant drug that is effective primarily against gram-positive bacteria is preferred. Several drugs fit these criteria (see Table 86-3). First-generation cephalosporins have been clinically most effective in this regard. Table 86-4 lists dosages of recommended drugs.

The next decision is route of administration, which is dictated by clinical presentation and disease progression. Treatment in patients with minimal to no neurologic dysfunction should begin with the appropriate oral antimicrobial drug. Parenteral therapy should be the initial step in dogs with moderate neurologic dysfunction, including ataxia and paresis. In rare instances, initial therapy may include relieving extradural cord compression with surgical decompression. Analgesics may be needed in dogs with intense hyperesthesia early in the course of treatment. For instance, with acute and rapidly progressive severe neurologic dysfunction, regardless of length of onset, IV administration of antibiotics is needed for 5 to 7 days, followed by a course of oral administration. In more slowly progressive situations, a single loading dose of parenterally administered antibiotics may be followed by oral

treatment. The minimal length of oral treatment is 6 to 8 weeks, regardless of favorable patient response in the early period. If *B. canis* titers come back positive, switching to a combined regimen of tetracyclines and aminoglycosides is advisable (see Chapter 40). *Brucella* test–positive dogs should always be neutered before treatment.

In all cases of bacterial diskospondylitis, improvement should begin within 3 to 5 days after initiation of therapy. If no response is noted and results of cultures of blood and urine are negative, the class of antimicrobial may be switched. In addition, attempts at surgical curettage of the lesion may be considered to obtain a direct bone culture.

The patient should be closely monitored over the first few days after institution of antimicrobial therapy and then evaluated at 2-week intervals once improvement is noted. Followup radiography for monitoring patient progress is controversial. Radiographs have been recommended as frequently as every 2 weeks, but subtle changes are difficult to interpret. A more pragmatic evaluation routine is to obtain radiographs 1 month after initiation of treatment and once again after cessation of therapy.[17] Therapy usually continues at least 2 to 4 months. Resolution of clinical signs occurs well before radiographic improvement. Resolving lesions are characterized by decreased osteolysis and osteoproliferation and new bone formation with intervertebral bridging. Radiographs are usually more of a benefit to document cases of aggressive, spreading infections that are not responsive to treatment.

In animals with complete paralysis, intensive, aggressive, parenteral antibiotic therapy must be instituted. If signs do not improve dramatically in 24 to 72 hours, changing of the antimicrobial agents or possible decompressing of the spinal cord and stabilizing of the vertebral column may be necessary. If vertebral fracture or dislocation occurs, surgical intervention is mandatory, and the prognosis is guarded. If a single disk is affected, based on neurologic and myelographic findings, and paralysis is severe, surgery might be recommended. However, if multiple lesions are causing compression, surgical intervention, including decompression, may not be feasible or advisable *unless* the goal of surgery is biopsy for microbiologic culture and susceptibility testing.[17] Cases of fungal diskospondylitis usually involve *Aspergillus terreus* infections in German shepherd dogs (see Chapter 64). The dogs usually have complicating signs of systemic infection and respond poorly to treatment.

OTITIS MEDIA AND OTITIS INTERNA

Clinical signs of otitis media and otitis interna usually reflect neurologic rather than musculoskeletal disease.[64] However, these conditions are discussed with musculoskeletal infection because the infection is a form of osteomyelitis in bone of the middle ear and the bony labyrinth of the inner ear. Therapeutic considerations are based on principles for treating osteomyelitis. In contrast, otitis externa is considered as an integumentary infection (see Chapter 85).

Anatomy

Knowledge of the anatomic interrelations of the compartments of the ear is important in understanding the pathogenesis of otitis media and interna and its treatment (Fig. 86-9). Both middle and inner ears are housed in the petrous temporal bone. The middle ear is separated from the horizontal portion of the external ear canal by the tympanic membrane. Together with the incus and stapes, the malleus connects the tympanic membrane to the oval window of the inner ear. The auditory ossicles are situated in a small dorsal concavity of the middle ear, the epitympanic recess. The larger, air-filled tympanic bulla forms the remainder of the middle ear and contains the round foramen and the aural opening of the auditory

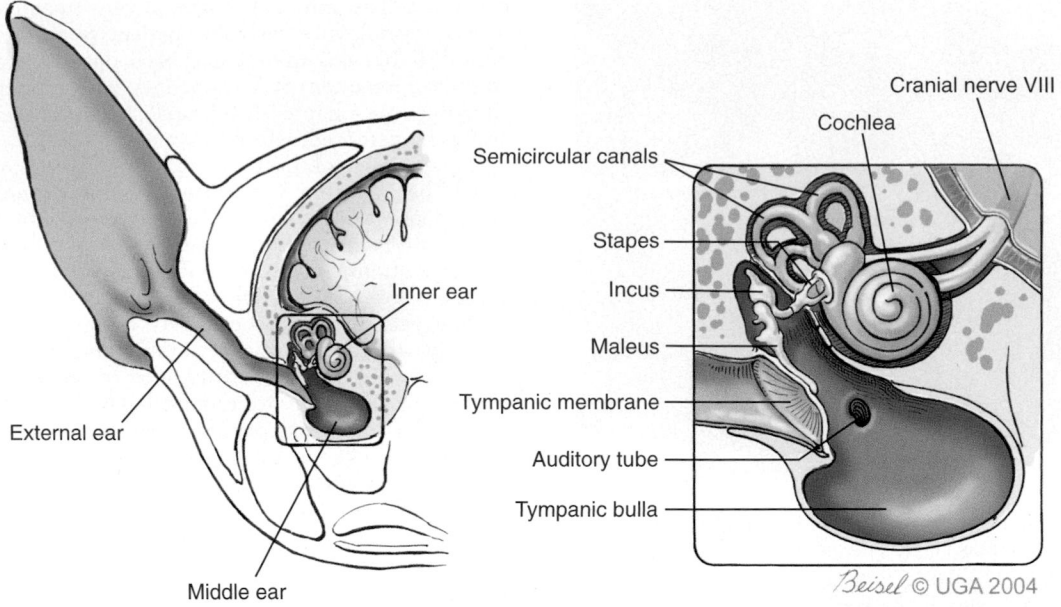

Fig 86-9 Diagram of the middle and inner ear of the dog with clinically relevant structures. The middle ear behind the tympanic membrane contains the semicircular canals and auditory structures involved in sound conduction. The inner ear contains the sensor organs of hearing (the cochlea) and balance (the utricle and saccule). (Courtesy University of Georgia, Athens, Ga.)

tube. The osseous bulla is a major site of localization of infection and a concern for therapeutic intervention. The aural opening is covered by the secondary tympanic membrane and communicates with the cochlea of the inner ear. The cochlea contains the peripheral sense organs of hearing. In addition to the auditory cochlea, the inner ear consists of semicircular canals and the utricle and saccule of the vestibule. These structures are involved with balance.[64]

Etiology and Pathogenesis

Otitis media and otitis interna in dogs and cats are usually caused by extension of otitis externa. Accordingly, *S. intermedius*, *P. aeruginosa*, *Proteus*, and *Streptococcus* are the most common bacterial pathogens, and fungi such as *Malassezia* and *Candida* may occasionally be isolated (see Chapter 85). Less frequently, otitis media and interna result from ascension of bacteria from the oral cavity through the auditory tube. Conversely, infections originating in the middle ear may reach the oral cavity through this same route. Rarely, hematogenous spread of blood-borne bacteria or fungi to the middle and inner ears has been observed. *Cryptococcus neoformans*, which often causes upper respiratory tract granulomas, has been associated with otitis media and interna in cats[7]; however, it can also cause vestibular dysfunction as a result of meningoencephalitis. Cavalier King Charles spaniels have a primary secretory otitis that may predispose them to develop otitis media.[107,114] Cats may have otitis externa as the nidus of otitis media and interna; however, cats also develop inflammatory polyps within the middle ear.[66,84] These polyps are often associated with bacterial infections; yet the order of occurrence or the association between these findings is not understood.[40] Polyps of cats did not contain feline calicivirus or herpesvirus-1 with polymerase chain reaction (PCR) evaluation.[124] Inflammatory polyps of the middle ear also occur in dogs, and they may be a cause of otitis externa or interna.[99] As with people, congenital palatine defects have also been associated with a higher prevalence of otitis media in dogs in cats.[55]

Clinical Findings

Clinical signs of simple otitis media are similar to those of otitis externa. Aural hyperesthesia is exhibited by head shaking or cocking, pawing of the involved ear, and discomfort on manipulation of the animal's pinna, auditory canal, or face. With unilateral involvement, sound localization may be impaired; and with bilateral disease, deafness is usually apparent. If the infection ascends via the eustachian tube, which is usually the case with chronic upper respiratory tract infections or congenital palatine defects, signs of external ear disease are usually absent. When the infection has followed otitis externa, the external ear canal is inflamed and usually contains debris. On otoscopic examination, the tympanic membrane may be absent or obscured by debris. When visible and intact, the membrane is usually discolored and often bulges outward. Occasionally, a fluid line is observed, indicating the presence of serum or exudate in the middle ear. Some animals may subsequently have evidence of facial nerve paralysis and Horner's syndrome because of the involvement of the facial nerve and ocular branch of the sympathetic trunk, respectively, as they pass through the middle ear.[64] Horner's syndrome can also be seen in cats with middle ear polyps.[40] Cats with middle ear polyps also show signs of obstruction of the nasopharynx in addition to vestibular manifestations. Signs of nasopharyngeal irritation include hypersalivation, coughing, and difficulty swallowing. Cavalier King Charles spaniels with otitis media show signs of cervical or cranial hyperesthesia or, eventually, vestibular dysfunction.[114]

With chronicity, the likelihood that the causative organism of otitis media will spread to the inner ear is increased. In these cases, evidence of peripheral vestibular disease occurs (Fig. 86-10). Clinical signs include head tilt toward the affected side, horizontal nystagmus with the fast component in a direction opposite the involved side, and asymmetric ataxia demonstrated variably by falling, rolling, and circling in the direction of the lesion. Most affected animals also have clinical evidence of otitis, both media and externa. When concomitant external ear disease is absent in either dogs or cats and only vestibular peripheral nerve dysfunction is noted, idiopathic peripheral vestibular disease or ascending infection from the oropharynx should be considered. If evidence exists of central vestibular disease (postural reaction involvement, vertical or variable direction nystagmus, involvement of cranial nerves other than facial, or mental depression), extension to the brain stem or subarachnoid space may have occurred or meningitis is the primary problem with involvement of the eighth cranial nerve.

Nystagmus and ataxia usually resolve despite the occasional irreversible destruction of the peripheral vestibular sense organs or nerves. Reasons why these signs resolve are not clear. However, affected animals probably compensate through accommodation of the vestibular system and reliance on other sensory modalities such as vision and conscious proprioception. Head tilt may remain, but this is usually a cosmetic rather than a functional handicap.[64] In the dark, and after anesthesia or various other stress factors, the head tilt or imbalance may be noticeably worse.

Diagnosis

Animals with clinical evidence of otitis media and interna should be anesthetized so that an otoscopic examination can be completed and radiographs taken. If the tympanic membrane is obscured by debris, the external ear canal should be gently flushed with a sterile saline or lactated Ringer's solution. Although dilute chlorhexidine or aqueous povidone-iodine solutions have been advocated, these should be used with caution because they can be detrimental to deeper tissues if the tympanic membrane is ruptured (see Otitis Externa, Chapter 85). The external canal is then suctioned and dried. Although the external ear canal should be examined by conventional otoscopy, video otoscopy provides

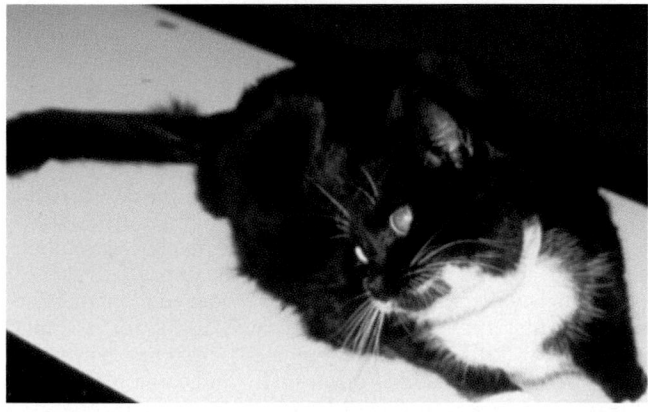

Fig 86-10 Cat with head tilt as a result of otitis media and interna. (University of Georgia, Athens, Ga.)

the best views of the tympanic membrane because of enhanced illumination and magnification. Cleaning and removal of debris can be done with more accuracy. If observed changes suggest middle ear disease, both open-mouth and lateral radiographs of the tympanic bullae should be taken. Radiographically, fluid accumulation will be reflected by increased density within the affected bullae. Radiographic examination of the tympanic bulla has low sensitivity because of difficulties in accurate positioning and the extent of bony involvement that must occur to be visible (Figs. 86-11 and 86-12). Cats with nasopharyngeal polyps often have chronic changes in the osseous bulla visible with radiographs. Radiography is more insensitive in early disease when inflammation or some effusion can be present without notable changes. In advanced cases, radiographic evidence exists of osteomyelitis of the bulla and, on rare instances, the adjacent temporomandibular joint. If available, CT offers a more definitive means of identifying these changes.[12] Even though changes found with CT may not be specific for the type of process involved, neoplastic versus inflammatory processes can usually be determined.[12] CT can be used to assess whether middle or inner ear involvement is present and whether the process involves intracranial or adjacent structures. Otolithiasis has also been detected using CT in dogs with chronic otitis.[134] MRI is more sensitive than CT is in detecting lesions early in the course of disease because most dogs and cats with clinical evidence of central vestibular disease have visible lesions with this modality.* With MRI, meningeal enhancement can be visualized in dogs and cats when a peripheral otitis media spreads into the central nervous system.[79,113] Reports indicate that ultrasonography is accurate in detecting fluid within the tympanic bulla of cadavers,[30] and although it was not as accurate as CT but more so than radiography, it is more available and less expensive.

Therapy

Choice of treatment for otitis media and interna depends on the stage of the disease. In acute cases, and if concurrent chronic otitis externa is not present, systemic administration of a broad-spectrum antibiotic, such as a first-generation cephalosporin or amoxicillin-clavulanate, has been recommended for a minimum of 14 days.[18] However, courses of 5 days have been found to be equally effective in human patients with acute otitis media[65] and might be considered for treating dogs and cats. In acute cases, antihistamines may be

*References: 2, 35, 48, 49, 89.

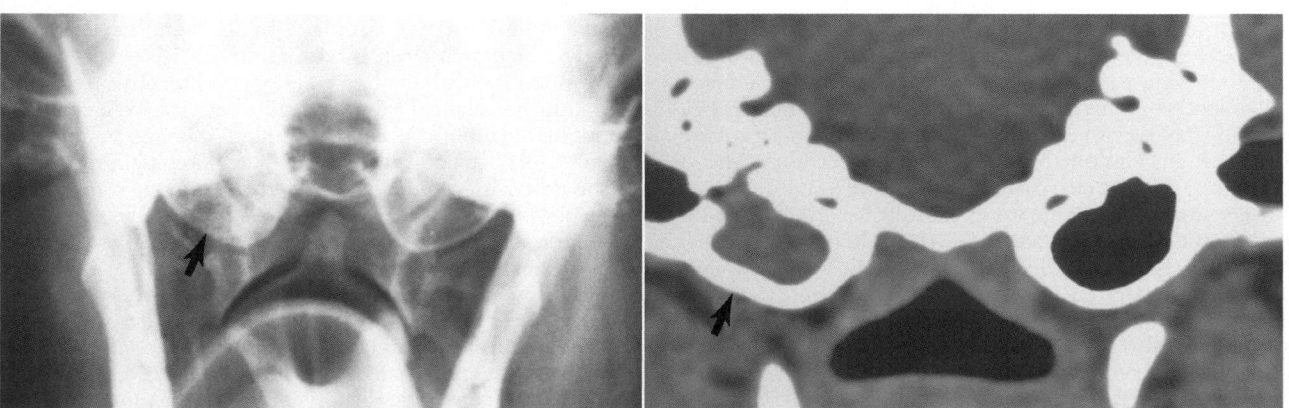

Fig 86-11 A, Osseous bullae radiograph via open-mouth view of dog with visible increased density and thickening of one tympanic bulla *(arrow)*. B, CT image of dog with thickened tympanic bulla and increase fluid density within *(arrow)*. (Courtesy University of Georgia, Athens, Ga.)

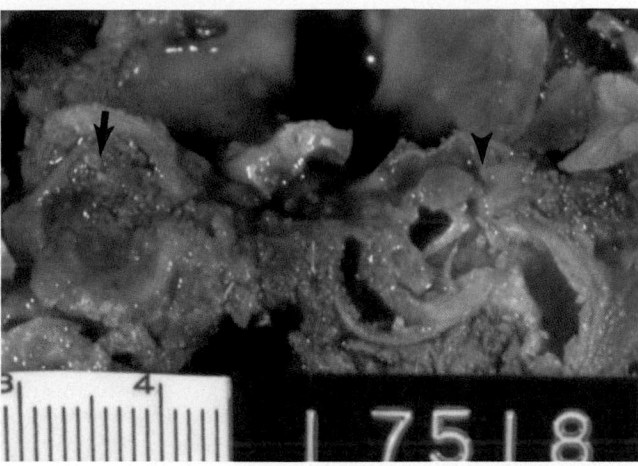

Fig 86-12 Necropsy specimen from a cat with otitis media on one side *(arrow)* and normal bulla on the other *(arrowhead)*. (Courtesy University of Georgia, Athens, Ga.)

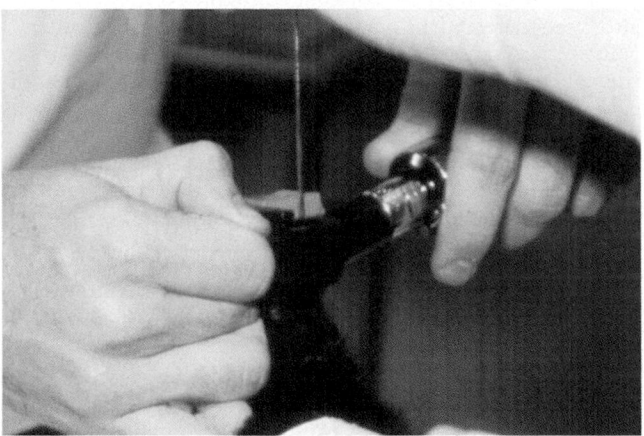

Fig 86-13 Myringotomy procedure on a cat performed through an otoscope. (Courtesy University of Georgia, Athens, Ga.)

beneficial to help relieve the swelling within the bony labyrinth, and low antiinflammatory doses of glucocorticoids might be considered for a single administration. Chronic otitis media is difficult to resolve with antibacterial therapy alone, given that resistant bacteria are often involved, and the bullae may become impacted with necrotic debris. Most dogs and cats with otitis media and interna usually also have chronic otitis externa and will benefit from myringotomy or ventral bulla osteotomy. Alternatively, in very chronic cases, total ear canal ablation with a concurrent bulla osteotomy may be necessary. If the tympanic membrane is intact, myringotomy should be accomplished using anesthesia at the time of otoscopic examination and radiography. Either a blunted 17-gauge needle or myringotomy knife is used for the procedure (Fig. 86-13). The needle allows simultaneous collection of fluid for culture and flushing. The needle is passed along the ventral horizontal ear canal so that it penetrates the ventral aspect of the pars tensa. Performing the procedure in this manner helps prevent iatrogenic damage to the auditory ossicles. After fluid has been withdrawn for bacterial culture and cytologic evaluation, the middle ear is repeatedly but gently flushed until the fluid recovered by suction is clear of debris and blood, and an antibiotic is then instilled. Selection of the antibiotic is based on prior culture results of the external ear. The antibiotic should be changed if followup culture

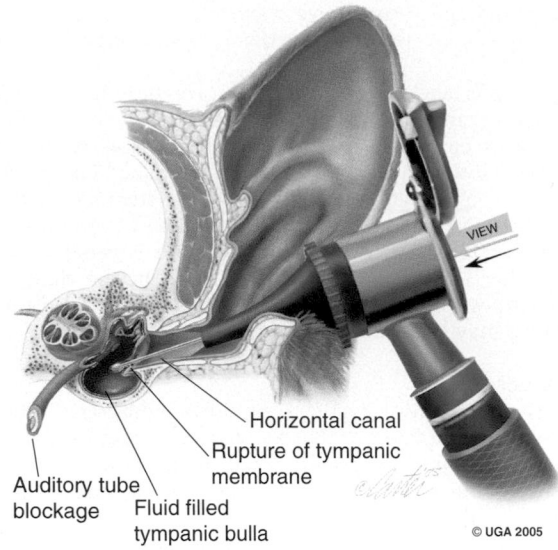

Fig 86-14 Myringotomy can be performed through an otoscope. Once the horizontal canal is entered, proper placement of an otoscope is needed for a myringotomy using a sharp probe. If a catheter is used, then the middle ear cavity can be gently flushed to dislodge inspissated debris as seen in the arrow in Fig 86-12. (Courtesy University of Georgia, Athens, Ga.)

results of middle ear fluid indicate unresponsiveness. When culture and susceptibility results are unavailable, a broad-spectrum antibiotic should be chosen (see Tables 86-3 and 86-4). Aminoglycosides might be avoided because they potentially impair auditory or cochlear nerve function, if these have not already been lost (see Aminoglycosides, Chapter 34). Cats treated by instillation of 3- or 30-mg/ml gentamicin solution into the middle ear developed vestibular dysfunction after a median time of 19 or 5 days, respectively.[92] Antibiotics should be applied topically for 10 to 14 days.

Animals with cytologic or cultural evidence of yeast infection should receive a topical antifungal agent for a similar period (see Otitis Externa, Chapter 85). Systemic antibiotics or antifungal agents are not usually indicated unless the disease is recurrent or establishment of drainage through the external ear is impossible. Animals with nystagmus and vertigo from acute otitis interna also may benefit from antihistamines or benzodiazepines.

Many dogs and cats with otitis media respond to a single session of middle-ear irrigation together with daily cleaning and topical antibiotic application. This approach is particularly effective in animals with recent onset because the inner ear often is either unaffected or only minimally affected. Care should be taken during irrigation because excessive trauma during cleaning can cause complete damage to middle and inner ear structures. Aminoglycoside-containing solutions should be used judiciously when the tympanic membrane is damaged because repeated flushing of dilute gentamicin-containing solutions in the middle ear of cats resulted in vestibular dysfunction.[92] Some animals with clinical evidence of otitis interna may respond rapidly after myringotomy, suggesting that the clinical signs are associated with either increased pressure within the bony labyrinth or reversible inflammation of the sensory end organs. Animals that fail to respond or have a chronic repetitive history and radiographic evidence of osteomyelitis are candidates for bulla osteotomy. This procedure allows for removal of proliferative tissue and more complete drainage. Operative techniques for this procedure can be found elsewhere.[40] Ventral bulla osteotomy is the treatment of choice for cats with inflammatory polyps. Canine inflammatory polyps should also be treated by surgical removal.[99] Lateral bulla osteotomy is often used with total ear canal ablation. Postoperative wound contamination is frequent during this procedure, and prophylactic antimicrobial therapy is indicated.[126]

The greatest danger of otitis media and interna is extension of the infection to the meninges and central nervous system along the cranial nerves. The danger is usually avoided if proper treatment is initiated early. Collection and evaluation of CSF should be done when the animal is anesthetized for the myringotomy procedure if neurologic signs suggest intracranial involvement.

JOINT INFECTIONS

Inflammatory joint disorders are defined as and characterized by inflammation in the synovial membrane and fluid. Systemic signs are variable and may include lethargy, fever, and leukocytosis. The causes of inflammatory joint diseases in dogs and cats are diverse and include both infectious and noninfectious disorders. This section focuses only on infectious arthropathies.

Etiology

Infectious inflammatory arthritis may be caused by bacteria, mycoplasmas, rickettsiae, spirochetes, fungi, and viral agents (see Table 86-2). Bacteria are the most common infective agents. Bacterial contamination occurs by either direct inoculation (surgery, penetrating wound, or extension from surrounding tissues) or hematogenous seeding of a distant infective nidus. Postoperative infection has been especially common following surgery of the stifle joint of dogs.[75] Dogs with preexisting chronic osteoarthritis that have joint surgery are more likely to develop complications of postoperative infection.[75] With direct inoculation by penetrating or surgical wounds, *Staphylococcus* and *Streptococcus* are the most common isolated agents.[10] Direct inoculation induces a monoarticular septic arthritis. If polyarthropathy is diagnosed, hematogenous spread of bacteria directly or immune-mediated disease secondary to a chronic distant infection should be considered. Hematogenously spread bacterial arthritis is uncommon in the dog and cat and is usually limited to neonates or debilitated patients. Young puppies and kittens may develop suppurative bacterial polyarthritis as a result of congenital or neonatal exposure. *Streptococcus canis* has been most commonly incriminated (see Chapter 35). Immunodeficient shar peis or Akitas may develop chronic polyarthritis (see Chapters 95 and 100). The most common distant sites of infection include skin, heart, lungs, prostate, anal sacs, umbilicus, and digestive tract.[9,10] Polyarthropathies of an infectious nature, other than bacterial, are being recognized more and more with the overall improvement of diagnostic abilities. Diseases such as ehrlichiosis, Rocky Mountain spotted fever, and Lyme borreliosis have been associated with polyarthropathies.[25,106,116,117] *Mycoplasma*-induced polyarthritis occurs in cats.[24] Fungal, viral, and protozoal (leishmaniasis) arthritis are rare and are usually signs of systemic disorders.[8] Reactive arthritis is a term used in human medicine to describe idiopathic progressive inflammatory arthritis, which may follow mucosal or other systemic infections; however, no organisms can be detected by conventional culture methods. PCR has been used to detect *Chlamydia trachomatis* and *Borrelia burgdorferi* DNA sequences in some of these patients, few of which have measurable antibody titers to the organism.[110] Similar testing is in animals to determine if any of such relationships exist. See the respective chapters for specifics on diagnosis and treatment of each infection.

Pathogenesis

Polyarthritis secondary to infectious diseases can result either from systemic spread of organisms to the joints, with subsequent inflammatory reactions, or from development of immune complexes that circulate systemically, eventually depositing in joint tissues with resultant immune complex–mediated injury. If the organisms involved in the primary disease cannot be recovered from the joints, this failure suggests an immune complex–mediated cause for the polyarthritis rather than a direct spread of microorganisms. Canine idiopathic erosive polyarthritis (CIEP) is a chronic symmetric erosive disease affecting the distal joints of the limbs[104] that is similar to rheumatoid arthritis in people and is thought to be noninfectious. Antibacterial therapy has little effect on the course of disease, and immunosuppressive and antiinflammatory therapy is only temporarily effective in controlling progression of the disease. This condition should be differentiated from bacterial polyarthritis, which generally takes a more rapidly advancing course and tends to be nonerosive in the early stages of illness. CDV has been incriminated as a cause of CIEP because increased levels of CDV antibodies have been found in the synovial fluid of affected dogs.[76] See Chapter 3 for a further discussion of Canine Distemper in this disease.

After direct bacterial invasion, an acute inflammatory response occurs within the joint. A complex set of interactions occurs between host defenses and various bacterial components, including enzymes, exotoxins, and endotoxins. Synovial fluid levels increase, causing higher intraarticular pressure, ischemia, and release or activation of cartilage matrix–damaging enzymes. Cartilage damage occurs quickly and is irreversible. Glycosaminoglycan depletion occurs within the first 5 days followed by cartilage softening and fissuring. This sequence of events leads to the mechanical weakening of the subchondral bone, as well as the cascade of changes within the synovial fluid, articular cartilage, and cartilage matrix.

Arthritis can develop in infectious diseases in the absence of detectable organisms in synovial tissues. Immune complex deposition in joints usually occurs in more chronic, persistent infections. Circulating antibody levels increase, resulting in formation of soluble antigen-antibody complexes that circulate from the site of infection and deposit in joints. Furthermore, after recovery from infections, when organisms enter synovial tissues by local spread or hematogenous means, persistent inactivated antigens or bacterial fragments may perpetuate the inflammatory process. Antibacterial therapy may also produce cell wall–free bacteria (L forms) that are difficult to detect and that can persist, causing continued inflammation (see Chapter 32).

Clinical Findings

Monoarthropathies cause an acute limb lameness and have been most common in medium- and large-breed male dogs.[10] The affected joint is usually swollen, warm, and often painful. Systemic signs, including fever, anorexia, and lethargy, are uncommon or variable. Most signs follow some type of insult to the affected joint. In cases of polyarthropathies, secondary to hematogenous spread, systemic signs along with joint abnormalities often occur. Onset of illness may be the classic acute form or the more chronic, local, and low grade. Lameness may vary from mild to severe; however, swelling is usually visible in the joints distal to the shoulder and hip (Fig. 86-15).

Diagnosis

In most cases, clinical signs allow a presumptive diagnosis. However, the definitive diagnosis is based on evaluation of synovial fluid obtained via arthrocentesis (Fig. 86-16 and Table 86-5). The synovial fluid will have increased turbidity and a

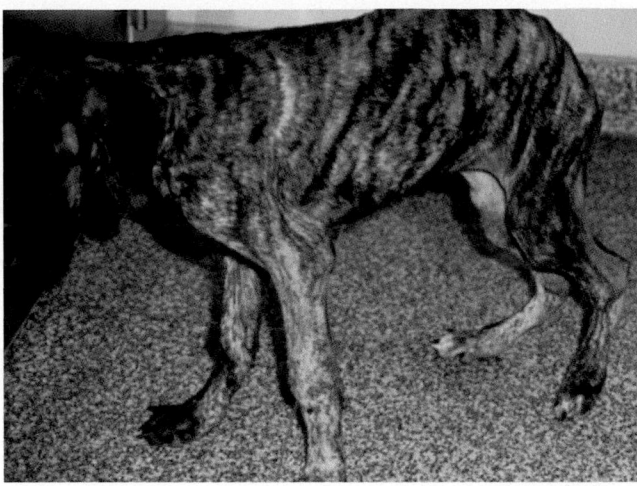

Fig 86-15 Dog with multiple swollen joints as a result of *Streptococcus canis* bacteremia. (Courtesy University of Georgia, Athens, Ga.)

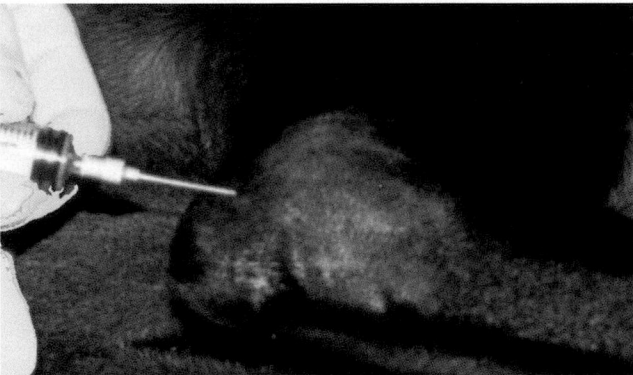

Fig 86-16 Joint aspiration of the elbow in a dog with suppurative arthritis. (Courtesy University of Georgia, Athens, Ga.)

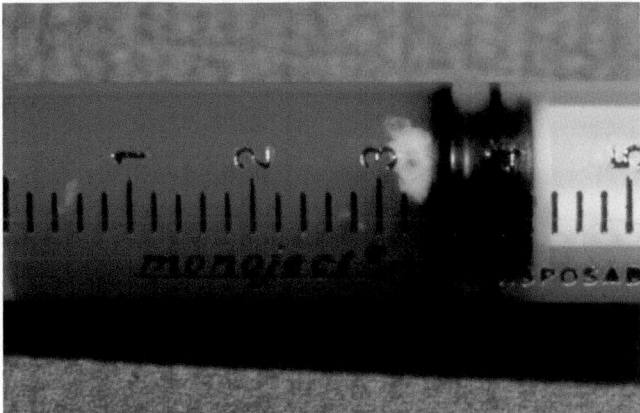

Fig 86-17 Turbid brown fluid obtained in large volume from the joint of the dog in Fig. 86-16. (Courtesy University of Georgia, Athens, Ga.)

Table • 86-5

Procedure for Arthrocentesis

Materials
   1-1.5 inch, 22-gauge needles
   3-ml syringe
   Sterile tube with EDTA anticoagulant
   Sterile gloves
   Clippers and 70% alcohol solution
   Blood culture bottles
   Glass slides
   Cytologic stain: Wright's, Giemsa, or Dif-Quik
Method
   Sedate or anesthetized the animal for immobility.
   Palpate the joint space using flexion and extension.
   Clip atraumatically over the intended area.
   Prepare the area with alcohol.
   Using gloved hands, palpate the site of penetration.
   Insert the needle slowly, with the syringe attached.
   Apply slight negative pressure when advancing or still.
   Release pressure when withdrawing.
Specimen Handling
   Clean the top of culture bottles or tubes with alcohol.
   Change needles and inoculate fluid directly into sterile EDTA.
   Put another aliquot in blood culture bottle for culture enrichment.
   Save a third aliquot or the balance in EDTA for cytology.

EDTA, Ethylenediaminetetraacetic acid.

poor mucin clot and may have an abnormal color (Fig. 86-17). Both numbers and types of leukocytes should be determined with respect to the number of erythrocytes, which usually suggest iatrogenic blood contamination. Cytologic examination will reveal increased total white blood cell counts with a shift in the cell population to polymorphonuclear leukocytes (Table 86-6). Estimates of synovial leukocyte counts have been made by comparing the number of leukocytes on a smear of fluid with the number of leukocytes in a corresponding blood smear with a known count.[135] Unfortunately, leukocyte estimates from synovial smears are inaccurate by generally overestimating counts. Hemocytometer or electronic particle counters should be employed wherever available and when sufficient volumes of fluid are obtained for counting methods.[51] Bacteria may be visualized; however, in many septic joints, no organisms are detected. Suppurative inflammation can indicate either infectious or immune-mediated disease given that neutrophils are often not degenerate in septic arthritis.[51,75] Direct synovial fluid culture samples should be taken, before antibacterial administration, to help determine if infection is present. These cultures do not always yield bacterial growth, even when bacteria are seen micro-

scopically. Thus inoculation of blood culture media with the synovial fluid sample should also be done to improve the chances for bacterial growth. These blood culture media samples should be allowed to incubate for 24 hours at 37° C before they are placed on culture media.[81] Blood cultures are indicated when suppurative joint infections are found because the offending organism may have originated from bacteremia or may have spread to the blood after establishing infection in the joint. In cats, L-form– and feline syncytium–forming viral-associated arthritis cause erosive lesions, whereas mycoplasmal-, caliciviral-, feline infectious peritonitis viral-,

Table • 86-6

Synovial Fluid Composition in Infectious Arthritis

PARAMETER	REFERENCE VALUES	BACTERIAL POLYARTHRITIS
Consistency	Clear, ropy strand 2.5-5.0 cm long, dripped from syringe	Cloudy, white or tan, less viscosity and more watery
Total protein	<3 g/dl	
pH	7-7.8	
Glucose	Same as blood	Reduced from blood
Cell count	<3000 cells/µl	>5000 cells/µl
Cell type	Mononuclear (PMN < 10%)	PMN > 30%

PMN, Polymorphonuclear neutrophils.

and borrelial-associated arthritis cause nonerosive lesions.[24] Negative culture results from a joint with changes typical of infective arthritis may be caused by an anaerobe that is difficult to culture. Controversy exists as to whether culture of joint capsule is more sensitive in detecting infection compared with synovial fluid culture. When synovial fluid or joint capsule biopsy material is directly inoculated onto blood agar plates, the tissue sample yields the highest rate of cultivation.[10] Culture of joint fluid was more productive than that of synovial biopsy when specimens were first inoculated into blood culture medium.[81] Therefore if arthrotomy is not indicated as part of the clinical management, then joint fluid should be inoculated directly into blood culture medium at the time of collection. For handling specimens for anaerobic culture, see Chapters 33 and 41. Culture of biopsied synovial tissue may be more sensitive than that of synovial fluid.

Hematologic and biochemical abnormalities may indicate systemic inflammatory or infectious diseases associated with arthritis. Inflammatory leukograms may be associated with systemic infections or may be seen secondary to the inflammation of an infected joint. Thrombocytopenia may be observed in animals with bloodstream infections or rickettsial diseases. Biochemical features of bacteremia may include increased serum alkaline phosphatase activity, hypoalbuminemia, and hypoglycemia. Proteinuria can be associated with glomerular diseases that may result from the same diseases causing immune complex or embolic polyarthritis.

Radiographs can also be of some use; however, early signs are usually too nonspecific to allow a diagnosis. By the time substantive radiographic signs appear, severe loss of bone mineral, intraarticular cartilage erosion, and cartilage matrix breakdown occur. Early signs include joint effusion and associated periarticular soft-tissue swelling. Later signs include joint surface pitting or irregularities and subchondral bony lysis. Nuclear scintigraphy can provide supportive data earlier than conventional radiography can; however, it is impractical in most practice settings.

Therapy

Goals of treatment are eradication of the causative agent and preservation of the articular cartilage. Regardless of the cause, infectious arthritis warrants aggressive early treatment. In animals with monoarthropathy, treatment should include the adequate drainage of suppurative material, débridement of the accessible necrotic tissue, removal of any foreign implants including suture material, and copious lavage of the joint. A

further benefit of drainage in the immature patient is decompression of the joint to avoid further vascular embarrassment of the epiphysis. Initial antimicrobial therapy centers on parenteral bactericidal antibiotics.

Adequate drainage and débridement of the joint are best accomplished by arthrotomy. Needle aspirations are difficult and do not provide for adequate débridement, drainage, or extensive lavage. In acute infections, primary closure of the joint after copious lavage is usually adequate. In more advanced cases, partial closure or application of a drainage system may be considered. Both of these methods require intensive postsurgical management. Drainage, lavage, curettage, and inspection of joint surfaces have been achieved with minimal invasion using arthrocentesis and arthroscopy.[41] Use of indwelling drains is generally not advised because they may act as a source of ascending infection for the joint.

Choice for antimicrobial therapy should be based on culture and susceptibility results. Initially, before obtaining culture results or in cases with negative results, antimicrobial choices should be based on the empirical criteria (see Tables 86-3 and 86-4). The drug should be bactericidal, active against β-lactamase–producing *Staphylococcus*, parenterally administered, and broad spectrum. Initially, antibiotics should be given IV for 48 to 72 hours and then orally for a minimum of 21 days. In more advanced cases, the antibiotic should be administered for at least 6 to 8 weeks. Posttreatment joint aspiration for cytology and culture should be considered in all cases.

Passive flexion and extension of the affected joint are advisable as soon as the patient tolerates the procedure. Exercise should be restricted to walks on a leash during the antimicrobial treatment period. For an additional 6 to 10 weeks, exercise should be increased gradually, but the dog should always be on a leash. Alternatively, or in addition, swimming is an excellent mode of physical therapy and can be encouraged as soon as all skin incisions or wounds are healed.

The prognosis is determined primarily by the amount of destruction of the articular cartilage and is difficult to estimate. Clinical evaluation over the next 1 to 2 months with radiographs on the second visit may begin to define the amount and severity of changes that have occurred; however, degenerative changes to the point at which the patient is showing clinical signs may take months.

Distinguishing infectious polyarthropathies from immune-mediated causes is warranted because immunosuppression can lead to disastrous consequences if systemic infections are present. A further problem is that infectious processes may be responsible for inciting immune-mediated joint diseases through the deposition of immune complexes or persistence of foreign antigens, or both, in synovial tissues. Nevertheless, immunosuppression is often reserved as a final modality in cases in which infection cannot be definitively incriminated. Because of the high frequency of tetracycline-susceptible organisms that cause polyarthritis, such as *Borrelia, Ehrlichia, Mycoplasma,* and L-forms, these drugs are often instituted as first treatment. Caution should be taken in attributing a favorable clinical response to an infection because tetracyclines are known to reduce their inflammatory effects (see Tetracyclines, Chapter 34).

Treatment of polyarthropathies associated with hematogenous bacterial agents is far more difficult for complete resolution. In these cases, diagnosis of the cause of the septic event must be addressed simultaneously with management of joint infection. Multiple arthrotomies are not feasible in most cases, and needle aspiration may be the only viable option for removal of a portion of suppurative material. Antibiotic therapy is the mainstay of treatment and should be aggressive, as described previously. Followup evaluation, physical therapy, and prognosis are also similar to those described for single joint treatment.

INFECTIOUS MYOSITIS

Inflammatory response in muscle can have infectious and non-infectious causes. Infectious inflammatory myositis can be divided into generalized or local disease. Most generalized infections are polymyopathies and are polysystemic. Muscular complications are part of the overall disease. In contrast, localized infectious myositis is usually a component of trauma-induced injury to the soft tissues of a confined region in which the regional musculature is involved. Noninfectious myopathies are usually classified as immune mediated; however, an underlying infectious agent may have provoked an antigenic response against the muscle.[38] Classic examples of this syndrome in people are viral infections, which incite an immunologic attack against muscle. In either case, in this chapter, discussion is limited to the management of muscle inflammation directly caused by infectious agents.

Polymyositis
Etiology
Infectious polymyopathies can be caused by bacteria, viruses, and protozoa (see Table 86-2). Examples of these polymyopathies include feline immunodeficiency virus infection, clostridial and spirochetal infections, hepatozoonosis, toxoplasmosis, and neosporosis.[5,27,32,98]

Clinical Findings
Clinical signs vary depending on potential infective agents. The site of infection can also markedly influence the observed abnormalities. Generalized inflammatory myopathies are characterized by signs such as weakness, stilted gait, muscle atrophy, dysphagia, dysphonia, trismus, and in dogs a megaesophagus. A puppy with myocarditis from parvovirus infection has signs that are far different from those in a cat with generalized toxoplasmosis or a dog with tetanus. Neosporosis of puppies may have less painful muscular involvement, which is exhibited clinically as paresis, paralysis, and rigid contracture of the affected area. Leptospirosis, hepatozoonosis, or toxoplasmosis may cause significant generalized muscle pain.[96] Associated neural tissue inflammation may be present in some diseases, which amplifies clinical paresis. With acute inflammation, swelling of the affected muscle regions also occurs. This condition is also seen in localized disease. Chronic disease is characterized by atrophy, fibrosis, and contracture.

Diagnosis
Polymyositis is determined based on clinical signs, elevated serum muscle enzyme (creatine kinase [CK] and aspartate aminotransferase) activities, and electromyographic (EMG) changes. The short half-life of CK allows serial measures to determine whether the disease is progressing or elevations are artifactual. CK activity is increased in active inflammation or necrosis of muscle. Artifactual elevations occur from traumatic venipuncture, hemolysis, or high serum bilirubin, endurance, extended recumbency, and surgical procedures.[94] Ultrasonography, computed axial tomography, or MRI can be used as a noninvasive means to localize the location and severity of muscle inflammation for further testing. EMG findings can include continuous insertional discharges, high-frequency discharges, and normal nerve-conduction velocities. Biopsy of the muscle can often provide valuable information. Histologic evidence of necrosis and inflammation confirms polymyositis but may not provide the specific cause. Biopsy samples can identify the source of the myositis, if infectious agents, such as

Hepatozoon schizonts, *Toxoplasma* or *Neospora* tachyzoites, or clostridial organisms, are seen in the tissue.[5,32,73,98] Serial serologic titers can provide valuable information in toxoplasmal and leptospiral infections. Additional information on most aforementioned organisms can be found in the chapters specifically dedicated to these infectious agents.

Therapy
Therapy should be directed toward the specific agent. For example, toxoplasmosis is treated with clindamycin. Initial treatment should be parenteral for the first week if the animal is severely affected. Only after clinical improvement is seen should oral administration be used. Antimicrobial treatment for myositis is usually continued for a minimum of 6 to 8 weeks. Supportive care is of equal importance in these cases because a protracted time frame of weeks occurs for the resolution of signs. For further information on the treatment of specific infections, consult Tables 86-3 and 86-4 and respective chapters. When infectious agents are not found and immune-mediated polymyositis is suspected, immunosuppressive therapy may be required.

Localized Myositis
Localized infectious myopathies are not commonly diagnosed because they are usually part of extending soft-tissue infections. These focal infections are the result of trauma, either blunt in nature or a penetrating wound such as a bite. Common bacterial agents include the normal skin flora (usually *S. intermedius*), oral flora, and occasionally *Clostridium perfringens*.[73,108] Certainly other bacteria should be considered with penetrating wounds, and cultures are advised. Clinical signs include fever and local or regional pain. Swelling with crepitus may be noted in cases of gas formation. Fistulation with drainage of foul-smelling discharge will also be apparent with anaerobic infections. Necrotizing fascitis and myositis, characterized by rapid spreading discoloration of overlying skin, fever, marked hyperesthesia, and progressive lower motor neuron paralysis are features of toxigenic gram-positive bacterial infections (see Streptococcal Toxic Shock Syndrome and Necrotizing Fascitis, Chapter 35). Leukocytosis, predominantly neutrophilia, and high CK activity are common. Radiographs are not generally beneficial in detecting localized swellings of soft tissues unless underlying osteomyelitis or diskospondylitis is present. Swelling and fluid accumulation can best be detected by fistulography, ultrasonography, and MRI.[118] Drainage of any purulent material, surgical removal of the necrotic muscle, and lavage of the region are performed when possible with intrasurgical parenteral and subsequent antimicrobial therapy. Empiric therapy should be based on the type of wound and the most likely contaminant. In most instances, use of an agent that has gram-positive and anaerobic antibacterial activity is a good first choice. Penicillin and derivatives, metronidazole, and clindamycin are recommended for anaerobic infections.

SUGGESTED READINGS*

1. Adamo PF, Cherubini GB. 2001. Discospondylitis associated with three unreported bacteria in the dog, *J Small Anim Pract* 42:352-355.
14. Bradley WA. 2003. Metaphyseal osteomyelitis in an immature Abyssinian cat, *Aust Vet J* 81: 608-611.
31. Dickie AM, Doust R, Cromarty L, et al. 2003. Comparison of ultrasonography, radiography and a single computed tomography slice for the identification of fluid within the canine tympanic bulla, *Res Vet Sci* 75:209-216.

*See the CD-ROM for a complete list of references.

36. Edwards R, Harding KG. 2004. Bacteria and wound healing, *Curr Opinion Infect Dis* 17:91-96.
38. Evans J, Levesque D, Shelton GD. 2004. Canine inflammatory myopathies: a clinicopathologic review of 200 cases, *J Vet Intern Med* 18:679-691.
51. Gibson NR, Carmichael S, Li A, et al. 1999. Value of direct smears of synovial fluid in the diagnosis of canine joint disease, *Vet Rec* 144:463-465.
55. Gregory SP. 2000. Middle ear disease associated with congenital palatine defects in seven dogs and one cat, *J Small Anim Pract* 41:398-401.
68. Lindsey MJ. 2000. Metaphyseal osteomyelitis, *Vet Rec* 146:28.
75. Marchevsky AM, Read RA. 1999. Bacterial septic arthritis in 19 dogs, *Aust Vet J* 77:233-237.

89. Owen MC, Lamb CR, Lu D, et al. 2004. Material in the middle ear of dogs having magnetic resonance imaging for investigation of neurologic signs, *Vet Radiol Ultrasound* 45:149-155.
101. Pumarola M, Moore PF, Shelton GD. 2004. Canine inflammatory myopathy: analysis of cellular infiltrates, *Muscle Nerve* 29:782-89.
118. Struk DW, Munk PL, Lee MJ, et al. 2001. Imaging of soft tissue infections, *Radiol Clin North Am* 39:277-303.
131. Whittem TL, Johnson AL, Smith CW, et al. 1999. Effect of perioperative prophylactic antimicrobial treatment in dogs undergoing elective orthopedic surgery, *J Am Vet Med Assoc* 215:212-216.

CHAPTER • 87

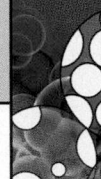

Cardiovascular Infections

Clay A. Calvert and Michelle Wall

BACTEREMIA

Bacteremia indicates the presence of bacteria in the blood, and although a presumptive diagnosis can be offered on the basis of clinical findings, it can be proven only by positive blood culture results. The term *septicemia* implies "toxemia" and associated inflammation along with pulmonary, cardiovascular, hepatic, and intestinal dysfunction.

Etiology

Bacteria normally are excluded from the blood stream by host defenses. On occasion, they do circumvent these barriers, gain access to the blood, and cause a transient bacteremia, a condition that is often unnoticed in clinically healthy individuals. For example, portal and systemic bacteremia (predominantly caused by gram-negative organisms) is found in clinically healthy dogs and is magnified in dogs with hepatic disease and portal hypertension.[87] The liver generally clears the bacteremia coming from the microflora-laden intestinal tract. However, bacteremia, particularly in the presence of immunosuppression, can lead to disastrous and overwhelming infection. Overwhelming bacteremia leads to sepsis, which often leads to decreased organ perfusion characterized by tachycardia, hypotension, gastrointestinal (GI) damage, liver dysfunction, lactic acidosis, and oliguria.

Any heavily colonized mucous membrane surface or localized site of infection can serve as a source for direct bacterial extension into the lymphatics or blood vessels. Many procedures in hospitals circumvent or alter host defense mechanisms. The use of intravenous (IV) and bladder catheters or respiratory, GI, and percutaneous endoscopic biopsies and surgery allow a direct means by which bacteria may gain access to body sites that are normally protected against such invasion. Commonly used medical treatments such as immunosuppressive agents, cytotoxic drugs, and radiation therapy diminish host defense mechanisms. Thus modern medicine and surgery provide the conditions for opportunistic bacterial infections to occur.

Bacteremia often leads to sepsis and may lead to septic shock. If treated quickly and aggressively, septic shock may be reversible; if not, it quickly becomes irreversible.[56] Bacterial virulence and the likelihood of septic shock depend on the presence of cell capsules isolating cell wall antigens from host inflammatory cells; microbial enzyme production facilitating rapid tissue penetration; and concentration of bacteria in the blood stream, which is related to size of the inoculum and duration of bacteremia.[133,163]

Treatment outcome is related to whether irreversible changes have occurred. Often bacteremia in dogs and cats is diagnosed when it is in an advanced state. The release of mediators of septic shock, such as endotoxin, exotoxin, tumor necrosis factor (TNF), and some interleukins (ILs), is associated with hypotension, hepatic failure, and breakdown of the GI mucosa-blood barrier, all of which are associated with high mortality. Prevention of bacteremia, identification of high-risk patients (e.g., patients receiving chemotherapy, patients who are otherwise immunosuppressed or debilitated, patients undergoing invasive procedures), and early recognition of sepsis are critical to reducing overall mortality.

Epidemiology

It is safe to assume that the incidence of bacteremia in dogs and cats is significantly underestimated, particularly in referral and emergency hospitals. Affected dogs and cats can be any age, breed, or gender.

Although bacterial prostatitis has been identified in some bacteremic male dogs, a causal relationship is difficult to prove. Nonetheless, the prostate gland should be suspected as a potential nidus of bacteremia in intact male dogs.[34,56] Chronic seeding of the blood stream by sites of infection such as bone, gingivae, and the prostate gland potentially predisposes them to bacterial endocarditis.[31,34] Bacteruria is either a source or a consequence of bacteremia.

Various factors influence the relative frequency of etiologic agents among different hospitals. Surgical and trauma practices may experience a higher prevalence of gram-negative and anaerobic infections. The site of local infection and prior antibiotic therapy and whether the infection is nosocomial or community acquired determine the most likely offending microbes. The percentages of isolation of various organisms from dogs and cats with bacteremia and bacterial endocarditis are summarized in Table 87-1. Because the recognized prevalence of bacteremia in cats has not equaled that of dogs, most of the discussion that follows concerns the disease in dogs. A discussion of endocarditis in cats follows the information on specific bacteria identified in dogs.

Staphylococci

Coagulase-positive staphylococci are among the most commonly isolated pathogens. Staphylococci can survive in the environment and be cultured from dried clinical material after several months. They are relatively heat resistant. Staphylococci are found in the nasopharynx and skin and can contaminate any site on the skin and mucous membranes. Multiplying staphylococci can overcome local phagocytic defenses and gain access to the lymphatics and blood stream. Staphylococcal bacteremia can lead to metastatic infections in the heart, lungs, and bones (see Chapter 36). Staphylococci secrete numerous enzymes and toxins that are implicated in their pathogenesis. Catalase can inhibit polymononuclear (PMN) free oxygen-radical–killing activity, and their toxins damage cell membranes and cause cell lysis. Manifestations of their infection vary from trivial, as in some pyodermas, to overwhelming sepsis. Coagulase-positive *Staphylococcus intermedius* (see Etiology, Chapters 36 and 85) have been common bacteria isolated from blood cultures of dogs with bacteremia alone, diskospondylitis, and endocarditis.[31,34] Common sources for blood stream infection include abscesses, pyoderma, and wound infections. Staphylococci tend to spread from localized abscesses, wounds, and deep pyodermas into the blood stream by invading blood vessels and producing septic thrombi or lymphatics and incompetent lymph nodes. Metastatic foci of infection are common and often involve the spleen, kidneys, bones, joints, or heart valves.

Only a small percentage of local infections caused by *S. intermedius* gain access to the blood stream.[40] Nonetheless, enzymes such as staphylokinase, hyaluronidase, and protease can enable tissue invasion. Sepsis can result from enterotox-

Table • 87-1

Frequency of Isolation of Bacteria from Positive Blood Culture[a]

BACTERIA	CANINE INFECTIVE ENDOCARDITIS (n = 58)[31,167,24,43,156,173]	CANINE BACTEREMIA (n = 73)[56,79]	FELINE INFECTIVE ENDOCARDITIS (n = 14)[183,115,53,36]	FELINE BACTEREMIA (n = 13)[56]
Gram Positive				
Staphylococcus intermedius or coagulase-positive species	6-33	11-36	20	—
Streptococcus spp.	12-26	18-21	20	0
Enterococcus species	0	4	—	0
Corynebacterium spp.	19	3	—	—
Erysipelothrix tonsillarum	Rare	0	—	0
Gram Negative				
Escherichia coli	6-30	18-71	20	14
Salmonella spp.	0	11-13	—	29
Enterobacter cloacae	0	3-8	—	0
Klebsiella pneumoniae	0	6-28	—	14
Pseudomonas aeruginosa	Rare	6-7	—	0
Proteus species	0	14	—	—
Pasteurella species	0	3	—	0
Moraxella species	0	2	—	0
Bartonella species	28	—	40	—
Bordetella avium-like	Rare	—	—	—
Anaerobic				
Clostridium perfringens	0	20	—	0
Propionibacterium acnes	6	0	—	14
Bacteroides spp.	0	4	—	14
Fusobacterium species	6	6	—	0
Multiple Species	0	53	—	0

[a]Values are expressed as a percentage of those cases in which organisms were isolated or detected by genetic means and represent a compilation of the cited references. The percentage of dogs for which negative isolation results were obtained is not included.

ins that bind to T cells and macrophages, stimulating the production of cytokines. One of the targets of *S. intermedius* is the endothelial cell.[40] Organisms bind to and are internalized by endothelial cells, where cytolysins are released that can disrupt the endothelium and allow access to tissue. They can survive inside of endothelial cells and phagocytic cells. This may explain their propensity to cause recurrent and refractory bacteremia.

S. intermedius is normally present on canine hair and skin, and an association of cutaneous infections with staphylococcal bacteremia in dogs is to be expected. These microbes also may gain entry into the blood stream of dogs from foci such as osteomyelitis, diskospondylitis, septic arthritis, aspiration pneumonia, and genitourinary infection.

Most *S. intermedius* strains produce a β-lactamase that induces resistance to penicillin G and ampicillins. Stability of the β-lactam ring of methicillin is high and varies for cephalosporins. Staphylococci can become resistant to all β-lactam antibiotics and all cephalosporins. Resistance is increasing to quinolones, aminogycocides, and macrolide antibiotics, such as clindamycin, as their indiscriminate use increases.

The coagulase-negative *Staphylococcus epidermidis* may be cultured from blood specimens but are often not fully identified in clinical microbiology laboratories. The majority of these are either contaminants or of no clinical importance. However, significant coagulase-negative staphylococcal bacteremia can occur in immunocompromised patients with indwelling IV catheters or profound neutropenia.

Intact skin and mucous membranes provide defense against staphylococcal invasion. When these defenses are breached, blood invasion can arise from any site but most often from localized skin or soft tissue infections, surgical wounds, and catheters. Various conditions may predispose animals to staphylococcal bacteremia. Debilitation resulting from malignancies, renal failure, diabetes mellitus, and liver disease are examples, as are compromise of immune protection by glucocorticoids, cytotoxic drugs, and other immunosuppressive agents.

A devastating complication of staphylococcal bacteremia is valvular endocarditis. Septic embolization of the kidneys and other organs may occur with chronic staphylococcal bacteremia and is consistently present with valvular endocarditis of the left side of the heart. Renal infarcts can be detected by excretory urograms and ultrasonograms. Proteinuria and pyuria are often present, and immune complex glomerulonephritis may be an additional complication. Other sites of septic embolization or abscess formation are the spleen, brain, joints, and lungs, including pulmonary arterial thromboembolism.

Disseminated intravascular coagulation (DIC) is another sequela of staphylococcal bacteremia, but its incidence is probably less than that associated with gram-negative bacteremia. Prolonged activated coagulation time, prothrombin time (PT), and activated partial thromboplastin time (APTT); thrombocytopenia; decreased plasma fibrinogen; and the presence of fibrin degradation products and D-dimers are consistent with the diagnosis. *Staphylococcus aureus* bacteremia in people occasionally triggers a septic shock syndrome *(toxic shock)*, which can be virtually indistinguishable from gram-negative bacillary endotoxic shock.

Streptococci

Systemic streptococcal infections are common in dogs and cats (see Chapter 35). Streptococcal bacteremia can originate from cutaneous sites and the upper respiratory tract. Streptococcal pneumonia may be associated with a high incidence of subsequent bacteremia. In bacteremic dogs with various underlying illnesses, blood culture results may be positive for hemolytic *Streptococcus canis* and non–β-hemolytic *Streptococcus viridans* and enterococci. Most β-hemolytic streptococci

enter the blood stream via the skin, whereas non–β-hemolytic streptococci usually enter via breaks in the mucous membranes. Non–β-hemolytic streptococci are normal skin commensals and occasionally may contaminate improperly collected blood culture specimens.

Group A streptococci *(Streptococcus pyogenes)* are enveloped in a hyaluronic acid capsule that retards phagocytosis by PMNs and macrophages. Toxins produced by *S. pyogenes* are pyrogenic, are cytotoxic, and enhance the susceptibility to the effects of endotoxin.[49] Group B streptococci can cause sepsis in dogs and cats and have been incriminated as a cause of bacteremia and death in the "fading puppy" syndrome. In people, bacteremia caused by group D streptococci (enterococci), including *Streptococcus faecium* and *Streptococcus faecalis*, usually originates from the urinary tract but also can develop after manipulation of the lower bowel. Enterococcal bacteremia, which has been reported in dogs, is especially serious because enterococci are resistant to many antibiotics.

Gram-Positive Aerobic Bacilli

Diphtheroids, a heterogenous group of bacteria including the genus *Corynebacterium*, are often interpreted as contaminants when isolated from blood culture because they normally inhabit skin and mucous membrane surfaces. *Corynebacterium* accounts for a minority of cases of bacteremia in dogs and has rarely been associated with endocarditis. *Bacillus* species are frequent blood culture contaminants. However, in the immunocompromised host, *Bacillus cereus* and *Bacillus subtilis* can gain access to the blood stream. *Corynebacterium* and *Bacillus* should be isolated from multiple blood cultures before diagnosing bacteremia as a result of these agents. *Erysipelothrix tonsillarum* strains have been isolated from the heart valves of dogs with endocarditis[173] (see Chapter 35).

Gram-Negative Bacilli

The term *gram-negative bacteremia* is typically applied to bacteremia caused by the Enterobacteriaceae and Pseudomonadaceae. Bacteremias resulting from gram-negative agents, such as *Pasteurella, Brucella, Bartonella,* and *Salmonella* species, which can also produce similar clinical manifestations, are usually considered discrete clinical entities. *Salmonella enteritidis* was the most common organism isolated from bacteremic cats in one study.[56] Gram-negative bacillary bacteremia usually represents a serious opportunistic infection that has developed subsequent to significant depression of host defenses. Gram-negative bacteremia is often associated with high mortality, and the number of such infections has increased along with the use of invasive medical devices and immunosuppressive therapy for malignancies and inflammatory diseases.

Gram-negative bacilli are ideally suited for opportunistic infections. Ubiquitous in the environment, they are major components of the fecal flora, are normal skin inhabitants, and are present in all hospital environments. They tend to be relatively resistant to moisture, drying, and some disinfectants. Some may persist and multiply in water. These agents tend to develop antibiotic resistance to a greater degree than gram-positive bacteria. Although antibiotic exposure per se does not induce resistance, it does provide a selective reproductive advantage to bacteria that are resistant.

Of bacteria of the family Enterobacteriaceae, *Escherichia coli* is the most common blood-stream isolate from animals. *E. coli* is abundant in the lower GI tract, which often serves as a reservoir for infection of other body sites. The urinary tract is another source. Oropharyngeal and fecal colonization with gram-negative bacilli may increase progressively in seriously ill hospitalized patients as their clinical status deteriorates. Gram-negative bacteria not only gain access to the blood from extravascular foci but also may originate from IV and urinary catheters and from septic thrombophlebitic conditions. In extravascular infections, bacteria often gain access to the blood via lymphatics or invasion of small blood vessels within a site of infection. Other sources for blood stream invasion include drainage tubes, contaminated IV fluids, and contaminated aerosolization devices; disrupted mucosal barriers (e.g., after dental procedures or endoscopic examinations); and decubital ulcers. In contrast to staphylococcal bacteremia, gram-negative bacteremia in dogs and cats seldom is associated with septic thrombosis and metastatic abscess formation but is often rapidly progressive and likely to result in endotoxemia (see Chapter 38).

Although common in the environment and occasionally present on mucosal surfaces, *Pseudomonas* species have rarely been isolated from deeper tissues of healthy patients. They have been more common in otitis externa, dermatitis, cystitis, and respiratory infections of dogs. Because *Pseudomonas* organisms are opportunists, their rapid colonization with subsequent development of bacteremia is much more likely to occur after disruption of host defenses, especially cutaneous barriers (surgery, IV catheters, and burns) and depletion of neutrophils, as occurs in patients who are receiving chemotherapy for cancer.[44] Extensive antibiotic use or contaminated IV fluids may also predispose patients to *Pseudomonas* bacteremia. Most reported cases of *Pseudomonas* bacteremia in dogs have been nosocomial.[44]

Prevention is easier than treatment of gram-negative bacteremia. The use of IV and urinary catheters should be limited to instances in which they are absolutely necessary. They should be inserted and maintained under scrupulously sterile conditions and removed or changed within 3 to 5 days. Strict aseptic precautions in the management of wounds, use of tube drainage systems, prevention of decubitus, and limitation of prophylactic antibiotics are all important in preventing opportunistic infections for all patients, particularly those with weakened immune systems.

Anaerobic Bacteria

Anaerobic bacteria, particularly anaerobic gram-negative rods, are considered to be serious pathogens. Development of anaerobic blood stream infections may be encouraged by the presence of periodontal disease, deep abscesses, granulomas, peritonitis, osteomyelitis, septic arthritis, and septic pleural effusion (see Chapter 41). *Clostridium perfringens* is the most common canine isolate, whereas *Bacteroides* and *Fusobacterium* are commonly isolated from cats. A mechanically correctable lesion (abscess, perforated bowel, necrotic tissue) is often the source of anaerobic bacteremia. *Bacteroides* may enter the blood stream via intraabdominal sources, such as GI and genital inflammatory diseases. *Fusobacterium* bacteremia often originates from infections of the respiratory tract. Characteristics of anaerobic bacteremia include fever, thrombophlebitis, and icterus, particularly with *Bacteroides* bacteremia. Sequelae to anaerobic bacteremia include metastatic abscess formation and endocarditis. Clostridial bacteremia tends to have a relatively insidious clinical course without obvious signs of sepsis, although septic shock occurs occasionally.

Polymicrobial Bacteremia

Blood stream infection with multiple species of bacteria occurs in up to 20% of dogs and 30% of cats with positive blood culture results. Anaerobic bacteria, especially *Bacteroides* and *Clostridium*, are often components of polymicrobial infection in dogs. Clinical implications of polymicrobial compared with monomicrobial bacteremia are not clearly established, and higher mortality rates have not been observed in dogs or cats. Factors that can predispose patients to polymicrobial bacteremia include neutropenia, GI and urogenital tract obstruction and infection, bowel perforation and surgery, and prostatic surgery.

Pathogenesis

Bacteremia develops as a normal but transient phenomenon whenever bacteria-laden mucosal surfaces, such as the nasopharynx and the GI and genital mucosae, are traumatized. Transient bacteremia is usually low grade, with 10 or fewer colony-forming units per milliliter; bacteremia is normally cleared within 1 hour by normal host defenses. Complement-mediated bactericidal activity is highly efficient at eliminating low-grade bacteremia. Serum-resistant gram-negative aerobic bacilli such as *E. coli* can escape this bactericidal protection. Clinically important bacteremia may occur when the blood stream is seeded with high numbers of bacteria via venous and lymphatic drainage from sites of infections. Fluid accumulation, high tissue pressure, surgical or physical manipulation of abscesses, areas of cellulitis, or other infected tissues all favor lymphatic and venous spread of bacteria to the systemic circulation. In most healthy individuals, bacteria are removed from the blood stream rapidly and effectively through phagocytosis by fixed tissue macrophages in the spleen and liver. Persistent bacteremia ensues when bacteria multiply at a rate that exceeds the mononuclear phagocyte system's ability to remove them. Serum from healthy patients is bactericidal, largely because of the presence of numerous humoral defense factors, including specific antibacterial antibodies of the IgM and IgG classes as well as complement proteins, properdin, and fibronectin. Bacterial capsules and other virulence factors may delay clearance of bloodborne bacteria, whereas bacteria that activate complement via the alternate (antibody-independent) pathway are cleared rapidly.

Sources of Infection and Risk Factors

Although not always identified, the most common sources of bacteremia include infections of the GI and genitourinary tracts, skin and wounds, respiratory tract, abdomen, and biliary tract. IV catheter-associated infections also occur.[31,34] Bacteremia can be a complication of parenteral nutrition, and the catheter should always be considered a source of infection. Infection often begins locally in the catheter wound when the patient's cutaneous flora invade the tract during catheter insertion and thereafter. Hub contamination is also a source of infection. Catheter-related bacteremia is confirmed when catheter and blood culture results yield the same microbe. The most common organisms are staphylococci. Catheters should always be removed and cultured immediately if bacteremia is suspected.

Catheter-related bacteremia originates from the migration of bacteria from the venipuncture into the catheter tract and along the external surface of the catheter to the intravascular tip, which becomes colonized.[88] In addition, contamination of the hub can allow migration within the catheter lumen. Teflon and polyurethane are more resistant to bacterial colonization than polyethylene or polyvinyl chloride. Some bacteria, such as staphylococci, can bind to host fibronectin that is deposited on catheters. Peripheral venous catheters have a lower risk of blood stream infection than central venous catheters.[88] Catheters impregnated with chlorhexidine or silver sulfadiazine are resistant to infection. Sterile gloves should be worn during catheter placement, and the area should be sterile. Insertion and maintenance of IV catheters by inexperienced staff members increase the incidence of catheter-related bacteremia.

In cats with bacteremia, underlying predisposing causes included pyothorax, septic peritonitis, GI tract disease, pneumonia, endocarditis, pyelonephritis, osteomyelitis, pyometra, and bite wounds.[22]

Various factors (Table 87-2) have been cited as predisposing patients to developing bacteremia. When considering mortality from bacteremia and sepsis, the single most important factor influencing outcome after infection is the severity of the patient's underlying disease. Death from bacteremia is much less likely to occur if the animal was healthy before the bacteremia developed.

Neutropenic patients are very susceptible to sepsis. Cancer chemotherapy-neutropenia is particularly dangerous because the destruction of GI crypt epithelial cells is usually a concomitant problem. Enteric bacteria gain access to the blood via the damaged mucosal barrier, and the neutropenia renders phagocytosis of these bacteria ineffective. To complicate matters, fever may be absent or minimal in a bacteremic patient because neutrophils are a component of the inflammatory process. The febrile neutropenic patient is a medical emergency. Patients who have had a splenectomy are also predisposed to bacterial sepsis because the spleen is an important component of the host's defense mechanisms.

Time Course

Relating the time course of bacteremia to the infecting organism is not always possible. Peracute bacteremia, which develops over several hours, often in debilitated or immunosuppressed patients, may be the result of either gram-positive or gram-negative infection. Acute bacteremia develops over 12 to 24 hours and is usually the result of gram-negative or staphylococcal infection. Subacute bacteremia develops and persists for several weeks or longer and is often the result of gram-positive but occasionally anaerobic infections. Chronic bacteremia, lasting weeks to months, may result from infections with microorganisms of low toxicity (e.g., *Brucella canis* and *S. intermedius*); sequestration of bacterial colonies on heart valves or in bone; abscess formation in the liver, spleen, kidneys, or muscles; or partial response to antibacterial therapy.

Secondary arthropathies, glomerulopathies, embolic abscesses or thrombi, and splenomegaly are more often associated with infective endocarditis (IE) than with bacteremia alone (Fig. 87-1; Table 87-3). Metastatic infection can result in life-threatening complications. Virtually all dogs with IE of the left side of the heart experience multiple continuous embolizations and renal infarctions, which may lead to renal failure. Subacute and chronic bacteremia can result in sustained antigenic stimulation of the immune system and increased circulating immunoglobulin. Circulating immune complexes (CICs) may be deposited in many tissues, leading to development of polyarthritis, myositis, vasculitis, and glomerulonephritis. Young, growing animals may develop metaphyseal embolization with resultant hypertrophic osteodystrophy.[166] In people, bacteremia has been found to result in hemolysis, presumably because of modified erythrocyte antigens that develop as a result of the circulating organism. A similar association of bacteremia with immune-mediated hemolytic anemia was not found in dogs.[128] Bacteria such as intraerythrocytic *Bartonella* species and hemotrophic mycoplasmas can induce hemolytic anemia (see Chapters 54 and 31, respectively), as do many protozoan erythroparasites.

Clinical Findings

Dogs

Dogs with bacteremia usually display some combination of lethargy, anorexia, GI disturbances (such as vomiting and diarrhea), fever, lameness, and myalgia (see Table 87-3). The presence of lameness (which may be intermittent), joint pain, muscle pain, and stiffness may suggest either immune-mediated disease or septic embolization of various tissues. Either infective or, more likely, immune-mediated arthritis may develop, and bilaterally symmetric joint involvement is more typical of immune-based arthritis. Lumbar or abdominal pain that is elicited by palpation suggests the possibility of renal or splenic inflammation secondary to septic embolization, infarction, abscess formation, or diskospondylitis. Diskospondylitis can also result in paresis or paralysis, depending on the location and degree of spinal cord compression (see Musculoskeletal Infections, Chapter 86). In younger animals, metaphyseal osteomyelitis causing malaise, fever, anorexia, swollen limbs, and reluctance to move has been observed. Occasionally, erosion of an artery occurs after septic embolization, and hemorrhage results. Vasculitis and thrombophlebitis

---

Table • 87-2

Factors Predisposing Dogs and Cats to Bacteremia

Specific Infectious Diseases
Ehrlichiosis (see Chapter 28)
Feline immunodeficiency virus infection (see Chapter 14)
Feline leukemia virus infection (see Chapter 13)
Canine parvoviral enteritis (see Chapter 8)
Feline panleukopenia (see Chapter 10)

Nidus of Infection
Abscesses (see Chapters 52 and 53)
Burns (see Chapter 55)
Colitis (see Chapter 89)
Gingivitis (see Chapter 89)
Stomatitis (see Chapter 89)
Pyoderma (see Chapter 85)
Urogenital infections (see Chapter 91)
Penetrating wounds (see Chapters 53 and 55)
Bowel injuries (see Chapter 89)
Musculoskeletal infections (e.g., osteomyelitis; see Chapter 86)

Immunodeficiencies (see Chapter 95)
Diabetes mellitus
Glucocorticoids
Cytotoxic drugs
Phagocytic defects
Hepatic failure
Renal failure
Solid tumors
Hematologic malignancies
Splenectomy
Old age
Shock
Congenital heart defects

Iatrogenic Manipulations
Dental prophylaxis (see Chapter 89)
Oral, abdominal, urogenital, or perianal surgery (see Chapter 55)
Invasive or protracted surgery (e.g., spinal, orthopedic; see Chapters 55 and 86)
Endoscopic procedures (see Chapter 55)
IV catheterization
Antimicrobial therapy (narrow spectrum or low dose)
Immunosuppressive therapy
Urogenital tract manipulations (see Chapter 91)

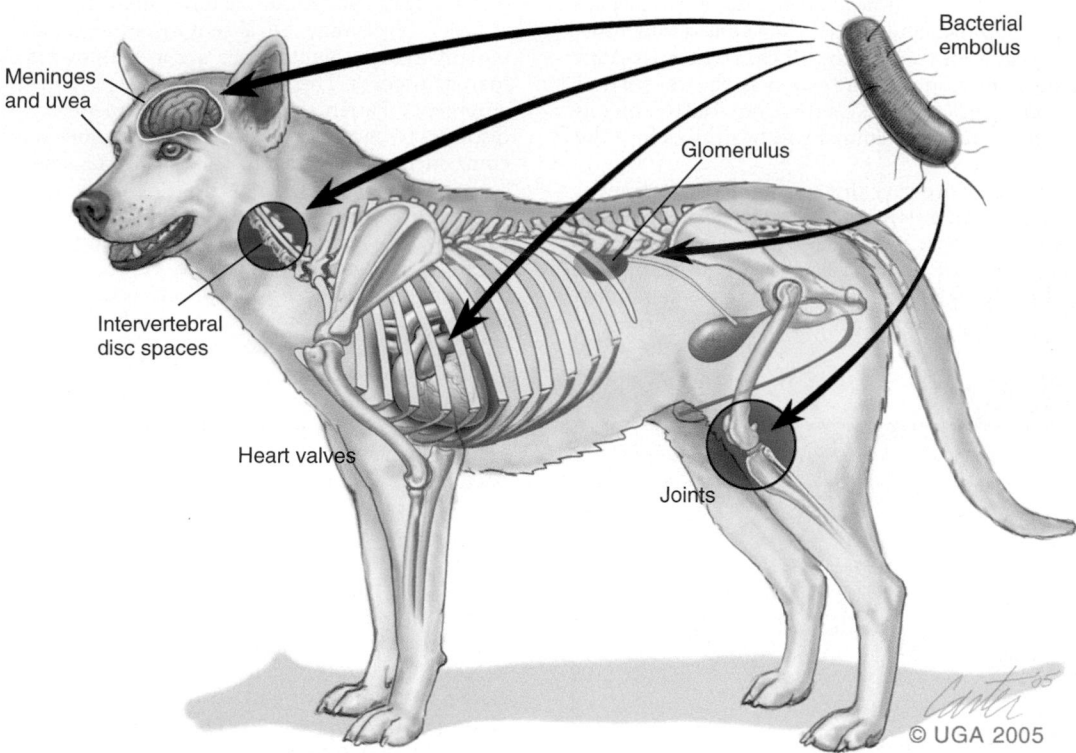

Fig 87-1 Sites of predilection for bacterial embolization in bacteremia are responsible for clinical illness that ensues. (Courtesy of University of Georgia, Athens Ga.)

Table • 87-3

Clinical Signs in Dogs with Bacteremia or Bacterial Endocarditis

CLINICAL SIGNS	BACTEREMIA ALONE (n = 77)	INFECTIVE ENDOCARDITIS (n = 45)
Fever (> 39.4° C [102.9° F])	75	70
Lameness: total	19	34
Lameness: shifting	6	18
Vomiting	17	35
Heart murmur	6	74
Ventricular arrhythmia	5	27

may produce hyperesthesia and lameness, with or without swelling of an extremity.

Organ failure in bacteremic septic patients can quickly lead to septic shock. In the dog, the GI tract, liver, kidneys, and lungs (in this order) are most affected. Mucosal sloughing, characterized by vomiting and bloody diarrhea, often with mucosal remnants, is commonly seen with advanced sepsis. Hepatic failure is characterized by vomiting, anorexia, ascites, and icterus. Oliguria is usually the result of hypotension and shock. Splenic inflammation may lead to splenomegaly or abdominal discomfort. Endocarditis is associated with cardiac manifestations of a heart murmur with or without arrhythmias.

Cats

In cats with bacteremia, with or without endocarditis, signs were anorexia, pyrexia, and shifting leg lameness.[36] Heart murmurs are found in those with endocarditis. In the cat, respiratory failure can occur early in the course of sepsis. In some cats, endocarditis may be more gradual, permitting the infected valves to become dystrophic.[115,138] With valvular lesions, although signs of sepsis have varied, cats invariably develop signs of right- or left-side congestive heart failure (CHF).

Diagnosis
Clinical Laboratory Findings

Dogs The leukograms of dogs with bacteremia alone and with bacterial endocarditis are similar.[34] A neutrophilic leukocytosis with an appropriate left shift and monocytosis are present in most dogs with gram-positive or anaerobic bacteremia and in virtually all dogs with chronic IE at some point during the course of disease. Leukopenia and inappropriate left shift have been more common with bacteremia alone, usually in association with peracute and acute gram-negative infections.

A normocytic, normochromic, nonregenerative anemia and thrombocytopenia are common with subacute or chronic bacteremia in dogs or cats.[22,34] With sepsis, hemoconcentration occurs after fluid losses from the intravascular space. Serum total solids tend to decrease because of the loss of protein from the intravascular compartment.

Serum chemistry abnormalities are common.[34] Hypoalbuminemia (less than 2.5 mg/dl), a twofold or greater elevation of alkaline phosphatase (ALP) activity, and hypoglycemia (less than 80 mg/dl) are consistent with bacteremia. Hyperglycemia occurs during the early phase (hyperdynamic phase) of septic shock.

The liver is an important site of removal of bacteria from the blood. Increased serum ALP activity is associated with gram-positive and gram-negative infections, and bacterial toxins are associated with impaired bile metabolism and cholestasis. Hyperbilirubinemia, bilirubinuria, and icterus can also occur (reactive hepatopathy of sepsis, see Chapter 90).

Hypoalbuminemia is a common manifestation of most types of bacteremia.[34] Subacute and chronic bacteremia may result in transcapillary leakage as a result of immune-mediated or embolic vasculitis or bacterial toxins. Sepsis also has been associated with reduced hepatic synthesis of albumin, and as many as 50% of bacteremic dogs may have increased bromsulphalein retention, suggesting either reduced hepatic function or reduced hepatic arterial blood flow. Bile acid levels may also be increased, suggesting hepatic insufficiency. Hypocalcemia is often observed and usually attributed to hypoalbuminemia.

The mechanism of hypoglycemia involves the effects of bacteria or bacterial toxins on the intermediary metabolism of glucose. In contrast, hyperglycemia has been correlated with a higher postoperative mortality in dogs than normoglycemia or hypoglycemic septicemic dogs.[33] This finding may be related to the fact that hyperglycemia has been seen in patients with early, severe septicemia, and hypoglycemia develops in more chronically affected cases.

Hypercoagulability leading to DIC is a common sequela of bacteremia. Evidence of DIC (low fibrinogen, prolonged PT and APTT, and increased fibrinogen degradation products) is consistent with advanced sepsis wherein major organ failure, including cardiovascular collapse, may be imminent.[93,107,119]

Septic patients often have a metabolic acidosis with respiratory compensation. The carbon dioxide tension can decrease severely to compensate for acidemia, but hypoxemia is uncommon in conscious patients.

Blood lactate levels are often increased in septic patients. Hemoconcentration and shock cause decreased oxygen delivery to the tissues, resulting in anaerobic metabolism. Cellular oxidative respiration is inhibited by an endotoxin or a mediator.[162] Furthermore, septic patients tend to be in a hypermetabolic state, requiring increased oxygen delivery to tissues.

Proteinuria, occult hematuria, and pyuria may occur in association with bacteremia or, more commonly, with bacterial endocarditis in which renal infarction, glomerulonephritis, and renal microabscess formation are common sequelae. Proteinuria with acellular urinary sediment suggests glomerular or tubular renal proteinuria and may occur with renal injury from immune-complex deposition caused by bacteremia. Urinary tract infections may be either a cause or a result of bacteremia, and urine cultures should be submitted regardless of whether abnormalities are detected on urinalysis.

Test results for immune-mediated diseases, such as antinuclear antibody titer (ANA), rheumatoid factor (RF), and lupus erythematosus cell preparation, occasionally are positive in bacteremic patients, particularly those with IE.

Bacteremia is only occasionally diagnosed by direct microscopic examination of leukocytes in blood smears. Direct Gram's stains of peripheral blood are usually unrewarding because the number of microorganisms present is often much lower than the 10^5 ml necessary for detection. Wright stains of buffy coat smears may increase the rate of detection. Acridine orange is more sensitive than Gram stain, because organisms can be detected at 10^4/ml concentrations. Slides must be handled carefully to prevent inadvertent contamination, which may be revealed as extracellular bacteria.

A simple method of performing leukocyte smears involves placing one drop of freshly collected, nonclotted venous blood on a clean glass coverslip and incubating it in a moist Petri dish for 25 minutes at 37° C (98.6° F). The clot on the coverslip is gently washed off with normal (0.9%) saline, and the coverslip with attached leukocytes is immersed in fixative (methanol or glutaraldehyde) before Giemsa staining and microscopic examination.

Cats In the most severe cases, cats have had prehepatic jaundice, associated with erythrocyte destruction, and neu-trophilia with a left shift. In cats, neutrophilia with a left shift is common.[22] Cats with sepsis often exhibit hypoxemia, hypercapnia, and metabolic acidosis. In addition, they often have hypoalbuminemia, low serum ALP activity, and hyperbilirubinemia.[22]

Blood Culture

The definitive diagnosis of bacteremia requires compatible clinical signs and laboratory data and the isolation of the offending microbe from blood cultures. Primary or secondary sites of infection, urine, and, although rarely, joint fluid may also contain the organism. Preferably, the bacteria should be isolated from more than one blood sample. In addition, a source of infection should be sought and attempts made to isolate an organism from that site. Negative blood culture results in bacteremic patients can occur as a result of prior antimicrobial therapy, chronic low-grade infections such as diskospondylitis and endocarditis, intermittent shedding of the organism, causative agents other than bacteria, uremia, and right-sided endocarditis.

When an etiologic diagnosis is established with positive blood culture results, more appropriate and effective antibiotic therapy can be used. Low blood culture yields are a frequent complaint but probably reflect the effects of poor selection on the part of the clinician of proper blood culturing techniques (e.g., timing, volume, number of specimens) and inadequate laboratory processing (e.g., improper handling techniques, failure to culture for anaerobes). By adhering to recommended guidelines for obtaining and processing blood culture specimens, the diagnostic yield from blood cultures can be rewarding.

Although empiric multiple-antibiotic therapy often has been instituted in critically ill patients before obtaining culture results, the effort and expense required for blood culture have been justifiable because improper treatment may increase mortality from bacteremia. Furthermore, prior administration of antimicrobials appears to slow but not prevent bacterial isolation.[56]

Indications Blood cultures are indicated in acutely ill patients with fever; leukocytosis, especially with a marked left shift; neutropenia; and unexplained tachycardia, hypoglycemia, circulatory collapse, tachypnea or dyspnea, anuria or oliguria, icterus, thrombocytopenia, or DIC. Complementary cultures of urine and any other obvious sites of possible infection should also be obtained.

Bacteremia is usually continuous, although low level. Intermittent bacteremia usually reflects established infections extrinsic to the blood stream. Samples should be taken from either a freshly placed, meticulously maintained jugular catheter or from several veins.[32,56] Duration of antimicrobial therapy is an important factor in the detection of bacteria.[84] Therapy for only 2 to 3 days may not interfere; however, longer courses of therapy require the use of antibiotic removal devices or discontinuation of therapy before sampling. Suppression of bacteremia often persists longer than antibiotic blood levels.

One of the most critical factors is taking an adequate sample volume, because the concentration of organisms in bacteremic specimens is small. In addition, multiple sample collections have been recommended in an attempt to detect an intermittent bacteremia. For dogs and cats, it has been suggested that at least three blood cultures be obtained over 24 hours.[31,33] In the case of critically ill, acutely septic patients, the three blood cultures should be obtained over 30 to 60 minutes before instituting antimicrobial treatment. However, for small animals, this may be too much blood. Taking larger volumes as recommended for human patients is often difficult in dogs and cats. The idea that bacteremias are intermittent or are correlated with fever spikes has also not been well substantiated. Therefore taking at least two specimens of sufficient volume from different vascular sites within a 10-minute interval may be sufficient to determine whether bacteria are present in the blood and whether positive blood culture results are a result of true bacteremia or contamination during collection. At least 5 to 10 ml of blood should be collected for each culture, because the chances of obtaining a positive result are directly related to the volume of blood cultured. The concentration of organisms is relatively low (fewer than five per milliliter) in the blood of most patients. It is recommended that as large a volume as practical be taken to maximize the chance of culturing an offending organism. A minimum of 20 ml is taken from large dogs, 10 ml from intermediate-size dogs, and 5 ml from cats and smaller dogs. If possible, a second specimen should be taken from a second venipuncture site within a short interval of the first. A blood-culture broth ratio of 1:10 must be maintained to counteract the bactericidal activity of serum. Anticoagulant and antiphagocytic effects of broth additives are diminished if dilution of blood in media is less than 1:8. Therefore the proper size blood culture bottle should be used for the intended blood sample volume.

Technique   Before venipuncture, thorough skin antisepsis, as for surgery, is the most effective means of avoiding culture contamination (Fig. 87-2, *A*).[89] Small numbers of bacteria may persist inside hair follicles and sweat and sebaceous glands, which may be penetrated by the needle. If the vein must be palpated after skin disinfection, a sterile glove should be worn. To minimize the risk of contamination, blood samples should not be drawn through an indwelling IV-catheter unless it is a recently and appropriately placed jugular catheter. Arterial blood specimens offer no advantage over venous blood specimens. Finding the same organism at two different surgically prepared sites reduces the likelihood that the organism is a contaminant, especially when sampling intervals are close.

The culture bottle diaphragm is disinfected with alcohol or iodine before sample inoculation (Fig. 87-2, *B*). Blood is inoculated immediately and directly into culture media using a syringe and new needle or a blood transfer set (Fig. 87-2, *C*). Only commercial culture bottles packed under vacuum and fitted with rubber diaphragms should be used for routine

blood cultures to minimize the risk of contamination (Table 87-4). Air must not be allowed to enter into vacuum bottles during blood injection. The blood should be dispersed in the culture medium by gently inverting the bottle 2 or 3 times. Blood culture bottles should be inoculated and can be maintained at room temperature to avoid killing temperature-sensitive bacteria; however, incubation at 37° C is often used in the laboratory.

Half of each blood sample should be inoculated into an aerobic broth culture medium and the other half into an aerobic broth. These media should be capable of supporting growth of fastidious bacteria and when appropriate should contain a resin to remove antibiotics.

For catheter-related bacteremia, the catheter should be removed aseptically with a sterile forceps after local antisepsis of the insertion site with a swab soaked with 70% alcohol. A blood sample can be taken at the same time for culture. After removal of the catheter, the distal segment should be cut off and placed in a sterile, dry tube to be sent to the laboratory.

Liquid Media   Commercial multipurpose nutrient broth media, such as tryptic soy broth, trypticase soy broth, Columbia broth, and brain-heart infusion broth (Difco Laboratories, Detroit, Mich.) are all suitable for *qualitative* recovery of aerobic and anaerobic bacteria. Thioglycolate and thiol broth (Difco), intended for anaerobic blood culture only, should not be relied on for multipurpose cultures because aerobic (especially *Pseudomonas*) and facultative anaerobic bacteria are not reliably isolated. Most liquid media are bottled under vacuum with carbon dioxide added and usually are suitable to support the growth of clinically important anaerobes. The use of special anaerobic broth is rarely necessary.

Most commercial blood culture media contain 0.025% to 0.05% sodium polyanethol sulfonate (SPS), a polyanionic anticoagulant that also inhibits complement and lysozyme activity, interferes with phagocytosis, and inactivates therapeutic serum levels of aminoglycosides. Dilution of blood with liquid media is essential to neutralize serum and cellular antimicrobial properties. Even at 1:10 dilutions, serum may be bactericidal to coliforms, an effect that is counteracted by the addition of SPS. However, SPS is inhibitory to mycoplasmas

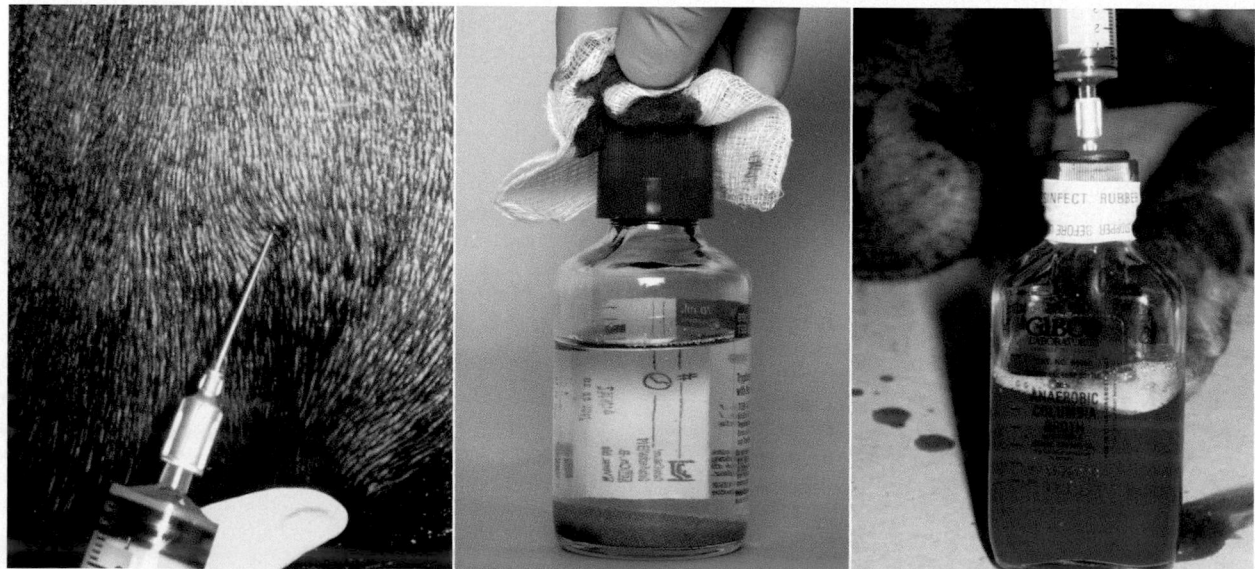

A,B   C

Fig   87-2   Blood culture method. **A,** Blood specimen is taken from jugular vein after surgical preparation. **B,** Top of bottle containing liquid blood culture medium is disinfected with povidone iodine solution. **C,** Blood is placed in culture media after changing to new needle. (Courtesy University of Georgia, Athens, Ga.)

Table • 87-4

Commercially Available Blood Culture Systems

INDICATED USE	COLLECTION MEDIA	MANUFACTURER
Aerobic and anaerobic	BBL SEPTI-CHEK with trypticase soy broth	Becton Dickinson Microbiology Systems, Franklin Lakes, N.J.
Pediatric patients	BBL SEPTI-CHEK with brain heart infusion	Becton Dickinson Microbiology Systems, Franklin Lakes, N.J.
Antimicrobial therapy	BBL SEPTI-CHEK with resins culture bottle	Becton Dickinson Microbiology Systems, Franklin Lakes, N.J.
Centrifugation lysis	ISOLATOR SYSTEM	Wampole Laboratories, Princeton, N.J.

and should not be in media intended for their isolation. Dilution of blood in culture broth usually lowers therapeutic concentrations of antibiotics to noninhibitory levels. When high levels of lactam antibiotics are present in blood before culture, β-lactamase can be added to the culture media. Para-amino benzoic acid, available in some commercial blood culture media, competitively antagonizes the actions of sulfonamides and increases the blood culture yields from patients receiving sulfonamide drugs.

Bacterial growth can be suppressed in blood culture vials containing blood from patients receiving antibiotics. Anionic and cationic resins have been incorporated into blood collection vials for antibiotic removal before broth culture. The effectiveness of removal varies.[47,161]

In the laboratory, culture bottles are examined daily for evidence of microbial growth, which includes turbidity, hemolysis, gas production, or colony formation. In aerobic culturing, the broth should appear turbid within 24 hours of inoculation. In 95% of all instances wherein bacteria are isolated from blood culture media, isolation occurs within 7 days. Longer incubation may be necessary for specimens from patients who previously received antibiotic therapy or those with endocarditis caused by fastidious organisms such as *Bartonella* (see Chapter 54). In addition to visual inspection, routine (blind) subcultures onto solid culture media usually are performed for antimicrobial susceptibility testing between 7 and 14 hours after blood collection and again after 48 hours of incubation.

Lysis-Centrifugation Although broth-based blood culture methods are sensitive, they provide no quantitative information about the number of microorganisms present. In contrast, inoculation of blood on solid agar allows for colony enumeration. Direct plating of freeze-thawed specimens of anticoagulated blood improves the sensitivity by freezing intracellular and phagocytized organisms. Only small volumes (1 ml) of blood can be directly plated. Lysis-centrifugation methods, with commercially prepared tubes (e.g., Wampole Isolator-tubes, Carter-Wallace Inc., Cranbury, N.J.), allow for lysis of cellular elements followed by microbial concentration through centrifugation. These methods may also shorten the time to isolation of bloodborne organisms, but they are associated with an increased risk of bacterial contamination. Lysis methods also enhance the ability to recover intracellular

organisms such as *Brucella, Mycobacterium, Histoplasma,* and *Bartonella.*

Interpretation of Results   It may be difficult to determine whether a positive culture result signifies actual bacteremia or simply indicates contamination. Contamination is best distinguished from bacteremia if multiple blood specimens are cultured. Knowledge of the normal canine and feline bacterial skin flora is helpful in interpreting blood culture results. Coagulase-negative staphylococci, β-hemolytic streptococci, *Micrococcus* species, and *Acinetobacter* species are normal skin commensals on the dog. *S. intermedius* is normally present on canine hair, whereas *Micrococcus* organisms, β-hemolytic streptococci, and *Acinetobacter* species are normally present on feline skin. Recovery of diphtheroids, *Bacillus* species, and coagulase-negative staphylococci usually signifies contamination unless they are isolated from multiple specimens. Non-hemolytic streptococci and β-hemolytic streptococci from single cultures are also of uncertain significance. In all cases the significance of positive blood culture results should be interpreted in light of the patient's clinical status and the potential sources for bacteremia. Because of the high prevalence of *Bartonella* organisms in the blood of clinically healthy cats, the only way to confirm the endocarditis is by using immunologic stains or performing a postmortem culture of valvular tissues.[19]

Urine Culture

Culture of urine has been commonly used to detect organisms associated with bacteremia and diskospondylitis. The presumption has been that these positive culture results represent the source of infection. In contrast, bacteriuria is likely a consequence of bloodborne bacteria reaching the kidney and being filtered by the glomerulus and from damage entering the renal tubule and urine. Bacteria are found in urine within minutes of IV infusion. Bacteremic animals with positive results for urine culture usually have no lower urinary tract signs, suggesting that the infection did not come from ascending infection.

Therapy

IV access lines are essential to the management of the bacteremic patient, not only for fluid and antibiotic administration but also for blood sampling. A urinary catheter is helpful for monitoring urine output in patients at risk for septic shock. Core and toe-web temperature readings should be monitored to assess peripheral blood flow and vasoconstriction.

Blood cultures and bacterial antibiotic susceptibility tests are essential for the proper treatment of bacteremia. It is important to choose a bactericidal antibiotic that has good tissue penetration and to use high (when permissible) IV doses for the first 5 to 10 days. Antimicrobial therapy should then be continued subcutaneously (SC) or orally for at least 3 weeks after IV administration. Bacteremia in debilitated patients or those with deep-seated or long-standing infections should be treated with IV and SC antibiotics for several weeks.

Despite the primary concern with the infectious agent, concomitant disorders should not be overlooked. In fact, the severity of comorbid disease is as important in treatment outcome as the invading organism itself. The ability to treat or control concomitant disease effectively may exert a more favorable influence on outcome than the chosen antibiotic regimen. Sources of infection should be identified and managed. Urinary and IV catheters should be removed when sepsis is suspected, and potential sites of infection should be drained, debrided, and otherwise treated.

In critically ill patients, antibiotic therapy should be instituted before the return of blood culture results, although this

Table • 87-5

Choice of Antimicrobial Therapy for Bacteremia or Endocarditis

ORGANISM	CONDITION OR SITE	FIRST CHOICE[a]	SECOND CHOICE[a]
Staphylococcus intermedius	Pyoderma	1cep, 2cep, brp	amg, ticar-clav, vanc, quin
Escherichia coli	Bowel compromise, peritonitis	amg, tms, quin	3cep, ticar-clav
β-hemolytic *Streptococcus*	Genital, navel, and skin infections	pen, amp, 1cep, amp- clav	2cep, clin, ticar, ticar-clav
Bartonella spp.	Vector-transmitted infections	doxy	quin, rif, azith
Pseudomonas spp.	Chronic wounds, leukopenia, burns, tracheostomy	amg,[b] quin	carb, ticar, 3cep[c]
Anaerobes	Abscesses, oral cavity lesions, bowel compromise, body cavity exudates	pen, met, clin	amp-clav, chlor

[a]*amg*, Aminoglycoside; *amp*, ampicillin, amoxicillin; *amp-clav*, ampicillin-clavulanate, amoxicillin-clavulanate; *azith*, azithromycin; *brp*, β-lactamase–resistant penicillin; *carb*, carbenicillin; *1cep*, first-generation cephalosporins; *2cep*, second-generation cephalosporins; *3cep*, third-generation cephalosporins; *chlor*, chloramphenicol; *clin*, clindamycin; *doxy*, doxycycline; *ery*, erythromycin; *met*, metronidazole; *pen*, penicillin; *quin*, fluroquinolone; *rif*, rifampin; *ticar*, ticarcillin; *ticar-clav*, ticarcillin-clavulanate; *tms*, trimethoprim-sulfonamide; *vanc*, vancomycin.
[b]May combine aminoglycoside with ticarcillin or carbenicillin for maximum efficacy.
[c]Only certain cephalosporins in this group, such as ceftazidime, are effective against *Pseudomonas* species.

approach has inherent shortcomings, such as selection for microbial resistance. Subsequent therapeutic adjustments may be made on the basis of culture results. If administered at all, bacteriostatic antibiotics should conclude rather than initiate treatment.

On the basis of predisposing infections or other factors, time course of infection, and known patterns of associated bacteria and their antimicrobial susceptibilities, the antibiotics most likely to be effective can be predicted (Table 87-5). This knowledge is important when blood culture results are negative and in critically ill patients before the return of blood culture results. Subsequently, appropriate adjustments in therapy may be necessary. In dogs and cats, staphylococci and streptococci are the most commonly encountered gram-positive pathogens, whereas the Enterobacteriaceae, such as *E. coli* and *Klebsiella*, and *Proteus*, and *Pseudomonas* organisms, are the most common gram-negative offenders.

Bactericidal rather than bacteriostatic antibiotics have been shown to result in higher concentrations of circulating endotoxin because bacteria die quickly in animals with experimental gram-negative bacteremia. However, in clinical practice, this does not translate into a clinically relevant syndrome in dogs.

Patients with bacteremia must be closely monitored (see also Endotoxemia, Chapter 38). Although clinical and hematologic evidence of improvement often occurs initially, relapse is common. Acquired antimicrobial resistance may develop rapidly. Clinical signs of resurging bacteremia include fever, which may be transient, deterioration of mucous membrane color, increasing capillary refill time, increasing rectal to toe-web temperature differential, decreasing blood pressure, and tachycardia. Detection of these signs of early deterioration indicates a need for intensification of therapy, including adjustments of antibiotic administration. It also should prompt a search for a persistent focus of infection (e.g., abscess, catheter) that may be treatable.

Antibiotics

For additional information on specific drugs discussed next, see Chapter 34 and the Drug Formulary, Appendix 8. The penicillin family of antibiotics includes the narrow-spectrum penicillin G; intermediate-spectrum ampicillin; and the extended-spectrum carbenicillin, ticarcillin, ticarcillin-clavulanate, and piperacillin (Table 87-6). A common misconception is that ampicillin is a broad-spectrum antibiotic. Most coagulase-positive staphylococcal isolates are resistant to penicillin and ampicillin, and these are poor empiric choices for serious and life-threatening infections. Penicillin G should be restricted to streptococcal and some anaerobic infections.

The extended-spectrum penicillins—carbenicillin, ticarcillin, ticarcillin-clavulanate, and piperacillin—are useful agents when antibiogram results indicate their effect against a highly resistant microbe. These antibiotics have a spectrum that includes that of ampicillin plus extended gram-negative activity, including activity against *Pseudomonas* and *Proteus* species. Ticarcillin is more potent than carbenicillin, and piperacillin is active against many anaerobes. With the exception of ticarcillin-clavulanate, these penicillins lack resistance to β-lactamase produced by staphylococci.

The first-generation cephalosporins are useful in the treatment of potentially life-threatening infections because of their activity against *Staphylococcus* and *Streptococcus* species, as well as a greater spectrum of activity than ampicillin against gram-negative bacteria. These antibiotics include cephalothin, cefazolin, and cephapirin but like many antibiotics are not effective against enterococci and *Pseudomonas* species and are susceptible to the β-lactamase activity of *Bacteroides fragilis*. Second- and third-generation cephalosporins (such as cefoxitin and cefotaxime, respectively) are generally effective against gram-negative bacteria that are resistant to the first-generation family. Cefoxitin is effective for resistant anaerobes, and cefotaxime is effective for bacterial infections involving the central nervous system (CNS) and gram-negative infections with demonstrated resistance to aminoglycoside and fluoroquinolone antibiotics. Cephalosporins are also useful when the nephrotoxic aminoglycosides are contraindicated. The third-generation cephalosporins, with the exception of ceftazidime, are generally ineffective against *Pseudomonas*. Cost is often a factor limiting the administration of the third-generation family.

Ceftiofur is a near third-generation cephalosporin that has an antibacterial spectrum similar to that of cefotaxime, but it has a longer half-life[28,175] and is less expensive (see Drug Formulary, Appendix 8). Ceftiofur is variably effective against *S. intermedius* and ineffective against *Pseudomonas* and *Bordetella* species. In addition, its anaerobic spectrum is narrow, and

Table • 87-6

Antimicrobial Dosages for Bacteremia with or without Endocarditis in Dogs and Cats

DRUG[a]	SPECIES	DOSE[b]	ROUTE	INTERVAL (HOURS)	DURATION (DAYS)[c]
Penicillin	B	$20–40 \times 10^3$ U/kg	IV	4–6	7–14
Imipenem	B	10 mg/kg	IV	8	7–14
Carbenicillin	B	40–50 mg/kg	IV	6–8	7–14
Piperacillin	B	30 mg/kg	IV	6	7–14
Ampicillin	B	20–40 mg/kg	IV, SC	6–8	7–14
Amoxicillin-clavulanate		20 mg/kg	PO	12	Follow-up
Ticarcillin	D	30–50 mg/kg	IV, SC	6–8	7–14
Ticarcillin-clavulanate	D	20–50 mg/kg	IV	6–8	7–14
	C	40 mg/kg	IV	6	7–14
Cefazolin (first generation)	B	20–30 mg/kg	IV, SC	8	7–14
Cefapirin (first generation)	B	15–30 mg/kg	IV, SC	8	7–14
Cefoxitin (second generation)	B	20 mg/kg	IV	8	7–14
Cefuroxime (second generation)		15 mg/kg		8	
Cefotaxime (third generation)	B	20–80 mg/kg	IV	8	7–14
Ceftiofur (third generation)		2.2–4.4 mg/kg	SC	12	Follow-up
Gentamicin[d]	B	4–6 mg/kg	IV	24	7–14
Amikacin[d]	B	7–10 mg/kg	IV	24	7–14
Trimethoprim—sulfonamide	D	15 mg/kg	IV	8–12	7–14
	R	30 mg/kg	SC, PO	12–24	Follow-up
Metronidazole	B	8–15 mg/kg	IV, PO	8	5–7
Clindamycin	B	10 mg/kg	IV	8–12	7–14
	B	10–11 mg/kg	PO	12	Follow-up
Chloramphenicol	D	15–25 mg/kg	IV	6–8	7–14
	C	10–15 mg/kg	IV	6–8	4–7
Ciprofloxacin[e]	B	10–15 mg/kg	PO	12	14
Enrofloxacin[e]	D	5–7 mg/kg	IV	24	4–7
	D	5–15 mg/kg	PO	24	Follow-up
	C	5 mg/kg	PO	24	Follow-up
Azithromycin	B	5–10 mg/kg	PO	12	Follow-up

B, Dog and cat; *D*, dog; *C*, cat; *IV*, intravenous; *SC*, subcutaneous; *PO*, by mouth.
[a]For additional information about the drugs listed, see Appendix 8.
[b]Dose per administration at specified interval.
[c]After the animal is stabilized, subcutaneous or oral therapy should be continued when possible for periods of 3 to 6 additional weeks (see text).
[d]Renal function and urinalysis must be closely monitored for signs of nephrotoxicity at this dosage and frequency. Reduce dose to 1–2 mg/kg every 8 hr if renal compromise is anticipated.
[e]For dosages of other quinolones, see Chapter 34 and the Drug Formulary, Appendix 8.

inadequate data have been collected concerning its effect on streptococcal species. In vitro activity against *Fusobacterium* is generally good, but it is poor against *Bacteroides* species.

Aminoglycosides are highly effective against *Staphylococcus* and many gram-negative bacteria. They are not effective against anaerobes and many streptococci and have limited activity in necrotic tissue and acid pH milieu. The primary limitation of gentamicin, amikacin, and tobramycin is nephrotoxicity, therefore other agents are required for extended antibiotic therapy. The incidence of gentamicin-associated acute renal failure has increased markedly since 3-times-daily administration has been used for systemic infections. Dehydration and sodium and potassium depletion predispose patients to nephrotoxicosis, as does administration for longer than 5 to 7 days. Aminoglycosides demonstrate more rapid bactericidal action for severe sepsis than do the penicillins and cephalosporins. They also invoke postantibacterial effects (i.e., bactericidal action after the serum concentration has decreased below the minimum inhibitory concentration).

Fluoroquinolones are often a good choice instead of the third-generation cephalosporins for gram-negative bacteremias not involving the CNS. The fluoroquinolones are very useful for the treatment of bacteremia, having bactericidal action at achievable concentrations. Like the aminoglycosides, they exhibit postantibacterial effects. They are effective against *Pseudomonas* and Enterobacteriaceae but are generally ineffective against anaerobes and enterococci. Efficacy against streptococci is limited. Ciprofloxacin is approved for IV administration in humans, and enrofloxacin solution has been diluted and given slowly IV to dogs. Enrofloxacin should not be injected into sodium containing fluid bags, IV lines, or IV catheters. A combination of enrofloxacin plus clindamycin may be as effective as and less toxic than ampicillin, gentamicin, and metronidazole for life-threatening sepsis caused by unknown bacteria. However, clindamycin is a bacteriostatic antibiotic.

In general, first-generation cephalosporins and β-lactamase resistant penicillins are effective in vitro against grampositive bacteria, whereas aminoglycosides, first-generation cephalosporins, and fluoroquinolones are effective against gram-negative agents. Thus a combination of an aminoglycoside, such as gentamicin or amikacin, with ampicillin, ticarcillin, piperacillin, or first-generation cephalosporin is a good choice for immediate treatment of life-threatening bacteremia in the absence of laboratory identification of an organism or its antibiotic susceptibility. The combination of first-generation cephalosporins and aminoglycosides, however, is not very effective against anaerobic bacteria. When an anaerobic infection is suspected, clindamycin, metronidazole, or cefoxitin is recommended. Despite in vitro susceptibility testing, trimethoprim-sulfonamide is a poor choice for anaerobic infections. Penicillin formerly was the preferred drug for anaerobic bacteremia. However, those infections caused by *Bacteroides* species are becoming increasingly resistant to penicillins and first-generation cephalosporins.

A highly effective triple therapy for dogs with sepsis, particularly for intraabdominal infections, is a β-lactam drug (ampicillin, ticarcillin, piperacillin, or first-generation cephalosporin) with an aminoglycoside and metronidazole. The combination of enrofloxacin and clindamycin is also effective and suggested when renal function is impaired.[56] Another nonaminoglycoside regimen is referred to as the *double β-lactam regimen*.[88] The regimen may consist of the combination of either ampicillin plus the third-generation cephalosporin ceftazidime or a second-generation plus a third-generation cephalosporin.

The advent of β-lactam antibiotics with broad-spectrum activity that achieve high serum bactericidal levels has made monotherapy an option for empirical treatment. The third-generation and "fourth-generation" cephalosporins and the carbapenems are candidates. Although ceftazidime has been used, it may be ineffective against some gram-negative and anaerobic isolates. Cefepime overcomes some of these limitations. Imipenem has the broadest spectrum of activity of any antibiotic and is effective against many anaerobes.

For cats, an antimicrobial spectrum encompassing gram-negative and anaerobic bacteria, such as *Bacteroides* species and *Propionibacterium* spp., is recommended. Piperacillin or clindamycin plus a first-generation cephalosporin are recommended.

To ensure adequate serum antibiotic concentrations, the upper limit of the usual dosage range of antimicrobial drugs is recommended (see Table 87-6). Parenteral treatment is desirable for 5 to 10 days, although this approach is not always practical. SC administration of ampicillin, cephalothin, ceftiofur, or clindamycin may be substituted for the IV route after 5 to 10 days of IV treatment. Except in animals with endocarditis or other internal sources of infection, such as bone, lung, and prostate gland, most properly treated bacteremic episodes are short lived. Ideally, oral antibiotic therapy should be instituted only after 5 days of IV therapy and even then only after clinical and hematologic normalization have been documented.

Combination antibiotic therapy is often provided for gram-negative infections because they may be associated with rapid progression and high mortality. Although clinical evidence supports the use of carbenicillin or ticarcillin with aminoglycosides for *Pseudomonas* and *Proteus*, these drugs must be given separately because of known in vitro incompatibilities. Amikacin, unlike tobramycin and gentamicin, is not inactivated in vitro by penicillins. Administration of some antibiotics such as aminoglycosides, cephalosporins, metronidazole, and enrofloxacin is recommended by infusion in a compatible solution over 30 to 60 minutes.

The Febrile Granulocytopenic Patient

The risk of bacterial infection increases substantially when the neutrophil count is less than 500/μl, although monocytes may compensate for neutropenia to an extent.[17,81] The lungs, oropharynx, urinary tract, and gut are frequent sources of infections in neutropenic patients. Some of the signs of infection are diminished in neutropenic patients because the cells that mediate the inflammatory response are absent. This may manifest as reduced pulmonary infiltrates with pneumonia, relatively nonpurulent exudates, and absence of pyuria with urinary tract infections. Furthermore, localized infections can quickly disseminate. In fact, patients with signs consistent with sepsis and neutropenia can present a diagnostic challenge as the clinician attempts to determine whether the neutropenia antedated the sepsis or is a response to overwhelming inflammation. An increase in band neutrophils that is higher than 20%, called *bandemia*, suggests appropriate granulocytopoietic activity.[17,81] Sepsis, especially gram-negative, causes accelerated platelet destruction, possibly as a result of binding of bacterial immune complexes to the platelet.[99]

When a new fever develops in a neutropenic patient, an empirical bactericidal, broad-spectrum antibiotic regimen should be quickly implemented as soon as blood culture specimens are obtained. Bacteremia in neutropenic patients can disseminate quickly and may prove rapidly lethal.[97] The majority of these patients do not have an obvious source of infection. Blood cultures (preferably three sets) should be performed. If a catheter is in place, a culture should be obtained through it if possible, the catheter removed, and the tip cultured. Gram-positive bacteria, especially staphylococci, are the most common causes of catheter-related infections.[136] Even subtle indications of inflammation must be considered as potential sites of infection in the face of granulocytopenia.

The appropriate role for quinolones in neutropenic patients has yet to be fully defined.[88] Because of their relatively poor activity against some gram-positive microbes, they should not be used alone for empirical therapy.

The combination of β-lactams with β-lactamase inhibitors (clavulanate and sulbactam) has produced powerful antibiotics such as ticarcillin plus clavulanate, which can be combined with an aminoglycoside for the empiric treatment of neutropenic, febrile patients.[88]

Prognosis

Many factors influence the natural course of bacteremia, including adequacy of therapy, severity of bacteremia, source of infection, delay before treatment, and presence of concomitant disorders, as well as the age and prior health status of the patient. The prognosis is better when abscesses, cellulitis, skin and wound infections are the sources of bacteremia than when gram-negative bacteria and endotoxemia are present. Mortality of bacteremic dogs with hypoalbuminemia, high serum ALP, and hypoglycemia is significantly higher than that of dogs without or with only one of these abnormalities.[34] Late relapse and death have occurred in some dogs when bacteriostatic antibiotics were chosen for treatment. Premature termination of antibiotic therapy may also result in relapse and death in bacteremic dogs, particularly those associated with antimicrobial-restricted sites, pneumonia, abscesses, and cellulitis. Relapse after IV antibiotic therapy that was maintained for only 1 to 2 days followed by oral antibiotics is common. Oral antibiotic therapy alone is dangerous when relied on either as initial treatment or after only a few days of IV antibiotic treatment.

The indiscriminate use of glucocorticoids (even with antibiotics as prophylaxis) is detrimental to bacteremic patients. One reason that glucocorticoids are administered to bacteremic dogs is the similarity in clinical manifestations of bacteremia and immune-mediated diseases.

Aspirin has been shown to reduce the virulence of staphylococcal endocarditis in people.[83] *S. aureus*, a nonmotile organism, has the affinity to bind substrates such as damaged heart valvular surfaces. The interaction of platelets and proteins facilitates this binding. Acetylsalicylic acid has been used in vitro and in vivo in experimental infections to reduce bacterial vegetations. Clinical studies are still needed, but the possibility of reducing bacterial adherence may be important as a prevention or therapy of endocarditis along with antimicrobial drugs.

Prophylactic antibiotic treatment usually is ineffective unless it is used when surgical or dental procedures (see Chapters 55 and 89) are performed or when the type of bacteria and its susceptibility are known. Bacterial resistance to frequently administered antibiotics is common. Thus effective prophylactic antibiotic therapy may require combinations of antibiotics. Even then, the tendency to select for resistant bacteria increases. In human medicine, antimicrobial treatment is recommended as a prophylaxis for endocarditis in patients undergoing dental procedures with underlying cardiac valvular defects.[77] Use of bactericidal antibiotics such as amoxicillin within 1 hour before the procedure is recommended (see Oral Infections, Chapter 89).

SEPSIS

Sepsis is defined as the systemic inflammatory response syndrome that occurs during infection (see also Chapter 38).[21] Sepsis occurs when bacteria proliferate at a nidus of infection and either invade the circulation or remain local and release inflammatory mediators such as exotoxins and teichoic acid from staphylococci and endotoxins from gram-negative bacteria. Endotoxin produced by gram-negative bacteria is composed of lipid, polysaccharide, and protein, and it is the lipid portion that is responsible for toxicity. These microbe-derived products can stimulate the release of endogenous host-derived factors from plasma protein precursors, monocyte macrophages, endothelial cells, and neutrophils.[68,102,103,184] It has been thought that the theory was that sepsis represented an uncontrolled inflammatory response.[180] However, sepsis not only is caused by an immune system gone awry but also may be associated with an immune system that becomes compromised and unable to eradicate pathogens as sepsis worsens. Bacterial sepsis is associated with hepatic, intestinal, renal, pulmonary, and cardiovascular dysfunction; hypothermia; oliguria; respiratory failure; and lactic acidosis. When sepsis results in systemic arterial hypotension, the syndrome is referred to as *septic shock*. The cause of death in septic patients is not clearly defined. Potential causes include refractory shock, respiratory distress syndrome, renal failure, and hepatic failure. Although myocardial depression occurs, cardiac output is usually preserved because of cardiac dilation and sinus tachycardia.[149]

Incidence

Sepsis in dogs and cats is common. Advances in veterinary care have contributed to the incidence through the increase use of cytotoxic and immunosuppressive drug treatments, invasive procedures, extensive surgery, and the widespread use of IV catheters.

Bacteria

Gram-positive and gram-negative bacteria can cause septic shock. Staphylococci, streptococci, and *E. coli* are probably the most commonly involved microbes. Rickettsemia can probably produce a similar syndrome. Any infectious site can lead to sepsis, and frequent causes are abscesses, deep pyodermas, infected wounds, cellulitis, prostate infections, pneumonia, peritonitis, and infected surgery sites. Sites of infection are more difficult to identify in neutropenic and immunosuppressed patients because inapparent infections can lead to blood stream incursion. Not only are nosocomial infections common in intensive care facilities because of the concentration of sick patients and bacterial contamination but also because bacteria causing nosocomial infections are often antibiotic resistant.

Pathogenesis

Numerous factors can initiate the pathway leading to sepsis. Exotoxins are produced by staphylococci, *Pseudomonas aeruginosa*, and others. Structural components of microbes such as teichoic acid antigens from staphylococci, the polysaccharide capsule of some streptococci, and the lipopolysaccharide (LPS) associated with the cell membrane of gram-negative organisms can initiate the toxic septic cascade.[68,102,104,184] LPS can be bound by a binding protein, which stimulates monocytes and macrophages to produce cytokines, such as TNF and ILs, that play a major role in the response to infection or endotoxin. Endotoxins interact with macrophages, neutrophils, and vascular endothelia by binding to cell receptors, causing a release of mediators of sepsis, the magnitude of which is directly related to the endotoxin concentration.[23,133] Endotoxin can activate the complement cascade, which can lead to vasodilation, increased vascular permeability, platelet aggregation and activation, and neutrophil aggregation. Subsequently, increased bradykinin levels also contribute to vasodilation and hypotension. Some cytokines cause the release of arachidonic acid metabolites from endothelial cells and leukocytes, which can cause vasodilation, platelet aggregation, and neutrophil activation. LPS activation of factor XII leads to extrinsic and intrinsic coagulation pathway activation, which can lead to DIC.

Numerous trials of antiinflammatory treatments using glucocorticoids, antiendotoxin antibodies, TNF antagonists, IL-1-receptor antagonists, and others have failed to demonstrate a positive influence on survival and have thus called into question whether uncontrolled inflammation exerts a negative influence on survival.[69,134,180,185] The animal studies suggesting sepsis is attributable to hyperinflammation used large doses of endotoxin or bacteria, which invoked levels of circulating cytokines, such as TNF, that are much higher than levels encountered clinically.[52,139,144,159,178] Initially, sepsis is associated with increases in inflammatory mediators; but as sepsis persists, a shift toward an antiinflammatory immunosuppressive state occurs.[108,140]

Macrophages and activated CD4 T cells can secrete inflammatory cytokines such as TNF-α, interferon (IFN)-α, and IL-2.[145] Other mediators, arising principally from neutrophils, platelets, and vascular endothelia, include leukotrienes, prostaglandins, and platelet-activating factors.[23,153,169] All of these mediators interact with inflammatory cells, vascular endothelia, and platelets in a complex way to modulates immune function.[23] Cytokines such as IL-4 and IL-10 are also secreted by CD4 T cells but contribute to antiinflammatory immunosuppression.[145]

Inflammatory mediators exert a negative impact on cardiovascular, pulmonary, GI, vascular, and hematologic integrity. TNF has been associated with hypotension and respiratory dysfunction. IL-1 causes fever, neutropenia followed by neutrophilia, and pulmonary vascular sequestration of granulocytes.[16] Platelet-activating factor causes platelet activation and aggregation; neutrophil activation, aggregation, and chemotaxis; increased vascular permeability; and GI ulceration. Thromboxane, a product of the prostaglandin cascade, is associated with vasoconstriction and platelet aggregation.[23,143] Leukotrienes are chemotactic and increase vascular permeability.[153] Cytokines and other inflammatory mediators also invoke secondary mediators of sepsis such as vasopressin, angiotensin II, catecholamines, histamine, and serotonin.[80] Organ failure associated with septic shock is the result of hypoxia, free-radical and lysozyme damage, thrombosis, and necrosis.[39,80,134,180,185]

It was believed that death of many cell types occurred in septic patients. However, this has been shown to be false. The two cell types that do undergo accelerated death in septic patients are lymphocytes and GI cells. Sepsis probably accelerates apoptosis of these cell types, which normally undergo a rapid turnover rate via that process. Drugs that block apoptosis of lymphocytes and GI cells have been shown to improve survival in animal models,[86,141] although no such drugs are currently clinically available.

Clinical Manifestations

Patients may have signs related to a primary focus of infection. A careful history, physical examination, imaging studies, and laboratory data often permit identification of the infection focus. Debilitated, immunosuppressed, and neutropenic patients are more challenging in this regard. Although the exception to the rule, patients with sepsis, particularly debilitated, uremic, or immunosupressed patients, may not develop a fever. This lack of an acute-phase response may reflect advanced sepsis immunosupression and may be associated with a worse prognosis. However, in most patients one or more signs of systemic inflammatory response are present. These include fever, tachycardia, tachypnea, and an inflammatory leukogram. Septic shock is characterized by hypotension, lactic acidemia, and progressive organ dysfunction. Multiple organ dysfunction syndrome includes tissue hypoperfusion (oliguria, lactic acidosis, cool extremities), renal failure (oliguria), hepatic failure (hyperbilirubinemia), and respiratory distress syndrome. DIC and respiratory distress syndrome are terminal events.[68,103,104,184]

Therapy

At least three approaches to treating sepsis exist. First, a nidus of infection, if present and identified, should be treated by surgery, offending foreign bodies or catheters removed, and high-dose, IV bactericidal antibiotics administered (see Bacteremia Therapy and Therapy, Chapters 37 and 38). Second, cardiovascular, respiratory, and organ dysfunction physiology may be reversible. Third, it may be possible to manipulate the toxic mediators of sepsis.[68,103,104,184]

Early aggressive fluid therapy to maintain cardiac output is vital to survival. Reversible septic shock in patients with adequate intravascular volume is often associated with brick-red mucous membranes, tachycardia, high cardiac output, and normal or low blood pressure. Hypodynamic shock occurs in patients with decreased intravascular fluid volume, and affected individuals tend to be pale, cold, tachycardic, and hypotensive. Rescue with rapid, aggressive fluid therapy is possible, unless irreversible shock (elevated blood lactate concentration, hepatic failure, oliguria, hypotension, cold extremities) has developed. Patients with irreversible shock cannot be stabilized by fluid therapy because of massive fluid leakage through permeable endothelium, vasodilation, and possibly myocardial failure.[45] Rapid restoration of organ perfusion and tissue oxygen delivery are essential for the management of the patient in septic shock (see also Endotoxemia, Chapter 38). Rapid fluid therapy (crystalloid fluid, colloid-crystalloid mixture, or hypertonic solution[7]) is required to raise the central venous pressure within 15 minutes. Aggressive volume resuscitation is initiated at 10 ml/kg/hour for 1 to 2 hours. Colloid is recommended if the serum albumin is less than 2 g/dl or crystalloid in all others. High volumes of fluids are required for the treatment of septic shock, and crystalloid fluid volumes can be decreased by the addition of a colloid. Hetastarch 120 or dextran 70 is usually administered for this purpose. At high dosages, both can prolong clotting times by decreasing platelet function and fibrin clot strength, though this is rarely clinically significant. Another treatment for cardiovascular support is the administration of hypertonic solutions. Hypertonic saline and glucose-insulin-potassium solutions are the two most often administered hypertonic solutions (Table 87-7). Glucose-insulin-potassium improves cardiovascular function and helps prevent hypoglycemia. Insulin therapy may exert a favorable influence on survival.[178]

Table • 87-7

Fluid Therapy in Septic Shock

FLUID	VOLUME	COMMENTS
Hypertonic saline Glucose-insulin potassium	4 ml/kg 10% volume bolus, remainder infused over 4-5 hr (1 g glucose, 1 U insulin, 0.25 mEq K/kg in 250 ml of lactated Ringer's solution or 0.45% saline-5% glucose)	Once May be repeated as needed
Colloids Hetastarch 120, Dextran 70	Maximum: 20 ml/kg for first 24 hr, then 10 ml/kg/ 24 hr	Constant rate infusion, or intermittent infusions over 4—6 hr

After the hypertonic solutions are administered, crystalloid administration is continued. Serum albumin, potassium, and erythrocyte concentrations decrease after aggressive fluid therapy, and peripheral edema is a common sequela.

Rapid-acting, powerful inotropes, such as dopamine and dobutamine (3 to 5 µg/kg/min) are indicated if fluid therapy fails to establish or maintain adequate tissue oxygen perfusion. If hypotension persists, a dobutamine infusion rate is increased to as high as 20 µg/kg/min. Monitoring of heart rate and rhythm, core-to-toe-web temperature differential, central venous pressure, and urine output is important. The mean systolic blood pressure should be improved and be greater than 75 mm Hg.

DIC often develops during sepsis. Anti-DIC prophylaxis is recommended if the clotting time and platelet count are mildly deranged. Synthetic colloids can help, but if crystalloids only are administered, low-dose heparin (75 to 100 U/kg SC every 8 hours) is suggested to inhibit coagulation and maintain blood flow in the microcirculation.[169] Plasma transfusion provides clotting factors and antithrombin III, which helps prevent and control DIC. Acute and end-stage DIC is more difficult to treat, requiring more intense heparinization along with coagulation factor replacement. Anemic patients should receive whole blood or packed erythrocyte transfusions.

A balance between oxygen consumption and oxygen delivery should be maintained. Adequate oxygenation is critical and supplemental oxygen should be a routine component of treatment. Oxygen therapy can be administered by a cage, a mask, or an intranasal catheter.

In the future, treatments that inhibit or potentiate the action of mediators may become useful. High-dose glucocorticoid administration can inhibit mediator release in some animal models of endotoxemia, but in clinical practice the use of these agents at supraphysiologic dosages is detrimental.[48] Because severely septic patients may have relative adrenal insufficiency, physiologic dosages are beneficial.[5]

Recombinant activated protein C, an anticoagulant, may be a useful treatment. It inactivates factors Va and VIIIa, thereby preventing thrombin formation.[117] Inhibition of thrombin formation reduces inflammation by inhibiting platelet activation, neutrophil recruitment, and mast cell degranulation. Activated protein C prevents inflammation by blocking not only the production of cytokines by monocytes but also cell adhesion. Hemorrhage is a potential adverse effect of activated protein C.

Plasma may be valuable in the treatment of sepsis. Plasma and polyvalent immunoglobulin infusion may provide protective antibodies against virulent proteins and superantigens. Enhancement of neutralization of a wide variety of superantigens and opsonization of bacteria may be provided. Plasma protease inhibitors, α-2-macroglobulin and α-1-protease inhibitor, are useful in patients with pancreatitis-related sepsis because they bind with circulating digestive enzymes.

Pentoxifylline (10 mg/kg, given every 8 hours) and its metabolites improve blood flow and microcirculation tissue oxygen delivery by decreasing blood viscosity and increasing the flexibility of erythrocytes and leukocytes. Furthermore, neutrophil adhesion and activation may be decreased. Another potential benefit of pentoxifylline is its ability to scavenge oxygen-free radicals. Pentoxifylline also inhibits the complement cascade and cytokine production.

Pentoxifylline serum concentrations are increased by concomitant administration of theophylline, cimetidine, and fluoroquinolones. Renal impairment may also lead to toxicity by reducing pentoxifylline clearance. Toxic effects include nervousness, tremors, and seizures. Adverse effects of pentoxifylline that may be encountered at therapeutic serum concentrations include dyspnea, epistaxis, nasal congestion, and angioedema. Bleeding tendencies are enhanced by pentoxifylline administration.

In patients with a hyperinflammatory response, strategies to block the action of cytokines, such as TNF-α and IL-1-β, may decrease cell injury.[185] Monoclonal antibodies to TNF and an IL-1 receptor antagonist are being developed for use in humans.[185] However, antiinflammatory drugs, including those that block TNF and IL-1 receptors, used in neutropenic patients and in those in an advanced stage of sepsis when the patient is immunosuppressed may be detrimental.[68,141,185] Rather, immune stimulation with agents such as IFN-γ can enhance macrophage function and may be beneficial.[55,134,140,145]

The pathogenesis of sepsis is complex and interdependent. Manipulation of the inflammatory response awaits the accurate recognition of stages of the septic cascade. Recognition of the components that represent the body's appropriate compensatory response to sepsis that have salutary effects, markers of harmful hyperinflammation, and the terminal immunosuppressive stage when immune stimulation may be beneficial, must be standardized. Furthermore, rigorous trials will be required before mediator inhibition can become an accepted component of therapy for sepsis.

INFECTIVE ENDOCARDITIS

Endocarditis denotes inflammation of the endocardial surface of the heart.[31] IE, also referred to as *vegetative endocarditis* or *bacterial endocarditis*, is the invasion by an infectious microbe of the endothelial surface of the heart, usually the valves. It is not known if infective microbes colonize microscopic sterile lesions or directly invade normal endothelium.

Pathogenesis

When infectious microbes colonize a heart valve, they not only produce proliferative lesions (vegetations) but also destroy valvular tissue. The vegetations vary in size and shape, from small warty nodules to large, cauliflower-like masses (Fig. 87-3). The vegetations comprise three layers[1]: a large inner layer of platelets, fibrin, erythrocytes, leukocytes, and bacte-

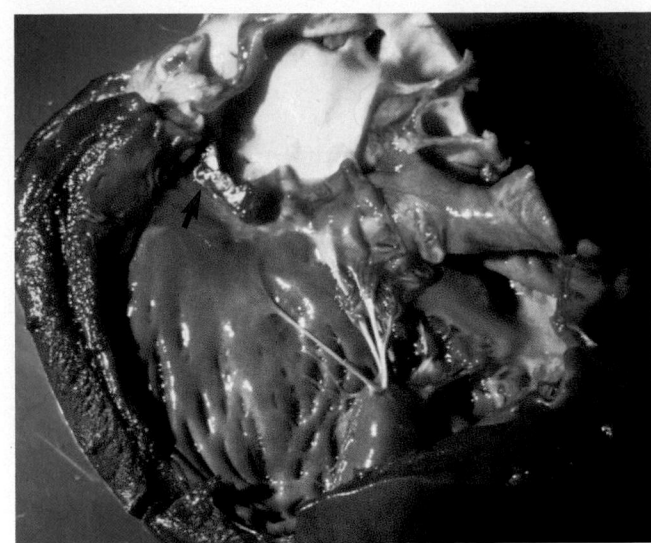

Fig 87-3 Aortic valve of dog with IE. One of the valve leaflets was pale, was cauliflower-like, was firm on palpation, and appeared to be calcified. (Courtesy University of Georgia, Athens, Ga.)

ria[2]; a middle layer of bacteria; and an outer layer of fibrin.[3] The bacterial colonies are found beneath the surface of the vegetation, and infiltration by phagocytic cells is minimal. This protected environment allows extremely high bacterial concentrations to develop. Deep within the fibrin-platelet matrix, bacteria often are in a state of reduced metabolic activity.

Bacteremia, Adherence, and Infectious Endocarditis

Bacteremia, either transient or permanent, must occur for IE to develop.[34] Surface changes may occur that result in deposition of platelets and fibrin that lead to a sterile vegetation. Bacteria must then reach this site, adhere to it, and then colonize. Certain bacterial strains are more capable of adhering and colonizing with a relatively low inoculum. Opossums and pigs can develop IE without prior valve damage,[177] and the same may be true of dogs. The most common bacteria of IE, streptococci and coagulase-positive staphylococci, adhere more quickly to the normal aortic valve than bacteria that uncommonly cause IE. Furthermore, the propensity to cause IE varies with the serotype of *S. aureus* in experimental models.

Organisms causing IE must be capable of adhering to a platelet-fibrin matrix. Production of adherence factors by bacteria facilitates the development of IE. Such factors include dextran and fibronectin-binding protein. Some strains of bacteria have been found to be potent stimulators of platelet aggregation, especially IE-producing streptococci and staphylococci. Clumping factor produced by coagulase-positive staphylococci favors attachment to fibrinogen and platelet-fibrin clots.[130] Culmination in IE involves the endothelium, hemostatic mechanisms, the host's immune system, surface properties of the microorganisms, and peripheral events that initiate bacteremia (Table 87-8). That the intact endothelium is resistant to infection can be deduced from the relative infrequency of IE compared to the known frequency of microbiemia.[33,34] Although phagocytic cells remove microbes from the blood, platelet-fibrin depositions may occur spontaneously, and at these sites microorganisms may adhere and initiate IE before the immune system can obliterate the infection. Adherence of coagulase-positive staphylococci to platelets is an important virulence factor. Furthermore, aspirin reduces *Staphylococcus*-induced platelet aggregation and adherence to fibrin.

Table • 87-8

Pathogenesis of Clinical Signs of Infectious Endocarditis

Valvular insufficiency and congestive heart failure
Bacteremia
Septic embolization and organ infarction
Metastatic infection and myocarditis
Immunopathologic sequelae and immune complex deposition
Glomerulonephritis
Uveitis
Polyarthritis
Meningitis

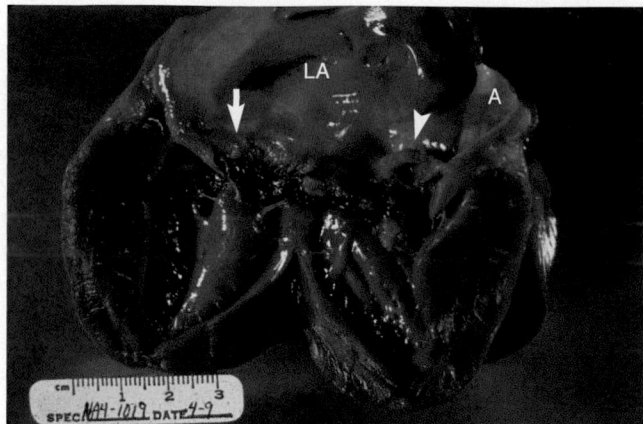

Fig 87-4 Opened left side of heart of dog with combined mitral *(arrow)* and aortic *(arrowhead)* valve bacterial endocarditis. Subendocardial hemorrhage is shown adjacent to portions of mitral valve. *LA*, Left atrium; *A*, aorta. (Courtesy University of Georgia, Athens, Ga.)

When staphylococci adhere to damaged valves, tissue thromboplastin is generated, which locally activates the clotting cascade, generating thrombin production. Thrombin elicits the secretion of a low molecular-weight protein with antimicrobial properties. Bacteria that are resistant to this factor are more likely to cause endocarditis. Once lodged on heart valves, bacteria must elude local defenses, including platelet microbicidal proteins and leukocytes if they are to survive. The presence of bacteria stimulates thrombosis mediated by thromboplastin generated from leukocytes adhering to fibrin.[12,104,172] Chronic, low-grade microbiemia increases the risk of IE.[32] Infective microorganisms in the blood must be capable of adhering to a platelet-fibrin matrix. Not only are leukocytes within this matrix unable to phagocytize bacteria, but the bacteria are very concentrated. Very few granulocytes are within the vegetation, and layers of fibrin, platelets, and erythrocytes protect the microorganisms.

The progression of the valvular lesion varies with the properties of the infecting organism. Some highly virulent organisms cause rapid necrosis and degeneration of the valve and more acute signs of heart failure. Other organisms of lower virulence produce a more gradual valvular injury and progressive cardiac signs. These organisms, such as *Bartonella*, often produce slowly enlarging vegetative lesions that increase in size over weeks or months and may become hardened or calcified. Resolution of an established endocardial proliferation is difficult because the colonies of bacteria are entrapped in an avascular coagulum of platelets, inflammatory cells, and fibrin that impedes antimicrobial drugs or immune defenses.

Valve Involvement

Heart valves are subject to constant trauma as they open and close. The incidence of IE appears to be directly related to the force placed on each valve. Lesions are generally located where high pressure and velocity of blood flow occurs. Prior valve or endocardial damage is one of the most important risk factors in the development of infection. The aortic valve is most commonly infected, followed in frequency by the mitral valve (Fig. 87-4). The tricuspid and pulmonic valves are seldom involved.[31-34] In a study of 45 dogs, 22 had aortic, 16 had mitral, 1 had both aortic and mitral, and 1 had tricuspid valve involvement.[31] The higher frequency of individual valves parallels the higher rate and pressure of blood flow in those regions.

Epidemiology

The prevalence of IE is much lower than dilated cardiomyopathy and myxomatous mitral valve degeneration. The incidences at two referral institutions were both approximately five cases per year.[31] Typically, affected dogs are 4 to 8 years old and medium or large sized; less than 10% weigh less than 10 kg.[31] Affected dogs are seldom younger than 2 or older than 10 years of age. German shepherds, boxers, golden retrievers, Labrador retrievers, and rottweilers may be overrepresented.[31] Males are affected more often than females; a 2:1 ratio, possibly a result of chronic bacterial prostatitis, has been reported.[31]

Vegetative endocarditis has been described in cats.* Organisms have included gram-positive and gram-negative bacteria, including *Bartonella* species (see Table 87-1). Evidence of concurrent disease has been found in some cats with endocarditis, including feline infectious peritonitis, thoracic lymphoma, mammary carcinoma, and megacolon.[36]

Predisposing Factors

Numerous factors predispose individuals to the development of microbiemia and IE. However, a common misconception is that IE is associated with structural heart disease. Mitral valve prolapse in humans is a common preexisting heart disorder in patients with IE. However, mitral valve prolapse is common, and the percentage of patients that develop IE is small. The risk of IE in patients with prolapse and regurgitation is fivefold to eightfold higher. Dogs with the highest incidence of myxomatous mitral valve degeneration (old, small-breed dogs) have a very low incidence of IE. Furthermore, IE is seldom associated with congenital heart diseases in dogs, with the exception of subvalvular aortic stenosis (SAS).[31] With SAS, turbulent, high-velocity blood flow in the outflow tract may produce micro-trauma on the valve leaflets and facilitate microbe colonization. Boxers, rottweilers, and golden retrievers have relatively high incidences of IE and SAS.[31,97] Less than 10% of dogs with SAS develop IE, and possibly less than 10% of dogs with IE have SAS.[31,97] Establishing or eliminating an ultrasound diagnosis of SAS with aortic valve IE is occasionally difficult because the vegetation may obscure the SAS lesion.

Predisposing factors for microbiemia include procedures involving the gingiva, oropharynx, GI tract, or infected tissues.[34] Endothelial damage can be produced by IV catheters. Portals of entry for microbes are also provided by wounds, biopsy sites, surgery, and urinary catheters. Although

*References 35, 36, 53, 115, 138, 164, 183.

gingivitis and stomatitis may be associated with bacteremia and bacterial endocarditis, dogs with the highest prevalence of oral infections (old, small-breed dogs) seldom develop IE.[31] Hypercoagulability associated with malignancies, DIC, hypercortisolemia, or immune-mediated diseases may predispose an individual to IE. Any abnormality that either is associated with chronic bacteremia (gingivitis, urinary or prostatic infection, pyoderma, and wounds) or impairs host defenses (such as neoplasia, diabetes mellitus, hyperadrenocorticism, exogenous glucocorticoids, or other immunosuppressive therapies) increases the risk of IE.[33,34] The source of infection may be suspected but is proven in less than 50% of dogs with IE.[31,33,34]

Damaged endothelium exposes the extracellular polysaccharide dextran, which facilitates the attachment of some bacterial species. Because of the limited species of microbes that account for the vast majority of IE cases, it can be deduced that certain organisms (such as coagulase-positive staphylococci and some streptococci) have an increased ability to colonize the endocardium. Fibronectin can be produced by endothelial cells and platelets in response to vascular injury, and receptors for fibronectin are present on the surface of some bacteria, including coagulase-positive staphylococci and some streptococci. Fibronectin can facilitate the adherence of some bacteria, including staphylococci, to intact endothelium.

Glucocorticoids

Dogs affected with IE often have a history of receiving glucocorticoids.[31] In some instances, glucocorticoids were administered in the weeks preceding the development of IE as a component of treatment for illness that was associated with unrecognized bacteremia, for the treatment of skin disease, or for the treatment for presumed immune-mediated disease. Dogs receiving glucocorticoids have shorter survival rates than nonrecipients.[31]

Infective Microbes

The vast majority of IE cases are the result of bacteria. Rickettsial agents are occasionally identified, but fungal IE is rare in dogs.[31,32,34] Although the range of microbial species capable of causing IE is large, only a few species account for most infections. Greater than 50% of infections in dogs are the result of coagulase-positive staphylococci and streptococci.[31,34,174] The association of streptococci and IE may be more closely related to the frequency with which they enter the blood stream and their ability to adhere to normal endocardium than their innate virulence. *S. intermedius* is the leading cause of IE in dogs. Although many species of gram-negative bacteria are cable of causing IE, they account for a small proportion of the total.

The prevalence of IE caused by anaerobic bacteria is unknown but as in humans is probably low. In humans, an important subgroup of cases are caused by a group of nutritionally fastidious gram-negative bacilli, *Hemophilus aphrophilus*, *Actinobacillus actinomycetemcomitans*, *Cardiobacterium hominis*, *Eikenella corrodens*, and *Kingella kingae*—a group often referred to by the acronym *HACEK*. Similarly, other fastidious agents such as *Brucella* species, *Bartonella* species, *Tropheryma whipplei*, *Coxiella burnetii*, and *Chlamydia* species have been incriminated as causative agents in culture-negative IE cases in humans.[127]

Bartonella species have been identified as an important cause of IE in dogs and cats (see Chapter 54). The prevalence of *Bartonella*, as well as other exotic organisms, is probably geographically variable. *Bartonella vinsonii* ssp. *berkhoffii*, *Bartonella clarridgeiae*, and a *Bartonella clarridgeiae*-like organism have been identified as a cause of endocarditis of dogs.[24,42] Additionally mitral valve endocarditis in a dog was caused by *Bartonella washoensis*.[43] *Bartonella henselae*, *Bartonella eliza-*bethae, and *Bartonella clarridgeiae* have been associated with systemic diseases and detection of *Bartonella* or their genomic DNA in blood of dogs.[74, 98,125,148]

Factors predisposing to fungal infections in humans, such as prosthetic valve replacement, IV drug abuse, chronic immunosuppressive therapy, and chronic broad-spectrum antibiotic usage are less common in dogs. In humans, *Candida* and *Aspergillus* species account for most cases of fungal IE.

Pathophysiology

Aside from the constitutional signs of infection, which are mediated by cytokines, the clinical manifestations of IE are the result of valvular destruction, embolic phenomena, and immune-complex disease. CHF is the usual outcome in dogs with aortic valve IE (see Table 87-8).[34]

Embolization leads to organ infarction and metastatic infection.[31] Embolization is a frequent cause of clinical signs and clinical deterioration. Even in the absence of clinical evidence, dogs always develop systemic emboli, and the kidneys are almost always infarcted. Emboli are usually present in many organs and tissues.[31,34]

Persistent bacteremia stimulates cell-mediated and humoral immune systems. CICs containing IgG, IgA, IgM, and complement may be deposited subendothelially along glomerular basement membranes, in joint capsules, and in blood vessels, leading to glomerulonephritis, arthritis, and vasculitis. Nonspecific antibodies can result in an increase in γ globulins and RF. Antiendocardial antibodies might be produced. Clinical signs of IE frequently mimic those of immune-mediated disorders, and positive immune-test results, such as Coombs' tests and ANA tests, can result from antigen-antibody-complement interactions.[31] RF, ANA, and CICs contribute to the development of polyarthritis, renal disease, and myocarditis.

Clinical Findings

IE shares many clinical features with nonendocarditis microbiemia. The manifestations of IE can mimic vasculitis, DIC, brucellosis, glomerulonephritis, malignancies, and immune-mediated diseases. Clinical findings in patients with possible endocarditis tend to be either sensitive or specific. For example, a diagnosis of IE based on fever and heart murmur would be sensitive but not very specific. On the other hand, the finding of an echocardiographic typical aortic valve lesion is specific.

Clinical signs associated with IE can be related to virtually any organ system. Fever is usual but is often not high grade. Fever is most likely to be absent in patients with chronic IE, with CHF, with renal failure, that are old, and that are receiving antibiotic treatment. Sequelae of IE include CHF, renal failure, proteinuria, splenomegaly, splenic abscess, musculoskeletal pain and weakness, kidney embolization, and signs consistent with embolism of the CNS.

Clinical signs and diagnostic abnormalities associated with IE are often nonspecific and frequently include extracardiac manifestations. The interval between the initiating bacteremic event and diagnosis of IE is usually uncertain, and a predisposing factor is not always evident.[31] Occasionally, a history of an illness exists that in retrospect may have initiated bacteremia 1 to 3 months before the diagnosis of IE.[31] Affected dogs may have signs of systemic infection, including fever and leukocytosis. Septic or sterile embolization or infarction, metastatic infections, and organ failure are responsible for many of the clinical signs.[31,34] These clinical signs are diverse and misleading—IE has frequently been called *the great imitator*. Owners variably report lethargy, depression, weakness, anorexia, weight loss, lameness, neurologic signs, and signs consistent with CHF. Often, fever is absent at the time of diagnosis because the bacteremia is low grade or because of previous therapy with antibiotics, glucocorticoids, or nonsteroidal antiinflammatory drugs.[31,34]

Heart Murmurs

Cardiac sequelae include valvular insufficiency because infection destroys the valvular tissue and interferes with function. The severity of destruction varies with chronicity and the virulence of the organism. IE is a cause of an aortic regurgitation murmur, and the aorta is the most commonly infected valve. Systolic murmurs result from mitral regurgitation or systolic flow turbulence generated by aortic valve vegetation. A murmur of recent onset, especially with a diastolic component, in the presence of fever is very suggestive of IE.[31] The femoral pulses associated with mitral valve IE are typically normal, although they may be weak if left-sided CHF is present.[31] The femoral pulses associated with aortic valve IE may be normal. However, they may be hyperdynamic and bounding because the systolic pulse pressure with aortic regurgitation is increased because of volume overload and resultant increased stroke volume, and the diastolic pressure is low because of arterial blood runoff back into the left ventricle during diastole. Thus not only may the diastolic pressure be low, but the systolic pressure wave duration may be shortened.

Lameness

Lameness is an occasional finding rarely caused by septic emboli but is usually the result of immune-mediated arthritis.[31] Synovial tissue may contain IgG, IgM, and complement, indicating an immune basis for the arthropathy.

Organ Failure

The affected dog may show signs consistent with CHF, usually on the left side, including coughing, dyspnea, pulmonary crackles (pulmonary edema), shortness of breath, weakness, or collapse.[31] CHF is most frequently associated with aortic valve IE. When the left side of the heart appears radiographically to be a normal size but pulmonary edema is present, the clinician should consider IE, because dramatic heart enlargement may not have time to develop in cases of acute IE. The index of suspicion of IE rises in dogs that have no history of a heart murmur or are not prone to cardiomyopathy or myxomatous valvular degeneration.[31]

Renal failure is another complication that may detract from recognition of IE. Renal failure is usually due to chronic infarction and glomerulonephritis.[31,33]

Polysystemic Signs

The constitutional signs of IE can mimic those of any polysystemic disease.[31] Many differential diagnoses must be considered, including immune-mediated diseases, rickettsial infections, bacteremia alone, sequelae of neoplasia, causes of CHF, and causes of renal failure.[24,31,33,34] Localized signs, such as lameness, edema, and pain often arise from complications of infection.[31] To avoid overlooking IE, the possibility should be investigated when one or more of the elements of endocarditis exist: (1) an unexplained fever, (2) a heart murmur of recent onset, (3) a source of infection, and (4) embolic phenomena.

Systemic Embolization

Embolization is a constant and important complication of IE but is often undetected before death. The presence of infection-related antiphospholipid antibodies may be a risk factor for embolic events. The kidneys consistently exhibit old and new infarcts that contribute to proteinuria and renal failure (Fig. 87-5, A). Other organs that may be infarcted include spleen (Fig. 87-5, B), brain (Fig. 87-5, C), and intestinal mucosa (Fig. 87-5, D). Pathologic kidney symptoms are con-sistently found in dogs with IE; infarction, glomerulonephritis, and abscess are the three pathologic processes, abscesses being least common. The liver and iliac or mesenteric arteries may be embolized. Splenic septic abscesses may contribute to persistent fever and leukocytosis.

Diagnosis

The diagnosis of IE requires integration of clinical and laboratory data. The most important criteria for the diagnosis of IE are (1) multiple positive blood culture results of usual culprit microbes, such as *S. intermedius* or streptococci; (2) typical electrocardiogram (ECG) findings, such as oscillating valvular mass; and (3) a murmur of recent onset, especially if it is diastolic. Clinical findings supportive of the diagnosis of IE include fever, an inflammatory leukogram, embolic phenomena, evidence of glomerulonephritis, and positive results for immune tests such as for RF and ANA. IE shares many clinical features with nonendocarditis microbiemia. The manifestations of IE also can mimic vasculitis, DIC, rickettsemia, brucellosis, glomerulonephritis, malignancies, and immune-mediated diseases. The advent of ECG has greatly facilitated the diagnosis. Because the aortic valve is usually involved, if IE is suspected ultrasonographic recognition is seldom difficult. Diagnosis of mitral valve IE is more difficult because the lesions of myxomatous degeneration can resemble those of IE. It should be recognized that those dogs with the highest incidence of myxomatous degeneration of the mitral valve (old, small-breed dogs) seldom are affected with IE. Signalment, clinical findings, femoral pulse characteristics, confirmation of bacteremia, and a murmur of recent onset, especially a diastolic murmur, are important to the diagnosis of IE if ECG is not available (Table 87-9).

Clinical Laboratory Findings

Hematologic findings of systemic inflammation are often absent. This may be a result of prior antibiotic or steroid administration or chronic, low-grade bacteremia.[31,34] Hematologic abnormalities include anemia, usually normocytic-normochromic and nonregenerative; thrombocytopenia; an inflammatory leukogram; and monocytosis. Left shift of the leukogram may be absent, mild, or moderate depending on the chronicity. Proteinuria, microscopic hematuria, casts, and bacteruria are variably present on urinalysis. Although an inflammatory leukogram does not always result, monocytosis is present in 90% of cases.[31,34] In some instances, mature neutrophilia and monocytosis indicate low-grade, chronic inflammation. Thrombocytopenia can be attributed to systemic vasculitis and immune or coagulatory consumption.[31,34]

A septic triad of low serum albumin concentration, high serum ALP activity, and low blood glucose levels can be seen in dogs with bacteremia and endocarditis. The high serum ALP activity is likely a result of the effect of bacterial toxins on biliary flow and excretion; icterus may be found in severe instances. The hypoglycemia is caused by effects of bacteria or their toxins on glucose metabolism.

Azotemia may be prerenal or caused by infarction and glomerulopathy. With embolization, the urine often contains protein, blood, casts, bacteria, or all of these.[31,33] Urine culture is recommended, not only because bacteria are filtered from the blood into the urine but also because the urinary tract may be a source of infection.[31,33] Patients with glomerular disease have proteinuria; however, the urinary sediment does not contain cells.

The presence of bacteria in endocardial vegetations stimulates the humoral immune system to produce nonspecific antibodies. This can result in an increase in γ-globulins, and antiendocardial antibodies may be produced. CICs are produced, and their concentrations correlate with extracardiac manifestations such as arthritis, splenomegaly, and glomeru-

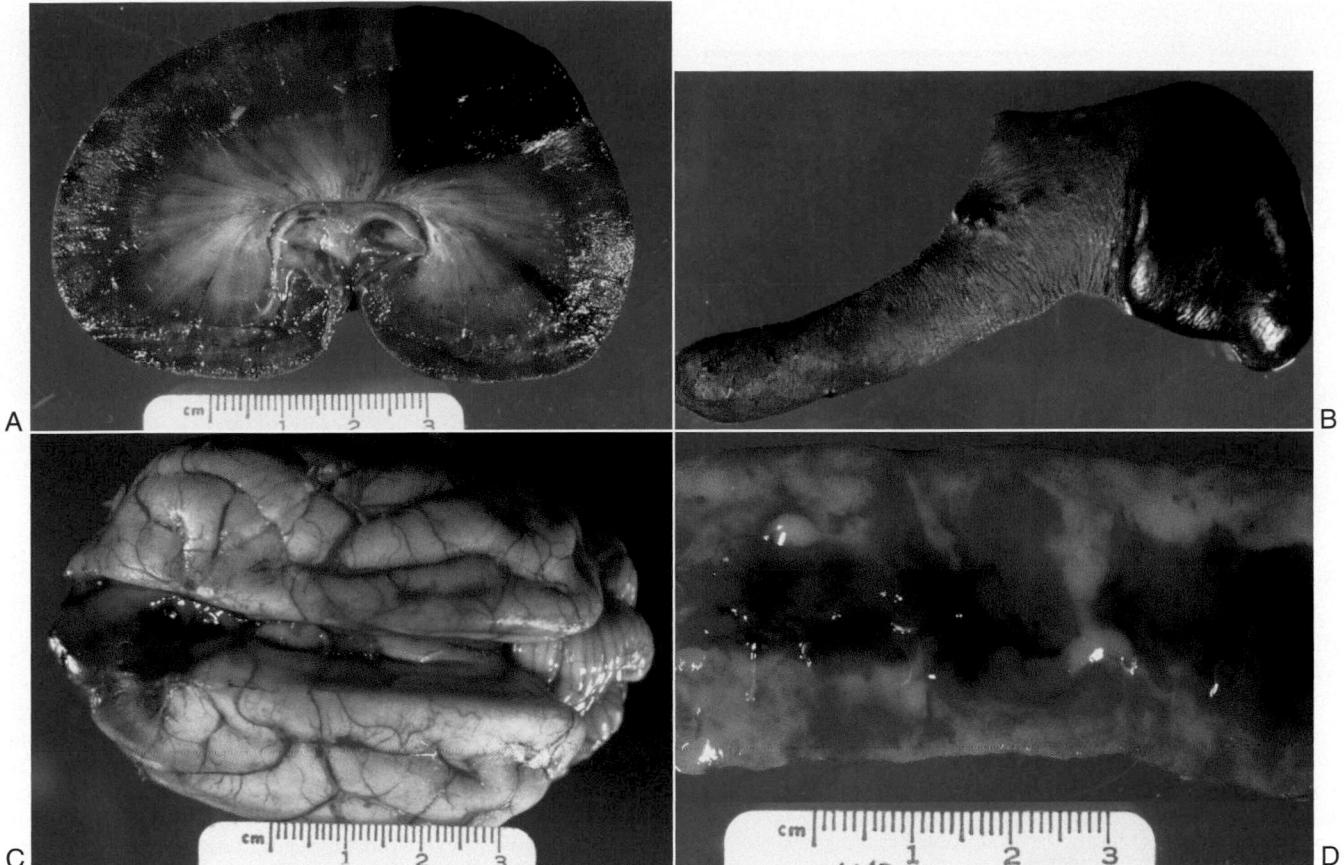

Fig 87-5 Organs from dog with aortic endocarditis and infarcts in various organs. **A,** Wedge-shape triangular infarct in kidney. **B,** One end of spleen. **C,** Left side of forebrain. **D,** Intestinal mucosa. (Courtesy University of Georgia, Athens, Ga.)

lonephritis. RF (anti-IgG IgM antibody) develops in some patients with IE, and the titers decrease with antibiotic therapy. ANAs may also develop and may contribute to fever, pain, and musculoskeletal symptoms. Opsonic (IgG), agglutinating (IgG, IgM), and complement-fixing (IgG, IgM) antibody synthesis are typical.

Identification of Bacteremia

Blood cultures should always be performed in an attempt to identify the offending organisms, but they lack sensitivity and specificity.[32,34,56] Performed properly, positive blood culture results are often obtained[31-33] (in the authors' experience, in approximately 30% to 50% of patients). Decreased sensitivity may be explained by improper laboratory techniques, the failure to culture for anaerobes, low bacterial concentrations in blood, endogenous bactericidal factors (complement and phagocytes), intermittent shedding of the organism, chronic IE with encapsulated vegetative lesions, or infections with fastidious slow-growing organisms such as *Bartonella*.[24,25,33,56]

The term *culture-negative IE* refers to active IE cases with multiple negative culture results. Many such cases are the result of antibiotic treatment that is sufficient to suppress bacteremia but not sterilize the vegetation. Other causes are *Bartonella* species, slow-growing bacteria such as HACEK, some streptococci, *Mycobacterium* species, nutritionally fastidious microbes requiring special procedures or supplemental media, and anaerobic microbes.[84,181]

Many negative blood culture results in humans with IE are caused by infection with *Bartonella* species, which are fastidious, gram-negative organisms.[26] The prevalence of *Bartonella*-IE is being recognized with increasing frequency in dogs and

cats as newer culture methods and the polymerase chain reaction (PCR) have been used. *Bartonella* organisms reside within the erythrocytes of their reservoir host and are present in low numbers in inadvertent hosts, making them difficult to isolate from blood cultures because special techniques are recommended.[24-26] *Bartonella* species can occasionally be isolated by prolonged incubation and subculture in broth media onto endothelial cell tissue.[57,106,168] Tissue culture methods may be required for obligate, intracellular organisms, such as *Coxiella* species, and for *Chlamydia*. Extraction of nucleic acid from blood and subsequent PCR amplification has been beneficial in the early diagnosis of bacteremia and confirmation of infection with fastidious or unculturable agents.[25,26] Because some anaerobes and members of the HACEK group are slow growing, holding cultures for 4 weeks may increase the recovery rate. In postmortem or surgical specimens, PCR of infected valvular tissue has greatly enhanced the detection and identification of organisms causing endocarditis in people that is blood-culture negative.[155]

Special Diagnostics

The diagnosis of IE requires integration of clinical and laboratory findings. Arrhythmias, usually atrial or ventricular premature contractions, are present in at least 50% to 75% of documented cases, seldom life threatening, and best evaluated by long-term continuous ECG monitoring, either cage side or by Holter recording. Other less common ECG abnormalities include bundle branch blocks and atrioventricular blocks. Radiographic interpretation may reveal chamber enlargements or no abnormalities. Chamber enlargement, most commonly left atrial, is usually present when IE is chronic.[31] If

Table • 87-9

Criteria for the Antemortem Diagnosis of Infective Endocarditis

Without Echocardiographic Examination
All of the following criteria should be met:
A murmur of recent onset
Positive blood culture results (preferably with more than one of the same microbe)
Clinical findings and laboratory data consistent with bacteremia and endocarditis

With Echocardiographic Examination
Aortic valve: Echocardiographic appearance is pathognomonic.
Mitral valve: Echocardiographic appearance is suggestive of endocarditis.

Supportive Clinical Findings
Signalment
Murmur of recent onset
Weak or hyperdynamic pulse
Fever
Limb edema
Joint swelling
Lameness
Limb ischemia
Limb hyperesthesia
Inflammatory leukogram
Positive blood culture results

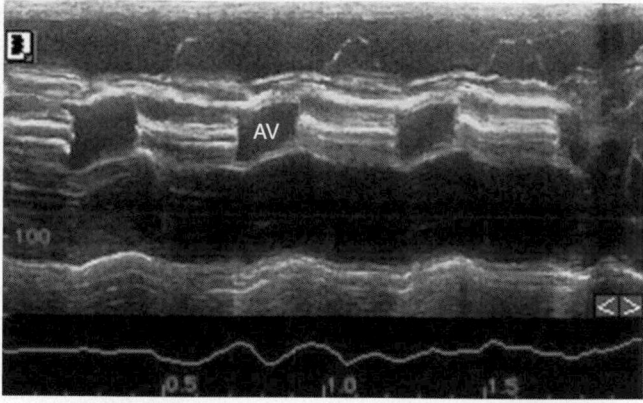

Fig 87-6 M-mode echocardiogram of thickened aortic valve *(AV)*. This echocardiographic image is typical of aortic valve vegetations.

overt or impending left-sided CHF is present, pulmonary edema, distention of the pulmonary veins, or both are present.[31]

ECG is the best diagnostic tool but is neither 100% sensitive nor 100% specific. Modern, two-dimensional equipment can detect small lesions. Detection of an echogenic oscillating vegetative mass on the aortic or mitral valve is a strong indication of the presence of IE. Both the M-mode and two-dimensional appearance of aortic valve vegetations is virtually pathognomonic for IE (Fig. 87-6). Echoes from vegetations on the mitral valve are usually on the cranial (anterior) leaflet but are not pathognomonic (although in some cases, the lesion is so large, is oscillating, or both that IE should be suspected). Operator skill and experience, as well as image quality, influence interpretation. Furthermore, results must be considered in the context of other clinical and laboratory findings. A false-positive test interpretation is most commonly attributable to mitral valve myxomatous degeneration. The clinician should always take into consideration the signalment and the history of the dog in question. The signalment associated with IE is largely different from that of dogs with advanced myxomatous degeneration. The presence of a new heart murmur is of special importance if the breed or age of the patient is not characteristic of dogs affected by myxomatous valvular degeneration.

Chamber enlargements and altered contractility may be evident.[31] Decreased contractility is typical of the high-pressure volume overload of advanced aortic valve IE but not of the low-pressure volume overload of mitral valve IE. Decreased contractility may also be related to chronicity of volume overload. Diastolic fluttering of the anterior (cranial) mitral valve leaflet is indicative of aortic insufficiency and therefore suggestive of IE. This fluttering is the result of the jet of aortic regurgitation striking the anterior (cranial) mitral valve leaflet when it is open in diastole. Color flow imaging is used to identify hemodynamic consequences of IE, such as valvular regurgitation or left ventricular outflow tract turbulence (Fig. 87-7, *A* and *B*). Doppler interrogation of aortic regurgitation is used to confirm the severity (Fig. 87-7, *C* and *D*). The spectral display of severe aortic regurgitation is characterized by a rapid deceleration of regurgitant velocity during diastole. A steep slope of regurgitation indicates a large regurgitant volume. Severe aortic regurgitation is incompatible with survival.

Therapy

Antibiotics and Other Drugs

Within the vegetation, organisms are protected, become metabolically dormant, and are less vulnerable to the killing activities of antimicrobials.[32] Prolonged parenteral administration of one or more bactericidal antibiotics is recommended. The goal of treatment is to kill the organism and minimize and manage the consequences of infection. Therapy ideally is based on blood culture antibiogram results, but treatment is usually initiated before results are received.[181,182] In spite of in vitro antibiotic susceptibility, complete eradication takes weeks to achieve. The difficulty of cure is a result of impaired host defense in a tightly encased fibrin meshwork in which the bacterial colonies are relatively free from phagocytes. Furthermore, the bacteria within these vegetations reach tremendous concentrations. At these high populations the bacteria may be in a state of reduced metabolic activity and cell division. They are less susceptible to antibiotics requiring cell wall synthesis and division for maximum activity.

Antimicrobial therapy should be bactericidal, and antibiotic serum concentrations should be high (Table 87-10), because antibiotics reach the central areas of avascular vegetations by passive diffusion. High concentrations are needed, therefore parenteral treatment is preferred to oral therapy. The fluoroquinolones may penetrate better into vegetations than some cephalosporins.[46] Antibiotic combinations should rapidly produce a bactericidal effect, such as those produced by the synergism of a penicillin plus an aminoglycoside. High serum concentrations are mandatory, and antibiotic serum concentrations should be maintained at the high end of the therapeutic range for at least 1 month. At least 1 to 2 weeks of IV antibiotic therapy is recommended, which is followed by SC administration for several weeks if possible; then oral bactericidal antibiotics should be continued for several months (see Table 87-5). When switching from parenteral to

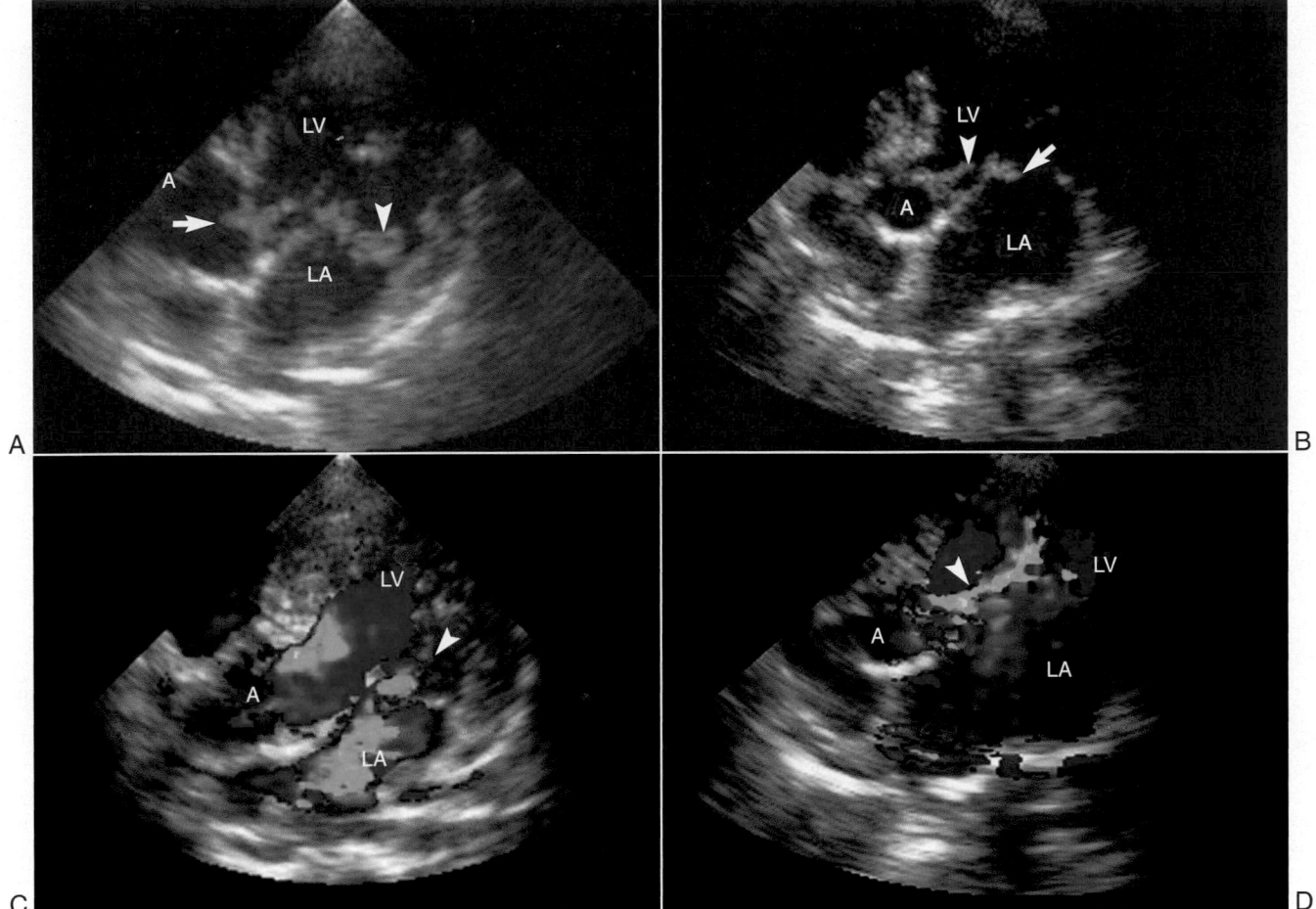

Fig   87-7 Two-dimensional echocardiogram in left apical, long axis, two-chamber imaging plane. **A,** During systole, aortic valve leaflet thickened by vegetation *(arrow)* is opened into aorta *(A)*. Vegetations are also seen on mitral valve leaflets *(arrowhead)*, which reside between left atrium *(LA)* and left ventricle *(LV)*. **B,** In diastole, vegetative aortic valve is closed, and portion of vegetation is protruding *(arrowhead)* into left ventricle *(LV)*. Open cranial (anterior) mitral valve leaflet is also thickened by vegetation *(arrow)*. **C,** Color-flow Doppler imaging in systole demonstrating turbulent mitral regurgitation *(arrowhead)*. **D,** Color-flow Doppler imaging in diastole demonstrating turbulent jet of aortic regurgitation *(arrowhead)*. *LA,* Left atrium.

Table • **87-10**

Principles of Antibiotic Therapy of Infective Endocarditis

1. Use bactericidal antibiotics.
2. Ensure high antibiotic serum concentrations by administering high dosages intravenously (IV).
3. Continue IV antibiotic administration for at least 1 to 2 weeks.
4. When IV administration of antibiotics is no longer practical, replace with subcutaneous (SC) administration.
5. Continue antibiotic therapy for at least 2 to 3 months.
6. Use oral antibiotics only after at least 1 month of IV and SC administration.

oral therapy, the oral bioavailability of the drug should be considered, and higher oral than parenteral doses should be used. For example, absorption of the oral penicillins and cephalosporins is lower, and levels can only be obtained by increasing the dosage. Lipid-soluble drugs such as clindamycin achieve a similar peak serum concentration by oral or parenteral dosing.

The most common infective bacteria are known, and their antimicrobial susceptibility patterns are somewhat predictable and the same as those associated with bacteremia alone (see Table 87-5). The choice for SC antibiotic administration should ideally be based on an antibiogram, but if blood culture results are negative or cultures not performed, ceftiofur, azithromycin, or ticarcillin may be used.

IE caused by anaerobes is uncommon in humans, but mortality is high. Penicillin, metronidazole, ticarcillin-clavulanate, or imipenem are good choices. Clindamycin is not recommended in humans because of its lack of bactericidal action. The HACEK organisms are sensitive to newer third-generation cephalosporins (ceftriazone or cefotaxime), which are the antibiotics of choice.[181]

P. aeruginosa-endocarditis is usually responsive to the combination of tobramycin and either extended-spectrum penicillin (ticarcillin, piperacillin) or ceftazidime.

Bacteriostatic antibiotics are generally ineffective in the treatment of IE. Failure to control the infection and latent relapses are common. An apparent response to tetracycline, erythromycin, or clindamycin should not be interpreted as indicative of successful treatment.

Table • 87-11

Supportive Therapy for Infectious Endocarditis

DRUG[a]	SPECIES	DOSE[b]	ROUTE	INTERVAL (HOURS)	DURATION (DAYS)
Enalapril or benazepril	B	0.25 mg/kg	PO	12—24	prn
	D	0.5 mg/kg	PO	12—24	prn
Spironolactone	D	1—2 mg/kg	PO	12	prn
Digoxin	D	0.005—0.01 mg/kg	PO	12	prn
	C	0.008—0.01 mg/kg	PO	24	prn
Pimobendan	D	0.3 mg/kg	PO	12	prn
Furosemide	D	0.5—2.0 mg/kg	PO	12	prn
	C	1—4 mg/kg	PO, SC, IV	12	prn
Amlodipine or felodipine	D	0.1 mg/kg	PO	12	Varies[c]
	C	0.625 mg/cat	PO	24	prn

B, Dog and cat; D, dog; C, cat; PO, by mouth; SC, subcutaneous; IV, intravenous; prn, as needed.
[a]For additional information about the drugs listed, see Appendix 8.
[b]Dose per administration at specified interval.
[c]Should be titrated every 4 to 7 days to a maximum of 0.4 mg/kg every 12 hours PO.

Supportive therapy is always a component of treatment (Table 87-11). Acid-base, fluid, and electrolyte balance must be addressed. Nutritional support may be an important component of therapy and may be maintained by either parenteral or tube alimentation. The consequences of valvular destruction must be addressed. Although a positive influence on disease progression is unproven, angiotensin-converting enzyme (ACE) inhibition is usually recommended if unequivocal left atrial or left ventricular enlargement develops. Enalapril or benazepril are common choices. Spironolactone, an aldosterone antagonist, may be added to the regimen as cardiac enlargement progresses. A diuretic and possibly digoxin should be used if CHF is overt. Furosemide is the diuretic of choice. A serum digoxin concentration should be obtained after 7 days of treatment from a sample drawn at 6 hours after the morning dosage. For most laboratories, a desirable serum digoxin concentration is 1 to 1.5 ng/ml. Pimobendan is probably a better choice than digoxin. In addition to superior therapeutic index and inotropic action, it also has arteriolar dilating activity.

Augmented afterload reduction may be a useful adjunct to ACE inhibition. Adjuvant afterload reduction (arteriolar dilation) may result in reduction of aortic or mitral regurgitant volume. When the total peripheral arteriolar resistance is decreased by increasing the total arteriolar cross-sectional area, the change in relative resistance to systolic and diastolic blood flow facilitates increased forward stroke volume and decreased aortic regurgitation. Systemic blood pressure should be monitored as adjuvant afterload reduction is initiated and up titrated. Amlodipine and felodipine are effective afterload reducers (see Table 87-11). Indirect blood pressure monitoring is important, although it is subject to inaccuracies. Dogs that subsequently developed signs of hypotension have consistently had lower indirect blood pressures compared with pretreatment and during early-dose titration. Up titration should be stopped if the systolic blood pressure is less than approximately 110 mm Hg or if the mitral regurgitation velocity measured by Doppler ultrasound is 4.5 to 5 m/s. This velocity range correlates with a systolic systemic blood pressure between 100 and 120 mm Hg. If clinical signs of hypotension (lethargy, trembling, weakness, anorexia) occur, amlodipine should be withdrawn for 24 hours and then reinstituted at the previous lower dosage. Severe hypotension is seldom encountered but requires IV fluid administration.

Anticoagulant Therapy
Anticoagulant therapy has not been shown to prevent embolization and may increase the risk of hemorrhage.[176] The role of aspirin in preventing embolization is being evaluated.[104] Studies confirm the use of aspirin in reducing the size of vegetations and microbial density within vegetations.[136] Aspirin may reduce bacterial dissemination and embolic events.[104]

Prognosis
The prognosis for long-term survival is poor.[31-34] Early diagnosis followed immediately by aggressive antibiotic therapy is critical for long-term survival, especially when the aortic valve is infected. Unfortunately, early diagnosis is difficult, and valvular damage is often advanced by the time of diagnosis. Aortic valve endocarditis is associated with a grave prognosis, for animals with this condition develop left-sided CHF, often within 1 to 3 months and almost always within 6 months of diagnosis. The trend in treating human patients with aortic valve endocarditis is to perform early valve replacement therapy.

Prevention
Chemoprophylaxis is controversial, for the risk-benefit ratio and economic rationale can be questioned, and clinical studies supporting efficacy are limited. The prophylactic use of antibiotics before medical procedures that cause bacteremia does not reduce the incidence of IE; this is not surprising because only a small proportion of all cases are attributable to such procedures. Chemoprophylaxis, even if effective, is not applicable to the majority of cases. However, the mortality associated with IE warrants chemoprophylaxis in patients at increased risk.

It is recommended to use prophylactic antibiotics when dental scaling, dental extractions, or surgery are performed in dogs with congenital heart diseases. Such procedure-focused chemoprophylaxis should not be initiated several days before the procedure because of the potential to select for antibiotic resistant organisms. Rather, it should be administered just before and after the procedure (see Chapter 89). For oral and dental procedures in patients that are at increased risk, ticarcillin or a first-generation cephalosporin, administered IV 1 hour before and repeated 6 hours after the procedure, is reasonable. Incision and drainage of infected skin are associated with coagulase-positive staphylococci, and either a first-generation cephalosporin, ticarcillin, or ticarcillin-clavulanate is a good choice for prophylaxis. Maintenance of oral hygiene is a more important preventive than procedure-focused chemoprophylaxis.

The male urinary tract is suspected to be a common source of chronic bacteremia, therefore castration can be viewed as a prophylactic measure because it reduces the risk of bacterial prostatitis.

INFECTIOUS MYOCARDITIS

Myocarditis (inflammation of the myocytes, interstitium, and vasculature) may result from primary or secondary causes. Active and chronic myocardial disease may be associated with infectious diseases of dogs (Table 87-12), and the relevant chapters should be consulted for additional information. Myocarditis secondary to infectious agents may be subclinical if the inflammation is focal and limited. Severe or diffuse myocarditis results in fever, malaise, weakness, cardiac

Table • 87-12

Infectious Causes of Myocarditis

Viruses
Canine distemper virus (neonate; see Chapter 3)
Canine parvovirus (prenatal, neonate; see Chapter 8)
Canine herpesvirus (see Chapter 5)
West Nile virus (see Chapter 26)

Rickettsiae
Rickettsia rickettsii (see Chapter 29)

Bacteria
Numerous genera
Borrelia burgdorferi (see Chapter 45)
Bartonella henselae (see Chapter 54, Cat)
Bartonella vinsonii ssp. *berkhoffii* (see Chapter 54, Dog)

Algae
Prototheca species (see Chapter 69)

Fungi
Cryptococcus neoformans (see Chapter 61)
Coccidioides immitis (see Chapter 62)
Aspergillus terreus (see Chapter 64)
Paecilomyces varioti (see Chapter 67)

Protozoans
Trypanosoma cruzi (see Chapter 72)
Toxoplasma gondii (see Chapter 80)
Hepatozoon americanum (see Chapter 74)
Neospora caninum (see Chapter 80)

Unknown
Transmissible myocarditis-diaphragmitis of cats

arrhythmia, and CHF. CHF caused by necrotizing myocarditis can be a lethal complication of neonatal canine parvovirus infection,[1,135] but it is rare because of the widespread existence of immune dams. PCR for viruses in paraffin-embedded myocardium from dogs with dilated cardiomyopathy and myocarditis have been screened for presence of canine parvovirus, adenovirus types 1 and 2, and herpesvirus.[122] Only adenovirus 1 nucleic acid sequences were detected in the heart of one dog. Natural West Nile virus infection in canids has been associated with myocarditis that accompanies the encephalitis.[30,111] Myocarditis, the feline panleukopenia virus genome, or both were detected in cats with idiopathic hypertrophic, dilated, and restrictive cardiomyopathy, suggesting a possible role of viral infection and inflammation in the pathogenesis of cardiomyopathy in this species.[124] Results were negative for herpesvirus, calicivirus, and coronavirus. In people, coxsackievirus B3 was detected in the heart muscle of approximately 50% of people with dilated cardiomyopathy.[51,66,92,95] The presumption is that injury by this cardiotropic virus leads to the production of autoantibodies specific for heart muscle and infiltrates of immune cells. Chlamydial infections have also been associated with myocarditis as they have been with endocarditis in people. Chlamydial infections lead to the activation of autoaggressive lymphocytes reactive to heart-specific antigens because of molecular mimicry with bacterial antigens.[151] Neither of these human pathogens has been incriminated as a cause of myocarditis in dogs or cats; however, a similar mechanism of autoimmune myocarditis may be triggered by myocardial infection.

Suppurative myocarditis that resulted in syncope was found in two sibling boxer puppies and was associated with *Citrobacter koseri* infection.[37] As a saprophyte the organism is considered to be an opportunist, and concurrent immunosuppression, possibly by parvovirus infection, was suspected in the dogs. Similar to their propensity to cause endocarditis, *Bartonella* species have been identified as the cause of myocarditis and endocarditis in dogs and cats (see Chapter 54). Cardiac arrhythmias, endocarditis, or myocarditis was identified in dogs with weight loss, syncope, collapse, or sudden death, often without fever.[24] Cats experimentally or naturally infected with *B. henselae* or *B. clarridgeiae* have had lymphocytic myocarditis histologically in association with inflammation of other organs, including concurrent endocarditis.[101]

Dogs infected with *Trypanosoma cruzi* develop granulomatous myocarditis that can cause heart failure and heart rhythm disturbance.[10,114] *Neospora caninum* and *Borrelia burgdorferi* can infect the myocardium, but the disease is usually mild and overshadowed by clinical signs associated with other organ or system involvement. However, sudden death has occurred as a result of *Neospora* myocarditis.[142]

The diagnosis of myocarditis is usually made when ventricular tachyarrhythmias, with or without ST segment changes, are detected in patients with evidence of systemic diseases. The interpretation of elevated levels of the myocardial fraction of serum muscle enzymes such as creatinine kinase (CK), lactic dehydrogenase, and aspartate aminotransferase has not been evaluated in dogs. Specific serologic testing is available for some of the underlying diseases. Therapy is directed at the primary infectious agent, control of cardiac arrhythmia, and treatment of CHF.

TRANSMISSIBLE MYOCARDITIS-DIAPHRAGMITIS OF CATS

Transmissible myocarditis-diaphragmitis is a sporadic disease, primarily affects adult cats, and occurs most commonly in the summer months. It has been reported in California and Florida.[78,150]

Although the disease can be experimentally transmitted between cats, the organism has not been identified.[150] A viral agent may be involved, and the disease resembles coxsackievirus B infection of people and other animals.[110] Clinical signs in cats include transient fever occurring 9 to 30 days after inoculation and usually lasting for 1 to 3 days. Some cats have a second fever spike. Lethargy, rough hair coat, and anorexia correlate with the fever. Hematologic and biochemical abnormalities are absent except for high serum CK activity in some cats. Gross necropsy findings during the febrile period are pale foci surrounded by hemorrhage in the ventricular myocardium and diaphragm. Gross lesions were absent in cats that had recovered. Myonecrosis and cellular infiltration predominantly composed of neutrophils but occasionally including macrophages have been found in heart and diaphragmatic muscle. In acutely infected cats, lymphoid tissues showed reactive changes and mild neutrophilic-histocytic infiltrates in the liver and renal interstitium.

Evidence in people shows that viral myocarditis may result in development of chronic inflammatory heart disease and dilated cardiomyopathy. Whether this infection in cats has any relationship to some cases of feline cardiomyopathy remains to be determined.

INFECTIOUS PERICARDIAL EFFUSION

Etiology

Many causes have been attributed to pericardial effusion in dogs and cats (Tables 87-13 and 87-14). Pericarditis (inflammation of the fibrous and serous layers of the pericardium) caused by infectious agents is uncommon but can be a sequelae of the bacteremia of staphylococci, streptococci, and *E. coli*. Pericarditis may result from local (pleural or pulmonary) infections, secondary to trauma, or from hematogenous spread of microorganisms.[70] Anaerobic bacteria and *Actinomyces*, *Nocardia*, *Mycobacterium*, and *Aspergillus* species are most likely to spread from pleural infections or migrating foreign bodies (see Chapters 41, 49, 50, and 64). Hematogenous infections of the pericardium can occur when infectious organisms embolize in the myocardial or pericardial vasculature. Bacteremias and viral infections, such as feline infectious peritonitis (see Chapter 11), can cause effusive pericarditis. Many viruses have been associated with pericarditis in people. Idiopathic pericardial effusion (IPE) in dogs is characterized by a hemorrhagic effusion but no identifiable cause. PCR was used to screen 10 IPE effusions for the presence of nucleic acid from coxsackie virus B, influenza type A virus, adenovirus type 2, parvovirus B19, cytomegalovirus, *B. burgdorferi*, and *Chlamydia pneumoniae*.[187] One specimen had positive tests results for influenza type A virus, and another tested positive for cytomegalovirus.

Pericarditis may be effusive or constrictive, but in the dog and cat it is almost always effusive. Effusions of infectious pericarditis are either modified transudates or exudates and usually serosanguineous or bloody.

Clinical Findings

The infectious nature of the underlying agent and the severity of pericardial effusion determine the findings of the patient's history. A recent history of fever and an inflammatory leukogram is occasional. Weight loss, weakness, dyspnea, and abdominal effusion are variable signs. Fever is an inconsistent finding, varying with the infectious agent and time course of the disease. As the severity of the pericardial effusion worsens, dyspnea, weakness, and abdominal effusion become pronounced.

The principal physical findings reflect external cardiac compression. As the effusion becomes more extensive, the intrapericardial pressure rises to or exceeds right atrial diastolic pressure. Intracardiac pressure increases, ventricular diastolic filling is impaired, and stroke volume is reduced. The central venous pressure is increased, and venous return to the right atrium is impaired, resulting in signs of right-sided heart failure. Jugular pulses and distention of the jugular veins are often present. Subsequently, increased venous pressure can lead to pleural and abdominal effusions. The triad of increased central venous pressure, as with evident jugular pulses, weak peripheral arterial pulses, and muffled heart sounds, is suggestive of pericardial effusion but can also occur with dilated cardiomyopathy.

When the effusion is severe, the heart and lung sounds are not clearly audible. Mucous membrane color is often pale, and the peripheral pulses are weak because of decreased cardiac output. A reflex tachycardia is often present.

Diagnosis

Thoracic radiographs are always abnormal when pericardial effusion is severe enough to produce cardiovascular impairment. However, because the pericardial and cardiac silhouettes cannot be distinguished by simple radiographs, the size of the heart and the severity of effusion cannot be accurately determined. In some cases, pleural effusion may partially obscure the pericardial-cardiac silhouette.

Massive effusion is characterized by a greatly enlarged, round cardiac silhouette in which the borders are smooth

Table • 87-13

Causes of Pericardial Effusion in 42 Dogs

CAUSE	NUMBER OF DOGS WITH SIGNS
Neoplastic	24 (57%)
Idiopathic hemorrhagic	8 (19%)
Cardiac	6 (14%)
Traumatic	2 (5%)
Uremic	1 (2%)
Infectious	1 (2%)

Data from Berg RJ, Wingfield W. 1994. Pericardial effusion in the dog: a review of 42 cases, *J Am Anim Hosp Assoc* 20:721–730.

Table • 87-14

Causes of Pericardial Effusion in 84 Cats

CAUSE	NUMBER OF CATS WITH SIGNS
Cardiac	20 (24%)
Feline infectious peritonitis	16 (19%)
Neoplastic	13 (15%)
Infectious (other than feline infectious peritonitis)	12 (14%)
Renal failure	9 (11%)
Coagulopathies	7 (8%)
Miscellaneous	5 (6%)
Iatrogenic	2 (2%)

Data from Rush JE et al. 1987. Retrospective study of pericardial disease in cats, *Proc Am Coll Vet Intern Med* 5:922; Harpster NK. The cardiovascular system. In Holzworth J (ed). 1987. p 820. *Diseases of the cat: medicine and surgery*. WB Saunders, Philadelphia, PA.

without the normal protrusions produced by the chambers. The silhouette is flattened where it contacts the thoracic walls. The parenchymal lung fields are not affected unless the lungs are the primary source of infection. The lobar arteries may appear small because of decreased right ventricular output.

ECG changes may be present, particularly when the degree of effusion is severe. Low-voltage complexes, electrical alternans, and ST segment changes may be present. ECG is an accurate means of determining the presence and severity of effusion and cardiac function. In many cases, two-dimensional ultrasound examination is helpful in the detection of intrapericardial masses.

Pericardiocentesis is performed immediately if severe cardiovascular impairment has occurred secondary to severe effusions. Otherwise, pericardiocentesis is performed after radiographic, electrocardiographic, and ECG examinations.

Cytologic analysis and microbial culture of the effusion should always be performed. Infectious pericardial effusion is either serosanguineous or (more often) bloody. The protein content is greater than 2.5 mg/dl and is often in excess of 3.5 mg/dl. Neutrophils and to a lesser extent, erythrocytes, are the predominant cell types. Macrophages and reactive mesothelial cells are usually present, especially when the effusion is chronic. Erythrophagia and hemosiderocytes may be observed. Degenerate neutrophils and infectious agents may be detected. When the latter are absent, hemorrhagic effusions caused by neoplasia, idiopathic benign (hemorrhagic) pericardial effusion, and infectious pericarditis cannot be distinguished by cytology. The presence of pyrexia, an inflammatory leukogram, or other biochemical data associated with bacteremia or sepsis are variably and inconsistently associated with infectious pericarditis.

Therapy

If the cause of a systemic infection is evident, aggressive antimicrobial therapy is indicated as soon as appropriate samples for culture are procured. In some cases the infectious nature of the effusion is not appreciated until the results of cytology and culture are obtained.

Continuous drainage via surgical intervention or an indwelling pericardial catheter along with antimicrobial therapy is appropriate but usually not necessary. Usually, pericardiocentesis, which may have to be repeated, plus aggressive antibiotic treatment is curative in dogs. When bacterial pericarditis is discovered latently via pericardial fluid culture, and pericardiocentesis must be repeated, an appropriate nonmyocardiotoxic antibiotic can be injected into the pericardial sac in an attempt to reach higher therapeutic concentrations.

Constrictive pericarditis-epicarditis may occur and is recognized at surgery. Although a pericardectomy can be performed, extensive fibrin deposition on the epicardium is difficult to remove. Stripping of the epicardium is tedious and associated with complications, such as tearing of the myocardium and heart rhythm disturbances.

Bacterial infection, although producing fibrinous pericarditis and epicarditis, can often be treated successfully once the pericardium is removed. Antimicrobial therapy should involve broad-spectrum, bactericidal drugs administered IV at high dosages when feasible and should always be guided by antimicrobial susceptibility results.

INFECTION AND CORONARY VASCULAR DISEASE

Serologic studies, pathologic changes, and animal studies have provided evidence of an association between *Chlamydia pneumoniae* infection in people and coronary artery disease, atherosclerosis, and myocardial infarction.[123] No such associations have been made in dogs and cats, and these pathologic changes are not as frequently observed as they are in humans.

SUGGESTED READINGS*

1. Agungpriyono DR, Uchida K, Tabaru H, et al. 1999. Subacute massive necrotizing myocarditis by canine parvovirus type 2 infection with diffuse leukoencephalomalacia in a puppy. *Vet Pathol* 36:77-80.
13. Bellhorn T, Macintire DK. 2004. Bacterial translocation. *Compend Cont Educ Pract Vet* 26:229-235.
29. Brown VA. 2004. Aortic valvular endocarditis in a dog. *Can Vet J* 45:682-684.
37. Cassidy JP, Callanan JJ, McCarthy G, et al. 2002. Myocarditis in sibling boxer puppies associated with *Citrobacter koseri* infection. *Vet Pathol* 39:393-395.
41. Chomel BB, Kasten RW, Sykes JE, et al. 2003. Clinical impact of persistent *Bartonella* bacteremia in humans and animals. *Ann N Y Acad Sci* 990:267-278.
113. MacDonald KA, Chomel BB, Kittleson MD, et al. 2004. A prospective study of canine infective endocarditis in Northern California: 1999-2001 emergence of *Bartonella* as a prevalent etiologic agent. *J Vet Intern Med* 18:56-64.
125. Mexas AM, Hancock, SI, Breitschwerdt EB. 2002. *Bartonella henselae* and *Bartonella elizabethae* as potential canine pathogens. *J Clin Microbiol* 40:4670-4674.
127. Millar BC, Moore JE. 2004. Emerging issues in infective endocarditis. *Emerg Infect Dis* 10:1110-1116.
152. Peterson PB, Miller MW, Hansen EK, et al. 2003. Septic pericarditis, aortic endarteritis, and osteomyelitis in a dog, *J Am Anim Hosp Assoc* 39:528-532.
179. Wall M, Calvert CA, Greene CE. 2002. Infective endocarditis in dogs. *Compendium* 24:614-625.

*See the CD-ROM for a complete list of references.

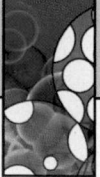

CHAPTER • 88

Bacterial Respiratory Infections

Craig E. Greene and Carol Norris Reinero

The respiratory system is divided into the upper and lower tracts and the pleural cavity. The upper respiratory tract consists of the nasal passages, nasopharynx, pharynx, larynx, and extrathoracic trachea. The lower respiratory tract consists of the intrathoracic trachea, bronchi, and alveoli. Specific diseases caused by viruses, fungi, protozoa, rickettsiae, *Mycoplasma*, and certain bacteria such as *Actinomyces* and *Nocardia* that infect primarily the respiratory system are covered in other chapters. This discussion focuses on bacterial infections of the respiratory system produced by invasion of normal microflora, by specific bacterial pathogens, or after impairment of normal host defense mechanisms. The normal microflora of the respiratory tract are discussed because these organisms frequently become involved in both upper and lower respiratory tract infections.

NORMAL BACTERIAL FLORA

Upper Respiratory Tract

Surveys of the bacterial microflora of the nasal cavities, tonsils, and pharynx of clinically healthy dogs and cats have found many types of aerobic and facultative anaerobic bacteria (Tables 88-1 and 88-2). Greater numbers of organisms are routinely cultured from the rostral than from the caudal nasal cavity. Because of marked individual variations, expecting to find the same organisms as flora of the nasal cavity and pharynx in each animal is not possible, but the presence of a certain range of flora can be predicted.

Lower Respiratory Tract

Bacteria are prevented from entering the lower respiratory tract by filtration of inspired air in the nasal turbinates, sneezing or coughing of inhaled particulate matter, and mucociliary clearance mechanisms. Despite these barriers, the normal tracheobronchial tree and lung are not continuously sterile. Airways down to the first bronchial division are contaminated with low numbers of organisms in clinically healthy animals. Studies using guarded culture swabs or tissue samples of the lower trachea of clinically healthy dogs have found some bacteria in 40% to 50% of samples (Table 88-3). Small numbers of bacteria (fewer than 2×10^3 colony-forming units [CFU]/ml) are also frequently cultured from the lower airways of healthy cats (Table 88-4). Oropharyngeal bacteria are aspirated and may be present for an unknown interval in the normal tracheobronchial tree and lung. Aerobic bacteria were isolated from 37% of lung tissue samples, whereas only 10% of dogs examined had no growth from cultures of multiple samples of their lung.[75] Most of the bacteria cultured from the trachea and lungs are identical to those found in the pharynx of these same dogs. This bacterial population has the potential to cause or complicate clinical respiratory infection and clouds interpretation of airway and lung cultures. Finding large (more than 10^5 CFU/ml) concentrations of bacteria or cytologic evidence of inflammatory cells in tracheobronchial washings makes their presence of more concern to the clinician.

UPPER RESPIRATORY TRACT INFECTIONS

Bacterial Rhinitis

Primary bacterial rhinitis is rare in the dog and cat. Bacterial rhinitis is commonly secondary to nasal trauma, allergic rhinitis, or inhalation of foreign material; reflux of liquids or food into the nose caused by pharyngeal, esophageal, or gastric dysfunction; viral, fungal, or parasitic infections; neoplasia; dental disease; oronasal fistula; and bacterial bronchopneumonia. One of the author's (CEG) beliefs asserts that once primary inflammation and mucosal injury begins, commensal microflora can proliferate as a secondary result, leading to chronic inflammatory rhinitis. This disease has been termed idiopathic lymphoplasmacytic or neutrophilic rhinitis, depending on the histopathologic findings.[67,147] It is characterized by chronic recurrent nasal discharge, fluid accumulation in the nasal passages and nasal sinuses, and eventual turbinate and bony loss (Fig. 88-1). This low-grade, progressive osteomyelitis likely develops because of the large number of bacterial flora residing within the nasal passages and the thin epithelial barrier over the fragile turbinate bones. Once it begins, the osteomyelitis becomes more difficult to control because infected necrotic bone acts as a sequestrum for continued osteomyelitis that becomes progressively more difficult to control with systemic or topical antimicrobials. Fungi such as *Alternaria* (see Chapter 67), *Aspergillus* and *Penicillium* (see Chapter 64), and *Cryptococcus* (see Chapter 61) may also colonize and produce disease in airways affected by bacteria or other processes while also producing nasal or disseminated disease in otherwise immunocompromised dogs and cats.

Clinical signs of bacterial rhinitis include sneezing, mucopurulent nasal discharge, ocular discharge secondary to nasolacrimal duct obstruction, and cough with gagging or retching. Epistaxis occurs infrequently with bacterial rhinitis but may be associated with underlying disease such as fungal rhinitis or neoplasia. Pawing at the face or nose indicates severe nasal irritation, often caused by foreign bodies lodged in the nasal cavity. Ulceration of the external nares and accumulation of crusted exudate occur in severe or chronic cases. Depigmentation of the external nares can also occur with chronic bacterial rhinitis as a result of the epithelial ulceration; however, it has been more commonly reported as a feature of nasal aspergillosis in dogs (see Chapter 64). Stenotic nares are seen in brachycephalic breeds and cats with long-standing rhinitis that develop infection at an early age in life. This nasal deformity is caused by damage to nasal bones and is similar to atrophic rhinitis in swine. For a discussion of nasopharyngeal polyps in cats, see otitis media and otitis interna in Chapter 86, Musculoskeletal Infections.

Because primary bacterial rhinitis is uncommon, a thorough search for underlying problems should be performed. Cryptococcal antigen testing of serum is helpful before invasive diagnostics because it will detect this disease before an anesthetic workup or invasive diagnostic tests (see Chapter 61). Diagnostic techniques include skull and nasal radiographs, endoscopic examination of the nasal passages, thor-

Table • 88-1

Bacterial Isolates from Nasal Swabs of Clinically Healthy Animals[a]

DOGS[124,22,4]	CATS[102]
Gram-Positive Aerobic or Facultative	
Staphylococcus (coagulase negative)	Streptococcus
Streptococcus (α- and nonhemolytic)	Staphylococcus
Corynebacterium	Corynebacterium
Bacillus	Micrococcus
Staphylococcus (coagulase positive)	
Streptococcus (β-hemolytic)	
Gram-Negative Aerobic or Facultative	
Neisseria	Pasteurella multocida
Escherichia coli	Escherichia coli
Enterobacter	Pseudomonas aeruginosa
Pasteurella multocida	Proteus
Moraxella	Klebsiella
Proteus	Enterobacter
Pseudomonas aeruginosa	Bordetella bronchiseptica
Alcaligenes	Moraxella
Bordetella bronchiseptica	Mycoplasma
Obligate Anaerobes	
Clostridium	

[a]Bacteria are listed in approximate order of frequency of isolation.

Table • 88-2

Bacterial Isolates from Tonsillar and Pharyngeal Swabs of Clinically Healthy Dogs[a,124,22,4,6,15,83,5]

Streptococcus (α- and nonhemolytic)	Proteus spp.
Staphylococcus (coagulase negative)	Pseudomonas spp.
Neisseria spp.	Corynebacterium spp.
Escherichia coli and Enterobacter spp.	Staphylococcus (coagulase positive)
Pasteurella multocida	Clostridium spp.
Bacillus spp.	Bacteroides spp.
Streptococcus (β-hemolytic)	Propionibacterium spp.
Alcaligenes spp.	Peptostreptococcus spp.
Klebsiella pneumoniae	Fusobacterium spp.

[a]Bacteria are listed in approximate order of frequency of isolation.

Table • 88-3

Bacterial Isolates from Tracheal Swabs and Lungs of Clinically Healthy Dogs[83,75]

Staphylococcus (coagulase positive and negative)	Enterobacter aerogenes
Streptococcus (α- and nonhemolytic)	Acinetobacter spp.
Pasteurella multocida	Moraxella spp.
Klebsiella pneumoniae	Corynebacterium spp.

Table • 88-4

Bacterial Isolation from Lower Respiratory Tract of Cats

CLINICALLY HEALTHY[a,62,105]	CHRONIC BRONCHIAL OR LOWER AIRWAY DISEASE[b,37,88,101,45,7,21,79]
Gram Positive	
Staphylococcus spp.	Staphylococcus spp.
Streptococcus spp.	Corynebacterium spp.
Micrococcus spp.	Streptococcus spp.[c]
	Bacillus spp.
	Enterococcus spp.
Gram Negative	
Escherichia coli	Escherichia coli[c]
Pasteurella multocida	Pasteurella multocida[c]
Pseudomonas aeruginosa	Moraxella spp.
Klebsiella spp.	Enterobacter spp.
Enterobacter spp.	Eugonic fermenter-4
Proteus spp.	Pseudomonas aeruginosa
Haemophilus felis	Bordetella bronchiseptica
	Salmonella typhimurium
	Bergeyella zoohelcum
Other	
	Mycoplasma spp.
	Mycobacterium spp.
	Fusobacterium spp.
	Peptostreptococcus spp.

[a]Collected by bronchoscopic alveolar lavage. Organisms isolated from the upper respiratory tract are found in lesser concentrations in the lower airways down to first bronchial division of healthy cats. Colony counts under 2×10^3 CFU/ml. No anaerobic bacteria or Mycoplasma isolated in healthy cats.
[b]Collected by endotracheal tube bronchial lavage, transtracheal lavage.
[c]Animals with these isolates have been septicemic, either as a cause or effect.[7]

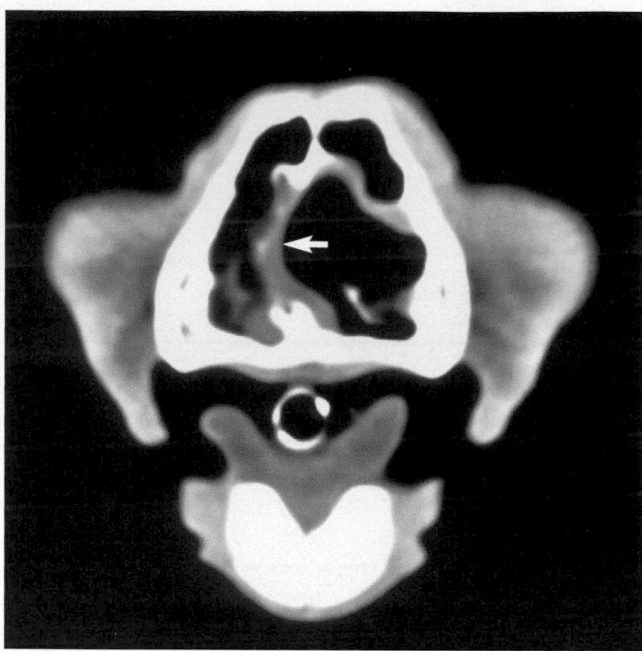

Fig 88-1 Computerized tomographic scan from a cat with severe turbinate loss and deviated nasal septum *(arrow)* within the nasal passages. (Courtesy University of Georgia, Athens, Ga.)

ough oropharyngeal examination, cytologic examination of exudate, and biopsy. These techniques are usually performed with the patient under general anesthesia.[118]

The radiographic features of chronic rhinitis are increased density of the nasal cavity as a result of excessive secretion accumulation. The turbinates are rarely destroyed, and the vomer bone is intact unless the disease is advanced. The frontal sinuses usually do not have increased density. Oblique views of the skull should be taken to evaluate the upper dental arcade. Dental film is ideal for evaluating infection of the tooth roots and the nasal sinuses of cats.

Computed tomography (CT), available at referral centers, has been shown to be superior to nasal radiography for evaluating the nasal cavities and frontal sinuses and in discriminating between cavitated and mass lesions.[118] Compared with radiography, CT is more sensitive in localizing and determining the extent of nasal disease.[23,120] The potential of rhinoscopy to detect significant abnormalities depends on the instrument and the amount of exudate or hemorrhage obscuring the field of view. Radiography or CT should be performed before rhinoscopic examination because nasal bleeding induced by rhinoscopy can obscure lesions on nasal imaging and because prior localization of the lesion is useful in guiding the rhinoscopist to the area of interest (e.g., the site of a foreign body or dental infection). Rhinoscopy is invaluable in the evaluation of neoplasia, inflammatory rhinitis, aspergillosis, and foreign bodies.[130] Purulent exudate and friable, hyperemic mucosa with or without ulceration are seen in bacterial rhinitis.

Without resorting to surgical biopsy, cytologic specimens can be obtained by flushing, swabbing, brushing, fine-needle aspiration, and impression smears of obtained tissue fragments.[17] With bacterial rhinitis, cytologic specimens of lesions or exudates will demonstrate with septic, purulent exudates. Cytologic evaluation may be helpful in assessing if inflammatory versus neoplastic processes are causing nasal disease; however, superficial inflammation can often overlay deeper neoplastic disease that can be missed by cytologic evaluation

alone. Therefore the observed inflammation may often be a secondary phenomenon. Furthermore, cytologic evaluation detects only acute inflammatory responses and misses chronic inflammatory changes found with corresponding histopathologic evaluation.[85] Bacterial cultures are difficult to interpret because they often yield a mixed population similar to that of the normal nasal flora and are not routinely recommended. Occasionally, a pure culture of a pathogen is helpful in choosing an appropriate antimicrobial based on susceptibility testing. However, the isolation of a predominant organism from such a contaminated site may indicate only that it is the most vigorous in its in vitro growth at the conditions implemented. Therefore cultures of the nasal area can often be misleading. Because of the rarity of primary bacterial rhinitis, clinicians must be cautious about over-interpreting bacterial cultures obtained from swabs, lavages, or biopsies of the nasal passages and realize that bacterial growth is likely secondary to an underlying problem that needs to be addressed before the bacterial infection will completely resolve.

Histopathologic specimens can be obtained by fluid flushes, punch biopsy, traumatic catheterization, and endoscopic biopsy forceps. In cats, the correlation of gross rhinoscopic mucosal abnormalities with histologic evidence of inflammation has been weak[67]; therefore histologic evaluation of biopsy specimens is essential, whether or not lesions are seen via rhinoscopy. Biopsy of nasal turbinates and mucosae may be helpful in identifying nasal diseases associated with bacterial rhinitis.

Bacterial rhinitis will often resolve without specific antibacterial therapy if the underlying problem, such as a foreign body, oronasal fistula, or dental disease, is corrected. In some patients, signs of rhinitis are temporary and may improve without treatment. Persistent or recurring signs require a further diagnostic workup. Although broad-spectrum antibacterials may appear to have a short-term benefit, the majority of patients will relapse with clinical signs of nasal disease until the underlying problem has been identified and addressed. Once significant bacterial osteomyelitis has developed, the process can be self-perpetuating. Therefore a complete nasal workup is strongly advised. Other nonspecific adjuncts to therapy include nebulization or vaporization, which helps mobilize secretions in the clogged nasal passages and soothes irritated mucous membranes, and sympathomimetic nasal decongestants, such as phenylephrine and oxymetazoline, in patients with copious serous or mucoid nasal discharges. However, nasal decongestants are contraindicated in patients with thick tenacious, mucopurulent nasal discharges because the exudates may become more viscous and difficult to expel. Glucocorticoid-responsive rhinitis associated with lymphoplasmacytic infiltrates of nasal mucosa, which may mimic bacterial rhinitis, has been described in the dog. The decision to institute glucocorticoid therapy is made after all other causes of nasal discharge have been ruled out and no evidence of a primary infectious process has been found during diagnostic evaluation.

Chronic Sinusitis

Chronic bacterial sinusitis is uncommon in the dog, although mucous accumulation does occur when nasal diseases occlude normal drainage of the frontal sinus through the sinus ostium. Chronic sinusitis in cats occurs as a result of mucosal and bone damage secondary to feline viral respiratory infections (see Chapter 16). Severe mucosal ulceration and turbinate destruction allow secondary bacterial infection of the nose and frontal sinuses. This syndrome is often called the "chronic snuffler" because the clinical signs in cats include chronic snorting and snuffling breathing, purulent nasal discharge, and sneezing. Many young cats with this syndrome are infected with feline leukemia virus (see Chapter 13), which may influence their response to treatment. Acute sinusitis often accompanies a large number of inflammatory conditions of the upper respiratory tract caused by inhaled irritants, allergens, and viral agents. In chronic cases, a wide variety of aerobic and anaerobic bacteria may be involved, similar to the situation found in people.[39] Although the relationship of these organisms to the pathogenesis of this infection is not completely understood, antimicrobial treatment should be based on broad-spectrum antimicrobial therapy.

Treatment of bacterial sinusitis is often frustrating because the underlying pathogenesis of the disease syndrome is poorly understood, and many patients fail to respond to all forms of symptomatic therapy. A course of broad-spectrum antibacterial (anaerobic and aerobic) therapy with good penetration into bone and secretions is recommended. Furthermore, given that opportunistic fungal infections are also involved, therapy against these organisms should be considered (see Nasal Aspergillosis and Penicilliosis, Chapter 64). The nasal cavity can be vigorously flushed with saline with or without antiseptic solutions to remove the exudate and inhibit bacterial growth. Drug penetration into the normal canine sinus is poor for the few antibacterials that have been evaluated and is probably similar in cats. Drug penetration will obviously increase with inflammation, but actual levels are unknown. Broad-spectrum antibacterials are used for prolonged periods (2 to 4 months) after bacterial culture and susceptibility testing. Nasal decongestants may be helpful in individual cats, but they can exacerbate the problem by drying the exudate. Surgical turbinectomy and sinus trephination may be helpful in establishing drainage of these areas and removing inspissated pockets of exudate. Nasal flushing and systemic antibacterials can be used subsequently to surgical intervention. More aggressive surgical approaches have included sinus obliteration and reconstruction of apertures into the frontal sinuses.

Tonsillitis and Pharyngitis

Tonsillitis is usually bilateral but may occasionally occur as a unilateral disease when a foreign body is trapped in the tonsillar crypt. Primary tonsillitis usually occurs in young, small-breed dogs that exhibit clinical signs of malaise, gagging cough with retching, fever, and inappetence. Inspection will often reveal a bright-red tonsil with an associated pharyngitis (Fig. 88-2). Punctate hemorrhages on the tonsil and purulent exudate in the tonsillar crypt may also be visible. The tonsil will be friable and will easily bleed on manipulation. Tonsillitis is not always associated with gross enlargement of the

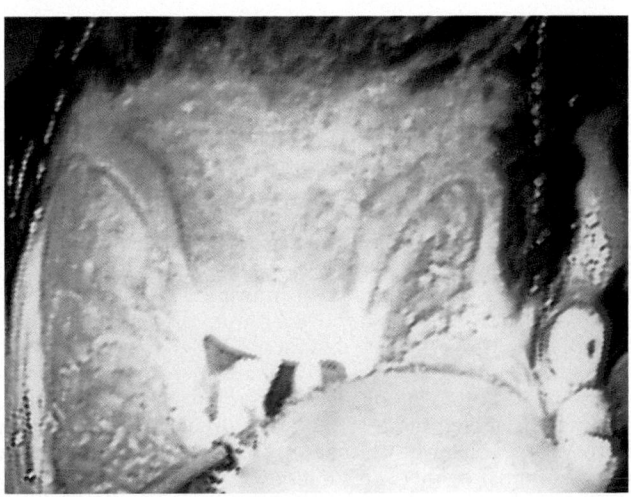

Fig 88-2 Tonsils are protruding and hyperemic in a dog with tonsillitis. (Courtesy University of Georgia, Athens, Ga.)

tonsil; in fact, the benign appearance of the tonsil in some cases may be in sharp contrast to the severity of clinical signs. Specific bacteria associated with primary tonsillitis have not been studied.

Tonsillitis most commonly occurs secondarily to a preexisting disease process. Primary diseases commonly associated with a secondary tonsillitis include chronic vomiting or regurgitation, chronic gingivitis or periodontitis, tracheobronchitis, and nasopharyngeal irritation caused by rhinitis.

Inflamed swollen tonsils are not an absolute indication for treatment. Elimination of preexisting problems usually results in resolution of the tonsillitis. If clinical signs are severe or persistent, then broad-spectrum antibacterial therapy for 10 to 14 days should be considered. Tonsillectomy is indicated when primary tonsillitis is a recurrent problem or hyperplastic tonsils protrude from the crypts, causing mechanical interference with breathing and swallowing.

Primary pharyngitis is uncommon but may occur concurrently with tonsillitis. Pharyngitis is usually a secondary problem as part of a widespread oral or systemic disease. Pharyngitis often accompanies viral or bacterial upper respiratory tract infections, pharyngeal foreign bodies, and retropharyngeal abscesses. Treatment is aimed at underlying diseases, such as removal of foreign bodies or surgical drainage of abscesses. Broad-spectrum antibacterial therapy may be used for 7 to 14 days.

Laryngitis

Laryngitis usually occurs as part of a widespread viral or bacterial respiratory infection such as canine tracheobronchitis or feline rhinotracheitis. Other common causes of acute noninfectious laryngitis are trauma to the larynx during endotracheal intubation and prolonged barking or dyspnea. Treatment is aimed at the coexisting infectious problem.

LOWER RESPIRATORY TRACT INFECTIONS

Tracheobronchitis

Canine infectious tracheobronchitis ("kennel cough") is a highly contagious respiratory disease of dogs and is characterized by coughing. This syndrome is associated with a wide variety of viral, mycoplasmal, and bacterial agents. The diagnosis is usually made based on history and physical examination alone. Chapter 6 discusses this syndrome in detail. *Bordetella bronchiseptica* is the bacterial pathogen that can be a primary respiratory pathogen in dogs without accompanying viral or *Mycoplasma* infection.[8,70,82] In cats, controversy exists about whether *B. bronchiseptica* is a primary or secondary pathogen, and although the organism has been associated with tracheobronchitis, conjunctivitis, rhinitis, and pneumonia, many culture-positive cats are clinically healthy (see Chapter 16). Of interest, an association between elevated culture positivity in cats (usually displaying minimal clinical signs) and contact with dogs with kennel cough has been identified, leading to speculation of interspecies transmission and the role cats may serve in maintaining the organism in the environment.[10,40] Human infections with *B. bronchiseptica* have been reported,[40] although the organism has a preference for infecting animals, and *B. pertussis* and *B. parapertussis* cause whooping cough in people (see Public Health Considerations, Chapter 6).[100,148] When human infections with *B. bronchiseptica* occur, they are often acquired through animal contact.

Widespread resistance of *B. bronchiseptica* isolates to cephalosporins and ampicillin has been reported[40]; therefore routine, indiscriminant use of antibiotics for all dogs with kennel cough should probably be avoided to minimize antibiotic resistance. If antibiotics are administered, those not active against *B. bronchiseptica* (see previous discussion) and those achieving low concentrations in airway tissues and fluids (e.g., amoxicillin-clavulanate and gentamicin administered parenterally) should be avoided.[70]

Chronic Bronchial Disease

The role of primary bacterial infections in initiating chronic bronchitis has not been determined. More commonly, chronic inflammation of the lower airways results in secondary bacterial infection. Severe bronchiolitis obliterans and organizing pneumonia has been observed in a dog.[110] Although infectious agents can cause this syndrome, toxic or irritant causes have been suspected. Bronchitis and bronchiolitis has been reported in a cat caused by cilia-associated respiratory bacillus-like organisms.[113] These silver-staining organisms were found in close parallel arrangement in association with mucosal cilia and the presence of airway inflammation. In dogs, chronic bronchitis leads to bronchiectasis. Bronchiectasis is more prevalent in certain breeds such as the American cocker spaniel, West Highland white terrier, miniature poodle, Siberian husky, English springer spaniel, and dogs over 10 years of age.[56]

Clinical signs of chronic bronchial disease in dogs are a chronic cough of 2 months or longer without signs of respiratory distress or tachypnea. Unlike pneumonia, constitutional signs of inappetence, weight loss, nasal discharge, or mental depression are usually absent. Thoracic radiographic abnormalities are either absent or consist of interstitial or peribronchial infiltration, or both. Cytologic abnormalities of increased airway mucus without hemorrhage have been characterized by increased neutrophils with occasional degenerate, occasional bacteria, and increased eosinophils in some dogs.[56] Culture results of airway washings usually yield a low number of a variety of bacterial agents. Quantitative bacterial cultures of bronchoalveolar lavage fluid are recommended to differentiate between airway colonization and infection. In dogs, chronic bronchitis is not commonly associated with clinically relevant bacterial growth when quantitative bacterial cultures and cytologic examination of lavage fluid is performed.[108] The role of infection in feline bronchial disease is poorly defined. Culture results of tracheal and bronchial exudates of clinically healthy cats often reveal a mixed pattern of low numbers of organisms (fewer than 5×10^3 organisms/ml), which probably reflect airway contamination rather than infection when greater than 10^5 organisms/ml is expected (see Table 88-4).[101] The role of *Mycoplasma* is intriguing because these organisms can be isolated in airway washings from cats with chronic bronchial disease[21,105] but not in those from healthy cats.[105] *Mycoplasma* degrade neural endopeptidase and prolong the effect of substance P, a potent bronchoconstrictor,[125] which may be involved in feline asthma, although this has yet to be proven. Bacterial infection may damage airway epithelium, resulting in chronic inflammation. In rare cases, cycles of repeated infection and inflammation in cats can lead to bronchiectasis and emphysema as a sequelae.[97] Bronchiectasis in dogs, as a result of and a contributor to infection, has also been described.[53,108]

Bacterial Pneumonia
Etiology

Many infectious agents cause pulmonary parenchymal inflammation (Table 88-5) (Fig. 88-3, *A* and *B*). This section focuses on bacterial infections; information on other infections can be found in their respective chapters. Bacteria enter the lower respiratory tract primarily by inhalation or aspiration of aerosols, oropharyngeal flora, foreign materials, or gastroesophageal contents; by local extension; or by hematogenous spread of extrapulmonary infections. Normal clearance mechanisms are generally effective unless the inoculum is greater than 10^7 organisms/ml or gastric acid is aspirated concurrently. Whether a respiratory infection will develop after bacterial

Table • 88-5

Infectious Agents Causing Pneumonia in Dogs or Cats

AGENT	CHAPTER
Viruses	
Canine distemper virus	3
Canine adenovirus-2	4
Canine herpesvirus	5
Canine parainfluenza virus	6
Feline rhinotracheitis virus	16
Rickettsia	
Ehrlichia canis	28
Rickettsia rickettsii	29
Bacteria[a]	
Bordetella	6, 16
Mycoplasma	32
Streptococcus	35
Escherichia coli	37
Klebsiella	37
Pseudomonas mallei	37
Yersinia pestis	47
Mycobacteria	50
Pasteurella	53
Eugonic fermenter-4	88
Fungi	
Blastomyces	59
Histoplasma	60
Cryptococcus	61
Coccidioides	62
Aspergillus	64
Penicillium	64
Protozoa	
Acanthamoeba	79
Toxoplasma	80

[a]See Tables 88-4 and 88-6 for additional isolates.

colonization depends on the complex interplay of many factors, including size of the inoculum, virulence of the organism, and resistance of the host. Clinical conditions that predispose the animal to bacterial pneumonia include preexisting viral, mycoplasmal, or fungal respiratory infections; regurgitation, dysphagia, and vomiting; reduced levels of consciousness (stupor, coma); severe metabolic disorders (diabetic ketoacidosis, uremia, hyperadrenocorticism); thoracic trauma or surgery; immunosuppressive therapy (anticancer chemotherapeutic agents, glucocorticoids); immunodeficiency diseases; neoplasia; and functional or anatomic disorders (tracheal hypoplasia, primary ciliary dyskinesia).

For aspiration pneumonia, risks are increased by recumbency or sedation, nasogastric or endotracheal intubation, debilitation, and esophageal or neuromuscular paralysis. Other factors are mechanical ventilation, concurrent illness, old age, and abdominal or thoracic surgery.[66]

Bacterial pneumonia is more common in the dog than it is in the cat. Of the primary bacterial pathogens, *B. bronchiseptica* appears to be the most common organism implicated in canine pneumonia. *Streptococcus zooepidemicus* may also be a

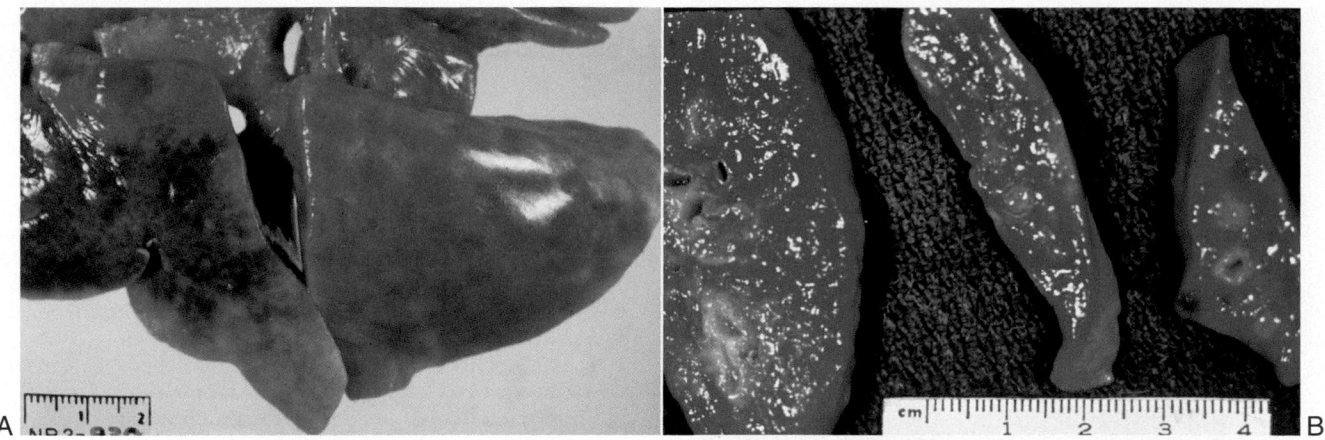

Fig 88-3 Lungs from dogs with bronchopneumonia. Surface **(A)** and cross section **(B)** of lung lobes showing inflammation and exudation. (Courtesy Veterinary Pathology, University of Georgia, Athens, Ga.)

primary pathogen (see Group C Streptococcal Infections, Chapter 35). Most isolates in dogs with pneumonia are thought to be opportunistic invaders, the most common of which are staphylococci, streptococci, *Escherichia coli*, *Pasteurella multocida*, *Pseudomonas* spp., and *Klebsiella pneumoniae* (Table 88-6).[132] A single pathogen is isolated in the majority of cases, but mixed infections are common. Gram-negative isolates predominate in both single and mixed infections.

Less is known about bacterial pneumonia in cats, in part, because cats with pneumonia may not show clinical signs and may lack abnormalities on hemograms and thoracic radiography.[79] In fatal pneumonia of cats, the bacterial species isolated included *Streptococcus canis*, *P. multocida*, *E. coli*, *Fusobacterium* spp., *Pseudomonas* spp., *Bacillus* spp., *Enterobacter cloacae*, *Enterococcus* spp., β-hemolytic *Streptococcus*, *B. bronchiseptica*, Eugonic fermentor-4a, *Peptostreptococcus* spp., and *Porphyromonas* spp.[79] As in dogs, single isolates were most common, but mixed infections were also seen.

B. bronchiseptica This upper respiratory tract inhabitant is the most common bacterial agent associated with tracheobronchitis in dogs and can cause pneumonia and bacteremia (Figs. 88-4 and 88-5). *B. bronchiseptica* can be a significant cause of pneumonia and mortality in kittens.[142,146] However, in a recent study evaluating bacterial growth from lower airway cultures in 133 client-owned cats with respiratory disease, *B. bronchiseptica* was not found to be a significant pathogen.[128] For further information on lower respiratory tract disease caused by this organism in dogs and cats, see Chapters 6 and 16, respectively.

Streptococcus As facultatively anaerobic gram-positive cocci, they are isolated from tracheal washings in 14% to 47% of dogs with pneumonia. Although less pathogenic α-hemolytic strains have been isolated, the predominant pathogens are β-hemolytic, with groups C and G being most important in dogs and cats (see also Chapter 35). Some virulence factors identified for hemolytic group A streptococci, which affect people, are capsular polysaccharides, surface protein A, and pneumolysin, a toxin that inhibits cilia, disrupts the alveolar capillary barrier, and interferes with neutrophil chemotaxis and lymphocyte function. Some of these factors are probably important in animal infections. In addition, nonvirulence products include neuraminidases that promote attachment, immunoglobulin proteases, adhesins, erythrogenic toxins, hyaluronidases, streptokinases, and streptolysins.[14]

Once streptococci reach the alveoli, development and progression of pneumonia depend on virulence factors of the

Table • 88-6

Bacteria Isolated in Tracheal Aspirates from Dogs with Bacterial Pneumonia[a]

BACTERIA	RANGE (%)
Gram Negative	
Escherichia coli	17-43
Klebsiella	3.9-23
Bordetella	3-23
Pseudomonas	4.9-33
Pasteurella	0-45
Enterobacter	0-5
Acinetobacter	0-7
Moraxella	2-26
Other gram-negative rods	4.4-12
Gram Positive	
Staphylococcus	5.4-27
Streptococcus	13.8-47
Nonhemolytic	0-13
α-Hemolytic	3-30
β-Hemolytic	0-16
Corynebacterium	0-5
Mycoplasma[b]	2.9-100
Anaerobes[c]	
Total	18.7
Bacteroides	23.7
Clostridium perfringens	5.3
Eubacterium	2.6
Fusobacterium	15.8
Peptostreptococcus	23.7
Prevotella	5.3
Porphyromonas	15.8
Propionibacterium	2.6

[a]Data taken from reference 27, 30 dogs; reference 52, 30 dogs; reference 132, 42 dogs; reference 59, 105 dogs; reference 64, 48 dogs; reference 3, 203 dogs.
[b]From pharyngeal isolates *Mycoplasma* are isolated 85.7% to 100% of the time, representing normal microflora; from transtracheal washings (34% to 69%); and from bronchiolar washings (7.1% to 26.9%). Data from references 64 and 114.
[c]A range is not listed because data are from one study of 203 dogs.[3]

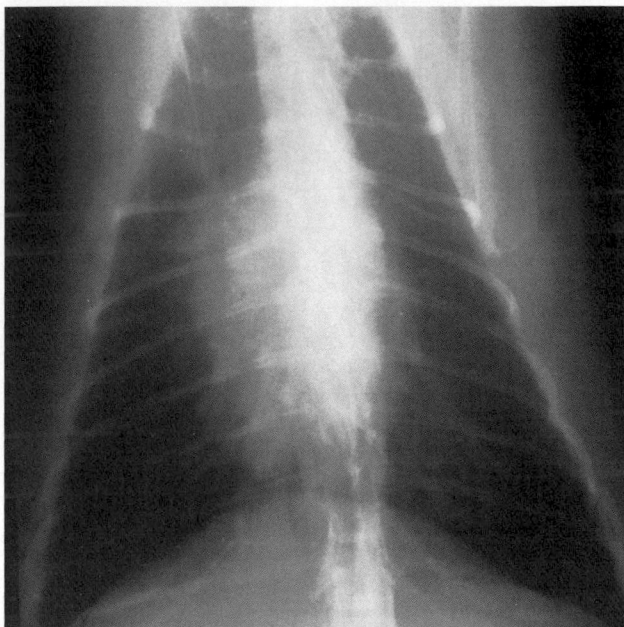

Fig 88-4 Radiograph of a cat with pneumonia caused by *B. bronchiseptica*. (Courtesy University of Georgia, Athens, Ga.)

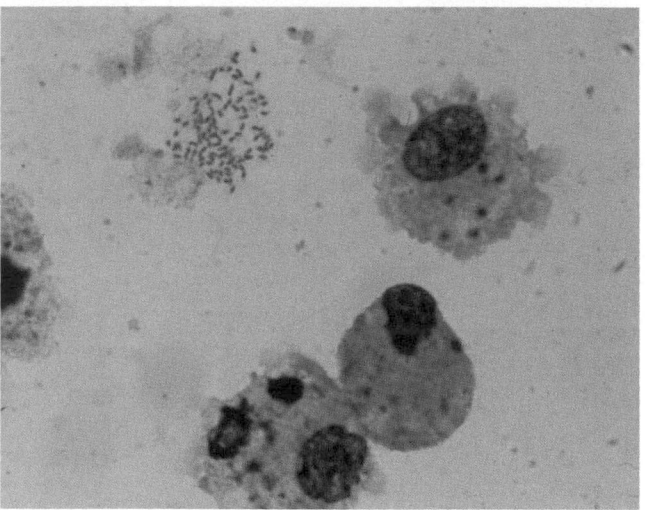

Fig 88-5 Cytology of endotracheal wash from cat with *B. bronchiseptica* pneumonia (Wright, ×1000). (Courtesy University of Georgia, Athens, Ga.)

offending agent. With the most virulent strains, vascular leakage and edema are mediated by pneumolysin and hyaluronidase. This fluid exudation facilitates spread of organisms throughout lung lobes. Less virulent strains damage some type 1 epithelial cells, whereas more virulent strains denude large areas of the epithelial surface from the basement membrane. More extensive epithelial loss results in type 2 pneumocyte proliferation and fibroplasia, leading to permanent pulmonary scarring.

Severe pneumonia with high mortality associated with group C streptococci has been reported in dogs, usually secondary to concurrent viral infection. Many persistent streptococcal pneumonias occur in dogs with concurrent immunodeficiencies. Streptococcal pneumonias may be associated with hematogenous spread of infection to meninges, joints, kidneys, heart valves, spleen, lymph nodes, and other organs.

E. coli These facultatively anaerobic bacilli are commensal flora of predominantly the lower gastrointestinal (GI) tract and are isolated from 17% to 43% of transtracheal washes from dogs with pneumonia. As gram-negative organisms, they contain endotoxin and can form antiphagocytic polysaccharide capsules and cell-injurious exotoxins. They also form fimbrial adhesins to bind to respiratory epithelial cells and siderophores, which allow them to compete for iron from the bound iron in host tissues and secretions.

E. coli usually enters the lower respiratory tract through aspiration from colonized nasal and oropharyngeal areas. In addition, bacteremic spread from the genitourinary or GI tract is possible but less frequently documented in dogs. Pneumonia has also occurred in dogs secondary to viral infections with long-term antibiotic or glucocorticoid therapy or with myelosuppressive or immunodeficiency diseases.[71] Persistent pneumonias have involved mixed infections with other organisms in dogs with immunodeficiencies. Complications of *E. coli* pneumonia are dissemination of infection to other organs such as the meninges, joints, uveal tracts, or glomeruli; disseminated intravascular coagulation; and endotoxin-induced lung injury, resulting in acute respiratory distress.

Pasteurella These facultatively anaerobic coccobacilli are isolated in up to 45% of transtracheal washings from dogs with pneumonia. *Pasteurella* are among the indigenous microflora of the nasopharynx and large airways of dogs and cats (see also Bite Infections, Chapter 53). Concurrent viral infections and other stresses to the host lead to proliferation and subsequent migration of *Pasteurella* to lower airways. Reduced defense mechanisms lead to impaired bacterial clearance from the lung, with resultant pneumonia. *Pasteurella* form adhesin, promoting their epithelial attachment, and polysaccharide capsule, which interferes with phagocytosis. Exotoxin production has not been documented as a feature of *Pasteurella* infections in dogs and cats, as is the case in other animals. However, gram-negative bacterial endotoxin decreases the quantity and increases the surface tension of pulmonary surfactant, altering pulmonary mechanics and gas exchange. Bacterial proliferation results in an influx of inflammatory cells and cytokine mediators, resulting in fibrinopurulent exudation typical of *Pasteurella* pneumonia. Once they develop, such pneumonias may be slow to resolve, and abscesses or pleuritis may develop.

Eugonic Fermenter-4 Group eugonic fermenter-4 (EF-4) is a collection of unclassified bacterial strains designated by the Centers for Disease Control and Prevention, Atlanta, Georgia. These bacteria, ecologically and culturally similar to *Pasteurella* spp., have been isolated as commensal and opportunistic flora from the oral cavity of dogs and cats (see Table 89-1) and from local infections in people as contaminating organisms of dog and cat bite wounds (see Chapter 53). The precise means by which EF-4 organisms produce respiratory, local, or systemic infections is unknown. Localized infections in dogs and cats have involved primarily cranial infections such as keratitis, retrobulbar abscess, otitis, sinusitis, and stomatitis. Infections probably arise as a result of contamination from the oropharyngeal area. Gingivitis has commonly been recognized in cats that develop EF-4 infection.[79,143] When pneumonia develops, inhalation or hematogenous dissemination of the organism from an oral site is suspected. Concurrent immunosuppression may be important for the organism to colonize other regions of the body.

Both domestic[36,65,84] and exotic[38,76,109] cats and domestic dogs[84,138] have been affected.[25] Anorexia, hypersalivation, and dyspnea have been the main clinical signs of respiratory infection. Sudden death, with or without premonitory signs, has been noted in some cases. Abdominal distention from exudative peritonitis was noted in one puppy. An epizootic outbreak of fatal pneumonia was identified in a closed research colony of cats.[143]

Diagnosis has been made primarily by culture of the abscess wounds at necropsy. The organism can be cultivated on blood agar, incubated aerobically or anaerobically, and classified by its biochemical reactions. In a few cases in cats, premortem leukopenia and nonregenerative anemia have been found. Multifocal nodular abscess formation is the typical pathologic finding in the lungs. The lesions are grossly indistinguishable from multifocal neoplasms or granulomas. Extrapulmonary lesions have included similar multifocal abscesses in the liver, peritoneal cavity, and lymph nodes. The abscesses are histologically characterized by neutrophilic and mononuclear infiltrates sometimes surrounding visible colonies of gram-negative bacteria.

Therapy for this type of infection is unknown but can be expected to be similar to that for plague (see Chapter 47 and Table 47-1).

Bergeyella (Weeksella) zoohelcum This organism, which is a microfloral resident of the oropharyngeal region of dogs and cats, has been linked to respiratory infection in a cat.[33] A 9-month-old cat developed oculonasal discharge that did not respond to therapy with amoxicillin-clavulanate or doxycycline. Weight loss and lower respiratory tract signs of anorexia, dyspnea, and harsh ausculted lung sounds were present. Temporary improvement was observed with treatment of marbofloxacin and prednisolone; however, the cat became anorectic and was euthanized. Of the antibacterials used for treatment, in vitro susceptibility testing of the organism indicated resistance only to tetracyclines. Necrotizing upper and lower respiratory tract infection was found. Infections by this organism have been primarily in people with infected bite wounds caused by dogs or cats (see Chapter 53).

Pathogenesis

Bacteria enter the distal airways and alveoli and elicit phagocytosis by resident alveolar macrophages, as well as neutrophilic recruitment. Virulence of organisms is important in their colonization and persistence in respiratory tissues. Adherence of organisms occurs through specific binding of ligands or adhesins to complementary receptors on mucosal surfaces. Bacterial pili are adhesive structures, whereas cell surface glycoproteins, glycolipids, and proteoglycans are the cell receptors.[19,112] In addition to attachment of organisms to respiratory surfaces, failure of host defenses such as mucociliary clearance is a primary mechanism that contributes to infections of the upper respiratory tract and bronchi. The mucosal surface is covered by a thin mucous layer that is propelled toward the larynx at up to 1 cm/minute by ciliated epithelial cells. Mucus reaching the larynx is usually swallowed or sometimes expectorated. Some pathogenic bacteria, such as *Pseudomonas aeruginosa, B. bronchiseptica, Mycoplasma pneumoniae,* coagulase-positive staphylococci, and β-hemolytic streptococci, interfere with ciliary movement or affect respiratory epithelial function.[63] Some organism by-products act on neutrophils, which produce ciliastatic hydrogen peroxide. Viruses such as canine distemper virus, canine parainfluenza virus type 2, and canine adenovirus-2 damage ciliated epithelial cells, resulting in decreased mucociliary clearance and secondary bacterial infections.

Mucociliary clearance requires functional cilia and appropriate levels and consistency of mucus, which is formed of glycoproteins, glycolipids, and other proteins. Two active ion transport mechanisms adjust the level of periciliary fluid to maximize the mucociliary clearance.[13] Bacterial infection makes mucus more voluminous, less compliant, and more difficult to propel the embedded bacteria, which remain stationary.[47,126]

Bacterial pneumonia after aspiration of contaminated materials occurs frequently as a nosocomial event from intubation associated with surgery or after recovery from anesthesia. Disorders that predispose patients to aspiration are swallowing impairment, laryngeal paralysis, megaesophagus, hiatal hernia, and regurgitation or vomiting from any cause. Conditions such as periodontal disease and intestinal stasis also increase the bacterial load in aspirated GI secretions.

Clinical Findings

History and clinical signs of canine bacterial pneumonia include cough (usually moist, productive), variable fever, dyspnea, serous or mucopurulent nasal discharge, inappetence, depression, weight loss, and dehydration. Auscultation usually reveals abnormal lung sounds, including increased intensity of bronchial breath sounds, crackles, and wheezes. Other physical examination abnormalities include tachypnea, weakness, exercise intolerance, and productive coughing. Aspiration pneumonia should be suspected in any animal that develops these signs while hospitalized or after episodes of vomiting or regurgitation.

In contrast to dogs, cats with pneumonia often lack clinical signs, especially cough. In a study of cats with fatal infectious pneumonia (of which 54% were bacterial in origin), 36% lacked clinical signs referable to the respiratory tract.[79] Of the cats displaying respiratory signs, tachypnea or dyspnea and nasal discharge were most common; cough was present only in 8%. Systemic signs of illness (anorexia, lethargy, and fever) were absent in 41% of these cats, despite histologic evidence of disseminated infectious disease in 74%. A high index of suspicion for pneumonia is required in cats, especially if evidence of infection exists in other organs. In a review of 21 cases of lower respiratory tract infection in cats that were not all fatal, signs were chronic cough (11), acute cough (6), dyspnea (2), anorexia (1), and neurologic signs (1).[45]

Diagnosis

In dogs, the diagnosis of bacterial pneumonia is suspected based on history and physical examination and is confirmed by hematologic findings, thoracic radiography, and microbiologic and cytologic examination of material from the tracheobronchial tree or lung. A neutrophilic leukocytosis with a left shift is frequently found on a complete blood count (CBC), but may be present in a low percentage of dogs. Arterial blood gas values correlate well with the degree of physiologic disruption in patients with bacterial pneumonia and are sensitive monitors of progress during treatment. Thoracic radiographs reveal an alveolar pattern characterized by increased pulmonary density in which margins are indistinct and in which air bronchograms may be seen (Fig. 88-6). A patchy or lobar alveolar pattern will be present in a cranial ventral lung lobe distribution.

In cats with infectious pneumonia, clinical signs, results of a CBC, and findings on thoracic radiography may not be abnormal.[79] When hematologic abnormalities are present, leukocytosis or leukopenia, neutrophilia, and left shift have all been reported. Thoracic radiographic abnormalities can include pulmonary infiltrates characterized by mixed bronchointerstitial or bronchoalveolar patterns or alveolar or interstitial patterns. Interstitial patterns are more typically a result of chronic bronchitis (see later discussion) or, as is the case in cats, caused by pulmonary fibrosis.[24] Although infections with certain pathogens may result in pulmonary fibrosis, the idiopathic form may be caused by a metabolic defect in type II pneumocytes.[145]

The definitive method of establishing a diagnosis of bacterial pneumonia is to obtain aspirates, washings, or brushings for microbiologic and cytologic examinations. Multiple procedures that bypass the oropharynx have been recommended to obtain these specimens. Blood cultures can also be helpful in identifying the etiologic agent causing bacterial pneumonia. In cases in which radiography, cytology, and culture fail to provide a definitive diagnosis (generally when secondary bacterial infections complicate an underlying interstitial lung disease or neoplastic process), histologic examination of the lung may be necessary.[95,96] Thoracic surgery may also be necessary for removal of a nidus of infection, for example, with foreign body pneumonia.

Transtracheal Aspiration Because animals are unable to expectorate sputum, and because it bypasses the oropharyngeal area, the method of transtracheal washing and aspiration is safe, simple, and clinically valuable for obtaining tracheobronchial and pulmonary material for culture and cytologic examination. The technique is well tolerated by most large dogs and requires only minimal restraint of the unanesthetized patient. Small dogs and cats tolerate endotracheal washings better.

Materials needed to perform transtracheal aspiration are listed in Table 88-7. Sedation is not required in most dogs, with the exception of the hyperexcitable miniature and toy breeds, for which narcotics are the drugs of choice. The animal is allowed to sit or is placed in sternal recumbency with its neck extended. The area of the larynx is clipped and scrubbed as for surgery. The cricoid cartilage, identified by palpating the tracheal rings from the midcervical region toward the larynx, is the first prominent ventral ridge at the larynx. Cranial to the cricoid cartilage and between the thyroid cartilages is the cricothyroid ligament. From 0.5 to 1 ml of 2% lidocaine is injected subcutaneously over the cricothyroid ligament. The needle and catheter are then directed caudoventrally through the skin and cricothyroid ligament into the larynx in a single motion (Fig. 88-7, *A*). In larger dogs, the catheter can be inserted into the lower regions of the trachea between cartilage rings to facilitate recovery of flushing solutions. The catheter is passed into the trachea, and the needle is withdrawn from the larynx (see Fig. 88-7, *B*). The needle guard is

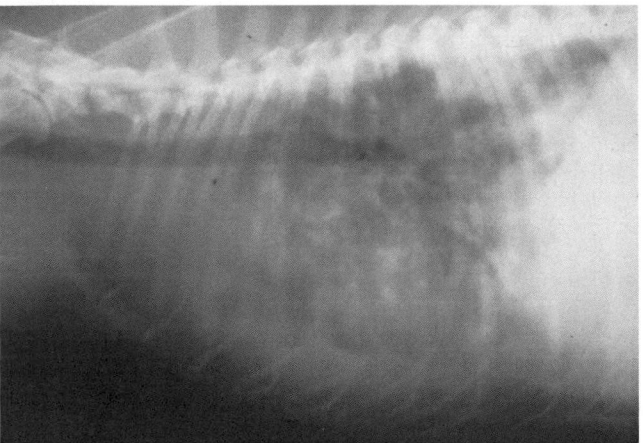

Fig 88-6 Radiograph of lung of dog with severe bronchopneumonia. (Courtesy University of Georgia, Athens, Ga.)

Table • 88-7
Materials Required for Performing Transtracheal Aspiration
16-gauge × 12-inch through-the-needle IV catheter[a] or 19-gauge × 8-inch through-the-needle IV catheter[b] (for small dogs and cats) Clippers Surgical scrub 1 ml of 2% lidocaine 20-ml syringe Sterile water or saline (nonbacteriostatic) Surgical gloves (optional when using a through-the-needle catheter)

[a]BD Intracath™, 16 gauge, 12 inch; Bard Biomedical, Murray Hill, N.J.
[b]BD Intracath™, 19 gauge, 8 inch; Bard Biomedical, Murray Hill, N.J.

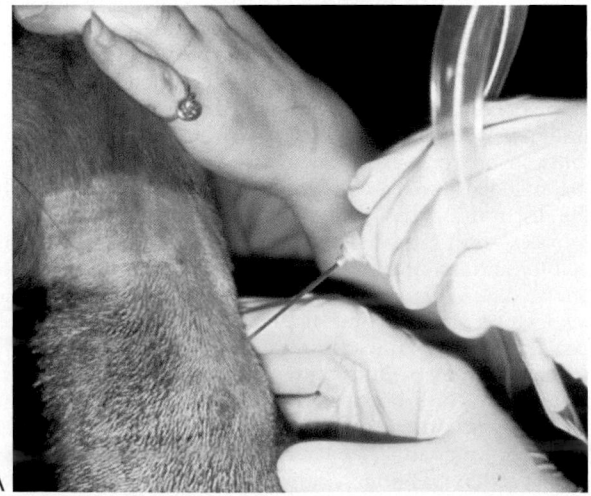

A

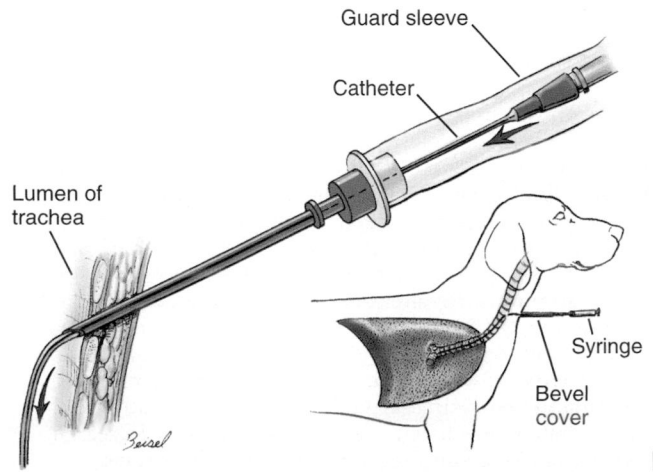

Guard sleeve
Catheter
Lumen of trachea
Syringe
Bevel cover

B

Fig 88-7 **A,** Placement of catheter for transtracheal wash at area of surgical preparation. **B,** Diagram showing position of catheter in the trachea. (Courtesy University of Georgia, Athens, Ga.)

then applied to prevent the catheter from being cut by the needle. Paroxysms of coughing can be expected as the catheter is passed into the trachea.

A syringe generally containing up to 15 to 20 ml of sterile, nonbacteriostatic saline is attached to the catheter and injected. As the animal coughs, suction is applied with the syringe. Resistance suggests that tenacious secretions are being collected in the catheter. If only air is aspirated, the syringe is disconnected, the air is expelled, and another 15 to 20 ml of fluid is injected and reaspirated. This procedure is repeated until respiratory secretions, which will appear as a cloudy fluid, are aspirated into the syringe. Up to 1 ml/kg of solution can be safely injected into the airway during a single flush without causing significant respiratory insufficiency. The largest amount of aspirate will be collected when the animal is coughing. When the specimen has been obtained, the syringe is detached and capped to prevent contamination. The catheter is removed and a light bandage is applied to prevent subcutaneous hemorrhage or emphysema. The specimen is mixed in the syringe and divided into aliquots for cytologic and microbiologic examination (see later discussion).

Although complications from transtracheal washing and aspiration are uncommon, the procedure is not without risk. As is the case with the majority of invasive diagnostic procedures, risk is significantly decreased with experience. The procedure is considerably more difficult in cats and small dogs than it is in larger dogs. Transtracheal washing should not be attempted in the fractious or uncooperative patient without adequate chemical and manual restraint.

The most common complication associated with transtracheal washing is subcutaneous emphysema, which occurs when persistent coughing or dyspnea causes air to leak from the puncture site into the cervical subcutaneous tissues. Other complications include endotracheal hemorrhage, tracheal laceration, cardiac arrhythmia, and infection at the puncture site.

Endotracheal Wash This technique involves general anesthesia and short-acting barbiturates. After endotracheal intubation with a sterilized endotracheal tube, a polypropylene urinary catheter is passed down through the lumen to the level of the carina. Two or more 10- to 15-ml aliquots (up to 5 ml/kg/aliquot in cats and small dogs) of sterile 0.9% saline solution are administered through the catheter, each followed immediately by aspiration attempts. Several advantages have been noted: washings can be obtained without producing tracheal injury and minimal equipment is needed, and it is technically simpler to perform in cats and small dogs. Disadvantages are oropharyngeal contamination, as is the case for bronchoscopy (see later discussion), and airway visualization is not possible.

Bronchoalveolar Lavage: Blind Technique This technique is performed using general anesthesia with or without the aid of an endoscope.[58] A blind technique can be used without an endoscope by positioning the animal in lateral recumbency and placing a single-lumen endotracheal tube just rostral to the carina. The cuff is inflated, and a syringe adaptor is connected to the end of the tube. Aliquots (5 ml/kg) of warmed sterile 0.9% saline are infused via syringe. Immediately after each aliquot, mild suction is applied to the syringe. The animal is tilted with its head lowered and caudal end elevated to assist in fluid recovery. The syringe is immediately disconnected after the fluid is taken, and 100% oxygen is given through the endotracheal tube for 5 minutes. Alternatively, in cats and small dogs, a 7-French polypropylene catheter can be introduced through the endotracheal tube until it is wedged (i.e., until gentle resistance is felt). Saline is lavaged through a syringe attached to the polypropylene tube and gently reaspirated.

Bronchoalveolar Lavage: Bronchoscopic Technique Tracheobronchoscopy is valuable for direct visualization of the airways and for obtaining brush catheter specimens for cytologic and microbiologic examination. The procedure requires that the patient be maintained under general anesthesia, which may be of concern in those with bacterial pneumonia. Intravenous anesthetic agents and a speculum will allow a thorough tracheobronchial examination with a rigid bronchoscope passed through the mouth. Brush catheters and suction cannulas may be passed through the lumen of the rigid bronchoscope to obtain specimens.

The transoral approach with a flexible fiberoptic bronchoscope inserted through an endotracheal tube is preferred. The patient is anesthetized, using standard procedures, intubated, and maintained on inhalation anesthesia or an intravenous anesthetic. An endotracheal tube T-adapter allows oxygen and anesthetic gas to flow without leakage to the patient while allowing placement of the flexible endoscope through the endotracheal tube. This technique is successful in moderate- to large-sized dogs during lengthy procedures. Small dogs and cats are given an intravenous anesthetic, and a flexible or small-diameter rigid fiberoptic endoscope is passed directly into the trachea and wedged in a terminal bronchus. During wedge lavage in cats and small dogs, oxygen may be infused alongside the bronchoscope through a 5-French diameter tube. Brush catheters are passed through the biopsy channel of the endoscope to obtain specimens.

Because of contamination from the oropharynx, bacterial cultures obtained with sterile, open-end, brush-in-catheter systems passed through the endoscope have been considered unreliable in the past. A commercially available catheter (Microbiology Specimen Brush, Microvasive Inc., Milford, Mass.) that enhances the ability to obtain reliable cultures of lower airway secretions through a bronchoscope has been developed. This system consists of a sterile brush contained within a telescoping double catheter occluded by a polyethylene glycol plug. This system is passed through the instrumentation channel of the bronchoscope. The brush is extended into the secretions to be cultured and then retracted into the inner catheter. The entire brush-in-telescope, double-catheter system is removed from the endoscope. The brush is advanced out of the catheter where the wire is transected with sterile scissors. The brush is placed in trypticase soy broth. The only disadvantage is the expense of a catheter system that can be used only once.

The advantages of tracheobronchoscopy are numerous when compared with other diagnostic techniques. Endoscopy allows the direct visualization of the tracheobronchial tree and the lesions associated with bacterial pneumonia, thereby allowing a better assessment of the patient's clinical status and prognosis. The cytologic preparations collected by bronchoalveolar lavage through the endoscope are superior to those obtained by transtracheal washing because cells and proteinaceous materials are obtained from the deeper portions of the lungs.[57] Quantitating bacteria obtained by airway washings is needed to distinguish lower airway contamination from actual infection. Bronchoalveolar lavage (BAL) quantitative cultures and quantitating intracellular bacteria on Gram-stained BAL cytologic specimens has been useful in identifying lower respiratory tract infections in dogs.[108] In this procedure, 10 to 25 ml of sterile saline were flushed into and withdrawn through the biopsy channel of a freshly rinsed bronchoscope with its tip wedged in the airway at the site of visible inflammatory changes. Bacterial colony counts of at least 1.7×10^3 CFU/ml of BAL fluid were considered significant. Correspondingly, more than two intracellular bacteria, visualized after examining 50 microscopic fields, was also considered indicative of lower airway infection. Dogs with chronic bronchitis had no evidence of bacterial infection using these criteria. When indicated, transbronchial biopsy specimens may also be taken, although these are not without risk.

Fine-Needle Lung Aspiration Transthoracic fine-needle aspiration can be used to procure material for microbial culture and cytologic examination directly from the lung. Fine-needle aspiration may be more beneficial than lavage is (especially tracheal washings and blind BAL) when focal lesions are present and should be considered before employing more aggressive diagnostics, such as a thoracotomy. The fine-needle aspiration techniques (blind, ultrasound-guided, or fluoroscopically guided), indications, contraindications, and complications have been reviewed elsewhere.[32] The fine-needle method has much less risk compared with transthoracic "true-cut" needle biopsy, which can cause severe pulmonary hemorrhage or pneumothorax. Using the fine-needle method, specimens can generally be classified as being neoplastic, inflammatory, or nondiagnostic. The recommended size of the needle is 25 or 27 gauge and 1.5 inches in length. The needle is advanced into the lung and moved in and out several times before gentle suction is applied with a 6-ml syringe.

Cytologic and Microbiologic Examination Preparation of material for cytologic evaluation can be done using several methods. Visible strands of exudate may be teased onto a microscope slide, smeared, and stained. Small quantities of material can be centrifuged and smears made of the sediment. New methylene blue wet mounts and Wright-Giemsa's or Gram's stain of air-dried smears can be used for identification of cellular elements and bacteria. Bacterial infections are associated with degenerate neutrophils and intracellular bacteria; excess mucus, proteinaceous material, and activated alveolar macrophages may be present. Bacteria are demonstrable only in fraction of washings from pneumonic animals, and their absence in cytologic specimens, especially if the patient has been placed on antibiotic therapy, does not rule out bacterial pneumonia.

All collection methods of airway washings can be associated with pharyngeal contamination. This explanation answers the question as to why many lower airway washings contain artifact, resident nasopharyngeal microflora. Pharyngeal contamination is detected by the presence in cytologic preparations of squamous epithelium or *Simonsiella (Caryophanon)*, a characteristic genus of oral bacteria, which appears as "stacked coins."

Because of the delay in bacterial culture, the organisms are classified as being rods or cocci or other recognizable bacterial or fungal elements. Anaerobes, *Actinomyces*, and *Nocardia* are often larger, pleomorphic, or filamentous. Acid-fast staining will help detect *Nocardia* or *Mycobacterium*. Additional staining may identify specific yeast or filamentous fungi (see Chapter 56). Mycoplasmas may be obtained if special media is used (see Chapter 32).

Bacteriologic Culture An aliquot of aspirated material can be cultured directly for aerobic and anaerobic bacteria. Gram-negative organisms are most commonly cultured, whereas gram-positive and anaerobic bacteria and *Mycoplasma* are less commonly isolated. Secretions that coat the distal end of the catheter can be cultured if the amount of aspirated material is minimal. Sensitivity of transtracheal washing and aspiration for recovery of bacteria is good, but because larger airways may contain low levels of microflora, specificity for infection rather than contamination cannot be determined. For BAL specimens, quantitative cultures are recommended in conjunction with examination of a Gram-stained specimen to enhance diagnostic sensitivity and specificity.[108] Clinically relevant bacterial growth in BAL spec-

imens from dogs are over 1.7×10^3 CFU/ml of BAL fluid. Bacterial infection can also be diagnosed with microscopic examination of 50 fields on a Gram-stained slide revealing more that two intracellular bacteria.[108] False-negative results may be obtained if antimicrobial therapy has not been discontinued for at least 1 week before sampling.

Blood Cultures Blood cultures have been recommended in people with bacterial pneumonia to help isolate the infectious agent. Documented bacteremia is also thought to be a poor prognostic finding. No studies in animals have been done that document the value of blood cultures in establishing a prognosis or isolating the bacterial agent in cases of pneumonia. Up to 50% of dogs with experimentally induced streptococcal pneumonia have been blood culture positive within 48 hours of onset of clinical signs.[90] Cats with histologically confirmed infectious pneumonia most commonly developed pneumonia from hematogenous spread; however, blood cultures were not performed in these cats.[79]

Pulmonary Biopsy Histopathologic evaluation of pulmonary tissue is the ultimate test to determine the underlying process within the lung parenchyma (Figs. 88-8 and 88-9). This assessment must be coupled with culture or histochemical tests to determine causative agents. Histopathology is most helpful in resolving causes of interstitial pneumonic processes because washings can frequently be productive in the alveolar diseases.

Aspiration Pneumonia

Aspiration of different materials can result in chemical pneumonitis, anaerobic abscesses, or classic bacterial pneumonia.[68] Inflammation in the lung that follows aspiration of gastric contents is more appropriately termed chemical pneumonitis. Fever, dyspnea, alveolar exudation, and pulmonary interstitial or alveolar infiltration are observed clinically. Bacteria are not always a feature of this syndrome because acidic gastric contents have low bacterial content. Inflammatory changes generally subside after 24 to 36 hours; however, if gastric pH has been increased by antacids or H2-receptor antagonists, or if small intestinal obstruction or bacterial overgrowth exists, then bacterial loads can be increased. If oral cavity contents are inhaled, then the term aspiration is better referred to as anaerobic pneumonitis because the oropharyngeal microflora

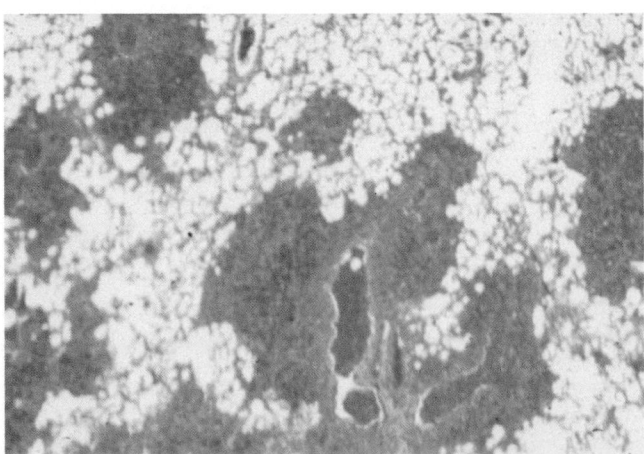

Fig 88-8 Bacterial bronchopneumonia postdistemper showing inflammatory infiltrates in alveoli (H and E stain, ×40). (Courtesy Veterinary Pathology, University of Georgia, Athens, Ga.)

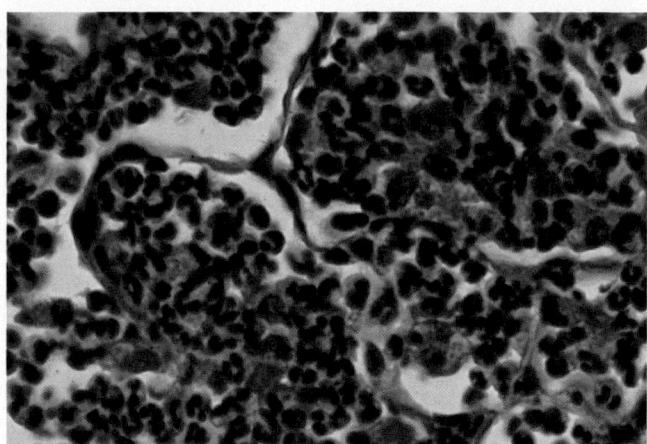

Fig 88-9 Histopathologic appearance of lung from dog with suppurative bronchopneumonia showing neutrophilic infiltrates in alveolar spaces (H and E stain, ×400). (Courtesy Veterinary Pathology, University of Georgia, Athens, Ga.)

is composed of a large number of microaerophilic and anaerobic organisms, which may lead to pulmonary abscesses.[68]

Pulmonary Abscess

Pulmonary abscesses—necrotic areas of lung parenchyma containing purulent material usually produced by pyogenic infection—are uncommon in dogs and cats. Most of these abscesses arise from aspiration of oropharyngeal or gastric contents and are termed primary lung abscess. Secondary lung abscess results from a primary underlying process such as bronchial obstruction, septic or heartworm thromboembolism, airway parasite, foreign body, bullous emphysema, tuberculous cavity, or neoplasia. Obligate anaerobic bacteria are identified more frequently than aerobic bacteria are, but mixed infections are common. *Mycoplasma* spp. have also been recovered in cats.

The clinical signs in pulmonary abscess formation depend on the cause but closely resemble those of chronic bacterial pneumonia. Clinical findings include weight loss, chronic fever, cough, and hemoptysis. Hematologic findings include leukocytosis with a left shift, anemia, and rarely hypoproteinemia. An abscess will usually appear on a thoracic radiograph as an ill-defined pulmonary nodule or mass with or without cavitation. Radiographically, abscesses are often indistinguishable from granulomas, traumatic bullae, tumors, and pneumatocysts. If the lesion is close to the chest wall, ultrasound can be used to visualize the abscess, which will appear fluid filled. Cytologic examination of brushings or lavage fluid is consistent with a septic or nonseptic purulent exudate. Ultrasound-guided, fine-needle aspiration is not recommended for lesions suspicious for an abscess because of the risk of spreading the infection to the pleural cavity.

Therapy of Lower Airway Infections

Compared with treatment of upper airway infections, lower respiratory tract infections must be treated more aggressively. Systemically effective antimicrobials must be used. Drug penetration into consolidated lung tissues is more effective systemically than it is by topical (i.e., aerosol) means.

Antibiotics

Drug dosages for airway infections are summarized in Table 88-8. Specific information on each drug is available in the Drug Formulary, Appendix 8. Oral or parenteral antibacterials are the principal therapies for lower respiratory tract bacterial infections. Expecting any single antibacterial to be routinely effective against the wide variety of organisms causing bacterial pneumonia is unrealistic. The most important criterion for selection of an antibacterial is identification of the bacterial organism. Substantially more patients recover if antibacterial therapy is administered according to culture results and in vitro susceptibility testing than not.[132] Morphologic characteristics of bacteria on a Gram-stained slide can aid in antibiotic choice until the results of bacterial culture and susceptibility have become available.[108] Cocci are usually staphylococci or streptococci. Rods are usually members of the family Enterobacteriaceae, which are most unpredictable with respect to antibacterial agents (Table 88-9).

Penetration of antimicrobial drugs into airway secretions and pulmonary tissues is favored by high lipophilicity and low molecular weight. Drugs enter normal bronchial secretions at a fraction of their serum concentrations. Trimethoprim, clindamycin, fluoroquinolone, erythromycin, and doxycycline enter in highest proportions. Penicillins have the lowest penetration; cephalosporins and aminoglycosides have intermediate distribution. With inflammation, penetrance is increased, but antibiotic distribution through the airway may be impaired in exudates.

The aminopenicillanic derivatives have a broader spectrum than penicillin, including activity against gram-positive, many gram-negative, and some anaerobic bacteria. *E. coli*, *Proteus*, *Klebsiella*, and *Pasteurella* are usually susceptible. Resistance is often present in *Enterobacter*, *Serratia*, and *Pseudomonas*. Resistance can be overcome in some instances by using a β-lactamase inhibitor such as clavulanate or sulbactam. Fluoroquinolones or aminoglycosides are recommended if resistant gram-negative infections are suspected. If cytologic information is not available, initial treatment with amoxicillin-clavulanate is recommended. Later therapy should be based on the susceptibility spectrum indicated by cultural results.

With severe clinical signs, respiratory distress, or evidence of bacteremia, intravenous therapy is recommended until the patient stabilizes. Levels of antibacterials in airway secretions after oral or parenteral administration are much lower than serum levels. Systemic antibacterials therefore should be administered in high doses for long periods so that maximum concentrations are reached in lung tissues and airway secretions.

For usually self-limiting tracheobronchitis, antibiotics are not usually indicated unless clinical signs persist for longer than 2 weeks, the dogs have a concurrent respiratory disease (e.g., collapsing trachea), or systemic signs of illness become evident. Of antibiotics administered for *B. pertussis*, high percentages of isolates are resistant to ampicillin and the first- and third-generation cephalosporins, with intermediate resistance to amoxicillin-clavulanate.[40] Macrolides (e.g., erythromycin, clarithromycin, azithromycin), fluoroquinolones, tetracyclines, chloramphenicol, and sulfonamides reach concentrations in airway tissues and secretions and should be considered as drugs of choice based on susceptibility testing.[70] For lower respiratory tract infections, treatment is generally recommended for at least 1 week beyond resolution of clinical illness or at least a 2-week minimum. With chronic bronchitis, or with bronchiectasis, treatment may be longer, or repeated cycles of antibiotic therapy may be indicated when a clinical relapse occurs.

Particularly severe or resistant gram-negative or anaerobic bacterial pneumonia must be treated parenterally with drugs such as the extended-spectrum penicillin, ticarcillin, combined with clavulanate. The combination is effective against gram-negative bacteria and anaerobes, as are imipenem-cilastatin or second- or third-generation cephalosporins. Aminoglycosides are effective against gram-negative organisms. Pneumonia secondary to bacteremia is often caused by

Table • 88-8

Recommended Dosages of Antibacterial Drugs for Respiratory Disease

DRUG[a]	SPECIES	DOSE[b]	ROUTE	INTERVAL (HOUR)
Amikacin	B	5.0—7.5 mg/kg	IV, IM, SC	12
	B	15 mg/kg	IV, IM, SC	24
Amoxicillin	B	15—20 mg/kg	PO, IM, SC	8
Amoxicillin-clavulanate	B	15 mg/kg	PO PO	8
	B	20 mg/kg		12
Ampicillin	B	22—30 mg/kg	PO, IV, SC	8
Ampicillin-sulbactam	D	20 mg/kg	IV, IM	6—8
Carbenicillin	D	10—30 mg/kg	IV, IM	6—8
Cefazolin (1st)	B	10—30 mg/kg	IV, IM, SC	6—8
Cefotaxime (3rd)	B	25—50 mg/kg	IV, IM	6—8
Cefotetan (2nd)	B	25—30 mg/kg	IV, SC	8
Cefoxitin (2nd)	B	10—20 mg/kg	IV, IM	6—8
Ceftiofur (3rd)	B	4.4 mg/kg	SC	12
Cephalexin (1st)	B	22—44 mg/kg	PO	8
Cephradine (1st)	B	22—44 mg/kg	IV, SC	8
Chloramphenicol	D	50 mg/kg	PO, IV, SC	8
	C	50 mg total	PO, IV, SC	12
Clindamycin	D	10 mg/kg	PO, SC	12
	C	10—15 mg/kg	PO, SC	12
Doxycycline[c]	B	5—10 mg/kg	PO	12
Enrofloxacin[d]	B	5—11 mg/kg	PO, SC, IV[e]	12
Gentamicin[f]	B	2 mg/kg	IV, IM, SC	8—12
	B	8 mg/kg	IM, IV	24
Imipenem-cilastatin	B	3—10 mg/kg	IV, IM	8
Kanamycin[f]	B	5—7.5 mg/kg	IV, IM, SC	8
Piperacillin	B	25—50 mg/kg	IV	8
Tetracycline	D	22 mg/kg	PO	8
Ticarcillin	B	40—75[e] mg/kg	IV	6—8
Ticarcillin-clavulanate	B	30—50[e] mg/kg	IV	6—8
Tobramycin[f]	B	2 mg/kg	IV, IM, SC	8
Trimethoprim-sulfonamide	B	15 mg/kg	PO, SC	12

B, Dog and cat; D, dog; C, cat; IV, intravenous; IM, intramuscular; SC, subcutaneous; PO, by mouth.
[a]For more information on all drugs, see Drug Formulary, Appendix 8.
[b]Dose per administration at specified interval. Duration is for at least 1 week after clinical response is noted. Responses should be noted within 3 to 5 days, and therapy should continue for at least 14 days.
[c]Also can substitute minocycline.
[d]Also can substitute ciprofloxacin.
[e]Highest levels for treating *Pseudomonas*.
[f]Potentially nephrotoxic. Must monitor urine sediment and serum urea concentration.

gram-negative sepsis in immunocompromised people or animals. If clinical improvement occurs and blood culture results are negative after 4 days, parenteral therapy can be discontinued and oral therapy begun. Antibiotic therapy should be continued at least 1 week past the resolution of all clinical and radiographic signs of pneumonia.

Damage to the lung with aspiration pneumonia is not always caused by the development of bacterial pneumonia; damage from gastric acid can cause a chemical pneumonia, and inhaled food can lead to inflammation and airway obstruction. Compromise of local host immune defense mechanisms may predispose the patient to secondary bacterial infections well after the initial noninfectious pneumonia has been initiated. Routine antibiotic use is therefore controversial. Because of the concern of developing bacterial resistance with indiscriminant antibiotic use, antimicrobials should ideally be delayed until secondary bacterial infection can be documented or until the animal fails to respond appropriately to

other therapy for this condition (see later discussion). When infection plays a role in aspiration pneumonia, a multiplicity of aerobic and anaerobic organisms can be involved and combination antibiotic therapy may be required. Culture and susceptibility results should guide selection of the antibiotic. Prevention of aspiration pneumonia involves identifying predisposing risk factors and addressing them directly (e.g., megaesophagus, prolonged anesthesia, neurologic deficits). Aspiration can be avoided by keeping the patient's body positioned in sternal recumbency or by keeping the cranial part elevated and minimizing gastric volume by frequent feedings or keeping feeding tubes in the small bowel (i.e., jejunostomy tubes) rather than the stomach or esophagus. To prevent aspiration and infection during anesthesia, aspiration of oropharyngeal secretions, maintenance of a cuffed endotracheal tube, close monitoring during anesthetic recovery, and avoidance of cross-contamination between patients by using sterilized equipment are recommended.

Table • 88-9

Antimicrobial Therapy for Lower Airway Bacterial Infections[a]

Gram-positive cocci	Ampicillin, amoxicillin, chloramphenicol, gentamicin, trimethoprim-sulfonamide, first-generation cephalosporins
Gram-negative rods	Amikacin, chloramphenicol, gentamicin, trimethoprim-sulfonamide, fluoroquinolones, second- and third-generation cephalosporins, ampicillin-sulbactam, imipenem-cilastatin, piperacillin, ticarcillin, carbenicillin
Pasteurella	Ampicillin, gentamicin, trimethoprim-sulfonamide, enrofloxacin
Bordetella	Tetracycline, gentamicin, chloramphenicol, trimethoprim-sulfonamide, tylosin, kanamycin, fluoroquinolones, amoxicillin-clavulanate, azithromycin
Anaerobes	Ampicillin- or amoxicillin-clavulanate, penicillin, second- or third-generation cephalosporins, clindamycin, metronidazole,[b] ticarcillin, carbenicillin
Mycoplasmas	Doxycycline, chloramphenicol, gentamicin, fluoroquinolones, tylosin, clindamycin

[a]Consult Drug Formulary, Appendix 8, for appropriate dosages and further information on each drug.
[b]Despite in vitro efficacy, metronidazole does poorly in treatment of anaerobic pulmonary infections because of the high oxygen tension in these tissues.

Pulmonary abscesses are seen with airway obstruction from severe infection, certain bacteria, such as *Actinomyces* or *Nocardia*, or from foreign material. Lung abscesses are usually initially treated without drainage but with long-term antibacterial therapy. Choice of antibacterials should be based on culture and susceptibility findings. Response to antimicrobial therapy may be temporary or incomplete, and relapse of fever and coughing can occur once treatment is discontinued, even after months of such treatment. Furthermore, evidence of a persistent pattern of alveolar consolidation may be apparent in thoracic radiographs. Bronchoscopy can be used to localize affected lobes and, if performed early, can be used to remove foreign material such as plant awns. With long-standing occlusion, scarring, and abscess formation, thoracotomy and lobectomy are indicated. Lobectomy is most effective in resolving pneumonias, and postoperative complications are least in pneumonias that are localized to individual lobes.[91]

Systemic Hydration

Maintenance of normal systemic hydration is an important therapeutic objective in patients with bacterial pneumonia. Dehydration hinders mucociliary clearance and secretion mobilization because normal respiratory secretions are more than 90% water.

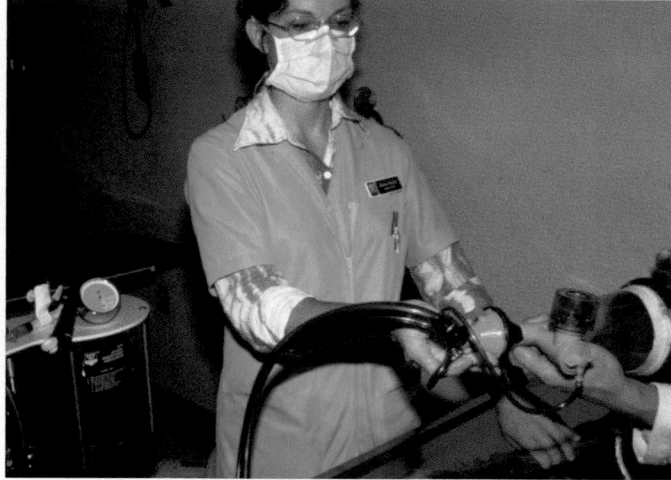

Fig 88-10 Nebulization of antimicrobials for a dog with pneumonia. Note protective mask during therapy. (Courtesy University of Georgia, Athens, Ga.)

Airway Hydration

Airway hydration can be directly addressed using aerosol therapy to mobilize secretions by adding water to the mucociliary blanket. A nebulizer that produces particles between 0.5 and 3.0 µm ensures that water is deposited in the lower airways. Water vaporizers or humidifiers are inadequate because the water particulate size is larger and droplets are generally deposited in the nasal cavity. For nebulization, the animal is placed in an enclosed chamber, and a bland aerosol (normal saline) is nebulized into the chamber. Physiotherapy should always be performed immediately after aerosolization to enhance secretion clearance. Methods include increased cough frequency by chest wall coupage or tracheal manipulation, mild forced exercise, and postural drainage. The animal should be nebulized two or three times daily for 20 minutes per treatment. Because bronchoconstriction may develop, pretreatment with bronchodilators can be considered.

Antibiotics can also be administered by nebulization for dogs with infectious tracheobronchitis (Fig. 88-10). A recent study showed gentamicin at an average dose of 6.9 mg/kg diluted 1:2 with sterile saline given via an aerosol significantly decreased cough.[86] Routine intratracheal or aerosol administration of antibacterials is not recommended in pneumonia. With severe alveolar consolidation in pneumonia, airway penetration of antimicrobials is inferior to systemic administration. Furthermore, people performing the procedure must take precautions to avoid inhaling the aerosolized drugs or avoid contact of the aerosols with their exposed mucous membranes.

Supportive Therapy

Animals with severe tachypnea, dyspnea, or marked hypoxemia (arterial oxygen tension under 60 mm Hg) require oxygen therapy. The early period of highest mortality with bacterial pneumonia corresponds to the period of greatest hypoxemia. The oxygen should be humidified to prevent drying of respiratory membranes. Oxygen can be administered in a cage, by intratracheal cannula or nasal catheter, or in intubated patients (with or without a mechanical ventilator). Drugs such as antitussives, diuretics, and antihistamines that inhibit mucokinesis and exudate removal from the respiratory tract are contraindicated with bacterial pneumonia. The use of systemic bronchodilators such as theo-

Table • 88-10

Prevalence Range of Bacteria Isolated from Canine and Feline Pyothorax[a,34,140,116,139,111]

ORGANISM	DOGS	CATS
Anaerobes		
Actinomyces spp.	9-46	0-15
Bacteroides spp.	6-33	7-24
Fusobacterium spp.	3-35	0-17
Peptostreptococcus spp.	8-27	0-20
Propionibacterium spp.	2	0
Prevotella spp.	6-23	9
Porphyromonas spp.	9	12
Clostridium spp.	3	1-38
Eubacterium spp.	3	0
Filifactor villosus	0	4
Fibrobacter succinogenes	0	4
Unidentified gram-negative rods	0-4	7-8
Unidentified gram-positive rods	3	2
Aerobes		
Actinomyces	9-19	0-15
Pasteurella	11-31	40-62.5
Escherichia coli	9-54	0-4
Proteus	3	0
Pseudomonas	4	0
Klebsiella	4	0
Enterobacter	7	0
Actinobacillus	0	4
Corynebacterium	11	0
Capnocytophaga canimorsus	4	0
Acinetobacter	0-4	4
Nocardia	4-22	0-7
Staphylococcus	3-4	0-4
Streptococcus	6-11	0
Enterococcus spp.	8	4
Unidentified filamentous	3	0
Unidentified nonfilamentous	0-8	4-18
Mycoplasma	4	0

[a]Fungi such as *Aspergillus*, *Blastomyces*, *Candida*, and *Cryptococcus* have been isolated from canine and feline pyothorax; however, no data are available.

phylline in animals with evidence of bronchoconstriction must be done with caution if chloramphenicol or fluoroquinolones are being used concurrently because these drugs increase the serum theophylline concentration. Terbutaline can be given at 0.01 mg/kg subcutaneously for emergency treatment of bronchospasm and acute respiratory distress. Cyproheptadine (2 mg, given orally, twice daily) has been administered in cats with bronchoconstriction that do not tolerate terbutaline.[103]

PLEURAL INFECTIONS

Purulent pleuritis, pyothorax, and thoracic empyema describe septic processes of the pleural cavity resulting in exudate accumulation.

Etiology

Pleural infections are almost always polymicrobic in nature, a factor evident when comparing the cytologic findings and culture results. A high incidence exists of obligate anaerobic bacteria as sole pathogens or in combination with aerobic-facultative and other anaerobic bacteria. Obligate anaerobic bacteria and gram-positive filamentous organisms such as *Nocardia* and *Actinomyces* are most commonly isolated from dogs with pyothorax (see Chapter 49). Isolation of *Actinomyces* has commonly been associated with grass-awn, foreign-body migration. *Actinomyces* and *Nocardia* have a filamentous appearance; however, these may be confused with *Filifactor villosus*, an anaerobic rod isolated from pyothorax in dogs and cats.[78,140] The most common aerobic organism isolated in feline pyothorax is *Pasteurella*, although anaerobes are frequently cultured as well.[139,140] Other bacterial, fungal, and yeast organisms isolated from pleural exudate of the dog and cat are summarized in Table 88-10. Sources of bacterial pleural infections are not identified in most cases but include penetrating thoracic wounds (e.g., bite wounds); migrating foreign bodies (grass awns); esophageal perforation; hematogenous spread; lung parasites; extension from cervical, lumbar, mediastinal, or pulmonary infections; and iatrogenic causes.[139] Grass awns enter the oral cavity when animals are breathing hard during field training. The awns are barbed so that only antegrade movement is possible. They migrate down the bronchial tree carrying commensal microflora from the oropharyngeal cavity into the lung parenchyma. The awns exit the visceral pleura and enter the pleural cavity where they can cause pyothorax or migrate up the diaphragmatic crura to the sublumbar vertebrae.

Clinical Findings

Pyothorax most commonly occurs in young adult medium- to large-breed dogs, especially of working and sporting breeds.[34] The link with these breeds is thought to be associated with grass-awn inhalation during vigorous exercise. Risk factors for cats include young age and being part of a multiple-cat household but not male gender or indoor or outdoor status, as was previously reported.[139] Clinical signs result from restrictive respiratory disease, including increased respiratory rate, shallow respirations, dyspnea, and orthopnea. Other signs include depression, exercise intolerance, cough, lethargy, anorexia, weight loss, and fever. Physical examination reveals muffled heart sounds, decreased breath sounds, and hyperresonant (dull) percussion sounds, especially over the ventral portions of the thorax. Chronic or severe infections may result in a dehydrated, debilitated, collapsed, or hypothermic patient. Approximately one third of cats with pyothorax may develop signs of sepsis or systemic inflammatory response syndrome (SIRS) (see Chapter 38). Signs in cats with SIRS include rectal temperature above 39.7° C (103.5° F) or below 37.8° C (100.0° F); heart rate above 225 beats/minute or below 140 beats/minute; respiratory rate above 40 breaths/minute; and white blood cell count over 19,500/μl or below 5000/μl, or band neutrophils above 5%.[139] In cats, hypersalivation and bradycardia are associated with a worse clinical outcome.[139]

Diagnosis

A diagnosis of pyothorax is confirmed by hematology, thoracic radiography, and thoracocentesis with cytologic evaluation and culture of pleural fluid. Neutrophilic leukocytosis with or without a left shift is the most common hematologic finding; however, in one report, only 56% of affected dogs and 36% of cats had this abnormality.[34] Leukogram results do not correlate with the severity of the underlying infection, however, and leukocyte counts within or lower than the reference range are found with some frequency. Biochemical abnormalities in some animals can include hypoalbuminemia, hyperglobulinemia, elevated hepatic enzyme activities, hyperglycemia or hypoglycemia, and azotemia.[34] Radiographic signs of free pleural fluid include increased hazy density of the lung fields (ventral portions of lung fields on lateral view), which obscures the cardiac silhouette; retraction of the lobar borders from the chest wall; visibility of the interlobar fissures; and rounding or filling of the costophrenic angles.

Cytologic evaluation of pleural fluid is usually consistent with septic or nonseptic exudates (Table 88-11). Degenerate neutrophils and mixed populations of bacteria are often observed. Cytomorphology of the neutrophil is most helpful for determination of whether pleural fluid should be cultured and for interpretation of the results of culture. Aerobic and anaerobic cultures of pleural fluid should be made, if available, regardless of whether bacteria are seen cytologically. Neutrophil degeneration may be observed in severe cases; however, the level of the neutrophil concentration can vary and does not always correlate with the severity of infection.

Therapy

Treatment of pyothorax should be prompt and aggressive. Initial goals include relief of respiratory embarrassment via thoracocentesis, appropriate fluid therapy, supportive care, and systemic antibacterials. If the animal dies during therapy, this often happens in the initial 48-hour management period of drainage and stabilization.[34] Drainage of pleural exudates and lavage are essential, as is the case for any accumulation of pus. Disadvantages of delay in pleural lavage are incomplete resolution of signs and formation of loculated abscesses and fibroses, which will necessitate later thoracotomy. Pleural drainage and lavage are achieved by tube thoracostomy. Advantages of closed chest drainage and lavage include avoiding frequent needle thoracocentesis, facilitating pleural fluid sampling to monitor therapeutic response, and allowing direct instillation of isotonic lavage fluid (+/− additives) into the pleural space (see later discussion). Disadvantages include maintaining drain placement and patency and risking pneumothorax and chest wall infection. Mortality appears to be higher in patients treated with multiple thoracocentesis and antibacterials than it is in those treated with tube thoracostomy alone. The average length of chest tube drainage is 3 to 7 days.

For tube placement, the patient is first given fluid therapy, and specimens for cytologic and microbiologic examination can be withdrawn for analysis by needle aspiration. After sedation with local anesthetic infusion or general anesthesia, a tube is placed in the intercostal space by tunneling under the skin a few interspaces and penetrating the pleura with the tube by hemostat or stylet. After fluid removal, radiographs should be taken to assess whether drainage is complete, especially on the contralateral side. If removal is incomplete, another tube may be required. The tubes are clamped and wrapped to prevent inadvertent air leakage into the pleural space. When available or practical, one-way continuous suction or intermittent suction every 2 hours may be applied. Fluid is infused through the tip of an intravenous administration set wedged firmly into the lumen of the tube's orifice. The clamp is used to control infusion rate. Fluid volumes for infusion are usually 100 ml for small dogs and cats, 500 ml for intermediate-sized dogs, and 1000 ml for large dogs. Lavage is continued for up to 7 days or until the removed fluid is clear of pus. This time interval can be as long as 21 days.[34] Cytologic improvement is exhibited by decreasing cell count, with loss of degenerative changes in neutrophils, and absence of bacteria.

Although no scientific studies in dogs or cats evaluating the effect of saline lavage (with or without heparin or streptokinase) have been done, empirical data in dogs and cats and studies in the human literature suggest that under some circumstances, lavage may facilitate removal of accumulated pus and bacteria and break down clots and fibrin bands. Heparin levels within the infusate have not been studied, and in all likelihood, it is rapidly absorbed in the systemic circulation giving only temporary anticoagulation. Therefore subcutaneous administration (100 IU/kg) given every 8 hours may provide a more sustained and constant effect during the course of lavage treatment. Instilling proteolytic enzymes such as streptokinase to infusate when treating dogs has been associated with increases in body temperature,[60] presumably as a reaction to the foreign protein. The benefit of such enzymes has not been substantiated, and the cost is significant; therefore they are not recommended. The intermittent approach involves at least twice-daily instillation of intravenous saline into the pleural space with mild coupage followed by immediate removal of whatever fluid can be obtained (Table 88-12). Addition of antimicrobial agents to the lavage fluid is controversial, as is the case for most absorbable antimicrobials; this is just another means of parenteral administration. In one report, the mean lavage time of lavage was 6.3 days (range of 2 to 21 days) without added antimicrobials to a mean of 4.8 days (range of 4 to 6 days) with them added.[34] Ampicillin (5 mg/kg) or amoxicillin-clavulanate (7 mg/kg) or metronidazole (4 mg/kg), alone or in combination, were used as intrapleural drugs.

Systemic antimicrobial therapy can be considered concurrently, but it is *ineffective* without lavage or drainage of the infected pleural cavity (see Table 88-8). No single antibacterial agent will inhibit the wide variety of facultative and

Table • 88-11

Characteristics of Pleural Fluid from Pyothorax

PARAMETER	REFERENCE CHARACTERISTICS	PYOTHORAX
Physical characteristics	Color: clear, transparent	Color: variable yellow to reddish-brown, opaque, flocculent; sometimes granules can be odorous
Cells	<500/μl	>7000/μl
Protein	<1.5 g/dl	>3 g/dl
Specific gravity	<1.017	≥1.025
Biochemistry of fluid	LDH activity and glucose concentration in reference blood range	LDH activity increased; glucose concentration decreased compared with blood[a]

LDH, Lactic dehydrogenase.
[a]These changes have been presently been documented in cats and people.

Table • 88-12

Comparison of Methods of Managing Pyothorax

METHOD	ADVANTAGES	DISADVANTAGES
Systemic antimicrobial therapy	Inexpensive and noninvasive	Does not allow for drainage of fluid or necrotic debris. Reduced efficacy of resolving intrapleural infection caused by poor antimicrobial penetration into exudates.
Repeated thoracentesis, without lavage	Inexpensive, available to most practices	Higher risk of pulmonary trauma from repeated puncture, causing hemorrhage or pneumothorax. Does not flush out loculated material, and may leave nidus.
Periodic lavage via indwelling tubes	Less monitoring, more convenient for practice. Can instill lavage solutions and reach loculated areas. Easier to monitor appearance of chest fluid by repeated sampling.	May develop thoracic wall infection or fistula. Animal must be collared or drain wrapped (or both) to prevent its removal.
Continuous suction via indwelling tubes	Less daily lavage needed once therapy has been initiated.	High expense of continuous-suction apparatus. Same problems as for Periodic Lavage above, and continuous suction does not reduce time period for lavage treatments. Requires constant 24-hour monitoring of suction equipment.

obligate anaerobic bacteria associated with pyothorax.[140] Penicillin or penicillin derivatives are often given because they are effective against obligate anaerobic, *Pasteurella*, and *Actinomyces* infections.

Systemic antibacterial therapy should be continued for at least 4 to 6 weeks. Regardless of the anaerobic or facultative anaerobic bacteria that are cultured, the regimen should always contain drugs effective against anaerobes. Lack of significant improvement in fluid consistency during lavage, formation of lung abscesses, repeated blockage of drainage tubes, recurrent pneumothorax, mediastinal masses, or radiographic evidence of fluid encapsulation are indications for surgical exploration or lobectomy. Surgical exploration allows for detection of foreign bodies, which are often incriminated as causing pulmonary infections and are often involved in persistent pulmonary abscesses that rupture, leading to pyothorax. Although surgical exploration is expensive, reports suggest that dogs having surgical exploration and débridement have a better outcome following treatment compared with pleural lavage alone.[116]

Radiographic monitoring is essential during treatment and followup of pleural infections. Radiography has limitations in evaluating the type and extent of lung lesions in the presence of fluid. When finances are not limited, CT or mirror resonance may be more valuable in initially assessing the need for early surgical intervention. Ideally, radiographic reevaluation should be performed after the fluid is initially removed, when the chest tube is removed, immediately before discontinuing antibiotics, and 1 to 2 weeks after discontinuing antibiotics to monitor for subclinical recurrence of disease.

SUGGESTED READINGS*

21. Chandler JC, Lappin MR. 2002. Mycoplasmal respiratory infections in small animals: 17 cases (1988-1999), *J Am Anim Hosp Assoc* 38:111-119.

24. Cohn LA, Norris CR, Hawkins EC, et al. 2004. Identification and characterization of an idiopathic pulmonary fibrosis–like condition in cats, *J Vet Intern Med* 18:632-641.

32. DeBerry JD, Norris CR, Samii VF, et al. 2002. Correlation between fine-needle aspiration cytopathology and histopathology of the lung in dogs and cats, *J Am Anim Hosp Assoc* 38:327-336.

34. Demetriou JL, Foale RD, Ladlow J, et al. 2002. Canine and feline pyothorax: a retrospective study of 50 cases in the UK and Ireland, *J Small Anim Pract* 43:388-394.

40. Foley JE, Rand C, Bannasch MJ, et al. 2002. Molecular epidemiology of feline bordetellosis in two animal shelters in California, USA, *Prev Vet Med* 54:141-156.

45. Foster SF, Martin P, Allan GS, et al. 2004. Lower respiratory tract infections in cats: 21 cases (1995-2000), *J Feline Med Surg* 6:167-180.

46. Foster SF, Martin P, Braddock JA, et al. 2004. A retrospective analysis of feline bronchoalveolar lavage cytology and microbiology (1995-2000), *J Feline Med Surg* 6:189-198.

67. Johnson LR, Clarke HE, Bannasch MJ, et al. 2004. Correlation of rhinoscopic signs of inflammation with histologic findings in nasal biopsy specimens of cats with or without upper respiratory tract disease, *J Am Vet Med Assoc* 225:395-400.

116. Rooney MB, Monnet E. 2002. Medical and surgical treatment of pyothorax in dogs: 26 cases (1991-2001), *J Am Vet Med Assoc* 221:86-92.

139. Waddell LS, Brady CA, Drobatz KJ. 2002. Risk factors, prognostic indicators, and outcome of pyothorax in cats: 80 cases (1986-1999), *J Am Vet Med Assoc* 221:819-824.

*See the CD-ROM for a complete list of references.

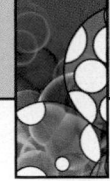
Gastrointestinal and Intraabdominal Infections

Craig E. Greene

This chapter discusses bacterial and fungal infections of the GI tract, which cause alterations in native microflora. For specific infections regarding enteropathogenic viral, bacterial, fungal, or protozoal pathogens, see the respective chapters in this book.

ORAL CAVITY

Oral Microflora

The resident microbial flora of the canine and feline oral cavity are composed of a wide variety of aerobic bacteria and facultative and obligate anaerobic bacteria (Tables 89-1 and 89-2). In most studies, *Streptococcus* and *Actinomyces* are the most frequently reported bacteria that are not obligate anaerobes. The frequency with which individual species are isolated depends on culture methods, sampling sites, and breed and individual differences. From a clinical standpoint, bacterial culture of specimens from the oropharyngeal region is meaningless because of the diversity of commensal organisms and the lack of accurate quantitative methods. However, antimicrobial agents used in treating oral infections such as gingivitis and stomatitis should be chosen with the composition of the resident microflora in mind. Organisms found in bite-inflicted and soft-tissue wound infections (see Chapter 53), pleural (see Chapter 88), and peritoneal infections (see Intraabdominal Infections later) reflect the composition of the oral microflora.

Gingivitis and Periodontitis

Inflammation and recession of perialveolar gum margins are common findings in dogs and cats.[203] They are initially caused by excessive accumulation of dental plaque resulting from deposition of by-products from breakdown of food and saliva by normal resident microflora. Plaque is an organic matrix of salivary glycoproteins and polysaccharides adhering to the tooth surface that provides sites for oral bacteria to proliferate. Microflora involved with supragingival and subgingival plaque in healthy mucosal sites in dogs are resident streptococci and *Actinomyces* species.[119,120] At first, these gram-positive, nonmotile aerobic cocci and bacilli predominate. These bacteria produce a glycopolysaccharide referred to as a *glycocalyx*, which facilitates the attachment of other bacteria. This biofilm is further consolidated into a film, or plaque. Plaque accumulation results in inflammation of the gums. Plaque can become mineralized, resulting in calculus (tartar). As periodontal inflammation progresses with associated calculus formation, gram-negative motile, obligate anaerobic rods and spirochetes proliferate (Fig. 89-1).[213,346] Pups have very few *Porphyromonas* species in their dental plaque; however, their numbers increase as the pup matures and inevitable periodontal disease develops.[141] Early bacterial damage occurs in the gingival epithelial tissues with penetration of the interdental retes. Proliferating spirochetes may disrupt the inter-

cellular junctions, creating a portal of entry for other bacteria.[213] Periodontal pathogens destroy the integrity of the dentition and oral mucosae and can also cause bacteremia or distant tissue embolization. Many of these bacteria possess proteolytic enzymes that allow them to colonize and invade periodontal tissues. Unfortunately, periodontal disease is irreversible, and damaged gum tissue cannot be restored to health. In people, periodontitis, which results from bacterial proliferation in the gingival sulcus, has been associated with an increased population of *Porphyromonas (Bacteroides) gingivalis*.[98] In comparison, microflora from anaerobic plaque and gingival crevices of dogs with periodontal disease are *P. gingivalis*; *Porphyromonas* species isolates; *Prevotella* and *Wolinella* species that are pigmented, gram-negative rods; *Actinobacillus actinomycetemcomitans*; and *Clostridium* and *Fusobacterium* species. Reduced numbers of streptococci, enterococci, and staphylococci are found compared with normal flora (Table 89-3).[140,141] In cats, differences in the microflora between clinically healthy animals and those with gingivitis have not been appreciated (see Table 89-2). *P. gingivalis* is the most likely periodontal pathogen associated with progressive periodontal disease in cats.[224-227] Salivary microflora, which differs from plaque microflora, remain relatively constant in the presence of periodontal disease.

Calculus is mineralized dental plaque that adheres to tooth surfaces, facilitating additional plaque formation and periodontal inflammation. Complete removal of all supragingival and subgingival calculi is essential in control of periodontal disease. Long-term intermittent periodontal care for dogs is highly recommended because it slows the progression of gingival recession and depth of periodontal crevices that develop in dogs not receiving dental hygiene.[137] Gingival hypertrophy and alveolar abscess formation are sequelae of calculus formation. The type of microflora present, the diet, and the animal's chewing habits may be important in the formation of calculus.[337] Advancing age is a predisposing factor in dogs.[126] Leukopenia and bacteremia occasionally develop as secondary effects.[189]

Although bacterial pathogens are important in periodontitis, antimicrobial therapy alone does not eliminate progression of disease. Proinflammatory cytokines, such as tumor necrosis factor (TNF) and interleukin-1 (IL-1), have been important in the progression of periodontal disease in experimental animals.[56,91] Cats with more severe periodontal disease have greater serum antibody titers to *Prophyromonas salivosa* and *P. gingivalis* than those with less severe periodontal disease.[193,223,227,228] Inhibition of IL-1 and TNF with specific blockers has been beneficial in inhibiting inflammation and preserving bone in the periodontal tissues. Other antiinflammatory drugs such as metalloproteinase matrix (e.g., tetracyclines) and prostaglandin inhibitors such as nonsteroidal antiinflammatory drugs (NSAIDs) have been beneficial in this regard. These findings support the concept that periodontal tissue loss is caused by an exaggerated host response to certain species of bacteria with the ability to grow on the tooth

Table • 89-1

Microflora Most Commonly Isolated from the Oral Cavities of Clinically Healthy Dogs

ORGANISM	SITES
Aerobic and Microaerophilic Anaerobic	
Gram-Negative	
Neisseria	B
Escherichia coli	B
Pasteurella	B
Pseudomonas	B
Proteus	T
Moraxella	N
Acinetobacter	N
Capnocytophaga	N
EF-4	N
Bergeyella (Weeksella) zoohelcum	N
Gram-Positive	
Actinomyces	N
Nonhemolytic streptococci	B
β-Hemolytic streptococci	B
Staphylococcus epidermidis	B
Staphylococcus intermidius	B
Corynebacterium	N
Lactobacillus	B
Bacillus	U
Obligate Anaerobic	
Bacteroides	U
Fusobacterium	U
Propionibacterium	U
Peptostreptococcus	U
Bifidobacterium	U
Clostridium	U
Veillonella	U
Eikenella corrodens	N
Simonsiella	N
Other	
Candida	T
Mycoplasma	T

B, Tonsillar and nontonsillar; *T*, tonsillar; *N*, nontonsillar, supragingival scrapings; *U*, unspecified sites.

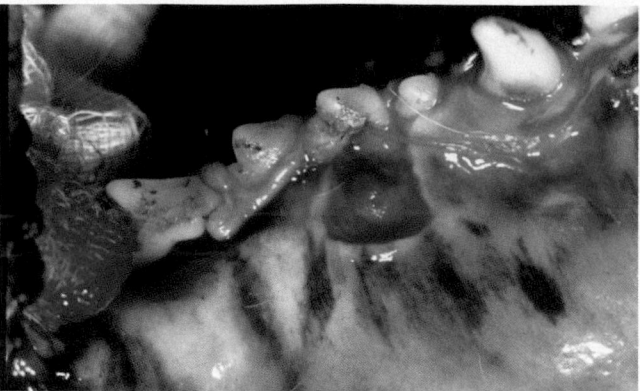

Fig 89-1 Accumulation of dental tartar and resulting perialveolar gingivitis in cat. (Courtesy University of Georgia, Athens, Ga.)

surface and in periodontal structures and a triggering of an inflammatory cascade.

Adjunctive management methods such as providing hard diets, regular tooth brushing, and oral hygiene chews have been shown to reduce the incidence of calculus accumulation.[88-90,137,251] Treatment includes the extraction of severely affected teeth, debriding necrotic or proliferative gum margins, and scaling calculi from the remaining involved dental surfaces.

Systemic antimicrobials such as tetracycline, metronidazole, and tinidazole and topical chlorhexidine have been evaluated for treatment of periodontitis in experimentally affected dogs.[253] Clindamycin treatment for 5 days after dental prophylaxis reduced subsequent oral odor and dental plaque formation when dogs were monitored for up to 70 days.[335] Treatment of clinically healthy beagle dogs with clindamycin for 14 days reduced the amount of gingival crevicular fluid, dental plaque, and gingivitis.[366] (For drug dosages, see Table 89-4 and the Drug Formulary, Appendix 8.) Tetracycline and metronidazole have been beneficial in reducing dental calculus or preventing its reformation when they have been given with or without mechanical cleansing. After 1 year of tetracycline therapy, dogs with periodontal disease had less alveolar bone resorption than untreated controls.[359]

Perioceutics are pharmaceutical formulations that are placed into periodontal pockets to allow for sustained antimicrobial activity against periodontal pathogens. They are used as an adjunct to scaling and cleaning the dental surfaces. These perioceutics, consisting of tetracyclines and having antibacterial and anticollagenase activity, are delivered into the periodontal pocket via a blunt cannula. Once there, the polymer gels coagulate, allowing for sustained release of the drug for up to 13 weeks.[42,165] Dogs with periodontal disease, having dental cleaning followed by doxycycline polymer applied to their gingival crevice, had less periodontal disease than untreated animals after 12 weeks of monitoring.[115,122,367] In addition to a reduction in the depth of alveolar pockets, a reduction in aerobic microaerophilic and anaerobic bacterial microflora and proteolytic enzymes, such as collagenase, have been observed.[367] Topically applied polymers containing doxycycline (Heska, Fort Collins, Colo.; Pharmacia Animal Health, Piscataway, N.J.) or minocycline (Sunstar Inc., Takatsuki, Japan) are available for treatment and control of periodontal disease in dogs. Metronidazole therapy has had similar beneficial effects.[229] Tinidazole had good efficacy against *P. gingivalis*–like bacteria, which are periodontal pathogens.[276] Flushing dental surfaces once daily with 0.1% to 0.2% chlorhexidine[106] or alternate-day brushing[281] may delay accumulation of calculi. Unfortunately, chlorhexidine may stain teeth light blue, but a commercial product formulated especially for dental purposes (Nolvadent, Fort Dodge Labs, Fort Dodge, Iowa) does not stain. Monoperoxyphthalic acid applied before chlorhexidine was used resulted in less dental staining.[40] Daily application of chlorhexidine gel was effective in reducing reoccurrence of dental plaque in dogs.[118] With twice-daily applications, nisin, an antimicrobial peptide, was as effective as chlorhexidine in preventing calculus in dogs.[134] Numerous cleansers and brushes have been developed for daily brushing of dogs' teeth, and they warrant consideration when a dog has a tendency to form calculi. Special diets are also available that may help to reduce calculus formation. Daily feeding of a commercial dental food significantly reduced plaque and gingivitis by 39% and 36%, respectively, compared with daily feeding of a control dry food diet.[185]

Table • 89-2

Facultative and Obligate Anaerobic Flora of Feline Gingival Margins

ORGANISM	CLINICALLY HEALTHY (PERCENTAGE OF ALL ISOLATES)[194]	CLINICALLY HEALTHY (PERCENTAGE OF ALL ISOLATES)[99]	GINGIVITIS (PERCENTAGE OF ALL ISOLATES)[99]
Aerobic and Facultative			
α-Hemolytic streptococci	NC	82[a]	NC
Enterococci	NC	50	NC
Corynebacterium	NR	75	NC
Bergeyella (*Weeksella*) *zoohelcum*	NR	75	NC
Pseudomonas	NC	69	NC
Moraxella	NC	62	NC
Flavobacterium	NR	46	NC
Nocardia	NC	50	NC
Actinomyces	12[b]	42	NR
Pasteurella multocida	9.3	72	NR
Other bacteria	NC	<10[c]	NC
Anaerobic			
Propionibacterium	6	NR	NR
Bacteroides	36.7[d]	7–57[e]	2–31
Fusobacterium	19.3[f]	11	20
Clostridium	8.7[g]	<10[h]	3
Wolinella	4.6[i]	NR	NR
Peptostreptococcus	3.3	<10	14

NR, Not reported; *NC,* no attempted culture.
[a]Includes *Micrococcus* spp., *Streptococcus sanguis, Streptococcus mutans,* and *Streptococcus mitis.*
[b]*A. viscosus, A. hordeovulneris,* and *A. denticolens.* In one other study, *Lactobacillus fermentum* and *Veillonella parvula* were also isolated.[75]
[c]Includes *Streptococcus epidermidis, Alcaligenes* spp., *Actinobacter* spp., *Achromobacter* spp., and group G β-hemolytic streptococci.
[d]*B. tectum, B. fragilis, B. heparinolyticus, B. salivosus, Porphyromonas gingivalis,* and other *Bacteroides* pigmented group members, including *Prevotella* spp. and *B. gracilis.*
[e]Includes *B. asaccharolyticus, B. melaninogenicus, B. oralis, B. fragilis,* and *B.* unspeciated.
[f]*F. alocis, F. nucleatum, F. russii,* and *F.* unspeciated.
[g]*C. villosum* and *C. novyi.*
[h]*C. perfringens.*
[i]*W. recta, W.* nonmotile

Table • 89-3

Percentage Distribution of Gingival Microflora from Dogs with Healthy or Diseased Gingival Tissues [119,120,169,338]

VARIABLE	HEALTHY DOGS[a]	GINGIVITIS DOGS[a]	PERIODONTITIS DOGS[a]
Aerobic and Facultative Organisms	**36.5**	**27**	**3.8**
Streptococcus: esculin-positive[b]	ND	5.8	3.2
Streptococcus: esculin-negative[c]	ND	6.45	23.2
Actinomyces[d]	ND	41.9	13.0
Other aerobes and microaerophiles	17–30	ND	7-15
Anaerobic Organisms	**48**	**70**	**95**
Gram-positive cocci	3	7	5-12
Bacteroides[e] group (nonpigmented)	16	ND	19
Bacteroides[f] group (pigmented)	6	15	20-34
Fusobacterium[g]	7	25	10-40
Gram-positive *bacilli*	5	10	6-25
Spirochetes	+	++	+++

[a]Supragingival and subgingival collection sites. Values are percentages of isolates. *ND,* Not determined. Referring to relative prevalence and frequency of isolating these organisms: +, low; ++, intermediate; +++, high.
[b]Esculin-positive, streptococci (*S. faecalis,* group D streptococci, enterococci).
[c]Esculin-negative, streptococci (*S. mitis;* includes facultative and anaerobic spp.).
[d]Includes aerobic and facultative spp.
[e]Nonpigmented *B. fragilis* group.
[f]Pigmented group containing *Porphyromonas,* including *P. asaccharolyticus, P. gingivalis, P. endontalis, P. canoris,* and *P. circumstantaris; Prevotella,* including *P. intermidia, P. loescheii, P. melaninogenica,* and *P. denticola; Bacteroides nodosus* (*Dichelebacter nodosaus*); and *Wolinella* (*Campylobacter*) *curus* and *Wolinella* (*Campylobacter*) *rectus.*
[g]*F. necrophorum* (subsp. *Funduliforme* and *Necrophorum*); *F. pseudonecrophorum; F. nucleatum* (subsp. *animalis, fusiforme, nucleatum, polymorphum,* and *vincentii*).

Table • 89-4

Systemic Therapy for Oral Infections

DRUG[a]	SPECIES	DOSE[b]	ROUTE	INTERVAL (HOURS)	DURATION (DAYS)
Gingivitis-Stomatitis					
Metronidazole[c]	D	10—15 mg/kg	PO	12	10-28
	C	8 mg/kg	PO	12	7-14
	C	5—10 mg/kg	PO	8	7-14
Tinidazole	D	15 mg/kg	PO	12	7-14
Tetracycline	D	20—40 mg/kg	PO	12—24	14-21
Clindamycin	B	5—10 mg/kg	PO	12	7-10
Enrofloxacin	D	5 mg/kg	PO	24	7-14
Ampicillin (amoxicillin)	B	20 mg/kg	PO	12	14-21
Amoxicillin-clavulanate	B	15—20 mg/kg	PO	12	14-21
Metronidazole	D	15	PO	12	14-21
Ketoconazole	B	5—10 mg/kg	PO	12	7-10
Dental Prophylaxis					
Ampicillin, amoxicillin	B	10—20 mg/kg	IV, SC	Varies[d]	1
Amoxicillin-clavulanate	B	12.5 mg/kg	SC, PO	Varies[d]	1
Chloramphenicol	B	15—25 mg/kg	IV	Varies[d]	
Clindamycin	B	5 mg/kg	IV, SC, PO	Varies[d]	1
Metronidazole	B	10—20 mg/kg	IV, PO	Varies[d]	1
Enrofloxacin	B	5 mg/kg	SC, PO	Varies[d]	1
Gentamicin	B	2 mg/kg	IV, SC	Varies[d]	1
Cephapirin	B	20 mg/kg	IV	Varies[d]	1

D, Dog; *C*, cat; *B*, dog and cat; *IL*, intralesional; *PO*, by mouth; *IV*, intravenous; *SC*, subcutaneous.
[a]For additional information, see Drug Formulary, Appendix 8.
[b]Dose per administration at specified interval.
[c]Metronidazole and spiramycin are available in combination (Stomorgyl) outside the United States for treatment of oral infections.
[d]Only given once just before or during anesthesia for dental procedures. In general, the desired spectrum is used to treat anaerobic bacteria. For gram-negative facultative anaerobes in severe pyorrhea, combine whatever drug is chosen with the aminoglycoside (gentamicin) or fluoroquinolone (enrofloxacin).

In cats with naturally occurring periodontal disease, clindamycin, doxycycline, or spiramycin-metronidazole, but not amoxicillin-clavulanate, reduced the numbers of *P. gingivalis*.[226] Furthermore, improvement was observed in the degree of periodontal inflammation. This occurred despite the fact that all isolated organisms showed susceptibility to all the tested drugs. These drugs should probably be selected for adjunctive treatment along with mechanical debridement in cats. The use of special diets supplemented with dental chews may be effective in reducing calculus formation on cat teeth.[135,138] Cats were fed either a dry diet only or a dry diet supplemented with dental chews. A two-period, crossover design was used, and the test phase lasted 4 weeks. Results indicated that the daily addition of dental chews to a dry diet was effective in reducing plaque and calculus accumulation and the severity of gingivitis. Dental brushing has also been helpful in the prevention of periodontal disease in cats.[135,138] Daily application of zinc ascorbate gel has also been effective in decreasing bacterial growth, plaque formation, and gingivitis in cats when it was used following dental prophylaxis.[41]

Systemic complications of periodontal disease, including cerebral and myocardial infarction and early mortality, have been linked in people. Similar relationships to heart, liver, and kidney disease have been made in dogs.[52] Ophthalmic manifestations can occur from dental disease because of the close proximity of the caudal maxillary teeth and the orbit (Table 89-5).

Gingivitis in Kittens

A syndrome of gingival hypertrophy and associated plaque formation has been observed in Abyssinian and Persian kittens around the time of eruption of their adult teeth.[355] It may be caused by inborn immunodeficiency with secondary proliferation of gingival and plaque-forming bacteria. Treatment involves gingival tissue debridement, plaque removal, and frequent dental prophylaxis. Systemic antibacterial therapy may temporarily halt the progression, but it cannot be used indefinitely. Fortunately, most cats have a reduction in the severity of proliferation as they mature.

Bacteremia and Dental Disease

Bacteremia associated with dental manipulations may be clinically nonsymptomatic, cause acute septicemia, or subsequently result in bacterial endocarditis or localized embolic tissue infections (see Chapter 87).[254] The severity of bacteremia frequently correlates with the degree of periodontitis present. In people, use of antibiotic prophylaxis during dental procedures in patients predisposed to infective endocarditis is widely accepted.[103] In cats with periodontitis undergoing dental scaling and extraction, 36% had positive blood culture results at the time of the dental procedures.[109] Bacteria most commonly isolated were *Propionibacterium acnes*, *Pasteurella multocida*, and *Staphylococcus epidermidis*. None of the cats became ill after the dental procedures. Positive blood culture results of resident microflora have also been found in up to 40% of dogs with periodontal disease undergoing dental

Table • 89-5

Ophthalmic Manifestations of Dental Infections

Orbital Cellulitis
Exophthalmos, reduced retropulsion
Protrusion of membrana nictitans
Pain on opening mouth
Chemosis
Conjunctival hyperemia
Fever, anorexia
Oral mucosal swellings

Periapical Abscess
Infraorbital swelling and drainage
Alveolar mucosal swelling

Conjunctival Signs
Hyperemia, chemosis
Chronic mucopurulent conjunctivitis

Nasolacrimal Signs
Chronic unilateral nasal discharge
Lacrimal fistula

Neuroophthalmologic Signs
Deficits in cranial nerves II, III, IV, and VI; lacrimal nerve; and
ciliary nerve. Optic neuritis; retinal degeneration;
blindness; ophthalmoplegia; anisocoria; reduced tear
production; Horner's syndrome

Uveitis, Endophthalmitis
Scleral congestion, ocular swelling, miosis, aqueous flare,
photophobia, blindness

Modified from Ramsey DT, Manfra Marreta S, Hamor RE, et al.
1996. Ophthalmic manifestations and complications of dental
disease in dogs and cats. *J Am Anim Hosp Assoc* 32:215-224.

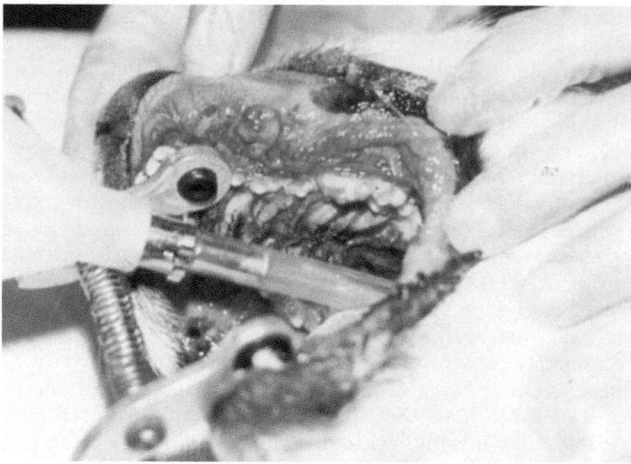

Fig 89-2 Diffuse necrotizing ulcerative gingivostomatitis in dog. (Courtesy D.W. Scott, Cornell University, Ithaca, N.Y.)

scaling and tooth extraction, and none showed clinical evidence of bacteremia.[108] Dental procedures should not be performed at the same time as other surgical procedures, because surgical wounds have been infected by bacteria released when simultaneous dentistry is performed. Oral microflora may establish themselves in tissue injured or devitalized by routine surgical procedures, sutures, or foreign implants. When dentistry is performed, prophylactic administration of antimicrobial drugs has been recommended (see Table 89-4). Routine use of antimicrobials for dental procedures should be mandatory in immunocompromised animals. Amoxicillin is the drug of choice for people undergoing dental cleaning; because of the risk of infection with viridans group streptococci, intravenous (IV) administration of aqueous penicillin during ultrasonic dentistry in dogs did not alter the prevalence of bacteremia before or after dental manipulation.[27] In dogs and cats, pretreatment with clindamycin at 5.5 mg/kg for 5 days decreased plaque and reduced aerosolization of bacteria during ultrasonic teeth cleaning.[369] Ampicillin (amoxicillin) has been recommended empirically beginning 1 hour before dental procedures.[128] On the basis of in vitro susceptibility testing, chloramphenicol, cephalosporin, erythromycin, or gentamicin have also been recommended. With the exception of erythromycin, all can be given parenterally while the animal is anesthetized. Gentamicin should never be administered alone because it is relatively ineffective against anaerobic bacteria. For these reasons, ampicillin (amoxicillin), chloramphenicol, clindamycin, metronidazole, or cephalosporin with

or without gentamicin or fluoroquinolone (although rarely) is recommended for dental prophylaxis. Prerinsing the oral cavity with chlorhexidine solutions can also be performed just before the sealing and cleaning procedure. Appendix 8 and Table 89-4 should be consulted for drug information and appropriate dosages. Therapy should begin no earlier than 4 hours before the dental procedure and preferably should be continued throughout the procedure by IV infusion. The most critical period is during the procedure. Drug administration should be terminated no longer than 12 hours after the procedure because no additional benefits are gained, and the risk for antibiotic-resistant bacteria causing infections increases.

Because of the large numbers of bacteria in the mouth and especially the gingival crevices, public health considerations are important. Face masks and ocular shields should always be worn by people who clean animals' teeth. In addition, biofilms that form on the inside surface of water lines of ultrasonic scalers may harbor *Legionella* species, which might produce acute pneumonia in susceptible individuals.[358]

Gingivostomatitis and Pharyngitis

In people, *necrotizing ulcerative gingivostomatitis (NUG)*, or "trench mouth," is a syndrome with multiple causes, is characterized by oral ulcerations and secondary infections, and may be observed in dogs or cats (Fig. 89-2). NUG may be a manifestation of systemic or immunosuppressive illness. Opportunistic overgrowth of oral microflora occurs in many diseases when immune defenses are impaired or oral ulcerations develop.[264,316] Similar to periodontitis, motile (predominantly anaerobic) bacteria, including spirochetes, often proliferate and may invade tissues before the development of necrotic lesions.[259] The causes of NUG in dogs and cats are equally diverse and include many acquired immunosuppressive conditions, such as diabetes mellitus, persistent neutropenia, feline leukemia virus (FeLV) and feline immunodeficiency virus (FIV) infections, and canine Cushing's disease. Exogenous glucocorticoid administration in dogs also increases their susceptibility to NUG.[213] The condition is common in Maltese terriers.[114] A virus antigenically related to feline calicivirus (FCV) was found to cause transient gingivitis and glossitis in a dog.[69] FCV appears to be especially prevalent in affected cats. As in people, psychologic and physical stresses may be involved in some animals. Bristles of plant awns can induce a similar syndrome when they become embedded in gingival tissues.[210] Fungal stomatitis can result from infection with *Candida* species. Candidiasis can be associated with diffuse oral inflammation, especially on the tongue and at mucocutaneous junctions. (See Chapter 65 for additional information concerning its diagnosis and treatment.)

Cats subclinically infected with FCV and feline herpesvirus (FHV-1) may develop oral ulceration with or without respiratory signs after stress or immunosuppression, such as with concurrent FIV infection. Stress also appears to reduce the amount of fibronectin, a receptor protein, on epithelial cells for gram-positive organisms. Thus overgrowth with gram-negative bacteria may develop. Hard, dry cat food also appears to have a role in exacerbating palatine ulceration in cats with acute FCV infection.[157] Proliferative stomatitis (see following discussion of feline lymphocytic plasmacytic gingivostomatitis) has been associated with persistent FCV infection, occasionally as a result of concurrent FIV infection.[167,320,344] The prevalence of FeLV infection in affected cats with stomatitis is lower than that of FIV. As a common but poorly understood syndrome with diverse causes, NUG often has uniform histopathologic features of lymphoplasmacytic infiltration.[344]

The pattern of oral ulceration may be helpful in determining its underlying cause (Table 89-6). Regardless of its cause, oral ulceration has a particular clinical syndrome characterized by reluctance to eat, hypersalivation, halitosis, and evidence of pain on opening the mouth. Hemorrhage may occur spontaneously or after oral manipulation. Although rare, systemic signs may include fever, lymphadenomegaly, and depression. Ulcers may be distributed throughout the oral cavity but are usually concentrated on the dental, labial, and gingival surfaces. Ulcers may be covered by a pseudomembranous exudate. White pseudomembranous plaques can be found in cases of candidal stomatitis. In many neutropenic cats infected with FeLV, the ulcers characteristically have minimal exudation; some can progress rapidly, with sloughing of large portions of the caudal oropharynx or larynx.

Diagnosis

Diagnosis of persistent stomatitis-pharyngitis in animals first involves examination for excessive accumulation of dental

Table • 89-6

Comparison of Ulcerative Lesions in Oral Cavities of Dogs and Cats

CAUSE	SPECIES	LESION LOCATION	THERAPY
Excessive licking (eosinophilic ulcer)	C	Upper incisor or carnassial area of lip, near philtrum, roof of mouth (hard palate)[a]	Intralesional or systemic glucocorticoids
Autoimmune diseases, bullous pemphigoid	D	Roof of mouth, lips, cheeks—often symmetric; other mucocutaneous regions, footpads	Systemic glucocorticoids
Irritants, uremia	B	Tip of tongue	Systemic antibacterials, amputation
Viral (parvoviral, see Chapters 8 and 10), rickettsial (Rocky Mountain spotted fever, see Chapter 29)	D	Multifocal lingual	Systemic antibacterials, antirickettsials
Maltese terrier stomatitis	D	Ulcerative lesions, lateral tongue and buccal mucosae	Systemic antibacterials
Dental tartar, periodontal disease	B	Periodontal regions (gingival margins), fusospirochetal proliferation	Systemic antibacterials, tartar removal, tooth extraction, chlorhexidine rinses, hard food diets
Herpesvirus (see Chapter 16)	C	Tongue, palate, multifocal	Systemic antibacterials
Calicivirus (see Chapter 16)	C	*Acute:* tongue, palate, multifocal *Chronic:* fauces (glossopharyngeal reflection, upper last molar region; occasionally extends rostrally; occasionally roof of mouth [hard palate])[b]	Systemic antibacterials, soft food diets, intralesional or systemic glucocorticoids, occasional molar extraction
Immunosuppression, hyperadrenocorticism, leukopenia, feline leukemia virus, feline immunodeficiency virus (see Chapters 13 and 14), Abyssinians, Persians	B	Periodontal region, may spread to gums and cheeks[c]	Systemic antibacterials, low-dose oral interferon, oral lactoferrin

C, Cat; D, dog; B, dog and cat.
[a]Eosinophilic infiltration on biopsy.
[b]Lymphocytic-plasmacytic infiltration on biopsy and polyclonal hyperglobulinemia are typical. Feline immunodeficiency virus coinfection can exacerbate.
[c]May be observed as an idiopathic syndrome in young cats. See text discussion of gingivitis in kittens. Retroviral infections are occasionally associated with a rapidly spreading gingival necrosis.

tartar. Systemic or underlying diseases are usually apparent from the results of urinalysis and routine hematology, biochemistry, and FeLV and FIV testing. Neutropenia or neutrophil function defects are a common underlying cause of oral ulceration. Results of bacterial culture and susceptibility testing are useless because most isolated organisms are merely commensals proliferating in already damaged tissues. Clinical features should be correlated with cytologic and histologic findings. Lymphoplasmacytic infiltration may be present in chronic inflammation from many different causes but has been most commonly associated with chronic stomatitis in cats.

Underlying disease processes and other causes of NUG should be eliminated or treated when they are encountered. Plant awns or foreign material embedded in the gums can be scraped away with a scalpel when the gum margins are debrided. Symptomatic therapy of stomatitis includes changing the diet to soft or bland foods to encourage eating and lessen the mechanical irritation of ulcers. With chronic, nonhealing ulcers, it is often beneficial to remove dental tartar and normal or diseased teeth in affected regions of the mouth.[19] Some lesions that arise adjacent to or later involve the tonsillar crypt may originate as or later develop into squamous cell carcinomas.

Therapy

Topical therapy such as swabbing and flushing of teeth, gums, and lesions throughout the oral cavity with 1% hydrogen peroxide has been recommended for gingivitis and stomatitis; however, excessive use of peroxide may cause vomiting. Astringents or disinfectants have also been advocated but can be irritating and distasteful. Cauterization with silver nitrate or dilute acid solutions also has been recommended but may interfere with healing and epithelization. Administration of vitamins B and C has been recommended on an empiric basis without adequate documentation of efficacy.

Systemic therapies for stomatitis are summarized in Tables 89-4 and 89-7. Topical or systemic antimicrobial therapy appears to hasten the resolution of NUG significantly, perhaps by inhibiting the overgrowth of anaerobic and spirochetal bacteria that colonize and impair healing of ulcerated lesions in the oral cavity. Oral administration of lactoferrin, an iron-chelating agent, was effective in treating intractable stomatitis in cats with and without FIV infections. (For dosages and other information, see Table 98-7 and Drug Formulary, Appendix 8.[280]) Improvement was presumably a result of its antibacterial effects. Candidal stomatitis is best treated by topical application of antifungal drugs, such as clotrimazole and nystatin (see also Table 57-3), or with systemic ketoconazole. Historically, tetracycline, chloramphenicol, ampicillin, and penicillin solutions have been applied topically for bacterial stomatitis, although the first two drugs may cause anorexia in cats. Systemic antibiotic therapy directed primarily against anaerobic bacteria appears to be more efficacious in treating stomatitis. Relapses may occur in some cases after termination of antimicrobial therapy, and a repeated course of therapy may be required.

Glucocorticoid therapy may be needed if an autoimmune disease such as pemphigus is suspected; however, the immunosuppression induced by glucocorticoids can itself cause or exacerbate some cases of NUG.

Feline Lymphocytic Plasmacytic Gingivostomatitis

Faucitis is characterized by vesicular, ulcerative, and later, proliferative lesions in the mucosa, usually accompanied by lymphoplasmacytic or eosinophilic infiltrations in the tissue of the caudal pharynx at the glossopharyngeal arch (fauces).[154,320] Faucitis frequently appears among a number of cats within a household and tends to be recurrent after the initial treatment or is unresponsive to treatment. In chronic stages, proliferation of granulation tissue forms large masses in the caudal pharynx (Fig. 89-3). FCV has been isolated in a high percentage of cats with this syndrome compared with clinically healthy cats or those with oral ulcers at other locations. Cessation of FCV shedding was associated with resolution of chronic gingivostomatitis in one cat.[1] It is likely a hypersensitivity phenomenon to persistent FCV infection. Coinfections with FIV or FeLV result in the most severe lesions. CD8 cells, representing cytotoxic and suppressor T cells, have been in the high reference range for all cats. In one study, cats with chronic gingivostomatitis were more likely to shed FCV and FHV-1 together than either virus alone.[188] Compared with nondiseased cats, affected cats showed a significant increase in the relative mRNA expression of IL-2, IL-4, IL-6, IL-10, IL-12 (p35 and p40), and IFN-γ. These results suggest the normal feline oral mucosa is biased towards a predominantly (Th)

Table • 89-7

Adjunctive Drug Therapy for Feline Ulcerative Gingivostomatitis

DRUG[a]	DOSE[b]	ROUTE	INTERVAL (HOURS)	DURATION (DAYS)
Prednisone, prednisolone	0.5-2 mg/kg	PO	12 hours	7-14 days
Triamcinolone	4 mg total	PO	24-48 hours	28 days
Methylprednisolone acetate	2 mg/kg	IM	7-30 days	3-12 months
	0.5-1 mg/kg	IL[c]	Once	28 days
Triamcinolone acetonide	0.1–0.2 mg/kg	IL[c]	Once	28 days
Aurothioglucose	1 mg/kg	IM	7 days[d]	prn
Thalidomide	50 mg	PO	24 hours	330 days[e]
Cyclosporin	7.5 mg	PO	12 hours	28 days[f]
Lactoferrin powder	200 mg	Topical	24 hours	330 days[g]

PO, By mouth; *IM*, intramuscular; *IL*, intralesional.
[a]See Drug Formulary, Appendix 8.
[b]Dose per administration at specified interval.
[c]Injection under anesthesia as a last resort.
[d]Give every 7 days until improvement, then once every 14 to 35 days as needed.
[e]Dose reduced to every other day after this time and than gradually discontinued.
[f]After this time and clinical resolution, therapy should be tapered to the lowest dose and frequency that is effective in maintaining remission.
[g]Drug given for 4 consecutive days of each week after this time.[1]

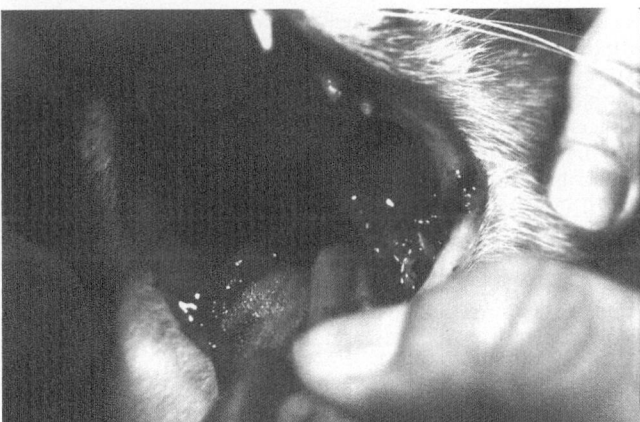

Fig 89-3 Necrotic ulcerative and proliferative gingivostomatis in cat. (Courtesy University of Georgia, Athens, Ga.)

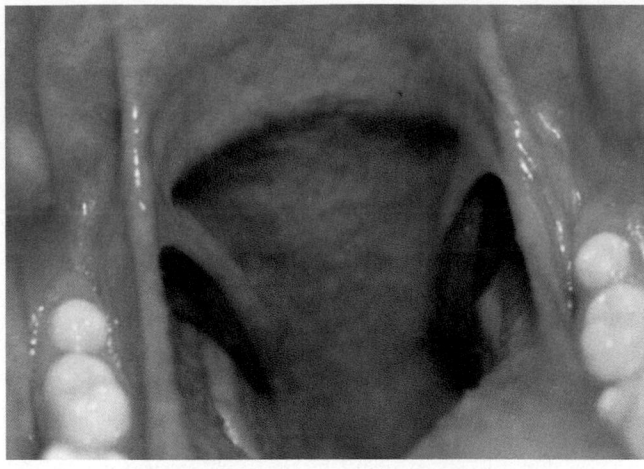

Fig 89-4 Bilateral tonsillar enlargement in dog caused by suppurative tonsillitis. (Courtesy University of Georgia, Athens, Ga.)

type 1 profile of cytokine expression and that during the development of lesions seen in feline chronic gingivostomatis, a shift in the cytokine profile from a type 1 to a mixed type 1 and type 2 response occurs.[111] Hyperproteinemia and polyclonal hyperglobulinemia are often present in cats affected with chronic stomatitis (faucitis) and lymphoplasmacytic infiltration. Monoclonal gammopathy may occur in some cats.[195] Cats with chronic gingivostomatitis have higher serum concentrations of IgG, IgM and IgA, likely reflective of chronic antigenic stimulation.[110] The release of high concentrations of serum immunoglobulins may facilitate local inflammation in the tissues. Lower salivary IgA may be caused by destruction by bacterial proteases or suppressed secretion. The lower concentration may predispose these cats to persistent oral bacterial infections. Specimens for FCV isolation can be taken by rubbing sterile swabs on the gums, soft palate, and oropharynx (especially palatine tonsillar region) and placing them directly into viral transport or culture media (see Chapter 1).

Although dentistry may reduce pain and discomfort, it is not by itself sufficient in controlling faucitis in many cats.[344] Similarly, antibiotic therapy results in improvement; however, the response is temporary. In some cats, removal and biopsy with histologic examination of chronic proliferative lesions may be required. Topical application of an astringent paste containing choline salicylate and cetalkonium chloride (Bonjela Gel, Reckett and Coleman Pharmaceuticals, United Kingdom) has been used as adjunctive therapy to reduce the proliferative lesions.[199] A cat that had recovered was treated with thalidomide, lactoferrin powder, and an additive-free diet containing fat-soluble vitamins.[1] However, clearing of the viral carrier state in this cat may have been coincidental. Treatment of periodontal disease, such as scaling, polishing, and extracting of teeth in areas of severe inflammation, is beneficial. Because faucitis is likely a hypersensitivity phenomenon related to FCV, immunosuppression, rather than immunostimulation, is the most beneficial.

Administration of antiinflammatory and immunosuppressive drugs has provided the most relief (see Table 89-7). Prednisone or other glucocorticoids may be administered when antimicrobial therapy is being discontinued in an attempt to break the cycle of recurrent chronic stomatitis or faucitis in cats. Reduction in serum immunoglobulin concentration has been observed in cats that were treated for at least 3 months with 0.5 mg/kg methylprednisolone.[110] Another systemic treatment with variable success has been parenteral administration of gold salts (aurothioglucose). In cats with refractory

faucitis, therapy with hypoallergenic diets, progesterones, or intralesional injections of repositol (water-insoluble) glucocorticoids using general anesthesia may be attempted as a last resort.

Cyclosporin has been effective in treating cats with faucitis. Over time the dosage is tapered to the lowest level that is clinically beneficial. Within 2 weeks of initiating treatment, reduction in gingival and buccal erythema subsides, and a reduction in ulcers, granulation tissue, and faucitis occurs. Appetites improve, and hypersalivation subsides.

Tonsillitis

Chronic tonsillar inflammation is most commonly recognized in dogs and is usually accompanied by pharyngeal irritation initiated by foreign bodies, chronic gingivitis or periodontitis, chronic coughing, persistent vomiting or gastroesophageal reflux of acid, and licking of infected sites, such as lesions caused by anal sacculitis. Dogs may have inappetence, hypersalivation, or sneezing and oculonasal discharge; they may scratch at their ears or repeatedly shake the head. Fever and malaise do not usually accompany tonsillitis unless it is secondary to underlying systemic infection or neoplasia.

Diagnosis is based on a thorough oral examination, which usually requires sedation. The pharyngeal mucosa is reddened, and tonsils are enlarged and frequently protrude from the crypts as the tongue is pulled rostrally (Fig. 89-4). Organisms cultured from inflamed tonsils have been *E. coli* and *Staphylococcus*, *Streptococcus*, *Pseudomonas*, *Pasteurella*, and *Enterococcus* species. However, these same organisms are also resident microflora, making diagnosis of primary bacterial tonsillitis questionable. Canine tonsillitis also has been associated with *Listeria monocytogenes* infection in two dogs.[173] Whether this organism can colonize the tonsils nonsymptomatically is uncertain. In general, culture of tonsils is unnecessary, and antibacterial therapy with amoxicillin, tetracycline, or trimethoprim-sulfonamide is recommended. Low antiinflammatory dosages of glucocorticoids have temporarily reduced the severity of clinical signs in conjunction with antimicrobial therapy.[36] Surgical removal of the tonsils, followed by histologic examination, is usually the best course of action when antibacterial therapy has been ineffective or transiently curative. Chronic tonsillar enlargement, if not corrected by surgery, usually serves as a nidus for continual infection and occasionally for chronic bronchitis (see also Tonsillitis and Pharyngitis, Chapter 88).

ESOPHAGUS AND STOMACH

The oral cavity and ingested material are the primary sources of microorganisms that colonize the proximal portions of the gastrointestinal (GI) tract (Fig. 89-5). The esophagus and stomach contain a transient population of organisms after saliva or food is swallowed. Once the stomach has been emptied of food, the low pH usually destroys most of the bacteria that remain. Those that persist during the fasting period are strains adapted to survival at low pH (Table 89-8). Esophagitis in dogs and cats is usually the result of trauma from ingestion of foreign bodies, irritation from ingested chemicals or drugs such as doxycyline, or from recurrent reflux of gastric acid from the stomach.[107] The oral cavity, esophagus, stomach, and proximal small intestine are colonized primarily by gram-positive aerobic and anaerobic bacteria, which are usually susceptible to penicillin or its derivatives. This susceptibility is the rationale for the clinical use of such drugs in treating ulcerations and perforations and for antimicrobial prophylaxis involving surgery of these portions of the GI tract.

Exudates from abscesses or cellulitis that develop after perforating lesions of the oral cavity or upper GI tract should be collected with sterile syringes that are capped or sealed imme-diately after collection. The latter method increases the chances of detecting anaerobic bacteria, although cultures must be performed soon after specimen collection (see Chapters 33 and 41). Various organisms, including gram-positive and gram-negative rods and cocci, yeasts, and spirochetes, have been found in the stomach of most normal dogs.[334] Nontoxi-genic *Clostridium perfringens* was found in the gastric contents of normal dogs and those with acute gastric dilation. The type and prevalence of organisms in clinically healthy dogs did not differ from those in dogs with acute gastric dilation. Bacteremia from bacterial translocation was studied in dogs with naturally occurring gastric dilation.[360] Approximately 40% had positive jugular venous blood culture results; however, they were comparable to those of clinically healthy dogs. Gram-negative rods were the most frequently cultured organisms. Culture of abdominal organs including the liver, mesenteric lymph node, and stomach also yielded a low rate but comparable degree of isolates. These results indicate that bacterial proliferation or dissemination is not an important feature of gastric dilation-volvulus. Because the stomach has a highly acidic environment and relatively low concentrations of resident microflora relative to other portions of the GI tract, bacterial gastritis is less frequent. However, numerous factors can

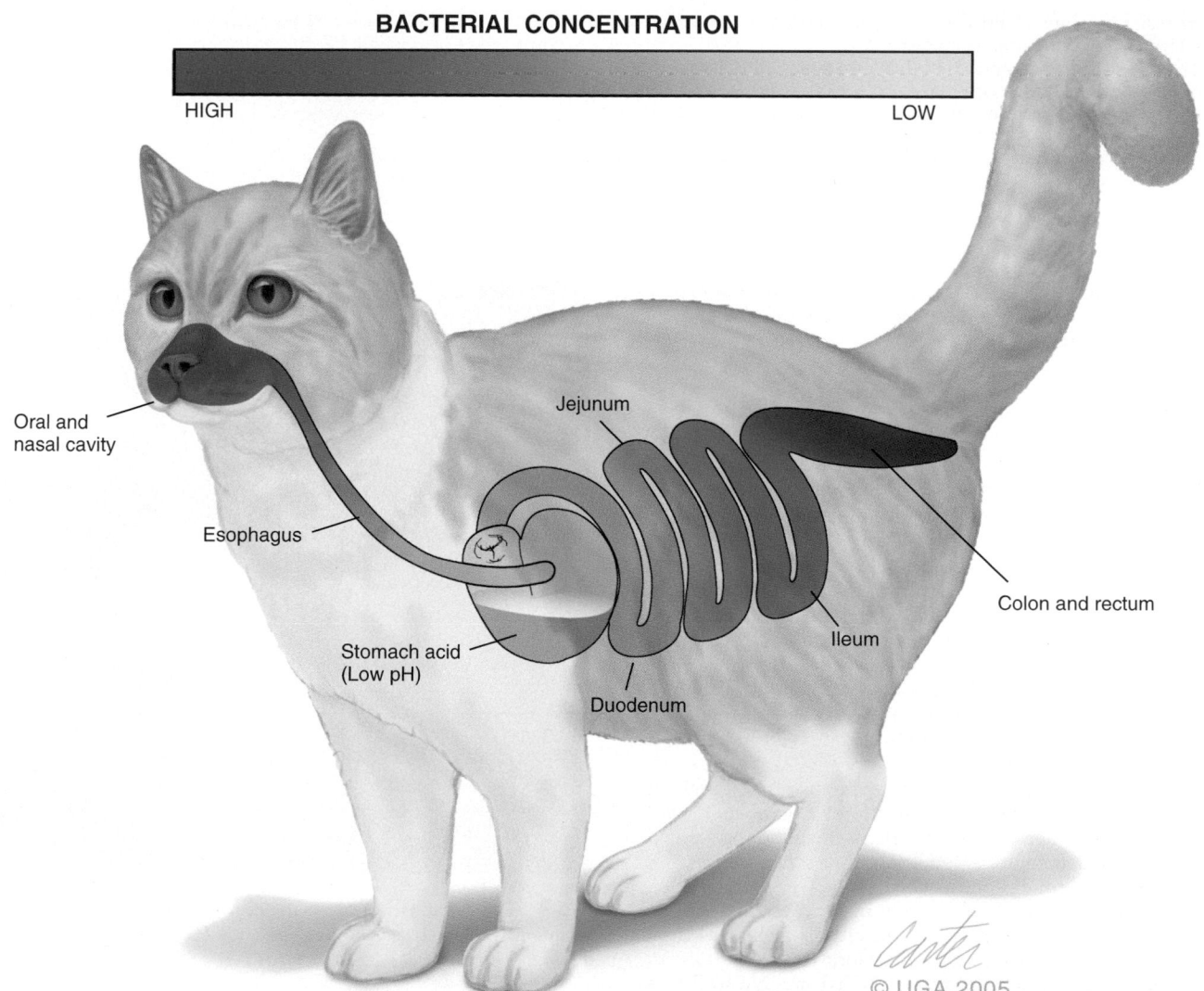

BACTERIAL CONCENTRATION

HIGH   LOW

Oral and nasal cavity

Jejunum

Esophagus

Colon and rectum

Stomach acid (Low pH)

Ileum

Duodenum

© UGA 2005

Fig 89-5 Relative concentrations of microorganisms throughout the intestinal tract are depicted in a cat. Highest concentrations are found in the oral cavity and colon. Lowest concentrations are in the stomach from the influence of high acidity. (Courtesy University of Georgia, Athens, Ga.)

Table • 89-8

Major Microflora of the GI Tract of Dogs and People[a]

VARIABLE	ORAL CAVITY[b]	STOMACH[c]	SMALL BOWEL PROXIMAL[d]	DISTAL	CECUM/COLON	FECES
Total Counts[d]						
Fasting	10^7	10^1-10^2	10^1-10^2	10^3-10^7	10^9-10^{10}	10^{10}-10^{11}
Postprandial	10^7	10^4-10^5	10^2-10^3	10^3-10^7	10^9-10^{10}	10^{10}-10^{11}
Aerobic Organisms						
Gram-positive[e]	+	$10^{0.4}$-10^1	$10^{0.4}$-10^2	$10^{1.4}$-10^3	10^4-10^9	10^4-10^9
Gram-negative[f]	+	10^1-10^2	10^2	10^2-10^6	10^7-10^8	10^7-10^8
Anaerobic Organisms						
Gram-positive[g]	+	$10^{0.3}$-10^2	$10^{0.1}$-10^3	10^2-10^6	10^7-10^9	10^7-10^{10}
Gram-negative[h]	+	—	+	10^1	10^6-10^{10}	10^6-10^{10}
Other Organisms						
Spirochetes	+	+	+	+	+++	0
Mycoplasma	+	—	—	—	—	—
Yeasts	+	—	—	—	10^5	+

+, Present but absolute quantity uncertain; +++, present in large numbers; —, absent or data not available; 0, normally absent.
[a]Data derived from studies in people and dogs.
[b]See Table 89-1 for information concerning frequency of isolation.
[c]All values listed are for fasting animals except in entries in which the postprandial state is indicated.
[d]Values expressed as organisms per milliliter or gram of intestinal contents.
[e]*Streptococcus, Staphylococcus, Bacillus,* and *Corynebacterium.*
[f]Enterobacteriaceae (primarily *Escherichia coli, Enterobacter,* and *Klebsiella*), *Pseudomonas, Neisseria,* and *Moraxella.*
[g]*Clostridium, Lactobacillus, Propionibacterium,* and *Bifidobacterium.*
[h]*Bacteroides, Fusobacterium,* and *Veillonella.*

allow for proliferation of gastric helicobacters and associated gastritis (Fig. 89-6). (For a discussion of Gastric *Helicobacter* Infections, see Chapter 39.)

SMALL INTESTINE

Microflora

Concentrations of bacteria in the proximal small bowel are relatively low because of the influence of gastric acid and bile, but they gradually increase toward the ileocecal region (see Table 89-8 and Fig. 89-5). Numbers of microorganisms in the distal small bowel or the large bowel are not affected by feeding and remain relatively constant after meals. Increased numbers of resident organisms may be found in the stomach and upper small intestine, or pathogenic organisms may proliferate when normal bowel defenses are impaired. Excessive use of antacids, obstruction or stasis of intestinal or bile flow, or decreased mucosal or IgA secretions can result in bacterial overgrowth in the small intestine.

The normal microflora of the small intestine plays an important role in preventing colonization by pathogenic bacteria by competing for available nutrients, maintaining oxygen levels, and producing antibacterial substances. In addition, the normal intestinal microflora assist the body in metabolizing bile acids and drugs and have a role in synthesizing volatile fatty acids and vitamins. Puppies and kittens lacking normal microflora at birth derive their microflora from exposure to their dam and littermates or from their environment by 2 to 3 weeks of life.[139] The organisms become established beginning on the first day of life and gradually shift from a predominance of aerotolerant forms to anaerobic species.[33] Organisms that initially colonize the intestinal tract (which may vary between individuals) permanently colonize the intestinal tract and have

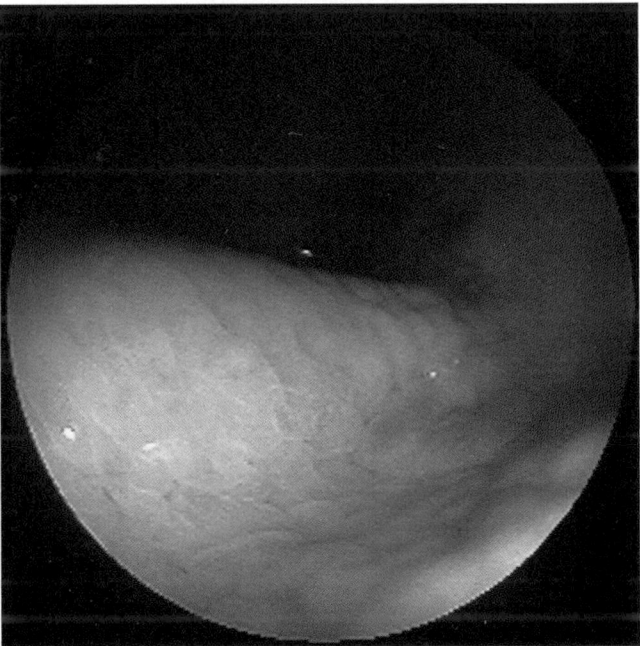

Fig 89-6 Endoscopic appearance of gastric mucosal swelling in dog with *Helicobacter*-induced gastritis. (Courtesy University of Georgia, Athens, Ga.)

a somewhat stable composition throughout the life of the individual. Changes in diet, nutritional status, and physiologic state of the host may influence the proportions of residing bacteria. High-meat diets ingested by most carnivores result in a predominance of streptococci and *C. perfringens* and a suppression of *Lactobacillus* species. Upper intestinal bacterial concentrations in carnivores such as the dog and cat are much higher than those in people, presumably relating to dietary differences in these species. Lactose in the diet of nursing animals contributes to acidification of the colonic contents, with a resultant increase in *Enterobacter* organisms and a decrease in *E. coli* and *Bacteroides* species.

Greater knowledge of the composition of the intestinal microflora of dogs and cats has been gained because of improved techniques for culture of anaerobic bacteria. Anaerobes are known to make up a majority of the intestinal microflora, greatly outnumbering aerobes (see Tables 89-8 and 89-9). The duodenum and upper jejunum primarily harbor gram-positive bacteria, including streptococci and lactobacilli. Anaerobes and gram-negative organisms predominate in the distal portions of the small bowel and colon. The maximum numbers of microorganisms are found in the cecum, colon, and feces.

Research studies using molecular-based methods for determining bacterial profiles in the Labrador retriever gut have exposed the limitations of traditional culture methods.[96] The classical cultural approach failed to reflect the diversity present in dog feces, and many of the isolates remained unclassified. Furthermore, agars designed for anaerobic isolation have poor recovery efficiencies. Thus future studies using molecular methods may help to better characterize resident enteric microflora and its alterations in disease.

Quantifying organism numbers is important in determining whether bacterial overgrowth may be occurring. In contrast to cats with GI illness, clinically healthy cats have much higher concentrations of bacteria in the duodenal or proximal

jejunal region (Table 89-10).[158,161] The most common anaerobes in cats were *Bacteroides*, *Eubacterium*, and *Fusobacterium*, whereas *Pasteurella* species were the most common among aerobic flora. In another study on cats,[233] in which similar numbers of bacteria were found, the most common anaerobes were *Clostridium*, *Fusobacterium*, and *Bacteroides* species. The most common aerobes were gram-negative rods, streptococci, enterococci, and staphylococci. In studies on healthy dogs, results of quantifying proximal small intestinal bacteria have varied, with some showing numbers of $<10^5$ per ml[342] and others having populations comparable to those in cats.[21,50,289]

The composition and distribution of the normal fecal flora can be altered by disease, such as diarrhea.[139] Decreased transit time of intestinal contents and evacuation of fluid feces result in decreased numbers of lactobacilli with concomitant increased numbers of *Bacteroides* organisms and members of the Enterobacteriaceae. Organisms such as *Enterobacter* species, which normally reside in the small intestine, may appear in the feces of dogs with diarrhea. The concentration of many anaerobes is reduced in the feces during diarrhea because these organisms normally require intestinal stasis and low oxygen tension for growth.

Intestinal Immunity

The GI tract is lined by a one cell layer of absorptive epithelium. Cells migrate up the villus to be shed in the intestinal epithelium. Lymphoid cells can be found as single cells in the lamina propria or as intraepithelial lymphocytes. Lymphoid follicles are located throughout the intestine as Peyer's patches. Mucosal lymphoid B cells produce secretory IgA.

Table • 89-9

Duodenal Microflora of Clinically Healthy Cats

	ENDOSCOPY[a]		NEEDLE	
	JOHNSTON ET AL, 1999	PAPASOULIOTIS ET AL, 1998	JOHNSTON ET AL, 1999	PAPASOULIOTIS ET AL, 1998
Aerobic and Microaerophilic Organisms				
Gram-negative				
Neisseria	$10^{3.78}$	ND	$10^{3.6}$	ND
Escherichia coli	ND	10^{2-6}	ND	$10^{2.5-6.7}$
Moraxella	ND	$10^{2-5.4}$	ND	$10^{2-6.6}$
Pasteurella	$10^{3.78-3.95}$	ND	$10^{3.6-6}$	ND
Gram-positive				
Staphylococci	$10^{3-3.3}$	$10^{2-7.4}$	10^{3}	$10^{2-4.9}$
Corynebacteria	$10^{3-4.32}$	10^{2-6}	$10^{3.7-6}$	$10^{2-4.9}$
Streptococci	$10^{3-4.8}$	$10^{2-8.3}$	ND	$10^{2-7.7}$
Anaerobic Organisms				
Gram-negative				
Fusobacterium	ND	$10^{2.3-6.6}$	ND	$10^{2-5.7}$
Bacteroides	$10^{3-5.48}$	$10^{2.3-6.8}$	$10^{3.3-5.93}$	$10^{2-7.7}$
Lactobacillus	$10^{3-5.5}$	ND	$10^{3.48-6.23}$	ND
Gram-positive				
Clostridium	$10^{3-4.28}$	$10^{3-7.5}$	$10^{3-3.95}$	$10^{2-7.3}$

ND, Not determined.

From Johnston KL, Lamport A, Ballèvre O, et al. 1999. A comparison of endoscopic and surgical collection procedures for the analysis of the bacterial flora in duodenal fluid from cats. *Vet J* 157:85-89; Papasouliotis K, Sparkes AH, Werrett G, et al. 1998. Assessment of the bacterial flora of the proximal part of the small intestine in healthy cats, and the effect of sample collection method. *Am J Vet Res* 59:48–51.
[a]Data from direct aspiration of contents without dilutional flush.

Table • 89-10

Duodenal Microflora from Healthy Cats and Cats with Gastrointestinal Disease

	CLINICALLY HEALTHY[a]		GASTROINTESTINAL ILLNESS[a,b]	
	RANGE	MEDIAN	RANGE	MEDIAN
Total	$10^{3.3-3.1}$	$10^{5.65}$	$10^{0-7.70}$	$10^{5.08}$
Aerobic	$10^{2.7-7.7}$	$10^{4.95}$	$10^{0-7.70}$	$10^{3.84}$
Microaerophilic	10^{0-6}	$10^{3.99}$	$10^{0-7.45}$	10^{0}
Anaerobic	$10^{0-8.05}$	$10^{5.21}$	$10^{0-7.45}$	$10^{4.78}$

From Johnston KL, Swift NC, Forster-van Hijfte M, et al. 2001. Comparison of the bacterial flora of the duodenum in healthy cats and cats with signs of gastrointestinal tract disease. *J Am Vet Med Assoc* 218:48–51.
[a]Samples were collected via endoscopy.
[b]Cats had signs of chronic weight loss, diarrhea, or vomiting. Ill cats had significantly lower numbers of *Pasteurella* spp., *Bacteroides* spp., and *Lactobacillus* spp. than healthy cats.

Probiotics

Microorganisms added to the food for their beneficial effects are called *probiotics*. Enterococci, lactobacilli, and bifidobacteria—normal colonic inhabitants—have often been administered after antimicrobial treatment, intestinal infections, weaning, stress, or dietary changes in an attempt to reestablish enteric microbial flora. Many of these microorganisms become transient constituents of the enteric microflora. In people, these bacteria have been administered in the form of yogurt, cheese, and milk products, and efforts have been made to include these in canine and feline diets. Theoretical benefits of probiotic food additives are antagonism of enteropathogens, reestablishment of enteric microflora flora after antimicrobial treatment, and the decrease in host reactivity to food antigens. In dogs, *Enterococcus faecium* SF68 has shown to provide the most benefit in enteric immunostimulation, and it is free of virulence factors and transferable antimicrobial resistance factors. Dogs fed *E. faecium* SF68 had stimulation of the mucosal immune system with production of polyclonal IgA secretion.[20] Furthermore, young pups fed a dry food supplemented with *E. faecium* SF68 also had a greater immune response to canine distemper vaccine than those not supplemented.[20] Probiotics have had some effects in inhibiting gastric helicobacters as an alternative or adjunctive treatment with antimicrobials.[74] Probiotics appear to be helpful in the prevention and treatment of antimicrobial-associated diarrhea in people[241] and in experimental colitis in animals.[283] In dogs receiving certain diets, feeding of *E. faecium* SF68 or *Lactobacillus acidophilus* resulted in a decrease of *C. perfringens* concentration in the stool.[20,307,309] These findings suggest that probiotics can be used to help reduce the anaerobic population of bacteria in the colon in lieu of antimicrobial therapy. This modality might be beneficial in treatment of inflammatory bowel disease (IBD), small intestinal bacterial overgrowth (SIBO), or dietary hypersensitivities. Commercial pet foods that claim to contain bacterial species had very low numbers of organisms and often did not contain the species noted on the label.[339] Not only may these misrepresented products be ineffective, but enteric flora is reestablished spontaneously and immediately after antimicrobial agents are discontinued. Furthermore, use of supplemental yeast in an attempt to reestablish the intestinal microflora may have caused intestinal colonization by these fungi in a dog with chronic diarrhea.[214] Intestinal flora may have an important role in the pathogenesis of IBDs. Probiotic supplementation, containing organisms such as lactobacilli and bifidobacteria, has been the most beneficial in clinical trials in people.[105] Lactobacilli may be best adapted to pet food because they can ferment starch.[166] Probiotics containing *L. acidophilus* have been incorporated into dry dog food and have survived intestinal transit in dogs to eventually reside in the colon.[9] Additional studies are needed to determine whether these supplements are effective in people and animals.

Prebiotics

Prebiotics are undigested foods that alter the replication of specific enteric bacteria in an attempt to alter fecal consistency or digestive function. Fructooligosaccharides (FOSs) are polymers of glucose that have been added to commercial diets as a source of soluble fiber. They occur naturally in plants or are synthesized from fermentation. Other natural sources rich in soluble fiber are oat bran or wheat pulp. FOSs are not digested by the mammalian small intestine, and they reach the colon intact. There they are fermented by anaerobic bacteria such as *Bifidobacterium* spp. or lactobacilli into short-chain fatty acids such as acetate, propionate, and butyrate. These organisms proliferate and inhibit growth of other potentially pathogenic microbes such as *Clostridium* species and *E. coli*. The effects of prebiotics on the intestinal microflora and immune parameters of dogs and cats are reviewed in Table 89-11 and other sources.[306]

Bacterial Translocation

The GI tract is a known reservoir of microorganisms, which under certain circumstances can spread by portal blood vessels or intestinal lymphatics to extraintestinal sites, including the mesenteric lymph nodes, liver, spleen, pancreas, and to other organs by systemic circulation. The inability to culture bacteria in the blood of affected animals may be explained by the fact that many organisms or their toxins first interact with immune cells in the gut-associated lymphoid tissue and then the mesenteric nodes, rather than immediately entering the systemic circulation. Rather than the bacteria entering the circulation, it may be their cytokines or toxins that enter the lymphatic or systemic circulation, leading to multisystemic inflammatory responses. Furthermore, mesenteric nodes drain into the thoracic duct, which can bypass the mononuclear phagocyte system or Kupffer cells in the liver and allow bacteria or their by-products to go directly to the lungs and systemic circulation. This can result in more virulent systemic inflammatory response syndrome or multiple organ dysfunction syndrome. (See endotoxemia, Chapter 38, for an additional discussion of diagnosis and treatment of these syndromes.) Table 89-12 summarizes the bacterial species iso-

Table • 89-11

Summary of Prebiotic Use in Diets of Dogs and Cats and Effects on Intestinal Microflora and Immune Parameters

PREBIOTIC	SUBJECTS AND/OR DIETS	EFFECT ON MICROFLORA OR IMMUNITY
Lactosucrose[318]	Adult dogs; 1.5 g/day for 14 days	Fecal bifidiobacteria increased and clostridia decreased from baseline
Short-chain fructooligosaccharides (scFOS)[353]	IgA-deficient German shepherd	Decreased aerobic and anaerobic bacteria in tissue and aerobic bacteria in duodenal/jejunal fluid samples compared with controls
Mannanoligosaccharides (MOS)[229a]	Adult beagle dogs; control diet (no MOS) or 1, 2, or 4 g MOS/kg	No difference in plasma protein or IgG
	Border collie pups; control diet (no MOS) vs. 2 g/kg MOS and vaccinated	Increased neutrophil activity
scFOS and inulin[265]	Dogs; either soy or soy and scFOS	Decreased fecal clostridia and increased bifidobacteria
Different fiber sources[132]	Beet pulp, scFOS, cellulose, or fiber blend	Supplemented with scFOS: greater number of aerobes in distal colon but not other regions
Oligofructose (OF), MOS, xylooligosaccharides (XOS)[303]	Ileal cannulated healthy adult dogs	Decreased fecal *Clostridium perfringens* in dogs fed MOS
scFOS[351]	Healthy beagle dogs	Ineffective in altering fecal flora, although disparity of fecal flora makes benefit difficult
OF[22]	Adult dogs; diet with or without 1% OF	Increased total fecal anaerobes, aerobes, lactobacilli, streptococci, clostridia, bifidobacteria
ScFOS, *Lactobacillus acidophilus* (LAC), or both[307]	Adult dog groups; sucrose plus cellulose, FOS plus cellulose, sucrose plus LAC, FOS plus LAC	FOS: lower *C. perfringens;* LAC: more effective in combination with FOS than alone
scFOS, MOS, or both[308]	Adult dog groups; control, scFOS, MOS, FOS plus MOS	*MOS vs. control dogs:* MOS dogs—lower fecal aerobes, greater *Lactobacillus,* greater concentration of plasma lymphocytes, and serum IgA; scFOS plus MOS dogs—higher ileal IgA
MOS and scFOS[309]	Adult dogs; MOS plus scFOS vs. sucrose placebo	Increased fecal aerobes, bifidobacteria, and *Lactobacillus;* increased ileal *Lactobacillus* concentrations; no effect on ileal IgA
MOS, transgalactosylated oligosaccharides (TOS), lactose, lactulose[365]	Dogs; MOS and other carbohydrates	MOS: decreased fecal pH and ammonia excretion but decreased nutrient digestibility
scFOS[77]	Adult dogs; ileal cannulated with four doses scFOS	ScFOS: increased ileal aerobes and decreased *C. perfringens* concentrations
Chicory, MOS, or both[97]	Geriatric dog groups; control, chicory, MOS, chicory and MOS	Either chicory or MOS alone: increased fecal bifidobacteria concentrations, and MOS alone decreased fecal *Escherichia coli* concentrations; some changes in neutrophils and lymphocyte subtypes
Lactosucrose[317]	Cats; lactosucrose for 14 days, checked feces at 7 and 14 days	Decreased fecal ammonia and decreased lecithinase-positive clostridia, fusobacteria, lecithinase-negative clostridia, staphylococci, and Enterobacteriaceae and increased lactobacilli, with all bacterial concentrations returning back to baseline 7 days after diet no longer fed
Fructooligosaccharides (FOS)[297]	Control diet for 8 weeks followed by FOS for 12 weeks	No decline in duodenal bacterial numbers, although marked variations in microflora; increased fecal lactobacilli and *Bacteroides* and decreased *E. coli* and *C. perfringens*
Chicory[234]	Control diet for 15 days followed by various chicory concentrations for 15 more days	Increased fecal bifidobacteria and lactobacilli when fed higher chicory concentrations

Table • 89-12

Bacterial Species Isolated from Lymph Node Tissues of 26 of 50 Clinically Healthy Bitches After Ovariohysterectomy

BACTERIAL SPECIES	NUMBER OF DOGS WITH ISOLATES
Staphylococcus intermedius	5
Nonhemolytic Streptococcus species	4
Bacillus species	5
Escherichia coli	6
Salmonella species	3
Pseudomonas species	2
Enterococcus species	2
Clostridium sordelli	1
Micrococcus species	1
Lactobacillus species	1
Propionibacterium acnes	1

Data from Dahlinger J, Marks SL, Hirsh DC. 1997. Prevalence and identity of translocating bacteria in healthy dogs. *J Vet Intern Med* 11:319-322.

lated from mesenteric lymph nodes of 26 of 50 clinically healthy bitches having ovariohysterectomies.[49] Corresponding peripheral venous and portal venous blood cultures yielded a gram-positive coccus and a coagulase-negative *Staphylococcus* species from the peripheral blood of one dog. Mesenteric lymph node culture needs additional evaluation in ill dogs before conclusions can be drawn about its clinical usefulness.

Bacterial overgrowth in the bowel can contribute to bacterial translocation. Use of antacids in certain patients may cause proximal gut colonization because of the reduction in gastric acid normally entering the small intestine. Conditions of reduced perfusion of splanchnic ischemia that can result from systemic hypotension or hemorrhagic shock can cause mucosal breakdown and gastric or intestinal compromise or ulceration. Bacterial translocation occurs in conditions associated with decreased peristalsis such as intestinal ileus or obstruction, blind loop syndromes, or hyperosmolar enteral or low-fiber diets. Administration of vasopressors, glucocorticoids, or NSAIDs can result in reduction in GI mucus production, a normal protective defense of the bowel against bacteria. Antimicrobial therapy that inhibits anaerobic GI microflora can lead to proliferation of more virulent gramnegative enteric bacteria. Conditions associated with bacterial translocation migration are intestinal resection, abdominal trauma, burns, abdominal radiation therapy, and obstructed biliary disease.[23] In humans, laparoscopic pneumoperitoneum, used for diagnosis of peritonitis, did not cause hematogenous translocation of enteric bacteria.[43] (For an additional discussion of this problem relative to abdominal surgical intervention, see Chapter 55.)

Clinical manifestations of bacterial translocation can be melena or vomiting of blood or severe ileus, decreased mentation, cardiac arrhythmias, systemic hypotension, cyanosis, reduced urinary output, tachycardia (often bradycardia in cats), and hypothermia. Laboratory abnormalities can include leukopenia or leukocytosis, elevated serum bilirubin or alanine transaminase (ALT) activity, azotemia and hypercreatinemia, thrombocytopenia, prolonged coagulation times, and low PaO_2 (arterial oxygen pressure) and elevated PCO_2 (carbon dioxide pressure) values.

Treatment involves increasing perfusion of the bowel and systemic circulation through the use of crystalloids or colloids. Oxygenation is accomplished by increasing inspired oxygen through nasal or cage oxygen. Infusion of whole blood, packed erythrocytes, or polymerized hemoglobin solutions can be used to increase the oxygen-carrying capacity. Blood pressure and tissue perfusion can be increased by infusion of sympathomimetic drugs such as dobutamine or dopamine. (For additional information and dosages, see Chapter 38.)

Prevention of bacterial translocation involves antimicrobial prophylaxis. For the GI tract, antimicrobials should be considered during manipulative procedures in which intraabdominal contamination is expected or occurs. In animals with anorexia or that are fasting for more than 3 days, enterocyte and villous atrophy can occur, resulting in altered absorption, secretion, and permeability. Forced or premature enteral intake can be associated with complications related to ileus such as diarrhea and bowel distention. Parenteral feeding can help maintain an animal's nutritional status; however, it is expensive and may cause thromboembolism. When initiating feeding, solid rather than liquid diets may help prevent bacterial translocation.[18] Insoluble fibers and nondigestible carbohydrates are also important in this regard. Glutamine has been considered an important nutrient in the integrity and replication of lymphoid and gut epithelial cells. It is an essential amino acid that has reduced mucosal inflammation when it is applied topically. Glutamine-enriched enteral diets or solutions have been beneficial in rodents but not in methotrexate-treated cats.[202] Additional studies are needed to determine whether this therapy is beneficial.

Oxidation is an important inflammatory mechanism and contributes to IBD through the production of free radicals. Supplementation with dietary oxidants is recommended, although specific documentation of efficacy does not exist. Fat restriction helps to prevent inflammatory responses in the bowel. Assimilation of dietary fat is a difficult digestive process and it should be restricted to no more than 20% calories. This is especially important when lymphangiectasia develops during IBD as a result of intestinal lymphadenitis. The addition of dietary n-3 polyunsaturated fatty acids (PUFAs) provides potential antiinflammatory activity by interfering with the arachidonic acid pathway. Concurrent antioxidant treatment helps to inhibit any oxidation of the PUFAs.

Pathophysiologic Mechanisms of Infectious Diarrhea

Enteropathogenic organisms, unlike resident and nonpathogenic transient microflora, have acquired means of overcoming the host defense mechanisms and the inhibitory properties of the normal microflora. Adherence factors (e.g., somatic pili) that permit intestinal pathogens to establish infection also allow them to attach to, multiply on, and colonize the intestinal mucosa. Some pathogenic bacteria that cause diarrhea remain on the mucosal surface and produce potent enterotoxins that disrupt fluid flux across the intestinal mucosa. Others are able to penetrate intact epithelial cells, producing inflammatory damage in the underlying mucosa. Enteric viruses damage the intestine by replicating within and destroying selected populations of epithelial cells. Various mechanisms by which microorganisms produce intestinal injury are covered in the following sections.

Normal Function of Intestinal Villi

Intestinal epithelial cells are produced by germinal epithelium located in the intestinal crypts (Fig. 89-7). Younger, undifferentiated, and primarily secretory epithelial cells, produced by the germinal epithelium of the intestinal glands (crypts), migrate up the intestinal villus as the older, differentiated, absorptive cells at the tip eventually slough into the intestinal lumen. Most of the absorptive process is confined to the differentiated cells at the villous tip, which also produce locally

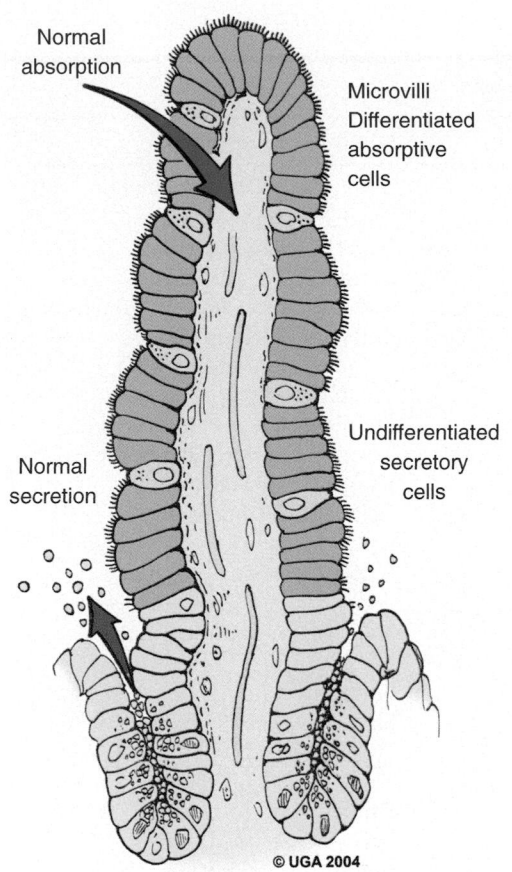

Fig 89-7 Structure of normal intestinal villus. (Courtesy University of Georgia, Athens, Ga.)

active intestinal enzymes that aid in the digestive process. The preponderance of intestinal secretion is confined to specialized goblet cells and undifferentiated cells that line the sides and depths of the crypts.

Noninvasive Enterotoxigenic Organisms

After attachment to the intact epithelial surface, noninvasive organisms produce powerful heat-labile exotoxins that bind to surface receptors on the small intestinal epithelial cells. Toxin acts at the cellular level to stimulate adenyl cyclase and other unknown mechanisms to increase intracellular cyclic adenosine monophosphate (AMP) (Fig. 89-8, *A*). The net effect of cyclic AMP is to increase secretion of chloride and to decrease absorption of sodium by intestinal epithelium, resulting in loss of large quantities of water and electrolytes in feces in the absence of morphologic injury to intestinal mucosa.

Many bacterial species that infect dogs and cats not only produce enterotoxin-induced diarrhea after initial colonization but also produce mucosal invasion (Table 89-13; see Chapters 37 and 39). Strains of some species, such as *E. coli*, can produce diarrhea by either mechanism. Several enterotoxin-producing strains of bacteria such as *Staphylococcus* species, *C. perfringens*, and *E. coli*, which commonly cause food-borne diarrhea and acute gastroenteritis, are harbored in the colons of clinically normal dogs and cats.[93] Presumably, the bacteria and toxin cause clinical illness only after being ingested or during bacterial overgrowth or intestinal stasis, when they proliferate in the small intestine. Enterotoxigenic *E. coli* have been recovered from dogs with acute diarrhea, but their importance as a primary cause of illness has been uncertain (see Chapter 37). Similar isolation of enteropathogenic strains has been made from cats.[242] *Clostridium difficile*, a bacterium associated with diarrhea in people and animals, produces an enterotoxin and a cytotoxin, which induces diarrhea and frequently mucosal ulceration and hemorrhage.

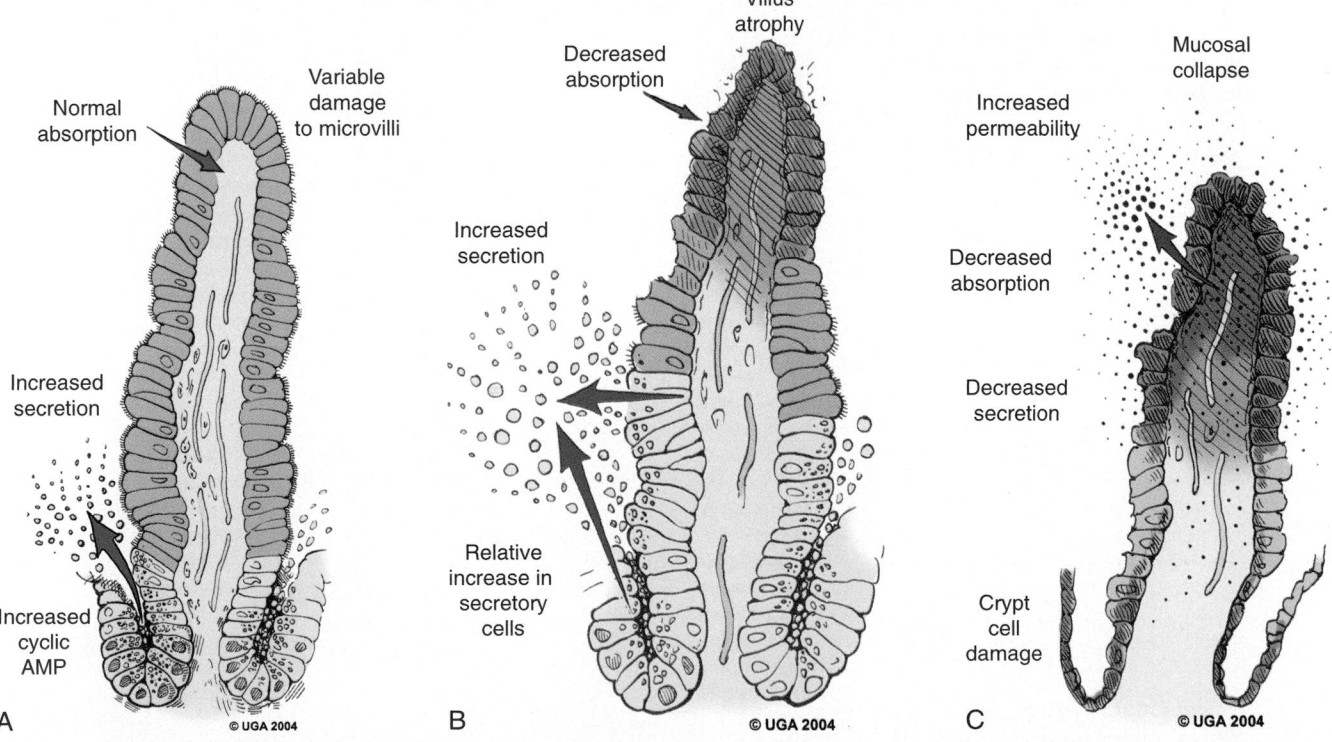

Fig 89-8 Pathogenesis of infectious diarrhea. **A,** Noninvasive enterotoxigenic bacteria (e.g., vibrios, staphylococci, and clostridia) primarily stimulate cyclic adenosine monophosphate (AMP). **B,** villous atrophy results from selective infection of apical epithelial cells with certain viruses (e.g., coronaviruses and rotaviruses). **C,** Intestinal gland degeneration and mucosal collapse occur when viruses (e.g., parvoviruses) damage germinal intestinal gland epithelium. (Courtesy University of Georgia, Athens, Ga.)

Table • 89-13

Mechanism and Site of Enteropathogenic Microorganisms[a]

MECHANISM AND ORGANISM	SITE OF ACTION[b]
Enterotoxin Production	
Vibrio cholerae (people)	Small intestine
Vibrio parahaemolyticus (people)	Small intestine
Staphylococcus (see Chapter 36)	Stomach, small intestine
Escherichia coli (see Chapter 37)	Some strains in small intestine, colon
Clostridium perfringens (see Chapter 39)	Colon
Clostridium difficile (see Chapter 39)	Colon
Yersinia enterocolitica (see Chapter 39)	Colon
Campylobacter jejuni, Campylobacter coli (see Chapter 39)	Small intestine, colon
Salmonella typhimurium (see Chapter 39)	Small intestine in initial stages, colon
Brachyspira pilosicoli	Small intestine colon
Entamoeba histolytica (see Chapter 78)	Colon, liver
Bacillus cereus (see Chapter 87)	Small intestine in initial stages
Klebsiella pneumoniae (see Chapter 88)	Small intestine
Enteroadherence	
Enterococci (see Chapter 35)	Small intestine, colon
E. coli (see Chapter 37)	Small intestine
Giardia (see Chapter 78)	Small intestine
Mucosal Invasion	
E. coli (see Chapter 37)	Some strains in colon
Salmonella (see Chapter 39)	Ileum in later stages
Shigella (see Chapter 39)	Colon
Campylobacter (see Chapter 39)	Small intestine
Helicobacter (see Chapter 39)	Stomach, small intestine, colon[b]
Balantidium coli (see Chapter 78)	Colon
E. histolytica (see Chapter 78)	Colon
Neospora caninum (dog, see Chapter 80)	Small intestine, colon
Toxoplasma gondii (cat, see Chapter 80)	Small intestine, colon
Coccidia (see Chapter 81)	Small intestine
Cryptosporidium (see Chapter 82)	Small intestine, colon
Cyclospora (see Chapter 82)	Small intestine
B. cereus (see Chapter 87)	Small intestine in later stages
V. parahaemolyticus	Small intestine in later stages
Submucosal Invasion	
E. coli (see Chapter 37)	Small intestine
Salmonella (see Chapter 39)	Small intestine
Shigella (see Chapter 39)	Small intestine and colon
Histoplasma (see Chapter 60)	Colon
Aspergillus (see Chapter 64)	Colon
Candida (see Chapter 65)	Colon
Pythium (see Chapter 67)	Stomach, small intestine, colon
Mucor, Absidia, Rhizopus (see Chapter 67)	Stomach and small intestine
Prototheca (see Chapter 69)	Colon
Villous Atrophy	
Coronaviruses (dog, see Chapter 8; cat, see Chapter 11)	Small intestine
Rotaviruses (dog, see Chapter 8; cat, see Chapter 12)	Small intestine
Reoviruses (cat, see Chapter 12)	Small intestine
Crypt Degeneration	
Canine parvovirus (see Chapter 8)	Primarily small intestine
Feline panleukopenia virus (see Chapter 10)	Primarily small intestine

[a]Host species affinities, where cited, appear in parentheses.
[b]Site depends on species. See relevant chapter for evidence of pathogenicity for dogs and cats.

Enteroadherent Organisms

Some organisms, notably adherent streptococci classified as enterococci, have been reported to be present on the intestinal epithelial surfaces of dogs and cats with diarrhea (see Table 89-13; see also Enterococcal Infections, Chapter 35, and the respective chapters for other organisms). Microscopically, diffuse colonization of intestinal enterocytes with mild inflammatory changes has been observed.[44,152] Bacterial attachment has not usually been seen in the upper small intestine.

Mucosal-Invading Organisms

After invasion of the mucosa, some bacteria produce hemorrhagic (dysenteric) stools (see Table 89-13). Two bacterial genera that classically produce dysentery are *Salmonella*, which usually has an affinity for the ileum, and *Shigella*, which has an affinity for the ileum and the colon. After they penetrate submucosal tissue, both produce a marked inflammatory response characterized by the influx of neutrophils. *Shigella* species and many strains of *Salmonella* are phagocytized and killed, although some may persist, causing a chronic carrier state (see Chapter 39).

Submucosal-Invading Organisms

The same organisms that invade mucosally can penetrate deeper into submucosal tissues (see Table 89-13). Host defenses are usually impaired, and systemic spread may occur. Submucosal invasion is characterized by hemorrhagic diarrhea, increased fecal leukocytes, leukopenia, leukocytosis, or leukopenia with a left shift and positive blood culture results. Clinical evidence of bacteremia is manifest by fever, hemorrhagic diarrhea, and shock. Fungal or protozoal pathogens or opportunists may also invade the submucosal layers, producing chronic granulomatous enterocolitis.

Villous Atrophy

The well-differentiated apical absorptive cells of the intestinal villus are responsible for producing digestive enzymes that act locally at the intestinal brush border. Reoviruses, rotaviruses, and coronaviruses have a selective affinity for replication within and destruction of these cells, resulting in villous atrophy (Fig. 89-8, *B*). Impaired absorption and digestion are characteristic of this type of diarrhea. A relative increase in intestinal secretion is usually associated with terminal villous atrophy because of continued replication of the undifferentiated germinal crypt epithelial cells, which have more secretory than absorptive functions.

Intestinal Crypt Degeneration

Because canine and feline parvoviruses require rapidly dividing cells for replication, they selectively damage mitotically active intestinal gland epithelium so that absorptive cells at the tips of the villi are not replaced, which leads to intestinal gland degeneration and eventual mucosal collapse (Fig. 89-8, *C*). The primary defect is in absorption; however, secretory processes are also inactivated. Damage to the mucosal barrier in most cases also results in an influx of inflammatory cells and increase in vascular permeability, with the eventual exudation of serum proteins.

Diagnosis of Acute Infectious Gastroenteritis

Collection of fecal samples for culture of aerobic bacteria is easier when commercially prepared, sterile, cotton-tipped applicators are used. These are supplied with transport media or enrichment broth in which the swab is placed immediately following specimen collection (see Chapter 33). Additional care can be taken to clean the anus with 70% alcohol or dilute organic iodine solution before inserting the cotton-tipped applicator. When organisms such as *Salmonella, Shigella, Helicobacter,* or *Campylobacter* are suspected, the laboratory can be notified because selective media or special cultural conditions may improve yield (see Diagnosis, Chapter 39).

Cytologic examination of fecal mucus or exudate can be an effective way to determine the integrity of the bowel mucosa. Infectious processes that cause damage to mucosal surfaces result in the appearance of large numbers of neutrophils and macrophages in feces. Diarrhea caused by parvoviruses and invasive bacteria can be distinguished by the presence of these inflammatory cells and erythrocytes.

Like cultures of specimens from the oral cavity, cultures of feces or other intestinal contents yield ambiguous results. Disturbances in the composition of microflora are not detected unless quantitative cultures are performed. Primary pathogens such as *Salmonella* and *Shigella* require selective media if they are to be isolated. Enterotoxigenic strains of bacteria require specific identification techniques that are not routinely available to most veterinarians.[243] Finding a potentially pathogenic organism is not the same as identifying the cause of diarrhea, because the prevalence of subclinical carriers of *Salmonella, Campylobacter,* and other enteropathogenic bacteria in dog and cat populations is high (see Chapters 37 and 39). Cultures should always be performed when zoonotic exposure to these pathogens is suspected.

Therapy for Acute Infectious Gastroenteritis

Antimicrobials

Antibacterial therapy is indicated in selected instances of intestinal disease, and it is usually combined with supportive care such as dietary modification, fluid therapy, motility modification, and antiemetics. Antimicrobials should be used when episodes of diarrhea or vomiting are accompanied by signs of systemic illness, including fever, depression, and impending shock, and the presence of leukopenia or leukocytosis with a marked left shift. These findings indicate that absorption of microbes or more likely, their toxins, has occurred.[231] In some instances, routine use of antimicrobials may be harmful, altering the composition and number of intestinal microorganisms that normally serve to inhibit the growth of pathogenic varieties or the induction of resistant strains. The choice of drugs depends on knowledge of the susceptibilities of the usual pathogens and the normal intestinal flora (see Drug Formulary, Appendix 8).

Antimotility Drugs

Antimotility agents have been routinely used in the treatment of infectious diarrhea. However, slowing intestinal transit may be counterproductive because diarrhea is a defense mechanism that eliminates harmful microorganisms and their toxins. Antimotility drugs have resulted in increased morbidity and persistence of infection in bacterial enteritis (see Salmonella Therapy, Chapter 39).

Fluid Therapy

Fluid therapy is probably one of the most important treatments of symptoms of the diarrheic animal. Fluids should be given IV when severe shock and hypotension, semicoma, or persistent vomiting or ileus accompanies the diarrheic episode. Less affected animals with these complications should receive subcutaneous (SC) fluids. The majority of animals with acute nonhemorrhagic diarrhea without vomiting can be treated with specific oral fluid preparations.[212] Oral fluid therapy is based on the observation that glucose is actively absorbed by the normal small bowel and sodium is carried with it in an approximately equimolar ratio. Hypertonic oral antidiarrheal fluid replacement solutions can be prepared that contain sodium and glucose in an equimolar ratio, in addition to bicarbonate and potassium in a composition similar to that of the fluid lost in diarrheic stool (Table 89-14). In most situations, amino acids commercially marketed

Table • 89-14

Chemical Composition of Various Orally Administered Rehydration Solutions for Infectious Diarrhea

FLUID (MANUFACTURER)	Na⁺ (mEq/L)	K⁺ (mEq/L)	Cl⁻ (mEq/L)	HCO₃⁻ (mEq/L)	CARBOHYDRATE (g/L)[a]	AMINO ACIDS (mmol/L)[b]	ENERGY (kcal/L)	OSMOLARITY (mOsm/L)
Body Fluids								
Normal plasma[c]	142	4.5	105	25	1	ND	ND	300
Cholera stool[c]	140	13	104	44	ND	ND	ND	ND
Replacement Fluids								
World Health Organization oral rehydration solution (WHO ORS)[c] (Jianas Bros, Kansas City, Mo.)	90	20	80	30	20	0	80	310
WHO ORS reduced osmolarity 2002[c]	75	20	65		13.6	0	54	245
Rehydrate solution (Ross, Columbus, Ohio)	75	20	65	30[d]	25	0	100	310
Pedialyte RS (Ross, Columbus, Ohio)	75	20	ND	ND	25	0	100	285
Ceralyte-90	90	20	ND	30	40	0	165	260
Gastrolyte Oral (Novum Pharma, Noordwijk, Holland)	90	20	80	30[d]	20	0	80	ND
Ion-Aid (Merial, Duluth, Ga.)	89	28	ND	0	24	125	559	480
Entrolyte (Pfizer, Providence, R.I.)[e]	105	26	51	80	23	63	399	490
Resorb (Pfizer, Providence, R.I.)[e]	80	30	27	0[f]	22	0	88	315
HY-SORB (BASF, Charlotte, N.J.)	120	10	70	40	56	0	224	ND
Biolyte (Pharmacia and Upjohn, Kalamazoo, Mich.)	184	31	104	111	68	0	272	ND
Rice-based (homemade)[g]	90	20	ND	30	50	ND	100	200
Maintenance Fluids								
Pedialyte (Ross, Columbus, Ohio)	45	20	35	30[e]	25	0	100	250
Infalyte (Bristol-Myers Squibb Princeton, N.J.)	50	25	40	50	13	0	50	200
Enterim-5 (Schering-Plough, Union, N.J.)	90	20	80	ND	31	0	521	ND
Supplementation								
Gatorade (Pepsico)[h]	21	3	11	3[f]	20	0	336	330
Apple juice[i]	1.7	26	0	0	ND	0	ND	ND

ND, No data, do not use in cases of GI obstruction or moribund animals; Na⁺, sodium; K⁺, potassium; Cl⁻ chloride; HCO₃⁻, bicarbonate.
[a]Multiply by 5.5 to get millimoles per liter of glucose.
[b]Supplied primarily as glycine.
[c]Data from Pierce NF, Hirshorn N. 1977. Oral fluid—a simple weapon against dehydration and diarrhea. How it works and how to use it, *WHO Chronicle* 31:87–93; Sack RB, Cassells SJ, Mitra R, et al. 1970. The use of oral replacement solutions in the treatment of cholera and othr severse diarrheal disorders, *Bull WHO* 43:351-360;[61] Commercially available as ORS (Jianas Bros Kansas City, MO.). These solutions also contain 10 mmol/L of citrate.
[d]Anion supplied as citrate instead of bicarbonate.
[e]Data from Lewis and Phillips. 1980. New information on fluid therapy for diarrheic calves, *Norden News* 55:4-8.
[f]Buffering capacity supplied as citrate.
[g]Can be prepared from precooked instant rice cereal (Gerber rice cereal for babies Fremont, Mich.).
[h]Stokely-Van Camp, Indianapolis, Ind., personal communication, December 1982.
[i]Data from Dupont and Pickering. 1979. pp 247-267. *Infections of the gastrointestinal tract.* Plenum Medical, New York, NY.

for veterinary use such as glycine have been added to facilitate absorption. Solutions containing glucose or sodium, either alone or in an imbalanced ratio of a decreased concentration, are *not* effective in reversing fluid and electrolyte flux across the intestinal mucosa. Similarly, polyionic, isotonic fluids such as lactated Ringer's solution, Pedialyte (Ross Laboratories, Columbus, Ohio), and Gatorade (Pepsico, Purchase, N.Y.) are helpful only for oral fluid maintenance or electrolyte supplementation and do little to stop ongoing or existing losses. Oral antidiarrheal solutions are effective only when the integrity of the intestinal mucosa is intact. This can be assessed in practice by looking for gross and microscopic evidence of blood and leukocytes in stools.

Promoted by the World Health Organization (WHO) for treating human cholera, an oral rehydration solution (ORS) called *WHO ORS* can be made by veterinarians or their clients (Table 89-15). The ingredients can be mixed and stored in a powdered state and reconstituted when necessary. Unused portions can be stored in a refrigerator for several days or weeks. Efforts to improve the original solution have resulted in reduced osmolarity (e.g., sodium ranges of 60 to 75 mEq/L and glucose ranges of 75 to 90 mmol/L).[61] WHO ORS is voluntarily accepted by most dogs and some cats, although some animals require gavage by syringe or stomach tube. The volume of WHO ORS to be administered depends on the circumstances, but a range of 50 to 100 ml/kg/day according to the fluid losses is usually given until the diarrhea stops. Vomiting, which may occur when use of these hypertonic solutions begins, can usually be obviated by giving small amounts more frequently. Although they facilitate fluid absorption, large volumes of hypertonic fluids may cause a transient increase in stool water volume because of residual unabsorbed electrolytes in the feces. Hypertonic oral fluids can also cause serum hyperosmolality and hyperosmolar coma when adequate volumes of water or isotonic fluids are not provided orally. Parenteral isotonic fluid therapy may have to be given concurrently with hypertonic fluids in small or young animals.

Protectants and Adsorbents

Protectants and adsorbents such as kaolin and pectin are limited because they are relatively ineffective in absorbing toxins produced by enteropathogenic bacteria. Kaolin (hydrated aluminum silicate) is a potent coagulation activator and may be of some benefit in treating diarrhea associated with mucosal disruption and hemorrhage. Pectin is a polymeric carbohydrate that is thought to act as an adsorbent; however, large amounts may produce diarrhea. Kaopectate should be used with caution in cats because it now contains salicylate.

NSAIDs such as aspirin have been shown to be beneficial in the management of infectious diarrhea. Clinical studies in people and experimental studies in dogs and cats have shown that salicylates interfere with the mechanism of enterotoxin-induced intestinal hypersecretion, presumably by blocking production of cyclic AMP and prostaglandin synthesis. Subsalicylate preparations (Pepto Bismol, Norwich Eaton Pharmaceuticals, Norwich, N.Y.) that are commonly provided in the treatment of diarrhea are thought to work in a similar manner. Additional studies have shown that bismuth subsalicylate has antibacterial activity because of the binding and killing of exposed pathogenic bacteria. Administration at a dose of 0.25 ml/kg every 4 to 6 hours early in the course of disease may be helpful in treating diarrhea that results from the mechanism of increased secretion.

Infectious Small Intestinal Disorders

Numerous defined syndromes attributed to alterations in intestinal microflora have been described and are discussed in the following sections. In many instances, the pathophysiologic mechanisms are not completely elucidated.

Neonatal Colibacillosis

Neonatal colibacillosis caused by *E. coli* has been described in many species, including dogs[32,79] and cats[242] (see Chapter 37). Characteristically, puppies are affected within the first week of life and have a high mortality rate. They show acute depression, weakness, hypothermia, cyanosis, and central nervous system signs before death. Older puppies that survive for several weeks may have persistent diarrhea, abdominal discomfort, weight loss, and dehydration. Gross necropsy findings include hemorrhagic lesions on serosal surfaces of all body cavities and throughout the GI mucosa. Septicemia can be confirmed by bacterial culture from the blood or from many organs. Histologic examination reveals gram-negative bacilli in many tissues of septicemic newborns.

The cause of *E. coli* septicemia in newborn puppies may be associated with their immunologic incompetency rather than the virulence of a particular strain of organism. Enterotoxic, attaching, and effacing bacterial strains of *E. coli* exist. Furthermore, intestinal epithelial cells of newborn puppies are highly and nonselectively permeable to various proteins (including bacteria), which are absorbed by pinocytosis. Exposure to *E. coli* before colostrum ingestion or the failure to obtain sufficient colostrum may further predispose newborn puppies to infection. *E. coli* is also able to cross the intestinal epithelial barrier 48 to 72 hours after birth, after which the cells also cease to absorb immunoglobulins. Puppies appear to be completely resistant to intestinal exposure to *E. coli* at 2 weeks of age. Enteropathogenic *E. coli* may cause disease in animals of any age.

Table • 89-15

Composition of World Health Organization Oral Rehydration Solution (WHO ORS)

DRY INGREDIENTS[a]	AMOUNT IN GRAMS (TEASPOONS)	SUBSTITUTES
Sodium chloride (table salt)	3.5 (0.64)	None
Sodium bicarbonate (baking soda)	2.5 (0.55)	None
Glucose powder (dextrose)	20.0 (6.0)	Sucrose (table sugar): 40.0 g (8 tsps) or equivalent amount of honey or corn syrup
Potassium chloride	1.5 (0.31)	Apple juice: 0.47 liter (1 U.S. pint)

g, Grams; *tsps*, teaspoons
Data modified from World Health Organization: Treatment and Prevention of Dehydration in Diarrheal Diseases, Geneva, WHO, 1976; Gangarosa EJ. 1977 Recent developments in diarrheal diseases, *Postgrad Med* 62:113–117; and Pierce NF, Hirschhorn N. 1977. Oral fluid—a simple weapon against dehydration in diarrhea. How it works and how to use it. *WHO Chron* 31:87–93, 1977.
[a]In 1 liter of water (1.05 U.S. quarts).

Klebsiella pneumonia has also been associated with enteritis and septicemia in young dogs[260] (see Chapter 37).

Small Intestinal Bacterial Overgrowth

SIBO in people is a syndrome characterized by increased proximal small intestinal bacterial concentrations leading to macrocytic anemia, steatorrhea, and weight loss. Reduced gastric acid, impaired peristaltic motion, and ileocecal valve dysfunction can all lead to increases in the load of small intestinal bacteria. Collection and culturing methods to confirm this disorder are critical to enable cultivation of anaerobes. Levels of 10^5 colony-forming units/ml of anaerobic bacteria are high in people; however, dogs and especially cats have much higher concentrations. Furthermore, levels of cobalamin and folate in serum are not consistently predictable and can be affected by amounts of these nutrients in the diets or other supplements.

SIBO in animals is a syndrome of bacterial proliferation in the upper intestinal lumen accompanied by chronic or recurrent small bowel diarrhea. It has been most commonly observed in German shepherd dogs.[13,17] Causes for SIBO in this and other breeds are impaired motility or obstruction of the GI tract, secretory IgA deficiency, and reduced gastric or pancreatic secretion. Dogs with SIBO are typically between 5 months and 2 years of age. They are usually bright and alert but show variable weight loss, which becomes apparent with time, and they consistently pass foul-smelling, watery feces for months. Results of quantitation of bacteria in duodenal secretions from affected animals have revealed increased numbers of *E. coli* and enterococci, typically normal flora of this site, and proliferation of anaerobes such as clostridia, which are unusual inhabitants.[17] Duodenal bacterial overgrowth also occurs in German shepherd dogs with pancreatic exocrine insufficiency (PEI). Furthermore, similar clinical features of PEI and bacterial overgrowth make these syndromes difficult to differentiate. Bacterial overgrowth in the jejunum has developed in dogs after surgical reconstruction of the biliary tract.[363]

Although disordered motility and hypochlorhydria are possible causes of SIBO, a secretory IgA immune deficiency is considered most important (see Chapter 95).[13,343,353,354] Histochemical analysis suggests that German shepherd dogs have defective synthesis or secretion of IgA despite the presence of IgA-committed plasma cells.[13] Duodenal biopsies from German shepherd dogs with IBD or SIBO had greater levels of expression of mRNA for inflammatory cytokines, IL-2, IL-5, IL-12p40, TNF-α, and transforming growth factor-β1 (TGF-β1) messenger ribonucleic acid (mRNA) expression than control dogs, but no significant differences between dogs with IBD or SIBO were found.[85] Furthermore, antibiotic treatment in five dogs with SIBO resulted in reduced TNF-α and TGF-β1 mRNA expression. Such alterations in cytokine mRNA expression suggest heightened immune responses within the duodenal mucosa in German Shepherd dogs with either SIBO or IBD.

Anaerobic bacterial overgrowth in the proximal small intestine leads to increased breath-hydrogen concentration in most dogs and variably increased serum folic acid concentration.[353] Increased serum folate results from increased synthesis of this compound by the large numbers of intestinal bacteria, with greater amounts available for absorption. In addition, reduced serum B_{12}, found in up to 25% of these dogs, is thought to be caused by bacterial binding of the vitamin within the intestine, preventing its absorption. Steatorrhea is usually mild or absent unless concurrent PEI is present. Xylose absorption has been variably reduced in affected dogs, presumably as a result of bacterial use of xylose in the proximal small bowel, thereby decreasing the amount being absorbed. In some cases, abnormal xylose absorption may be corrected by prior administration of antibiotics. Differential sugar absorption testing has been used to confirm the presence of SIBO and monitor the response to treatment.[269] Serum trypsinlike immunoreactivity and absorption of bound para-aminobenzoic acid have been within reference ranges unless concurrent PEI is present. Minimal histologic abnormalities have been found in affected dogs, and the activities of some brush border intestinal enzymes have been altered depending on whether anaerobic or aerobic bacteria predominate and whether PEI is present.[15,16,357] Chronic SIBO may result in protein-losing enteropathy, which can be controlled by antimicrobial therapy.

Although difficult to perform in routine practice, quantitative culture of duodenal or proximal jejunal fluid from dogs with overgrowth shows bacterial counts greater than 10^5 organisms per milliliter.[50,57] Proliferating organisms in dogs often consist of small intestinal microflora such as *E. coli*, *Enterobacter*, *Enterococcus*, and *Lactobacillus*, but occasionally unusual species for the location, such as clostridia, predominate.

When possible, underlying causes of SIBO should be determined and eliminated. Response to antimicrobial therapy supports the diagnosis (Table 89-16). Oxytetracycline and tylosin are recommended for dogs and metronidazole for cats.[356] Because of the development of overgrowth in some dogs with PEI, antimicrobial therapy may be required in those that do not respond to enzyme supplementation alone. In addition, a bland diet, such as boiled rice with cottage cheese or chicken or specialized diets (I/D, Hills Foods, Topeka, Kan.) have often been recommended during the treatment period to obtain more consistent responses. Increased-fiber diets actually reduced transit time and intestinal bacterial populations. Feeding IgA-deficient dogs with SIBO FOSs reduced bacterial populations in their proximal small intestines.[353]

Inflammatory Bowel Disease

IBD can be attributed to various pathogenic or opportunistic enteric microorganisms (Table 89-17); however, in other cases, specific organisms cannot be incriminated despite chronic inflammatory enteric disease. In this latter idiopathic IBD, resident microflora may become secondarily involved in perpetuating the inflammatory process. IBD is suspected to be caused by an immune hypersensitivity derangement resulting in immunoreactive or autoreactive intestinal injury. In humans, IBD can involve any part of the GI tract (e.g., Crohn's disease) or be regional (e.g., ulcerative colitis). Care must be taken when extrapolating pathogenesis from the human disease. The clinically healthy intestinal tract is exposed to a large variety of foreign dietary and microbial antigens. It develops immunologic tolerance through a complex interaction of the gut-associated lymphoid tissue (GALT). Recognition of antigens outside of this group can trigger an inflammatory response. With dietary proteins, soluble antigens tend to evoke less of a secretory antibody response compared with insoluble ones. Clinical observations and animal models incriminate luminal bacteria or their products in the initiation and perpetuation of the disease. Outside of dietary antigens, the ability to recognize pathogens is genetically conserved and is based on Toll-like receptors (TLRs) in the intestinal cell membrane. In the healthy intestine, TLR expression is low. Should microbial antigens such as lipopolysaccharide, lipoteichoic acid, or peptidoglycan be detected, a sequence of inflammatory cascades occurs. Transcription factor (NF-kB) induces gene transcription of inflammatory cytokines such as IL-1, IL-6, IL-8, IL-12, and CD80/CD86. A key factor in the pathogenesis of IBD is disruption of the mucosal barrier and associated chronic inflammation. The production of antibodies against self-antigens in immune cells such as granulocytes and mast cells and against cell wall components of bacteria

Table • 89-16

Antimicrobial Therapy for Bacterial Overgrowth, Lymphoplasmacytic Enteritis, and Enteropathogenic Bacteria

DRUG[a]	USE	SPECIES	DOSE (mg/kg)[b]	ROUTE	INTERVAL (HOURS)	DURATION (DAYS)
Tylosin	SIBO, LPE, EPB	B	10-15	PO	12	7-14
Tetracycline[c]	SIBO	B	20	PO	8	28
Metronidazole	SIBO, LPE	D	15	PO	12	7-14
		D	10	PO	8	7-14
		C	30	PO	24	7-14
Sulfasalazine[d]	LPE	D	12.5	PO	6	21-28
		D	10-30	PO	8	21-28
		C	250 mg total	PO	24	14-21
		C	20	PO	24	14-21
Prednisolone	LPE	B	0.5-2	PO	12	14-21
Azathioprine	LPE	D	1-2.5[e]	PO	24	14-21
		C	0.3	PO	48	14-21
Erythromycin	EPB	D	10	PO	8	7-14
Enrofloxacin	EPB	D	5	PO	12	7-14
		C	5	PO	24	7-14
Gentamicin	EPB	B	5	IV, IM, SC	24	7
Trimethoprim-sulfonamide	EPB	B	15	PO, SC	12	7-14

SIBO, Small intestinal bacterial overgrowth; *LPE*, lymphoplasmacytic enteritis; *EPB*, enteropathogenic bacteria (see Chapter 39); *B*, dog and cat; *D*, dog; *C*, cat; *PO*, by mouth; *IV*, intravenous; *IM*, intramuscular; *SC*, subcutaneous.
[a]See Drug Formulary, Appendix 8, for additional information on each drug.
[b]Dose per administration at specified interval.
[c]Or oxytetracycline.
[d]Azulfidine.
[e]Dose also expressed as 40 mg/m^2 based on body surface area.

may perpetuate a chronic inflammatory process. Chronic inflammation with or without altered host immunity may lead to invasion by enteric organisms as a secondary complication. Microbial flora in the intestinal tract, including bacteria and yeasts, are therefore pathogenic elements in the disease progression. To develop, this disease likely involves an interaction between enteric microorganisms in hosts having a particular immunologic and genetic composition. Chronic exposure of GALT to ingested or endogenous microfloral antigens or toxins may be responsible.

Immunohistochemical studies suggest that IgG is the major antibody in the immune response in the lamina propria of affected dogs.[206] A disordered imbalance of cytokines in IBD also exists. Increased numbers of B and T cells are found in the intestinal wall of dogs with IBD, indicating a chronic cellular immune reaction.[302] Immunohistochemical studies of the intestinal mucosa from dogs with various diarrheal disorders and control dogs have indicated alterations of immune elements.[84] Compared with controls, dogs with antibiotic-responsive diarrhea had increased numbers of lamina propria IgA$^+$ plasma cells and CD4+ cells. More marked alterations were noted in dogs with IBD, with significant increases in lamina propria IgG+ plasma cells, T cells (CD3+), CD4+ cells, macrophages, and neutrophils but reduced mast cell numbers. Compared with controls, dogs with IBD had increased intraepithelial CD3+ T cells. However, when compared with controls, dogs with adverse food-induced diarrhea had unchanged lamina propria and epithelial populations. The altered mucosal immune cell populations observed in dogs with antibiotic-responsive diarrhea or IBD may reflect an underlying immunologic pathogenesis in these disorders.

Numerous nutritional derangements occur in IBD that result in metabolic abnormalities. Hypomagnesemia develops through a combination of anorexia, fluid diuresis, and malabsorption. Cobalamin deficiency develops, especially in older cats with various GI diseases and pancreatic insufficiency.[290] These cats, which can develop villus atrophy or megaloblastic anemia, may benefit from parenteral cobalamin administration.[288] Microcytic hypochromic anemia can also be observed, as a sign of chronic blood loss or inflammatory sequestration of iron.[258] Anemia and malabsorption, especially in cats, may also result from the B$_{12}$ deficiency associated with IBD and other malabsorptive enteric and pancreatic diseases.[290] Thrombocytopenia has also been documented.[255] Before evidence of hypoalbuminemia, fecal α-1 proteinase inhibitor (α-1PI) was increased in the stool of dogs with histopathologic changes in their enteric mucosa, a fact that may be helpful in early detection of protein-losing enteropathy.[217]

Idiopathic *IBD*, previously termed "lymphocytic-plasmacytic enteritis," is a frequent cause of GI illness in dogs[268,313] and cats.* It is characterized by diffuse mucosal infiltration of lymphocytes, plasma cells, eosinophils, and neutrophils.[47] Variants of IBD are eosinophilic and granulomatous infiltrations. IBD may or may not involve the stomach and colon. In cats, it has been observed in association with cholangiohepatitis and pancreatitis.[340]

In contrast to SIBO, no dog breed is predisposed to this syndrome, and affected animals are usually older than 2 years. The disease generally affects older purebred cats. Chronic or intermittent intractable diarrhea with occasional vomiting is noted in dogs. Stools may vary in consistency, but gross evidence of hemorrhage is often lacking in dogs with small bowel inflammation. With long-standing and severe disease, weight

*References 58, 112, 142, 311, 312, 319, 349, 361.

Table • 89-17

Microorganisms Causing Chronic Inflammatory Bowel Diseases in Dogs and Cats

TYPE OF BOWEL DISEASE	MICROORGANISMS
Suppurative	
Bacterial	*Salmonella* spp. (see Chapter 39), toxigenic *Escherichia coli* (see Chapter 37), *Yersinia* spp. (see Chapter 39)
Lymphoplasmacytic	
Viral	FCV-associated gingivostomatitis (see Chapter 16), immunosuppression induced by FIV (see Chapter 14) or FeLV (see Chapter 13)
Bacterial	*Helicobacter* spp. (see Chapter 39), *Campylobacter* spp. (see Chapter 39), *Clostridium perfringens* (see Chapter 39), resident microflora (overgrowth, SIBO)
Protozoal	*Cryptosporidium* spp. (see Chapter 82)
Granulomatous	
Viral	Feline coronavirus (see Chapter 11)
Bacterial	*Mycobacterium* spp. (see Chapter 50)
Fungal	*Histoplasma* spp. (see Chapter 60), *Cryptococcus* spp. (see Chapter 61), *Zygomycetes* spp. (see Chapter 67), *Pythium* spp. (see Chapter 67)
Algal	*Prototheca* spp. (see Chapter 68)
Protozoal	*Leishmania* spp. (see Chapter 73), *Toxoplasma* spp. (see Chapter 80)

FCV, Feline calicivirus; *FIV,* feline immunodeficiency virus; *FeLV,* feline leukemia virus; *SIBO,* small intestinal bacterial overgrowth.

loss develops. Dogs with lower bowel involvement have the greatest prevalence of increased frequency of defecation and hematochezia and mucus in their stool.[47] In contrast, vomiting and weight loss are major signs in affected cats; vomiting is often unrelated to eating and may occur in sporadic episodes.[361] Diarrhea is less common and variable and can have a small- or large-bowel origin. Some cats have colonic localization with signs of large-bowel diarrhea with hematochezia.[58] Appetite may be reduced, corresponding to the episodic nature of vomiting and diarrhea. Some dogs and cats with significant weight loss have voracious appetites similar to those in PEI. Thickening or discomfort may be found on pal-

pation of the intestine. Hepatomegaly has been observed in some cats. Edema, hydrothorax, or ascites may be found in animals with severe hypoproteinemia.

Neutrophilia, occasionally with a left shift, or a stress leukogram and hypoproteinemia are seen in dogs with moderate to severe disease. Cats may have high serum activities of ALT and alkaline phosphatase (ALP).[112] Clinical laboratory evaluation for malabsorption or maldigestion is generally within reference ranges. Measurement of nonspecific markers of inflammation has been used in human medicine to determine whether chronic bowel inflammation is occurring. Blood parameters such as acute phase reactants, C-reactive protein (CRP), and erythrocyte sediment rates are increased. Similarly, CRP was increased in affected dogs, which paralleled the laboratory and histologic severity of illness.[148,153] As another measure of bowel inflammation, high concentrations of IgG and nitrates can be detected in colonic lavage analytes.[101] In dogs with IBD, serum antibody reactivity to perinuclear cytoplasm of neutrophils (pANCA) and *Saccharomyces cerevisiae* (ASCA) has been more prevalent than in clinically healthy dogs and those with other types of acute diarrhea or chronic non–IBD-associated diarrhea.[4] The ASCA result was more inconsistent, perhaps because of the dietary differences among dogs, whereas that for pANCA had a low level of sensitivity, making it less valuable as a screening blood test. In addition, tests for absorption of inert sugars show altered values in dogs with IBD.[294] Contrast radiographic findings vary and have low yields. Intestinal biopsy by endoscopy or exploratory laparotomy is the *only* means of definitive diagnosis. Biopsies of mesenteric lymph nodes should be taken if the nodes are enlarged.

Caution should be taken when interpreting biopsy reports of mild lymphoplasmacytic infiltrations in the intestinal mucosae. Pathologists may vary in their interpretations of mild infiltrates, which may be found in intestinal biopsy specimens of clinically healthy animals.

In cats, lymphoplasmacytic infiltrates, crypt distortion, villous blunting and fusion, and fibrosis have been most commonly seen in cats with moderate or severe IBD.[8] Clinicopathologic findings of some cats have included anemia, leukocytosis or leukopenia, hypocholesterolemia, and hyperproteinemia or hypoproteinemia. Abnormalities are not apparent on abdominal radiography; however, contrast studies using barium can reveal radiographic abnormalities in a few cats. Ultrasonographic abnormalities, which are present in a majority of cats, include poor intestinal wall layer definition, focal thickening, and large mesenteric lymph nodes with hypoechoic changes consistent with IBD. Endoscopic observation can reveal gross findings (e.g., erythema, plaques, mucosal friability) consistent with bowel inflammation in only about half of the cases.

Therapy for IBD is very similar to that for chronic colitis. Bacterial overgrowth may be involved, especially in longstanding cases, and should be addressed in some treatments. Hypersensitivity to enteric organisms or food ingredients may be associated with the pathogenesis, and hypoallergenic diets are recommended for initial treatment. Elimination diets, in which offending foods can be identified, are helpful in many dogs and cats affected with IBD having regional involvement and lymphoplasmacytic, eosinophilic, or mixed cellular infiltrates.[39] Theoretically, protein hydrolysate diets provide less antigenic stimulation to the intestinal immune system and have offered empiric improvement in animals with IBD. Presumably, less antigenic stimulation reduces intestinal inflammation, resulting in improved mucosal integrity.

Increased fiber may benefit animals with IBD. Fermentable fibers affect intestinal flora by causing increases in favorable microflora species. Probiotics are microbial preparations that colonize the host and alter the composition of intestinal microflora.

Because immune-mediated and infectious causes may be involved, antimicrobial (metronidazole, tylosin, sulfasalazine) and antiinflammatory or immunosuppressive (glucocorticoid or azathioprine) therapies are recommended if dietary management fails or cannot be implemented (see Table 89-16). When the diagnosis is uncertain, antimicrobial therapy should be instituted first because of potential complications of immunosuppression of dogs with bacterial overgrowth. Protein and energy malnutrition may result from decreased absorption. Iron and B_{12} deficiency can develop in dogs and cats.[39] Doses of B_{12} for both species are 500 µg SC daily for 4 to 5 weeks. Some discomfort can result because of local irritation. Vitamin K supplementation may be needed, especially in cats with a coagulopathy. Administration of other parenteral water-soluble vitamins and fat-soluble vitamins is also indicated for patients that have poor body condition. Low serum magnesium levels have also been identified in some dogs and cats with primary intestinal disease.[204,323] Response to therapy varies and is unpredictable. Although some animals show improvement after therapy is instituted and have prolonged remissions, others relapse or do not respond at all. Hypoalbuminemia at the time of diagnosis has been associated with a poor response to therapy.[47]

Hemorrhagic Gastroenteritis

Hemorrhagic gastroenteritis (HGE), a syndrome characterized by the sudden onset of vomiting and production of profuse, mucoid, bloody diarrhea, was primarily described in small house dogs between 2 and 4 years of age.[34] The syndrome is also marked by hematologic findings that include relative polycythemia, with a normal or low plasma protein concentration, and coagulation test results suggestive of disseminated intravascular coagulation (DIC) and occasionally, acute oliguric renal failure.

The pathogenesis of the syndrome of acute HGE is unknown, but many clinical and laboratory findings are similar to those produced in dogs by experimental administration of bacterial endotoxin or enterotoxins with resultant DIC (see Chapters 37 and 38). Whether a cause or an effect, DIC may explain many of the clinical features that have been observed in dogs. Allergic, hereditary, autoimmune, and infectious causes for HGE have been proposed. This syndrome has features that are very similar to those produced in bacterial translocation. The high prevalence of HGE in certain breeds, such as schnauzers and miniature poodles, has been explained by their hereditary predisposition to such causative factors. Dogs have been reported to develop hemolytic-uremic syndrome as well, which may be related to enterotoxigenic bacteria.[127] The influence on microbial flora of the highly digestible meat-based protein diets commonly fed to well-cared for house dogs should be examined. Diagnosis of the syndrome of HGE is based on historical, clinical, and laboratory findings. Treatment is essentially similar to that for endotoxemia (see Chapter 38). Rehydration and diuresis with polyionic isotonic fluids are the most important components of treatment. Antimicrobial therapy for enteropathogens is recommended because of the damaged mucosal integrity (see Table 89-16). Some enteropathogenic bacteria, including members of the genera *Clostridium*, *Escherichia*, and *Salmonella*, can also cause similar appearing, acute hemorrhagic diarrhea (see Chapters 37 and 39).[7,325]

LARGE INTESTINE

Microflora

The cecum and colon are the richest sources of intestinal microflora, and a single gram of feces contains up to 10^{11} organisms,[44] approximately 100 times the human population of the world. Organisms that inhabit the lower bowel are primarily gram-negative aerobes and spore-forming and non–spore-forming anaerobes (see Table 89-8 and Table 89-18). Anaerobic bacteria, which usually comprise more than 90% of the colonic microflora, include clostridia, lactobacilli, and *Bifidobacterium* and *Bacteroides* organisms. Aerobic or microaerophilic bacteria primarily consist of streptococci, members of the Enterobacteriaceae, and spirochetes. In cats that were older than 9 years, fecal *C. perfringens* concentrations were higher and bifidobacteria and lactobacilli concentrations were lower.[235] Cats fed high-protein cat food had a significantly higher fecal *C. perfringens* concentration than those fed dry cat food.[236]

Acute Colitis

Numerous acute inflammatory diseases of the colon have been described in dogs and cats. Colitis, whether acute or chronic, usually involves the microflora as a secondary phenomenon. As with stomatitis, many cases of acute colitis in dogs and cats can be associated with the stressful circumstances or immunosuppressive diseases. Acute colitis has been reported in cats experimentally infected with panleukopenia virus, although the colonic lesions were milder than those in the small intestine.[286] One case of mycotic colitis in a cat was assumed to be a sequela to panleukopenia virus infection.[28] Acute ulcerative colitis of undetermined cause has also been recognized in young cats.[68,179,329]

Table • 89-18

Colonic Bacterial and Fungal Microflora

MICROFLORA	CONCENTRATION[a]
Microaerophilic Aerobes	
Gram-negative	
Escherichia coli	10^7–10^8
Enterobacter species	ND
Klebsiella species	10^7–10^8
Proteus species	ND
Pseudomonas species	ND
Gram-positive	
Staphylococcus species	$10^{4.7}$
Streptococcus species	10^8–10^9
Lactobacillus species	10^8–10^9
Ruminococcus species	ND
Corynebacterium species	$10^{8.7}$
Obligate Anaerobes	
Bacteroides species	10^8–10^{10}
Bifidobacterium species	$10^{6.6}$
Fusobacterium species	ND
Veillonella species	$10^{5.9}$
Eubacterium species	ND
Bacillus species	$10^{5.4}$
Clostridium species	10^7–$10^{9.1}$
Spirochetes	ND
Yeasts	10^5

[a]Organisms per milliliter of contents. *ND*, No data.
Data from Strombeck DR. 1996. *In* Guilford WS, Center S, Strombeck D, et al (eds), *Strombeck's small animal gastroenterology.* WB Saunders, Philadelphia, PA.

Antimicrobial Drug–Associated Pseudomembranous Colitis

Antimicrobial drug-associated pseudomembranous colitis syndrome can be caused by species of *Clostridium* (especially *C. difficile*) and staphylococci in people. Suppression of normal flora by antimicrobial agents, immunosuppression, or nosocomial acquisition is a possible predisposition. Although this syndrome has been well documented in people and horses, especially those given macrolides, it is not well recognized in dogs and cats. Carriage of *C. difficile* with a proportion of toxigenic strains has been documented in cats housed in a veterinary teaching hospital.[197] Cats with toxigenic strains had at least one risk factor, and half of the cats had diarrhea. Treatment for this disease in people involves vancomycin or metronidazole. (For an additional discussion of clostridial colitis, see Chapter 39.) Antibiotic-associated colitis caused by an imbalance in colonic microflora (presumably, proliferation of streptococci and *Pseudomonas* organisms) was suspected in a dog treated with enrofloxacin and ampicillin.[350]

Spirochetal (Brachyspira pilosicoli) Diarrhea

Spirochetes have been recognized in the colonic crypts and feces of clinically healthy dogs for decades. In addition, numerous reports have been made of spirochetes causing diarrhea in dogs and cats.[92] Their role in disease has been debatable, and several reasons explain this discrepancy. A diverse group of related spirochetes are known to be a part of the normal microflora throughout the GI tract of dogs and cats, with the greatest numbers in the oral cavity, cecum, and colon. Because spirochetes are not demonstrable by hematoxylin-eosin (H and E) staining, they have been overlooked in biopsy specimens by pathologists. Historically, confusion is also associated with histologic examination of spiral helicobacters (see Chapter 39). Scanning or transmission electron microscopy (EM) and special staining procedures can help to confirm the presence of spirochetes, which are usually attached to the intestinal epithelia at the base of crypts. Intestinal spirochetosis caused by *Brachyspira (Serpulina) pilosicoli* has been documented in people as an enteric disease with potential zoonotic implications.[64] This organism was a resident spirochete in the large intestine and feces of nonhuman primates, dogs, pigs, and birds. Dogs might be one of several animal reservoirs for these infections in people. Clinical illness has also been produced in swine with *S. pilosicoli*, and it may be responsible for illness in other immunocompromised animals.[293] In addition, a second spirochete, *Serpulina canis*, has been identified as a nonpathogenic commensal because it has primarily been isolated from clinically healthy dogs.[64]

Because of intestinal adherence, spirochetes are not shed in formed feces of dogs and cats. During large-bowel diarrheal episodes, especially in pups, they dislodge from the epithelia and appear in large numbers in feces. Spirochetes in stool cannot be incriminated as the cause of diarrhea, despite their close relationship with *Serpulina (Treponema) hyodysenteriae*—the cause of swine dysentery[63]—and spirochetes from people with diarrhea.[176,178] An specific-pathogen–free beagle pup with a history of chronic diarrhea and concurrent giardiasis had suspected colonic spirochetosis.[62,63] Spirochetes were attached to the lamina propria in areas of superficial mucosal erosions, similar to those in swine and human intestinal spirochetosis. Treatment recommended for intestinal spirochete infections has often centered around tylosin; however, studies have shown increasing genetic resistance of canine intestinal spirochetes to this antimicrobial agent.[244]

Anaerobiospirillum Species Ileocolitis

Ileocolitis caused by *Anaerobiospirillum* species was found in six cats. Acute diarrhea, with or without vomiting, was found in two cats; in addition, one cat had chronic diarrhea, another had anorexia and lethargy, and two cats did not have signs of GI illness.[53] The presence of an *Anaerobiospirillum* species was demonstrated on the basis of ultrastructural morphology of spiral bacteria associated with intestinal lesions and polymerase chain reaction (PCR) amplification of a genus-specific 16S ribonucleic acid (rRNA) gene from affected tissues from each cat. The colons of three clinically healthy cats without lesions and one cat with mild colitis not associated with spiral bacteria were negative for *Anaerobiospirillum* species in the same assay. (For additional information on enteric spiral bacterial infections in dogs, see *Anaerobiospirillum* Infections, Chapter 39.)

Histocytic Colitis

The colitis that occurs in boxers, French bulldogs, and occasionally in other breeds (e.g., one time in a Mastiff, an Alaskan malamute, an English bulldog, and a Doberman pinscher) and begins at a young age is characterized by large-bowel diarrhea including hematochezia, increased frequency of defecation, and tenesmus.[131,301,315] One report of the disease in a cat has also been made.[328] The lesions are typically granulomatous and associated with infiltrates of periodic acid-schiff (PAS)-positive histocytes. It may be a secondary result of chronic ulceration and a reaction to intestinal microflora. Immunohistochemical studies have described increased numbers of CD3+ T cells, IgG3+ and IgG4+ plasma cells, major histocompatibility complex class II+ cells, L1+ macrophages, and neutrophils, as well as decreased numbers of goblet cells in the colonic lesions.[84] Although organisms have not been confirmed in lesions and are difficult to visualize by light microscopy, EM and other observations have suggested that organisms such as enteroadherent bacteria, cell-wall deficient mycobacteria, or *Mycoplasma*, *Chlamydia*, or *Bartonella* species have been involved. This situation is reminiscent of one related to Whipple disease in people, in which a new actinomycete bacillus—*Tropheryma whipplei*—related to other soil bacteria was finally discovered. In Whipple disease, macrophages containing PAS-positive granules, presumably from staining of bacilli and their remnants, are found within the lamina propria of the small intestine.[75] Empirically, histocytic colitis has been successfully treated with a combination of clavamox, metronidazole, spiramycin, and enrofloxacin. However, enrofloxacin has also been used as the only antimicrobial to control this disease,[51,131] indicating that a yet-to-be-identified quinolone-susceptible microorganism is likely responsible for the disease (Table 89-19). Remarkably, histologic abnormalities of cellular infiltration resolved in dogs beginning the first week of treatment, and diarrhea usually resolves within 12 days of instituting treatment. The duration of treatment has ranged from 1 to 21 months, and the length can only be established by stopping therapy to determine whether clinical signs recur. Treated and recovered dogs have been off therapy for up to 14 months without relapse of signs even though PAS-positive macrophages persisted in their colonic biopsy specimens.[131] This response to the quinolone administration suggests that an undetermined microorganism may be responsible for this syndrome, or quinolones may have an unknown immunomodulatory effect on this condition. Granulomatous inflammation of the bowel can also develop in animals with feline infectious peritonitis, prototlecosis, mycobacteriosis, and zygomycosis and pythiosis (see Chapters 11, 50, and 67, respectively).

Chronic Colitis

Chronic idiopathic colitis is a common syndrome recognized in dogs, characterized by intermittent diarrhea with hematochezia and tenesmus, weight loss, occasional vomiting, and abdominal pain. As a syndrome, it does not appear to be as important as it is in cats. Fever is not a consistent finding with

Table • 89-19

Therapy for Colitis

DRUG[a]	SPECIES	DOSE[b]	ROUTE	INTERVAL (HOURS)	DURATION (DAYS)
Antimicrobials					
Sulfasalazine (Azulfidine)	D	12.5 mg/kg	PO	6	21—28
	D	10—25 mg/kg	PO	8	21—28
	C	5—10 mg/kg	PO	8	14—21
	C	25 mg/kg	PO	24	14—21
Chloramphenicol	D	25 mg/kg	PO	8	14—21
	C	15—25 mg/kg	PO	8	7—14
Metronidazole	B[c]	10—20 mg/kg	PO	12	14—21
	B[c]	7.5—10 mg/kg	PO	8	14—21
	B[c]	30 mg/kg	PO	24	14—21
Tylosin	D	10—25 mg/kg	PO	8	14—21
Enrofloxacin[d]	D	5 mg/kg	PO	12	21—90
Amoxicillin-clavulanate	D	12.5 mg/kg	PO	12	21—28
Spiramycin	D	500 mg[e]	PO	24	21—28
Motility Modifiers					
Clidinium and chlordiazepoxide[f]	D	0.1 mg/kg	PO	6—12	prn
Diphenoxylate	D	0.5—1 mg/kg	PO	8—12	prn
Loperamide	D	0.1 mg/kg	PO	6	prn
Diazepam	B	5 mg total	PO	8—12	prn

D, Dog; *C*, cat; *B*, dog and cat; *prn*, as needed; *PO*, by mouth; *prn*, as needed.
[a]See Drug Formulary, Appendix 8 for additional information on each drug.
[b]Dose per administration at specified interval.
[c]Most cats get one fourth of a 250-mg tablet per day.
[d]Recommended for histiocytic ulcerative colitis of boxers and other dogs.
[e]75,000 units/kg in equivalent dosage.
[f]Librax, Roche Products Inc., Marrati, P.R.

large-bowel inflammation. Chronic ulcerative colitis does not appear to be associated with primary bacterial pathogens but probably results from stress, debilitation, or immunosuppression in conjunction with an immune imbalance. Comparison of cell populations among dog groups indicated that IgA- and IgG-containing cells and CD3+ T cells were significantly more numerous in the colonic mucosa of dogs with lymphocytic-plasmacytic colitis (LPC).[149] Chronic colitis has also been identified in dogs with perianal fistulas.[143] Semiquantitative reverse transcriptase PCR (RT-PCR) was performed using specific primers on RNA isolated from the colonic mucosa of healthy dogs, dogs with clinical signs of large intestinal disease but normal histopathologic signs in the colon, and dogs with LPC.[257] In comparison with healthy colonic mucosa and the mucosa of dogs with large intestinal diarrhea but normal histopathologic signs, canine LPC was associated with overexpression of IL-2. Higher levels of TNF-α mRNA were also seen in the mucosa of dogs with LPC than those with healthy mucosa. These results suggest that LPC is associated with activation of CD4+ T-helper lymphocytes and increased production of T-helper-1-type cytokines. That the lesions are invaded by intestinal microflora after mucosal disruption may explain the apparent beneficial effect of antibiotics and the occasional deleterious effect of glucocorticoids in treating this disease.

Older cats appear to be affected by a chronic ulcerative colitis similar to that of dogs.[348] Cats infected with FeLV or FIV can develop chronic ulcerative colitis, presumably as an immunosuppressive phenomenon. LPC, a chronic IBD, has been described in cats with chronic large-bowel diarrhea.[220]

Acute or chronic colitis should be suspected in any animal with large-bowel diarrhea. A stained fecal smear and rectal scraping and a parasite examination are helpful in eliminating parasitism, neoplasia, and algal and fungal disorders as causes of the diarrhea and in many cases, they help to confirm a diagnosis. A presumptive diagnosis of colitis should be confirmed by colonoscopy and biopsy (Fig. 89-9).

Increased fiber may benefit animals with colonic inflammatory diseases as a result of enhanced motility, increased fluid and electrolyte absorption, or dilution of luminal toxins. Either fermentable (soluble) or nonfermentable (insoluble) fiber can be considered. Soluble fiber, such as that found in oat bran, is fermented into short-chain fatty acids (acetate, butyrate, propionate) that facilitate the colonic mucosae and reduce pathogenic microbial growth.[80] Diets containing insoluble fiber from wheat bran or other cellulose are often beneficial because they solidify the stool and absorb free water. FOS-containing diets have been used in cats to increase fecal numbers of lactobacilli and *Bacteroides* and decrease numbers of *E. coli* and clostridia.[297] Their overall benefit for clinical use in colonic inflammatory diseases has not been evaluated.

The antibiotics that have been useful in treating canine and feline ulcerative colitis are primarily those that are effective against anaerobic bacteria (see Table 89-19). Metronidazole, tylosin, and sulfasalazine have been most commonly used (see Drug Formulary, Appendix 8). Without antimicrobial and adjunctive therapy, lesions usually do not resolve spontaneously. Additional measures include dietary management, which is often attempted first in dogs and cats. Food should be withheld for 24 to 48 hours, and the animal should start on a bland diet, receiving multiple, small feedings. A nonallergenic,

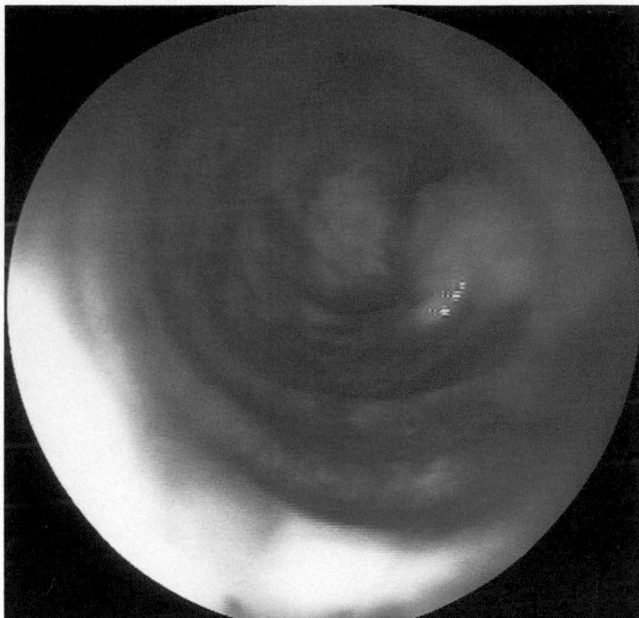

Fig 89-9 Colonic mucosal swelling and hemorrhage in dog with ulcerative colitis. (Courtesy University of Georgia, Athens, Ga.)

low-fat diet, such as boiled rice, meat, and potatoes, is satisfactory.[256] For dogs, prescription diets (I/D or D/D, Hills, Topeka, Kan.) are indicated. Drugs that have been most effective in dogs and cats include oral sulfasalazine, oral chloramphenicol, and oral metronidazole. In addition to its antibacterial effect, sulfasalazine inhibits intestinal hypersecretion by interfering with leukotriene and prostaglandin synthesis. After several weeks of therapy, the dosage should be reduced, and in animals requiring long-term therapy, the minimum effective dose should be determined. Cats with LPC have responded to sulfasalazine with or without concurrent metronidazole and glucocorticoid therapy or to dietary management of lamb and rice or a prescription diet (c/d DIET, Hills, Topeka, Kan.).[220] Omega-3 fatty acids have been added to commercial diets for IBD because of their antiinflammatory effects. Glucocorticoids should be provided at antiinflammatory doses with caution and only if relapses have occurred after clinical improvement has been noted with antimicrobial therapy. When stress is suspected to be a problem or diarrhea is incessant, clidinium and chlordiazepoxide, diphenoxylate, loperamide, or diazepam may be added to the regimen. Because colonic motility is already depressed in dogs with colitis, there is no need for routine anticholinergic or opiate drugs unless given for relief of acute straining. Antispasmodic drugs, such as diphenoxylate and loperamide, must be used with caution in invasive bacterial infections of the bowel because of the increased risk of sepsis or toxemia. In acute experimental colitis in dogs, drugs such as desferrioxamine, verapamil, and disulfiram, which are oxygen free-radical scavengers, were effective in preventing mucosal ulceration.[168]

INTRAABDOMINAL INFECTIONS

Pancreatitis

Pancreatic infection with bacteria develops in less than 10% of humans with acute pancreatitis but in up to 40% of those with severe pancreatitis. Bacterial contamination may arise from hematogenous spread from the systemic circulation, duodenal reflux up the pancreatic duct, contamination from the biliary tree, or bacterial translocation from the lower

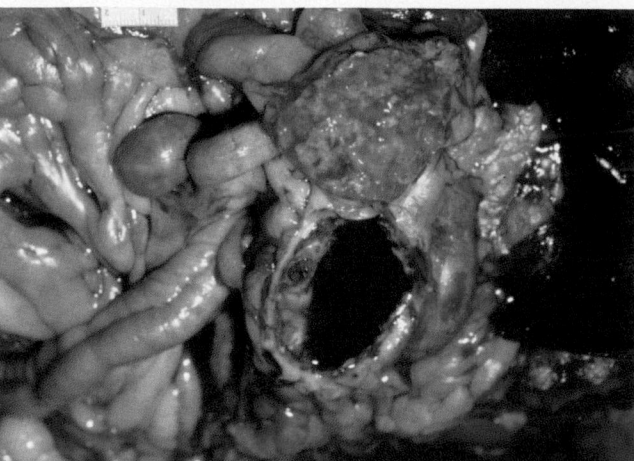

Fig 89-10 Pancreatic abscess from dog. (Courtesy University of Georgia, Athens, Ga.)

bowel via the portal circulation. With necrotizing pancreatitis, structural and functional hemodynamic alterations in the bowel cause bacterial translocation from the intestine to the diseased pancreatic tissue. The goal of antibiotic prophylaxis is to reduce mortality by decreasing or delaying pancreatic colonization and systemic circulation of translocated bacteria.[291] Common enteric organisms are usually involved, causing secondary infection of acutely inflamed or necrotic pancreatic tissue (Fig. 89-10). People with severe acute necrotic pancreatitis who receive prophylactic antibiotics IV have a lower mortality rate than those who do not.[123] Routine broad-spectrum prophylactic antibiotic use has altered the colonizing organisms from predominantly gram-negative coliforms to gram-positive organisms without altering the rate of β-lactam resistance or fungal infection.[133] Even though pancreatic infections cannot be eliminated, treatment with a broad-spectrum antibacterial agent with adequate pancreatic tissue penetration reduces the morbidity and mortality of people with necrotizing pancreatitis.[285] Although similar associations between bacterial infection have not been determined for a majority of pancreatic infections in dogs and cats, veterinarians commonly use antibacterial drugs when treating this disease. In this event, similar recommendations might be considered for treating dogs and cats, especially those with severe pancreatic necrosis. Unfortunately, no pathognomonic features have been observed that distinguish acute necrotizing from chronic nonsuppurative pancreatitis in cats.[76] In cats, experimental inoculation of pancreatic ducts with *E. coli* resulted in infection with concurrent pancreatitis, whereas bacteria were cleared in cats with healthy pancreatic tissue.[345] Antimicrobial therapy with cefotaxime (50 to 100 mg/kg, given intramuscularly (IM) every 8 hours) was started 12 hours after inoculation. Infection developed in 73% of animals receiving no antibiotics and in none of the cats receiving antibiotics. In one report of natural infection, *Enterococcus hirae* enteropathy was associated with ascending cholangitis and pancreatitis in a kitten.[175]

In dogs with intestinal colonization by genetically labeled *E. coli*, organisms had spread to the pancreas and mesenteric lymph nodes after experimentally induced pancreatitis.[164] Secondary ischemic damage to jejunal and ileal mucosa was noted in affected dogs and was probably responsible for portal venous bacteremia. In dogs with acute experimental pancreatitis, significant differences in bioactive levels were found between antibiotics in pancreatic tissue.[324] Ampicillin, gentamicin, and cefazolin reached therapeutic levels in blood but not in normal or inflamed pancreatic tissue. Of other drugs tested, clindamycin, metronidazole, and chloramphenicol achieved penetrance in normal and inflamed pancreas. Cefotaxime has been shown to reach effective therapeutic levels in feline pancreatic tissue.[345] From these results, lipid-soluble drugs appear to have the best penetration in pancreatic tissue. Other drugs or combinations used in people are imipenem-cilastatin, quinolone combined with metronidazole, and an extended-spectrum penicillin (see Table 89-20 and the Drug Formulary, Appendix 8).

Peritonitis and Intraabdominal Abscesses

Etiology and Clinical Findings

Peritonitis and intraabdominal abscess formation are frequent complications of intestinal perforation caused by postsurgical wound dehiscence of the GI tract, foreign bodies (Fig. 89-11), severe ulcerative enteritis, penetrating abdominal wounds, and rupture of abscesses of intraabdominal organs.[129,130,321] Anaerobes are the predominant organisms in the generation of adhesions or abscesses or pyoabdomen. Infection of ascitic fluid may occur from hematogenous, lymphogenous, and transmural migration from the GI or genitourinary tract. Animals with peritonitis may become depressed, weak, and hypotensive after a GI illness or abdominal wounds. Fever and abdominal distention and pain are variable findings. Anaerobic bacteremia is a frequent complication.

Table • 89-20

Parenteral Antibacterial Penetration into Pancreatic Secretions and Tissues[a,123,164,250,324,345]

Pancreatic Secretions
Mezlocillin
Cefotaxime
Chloramphencol
Quinolones
Clindamycin
Metronidazole
Doxycycline

Normal Pancreatic Tissue or with Chronic Pancreatitis
Mezlocillin
Piperacillin
Cefotaxime
Ceftazidime
Imipenem-cilastatin
Quinolones
Metronidazole

Pancreatic Tissue with Acute Pancreatitis (Tissue)
Mezlocillin
Cefotaxime
Ceftazidime
Ceftizoxime
Imipenem-cilastatin
Quinolones
Metronidazole

Ineffective
Ampicillin
Azlocillin
First-generation cephalosporin
Second-generation cephalosporin
Aminoglycosides

Diagnosis

Peritonitis should be suspected when a severe, inappropriate left shift in the leukogram is found. Hypoproteinemia and hypoalbuminemia (2.5 g/dl) correlate with an increased risk of leakage after intestinal anastomosis and resultant peritonitis.[247] Radiography may be misleading in early or localized disease. Confirmation of intraabdominal sepsis is best achieved through abdominal paracentesis. Radiographs should always precede paracentesis because pneumoperitoneum that may result can be confused with that caused by bowel perforation. Ultrasound may also be helpful before diagnostic paracentesis because it can detect small pockets of abdominal fluid for collection. In addition, it is very helpful in detecting ingested and perforating wooden foreign bodies that appear hyperechoic with shadowing.[237] Focal bowel ischemia and associated localized peritonitis have been also detected with ultrasound.[332]

Abdominal Paracentesis and Diagnostic Peritoneal Lavage

For abdominal paracentesis and diagnostic peritoneal lavage (DPL), the animal is placed in lateral recumbency. The skin of the midline ventral abdomen is clipped free of hair and prepared as for surgery from the umbilicus to the inguinal region. An 18-gauge, 1-inch needle fitted to a 20-ml syringe can be used to make the tap. The needle is inserted at the level of the umbilicus. The needle is first inserted without a syringe attached to determine whether fluid flows freely. The needle can be rotated on its long axis to free any tissue that may have occluded the tip. If no fluid is obtained, a 3- to 6-ml syringe is attached, and gentle suction is applied. Plastic IV catheters or metal teat cannulas are less likely than metal needles to penetrate intraabdominal structures accidentally, and they allow sampling at greater depths. Over-the-needle catheters, into which several side ports have been incised, may increase the likelihood of fluid collection.[333] The use of needles and IV catheters is frequently unrewarding because of occlusion, too small a volume of abdominal fluid being recovered, and localization of the inflammatory process. Multiple collection attempts in each of the four abdominal quadrants are recommended. DPL should be attempted if no material can be aspirated.[25,26] For this procedure, peritoneal dialysis catheters or cutting fenestrated openings in flexible Teflon vascular catheters facilitates administration and withdrawal of fluid. Animals often require additional sedation for this procedure. DPL is performed by inserting the large catheter through the

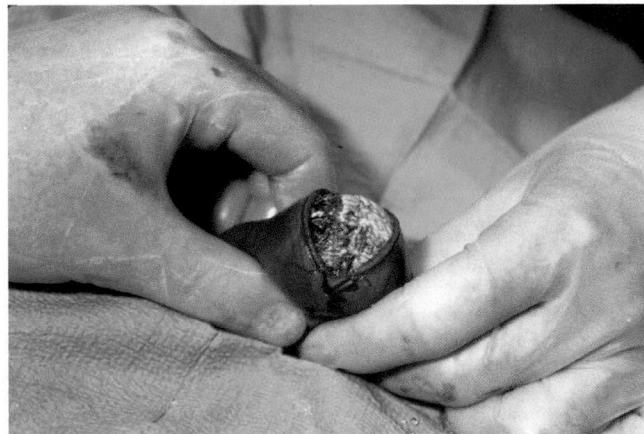

Fig 89-11 Intestinal foreign body removal from dog via enterotomy can result in contamination of surgical site and intraabdominal infection. (Courtesy University of Georgia, Athens, Ga.)

caudal ventral abdominal wall in the direction of the pelvic canal. A negative aspiration is followed by rapid (2- to 5-minute) infusion of warmed isotonic saline through an IV drip set at a volume of 20 ml/kg. After the animal has been gently rotated, the fluid can be removed by placing the still-connected fluid bottle on the floor to allow gravity drainage. Caution should be exercised in interpreting specimens obtained by DPL because they are diluted by the infused fluid. A portion of the fluid that runs back into the bottle should be analyzed for protein concentration and examined cytologically. If an inflammatory exudate is detected, an aliquot should be submitted for culture. The presence of degenerative neutrophils with nucleated cell counts greater than 9000 cells/µl, intracellular bacteria, or organic debris indicates bacterial peritonitis. In bile peritonitis, mucinous material may be found in the abdominal fluid.[230] A portion of the fluid should be kept in a sealed syringe to preserve anaerobes during transport to the laboratory. Immediate inoculation of an aliquot of fluid into a blood culture bottle improves the isolation rate of aerobic bacteria, even compared with centrifugation-lysis methods.[287] Rare complications of paracentesis include introduction of contaminants, spread of infection from an abscess, laceration of a hollow viscus, or intraperitoneal bleeding.

Although cytologic examination is most helpful in determining whether septic peritonitis is present, toxic neutrophils or intracellular bacteria are not always consistently found. Simultaneous measurement of pH, bicarbonate, lactate and glucose concentrations in peritoneal fluid and blood has been evaluated as means of distinguishing septic peritonitis.[29] A glucose concentration difference of 20 mg/dl between blood (higher) and peritoneal fluid (lower) was a reliable means of differentiating septic from nonseptic effusions. In some of the dogs a blood-to-fluid lactate difference was evaluated, and a difference of 2.0 mmol/L was helpful. In additional studies, dogs with septic abdominal effusions had absolute peritoneal fluid concentrations greater than 2.5 mmol/L and a peritoneal fluid lactate concentration higher than that of blood.[180] However, this same method was not accurate in detecting septic peritoneal effusions of cats. DPL was also helpful in identification of blastomycosis in a dog with peritoneal involvement.[221]

Therapy

Antibiotic therapy is important in the management of intraabdominal infections (Table 89-21).[11] Mixed infections caused by indigenous flora are associated with GI leakage. With gastric leakage, lower concentrations of bacteria result in lower prevalence of infection, unless microbial overgrowth develops from decreased gastric acid output and gastric motility or from gastric ulcers or malignancies.[222] With biliary leakage, contamination rates are intermediate. With lower small intestinal and colonic leakage, infection is certain. Organisms in all cases are a mixture of facultative anaerobic bacteria, usually Enterobacteriaceae, and obligate anaerobes.

A combination of surgical drainage and antimicrobial therapy is required for treating most cases of intraabdominal infections. The use of either primary closure or open peritoneal drainage for treatment of septic peritonitis appears to be equivocal with survival rates that have ranged between approximately 50% and 70%.[299,174] Dogs with open drainage were more likely to require plasma transfusions and placement of a jejunostomy tube because of protein loss than those treated with primary closure. Closed-suction drainage has been beneficial in treating animals for which primary closure is used.[216] Therapy to treat facultative enteric gram-negative bacteria (e.g., E. coli) and anaerobes (e.g., Bacteroides fragilis) is essential when leakage occurs from the small intestine, cecum, or colon. Aerobes (e.g., E. coli) are important in producing bacteremia and early mortality in intraabdominal infections, whereas the obligate anaerobes, which outnumber them, are instrumental in leading to adhesions, abscess for-

mation, and pyoabdomen. Drugs such as aminoglycosides have been recommended because of their effect on gram-negative bacteria.[124,155] In animals with experimentally induced intraabdominal sepsis, the administration of aminoglycosides alone greatly reduces the mortality associated with gram-negative sepsis, although the prevalence of postoperative adhesions and abscess formation are unaffected. Under similar experimental circumstances, the use of drugs effective against anaerobic bacteria such as clindamycin resulted in death from gram-negative septicemia, even though the prevalence of intraabdominal abscesses was reduced. This finding indicates that antimicrobial drugs or combinations used in treating intraabdominal sepsis must be effective against aerobic and anaerobic intestinal flora to decrease mortality and abscess formation after peritonitis. Animals with severe bacterial peritonitis may be sensitive to the nephrotoxicity associated with aminoglycosides. Regimens in which a third-generation cephalosporin such as cefotaxime is substituted for the aminoglycoside or metronidazole is substituted for clindamycin give similarly favorable results. Combinations in which a parenteral quinolone is substituted for an aminoglycoside are also possible for dogs. Parenteral amoxicillin-clavulanate offers an effective combination in available areas outside the United States. In humans for whom cost is not a factor, single-agent regimens include a ß-lactam and ß-lactamase inhibitor combination (e.g., ampicillin-sulbactam, ticarcillin-clavulanate, or piperacillin-tazobactam), or a carbapenem (ertapenem, meropenem, or imipenem-cilastatin).[292] The combination regimens recommended for use in humans include a second- or third-generation cephalosporin (cefazolin or cefuroxime) plus metronidazole, a quinolone plus metronidazole, or aztreonam plus metronidazole.[292] Based on expense and the risk of inducing resistant bacterial strains that might transfer from animals to people, these combinations should be restricted in animal use. A summary of antimicrobial drug combinations recommended for abdominal sepsis in dogs and cats is presented in Table 89-21.

Antimicrobial Prophylaxis

To reduce postoperative complications, antimicrobial agents can be administered to animals without established infections when they undergo abdominal surgery in which spillage of ingesta is anticipated. Preoperative and intraoperative administration of cephalosporins or penicillin derivatives combined with aminoglycosides has been effective in reducing the complications of intestinal leakage and peritoneal contamination in people. However, total sterilization of the bowel before surgery is impossible in a conventional environment. Bowel sterilization has been achieved only experimentally in dogs that have been kept in a germ-free environment, fed sterilized food, and given combination therapy with large dosages of nonabsorbable antibiotics.[331] Even with these elaborate procedures, decontamination was incomplete, and the microflora was reestablished within 1 week after termination of therapy. Administration of prophylactic antimicrobial therapy for GI surgery should begin 12 to 24 hours before the operation and terminate on the day of surgery if the bowel contents are not spilled. One week of therapy is indicated if contamination occurs during the surgical procedure.

Granulocytic colony-stimulating factor (G-CSF) has been administered before experimental peritonitis in mice.[330] Compared with antibiotics alone, antibiotics in combination with G-CSF improved survival, decreased splenic bacterial colony-forming units, and increased IL-10.

Management of Surgical Contamination

Postoperative peritonitis can have a higher risk of complications than naturally acquired forms of peritoneal inflammation.[261] An advantage is that spillage can be anticipated, and a knowledge of the normal enteric flora can assist in appropri-

Table • 89-21

Antimicrobial Therapy for Intraabdominal Infections

DRUG[a]	SPECIES	DOSE[b] (mg/kg)	ROUTE[c]	INTERVAL (HOURS)	DURATION (DAYS)
Pancreatitis					
Cefotaxime	C	50—100	IV, IM, SC	8	3—5
	D	20—80	IV, IM, SC	8	3—5
Clindamycin	B	5—11	IV, SC, PO	8—12	3—5
Metronidazole	B	7—15	IV, PO	8—12	3—5
Chloramphenicol	D	25—50	IV, IM, SC, PO	8	3—5
	C	50	IV, IM, SC, PO	12	3—5
Intraabdominal Sepsis					
Combination of					
Clindamycin	B	5—11	IV, SC, PO	8—12	5—7
or					
Metronidazole	B	10—15	IV, SC, PO	8—12	5—7
or					
Amoxicillin	B	20—25	IV, IM, SC, PO	8	5—7
combined with					
Gentamicin	B	4.4	IV, SC	12	5—7
	D	8—12	IV, SC	24	5—7
or					
Cefotaxime[d]	C	50—100	IV, SC	8	5—7
	D	20—80	IV, SC	8	5—7
or					
Enrofloxacin[e]	D	5—10	SC, PO, IV[f]	12	5—7
	B	5	SC, PO	24	5—7
Single agent					
Ticarcillin-clavulanate	B[g]	30—50	IV	6—8	5—7
Piperacillin-tazobactam	B[g]	50	IV, IM	4—6	5—7
Ampicillin-sulbactam	B[g]	20	IV, IM	6—8	5—7
Imipenem-cilastatin	B[g]	3—5	IV	8	5—7

C, Cat; D, dog; B, both, IV, intravenous; IM, intramuscular; SC, subcutaneous; PO, by mouth.
[a]See Drug Formulary, Appendix 8 for additional information on these drugs.
[b]Dose per administration at specified interval.
[c]Oral route recommended for pancreatitis and only in intraabdominal sepsis when animals are not vomiting.
[d]Or other third-generation cephalosphorin.
[e]Or other fluoroquinolone.
[f]Must be diluted 10-fold before IV administration, and then given very slowly over 10 minutes.
[g]Extrapolation of human dose with limited studies in dogs and cats.

ated choice of prophylaxis to use. Spillage of intestinal contents during experimental surgery in dogs has been best controlled by rinsing the peritoneal cavity with an irrigation solution of neomycin (500 mg), polymyxin (500,000 U), and bacitracin (50,000 U) mixed in 1 L of saline.[246,331] Similar broad-spectrum antimicrobial activity can be achieved by rinsing the peritoneal cavity with organic iodine solutions diluted 1:10 to 1:20 with physiologic saline. Intraabdominal instillation of povidone-iodine solutions can cause peritonitis and hepatotoxicity in dogs.[218] Dosages of 3.5 ml/kg of a 10% solution caused neutrophilic leukocytosis, increased hepatic enzyme activity, icterus, and death. Lower dosages (2 ml/kg) had fewer side effects. Although beneficial when given with antimicrobial therapy or drainage, saline alone to rinse the abdominal cavity has been less successful in preventing infection, despite its diluting effect on the spilled material (see Halogens, Chapter 94).

Management of Established Peritonitis

Antimicrobial therapy is essential for animals with acute septic peritonitis. Broad-spectrum antimicrobial therapy is less important than lavage in the management of established peritonitis. This procedure involves the placement of intraabdominal tubes and daily infusion and removal of isotonic saline solutions. Antimicrobial agents can be placed in the infusion fluid to reach higher concentrations than when they are given orally or parenterally. Only small amounts of many systemically administered antibiotics reach the peritoneal cavity, whereas most of the drug introduced into the abdominal cavity enters the systemic circulation.

Open peritoneal drainage has usually been successful for treatment of established generalized peritonitis in dogs and cats.[48,94] The technique involves exploratory laparotomy, surgical correction of the cause, lavage of the abdominal cavity, and incomplete closure of the ventral midline incision with supportive wraps. The abdominal cavity is treated like one large abscess that can drain through the open incision. When the bandage is changed, additional lavage is performed. Complications are loss of fluids, proteins, and electrolytes. Absorbent abdominal pads are applied under a supportive wrap to draw fluid away from the incision. This method is reserved for advanced cases of septic peritonitis in which all the tissues cannot be debrided and sepsis is expected from residual intraabdominal inflammation. Closure of the peritoneal cavity was usually done 3 to 4 days after surgery. Antimicrobial therapy was continued until the time of final closure.

Aminoglycosides, such as gentamicin given IM, and cephalosporins given orally or IM result in minimal peritoneal concentrations. Higher concentrations, should they be desired, might be added in restricted therapeutic doses to the peritoneal lavage fluid. When given orally, metronidazole, a relatively effective drug for anaerobic infections, reaches a higher concentration than most other antimicrobial agents in peritoneal effusions.[81]

SUGGESTED READINGS*

4. Allenspach K, Luckschander N. 2004. Evaluation of assays for perinuclear antineutrotrophilic cytoplasmic antibodies to *Saccharomyces cerevisiae* in dogs with inflammatory bowel disease. *Am J Vet Res* 65:1279-1283.

8. Baez JL, Hendrick MJ, Walker LM, et al. 1999. Radiographic, ultrasonographic, and endoscopic findings in cats with inflammatory bowel disease of the stomach and small intestine: 33 cases. 1990-1997. *J Am Vet Med Assoc* 349-354.

39. Cave NJ, Marks SL. 2004. Mechanisms and clinical applications of nutrition in inflammatory bowel disease. Proceedings of the 2003 Nestle Purina Nutrition Symposium. *Suppl Compend Cont Educ Pract Vet* 26:51-57.

51. Davies DR, O'Hara AJ, Irwin PJ, et al. 2004. Successful management of histiocytic ulcerative colitis with enrofloxacin in two boxer dogs. *Aust Vet J* 82:58-61.

53. De Cock HE, Marks SL, Stacy BA, et al. 2004. Ileocolitis associated with *Anaerobiospirillum* in cats. *J Clin Microbiol* 2752-2758.

61. Duggan C, Fonatine O, Pierce NF, et al. 2004. Scientific rationale for a change in the composition of oral rehydration solution. *JAMA* 291:2628-2635.

131. Hostutler RA, Luria BJ, Johnson SE, et al. 2004. Antibiotic-responsive histiocytic ulcerative colitis in 9 dogs. *J Vet Intern Med* 18:499-504.

147. Jergens AE. 2002. Feline inflammatory bowel disease—current perspectives on etiopathogenesis and therapy. *J Feline Med Surg* 4(3):175-178.

148. Jergens AE. 2004. Clinical assessment of disease activity for canine inflammatory bowel disease. *J Am Anim Hosp Assoc* 40:437-445.

165. Kelly HM, Deasy PB, Ziaka E, et al. 2004. Formulation and preliminary in vivo dog studies of a novel drug delivery system for the treatment of periodontitis. *Int J Pharm* 274(1-2):167-183.

180. Levin GM, Bonczynski JJ, Ludwig LL, et al. 2004. Lactate as a diagnostic test for septic peritoneal effusions in dogs and cats. *J Am Anim Hosp Assoc* 40:364-371.

183. Lin HC. 2004. Small intestinal bacterial overgrowth. A framework for understanding irritable bowel syndrome. *J Am Med Assoc* 292:852-858.

*See the CD-ROM for a complete list of references.

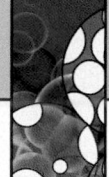

CHAPTER • 90

Hepatobiliary Infections

Sharon A. Center

ANTIBACTERIAL DEFENSE

Bacteriologic studies of portal vein blood of the mature dog have shown that alimentary flora commonly circulates to the liver.[22,24] Although unproven, the suspicion is that this activity also occurs in the cat. Enteric organisms delivered to the liver in the healthy animal are extracted by the hepatic Kupffer cells and either killed or excreted in bile. Liver disorders associated with ischemic injury, impaired hepatic artery perfusion, reduced macrophage function, and cholestasis can be complicated by infections derived from this normal enteric flora.[16]

SUSCEPTIBILITY TO INFECTION

Given the dual blood supply and strategic location of the liver, its exposure to substances derived from the splanchnic and systemic circulations is considerable (e.g., gut-derived particulate debris, toxins, microorganisms, immunoreactive substances). The hepatic Kupffer cells (hepatobiliary macrophages) play an essential role in the innate immune response to bacteria and their by-products entering from the portal system. These cells also protect against systemic bacteremia by cleansing blood delivered through the hepatic artery. Hepatoprotection against systemic toxicity and infections can become compromised when the liver is injured in a variety of ways. The integrity of the hepatic reticuloendothelial system (RES), which influences systemic susceptibility to enteric bacterial translocation (i.e., is associated with hemorrhagic and endotoxic shock, trauma, and bowel ischemia), is compromised in chronic liver disease, portal hypertension, portosystemic shunting, and cholestasis.[120] Consequently, patients with liver disease have increased risk for hepatic infection with or without polysystemic complications. In addition, the expansive sinusoidal endothelium of the liver provides a site for invasion by vasculotropic organisms.

Substantial host-dependent differences exist in hepatic clearance of blood-borne particulates. In dogs, 60% to 90% of hematogenously borne bacteria and particulates are removed by the liver and spleen, giving them an inherent propensity for hepatobiliary infections.[40,180] Comparatively, the cat appears to target pulmonary macrophages preferentially. Failure of hepatic Kupffer cells to function properly can shift the burden of RES function to other organs, such as the spleen, lungs, and lymph nodes, as has been shown in dogs with chronic liver disease associated with acquired portosystemic shunting and in dogs with congenital portosystemic vascular anomalies (PSVA).[78,95] Humans with cirrhosis have an increased incidence of bacterial infections; similar data is unavailable for the dog and cat. Current belief asserts that the predominant perfusion of hepatic sinusoids with portal venous blood, a low-flow low-pressure system, rather than arterial blood, facilitates efficient bacterial removal by the RES because slower flow permits greater opportunity for phagocytosis.[85,140] Given that hepatic arterial perfusion compensatively increases when portal flow is compromised (for example, chronic liver disease with portal hypertension and portosystemic shunting or PSVA or hepatofugal circulation), change in sinusoidal blood flow may thwart efficient phagocytosis.

ENDOTOXIN

Endotoxin, or lipopolysaccharide (LPS), is derived from enteric microorganisms and is a normal constituent in portal venous blood. These glycolipids represent a portion of the outer bacterial cell membrane of gram-negative bacteria and are largely derived from organisms colonizing the colon.[162] Normally, hepatic Kupffer cells efficiently clear endotoxin such that the liver attenuates systemic exposure. Endotoxin extraction is enabled by high-affinity LPS receptors on Kupffer cells and LPS-binding glycoproteins on hepatocytes that facilitate transfer to Kupffer cell receptors. On exposure to endotoxin, Kupffer cell activation initiates a series of signals eventuating in production of proinflammatory cytokines. Consequently, increased hepatic exposure to endotoxin can exacerbate ongoing liver injury and produce changes in liver enzymes reflecting inflammation.

Certain changes in liver function or perfusion can increase hepatic and systemic exposure to endotoxin. In fact, endotoxemia in the absence of overt sepsis is a common finding in cirrhotic humans. Although higher levels of endotoxemia are associated with hepatic failure, hepatic encephalopathy, and death, it is unclear whether detectable systemic endotoxin levels reflect normal exposure left unchecked by the dysfunctional liver, relevant systemic abnormalities, increased enteric uptake (i.e., enhanced enteric endotoxin translocation), or if they play a causal role in liver disease or merely represent an epiphenomenon. Because enteric bile acids bind and inactivate endotoxin, patients with extrahepatic bile duct occlusion (EHBDO) or severe cholestasis having impaired enterohepatic bile acid circulation may experience increased enteric endotoxin uptake and hepatic exposure.[155] Dogs with experimentally induced chronic liver disease (chronic administration of dimethylnitrosamine) with acquired portosystemic shunts develop measurable portal, hepatic, and caudal vena caval venous endotoxemia.[79] Dogs with PSVA (n = 10), medically stable at the time of laparotomy for vascular ligation, also had detectible endotoxemia in portal and peripheral venous samples (mean ± SD, 28.0 ± 16.9 versus 19.6 ± 7.0; median [range], 20 [12 to 40] versus 17 [8 to 30]). In the PSVA dogs, shunt ligation attenuated peripheral endotoxemia at postoperative sampling (at 5 to 13 months).[135] Small patient numbers precluded achieving significant differences (p

= 0.06, six dogs studied postoperatively). These observations in clinically relevant conditions suggest that systemic endotoxemia is a real phenomenon in dogs and, by inference, suggest increased systemic exposure to enteric microbes and their by-products in the circumstance of hepatofugal circulation. However, systemic response to endotoxemia, the presence of bacteremia, or evidence of altered oxygen utilization in portal blood have not been shown in dogs with PSVA.[169]

ROLE OF KUPFFER CELLS

Hepatic Kupffer cells comprise the largest compartment of tissue macrophages in the body, representing 80% to 90% of the total fixed macrophages and approximately 35% of the nonparenchymal liver cells.[70] Residing mainly within the lumen of the hepatic sinusoids and adherent to endothelial cells by long cytoplasmic processes, Kupffer cells are most numerous in the periportal area where they offer first-line defense against bacteria, endotoxin, and microbial debris entering from the alimentary canal.[57] Kupffer cells possess both F_C and C_3 receptors and phagocytize a wide variety of opsonized and nonopsonized particulates.[100] Similar to other mononuclear phagocytes, Kupffer cells also have the capacity to function as antigen-presenting cells, for induction of T lymphocytes, and on activation, can release superoxide radicals, hydrogen peroxide, nitric oxide, hydrolytic enzymes, and eicosanoids (prostaglandins and leukotrienes), which can aid in antigen destruction. They also release a large number of different immunoregulatory and inflammatory cytokines, including interleukin (IL)-1, IL-6, tumor necrosis factor (TNF)-α, platelet-activating factor, transforming growth factor-β (TGF-β), and interferon (IFN)-γ. A heterogenous population of Kupffer cells resides in different lobular zones. Cells associated with the portal triad (zone 1) are larger, more phagocytic, and generate greater amounts of TNF-α, IL-1, prostaglandin E, and lysosomal enzymes. Smaller cells are associated with zone 3 where more nitric oxide and superoxide are produced; these exhibit greater cytotoxic activity to certain stimuli and are more easily activated.[52] Nitric oxide released by Kupffer cells mediates a wide variety of physiologic events, including (but not restricted to) vasodilation, neutrophil chemotaxis, and adhesion of neutrophils to vascular endothelium in response to bacteria or endotoxin.[70] As potent inducers of inflammatory cytokines, Kupffer cells are implicated in the pathologic events leading to liver injury.[162] Inflammatory mediator release from Kupffer cells is enhanced after *priming* by endotoxin exposure in *reactive* hepatobiliary processes. Later, during the course of infection, other cells including hepatocytes, T lymphocytes, and immigrating phagocytes (monocytes and neutrophils) contribute cytokines to the inflammatory process. Certain bacteria undergo initial physical attachment to Kupffer cell surface receptors (macrophage scavenger receptors) and are subsequently cleared from the sinusoidal circulation. These receptors have a high affinity for a broad range of polyanionic ligands, including lipoteichoic acid, a component of gram-positive bacteria.[52,131] However, some organisms are not efficiently cleared by Kupffer cells (e.g., *Pseudomonas aeruginosa*, *Morganella morganii*, and *Serratia marcescens*) caused by cell surface composition or increased hydrophobicity, or both.[69]

ROLE OF NEUTROPHILS

Routine, uneventful removal of bacteria, endotoxin, and particulate and antigenic debris acquired from the portal venous circulation occurs in part in collaboration with infiltrating neutrophils. Immigrating neutrophils contribute an early bactericidal influence important for bacterial pathogen clearance.[69] While providing this ancillary defensive role, neutrophil participation also may impart self-injury. Neutrophil accumulation in hepatic sinusoids, a distinguishing feature of endotoxemia and sepsis, fosters the production, release, and accumulation of toxic metabolic products and degradative enzymes (reactive oxygen intermediates and proteolytic enzymes) from themselves, as well as from neighboring Kupffer cells. This involvement of neutrophils in response to endotoxin exposure confuses histologic interpretation of hepatobiliary lesions, erroneously suggesting in some cases the actual presence of an infectious organism. This response may contribute to the lesion characterized as *reactive hepatitis*, commonly described in liver biopsies from veterinary patients with inflammatory bowel disease (IBD). Neutrophil associated tissue injury is normally limited by neutrophil apoptosis and phagocytosis by hepatic Kupffer cells on infection control or toxin elimination. Dysregulation of these mechanisms can propagate chronic liver injury and inflammation.

BILE: PROTECTION FROM INFECTION

Hepatobiliary production of bile and IgA contribute importantly to the health of the biliary and gastrointestinal (GI) systems. Secretory IgA (S-IgA) is the major immunoglobulin in bile; IgG and IgM are present in much smaller amounts. IgA binds to a secretory component, made in the liver, forming an S-IgA complex, which assists in maintaining mucosal integrity by binding infectious agents (e.g., bacteria, viruses). Bile and IgA both influence enteric bacterial populations (type, number of organisms, and enterocyte adherence). Normal physiologic choleresis (bile flow) routinely cleanses biliary pathways. The normal biliary-entero-bacterial cycle permits rapid elimination of bacteria achieving entrance to the biliary tree, and local IgA production protects against epithelial invasion.[20,154] Bile salts contribute an antibacterial influence synergistic with IgA binding, limiting enteric and biliary bacterial translocation. Normally, tight junctions between hepatocytes resist bacterial entry into canalicular bile. Along with the high competence of the extrahepatic biliary structures, normal pressure differentials in the biliary system limit retrograde access of enteric organisms to the hepatobiliary system. However, development of EHBDO or substantial cholestasis of any cause can interrupt these mechanisms, increasing host susceptibility to infection.[154]

BACTERIAL FLORA OF THE HEPATOBILIARY SYSTEM

The sterility of the portal venous circulation, hepatic tissue, and bile in health has been investigated for more than 50 years. Although older studies suggest that liver tissue is commonly contaminated, especially with *Clostridium* spp., more recent work is contradictive.[38,49] In the absence of biliary tree obstruction or choleliths, gallbladder and bile are now thought to be normally sterile.[155] Improved methods of collecting samples (reducing cross-contamination) has been suggested to explain disparate observations.

Normally, enteric organisms delivered to the liver are extracted and killed by neutrophils and hepatic Kupffer cells. Remaining organisms are thought to be excreted in bile. Clearly, even in normal animals, portal venous translocation of large bacterial inocula result in hepatic sinusoidal bacterial exposure and bacterobilia.[162] In the diseased liver (e.g., perfusion abnormalities, impaired macrophage function, cholestasis), survival of infectious agents may be permissively affected by loss of normal protective mechanisms already discussed.[20] Consequently, diseases of the biliary tract and liver may be complicated by the presence of pathogenic bacteria (in bile [bacteriobilia] or liver tissue) as a secondary phenomenon. Positive bacterial culture results from liver tissue and bile from animals with chronic liver disease in the author's hospital supports this contention.

CIRCUMSTANCES INCREASING THE RISK OF HEPATOBILIARY INFECTION

The liver plays a key role in providing protective responses during gram-negative sepsis. Consequently, a variety of liver diseases place the host at increased risk for infection. Enhanced pathogenicity of gram-negative sepsis has been demonstrated in experimental cirrhosis in animal models.[77] An important point to acknowledge is that bacterial organisms commonly found in bile, gallbladder, or liver tissue, in disease, are nearly always enteric in origin. Greatest risks for infection and postoperative sepsis exist for EHBDO and chronic liver disease associated with portal hypertension, compromised hepatic perfusion or Kupffer cell function, or both, and conditions promoting enteric bacterial translocation.

Along with reduced mechanical cleansing of the biliary tree, impaired biliary IgA production or delivery, enhanced translocation of gut flora into the splanchnic circulation, impaired Kupffer cell activation and phagocytosis, reduced humoral immunity, compromised neutrophil rolling, migration, or adherence in hypertensive splanchnic vasculature (but not in hepatic sinusoids), disruption of tight junctions between hepatocytes, and increased access to hepatic lymph, each facilitate infection.* Cholestasis also imposes an immunosuppressive effect by reducing in vitro lymphocyte transformation testing. This activity relates to high plasma, tissue, and bile concentrations of dihydroxy bile acids.[155]

INFLUENCE OF CHOLESTASIS ON HEPATOBILIARY INFECTIONS

Any disorder invoking cholestasis can compromise protective mechanisms normally derived from bile and normal choleresis. EHBDO provokes numerous changes facilitating hepatobiliary and systemic bacterial infection. Animal models of EHBDO, including dogs and cats, convincingly demonstrate that impaired enteric bile flow favors small intestinal bacterial overgrowth (SIBO) and enteric-bacterial translocation.[34] Cessation of enteric bile delivery (bile salts and s-IgAs) curtails the normally suppressive influence of bile salts on the endogenous bacterial population and s-IgA on bacterial mucosal adherence. Defective RES function, altered sinusoidal fenestra in the area of the peribiliary plexus (permitting greater access to bacterial organisms), reduced enteric mucosal integrity, and impaired endotoxin clearance or inactivation augment the opportunity for enteric bacterial and endotoxin translocation to mesenteric lymph nodes, liver, and the systemic circulation. Given that the liver is metabolically compromised in cholestasis and the RES dysfunctional, a heightened risk of hepatobiliary infection is achieved. In this circumstance, development of cholangitis by any route (ascending, hematogenous, or lymphatic) is favored.[155] Inadequate RES function and liberalized portal bacteremia increases the risk for systemic bacteremia and endotoxemia.[128] Although biliary decompression ameliorates jaundice, chronic damage to the biliary tree causing functional changes reverse slowly, and certain functionality is never fully restored. Immune dysfunction in cholestatic liver injury derives from inadequate or inappropriate antigen processing by the RES, cytokine production by Kupffer cells, or abnormal Kupffer-

*References: 47, 88, 133, 138, 139, 141, 143, 165, 167, 172, 174.

Table • 90-1

Organisms Associated with Suppurative or Pyogranulomatous Hepatobiliary Inflammation and Abscesses in Dogs and Cats[a]

Aerobic Cultures (Positive Cultures: n = 108)	Anaerobic Cultures (Positive Cultures: n = 49)[a]
n = 5 each[a]	**n = ≥6 each[a]**
Escherichia coli	Clostridium perfringens,
Streptococcus group	Clostridium sp.
D enterococci	Propionibacterium acnes
Staphylococcus aureus	Bacteroides
Staphylococcus	melaninogenicus
intermedius	**n = 3 each[a]**
Enterococcus	Actinomyces
Staphylococcus	Peptostreptococcus
epidermidis	**n = 1 each[a]**
Enterobacter aerogenes	Corynebacterium spp.
Streptococcus β-hemolytic	Fusobacterium
n = 3 or 4 each[a]	Anaerobic streptococci
Pseudomonas aeruginosa	Bacillus
Enterobacter agglomerans	**Additional Microbes**
Citrobacter freundii	**Reported Elsewhere**
n = 2 each[a]	**(Case Reports)**
Acinetobacter calcoacetius	Bacillus piliformis
Pasteurella multocida	Francisella tularensis
Pseudomonas fluorescens	Listeria monocytogenes
Nocardia	Eugenic fermenter-4
Klebsiella pneumoniae	bacilli
Bacillus spp.	**Other noncultured**
Serratia marcesens	**infectious agents**
n = 1 each[a]	**proven based on**
α—hemolytic	**antibody titers,**
Streptococcus	**histopathology, or**
Bordetella bronchiseptica	**molecular testing**
Campylobacter jejuni	**(or any combination)**
Candida sp.	**and response to**
Enterococcus	**treatment)**
hermanniensis	Leptospira serovars[a]
Lactobacillus sp.	Borrelia burgdorferi[a]
Moraxella phenylpyruvica	Ehrlichia sp.[a]
Morganella morgani	Rickettsia
Proteus sp.	rickettsii[a]
Pseudomonas fluorescens	Toxoplasma[a]
Salmonella	Babesia sp.
	Trematodes (cats)[a]

[a]In order from most to least common. Data acquired from case records, 1985–2001, Companion Animal Hospital, College of Veterinary Medicine, Cornell University, Ithaca, N.Y.

hepatocyte interactions. Chronic down regulation of Kupffer cell vigilance against endotoxin increases risk for endotoxemia during episodes of heightened exposure (e.g., hemorrhagic gastroenteritis). Hepatofugal portal circulation reduces hepatic delivery and extraction of substances in the portal splanchnic vasculature, causing increased systemic exposure to immune complexes, enteric bacteria, and antigens. Impaired bacterial opsonization reduces appropriate macrophage bacterial clearance and heightens risk of infection. Dysregulation of inflammatory cascades, crucial to wound healing, may increase postoperative complications, including wound dehiscence and infections that compromise surgical recovery.[155]

Experimental models have clarified the significance of enteric portal bacteremia. Infusion of 10^5 to 10^7 bacteria into the splenic vein of normal cats results in a significant reduction in bile flow and the appearance of bacteria in bile within 30 minutes. However, in the presence of EHBDO, modest bacterial inocula (10^3) cause bacterobilia within the same time frame. Bacteria enter sinusoidal blood where some are phagocytized (Kupffer cells and neutrophils), but ultimately, viable organisms enter bile.[167] Although mechanical obstruction of the biliary tree clearly augments bacteriobilia, also apparent is that any cause of cholestasis may impart this influence. Given that hematogenously dispersed gram-negative organisms impart a cholestatic response in both dogs and cats, this activity likely augments their risk for hepatic infection. This phenomenon may explain why bacterial organisms are unexpectedly cultured from liver tissue and bile in animals with illnesses thought not to be primarily bacterial in origin (Table 90-1).

TRANSMURAL PASSAGE OF ENTERIC ORGANISMS

The idea that translocation of bacteria and endotoxin from the GI tract may initiate or exacerbate infection has been increasingly accepted as the so-called gut hypothesis of sepsis and multiple organ failure.[45] Increased vulnerability of the jaundiced host to gut-barrier breakdown and bacterial translocation has been confirmed by many experimental studies and is strongly supported by clinical observations in veterinary patients. Diseases involving the biliary tract especially thwart protective mechanisms, leading to bacteriobilia.[164]

Study of dogs undergoing routine ovariohysterectomy proves that enteric bacterial translocation occurs even in normal dogs.[37] In this study, bacteria was verified in 52% of 26 dogs by positive results of culture of a single mesenteric lymph node; the number of bacteria cultured varied from 50 to 10^5 organism/g of tissue. Organisms isolated, in decreasing prevalence, were Escherichia coli (n = 6), Bacillus (n = 5), non-hemolytic Streptococcus (n = 4), Salmonella (n = 3), coagulase-negative Staphylococcus (n = 2), Enterococcus (n = 2), and one each with Staphylococcus intermedius, Clostridium sordelli, Micrococcus spp., Pseudomonas spp., Lactobacillus spp., and Propionibacterium acnes. However, no bacteria were isolated from a single portal blood specimen.[42]

Translocated enteric bacteria and endotoxin invoke Kupffer cytokine secretion, neutrophil chemotaxis, vascular adhesion, and degranulation, as well as proinflammatory changes in sinusoidal endothelial cells and hepatic stellate cells (the source of connective tissue in chronic liver disease), leading to fibrosis. Tissue injury derives from products of activated Kupffer cells and neutrophils, including reactive oxygen species, cytokines, and proteases, along with reactions involving complement and coagulation system activation. Gut-derived bacteria or endotoxin may provoke development of the sepsis syndrome in the absence of clinically proven microbiologic infection. Although compromised gut-barrier function is believed to be relevant to sepsis in the jaundiced patient, correlation of plasma endotoxin concentrations with morbidity and immunosuppression is inconsistent and quite variable as a result of differences in regional blood sample collection, methods employed to detect endotoxin, units of expression, and inconsistent use of endotoxin standards and expression units.[67,138]

Enteric translocation of bacteria and subsequent hepatobiliary invasion is enhanced in the presence of (1) bowel disease (direct mucosal injury), (2) altered gut flora with gram-negative microbial overgrowth (SIBO), (3) portal hypertension, (4) splanchnic hypoperfusion, (5) hepatofugal portal circulation, proven in dogs with acquired and congenital portal shunting, (6) local or systemic immunosuppression, including impaired macrophage function, (7) altered gut motility (slow transit time documented in cirrhosis), and (8) absence of enteric bile (bile acids, IgA, mechanical cleansing function of bile in the biliary tree). In human and animal models with chronic liver disease, reduced enteric transit rate has been shown to increase the risk of SIBO and enteric bacterial translocation.[134] Contributing factors include portal hypertension, acquired varices, gastroduodenal vascular ectasia associated with portal hypertensive gastroenteropathy, and oxidative damage in the bowel (with or without coexistent IBD).[30,151,182] An increased propensity for enteric translocation of bacteria in EHBDO has been proven in dogs and cats.[29,167] The clinical impact of cholestasis on enteric translocation is exemplified in humans in whom postoperative infectious complications following EHBDO decompression are reduced by preoperative internal biliary drainage.[106,175]

BACTERIOBILIA

Bacteriobilia may be clinically silent until biliary obstruction leads to systemic sepsis by biliary-venous reflux. Increased pressure in the biliary system (at least 25 cm water), causing retrograde flow of bile (regurgitation) into hepatic sinusoids is a proven prerequisite for infection. The importance of mechanical disruption of bile flow is well exemplified by the long-term follow-up of humans with choledochoduodenostomy in which retrograde invasion of the biliary tree by bacteria is the rule. These patients do not develop septic cholangitis as long as mechanical obstruction to bile flow is avoided. Furthermore, clinical and experimental evidence suggests that infection is most likely when obstruction is incomplete or intermittent and is seemingly potentiated by the presence of a foreign body such as a cholelith.[48]

Once enteric organisms gain access to bile, they may dehydroxylate and deconjugate bile acids, generating membranocytolytic forms (e.g., chenodeoxycholate yielding lithocholate) capable of provoking cholestasis, oxidant cell injury, immunotargeting of biliary epithelium or hepatocytes, and cell death by cytolytic necrosis or apoptosis. This activity is thought to greatly facilitate tissue injury in cats with cholangiohepatitis.

Unfortunately, the bacterial flora in bile is not accurately represented by detection of systemic bacteremia or urinary tract organisms. Anaerobic bacteria are infrequently found in blood, as compared with bile, and *E. coli* is found far more commonly in bile. Consequently, no easy and practical screening method exists for detecting bacteriobilia. Despite many experimental studies of bacterial translocation that show compelling evidence supporting this infectious pathomechanism, exactly which clinical patients besides those with EHBDO have greatest risk has not been clearly defined in either human or veterinary patients.

Cytologic evaluation of bile with a Wright-Giemsa's stain discloses a rich blue amorphous material. Identification of multilobular nuclear remnants (released from degenerating neutrophils) may be the only evidence of inflammation. However, with sepsis, bacterial organisms are commonly seen, sometimes in the absence of well-defined inflammatory cells.

RISKS INCREASING POSTOPERATIVE SEPSIS

Given that mechanical resolution of EHBDO allows acute mobilization of *sequestered* bacteria, a sudden appearance of bacteria in bile is realized. Failure to provide adequate antibiotic coverage during this transition increases risk of postoperative infection and sepsis in patients with biliary tree infection and EHBDO undergoing surgical investigation and correction. An important point to remember is that surgical trauma augments the risk imposed by reduced gut-barrier function in patients with cholestasis or severe hepatobiliary dysfunction.[46,132] Presurgical internal drainage of the biliary tree in humans with EHBDO has been shown to reduce postoperative septic complications. Modifying the enteric microbial population with antibiotics (e.g., fluoroquinolones, neomycin, tobramycin) or using certain probiotics (Lactobacilli combined with antioxidants) also has reduced septic complications in humans and animal models with cholestatic liver disease. Treatment of cirrhotic humans with ciprofloxacin reduces spontaneous bacterial infections with enteric organisms.[142] Restoration of biliary-enteric communication improves RES function and restores protective mechanisms lost to cholestasis, reducing the risk of systemic and biliary tree infection.[155]

INNOCENT BYSTANDER EFFECTS ON THE HEPATOBILIARY SYSTEM

Despite the immense potential for exposure of the liver to infectious organisms, increased liver enzyme activity and hepatic dysfunction in infectious disease more commonly reflect secondary effects of systemic infection rather than specific hepatic involvement.[116,123] Pyrexia, anoxia, nutritional deficits, released toxins, and inflammatory mediators each contribute to clinicopathologic abnormalities. "Innocent bystander" injury from pathologic conditions initiated elsewhere in the body can lead to inappropriate diagnostic emphasis on the hepatobiliary system. Occasionally, a self-perpetuating form of chronic active hepatitis may develop as a complication of infection with bacterial or viral agents. Examples include chronic hepatitis in dogs after infection with leptospirosis or canine adenovirus-1.[13,64] An emerging role of *Helicobacter* spp. in humans with cholestatic liver disease, cholecystitis, and neoplasia of the biliary tree suggests that a relationship may also exist between this organism and liver disease.[58,102,121] Isolation of *Helicobacter canis* from a single dog with multifocal necrotizing hepatitis has been reported; organisms were observed using a silver stain at the periphery of necrotizing lesions.[59] Bacteria were concentrated between adjacent hepatocytes in bile canaliculi and observed in the lumen of bile ducts. Organisms were cultured and phenotypically and molecularly identified as being different from *H. canis*. Detection of *Helicobacter* DNA using polymerase chain reaction (PCR) and amplicon sequencing from archived formalin-fixed liver tissue from 2 out of 29 cats with cholangiohepatitis and a cat with PSVA included in a control group was reported in a scientific abstract.[71] Based on comparisons to published sequence homology, *H. nemestrinae—H. pylori* and a combination of *H. nemestrinae—H. pylori*, and *H. felis—H. cinaedii* in the two cats with cholangiohepatitis and *H. bilis* in the PSVA cat were identified. In no case were organisms identified by silver stains or immunocytochemistry.

SYSTEMIC INFECTIONS

Sepsis and Endotoxemia

Hepatic dysfunction and cholestatic liver injury have been documented in people and in numerous animal models as a result of systemic bacterial infection and endotoxemia.[49] Intrahepatic cholestasis induced by severe extrahepatic bacterial infection has been experimentally modeled in dogs and cats and observed clinically in these species.[167,171] Response of the liver to systemic infection has been studied in dogs experimentally infused with endotoxin or live gram-negative bacteria, or both.[55,72-74] Acute morphologic changes include dilation and congestion of sinusoids and hepatic veins, central (zone 3) and midzonal (zone 2) hepatocellular necrosis, fatty or vacuolar degeneration (not glycogen associated), acute diffuse influx of inflammatory cells (neutrophils and monocytes), and microabscess formation. Kupffer cell hyperplasia is occasionally described, and canalicular stasis (microscopically evident "bile plugs") has also been described with chronicity. Considerable hepatocellular dysfunction can cause a shift to anaerobic metabolism, impair gluconeogenesis, and mobilize lipid from adipose stores. In dogs, acutely increased serum triglyceride, nonesterified fatty acids, and cholesterol concentrations reflect a metabolic shift to fatty acid oxidation.[72] If this activity also occurs in cats, peripheral fat mobilization might augment development of hepatic lipidosis. In fatty liver modeled in the choline-deficient rat, impaired RES function increases host susceptibility to endotoxemia.[122] Although it is not known if this is also true in cats with hepatic lipidosis, the common occurrence of a more primary disease causing anorexia and subsequently the lipidosis syndrome warrants consideration that IBD or constipation might potentiate endotoxemia in these patients.

Logically, animals with compromised liver function or cholestasis experiencing gastroenteric hemorrhage have an increased risk for endotoxemia, as is shown in humans. These patients should be treated with broad-spectrum antimicrobials appropriate for enteric opportunists. Unfortunately, a risk exists that aggressive antimicrobial treatment for gram-negative organisms may intensify endotoxin release and related clinical signs (as suggested by some in vitro and in vivo work). This risk relates to the type of antibiotic action and whether the microbial cell wall remains intact.[41,81,83] For β-lactam antibiotics, endotoxin-enhancing properties relate to the affinity of the penicillin-binding proteins (PBP) in the bacterial cell wall. Antibiotics with highest affinity for these proteins (PBP-2) initiate bacterial transformation to rounded spheroplast forms without cell lysis or endotoxin release. Antibiotics with highest affinity for the penicillin-binding proteins (PBP-3) convert bacteria to long-filament forms, with substantial endotoxin release. Antibiotics with high affinity for both receptors have an intermediate effect. In addition to endotoxin-induced hepatic injury, patients with obstructive jaundice, cirrhosis, or following extensive hepatic mass excision have greater susceptibility to endotoxemia caused by impaired Kupffer cell function and hepatic perfusion and greater enteric microbial translocation.

Tick-Borne Diseases

Ticks transmit a variety of organisms, including protozoal, bacterial, and rickettsial organisms. The most common agents encountered in dogs that may have clinical evidence of liver involvement (increased liver enzymes and less consistently hyperbilirubinemia) include *Ehrlichia* sp., *Rickettsia rickettsii* and *Borrelia*. Pathomechanisms of rickettsial agents easily explain their apparent hepatic involvement in systemic infection because these organisms may infect either hepatocytes or endothelial cells. Considering the extensive endothelial network in the liver, organisms with endothelial tropism may involve the liver as an innocent bystander. In humans, hepatic involvement in ehrlichial infection occurs in over 80% of patients causing mild transient increases in transaminase activity.[51] Rarely, cholestasis and liver failure may occur, but in most cases, signs of liver injury resolve with appropriate antimicrobial therapy. A similar phenomenon may also occur in dogs. Liver injury is related to proliferation of organisms in hepatocytes and by stimulation of immunologic and nonspecific inflammatory mechanisms. In humans, lesions vary from

focal hepatic necrosis to granulomas and cholestatic hepatitis associated with a mixed portal infiltrate, sinusoidal lymphoid cell infiltrate, and reactive Kupffer cells.[51,118] Vasculotropic *Rickettsia* such as the organism causing Rocky Mountain spotted fever can involve hepatic endothelium, leading to mild or moderate increases in hepatic transaminase activity, hepatocellular apoptosis, and less commonly, cholestasis. In humans, cholestasis often reflects pancreatic infection and vasculitis, leading to common bile duct entrapment.[178,181] Hemolysis also may contribute to hyperbilirubinemia.[181] Similar effects likely occur in dogs but have not been well characterized. Systemic borrelial infections in humans, early in the course of disease, can also be associated with clinical evidence of hepatic infection (high liver enzyme activity). In dogs, this association has also been observed clinically and confirmed by liver biopsy in two ill dogs (several weeks of illness) observed by the author. Histologic lesions were consistent with lobular dissecting hepatitis in one dog and a mixed multifocal inflammatory reaction causing focal pyogranulomas in the other. Experimental work with *Borrelia* suggests that organisms are rapidly extracted by Kupffer cells following systemic dispersal and killed by nonopsonic phagocytosis (in vivo and in vitro).[144] Considering the complicated immunopathogenesis of *Borrelia* infections, aberrant immune response, humoral immune activity, cytokines, and cell-mediated immune events likely invoke liver injury.[80] Experimental work with the *Borrelia* suggests direct hepatic invasion by the spirochete in conjunction with cellular and humoral immunologic mechanisms.[181]

Leptospirosis

During the last 15 years, retrospective clinical reports of leptospirosis in dogs in North America and additional reports from other continents have been published, owing to increased disease recognition and diagnostic surveillance (see Chapter 44). A retrospective report of cases managed in the author's hospital documented hepatic involvement in 22 out of 36 (61%) dogs based on increased liver enzyme activity.[12] Approximately 17% became hyperbilirubinemic, although some of these dogs had evidence of microangiopathic anemia as a complicating factor. Increased serum alkaline phosphatase (ALP) activity was most common (60% of dogs with high liver enzymes) and was evident either on initial blood work or developed after initiation of treatment (antimicrobial therapy). High transaminase activity in some dogs reflected muscle injury, substantiated by concurrently high creatine kinase activity. Rise in liver enzyme activities and evidence of cholestasis during the first week of treatment is thought to reflect hepatocellular or vascular injury derived from released bacterial toxins or immunologic responses. An association between infection with *L. pomona* and high liver enzymes has been appreciated. Other retrospective and experimental studies of leptospiral infection in dogs confirm that increased ALP activity is the most common indicator of hepatic involvement.* Evidence of liver injury in the absence of renal involvement seems uncommon but may occur. Hepatic lesions in a small number of necropsied dogs were characterized by marked hepatic venous and sinusoidal congestion, severe perivenous edema, and a predominantly neutrophilic multifocal inflammatory reaction. Association between leptospiral infection and chronic hepatitis also has been recognized.[13]

Clinical Findings of Hepatobiliary Involvement in Infectious Disorders

Hepatomegaly, splenomegaly, fever, icterus, and lethargy are common clinical signs. The hemogram may depict a leukopenia, degenerative left shift, and nonregenerative anemia.

*References: 12, 76, 86, 89, 137.

Markers of an acute phase response including hyperglobulinemia and hyperfibrinogenemia, a negative acute phase response of hypoalbuminemia, and hypoglycemia may develop rapidly. These changes are accompanied by variable increases in the serum activity of liver enzymes, notably alanine aminotransferase (ALT) and aspartate aminotransferase (AST). In the dog, ALP activity consistently increases after several days, and hyperbilirubinemia occurs in dogs and cats after 36 to 48 hours. Certain bacterial organisms can directly induce jaundice without causing substantial hepatic injury; however, generally, the development of jaundice portends a poorer prognosis. Disseminated intravascular coagulation (DIC), acute renal failure, and myocardial dysfunction may develop in terminal cases.

Therapy

The cornerstone of treatment is the provision of adequate fluid therapy, including colloids, parenteral antibiotics effective against involved organisms, glucose supplementation in the event of hypoglycemia caused by the sepsis syndrome or hepatic failure, and identification and correction of associated conditions (see Endotoxemia, Chapter 38). Widespread interest in and documentation shows that oxidant and perioxidative injury is an important pathomechanism in necroinflammatory. Cholestatic liver disease, as well as in infectious disease, and the recent documentation of antioxidant depletion in companion animals with spontaneous liver diseases warrant provision of adequate nutritional and vitamin support and antioxidant supplementation.[28] Maintaining a positive nitrogen balance is important for cell repair and hepatic regeneration. Antioxidant supplementation in the form of thiol donors, that is, nutritionally as cystine, cysteine, or methionine or by supplementation with N-acetylcysteine or S-adenosylmethionine (SAMe), along with α-tocopherol (vitamin E) for biomembrane protection, is recommended.[28]

SPECIFIC HEPATOBILIARY INFECTIONS

Bacterial infections restricted to the hepatobiliary system are relatively uncommon. These infections may assume the form of multifocal microabscess formation, diffuse suppurative cholangitis-cholangiohepatitis, cholecystitis, choledochitis, ill-defined hepatic inflammation (as is the case in chronic hepatitis), or they may be associated with discrete, focal suppuration, and necrosis involving large abscesses. Conditions predisposing the patient to hepatobiliary infections are summarized in Table 90-2.

Pyogenic Abscess

Unifocal pyogenic hepatic abscesses are rare but may develop consequent to a significant number of disorders (see Table 90-2).* Most common causes include trauma, extension of sepsis from adjacent viscera or the peritoneal cavity, hematogenous distribution, ascending biliary tract infection, or ischemia associated with liver lobe torsion or a neoplastic mass that has outgrown its blood supply. In humans, dental infection is an important occult cause commonly overlooked; this also may be true in animals. Patients with solitary abscesses may have no discernible underlying or predisposing condition, whereas those with multiple abscesses usually have some other disease in the abdominal cavity or disorder producing bacteremia. Because of the dynamics of the portal circulation delivering splanchnic blood first to the right liver lobes, focal abscess formation is most common on that side in humans. Despite observation that portal blood also first disseminates here in

*References: 16, 54, 73, 75, 94, 104, 114, 153.

Table • 90-2

Conditions Predisposing to Hepatobiliary Infections[a]

Obstructed Bile Flow
  Extrahepatic bile duct occlusion
  Disease of the gall bladder:
    Dysmotility
    Cholelithiasis
    Cystic duct occlusion
    Cholecystic neoplasia
  Parenchymal cholestasis
    Destruction of intrahepatic bile ducts: ductopenia (e.g., certain cats with chronic cholangitis, cholangiohepatitis)
    Microcholelithiasis (intrahepatic bile ducts)
  Pancreatitis
Impaired Hepatic Perfusion +/− Oxidant Injury
  Chronic necroinflammatory liver disease: chronic hepatitis, chronic cholangiohepatitis
  Cirrhosis
  Copper storage hepatopathy
  Acquired portosystemic shunting
  Congenital portosystemic shunting
  Liver lobe torsion
  Hepatic neoplasia
    Primary: development of a necrotic center
      Hepatocellular carcinoma, hepatoma
    Metastatic:
      Lymphosarcoma, adenocarcinoma, malignant histiocytosis
    Portal venous thrombosis
  Pancreatitis
  Trauma: automobile accident, bite wounds, penetrating wounds
Compromised Immunocompetence
  Hyperadrenocorticism
  Diabetes mellitus
  Severe hypothyroidism
  FIV, FeLV infection
  Treatment with immunomodulatory drugs:
    glucocorticoids, azathioprine, methotrexate, chemotherapy
  Amyloidosis
Increased Translocation of Enteric Organisms
  Inflammatory bowel disease
  Enteric neoplasia: lymphosarcoma, adenocarcinoma
  Chronic liver disease
  Extrahepatic bile duct occlusion
  Reduced bowel motility
Pancreatitis
Neonatal
  Omphalitis
Visceral larval migrans
  Toxocara
Iatrogenic
  Extension from a feeding device
  Surgical infection

FIV, Feline immunodeficiency virus; *FeLV*, feline leukemia virus.
[a]Disorders in dogs and cats with culture positive hepatobiliary infections.

dogs, lateralization to the right side does not appear to occur in this species. Lethal hepatic abscesses derived from omphalogenic infections have been reported in neonates in which *Staphylococcus* appears to be the most common isolate.[75]

In most cases, hepatic abscesses are linked to portal bacteremia or extension from biliary tract infections; impaired tissue perfusion increases the risk of infection.[16,94] Portal thromboembolism related to enteric and mesenteric disease processes, liver lobe or splenic torsion, or necrosis of tumor tissue are likely causes. Immunocompromised patients have the greatest risk. In humans, polymicrobial infections and anaerobic bacteria are isolated from approximately 50% of large solitary abscesses.[112] Organisms retrieved from cultures of liver and bile from dogs and cats with suppurative hepatic inflammation and abscesses are given in Table 90-1. Approximately 50% of these organisms were polymicrobial, at least on morphologic (cytologic) evaluation. Infections with gram-negative organisms are complicated by LPS. Some organisms (e.g., *Pseudomonas aeruginosa*) produce exotoxins that induce clinical signs of illness. Purified exotoxin A associated with *P. aeruginosa* is highly lethal for animals, producing shock in dogs. This toxin inhibits hepatic protein synthesis and impairs lymphocyte response to mitogens.[152]

Multifocal microabscess formation also may occur in conjunction with a variety of organisms causing systemic infection; examples include *Listeria, Salmonella, Brucella, E. coli, Yersinia pseudotuberculosis, Bacillus piliformis, Actinobacillus lignieresii, Actinomyces, Nocardia,* and *Pasteurella.*

Clinical Findings

As an isolated focus of infection, hepatic abscess formation may provoke only vague clinical signs, including fever, lethargy, anorexia, vomiting, diarrhea, trembling, weight loss, and rarely, polyuria, and polydipsia. Physical examination usually discloses fever and abdominal tenderness, tachycardia, tachypnea, dehydration, and, less commonly, bleeding tendencies (surface hemorrhages, retinal hemorrhages), hepatomegaly, or a cranial abdominal mass effect, as well as suspicion of abdominal effusion. Early diagnosis may be difficult. Animals with systemic infections usually show signs commensurate with other organ system involvement, with the hepatobiliary system a secondarily and less overtly affected site.

Diagnosis

Most patients develop a neutrophilic leukocytosis inconsistently associated with a left shift, toxic neutrophils, and monocytosis. Some patients become thrombocytopenic (severe to mild) and demonstrate a nonregenerative anemia. Increased serum ALT (1.1 to 50 times high normal), AST (1.1 to 18 times high normal), and ALP (1.2 to 21 times high normal) activities and hyperglobulinemia are common. Hyperfibrinogenemia with an associated hyperglobulinemia represents an acute-phase response. Hyperbilirubinemia is inconsistent and usually mild. The sepsis syndrome is exhibited by hypoglycemia and high lactate concentrations.[55] Studies in dogs confirm that lactic acidosis derives from increased splanchnic lactate production and reduced hepatic lactate extraction.[33] Gram-negative bacterial abscess formation often evokes laboratory features of endotoxemia. Septic peritonitis follows abscess rupture. Blood cultures are more likely to be positive in patients with multiple abscesses and rarely disclose anaerobic organisms.

Ultrasound (US) provides the best chance for early diagnosis of unifocal hepatic abscess formation and is capable of disclosing focal lesions that are 0.5 cm or larger. In humans, US is considered the diagnostic modality of choice because of high utility in both detecting and serially monitoring lesions.

US imaging also may disclose evidence of multiple *miliary* abscesses overlooked by more sophisticated imaging modalities (e.g., computerized tomography [CT], contrast-enhanced imaging).[171] US appearance of hepatic abscesses is variable and may appear as anechoic masses having irregular margins, as lesions with a well defined rim, or it may contain variable and complex internal echoes (Figs. 90-1 and 90-2, A and B). The presence of a gas-associated anechoic (fluid) compartment highly suggests infection; gas appears echogenic with or without acoustic shadowing depending on its amount and distribution. Overall echogenic patterns associated with hepatic abscesses have been described as (1) *hypoechoic lesions,* consistent with liquefaction necrosis, (2) *heteroechoic lesions,* reflecting an irregular hyperechoic abscess rim surrounding a liquefied hypoechoic center, or (3) *hyperechoic lesions,* representing a highly cellular "cellulitis" or pyogranulomatous reaction, caseation, dystrophic mineralization, or an emphysematous foci.[82,114] Rarely, a target lesion similar in appearance to hepatic neoplasia (especially carcinoma) may be observed. An important rule-out diagnosis is fluid collection in benign cystic structures; these are comparatively free of internal echoes and are associated with well-defined walls, usually generating excellent sonographic transmission. Unfortunately, US images of hepatobiliary abscesses may be compromised by intestinal ileus in which enteric gas compromises the imaging "window." Plain radiographs usually have limited value in diagnosing hepatic abscess formation. Exceptionally, radiographs may disclose loculated hepatic gas, free abdominal gas, focal mineralization, mass lesions, or reduced peritoneal detail, reflecting peritonitis or effusion, or both (Fig. 90-3). Miliary abscess formation cannot be distinguished from other multifocal hepatic parenchymal lesions based on US or radiographic imaging. Thoracic radiographs may reveal evidence of pneumonia, reflecting increased pulmonary exposure to infectious organisms. The presence of sternal lymph node enlargement may signal abdominal inflammation or infection because this lymphatic pathway drains the abdominal structures.

Although blood and urine cultures may identify causal organisms, these cultures are unreliable. More direct diagnostic sampling is achieved by lesion aspiration. Cytologic examination of aspirated material should be initially completed

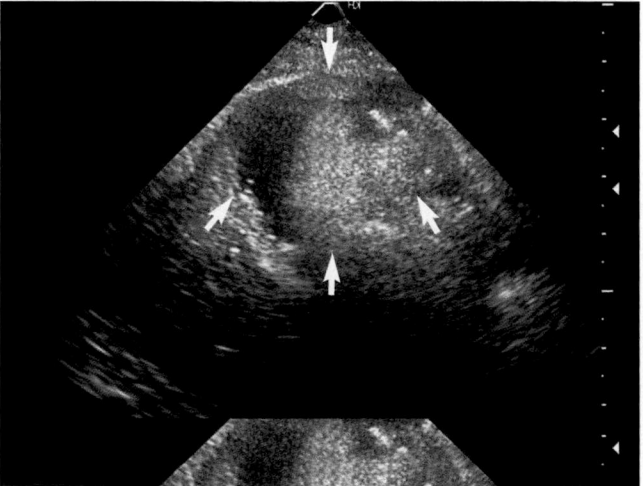

Fig 90-1 Ultrasonographic image of a hepatic abscess showing a hyperechoic rim and heterogenous interior echogenicity *(between arrows).* The image reflects solid or complex mass structure associated with hemorrhagic, cellular, or edematous fluid or caseation. The gross appearance of this abscess is shown in Fig. 90-2, **A** and **B.**

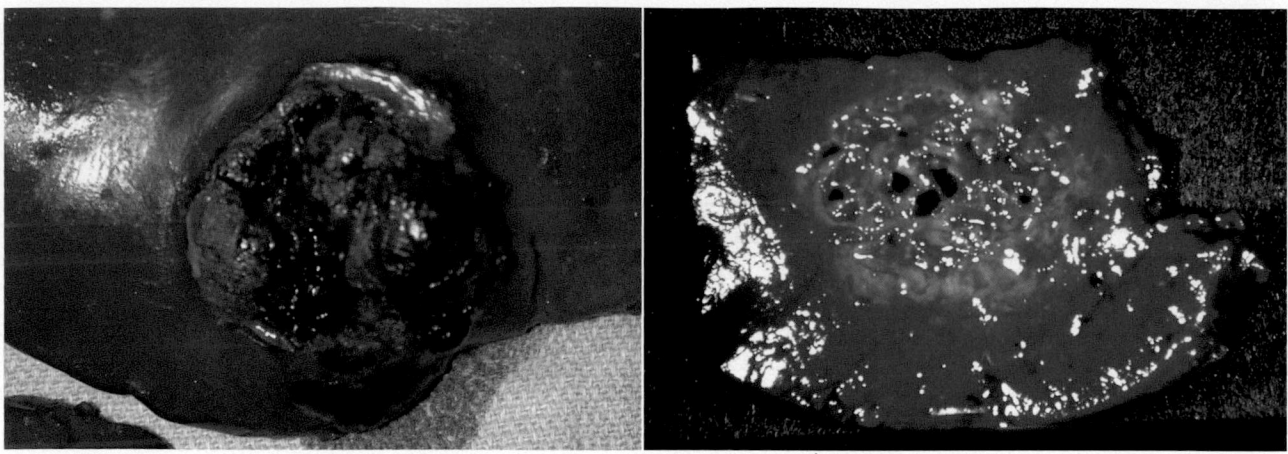

Fig 90-2 Gross appearance of the hepatic abscess demonstrated in Fig. 90-1. **A,** Lesion on surface of the liver. **B,** Lesion on cut surface. A polymicrobial infection was proved to involve *Bacteroides.*

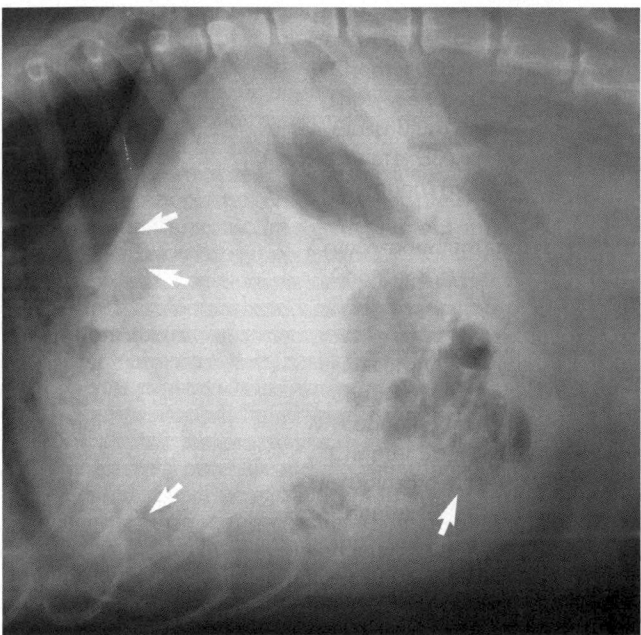

Fig 90-3 Radiograph demonstrating pneumoperitoneum associated with emphysematous hepatic abscesses *(arrows)* and pneumoperitoneum from a mature dog. Central necrosis of a large hepatic adenoma was the underlying disease. A clostridial organism was suspected based on Gram stain characteristics and was subsequently confirmed by anaerobic bacterial culture.

using a modified Wright-Giemsa's stain (Diff Quik). Identified microorganisms are subsequently characterized by Gram staining. Although exceedingly useful, diagnostic and therapeutic abscess aspiration is associated with a risk of peritoneal contamination, requiring forethought as to the need for emergency laparotomy. Anaerobic and aerobic cultures of abscess contents should always be submitted. Polymicrobial infections nearly always involve an anaerobic organism; approximately 50% of solitary hepatic abscesses in dogs appear to be polymicrobial. Because anaerobes are difficult to culture, they should be suspected and treated when cytologic evaluation discloses a polymicrobial population. Furthermore, therapy should continue even if no organisms are cultured or only a few aerobic organisms are grown. When causal factors remain illusive,

hepatic biopsy may be indicated in a search for underlying neoplasia or other primary hepatic processes permissive to infection.

Therapy

Successful management of multifocal microabscess formation in 60% of treated human cases is accomplished when only intravenous (IV) antibiotics are used.[117] Successful outcome usually requires early diagnosis, aggressive abscess drainage (needle-catheter or surgical drainage), lobectomy, or any combination of these, and long-term administration (minimum of 6 to 8 weeks) of an appropriate antibiotic. Needle or catheter drainage procedures have received increased attention as a therapeutic option for successful management of single (or few) abscesses owing to the wide availability and high sensitivity of US imaging.[36,114,153] Aspiration using an 18-gauge needle (superficial abscess) or 22-gauge spinal needle (deep abscess) or via a drainage catheter placed by guide-wire technique may be performed with the intent of removing all liquefied suppuration (large syringe, three-way valve, and collection reservoir prepared in anticipation). Flushing the abscess cavity with sterile saline is recommended if physically possible after evacuation. Reappraisal for potential peritoneal contamination by US imaging is recommended within 24 to 48 hours. Response to therapy is monitored with serial US images, body temperature, and measurement of liver enzymes. In human medicine, bedside US imaging and abscess drainage (n = 886 cases) by the managing clinician have been proven to be advantageous and safe.[36] Aspiration drainage by clinician-operated US technique met or exceeded information and treatments afforded by imaging specialists or alternative imaging modalities (e.g., fluoroscopy, CT imaging).[36]

US-guided abscess aspiration as a primary mode of abscess treatment has been successfully applied to veterinary patients. This approach is recommended for several reasons: (1) as a method of confirming the diagnosis, (2) to provide time for patient stabilization before surgical exploration for liver lobe resection, and (3) because it is successful as a solitary means of therapy in a subset of patients. Major factors arguing against this technique include unsafe access (i.e., abscess immediately adjacent to large vascular structures in the porta hepatis or main biliary structures) and lesion depth exceeding aspiration needle length. When aspirating a suspected hepatic abscess, the clinician must always anticipate a need for immediate surgical intervention in the event of abscess rupture into the peritoneal cavity. Given that primary hepatic tumors comprise an important underlying cause of hepatic abscess formation in older dogs, these lesions must always be considered. Unfortunately, although these lesions require resection, they may not be diagnosed until tissue is resected and examined histologically.

The duration of antimicrobial treatment remains empirical, being based objectively on perceived patient response. In humans, certain organisms (e.g., *Actinomyces*) are routinely treated for a minimum of 3 months.[156] Because polymicrobial infections involving anaerobes are relatively common, antibiotics effective against both aerobic and anaerobic organisms should be initially administered. Anaerobes may act synergistically with other pathogens, altering the course of infection and the prevalence of other pathogens caused by microniche modification. In this circumstance, infection control and bacterial eradication may become more difficult, requiring a longer course of treatment. Anaerobes can enhance virulence of other bacteria by inhibiting phagocytosis (i.e., impairing opsonization, neutrophil chemotaxis) and by locally interfering with the efficacy of antibacterial therapy.[102,154,155] *Bacteroides fragilis* is one of the worst offenders, producing β-lactamases, which can overwhelm the function of β-lactamase inhibitors.[106]

Good initial therapy for hepatic abscess formation is achieved with a combination of a penicillin and a fluoroquinolone or an aminoglycoside. Metronidazole or clin-

damycin can be substituted for penicillin to provide an anaerobic spectrum (see Therapy sections and Tables 90-3, 90-4, and 90-5). Fluoroquinolones provide broader gram-positive coverage compared with aminoglycosides and are thought to have better penetration across an abscess wall. First-generation cephalosporins, potentiated sulfonamides, and aminoglycosides are uniformly ineffective against anaerobes.

Treatment of hepatic microabscesses requires extensive supportive care and long-term administration of a tailored antibiotic regimen specifically targeting involved pathogens along with identification and management of the underlying cause. Disseminated sepsis should initiate a search for an underlying condition compromising immune defense (see Table 90-2).

Granulomatous Hepatitis
Granulomatous hepatic inflammation is an uncommon diagnosis characterized by multiple discrete, sharply defined nodular infiltrates consisting of macrophage aggregates (and sometimes epithelioid cells) surrounded by or intermixed with (or both) lymphocytes and plasma cells. Lesions may be focal, multifocal, or diffuse. Underlying causes include metazoal (e.g., schistosomiasis, dirofilariasis), fungal (e.g., histoplasmosis, paecilomycosis), protozoal (e.g., visceral leish-

Table • 90-3

Guidelines for Selection of Initial Antimicrobials for Anaerobic Hepatobiliary Infections Based on Gram Stain Characteristics[3,9,45]

ANTIMICROBIAL	GRAM-NEGATIVE RODS (NON-SPORE-FORMING)	GRAM-POSITIVE RODS (SPORE-FORMING)	GRAM-POSITIVE RODS (NON-SPORE FORMING)		GRAM-POSITIVE COCCI
	Bacteroides	*Clostridium*	*Propionibacterium*	*Actinomyces*	*Peptostreptococcus*
Penicillin G	–	+++	+++	+++	+++
Penicillin and β-lactamase inhibitor	– to ++	+++	+++	+++	+++
Ticarcillin	+++	+++	+++	+++	+++
Imipenem	+++	+++	+++	++	+++
Cephalosporins					
Cephalothin (first generation)	–	–	+++	++	–
Cefoxitin (second generation)	– to ++	– to +++	– to++	– to ++	+++
Cefotaxime (third generation)	–	– to +++	– to ++	– to ++	+++
Metronidazole	+++	+++	+++	–	++ to +++
Clindamycin	++ to +++	+++	+++	++	+++
Chloramphenicol	+++	+++	+++	++	+++
Tetracycline	– to +	– to ++	– to ++	–	–
Doxycycline	– to +	– to ++	– to +++	–	–
Fluoroquinolones	–	– to ++	NA	–	– to ++
Aminoglycosides[a]	–	–	–	–	–
Trimethoprim-sulfonamide[b]	–	–	NA	NA	–
Vancomycin	–	+++	+++	++	+++

NA, Not available; –, not effective; +, slight efficacy; ++, effective; +++, very effective.
[a]Aminoglycosides require transport enzyme systems to gain entrance to the interior of the bacteria; these are lacking in anaerobes.
[b]Sulfonamides are usually not effective despite in vitro sensitivity testing results. Tissue necrosis and suppuration commonly associated with anaerobic infections result in competitive inhibition of sulfonamide activity.

Table • 90-4

Guidelines for Selection of Initial Antimicrobials for Aerobic Hepatobiliary Infections Based on Gram Stain Characteristics[3,4,9,50,145,146]

VARIABLE	GRAM-POSITIVE COCCI			GRAM-NEGATIVE RODS				
	Staph.	Strep.	Enteroc.	E. coli	Past.	Enterob.	Pseud.[a]	Kleb.
Penicillin G	− to +	+++	−	− to ++[b]	+++	−	−	−
Penicillin and β-lactamase inhibitor	+ to +++	+++	− to ++[b]	− to ++[b]	+++	−	−	−
Extended-Spectrum Penicillin								
Ticarcillin	− to +	+++	++[b]	− to ++[b]	+++	+++[b]	− to +++[b]	−
Ticarcillin and β-lactamase inhibitor	− to +++	+++	++[b]	− to ++[b]	+++	+++[b]	− to +++[b]	− to +++[b]
Imipenem/cilastatin	− to +++	+++	+++	+++[b]	+++	+++[b]	+++[c]	+++[b]
Cephalosporins								
Cephalothin (first generation)	− to +	+++	−	++	+++	−	−	+++
Cefoxitin (second generation)	− to +	+++	−	++	+++	− to ++	−	+++
Cefotaxime (third generation)	− to ++	+++	−	+++	+++	+++	− to ++	+++
Metronidazole	−	−	−	−	−	−	−	−
Clindamycin	− to +++	++	−	−	−	−	−	−
Chloramphenicol	− to +	+++	−	+++	+++	− to ++	− to ++	− to +++
Tetracycline	−	NA	−	−	++ to −	−	− to ++	−
Doxycycline	−	− to +++	−	−	+++	−	− to ++	−
Fluoroquinolones	− to +	− to +	− to +	+++	+++	+++	++[c]	+++
Aminoglycosides[d]	− to +	−	− to +	+++	+++	+++	NA	+++
Trimethoprim-sulfonamide[e]	− to +	− to +	− to +	− to +++	NA	++	−	+++
Vancomycin	− to +++	+++	+++					

Staph., Staphylococcus; Strep., Streptococcus; Enteroc., Enterococcus; E. coli, Escherichia coli; Past., Pasteurella; Enterob., Enterobacter; Pseud., Pseudomonas; Kleb., Klebsiella; NA, data not available; −, not effective; +, slight efficacy; ++, effective; +++, very effective.
[a]*Pseudomonas* may require parenteral third-generation cephalosporins, antipseudomonal penicillins: ticarcillin, carbenicillin, ticarcillin clavulanate, or lastly, a fluoroquinolone.
[b]Synergistic with aminoglycosides.
[c]Not used for *Pseudomonas fluorescens* infections.
[d]Aminoglycosides require transport enzyme systems to gain entrance to the interior of the bacteria; these are lacking in anaerobes.
[e]Sulfonamides are usually not effective despite in vitro susceptibility testing results. Tissue necrosis and suppuration commonly associated with anaerobic infections result in competitive inhibition of sulfonamide activity.

maniasis, toxoplasmosis), bacterial (e.g., infections with mycobacteria, *Nocardia*, *Bartonella*, *Brucella*, *Borrelia*, *Propionibacterium acnes*), and viral (e.g., feline coronavirus [feline infectious peritonitis virus] infections; visceral larval migrans *(Toxocara migration);* and noninfectious disorders (drug reactions, lymphangiectasia, histiocytosis or histiocytic neoplasia, lymphosarcoma, and immune-mediated inflammation). These disorders may be associated with a positive antinuclear antibody test.[26] Causal factors have remained elusive in at least 50% of cases; however, with increased molecular surveillance for infectious origins, more definitive diagnoses are anticipated.

Clinical signs may remain vague. In patients with diffuse hepatic involvement, signs may involve profound hepatomegaly, causing discomfort, icterus, and (later) ascites. Laboratory features include hyperbilirubinemia, high serum ALP, and more variable transaminase activity. In patients with diffuse severe parenchymal involvement, hepatic failure is indicated by subnormal cholesterol and urea concentrations and prolonged coagulation times. Although hepatomegaly is associated with severe diffuse parenchymal involvement, chronic disease may lead to a reduced liver size. Change in hepatic size is usually evident radiographically. The US image may appear normal or disclose a diffusely or irregularly hyperechoic hepatic parenchyma and regional hypoechogenicity. Splenomegaly and mesenteric lymphade-

nopathy are common, followed later by peritoneal effusion. Histopathologic lesions vary in zonal distribution, severity, and cell involvement, depending on the underlying cause.[31]

Infectious causes require specific targeted therapy. In idiopathic cases in which an immune-mediated mechanism is surmised, lesions may abate with glucocorticoid or other immunosuppressive therapies (e.g., azathioprine, cyclosporin, methotrexate). However, immunosuppression requires vigilant monitoring for opportunistic pathogenicity of undetected infectious agents. Molecular techniques for detecting infectious causes has been widely used and applied successfully in human medicine. Recently, PCR analysis detected *Bartonella* spp. infection from two dogs with hepatic disease, one with blatant pyogranulomatous inflammation and the other unexpectedly (Doberman pinscher with chronic hepatitis used as a disease control).[63] Hepatosplenic *Bartonella* infection in humans is thought to be widely under-diagnosed when it is associated with multinodular lesions involving either bacillary angiomatosis or peliosis hepatica (the latter lesion has been reported in an infected dog) or a necrotizing granulomatous reaction.[43,93,129]

Feline Hepatobiliary Infections
Cholangitis-Cholangiohepatitis
The cholangitis-cholangiohepatitis syndrome (CCHS) is the most common necroinflammatory hepatobiliary disorder of

Table • 90-5

Dosages of Drugs for Treatment of Hepatobiliary Infections and Modifications for Hepatic Insufficiency or Jaundice

DRUG[a]	DOSE[b]		ROUTE	INTERVAL (HOURS)	TOXICITY WITH ACCUMULATION[c]
	STANDARD	LIVER-IMPAIRED			
Antimicrobials					
Penicillin G	20,000—40,000 U/kg	—	IV, IM, SC	4	Low
Amoxicillin-clavulanate	10—20 mg/kg	—	PO	12	Low
Ticarcillin	15—25 mg/kg over 15 min then CRI	—	IV, IM, SC	IV loading then CRI or discrete dosing at 6—8	Low
	7.5—15 mg/kg/hr or 40—80 mg/kg	—	IV, IM, SC	IV loading then CRI or discrete dosing at 6—8	Low
Imipenem	5—10 mg/kg	—	IV / IM	6—8	Low
Cephalosporins					
1st generation	10—30 mg/kg	—	PO, IV, IM, SC	8	Low
2nd generation	10—20 mg/kg	—	IM, IV	8	Low
Ceftazidine	30—50 mg/kg	—	IV	8—12	Low
Metronidazole	15 mg/kg	7.5 mg/kg	PO	12	Neurotoxic
Clindamycin	10—16 mg/kg	5 mg/kg	SC	24	Anorexia, vomiting, diarrhea
	5—10 mg/kg	5 mg/kg	PO	12	Anorexia, vomiting, diarrhea
Chloramphenicol (rarely indicated)	D: 25—50 mg/kg	12—25 mg/kg	PO, IV, IM, SC	8	Myelosuppression
	C: 16—22 mg/kg	8—11 mg/kg	PO, IV, IM, SC	8	Myelosuppression
Tetracycline	10—20 mg/kg	—	PO	8	Potential hepatotoxic
Doxycycline	2.5—5 mg/kg	—	PO	12	Low
Enrofloxacin	D: 2.5—5 mg/kg	—[d]	PO, IM, SC	12	Drug interactions, seizures
	C: 2.5 mg/kg/day	—[d]	PO, IM, SC	24	Drug interactions, seizures
Gentamicin	6—8 mg/kg	—	IV, IM, SC	24	Nephrotoxic, ototoxic; therapeutic monitoring
Amikacin	10—15 mg/kg	—	IV, IM, SC	24	Nephrotoxic, ototoxic; therapeutic monitoring
Trimethoprim-sulfonamide	30 mg/kg	15 mg/kg	PO, SC	12—24	Cholestasis, immune complex disease
Vancomycin	15—20 mg/kg	—	IV (slowly over 30—60 min)	8—12	Nephrotoxic, painful IM; therapeutic monitoring recommended esp. cats.

Table • 90-5

Continued

DRUG[a]	DOSE[b]		ROUTE	INTERVAL (HOURS)	TOXICITY WITH ACCUMULATION[c]
	STANDARD	LIVER-IMPAIRED			
Supportive Therapy					
B-Vitamins	2 ml/liter fluid therapy	—	IV	Each fluid allocation	Low
Vitamin K$_1$	0.5–1.5 mg/kg	—	SC	12[e]	Anaphylaxis if IV, hemolysis if too great a dose: heinz bodies
Vitamin C (avoid if high liver tissue Cu or Fe concentrations in biopsy)	100–500 mg total	—	PO, IV	24	Low, may augment hepatic oxidative injury associated with transition metals (Cu & Fe)
Vitamin E	10–15 U/kg		PO	24	Low
Ursodeoxycholic acid	7.5 mg/kg	—	PO	12	Pruritus[f]
Crystalloids	66 ml/kg	—	IV, SC	24	Edema, hypertension
Hetastarch	D: 10–20 mg/kg	—	IV	24	Hypertension
	C: 10–15 mg/kg	—	IV	24	Hypertension
Desmopressin acetate DDAVP	1–5 µg/kg 20 min before effect, lasts only 2 hr	—	IV	1 time treatment Also use as pretreatment for blood donor to increase vWF & Factor VIII	High dose may augment water retention and aggravate edema or ascites, rarely a problem

CRI, Constant rate infusion; *D*, dog; *C*, cat; *DDAVP*, deoxy-d-arginine vasopressin; *vWF*, vonWillebrand's factor
[a]For further information on antimicrobial drugs, see Drug Formulary, Appendix 8.
[b]Dose per administration at specified interval.
[c]For additional information on toxicity, see Drug Formulary, Appendix 8.
[d]Data on dose reduction not established.
[e]Use for 1–3 doses, then dose every 7–10 days. Too frequent administration or too high a dose will cause Heinz body hemolytic anemia in cats.
[f]Avoid use until complete biliary obstruction is relieved.

the domestic cat.[24,61,87] Inflammation involving intrahepatic bile ducts (cholangitis) is frequently associated with chronic interstitial pancreatitis possibly because of the anatomic proximity of these tissues (anatomic fusion of the common bile and pancreatic ducts), because of shared epitopes on epithelial cells of these ductular structures, or because of a common, as of yet unidentified, infectious organism. Concurrent presence of IBD and interstitial nephritis is also clinically recognized. Cholangiohepatitis as a classification exists when cholangitis extends to involve surrounding hepatic parenchyma. CCHS may be suppurative or nonsuppurative; cats with suppurative disease are more acutely and severely ill. Although some researchers have postulated that suppurative inflammation may progress to nonsuppurative disease, this has not been confirmed. CCHS has been detected in cats infected with a variety of agents, including trematodes, *Toxoplasma* (see Chapter 80), an organism resembling *Hepatozoon canis* (see Chapter 74), gram-negative intestinal bacteria, *Clostridium piliforme*, formerly *Bacillus piliformis* (see Chapter 39) (Fig. 90-4), *Bartonella* (experimentally), and recently, *Heli-*

cobacter DNA found in archived formalin-fixed tissue from two cats.[71] Given that a general unifying infectious cause of CCHS has not been discovered, most cats are classified as having idiopathic disease if infectious agents are not identified cytologically or cultured from liver and bile samplings. Although infectious agents may initiate inflammation, the process appears to involve chronic and self-perpetuating immunologic and oxidative tissue injury. However, some cats with nonsuppurative CCHS have had positive bacterial cultures from liver tissue and bile.

Suppurative Cholangitis
Suppurative cholangitis occurs least commonly.* Most cats are middle aged or younger, predominantly male, and have only a short duration of clinical illness (under 5 days). Fewer than 50% of patients have hepatomegaly, and most are jaundiced, febrile, lethargic, dehydrated, and exhibit abdominal pain. Vomiting or diarrhea occurs in approximately 50% of cases.

*References: 22, 24, 55, 61, 79, 84.

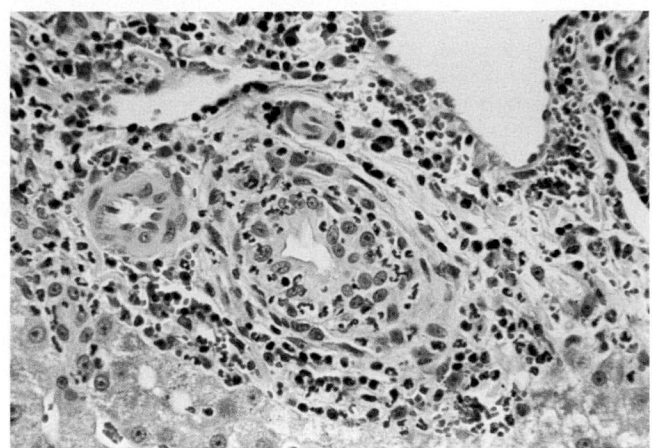

Fig 90-4 Photomicrograph of hepatic tissue from a cat with suppurative cholangiohepatitis. Even though the suppurative nature of the inflammation is recognizable, infectious organisms could not be seen (H and E stain, × 600). Bacterial organisms were clearly evident on an impression cytologic imprint.

Most cats with suppurative CCHS have underlying disorders of the biliary system, causing bile stasis (cholestasis), including EHBDO, cholelithiasis, cholecystitis, choledochitis, or periductal pancreatic and biliary duct fibrosis derived from ascending infection, pancreatitis, trematode infection, immune-mediated mechanisms (presumed) or congenital biliary tract malformation (polycystic liver disease). Inflammatory bowel disease is a common concurrent problem and is thought to contribute to infection. Culture of tissue, bile, and choleliths have disclosed infections with, in descending order of frequency, *Enterococcus*, *E. coli*, *Enterobacter*, *Staphylococcus* spp., α-hemolytic *Streptococcus*, *Klebsiella*, *Acinetobacter*, *Citrobacter freundi*, *Pseudomonas*, *Actinomyces*, *Clostridium perfringens*, *Clostridium* spp., and *Bacteroides*. Unfortunately, a positive result on bacterial culture does not define a causal relationship because cholestasis predisposes to infection by opportunists translocated from enteric flora, ascending the biliary tree, or hematogenously dispersed. Most cats have intermittent vomiting and diarrhea, which circumstantially may coincide with portal bacteremia or reflux of enteric flora into biliary or pancreatic ducts.

Suppurative cholangitis is characterized by a neutrophilic infiltrate around and within intrahepatic bile ducts and associated periductal edema, hepatocellular cholestasis (canalicular bile plugs), and eventually, with chronicity of greater than several weeks, a circumferential periportal fibrolamellar mantle.

Nonsuppurative Cholangitis
Nonsuppurative cholangitis is the most common form of CCHS, occurring in middle-aged to older cats. This form of disease is associated with variable clinical signs and slow, insidious progression. No sex or breed predisposition has been found, feline leukemia or feline immunodeficiency virus infection is not a predisposing factor, most cats are ill for more than 3 weeks, and many are ill for greater than 2 months or for several years. Intermittent anorexia, vomiting and diarrhea, weight loss, cyclic fever, hepatomegaly, and jaundice occur in 70% of cats. Most cats are not consistently lethargic, and chronic disease may lead to polyphagia, apparently associated with maldigestion induced by impaired bile flow and chronic IBD. Common concurrent chronic disorders include IBD, fibrosing pancreatitis, and cholecystitis. In some cats, a history of EHBDO or prior suppurative CCHS exists, which may

have initiated the disease process (presumably). However, in some cats, chronic CCHS is the only identified disorder. Importantly, some of these cats develop hepatobiliary infections possibly as a consequence of immunosuppressive therapy or overlooked primary infectious origins. Some of these cats progress to develop biliary tree neoplasia (adenocarcinoma).

Retrospective and prospective evaluation of affected cats in the author's hospital suggests several different histologic categories included in the morphologic description of nonsuppurative CCHS: (1) *lymphoplasmacytic cholangitis*, (2) *lymphocytic cholangitis*, (3) *lymphoproliferative disease* (low-grade lymphosarcoma confined to the liver), and (4) a *sclerosing cholangitis* form associated with destruction of small to medium sized bile ducts.[22,24] Discussion of each subset is beyond the scope of this chapter. Histologically, nonsuppurative inflammation is characterized by bile duct hyperplasia, periportal and periductal fibrosis, lymphoid or lymphoplasmacytic aggregates in the portal triads, and (with chronicity) biliary cirrhosis. Duct destruction in certain cats leads to "ductopenia" or a sclerosing cholangitis category characterized by obliteration of small and medium-sized bile ducts proven by application of an epithelial specific immunocytokeratin stain. The least common type of portal inflammation in cats is characterized by portal lymphocytic or lymphoplasmacytic infiltrates lacking an apparent involvement of bile ducts; these are more appropriately described by the term *lymphocytic portal hepatitis*.[61]

Clinical Laboratory Findings
Suppurative cholangitis is usually associated with a moderate-to-severe neutrophilic leukocytosis, which may be accompanied by a left shift with or without toxic changes. Nonsuppurative cholangitis may be associated with a mild nonregenerative anemia, normal leukogram, neutrophilic leukocytosis, or lymphocytosis. Variable magnitudes of increased serum activities of ALT, AST, ALP, and γ-glutamyltransferase (γ-GT) develop, depending on the duration and degree of tissue inflammation and cholestasis. Hyperglobulinemia and prerenal azotemia are common on initial presentation of overtly ill animals. Hyperbilirubinemia is more consistent in cats with nonsuppurative cholangitis and has an insidious onset and cyclic nature. In the anicteric cat, detection of bilirubinuria is a sensitive measure of impending hyperbilirubinemia. Measurement of serum bile acids can also detect cholestasis before overt hyperbilirubinemia. Abnormal coagulation test results and bleeding tendencies responsive to vitamin K_1 are observed in severe CCHS accompanied by anorexia of several days' duration, EHBDO, or intrahepatic ductopenia. Radiography is fairly unrewarding, although dystrophic mineralization is sometimes observed in cats with chronic intrahepatic bile duct inflammation and infection, when radiodense choleliths exist, or when unexpected hepatomegaly is confirmed. Hepatic US may fail to disclose altered liver echogenicity, may reflect diffuse hyperechogenicity (a result either from fibrosis, inflammation, or development of hepatic lipidosis), or disclose a heterogenous multifocal pattern. Mineralization of intrahepatic bile ducts is rarely observed. Thickening of biliary structures and evidence of EHBDO may be found. Abdominal effusion is rare in cats with CCHS unless suppurative inflammation and infection exist or severe portal hypertension caused by extensive periportal fibrosis has developed.

Therapy
Surgical exploration is necessary for definitive diagnosis of necroinflammatory hepatobiliary disorders in the cat because it allows visual and mechanical inspection of the biliary tree, sampling of multiple tissues (biopsy of liver, gut, pancreas, and

mesenteric lymph nodes), and collection of samples (tissue, bile) for aerobic and anaerobic bacterial culture. If the common bile duct is occluded, a biliary diversion can be implemented or inspissated bile removed. Hydrocholeresis can be used to improve bile flow postoperatively in these cats through administration of ursodeoxycholic acid. Surgical biopsies provide better intestinal samples as compared with endoscopically retrieved samples and have the advantage of permitting biopsy of jejunum and ileum in addition to duodenum and stomach, as well as safe pancreatic sampling, bile aspiration, and collection of liver biopsies from several different liver areas in a short period. Biopsy of several liver lobes is recommended because differential liver lobe involvement has been shown in patients with high liver enzymes (i.e., minimal involvement in one liver lobe with concurrent severe involvement in another).

A therapeutic strategy is formulated after examination of the liver and bile for sepsis. Aggressive antibiotic therapy is implemented if infection is suspected while aerobic and anaerobic bacterial culture results are pending. Hepatic tissue should be submitted for routine histologic evaluation and reviewed for infectious agents with special stains or immunohistochemistry or subjected to PCR-amplification techniques for unusual organisms. If flukes are considered a possibility, feces should be examined preoperatively and bile collected intraoperatively for trematode egg detection.

Management of CCHS requires long-term supportive care, including fluid therapy, nutritional support by feeding appliance if necessary (esophagostomy or gastrostomy is preferred in most cases) with a balanced feline ration, supplemental water-soluble vitamins (two times normal dosing), antibiotics tailored to the involved infectious organisms, ursodeoxycholic acid for its immunomodulatory-antifibrotic-choleretic and hepatoprotective effects, and, in cases of nonsuppurative CCHS in which no infectious agent has been detected, immunomodulation (antiinflammatory doses of prednisolone are customary).[22,24] Suppurative cholangitis should be treated with antibiotics for at least 6 to 8 weeks. Periodic reevaluation (every 2 to 3 weeks) using physical assessment, hemogram, liver enzyme activities, and bilirubin concentration, is used to monitor patient response. Assessments are based on patient physical status, including body weight and condition, absence of fever, resolution of leukocytosis and jaundice, and reduced liver enzyme activities. Reevaluation of a liver biopsy is desirable but often cannot be justified. In some cases, an US-guided hepatic and bile aspiration permits reevaluation of infection (cytology and cultures). Aspiration of hepatic parenchyma may also disclose developing hepatic lipidosis and initiate further metabolic and nutritional supportive efforts and restriction of glucocorticoids. Some cats with nonsuppurative CCHS appear to be glucocorticoid intolerant, developing hepatic lipid vacuolation or becoming diabetic.

Cats with nonsuppurative cholangitis should be prophylactically treated with antibiotics for possible infectious causes until culture results, antibody titers, cytology of impression smears, and histopathology rule out an infectious cause or decrease it from consideration. If peribiliary fibrosis is observed and culture and titer results deny infectious agents, prednisolone is given initially at a dose of 2.0 to 4.0 mg/kg, orally, once per day. This dose is tapered after the first 1 to 4 weeks depending on patient drug tolerance and clinical response. Chronic administration of antiinflammatory and chemotherapeutic drugs is necessary to control severe nonsuppurative CCHS. Given that hepatic glutathione concentrations have been shown to be low in cats with CCHS, antioxidants are now routinely recommended in the form of (1) S-adenosylmethionine (Denosyl-SD4 [Nutramax Laboratories, Inc., Edgewood, Md.] 200 mg/cat per day) and (2) α-tocopherol (vitamin E; 10 IU/kg/day), along with a daily source of water-soluble vitamins because deficiency of certain B vitamins can limit important metabolic pathways that may facilitate antioxidant function and development of hepatic lipidosis. The adequacy of vitamin B_{12} is appraised in all cats with CCHS because this vitamin undergoes enterohepatic circulation and is known to be seriously compromised in cats with substantial gut disease (infiltrative disease such as lymphoma or severe IBD and enteric lamina propria fibrosis). An important subset of cats with hepatic lipidosis exhibits vitamin B_{12} deficiency, possibly lending to both glutathione deficiency and inadequacy of l-carnitine, dependent on adequate methylation reactions (influenced by SAMe availability and vitamin B_{12}). In cats with the sclerosing CCHS form of disease, methotrexate is used by the author at a total dose of 0.4 mg, given every 8 hours per day once weekly, along with folinic acid (folate) at 0.25 mg/kg and the other medications described previously.[22,24] Most of these cats also receive chronic low-dose metronidazole (7.5 mg/kg, orally, every 12 hours) for its immunomodulatory effect useful in managing IBD (typically a coexistent problem), as well as its excellent protection against anaerobic bacterial organisms that may opportunistically complicate the illness.

Cholecystitis and Extrahepatic Bile Duct Occlusion

Septic inflammation of the bile ducts and gallbladder can develop in dogs and cats as a distinct entity.[56] With chronicity, many of these patients eventually develop EHBDO or a ruptured biliary tree (bile peritonitis). Bile peritonitis is discussed in another section. Although the pathogenesis of acute cholecystitis is not clearly understood, a variety of associated causes are implicated, including any disorder causing obstruction of the biliary tree, gallbladder dysmotility, septicemia, or ascending bacterial invasion of the biliary structures.[22] Acute cholecystitis can be experimentally created by introducing pepsin, activated proteolytic pancreatic enzymes, neutrophils, or bacteria into the bile duct.[65,158] Such spontaneous reflux of initiating agents up the shared bile duct may occur in the cat, especially considering ductal pressure changes invoked by the vomiting reflex. Cholelithiasis and choledocholithiasis may each be associated with septic and nonseptic cholangitis, cholecystitis, and choledochocystitis (gallbladder and duct inflammation) in both dogs and cats.[92] In dogs, old, small- to medium-sized breed females are more commonly afflicted with cholelithiasis, especially if an underlying disorder of lipid metabolism exists (e.g., hereditary defect of lipoprotein metabolism, hypothyroidism). Bile stasis, biliary inflammation and infection, altered bile composition (increased cholesterol or bilirubin concentrations), or biliary mucosal irregularity associated with neoplasia or cystic mucinous hyperplasia can promote biliary lithiasis or gallbladder mucocele formation. The slow, insidious onset of duct occlusion by choleliths or slow-growing neoplasia augments development of biliary infection. E. coli is a common isolate from biliary tissue and bile in animals with cholecystitis. Aerobic bacterial culture results of bile from dogs with gallbladder mucoceles have been positive[10]; however, microscopic abnormalities did not suggest primary biliary tract infection, and bacterial colonization may likely be secondary to biliary stasis. Chronic cholecystitis also has been associated with Salmonella (dogs) and Pasteurella (cats). Acute cholecystitis has been reported in dogs with Campylobacter (likely Helicobacter) infections (see Chapter 39). Although still controversial, the pathologic role of Helicobacter in certain forms of biliary tree disease in humans and animal models is expanding.[102] Most diagnoses are based on PCR detection of Helicobacter DNA, and whether this represents enterohepatic circulation of DNA in bile, transient colonization, or colonization with pathogenicity remains arguable.[102] Given that conditions such as biliary infection, cystic duct occlusion, EHBDO, and acute cholecystitis are known to decrease bile pH significantly, markedly, researchers have suggested that Helicobacter spp. may opportunistically appear in patients with more primary hepatobiliary disorders.

In human and in experimental animal models, the general belief holds that bacteria play an important role in the formation of pigment gallstones. Glucuronidases produced by certain Enterobacteriaceae can deconjugate bilirubin diglucuronide, resulting in precipitation of calcium bilirubinate, which may culminate in stone formation.[170] Other organisms may interact with bile through production of hydrolyzing enzymes, perpetuated inflammation (foreign body effect), and provision of nucleating proteins such as immunoglobulins or debris derived from bacteria, mucus, or cells that can act as a nucleation nidus.

Clinical Signs

Infections involving the bile ducts and gallbladder generate clinical signs of infection and EHBDO. These signs include fever, anorexia, vomiting, abdominal tenderness, hepatomegaly, jaundice, and (with EHBDO) acholic feces and bleeding tendencies. Clinical signs can be persistent, intermittent, or episodic.

Diagnosis

Cholecystitis is frequently associated with clinicopathologic abnormalities typical of EHBDO and severe CCHS in cats. A nonregenerative anemia attributable to chronic inflammation may develop. A strongly regenerative anemia may reflect substantial enteric hemorrhage derived from gastroduodenal ulcers associated with gastroduodenal vascular ectasia, portal hypertensive gastroenteropathy compromising mucosal perfusion and repair, and co-existent IBD. Portal hypertension derives from biliary cirrhosis, which is a predictable sequela to complete EHBDO after 6 weeks. A marked leukocytosis with a left shift is common. Liver enzyme activities, especially ALP and γ-GT, are markedly increased (5 to 10 times reference values). Severe cholestasis is common, with hyperbilirubinemia reaching as much as 20 times reference values. Serum concentrations of total cholesterol usually increase two to four times reference values in complete EHBDO. Prolonged coagulation times may develop as a result of vitamin K_1 deple-

tion or DIC. Lack of an enterohepatic circulation of vitamins B_{12} and K_1 (and possibly folate) are seemingly more problematic for cats. Septic bile peritonitis may prevail if the biliary system ruptures subsequent to necrotizing cholecystitis. Abdominocentesis yielding yellowish-orange fluid containing bile with or without bacteria indicates the need for abdominal lavage and surgical intervention. Abdominal radiographs may disclose the presence of abdominal effusion and, in exceptional cases, radiodense mineralized choleliths (Fig. 90-5). Although many choleliths are radiopaque in cats and dogs, a considerable subset of cats have radiodense choleliths identifiable on good quality survey abdominal radiographs.

US images provide important diagnostic information, revealing changes consistent with EHBDO as early as 72 hours of onset. Initial changes include thickening and distention of biliary structures, obstruction-induced tortuosity of the common duct, and choleliths, reflecting acoustic shadows in the gallbladder (Fig. 90-6).[121,176] Choleliths within the common or cystic ducts are less easily imaged because of adjacent enteric gas. Care must be taken to avoid confusion caused by commonly visualized gallbladder "bile sludge" or "sediment" observed in anorectic patients. Gravitational mobility can be used to evaluate bile fluidity. The "kiwi fruit" sign indicative of a biliary mucocele also may be disclosed (Fig. 90-7). A bi- or trilaminar appearance of the gallbladder wall associated with a heterogenous or kiwi fruit sign suggests a biliary mucocele associated with necrotizing cholecystitis and a need for emergency cholecystectomy, biliary diversion, common duct repair, or any combination of these measures (Fig. 90-8). US evaluation may also disclose pericholecystic effusion and guide accurate needle sampling for cytologic and culture analyses.

Cholecystocentesis

Diagnostic sampling of bile may be useful in certain cases in which infection of the biliary tree or cholecystitis is considered possible.[177,147] This procedure is ill advised in the presence of suspected EHBDO or US changes indicative of necrotizing cholecystitis. Sampling of bile can be safely achieved by US guidance using a transhepatic approach. The transhepatic approach provides some degree of compression on the site of gallbladder puncture limiting bile extravasation. Nevertheless, sampling should be completed with the intent of removing as much liquid bile as possible to reduce subsequent leakage. Sampling by US guidance is done using a 22-gauge spinal needle, a 3-way valve, extension tubing, syringe, and receptacle; sterile

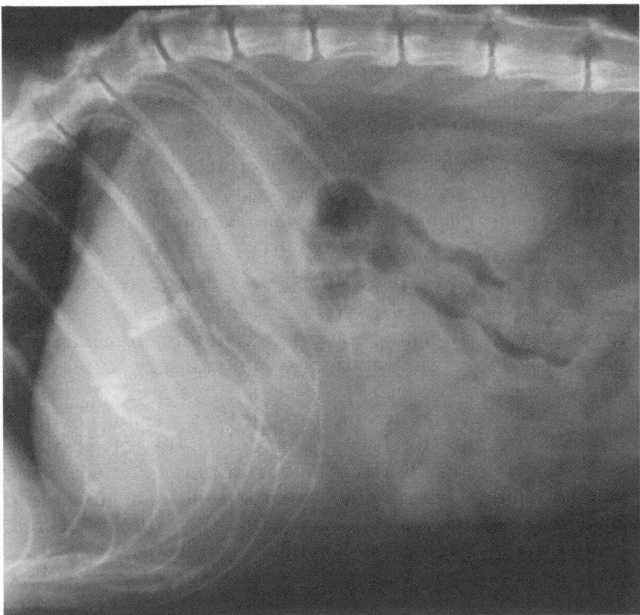

Fig 90-5 Radiograph showing radiodense choledocholithiasis within the intrahepatic biliary tree in a mature cat that 2 years previously underwent cholecystotomy for cholelith removal. Chronic cholangitis, biliary infection, and sludged bile were contributing causes of cholelith development.

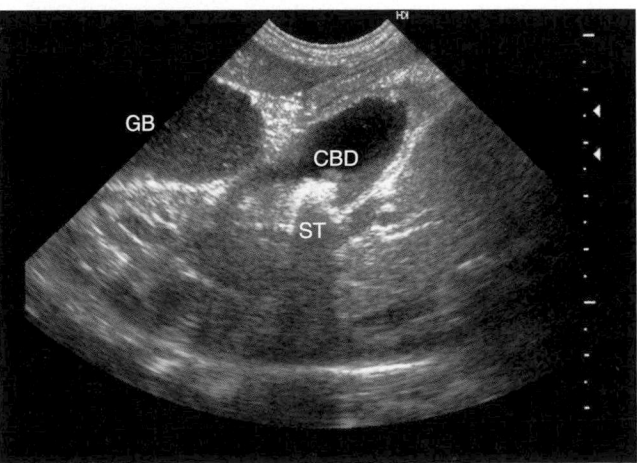

Fig 90-6 Ultrasonographic image showing a mineralized cholelith with acoustic shadowing in a cat with suppurative CCHS (*GB*, gallbladder; *CBD*, distended common bile duct; *ST*, stone).

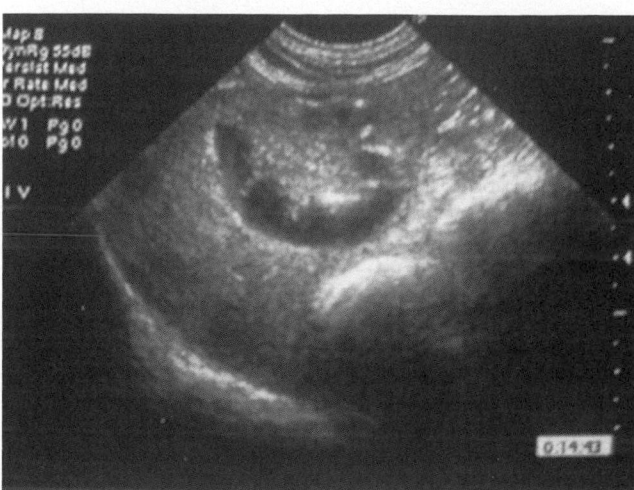

Fig 90-7 Ultrasonographic image showing the "kiwi fruit" sign, consistent with the presence of a biliary mucocele. A biliary mucocele is composed of thick tenacious mucous and biliary debris entrapped in a dysfunctional gallbladder. This phenomenon can lead to necrotizing cholecystitis complicated by infection.

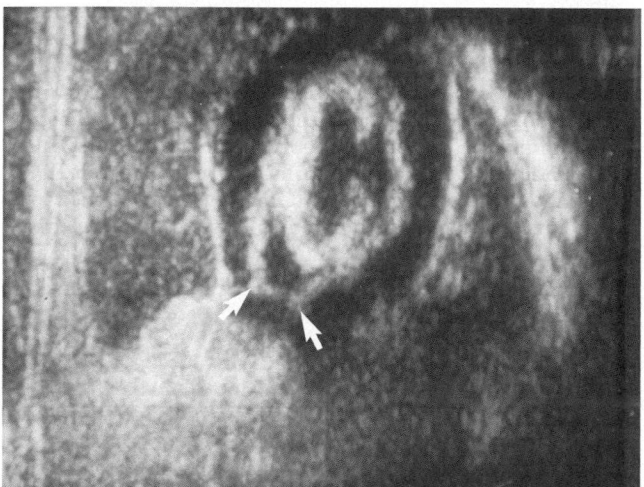

Fig 90-8 Ultrasonographic image of the gallbladder in a dog with necrotizing cholecystitis. Notice the laminar appearance of the gallbladder wall *(arrows)*, consistent with edema and tissue necrosis, obvious on histologic section.

tubes for collecting culture specimens should be available. Penetration of the gallbladder is accomplished using a rapid thrusting motion rather than slow-dull pressure because the latter technique may induce a vasovagal response that can lead to pathologic bradycardia, hypotension, and asystole (see later discussion under Cholecystitis). During exploratory laparotomy or laparoscopy, direct gallbladder puncture for bile collection should also be completed with the intent of emptying the gallbladder to reduce postsampling leakage. US evaluation of the biliary tree 24 to 48 hours after nonsurgical transhepatic sampling is advised to monitor for the presence or extent of focal bile accumulation, especially if biliary sepsis is found on cytologic evaluation of the aspirated bile.

Therapy
Treatment of septic cholecystitis includes prolonged administration of antibiotics effective against involved aerobic and

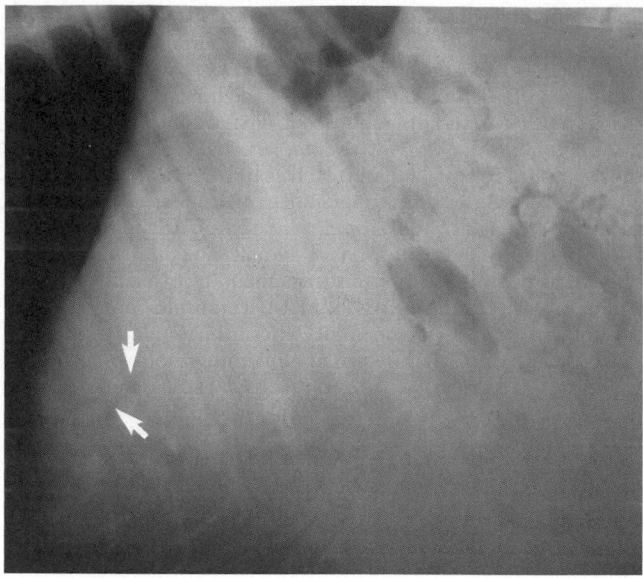

Fig 90-9 Radiograph demonstrating emphysematous cholecystitis observed in a dog with diabetes mellitus *(arrows denote gas in gallbladder)*.

anaerobic bacteria. Selection of antibiotics that achieve good systemic concentration is important. Laparotomy is necessary to confirm the diagnosis, to identify etiologic factors, and to perform cholecystectomy or biliary diversion, or both (e.g., biliary decompression, provision of an alternate route of bile drainage, cholecystoenterostomy, choledochoenterostomy). The need for cholecystectomy is determined by the surgeon and is advised when even a small portion of the gallbladder wall appears devitalized or when neoplasia is suspected. Emergency laparotomy is essential if biliary rupture or septic bile peritonitis is detected. Management of bile peritonitis is discussed later. Hydrocholeresis in conjunction with appropriate antibiotics is used on a long-term basis to diminish bile stasis, after biliary obstruction is resolved. See General Treatment Considerations.

Emphysematous Cholecystitis
Emphysematous cholecystitis is an uncommon and life-threatening condition diagnosed in dogs with and without diabetes mellitus.[18,73,104,105] Diagnosis in the cat is rare. The most commonly recognized precipitating factor is cystic duct obstruction. Ischemia of the gallbladder wall as a result of tense gallbladder distention potentiates an environment conducive to invasion by gas-producing anaerobes. Accessed bacteria can proliferate in the gallbladder wall and spread within adjacent tissues or shared microvasculature. Left untreated, the gallbladder may rupture and organisms spill into the abdominal cavity, leading to pneumoperitoneum and septic peritonitis (Fig. 90-9).

Clinical Findings
Clinical signs associated with emphysematous cholecystitis include abdominal tenderness, fever, jaundice, anorexia, and vomiting. Neutrophilic leukocytosis with a left shift and toxic changes; hyperbilirubinemia; increased serum ALP, γ-GT, ALT, and AST activities; and prerenal azotemia are common. A tympanic abdomen may follow gallbladder rupture. Initial radiographic features may consist only of poorly defined gas infiltrates in the gallbladder wall. Over time, this activity may expand to fill the gallbladder lumen and progressively involve pericholecystic tissues. A sufficient volume of gas for radiographic detection usually accumulates within a few days of

overt clinical signs; radiography, however, is insensitive for an early pivotal diagnosis. US may disclose small amounts of gas in the gallbladder wall as an echogenic line. Large amounts of gas may prevent visualization of the gallbladder wall, casting a distinct acoustic shadow. Unfortunately, US may not clearly differentiate whether gas localizes to the gallbladder wall or extends into the surrounding tissue.[92] Rarely, small amounts of gas may be detected within intrahepatic bile ducts. Conditions other than emphysematous cholecystitis compromising US visualization of the gallbladder include the presence of a porcelain gallbladder (mineralized wall), a contracted gallbladder filled with choleliths, and duodenal ileus (gas-filled intestines that may be overcome by intercostal positioning of the probe or imaging of patient in standing posture). The most common bacteria isolated from humans and dogs with emphysematous cholecystitis are *Clostridium* spp. (Fig. 90-10).

Therapy

Management of emphysematous cholecystitis involves cholecystectomy combined with prolonged administration of antibiotics effective against anaerobes, but even then, the prognosis is poor. Only rarely have patients with emphysematous cholecystitis survived without surgical intervention. Medical and surgical treatment for septic peritonitis is usually needed.

Bile Peritonitis

Bile peritonitis is a serious complication of biliary tree infection, inflammation, ischemia, or trauma. The toxicity of bile on tissues and hypovolemic shock associated with the pooling of fluid in the peritoneal cavity are responsible for most clinical signs. Pleural effusion of a similar composition may also accumulate.[8] Bacterial contamination of biliary ascites may spontaneously develop and is the usual cause of death.[19,22,124] Bile-induced permeability changes in the intestinal wall promote passage of enteric flora into the peritoneal effusion. Anaerobic organisms (*Clostridium* spp.) have also been shown to spontaneously invade experimentally created biliary ascites in dogs.

Clinical Findings

Animals with bile peritonitis usually have histories of anorexia, vomiting, abdominal tenderness and distention, fever, and lethargy. Most patients are overtly jaundiced. However, some animals with aseptic bile peritonitis can be relatively free of clinical signs because of omental and adhesion loculation of spilled bile. Animals with septic peritonitis may develop emphysematous peritonitis subsequent to growth of gas-producing bacteria; this condition may progress, causing a tense and tympanic abdomen (see Fig. 90-3).

Diagnosis

Hematologic abnormalities typically include a left-shifted neutrophilic leukocytosis with toxic changes. Some patients have a degenerative left-shifted leukon, representing systemic sepsis and peritoneal leukocyte migration. However, some patients with walled-off abdominal infection show no hematologic features. Biochemical abnormalities typically reflect the underlying disease process involving biliary structures. Increased serum activities of liver enzymes and moderate to severe hyperbilirubinemia are typical. Hypercholesterolemia develops if EHBDO precedes biliary tree rupture. Progressive hypoalbuminemia reflects sequestration of a protein-rich abdominal effusion. Prerenal azotemia reflects systemic volume contraction and reduced renal perfusion and may indicate endotoxemia. Prolonged hypovolemia or hypotension may provoke acute renal failure.

Abdominal radiography typically discloses a diffuse loss of visceral detail. Careful evaluation for free abdominal gas or gas within the biliary structures is essential because anaerobic bacterial infection is indicated. Cholangiography or cholescintigraphic studies are rarely indicated. Cholangiography may not delineate the site of biliary rupture because of competition between iodinated imaging agents and bilirubin, as well as reduced flow within the biliary tree. Cholescintigraphy using an iminodiacetic analog can provide a noninvasive method of documenting the site of bile leakage, but this too lacks practicality, can be done only in selected centers, and does not reliably indicate the anatomic site of bile leakage.[98]

Abdominocentesis reveals a yellowish-orange or golden-green effusion. Cytologic evaluation usually discloses a modified or exudative effusion with many neutrophils, macrophages, erythrocytes, and variable numbers of bilirubin crystals (Fig. 90-11). Given that yellow discoloration of effusion is expected in a jaundiced animal, effusion color alone cannot be used as definitive evidence of bile peritonitis. The presence of bile "crystals" and a very high fluid bilirubin concentration in relation to serum are useful in confirming the diagnosis. The presence of bacteria is confirmed using a Wright-Giemsa's or new methylene blue stain. Thereafter, Gram stain elucidates bacterial morphology and the presence of sporulated anaerobes, which can greatly facilitate initial antimicrobial selection. Aerobic and anaerobic cultures of

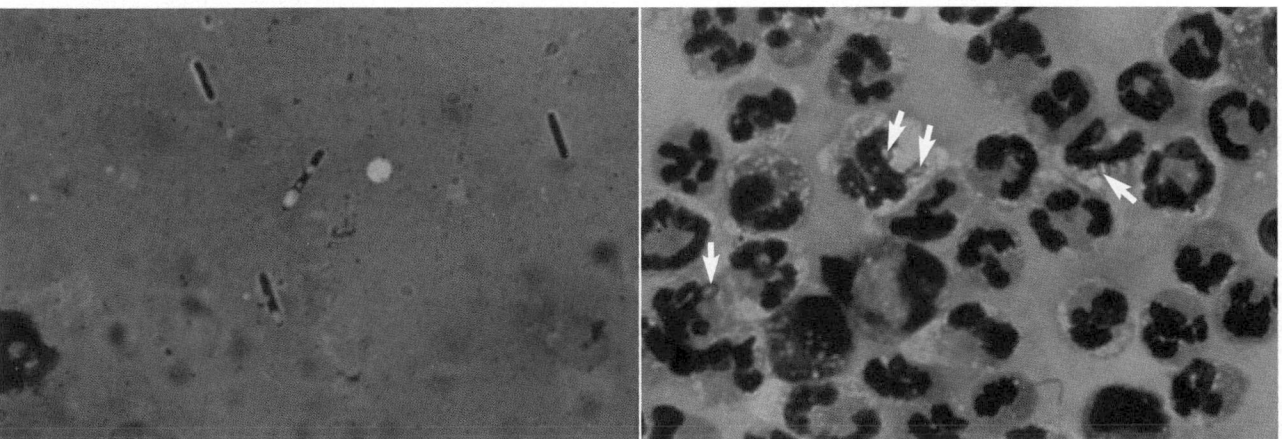

Fig 90-10 A, Sporulating *Clostridium* spp. found in the abdominal effusion. **B,** Free spores *(arrows)* from a dog with an emphysematous hepatic abscess, pneumoperitoneum, and septic peritonitis (Wright-Giemsa, ×680). Same dog as that shown in Fig. 90-3.

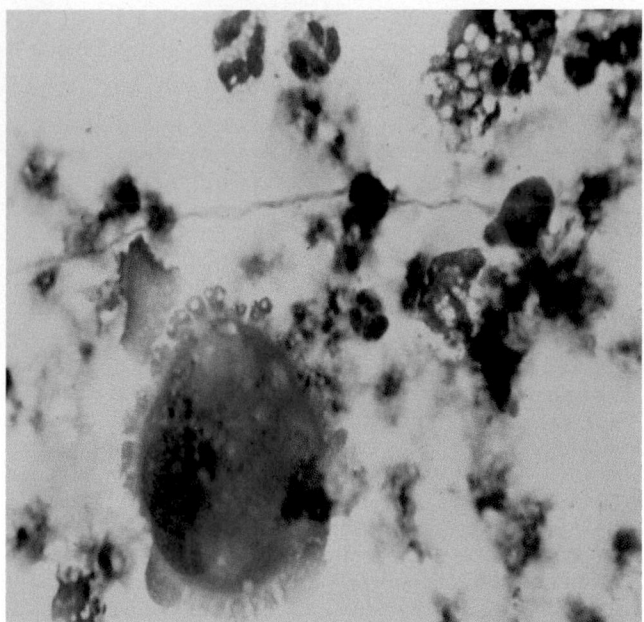

Fig 90-11 Photomicrograph showing cytologic features of an abdominal effusion observed in a dog with septic bile peritonitis. Neutrophils, macrophages, erythrocytes, intracytoplasmic large Gram stain positive rod-form bacteria, and golden bilirubin crystals were observed (Wright-Giemsa, ×680).

abdominal effusion should be collected and immediately submitted when bile peritonitis is suspected, irrespective of whether bacteria have been observed. Antimicrobial therapy is indicated when this diagnosis is considered probable.

Therapy
Surgical intervention is indicated whenever bile peritonitis is suspected. The presence of sepsis makes the situation urgent. Before general anesthesia and laparotomy, the patient must receive aggressive supportive care, including colloid administration to reinstate deficient oncotic pressure, vitamin K_1 to ensure its repletion, blood-component therapy to correct acute symptomatic bleeding tendencies, and IV antimicrobials targeting enteric aerobes and anaerobes derived from transmural enteric translocation. Whether colonic lavage with nonabsorbable antimicrobials should be routinely enacted remains controversial. Experimental and clinical evidence in humans suggests that this procedure may reduce enteric bacterial translocation that predisposes the patient to endotoxemia and septicemia. Neomycin given at 22 mg/kg as a retention (high) enema may be used up to every 8 hours. At surgery, visual inspection of visceral structures usually reveals the site of biliary rupture and provides information essential for an appropriate operative approach. If the gallbladder appears inflamed or devitalized, a cholecystectomy is necessary. If a portion of the common bile duct is damaged, a biliary diversion such as a cholecystoduodenostomy or cholecystojejunostomy may be needed. If the cystic duct is damaged, cholecystectomy is usually done; alternatively, placement of a T tube, or choledochoenterostomy, may be implemented. A careful and systematic inspection of the biliary tree with appraisal of its patency and bile fluidity is essential. Choleliths or mass lesions, as well as inspissated bile or biliary mucoceles, must be removed. Biliary mucoceles are firm conglomerations of bile that lead to necrotizing cholecystitis (more common in hyperlipidemic dogs such as Shetland sheepdogs and Schnauzers with hereditary hyperlipidemia); these are associated with a unique kiwi fruit appearance on abdominal US; these also require cholecystectomy (see Fig. 90-7). Biopsy specimens

optimally should be collected from adjacent and distant portions of the hepatic parenchyma, as well as from representative portions of the diseased biliary system. Parenchymal samples collected from tissues located distal to the biliary structures clarify the presence of diffuse and preexisting hepatobiliary disease. Samples should be evaluated for cytologic and histopathologic features and submitted for both aerobic and anaerobic bacterial culture. During surgical manipulations, remaining vigilant for an induced vasovagal crisis derived from iatrogenic pressure on main biliary structures is important. Vasovagal crisis is characterized by hypotension, bradycardia, and asystole, and correction requires elimination of vagal stimulation (relief of biliary tree pressure or manipulation) and administration of atropine. A similar response may be noted during cholecystocentesis when slow penetration of the gallbladder occurs before needle puncture.

Peritoneal sepsis may be apparent at laparotomy by discovery of a notable fetid odor when the abdomen is first opened. Before abdominal closure, peritoneal lavage with sterile saline is recommended in all cases of bile peritonitis to diminish chemical peritonitis and to remove bacterial organisms mechanically. Appropriate antibiotics should be continued for 4 to 6 weeks postoperatively. Repeated administration of blood components or synthetic colloids may be necessary to correct for bleeding tendencies and to maintain plasma oncotic pressure during surgery and during the immediate postoperative interval because of prodigious loss of plasma proteins and fluid into the abdominal cavity. In cases in which surgery is delayed, abdominal lavage should be aseptically performed to assist in eliminating bile (causing chemical peritonitis) and infectious organisms.

General Treatment Considerations
Supportive Care
Fluids, Electrolytes, Oncotic Support, and Blood Component Therapy Initial management of the animal with hepatobiliary infection involves provision of fluid therapy and correction of electrolyte abnormalities. Polyionic crystalloid fluids are given to correct dehydration deficits, to cover contemporary losses, and to provide for maintenance needs. A commercially available colloid (hetastarch, Hespan® [Bristol Myers Squibb, New York, N.Y.], or generic) may be used to reinstate colloid oncotic pressure; however, its use may promote bleeding tendencies because of effects on platelet aggregation. The author prefers using hetastarch rather than dextran-70 in veterinary patients with liver disease (subjectively, fewer complications with bleeding tendencies). Blood-component therapy may be essential during the first several days in treating patients with chronic EHBDO or severe diffuse parenchymal cholestasis, as well as intraoperatively in patients undergoing surgical resolution of bile peritonitis and cholecystectomy. If present, hypoglycemia is ameliorated with fluids supplemented to a 2.5% or 5.0% dextrose concentration, as necessary. If hypoalbuminemia, hepatic insufficiency, ascites, or a tendency for sodium retention exists, attention must be given to avoid sodium loading (use solutions with lowest sodium content, or prepare a mixed solution combining 5.0% dextrose in water mixed 1:1 v/v with a balanced polyionic fluid). Judicious supplementation with potassium chloride (use the conventional sliding scale for potassium administration) is important, as well as monitoring serum phosphate and administration of potassium phosphate if serum phosphate is less than 2.0 mg/dl (using a constant rate infusion, provide 0.02 to 0.06 mmol/kg/hr). Close monitoring to ensure repletion of potassium and phosphate is important because subnormal electrolyte concentrations can have dire metabolic and physiologic complications in the patient with liver disease. Low potassium can promote hyperammonemia, anorexia, weakness, enteric ileus, and hyposthenuria that can aggravate electrolyte wasting. Hypophosphatemia can lead to

metabolic encephalopathy, anorexia, vomiting, diarrhea, weakness, ataxia, hemolysis, rhabdomyolysis, and bleeding tendencies (platelet dysfunction). Careful sequential monitoring of electrolytes is important to avoid over-supplementation with either electrolyte. Potassium should never be given IV at a rate exceeding 0.5 mEq/kg/hour.

Bleeding Tendencies Vitamin K_1 should be administered by subcutaneous injection in patients with jaundice, whether caused by EHBDO or chronic diffuse cholestasis and whether patients are displaying bleeding tendencies. Vitamin K supplementation has particular relevance in patients with overt bleeding or prolonged coagulation times (see Table 90-5). Coagulation assessments include a thorough physical assessment for bleeding tendencies (including careful inspection of retina, oral cavity, prepuce and penis, vulvar mucosa, as well as more easily inspected cutaneous surfaces), bench coagulation tests (prothrombin time and activated partial thromboplastin time assessments), and a buccal mucosal bleeding time (longer than 5 minutes is abnormal). Unfortunately, routinely evaluated clotting tests are relatively insensitive for detecting clinically relevant bleeding tendencies. The author prefers using the PIVKA (proteins invoked by vitamin K antagonism) clotting test to most routinely performed bench assessments because PIVKA clotting times have higher sensitivity for detecting compromised clotting.[26,27] Increased PIVKA clotting times appear to develop rapidly in cholestatic liver disorders treated with long-term oral antimicrobials, possibly because of synergistic influences, including suppression of enteric microbial vitamin K synthesis, impaired enteric vitamin uptake (caused by lack of sufficient alimentary bile), and compromised hepatic rejuvenation of active vitamin K. Cats appear to have increased risk.[25]

Bleeding tendencies may be recognized before or appear only during invasive procedures (surgery, tru cut needle biopsy, catheterizations). Treatment requires initiating fresh, compatible blood transfusion and may benefit from administration of synthetic vasopressin (desmopressin, DDAVP® [Aventis, Bridgewater, N.J.], or generic; 1 to 5 μg/kg, subcutaneously, 30 minutes before tissue injury, a one-time-only therapy). Fresh whole blood rather than stored frozen plasma is usually better for patients with compromised liver function because of the possibility that thrombocytopenia or acquired thrombopathia may contribute to bleeding tendencies and because ammonia may accumulate in stored blood products. Pretreatment of a blood donor with DDAVP may augment von Willebrand's factor concentration in the collected product. Although DDAVP has been observed to reduce pathologic hemorrhage in humans and companion animals with severe liver disease, the mechanism remains ill defined and is clearly more complex than simple elaboration of von Willebrand's factor from vascular endothelium and increasing factor VIII.[91,110]

Nutritional Support Nutritional support of the patient with hepatobiliary infections requires provision of a nutritionally and calorically adequate diet. These animals should not be initially placed on a protein-restricted diet unless overt signs of hepatic encephalopathy or hyperammonemia (ammonium biurate crystalluria) exist. Avoiding a negative nitrogen balance is important in the patient with hepatobiliary disease and sepsis because this precaution protects tissues from catabolism, provides nitrogen for tissue regeneration and repair, and protects cats from developing hepatic lipidosis. Anorexia is managed whenever possible using enteric modes of feeding (e.g., nasogastric, esophageal, or gastric intubation). The use of appetite stimulants cannot be endorsed (e.g., benzodiazepines, cyproheptadine) because these drugs are inconsistent in effect and are generally unreliable in establishing adequate energy intake. Furthermore, in the circumstance of hepatic insufficiency, benzodiazepines are contraindicated.

Although enteral feeding was found to enhance SIBO in dogs with EHBDO, the prerequisite for correction of biliary tree occlusion in patients makes this complication less important.[34,35] In patients with uncorrectable biliary occlusion (e.g., cats with intrahepatic ductopenia caused by chronic CCHS), chronic antimicrobial therapy may assist in protecting the patient against the complications induced by SIBO. Use of ursodeoxycholate will not solve this problem because this bile acid has limited physiologic influence on nutrient assimilation compared with the natural primary bile acids. Patients with active pancreatitis may require enteral feeding via a weighted jejunostomy tube or temporary support with total parenteral alimentation (TPN). Use of partial parenteral nutrition (PPN) or TPN may be necessary if vomiting is persistent despite administration of metoclopramide (0.2 to 0.4 mg/kg, subcutaneously or intramuscularly, every 8 hours or IV constant-infusion drip of 0.01 to 0.02 mg/kg/hr) or ondansetron (0.1 to 1.0 mg/kg every 12 to 24 hours). Although PPN can be given through a peripherally placed long-line catheter, its use is restricted to a 5- to 7-day interval. This interval may importantly limit the extent of lean body mass catabolism during the initial treatment phase. However, after the first week, transition to an enteral feeding method is recommended. TPN requires placement of a committed central catheter, is costly, requires close monitoring, increases the risk of iatrogenic hemorrhage and septicemia, and may result in enteric changes permissive to transmural microbial translocation. Therefore other modes of nutritional support are more practical, are associated with fewer iatrogenic effects, and are advised.

Caloric intake should achieve at least 70 to 90 Kcal/kg/day optimal body weight in cats and for dogs should at least meet values for resting energy requirements ($99 \times$ body weight $[kg]^{0.67}$, $70 \times$ body weight $[kg]^{0.75}$ or $30 +$ weight $[kg] + 70 \times$ body weight $[kg]$). Although adding an illness factor (a constant that estimates energy needs above resting energy requirements) is commonly recommended, these factors have been empirically devised (1.2 to 1.6 times resting energy requirements for illness).

Vitamins, Antioxidants, and Conditionally Essential Nutrients Water-soluble vitamins should be provided at a doubled conventional daily dose, whether the patient is eating or not, because they are necessary for intermediary metabolism. Antioxidants in the form of vitamin E and thiol donors (N-acetylcysteine, 140 mg/kg IV; dilute 10% solution 1:1 in saline, administer through a 0.2 mm filter; subsequent dosing at 70 mg/kg IV up to every 6 hours; or S-adenosylmethionine 20 mg/kg enteric-coated tablets on an empty stomach, orally, once a day) may be advantageous. This dosage has not been proven but is supported by disease modeling. Furthermore, research shows that spontaneous necroinflammatory and cholestatic liver disease in the dog and cat are associated with a risk of low hepatic glutathione (GSH) concentrations. (GSH is the major intracellular thiol antioxidant with pivotal importance in the liver, which provides GSH precursors for use elsewhere in the body.)[28] Supplementation with L-carnitine has been shown to facilitate hepatocellular regenerations in the circumstance of severe hepatotoxicity; in this capacity, increased facilitation of fatty acid oxidation may assist in cell recovery and repair.[29] Comparable studies in the dog and cat have not been undertaken, although L-carnitine has been proven to increase the metabolic utilization of fatty acids for energy production in healthy cats.[25]

Antibiotics

Antibiotics for hepatobiliary infections should possess relevant activity against enteric organisms commonly cultured from liver tissue and bile (see Tables 90-1 to 90-6).* Culture

*References: 3, 4, 9, 50, 145, 146, 160, 161.

and susceptibility of involved organisms remains the best measure for correct antibiotic selection. Cytologic evaluation of each sampled tissue and bile may importantly contribute to identification of infectious agents because a positive culture result may be denied by prior antibiotic therapy or mechanistic factors interfering in organism growth in vitro. Using a simple Wright-Giemsa's staining procedure, infectious organisms that are difficult to visualize on routinely prepared histologic specimens may be readily apparent. Bacterial mor-

†References: 3, 4, 9, 24, 50, 145, 146.

Table • 90-6

Achieved Biliary Concentrations of Certain Antimicrobial Agent in the Absence of Major Bile Duct Occlusion[a,3,107]

ANTIMICROBIAL AGENT	RATIO OF ANTIBIOTIC BILE/SERUM
Aminoglycosides	
Amikacin	0.3
Gentamicin	0.3—0.6
Kanamycin	1
Streptomycin	0.4—3.0
Cephalosporins	
Cefazolin (first generation)	0.3—3.0
Cephalothin (first generation)	2.2
Cefoxitin (second generation)	2.8
Ceftriaxone (third generation)	2—5
Penicillins	
Natural Penicillin	
Penicillin G	5.0
Penicillinase resistant	
Oxacillin	>1.0
Nafcillin	>100
Aminopenicillins	
Ampicillin	1.0—30
Amoxicillin	1—30
Amoxicillin, clavulanate	1—30
Antipseudomonal Penicillins	
Piperacillin	10—60
Mezlocillin	10—60
Ticarcillin	NA
Imipenem	Minor
Tetracyclines	
Tetracycline	2—32
Doxycycline	2—32
Miscellaneous	
Chloramphenicol	0.2—1
Clindamycin	2.5—3
Ciprofloxacin	2.8—4.5
Erythromycin	8—25
Metronidazole	1
Trimethoprim/sulfonamide	1—2/0.4—0.7
Vancomycin	0.5

[a]Data derived from experimental literature and from work in human beings.

phology, including Gram stain characteristics, assists in selecting the initial course of antimicrobial therapy (see Tables 90-2 to 90-4).[†] Satisfactory and clinically effective biliary excretion of many antibiotics is achieved in an unobstructed biliary system.[163,164] Although selection of an antimicrobial having good penetration into the biliary tract seems logical (Table 90-6),[145,170] the achieved systemic activity may be most important. Preventing bacteremic dissemination from the biliary tree to the systemic circulation requires that serum antimicrobial concentrations achieve effective plasma levels against involved microorganisms, especially aerobes. Antibiotics with good serum but poor biliary concentrations have proven efficacy in this scenario, preventing both systemic dispersal and infection of surgical wounds. Use of antibiotics achieving lower relative serum and yet good biliary levels may not afford comparable protection.[90] Such drugs may not achieve effective concentrations in bile in the face of cholestasis, particularly considering that the minimum inhibitory concentration of an antibiotic for a particular microorganism may be many fold higher in bile versus serum. Although antibiotic prophylaxis cannot likely prevent bacterial invasion in the face of bile stasis, antibiotics protecting against systemic infection are essential before surgical manipulations in which bacteremia, local trauma, and infection are unavoidable.[163] Although antibiotics administered during EHBDO do not attain therapeutic concentrations in bile because of the cessation of bile flow, it has been proven in animal models and humans with EHBDO that achieving a critical therapeutic plasma concentrations of an effective antimicrobial before surgical manipulations protects against septicemia and endotoxemia. To eradicate biliary tree infection in EHBDO successfully, bile flow must be reinstated by removing the obstruction or by creating a biliary-enteric anastomosis. This augments removal of infectious organisms by the responsive choleresis concurrent with delivery of the antimicrobial into the biliary compartment. Immunocompromised patients and those with uncorrectable diffuse disease involving the intrahepatic biliary tree (e.g., certain cats with cholangitis causing destruction of small to medium sized bile ducts) will maintain a chronic predisposition for hepatobiliary infection.

In the absence of culture and susceptibility, or morphologic features of involved organisms, antimicrobial treatments should cover aerobic and anaerobic enteric opportunists. A combination of drugs is required. β-lactamase–resistant penicillin, clindamycin, or metronidazole is given IV as a good first-choice antibiotic for anaerobic organisms. The dose of clindamycin and metronidazole is adjusted for cholestasis and severe hepatic dysfunction; see later discussion. One of these drugs is used in combination with either an aminoglycoside or a fluorinated quinolone (e.g., enrofloxacin, orbifloxacin) to achieve efficacy against aerobic gram-negative organisms. Aminoglycosides should not be given until the patient's hydration status and prerenal azotemia are corrected. Aminoglycoside nephrotoxicity should be monitored by examining urine sediment for granular casts on at least an alternate-day schedule.

Antibiotics that require extensive hepatobiliary activation, biotransformation, or excretion or those that have been associated with adverse effects on the hepatobiliary system are considered poor first-choice selections when liver function is compromised. These drugs include hetacillin, tetracycline, doxycycline, lincomycin, erythromycin, sulfonamides, trimethoprim-sulfonamide, and chloramphenicol. Severe jaundice argues against using antibiotics excreted predominantly in bile and that undergo enterohepatic circulation; examples include chloramphenicol, erythromycin, doxycycline, rifampin, clindamycin, and nafcillin. Use of such drugs in the face of reduced liver function, especially overt jaundice, necessitates reduction of conventional dosing usually by as

Table • 90-7

Influence of Hepatic Disease on Disposition of Selected Antimicrobials in Humans with Severe Hepatic Disease, Insufficiency[3,9]

ANTIBACTERIALS	PLASMA CLEARANCE	VOLUME OF DISTRIBUTION	HALF-LIFE
Amikacin	–	↑ 200%	No change
Ampicillin	No change	↑ 46%–200%	↑ 30%–45%
Carbenicillin	–	–	↑ 90%
Cefoperazone	↓ 0–40%	↑ 150%	↑ 200%
Cefotaxime	↓ 30%–40%	–	Increased
Chloramphenicol	↓ 65%–70%	↓ 20%	↑ 130%–150%
Clindamycin	↓ 25%–60%	↓ 40%	↑ 15%–40%
Erythromycin	↓ 30%	↑ 50%	↑ 60%–65%
Gentamicin	–	No change	↑ 85%
Metronidazole	No change	No change	↑ 40%–150%
Mezlocillin	↓ 50%	–	↑ 170%
Norfloxacin	No change	–	No change
Pefloxacin	↓ 70%	↓ 20%	↑ 255%
Vancomycin	↓ 70%	No change	↑ 130%

much as 50% (Table 90-7).[3,9] Consultation with a comprehensive pharmaceutical reference is recommended before adjusting drug doses.[4,146] Tetracyclines are best avoided unless specific therapy is indicated (e.g., rickettsial infections, clearing leptospirosis) because of their inhibitory influence on egress of triglycerides from the hepatocyte (promotes hepatic lipid accumulation in all species studied) and because tetracyclines have experimentally induced hepatic encephalopathy in dogs with portosystemic shunts. When circumstances warrant using *contraindicated* drugs, Table 90-6 should be consulted for cases in which recommendations have been derived from multiple references pertinent to humans, considering the lack of information for animals.

Prophylactic treatment with a best-guess antimicrobial combination is recommended for biliary obstruction and known or suspected bacterial infection, both before and during surgery. Given that this approach diminishes the ability to culture involved organisms from surgical specimens, presurgical hepatic-bile aspiration and preparation of bile and tissue imprints for cytologic evaluation (including Gram staining) becomes imperative. Antibiotic administration is necessary until biliary tree obstruction and cholestasis have been eliminated (e.g., when EHBDO or specific infection of the biliary tree has been resolved) or may be continued as part of chronic medical therapy.

Bacterial enteric translocation is known to be reduced by long-term administration of antibiotics suppressing aerobic intestinal flora. In humans, fluorinated quinolones are used most often for this purpose in cirrhosis. Predisposition to enteric bacterial translocation during surgery (e.g., cholestasis, chronic liver disease) is also diminished in humans by orally administered neomycin, fluoroquinolones, polymyxin B, or tobramycin. This effect has not been studied in veterinary patients.

Probiotics and Nondigestible Carbohydrates

An alternative nonantibiotic approach, *microbial interference therapy*, is receiving greater attention in human medicine owing to the increasing appearance of antibiotic-resistant enteric microorganisms. Such therapy involves maintaining or restoring health by introducing live nonpathogenic microorganisms from a probiotic to ostensibly *stabilize* the balance of intestinal flora. This concept is based on experimental work indicating that certain probiotics can reduce intestinal bacte-

rial overgrowth, improve local immunologic host defenses, increase enteric and splanchnic neutrophil phagocytic function, inhibit enterovirulence of natural gut microbes, and reduce enteric bacterial translocation (modeled in rodents). Consequently, probiotics are claimed to reduce the risk of spontaneous infection in patients with chronic liver disease associated with portal hypertension, ascites, and cholestasis.

Bacteria considered host beneficial include bifidobacteria, eubacteria, and lactobacilli; and when these are combined with a fermented carbohydrate, they are referred to as *liver probiotics*. Whether they provide a reliable benefit remains controversial. Lactobacilli are considered an integral part of normal enteric microecology and have received the greatest investigation. These organisms have been capitalized on for their demonstrated effects on local enteric flora, immune response, and host metabolism. Adherence of lactobacilli to enterocyte receptors can induce expression of genes coding for variants of intestinal mucins that inhibit adherence of enteropathogens (e.g., *E. coli*).[105] They also produce antimicrobial effects through production of bacteriocin and metabolic end products, demonstrated in animals and humans. However, an important point to recognize is that different lactic acid bacterial strains have very different probiotic effects such that results obtained with a single strain cannot be universally expected for all others. Although use of probiotics to reduce opportunistic gram-negative and anaerobic enteric microorganisms is widely proposed, benefits remain controversial, and a risk of probiotic organisms achieving opportunistic hepatic or systemic infections exists.[136,148]

Experimental evidence and limited information in humans with liver disease suggest that certain probiotics may have a prophylactic and therapeutic effect on hepatic encephalopathy and predisposition of patients with acute hepatic failure or necrosis to endotoxemia or sepsis. They also may beneficially modulate enteric inflammation co-existent with liver disease. Nondigestible carbohydrates that serve as fermentable microbial energy substrates are commonly used to ameliorate clinical signs of hepatic encephalopathy. These substances encourage bacterial nitrogen fixation, acidify the colonic lumen, modulate mucosal and microbial protease activity, and produce a cathartic effect (from osmotic solute production) useful for controlling SIBO and eliminating enteric toxins and ammonia, contributing to hepatic encephalopathy. They may also ameliorate endotoxemia through modifying the enteric microbial ecosystem, reducing the enteric bacterial pool size, or through a direct antiendotoxic effect.[37,103,149] In this regard, lactulose is the prototype nondigestible carbohydrate.[45] Oral or rectal administration of lactulose has been proposed as an alternative means of modulating bowel flora, which may reduce postoperative sepsis. Probiotics combining the benefit of a poorly digested carbohydrate (by the mammalian host) and a *beneficial* microbial organism also are available. Many of these probiotics *likely* provide a variety of effects, but none have proven efficacy.[37] Based on experimental work, combined administration of a probiotic and antioxidants may significantly alter pathologic changes, encouraging enteric bacterial translocation, by altering the concentration of enterobacteria and enterococci in the lower bowel, reducing peroxidative bowel wall damage, and reducing endotoxin translocation. Increased intestinal oxidative damage and bacterial translocation are observed in rats with prehepatic portal hypertension and EHBDO. Oxidative bowel damage is associated with slow enteric transit time in several experimental models and has been implicated as a cause of SIBO in cirrhotic humans.[30,130] Proclivity for enteric bacterial translocation (using this model) is reduced with a variety of antioxidants, including vitamin C, vitamin E, allopurinol (50 mg/kg twice weekly), and glutamine (1 gm/kg per day) as a means of promoting enterocyte metabolism and cell size.[32,150,151]

Surgery

Laparotomy may be required to alleviate the source of hepatobiliary sepsis. Surgical intervention becomes imperative when hepatobiliary abscesses cannot be effectively managed by US-guided drainage and antimicrobial therapy and in the circumstances of septic peritonitis, bile peritonitis, or major bile duct occlusion. Hepatic or bile aspirate or biopsy is the only definitive method of confirming an infectious process. Biopsy of the liver and involved biliary structures is required for definitive diagnosis of underlying disease. At surgery, the abdominal viscera should be inspected for a primary disease process. Mesenteric and hepatic lymph nodes should be visualized and biopsy specimens taken for histologic evaluation and culture, especially if a primary diagnosis remains uncertain. Liver specimens from one or more sites should be sampled to ascertain disease local to the obvious disease process and to determine whether diffuse liver disease preceded or evolved from the current condition. If entire lobes of liver appear involved in an abscess or appear necrotic, they should be resected. Infarcted or devitalized areas should be manipulated minimally before resection. Venous outflow from such tissue should be ligated as early in resection as possible to avoid systemic dispersal of noxious substances (e.g., endotoxin, bacterial products, infectious organisms). The biliary tract should be evaluated for patency by gentle compression of the gallbladder and bile fluidity and flow determined. The gallbladder and major bile ducts should be carefully palpated for choleliths, intraluminal or mural masses, and sludged bile. If abnormalities are detected, a cholecystotomy should be done, a biopsy of the gallbladder taken, and any abnormalities inspected and removed. Biliary mucocele requires gallbladder resection and removal of tenacious bile from the cystic and major bile ducts. Extrahepatic bile ducts should be flushed with sterile saline using a soft catheter to remove choleliths and sludged bile, taking care to avoid peritoneal contamination. In some cases, sludged bile may require mechanical removal using forceps or a curette. Cholecystectomy is necessary if the gallbladder wall appears devitalized or involves a suspected neoplasm.

Samples of tissue and bile should be cultured for aerobic and anaerobic organisms. Bile for culture and cytology should be collected by fine-needle (22-gauge) aspiration into a syringe. The needle should enter the gallbladder at an oblique angle to reduce postaspiration bile leakage. Using a large syringe and aspirating the entire volume of bile minimizes postaspiration bile leakage. If cholecystitis or cholangitis is suspected, biopsy and culture of a portion of the gallbladder wall and liver increases the chance of identifying the infectious agent. Choleliths also should be submitted for culture.

Cytologic smears should be made from each tissue biopsied and from bile to permit morphologic characterization of infectious agents and to achieve early recognition of neoplasia. Strict attention must be paid to the methods of handling and transporting specimens for anaerobic bacterial cultures (see Chapter 33). Gram staining of tissue and bile imprints guides selection of initial antibacterial therapy. Cytologic evaluation serves as an important quality control indicator of transport and culture procedures. If organisms are identified on smears made at surgery and yet are not grown, transport or culture methods were probably inadequate unless antimicrobial therapy is a complicating factor. If trematode infection is possible, bile and feces should be examined cytologically for trematode eggs. Hepatic tissue should always be submitted for routine histologic evaluation, and the pathologist should be prompted to examine tissues for infectious agents with special stains.

Hydrocholeresis

After establishing patency of the biliary tract, hydrocholeresis can improve bile flow in patients with resolved extrahepatic cholestasis, cholelithiasis, or inspissated bile. Hydrocholeresis also improves mechanical removal of infectious organisms involved in diffuse septic cholangitis. Resolution of bile stasis assists in clearing biliary infection and reduces the potential for further stone formation. Ursodeoxycholic acid (see Table 90-5) is used as a long-term therapeutic agent in patients with persistent cholestatic liver injury. Choleresis is provided in conjunction with maintaining adequate patient hydration, which optimizes the hydrocholeretic response. In addition to choleresis, ursodeoxycholic acid also provides a large number of advantageous effects beneficial to chronic cholestatic and necroinflammatory liver disorders (i.e., it has immunomodulatory, cytoprotective effects for the hepatocyte and biliary epithelium, a choleretic influence, antiendotoxic, antioxidant, and antifibrotic effects, and importantly, attenuates accumulation of membranocytolytic bile acids in bile, hepatic tissue, and plasma).

SUGGESTED READINGS*

39. Cole TL, Center SA, Flood SN, et al. 2002. Diagnostic comparison of needle and wedge biopsy specimens of the liver in dogs and cats, *J Am Vet Med Assoc* 220:1483-1490.
53. Eich CS, Ludwig LL. 2002. The surgical treatment of cholelithiasis in cats: a study of nine cases, *J Am Anim Hosp Assoc* 38:290-296.
96. Konno K, Ishida H, Naganuma H, et al. 2002. Emphysematous cholecystitis: sonographic findings, *Abdom Imaging* 27:191-195.
111. Mayhew PD, Holt DE, McLear RC, et al. 2002. Pathogenesis and outcome of extrahepatic biliary obstruction in cats, *J Small Anim Pract* 43:247-253.
127. Owens SD, Gossett R, McElhaney MR, et al. 2003. Three cases of canine bile peritonitis with mucinous material in abdominal fluid as the prominent cytologic finding, *Vet Clin Pathol* 32(3):114-120.

*See the CD-ROM for a complete list of references.

147. Savary-Bataille KC, Bunch SE, Spaulding KA, et al. 2003. Percutaneous ultrasound-guided cholecystocentesis in healthy cats, *J Vet Intern Med* 17(3):298-303.

159. Sterczer A, Gaál T, Perge E, et al. 2001. Chronic hepatitis in the dog—a review, *Vet Q* 23:148-152.

177. Vörös K, Sterczer A, Manczur E, et al. 2002. Percutaneous ultrasound-guided cholecystocentesis in dogs, *Acta Vet Hung* 50(4):385-393.

179. Watson PJ. 2004. Chronic hepatitis in dogs: a review of current understanding of the etiology, progression, and treatment, *Vet J* 167(3):228-241.

CHAPTER • 91

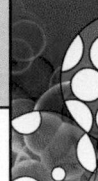

Genitourinary Infections

Jeanne A. Barsanti

Bacterial infections of the urogenital system are among the most frequently encountered infections in small animal practice. Urinary tract and genital infections can occur separately or concomitantly. Infections range in severity from asymptomatic to life threatening. *Escherichia coli* is the most common agent associated with these infections. Infections with other types of organisms, especially fungi, are found but are much rarer than those caused by bacteria.

NORMAL FLORA

The vagina, vestibule, prepuce, and distal urethra have a normal microflora. The clinical importance of this microflora is twofold: first, it must be considered when the results of cultures of urine, semen, and preputial and vaginal discharges are interpreted; second, the normal microflora is thought to be an important factor in host defense against pathogenic organisms. The oral and anal flora of neonatal puppies correlate with the flora from the milk, vagina, and oral cavity of their dams. The flora of puppies from different dams vary with the dam.[183]

Bacteria are not normally found in the upper urinary tract, bladder, proximal urethra, or prostate gland.[16,108] Bacteria are not normally found in the uterus, except during proestrus and estrus.[46,59,275]

Dogs

In healthy male dogs, commensal organisms cultured from the distal urethra and prepuce include gram-positive and gram-negative organisms (Tables 91-1 and 91-2).[14] Mycoplasmas are found in the distal urethra and the prepuce and have also been isolated from the canine prostate. When sampling the prepuce, usually more than one organism is recovered; however, only a single species is obtained in about 20% of preputial and semen samples.[37] The prostatic fraction of a cleanly collected ejaculate from healthy, fertile stud dogs is usually sterile (70% of samples).[37]

The normal flora of the vagina includes the same types of bacteria (Table 91-3).[14,36,183] Aerobic and anaerobic organisms live in the vagina normally.[183] Although the same types of organisms are found throughout the vagina, the nearer they are to the cervix, the lower the number of organisms.[200] Two or more bacterial species are usually recovered from vaginal cultures; however, 18% of vaginal cultures from healthy bitches contain only one organism, and repeated cultures from most dogs yield a pure culture on at least one occasion.[36]

Mycoplasmas can also be isolated from the vagina of healthy bitches.[36,61,162] Changes in the microflora occur with stages of the estrous cycle, but the change is primarily in the frequency of organism isolation rather than the type of organism found.[36] Few changes are associated with neutering.[107,162,200] *Staphylococcus* species have been isolated more frequently from prepuberal and postpartum bitches than from postestrual bitches.[36,200] The same organisms are found in the uterus during proestrus and estrus as are found in the vagina, with the exception that mycoplasmas were not found in the uterus.[275]

Treatment with either ampicillin or trimethoprim-sulfamethoxazole altered the normal microflora of the vagina in healthy bitches.[254] The normal microflora was suppressed in only two of five ampicillin-treated dogs. In three ampicillin-treated dogs and in all dogs treated with trimethoprim-sulfamethoxazole, bacteria sensitive to the antimicrobial tended to be eradicated, whereas resistant bacteria remained or appeared. Thus the use of these antimicrobial agents to "sterilize" the vagina before mating is irrational and ineffective. Commensal bacteria are occasionally transferred between dog and bitch during mating.[36,37] This transfer does not affect the fertility of either the male or the female.

Cats

Aerobic bacteria are those most commonly isolated from the vagina of healthy intact female cats (Table 91-4). *E. coli*, staphylococci, and streptococci are most common.[110] Anaerobic bacteria are rarely isolated from the vagina.[110] Pure growth of a single organism was common in normal cats and should not be considered indicative of disease when cytology is normal.[110] Vaginal cultures from normal cats can be negative.[110] The bacterial population of the vaginas of cats was not influenced by mating or administration of progestins.[110] Relative numbers of vaginal organisms were greater in young cats (younger than 1 year) and pregnant cats.[46] Although one study showed more profuse growth from cats in estrus,[16] another study showed no effect of estrus on number of bacteria, but an effect was found on type of bacteria, with estral cats having more bacteria that belonged to the family Pasteurellaceae.[110] Although one study found bacteria in 2 of 29 uterine cultures, both from cats in estrus,[46] a more recent study found no bacteria in the uterus of 66 adult female cats, nine of which were in estrus.[110]

Aerobic bacteria are those most commonly found in the prepuce of intact male cats (Table 91-5) with Pasteurellaceae,

Table • 91-1

Bacteria Isolated from the Distal Urethra of Clinically Healthy Male Dogs[20]

Staphylococcus intermedius
Staphylococcus epidermidis
Corynebacterium spp.
Escherichia coli
Flavobacterium spp.
Haemophilus spp.
Klebsiella spp.
Streptococcus canis
Streptococcus viridans
Mycoplasma spp.
Ureaplasma spp.

Table • 91-2

Bacteria Isolated from the Prepuce of Clinically Healthy Male Dogs[14,37,162]

Staphylococcus intermedius
Staphylococcus epidermidis
Corynebacterium spp.
Escherichia coli
Flavobacterium spp.
Haemophilus spp.
Klebsiella spp.
Moraxella spp.
Acinetobacter spp.
Mycoplasma spp.
Ureaplasma spp.
Proteus spp.
Pasturella spp.
Bacillus spp.
Streptococcus spp.
Streptococcus equisimilis
Streptococcus canis
Streptococcus viridans
Streptococcus faecalis
Enterococcus spp.
Pseudomonas spp.

Table • 91-3

Bacteria Isolated from the Vagina of Clinically Healthy Bitches[14,36,107,183,254]

Staphylococcus intermedius
Staphylococcus epidermidis
Streptococcus viridans
Streptococcus canis
Streptococcus faecalis
Enterococcus spp.
Streptococcus zooepidemicus
Streptococcus spp.
Escherichia coli
Pasteurella spp.
Proteus spp.
Haemophilus spp.
Acinetobacter spp.
Prevotella spp.
Clostridium spp.
Moraxella spp.
Micrococcus spp.
Neisseria spp.
Bacteroides spp.
Bacillus spp.
Enterobacter spp.
Klebsiella spp.
Flavobacterium spp.
Citrobacter spp.
Mycoplasma spp.
Ureaplasma spp.
Corynebacterium spp.
Pseudomonas spp.
Fusobacterium spp.
Peptostreptococcus spp.

Table • 91-4

Bacteria Isolated from the Vagina of Clinically Healthy Queens[16,110]

Escherichia coli
Staphylococcus spp.
Streptococcus spp.
Pasteurellaceae family members
Bacteroides spp.
Lactobacillus spp.
Corynebacterium spp.
Haemophilus spp.

E. coli, staphylococci, and streptococci being most common.[110] In contrast to female cats, anaerobic bacteria were isolated from 41% of male cats.[110] Anaerobic species were Bacteroides spp., Fusobacterium spp., and anaerobic streptococci. The mean number of bacterial spp. isolated from the prepuce of male cats was 1.8 per cat, compared with 1.1 per cat in vaginal samples.[110] Pure cultures from the prepuce were uncommon, and negative culture results were not found.[110]

URINARY TRACT INFECTIONS

Etiology

Urinary tract infection (UTI) refers to microbial colonization of the urine or of any urinary tract organ, except the distal urethra, which has a normal bacterial flora. Infection of the urinary tract may affect more than one organ or may be local-ized to the upper tract (kidney and adjacent ureter; bacterial pyelonephritis) or to the lower tract (bladder and adjacent urethra; bacterial cystitis; bacterial urethrocystitis). Infections of the lower urinary tract in intact male dogs are considered to concomitantly affect the prostate gland (bacterial prostati-tis). Infection of one part of the urinary tract increases the likelihood that the rest of the tract will become infected.[188,189]

It has been estimated that 14% of all dogs develop a UTI during their lifetime.[156] Bacterial UTIs are most common in female spayed dogs, followed by male castrated dogs and

Table • 91-5

Bacteria Isolated from the Prepuce of Clinically Healthy Male Cats[110]

Escherichia coli
Staphyloccus spp.
Pasteurellaceae family members
Streptococcus spp.
Corynebacterium spp.
Simonsiella spp.
Moraxella or Brahamella spp.
Bacteroides spp.
Fusobacterium spp.

Table • 91-6

Major Host Defenses Against Urinary Tract Infection[205]

Normal micturition
Normal anatomy
Intact mucosal defense
Surface glycosaminoglycans
Cell exfoliation
Normal microflora
Local antibody production
Epithelial cell antimicrobial properties
Antimicrobial properties of urine
Hyperosmolality concentration
Tamm-Horsfall mucoprotein
Systemic immunocompetence

intact female dogs.[47] In dogs, UTIs are least common in intact males.[47] In a large study over a long period, 3.9% of female dogs and 2.9% of male dogs examined in one teaching hospital had positive urine culture results, although some dogs had their urine cultured only if the urinalysis was abnormal, which would lower the infection rate because some dogs with a UTI documented by culture have normal urinalyses.[161] Infection rate in 85 asymptomatic, adult, intact male dogs was 9%.[38] Half of these dogs had the same organism isolated by direct aspiration of small prostatic cysts.[38]

More than 70% of UTIs in dogs are caused by a single bacterial species.[161] In complicated infections secondary to anatomic or functional abnormalities of the urinary tract, infection with multiple organisms becomes more likely. The most common gram-negative organisms are E. coli, Proteus, Klebsiella, Pseudomonas, and Enterobacter. E. coli is by far the most common urinary tract pathogen, causing 37% to 45% of UTIs.[47,161,215,243a] In fact, most E. coli infections in dogs involve the urinary tract.[201] Certain E. coli isolates from canine UTIs are indistinguishable from certain human extraintestinal E. coli infections, even using highly sensitive typing methods.[128] In comparison with human urinary isolates, canine E. coli were more likely to be antibiotic resistant and to have a higher R-plasmid transmissibility rate.[195] Gram-positive organisms (Staphylococcus, Streptococcus, Enterococcus) account for 25% to 30% of naturally occurring UTIs.[47,161,215,285] Infection with Staphylococcus or Proteus is often associated with struvite calculi because of alkalinization of the urine by the organisms' metabolism of urea. Urinary tract infections due to methicellin-resistant Staphylococcus aureus have been reported and are of concern to human public health.[275a] The most common eight species just listed account for 93% of all UTIs.[161] Although mycoplasmas have been reported as causes of UTIs in dogs, their significance remains obscure because most of the reported cases were complicated by multiple disease processes.[118] In the largest study of UTIs in dogs, 35 bacterial genera and 4 species of fungi were identified as causing UTIs.[161] Occasionally, cases involving more unusual bacterial organisms are reported, such as Arcanobacterium (Actinomyces) pyogenes,[34,161] Corynebacterium urealyticum,[161,255] and Clostridium species.[87,161]

UTIs are less common in cats than in dogs. Numerous studies have shown that young adult cats having signs of lower urinary tract problems (dysuria with hematuria) rarely have bacterial UTIs.[19,142] However, bacterial UTIs may develop secondary to urinary catheterization or urinary tract surgery, such as perineal urethrostomy, in cats with urethral obstruction.[18,56,91] UTIs are more common in cats older than 10 years.[23] When bacterial infection occurs in cats, the organisms most frequently involved are the same as those in dogs, except Pasteurella organisms are more commonly reported in cats.[285]

Viruses and mycoplasmas have been considered as potential causes of lower urinary tract signs in cats. Investigators have been unable to find evidence of viral infections in clinical cases, and experimental viral infections have not induced clinical signs in cats.[139-141] Mycoplasma felis and Mycoplasma gateae could not survive in osmotic conditions present in normal feline urine, although a Ureaplasma species could.[41] However, ureaplasmas were not isolated from any cats with signs of lower urinary tract diseases.[142]

Yeast and fungi in urine can indicate contamination of the sample. However, fungi in properly collected (cystocentesis) and promptly examined urine samples are abnormal. A positive culture of urine collected by cystocentesis is needed to confirm the diagnosis of a fungal UTI. Fungal UTIs caused by Trichosporon domesticum, Candida species, or Aspergillus species usually have been associated with abnormalities in host defenses, antibiotic usage, and urogenital diseases.[2,216,233] Systemic mycotic agents (e.g., Blastomyces, Cryptococcus) may be found in urine in animals with systemic infections caused by these organisms and may cause UTIs.[191]

Pathogenesis

UTIs are usually caused by bacterial organisms that are constituents of the microflora of the intestinal or lower urogenital tracts. Dogs with a UTI associated with E. coli or Proteus mirabilis were likely to carry the same organism in their intestinal tracts and prepuce or vagina.[84,128,166] The usual method of infection of the bladder involves organisms ascending the urethra.[247] Pyelonephritis is believed to be most commonly caused by ascending infection from bladder urine. The renal cortex is much more resistant to infection than the renal medulla, decreasing the likelihood of hematogenous infection.[174,236]

Development of a UTI indicates an alteration in the host and bacterial flora relationship.[205] To accomplish infection, bacteria must attach to and colonize the mucosa of the urethral orifice and transport themselves up the urethra, adhering to the uroepithelium. Both host defense mechanisms and bacterial virulence properties are important in determining whether infection occurs, as well as which part of the urinary tract is affected (Table 91-6).

Host Factors

The inflammatory response in a UTI involves three steps: the bacteria stimulate uroepithelial cells to produce inflammatory mediators, these mediators direct inflammatory cells to the site of infection, and the local inflammatory response determines if the infection is eliminated or if tissue damage results. Thus the host response is important in determining the degree of clinical signs and severity of tissue injury.[257] Neutrophils that migrate from blood vessels through tissue and cross the epithelial cell layer to enter the urinary space result in pyuria. In humans, as in dogs and cats, many UTIs are asymptomatic and not accompanied by pyuria. Such occult infections are associated with diabetes mellitus and hyperadrenocorticism in dogs but occur in dogs and cats without these diseases as well. The reasons for this are not understood, but one idea in humans is that these affected individuals are genetically different from those that develop symptomatic infections in regard to their host response.[257] The genetic characteristics of a host organism have also been investigated in relation to susceptibility to UTIs and may be important in pathogenesis in some populations.[81,236,257] For example, the vaginal epithelial cells of women with recurrent UTIs demonstrate more bacterial adherence in vitro than epithelial cells from women without UTIs.[236]

Important host factors in resistance to infection are normal, frequent emptying of the urinary bladder, the presence of the normal flora, the age and sex of the host, characteristics of urine, and normal urinary tract anatomy, including normal urinary tract epithelium with its glycoprotein coat, and immunologic responses.[196,236] The importance of host factors is shown by the fact that many E. coli isolated from canine UTI have no detectable urovirulence factors.[65]

Structural, functional, or metabolic abnormalities predispose to UTIs (Table 91-7).[193,236] Such abnormalities include obstructive lesions; metabolic diseases such as diabetes mellitus, hyperadrenocorticism, and renal failure; instrumentation or catheterization or abnormal voiding, particularly with neurologic diseases; and anatomic abnormalities. UTIs have been found in more than 40% of dogs with hyperadrenocorticism and 40% of dogs with diabetes mellitus.[74] Lower urinary tract obstruction with secondary vesicoureteral reflux of infected urine is a contributing factor to the development of pyelonephritis, as are anatomic abnormalities such as ectopic ureters.[237] Approximately 17% of dogs with ectopic ureters were found to have pyelonephritis.[111] Other anatomic abnormalities associated with a chronic UTI include persistent urachus, other bladder diverticuli, perivulvar dermatitis, a recessed vulva, and vestibulovaginal stenosis.[155,165] A study found that surgical therapy for a recessed vulva was unsuccessful in resolving a UTI if severe vestibulovaginal stenosis (defined as a ratio of less than 0.2 between the height of the vestibulovaginal junction to the maximal height of the vagina on a lateral positive-contrast cystourethrovaginographic view) was present.[51]

Bacteria adhere poorly to normal bladder epithelium because of the presence of a glycosaminoglycan coating.[51] This coating, which can be replaced within 24 hours if injured, is extremely hydrophilic, so a layer of water forms at the surface. This aqueous layer provides a barrier between the transitional epithelium and the urine, explaining in part why bladder epithelium can tolerate constant exposure to a substance as irritating as urine. Infection is more likely to occur if this surface coating is damaged as by uroliths, neoplastic transformation, or exposures to chemical irritants such as cytoxan. The kidney has no natural barrier against bacterial adherence.[236]

Bladder epithelial cells exfoliate in response to infection and are cleared with the flow of urine, an important defense mechanism. The bladder epithelium normally has a slow turnover rate of approximately 40 weeks in humans and mice.[181] In humans with a UTI, large numbers of exfoliated bladder epithelial cells are often found.[181] Although this exfoliation is considered a host defense mechanism, it is also a way for bacteria to be spread into the environment and may also expose underlying epithelial cells to infection. This might allow bacteria to enter a more sheltered environment where they could persist. It has been shown in mice that uropathogenic E. coli can survive in low levels in bladder tissue for weeks to months in a quiescent state, protected from antimicrobial therapy.[181]

The antibacterial effects of urine include osmolality, urea concentration, and organic acid concentration.[236] Variations in pH (with urine being markedly acidic, having a pH of 5) and specific gravity (with urine being markedly concentrated) have an inhibitory effect on bacterial growth. The ability of cats to highly concentrate their urine may be one explanation for the low incidence of bacterial UTIs in young cats. Urine that is less acidic and not well concentrated supports multiplication of urinary tract pathogens almost as well as nutrient broth.[133]

Specific serum and urine antibody responses accompany acute pyelonephritis in experimental models. These antibodies can be synthesized locally within the kidney and may enhance bacterial opsonization and ingestion by phagocytic

Table • 91-7

Terms Used to Categorize Urinary Tract Infections

BY LOCATION
Pyelonephritis: Kidney
Cystitis: Bladder
Urethritis: Urethra
Prostatitis: Prostate

BY COMPLEXITY
Simple-uncomplicated: No underlying structural or functional abnormality is suspected or found
Complicated: Infection associated with structural or functional abnormalities within the urinary tract or with impaired immunocompetence:
  Urinary obstruction
  Incomplete bladder emptying
  Anatomic abnormalities
    Congenital (urachal diverticula, ectopic ureters, vestibulovaginal stenosis)
    Acquired (excessive perivulvar skin-folds)
  Surgical diversion procedures
  Urolithiasis
  Indwelling urinary catheters
  Neoplasia, polyps
  Cytotoxic drugs (cyclophosphamide)
  Hyperadrenocorticism or glucocorticoid therapy
  Diabetes mellitus
  Renal failure

BY RESPONSE TO THERAPY
Persistent: Bacteriuria with the same organism that continues during therapy with appropriate antimicrobial agents
Relapsing: Infection with the same microorganism that recurs within several weeks of cessation of antimicrobial therapy
Reinfection: Infection with initial microorganism that responds to therapy but is then followed by infection by a different organism weeks to months after cessation of therapy
Superinfection: Infection with new organisms that develops during therapy for the initial infecting organism; usually associated with an indwelling catheter, severe anatomic abnormalities, or surgical diversion techniques

cells; however, their importance is debated.[236] The role of urinary immunoglobulins in preventing infection of the bladder is even more unclear.[236] The urinary tract mucosa produces secretory IgA, which is thought to have a role against the entry of pathogens—probably by interfering with bacterial adherence, although absence of its production does not lead to increased UTI susceptibility.[264] Evidence is lacking for a protective role for cell-mediated immunity in UTIs.[236]

It is clear from UTI research that minor weaknesses in host defenses necessitate more virulent organisms to induce disease. Normal host defenses clear some infections spontaneously, and some require minimal antimicrobial therapy. The more severe the host defense abnormality, the more prone the host is to infection, even with less virulent organisms, and to severe infections that require precise and extensive therapy.[236]

Bacterial Virulence Factors

Uropathogenic *E. coli* are a genetically heterogeneous group of *E. coli* that differ from nonpathogenic *E. coli* by the presence of virulence genes.[181] It has been found that uropathogenic *E. coli* typically carry large blocks of genes called pathogenicity-associated islands (PAIs), which are not found in fecal isolates.[95] PAIs code for virulence factors such as hemolysin, adhesins, iron acquisition systems, fimbriae, and toxins.[95] The presence of PAIs allows virulence genes to be easily spread among bacterial populations by horizontal gene transfer.[196]

The type of virulence genes present in a certain strain appears to determine the site of infection (lower versus upper tract) and the severity of the infection.[196] One genetic type of uropathogenic *E. coli* can change virulence properties depending on host response during infection.[181] Current studies are attempting to determine whether *E. coli* isolates that cause cystitis are distinct from those that cause pyelonephritis in genetic profiles or whether the host response determines the way the genes operate.[95] *E. coli* from UTIs in dogs have been found to have varying propensities to cause pyelonephritis and renal damage in mice based on urovirulence factors.[289] Even though bacterial virulence factors are very important, the severity of the tissue injury also depends on the inflammatory reaction of the host.

Uropathogenic *E. coli* are usually thought of as extracellular pathogens because they are cultured from the urine. Observations have found that these organisms are not always extracellular.[238] Piliated type 1 *E. coli* are able to enter bladder epithelial cells. Usually, this triggers the epithelial cell to undergo apoptosis and exfoliate. However, some *E. coli* seem to be able to persist intracellularly in some hosts by moving to other superficial cells or deeper epithelial cells.[181,238] Thus infection can persist even though bladder urine is sterilized by antimicrobial therapy. Many recurrent infections are relapses with the same bacterial strains. The ability of *E. coli* to persist intracellularly is a possible explanation for some cases of recurring UTIs.[238]

Catheter-Induced Urinary Tract Infections

One important iatrogenic cause for UTIs is urinary tract catheterization. Bacteria, especially *E. coli* and *Klebsiella*, establish periurethral colonization, and these bacteria are inoculated into the bladder during intermittent catheterization.[239] Even a single catheterization can cause a UTI in female dogs.[51] In people, the risk of a UTI with intermittent catheterization is 1% to 3% per insertion, so if a catheter must be inserted several times a day, most people become infected after a few weeks.[232] Risk of infection is greater if the catheter is left in place (indwelling).[15,51,163,232] Bacteria can readily ascend either around or through the catheter. Closed, sterile systems can prevent bacterial access within the catheter lumen, which is the most rapid route of entry, but no method

to date has effectively prevented access up the extraluminal side of the catheter.[192,224,226]

Biofilm formation on the catheter is important in the development of infection when catheters are indwelling. Certain uropathogenic *E. coli* can promote biofilm formation on abiotic surfaces.[196] Biofilms consist of host materials including Tamm-Horsfall protein and crystals and bacterial products including bacterial polysaccharides, bacterial glycocalyces, and living bacteria.[58,252] A biofilm can be deposited within hours of catheter insertion.[58] Bacteria embedded in the biofilm are less susceptible to antimicrobial agents. Once infections become established on a urinary catheter, they are difficult to treat successfully, and the catheter must be removed.

Consequences of bacteriuria arising from indwelling catheterization include pyelonephritis, bacteremia, prostatitis, and epididymitis. Of people with catheter-associated UTIs, 1% to 4% developed bacteremia, and fatality rates as a result varied from 13% to 30%, depending on the study.[58] The risk factors for UTI-related bacteremia in people are unclear.[232] Many catheter-induced infections are asymptomatic. In one study in children, *E. coli* caused the majority of symptomatic infections.[239] Interestingly, the same *E. coli* clones were associated with symptomatic and asymptomatic infections.[239]

Clinical Findings

Asymptomatic Bacteriuria

UTIs in dogs and cats are often asymptomatic.[157] For example, 95% of dogs with diabetes mellitus or hyperadrenocorticism and a UTI had no UTI symptoms.[74] Because of the lack of historical and physical signs, such infections are difficult to localize to the upper or lower urinary tract. In one study, 6 of 12 clinically nonsymptomatic female dogs with UTIs had infection localized to one or both kidneys, whereas 6 had bladder infections.[160] Despite the absence of clinical signs, three of the dogs with renal infection and three of the dogs with bladder infection had mild to moderate inflammation in the infected organ. Animals with few historical signs have had severe tissue injury, such as renal or prostatic abscess formation. Duration of nonsymptomatic infection or other host factors may be important in determining the degree of tissue injury. This situation emphasizes the importance of routine analysis of cystocentesis-collected urine in health screening.

Pyelonephritis

Pyelonephritis is rarely responsible for renal failure in the absence of other underlying kidney disease, such as urolithiasis. However, in humans, renal infection may induce inflammation that impairs renal function transiently and leads to scarring.[24,131] In the early stage of acute renal injury caused by infection, renal tubular cells produce local inflammatory mediators such as cytokines and nitrous oxide, which recruit macrophages and neutrophils. In association with bacterial virulence properties, this leads to renal injury.[131] Dogs can have pyelonephritis for years without developing progressive renal failure.[246] Pyelonephritis has been diagnosed in association with renal dysplasia in juvenile dogs, but the cause-effect relationship is difficult to establish in spontaneous cases.[1]

Dogs with acute bacterial pyelonephritis may be systemically ill with fever, depression, anorexia, renal pain, and leukocytosis. Gastrointestinal (GI) signs, particularly vomiting, may be seen. In humans, GI signs have been attributed to a secondary paralytic ileus.[259] All signs are inconsistent and in experimentally induced disease, transient (lasting less than 5 days).[16] Clinical signs in cats with pyelonephritis include fever, lethargy, anorexia, renal pain, and vomiting.[261] Chronic pyelonephritis may be asymptomatic or associated with polyuria and secondary polydipsia. Polyuria can occur before the onset of renal lesions and can resolve with eradication of infection.

Diseases reported to develop secondarily to pyelonephritis include septicemia,[246] diskospondylitis,[274] and distal renal tubular acidosis.[273]

Cystitis and Urethritis

The bladder and proximal urethra are so closely associated that inflammation in one is thought to affect the other. Infection of the distal urethra unassociated with infection in the rest of the lower urinary tract is uncommon unless an anatomic abnormality exists.

Urethrocystitis is characterized by dysuria (straining) and pollakiuria (frequent voiding of urine). The urine is often cloudy and hemorrhagic and may have a foul odor. Gross hematuria at the end of urination suggests that the blood is from the bladder. Gross hematuria at the beginning of urination or a urethral discharge may be associated with urethral or prostatic disease. Prostatic disease is a more common cause of a urethral discharge independent of urination than is urethral disease in dogs. Signs of systemic illness, such as fever and leukocytosis, are not associated with bacterial urethrocystitis. The bladder may be painful on abdominal palpation, and with chronic infection, the wall becomes thickened.

Diagnosis

Culture of bladder urine collected by cystocentesis is the preferred method by which UTIs are confirmed. Samples of urine for urinalysis and culture should be collected before initiation of antimicrobial therapy. If antimicrobial therapy was initiated on the basis of clinical signs and the diagnosis of a UTI is in doubt, it should be discontinued for 3 to 5 days before urine culture to minimize inhibition of bacterial growth.[203] Although a urinalysis can screen for UTI, the visualization of bacteria on a urine sediment examination does not consistently correlate with culture results.[173] UTIs without pyuria are common also, especially in dogs with diabetes mellitus[74,173] and hyperadrenalcorticism.[74]

The presence of bacteria in urine collected from the bladder confirms UTI but does not identify the specific area of the infection. The bacteria could be originating from the kidneys, bladder, prostate gland, or all of these. Diagnostic tests in addition to history and physical examination, which help narrow the location of the infection to an anatomic site in the urinary tract, include radiography, ultrasonography, and prostatic fluid evaluation. No convenient, reliable, noninvasive means to distinguish bladder from renal infections exists.[252]

Because of the difficulty in identifying the location of a UTI in an anatomic site in the urinary tract, UTIs are also subdivided on the basis of response to antimicrobial therapy (see Table 91-7). The extensiveness of the diagnostic evaluation required on each case varies with response to initial antimicrobial therapy as well as severity of illness (Table 91-8).

Urine Collection

Because the distal urethra, vagina, and prepuce have a normal bacterial flora, the method of urine collection is important for accurate assessment of the results of urinalysis and urine culture. When a urine sample is collected, the method of collection should be recorded.

Cystocentesis Cystocentesis is the preferred method of urine collection for culture because lower genitourinary tract contamination is avoided. Any bacteria present in such samples are indicative of infection unless inadvertent bowel penetration or skin contamination occurs. Because of the possibility of inadvertent contamination, diagnosis is more certain if urine is cultured quantitatively, with evaluation of the number of organisms found, as well as qualitatively, to identify the infecting species. For a laboratory to do a quantitative culture, a small volume of urine must be submitted. Sterile swabs dipped in urine are not suitable.

Before cystocentesis is performed, a small area of skin around the site of needle insertion should be clipped free of hair and cleansed. The bladder should be palpated and immobilized against the pelvis with one hand. In animals in which the bladder is not palpable, cystocentesis can be performed using ultrasound guidance. A 21-gauge or smaller needle is inserted into the bladder at an oblique angle, and urine is withdrawn into a syringe. The palpating hand releases pressure on the bladder, and negative pressure on the syringe is discontinued. The needle is withdrawn.

Cystocentesis is performed with the animal in the position in which it seems most comfortable (standing, lying down, or suspended by the front or rear limbs; Fig. 91-1). The only serious potential complication is leakage of urine from the

---

Table • 91-8

Guidelines for Diagnostic Tests and Therapy for Urinary Tract Infections

CLINICAL CLASSIFICATION	DIAGNOSTIC TESTS	THERAPY
Simple cystitis or nonsymptomatic, initial episode	Urinalysis, urine culture	Antimicrobial agent for 10 days in cats and female or neutered male dogs, 21 days for intact male dogs
Relapsing or persistent	Urinalysis, urine culture, radiography, ultrasonography, prostatic fluid examination in intact males	Antimicrobial agent for 6 weeks, treatment of any underlying disease process
Reinfection	Urinalysis, urine culture	Therapy as for simple cystitis, but consider prophylactic therapy if reinfections are frequent
Suspect pyelonephritis	Urinalysis, urine culture, complete blood count (CBC), blood urea nitrogen, serum creatinine, excretory urography, nephrosonography	Antimicrobial agent for 4 weeks, longer if chronic
Suspect prostatitis	Urinalysis, urine culture, CBC, prostatic ultrasonography, prostatic fluid examination	Antimicrobial agent for 4 weeks, 6 weeks if chronic

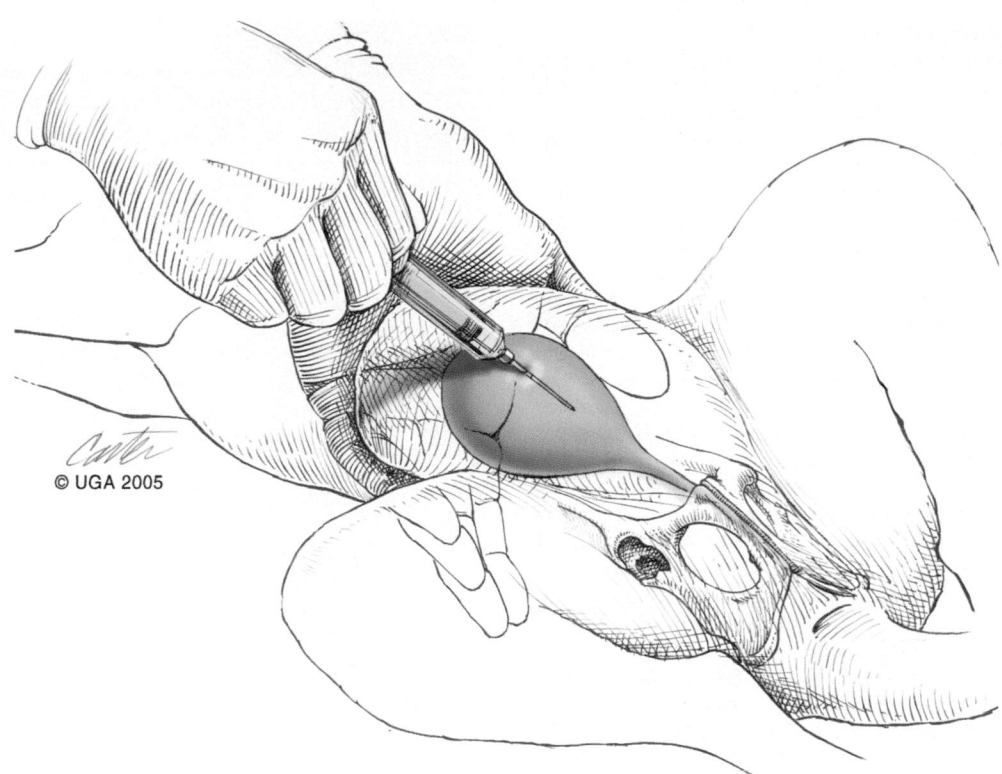

© UGA 2005

Fig 91-1 Cystocentesis with animal in dorsal recumbency. The palpating hand is positioned to hold bladder back against pelvic brim. (Courtesy University of Georgia, Athens, Ga.)

puncture hole in the bladder. This is rare, unless the bladder is distended because of an inability to voluntarily void urine. Animals that are unable to urinate because of distended bladders should have their bladders emptied as soon as possible after cystocentesis. Cystocentesis can cause a mild degree of hematuria to be detected on urinalysis.

Catheterization If the bladder is not palpable or cystocentesis fails, urine from male dogs should be collected for culture by catheterization. Catheterization should always be performed as aseptically and gently as possible. The prepuce should be retracted and the penis cleansed and dried. A sterile, disposable catheter should be used. The catheter should be passed using only sterile instruments or gloves. This method of catheterization introduces only low numbers of bacteria (less than 10^3 per milliliter) into urine.[32,48]

In contrast, catheterization of female dogs, even when being vigilant about using aseptic technique, introduces bacteria approximately 50% of the time; occasionally, large numbers (10^5 per milliliter) of organisms are introduced.[48] Experimentally, introduction of large numbers of bacteria into the bladders of normal female dogs by catheterization does not usually result in a persistent UTI unless a complicating factor, such as a foreign body in the bladder, is present.[32] However, because of the difficulty in distinguishing infection from contamination and because of the small risk of inducing a UTI, catheterization is not an adequate substitute for cystocentesis in female dogs. Diuretics such as furosemide (1 mg/kg given subcutaneously [SC]) to distend the bladder for cystocentesis are preferable to evaluate a UTI, although the effect on specific gravity must be noted.

In normal cats, catheterized samples have fewer than 10^3 bacteria per milliliter in males and females.[153] However, unsedated cats may be difficult to catheterize without causing trauma. As in female dogs, diuretics may be needed to distend the bladder so that cystocentesis can be accomplished.

Samples may be obtained through an indwelling urinary catheter for quantitative culture. In people, low numbers of organisms in samples obtained from indwelling urinary catheters usually progress within days to high concentrations of bacteria unless the catheter is removed.[232] Culture of the tip of an indwelling urinary catheter on its removal is much less accurate in identifying infection than is urine culture.[245a]

Midstream Collection Collection during voluntary voiding in normal dogs has been found to introduce bacteria in large numbers (occasionally greater than 10^5 bacteria per milliliter).[48] Because of the chance of significant contamination during voiding, midstream collection should not be used to obtain urine for culture from dogs.

Midstream-collected urine occasionally is used for culture in severely dysuric cats in which the bladder may not fill sufficiently for successful cystocentesis, even after administration of diuretics. In these cases, urine should be expressed as cleanly as possible into a sterile container. The urine should be cultured quantitatively.

Handling of Urine Samples

Once urine is collected for culture, it must be handled properly to prevent changes in bacterial numbers. Specimens should be refrigerated and cultured within 6 hours.[207] However, tubes with preservatives maintain types and numbers of bacteria in urine for up to 72 hours with refrigeration.[4] Before culture, urine should not be incubated, kept at room temperature, or frozen. Storage at room temperature for 2 hours or longer causes increased bacterial numbers.[133]

If a veterinary practice cannot deliver urine samples to a laboratory in a timely manner, it can use calibrated loops to inoculate blood agar plates.[203] The plates are incubated at 37° C for 24 hours. If bacteria grow, the plates or swab cultures from the plates can be sent to a commercial laboratory for species identification and antimicrobial susceptibility tests.

Interpretation of Urinalysis

To evaluate a dog or cat for infection, a complete urinalysis, *including* a sediment examination, must be performed. Findings on a urine dipstick that may indicate infection are positive occult blood and protein, but these also indicate hemorrhage, which has many causes. Infection can also occur without hemorrhage and can be associated with a normal dipstick evaluation. Dipstick leukocyte assays and dipstick assays for bacteria are inaccurate in companion animals.[135,265]

Findings on a urine sediment examination that suggest a UTI are pyuria, hematuria, and bacteriuria. Of these, the most specific is bacteriuria. Bacteriuria on urinalysis of a cystocentesis sample with a negative urine culture result can occur as a consequence of nonviable microbes, contamination of the sample, improper handling or culture of the sample, or misinterpretation of brownian movement or amorphous debris as bacteria on the urinalysis. False-negative results are possible because large numbers of organisms must be present to be consistently visualized. In one study of dogs with hyperadrenocorticism or diabetes mellitus, 31% had no bacteria visualized on urinalysis despite positive urine cultures.[74] Correlation of Gram-stained smears of canine urine with culture results was good,[197] whereas that of unstained smears was poor.[48,173,227] In human urine, Gram-stained smears were positive in 80% of samples with 100,000 or more bacteria per milliliter but in only 20% of the samples with fewer bacteria.[133]

Pyuria is defined as greater than 3 white blood cells (WBCs) per high-power field (hpf; 40× objective) on cystocentesis samples and greater than 8 WBCs/hpf on catheterized or voided urine samples.[203] Pyuria is not always present in association with bacteriuria, thus the absence of pyuria cannot be used as evidence of absence of bacteriuria.[133] Pyuria without bacteriuria indicates inflammation, and a culture of urine is indicated to determine whether infection is the cause of the inflammation. Bacteria are more difficult to detect than WBCs on urine sediment examination. Infection with minimal tissue invasion may not induce pyuria, and the magnitude of the WBC response seems to vary markedly, even in the same animal.[157] Pyuria was only found in 60% of dogs with UTIs and hyperadrenocorticism or diabetes mellitus.[74] A UTI without pyuria was also common in another study of diabetic dogs.[173]

Nineteen percent of dogs with UTIs and either diabetes mellitus or hyperadrenocorticism had neither pyuria nor bacteriuria on urinalysis.[74] Urine cultures should be routinely performed in dogs with these diseases and in dogs treated with glucocorticoids.

Interpretation of Urine Culture Results

Dogs and Cats The definitive test for UTIs in dogs and cats is isolation of bacteria from a properly collected cystocentesis sample (Table 91-9). Most UTIs involve a single bacterial species, present in high numbers (more than 100,000/ml).[157] Urine culture that results in isolation of multiple types of bacteria or low (fewer than 1000/ml) numbers must be assessed carefully. Artifactual contamination of urine with intestinal contents leads to the presence of multiple bacterial species. Contamination from the skin or in the laboratory leads to fewer organisms. Multiple types of bacteria may be isolated in UTIs and are secondary to indwelling catheters or marked anatomic abnormalities.

Dogs In male dogs, more than 10^4 bacteria per milliliter in a catheterized sample indicates infection (see Table 91-9). Fewer than 10^3 bacteria per milliliter suggests contamination. Intermediate numbers may indicate either contamination or infection. Other case information such as history, physical examination, urinalysis results, and degree of potential contamination during catheterization can help guide a decision about whether infection exists when culture results are inconclusive. Midstream or expressed urine samples and catheterization of female dogs should not be used for culture because of the likelihood of contamination.

Cats In samples of urine obtained by catheterization, bacterial counts greater than 10^3 per ml are considered indicative of infection in male and female cats (see Table 91-9).[153] If midstream samples must be used in a dysuric cat, greater than 10^5 bacteria per milliliter suggests infection if contamination during collection was minimal. Even counts greater than 10^5 bacteria per milliliter would not confirm infection, because counts this high were found in a small number of urine specimens from cats with negative culture results by cystocentesis.[153] Urinalysis results should be correlated with culture results when making a final determination about whether the bacteria are a result of infection or contamination.

Bacterial Pyelonephritis

Bacterial pyelonephritis may be suspected on the basis of history and physical examination as discussed previously or because the UTI is persistent or recurring (see Table 91-7). The diagnosis of bacterial pyelonephritis is supported by laboratory tests, radiography, excretory urography, and nephrosonography. The diagnosis can be confirmed only by culture of urine obtained by pyelocentesis or culture of tissue obtained by renal biopsy. Treatment is often based on a presumptive diagnosis using urinalysis, urine culture, and excretory urography or ultrasonography. Definitive diagnosis is usually sought if the case is difficult or unusual, the renal pelvis is easy to image by ultrasound, or anesthesia or surgery is to be performed for another reason, such as to remove nephroliths.

Laboratory Findings A complete blood count (CBC) may show a neutrophilic leukocytosis with or without a left shift in acute or complicated chronic pyelonephritis, especially with renal abscess formation or ureteral or renal pelvic obstruction. An inflammatory leukogram may also indicate bacteremia secondary to acute pyelonephritis or complicated, chronic pyelonephritis. A normal CBC result does not eliminate the possibility of pyelonephritis.

Abnormalities in renal function (abnormal creatinine clearance, inadequate urine concentrating ability in spite of

Table • 91-9

Criteria for Determining Infection in Urine Specimens Based Upon Method of Collection

CULTURE METHOD	CONTAMINATION (bacteria/ml)	INFECTION
Midstream voided	$<10^5$	Cannot distinguish in dogs $>10^5$ in cats[a]
Catheterization	$<10^3$ in male dogs, any number in female dogs	$>10^4$ in male dogs
	$<10^3$ in cats	$>10^3$ in cats any number with indwelling catheters
Cystocentesis	$<1000^b$	$>10^3$

[a]Small numbers of clinically healthy cats had 10^5 bacterial/ml by this collection method.
[b]Any bacteria in bladder urine suggest infection, but low numbers may occur with contamination from the skin or in processing since most UTI are associated with high numbers of bacteria.

demand, azotemia) in association with a UTI suggest that the UTI may be of renal origin. However, additional tests are indicated because the UTI may be a lower tract infection if an animal has a decreased concentrating ability caused by renal disease with a noninfectious origin.

As mentioned, urinalysis may reveal hematuria, pyuria, and bacteriuria, but these are not specific for pyelonephritis. Consistently low urine specific gravity readings should increase the suspicion of pyelonephritis. Concentrated urine (with a specific gravity of greater than 1.035) does not rule out pyelonephritis because the infection may be unilateral. The degree of concentrating defect depends on how diffusely and severely the renal medulla is affected. The presence of leukocyte casts suggests renal infection; however, such casts are rarely seen.[205] In a very small study, two dogs with pyelonephritis had much higher concentrations of urinary N-acetyl-ß-D-glucosaminidase than four dogs with lower UTIs, suggesting that this test might be useful in differentiating dogs with pyelonephritis from those with a lower UTI.[235]

Survey Abdominal Radiography   An abnormality in renal size or contour may be seen with pyelonephritis. Normal renal size is determined by comparing the kidneys to the second vertebral body (L2); canine kidneys are 2.5 to 3.5 times L2, and feline kidneys are 2.4 to 3 times L2.[73] Most textbooks state that acute pyelonephritis is associated with renomegaly; however, this has not been reported in experimentally induced infections in dogs. Renomegaly may be noted with renal abscess formation. Unilateral renomegaly was found in a cat with pyelonephritis without abscessation.[261] With chronic pyelonephritis without abscess formation, renal size decreases and renal contour may become irregular,[16] changes that are nonspecific for pyelonephritis. Survey abdominal radiographs help to detect radiopaque nephroliths. The concurrent findings of UTI and nephroliths are suggestive of pyelonephritis.

Excretory Urography   Signs suggestive of pyelonephritis are decreased opacity of the vascular nephrogram, decreased opacity and blunting of the pelvic recesses, and renal pelvic and ureteral dilatation (Fig. 91-2).[12] In animals with experimental infections, the size of infected kidneys progressively decreased over weeks.[16] Absence of these findings does not rule out renal infections, especially in acute cases (those lasting 10 days or less).[16,189]

Nephrosonography   The major sonographic findings in pyelonephritis are pelvic dilatation (pyelectasis) and proximal ureteral dilatation (ureterectasis) and a hyperechoic line within the renal pelvis or proximal ureter.[189] Other common findings are a generalized hyperechoic renal cortex, focal hyperechoic areas within the medulla, focal hyperechoic or hypoechoic areas in the renal cortex, and poor corticomedullary differentiation.[189] These abnormalities were found within 2 days of inducing infection.[189] Some of these findings, such as a hyperechoic renal cortex, are nonspecific and common with most types of renal disease, and occasionally are normal. Others such as pyelectasis can be seen with other conditions such as hydronephrosis and can occur during fluid diuresis. Fluid diuresis induced pyeloectasis in 70% of dogs, and was asymmetric in most of the animals.[117] However, diuresis did not induce ureterectasis.[117] The combination of suggestive ultrasonic findings in a case with UTI and appropriate clinical signs or relapsing infections are highly suggestive of pyelonephritis. As with excretory urography, a normal nephrosonogram does not rule out pyelonephritis.[189]

Using ultrasonography to examine the kidneys has many advantages. No ionizing radiation or contrast agent is required, it is unaffected by renal dysfunction, and it is safe in animals with azotemia. However, performance and evaluation of ultrasound examination are operator dependent, and the accuracy

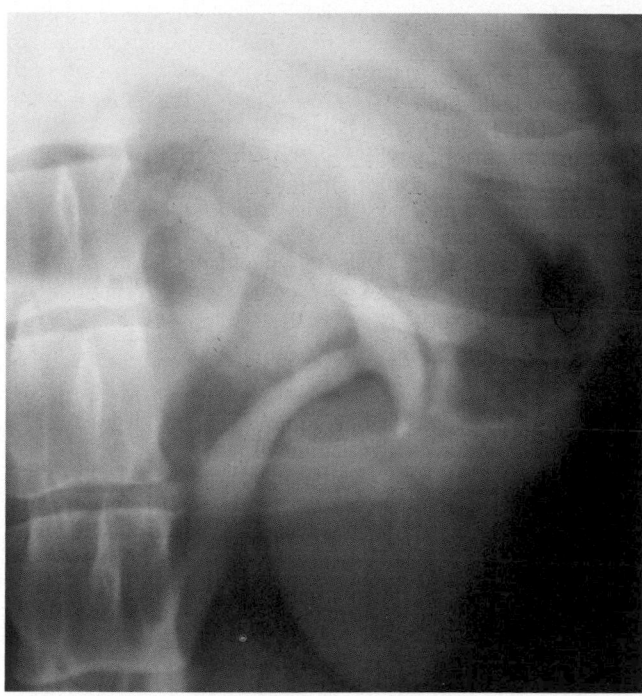

Fig   91-2   Excretory urogram showing dilation of renal pelvis with lack of opacification (blunting) of pelvic recesses and dilation of proximal ureter. These signs are consistent with pyelonephritis.

of the outcome is directly related to the skill of the examiner. The animal's body size and lack of cooperation may also limit the value of ultrasonography.

Pyelocentesis   Percutaneous nephropyelocentesis allows collection of urine for cytology and culture directly from the renal pelvis.[159,237,261] Two different methods have been described. In one, the renal pelvis is visualized by means of excretory urography and fluoroscopy and dilated by application of an abdominal compression band. A 20-gauge disposable arterial needle is then directed through the skin of the lateral flank into the dilated renal pelvis. A positive culture result confirms renal pelvic infection. In the other, ultrasound is used to guide a 21-gauge needle into the renal pelvis.[261] Pyelocentesis is not commonly used.

Renal Biopsy   Renal biopsy is rarely performed to confirm a diagnosis of pyelonephritis, because the lesions are often focal and medullary, thus they may be missed on renal biopsy samples, which are usually only a small, cortical sample. If surgery is performed for another purpose, such as nephrolith removal, culture of urine from the renal pelvis and culture and histologic examination of renal tissue samples should be performed to confirm a diagnosis of bacterial pyelonephritis.

Bacterial Cystitis-Urethritis

The diagnosis of acute bacterial cystitis is usually based on history and clinical signs and on confirming a UTI by urinalysis and urine culture. In cases of relapsing or persistent UTIs, a complicated infection should be suspected (see Table 91-7). In these cases, imaging of the bladder is important.

Emphysematous cystitis is characterized by gas-filled vesicles in the bladder wall and often gas bubbles in the bladder lumen. Gas formation is due to infection with gas-producing bacteria, using glucose, protein, or tissue carbohydrates as substrates. Emphysematous cystitis is usually diagnosed radiographically or ultrasonically, although it may be suspected by the sound of air being voided during urination or by the palpation of crepitus within the bladder on physical examination. Although diabetes mellitus may predispose an animal to emphysematous cystitis, this type of cystitis also occurs in animals without diabetes. Because of bacterial fermentation, the absence of glucosuria does not exclude a diagnosis of diabetes mellitus, which should be determined by measurement of blood glucose.[219] In animals without diabetes, urine proteins are suspected to be the substrate for gas formation.[219] Cases in animals without diabetes are usually complicated,[56] and the usual infecting organism is *E. coli*,[56,219,286] although infections with other organisms including anaerobes have been reported.[87]

Polypoid cystitis is a rare disease of the bladder, in which the bladder mucosa develops villuslike sessile projections or folds. It has been reported to be related to chronic inflammatory diseases of the bladder, including chronic UTIs and urolithiasis. Affected dogs are most commonly female and show hematuria and recurrent UTIs.[171] Although many bacterial species have been involved, *Proteus* species are most common.[171] It is unknown whether the polyps predispose animals to UTIs or the chronic UTI results in polyp formation.

In dogs with urolithiasis and a positive urine culture, the same organism was cultured from bladder mucosal samples and uroliths, leading to the conclusion that urine cultures were sufficient in such cases.[97] However, in dogs with urolithiasis and a negative urine culture, a bacterial organism was cultured from the bladder mucosa or the urolith in 18.5% of cases.[97] Thus when a urine culture is negative in a dog with uroliths, an aerobic culture of a bladder mucosal sample and the urolith should be performed.

Survey Radiography　Most uroliths can be detected on good-quality survey abdominal radiographs. Urolithiasis and emphysematous cystitis are the only bladder problems that are able to be diagnosed by survey radiographs.

Ultrasound and Contrast Cystography　Ultrasound of the bladder is an excellent diagnostic technique because of the bladder's superficial location and the excellent acoustic properties of fluid. However, an empty bladder is difficult to assess by ultrasound, whereas bladder size can be manipulated during contrast cystography. On cystography and ultrasound, increased bladder wall thickness suggests chronic inflammation (Figs. 91-3 and 91-4). Bladder wall thickness does vary with the degree of bladder distention. Mean bladder wall thickness in dogs is 2.3 mm with minimal distention (0.5

ml/kg) and 1.4 mm with moderate distention (4 ml/kg).[154] Bladder wall thickness in cats is about 1.7 mm.[154] Polyps (polypoid cystitis) can be visualized with ultrasound or cystography. Inflammatory polyps are usually located in the cranioventral bladder wall.[171] Although the most typical location is different than transitional cell carcinoma (bladder neck and trigone), mass lesions in the bladder require biopsy for differentiation of inflammatory conditions from neoplasia.[179,171] This differentiation is important because polypoid cystitis can resolve with appropriate antimicrobial therapy. Polyp removal also seems beneficial.[171] A urachal diverticulum or other diverticulum may predispose animals to developing chronic lower UTIs and is visualized with bladder ultrasound or contrast cystography.[165]

Biopsy　Biopsy of the bladder wall should be performed in difficult cases.[115] Biopsy specimens should be cultured for bacteria as well as processed for histologic evaluation. Gram stain may be helpful in examining bladder tissue for bacteria.[115]

Therapy
Urine Concentration of Antimicrobial Agents
The major difference between therapy for UTIs and infections in other organ systems is that most antimicrobials are present in urine in high concentrations as a result of renal excretion (Table 91-10).[144,249] Because most antimicrobial disks contain serum concentrations, routine antimicrobial susceptibility results should be considered only as rough guidelines for treatment of UTIs. If the infecting organism is reported to be susceptible to an antimicrobial agent, that agent is likely to be effective if it is excreted in active form by the kidney and renal function is normal. Furthermore, an antimicrobial to which the organism is reported to be resistant may also give good results in vivo because of significantly higher concentrations in urine than serum in animals that can concentrate their urine.

Another method of choosing an effective therapeutic agent for UTIs is to determine the minimum inhibitory concentration (MIC) of antimicrobials for the infective agent. The MIC is defined as the least amount of an antimicrobial agent that

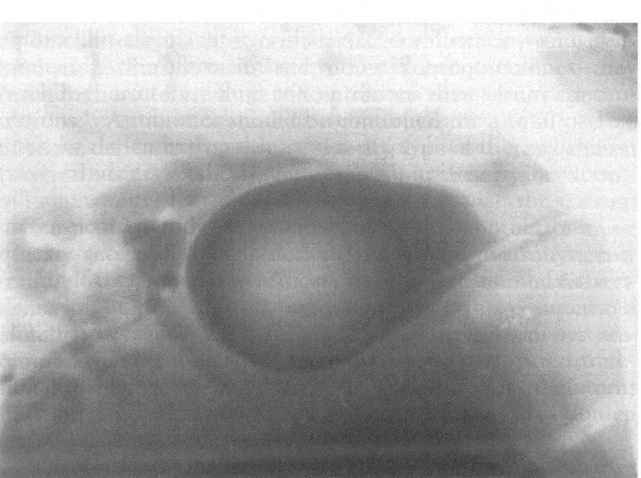

Fig 91-3　Double-contrast cystogram showing thickened bladder wall at outer edges of air-filled bladder.

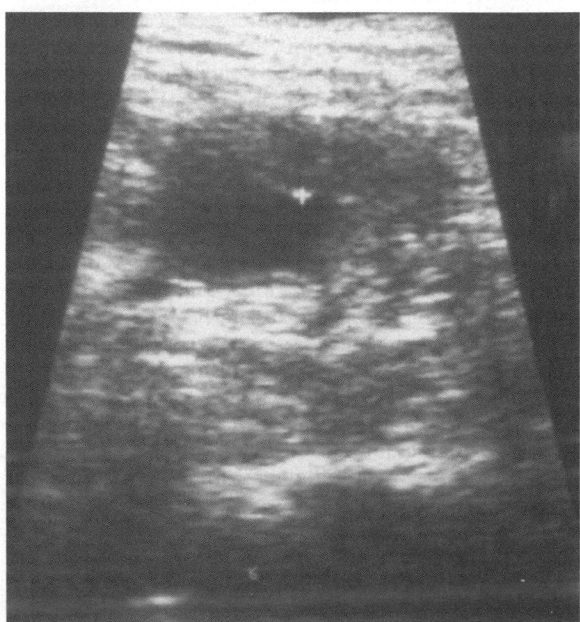

Fig 91-4　Ultrasound examination showing thickened bladder wall. Two crosses denote outer and inner margins of wall. (Courtesy University of Georgia, Athens, Ga.)

Table • 91-10

Mean Urine Concentrations of Antimicrobial Agents Used in Management of Canine Urinary Tract Infection[a]

DRUG[b]	DOSAGE (mg/kg)[c]	ROUTE	INTERVAL (HOURS)	MEAN URINE CONCENTRATION (μg/ml)
Ampicillin	22	PO	8	309
Amoxicillin	11	PO	8	201.5
Chloramphenicol	33	PO	8	124
Nitrofurantoin	4.4	PO	8	100
Trimethoprim-sulfonamide	13	PO	12	26/79[d]
Gentamycin	2	SC	8	107
Amikacin	5	SC	8	342
Cephalexin	8	PO	8	225
Enrofloxacin	2.5	PO	12	40
Tetracycline	18	PO	8	138

PO, By mouth; SC, subcutaneous.

Most data determined by and supplied courtesy Gerald Ling, University of California, Davis, Calif.

[a]Values were determined in hydrated dogs with normal renal function. To determine the efficacy of a drug, multiply by 4 the minimum inhibitory concentration (MIC) of the bacteria isolated. If the total is less than the mean urine concentration for that drug, the drug has a 90% to 95% chance of being effective.

[b]See Drug Formulary, Appendix 8 for additional information on each drug.

[c]Dose per administration at specified interval. (For duration, see Table 91-8.)

[d]Mean concentration of trimethoprim in urine is 26, and mean concentration of sulfonamide is 79.

Table • 91-11

Type of Organism Most Likely to Cause Initial Urinary Tract Infection and Initial Antibiotic Choice

URINE pH	BACTERIAL CHARACTERISTICS	LIKELY ORGANISM[a]	INITIAL ANTIBIOTIC CHOICE[b]
Acidic	Rods	*Escherichia coli*	Trimethoprim, enrofloxacin
	Cocci	*Enterococcus* or *Streptococcus*	Ampicillin,[c] amoxicillin
Alkaline	Rods	*Proteus mirabilis*	Ampicillin, amoxicillin
	Cocci	*Staphylococcus* spp.	Cephalexin, amoxicillin-clavulanate

[a]Based on urine pH and bacterial characteristics on urine sediment examination.

[b]May need to be modified after the causative organism and its antibiotic susceptibility are determined by urine culture.

[c]Enterococci may often show antibiotic resistance.

causes complete inhibition of growth of the infecting bacteria under standardized conditions. MIC is most accurately measured by microdilution analysis with varying antimicrobial concentrations but can be estimated from the diameter of the zone of inhibition of Kirby-Bauer plates.[7] Rather than absolute susceptibility or resistance, the concentration of antimicrobial that inhibits the growth of the organism is reported. MIC is then compared with the concentration reached by that antimicrobial in urine. If the mean urine concentration exceeds the MIC by at least 4 times, the antimicrobial agent should be effective (see Table 91-10). In renal parenchymal and prostatic infections, special considerations apply to antimicrobial penetration, which is discussed in the Bacterial Pyelonephritis and Prostatitis sections, respectively.

Antibiotic Choice

Determination of organism type and its in vitro antimicrobial susceptibility is the optimal way to determine therapy for a UTI. However, clinicians usually begin therapy pending culture results. By examining urine pH and whether the organisms in the urine are rods or cocci on urine sediment examination, clinicians can make an educated guess about the type of organism present and a reasonable first choice of

antimicrobial agent (Table 91-11). With recurrent UTIs, clinicians should compare the findings from the current urinalysis with those from prior urinalyses and urine cultures to determine the most likely causative organism and its susceptibility, pending culture results. On the basis of MIC determinations for common urinary tract pathogens, usually effective antimicrobials have been determined (Table 91-12).

Fluoroquinolones are often used to treat UTIs because they are bactericidal with high urine concentrations and effectively treat the most common causative organisms.[47,201] Several fluoroquinolones are available for veterinary use, including enrofloxacin, marbofloxacin, orbifloxacin, and difloxacin. Enrofloxacin is metabolized to ciprofloxacin. A small proportion of cats develop irreversible blindness after treatment with fluoroquinolones. Risk factors include older age, intravenous (IV) administration, high doses, and prolonged courses of treatment.[280] Considering the risk of blindness, fluoroquinolone use for UTIs in cats should be limited to those cases in which urine culture indicates a need for this class of drugs. Other drugs to which *E. coli* is often sensitive include aminoglycosides and trimethoprim-sulfonamide. Aminoglycosides are rarely used to treat UTIs because of the risk of nephro-

Table • 91-12

Antimicrobials for Genitourinary Infections Based on Causative Bacteria[156,229,64,202,206,243,23]

IDENTIFIED ORGANISM[a]	ANTIMICROBIALS RECOMMENDED
Escherichia coli	Trimethoprim-sulfonamide, amoxicillin-clavulanate, fluoroquinolone, chloramphenicol
Staphylococcus	Amoxicillin-clavulanate, first-generation cephalosporins
Streptococcus or Enterococcus	Ampicillin, amoxicillin
Proteus	Ampicillin, amoxicillin
Pseudomonas[b]	Tetracycline, fluoroquinolone
Klebsiella[b]	First-generation cephalosporins, trimethoprim-sulfonamide, amoxicillin-clavulanate, fluoroquinolone
Enterobacter	Trimethoprim-sulfonamide, fluoroquinolone

[a]Highly antibiotic-resistant UTIs can be a problem with any of these organisms, especially in animals that have received antimicrobial therapy. For this reason, this table provides general guidelines only. Identification of the organism and its susceptibility is important in each clinical case for appropriate antimicrobial selection. In highly resistant gram-negative infections, quinolones, third-generation cephalosporins, and extended-spectrum penicillins may be needed.

[b]Pseudomonas and Klebsiella infections are the most difficult for which to predict susceptibility. Although these organisms are usually susceptible to aminoglycosides, aminoglycosides are not usually used because of nephrotoxicity. Repeated urine evaluations during and after therapy are essential to determine treatment efficacy in infections with these organisms.

toxicity.[201] Drugs with the poorest efficacy against E. coli include the penicillin derivatives, tetracyclines, and first-generation cephalosporins.[201]

UTIs in humans are becoming increasingly antibiotic resistant, especially to certain drug classes.[93,94,172,252] In uncomplicated, community-acquired UTIs in women, one in three bacterial isolates are resistant to ampicillin, and approximately 20% are resistant to trimethoprim-sulfonamide.[93,43a] Up to 45% of E. coli that cause UTIs are resistant to ampicillin, and up to 31% are resistant to trimethoprim-sulfonamide.[172]

An increase in fluoroquinolone resistance in bacteria, especially among E. coli, isolated from canine UTIs has been documented in some studies[47,49] but not others.[201] Increased fluoroquinolone use was correlated with increased resistance.[49] Resistance to multiple other drugs commonly used to treat UTIs accompanies enrofloxacin resistance.[49] Pseudomonas aeruginosa and Enterococcus species isolated from canine otitis and UTIs became rapidly resistant to enrofloxacin in vitro.[40] Klebsiella, Proteus, Streptococus, E. coli, and Staphylococcus were less likely to develop resistance in this study.[40] Canine UTIs caused by Staphylococcus were increasingly antibiotic resistant, especially to ampicillin and penicillin.[202] A study found that resistance correlated with drug usage.[215] In this study, resistance of Staphylococcus aureus and Staphylococcus intermedius infections to ampicillin decreased but markedly increased to the fluoroquinolones as usage of these drugs either declined

(ampicillin) or increased (fluoroquinolones). Another study found that antibiotic resistance is common in canine UTI and develops in response to treatment, especially with trimethoprim-sulfa. Antibiotic resistance could also be lost when antibiotics are discontinued.[65] Based on all these studies, it is optimal to base UTI therapy on culture and susceptibility to improve therapy efficacy and avoid inappropriate antimicrobial use.

A little used drug that may efficiently treat some resistant bacteria from UTIs is nitrofurantoin. Nitrofurantoin effectively treats gram-positive and gram-negative organisms, but it does not penetrate the prostate gland. Nitrofurantoin should be given only as the macrocrystalline formulation to decrease adverse GI effects and maximize efficacy.

Although selection of an antimicrobial agent by organism identification and susceptibility testing usually correlates with success of therapy in vivo, the correlation is not 100%. Various factors such as GI absorption, location of infection, renal function, polyuric state, and urine characteristics influence antimicrobial urine concentrations. The only way to be certain that the chosen drug is effective is to reexamine the urine during and after therapy. Urine should be recultured, or the sediment should be examined cytologically after a few days of therapy. If the antibiotic eliminates bacteria within a few days, the drug's efficacy against that bacterial species is confirmed. However, a longer course of therapy is necessary to eliminate the organism from infected bladder, renal, or prostatic tissues.

Whenever any antimicrobial is dispensed, adverse reactions are possible. One client survey found the highest rate of adverse reactions in dogs to be with erythromycin (52%, with the most common reaction being vomiting) and the lowest to be with amoxicillin (7.5%).[145] Even though reports have been made of serious toxicity with trimethoprim-sulfadiazine, this drug had a relatively low percentage of adverse reactions (18%, with the most common reactions being anorexia, lethargy, and polyuria-polydipsia), despite being the most commonly prescribed drug in the survey.[145] An approximately 15% incidence of keratoconjunctivitis sicca (KCS) was found with trimethoprim-sulfadiazine; dogs weighing less than 12 kg were at greater risk.[25] Enrofloxacin should not be given to immature dogs, to dogs prone to seizures, or to uremic animals without dosage modification.[5,206,242] As noted previously, caution should be used when giving enrofloxacin to cats.

Therapy for Different Types of Bacterial Urinary Tract Infections

Optimal duration of therapy for different types of UTIs in dogs and cats has not been determined by clinical studies. The recommended duration of therapy varies with anatomic location and severity of the infection. It also varies according to whether the infection is complicated and whether the infection is an initial infection, relapsing, or persistent (see Tables 91-7 and 91-8). Because of these differences, it is best to classify a UTI by as many characteristics as possible. For example, an uncomplicated initial cystitis requires much less intensive diagnostic and therapeutic efforts than a complicated, relapsing pyelonephritis. In humans, a first infection is typically caused by an organism, usually E. coli, that is sensitive to many different antimicrobial agents.[193] However, recurrent infections are likely to be caused by organisms with increasing levels of antimicrobial resistance. This same situation is apparent in some dogs.[243a]

Asymptomatic Bacteriuria A diagnostic effort should be made to determine whether an underlying cause of immunosuppression exists, such as glucocorticoid therapy or hyperadrenocorticism. Asymptomatic infections should be treated based on urine culture results (see Table 91-8). A urine culture should be repeated approximately 1 week after concluding therapy. If the infection remains, a diagnostic effort should be made to identify the tissue source (kidney, bladder, prostate) and any underlying disease (urolithiasis, neoplasia, congenital defect).

Acute Pyelonephritis Antibiotic therapy should be started on the basis of urinalysis and pending culture results (see Tables 91-8 and 91-11). Although aminoglycosides have excellent renal tissue penetrance, nephrotoxicity makes their administration risky. Other drugs that can diffuse into renal tissue are preferred (Table 91-13).[16] Nitrofurantoin should not be given in acute pyelonephritis because it is ineffective for bacteremia, which may accompany acute pyelonephritis.[52]

If the animal is systemically ill, initial therapy should consist of parenteral antibiotics as well as IV fluid support. Parenteral therapy should be continued until response is indicated by normalization of body temperature and appetite. In children, the standard protocol is 3 days of IV antibiotics. Longer courses of parenteral antibiotics did not reduce the incidence of renal scarring or the incidence of recurrent infections.[24]

If the organism is reported to be resistant to the initially chosen antimicrobial but the animal is better clinically, a urinalysis should be checked before changing therapy to determine whether the drug is efficacious in vivo. If the drug is not efficacious, therapy should be changed. If the drug is efficacious, initial therapy should be continued for 3 to 4 weeks, with follow-up cultures 1 to 2 weeks after the conclusion of treatment. Urine cultures should be performed monthly for several months to detect recurrence (Table 91-14).

Chronic Pyelonephritis Antibiotics with the ability to penetrate renal tissue are preferred if the causative organism is susceptible to one of them (see Table 91-13). Sulfonamides do not reach effective intrarenal concentrations, so only the trimethoprim component of trimethoprim-sulfonamide is effective for treating renal infections.[26] Nitrofurantoin can be used for chronic renal infections but not in animals with renal dysfunction.[52] Efficacy of the chosen antimicrobial agent should be checked by urinalysis and urine culture after the first 2 weeks of therapy. If the urine is not sterile at this point, therapy should be changed. If the urine is sterile, the antimicrobial agent should generally be continued for at least 6 weeks. Urine cultures should be repeated on a periodic basis after finishing therapy (see Table 91-14). Pyelonephritis is very difficult to cure in dogs and cats.

Nephrectomy may be necessary if renal abscess formation is present. The remaining kidney must be able to maintain renal function. Crude indicators of adequate renal function are normal serum urea nitrogen, normal serum creatinine, concentrated urine, normal radiographic and ultrasonographic appearance, normal excretion of dye on excretory urography, and normal appearance at surgery. One needs to recognize that all these tests are insensitive, and normal findings do not confirm normal function.[89] Renal scintigraphy has been recommended to more thoroughly assess individual kidney function before surgery.[89] Even with this test, 9 of 21 dogs undergoing nephrectomy became azotemic, albeit mildly so, after nephrectomy.[89] At the time of surgery, urine should be collected from the renal pelvis or ureter of the remaining kidney and cultured for bacteria to direct future therapy and provide a more accurate prognosis to the owner.

Initial Episode of Acute Cystitis Acute, uncomplicated bacterial cystitis in female dogs, neutered male dogs, and cats should be treated for 7 to 14 days (see Tables 91-8 and 91-11). Because clinical signs often improve within 48 hours, the client must be instructed to give all medication as directed. One week after therapy is concluded, a urine sample should be collected for culture to ensure efficacy. Such a follow-up is important to prompt an early search for an underlying predisposing cause for treatment failure, such as uroliths, pyelonephritis, abnormal bladder or urethral function, renal failure, urinary tract neoplasia, or hyperadrenocorticism. Whenever one part of the urinary tract is infected, the entire tract is at risk; pyelonephritis may be present with the cystitis.

In intact male dogs, prostatitis often occurs in conjunction with cystitis, necessitating longer therapy (see Table 91-8). Reexaminations should include evaluation of prostatic fluid as well as urine. Drugs with prostatic penetrance are preferred (see Table 91-13). However, one study found no difference in clinical response to ampicillin (little prostatic penetrance) and trimethoprim-sulfonamide (good prostatic penetrance) in UTIs in intact male dogs.[156]

Reinfections In some dogs, acute cystitis recurs frequently because of different organisms. The causative organism must be determined by urine culture in each instance of infection to differentiate reinfection from relapse (see Table 91-7). Reinfection suggests a problem with host defenses (see Table 91-6). A careful history should be taken and complete physical examination performed to determine whether micturition and urinary tract anatomy are normal. Hyperadrenocorticism and glucocorticoid therapy are predisposing causes of reinfections. Some bitches have recurrent cystitis with no other discernible abnormalities.

Each episode of reinfection is treated individually. If infections recur frequently (more than three to four episodes per year), low-dose, prophylactic therapy can be provided (see Prophylactic Therapy).

Complicated Cystitis Cystitis is considered complicated if it is associated with an underlying risk factor such as urolithiasis or diabetes mellitus (see Table 91-7). Complicated bacte-

Table • 91-13

Antimicrobials for Genitourinary Infections Based on the Site of Infection

SITE	ANTIMICROBIAL AGENT
Kidney	Trimethoprim, quinolones
Prostate	Trimethoprim, quinolones, erythromycin, clindamycin
Uterus	Quinolones, trimethoprim
Mammary gland	Ampicillin, amoxicillin-clavulanate, cephalosporin (first generation)

Table • 91-14

When Urine Cultures Should be Repeated to Ensure Efficacy of Urinary Tract Infection Therapy

NONCOMPLICATED	COMPLICATED
1 week after conclusion	1 week after conclusion
	Monthly for 3 months
	Then at 6 months
	At 9 months
	At 12 months
	At 18 months
	At 24 months

rial cystitis requires resolution of underlying factors and protracted treatment. Removal of polyps may improve the chance to resolve chronic UTIs in dogs with polypoid cystitis.[171] Episioplasty was beneficial in resolving chronic bacterial cystitis in dogs with excessive perivulvar skin folds.[155]

Urine should be recultured or checked by sediment examination 3 to 7 days after therapy begins. If the urine is sterile, that antimicrobial agent should be continued for 3 to 6 weeks. If it is not sterile, another antimicrobial should be chosen. Culturing should be repeated after approximately 7 days of treatment until an effective agent is found. Urine should be recultured 4 to 7 days after the conclusion of therapy (see Table 91-14).

Relapsing or Persistent Urinary Tract Infections Treatment is considered ineffective and a UTI persistent when bacteria can be isolated from urine during therapy, even if the bacterial count has been reduced. Repeated isolations of the same organism within several months of therapy and after a negative culture result at the conclusion of therapy indicates a relapse. When no culture has been performed during or within a week of concluding therapy, it is not possible to differentiate between a persistent infection and a relapse. Potential causes of failure of antimicrobial therapy include selection of an ineffective drug or administration of a subtherapeutic dose of a drug, poor owner compliance with administration of the drug, bacteria in tissue sites impenetrable to the antimicrobial chosen, bacteria acquiring resistance to the antimicrobial agent, host factors including failure to absorb the drug, and failure to eliminate an underlying condition. Whether a relapsing or persistent UTI, all these factors should be considered. A diagnostic investigation should be undertaken to determine the site of tissue infection and any underlying disease process that is causing the infection to be complicated (see Tables 91-7 and 91-8). Any underlying factors discovered should be treated.[243a] For example, surgical correction of vestibulovaginal stenosis resulted in resolution of UTIs for at least 5 months in four dogs that had an average chronic UTI duration of almost 2 years.[147]

Antimicrobial therapy should be continued at least 6 weeks (see Table 91-8). Urine cultures should be evaluated during and after therapy (see Table 91-14). If antimicrobial therapy eliminates bacteriuria during therapy but bacteriuria recurs with discontinuation of therapy, a longer course of therapy (4 to 6 months) should be considered. When providing antimicrobials for this duration, consideration must be given to side effects. Prolonged use of drugs with significant potential side effects should be avoided. The risk of KCS and other toxicities with trimethoprim-sulfonamide should be conveyed to the owner (see Drug Formulary, Appendix 8). Tear tests should be performed before prolonged therapy with trimethoprim-sulfonamide.

In a study of multidrug-resistant infections, one small study of four dogs with cystitis suggested that local administration of an EDTA-Tris solution (250 mmol/L EDTA and 50 mmol/L tromethamine at a pH of 8) once a day for 7 days in conjunction with a parenterally administered cephalosporin, fluoroquinolone, or aminoglycoside was effective.[71] The infecting organisms in this small study were P. aeruginosa, E. coli, or P. mirabilis.

Suppressive Therapy If the patient experiences relapses each time antimicrobial therapy is stopped, suppressive therapy can be tried to prevent extension of the infection and control symptoms.[237] Once the urine is sterile from full-dose therapy, suppressive therapy begins. A single dose per day of an antimicrobial is administered, preferably when the animal is to be confined (usually evening) so that urination is prevented for several hours. Drugs to consider for suppressive therapy are trimethoprim, nitrofurantoin, cephalexin, and enrofloxacin. Risks include antimicrobial toxicity and induction of bacterial resistance. Urine should be cultured monthly during suppressive therapy to ensure that the drug remains effective.

Urinary Tract Infection Associated with Catheterization
Treatment of UTIs developing during indwelling urinary catheterization should be delayed until the catheter is removed unless systemic signs of infection develop. When the urinary catheter is removed and the animal is again urinating normally, urine should be cultured and appropriate antimicrobial therapy started if infection is found. Treatment should continue for 10 days, with reculture of urine approximately 1 week after therapy is discontinued.

Catheter-induced infections may involve more than one bacterial species with different antimicrobial susceptibility patterns. In these cases, one species is treated first. Urine is reevaluated after treatment, and if infection persists with another species, that infection is treated. Except for combinations such as trimethoprim-sulfonamide, simultaneous administration of two or more antimicrobial agents is generally avoided when treating UTIs.

Fungal Urinary Tract Infections
Fortunately, fungal UTIs are rare because they are difficult to treat. If the animal is asymptomatic, as many are, the only treatment required is to eliminate or control the underlying factors compromising host immunity.[170,216] Such factors include indwelling urinary catheters, anatomic abnormalities, diabetes mellitus, and antibacterial therapy.

If the animal is symptomatic, antifungal therapy can be provided in conjunction with control of underlying factors, although reports of results of therapy are scarce in the veterinary literature. Treatment with itraconazole or ketoconazole is not recommended because they are not excreted in therapeutic concentrations in urine.

The most common organism for which therapy is reported is Candida. Susceptibility of Candida species was found to change on exposure to antifungal agents and be unpredictable, with some species being susceptible to several drugs and other species being highly resistant.[216] 5-Fluorocytosine was used successfully, in addition to correction of a urethral stricture, in one cat with candidal urethrocystitis.[83] Fluconazole (FCZ) was used most often in one retrospective study and is considered to be the azole of choice due to its excretion in urine in active form.[216] However, only one case was documented to resolve with this therapy, and it failed in five cases.[216] FCZ was successful in treating aspergillus cystitis in a cat at a dose of 7.5 mg/kg every 12 hours orally for 10 weeks.[2] Use of intravesicular clotrimazole was used successfully in one dog[75] and on one cat[262a] with candidiasis. These reports underline the importance of following up a treated case with repeated urinalysis and urine culture during and after therapy to document resolution of infection.

Prophylactic Therapy
Prophylactic therapy is defined as the administration of antimicrobial drugs to prevent establishment of infection in uninfected sites.[281] In relation to the urinary tract, such therapy is provided to prevent bacterial reinfections in animals that have a history of frequent reinfection (greater than 3 to 4 times a year), to prevent sepsis during surgery in animals with UTIs, and to prevent bacterial UTIs from urinary tract manipulation and catheterization. Prophylaxis is effective only if the antimicrobial drug is present at the time of bacterial inoculation.[281] Prophylaxis with drugs is not as important as aseptic technique in preventing infections related to medical procedures.

Reinfections

Before beginning prophylactic therapy, infections should be treated until urine is sterile. Drug choice is based on the susceptibility of the most recent isolate.[157] The chosen drug is given once just before a 6- to 12-hour period when urine will be retained in the bladder, such as at night in house dogs. The dose is one half to one third of the usual total daily dose. Therapy is continued for 6 months. Urine should be cultured every 4 weeks to ensure UTIs are prevented. If the urine remains sterile for 6 months, prophylactic therapy can be discontinued and the animal monitored for reinfection (see Table 91-14). If reinfections do occur, each is eliminated with full-dose therapy, and prophylactic therapy is reinstituted. Potential adverse effects of prophylactic therapy include induction of antimicrobial resistance and drug toxicity. All urine samples for culture should be collected by cystocentesis in animals receiving prophylactic therapy, because they may be more susceptible to induction of infection when catheterization is performed.[157]

Perioperative Therapy

If surgery is to be performed on an animal with a urogenital infection, antibiotics should be administered before and during surgery to reduce the possibility of sepsis. If the animal's condition permits, determination of the causative organism and its susceptibility before surgery is recommended.

Urinary Tract Manipulation

To prevent introduction of UTIs in animals without infection, short-term administration of a broad-spectrum antimicrobial may be helpful during urinary tract procedures such as cystoscopy, urethroscopy, contrast urethrocystography, electrodiagnostic procedures, urohydropulsion, and prostatic massage.[29] Its use for 24 to 72 hours, beginning a few hours before the procedure, should be sufficient. Drugs to consider include amoxicillin-clavulanate, trimethoprim-sulfonamide, macrocrystalline nitrofurantoin, a first generation cephalosporin, or enrofloxacin.

A single administration of amoxicillin or a cephalosporin may act as a preventative if a catheter is passed only once into the urinary bladder. However, a single episode of catheterization rarely results in a UTI and usually does not warrant antimicrobial therapy. With repeated, intermittent urinary catheterization, antibiotic prophylaxis is also not indicated. In children with intermittent catheterizations, antimicrobial prophylaxis was not associated with a lower rate of bacteriuria, reduction of periurethral colonization by bacteria, or a lower rate of symptomatic UTI.[239] In adults with intermittent catheterizations, the incidence of UTIs was reduced by bladder irrigation with a solution of neomycin and polymyxin (Neosporin G.U. Irrigant, Burroughs Wellcome, Research Triangle Park, N.C.) or by oral methenamine hippurate or nitrofurantoin.[52,251]

Indwelling Urethral or Cystic (Cystostomy Tube) Catheterization

The three following factors are most important in preventing UTIs in an animal with an indwelling urinary catheter: (1) aseptic catheter placement, (2) maintenance of a closed catheter system, and (3) minimization of the duration of catheterization.[163,272] The guiding rule should be to avoid catheterization when not required and when required, to terminate use as soon as possible. Appropriate indications for indwelling catheters are temporary relief of anatomic or functional obstruction, urinary incontinence in patients with periurethral wounds, urine output monitoring in critically ill patients, and in the preoperative and postoperative management of lower urinary tract trauma.

The most important risk factor for UTIs in closed-catheter systems is duration of catheterization.[232] In humans, lack of proper hand washing by health care personnel is largely responsible for transmission of nosocomial UTIs in catheterized patients.[232] It is recommended that individuals wear gloves when manipulating or emptying urine drainage bags and wash hands after contact with every patient. In men and women, intermittent catheterization is less conducive to infection than indwelling catheters.[232,251] This may also be true for male dogs but is less likely to be true for female dogs because the urethral orifice is intravestibular.

Antibiotics should generally not be given to prevent UTIs during indwelling catheterization because of potential adverse effects and development of drug resistance.[16,232] Although antibiotics may delay the onset of bacteriuria, they cannot prevent infection if the catheter remains in place, especially for 3 days or longer. Prophylactic use of an antimicrobial may reduce infection rates with short-term use (less than 3 days) of a closed, indwelling catheter system. However, even with short-term catheterization, urinalysis, urine culture, and treatment after catheter removal may be preferable to prophylactic antibiotics. Use of antiseptics such as methenamine are also not recommended.[232]

Instillation of antimicrobial agents into the bladder in people with indwelling catheters is of little benefit.[232] In general, the short contact time plus the necessity of disconnecting the closed catheter system to infuse the antimicrobial substance abrogates any beneficial effect. Constant unidirectional flow from the bladder to the drainage bag is best.[232] Placing antimicrobial agents into the drainage bag has not been found to be beneficial.[232] Placing lubricants or antibiotic creams at the urethral meatus was also of no benefit in humans.[232]

Glucocorticoids, even at antiinflammatory doses, should be avoided in animals with indwelling urinary catheters. In cats with indwelling urinary catheters, 5 mg/day of oral prednisolone predisposed the cats to developing bacterial pyelonephritis and did not reduce catheter-associated inflammation.[22]

A newer way to prevent symptomatic UTIs in people with indwelling urinary catheters is to inoculate such individuals with an E. coli strain associated with asymptomatic infection.[54] In 30 colonized people, the incidence of symptomatic UTIs was markedly reduced compared with the incidence in people not inoculated with this organism.

MALE GENITAL INFECTIONS

Organisms associated with genital infections in male dogs are the same as those associated with UTIs.[138] Anaerobes are occasionally associated with abscess formation. Fungal infections, especially with disseminated infections, are reported, but rarely.[116,132,283] A parainfluenza virus was isolated from the prostatic fluid of a dog; however, the dog was asymptomatic.[268] Genital infections in male cats are uncommon, with the exceptions of those being caused by scrotal injuries during fighting and associated with feline infectious peritonitis. For example, only one case of chronic bacterial prostatitis has been reported in cats.[231]

Prostatitis
Etiology and Pathogenesis
Prostatitis is an inflammatory disease of the prostate gland and is most commonly associated with bacterial infection (Fig. 91-5). E. coli is the most common infectious agent. Strains of E. coli causing prostatitis in men have been found to express urovirulence factors including cytotoxic necrotizing factor-1, hemolysin, and P fimbriation.[164] Although benign prostatic hyperplasia is the most common canine prostatic disease and the most common cause of clinical signs in dogs with prostatic disease, prostatitis is the second most common canine prostatic disease to cause clinical signs.[260] Prostatitis may be acute

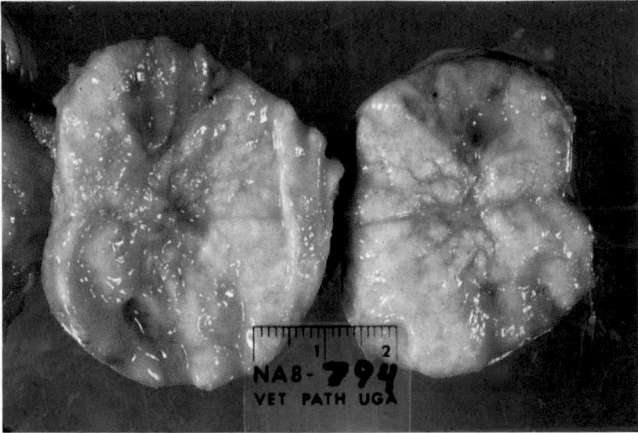

Fig 91-5 Gross appearance of purulent prostatitis in dog (Courtesy University of Georgia, Athens, Ga.)

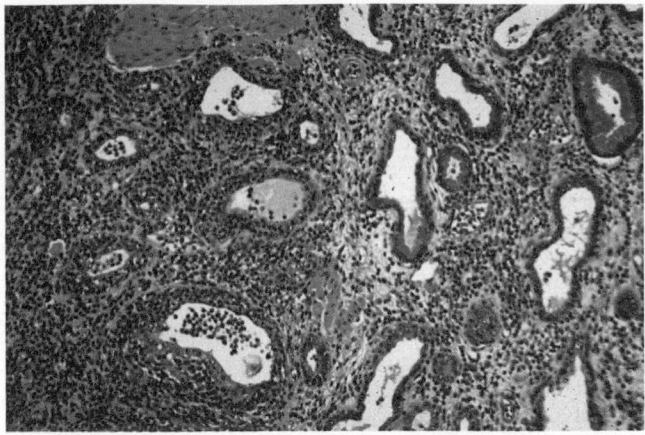

Fig 91-6 Microscopic appearance of purulent prostatitis in dog. (Courtesy Veterinary Pathology, University of Georgia, Athens, Ga.)

or chronic. Chronic infections are more common.[138] Prostatic cysts develop commonly with hyperplasia, and such cysts have been found in 14% of adult, male intact dogs.[38] Approximately 42% of such cysts are infected, and the same organism is usually found in the urine.[38] Abscesses develop when the infection is severe and encapsulation of purulent material occurs. Prostatic infections are mainly a problem in intact male dogs. If an infection is present before neutering, the infection may persist.

Of the male dog's genital organs, the prostate gland is the closest to the indigenous microflora of the distal urethra. Migration of bacteria up the urethra to the prostate is inhibited by urine flow during micturition, urethral pressure, characteristics of the urethral mucosa, normal secretion of prostatic fluid, and the antibacterial nature of normal prostatic fluid. The prostate gland can also produce IgA as a local response to bacterial infection. The higher prevalence of UTIs in castrated male dogs than in intact dogs may reflect the importance of prostatic defense mechanisms.[113]

The pathogenesis of prostatic infections is incompletely understood. Most infections are assumed to be secondary to migration of bacteria up the urethra, although spread via blood, urine, semen, and rectal flora (via direct extension or lymphatics) has also been postulated. The close anatomic relationship between the bladder, proximal urethra, and prostate gland is reflected in the high frequency with which all three are simultaneously infected. Prostatic fluid normally refluxes into the bladder, and urine can enter prostatic ducts during micturition. Whether prostatic infection usually precedes, follows, or develops simultaneously with bladder infection cannot usually be determined. Any condition that increases bacterial numbers in the prostatic urethra predisposes the animal to infection. Examples include urethral urolithiasis, neoplasia, trauma, stricture, or a lower UTI. Diseases that interfere with normal prostatic fluid formation and excretion also predispose the animal to infection. An example is squamous metaplasia of the prostate secondary to hyperestrogenism.[177,210]

Acute bacterial prostatitis and abscess formation may result in septicemia, which is responsible for the severity of clinical signs in some cases. Chronic prostatitis may be a sequela to acute infection or may develop insidiously. Bacteria are not always isolated from prostate glands showing histologic evidence of inflammation (Fig. 91-6). This has been found in human medicine, and some data suggest that prostatic infections can be the result of bacteria that are not detectable by conventional microbiologic culture.[62] Reflux of urine into the prostate gland, causing a chemical inflammatory response, may also be an underlying mechanism for culture negative prostatitis.[62] Abscess formation is thought to result from chronic infection and prostatic cyst infection. Abscesses may rupture, leading to peritonitis.

Clinical Findings

Signs associated with acute bacterial prostatitis include fever, depression, anorexia, urethral discharge, and pain on prostatic palpation. Vomiting is possible because of localized peritonitis. Less common signs are a stiff, stilted rear-limb gait and constipation from defecation avoidance because of pain. The size, symmetry, and contour of the prostate gland are normal unless it is enlarged as a result of hyperplasia.

Chronic bacterial prostatitis is usually not associated with signs of systemic illness, although some dogs may be more lethargic than normal.[138] A purulent or hemorrhagic urethral discharge may be present. In some dogs, the only indication of chronic bacterial prostatitis is recurrent UTI or mild hematuria. Chronic prostatitis should be considered in stud dogs with signs of infertility. The prostate gland is not painful on palpation, and infection alone does not affect prostatic size,[6] although some variation in consistency is associated with increased fibrous tissue.

The most common signs of prostatic abscess formation in dogs are fever, depression, and lethargy, associated with caudal abdominal pain.[180,279] The prostate is often enlarged and asymmetric, causing tenesmus and constipation. A constant or an intermittent urethral discharge, which is hemorrhagic, purulent, or both, may be present. Dysuria can occur as a result of interference with normal urethral function. Chronic partial urethral obstruction resulting from abscess formation can lead to a distended bladder, eventual detrusor dysfunction, and overflow urinary incontinence. About 10% of dogs have signs of septic shock (tachycardia, pale mucous membranes, delayed capillary refill, and weak pulse).[180] Icterus from hepatic compromise may be present. Rupture of a prostatic abscess can cause localized or diffuse peritonitis with signs of abdominal pain and vomiting. If the abscess is secondary to squamous hyperplasia from hyperestrogenism, other signs of hyperestrogenism such as pendulous prepuce, truncal alopecia, hyperpigmentation, and gynecomastia may be seen. In the one reported case of chronic prostatitis with abscess formation in a cat, the presenting sign was dyschezia caused by constipation resulting from encroachment on the colon by the enlarged prostate.[231] No signs of systemic disease were found in this cat.

Diagnosis

The main diagnostic techniques used to determine whether bacterial prostatitis is present are history and prostatic palpation, CBC, urinalysis and urine culture, prostatic fluid evaluation, ultrasonography, and prostatic aspiration and biopsy. Associated clinical signs and physical examination findings in conjunction with CBC and urinalysis and urine culture results are often sufficient to establish a tentative diagnosis of acute prostatitis. Additional tests are necessary in cases of chronic prostatitis to localize the site of infection to the prostate gland, because clinical signs are minimal. Prostatic ultrasonography with aspiration is necessary to confirm the presence of an abscess.

Laboratory Findings An inflammatory leukogram with or without a left shift is often associated with acute bacterial prostatitis and prostatic abscess formation.[279] The CBC is usually normal in dogs with chronic prostatitis without abscess formation.[21] Urinalysis and urine culture indicate UTIs in most but not all cases. In one study, four of five dogs with infected prostatic cysts had the same bacterial species isolated from urine cultures.[38]

Blood chemistry is usually normal with acute and chronic prostatitis but may be abnormal with abscess formation and bacteremia secondary to acute infection. Serum bilirubin concentration and liver enzyme activities (especially alkaline phosphatase [ALP]) may be increased.[279] Even in the absence of icterus, liver function tests such as bromsulphalein retention or bile acids may be abnormal. Hypoglycemia was found in 40% of cases with abscess formation.[180]

Prostatic Fluid Evaluation Prostatic fluid is usually not evaluated in dogs with acute prostatitis because affected dogs are often in too much pain to ejaculate and because of the difficulty in interpreting prostatic massage samples when a UTI is present. However, an ejaculate is usually essential for diagnosis of chronic prostatic infection. The prostatic fluid is the last and largest fraction of the ejaculate, after the sperm-rich fraction. When collecting the ejaculate, the dog is allowed to urinate and is then returned to a run or to a quiet environment. Any preputial discharge is removed from the sheath by gentle, minimal cleansing with moistened gauze sponges. The area is gently dried. The ejaculate is collected with a sterile funnel and tube; a large, sterile plastic syringe case; or a sterile urine cup. If a dog's semen cannot be collected after manual manipulation, the dog can be teased by an estrous bitch or an anestrous bitch to whose vulva p-methyl hydroxybenzoate (Eastman Kodak, Rochester, N.Y.) has been applied. Part of the ejaculate is used for cytologic study and part for quantitative culture. Quantitative culture is essential because of the normal flora of the distal urethra.

Both ejaculate cytology and culture results must be considered when determining whether an infection is present. Normal dogs occasionally have leukocytes and positive culture results. Bacteria number fewer than 10^5 per ml and are usually gram-positive. In dogs with bacterial prostatitis, the prostatic fluid is usually purulent and septic and may be hemorrhagic (Fig. 91-7). Quantitative culture of urine and prostatic fluid should yield significant numbers of the same organism. Dogs with experimental chronic bacterial prostatitis had greater than 1000 organisms per milliliter, but establishing a definitive number to distinguish infection from urethral or preputial contamination is difficult. High numbers of gram-negative organisms with large numbers of leukocytes indicate infection. Large numbers of gram-positive organisms with large numbers of leukocytes also indicate infection if preputial contamination did not occur. Lower numbers of gram-negative or gram-positive organisms must be correlated with clinical signs and ejaculate cytologic findings to determine their significance. If

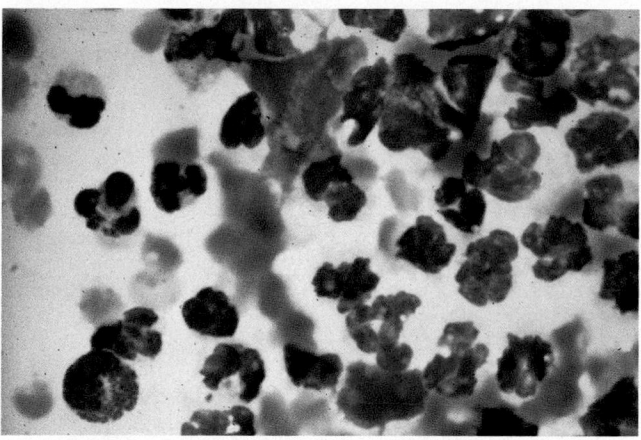

Fig 91-7 Microscopic appearance of purulent and hemorrhagic ejaculate from dog with prostatitis showing many erythrocytes and degenerate neutrophils. (Courtesy University of Georgia, Athens, Ga.)

results of culture and cytology are questionable, a second sample should be evaluated. The finding of macrophages in prostatic fluid correlated with prostatic infection in experimentally induced prostatitis in dogs.

For detection of chronic prostatitis, evaluation of prostatic fluid collected by ejaculation is preferred to fluid collected after prostatic massage. The results of prostatic massage in dogs with UTIs are difficult to interpret because of the large number of bacteria already in the urinary tract. To effectively use prostatic massage to diagnose bacterial prostatitis, a UTI must be controlled first with prior antimicrobial therapy. Prostatic massage in normal dogs yields only a few erythrocytes and transitional epithelial cells.

With prostatic massage, the dog is allowed to empty the bladder by normal voiding. A urinary catheter is passed to the bladder with aseptic technique. Residual urine volume should be measured as the bladder is emptied. The bladder is flushed several times with sterile saline to ensure that all urine is removed. The last flush of 5 to 10 ml is saved as the premassage sample. The catheter is then retracted distal to the prostate, as determined by rectal palpation, and the prostate is massaged rectally or abdominally for 1 to 2 minutes. After massage, sterile physiologic saline is injected slowly while the urethral orifice is occluded around the catheter to prevent reflux of the fluid. The catheter is slowly advanced to the bladder, with repeated aspiration in the prostatic urethra. The bulk of the fluid is aspirated from the bladder. The premassage and postmassage samples are examined by cytology and quantitative culture. It is important to compare the postmassage sample with the premassage sample to ensure that any abnormalities arose in the prostatic fluid and did not preexist in the bladder or urethra.

Radiography The only radiographic sign of acute prostatitis is an indistinct cranial prostatic border. This is not noted in all cases. Contrast radiography is not often performed in acute prostatitis, because the diagnosis can usually be made without it.

A change associated with some cases of chronic prostatitis is granular, parenchymal mineralization, but the prostate is often radiographically normal with chronic infection, and prostatic mineralization occurs more commonly with prostatic neoplasia.[73] Infection without abscess formation does not cause marked prostatomegaly. With abscess formation, the prostate is usually enlarged and irregular,[73] and the caudal abdomen may have poor contrast. The iliac lymph nodes may be enlarged. Radiography revealing gas within the prostate gland indicates emphysematous prostatitis from infection with gas-forming bacteria, most commonly *E. coli*.[129] Prostatic calculi may accompany bacterial prostatitis. These calculi are composed of bacteria, debris, and minerals.[262]

Radiography is important for detecting bone lesions caused by metastasis from prostatic neoplasia and detecting diskospondylitis caused by bacteremia from an associated UTI.[73] With chronic prostatitis, greater than normal urethroprostatic reflux may be noted on retrograde urethrography, but this is not specific and accompanies most other prostatic diseases. With abscess formation, periurethral asymmetry and narrowing of the prostatic urethra may be observed in addition to urethroprostatic reflux.[129] Urethroprostatic reflux is not present in all cases. The prostatic urethral lumen may appear undulant but is not distorted or destroyed.[16] A prominent colliculus seminalis is sometimes seen with squamous metaplasia of the prostate gland. The colliculus seminalis appears like a protuberance into the urethra; it is differentiated from a neoplasm by its smooth, round borders.

Ultrasonography Ultrasonography provides more information about prostatic internal structure than radiography. Ultrasonographic measurements have been shown to correlate with physical measurements.[6] Ultrasonography of the canine prostate gland has been most often performed transabdominally. A transrectal approach allows a higher resolution transducer to be placed closer to the prostate gland, resulting in a better image.[210] Ultrasonography is less sensitive in imaging the prostatic urethra; thus in dogs that are dysuric, urethrocystography should be performed in addition to ultrasonography.[73]

The normal prostate is uniformly hyperechoic compared with surrounding structures, with a small hypoechoic area in the center that is the prostatic urethra. Ultrasound alone should never be relied on to make a definitive diagnosis as there is considerable overlap in ultrasonographic appearance with different prostatic disease processes. In asymptomatic dogs, Doppler ultrasound could not differentiate between a normal prostate and one with inflammation.[190] Nevertheless, some ultrasonographic patterns are more typical of some diseases than others. Focal, multifocal, or diffuse hyperechogenicity has been associated with prostatic inflammation. Neoplasia tends to produce a complex combination of hyperechoic and hypoechoic areas with some unaffected parenchyma.[73] With abscess formation, the prostate gland is usually hyperechoic with parenchymal hypoechoic cavities (Fig. 91-8), irregular outlines, and asymmetric shapes.[167] The cavitary areas exhibit distal enhancement, suggestive of being fluid filled, but these cannot be distinguished from noninfected prostatic cysts, cavitary neoplasias, or hematomas.[73] Ultrasonography is useful in guiding aspiration of fluid-filled areas and biopsy of solid areas (see Needle Aspiration and Biopsy). In dogs with fluid-filled areas in the prostate, aspiration using ultrasound guidance is replacing collection of ejaculates and prostatic massage samples as a method for obtaining prostatic fluid.

Urethroscopy Urethroscopy of male dogs greater than 12 kg is usually possible using flexible endoscopic equipment.[262] The prostatic urethra can be visualized. It may be possible to verify that an exudate or a hemorrhage is entering the prostatic urethra and to exclude nonprostatic urethral lesions as a cause for a urethral discharge.

Needle Aspiration or Biopsy Diagnosis of prostatic disease can also be approached by needle aspiration or biopsy by the perirectal or transabdominal route, depending on the location of the prostate. Transrectal fine-needle aspiration with a Franzen needle guide (Precision Dynamics,

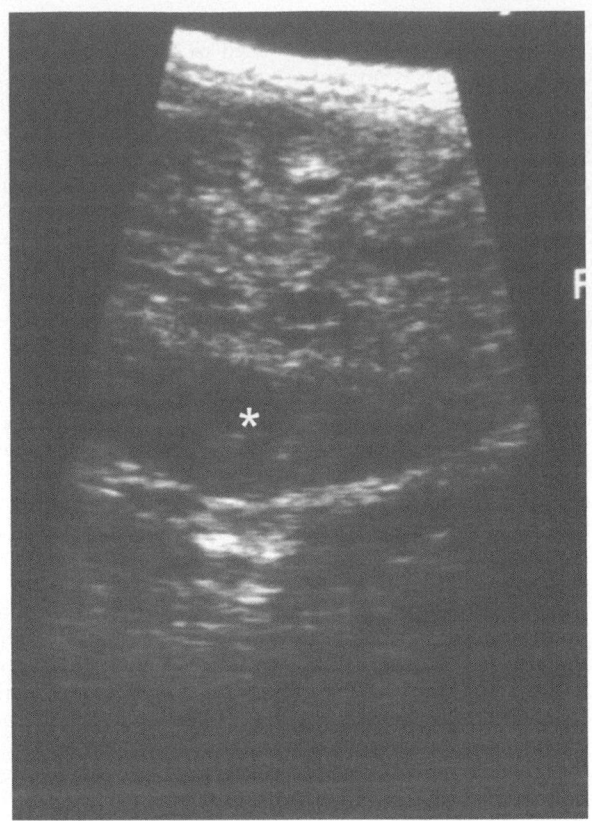

Fig 91-8 Ultrasound examination showing hypoechoic areas within hyperechoic prostate gland. Aspiration of largest hypoechoic area (*asterisk*) confirmed abscess formation. (Courtesy University of Georgia, Athens, Ga.)

Burbank, Calif.) and a 22-gauge needle has also been described.[210] Ultrasonography can guide the process. If the prostate contains fluid-filled spaces, they should be aspirated before a needle biopsy. If the prostate is solid, both aspiration and biopsy can be performed. If ultrasonography is not available, fine-needle aspiration should always be performed before needle biopsy because of the possibility of an occult abscess.

Before aspiration and biopsy, hair at the site should be clipped and the site prepared aseptically. If ultrasound guidance is used, the transducer should be covered with a sterile sleeve, and sterile acoustic gel should be used. Clean but not aseptic technique for prostatic aspiration resulted in conversion of a prostatic cyst to a prostatic abscess in one dog.[13]

Needle aspiration is performed with a 21-gauge, 1- to 2½-inch needle, depending on the size of the animal and prostate. The needle used in the perirectal approach should have a stylet (such as that on a spinal needle) and is guided by rectal palpation. The procedure can be performed in most dogs with mild tranquilization. Perirectal aspiration is best avoided in dogs with suspected abscesses, because bacteria may be seeded along the needle track. After aspiration of abscesses, some dogs have developed signs of localized peritonitis that required parenteral antibiotic therapy to resolve. Cytology should be performed on all aspirates. If pus is aspirated, aerobic and anaerobic bacterial cultures are indicated.

Prostatic biopsy can be performed perirectally or transabdominally or via a caudal abdominal surgical exposure. Nonsurgical biopsy procedures require tranquilization and local anesthesia. An automatic, spring-loaded biopsy device (Biopty gun, Radiplast AB, Uppsala, Sweden), with a 14- to 18-gauge needle makes the procedure less difficult. Closed biopsy can be directed by palpation or by ultrasonography. The only complication reported from blind prostatic biopsy is mild hematuria, although significant hemorrhage is possible in any blind biopsy procedure. The dog should always be monitored closely for several hours after biopsy. Biopsy samples can be cultured for bacteria as well as examined histologically.

Ultrasound-guided aspiration, biopsy, or both of the prostate resulted in an accurate diagnosis in 14 of 17 cases (82%) in one survey.[13] In the remaining cases, neoplasia was confirmed or suspected, but aspiration revealed hemorrhage or abscess formation. One difficulty with diagnosis by aspiration or biopsy is that the prostate may be affected by more than one disease process. This possibility necessitates that all the data about a clinical case be evaluated together. A diagnosis must be reconsidered if response to therapy is not as predicted. Biopsy samples should be collected if surgery is performed.

Therapy

Acute Bacterial Prostatitis In acute bacterial prostatitis, an antibiotic should be administered for 28 days (see Table 91-8). The choice of antibiotic can be based on urine culture results, because the organism in the urine probably originated from the prostate. Because the blood-prostatic fluid barrier is damaged in acute inflammation, a wide choice of antibiotics similar to that for UTIs may be considered for initial treatment (see Table 91-12). If the presenting signs are severe, the antimicrobial is initially given IV. Supportive therapy should be given as necessary for systemic illness. Once the dog's condition is stable, an oral antimicrobial with prostatic penetrance is preferred for the remainder of therapy (see Table 91-13). Because acute infections may become chronic, reexamination should be performed 7 days after antibiotic therapy is finished. This examination should include physical examination, urinalysis, urine culture, and prostatic fluid cytology and culture.

Chronic Bacterial Prostatitis Cases of chronic bacterial prostatitis are very difficult to treat effectively. One factor is the blood-prostatic fluid barrier. This barrier is related to the pH difference between the blood and prostatic interstitium and the prostatic fluid and the characteristics of the prostatic acinar epithelium. A drug's ability to enter prostatic fluid depends on its lipid solubility, its degree of ionization in plasma (ionization constant—pKa), its molecular size if it is water soluble, and its plasma protein-binding characteristics.[164]

The pH of the blood and the prostatic interstitium is 7.4, whereas the pH of normal and infected prostatic fluid in dogs is less than 7.4.[21] Most antimicrobial agents are weak acids or weak bases and ionized to varying degrees in biologic fluids. The degree of ionization is determined by the pKa of the drug and the pH of the fluid. Drugs with a pKa close to 7.4 are only slightly charged in serum, whereas those with a pKa higher or lower than 7.4 are charged in serum.[77] Because canine prostatic fluid is usually acidic, basic antibiotics (pKa greater than 7) such as erythromycin, clindamycin, and trimethoprim cross the barrier more readily than other antibiotics (see Table 91-13; Fig. 91-9).[17] In men, infected prostatic fluid is alkaline, thus drug efficacy in men cannot be directly extrapolated to dogs. Fluoroquinolones are more active in alkaline environments (pH greater than 7.4) for gram-negative bacteria and thus may be more effective in chronic prostatitis in men than in dogs.[42]

Lipid solubility is also an important factor in determining drug movement across the prostatic epithelium. Chloramphenicol, macrolide antibiotics, trimethoprim, and enrofloxacin are examples of lipid-soluble drugs that can cross the barrier effectively.[42,63] In general, diffusion of tetracyclines into

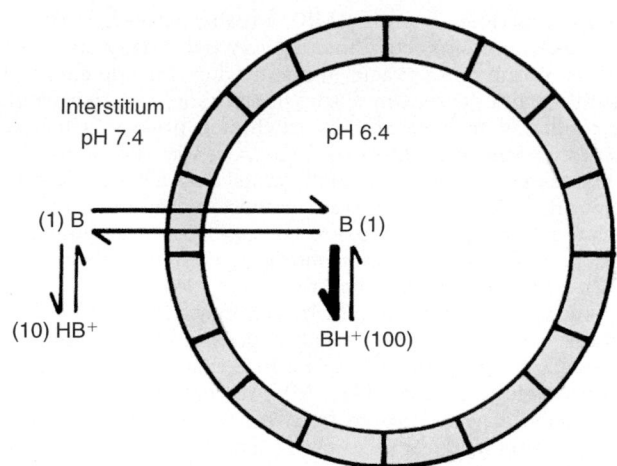

Fig 91-9 Diffusion into prostate of antibiotic that is a weak base (ionization constant [pKa] of 8.4) is shown at equilibrium. More acidic pH within prostate causes drug to become more ionized, hence it cannot leave prostatic fluid. Prostatic fluid-plasma ratio is 101:11 (B, basic drug [pKa greater than 7]; BH, HB, ionized drug). (From Barsanti JA, Finco DR. 1979. Canine bacterial prostatitis, *Vet Clin North Am* 9:679-699.)

canine prostatic fluid is minimal. Although clinical studies in men with prostatitis demonstrated efficacy of minocycline and doxycycline, these lipid-soluble drugs did not penetrate well into canine prostatic fluid. Drugs with low lipid solubility, such as penicillin, ampicillin, cephalosporin, and aminoglycoside, cannot cross into the prostatic acini.

Protein binding in plasma also determines the amount of drug that enters prostatic fluid. The more drug bound to protein, the less drug that is available to cross the prostatic epithelium. This factor is probably less important than lipid solubility or ionization, because biologic systems rarely reach equilibrium. Examples of drugs with significant protein binding are clindamycin and chloramphenicol.

In addition to a blood-prostatic barrier, chronic bacterial infections of the prostate gland may be difficult to cure because of the local microenvironment. One study of chronic prostatitis in rats showed that successful eradication of infection was not related to norfloxacin concentrations. This suggested that the bacteria were protected in microcolonies and biofilms in those rats that were not successfully treated.[62]

Recommendations for the treatment of chronic bacterial prostatitis are based on whether a gram-positive or gram-negative organism is the infective agent. If the causative organism is gram-positive, erythromycin, clindamycin, or trimethoprim can be given, depending on the organism's susceptibility. If the causative organism is gram-negative, trimethoprim or a quinolone, such as enrofloxacin, is best. Although trimethoprim is often combined with a sulfonamide drug, sulfonamides do not diffuse into the prostate gland.[9] Trimethoprim alone is considered as effective as the combination in men[77] and may have fewer side effects. Fluoroquinolones typically have a small molecular size, high lipid solubility, and low protein binding, which makes them useful in chronic prostatic infections. It has been suggested that the dose of enrofloxacin be determined by the degree of sensitivity of the infecting organism as determined by MIC.[262] If the organism has an MIC of 0.1 μ/ml, then a dose of 5 mg/kg once a day is appropriate. If the organism has an MIC of 0.1 to 0.5 μ/ml, then a dose of 10 mg/kg once a day is suggested. If the organism has an MIC of 0.5 to 1 μg/ml, then a dose of up to 20 mg/kg once a day may be needed. Because a higher maximum concentration is more important in efficacy than duration of time above the MIC, a higher once-daily dose is considered more effective than a lower twice-daily dose. Side effects of oral enrofloxacin in mature dogs include anorexia, vomiting, and depression. Other fluoroquinolones that would be predicted to have efficacy in chronic prostatitis include marbofloxacin and ofloxacin. Ofloxacin was shown to concentrate in the prostate gland of normal dogs after oral administration.[10] Ofloxacin was also administered by intraprostatic injection. The prostatic tissue concentration was similar to that of orally administered ofloxacin, even though a much lower dose was injected than that given orally.[10]

Antibiotic therapy should be continued for 6 weeks (see Table 91-8). If a UTI is present, urine should be reevaluated by culture during therapy to be sure that the administered drug has eliminated the UTI. After discontinuing antibiotics, urine should be recultured (see Table 91-14) to ensure that the infection has been eliminated, not merely suppressed. In men it has been noted that if chronic bacterial prostatitis is not eliminated with 6 to 12 weeks of therapy, longer courses of therapy do not increase the likelihood of cure.[77,164] In this situation in men, suppressive therapy for UTIs is recommended. The prognosis for cure in men is approximately 70% with 6 months of follow-up,[77,184] but success rates seem to decrease beyond 6 months because of recurrence.[185] Similar studies have not been performed in dogs, but the author's experience is that canine infections are similarly difficult to cure in intact dogs.

Castration is recommended as adjunctive therapy in dogs to control infection. Limited studies indicate that castration in dogs is beneficial in resolving prostatic infection.[50] Estrogens used as chemical castration are not recommended as therapy for prostatitis because estrogens can induce squamous metaplasia and thus predispose the dog to infection.[16] Estrogen therapy can also be associated with the rare complication of significant bone marrow toxicity. Whether other drugs that cause prostatic involution in dogs, such as flutamide or finasteride, would be useful in resolving prostatic infections in intact dogs has not been studied.

If the animal is not cured within 6 weeks of antimicrobial therapy and castration, suppressive therapy should be considered. The goal of suppressive therapy is to eliminate the UTI. It has been found in men that this regimen often results in symptomatic relief and little progression of infection within the prostate gland. Suppressive therapy involves indefinite treatment with a once-daily dose of the antimicrobial agent. Drugs chosen must be well tolerated and must be active against the infective agent at obtainable urine concentrations. In men the drugs of choice are trimethoprim, trimethoprim-sulfamethoxazole, a fluoroquinolone, or nitrofurantoin.[77] Long-term therapy with trimethoprim-sulfonamide in dogs can result in KCS, mild anemia because of folate deficiency, secondary hypothyroidism, and immune-mediated diseases.[16,90,282] Folic acid can be supplemented when administering trimethoprim-sulfonamide for longer than 6 weeks.

Prostatic Abscesses Prostatic abscesses require surgical drainage. Relatively small (smaller than 1.5 by 2.4 cm), infected prostatic cysts in asymptomatic dogs are often cured with ultrasound-guided drainage and antimicrobial therapy.[38] Some abscesses and symptomatic cysts in dogs whose owners have financial limitations have been managed with ultrasound-guided drainage and long-term antimicrobial therapy, but this therapy is unlikely to be curative.[221] Intracapsular prostatic omentalization is considered the surgical approach of choice.[279] Partial prostatectomy with an ultrasonic surgical aspirator has few complications and allows an equally rapid recovery, but the equipment is expensive.[221]

If prostatic enlargement has resulted in partial urethral obstruction, bladder and urethral function should be carefully assessed. Prolonged bladder distension may have resulted in bladder atony. An indwelling urinary catheter may be necessary to allow the detrusor muscle to recover. If the bladder wall has been chronically distended and infected, it may be irreversibly damaged.

Castration is recommended as adjunctive therapy. Castration without abscess drainage leads to reduction of prostatic tissue but continuation of the abscess pockets.

An affected dog should also be treated with antibiotics as described previously for chronic prostatitis. The antibiotic choice should be modified based on the results of culture and susceptibility and the presence or absence of bacteremia. IV antimicrobials should be provided when the dog is systemically ill and during surgery. If possible, surgery should be delayed until after culture results are obtained. The prostate gland should be reexamined by palpation and ultrasonography at monthly intervals until abscess resolution is confirmed. In one survey, 31% of dogs with a successful surgical outcome had a UTI recurrence within 1 year.[221] These dogs are usually asymptomatic, so detection of such recurrences requires urinalysis and urine culture, not just questioning of the owner about the presence of clinical signs.

Polyuria and polydipsia, similar to those expected with nephrogenic diabetes insipidus, have been noted in a few dogs with prostatic abscesses.[99] These problems resolved within 1 month after surgery. Evidence of hepatopathy also resolved postoperatively. It is assumed that these signs are caused by secondary septicemia or endotoxemia.

If the owners decline surgery, the dog can be managed with long-term suppressive antibiotic therapy after the UTI is controlled with at least 6 weeks of standard, full-dose therapy. The owners must realize that the abscess will persist and may result in a life-threatening infection.

Epididymitis and Orchitis
Etiology
Bacterial infection is the most common cause of epididymo-orchitis, which is relatively uncommon, especially in cats.[114] As in UTIs, E. coli is a common causative organism. Brucella canis infection should always be a consideration in dogs. Infection may be secondary to trauma (such as a bite wound) or may result from breeding a healthy male with an infected female, hematogenous spread of a systemic infection, or spread from a urinary tract or prostatic infection. Infection with feline infectious peritonitis virus has been reported as a rare cause of orchitis in cats.[76,246] In both reported cases, orchitis was the initial presenting problem, and then the disease progressed to its systemic form.

Clinical Findings
Any age or breed of dog may be affected, although dogs younger than 2 years were most common in one small series of cases.[217] Both the testicle and epididymis may be involved, and the infection may be unilateral or bilateral (Fig. 91-10). Clinical signs in acute infections include pain (which may manifest as rear-limb lameness), heat, and swelling, which is doughy to firm in consistency. The dog often licks the edematous scrotum, which may cause dermatitis. Systemic signs such as fever vary. With chronic infections, fibrosis produces increased firmness and contracture. Localized areas of abscess formation may feel soft.

Diagnosis
Orchitis or epididymitis is usually strongly suspected on the basis of physical examination. Diagnostic tests should include CBC, urinalysis, urine culture, and brucellosis testing. The CBC may show leukocytosis if the inflammation is active. Urinalysis and urine culture determine whether the animal has an associated UTI. If a UTI is confirmed, the responsible

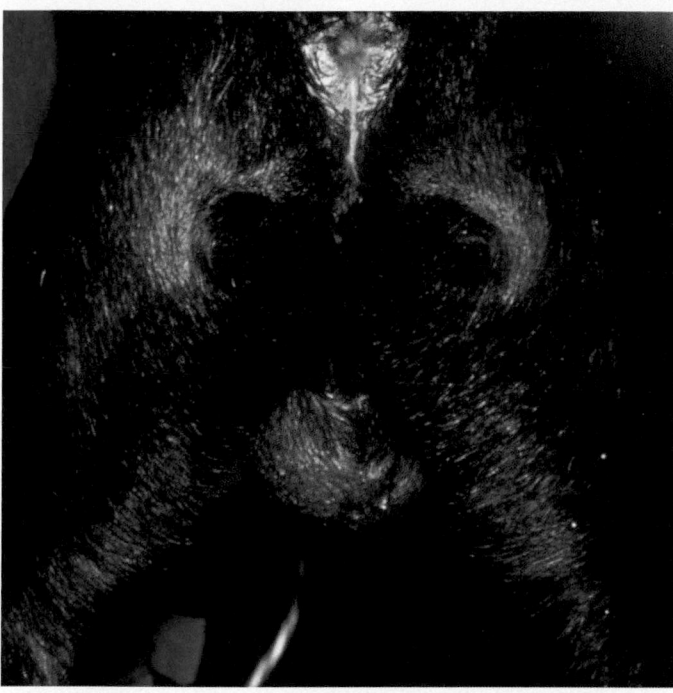

Fig 91-10 Dog with unilateral epididymitis-orchitis. (Courtesy University of Georgia, Athens, Ga.)

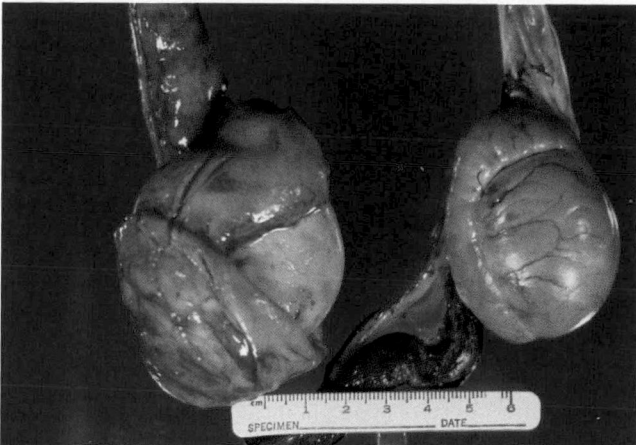

Fig 91-11 Unilateral *E. coli* epididymitis in a dog. Epididymis is enlarged on left, and both testicles are shrunken from atrophy caused by increased temperature in scrotal sac. (Courtesy University of Georgia, Athens, Ga.)

organism is assumed to be the cause of the epididymitis-orchitis. In dogs with brucellosis, urine may contain the organism, although usually only in low numbers (fewer than 1000 per milliliter).[44] Although semen is a more productive *Brucella* culture sample, handling it has greater public health risk (see Chapter 40).

If the dog does not have a UTI and will ejaculate, cytologic examination and quantitative culture of semen should be performed. With semen, the cytologic finding of bacteria and neutrophils and the culture of more than 10^5 gram-negative organisms per milliliter suggest infection. Because of the urethral microflora, quantitative cultures are mandatory for assessment of results.

If the urine is not infected and semen cannot be collected, aspiration of the testicle or epididymis with a 21- to 23-gauge needle and a 12-ml syringe can be performed for cytology and culture. Before the aspiration, dogs are usually sedated, depending on their nature, and the scrotal skin should be cleansed. Ultrasonography can guide the aspiration to abnormal areas of the epididymis or testicle. In one study, no adverse effects from aspiration were noted.[53]

Ultrasonography can also be used to determine whether a palpable abnormality in the scrotal contents is testicular, epididymal, or both or is outside the testicles and epididymides. A cause of swelling can be defined as being caused by fluid or a solid mass.[68,129] It may be possible to differentiate an inflammatory disease from testicular torsion, traumatic rupture, or neoplasia.[217] Ultrasonographic findings associated with acute epididymitis-orchitis include a diffuse, patchy, hypoechoic pattern; testicular enlargement, epididymal enlargement, or both; and occasionally, extratesticular fluid.[217]

Therapy
Bilateral orchidectomy is the treatment of choice for orchitis and epididymitis. If the dog is a valuable sire and the condition is unilateral, the testicle and epididymis on the affected side should be removed to save the other from thermal degeneration (Fig. 91-11).[68,136] If unilateral orchidectomy is performed, the owner should be advised that a subclinical infection of an apparently normal testicle and epididymis or a concurrent prostatic infection could cause future problems for the dog.

Antibiotics should be given regardless of whether surgery is performed. Isolation of the causative organism and antimicrobial susceptibility testing should guide therapy. Therapy should be continued for at least 2 weeks. While culture results are pending, an antibiotic such as enrofloxacin, chloramphenicol, or trimethoprim-sulfonamide should be started. Adjunctive soaks in cool water may help to reduce testicular degeneration from the hyperthermia of inflammation.

Balanoposthitis
Balanoposthitis is usually caused by bacteria that are normally present in the prepuce (see Table 91-2). Herpesvirus infections and blastomycosis also have caused balanoposthitis.

Mild balanoposthitis is so common that it is considered normal in male dogs. It is characterized by a purulent exudate within or dripping from the prepuce, with variable degrees of inflammation of the preputial mucosa. The animal has no signs of systemic illness. Dogs usually are asymptomatic, but some lick the prepuce.

No specific diagnostic test exists for balanoposthitis except cytologic examination of preputial exudate. Bacteria and large numbers of degenerate and nondegenerate neutrophils are seen. A culture of pus is difficult to interpret because of the abundant normal flora. Culture is not required for successful management of most cases.

Balanoposthitis is not a serious medical problem but may be an annoyance to the owner. Cleansing antiseptic douches or local antibacterials may be of benefit. Neutering affected animals may help reduce the amount of secretion produced.

FEMALE GENITAL INFECTIONS

Organisms associated with genital infections in female dogs are the same as those associated with UTIs.[16] *E. coli* is consistently the most common organism associated with pyometra.

Vaginitis
Etiology
Inflammation of the vagina can be a result of bacterial or viral infections, immaturity, or irritation from urine, foreign mate-

rial, neoplasia, trauma, or anatomic abnormalities such as a recessed vulva or vaginal stenosis. Bacterial infection can be a secondary result of these irritations. Vaginitis is more common in bitches than in queens and is most common in young dogs, with affected dogs being an average age of 7 months.[182] Juvenile or puppy vaginitis is common in otherwise normal, healthy prepubertal bitches and resolves spontaneously with physical maturity in most. Vaginitis in the young dog (younger than 1 year) is more likely a problem related to immaturity than to a bacterial infection.[121]

Bacterial organisms recovered from bitches with vaginitis are the same organisms found in the normal flora, although the numbers of bacteria may be higher in mature dogs with vaginitis.[121,267] Isolation of a single bacterial species occurs in about 25% of bitches with vaginitis; *E. coli*, *Streptococcus*, and *Staphylococcus* are the most common.[35] Although infection with *Coxiella burnetii* is rare in cats, the organism can cause abortion with associated vaginal discharge. Because *C. burnetii* is a significant public health hazard, care should be taken when assessing vaginal discharges in cats (see Chapter 29).[209]

Viral infections of the canine or feline vagina are uncommon. Herpesviruses (canine herpesvirus, feline rhinotracheitis virus) cause vesicular lesions and erythema when inoculated intravaginally.[106,112] Although genital tract infection readily occurs after experimental inoculation, genital herpesvirus infection is an uncommon clinical entity.[218] Vaginal lymphoid follicular hyperplasia, which could result from any inflammatory process, may be mistaken for vesicle formation. Confirmation of genital herpesvirus infection should include viral isolation and histologic examination of the vesicular lesions (see Chapter 5).

Clinical Findings

The most common historical and physical finding associated with vaginitis is the presence of a vulvar discharge in an otherwise healthy animal. The discharge is mucus, mucopurulent, or purulent, varying in color from cloudy white to yellow to green.[121] The presence of blood in the discharge is rare.[121] The discharge may attract male dogs and may cause the affected dog to lick the vulvar area. The perineal hair may be discolored by saliva and exudate. Pollakiuria occurs in about 10% of affected bitches.[121] Signs of systemic illness are not expected. Vaginal discharge must be related to the stage of the estrous cycle as a serosanguineous discharge is normal in proestrus, a mucoid discharge is normal is diestrus, and a dark brown or green discharge is normal for up to 6 weeks postpartum. Vaginal discharges may also be caused by a uterine disease such as metritis or pyometra or may be urine in incontinent dogs. A complete physical examination including digital rectal and vaginal examinations should be performed in all animals with an abnormal vaginal discharge.

Diagnosis

The diagnosis of vaginitis is strongly suggested by the history, presence of vaginal discharge on physical examination, and vaginal cytology. This approach is sufficient for dogs younger than 1 year without UTI signs. In older dogs, especially those with chronic vaginitis, vaginoscopy, as well as urinalysis and urine culture, should be performed. A CBC and abdominal imaging (radiography or ultrasonography) may be needed to exclude the possibility of uterine disease. The most important diagnostic considerations are whether the vulvar discharge is abnormal and whether the inflammatory process is confined to the vagina.

Cytologic evidence of inflammation (neutrophils, possibly lymphocytes and macrophages in chronic cases) with or without bacteria is expected from animals with vaginitis.[218] Vaginal cytology must be interpreted with regard to the stage of the estrous cycle. WBCs are often numerous during the first few days of diestrus. This normal phenomenon can be distin-

guished from inflammation because the number of WBCs declines markedly in 24 to 48 hours of diestrus, whereas it persists with vaginitis. A vulvar mucoid, green to brownish discharge is normal during the early postpartum period in the bitch and queen. A hemorrhagic vulvar discharge is normal during proestrus and estrus in the bitch.

CBCs are normal in dogs with vaginitis.[121] In one study, UTIs were found in approximately 20% of mature bitches with vaginitis.[121] UTIs were not found in puppies with vaginitis, but urine from only a few puppies was examined.[121] At least a urinalysis and optimally a urine culture are indicated in mature dogs with vaginitis and puppies with signs of pollakiuria.

The results of vaginal cultures must be interpreted cautiously, because the most common pathogens of the vagina and uterus are *E. coli*, *Streptococcus*, and *Staphylococcus*, which are also commensal organisms (see Table 91-3). To avoid contamination from the skin and the vestibule, samples for bacterial culture from the cranial vagina should be obtained with a guarded swab or through a sterile speculum. Bacterial cultures do *not* confirm the diagnosis of vaginitis, because some bacterial growth *is* expected. Heavy growth of a single organism is a more convincing sign that the organism could be causing the clinical signs.

Vaginoscopy helps determine the source of the discharge and the nature and extent of vaginal lesions. Sedation or general anesthesia is usually necessary for a thorough examination. With vaginitis, the vaginal mucosa is hyperemic, and exudate in the vaginal lumen is present. Ulcers or lymphoid follicles may be seen (Fig. 91-12). The inciting cause of the vaginitis may be identified (Table 91-15). Vaginal cultures are easily obtained during vaginoscopy. Vaginal biopsy samples are taken when discrete lesions are seen.

Therapy

Treatment of puppy vaginitis is either none or conservative (perivulvar cleaning only), because the condition subsides with or without therapy in most cases.[121] Some recommend that the affected animal be allowed to experience an estrous cycle to increase the chance of spontaneous recovery[267]; however, the majority of young bitches recover before experiencing an estrous cycle.[121,123] Estrogen in the maturing bitch induces antibacterial activity in the vaginal mucosa, which

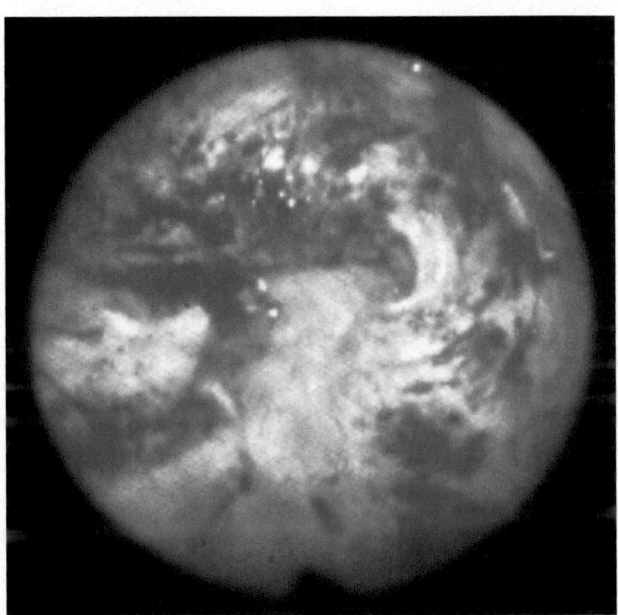

Fig 91-12 Vaginal inflammation visible through endoscope. (Courtesy University of Georgia, Athens, Ga.)

Table • 91-15
Underlying Causes of Vaginitis
Atresia
Strictures
Septa
Neoplasia, granuloma
Clitoral hypertrophy
Foreign objects
Urinary incontinence
Urinary tract infection

may facilitate recovery. The recommendation is that young bitches with clinically significant vaginitis not undergo ovariohysterectomy until they have experienced estrus or the vaginitis has resolved.[123,218] Although most cases of juvenile vaginitis resolve, about 20% of puppies have a recurrence.[183]

Most mature bitches with vaginitis have a predisposing abnormality (see Table 91-15).[121,123] Recovery from vaginitis requires correction of the underlying disorder. One study found that vaginitis associated with a recessed vulva resolved with vulvoplasty.[98] Surgical correction of vestibulovaginal stenosis resulted in resolution of chronic vaginitis in two dogs.[147]

In mature bitches with no underlying abnormality, vaginitis, even if chronic, resolves spontaneously in 75% of cases, although a full recovery may take months.[123] The remaining 25% of cases are frustrating for owners and veterinarians because no current therapy is consistently effective.[121] In intact bitches, an ovariohysterectomy does not improve clinical signs of vaginitis.[121]

The relative efficacy of various treatments for vaginitis has yet to be investigated in small animals. Antiseptic douches, instillation of antibiotic suppositories, ointments, or solutions, and systemic antibiotic therapy have been tried.[14] Solutions that alter pH, such as vinegar (0.25%) or most commercial douches, may discourage the overgrowth of vaginal bacteria. Douching should not be performed during proestrus or estrus.[123] Many owners are unable to douche their pets effectively.

Systemic antibiotics may diminish clinical signs in mature bitches with chronic vaginitis. The antimicrobial should be chosen on the basis of urine and cranial vaginal cultures. Antibiotics usually provided are ampicillin, trimethoprim-sulfonamide, amoxicillin-clavulanate, cephalosporin, and chloramphenicol.[123] Although in one study, ampicillin did not concentrate in the vaginal secretions of bitches, it did eradicate susceptible bacteria within 24 hours in healthy bitches.[254] Trimethoprim, which was shown to concentrate in vaginal secretions, did not eradicate all in vitro susceptible organisms in healthy bitches.[254] During therapy with either ampicillin or trimethoprim-sulfonamide, organisms were still present in the vaginal secretions of 8 of 10 bitches, and additional organisms emerged.[254]

If vaginitis is concurrent with pregnancy, the possible teratogenic or abortifacient effects of therapy must be considered. If vaginitis occurs in proestrus or estrus and the bitch is scheduled for breeding, the possibility of transmission of infection to the stud and the effects of therapy on sperm survival should be considered.

Metritis

Etiology and Pathogenesis

Metritis usually refers to acute ascending bacterial infection of the uterus.[168] Metritis may follow abortion, dystocia, obstetric manipulation, retention of fetal or placental parts, or normal parturition. Rarely, metritis may occur after natural or artificial insemination. The most common causative organism is *E. coli*. Chronic metritis occurs but is rarely described in the literature in dogs and cats.[85]

Many organisms cross the canine placenta and infect fetuses but do not infect the uterus per se. However, they may be transiently recovered from uterine or vaginal cultures of parturient or periparturient bitches. These organisms include canine herpesvirus, adenovirus, distemper virus, *B. canis*, and *Toxoplasma gondii*.[137] Experimental, intrauterine inoculation of *Mycoplasma canis* can cause uterine disease in bitches,[61] but the role of mycoplasmal infection in spontaneous disease is uncertain (see Chapter 32). In cats, feline leukemia virus, panleukopenia virus, and herpesviruses can be transmitted to the fetuses of viremic queens.

Clinical Findings

Animals with acute metritis are depressed, anorectic, febrile, and tachycardic and have a fetid, septic, purulent vaginal discharge. Signs usually develop within 1 week of parturition. Dehydration, sepsis, and endotoxemia can occur. Neonates of affected dams are usually neglected and crying from hunger as milk production declines.

Diagnosis

A presumptive diagnosis is based on the history and physical findings. Cytology and bacterial culture and susceptibility should be performed on the discharge. Cytology shows a hemorrhagic, septic, purulent exudate. Cytologic evidence of endometrial cells or uteroverdin indicates uterine involvement, but these are not consistently present. A neutrophilic leukocytosis is often evident on a CBC.[30] Abdominal radiography, uterine ultrasonography, or both should be performed to locate fetal remnants and assess the integrity of the uterus. In contrast to pyometra, the uterus is normal or minimally enlarged with metritis on survey abdominal radiographs.[82] Ultrasonographic diagnosis of metritis is not very accurate because the changes are subtle. The uterus may be slightly enlarged, and echogenicity may be abnormal.[288]

Therapy

IV fluids should be administered if needed to maintain normal hydration. A systemic, broad-spectrum antimicrobial should be given, pending the uterine culture results. An antimicrobial that is usually effective against *E. coli* should be chosen (see Tables 91-12 and 91-13). Antibiotic therapy is reassessed when the culture results are returned. Therapy should continue for 7 to 10 days if the uterus is removed and 2 to 4 weeks if it is not. Neonates are usually hand reared until the mother is sufficiently recovered to care for them.

A decision must be made about whether therapy of the infected uterus should be surgical or medical on the basis of the severity of the illness and the owner's desire to maintain the animal's reproductive capability. An ovariohysterectomy should be performed if the uterus has ruptured. An ovariohysterectomy or a hysterotomy with lavage is necessary if placental or fetal tissues are in the uterus.

Medical management involves stimulating the evacuation of the uterine contents. If the animal is within 24 hours of parturition, oxytocin can be administered at 0.5 to 1 U/kg, with a maximum of 20 U intramuscularly once or twice.[92] Natural prostaglandin $F_{2\alpha}$ (PGF$_{2\alpha}$ Lutalyse, Upjohn Company, Kalamazoo, Mich.) can be given any time postpartum at a dose of 0.1 mg/kg SC once a day for 2 to 3 days.[124] Adverse effects include vomiting, panting, restlessness, vocalization, and change in pupil size. Neither oxytocin nor PGF$_{2\alpha}$ affects lactation or neonatal health.[124] Intravaginally administered PGF$_{2\alpha}$ (150 µg/kg every 12 to 24 hours) was also found to be effective in conjunction with antibiotics.[85]

Intrauterine infusion of antiseptic or antibiotic solutions is of questionable value. The canine cervix is difficult to cannulate, therefore most infusions via the vagina are probably intravaginal rather than intrauterine. Intrauterine infusion of nitrofurazone may actually decrease subsequent fertility in some species.[168] Surgical placement of drains within the uterus and subsequent flushing is usually not successful.[100]

Pyometra

Etiology and Pathogenesis

Pyometra is an inflammatory disease of the uterus associated with intraluminal accumulation of pus. Pyometra involving the uterus masculinus of hermaphrodites also occurs in dog and cats.[240] Unlike metritis, which is usually a periparturient disease associated with infection or uterine trauma, pyometra is secondary to uterine pathologic signs induced by progesterone over successive heat cycles or by exogenous therapy.[100] The sustained influence of progesterone causes cystic endometrial hyperplasia, fluid accumulation within the endometrial glands and uterine lumen, suppressed leukocyte activity in the uterus, and decreased myometrial activity. The uterine disease and decreased contractility favor secondary ascending bacterial infection. E. coli is the most common causative organism, in part because E. coli binds to the endometrium more effectively during the luteal phase of the estrous cycle.[80] Because progesterone initiates the sequence of events leading to pyometra, pyometra occurs during the luteal phase of the cycle in dogs (diestrus) or after the administration of progestins.[270] The disease does not develop during pregnancy, and nulliparous bitches have a moderately higher risk than primiparous and multiparous dogs.[82,194]

Despite the commonly accepted pathogenesis discussed, it is clear that not all bitches with cystic endometrial hyperplasia develop pyometra, thus the relationship of cystic endometrial hyperplasia to pyometra is not accepted by all.[57,80] Some believe that pyometra is an age-related disease, and others emphasize bacterial infections, particularly with E. coli, as primary causes, with coincidental cystic endometrial hyperplasia.

Pyometra occurs most frequently in dogs. In one study, affected dogs tended to be middle-aged or older, with an average age of onset of 9 years, but administration of estradiol cypionate induced pyometra in young dogs.[194] In this study, no significant increased risk was found with a single treatment of medroxyprogesterone acetate therapy. Repeated administrations would be expected to increase risk. Potential reasons for an increased risk with estrogen therapy are that the cervix may be relaxed for a longer time, and estrogen enhances the effects of progesterone on the uterus.[194] The risk of a female dog younger than 10 years of age developing pyometra was 2% per year. The risk increased with age, so dogs of 8 to 10 years had a risk of 6% per year.[66] By 10 years of age, 23% to 24% of bitches developed pyometra.[66] The risk also varies by breed, with collies, rottweilers, Cavalier King Charles spaniels, and golden retrievers having a higher risk.[66,194] Breeds with lower risk include dachshunds and mongrels. Fifteen percent of beagles older than 4 years of age develop pyometra.[82]

The lower incidence of pyometra in cats is attributed to the fact that cats are induced ovulators and thus not under the influence of progesterone for as long a period as dogs. However, a correlation between the presence of corpora lutea and pyometra has also been found in cats. Pyometra occurs after nonfertile matings, drug-induced ovulation, and treatment with progestins.[16,290] Some cats have been found to be in the luteal phase of the ovarian cycle, even though they were isolated from male cats and received no therapy, suggesting that the luteal phase must be able to be induced by other factors as well.[150,151] Progesterone is not the only factor involved in cats, because some affected cats are in the follicular phase of the ovarian cycle.[151,213] The ages of affected cats

in different surveys have varied from 3 to 6 years of age,[55,151,278] to older than 5 years,[213] to an average age of 7 years.[127] In queens, no correlation was found between development of pyometra and age at first breeding, age at first queening, or number of litters produced.[213]

E. coli is the most common organism isolated, being the single agent in most cases.[60,79,143,152,214,222] E. coli infection causes the morbidity and mortality associated with pyometra. The blood concentrations of endotoxin in dogs with pyometra are higher than control animals and the level correlated with the severity of the disease.[198]

E. coli is thought to ascend into the uterus from the vagina when the cervix is open during proestrus and estrus. E. coli isolates from dogs that suffer from pyometra have been biochemically compared with corresponding fecal isolates. Strains from infected uteri were biochemically similar to fecal isolates from the same dog, confirming the hypothesis of fecal contamination of the genitourinary tract.[80] E. coli strains isolated from bladder urine and from the uterus in the same dog have been found to be identical.[96] Even though some uterine cultures from the same dog seemed to contain multiple types of E. coli based on characteristics in culture, all the organisms from the same dog were identical based on pulsed-field gel electrophoresis.[96] Even though E. coli strains in the same dog were identical, E. coli strains from different dogs were different, indicating that these E. coli strains are not spread among animals.[96]

E. coli strains that cause pyometra are less diverse than fecal E. coli, suggesting the clustering of virulence properties, similar to those in E. coli that cause UTIs. E. coli isolated from dogs with pyometra have virulence factors similar to uropathogenic E. coli, suggesting that the pathogenetic mechanisms of E. coli infection in pyometra and UTIs are similar.[45]

Other organisms occasionally isolated from uteri with pyometra are streptococci, staphylococci, Proteus species, Klebsiella species, Serratia marcescens, Salmonella species, and P. aeruginosa.[152,222] Aerobic and anerobic cultures of purulent material from bitches with pyometra may be negative,[60,143] suggesting that some animals may not have an infection. However, antimicrobial therapy has been used before obtaining a culture in most of these cases.

Dogs with pyometra have been found to have an impaired lymphocyte response to mitogens, the degree of which corresponds with severity of illness.[69] Sera from affected dogs had higher concentrations of immunoglobulins and circulating immune complexes.[69]

Clinical Findings

Affected dogs and cats are usually presented 2 months after estrus or breeding or have been given estrogens or progestogens. In dogs, owners may note vulvar discharge (generally purulent), lethargy, vomiting, and polyuria-polydipsia.[244,278] Affected dogs lose weight.[82] In cats, vaginal discharge (mucopurulent to hemorrhagic) and abdominal distention are the most common signs.[55,213] Nonspecific signs of illness such as anorexia, weight loss, an unkempt appearance, lethargy, and vomiting are seen in some cats.[126,290] Polyuria and polydipsia are seen less commonly in cats than in dogs.[126] The signs in the most severely affected animals are related to a systemic inflammatory response syndrome (sepsis, septic shock).[80]

Uterine enlargement is found on physical examination. Fever is not common.[127,244,278] The mean body temperature in 55 affected dogs was 102.7° F (39.3° C).[104] Open pyometra (with the cervix open and draining) is more common than closed pyometra.[104,175,244,278] Approximately one third of affected cats are dehydrated.[126] Septicemia or endotoxemia may develop at any time, in which case animals may have tachycardia, tachypnea, poor peripheral perfusion, and a subnormal body temperature. Animals with closed-cervix pyometra are at greater risk for developing septicemia and endotoxemia.[120,186]

Diagnosis

The diagnosis is established by the history, stage of the estrous cycle, physical examination, and laboratory and radiologic imaging abnormalities. A CBC, biochemical profile, and urinalysis are essential for detecting the metabolic abnormalities associated with septicemia or toxemia and to evaluate renal function and the possibility of a concurrent UTI. Urine collection should be done carefully, because of the risks of perforating the enlarged uterus during cystocentesis or introducing the organisms from the reproductive tract into the bladder during catheterization.

Results of vaginal cytology show degenerate neutrophils and bacteria.[16,55] Endometrial cells may also be found.[199] It is very important to obtain a sample of uterine fluid for bacteriologic culture to direct antimicrobial therapy. With open-cervix pyometra, the sample should be obtained from the cranial vagina using a guarded culture swab or at surgery. With closed-cervix pyometra, the sample is obtained at surgery.

Laboratory abnormalities are most severe in animals with closed-cervix pyometra. Leukocytosis with a left shift is often present,[55,213,278] but approximately 25% of dogs with pyometra had normal WBC and differential counts in one survey.[244] Leukopenia with a degenerative left shift and neutrophil toxicity may be found in animals with septicemia. Anemia is mild when present and is nonregenerative, associated with the systemic inflammatory response.

Hyperglobulinemia and hyperfibrinogenemia are attributed to inflammation (acute-phase reaction), as is mild hypoalbuminemia.[80] Increased serum concentrations of ALP, bilirubin, and cholesterol are attributed to cholestasis associated with the systemic inflammatory response rather than with primary hepatocyte injury. Alanine aminotransferase concentrations are usually normal. Liver biopsies in affected dogs confirm lack of hepatocellular necrosis.[80] On rare occasions, the sodium-potassium ratio is between 20 and 24.[230]

Azotemia is detected in approximately 15% to 30% of cases.[16,80] More precise measurement of the glomerular filtration rate has confirmed that it varies in dogs with pyometra.[103] The cause of azotemia may be prerenal, renal, or both. Inappropriately low specific gravities in animals with dehydration azotemia, or both are common in bitches with pyometra.[104] Reduced urine concentrating ability is thought to be a result of endotoxin-induced unresponsiveness to antidiuretic hormone and to renal tubular injury. Tubular disease is the most consistent pathologic finding.[103,253] Proteinuria is common on urinalysis. Proteinuria may be the result of inflammation with an associated UTI or the result of tubular injury; proteinuria may also be a result of glomerular lesions characteristic of immune complex deposition, which are found in some bitches with pyometra. In one small study, the urinary NAG index on admission was above normal in two bitches that developed azotemia after ovariohysterectomy, whereas in two other dogs, it was not.[235] This suggests that this test might predict which dogs are at risk of renal failure from therapy for pyometra.

Concurrent UTIs are detected in 25% to 69% of affected bitches.[104,244] The organism in the urine is the same as that in the uterus.[104,241]

The most important diagnostic consideration is differentiating pyometra from pregnancy with associated vaginitis. Abdominal radiography confirms the presence of uterine enlargement in most but not all dogs with pyometra (Fig. 91-13). In 10% of cats with pyometra, the uterus appeared to be normal on survey abdominal radiographs.[150] The cause of uterine enlargement on survey abdominal radiographs cannot be determined until pregnancy can be confirmed by the presence of calcified fetal structures at approximately 42 to 45 days of gestation.

Ultrasonography is useful in differentiating fetal structures, solid masses, and luminal fluids. A large, fluid-filled uterus with no fetuses is characteristic of pyometra (Fig. 91-14).[55,223] The enlargement of the uterus is usually uniform, but in some cases, the area of enlargement is focal or segmental.[266] In pregnant dogs, fetal heartbeats may be seen by ultrasonogram as early as 17 to 20 days after breeding, and fetal structures are readily identifiable by 28 days.[175,31] Because pyometra occurs more than 28 days after estrus, ultrasonography is the most diagnostic test in differentiating pregnancy from pyometra.

Therapy

Treatment should be prompt and aggressive because rapid deterioration can occur in animals with pyometra. The sooner that definitive therapy begins, the more quickly dogs recover.[82] Therapy consists of administration of IV fluids and an appropriate antibiotic and evacuation of uterine contents.

Fluid Therapy Fluid therapy should be prompt and continued throughout surgical or medical management to ensure adequate tissue perfusion. If the dog is hypotensive or dehydrated, these conditions should be reversed with fluid therapy before inducing anesthesia and should be accomplished within 1 to 4 hours.

Different types of fluid therapy have been evaluated in small numbers of dogs with septic shock secondary to pyometra. In one study, hypertonic saline with dextran 70 was compared with an eightfold higher volume of isotonic saline.[70] The hypertonic saline with dextran significantly increased the mean arterial pressure (range of mean [rom] approximately 60 to 90 mm Hg) and urine output, whereas isotonic saline did not. Most other parameters measured were not significantly different between groups. Cardiac output and index increased in both groups. Oxygen consumption and extraction and degree of acidosis did not improve with either therapy. Two dogs in the isotonic saline group died of renal failure within 2 weeks after surgery. However, comparative data on renal function between the groups before therapy were not provided in the article. This study used infused lactated Ringer's solution before and after the administration of the test fluids, which were administered just before the ovariohysterectomy.

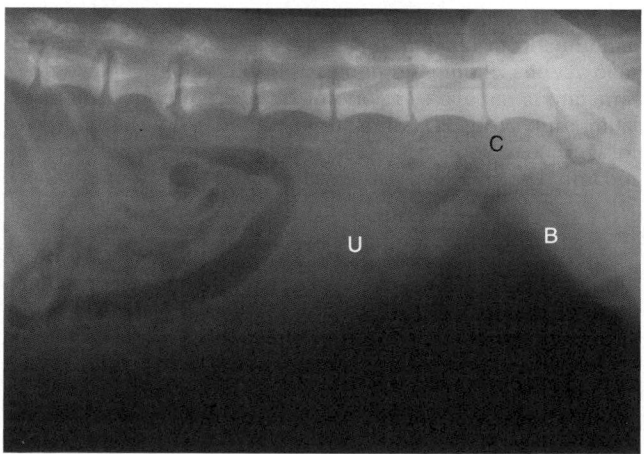

Fig 91-13 Radiographic examination of dog with pyometra showing enlarged, fluid-filled uterus (U) in caudal ventral abdomen. Note relationship to colon (C) and bladder (B). (Courtesy University of Georgia, Athens, Ga.)

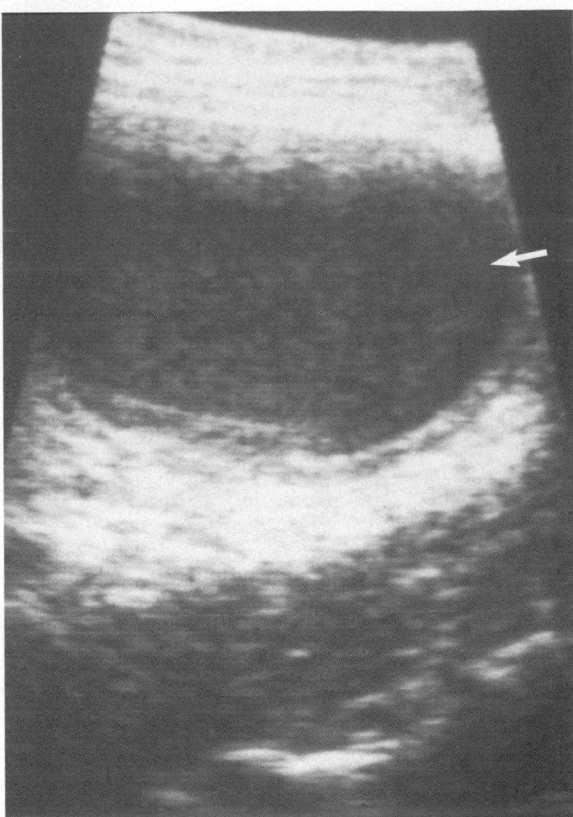

Fig 91-14 Ultrasound examination of fluid-filled uterus *(arrow)* confirmed at surgery to be pyometra. (Courtesy University of Georgia, Athens, Ga.)

Antimicrobial Therapy Antimicrobial therapy should be chosen on the basis of culture and susceptibility testing of the uterine exudate. This is important because almost 40% of *E. coli* isolated from the uteri of dogs with pyometra were resistant to two or more drugs, and 4% were resistant to 12 or more antimicrobial drugs.[277]

Because antibiotic therapy should begin immediately, an antibiotic generally effective against *E. coli* should be administered (see Table 91-12) until culture results are available. In one survey, *E. coli* isolated from bitches with pyometra were most commonly susceptible to enrofloxacin, trimethoprim-sulfonamide, chloramphenicol, and aminoglycosides.[152] In another report, *E. coli* from uteri showed susceptibility to amoxicillin-clavulanate, cephalexin, enrofloxacin, and gentamicin.[287] Enrofloxacin and other fluoroquinolones may reach higher uterine fluid concentrations than serum concentrations.[42] Antibiotics should be continued for a total of 1 to 3 weeks, depending on disease severity, type of therapy chosen (surgical versus medical), and response to therapy.

Surgical Therapy Evacuation of uterine contents is most quickly accomplished surgically (i.e., with an ovariohysterectomy). If the animal is in critical condition, the animal has evidence of uterine rupture or peritonitis, or the pyometra is closed (no vaginal discharge), an ovariohysterectomy is recommended. An ovariohysterectomy can be performed traditionally or by laparoscopy.[178] The large and often friable uterus must be handled carefully to avoid spillage into the abdomen (Fig. 91-15).

The prognosis for recovery from pyometra is good after surgery. Intraoperative and immediate postoperative death occurs in 5% to 8% of cases.[126,278] If the uterus ruptures, the mortality increases to 50%. Severely azotemic dogs (with a blood urea nitrogen level of greater than 150 mg/dl) also have

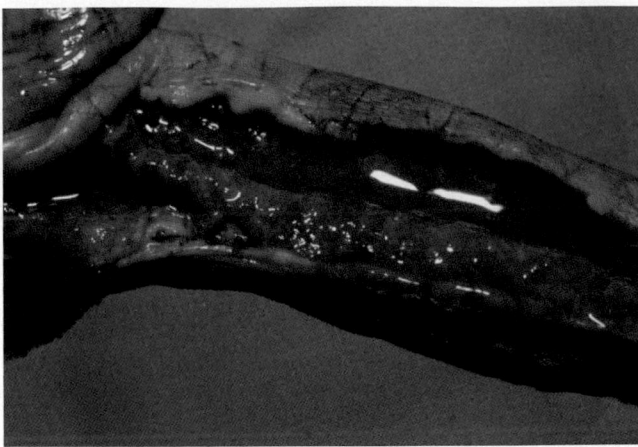

Fig 91-15 Gross view of pus-filled uterus at necropsy from dog with pyometra. (Courtesy University of Georgia, Athens, Ga.)

poor prognoses. Postoperative complications in dogs with pyometra include intracranial thromboembolism, septicemia, and osteomyelitis secondary to septicemia.[278]

Medical Therapy to Evacuate Uterine Contents An ovariohysterectomy may be unacceptable to owners who would like to preserve their animal's reproductive ability. In animals that are not systemically ill and have open-cervix pyometra, prostaglandin therapy is a reasonable alternative for owners who would like to breed the dog again and understand the limitations and side effects of medical therapy. Prostaglandin therapy causes contraction of the myometrium and relaxation of the cervix. The beneficial effects of prostaglandins are a result of evacuation of uterine contents rather than from changes in the endometrium or ovarian function. Only naturally occurring prostaglandin should be used, because synthetic prostaglandin is much more potent, and a safe dose has not been established for dogs and cats.[55]

Naturally occurring PGF_{2a} is given at a dose of 0.1 to 0.25 mg/kg SC once or twice per day for 3 to 7 days until the uterine diameter decreases, vaginal discharge stops, and a normal leukogram is obtained.[16,31] Much lower doses (0.025 to 0.03 mg/kg twice a day to effect, generally for 5 to 8 days) are also reported to be successful and have fewer side effects.[80,248] Intravaginal administration at 0.15 mg/kg every 12 to 24 hours was also reported to be successful in 13 of 15 dogs and had no side effects.[85] Immediately after infusion, the dogs' hindquarters were raised for 3 to 5 minutes. Efficacy of these different dose regimens has not been compared prospectively.

Clinical improvement is not generally apparent for the first 48 hours after starting therapy, reinforcing the thought that medical therapy is not appropriate for dogs with sepsis or toxemia. Adverse reactions to prostaglandin therapy are dose related and include restlessness, pacing, hypersalivation, vocalization, panting, vomiting, diarrhea, abdominal discomfort, tachycardia, mydriasis, and fever. These signs usually resolve within 1 hour of therapy.[55] Because vomiting is common, dogs should not be fed for 3 hours before therapy with higher dosage regimens.[92] With injectable drugs, starting at a lower dosage and increasing the dose each day may reduce the severity of adverse effects because adverse reactions tend to diminish in severity and duration with repeated administrations.[55] Because adverse effects are common, hospitalization during high-dose therapy is recommended.

All medically treated dogs should be rechecked 2 weeks after therapy. If uterine enlargement, which occurs in approximately 33% of treated dogs,[92] is still evident, therapy should be repeated. A prolonged vaginal discharge should prompt reevaluation of the choice of antibiotics.

When prostaglandin therapy is used, the animal should be bred during the next estrus.[175] PGF$_{2a}$ is usually successful in treating open-cervix pyometra in dogs and cats (with 93% to 100% resolution of clinical signs; 55% to 87% for subsequent pregnancy).[55,127] However, recurrence of pyometra can occur.[127] PGF$_{2a}$ is less successful in dogs with closed-cervix pyometra (with only about a 25% to 34% success rate).[127,175] No reports have been made of successful medical management of closed-cervix pyometra in the queen.

The antiprogestin RU46534 (Aglépristone [Virbac Laboratories, Carros, France as Alizine]) has also been used for medical treatment of pyometra.[109] A dose of 10 mg/kg was used in 31 bitches on days 1, 2, and 7. No side effects were observed. Antimicrobial therapy was also given. Treatment was successful in 21 bitches with serum progesterone concentrations greater than 3.2 nmol/L, which was indicative of diestrus. During a mean observation period of 14 months, pyometra recurred in one successfully treated dog. Two bitches were successfully bred. The same dose and frequency of therapy was used in four cats, had no side effects, and resolved pyometra in all four animals.[102]

Mastitis
Etiology
The usual cause of mastitis is bacterial infection. *Staphylococcal* species are the most common[130]; *E. coli* and *Streptococcus* species are the second and third most common.[130] Damp or unsanitary conditions and possibly trauma, such as by offspring, are potential predisposing causes.

Clinical Findings
Mastitis is most common in postpartum dogs but may also occur in late pregnancy and in pseudopregnancy.[119,130] It is uncommon in queens.[119] Mastitis may develop any time during lactation and until approximately 1 week after weaning.[149] Heavily lactating bitches are more likely to develop postweaning mastitis, especially if food intake is not restricted during the early weaning period.[149]

Mastitis may be localized, be diffuse within one gland, or involve multiple glands. The classic clinical signs of acute mastitis are mammary gland heat, pain, redness, and swelling, which may be edematous or firm. Crepitus may also be noted.[269] If the dog has septic mastitis, signs include fever, anorexia, weakness, dehydration, and neglect of offspring. Shock may ensue with signs of vomiting, profound depression, tachycardia, and marked fever.[269] Mastitis is usually acute; abscesses or gangrenous changes may occur secondarily. The only sign in dogs with subclinical or chronic mastitis is failure of puppies to thrive.

Diagnosis
Diagnosis is usually based on physical findings and examination of milk. A hemogram may show a neutrophilic leukocytosis. Reactive thrombocytopenia, possibly secondary to disseminated intravascular coagulation, was found in one animal with gangrenous staphylococcal mastitis.[101] Milk may appear normal or abnormal. Cytology of the milk confirms septic, purulent inflammation. Bacterial culture and susceptibility of milk are recommended to determine the causative organism and the most efficacious antimicrobial therapy. A reported case involved a highly antibiotic resistant organism despite no prior antibiotic therapy. In this case, obtaining a culture on the day of admission prompted early appropriate therapy and recovery.[269]

Therapy
In acute mastitis, therapy includes systemic, broad-spectrum antibiotics, warm packs, a clean environment, frequent milking of affected glands, and fluid therapy if dehydration is present. When choosing an antibiotic, the clinician must con-sider the susceptibility of the responsible organism, this drug's ability to reach the milk, and the effects on nursing neonates. Because of potential bacterial resistance, culture and susceptibility testing should be used to direct therapy. Initial drugs of choice pending culture results include amoxicillin-clavulanate, first-generation cephalosporins, macrolides, or trimethoprim-sulfonamide because of efficacy and low incidence of side effects in the mother and puppies.[31] Antibiotic therapy should be continued for several days after mastitis resolves. Most animals require therapy for approximately 1 week.[122]

Occasionally, a severely abscessed gland may require surgical drainage. This should be done carefully because hemorrhage is a potential complication.[149] Abscessed or ruptured glands should be debrided of devitalized tissue and allowed to drain, with at least twice-daily flushing of an antibacterial solution. In this situation, the puppies should be removed from the mother and hand raised.

Whether offspring need to be removed from the dam if she is ill is not known, but they are often removed because the dam is in pain. If the mother is not systemically ill, offspring do not need to be removed.[149] Affected animals often have decreased milk production, so supplemental feeding of offspring may be required. Transient diarrhea may occur in neonates ingesting milk that contains antibiotics.[31]

In chronic mastitis, macrolides have been recommended pending culture and susceptibility results. This choice is based on milk's acidity, which leads to ion trapping of basic antimicrobial agents, and on the lipid solubility of macrolides.

Prognosis
Mastitis usually resolves with appropriate therapy, and future mammary gland function is not affected unless abscess formation or gangrene has required surgical therapy. The condition may recur with future pregnancies.

SUGGESTED READINGS*

47. Cohn LA, Gary AT, Fales WH, et al. 2003. Trends in fluoroquinolone resistance of bacteria isolated from canine urinary tracts. *J Vet Diagn Invest* 15:338-343.

75. Forward ZA, Legendre AM, Khalsa HDS. 2002. Use of intermittent bladder infusion with clotrimazole for treatment of candiduria in a dog. *J Am Vet Med Assoc* 220:1496-1498.

88. Gobello C, Castex G, Klima L, et al. 2003. A study of two protocols combining aglepristone and cloprostenol to treat open cervix pyometra in the bitch. *Theriogenology* 60:901-908.

105. Heiene R, van Vonderen IK, Moe L, et al. 2004. Vasopressin secretion in response to osmotic stimulation and effects of desmopressin on urinary concentrating capacity in dogs with pyometra. *Am J Vet Res* 65:404-408.

128. Johnson JR, O'Bryan TT, Low DA, et al. 2000. Evidence of commonality between canine and human extraintestinal pathogenic *Escherichia coli* strains that express papG allele III. *Infect Immun* 68:3327-3336.

130. Jung C, Wehrend A, Konig A, et al. 2002. Investigations about the incidence, differentiation and microbiology of canine mastitis. *Praktischer Tierarzt* 83:6, 508-511.

173. McGuire NC, Schulman R, Ridgway MD, et al. 2002. Detection of occult urinary tract infections in dogs with diabetes mellitus. *J Am Anim Hosp Assoc* 38:541-544.

216. Pressler BM, Vaden SL, Lane IF, et al. 2003. *Candida* spp. urinary tract infections in 13 dogs and 7 cats: predisposing factors, treatment, and outcome. *J Am Anim Hosp Assoc* 39:263-270.

*See the CD-ROM for a complete list of references.

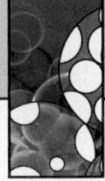

CHAPTER • 92

Bacterial Infections of the Central Nervous System

Marc Kent

ETIOLOGY

Central nervous system (CNS) inflammation is described as encephalitis, myelitis, and meningitis based on whether the process affects the brain, spinal cord, and meninges, respectively. Inflammation in the CNS may be the result of an infectious process, immune-mediated inflammation in the absence of infection, neoplasia, trauma, or infarction. The underlying pathogenesis of immune-mediated disease is often unknown. Granulomatous meningoencephalitis (GME) is a classic example of an immune-mediated process without a determined cause.[19] Other immune-mediated diseases preferentially affect certain breeds. Breed-specific inflammatory disease has been identified in the pug dog,[38] Maltese terrier,[169] Yorkshire terrier,[179] Pekingese,[28] and greyhound.[25] Other immune-mediated diseases such as steroid-responsive meningitis arteritis (SRMA) typically affects young patients, usually under the age of 2 years.[116] See Chapter 84 for more information on the inflammatory diseases described previously. Alternatively, immune-mediated disease is sometimes categorized based on the principle inflammatory reaction, GME,[19] or eosinophilic meningoencephalitis.[160] Chemical meningitis can be induced by the subarachnoid injection of contrast agents as is seen with myelography.[29] Finally, some neoplasms such as meningioma have been associated with an inflammatory response.[10,30]

Infectious diseases that affect the CNS include viral, protozoal, fungal, rickettsial, and bacterial organisms. Some viruses (canine distemper virus [CDV; Chapter 3] and rabies virus [Chapter 22]) are neurotropic, as are some protozoans such as systemic amoeba infections (Chapter 79) and *Toxoplasma gondii* and *Neospora caninum* (Chapter 80). These disorders produce primarily parenchymal inflammation.[171] Others agents that are nonneurotropic become microembolized in the meningeal vasculature as a result of their systemic spread to many tissues. In this somewhat immunoprivileged site, they cause disease as a consequence of their induction of vasculitis and meningitis with secondary parenchymal injury, for example, feline infectious peritonitis virus (FIPV; Chapter 11), *Ehrlichia* and *Anaplasma* (Chapter 28), *Rickettsia rickettsii* (Chapter 29), *Blastomyces dermatitidis* (Chapter 59), *Cryptococcus neoformans* (Chapter 61), and *Coccidioides immitis* (Chapter 62). The main focus of this chapter is on bacterial infections of the CNS. Bacteria by their nature are nonneurotropic. They cause infection by producing meningitis or abscess formation. Bacterial meningitis is an inflammatory response to bacterial invasion of meninges and cerebrospinal fluid (CSF). Such infections can rapidly disseminate and, based on the virulence of the pathogen, lead to serious illness and death.[109] Bacterial meningitis, which can be localized or diffuse, occurs when pathogenic organisms overcome (or elude) host defense mechanisms and reach the subarachnoid CSF. Meningitis typically causes diffuse or multifocal lesions in dogs and cats, although the clinical signs may

not reflect the diffuse nature of the disease.[178] Brain abscesses, which result from a focal pyogenic infection, appear to result from contiguous spread of infections, such as progression of otitis interna, more than from hematogenous spread of organisms. Brain abscesses are uncommon in the dog and cat.[23,115] This finding may be caused in part by the inability of the CNS to form scar tissue, which restricts the spread of pyogenic infections in other tissue. Because epidural abscess develops outside the parenchyma of the CNS, true abscess formation can occur.[44,121] This condition is much less common compared with meningitis. In people, staphylococci or streptococci are the most commonly implicated agents, and skin infections are a frequent source. In the report of this condition in two dogs, both affected animals were young Irish wolfhounds, but a predisposition is uncertain.[44] Spinal epidural abscesses are more common than cranial epidural abscesses because of the greater available space in the spinal canal.

The veterinary literature details numerous examples of isolated cases and a few retrospective reviews of a limited number of cases of bacterial CNS infections.[35,130,147,178] Consequently, much of the information regarding bacterial CNS infections in veterinary patients must be gleaned from experimental studies and the literature pertaining to cases in people. In humans, bacterial meningitis is caused by several distinct microorganisms that demonstrate neurotropism. These microorganisms include *Haemophilus influenzae* type b (Hib), *Neisseria meningitidis*, and *Streptococcus pneumoniae* serotype C.[94] In the last 15 years, the epidemiology of bacterial meningitis in people has changed dramatically. Hib infection has virtually disappeared as a result of immunizations, a decrease in *N. meningitidis*, and a slight increase in *S. pneumoniae* infections.[155] In addition, occurrence of clusters of cases of bacterial meningitis and septicemia in adolescents has increased as a result of contact in schools and universities.[58] Several risk factors have been identified in human cases. Age, socioeconomic factors, and cigarette smoking have all been associated with bacterial meningitis.[58]

In contrast to people, bacterial meningitis in veterinary patients does not seem to be caused by microorganisms with a predilection for the nervous system. Consequently, bacterial CNS infections in small animals are relatively uncommon. A wide variety of bacterial organisms have been reported in small animals. These organisms have included *Staphylococcus* spp., *Streptococcus* spp., *Pasteurella* spp., *Escherichia coli*, *Klebsiella* sp., *Proteus* spp., *Salmonella* spp., *Actinomyces* spp., and *Nocardia* spp.* Anaerobes, such as *Prevotella oralis*, *Fusobacterium* spp., *Bacteroides* spp., *Peptostreptococcus* spp., *Eubacterium* spp., *Flavobacterium breve*, and *Propionibacterium* sp., have been identified in the CNS.[†]

---

*References: 23, 24, 43, 45, 68, 72, 75, 90, 119, 130, 139, 147.
†References: 3, 23, 45, 64, 130.

PATHOGENESIS

Infection in the CNS requires numerous interactions between the pathogen and the host immune system. Bacterial organisms can spread to the CNS in a wide variety of ways. The most common route of infection is through hematogenous spread from a distant focus. Other less common routes into the CNS include direct penetration (blunt trauma, bite wound, or penetrating objects), contiguous spread (nasal cavity, paranasal sinuses, and otitis media and interna), and invasion along nerves and nerve roots (Table 92-1). In people, the first step in the pathogenesis of hematogenously spread infections involves mucosal colonization by bacteria, then evasion of local host mucosal defenses, and eventually entrance into the intravascular space. This process has been well defined in people.[98] Bacteria such as *S. pneumoniae, N. meningitidis,* and *H. influenzae* are known to secrete proteases, which degrade mucosal IgA, allowing for colonization.[188] Once beyond the mucosal barrier, bacteria can enter the subepithelial vasculature. Systemic infections, which may ultimately lead to CNS bacterial infections, arise from splenic abscesses, pleuritis, lung abscesses, vegetative endocarditis, bite wounds, urinary tract infections, pneumonia, infected cranial sinuses, and middle ear infections.* Intravascular survival depends on the ability of bacteria to circumvent immune system activation. The ability to evade major host defenses against bacteremia, complement activation, circulating antibodies, and neutrophil phagocytosis has been attributed to bacterial capsular polysaccharides.[98] To gain entry into the CNS from the vascular space, pathogens must traverse a final impediment.

This last obstacle is composed principally of two barriers: the blood-brain barrier (BBB) and the blood-CSF barrier.[126] The BBB is formed primarily by the brain endothelium. The brain endothelium is unique in that it lacks the fenestrae found in other capillary beds (Fig. 92-1). Brain endothelial cells are interconnected by tight junctions composed of zona occludens and zona adherens. These tight junctions form a seal at the apical region of brain endothelial cells that result in the lack of permeability of the BBB, effectively segregating the brain from the vascular space. Of note is that the development and maintenance of this aspect of the BBB depends on astrocytes, perivascular microglia, and the basal laminae.[1] In addition, the endothelial cells in the brain are relatively devoid of pinocytotic vesicles, suggesting little transcellular movement of substances. An analogous barrier is constructed between adjacent epithelial cells of the choroids plexus, making up the blood-CSF barrier, which prevents entry into the CSF.[126] For pathogens to cross the BBB, they must first adhere to the brain endothelium or the epithelium of the choroids plexus. For *E. coli* K1, fimbrial components have been identified that preferentially bind brain endothelial cells.[170] Attached to the endothelium, pathogens can traverse the BBB through paracellular pathways, transcellular transport, or intracellularly within white blood cells as they undergo diapedesis. Bacteria traversing the BBB can lead to infection of the CNS parenchyma, resulting in encephalitis or myelitis; the leptomeninges via blood vessels of the pia mater, causing meningitis; or entering across the choroid plexuses, leading to ventriculitis.[136] Regardless of the site of penetrance, infection can disseminate through the brain parenchyma to the CSF or from the CSF to the brain parenchyma because the extracellular fluid in the brain is contiguous with the CSF.

Alternatively, the BBB can be circumvented by direct penetration. Normal anatomic structures such as the vertebral column, calvaria, and meninges help protect the nervous system. However, with blunt impact trauma or penetrating objects, this aspect of the protective barrier around the CNS

*References: 6, 49, 89, 109, 162, 178.

Table • 92-1

Source and Localization of Nonneurotrophic Infections of the Central Nervous System

POINT OF ENTRY	USUAL LOCATION OR TYPE OF INFECTION
Hematogenous	Diffuse subarachnoid infection
	Focal parenchymal abscess or granuloma
Spinal cord	Diffuse subarachnoid infection
Paranasal sinuses	Frontal lobes
	Focal epidural abscess
	Diffuse epidural empyema
Petrous temporal bone (otitis media)	Temporal lobe (cerebrum)
	Cerebellum
	Brain stem (cerebellopontomedullary junction)
Cranial nerves	Basilar meninges
	Most frequently cranial nerves VII and VIII

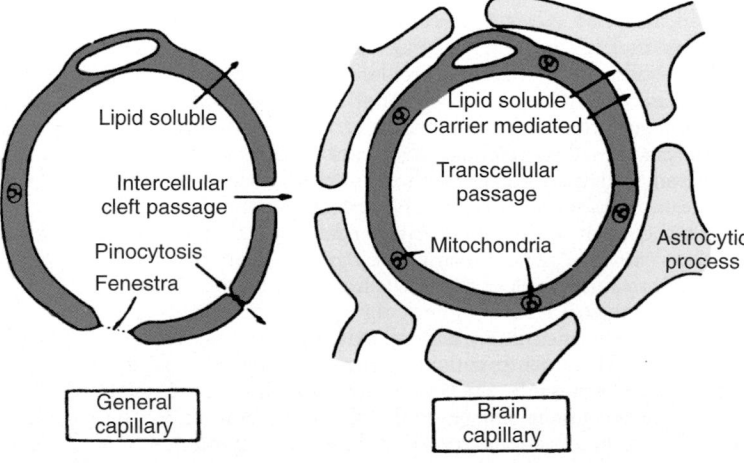

Fig 92-1 Comparison of features of systemic capillaries and the capillary endothelial cells of the brain. (From Oldendorf WH. 1977. The blood-brain barrier, pp 177-190. *In* Bito LL, Dauson H, Fenstermacher JD [eds], Experimental eye research, Supplement, vol 25: the ocular and cerebrospinal fluids. Academic Press, New York, NY. Reprinted with permission).

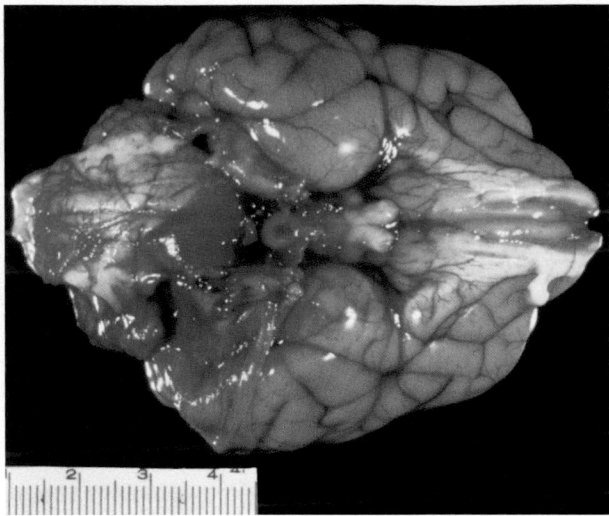

Fig   92-2   Ventral surface of brain showing cerebellopontine angle abscess that began as a result of otitis interna spreading from the infected petrous temporal bone.

tissue can be overcome. Microorganisms can also enter the CNS during infections in adjacent structures containing penetrating nerves. Nasal aspergillosis can result in significant osteolysis of the nasal turbinates and cribriform plate,[157] which may allow for direct invasion into the brain. Encephalopathy and suppurative meningoencephalitis have been reported secondary to topical treatment of nasal aspergillosis in the dog.[110] Similarly, otitis interna and media can invade the adjacent brain stem, usually along cranial nerves VII and VIII, which penetrate the petrous temporal bone on their course to the brain stem, producing meningitis, with or without abscess formation of the neuroparenchyma (Fig. 92-2).[166] Although hematogenous spread predisposes the patient to meningitis or parenchymal infarction, or both (see Fig. 87-5,C), contiguous spread into the CNS along nerve access often causes subdural abscesses.[185] Despite the close proximity, diskospondylitis rarely progresses to invade the adjacent spinal cord parenchyma.[52] Spinal empyema has been reported in the dog.[44] Microorganisms can also invade the CNS by traveling within axons from peripheral nerves. In ruminants, *Listeria monocytogenes* likely gains access to the CNS along axons of the trigeminal nerve.[171] Concurrent CNS and sinonasal infections with *C. neoformans* has been documented.[13] Whether CNS involvement is related to direct penetration through a damaged cribriform plate, the result of extension along the olfactory nerves, or through hematogenous spread is unclear.

Once inside the BBB, the host defenses are severely limited. The CSF is largely devoid of complement, opsonizing proteins such as immunoglobulins and neutrophils, which, in part, allow for bacterial replication to occur largely unchecked.[98] With increased bacterial replication and autolysis, concentrations of the bacterial cell wall products, lipopolysaccharides, teichoic acid, and peptidoglycans are increased, which stimulate the host inflammatory response.[98] Unlike in extraneural sites, in CNS infections, the damage is largely the result of the inflammatory response rather than the pathogen itself.[174] The inflammatory response involves the production numerous cytokines and chemokines (tumor necrosis factor-α [TNF-α], interleukin [IL]-1, IL-6, IL-8, and IL-10), matrix metalloproteinase (MMP), reactive oxygen species (ROS), and nitric oxide synthetase (NOS).[98] Cytokines and chemokines are small proteins that are crucial in the development and modulation of inflammation. In general, cytokines are factors that bind to cell membrane

receptors and modulate leukocyte function, whereas chemokines bind to transmembrane receptors and function as chemoattractants.[26] Many different cells possess the capability of producing these various proinflammatory molecules. Brain cells such as endothelial cells, ependymal cells, resident macrophages, astrocytes, and glial cells can express cytokines in response to stimuli in bacterial meningitis.[152] Among the cytokines, IL-1 and TNF-α, play a crucial role early in the inflammatory process in the CNS.[133] In bacterial meningitis, IL-1 and TNF-α concentrations increase early in the disease course. Both IL-1 and TNF-α induce the generation of IL-6, IL-8, and IL-10. IL-6 induces the release of acute-phase reactants, fever, and leukocytosis. IL-8 is important in mediating neutrophil chemotaxis, adhesions, and migration into the subarachnoid space. IL-10 is largely antiinflammatory, causing a reduction in the levels of IL-1, IL-6, IL-8 and TNF-α. TNF-α also causes the production of MMPs. Metalloproteinases are a family of proteinases that help break down the extracellular matrix, thereby allowing for the migration of leukocytes. MMP-8 and MMP-9 are elevated in meningitis and contribute to the breakdown of the BBB.[152] ROS and NOS also play prominent roles in the inflammatory process. As a result of their free radical actions, ROS are cytotoxic. The brain is particularly sensitive to free-radical injury owing to a lack of antioxidants, relative high oxygen consumption, and high concentration of unsaturated fatty acids.[98] Nitric oxide (NO) also plays a substantial role in perpetuation of inflammation, the alterations in cerebral vascular perfusion, and the production of peroxynitrite, a potent free radical responsible for lipid peroxidation.[152]

As the inflammatory process progresses, breakdown of the BBB continues. With diminished functionality of the BBB, leukocytes and other soluble mediators of inflammation can cross the damaged barrier and positively feed back on the inflammatory reaction.

Meningeal inflammation is largely responsible for the clinical signs seen in meningitis more than the direct effects of organisms. The direct toxic effects of a pathogen contribute to neuronal injury; however, the indirect effects of the inflammatory mediators are more important factors in neuronal loss. Experimental models and autopsy findings in humans reveals two distinct histologic forms of injury: extensive cortical damage and selective injury to the dentate gyrus of the hippocampus.[84] TNF-α may be responsible for apoptotic loss of neurons in the hippocampus.[173] ROS and NO likely cause the ischemic injury to the cortex through their regulation of cerebral blood flow.[173] Excitatory amino acids such as glutamate also contribute to neuronal loss.[97] In addition, the production of cytokines and other proinflammatory molecules results in endothelial damage, disrupting the BBB and allowing plasma components and leukocytes to traverse into the CNS, which plays a part in the development of vasogenic edema.[173] If the endothelial damage is severe enough, thrombosis can occur, producing ischemia and necrosis. Additionally, cerebral edema contributes to intracranial hypertension, which alters autoregulation of the cerebral vasculature and cerebral perfusion, ultimately contributing to ischemia and neuronal loss.[7]

Ependymal inflammation from bacterial meningitis may lead to obstructed CSF flow with secondary hydrocephalus,[43] a phenomenon also found with FIPV meningoencephalitis of cats (see Chapter 11) and parainfluenza virus meningoencephalitis of dogs (see Chapter 7).

CLINICAL SIGNS

Extraneural Signs

Patients with CNS infections can show a wide variety of clinical signs, ranging from those indicative of both systemic and neurologic dysfunction to those strictly referable to the CNS.[178] If the primary source of infection is located in another organ system, clinical signs may reflect dysfunction of that particular organ. Thorough ocular, funduscopic, and otoscopic examinations should be performed on every patient suspected of having meningitis. The optic nerves are a direct extension of the diencephalon. Abnormalities such as papilledema, optic neuritis, chorioretinitis, retinal hemorrhages, and uveitis can be seen with inflammatory CNS disease.[159] Similarly, the ear canal can provide a portal of entry of organisms into the CNS. Fever may result from the inflammatory process or the consequence of components of bacterial cell walls. Alternatively, elevated body temperature (hyperthermia) may be secondary to muscular activity, seizures, or environmental factors. Severe systemically affected patients may have signs consistent with shock, hypotension, and disseminated intravascular coagulation.[115] Abnormalities in the cardiac rate, rhythm, or a newly diagnosed murmur may be supportive of bacterial endocarditis as the primary source of sepsis. Additionally, bradycardia with concurrent systemic hypertension (Cushing's reflex) may be the consequence of intracranial hypertension.[7] Nausea and vomiting can also occur with meningitis.[115] In advanced disease, with severe brain edema or mass effect, brain herniation with acute respiratory insufficiency may be seen.

Neural

As with all other aspects in neurology, the key to accurate diagnosis relies heavily on a precise neuroanatomic diagnosis. Classically, infectious diseases of the CNS have been associated with multifocal neurologic signs.[123] However, focal signs do not exclude the possibility of infection. Hyperesthesia is a cardinal feature of inflammatory or compressive diseases involving the meninges. In the cranial region, hyperesthesia may be demonstrated by compression of the cranial vault across the temporalis muscles or by opening the jaw. Photophobia or nuchal rigidity may also be present. Two thirds of patients with inflammatory disease processes of the CNS have focal neurologic deficits.[178] Focal inflammation of cranial or spinal nerves occurs in the subarachnoid space as the roots of these nerves enter and exit the CNS and are bathed by CSF. Focal signs of hyperesthesia, lower motor neuron dysfunction, or involuntary twitching of muscles may occur. Depending on the anatomic site affected, inflammation of the meninges, parenchyma of the brain, or of the spinal cord is termed meningitis, encephalitis, or myelitis, respectively. Similarly, inflammation in the CSF is referred to as meningitis. Prosencephalic (cerebrum and thalamus) lesions may alter mentation, cause seizures, and result in abnormal postural reactions with a preservation of gait. Brain stem lesions can also alter mentation. Moreover, brain stem lesions frequently result in cranial nerve deficits and gait abnormalities. Signs associated with spinal cord lesions depend largely on the level at which the spinal cord is affected. In general, proprioceptive ataxia and paresis are the hallmarks of spinal cord dysfunction. Further assessment of reflexes helps localize the affected spinal cord segments. Spinal meningeal inflammation may result in paraspinal discomfort, paraspinal muscle rigidity, and decreased vertebral.[162]

DIAGNOSIS

CSF analysis and culture are the sole methods of providing a definitive diagnosis of CNS bacterial infection. Because of the BBB, the absence of fever or leukocytosis does not eliminate meningitis from consideration. However, establishing a definitive diagnosis is complicated by the difficulty in identifying an underlying etiologic agent. Ancillary laboratory tests such as a complete blood count (CBC), biochemical profile, and urinalysis provide a minimal database. When present, abnormalities in the CBC, leukocytosis (neutrophilia with or without a left shift), or leukopenia largely reflect a systemic inflammatory response rather than provide a specific diagnosis. Biochemical profile abnormalities may provide insight into a possible source of sepsis or concurrent disease process. Alternatively, results of these tests may be within reference limits.[178]

In postoperative neurosurgical patients, distinguishing surgically induced bacterial infections of the meninges from irritant meningitis caused by contrast agents, surgical trauma, and lavage performed at the time of surgery can be difficult. In people, an overlap exists of CSF test results for patients with chemical meningitis and infectious meningitis determined by bacterial isolation or identification.[21] Therefore administration of antibacterials may rely instead on detecting surgical wound infections, additional neurologic signs such as mental changes or seizure disorders, high rectal temperatures, or otorrhea or rhinorrhea.

Cerebrospinal Fluid Evaluation

Given the close physical relationship that exists between the CSF and CNS parenchyma, disease affecting the parenchyma may be reflected as changes in the CSF. Furthermore, the CNS has limited ways to respond to disease. Therefore most disease processes in the CNS result in inflammation. As a consequence, even using CSF analysis, definitive diagnosis may be difficult, if not impossible, to obtain in at least one third of patients with inflammatory CNS disease.[178] Despite this problem, CSF analysis is necessary for determining that inflammatory CNS disease is present and obligate for the diagnosis of bacterial CNS disease.

Technique

CSF is often obtained from the cerebellomedullary cistern (CMC). Additionally, CSF can be collected from the dorsal or ventral subarachnoid space at the L5-L6 intervertebral spaces. Alternatively, CSF can also be obtained from the L6-L7 intervertebral space in some patients. In cases of hydrocephalus, CSF can also be collected from the lateral ventricles.[122] One ml per 5 kg of body weight can safely be taken from patients.[32]

Obtaining CSF for analysis does require general anesthesia, and all patients must be intubated to prevent obstruction of the airway during patient positioning. Normal endotracheal tubes are adequate; however, in certain circumstances, wire-reinforced endotracheal tubes provide added insurance that the airway will remain patent during the procedure.

Little specialized equipment is needed for collecting CSF. In general, a 22-gauge, 1.5- or 2.5-inch spinal needle is used. For small patients (cats and dogs under 5 kg), a 23-gauge, 0.5-inch scalp-infusion needle ("butterfly needle") is used, which allows for better control. Sterile surgical gloves are worn by the person performing the procedure. CSF should be collected in sterile containers without preservatives such as ethylenediaminetetraacetic acid (EDTA). EDTA can artificially lower cell counts and alter protein measurements.[31]

When obtaining CSF from the CMC, the patient is positioned in lateral recumbency on a stable, flat surface. For *right-handed individuals*, patients are placed in right lateral recumbency to allow landmarks to be palpated by the left hand and manipulation of the spinal needle with the right hand. The hair on the dorsum of the patient's neck from approximately the caudal aspect of the pinnae to the level of the second or third cervical vertebrae is shaved and surgically prepared.

With the patient in right lateral recumbency, the head is flexed to a 90-degree angle with respect to the axis of the vertebral column.[62] The axis of the head must remain straight (parallel to the table) to ensure that the vertebral column is not rotated. Positioning is done by an assistant who is situated across the table from the person performing the procedure. Once proper positioning is attained, the assistant should be instructed not to move the patient until the spinal needle is withdrawn from the skin when the procedure is completed.

CSF from the CMC is obtained by inserting a needle between the occipital bone of the calvaria and the dorsal lamina of the first cervical vertebra. Landmarks for this site include the external occipital protuberance and the cranial aspect of the wings of the atlas.[42] An imaginary line is drawn from the external occipital protuberance caudal along the midline. Similarly, a second imaginary line is drawn between the cranial aspects of the wings of the atlas. These lines bisect at approximately the level of needle insertion. The needle is inserted parallel to the surface of the table and directed perpendicular to the long axis of the vertebral column (Fig. 92-3).

The needle is advanced by holding it at the hub with one hand and is held steady along the shaft of the needle by the other hand. The needle is held continuously throughout the procedure. The needle is advanced slowly, approximately 1 to 2 mm at a time, after which the stylet is removed to observe for flow of CSF. If no flow is seen, the stylet is replaced and the needle is slowly advanced again. As the needle passes through tissue, sudden loss of resistance results in a "pop". After each pop, the stylet is withdrawn to observe for CSF flow. If CSF is not observed, the stylet is replaced and the needle is advanced again. If bone is struck, the needle may be withdrawn slightly, angled either cranial or caudally, and then advanced again. Although this "walking" of the needle can be successful, in many cases, the needle must be withdrawn completely and repositioned for another attempt. Alternatively, the stylet can be withdrawn from the needle once the needle has penetrated the skin. This action enables the person performing the procedure to see flow of CSF immediately on entry into the subarachnoid space. This method also provides an added measure of safety in performing the procedure; however, it can result in significant blood contamination, which may alter CSF analysis.

The depth at which CSF is obtained at the CMC varies between individuals. In cats and small dogs, this distance can be small; therefore extreme care should be taken when collecting CSF from small patients. In overweight patients, landmarks can sometimes be difficult to palpate.

For collection of CSF from the lumbar subarachnoid space, an area of skin is clipped several inches wide along the dorsum from approximately the level of L4 through the sacrum and surgically prepared. The patient is placed in lateral recumbency, and the vertebral column is flexed by positioning the pelvic limbs cranially. As with CMC punctures, care must be taken to make sure that the vertebral column is parallel to the table. Rotation of the axis of the vertebral column will result in misdirection of the needle. The spinous processes are palpated to identify the appropriate interspace. Landmarks for lumbar puncture include the spinous process of L7 and the smaller spinous process of the sacrum, both of which are palpable between the tuber coxae of the pelvis. Once the L7 spinous process is identified, the L5-L6 intervertebral space lies between the spinous processes of L5 and L6 vertebrae. In large dogs and in overweight patients, the spinous process of L7 and the sacrum may not be palpable. In these cases, the first spinous process cranial to the tuber coxae is usually L6. Generally, the L6 spinous process is larger than the L7 spinous process. Occasionally, radiographs are needed to establish landmarks.

The needle is handled as previously described. The needle is inserted through the skin at the level of the cranial aspect of the L6 spinous process (for the L5-L6 intervertebral space) on the midline and advanced perpendicularly toward the vertebral column. If bone is struck, the needle is adjusted cranially or caudally to reach the intervertebral space. Resistance is felt as the needle is advance through the interarcuate ligament. The pelvic limbs and tail may twitch as the needle passes through the dura mater. As with CMC collection, the

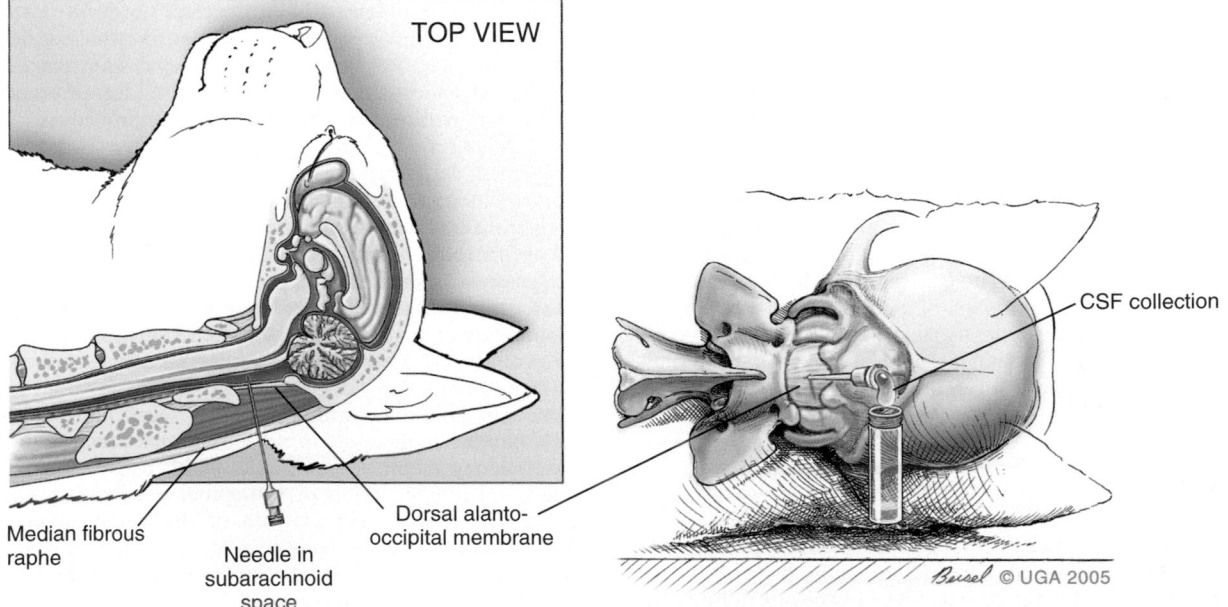

Fig 92-3 One landmark for cerebrospinal fluid collection is the intersection of a line drawn transversely between the wings of the atlas on the cranial aspect and along the dorsal midline drawn through the occipital protuberance (Courtesy of University of Georgia, Athens, Ga.)

stylet is periodically removed to observe flow of CSF. If flow is not appreciated, the stylet is replaced and the needle advanced. Lumbar subarachnoid pressure is lower than it is at the CMC; therefore CSF flow may be slower, and the needle that is used is often longer than that used for CMC punctures. Consequently, more time should be allowed to observe for CSF flow. In both instances, once the sample is obtained, the needle is withdrawn without replacing the stylet.

Complications

Blood contamination is often encountered. If the CSF flows readily, mild blood contamination may clear with additional drops or by replacing the stylet and waiting 1 minute before collecting additional, less contaminated CSF. Correction factors have been used to predict the leukocyte count in blood-contaminated samples. These correction formulas are inaccurate.[192] Moreover, mild blood contamination does not significantly alter the number of leukocytes in CSF samples.[73,192] If substantial blood or "pure" blood is encountered, the needle is withdrawn without replacing the stylet and a new needle is used for another attempt. Many times, obtaining pure blood means that the needle was misdirected laterally.

More serious and devastating complications include penetration of the needle into the CNS parenchyma and brain herniation. With lumbar punctures, needle penetration into the nervous tissue is often unavoidable because, in many cases, CSF cannot be collected from the dorsal subarachnoid space. However, at the level of the low lumbar vertebral column, this problem rarely results in clinical deficits. In stark contrast, injury at the level of CMC can be devastating. In cases with confirmed or suspected intracranial hypertension, CSF collection can result in brain herniation.[82] By removing CSF, a pressure gradient is created whereby intracranial contents can shift from an area of high pressure to one of lower pressure (i.e., the site of CSF collection). Brain herniation can result in alterations in mentation, pupil size and symmetry, abnormal nystagmus, tetraparesis, and abnormalities in respiration and cardiac rhythms, apnea, and death. Brain herniation can also be clinically silent. Herniation has been associated with anesthesia and CSF collection.[91] Care should be exercised when considering CSF collection in patients with suspected or confirmed intracranial disease or intracranial hypertension.

Cerebrospinal Fluid Analysis

After collection of CSF, analysis should consist minimally of the following tests: gross visual inspection; total cell count, as well as leukocyte and red blood cell counts; differential white blood cell count; and total protein analysis. Further biochemical, microbiologic, and serologic testings should be performed based on the results of the aforementioned tests. Normal CSF contains a relatively low protein concentration and is therefore hypotonic. As a result, cell lysis can occur quickly. Consequently, analysis should be performed quickly after collection, ideally within 30 minutes of collection.[32] If analysis cannot be performed immediately, several techniques can be used to prevent in vitro cell degeneration. Refrigeration can slow degeneration for several hours; however, several improved methods of preserving cellular morphology have been developed. The addition of an equal volume of bovine albumin to the CSF sample preserves cell morphology for up to 4 hours.[134] Alternatively, an equal aliquot of serum from the patient can be mixed with its CSF, which preserves cell morphology and provides accurate cell counts for up to 48 hours.[15] Precise measurements of the amount of CSF and the amount of serum mixed together are needed to calculate final cell counts. A separate aliquot of CSF, not diluted with serum or bovine albumin, is needed for measuring protein content. Mixing CSF with either 40% ethanol or 10% formalin has also been suggested to help preserve cell morphology.[88]

Normal CSF is clear and colorless. In general, turbidity or cloudiness becomes grossly visible with nucleated cell counts greater than 500 cell/µl. Other authors have suggested that turbidity is seen with nucleated cell counts greater than 200 nucleated cells/mm³ and 400 erythrocytes/mm³.[32] Blood contamination or recent hemorrhage into the subarachnoid space will result in a pink to red discoloration of the CSF. Most often, blood contamination is iatrogenic as a consequence of the needle puncture rather than an underlying disease. Xanthochromia, a yellow-orange color in the supernatant, is usually an indication of previous hemorrhage caused by the breakdown of hemoglobin into bilirubin. In some instances, prolonged hyperbilirubinemia can cause xanthochromia. High CSF-nucleated cell counts and protein concentrations are indicative of neurologic disease, even if a moderated number of erythrocytes are present from iatrogenic blood contamination.[73]

Normal CSF contains a leukocytes in the range of 0 to 6 cells/µl in dogs and 0 to 2 cells/µl in cats, composed primarily of mononuclear cells and little to no red blood cells.[32] Further characterization of mononuclear cells is sometimes difficult because of the morphologic alteration induced in leukocytes as a result of preparation techniques.[79] An elevation in CSF nucleated cell count is called pleocytosis. Performing differential cell counts is important even in cases that have total cell counts within normal ranges.[33] One fourth of low cellularity samples were cytologically abnormal with cytocentrifuge preparations, with the most common abnormalities being increased phagocytocytic activity, neutrophils, and reactive lymphocytes.[33]

In general, cell-concentration techniques are needed to improve cytologic evaluation of CSF given that most samples have low cellularity. The most accurate method is cytocentrifugation whereby CSF is spun at 1500 g for 10 minutes in a conventional centrifuge[60] or 100 g for 10 minutes in a cytocentrifuge (Cytospin, Shandon Southern Instruments, Sewickley, Penn.).[33] Sedimentation procedures can also be employed whereby CSF is mixed with serum and allowed to sediment for 1 hour. In this procedure, larger amounts of CSF are required. Various techniques can be used whereby an aliquot of CSF is allowed to sediment on a glass slide, which is then air dried and stained for interpretation.[36,79] Another method for CSF cytologic analysis uses membrane filtration; however, this method is more technical and requires different staining techniques (trichome or hematoxylin) and results in poor morphologic preservation of cells.[141]

The hallmark of bacterial CNS infections is a neutrophilic pleocytosis. Toxic changes can be appreciated with cytologic evaluation of neutrophils in CSF. Occasionally, intracellular bacteria can be seen within neutrophils or other phagocytic cells. However, the significance of organisms observed outside of leukocytes (free, nonphagocytosed) in the CSF should be interpreted with caution. Free organisms can be the consequence of in vitro contamination. The implication of free organisms should be defined based on cytologic evidence of infection and clinical signs. Alternatively, repeat CSF analysis can be performed to validate the existence of bacterial organisms in CSF. Unfortunately, neutrophilic pleocytosis is not specific for bacterial disease. SMRA can result in a pronounced pleocytosis composed mostly of neutrophils.[116] Many of these patients will also have fever and cervical hyperesthesia, mimicking the signs of bacterial meningitis.[116] Acute viral meningoencephalitis as a result of CDV infection can cause necrosis, resulting in a occasional marked neutrophilic pleocytosis.[186] Dogs with CDV infections may have systemic signs of illness, including gastrointestinal and respiratory signs. In cats, infection with FIPV usually results in a mixed pleocytosis; however, some cases have CSF inflammatory reaction composed predominantly of neutrophils.[87] Cats infected with FIPV may also show systemic signs and clinicopathologic changes such as fever, anemia, and hyperglobulinemia. Aberrant *Cuterebra* larval migration through the CNS can also cause a neutrophilic response in the CSF.[56] Prodromal signs often include upper respiratory signs and abnormal body temperature (hyperthermia or hypothermia). Meningioma in the dog has also been associated with neutrophilic pleocytosis, although relationships between patterns of CSF changes and specific histologic tumor types cannot be made.[10] Typically, dogs with intracranial neoplasia are older than 5 years and have progressive signs related to focal deficits. Myelography can also cause a change in CSF cytology consisting of primarily a neutrophilic pleocytosis (Table 92-2).[29,191]

Mononuclear pleocytosis composed of lymphocytes and monocytes is typically seen in viral encephalitis such as that caused by CDV,[19,92,177,186] and GME.[9,19,147,176] The breed-specific inflammatory diseases such as those affecting the pug dog,[38] Maltese terrier,[169] and Yorkshire terrier[46,149,179] have been associated with a mononuclear pleocytosis. In protracted cases of SRMA, a mononuclear pleocytosis can be observed.[34,180] In bacterial CNS infections, the predominant inflammatory cell type in CSF may change from a neutrophilic to a mononuclear pleocytosis following treatment.[52] CNS infections with *Ehrlichia* spp. can also cause mononuclear pleocytosis.[70,112] *Anaplasma* is more likely to cause neutrophilic pleocytosis.[106]

Mixed inflammatory pleocytosis is a common finding. The cell population may consist of varying numbers of lymphocytes, monocytes, neutrophils, and eosinophils. Many infectious diseases will have a mixed inflammatory reaction in the CSF. Infections with FIPV[87] and CDV have both been associated with a mixed pleocytosis.[147] *T. gondii* and *N. caninum* infections can result in a mixed inflammatory response.[40,66,76,143] Degenerative CNS disease can provoke a mixed inflammatory response.[186] Intervertebral disk disease may have mixed pleocytosis.[186] Mixed inflammation has also been seen with neoplastic disease of the CNS.[10,30]

Eosinophilic pleocytosis is a rare finding. Occasionally, CNS cryptococcosis has been associated with eosinophilic pleocytosis.[14] *T. gondii* infections may invoke an inflammatory reaction in which eosinophils predominate.[160] Eosinophilic meningoencephalitis can also be idiopathic.[12,160] Eosinophils can be part of the mixed inflammatory response seen in aberrant *Cuterebra* larval migration through the CNS.[56,69]

CSF protein analysis should also be performed. Several methods can be used to quantitate CSF protein.[79] Normal CSF protein concentration varies depending on the site of collection.[8] CSF from the CMC normally has a protein content of less than 30 mg/dl, and CSF obtained from lumbar puncture can have protein content up to 45 mg/dl.[32] The Pandy reaction and Nonne-Apelt test are semiquantitative methods of assessing CSF immunoglobulin concentrations.[79]

Elevations in CSF protein concentrations may be the result of disruption of the BBB and secondary transudation of serum proteins, intrathecal immunoglobulin production, necrosis of the CNS parenchyma, or alteration in the flow of CSF through the ventricular system and subarachnoid space.[32] Severe blood contamination can also increase CSF protein concentration. An increased CSF protein measurement with a normal cell count is referred to as albuminocytologic dissociation. This pattern has been associated with primary brain tumors in dogs.[10] In addition to CSF total protein content, the specific components of CSF, albumin, and globulin fractions can be evaluated. The constituents of canine CSF have been reported from normal dogs[93,165] and from dogs with CNS disorders.[163,164,181]

Numerous other elements of the CSF have been evaluated. CSF glucose concentrations are normally 60% to 80% of the serum glucose concentrations. In humans, CSF glucose concentrations are generally less than 40 mg/dl.[193] The exact relationship between serum and CSF glucose concentrations has not been established in veterinary medicine. In the limited number of cases in which CSF glucose has been evaluated, CSF concentrations have been lower than serum, ranging from 10 to 100 mg/dl.[24,72,75] CSF lactate values have been increased in the CSF of people with bacterial meningitis because of a metabolic shift toward anaerobic metabolism.[98] Enzymes such as creatine kinase, lactate dehydrogenase, alanine aminotransferase, and aspartate aminotransferase activities have been documented with various CNS disorders in veterinary medicine; however, correlation with specific diseases can not be made.[32]

Microbial Culture and Susceptibility Testing

Microbial culture and susceptibility testing are of great importance in defining specific antimicrobial therapy. Samples should be collected in sterile containers that lack preservatives. Both aerobic and anaerobic cultures of CSF should be performed in cases of suspected bacterial CNS infections. Bacteria are often in low concentrations in CSF; therefore enrichment media may be helpful in supporting bacterial growth. However, in humans, broth cultures are more likely to result in false positive growth from bacterial skin contaminants.[193] In veterinary medicine, cultures are often negative in cases of bacterial CNS disease, which may be the consequence of a low concentration of bacteria in CSF, improper sample preparation, or improper culture technique.[52] CSF may also suppress bacterial growth, either as a result of specific inhibitors or from a lack of nutrients to support growth.[2] Care must also be exercised when interpreting drug sensitivities using qualitative methods (disk diffusion) because breakpoints are derived from drug concentrations obtainable in serum and not CSF.[120]

Gram staining may help identify organisms. Gram staining has a sensitivity of 60% to 90% and a specificity approaching 100% in people with bacterial CNS infections.[193] Similarly, blood cultures identify the causative organism in 80%, 90%, and 94% of humans with *S. pneumoniae*, *N. meningitidis*, and *H. influenzae*, respectively.[193] Blood cultures were positive in one of three dogs evaluated.[130]

Immunologic Testing

The identification of specific antibodies or antigens within the CNS is helpful in establishing the diagnosis of some viral, fungal, protozoal, and rickettsial infections. Unfortunately, such tests are not available to establish the presence of bacterial disease in veterinary patients. The finding of antibodies in the CSF that are directed against specific pathogens does suggest intrathecal production of IgG molecules. However, serum immunoglobulins can enter the CSF in the presence of meningeal inflammation unrelated to an infection. Therefore, though provocative, the finding of antibodies in the CSF does not definitively establish an etiologic diagnosis. With meningeal inflammation, both albumin and IgG contents are increased in CSF from a loss of integrity of the blood-CSF barrier or BBB, which allows for secondary transudation. Increased albumin content in the CSF lends support to leakage of serum proteins across a disrupted barrier. Mathematical formulas relating serum albumin and globulin with that in the CSF can also assist in identifying local production of immunoglobulin. Unfortunately, such formulas as albumin quotient and CSF IgG index do not provide specific information regarding the cause. The concurrent measurement of serum and CSF antibody titers paired with those directed against another pathogen not known to infect the CSF and for which the patient has already developed measurable antibodies (e.g., canine parvovirus) can support a causality.[61] This procedure is often used in the diagnosis of CDV and other

Table • 92-2

Representative CSF Changes Seen in Various CNS Inflammatory Diseases of Dogs and Cats[32,51,135,178]

DISEASE (CHAPTER)	WBC[a,b] COUNT	WBC TYPE	TOTAL PROTEIN CONCENTRATION (mg/dl)[c]	ALBUMIN PROPORTION	GLOBULIN PROPORTION	CSF ANTIBODIES DETECTED	ORGANISMS SEEN
Bacterial meningitis (92)	++ (+++)	PMN (mixed)	++ (+++)	++	++	Varies	Yes (Varies)
Steroid-responsive meningitis/arteritis (84)	+++ (++)	Mixed (mono)	+++(++)	++	+(++)	No (IgA)	No
Tumor (e.g., meningioma)-associated pleocytosis[d]	+ (++)	PMNs (mixed)	+ (++)	+ (++)	WNL	No	No
Granulomatous meningoencephalitis (84)	++ (+++)	Mixed—PMN, mono	++ (+++)	++	++	No	No
Feline infectious peritonitis (11)	+++ (++)	Mixed—PMNs, some mono	+++	++	++	Yes (?)	No
Fungal meningoencephalitis (59-62, 67)	++	Mixed—PMN, eos, mono	++	++	+ (++)	Varies	Varies
Protozoal meningoencephalitis (72, 75, 77, 79)	+	Mixed—PMN, eos, mono	+ (++)	+	+ (++)	Variable	Rarely
Ehrlichiosis (28)	+ (++)	Mono	+	+	+	?	Varies
Rocky Mountain spotted fever (29)	+	Mixed (neutro)	+ (WNL)	+	+	?	No
Eosinophilic meningitis	+ (++)	Eos	+	+	+	No	No
Canine distemper (3)							
Inflammatory	+	Mono (lymph)	+	WNL	+	Yes	No
Noninflammatory	WNL (+)	Mono (lymph)	WNL	WNL	WNL (+)	No (varies)	No
Other viral encephalitis (7, 26)	+	Mono	+ (++)	WNL	+	?	No
Necrotizing encephalitis in Yorkshire terriers (84)	+	Mono	+	+	+	No	No

CSF, Cerebrospinal fluid; WBC, white blood cell; PMN, polymorphonuclear neutrophils; mono, monocytes (lymphocytes, plasma cells, monocytes, and macrophages); mixed, mononuclear cells, neutrophils, and eosinophils; eos, eosinophils; neutro, neutrophils; lymph, lymphocytes; WNL, within normal limits; +, mild elevations; ++, moderate elevation; +++, marked elevation; ?, uncertain

[a]Symbols in parentheses indicate less frequent variations; for example + (++) indicates that typically the test results are mildly elevated but in some patients are moderately elevated.

[b]WNL for WBC count, <4/µl; +, 5–80/µl; ++, 81–500/µl; +++, > 500/µl.

[c]WNL for Total Protein Concentration, < 25 mg/dl; +, 25–100 mg/dl; ++, 100–300 mg/dl; +++, > 300 mg/dl.

[d]For neoplasia, typically protein increase is greater than that of leukocytes (albuminocytologic dissociation); for lymphoma in subarachnoid space, greater number of cells are present of mononuclear variety.

infections. See Diagnosis in Chapters 3, 45, 80, and 84. In the case of CNS *Cryptococcus*, a specific latex-agglutination test identifying intrathecal antigen has been developed that can provide a specific and accurate diagnosis (see Chapter 61).

Polymerase Chain Reaction

This method, which is in the early stage of evaluation of CNS pathogens, has been used to detect various infectious agents in inflammatory disorders in humans and has included primers directed at specific bacterial pathogens expected in meningitis.[101] Given that cultivation of CSF has been frequently unrewarding, this method might be considered as a way to detect bacterial or other pathogens in the CSF from animals having inflammatory CSF analysis results. In human meningitis, bacterial pathogens such as *Neisseria* or *Haemophilus* are so specific having a predilection for the CNS that latex-agglutination and polymerase chain reaction tests that allow for the detection of specific bacterial antigens and nucleotides, respectively.[131]

Radiologic Imaging

Given that most cases of bacterial meningitis in veterinary patients are the result of hematogenous or contiguous spread of organisms, thorough screening of suspected cases is warranted. In addition to the minimal database, chest radiographs, and abdominal imaging, abdominal radiography or ultrasonography should be performed. Cultures of other bodily fluids, blood, and urine may be helpful in identifying bacteria. In patients with newly diagnosed heart murmur, echocardiography should be performed to investigate the possibility of bacterial valvular endocarditis.

The most sensitive methods of imaging the CNS are magnetic resonance imaging (MRI) and computed tomography. All patients with clinical indications of parenchymal disease, encephalitis, or myelitis, or those with focal neurologic deficits, should undergo advanced imaging procedures. Patterns of meningeal enhancement with MRI have been reported.[99,113] Inflammatory lesions generally appear less intense with T1-weighted imaging and more intense with T2-weighted imaging. Although advanced imaging procedures provide a sensitive method for detecting disease, findings are often not specific enough to allow for definitive diagnosis. Despite this disadvantage, imaging may provide information regarding the possibility of surgical intervention for drainage of infective material in focal disease.

THERAPY

Treating bacterial CNS infections presents unique challenges. The mainstay of treatment revolves around the administration of appropriate antimicrobials based ideally on antibiotic susceptibility testing. In many cases, this information is unavailable, and treatment needs to be instituted empirically based on clinical suspicion. For successful treatment, an understanding of both the pharmacokinetic and the pharmacodynamic properties of the various antibiotics is essential. Pharmacokinetics is the study of the drug concentration in serum and the site of action of the drug, and pharmacodynamics refers to the relationship between drug activity and concentration. Drug kinetics in the nervous system is very different than it is elsewhere in the body, largely because of the BBB. Numerous factors influence drug penetration in the CNS. The major factor limiting penetration into the CNS is lipid solubility.[103] Lipophilic drugs reach higher concentrations in the brain because they are able to penetrate by diffusion into the BBB (Table 92-3).[146] Hydrophilic drugs such as β-lactams are weak acids that, at physiologic pH values, are ionized and therefore hydrophilic, which limits their penetration into the CNS.[53] Quinolones, rifampin, and metronidazole are lipid soluble and more easily enter the CNS.[4] Molecular size also influences drug penetration, with large macromolecules being more effectively excluded from entering the CNS. In a similar fashion, the degree of protein binding also inhibits

Table • 92-3

Antimicrobial Drugs Penetrating Blood-Brain Barrier and Blood–Cerebrospinal Fluid Barrier

DRUG ACTION	GOOD PENETRATION C_{CSF}/C_{serum} (%) > 35	INTERMEDIATE PENETRATION C_{CSF}/C_{serum} (%) > 12 and <35	POOR PENETRATION C_{CSF}/C_{serum} (%) ≤ 12
Microbiocidal drugs	Trimethoprim-sulfonamide Metronidazole Ofloxacin	Methicillin Oxacillin Carbenicillin Ticarcillin Piperacillin Ceftazidime Cefepime Imipenem Ceftizoxime Aminoglycosides Moxalactam Trovafloxacin Ciprofloxacin	Penicillin Ampicillin Cefotaxime Ceftriaxone First-generation cephalosporins Clindamycin Daptomycin
Microbiostatic drugs	Chloramphenicol Sulfonamides Doxycycline Fluconazole Pyrazinamide Isoniazid	Tetracyclines Flucytosine Rifampin	Amphotericin B Erythromycin Ketoconazole Itraconazole

C_{CSF}/C_{Serum}, Concentration cerebrospinal fluid over concentration serum, expressed as a percentage.

Table • 92-4

Recommended Antimicrobials for Specific Agents or Settings[2,63]

ORGANISM	FIRST CHOICES	SECOND CHOICE
Gram-positive bacteria		
Staphylococcus	Nafcillin	Vancomycin, vancomycin + rifampin, ampicillin, trimethoprim-sulfonamide
Streptococcus	Penicillin, ampicillin	Ceftriaxone, vancomycin
Actinomyces	Ampicillin	Minocycline
Gram-negative bacteria	Cefotaxime + ampicillin	Gentamicin + ampicillin, gentamicin + ceftriaxone
Pseudomonas	Ceftazidime + aminoglycoside[a]	Piperacillin + aminoglycoside,[a] carbenicillin + gentamicin[a]
Pasteurella	Ampicillin	Trimethoprim
Brucella	Minocycline	Gentamicin[a]
Salmonella	Ceftriaxone	Ampicillin, chloramphenicol
Enterococcus	Ampicillin	Minocycline
Bacteroides	Metronidazole	Chloramphenicol, piperacillin

[a]Fluoroquinolone can be substituted.

penetration into the CNS. Because most antibiotics are, in part, bound to albumin, only the unbound portion is available to cross the BBB. Highly protein-bound antibiotics are hydrophobic and are very large molecules, both of which hinder entry into the CNS. Lastly, the choroid plexus contains an energy-dependent pump that moves agents out of the CNS. This efflux system is responsible for approximately 70% of the elimination of penicillin, and other drugs such as the quinolones are eliminated to a lesser degree.[4]

Although these factors influence the ability of a drug to penetrate the BBB, in many disease states, the functionality of the BBB is altered. With inflammation, a disruption of the BBB tight junctions occurs, which effectively allows entry of the drug and which, under normal states, would be excluded.[128] Many antibiotics will reach concentrations 5 to 10 times higher when the BBB is disrupted.[154] Of importance is that, as inflammation subsides, the BBB also returns to normal function, limiting again antibiotic penetration.[103] Similarly, other factors may influence drug activity in meningitis. These factors include changes in pH, which may reduce or inactivate the antimicrobial effects of antibiotics such as aminoglycoside; increased protein content in CSF with inflammation, resulting in binding of free (active) drug; and slower growth rates of bacteria.[154]

Antimicrobial Therapy

Because the CSF is devoid of complement and opsonizing proteins, essentially an ineffective immune system, it is imperative that antibiotic reach the CNS in bacteriocidal concentrations to eradicate an infection.[154] Unlike extraneural infections in which the host can rely, in part, on the immune system to participate in removing microorganisms, the CNS cannot. Antibiotics can be divided based on their patterns of bactericidal activity in body fluids. Some antibiotics demonstrate increased bactericidal activity with increasing concentrations and are referred to as concentration-dependent drugs. Aminoglycosides and quinolone antibiotics fall into this category. Other antibiotics show no increases in bactericidal activity with increasing concentrations. Instead, these drugs demonstrate increases in bactericidal activity with increasing time over which the concentration remains above the minimum inhibitory concentration (MIC) of the organism (T > MIC). Antibiotics such as the β-lactams fall into this group. Knowledge of an antibiotic's bactericidal activity, concentration dependent versus concentration independent, influences

dosing intervals. Additionally, bacteriostatic and bacteriocidal antibiotics should not be used together because the combination may be antagonistic.[154] Refer to Chapter 34 for a more complete discussion of the drugs covered in this chapter.

Information in the veterinary literature describing the treatment of bacterial meningitis is limited. Compounding this lack of data is the fact that most of the experimental animal models are designed to evaluate pathophysiologic sequelae and therapeutic regimens related to specific pathogens encountered in human medicine. Despite this lack of information, some generalizations regarding specific antibiotics can be made. Recommended antimicrobial agents used to treat specific infectious agents are presented in Table 92-4. Dosing regimens for specific antimicrobials are presented in Table 92-5.

Drug Administration

Of critical importance in the successful treatment of bacterial meningitis is obtaining CSF antimicrobial concentrations above the minimum bacteriocidal concentration (MBC) for the infecting organism. Dosing regimens should be chosen that maintain CSF concentrations well above MBC for the greatest time period. To ensure success, concentration of 10 to 30 times the MBC should be achieved.[172] Given that CSF concentrations are a reflection of serum concentrations, intravenous (IV) administration is advocated for at least 3 to 5 days, and then oral administration can be used. If possible, repeat CSF analysis, as well as culture and susceptibilities, should be performed before discontinuing antibiotic therapy to ensure eradication.

Increased BBB permeability that occurs in inflammatory CNS diseases also increases the permeability to antibacterial drugs. Antibacterials are not metabolized in the CSF and therefore their concentrations are based on the balance between drug penetration and elimination. Drugs enter the CSF predominantly via passive diffusion down a concentration gradient; the main determinant is high lipid solubility. Lipoidal drugs such as quinolones or rifampin cross intracellularly and reach peak concentrations rapidly, and water-soluble β-lactams must cross intercellularly, and transport is delayed or reduced unless tight junctions between cells are compromised. Concentrations in CSF lag behind those in serum and therefore can be predicted only by repeated CSF concentration measurements for which data is largely unavailable. Meningeal inflammation not only increases permeability,

Table • 92-5

Antimicrobial Drug Dosages for CNS Bacterial and Fungal Infections of Dogs and Cats[a]

DRUG[b]	DOSE[c]	ROUTE	INTERVAL (HOURS)
Penicillin (aqueous)	$10-22 \times 10^3$ U/kg	IV	4—6
Ampicillin	5—22 mg/kg	IV	6
Carbenicillin	10—30 mg/kg	IV, IM	4—6
Oxacillin (or cloxacillin)	8.8—20 mg/kg	IV, PO	4—8
Trimethoprim-sulfonamide[d]	15—20 mg/kg	IV, PO	8—12
Gentamicin[c]	2 mg/kg	IV, IM	8
Chloramphenicol	10—15 mg/kg	PO	4—6
Cephalexin	20 (10—30) mg/kg	PO	8
Cephapirin	20—30 mg/kg	IV, IM	8
Amphotericin B[d]	0.15—0.50 mg/kg	IV	48
Flucytosine	50 mg/kg	PO	8
Rifampin	10—20 mg/kg	PO	8—12
Metronidazole	10—15 mg/kg	PO	8
Cefotaxime	6—40 mg/kg	IM, IV	4—6
Enrofloxacin[e]	5—10 mg/kg	PO	12

IV, Intravenous; *IM,* intramuscular; *PO,* by mouth.
[a]See discussion of drug administration for recommended duration of therapy and precautions. See respective chapters for dosages in treating viral, protozoal, and some fungal infections.
[b]For further information on those drugs, see Drug Formulary, Appendix 8.
[c]Dose per administration at specified interval.
[d]Potential for renal toxicity is greatest in cats and young or dehydrated dogs. Closely monitor renal functions and use lowest dosage under these circumstances.
[e]Other fluoroquinolones such as orbifloxacin or marbofloxacin can be substituted.

but also inhibits the elimination pump so that concentrations can be unpredictable over time. With successful antibacterial treatment, inflammation is reduced and the BBB integrity improves. Further penetration of ionic drugs becomes more difficult, which is important in considering followup or long-term therapy in which the initial response to treatment is beneficial. Fortunately, many antibacterials, with the exception of some tested quinolones, have prolonged antibacterial effects and longer half-life in the CSF as compared with serum.[103]

Aminoglycosides

Aminoglycoside antibiotics demonstrate concentration-dependent bactericidal activity. In addition, they display a prolonged postantibiotic effect, a period during which continued inhibition of microbial growth despite concentrations below MIC occurs. Both of these properties form the rationale for once-daily dosing. However, the penetration of aminoglycosides remains poor even in the presence of significant meningeal inflammation.[4]

Cephalosporins

Largely because of their low lipophilicity, cephalosporins poorly penetrate through the BBB, achieving relatively low CSF concentrations.[102] However, third-generation cephalosporins (moxalactam, ceftriaxone, cefotaxime) can cross inflamed meninges.[94] The concentration achieved by most agents varies inversely with the protein binding of the drug. In addition to the high penetration of cephalosporins, the MBC of cephalosporins for many pathogens can be low so that CSF concentrations can be achieved at levels several times higher than MBC. To achieve greater CSF concentrations, higher doses can be administered safely for longer periods given the low toxicity. Cephalosporins demonstrate time-dependent bactericidal activity. Consequently, dosing regimes that result in CSF con-

centrations above MIC for the longest time period should be used. For these reasons, third-generation cephalosporins are currently recommended as the drug of choice for empirical therapy of bacterial meningitis in people with common meningeal microbial pathogens.[129]

Chloramphenicol

Chloramphenicol has been generally classified as a bacteriostatic antibiotic; however, in concentrations achievable in tissues and body fluids, it has been shown to be bactericidal.[132] Chloramphenicol reaches high CSF concentration (45% to 90% of serum) regardless of meningeal inflammation.[54] This drug also appears to concentrate in the CNS, reaching levels that exceed those in serum; however, large doses are required for bactericidal effects in the CNS.[125] Despite these pharmacodynamic properties, a high relapse rate occurs with this drug, suggesting it is not bactericidal at doses used in dogs and cats.[125] Consequently, this drug should not be used as a first choice.

Clindamycin

Clindamycin does not readily cross the BBB.[11,109] Although this drug achieves clinically useful concentrations in most tissues, a notable exception is the CSF, even with inflamed meninges.[50] Brain tissue concentrations may be higher than CSF concentrations because of the lipid solubility of clindamycin.[168] Usage of clindamycin is limited to specific protozoal infections in the nervous system.

Fluoroquinolones

As a whole, quinolones are moderately lipophilic, exhibit low to moderate binding to serum proteins, and have a relatively low molecular weight and therefore achieve good penetration into the CNS.[4] The pharmacodynamic effects of quinolones in CSF are different with respect to other sites in the body because they have a short postantimicrobial effect and need to continue to exceed the bactericidal concentration to achieve maximal effect.[103] Quinolones are used primarily for gram-negative aerobic infections. They can also be considered a safe alternative to aminoglycosides.

Penicillins

Generally, penicillins tend to have low penetration into the CNS, but with meningeal inflammation, concentrations are greater. CSF concentrations are approximately 1% to 2% of serum concentrations without meningeal inflammation; however, concentrations increase to 18% to 21% with meningeal inflammation.[71,142] As stated earlier, an efflux pump can be used to eliminate penicillins from the CSF, which limits achievable concentrations.[4] Ampicillin is the exception to these properties in that significant CSF concentrations can be obtained regardless of the state of the meninges.

Metronidazole

Metronidazole exhibits good penetration into the CSF and brain abscesses[50] and demonstrates bactericidal activity against anaerobes. Metronidazole penetrates the CSF more completely than does any other single agent, with reports of CSF levels approaching 90% of those in serum.[4] Metronidazole is used primarily to treat anaerobic infections.

Trimethoprim-sulfonamides

Trimethoprim-sulfonamides penetrate both the normal and the inflamed meninges at therapeutic levels. Recommendations are that animals that respond to ampicillin be switched to this drug for extended therapy. This drug has not been used as a first-line medication likely as a result of a lack of availability of a parenteral formulation.

Glucocorticoid therapy

Increasingly clear is that the majority of injury to the CNS in bacterial meningitis is related to the host immune system rather than the infectious organisms. In fact, the host response is accentuated at the time bactericidal antibiotics treatment is initiated, organisms are lysed, and an abrupt release occurs of inflammatory cell wall components, lipopolysaccharides, and outer membrane vesicles from the organisms.[39] Studies in animals have shown that bacterial lysis, induced by treatment with antibiotics, leads to greater inflammation in the subarachnoid space, which may contribute to an unfavorable outcome.[41] Steroids have antiinflammatory effects. They inhibit the transcription of mRNA for TNF-α and IL-1 and the production of prostaglandins and platelet activating factor, reduce vasogenic cerebral edema, and reduce the production of inducile NOS.[48] Consequently, the use of adjunctive glucocorticoids have been advocated in the treatment of bacterial meningitis. Current recommendations for dexamethasone therapy include 0.15 mg/kg administered 15 to 20 minutes before starting antibacterial therapy and thereafter every 6 hours for 4 days or at 0.4 mg/kg every 12 hours for 2 days.[145] The beneficial effects of glucocorticoids were not seen if steroid use was delayed for 12 to 24 hours after the first antimicrobial dose.[78] In addition to the side effects of glucocorticoids, some concern has surfaced that steroids may reduce the penetration of antibiotics into the CSF by restoring the BBB.

Importantly, glucocorticoid use has been studied in the setting of important pathogens for humans, particularly Hib. Therefore extrapolation to veterinary medicine must be done with caution given than bacterial meningitis in veterinary patients can involve alternate primary sources, a different time course often with relapses.[114] Empiric glucocorticoid therapy before diagnostics remains contraindicated. Glucocorticoids can alter diagnostic test results such as CSF interpretation. In addition, although many patients may benefit from their use, patients with viral, fungal, protozoal, and rickettsial meningoencephalitis may be adversely affected. Glucocorticoids may reduce the permeability of the BBB in meningitis and therefore decrease the penetration of hydrophobic antibiotics into CSF.[153]

Supportive Therapy

Supportive care can be divided into systemic- and brain-specific therapy. Systemic therapy is aimed at correcting metabolic abnormalities. Hydration is an important aspect of treatment. In hydrated patients that are able to drink, access to water may be all that is needed. However, in dehydrated patient or those unable to drink, fluid therapy should be aimed at the restoration and maintenance of normal hydration and intravascular fluid volume. Overhydration should be avoided because it can potentiate cerebral edema. Experimentally, fluid therapy did not worsen brain edema.[175]

Hyperthermia can be treated in a wide variety of ways, ranging from adjusting the environmental temperature with air conditioning or fans, to administering IV fluids at room temperature, to more active processes such as applying alcohol to the foot pads or placing ice packs on the patient. Unless body temperature becomes dangerously high, pharmacologic treatment of fever should be avoided because the resolution of a fever may be used as an indicator of successful antimicrobial therapy. Patients with clinical and biochemical findings indicative of a systemic inflammatory response should be treated for sepsis (see Chapter 38).

Analgesia should be provided to patients with cervical hyperesthesia. The clinician must balance patient discomfort with the ability to critically judge therapeutic success and patient assessment. Care should be exercised when administering analgesics to patients with altered mentation given that some opioid analgesics can cause sedation.

Brain-specific therapy is aimed at ameliorating intracranial hypertension and seizures. Some indications of intracranial hypertension include altered mentation (obtundation, somnolence, stupor, and coma), bradycardia with systemic hypertension, papilledema, and head pressing. Mannitol is an osmotic diuretic that can be used to reduce intracranial pressure. Mannitol can be administered at a dosage of 1 to 2 g/kg of body weight IV for 5 to 10 minutes.[7] The effect is potentiated by the co-administration of furosemide at 0.7 mg/kg of body weight IV, 15 minutes after administering mannitol.[137]

In patients with seizures, anticonvulsants should be given. Phenobarbital is a safe and effective anticonvulsant medication. In general, phenobarbital is initiated at 2 to 4 mg/kg of body weight, but it can be given to a total dose of up to 16 mg/kg in circumstances such as status epilepticus.

General nursing care should be dictated by patient needs. Recumbent patients should be placed on soft-padded bedding and frequently turned to alternate recumbent positions. Assistance with bladder and bowel evacuation should be done with patients that are unable to perform these functions. Physical therapy has been described elsewhere.[105]

Prognosis

Ultimately, the prognosis depends on a timely, accurate diagnosis and implementation of appropriate therapy. Despite advances in human medicine, the mortality rate in people with bacterial meningitis ranges from 5% to 40% of patients, with 30% of survivors having permanent neurologic deficits.[86,189] These lasting consequences are divided into three categories: loss of hearing, obstructive hydrocephalus, and brain parenchymal damage as evidenced by sensory motor deficits, cerebral palsy, learning deficits, cortical blindness, and seizure disorders.[173] Several factors have been identified in people with bacterial meningitis. The degree of impairment of consciousness was correlated with prognosis, and seizures were not.[94] The age of the patient plays a role in prognosis, with children under 1 year and adults over 40 years having a worse prognosis.[94] Biochemical parameters such CSF leukocyte count, CSF glucose concentration, and the time required to sterilize the CSF have all been evaluated in humans with bacterial meningitis.[81] Additionally, CSF concentrations of IL-1 and TNF-α correlate with prognosis.[118,187] Although prognosis has not been well established in veterinary patients, similar aspects are likely to play a role in the prognosis.

SUGGESTED READINGS*

37. Cook LB, Bergman RL, Bahr A, et al. 2003. Inflammatory polyp in the middle ear with secondary suppurative meningoencephalitis in a cat, *Vet Radiol Ultrasound* 44:648-651.
39. Coyle PK. 1999. Glucocorticoids in central nervous system bacterial infection, *Arch Neurol* 56:796-801.

*See the CD-ROM for a complete list of references.

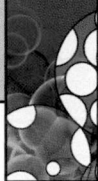

CHAPTER • 93

Ocular Infections

Jean Stiles

EXTRAOCULAR INFECTIONS

Normal Flora

Despite the fact that all dogs probably have indigenous bacteria in their conjunctival cul-de-sac, positive isolation rates of between 46% and 91% in clinically healthy dogs have been reported (Table 93-1). Variables in the type of and frequency of isolate may be a result of geography, culturing technique, breed, and season. Fungi are isolated from 10% to 22% of dogs.[42,100]

In contrast to dogs, cats have a relatively lower rate of cultivable bacteria in their conjunctival sac.[33] Bacteria or mycoplasmas have been isolated from 34% of the conjunctival samples and from 25% of the samples from the lid margins. In one study of 50 cats, no organisms were isolated from 42% of the cats, bacteria were isolated from the conjunctiva of 34% of the cats or 47% of the eyes, and 26% of the cats or 14% of the eyes had fungal isolates from the conjunctiva (Table 93-2). No anaerobes were isolated.[40]

Ocular Surface and Adnexa

Most surface bacterial infections are not strictly primary; other debilitating conditions often potentiate the pathogenicity of organisms that are indigenous to the ocular surface. Other local nidi of infection, such as in the lacrimal sac and meibomian glands or structures adjacent to the eye (ears, lip-folds), should be sought and corrected to overcome persistent or recurring infection. Control of the normal ocular flora is maintained by rinsing of the ocular surface with tears and blinking, which pushes the tears into the nasolacrimal (NL) system. Tears also contain IgA and other antibacterial substances such as lactoferrin. Competitive interactions among the indigenous flora keeps the numbers of organisms lower, whereas disrupting this balance may cause an overgrowth of one species. Conditions debilitating to the ocular surface, such as reduced tear secretions, ultraviolet (UV) radiation, immune suppression (e.g., with diabetes mellitus or Cushing's disease), and trauma creating breaks in the epithelial barrier, may allow indigenous bacteria to adhere and possibly overgrow to produce disease. To become established, bacteria must adhere, replicate, and then invade the tissue. Invasion subsequently incites inflammation. Tissue damage with infection produces a combination of toxins from the organism and enzymes such as collagenase, elastase, and cathepsins liberated by the neutrophilic response.[102] Bacteria, such as *Pseudomonas aeruginosa*, that have various proteolytic enzymes typically produce rapidly progressive corneal ulcers.

Blepharitis in Dogs

Blepharitis, or inflammation of the eyelids, may develop secondary to bacterial, fungal, or parasitic agents. Blepharitis can develop with other dermatologic diseases, with other ocular diseases such as conjunctivitis, or as a sole clinical presentation. Clinical features of blepharitis include eyelid swelling, erythema, skin ulceration, chalazia (granulomatous foci of inflammation along meibomian glands), and pruritis.

Staphylococcus species can cause a primary blepharitis and may also generate a hypersensitivity reaction. Pruritis may lead to self-trauma, exacerbating the blepharitis. Bacterial infection of the eyelids may also occur with keratoconjunctivitis sicca (KCS) or atopy.

Treatment of bacterial blepharitis should include cleansing the skin with dilute povidone iodine solution and rubbing a broad-spectrum ophthalmic antibiotic into ulcerated skin as well as placing it in the eye 3 to 4 times daily. If skin is very inflamed, an antibiotic with dexamethasone is indicated. Severe cases may require systemic antibiotic therapy such as cephalosporins and possibly antiinflammatory doses of oral glucocorticoids. Any underlying condition that can be identified should also be addressed.

Canine juvenile pyoderma develops occasionally in puppies ages 3 to 16 weeks. Early reports suggested a hypersensitivity reaction to *Staphylococcus* species, although the cause is considered unknown. Pustules and granulomatous inflammation are present in the eyelids and face. In some cases the pinna and regional lymph nodes are also affected. Rarely, joints may also be involved.

The condition responds quickly to administration of systemic glucocorticoids, suggesting an autoimmune disease. Diagnosis is based on age, history, and clinical presentation. Prednisolone (2 mg/kg/day) should be administered for 2 to 3 weeks. Lesions typically improve within a few days of beginning therapy. A systemic antibiotic such as a cephalosporin is indicated if skin has become secondarily infected with bacteria.

Table • 93-1

Frequency of Bacterial Isolation from the Conjunctival Sacs of Clinically Healthy Dogs[7,41,51,118]

ORGANISM	ISOLATION (PERCENTAGE)[a]
Staphylococcus (Total)	57—70
Coagulase-positive	24—45
Coagulase-negative	46—55
Streptococcus (Total)	6—43
Nonhemolytic	12—51
α-Hemolytic	4—34
β-Hemolytic	2—7
Corynebacterium (Total)	30—75
Undifferentiated	11
C. pseudodiphtheriticum	9
C. xerosis	13
Neisseria (Total)	26
Undifferentiated	4
N. catarrhalis	9
N. pharyngis	4
N. sicca	3
N. caviae	3
N. lactamicus	3
N. flavescens	3
Pseudomonas (Total)	14
Moraxella (Total)	7
Bacillus (Total)	6—18

[a]Percentages are based on the numbers of animals from which organisms were isolated.

Table • 93-2

Bacterial and Fungal Isolates from Clinically Healthy Cats[33,40]

LOCATION	ORGANISM	PERCENTAGE[a]
Conjunctiva	*Staphylococcus* spp.	27
	Corynebacterium spp.	1.3—5
	Bacillus spp.	3—5
	Streptococcus spp.	2—2.5
	Mycoplasma	0—5
	Fungal isolates	13
Lids	*Staphylococcus* spp.	23—28
	Streptococcus spp.	0—2
	Bacillus spp.	2—5
	Corynebacterium spp.	1.6

[a]Percentages are based on the numbers of animals from which organisms were isolated.

Blepharitis in Cats

Blepharitis in the cat is less common than in the dog. Cats appear relatively resistant to bacterial blepharitis, except when they have a traumatic injury and resulting bacterial invasion. This type of injury most commonly occurs in cat fights and may involve the head and eyelids. Abscesses near the eyelids should be opened as they would be elsewhere and appropriate systemic antibiotics administered.

Conjunctivitis in Dogs

Bacterial conjunctivitis may be a primary condition or secondary to another ocular condition such as KCS, distemper virus, a parasitic invasion, or the presence of a foreign body. Primary bacterial conjunctivitis typically occurs for unknown reasons and in some cases is secondary to an insult that is no longer apparent or is merely an overgrowth of normal conjunctival flora. The symptoms are purulent discharge with mild to moderate discomfort. Diagnosis should be based on cytologic examination of the exudate and identification of bacteria and neutrophilic inflammation. KCS should be ruled out based on a normal Schirmer tear test. Bacterial overgrowth is common when tear production is low, and the underlying problem of KCS must be addressed. Culture is typically not warranted for bacterial conjunctivitis unless response to therapy is poor. A complete ocular exam, including a Schirmer tear test, fluorescein staining of the cornea, fluorescein evaluation of NL duct patency, and a search for a foreign body in the conjunctival sac and behind the third eyelid, should be performed. Therapy should include a broad-spectrum topical antibiotic such as bacitracin-neomycin-polymixin B every 6 hours until resolution.

Viral conjunctivitis in dogs has been associated most often with distemper virus. The first signs of distemper are bilateral conjunctivitis with a discharge that progresses from serous to mucopurulent. The virus may also invade lacrimal tissue, causing an adenitis that results in KCS. In this situation the cornea may become ulcerated and possibly even become perforated. KCS typically resolves over several weeks in dogs that recover from distemper. Early diagnosis of dogs with distemper may be possible by fluorescent antibody stains of conjunctival epithelial cells obtained from a scraping.

Therapy should include cleansing of eyes, application of a broad-spectrum topical antibiotic to help prevent secondary bacterial infection, and if KCS is present, topical cyclosporine and artificial tears.

Conjunctivitis in Cats

Bacterial conjunctivitis in cats is unusual, with the exception of infection with *Chlamydophila felis*, which is a common cause of conjunctivitis in cats (see Chapter 31). The typical clinical picture is unilateral conjunctivitis with involvement of the second eye a few days later. The clinical presentation is indistinguishable from conjunctivitis caused by feline herpesvirus-1 (FHV-1), and the two organisms may be present simultaneously. Diagnosis is based on seeing the typical elementary body in the cytoplasm of conjunctival epithelial cells (Fig. 93-1) or obtaining a positive fluorescent antibody (FA) test result on a conjunctival scraping. *C. felis* can also be cultured but requires special transport media. Elementary bodies are often few in number and the numbers diminish with chronicity, making them easy to miss. In an experimental study of chlamydial conjunctivitis, infection with feline immunodeficiency virus (FIV) prolonged the duration of clinical signs and led to chronic conjunctivitis.[86] Conjunctivitis caused by *Chlamydophila* should be treated with topical tetracycline applied to both eyes 4 times daily until resolution and then an additional 1 week. Oral doxycycline at 10 mg/kg/day was found to be superior to twice-daily topical fusidic acid or chlortetracycline in one experimental study.[103] Treatment with oral doxycycline may also be advisable to clear the GI tract of infection.[86] The potential of this organism to infect people is uncertain; however, washing hands after treating an affected cat is advised.

Mycoplasma felis has been variably implicated as a cause of conjunctivitis in cats (Fig. 93-2). Some studies have recovered *Mycoplasma* species as normal flora from feline conjunctiva, whereas others have not. Similarly, experimental infections of healthy, young cats have produced conjunctivitis in some

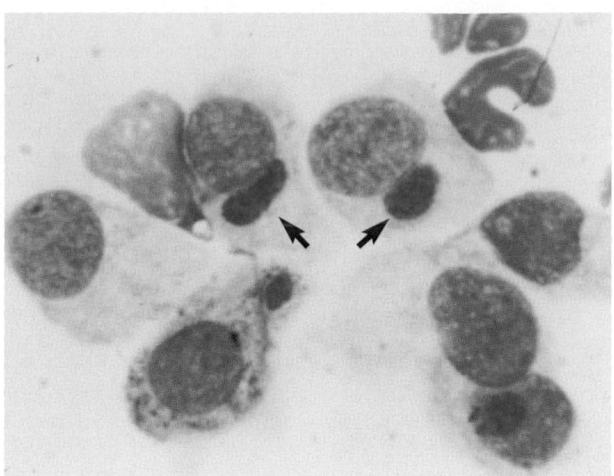

Fig 93-1 Intracytoplasmic *C. felis* inclusions in conjunctival epithelial cells of a cat with conjunctivitis (Giemsa stain, ×330).

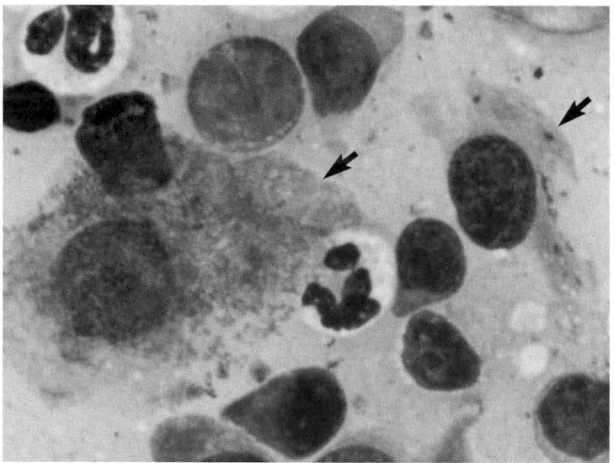

Fig 93-2 *Mycoplasma* organisms within conjunctival epithelial cells in a cat with conjunctivitis (Wright stain, ×330).

studies[50] and not in others. *Mycoplasma* organisms may require a stressor such as FHV to cause disease. *Mycoplasma* species are sensitive to many topical antibiotics, including tetracycline.

FHV-1 is a frequent cause of ocular disease in cats.[2,106,107,120] Young cats with respiratory tract disease generally have conjunctivitis with marked conjunctival hyperemia, chemosis, and serous to purulent ocular discharge (Fig. 93-3). The condition is usually self-limiting and resolves in 1 to 2 weeks. In severe cases of herpesvirus conjunctivitis, the risk of symblepharon is high. Symblepharon, or adhesions of the conjunctiva to itself or the cornea, may lead to permanent visual impairment, and an attempt to break these adhesions early should be made. After application of topical anesthesia, a cotton-tip swab can be used to break adhesions and strip off cellular debris and fibrin. This process may need to be repeated frequently until the conjunctivitis has resolved. In severe conjunctivitis a topical antiviral such as trifluridine should also be used at least 4 times daily. In addition to general supportive care, the eyes should be cleansed frequently and a broad-spectrum topical antibiotic applied to minimize secondary bacterial infection as the conjunctival surface sloughs. Once infected, cats become

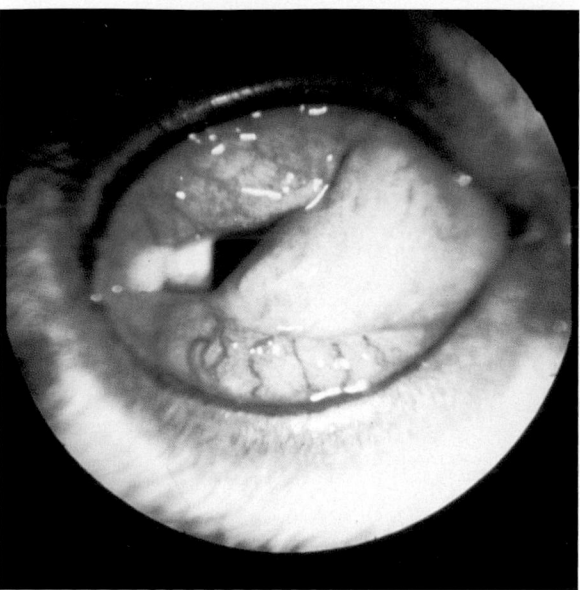

Fig 93-3 Acute conjunctivitis secondary to feline herpesvirus. Note severe chemosis and conjunctival hyperemia.

latent carriers of FHV-1 and may have recurrences of ocular disease, including conjunctivitis and corneal ulcers. Many cats have transient episodes of conjunctivitis, with conjunctival hyperemia, serous or purulent ocular discharge, and blepharospasm. Most cases are self-limiting and do not require treatment. If a topical antibiotic is used, tetracycline is the most appropriate choice because of its efficacy in treating *C. felis* and *M. felis*, which are common feline conjunctival pathogens that may contribute to conjunctivitis in addition to FHV-1. *Hartmannella vermiformis*, an amebic endosymbiont that contains the *Chlamydia*-like agent *Neorickettsia hartmannellae*, has been isolated in greater prevalence from cats with keratitis or conjunctivitis than from clinically healthy cats.[121]

Cats may develop chronic conjunctivitis or proliferative keratitis associated with FHV-1.[17,104] Laboratory diagnostic tests, such as virus isolation from the conjunctiva and conjunctival scrapings for fluorescent antibody testing, to prove FHV-1 as a cause of conjunctivitis in cats are frequently negative, making the diagnosis uncertain.[85] Identification of FHV-1 DNA in conjunctiva or the cornea by the polymerase chain reaction (PCR) is a more sensitive test than virus isolation or FA testing, although a high percentage of clinically normal cats have positive tests for viral DNA by PCR.[108,116] Treatment with an ophthalmic antiviral medication such as trifluridine can be used in cats with chronic conjunctivitis, although results vary. Treatment for KCS in cats with FHV-1 conjunctivitis can include topical 0.2% cyclosporine ointment in addition to antiviral therapy. Recombinant interferon (IFN) has also been administered to cats with chronic FHV-1–related ocular disease, although no studies have documented its effectiveness. Oral (see Chapter 2) and topical administration of IFN have been used.[76,111,112] Topical administration is discussed in the later Keratitis in Cats section.

Treatment with oral lysine has been shown to be efficacious in reducing the severity of FHV-1–induced conjunctivitis in an experimental setting.[47,110] Cats receiving 500 mg of oral L-lysine twice daily had less severe conjunctivitis than cats receiving placebo, although the length of disease and isolation of virus did not differ between the groups. Kittens with FHV-1–related disease may benefit from administration of 250 mg oral lysine twice daily. Adult cats with frequent recurrences of

FHV-1–related disease can be treated long term with 500 mg of oral lysine twice daily. Lysine should be given with food to avoid gastric upset.

Keratitis in Dogs

Infectious keratitis in dogs develops after a corneal ulceration or traumatic wounding. Bacterial flora inhabiting the ocular surface are those most likely to invade a corneal wound. Ulcerative keratitis and corneal abscesses are the two bacterial corneal diseases of concern. *Staphylococcus* and *Streptococcus* species are especially common, although infections with gram-negative bacteria may also develop.

Bacterial keratitis usually incites a visible neutrophilic response, characterized by a yellow to white cellular infiltrate within the cornea. Vascular growth into the cornea also occurs but usually does not begin for several days after injury and infection. Vessels originate from the limbus and grow at a rate of approximately 1 mm/day toward the site of infection. Rapid corneal destruction may occur with infectious keratitis. Invading bacteria and neutrophils may release proteases and collagenases, which contribute to corneal melting. Increased cyclooxygenase-2 expression has been documented in all corneal layers of dogs with keratitis, indicating that antiprostaglandin therapy may be a potential treatment for inflammatory keratitis.[101] Fungal keratitis, which can be indistinguishable from bacterial keratitis, is less common but can be caused by penetrating injuries with plant material or prolonged topical treatment with antibacterial or glucocorticoid therapy. White or brown infiltrates in the cornea are more likely to be caused by fungal growth. Fungal keratitis manifests as ulcerative keratitis, interstitial inflammation, or eventually iris prolapse because of damage to Descemet's membrane and corneal perforation.

Diagnosis of infectious keratitis is based on clinical findings, cytology, and culture. Fluorescein staining is used to detect epithelial ulceration. All corneal ulcers that are progressive or involve the stroma should be cultured. A mini-tip culturette with a moistened tip should be gently swabbed over the ulcer bed. After application of topical proparacaine, a flattened spatula or the blunt end of a scalpel blade should be used to gently scrape the ulcer edge for a cytology sample. Healthy corneas have noncornified epithelial cells. Keratin debris, an occasional bacterium, and mucus may also be observed. With bacterial keratitis, neutrophils are the predominant cell type, and bacteria may be either numerous or few or not visualized on cytology. Antibacterial treatment should be instituted to prevent the colonizing bacteria from causing more damage to the cornea. The initial decision about therapy should be based on whether cocci or rods have been identified. Culture is more sensitive than cytology for detecting bacteria and is the only way to confirm the species type and its antibacterial susceptibility. Until culture results are known, the broadest spectrum of antibacterial drugs possible should be used. Often, this means combination therapy, such as a topical fluoroquinolone and cefazolin. To achieve broad-spectrum bactericidal activity, commercial antibiotics can be fortified, and injectable antibiotics can be used with artificial tears or saline to create topical formulations (Tables 93-3 and 93-4). Frequency of application is critical. In a rapidly progressive corneal ulcer, topical antibiotics should be applied every 1 to 2 hours.

Systemic antibiotics are usually not indicated unless the cornea has a penetrating wound. Fungal keratitis is also treated with topical medication because systemic drug penetration of ocular tissues is poor (Table 93-5). Topical atropine can be used 2 to 4 times daily if miosis is present, although it should not be used in dogs with KCS or glaucoma. The use of topical agents to halt the proteolytic destruction of the cornea may be beneficial. Autogenous serum, acetylcysteine, or sodium ethylenediaminetetraacetic acid applied topically several times daily have all been advocated. The author favors autogenous serum because it is readily available and not irritating, although it must be handled and maintained using a sterile technique. Serum should be refrigerated and replenished every 48 hours.

If fungal keratitis is documented or suspected, it should be treated with a topical antifungal agent every 2 to 3 hours (see Table 93-5). Although natamycin is the only approved ophthalmic antifungal agent, other agents such as silver sulfadiazine have proven effective and safe for topical ocular use.[81]

Deep corneal ulcers in danger of perforating respond best to surgical therapy, such as placement of a conjunctival flap.

Ocular discharge should be cleansed frequently to remove neutrophils and their proteolytic enzymes. If tear production is inadequate, topical cyclosporine every 12 hours and artificial tears several times daily should be administered to supplement and stimulate lacrimation. Closing the lids or placing a third eyelid flap should be avoided. These procedures limit drug contact with the cornea, impair discharge drainage, increase the temperature of the environment—thus promoting bacterial growth, fungal growth, or both—and prevent visualization of the ulcer's progress.

Systemic antiinflammatory agents can be beneficial as analgesics and to aid in the treatment of uveitis associated with deep corneal ulcers. Oral carprofen at 2 mg/kg every 12 hours is well tolerated by most dogs but is not recommended for cats.

Keratitis in Cats

Bacterial keratitis in cats may occur secondary to corneal ulcers (including those initiated by FHV-1) or traumatic wounding. Appearance, diagnosis, and treatment are the same as for the dog.

Corneal ulceration and keratitis from FHV is very common and begins with invasion of the corneal epithelium by the virus.[106] The most common corneal abnormality is punctate or linear epithelial erosions (Fig. 93-4), which may enlarge to form geographic ulcers. Conjunctivitis usually accompanies corneal ulcers.[104] Mechanical debridement of loose epithelium to remove virus and treatment with a topical antiviral agent have been the most successful therapies, although many of the ulcers heal without antiviral agents. Grid keratotomies should not be performed in cats because this treatment modality appears to increase the risk of corneal sequestration.[60] Antiviral agents such as trifluridine are virostatic and should be given at least 4 times daily until the ulcer heals and for approximately 1 week afterward.

Stromal keratitis is one of the most serious manifestations of FHV-1 corneal infection and is thought to primarily be a result of an immune reaction to the virus. Clinically healthy cats without apparent infection may harbor the virus in a latent or an active form in their corneas or trigeminal ganglia.[116] Experimentally, subconjunctival dexamethasone caused cats infected with FHV-1 to develop stromal keratitis.[82] Stromal keratitis may develop with or without a corneal ulcer. Vascularization and cellular infiltrate of the deeper layers of the cornea, often accompanied by chronic discomfort, are typical symptoms (Fig. 93-5). Antiviral agents alone usually do not improve the keratitis. Topical antiinflammatory agents, such as glucocorticoids, nonsteroidal topical agents, or cyclosporine, may help the inflammatory response but could exacerbate the viral infection. Antiinflammatory agents should be used only in conjunction with an antiviral agent. Topical glucocorticoids may predispose cats to the development of corneal sequestration. Topical IFN has been used in humans with herpetic keratitis and may be beneficial in cats,[76,111,112] although controlled studies are lacking. Lyophilized recombi-

Table • 93-3

Commercially Available Ophthalmic Antibacterial Agents

GENERIC NAME	TRADE NAME	CONCENTRATION SOLUTION (PERCENTAGE)	OINTMENT
Individual Agents			
Bacitracin	AK-Tracin	NA	500 U/g
	Available generically		
Chloramphenicol	AK-Chlor	0.5%	NA
	Chloromycetin	0.16%	10%
	Chloroptic	0.5%	10%
	Available generically	0.5%	NA
Ciprofloxacin hydrochloride	Ciloxan	0.3%	0.3%
Erythromycin	Available generically	NA	0.5%
Gentamicin sulfate	Gentamicin	0.3%	0.3%
	Genoptic	0.3%	0.3%
	Gentacidin	0.3%	0.3%
	Gentak	0.3%	0.3%
	Available generically	0.3%	0.3%
Norfloxacin	Chibroxin	0.3%	NA
Ofloxacin	Ocuflox	0.3%	NA
Sulfacetamide sodium	AK-Sulf	10%	10%
	Bleph-10	10%	10%
	Sulf-10	10%	NA
	Available generically	10%	10%
Tobramycin sulfate	Tobrex	0.3%	0.3%
	Aktob	0.3%	0.3%
	Tomycin	0.3%	NA
	Available generically	0.3%	NA
Mixtures			
Polymyxin B-bacitracin—Zinc	AK-Poly-Bac	NA	10,000 U
	Polysporin		500 U/g
	Available generically		
Polymyxin B-neomycin bacitracin	AK-Spore	NA	10,000 U
	Neosporin		3.5 mg
	Available generically		400 U/g
Polymyxin B-neomycin-gramicidin	AK-Spore	10,000 U	10,000 U
	Neosporin	1.75 mg	3.5 mg
	Available generically	0.025 mg/ml	NA
Polymyxin B-oxytetracycline	Terramycin	NA	10,000 U
	Terak		5 mg/g
Polymyxin B-trimethoprim	Polytrim	10,000 U	NA
	Available generically	0.1%	NA

NA, Not available.
Modified from Whitley RD. 2000. Canine and feline primary ocular bacterial infections. *Vet Clin North Am* 30(5):1151–1167.[122]

Table • 93-4

Fortified and Noncommercial Topical Antibiotic Solution Preparation

Gentamicin (fortified)

Gentamicin injectable (50 mg/ml)	6 ml
Artificial tears	<u>24 ml</u>
TOTAL	30 ml

Final concentration = 10 mg/ml (1% solution)

or

Add 2 ml of injectable gentamicin (50 mg/ml) to the 5-ml bottle of commercial ophthalmic gentamicin solution (0.3%)
Final concentration: 14 mg/ml (1.4% solution). Shelf-life: 30 days

Amikacin

Amikacin injectable (250 mg/ml)	4 ml
Artificial tears	<u>26 ml</u>
TOTAL	30 ml

Final concentration = 33 mg/ml (3.3% solution)

or

Remove 2 ml from a 15-ml squeeze bottle of artifical tears and discard
Add 2 ml of injectable amikacin (50 mg/ml)
Final concentration: 6.7 mg/ml (0.67% solution). Shelf-life: 30 days

Ampicillin

Mix 125-mg vial ampicillin with sterile saline or artificial tears to a concentration of 20 mg/ml

Cefazolin

Remove 2 ml from a 15-ml squeeze bottle of artificial tears and discard
Reconstitute a 500 or 1000 mg vial of cefazolin with sterile saline to a concentration of 250 mg/ml
Add 500 mg of the reconstituted cefazolin (2 ml) to the bottle of artificial tears
Final concentration: 33 mg / ml (3.3% solution). Shelf-life: 14 days. Keep refrigerated

Cephalothin

Remove 6 ml from a 15-ml squeeze bottle of artificial tears and save
Add the 6 ml of tear solution to a 1000 mg vial of cephalothin
Add the entire 1000 mg of the reconstituted cephalothin (6 ml) to the bottle of artificial tears.
Final concentration: 67 mg/ml (6.7% solution). Keep refrigerated

Ticarcillin

Reconstitute a 1-g vial of ticarcillin with 10 ml of sterile saline
Add 1.0 ml (100 mg) of this solution to a 15-ml squeeze bottle of artificial tears.
Final concentration: 6.7 mg/ml (0.67% solution). Shelf-life: 4 days. Keep refrigerated

Tobramycin (fortified)

Add 1.0 ml of injectable tobramycin (40 mg/ml) to a 5-ml bottle of commercial ophthalmic tobramycin solution (0.3%)
Final concentration: 9.2 mg /ml (0.92% solution). Shelf-life: 30 days.

Vancomycin

Remove 9 ml from a 15-ml squeeze bottle of artificial tears and discard
Reconstitute a 500-mg vial of vancomycin with 10 ml of sterile saline
Add the entire 500 mg of reconstituted vancomycin (10 ml) to the bottle of artificial tears
Final concentration: 31 mg/ml (3.1% solution). Shelf-life: 4 days. Keep refrigerated

Adapted from Whitley RD. Canine and feline primary ocular bacterial infections, *Vet Clin North Am* 30(5):1151–1167, 2000, with permission.[122]

Table • 93-5

Commercially Available Ophthalmic Antifungal Agents

GENERIC NAME	CONCENTRATION AND FORMULATION	MYCELIAL	YEASTS
Polyenes			
Natamycin	5% suspension	*Aspergillus, Fusarium*	—
Amphotericin B	0.15% suspension[a]	*Aspergillus* variable efficacy	Numerous, *Candida*
Azoles			
Miconazole	Vaginal cream or compounded[a]	*Aspergillus, Fusarium, Alternaria, Penicillium*	*Candida*
Ketoconazole	2% solution[a]	*Aspergillus, Fusarium, Candida, Curvularia*	*Candida*
Itraconazole	1% in 30% DMSO compounded[a]	*Aspergillus, Pseudallescheria*	*Candida*
Fluconazole	0.2% solution[a]	*Aspergillus*	*Candida*
Voriconazole	1% solution[a]	*Aspergillus, Fusarium, Penicillium, Scedosporium*	—
Other			
Silver sulfadiazine	1% cream	*Aspergillus, Fusarium*	*Candida*
Disinfectants			
N-acetylcysteine	10% solution	*Aspergillus, Fusarium*	—
Chlorhexidine	0.2% solution	Various species	Variety
Povidone iodine	1 : 10 to 1 : 50 solution	Various species	Variety

DMSO, Dimethylsulfoxide.
Modified from Whitley RD. 2000. Canine and feline primary ocular bacterial infections. *Vet Clin North Am* 30(5):1151–1167.[122]
[a]Not available commercially for ophthalmic use. Must use existing parenteral or topical solutions or make by compounding pharmacy.

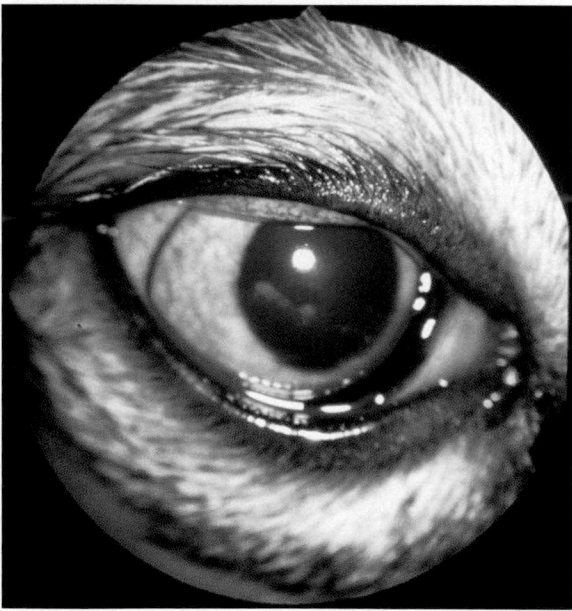

Fig   93-4   Linear epithelial ulcer caused by feline herpesvirus. Note chemosis from dorsal conjunctiva.

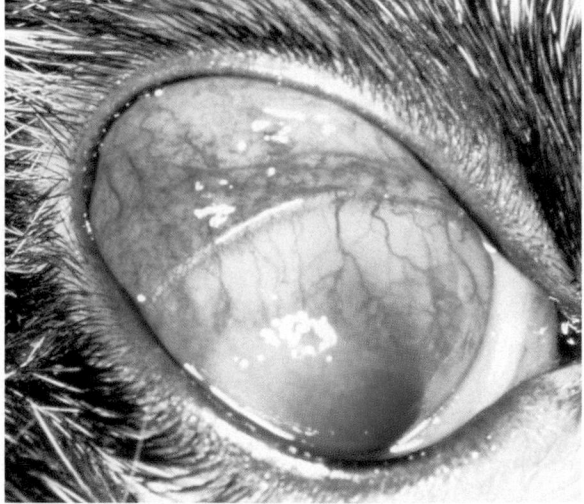

Fig   93-5   Corneal stromal keratitis in cat. Note corneal vascularization, edema, and conjunctivitis.

nant α-IFN can be reconstituted in saline and used as a topical drop. The dosage for cats is typically one drop every 6 hours of a solution ranging from 100 to 2500 U/ml, whereas in humans up to 10^6 U/ml have been used. Oral IFN can also be used and is discussed in Chapter 2. Lysine for ocular herpetic disease is discussed under feline conjunctivitis.

Corneal sequestration is a common disorder in cats, particularly Persians and Himalayans, and may follow chronic corneal ulcers or keratitis caused by FHV-1 (Fig. 93-6). It has been noted to occur after topical glucocorticoid treatment in FHV-1 experimentally infected cats, and in cats receiving grid keratotomies.[60,83] The condition is characterized by an area of corneal degeneration with a brown to black discoloration. The lesions vary from pinpoint sequestra to those that occupy more than half the cornea; vascularization may be intense or absent; and ocular pain ranges from none to marked. Like

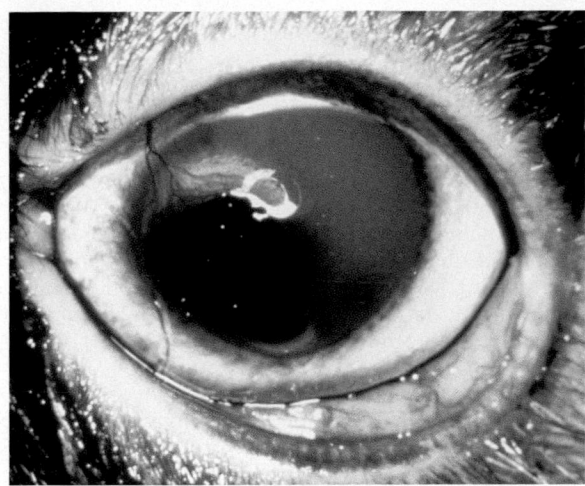

Fig 93-6 Corneal sequestrum in a cat. Note corneal blood vessels.

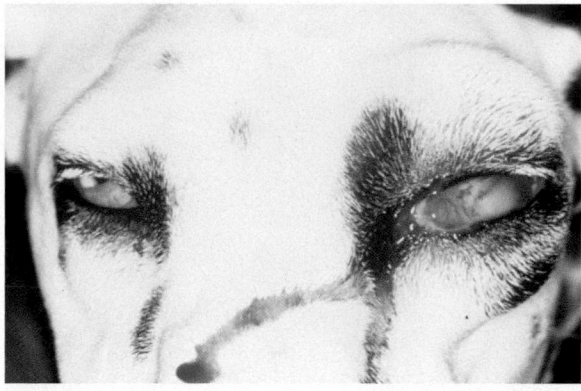

Fig 93-7 Orbital abscess in dog. Note severe periorbital swelling. (Courtesy Kirk Gelatt, Gainesville, Fla.)

stromal keratitis, sequestra can be one of the most serious and potentially blinding sequela of FHV-1. Most ophthalmologists recommend keratectomy followed by a graft (corneal or conjunctival) as the therapy for sequestra.

Dacryocystitis in Dogs and Cats

Dacryocystitis, or inflammation of the NL system, is usually associated with a bacterial infection. NL foreign bodies such as plant material are frequently the inciting cause. Dacryocystitis is more uncommon in cats than dogs. Clinical manifestations of dacryocystitis include conjunctival hyperemia, especially of the ventral conjunctival sac, purulent ocular discharge, and epiphora. Blepharospasm may or may not be present. Pain, purulent exudate, or both from the lacrimal puncta occasionally can be elicited by pressing on the skin near the medial canthus. Swelling or draining tracks in the skin near the medial canthus may also occur.

The diagnosis is confirmed by NL flushing with culture of any purulent debris recovered. Dacryocystorhinography may be necessary to identify foreign bodies or cystic structures within the NL system. If foreign bodies cannot be flushed from the system, surgical removal via a dacryocystotomy may be required.

After NL flushing, a broad-spectrum antibiotic solution such as polymixin-B-neomycin-gramicidin should be used 4 to 6 times daily. Systemic antibiotics are not indicated if the infection is confined to the NL system. Repeated flushings may be needed to maintain patency. The NL duct can also be cannulated with Silastic tubing to establish and maintain patency. Stricture of the NL duct may occur with dacryocystitis leading to chronic epiphora.

Orbital Infections in Dogs and Cats

Orbital disease caused by bacterial infection generally has a fairly rapid onset compared with the slow progression of clinical signs seen with orbital neoplasia. Typical clinical signs of orbital abscess and cellulitis include periorbital swelling, exophthalmos, elevation of the nictitating membrane, conjunctival hyperemia, and pain on palpation of periorbita or when opening the mouth (Fig. 93-7). Swelling of the oral mucosa behind the last molar is evident in some animals.

Bacterial infection of the orbit is common, especially in dogs, although fungal infections have also been reported in both dogs and cats.[52,126] Infectious agents may gain access to the orbit by several routes, including through the oral mucosa behind the last molar, from the frontal sinus through break-

down of medial orbital bone, from tooth root abscesses in which bacteria dissect through soft tissue planes, from penetrating wounds or foreign bodies of the skin or oral cavity, and through hematogenous spread from distant sites of infection.

Orbital bacterial abscesses are best diagnosed with ultrasonography, in which the abscess appears as a hypoechoic area posterior to the globe (Fig. 93-8). A fungal granuloma would appear hyperechoic and could not be readily differentiated from neoplasia. Computed tomography or magnetic resonance imaging are more helpful for delineating infections that involve the respiratory system and orbit simultaneously, which is more likely in fungal infections.

Drainage of orbital abscesses should be established when possible. Because only soft tissue separates the oral cavity from the ventral orbit in the dog and cat, an incision through the tissue behind the last molar can be used to access the orbit. A small mosquito forceps should be advanced into the orbit, using blunt probing—not grasping—to attempt to hit the abscess. Any purulent material should be cultured for aerobic and anaerobic bacteria and submitted for cytologic evaluation. Pending culture results, broad-spectrum systemic antibiotic therapy such as clindamycin and a penicillin or cephalosporin should be instituted.

The prognosis for bacterial orbital abscesses is generally good, whereas the prognosis for orbital fungal infections is more guarded.

Diagnosis

The decision to perform cultures from the ocular surface should be made early in the examination before various eye drops have been administered and manipulations performed. The use of a moist or calcium alginate swab improves the recovery rate.[51,118] Because the volume of material collected is usually small and subject to drying, swabs should be inoculated quickly onto appropriate media or placed in transport media.

Cytologic examination of conjunctival and corneal scrapings is an important and rapid diagnostic aid. Topical proparacaine should be applied and the appropriate surface scraped with a small, flat spatula or the blunt end of a scalpel blade. Excessive ocular discharges should be removed before scraping. Collected material should be gently spread onto glass slides and air dried. Multiple slides should be prepared, because some slides may not have adequate numbers of cells. The slides can be stained with a modified Giemsa or Wright's stain for cytologic evaluation and a Gram stain to evaluate the type of bacteria that might be present. Slides can also be made for examination by indirect FA for distemper virus, FHV, and *C. felis*.

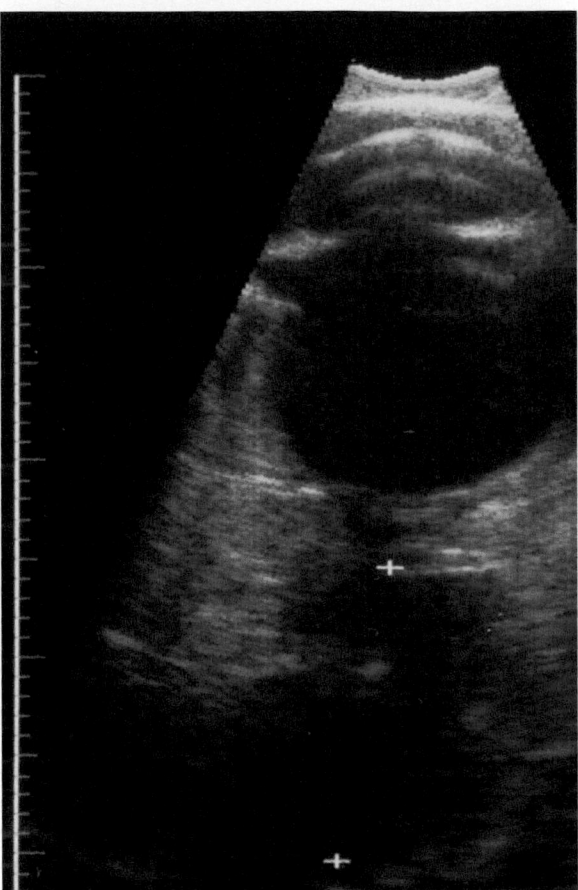

Fig   93-8   Ultrasound image of retrobulbar abscess in a cat. Markers delineate a hypoechoic structure posterior to globe.

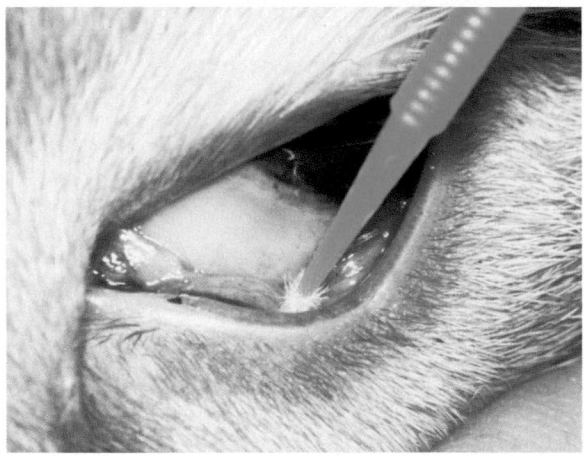

Fig   93-9   Nylon bristle brush used to obtain conjunctival cytology specimen.

An alternate technique is to roll a small, nylon bristle-brush applicator (Microbrush, Grafton, Wisc.) over the appropriate surface and then roll it onto a slide (Fig. 93-9). Preparations made with this method have fewer cells that are dispersed better on the slide and have less crushing artifact.[117,127] This method is less traumatic and easier to perform on cats and small dogs with tight lid-globe conformations.

Small snip biopsy specimens of the conjunctiva can be readily obtained using topical anesthesia for the animal. These small pieces of tissue should be spread out on a piece of paper before they are placed in fixative.

INTRAOCULAR INFECTIONS

Intraocular bacterial infections may be exogenous or endogenous in origin. The source of an exogenous infection from a penetrating ocular injury may be obvious from the history and appearance of the eye, but it may be an inapparent injury, such as a self-sealing cat claw injury through the conjunctiva and sclera. Exogenously induced infections are usually unilateral, whereas endogenous infections are often bilateral.

Local Injury

All recent perforating ocular injuries should be considered septic and treated intensively with bactericidal broad-spectrum antibiotics, topically and systemically, until susceptibility data are obtained. Topical fluoroquinolones, especially ofloxacin, have excellent corneal penetration and achieve therapeutic levels in the anterior segment against a wide variety of bacteria.[128] In suspected or confirmed bacterial endophthalmitis, a topical fluoroquinolone should be used every 1 to 2 hours. Topical antiinflammatory therapy is also indicated and may include frequent prednisolone acetate or a nonsteroidal agent such as flurbiprofen. Systemic broad-spectrum antibiotic therapy as well as systemic antiinflammatory therapy should also be administered.

Most active intraocular inflammations associated with perforating injuries should have centesis performed. Anterior chamber centesis for cultures and cytology is safe and may yield specific information to guide future therapy. Aqueous centesis is not as reliable as vitreous centesis in demonstrating bacterial growth in endophthalmitis; consequently, negative culture results from an aqueous sample are not definitive evidence of sterile inflammation.[37] Sepsis is indicated on oculocentesis by degenerate neutrophils and bacteria. Nondegenerate neutrophils may indicate a sterile purulent inflammation such as phacoclastic uveitis (phacoanaphylaxis, lens-induced inflammation) caused by lens capsule rupture.

Systemic Disease

The eye is often a target organ for systemic infectious agents. The ocular disease may be the primary complaint, with the systemic disease being unidentified or overlooked. It is important to recognize the systemic involvement to give an accurate prognosis and provide adequate therapy. Conversely, animals with systemic disease should have ocular examinations, which may provide rapid diagnostic clues and prognostic information. Most infectious agents access the eye via the uveal or vascular tunic. Typically, infectious agents or immune complexes become established in the uvea, producing a posterior uveitis or chorioretinitis, an anterior uveitis, or if overwhelming, endophthalmitis or panophthalmitis.

Canine Distemper

Ocular signs of distemper (see Chapter 3) usually include bilateral conjunctivitis with a discharge that progresses from serous to mucopurulent. The palpebral conjunctiva is primarily involved. Lacrimal adenitis may result in reduced tear production, which in turn results in more profound signs of conjunctivitis, corneal ulceration, and pain. The dry eye usually resolves if the animal recovers from systemic infection. Occasionally, conjunctival or lacrimal involvement has such mild systemic signs that distemper is not suspected.

Distemper virus often produces a multifocal, nongranulomatous chorioretinitis that does not usually cause blindness. The prevalence of chorioretinitis is unknown but probably varies, as do the neurologic signs, with strain of virus and

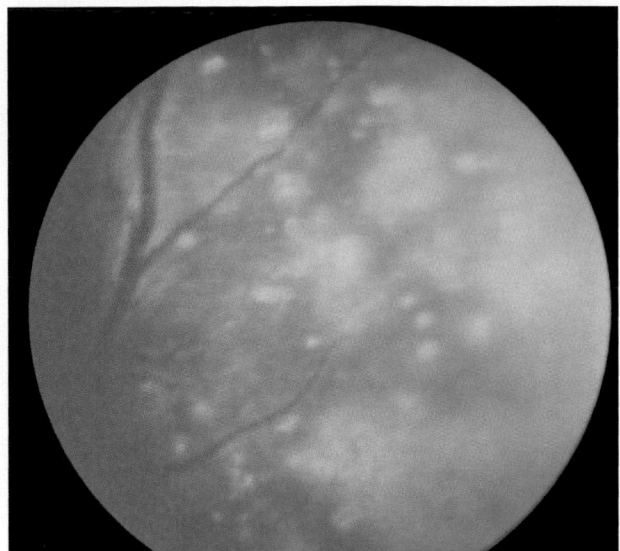

Fig 93-10 Multifocal acute distemper lesions in nontapetum of dog. Active lesions are recognized by their white cellular infiltrates with hazy borders.

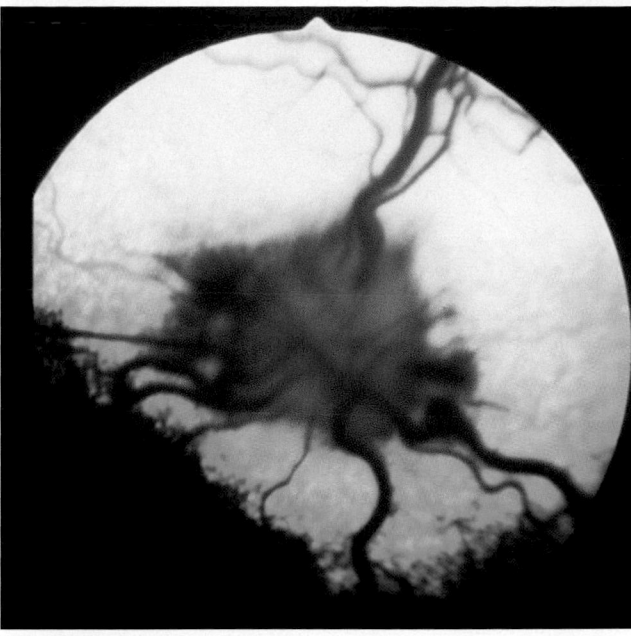

Fig 93-11 Acute optic neuritis characterized by elevated disc, peripapillary hemorrhages, and loss of vision. Distemper is one cause for this syndrome.

immune competency of the host. Dogs with neurologic forms of distemper had an overall prevalence of chorioretinal lesions of 41%, but 83% of the dogs with chronic leukoencephalopathy syndromes had chorioretinal lesions.[115] Occasionally, chorioretinitis is diffuse and blinding and may mimic the genetic syndrome of progressive retinal atrophy. Acute focal lesions in the tapetum or nontapetum have gray to white, hazy or ill-defined borders (Fig. 93-10).[36] Chorioretinal scars resulting from distemper virus have sharply demarcated borders, are hyperreflective in the tapetum, and are depigmented in the nontapetum. Histologically, retinal changes are characterized by degeneration of the retina with perivascular cuffing in some instances. Lesions may be focal or diffuse degeneration of ganglion cells, proliferation of retinal pigment epithelium, atrophy of photoreceptors, disorganization of retinal layers, focal gliosis, and distemper inclusion bodies in glial cells.

The most serious clinical ocular problem associated with distemper is optic neuritis.[35] Optic neuritis is characterized by an acute onset of bilateral blindness and mydriasis. If inflammation extends rostrally to the optic papilla, ophthalmoscopic signs of peripapillary hemorrhages and edema, retinal vascular congestion, and elevation of the papilla are observed (Fig. 93-11).[35] If the neuritis remains retrobulbar, the diagnosis is made by exclusion (e.g., blind eyes with mydriasis and normal retinal function as tested by electroretinography). The optic neuritis may be isolated, prodromal, or concurrent with other neurologic distemper signs. Distemper-associated blindness also may occur with inflammation of the occipital cortex or optic radiations, but pupillary reflexes are usually normal under such circumstances. Optic neuritis may occur with other central nervous system (CNS) inflammatory conditions such as granulomatous meningoencephalitis (see Chapter 84).

Ocular signs are suggestive but not definitive for distemper. Acute lesions of chorioretinitis usually correlate well with concurrent systemic disease, but chorioretinal scars do not. Finding distemper inclusions or positive immunofluorescence on a conjunctival scraping may be of diagnostic help early in the course of systemic disease (5 to 21 days after inoculation), but a negative finding is inconclusive. Distemper should be considered in any animal with acute optic neuropathy or an acute onset of KCS.

Because no specific antiviral therapy is available, treatment is primarily symptomatic. Acute optic neuritis or severe chorioretinitis should be treated with systemic antiinflammatory dosages of glucocorticoids. Dry eye should be treated with topical cyclosporine twice daily and artificial tears. Corneal ulcers should also be treated with a topical broad-spectrum antibiotic several times daily.

Infectious Canine Hepatitis
Canine adenovirus-1 (CAV-1) infection has been estimated to produce ocular lesions in approximately 20% of dogs recovering from natural infections, whereas a 0.4% or less prevalence has been noted in CAV-1-vaccinated dogs (see Chapter 4). The universal use of CAV-2 for immunization has made the postvaccinal reaction of corneal edema and uveitis much less common. The lesion, considered to be an immune complex Arthus reaction, occurs 10 to 21 days after vaccination and requires about an equal time to resolve. The condition is bilateral in 12% to 28% of the cases. The Afghan hound has been reported to have an increased prevalence,[19] and other sight hounds and Siberian huskies may have similarly high frequencies of ocular reactions to CAV-1.

The most visible ocular lesion is stromal corneal edema resulting from inflammatory damage to the corneal endothelium (Fig. 93-12). Occasionally, a dog has signs of uveitis (blepharospasm, miosis, hypotony, and aqueous flare) 1 to 2 days before the corneal edema is evident. Corneal edema may be focal or generalized and is usually transient. In some instances, the edema is permanent or may require several months to clear. A marked hypotony combined with altered corneal rigidity may result in a keratoconus. Glaucoma, the most significant sequela of uveitis, may be missed in the early stages because of the preexisting corneal edema and conjunctival hyperemia. Uveitis associated with vaccination is usually diagnosed by the typical ocular lesions combined with the history of recent vaccination in a puppy or young (younger than 2 years of age) dog. Other causes of corneal edema, such as congenital pupillary membranes, glaucoma, or corneal ulceration, should be ruled out. Therapy is similar to that for other

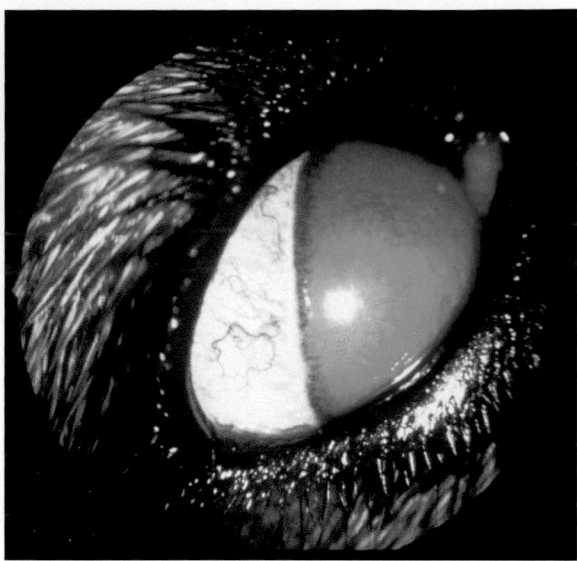

Fig 93-12 Diffuse corneal edema induced by vaccination with canine adenovirus-1 live vaccine.

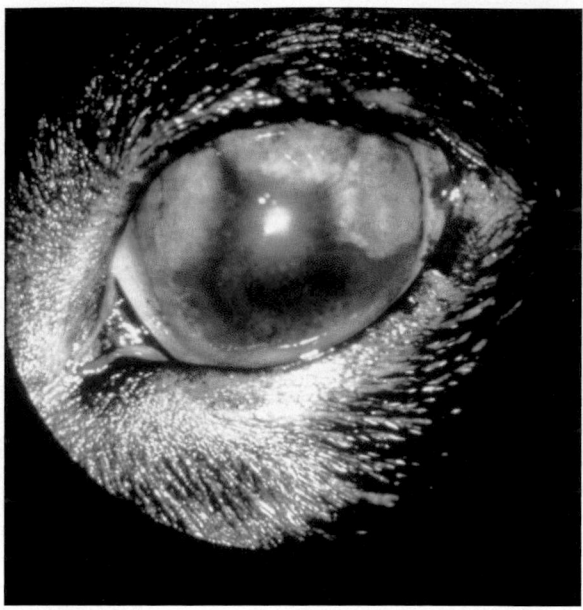

Fig 93-13 *E. canis*–induced anterior uveitis with hyphema. Iris bombe is present.

forms of nonseptic anterior uveitis—specifically, topical prednisolone acetate 4 to 6 times daily and atropine to achieve mydriasis. Oral carprofen may also be helpful.

Canine Herpesvirus Infection

Canine herpesvirus (CHV) infection (see Chapter 5) in the adult dog has produced only a transient conjunctivitis and vaginitis of 4 to 5 days duration. Occasional dendritic corneal ulceration patterns are seen in the dog, but their cause has not been determined. Neonatal CHV infection produces a bilateral panuveitis with keratitis, synechiae, cataracts, retinal necrosis and disorganization, retinal atrophy and dysplasia, and optic neuritis and atrophy.[1]

Rickettsial Agents of Dogs

Ehrlichiosis Ocular lesions occur frequently in dogs with ehrlichiosis caused by *Ehrlichia canis*, although the ocular abnormalities may vary in severity and do not develop in every patient (see Chapter 28). The most typical lesions include unilateral or bilateral anterior uveitis characterized by one or more of the following: conjunctival and episcleral hyperemia, miosis, aqueous flare, hypopyon, keratic precipitates, hyphema, synechiae, and hypotony. Glaucoma may occur secondary to chronic anterior uveitis (Fig. 93-13). Signs of posterior segment inflammation may include chorioretinitis as evidenced by inflammatory cell infiltrate under and within the retina, serous retinal detachment, retinal hemorrhage, and optic neuritis. Optic neuritis may be evidenced by a swollen optic disk and peripapillary hemorrhages. Anterior uveitis has also been seen in dogs naturally infected by *Ehrlichia chaffeensis*.[8] In an experimental study of dogs infected with *E. canis*, *E. chaffeensis*, or *Ehrlichia ewingii*, histologic examination of eyes showed uveitis only in dogs infected with *E. canis*.[91] The lymphocytic inflammatory infiltrate was most intense in the ciliary body, becoming less intense in the choroid, iris, and retina, respectively.

The granulocytic ehrlichial agents *E. ewingii* and *Anaplasma phagocytophilum* have not been as extensively studied as *E. canis*. However, it appears that they may also be capable of inciting ocular inflammatory disease in dogs.[105] They cause polyarthritis and meningitis in dogs and would be expected to cause uveitis. Inflammation at these sites is characteristic of depositing immune complexes or bloodborne agents such as rickettsiae (see Chapter 28). More information is needed to define the pathogenesis of these agents, but serum antibody titers that include these agents should be measured in dogs being evaluated for tickborne disease.

Thrombocytic Ehrlichiosis *Anaplasma platys (Ehrlichia platys)*, the agent of canine infectious cyclic thrombocytopenia, is common, particularly in the southern states. Based on serologic evidence, dogs in Florida and Louisiana have a high rate of infection.

Uveitis with *A. platys* infection has been only infrequently reported.[8,44] It is possible that uveitis occurs more commonly than the literature suggests and is missed. If the organism is not detected within platelets on a blood smear, an antibody test for *A. platys* may not be requested for a dog with uveitis. Likewise, if platelet numbers are not dramatically low, infection with *A. platys* may not be suspected.

Rocky Mountain Spotted Fever Ocular lesions are frequently associated with Rocky Mountain spotted fever (RMSF) caused by *Rickettsia rickettsii* and primarily arise as a consequence of vasculitis (see Chapter 29). Lesions include conjunctival hyperemia, subconjunctival hemorrhage, hyphema, anterior uveitis, iris hemorrhage, retinal hemorrhage, retinal edema, and retinal perivascular inflammatory cell infiltrate (Fig. 93-14). Fluorescein angiography in experimentally infected dogs demonstrated increased retinal vascular permeability beginning on day 6 after infection and 2 days after the onset of pyrexia.[22] Venules were found to be affected twice as frequently as arterioles, and smaller vessels were affected more frequently than larger primary vessels. Retinal vascular lesions in this study paralleled the progression of fever, leukopenia, thrombocytopenia, and prolongation of activated partial thromboplastin time during the second week after infection.

It is critical to examine the fundus of dogs confirmed or suspected to have RMSF, because the anterior segment may be normal, although iris hemorrhage and hyphema develop as well. Lesions tend to be bilateral in affected dogs but may not be symmetrical. Nystagmus may occur in dogs that have vestibular disease associated with RMSF.

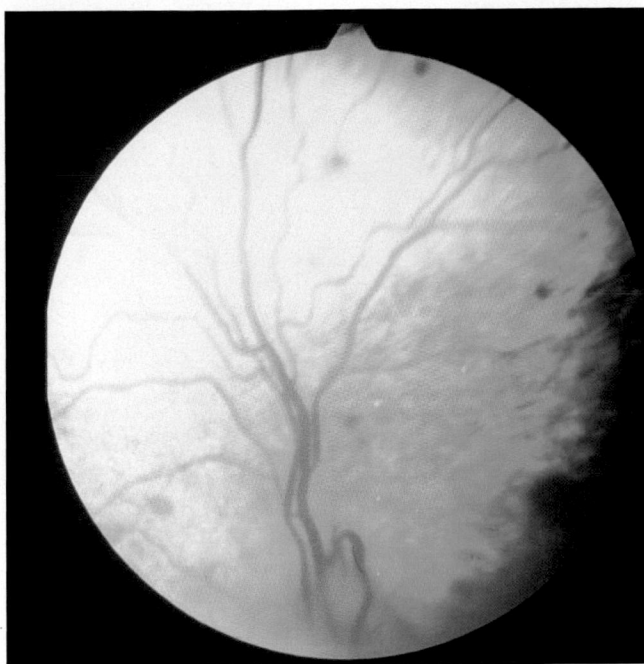

Fig 93-14 Multifocal retinal hemorrhages in a dog with Rocky Mountain spotted fever.

The ocular signs of RMSF may overlap with those of canine ehrlichiosis. Although ocular hemorrhages are the most common ophthalmic sign of RMSF, hemorrhage may also occur with ehrlichiosis. Although exceptions occur, intraocular hemorrhages and inflammatory cell infiltrates tend to be less dramatic in RMSF than ehrlichiosis.[45]

Therapy for Rickettsial Disease Treatment of ocular signs of canine ehrlichiosis must include antiinflammatory therapy in addition to appropriate systemic antimicrobial therapy (see Chapter 28). Appropriate topical glucocorticoid preparations for treating anterior uveitis include 1% prednisolone acetate and 0.1% dexamethasone. Frequency is dictated by the severity of the uveitis, but administration every 6 hours is typically the minimum desirable frequency. Choroiditis or other posterior segment disease must be treated by the systemic route and should include an antiinflammatory dose of oral prednisolone. In addition to treating posterior segment ocular disease, oral glucocorticoids are helpful in reducing other immune-mediated consequences of ehrlichiosis, such as vasculitis and the production of antiplatelet antibodies that result in worsening thrombocytopenia.

Ocular lesions in dogs infected with RMSF may resolve quickly with appropriate systemic antibiotic therapy if they include only small retinal hemorrhages. If more severe uveitis occurs, systemic and topical glucocorticoid therapy as described for ehrlichiosis should be instituted.

Canine Brucellosis

Brucella canis has been documented as a cause of unilateral or bilateral anterior uveitis and endophthalmitis and is often accompanied by intraocular hemorrhage. Ocular involvement is often severe and blinding (see Chapter 40).[48] A retrospective study of the prevalence of ocular lesions among dogs examined for brucellosis at veterinary schools in the United States and Canada found that 38 of 313 (14.2%) dogs had ocular involvement.[119] Testing for *B. canis* should be performed in dogs with unexplained uveitis or ocular hemorrhage. Therapy consists of systemic antibiotics as well

as topical prednisolone acetate for anterior uveitis. The prognosis for uveitis associated with brucellosis is guarded.

Lyme Borreliosis in Dogs

Lyme disease, or borreliosis, produced by the spirochete *Borrelia burgdorferi* may cause ocular lesions in humans, horses, and dogs (see Chapter 45). An increasing number of humans is being diagnosed with ocular Lyme disease.[79,95] The most common ocular manifestation appears to be uveitis, but neuroophthalmic disorders and surface inflammations such as episcleritis and keratitis have also been reported. Ocular manifestations are more likely to be seen in late-stage disease.

A single case report describes isolation of *B. burgdorferi*, which was isolated from the eye of a pony with uveitis.[10] However, such documentation is lacking in dogs. In a retrospective review of 132 dogs seropositive by indirect FA, five had the primary symptom of ocular lesions. Ocular lesions reported were conjunctivitis, anterior uveitis, corneal edema, retinal petechia, chorioretinitis, and retinal detachment.[16] Follow-up with Western blot was not performed. In this study 24 dogs, were also seropositive for *E. canis*, although information was not provided as to whether dogs with ocular disease were positive for ehrlichiosis, thus it is impossible to ascribe the ocular lesions to borreliosis. Although it is highly likely that Lyme disease can cause ocular disease in infected dogs, more definitive information is needed to document the condition. Diagnosis and treatment of systemic borreliosis are discussed in Chapter 45. Ocular disease should also be treated with topical prednisolone acetate 4 to 6 times daily for anterior segment inflammation and oral prednisolone at a dose of 1 to 2 mg/kg/day for posterior segment inflammation.

Leptospirosis in Dogs

Leptospirosis, a spirochete bacterial infection, can affect any organ but has been primarily associated with renal disease in the dog (see Chapter 44). Leptospires incite vasculitis and endotheliitis, making the eyes a potential target organ. Although leptospires have been found in the eyes of infected dogs, the paucity of reports of uveitis associated with canine leptospirosis in the literature probably does not reflect the true incidence of disease.[30] Leptospirosis is considered a major cause of uveitis in horses and has also been reported in humans. In these species the development of uveitis often occurs months after acute infection. This likely represents a delayed hypersensitivity reaction between cell-bound antibodies and persistent leptospiral antigens in the eye. This delayed response has not been reported in the dog. The author has seen dogs with anterior uveitis, as well as chorioretinitis with retinal detachment, and high serum titers against serovars canicola, grippotyphosa, pomona, and bratislava.

Treatment should consist of appropriate systemic antibiotic therapy. Anterior uveitis should be treated with frequent topical prednisolone acetate, whereas chorioretinitis with or without retinal detachment should be treated with oral prednisolone at a dose of 1 to 2 mg/kg/day.

Neosporosis in Dogs

Neospora caninum is a protozoal parasite that is morphologically similar to *Toxoplasma gondii* (see Chapter 80). Transplacental transmission has been documented, and reports in the dog have primarily involved infections in neonates and puppies younger than 6 months of age. Although puppies die or are euthanized because of neuromuscular signs, ocular lesions are present in many cases. The ocular lesions are primarily a retinitis with extension into the choroid (retinochoroiditis). A mild anterior uveitis was also reported.[28]

Leishmaniasis in Dogs

The dog is a reservoir host for the protozoal organism *Leishmania donovani* in endemic areas of the Mediterranean, Africa, and Asia (see Chapter 73). Most documented cases in North America have been in dogs imported from endemic areas, but reports involving a closed research colony of English foxhounds in Ohio and Oklahoma indicated that once introduced, the agent can be transmitted in the United States.[113] Leishmaniasis was diagnosed in a Maryland poodle that had not traveled outside the United States.[31]

Ocular and periocular lesions associated with leishmaniasis developed in 25% of 105 dogs in a study.[94] In 15% of the dogs in the study, ocular lesions were the only clinical sign. Clinical ocular disease, in decreasing order of frequency, included anterior uveitis, conjunctivitis, keratoconjunctivitis, periocular alopecia, diffuse blepharitis, posterior uveitis, orbital cellulitis, and a solitary eyelid nodule.

The diagnosis is made by histopathologic identification of the organism, serologic testing, PCR testing, or all of these. In dogs with conjunctivitis, scraping and cytologic examination have revealed the organism in some cases. The inflammation is mononuclear, and the organism is found within histiocytes.

Therapy is discussed in Chapter 73. In addition to systemic antiprotozoal therapy, keratoconjunctivitis or uveitis should be treated with topical prednisolone acetate several times daily. Blepharitis can be treated with a topical ophthalmic antibiotic-dexamethasone ointment that is rubbed into the skin several times daily, whereas posterior uveitis should be treated with oral prednisolone at a dose of 1 to 2 mg/kg/day.

Other Bacterial Infections of Dogs

Septicemias caused by various bacteria may affect the eyes. Infections such as bacterial endocarditis, urinary tract infection, pyometra, and dental infection may cause uveitis through hematogenous spread of bacteria to the eye. Simultaneously cleaning teeth and performing intraocular surgery should be avoided to minimize the risk of bacteria localizing in injured ocular tissue. Contagious bacterial infections such as tuberculosis and salmonellosis may also manifest with ocular lesions.

Mycoses of Dogs and Cats

The systemic mycoses in North America are frequently associated with a granulomatous posterior uveitis. Anterior uveitis accompanies chorioretinitis in a large number of cases. With the exception of cryptococcosis, systemic fungal infections are less common in the cat than the dog; however, when they develop, ocular lesions are often present. In many animals, the ocular signs are the primary symptom.

In indigenous regions of the Mississippi and Ohio Rivers and the central Atlantic states, *Blastomyces dermatitidis* is common in dogs (see Chapter 59). Ocular involvement occurs in up to 52% of the cases.[6] Ocular lesions are from chorioretinitis, which may vary from a focal granuloma in the fundus to widespread subretinal infiltrates of organisms and granulomatous inflammation (Fig. 93-15).[11] Anterior uveitis is common with extensive posterior segment disease, although the organism is not usually found in these tissues or in aqueous humor aspirates; however, in cases with endophthalmitis and granulomas in the anterior segment, the organism is widespread within the eye (Fig. 93-16). Secondary glaucoma is a frequent complication.

Histoplasma capsulatum infection develops most commonly in the Ohio, Missouri, and Mississippi River valleys but has been reported in many states in North America (see Chapter 60). As evidenced by published reports, ocular involvement with histoplasmosis is relatively rare in dogs.[48] In the cat, systemic histoplasmosis causes nonspecific clinical signs such as weight loss, anorexia, fever, and anemia. Ocular

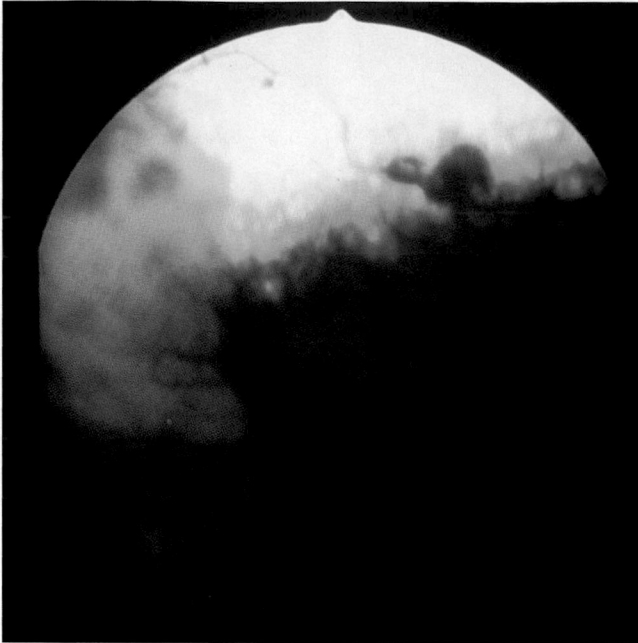

Fig 93-15 Large subretinal granuloma and retinal hemorrhage in a dog with blastomycosis.

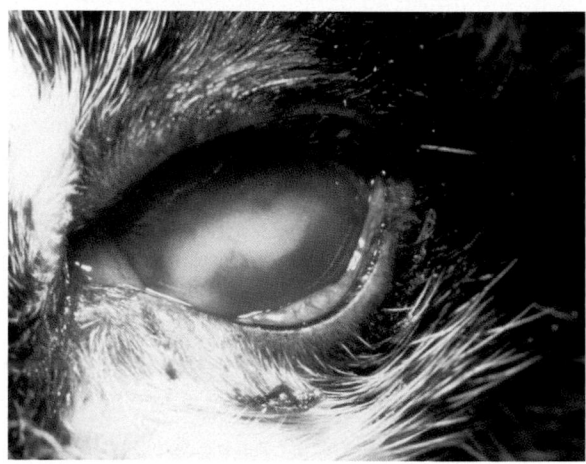

Fig 93-16 Endophthalmitis caused by blastomycosis in a cat. Note granuloma in anterior chamber. (Courtesy Sheryl Krohne, West Lafayette, Ind.)

lesions occur in a fairly high percentage of affected cats and include granulomatous chorioretinitis, retinal detachment, anterior uveitis, and secondary glaucoma.[43]

Coccidioides immitis is endemic in the southwestern United States, Mexico, and Central and South America (see Chapter 62). Ocular lesions are similar to those of blastomycosis, namely granulomatous chorioretinitis, retinal detachment, anterior uveitis, and secondary glaucoma. Organisms are found predominantly in the choroid. Limited data exist regarding the prevalence of ocular lesions in dogs and cats with coccidioidomycosis. Ocular lesions may be the presenting sign in up to 42% of dogs, and in 80% of dogs the lesions are unilateral.[4] One study found that 13% of 48 cats had ocular lesions.[46]

Cryptococcus neoformans is the most commonly reported feline mycotic infection and enters the body through the respiratory tract (see Chapter 61). This mycotic infection is

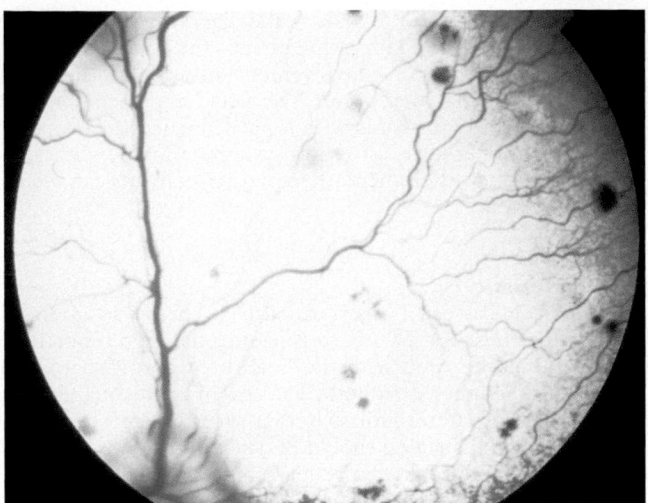

Fig 93-17 Multifocal subretinal granulomas in a dog with cryptococcosis. Larger lesions are producing small bullous detachments.

common in dogs as well. Chorioretinitis with granulomatous inflammation and retinal detachment is the most common manifestation; anterior uveitis is less common. The appearance of chorioretinal lesions is often somewhat different than the other mycotic infections. Tapetal lesions are usually dark gray in color, in contrast to the whitish appearance of most fungal granulomas (Fig. 93-17). Optic neuritis may also develop, particularly if the CNS is involved. A feline case of adnexal cryptococcus without intraocular or systemic lesions has been described.[73]

Bilateral granulomatous chorioretinitis or endophthalmitis should suggest the possibility of systemic mycoses. Associated systemic signs of fever and respiratory, skeletal, dermatologic, or CNS involvement are often present. The specific diagnosis is often made by finding the organism in tissue aspirates. Vitreal centesis in an eye with endophthalmitis may be the best method of diagnosis if other sites are unyielding.

Therapy for ocular involvement with the systemic mycoses includes appropriate systemic antifungal therapy as discussed in Chapter 57. In many instances the ocular inflammatory reaction continues to worsen with systemic therapy because of the immune reaction to the dying organisms. The use of oral prednisolone at a dose of 1 to 2 mg/kg/day has been extremely valuable in halting this vision-threatening inflammatory response. Oral prednisolone should be continued until fundic lesions completely resolve, which may take several weeks to months.[59] If anterior uveitis is present, topical prednisolone acetate should be used several times daily, tapering once the overall disease is in remission.

Enucleation of blind eyes has been proposed as a means of eliminating a nidus of infection that may cause relapses. Although it is justifiable to remove a blind, painful eye (such as one with glaucoma), no rationalization can be made for removing an eye that has been affected by blastomycosis but is comfortable.

Protothecosis in Dogs and Cats
Prototheca species are ubiquitous algae in soil and water and occasionally pathogenic in dogs and cats (see Chapter 69). More than 50% of affected dogs have ocular involvement,[78] whereas ocular lesions have not been reported in cats. Most dogs with ocular lesions also have systemic signs such as diarrhea, but in some instances the systemic signs are inapparent or missed. Lesions include a granulomatous posterior uveitis, often with retinal detachment, that is similar in appearance to

those associated with fungal infections like blastomycosis. Anterior uveitis is often present as well. Definitive diagnosis is usually made by finding the organism in aspirates, urine sediment, or biopsy samples. Vitreous centesis often yields the organism in dogs with ocular protothecosis. No efficacious therapy has been reported.

Toxoplasmosis in Cats and Dogs
Generalized toxoplasmosis has been associated with ocular inflammation in cats and dogs (see Chapter 80). The most prominent lesion is choroiditis with extension into the retina.[20] These lesions typically appear as multifocal dark gray infiltrates in the tapetal fundus and fluffy white infiltrates in the nontapetal fundus. Anterior uveitis also occurs, and *T. gondii* bradyzoites and tachyzoites have been identified histopathologically in the iris and ciliary body of systemically affected cats.[28]

The ability of *T. gondii* to cause ocular disease without systemic disease is poorly understood. The fact that many cats have positive serum antibody titers to *T. gondii*, particularly IgG, makes it difficult to correlate uveitis alone with toxoplasmosis. It is possible that *T. gondii* may incite an immune-mediated uveitis without systemic disease. Several mechanisms have been proposed, including homing of activated immune cells to ocular tissues, molecular mimicry, circulating antigens or immune complexes from nonocular sites of parasite replication, and a nonspecific increase in immune response.[20,23] In kittens experimentally infected in utero or in the early neonatal period, chorioretinitis and anterior uveitis developed without other evidence of clinical illness.[97]

Serologic testing for *T. gondii* should include IgM and IgG. IgM increases and decreases for 3 months after infection, whereas IgG stays elevated for years. Cats coinfected with FIV and *T. gondii* may develop a positive IgM titer, whereas the IgG titer remains negative.[65]

T. gondii-specific antibodies can be measured in aqueous humor. Antibody levels can be compared with serum levels through use of the Witmer-Goldman coefficient, or C-value. C-values of greater than 8 suggest intraocular antibody production and may be more helpful than serum titers alone in diagnosing ocular toxoplasmosis. Aqueous humor can also be evaluated by PCR for the presence of *T. gondii* DNA.[74]

Treatment of ocular toxoplasmosis in cats and dogs should include clindamycin at a dose of 12.5 mg/kg every 12 hours for 21 to 30 days.[64] The uveitis should also be treated with antiinflammatory agents such as topical prednisolone acetate or a nonsteroidal ophthalmic preparation several times daily for anterior uveitis. Chorioretinitis should be treated with oral prednisolone at a dose of 1 to 2 mg/kg/day until resolution.

Feline Immunodeficiency Virus
Ocular inflammation has been associated with FIV in experimentally and naturally infected cats (see Chapter 14). Anterior uveitis is the most commonly reported ocular abnormality. Conjunctivitis, pars planitis, and chorioretinitis have also been reported. Ocular inflammation may be caused by direct viral damage to tissue, initiating immune-mediated disease, or allowing opportunistic infections to develop.[125] Other common feline pathogens, such as herpesvirus, *C. felis*, and *T. gondii*, that can cause ocular disease should be considered in FIV-positive cats. In an experimental study of chlamydial conjunctivitis, coinfection with FIV markedly prolonged the duration of clinical signs and led to chronic conjunctivitis.

Serologic evidence of coinfection with *T. gondii* was present in 28 (57%) of 49 FIV-positive cats in one study.[90] Approximately 43% of cats coinfected with FIV and *T. gondii* had positive *T. gondii*–specific IgM serum antibody titers without a positive *T. gondii*–specific IgG titer.

If another infectious disease can be identified in an FIV-positive cat, it should be treated as specifically as possible. Uveitis caused by FIV can be expected to be a chronic problem. Treatment should be symptomatic and include topical antiinflammatory agents such as prednisolone acetate or a nonsteroidal agent such as flurbiprofen. For long-term use, a topical nonsteroidal drug is preferred because of the risk of exacerbating ocular herpesvirus with glucocorticoids. Oral prednisolone may be required for chorioretinitis. The author's experience in treating pars planitis has been poor.

Feline Infectious Peritonitis Virus

The most common ocular manifestation of infection with feline infectious peritonitis virus (FIPV) is bilateral granulomatous anterior uveitis, often accompanied by chorioretinitis (see Chapter 11). Frequently, large keratic precipitates and a fibrinous exudate are found in the anterior chamber (Fig. 93-18). The nature of the disease is a vasculitis, and it is common to see a pyogranulomatous exudate sheathing the retinal vessels (Fig. 93-19). Retinal hemorrhages and detachments may also develop.

Ocular disease is more common with the noneffusive, or dry, form of FIPV infection and may be the initial presenting sign. Diagnosis of FIPV-associated ocular disease is difficult because of the nonspecific nature of available coronavirus serum antibody tests. Rising serum antibody titers in the presence of characteristic ocular lesions is suggestive.

Because no effective treatment exists for FIPV infection, treatment of ocular disease is symptomatic. Topical glucocorticoids such as prednisolone acetate should be used several times daily for anterior uveitis. Systemic prednisolone should be used for chorioretinitis. Ocular disease may be temporarily ameliorated, but it usually recurs if the systemic disease worsens.

Feline Leukemia Virus

The predominant ocular manifestation of feline leukemia virus infection is lymphosarcoma (see Chapter 13).[9] The uveal tract is a common site for metastasis of neoplastic lymphocytes via hematogenous spread. Cats with ocular lymphosarcoma may initially show signs of mild uveitis, including miosis, aqueous flare, and keratic precipitates. As the disease progresses, the iris becomes greatly thickened and distorted with the infiltration of tumor cells. Glaucoma is a common sequela because tumor cells infiltrate the iridocorneal angle. Aqueous

centesis may be helpful in making the diagnosis, because neoplastic lymphocytes readily exfoliate into the aqueous humor. In addition to intraocular involvement, invasion of the orbit by lymphosarcoma may occur. Aggressive treatment of cats with ocular lymphosarcoma with topical glucocorticoids, such as prednisolone acetate, as well as systemic therapy with glucocorticoids and other chemotherapeutic protocols can result in improvement.

Diagnosis

Aqueous Centesis

Aqueous centesis can be performed using heavy sedation or general anesthesia. A 27- to 30-gauge needle on a tuberculin syringe should be used with the "seal" broken so that movement of the plunger is smooth. The site of centesis is usually at the dorsal or lateral limbus because it is the most accessible. Topical proparacaine should be used even with sedation. A cotton-tip swab soaked in proparacaine and held at the site of centesis for 60 seconds before insertion of the needle facilitates the procedure. Forceps applied to the conjunctiva close to the limbus should be used to fixate the globe and apply counter pressure to the needle. The needle enters the cornea just rostral to the limbus and parallel to the plane of the iris (Fig. 93-20). The operator must be careful to avoid the iris, lens, and corneal endothelium. The procedure may be more hazardous in the diseased cornea because the needle point is obscured, and the increased corneal thickness results in a longer, beveled tract before the needle enters the anterior chamber. Unless the anterior chamber is collapsed, the volume that can be removed from the dog is about 0.3 ml and from the cat is about 0.5 ml. A culture swab is saturated with a portion of the aspirated aqueous, and the remaining aliquot is prepared for cytology by centrifugation. If fibrin is present or iris adhesions of less than a few days' duration are present, 25 μg of tissue plasminogen activator (tPA) may be injected to dissolve clots and break synechiae.[72]

Vitreous Centesis

Centesis of the vitreous cavity has more potential complications than aqueous centesis and is usually reserved for eyes that have lost considerable visual function. Choroidal

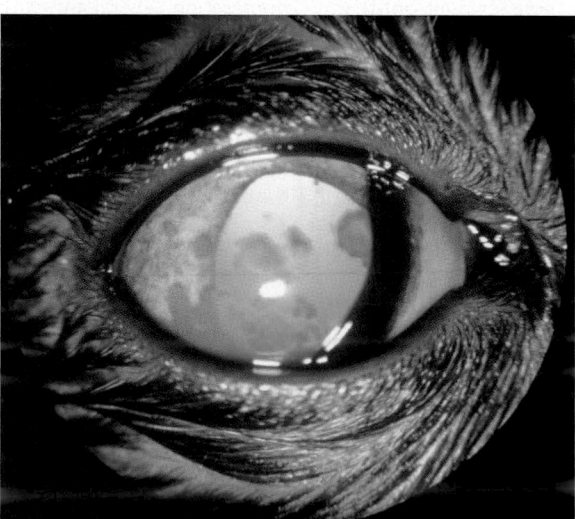

Fig   93-18 Anterior uveitis with large keratic precipitates in a cat with feline infectious peritonitis.

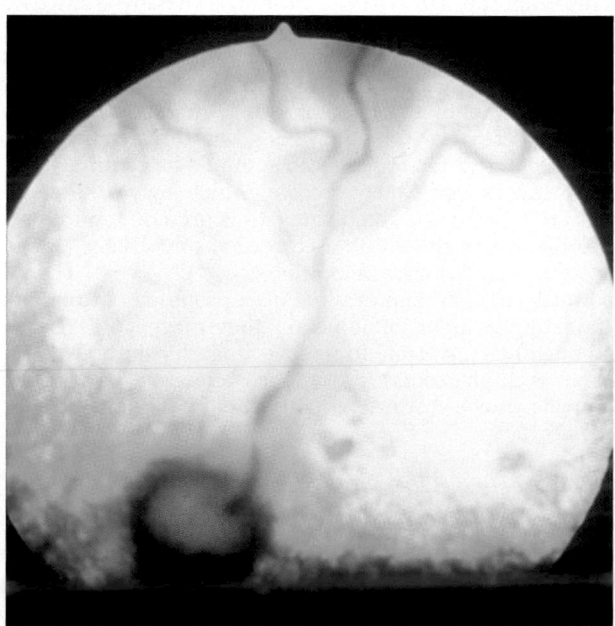

Fig   93-19 Chorioretinitis and retinal perivascular sheathing in a cat with feline infectious peritonitis.

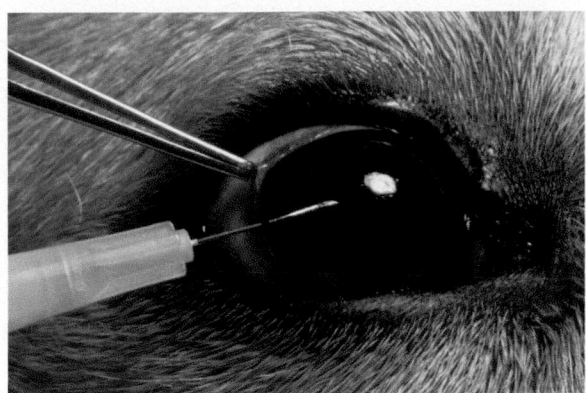

Fig 93-20 Aqueous centesis in a dog. A 27- to 30-gauge needle enters at limbus, avoiding iris and corneal endothelium.

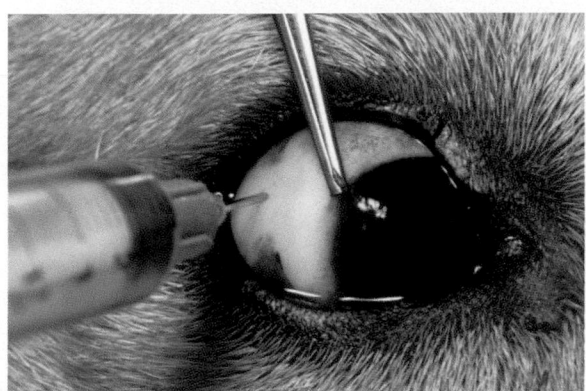

Fig 93-21 Vitreous centesis in a dog. Needle enters 6 mm posterior to limbus and is directed slightly posterior and toward center of globe.

hemorrhage and retinal tears are the two most likely complications. A 25- to 22-gauge needle with a 3-ml syringe should be used. The site of entry is 6 mm caudal to the limbus in the dorsolateral quadrant. Forceps are used to apply counter pressure, and the needle point is aimed posteriorly away from the lens and toward the center of the vitreous cavity (Fig. 93-21). The needle should be short (0.5 inch) so that it does not inadvertently pass completely across the vitreous humor and tear the opposite retina. Approximately 0.5 ml of vitreous humor can be removed for culture and cytology. If fluid cannot be obtained, minor positioning changes of the needle point should be attempted.

Therapy

The therapeutic routes available for treating ocular infections and inflammations are topical, subconjunctival, intraocular, and systemic. The routes selected depend on the location, severity of the infection, and the drug being administered. The eye has three barriers to drug penetration: the intact cornea for topical penetration and the blood-aqueous and blood-retinal barriers for systemic drug penetration. In general, drugs with a differential solubility in water and lipids and small molecular size are better able to penetrate these barriers. Inflammation or ulceration weaken these barriers to variable degrees and allow better penetration. The ability of antibiotics to penetrate into the normal eye varies by drug and route (Table 93-6).[53] The vitreous humor is a large, rather inert structure, resulting in low drug levels by any route of drug administration except direct intravitreal injection, in which the vitreous humor acts as a depot for the relatively slow release of the drug.

Topical

Depending on the drug and whether the cornea is intact, topical therapy may provide adequate drug levels only on the surface or as deep as the iris and ciliary body. Epithelial defects of 25% to 50% increase drug penetration into the corneal stroma and aqueous by nine times, but larger defects do not produce an additional increase.[56] Other variables influencing drug concentrations via topical administration are the frequency of application, drug contact time, and drug concentration. Solutions are generally easier to apply to a painful eye and therefore are preferred in terms of compliance. To a point, a higher drug concentration increases the absorption. However, concentrated drugs may increase reflex lacrimation and become diluted by osmotically drawing fluid from the tissues.

When solutions are used, one drop (about 30 to 50 µl) of a preparation is adequate. Multiple or rapidly repeated instillations of the same or different preparations simply increase the rate of loss via the NL duct or mutually dilute each preparation, thereby reducing the availability of each drug. Waiting an interval of at least 5 minutes between instillation of multiple drugs is preferred to allow reflex tearing to subside and prevent dilution of the previous drop.

Treatment of routine surface infections of the conjunctiva or prophylactic antibacterial therapy of corneal ulcers should include topical broad-spectrum antibiotics such as neomycin-polymyxin-bacitracin that are not applied systemically. This rationale is based on minimizing bacterial resistance to antibiotics that are beneficial in systemic therapy and avoiding sensitization of a patient by a topical antibiotic that might have potential in systemic therapy.

Reports have begun to emerge of anaphylactic reactions in cats after administration of topical bacitracin-neomycin-polymixin B preparations.[96] Most cases have been fatal, thus it would be best not to use this formula in cats.

Subconjunctival

Subconjunctival administration of antibiotics or antiinflammatories is used primarily for anterior segment disease and can achieve therapeutic intraocular levels of medication. The major limitations of subconjunctival injections are drug irritation and ocular manipulation. The means by which a subconjunctivally injected drug reaches the interior of the eye are controversial, but direct diffusion through the sclera, which has no epithelial barrier as the cornea does, and leakage through the needle hole with topical absorption have been demonstrated. Except for long-acting drugs, most others must be readministered at 12- to 24-hour intervals to maintain therapeutic levels. Typically a single injection of a subconjunctival drug is administered, followed by topical agents, systemic agents, or both.

Drugs should be injected under the bulbar conjunctiva, not the palpebral conjunctiva. The dorsal 12 o'clock position is easiest to access. Adequate topical anesthesia is required. A proparacaine soaked cotton-tip swab should be held at the injection site for at least 60 seconds, followed by slow injection of drug with a 25-gauge needle. In many animals, this can be accomplished without sedation, although sedation may be required in some. In dogs and cats a volume of 0.2 to 0.5 ml can be administered, creating a bleb that resolves in a few hours.

Whereas significant posterior segment levels of drugs can be obtained when injecting near the equator of the globe, the subconjunctival route is *not* adequate for bacterial infections of the vitreous or optic nerve. Subconjunctival dosages vary by antibiotic (see Appendix 9).

Table • 93-6

Intraocular Penetration of Antibacterial Agents in the Uninflamed Eye

AGENT	PENETRATION BY ROUTE		
	SYSTEMIC	TOPICAL	SUBCONJUNCTIVAL
Penicillin	Poor	Poor	Good
Ampicillin	Poor	Poor	Good
Methicillin	Good (multiple dose)	NA	Good
Erythromycin	Poor	Good	Good
Cephalosporins	Poor	Poor	Good
Enrofloxacin	Good	NA	NR
Gentamicin	Poor	Poor	Good
Tobramycin	Poor	Poor	Good
Lincomycin	Good	NA	NA
Neomycin	NA	Poor	NA
Choramphenicol	Fair	Good	Good
Tetracycline	Poor	Good	NA
Doxycycline	Good	NA	NA
Bacitracin	NA	Poor	Poor
Polymyxin B	NA	Poor	NA
Trimethoprim-sulfadiazine	Good	Good	Good
Sulfonamides (in general)	Good	Good	Good
Ciprofloxacin	Good	Good	NR
Ofloxacin	NA	Good	Good

NA, Not available in a form for route of administration; *NR*, not recommended due to retinal toxicity.

Intraocular

Intracameral or intraocular injection of antibiotics is a heroic and an extremely effective means of obtaining high levels of intraocular antibiotics for the treatment of bacterial endophthalmitis. If vision is to be preserved, the decision to use the intracameral route must be made early to avoid rapidly devastating inflammation to delicate intraocular structures. Because culture and susceptibility testing results are not available for a few days, a broad-spectrum bactericidal antibiotic is usually administered.

The use of intravitreal vancomycin is common in human medicine for the treatment of bacterial endophthalmitis following injury or intraocular surgery. Dosages of 1 mg (0.1 ml) of vancomycin have been injected into the vitreous, along with 2.25 mg (0.1 ml) ceftazidime or 0.4 mg (0.1 ml) amikacin.[34,38,99] Typically, vancomycin is also administered intravenously. The intracameral injection of the drug combination can be repeated 3 to 4 days later.

Systemic

The systemic route of therapy is indicated in cases of chorioretinitis and optic neuritis, because topical or subconjunctival application does not result in therapeutic levels of drug in these tissues. Many drugs are unable to cross the blood-retinal or blood-aqueous barrier, although some agents have good ocular penetration (see Table 93-6). However, in animals with inflammation, most drugs administered systemically do penetrate the eye. Antiinflammatory agents such as prednisolone, carprofen, and aspirin reach therapeutic levels in inflamed ocular tissue. Likewise, most antibiotics reach therapeutic intraocular levels when the blood-aqueous and blood-retinal barriers are disrupted by inflammation. Of the systemically administered antifungal azole compounds, fluconazole penetrates the eye and CNS best. Itraconazole has also been effective in many animals for treating systemic mycoses such as blastomycosis with ocular involvement.

In some cases, administration of a systemic medication may have an adverse effect on the eye. Systemic fluoroquinolones penetrate normal ocular tissue and have the potential to damage the retina. Some cats receiving systemic enrofloxacin (oral or injectable) have developed acute retinal degeneration and permanent blindness.[39,123] This has been most notable in cats receiving greater than the recommended dose of 5 mg/kg/day. However, even lower doses may cause retinal degeneration in some cats, particularly older or debilitated animals, and all systemically administered fluoroquinolones should be viewed as potentially retinotoxic.

Adjunctive

In addition to specific antimicrobial therapy, standard nursing care involves cleansing of the ocular surface and lids with warm, moist swabs or using hot packing if lid and orbital swelling is evident. Systemic nonsteroidal agents such as carprofen or aspirin (for dogs only) are analgesic and lessen the inflammatory reaction. Topical atropine minimizes ocular pain from ciliary muscle spasms and helps prevent synechia; however, atropine should not be used if KCS, glaucoma, or iridocorneal angle compromise are present. Injection of 25 μg of tPA into the anterior chamber is an effective and dramatic means of breaking down adhesions and dissolving fibrin clots if given within 3 to 7 days of formation. Once the clot is organized, the efficacy is lost. If active or recent bleeding has occurred in the eye, intraocular rebleeding may occur after injection of tPA. Injections may be repeated if necessary. Injection of tPA into the vitreous humor is not as safe because of retinal toxicity.

SUGGESTED READINGS*

54. Helps C, Reeves N, Egan K, et al. 2003. Detection of *Chlamydophila felis* and feline herpesvirus by multiplex real-time PCR analysis. *J Clin Microbiol* 41:2734-2736.

69. Maggs DJ, Nasisse MP, Kass PH. 2003. Efficacy of oral supplementation with L-lysine in cats latently infected with feline herpesvirus. *Am J Vet Res* 64:37-42.

91. Panciera RJ, Ewing SA, Confer AW. 2001. Ocular histopathology of ehrlichial infections in the dog. *Vet Pathol* 38:43-46.

94. Pena MT, Roura X, Davidson MG. 2000. Ocular and periocular manifestations of leishmaniasis in dogs: 105 cases (1993-1998). *Vet Ophthalmol* 3:35-41.

97. Powell CC, Lapin MR. 2001. Clinical ocular toxoplasmosis in neonatal kittens. *Vet Ophthalmol* 4:87-92.

103. Sparkes AH, Caney SM, Sturgess CP, et al. 1999. The clinical efficacy of topical and systemic therapy for the treatment of feline ocular chlamydiosis. *J Feline Med Surg* 1:31-35.

110. Stiles J, Townsend WM, Rogers QR, et al. 2002. Effect of oral administration of L-lysine on conjunctivitis caused by feline herpesvirus in cats. *Am J Vet Res* 63:99-103.

116. Townsend WM, Stiles J, Guptill-Yoran L, et al. 2004. Development of a reverse transcriptase-polymerase chain reaction assay to detect feline herpesvirus-1 latency-associated transcripts in the trigeminal ganglia and corneas of cats that did not have clinical signs of ocular disease. *Am J Vet Res* 65:314-319.

119. Vinayak A, Greene CE, Moore PA, et al. 2004. Clinical resolution of *Brucella canis*-induced ocular inflammation in a dog. *J Am Vet Med Assoc* 224:1804-1807.

*See the CD-ROM for a complete list of references.

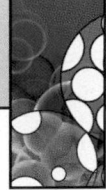

CHAPTER • 94

Environmental Factors in Infectious Disease

Craig E. Greene

MEANS OF TRANSMISSION

The reservoir of an infectious disease is the natural habitat of its causative agent. Organisms such as *Clostridium* and *Salmonella* can survive and multiply in inanimate reservoirs such as soil and water. Animate reservoirs, known as carriers, can be clinically or subclinically infected with and shed microorganisms that cause disease. Reservoirs and carriers are distinguished from the source of infection, which can be any vertebrate, invertebrate, inanimate object, or substance that enables the infectious agent to come into immediate contact with a susceptible individual. In many cases, the source is the reservoir.

The transmissibility or communicability of an infection refers to its ability to spread from infected to susceptible hosts. *Contagion* and *transmissibility* have been used interchangeably; however, the former implies spread after intimate contact. Transmission can occur between members of the same population (horizontal) or succeeding generations through the genetic material (vertical). Spread of infection to offspring by the placenta, from genital contact at birth, or in the milk is actually horizontal transmission. Not all infectious diseases are transmissible (e.g., systemic mycotic infections originate from soil rather than spreading between individuals).

Direct contact transmission is probably the most frequent and important means of spread of infection. This transmission involves direct physical contact or close approximation between the reservoir host and the susceptible individual. Venereal transmission of *Brucella canis* between dogs and bite transfer of feline immunodeficiency virus (FIV) between cats are examples of direct physical contact transmission. Aerosol droplets from respiratory, fecal, or genitourinary secretions of dogs and cats generally do not travel farther than 4 or 5 feet; therefore droplet spread can be considered a form of direct transmission. The spread of infection under such circumstances can usually be limited, as long as fomite transmission is prevented, by ensuring adequate distance between affected and susceptible animals.

Vehicle, or indirect, transmission involves the transfer of infectious organisms from the reservoir to a susceptible host by animate or inanimate intermediates known as vehicles or fomites. Indirect transmission is dependent on the ability of the infectious agent to survive temporarily adverse environmental influences. The most common animate fomites involved in indirect transmission in veterinary practice are human hands. Inanimate fomites can include anything by which an agent indirectly passes from infected to susceptible individuals, such as food dishes, cages, and surgical instruments. Canine and feline parvoviruses are often spread in this manner because of the short shedding period in infected animals and the relatively long period of environmental persistence of these viruses.

Common-source transmission involves the simultaneous exposure of a significant number of individuals within a population to a vehicle contaminated by an infectious agent. The vehicles of common-source infections are usually blood products, drugs, food, and water. Food-source outbreaks of *Salmonella* gastroenteritis have been observed in small animal practice.

Airborne spread of infection depends on the ability of resistant microorganisms to travel for relatively long distances or to survive in the environment for extended periods until they encounter susceptible hosts. Freshly aerosolized particles containing microbes rarely remain airborne for more than 1 minute unless they are smaller than 5 μm in diameter. Droplet nuclei, which are desiccated aerosolized particles containing resistant microbes, may also be carried alone or on dust particles by air currents for extended periods and distances. Resistant respiratory pathogens such as *Mycobacterium tuberculosis* and *Histoplasma capsulatum* are commonly spread by this means. In human hospitals, nosocomial infections with *Staphylococcus aureus*, *Bordetella pertussis*, and *Streptococcus pyogenes* can be spread by these means.[163] *S. aureus* infections have been a concern because antimicrobial-resistant strains of *S. aureus* have been transmitted from people to dogs and cats (see Chapters 35 and 99).

Vector-borne disease may be considered a specialized form of vehicular or indirect contact spread whereby invertebrate animals transmit infectious agents. Vectors are generally arthropods that transmit infection from the infected host or its excreta to a susceptible individual, to its food and water, or to another source of immediate contact. Vectors such as flies may transfer organisms externally, or mechanically, on their feet or internally within their intestinal tracts. The ability of organisms to survive in the vector without further propagation has been demonstrated with *Shigella* and *Salmonella* infections. Propagative transmission means that the infectious agent multiplies in or on the vector before transfer. Transmission of the plague bacillus, *Yersinia pestis*, by fleas occurs in this manner. Transovarial transmission results when the vector transfers the organism to its progeny, as in the case of ticks transmitting *Rickettsia rickettsii*, the agent of Rocky Mountain spotted fever. Transtadial transmission, the transfer of infection only between molting stages in the life cycle of the vector, occurs in canine ehrlichiosis. True biologic (developmental or cyclopropagative) transmission by arthropod vectors involves an obligate developmental stage in the life cycle of the vector. Some of the protozoal pathogens of the dog and cat (e.g., *Hepatozoon*, *Trypanosoma*, *Leishmania*) have a developmental life cycle in the vector.

A pathogenic organism must evolve a mechanism that enables it to spread from one infected animal via the reservoir or carrier to other animals to perpetuate the cycle of infection. Generalized spread of the infection to many body tissues results in contamination of many body secretions. Acute localized respiratory and gastrointestinal (GI) infections usually result in heavily contaminated secretions or excretions, such as aerosols produced during coughing and sneezing or diarrhea and vomitus, respectively. Genitourinary infections are transmitted in urine, uterine or vaginal discharges, and semen. Occasionally, infectious organisms may be shed from open, draining wounds.

Clinical illness is not always encountered in animals that are shedding. Many subclinical carriers exist; they are usually in the chronic or convalescent stage of disease. Latent carriers may shed organisms intermittently in association with reactivation of infection. Infection potential, however, generally varies inversely with the length of time over which a disease is communicable. Acute, severe illnesses are usually associated with highly contagious secretions because transmission occurs over a short time.

ENVIRONMENTAL CONTROL OF MICROBES

The health of both humans and domestic animals depends on the ability to control microorganisms that cause or have the potential to cause disease. Destruction of the organisms occurs when the microenvironment is changed adversely by physical or chemical means. Several levels of microbial disinfection are recognized (Table 94-1). Good decontamination always requires initial cleaning to remove organic residues and debris. With prior cleaning, most of the organisms are removed and disinfectants are more effective.

Sterilization is the process by which microorganisms are destroyed by chemical or physical means. All life forms, including heat-resistant spores, are killed. Sterility is an absolute condition; no partial sterilization process is possible.

Table • 94-1

Levels of Microbial Disinfection

LEVEL OF DISINFECTION	DESCRIPTION
High	Free of all microorganisms, including spores; equivalent to sterilization
Intermediate	Free of all vegetative bacteria, fungi, and most viruses
Low	Free of most vegetative bacteria, fungi, and enveloped viruses

Disinfection is the destruction of most pathogenic microorganisms, especially the vegetative forms, but not necessarily bacterial spores. Although disinfection may be brought about by physical agents, as well as chemical agents, a disinfectant is usually a chemical used on inanimate objects. Antisepsis, a special category of disinfection, is the inhibition or destruction of pathogenic microbes on the skin and mucous membranes. The assumption holds that all pathogenic vegetative microbes are destroyed; however, resident flora may persist. Importantly, the antiseptic must not be toxic to animal tissues. To reduce tissue toxicity, chemicals must be either diluted or applied for a shorter period than would be necessary to produce sterility.

Sanitation is the reduction of the number of bacterial contaminants to a safe level. A sanitizer is not concentrated enough, nor is it in contact with the organisms long enough, to effect disinfection.

In practice, in the absence of bacterial spores, sterilization and disinfection produce identical results. However, when spores are present, only the harshest of measures can ensure sterility. Unless the item to be treated can withstand sterilization procedures via autoclave or ethylene oxide (EO), either physical or chemical disinfection must be relied on to reduce the number of microorganisms to a safe level.

Protozoal cysts, mycobacteria, and bacterial spores are highly resistant to disinfection and sanitation. Prions, the proteinaceous agents that cause transmissible degenerative encephalopathies (see Chapter 84), are the most resistant infectious agents known. Some loss of infectivity of prions occurs at 100° C; however 130° C for 30 to 60 minutes is required for their inactivation. Prions are not affected by sterilizing levels of radiation, formalin, nonpolar organic solvents, burial for years, or passage through 0.1-μm filters. Their infectivity is destroyed by 1 M sodium hydroxide at 55° C or sodium hypochlorite (household bleach) diluted 1:1.

Physical Agents
Heat
Use of either moist or dry heat is one of the oldest physical controls of microorganisms. Of the two, moist heat, especially under pressure, is more efficient, requiring shorter exposure at a lower temperature than is needed for disinfection by dry heat. When used correctly, steam under pressure is the most efficient means of achieving sterility. The recommended temperature-pressure–exposure time to produce sterilization with an autoclave is 121° C at 15 pounds per square inch (psi) for 15 minutes or 126° C at 20 psi for 10 minutes. Steam heat is also most effective for eliminating resistant protozoal cysts, such as *Toxoplasma* and coccidia. Hot-air ovens are the most common dry-heat sterilizers, but to be effective, they must provide a consistent heat source. Dry-heat sterilization can be assumed if objects are maintained at 160° ± 10° C for a

minimum of 1 hour but preferably 2 hours. Microwave oven sterilization times of dry materials are similar to those of dry ovens once the sterilization temperature is reached. The only advantage of the microwave is the shorter time it takes to achieve these temperatures. Dry heat is recommended for sterilizing cutting instruments and glassware or items that might be damaged by moisture, such as glass syringes and reusable needles.

Radiation

Ionizing or high-energy radiation can be produced by radioactive elements, which are sources of γ-rays, or by a cathode-ray tube that produces x-rays. γ-rays and x-ray radiations induce ionization of the vital cell components, especially nuclear DNA. Because of the cost and dangers of handling this equipment, this type of microbial control has found practical application chiefly in the industrial field. Pharmaceuticals, plastic disposables, and suture materials are generally sterilized by the manufacturer by means of ionizing radiation. Foodstuffs can be sterilized or disinfected of pathogenic microbes by using ionizing radiation. This process is safe and efficient but has met with resistance by the public. An unfounded misconception exists concerning residual radioactivity in treated foods. Nonionizing, or low-energy, radiation in the form of ultraviolet (UV) light has found practical application in the destruction of airborne organisms. Because low-energy rays do not penetrate well, they are used primarily as surface-active agents. The bactericidal range of UV light is 240 to 280 nm. UV lamps usually produce radiation in the range of 254 nm and work at maximal efficiency at temperatures of 27° to 40° C. They depend on air convection currents to circulate air-

borne organisms. Germicidal lamps must be positioned above eye level to prevent retinal burns. For best efficiency, the lamps can also be placed in air conditioning or heating ducts. (See Air-Borne Contaminants, under Prevention of Nosocomial Infections.)

Chemical Agents

Biocides (germicides) denote chemical agents having antiseptic, disinfectant, or preservative properties. In addition to the environmental control of infection, many of these agents are used to preserve food, pharmaceuticals, and medical supplies. Typically, biocides lack selective toxicity to microorganisms. The antimicrobial properties of various chemical disinfectants are summarized in Table 94-2. Table 94-3 describes the uses of the compounds to disinfect hospital equipment.

Alcohols

Ethyl and isopropyl alcohol are rapidly bactericidal against vegetative bacteria but have little effect against spores. Alcohols can be virucidal, provided that exposure time is adequate. Ethyl alcohol is more effective against the nonenveloped viruses than is isopropyl alcohol, whereas the reverse is true for the enveloped viruses. Ethyl alcohol is effective against *Proteus* and *Pseudomonas*, whereas isopropyl has a broader antibacterial spectrum. Alcohol is effective only as long as it remains in contact with the item to be disinfected. Because it evaporates readily, repeated applications may be needed to ensure adequate effect. Alcohol is applied primarily on viable tissues as an antiseptic agent but only on intact skin. Alcohols inactivate hexachlorophene but are used as a diluent for iodine to enhance its disinfection properties. Alcohol has often

Table • 94-2

Antimicrobial Properties of Common Classes of Chemical Disinfectants

CLASS OF DISINFECTANT	BACTERIA				FUNGI	VIRUSES	
	GRAM POSITIVES	GRAM NEGATIVES	ACID FAST	SPORES		ENVELOPED	NONENVELOPED
Alcohols							
Ethyl	+	+	+	−	−	+	+
Isopropyl	+	+	+	−	−	+	−
Halogens							
Chlorine (hypochlorite)	+	+	+	+	+	+	+
Iodine	+	+	+	±	+	+	±
Chlorine dioxide	+	+	+	+	+	+	+
Aldehydes							
Formaldehyde	+	+	+	+	+	+	+
Glutaraldehyde	+	+	+	+	+	+	+
Ortho-phthalaldehyde	+	+	+	+	+	+	+
Phenolics	+	+	+	−	+	+	±
Potassium monopersulfate	+	+	+	+	+	+	+
Surface-Active Compounds							
QUATs (cationic)	+	±	−	−	+	±	−
Amphoterics (anionic)	+	±	+	−	+	±	−
Biguanides	+	+	−	−	−	?	?
Ethylene oxide	+	+	+	+	+	+	+

+, Effective; ±, somewhat effective; −, not effective; ?, effectiveness not known; *QUATs*, quaternary ammonium compounds.

Table • 94-3

Treatment Time Required for Chemical Disinfection of Hospital Equipment

EQUIPMENT	TYPE OF DISINFECTION[a]	DISINFECTANT[b]	EXPOSURE TIME
Objects with smooth hard surfaces	H	17	3—12 hrs
	H	18—10	15—18 hrs
	H	11	5 hrs
	I	1—3, 6, 8—10, 12	30 min
	L	1, 4, 7, 13, 14—16	10 min
	L		5 min
Rubber tubing (completely filled) and catheters	H	17	3—12 hrs
	I	6, 10, 12	30 min
	L	7, 13, 14—16	10 min
Polyethylene tubing (completely filled) and catheters	H	17	3—12 hrs
	H	8—10	15—18 hrs
	I	1, 2, 6, 10, 12	30 min
	L	1, 7, 13—16	10 min
Thermometers (wiped thoroughly clean)	H	8—10	10—12 hrs
	I	2, 5, 10	30 min
	L	6	10 min
Lens instruments	H	9—11	10—12 hrs
	I	9, 10	30 min
	L	7, 13—16	10 min
Hinged instruments (free of organic material)	H	9, 10	10—12 hrs
	I	2, 8—10	20 min
	I	6, 12	30 min
	L	8—10	10 min
	L	1, 7, 13—16	20 min
Inhalation, anesthetic, and endoscopic equipment	H	9, 11	10 hrs
	H	17	3—12 hrs
	I	2, 10	20 min
	L	1, 14—16	20 min
	L	10, 11	5 min
Housekeeping (floors, furnishings, and walls)	I	3, 6, 12	20 min
	L	4, 7, 13—16	10 min

[a]H, High-level disinfection (free of all microorganisms; equivalent to sterilization); I, intermediate-level disinfection (free of all vegetative bacteria, fungi bacilli, and most viruses); L, low-level disinfection (free of vegetative bacteria, fungi, and most enveloped viruses).
[b]1, 70%–90% ethyl or isopropyl alcohol; 2, 70%–90% ethyl alcohol; 3, hypochlorite (1000 ppm); 4, hypochlorite (100 ppm); 5, 0.2% iodine + alcohol; 6, iodophors (500 ppm); 7, iodophors (100 ppm); 8, 20% formalin + alcohol; 9, 20% formalin aqueous; 10, 2% activated glutaraldehyde aqueous; 11, 0.13% activated glutaraldehyde + phenate complex; 12, 2% phenolic aqueous; 13, 1% phenolic aqueous; 14, quaternary ammonium compounds; 15, amphoterics; 16, chlorhexidine; 17, ethylene oxide.

been used as a rinse for povidone-iodine or chlorhexidine in skin decontamination. Because water is essential for the antimicrobial action, absolute (100%) alcohol has no disinfecting qualities. Concentrations found to be most bactericidal are between 50% and 95% by volume. The two most widely employed concentrations are 70% and 85%. The alcohols are inactivated by organic soil, and they are ineffective if diluted to less than 50%. Alcohols are not effective for cold sterilization of instruments, and they dissolve lens-mounting cements, blanch asphalt tiles, and harden plastics on long-term exposure.

Halogens

These compounds are ineffective or unstable in the presence of organic material, soap, or hard water. Halogens are active against a wide variety of viruses and resistant bacteria, such as *Proteus* and *Pseudomonas*. Table 94-4 summarizes the disinfectant activity of chlorine and iodine, which are described in greater detail.

Household bleach, a 5.25% sodium hypochlorite solution diluted to a maximum of 1:30 (vol/vol), is a common form of chlorine for disinfection. Bleach is sold with a pH of 12 to prolong its shelf life. To increase its germicidal activity, especially against spores, the bleach is diluted with water to increase the available chlorine and acetic acid to change the pH of the solution to 7.0.[151] Increasing the temperature of the solution decreases the exposure time needed. Other than aldehydes, this chemical is one of the few that will inactivate parvoviruses. Dilution and acidifying bleach solutions reduces their stability, and bleach is also deactivated by light. Therefore bleach should be kept in opaque containers and diluted fresh daily.

Chlorine dioxide, a halogen, is superior to chlorine in the destruction of bacteria, including spores and viruses. It has high solubility and no odor, and it is unaffected by pH in the range of 4 to 10 and is nonreactive with ammonia compounds. Unlike bleach, chlorine dioxide is noncorrosive even at high chlorine concentrations. It must be generated from on-site

Table • 94-4

Disinfectant Activity of Chlorine and Iodine[7,188]

CHEMICALS	CONCENTRATION (mg/L)	TEMPERATURE (°C)	TIME (min)
Chlorine			
Gram-negative bacteria	0.1	5	0.16
Campylobacter	0.3	25	0.5
Giardia cyst	2.5	60	5
Cryptosporidium oocyst	10	20	720
Bacillus anthracis spores	2.3	22	60
Unenveloped virus		5	30
Iodine			
Gram-negative bacteria	1.3	2–5	1
Giardia cyst	4	5	120
Unenveloped virus	0.5	5	30

synthesis or can be ordered in a stabilized form. Chlorine dioxide has high penetration of environmentally resistant bacterial biofilms and has been used to treat air conditioning cooling systems to remove pathogenic bacteria.

Iodine is only slightly soluble in water; therefore disinfectant solutions are made by dissolving it in alcohol or combining it with organic compounds. Iodine is sporicidal, fungicidal, protozoacidal, and somewhat virucidal, depending on exposure time and concentration of free iodine. Destruction of bacterial spores requires moist contact for more than 15 minutes. Unlike chlorine, iodine exerts its effect over a wide range of pH.

Iodophors are iodine solutions complexed with surfactants or polymers, which help increase the contact of the iodine with the surface to be disinfected while limiting the concentration of free iodine. The advantages of iodophors over iodine are that they are nonstaining and produce minimal tissue damage. Organic matter may reduce their activity, especially with dilute solutions, but the effect is less marked than it is with hypochlorites. Rinsing with alcohol will reduce these solutions' residual antibacterial activity. Povidone-iodine is a complex of polyvinylpyrrolidone and iodine (Betadine solution, Purdue Frederick, Norwalk, Conn.). Such iodine compounds have been used for presurgical preparation, topical wound therapy, and joint or body cavity lavage. Solutions of 10% (undiluted) to 1% (1:9) povidone-iodine have been applied for skin and wound disinfection. Dilutions (1:4 to 1:100) of 10% stock solution result in increased bactericidal activity owing to increased concentrations of free iodine more so than in the undiluted stock solution. A 1:50 dilution of povidone-iodine is recommended as an ocular surface disinfectant in presurgical situations.[125,126] A 7.5% scrub containing an anionic detergent damages tissues and should be used only on intact skin. Bacterial concentrations are reduced on canine skin for up to 1 hour after scrub application.[125] Polyhydroxydine is a potent iodine-containing wound and skin antiseptic (Xenodine, Squibb Animal Health Division, Princeton, NJ.). It has been effective in treating canine wounds when used undiluted (100%) or as a 1:9 dilution (10%). As long as the iodophor solution maintains its color, it is effective.

Systemic absorption of iodine may result in transient reduction in serum thyroxine or bicarbonate concentrations. Contact dermatitis that persists for several hours may occur in dogs.[125-127,142] The skin irritation may lead to inactivation of the iodine through weeping proteins and increased

postsurgical infection. Iodophors are also damaging to deeper tissue fibroblasts and must be diluted to 0.001% to be applied as wound or body cavity rinses.[98] Concentrations of 0.5% to 1% have been effective but may be too strong for lavage of contaminated peritoneal cavities. Peritoneal lavage with 10% povidone-iodine can be fatal to dogs if 8 ml/kg is infused with intact peritoneum or 2 ml/kg with peritonitis. Concentrations of greater than 0.1% should not be used in joint irrigation.

Aldehydes

Aldehydes have been employed as gaseous sterilants, as well as chemical disinfectants. The exposure time needed for formaldehyde to effect sterilization is long because the gas does not penetrate well and has been replaced by more efficient gases. A 100% formalin solution is approximately 40% formaldehyde in water. A 20% formalin solution (8% formaldehyde) is a high-level disinfectant (sporicidal), and its biocidal activity can be increased by the addition of 70% alcohol, but the solution is irritating to tissues and mucous membranes.

Glutaraldehyde is chemically related to formaldehyde but is more reactive, even in the presence of organic materials, soaps, and hard water. A 2% aqueous alkaline solution is equivalent to 20% formalin in alcohol in biocidal activity. The alkaline solution is much more biocidal but less stable. Stability is maintained for approximately 2 weeks at pH 7.5 to 8.5. At the dilution at which it is used, glutaraldehyde is slightly irritating to the skin and mucous membranes and very irritating to the eyes. Both glutaraldehyde and formalin are high-level disinfectants for cold sterilization of instruments that are unable to withstand steam or EO gas, including lens instruments, such as endoscopes, and plastic tubing and catheters. After disinfection, items should be rinsed thoroughly with sterile distilled water. A glutaraldehyde-phenate complex (Sporicidin, Sporicidin International, Washington, DC) has been shown to be as effective at 1:16 dilution as is undiluted glutaraldehyde and as stable and less irritating.

Ortho-phthalaldehyde (OPA), a clear pale liquid of pH 7.5, and a working solution contains 0.55% OPA. Unlike glutaraldehyde, OPA is stable over pH of 3 to 9 and is more potent compared with glutaraldehyde, even against mycobacteria. Furthermore, OPA requires no activation and is not a tissue irritant. OPA is compatible with many materials; however, it stains proteins gray, including unprotected skin, and must be handled with protective clothing. High-level disinfection at 20° C varies from 5 to 12 minutes, depending on the country.

Phenolics

Phenolics are good housekeeping disinfectants because they remain stable when heated and, after prolonged drying, will redissolve on contact with water. They remain active in the presence of organic soil, soap, and hard water and are usually the disinfectant of choice in treating fecal contamination, such as with *Salmonella*. Phenolics must be thoroughly rinsed from areas contacted by cats because of greater toxicity in this species, and they are irritating to the skin and mucous membranes.

Hexachlorophene, a phenolic derivative commonly formulated with hand soap, is used as a degerming agent for the skin and mucous membranes because it causes little tissue irritation. Used only once, hexachlorophene is no more effective than soap is in eliminating microorganisms. Hexachlorophene takes longer than chlorhexidine or povidone-iodine to be effective. Its activity is reduced by organic material, and it is inactivated by alcohol. Hexachlorophene is also neurotoxic when absorbed from the skin, and it should be avoided over extensive areas and in neonates and animals with severely abraded skin.

Diphenol hydroxybenzene complex (Citricidal® Nutribiotic Co., Lakeport, Calif.), a quaternary compound from grapefruit seed bioflavonoids, is a nontoxic, biodegradable, noncorrosive disinfectant. This compound comes as a liquid or powder concentrate and was virucidal for enveloped viruses such as feline herpesvirus but was not effective against feline calicivirus or feline parvovirus.[51]

Hydrogen Peroxide

This common irrigant has been advocated for flushing directly into contaminated or infected wounds. Because its lack of antibacterial activity and potential cytotoxicity, hydrogen peroxide is recommended as an initial flush in wounds for its effervescent action and increased oxygenation, which retard anaerobic bacteria. It works best as a disinfectant for nebulizer and anesthetic equipment.

Potassium monopersulfate, a water-soluble complex salt, is an oxidizing disinfectant that can be used in a wide variety of environmental cleaning purposes and in oral hygiene solutions. Potassium monopersulfate has been commonly used for nonchlorine oxidation and disinfection of swimming pools and spas. A 1% solution is not corrosive for finer surgical instruments. The chemical is highly bactericidal and virucidal and has efficacy against resistant organisms such as foot-and-mouth disease virus.

Surface-Active Agents

These agents are chemicals that alter the surface tension of the organism and are classified as cationic or anionic. The quaternary ammonium compounds (QUATs) are cationic detergents that have been used for disinfection and antiseptic purposes, although their activity as disinfectants may have been overrated. They are inactivated by organic material, soap, and hard water. They should not be used in preparation of skin for surgery because they are inactivated by detergents in surgical scrubs. QUATs are algicidal, fungicidal, bactericidal, and virucidal (against some enveloped viruses) at medium concentrations. Virucidal activity of newer QUATs such as dodecyl dimethyl ammonium chloride or *N*-alkyl dimethyl benzyl ammonium chloride is incomplete against viruses (even herpesviruses) in contrast to the claims of manufacturers.[91] When properly used, QUATs are effective bactericides against both gram-positive and gram-negative bacteria; however, they display greater activity against gram-positive organisms. They have an unusual ability to kill *Giardia* cysts

at refrigerator and room temperatures (see Prevention, Chapter 78). QUATs are ineffective against myobacteria, *Proteus*, *Pseudomonas*, bacterial spores, and nonenveloped viruses even at high concentrations. When the temperature is increased from 20° to 37° C, the concentration of the solution can be reduced by one half. Benzalkonium chloride is the most common compound of this group.

As an environmental or skin disinfectant, concentrations of 0.001% to 1% benzalkonium chloride are generally used. Benzalkonium chloride has also been employed in medicine as an antiseptic and in flushing infected wounds at very low (no more than 0.007%) concentrations. QUATs are thought to form a film over the skin, with the inactive part of the compound directed toward the skin, possibly trapping bacteria but not killing them. The germicidal part is directed toward the environment, preventing further contamination. Degerming the skin with a more effective antiseptic before applying a QUAT may overcome the problem. Care must be taken not to allow undiluted QUATs to contact exposed tissues. Chemical burns occurred after applying undiluted (10% to 17%) benzalkonium chloride on skin surfaces or 0.1% to 0.5% on conjunctivae or mucosae of dogs and cats. Cats also developed oral and esophageal ulcerations after licking treated skin areas, and oral ingestion should be avoided. Concentrations as low as 0.002% to 0.007% must be used on wounds, but other agents such as chlorhexidine or povidone-iodine are preferred.

Anionic surfactants or amphoterics, organic acids that have the detergency of anionic compounds, are effective against both gram-negative and gram-positive bacteria and are reported to be fungicidal but not sporicidal. Unlike QUATs, they are effective against *Proteus* and *Pseudomonas*. Amphoterics are effective in one application and are not inactivated by serum or hard water, although soaps and detergents affect them adversely. Similar to QUATs, amphoterics leave a film on the skin that will block the transfer of organisms from unwashed to washed hands. Amphoterics are nontoxic to tissues and noncorrosive to moist surfaces, and they have a deodorizing ability. They can greatly reduce the total number of bacteria on hospital floors.

Biguanides

Chlorhexidine, the most common disinfectant of this class, has gained popularity for surgical skin preparation and as a wound antiseptic because of its low tissue toxicity.[126] It is effective against *Proteus*, *Escherichia coli*, staphylococci, and *Pseudomonas*. In the skin, chlorhexidine binds to stratum corneum, giving up to 2 days residual activity after a single application. It has been shown to be an effective and nonirritating antiseptic for irrigating canine wounds. Concentrations of chlorhexidine of 0.5% in water, saline, lactated Ringer's solution, or alcohol have been shown to reduce bacterial contamination in canine wounds or as a surgical antiseptic, but they retard granulation tissue formation and epithelization. Lower concentrations of chlorhexidine (0.05% to 0.1%) were less antiseptic but can be used as a lavage for tissues or joints and did not inhibit wound repair. Chlorhexidine has not been effective in treating dermatophytosis (see Chapter 58). Because of irritation, even low concentrations should never be placed in the eye or in the ear canal with a damaged tympanum, although use with a damaged tympanum has been shown to be safe in dogs.[98] These compounds retain some activity in the presence of organic material and hard water but are inactivated by soaps. They are more effective at an alkaline pH.

Surfacine® (Surfacine Development Co., Tyngsborough, Mass.) is composed of a water-insoluble antimicrobial, silver iodide, and a surface coating of a polyhexamethy enebiguanide. The biguanide is attracted to the lipid in the bacterial cell outer membrane and transfers and accumulates the silver halide into the organism, causing bacterial cell death. Animate or inanimate surfaces can be treated with this solution followed by drying leading to a persistent antimicrobial activity.[148] It is not toxic to mammalian cells and can be applied to inanimate and animate surfaces without prior surface treatment.

Ethylene Oxide

When properly applied, this gas is the most effective chemical sterilant. As with other chemical disinfectants, EO is subject to limitations imposed by temperature, moisture content, concentration, and exposure time. Recommendations are that routine sterilization be performed at 30° to 55° C. If the temperature is not properly maintained, the gas may condense; or if the exposure time is too short, sterility failures can occur. Most EO sterilizers in hospitals are designed to produce 50% to 60% relative humidity; it must not fall below 30% or sterility failure will occur. Biologic indicators are available that monitor the efficacy of EO sterilization.

EO sterilization is not recommended for some plastics and pharmaceuticals or for animal feeds and beddings. The gas reacts with or is absorbed by these items. Solutions in sealed glass containers cannot be sterilized because the gas cannot penetrate glass. Instruments and other items should be clean, dry, and as free of contamination as possible before EO sterilization. Items are placed in semipermeable plastic wraps. After the sterilization process, articles must be aerated to allow the residual gas to dissipate because the absorbed gas is irritating to skin and mucous membranes. In in vivo and in vitro studies, ethylene oxide has been effective in inactivating feline leukemia virus (FeLV) infection in bone allografts for transplantation.[29,30] Recommended routine aeration procedures are as follows: at room temperature, 48 to 168 hours, depending on the items sterilized and their use or with forced-air cabinets, 8 to 12 hours, depending on the cabinet temperature.

Hydrogen Peroxide Plasma

Temperature-sensitive equipment can also be sterilized using hydrogen peroxide plasma sterilizers. This gas vapor is able to sterilize equipment in times of up to 72 minutes. Devices with small lumens can be effectively treated in this manner. This process leaves no toxic residues and can be used for endoscope or other immersible instruments.

NOSOCOMIAL INFECTIONS

Nosocomial (hospital-acquired) infections can arise endogenously from the spread of indigenous microflora or exogenously from contact with organisms on external sources (Table 94-5). Exogenous sources of infection commonly include other animals and fomites such as human hands, rodents, arthropods, food dishes, catheters, and hospital cages. Transmission can occur by airborne, contact, or vehicle routes. Many nosocomial infections result from opportunistic spread of the normal microflora rather than newly acquired agents. The prevalence rate of nosocomial infections in humans and probably veterinary hospitals is 5% to 10% of hospitalized patients.

Not all infections that develop in the hospital environment are nosocomial in origin. Infections that are present or incubating at the time of admission are excluded. Moreover, nosocomial infections may not become clinically evident until after the patient has been discharged from the hospital. Hospitalized animals are more prone to infection because of increased exposure to pathogens, concurrent immunosuppressive illness, and the increased stress imposed by technologic advances in medical practice (Table 94-6). Excessive antimicrobial therapy may increase the risk of colonization with

Table • 94-5

Nosocomial Opportunistic Infections in Companion Animal Veterinary Hospitals

ORGANISM(S)	OUTBREAK CIRCUMSTANCES
Klebsiella spp.	Intensive care infection in 23 dogs and 1 cat. Most common in surgical wounds, urinary tract and blood.[69]
Serratia marcescens	Contaminated IV catheters and respiratory and genitourinary tracts and skin of hospitalized animals as a result of contaminated benzalkonium chloride.[60]
Enterobacter cloacae	Contaminated cleansing solution causing infection in four dogs and a cat.[12]
Staphylococcus intermedius	Methicillin-resistant infection in 11 dogs following postsurgical or traumatic wounding or with recurrent pyoderma.[181]
Acinetobacter baumannii	Nosocomial infection in 17 dogs and 2 cats an intensive care unit over 2.5-year period. Isolates were made from the urine, indwelling catheters.[63]
Acinetobacter baumannii, Enterococcus faecalis, Enterococcus faecium, S. intermedius	Surgical wounds and other wound infections, urinary infections. One *A. baumannii* isolate was transferred to an equine patient in the same hospital.[20]
Serratia spp., *Acinetobacter anitratus, Citrobacter freundii, S. intermedius, Klebsiella* spp., *Escherichia coli*	IV catheter in dogs with parvoviral enteritis. Organisms were variably drug-resistant. Only one dog developed signs of catheter-related infection.[99]
E. coli	Hospital-acquired infections in intensive care and other wards and also found in environment of the hospital.[152]

IV, Intravenous.

antimicrobial-resistant pathogens. Nosocomial pathogens are either naturally resistant to antimicrobial drugs or develop resistance during hospital therapy. Attention to hand hygiene (Table 94-7), alcohol-based hand disinfectant (rubs), or use of gloves are ways that antimicrobial resistance has been controlled in human hospitals.[186] Of the disinfectants, alcohols have the most rapid microbicidal activity of all antiseptics. Furthermore, alcohol-based hand rubs have excellent spread-

Table • 94-6

Factors Associated with Increased Nosocomial Infection Risks

Exposure to Pathogens
Enterotomy with spillage
Dental procedures
Airway catheterization or endoscopy
Retrograde urinary or gastrointestinal endoscopy
Contaminated blood product transfusions
Vaccine-induced illnesses

Concurrent Immunosuppression
Cytotoxic chemotherapy
Glucocorticoid therapy
Irradiation
Splenectomy

Technological Advances
Antimicrobial therapy—causing resistance
Indwelling tubes or catheters
Orthopedic implants

Table • 94-7

Methods for Hand Disinfection[122,123]

Hand Washing
1. Completely wet hands and wrists in a running stream of warm water.
2. Keep hands lower than elbows to avoid recontamination.
3. Apply soap over front and back of hands.
4. Rub all surfaces of hands, and interlace fingers and lather for 15 minutes.
5. Thoroughly rinse hands in clear running water.
6. Turn off faucets with a paper towel.
7. Dry hands thoroughly with new disposable paper towels.

Hand Disinfectants
1. Place hand disinfectant dispenser in a readily available place on each animal cage.
2. Squeeze the disinfectant on hands, and rub all surfaces.
3. Let disinfectant dry thoroughly before handling objects.

ing quality and rapid evaporation. They are not irritating to the hands after repeated use as is a complication of frequent hand washing. Health care workers complied best with hand disinfection when dispensers containing alcohol-based hand rubs were available at each patient.[22] In the veterinary hospital ward or intensive care, dispensers can be suspended on the outside of each cage or run to facilitate hand hygiene. These measures reduce the spread of pathogenic organisms between animals and the zoonotic risk of infection.

Development of Antibacterial Resistance

Microorganisms have evolved means of overcoming the effects of antimicrobial drugs. Most resistance mechanisms are under genetic control. Spontaneous chromosomal mutations are relatively rare in bacterial populations; extrachromosomal transfer of genetic material or plasmids is more important.

Plasmid transfer occurs most frequently during bacterial conjugation, although alterations in bacterial nucleic acid may also occur through bacteriophages (via transduction), acquisition from naked nucleic acid (via transformation), or exchange between bacterial and host DNA (via translocation). Plasmid transfer also commonly occurs between bacteria of different genera.

Genetic acquisition of bacterial resistance to antimicrobials may be demonstrated in a wide variety of ways, including changes in permeability to the drug, in receptors for the drug, or in metabolic pathways. Plasmid resistance is frequently associated with cross-resistance among a large number of structurally related antimicrobials.

The prevalence of antibiotic resistance commonly increases in proportion to the frequency of use. Resistance often develops with streptococci, staphylococci, *E. coli*, *Salmonella*, *Proteus*, and *Klebsiella*. Suppression of normal enteric flora and proliferation of antimicrobial-resistant strains occur with partially absorbed antimicrobials or those that are excreted in the bowel in active form, such as tetracycline, chloramphenicol, ampicillin, metronidazole, furazolidone, amoxicillin, and cloxacillin. Antibiotic resistance in fecal coliform bacteria has been documented in domestic pets in association with the increased use of antibacterial drugs in such animals. Heightened antibacterial resistance among pets in rural environments was correlated with the increased use of antibiotics in livestock feeds. These findings should caution veterinarians against indiscriminate administration of antimicrobials. Moreover, similar resistance patterns have been identified in human contacts of both types of animals.

Antimicrobial resistance in human medicine has been shown to be more of a problem in hospitalized patients, in whom antibiotic usage is widespread, than it is among patients in general.[158] Similar findings probably exist in veterinary practices. Transmission of opportunistic multidrug-resistant pathogens has been observed in veterinary teaching hospitals.[20] *Acinetobacter baumannii*, *Enterococcus faecalis*, *Enterococcus faecium*, and *Staphylococcus intermedius* were involved (see Table 94-5). The drug-resistant *A. baumannii* infection was traced to a contaminated intensive care unit in a veterinary teaching hospital.[63] The *S. intermedius* strains were not similar, suggesting that they were a result of infection of resident organisms in individual hosts. This contrasts with nosocomial and community-acquired infections with drug-resistant *S. aureus* between humans and from humans to dogs, which likely represents an anthropozoonosis. Several different strains were found; however, identical typing in some indicated spread among the hospitalized animals. Localized and systemic infections were found. All animals had intravenous (IV) or other types of indwelling catheters or tubes placed during their hospital stays. Surveillance and improved practices will be required in intensive care units to reduce the future risk of such events. Unfortunately, the development of new antibacterial drugs has just barely kept ahead of evolving resistance patterns. Widespread or indiscriminate usage of gentamicin, trimethoprim-sulfonamide, and fluoroquinolone by veterinarians may threaten the efficacy of these antibiotics in the near future. The availability of a large number of antibacterial drugs should not give the veterinarian a sense of security because many drugs have become obsolete as a result of evolving bacterial resistance.

Development of bacterial resistance can be prevented by certain adjustments during antimicrobial therapy. Measures include restricted prophylactic drug therapy, fully effective doses at adequate intervals, narrow-spectrum antibacterials specific for the isolated organisms, isolation of animals receiving long-term antibacterial therapy, selection of antibacterials against which the isolated organisms are not prone to develop resistance, changing of antibacterials after an effective treatment period, restriction of indiscriminate use of antibacterial drugs, and topical or local rather than systemic therapy whenever possible.

Biofilms

Microorganisms adhere to inert or living tissues by producing extracellular polymers that allow for adhesion and produce a structural framework for their support and protection. These microbial biofilms develop in all types of indwelling or external medical devices within the hospital environment (Table 94-8).[43,44] Biofilms are a health risk because organisms involved are often highly resistant and have ready access to the body via the implant site (Table 94-9). The resistance occurs because antimicrobial agents must diffuse into the matrix, the organisms in biofilms have reduced metabolic requirements and growth rates, and the immediate environment provides further conditions protecting the organism. Plasmid resistance can also be shared between bacteria within a biofilm. The extracellular matrix of a biofilm is composed of polymeric compounds that are primarily polysaccharides surrounding the microorganisms in sheets or strands of amorphous material. Bacteria colonize indwelling medical devices such as catheters shortly after they are implanted. The rate of bacterial cell adherence depends on the property of the body fluids bathing the device, the rate of fluid flow over the surface and the composition of the biosynthetic device.

Conditions Associated with Nosocomial Infections

In human and probably veterinary hospitals, the most common nosocomial infections are urinary tract infections, followed by pneumonias, surgical site infections, and bac-

Table • 94-8

Indwelling Devices Associated with Biofilm Formation

Intravenous catheters
Urinary catheters
Peritoneal dialysis catheters
Endotracheal tubes
Feeding tubes
Contact lenses
Cardiac pacemakers
Prosthetic joints

Table • 94-9

Bacteria Commonly Associated with Biofilms

Gram Positive
Streptococcus viridans
Staphylococcus epidermidis
Staphylococcus aureus
Enterococcus faecalis

Gram Negative
Escherichia coli
Pseudomonas aeruginosa
Klebsiella pneumoniae
Proteus mirabilis

teremias.[54] For surgical and wound related infections, see Chapter 55.

Urinary Catheterization

This procedure is probably the most common cause of nosocomial infection in veterinary practice. Fluid washout from urine flow is a primary defense mechanism of the urinary tract. Catheters upset this barrier by permitting entry of organisms at the urethral meatus and catheter junction. The distal urethra and prepuce or vagina are normally inhabited by commensal organisms. When catheters are left in place, these bacteria can migrate in retrograde fashion and infect the rest of the urinary tract, which is normally sterile, generally occurring in 1 to 3 days. Transient bacteremia also may occur after manipulation of urinary catheters in infected patients. To prevent infection, the external genitalia must be thoroughly cleansed, after which catheterization must be performed under strict aseptic conditions. A short-term, repeated, nontraumatic catheter is preferable to placement of a long-term indwelling catheter. Prophylactic topical or systemic antimicrobial therapy does not reduce the prevalence of infection unless the catheter is left in place for fewer than 4 days. Treatment with prophylactic antibacterial drugs may increase the risk of urinary or systemic infection with resistant bacteria or with fungi such as Candida[81] (see Indwelling Urinary Catheters, Chapter 91, and Candida infections, Chapter 65). Antimicrobial therapy should not begin until the catheter is removed. At this time, the urine can be cultured, the sediment examined, and the animal started on therapy, which should be modified when the culture results are received. Antimicrobial therapy instituted while the catheter is in place merely selects for resistant infections. Periodic instillation of a disinfectant such as hydrogen peroxide into closed urinary drainage systems has not been effective in preventing catheter-associated bacteriuria in people.

Intravenous Catheterization

IV infusions are both essential and lifesaving in veterinary practice. Since the development of flexible plastics, IV catheters are maintained in the patient for longer periods; however, the possibility that the infusion system can become contaminated is greater. The improper use of indwelling catheters has resulted in a high prevalence of nosocomial bacteremias and some fungemias.[81] IV catheter–related infections are more common than is realized in veterinary practice. Organisms originate from contaminated infusates, the patient's skin, or from health care personnel. Although uncommon, infusion bottles, bags, or administration sets can become contaminated from hairline cracks produced during the manufacturing process. Organisms may enter infusion systems when the administration set is inserted into the bottle, allowing the influx of room air when the vacuum is released or when medicaments are added. Organisms can also be introduced at the connection of the infusion set with the hub of the IV catheter. Antimicrobial lock solutions have been used to reduce the frequency of associated infections.[3]

Finally, and most commonly occurring, is the migration of skin organisms at the insertion site into the cutaneous catheter tract and subsequent colonization of the catheter tip. Bacteria have a greater chance of gaining access when skin preparation is inadequate before catheter insertion because bacterial microflora density at the catheter insertion site is a major risk factor. Povidone-iodine has been the most widely used antiseptic for cleansing IV catheter sites, although cleansing with 70% alcohol or 2% chlorhexidine gluconate scrub has been comparable. A 2% tincture of chlorhexidine preparation has become available and needs further evaluation. In dogs, a 1-minute, 4% chlorhexidine gluconate scrub produced lower cutaneous bacterial counts than no disinfection when measured before catheter insertion or before withdrawal.[28]

Uncleaned legs also had more microscopic dermatitis when the catheter was placed for 77 hours. Thrombus formation and phlebitis was observed microscopically in all dogs regardless of skin management. Interestingly, no difference was observed in the colonization rate of the catheter tip between the two groups. Catheter colonization rates are likely high as dogs with parvovirus infections had a 22% rate of bacterial isolation.[99] Organisms were generally gram-negative, multidrug resistant, and were of environmental or GI origin. Colonization rate of catheters from dogs in the same veterinary hospital with other conditions was not available.

Although they can enter the lumen of the catheter at the hub, bacteria usually enter the IV infusion system at the site of penetration of the catheter tip by migrating between the catheter and skin surfaces. The prevalence of local infection is greatly increased when IV cutdown sites are used and catheters are in place for longer than 24 to 48 hours. Organisms producing localized infection at the catheter site can be infused systemically during the administration of fluid or during flushing of clogged catheters. Bacteria can also migrate in retrograde fashion, even against gravity flow, from the contaminated catheter to the infusion bottle.

Organisms such as coagulase-negative staphylococci have been shown to adhere to plastic catheters with subsequent replication and production of catheter-associated infections.[71] Some investigators believe that the slime-producing strains of bacteria are more effective in catheter colonization. Inserted catheters readily develop biofilms containing large numbers of organisms.[43,44] This layer may offer a physical barrier to host defenses or antibiotics in eliminating the bacteria. Several measures have been investigated to reduce biofilm formation given that the number of organisms in the catheter tip is directly related to the occurrence of bacteremia. Adding antimicrobial solutions to the heparin flush solutions (using antibacterial-impregnated catheters), sterile placement technique, and local application of antibacterial ointments at catheter insertion sites have been beneficial in reducing catheter-associated contamination.[32,43,44] Changing catheters is also important because biofilms become more resistant to antimicrobial therapy with time. If organisms with acquired resistance are present in the biofilm, the chance of transfer of resistant plasmids to other colonizing organisms can increase with time as long as the catheter is in place. Results from in vitro studies reveal that polyvinyl chloride or polyethylene catheters are less resistant to the adherence of microorganisms than are catheters made of Teflon® (Dupont, Wilmington, Del.), silicone elastomer, or polyurethane.[6]

With the intent of preventing bacterial migration along the external IV catheter surface, IV catheters have been made with silver-chelated collagen cuffs or silver impregnation (Table 94-10).[34] Although these systems have had variable efficacy in people, animal studies have not been conclusive. In contrast, silver iontophoretic catheters and those coated with silver sulfadiazine-chlorhexidine have been effective in preventing IV catheter–related infections in animal studies.[34] Silver coating of medical devices or topical silver creams applied to the point of catheter insertion may have benefit in reducing infection rates; however, systemic silver toxicity has been reported in people when leaching of surfaces occurs.

To help reduce the prevalence of IV catheter–related infections, tunneling under the skin before the venous penetration site has been used. Keeping such sites free of moisture or contamination is still important in maintaining sterility and avoiding moisture on, or contamination of, the end-cap or penetration site (Fig. 94-1).[42]

Organisms of the family Enterobacteriaceae, such as *Klebsiella*, *Enterobacter*, and *Serratia*, as well as *Citrobacter*, proliferate readily at room temperature in 5% dextrose and can

Table • 94-10

Silver Coatings For Prevention of Catheter-Associated Infections[45a]

CENTRAL VENOUS CATHETERS	PROVEN BENEFIT IN ANIMALS
Silver-chelated cuff	Unknown
Silver alone	Unknown
Silver iontophoretic	Effective
Silver sulfadiazine-chlorhexidine	Effective
Silver sulfadiazine	Not effective
Silver-benzalkonium chloride	Unknown
Peritoneal Catheters	
Silver alone	Effective
Silver ring	Unknown
Surgical Devices	
Silver-coated external fixation pins	Not effective
Silver-coated sutures	Unknown

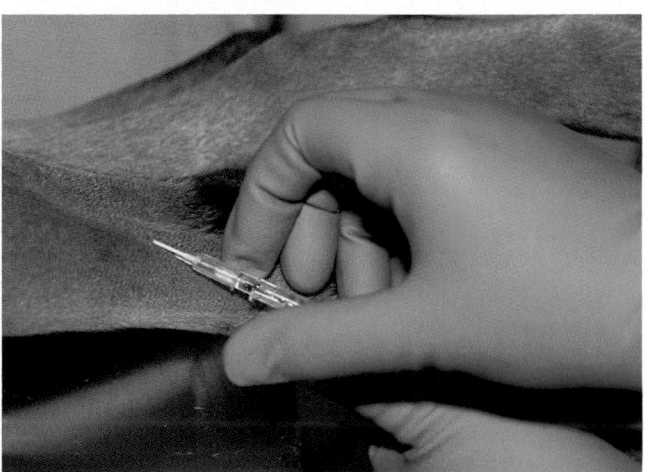

Fig   94-1 Placement of catheter with wrapping of the limb to prevent motion or protection from soiling or moisture. (Courtesy University of Georgia, Athens, Ga.)

reach concentrations of 10^5 and 10^6 organisms/ml without producing obvious clouding of the solution. Many other common contaminants, such as *Staphylococcus*, *Pseudomonas*, *E. coli*, and *Proteus*, do not survive or proliferate in 5% dextrose, although *Candida* can grow very slowly. *Serratia marcescens* has been incriminated as a common cause of medical device–related infections in small animal and human medical practice.[124] Benzalkonium chloride solutions should not be used for skin preparation because these antiseptic solutions can support the growth of *S. marcescens* and other microorganisms. In one instance, this organism was isolated from alcohol-soaked cotton balls used for skin decontamination.[83] *Pseudomonas* can grow in distilled water, normal saline, and even iodophors.[71] *Candida* grow well in protein hydrolysates, whereas *Candida* and *Malassezia* proliferate in lipid emulsions.

Lactated Ringer's solution, normal saline, other isotonic fluids, and hypertonic saline solution have been less commonly incriminated as the sources of nosocomial bacteremia than have dextrose solutions; however, they can support the growth of a variety of organisms. Parenteral hyperalimentation fluids and other hypertonic solutions readily support the growth of *Candida*. Blood products, even when stored at refrigerated temperatures, can become contaminated and support the growth of cold-growing microorganisms such as *Pseudomonas* and some coliforms such as *S. marcescens*. *S. marcescens* was responsible for contaminating feline blood units.[83] Bacterial growth in the blood units caused slight brown discoloration of the blood.

Clinical signs of catheter-associated infection include localized swelling and warmth at the insertion site and venous cording. The systemic spread of infection is characterized by fever, hypotension, tachycardia, and GI and central nervous system signs. Overwhelming infections associated with endotoxemia are more likely to occur when gram-negative organisms are involved and in immunosuppressed patients. Clinical signs in such cases are shock, collapse, coma, and death. In cats receiving blood contaminated with *S. marcescens*, vomiting, collapse, diarrhea, icterus, panting, fever, and death were variable findings.

Diagnosis of IV infusion–associated infection is frequently made when the clinical signs improve suddenly after terminating fluid therapy. However, because bacteremia may seed many organs, clinical signs can persist after the infusion is discontinued. Culture or Gram's staining of catheter tips has been recommended and is a more rapid and practical means of determining presence of infection. After removal, the IV or intracutaneous segment of the catheter is rolled across an agar plate, and the resultant colonies that grow are counted. A count greater than 15 colony-forming units is often associated with bacteremia.[71] However, this finding alone may not always confirm the presence of bacteremia. When blood cultures are performed, isolated organisms should correspond to those found at the catheter site. Pseudobacteremia may also occur when the infected catheter site locally seeds the venous effluent being sampled. At least two to three blood samples should be taken from different sites at intervals of at least 10 minutes once the catheter has been removed. Once catheter-related infection is suspected and the catheter tip or blood cultures are taken, the offending catheter should be removed. The animal should be started on antimicrobial therapy. Most infections can be eliminated with a 10- to 14-day course of antibacterials if the appropriate drug is selected.

IV catheter–associated infections can be prevented with adequate precautions (Table 94-11). Adequate skin preparation and antisepsis at the collection sites are essential. Hands should be washed before catheter placement. A large area of fur at the catheter site should be removed by careful clipping to avoid microabrasions of the skin. Gentle mechanical cleansing of the skin with an iodophor or with soap and water for 2 to 5 minutes should be followed by alternate disinfection using 70% alcohol and 1% to 2% tincture of iodine or iodophor solutions or, preferably, 2% chlorhexidine-

Table • 94-11

Recommended Procedures to Reduce the Risk of Intravenous Catheter–Related Infections

CONTROL MEASURE	RECOMMENDATIONS	BENEFIT OF REDUCING INFECTION
Catheter site	Peripheral veins versus jugular or femoral	Unknown
Catheter material	Teflon® or polyurethane versus polyvinyl chloride or polyethylene	Yes
Hand hygiene	Washing hands before catheter placement and each time it is handled. Wearing clean gloves is superior and acceptable versus sterile gloves.	Yes
Skin preparation	Povidone iodine (10%), chlorhexidine gluconate (2%–4%), tincture of chlorhexidine (2%)	Yes
Catheter dressing replacement	Transparent or gauze, the latter if leaking blood. Replace dressing if damp, loosened, or soiled.	Unknown
In-line filters	Use to reduce phlebitis but not infection.	No
Antimicrobial impregnation	Chlorhexidine-silver sulfadiazine superior but very expensive for veterinary use.	Yes
Topical antimicrobial ointment	Povidone iodine reduces bacterial but not fungal contamination or antimicrobial resistance.	No
Anticoagulants	Heparin flush	No
Catheter replacement timing	Replace no more frequently than 72–96 hrs because bacterial colonization and phlebitis increases.	Yes
Administration set replacement	Replace intravenous tubing no more frequently than 72 hrs unless blood or lipids, in which case 24 hrs replacement is recommended.	Yes
Hang time for parenteral fluids	No timing of intravenous fluids; lipid emulsions should limit to 24 hrs and blood products for 4 hrs.	Yes
Tunneled catheters	Used for central venous catheters or when placed longer than 96 hrs.	Yes

Based on recommendations for humans as published in O'Grady.[121] Guidelines for the prevention of intravascular catheter-related infections, *Clin Infect Dis* 35:1281–1307, and *MMWR* 2002, 51:1–26; Slaughter SE. 2004. Intravascular catheter–related infections, *Postgrad Med* 116:59–66.

gluconate.[102] Iodine-containing antiseptics are effective against most bacteria and fungi, with the exception of spores. Tincture of iodine preparations, superior to iodophors for the final application, is frequently too irritating for repeated application.

To restrict movement, catheters should be firmly stabilized with adhesive tape. A small amount of a broad-spectrum antimicrobial ointment, such as one containing organic iodine or neomycin-bacitracin-polymyxin, should be applied at the point of catheter penetration through the skin, and the site should be covered with a sterile occlusive dressing. If only tape is to be used, it must be sterile. The date and time of catheter insertion should be recorded. No catheter should be left in place longer than 72 hours. If the catheter must remain in place for longer periods, the IV site should be inspected and dressed with a new sterile dressing at 48- to 72-hour intervals. Disconnecting the IV catheters for sampling or administering medicines should be minimized. Concurrent administration of antibiotics does little to prevent IV catheter–associated infection but causes the development of an antimicrobial-resistant infection.

When long-term IV catheterization is required, special catheters such as the Broviac or Hickman type (C. R. Bard, Inc., Murray Hill, NJ.) should be considered.[19,71] These catheters have been designed to reduce migration of bacteria toward the implanted portion by a built-in cuff and subcutaneous tunneling of the proximal portion. These catheters are made of more flexible and nonreactive silicone, which is less irritative and thrombogenic, reducing the chance for a nidus of infection. Unfortunately, these catheters do not overcome the less common hematogenous seeding of bacteria on the catheter tips, which may occur from distant sites of infection.

When a small volume or slow infusion rate is required, multiple small infusion bottles are preferred to one large bottle. The rationale is that should the system become contaminated, the time for microorganism multiplication is minimized. Infusion bottles should be checked for turbidity and vacuum, and infusion bags should be squeezed before use to detect leaks. Infusion filters 0.22 μm in diameter are available to restrict the flow of microorganisms through the fluid catheter into the patient; however, they will not prevent passage of endotoxins and pyrogenic factors. Drugs should be added to infusion fluid containers in uncontaminated surroundings after proper disinfection of the site of addition to the infusion fluid. Technologic advances have been made with catheters to prevent bloodstream infections in humans. Iodinated alcohol solutions within catheter hubs,

Table • 94-12

Polymicrobial Infections and Sites in Dogs and Cats

DISEASE	AGENTS	COMMENTS
Gastroenteritis or intraabdominal infection	Gram negatives and anaerobes	Usually, give at least two drugs simultaneously to cover both spectra; however, can consider third-generation cephalosporins or penicillins.
Stomatitis, periodontitis	Gram positives and anaerobes	Treat anaerobic flora with drugs such as clindamycin, metronidazole.
Chronic otitis externa	*Staphylococcus, Pseudomonas, Proteus*	May need bone-penetrating or central nervous system—penetrating antibacterial.
Chronic rhinitis with osteolysis	Variety of opportunistic nasal flora including *Aspergillus*	Systemic antibacterials may offer temporary improvement; may need curettage or topical infusions (or both) of antifungal drugs for recurrent cases.
Canine tracheobronchitis	Viruses and bacteria	In dogs, antibiotics not usually used; more widely used in cats. Usually a single broad-spectrum drug is used.
Pyothorax	Variety of anaerobic bacteria and some facultative anaerobes	Requires drainage and lavage; critical for recovery.
Aspiration pneumonia	Aerobic and anaerobic bacteria	Usually, coverage with two antimicrobials.
Necrotizing fascitis	Gram-positive streptococci or staphylococci and anaerobes	Clindamycin of choice but may need surgical drainage or amputation.
Indwelling catheter- or tube-related infections	Variety of organisms in biofilms; see intravenous catheter infections	Recommended not to treat until device is removed.
Abscesses or necrotic soft-tissue infections	Variety of organisms, including anaerobes	Drainage is critical along with antimicrobial therapy.
Osteomyelitis	Variety of organisms, especially if the result of a compound fracture	Drainage and curettage along with antimicrobials that penetrate biofilms.
Burns	Variety of organisms from the environment	Always handle with gloves; use shower hydrotherapy versus whirlpools; and when extensive, use skin grafts.

chlorhexidine-silver-sulfadiazine or antibiotic-impregnated catheters, and antibacterial-impregnated sponges have all been evaluated.[113]

Polymicrobic Infections

Many polymicrobic infections arise from opportunistic growth and invasion by normal flora or organisms in biofilms in the environment. Because of their persistence, antimicrobial resistance, and collective experience, microorganisms in the biofilms have been exposed to many more antimicrobial insults than those that are solitary, and biofilm inhabitants may be more resistant to treatment and disinfection. For polymicrobic infections to occur, a complex interaction must take place between two or more microorganisms, allowing them to live in close association. For example, infections of the skin or mucosal surfaces, infection, underlying damage to the epithelium can lead to colonization and potential invasion by a variety of surface bacteria or fungi. A list of common sites and types of polymicrobic infections is in Table 94-12. Opportunistic commensal or environmental fungi such as *Candida* often interact with bacteria in these sites producing co-infections. Polybacterial disease is common in osteomyelitis, abscesses, vaginitis, periodontal diseases, chronic rhinitis with osteolysis, and necrotic soft-tissue infections.

Respiratory Infections

The upper respiratory tract passages have anatomic defense mechanisms that prevent most inhaled particles from reaching the lower airways. However, invasive procedures such as tracheostomy, fiberoptic endoscopy, transtracheal catheterization, nebulization, and endotracheal intubation bypass these defense mechanisms and expose the respiratory tract to increased numbers of organisms, especially gram-negative organisms. The occurrence of nosocomial pneumonias was *much* higher in endotracheally intubated human patients receiving histamine H_2-receptor antagonist. Retrograde contamination of the oropharynx with gram-negative bacteria from the stomach was thought to be responsible.

Decreased respiratory clearance function has also been associated with an increased risk of nosocomial respiratory infections. Decreased clearance activity can occur with CNS depression, neuromuscular paralysis, chronic obstructive lung disease, and impairment of pulmonary alveolar macrophage function. Inhalation anesthesia, nebulization, humidification, and ventilatory support increase the risk of nosocomial infection resulting from cross-contamination. Appropriate disinfection protocols for the equipment in these procedures are discussed later (see Prevention of Nosocomial Infections).

Gastrointestinal Infections

Enteric pathogens, such as parvoviruses, coronaviruses, *Salmonella*, and *Giardia*, may spread among dogs or cats in a veterinary hospital or animal-holding facility. Outbreaks are usually the result of poor sanitation, inadequate disinfection, and crowding of animals. Wards, treatment areas, waiting rooms, cages, exercise runs, thermometers, and feeding utensils are all sources of infection. All outbreaks of gastroenteritis among recently hospitalized patients should be investigated as to the cause and possible source of infection. Fecal examinations and cultures for protozoa and parvovirus should be performed when economically feasible.

Prevention of GI infections requires intense cleaning and disinfection procedures. All feces within the hospital should be removed as soon as possible, and the contaminated surface should be thoroughly disinfected with a diluted (1:32) chlorine bleach solution. Smooth, impervious floor and cage surfaces will facilitate disinfection and cleaning. Crowding of animals in waiting rooms and in hospital wards should be avoided. Use of gloves and hand washing should be enforced. Hospitalized animals should not be moved from cage to cage, but each should be assigned to one cage. Animals having episodes of acute vomiting or diarrhea either before or after being admitted to the hospital should be isolated.

Decubital Ulcers

These types of ulcers are the most common nosocomial skin infections to develop in incapacitated animals maintained in immobile or recumbent positions on unpadded surfaces. Abrasion and continuous pressure over bony surfaces cause devitalization of skin and secondary bacterial invasion. Immunosuppressed animals may develop septicemia as a result of decubital sores. *Pseudomonas* commonly contaminates these wounds. Identification of the invading microorganism and antibacterial therapy are usually of little benefit unless the primary cause is eliminated. Prevention is easier than cure; it involves frequent turning of recumbent patients and placing padding in their cages. Open drains in whirlpool or other baths used for rehabilitation of recumbent patients have been found to harbor *Pseudomonas* and cause outbreaks of nosocomial infection.[15] In such instances, *Pseudomonas* can persist in biofilms within the plumbing system despite the use of disinfectants such as chlorine or bromine.

Prevention of Nosocomial Infections

Most nosocomial pathogens, whether acquired endogenously or exogenously, do not produce disease by themselves. The risk of nosocomial infections is greatest for immunocompromised or surgery patients and for newborns. Prevention of these infections can be achieved only by strict monitoring of the known predisposing causes. Attempts should be made to reduce the contact of high-risk patients with potential pathogens by segregating them from the general hospital population or minimizing their hospital stay. Additional measures include placing indwelling catheters only when necessary, minimizing surgical procedures, and practicing routine disinfection. Chemical disinfection procedures in veterinary hospitals are reviewed in the following section and are summarized in Table 94-3. Other procedures to control the threat of nosocomial infections are listed in Table 94-13.

Antimicrobial Prophylaxis

Prophylactic antimicrobial drugs are controversial. The unnecessary use of antibiotics has caused justifiable concern because of the increased prevalence of resistant microorganisms. Antibiotics alter the patient's microflora and allow infection by resistant bacteria. For many years, microflora were thought to be responsible for bacterial superinfections after prophylactic administration of antimicrobial drugs; however, invasion

---

Table • 94-13

Practices to Reduce the Nosocomial Threat of Infections in the Hospital

Use of gloves when touching any body fluid, secretions, or excretion

Hand washing or hand disinfection before and after handling each patient

Face or eye shields and mask during procedures likely to generate aerosols

Disinfection of environmental surfaces or inanimate objects contaminated with body fluids using 1:100 dilution of household bleach

Soiled linens placed in leak-proof bags; can be decontaminated in an autoclave or incinerated; can be laundered in a normal hot-water cycle with bleach

by exogenous-resistant organisms is more likely. Prolonged antibiotic administration may not lessen an animal's susceptibility to infection but may merely alter the microbial flora that causes the problem.

Certain justifications exist for instituting treatment with antimicrobial drugs before documenting that an infectious process exists. Immunosuppressed hosts that have been exposed to disease may require antimicrobial therapy; however, most clinicians would argue that close monitoring of the patient should be followed by IV administration of antimicrobials only if fever or other signs of infection appear. High-risk conditions associated with immunosuppression and with secondary infection include diabetes mellitus, persistent neutropenia, Cushing's disease, immunosuppressive or cancer chemotherapy, and chronic bronchopulmonary disease. Traumatic or contaminated wounds and burns may require topical or systemic chemotherapy. For information on antimicrobial prophylaxis in wounds, burns, and surgical procedures, see Chapter 55.

Isolation Precautions

Restricting animal movement and contact within a veterinary hospital is important in controlling spread of nosocomial infections. As a general rule, animals entering the hospital should be currently vaccinated (see Chapter 100) or should be vaccinated if their status is uncertain. Any animal infested with ectoparasites should be dipped on admission if its condition permits. Immunosuppressed patients should not be housed in the hospital or, if admitted, should be moved to a separate area. If an infection is identified in an animal, four categories are proposed for which isolation precautions are indicated (Table 94-14).

Class 1 infections have little chance of spread between individuals, and the zoonotic potential is low. Systemic mycotic and algal infections are contracted primarily by environmental exposure. Systemic herpesvirus infection is a threat only to young neonates, and dogs showing only neurologic signs with canine distemper are unlikely to spread disease. No additional precautions are needed, and routine cage cleaning, hand washing, and disinfection of hospital equipment are all that is necessary.

Class 2 infections are of greater risk of transmission compared with class 1. Close contact is required between animals with papillomatosis or FeLV or feline infectious peritonitis. Many of these infections can be spread by contact with infected body fluids. Most other infections in this group are vector transmitted so that proper arthropod control will minimize the risk of spread from infected individuals. Most of the organisms cannot survive outside the host and are susceptible to routine disinfectants.

Class 3 infections are spread by close or direct contact with infected individuals or their excreta, but the risk of transmission via body fluids and excreta can be minimized by sanitary measures. These animals can be admitted to the general hospital population, but they should remain in their cages so as to restrict the contact of their urine and feces with other animals. Their cages should be identified as to the particular illness. Hand washing and cage cleaning must be critically practiced between animals, and feces or diarrhea, urine, and vomitus should be removed immediately. Dilute (1:30) bleach for viruses and phenolic compounds for bacteria should be used for disinfection. *Toxoplasma* and *Cryptosporidium* oocysts are inactivated by 10% ammonia solutions or by boiling water or steam cleaning. *Giardia* cysts are most susceptible to some dilute (1:100 or greater) QUAT disinfectants.

Animals with *Class 4* infections should be strictly isolated in a separate ward and should not be admitted to the general animal population. Infections in this category have a high degree of zoonotic risk, with potentially serious complications, or they are rapidly spread between susceptible animals. Animals with upper respiratory tract infections are preferably not admitted to the hospital and should be treated as outpatients. These highly contagious diseases are spread by air or contact. The animal's body exudates or secretions are highly infectious or the organisms are too resistant to enable control of spread. Persons handling these animals should wear protective outer garments, shoe covers, and rubber gloves. Contaminated wastes from these areas should be double-bagged in plastic and disposed of separately. Cages should be thoroughly disinfected once the animal is discharged. If the patient had *Salmonella*, the treated cage surface should have negative culture results before being used again.

Hands Hands are the most common reservoirs or fomites for microorganisms associated with nosocomial infection, and hand disinfection is probably the *single most important* and immediate way of reducing its hospital-acquired infections (Table 94-15). Alcohol hand rinses have become widely available for hand hygiene purposes. They have rapid and broad-spectrum microbicidal activity with little risk of emerging resistance.[97] Alcohol hand rinses should be used immediately before and after contacting patients or handling contaminated fomites. Because frequent hand washing of skin can cause dermatitis and secondary bacterial colonization, its recommended use has become more limited. In the cases in which washing is needed, hands should be washed routinely with water and mild, noncaustic soap or detergent after handling blood, secretions, and excretions or before surgical procedures and gloving. The mechanical effect of soap and water cleansing is most important in reducing the numbers of transient bacteria on the skin surface (Fig. 94-2). Frequent use of antiseptics should be avoided because they can burn or dry the skin. Preexisting dermatitis will result in the persistent carriage of large numbers of microorganisms, which negates the effect of hand washing. Bar soaps, allowed to dry between uses, appear to have a lower prevalence of contamination than liquid soaps. Liquid soap canisters can become contaminated and must be routinely emptied, cleaned, and disinfected before being refilled.

Iodine-containing soaps are superior as scrubbing agents before surgery; however, they may produce dermatitis in sensitive individuals. A comparison of the available hand-washing soaps and antiseptics appears in Table 94-16. Hand-washing sinks and bathing tubs in all areas of a veterinary hospital can be disinfected with chlorine bleach to reduce contamination with organisms such as *Pseudomonas*. Rubber gloves may be used as an adjunctive means of reducing spread of infection when hand washing must be done so frequently as to prove impractical or irritating to the skin.

Airborne Contaminants

These contaminants can be reduced by having impervious floor coverings and using wet mops or filtered vacuums throughout the hospital. Air conditioning systems should be electronically filtered if possible and should be designed to reduce turbulent airflow. The best ventilation systems have air inlets near the ceiling and air outlets near the floor, allowing air to travel downward toward the heavily contaminated floor region. Air exchange rates of 6 to 10 times per hour have been shown to reduce the number of airborne microorganisms efficiently in animal-holding facilities while producing minimal air turbulence. Electronic purification and reduction in airborne bacteria can be achieved with installation of ozone-producing devices that are mounted in a given room or in the supply air plenum (Aqua-Mist Inc, Winston-Salem, NC.). A UV radiation decontamination device that is effec-

Table • 94-14

Classification and Guidelines for Management of Infectious Diseases Based on Risk of Nosocomial or Laboratory Exposure and Zoonotic Transmission

TRANSMISSION	DISEASE	PRECAUTIONS FOR HANDLING
Class 1. Acquired from the Environment or Limited Shedding or Susceptibility Period		
Soil reservoir, vector transmitted, blood transfusion	Histoplasmosis,[a] cryptococcosis,[a] coccidioidomycosis,[a] blastomycosis, prototheocosis, neurologic canine distemper, haemobartonellosis, ehrlichiosis,[a] anaplasmosis,[a] trypanosomiasis,[a] borreliosis,[a] RMSF,[a] leishmaniasis,[a] nontuberculous mycobacteriosis[a]	No need for isolation. Transmission risk is low unless insect vectors are present. Some infections can spread to people or other animals if inadvertent inoculation of body fluids or tissues occurs. Always use gloves when performing procedures. Mycotic agents pose a high risk from laboratory cultivation of mycelial phases.
Dermal or transcutaneous contact	Dermatophytosis,[a] sporotrichosis,[a] dermatophilosis, L-form infection	Use gloves and protective clothing when handling animal and body fluids. Disinfect all instruments contacting animals. House animal separately, and disinfect surfaces with halogens.
Class 2. Close Contact or Vector Transmission Required of Environmentally Nonresistant Organisms		
Bite transmitted	Rabies, *Babesia gibsoni* infection	Animals should be quarantined separately. With zoonoses, such as rabies, no direct human contact should occur without protective equipment.
Class 3. Zoonotic Potential with Direct Transmission to People		
Close salivary or genital contact for transmission, urinary transmission; zoonotic spread through mucosae or cuts in skin	Leptospirosis,[a] feline leukemia, canine herpesvirus infection, canine viral papillomatosis, canine brucellosis[a]	Provide no-contact housing. Disinfect hands between handling of patients. Wear protective clothing when handling urine or genital secretions from animals with zoonoses.
Fecal-oral transmission, low contagion; risk of spread enhanced by diarrheic feces	Giardiasis,[a] cryptosporidiosis,[a] salmonellosis,[a] campylobacteriosis,[a] feline coronavirus infections, toxoplasmosis[a]	Animal should remain in a designated cage. Clean and disinfect all cages and litter boxes, and dispose of all feces in sanitary containers. Protective clothing is recommended because most are zoonoses.
Class 4. Transmission by Infected Body Secretions with Organism of Moderate Environmental Resistance and Zoonotic Potential		
Aerosol transmission, high contagion	Feline herpesvirus infection, calicivirus infection, bordetellosis,[a] tuberculous mycobacteriosis,[a] canine respiratory viruses, canine distemper, feline chlamydiosis, plague,[a] tularemia[a]	House in separate facilities if infection is acute and active. Wear protective clothing, including headgear, when handling patient with zoonoses, and wash hands between patients.
Fecal-oral transmission, high contagion	Canine parvoviral infection, feline panleukopenia, canine distemper (multisystemic), infectious canine hepatitis	Strict isolation in separate facility. High risk of transmission and severe often fatal disease.

[a]Zoonotic potential with direct transmission to people.

Table • 94-15

Indications for Hand Hygiene in the Veterinary Hospital[a]

Hand Washing or Disinfection

1. At the times of arrival or leaving the hospital
2. Between direct contact with each patient
3. After touching likely contaminated inanimate objects (catheters, drapes, cages, soiled surgical or bedding linens)
4. After handling patients likely colonized with multiple or resistant bacteria
5. Before preparing food or medications for patients
6. After removing gloves because of potential leak
7. After inadvertent contact with urine, feces, blood, or other body fluids or secretions
8. After personal body functions, including urination, defecation, sneezing, coughing, or nose blowing

Wearing Latex Gloves

1. Before and after handling open wounds
2. Before performing surgical, endoscopic procedures, or placing indwelling catheters
3. Before handling particularly susceptible patients (immunosuppressed or with indwelling tubes or catheters)
4. Gloves should not be rinsed before removing because of potential leaks

[a]Adapted from recommendations from Osborne CA. 2000. Are your patients in safe hands? *DVM Newsmagazine* Mar-Apr: 24–26 and other sources.

tive in inactivating environmentally resistant organisms, such as *P. aeruginosa* and *Mycobacterium tuberculosis*, in air ducts is commercially available (Sterilite, AB-medica, Milan, Italy).[2]

Surgical Equipment

Surgical equipment should be appropriately sterilized with steam autoclaves or EO rather than cold disinfection, and it should be stored in dust-free, enclosed cabinets. Cold disinfection should be avoided when possible because it may be associated with the increased risk of infections from soil saprophytes such as *Clostridium tetani*. All surfaces in operating rooms that do not come in contact with the patient should be routinely disinfected with phenolic compounds. Floors can be washed with disinfectants and wet mopped or polished. Wet

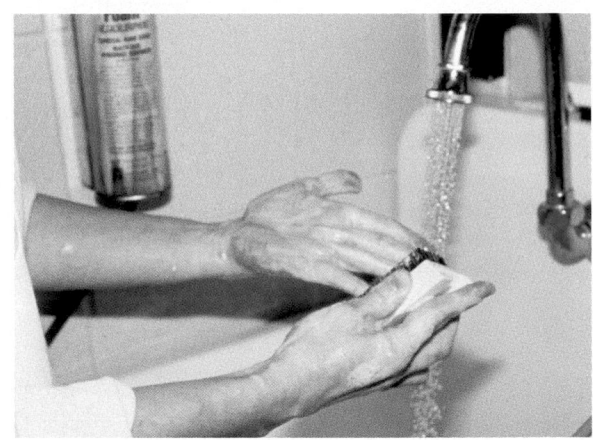

Fig 94-2 Proper hand-washing technique using soap and water. (Courtesy University of Georgia, Athens, Ga.)

Table • 94-16

Comparison of Commonly Used Topical Soaps and Antiseptics

AGENT	ADVANTAGES	DISADVANTAGES
Hand soap	Noncaustic, inexpensive	Liquids and moist bars support bacterial growth
Hexachlorophene (phenolic)	Good for *Staphylococcus*	Must use daily, central nervous system toxicity with absorption, minimal effect on gram-negative bacteria and fungi
Benzalkonium chloride (QUAT)	Inexpensive	Ineffective, harbors opportunistic bacteria (e.g., *Serratia*)
Alcohol	Relatively inexpensive, need 70% aqueous, ethanol Superior, rapid microbial killing, added moisturizers reduce irritation	Volatile, flammable, drying, bacterial resistance common
Iodine (halogen)	Good for viruses, fungi, and vegetative and sporulated bacteria; most effective as tincture; sustained germicidal action	Irritating, hypersensitivity, stains skin, drying
Iodophors (halogen)	Water soluble, low irritation, less staining	Reduced potency compared with iodine, drying

QUAT, Quaternary ammonium compound.

mops or vacuums with filtered exhaust elements can pick up excess disinfectant and loosening debris. Built-up disinfectant films can be removed with a solution of 0.12 L (one half cup) of vinegar in 3.8 L (1 gallon) of water. Dry mops and brooms should never be used to clean hospital floors because they disseminate microorganisms in dust. Personnel should wear facemasks to minimize aerosol contamination in surgery areas. Hand washing and gloving for surgery are superior to hand washing alone in minimizing the spread of skin microflora to the patient. Antisepsis of the skin at the incision site is similar to that in preparing IV catheter sites, but a final application of tincture of iodine or iodophor solution takes place just before the animal is draped.

Anesthesia and Nebulizer Equipment

Anesthesia and nebulizer equipment should be washed with water and detergents. This equipment may be heat sensitive, and it may need to be sterilized with EO gas or soaked in 2% glutaraldehyde for 30 minutes, followed by aeration or sterile water rinse, respectively. All equipment should be completely dry before it is used. Solid rubber facemasks that can withstand heat disinfection may be flash autoclaved at 56° C for 3 minutes.

Rubber anesthesia circuits can be disinfected by immersion in 80° C water for 15 minutes. Soda lime canisters should be completely emptied and disinfected by similar means when needed.

Nebulizers and humidifiers can be disinfected by flushing hydrogen peroxide (20% by volume in water) through the system. Acetic acid at a concentration of at least 2% has been used, but it is somewhat ineffective against the more resistant gram-negative bacteria. Chlorhexidine (0.02%) is better for this purpose, especially at a temperature of 50° C. Temperature-controlled nebulizers that can be maintained at 45° C have the lowest prevalence of contamination. Periodic disinfection of nebulizer chambers with chlorine bleach or sterilization with EO gas is also recommended.

Endoscopic Equipment

Endoscopic equipment should be cleaned with soap and water as soon as possible after each use to remove gross soil, rinsed thoroughly with clean water, then rinsed with a disinfectant solution. Iodophors and bleach are corrosive to metal parts. Flexible endoscopes should be effectively disinfected or sterilized between uses whenever possible, particularly if they are employed to examine normally sterile areas such as the respiratory and genitourinary tracts. Nosocomial outbreaks of *Pseudomonas* infections has been associated with incomplete cleaning of the biopsy channel of flexible bronchoscopes.[170] Flexible endoscopes can be sterilized by soaking in alkaline glutaraldehyde for 10 minutes and then rinsed with sterile water. Automated endoscope-reprocessing systems have also been developed that use performic acid as a sterilant.[149] Sterilization can be achieved with EO gas, but many endoscopes cannot withstand the 63° C aeration temperature that is commonly used and require more prolonged aeration at lower temperatures. Unlike rigid metal endoscopes, most flexible endoscopes cannot tolerate sterilization by steam autoclaving.

Cages

Animal-holding facilities must receive adequate disinfection. Mere cleansing of cages with liquid disinfectants between uses is insufficient. High-pressure cleaning will help remove organic residue (Fig. 94-3). Steam cleaning on a monthly basis is the most effective means of ward and cage sanitation. Transient washing at 82° C is considered optimal for cage disinfection except against spores of *Bacillus*, which can be killed if the washing is prolonged for a minute or more. Lower tem-

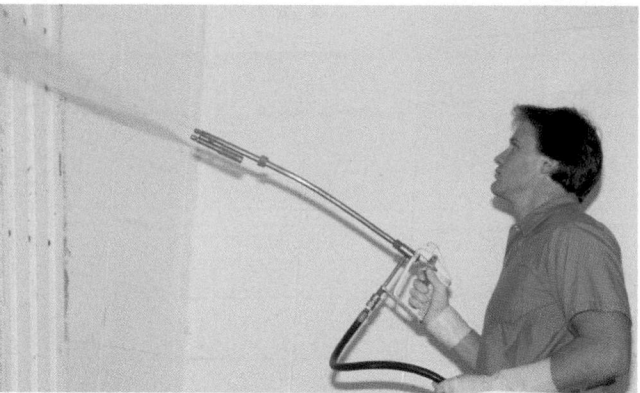

Fig 94-3 Spraying walls with water as a cleaning practice to reduce dust and debris that can harbor microorganisms. (Courtesy University of Georgia, Athens, Ga.)

peratures may be effective in destroying vegetative bacteria (Table 94-17).

Clothes and Dishes

Disinfection of these articles requires higher temperatures that can be achieved with automatic clothes washers, and dishwashers are preferred to manual rinsing (see Table 94-17). At high temperatures, most organisms will be killed; bacterial spores are the exception. Low-temperature (22° C) washing using laundry chemicals and bleach followed by drying is as effective as high-temperature (71° C) washing is for eliminating pathogenic bacteria.

CONTROL OF FREE-ROAMING ANIMALS

Free-roaming animals constitute a major reservoir for infectious diseases. Trapping, neutering, and returning animals to their environment has been done for free-roaming cats in many areas.[128,154] Zoonotic diseases transmitted by free-roaming cats include plague, rabies, toxoplasmosis, *Bartonella henselae* infection, and *Salmonella typhimurium* infection. Feral cats can also transmit these and other nonzoonotic infections such as FeLV and FIV to native wild felids. Animals should be identified, and many female cats are pregnant during the course of infection. Euthanasia of debilitated cats is usually required.

Quarantine to Reduce Spread of Exotic Infections

Restricting travel of infected dogs and cats is essential in some regions to control the spread of infections to nonendemic areas. The rapid speed and long distance of current international transportation of animals has a high risk of spreading infectious agents. Even quarantine may be insufficient to stop the entry of some persistent infections. Dogs infected with *Babesia*, *Ehrlichia*, and *Leishmania* have been detected in those imported into the United Kingdom under its new "Pet Travel Scheme" or conventional quarantine.[162] This system replaces the 6-month quarantine for some specified countries and rabies-free islands. A shortened quarantine period may facilitate the movement of animals into the general population and the potential of establishing an endemic focus, should suitable vectors or reservoir animal hosts be available.[167] In contrast, 6-month quarantine periods may have some psychologic effects on pets and their owners.[143] Future efforts to implement genetic screening for insidious exotic infectious agents may allow for more rapid detection of containment of infectious diseases and reduce the need for extended quarantines. Table 94-18 summarizes some infectious diseases of dogs

Table • **94-17**

Susceptibility of Bacteria to Heat Disinfection

PROCEDURE	ORGANISMS KILLED	TEMPERATURE °C	°F	TIME	COMMENTS
Dishwashing					
Automatic wash	Most vegetative bacteria	60	140	20 sec	Add detergent
Sterilization	All vegetative bacteria, most spores	82	180	10 sec	Add detergent
Manual wash	Some vegetative bacteria	43–49	110–120	10–20 sec	Add detergent
	All bacteria but spores	76.5	170	30 sec	Add disinfectant
Cage Cleaning	Gram-negative rods, gram-positive cocci	49	120	2–4 min	Steam or hot water
	Gram-negative rods	40–60	120–140	Instantaneous	Steam or hot water
	Gram-positive cocci	71	160	2–4 min	Steam or hot water
	All but *Bacillus* spores	82	180	Instantaneous	Steam or hot water
	Bacillus spores[188]	100	212	5 min	Steam or hot water
Anesthetic Tube Cleaning					
Mild disinfection	Most vegetative bacteria	55	132	3 min	Hot water
Pasteurization	All bacteria but spores	80	176	15 min	Hot water
Clothes Washing					
(Automatic)	All bacteria including spores	>71	>160	25 min	Add detergent and bleach to increase cidal activity
Heat Inactivation (dry heat)					
	Gram-negative rods	60	140	5 min	No organic material
		65	149	3 min	
		70	158	1 min	
	Unenveloped viruses	56–60	133–140	20–40 min	No organic material
		80	176	1 min	
	Foot-and-mouth disease virus[39]	50	122	2 days	No organic material
		80	176	3.75 min	No organic material
	Cryptosporidium	64	147	2 min	No organic material
		72	162	1 min	No organic material
	Giardia	70	158	10 min	No organic material
	Bacillus spores[188]	150	302	10	No organic material

and cats that require screening or quarantine for international travel.

VECTOR-BORNE INFECTIONS

Fleas

The host is essential in the maintenance and propagation of fleas in the environment. After feeding on the host, mating occurs, and the female begins to lay eggs within 24 hours. Forty or more eggs are laid per day, and they drop off in the host's environment. Fleas must be permanently associated with the host for survival. Use of insecticides and insect growth regulators with convenient formulations have allowed for control of fleas because of enhanced efficacy and improved owner compliance. Tables 94-19 and 94-20 summarize control measures for vectors of infectious diseases of dogs and cats.

Ticks

A large number of infectious agents, including viral, bacterial, and protozoa, are transmitted by ticks (Table 94-21). Most are three-host ticks in which each stage feeds on a different stage after molting. Most ticks of medical importance to dogs and cats are hard bodied, belonging to the family Ixodidae. These ticks have a hard dorsal back plate known as a scutum. The larval tick hatches from the egg within days to months, depending on environmental temperature and humidity. The tick can be recognized by having six legs and generally feeds on small rodents or birds because it remains on or close to the ground or on short vegetation. After feeding on the host for several days and becoming engorged, it drops off and molts into an eight-legged nymph. Nymphs find a suitable host, feed to engorgement, and then fall off to molt into the adult tick. Nymphs and adults generally feed on successively larger hosts. Ticks require feeding for reproduction and development. They seek (quest) for hosts during time periods when environmental temperature and humidity are suitable for this process. Once on the host, ticks crawl on the host to find a suitable place to attach. After they penetrate the epidermis and insert their hypostome, they secrete a cement-like substance that affixes them to the host. They do not feed until after 24 to 36 hours after attachment. Females, larvae, and nymphs slow feed

Table • 94-18

Organisms Persisting in the Host That Require Potential Screening or Quarantine for International Transport

ORGANISM (CHAPTER)	SCREENING METHOD	VECTOR	GEOGRAPHIC DISTRIBUTION
Rabies virus (22)	RFFIT or FAVN http://www.vet.ksu.edu/depts/rabies/	Mammalian carnivore by bites, rarely aerosols	Worldwide except some insular and peninsular nations
Ehrlichia canis (28)	Single IgG titer	Rhipicephalus sanguineus	Worldwide except some insular nations
Brucella canis (40)	Single IgG titer	Venereal, aerosols	Americas; foci in other areas
Leptospira spp. (44)	Agglutination titers with high values	No vectors	Worldwide and focused in temperate and tropical regions around water sources
Lyme borreliosis (45)	C6 protein-specific IgG assay or PCR of connective or other tissue	Ixodes spp. (ticks)	Worldwide with specific foci in vector habitat
Yersinia pestis (47)	Cytology and culture	Fleas	Wordwide with specific foci
Leishmania spp. (73)	Single IgG titer as a screen[a] Identification of organism by cytology, biopsy, culture, or PCR in blood, body fluids, or tissues	Phlebotomine sandflies	Worldwide with specific foci
Babesia spp. (77)	Serology as a screen[a]; cytology of blood smears or PCR of blood cells	Various ticks, dog bites, transfusions, venereal, congenital	Worldwide; however, certain foci and variable by species
Trypanosoma cruzi (72)	Single IgG titer as screen[a]; identification of organism by cytology or biopsy of blood or tissues	Reduvid bug	Americas in certain foci
Trypanosoma spp. (72)	Cytology of blood smears	Tse tse fly	Africa in certain foci
Hepatozoon canis (74)	Organism identification in blood smears; antibody titer performed	Rhipicephalus sanguineus	Worldwide foci in certain areas
Hepatozoon americanum (74)	Organism identification in muscle biopsy, rarely in blood smear	Amblyomma maculatum	Gulf Coast of North America
Cytauxzoon felis (76)	Organism identification in blood smears or as schizont in tissues	Dermacentor variabilis	Lower Eastern United States

RFFIT, Rapid fluorescent-focus inhibition test, FAVN, fluorescent antibody virus neutralization; PCR, polymerase chain reaction.
[a]Cross-reactivity within and between genera of protozoans can make this screening unreliable and may indicate transient infection or vector exposure; however, the presence of a antibody titer to one of these infections indicates further documentation should be considered.

for a range of 2 to 14 days, with the females feeding for the longest period. Male ticks feed briefly, if at all. In females that mate, a rapid feeding phase of engorgement occurs within the last day of attachment. While feeding, blood is consumed by the tick as its salivary gland secretions enter the host. These secretions contain biologically active compounds that serve as anticoagulants and antiinflammatory agents to help the tick avoid host immune mechanisms. Infectious agents harbored by the tick can be inoculated into the host during the feeding period.

Ticks can be removed manually using tweezers or forceps taking care using constant traction without twisting. Care should be taken so that mouthparts are not left embedded because foreign body inflammation will persist. Prevention involves periodic use of acaricides (see Tables 94-19 and 94-20).

Rhipicephalus sanguineus is one of the most ubiquitous tick species in the world. All three stages will feed on dogs, making it a domiciled pest wherever dogs are housed. As a result, the tick can be transported with dogs and establish infections in quarantine facilities and transmit infections to exposed dogs.

Although previously not found in the United Kingdom, live ticks have escaped detection and have been capable of propagating,[11] which may be caused by the change away from the 6-month quarantine as a result of reciprocity in the European Union. Live *R. sanguineus* have also been found in dogs living only in the United Kingdom that were exposed to automobiles or quarantine stations that housed imported dogs.

Sandflies

Flies of the genera *Lutzomyia* and *Phlebotomus* are important in the transmission of leishmaniasis. Control of these vectors should involve spraying the environment, most commonly with pyrethrin-based insecticides. Safer topical insecticides should also be applied to the skin and clothing of the human inhabitants and on animal fur. Because the dog is considered a potential reservoir in some countries, topical therapy or avoidance of vectors, which often feed at night, is essential in reducing the public health risk.[1]

Table • 94-19

Control Measures for Vectors of Infectious Diseases of Dogs and Cats

INSECT OR ARACHNID	AGENTS TRANSMITTED	CONTROL MEASURES	RECOMMENDED INSECTICIDES, REPELLENTS, GROWTH REGULATORS
Flies	*Leishmania* spp., *Anaplasma* sp., *Bacillus anthracis*, *Francisella tularensis*	Hair clipped around wound Pick larvae out of wound Sanitation Elimination of larval food Use of screens with small mesh size Use of light traps, baited jar traps	Host—DEET Environment—chlorpyrifos
Mites	*Rickettsia tsutsugamushi*	Skin scrape to detect Control environment and maintain sanitation	Amitraz, phthalimide dip, selamectin, ivermectin
Fleas	*Yersinia pestis*, *Rickettsia felis*, *Francisella tularensis*, *Rickettsia typhi*	Sanitation Treat infested animals with appropriate flea control Treat outdoors with sprays and elimination of rodents Treat indoors with use of vacuum and baseboards	DEET, permethrin, fipronil, imidacloprid, lufenuron, selamectin, nitenpyram, methoprene, pyriproxyfen, organophospates
Ticks	*Ehrlichia* spp., *Borrelia* spp., *Francisella tularensis*, *Hepatozoon* spp., *Rickettsia rickettsii*, *Cytauxzoon felis*, *Anaplasma phagocytophilum*, *Babesia* spp.	Remove leaf litter, landscape barriers, deer fencing, bait box placement, host treatment, biologic control (chitin-synthesis inhibitors)	DEET, fipronil, organophosphates, amitraz, permethrin, selamectin
Mosquitoes	Equine encephalomyelitis, West Nile virus	Avoiding infested habitats Wearing protective clothing Using insect repellent Draining of swamps Cleaning ditches Treating of streams and ponds Management and cleaning of storm water—retention structures	DEET, citronella, Skin-So-Soft Bath Oil®

Table • 94-20

Some Chemicals Used in the Control of Arthropod Vectors of Infectious Diseases of Dogs and Cats

CHEMICAL (BRAND NAME, COMPANY; PREPARATION)	AFFECTED VECTOR	DOSE (DURATION)	SPECTRUM
Organophosphates (Paramite™, Vet-Kem; topical sponge-ons)	*Ixodes scapularis* eliminated rapidly with environmental damage[189]	11.6% active ingredient; 1 oz/gal of water (kills adult fleas 16 days)	Ticks, fleas, mites (adulticide)
Amitraz (PREVENTIC™ collars, Virbac; impregnated collar)	*I. scapularis* did not transmit *Borrelia burgdorferi* 7 days after collar placed[52]	9% amitraz (one collar effective for 3 mos)	Ticks, mites (preventative: inhibits mouth parts)
Permethrin (Proticall®, Defend®, EXspot®, Schering-Plough; topical spray and spot-on)	*I. ricinus*,[140] *I. scapularis*, *Rhipicephalus sanguineus*, *Dermacentor variabilis*, *Ctenocephalides* spp.	1 cc/30 lb (effective against *Ixodes*, *C. felis* 4 wks, *Dermacentor* 3 wks)	Ticks, fleas (adulticide)
Fipronil (Frontline®, Merial; topical spray and spot-on)	*Ctenocephalides felis*, *Ixodes*, *Dermacentor*, *R. sanguineus*, *Amblyomma*, *Haemophysalis*,[161] *Otodectes*[40]	Contains 9.7% fipronil 7.5—15 mg/kg (every 30 days but can control fleas for up to 3 mos)	Ticks, fleas (adulticide, ovicide, larvicide)
Permethrin-imidacloprid (K9Advantix®, Bayer; topical spot-on)	*R. sanguineus* 98.5% efficacy after 3 days,[93] *D. variabilis*, *Ctenocephalides* spp., *I. ricinus* (product insert)	8.8% imidacloprid, 44.0% permethrin (every 30 days, kills ticks up to 4 wks)	Fleas, ticks, mosquitoes (adulticide, larvicide)
Imidacloprid (Advantage®, Bayer; topical spot-on)	*Ctenocephalides* spp. (product insert)	9.1% imidacloprid 10—20 mg/kg (every 30 days) <10 lb = 0.4 ml tubes, 11—20 lb = 1.0 ml, 21—55 lb = 2.5 ml, >50 lb = 4.0 ml	Fleas (adulticide, larvicide)
Lufenuron (Program®, Sentinel®, Novartis; oral)	*C. felis* on cats treated with 30 mg/kg produced nonviable eggs for 14 days; larvacidal activity for 32 to 44 days (product insert)	Injectable: 10 mg/kg (every 6 mos); oral suspension: 30 mg/kg (every 30 days); tablet: 10 mg/kg (every 30 days)	Fleas (larvicide, ovicide)
Lufenuron/milbemycin oxime (Program Plus®, Novartis; oral)	*C. felis*, *Dirofilaria immitis*, *Ancylostoma caninum*, *Toxocara canis*, *Trichuris vulpis* (product insert)	0.5 mg/kg milbemycin oxime, 10 mg/kg lufenuron every 10 days	Fleas (larvicide, ovicide); anthelmintic
Nitenpyram (Capstar™, Novartis; oral)	*C. felis*[161]	2—4 mg/kg (daily)	Fleas (adulticide)
Selamectin (Revolution™, Pfizer; topical spot-on)	*R. sanguineus*, *D. variabilis*,[140] *Ctenocephalides* spp., sarcoptic ascariasis[40]	Dog: 6 mg/kg (every 30 days)	Fleas, ticks, mites (adulticide, larvacide, ovicide)
Permethrin/methoprene (Zodiac FleaTrol®; topical spot-on)	*Ctenocephalides* spp. (product insert)	Permethrin 45%; methoprene 2.9% (every 30 days)	Fleas (ovicide)

Compiled from Elfassy OJ, Goodman FW, Levy SA, et al. 2001. Efficacy of an amitraz-impregnated collar in preventing transmission of *Borrelia burgdorferi* by adult *Ixodes scapularis* to dogs, *J Am Vet Med Assoc* 219:185–189; Endris EG, Cooke D, Amodie D, et al. 2002. Repellency and efficacy of 65% permethrin and selamectin spot-on formulations against *Ixodes ricinus* ticks and dogs, *Vet Ther* 3:64–71; Shaw SE, Birtles RJ, Day MJ. 2001. Arthropod-transmitted infectious diseases of cats, *J Feline Med Surg* 3:193–209; Demanuelle TC. 2000. Modern flea eradication: the best of the old and the new, *Vet Med* 95:701–704; Wilson ME. 2002. Prevention of tick borne diseases, *Med Clin N Am* 86:219–235; Kidd L. 2003. Transmission and prevention of tick-borne diseases in dogs, *Compend Cont Educ Pract Vet* 25: 742–747; FAN: http://www.fluorideaction.org/pesticides/lufenuron.fipronil.pets.htm.

Table • 94-21

Tick Vectors of Infectious Diseases of the Dog or Cat

SPECIES	INFECTIOUS DISEASE TRANSMITTED	MORPHOLOGY	PREFERRED HOSTS	GEOGRAPHIC DISTRIBUTION
Amblyomma americanum	Ehrlichia chaffeensis, E. ewingii, Borrelia lonestari, Francisella tularensis	Single white spot dorsal on female, males have white or yellow lines on scutum; long palps and hypostome, eyespots and festoons	L, N: ground birds, deer, canids, felids, rodents, people A: canids, herbivores	Fig. 28-3 Southern, Midwestern, and Eastern United States
Amblyomma maculatum	Hepatozoon americanum	Multiple black stripes on male scutum. Single black stripe on female scutum. Long palps and hypostome, eyespots and festoons.	L, N: small rodents, ground-dwelling birds, dogs A: canids, felids, herbivores	Fig. 74-10 Southeast and Midwestern United States
Dermacentor andersoni	R. rickettsii, F. tularensis	Second segment of palpi not laterally produced, mouthparts as long as basis capituli festoons present	L, N: voles, mice, canids, opossum, rabbit, raccoon A: canids, carnivores, herbivores	Fig. 29-3 Northwest United States
Dermacentor variabilis	Cytauxzoon felis, F. tularensis, Rickettsia rickettsii	White markings covering scutum, festoons on the posterior abdomen, and short palpi	L, N: voles, mice, canids, felids, opossum, rabbit A: felids, canids, herbivores	Fig. 29-3 Eastern and Midwestern United States, small strip along California coast
Ixodes pacificus	Anaplasma phagocytophilum, E. chaffeensis, B. burgdorferi	Anal groove in front of anus, palpus longer than hypostome; narrow basis capituli	L, N: lizards, small rodents, birds A: canids, herbivores	Fig. 45-2,B Northeast, Southeast, Western Coast of United States
Ixodes scapularis	A. phagocytophilum, Babesia microti, Borrelia burgdorferi	Anal groove in front of anus, palpus longer than hypostome; narrow basis capituli	L, N: rodents, birds, lizards, felids, squirrels A: felids, canids, herbivores	Fig. 45-2,B Northeast, Southeast, Western Coast of United States
Ixodes ricinus	Borrelia burgdorderi, A. phagocytophilum	Anal groove in front of anus, palpus longer than hypostome; narrow basis capituli	L, N: small rodents, birds A: large animals	Fig. 45-4 Europe, Mediterranean
Ixodes persulcatus	Borrelia burgdorferi	Anal groove in front of anus, palpus longer than hypostome; narrow basis capituli	L, N: small rodents, birds A: large animals	Fig. 45-4 Eurasia
Rhipicephalus sanguineus	Anaplasma platys, Babesia canis, Babesia gibsoni, Ehrlichia canis, Bartonella vinsonii subsp. berkhoffii	Festoons on the posterior abdomen	L, N: canids, rodents, rabbit A: canids	Worldwide

L, Larval ticks; N, nymphal ticks; A, adult ticks.

SUGGESTED READINGS*

20. Boerlin P, Eugster S, Gaschen F, et al. 2001. Transmission of opportunistic pathogens in a veterinary teaching hospital, *Vet Microbiol* 82:347-359.
32. Crnich CJ, Maki DG. 2004. Are antimicrobial-impregnated catheters effective? Don't throw out the baby with the bathwater, *Clin Infect Dis* 38:1287-1292.
40. Demanuelle TC. 2000. Modern flea eradication: the best of the old and the new, *Vet Med* 95:701-704.
46. Dryden MW, Broce AB. 2002. Integrated flea control for the 21st century, *Suppl Compend Contin Educ Pract Vet* 94:36-40.
51. Eleraky NZ, Potgieter LND, Kennedy MA. 2002. Virucidal efficacy of four new disinfectants, *J Am Anim Hosp Assoc* 38:231-234.
55. Endris RG, Cooke D, Amodie D, et al. 2002. Repellency and efficacy of 65% permethrin and selamectin spot-on formulations against *Ixodes ricinus* ticks on dogs, *Vet Ther* 3:64-71.
63. Francey T, Gaschen F, Nicolet J, et al. 2000. The role of *Acinetobacter baumannii* as a nosocomial pathogen for dogs and cats in an intensive care unit, *J Vet Intern Med* 14:177-183.
94. Kritchevsky SB, Braun BI, Wong ES, et al. 2001. Impact of hospital care on incidence of bloodstream infection: the evaluation of processes and indicators in infection control study, *Emerg Infect Dis* 7:193-196.

99. Lobetti RG, Joubert KE, Picard J, et al. 2002. Bacterial colonization of intravenous catheters in young dogs suspected to have parvoviral enteritis, *J Am Vet Med Assoc* 220:1321-1324.
109. McEwen SA, Fedorka-Cray PJ. 2002. Antimicrobial use and resistance in animals, *Clin Infect Dis* 34(Suppl 3):S93-S106.
113. Mermel LE. 2001. New technologies to prevent intravascular catheter-related bloodstream infections, *Emerg Infect Dis.* 7:197-199.
116. Nichols RL. 2001. Preventing surgical site infections: a surgeon's perspective, *Emerg Infect Dis* 7:220-224.
152. Sanchez S, McCrackin Stevenson MA, et al. 2002. Characterization of multidrug-resistant *Escherichia coli* isolates associated with nosocomial infections in dogs, *J Clin Microbiol* 40:3586-3595.
162. Shaw SE, Lerga AI, Williams S, et al. 2003. Review of exotic infectious diseases in small animals entering the United Kingdom from abroad diagnosed by PCR, *Vet Rec* 152:176-177.
169. Slaughter SE. 2004. Intravascular catheter-related infections, *Postgrad Med* 116:59-66.
181. Tomlin J, Pead MJ, Lloyd DH, et al. 1999. Methicillin-resistant *Staphylococcus aureus* infections in 11 dogs, *Vet Rec* 16:60-64.

*See the CD-ROM for a complete list of references.

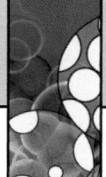

CHAPTER • 95

Immunodeficiencies and Infectious Diseases

Urs Giger and Craig E. Greene

Immunodeficiencies are a large heterogeneous group of hereditary and acquired disorders of host immunity that can be associated with an increased risk of infection (Table 95-1).[40,77,92,102] They can arise through disturbances in antigen-specific defense mechanisms mediated by lymphocytes, the nonspecific defense system (which includes phagocytes, plasma proteins, and physical barriers), or both. Although the exact pathogenesis of many canine and feline immunodeficiencies remains unknown, the molecular defects for some forms have been elucidated. Because many effective preventive and therapeutic measures are now available to control infectious diseases in individuals with intact host defense mechanisms, animals with persistent, antimicrobial-unresponsive infections likely suffer from an immunodeficiency disorder. A few hereditary immunodeficiency disorders are prevalent within certain breeds of dogs and cats, whereas others have been described once and may currently exist only in research animal colonies.

Some major clinical features suggest that a patient has an impaired immune system (Table 95-2). Specific organisms and medical conditions often implicated in immunocompromised hosts are listed in Table 95-3. A definitive diagnosis often requires specific immune testing in addition to routine laboratory tests, and therapeutic interventions are limited. Immun-

odeficiencies can be divided into primary or secondary forms depending on whether they are inherited or acquired.

PRIMARY OR HEREDITARY IMMUNODEFICIENCIES

Many genetically determined immune defects have been described in the dog, whereas only a few are known in cats. They occur rarely and are summarized in Table 95-4; some are discussed next in more detail in the Specific Primary or Inherited Immunodeficiencies section of this chapter. They can be broadly classified according to defects of the specific or nonspecific immune system as well as combinations thereof.[72] The nonspecific immune system, also known as *innate* or *natural immunity*, should be functional at birth and available on short notice to protect the host from invasion by all sorts of organisms. It includes physicochemical barriers, phagocytes, complement and other plasma proteins, and natural killer cells. Congenital barrier defects particularly involve the skin and mucous membrane surfaces and are associated with infections of particular organs. The Ehlers-Danlos syndrome, causing fragile, hyperextendable skin in many dogs and cats as well as the myxedematous skin and immunodeficiencies of Shar-peis,

Table • 95-1

Features of Immunodeficiency Diseases Based on the Underlying Defect

DEFECT	SUSCEPTIBILITY TO SPECIFIC INFECTIONS	DIAGNOSTIC TESTS TO CONFIRM DEFECT
Physical barrier		
Ciliary dyskinesia	Respiratory infections	Electron microscopy of cilia
Ehlers-Danlos syndrome	Skin injury and infections	Histopathology and electron microscopy of skin
B cell	Pyogenic bacteria, *Giardia* spp.	Globulin, serum electrophoresis, tetanus antibody response
T cell	Bacterial sepsis, mycobacteria, *Candida* and *Pneumocystis* spp.	Thymic radiographs, skin testing delayed hypersensitivity, CD4 and CD8 lymphocytes
Granulocyte	Bacteria; streptococci; *Pseudomonas*, *Candida*, *Nocardia*, and *Aspergillus* spp.	Neutrophil count, phagocytosis assays
Complement	Pyogenic bacteria	CH_{50} assay

Table • 95-2

Major Clinical Signs of Immunodeficiency Disorders

1. Recurrent infections, chronic and protracted course of infection, or both
2. Infection with common nonpathogenic (opportunistic) or aberrant infectious agents
3. Severe and often atypical infectious disease manifestations
4. Delayed, incomplete, or lack of response to antimicrobial therapy
5. Adverse reactions to modified-live virus vaccines

Table • 95-3

Organisms and Medical Problems Commonly Implicated in Immunocompromised Hosts

Opportunistic Organisms

Viruses: Feline herpesvirus, feline infectious peritonitis virus, feline calicivirus, canine papillomavirus, canine herpesvirus

Mycoplasma: *Mycoplasma haemofelis*

Bacteria: *Citrobacter* spp., *Escherichia coli*, *Enterobacter* spp., *Klebsiella pneumoniae*, *Mycobacterium* spp., *Nocardia asteroides*, *Proteus* spp., *Pseudomonas aeruginosa*, *Serratia marcescens*, *Staphylococcus intermedius*

Fungi: *Aspergillus* spp., *Candida* spp., *Cryptococcus* spp., *Histoplasma* spp., *Blastomyces* spp., *Coccidioides* spp., *Mucor* spp.

Protozoa: *Pneumocystis* spp., *Toxoplasma gondii*, *Neospora caninum*, *Cryptosporidium* spp., *Giardia* spp., *Tritrichomonas* spp., *Isospora* spp.

Metazoa: *Demodex canis*, *Otodectes notoedres*

Medical Problems

Recurrent skin infections
Recurrent mucosal infections
Neonatal sepsis and mortality
Reactive amyloidosis
Vasculitis, arteritis, polyarthritis
Recurrent bacteremia
Granulomatous infections
Chronic hypersensitivity reactions
Autoimmune diseases
Persistent intracellular rickettsial or bacterial infections
Disproportional leukocytosis
Persistent lymphopenia

predisposes the animals to pyoderma, whereas ciliary dyskinesia in dogs increases the susceptibility to rhinosinusitis and pneumonia. Disorders of the phagocytic system involve defects of neutrophils and monocytes as well as the complement system and can lead to pyogenic and granulomatous infections. The granulomatous reaction can occur when neutrophils malfunction and mononuclear cells are recruited. A wide variety of pyogenic bacteria (e.g., staphylococci, *Escherichia coli*, *Klebsiella*, *Enterobacter*) are usually involved, most of which are normal microflora or pathogens of relatively low virulence. Recurrent infections of the skin, respiratory tract, and oral cavity are common, and intermittent bacteremia and overwhelming sepsis are also seen. Multisystemic amyloidosis, vasculitis, and immune complex disease are complications that can occur as a result of chronic recurrent or persistent infection. Cyclic hematopoiesis and leukocyte adhesion deficiency (LAD) are examples of quantitative and qualitative phagocytic defects, respectively.

The specific immune system can be divided into humoral and cell-mediated immune systems and includes B and T lymphocytes, immunoglobulins, and cytokines.[72] Deficiencies of B lymphocytes or humoral immunity affect the production of immunoglobulins and lead to increased susceptibility to pyogenic bacterial infections. Deficiencies of T lymphocytes or cell-mediated immunity (CMI) are associated with viral and fungal infections, but intracellular bacterial infections may also occur. Animals with cellular immunodeficiencies may have smaller thymic and tonsillar tissues as well as intestinal

and peripheral lymph nodes and decreased numbers of circulating lymphocytes.

The degree of immunodeficiency varies greatly between defects. Infections may be systemic or restricted to a particular organ system like the skin or respiratory tract. Some immunodeficiencies lead to overwhelming infections and

Table • 95-4

Primary or Hereditary Immunodeficiencies of Dogs and Cats[a]

DISEASE (SYNONYMS)	INHERITANCE[b]	BREEDS	DEFECT	CHARACTERIZATION
Dogs				
Ciliary dyskinesia[48,68,81,142] (immotile cilia syndrome)	AR	Many breeds[b]	Functional and morphologic cilia abnormalities	Rhinosinusitis, bronchopneumonia with bronchiectasis, situs inversus
Complement component 3[14,248,249] (C3 deficiency)	AR	Brittany spaniel	C3 deficiency	Pyogenic infections, lack of C-mediated phagocytosis in colony of dogs with neuromuscular disease
Neutrophil Defects				
Bactericidal neutrophil defect[17]	U	Doberman pinscher	Unknown	Upper respiratory infections, reduced bactericidal activity, ciliary dyskinesia not excluded
Cyclic hematopoiesis[126,151] (cyclic neutropenia)	AR	Collie (gray)	Hematopoietic growth factor defect	Severe neutropenia every 12—14 days, reactive amyloidosis
Chronic idiopathic neutropenia[138]	U	Rottweiler	G-CSF deficiency	Recurrent fever, sepsis, polyarthritis, pyoderma
Leukocyte adhesion deficiency[c]	AR	Irish setter, Red and white setter	CD11/18 deficiency β chain (CD18) deficiency	Severe leukocytosis, infection with limited pus formation, lack of neutrophil adhesion
Pelger-Huët anomaly[16,140]	AD	Australian shepherd, foxhound, others	Unknown	No immunodeficiency, hyposegmented granulocytes
Selective cobalamin malabsorption[86,87,187]	AR	Giant schnauzer, border collie, beagle, Australian shepherd	Ileal cobalamin receptor defect	Weight loss, inappetence, leukopenia with hypersegmentation megaloblastic bone marrow, methylmalonic aciduria
Cell-Mediated Immune Defects				
Increased susceptibility to avian mycobacteriosis[41,56,107,227]	U	Basset hound	Possible RAMP deficiency	Systemic avian tuberculosis (see Chapter 50), toxoplasmosis and neosporosis
Increased susceptibility to Pneumocystis pneumonia[15,39,70]	AR	Dachshund	Unknown	Pneumocystis pneumonia (see Chapter 68)
Susceptibility to fungal and rickettsial infections; pyoderma[29,50,173,210,250]	U	German shepherd	Possible macrophage or T-cell defect	Severe ehrlichiosis (see Chapter 28), Rocky Mountain spotted fever (see Chapter 29), disseminated aspergillosis (see Chapter 64), deep pyoderma
X-linked severe combined immunodeficiency (X-SCID)[d]	XR	Basset hound, Cardigan Welsh corgi	Common gamma chain of IL-2 and other cytokines	Severe bacterial and viral infections, no IgG and IgA, deficient lymphocyte blastogenesis
Severe combined immunodeficiency (SCID)[d]	AR	Jack Russell terrier	DNA-protein kinase catalytic subunit	Severe serum immunoglobulin deficiency, hypoplasia of lymphoid tissues
Combined immunodeficiency[206]	U	Shar-pei	T-cell and B-cell defects, low IL-6 and IL-2	Skin, respiratory, and gastrointestinal infections
Immune vasculitis, amyloidosis[e]	U	Shar-pei	Elevated IL-6	Arthritis, amyloidosis, renal failure, hepatic rupture, hypoproteinemia

Table continued on the next page

Table • 95-4

Continued

DISEASE (SYNONYMS)	INHERITANCE[a]	BREEDS	DEFECT	CHARACTERIZATION
Lethal acrodermatitis[123]	AR	Bull terrier	Zinc metabolism defect	Zinc deficiency, hyperkeratosis
Increased susceptibility to parvoviral infection	U	Rottweiler, Doberman pinscher	Unknown	Parvovirus infection (see Chapter 8)
Vaccine-exacerbated immune disturbance[66]	U	Akita	Unknown	Variable meningitis, polyarthritis, amyloidosis (see Chapter 100)
Thymic abnormalities and dwarfism[211, 212]	U	Weimaraner	Unknown	Reduced growth, thymosin responsive
Humoral Immune Defects				
Recurrent infections[41,56,107,227]	U	Weimaraner	Reduced IgG	Pyoderma, severe abscess, bleeding tendency (HOD, see Chapter 100)
Selective IgA deficiency[73,89,97,175,247]	U	Beagle, Shar-pei, German shepherd	IgA deficiency	Respiratory and GI infections
Cats				
Hypotrichosis congenital and thymic atrophy[25]	AR	Birman	Unknown	Nude kittens, neonatal death, no thymus
Leukocyte granulation[115]	U	Birman	Unknown	No immunodeficiency, acidophilic granules
Pelger-Huët anomaly[141]	AD	Domestic shorthair	Unknown	No immunodeficiency, hyposegmentation
Chédiak-Higashi syndrome[37,135]	AR	Persian	Unknown	No immunodeficiency, large granules in phagocytes, bleeding tendency
Reactive (AA) amyloidosis[62,63,108]	U	Abyssinian	Unknown	Reactive (AA) amyloidosis, renal failure
Feline GM1 gangliosidosis[42]	U	Domestic shorthair	Unknown	Premature thymic involution

G-CSF, granulocyte colony-stimulating factor, HOD, hypertrophic osteodystrophy RAMP, resistance-associated macrophage protein. AR, Autosomal recessive; U, unknown; XR, X-linked recessive; AD, autosomal dominant.
[a]For additional references, see Reference 102. In addition to the listed syndromes, bone marrow dyscrasias have been described in miniature and toy poodles and transient hypogammaglobulinemia in Samoyeds, but less is known of these disorders.
[b]For example, springer spaniel, old English sheepdog, English setter, West Highland white terrier, pointer.
[c]References 57, 93, 203, 232, 233, 235.
[d]References 60, 77, 78, 114, 122, 219–222.
[e]References 64, 125, 149, 162, 207, 208, 229.

death within the first few days to weeks of life, whereas others, such as morphologic leukocyte changes, are not consistently associated with any noticeable predisposition to infection. Chédiak-Higashi syndrome in smoke-colored Persian cats is characterized by abnormally large eosinophilic granules in polymorphonuclear leukocytes. It causes no immunodeficiencies but does cause a bleeding tendency resulting from a platelet storage pool disease.[171] Similarly, Birman cats with acidophilic granulation of neutrophils and dogs and cats with various lysosomal storage diseases (e.g., mucopolysaccharidosis, gangliosidosis, mannosidosis) have granulation or vacuolation of leukocytes without being immunocompromised. The Pelger-Huët anomaly, which is characterized by hyposegmentation of granulocytes, causes no immunodeficiency, despite the fact that the leukograms of affected dogs and cats reveal the most severe left shift with a normal leukocyte count. In foxhounds, in vitro chemotactic response of these neutrophils

was diminished, whereas in basenjis no functional abnormalities have been found.[16,139-141]

Although an increased susceptibility to opportunistic infections develops, the type of infection varies depending on the type of defect within the immune system. A few immunodeficiency disorders predispose animals to a restricted group of unusual infectious agents. Some male dachshunds appear predisposed to *Pneumocystis* pneumonia, and German shepherd dogs may be prone to systemic aspergillosis or rickettsioses. Doberman pinschers and Rottweiler dogs are more likely to develop parvoviral disease. Golden and Labrador retrievers that had high serum antibody titers to *Borrelia burgdorferi* were more likely to have glomerulonephritis.[47] Basset hounds and miniature schnauzers have an increased susceptibility to systemic avian mycobacteriosis, toxoplasmosis, and neosporosis. Foxhounds appear to be predisposed to developing leishmaniasis. Great Danes and Dobermans may

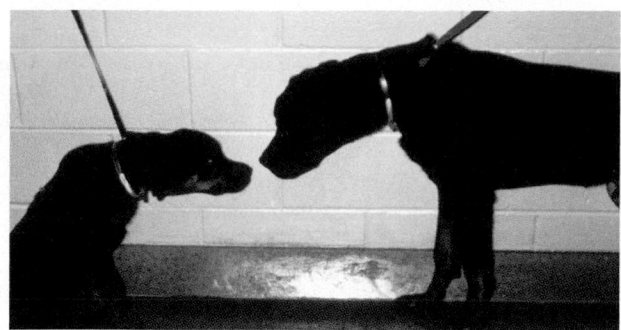

Fig 95-1 Two littermate Rottweiler pups. Pup on left has stunted growth from chronic recurrent infections. (Courtesy University of Georgia, Athens, Ga.)

be more susceptible to cryptococcal infections.[157] A genetic predisposition to demodicosis has been proposed in various canine breeds and families. Feline infectious peritonitis has also been suggested to have a genetic basis (see Chapter 11). The mechanisms predisposing particular animals to specific infections remain unknown in many breeds.

The previously mentioned key signs of infection (see Table 95-2) develop in animals with a primary immunodeficiency generally early in life. Despite receiving colostrum, clinically affected animals may have illness during the neonatal to juvenile period and may develop recurrent and overwhelming infections that lead to severe debilitation and death before 1 year of age. Several animals, but typically not all, in a litter may be affected, whereas the parents are usually healthy. A genetic predisposition to infection is rarely noted after 1 year of age (e.g., avian tuberculosis in basset hounds). Furthermore, animals with primary immunodeficiencies may have other special clinical manifestations. Hypersensitivity reactions may occur and reflect an overall dysregulation of the immune system caused by a lack of one or more components or a chronic antigen stimulation from inadequate clearance of infections. Chronic systemic infections may also hamper the growth rate (Fig. 95-1). Characteristic coat color dilutions and increased tendency for surface bleeding are seen in collies with cyclic hematopoiesis, Persian cats with Chédiak-Higashi syndrome, and Weimaraners with an incompletely defined immunodeficiency.

The mode of inheritance of primary immunodeficiencies has not yet been determined in all cases. Autosomal recessive transmission, with affected males and females born to healthy parents, is usual, but a few exceptions exist. The Pelger-Huët anomaly is inherited as an autosomal dominant trait. A severe combined immunodeficiency from different mutations in the common γ-chain interleukin-2 (IL-2) receptor in basset hounds and Cardigan Welsh corgis is an X-linked recessive disorder, so only males are affected, and the dams and half of the female littermates are carriers. Thus the breed, gender, age of onset, type of infections, and other special characteristics may suggest a particular immunodeficiency.

SECONDARY OR ACQUIRED IMMUNODEFICIENCIES

All components of the immune system of animals with secondary immunodeficiencies are initially intact and functional but become transiently or permanently impaired during or after an underlying disease condition or exposure to certain agents. Thus secondary immunodeficiencies occur much more commonly than primary forms. They are associated with organ impairment and entrance of infectious agents into the body.

This infection may cause additional damage to the particular organ or lead to systemic infectious diseases. Various barrier disturbances lead to surface infections, such as respiratory tract, urogenital, and gastrointestinal infections and dermatitis. Furthermore, certain infections, particularly viral diseases in cats, directly impair the immune system, predisposing the animals to secondary bacterial, fungal, or protozoal infections. For example, cats infected with the feline immunodeficiency virus (FIV) harbor more diverse fungal microflora on the hair and mucosal surfaces than noninfected cats,[218] which may predispose the FIV-infected cats to a greater prevalence of secondary fungal infections.

Puppies and kittens are particularly vulnerable to infections because of their incompletely developed immune systems. Colostrum intake during the first day of life transfers maternal immunoglobulins and provides protection during the first few weeks of life in small animals. Although colostrum deprivation has been shown in large animals to result in major neonatal losses, neonatal kittens and puppies kept in high-quality catteries or kennels do not seem to be predisposed to infections. However, a transient hypoglobulinemia after the decline of maternal antibodies in the plasma and before the immunocompetency of 2- to 4-month-old animals may increase the susceptibility to various infections.[217] Similarly, older animals may again become immunocompromised. Various drugs and chemicals as well as nutritional deficiencies may drastically impair the production and function of leukocytes. Known secondary immunodeficiencies in companion animals are listed in Table 95-5, and some are discussed in detail at the end of this chapter.

DIAGNOSTIC STUDIES

Although an immunodeficiency may be suspected on the basis of clinical evidence, specific laboratory tests are generally required to reach a definitive diagnosis.[90] A minimum database of information, including results of a complete blood count, serum chemistry screen, and urinalysis, should always be obtained and may suggest a specific disorder. The differential leukocyte count is the most important test result. Leukopenia in the presence of an active bacterial infection is by far the most feared condition. It should be noted that generally, some breeds have low white blood cell counts. Neutropenia may be transient, as it is with cyclic hematopoiesis every 12 to 14 days, or persistent, as it is in animals with cobalamin deficiency or overwhelming infections (sepsis). Lymphopenia may be observed in dogs with a T-cell or severe combined immunodeficiency. Although leukocytosis is expected during periods of infection, defects in leukocyte adhesion and egress from blood circulation at sites of infection may be associated with disproportionately high leukocytosis for the degree of infection as with hereditary LAD and glucocorticoid usage. Dachshunds with *Pneumocystis* pneumonia also have very marked leukocytosis. The erythrocyte count may be in the normal range even if the animals have active infections and during periods of treatment and remission. Careful review of a blood smear may reveal leukocyte abnormalities such as granulation and vacuolation resulting from lysosomal storage diseases or Chédiak-Higashi syndrome,[135] acidophilic granulation of leukocytes in Birmans,[115] phagocytized microorganisms, or toxic leukocyte changes that suggest overwhelming infections.

Serum globulin concentrations are generally higher during chronic infections. Low or normal globulin levels in infected animals may suggest major external losses or diminished production from a humoral (B-cell) immune defect. Indeed, specific immunoglobulin deficiencies have been recognized in dogs. Serum protein electrophoresis may identify a γ-globulin

Table • 95-5

Secondary or Acquired Immunodeficiencies

Age Related	Barrier Impairment	Physical, Chemical, or Drug-Induced[67]
Colostrum deprivation	Burns	Whole body irradiation
Neonatal hypothermia	Invasive or indwelling catheters	Myelosuppressive drugs
Transient hypoglobulinemia	Endoscopic devices	Cytotoxic agents
(between 2–6 mos)	Splenectomy	Chloramphenicol
Weakened immune system in very	Centesis	Barbiturates
young and old[100,215,217]		Griseofulvin
		Estrogens (dogs and ferrets)
Organ Disorders	**Immunosuppressive Co-Infections**	Immunosuppression
Hyperadrenocorticism	Feline leukemia virus (FeLV)[116,136,155]	Glucocorticoids[61]
Diabetes mellitus	Feline immunodeficiency virus*	Infectious agents—*Ehrlichia canis, FeLV*
Hepatic insufficiency	Feline and canine parvovirus	Anesthetic agents
Skin diseases	Canine distemper virus	Antibacterial- or antacid-induced
Pulmonary diseases	Canine retrovirus[13,174,193,223,224]	alteration of intestinal microflora
Gastrointestinal diseases	Demodicosis[6]	
Malnutrition	Ehrlichiosis	**Nutritional Disorders**
Systemic lupus erythematosus	Protracted bacterial infections	Vitamin A deficiency
Chronic hemolytic anemias		Vitamin E deficiency
Dysproteinemias		Protein-caloric restriction
Cancer		Zinc deficiency
Hemopoietic neoplasia		

*References: 5, 22, 49, 116, 159, 204, 205, 230, 253

deficiency, but immunoelectrophoresis is required to detect the class and degree of immunoglobulin deficiency. Maternal immunoglobulins can only be absorbed during the first day of life and influence the values during the first few weeks. IgM can be synthesized very early in life, whereas the development of IgA may be delayed for months. Thus it is important to compare values with data from age-matched controls. Titers against specific antigens can be measured, followed by evaluation of the antibody response to vaccination against particular agents. However, despite the antibody titer level, cellular immunity is not being assessed. Biopsy specimens of lymph nodes may reveal disorganization with loss of germinal centers and normal paracortical lymphocytes. Decreases in plasma cell populations may also be evident.

T-cell or combined immunodeficiencies cause defective CMI responses. The animal may have prolonged allograft rejection times and decreased delayed-type hypersensitivity to skin testing with viral vaccines, tuberculin, or dinitrochlorobenzene (DNCB).[186] Reduced in vitro lymphocyte stimulation results may also be caused by a primary lymphocyte defect or the infection.

The identification of the agents infecting an animal is important for diagnostic as well as therapeutic reasons. (Appropriate cultures of tissues, body fluids, and excretions for microorganisms and antigen and serologic blood tests are addressed in the chapters on specific infectious agents.) Antibody titers may also be used to assess a response to vaccines and humoral immunity. For instance, Rottweilers appear to respond late to parvovirus vaccines and have an increased susceptibility to the infection.

Gross and microscopic histopathology and cytology may reveal certain microorganisms but are most helpful in characterizing the architecture, morphology, maturation, and function of the immune system, such as of the leukocytes, bone marrow, lymph nodes, thymus, and spleen, as well as other barrier systems. In ciliary dyskinesia, morphologic abnormalities of cilia may be identified by electron microscopy, but functional studies by imaging techniques or on respiratory epithelial biopsy specimens are also indicated.

For additional characterization of the immunodeficiencies, special leukocyte studies are often required. Surface marker studies by fluorescent-assisted cell sorters or flow cytometers can differentiate between T- and B-cells, determine T- and B-cell ratios, and determine the presence or absence of leukocyte adhesion proteins (CD11/18) or IL-2 receptors. Lymphocyte function studies include lymphocyte stimulation and plaque-forming assays for in vitro immunoglobulin production. Phagocyte function studies assess leukocyte adhesion, migration, chemotaxis, phagocytosis, "respiratory burst," and bactericidal activity. All functional assays should be performed on fresh blood cells and compared simultaneously with an age- and breed-matched control. Furthermore, in vitro lymphocyte functions are generally impaired and phagocyte functions are enhanced during periods of active infection. Whenever possible, it is advisable to control the infection before studying leukocyte function.

TREATMENT AND PREVENTION

Successful control of infection in immunodeficient animals depends on the underlying disease as well as the type and severity of the immune defect. In immunocompromised patients, early and aggressive antimicrobial therapy is indicated even for mild infections with nonpathogenic agents. Because of the immunodeficient host's potential inability to kill bacteria, bactericidal antibiotics are recommended until bacterial infections are controlled. If the underlying disorder causing a secondary immunodeficiency can be corrected, the infection is often easily controlled. The underlying disorder should be treated and triggering agents such as drugs eliminated immediately.

No practical treatments for primary immunodeficiencies exist. Immunocompromised animals with infection generally have a guarded to poor prognosis. Despite aggressive antimicrobial therapy, their infections are difficult to control, leading to overwhelming infections, protracted courses, and recurrences. Some leukocyte defects cause death before 1 year of age, whereas others may not lead to a markedly increased predisposition to infection. In experimental studies, bone marrow transplantation corrected several leukocyte defects.[111,152] Granulocyte colony-stimulating factor (GCSF) has been used to increase neutrophil numbers and treat chemotherapy-induced and cyclic neutropenia (see Chapter 2).

Fresh whole blood may be transfused repeatedly to animals with overwhelming infections and neutropenia or neutrophil dysfunction, but the effect is very transient. Plasma transfusions or immunoglobulin injections may temporarily support animals with humoral immunodeficiencies. However, these products should not be used in animals with complete IgA deficiency because they may experience anaphylactic reactions to the foreign IgA protein. No commercial canine γ-globulin is available, and the human γ-globulin preparations are exorbitantly expensive and may cause allergic reactions upon repeated use. No data support their use in immunodeficient infected small animals, although they have been successfully treated immune-mediated diseases. Nonspecific immunostimulators have not been documented as being beneficial in animals with cell-mediated immunodeficiencies. However, immunocompromised animals with active infections should not be vaccinated. Furthermore, the use of modified live virus (MLV) vaccines should be avoided in animals with inherited or acquired T-cell defects, because they may develop clinical disease from the vaccine virus.

Owners must consider the potential zoonotic risks involved with keeping an immunodeficient animal with infections that may be contagious to humans, particularly immunosuppressed humans (see Chapter 99).

SPECIFIC PRIMARY OR INHERITED IMMUNODEFICIENCIES

Dogs

Primary Ciliary Dyskinesia

Primary ciliary dyskinesia, also known as *immotile cilia syndrome*, is caused by various functional and ultrastructural ciliary abnormalities, including lack of outer or inner dynein arms, abnormal microtubular pattern, random ciliary orientation, and electron-dense cores in the basal body. Because of impaired mucociliary clearance, affected animals have recurrent bacterial rhinitis, sinusitis, and bronchopneumonia with bronchiectasis. Poorly motile or immotile live sperms lead to male infertility, and although evidence is lacking, dysfunction of ependymal cilia may cause hydrocephalus. Otitis media may also occur. The lack of coordinated cilia motility during embryogenesis is responsible for the 50% prevalence of concurrent situs inversus in some forms of primary ciliary dyskinesia. The clinical triad of rhinosinusitis, bronchiectasis, and situs inversus is known as *Kartagener's syndrome*.[68,177,201]

Primary ciliary dyskinesia is inherited by an autosomal recessive trait. It represents a heterogeneous group of defects that have been described in more than a dozen breeds.[244] Clinical signs typically begin at a young age, and recurrent respiratory infections lead to death or euthanasia before 1 year of age. However, a few dogs have remained nonsymptomatic for months to years.[81] A diagnosis is reached by documenting an absence of ciliary clearance of a microaggregated albumin that is labeled with technetium 99m (Tc 99m) and placed through

a catheter into the nasal cavity or the tracheal bifurcation and by tissue biopsy of ciliated mucosae with ultrastructural analysis and in vitro motility studies.[33,48] Induction of ciliogenesis can also be determined by use of in vitro cell culture.[33]

Rhinitis and Bronchopneumonia in Irish Wolfhounds

Chronic recurrent respiratory infections have been observed in related Irish wolfhounds from Europe and Canada.[34,142] In puppies the disease begins with a serous rhinitis that later becomes catarrhal to hemorrhagic with turbinate ulceration and destruction. Pneumonia and generalized lymphadenomegaly are apparent in later stages. Although the disease is responsive to antimicrobial treatment, it may progress in intervening periods. Although a familial relationship exists, the exact mode of inheritance and the underlying defect are uncertain. A primary ciliary dyskinesia has been identified in some wolfhounds[24] but has not been a consistent feature of the disease. Serum IgA levels were reduced in some dogs, but bronchoalveolar lavage fluid had high IgA concentrations in tested dogs, which may relate to their inflammatory response to infection.[34]

Neutrophil Bactericidal Defect with Respiratory Infection in Doberman Pinschers

Neutrophil dysfunction was described in a family of Doberman pinschers in which a young animal had chronic recurrent respiratory tract infections.[17] Oxygen radical formation and bactericidal activity of neutrophils were reduced despite normal phagocytosis of bacteria. The specific defect has not yet been identified, and primary ciliary dyskinesia has not been completely ruled out. The ciliary morphology appeared normal, but no functional studies have been performed. Affected Doberman pinschers develop clinical signs of upper respiratory tract infections at a few weeks of age. They respond to antibiotics, but the prognosis is guarded.

Cyclic Hematopoiesis

Cyclic hematopoiesis is characterized by a periodic production and maturation defect of hematopoietic cells in the bone marrow.[178] In affected dogs, all blood cell counts cycle precisely at a 12- to 14-day interval, whereas in human patients the cycle is 21 days. Because of the short half-life of granulocytes, severe neutropenia (fewer than 1000 per microliter) is seen every 12 to 14 days and lasts for 3 to 4 days, thus the synonym *cyclic neutropenia syndrome*. Serial blood counts are used to reach a definitive diagnosis. During periods of severe neutropenia, dogs are highly susceptible to bacterial infections. Clinical symptoms appear at 6 to 8 weeks of age with regularly recurring bacterial infections (Fig. 95-2). The chronic exposure leads to systemic amyloidosis, and death may be result from organ failure (of the kidney and other organs) and sepsis before 1 year of age. Furthermore, gingival bleeding may occur from an associated platelet storage pool disease. Affected collies have a silver gray or light beige to tan coat color, and secondary hormonal cycling has been observed.[126,151]

Cyclic hematopoiesis was the first reported canine immunodeficiency observed and has only been clearly described in collies that are hypopigmented, hence the term *gray collie syndrome*. It is inherited as an autosomal recessive trait, but no clinical case has been reported since the 1970s. The basic mechanism for the defect is still being determined. Experimentally, bone marrow transplantation completely corrects this syndrome, including the coat color dilution. Furthermore, administration of lithium carbonate at extremely high and otherwise toxic doses is known to induce leukocytosis and ameliorates the cyclic neutropenia in affected animals. Similarly, injections of GCSFs, alone or in combination with steel factor, abolish the cycling, suggesting a signaling defect in the proliferation and maturation of hematopoietic cells. Mutations in a leukocyte elastase have been identified in humans with a similar syndrome.[178] However, the defect in dogs is associated with a homozygous mutation of the gene encoding the dog adaptor protein complex 3 β-subunit that directs trans-Golgi export of transmembrane cargo proteins to lysosomes.[11,129]

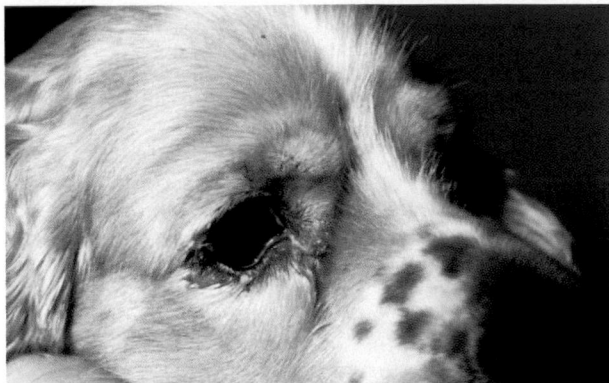

Fig 95-2 Chronic recurrent conjunctivitis, one of primary manifestations of recurrent infection in young cocker spaniel with cyclic hematopoiesis. (Courtesy University of Georgia, Athens, Ga.)

Leukocyte Adhesion Deficiency

LAD has previously been described as *canine granulocytopathy syndrome* in Irish setters and is also known as *canine leukocyte adhesion deficiency (CLAD)*.[203] It is known to be caused by the absence of a family of three leukocyte integrins.[57,93,233,235] These proteins are heterodimers (CD11a-c/CD18) with a specific α-chain (CD11a-c) and a common β-chain (CD18). In LAD, the β₂-subunit is missing (CD18 deficiency), resulting in a lack of surface expression and function of all three leukocyte integrins. The CD11b/18 is the most critical integrin because is the CR3 receptor that binds C3bi and ICAM-1 of activated endothelium, thereby mediating tight adhesion leukocytes. Because of this deficiency, granulocytes are unable to marginate, migrate randomly or by chemotaxis, and kill microorganisms, resulting in an impaired inflammatory response despite marked leukocytosis (Fig. 95-3, *A*). Furthermore, the in vitro lymphocyte stimulation response is reduced. A single missense mutation substituting a cystine with a serine has been identified in affected Irish setters, and the same mutation has been found in red and white setters.[57,84,131-133] Hematopoietic stem cell transplantation of CD18+ donor cells reverses the defect.[8]

Affected dogs have a severely increased susceptibility to bacterial and fungal infections. Signs of pyogenic infections develop during the first weeks to months of life, are often recurring, and are poorly responsive to antibiotics. Omphalophlebitis and gingivitis are often the first infections and might be followed by pyoderma, pododermatitis, thrombophlebitis, pneumonia, pyometra, osteomyelitis (especially

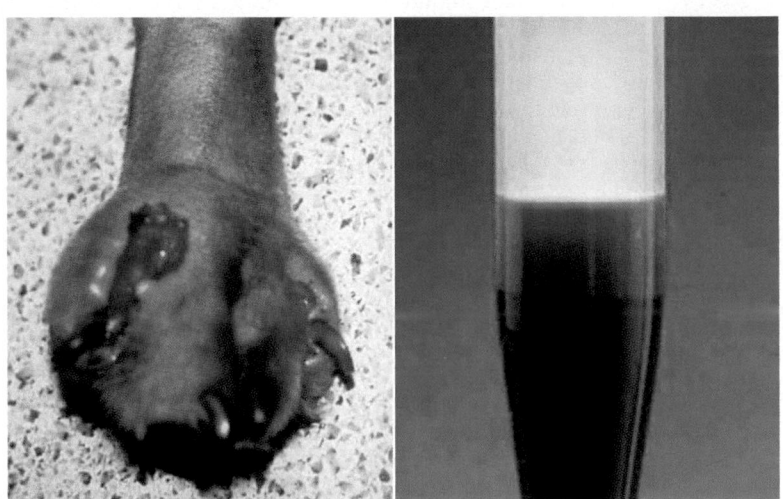

Fig 95-3 Leukocyte adhesion deficiency in Irish setter. **A,** Lack of pus formation. **B,** Severe leukocytosis (180,000 cells/μl) as seen in visible buffy coat. **C,** Decreased neutrophil adhesion to plastic in control dog and affected dog. (Courtesy Teaching File, University of Pennsylvania, Philadelphia, Pa.)

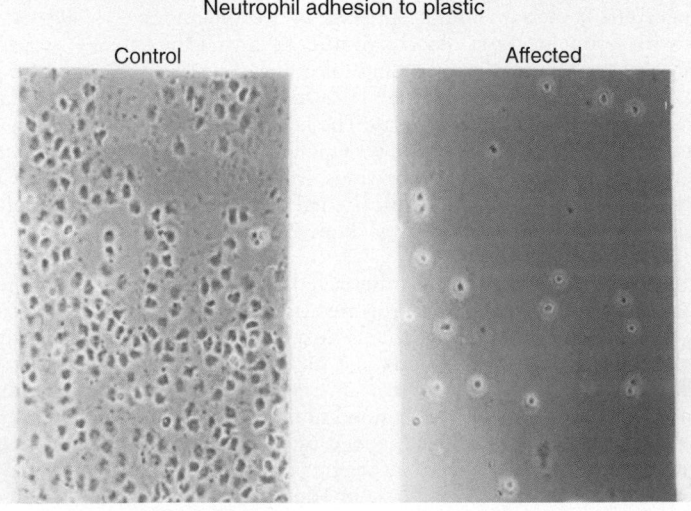

Neutrophil adhesion to plastic

Control

Affected

craniomandibular and metaphyseal), and fatal sepsis. Pups are often stunted or have poor body condition.[43,232] The sites of infections exhibit only minimal inflammation and pus formation despite a most severe persistent leukocytosis of 25,000 to 500,000/µl (see Fig. 95-3, B). Regional lymphadenomegaly and poor wound healing are commonly noted. Long-term therapy with bactericidal antibiotics is required to keep affected animals alive.

LAD has been reported in Irish setters worldwide and is an autosomal recessive disease. The defect also has been documented in red Holstein cattle and in humans.[131] The diagnosis is currently made by mutation-specific DNA testing,[84,132,133] whereas in the past, demonstration of a lack of neutrophil adherence to glass, plastic, or wool and deficiency of leukocyte glycoproteins CD11/CD18 by flow cytometry analysis were used (see Fig. 95-3, C). A polymerase chain reaction (PCR) test is also available[239] (see Appendix 6). Laboratories are available that can perform these assays commercially (see Appendix 5 for commercial laboratories). The same LAD mutation appears to be widespread in Irish setters and Red and White setters.[84,124,133] Carrier dogs can be detected by genetic testing.[57] Mixed chimeric hematopoietic stem cell transplantation from a histocompatible littermate has been shown to reverse the clinical signs of illness in an affected dog.[44] At times, donor recipients were immunosuppressed with cyclosporine and mycophenolic acid mofetil during the 2 months after transplantation.

Complement C3 Deficiency

A C3 deficiency was found in a colony of Brittany spaniels with spinal muscular atrophy.[14,248,249] C3 is a key factor of the complement system required in opsonizing bacteria. Affected dogs have defective chemotaxis and bacterial phagocytosis from a complete deficiency of C3 (0.1%) and less than 1% plasma complement activity. The immunodeficiency is generally mild and animals live until adulthood, but serious infections may occur, including pneumonia, pyoderma, sepsis, pyometra, and septic arthritis. Affected dogs may develop renal failure with amyloidosis. This is an inherited autosomal recessive disorder, and a diagnosis can be reached by documenting a lack of serum complement activity.

Selective Cobalamin Malabsorption

Chronic neutropenia and megaloblastic anemia have been described in giant schnauzers, beagles, Australian shepherds, and border collie pups.[85,87,187] Affected animals fail to thrive and show signs of lethargy, inappetence, and cachexia but are only rarely predisposed to infection accompanied by fever, lameness, or diarrhea. Blood smears show neutropenia with hypersegmented neutrophils. Affected animals have low serum cobalamin concentrations and methylmalonic aciduria. A cobalamin ileal receptor defect was documented in affected giant Schnauzers.[87] Treatment with parenteral administration of cobalamin once or twice monthly is highly effective.[85]

Hereditary Neutropenia in Border Collies

Chronic neutropenia and recurrent bacterial infections has been found in certain lines of border collies in Australia and New Zealand.[2] This suspected autosomal recessive defect is characterized by stunted growth in pups by 2 weeks of age and fever, anorexia, diarrhea, and lameness by 2 months of age. Metaphyseal osteomyelitis is seen radiographically, and neutropenia (fewer than 3×10^9 cells/µl) is consistently found. Bone marrow cytology shows granulocytic hyperplasia with a shift to the right, suggesting that the developing cells cannot enter the systemic circulation. Fasting hypercholesterolemia is also observed. Pups respond poorly to antimicrobial therapy and eventually succumb to systemic infections.

Common Variable Immunodeficiency in Miniature Dachshunds with Pneumocystosis

Certain lines of miniature dachshunds are predisposed to developing *Pneumocystis* pneumonia by 1 year of age (see Chapter 68). This predisposition also occurs in Cavalier King Charles spaniels; however, additional immunologic studies in those dogs are not available. Affected miniature dachshunds have hypogammaglobulinemia, with decreased IgA, IgG, and IgM; decreased lymphocyte transformation to phytohemagglutinin and pokeweed mitogens; and absence of B cells and presence of T cells in lymphoid tissues (stained by CD3 and CD79a cell markers).[146]

Miscellaneous Defects in Dogs

Increased susceptibility to avian mycobacteriosis has been recognized in basset hounds and miniature schnauzers (see Chapter 50). The underlying defect is unknown, but it may represent a defect in the resistance against mycobacterial protein. Similarly, English and American foxhounds in the United States are commonly infected with leishmaniasis[88,188] and pit bulls and greyhounds with babesiosis (see Chapter 77), thus a genetic predisposition is suspected. Although the Pelger-Huët anomaly has been observed in dogs, it has not been associated with clinical illness.[139]

German Shepherd Infections

German shepherds are more severely infected with *Ehrlichia canis* (see Chapter 28), *Rickettsia rickettsii* (see Chapter 29), and *Aspergillus* spp. (see Chapter 64). Some German shepherd dogs also are predisposed to pyoderma.[29,50] These predispositions may involve separate defects that have yet to be undefined. Affected dogs have pruritus with a deep pyoderma over the lumbosacral region, which may spread to other regions.[210] Coagulase-positive *Staphylococcus intermedius* is most commonly cultured. Proposed mechanisms for this susceptibility include hypothyroidism, cell-mediated immunodeficiency associated with serum inhibitors or defective helper T cells, and bacterial hypersensitivity reactions to staphylococci.[29,50,52,250] Although the inciting causes may be multivariate, the condition responds favorably to long-term administration of systemic antimicrobials. A German shepherd with familial cutaneous vasculopathy developed demodicosis after recovery from its vascular lesions.[80]

X-Linked Severe Combined Immunodeficiency

X-linked severe combined immunodeficiency (X-SCID) is characterized by a failure of humoral immunity and CMI.[72,75,78] It develops in various animal species when lymphocyte precursors fail to differentiate into mature lymphocytes because of mutations within recombinase-activating genes 1 and 2 or within the genes encoding DNA-dependent protein kinase (DNA-PK). It also develops when differentiated lymphocytes are incapable of completing signal transduction pathways because of defects in cell surface receptors for ILs.[197] In dogs, defects in the γc chain lead to deficiency of several cytokine receptors (IL-2, IL-4, IL-7, IL-9, IL-15, and IL-21).[74] Although profound deficiencies are found in T-cell function, some B-cell activities are preserved.[110] For example, canine X-SCID B cells are capable of producing IgM but do not class-switch to the production of IgG after mitogen stimulation. The shared usage of a γc chain by these cytokines explains the profound immunologic abnormalities and the impaired IgG response.[189] The ability of lymphocytes to bind to IL-2 and proliferate is severely impaired, and the development of thymocytes is drastically reduced, with an increased proportion of CD4-/CD8-thymocytes.[221,222] Serum IgG and IgA concentrations are low, but IgM values are normal.[122] Because of the X-chromosomal recessive mode of inheritance, male dogs are affected, whereas females (the dams and some

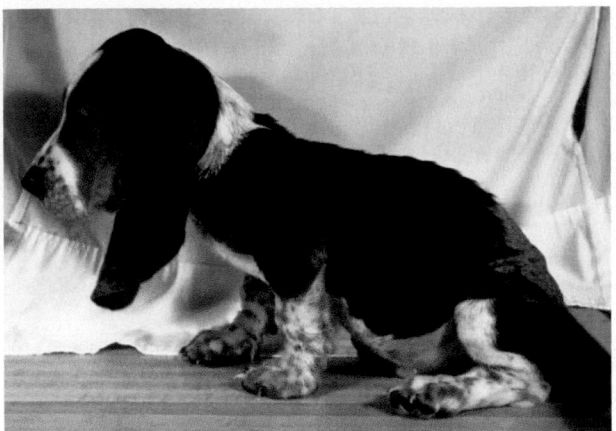

Fig 95-4 Basset hound puppy showing pyoderma and demodicosis from X-linked severe combined immunodeficiency. (Courtesy Peter Felsburg, University of Pennsylvania, Philadelphia, Pa.)

littermates of those affected) are carriers. The gene defect for this disease in dogs and people is on the proximal short arm of the X chromosome (Xq13). Two molecular mechanisms cause SCID in dogs. Jack Russell terriers have a mutation within the DNA-PKcs gene, whereas the Cardigan Welsh corgi and the basset hound have defects in the gene encoding the gamma chain that is common to the receptors for IL-2, IL-4, IL-7, IL-9, IL-15, and IL-21.[197] Bassets with X-SCID have a deletion of four base pairs, which produces a frame shift and subsequent premature stop codon in exon 1.[114] Affected Cardigan Welsh corgis have a cytosine insertion, resulting in a premature stop codon.[113,199,220] Because of the variable genetic defect, the clinical spectrum of disease manifestations can differ among affected genetic lineages of dogs.

After the decline of maternal immunity, affected male dogs develop bacterial skin, gastrointestinal (GI), and respiratory infections (Fig. 95-4). Puppies fail to thrive and grow, and they die within a few months. The most characteristic clinical features are a lack of lymph nodes, tonsils, Peyer's patches, and thymus. Basset hounds develop vaccine-induced distemper when the dam has a loss of immunity. If they survive, they are poor doers and die by 5 to 6 months of age. Corgis have reduced serum γ-globulin concentration and often die by 5 months of age because of infections acquired from the environment or vaccinations. They can survive in germ-free environments; however, an increased prevalence of leukemia has been observed.[77] A diagnosis is reached by histopathology, immunologic testing, or a PCR-based test to identify the specific mutation in bassets and corgis; however, these mutations appear to have been eliminated from breeding populations other than those in research colonies.

Bone marrow transplantation from unaffected littermates was effective in reestablishing normal T- and B-cell function in affected dogs.[76,109,111]

Autosomal Recessive SCID of Terriers

Affected Jack Russell terriers succumb to opportunistic and vaccine-induced infections within 2 to 4 months of age.[170] They experience severe lymphopenia, agammaglobulinemia, thymic dysplasia, and peripheral lymphoid aplasia. A faulty V(D)J recombination and complete deficiency of DNA-PK activity result from a reduced expression of the DNA-PK catalytic subunit.[10,170] This defect is different from the X-linked disease in bassets and corgis but similar to the C.B-17 SCID mice and Arabian SCID foals.[196]

Selective IgA Deficiency

Various forms of selective IgA deficiency have been described in several breeds, including beagles,[72,97] Shar-peis,[175] German shepherd dogs,[247] and others,[182] but the mode of inheritance remains unknown. The defect may be either an inherited primary defect of certain breeds or may arise secondary to pathologic changes within the intestinal mucosae. Serum IgA concentrations may be completely absent or markedly reduced and only very slowly developing over the first year of life. Complete deficiencies are found in Shar-peis, and partial deficiencies have been found in German shepherds.[54] Thus serum IgA concentrations need to be compared with those of age-matched controls. Reduced concentrations of IgA have been found in duodenal explant cultures of some German shepherd dogs that had serum IgA values within reference limits.[89] Therefore this measurement may be more reliable than serum concentrations. The serum IgG and IgM concentrations are consistently within reference values. Reduced secretory IgA concentrations have also been found in bronchial secretions of affected dogs.[182] Affected juvenile dogs are predisposed to mucocutaneous infections such as chronic recurrent respiratory infections involving parainfluenza and *Bordetella bronchiseptica*, gastroenteritis, pyoderma, and otitis. IgA-deficient dogs may have a positive rheumatoid factor, anti-IgA antibodies, or both and may develop allergies and autoimmune diseases. IgA deficiency in German shepherds is not linked to their predisposition to develop disseminated aspergillosis.[53] Although affected dogs have large polyclonal increases in serum IgG concentration, it is not directed against *Aspergillus terreus*.

Immunodeficiencies in Weimaraners

At least two distinct syndromes of immunodeficiency have been observed in Weimaraners. In one syndrome, which has been reported only once, growth hormone deficiency has been associated with wasting and thymic hypoplasia.[211,212]

The second syndrome, which is similar to the common variable immunodeficiency syndromes described in humans, involves recurrent bacterial infections and inflammatory conditions in young Weimaraners, which often become systemic.[40,56,79,107,227] Some dogs may outgrow their condition and not show signs later in life. Clinical signs of those with recurrent disease generally start at a few months to 3 years of age and are characterized by lethargy, anorexia, intermittent fever, lymphadenomegaly, pyogranulomatous disease, large abscesses in muscle, stomatitis, osteomyelitis, surface bleeding, and coat color dilution. Some dogs have diarrhea or vomiting. Hyperesthesia of long bones or joints (Fig. 95-5), swelling at injection sites, and recurrent urinary infections or pyoderma have also been observed. Signs in many Weimaraners are precipitated at the time of their early vaccination series and are characteristic of hypertrophic osteodystrophy (HOD). These dogs respond most favorably to antiinflammatory doses of glucocorticoid therapy, and the syndrome may be caused by MLV distemper vaccines (see Chapters 3 and 100). Some dogs later develop polyarthritis or meningitis. Although the dogs respond favorably to antibacterial therapy, glucocorticoid therapy, or both, recurrence of systemic inflammatory disease can occur. Although an immunologic deficiency is suspected, inconsistencies exist in the immunologic studies performed on these dogs. Neutrophilia, which is often marked with a left shift, has been observed. Decreased neutrophil phagocytosis of opsonized bacteria and chemiluminescence as well as slightly low serum IgG and IgM concentrations have been reported in some dogs with increased amounts of circulating immune complexes (CICs).[41] In other reports, reduced serum IgG, IgA, and IgM have been observed with no increase in CICs.[79] The lack of CICs in most reports suggests that primary decreased production rather than secondary immunoglobulin

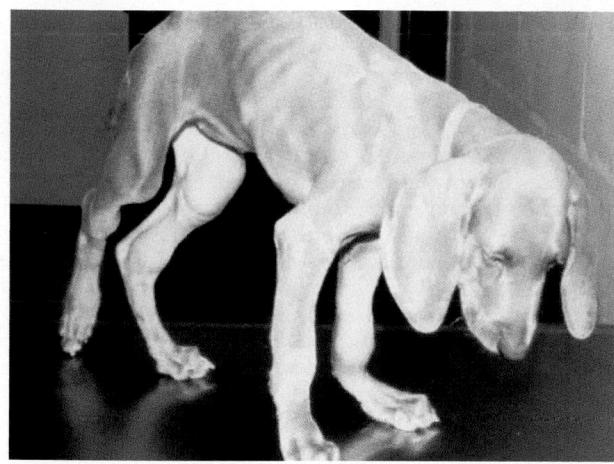

Fig 95-5 Weimaraner puppy, with lameness from immunodeficiency. (Courtesy Teaching File, University of Pennsylvania, Philadelphia, Pa.)

consumption is responsible for the defect. No specific diagnostic tests are currently available. Despite antibiotic and supportive therapy (draining of abscesses), the prognosis remains guarded. Some Weimaraners also appear to have an increased tendency to develop HOD, which has been associated with a postvaccination reaction (see Chapter 100). Whether this predisposition is only involved with this reported immunodeficiency syndrome is uncertain, although similar postvaccination complications have been frequently noted in these immunoglobulin-deficient dogs.[79]

Immunodeficiencies in Shar-peis

In addition to the severely abnormal skin structure, which leads to a barrier failure, two distinct syndromes have been characterized in the Shar-pei dog—one involving combined antibody and CMI defects and the other involving renal amyloidosis and swollen joints.

The *combined immunodeficiency syndrome* may have been confused with the selective IgA deficiency described in this breed (see previous Selective [IgA] Deficiency section). Dogs 7 months to 7 years of age develop recurrent infections involving respiratory, skin, and GI systems.[206] Chronic bronchitis, gastroduodenal or colonic ulceration, diarrhea and vomiting, adult-onset pyoderma, demodicosis, and bacterial and fungal otitis develop. In addition, the dogs have are predisposed to developing GI neoplasia, lymphoma, and other malignancies. Single or multiple immunoglobulin class deficiencies are observed in dogs, with IgM deficiency and decreased IL-2 synthesis predominating. Dogs with GI signs or malignancy usually had reduced IgM. Decreased lymphocyte stimulation test results were found in most of the dogs, suggesting a combined T- and B-cell defect.[206] In addition, peripheral blood mononuclear cells had reduced IL-6 synthesis.

Recurrent fever of unknown origin and swelling of the tibiotarsal joints are the symptoms of another immune-based syndrome in Shar-peis, known as *Shar-pei fever* or *Shar-pei hock*.[64,162,208] The lameness can be monoarticular or involve multiple joints, usually affecting the tibiotarsal joints and occasionally the carpus. Predominant mononuclear cell polyarteritis and cellulitis, with or without synovial inflammation, can develop. Clinical signs of renal failure—a result of amyloid deposition in the kidney—and the nephrotic syndrome (proteinuria, hypercholesterolemia, and hypoproteinemia) eventually develop. Although a majority of the dogs have amyloid deposition in the renal medulla, glomerular involvement from amyloid or membranous glomerulitis occurs in only 60% to 80% of affected dogs.[64] Polydipsia, polyuria, weight loss, dehydration, ascites, and peripheral edema may occur. Thromboembolism may be a sudden complication in some dogs with the nephrotic syndrome. Radiographic changes are soft tissue swelling with periarticular bone erosion and bone production. Recurrent fever, joint pain, and swelling often resolve within 24 hours.[162] Postpartum metritis has developed in intact females and may be another inflammatory feature of this illness.[64] Hyperglobulinemia and increased levels of IL-6 are found in affected dogs.[207] This syndrome is similar to familial Mediterranean fever, a human hereditary disorder characterized by polyserositis and reactive amyloidosis. Treatment with colchicine early in the course of disease may reduce amyloid deposition in people and has been proposed for affected dogs.

Lethal Acrodermatitis in Bull Terriers

Also known as *zincers* among bull terrier breeders, the lesions of lethal acrodermatitis are similar to those of zinc deficiency in dogs. This syndrome is characterized by hyperkeratosis and parakeratosis and thymus and lymph node hypoplasia, leading to increased susceptibility to infection and failure to thrive.[123,166] Growth retardation, hard and cracked footpads, pyoderma around body orifices, and aggressive to unresponsive behavior are hallmark features at a few weeks of age. The disease symptoms resembles zinc deficiency but are unresponsive to zinc therapy. Thus affected dogs die or are euthanized before 6 months of age. Affected dogs have lower plasma IgA concentrations than clinically healthy dogs.[165]

Immunodeficiencies in Related Rottweiler Dogs

In one study, a litter of Rottweiler pups either died before 6 months of age from systemic inflammatory disease or subsequently developed chronic inflammatory skin disease.[51] Serum IgA and IgG concentrations were low. Secondary lymphoid tissues had reduced numbers of CD3+ T cells, although some were found within foci of B-cell follicles. Irregularities were found in plasma cell development, and plasma cells were absent from all mucosal and cutaneous sites. In inflammatory lesions, macrophages expressing major histocompatibility complex (MHC) class II molecules were present. Related unaffected dogs had reduced serum IgA concentrations; however, the spectrum of the defect in affected dogs suggests a more complex underlying defect. Rottweilers are more susceptible to parvovirus infection, oral papillomatosis, and nasal and systemic fungal infections; however, it is uncertain whether these abnormalities are interrelated.

Susceptibility to Parvovirus Infection

Numerous purebred dogs have an increased prevalence rate of parvovirus infection. The breeds include Doberman pinschers, Rottweilers, American pit bulls, and Dalmatians, among others (see Chapter 8). The reason for this apparent susceptibility is unknown.

Akita Polyarthritis

Akita polyarthritis has been observed in related Akita dogs and is exacerbated by MLV vaccines (see Chapter 100).

Cats

Hypotrichosis Congenita with Thymic Aplasia

Hypotrichosis congenita with thymic aplasia is a defect that is characterized by the birth of nude athymic kittens with severe immunodeficiencies, kittens that are similar to the well-known nude mice in laboratories. This lethal syndrome has been recognized in the Birman breed and is an autosomal recessive inherited disorder (Fig. 95-6).[25] One author has observed a syndrome of unknown cause in ragdoll kittens

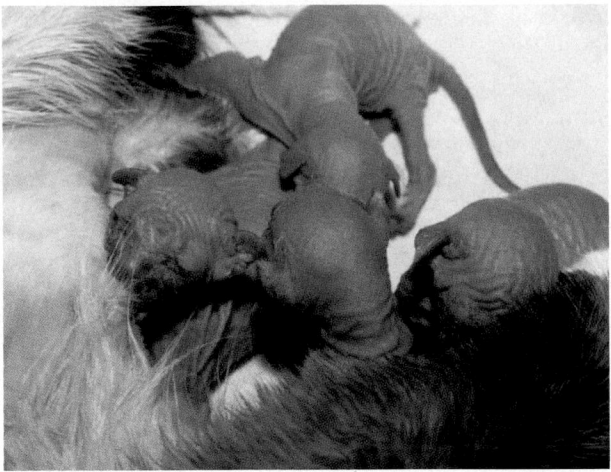

Fig 95-6 Nude Birman kittens with congenital hypertrichosis with thymic atrophy. (Courtesy Margret Casal, University of Pennsylvania, Philadelphia, Pa.)

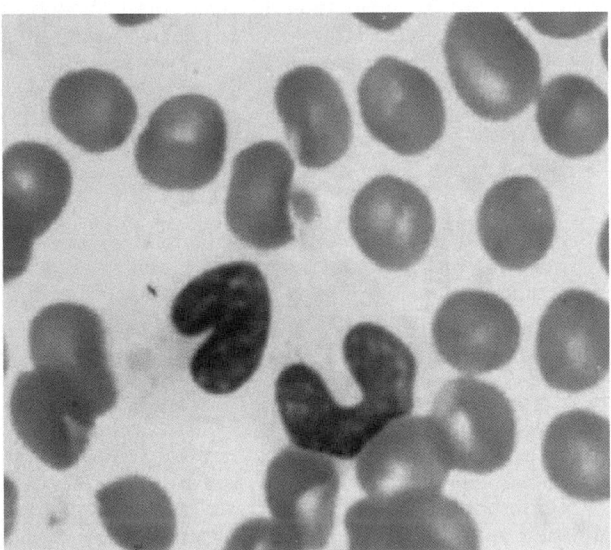

Fig 95-7 Pelger-Huët anomaly in cat with hyposegmentation of nucleus. Despite morphologic changes, no clinical immunodeficiency was observed. (Courtesy Teaching File, University of Pennsylvania, Philadelphia, Pa.)

characterized by fatal infections in the neonatal to weaning period. Use of MLV panleukopenia vaccine may have accelerated their death. Some kittens died of panleukopenia at a younger age. By weaning, others developed numerous systemic fatal infections. Thymic, splenic, and lymphoid hypoplasia were observed in these affected kittens.

Other Defects

Neutrophil abnormalities have been observed in Birman cats with leukocyte granulation,[115] Persian cats with Chédiak-Higashi syndrome,[135,171] and domestic short-haired cats with the Pelger-Huët anomaly (Fig. 95-7).[139] Clinical immunodeficiencies with these defects have not been recognized. Loss of thymic mass has been observed in cats with GM1 gangliosidosis.[42] Other purebred cats have had more problems with viral respiratory (see Chapter 16) and coronavirus (see Chapter 11) infections, but specific defects have not been elucidated.

Reactive Amyloidosis in Abyssinians

Abyssinians are predisposed to developing reactive AA amyloidosis in many organs, but clinical signs are caused by renal dysfunction. A genetic basis is suspected, but the mode of inheritance is uncertain. This syndrome is similar to amyloidosis in Shar-pei dogs and familial Mediterranean fever in people. Splenic inflammatory diseases, often related to secondary infections from immunodeficiencies, are responsible for the amyloid deposition in reactive amyloidosis. However, in some affected cats, concurrent inflammatory disease is not detected.[63] Generalized amyloidosis has also been observed in Siamese and oriental cats, but clinical features and amyloid protein composition differ.[179,237] Reactive amyloidosis has also been detected in Siberian tigers (*Panthera tigris altaica*)[214] and cheetahs (*Acinonyx jobatus*)[190]; it may represent a genetically based increased susceptibility to infectious disease.

SPECIFIC SECONDARY OR ACQUIRED IMMUNODEFICIENCIES

Acquired or secondary immunodeficiencies can develop at any time as a result of an interference with host defense mechanisms. Immune defects secondary to many infectious diseases, metabolic disturbances, intoxications, and drug therapies[35,172] have been reported (see Table 95-5).

Infectious Diseases

Canine Distemper

Disseminated viral infections that involve replication in and damage to lymphoid tissue, such as canine distemper, are associated with depression of CMI. Persistent immunodeficiencies caused by canine distemper virus (CDV) usually develop when infection develops prenatally or within the first weeks of neonatal life, when full immunocompetence has not been established. Affected dogs frequently are stunted and may develop chronic infections with protozoans such as *Giardia* and with *Mycoplasma (Haemobartonella)*. They can also be expected to be more susceptible to infection with viral and fungal pathogens, and they frequently have pronounced lymphopenia and hypogammaglobulinemia. Persistent suppression of CMI in neonatal puppies can be detected by decreased lymphocyte stimulation test results and decreased synthesis of T-cell–dependent antibodies (IgG and IgA). IgM levels are also reduced if thymic hypoplasia results from early in utero infection. Transient depression of CMI has been reported in older neonates that are infected with virulent CDV. Some of this suppression has been shown to be caused by lymphocyte immunoregulatory factors in serum. Depression of immunoresponsiveness after vaccination is minimal if it occurs at all (see Chapter 3).

Canine Parvovirus Infection

Canine parvovirus has an affinity for replicating in rapidly dividing cells and produces severe lymphopenia and immunosuppression in neonates (see Chapter 8). An increased risk of secondary infections, including greater susceptibility to encephalitis induced by canine distemper vaccine, has been reported in 3-week-old pups (see Chapter 100). Lymphocyte stimulation assay results were depressed in adult mongrel dogs that were shedding canine parvovirus in the feces.[185] Because of the concurrent leukopenia and intestinal mucosal disruption, parvovirus-infected dogs are at increased risk for developing secondary infections. Pups recovering from parvoviral infection have had a higher prevalence of urinary tract infections than age-matched control pups. Bacterial septicemia and disseminated candidiasis have been reported in animals with parvovirus.

Canine Ehrlichiosis

Depression of in vitro lymphocyte stimulation and skin hypersensitivity with DNCB have been reported in dogs with ehrlichiosis several months after the initial infection, when hyperglobulinemia develops. The depression does not appear to alter the course of infection, although certain breeds (e.g., German shepherds) have more severe illness and greater CMI depression before and after infection than other breeds. No increased susceptibility to infection has been documented in dogs with acute ehrlichiosis as yet; however, they are susceptible to pyogenic infections during the chronic neutropenic phase of the disease (see Chapter 28).

Canine Leishmaniasis

Dogs with leishmaniasis are prone to developing secondary infections, presumably because their immune system is preoccupied with defending the body against a persistent intracellular organism. Generalized demodicosis has been described in dogs with leishmaniasis.[176] Immunoreactive CD3 lymphocytes were sparse in lesions, whereas MHC II class macrophage expression was abundant. Cell-mediated immunosuppression was suspected as a secondary complication.

Canine Demodicosis

Dogs with generalized demodicosis have decreased in vitro lymphocyte stimulation, T-lymphocyte deficiency, and random neutrophil movement.[6,206] Serum proteins with apparent immunoregulatory roles are responsible for the findings. No increased susceptibility to infection has been documented in vivo, although many dogs do develop severe secondary pyoderma. Secondary bacterial infection rather than the mite Demodex canis has been thought to be responsible for the suppressed immune response, because neutrophilic chemotactic movement has been decreased in bacterial (staphylococcal) pyoderma in dogs. Histologically, mural folliculitis is a consistent lesion of active demodicosis. Histochemical studies indicate a preponderance of CD3+ and CD8+ infiltrating lymphocytes and a low CD4+/CD8+ ratio in follicular lesions and peripheral blood.[26,29] These cytotoxic lymphocytes may induce the inflammatory lesions or be a deleterious response in dogs that develop this disease. Compared with dogs with localized demodicosis or clinically healthy dogs, those with generalized demodicosis had lower messenger ribonucleic acid (mRNA) expression of for interferon-γ and tumor necrosis factor-a (TNF-α) and higher expression of IL-5 and transforming growth factor-β. As in other studies of Demodex and pyoderma with successful antimicrobial therapy for pyoderma or antiparasitic treatment of demodicosis, the test results return to reference ranges with clinical improvement.

Feline Panleukopenia

Feline panleukopenia virus has a predilection for rapidly dividing cells and produces permanent cell-mediated immunosuppression and thymic atrophy in kittens infected in utero. Lymphoid depletion, mild depression of in vitro lymphocyte function, and neutropenia are characteristic in neonatally infected cats, which may have a transiently increased susceptibility to infection. Overwhelming sepsis from gram-negative enteric microflora, which accompanies feline panleukopenia, may be related to the immunosuppression caused by the virus (Fig. 95-8) (see Chapter 10).

Feline Leukemia Virus Infection

Immunodeficiencies in feline leukemia virus (FeLV) infection often develop before malignant transformation of T lymphocytes. A reduction in CD4+ and CD8+ lymphocyte subset ratios has been shown to develop in FeLV-infected cats, as it

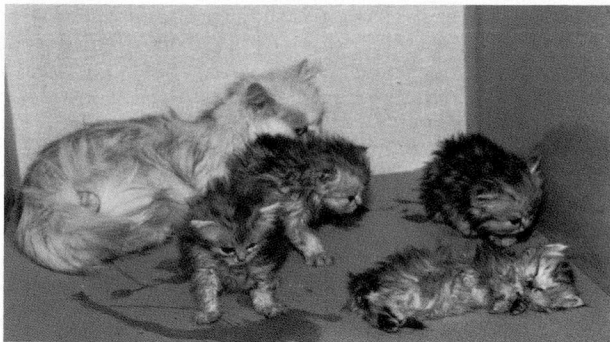

Fig 95-8 Queen and her litter of kittens, which were dying of panleukopenia. Kittens had thymic atrophy and neutropenia associated with neonatal infection with a parvovirus. (Courtesy University of Georgia, Athens, Ga.)

does in cats infected with the feline immunodeficiency virus (FIV).[116] FeLV-infected cats have impaired T-cell–mediated immunity as characterized by reduced in vitro lymphocyte stimulation, prolonged retention of cutaneous allografts, and impaired response to delayed hypersensitivity skin testing. Secondary hyperglobulinemia and complement depletion have also been found. Immune complex formation may also interfere with lymphocyte function, because immune complex removal has improved the clinical condition of infected cats. Infected cats that do not develop neoplasia have a high mortality rate and increased susceptibility to concurrent infection with other organisms, such as commensal bacteria, pathogenic fungi, Mycoplasma (Haemobartonella) spp., and feline infectious peritonitis (FIP) virus. Certain forms of FeLV infection also result in severe neutropenia, which increases the risk of secondary bacterial infection. Persistent neutropenia may also develop in some cats latently infected with FeLV. A panleukopenia-like syndrome can develop in cats that are coinfected with FeLV and FIV (see Chapter 13).[155]

Feline Immunodeficiency Virus Infection

Cats naturally affected with FIV develop fever, variable neutropenia, and chronic infections of the skin and mucosal surfaces (see Chapter 14). Experimentally inoculated cats develop generalized peripheral lymphadenomegaly and transient neutropenia followed by a disease-free period. Alterations in the phenotype of CD8+ and other blood lymphocytes eventually leads to immunodeficiency.[216] In natural circumstances, opportunistic infectious agents, which are normally controlled by CMI, are also involved in producing disease. Calicivirus, FIP, Toxoplasma spp., and systemic fungi are notable examples.[49,205] Compared with uninfected cats, Cryptococcus neoformans and Candida albicans are isolated more frequently from the oropharyngeal mucosa of FIV-infected cats, and Microsporum canis are isolated more frequently from skin.[159] Defective natural killer cell cytotoxic activity has been detected.[253] Incidental and opportunistic infections may accelerate the development of acquired immunodeficiencies in infected cats.[204] During therapy, FIV-infected cats that were treated with the protease inhibitor TL-3 were protected from developing central nervous system (CNS) signs or the progression of already evident CNS signs.[121] Cats with FIV must be vaccinated with killed vaccines (see Chapter 100).

Retroviruses Isolated from Diseased Dogs

Anorexia, depression, and multiple lymphadenomegaly have been described in a Rottweiler. A cell line from this dog contained an identifiable C-type retrovirus.[13] Retroviral elements have been isolated from cells derived from canine lymphosarcoma and endogenous sequences from normal canine cells.[223,224] A new canine lentivirus has been isolated from the buffy coat of a leukemic dog.[193] Clinically healthy dogs have also had positive PCR blood test results for FIV, although the accuracy of these assays has been questioned.[12] Whether canine retroviruses cause clinical illness in dogs remains to be determined.

Overwhelming Bacteremia

Severe endotoxemia or sepsis has been shown to impair CMI in dogs and decrease neutrophil bactericidal function (see Chapter 38). Neutrophilic phagocytosis was markedly deficient in a dog with systemic β-hemolytic streptococcal infection.[32] Sera from dogs with pyometra inhibited lymphocyte activity.[69] It also contained higher concentrations of immunoglobulins and CICs.

Hemophagocytic Syndrome

Pathologic proliferation of the mononuclear phagocyte system can either result from infectious diseases or contribute to immunologic dysfunction and signs of debilitation, weight loss with anorexia, and relapsing fever in dogs or cats.[225,243] Splenomegaly and hepatomegaly may be apparent. Viral or neoplastic diseases are commonly considered to be contributors to this syndrome. In dogs, parvovirus infection or lymphoid or myelomonocytic leukemia has been described. Immune aberrations are suspected to be responsible. The outcome of animals with this condition is guarded; in one dog, disseminated intravascular coagulation was reported as a complicating factor.[225]

Metabolic Disturbances

Many biochemical processes that occur in noninfectious disease states interfere with normal immune mechanisms. Failure of neonates to ingest colostrum and dysproteinemia are both associated with impaired humoral antibody function. Decreased complement concentration has been noted with endotoxemia, immune-mediated hemolysis, and malnutrition. Age has a marked influence on CMI. Newborn puppies and kittens experience a hypothermic state during the first week of life that suppresses T-cell function. A decline in CMI, which also develops in older dogs and cats, may explain their increased susceptibility to infectious and neoplastic disorders. Lymphocyte stimulation by various mitogens is depressed in older dogs, and male dogs were more profoundly affected. A decline in B-cell percentages was also noted.[100] Proper nutrition is also an important determinant of immunoresponsiveness. Protein and caloric restriction has resulted in premature thymic atrophy and decreased cell-mediated, humoral, and phagocytic responses in animals. In contrast, overfed, obese dogs have been more susceptible to infections and severe clinical illnesses.

Vitamin E and selenium deficiencies in dogs have been associated with decreased in vitro lymphocyte responsiveness, decreased serologic response to vaccination, and increased susceptibility to infection with opportunistic pathogens. The deficit can be accentuated by excessive intake of polyunsaturated fats (strong oxidants that counteract the effects of vitamin E). Vitamin E deficiency causes the animal to produce a suppressor serum factor capable of decreasing lymphocyte responsiveness to antigenic stimulation. Increased incidence of distemper infection has been noted in a kennel of dogs that

Table • 95-6

Acquired Defects in Phagocyte Function

DISEASE	MECHANISM	SITE OF INFECTION	INFECTING ORGANISMS	PREDISPOSING FACTORS
Uremia	Decreased phagocytosis	Catheter sites, lungs, urinary tract, blood	Staphylococci, aerobic gram-negative organisms	Peripheral vascular disease
Diabetes mellitus	Increased adherence, variable chemotaxis, decreased phagocytosis and respiratory burst	Lungs, urinary tract, catheter sites, eyes, bone	Staphylococci, Enterobacteriaceae, filamentous fungi	Hyperglycemia, total parenteral nutrition, skin ulcers, urinary catheterization
Hepatic cirrhosis	Increased adherence with decreased chemotaxis and phagocytosis	Urinary tract, lungs, blood, soft tissues	Staphylococci, Enterobacteriaceae, other enteric organisms	Urinary catheterization
Systemic lupus erythematosus	Increased adherence, decreased chemotaxis, decreased phagocytosis	Lungs, blood	Gram-positive bacteria, mycobacteria, opportunistic organisms	Immunosuppressive therapy
Burns	Decreased chemotaxis and phagocytosis	Wounds, urinary tract, blood, lungs	Staphylococci, aerobic gram-negative organisms, yeasts	Extensive burns, age extremes
Traumatic injuries	Decreased chemotaxis and phagocytosis	Wounds, urinary tract, blood, lungs	Staphylococci, aerobic gram-negative organisms	Old age

Modified from Engellich G, Wright DG, Hartshorn KL. 2001. Acquired disorders of phagocyte function complicating medical and surgical illnesses. *Clin Infect Dis* 33:2040–2048.

Table • 95-7

Causes of Neutropenia

Pathologic Demand
 Sepsis
 Peritonitis
 Pyometra

Drug Associated
 Cisplatin
 Cyclophosphamide
 Diethylstibesterol
 Phenobarbital
 Vincristine and L-asparaginase[184]
 Antipsychotics[150]

Primary Bone Marrow Failure
 Myelopthesis
 Plasma cell neoplasia
 Myelodysplasia
 Aplastic marrow

Infectious Agents
 Dogs: Ehrlichia canis infections
 Cats: Feline leukemia virus (FeLV) and feline
  immunodeficiency virus (FIV) infections
 Dogs and cats: Parvoviral infections, histoplasmosis

Immune Mediated
 Inherited granulocyte colony-stimulating factor
  deficiency [138]

---

developed "brown fat disease" as a result of a diet deficient in vitamin E.

Vitamin A deficiency can cause immunosuppression and opportunistic infections similar to those associated with vitamin E deficiency. In areas of the world where vitamin A deficiencies exist, human measles virus infection has a high mortality. A similar phenomenon might be expected to occur in dogs with canine distemper. Zinc deficiency during prenatal and neonatal periods can result in impaired CMI responses and thymic atrophy. Immunosuppression caused by dietary deficiencies can be relieved by adequate supplementation.

Depressed phagocyte function has also been reported in humans with diabetes mellitus, systemic lupus erythematosus, and renal failure (Table 95-6). Similarly, poorly regulated or untreated diabetic dogs had weaker neutrophil adherence than controlled diabetic and nondiabetic dogs. Diabetic dogs have an increased prevalence of urinary tract infections[134] and hepatic abscesses.[104] Any cause of permanent neutropenia, such as bone marrow aplasia, significantly impairs phagocyte function. Intestinal lymphangiectasia is associated with depressed CMI because of lymphocyte loss. Immunosuppression can be induced during treatment of immune-mediated diseases. Glucocorticoids, cytotoxic drugs, and cyclosporine are the most potent agents that can lead to secondary infections. Endogenous or exogenous hyperadrenocorticism is associated with a high prevalence of urinary tract infections. Use of gold salts, danocrine, or immunoglobulins to treat immune-mediated diseases has the most sparing effect on host

immunocompetence. Splenectomies in humans are associated with a high risk of bacterial and protozoal infections; in dogs and cats, reactivation of babesiosis and haemobartonellosis is most notable.

Neutropenia

Neutrophils are important in a host's defense against bacteria. Neutropenia increases the risk of bacterial infection. Decreased production and increased use are basic mechanisms and can be subdivided into additional categories (Table 95-7).[18,19,71] As mentioned previously, numerous infectious agents can result in neutropenia. Myelosuppression can be caused by cytotoxic drugs or infectious agents. Immune-mediated neutropenia has also been observed in dogs and cats.[156,168,194] Animals with neutrophil deficiencies develop recurrent bacterial infections and have resolution of clinical signs after antibacterial administration but no increase in neutrophil counts. The prevalence of infection in animals with immune-mediated neutropenia is generally low compared with that in animals with cobalamin deficiency. Despite the circulating neutropenia, animals have adequate or high numbers of proliferating neutrophil precursors in the bone marrow. If antibody is directed against neutrophil precursors, precursors may be few or absent. No test exists to measure antineutrophil antibody, and diagnosis is usually made by a favorable response of increasing numbers of circulating neutrophils after institution of treatment. Rapid increases in neutrophil numbers, usually within 48 hours, are observed after immunosuppressive doses of glucocorticoids are given.

SUGGESTED READINGS*

9. Bauer TR Jr, Gu YC, Creevy KE, et al. 2004. Leukocyte adhesion deficiency in children and Irish setter dogs. *Ped Res* 55:363-367.

12. Bienzle D, Reggeti F, Wen X, et al. 2004. The variability of serological and molecular diagnosis of feline immunodeficiency virus infection. *Can Vet J* 45:753-757.

36. Cohn LA, Rewerts JM, McCaw D, et al. 1999. Plasma granulocyte colony-stimulating factor concentrations in neutropenic, parvoviral enteritis-infected puppies. *J Vet Intern Med* 13:581-586.

44. Creevy KE, Bauer TR, Tuschong LM, et al. 2003b. Mixed chimeric hematopoietic stem cell transplant reverses the disease phenotype in canine leukocyte adhesion deficiency. *Vet Immunol Immunopathol* 95:113-122.

74. Felsburg PJ, Hartnett BJ, Gouthro TA, et al. 2003. Thymopoiesis and T cell development in common gamma chain-deficient dogs. *Immunol Res* 27:235-246.

79. Foale RD, Herrtage ME, Day MJ. 2003. Retrospective study of 25 young Weimaraners with low serum immunoglobulin concentrations and inflammatory disease. *Vet Rec* 153:553-558.

121. Huitron-Resendiz S, De Rozières S, Sanchez-Alavez M, et al. 2004. Resolution and prevention of feline immunodeficiency virus-induced neurological deficits by treatment with the protease inhibitor TL3. *J Virol* 78:4525-4532.

197. Perryman LE. 2004. Molecular pathology of severe combined immunodeficiency in mice, horses, and dogs. *Vet Pathol* 41:95-100.

239. Verfaillie T, Verdonck F, Cox E. 2004. Simple PCR-based test for the detection of canine leukocyte adhesion deficiency. *Vet Rec* 154:821-823.

*See the CD-ROM for a complete list of references.

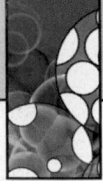

CHAPTER • 96

Fever

Katharine F. Lunn

Fever is a common clinical finding in patients with infectious, parasitic, inflammatory, immune-mediated, or neoplastic disease. In many of these patients, fever is accompanied by other more specific or localizing clinical signs, and the cause of the fever is determined with simple diagnostic tests. In some cases, the cause of the fever is not readily apparent, but it resolves spontaneously or in response to empirical therapy, often with antibiotics. In a small subset of patients, the cause of fever is not easily determined and not therapeutically responsive, and the problem becomes persistent or recurrent. Such cases of fever of unknown origin (FUO) present a particular diagnostic challenge in both human and veterinary medicine.[32,60] This chapter outlines the pathophysiology of fever and presents an approach to the small animal patient with FUO.

PATHOPHYSIOLOGY OF FEVER

Body temperature is determined by the set-point of the hypothalamic thermoregulatory center. Thermoregulation depends on sensory information from external and internal thermoreceptors and on physiologic and behavioral effector mechanisms that control heat production and heat loss. Body heat is lost through the skin and the respiratory tract and can be gained by transfer from the environment or generated by muscle activity or body fat catabolism. Body temperature is decreased by panting, cutaneous vasodilation, seeking shelter, and remaining inactive (Fig. 96-1, A). In a cold environment, body temperature is maintained by shivering, postural changes, piloerection, and cutaneous vasoconstriction (see Fig. 96-1, B). In a normal animal, these mechanisms balance heat loss and heat gain and keep the body temperature as close as possible to the normal hypothalamic set-point (Fig. 96-2, A).

Hyperthermia refers to any increase in body temperature above normal. In true fever, the hypothalamic set-point is elevated, and body temperature is increased by enhanced heat production and conservation. Heat gain and heat loss mechanisms now act to maintain body temperature at the new set-point (see Fig. 96-2, B). In nonfebrile hyperthermic conditions, the hypothalamic set-point is *not* altered, and elevated body temperature is the result of increased and unregulated heat gain or heat production or impaired heat loss (see Fig. 96-2, C). Examples of nonfebrile causes of hyperthermia include heat stroke, exercise-induced hyperthermia, malignant hyperthermia, seizure activity, and hypermetabolic disorders. Hyperthermia of this type can progress to multiorgan-dysfunction syndrome caused by an interplay among circulatory disturbances, hypoxia, increased metabolic demand, cytotoxicity of high temperature, and activation of inflammatory and coagulation cascades.[7]

Fever is mediated by the action of pyrogens. Exogenous pyrogens (infectious agents and their products, tumors, drugs, and toxins) stimulate inflammatory cells to release endogenous pyrogens (cytokines such as interferons, interleukin [IL]-1 and -6, and tumor necrosis factor [TNF]-α) that use the cell-signaling apparatus gp130. Exposure to these cytokines leads to induction of cyclooxygenase 2 activation of the arachidonic acid cascade, with enhanced synthesis of prostaglandin E_2 (PGE$_2$). PGE$_2$ is synthesized by hypothalamic vascular endothelial cells and acts on thermoregulatory neurons to raise the hypothalamic set-point. The thermoregulatory set-point is located in a rich vascular network called the organum vasculosum laminae terminalis in the preoptic-rostral hypothalamus that possesses little if any blood-brain barrier. Endothelial cells within this area are thought to release arachidonic metabolites themselves, and then metabolites of cyclooxygenase such as PGE$_2$ are thought to diffuse the short distance to the hypothalamic neurons and induce fever. PGE$_2$, which itself is not neurally active, may induce production of cyclic adenosine monophosphate (cAMP) or other neurotransmitters, which, in turn, raises the temperature set-point of the body. Additional evidence suggests that the thermoregulatory center may also be stimulated via vagal fibers that respond to release of cytokines locally released in tissues.[58] The pathogenesis of fever is summarized in Figure 96-3.

FEVER OF UNKNOWN ORIGIN

FUO in both human and veterinary medicine can be most usefully defined as fever that does not resolve spontaneously in the period expected for self-limited infection and the cause of which cannot be ascertained despite considerable diagnostic effort.[2] In veterinary medicine, this diagnostic effort typically includes a complete history and physical examination, complete blood (cell) count (CBC), chemistry, urinalysis (UA), and radiography. Also common is for veterinary patients to receive antibiotic therapy to address possible bacterial infection before it is determined that the origin of the fever is unknown.[16]

Etiology of Fever of Unknown Origin

Although fever is frequently associated with infectious diseases, the same response can be elicited by many inflammatory, immune, or neoplastic disorders. Because the list of differential diagnoses for FUO is extensive, grouping these causes into broad categories based on the underlying disease process is useful. Table 96-1 shows the causes of FUO divided into infectious and parasitic diseases, Table 96-2 summarizes inflammatory and immune-mediated causes of FUO, and neoplastic and miscellaneous causes are listed in Table 96-3. In the human medical literature, the causes of FUO are typically distributed as follows: 30% to 40% are infectious, 20% to 30% are neoplastic, 10% to 20% are rheumatologic, 15% to 20% are miscellaneous, and 5% to 15% are undiagnosed. Broadly similar distributions have been reported in veterinary patients, but variation can be found among reported case series.[46] This variation may be cause by both the particular clinical interests of the authors and their geographic locations. Published case series are also exclusively or predominantly canine.[23,46]

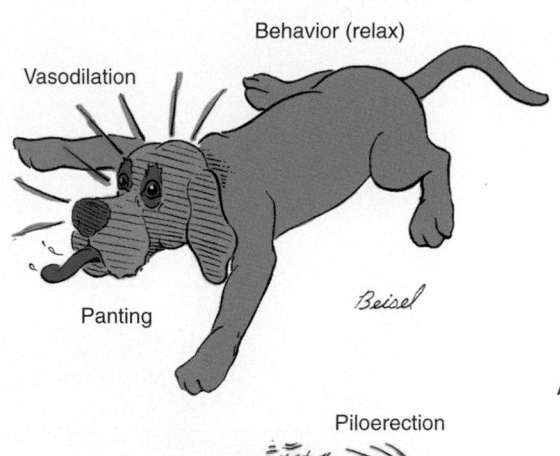

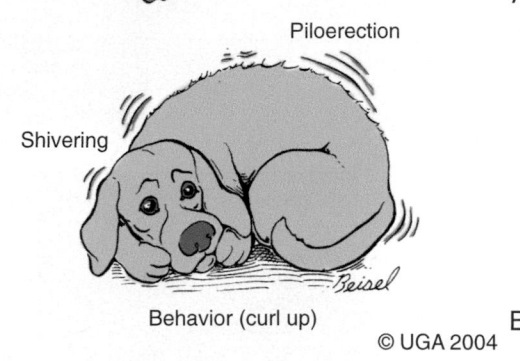

Fig 96-1 Behavioral mechanisms of decreasing body temperature (**A**) and increasing body temperature (**B**). (Courtesy University of Georgia, Athens, Ga.)

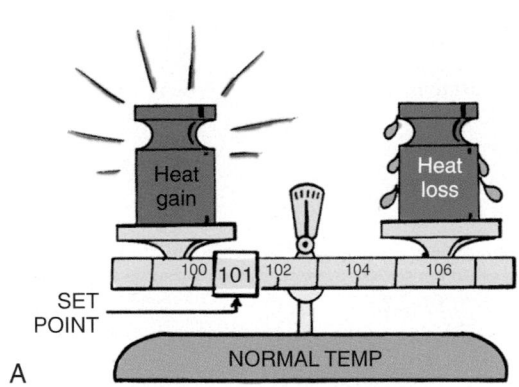

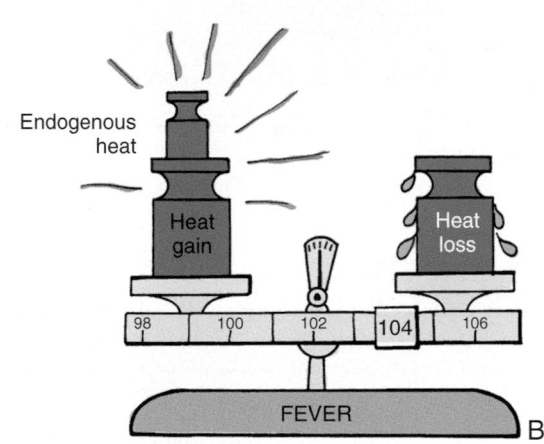

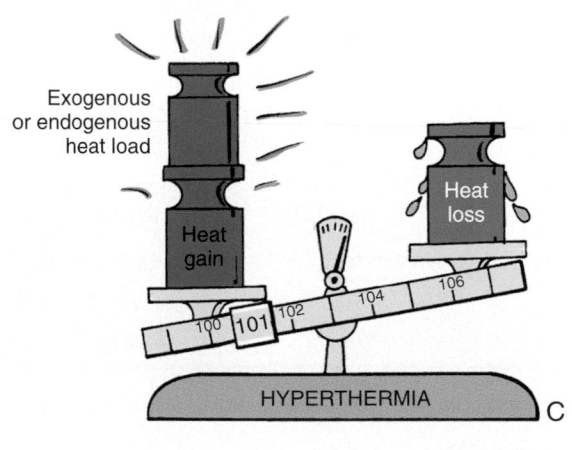

Fig 96-2 **A,** Temperature regulation in the normal animal showing a thermal set-point of 38.3° C (101° F) with balanced heat gain and heat loss mechanisms. **B,** Mechanism of fever involves a rise in set-point to 40° C (104° F), which increases endogenous heat production and conservation while maintaining a balance between heat gain and heat loss. **C,** Mechanism of hyperthermia, in contrast to that of fever, involves an increase in heat load on a normal set-point. Increased heat gain can be from exogenous (environmental) or endogenous (muscle activity) sources. (Courtesy University of Georgia, Athens, Ga.)

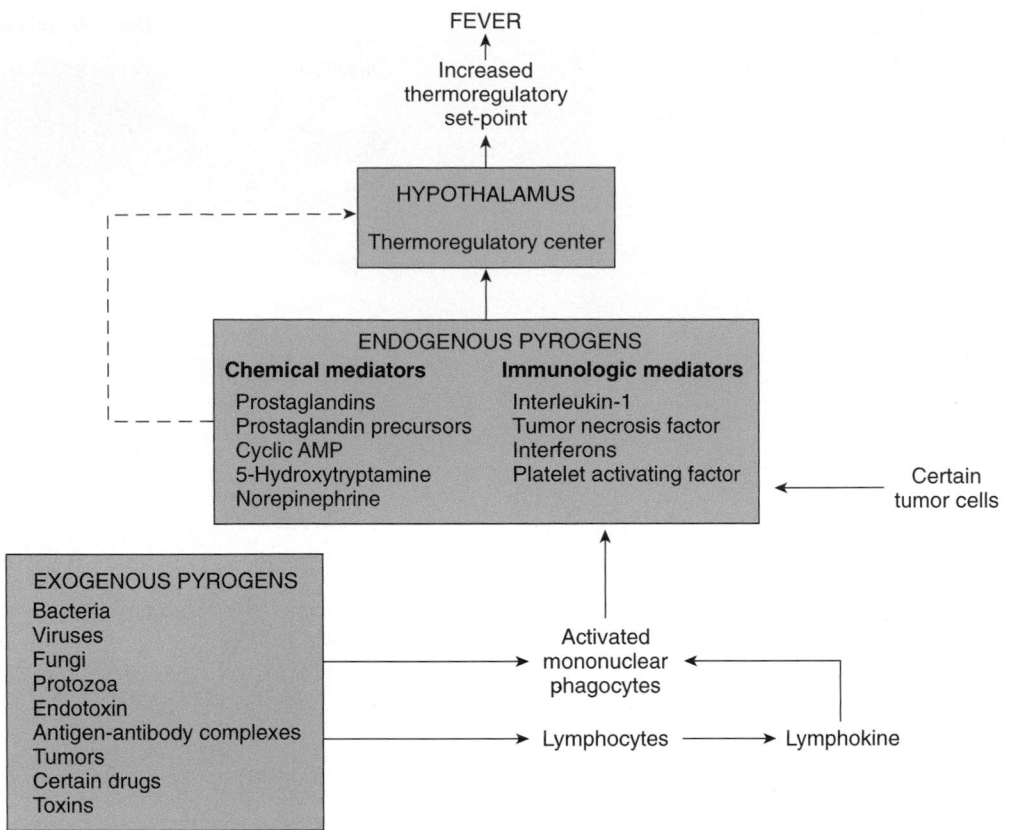

Fig 96-3 Pathogenesis of fever. (*AMP*, Adenosine monophosphate.)

Table • 96-1

Infectious and Parasitic Diseases Associated with Fever of Unknown Origin

TYPE OF INFECTION	EXAMPLES
Systemic bacterial	Infective endocarditis (D), bacteremia from inapparent focus (B)
Localized bacterial	Infective endocarditis (D), pyelonephritis (B), prostatitis (D), stump pyometra (B), pyothorax and lung infections (B), pancreatitis (D), hepatic abscess or cholangiohepatitis (B), peritonitis (B), septic meningitis (B), septic arthritis (B), osteomyelitis (B), diskospondylitis (B), tooth root abscess (B), other abscesses or cellulitis (B)
Specific bacterial	Leptospirosis (D), Lyme disease (D), brucellosis (D), mycobacterial infection (B), bartonellosis (B), plague (C), L-form infections (B)
Viral	Feline leukemia virus infection (C), feline immunodeficiency virus infection (C), feline infectious peritonitis (C), feline calicivirus infection (C), canine distemper virus infection (D)
Rickettsial and mycoplasmal	Ehrlichiosis (B), anaplasmosis (D), hemotrophic mycoplasmosis (B), mycoplasmal infections (B)
Fungal	Blastomycosis (B), cryptococcosis (B), coccidioidomycosis (B), histoplasmosis (B)
Protozoal	Toxoplasmosis (B), neosporosis (D), hepatozoonosis (B), babesiosis (B), leishmaniasis (B)

D, Predominantly dog; *C*, Predominantly cat; *B*, both dog and cat.

Table • 96-2

Inflammatory and Immune-Mediated Diseases Associated with Fever of Unknown Origin

TYPE OF DISEASE	EXAMPLES
Immune-Mediated	Systemic lupus erythematosus (D, rare in C), idiopathic immune-mediated polyarthritis (B), rheumatoid arthritis (D), polymyositis (B), steroid-responsive meningitis-arteritis (beagles, boxers, Akitas, Bernese Mountain dogs, German shorthaired pointers), vasculitis (B)
Inflammatory	Nodular panniculitis (B), lymphadenitis (B), steatitis (D), pancreatitis (C), inflammatory bowel disease (B), granulomatous diseases (B), hypereosinophilic syndromes (B)

D, Predominantly dog; *C*, predominantly cat; *B*, both dog and cat.

Table • 96-3

Neoplastic and Miscellaneous Diseases Associated with Fever of Unknown Origin

TYPE OF DISEASE	EXAMPLES
Solid tumors	Several, including hepatic tumors, gastric tumors, lung tumors, bone tumors, metastatic disease, and any necrotic tumor (B)
Hematopoietic tumors	Lymphoma (B), leukemia (B), myeloma (B), malignant histiocytosis (B)
Miscellaneous	Metaphyseal osteopathy (D), panosteitis (D), portosystemic shunt (B), pansteatitis (C), drug reaction (B), Shar-pei fever (D)

D, Predominantly dog; *C*, predominantly cat; *B*, both dog and cat.

Infection, immune-mediated disease, and neoplasia are the most common causes of FUO in the dog, whereas FUO in cats appears most likely to be infectious in origin.[41]

Fever is rarely an isolated finding in these cases, given that the cytokines induce a large number of complex immunopathologic events. These events include increases in total or relative numbers of circulating immature neutrophils and an increase in synthesis of a wide variety of acute-phase proteins from the liver. Other synthesized proteins are antiproteases, complement components, fibrinogen, ceruloplasmin, ferritin, and haptoglobin. In addition, even larger amounts of C-reactive protein and serum amyloid A protein are produced.[19] This production occurs despite a dramatic reduction in the synthesis of albumin, lipoprotein lipase, and cytochrome P_{450}

by the liver. The presence of fever and concomitant changes in these serum proteins is referred to as an acute-phase response to infection. The ability of cytokines to suppress or alter gene expression for synthesis or suppression of commonly produced protein molecules accounts for the altered lipid, protein, and drug metabolism observed in patients with chronic infectious or inflammatory disease states. It may also result in the deposition of amyloid proteins in the syndrome known as reactive AA amyloidosis.

IL-1 and TNF also have dramatic effects on endothelial cells, causing the synthesis of prostaglandin I_2 (PGI_2, prostacyclin) and PGE_2. These arachidonate metabolites caused increased blood flow. IL-1 and TNF also stimulate the plasma membrane of endothelial cells by increasing the expression of intercellular adhesion molecule 1 so that they become more adherent and attract neutrophils, monocytes, and lymphocytes. IL-1 and TNF increase procoagulant activity on the endothelial cell surface at the same time that they induce plasminogen activator inhibitor. These effects lead to activation of factor VIII and thrombin and platelet aggregation in the initiation of coagulation. These events are similar and involve the same pathways as those in the body's response to endotoxin (see Chapter 38).

Development of a Diagnostic Plan for Fever of Unknown Origin

Although some patients with FUO may have uncommon infectious, inflammatory, or neoplastic diseases, many patients are ultimately found to have an unusual or early manifestation of a common disorder.[2] Therefore the clinician must approach these cases in a systematic fashion that allows for the detection of any potential cause of fever while avoiding unnecessary testing and minimizing patient discomfort. A diagnostic plan for FUO may be based on consideration of the disease process, as outlined in Tables 96-1, 96-2, and 96-3. A complementary approach is summarized in Table 96-4 in which the causes of FUO are grouped according to anatomic or body system location. This approach is helpful in selecting diagnostic tests, particularly when localizing clinical signs are absent or subtle. By combining a disease process and anatomic approach, the clinician can develop a comprehensive diagnostic plan for any FUO patient.

In addition to appropriate diagnostic tests, the diagnostic plan should follow a sequence that is both logical and flexible. The typical diagnostic plan will begin with tests that are safe, simple, inexpensive, and easy to interpret. A staged approach can be used to guide the selection of diagnostic tests, and examples are outlined in Table 96-5.

The results of stage 1 tests in the FUO patient will then determine the tests to be performed at the next stage. If the fever has not been localized, more specialized procedures can also be introduced.

Stage 2 test results again require the repetition of earlier tests and introduce the need for advanced imaging and more invasive procedures. Ideally, the selection of these tests will be based on abnormalities detected in stages 1 and 2.

An important aspect of stage 3 test results in the FUO patient is the need to repeat the early, less invasive, and inexpensive tests frequently enough to detect new changes. The key is not to rigidly follow a predetermined and fixed diagnostic plan but rather to review and modify the plan as new results become available. For example, if repeated CBCs demonstrate developing pancytopenia, a bone marrow aspirate and biopsy should be performed early in the diagnostic plan and not reserved for stage 3.

Client Communication

The management of the FUO patient demands flexibility, dedication, and patience from both the clinician and the client. By definition, patients with FUO will already have undergone

Table • 96-4

Causes of Fevers of Unknown Origin Grouped by Body System or Region

BODY SYSTEM OR REGION	APPROPRIATE DIAGNOSTIC TESTS	EXAMPLES
Blood and hematopoietic	CBC, blood film evaluation, bone marrow aspirate, urinalysis, ophthalmic fundic exam, bone marrow biopsy, serum protein electrophoresis, FeLV and FIV tests, other serology, blood culture	Leukemia, myeloma, bacteremia, drugs, ehrlichiosis, granulocytopathy, hypereosinophilic syndromes, hemotrophic mycoplasmosis, metastatic neoplasia, walled-off hematomas
Lymphoid	Lymph node palpation, lymph node cytology and culture, lymph node biopsy, lymphangiography	Lymphoma, lymphadenitis, lymphangitis
Cardiovascular	Auscultation, radiography, angiography, electrocardiography, echocardiography, vascular biopsy, pericardiocentesis, blood culture	Endocarditis, pericarditis, vasculitis
Respiratory	Radiography, transtracheal or endotracheal wash, fine-needle aspiration, biopsy, ultrasonography, bronchoscopy, bronchoalveolar lavage, CT, thoracoscopy	Bronchial foreign body, fungal or bacterial pneumonia, neoplasia, pulmonary embolism
Nervous system	Fundic and neurological examination, radiography, myelography, CT, MRI, nerve or muscle biopsy, CSF analysis	Toxoplasmosis, fungal infection, steroid-responsive meningitis-arteritis, FIP
Musculoskeletal	Radiography, arthroscopy, blood culture, arthrocentesis, synovial membrane biopsy, bone biopsy, RF, ANA	Immune-mediated polyarthritis, myositis, panosteitis, diskospondylitis
Gastrointestinal	Radiography, barium contrast studies, ultrasonography, rectal examination, fecal cytology, rectal cytology, fecal culture, oral and dental radiographs, lipase and amylase activities trypsin-like immunoreactivity, endoscopy, laparoscopy, exploratory surgery, biopsy	Neoplasia or abscess anywhere in GI tract, pancreatitis, inflammatory bowel disease, fungal disease, portosystemic shunt, hepatobiliary, gastric, or splenic inflammation
Urogenital	Urinalysis, urine culture, prostatic wash and ejaculate cytology and culture, radiography, ultrasonography, IV pyelography, cystography, cystoscopy, vaginoscopy, cytology, biopsy	Prostatitis, stump pyometra, pyelonephritis, orchitis
Endocrine	Biochemical profile, thyroid hormone	Hyperthyroidism
Pleural or peritoneal cavity	Radiography, ultrasonography, fluid analysis, cytology, microbial culture, biopsy	Pyothorax, FIP, peritonitis, neoplasia
Skin	Physical examination, cytology, biopsy, microbial culture, fistulography	Abscess, fungal infection, nodular panniculitis, vasculitis, actinomycosis, nocardiosis, mycobacteriosis

ANA, Antinuclear antibody; *CT,* computed tomography; *MRI,* magnetic resonance imaging; *RF,* rheumatoid factor; *CBC,* complete blood cell count; *FeLV,* feline leukemia virus; *FIV,* feline immunodeficiency virus; *IV,* intravenous; *CSF,* cerebrospinal fluid; *FIP,* feline infectious pertonitis; *GI,* gastrointestinal.

several basic diagnostic tests, and some may have received one or more courses of antibiotic therapy. Clients may be frustrated by the failure to reach a diagnosis or the continuation of the patient's clinical signs. Good client communication is vital to the successful resolution of the FUO case. The clinician should explain that many diagnostic tests, including repeated tests, may be necessary to reach a diagnosis and that the process may be time consuming cIind expensive. However, clients should also be reassured that a diagnosis is reached in most cases, that many causes of FUO may be treatable or even curable, and that the fever itself is rarely harmful to the patient.

History

The patient history should include details of geographic location and environment, travel history, lifestyle (e.g., indoor versus outdoor, history of hunting), and exposure to ticks or other vectors. All of these factors will influence exposure to specific microorganisms. The medical history should cover diet, vaccination, heartworm and other parasite treatment and prevention, the administration of any other medications, and previous medical or surgical problems. The response to past therapies used for the fever problem should be noted. Clients should be questioned about the patient's urination and defecation habits and the presence of clinical signs such as lame-

Diagnostic Plan for Fever of Unknown Origin[a]

1. History
   a. Detailed
   b. Additional questions for other medical problems
2. Physical examination
   a. System by system complete exam
   b. Fundic examination
   c. Neurologic examination
3. Laboratory testing
   a. CBC, blood smear
   b. Biochemical profile
   c. Additional biochemistry: bile acids, lipase, amylase, CK, T_4
   d. Complete urinalysis including sediment
4. Radiologic imaging
   a. Thoracic and abdominal radiography
   b. Abdominal ultrasonography, if other results negative
   c. Echocardiography, if murmur
   d. Spinal survey series
   e. Long bone or joint survey
   f. Dental radiography
   g. Contrast radiography as indicated by system
   h. Computerized axial tomography
   i. Magnetic resonance imaging
   j. Nuclear scintigraphy scans
5. Cytologic evaluation
   a. Evaluation of any enlarged lymph nodes or masses
   b. Synoviocentesis, especially with hyperesthesia
   c. Bone marrow evaluation
   d. Bronchoscopy with bronchoalveolar lavage
   e. CSF analysis, especially with hyperesthesia
6. Serologic testing
   a. For persistent pathogens
      i. Dogs — *Ehrlichia, Brucella, Bartonella, Neospora*
      ii. Cats — FeLV, FIV, FCoV, *Toxoplasma*
      iii. Other persistent infections as indicated
   b. Immunopathologic diseases
      i. ANA, RH, and LE tests
      ii. Anti-platelet, anti-erythrocyte, anti-leukocyte tests
7. Bacteriologic testing
   a. Urine, blood, or joint-fluid cultures
   b. Fecal cultures
8. Tissue biopsy
   a. Bronchoscopy or thoracoscopy with biopsy
   b. Exploratory laparotomy with biopsy buffet
9. Therapeutic trial
   a. Selected antibacterial drugs
   b. Antifungal drugs

CBC, Complete blood (cell) count; *CK*, creatinine kinase; T_4, thyroxine; *CSF*, cerebrospinal fluid; *FeLV*, feline leukemia virus, *FIV*, feline immunodeficiency virus, *FCoV*, feline coronavirus; *ANA*, antinuclear antibody; *RF*, rheumatoid factor; *LE*, lupus erythematosus

[a]Fever is not harmful. Many diagnostic tests are needed and may have to be repeated or this list recycled. Tests listed lower under each section generally have higher cost or risk, or less immediate indication and should be considered with successive work-ups. With persistence, a diagnosis is often made and there is a favorable response to treatment.

ness; neck, back, or abdominal pain; skin lesions; masses or swellings; weakness; exercise intolerance; coughing; nasal discharge; and dyspnea.

Physical Examination

All body systems should be examined in detail, and a complete physical examination should be repeated at each hospital visit for outpatients. Inpatients should be examined twice daily. The physical examination should include careful cardiac auscultation and regular examination of the oral cavity and rectum, bones and joints, lymph nodes, and skin. Repeated ocular examinations should not be overlooked because they may provide evidence of infectious, inflammatory, or neoplastic disease. Given that fever can often wax and wane in FUO, the pattern of fever in an individual patient should be determined by serial measurement of body temperature. This measure is not of any value in elucidating the underlying cause, but it is important in monitoring the response to any subsequent therapy.

Complete Blood Count and Serum Chemistry Profile

The problem of fever is often accompanied by neutrophilia or a stress leukogram, and serum chemistry tests are frequently nonlocalizing in FUO patients. However, any abnormalities detected on these tests should be used to direct further testing. The CBC should always be accompanied by examination of a blood smear so as to determine blood cell morphology and look for microorganisms. Automated CBCs should be verified by manual counts.

Urinalysis and Urine Culture

Because FUO may be associated with focal urogenital infections (e.g., prostatitis, pyelonephritis), UA and urine culture are mandatory in the evaluation of fever patients. Urine samples should be obtained by cystocentesis and submitted for bacterial culture and susceptibility testing, regardless of the appearance of the urine sediment.

Radiography

Thoracic and abdominal radiographs should be obtained during the first stage of evaluation of the FUO patient. These radiographs are simple to obtain and may provide early evidence of neoplastic disease or suggest infectious disease such as bacterial or fungal pneumonia. In the second or third stages of diagnosis, long bone, joint, vertebral, and dental radiographs should be considered. Contrast radiographs (e.g., intravenous [IV] pyelography, barium series, cystography, myelography, fistulography) may be indicated in some cases.

Ultrasonography

Abdominal ultrasonography can be used to look for potential sources of fever in organs such as the liver, spleen, pancreas, gastrointestinal (GI) tract, urinary tract, prostate, uterus, lymph nodes, and adrenal glands. Other regions that can be investigated by ultrasonography include the thorax (particularly in the presence of effusions or masses), the retrobulbar area, and any other peripheral mass lesion or swelling. Ultrasonography is particularly useful in facilitating the minimally invasive acquisition of fine-needle aspirates or biopsies.

Echocardiography

Ultrasonographic examination of the pericardium, myocardium, endocardium, heart valves, and great vessels is essential in the evaluation of the patient with FUO and a heart murmur, particularly if the murmur is of recent onset. These findings are suggestive of infective endocarditis, particularly if a source of infection (e.g., gingivitis, prostatitis, an IV catheter) is also present. Although echocardiography is not 100% specific or sensitive for the diagnosis of infective endocarditis, the finding of vegetative aortic valve lesions is considered to be pathognomonic.[73] Mitral valve lesions can suggest a diagnosis of infective endocarditis if present together with other supportive findings. Therefore the results of echocardiography should be interpreted in light of the patient's signalment, clinical signs, and blood culture results. Infective endocarditis is much more common in dogs than it is in cats, and middle-age dogs of medium to large breeds (e.g., German shepherd dogs, boxers, golden and Labrador retrievers) appear to be over-represented.[73]

Computed Tomography and Magnetic Resonance Imaging

These advanced imaging modalities are now available to many clinicians in referral hospitals. These assessments should be regarded as third stage tests in the evaluation of the FUO patient and used when clinical signs have been localized to a particular body system. For example, computed tomography is useful for detecting certain pulmonary lesions and for examining the nasal cavity, tympanic bullae, and pharynx. Magnetic resonance imaging is often used in evaluation of the central nervous system (CNS).

Aspirates and Biopsies

Fine-needle aspirates are usually simple and safe to obtain, and touch preparations or impression smears can also be made from ulcerated lesions or discharge material. Cytologic examination of these samples is relatively inexpensive and, depending on the skill of the clinician, can sometimes be performed in-house. For example, if blastomycosis is suspected, repeated aspirates from lymph nodes or skin nodules can be examined for *Blastomyces* organisms because they are relatively easy to identify. Aspirates can also be obtained from lymph nodes, abnormal fluid accumulations, and from masses or abnormal organs detected with imaging such as ultrasound or radiography. Examples include aspiration of consolidated lung lesions, splenic aspirates if unexplained splenomegaly is detected, and aspiration and analysis of exudates and effusions. Aspirates of fluids such as pleural, pericardial, or peritoneal effusions; cerebrospinal fluid (CSF); synovial fluid; or bile should also be submitted for bacterial and other cultures. Aspiration of peripheral lymph nodes, even if palpably normal, is recommended in the second stage of diagnostic testing if the source of the fever has not been localized.

Specialized techniques such as CSF sampling, bronchoalveolar lavage, transtracheal or endotracheal lavage, prostatic wash and ejaculation, bone marrow aspiration, and arthrocentesis are used to obtain cytology and culture samples from specific locations. The use of bone marrow aspiration and arthrocentesis are discussed later in this chapter.

Tissue biopsies are often obtained in the second or third stages of the diagnostic evaluation, when the source of the fever has been localized to a specific organ or tissue. However, in some cases, specific localizing signs may be absent. When biopsies are obtained with an invasive procedure, for example exploratory laparotomy, obtaining tissue from multiple sites and in sufficient quantities is important to allow histopathology, special stains for infectious agents, and culture for organisms such as aerobic and anaerobic bacteria, mycobacteria, and fungi. If necessary, the diagnostic laboratory should be contacted in advance to discuss optimal tissue handling, preservation, and transport. Biopsies may also be obtained with techniques such as thoracoscopy, laparoscopy, endoscopy, or arthroscopy, or they can be obtained percutaneously, sometimes with guidance from ultrasound or radiography.

Bone Marrow Cytology and Histology

Bone marrow disease is a relatively common cause of FUO. Reported examples include myelodysplasia, lymphoid leukemia, myeloma, and disseminated adenocarcinoma.[23,32]

Bone marrow aspiration is indicated in the early stages of diagnostic testing if CBCs show unexplained cytopenias. Pancytopenia requires the evaluation of both cytology of a bone marrow aspirate and histopathology of a core biopsy. In cats, bone marrow cytology slides should also be reserved for feline leukemia virus fluorescent antibody testing. Bone marrow aspiration is indicated in the third stage of the diagnostic plan if the FUO has not yet been localized.

Arthrocentesis

Immune-mediated polyarthritis is a common cause of FUO in published canine case series.[23,46] The condition may be idiopathic (nondeforming and nonerosive), or it may be caused by rheumatoid arthritis or associated with other immune-mediated disorders such as systemic lupus erythematosus or steroid-responsive meningitis-arteritis. Occasionally, nonerosive immune-mediated polyarthritis can be secondary to chronic infectious disease, GI disease, or neoplasia.[61] Immune-mediated polyarthritis is also seen in cats and occurs as both a chronic periosteal-proliferative form and a less common erosive form.[61]

Lameness, joint swelling, and periarticular pain may wax and wane or be apparently absent in patients with immune-mediated polyarthritis. Therefore arthrocentesis should be performed in the second stage of evaluation of canine patients with FUO. Samples should be obtained from both carpi, both tarsi, and both stifles. The fluid should be examined for color, clarity, and viscosity and submitted for cytology. Bacterial and mycoplasma culture should also be performed if sample size is large enough.

Dogs with FUO and evidence of spinal pain may have concurrent immune-mediated polyarthritis and steroid-responsive meningitis-arteritis.[76] Therefore arthrocentesis is also recommended in all dogs in which this form of meningitis is suspected.

Blood Culture

Blood cultures are indicated in all patients with unexplained fever and are particularly indicated in the presence of a cardiac murmur; back, bone, or joint pain; or neutropenia. Peracute bacteremia associated with sepsis is usually caused by gram-negative organisms such as *Escherichia coli*. Subacute or chronic bacteremia is usually associated with a persistent focus of infection such as infective endocarditis or diskospondylitis.[11] More than one half of all canine infective endocarditis cases are caused by infection with coagulase-positive staphylococci and streptococci. Organisms implicated in diskospondylitis include *Staphylococcus intermedius*, *Streptococcus canis*, *Brucella canis*, and *E. coli*. In some cases, these organisms may be seeded from other locations such as the skin or urogenital tract.

Few prospective studies have been done of blood culture techniques in veterinary patients, although this subject has been extensively reviewed in the human study literature.[56] In human medicine, the likelihood of obtaining a positive culture result is directly correlated with the volume of blood drawn, regardless of whether the blood is obtained as a single blood culture set or divided into several sets over a 24-hour period. In one study, the yield from a 30-ml blood sample was found to be 62% more than that from a 10-ml sample. However, the sensitivity of blood cultures is also improved by obtaining more than one set. For example, in a study of bacteremic people, 91.5% of bacteremic episodes were detected by the first blood culture set, and 99.3% were detected by the first two sets. Increasing the number of blood culture sets will also increase the specificity of the test because contaminants are unlikely to be present in all sets.

In dogs and cats, blood culture techniques should focus on the collection of adequately large volumes of blood, with less emphasis on the timing or periodicity of the collections. The total volume of blood that can safely be obtained will depend on patient size. If size allows, more than one blood culture set should be obtained to increase the sensitivity and specificity of the test. Samples for blood culture should be obtained by venipuncture, not from intravascular catheters, and the operator should prepare the site using aseptic techniques and should wear sterile gloves for the venipuncture. The blood sample should be immediately and aseptically inoculated into both aerobic and anaerobic blood culture bottles. Bottles of different sizes are available and should be selected to give the optimum ratio of blood-to-culture medium (see Diagnosis under Cardiovascular Infections, Chapter 87). Blood culture bottles containing resins may be used for patients receiving antibiotic therapy.[46]

Serology

Serologic tests available for the diagnosis of infectious disease include assays for specific antibodies or antigens, as well as molecular tools such as Western blotting and polymerase chain reaction. Consideration of the signalment, clinical signs, geographic location, and possible vector exposure of the patient should direct selection of the most appropriate tests. Vaccination history, timing of the samples, local disease prevalence, sensitivity, specificity, and positive and negative predictive value must be considered when interpreting the results of any serodiagnostic test.

Serologic tests are also available for the diagnosis of certain immune-mediated diseases. For example, the Coombs' test detects antibodies against erythrocytes and is used in the diagnosis of immune-mediated hemolytic anemia. However, patients with this disorder are likely to have concurrent localizing clinical signs and are unlikely to present with FUO. Antinuclear antibody (ANA) can be detected in patients with systemic lupus erythematosus. However, diagnosis of this uncommon multisystem disorder requires the demonstration of multiple clinical and immunologic abnormalities and should never be based on elevated ANA alone.[13,14] In addition, ANA can be elevated in some normal dogs and in association with other medical conditions. Rheumatoid factor has been found to be of poor sensitivity and specificity in the diagnosis of canine rheumatoid arthritis.[61] This disorder is more appropriately diagnosed by a combination of radiographic changes indicating an erosive polyarthritis together with joint fluid analysis and possibly synovial membrane biopsy.

In summary, extensive arrays of wide-ranging serodiagnostic tests are not recommended in the investigation of FUO, and the use of *immune panels* is particularly discouraged. Ideally, serologic tests should be used to investigate a diagnosis that is suspected based on other findings.

Nuclear Medicine

Nuclear medicine has provided several techniques that can be used to visualize infection or inflammation in human patients.[65] Scintigraphic imaging can demonstrate many of the steps involved in the inflammatory process and can therefore potentially localize some causes of FUO. For example, leukocyte infiltration of tissues can be visualized with indium-111 or technetium 99m–labeled neutrophils. The latter approach has been used experimentally to localize abscesses in dogs[21] but has not been applied to clinical cases. Other techniques in nuclear medicine include the use of radiolabeled human immunoglobulin, or gallium-67, which binds to transferrin in the blood, to nonspecifically demonstrate areas of increased fluid extravasation associated with enhanced vascular permeability in inflammation. Radiolabeled interleukins have also been used to localize inflammatory cells, and bacterial infection can be detected with labeled antibiotics such as technetium 99m-ciprofloxacin. A recent development in human

medicine is the use of positron emission tomography with fluorine-18 fluorodeoxyglucose. This substance accumulates in areas of increased glucose metabolism such as tumors and inflammatory lesions.

Tissue Biopsy

Specimens can be obtained percutaneously, with or without imaging, or by direct surgical collection. Generally, the organs biopsied are indicated by the suspicions of the clinician; however, in undiagnosed fevers, multiple organ biopsies are often taken via exploratory laparotomy. Samples are placed in fixatives for routine histopathology; however, samples should also be submitted or saved fresh frozen for cultivation of organisms or nucleic acid testing based on the results of the histologic examination. Special stains for fungal or rickettsial agents must be used in some cases in which these agents are suspected based on initial findings.

THERAPY OF FEVER

Trial Therapy

In many cases, the investigation of the FUO patient will achieve a definitive diagnosis, and treatment of the underlying cause will lead to resolution of the fever and other clinical signs. However, in some cases of true FUO, a diagnosis is not reached, and in other cases, diagnostic testing is discontinued because of client or patient factors. In these cases, therapeutic trials are undertaken in the absence of a definitive diagnosis. Antibiotic, antifungal, or corticosteroid therapy are often used in therapeutic trials.

The goals of a therapeutic trial should be to confirm a presumptive diagnosis indirectly, control or cure the underlying disease, and resolve the patient's clinical signs, without inducing intolerable side effects or exacerbating an undiagnosed disease.

A therapeutic trial should be planned and monitored as rigorously as the diagnostic plan. It is important to begin with a tentative diagnosis, select safe and appropriate therapies, and implement a careful monitoring program, using predetermined criteria for success or failure of the therapeutic trial. Medication should be used at appropriate doses, and the duration of therapy should be sufficient to detect both the presence and absence of a response, particularly because fever can wax and wane independent of therapy.

Good client communication is essential in developing and monitoring a therapeutic trial, and clients should understand the risks of such an approach. Such risks include the continued progression of an undiagnosed disease if an ineffective therapy is used, development of medication side effects or toxicities, and the possibility of exacerbating an underlying infectious disease if immunosuppressive therapy is used. Clients should also understand that some medications, such as antifungals, can be expensive. A therapeutic trial is unlikely to be helpful if the client abandons the plan because of expense, side effects, or lack of immediate response to treatment.

Many causes of FUO are inflammatory or immune mediated; therefore glucocorticoids are commonly used in patients with FUO in the absence of a specific diagnosis. This approach can be dangerous if infectious disease has not been ruled out first. If glucocorticoid therapy is used in this way, the patient should be monitored closely for exacerbation or development of new clinical signs. The indiscriminate use of glucocorticoids may also interfere with future diagnostic testing or future more specific therapies. This practice is a particular concern for patients with neoplasia such as lymphoma. Glucocorticoids can also have nonspecific antiinflammatory effects and may improve the patient's clinical signs without addressing the primary cause of the fever. This characteristic is also true of some antibiotics, such as metronidazole or doxycycline.

Empirical antibiotic therapy is commonly used in small animal patients with fever, often with a successful outcome. Ideally, such therapy should be based on culture and susceptibility testing, although this is not always feasible. In trial therapy for FUO patients, antibiotics should be chosen based on a tentative but specific diagnosis, with consideration of spectrum of activity, and an understanding of pharmacokinetics. A significant risk of indiscriminate antibiotic therapy is that it contributes to antibiotic resistance in bacterial populations,[35] which may also be true for other antimicrobial agents.

When a systemic mycosis is suspected, often based on typical radiographic or ocular lesions, but cannot be confirmed, trial therapy with antifungal agents may be attempted. Fever may resolve within days, but fungal lesions may respond slowly to therapy; hence trial therapy with antifungals can take several weeks.

Antipyretic Therapy

If elevated body temperature is the result of nonfebrile factors such as heat stroke or prolonged seizure activity, physical methods of cooling should be employed. Examples include the use of fans and cool water baths and administration of cooled fluids via IV or by colonic or gastric irrigation. These methods are seldom needed for the true FUO patient because body temperature rarely exceeds 41.1° C (106° F) in these cases. Also important to remember is that fever is a *regulated* elevation in body temperature; therefore any attempts to physically cool the patient will be working against the body's own thermoregulatory mechanisms. Fever is also a protective adaptive response to the effects of infection and can have beneficial effects. External cooling is the treatment of choice for hyperthermia in which core temperature exceeds the thermoregulatory set-point. Thus when external cooling is used to treat hyperthermia, no opposition of regulatory process takes place in an attempt to increase heat gain, as is the case with fever.

Body temperatures above 41.1° C (106° F) can lead to CNS damage, disseminated intravascular coagulation, metabolic derangements, and even death. Fevers of 39.5° to 40.8° C (103° to 105.5° F) are more typically seen in FUO patients and may be associated with nonspecific signs such as anorexia, lethargy, arthralgia, and dehydration. Dehydration is caused by reduced water intake and increased sensible and insensible losses in the fever patient. IV fluid therapy can correct these conditions in the debilitated patient. In some conditions, attempts to lower the body temperature by cooling and antipyretic drugs might be considered. In patients with concomitant reduced cardiac output, systemic vascular hypertension, or extreme obesity may benefit. If quality of life is significantly affected by the fever, or if body temperatures are in excess of 41.1° C (106° F), antipyretic medications should be considered in patients with FUO. Table 96-6 lists the dosages and potential adverse effects of acetaminophen and several nonsteroidal antiinflammatory drugs that may be effective in reducing fever. These medications inhibit cyclooxygenase and therefore act centrally to reduce the hypothalamic set-point.

Table • 96-6

Doses of Antipyretic Agents Used in Dogs and Cats

DRUG	SPECIES	DOSE (mg/kg)[a]	ROUTE	INTERVAL (HOURS)	ADVERSE EFFECTS AND PRECAUTIONS
Acetaminophen (Paracetamol)	D	10-20	PO	12-24	Hepatotoxicity if overdosed. Do not use in cats.
Aspirin	B	D: 10 C: 10	PO	D: 8-24 C: 48-72	May cause GI irritation or bleeding; avoid if GI ulcer present. Reduces platelet aggregation. Caution with severe liver or renal disease. Dose carefully in cats due to prolonged half-life.
Carprofen	B	2	PO, IV, SC, IM	12	Mild GI irritation. Avoid if bleeding disorder. Idiosyncratic hepatotoxicity reported in dogs. Limit to 2-day duration in cats as safety unknown.
Ketoprofen	B	1	PO	24	May cause GI irritation or bleeding; avoid if GI ulcer present. Reduces platelet aggregation. Potentially hepatotoxic or nephrotoxic. Injectible available. Limit to 5-day duration in cats.
Meloxicam	B	0.1	PO	24	As above. Not currently approved for veterinary use in the USA.

D, Dog; *C*, cat; *B*, dog and cat; *GI*, gastrointestinal; *USA*, United States of America: *PO*, by mouth; *IV*, intravenously; *IM*, intramuscularly; *SC*, subcutaneously.
[a]Dose per administration at specified interval.

Many antipyretic drugs can potentially cause GI irritation, ulceration, or bleeding, and they should not be used concurrently with glucocorticoids. Hepatotoxicities and exacerbation of bleeding tendencies are also possible side effects. The risk of nephrotoxicity is increased if these medications are used in patients with preexisting renal disease, hypotension, hypovolemia, or concurrent administration of nephrotoxic medications. Nonsteroidal antiinflammatory drugs should be used cautiously in elderly or debilitated patients. However, if used carefully, these medications can relieve discomfort while allowing continued diagnostic testing of the patient with FUO.

SUGGESTED READINGS*

9. Breitschwerdt EB, Abrams-Ogg ACG, Lappin MR, et al. 2002. Molecular evidence supporting *Ehrlichia canis*-like infection in cats, *J Vet Intern Med* 16:642-649.

23. Dunn KJ, Dunn JK. 1998. Diagnostic investigations in 101 dogs with pyrexia of unknown origin, *J Small Anim Pract* 39:574-580.

27. German AJ, Foster AP, Holden D, et al. 2003. Sterile nodular panniculitis and pansteatitis in three weimaraners, *J Small Anim Pract* 44:449-455.

55. McCarthy PL. 2004. Fever without apparent source on clinical examination, *Curr Opin Pediatr* 16:94-106.

60. Øvrebø Bohnhorst J, Hanssen I, Moen T. 2002. Immune-mediated fever in the dog. Occurrence of antinuclear antibodies, rheumatoid factor, tumor necrosis factor and interleukin-6 in serum, *Acta Vet Scand* 43:165-171.

76. Webb AA, Taylor SM, Muir GD. 2002. Steroid-responsive meningitis-arteritis in dogs with non-infectious, nonerosive, idiopathic, immune-mediated polyarthritis, *J Vet Intern Med* 16:269-273.

*See the CD-ROM for a complete list of references.

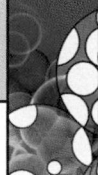

CHAPTER • 97

Prevention and Management of Infectious Diseases in Multiple-Cat Environments

Janet Foley

Multiple-cat environments contain at least five cats and include multiple-cat homes, breeding catteries, pet stores, research catteries, shelters, foster or rescue homes, veterinary hospitals, groomers and boarding facilities, and feral cat colonies. Cats in multiple-cat environments are usually infected with different pathogenic microorganisms because infectious disease (ID) prevalence often is correlated with animal density and population size and because caretakers of multiple-cat households often have limited resources for disease control. Many of the important cattery infections are chronic, difficult to treat, or both, thus efficient management and disease prevention are paramount for success in multiple-cat husbandry.

Some degree of exposure to infectious agents is inevitable, given the ubiquitous nature of viruses such as feline herpesvirus (FHV) and feline calicivirus (FCV) and the environmental persistence of others such as feline panleukopenia virus (FPV). IDs may be transmitted directly by immediate or close contact between reservoir and susceptible hosts, indirect transmission including through inanimate vehicles (fomites), air or droplets, or various mechanical or biologic vectors. Whether infection becomes important in a cattery depends on host, environment, and pathogen attributes. Pathogen attributes include virulence, dose, and route of pathogen inoculation. Virulence is not under the control of the cattery manager, but dose and route of infection may be. Environment and host contributors to IDs also are important targets for minimizing IDs. This chapter reviews management strategies in catteries, major cattery infectious syndromes, and special cases of multiple-cat environments.

GENERAL MANAGEMENT STRATEGIES

Management of IDs in catteries should emphasize preventive medicine (Fig. 97-1). Colony immunity—the resistance of a group of animals to invasion and spread of an infectious agent—should be maximized, as should the *colonization resistance* (CR) of each individual. CR is the innate and acquired capability of an animal to resist ID and includes behaviors (such as avoiding filth), physical barriers (mucus, epithelium, fur), physical and chemical attributes of the host (low gastric pH, intestinal peristalsis, urine flow, mucociliary escalator), classical immunity, and normal flora. Animals with impaired CR (e.g., cats with feline immunodeficiency virus [FIV], geriatric or immunosuppressed cats, cats receiving antibiotics) not only are more susceptible to disease but also reduce colony immunity.

Ideally, a preventive management program should be implemented by a team consisting of at least a veterinarian and cattery manager who are familiar with the physical structure of the cattery, cattery staff and operations, and other details. Effectively managing a cattery to decrease risk of infection includes (1) minimizing population and individual risk factors for ID and (2) *movement control*, which is the regulation of access to other cats and fomites that could transmit infection.

Isolation and Quarantine

Cats that appear healthy but could be incubating IDs should be in quarantine for at least 10 days and preferably 3 weeks.

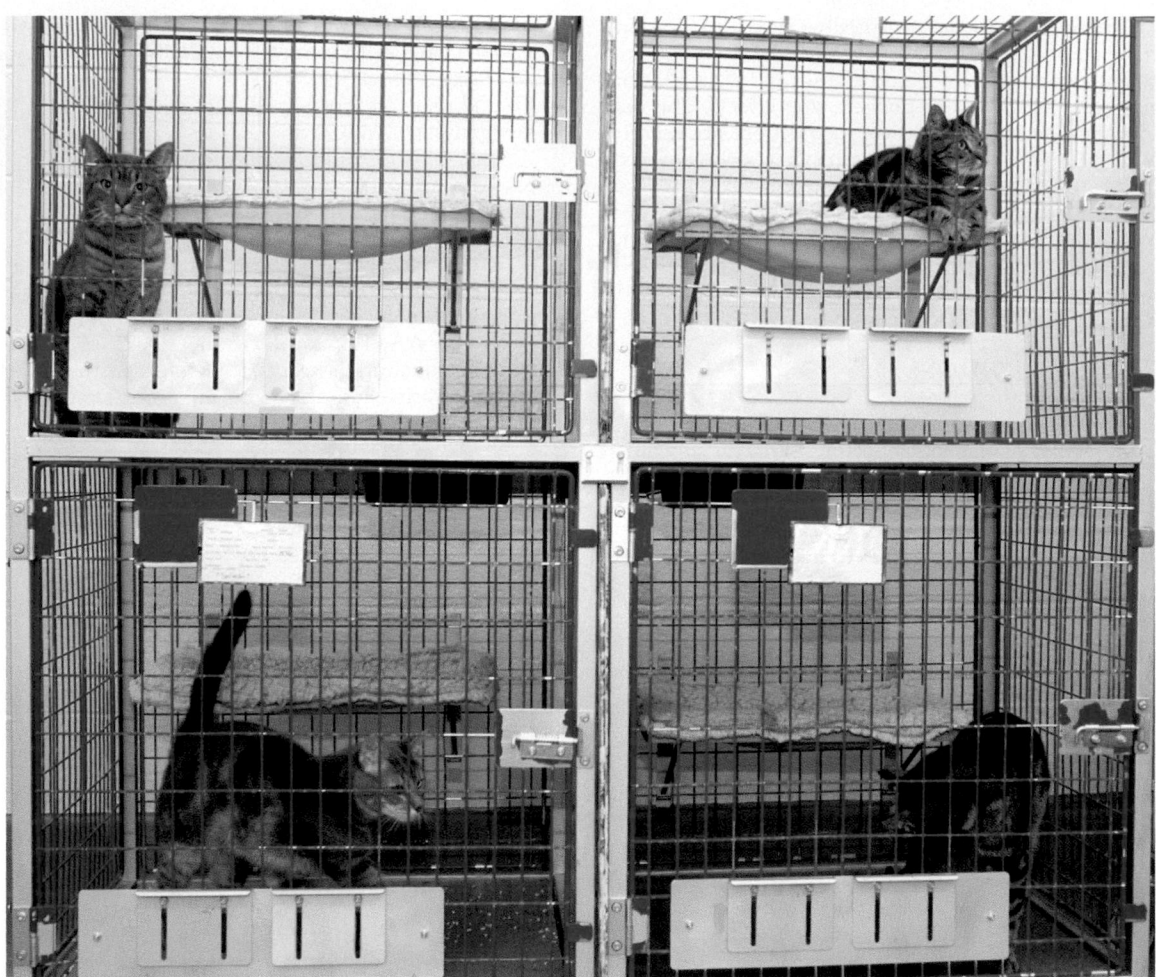

Fig 97-1 Good husbandry is vital to an effective preventive medicine program.

During quarantine, the cats should receive well-cat care treatments (e.g., vaccinations, antiparasite treatments) and be observed daily by someone qualified to perform physical examinations and detect clinical signs of ID. When the quarantine period is over, it is presumed that the cat is clinically healthy. At that time, it should be allowed to interact with or be caged near other well cats in a way that minimizes stress and facilitates cleaning and cattery management.

Cats showing signs of ID must be isolated—but not in the quarantine area because it would result in infection of the quarantined cats. In a veterinary clinic or shelter, isolation needs and areas are obvious. In a cattery or home, a cat could be isolated in a bathroom; however, it is very difficult for owners to avoid carrying infections on their clothing, shoes, and skin from a sick cat to other cats. A cat with dermatophytosis, an upper respiratory infection (URI), diarrhea, or other contagious illness should not be isolated in the same house as healthy cats; they should be moved to a separate building or a veterinary clinic that will accept them. To ensure that IDs are not tracked throughout a cattery, a specific order of care should be followed: (1) feed and clean well cattery cats, (2) feed and clean quarantine cats, and finally, (3) feed and clean isolation cats. In a large facility, isolation cats should be handled by someone who is not also handling the well cats. Only if absolutely necessary should a caregiver attend to well cats after attending to cats in isolation, and then *only* if the

caregiver has changed clothes and shoes and washed all exposed skin. If the facility is a shelter, a clinic, or another facility that does not keep cats longer than an average of 3 weeks, then cats remain in effective quarantine or isolation at all times.

In some situations, such as high-volume shelters, quarantining animals is impossible. In such cases, the next best option may be cohort admission. One method of cohort admission is to fill cages consecutively according to the date each animal enters a shelter and ensure that cats have no contact with contaminated elements in the environment *(all-in-all out)*. In shelters or clinics with too many sick animals, the isolation area must be expanded. Isolation expansion is contrary to the common practice of allowing sick animals to comingle with well animals ready for adoption. Mildly ill animals may still be adoptable; potential owners should be allowed to view mildly ill animals in an isolation area.

Risk Factors for Disease

Risk factors for disease should be systematically evaluated and corrected if possible. Risk factors include environmental factors and population characteristics. The two most important cattery risk factors are (1) overall cat numbers and (2) density, or the number of cats per unit space. Other intrinsic environmental risk factors include caging strategies, stresses (e.g., dogs, noise, unstable social structures), rate of new cat introduction, sanitation, air flow and quality, well-cat programs, insect and vermin control, and season and climate. Population risk factors include population age composition, inbreeding status, breeds housed in the cattery, and presence of concurrent diseases.

Cat Numbers and Density

Cat numbers and density should be kept as low as possible, with an emphasis on minimizing the proportion of kittens and immunocompromised cats. Caging in stable cat groups should allow for some social interactions but not fighting. Cages should provide plenty of opportunities for cats to hide, vertical space, natural light and air, and windows through which cats can look. The details of group housing cats are too numerous to discuss thoroughly in this chapter but have been reviewed in other excellent sources.[24]

Cages for individual cats should be more than sterile boxes because the increased susceptibility to disease caused by stress outweighs the reduction achievable by ease of cleaning. Environmental enrichment (hiding places, vertical spaces, and things to look at and play with) is very important (Fig. 97-2). Cages should not extend all the way to the ground (with bottom cages being at least a foot off the ground), and sick cats should never be housed above well cats; sick cats should be in isolation. *All* components of the cattery should be either disposable or completely disinfectable, precluding items such as carpet-covered scratching posts, carpeted floors, and porous wood structures. Any potentially nondisposable items should be kept in closed rooms and decontaminated or disposed of when the group of cats has finished with them.

Sanitation

Sanitation is important but often improperly handled. The main sources of ID are not cages—they are cats and contaminated, uncleanable environment components (such as carpet). Cleanliness is essential in a cattery. If a cattery has dirty litter boxes, litter scattered around, or a smell of ammonia in the air, it is not clean. When a cage, bowl, tray, or litter box is introduced to a cat, it should be new or should have been cleaned with 1:10 diluted bleach with at least 10 minutes of contact time. For routine cleaning, cages and bowls should be kept clean and litter changed every day. Everything in the cattery should be scrubbed and sanitized weekly, which frees the cattery managers from bleaching all bowls and litter boxes daily and leaves them more time to improve the cats'

behavioral welfare, manage isolation and quarantine, and enjoy the cats.

Air Flow and Quality

Air flow and quality are significant factors, but their importance is overrated. The advantages of increasing air turnover from 10 to 15 changes per minute are not enormous, but the increase in expense is. In general, the greater the population density, the greater the need for increased number of air changes per hour. In homes, by far the most efficient way to achieve quality air is to open windows or have indoor-outdoor catteries. Most cats do not need air conditioning as long as they have fresh water, protection from rain, and shade. In cold weather, cats need heat.

Population Risk Factors

Population risk factors for ID include population age composition, inbreeding status, breeds housed in the cattery, and presence of concurrent diseases. Many of the risk factors that increase the likelihood of endemic or epidemic disease in catteries are also factors increasing risks to individual cats. Individual cats are more prone to infectious disease if they are very young, especially if they are colostrum deprived or very old, if they are stressed or on inadequate nutrition, or if they are already incubating an infection. In cats, inbreeding per se is not a risk factor, but being a member of a more susceptible pedigree may be.

Well-Cat Programs and Vaccinations

Well-cat programs and insect control minimize individual risk factors for ID, maximize colony immunity, and provide a systematic opportunity for cats to be evaluated and either treated or removed from the population if they are not well. Routine screening of cats should be performed *at least* annually by a veterinarian, preferably at the cattery, and should include a complete physical examination of all cats and vaccination boosters for the respiratory viruses and any other disease that may be a problem in the cattery.

The veterinarian and cattery manager should inspect the animals and premises for arthropods. Fleas transmit tapeworms and diseases such as bartonellosis, and all arthropods promote allergic reactions and dermatopathy. Cats can be infested with lice, ear mites, and mange mites. Catteries should have zero tolerance for arthropods. If any arthropods are seen during a routine inspection, the entire premises should be cleaned and treated with an approved pesticide, and every cat should receive treatment for ectoparasites. Monthly antiarthropod treatment should be provided if needed to ensure that no cats are infested.

Vaccinations have four primary disadvantages: (1) some vaccines cause mild disease or transient immunosuppression; (2) parenteral, adjuvanted vaccines can trigger vaccine-associated sarcoma; (3) vaccines induce antibodies that could interfere with testing for the disease; and (4) use of vaccines may lead to a false sense of security that cats are adequately protected and other preventive management practices can be neglected. Although disadvantages exist, colony immunity is increased with the appropriate use of vaccines. Vaccine programs may be different for each different cattery. During primary vaccination, killed virus (KV) vaccines must be given at least 2 times (at least 2 to 4 weeks apart) before effective immunity is produced and thus are inappropriate in catteries with high turnover rates. KV vaccines may be advantageous in facilities where vaccine-associated diseases are unacceptable (e.g., in research catteries) and where it is important that no vaccine-induced antibodies are produced. Traditional modified live virus (MLV) vaccines use high-passage virus to give animals a mild infection. The protective effects develop more quickly than they do with KV vaccine, but respiratory vac-

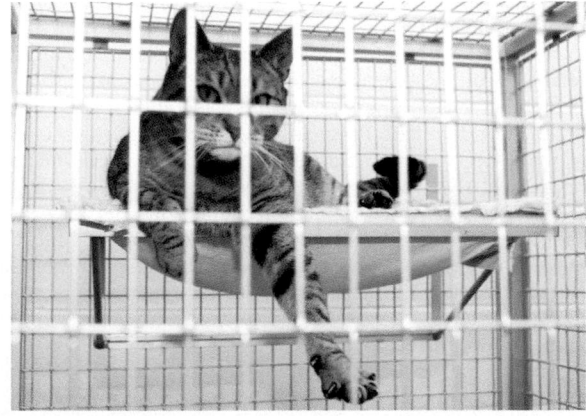

Fig 97-2 Hammocks provide cats with a peaceful environment.

cines may cause a mild URI. High-antigen mass (HAM) vaccines have lower passage, less attenuated virus strains than traditional MLV vaccines. These vaccines have are supposed to be able to overcome maternal antibody interference with vaccine efficacy. Because HAM vaccines are given mucosally, it is hoped that a local mucosal antibody (IgA) may be produced that could block the attachment of the virus to receptors, thus aborting an infection if the animal were exposed. Advantages of HAM vaccines include protection from vaccine-associated sarcomas, earlier protection than MLV vaccines, and possible protection for young kittens despite the presence of maternal antibodies. The major disadvantages are mild, temporary vaccine-induced immunosuppression and morbidity.

Morbidity and Mortality

It is important to diagnose causes of mortality and morbidity in a cattery to better plan and implement medicine programs. Necropsies should be performed after deaths, especially in breeding and research catteries. When infectious causes are suspected, laboratories should be advised of tentative diagnoses before the necropsy, if possible. It is impractical to submit samples from every sick cat for diagnosis, but spot-checking is very helpful, particularly during an apparent outbreak.

IMPORTANT INFECTIOUS SYNDROMES IN CATTERIES

Respiratory Disease

Etiology

Respiratory tract disease (upper, and less commonly lower, respiratory tract infection) is the most prevalent and easily recognizable infectious problem in catteries, and it is also the most difficult problem to manage.[12] The five most important pathogens in feline URIs, in increasing order of importance, are Bordetella bronchiseptica, Chlamydophila felis, Mycoplasma spp., FCV, and FHV (see Chapter 16).

B. bronchiseptica, a nonenteric gram-negative bacterium, contributes to mild respiratory tract infections, often in association with respiratory viruses.[3,54] If the bacterium is protected and kept moist, it can survive in the environment for weeks. Cats may have mild primary bordetellosis with conjunctivitis and mild oculonasal discharge or have Bordetella pneumonia. FCV is an RNA virus with a high rate of mutation and is antigenically and genetically diverse.[27,50] The infection is transmitted by aerosol, and the virus is introduced into cats through oral and nasal routes. Respiratory shedding of virus occurs for at least 10 to 14 days and commonly occur for months in shelters and kittens. FCV infection can cause conjunctivitis and rhinitis with serous ocular discharge, vesicular stomatitis and faucitis (aphthous stomatitis), pneumonia, transient fever and limping, and immune-complex polyarthritis and gingivitis. A very pathogenic series of FCV infections were reported in which cats developed facial and limb edema, apparently caused by vasculitis secondary to FCV, comparable to the hemorrhagic fever syndrome observed in rabbit hemorrhagic calicivirus infections.[46] FHV is an enveloped DNA virus that only infects felids.[37] Kittens often acquire the infection at a very young age, because parturition efficiently induces recrudescence of the virus. Later in life, transmission of the FHV requires intimate contact between cats. After infection, the virus persists in the trigeminal nerve with periodic or chronic activation that manifests in classical URI clinical signs, especially during stressful periods or immunosuppressive events. Disease signs may include conjunctivitis, anterior uveitis, serous ocular discharge with secondary bacterial infection and mucopurulent discharge, or keratitis with or without dendritic ulceration. Ulcerative and necrotizing nasal dermatitis resembling shingles has been described in some cats with FHV infection.[21] Occasionally, URI signs in cats are caused by infection with C. felis, an obligate intracellular bacterium. The reservoir for the feline pathogen is feline conjunctival and genital mucosa (and possibly gastrointestinal [GI]). Chlamydial disease in cats often is acquired shortly after weaning. The typical sign is conjunctivitis, which is often unilateral. Mycoplasma spp. are degenerate, obligative parasitic bacteria with no cell wall, reduced genomes, and minimal ultrastructure. The reservoir for mycoplasmas is respiratory and genital mucosa, and transmission is via the aerosol route. Feline diseases attributed to mycoplasmas include URIs, conjunctivitis, and arthritis. Many people remain unconvinced that mycoplasmas are primary URI pathogens in cats, given that they commonly are recovered from clinically healthy cats.

Clinical Findings

Some or all cats with URIs show signs of conjunctivitis, anterior uveitis, ocular or nasal discharge, gingivitis, faucitis, stomatitis, glossitis, fever, and lymphadenomegaly. Vesicular stomatitis and faucitis are suggestive of FCV infection. Lameness and joint pain suggest infection with Mycoplasma organisms or FCV. A greenish colored or tenacious ocular or nasal discharge indicates bacterial contamination in the site but does not help identify the underlying pathogen. A cough suggests bronchitis (allergic or infectious) or pneumonia. Although far less common, a cat with a cough may have cattery cough (i.e., B. bronchiseptica tracheitis). Keratitis and corneal ulceration suggest FHV infection. Chronic sinusitis, often with turbinate destruction, may be from infection with either FHV or FCV followed by secondary bacterial infection. Fever develops most commonly with FHV or FCV infections. Cats with serous or purulent ocular discharge, nasal discharge, or both without the other more specific diagnostic signs could be infected with more than one of the URI pathogens.

Diagnosis

Rapid laboratory confirmation of the etiologic agent is unlikely. Possible tests include cytology of conjunctival cells, bacterial, viral, and mycoplasmal culture, and the polymerase chain reaction (PCR). URIs are managed in a cattery by minimizing their impact. Infected and exposed cats may have recurring disease, and few catteries (except specific pathogen-free [SPF] research catteries) are free of URIs. Chronically symptomatic cats can be identified during quarantine when the stress associated with the move often induces recrudescence of chronic or latent disease and should be excluded from the cattery. Unfortunately, some of the MLV vaccines (often given before or during quarantine) induce mild to moderate URIs that are clinically indistinguishable from disease caused by field-strain pathogens. Commercial vaccines are available for feline bordetellosis, FCV, FHV, and C. felis. Pregnant queens should be vaccinated only with KV vaccines. Some catteries use partial doses of intranasal (HAM) vaccines to protect kittens as young as 1 to 2 weeks old. This practice can be dangerous because HAM vaccines induce mild, transient immunosuppression. Cats in well-managed breeding catteries should have excellent maternal-induced immunity, particularly if colostrum intake is ensured in all neonates. Innate resistance of every cat should be maximized.

As mentioned previously, the fraction of the cattery that consists of susceptible cats (immunosuppressed, geriatric, or young cats) should be minimized. Environmental decontamination for URIs should consist of frequent cleaning rather than sterilization because the primary reservoirs for URIs are other cats. Most URI pathogens are susceptible to many commonly used cattery disinfectants.

Therapy

Individual cats with URIs should receive nursing care and fluids if needed and be encouraged to eat. Antibiotics should be reserved for cats that have green, purulent discharge; may be septic; or are strongly suspected of being infected with *Chlamydophila*, *Mycoplasma*, or *B. bronchiseptica* organisms. For purulent discharge, a good, broad-spectrum drug with activity against pathogenic staphylococci is appropriate, such as cephalexin or amoxicillin-clavulanate. For possible sepsis, drugs with excellent broad and enteric spectra should be included, such as amoxicillin- or ticarcillin-clavulanate, enrofloxacin, or a penicillin with an aminoglycoside. The drug of choice for *B. bronchiseptica*, *Mycoplasma* spp., and *C. felis* is doxycycline, although acceptable substitutes may include enrofloxacin and azithromycin for mycoplasmas and *C. felis* and trimethoprim-sulfamethoxazole for *B. bronchiseptica*. *B. bronchiseptica* isolates often are resistant to multiple drugs.[9] Cats with suspected *C. felis* or *Mycoplasma* spp. infection may be candidates for topical ophthalmic antibiotics and usually improve clinically within a few days. It is *not* appropriate to treat all affected cats with antibiotics because most are infected with viruses, and antibiotic use adversely affects normal flora, increases susceptibility to additional infections, and promotes antibiotic resistance.

No specific drugs are used to treat FCV, but several drugs may mitigate infection with FHV, including idoxuridine (Herplex®Allergen, Inc., Irvine, Calif.), trifluridine (Viroptic®, King Pharmaceuticals, Bristol, Tenn.), and vidarabine (Vira-A®, Parke Davis, Morris Plains, N.J.), all given topically 5 to 7 times a day (see Chapter 2). Acyclovir is an excellent systemically active drug used to treat human herpesvirus infection but is ineffective against FHV. Lysine occasionally is used to treat human and feline herpesvirus infections, with the justification that it antagonizes use of arginine in herpesvirus protein synthesis if dietary arginine is restricted. However, restriction of arginine is not safe for cats; nevertheless, some clinicians report that lysine treatment improves the clinical status of some cats with FHV infection. α-Interferon has direct antiviral properties and has been used with some success in FHV infection but is only available as a recombinant human protein, to which cats quickly become resistant (see Chapter 16).

Gastrointestinal Disease

Etiology

Stress, diet change, and a few primary pathogens can instigate diarrhea and vomiting, but many opportunistic organisms also accompany primary pathogens or other bowel disruptions. The complicated etiology makes management difficult. The major primary GI pathogens in catteries are FPV, *Salmonella enterica* serotypes, *Campylobacter* spp., *Giardia lamblia*, *Cryptosporidium parvum*, and *Tritrichomonas fetus*.

Clinical Findings

FPV (a parvovirus) is a small DNA virus that produces life-threatening diarrhea, vomiting, and immunosuppression (see Chapter 10). FPV has prolonged environmental persistence, is resistant to most chemical disinfectants, and has a tropism for rapidly dividing cells such as epithelial cells of the GI tract, white blood cell precursors in bone marrow, and cerebellar Purkinje's cells in neonatal or very young kittens. The incubation period of FPV can be between 3 days and 2 weeks but is usually 5 to 7 days. Animals younger than 6 months are most likely to develop severe disease, whereas adult animals may have mild disease that is indistinguishable from diarrhea of any other cause. Infection with FPV manifests as vomiting

and diarrhea that lead to dehydration. Infection is usually accompanied by immunocompromise from loss of white blood cells as the infection targets the bone marrow precursors, which can predispose the animal to septicemia, shock, and death. In the neurologic form of feline panleukopenia, damage to the Purkinje's cells results in poor gross motor control from the cerebellum, although other peripheral nerves and the cerebrum remain intact.

S. enterica ser *typhimurium* is a zoonotic enteric bacterium with a broad host range including humans, birds, rodent, cows, pigs, horses, dogs, and cats. Cats with salmonellosis may be nonsymptomatic, diarrheic, or systemically ill. Hematologic values in cats are sometimes suggestive of panleukopenia with neutropenia that has a severe left shift. *Salmonella* endotoxin creates a massive disruption of the host inflammatory mechanisms, resulting in release of acute-phase proteins from liver, fever, vasodilation, increased vascular permeability, thrombosis, reduced organ perfusion with blood, reduced blood pressure, disseminated intravascular coagulation, shock, and death (see Chapter 39). *Campylobacter* organisms are zoonotic gram-negative, motile, curved, rod-shape bacteria. Many organisms are common in juvenile or stressed animals and results in a range of clinical signs from no symptoms in carriers to severe diarrhea. *Campylobacter upsaliensis* has been associated with bloody diarrhea outbreaks in day care centers for children and in groups of dogs and cats.[97a,105a,190a] Often, diarrhea associated with campylobacteriosis is self-limiting, but debilitated, dehydrated, or very young animals may die of the infection without extensive nursing care (see Chapter 39).

G. lamblia is a flagellate protozoan, which in addition to the apicomplexans *Cryptosporidium felis* and *Cryptosporidium parvum*, is a primary pathogen (see Chapters 78 and 82).[25] *C. parvum* has a wide host range including wild mammals, cattle, dogs, and cats. Diarrhea is most severe in young and immunosuppressed animals. *T. fetus* also is a flagellate, is better known as a parasite in cattle, and superficially resembles *G. lamblia* in fresh feces. Cases have been reported in cats with severe, watery diarrhea.[12] The infection is spread directly from cat to cat.

Numerous GI opportunists may exacerbate clinical diarrhea, including the enteric *Helicobacter* spp. (*colifelis*, *canis*, *hepaticus*, *bilis*, *pullorum*, *fennelliae*, and *cinaedi*); *Clostridium difficile* (a zoonotic anaerobe associated with severe disease [see Chapter 39]); and *Isospora* spp. Human pseudomembranous colitis is a nosocomial infection with underlying disease, antibiotic usage, or both, and *C. difficile* in cats probably is as well. *Isospora* spp. in small numbers are exceptionally common in kittens. The life cycle is complex and includes sexual and asexual stages. GI cells become damaged when the *Isospora* progeny emerge. The number of asexual reproductive cycles appears to be programmed; only two or three occur in any one host individual, and infection is self-limiting. The disease associated with large numbers of *Isospora* is profuse, watery diarrhea, often with concurrent bacterial infection (see Chapter 81).

Diagnosis

Testing for GI pathogens can be difficult, because some animals with primary pathogens lack clinical signs, and the presence of opportunists is difficult to interpret. Exhaustive testing is expensive, is difficult, and often fails to identify a specific cause. Severe, life-threatening disease is suggestive of FPV infection in which clinical evaluation might reveal dehydration and bowel fluid and gas distension; if the animal is septic or in shock, signs may include pale mucous membranes, delayed capillary refill time, and increased heart and respiratory rates. Laboratory tests to evaluate diarrhea start with the complete blood cell count (CBC). Most viruses cause mild to moderate reduction in white cell counts, whereas FPV infection causes severely depauperate or almost no white blood cells, reflecting the viral infection in the bone marrow.

Some of the commercially available fecal enzyme-linked immunosorbent assays (ELISAs) designed for the detection of parvovirus antigen in canine feces can be used for cats. Because the tests are antigen ELISAs, they are positive only when virus is in the sample. Some false-positives result occasionally because of vaccinations, thus cats should not be diagnosed with parvovirus enteritis unless they have appropriate clinical signs or a very low CBC. Bacteria involved in vomiting and diarrhea can be evaluated by a Gram stain of feces followed by aerobic, microaerophilic, and anaerobic culture. Aerobes including *Salmonella* spp., *Escherichia coli*, and *Yersinia enterocolitica* may be identified using standard microbiologic techniques. *Campylobacter* and *Helicobacter* organisms generally must be cultured in reduced oxygen, because they have only a small amount of superoxide dismutase and cannot tolerate more than about 10% oxygen; room air has about 20% oxygen. Routine microaerophilic culture on selective agar often is conducted at elevated temperatures (e.g., 42° C) and may miss less thermotolerant strains. However, the majority of pathogenic *Campylobacter* spp. are detected and additional infections identified if fecal Gram stains are performed, especially if carbol fuchsin is used as a counter stain. To identify a clostridial infection, an anaerobic culture can be performed on selective media, and immunologic assays can be used to detect *C. difficile* toxin A. *Helicobacter* spp. may be much more difficult or impossible to culture.

Fastidious helicobacters and campylobacters may be evaluated using biopsy and molecular techniques. PCR is a relatively new test that identifies nucleic acids specific to a microorganism (commonly used for parvoviruses and feline enteric coronavirus [FECV]) and can be used to test any tissue in which virus is suspected, including feces, gut, bone marrow, respiratory secretions, and the cerebellum and brain.

Thorough parasite evaluation includes direct microscopic examination of fresh feces, flotation, and ELISA or fluorescent antibody (FA) testing. *Giardia*, *Tritrichomonas*, and coccidia organisms can be seen in fresh feces in saline. Fecal flotation is a standard procedure for identifying parasites but often reveals parasites that are not contributing to the diarrhea. Failure to find *Isospora* oocysts on flotation or direct smear does not rule them out as contributing to the diarrhea, because the test has low sensitivity in early infection. *Cryptosporidium* and *Giardia* spp. in feces may be more easily detected with ELISA or FA, but FA testing requires a fluorescent microscope, and the ELISA generally is available as a send-out test to a commercial laboratory (see Chapter 78 and Appendices 5 and 6). However, these tests markedly improve sensitivity for detection of *Cryptosporidium* organisms.

Cattery management of GI disease should include surveillance and outbreak investigations to clarify the status of infection in the colony and prevention of new cases through support of CR and blocking disease transmission. Surveillance should include regular quantification of GI disease present, including number of cases for which specific pathogens are identified. Animals can best resist GI infections when they are otherwise healthy and well nourished, not stressed, have intact normal bacterial flora, and have been appropriately vaccinated. Problems arise in high-density catteries with high turnover of animals, highly susceptible animals, and changes in diet. It is important to ensure that kittens receive colostrum. Even if vaccinations are given to all incoming animals, they have no effect on most of the GI pathogens. Kittens may not be protected because of maternal antibody interference and immunologic immaturity, and no cats are be protected immediately after being vaccinated. The avail-

able vaccines for GI pathogens include FPV and *Giardia*. FPV vaccine is available as KV, MLV-traditional, and MLV-HAM.

It is better to perform less-frequent but thorough disinfections than daily cursory disinfections, although spot cleaning should be performed every day. Because many GI pathogens are difficult to kill, the environment should be as dry as possible, exposed to ultraviolet light, and decontaminated with bleach. To prevent the casual spread of GI pathogens, bleach foot baths should be set up at or built into entrances to catteries or shelters. If possible, a 14-day quarantine is helpful. If the facility has an inadequate amount of space and holding time for a functioning quarantine, the next best option is cohort admission.

Therapy

In cases in which specific diagnostic tests are not run or results are all negative, empiric treatment of diarrhea may be advised, including antibiotics, motility modulators, a bland diet, or antiinflammatory agents. Each has drawbacks. Antibiotics may adversely affect normal flora. Drugs to reduce gut motility and diarrhea increase retention time of all luminal contents, including pathogens that can exacerbate the disease. Bismuth subsalicylate should be used carefully in cats because they have very low tolerance for salicylic acid. Even a bland diet can be counterproductive if the animals will not eat it.

Treatment for parvovirus includes nursing care, management of hydration and electrolyte status, prevention and management of secondary bacterial infection and septicemia caused by loss of white blood cells, and facilitation of the recovery of the bone marrow. Other GI infections generally have a better prognosis than parvovirus if identified and treated appropriately. Treatment of many parasitic infections is straightforward. Metronidazole and fenbendazole are the drugs of choice for *Giardia* organisms (see Table 78-3). However, treatment failure is common, particularly in Abyssinians, Bengals, and some other purebred cats. If treatment fails, the feces should be reevaluated to determine whether the protozoa are *Tritrichomonas* spp. that have been misdiagnosed as *Giardia*, and additional diagnostics should be performed to identify other underlying diseases that might be present. *Cryptosporidium* organisms are considered self-limiting; if treatment is necessary, paromomycin and azithromycin might be considered, although both have low to moderate efficacy. Treatment of *Tritrichomonas* organisms is quite difficult. Metronidazole and paromomycin have been used; however, neither is very effective, and paromomycin is toxic in cats. Coccidiostatic drugs such as sulfadimethoxine can reduce the number of asexual progeny being produced by the organism so that the host's epithelium can repair itself. Often animals with severe coccidiosis respond better to treatment when they also receive metronidazole, clindamycin, or ampicillin.

Primary bacterial pathogens should be treated with antibiotics appropriate to the bacterium (see Tables 39-2, 39-6, and 39-10). For *Campylobacter* spp., good choices include erythromycin, tetracycline, enrofloxacin, and tylosin. Triple therapy is helpful for severe or refractory cases, including bismuth subcitrate or subsalicylate (caution in cats), ampicillin, and metronidazole. The author has found it helpful to substitute enrofloxacin for ampicillin in some animals. Older literature indicates that patients receiving antibiotics for *Salmonella* spp. may become carriers. With modern antibiotics, the greater concern is the evolution of resistant strains, although most infections can be eradicated with chloramphenicol, enrofloxacin, tetracycline, or trimethoprim-sulfonamide drugs, provided the bacteria are susceptible. Adjunctive therapy should include fluids as needed and possibly lipopolysaccharide hyperimmune serum. If opportunistic bacteria are detected, an additional evaluation for underlying diseases should be performed and the diseases treated if possible. Many animals have self-limiting opportunistic infections; antibiotics only serve to scour the gut of normal flora and increase the likelihood of additional problems. If an animal is diagnosed with a *C. difficile* infection, it is particularly important to address the underlying disease and decontaminate the environment. The two best drug choices are metronidazole and vancomycin, because many isolates are resistant to metronidazole. Public health veterinarians may be concerned justifiably about the use of vancomycin in shelter animals.

Dermatophyte Infections

Dermatophytes are molds in the Ascomycota; 95% of all cat cases of dermatophytosis are caused by *Microsporum canis*.[40] The conidia gain access to keratinized epithelium, often through a defect in the stratum corneum, then germinate, and mycelia enter cornified strata. As arthroconidia develop in tissue, clinical signs develop because of fungal products such as elastase, collagenase, and keratinase and as a result of allergic responses to the fungi. The incubation period for ringworm is between 4 days and 4 weeks. Infection finally may be resolved by cell-mediated immunity in weeks or months, although some carriers remain chronically infected. Severe or chronic disease prevalence is higher in geriatric cats and those younger than 1 year, as well as Persian cats, cats that have FIV and feline leukemia virus (FeLV) infections, are pregnant or lactating, are malnourished, are taking antiinflammatory drugs, or that have cancer or are stressed. Ringworm is zoonotic.

Accurate diagnosis of ringworm is critical because ringworm contamination can rapidly get out of control. Unfortunately, many shelters euthanize affected cats because they cannot contain ringworm. Classically, the condition is characterized by a circular, inflamed lesion with stratum corneum hypertrophy from which hair is lost and crusting develops. Severe ringworm may be confused superficially with mange, whereas mild cases may be subtle, with small areas of hair loss or a few crusts. The most common locations include the face, ears, feet, and tail. Examination with a Wood's lamp reveals *bright* green fluorescence in about 50% of affected animals. Microscopic examination for ringworm is performed on hairs plucked from the periphery of suspect lesions. Hair is cleared of keratin by suspending it in 10% to 20% potassium hydroxide (KOH). The slide is then gently heated for 15 to 20 seconds or allowed to stand for 30 minutes at room temperature before being examined. Infected hairs appear swollen and frayed, with loss of normal structure. Arthroconidia and hyphae occasionally can be seen.

Fungal culture is the most reliable method of assessing the presence of ringworm. Samples are collected by plucking hair from the edge of the lesion or running a new toothbrush through the coat. The hairs or toothbrush tines are placed onto an appropriate agar such as dermatophyte test medium (DTM) or rapid sporulation medium (RSM) that contain antibiotics and antifungal drugs to discourage growth of contaminants, although some nondermatophytes do grow. DTM contains phenol red, which turns red in the presence of alkaline metabolites produced primarily by dermatophytes and a few saprophytes. Bromothymol blue in RSM turns blue-green in the presence of dermatophytes. Plates incubated in air at room temperature for days to a few weeks, should be observed for visible fungal mycelia and color change daily. When candidate dermatophytes are observed, hyphae should be examined under the microscope for the characteristic conidia (most easily seen on RSM) to confirm the diagnosis. This step, which commonly is skipped, is essential. The morphology and presence of macroconidia and microconidia are essential for confirming and identifying dermatophytes; their characteristics are described in the package insert with the culture plates or in various microbiology texts.

In addition to controlling infection in the environment, colony management of ringworm should incorporate the assumption that infected animals periodically enter the facility, and minimizing movement and contact are important. Ringworm-positive and possibly affected animals should be isolated, especially from cats with URIs. Staff members should wear gloves, smocks or coveralls, and boots or shoe covers while working with affected cats. After contact with ringworm-positive cats, staff members should not have contact with well cats until they have showered and changed clothes. Affected animals should not be allowed into the main facility until several weeks after their apparent clinical recovery and culture results have been negative for 2 weeks. Ringworm is very viable in the environment. Grooming instruments and fomites such as toys should be disposable or able to be decontaminated. Dermatophytes are susceptible only to prolonged contact (preferably overnight) with strong bleach. Washable items can be cleaned in a dishwasher if it has a water temperature at least 43.3° C (110° F).

Many cats spontaneously recover in about 3 months. Topical treatment reduces contamination of the environment and arguably does not reduce the clinical severity or accelerate recovery.[41] Clipping, which should be performed *gently* with a #10 blade, removes infected hairs from the animal and therefore environment. A lime-sulfur dip (4%) used twice weekly is relatively effective and safe if patted on rather than rubbed into the coat. Creams, ointments, and azole-containing shampoos have disappointing results.

The drawbacks to systemic therapy are the high cost, toxic side effects, long course of treatment required, and lack of efficacy in reducing clinical severity or speeding recovery. Griseofulvin is fungistatic, less expensive than itraconazole, and more likely to cause vomiting, diarrhea, and bone marrow suppression. Itraconazole does not efficiently resolve ringworm in cats, and its adverse effects include hepatic disease and vasculitis. Daily oral lufenuron therapy has been reported as an effective treatment for ringworm, although some trials have not documented improved recovery. Vaccinating affected cats with a killed *M. canis* vaccine is intended to speed recovery. (See Chapter 58 for additional information about this disease.)

Retroviral Infections

The retroviruses—FeLV and FIV—are insidious, feline-specific infections that can predominate densely housed populations of cats unless preventive management strategies are implemented.[44] FeLV is transmitted through direct contact with urine, saliva, milk, and blood of infected cats or through in utero exposure. Neither FeLV nor FIV can persist in the environment. After exposure, many cats eliminate the infection and become immune. If the virus is not eliminated, infection may persist for months to a few years until the cat develops neoplasia, disregulated blood cell production, immunosuppression, or one of many rare and bizarre FeLV-associated syndromes such as cutaneous horns, immune complex nephritis or arthritis, or both. Because signs of FeLV infection can be vague (e.g., weight loss, vomiting, lack of energy) and because of the long latent period during which cats can be infectious but not symptomatic, it is critically important to screen cats before entry into a multiple-cat environment and to maintain an FeLV-free colony. Most FeLV infections are identified by ELISA, which detects the p27 antigen that is present in viremic cats. After exposure to FeLV, a cat has positive test results in blood within days to a week and if able, eradicates the virus within about 2 weeks. To ensure without a doubt that the virus has been eliminated, healthy cats should be retested in 4 to 6 weeks. If a cat has a positive result at that point, they should be considered chronically infected.

If effective screening tests are performed, it is unlikely that cats with FeLV will be introduced, but good husbandry practices should be in place to prevent viral transmission in the event that an FeLV-infected cat is missed. FeLV-positive cats should be isolated or kept only with other infected cats. Some safe commercial vaccines against FeLV infection can be given yearly. Expert opinions differ about the vaccine's effectiveness. Certainly, most vaccinated cats do not develop FeLV infection, but neither do most otherwise well adult cats.

FeLV is a fatal infection; at best, cats do well clinically for months to a few years. The only goals for treatment are to keep virus levels as low as possible, reduce the impact of FeLV-associated disorders, and maximize quality of life. Treatment usually fails within a few months. If managers opt to treat FeLV-positive cats, they should be well educated about preventive management to protect healthy cats do not acquire the infection and about quality of life of infected cats so that euthanasia can be performed at an appropriate time. (For additional information about FeLV infection, see Chapter 13.)

FIV is a lentivirus that is closely related to the human immunodeficiency virus (HIV; see Chapter 14). The main routes of FIV transmission are via biting and breeding. Cats can live together in one home without transmitting the disease, although biting tends to be most common during initial introductions. After infection, the cat develops a high level of viremia followed by host immune-induced significant reductions in circulating virus load. Over time (5 or more years), progressive immunocompromise develops—manifest as *feline acquired immunodeficiency syndrome (AIDS) related complex*—with secondary oral disease, severe URIs, hemotropic mycoplasma infection, neoplastic disease, and other conditions, followed by true AIDS.

The screening test for FIV is an antibody ELISA. PCR for FIV is not sensitive enough for diagnostic use, although real-time PCR shows promise. Because ELISA gives some false-positive results, infection can be confirmed with a Western blot. Maternal antibodies may interfere with FIV testing in kittens, but false-positive test results rarely occur at 4 months of age and are very unlikely by 6 months.

The decision about how to manage FIV in a cattery is difficult because although infected cats have an excellent quality of life for years, they have a contagious, fatal infection. If a manager can prevent transmission, affected cats can be kept in a multiple-cat environment if they are well nourished, protected from stress and other infectious diseases, and are treated for secondary conditions. Antiretroviral drugs have been researched extensively, but no cure for FIV infection exists. Because even moderately immunosuppressed cats are more susceptible to infection, FIV-positive cats may contribute disproportionately to the load of infectious organisms in a multiple-cat environment, increasing risks for other cats. Cats with FIV should be housed only with other cats with FIV and should not be housed with FeLV-positive cats. A vaccine for FIV exists, and new technologies are actively being researched that will probably result in additional vaccines within a few years. Unfortunately, widespread use of vaccine will make screening difficult because vaccinated cats will have positive ELISA results.

Feline Enteric Coronavirus and Feline Infectious Peritonitis

FECV is a ubiquitous, clinically silent feline coronavirus (FCoV) infection found in virtually all cats in endemic multiple-cat environments.[7] The virus localizes in GI villous tip epithelium and produces mild pathologic lesions with minimal if any detectable clinical signs (see Chapter 12). The virus is spread directly among cats through exposure to infected feces. The significance of FECV in cats is that mutant forms of FECV known as *feline infectious peritonitis virus (FIPV)* arise frequently in cats and may acquire the ability to enter and replicate within feline macrophages.[48] When accompanied by a particular feline immune response, this can result in feline infectious peritonitis (FIP; see Chapter 11). FIP is the cat's immune-mediated response to the infection; immune complexes are formed, and immunologic reactions lead to the characteristic pathologic and clinical abnormalities. In noneffusive FIP, granulomatous masses form on kidneys, on mesenteric lymph nodes, on liver, in the brain and eyes, or all of these and may lead to organ failure. Cats with effusive FIP develop a high-protein, yellow-colored effusion fluid in their chest or abdomen, causing dyspnea or abdominal distention.

The diagnosis of FIP is based on a composite of history, signalment, clinical observations, physical examination, and laboratory findings. FIP is most common in 1- to 3-year-old cats from multiple-cat households and shelters. Cats typically have symptoms of a cyclic nature, antibiotic-unresponsive fever, lethargy, and failure to grow.[8] CBC abnormalities include elevated total protein (mainly globulin) and mild neutrophilia and lymphopenia. Because FECV and FIP virus (FIPV) antibodies *completely* cross-react, the diagnosis of FIP by antibody tests in a healthy cat cannot be made. These antibody detection tests should be appropriately termed *FCoV antibody tests* rather than FIPV antibody tests. Because of its extremely high sensitivity and the lack of discernable differences in the viral genomes, PCR that detects viral RNA *cannot* differentiate between FIPV and FECV, although a positive PCR in tissues from some anatomic locations such as the brain (which is not invaded by FECV) strongly suggests FIP. Newer experimental mRNA-detection methods show some promise in making this distinction (see Chapter 11). The only way to confirm a diagnosis of FIP is to identify the FIPV in biopsies or at necropsy—if necessary, by using an FCoV-specific immunohistochemical stain. Finding large quantities of FCoV by immunofluorescence in tissues outside the enteric lumen is typical of FIP.

Virtually every cat with FIP dies. Given the infection's immune-mediated pathogenesis, immunosuppressive drugs may slow disease progression but do not result in a cure. Cats should receive broad-spectrum antibiotics and nursing care for as long as they are comfortable. Once the disease becomes debilitating and weight and appetite decline, the cat should be euthanized. Very little can be done to effectively prevent FIP in multiple-cat environments. Cats acquire FIP directly from other cats via fecal-oral spread of FECV and resultant mutation of the FECV within the individual cat's gut. If cats are exposed to FECV, the risk that FIP may develop *always* exists; FECV can only be eradicated in very small groups of cats (less than four *per building*). In multiple-cat groups, 40% to 60% of the cats shed virus in their feces at any given time, and virtually all cats have seropositive FCoV test results. The available FIP vaccine is not very effective in protecting cats from FIP or FECV, but it appears safe. It must be given before FeCV exposure to have any efficacy. Prevention of FIP should focus on keeping cats as clinically healthy as possible and efficiently diagnosing existing infections.

SPECIAL SITUATIONS

Veterinary Hospitals

Veterinary hospitals are unique multiple-cat environments characterized by high turnover, high proportions of ill cats, and often, multiple species. The missions of a veterinary hospital with respect to cats usually include well-cat preventive care, ill-cat care, possible boarding, and possible management of in-house cats (e.g., residents, blood donors). Preventive management in a hospital should rely on movement control and routine disinfection. All surfaces exposed to cats (e.g., floors, cages, examination tables) should be washed daily with soap and water and disinfected with bleach after each cat contact. The movement of obviously infectious cats should be highly restricted and if hospitalized, such cats should be housed in isolation wards and managed by staff members who do not interact with well cats until they have changed their clothes and, preferably, showered. Most veterinary hospitals have little need for a routine, incoming-cat quarantine procedure.

Boarding and Grooming Catteries

The mission of boarding and grooming facilities generally includes well-animal management. The first step in movement control is to ensure that sick or infectious cats are not admitted and are routed to a veterinary hospital. This step requires a vigilant, well-trained staff. If cats are boarded for prolonged periods, they should be quarantined initially. For all cats that are entering or leaving the facility, movement control should preclude contact of cats with each other and fomites. Cages and all equipment must be cleaned and disinfected between each cat contact. Kitten boarding and grooming should be minimized, and all incoming cats should have current vaccinations.

Shelters

Various shelter types with various missions exist, ranging from animal control facilities that accept all cats and have high turnover to *no-kill* and other animal shelters with random-source intake but low turnover and some long-term residents. In some animal *sanctuaries*, admission is severely restricted, and cats may stay for life. Most shelters have a high prevalence of infectious disease because of concurrent debilitating factors (e.g., stress, poor nutrition, inadequate well-cat care), numerous circulating infections, crowding, inadequate sanitation, and inadequate vaccinations. Optimal practice of shelter medicine is a very complicated subject; appropriate use of quarantine, movement control, and isolation are extremely important. Cats should receive vaccinations for the common diseases on entry. Medical and well-cat preventive care should be performed in consultation with an in-house veterinarian. It is unfortunate that the majority of sick cats in shelters acquire their infections from the shelter, a fact that should prompt shelter managers and veterinarians to make preventive colony management a top priority.

Retail Outlets

Retail pet stores share some characteristics of shelters in that they may have high turnover, constant visitation from the public, noise, and stress. The control of infectious diseases in pet stores is exacerbated by the high prevalence of kittens in the population. However, retail stores have considerable control over the incoming population—if they choose to exercise it. Kittens that are shipped from distant sources shortly after weaning are *very* stressed and susceptible to disease. Stores should only accept fully vaccinated kittens older than 3 months of age from highly reputable sources. Shipping must be humane and as stress-free as possible. All incoming cats should be screened at intake by a medically knowledgeable staff person (preferably a veterinarian or veterinary technician) and placed either in quarantine or isolation. Any money saved by skipping this step results in a far greater expense later when the cats become ill and the clients become dissatisfied. Cats in isolation should be under the care of a veterinarian. Cats in quarantine may be available for purchase but should not be mixed with cats that have completed quarantine or with possibly infected fomites, including the public. Obviously, humane and stress-free environments with minimal exposure to noise, excellent sanitation and nutrition, and gentle handling also minimize infectious disease.

Research and Specific Pathogen-Free Catteries

In many ways, infectious disease control in SPF catteries is easier than in other multiple-cat environments. If incoming cats are quarantined individually or in small groups they can be tested and denied entry unless they are nonsymptomatic and free of antibodies (or antigen) for FeLV, FIV, FECV, FHV, FCV, and FPV. Commercially available SPF cats often are infected with FECV and multiple GI pathogens, including *G. lamblia*, *C. parvum* and *C. felis*, and *Campylobacter* spp., producing infections that often are asymptomatic and difficult to eradicate. Obtaining completely disease-free cats may require cesarean delivery of kittens and housing in small, contained, sterile facilities. These miscellaneous opportunistic infections may be most intolerable in research programs with immunosuppressed animals, but it is disconcerting how many endemic, ineradicable infections are common in even well-managed, multiple-cat environments. It is also amazing how well most cats tolerate them.

SUGGESTED READINGS*

7. Foley JE, Poland A, Carlson J, et al. 1997a. Patterns of feline coronavirus infection and fecal shedding from cats in multiple-cat environments. *J Am Vet Med Assoc* 210:1307-1312.

9. Foley JE, Rand C, Bannasch MJ, et al. 2002. Molecular epidemiology of feline bordetellosis in two animal shelters in California, USA. *Prev Vet Med* 54:141-156.

12. Gaskell R, Gaskell C. 1997. Respiratory disease. *Vet Q* 19:S48.

24. Kessler M, Turner D. 1999. Socialization and stress in cats *(Felis silvestris catus)* housed singly and in groups and in groups in animal shelters. *Animal Welfare* 8:15-26.

*See the CD-ROM for a complete list of references.

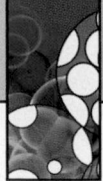

CHAPTER 98

Prevention and Management of Infection in Kennels

Dennis F. Lawler

Dog kennel populations can be described as stable or transient and can be defined further by their purpose. Relatively stable adult canine populations are found in kennels that support purebred interests (breeding or performance), in those that produce puppies for commercial pet channels, in research kennels that maintain long-term residents, and in multiple-pet households. Transient populations are usually associated with veterinary hospitals, grooming and boarding facilities, community shelters, retail outlets, suppliers that acquire and condition dogs for resale, and research kennels that do not maintain long-term residents. Shelters that do not euthanize have characteristics of both stable and transient kennels. Additionally, characteristics of both stable and transient populations can be noted in breeding and performance kennels if bidirectional transport of dogs constitutes a substantial and ongoing portion of routine activities.

ALL KENNEL POPULATIONS

General Characteristics

Regardless of their intended purpose, all kennel populations share general features, including close proximity of residents, some means of confinement, a system for sanitation and husbandry, a level of health care, and environmental effects (Fig. 98-1). Yet, each facility possesses unique features that influence occurrence of infectious diseases. For example, in most geographic areas, nearly all dogs housed in kennels are exposed to the same environmentally stable agents, such as canine parvovirus (CPV; see Chapter 8). However, kennels that produce many litters of puppies are likely to experience greater incidence of clinical CPV infection because of environmental contamination and sequential passage to susceptible younger litters.

Clinical diseases caused by more labile agents are influenced by interactions between environmental stressors and the natural biology of the agents. Seasonal tracheobronchitis in crowded boarding kennels is one important example of the latter (see Chapter 6). Another important example relates to bacterial infections of the female reproductive system in breeding kennels. A slight increase in mastitis or metritis might be expected—and should be anticipated—in association with seasonally increased humidity. When such events become frequent, other management errors are likely contributory. Most common among these errors are inadequate clipping of hair from mammary glands before lactation, infrequent or inadequate removal of feces (particularly from pens housing litters), inadequate flushing of pens during cleaning (and poor general sanitation practices), poorly trained caretakers, and failure to examine lactating bitches with sufficient frequency.

One underlying characteristic of all kennel populations is frequently problematic and can be the most difficult to address: the nature of human decision making. Increased population susceptibility to infections is the usual outcome of the more common management errors that are made by kennel operators. These errors include (1) overcrowding of facilities,

(2) inattention to basic principles that relate to movement of dogs within and among populations, (3) improper environmental management, and (4) poor breeding stock selection in production environments.

Regardless of the type of facility, most kennel operators are aware that some means of vaccination and parasite control are necessary. However, appreciating the level of planning and the expenditure that accompanies effective prevention may be difficult. Too often, greater effort and financial loss will ultimately associate with problem solving, absent of established prevention based on education and forethought. Most frequently, then, it is in the application of routine preventive practices, and also in the mechanisms of problem solving, that the assistance of experienced professionals becomes critical. In all environments, planned preventive management is far more efficient and cost effective compared with purely therapeutic or reactive management. In this respect, training staff members thoroughly in environmental hygiene and personal protection is particularly important because of the zoonotic aspect of many infections agents.

Transmission

Transmission of infectious agents can be direct through immediate or close contact between reservoir hosts and susceptible subjects. Microorganisms can also spread by inanimate vehicle (fomite), by air or droplet, or by various mechanical or biologic vectors.[6] Host factors that influence expression of infection as clinical disease include age, inbreeding coefficient, nutritional status, and general health. Organism factors include virulence and dose of the infecting strain and route of inoculation. Variable but unique environmental factors (season, crowding, ventilation, sanitation) influence the interaction among source, organism, and host and often strongly influence the outcome.[16,17] Recognizing the nature of these interactions in individual kennels is an extremely important part of developing effective preventive management strategies that are tailored to each facility.

Disease Management

Depending on logistic and economic circumstances, the goal may be to prevent one or more diseases (i.e., disease does not occur) or to maintain acceptable suppression (i.e., disease occurs with control of morbidity and mortality). The key factor is interrupting transmission of microorganisms, and the essential element is knowing the biology or life cycles of target infectious agents. An important point to realize is that target organisms may change with the seasons and may change over time for various reasons. The latter is particularly critical in facilities that have unstable populations. In all cases, management procedures that need to be considered include vaccination and parasite control, ongoing surveillance, disinfection practices, training of staff in procedures to minimize transmission, traffic patterns within the facility, changes in the population, and genetic supervision of breeding kennels. Long-term successful management is possible only if major target organisms have been identified and all aspects of the preventive process have been addressed.

The sanitary state of the kennel influences occurrence of infectious disease directly by providing or preventing access to concentrations of microorganisms and indirectly by modulating stress. Disinfection alone is not a substitute for good overall management. In many cases, kennel operators simply wish to know which disinfectant should be purchased (see Chapter 94). However, the nonspecific effectiveness of chemical disinfection depends substantially on the intended environment and manner of use.[1,10,11,15] The primary goal of environmental management is to maintain surroundings that harbor the lowest possible number of infectious agents and that reduce stress as much as possible.

Disinfection and effective parasite control are essentially impossible in kennels with dirt flooring, especially in warm, humid climates or during wet seasons. Increased environmental microorganism load can compromise reproductive or work performance, and additional parasite burden can be devastating for puppies. Facilities that use grass surfaces ultimately face the same problems unless these areas can be rotated regularly; the household is the lone possible (but not universal) exception.[1,11]

Gravel runs provide drainage and are not prohibitively expensive, and sanitation can be managed reasonably well for small numbers of dogs if preventive health care is adequate. For larger facilities, gravel maintenance and disease control require more effort. Digging by dogs is followed by accumulation of standing water, providing a reservoir for infectious agents such as enteropathogenic bacteria and possibly flagellate parasites. Chemical disinfection is more difficult because of the large surface area provided by several inches of gravel and because large amounts of organic material accumulate readily, reducing the effectiveness of many disinfectants. Weed control and removal of wasted feed must be aggressive to control external parasites and rodents. Regular worming schedules should be implemented and monitored frequently with fecal examinations. Scrupulous daily removal of feces is imperative. Complete replacement of gravel materials at intervals may solve these problems but adds greatly to investments of time, money, and labor.[1,11]

Concrete pens are more expensive to construct, but sanitation and disease control can be managed more effectively. A surface that is slightly roughened (to minimize injuries) and gradually sloped for drainage can be disinfected regularly and kept clean daily without difficulty. Cracks and other damage need to be repaired as they occur. Environmental management programs designed to maximize effectiveness of disinfecting agents in individual kennels still must be based on knowledge of primary target disease agents, but broadly applicable general principles of sanitation greatly facilitate this process (Table 98-1).[1,11]

Pens of any design should be dry and sheltered from prevailing winds during inclement weather, and puppies should not be allowed to become wet or chilled. Rapid changes in temperature and humidity can facilitate development of infectious diarrhea and respiratory disease, especially when the environment is crowded or when young dogs are present. Increased stress and easier transmission of infectious organisms are the most likely explanations for disease outbreaks.

Cages should be cleaned and disinfected daily and between occupants. Periodic steam cleaning is helpful when available.[6] In the absence of steam cleaning or power spraying capability, frequent and copious flushing of pens with water is an important adjunct to a sanitation program. Animals should not be placed in wet cages or pens because of the risk of injury or direct exposure to disinfectant. For the same reason, caretakers need to be trained thoroughly in proper application of disinfectant chemicals, in the necessity for aggressive sanitation,

Table • 98-1

General Principles of Environmental Management in Kennels

1. Regular cleaning and disinfecting schedule should be established.
2. Surfaces should be cleared of wastes and other organic material before disinfectants are applied. Organic materials compromise the effectiveness of many disinfectants.
3. Disinfectants and other cleaning products such as soaps should be combined only by, or on direction of, the manufacturer. Inappropriate combinations can cause loss of effectiveness. Manufacturer's directions for product use should be followed exactly. Dogs should be removed from pens that are being disinfected and reintroduced when pens are dry.
4. Many products are more effective in hot water and less effective in hard water or when combined inappropriately with other agents. Municipal water supplies are usually safe for drinking, but wells, ponds, and other nonstandard water sources should be monitored for bacterial and protozoal (i.e., *Giardia*) contamination, as well as for mineral content.
5. Bedding should be clean and dry. Access by insects, rodents, and birds should be prevented. Bedding should be changed as often as needed to maintain sanitation. Some litters of puppies may require multiple changes daily.
6. Feed should be stored in containers that prohibit access by insects, birds, and rodents (i.e., metal cans with tight-fitting lids). Great caution must be used with home-formulated feeds, especially in large kennels, from nutritional and disease perspectives.
7. Fecal waste should be disposed of daily, and waste containers should be disinfected frequently. Fecal wastes should not be disposed of within animal areas.
8. Equipment such as heating and cooling systems and vacuums should be cleaned and serviced regularly by qualified persons to avoid creating habitats for microorganisms.
9. Stored equipment, debris, weeds, and other items not critical to kennel function should not be allowed to accumulate.

and in personal safety. Animal handling should ordinarily be done on an age-priority basis, such as youngest first and progressing through older groups.

Nutrition

Population nutrition is a challenge because effective feeding management in group environments requires consideration of the type of kennel, individual housing, seasonal influences, ambient temperature, amount of work or exercise, and environmental stressors such as crowding, exposure to sudden weather changes, and burden of infectious agents. Energy requirements are increased by lower ambient temperatures, work, exercise, gestation, lactation, and environmental stressors and tend to be decreased by inactivity and higher ambient temperatures. Each dog is part of the population, but each dog is an individual in terms of health, temperament, and nutri-

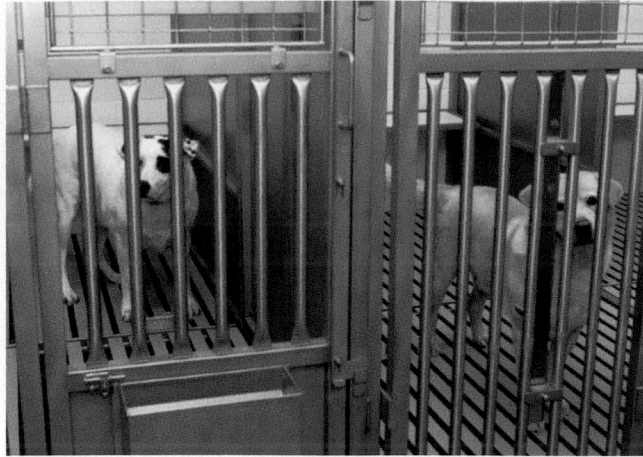

Fig 98-1 Functional kennels should provide a comfortable environment for dogs and provide for ease in sanitation and husbandry.

tional requirements. Nutritional needs of individuals can vary widely in the same facility, among breeds, within the breed, and even among siblings. Therefore dogs in populations need to be fed as individuals and according to their apparent (and often changing) needs, which requires a consistent level of oversight.

Nutritional fads and extremes should always be avoided. Anecdotal reports of effects of unusual diets or supplements should be regarded suspiciously until results of controlled studies can be produced. Nutritional supplementation adds considerably to overhead costs and is seldom necessary or particularly effective if basic feeding practices are sound. In studies of growing puppies that were supplemented with vitamin-mineral combinations or excessive protein, no beneficial effects on immunologic measures were found.[14] Good-quality, nutritionally complete and balanced commercial products should be chosen for applicable life stages, and manufacturers' claims should be supported by feeding studies and not simply by analytical results based on National Research Council guidelines.

A study of long-term caloric restriction in dogs demonstrated that reduced intake (25% less food) over the lifetime of 24 Labrador retrievers, as compared with 24 control-fed pair mates, resulted in a significantly longer (15%) median life span. Along with this outcome were associated a significant number of favorable morphometric changes that included lower body weight, body fat mass, and body condition scores, as well as longer maintenance of lean body mass into late life. Physiologically, variables that measure insulin-glucose metabolism were influenced favorably, along with time of expression of numerous diseases of later life, such as osteoarthritis.[10,8,9] No increase in the incidence of infections was noted in the food-restricted group of dogs, although the research environment was managed aggressively with respect to sanitation and preventive health care.

The importance of this research, in addition to the obvious question of maintaining lean body mass and avoiding any degree of obesity, is that it further underscores the need to be conscious of the individuality of dogs in group environments. Some problems of late life, such as effects of osteoarthritis, are actually initiated relatively early. For example, in the food-restriction study, several of the control-fed dogs had evidence of osteoarthritis by early adulthood. These individuals tended to have more severe clinical signs of osteoarthritis during middle and late life. Among food-restricted dogs, osteoarthri-

tis of multiple joints occurred less often, was generally less severe, and was associated with much later occurrence of clinical signs.[9] The risk of infections in these compromised individuals is likely to become proportionately greater as other management and sanitation practices become progressively less adequate or essentially neglected.

STABLE KENNEL ENVIRONMENTS

Breeding Kennels
Isolation
Stable facilities usually have low adult population turnover and therefore offer opportunity for point-of-entry control of infectious diseases. Entering dogs in larger breeding kennels should be isolated for approximately 4 weeks for observation, worming, vaccination, and selected surveillance laboratory procedures. (See Appendix 5 and respective chapters for testing for specific microorganisms and preferred diagnostic and screening procedures.) Brucellosis testing should always be done before departure from the source kennel and repeated one or more times at 30-day intervals in the destination kennel (see Chapter 40). Isolation should occur outside of usual traffic patterns. Isolated dogs should be cared for after other residents or by different personnel. When this practice is not possible, hand washing, clothing change, and separate footwear may be indicated if the risk of introducing new infectious agents is high.[1]

In smaller kennels where time, space, and funding do not permit isolation, careful evaluation of the infectious disease status of the source kennel should precede entry to the destination kennel. Vaccinations, parasite checks, and other surveillance procedures should be completed 2 to 4 weeks before entry, and veterinary examination also should be completed before entry.

Inbreeding
Inbreeding is frequently practiced to concentrate traits that are perceived as being superior. However, excessive emphasis on aesthetic desirability (such as coat color or conformation or on any individual trait) can be hazardous. Excessive inbreeding can be associated with immunocompromise and increased susceptibility to infection (see Chapter 95),[3] which may explain in part why certain breeds seem to have disproportionate susceptibility to diseases such as CPV infection. In fact, one important signal that excessive inbreeding may be occurring in a production facility is a general increase in the frequency of infections and especially increased severity of infections that ordinarily occur as relatively minor problems. Declining reproductive efficiency may also be observed consequent to excessive inbreeding, resulting in smaller litters and greater neonatal mortality.[13] Another indicator of excessive inbreeding is increased incidence of behavioral disorders among breeding kennel residents or offspring. That abnormalities in all of these areas will occur simultaneously is not obligatory, but eventually all appear if excessive inbreeding or poor choices of breeding stock are practiced over time.

Age
Advanced age represents a theoretical risk factor for infections because of naturally declining immune function.[5] However, practical experience in kennels that are managed well has shown that occurrence of, and death from, infectious diseases does not increase with advancing age if other management factors are controlled well. Longitudinal evaluation of immune functions were conducted as a part of lifetime evaluation of the effects of restricted food intake.[4] These studies demonstrated age-related decline of absolute numbers of total

lymphocytes, T cells, CD-4 lymphocytes, and CD-8 lymphocytes in males and females.[4] This experimental population of 48 dogs was part of a much larger colony, and despite decline in some measured immune functions, neither control-fed nor calorie-restricted dogs appeared clinically to be differentially susceptible to infections.[4] Therefore maintaining older dogs in stable, well-managed populations seems to pose no significant infectious risk to individuals or to the kennel, provided that other aspects of genetic, environmental, and nutritional management are done properly.

Poorly managed breeding kennels may experience increased neonatal mortality from bacterial infections. In these facilities, however, increased neonatal mortality resulting from hypoxia also may be observed through careful necropsy practices because outcomes of poor management practices usually occur in multiples. The highest risk for infection in most kennels occurs after weaning as a consequence of the relationship of maternal antibody decline to exposure to infectious organisms by animal or environmental contact.[7] Deficient vaccination and parasite control, environmental mismanagement, and poor breeding selection policies become evident, but recognizing these contributing factors is more difficult in kennels that retain few puppies past the immediate postweaning period.

Information about problems that occur at destination kennels may be necessary when planning corrective strategies in some source kennels, but multiple-source or poorly managed destination kennels can present interpretive dilemmas. In the latter instances, evaluation of multiple facilities may be necessary.

Health Maintenance

Vaccination and parasite control need to be individualized by kennel because the biologic and environmental factors that interact to influence occurrence of infectious diseases can result in varying patterns of morbidity and mortality.

Identifying and targeting offending infectious microorganisms do not differ procedurally from individual clinical presentations, but population-based problems almost always occur in magnitude commensurate with population size, density, and stress. Investments in determining the type and extent of specific infectious disease prevalence are worthwhile. Clinical signs and response to empiric therapy alone should not be used as criteria for designing or modifying management programs. Most kennel populations harbor several infectious agents that induce clinical disease variably and often in cyclic fashion. Transmission can be interrupted effectively when all offending agents are identified and when their seasonal and environment-based influences are understood.

Mortality

Veterinarians are sometimes reluctant to recommend postmortem examination, and clients may be reluctant to agree. However, in breeding kennels, causes of mortality must be identified. Most puppy mortalities occur as stillbirths (30%) or during the 0- to 3-day neonatal period (50%).[12] Variations in this expected pattern should prompt investigation. Neonates react in limited scope to dissimilar insults, whether infectious, physiologic, environmental, or genetic (anatomic or metabolic) in origin. When infectious causes are suspected, consulting laboratories should be advised of tentative diagnoses before necropsy, if possible. Tentative diagnoses can be established through review of clinical signs in pertinent literature and should be supported by further review at the time of gross necropsy so as to ensure that proper samples are taken. Appropriate procedures must then be followed for taking correct diagnostic samples, given that these can vary among infectious agents. Successful diagnosis depends absolutely on proper sample preservation, shipping, and processing.[1] (See Chapters 1, 33, 56, 70, and Appendix 5 for pertinent information.)

Increased morbidity and mortality in specific age groups within populations should increase suspicion for genetic or infectious causes. However, clinical findings should be considered in light of overall kennel health and management status because transmission of infectious agents has an environmental component. For example, increased incidence of viral enteritis among puppies may reflect overproduction and crowding with successive litters such that the environment facilitates transmission from older to younger puppies. Alternatively, the number of litters that are present simultaneously may be managed well, but inattention to proper sanitation or traffic patters may facilitate transmission. Patterns of morbidity and mortality, established over time, can be used along with specific diagnoses to develop preventive strategies. However, these efforts will be successful only of all possible contributing factors are considered and addressed.

Research and Performance Kennels

In research and performance kennels that maintain long-term residents with minimal reproductive activity, isolation on entry, parasite control, vaccination, and surveillance should be practiced aggressively, as is the case for breeding kennels. The intensity of the control program is usually less than it is in production kennels with high puppy populations, although the size and density of the adult population do influence stress and ease of transmission of infectious agents.

In research kennels, valid interpretation of experimental data depends absolutely on having a complete health database. Careful attention should be given to the type of research that is in progress and the potential for undiagnosed infections to compromise experimental data. For example, nutritional or gastrointestinal research should be accompanied by aggressive monitoring for enteric viral, bacterial, and parasitic agents. Cardiovascular research necessitates continuing evaluation for bacterial diseases, especially those that have systemic potential. The quality and outcome of studies involving immunity, such as vaccine research, depend on documenting that only the experimental agent is introduced (i.e., potentially interfering infectious agents are surveyed and not found), on knowing the status of control subjects with respect to the experimental agent, and on knowing the immunocompetence of dogs in control and test groups. The last point relates at least partially to degree of inbreeding, and therefore knowledge about source kennels can be extremely important to data interpretation.

Specific-pathogen–free dogs can be purchased for research kennels; however, in many circumstances, these dogs originate from more transient types of kennels. When new diseases are recognized in destination kennels, investigation of the status of source kennels can facilitate early diagnosis, which in turn supports rapid implementation of control measures to minimize further transmission. At times, alternate-source kennels may need to be sought, but accurate records are essential to support exclusion of problem sources on factual grounds only.

Giardiasis and nocardiosis are relatively common problems in performance kennels. Both conditions are consequences of the purpose of the kennel. Population concentration and movement of dogs among kennels tend to facilitate transmission of *Giardia*, and drinking from field water sources presents ready sources of infection and reinfection. Environmental sanitation is helpful in reducing clinical disease associated with *Giardia* cysts in the kennel. Use of quaternary ammonium disinfectants and flushing the kennel with a power sprayer should help reduce the cyst burden in the environment. Infection of sporting dogs with *Nocardia*, an opportunist organism, likely occurs during field training, hunting, or competition. Vigilance for clinical signs is important in sporting kennels (see Chapters 49 and 78).

Households

Extensive evaluations are less the custom for entry of new pets into multiple-pet households. Vaccination and parasite control should be current before entry, and physical examination should be conducted for external parasites. Sanitation should be strict with respect to fecal wastes, but the home environment usually limits use of disinfectant chemicals. When two or more dogs in the same household have similar clinical signs, an important point to remember is that proximity often means common exposure to infectious agents. However, individual characteristics, such as behavior, age, or immune status, also may influence clinical expression. Clinical illness in one dog in a multiple-dog or a multiple-pet household does not rule out group exposure.

Practicing clinicians should remember also that a neighborhood or a community represents a population as well, albeit less dense compared with a kennel environment. Nonetheless, clinicians in community practice often recognize temporally associated, similar clinical signs among pets that are owned by different households in a geographic area. These occurrences often tend to be treated symptomatically, especially if the clinical signs are not severe. Although this approach might represent practical clinical medicine, it does result in missed opportunity for specific diagnosis. Progress in community practice would be facilitated by increased attempts at specific diagnosis, and this information would be helpful in recognizing seasonal or other circumstantial influences on clinical expression of disease caused by some organisms. With specific diagnosis, more directed attempts at prevention become possible, and recognition of potential zoonoses is facilitated.

TRANSIENT ENVIRONMENTS

Management of infectious diseases in transient environments is much more difficult. Maintenance is short term, and sources usually are random. Residents are often stressed by illness, inappetence, or anxiety. This combination of population and environmental factors allows multiple simultaneous introduction of infectious agents to a transient and susceptible population. In all transient facilities, sanitation should therefore be extremely strict. In addition, admissions to these environments should be limited to individuals that are currently vaccinated, except in those populations that are composed largely of unowned pets. In the latter instance, strict sanitation, temporary isolation where possible, and vaccination on entry are important management factors. In transient environments, sanitation procedures, traffic patterns, waste disposal, hygiene procedures that limit dissemination of microorganisms and parasites, and recognition of clinical signs of illness should be part of personnel training. Procedures should be written and reviewed frequently for updating. Veterinary consultation is a necessary and very important part of disease management in transient populations.

Veterinary Hospitals

Disinfectants are important because of the high frequency of presentation of animals with infectious diseases and the risk of transmitting to other hospitalized patients or establishing nosocomial infection patterns.[6] Disinfectants should be chosen for broad-spectrum activity unless specific agents are being targeted (see Chapter 94).[1,11,15] Hospital personnel should be taught to clean and disinfect table surfaces and equipment between patients, to wash hands after each hospitalized or boarded patient is handled, to wear protective gloves when handling patients that are known or suspected to be infectious, and to recognize clinical signs of major internal and external infections. The outdoor area of the hospital should be cleaned and disinfected regularly to prevent exposure of patients by environmental contamination.

Patients with potentially contagious diseases should be isolated as well as possible, with rapid removal of wastes from animal areas. Careful attention to fomite transmission of environmentally stable and unstable agents is needed because transmission distances are usually very short. Special care should be taken to protect individuals that might be immunodeficient.[3]

Thorough vaccination programs should be pursued with all clients individually and through community education by local veterinary associations. Current vaccinations should be required for elective surgery and boarding patients and updated before admission. Every entry, whether inpatient or outpatient, should be checked carefully for external parasites and for signs of dermatophytosis (see Chapter 58).

Grooming and Boarding Kennels

Population turnover is high and constant; residence is usually very brief. Separation anxiety, close proximity or crowding, and poor ventilation often facilitate transmission of infectious agents by direct, aerosol, and fomite routes. Some opportunity for control is afforded by the fact that dogs and cats in these kennel populations are nearly always owned pets. Appropriate vaccinations can be required before entry, and entry also should be accompanied by brief screening for external parasites or dermatophytosis and by examination of the haircoat to detect signs of diarrhea or excess respiratory or ocular secretion. Veterinarians should play active roles in helping to establish policies for vaccination requirements, preentry parasite control, screening for signs of general health, and training of personnel.

Grooming and other equipment that is used in common among dogs should be kept meticulously clean and disinfected after each use. Disposable feeding bowls can work well for controlling spread of infections in some facilities, but expense and potential for some residents to shred and swallow disposable equipment needs to be considered. Operators of grooming and boarding facilities should be trained to recognize external parasites such as fleas, ticks, and lice and to note clinical signs suggesting sarcoptic mange and dermatophytosis. In addition, all personnel involved should understand how these diseases, as well as major viral and bacterial diseases, are transmitted.

Shelters

Most shelters house random-source populations with high turnover and high incidence of infectious diseases. Point-of-entry control is essentially impossible, except for individuals that have obvious clinical signs on entry. Crowding occurs frequently and represents a circumstance that is sometimes unavoidable. However, crowding does greatly increase risk for repeated introduction and rapid transmission of infectious diseases.

All clinically healthy dogs should be vaccinated and wormed. Intranasal vaccines for respiratory diseases should be provided. Unhealthy animals should be segregated for triage. Those that have severe clinical signs of infection, and especially those with high potential for transmission and low potential for survival, should be euthanized unless they can be isolated effectively for treatment.[2] Animal control officers should be trained to recognize general clinical signs that suggest infection so that accidental introduction of infectious agents is minimized. In large shelters, daily veterinary attention is essential. In smaller shelters, all supervisors should understand disease-control policies, and veterinary consultation should be available at all times.

Retail Outlets

Residents of retail outlets are usually young puppies that are shipped from distant sources shortly after weaning. Residence is short term, and stress associated with weaning, shipping, anxiety, and anorexia is significant. Some level of direct or indirect contact with other species frequently occurs.

Point-of-entry control is possible but must be based on accurate individual diagnosis (either in-house or after sale) and records that clearly establish source and means of transportation. Control is established by working with suppliers and their veterinarians to implement improved breeding programs. Preshipping management changes may also be needed, as well as improved means of transportation, adjusted allowable population density at the destination kennel, revised management procedures at the source and the destination outlet, and use of different suppliers, if necessary. Each work shift should have at least one employee trained to recognize clinical signs of viral, bacterial, parasitic, and dermatophyte infections. Species segregation should be strict.

Research Kennels

Research kennels that maintain short-term residents must understand the conditioning or health programs that suppliers use and must have aggressive and thorough in-house veterinary service. If residence duration is sufficiently short, time for development of clinical signs of infectious diseases may be insufficient. Negative effects on research protocols and their results may therefore be unrecognized. In general, the princi-

ples that apply to influence of infectious diseases on research projects in long-term facilities also apply to transient research populations.

Suppliers

Suppliers usually work with adult dogs from random sources and have varying conditioning programs. At a minimum, these measures should include careful examination, vaccination, parasite control, and behavioral evaluation. Facilities are usually too small and residence terms too short to permit effective isolation of all new entries. Operators should be trained therefore to recognize general signs of internal and external infectious diseases. The ability to conduct routine screening of feces for intestinal parasites is also helpful and can usually be done at minimal expense.

SUGGESTED READINGS*

4. Greeley EH, Ballam JM, Harrison JM, et al. 2001. The influence of age and gender on the immune system: a longitudinal study in Labrador retriever dogs, *Vet Immunol and Immunopath* 82:57-71.
9. Kealy RD, Lawler DF, Ballam JM, et al. 2000. Evaluation of the effect of limited food consumption on radiographic evidence of osteoarthritis in dogs, *J Am Vet Med Assoc* 217:1678-1680.
15. Lemarie RJ, Hosgood G. 1995. Antiseptics and disinfectants in small animal practice, *Compend Cont Educ Vet Pract* 17:1339-1351.

*See the CD-ROM for a complete list of references.

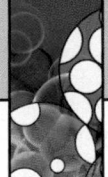

CHAPTER • 99

Immunocompromised People and Shared Human and Animal Infections: Zoonoses, Sapronoses, and Anthroponoses

Craig E. Greene and Julie K. Levy

IMMUNODEFICIENCIES IN HUMANS

Immunodeficiencies in people have various physiologic and pathologic causes (Table 99-1). Genetically induced deficiencies cause an increased susceptibility to numerous pathogens, which vary according to the type and penetrance of the defect.[119] Age is one determinant; for example, fetuses, neonates, and young children have underdeveloped immune systems. Similarly, frail older adults, especially those in nursing homes or hospitals, have apparent increased risks of developing infections. In addition to having physical disabilities and altered resistance, they may also be cognitively impaired.[199] Invasive fungal infections are an increasing problem in older adults.[99] A closed institutional environment favors more intense exposure to microorganisms because of limited ventilation and frequent close contact with other individuals. When

pets are brought to these facilities, they are often a source of infections for residents of these facilities.

Concurrent factors such as other illnesses, pregnancy, burns, or indwelling tubes, catheters, or implants increase the risk of infection by breaching natural barriers to infectious agents. Immunodeficiency is also a result of cancer chemotherapy and leukopenic disorders and may be the result of congenital or hereditary defects in the immune system. The most rapidly advancing cause of immunodeficiency in people is the acquired immunodeficiency syndrome (AIDS) resulting from infection with the human immunodeficiency virus (HIV).

Approximately 1,039,000 to 1,185,000 people in the United States are infected with HIV, and approximately 25% do not know they are infected.[63a] Up to 50% own companion animals,[47,166] as is typical for the population at large.[194]

Table • 99-1
Characteristics Associated with Immunocompromised People
Susceptible Individuals by Age
Fetuses, infants, preschoolers, older adults
Health Issues
Hospitalizations, concurrent illnesses, organ transplantation, diabetes mellitus, chronic renal failure, pregnancy, burns, leukopenia, congenital immunodeficiencies, hepatic cirrhosis, malnutrition, splenectomy
Therapeutic Agents
Cancer chemotherapy, immunosuppressive therapy, antirejection therapy
Medical Instrumentation and Procedures
Catheters, indwelling tubes, synthetic implants, splenectomy
HIV Infection
AIDS complex

HIV, Human immunodeficiency virus; *AIDS,* acquired immunodeficiency syndrome.

Approximately 132 million pet dogs and cats live in the United States.[1] The estimated prevalence of companion animals in all United States households is 60%, 38.2% of which are dogs, 30.5% cats, 5.7% birds, and 2.8% horses. Although more households have dogs, the total number of cats is greater than that of dogs. The psychological benefits that these companion animals provide are great, and the risk for acquiring infections from animals is low. Nevertheless, certain precautions that are taken while handling and caring for pets reduces any inherent risks. The information in this chapter emphasizes documented AIDS-related zoonoses, although people with immunodeficiencies from any cause should use similar guidelines when handling their pets. Furthermore, because zoonoses can develop in immunocompetent people, many of the principles and practices can be used by anyone with pets.

ZOONOTIC RISK

In the strict sense, *zoonoses* are defined as infectious diseases naturally transmitted from living animals to humans.[89] Based on their animal reservoir hosts, they can be *synanthropic* with an urban or a domestic animal cycle or *exoanthropic* with a feral or wild animal cycle. Immunocompromised people who own pets are at greater risk of contracting directly transmitted zoonotic infections than those without pets (Table 99-2). Inhalation or ingestion of infectious body secretions and excretions are the common means by which many zoonotic infections may be transmitted directly. However, transmission can occur percutaneously through contamination of preexisting skin wounds or by bites or scratches. Spread can also occur after contact of mucosae with vehicles or fomites such as contaminated utensils or food or water. Vector transmission via arthropod-borne transmission also occurs in some infections of dogs and cats, and people can become infected when these vectors feed on them. In some cases, dogs and cats

can bring vectors that are already infected with an organism closer to people. Once infected, spread of true zoonoses among humans is uncommon. Some zoonotic infections can be highly severe or fatal because people are inadvertent hosts.

Sapronoses are infections of people and animals that are maintained in nature by replication of the organism in soil, water, or vegetation or in the decay of dead animals or animal excreta. With these zoonoses, people and animals acquire infections simultaneously and independently of each other. Sapronoses were previously but inaccurately called "sapro-zoonoses," but they are not truly acquired by people from living animals (see Table 99-2).

Anthroponoses are infections in which the source, replication, and primary means of transmission occur in humans. Some of these infections can affect animals such as dogs and cats (see Table 99-2).

The importance of zoonotic diseases has become more apparent because of the AIDS epidemic in humans. In fact, the appearance of unusual zoonotic infections in people was one reason that AIDS was first recognized. The increasing incidence of zoonotic infections in immunosuppressed people makes it imperative that veterinarians know the most updated information about these diseases. Compared with veterinarians, most physicians are not as well trained in zoonoses and their advice, when given, is often to give up their pets.[4,66] Veterinarians may be in a better position to advise immunocompromised people about the relative risk of pet ownership and provide them with accurate information on precautionary measures. No significant difference was found in the type of opportunistic infections in people with AIDS, regardless of whether they owned a pet.[47] Although veterinarians are among the best educated concerning animal infections, few have taken an active role in educating their immunodeficient pet owners.[4,166] People with AIDS who have questions about their pets most frequently consult physicians, nurses, and community health personnel, many of whom give conflicting advice, whereas very few consult their veterinarians.[4,47,65] Many people with AIDS have misconceptions about zoonoses and have received misleading or no information concerning the transmission risks.[47] Surveys have shown that more than 60% to 90% of people infected with HIV have been advised by human health professionals to give up their pets, whereas only 5% have followed this advice.[25,166] The latest guidelines from the United States Public Health Service and the Infectious Disease Society of America indicate that rather than give up their pets, immunocompromised people can take simple precautions to prevent infection.[7,11,95,113]

At first glance, the risk of acquiring animal infections may seem to dominate the medical literature and media reports, but only a relatively small fraction of infections in people can actually be attributed to pet contact. People with immunosuppression are at increased risk for acquiring all types of infections, including zoonoses. People are more likely to acquire infections from other people than from animals. Furthermore, some of the highly publicized zoonoses in AIDS patients such as toxoplasmosis are caused by reactivation of a previously acquired infection and are not related to pet exposure. The Internet is a tremendous resource for information on zoonotic diseases. Table 99-3 lists important Web sites for health care workers associated with immunocompromised individuals.

OCCUPATIONAL AND ENVIRONMENTAL RISKS

Veterinarians and animal health workers may be at greater risk for acquiring zoonoses. People who work in allied professions

Table • 99-2

Means of Zoonotic Infection Transmission[a]

Zoonoses from Dogs and Cats

Bite or saliva: Rabies (see Chapter 22), pasteurellosis (see Chapter 53), capnocytophagiosis (see Chapter 53), helicobacteriosis (see Chapter 39), mycoplasmal infection (see Chapter 31), tularemia (see Chapter 48), bordetellosis (see Chapters 6, 88, and 100)

Scratch or close physical contact: Dermatophytosis (see Chapter 58), bartonellosis (see Chapter 54), tularemia (see Chapter 48), sporotrichosis (see Chapter 63), *Malassezia pachydermatis* infection (see Chapter 58), *Chlamydophila felis* infection (see Chapter 30)

Aerogenic: Plague in cat (see Chapter 47), tularemia (see Chapter 48), bordetellosis (see Chapters 6 and 88), coxiellosis (see Chapter 29), rhodococcosis (see Chapter 35)

Feces: Toxoplasmosis (see Chapter 80), cryptosporidiosis (see Chapter 82), campylobacteriosis (see Chapter 39), enteric yersiniosis (see Chapter 39), helicobacteriosis (see Chapter 39), salmonellosis (see Chapter 39), giardiasis (see Chapter 78), ancylostomiasis, toxocariasis

Urine or genital secretions: Canine brucellosis (see Chapter 40), leptospirosis (see Chapter 44), coxiellosis (see Chapter 29)

Shared Vector-Acquired Zoonoses

Ehrlichiosis (see Chapter 28), Rocky Mountain spotted fever and *Rickettsia felis* infection (see Chapter 29), tularemia (see Chapter 48), plague (see Chapter 47), borreliosis (see Chapter 45), bartonellosis (see Chapter 54), dipylidiasis

Zoonoses from Other Animals

Rhodococcus equi infection (horse), *Mycobacterium marinum* infection (fish), psittacosis (birds), salmonellosis (reptiles and amphibians), *Mycobacterium bovis* (cattle), cowpox (cattle)

Sapronoses (Environmentally Acquired Infections)

Pneumocystosis (see Chapter 68), microsporidiosis (see Chapter 75), *Mycobacterium avium*-complex infection (see Chapter 50), infection with rapid-growing mycobacteria (see Chapter 50), cryptococcosis (see Chapter 61), coccidioidomycosis (see Chapter 62), histoplasmosis (see Chapter 60), blastomycosis (see Chapter 59), aspergillosis (see Chapter 64), anthrax (see Chapter 35), listeriosis (see Chapter 35)

Anthroponoses (Infections Transmitted from Humans to Dogs and Cats)

General: Group A streptococcal infections (see Chapter 35), *Mycobacterium tuberculosis* infection (see Chapter 50), methicillin-resistant staphylococcal infections (see Chapter 36), *Streptococcus pneumoniae* infection (see Chapter 35), *Entamoeba histolytica* infection (see Chapter 78)

Unique to people: Cytomegalovirus disease, herpes simplex virus disease, varicella-zoster virus infection, human papillomavirus infection, hepatitis B infection, influenza virus infection

Overgrowth or invasion by indigenous microflora: candidiasis, bacteria associated with sepsis

[a]Predominantly dog and cat, unless otherwise indicated.

involving animal products for food or fiber are also at risk, as are those on farms or who visit zoological gardens where animal contact is allowed. In the zoological gardens, almost all exposures involved domestic herbivores and infections with fecalborne pathogens such as *Campylobacter, Giardia, Salmonella,* and *Cryptosporidium* spp.[21] In a study of veterinarians in South Africa, those in farm practice were 3 times more likely to have contracted a zoonotic disease than those working in other veterinary fields.[78] Urban zoonoses can be caused by members of the genera *Bartonella, Coxiella, Ehrlichia,* and *Rickettsia* (Table 99-4). These diseases have synanthropic cycles in which vertebrate hosts and their associated arthropod vectors can survive in metropolitan regions. Increasing population densities, encroachment on sylvan cycles of infection, increased homelessness, greater numbers of immunosuppressed people, and poor hygiene in economically disadvantaged inner city environments are all responsible for this development.[46] In one study in northern Florida, the prevalence of zoonotic infections such as toxoplasmosis or bartonellosis among feral and pet cats was equivocal,[109]

making feral cats appear to pose no greater risk to people than owned pet cats. In another report, feral and pet cats from one county in rural North Carolina had similar prevalence rates of infection with *Cryptosporidium* spp., *Giardia* spp., and *Toxocara cati.* However, a statistically higher seroprevalence of *Bartonella henselae* and *Toxoplasma gondii* antibodies was found in feral cats,[136] presumably because of greater exposure to outdoor vectors of these diseases. These studies seem to refute the common conception that feral cats have poor health and are poor choices as pets, especially for immunocompromised people. A more important criterion appears to be whether the potential pet frequents outdoor environments.

BENEFITS OF PET OWNERSHIP

Pets offer important physiologic and psychological benefits for people, especially for those who are ill (Table 99-5). Important friendships exist between people and their pets. Although

Table • 99-3

Resources for Pet Owners Infected with Human Immunodeficiency Virus Infection and for Health Care Workers

Local Groups by State or Country
- **Centers for Disease Control and Prevention (CDC):** Specific information on selected local support organizations listed by state or country[a]:
  http://www.cdc.gov/healthypets/resources/local_organizations.htm
- **CDC National Aids Hotline:** Specific information on selected local support organizations listed by state or country[a]: (800) 458-5231.

International Organizations
- **Office of International Epizooites (World Organization for Animal Health):** http://www.oie.int/eng/en_index.htm
- **Food and Agriculture Organization of the United Nations:** http://www.fao.org
- **World Health Organization:** http://www.who.int/en/

Other Organizations
- **Pet Owners with HIV/AIDS Resource Service, Inc.:** http://www.thebody.com/powars/powars.html or (212) 246-6307
- **Companion Animal Parasite Council:** http://capcvet.org, (877) CAPC-ORG, or e-mail a request to info@capcvet.org
- **Delta Society:** 875 124th Ave NE, Ste 10, Bellevue, WA 98005; (425) 226-7357; or e-mail info@deltasociety.org for information on service dogs
- **Department of Environment, Food, and Rural Affairs (United Kingdom):** for reports on zoonotic diseases, www.defra.gov.uk/animalh/diseases/zoonoses/reports.htm

General Resources
- **California Veterinary Medical Association:** 5321 Madison Ave, Sacramento, CA 95841; (916) 344-4988
- **Center for Animals in Society:** University of California, Davis, CA 95616; (916) 752-3602
- **The Latham Foundation:** 1826 Clement Ave, Alameda, CA 94501; (510) 521-0920
- **American Animal Hospital Association:** P.O. Box 150899, Denver, CO; (303) 986-2800
- **American Veterinary Medical Association:** 1931 N. Meacham Rd, Suite 100, Schaumburg, IL 60173; (800) 248-2862
- **Delta Society:** 321 Burnett Ave, S, 3rd Fl, Renton, WA 98055, (205) 226-7357 or (800) 869-6898

Additional Internet Resourses
- **CDC Healthy Pets, Healthy People:** Resource for organ transplant patients, infants and young children, and pregnant women, http://www.cdc.gov/healthypets/extra_risk.htm
- **CDC:** Guidelines for hand hygiene, http://www.cdc.gov/od/oc/media/pressrel/fs021025.htm
- **American Association of Feline Practitioners:** Guidelines for zoonotic diseases in cats, http://www.aafponline.org/pdf/zoonoses_guidelines_1003.pdf
- **AORN:** Precautions for handling patients with MRSA infection, http://www.aorn.org/journal/2001/sepci.htm
- **Pets are Wonderful Support (PAWS):** San Francisco, Calif.: http://www.pawssf.org, (415) 241-1460; Los Angeles, Calif.: http://www.pawsla.org, (213) 876-7297; affiliates located in other major cities
- **PETS-DC:** Washington, DC. http://www.petsdc.org or (202) 234-7387
- **Pets are Loving Support for People with AIDS (PALS):** Atlanta, Ga.: http://www.palsatlanta.org, (404) 876-7257

Recommended Brochures for Affected Clients
- **PAWS:** Questions You May Have About Toxoplasmosis and Your Cat. PAWS of San Francisco, Calif.
- **PAWS:** Safe Pet Guidelines: Toxoplasmosis and Your Cat, Cat Scratch Disease, Zoonoses and Your Bird. PAWS of San Francisco, Calif.
- **American Animal Hospital Association:** Pet Owner Guidelines for People with Immunocompromised Conditions. For AAHA members: (800) 252-2242, ask for Member Service Center.
- **CDC Division of HIV/AIDS Prevention:** A Guide for People with HIV Infection. http://www.cdc.gov/hiv/pubs/brochure/oi_pets.htm

[a]Includes Arizona, California, Connecticut, Delaware, District of Columbia, Florida, Georgia, Hawaii, Illinois, Massachusetts, Michigan, Minnesota, Missouri, New Jersey, New Mexico, New York, North Carolina, Pennsylvania, Tennessee, Texas, Washington, Australia, and Canada.

Table • 99-4

Urban or Suburban Zoonoses Associated with Dogs or Cats

ORGANISM	METHOD OF TRANSMISSION TO PEOPLE	VECTOR	ANIMAL RESERVOIR
Rabies (see Chapter 22)	Bites (dogs or cats) or aerosol (bats), wildlife	None	Feral dogs (not in United States), wild carnivores
Ehrlichia chaffeensis (see Chapter 28)	Tick bites	*Amblyomma* spp.	Deer, (raccoon, opossums, dogs uncertain)
Rickettsia rickettsii (see Chapter 29)	Tick bites	*Dermacentor* spp.	Rodents, dogs
Rickettsia felis (see Chapter 29)	Flea or tick bites	*Ctenocephalides* spp., ticks (uncertain)	Opossums, cats, dogs (uncertain)
Rickettsia typhi (see Chapter 29)	Flea bites	*Xenopsylla* spp., *Ctenocephalides* spp.	Rats, cats, opossums
Coxiella burnetti (see Chapter 29)	Aerosol	Ticks	Herbivores, cats
Leptospira spp. (see Chapter 44)	Contact between mucosae or broken skin and contaminated water	None	Rodents, dogs
Borrelia burgdorferi (see Chapter 45)	Tick bites	*Ixodes* spp.	Rodents, deer
Bartonella henselae (see Chapter 54)	Scratches or bites by cats (common) or dogs (rare) or by flea bites (uncertain)	*Ctenocephalides* spp.	Cats
Toxoplasma gondii (see Chapter 80)	Ingestion of animal tissues or cat feces	Cockroaches	Herbivores (tissues), cats (feces)

Table • 99-5

Benefits of Pet Ownership

- **Encourages Physical Activity**
- **Provides Companionship**
- **Provides a Stabilizing Force**
  - For those with psychological issues and emotional problems
  - For those with physical handicaps

- **Relieves Stress**
  - Provides warmth, contact, and comfort
  - Lowers blood pressure

- **Helps Marital Relationships**
- **Assists with Duties**
  - By herding
  - By tracking
  - By assisting those with handicaps

Additional references and contacts: Becker M. 1999. Pets keep people healthy. *Vet Econ.* special ed 1999:40-47; Delta Society, (800) 869-6898, www.deltasociety.org, accessed 3/10/05; American Association of Human-Animal Bond Veterinarians, http://aahabv.org, accessed 3/10/05; Center for the Human-Animal Bond, Purdue University School of Veterinary Medicine, (765) 494-0854, http://www.vet.purdue.edu/chab/, accessed 3/10/05.

illness and disability often alienate homebound people with AIDS from their family, friends, and acquaintances, pets provide continued companionship and help their owners overcome the deleterious effects of loneliness.[38,161a]

Pets also provide pleasure, protection, and a sense of worth.[38] It may be more detrimental to the well-being of isolated immunocompromised people to lose their pet companions than to risk acquiring a zoonotic infection.

SUPPORT GROUPS

Immunodeficient people may develop emotional and physical limitations that prevent them from adequately caring for their pets. Extended, unanticipated hospitalizations and physical or financial limitations are often present. In addition, needs for preventive and disease-related veterinary care and feeding are expected. Veterinarians can advise their clients about the relative risks of and precautions to contain zoonoses and direct them to support groups to help them with home pet care. Veterinarians can also assist by channeling donations of money and offering their time and professional expertise to these local groups. Veterinarians can discretely demonstrate their willingness to participate in a zoonoses prevention program by having signs or brochures in their waiting room. They must recognize that the increased cost of surveillance and treatment to prevent zoonoses increases the financial obligation for the client. In addition to home pet care, support groups can provide speakers, slide shows, newsletters, and brochures concerning pet care, zoonoses, and personal hygiene. They can provide assistance with screening suitable pets, financing pet health care, and educating pet assistants for routine care and emergencies. Numerous organizations are available to help with these needs. Pets Are Wonderful (PAWS), which originated in San Francisco, and Pet Owners With AIDS/ARC Resource Services, which is based in New York City, are nonprofit volunteer organizations dedicated to providing information and at-home support for immunocompromised people who want to keep their pets. PAWS publishes *Safe Pet Guidelines*, a brochure from their San Francisco office that gives immunocompromised pet owners background information on keeping their pets and themselves healthy. A list of a national network of support organizations and brochures is provided in Table 99-3.[76,159]

PET ADVISEMENT

Although veterinarians generally are better prepared to answer questions about animal diseases and human risks than physicians, few patients view them as the primary providers of this information. Paradoxically, physicians seem to be uncomfortable discussing zoonotic with their clients and view the veterinarian as playing a more important role in this service. Surprisingly, veterinarians and physicians rarely communicate with each other about this topic; physicians' perceptions of relative risk did not match data on known disease transmission.[73,127]

DISEASES

More than 250 organisms are known to cause zoonotic infections, and approximately 30 to 40 involve companion animals. Of these, a selected few have been reported with greater frequency in people with immunodeficiency and AIDS (see Table 99-2).[5] The appearance of a few of these infections (cryptosporidiosis, *Mycobacterium avium*-complex infection, cryptococcosis, salmonellosis, toxoplasmosis) has been used to define the onset of AIDS in people with HIV infection. Some of the AIDS-related zoonoses are acquired directly from companion animals, and others are probably acquired from environmental exposure rather than from pets. The zoonoses described in the next section only include those that have been associated with exposure of immunodeficient people to companion animals. Most of the zoonoses, with the exception of infections caused by *B. henselae* or zoophilic dermatophytes, are more commonly acquired from the environment or other vectors or hosts than from dogs or cats. Nevertheless, pet ownership does pose a risk to immunocompromised people and should always be considered.

Spread by Bites and Through Saliva

Bites are among the most common source of zoonoses, and immunocompromised people have the greatest risk of developing a systemic infection as a result of bite wound injuries (see Chapter 53). Numerous organisms such as *Capnocytophaga* and *Pasteurella*, which represent oropharyngeal flora, are frequently found in bite infections. In addition, many other aerobic and anaerobic bacteria have been isolated. Whenever people are bitten, especially those who are immunocompromised, they should be advised to immediately seek medical attention for their injuries.

Rabies

Virtually any mammal can transmit rabies; however, in many parts of the world, pets are not commonly involved in transmission, likely because of previous postexposure prophylaxis

(people) and vaccination (dogs and cats). In areas where vaccination of domestic dogs is mandatory, wild animals are the major reservoir species for human exposure. In these areas, such as the United States, the annual incidence of rabies in cats has exceeded that of dogs, and cats are the most common domestic animal to have rabies.[92a,103] Despite this fact, most recent human cases have been associated with exposure to bats. In parts of the world where uniform vaccination of dogs has not been implemented, the risk of people acquiring rabies from feral domestic dogs is high. Despite the fact that cats do not frequently transmit rabies to people, they should be vaccinated because the financial, psychological, and health implications of exposure are disruptive. The incidence and prevalence of infection in a given area depend on geographic factors. Not all exposed people need postexposure prophylaxis; this has to be determined on an individual basis (see Chapter 22).

Capnocytophagiosis

Capnocytophaga (formerly DF-2) is a risk to immunosuppressed people who develop more severe systemic complications. *Capnocytophaga* and *Pasteurella* spp. are the most documented bacterial species involved in systemic complications from bite wounds (see Chapter 53). Splenectomy, chronic obstructive pulmonary disease, alcoholism, old age, or other immunosuppressive diseases are associated with an increased risk of fatal sepsis from these bacteria. Signs are acute severe cellulitis and bacteremia, which may develop within 24 to 48 hours of the bite. Cats and dogs should not be allowed to lick open cuts or wounds.

Pasteurellosis

Although cats statistically are associated with fewer bites than dogs, the severity of *Pasteurella* infection is greater than infection by other organisms cultured from their saliva. This is likely because of the virulence of *Pasteurella multocida*, which is carried in the oropharyngeal and nasal regions in a high percentage of cats. (For additional information on aerobic and anaerobic organisms associated with cat bites, see Chapter 53.) Although *Pasteurella* is virulent in its own right, the immunocompetence of the bitten individual is also an important factor in the final outcome.

Infection with Mycoplasma and Other Bite-Inoculated Organisms

Various organisms including anaerobic bacteria can be inoculated into bite wounds from dogs or cats. (See Chapter 53 for an extensive discussion of the public health risks.) Bites or scratches should always be washed immediately with soap and water. All people, especially those who are immunocompromised, should be advised to consult with a physician immediately.

Helicobacteroisis

Helicobacter infections occur in people and their pets; however, many host-adapted species are involved. *Helicobacter pylori*, a primary human gastric commensal and pathogen, has been isolated in a laboratory cat colony in association with human exposure; however, it is considered unusual and natural infections are unlikely. Epidemiologic studies do not show an association between cat ownership and *H. pylori* infection in people.[187] The presence of *Helicobacter heilmanni*, an animal pathogen, was found in a human with gastric erosions and in his two cats.[54] Genetic analysis showed that the human and feline strains were closely related and that more than one strain can concurrently infect a person. One isolate from cats and humans was identical, suggesting zoonotic or anthroponotic spread.

Oral-oral transmission is the primary means of gastric helicobacter spread between animals and people, so contact with the oral cavity or saliva of pets should be avoided. Humans are most likely to acquire this infection from other people because they are the reservoirs for *H. pylori* and other human strains. Precautions to prevent infection should be taken, such as not sharing feeding utensils with people or pets. (For additional information on the zoonotic risks, see Chapter 39.)

Blastomycosis

Blastomycosis is a systemic mycosis caused by a dimorphic fungus and develops in dogs and people that live in endemic areas. Although it is usually acquired from inhalation of spores from mycelia in the soil, localized infections can develop as a result of inadvertent transdermal inoculation of yeasts while handling body tissues or exudates of animals. Localized infections have developed in animal health workers after accidental needle punctures and lacerations at necropsy and in others after being bitten by a dog[72,148] (see Chapter 59).

Spread by Scratch or Close Physical Skin or Mucosal Contact

Bartonellosis

Bartonellosis is caused by a group of small gram-negative bacteria that infect people and animals. A few of the species involve infections in cats and dogs. The immune system of the host is as important as the organism in determining the outcome of infection. *B. henselae* causes various illnesses, including cat-scratch disease or regional pyogranulomatous lymphadenitis, neuroretinitis, Parinaud's oculoglandular syndrome, and aseptic meningitis (see Chapter 54). In contrast, immunodeficient people can also develop bacteremia, aseptic meningitis, peliosis hepatis, and bacillary angiomatosis. *B. henselae* and *Bartonella clarridgeiae* can be isolated from clinically healthy cats, and exposure to cats is associated with many of these diseases in people. Cat ownership was associated with an increased risk of *B. henselae* seropositivity and with cognitive decline in individuals infected with HIV.[159a] The organism has also been isolated from clinical healthy and diseased dogs.[44,79,123] *B. henselae* infection has been identified as a cause of fever of unknown origin in children.[92] Other *Bartonella* spp. have been isolated from people, dogs, and cats, but a direct zoonotic association has been made only for *B. henselae* and *B. clarridgeiae*. *B. henselae* has adapted to live in feline erythrocytes and has probably coexisted with cats for millenia. *B. henselae* has been isolated from the blood of African lions[146] and using the polymerase chain reaction (PCR), it was demonstrated to be detectable in the dental pulp of stray cats that had been buried for 1 year[1b] and in 800-year-old feline museum specimens.[183a]

Fleas have been associated with transmission of infection between cats and humans. Eliminating and controlling fleas is essential for reducing the spread of infection among cats. Because the means of transmitting infection from cats to people is uncertain but possibly involves flea excreta, cat bites or scratches should not be rubbed with uncleaned hands and should be washed immediately. Hands should always be washed immediately after handling known or suspected flea-infested cats. Dog or cat bites might be directly contagious because oral secretions may contain blood in animals with gingival hemorrhage. No absolute recommendation can be made for serologic or blood-culture screening of all cats because treatment efficacy is questionable and the potential exists for inducing antimicrobial resistance. Testing of cats to determine whether they are infected is not generally advised unless they are clinically symptomatic. Because of the high rate of infection in cats, the asymptomatic nature of infection, and the chance of inducing antimicrobial resistance, routine treatment of identified infected cats should be questioned. Because immunity can develop in cats to specific strains, resulting in clearing of infection with time, kittens (younger than 6 months old) are more susceptible to infection, and they have a much higher rate of exposure within a given environment (see Chapter 54). Declawing is not recommended; however, nails can be clipped to reduce the chance of their lacerating the skin. Behavior that invokes biting or scratching should be avoided. To prevent bartonellosis or other infections, cats should never be allowed to lick exposed cuts or wounds. Immunocompromised people are also at risk for becoming infected with other *Bartonella* spp. through vectors that feed on other domestic animals or wildlife species.

Immunocompetent hosts infected with *Bartonella* are not usually treated unless they have one of the bacteremic forms of the disease or are temporarily immunosuppressed. The most effective antimicrobials have included doxycycline, azithromycin, erythromycin, or rifampin.

Chlamydophila felis

Chlamydophila felis has been identified as a cause of conjunctivitis in cats and has been incriminated in infections in humans. Fewer than 10 cases have been reported of zoonotic transmission to people with a range of upper and lower respiratory tract infections. Unfortunately most of these claims were made before the availability of genetic identification and the reclassification of the genus *Chlamydia*, separation of the species *Chlamydia psittaci*, and the recognition of *C. felis*.[31] In almost all instances, the reports were ambiguous with only circumstantial evidence, and the claims were not supported by simultaneous isolation and genetic comparison of the organism from the people and the incriminated cats. In one instance[84] a definitive genetic comparison was made in which chronic conjunctivitis in an immunocompromised human was attributed to *C. felis*. In another report[107] of 15 people with chronic follicular conjunctivitis, PCR and genetic analysis were used to identify human *Chlamydia pneumoniae* and avian *C. psittaci*, which predominated, and two of the cases involved a mammalian strain. Both of the people with the mammalian strain had kittens with conjunctivitis; however, no isolation or comparison of organisms was performed from the cats. Based on the scarcity of reports and the frequency of isolation of this *C. felis* from cats with upper respiratory illness, the zoonotic transmission must be uncommon, especially in immunocompetent people. This is also true in comparison to the higher rate of zoonotic transmission of *C. psittaci* infection from birds.

Sporotrichosis

Sporotrichosis is a disease caused by the saprophytic dimorphic fungus *Sporothrix schenckii* and is found worldwide in soils rich in organic matter. Dogs and cats can be affected with cutaneous, lymphatic, or disseminated forms (see Chapter 63). Humans can be affected by puncture wounds; however, they can be infected by cats through close contact and presumably through small wounds caused by claws or teeth contaminated with the organism.

Malassezia pachydermatis *Infection*

Malassezia pachydermatis, a commensal yeast of animals including dogs and cats, has been identified as a cause of nosocomial infection of infants in intensive care units in hospitals.[41,192] Health care workers transmitted the infection and likely became infected by their pet dogs at home. Isolates from the infants and those of the workers' dogs had matching genotypes. Improving handwashing stopped the spread of this infection (see Chapter 58).

Dogs with and without inflammatory skin disease and their respective owners were sampled in pairs for culture and PCR to detect *M. pachydermatis*.[126] Fungal culture was found to be insensitive, but perhaps it was more clinically relevant than PCR because it detected higher prevalence of organisms on people with clinically diseased pets. PCR methods did not detect a difference in the rate of carriage between the two groups of people. Perhaps higher concentrations of organisms on diseased skin facilitate the less sensitive culture method. It is presumed that both groups of people became contaminated from contact with dogs with or without dermatitis. This study reinforced the theory that *M. pachydermatis* is a commensal on canine skin. Health care workers in intensive care units or those who care for immunocompromised people must have thorough handwashing techniques.

Dermatophytosis

Infection in pet animals is caused by two zoophilic fungi—*Microsporum canis* and *Trichophyton mentagrophytes*—and cats and dogs, respectively, are their inapparent carriers. Cats infected with feline immunodeficiency virus (FIV) harbor more diverse fungal genera, such as *Malassezia*, than uninfected cats.[161] People develop classic lesions with circular alopecia, scaling, crusting, and ulceration. Topical therapy of lesions in people is often rewarding, but topical and systemic therapy of pets and environmental decontamination and cleanliness are often needed to prevent recurrence (see Chapter 58).

Cowpox Infection

People with immunodeficiencies are especially susceptible to cowpox infections transmitted from cats (see Chapter 19).

Retroviral Infections

Veterinarians are exposed to feline retroviruses such as feline leukemia virus (FeLV), FIV, and feline foamy virus (FeFV) during the course of their work (see Chapters 13, 14, and 17). Blood samples from 204 veterinarians, laboratory scientists, and other people with occupational exposure to cats, were tested for antibodies to FIV, FeLV, and FeFV and for FeLV provirus by PCR.[36] The subjects reported a mean of 17.3 years of exposures to cats and high-risk exposures such as cat bites and scratches and injuries with sharp instruments. Neither serologic nor molecular evidence of exposure in these individuals was found. Nevertheless, people, especially those who are immunocompromised, should be cautious when handling secretions of these animals because immunocompromised cats are often coinfected with opportunistic pathogens that may have zoonotic risks.

Aerogenic Spread

Bordetellosis

Infections caused by *Bordetella bronchiseptica* have been reported in immunocompromised people.[57,196] This commensal bacterium of animals has pathogenic potential, and bordetellosis has been reported in people with close animal contact, including contact with dogs or cats[57,77] (see Chapters 6, 16, and 88). The infection usually involves the respiratory tract; however, it may become disseminated. Although bordetellosis is uncommon, even in immunocompromised individuals, it has been recommended that immunocompromised people, their pets, or both should avoid contact with animals in dog kennels, catteries, or animal shows, where the infection is more prevalent. Swine and rabbits are another major source of infection, so contact should be avoided. If necessary, vaccination of an immunocompromised person's pets may be considered to help control the spread of an outbreak of infection; however, the vaccination procedure should be carefully monitored because immunosuppressed people may also become infected with the organism used in the modified live intranasal vaccine. Young children and infants have been infected in this way (see Chapter 100).[134,150] Therefore such individuals should not restrain their pets during the vaccination; ideally, they should not be in the room when the vaccine is being administered.

Coxiellosis

Serologic evidence of *Coxiella burnetii* infection is much higher in veterinarians who remove bovine placentas without wearing gloves than in those who do.[134] Because coxiellosis has developed in people who have been exposed to parturient cats (see Chapter 29), protective gloves and garments, including masks and protective eyewear, should be worn when performing procedures involving the genital tissues or secretions of parturient or aborting animals.

Plague

Yersinia pestis is a bacterium of rodents that is transmitted by their fleas. Many reports have been made of infected cats that have infected people, presumably through direct contact. Cats can also play a role in human infections because they can harbor infected fleas and bring them into close contact with people. Cats develop plague, presumably through contact with infected fleas or rodents. People become infected from cats either aerogenously, which causes a pneumonic form of illness, or by percutaneous inoculation, which causes regional lymphadenomegaly (see Chapter 47). Although cats are more susceptible, dogs pose a risk to humans by transporting infected fleas or the carcasses of their flea-infested prey into the home.[124]

Tularemia

Francisella tularensis is an endemic organism found in many parts of the world (see Chapter 48). People can become infected in various ways and because of the virulence of the organism, even immunocompetent hosts are susceptible. Cats are the most common domestic animal vector for human infection. The cats become infected by insect bites or ingesting infected prey. People can become infected from tick bites or from cats through bites, scratches, or aerosols. Preventing cats from hunting and controlling insect vectors are the primary means of reducing infection risk.

Rhodococcus *Infections*

Rhodococcus equi, a soil saprophyte, has been isolated from patients with AIDS who have respiratory infections and have been exposed to the bacteria through horses or farm animals or environmental exposure to the soil. The organism is found in greatest numbers in soil contaminated by herbivore manure. Clinical signs are usually related to pneumonia with pulmonary abscess formation. Dogs owned by a nurse who worked in a respiratory unit in a hospital were determined to be the source of a *Rhodococcus bronchialis* infection in a hospitalized patient.[152] The organism was found in the patient's wounds and on the hands, scalp, and mucous membranes of the nurse, as well as on the skin of her two dogs. (See Chapter 35 for additional information on *Rhodococcus* infections.)

E. coli *Infections*

Severe peracute hemorrhagic pneumonia was documented in dogs in a research facility.[83] Two of the isolates were serotype 06 and two were 04. Isolates from all four dogs were positive for the virulence factors α-hemolysin and cytotoxic necrotizing factor 1 and for the adhesin factor class-III papG allele. Although no zoonotic transfer was documented, this class of extraintestinal pathogenic *E. coli* is becoming more frequently implicated as a cause of extraintestinal infection in animals and people and may represent a zoonotic risk to humans who work with research dogs.

Fecal-Oral Spread

Enteric organisms of zoonotic risk can be detected in the feces of clinically healthy dogs and cats.[83a,86,165] In most cases, the organisms do not cause additional problems unless the animal develops diarrhea. In this case, the increased frequency of bowel movements and fluidity of the stool promotes spreading and environmental contamination. A concern is that protozoa such as *Toxoplasma*, *Giardia*, and *Cryptosporidium* spp. can become established in freshwater and saltwater environments and in the animals that inhabit them.[63] Data suggest that *Toxoplasma gondii* oocysts can sporulate in sea water and can remain infectious for several weeks. Areas of freshwater runoff into the ocean have the highest risk of causing contamination. Survival of the organisms in the water can result in widespread dissemination and establishment of infection in invertebrates and vertebrates.

Toxoplasmosis

Toxoplasmosis has been an extremely publicized zoonotic disease, partly because it is acquired from pets, partly because of the training in animal diseases received by physicians. Approximately 30% of childbearing women in the United States have antibodies to *T. gondii* and are protected against congenital transmission. If one of the remaining 70% of the women should become pregnant and infected during pregnancy, the probability that the fetus will be infected is 20% to 50%. The most severe complications in the fetus occur between the second and sixth months of gestation.

Toxoplasmosis occurs in 10% of patients with AIDS and is thought to be responsible for at least 30% of central nervous system (CNS) complications.[65] Most cases of CNS toxoplasmosis are a result of reactivation of quiescent infections rather than of recent exposure. *Toxoplasma* antibody seroconversion is unusual in adults with HIV and appears unrelated to cat exposure.[185] Although it can be acquired by ingestion of oocysts shed by infected cats, infection in people living in industrialized countries is usually caused by ingestion of undercooked meats, especially goat, mutton, or pork. Actually, the overall risk of becoming infected by cats in the household is comparatively low, although young children can contract infection from soil exposure in rural environments.[185] Isolated outbreaks of disease have also been reported after handling or inhaling soil or dust contaminated by cat feces or contaminated water supplies.[13] Typically, cats shed oocysts for no longer than 2 weeks after their first exposure to the organism and generally do not shed them again. This is true even when they are receiving high exogenous doses of glucocorticoids or have immunosuppressive diseases such as FIV AIDS. Therefore cats that have positive serologic test results for antibodies to *T. gondii* either as IgG or IgM will likely not shed again because the first shedding period is generally finite. However this serologic testing should be done early in the course of pregnancy if it is to be predictably useful. However, pregnant women rarely become infected from their own cats, so serologic testing is not more helpful than taking general precautions against exposure. However, children who acquire a cat before 15 years of age and who are from rural backgrounds have a likelihood of being seropositive for *T. gondii*, and higher titers are associated with owning greater numbers of cats.[143] This finding suggests that the children were exposed to the organism through the soil around their households. Oocysts must sporulate to be infectious, a process that takes 1 to 5 days. Because the feces do not remain on the fur and oocysts do not appear to sporulate on the fur, handling of cats is an unlikely source of infection (see Chapter 80). One report has been made of an epidemic of toxoplasmosis in humans that was traced to soil contamination by cat feces.[174] In an indoor riding arena, cats defecated and contaminated the soil. Dust generated by exercising horses generated airborne particles, which were presumably inhaled by the riders, resulting in clinical disease.

Because of their environmental resistance, oocysts can enter the freshwater and marine water supplies and cause disease in people or animals that ingest contaminated water or invertebrates harboring these organisms. Outbreaks have been associated with contamination of municipal water supplies by oocysts from feral or wild felids,[22,28,34] and evidence exists of widespread infection among marine mammals.[55]

Immunosuppressed people should wear gloves and wash their hands after contact with soil or raw meat. Cat litter boxes should be changed daily, preferably by an immunocompetent person who is not pregnant. Hands should be thoroughly washed after changing the litter box or gardening or after other contact with the soil. All raw fruits and vegetables should be washed well before being eaten. Cats should be kept inside and fed only commercial diets or well-cooked table food. Patients do not have to be advised to part with their cats or have them separately tested for toxoplasmosis, either serologically or by fecal examination. Cats can be treated with effective drugs to reduce or clear oocyst shedding. Cats that have serologic positive test results (especially a measurable IgG titer) are likely protected from oocyst shedding because it is transient and generally occurs after the very first exposure.

Pet owners and physicians should be reminded that consumption of undercooked meat is the predominant way humans become infected with toxoplasmosis. Wearing gloves and using precautions during cooking are important to ensure that raw meat does not contact cutting boards or foods that are to be eaten raw, such as salads. Surface water can also be contaminated by oocysts; filtering or boiling water is the only effective way to eliminate the risk. All people with HIV or who are pregnant should be tested for IgG as early as possible so that they can be educated about any potential complications or risks and predict whether they are already infected. (See Chapter 80 for additional information on preventing this infection.)

Cryptosporidiosis

Cryptosporidiosis is an intestinal infection caused by a ubiquitous, relatively non–host-specific coccidian parasite of vertebrates and can be acquired from young domestic herbivores (i.e., calves, lambs, kids, piglets) or less commonly from pets (see Chapter 82). *Cryptosporidium parvum*, the least host-specific species, has been identified in many mammals including humans, dogs, and cats. Other species, such as *Cryptosporidium canis* and *Cryptosporidium felis*, are predominant strains in dogs and cats, respectively; however, they also have been found to infect humans with HIV that develop diarrhea, and thus must be considered to be zoonotic.[37, 62,144] In one study of people with HIV with and without cryptosporidiosis, pets were not a major risk factor for infection.[67] *C. felis* was identified as an unusual species of *Cryptosporidium* isolated from people with HIV in Portugal; however, in only one instance was the infection associated with kittens in the home.[114] Kittens, especially those with diarrhea or concurrent immunosuppressive infections with FeLV or FIV, or puppies are more likely to have clinical illness characterized by diarrhea and shedding of organisms. Organisms can be found in the feces of animals with or without diarrhea.[86,121,158,165] Healthy mature animals are often clinically unaffected. Human-human transmission occurs without animal reservoirs, and outbreaks have been noted in daycare centers and family groups. The usual source of outbreaks from environmental exposure is raw sewage or contaminated water sources. Water runoff from land with grazing animals, animal-holding facilities, or sewage treatment facilities can contaminate surface water supplies. Oocysts are highly resistant and can remain infectious under cool, moist conditions for many months as long as they do not freeze. They can survive in freshwater and saltwater and in water that has been chemically treated in swimming pools. Chlorination of water does not kill these parasites, and filtration systems for municipal water must be extremely efficient to eliminate these organisms.[24] Boiling water for 1 minute will kill them. *Cryptosporidium* oocysts can be found in 90% of untreated municipal water supplies and in 30% of treated systems that draw their water from lakes and rivers. As a result, most people do not become infected with this organism because of exposure to their pets; approximately 15% of patients with AIDS develop this complication.[32]

Newborn and young pets may transmit this infection; stray animals or any pets with diarrhea should not be adopted. Infected dogs and cats with diarrhea have transmitted infection to people.[75] Puppies or kittens younger than 6 months should have their stools examined by a veterinarian for *Cryptosporidium* oocysts. Stools can be examined with acid-fast staining or immunoassay methods (either by enzyme-linked immunosorbent assay or fluorescent microscopy), which greatly increase the likelihood of finding organisms compared with conventional microscopic methods. Unfortunately, without using molecular techniques, it is impossible to distinguish the public health risks of particular strains because not all of the strains found in animals infect people. For this reason, it would be better to be overly cautious when the organisms are found. In addition, immunosuppressed people should avoid exposure to calves and lambs and should not drink untreated water directly from lakes or rivers.

Immunocompetent people show signs of abdominal pain and self-limiting diarrhea for 5 to 10 days. Immunodeficient individuals have severe, watery, debilitating, chronic diarrhea that is refractory to therapy. Oocysts in feces are small (2 to 4 μm) and are difficult to see without concentration procedures and special staining.

Treatment is more difficult than that for other intestinal protozoa, so avoiding infection is the best plan. Immunosuppressed individuals should avoid direct contact with infected adults and should not handle diaper-age children without wearing gloves. Good hygiene while caring for infants or young children, especially those who are in daycare or nursery facilities, is essential. Immunosuppressed individuals should not share a room or bathroom with people known to be infected. Drinking contaminated tap or surface water (e.g., from lakes or rivers, the ocean, certain chlorinated pools, or ornamental water fountains) or contacting contaminated surface water during recreation or by eating contaminated raw foods may also result in cryptosporiosis. Some municipal water supplies are contaminated, so water may need to be boiled for at least 1 minute, or submicron water filters may be needed. The safety of commercial beverages, including bottled waters, may vary; however, those that are pasteurized are generally safe. Immunosuppressed people should not eat raw oysters.

Giardiasis

The cause of giardiasis, *Giardia duodenalis* (synonyms *intestinalis* and *lamblia*), is a ubiquitous protozoal enteropathogen found in the intestinal tracts of vertebrate animals and people. Molecular techniques have been used to reveal that *G. duodenalis* has different phenotypic and genotypic strains; transmission between different host species occurs in some human outbreaks with less adapted genotypes, whereas in others, human adapted strains are responsible for clinical illness in people.[175] Human infections involve strains from Assemblages A and B, with each having their own groups of preferred animal hosts. Dogs and cats can become infected with Assemblage A, whereas only dogs are infected with Assemblage B.

Species-specific assemblages also exist for dogs (Assemblages C and D) and cats (Assemblage F). No documented cases of giardiasis acquired from cats have been reported, but the same Assemblage B has been found to infect dogs and people. Infected dogs and cats should be a presumed health risk. No guarantee can be made that infected animals can be effectively cured, and no evidence suggests that once cured they are completely protected from reinfection. (For additional information on the genetic assemblages, treatment, and prevention of *Giardia*, see Chapter 78.) Waterborne outbreaks of giardiasis occur frequently and are a major health concern. Results from genetic analyses of strains involved in waterborne outbreaks suggest that water sources become contaminated with *Giardia* from wildlife or livestock. Outbreaks can occur when several people ingest contaminated water, and the infection can subsequently spread among individuals.[175] Zoonotic incidents involving dogs and cats are not usually waterborne and are more likely to result from direct fecal contamination.[175] Although *Giardia* organisms are probably the most prevalent enteric parasite of dogs and cats, infection is often subclinical and cyst excretion is intermittent[117,178] Young (younger than 6 months old) animals and those with diarrhea should be avoided as pets. Pets being considered for adoption can be screened for *Giardia* infection, and treatment can begin if needed. With or without use of protective gloves, hands should be washed after handling fecal material from infants, children, or animals in daily life. Boiling or filtering drinking water for people and pets eliminate the risk of infection from a contaminated water supply.

Outbreaks involving human-human transmission often involve people in group environments where hygiene may be poor such as in some daycare centers or communal groups of economically disadvantaged individuals. The primary sign of infection in immunocompetent people is watery, foul-smelling diarrhea with flatus, and abdominal distention or asymptomatic shedding can occur. Immunocompromised hosts, which can include infants, older adults, or people with AIDS, have a greater risk of infection and may develop chronic diarrhea with malabsorption. Diagnosing the infection in people may be difficult because the chance of finding the parasite from as many as three stool examinations is no greater than 50%.[160] Therefore treatment is often empiric (see Chapter 78).

Salmonellosis

Salmonellosis develops in approximately 5% of patients with AIDS. Foodborne exposures from contaminated meat account for many infections, but a few pet-related exposures have involved turtles. Severe recurrent diarrhea and bacteremia are common in patients with AIDS. Compared with the prevalence of infection in cold-blooded animals, dogs and cats are rarely colonized with these organisms. Therefore, immunocompromised people should avoid having reptiles and amphibians as pets. Multiple drug resistant *Salmonella typhimurium* DT104 has been isolated from dogs and cats, and cases in people have been identified in association with cats and dogs.[85] Young, debilitated, coinfected, or otherwise immunocompromised dogs and cats are more likely to harbor and shed these organisms. Housing and management of animals can be important in the overall carriage rate of *Salmonella*. In one study 54% of group-housed cats, 8.6% of diseased cats, and 0.36% of clinically healthy pet house cats had *Salmonella* organisms in rectal swab specimens.[182] Acquired antimicrobial resistance genes were found in these isolates. Environmental surveillance in a veterinary teaching hospital has shown that surfaces in hospitals are frequently contaminated.[33] This contamination can be a potential reservoir for infection for hospital personnel or animals and pet owners. Cases of multiple drug resistant *Salmonella* organisms have been associated with infections in small animal practices with inadequate hygiene.[10,42,108,184] Immunocompromised people, children, and older adults who become exposed are highly susceptible to infection and clinical illness. (For additional information on the epidemiology and prevention of infection in dogs and cats, see Chapter 39.)

Campylobacteriosis and Helicobacteriosis

Campylobacteriosis is caused by a microaerophilic group of gram-negative, curved, motile rods that are commensal flora of animals. Although *Campylobacter jejuni*, *Campylobacter coli*, and *Campylobacter upsaliensis* have been most commonly isolated from dogs and cats,[82] *C. upsaliensis* has been associated with enteritis in people, and it is suspected that dogs may be an important source of human infection.[69] *C. jejuni* is frequently isolated from dogs and cats (especially younger than 1 year of age) recently acquired from pet stores, kennels, animal shelters, or pounds. Pups and kittens with diarrhea have been most commonly associated with human infections. Uncooked meat, especially poultry, is probably a more common source of infection for people. Fecal-oral, foodborne, and waterborne modes of transmission are the principal avenues for infection. A contaminated water supply, possibly as a result of migrating waterfowl or herbivores, may be a source of infection for outdoor pets. Children younger than 5 years with a newly acquired puppy have the highest prevalence of infection.[156] Signs of infection in people are intense abdominal discomfort, bloody diarrhea, fever, tenesmus, and fecal leukocytosis. Immunosuppressed individuals with AIDS develop recurrent diarrhea, dehydration, and bacteremia.

Recommendations for reducing infection among immunocompromised people include avoiding animals with diarrhea and pets younger than 1 year of age. Veterinarians should culture feces of newly acquired animals for *Campylobacter* organisms. Washing hands after handling pets and especially before eating is the most important precaution. Feeding raw meat to pets should be avoided; only commercial diets or cooked foods (greater than 180° F for poultry and 165° F for red meats) should be used. Keeping pets indoors is the most reliable way to help control pet exposure to contaminated environmental sources. Precautions should be taken to prevent the risk of inducing antimicrobial resistant strains by not treating subclinically infected animals. Subclinically infected pets should not be considered for adoption by immunocompromised people.

A wide variety of related, potentially zoonotic *Helicobacter* species exist in domestic and wild animals. For a further discussion of these organisms, see Chapter 39.

E. coli *Infections*

Attaching and effacing *E. coli* strains that belong to a variety of serotypes have been isolated from the feces of dogs, cats, and other animals with and without diarrhea.[101b,131] The virulence factors found in these strains were similar to those found in human strains, suggesting that they may transmit back and forth between people and dogs.

Urogenital Spread

Leptospirosis

Leptospirosis is caused by several serovars that can infect a wide variety of animals and are shed in the urine into the water supply or moist environments. People become infected by contact of mucous membranes with contaminated water or through cuts or abrasions on the skin. In a similar manner, people who inadvertently come into contact with fresh urine from infected animals is a potential source of transmission. However, once treatment with proper antibacterial drugs is instituted, the urine of infected dogs is no longer infectious. Most disinfectants kill the spirochete quickly; as a precaution, disinfectant should be applied on urine in cages or runs before they are cleaned. An outbreak of leptospirosis in dog handlers at Lackland Air Force Base in Texas received attention because

of the possibility that the dogs were the source of infection; however, contact with rodents or contaminated ground water was not excluded (www.veterinarypartner.com, accessed 02/25/05). Additional studies are needed to determine whether the dogs and people were infected with the same serovar (see Chapter 44).

Brucellosis

Brucella canis is a venereally transmitted organism that is harbored intracellularly by dogs. People usually become infected through contact with the organism in female genital secretions or from laboratory culture. Infection requires a threshold dose, and the number of organisms usually in urine is lower than that in vaginal discharges. Animals with this disease should always be neutered to help reduce the public health risk should they be kept as pets. The zoonotic risk of a neutered animal is low; however, concerns about keeping an infected animal in the household with an immunocompromised person may be valid. (See Chapter 40 for a discussion of the public health risk with this infection.)

Coxiellosis

Q fever is primarily an occupational hazard in people who are in contact with domestic livestock, such as goats or cattle, or workers in animal health or slaughter facilities. Cases sporadically occur in urban areas after people are in contact with infected dogs or cats. Parturient cats have been the most important source of these infections. People become infected from aerosols from placental tissues. Pneumonia is the primary clinical sign in infected humans (see Chapter 29).

E. coli *Infections*

Virulent pathogens causing genitourinary infections in dogs and cats could conceivably be pathogenic for humans who have close contact with these animals. Phylogenetic background and virulence genotype of isolates from dogs with urinary tract infections (UTIs) were compared with extraintestinal isolates from people.[93] Although similarities were found between individual canine and human isolates representative of five clonal groups, no clinical significance was found in people harboring these similar strains. Nevertheless, this suggested that dogs might serve as a source for potentially virulent human infections. Similarly, virulence markers have been used to document extensive similarities among *E. coli* isolates in two adult humans and a cat, including a strain that caused UTI in one female household member.[130] Although humans and pets sometimes carry the same fecal strain, this report documents the ready spread of *E. coli* over time and its ability to cause an extraintestinal infection rather than mere commensal colonization. The ability of animal bacteria to colonize people makes antibacterial therapy choices more critical to avoid resistant strains.

Vectorborne Infections

Numerous insects transmit infections to people. The mammalian reservoirs of these infections are often wildlife species; dogs and cats are not usually the direct source of infections for people. Instead, they act as sentinels for infection or they bring the shared vectors closer to humans. Sufficient tick attachment duration is important in the successful transmission of many of these diseases.[98] Therefore good ectoparasite control for people and pets can help to reduce the threat of infection.

West Nile Virus Infection

Antibody reactive to West Nile virus has been found in sera of 26% of 116 dogs and 9% of 138 cats tested in Louisiana during the 2002 outbreak of this disease in the United States caused by this virus.[101a] Outdoor-only, family-owned dogs had a 19 times higher prevalence rate compared to that of indoor-only, family-owned dogs. Stray dogs had twice the odds of seropositivity as compared to that of family-owned dogs. Family dogs not receiving heartworm preventative had twice the level of positive results as those dogs receiving heartworm preventative.

European Tickborne Encephalitis

European tickborne encephalitis is an arboviral infection in Europe that is transmitted by *Ixodes* ticks (see Chapter 26) and mirrors the geographic range of borreliosis. People and dogs can become clinically ill with this virus infection.

Borreliosis

Tick transmission is a required component of *Borrelia burgdorferi* virulence (see Chapter 45). Therefore as with most arthropod-borne infections, animals do not directly transmit the disease. However, animals share the same environment as people and act as sentinels for infection. Pets may bring the vector into contact with people; however, unless refeeding occurs, handling of ticks by people is not a major risk.

Rocky Mountain Spotted Fever

Unlike some of the other tickborne diseases, engorged ticks that are feeding on pets are highly infectious for people if hemolymph of infected ticks contacts broken skin or mucous membranes. People must be very cautious when removing and disposing of ticks from animals. Unfortunately, because of its diverse clinical manifestations, diagnosis of Rocky Mountain spotted fever in dogs and people can be delayed, possibly leading to death. Simultaneous infections in dogs and their owners are not uncommon.[58,137] Because dogs can serve as sentinels for disease, a high index of suspicion by veterinarians and good communication with people and their physicians can help prevent infection (see Chapter 29).

Rickettsia felis and Rickettsia typhi Infections

Numerous rickettsial species have been isolated from cat fleas (*Ctenocephalides* species). Dogs and cats may be subclinically infected; however, rickettsial diseases in people are indistinguishable from typhus (see Chapter 29).

Ehrlichiosis and Anaplasmosis

Ehrlichiosis and anaplasmosis are maintained in wildlife hosts and transmitted by bites of infected ticks. Transmission may require at least 36 hours of tick attachment.[98] *Ehrlichia chaffeensis*, *Ehrlichia ewingii*, and *Anaplasma phagocytophilum* infect people and animals. Circumstantial evidence suggests that exposure to deer blood during dressing of carcasses may be a direct means by which *A. phagocytophilum* is zoonotically transmitted.[16,173] Humans and domestic animals such as dogs are incidental hosts and are not reservoirs of infection. Furthermore, infection transmission between domestic animals and people is unlikely (see Chapter 28).

Anthroponoses

Methicillin-Resistant Staphylococcal Infections

Methicillin-resistant strains of *Staphylococcus aureus* (MRSA) are important nosocomial pathogens in human hospitals. *S. aureus* is a human-adapted commensal and opportunist. The organisms are usually harbored by people, and medical health workers can be come colonized and inadvertently transmit the infection to human patients. Similarly contamination of the veterinary hospital environment can occur as a result of human contact, and organisms can be transmitted to hospitalized animals.[188] MRSA infections have been identified in dogs.* Methicillin resistance in staphylococci is mediated by the *mecA*

*References 40, 70, 87, 177, 181, 189.

gene, which encodes the penicillin-binding protein 2a (PBP2a). In one study of various domestic animals,[180] all but one of the MRSA isolated from animals, as detected by the *mecA* gene, had distinct nucleic acid compositions when compared with human isolates. The MRSA that were found were from dogs, indicating that dogs may carry more MRSA than other species. Unfortunately, the MRSA were also highly resistant to multiple antibacterial drugs. In another instance, a cat kept in a rehabilitation geriatrics ward for pet-facilitated therapy was incriminated in a staphylococcal infection in hospitalized patients. Presumably, the infections result from animal health workers or owners transmitting their resistant strains to a pet. The concern is that these organisms can be transmitted from the animal to other people who might be immunocompromised or who have other medical conditions that would be complicated by these highly resistant organisms. Judicious use of antimicrobials by veterinarians and strict personal hygiene, especially hand protection and washing, can help reduce the chance of the infection spreading among animal health workers in veterinary practices. Because of the high risk and ready spread of these organisms through close contact or fomite transmission, additional precautions may need to be taken by workers in the paraprofessional pet industry, such as those in grooming, boarding, and breeding facilities.

The most common dermal isolate from dogs is *Staphylococcus intermedius*. Most strains of *S. intermedius* have predictable and more narrow antimicrobial susceptibilities than *S. aureus*. Reports of this organism infecting people are uncommon; however, in one instance, *S. intermedius* infected a postsurgical wound site of a person after a dog frequently licked the wound.[101] A newly recognized isolate from dogs, *Staphylococcus schleiferi*, has a much broader host range, which includes dogs, and a wider antimicrobial resistance pattern, including that of methicillin.[87,94] That *S. schleiferi*, unlike *S. intermedius*, has been isolated more frequently from human infections is concerning to medical professionals. Additional documentation of this infection in people is necessary, and it may be both a zoonotic and anthropozootic problem. (For precautions in handling patients with MRSA infections, see *www.aorn.org/journal/2001/sepci.htm*; accessed 2/25/05.)

Group A Streptococcal Infections

When initially reported, dogs were incriminated as persistent reservoirs of group A streptococcal infections in people (see Chapter 35). However, crude antimicrobial susceptibility testing was done, and genetic subtyping of strains is needed to definitely document the epidemiology of infection. Nevertheless, households with high prevalence rates of this infection also have a higher rate of exposure to the organisms through pets. However, compared with the infection in people, the infection is transient in animals; the possibility of other humans in the household being more efficient reservoirs should be considered. Studies have shown that other household members are likely to be colonized with the bacteria when a child is symptomatic.

Human Urinary E. coli Spread to Pets

Household pets have been proposed as potential reservoirs of *E. coli* that cause UTIs in humans (see previous section); however, it is uncertain whether human strains spread to pets, which might act as reservoirs or amplification hosts. In one study,[157] *E. coli* from women with UTIs were compared with those isolated from dog fecal specimens and from 76 healthy human volunteers. Antibacterial resistance was more common and extensive among isolates from women with UTIs than in the other groups. The data from this report suggested that dogs might acquire resistant strains from infected people, but dog fecal strains were not likely to be sources for human UTIs.

Mycobacterium tuberculosis *Infection*

Tuberculosis in dogs can be caused by *Mycobacterium tuberculosis* acquired from infected people,[61,80] because people are the natural reservoir for this organism. In one report of a person with tuberculosis, the person's dog often sat in the person's lap and licked the owner's face, which may have been responsible for the transmission.[61] Although intradermal skin testing has been used, definitive antemortem diagnosis of tuberculosis in dogs or cats is difficult without special culture and histopathologic confirmation of the granulomatous lesions. Because of the uncertainty of whether this infection in animals can be transmitted back to people, treatment of pets is not usually recommended (see Chapter 50).

Streptococcus pneumoniae *Infection*

One report has been made of transmission of *Streptococcus pneumoniae* from a human to a cat (see Chapter 35).

Avian Influenza

It is hypothesized that all mammalian influenza virus infections arise from an avian reservoir. Aquatic birds are the reservoirs of all types of influenza A viruses. The viruses replicate in the digestive tract of the birds but cause no clinical illness. The viruses can enter the food supply through fecal contamination of the carcasses, which are then ingested by people or other animals such as pigs or horses, or through contamination of water supplies. Similarly other birds, wild and domestic, can become infected as a result of the migratory patterns of the water fowl. In Asia, where pigs and fowl are raised together, cross-contamination with virus is likely. This mixing of the two strains can result to genetic recombination of the isolates with major antigenic shift and new infecting strains within a given host species (see Chapter 25). This crossover of viral replication from birds to mammals such as people, dogs, and cats is especially prevalent in the Orient. The live-bird markets and spread of infection to swine housed in close proximity are thought to be the important starting point for these pandemics. The newly adapted strains can spread simultaneously in people and their pets; however, clinical illness in infected dogs or cats has generally been limited or subclinical. In the most recent pandemic in October 2004, which was caused by the H5N1 strain, clinical illness was fulminant in tigers and leopards in Thailand and many either died or were culled because of severe clinical signs and risk of infecting other animals and people[100,176] The outbreak appeared to be caused by the feeding of raw infected chicken to the exotic cats. Gross necropsy findings included severe pulmonary consolidation and multifocal hemorrhages throughout other organs.[100] Diffuse fibrinous pneumonia and multifocal encephalitis were observed. This strain of virus appears to be highly pathogenic for tigers, leopards, and domestic cats and may spread among them.[104] Additional studies on the potential for cats to transmit this virus to people is needed. In Austria, the seroprevalence of antibodies to influenza virus H1N1 was higher among veterinarians than in the general population.[134] Immunocompromised people should be especially wary because mortality from influenza is highest in immunocompromised individuals. (For additional information on influenza in dogs or cats, see Chapter 25.)

Ebola Virus Infection in Dogs

Ebola virus, a member of the family *Filoviridae*, causes fulminant hemorrhagic fever in human and nonhuman primates. During the 2001 to 2002 outbreak of Ebola virus in Gabon, Africa, dogs were observed feeding on animal carcasses. Serum samples containing Ebola virus-specific IgG were more prevalent (25.2 %) from dogs in the virus-epidemic area than levels from dogs from nonepidemic areas of Gabon (15.2%) or France (2%).[2a] Within the epidemic-area villages, villagers consumed meat from infected animal carcasses found in the forest and subsequently served as the source of infection for others in the village. The prevalence rate in dogs from these villages with an animal source and subsequent human infection was as high as 31.8%. Neither Ebola virus antigens nor nucleotide sequences or cultivated virus were detected in any of the seropositive or seronegative dog blood samples. Clinical signs were not observed in exposed dogs, suggesting that asymptomatic or mild Ebola virus infection occurs in dogs. Whether they could serve as a source of infection for people is uncertain. However, handling dogs that have been exposed to infected carcasses could pose some risk for people. This may help to explain infection among people who had not been associated with other infected humans. The prevalence of infection in Gabon dogs outside epidemic areas may relate to contact with infected small terrestrial animals, bats, or birds.

Zoonoses from Other Animals

Nipah Virus Infection

Outbreaks of encephalitis in people in Malaysia have been linked to a new paramyxovirus that affects pigs and other domestic animals (see Chapter 18). It has been associated with death in pigs on affected farms, and close contact with pigs was considered the primary source of infection.[138] However, death of infected dogs and cats was also identified as a risk factor for some of the affected people without direct pig exposure. Transmission from these animals to their human owners could not be excluded. Additional work will be needed to determine the risk of potential transmission through these pets.

Psittacosis

Psittacosis is an endemic infection of birds worldwide caused by *Chlamydia psittaci*. It may be transmitted by direct contact with birds or indirectly through their feces or feathers. Infected birds may remain carriers. Animal care workers have a high risk of becoming infected.[71] Affected people develop pneumonia with various systemic manifestations, including arthralgia and myalgia. The risk of infection has been greatly reduced through the introduction of tetracycline in poultry feeds; however, this practice produces antimicrobial-resistant strains and does not reduce the prevalence of infection in pet birds. Dogs and cats may become infected with the strains from birds, as can people (see Chapter 30). The risk of this infection does not appear to be any greater for immunocompromised people than it is for those who are clinically healthy.

Listeriosis

Listeriosis is caused by a saprophytic gram-positive bacillus and occurs most commonly in pregnant women, the old or very young, those taking immunosuppressive drugs, or those with AIDS. The organism can be isolated in the environment from soil, and humans may contract it from contaminated meat or vegetables (see Chapter 35).

Sapronoses

Mycobacteriosis

Although people and pets become infected with *Mycobacterim avium* complex (MAC) organisms, the infections are related to common environmental exposure rather than spread among animals or human hosts (see Chapter 50). Treatment of MAC infection is possible. Nevertheless, in households with immunocompromised people, a decision to remove an infected pet is understandable. *Mycobacterium marinum* infection is acquired by immunosuppressed people who clean fish aquariums or are exposed to other aquatic environments.

Cryptococcosis

Cryptococcosis is a fungal disease that has been identified as a respiratory illness in people with AIDS. Immunocompetent people are subclinically infected. As with the other systemic mycoses, the organisms are acquired from contact with contaminated soil. Pigeon and other bird droppings enrich the soil and transport organisms into new areas. Areas with large congregations of birds should be avoided. Although cats and occasionally dogs develop cutaneous infections, aerosols from these lesions do not infect people in the immediate environment (see Chapter 61).

Other Mycoses

Numerous fungal infections such as histoplasmosis (see Chapter 60), coccidioidomycosis (see Chapter 62), zygomycosis (see Chapter 67), and aspergillosis (see Chapter 64) are acquired by people and animals from the environment. They often affect immunocompromised individuals, and heavy levels of exposure can overwhelm the remaining immune defenses. With the exception of blastomycosis, sporotrichosis, and dermatophytosis, people do not become infected directly by their pets.

Microsporidiosis

Microsporidiosis has been reported with increasing frequency as a cause of chronic watery diarrhea in human patients with AIDS. Before the beginning of the AIDS epidemic, very few cases had been reported.[65] The protozoan parasites are a heterogenous group in the phylum Microspora (see Chapter 75). Although various microsporidia infect animals, none of the infections in humans (primarily *Enterocytozoon bieneusi*) has been definitively traced to household pets or any animal reservoir.[53] In one report, a child seroconverted after being exposed to a litter of puppies infected with *Encephalitozoon cuniculi*.[118] A wide variety of environmental exposures exist, and numerous species of farm animals, monkeys, rodents, rabbits, and fish have become infected. The premise that pets are involved has not been well substantiated. Because of the ubiquitous nature of microsporidians, no specific precautions other than careful handwashing and food washing can be justified.

Other Zoonoses

Numerous other zoonoses have not been documented with any greater frequency in immunosuppressed individuals than in the general population. The references at the end of this chapter and the Public Health Considerations sections in other chapters in this book should be consulted for a more extensive review of all companion-animal–associated zoonoses.

RECOMMENDATIONS

According to guidelines established by medical experts,[7] human health care providers should advise people infected with HIV of the potential risk posed by pet ownership. However, those giving advice should be sensitive to the possible psychological benefits of pet ownership and should not routinely advise people infected with HIV to part with their pets. Table 99-3 lists Internet addresses for the Centers for Disease Control and Prevention's (CDC) Healthy Pets, Healthy People program, which offers guidelines for safe pet ownership by people infected with HIV, patients who have had organ transplants, and young children. In regards to infection, handling pets is no more risky for an immunosuppressed person than is contact with other people or the environment. In fact, zoonotic diseases are more likely to be acquired from another infected human than a clinically healthy, parasite-free adult dog or cat.[66,167] Simple hygienic measures taken by immunosuppressed owners greatly reduces the risk of exposure to zoonoses (Table 99-6). For additional information on hand hygiene, see Chapter 94. (See Table 99-3 for the online CDC guidelines for hand hygiene.) Factors that can cause

animals to become greater risks include some of the unique organisms they can harbor and the lack of sanitary behavior often practiced by animals. Owners can often institute routines in their own behavior that will make it unlikely that they will contract a disease from their companion animals. Veterinarians can institute certain screening procedures to identify potential zoonoses and initiate treatment or prevention protocols if indicated (Table 99-7). (For information on reducing the risk of transmitting zoonotic agents in animal health or housing facilities, see Table 99-8, and for additional hygiene recommendations, see Chapter 94.)

Screening

In general, precautions should be taken if an immunosuppressed person decides to acquire a pet for companionship or when a pet is being used to provide companionship for people in hospitals or nursing homes. In a survey of American and Canadian animal-assisted therapy programs, 94% used dogs or cats.[186] Two thirds of these animals visited older adults in nursing homes, one fourth were taken to schools, and another one fourth were taken to hospitals. Although unfounded, the major zoonotic concerns were rabies, ringworm, and external parasites.[186] Less than half of the therapy groups consulted veterinary professionals, and only 10% had written guidelines for zoonoses transmission. Although the benefits of animal-assisted therapy are many, guidelines should be developed to reduce risk of zoonotic disease transmission in health care environments.[29a,56a,101a]

In dogs and cats, infectious diseases, including zoonoses, are more frequently a problem when they are puppies or kittens, and the general guidelines for obtaining a new pet include looking for one older than 1 year old. Exotic or wild animals are not as tractable, may cause injuries, and may harbor unusual parasites or infections. Furthermore, stray animals or animals being housed in areas of high-population densities, such as humane shelters, pet-breeding facilities, pounds, puppy or kitten mills, or crowded pet stores may have a greater chance of harboring pathogens. Acquiring a new adult pet from a single-pet household may be the best option. Any newly acquired pet should be thoroughly examined by a veterinarian before being introduced to a household. It should be clinically healthy and have no evidence of illness (especially diarrhea) or immunosuppression. All animals should be examined by a veterinarian for *Cryptosporidium*, *Salmonella*, and *Campylobacter* organisms (see Table 99-7 and respective chapters).

Handling

Immunosuppressed people should wash their hands frequently during the day and consistently after handling their pets or their pets' excretions. Handwashing is especially important before eating, smoking, performing dental hygiene, and putting in corrective lenses. The pet should be kept indoors and its environment should also be kept clean and free of dirt, uneaten food, and excrement.

Health Care

Newly acquired pets should receive their vaccinations and routine anthelminthic therapy for roundworms and hookworms. Serologic testing for FeLV and FIV is recommended for cats. Although FeLV and FIV pose no chance of infecting people, cats affected with these immunosuppressive viruses are more likely to develop other infectious diseases. Measuring IgG toxoplasmosis titers might help determine prior exposure in cats but is not definitive and is not predictive of risk because most people are not infected by their own cats. Younger kittens are more likely to be seronegative and are may shed oocysts after their first exposure to *T. gondii*. IgG seropositivity indicates prior exposure and minimal risk, because cats rarely reshed oocysts after initially being infected

Table • 99-6

Guidelines for People with Immunodeficiencies: Reducing the Public Health Risk Posed by Their Dogs and Cats

Pets can have zoonoses, or infections that also develop in people. People with an immunodeficiency are more susceptible to developing infections. In some instances, zoonoses can spread to people from pets and in other instances, people contract these infections from the same sources, which include contaminated food, soil, water, or other people. No evidence proves that pets can become infected with or transfer the human immunodeficiency virus from one person to another. People do not need be advised to part with their pets if they are willing to take simple precautions.

Selection
The energy level of the pet should match that of the owner. Choosing a young (younger than 6 months old) puppy or kitten poses a greater risk of infection because of their increased susceptibility to infections. Pets older than 1 year of age and in good health are best. Likewise, stray, exotic, wild, ill, or debilitated animals are more likely to carry zoonotic infections. Potential sources of pets that have poor hygiene, unsanitary facilities, and crowded conditions should be avoided. A veterinarian can give advice on pet selection, screen the animal for infectious agents, and begin a vaccination and parasite control program. Immediate veterinary attention should be sought if a new pet becomes ill. New pets with diarrhea or parasite infection or infestation should not be considered for adoption. Should the owner or the pet become ill, friends and local support groups can help care for the pet.[a]

Feeding
Pets should be fed commercial rations or pelleted feeds. If pets are fed meat, it should be cooked until it is no longer pink (and to greater than 176° F [80° C]). Only pasteurized dairy products should be used. Restrict the pet's access to carrion and prevent the pet from hunting; preventing cats from hunting usually requires them to be kept indoors. Pets can drink tap water but should never drink from the toilet. Pet foods should be protected from contamination by vermin.

Recreation
Although declawing of cats is not advised, owners should avoid activities that would result in bites or scratches from pets. Should bites or scratches occur, they should be flushed and washed with water and antiseptic soaps promptly. Animals should never be allowed to lick open wounds or mucous membranes.

Personal Hygiene
Pets' mouths contains organisms that might infect their owner should they enter the owner's body through open wounds or by biting or scratching. Activities that might induce biting or scratching or result in exposure to their saliva, such as licking the face or wounds, should be avoided. Feeding utensils should not be shared with pets. Gloves should be worn when giving pets oral medications or brushing their teeth. As a general rule, hands should be washed after handling pets. Bite or scratch sites should be washed promptly and medical attention sought immediately for any bite injuries. Contact with pets' excreta (urine, feces, vaginal or seminal discharges) should be minimized. Gloves and a face mask should be worn when cleaning the litter box or diarrhea or urine from the pet, or perhaps others can help. Hands should then be washed, even if gloves were worn. Litter boxes should be emptied daily; liners make this job easier and minimize exposure. The litter box should be kept out of food preparation or eating areas. Scalding water is the best method for disinfecting litter boxes. Household bleach is effective against many viruses and bacteria; however, ammonia should be used to decontaminate litter boxes with *Toxoplasma gondii* (see Chapter 80). Sandboxes should be covered and gloves worn while gardening. Water from the environment for consumption should be filtered or preferably boiled.

Parasite and Transport Host Control
The veterinarian can assist in controlling diarrhea or external parasites, such as fleas or ticks, which may transmit zoonotic infections to people. Gloves should be worn when removing ticks from the pet. Testing for and treating intestinal parasites is also warranted because they can cause diarrhea and in some cases can infect people. Flies and cockroaches should be controlled because they can transfer infectious agents among hosts.

Disease Testing and Vaccination
The stools of dogs and cats can be checked for *Cryptosporidium* oocysts (see Chapter 82). Feces can also be cultured for *Salmonella* and *Campylobacter* (see Chapter 39) organisms, especially if the pet has diarrhea. Cats can be tested for and treated for *Bartonella* infection, although the need for this controversial (see Chapter 54). Serologic testing for *Toxoplasma* may reveal the public health risk of a cat, although it is not generally advised (see Chapter 80). Cats should receive their primary immunizations and periodic boosters. It is extremely important that they be vaccinated for rabies.

Recommendations compiled from various sources, including Angulo FJ, Glaser CA, Juranek DD, et al. 1994. Caring for pets of immunocompromised persons. *J Am Vet Med Assoc* 205:1711-1718; Anonymous. 1995. Centers for Disease Control and Prevention. USPHS/ISDA guidelines for the prevention of opportunistic infection in persons infected with HIV: a summary. *MMWR* 44:1-34; Anonymous. 1997. USPHS/IDSA guidelines for the prevention of opportunistic infections in persons infected with human immunodeficiency virus: disease specific recommendations. *Clin Infect Dis* 25:S313-S335; Glaser CA, Angulo FJ, Rooney JA. 1994. Animal associated opportunistic infections among persons infected with the human immunodeficiency virus. *Clin Infect Dis* 18:14-24; Goldstein EJC. 1991. Household pets and human infections. *Infect Dis Clin North Am* 5:117-130.

[a]A veterinarian can provide the names of assistance programs that can provide in-home pet care, change litter boxes and walk dogs, provide home flea control, provide care for or give medication to pets if the owners are hospitalized or ill, bathe pets, provide foster care and adoption options, and deliver pet food.

Table • 99-7

Veterinary Guidelines for Handling Dogs and Cats: Controlling Directly Transmitted Zoonoses Most Commonly Affecting Immunocompromised People

DISEASE AND PET	DIAGNOSIS	TREATMENT	PRECAUTIONS
Toxoplasmosis: C (see Chapter 80)	NR: fecal exam—oocysts rarely found; serology—cannot predict oocyst shedding; seropositive generally protected because of previous exposure	NR: clindamycin—reduces oocyst shedding; bathing—feces not often on fur	R: litter box hygiene—daily cleaning by immunocompetent assistant; preventing cat from hunting or eating raw meat
Giardiasis: C, D (see Chapter 78)	R: test pups, kittens, diarrheic pets; zinc sulfate method	R: metronidazole, albendazole, fenbendazole	R: litter box hygiene; handling feces with gloves
Cryptosporidiosis: C, D (see Chapter 82)	R: acid-fast or direct FA staining of feces	R: paromomycin; untreated may shed for 2 weeks	R: litter box hygiene; handling feces with gloves
Campylobacteriosis, helicobacteriosis: C, D (see Chapter 39)	R: fecal culture NR: culture stomach contents or biopsy, histopathology with silver stains	R: I—erythromycin, chloramphenicol R: G—metronidazole, ampicillin, bismuth subsalicylate	R: preventing ingestion of raw meat
Salmonellosis: C, D (see Chapter 39)	R: fecal culture, selective media	NR: fluoroquinolones	R: preventing hunting and carrion or raw meat ingestion; if positive, temporarily removing animal from household
Bartonellosis: C (see Chapter 54)	R: blood culture or PCR if screening a cat or dog, respectively, is under consideration NR: antibody testing	R: fluoroquinolones, doxycycline, rifampin, azithromycin	R: strict flea control, screening or avoiding kittens, avoiding bites or scratches and washing immediately if they occur
Bordetellosis: C, D (see Chapters 6, 16, and 88)	NR: endotracheal wash and culture	R: tetracyclines	R: avoiding exposure to boarding kennels, dog shows, and congregated dogs; vaccinating if exposure likely

NR, Not recommended; *R,* recommended; *FA,* fluorescent antibody; *C,* cat; *D,* dog; *I,* intestinal *Campylobacter* organisms; *G,* gastric *Helicobacter* organisms; *PCR,* polymerase chain reaction.

(see Chapter 80). To reduce the risk of zoonotic transmission of parasites and enhance the health of pets, the Companion Animal Parasite Council recommends year-round treatment with broad-spectrum heartworm anthelmentics with activity against roundworms and hookworms and preventive flea and tick products for the life of the pet (see Table 99-3 for the Internet address). Yearly physical examinations and fecal parasite examinations are indicated to maintain the health of the pet, and vaccinations should be administered as appropriate for the lifestyle of the pet (see Table 100-9). Illness in any pet should be an important reason to seek immediate veterinary care.

Grooming

The animal's hair coat and skin should be kept in good condition by occasional baths if needed and regular brushing and trimming of matted fur. Nails of dogs and cats should be trimmed frequently to reduce the chance of scratch injuries. If cats scratch when handled, declawing should be considered. Fleas should be managed with monthly flea preventatives and intensive environmental treatment in the area that the animals

frequent (see Chapter 94), including indoor floors and carpets, especially where they sleep, their sheltered roaming areas, and those areas frequented by other contact animals. Environmental treatment using flea bombs or sprays should include larvicidal growth inhibitors as well as adulticide compounds. Newer oral or topical products that interfere with flea development and reproduction are warranted. More effective control of fleas in the environment may require a professional exterminator.

To control ticks, routine daily checking of pets or checking immediately after leaving tick-infested areas is indicated. Use of amitraz collars and topical fipronyl may be indicated in areas of heavy tick infestation. Any attached ticks should be removed with rubber gloves or tweezers, and hands should be washed after removal. Ticks should not be removed or crushed with bare, exposed hands. For further information on tick removal and prevention, see Chapters 29 and 45. Flies, cockroaches, and vermin may also transport infectious organisms. Pets should be restricted from areas where rodents burrow, and measures should be taken to eliminate areas near the home where vermin may nest.

Table • 99-8

Reduce Risk of Transmitting Zoonotic Agents in Veterinary Hospitals or Animal Housing Facilities

MEANS OF SPREAD	RECOMMENDATIONS
General	Wash hands before and after contact with animals or their secretions or excretions. Wear gloves when any pathogens may be present or when in contact with tissue. Wash hands after removing gloves. (For instructions on hand washing see Table 94-7.) Avoid contact with inanimate objects in the facility until hands are cleaned. Eating, drinking, or storing food should never be done in areas where animals are kept or handled or where their biologic specimens are stored. In cases of known or suspected infection, special diagnostic procedures such as radiographic imaging or surgery should be postponed until the end of the day so that other animals do not come in contact with affected areas until they are decontaminated and clothing can be changed before the next day. All disinfectants applied to surfaces that are cleaned first to remove organic material should have at least 10 minutes of contact before being rinsed.
Bite or saliva	Wear gloves to examine oral cavities. Immediately rinse any bite wounds under water pressure, and apply disinfectant solution. Seek medical attention immediately.
Scratch or close contact	Disinfect scratches by rinsing them immediately in water, and apply disinfectant solution. Animal's bedding and carriers must go home with them. All cage papers, waste, and litter should be disposed of after each pet is discharged and the run or cage disinfected.
Aerogenic	No animals susceptible to a suspected infection should be housed closer than 1.3 meters to each other and never in adjacent cages. Always wear gloves and barrier clothing when handling such pets. Wash hands and change gown immediately after handling or medicating each affected pet. Disinfect surfaces in rooms where animals have had the opportunity to cough or sneeze.
Feces	Wear gloves and gown when handling patients. Diarrhea is especially infectious. If a highly contagious disease, such as *Salmonella* infection, is suspected, meet clients outside on their arrival, and coordinate their hospital entrance directly into an examination room or quarantine area that can be cleaned. Should the animal be admitted, it must be placed in an isolation area where appropriate barrier hygiene can be practiced. Using gloves, collect specimens with a syringe if they are liquid and a tongue depressor if they are solid.
Urine or genital	Wear gloves if wiping up urine with hands. Otherwise, use a mop soaked in dilute hypochlorite. Add disinfectant such as hypochlorite solution to urine before hosing or spraying cages or runs.
Transport Host (Vermin)	Use fumigants in rooms or buildings with major problems. Otherwise, use baits, sprays, and insect traps to control flies, cockroaches, and rodents.
Arthropod	Bathe and dip the animal or administer oral or topical insecticides, insect repellents, or growth regulators (see Table 94-20).
Sapronoses	Handling infected pets poses minimal risks, although precautions should be taken for certain diseases and by immunocompromised individuals. Avoid outdoor activities in areas where soil is disturbed. Wear masks and gloves when working outdoors under such conditions.
Anthroponoses	Be aware that human pathogens can spread to dogs and cats. Use hygiene, as outlined in previous sections, for preventing pet-person spread and to prevent spread of human infection to pets when a person is known to be or suspected of being infected.
Quarantine or isolation	Handling cases of highly contagious zoonoses, fatal zoonoses, or both requires isolated facilities. Isolation should be in a separate room with its own ventilation and cleaning facilities and in an area of the hospital where an ante room can be used for putting on barrier clothing such as gowns, masks, gloves, and protective footwear. Ideally, the area should have its own doorways into and out of the hospital. Disposable materials and animal waste leaving the area for decontamination should be sprayed with disinfectant and double bagged, with the outer bag also being sprayed with disinfectant. All reusable items that leave the area should be either autoclaved or washed and dried at high temperatures with automatic equipment. Reusable items should be washed, rinsed, and soaked in disinfectants after an animal vacates and before the item leaves the area. The facilities should be cleaned and disinfected routinely. A foot bath may be needed to prevent tracking of microorganisms. The animal should be bathed and then dipped in a dilute hypochlorite solution before leaving the area (see Chapter 94).

Excrement

Although pathogens such as *Salmonella*, *Cryptosporidium*, and *Giardia* are immediately infectious, *Toxoplasma* spp. require sporulation of the oocyst to be infectious. Therefore daily cleaning of feline litter boxes can prevent *Toxoplasma* infection. Immunosuppressed individuals should try to avoid direct contact with pet excretions and wear gloves when handling fecal material. When possible, diarrhea should be handled by others. Diarrheic stools are particularly challenging to remove without becoming exposed to pathogens they may contain. Feline litter boxes should be kept out of eating areas and be cleaned by an immunocompetent adult who is not pregnant. Creation of litter-box dust can be avoided by using bag liners and dust-free litters and by moistening litter before sealing bags. Although the litter box should be emptied outdoors or in well-ventilated areas to prevent inhalation, the litter should not be placed directly into the environment. The coccidian oocysts in a litter box can be disinfected once monthly by filling the box with boiling water or dilute (5% to 10%) household ammonia solutions for 10 minutes (see Chapter 80).

Dogs should be discouraged from coprophagia, and cat litter boxes should be isolated from other nonfeline pets. Within communities, animals should be restricted from defecating in playgrounds, parks, and walkways, or owners should remove their pets' excrement from public places.

Improved health education of children should be provided. Children should be educated not to practice geophagia or pica and to wash their hands after playing in soil. Those with aquatic or cold-blooded pets should wear rubber gloves for cleaning aquariums or terrariums. Diarrheic pets should not be exposed to the general household and should not contact young children of immunosuppressed members in a household. Animals with diarrhea should be bathed as needed to decontaminate their hair coat. Pet owners should be instructed to wear rubber gloves during cleaning of diarrheic or other stools and to use sodium hypochlorite (bleach) at a dilution of 1 ounce per quart of water for disinfection. Similar precautions can be recommended for handling other body fluids, including blood, urine, and saliva. Hands should be washed after the gloves are removed.

Oral Hygiene

Immunocompromised owners should be advised not to let pets lick them on the mouth and to practice good preventive dental hygiene for themselves and their pets. Routine dental prophylaxis with scaling or brushing is recommended for pets exposed to immunocompromised people. Veterinarians or other household members or assistants should assume these responsibilities. Saliva should be washed from hands or open wounds. Rubber gloves should be worn when oral medication is given to pets, or someone else should assume these responsibilities.

Bite wounds are probably the most common health risk faced by immunocompromised individuals. Pets that are aggressive in behavior or play should not be kept by immunocompromised people. People who are inadvertently bitten should immediately wash the wound with soap and water and rinse it with dilute organic iodine solutions or quaternary ammonium compounds as an alternative. A physician should promptly examine any injuries. Pets should not be allowed to lick human wounds. Children should be taught not to startle feeding or sleeping animals. Prophylactic antimicrobial therapy may be considered by physicians who know the patient's immunocompromised status.

Nutrition

The diet of pets is extremely important in limiting fecal-oral pathogens. Only commercial diets that have been cooked or pelleted should be fed. Raw or unprocessed meat or offal or unpasteurized dairy products should not be provided. Pets should be prevented from coprophagy, scavenging, hunting, and feeding on carrion or garbage. They may have to be leashed or confined or be supervised outdoors. Bells can be placed on cats' collars to reduce their success at hunting. Water from the tap should always be available to pets. Commercial bottled water should be provided if the tap water is unhealthy from inadvertent contamination with bacteria or protozoa. Access to outside surface water or toilet bowl water should be restricted.

SUGGESTED READINGS*

8. Anonymous. 2002. Guidelines for preventing opportunistic infections among HIV-infected persons—2002. Recommendations of the USPHS and the IDSA. *MMWR* 51:1-51.

14. Asano K, Suzuki K, Nakamura Y, et al. 2003. Risk of acquiring zoonoses by the staff of companion-animal hospitals. Kansenshogaku Zasshi 77:944-947.

37. Caccio S, Pinter E, Fantini R, et al. 2002. Human infection with *Cryptosporidium felis*: case report and literature review. *Emerg Infect Dis* 8:85-86.

42. Cherry B, Burns A, Johnson GS, et al. 2004. *Salmonella typhimurium* outbreak associated with veterinary clinic. *Emerg Infect Dis* 10:2249-2251.

56b. Duquette RA, Nuttall TJ. 2004. Methicillin-resistant *Staphylococcus aureus* in dogs and cats: an emerging problem. *J Sm Anim Pract* 45:591-597.

63. Fayer R, Lindsay D. 2004. Zoonotic protozoa in the marine environment: a threat to aquatic mammals and public health. *Vet Parasitol* 25:131-135.

78. Gummow B. 2003. A survey of zoonotic diseases contracted by South African veterinarians. *Tydskr S Afr Vet Ver* 74:72-76.

80. Hackendahl NC, Mawby DI Bemis DA, et al. 2004. Putative transmission of *Mycobacterium tuberculosis* infection from a human to a dog. *J Am Vet Med Assoc* 225:1573-1577.

83a. Harada T, Tsuji N, Otsuki K, et al. 2005. Detection of the *esp* gene in high-level gentamicin resistant *Enterococcus faecalis* strains from pet animals in Japan, *Vet Microbiol* 106:139-143.

85. Hendriksen SW, Orsel K, Wagenaar JA, et al. 2004. Animal-to-human transmission of *Salmonella typhimurium* DT104A variant. *Emerg Infect Dis* 10:2225-2227.

85a. Heuer OE, Jensen VF, Hammerum AM. 2005. Antimicrobial drug use in companion animals, *Emerg Infect Dis* 11:344-345.

101a. Kile JC, Panella NA, Komar N, et al. 2005. Serologic survey of cats and dogs during an epidemic of West Nile Virus infection in humans, *J Am Vet Med Assoc* 226:1349-1353.

101b. Krause G, Zimmermann S, Beutin L. 2005. Investigation of domestic animals and pets as a reservoir for intimin-(*eae*) gene positive *Escherichia coli* types, *Vet Microbiol* 106:87-95.

*See the CD-ROM for a complete list of references.

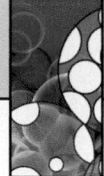

CHAPTER • 100

Immunoprophylaxis

Craig E. Greene and Ron D. Schultz

Immunoprophylaxis (vaccination) involves enhancement of a specific immune response in an animal in an attempt to protect it against infectious disease. This response can be actively induced through vaccines containing microorganisms, their components, or their metabolic by-products. Immunity can also be passively transferred by the administration of humoral or cellular factors obtained from a previously sensitized donor. Immunoprophylaxis also implies preexposure potentiation of the immune system, and it should be differentiated from immunotherapy, which is the attempt to increase nonspecifically the immune response in an already infected animal. See Chapter 2 for a discussion of immunotherapy and available treatments. Immunoprophylaxis is successful in the prevention of viral and bacterial diseases because the relatively small number of antigens needed to stimulate an immune response is present in these organisms. Fungal, protozoal, and metazoan pathogens and neoplasms contain more complex antigenic determinants and are often controlled with nonspecific immunotherapy. Nevertheless, vaccines are being developed for some of these infections of dogs and cats.

MATERNAL IMMUNITY

IgG from breast milk is transported across the intestinal epithelium into the circulation of the neonate. This action occurs in the duodenum and jejunum through membrane receptors on the intestinal epithelium that facilitate transport of IgG into the systemic circulation. This process is maximal at the time of birth (under 24 hours) but also occurs to a limited degree throughout the remainder of the nursing period. Animals that do not obtain these maternal-derived antibodies (MDAs) in large quantities during the early nursing period are at high risk for developing infectious diseases. As long as they circulate, MDAs absorbed into the circulation of the neonate feed back to inhibit endogenous IgG production; however, IgG synthesis will ensue again sometime after weaning. Over time, MDAs in the neonate naturally decay, causing a decline in the available protective antibody level until the animal is vulnerable to disease-causing organisms in the environment.

Although IgG concentration and absorption is important in the first few days of neonatal life, secretory IgA (S-IgA) is found in milk during the entire nursing period and becomes the primary defense against enteric and upper respiratory mucosal infections.[577] In the dam, antigens of pathogenic organisms to which her mucosae are exposed prime T cells for cell-mediated immune (CMI) responses. These antigens activate B cells that produce the immunoglobulin found in her mammary secretions. IgG and IgM are in high concentrations in the colostrum; however, low levels persist throughout the entire nursing period. S-IgA is present in breast milk throughout lactation. S-IgA is highly effective in inhibiting the adherence of pathogens at the mucosal surface, causing their immediate neutralization.

Antibody production in the neonate can be stimulated only when the circulating MDA levels decrease below a specific threshold. This level is not absolute but is determined by the ratio of MDA to the dose level of pathogenic or vaccine antigen. Usually, pathogenic organisms can *break through* a higher level of this *blocking antibody* than attenuated organisms in live vaccines. Increasing the dose (titer) of vaccine antigen allows for earlier immunization in the face of MDA. The level of MDA transferred to each neonate varies according to the titer of the dam, the number of nursing offspring, and the level of exposure of the dam to vaccine or the virulent agent.

PASSIVE IMMUNIZATION

Artificial (passive) transfer of specific antibodies or other immunoreactive substances from one individual to another has been classically used to treat a variety of infectious diseases in humans and animals. Use of passive immunization itself has been decreasing; however, it is beneficial in diseases in which serum antibody is protective; the host does not have the time or ability to mount an immune response; or antimicrobial chemotherapy is not available or effective. When given prophylactically or therapeutically, antibodies with specific organism-neutralizing activities can transfer specific protection from, or reduction in, numbers of infectious agents. Developing passive immunization protocols for opportunistic and nosocomial infections is even considered in human medicine.[582] Currently, passive immunization is used in small-animal veterinary practice in a few special instances. Various aspects of passive immunization are summarized in Table 100-1. Immunoglobulins have been used to prevent infections with canine distemper virus (CDV), canine parvovirus (CPV), feline panleukopenia (parvovirus) virus (FPV), canine herpesvirus-1 (CHV-1), and feline herpesvirus-1 (FHV-1) in exposed, susceptible neonates. Specific immunoglobulins are less effective in treating infections once they have become established. In addition, they have little role in the protection against organisms that can persist intracellularly in phagocytes or lymphoid cells.

Passive administration of serum or immunoglobulin has a beneficial role in protecting colostrum-deprived neonates (under 2 days of age) against certain diseases such as parvoviral infections. Active immunization must be avoided because of the risk of inducing disease with modified live vaccines and because of the weaker response to killed vaccines at this age. Antisera given to older kittens (under 8 weeks) that become inadvertently exposed to FPV provide protection much sooner compared with that produced after vaccination. Passive immunization may also temporarily benefit severely immunosuppressed dogs and cats receiving cancer chemotherapy that may become exposed to infectious agents during a course of hospitalization.

Immune sera may be of prophylactic or therapeutic benefit in treating litters of puppies that are clinically affected with

Table • 100-1

Comparison of Passive and Active Immunoprophylaxis

VARIABLE	PASSIVE	ACTIVE
Advantages	Immediate protection	Stronger protection
	Works for agents that are poor immunogens	Longer protection
		Anamnestic response
Disadvantages	Allergic reactions	Delayed response
	Hypersensitivity reactions	
	Delays ability to vaccinate	
	Short-lived protection	
	Transfer of disease more likely	
Indications	Exposed susceptible neonates	Unexposed susceptible neonates
	Colostrum-deprived neonates	Routine immunization
	Exposed immunosuppressed animals	Booster vaccinations

neonatal herpesvirus infections (see Therapy, Chapter 5). Serum, for treating CHV infection, should be prepared from recovered bitches that have previously had affected litters. Hyperimmune serum has been beneficial in treating parvovirus-infected cats and dogs within 4 days of experimental postinoculation (PI), which corresponded to the first day or two of clinical illness.[258,386] In a placebo-controlled study involving dogs presented to a teaching hospital with parvoviral infection, the efficacy of a preparation of specific canine lyophilized IgG was investigated.[344] Dogs receiving lyophilized IgG as adjunctive treatment had significantly decreased hospitalization time, reduced severity of disease, and reduced cost of treatment compared with dogs treated with conventional therapy alone. A commercial, multivalent, homologous hyperimmune immunoglobulin preparation (Stagloban® SHP, Hoechst Veterinär Gmb, Munich, Germany) containing a combination of high concentrations of antibodies against CPV, CDV, and canine adenovirus (CAV)-1 had been available in Germany for this purpose, although its manufacture has been discontinued. A commercial heterologous antisera produced in horses containing highly concentrated immunoglobulins is available in some European countries for treatment of cats (Feliserin® PRC, Impfstoffwerk, Dessau-Tomau, GmbH, Rodleben, Germany). This antisera contains a combination of antibodies against FPV, FHV-1, and feline calicivirus (FCV).

Increased levels of endotoxin and tumor necrosis factor have been observed in dogs with naturally occurring parvoviral enteritis.[429] Heterologous antiserum produced in horses for *Salmonella typhimurium* endotoxin is commercially available (Septiserum®, Immvac®, Columbia, Mo.), and it has shown benefit in treating endotoxemia in dogs associated with experimental parvoviral infection (see Chapters 8 and 38 and Drug Formulary, Appendix 8).[122] Passive immunization with heterologous (equine or human) antitoxin is used in the initial treatment of dogs and cats with tetanus (see Chapter 43). Monoclonal antibodies (MABs) have been provided as specific passive immunoprophylaxis for infectious agents, but because they are usually produced in rodents, tolerance is low to systemically administered foreign immunoglobulins.

The efficacy of passive immunization depends on many factors, including the antibody titer to the specific agent involved and volume administered, the relative importance of serum antibody in controlling the particular infection involved, and the timing of administration of antibody compared with exposure. Because of the large amounts of foreign protein that are administered, allergic reactions are more likely with passive immunization. Transfer of infectious agents is more likely with administration of serum when noncommercially prepared products are used. Unfortunately, the administration of immunoglobulins also delays the ability to stimulate active immunity in the host by vaccination. Large amounts of exogenously administered antibody may negate endogenous antibody production by tying up vaccine antigens or by direct feedback mechanisms that are not clearly understood. The duration of protection received from passively administered antisera is short lived (often 2 to 3 weeks). The amount received is finite and, as with all exogenous proteins, undergoes accelerated elimination from the body, especially if it originates from a different species.

Although not readily available commercially in many countries, canine and feline immune sera can be prepared in veterinary practices by sterile harvesting serum or plasma. Immune serum (or plasma) is derived from clinically healthy, pathogen-free individuals or from groups of animals that have recovered from the disease in question, whereas hyperimmune serum comes from animals that have been well vaccinated against specified infectious agents. Veterinarians who prepare their own serum must carefully screen donors for insidious blood-borne infectious diseases such as bartonellosis, hemotropic mycoplasmosis, feline leukemia virus (FeLV) or feline immunodeficiency virus (FIV) infections, canine brucellosis, leishmaniasis, babesiosis, or ehrlichiosis. If noncommercial sera harvested from donor cats are used, the time of protection is unknown and depends on the amount of antibodies administered. In cats, because of naturally occurring blood-group antibodies, ideally, the blood type of both donor and recipient should match, or if cross-matching is not performed, only type A cats should be used as donors.

The minimum amount of immune sera required to confer protection is unknown and will depend on the respective antibody concentration. Doses of adult dog serum given to colostrum-deprived pups have ranged from 22 to 40 ml/kg; however, the serum IgG concentrations at this dose have been lower than that afforded by naturally acquired colostrum.[52,453] Therefore higher range doses might be needed for pups unless they will be given an earlier initial vaccination series. The dose shown effective for cats, which was equal to that provided by nursing colostrum, is 5 ml of adult cat donor serum given subcutaneously (SC) or intraperitoneally (IP) at birth. This application is repeated again at 12 and 24 hours of age.[331] This dose is equivalent to 150 ml/kg based on the body weight of neonatal kittens. Careful attention must be paid to sterility during collection process, storage, and administration. Jugular venipuncture is preferred, and the area over the jugular vein should be shaved and prepared aseptically. Blood, at least double the amount of required serum, should be collected into sterile clotting tubes without additives. Serum can be stored frozen in single dose aliquots because IgG is a highly stable molecule; it can be stored up to a year if frozen (–20° C) promptly after collection.[331]

Usually, serum is given SC; IP routes are possible and sometimes more accessible for puppies and kittens. Oral administration of serum, either alone or in a milk substitute, is probably the most effective means of treating colostrum-deprived neonates in their first (under 24) hours of life. Immunoglobulins might be absorbed to a lesser degree for up to 72 hours. Any mucosal protection afforded by orally administered serum is only temporary because unstable serum IgG, IgM, and IgA are destroyed by proteolytic enzymes once the neonate develops improved digestive function and bacterial colonization. In contrast, because of its stability, natural S-IgA in the dam's milk offers continued protection against mucosal pathogens during the entire period that the animal is nursing. Other routes for serum administration in neonates are intramuscular (IM), SC, intramedullary, and IP. These products have also been used intranasally (IN) to treat neonates with infectious upper respiratory disease. Immune sera is not usually administered intravenously (IV) to small puppies or kittens because of the tendency to produce immunologic or coagulatory reactions in the recipient and because of the difficulty in cannulating a vein. If given IV, plasma anticoagulated with citrate is more desirable compared with serum.

MATERNAL IMMUNITY AND VACCINATION

Newborn pups and kittens have the inherent capacity to respond immunologically to numerous antigens at birth, but this response is slower and inferior compared with that of older animals. Under normal circumstances, protection against infection during these early weeks of life is afforded by passive transfer of immunoglobulins and small amounts of cellular material from the dam. The amount (2% to 18% of the total) of antibody transferred in utero from an immune dam protects colostrum-deprived puppies or kittens but makes them refractory to immunization for a period (Table 100-2). Subsequently, the immunoglobulin absorbed systemically from colostrum may give the neonate a titer that may almost equal that of the dam in some instances (Table 100-3). Over time, the MDA declines with each disease having a characteristic half-life for elimination (Table 100-4).[256] Antibody class is also important with respect to titer loss. Serum maternally derived IgA, IgM, and IgG in neonates are usually lost in the order given.

Table • 100-2

Effect of Maternal Immunity on Vaccination for Selected Canine Infectious Diseases

DISEASE[a]	MINIMUM TITER PREVENTING REPLICATION (METHOD DETERMINED)[b]		MINIMUM AGE (WEEKS)		
	VIRULENT VIRUS	VACCINE VIRUS	TO BEGIN VACCINATING COLOSTRUM DEPRIVED	TO BEGIN VACCINATING COLOSTRUM RECIPIENTS	TO STOP VACCINATING COLOSTRUM RECIPIENTS
Canine distemper[32,193]	1:20-1:30 (SN)	1:30 (SN)	2-3	6	12-14
Infectious canine hepatitis[75,76]	NR	1:5 (SN)	2-3	6	12
Canine parvoviral infection[455,456]	1:80 (HI)	<1:10 (HI)	4-5[c]	6-9	12-14[d]

SN, Serum neutralization (viral neutralization); NR, not reported; HI, hemagglutination inhibition.
[a]Numbers in this column refer to reference numbers cited at the end of this chapter or on the CD.
[b]Absolute titers will vary between laboratories.
[c]One product is licensed for 4 weeks of age; see text.
[d]Recommendation for high-titer lower passage ("potentiated") parvoviral vaccines; may need up to 20 weeks with "conventional" products; see text.

Table • 100-3

Comparison of Maternal Immunity for Selected Canine and Feline Infectious Diseases

DISEASE[a]	SERUM TITER OF NEONATE			HALF-LIFE MATERNAL ANTIBODY (DAYS)
	% OF DAM'S TITER		% OF NEONATE'S TITER	
	PRESUCKLE	POSTSUCKLE	OBTAINED IN UTERO/ COLOSTRUM	
Canine distemper[32,193]	3	77	4/96	8.4
Infectious canine hepatitis[75,76]	NR	92	NR/NR	8.6
Canine parvoviral infection[455,456]	5.7	60	10/90	9.7
Feline panleukopenia[510,512]	<1	97	1/99	9.6

NR, Not reported.
[a]Numbers in this column refer to reference numbers cited at the end of this chapter or on the CD.

Table • 100-4

Half-Life of Maternally Derived Immunoglobulins in Neonatal Dogs and Cats

DISEASE[a]	HALF-LIFE (DAYS)	USUAL DURATION OF PROTECTION AGAINST DISEASE (WEEKS)[b]
Canine distemper[193]	8.4	9-12
Canine parvovirus[456,457]	9.7	10-14
Infectious canine hepatitis[75]	8.4	9-12
Feline panleukopenia[510]	9.5	8-14
Feline leukemia[261]	15.0	6-8
Feline rhinotracheitis[c] [137,185,464]	18.5	6-8
Feline calicivirus infection[265,266]	15.0	10-14
Feline coronavirus infection[443]	7.0	4-6

[a]Numbers in this column refer to reference numbers cited at the end of this chapter or on the CD.
[b]The duration of maternal antibody protection against disease usually corresponds to the interval over which vaccines are ineffective.
[c]Feline herpesvirus-1 infection.

The absolute titer of MDA in the serum of a neonate depends on the quantity of immunoglobulin received during nursing and the absolute titer of the dam. The amount is also inversely proportional to the size of the litter. Titers may be increased by vaccination of the dam just before conception. In one instance, vaccination during pregnancy has also been shown to have benefit for protecting neonates (see later discussion, Feline Vaccination Recommendations, Feline Viral Respiratory Disease); however, caution should be exercised by avoiding the use of attenuated-live products. Titer values are so variable among individual animals that quantitative predictions cannot be made short of direct measurement of serum immunoglobulins of the dam or puppy. Commercially available enzyme-linked immunosorbent assay (ELISA) kits are available for semiquantitative measurement of antibodies to CPV with or without CDV (Immunocomb®, Biogal®, Kibbutz Gal'ed, Israel; TiterCHEK™ CDV/CPV, Synbiotics, San Diego, Calif.; see Appendix 6).[585] Repeated measurements (nomogram determinations) in neonates are usually impractical and expensive. Veterinarians usually use multiple vaccines, given at 2- to 4-week intervals, in an attempt to break through maternal immunity before exposure to virulent organisms (Figs. 100-1 and 100-2). Frequently given vaccines may also accelerate the depletion of the MDA present in the neonate's circulation. Attempts to overcome the interfering effects of MDA on vaccination have included antigenically related vaccines, such as measles for CDV; alternate routes, such as IN administration for canine or feline respiratory viruses or *Bordetella*; and different vaccine strains or types that are able

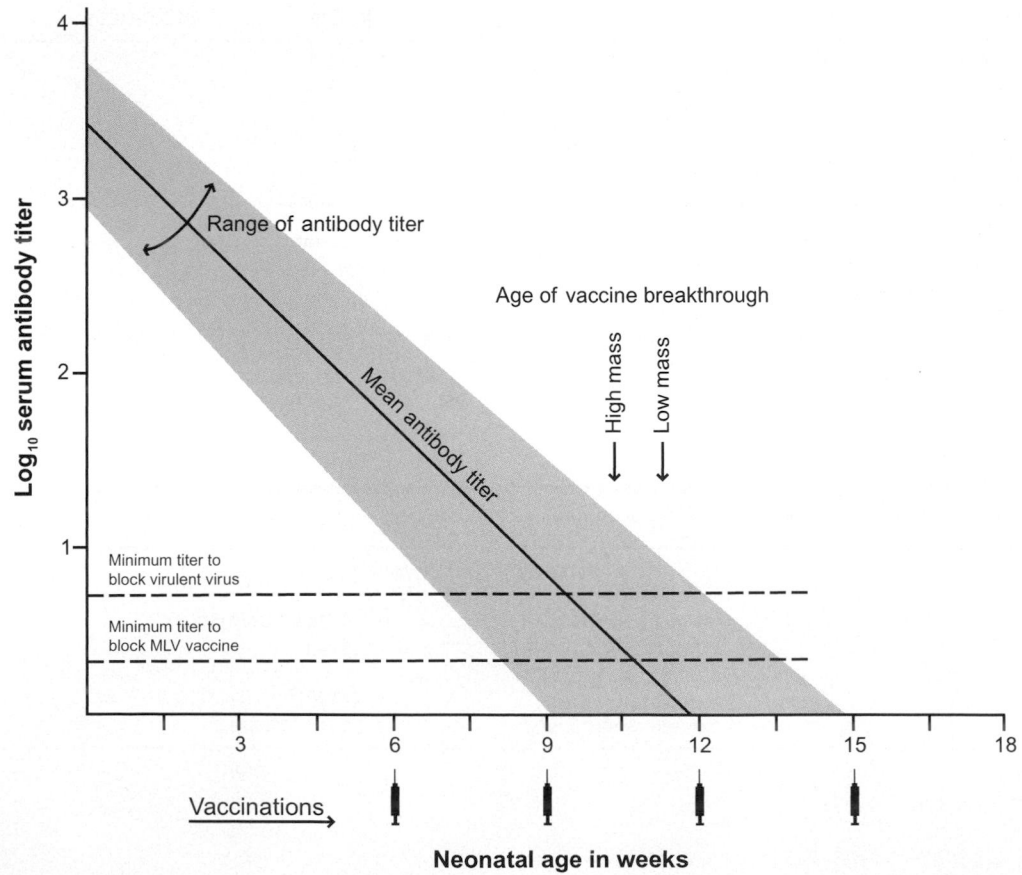

Fig 100-1 Elimination of maternal antibody in the neonate in relation to vaccination. At a critical period, the antibody titer may block a modified live virus vaccine but fail to protect against infection with virulent virus. Higher antigen mass or less-attenuated vaccines break through this maternal antibody barrier sooner than lower antigen mass or more attenuated products.

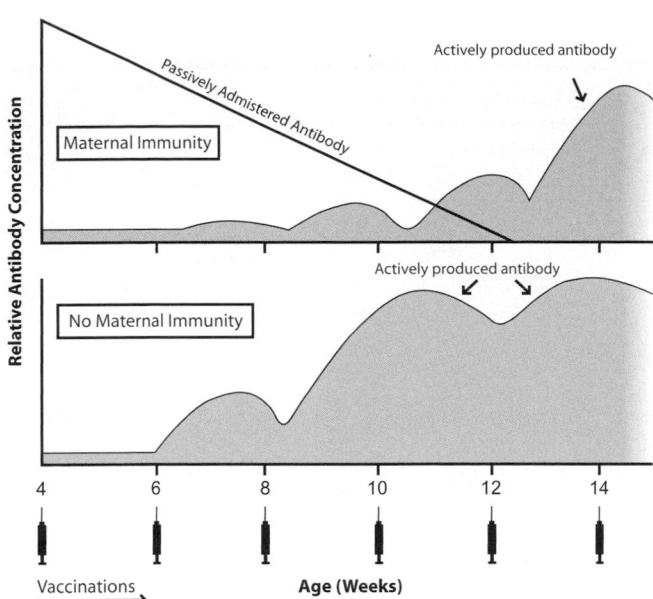

Fig 100-2 Comparison of response to sequential (2-week interval) vaccination in neonates with *(top)* and without *(bottom)* maternal antibody protection. The presence of maternal antibody delays the neonate's ability to produce successful active immunization.

to overcome maternal immunity at a younger age as with higher titer, lower passage CPV vaccine.

ACTIVE IMMUNIZATION

Vaccination, the production of an active immune response, involves stimulating the host with antigenic extracts or whole cultures of microorganisms. Clinical vaccination in small animals has been limited to diseases caused by viruses, bacteria, and some protozoa.

Types of Vaccines

Classic vaccines have generally been derived from whole organisms and are either live attenuated (modified live) or noninfectious or inactivated (killed). The advantages and disadvantages of these conventional whole-agent products are summarized in Table 100-5. To increase potency and remove nonessential, potentially allergenic proteins, newer vaccines are being developed. Live agents are being modified by genetic deletion or recombination or use of naked nucleic acids. Newer noninfectious vaccines are using subunit fractions of purified agents or synthetic peptides produced by genetic recombination or antiidiotypes (see later discussion). Table 100-6 compares these newer vaccines.

Live

Live whole agents in vaccines must be modified (attenuated) so that they retain immunogenicity and the ability to replicate in the intended host without producing illness. Attenuated vaccines stimulate CMI and long-lived humoral immune responses compared with noninfectious (inactivated or purified antigen) vaccines. T-cell stimulation is superior with attenuated products. Because they replicate in the host, initial antigenic content is of low importance; however, any factor that neutralizes or inactivates the vaccine will make it ineffective. Attenuation of agents is usually achieved by adapting them to unusual hosts, by subjecting them to prolonged storage, or by serial passage in tissue culture. Vaccines also have been developed by inoculating only partially attenuated strains of organisms at sites other than those of their tissue

tropism. Use of an alternate vaccination site has been used to produce parenteral vaccines against respiratory pathogens, such as for feline viral respiratory disease. The agents undergo limited replication at the alternative sites, but, unfortunately, they may produce a greater systemic response rather than local antibody response. Furthermore, inadvertent contact of these agents with respiratory tissues may cause disease (see later discussion, Postvaccinal Complications).

Quality control is an essential factor in the production of biologics to ensure that cell lines used in attenuating vaccine agents do not contain latent pathogens, especially in veterinary vaccine production, because this usually involves primary and secondary cell cultures (see Adventitious Agents under Postvaccinal Complications, later). Primary cell cultures are those derived from tissues harvested directly from an animal. Secondary cultures originate from further cultivation of primary cell lines. Both of these lines are at risk of containing pathogens. Established (continuous) cell lines employed for diagnostic virology, which have been adapted for stable growth in vitro, are usually too anaplastic for vaccine production. Unlike human vaccines, the primary or secondary cell lines for animals are usually produced from cells of the species for which the vaccine is intended. This practice increases the risk of contamination with potentially pathogenic, latent, or passenger organisms.

Live vaccines are usually lyophilized (freeze dried), which increases their stability and storage life span. Temperature is another important factor determining storage life span; vaccines should always be stored refrigerated at 4° C (39.2° F). Commercially prepared live vaccines usually contain excess antigen because some deterioration is expected.

Genetically altered recombinant vaccines involve removing genetic sequences that code for virulence factors while maintaining reproductive function. A gene-deleted FHV-1 vaccine has been developed experimentally.[305] This method allows for selective attenuation of a variety of infectious agents when existing modified live–agent vaccines are ineffective. Insertion of a genetic marker may also be desired when determining vaccinated versus naturally diseased animals is important. When antibody titers are being used to distinguish between natural and vaccine exposure, such as with FIV infection, a unique vaccine marker would be beneficial.

Live agent recombinant vector vaccines use vector agents that are nonpathogenic to the intended host. These expression vectors are organisms in which genetic code has been inserted to produce key immunogenic proteins on a sustained basis after inoculation of the host. Vector systems can also be genetically altered to elicit killer T-cell or cytotoxic T-lymphocyte activity. Protein epitopes can be targeted by vaccines that are important for the agent's attachment, replication, development, or spread within the host. Multiple genes may be inserted, including those for cytokines such as interleukin (IL)-2, which may enhance the immune response to the simultaneously generated immunogenic proteins.

Expression vectors have included poxviruses, simian virus 40, bovine papillomavirus, adenovirus, and herpesvirus.[31,609] Bacterial vectors such as *Salmonella typhimurium* and *Mycobacterium bovis* bacille Calmette-Guérin (BCG) and plants can also be used. All potentially pathogenic vectors must be attenuated for the host. Poxviruses such as vaccinia work well because of their large genome and wide host range. One potential problem with recombinant vector vaccines is that the host may mount an immune response to the vector. A recombinant vaccinia virus expressing FeLV gp70 envelope protein was not successful in producing antiviral antibodies in cats.[191] Instead, inoculated cats developed neutralizing antibody against the vaccinia virus. Experimental recombinant vaccinia virus products have been capable of inducing immune responses in dogs to human influenza virus, rabies virus, herpesvirus, and hepatitis virus.[25]

Table • 100-5

Comparison of Two Main Types of Conventional Whole-Agent Vaccines

	MODIFIED LIVE (ATTENUATED) VACCINE	NONINFECTIOUS WHOLE AGENT (INACTIVATED) VACCINE
Advantages	Rapid protection Prolonged protection Lower antigen mass needed Administer by natural routes Stimulates secretory antibody Better able to stimulate CMI Can administer locally (IN, PO) Better stimulator of interferon Overcome MDA interference One administration can protect Reduced allergenicity	No reversion to virulence Increased immunity with added adjuvants Stability in storage Safe in immunosuppressed animals
Disadvantages	Risk of adventitious agents Can produce vaccine-induced illness in immunosuppressed hosts Susceptible to inactivation Require more rigorous testing for potency and reversion to virulence Require multiplication in host Might revert to virulence No preservatives for storage	Primarily stimulates humoral immunity Minimum of 2 doses needed for maximum protection Increased risk of allergic complications Shorter duration of immunity than modified live vaccines Higher antigen mass needed Restricted to parenteral use Adjuvants frequently required More hypersensitivity reactions (local and systemic)
Indications	Outbreaks Production of mucosal immunity Routine vaccination	Pregnant animals Debilitated/immunosuppressed animals Colostrum-deprived neonates (passive immunization preferred)
Diseases for which used	Canine: Parvoviral enteritis Hepatitis Bordetellosis (IN) Parainfluenza Distemper Measles Feline: Panleukopenia Calicivirus infection Rhinotracheitis Infectious peritonitis (IN) Bordetellosis (IN) *Chlamydophila* infection	Canine: Lyme borreliosis Coronaviral enteritis Parvoviral enteritis Hepatitis Bordetellosis (parenteral) Leptospirosis Herpesvirus-1 infection Babesiosis Giardiasis Rabies Feline: Panleukopenia Calicivirus infection Rhinotracheitis FeLV infection Rabies FIV infection Giardiasis *Chlamydophila* infection

CMI, Cell-mediated immunity; *IN*, intranasal; *PO*, by mouth; *MDA*, maternally derived antibody; *FeLV*, feline leukemia virus; *FIV*, feline immunodeficiency virus

Table • 100-6

Comparison of Newer Types of Vaccines

TYPE[a]	PRODUCTION METHOD	ADVANTAGES/ DISADVANTAGES	EXAMPLES
Attenuated (Modified Live)			
Genetic deletion[305]	Selected genome removed to reduce virulence	A: Controlled attenuation D: Only certain organisms can be modified this way; costly to produce	Experimental: FHV-1[b] infection
Recombinant vector[115,481,559,561]	Genomic portion encoding for immunogen of pathogenic organism inserted into an avirulent "vector" organism	A: Stimulate immunity without disease-producing potential; may co-express immunomodulators or multiple agents simultaneously D: May produce persistent immunopathologic response; may spread environmentally; may produce genetic instability of vector or host; costly to produce; vector can be cytolytic	Experimental: oral and parenteral rabies; FIP, panleukopenia, feline leukemia, canine distemper, CPV infection[b]; Commercial: canine distemper Recombitek® CDV (Merial)[b]; Feline leukemia PureVax® and Eurifel® (Merial)[b]; Feline rabies PureVax® (Merial)
Nucleic acid (DNA, RNA)[263,473]	Naked genes encoding for antigen are inserted into a plasmid carrier	A: Triggers cell-mediated immunity; yields protein antigens in natural form; easy to manufacture D: Potential antinucleic responses; introduces foreign genes into host	Experimental: canine distemper Experimental: CPV infection
Noninfectious			
Purified subunit[311]	Organism propagated in vitro with purification of selected components; otherwise chemical synthesis of specific immunogenic proteins	A: Purified proteins; less allergenic; no postvaccinal illness D: Works primarily for humoral immune protection; costly to produce	Experimental: CPV-V$_2$ protein Commercial: bordetellosis (cell wall extract), Bronchicine® (Pfizer)[b]; feline leukemia, Leukocell® 2-(Pfizer)[b]; leptospirosis (envelope), Duramune® Max (Fort Dodge)[b]
Recombinant protein	Desired gene cloned into organism that produces it in vitro, followed by harvesting and purification	A: Highly purified immunogen; higher potency possible D: Primarily stimulates humoral immune protection	Commercial: feline leukemia, Leucogen® (Virbac)[b]; borreliosis, Recombitek® Lyme (Merial)[b]; borreliosis, Prolyme® and Nobivac® (Intervet)[b]
Antiidiotypes	Immunoglobulins produced against antigen-combining sites on immunoglobulin directed against the infectious agent	A: Highly specific immune response; stimulates cell-mediated immunity D: Foreign proteins potentially reactive	None

A, Advantage; *D*, disadvantage; *FHV*, feline herpesvirus-1; *FIP*, feline infectious peritonitis; *CDV*, canine distemper virus; *FeLV*, feline leukemia virus; *CPV*, canine parvovirus.
[a]Numbers in this column refer to reference numbers cited at the end of this chapter or on the CD.
[b]See Appendix 3 for more information on particular commercial products.

Commercially available oral rabies vaccines with poxviruses as vectors have been employed to protect wildlife. Canarypox has been an effective vector in vaccines for canine distemper, rabies, and feline leukemia.[207,559,561,562] Throughout the world, a canine canarypox virus–vectored distemper vaccine is commercially available for administration by injection (Recombitek CDV, Merial). Pups vaccinated with canarypox-rabies vaccine could be protected at a young age despite the negating influence of MDAs.[561] Parenteral canarypox-FeLV recombinant vaccine (Eurifel, Merial), expressing the envelope and *gag* genes, was protective against oronasal challenge with virulent FeLV.[207,561] A needle-free injection system (VET JET®, Bioject Medical Technologies, Tualatin, Ore.) is licensed to administer a similar product (PureVax, Merial) transdermally.[207,436] A recombinant baculovirus was used to express the VP2 capsid component of CPV, and the respective vaccine produced titers in dogs that were higher than those from commercially available inactivated vaccine.[115,122] A canine adenovirus 2–based CDV vaccine expressing the H and F antigens was effective, in the face of MDAs, in protecting pups against a challenge with virulent CDV.[160]

Various plant sources, *Agrobacterium tumefaciens* TL plasmid, cow pea mosaic virus, and potato virus C have been used as expression vectors for CPV-2 vaccination of dogs.[212,383,408]

Nucleic acids (RNA or DNA), when inoculated as naked or plasmid-containing molecules containing complete gene coding, can stimulate production of immunogenic proteins by the host without being permanently incorporated into the host cell genome. Thus, unlike attenuated vaccines, nucleic acids are noninfectious and have no risk of causing disease. Nucleic acid vaccines are stable, resisting extremes in temperature, making their storage and preservation more practical and less expensive. They can be used to develop broader antigenic subtypes and induce both humoral and CMI responses. DNA vaccines appear to be most effective in stimulating long-lasting cytotoxic T cells and variable antibody responses against expressed proteins. Direct IM or intradermal (ID) inoculation of DNA from pathogenic organisms is a promising method for vaccination against some diseases.[473] Practical limitations to use of these vaccines are that they may alter the genome of inoculated hosts and the numerous patent considerations on the technology used to create the final product. The nucleic acids are injected by inoculation devices, with or without substances such as liposomes or gold particles, which facilitate uptake by host cells. Second-generation DNA vaccines have been designed to contain genes encoding for cytokines or immunostimulatory molecules that act as biologic facilitators of the immune response. Without being able to deliver the genes and express them at sufficient levels at the correct site, the technology may not be commercially viable.[28]

Classical DNA vaccines are injected IM and have little ability to stimulate S-IgA responses. Formulations with microparticles, cationic lipids, protein polymers, or biodegradable microspheres allow for oral or IN delivery and result in significant S-IgA production at the mucosal sites.[536] Such DNA vaccines have been used in clinical trials in people, and unfortunately, they provide weaker responses as compared with conventional vaccines. Giving a combination of a DNA vaccine first, followed by a booster using a different type of vaccine for the same disease, can provide an accentuated immune response.

A CDV nucleic acid vaccine has been produced that causes expression of the nucleocapsid, fusion, and hemagglutinin proteins.[85] Three IM injections of 12-week-old dogs, at 4-week intervals, induced a humoral IgG response and protected dogs against challenge with virulent CDV. In subsequent studies, this vaccine was found to break through maternal immunity 2 weeks after birth because it was effective in priming the

immune system to subsequent vaccination after a conventional modified live virus (MLV) CDV vaccine at 9 weeks.[206]

Noninfectious

Noninfectious whole agent (inactivated or killed) vaccines are produced in a similar fashion to live vaccines. Because noninfectious vaccines fail to replicate in the host, the level of antigenic mass is a critical determinant in the efficacy of a particular product. Inactivated whole-agent products contain agents subjected to various forms of denaturation without destroying their immunogenicity. Heat and light treatments have been relatively ineffective because, in many cases, they destroy immunogenicity without complete inactivation. Chemical inactivation with formalin produces slight modification in antigenic composition of the product, reduction in immunogenicity, and severe irritation to the animal at the site of injection. Ethylenediamine and β-propiolactone are inactivating agents that overcome many of these disadvantages. Having greater antigenic mass and added adjuvants (see Adjuvants, later), inactivated vaccines have an increased tendency to produce local and systemic allergic reactions.

Noninfectious vaccines are stable and have no risk of producing vaccine-induced illness. They are sometimes considered safer for this reason. However, these vaccines do not mimic natural infection and therefore may not produce adequate mucosal immunity or CMI. In general, noninfectious vaccines must be given at least twice to produce an anamnestic response that equals one attenuated vaccination (Fig. 100-3). Full protection may not develop until 2 to 3 weeks after the last immunization. Despite this shortcoming, immunity that is stimulated by noninfectious products is commonly sufficient for clinical protection and routine use. After vaccination with noninfectious vaccines, many partially protected animals probably become infected when exposed to virulent agents. They develop a mild or subclinical infection that further boosts their immunity to the disease.

Purified subunit vaccines are composed of purified immunogenic components of infectious agents that are used in an attempt to increase the specificity and quantity of the

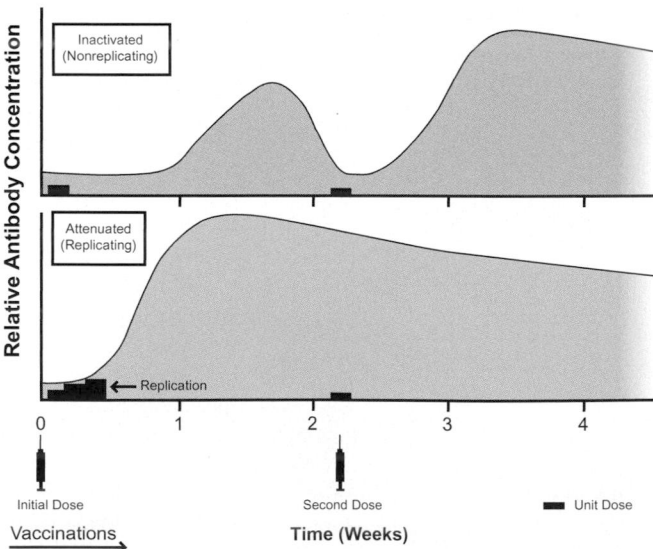

Fig 100-3 Comparison of antibody response after inoculation with noninfectious (*top*) and live attenuated (*bottom*) virus vaccine. One dose of the live attenuated virus vaccine continues to drive the immune response. Two doses of noninfectious vaccine are required to produce a similar effect. (Modified from Mims CA. 1977. *The pathogenesis of infectious disease*. Academic Press, New York, N.Y. Used with permission.)

immunogen while reducing its allergenicity. The components are recognized by the host immune system as foreign and elicit an antibody-based immune response. Examples of subunit vaccines are Pfizer Leukocell® 2 (Pfizer, New York, N.Y.) vaccine for FeLV, which is produced by harvesting cell-free supernatants from cell culture; parenteral lipopolysaccharide (LPS)-extracted cell wall *Bordetella* vaccine such as Bronchicine® (Pfizer, New York, N.Y.); and a purified outer membrane protein, leptospiral vaccine (Duramune® Max, Fort Dodge, Fort Dodge, Iowa).

Recombinant protein vaccines, developed using DNA technology, also allow for in vitro production of large quantities of immunogenic proteins by introducing coding into bacteria, yeasts, and continuous cell lines. These differ from recombinant vectors in that the preformed antigen is produced in large amounts ex vivo and then administered to the animal as a purified component. The FeLV vaccine (Leucogen®, Virbac, Carros Cedex, France; Nobivac®, Intervet, Boxmeer, The Netherlands) consists of synthetic glycoprotein for FeLV (gp70) subgroup A expressed in *Escherichia coli*.[362] Recombinant outer surface protein A (OspA) protein vaccines are also available for vaccination of dogs for Lyme borreliosis (Recombitek® Lyme, Merial, Iselin, N.J.; ProLyme®, Intervet, Millsboro, Del.). Synthetic antigens can be produced by identifying the antigenic or genetic determinants using MABs. Once the nucleotide and amino acid sequences have been determined, the protein can be synthesized. Unfortunately, many antigenically active peptides by themselves are weak antigens that require adjuvants. Recombinant subunit protein vaccines have a similar duration of immunity (DOI) as inactivated whole-agent vaccines, which is shorter compared with live attenuated products. A synthetic peptide VP2 has been effective in protecting dogs against CPV-2 infection.[311]

Adjuvants

Adjuvants have been added to noninfectious biologics in an attempt to increase their duration and amount of immunostimulation to a level comparable to that of MLVs. Adjuvants are helpful in accentuating the immune response to killed whole organism or purified antigens. They can prolong antigen exposure, enhance antigen presentation, and increase cytokine and immune responses.[335] By definition and in principle, adjuvants produce a heightened inflammatory reaction, which can sometimes be deleterious. Fever, anorexia, swelling, hyperesthesia, uveitis, arthritis, meningitis, and glomerulitis are potential complications of adjuvant used. Examples and properties of adjuvants used clinically and experimentally are listed in Table 100-7.

Adjuvants are basically of two types: vehicles and immunomodulating compounds. *Vehicles* can be composed of metallic salts, microparticles, copolymers, polysaccharides, oils, liposomes, emulsions, saponins, and immunostimulating complexes (ISCOMs). The type of adjuvant selected for a particular vaccine depends on the route of administration, the type of infectious agent, and the host being vaccinated.[535] Adjuvants for mucosal vaccines must withstand harsh environments and facilitate an IgA response. Liposomes and other lipid moieties such as ISCOMS or microparticles and nanoparticles are used to coat antigens at the same time they facilitate an immune response. For a further discussion of liposomes and ISCOMs, see the discussion under Immunotherapy in Chapter 2.

Vehicles maintain antigen at a specific site and intensify the body's reaction to the antigen. Purified subunit or recombinant products are poorly immunogenic without inclusion of an adjuvant. Emulsified water-in-oil (Freund's incomplete adjuvant) and mineral gels or metallic salt adjuvants such as aluminum hydroxide, aluminum phosphate, gold salts, and alum have been used.

Aluminum-based adjuvants are frequently associated with granulomatous reactions at vaccination sites. These reactions have been linked with sarcoma development in cats (see Postvaccinal Complications). The amount of aluminum can vary from 350 ppm for some FeLV vaccines to 800 ppm for some rabies products.[354] Highest levels are contained in rabies vaccines having a 3-year DOI. One-year vaccines have approximately one half as much adjuvant, and some 3-year vaccines are sold under separate labels as 1-year products. To reduce the amount of adjuvant load, 3-year intervals of vaccination are recommended where legally approved.

Immunomodulators, which are usually composed of mammalian proteins or microbial components, include substances such as muramyl dipeptides, copolymers, and saponins, which stimulate local secretion of cytokines. They may enhance CMI, provide for slowed antigen degradation and release, and stimulate the function of the mononuclear phagocyte system to produce IL-1. This cytokine stimulates T cells to release IL-2, which, in turn, potentiates cellular defense mechanisms. Some cytokines have been given directly in an attempt to boost the immune response (see discussion of cytokines under Immunotherapy in Chapter 2).

Saponins are plant-derived extracts that are glycosides with hydrophobic moieties. Quil A (Spikoside® Isotec AB, Luleå, Sweden) has been given alone and in combination with aluminum hydroxide in a variety of veterinary vaccines. Quil A stimulates both humoral immunity and CMI by enhancing recognition of both soluble and membrane-bound antigens. Quil A is also a component of ISCOMs. Combination of a modified live feline viral rhinotracheitis-calicivirus-panleukopenia (FVRCP) vaccine with an inactivated FeLV vaccine increased the serologic response in kittens compared with those given the MLV FVRCP vaccine alone.[208] Presumably, adjuvants in the FeLV vaccine were responsible.

Adjuvants have also been evaluated in stimulating protective immunity at mucosal surfaces.[334] Adjuvants such as cholera toxin β-subunits, muramyl dipeptides, saponins, and phorbol esters have been used. Combinations of antigens with these substances produce specific S-IgA responses.

Using modified bacterial toxins to deliver vaccine antigens allows for more specific stimulation of protective cytotoxic T-lymphocyte responses.[519] The inherent ability of these toxins to bind and enter host cells makes them excellent candidates for this purpose. For safety, the toxin's enzymatic activity must be inactivated before use. Besides cholera toxin, others from virulent bacteria such as *Bordetella pertussis*, *Pseudomonas*, *Bacillus anthracis*, and *Listeria monocytogenes* have been used.

One disadvantage of adjuvants is that they may evoke local tissue reactions, granulomas, or abscess formations at the site of injection. Systemic manifestations of polyarthritis, uveitis, and autoimmune reactions have been documented in vaccinated people. Another concern is the potential development of vaccine-associated injection-site sarcomas (see Postvaccinal Complications).

Antiidiotypic antibodies are immunoglobulins produced against antigen-combining sites on specific immunoglobulins directed against the infectious agent. The antiidiotypic antibody actually resembles the antigen itself and stimulates T cells in a manner similar to that of a vaccine. Although veterinary vaccines of this type are only in experimental stages, antiidiotypic vaccines have the advantages of being produced by genetic manipulation and are safe because they lack the risk of the infectious agents contaminating attenuated vaccines.

Alternative Routes

New immunization strategies have been developed that make the deliver of vaccines possible without the use of needles or syringes. Originally developed for DNA vaccination, transder-

Table • 100-7

Comparison of Vaccine Adjuvants[a]

ADJUVANT	COMPOSITION AND EXAMPLES	ADVANTAGES /EFFECTS	IMMUNE EFFECT	DISADVANTGES AND COMPLICATIONS
Metal salts	Aluminum hydroxide, gold salts	Safety	Stimulate Th2	Granulomas and potential neoplasia?
Oil emulsions	Oil-in-water and water-in-oil emulsions with surfactant	Strong response, can prolong antigen exposure	Humoral response	More granuloma and injection site inflammation
Liposomes	Vesicles of cholesterol and phospholipids	Safe	Humoral response and stimulate CTL	Weaker response without co-administered immunomodulators
Microparticles	Particles of biodegradable polymers such as cyanoacrylates	Long-term antigen release with dissolution	Humoral and CMI response, can use for topical administration	Microencapsulation may alter antigen properties
Saponins	Chemical extracts of the tree *Quillaia saponaria* (e.g., Quil A)	Relatively safe, currently used in many veterinary vaccines	Strong Th1, Th2, and CTL responses	Hemolysis with inadvertent IV administration
ISCOMs	Lipid moieties containing saponins, cholesterol and phospholipids	Relatively safe, used in a few veterinary vaccines, many preclinical trials	Strong Th1, Th2, and CTL responses	Toxic only at high doses
Copolymers	Nonionic hydrophobic petroleum-based polymers	Relatively safe	Humoral and some CTL responses	Local reactions since not biodegradable
Polysaccharides	High molecular-weight dextrans	Nonirritating locally	Block phagocytosis and slow antigen degradation	Systemic hypersensitivity reaction with repeated use
Proteins	Diphtheria or tetanus toxoid, bovine serum albumin, KLH	Relatively safe	Improve antigen recognition	Systemic hypersensitivity reaction with repeated use
Bacterial products	*Propionibacterium* spp., muramyl dipeptide, cholera toxins, LPS components, *Bacillus anthracis* toxin	Potent immunostimulants	Strong humoral and CRL responses	Can induce more severe sensitivity reactions
Cytokines	IFN-γ, IL-1, IL-2, GM-CSF, IL-12	Can direct specific immune response	Response depends on cytokine used	Often species specific in composition and effects; may promote autoimmune or hypersensitivity reactions
Complement derivatives	C3d fragment	Can direct specific immune response	Response depends on fragment used	Theoretical but unproven humoral hypersensitivity or autoimmunity

CTL, Cytotoxic lymphocytes; CMI, cell-mediated immunity; Th1, helper lymphocyte-1 (CMI); Th2, helper lymphocyte-2 (humoral); IV, intravenous; ISCOMs, immunostimulating complexes; KLH, keyhole limpet hemocyanin; LPS, lipopolysaccharide, IFN, interferon; IL, interleukin; GM-CSF, granulocyte-macrophage colony-stimulating factor.
[a]Adapted from information presented in Spickler AR, Roth JA. 2003. Adjuvants in veterinary vaccines: modes of action and adverse effects, J Vet Intern Med 17:273-281.

mal administration is achieved by using devices that generate high-pressure aerosols and inoculate the vaccine solution with minimal pain or apparent injury at the site of inoculation.[5] Lower vaccine volumes can be used with this technique. Transdermal needle-free inoculation is commercially available for animal vaccination, specifically FeLV vaccination in cats[207] (see Appendix 3), and is likely to expand as newer products are licensed.

Mucosal application is used for a large number of commercial immunogens. S-IgA, produced by mucosal-associated lymphoid tissue, is effective in local protection against mucosal infection or penetration by infectious agents. Commercially available vaccines for respiratory infections in dogs and cats and feline coronaviral (FCoV) disease in cats make use of this locally protective immune response. IN vaccines are commercially available, depending on the product. Alternate mucosal delivery methods are also being considered to reduce side effects of parenteral inoculation, stimulate local immunity, and increase effectiveness. Orally administered vaccines using microencapsulation or chimeric plant viruses are in development. The chimeric plant–virus vaccines are made by recombinant technology, and immunogenic protein genes are inserted into plant viruses that are often administered in food plants or grains by enteral routes (see previous discussion, Live Agent Recombinant Vector Vaccines).

When mucosal response to vaccine is evaluated, S-IgA should be used instead of serum IgA levels. Some secreted IgA does enter the blood following an immune response to a surface antigen exposure, and this adds to the total increase in blood IgA that is measured. Because of the ease of measuring serum IgA, vaccine manufacturers have often used this method as a means of determining protection; however, this method can be misleading.

Microencapsulation involves placing antigens into hydrogels or microspheres to protect orally administered antigens from gastrointestinal (GI) degradation. This approach sustains the antigenic stimulation and allows them to be exposed to the intestinal lymphoid tissues. Biodegradable microspheres are inert synthetic polymers (e.g., poly-D, L-lactide-co-glycolide) used to coat antigen and are similar to those used in absorbable suture material. Lipid microcarriers have been used to increase the immune response to topically applied vaccines. The type and size of the coating determine the duration of the antigenic stimulus. The primary and secondary waves of antigen release can be modified with coatings to simulate repeated vaccination after single-dose administration. Microspheres also have a potential usefulness in oral vaccines in that they protect against antigen degradation by gastric acid, allowing the antigens to reach intestinal lymphoid tissues in Peyer's patches. IP administration of adjuvanted vaccines may also have a regional effect on stimulating local intestinal lymphoid tissues.

Dermal vaccination involves administering vaccines in sprays and patches on the skin surface. Topical immunization has the potential to make vaccine delivery safer, with fewer reactions and better compliance.[439] The skin-associated lymphoid tissue include keratinocytes, Langerhans cells, and T lymphocytes within local nodes. Keratinocytes establish the physical barrier while producing a variety of cytokines when they are exposed to antigens. Langerhans cells, located at the basal layer of the epidermis, capture and process antigens. They migrate via efferent lymphatics to paracortical T-cell areas of draining nodes and present these to naïve T cells. Antigens applied onto bare skin penetrate the continuous stratum corneum via intracellular or intercellular routes. The skin barrier can be made more permeable by hydration. Topical administration of cholera toxin (CHT) onto hydrated skin can confer protection against lethal mucosal toxin challenge in animals.[195]

In addition to skin, the mucosal application of CHT or heat-labile enterotoxin, from gram-negative bacteria with other antigens, acts as an adjuvant. Adjuvants used to stimulate mucosal immunity (such as IL-1 or CHT) can induce both helper lymphocyte-1 (Th1) and helper lymphocyte-2 (Th2) immune responses, with mucosal delivery resulting in a predominant Th2 response. Vitamin D_3 precursor, 1α-dihydroxy D_3, is a strong mucosal adjuvant that directs trafficking of dendritic cells in mucosae and causes a predominant S-IgA response. With or without adjuvant, IN vaccination gives better IgA levels than do IM injections. A significant number of vaccines that incorporate these antigens are under development. Because the skin and mucosae of various animals are physiochemically different, current research involves finding efficient delivery systems that will allow consistent antigen delivery.[216]

CONTROVERSIES CONCERNING ANNUAL VACCINATION AND INDIVIDUALIZED PROTOCOLS

Despite their tremendous benefit, vaccines are not always innocuous. The practitioner must weigh the potential for adverse consequences and financial limitations with the potential risk of infection against the inherent protection provided by individual products.[466,533] Vaccine-induced illness has become a more significant concern given that its prevalence, although low, supercedes that of the diseases for which the vaccines are intended. Certain breeds and families of dogs have a higher prevalence of postvaccinal reactions (see Postvaccinal Complications, later). With routine standard protocols, some animals will be vaccinated too frequently or for diseases for which they have no risk or for which vaccines are of questionable benefit. There are other animals for which the risk of infection is so great that more frequent or earlier vaccination, or both, is needed. Use of multivalent vaccines is convenient and cost effective; however, at times, it may limit customization of vaccine schedules for animals when exceptions are needed.

Recent protocols and recommendations from veterinary organizations in North America and Europe have indicated that vaccination intervals of animals over 1 year of age should be increased beyond the annual basis.* The consensus of these groups asserts that no one schedule is optimal for all animals. Because of increased awareness of vaccine reactions, vaccination schedules must be individualized for each patient. Yearly boosters can no longer be recommended for all animals. Annual clinical examinations rather than vaccination should be emphasized for pets. A summary of these recommendations can be found in Tables 100-8 and 100-9.

Overvaccination

With current vaccines, a series of at least three injections for kittens and puppies, ending at 12 and 16 weeks, respectively, can be recommended. One year later, a booster can be given, but subsequent boosters can be given triennially.

Annual vaccination of dogs and cats is a convenient but arbitrary circumstance. However, concerns have been raised that annual vaccination of dogs and cats may be too frequent. In a survey of private practice veterinarians and their clients in the United States, more than 96% of veterinarians recommended annual vaccination for distemper, hepatitis and parainfluenza, and parvovirus infections.[407] Clients of these same veterinarians recognized that their dogs were receiving rabies (86%), distemper (84%), and parvovirus (84%) vacci-

*References: 123, 148, 184, 295, 480.

Table • 100-8

Recommended Booster Vaccination for Dogs Based on Lifestyle and Habits[a]

CANINE CLASSIFICATION	HABITS	FREQUENCY, BOOSTER TYPE
Kennel-group housing	In large animal holding facility such as a boarding or breeding kennel, humane society, laboratory research colony, or animal control housing	Annual: CDV, ICH, CPV, L, CPiV, Bd Optional: CHV, Bab, Gia, CCV, Lyme Triennial: R[b]
Outdoor enthusiast	Most of the time outdoors running unrestrained; unsupervised roaming and supervised or unsupervised hunting or fieldwork	Annual: CDV, ICH, CPV, L, CPiV, Bd, CCV,[c] Lyme[c] Triennial: R[b]
Outdoor socialite	Some of time outdoors; may contact other strange dogs on a periodic basis	Annual: L, CPiV, Bd,[c] R[b] Optional: CCV,[c] Lyme[c] Triennial: CDV, ICH, CPV, R[b]
Indoor socialite	Multiple-dog household, mostly indoors or confined but frequent contact with other known dogs through feeding, elimination, boarding, showing	Annual: L, CPiV, Bd, CCV[c] Triennial: CDV, ICH, CPV, R[b] None: Lyme
Indoor elitist	One- or two-dog household. Indoors mostly, but comes into contact with unknown dogs by occasional escapist activities	Triennial: CDV, ICH, CPV, R[b] Optional: L, CPiV, Bd[c] None: Lyme, CCV
Indoor pampered pooch	Strictly indoor, never comes into contact with other dogs; sits in the lap for hours at a time; rarely touches bare earth, a real couch potato	Triennial: CDV, ICH, CPV, R[b] None: L, CPiV, Bd, CCV, Lyme

CDV, Canine distemper; *ICH*, infectious canine hepatitis (canine adenovirus-2); *CPV*, canine parvovirus infection; *L*, leptospirosis; *CPiV*, canine parainfluenza virus infection; *Bd*, *Bordetella bronchiseptica* infection (bordetellosis [canine infections tracheobronchitis]); *R*, rabies; *CCV*, canine coronavirus infection; *Bab*, babesiosis; *Gia*, giardiasis; *CHV*, canine herpesvirus infection; *Lyme*, *Borrelia burgdorferi* infection (Lyme borreliosis).
[a]An annual booster is given the first year after the primary immunization series of all puppies. Use these guidelines for subsequent boosters. These guidelines could vary based on the animal's source, breed, age, reproductive status, geographic location, boarding and travel, recreational or work use, disease prevalence or past diseases, or particular vaccine efficacy or complications. As an alternative to triennial vaccination, antigens can be separated with some being given each year.
[b]Recommendations will be superseded by local public health laws. Rabies booster can be annual or triennial based on vaccine labeling.
[c]Use of this vaccine also depends on prevalence in a given region.

nations. Fewer realized that antigens for hepatitis (58%), parainfluenza infection (55%), and leptospirosis (53%) were included. Veterinary opinion, not public pressure, is responsible for the antigenic content and frequency of vaccines given to pets. Recommendations for annual revaccination boosters were established in the late 1960s as an educated guess by experts in the field.[254] The assumption was that annual vaccination would not hurt and would provide a means for a periodic preventative medicine program for animals.[502] In general, the trend has been to combine all vaccine antigens within a single product.

With some viral infections, such as those caused by CDV, CPV-2, CAV-2 in dogs, and FPV and FCV in cats, serum antibody lasts for years without revaccination or exposure to virulent virus. Although such sustained response was initially attributed to MLV vaccination, it has been observed with some killed vaccines such as those for FPV. Specific-pathogen–free (SPF) research kittens that were vaccinated at 8 and 12 weeks of age had persistent antibody titers and were completely protected against FPV challenge 7.5 years later.[514]

Protection against disease was not complete in that serum antibody titers declined beginning 3 to 4 years after vaccination, and clinical illness following FHV-1 and FCV challenge was 52% and 63%, respectively, less severe in vaccinated as compared with control cats. In another study,[312] SPF cats were challenged between 9 and 36 months after vaccination, with one of three IN or parenteral commercially available vaccines containing FHV-1, FCV, and FPV. Following challenge, all vaccinated cats were protected against virulent FPV that caused illness in all the control cats. Protection against clinical illness in FHV-1 and FCV challenge was partial as in the previous study. Similar extended DOI challenge studies have been published on components in multivalent canine vaccines.[1,192] (See Duration and Degree of Immunity, later.) Antigens for CDV, CPV, and CAV$_2$ stimulate strong immune protection and dogs have been immune to challenge infection, which caused clinical illness in controls, after a 3-year interval.

Parvovirus diarrheal epidemics beginning in the late 1970s and breakthrough of protection from this infection with conventional products helped instill more frequent and extended

Table • **100-9**

Recommended Booster Vaccination for Cats Based on Lifestyle and Habits[a]

FELINE CLASSIFICATION	HABITS	FREQUENCY, BOOSTER TYPE
Cattery-group housing	In a multiple-cat, high-density environment, cats in direct contact and sharing litter boxes; stray or feral cats are being admitted on a periodic basis	Annual: FHV, FCV, FPV, R[b], FeLV Optional: Gia, Bd, Chlam, FIP, FIV[d] Triennial: R[b]
Outdoor enthusiast	Most of the time outdoors; frequent contact with strange cats; multiple-cat open household, with new stray or feral cats being admitted	Annual: FHV, FCV, FPV Chlam,[a] R,[b] FeLV,[c] FIP[d], Optional: *Gia*, Bd, FIP, FIV Triennial: R[b]
Outdoor socialite	Some of time outdoors; may contact other strange cats; fewer than three other cats in household	Annual: FHV, FCV, FPV, R,[b] FeLV Optional: Chlam[c,d] FIP[c,d]
Indoor socialite	Multiple-cat household, mostly indoors or confined but frequent contact with other known disease-free cats when feeding, eliminating, boarding, showing	Optional: Chlam,[d] FeLV,[c,d] FIP[c,d] Triennial: FHV, FCV, FPV, R[b]
Indoor elitist	One- or two-cat household; indoors mostly, comes into contact with unknown cats by occasional escapist activities	Optional: R[b], FeLV,[c,d] FIP[c,d] Triennial: FHV, FCV, FPV, R[b]
Indoor window watcher	Strictly indoor, never comes into contact with other cats; sits at the window for hours at a time	Triennial: FHV, FCV, FPV, R[b] None: Chlam, R,[b] FeLV, FIP, Bd, Gia

FHV, Feline herpesvirus (feline rhinotracheitis virus [FRV]) infection; *FCV*, feline calicivirus infection; *FPV*, feline panleukopenia virus infection; *Chlam*, chlamydiosis; *R*, rabies; *FeLV*, feline leukemia virus infection; *FIP*, feline infectious peritonitis; *Bd*, *Bordetella bronchiseptica* infection (bordetellosis); *Gia*, giardiasis.

[a]Annual booster is given the first year after the primary immunization of all kittens. Use these guidelines for subsequent boosters. These guidelines can vary based on the animal's source, breed, age, reproductive status, geographic location, boarding or hunting and travel, disease prevalence or past diseases, and particular vaccine efficacy or complications. FeLV- and FIV-infected cats should only receive noninfectious vaccines. As an alternative to triennial vaccination, antigens can be separated with some being given each year.

[b]Recommendations will be superseded by local public health laws. Rabies booster is given annually or triennially based on vaccine labeling.

[c]Disease prevalence or serotesting, or both, will determine need for routine use.

[d]Annual vaccination recommended for this optional product.

vaccination protocols for pups and yearly boosters for adult dogs. Vaccination programs for cats changed in the 1980s as rabies outbreaks necessitated more widespread vaccination. The rabies vaccines changed to noninfectious adjuvanted products because of vaccine-induced disease that occurred with MLV products (see Vaccination, in Rabies, Chapter 22). In addition, a variety of noninfectious FeLV vaccines were introduced. These adjuvanted products have been suspected to be responsible for the increased prevalence of injection-site feline sarcomas (see later discussion). Despite documented adverse reactions to vaccines, the development of sarcomas in cats brought the concern regarding postvaccinal reactions and the questionable need for annual vaccination to the forefront.

On the side of the argument for annual vaccination, pets may be more stressed and exposed to unsanitary conditions in their natural environment than animals in the research laboratories where challenge studies are performed. Dogs and cats may come into direct contact with other animals. Protection elicited by one product may not be used to predict the immune response generated by another brand of vaccine containing the same antigens. Furthermore, serotesting pets each year to determine whether boosters are needed rather than administering them may be impractical, expensive, and inaccurate (see Vaccine Efficacy, later). Annual or periodic vacci-

nation allows for regular clinical examinations for detection and prevention of incipient illnesses. Up to 52% of dogs and cats brought to veterinary clinics for vaccination were found to have intercurrent disease, a factor that increased with advancing age.[34] Older dogs and cats have a noticeable decline in their immunity after 10 years of age.

Based on DOI studies on vaccine antigens, a compromise would be to extend booster immunizations every 3 years in adult animals for recommended (core) vaccines in dogs such as distemper, parvovirus enteritis, infectious hepatitis, and rabies and in cats for panleukopenia, viral respiratory infections, and rabies. Optional (noncore) vaccines in cats, which incidentally have shorter DOI intervals, are for feline leukemia, giardiasis *Chlamydophila* infection, and feline infectious peritonitis (FIP). In dogs, these noncore products are for Lyme borreliosis, giardiasis, and coronavirus and upper respiratory tract infections. If veterinarians elect to use revaccination intervals other than those indicated on the label, they should base their recommendations on the individual needs of the patient and sound immunologic principles.[254] In the future, labeling of vaccines may indicate the specifics of challenge studies rather than a recommended 1-year booster interval. Recommended guidelines for vaccination boosters for dogs and cats with various backgrounds are summarized in Tables 100-8 and 100-9, respectively.

Overvaccination has also been questioned in the vaccination of neonates. The onset and frequency of vaccination and number of vaccine antigens have intensified as a result of disease outbreaks and the licensing of multivalent vaccines. In general, vaccines should not be given to animals under 6 weeks of age, and for some diseases, the animals should be older. MDA breakthrough at younger ages would likely occur only if the animal was colostrum deprived, or if IN vaccination was used. The immune system of pups and kittens is compromised during the first 2 weeks of life because of hypothermia. MLV vaccines, especially those for parvoviruses, have the potential for damaging tissues with rapidly replicating cells during this developmental period. Once vaccination is initiated, by at least 6 weeks of age, the subsequent interval of vaccination in this primary series should never be more frequent than every 2 weeks, with a 3- or 4-week interval being more desirable. The 2-week interval must be considered when the prevalence of disease in the animal's environment is high. For noninfectious vaccines, with the exception of those for rabies, at least two vaccines must be given, even in the absence of MDA. Many components of combination vaccines are not required during the initial vaccination series. When their need is justified, optional components (e.g., for respiratory diseases, leptospirosis, borreliosis, feline leukemia, coronaviral infection) should be given later in the series. This application will help maximize the immune response and reduce the chance that allergic reactions will develop in animals when susceptibility to severe consequences is greater.

Vaccine Efficacy

Immunity after vaccination takes several days to develop, but it may last for years. After first-time or primary exposure to an antigen, the initial protection is usually provided by interferon (IFN) and later by an immunoglobulin response. The primary response is slower in onset than a secondary or an anamnestic response and initially is predominantly composed of IgM. A secondary response that follows reexposure to the antigen is characterized primarily by IgG.

Fortunately, veterinary vaccines, unlike their human counterparts, can be more extensively tested in the species for which they will be used, and appropriate challenge tests can be performed. The efficacy of a vaccine is determined by subsequently exposing vaccinated and unvaccinated animals to the same challenge dose and by measuring the incidence and severity of clinical disease that follows. Both humoral and CMI responses are important in protection from infection. Vaccines have an important role in stimulating both mechanisms. Unfortunately, humoral immune responses have often been measured after vaccination and thus equated with protection of an animal from infection. Some animals may actually be protected even in the absence of a serologic response. The significance of an absolute antibody titer is meaningful only when standardized serologic procedures are used and when this absolute titer is related to titers of protected animals following challenge infections. The correlation between antibody titers and protection from disease is good for self-limiting systemic infections such as with CDV, CPV, and FPV (Tables 100-10 and 100-11). Absolute titers may vary among laboratories and methodologies, making interlaboratory comparisons difficult.[205,532,570] For FHV, FCV, and FPV, serologic titers have been correlated with resistance to challenge.[312,514] In contrast, protection against many respiratory and GI mucosal surface infections is based on secretory rather than serum immune responses. Protection against persistent intracellular infections is more dependent on effective CMI. Challenge of the animal with a virulent agent is therefore a more reliable measure of vaccine efficacy. Cellular memory of past exposure to an antigen may persist long after serum antibody titers decline.

The development of tissue culture of viruses has greatly improved both the quality and the means of manufacturing veterinary vaccines. Commercial production, licensing, and marketing of biologics is rigidly controlled by the U.S. Department of Agriculture (USDA), the Ministry of Agriculture in the United Kingdom, the Bureau of Animal Health in Australia, the Department of Agriculture in Canada, and similar bureaus in other countries. Current testing guidelines include DOI, potency, and safety studies. Vaccines are evaluated for safety as demonstrated by tests for sterility, toxicity, and adventitious agents. Efficacy of products marketed in the United States is subsequently confirmed by challenge studies. The USDA has published procedures for evaluating efficacy of protection for many of the licensed veterinary vaccines (http://www.aphis/usda/gov/vs/cvb). Vaccine manufacturers are not required to test their products against those of competitors or evaluate them for interactions when their products are used in conjunction with those of other companies. Furthermore, they are not required to show challenge protection against infections produced by heterologous strains of the infectious agent under consideration. Generally, use of a vaccine from one manufacturer followed by boostering with another vaccine antigen is considered to be anamnestic. However, it should not be presumed that vaccines produced by different manufacturers, for the same antigen, are of equal efficacy. It cannot be assumed that the level and DOI will be identical for all brands. Differing strains are of especial concern for canine leptospirosis and borreliosis, and feline calicivirus, FeLV, and FIV infections.

After vaccines are studied in the laboratory on experimental animals, they are subjected to field testing by a limited number of practicing veterinarians before they are released for general usage. Many products had been initially marketed without complete knowledge of DOI or adverse side effects. Manufacturers are receptive to reports of complications encountered by practicing veterinarians and, in turn, keep the veterinary profession informed of continuing efficacy studies and potential complications (see Postvaccinal Complications, later). For a listing of available vaccines and manufacturers in the United States, see Appendix 3.

Duration and Degree of Immunity

DOI is important in determining the timing for booster vaccinations. With the exception of rabies vaccines, DOI of many marketed vaccines sold in the United States is not available because most challenge studies were performed 2 to 4 weeks after the last vaccination in a series. Manufacturers in the United States were under no legal obligation to demonstrate longer DOI for already-licensed antigens. In other countries, such as in Europe, vaccine licensing requires proof of DOI. Presently in the United States, USDA guidelines now require actual DOI challenge studies for vaccines containing "novel" antigens for which no other products are available such as *Borrelia* or FIV. Animals are held in isolation for the labeled period and are subsequently challenged or tested for serum antibody titers. Findings of longer-term studies must be comparable to challenge studies obtained a few weeks after vaccination. Although the minimum DOI must be determined, manufacturers are not obligated to establish the maximum duration. Table 100-12,*A* and 12,*B* summarizes the studied DOI for many vaccines used in dogs and cats.

The DOI or efficacy of a vaccine to withstand challenge infection is expressed in terms of *preventable fraction*, which accounts for the proportion of vaccinated animals that do not develop a disease after challenge compared with those unvaccinated animals that do develop the disease. The number represents the fraction of animals that were truly protected by the vaccine. The formula is calculated as follows:

Table • 100-10

Comparison of Canine Infections Prevented by Vaccination

CANINE DISEASE	TYPE INFECTION	PERSISTENCE	ORGANISM DETECTION METHODS[a]	PREFERRED ANTIBODY DIAGNOSIS	ANTIBODY MEASURES PROTECTION
Distemper	Self-limiting	CNS, retina	Direct FA: blood, conjunctival smear PCR: serum, urine, CSF	IgM-single; IgG fourfold change	Yes, VN preferred standard; Indirect FA and ELISA also used
Adenovirus-1 infection	Self-limiting	Occasionally liver	Direct FA: liver, kidney Cytology: intranuclear inclusions	IgM-single; IgG fourfold change	Yes, VN standard
Parvovirus infection	Self-limiting	None	ELISA: stool PCR: stool Direct FA: intestine	IgM-single; IgG fourfold change; Indirect FA preferred	Yes, HI standard; VN, ELISA also used
Leptospirosis	Self-limiting	Kidney, liver	Direct FA: tissues Immunoperoxidase: kidney	Agglutinin: single tentative Agglutinin: change best	Yes, neutralizing best Agglutination: short lived, low
Borreliosis	Self-limiting	Connective tissues	Direct FA: tissues PCR: tissues	C6 protein ELISA	OspA by immunoblot is best
Babesiosis	Persistent	Erythrocytes	PCR: whole blood Direct FA or cytology: smears	IgG: past exposure or active infection; ambiguous	No protection
Bordetellosis	Mucosal	Airway commensal	Direct FA: secretions or tissues	None	S-IgA, hard to quantify
Coronavirus infection	Mucosal	Intestinal mucosae	Direct FA: intestine	None	S-IgA, hard to quantify
Parainfluenza virus infection	Mucosal	Airway commensal	Direct FA: secretions or tissues	None	S-IgA, hard to quantify
Adenovirus-2 infection	Mucosal	Respiratory tract	Direct FA: airway secretions	None	S-IgA, hard to quantify
Herpesvirus-1 infection	Mucosal	Trigeminal and other neurons	Direct FA: mucosae during active infections	None	S-IgA, hard to quantify, virus latency
Giardiasis	Mucosal	Duodenum	Direct FA or immunoassay: stool	None	S-IgA, hard to quantify
Rabies	Persistent		Direct FA: CNS tissue	None	Yes, RFFIT, FAVN, neither infallible

CNS, Central nervous system; FA, fluorescent antibody; PCR, polymerase chain reaction; CSF, cerebrospinal fluid; VN, virus neutralization; ELISA, enzyme-linked immunosorbent assay; HI, hemagglutination inhibition; OspA, outer surface protein A; S-IgA, secretory IgA; RFFIT, rapid fluorescent focus inhibition test; FAVN, fluorescent antibody virus neutralization.
[a]Other than by isolation of the organism.

Table • 100-11

Comparison of Feline Infections Prevented by Vaccination

FELINE DISEASE	TYPE	PERSISTENCE	PREFERRED ANTIBODY DIAGNOSIS	ANTIBODY MEASURES PROTECTION
Panleukopenia	Self-limiting	None	IgM-single IgG-rise	Yes, VN preferred
Feline leukemia virus infection	Persistent intracellular	Lymphoid, myeloid	None, antigen used	Yes, VN standard; not available
Feline immunodeficiency virus infection	Persistent intracellular	Lymphoid	Yes-ELISA	No
Feline enteric coronavirus infection	Mucosal	None, occasional gut shedders	None	S-IgA
Feline infectious peritonitis	Persistent intracellular	Phagocytes	IgG-indirect FA	No
Feline calicivirus infection	Mucosal, generally	Airway commensal	None	S-IgA
Feline herpesvirus infection	Mucosal	Airway commensal	None	S-IgA
Bordetellosis	Mucosal	Airway commensal	None	S-IgA
Chlamydophila infection	Mucosal	Airway commensal	None	S-IgA
Rabies	Persistent		None	Yes, but not infallible

VN, Virus neutralization; ELISA, enzyme-linked immunosorbent assay; FA, fluorescent antibody; S-IgA, secretory IgA.

$$\frac{\text{Prevalence (\%) of disease in nonvaccinates} - \text{Prevalence (\%) in vaccinates}}{\text{Prevalence (\%) in nonvaccinates}}$$

Serologic Testing and Challenge Studies to Determine Efficacy or Duration of Vaccination Responses

The concern about overvaccination has renewed interest in the use of antibody measurements instead of annual vaccination. Testing an animal's serum antibody titer has been proposed as a measure of protection against infections; however, such interpretations have limitations. Serologic responses are monitored in some instances for extended periods, but, unfortunately, serum antibody titers do not represent an absolute measure of protection in all types of infectious diseases. Additionally, it cannot be assumed that an animal with low serum antibody titer is unprotected or that animals with high serum antibody titers are protected. Therefore serologic monitoring must be done with discretion.

The type of antibody measurement is important in determining whether an animal is susceptible to infection. For example, serum neutralization (SN) and hemagglutination inhibition (HI) titers correlate with resistance to parvovirus infection. ELISA kits have been developed to detect antibodies against infectious agents. However, discrepancies can be found between measured antibody titers and protection because ELISAs are generally more sensitive and may detect other classes of antibodies.[312] Only ELISAs that have been correlated with challenge studies should be used. Furthermore, failure to detect serum antibodies does not necessarily indicate that animals are not protected, especially if adult cats have been previously vaccinated.[312] However, to err on the side of caution, overvaccinating animals with low or no measurable antibody titers is not considered a problem. Serologic testing should never be used to determine the level of pro-

tection of immunosuppressed animals or neonates with MDAs.

The type of infection produced by an agent is important in determining whether antibody titers will correlate with protection. Organisms that spread extracellularly in body fluids during the course of infection are most susceptible to the effects of circulating antibodies. In these infections, adequate antibody titers can provide sterile immunity. When immunity is sterile, it provides complete protection against infection. In such instances, challenge with a virulent or attenuated infectious agent results in no replication of the organism and no change in the serologic titer. Serum antibody titer measurements may provide valuable insight into the degree of protection for extracellular spreading systemic infections such as with canine and feline parvovirus infections and infectious canine hepatitis (ICH) and canine distemper.*

The absolute values of titers for protection against these diseases vary depending on the laboratory and method used. Antibody titers of sufficient magnitude indicate presence of an immune response and correlate with sterile immunity against infection. Cut-off titers are determined by correlating challenge protection studies or low prevalence of infection with measured antibody titers in the population studied. The absolute value of cut-off titers for protection will vary depending on the laboratory and method used. One problem is that not all laboratory assays have been validated. Practitioners should carefully evaluate whether the assays they are requesting have been correlated with reference laboratories that have measured challenge protection.

For mucosal infections such as bordetellosis, canine coronaviral enteritis, and FCV and FHV-1 infections, S-IgA concentrations are more important than are serum antibody titers. For persistent intracellular infections, such as FIV and FeLV infections and FIP, CMI is critical. Antibody titers are best

*References: 312, 374, 504, 565, 575.

Table • 100-12A

Summary of Longer Term (>8 Weeks) Duration of Immunity Challenge Studies in Dogs

ANTIGEN: VACCINE[a,b]	AGE OF VACCINATES	POSTVACCINATION CHALLENGE		NUMBER OF INFECTED ANIMALS		PREVENTABLE FRACTION (%)
		INTERVAL	ROUTE	VACCINATES (%)	CONTROLS (%)	
Canine Distemper Virus						
Duramune Adult; United States only[192]	6-8; 9-11 wks	3 yrs	Intracranial	0/10 (0)	3/3 (100)	100
Galaxy DA2PPvL +Cv[1]	7-8, 10-11 wks	57 mos	IN, IV	1/10 (90)	9/9 (100)	90
Canine Adenovirus						
Duramune Adult; United States only[192]	6-8; 9-11 wks	3 yrs	IV	0/12 (0)	2/2 (100)	100
Galaxy DA2PPvL + Cv[1] (CAV-1)	7-8, 10-11 wks	56 mos	IV	0/10 (100)	8/8 (100)	100
Canine Parvovirus						
Duramune Adult; Unites States only[192]	6-8; 9-11 wks	3 yrs	ON	0/10 (0)[f]	2/2 (100)	100
Galaxy DA2PPvL + Cv[1]	7-8, 10-11 wks	55 mos	ON	0/10 (100)	9/9 (100)	100
MLV[74]	2-16 mos	24 mos	ON	0/5 (100)	5/5 (100)	100
	14 mos	12 mos	ON	0/7 (100)	5/5 (100)	100
Vovax®—killed[583]	NA	13 mos	Oral	0/3 (0)	3/3 (100)	100
Experimental—killed[465]	8-12; 10-14 wks	≥12 mos	Oral	2/10 (20)	4/4 (100)	80
***Leptospira* spp.**						
Eurican/Lepto Dog[569a]	NA	44 wks	Subconjunctival and IP	B: 10/10 (100) U: 2/10 (20) K: 0/10 (0)	B: 9/9 (100) U: 7/8 (88) K: 5/8 (63)	B: 0 U: 77 K: 63
Vanguard[10]	9, 12 wks	19 wks	Subconjunctival and IP	B and U: 1/6 (17)	B and U: 6/6 (100)	83
Dohyvac[10]	9, 12 wks	19 wks	Subconjunctival and IP	B and U: 2/4 (50)	B and U: 6/6 (100)	50
Nobivac[10]	9, 12 wks	19 wks	Subconjunctival and IP	B and U: 0/6 (0)	B and U: 6/6 (100)	100
Nobivac[293] (*L. canicola*)	9, 13 mos	27 wks	Subconjunctival and IP	B: 3/6 (50) U: 0/6 (0)	B: 6/6 (100) U: 6/6 (100)	B: 60 U: 100
		56 wks	Subconjunctival and IP	B: 6/6 (100) U: 1/7 (17)	B: 6/6 (100) U: 6/6 (100)	B: 0 U: 83
Nobivac[293] (*L. icterohemorrhagiae*)	9, 13 wks	27 wks	Subconjunctival and IP	B: 2/6 (33) U: 0/6 (0)	B: 6/6 (100) U: 2/6 (33)	B: 67 U: 100
		56 wks	Subconjunctival and IP	B: 2/6 (33) U: 0/6 (0)	B: 5/6 (83) U: 0/6 (0)	B: 60 U: 0
Borrelia burgdorferi						
Lymevax[87]	<18 mos	156 days	IP, SC, ID	2/10 (10)	9/14 (64)	84
Experimental subunit[87]	12, 16 wks	3 mos	Tick feeding	2/10 (20)	10/10 (100)	80

DA2PPvL+Cv, Distemper-adenovirus-parvovirus-parainfluenza-leptospira-coronavirus; *IN*, intranasal; *IV*, intravenous; *CAV-1*, canine adenovirus type 1; *ON*, oronasal; *MLV*, modified live virus; *IP*, intraperitoneally; *B*, blood culture; *U*, urine culture; *K*, kidney culture; *NA*, not available.
[a]See Appendix 3, Canine and Feline Biologics Manufacturers and Products Available Wordwide, for information on vaccines listed below.
[b]Numbers in this column refer to reference numbers cited at the end of this chapter or on the CD.

Table • 100-12*B*

Summary of Longer Term (>8 Weeks) Duration of Immunity Challenge Studies in Cats

ANTIGEN: VACCINE[a,b]	AGE OF VACCINATES	POSTVACCINATION CHALLENGE		NUMBER OF INFECTED ANIMALS		PREVENT-ABLE FRACTION (%)
		INTERVAL	ROUTE	VACCINATES (%)	CONTROLS (%)	
Feline Panleukopenia Virus						
Eclipse[313]	12-16; 16-20; 14-15 mos	30 mos	IP	0/12 (0)	4/4 (100)	100
Fel-O-Vax[514]	8; 12 wks	7.5 yrs	ON	2/9 (22)	6/8 (75)	71[c]
Heska Intranasal[313]	NA	9 mos	IP	0/14 (0)	10/10 (100)	100
Feline Herpesvirus						
Fel-O-Vax[514]	8; 12 wks	7.5 yrs	ON	?/9	8/8 (100)	52[d]
Feline Calicivirus						
Fel-O-Vax[514]	8; 12 wks	7.5 yrs	ON	?/9	7/7 (100)	63[d]
Feline Leukemia Virus						
Leukocell 2[218]	9-11; 12-14 wks	12 mos	ON	4/18 (20)	9/5 (60)	63
Eurofel FeLV[462]	Monovalent: 7-8; 10-12 wks	12 mos	ON	3/16 (19)	8/12 (82)	77
	Polyvalent: 7-9; 10-12 wks	12 mos	ON	2/10 (20)	8/12 (82)	76
Chlamydophila felis						
ML Psittacoid[300]	18-24 wks	12 mos	ON	5/20 (25)	10/10 (100)	75
		6 mos	ON	2/19 (11)	6/6 (100)	89
Fel-O-Vax[588]	9-11 wks	12 mos	ON	3/10 (30)	6/7 (86)	65
Feline Coronavirus[e]						
Intranasal MLV[158]	<12 mos (given 2 IN doses)	12-19 mos	Field exposure	13/300 (4)	18/309 (6)	33

IP, Intraperitoneally; *ON,* oronasal; *MLV,* modified live virus.
[a]See Appendix 3 for information on vaccines listed below.
[b]Numbers in this column refer to references cited at the end of this chapter on the CD.
[c]Based on viral shedding following challenge given that clinical signs were minimal in challenged cats.
[d]Based on calculation of clinical scores as calculated by the author of this study.
[e]For feline infectious anemia.

used to document these infections rather than as a measure of protection. These intracellular organisms can replicate in cells regardless of the concentration of extracellular antibodies. Serum antibody measurements have no relevance with respect to protection against these infections. However, cell-mediated immune responsiveness is difficult to measure objectively in a clinical setting.

Dogs

HI titers for CPV and SN titers for CDV were measured in 122 dogs ranging from age 1 to 13 years that were vaccinated between 271 and 1665 days prior.[374] These two assays are generally considered the gold standard of antibody measurement for the respective diseases. Twenty-five percent of the dogs had a less than protective CDV titer, and 27% had a less than protective CPV titer, showing that a majority of dogs are protected, even with a delay in annual revaccination. In another study, sera from 1441 dogs in the United States, ranging from 6 weeks to 17 years of age, were tested for indirect fluorescent antibodies (FA) to CPV and CDV.[575] In this study, positive

seroreactivity was correlated with protective HI and SN titers performed by a reference laboratory. The results indicated a high prevalence of antibody response to CDV (96.6%) and CPV (95.1%). Of the 468 dogs for which vaccine histories were available, the interval between testing and prior vaccination was 1 to 2 years for 281 dogs, 2 to 7 years for 142 dogs, and less than 1 year for 45 dogs. Dogs 2 years age or older were evaluated for their antibody titers to CDV, CPV, CAV-1, CAV-2, and canine parainfluenza virus (CPiV) before and after vaccination, with a delay of up to and beyond 48 months since a previous vaccination with the same vaccine used previously.[397] The percentage of dogs that had titers at or greater than the threshold values for being protected or that responded to revaccination with a greater than or equal to fourfold increase in antibody titer was 98.1% for CDV, 98.1% for CPV, 98.4% for CAV-1, 99% for CAV-2, and 100% for CPiV. Serum antibody titers to CDV, CPV, and CAV were measured in dogs from the south of England that had not been vaccinated for a range of 3 to 15 years.[48] Protective titers were found in 95% to CPV, 71% to CDV, and 82% to CAV. The high prevalence of titers to CPV was presumably caused by natural exposure in the environment. In a majority of dogs, a significant increase in antibody titers after booster vaccination with the three MLV antigens was not found, which suggests that the dogs were protected from infection with the MLV vaccines despite the variable delay in vaccine boosters. This finding is important because studies determining whether dogs or cats develop a greater than or equal to fourfold increase in antibody titer following vaccination show that the antibody titer had decreased sufficiently to allow the immune response to occur. Even though the antibody response had waned, life-long memory cell immunity is still present in these animals, and they will respond more rapidly than will the naïve animal. Unfortunately, the antibody blockade also explains why it is difficult to produce hyperimmune sera in dogs against infections in which antibody is protective, such as canine and feline parvoviral infection and canine distemper.

An MLV combination CDV, CPV, CAV-2, and CPiV vaccine was evaluated for DOI protection in pups given two vaccines at 7 to 8 and 10 to 11 weeks of age, with challenge 55 to 57 months after initial vaccination.[1] All vaccinates were protected against clinical disease following parvovirus and CAV-1 experimental challenge, and 90% were protected against CDV infection. None of the control animals were protected. This result would suggest at least a 4-year DOI for these core fractions of the vaccine. Similarly, a 3-year DOI challenge study has been conducted for a vaccine containing MLV combination distemper, adenovirus-2, and parvovirus-2.[192,315] Dogs were vaccinated at 6 weeks of age or less and 3 weeks later. Groups of dogs were challenged independently for each antigen 3 years later (intracerebrally for CDV and oronasally [ON] for CAV-1 and CPV-2). All vaccinates were protected against infection with CDV and CPV-2 while all controls were ill. In the CAV-1 challenge, only 25% of vaccinates showed mild illness while all of the controls were severely affected.

Cats

Information correlating serum antibody titers with protection against challenge infection is available for FPV, FHV-1, and FCV infections. With FPV, serum antibody titers measured by virus neutralization (VN) or ELISA can be used to measure resistance to infection. SPF laboratory kittens, vaccinated with inactivated products, were protected against challenge 7 years after the initial series.[514] Measured titers following vaccination, which have been correlated to challenge studies, have been used to predict protection.[312,514] In a serologic evaluation, cats 2 years of age or older were tested for antibody titers to FPV, FCV, and FHV before and after MLV vaccination with the respective antigens.[398] There had been a delay of up to 48 months or more since the last vaccination. The percentages of cats with titers at or above the threshold values, or responded to revaccination with an equal to or greater than fourfold increase in titer were 96.7% for FPV, 97.8% for FCV, and 88.2% for FHV. Notably, vaccine protection for FHV-1 and FCV is not complete; instead, it lessens the severity of infection on subsequent challenge.

A 12-month DOI study was conducted for FeLV vaccine in which kittens were vaccinated at 9 and 12 weeks of age.[218] The preventable fraction after challenge was 63%. Although VN antibodies were not increased following FeLV vaccination, they were increased following challenge with virulent virus in cats that were protected from infection. Other animals that did not develop VN antibodies after challenge became persistently viremic.

Rabies

Evidence for long-term immunity following rabies vaccination is based on challenge compared with serologic data. SN titers of 0.5 IU/ml have correlated with protection against challenge with virulent rabies virus in dogs and cats. This level is currently the cut-off titer for protection, as designated by the World Organization for Animal Health, Office of International Epizootics (see Chapter 22 and Table 99-3). The rapid fluorescent-focus inhibition test (RFFIT), a modified VN method, and the fluorescent antibody virus neutralization (FAVN) methods have supplanted the standard SN test as a measure of protection following rabies vaccination. See Appendix 5 for a list of some laboratories that perform these assays. Generally, many countries require a rabies immunization at least 3 to 6 months before importation with a minimum acceptable antibody titer and implantation with an identifying microchip. The required interval between vaccination and titer measurement varies among countries. A protective titer is a minimum of 0.5 IU/ml for the RFFIT or FAVN, and this value corresponds to a protective level determined with the SN titer. If the titer is insufficient, then a booster dose of vaccine with a followup titer is indicated. In the United Kingdom, the guidelines for importing pets involve the Pet Travel Scheme (PETS). A physical description of the animal and its vaccination history are available along with submitted serum. In a group of 1002 serum samples, 48 failed the blood test for importation, and all of these failures had received only their primary vaccination.[66] Subsequent analysis of failing animals at two laboratories showed that the failure rate for dogs was 4.12% and 5.16% and for cats was 2.85% and 2.67%. Significant differences in response rates were noted between the vaccine brand, between one or two doses of vaccine (dogs only), and between 4 to 5 weeks after vaccination. In cats, neutered animals had less risk of failing the serologic response. This finding suggests that animals that fail the criteria should be revaccinated with another product and the sampling be performed between 4 to 5 weeks after vaccination, should these criteria be suitable for the importing country. For cats, neutering may be of benefit if it is not of concern to the owner.

PETS was introduced as an alternative to quarantine for dogs entering the United Kingdom from rabies-free countries. Although quarantine was effective, animal welfare concerns were that isolation of animals was detrimental to the well being of pets and their owners. However, in addition to preventing rabies, the quarantine procedures have detected a large number of exotic diseases that might have entered the country unchecked.[359] For further information, see Quarantine to Reduce Spread of Exotic Infections, Chapter 94.

Effect of Age on Immune and Vaccine Responses

Dogs' and cats' immune systems are fully mature by 6 months of age. Therefore a booster vaccination is recommended after 1 year has lapsed from the primary immunization given during the early postnatal period. With some systemic extracellular spreading organisms, in which antibody is protective, such as CPV, CDV, and FPV infections, one vaccination may produce long-term immunity lasting many years and perhaps for the life of the animal.

Decline in the immune response to vaccination with advancing age may be a concern for the timing and frequency of inoculation of older dogs and cats. Aging is a multifactorial process, involving genetic control and a gradual decline of the immune, neuroendocrine, musculoskeletal, cardiac, and renal systems. In tissues, oxidative changes in cells and nucleic acids are responsible for many of these changes, and antioxidant nutrients may be beneficial in slowing this decline.[491]

Compared with mice and humans, relatively little is known about the effect of age on the immune system of dogs. Concentrations of IgA have been shown to be increased in serum and saliva of aged dogs.[188] No difference in the concentration of serum IgG was found between young and aged German shepherd dogs.[548] Older Labrador retrievers have decreased lymphocyte stimulation to mitogens and increased percentages in total T cells but a decreased percentage of CD4+ cells.[199,222] In dogs of various breeds, 32 young (3.15 ± 0.8 years) and 33 old dogs (12.1 ± 1.3 years) were vaccinated against distemper, parvovirus, and rabies.[241] No differences in postvaccination titers against any of the viruses between old and young dogs were noted. Whether such titers would persist after a 3-year vaccine interval is uncertain.

Few studies have been conducted concerning the aging of cats and their immune responses. Cats are considered young adults between 2 and 5 years of age, old adults at 7 to 8 years of age, and geriatric after 10 to 12 years of age. Geriatric cats had higher serum IgA and IgM but lower leukocyte counts and lower absolute values of T cells, B cells, and natural killer cells compared with young adult cats.[69] In geriatric cats, prevention of obesity by chronic restriction of caloric intake is correlated with a slowing of the aging process. However, within 4 days, acute nutrient deprivation in cats causes a reduction in lymphocyte stimulation, lymphocyte numbers, and lowered CD4+/CD8+ ratios.[172] Following reinstitution of feeding, older cats (over 8 years) took three times longer to return to previous values as compared with young felines. Monocyte-cell function, as expressed by phagocytic activity and major histocompatibility complex (MHC) class II expression, was reduced in old versus young clinically healthy cats during short-term nutrient deprivation.[522] Vaccine studies were conducted in a group of 28 aged cats that were fed a diet with or without enrichment (omega-6 or omega-3 fatty acids). Cats with the supplement had an enhanced T-cell response to a bacterial immunomodulatory drug but had a diminished CMI response, as well as a reduced response to a viral-directed vaccine challenge.[491] This finding suggests that diet manipulations of fatty acids may alter the immune response of aged cats and potentially their vaccine responsiveness.

Combination Vaccines

Commercial production of combined vaccines has made vaccination protocols less expensive and more convenient for both the veterinary professionals and pet owners. Interference testing, required for licensing, helps assure the veterinarian that antigens in multivalent products will produce immunity equal to individual antigens administered separately without risk of complications. Separate vaccine products may result in exposure to more extraneous proteins and allergenic components than the same antigens in combination; however, using combined antigen products may contain more total adjuvants than using products with only the desired components. Chemicals or adjuvants intended for one product may interfere with the effectiveness of another. As a general guideline, to prevent potential allergic or neoplastic complications, as few inactivated antigens as needed should be used during routine booster immunization. Veterinarians should administer these antigens as they believe necessary by profiling patients and giving the antigens as multivalent products when possible. The only disadvantage is that more than one multivalent combination vaccine may be needed in inventory.

Vaccination Failures

Vaccination does not equal immunization. Even with all factors taken into consideration, no vaccine stimulates an immune response in 100% of the population to which it is administered. Compared with the degree of severity of illness in unvaccinated animals, some licensed vaccines may reduce severity of clinical disease or the number of ill animals after challenge infection rather than provide complete protection. Even with vaccines that are highly protective, biologic variation is responsible for vaccine breaks in a low percentage of vaccinates. Protection of 70% of the population may be effective in reducing the prevalence of diseases when communicability is low, such as has occurred with rabies. However, vaccination is unacceptable in preventing rapidly transmitted diseases such as CPV enteritis. Depending on the disease, the acceptable efficacy of protection allowed for most vaccines is between 65% and 95%, meaning a certain percentage of animals will be unprotected in any vaccinated population. Unfortunately, from an individual animal standpoint, one vaccine break constitutes a failure.

Veterinarians are often blamed for animals developing disease after apparently adequate vaccinations. The animal was possibly incubating the disease before vaccination. Because of the high resistance of agents such as parvoviruses, acquisition of the infection can occur around the home environment. Puppies and kittens from animal shelters are often exposed to high levels of pathogens before vaccination. Other factors, however, are under direct control of the veterinarian. Many of these vaccine breaks may be caused by inattention to precautions that should have been taken during the vaccination procedure. Dogs and cats may contact high concentrations of pathogenic agents, such as parvoviruses, for the first time when they enter the veterinary hospital for vaccination. This exposure may occur in the hospital waiting room or ward area because of improper traffic flow or inadequate disinfection or isolation procedures for animals that are already infected. Vaccination of animals with existing mild illness or immunodeficiencies may not be contraindicated. In such situations, inactivated or other noninfectious products are recommended. For further information, see later discussion of Postvaccinal Complications and specific vaccine-induced illnesses, and see Chapter 95 concerning immunodeficiency disorders.

The many causes of vaccination failure in dogs and cats are summarized in Table 100-13. A few of the more pertinent features are discussed in this section. Not all vaccines will effectively immunize those patients to which they are given because of inherent host factors discussed previously, as well as difficulties with the vaccine or errors made in the process of administration. Vaccination in the presence of MDA is the most common cause of vaccine interference in young animals and has been discussed previously. Other potential causes are considered later in this text.

Care and handling of vaccines is important in the animal's immune response as inactivation of a live product negates the animal's immune response. Directions for proper storage and handling as indicated on the product label should be strictly followed. Directions given by the manufacturers for handling of vaccines should always be followed because of the labile and occasionally harmful nature of biologic products and the liability risk to the veterinarian. Refrigeration is essential for almost all biologics, and inadvertent freezing may damage many products and inactivate live agents. Sunlight is damaging to many vaccines because it inactivates many viruses and bacteria. Stock should always be rotated to ensure that vaccines are used before the expiration dates. If lyophilized products are used, vaccines should always be mixed with the diluents provided and administered soon after reconstitution.

Needle size and composition may be important in the immune response. For most vaccines in small animals, a 22-gauge, 1-inch needle is best. Theoretically, this size places the agent in the SC site with a minimal amount of leakage from the injected area. Vaccines marketed for individual use should never be mixed in the same syringe because of potential incompatibilities. In addition, injecting multiple vaccines at the same site in the animal is not advised. In one study, when individual vaccines were combined and given SC at one site, the antibody responses were inferior compared with the responses when antigens were given at separate sites.[108] For

Table • 100-13

Causes of Vaccination Failure

HOST FACTORS	VACCINE FACTORS	HUMAN ERROR
Immunodeficiencies	Rendered noninfectious during handling	Improper mixing of products
Maternal antibody interference	Improper storage	Exposed at time of vaccination visit
Age: very young or very old	Vaccines do not protect 100% of	Concurrent use of antimicrobials or
Pregnancy	population (biologic variation)	immunosuppressive drugs
Stress, concurrent illness	Disinfectant used on needles and syringes	Simultaneous use of antisera
Pyrexia, hypothermia	Wrong strain	Too frequent administration (<2-week
Incubating disease at time of	Excessive attenuation	interval)
vaccination	Overwhelming exposure	Disinfection of skin (uncertain)
Cytotoxic drugs or glucocorticoids		Wrong route of administration
Anesthesia (uncertain)		Delay between vaccines in initial series
Hormonal fluctuations		Omit booster vaccination
General debilitation, malnutrition		Concurrent surgery or anesthesia
Overwhelming exposure		

this reason, only licensed combination products, which have been screened for compatibility, should be administered, and different products should never be mixed. The potency of attenuated products requires that they replicate, and inadvertent inactivation will reduce their effectiveness.

Aseptic methods should always be used in rehydrating vaccines, complete doses should be used, and unused opened diluents should be discarded. Most vaccines have adequate particle numbers to overcome possible reductions in antigen mass or organism numbers that occur during handling and storage.

Serial numbers of vaccines and sites of vaccination should be entered in medical records to assist in tracking vaccine breaks or vaccine-induced illnesses. Used bottles or those containing expired biologics should be considered a biohazard and should always be disposed in a safe manner.

Splitting doses of vaccine is *never* advised. Some veterinarians split doses for smaller animals to reduce proportionally the amount of extraneous proteins that might cause allergic reactions (see discussion of type I immunologic complications, Postvaccinal Complications). Reducing antigen levels voids implicit warranties of the manufacturer and shifts the liability to the veterinarian should a break in protection occur. The only recognized reduction in vaccine dose that has been recommended is in the IN vaccination of neonatal kittens for upper respiratory tract disease. In this instance, a few drops are administered in the nostrils of each kitten rather than giving an entire dose.

Cytotoxic agents or glucocorticoids may be associated with a decreased response to vaccination, depending on the dose and duration of treatment. When glucocorticoids are given long term, alternate-day therapy is less likely to cause immunosuppression. Although glucocorticoids are less likely to interfere with booster vaccinations, they are not recommended when the primary immune response to a particular antigen is being elicited. Moderate doses of prednisolone were administered to previously unvaccinated 13-week-old puppies for a 3-week period before vaccination for CDV.[404] Doses of 1 or 10 mg/kg were given every 12 hours for the first week, once daily for the second week, followed by alternate-day therapy for the last week. The dogs were challenged with virulent virus 3 days after vaccination. Although in vitro lymphocyte stimulation testing showed a depressed response compared with that in control dogs, all vaccinated puppies receiving glucocorticoid therapy were immune to challenge.

Antibody responses to measles and CDV vaccination have also been studied in dogs that were more severely immunosuppressed with concurrent methotrexate and antithymocyte sera.[525] Dogs immunosuppressed before CDV vaccination developed vaccine-induced systemic illness and encephalitis and died. Dogs immunosuppressed after CDV vaccination and later challenged with virulent CDV resisted challenge, but they had no increase in neutralizing antibody titer.

Dexamethasone, at a daily dosage of 0.25 mg/kg (equivalent to 1.25 mg/kg prednisolone), was given to dogs before and after their first vaccination with rabies vaccine.[46] No difference was found in the serum antibody titer of treated dogs compared with untreated animals.

Tetracycline, alone or in combination with niacinamide, has been used as an effective treatment of some cases of immune-mediated skin disease in dogs. Treatment of dogs with this combination did not interfere with antibody responses following vaccination against canine distemper and parvovirus infection.[399]

Changes in *body temperature* may influence the immune response. Elevated rectal temperature, artificially induced by high environmental temperature and humidity, has been shown to inhibit the serologic response of 8- to 12-week-old puppies to canine distemper vaccination. Puppies with elevated rectal temperatures (39.8° C [103.6° F]) that were kept under these conditions developed clinical illness after subsequent challenge with virulent CDV, whereas those with lower rectal temperatures were protected.[589] The serologic response after vaccination for ICH was not affected by these conditions. Hypothermia is also known to decrease the measured in vitro CMI response of dogs, and probably cats, to vaccination.[507]

Anesthesia and surgery may have an indirect effect on concurrent vaccination. General anesthesia or surgery causes a suppression of the response in lymphocyte-stimulation testing, but the clinical significance of such results is probably minimal, and the serologic response is unaffected.[283] Vaccination before and after surgery had no effect on the humoral or CMI vaccine response to CDV or CPV-2 in dogs and did not predispose them to vaccine-induced illness.[390] However, vaccination while under anesthesia is not recommended in case a hypersensitivity reaction develops that may go undetected.

Inactivation of modified live vaccine is less commonly a cause of vaccine failure because of the current manufacture and lyophilization of vaccines, refrigerated storage, and use of heat-sterilized disposable syringes rather than chemically disinfected syringes. Vaccines should be injected into visibly clean skin sites. Topical disinfection of the injection site in animals is questionable inasmuch as the hair is not routinely clipped before this procedure. Should routine practices result in local contamination, this may interfere with the injection procedure. Little evidence has been found to show that topical disinfectants themselves will alter the viability of SC inoculated products.

Vaccine interference can occur whenever attenuated antigens are administered at too-frequent intervals. Administering several attenuated vaccines simultaneously is better than giving them 1 to 4 days apart because of the blocking effect that the first vaccine may have on the second. This interference may be related, in part, to the production of INF by infected cells. Whenever possible, modified live vaccines should not be administered in the presence of other infectious diseases for this reason. Postponement of vaccinations for at least 2 to 3 weeks after illness or before sequential vaccinations with the same or a different product has been shown to be sufficient to overcome this interference. Animals with preexisting fever, debilitation, or multisystemic illness should not be vaccinated because immunization may fail and vaccine-induced illness or further immunosuppression is possible. Some researchers have suggested that immunosuppression occurs with use of CPV-2 vaccine strains because they induce lymphopenia, lymphocyte depletion, and suppressed lymphocyte stimulation in response to mitogens, but these responses are likely just a reflection of the expected response to a live agent. In multivalent vaccines, product licensing requires that combined antigens produce the same degree of protection as when they are given separately. In some cases, especially in naïve animals, administering multiple antigens may interfere with the response to each antigen alone. For this reason, in addition to the potential for allergic reactions, the authors (CEG and RDS) do not recommend using *Leptospira* or inactivated coronaviral vaccines in pups younger than 9 weeks of age during their primary vaccination series.

Delayed completion of a primary vaccination series is another potential cause for vaccination failure. Many times, delayed completion is the result of poor client compliance or client relocation. Under such circumstances, a delay of longer than 2 to 3 months between vaccines or delayed presentation for the first visit, should be corrected by administering at least two injections, 2 to 3 weeks apart, even if animals are beyond the age of MDA interference. Should the brand or formulation (recombinant versus inactivated versus attenuated) of vaccine be significantly different, or should the vaccination status be unknown or uncertain, a similar protocol of two vaccinations should be followed. Multivalent combination products are recommended in older animals receiving their primary vaccination series. Whatever protocol is used, some veterinarians prefer to administer rabies vaccine on the last visit in the series to help ensure compliance.

In some circumstances, *the route of vaccination* is also critical in maximizing the immune response because MLV rabies, feline respiratory, and canine measles vaccines are more effective when given IM rather than SC. For MLV rabies vaccines, which have been discontinued in most countries, this discrepancy may be explained by the fact that vaccine virus replicates better in innervated muscle as opposed to less innervated subcutaneous tissue. For other products, the difference may be related to greater blood supply or better tissue environment. Unfortunately, IM, versus SC, vaccination is more painful and is associated with a higher risk of postvaccinal type I immunologic reactions (see Postvaccinal Complications, later).

LIABILITY RELATED TO VACCINATION

Since 1996, legal statues in the United States involving the USDA have freed vaccine manufacturers from liability regarding vaccine-induced complications, unless they are caused by improper manufacture of their vaccines. Veterinarians can no longer shift the liability of complications to the vaccine manufacturer. As a result, consumer claims regarding vaccines will be focused on veterinary malpractice or the failure of veterinarians to adhere to common standards. The question will be: did the veterinarian act in a manner comparable to what would be expected by a practitioner with equal experience and training? This is termed practicing according to a specific *standard of care*, and it applies to the decision concerning which vaccines to administer to each animal. Standard of care means what a practitioner of equal experience and training would deliver under similar circumstances. Only rabies vaccination is dictated by local public health laws. Several organizations have published recommendations regarding vaccine protocols for dogs and cats (Table 100-14). Although the standard for vaccination of dogs and cats is undergoing substantial reconsideration, the adoption of suggested guidelines by the veterinary community will have the greatest impact in determining the standard of care.

An important consideration with respect to future liability is the principle of *informed consent*. Veterinarians are expected to educate their clients concerning infectious disease risks for their pets, to inform clients of the risks and benefits of particular vaccines, and to handle and administer the products in accordance with the manufacturer's guidelines and commonly accepted standards of practice (Table 100-15). Veterinarians should obtain written informed consent from their clients. This consent means veterinarians should provide information to the client regarding the advantages, alternatives, and any risks of vaccines in lay terms. The final decision of the client is made to approve or disapprove of vaccination. The information can be provided as written guidelines for the practice that the client reads but should also be reinforced by commentary during the examination and vaccination process. Whether or not clients sign any statement that they were properly informed, the decision of the client and veterinarian regarding the pet's vaccination protocol should be recorded at the time of the visit. Spelling out the guidelines for future vaccination of the pet would seem appropriate at that time so that a plan can be followed with or without modification in the future. Given that no specific rules or guidelines exist, veterinarians are now subject to greater litigation than they were in the past. The medical record is an important tool to document the type of vaccinations given and information regarding the veterinarian's suggestions and owner's decisions. Information regarding vaccination needs should be altered on a yearly basis depending on the animal's individual health and environmental risks. At the time of each vaccination, the date, vaccine type, manufacturer, expiration date, and lot or serial number should be recorded. The site of administration should also be documented, and for cats, standard recommendations exist. Serologic results or prior adverse events should also be well documented. A signed consent form from a client that indicates awareness of discussed vaccine risks and suggested regimens is also judicious.

The manufacturers' responsibilities end with ensuring efficacy, purity, potency, and safety of their products. However, the number of animals that can be tested during preliminary trials is limited. Therefore safety is never absolute, and the veterinarian must consider balancing efficacy and the reduction of disease with the incidence of adverse events. Other than reporting of possibilities of anaphylactic reactions (see Type I hypersensitivity, later), vaccine labels have provided little

Table • 100-14

Contact Information for Veterinary Biologics and Adverse Event Reporting

PURPOSE	ORGANIZATIONS	CONTACT INFORMATION AND URL
Vaccine efficacy studies and adverse event reporting for the United States	U.S. Department of Agriculture (USDA), Animal Plant Health Inspection Service (APHIS), Center for Veterinary Biologics (CVB), Ames, Iowa	http://www.aphis/usda/gov/vs/cvb Phone: 800-752-6255
Data on diseases and vaccine challenge	Data on diseases and vaccine issues during the previous 2 years. Studies conducted at universities and efficacy data	http://www.ncbi.nlm.nih.gov/entrez/query.fcgi
Adverse event reporting for practitioners	United States Pharmacopeia (USP) Veterinary Reporting Program[a]	http://www.usp.org Phone 800-487-7776
Canine and feline vaccination guidelines	American Veterinary Medical Association (AVMA), including COBTA Report[295]	http://www.AVMA.org
Canine vaccination guidelines	American Animal Hospital Association (AAHA)[441]	http://www.aahanet.org Phone: 303-986-2800
Feline vaccination guidelines	American Association of Feline Practitioners (AAFP)[480]	http://www.aafponline.org Phone: 800-204-3514
Respective vaccine manufacturers	See Appendix 3	See Appendix 3

COBTA, Council on Biologic and Therapeutic Agents.
[a]This site is on limited funding and may no longer be supported in the future.
For further information on contact information for specific biologic manufacturers, see Appendix 3.

Table • 100-15

Standard of Care for Veterinarians with Respect to Vaccination

1. Did the animal need the vaccine?
   Consider: degree of contagion, severity of illness, permanence of immunity, waning antibody titer, prevalence of disease, outbreaks of illness, zoonotic risk.
2. Did the veterinarian select the proper antigen(s) for the patient?
   Consider: pet lifestyle and exposure risk, predisposing breed or immune factors, onset and duration of protection, potential side effects.
3. Was the proper product selected for the intended antigen?
   Consider: vaccine testing, challenge interval after vaccine and duration of immunity studies, field versus laboratory strain challenge, heterologous or homologous strain protection, academic institution opinions, age and breed of challenged animals, reported adverse reactions in field studies.
4. Was the vaccine given in a proper manner and location?
   Consider: use as prescribed by manufacturer, record site and route of administration, use aseptic means, justified interval of administration.
5. Was informed consent obtained from the client before vaccination?
   Consider: use of a permission form as documentation, education regarding disease particulars, not overstating vaccine safety, educating on risk of potential complications, educating on vaccine benefits and efficacy, outlining alternatives to vaccination, always having a written record of the consent.
6. Were adverse events monitored, documented, and reported?
   Consider: vaccinating earlier in the examination process to allow for adverse events before discharging the animal, reporting adverse events to manufacturer, to the U.S. Pharmacopeia or other reporting service, documenting any adverse reactions in the written record and taking precautions for avoiding them in the future.
7. Were mistakes made that increased the risk to the patient or liability of the veterinarian?
   Never doing the following: reducing a vaccine dose in an effort to minimize potential reactions, exaggerating claims relative to efficacy of a product, minimizing the potential for side effects of a particular vaccine, vaccinating for diseases for which a risk of infection cannot be justified, combining separate vaccine products before administration, vaccinating an animal that is clinically ill, vaccinating an animal with a known previous reaction without precautions.

information with regard to potential vaccine reactions. License requirements for newer products marketed in the United States have included listing of associated vaccine-related events. Because of differences in the timing of licensing, not all competitive products have the same level of safety information.

POSTVACCINAL COMPLICATIONS

The benefits of vaccination of dogs and cats for serious diseases outweigh the risk of complications. However, because the prevalence of these diseases has decreased through vaccination, the prevalence of vaccine reactions may supersede that of their use in disease prevention. Despite claims of many antivaccination advocates, epidemiologic analysis does not show a correlation between vaccination within the last 3 months and ill health in dogs.[138] In the United Kingdom, an Adverse Reaction Surveillance Scheme has been evaluating adverse vaccine reactions since 1985.[198] In the period from 1995 to 1998, a total of 3188 adverse reactions have been reported; however, of the 841 for which sufficient information was available (369 dog, 472 cat), only 64 (7%) reactions were deemed vaccine related, 149 (18%) possibly related, and 628 (73%) probably unrelated. Even if all 841 events were considered an annual occurrence, this is only 0.004% of the 6 to 8 million vaccines given in the United Kingdom annually. Although the prevalence of vaccine-induced reactions is low, some precautions may be in order for routine vaccination of animals with underlying disease or immune aberrations. Many immune-mediated and nonimmune complications are severe enough to restrict or eliminate the routine periodic use of particular vaccines in predisposed animals. Repeated annual revaccination of veterinary patients cannot always be justified with respect to all the components included in currently available combination products. Veterinarians should be aware of potential complications caused by each vaccine component so that particular antigens can be deleted from subsequent boosters if problems arise. They should consider educating clients, either verbally or in writing, of potential vaccine complications to facilitate early recognition and treatment. For vaccine guidelines and for reporting such reactions in the United States, see Table 100-14. For a summary of the immunologic and nonimmunologic complications described next, consult Table 100-16. For a summary of preventive measures to avoid vaccine-induced complications, see Table 100-17. For a list of manufacturers to report specific vaccine or drug reactions, see Appendix 3.

Immunologic Complications

Hypersensitivity reactions that are known to develop after vaccination in certain dogs and cats are types I, II, III, or IV hypersensitivities reactions, or any combination of these (see Table 100-16).

Type I

Type I reactions involve an interaction between cytophilic IgE and antigen, with resultant degranulation of circulating basophils and tissue mast cells releasing large amounts of heparin, chemotactants, prostaglandins, histamines, and biogenic amines into the systemic circulation. Anaphylaxis may occur after the use of any vaccine, although it is most commonly associated with the use of adjuvanted or multivalent products containing large amounts of foreign protein, such as inactivated rabies vaccine, canine coronavirus (CCoV) vaccine, FeLV vaccine, *Leptospira* bacterin, and parenteral *Bordetella* vaccine. Potentiated parvoviral products containing large amounts of antigen have also been incriminated. Foreign proteins, such as fetal bovine serum (FBS), used in cell cul-

ture, can cause type 1 hypersensitivity reactions. With the advent of inactivated and adjuvanted viral vaccines for rabies in cats and dogs, feline respiratory disease, FPV, and FeLV infections, an increasing prevalence of type I hypersensitivity reactions has been noted, especially in cats. Miniature dachshund pups and some of the other miniature breeds have a disproportionally high reaction rate. Ferrets have a similar tendency to develop this reaction, even when CDV or rabies vaccines are administered that are licensed for use in that species.[200]

In the dog, clinical signs include facial edema ("big head"), pruritus, hypotensive shock, weakness, dyspnea, and vomiting with or without diarrhea that can be hemorrhagic.[420] Local or systemic reactions may occur in young puppies within 1 to 24 hours after their second or third vaccination and may result in acute clinical signs described previously, as well as death. Puppies that survive such episodes should not be revaccinated with known allergenic components through the remainder of their initial vaccination series. For example, if the affected animals are allergic to leptospiral antigen, they should not be revaccinated with the leptospiral fraction until they are at least 16 weeks of age. At this time, the veterinarian should administer antihistamines as a precautionary measure before giving the vaccines. In addition, the patients should be hospitalized and monitored for 1 to 2 hours after the vaccine is given.

Cats show facial pruritus, hypersalivation, vomiting, diarrhea, dyspnea, collapse, and respiratory distress from acute pulmonary edema, usually within minutes to hours (under 24 hours) of vaccination. Diarrhea is usually watery but may become hemorrhagic if it is severe or persistent. Even with recovery, diarrhea may persist in some cats for several days thereafter. Respiratory distress, exhibited by dyspnea and cyanosis, is the most severe reaction. A majority of cats will respond favorably to 0.2 ml IV of 10-fold diluted epinephrine (1:10,000) and parenteral antiinflammatory doses of glucocorticoids, but those with severe progressive respiratory symptoms or hemoptysis usually die.

When anaphylaxis is a problem for an animal, the veterinarian is advised to (1) modify the vaccination schedule to reduce the number of antigens given simultaneously, (2) switch to MLV instead of inactivated adjuvanted products, and (3) use SC or IN (when available) rather than IM inoculations, which decrease the rate of uptake of the product into the systemic circulation. Syringe aspiration is essential before injecting any parenteral vaccine to determine whether a blood vessel has inadvertently been penetrated. Animals should be vaccinated early during the office visit to allow an adequate observation period. Clients should also be advised to keep their pets inside and under observation for at least 1 hour after arriving home following vaccination. Antihistamines (e.g., diphenhydramine, 1 mg/kg given SC or IM 15 minutes before vaccination) should always be given to these reactors before subsequent vaccinations, and vaccine antigens should be administered separately, when available, to allow identification of the problematic component. Measurement of antibody titers to certain infectious agents might determine whether and when revaccination is necessary (see Vaccine Efficacy, previously). Skin testing animals by ID inoculation of 0.1 ml of the suspected vaccine may also elicit a type 1 hypersensitivity to offending products. The site should be observed for at least 1 hour for development of urticaria (wheal), and saline and histamine controls should be used for comparison. Not all animals that develop a positive ID skin test result will have signs of hypersensitivity after vaccination. For example, many dogs develop an immediate hypersensitivity reaction to *Leptospira* antigen months or years after vaccination, but only a certain number of those dogs will develop a clinically relevant adverse reaction (anaphylaxis, facial edema, bloody diar-

Table • 100-16

Postvaccinal Complications Associated with Canine and Feline Biologics

TYPE OF PROBLEM	MECHANISM OF PRODUCTION	RESPONSIBLE VACCINES
Immunologic		
Type I	Immediate hypersensitivity; allergy, anaphylaxis	*Leptospira* bacterin; inactivated adjuvanted rabies, FeLV and respiratory vaccines
Type II	Cytotoxicity (hypersensitivity or autoimmunity):	
	Hemolytic anemia	MLV CPV vaccine
	Thrombocytopenia	MLV CDV vaccine
Type III	Immune complex (hypersensitivity):	
	Uveitis	MLV CAV-1 vaccine
	Generalized serum sickness	Passive immunization
Type IV	Cell-mediated (hypersensitivity or autoimmunity):	
	Granuloma	BCG immunotherapy
	Encephalitis	Nervous tissue-derived rabies vaccine
	Polyradiculoneuritis	Inactivated neonatal mouse brain rabies vaccine
Nonimmunologic		
Local reaction at injection site, cutaneous granulomas, or sarcomas (especially cats)	Adjuvants, preservatives, inactivators	Bacterins such as for *Bordetella* and *Leptospira;* inactivated adjuvanted viral vaccines such as for rabies and FeLV
Systemic fever and malaise	Local lymphoid replication of MLV products	Any MLV vaccine
Neurologic complications	Viral	MLV rabies and CDV vaccines
Abortion, infertility, congenital malformation	In utero or early neonatal infection	Any MLV vaccine during pregnancy Parvoviral vaccines during neonatal period
Clinical disease in vaccinates	Incomplete attenuation or local administration of attenuated vaccines	IN vaccines: Feline calicivirus, herpesvirus (IN or parenteral product); canine parainfluenza virus (mild) or canine *Bordetella* vaccine (mild)
	Feline limping	MLV caliciviral vaccine
	Polyarthritis in Akitas	Combined MLV or inactivated adjuvanted vaccines
	HOD and juvenile cellulitis	MLV CDV vaccine
Postvaccinal shedding	Virus localization	CPV-gastrointestinal, CAV-1 vaccine-renal, CAV-2 vaccine-respiratory
Postvaccinal encephalitis	Immunosuppressed animal or relatively unattenuated virus enters the nervous system when immune defenses are poor	CDV vaccine, measles vaccine, MLV rabies vaccine

CPV, Canine parvovirus; *CDV,* canine distemper virus; *CAV-1,* canine adenovirus-1 (hepatitis); *BCG,* bacille Calmette-Guérin; *CAV-2,* canine adenovirus-2 (respiratory); *MLV,* modified live virus; *HOD,* hypertrophic osteodystrophy; *FeLV,* feline leukemia; *IN,* intranasal.

rhea). Inbred atopic dogs have been shown to develop enhanced antipollen IgE responses when vaccinated with CDV, CAV-1, and *Leptospira* vaccines just before, but not after, exposure to pollen extracts.[173] In another study, vaccination of some dogs for rabies increased serum concentrations of total IgE and induced specific IgE for vaccine antigens, including those in tissue culture.[240] Aluminum adjuvant in the vaccine was suspected as the cause for the nonspecific increase. Despite the persistence of IgE in some dogs, none showed evidence of allergic disease after vaccination. However, because of this immunopotentiation, recommendations suggest that atopic dogs receive their booster vaccinations during nonallergic seasons or disease-free intervals.

Type II

Type II hypersensitivity, or autoimmunity resulting in cellular injury, has been suspected or reported after MLV vaccination in dogs. This reaction involves binding of antibody with or without complement with subsequent damage to host cells. Autoimmune hemolytic anemia (AIHA) and autoimmune nonregenerative anemias (autoimmunity to erythrocyte precursors) have been suspected to occur after MLV CPV vaccination in dogs. This phenomenon might also occur after natural infections but has rarely been reported. One-fourth of dogs studied with AIHA had been vaccinated with polyvalent products within 1 month of onset in one study.[134] The dogs with this association had lower platelet counts, increased trend

Table • 100-17

Contraindications to Routine Vaccination of Dogs and Cats

DISEASES OR CONDITION	VACCINES TO AVOID	RECOMMENDED ALTERATIONS
Genetic immunodeficiencies (see Chapter 95): Weimaraners and Akitas	MLV vaccines, especially Rockborn or Snyder Hill CDV	Inactivated or other noninfectious products. Onderstepoort or preferably recombinant CDV
Acquired immunodeficiencies (see Chapter 95): FIV, FeLV, cancer, chemotherapy, cytotoxic or myelosuppressive drugs[a]	Modified live vaccines	Inactivated or other noninfectious products
Immune-mediated diseases: uveitis, glomerulitis, polyarthritis, polyradiculoneuritis	Annual vaccination	Triennial rabies and minimize other antigens
Immune-mediated diseases: hemolytic anemia or thrombocytopenia	MLV parvoviral or combination vaccines	Triennial vaccination
Type I hypersensitivity vaccine reaction: dachshunds	Inactivated, adjuvanted vaccines, IM administration	Modified live vaccines (see text for additional precautions)
Mild or one-system disease, fever	Modified live vaccines	Control disease or use noninfectious vaccines
Pregnancy or lactation	Modified live vaccines	Inactivated or other noninfectious products
Vaccine-induced sarcoma	Inactivated, adjuvanted vaccines	Nonadjuvanted inactivated or noninfectious products, modified live vaccines, triennial vaccination
Chronic feline ulcerative gingivostomatitis and faucitis (see Chapter 89)	Inactivated adjuvanted calicivirus vaccine	Reduce vaccine booster frequency, or use modified live vaccines when necessary

MLV, Modified live virus; *CDV*, canine distemper virus; *FIV*, feline immunodeficiency virus; *FeLV*, feline leukemia virus; *IM*, intramuscular.
[a]Methotrexate, azathioprine, cyclophosphamide in dogs or cats; or extended use of chloramphenicol, sulfonamides, trimethoprim, dapsone, griseofulvin, or sulfadiazine in cats.

toward intravascular hemolysis and spontaneous microagglutination, and higher mortality compared with the other affected animals. The vaccine components may have induced autoantibody production or activated the immune system to destroy erythrocytes with preexisting surface autoantibodies. Other studies have not found this suspected association,[297] and although inciting controversy, the subject of vaccine-induced autoimmunity requires further study in dogs and cats.[435] Vaccines, as with certain drugs, infections, and other factors, are known to serve as triggers in development or exacerbation of autoimmune disease in genetically susceptible humans.[93] Killed products with bacterial antigens are most likely to serve as a nonspecific trigger because the immune enhancing effects of adjuvants and bacterial cell walls. Attenuated agents are thought to invoke the process through molecular mimicry in which "like antigens," those similar between antigens in the organism and host, cause immunologic cross-reactivity against certain host tissues.

Transient thrombocytopenia also was reported after MLV combination vaccines in dogs.[126,550] Thrombocytopenia, which developed in most vaccinated dogs, was mild (more than 100,000 and fewer than 200,000 platelets/μl) and subclinical. Despite transient thrombocytopenia, no change in platelet function was detected. Whether this form of thrombocytopenia is caused by autoimmune or infectious mechanisms is uncertain. Only animals with concurrent congenital or acquired bleeding tendencies may be expected to show hemorrhagic tendencies. Veterinarians may want to delay elective surgery on animals with known bleeding tendencies for a

2-week period after vaccination. Severe immune-mediated thrombocytopenia can also occur within 1 to 2 weeks after vaccination of some dogs. These animals have overt petechiae and hemorrhagic tendencies, with platelet counts less than 50,000/μl. Glucocorticoid therapy is usually required for several weeks thereafter to increase the platelet count, and subsequent boosters may have to be avoided or minimized to prevent a recurrence of the problem in affected dogs. Dogs with autoimmune disease disorders should probably have antibody titers evaluated in lieu of revaccination.

Type III

This hypersensitivity reaction, also known as serum sickness, is associated with immune complex formation and deposition and is responsible for the anterior uveitis that occurs in some dogs receiving the MLV CAV-1 vaccine and rarely with CAV-2 vaccines. This local type III, or Arthus, reaction results from virus-antibody complex formation within the eye (see Pathogenesis, Chapter 4). The process often resolves spontaneously unless secondary complications such as glaucoma develop.

Generalized serum sickness is the result of widespread immune complex deposition throughout the walls of the microvasculature of certain structures, such as the renal glomeruli, joints, and uveal tracts. Usually, this complication is seen only after the administration of large amounts of hyperimmune serum or globulin. Because passive immunization is used infrequently in dogs and cats, the prevalence of serum sickness is minimal, which has developed in a dog as a complication of *Propionibacterium acnes* immunotherapy (see Chapter 2).[329] Glomerulonephritis and amyloidosis can result from chronic or repeated antigenic exposure. One example would be vaccine-associated polyarthritis in Akitas (see Vaccine-Associated Disease in Young Akita Dogs, later). This finding is one reason why human beings are not given booster doses annually, as is the practice in veterinary medicine. Both amyloidosis and glomerulonephritis have been experimentally produced in animals after desensitization therapy protocols using repeated injections of large quantities of foreign antigen. Although concern exists, neither disease has been attributed to repeated administration of biologics in immunocompetent dogs or cats. See later discussion, and Chapter 95, for further discussion of vaccine-induced complications in immunodeficient dogs and cats.

Type IV

Cell-mediated, or type IV, hypersensitivity reactions can occur after BCG is used as an immunostimulatory compound (see Immunotherapy, Chapter 2). Large, exuding granulomas may develop at the site of injection. Historically, postvaccinal encephalitis was an allergic reaction that occurred after nervous tissue–derived rabies vaccinations were given.

Polyradiculoneuritis

Known as coonhound paralysis in dogs and Guillain-Barré syndrome in humans, polyradiculoneuritis is an immune-mediated inflammation of nerve roots that has been seen after a variety of vaccines were given to dogs and cats.[187,201,501] Coonhound paralysis is an immunologic disease caused by antigens in raccoon saliva that cross-react with the basic myelin protein of peripheral nerves to which dogs become exposed after direct contact with raccoons. As with other immune-mediated diseases, a genetic predisposition for coonhound paralysis exists. Although various vaccines can be incriminated, the highest frequency of polyradiculoneuritis has occurred after some lots of suckling mouse brain–derived inactivated rabies vaccines were used.[201] The central nervous system (CNS) of the newborn mouse, normally devoid of myelin, is well adapted to the production of large quantities of rabies virus needed to produce inactivated vaccine. Apparently, the nervous tissue of older mice was inadvertently used in production of the vaccine, or peripheral or cranial nerve myelin was accidentally included. This circumstance resulted in transient acute lower motor neuron (LMN) paralysis 1 to 2 weeks after vaccination in a proportion of dogs, similar to what is seen in experimental allergic neuritis.

Polyradiculoneuritis is similar whether it is caused by a vaccine or raccoon bite exposure. Rapid and progressive LMN weakness develops, usually beginning in the pelvic limbs and progressing forward. Pain sensation remains intact, and animals are hypersensitive to muscle palpation. Cranial motor nerve abnormalities such as facial paralysis may be observed. Occasionally, animals may have difficulties in swallowing and breathing or autonomic dysfunction that can lead to death.

The diagnosis of acute polyradiculoneuritis can be presumed based on marked diffuse muscle atrophy, preserved pain, and presence of hyperesthesia. When the equipment is available, electromyographic changes show fibrillation potentials characteristic of LMN denervation, and nerve conduction velocities are variably reduced, depending on the degree and location of myelin loss. Clinical improvement with demyelination alone begins within 2 weeks of onset of paralysis, and recovery to normal occurs in 1 to 2 more weeks. With axonal injury, recovery may be delayed for several months or may be incomplete. Subsequent exposure to the inciting cause may result in more severe and prolonged paralysis. Although glucocorticoid therapy has minimal effect on the course of this disease, one of the authors (CEG) has found that one dose of cyclophosphamide (50 mg/m²) given early in the course of illness may alleviate the severity of recurrent illness.

Local Reactions

Many complications have been associated with either local irritation or production of disease by canine and feline biologics. Local reactions after vaccination include pain, erythema, swelling, irritation, loss of hair, change of hair color, and abscess formation. Erythema, swelling, and irritation typically occur within 30 minutes to 1 to 2 weeks after inoculation. Onset of the other findings occurs within days to weeks. Pain can be caused by many components in the vaccine, such as stabilizers, high or low pH, high osmolality, adjuvants, or preservatives. Swelling is most frequently noted with the noninfectious products containing adjuvants or with the bacterial products owing to bacterial cell wall and foreign protein derived from the culture media. Parenteral *Bordetella*- and *Leptospira*-adjuvanted bacterins and adjuvanted-inactivated viral vaccines for rabies, FeLV, and feline respiratory diseases have most commonly been incriminated. Local reactions that enlarge or persist 2 to 3 months after vaccination should be evaluated by needle aspiration or biopsy, especially in cats because they may develop into injection site–associated sarcomas (ISS).

Contamination

Local and systemic inflammatory reactions have occurred from the inadvertent inclusion or growth of pyrogens in vaccines. Multidose vials contribute to this problem. *Pseudomonas*, other psychrophilic bacteria, and fungi can grow even during refrigerated storage. High amounts of endotoxin in early inactivated whole cell, parenteral *B. bronchiseptica* vaccines caused systemic manifestations in dogs, such as depression, shivering, tremors, and vomiting,[56] and produced local reactions and abscesses. Newer products with reduced levels of endotoxin have alleviated this complication as has the development and extensive use of modified live IN vaccines. Individual syringes and needles should be used for all vaccines given to dogs and cats. When insufficiently cleaned injection devices have been reused, inadvertent transmission of attenuated viruses has occurred.[356]

Adventitious Agents

Most viruses are grown in cell culture that must contain serum, which is almost always obtained from bovine fetuses. FBS has on several occasions been the source of contamination with viruses such as bovine viral diarrhea virus (BVDV), blue tongue virus, bovine parvovirus, and probably others. Vaccination of pregnant animals is not advised but is done under some circumstances. Blue tongue virus grew undetected in one killed commercial release of canine vaccine and caused abortions, cardiac failure, and respiratory distress in pregnant bitches vaccinated in the last trimester of gestation.[6,594] Necropsy findings were sanguineous pleural effusion, serous pericardial effusion, pulmonary congestion, splenomegaly, and enlarged mesenteric lymph nodes. Histologic features were multifocal vasculitis in parenchymal organs, interstitial pneumonia, multifocal myocardial edema, and myofiber degeneration.[156] No reported illness was found in nonpregnant dogs, and no lesions were present in the aborted pups.[58] The virus was isolated from maternal organs and from a repository of the incriminated lot of vaccine.

Mycoplasmas and mycoplasmal DNA detected by polymerase chain reaction (PCR) have been found in some commercial veterinary vaccines.[299] BVDV was found to contaminate an MLV multicomponent product, but no adverse reactions were reported from its presence. Parvoviruses, including bovine and porcine viruses, have been found as contaminants in vaccines.

Focal Cutaneous Granulomatous Reactions and Alopecia

Adjuvants used in noninfectious vaccines potentiate the immune response by creating a depot effect, which sequesters antigen and stimulates a sustained inflammatory reaction. Certain bacteria, especially gram-negative bacteria such as *B. bronchiseptica*, can serve as an adjuvant in multicomponent vaccines. As a result of certain adjuvants, firm dermal or subcutaneous nodules may form at sites where vaccines are given to dogs or cats.[225] These nodules typically regress after 2 to 6 weeks, but other vaccines such as certain FeLV and *Giardia* vaccines cause similar reactions. Such reactions have been more commonly reported after inactivated rabies vaccination of dogs and cats.[225] Vaccines may also produce visible hyperpigmented alopecic macules in the overlying dermis of breeds without undercoats, such as the poodle, Bichon Frisé, and Briard.[40] Nonadjuvanted products such as the recombinant canarypox rabies–vectored vaccine (Purevax®, Merial, Duluth, Ga.) do not cause this adverse reaction.

Histologically, the nodules created by adjuvanted rabies vaccine were characterized by a local nonsuppurative vasculitis with rabies antigen–specific fluorescence in the wall of the blood vessels. Central necrosis of tissue is surrounded by a granulomatous reaction with influx of macrophages and variable numbers of lymphocytes, plasma cells, and eosinophils. Lymphocytes are numerous, in many cases forming follicles. Globular gray-brown material within the necrotic zone and in macrophage cytoplasm represents residual vaccine adjuvant. Macrophages may transport this material to distant sites, perpetuating and disseminating the reaction. Dogs or cats exhibiting such reactions may be more likely to develop anaphylaxis on subsequent boosters should vaccine be inadvertently absorbed systemically at a rapid rate. Additionally, concern has been expressed that cats that are predisposed to inflammatory reactions may be more likely to develop vaccine associated ISS.[347]

Injection Site—Associated Sarcomas in Cats

ISS were reported initially in 1991; however, increased sarcomas at sites where vaccines are normally injected were observed at the mid to late 1980s following the introduction of killed aluminum-adjuvanted rabies and FeLV vaccines. These sarcomas have been presumed to originate at areas of persistent inflammation produced by these vaccines.[483a] Other sources of trauma in cats can also lead to sarcoma development.[130] Feline oncornavirus and papillomavirus infections do not appear to be involved in a cat's susceptibility.[143,286,288] However, sarcomas have been reported in cats following the use of other adjuvant-containing vaccines and other injectable products.[225] Injection of benzathine penicillin, parasiticides (lufenuron), or even reposital glucocorticoids or absorbable sutures have been associated with this reaction.* Deep-tissue sutures and penetrating injuries of the eye have resulted in sarcoma development in cats. Cats are the only species in which traumatic ocular sarcomas have been reported. The occurrence of ISS is not unique to the cat given that other species (e.g., dog, ferret, humans) had reportedly developed them at injection sites but at extremely lower frequency.[387,551]

The component thought to be associated with postvaccinal inflammation is the adjuvant.[346,352,354,508] However, anything that stimulates a strong inflammatory reaction might cause an ISS. The inflammatory reactions to deposited aluminum and other proprietary adjuvants cause tissue reactions. These reactions consist of proliferation of fibroblasts and myofibroblasts, as well as infiltration of lymphocytes and macrophages and other cells.[347] These cells, in turn, release multiple cytokines, growth factors, and other molecules,

which increase reactive oxygen species that, in genetically susceptible animals, may lead to transformation of certain cell types, resulting in a neoplastic disease. In addition to fibrosarcomas, cats have developed osteosarcomas, liposarcomas, rhabdomyosarcomas, chondrosarcomas, and malignant histiocytomas, among other neoplasms, at vaccination sites. Depending on the brand of vaccine used, in cats vaccinated with inactivated rabies vaccine, 80% to 100% develop local inflammatory reactions. Inflammatory reactions with the rabies vaccines were larger than that observed with FeLV vaccines. No local inflammation was evident at nonadjuvanted FeLV vaccine sites. Despite the common microscopic occurrence, the prevalence of these grossly visible and palpable swellings at 21 days postvaccination were reportedly as high as 11.8 out of 10,000 vaccine doses.[196] Some researchers believe that this inflammatory response is a prerequisite for sarcoma development, although this theory is controversial. These swellings usually subside within 3 months. Tumors usually arise between 3 months to 3.5 years after vaccination, with 1 year as a median time.

ISS likely result from hyperinflammatory responses in mesenchymal tissue at the site of inoculation. ISS can also originate at other sites, presumably as a result of migration of aluminum-containing macrophages. In such tumors, increased MHC class II and lymphocytes expressing CD11b and CD3 prevail.[80] Platelet-derived growth factor (PDGF) levels are increased in sarcomas. PDGF comes from macrophages and lymphocytes at the site of tissue injury and is a normal response to wound healing. In addition, in inflammatory tissues that become neoplastic, P53 (tumor-suppressor gene) is upregulated following DNA damage, resulting in tumor proliferation.[233] In cell culture, DNA damage is caused by all types of adjuvant-containing products but not with live feline respiratory vaccines.[381] Because of the DNA damage, and the difficulty of resecting malignant fibrosarcomas, once a tumor is removed, the chance of reoccurrence is 42%.

Compared with cats receiving adjuvanted-inactivated rabies vaccines,[345,508] reactions were less frequent or inconsistent after FeLV vaccination, especially with nonaluminum-adjuvanted and nonadjuvanted products. Nonadjuvanted rabies vaccines, especially the canarypox virus–vectored rabies product, produced little to no inflammatory changes when they were administered to rats,[347] cats, ferrets, and mink.[80] Postvaccinal inflammation occurs to the same degree whether the vaccine is given SC or IM; however, the location of the inflammation is in a deeper location with the latter route. Massaging a vaccine site changes only the shape, but not the volume, of the postvaccinal inflammation.[351] Sarcoma occurrence is not restricted to vaccines containing only aluminum salts adjuvants. Vaccines other than those for rabies or FeLV have also been incriminated[67] because anything that produces inflammation in the tissues of susceptible cats may result in development of ISS.

Although inflammation is common at most sites of adjuvanted-inactivated vaccine administration, ISS development is rare. A genetic susceptibility component among cats is suspected given that only a few cats develop sarcomas at sites of vaccination. Related cats have had more prevalent tumor development. Cytogenetic studies may provide more insight into this predisposition. Lymphocytes in ISS associated with vaccines are positive for PDGF and other proinflammatory cytokines.[226] The expression of C-jun, an oncogene coding for a protein (AP-1) that is associated with cellular oncogenesis in vitro in vaccine-associated ISS, is strong.[226] These sarcomas contain altered MAB reactivity to p53 nuclear protein, a critical regulator in the cell cycle.[80,233]

The estimated prevalence of occurrence in the United States based on biopsy submissions was 1 in 10,000 vaccinated cats, although it may be as high as 1 in 1000 vaccinated

*References: 64, 67, 153, 175, 196, 276, 330.

cats.* In an epidemiologic survey of practicing veterinarians, the estimated prevalence was 2.1 cases per 10,000 cat visits or 3.6 cases per 10,000 cats.[105] In the United Kingdom, where vaccination practices differ, where rabies and FeLV vaccines are less used, a range of incidence of 0.021 to 0.61 sarcomas for every 10,000 doses used was reported.[184,534] Repeated yearly boosters may increase the risk. Unnecessary vaccines or boosters are not advised. In a multicenter case-control study of ISS risk, no single vaccine brand or manufacturer within an antigen class was found to be associated with sarcoma formation.[276] Unfortunately, almost all vaccines administered to cats in this study contained an adjuvant or involved use of multi-dose vials; therefore the risk of these parameters could not be accurately determined. One important risk factor that was associated with sarcoma development was administration of cold vaccines.

Three methods for reducing the prevalence of sarcomas that involve the veterinarian, the owner, and the vaccine manufacturer have been suggested (Table 100-18). The site of sarcoma development has been most commonly in the interscapular area, presumably because this is a preferential location for veterinarians to inoculate cats. The interscapular area should be avoided because neoplasms in that location are difficult to remove, and drainage of inflammatory reactions is poor, resulting in sequestered adjuvants. Recommendations have been made to give vaccinations at specified sites to enable future tracking of reactions and at extremities where they can be more easily observed and removed. Rabies vaccine should be given SC in the Right rear leg as distal as possible on the extremity; feline Leukemia vaccine is given on the Left leg at a corresponding site. Other products are given on the trunk just on either side of midline. Despite the potential of sarcoma development, the public health benefits of continuing rabies vaccination outweighs any complication. However, the development of newer, safer rabies products will hopefully reduce the risk of ISS associated with vaccines. Restricting FeLV vaccination presents another acceptable alternative. Nonadjuvanted leukemia products can be used, animals not at risk should not be vaccinated, and animals at risk can be vaccinated twice as kittens, possibly again at 1 year of age, then *never* again without an increased risk of becoming persistently infected with FeLV. Noncore parenteral vaccines that are known to induce local granulomas should be given to cats only when it can be shown to be necessary and when it will provide a significant benefit.

Recommendations can also be made to monitor vaccination sites because early detection and removal of sarcomas offer the best chance for a cure (Table 100-19). After inoculation, the owner should monitor vaccine sites for a 12-week period. Most masses that develop within 3 weeks of vaccination are granulomas that will resolve in 1 to 2 months, although some will persist. Should the mass enlarge during the observation period, wide local excision should be performed. Removal of the early reactive granulomatous mass may reduce the overall immune response to the vaccine but more importantly will reduce the chance of sarcoma development. If the mass continues to enlarge past the 3-month period, progressive enlargement is probably related to a growing sarcoma. If this condition is suspected, the patient should be referred to a specialty practice for a needle or incisional wedge biopsy. Alternatively, only extremely wide and deep mass removal should be considered. Excisional biopsy (lumpectomy) alone after this period is rarely curative. Even wide surgical excision has often resulted in a 30% to 70% failure rate. Radical surgery combined with local irradiation has been advised.[94,291] Sarcomas are usually locally invasive;

*References: 155, 275, 330, 346, 373.

however, metastasis has been reported in up to 22% of cases.[154,234,489,494] Few cats receiving surgical therapy alone survive longer than 2 years. When the tumor is located on the limbs, the time to first recurrence was longer than that with tumors on the trunk. Although combined surgery and drug therapy, with or without radiation therapy, has been beneficial, many cats succumb despite this approach.[348] A review of the management of these tumors has been published.[373]

Systemic Illness

Systemic illness characterized by fever and malaise may also occur from self-limiting infection with modified live vaccine within local lymphoid tissues without systemic spread. This illness, which commonly does not last longer than 1 to 2 days after vaccination, often explains the transient anorexia and depression noted in recently vaccinated animals. Rarely are antiinflammatory drugs, antipyretics, or other supportive therapies indicated. MLV FPV vaccine resulted in severe clinical disease characterized by fever, diarrhea, and leukopenia in kittens infected 60 days before with FIV.[62] An IN trivalent vaccine containing MLV FPV was thought to cause viral enteritis in cats co-infected with *Salmonella*.[166] The vaccine has been reformulated; however, IN vaccination for FPV is not as effective as parenteral vaccination is against FPV and should not be relied on for primary vaccination. Thus parenteral FPV monovalent products should always be used in conjunction with IN FHV-1 and FCV vaccines, whether or not an IN vaccine contains MLV FPV.

Attenuated *Chlamydophila* products can cause systemic illness in a low number of cats within 1 to 3 weeks after vaccination. Clinical signs include fever (41° C [106° F]), lethargy, weakness, anorexia, and stiffness. Short-term therapy with glucocorticoids or analgesics may help alleviate these clinical signs.

Inadvertent parenteral inoculation of attenuated *B. bronchiseptica* and CPiV vaccine intended for IN use has caused localized pain and swelling, pyrexia, vomiting, mature leukocytosis, hypercholesterolemia, hypoalbuminemia, increased alkaline phosphatase and alanine aminotransferase activities, and hyperchloremia in an affected dog.[569] Diffuse hepatocellular necrosis was found with liver biopsy. In another case observed by one of the authors (CEG), the illness was fatal. Management of these local and systemic reactions and acute hepatic necrosis involves symptomatic therapy with daily application of warm compresses to the injection site, systemic antiinflammatory drugs as needed, and antibacterial drugs such as gentamicin, tetracycline, or trimethoprim-sulfonamide. Parenteral treatment with gentamicin, and SC fluids at the injection site, early in the course of illness is thought to be very important in management of this potentially fatal condition.

Neurologic Complications

Neurologic disease has been the most commonly documented postvaccinal reaction described in dogs and cats. This finding may be related to the overt nature of neurologic illness and to the decreased immunocompetence of the CNS against MLV agents. Rabies encephalomyelitis has been reported after vaccination with MLV vaccines. Most licensed rabies vaccines for dogs and cats throughout the world are noninfectious, although an MLV vaccine has been licensed in Europe. MLV rabies vaccines should never be used in exotic carnivores because of the uncertainty that exists with respect to species-related susceptibility to vaccine-induced disease. In fact, no MLV vaccines should be used in exotic carnivores unless it is absolutely necessary and it is known that they will not cause disease in the species.

Vaccine-induced rabies in dogs and cats after MLV vaccination begins with paralysis in the inoculated limb within 7

Table • 100-18

Practices That May Reduce the Occurrence of Postvaccinal Sarcomas in Dogs and Cats

VETERINARIANS

1. Profile pet and administer annual booster vaccines only for those agents for which pet is at risk for exposure. Vaccines used should be based on the needs of each patient. Do not overvaccinate.
2. Serotest, when applicable (see text), to determine if vaccines are needed.
3. Use MLV recombinant vector products, nonadjuvanted noninfectious, or IN, when available and effective.
4. Use SC vs IM route. Both can cause tumor formation; however, tumor development is detected earlier with SC.
5. Administer different vaccines at widely spaced sites, and use a consistent location for subsequent boosters.
6. Rabies right pelvic limb, leukemia left pelvic limb, and FHV-C-P on the lateral trunk or over the forelimb on either side
7. Do not administer vaccines at the interscapular space.
8. Massage vaccine sites immediately after inoculation to help disperse adjuvant (uncertain benefit).
9. Map and record these sites, vaccine brand, and serial numbers.
10. Advise owners of risk and need for monitoring vaccine sites. Inform them of risk of local and systemic vaccine reactions.
11. Reduce use of vaccines containing aluminum-based adjuvants.
12. Identify core vaccines (see text) and assess risk for noncore diseases before vaccinating.
13. Use single-dose rabies vaccines, and always mix well.
14. If multidose containers are used, mix them well before using to disperse adjuvants evenly.
15. Reduce use of combined multivalent products that compound the amount of adjuvants per dose.
16. Reduce the frequency and number of unnecessary vaccinations such as for FeLV.
17. Consider reducing the frequency of booster vaccines in adults. After the first annual booster, consider triennial boosters.
18. Bring vaccine to room temperature before using.[a]
19. Consider use of monovalent boosters and stagger these over annual visits rather than all antigens yearly.
20. Consider offering preventive health measures rather than vaccination for yearly visits.
21. Consider use of topically applied MLV vaccines for respiratory diseases in high prevalence areas.
22. Surgically remove swellings that persist at vaccine sites beyond 90 days.
23. Report all vaccine-associated sarcomas to the United States Pharmacopeia (http://www.usp.org; 800-487-7776).

OWNERS

1. Monitor vaccine sites for increased swelling.
2. Reduce animal co-mingling and improve sanitation to limit exposure and need for repeated boosters.
3. Return for annual physical examination regardless of need for vaccination.

MANUFACTURERS

1. Establish DOI for products for proper booster frequency.
2. Develop vaccines for nonparenteral routes.
3. Reduce, alter, or eliminate sarcoma-inducing adjuvants.
4. Develop and market monovalent vaccines.

VETERINARY ORGANIZATIONS AND ASSOCIATIONS

1. Work with local governments to ensure rabies vaccine requirements are compatible with existing licensed product recommendations and DOI.
2. Continue to update and publish guidelines regarding vaccine practices.
3. Support funding for studies to determine or document safety and efficacy of current vaccines.
4. Encourage manufacturers and governing agencies to institute consistent, effective, and readily available reports on vaccine-induced adverse events.

MLV, Modified live virus; *IN,* intranasal; *SC,* subcutaneous; *IM,* intramuscular; *FHV-C-P,* feline herpesvirus (feline rhinotracheitis virus [FRV])-calicivirus-panleukopenia; *FeLV,* feline leukemia virus; *DOI,* duration of immunity.
Recommendations from: The Feline Sarcoma Task Force, American Association of Feline Practitioners (Ref), and the Committee for Veterinary Medicinal Products, European Union (*Anon Vet Rec,* 2003).
[a]Kass PH, Spangler WL, Hendrick MJ, et al. 2003. Multicenter case-control study of risk factors associated with development of vaccine-associated sarcomas in cats. *J Am Vet Med Assoc* 223:1283-1292.

Table • 100-19

Postvaccinal Sarcoma Recommendations

Diagnostic Monitoring:

Site monitoring: record the location, shape, and size (in three dimensions) of all masses occurring at injection sites.

All masses occurring at injection sites are assumed malignant until proven otherwise.

Further diagnostics and management needed if the swelling:

Persists more than 3 months after vaccination

Enlarges to greater than 2 cm diameter

Increases in size after 1 month

If a mass displays any of the above criteria:

Perform diagnostic incisional wedge or needle (tru-cut) biopsy (not aspirates)

Therapeutic Plan:

Stage the tumor and screen the patient by performing a CBC, serum chemistry profile, urinalysis, and thoracic radiographic exam.

Additionally screen for FeLV and FIV, from a prognostic rather than etiologic concern.

Consult an oncologist for multimodal treatment planning.

When possible, use computed tomography or magnetic resonance imaging to evaluate the location and spread of tumor in the body.

Never perform a "lumpectomy" or "shell out" the tumor.

Even aggressive surgery is often incomplete, unless *very* early.

Radiation or chemotherapy may be needed in conjunction with surgery.

Submit the entire mass removed for histopathology.

Report all histopathologically confirmed vaccine-associated sarcomas to the product's manufacturer and the U.S. Pharmacopeia Veterinary Practitioner's Reporting Program, 12601 Twinbrook Parkway, Rockville, MD 20852. Voice phone 800-487-7776; fax 301-816-8532 or http://www.usp.org/prn.

Recheck the cat by followup physical examination every month for the first 3 months and every 3 months for at least 1 year.

CBC, Complete blood (cell) count; *FeLV,* feline leukemia virus; *FIV,* feline immunodeficiency virus.

Information was adapted from the recommendations of the Vaccine-Associated Feline Sarcoma Task Force.

to 21 days and progresses bilaterally, in an ascending fashion.[36,38,444] Affected cats have had progressive LMN paralysis with unusual extensor rigidity of the limbs. Pain sensation and reflex function were decreased in an ascending fashion. Progression to forelimb and intracranial involvement was more common in affected cats, whereas dogs usually recovered completely within 17 days to 2.5 months. Injection in the cervical musculature, closer to the brain, has been associated with a much greater prevalence of neurologic complications. A peculiar feature of the paralysis in some cats is a sign of hyperextended limbs rather than flaccid paralysis. Animals with vaccine-induced rabies do not represent a health hazard because the virus is attenuated and is not shed in the saliva. Because of the difficulty in distinguishing the vaccine virus from virulent virus, expert virologists and public health officials should be contacted for recommendations concerning disposition of an affected animal (see Chapter 22 and Appendix 4). Vaccine-induced rabies should not be a problem when inactivated vaccines are used unless they inadvertently contained live virus.

Encephalomyelitis has been reported after CDV vaccination in dogs, especially in very young pups or immunosuppressed dogs (see Canine Distemper, earlier, and Prevention, Chapter 3). Postvaccinal distemper has been reported after immunosuppression of dogs with cytotoxic chemotherapy (see previous discussion, Vaccination Failures, and Canine Distemper, later) and in association with virulent CDV infection (see Canine Parvoviral Enteritis, later). Atrophy of the Purkinje's cells and cerebellar dysfunction developed in three of six pups given MLV measles vaccine at 6 weeks of age[157]; however, this observation seems unusual in that measles virus does not generally replicate to any extent in the dog. MLV FPV vaccines and CPV vaccines should not be administered to animals younger than 4 to 5 weeks. Cerebellar degeneration and myocarditis may develop in kittens and puppies, respectively, from virulent parvovirus. MLV vaccine might also cause cerebellar disease in very young (under 3 weeks) immunosuppressed dogs or cats.[497] Cases of cerebellar hypoplasia from vaccinating pregnant cats or dogs with attenuated parvoviral vaccines are rare because most veterinarians are aware of this contraindication. Parenteral vaccination with one of the first licensed, attenuated CCoV vaccines was associated with disseminated vasculitis and meningitis in dogs that was similar to FIP in affected cats.[364,598] The authors have observed a modified live CDV Rockborn strain vaccine to cause an increased frequency of CDV postvaccinal encephalitis when it was added to a combination product that previously had a low or no postvaccinal complications.

Prenatal and Neonatal Infections

If MLV vaccines are given during pregnancy, vaccine infections can result in fetal malformation or death or infertility and abortion in the dam. Neonatal infection can also occur after the use of MLV CPV or FPV vaccines in puppies or kittens younger than 4 weeks. Although some vaccines may be safe, the general recommendation is to avoid giving MLV vaccines to pregnant females. Furthermore, unless specified on the label as safe for use in pregnant animals, noninfectious vaccines should not generally be given to pregnant animals because systemic allergic reactions might develop that might jeopardize the pregnancy.

Respiratory Disease

Clinical illness can develop as an expected postvaccinal event when IN vaccines are used for FCV, FHV-1, CPiV, CAV-2, and *B. bronchiseptica* infections. The mild clinical syndrome is usually self-limiting, but the organisms may produce respiratory tract inflammation, a carrier state, or may spread to other susceptible animals. In general, cats are more severely affected compared with dogs. The onset and level of secretory immune responses with IN vaccines are superior to those of parenteral vaccines. However, the clinical disease that these vaccines can produce has restricted their use by veterinarians because clients become concerned even when mild clinical signs are present. Parenteral MLV feline respiratory vaccines inadvertently or accidentally released into the environment or on the haircoat or aerosolized during administration can cause similar or more severe postvaccinal reactions because they are not attenuated as do the strains intended for IN inoculation. In some purebred catteries where genetic immunodeficiencies exist, the use of MLV respiratory vaccines may have to be avoided because of the potential of vaccine-induced respiratory disease. Feline chronic ulcerative gingivostomatitis and faucitis (see Chapter 89) are likely caused by hypersensitivity to persistent FCV infection. Routine annual boosters, especially of adjuvanted noninfectious products, are not recommended in affected cats. In some cases, one of the authors (CEG) has observed activation of oral ulceration after vaccine boosters of carrier cats.

Febrile Limping Syndrome of Cats

This problem is noted in kittens after the use of products containing attenuated FCV. The illness usually occurs in kittens younger than 6 months of age and within 21 days following a vaccination.[110,111] Animals are lame, anorectic, and febrile as early as 7 days after immunization. Pyrexia is commonly present, and some cats show concurrent signs of respiratory disease with or without oral ulceration. Kittens show a shifting-leg lameness and hyperesthesia that cannot be localized to a particular joint. The clinical signs resolve with symptomatic therapy of fluids, antibiotics, and analgesics; complete recovery is noted in 3 to 4 days. One theory suggests that vaccinated kittens may have been incubating field virus at the time of vaccination, which triggers a hyperimmune response and resultant immune-mediated polyarthritis. However, the more likely premise is that vaccine virus spreads to the joints from viremia following inoculation, with a subsequent inflammatory response. Similar lameness occurs in lower frequency in unvaccinated cats that become naturally infected with FCV.

Lethargy, mental depression, anorexia, and lameness have been reported in cats within 7 to 21 days following vaccination with attenuated *Chlamydophila* products. Because the clinical disease is mild and the reaction to vaccination is often more severe, the routine use of *Chlamydophila* vaccines is not recommended.

Vaccine-Associated Disease of Young Akita Dogs

Families of closely related Akita dogs have developed immune-mediated polyarthritis 3 to 29 days after receiving MLV vaccines and less frequently or less rapidly after receiving noninfectious vaccines[129,603] (see also Chapter 95). Such defects in their immunity are expected because Akitas are highly inbred from a relatively small gene pool. By 16 weeks of age, the dogs usually developed signs consisting of cyclic fever, joint pain, neutrophilic leukocytosis, and nonregenerative anemia. Elevated levels of hepatic enzymes, creatine kinase, and azotemia have been observed. Joint fluid analysis reveals nonseptic, purulent polyarthritis. Treatment with glucocorticoids helps alleviate the clinical signs, but relapses are frequent, and higher continuous doses of glucocorticoids may be needed. Unfortunately, long-term high doses of glucocorticoids may lead to iatrogenic hyperadrenocorticism. Dogs usually have to be euthanized by 2 years of age because of progressive systemic inflammatory disease, amyloidosis, and renal failure as a result of glomerular amyloidosis. The disease may be an immune-mediated disorder induced by an immunodeficiency with increased susceptibility to vaccine organisms or coincidental exposure to other environmental or commensal microflora. The condition shows many similarities to the syndrome of recurrent fever, polyarthritis, and renal amyloidosis in Chinese Shar-pei dogs (see Chapter 95).

Vaccine-Associated Hypertrophic Osteodystrophy and Juvenile Cellulitis, Especially Noted in Weimaraners

A syndrome has been observed after administration of combination vaccines, including MLV CDV, characterized by fever, limb swelling, radiographic changes typical of hypertrophic osteodystrophy (HOD), and variable systemic manifestations such as coughing from pneumonia, lymphadenomegaly, diarrhea, pyoderma, and oral ulceration.[128,221] Reactions usually develop after the second dose of vaccine given between 8 to 20 weeks of age.[127] Signs usually begin 1 to 27 days after vaccination, with a mean of 10.5 days. The most

commonly affected signalment has been young (2 to 5 months of age) Weimaraners, and less frequently, other large-breed dogs, and occasionally small-breed dogs. Typical cases of juvenile cellulitis have been associated with this syndrome.[357] In one of the author's (CEG) experience, some dogs with juvenile cellulitis may have radiographic evidence of HOD, even when concurrent dermal lesions are the predominant manifestation. The simultaneous occurrence of these two syndromes following CDV vaccination suggests that they may be related to infection with attenuated distemper vaccine virus in an immunocompromised host. However, infection with virulent CDV in dogs incompletely protected by vaccination cannot be excluded. Virulent CDV has also been associated with metaphyseal osteodystrophy in dogs (see Chapter 3), and primary immunodeficiencies have been established in Weimaraners that may make some dogs more susceptible (see Chapter 95). This syndrome usually occurs following the administration of the second dose of MLV CDV–containing vaccine in the puppy series. Leukocytosis is the main laboratory abnormality, although neutropenia has been observed. Low plasma protein and low levels of IgG and IgM have been observed. Treatment with antiinflammatory dosages of glucocorticoids (0.5 to 1.0 mg/kg/day prednisolone) over 1 to 3 weeks at a gradually reduced level is adequate to cause resolution of signs. This syndrome has occurred most commonly with vaccination with the Rockborn, Snyder Hill, and certain Onderstepoort strains of vaccines. Subsequent immunization of affected dogs or any vaccinations of Weimaraners, with less virulent Onderstepoort strain or recombinant canarypox virus–vectored distemper vaccine, is recommended (see Table 100-17). One alternative that appeared to reduce this reaction in Weimaraners was to separate the parvovirus from the distemper-adenovirus-*Leptospira* immunogens into an every-other 2-week interval.[221] Dogs in the group receiving the separated antigens reacted only after administration of the second distemper vaccine, and then only at that time. Pups given both distemper and parvovirus and the other immunogens in combination on a 4-week-interval schedule developed varying degrees of the HOD reaction after each dose in the vaccine schedule. Dogs that reacted to the vaccine did not develop measurable antibody titers, if at all, until after the immunization protocol was completed. They also had low levels of IgG before immunization.

Given that certain families of Weimaraners are prone to develop this reaction, they should be vaccinated differently; they should also be serotested 1 month after the vaccination series is complete to ensure successful immunization for CDV and CPV. An alternative vaccination method that may be tried if MLV CDV is causing the problems is to use only the canarypox virus–vectored CDV combination product because it contains no live CDV and is as effective as MLV CDV after 3 doses of vaccine given over a period of 9 to 12 weeks starting at 6 weeks of age. One other recommendation is to restrict the use of combined antigen products, such as with *Leptospira* bacterin, in these dogs during their primary vaccination series because they may suppress an already tenuous immune response.

Shedding of Vaccine Agent

Shedding of vaccine virus, which occurs with the IN MLV products, also occurs after administration of parenteral vaccines such as MLV canine-origin and feline-origin parvoviral vaccine (feces), CAV-1 vaccine (urine), and CAV-2 vaccine (respiratory secretions). This shedding may serve to vaccinate other susceptible animals of the same species that come in contact with infected secretions. However, caution must be exercised when mixed animal species are vaccinated, especially when exotic and wildlife species are in contact with a vaccinated animal that is shedding virus. Although the potential exists, reversion to virulence for the target species has not been demonstrated with any virus that is shed as a result of vaccination with commercially available veterinary vaccines.

Influence on Drug Disposition

A potential influence of vaccines or viral infections on drug disposition exists in that they induce IFN synthesis, which, in turn, inhibits hepatic enzyme systems. This factor might prolong the effects of drugs eliminated by oxidative metabolism, such as aminophylline, barbiturate, lidocaine, propranolol, chloramphenicol, tylosin, griseofulvin, and trimethoprim. However, no studies have been performed to demonstrate this potential effect.

False-Positive Test Results

Bovine serum or other proteins in cell culture can cause reactions that give false-positive ELISA results, especially when adjuvanted noninfectious products were used. These results have been found in serotests for antibody in the diagnosis of toxoplasmosis, FIP, and FIV infection after routine use of CHV, FCV, and FPV vaccines. Vaccines for feline respiratory disease or panleukopenia are often grown in Crandell-Reese feline kidney (CRFK) cells. To determine if cross-reactivity exists, kittens were vaccinated with either CRFK or feline renal tissue (FRT) extracts or with one commercially available product including either an intranasal or one of three parenteral vaccines.[313,314] Cats vaccinated with the CPFR or FRT extracts or parenteral vaccines had seroconversion and developed measurable serum antibodies to FRT. Cats vaccinated SC had greater antibody responses to CRFK cells than did those that were vaccinated IN. Whether this laboratory finding has a bearing on development of renal disease in cats is uncertain. Routine vaccination in research beagle dogs with multivalent and rabies vaccine was associated with an increase in species-specific tissue autoantibodies.[516] In beagles, the increase was in antibovine thyroglobulin antibodies, while in pet dogs, an increase was noted in anticanine thyroglobulin antibodies after vaccination. Whether these increases are an artifact of cross-reactivity or an indicator of stimulating thyroid autoimmunity is uncertain.

Immunosuppression

Some concern has been expressed regarding deleterious effects of attenuated vaccines on the immune response, especially during primary vaccination of naïve animals. To be effective, attenuated vaccine antigens have to produce transient infection themselves, which leads to immunologic activation and sometimes potential immunosuppression. Polyvalent vaccines can cause lymphopenia and suppress the response of lymphocytes to mitogens when testing is performed within the first week after vaccination. Individual antigen components do not cause this problem as frequently as do combined immunogens, and in one report in dogs, combined CDV and CAV antigens were incriminated.[449] When vaccine antigens are combined, they are required to have testing, which shows that the combination does not suppress the immune response to the same antigens given separately. Evidence suggests, however, that use of attenuated vaccine agents along with concurrent, potentially virulent infectious agents may lead to greater susceptibility to disease caused by either agent. One of the authors (RDS) has observed some dogs with localized demodicosis developed generalized disease 2 weeks after vaccination with combination products. Clinical salmonellosis and suspected concurrent parvoviral enteritis were observed in a cattery with endemic *Salmonella* infection after vaccination with IN modified live FPV, FHV, and FCV vaccine.[165] Vaccine-induced distemper encephalitis has been observed in MLV CDV–vaccinated 3-week-old pups that

were co-infected with virulent CPV (see Chapter 8). Under certain circumstances, inactivated vaccines have also been suspected to cause transient immunosuppression. When bacterins for *Leptospira* are used in combination early in the primary vaccination series of pups, they may reduce the serologic response to the viral antigens compared with that of pups not receiving them.

Human Health Risk to *Bordetella bronchiseptica* Intranasal Vaccine

B. bronchiseptica, a cause of respiratory disease in dogs and cats, can infect people as a zoonotic infection (see Chapters 6 and 16). Most cases of human infection with this organism have been in immunocompromised individuals. Young children, elderly, and human immunodeficiency virus (HIV)-infected people with acquired immunodeficiency syndrome (AIDS) have been most susceptible. Infections have usually involved the respiratory tract or contamination of surgical or traumatic wounds. The attenuated IN vaccine for *Bordetella* was suspected to cause respiratory infection in a 14-year-old boy.[44] A veterinarian inadvertently sprayed the face of a boy (while the boy was restraining his dog) with an aerosol that contained both CPiV and *B. bronchiseptica*. The boy developed a paroxysmal cough beginning 5 days after the event, and clinical signs persisted for 3 to 4 months. The boy was treated with antibiotics and recovered. No cultures were performed of his respiratory system; however, with subsequent investigation, two morphologically distinct isolates of *B. bronchiseptica* were cultivated from the vaccine. Because no other cases of respiratory illness were observed in the boy's school or family contacts, the infection was presumably caused by the vaccine. For this reason, veterinarians should reconsider the manner in which they administer IN vaccine to their patients. When possible, the animal should be restrained by hospital personnel rather than clients. If clients are present during administration, avoid having infants, pregnant females, elderly adults, or known immunosuppressed individuals within a distance of 2 to 3 meters. An alternative would be to have them leave the room, or the animal should be taken to another area to administer this product.

VACCINATION RECOMMENDATIONS FOR SPECIFIC DISEASES

The diseases to be discussed are those for which vaccines are commercially available. Specific chapters on each disease should be consulted for additional information. Overall recommendations for canine and feline immunization protocols are summarized in Appendices 1 and 2, respectively. Appendix 3 lists veterinary biologics available in many countries.

Vaccination of Exotic Carnivores

Many nondomestic carnivores are vaccinated for diseases of dogs and cats with commercially available canine and feline vaccines. In general, one of the authors (RDS) recommends that unless absolutely necessary, MLV products should not be used in exotic species because they may cause clinical illness, and in addition, a potential always exists for reversion of the attenuated strain to virulence in a foreign host. Only noninfectious rabies vaccines should be used in these animals. Oral recombinant-vectored vaccines are available for wildlife, and a parenteral rabies canarypox virus–vectored rabies product is available for cats. The killed and recombinant rabies products should be tested and used only after safety and efficacy can be demonstrated in the specific exotic species. Because of the risk of vaccine-induced distemper, a concern has been expressed for vaccinating nondomestic carnivores with MLV

Table • 100-20

Vaccination of Families of Terrestrial Carnivores and Their Susceptibility to Infectious Diseases of the Dog and Cat[a]

DISEASE	SUSCEPTIBILITY/WHETHER TO VACCINATE						
	CANIDAE[b]	FELIDAE[c]	PROCYONIDAE[d]	URSIDAE[e]	MUSTELIDAE[f]	VIVERRIDAE[g]	HYENIDAE[h]
Canine distemper[i]	+/+	−/−	+/+	+/−	+/−	?/±	?/?
Feline panleukopenia[i]	−/−	+/+	+/+	?/?	+/+	?/±	−/−
Infectious canine hepatitis[i]	+/+	−/−	−/−	+/−	−/−	−/−	?/±
Feline respiratory disease	−/−	+/+	−/−	−/−	−/−	−/−	−/−
Parainfluenza	+/+	+/−	?/?	?/?	?/?	?/?	?/?
Rabies	+/+	+/+	+/+	+/+	+/+	+/+	+/±
Leptospirosis	+/+	+/−	+/±	+/−	+/±	+/±	+/±

+, Yes; −, no; ±, optional; ?, uncertain.

[a]For reference sources, see Fowler ME, Theobald J. 1978. Immunity procedures, pp 613-617. *In* Fowler ME (ed), Zoo and wild animal medicine. WB Saunders, Philadelphia, PA; Appel MJ. 1987. Virus infections of carnivores. *In* Horzenik MC (series ed), Virus infections of vertebrates, vol 1. Elsevier, New York, NY; Appel MJ. 1988. Personal communication. Cornell University, Ithaca, NY; 1981. Susceptibility of various exotic animals to canine distemper and feline distemper viruses. Norden Laboratories, Lincoln, NE. Sedgwick CJ. 2005. Personal communication, Aromas, CA.

[b]Coyote, dingo, domestic dog, jackal, raccoon dog, wolf, red fox, gray fox. Only modified live virus (MLV) chicken tissue culture vaccines or noninfectious or vector-recombinant distemper vaccines should be used on the gray fox.

[c]Cheetah, lion, jaguar, margay, ocelot.

[d]Bassariscus, coati, kinkajou, raccoon, lesser panda. Only noninfectious or vector recombinant canine and feline distemper vaccines should be used on the lesser panda.

[e]Bears, giant panda. The giant panda, and some Bear species such as the American Black Bear, should recieve noninfectious vaccines for canine and feline distemper.

[f]Ferret, fisher, grison, marten, mink, otter, sable, skunk, wolverine, badger. Only MLV chicken tissue culture or mammalian cell vectored recombinant vaccines should be used on ferrets.

[g]Binturong, linsang, civet. The mongooses and meerkats are in the related family Herpestidae and should be treated similarly.

[h]Hyena.

[i]Noninfectious vaccines are preferred when available.

CDV vaccine; however, noninfectious whole viral products have been ineffective. Chicken embryo–derived CDV vaccines appear to be safer in this regard for species such as the domestic ferret, but they can cause disease in the black-footed ferret. The product of choice is the recombinant canarypox virus–vectored CDV vaccine that has been proven safe and effective in ferrets.[542] In the United States, the USDA-Animal and Plant Health Inspection Service (APHIS) has proposed allowing wolves and wolf-dog hybrids to be inoculated with the same vaccines used for dogs.[11] Similarly, proposals to give the same consideration to Bengal-cat hybrids have been offered. Vaccinating these animals creates legal and ethical issues for veterinarians and public health officials. In jurisdictions where these animals are not legal pets, they should not be vaccinated; however, veterinarians may decide to vaccinate in areas where ownership is allowed. The owner must receive notice, preferably in writing and as part of informed consent, that efficacy of vaccines is not proven in these animals. Susceptibility to canine and feline infections and recommendations for vaccinating wild or exotic carnivores are summarized in Table 100-20.

Vaccination Requirements for Transport of Animals

Interstate shipment of animals that are affected with or have recently been exposed to infectious diseases is prohibited within the United States. Each state has established guidelines that normally include a physical examination and current rabies vaccination. General information is available in the current regulations of the USDA (http://www.usda.gov), APHIS (http://www.aphis.usda.gov), Department of Agriculture in Canada (http://www.agr.gc.ca), Bureau of Animal Health in Australia (http://www.aahc.com.au), Ministry of

Agriculture in the United Kingdom (http://www.defra.gov.uk), and similar bureaus in other countries.

In the European Economic Community (EEC), animals may move between member countries provided they show no signs of disease, are identified by tattoo or microchip, are vaccinated using a World Health Organization–approved vaccine certified by an official veterinarian, and are accompanied by an animal passport clearly identifying the individual.[21]

Amendments have been added to regulate the importation of animals into rabies-free areas such as the United Kingdom and Ireland. An animal originating outside the EEC is required to have an import license and a minimum of 6-months post import quarantine in approved facilities. Animals from EEC member nations must originate from a registered holding facility and must have been born and kept in captivity from birth, with no contact with wildlife. The animals must be identified with a microchip and be vaccinated against rabies at least 6 months before shipping and be at least 12 weeks of age at the time of vaccination. After vaccination, an internationally agreed on serologic test such as the RFFIT or FAVN must demonstrate a protective rabies titer of at least 0.5 IU/ml. If the test is carried out after the first vaccination, it must be between the first and third months after vaccination. Further changes in this law are being considered.[22] For information regarding serologic testing and proof of rabies immunization for transport of animals, see previous section of Rabies and in Chapter 22.

Rabies Vaccination Recommendations for Dogs and Cats

Rabies vaccines have been extremely effective in reducing the prevalence of this disease in dogs. As a result, the incidence of human disease has decreased substantially, whereas the relative incidence of feline rabies has increased. The first vaccines for rabies, derived from nervous tissue of infected animals, evoked severe autoimmune reactions in the CNS. Subsequently, more purified, extraneurally produced MLV vaccines were cultivated in avian embryo and tissue culture media. Unfortunately, certain MLV vaccines produced postvaccinal rabies in dogs and cats (see previous discussion of Neurologic Complications). Because of this problem, the trend has been to switch from MLV to inactivated rabies vaccines. No MLV rabies vaccine is currently available in the United States, but a genetically attenuated MLV rabies vaccine has been licensed in Europe, and MLV vaccines are available in a large number of countries throughout the world (see Appendix 3). All MLV rabies vaccines must be given IM at one site in the thigh. MLV requires fixation to nerve endings to be effective, and these are more plentiful in muscle compared with subcutaneous tissue.

Inactivated rabies virus vaccines provide an adequate duration and level of protection but not necessarily comparable to that of MLV products. Inactivated rabies vaccines must contain high viral content, and adjuvants, such as aluminum hydroxide, need to be added. Combination products containing rabies antigen have been licensed for cats but one of the authors (RDS) believes strongly that rabies should be given only as a monovalent vaccine. These modifications, required to make inactivated rabies immunogenic, may be associated with a greater degree of allergic and neoplastic reactions, especially in cats (see Postvaccinal Complications, earlier). In general, inactivated rabies virus vaccines given IM often give stronger immune responses than those given SC, but the former is associated with more systemic allergic reactions. A canarypox virus–vectored recombinant feline rabies vaccine (Purevax Feline Rabies®, Merial, Athens, Ga.; see Appendix 3) that produces few local inflammatory reactions is effective in cats. The product is currently licensed only as a 1-year product.

For recommendations on rabies vaccines used in the United States, the *Compendium of Animal Rabies Vaccines* published by the National Association of State Public Health Veterinarians should be consulted (see Appendix 4). In summary, both dogs and cats should receive their first rabies vaccine no earlier than 3 months of age. Rabies vaccines are frequently given on the last visit of the neonatal vaccination series (Appendices 1 and 2). Subsequent boosters are administered 1 year later, then either 1 or 3 years later, depending on the age of the animal, the vaccine manufacturer's recommendation, and the local public health laws. Although inactivated vaccines generally require at least two vaccinations in a series 2 to 4 weeks apart to offer full protection, rabies vaccines can provide adequate protection with one dose. The current challenge procedure for licensing of rabies vaccines involves giving one dose at 12 to 16 weeks of age, then waiting 1 year with the 1-year rabies vaccine and 3 years with the 3-year products. The animals are then challenged to demonstrate protection. One-year products often become licensed as 3-year products by showing that they provide the same protection 2 years later as they did at 1 year. Triennial vaccination with a 3-year product provides the same protection as does yearly vaccination with a 1-year product. Using 3-year products is preferred because they provide the same protection and reduce the chance of an adverse reaction. Only a few states, cities, or local municipalities require that rabies vaccines be given more often than once every 3 years after the booster at 1 year. Because of the confusion it might cause in diagnosis and management, rabies vaccination is not recommended for wild animals that are kept as pets; however, when needed, only noninfectious or recombinant-vector products should be considered.

Rabies vaccination of cats is mandatory in some counties in the United States and discretionary in others. The vaccine requirements vary from annual to triennial. Unlike the situation in dogs, licensing is not tied to vaccination, and few county governments require that cats be licensed, even where mandatory feline rabies vaccination exists. Therefore as guided by the Council on Biologic and Therapeutic Agents report of the American Veterinary Medical Association, in many situations, veterinarians have the task of recommending rabies vaccination of cats to their clients based on the regional variation of disease, different feline lifestyles, risk of reaction of a particular breed, and preference of the owner and veterinarian.[296]

Canine Vaccination Recommendations
See Appendices 1 and 3.

Canine core vaccines
Since the 1970s and especially the 1980s, annual vaccination has been the routine practice for immunization of dogs. The prevalence of many diseases for which the vaccines were developed has been decreased significantly. Evaluation of early vaccines showed that not all pups maintained sterilizing antibody titers (protection from infection) to CDV after the initial series. However, it was not known at that time that CMI played an important role in protection from disease and that sterile immunity was not necessary for protection from disease. Therefore annual boosters were recommended because serologic testing was more difficult and costly compared with revaccination. However, the lowered frequency of infection and information on adverse reactions recently has prompted the question, *"Are we vaccinating too often?"* The too-frequent administration of boosters and potential for development of hypersensitivity or other reactions creates a medical dilemma. For this reason, veterinary scientists and professional veterinary groups have categorized vaccines into core vaccines and optional (noncore) vaccines, with individual customization based on the animal and its environment (see Appendix 1).[295,441] Components considered *core* vaccines for dogs are canine distemper, canine adenovirus, canine parvovirus type 2, and rabies virus; they are recommended for all dogs. Noncore vaccines are vaccines used to prevent or manage diseases such as infectious tracheobronchitis, leptospirosis, coronaviral enteritis, Lyme borreliosis, and giardiasis that are of lesser severity, for which less effective vaccines are available, or to which the pet may have limited exposure based on geographic or utilitarian factors. These products should be given only to animals at risk, and they often need to be given on an annual or more frequent basis based on potential for exposure.

Canine distemper (Also see Prevention, Chapter 3.) Immunity to CDV is based on humoral (antibody) and CMI responses. However, the magnitude of the antiviral antibody response in the host determines whether a dog is protected from infection or if it will develop the epithelial or neurologic form of the disease (see Chapter 3, and Serologic Testing, previously). Passive administration of serum antibodies to CDV can be used to protect animals from becoming infected (passive sterile immunity). Only MLV vaccines and live recombinant–vectored CDV vaccines are highly effective in protecting dogs against CDV. However, these vaccines are not homogenous with respect to the degree and duration of neutralizing antibodies that are produced following vaccination.[484] Noninfectious vaccine gives incomplete and short-lived protection from CDV and is not licensed in most countries. MLV vaccination can also cause false-positive test results for viral detection in serum up to 4 weeks after vaccination.[527]

Distemper vaccination is performed in combination with other antigens, mainly CAV, CPV-2, and CPiV, at 3- to 4-week intervals, beginning at 6 to 9 weeks of age. Most currently used

Table • 100-21

Distemper Viral Strains in Commercially Available Vaccines[a]

STRAIN	BRAND	MANUFACTURER	IMMUNITY	RISK OF POSTVACCINAL DISEASE
Rockborn MLV	Duramune®	Fort Dodge	+++	**
Snyder Hill MLV	Vanguard®	Pfizer	+++	**
Onderstepoort MLV	Progard®	Intervet	++	*
	Galaxy®	Schering-Plough		
	Duramune® Max	Fort Dodge		
Recombinant vector	Recombitek® CDV	Merial	++	–

MLV, Modified live virus; *CDV,* canine distemper virus; +++, more protective; ++, protective; **, possible; *, low likelihood; –, none.
[a]Refer to Appendix 3 for additional information on these vaccines and manufacturers.

vaccines are able to break through MDA by the time the animal is 12 weeks of age. Distemper vaccines differ in their ability to immunize and break through MDA, even among the recombinant and conventional MLV products,[472,484] but most are able to provide protection when given at or after 12 weeks of age. The Onderstepoort strain, which has been chicken-embryo adapted, later avian-cell adapted and later canine-cell adapted, are generally, but not always, less immunogenic than the canine cell–adapted Rockborn or Snyder Hill strains (Table 100-21) Improvements have made many of the MLV products comparable. Colostrum-deprived puppies should not be vaccinated with MLV distemper vaccine before 4 weeks of age. A canarypox virus–vectored vaccine may be considered at this age if a monovalent was available.

Measles vaccine (MV) in combination with distemper has been recommended as the first vaccination given to high-risk puppies between 4 and 6 weeks of age. MV creates a heterotypic immune response in the presence of a high concentration of MDA to CDV, at a time when vaccination with MLV distemper vaccine alone would fail. Four- to 6-week or older puppies will respond to measles antigen, whereas only 50% or less may respond to CDV antigen. MV does not typically produce a humoral response to CDV such as the CDV vaccine virus, but it does prime the immune system to prevent disease. Distemper antigen has been combined with measles (MV-CDV) by one vaccine manufacturer (Pfizer, New York, N.Y.) with the assumption that it would produce a superior homotypic response in those puppies whose maternal immunity is weak. MVs should not be given to bitches if they are going to be bred or if they are 12 weeks of age or older, otherwise MDA to MV will be present in their colostrum if they are bred and have a litter after the first heat. This transfer of MDA will interfere with the effectiveness of MV subsequently given to the pups. By 12 weeks of age, MDA will have waned sufficiently that distemper vaccine alone should be effective. One of the authors (RDS) has demonstrated in unpublished observations that the monovalent recombinant canarypox virus–vectored CDV vaccine (Recombitek®, Merial, Duluth, Ga.) will immunize puppies with high maternal CDV antibody titers and thus can provide early protection from CDV and at an age when some conventional MLV vaccines fail to provide protection. Furthermore, with at least two additional doses in the vaccine series, the antibody response will then be at levels equal to that provided by conventional MLV vaccines.

At least one dose, if not two doses, of MLV CDV or recombinant CDV vaccine should be given whenever dogs older than 12 weeks are presented for their first vaccination. One MLV distemper vaccine provides strong protection in the naïve animal, even in the absence of MDA; however, a second vaccine will ensure more lasting protection. After the primary series, dogs should be revaccinated 12 months later or at 1 year of age. Similarly, in humans, a second booster for measles during the primary vaccination series has been shown to provide more sustained and better protection than a single vaccine does when children are immunized beyond the waning of serum MDA.[114,182]

Vaccination of dogs with MLV CDV vaccine may even be effective in preventing disease when it is given within 3 to 4 days after initial exposure (not after onset of clinical signs) to virulent CDV (see Prevention, Chapter 3). MLV vaccine (monovalent product) should be given whenever exposure occurs, if the vaccination history is unknown. For animals older than 1 year, boosters for distemper need not be given more often than every third year. The evidence for this is supported by challenge studies with virulent virus and serologic testing following vaccination (see Table 100-12). In the absence of CDV, two-thirds of dogs tested had protective antibody titers from 8 to 10 years after vaccination.[425] One of the authors (RDS) has demonstrated that the DOI for CDV is a postvaccination minimum of 7 years as determined by challenge and up to 15 years by serology. With less protective vaccine strains, such as certain of the older Onderstepoort vaccines sold in Europe, immunity may wane with time (e.g., 3 or more years) in dogs that do not receive periodic boosters.[302] However, dogs over 2 years of age generally have better maintenance of their antibody titers than do younger animals.[484] Adequate VN titers developed in 90% of vaccinated dogs. Dogs were protected against infection when challenged up to 5 to 7 years after vaccination.[502] Some distemper breaks have occurred when less protective distemper vaccines had been used, revaccination had waned, or low environmental exposure suddenly increased (see Vaccination, Chapter 3).[47,140,194,219] As a systemic viremia that is susceptible to neutralizing antibody, distemper is one disease for which antibody titers are an effective means to determine susceptibility of a vaccinated animal to distemper. Seroconversion that occurs following vaccination indicates that the animal did not have sterile immunity and that the vaccine provided some additional booster protection.

Some concern has been expressed that outbreaks of CDV infection might be caused by poor immunity resulting from differences between field isolates and vaccine strains. Although genetic differences were found in naturally occurring strains,[50] cross-protection studies show similar protection, regardless of the isolate, and no variants have been reported that are antigenically different from the vaccine viruses. In Chicago, Illinois, an outbreak of distemper in dogs that were adopted into a community was traced to infected raccoons housed in the same animal control facility. A corresponding outbreak in the zoological garden was attributed to the wildlife outbreak and the wandering or raccoons onto zoo grounds. Analysis of the strains involved in epizootics of the zoological garden and dying raccoons over several years have shown genotypic and phenotypic variation of the viruses responsible for the outbreaks.[324] Limited cross-protection studies in dogs done by one of the authors (RDS) showed protection between strains, suggesting that management in the animal control facility was responsible for these outbreaks, although further studies and monitoring are needed.

Distemper can rarely develop in a vaccinated dog; however, when virulent virus is present at high levels and the dog has other concurrent illnesses, is immunosuppressed, or is a genetic-poor responder or nonresponder, disease may develop. Individuals in every breed can be found that are unable to develop an immune response that will protect the animal from disease when it is challenged with virulent virus. This animal is not immunosuppressed; instead, it is an animal whose immune system cannot recognize important immuno-determinants (HA and F antigens) of CDV. One of the authors (RDS) estimates approximately 1 in 1000 to 10,000 dogs are nonresponders for CDV. Given that this trait is genetic, it might be higher in certain breeds and will surely be higher in certain families of dogs. Attenuated distemper vaccines give the strongest immunity and long-term protection; unfortunately, these vaccines have the greatest risk of producing postvaccinal reactions. One of the authors (RDS) also estimates postvaccinal encephalomyelitis at approximately 1 case per 10,000 doses for the more virulent CDV vaccine strains. Distemper vaccine–induced encephalomyelitis, also termed inclusion body polioencephalitis, usually develops 7 to 15 days after vaccination in immunosuppressed dogs or with particular lots or strains of vaccine (see Chapter 3 and Postvaccinal Complications, previously). The illness, which can appear as an acute or more chronic progressive condition, is caused by a nonproductive CDV infection of neurons by vaccine virus.[406] As a result, the illness usually affects gray matter in the diencephalon, mesencephalon, and medulla oblongata, although cortical and spinal cord involvement has been observed.[92] Systemic signs are uncommon. Unlike conventional CDV infections, the CNS progression may subside, and dogs may survive with clinical improvement or residual neurologic deficits.[92] The Snyder Hill and Rockborn strains produce the strongest immunity but have the greatest risk of producing postvaccinal encephalitic disease. Care must be taken therefore to avoid vaccinating certain dogs for distemper with MLV vaccines, especially neonates younger than 3 months of age that have a known or suspected immunodeficiency disorder or are receiving immunosuppressive therapy. Care should also be taken in vaccination of exotic carnivores with MLV distemper vaccines because these can induce vaccine-induced encephalitis.[139] For further information on these topics, see Prevention, Chapters 3 and 8.

A recombinant canarypox virus–vectored distemper vaccine expressing H and F antigens (Recombitek® CDV, Merial, Athens, Ga.) is available (see Chapter 3) that is safe and effective for all animals, including immunocompromised pups and wild carnivores. A similar product has also been licensed for ferrets.[436,542] Initially, the duration of long-term immunity was uncertain with the recombinant vectors vaccines; thus yearly boosters have been recommended. However, studies by one of the authors (RDS) shows that when three doses of recombinant monovalent CDV product for ferrets are given at 2- to 4-week intervals to pups with high levels of blocking MDA, the antibody response is very high and above levels required for sterile immunity (greater than 1:20 VN titer). Furthermore, preliminary data from one of the author's

(RDS) unpublished studies suggest that the recombinant product might provide a minimum of 3 years DOI. Therefore the recommendation for vaccination with the recombinant distemper combination might be similar to that for MLV vaccines (see Appendix 1).

Infectious canine hepatitis (Also see Chapter 4.) Serum antibody against CAV-1, derived from MDA, passively administered serum, or produced following vaccination, is protective against this cytolytic, systemically spreading virus. Vaccination against this disease has brought about a dramatic reduction in the occurrence of this once widespread and potentially fatal illness. Few, if any, cases of hepatitis are seen in older animals (older than 6 months of age), which suggests long-term protection following MLV vaccination or recovery from natural infection. Vaccines containing MLV-CAV-1 were originally produced; however, in the 1970s, it was replaced with the safer, antigenically related CAV-2, and now most products contain this latter antigen. CAV-1 vaccines were evidently associated with more allergic uveitis than naturally occurring CAV-1 infection. Where CAV-1 antigen is found, it is generally an inactivated product. In areas where vaccination rates are high, ICH is rarely seen in domesticated dogs. Yet, although the disease is rare, a continual reservoir exists in wildlife and outbreaks or isolated cases can still occur when vaccination of puppies is delayed or incomplete. For this reason, CAV-2 is considered a core vaccine.

The shedding of MLV CAV agents and high viral stability has been responsible for inadvertent but beneficial vaccination of many dogs for this disease. However, regulations in many countries require that vaccine viruses are not shed. For this reason, inactivated CAV-1 and CAV-2 vaccines have been available in some parts of the world. Vaccination for ICH is usually performed in combination with that for distemper, CPiV, and CPV-2, beginning at 6 to 9 weeks of age. When using inactivated product, a booster dose must be given annually, whereas in many cases, the MLV products produce longer immunity of at least 3 years (see Table 100-12).

Canine parvoviral enteritis (Also see Prevention, Chapter 8.) Vaccination for CPV enteritis is essential because CPV is as contagious or is more contagious compared with CDV and is more stable in the environment. Exposure to virus is likely early in life, and as soon as pups are susceptible, they may become infected from a contaminated environment. Even before their first vaccination, pups from vaccinated dams can have virulent CPV in their stool, as demonstrated by PCR.[492] Before weaning, replication of enteric virus in pups is likely being suppressed by MDA protection in the sera and locally from their dam's milk.

One of the authors (RDS) has demonstrated that infectious virus survives for at least 1 year in sandy or clay soils. This information provided an explanation as to how the virus infected new litters of gray timber wolves (*Canis lupus*) in northern Wisconsin for a significant number of years after repopulation programs were put in place. The soil in the wolf den remained infected year after year. This finding means that more than 90% to 95% of dogs in a given population may have to be successfully immunized to prevent spread of infection.

Vaccines are produced from a variety of CPV-2 isolates and genotypes, but all are antigenically related. Both inactivated and MLV vaccines are available (Table 100-22). As with other diseases, MLV CPV vaccines offer a longer DOI and, more importantly, stimulate immunity much sooner than do killed vaccines. Postvaccinal shedding of vaccine virus occurs with MLV vaccines; however, it is of no clinical significance and may cause seroconversion in naïve contact animals and weak-positive parvovirus fecal-ELISA results[247] (see Chapter 8).

Table • 100-22

Comparison of Vaccines Available for Canine Parvovirus Infection[a]

VARIABLE	INACTIVATED VIRUS	MODIFIED LIVE VIRUS (CONVENTIONAL)	POTENTIATED
Recommended for use in pregnancy	Yes	No	No
Shedding of vaccine virus	No	Yes	Yes, consistent
Protects contacts of vaccinates	No	Variable	Frequently
Positive test results for fecal vaccine virus	No	3-5 days	5-7+ days
Prevents shedding of virulent virus	No	Yes	Yes
Relative magnitude of humoral response	Low	High	High
Relative particle mass of vaccine	High	Low	High
Breakthrough of maternal antibody			
Start vaccinating (weeks)	9	6-9	5-8
Generally protected (weeks)	18-20	16-18	12
Stop vaccination series (weeks)	18-20	16-18	12-14
Stop vaccination in problem breeds[b] (weeks)	16-22	16-22	16
Single dose protects naïve dog[c]	No	Yes	Yes
Selected examples of products	Adenomune, Parvocine (BioCor) Performer (Agri Labs) Vanguard (Pfizer) ImunoVax (RXV) Canlan (FD)	Parvocine Vanguard (Pfizer) Solo-Jec (Aspen) CPV/LP (Vaccicel) Adenomune (Biocor) Parvoid (Fort Dodge) Dohyvac (Fort Dodge) Parvodog (Merial) Enduracell (Pfizer) Tissuevax (Schering Plough) Parvigen (Virbac)	Progard, Nobivac (Intervet) Vanguard Plus (Pfizer) Recombitek (Merial) Galaxy (Schering-Plough) Duramune (Fort Dodge)[d] NeoPar (NeoTech) Kavak (Fort Dodge) Eurican; Primodog (Merial) Quantam (Schering Plough) Parvigen; Canigen (Virbac)

[a]Refer to Appendix 3 for complete information on products in this table.
[b]Rottweiler, Doberman pinscher, American Staffordshire terrier, German shepherd dog.
[c]Assuming no interference from maternal antibody.
[d]Originally formulated product protects similar to potentiated products.

Unfortunately, fecal-oral spread or topical administration of MLV does not provide suitable protection against CPV because it does not reach lymphoid tissue in sufficient concentration compared with parenteral administration. Protection during primary immunization can be provided by one MLV CPV-2 injection or two doses of killed vaccine. In themselves, killed vaccines may not provide as long-term immunity as does MLV; however, under field conditions, the provided protection allows the pup's immunity to be boosted by subsequent exposure to virulent virus. In contrast to inactivated vaccines, MLV vaccines provide a high level of antibody and sterile immunity that not only prevents disease, but also prevents infection or shedding after challenge with virulent virus. For this reason, dogs that are housed in large groups should be vaccinated with MLV vaccines because they will not shed virulent virus should an outbreak occur.

Vaccination for CPV enteritis might seem to be indicated earlier than 6 to 8 weeks of age when the prevalence of the disease is high or when puppies are colostrum-deprived. However, only inactivated products are generally recommended in puppies younger than 4 weeks because of potential damage by CPV-2 to rapidly dividing cells, such as those in the myocardium or cerebellum. MLV products are also not recommended in immunosuppressed or pregnant dogs. Severely immunosuppressed animals or exotic species may develop disease from CPV-2 vaccine virus and should be given only inactivated products. If previously unvaccinated very young or immunosuppressed pups are in high-risk environments and require immediate protection, immune sera (see Passive Immunization, earlier) should be considered.

A parenteral CPV-2 vaccine has been licensed in puppies 4 weeks of age or older, as a monovalent or bivalent product

(Progard® -CPv or -DPv and Nobivac® Puppy DP, Intervet, Millsboro, Del., and Boxmeer, The Netherlands, respectively). Ideally, bitches should be vaccinated with MLV CPV-2 products 2 months before breeding, and they should never be vaccinated with MLV while they are pregnant. If already pregnant with an uncertain level of antibody, the bitch can be given two doses of inactivated monovalent CPV-2 vaccine 3 to 4 weeks apart in the last trimester, but these products have not been approved for pregnant animals and vaccination-induced reactions can cause animals to abort or cause premature parturition.

Lack of vaccinations and incomplete vaccination series are important factors in the development of CPV enteritis. Vaccine breaks that occur with a seemingly *good* vaccine schedule in young dogs (younger than 2 years) are probably accounted for by MDA blockade. MDA may fall below protective levels, requiring earlier vaccination, in areas of high environmental contamination. Attenuated vaccine strains do not break through maternal immunity as effectively as virulent CPV resulting in a period of susceptibility. In the past, manufacturers claimed that their *conventional* CPV-2 vaccines would break through maternal immunity as early as 6 weeks of age with one dose. Generally, prevaccination titers were low in those litters reportedly protected at such young ages by conventional vaccines. Conventional products often failed to immunize pups until 18 to 20 weeks, even though MDA against a virulent virus was, in many cases, gone by 6 to 9 weeks of age.

Manufacturers have been able to overcome the susceptibility period when vaccines are ineffective by using more immunogenic strains, raising the virus titer per dose of vaccine, and lowering the serial passage, thus creating *potentiated* CPV-2 vaccines (see Table 100-22).[72,317-319] Increased immunogeneity of these newer CPV products developed since 1995 (see next paragraph) has provided immunity in the majority of pups vaccinated at 12 weeks of age or older. The high efficacy of the new products in these puppies has resulted in a recommendation to give a complete series of vaccinations, with doses given every 3 to 4 weeks until pups are at least 12 to 14 weeks of age.[372] No need has been found to vaccinate to the 18 to 20 weeks required by the conventional CPV-2 vaccines. The *window of susceptibility* is rarely greater than 2 weeks. In contrast, certain breeds of pups or pups born to bitches with very high antibody titers may not respond to conventional CPV-2 vaccines until up to 20 weeks of age. The remaining conventional products on the market are those manufactured for some of the feed stores and catalog sales (over-the-counter products) and by Pfizer Inc. (New York, N.Y.) as Vanguard®.

As with distemper, certain breeds appear to be more clinically susceptible to CPV-2 disease; and in some breeds, more low responders and nonresponders to the CPV-2 vaccines exist. The incriminated breeds include Doberman pinschers, American Staffordshire terriers, Rottweilers, and German shepherd dogs.[251] One of the authors (RDS) estimates the nonresponders to CPV-2 at 0.1% and the poor responders at 1% to 5%, with that number higher in certain breeds and lower in others.

Because of the large amount of virus excreted by infected dogs, vaccination alone is often inadequate in breaking the CPV infection cycle, especially in a shelter environment. Pups may need to be isolated from birth to 12 weeks from viral exposure to control an outbreak. Pups should be kept away from parks, boarding facilities, other litters, and shows until a dose of vaccine is given at or after 12 weeks of age. Simultaneous vaccination and infection with wild-type virus will generally result in disease, unlike CDV in which, because of a longer incubation period, the vaccine can be given up to 72 hours after infection and it can prevent disease.

Although combined vaccination with MLV CDV and CPV-2 vaccines has been rumored to cause immunosuppression, more controlled experimental studies have refuted these claims.[449,450,555,556] Despite the safety of combined CDV-CPV products, some breeders have expressed some concern about using multivalent products for the first vaccinations of pups. However, alternating these antigens in an initial vaccination series will leave a pup highly susceptible to infection with either virulent CDV or CPV, depending on which is omitted. Another argument posed by breeders has been to give the vaccines alternatively on a weekly basis; however, spacing MLV inoculations too closely may cause vaccine interference. Instead, vaccines should be given at a minimum interval of 2 weeks, although 3- to 4-week intervals are desired. Caution should be used when vaccinating pups suffering from CPV-2 illness. A potential problem with CDV postvaccinal encephalitis exists if neurotropic MLV CDV vaccines are administered (see Chapter 3). Therefore Onderstepoort CDV strain or recombinant CDV vaccines are recommended for use when concurrent CPV outbreaks are occurring.

Dogs that have recovered from subclinical infection with virulent virus or those that have been vaccinated and produced immunity to MLV vaccines have DOI that lasts at least 7 years. Cases of CPV-2 infection in susceptible older dogs are uncommon, and therefore older dogs may not require annual boosters for CPV. Annual vaccination programs have continued because of the use of multiple antigen vaccines. Revaccination of CPV-immune dogs does not often cause a significant (fourfold) increase in their antibody titer. This finding indicates that preexisting antibody has neutralized the vaccine virus before it could stimulate immune cells. Therefore periodic vaccination on an annual or triennial basis may not improve already-established immune protection for this disease. Similarly, producing hyperimmune sera by repeated vaccination of blood donors that might be used for treating CPV-susceptible pups would also be difficult. In a study of 106 dogs vaccinated against CPV-2 within the last 1 to 4 years, only one dog had a fourfold increase in antibody titer after revaccination because the dog had a low HI titer (lower than 1:160) before a booster vaccination.[502]

A shifting of antigenic determinants and genetic composition of CPV-2 began taking place in approximately 1981 with the CPV-2a strain and again in 1985 with the CPV-2b strain. Despite marketing claims to the contrary, excellent cross-protection exists between the old strains in the vaccine and the new field isolates. Molecular virology has shown that the most common viral type now isolated is CPV-2b (see Chapter 8). Similarly, immunodiagnostic tests based on MAB to original isolates are still sensitive in detecting newer strains of virus. Significantly, CPV-2b can infect and cause clinical illness in cats (see Feline Panleukopenia, later, and Chapter 10). This finding is in contrast to the original 1970's CPV-2 isolate, which was unable to even replicate in susceptible cats.

Immunity in the vaccinated animal is provided by IgG-neutralizing antibody. Passively acquired antibody from colostrum completely prevents infection for variable periods after birth. Serologic assays including ELISA, HI, VN, and indirect FA tests have been developed to detect this antibody. The ELISA is frequently used for diagnosis of virus in feces, and a variety of in-office kits are available (see Appendix 6). Antibody titers should be determined in selected laboratories that perform HI or VN tests. Measurement of serum antibody titers is a useful tool to determine need for vaccination against CPV infection. Absolute titers vary between laboratories, depending on the method used and test conditions. Each laboratory should provide reference values, and if a laboratory does not perform HI or VN, they should have quality assurance performed by outside reference laboratories testing many samples by HI or VN. An in-office ELISA has been developed, TiterCheck® (Synbiotics, San Diego, Calif.), which has been approved by the USDA and has been quality controlled with VN and HI.

CPV-1 infection The so-called *minute virus of canines* may cause illness in very young puppies and reproductive disease (e.g., embryonic death, abortions) (see Chapter 8). CPV-1 outbreaks have been associated with neonatal and in utero mortality. CPV-1 is not related antigenically to CPV-2, nor does a vaccine exist or much evidence that CPV-1 causes disease in a significant number of animals. The lack of immunologic cross-reaction also means that CPV-1 will not be detected by immunologic tests intended for CPV-2 in feces or tissues.

Noncore vaccines

Canine infectious tracheobronchitis (Also see Prevention, Chapter 6.) Infectious tracheobronchitis, also known as kennel cough or canine infectious upper respiratory disease (CIURD), is incited by a large number of viruses, bacteria, and mycoplasmas. Viruses can include CPiV, CAV-2, CDV, and CHV-1; secondary opportunistic bacteria such as *B. bronchiseptica*, *Streptococcus* spp., *Pasteurella* spp., and *Mycoplasma* spp. are often incriminated in complicating infections. Viruses such as CPV-2 can also be involved, especially by causing immunosuppression from co-infection. Multiple agents are often involved in an individual animal's illness. Because of the multiplicity of agents and short-term immunity to mucosal infections, prediction of protection following vaccination with CAV-2, CPiV, and *B. bronchiseptica* is impossible. Serum antibody titers to *B. bronchiseptica* increase to greater levels with parenteral vaccination rather than via IN route.[144] However, serum antibody levels play an uncertain role in predicting protection against infections of the respiratory tract or other mucosal surfaces. S-IgA and other local innate and specific immune mechanisms, which are difficult to measure, transiently increase following IN vaccination. These factors may be more important for protection against respiratory tract pathogens than systemic responses. However, challenge studies indicated better protection in pups that were sequentially vaccinated with one manufacturer's products using modified live IN and killed IM products during the primary vaccination series as compared with vaccination with either product alone.[141] Important to note is that the IM product used in this study is no longer licensed in the United States and has been replaced by a SC variety of different manufacture. Further studies on the use of SC products will be needed because they may not provide as strong a protection as afforded by IM injection. In contrast, in a large ongoing study in shelters by one of the authors (RDS) where 50% of the dogs receive parenteral vaccines and 50% receive IN vaccines, no significant differences have been seen between the vaccines and CIURD in any of the shelters. This result is not surprising given that this condition is a complex respiratory disease caused by many organisms that cannot be prevented by vaccines. Immunization against these infecting organisms can only help manage the disease and hopefully keep infected animals from developing severe pneumonia and possibly dying. Many dogs that are never vaccinated with kennel cough products resist the disease, as well as those vaccinated every 6 months to a year; thus probably even more factors are involved than those previously cited. These additional factors include genetics of the animal and anatomic differences among breeds or individuals. Severe kennel cough with death occurs regularly in racing greyhounds in spite of routine and constant vaccination with any and all commercial vaccines. However, if vaccines were not used, the morbidity and mortality rates may be even higher. Some of the mortality in greyhounds that occurs in spite of vaccination has been attrib-

uted to other respiratory pathogens such as equine influenza virus (see Chapter 25) and group D streptococci (see Chapter 35).

Available vaccines include avirulent live cultures, given IN, and whole-cell bacterins and antigenic extracts given parenterally. MLV CDV and CAV-2 viruses, both of which can cause respiratory tract infections, are included in routine parenteral vaccines, and CAV-2 is available in some IN vaccines (see Table 6-4 and Appendix 3). Modified live CPiV and killed *B. bronchiseptica* bacterin are available in some parenteral combinations. The DOI produced by respiratory vaccines against most primary respiratory pathogens, such as CPiV and *Bordetella*, has not been well established. One concern is that genetic differences exist between a number of field isolates and vaccine strains of *B. bronchiseptica*.[280,282,475] This finding may also help explain outbreaks of infection in vaccinated animals. In an attempt to obviate this problem, some vaccine companies have a variety of strains in their products, and the composition is periodically modified with current field isolates.

Parenteral canine respiratory vaccines usually do not produce protection until 2 to 3 weeks after the second vaccination. Originally, parenterally administered *Bordetella* bacterins contained large amounts of LPS (endotoxin), which produced fever, swelling, pain, or abscess formation at the site of injection. Newer parenteral products have modified whole cell or partially purified cell wall components that obviate some of the adverse reactions. Some reduction in efficacy and DOI has been associated with the purification process. Despite this disadvantage, administering parenteral products today is more convenient than are the older products that cause significant adverse reactions. Parenteral products produce higher serum IgG titers following vaccination.[144] However, this measure of protection is not as valid as is challenge infection. Parenteral products can be used for initial vaccination in the puppy series and subsequently in booster vaccinations. Vaccination with many parenteral products can begin at 6 to 8 weeks of age, depending on label recommendations. Because of the killed *Bordetella* component in parenteral vaccines, and to obtain adequate levels of S-IgA for all antigens, recommendations are that animals receive at least two doses 2 to 4 weeks apart for primary immunization.

IN vaccines, including both modified live CPiV and *B. bronchiseptica*, with or without CAV-2, have been developed in an attempt to increase the local immune response to vaccination (see Table 6-2 and Appendix 3) and to reduce the local and systemic adverse hypersensitivity-like reactions from parenteral products. IN vaccine may be used to boost immunity before anticipated exposure, or at the time of unanticipated exposure, to infected dogs. IN *Bordetella* vaccine has been shown to protect against clinical illness and to reduce the shedding of organisms after challenge exposure.[98] Most animals were protected against infection by 4 to 14 days after vaccination with a single dose. IN CPiV and *Bordetella* vaccines show some protection from challenge infection beginning 72 hours after administration.[197a] These vaccines can help prevent illness in a kennel outbreak or in pets before hospitalization or boarding. The clinical illness resulting from IN-administered canine respiratory vaccine is generally mild or unnoticeable compared with that of topically applied feline respiratory vaccines. Occasionally, vaccinated dogs will develop a persistent rhinitis or cough, and some immunosuppressed pups have had more severe lower respiratory tract infection. IN vaccines should never be used in dogs with preexisting respiratory tract disease.

Vaccines against canine ITB are recommended when an increased risk of respiratory infection is known or suspected. Naïve dogs should be vaccinated initially, with at least two parenteral or one IN vaccine at least 10 to 14 days before possible exposure at dog shows, kennels, or veterinary hospitals. With IN vaccines, the animal may be vaccinated immediately before exposure as a less desirable, but practical, alternative. Puppies as young as 3 to 4 weeks can be given IN vaccine because it is not affected by MDA as are parenteral products, and it has been shown to be safer at these early ages. Some of the products are also recommended as safe for pregnant bitches, but no reason has been found to use them in the pregnant animal. Annual or more frequent boosters are recommended in animals who are at high risk. Up to 10 months of protection has been demonstrated for some products. In many instances, individuals who show dogs do not use any kennel cough products, and they report no more or less kennel cough than do their colleagues that vaccinate every 3 to 6 months (personal communications with breed association members). That natural immunization would be very high in dogs that routinely go to dog shows should be expected.

Canine coronavirus infection (Also see Prevention of Coronaviral Infections, Chapter 8.) Immunity to canine coronavirus (CCV) infections generally involves S-IgA. S-IgAs have been difficult to measure for CCV vaccines in the clinical laboratory. Reproducing clinical disease with a variety of CCVs in susceptible experimental dogs is also impossible; thus vaccine efficacy cannot be reliably demonstrated. Serum antibody titers, which are easier to measure, indicate a systemic immune response to vaccine or indicate exposure to CCV, but they do not necessarily correlate with protection. S-IgA has been increased in challenged vaccinated animals compared with unvaccinated controls. A large number of products have been licensed in the United States for protection against this disease (see Appendix 3), and most are inactivated; however, one MLV vaccine has been developed. Inactivated and parenteral modified live CCV vaccines provide no or poor S-IgA response. Neither MLV or killed products administered parenterally to dogs prevent viral replication and fecal shedding after challenge infection.[437,467] Experimentally, MLV CCV vaccine given parenterally does prevent fecal shedding following challenge; however, the dogs still show seroconversion, indicating some replication in the host.[468] Regardless of which vaccine is used, dogs do not develop sterile immunity following vaccination as they do transiently following natural CCV disease.[502] Therefore vaccination with CCV will not prevent the increase in virulence of CPV-2.

CCV produces only mild and self-limiting clinical illness, primarily in pups younger than 6 weeks of age. The disease is in no way comparable to CPV-2 enteritis. Combined infections with CPV-2 and CCV can be more severe than with either infection alone; however, CCV vaccination does not prevent the CCV from enhancing the severity of CPV-2 infection. Thus vaccination against CPV-2 is the predominant determinant in viral enteritis protection. Vaccination against CCV is not generally recommended in either puppies or older dogs. Discontinuing CCV vaccination in shelters, commercial kennels, and in pet dogs has not lead to an increase in enteritis or any change in enteric disease prevention in the unvaccinated animals.

Complications have arisen during the development of CCV vaccines in the past. The first MLV vaccine for CCV was licensed in the United States in 1983; however, it was removed from the market because of a 5% rate of postvaccinal vasculitis and meningoencephalitis similar to the lesions of FIP.[364,598] Later, another manufacturer incorporated a new strain of modified virus into their vaccine. Unlike the previously marketed MLV CCV vaccine, the MLV vaccine strain produced no neurologic or systemic disease when administered alone. However, when it was placed in a combination product, it increased the neurovirulence of the CDV vaccine strain component, resulting in an increased risk of CDV vaccine–induced

encephalitis.[77] Thus marketing of the combination product with this CDV strain had to be discontinued.

A combination of *Leptospira* bacterins and inactivated CCV antigen in the same vaccine has caused some difficulties. Increased allergic reactions have been found when adjuvants are present. Because of antigen degradation, adjuvants are required when inactivated components, such as *Leptospira* or coronavirus antigens, are in formulated liquid diluent fraction, rather than the lyophilized fraction of the vaccine, and are being used in lieu of sterile water diluent. To overcome allergic complications with leptospiral antigen fractions, manufacturers have had to purify the leptospiral products to remove foreign proteins. Similarly, allergenicity seems less of a problem if *Leptospira* bacterins are administered at another site in the animal at the same time as a multiple-component vaccine. If allergic reactions are noted, combined inactivated CCV vaccines and *Leptospira* bacterins should be avoided.

Infection in young pups between 2 to 10 weeks of age with CCV is common, but disease is rare. The reason that CCV occasionally causes disease is not known. Research is needed to determine whether the disease is caused by a genetically distinct variant that is highly virulent or that certain dogs are susceptible to disease caused by CCV, or both. Isolates of CCV that have been associated with disease in a small number of dogs caused no disease when given to susceptible 2-week-old pups. Furthermore, a combination of MLV CPV-2 vaccine viruses and the CCV isolates caused no disease when given to susceptible pups.[501a] Dogs immunosuppressed with glucocorticoids and cytotoxic drugs appeared to be more susceptible to histologic changes in the GI tract when experimentally infected with some isolates of CCV. CCV should be considered a common inhabitant of the canine GI tract, similar to canine rotaviruses and reoviruses or *E. coli*. Under rare and unusual (and as yet poorly defined) circumstances, any or all of these infectious agents may cause some tissue pathology and disease. However, no indication exists that a vaccine will prevent that event; thus CCV vaccine is not recommended until it can be demonstrated that it prevents disease.

Canine herpesvirus infection A subunit vaccine consisting of herpesvirus glycoproteins is available in Europe for vaccination of pregnant dogs against CHV infection (Eurican® Herpes 205, Merial, Duluth, Ga.; see Chapter 5 and Appendix 3).[395,463] The vaccine is recommended just before breeding and a second one 1 to 2 weeks before anticipated parturition. Specific CHV MDA is passed in the colostrum to newborn pups, providing them with early neonatal protection. In breeding kennels, vaccine use was associated with higher rate of pregnancy and lower puppy mortality before weaning. The potential effect on a breeding establishment would be to increase birth weight and weaning rate and to reduce CHV-1 mortality in pups. Some evidence suggests a reduction in fetal death as demonstrated by higher litter size for vaccinated, as compared with unvaccinated, dams. Because the vaccine it is a subunit vaccine, no interference occurs with PCR or viral isolation methods.

Leptospirosis (Also see Prevention, Chapter 44.) Protection against *Leptospira* involves leptospirocidal or neutralizing antibodies to outer surface proteins or carbohydrates of the organism. Variations in the carbohydrate composition of the LPS are responsible for the variety of serovars[298] and less than complete heterologous protection afforded by current vaccines or recovery from prior infection with another serovar. Complete protection generally requires homologous vaccine antigen.

Serologic tests used to diagnose leptospirosis generally involve agglutinating antibodies that may not always correlate with protective immunity. Agglutination titers, determined by the microscopic agglutination test (MAT), measure IgM and some IgG levels and are better diagnostic measures of exposure or infection, rather than protection. MAT titers are generally low (no greater than 1:400) after vaccination. MAT titers of 1:100 or greater, which are considered protective following vaccination, are often not present to one or more of the vaccine serovars after primary immunization. When present after vaccination, MAT titers often decrease nonreactive (less than 1:100) within 2 to 3 months in pups receiving two doses and after 6 months in adult dogs vaccinated multiple times.[320]

ELISA antibodies have been measured on a limited basis for diagnostic purposes in which IgM and IgG can be specifically evaluated. ELISA-based antibodies are more sensitive for exposure to virulent or vaccine antigens and may last for periods beyond the protective period (see Chapter 44). Therefore these antibodies are not reliable in predicting protective immunity. More specific antibodies for protection are leptospirocidal titers; and although they are better indicators of immunity, they are difficult to measure. For these reasons, challenge experiments are needed to provide accurate information about duration of immunity.

A few manufacturers claim that their products provide varying degrees of protection from disease after challenge for up to 12 to 14 months. However, none of the present *Leptospira* vaccines consistently protect against infection, as measured by leptospiremia and shedding in urine, in dogs challenged with virulent organisms. In a short-term (1 month following vaccination) DOI study of 34 dogs comparing three commercially available vaccines, all control dogs shed spirochetes in their urine at various times for the first 3 weeks after challenge.[10] In contrast, vaccinates were generally protected against spirochetemia and challenge. A few vaccinated dogs had transient spirochetemia, and organisms could be detected in the urine of a few dogs, although control unvaccinated dogs were more severely affected.

In one long-term challenge study, three groups of dogs were vaccinated with a bivalent product for *Leptospira* and challenged via mucosal and IV inoculation.[293] Challenge was performed at 5, 27, and 56 weeks after vaccination. After challenge, all vaccinates were protected against renal shedding because organisms could be cultured from the urine of controls but not vaccinates. Histologic evidence of interstitial nephritis was found in the control but not vaccinated dogs. *Leptospira canicola* antigen was slightly more immunoprotective then that of *Leptospira icterohaemorrhagiae*. Protection against leptospiremia was complete at 5 weeks and partial at 27 weeks; however, 1 year after vaccination, 100% of dogs vaccinated for *L. canicola* and 33% of those vaccinated for *L. icterohaemorrhagiae* had transient spirochetemia. The vaccine was more consistently protective against urinary shedding of spirochetes after challenge for the three sampling times up to 56 weeks after vaccination. Based on the results for this one vaccine, efficacy of leptospiral vaccine seems poor for sterile immunity, and duration of strongest immunity is relatively short (approximately 6 months to 1 year) compared with that of some of the other vaccine antigens. Because these studies show a reduction in protection with time, a 1-year DOI with this vaccine would be a projected maximum.

As nonviable antigens, *Leptospira* products have to be administered at least twice over 2- to 3-week intervals to produce an initial immune response in a previously unvaccinated dog. Booster vaccination is recommended at yearly intervals but may be insufficient to maintain protective levels of immunity.

Leptospira bacterins for dogs most often contain inactivated whole bacteria or potentially purified cell wall antigens of *L. canicola* and *L. icterohaemorrhagiae*. Vaccination with these products is not recommended in animals younger than 9 weeks. In general, they are preferably administered at 12 weeks or older because of the allergenic nature of the vaccines. Anaphylaxis and other less-severe type I hypersensitivity reactions (e.g., facial edema, hives) may be present within 1 hour after the second or third vaccination in puppies given the initial series (see previous discussion of type I immunologic complications). A prior allergic reaction to a combination booster in any dog is probably enhanced by *Leptospira* bacterin; therefore, it should be eliminated or administered separately in subsequent vaccinations. Similarly, *Leptospira* bacterins should be avoided in miniature dachshunds and pugs, breeds that have a high rate of allergic reactions. Combination of *Leptospira* bacterins with noninfectious adjuvanted vaccines increases the risk of anaphylaxis. *Leptospira* bacterin is usually marketed in a liquid form and is usually used to reconstitute the lyophilized components in combination vaccines. The liquid formulation of *Leptospira* vaccine has adjuvants that are omitted when this fraction is lyophilized and incorporated with the other vaccine components. Sterile diluent provided by the manufacturer may be substituted for the *Leptospira* fraction when a reason exists to omit it. When using *Leptospira* bacterin alone is appropriate, the liquid portion of the vaccine should be administered.

All of the available products contain serovars *L. canicola* and *L. icterohaemorrhagiae*. Manufacturers market vaccines against *Leptospira grippotyphosa* and *Leptospira pomona* serovars, which have been associated with recent cases of canine leptospirosis. One quadrivalent *Leptospira* product (Duramune® Max 5+4L, Fort Dodge Animal Health, Fort Dodge, Iowa) is a partially purified outer membrane protein product (see Chapter 44 and Appendix 3). Other manufacturers are considering adding these latter serovars to their vaccines. A quadrivalent bacterin containing serovars grippotyhosa, pomona, icterohaemorrhagiae, and canicola (Vanguard Plus 5, Pfizer Animal Health, Exton, Pa.) is also available for this purpose. Newer subunit vaccines containing the immunogenic envelope of *Leptospira* are being evaluated to avoid the disadvantages of currently available products that cause adverse reactions. Leptospiral vaccines have been considered optional (noncore) by veterinarians in many areas because of the perceived rarity of the disease, short DOI, and risk of postvaccinal hypersensitivity.

When assessing the need for *Leptospira* vaccination, generally outdoor, sporting breeds, or large breeds (weighing more than 15 kg) are most affected during the summer or fall months.[203,586] Therefore these breeds should be targeted for this vaccine, preferably in the spring to help provide more complete protection over the problematic period of summer exposure. The highest risk factor for disease prevalence is in rural areas and urban areas that are encroaching on rural environments.[587] Dogs that visit rural areas also have a high inherent risk of exposure, which should not preclude vaccination of dogs that frequent buildings in urban areas with high rodent populations. One of the authors (CEG) is aware of a large number of cases of leptospirosis with serogroup *L. grippotyphosa* infection in dogs used for police surveillance in urban areas.

Lyme borreliosis (See also Chapter 45.) Serum antibodies are not completely protective against *Borrelia burgdorferi* because the organism not only has the propensity to alter its outer surface proteins during the course of infection, but also has the ability to encyst. Vaccination induces production of OspA antibodies that are expressed by the organism while it is attached to the midgut of its tick vector. Antibodies to OspA interfere with the organism in the midgut of the attached tick before it can infect the host. These antibodies must be present in the serum at the time of tick attachment to be protective.

Antibodies to OspA might be measured as an indicator of past vaccination and therefore might serve as a marker of some protection. Measurement of borrelicidal antibodies using live organisms gives a better indication of protection. Once the organism enters the host, outer surface protein C (OspC) antigens are predominantly expressed by the organisms.

Two commercial inactivated whole cell bacterins (Galaxy® Lyme, Schering-Plough, Union, N.J. and LymeVax®, Fort Dodge, Fort Dodge, Iowa) and two recombinant subunit OspA vaccines (RM Recombitek®, Merial, Duluth, Ga. and Prolyme®, Intervet, Millsboro, Del.) are available for protection against Lyme borreliosis (see Table 45-6 and Appendix 3). Studies by the various manufacturers have shown protection when dogs were challenged at times ranging from 156 to 366 days after the second vaccination. Vaccines protect dogs from spirochetemia and clinical limping episodes after challenge with virulent organisms compared with unvaccinated control dogs. Although the numbers of dogs have been small, these vaccines appeared to offer advantages for high-risk dogs (predisposed to tick exposure) in high-prevalence regions; it cannot be recommended for routine vaccination. The vaccine interferes with accurate interpretation of serologic titers for months to years unless immunoblotting is used (see Chapter 45) or with the SNAP® 3Dx® Test (Idexx Laboratories, Westbrook, Me.) when C6 antibody is detected. Concern has been expressed regarding immune-mediated complications such as hypersensitivity reactions or accentuating polyarthritis from Lyme vaccine.[336] These claims have not been adequately tested and might be less of a concern with recombinant OspA product. The human Lyme vaccine that was available for several years has been taken off the market because a small population of people with a certain human leukocyte antigen type developed nontreatable chronic arthritis. A similar problem may be present in vaccinated dogs, but additional studies are needed. Another concern is that the vaccines contain a limited number of strains that may not cross-protect against the known *Borrelia* spp. and serovars; however, further information is needed from field studies to show this is an issue of concern.

Despite the controversy that exists, *Borrelia* vaccines appear to be effective in challenge studies that have accompanied vaccine licensing. Because *B. burgdorferi* is virtually impossible to eradicate from tissues once infection is established,[549] and because antibodies against OspA should be present at the time of tick exposure, pups determined to be at risk in endemic areas should be vaccinated *before* they have the opportunity for natural exposure. *Borrelia* vaccines are recommended, depending on the product, for use beginning at 4 to 9 weeks of age during the primary vaccination series and consist of two to three inoculations, 3 weeks apart (see also Appendix 3 and Table 45-6). Revaccination of dogs at potential risk should *not* be postponed until booster age; instead, they should be vaccinated again at the beginning of the tick season. Concern has been expressed for both overdiagnosis and overvaccination for borreliosis in the veterinary community. If Lyme disease can be documented in dogs within a given geographic area, then this vaccine should be considered as one means of preventing the disease along with tick control measures. The vaccine should not be used outside these areas unless dogs will be traveling to endemic regions.

Giardiasis (See also Prevention for Giardiasis, Chapter 78.) Humoral immunity is important in the elimination of *Giardia* trophozoites from the host intestine. Increases in IgM, IgG, and IgA antibodies to surface and cytologic antigens of the parasite have been observed in the serum and GI mucosa between 10 to 17 days after infection.[422] However, certain hosts do not develop this humoral immune response, and CMI does not appear to be directly involved in immune clearance of the parasite. A *Giardia* vaccine has become commercially available in the United States for prevention of clinical illness and reduction of cyst shedding in dogs and cats (see Appendix 3). In challenge studies for licensing, pups were vaccinated SC at 3-week intervals. Placebo-inoculated dogs received only adjuvant. Challenge was at 6 months and 1 year. Vaccination reduced the duration and number of cysts shed and the severity of diarrhea. Control animals lost weight, while the vaccinated ones either maintained or gained weight. Trophozoites were abundant in the small intestine of control animals but absent in vaccinates. In one study of 13 dogs, vaccination of symptomatic dogs was associated with a resolution of clinical signs and termination of oocyst shedding.[423] However, no control dogs were used in that study. In another controlled field study to evaluate the vaccine for treatment of infected dogs, 20 dogs with antigen test–positive results for *Giardia* were divided in two groups and were given either *Giardia* vaccine or a saline placebo.[9] No significant differences were found in the vaccinated control groups with respect to antigen test–positive dogs over a 20-week period. To date, the vaccine has not been adequately tested in dogs in the field to determine its efficacy, and *Giardia* rarely causes clinically significant disease, even though infection is common. The American Animal Hospital Association Committee[441] places *Giardia* vaccine in the "Generally Not Recommended" category.

Babesiosis (See also Prevention, Chapter 77.) Serum antibodies are indicative of exposure but not protection in evaluating immune responses of the host to intraerythrocytic parasites such as *Babesia*. A commercial vaccine against *Babesia canis* infection (Pirodog®, Merial, Lyon, France) is available in Europe (see Appendix 3). This vaccine contains antigens derived from cell culture of *B. canis*. Vaccination does not prevent infection but it appears to prevent many of its pathologic consequences.

Leishmaniasis (See also Prevention, Chapter 73.) An experimental vaccine containing the fucose mannose ligand antigen of *Leishmania donovani* combined QuilA saponin was effective in protecting dogs against experimental field challenge.[51] Challenge was accomplished by placing dogs in highly endemic environments and evaluating them for the development of infection over 3.5 years. In challenged dogs, 25% of controls and 5% of vaccinates developed fatal clinical illness within the course of the experiment. A preventative fraction of 80% was calculated. Vaccines are not commercially available for this disease and further studies are needed to determine cross-protection among worldwide species of *Leishmania*.

Feline Vaccination Recommendations
(See Appendices 2 and 3.)

Core vaccines
Feline panleukopenia (Also see Prevention, Chapter 10.) Antibody titers can be used to predict protection against infection with FPV. VN or HI titers are the reference method to elucidate titers.

Both inactivated virus and MLV vaccines are effective in preventing this disease. In the absence of MDA interference, at least two doses of inactivated vaccine are required in kittens to equal the protection afforded by one dose of MLV vaccine. At least two MLV or three inactivated vaccine doses should be given at 3- to 4-week intervals to kittens in the initial series at 8 to 9 weeks of age. The second MLV vaccine ensures that an anamnestic response will occur if the first vaccine was blocked by MDA, which is usually negligible by 12 weeks of age.

Although FPV infection has been considered a disease of unvaccinated shelter kittens, it has been documented in *fading kittens* from well-vaccinated pedigree breeding catteries.[3] Virus was detected in the feces by CPV-2 and FPV ELISAs. Further studies indicated that the virus was FPV and not CPV-2 and that vaccine breaks were occurring because of exposure of kittens to large amounts of virus in a contaminated environment.

Both parenteral and IN MLV FPV vaccines are available. The IN vaccine (Feline UltraNasal® FVRCP, Heska, Fort Collins, Colo.) is combined with the FHV and FCV components. As with CPV infection, parenteral vaccination offers stronger protection than IN vaccination because replication in lymphoid tissues is stronger following parenteral administration of parvovirus vaccine. Systemic immune response and serum antibody titers are more important than S-IgA is in defense against systemic parvoviral viremia. However, IN vaccine may offer less risk of allergic or neoplastic complications, but MLV FPV has not been associated at a significant level with development of ISS; thus this should not be a consideration. Use of this combination IN vaccine was associated with an outbreak of panleukopenia in Persian kittens infected with *Salmonella* (see Chapter 10)[166] and with outbreaks of FPV in several shelters. This result may be associated with some virulence with the topically administered product and the possibility of MLV virus causing either disease or immunosuppression or because topical (IN or oral) vaccination is not as effective as SC or IM administration in protecting against this disease. The topically administered vaccine involved in this episode was withdrawn from the market and was reformulated to deliver a smaller volume and to decrease postvaccinal complications.

Genetic modification of the CPV-2 virus to the CPV-2a and CPV-2b strains has been associated with an adaptation of these genotypes to infect cats and potentially produce disease identical to feline panleukopenia (see Chapters 8 and 10 and prior discussion of canine parvoviral infection).[257,391,402,571] To date, experimentally reproducing clinical disease in susceptible cats has not been possible with some of the most highly virulent CPV-2b strains that regularly cause up to 100% mortality in susceptible puppies. In two studies, CPV-2b isolation rates of 3% to 10% were found in naturally infected clinically ill cats, while the remainder of isolates were FPV.[181,571] Feline FPV vaccines, canine CPV-2b vaccines, and killed mink enteritis virus (MEV) vaccines were all effective in preventing infection in cats challenged with virulent CPV-2b virus.[501a] In these studies, challenge with virulent virus was performed within 1 month or less following vaccination; however, longer DOI studies are needed following heterologous vaccination.

After homologous vaccination with FPV vaccine, antibody titers and challenge protection persist for at least 7.5 years even after two doses of killed FPV vaccine in kittens[514] (see Overvaccination, earlier). MLV vaccines provide longer immunity, probably life long. After the initial series in kittens and an annual booster 1 year later, vaccination can be done every 3 years or less to minimize the number of boosters. MLV vaccines would be recommended over inactivated virus products when FPV is a significant concern (e.g., shelters, catteries, pet shops). Inactivated virus vaccines are preferred if a risk of producing vaccine-induced illness exists or if vaccination is absolutely required in pregnant queens. Newborn kittens are immunologically responsive to FPV by 7 days of age; however, MLV vaccine must be avoided before 4 to 5 weeks of age because of its potential for producing cerebellar damage or clinical disease. Colostrum-deprived kittens in a low-risk environment (pet cats) can receive vaccinations between 2 and 4 weeks of age, but inactivated virus vaccines should be used at this age. Routine parenteral MLV vaccination of 4- to 6-week-old kittens is recommended in endemic catteries or shelters to reduce the prevalence of disease. Homologous hyperimmune serum can be administered to provide immediate protection to exposed unvaccinated kittens (see Passive Immunization, earlier). In a serologic study of feral cats by one of the authors (RDS), an unexpected finding revealed that 50% of the feral cats had never been infected with FPV, CPV-2, or MEV.[212a] This finding was unexpected because these parvoviruses are extremely stable in the environment and remain infectious for at least 1 year or longer.

Feline viral respiratory disease (Also see Prevention, Chapter 16.) Feline respiratory disease complex (FRDC) or upper respiratory infections in cats are common, especially in catteries, multiple-cat households, shelters, and pet shops. As in CIUDC, FRDC involves infectious agents mainly FHV-1, many serotypes of FCV, a variety of bacteria, *Chlamydophila*, and *Mycoplasma*, and is impacted by environmental factors (humidity, temperature, ventilation, gases), stress, and poor hygiene. Given that FRDC is rarely caused by only one of these factors, not surprisingly, vaccines cannot prevent disease in high-risk environments. Serum antibody titers were measured in SPF cats vaccinated with two doses of inactivated virus vaccine as kittens.[513] In this study, antibody titers began to decline by 3 to 4 years. The vaccines did not prevent cats from acquiring the infection (sterile immunity) but reduced the severity of clinical illness when they were challenged with FHV-1 or FCV 7.5 years after vaccination. Thus serologic assays may be used to measure evidence of immunologic memory but not equate with complete protection from these viruses.

FCV and FHV-1 vaccines are available as MLV and inactivated parenteral and as MLV IN products. IN products provide more rapid, superior local protection, and better breakthrough of MDA. Parenteral vaccination for respiratory infections produces a slower response to protection, usually requiring at least two doses of vaccine at a minimum of 3 to 4 weeks apart. In contrast, IN vaccine may provide protection within 48 hours in a susceptible cat but may typically produce a high incidence of mild contagious respiratory illness after vaccination, and viral shedding is common. Cats can become colonized with these attenuated strains of vaccine virus, which may provide them with a sort of premonition against infection with virulent strains.

Despite the rapid induction of S-IgA response afforded by the IN vaccine, veterinarians dislike the IN route of vaccination because of the high prevalence of vaccine-induced disease. Although IN vaccine has been recommended as a treatment for cats that suffer from chronic persistent respiratory infection, no studies have been conducted to document its effectiveness in resolving persistent infections. Parenteral products are less attenuated compared with IN vaccines. When giving parenteral vaccine, care should be taken to prevent accidental oronasal exposure of cats to aerosols or spilled vaccine. Following inhalation, postvaccinal respiratory disease may be more severe with parenteral products compared with IN products. A recommended method of administering IN vaccine to adult cats is to have an assistant raise the muzzle to 45 degrees. One hand of the administrator covers the eyes, and the other delivers the vaccine.[54]

Protection afforded against the development of respiratory diseases is usually incomplete and temporary, whether parenteral or IN vaccination is administered because of the transient persistence of S-IgA on mucosal surfaces. However, the response to reexposure can be more dramatic than that of unvaccinated animals because of immunologic memory. Regardless of the vaccine interval, vaccines do not prevent infection, latency of FHV-1, or all manifestations of disease. Cats that contract respiratory viruses after vaccination should have milder clinical illness than they would have had without vaccination but that is not always the case. Severe outbreaks have occurred, even in households, catteries, and shelters where all animals have been vaccinated.[574] Attenuated vaccine strains of FCV may colonize the vaccinated cat's respiratory tract in a persistent carrier state, and FHV-1 will become latent because vaccines cannot prevent latency with wild type FHV-1 strains.

For the last 30 years, the majority of FCV vaccines have been composed of a diverse serotype that cross-reacts with a majority of the field strains. However, the virus has a variable genetic profile that allows for the selection of field isolates with progressively greater resistance to host immunity. These vaccines can protect against clinical disease but do not provide sterile immunity.

When respiratory disease is endemic in closely congregated cats, kittens will likely be exposed and become ill early in life before successful immunization can be achieved. Colostric immunity to feline respiratory viruses is thought to last for not longer than 6 weeks, depending on the queen's titer and the virus (see Table 100-4). Early vaccination may protect kittens in congregated environments in which respiratory disease is endemic. IN FHV-1 and FCV vaccines can break through MDA earlier because of the reduced level of serum antibodies on mucosal surfaces. Early vaccination, before weaning, between 4 and 6 weeks of age with IN or parenteral vaccines, may be beneficial in controlling endemic respiratory disease in problem catteries, but they may also contribute to a carrier state and mild to moderate disease. When outbreaks occur at an earlier age, small doses of IN vaccine to 2- to 4-week-old kittens have been recommended to help stop or reduce disease in severe outbreaks.

Some breeders have vaccinated queens during pregnancy to increase protection against neonatal respiratory outbreaks; however, the value of this practice has been questioned. Nevertheless, in one study, vaccination during gestation was more beneficial than those given before conception in protecting against outbreaks of respiratory disease in kittens.[255] Kittens born to queens vaccinated during gestation had reduced morbidity and mortality rates from respiratory infections, without any adverse effects on reproductive performance. When vaccinating pregnant queens is necessary, they should be vaccinated with inactivated vaccines just before conception with the shortest time interval possible.

Parenteral inactivated respiratory virus vaccines are safe for debilitated cats, in kittens younger than 4 weeks that have been deprived of colostrum, and in pregnant queens, although protection is generally weaker than that provided by MLV products. With these exceptions, MLV vaccines should always be used to protect cats in case of an outbreak. IN vaccine may be preferred in certain cases, especially pet cats. Inactivated virus vaccines that contain adjuvants have a greater risk of producing allergic or neoplastic complications so that the frequency of their use as boosters should be reduced (see Postvaccinal Complications, earlier). Because chronic ulcerative gingivostomatitis may be a hypersensitivity reaction to persistent FCV carriage, repeated booster vaccination against respiratory viruses is not recommended in affected cats.

In studies conducted over several years by one of the authors (RDS), none of the products used against respiratory infection, regardless of number of vaccinations, type of vaccine, or route of delivery, prevented FRDC in a significant percentage (e.g., 30%) of cats. Also noted was that in high-stress, high-density shelters, the killed products were preferred because fewer cats were showing mild or moderate signs of disease. Also shown in a certain number of these shelters was that the cats were so suppressed that the MLV IN products caused disease that was severe enough to lead to euthanasia of a high percentage of the cats. In contrast, in low-stress, low-density cat shelters that can isolate incoming cats, the IN vaccines were better than the MLV parenteral, and the killed

products were the least effective. Ongoing studies will hopefully provide more information on the benefit, as well as the disadvantages, of these products in different environments. Results of these studies also suggest that vaccines against *Chlamydophila* and *B. bronchiseptica* provided no advantage and occasionally seemed to increase the severity of respiratory disease.

Several new serotypes of FCV initially isolated from cats in California were found that caused severe disease. These isolates have been confirmed in cats from the Midwest and East Coast and do not seem to be controlled by the current vaccines (see Chapter 16).

Noncore vaccines

Feline leukemia (See also Prevention, Chapter 13.) Protection against persistent infection with FeLV is dependent on humoral and cell-mediated mechanisms. Vaccinated kittens that develop measurable neutralizing antibodies to FeLV gp70 protein are protected from infection following challenge with virulent virus that readily infects unvaccinated kittens. Testing serum of cats for antibodies to gp70 protein might be used to determine which animals need to be vaccinated. However, antibody testing for FeLV is not routinely used and not readily available.

Prevaccination testing Only clinically healthy and FeLV-negative cats should be vaccinated. Low-risk groups for infection include cats from single-cat households, FeLV-negative catteries, and isolated environments (Table 100-23). Whether these individuals should be tested is usually based on the practitioner's decision or advice given to the client and the client's reaction to the cost involved. Although some expense and inconvenience is inherent in prevaccination testing of all cats, it is not always comparable to the cost to the client of the complete vaccination series. In this regard, it can be recommended that all cats of all ages be tested for FeLV viremia before vaccination. If testing and eliminating all persistently viremic cats were possible, eradicating FeLV would be possible. The ELISA results can usually be used as the criteria for response to vaccine. Vaccines do not benefit ELISA-tested viremic cats and therefore are not recommended. Because transient and especially persistently viremic cats are the only source of virus to infect susceptible cats, viremic cats should be isolated from other cats, especially those younger than 6 months of age. When the cat is established as persistently infected, every effort should be made to spay or neuter the cat if the owners plan to keep the cat rather than eliminate it from the household or cattery. Vaccination of every cat will fail to reduce the prevalence of FeLV infection or disease significantly because vaccination cannot prevent infections before 3 months of age, the time of greatest susceptibility to FeLV infections that lead to persistent viremia. Vaccines cannot provide immunity before 3 months because the earliest that the first vaccination can be given is 8 to 10 weeks, depending on the product, and no significant immunity occurs until 1 to 2 weeks after the second dose; thus 3 months or more would be required for protection if the most effective vaccines are used and probably longer with use of less effective products.

Persistent viremic cats should not be bred because infection in utero and at birth will ensure all or most of the kittens would be persistently viremic.

Vaccination should be recommended for all at-risk kittens during their initial vaccination series. Vaccination should be started in young (younger than 12 weeks) cats that are at the greatest risk for developing infection if they are exposed. Cats at high risk of infection include those in endemic multiple-cat environments, outdoor roaming or stray cats, or those in groups with unknown status. Although cats in that age group are 85% susceptible to infection following exposure, the risk

Table • 100-23

Recommendations for Testing for Feline Leukemia Virus and Feline Immunodeficiency Virus[a]

FeLV Viremia

1. General:
   a. FeLV status of *all* cats of *all* ages is desirable
   b. Positive cats should not be vaccinated
   c. Testing allows disease prevention and elimination
2. Timing:
   a. When cat is first acquired and before introduction
   b. If cat has never been tested before and is first presented
   c. Maternal antibody in young kittens does not interfere[b]
   d. Before *any* FeLV vaccination
3. Repeating:
   a. If serology results are positive or equivocal
   b. To confirm positive blood, saliva, or tear test results
   c. After two positive ELISA tests, perform indirect FA
   d. Discordant results: repeat ELISA and indirect FA
   e. Annual retest of high-risk cats, which includes those going outdoors; in open households; in closed households with test-positive cats

FIV Antibody

1. When:
   a. Test all cats older than 6 months of age
   b. Positive cats should not be vaccinated
   c. All vaccinated cats should be identified with microchip or tattoo
2. Timing:
   a. When cat is first acquired and before introduction
   b. When newly adopted
   c. Any previously untested cats
   d. After known exposure (2-3 mos for seroconversion)
   e. With unexplained fevers or recurrent infections
3. Repeating:
   a. ELISA is screen; indirect FA or immunoblot is more discriminating for positive results
   b. Passively acquired maternal antibody may cause false-positive results in kittens; retest after 6 mos of age
   c. Periodic retesting of at-risk cats (fighting, strays, unexplained wounds, routinely outdoors, mating to unknown male, known positive cat in household) recommended

FeLV, Feline leukemia virus; *FIV,* feline immunodeficiency virus; *ELISA,* enzyme-linked immunosorbent assay; *FA,* fluorescent antibody.
[a]For further information, consult American Association of Feline Practitioners/Academy of Feline Medicine, *Recommendations for Feline Retrovirus Testing* (6808 Academy Parkway East NE, Suite B-1, Albuquerque, NM 87109). Elston T, Rodano I, Flemming D, et al. 1998. Report of the American Association of Feline Practitioners and Academy of Feline Medicine Advisory Panel on feline vaccines, *J Am Vet Med Assoc* 212:227-241.
[b]Less than 10 to 12 weeks of age, false-negative results from maternal antibody suppression of viremia might occur, although this is controversial.

percentage drops to 15% after 6 months of age. Cats older than 1 year of age have substantial natural immunity.

If cats receive their initial vaccination 8 to 10 weeks of age or older, a prevaccination blood sample can be obtained at the time. This procedure saves the client an additional visit. If testing is not performed before vaccination, clients would become more concerned when their already-vaccinated cat later has a positive test result. Although some cats can be latently infected at the time of vaccination but remain undetected by FeLV testing until a later date, these cats may benefit from vaccination. The decision of whether and when to vaccinate cats with the currently available products rests with the practitioner. If the test result is negative, the vaccination series can be continued. If the result is positive, the series must be discontinued, and a second ELISA should be performed 4 to 8 weeks later. If the second test result is negative, the cat may be presumed to have recovered from natural infection, and the need for vaccination is minimal. If the second result is positive, an indirect FA test might be done; however, two positive ELISAs 2 months or more apart strongly suggests persistent viremia. An indirect FA test can determine whether the bone marrow is infected because most indirect FA–positive cats have a poor prognosis and remain persistently viremic. Persistently viremic cats are the major source of viral infection for contact susceptible cats (see Chapter 13). For general guidelines concerning FeLV and FIV testing, see Table 100-23.

Challenge studies Of the licensed FeLV vaccines, most contain noninfectious partially purified whole virus; one product is a genetically engineered subunit type; a final product is a canarypox virus–vectored recombinant vaccine. Varying types and quantities of adjuvant are present in some, but not all, vaccines (Table 100-24). Challenge studies of the vaccines, completed by their respective manufacturers using SPF cats, represent ideal laboratory conditions that may not be met in the field. Challenge studies vary tremendously with regard to age of vaccinates, route of challenge, type and dose of challenge strain, and the number of vaccinates and controls used. Manufacturers' licensing studies (see Table 100-24) may represent the best-case scenario for measured protection. Direct challenge models generally show higher degrees of protection than occur with natural-exposure challenge models, which may explain some of the discrepancies in various vaccine studies conducted between manufacturers and independent researchers. Natural exposure studies involve placing vaccinated and unvaccinated immunocompetent cats directly in an environment with FeLV-positive cats. For general guidelines on FeLV and comparative features of these products, see Table 100-24 and Appendix 3. For general guidelines concerning FeLV and FIV testing, see Table 100-23.

Number of vaccine doses As with other noninfectious products, antigen mass and repetitive vaccinations offer the best assurance of protective response. A reasonable recommendation is that all cats at risk be vaccinated with two doses as kittens. Based on manufacturer recommendations, cats receiving only one dose of FeLV vaccine in the initial series and not revaccinated within a 4- to 6-week period should have the vaccination series started over. Although studies on DOI are not available, subsequent annual revaccination with a single dose is recommended when need for ongoing protection is justified. Because of risk of sarcoma development and early age of susceptibility, continual revaccination has been questioned beyond the first year booster as stated previously. FeLV boosters are optional in older cats. Annual revaccination can be given to cats at very high risk of exposure. On the other hand, solitary cats should not receive vaccination beyond the primary series, if at all.

Table • 100-24

Comparison of Commercially Licensed Feline Leukemia Virus Vaccines[a]

VARIABLE	FEL-O-VAX®	FEVAXYN/ QUANTUM CAT®	LEUCOGEN/ NOBIVAC®[b]	LEUKOCELL-2®	EURIFEL FeLV®	PUREVAX®
Manufacturer	Fort Dodge	Schering-Plough	Virbac, Intervet	Pfizer	Merial	Merial
Composition						
Viral subgroups	A, B	A, B	A	A, B, C	*Env-A* and *gag* genes	*Env-A* and *gag* genes
Adjuvant	Yes, dual proprietary	Yes, aqueous proprietary	Yes, ALOA Quil A/ QS21	Yes, ALOH and Quil A	No	No
Formulation	Whole virus	Whole virus	Gp70 (p45) *env* Antigen purified subunit	Viral subunits from culture supernatant	Recombinant virus producing viral proteins	Recombinant virus producing viral proteins
Propagation	Genetically cloned feline cell line	Tissue culture cell line	Genetically produced in *Escherichia coli* plasmid	FeLV transformed lymphocytes	Recombinant canarypox vector	Recombinant canarypox vector
Licensing Studies						
Vaccine route	SC, IM	SC, IM	SC	SC	SC	Transdermal
Vaccine strain/ challenge strain	61E-A/61E-A	?/Rickard	Glasgow-1/ Glasgow-1	UCD-1[c]/ Rickard	NA/61E-A	NA/61E-A
Challenge route	IP	ON	IP	IN	ON	ON
Challenge immunosup-pression	Yes	Yes	No	Yes	No	No
Postvaccination challenge interval	2 wks	2 wks	2 wks	2 wks	2-3 wks and 1 year	4 wks
Latency examined[d]	Yes	Yes	No	Yes	Yes	No
Vaccinates persistently infected (%)	4 of 90 (4)	12 of 144 (8)	3 of 20 (15)	7 of 25 (28)	2-3 wk: 7 of 30 (23) 1 yr: 5/26 (19)	4 wk: 0 of 9 (0)
Controls persistently infected (%)	53 of 58 (91)	39 of 45 (87)	14 of 20 (70)	6 of 10 (60)	2-3 wk: 15 of 18 (83) 1 yr: 18 of 22 (82)	4 wk: 9 of 10 (90)
Preventable fraction (calculated efficacy; see text)	91-4/91 = 95%	87-8/87 = 91%	70-15/70 = 79%	60-28/60 = 53%	2-3 wk: 83-23/83 = 72% 1 yr: 82-19/67 = 77%	4 wk: 90-0/90 = 100%
Manufacturer publication[e]	517	236	90	213	462,559	207
Reported reaction rate	6%	1.4%	2%-6%	2%	Local: <2.2%; Systemic: <0.5%[f]	<2%

Table continued on the next page

Table • 100-24

Continued

VARIABLE	FEL-O-VAX®	FEVAXYN/ QUANTUM CAT®	LEUCOGEN/ NOBIVAC®[b]	LEUKOCELL-2®	EURIFEL FeLV®	PUREVAX®
Other Studies						
Literature and advertisements[d,g] vaccinates protected	91	91	85	>70	NA	NA
Independent studies preventable fraction[d,g]	85-100	90-100	52-93	5-100	NA	NA
Exposure routes	ON, IP, NE	ON	IP, ON	ON, SC, IP, NE	NA	NA
Latency examined in some studies	Yes	Yes	Yes	Yes	NA	NA
References for all studies[e]	242, 243, 326	445	260, 328	218, 260, 326, 458, 517, 564	NA	NA
Administration						
First, age (wks)	≥10	≥9	≥8	≥9	≥8	≥9
Interval to second (wks)	3-4	3-4	2-3	3-4	3-5	3
Recommended booster	Annual	Annual	Annual	Annual	Annual	Annual

ALOH, Aluminum hydroxide; *FeLV,* feline leukemia virus; *SC,* subcutaneous; *IM,* intramuscular; *?,* uncertain or not reported; *IP,* intraperitoneal; *ON,* oronasal; *IN,* intranasal; *NE,* natural exposure; *NA,* not available.
[a]Although the vaccines are listed here for comparative purposes, the conditions of testing for licensing and experimental studies have varied between products, making absolute comparisons difficult. For additional information on available vaccines and manufacturers, see Appendix 3.
[b]*Leucogen®* (Virbac Ltd) in countries outside the United States.
[c]UCD-1 is Kawakami-Theilen strain.
[d]Preventable fraction has not been calculated for all of these studies, making exact comparison of percentages difficult.
[e]Numbers in this row refer to references cited at the end of this chapter or on the CD.
[f]Data is on monovalent product only; however, a combination product which includes adjuvant had a local reaction rate of up to 17.3% and a systemic rate of up to 6% (http://www.emea.eu.int/vetdocs/vets/Epar/Eurifel/repFeLV.htm. Last accessed 02/27/05).
[g]Examining for latency is a more critical assessment of whether a cat is infected. Unfortunately, the time for examining for latency viremia after challenge varies among the studies, making exact comparison of percentages difficult.

Vaccination of high-risk cats Cats that are in contact with viremic cats are known as high-risk cats. Multiple-cat households, catteries, and research facilities allow for close contact and therefore greater risk that FeLV infection will be spread when a viremic cat is present. Outdoor and roaming or feral cats have a high chance for contacting other infected cats. This virus is highly labile and is not highly contagious, thus small amounts of virus in the environment are not a major source of infection. Because efficacy of vaccines is never 100% under natural circumstances, clients should be advised to avoid placing FeLV-vaccinated cats less then 6 months of age in the same environment with viremic cats. Similarly, in established FeLV-free populations, vaccination *should not* be a substitute for routine FeLV testing and elimination or quarantine of viremic cats. Because of the short period of residence compared with the time and expense to induce protective immunity, vaccination of all cats entering humane shelters cannot be justified. Testing and removal of all incoming viremic cats will be of much greater benefit in shelters. Studies that have claimed a reduction in FeLV in infected populations in which vaccination is instituted have been misleading. The initial prevalence of infection cannot be accurately compared with subsequent incidence data because vaccination has been coupled with removal of infected cats. Ironically, the prevalence of FeLV in the general cat population has not changed over the last 30 years; it was approximately 3% ± 1% then and is now. However, one factor that has changed is that the number of cats with leukemia and lymphoma that are FeLV-positive is much lower today than it was 30 years ago. The prevalence of FeLV-persistent viremia in the feral cat population is the same as that seen in the domestic cat population.

Vaccine safety Adverse reactions to FeLV vaccines have been primarily of an allergic or a neoplastic nature. Vaccines do not cause immunosuppression in uninfected cats or any change in the course of illness of an already viremic cat, nor does vaccination appear to activate latent infections. Vaccines are noninfectious products and will *not* produce FeLV infection or cause cats to have positive FeLV diagnostic test results. No data exist on the prevalence of allergic reactions, but IM is more likely than SC administration is to produce anaphylaxis because of the more rapid absorption of antigen. The amount and composition of adjuvants vary among the products (see Table 100-24 and prior discussion of Adjuvants). Precautions should be taken to limit the number of antigens given simultaneously to cats if such allergic reactions are noted. Limited safety studies have involved these vaccines in exotic cats. FeLV and rabies vaccines are associated with highest number of ISS. Reducing the number of boosters, through risk assessment, should decrease the risk of ISS in cats.

***Chlamydophila* infections** *Chlamydophila* vaccines are available as MLV or inactivated products for parenteral administration. Vaccines offer some degree of protection against clinical illness caused by *C. felis*, but immunity is not complete; exposed vaccinated cats develop milder clinical illness than do unvaccinated cats. MDA interference does not appear to be important with this vaccine, and no teratogenic effects are known. Kittens can be vaccinated as early as 3 weeks of age when neonatal conjunctivitis is a problem. Certain parenteral *Chlamydophila* vaccines have been shown to produce protective immunity for 6 to 12 months. Attenuated chlamydophilal vaccines have produced postvaccinal fever and malaise, and, as a result, some have had to be further attenuated. With combination products, vaccination for chlamydophilosis, although probably not essential, can be accomplished without much additional expense or inconvenience to cat owners. The overall low prevalence of chlamydophilal respiratory disease, or the potential for postvaccinal reactions, makes these products less essential or desirable on a routine basis. Nevertheless, inclusion of these products provides the potential for more complete protection. Should the disease be endemic, yearly boosters are recommended. A higher prevalence of feline chlamydophilosis has been observed in the United Kingdom, justifying routine vaccination. Routine vaccination against all of the feline respiratory diseases is often necessary in cats that are stressed or congregated in catteries, research facilities, and multiple-cat households.

Feline bordetellosis Feline respiratory disease can be complicated by bordetellosis. *B. bronchiseptica*, a commensal organism of the upper respiratory tract, has been isolated from cats with pneumonia and systemic manifestations. Disease is of most concern in catteries where significant numbers of clinically healthy cats and recovered cats carry the organism. Although experimental infections can produce mild disease, the importance of this problem in clinical settings is uncertain (see Feline Respiratory Disease, Chapter 16). A fimbrial antigen-based subunit vaccine (Nobivac® Bb Cat, Intervet, Boxmeer, The Netherlands) has been licensed only in The Netherlands. In the United States, a modified live IN vaccine (Protex®-Bb; Intervet, Millsboro, Del.), similar to vaccines used in dogs, is available (see Appendix 3).[596] This vaccine causes a mild self-limiting respiratory infection in cats and microscopic inflammation throughout the respiratory tract.[204] The vaccine should not be used in cats that are debilitated, immunosuppressed, or already showing clinical illness. The author (CEG) has also demonstrated spread of the organism from vaccinated to contact cats. In the cycle of natural exposure, the prevalence of this infection is highly variable and is usually restricted to multiple-cat environments. If this vaccine is used, it should be reserved primarily for unaffected cats in an environment where an outbreak has been documented. Compared with control cats, signs of disease in vaccinated cats were reduced but not eliminated following vaccination. In some shelter studies, cats that received this vaccine had more severe disease than seen when only FCV and FHV vaccines were given.

Feline infectious peritonitis (See also Chapter 11.) Protection against FIP involves both humoral and cellular mechanisms. In the early stages, S-IgA is important in reducing the replication of surface coronavirus, which, in turn, reduces the chances that mutant FIP virus (FCoV) will originate. An IN product has been available for vaccination for approximately 15 years (Primucell® FIP, Pfizer, Exton, Pa.). The vaccine consists of a temperature-sensitive restricted replicating mutant that reportedly produces local secretory antibody and sys-

temic CMI responses to FCoV. The IN vaccine is intended to produce local protection against viral replication, with subsequent mutation and invasion of the epithelial barrier, a prerequisite to the development of FIP. Previous use of parenteral vaccines caused sensitization of the humoral immune response and acceleration and precipitation of illness in vaccinates compared with controls (antibody-dependent enhancement). In certain studies, the IN vaccine was also reported to cause acceleration of disease.[511a] Initial concern by the manufacturer was expressed that high aerosol or IN viral challenge doses allowed virulent virus to gain entry into the body despite IN vaccination.[509,515] When such high-challenged doses were administered, animals developed antibody-dependent enhancement of disease. In contrast with lower oral–challenge doses, the vaccine was more protective. However, the amount of virus naturally infecting cats cannot be controlled, thus these studies may be misleading. In three controlled challenge studies reported by the manufacturer, preventable fractions ranged from 67% to 82%.[189] The perceived low prevalence of disease, prolonged incubation period, and required IN administration make the routine use of a vaccine for FIP questionable. However, the vaccine has been shown to be beneficial in controlled studies in which naïve animals (not infected with coronaviruses) are vaccinated before entering contaminated catteries.[158,460] In these studies, vaccinated animals had a lower subsequent incidence of FIP than did unvaccinated animals; however, the overall incidence rate of FIP in these cats was low. In another study in which SPF cats were housed with cats from an endemic cattery, no difference in disease incidence was found between vaccinated and unvaccinated SPF cats.[340] The vaccine is labeled for use in cats at 16 weeks of age or older, with a series of two inoculations being given 3 to 4 weeks apart. However, virtually all cats in endemic environments become infected immediately after weaning between 6 to 12 weeks of age. Cats having low or no antibody titer at the time of vaccination may benefit, while those already infected, which are a majority of cats over 9 weeks of age, that have a high FCoV antibody titer or infection may develop FIP despite vaccination.[158] Vaccination, when recommended in cats from environments in which FIP has been diagnosed, has not been shown to be beneficial. In one survey, owners of less than five breeding cats were more willing to vaccinate their cats as compared with larger professional cat breeders.[49] In addition to vaccination, other husbandry and control measures may be equally, if not more important, in reducing the prevalence of FIP-related illnesses in such catteries. This vaccine is not recommended by many feline vaccine experts, nor is it recommended by the American Association of Feline Practitioners (AAFP) in their most recent guidelines.[149]

Feline immunodeficiency virus infection (See also Chapter 14.). A commercial FIV vaccine has been licensed as an adjuvanted-inactivated whole-virus vaccine, containing subtypes A (Petaluma) and D (Shizuoka) strains, which induces a strong antibody response. In one challenge study, the type A (Dixon) strain that differed in genetic homology by 10% from the vaccine virus was used.[13] After challenge with this strain, the preventable fraction in vaccinated cats was a maximum of 82%. In other studies, the protection rate was lower. However, field isolates vary among subtypes; thus the preventable fraction in the field may be even lower.

A major disadvantage of the vaccine is that, because the definitive test for infection relies on detecting serum antibodies, those induced by the whole-virus vaccine cannot be distinguished from those produced by natural infection. Thus current diagnostic tests will no longer be of value in detecting infected cats.[332] Cats that were vaccinated, but not clearly identified with tattoos or microchips, might be considered as being infected with virulent virus. Furthermore, because some vaccinated cats might still become infected, the true infection status of known vaccinated cats cannot be determined. If a cat does not get tested before vaccination and is already infected when it is vaccinated, a similar problem might arise.

For this reason, cats should have negative antibody test results immediately before receiving the vaccine. If kittens have positive results, their antibody may be from MDA, which is usually gone by 12 weeks.[343] They should be retested at 12 to 16 weeks. A decline in antibody indicates MDA was present, but these kittens may already be infected from the queen; thus vaccination may be of no benefit.

Cats that have recently been bitten should not be vaccinated earlier than 60 days thereafter because this is the time period for seroconversion following natural infection. The AAFP has recommended that the currently available vaccine not be used until a suitable diagnostic test for infection can be developed.

Antibody titers are still the preferred means of diagnosis of FIV infection. PCR does not detect all viral subtypes and is not standardized, thereby leading to low test sensitivity and specificity.[45] Furthermore, PCR has not been evaluated for all strains of FIV, methods have not been standardized between laboratories, and the cost of a test, if developed, will be much higher than antibody measurements.

Feline giardiasis A licensed vaccine (GiardiaVax™, Fort Dodge, Fort Dodge, Iowa) containing inactivated, adjuvanted *Giardia lamblia* tachyzoites has been shown to provide some protection when given to kittens in two doses at a 3-week interval.[417] Vaccinated animals had greater body weight gain, less diarrhea, and reduced prevalence and quantity of cyst shedding as compared with control unvaccinated kittens. The vaccine is licensed for use in cats that are 8 weeks of age or older. In 16 young adult cats infected with *Giardia*, vaccination at weeks 4, 6, and 10 PI was not effective in eliminating the organism from infected cats.[540] The vaccine is similar to that marketed for use in dogs; however, the feline vaccine contains a different adjuvant. The vaccine causes significant injection-site reactions that are more severe than those seen with adjuvanted rabies. If ISS is a concern, use of this product would not be advised. Furthermore, little or no field data have been found to show that the product is needed; therefore it is not generally recommended.

Feline bartonellosis Cats are known reservoirs for *Bartonella* spp. that cause cat-scratch disease and related illness in people. Experimentally, *Bartonella henselae* vaccines have been protective in some studies to rechallenge infections (see Chapter 54). Although homologous protection has been demonstrated, cats can still be infected, albeit at lower levels of bacteremia, with heterologous strains and closely related species. This finding makes the possibility of a universal vaccine for this disease unlikely. Prevention is best accomplished through control of the flea vector.

Feline toxoplasmosis An experimental MLV *Toxoplasma gondii* vaccine was developed as an aid in the prevention of oocyst shedding by cats.[86] This vaccine consisted of tissue culture-propagated bradyzoites that have been purified. The vaccine was given orally with two doses at 3- to 4-week intervals, and it prevented oocyst shedding after challenge. This strain appears to be a phenotypically stable mutant, which does not produce oocysts (see Chapter 80). This vaccine is not available commercially.

NOSODES

Nosodes are homeopathic preparations of tissues from animals with the disease for which they are intended to prevent. They have also been recommended to be given immediately after exposure to an infectious agent. These alternative medical therapeutic preparations are claimed to protect animals as specific immunomodulators against a variety of infectious diseases. Their preparation consists of serial dilution with intervening agitation (succession, potentiation, vortexing) of tissues, discharges, or excretions from animals with corresponding diseases. Nosodes are administered orally. Clinical trials involving nosodes to prevent infectious disease[112,495] have not been well controlled. In a controlled CPV challenge of puppies, nosodes were not protective.[501a,604] Use of homeopathic nosodes to prevent serious infectious diseases is not advised.

SUGGESTED READINGS*

1. Abdelmagid OY, Larson L, Payne L, et al. 2004. Evaluation of the efficacy and duration of a canine combination vaccine against virulent parvovirus, infectious canine hepatitis virus, and distemper virus experimental challenges, *Vet Ther* 5:173-186.

23. Anonymous. 1998. 1998 Report of the American Association of Feline Practitioners and Academy of Feline Medicine Advisory Panel on Feline Vaccines, *J Am Vet Med Assoc* 212:241.

65. Burr H, Coyne M, Gay C, et al. 1998. Duration of immunity in companion animals after natural infection and vaccination, Publication SAB9824. Pfizer Animal Health, New York, NY.

123. Dittmann S. 2001. Vaccine safety: risk communication—a global perspective, *Vaccine* 19:2446-2456.

138. Edwards DS, Henley WE, Ely ER, et al. 2004. Vaccination and ill-health in dogs: a lack of temporal association and evidence of equivalence, *Vaccine* 22(25-26): 3270-3273.

141. Ellis JA. 2001. Effect of vaccination on experimental infection with Bordetella bronchiseptica in dogs, *J Am Vet Med Assoc* 218:367-375.

148. Elston T, Rodano I, Flemming D, et al. 1998. Report of the American Association of Feline Practitioners and Academy of Feline Medicine Advisory Panel on Feline Vaccines, *J Am Vet Med Assoc* 212:227-241.

184. Gaskell RM, Gettinby G, Graham SJ, et al. 2002. Veterinary products committee working group report on feline and canine vaccination, *Vet Rec* 150:126-134.

192. Gill M, Shrivas J, Morozov I, et al. 2004. Three-year duration of immunity for canine distemper, adenovirus, and parvovirus after vaccination with a multivalent canine vaccine, *Intern J Appl Res* 2:227-235.

196. Gobar GM, Kass PH. 2002. World wide web-based survey of vaccination practices, postvaccinal reactions, and vaccine site-associated sarcomas in cats, *J Am Vet Med Assoc* 220:1477-1482.

197a. Gore T, Headley M, Laris R. 2005. Intranasal kennel cough vaccine protecting dogs from experimental *Bordetella bronchiseptica* challenge within 72 hours, *Vet Rec* 156:482-483.

206. Griot C, Moser C, Cherpillod P, et al. 2004. Early DNA vaccination of puppies against canine distemper in the presence of maternally derived immunity, *Vaccine* 22:650-654.

218. Harbour DA, Gunn-Moore DA, Gurffydd-Jones TJ, et al. 2002. Protection against oronasal challenge with virulent feline leukaemia virus lasts for at least 12 months following a primary course of immunization with Leukocell™ 2 vaccine, *Vaccine* 20:2866-2872.

*See the CD-ROM for a complete list of references.

268. Jones PD, Kitchell BE. 2002. Vaccine-associated sarcomas in cats: applying the latest research to practice, *Vet Med* 97(1):34-44.

276. Kass PH, Spangler WL, Hendrick MJ, et al. 2003. Multicenter case-control study of risk factors associated with development of vaccine-associated sarcomas in cats, *J Am Vet Med Assoc* 223:1283-1292.

295. Klingborg DJ, Hustead DR, Curry-Galvin EA. 2002. AVMA Council on Biologic and Therapeutic Agents' report on cat and dog vaccinations, *J Am Vet Med Assoc* 21:1401-1407.

312. Lappin MR, Andrews J, Simpson D, et al. 2002a. Use of serologic tests to predict resistance to feline herpesvirus 1, feline calicivirus and feline parvovirus infection in cats, *J Am Vet Med Assoc* 220:38-42.

353. Macy DW. 2004. Quoted in: "Researchers probe vaccine-associated feline sarcoma," *J Am Vet Med Assoc* 224:813.

480. Richards J, Rodan I, Elson T, et al. 2001a. 2000 Report of the American Association of Feline Practitioners and Academy of Feline Medicine Advisory Panel on Feline Vaccines, *J Feline Med Surg* 3:47-72.

483a. Richards JR, Starr RM, Childers HE, et al. 2005. Vaccine-Associated Feline Sarcoma Task Force: Roundtable Discussion. The current understanding and management of vaccine-associated sarcomas in cats, *J Am Vet Med Assoc* 226:1821-1842.

513. Scott FW, Geissinger C. 1997. Duration of immunity in cats vaccinated with an inactivated feline panleukopenia, herpesvirus, and calicivirus vaccine, *Feline Pract* 25:12-19.

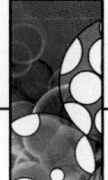

APPENDIX • 1

Recommendations for Core and Noncore Vaccinations of Dogs

Craig E. Greene, Gerryll Gae Hall, and Janet Calpin

			PUPPIES			
DISEASE (CHAPTER)	SEVERITY	ORGANISM SURVIVAL IN ENVIRONMENT	EXPOSURE RISK	VACCINE[a] EFFICACY	OVERCOME MATERNAL IMMUNITY[b,c]	PRIMARY PUPPY VACCINATION[b] (Optional)
Core Vaccines						
Canine distemper (3)	Potentially fatal	Labile: sunlight, dessication; high temperature inactivates	High	MLV: strongest, quickest protection Recombinant: lower	MLV: 12 Recombinant: 12	MLV: (6-8), 9-11, 12-14 Recombinant: (15-18)
Hepatitis (adenovirus) infection (4)	Potentially fatal	Stable: highly resistant; mos to yrs	High	MLV: high Killed (inactivated): lower	12	(6-8), 9-11, 12-14
Canine parvovirus infection (8)	Potentially fatal	Stable: highly resistant; mos to yr	High	MLV: strongest Killed: lower	MLV: 12 Killed: 18	(6-8), 9-11, 12-14, (15-18, especially if killed)
Rabies (22)	Fatal, zoonosis	Labile: persists in reservoir hosts	High	High: established by product	12	≥12; depends on product
Noncore Vaccines						
Canine parainfluenza virus infection (6)	Low	Labile: sunlight, dessication; high temperature inactivates	High in dense population	IN: good, partial protection Parenteral: low	IN: 6; Parenteral: 12	IN: ≥12 Parenteral: (6-8), 9-11, 12-14
Bordetellosis (6)	Low to moderate	Labile: persists in reservoir hosts	High with dense populations	IN: moderate Parenteral: low	IN: 2-3 Parenteral: 12	IN[d] & Parenteral: 9-11, 12-14
Canine coronavirus infection (8)	Mild	Stable: environment 2 mos	High in dense populations	Partial protection	12	(6-8), 9-11, 12-14
Leptospirosis (44)	Subclinical to fatal, zoonotic risk	Labile: wildlife and domestic reservoirs	Geographic and seasonal	Variable response, serovar specific	12	9-11, 12-14
Borreliosis (45)	Mild to moderate	Labile: tick reservoir	Geographic and seasonal	Effective if given prior to any tick exposure	Unknown	8-11, 12-14
Giardiasis (78)	Mild	Stable: high in unsanitary conditions	Variable	Reduce organism replication	Unknown	8-11, 12-14

		ADULTS		
DISEASE (CHAPTER)	SUBSEQUENT BOOSTERS	PRIMARY ADULT VACCINATION°	ESTABLISHED LONG-TERM DURATION OF IMMUNITY WITH CHALLENGE^e	COMMENTS/REACTIONS
Core Vaccines				
Canine distemper (3)	1 yr; thereafter 1-3 yrs depending on environmental exposure and vaccine type used	2 doses all products	MLV: ≥7 yrs sterile immunity (Rockborn and Snyder Hill strains); ≥5 yrs (Onderstepoort strain) Recombinant: ≥1 yr	Variable DOI of MLV products is based on vaccine strain. MLV products provide strongest protection but there is potential of postvaccinal encephalitis or hypertrophic osteodystrophy. DOI of recombinant products has not been established beyond 1 yr. Boosters could be extended to 3 yrs if primary vaccination series uses MLV product. Recombinant vaccines should not be used in previously unvaccinated dogs exposed to high population density and/or highly contaminated environments. Distemper/measles combination vaccine is only recommended for IM use in pups <12 wks for first vaccine if the environment is highly contaminated and routine distemper immunization beginning at 6-8 wks does not control vaccine breaks.
Hepatitis (adenovirus) infection (4)	1 yr; thereafter 3 yrs for MLV and 1 yr if only killed (inactivated) used	MLV: 1 dose Killed: 2 doses	MLV: ≥7 yrs sterile immunity Killed: 1 yr	CAV-2 vaccines have fewer adverse reactions compared to CAV-1, which can cause "blue eye" reaction. CAV-2 vaccines are preferred and are effective against infections causing tracheobronchitis and systemic infection by CAV-1. For these reasons, vaccines containing CAV-1 are not recommended.
Canine parvovirus infection (8)	1 yr; thereafter 3 yrs for MLV and 1 yr for killed unless as initial series	MLV: 1 dose Killed: 2 doses	MLV: ≥7 yrs sterile immunity Killed virus ≥mos	MDA blockade is strong. Potentiated products are most effective in overcoming this blockade. Cross protection between all strains CPV2, 2a, 2b, 2c exists. Killed vaccines do not break through MDA as well as MLV vaccines. Vaccinate to at least 16 wks with killed products and do not use them for animals housed in high density and/or highly contaminated environments. Killed vaccine may protect >1 yr as vaccinated animals have a likely risk of exposure to virulent virus or MLV virus in the environment which boosts their immunity.
Rabies (22)	1 yr; thereafter 1-3 yrs, see comments	1 dose all products	1 or 3 yrs	Adjuvanted vaccines have potential to cause allergic or neoplastic complications. State and local public health laws govern the frequency of administration.
Noncore Vaccines				
Canine parainfluenza virus infection (6)	1 yr for animals in high-risk environments; 3 yrs for others	IN: 1 dose Parenteral: 2 doses	IN and parenteral: up to 1 yr; however, no long-term studies available	Recommended for dogs in shelters, kennels, shows, large colonies, or breeding establishments. Use IN vaccine at least 1-2 wks prior to exposure for optimal protection. Natural resistance develops with increasing age.
Bordetellosis (6)	1 yr; thereafter IN at least 1 wk prior to anticipated	Killed injectable: 2 doses 2-4 wks	Natural infection: partial protection for 6-12 mos	MLV IN vaccine is recommended for dogs in shelters, kennels, shows, large colonies, or breeding establishments. Prevalence of postvaccinal illness is low and is characterized

DISEASE (CHAPTER)	SUBSEQUENT BOOSTERS	PRIMARY ADULT VACCINATION[a]	ESTABLISHED LONG-TERM DURATION OF IMMUNITY WITH CHALLENGE[e]	COMMENTS/REACTIONS
	exposure	apart MLV IN: 1 dose	Longest vaccine challenge study is 10 mos; most are ≤1 mo.	by rhinitis with persistent sneezing, cough, and nasal discharge. Should these signs persist, antimicrobial therapy is indicated. Avoid IN MLV in immunosuppressed animals. Purification of killed parenteral vaccine has reduced side effects of hypersensitivity but has also reduced potency. Alternating parenteral or IN vaccines, and using at least 3 doses in the initial series increases the primary immune response to challenge.
Canine coronavirus infection (8)	1 yr, if indicated	MLV: 1 dose Killed: 2 doses	Unknown, no long-term studies. Protection is partial.	Incidence is high in shelter, show, and breeding environments. Routine use is of questionable benefit. Disease is mild. Immunity is transient. Adverse reaction rates for vaccines are low, although adjuvants in killed products may increase reaction to leptospiral or high-titer CPV vaccines. MLV vaccine has no adjuvants and better breakthrough.
Leptospirosis (44)	1 yr, if indicated	Minimum of 2 doses, 2-4 wks apart	1 yr partial protection based on unpublished vaccine manufacturers' data. Protection against carrier state is variable.	Some products may cause anaphylaxis. Purification has been increased since combined with coronaviral products. Should not begin vaccination <9 wks of age because of increased rate of fatal complications in younger animals. Older animals are more consistently protected. Vaccines should include products with most commonly observed serovars.
Borreliosis (45)	1 yr, if indicated; thereafter preferably prior to tick season	2 doses 3-4 wks apart	1 yr based on vaccine licensing data; all companies have 1 yr licensing challenge data	Young (<24 wks) animals are more at risk. Where exposure rate is high, disease incidence is low. Side effects associated with vaccine are controversial. Subunit products are less reactive; however, whole-cell products may produce more consistent initial protection. Following at least 3 vaccines, especially subunit vaccines, immune response is more consistently protective.
Giardiasis (78)	1 yr, if indicated	2 doses 2-4 wks apart	1 yr based on vaccine licensing data; use in adults questionable	Animals vaccinated prior to exposure had reduced clinical signs of diarrhea and intestinal replication of organisms. Oocyst shedding was reduced. Disease is generally mild or subclinical, even in neonates.

MLV, Modified live virus; IN, intranasal; DOI, duration of immunity; IM, intramuscular; MDA, maternally derived antibodies; CPV, canine parvovirus; CAV, canine adenovirus.

References: Coyne MJ, Burr HH, Yule TD, et al. 2001. Duration of immunity in dogs after vaccination or naturally acquired infection, *Vet Rec* 149:509-515; Paul MA, Appel M, Barrett R, et al. 2003.

Report of the American Animal Hospital Association (AAHA) canine vaccination task force: Executive summary and 2003 canine vaccine guidelines and recommendations, *J Am Anim Hosp Assoc* 39:119-131; Klingborg DJ, Hustead DR, Curry-Galvin EA. 2002. AVMA Council on biologic and therapeutic agents' report on cat and dog vaccinations, *J Am Vet Med Assoc* 21:1401-1407.

[a]See Appendix 3 for vaccine types.
[b]Age in weeks.
[c]See Tables 100-2, 100-3 and 100-4 for details on maternal immunity transfer and vaccine blockade.
[d]Some IN vaccines are licensed for use as early as 2-3 weeks of age.
[e]See also Table 100-12A for specifics on long-term (≥8 wks) duration of immunity.

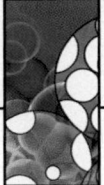

APPENDIX • 2

Recommendations for Core and Noncore Vaccinations of Cats

Craig E. Greene, Gerryll Gae Hall, and Janet Calpin

			KITTENS			
DISEASE (CHAPTER)	SEVERITY	ORGANISM SURVIVAL IN ENVIRONMENT	EXPOSURE RISK	VACCINE[a] EFFICACY	MATERNAL IMMUNITY WANE[b]	PRIMARY KITTEN VACCINATION[b] (OPTIONAL)
Core Vaccines						
Panleukopenia (10)	Potentially fatal	Stable: highly resistant; mos to yrs	High[c]	MLV: strongest Killed (inactivated): lower	12[c,d]	(6-8), 9-11, 12-14
Herpesvirus-1 infection (16)	Potentially fatal in young kittens	Fragile: short survival time	High[c]	MLV: strongest Killed: lower	12[c,d]	(6-8), 9-11, 12-14
Calicivirus infection (16)	Potentially fatal	Stable: moderately resistant; survives about 2 wks	High[c]	MLV: strongest Killed: lower	12[c,d]	(6-8), 9-11, 12-14
Rabies (22)	Fatal, zoonosis	Labile: persists in reservoir hosts	High	High: established by product	NA	≥12 depends on product; canarypox-vectored vaccine can be administered at 8 wks
Noncore Vaccines						
Chlamydophila felis infection (30)	Mild to moderate[d]	Labile: environmentally very unstable[d]	High in contaminated environment	MLV: low to moderate Killed: low	Unknown	9-11, 12-14
Bordetella bronchiseptica infection (16)	Low to moderate	Labile: persists in reservoir hosts	High in contaminated environment	IN: low[c]	IN: approximately 6 wks	≥8, 1 dose (label)
Feline infectious peritonitis (coronavirus infection) (11)	FECV infection: low FIP: fatal	Stable: persists in environment about 2 mos	FECV: high FIPV: low	IN: low	Approximately 6 wks	≥16, 2 doses 3-4 wks apart
Giardiasis (78)	Subclinical to severe[d]	Stable: high in unsanitary conditions	Variable	Reduces organism replication	Unknown	8-11, 12-14
Feline leukemia (13)	Fatal	Labile: 24-48 hrs at moist warm temperatures	Moderate to high with long-term exposure to a positive cat	−14% to 100% depending on study	Approximately 12 wks	9-11, 12-14
Feline AIDS (14)	High	Labile	Moderate to high with one exposure	0% to 82%	12[e]	9-11, 12-14

| DISEASE (CHAPTER) | SUBSEQUENT BOOSTERS | ADULTS | | COMMENTS/REACTIONS |
		PRIMARY VACCINATION ADULT[a]	ESTABLISHED LONG-TERM DURATION OF IMMUNITY WITH CHALLENGE[f]	
Core Vaccines				
Panleukopenia (10)	1 yr; thereafter 1-3 yrs depending on environmental exposure and vaccine type used	MLV: 1 dose Killed (inactivated): 2 doses	7 yrs sterile immunity[d] 30 mos[g] sterile immunity	Highly recommended for all cats. In most cats, protection derived following administration of booster vaccination 1 yr after primary vaccination is sustained for at least 3 yrs and probably longer. MLV vaccines should not be administered to pregnant queens or kittens <4 wks old. IN is less effective than parenteral because fewer virus particles reach lymphoid tissue.
Herpesvirus-1 infection (16)	1 yr; thereafter 1-3 yrs depending on environmental exposure and vaccine type used	MLV: 1 dose Killed: 2 doses	7 yrs[d] and 36 mos[g] with decrease in clinical signs	Highly recommended for all cats. MLV vaccines should not be administered to pregnant queens. IN is capable of inducing a local immune response in the face of high MDA titers. Can administer >2 wks of age. All vaccines reduce clinical signs of disease; they do not prevent infection.
Calicivirus infection (16)	1 yr; thereafter 1-3 yrs depending on environmental exposure and vaccine type used	MLV: 1 dose Killed: 2 doses	7 yrs[d] and 36 mos[g] with decrease in clinical signs	Highly recommended for all cats; MLV vaccines should not be administered to pregnant queens. IN is capable of inducing a local immune response in the face of high MDA titers. Can administer >2 wks of age. All vaccines reduce clinical signs of disease; they do not prevent infection. They do not induce protection from all isolates FCV.
Rabies (22)	1 yr; thereafter 1-3 yrs, see comments	1 dose all products	1 or 3 yrs	Highly recommended for all cats. Adjuvanted vaccines have the potential to cause allergic or neoplastic complications. One recombinant nonadjuvanted product available for 1-yr duration. State and local public health laws govern the frequency of administration.
Noncore Vaccines				
Bordetella bronchiseptica infection (16)	1 yr; thereafter IN at least 1 wk prior to anticipated exposure	MLV: 1 dose	3 wks following 1 dose at 4 wks of age (as per label) with decrease in clinical signs	Not recommended for routine use. Can be used in cats in large groups (shelters, catteries, shows, breeding establishments) where organism has been documented. Prevalence of postvaccinal illness is low, characterized by rhinitis with persistent sneezing, cough, and nasal discharge. Should these signs persist, antimicrobial therapy is indicated. Avoid IN MLV in immunosuppressed animals.
Chlamydophila felis infection (30)	1 yr; thereafter annually if indicated	MLV: 1 dose Killed: 2 doses	13-mos data available from manufacturers with decrease in clinical signs	Not recommended for routine use. Consider for use in in multiple-cat environments where *C. felis* infections associated with clinical disease have been documented. May cause transitory fever and lethargy. Antimicrobials are effective in controlling the clinical illness.

Continued

		ADULTS—cont'd		
DISEASE (CHAPTER)	**SUBSEQUENT BOOSTERS**	**PRIMARY VACCINATION ADULT**[a]	**ESTABLISHED LONG-TERM DURATION OF IMMUNITY WITH CHALLENGE**[f]	**COMMENTS/REACTIONS**
Feline infectious peritonitis (coronavirus infection) (11)	1 yr; thereafter annually if indicated	MLV: 2 doses, 3-4 wks apart	12-mos field exposure	Not recommended for routine use. At this time, there is insufficient evidence to support the conclusion that the vaccine induces clinically relevant protection.
Feline leukemia (13)	1 yr; thereafter annually if indicated	2 doses, 2-4 wks apart for all products	Killed-adjuvanted (some): 1 yr Recombinant-vectored: 28 days	Recommended for cats that are not restricted to a closed, indoor, FeLV-negative environment; most important for cats <16 wks old. Not recommended for cats >16 wks old with minimal to no risk of exposure to FeLV-infected cats.
Feline AIDS (14)	1 yr; thereafter annually if indicated	3 doses, 2-4 wks apart	Not available	Not recommended. Vaccinated cats will become seropositive as determined by the currently available, commercial antibody-based diagnostic tests. This may complicate existing testing guidelines and disease control strategies.
Giardiasis (78)	1 yr; thereafter annually if indicated	2 doses, 2-4 wks apart	1 yr based on vaccine licensing data; of questionable use in adults	Not recommended for routine use. Vaccination may be considered as a component of a comprehensive control program in multiple-cat environments in which infections associated with clinical disease have been documented.

MLV, Modified live virus; *IN*, intranasal; *FECV*, feline enteric coronavirus; *FIP(V)*, feline infectious peritonitis (virus); *AIDS*, acquired immunodeficiency syndrome; *MDA*, maternally derived antibodies; *FCV*, feline calicivirus; *FeLV*, feline leukemia virus.

References: Elston T, Rodan I, Flemming D, et al. 2001a. Report of the American Association of Feline Practitioners (AAFP) and Academy of Feline Medicine (AFM) advisory panel on feline vaccines. Part 1, *Compend Cont Educ Pract Vet* 23(2):116-126; Elston T, Rodan I, Fleming D, et al. 2001b. Report of the American Association of Feline Practitioners (AAFP) and Academy of Feline Medicine (AFM) advisory panel on feline vaccines. Part II. Feline vaccine liability and management, *Compend Cont Educ Pract Vet* 23:116-126; Lappin MR, Andrews J, Simpson D, et al. 2002. Use of serologic tests to predict resistance to feline herpesvirus 1, feline calicivuris and feline parvovirus infection in cats, *J Am Vet Med Assoc* 220:38-42; Klingborg DJ, Hustead DR, Curry-Galvin EA. 2002. AVMA Council on biologic and therapeutic agents' report on cat and dog vaccinations, *J Am Vet Med Assoc* 21:1401-1407. MacDonald K, Levy JK, Tucker SJ, et al. 2004. Effects of passive transfer of immunity on results of diagnostic tests for antibodies against FIV in kittens born to vaccinated queens, *J Am Vet Med Assoc* 225:1554-1557.

[a]See Appendix 3 for vaccine types.
[b]Age in weeks.
[c]See Klingborn et al. 2002, above.
[d]See Elston et al. 2001a and 2001b.
[e]See MacDonald et al. 2004.
[f]See Table 100-12B for specifics on long-term (≥8 wks) duration of immunity.
[g]See Lappin et al. 2002, above.

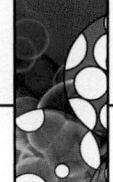

APPENDIX • 3

Canine and Feline Biologics Manufacturers and Products Available Worldwide

Gerryll Gae Hall and Craig E. Greene

USA MANUFACTURERS/ DISTRIBUTORS	ADDRESS	CUSTOMER (C) OR TECHNICAL (T) SERVICE PHONES
AGRI LABORATORIES LTD.	20927 State Route K, P.O. Box 3103, St. Joseph, MO 64503 www.agrilabs.com	C: 816-233-9533 T: 800-542-8916
ASPEN VET RESOURCES, INC.	3701-A NE Kimball Dr., Kansas City, MO 64161	C: 816-413-1444 T: 816-413-1444
BIOCOR ANIMAL HEALTH, INC.	2720 North 84th St., Omaha, NE 68134 or www.pfizer.com	C: 800-441-7480 T: 800-441-7480
BOEHRINGER INGELHEIM ANIMAL HEALTH, INC.	2621 North Belt Hwy., St. Joseph, MO 64506 www.boehringer-ingelheim.com/corporate/products/prod_animal.htm	C: 816-233-1385 T: 800-325-9167
DELMONT LABORATORIES, INC.	715 Harvard Ave., P.O. Box 269, Swarthmore, PA 19081 www.delmont.com	C: 800-562-5541 T: 800-562-5541
DURVET, INC.	100 S. E. Magellan Dr., Blue Springs, MO 64014 www.durvet.com	C: 800-821-5570 T: 800-821-5570
FORT DODGE ANIMAL HEALTH	9225 Indian Creek Pkwy., P.O. Box 25945, Overland Park, KS 66225-5945 www.wyeth.com/divisions/fort_dodge.asp	C: 800-685-5656 T: 800-533-8536
HESKA CORP.	3760 Rocky Mountain Ave, Loveland, CO 80538 www.heska.com	C: 800-464-3752 T: 800-464-3752
IMMVAC, INC.	6080 Bass Ln., Columbia, MO 65201 www.immvac.com	C: 573-443-5363 T: 573-443-5363
INTERVET, INC.	29160 Intervet Ln., P.O. Box 318, Millsboro, DE 19966 www.intervetusa.com	C: 800-441-8272 T: 800-992-8051
MERIAL LTD.	3239 Satellite Blvd., Duluth, GA 30096-4640 us.merial.com	C: 888-637-4251 (ext. 1) T: 888-637-4251 (ext. 3)
NEOTECH, LLC	10061 Hwy. 22, Dresden, TN 38225	C:877-636-8324 T: 731-364-5856
PFIZER ANIMAL HEALTH, INC.	Whiteland Business Park, 812 Springdale Dr., Exton, PA 19341 www.pfizer.com	C: 800-733-5500 T: 800-366-5288
RX VETERINARY PRODUCTS (FIRST COMPANION)	4869 East Raines Rd., Memphis, TN 38115	C: 800-338-3362 T: 800-338-3362
SCHERING-PLOUGH ANIMAL HEALTH CORP.	556 Morris Ave., Summit, NJ 07901-1330 www.spah.com/home.com www.MyVetOnline.com	C: 800-521-5767 T: 800-224-5318
VACCICEL	P.O. Box 847, 101 Greenbrair St., Belton, TX 76513	C: 254-939-7778 T: 254-939-7778
VIRBAC CORP.	3200 Meacham Blvd, Fort Worth, TX 76137 www.virbaccorp.com	C: 800-338-3659 T: 800-338-3659

SELECTED INTERNATIONAL MANUFACTURERS	ADDRESS	VOICE (V) PHONE OR FAX (F)
FORT DODGE	Global Headquarters: 9225 Indian Creek Pkwy., P.O. Box 25945, Overland Park, KS 66225-5945 Regional Offices: Australia, Thailand, Canada, Japan, and the Netherlands. For Latin America, Africa, Eastern Europe, Singapore, Soviet Republics and Middle East: us fax www.wyeth.com/divisions/fort_dodge.asp	V: 913-664-7301 F: 913-664-7062
INTERVET INTERNATIONAL	P.O. Box 31, 5830AA Boxmeer, Netherlands Regional Offices: Australia, Belgium, Brazil, Canada, Colombia, Denmark, Finland, France, Germany, Greece, Hong Kong, Hungary, Indonesia, Ireland, Italy, Japan, Malaysia, Mexico, Netherlands, Norway, Philippines, Poland, Portugal, Russia, South Africa, Spain, Switzerland, Thailand, Turkey, United Kingdom www.intervet.com	V: 31-485-587600 F: 31-485-577333
MERIAL LTD	3239 Satellite Blvd., Duluth, GA 30096-4640 Regional Offices: Argentina, Belgium, Brazil, Canada, Colombia, Denmark, France, Germany, Italy, Mexico, Netherlands, Portugal, Spain, United Kingdom, United States of America International Offices: Australia, Hong Kong, Japan, New Zealand, Singapore, South Africa, South Korea, Taiwan, Thailand corp.merial.com/main.html	V: 678-638-3000 F: 678-638-3000
PFIZER ANIMAL HEALTH	Global Headquarters: 235 E. 42nd St., New York, NY 10017 Regional Offices: Argentina, Belgium, Brazil, Chile, Colombia, Costa Rica (for Central America), Denmark, France, Germany, Italy, Japan, Korea, Mexico, Netherlands, New Zealand, Norway, Portugal, South Africa, Spain, Sweden, United Kingdom, Venezuela. www.pfizer.com	V: 212-733-2875 F: 212-733-2875
SCHERING-PLOUGH	Global Headquarters: 556 Morris Ave., Summit, NJ 07901-1330 International Offices: Africa and Middle East, Argentina, Australia, Belgium, Brazil, Canada, Central Eastern Europe, China, Colombia, Denmark, Finland, France, Germany, Greece, Ireland, Italy, Japan, Malaysia, Mexico, Netherlands, New Zealand, Norway, Paraguay, Philippines, Portugal, South Africa, Singapore, Spain, Sweden, Taiwan, Thailand, United Kingdom, Venezuela. www.spah.com/home.cfm	V: 908-298-4000 F: 908-473-3306
VIRBAC	Global Headquarters: 13 eme rue LID, BP 27, 06511 Carros Cedex, France Regional Offices: Australia, New Zealand, China, Japan, Thailand, Vietnam, Taiwan, Philippines, Korea, Brazil, Colombia, Costa Rica, Mexico, United States, Canada, Spain, Portugal, Italy, Germany, United Kingdom, Austria, Belgium, Netherlands, Hungary, Switzerland, France, South Africa www.virbac.com	V: 33-49-208-7100 F: 33-49-208-7165

BIOLOGIC PREPARATIONS			
ANTIGENS	ROUTE	COUNTRY (AS INDICATED)	MANUFACTURERS: PROPRIETARY NAMES

Canine and Feline Rabies Vaccines

Rabies *(see also Chapter 22 and Appendix 4, Compendium of Animal Rabies Control, 2005)*

I	SC, IM	USA, Canada	FORT DODGE: *Rabvac;* INTERVET: *PRORAB;* MERIAL: *Imrab;* PFIZER: *Defensor;* SCHERING-PLOUGH *Rabdomun*
I	SC, IM	Other countries	FORT DODGE: *Rai-Vac* (Latin America), *Rabvac, Trimune* (Latin America, Asia), *Dohyrab, Unirab* (Europe); INTERVET: *Nobivac* (Europe, Asia, South Africa, Latin America); MERIAL: *Rabisin* (France), *Imrab* (many); PFIZER: *Enduracell* (Europe), *Endurall, Defensor* (Latin America, Asia); SCHERING-PLOUGH: *Rabdomun* (many), *Tissuvax* (Brazil); VIRBAC: *Rabigen* (many)
VR	SC	USA, Canada	MERIAL: *PUREVAX Feline Rabies*

Rabies Combined Products

I	SC, IM	Other countries	INTERVET: *Nobivac;* MERIAL: *QUADRICAT, Eurican;* PFIZER: *Enduracell* (Europe), *Felocell* (Germany); SCHERING-PLOUGH: *Epivax, Fiovax* (Germany)
I	SC	Other countries	VIRBAC: *CANIGEN DHPPi/LR, FELIGEN RCP/R* (many)
VR	SC	USA, Canada	MERIAL: *PUREVAX Feline/Rabies*

Canine

Distemper *(see also Chapter 3 and Table 100-9)*

L	SC, IM	USA, Canada	AGRI LABS: *Champion Protector, Performer, Puppy Protector;* ASPEN: *Cooper's Best Companionvac, Solo-Jec;* BOEHRINGER: *Solo-Jec;* DURVET: *Canine Spectra;* FIRST COMPANION: *Imuno-Vax;* FORT DODGE: *Duramune Adult, Duramune Max, Puppyshot, Puppyshot Booster;* INTERVET: *Continuum, PROGARD;* PFIZER: *Vanguard, Vanguard Plus;* SCHERING-PLOUGH: *Galaxy*
L	SC, IM	Other countries	BIOCOR: *Paramune, Adenomune, Commander* (Latin America, Eastern Europe, Middle East); FORT DODGE: *Duramune* (Asia, Australia, Europe, Latin America, New Zealand), *Kavak, Canlan* (Europe), *Duramune* (Europe, Japan), *Galaxy, Duramune* (Asia, Latin America), *Protech, Duramune* (Australia, New Zealand), *Puppyshot, Puppyshot Booster* (Latin America); INTERVET: *Nobivac* (many); MERIAL: *Eurican* (Brazil, Europe, Japan, Latin America, South America); PFIZER: *Vanguard* (Asia, Australia, Europe, Latin America, New Zealand, South Africa), *Enduracell* (Europe), *Rescamune* (Japan); SCHERING-PLOUGH: *Quantum, Epivax, Tissuvax; Procyon* (many); VIRBAC: *CANIGEN* (many)
VR	SC only	USA	MERIAL: *Recombitek*
VR	SC only	Other countries	MERIAL: *Recombitek* (Latin America, Asia)

Measles *(see also Chapter 3)*

L	IM only	USA, Canada	PFIZER: *Vanguard* (combined distemper antigen)
L	IM only	Other countries	PFIZER: *Vanguard* (Asia, Latin America, New Zealand, South Africa)

Adenovirus 1 *(see also Chapter 4)*

L	SC, IM	USA	AGRI LABS: *Champion Protector, Performer, Puppy Protector;* ASPEN: *Cooper's Best Companionvac, Solo-Jec;* BOEHRINGER: *Solo-Jec;*
L	SC, IM	Other countries	BIOCOR: *Paramune, Adenomune* (Eastern Europe, Middle East, Latin America)

Adenovirus 2 *(see also Chapter 4)*

L	SC, IM	USA, Canada, Other countries	See Distemper L and VR, previously
L	IN	USA, Canada	FORT DODGE: *Bronchi-Shield III;* INTERVET: *Continuum RESP, PROGARD KC, Plus;* SCHERING-PLOUGH: *Intra-Trac 3*
I	SC, IM	USA	AGRI LABS: *Performer;* ASPEN: *Cooper's Best Companionvac;* FIRST COMPANION: *Imuno-Vax*
I	SC, IM	Other countries	Biocor: *Adenomune* (many)

Continued

BIOLOGIC PREPARATIONS—cont'd			
ANTIGENS	ROUTE	COUNTRY (AS INDICATED)	MANUFACTURERS: PROPRIETARY NAMES

Parainfluenza *(see also Chapter 6 and Table 6-2)*

L	SC, IM	USA, Canada, Other countries	See Distemper L and VR, previously
L	IN	USA, Canada	BOEHRINGER: *Naramune-2;* FORT DODGE: *Bronchi-Shield III;* INTERVET: *Continuum RESP, PROGARD KC, Plus;* SCHERING-PLOUGH: *Intra-Trac II, 3*
L	SC, IM	Other countries	INTERVET: *Nobivac Pi* (United Kingdom and others)
L	IN	Other countries	INTERVET: *Nobivac* (many); SCHERING-PLOUGH: *Intrac* (Europe)

Leptospira *(see also Chapter 44)*

I	SC, IM	USA, Canada	See Distemper L and VR, previously; FORT DODGE: *Duramune Max, LeptoVax 4;* INTERVET: *Continuum Lepto;* PFIZER: *Vanguard Plus 5 L4*
I	SC, IM	Other countries	See Distemper L and VR, previously

Parvovirus-2 conventional[a] *(see also Chapter 8 and Table 100-10)*

L	SC, IM	USA, Canada	AGRI LABS: *Champion Protector, Performer, Puppy Protector;* ASPEN: *Cooper's Best Companionvac, Solo-Jec;* BOEHRINGER: *Solo-Jec;* FIRST COMPANION: *Imuno-Vax;* PFIZER: *Vanguard;* VACCICEL: *CPV/LP*
L	SC, IM	Other countries	See Distemper L for combination; BIOCOR: *Adenomune* (Eastern Europe, Latin America, Middle East); FORT DODGE: *Parvoid* (Asia, Latin America), *Dohyvac* (Europe, Japan); MERIAL: *Parvodog, Canimid-P, Caniffa, EuricanPF* (many); PFIZER: *Enduracell* (Europe), *Rescamune* (Japan), *Vanguard* (Asia, Latin America); SCHERING-PLOUGH: *Tissuvax, Epivax* (many); VIRBAC: *Parvigen* (many), *Canigen* (Central America)
I	SC, IM	Other countries	BIOCOR: *Adenomune, Parvocine* (Asia, Eastern Europe, Latin America, Middle East); FORT DODGE: *Canlan* (Europe); PFIZER: *Vanguard* (Argentina, Brazil, Chile, Mexico)

Parvovirus-2 potentiated[a] *(see also Chapter 8 and Table 100-10)*

L	SC, IM	USA, Canada	DURVET: *Canine Spectra Parvo;* FORT DODGE: *Duramune Adult, Duramune Max;* INTERVET: *Continuum, PROGARD;* MERIAL: *Recombitek;* NEOTECH: *NeoPar;* PFIZER: *Vanguard Plus;* SCHERING-PLOUGH: *Galaxy*
L	SC, IM	Other countries	FORT DODGE: *Kavak* (Europe), *Duramune,* (Asia, Australia, Europe, Latin AmericaNew Zealand), *Galaxy* (Asia, Latin America,), *Protech* (Australia, New Zealand), *Puppyshot* (Latin America); INTERVET: *Nobivac* (many); MERIAL: *Primodog, Recombitek* (Latin America), *Eurican, Primodog* (Europe), *Eurican, Primodog* (many); PFIZER: *Vanguard* (Europe), *Vanguard HTLP* (Brazil, Thailand, Venezuela), *Vanguard Plus* (Asia, Latin America, South Africa, New Zealand); SCHERING-PLOUGH: *Quantum* (many); VIRBAC: *PARVIGEN; CANIGEN PUPPY 2b* (many)

Bordetella Canine *(see also parainfluenza earlier and Table 6-2)*

I	SC only	USA	AGRI LABS: *Performer Borde-Vac;* PFIZER: *BronchicineCAe*
I	SC, IM	Other countries	MERIAL: *Pneumodog* (France); PFIZER: *Coughguard B, Vanguard 5/B* (Asia, Latin America); VIRBAC: *Canigen KC*
L	IN	USA, Canada	BOEHRINGER: *Naramune-2;* FORT DODGE: *Bronchi-Shield III;* INTERVET: *Continuum RESP, PROGARD KC, Plus;* PFIZER: *Nasaguard B;* SCHERING-PLOUGH: *Intra-Trac II, 3*
L	IN	Other countries	FORT DODGE: *Bronchi-Shield III* (many); INTERVET: *Nobivac KC* (many); SCHERING-PLOUGH: *Intrac* (many)

Borrelia burgdorferi *(see also Chapter 45)*

I	SC, IM	USA, Canada	FORT DODGE: *LymeVax, Puppyshot + LymeVax, Puppyshot Booster + LymeVax*
I	SC, IM	Other countries	MERIAL: *Merilym* (Europe)
I	IM only	USA	SCHERING-PLOUGH: *Galaxy Lyme*
SR	SC only	USA	INTERVET: *Continuum Lyme, ProLyme;* MERIAL: *Recombitek Lyme*

			BIOLOGIC PREPARATIONS—cont'd
ANTIGENS	**ROUTE**	**COUNTRY (AS INDICATED)**	**MANUFACTURERS: PROPRIETARY NAMES**

Coronavirus *(see also Chapter 8)*

I	SC, IM	USA, Canada	FORT DODGE: *Duramune Cv-K*; INTERVET: *Continuum Corona, PROGARD-CvK*; PFIZER: *FirstDose CV, Vanguard, Plus*; SCHERING-PLOUGH: *Galaxy Cv*—feline origin; VACCICEL: *COR-1*
I	SC, IM	Other countries	FORT DODGE: *Duramune* (Asia, Europe, Latin America), *Kavak, Canlan* (Europe), *Dohyvac* (Europe), *Galaxy* (Latin America, Asia), *Puppyshot* (Latin America); INTERVET: *Nobivac* (many); PFIZER: *FirstDose, Vanguard* (Asia, Latin America); SCHERING-PLOUGH: *Tissuvax* (Brazil), *Procyon* (United Kingdom)
L	SC	USA, Canada	MERIAL: *Recombitek, Recombitek Canine Corona-MLV*
		Other countries	MERIAL: *Recombitek* (Latin America)

Endotoxin (Salmonella) *(see also Chapter 39)*

Ab	IV, SC	USA	IMMVAC: *SEPTI-Serum*
		Other countries	IMMVAC: *SEPTI-Serum* (Japan, Korea, Latin America, Taiwan)

Babesia *(see also Chapter 77)*

I	SC, IM	Other countries	MERIAL: *Pirodog* (Belgium, France, Italy, Spain, Switzerland); INTERVET: *Nobivac Piro* (Europe)

Giardia *(see also Chapter 78)*

I	SC, IM	USA	FORT DODGE: *GiardiaVax*
I	SC, IM	Other countries	FORT DODGE: *GiardiaVax* (Latin America)

Herpesvirus *(see also Chapter 5)*

I	SC	Other countries	MERIAL: *Eurican Herpes* (Europe, Latin America)

Staphylococcus aureus *(see also Chapter 36)*

I	SC	USA, Canada	DELMONT: *Staphage Lysate SPL*
I	SC	Other countries	DELMONT: *Staphage Lysate SPL* (Belgium, Brazil, New Zealand)

Feline Vaccines

Panleukopenia (see also Chapter 16)

L	SC only	USA, Canada	AGRI LABS: *Performer*; FIRST COMPANION: *Imuno-Vax 4*
L	SC, IM	USA, Canada	AGRI LABS: *Champion Protector*; DURVET: *Feline Focus*; FORT DODGE: *Fel-O-Guard Plus*; INTERVET: *PROTEX*; MERIAL: *PUREVAX*; PFIZER: *Felocell FPV, Felocell*; SCHERING-PLOUGH: *Eclipse*
L	SC, IM	Other countries	BIOCOR: *Rhinopan* (Eastern Europe, Latin America); FORT DODGE: *Feline 3* (Australia, New Zealand), *Dohycat, Katavac* (Europe), *Eclipse* (Latin America, Asia); INTERVET: *Nobivac Tricat* (many); MERIAL: *LEOCORIFELIN* (Europe), *Corifeline, QUADRICAT* (France), *Feliniffa* (South America); PFIZER: *Felocell* (Asia, Europe, Latin America, South Africa, New Zealand); SCHERING-PLOUGH: *Quantum, Fiovax* (Europe); VIRBAC: *FELIGEN RCP* (many)
L	IN only	USA	HESKA: *Feline UltraNasal: FVRCP Vaccine*
I	SC only	USA	FIRST COMPANION: *Imuno-Vax 3*
I	SC, IM	USA	FORT DODGE: *Fel-O-Vax*; Schering-Plough: *FVR C-P, Panagen*
I	SC, IM	Other countries	Fort Dodge: *Fel-O-Vax* (Asia, Australia, Europe, Latin America, New Zealand), *Pentofel; Fortvax; Dohycat* (Europe), *FPI* (Australia, New Zealand), *Eclipse* (Asia, Latin America); MERIAL: *Eurifel, QUADRICAT* (many); SCHERING-PLOUGH: *FVR C-P, Panagen* (Japan), *Quantum HCP* (many)

Rhinotracheitis (see also Chapter 16)

L	SC only	USA	See Panleukopenia L and I (SC only), previously
L	SC, IM	USA	See Panleukopenia L, previously; SCHERING-PLOUGH: *FVR C*
L	SC, IM	Other countries	FORT DODGE: *FR-FC, Feline 3, FPI* (Australia, New Zealand); INTERVET: *Nobivac Ducat* (Europe)
L	IN only[b]	USA	HESKA: *Feline UltraNasal: FVRC Vaccine*; PFIZER: *Felomune CVR*
I	SC, IM	USA	FORT DODGE: *Fel-O-Vax*
I	SC, IM	Other countries	See Panleukopenia I, previously

Calicivirus (see also Chapter 16)

L and I			See Rhinotracheitis, previously

Continued

ANTIGENS	ROUTE	COUNTRY (AS INDICATED)	MANUFACTURERS: PROPRIETARY NAMES
**BIOLOGIC PREPARATIONS—cont'd**			

Feline Infectious peritonitis virus (see also Chapter 11)

ANTIGENS	ROUTE	COUNTRY (AS INDICATED)	MANUFACTURERS: PROPRIETARY NAMES
L	IN	USA, Canada	PFIZER: *Primucell FIP*
L	IN	Other countries	PFIZER: *Primucell FIP* (Europe)

Chlamydophila *(see also Chapter 30)*

ANTIGENS	ROUTE	COUNTRY (AS INDICATED)	MANUFACTURERS: PROPRIETARY NAMES
L	SC only	USA	AGRI LABS: *Performer;* FIRST COMPANION: *Imuno-Vax 4*
L	SC, IM	USA, Canada	DURVET: *Feline Focus;* FORT DODGE: *Fel-O-Guard Plus;* INTERVET: *PROTEX;* MERIAL: *PUREVAX;* PFIZER: *Felocell;* SCHERING-PLOUGH: *Eclipse*
L	SC, IM	Other countries	BIOCOR: *Rhinopan* (Eastern Europe, Latin America); FORT DODGE: *Dohycat, Katavac* (Europe), *Eclipse* (Asia, Latin America); INTERVET: *Nobivac Forcat* (Netherlands); MERIAL: *Eurifel* (Europe); PFIZER: *Felocell* (Asia, Europe, Latin America, South Africa, New Zealand); SCHERING-PLOUGH: *Quantum*
I	SC, IM	USA, Canada	FORT DODGE: *Fel-O-Vax, Fel-O-Guard Plus*
I	SC, IM	Other countries	FORT DODGE: *Fel-O-Vax* (Asia, Australia, Europe, Latin America, New Zealand), *Pentofel, Fortvax* (Europe)

Bordetella Feline *(see also Chapter 16)*

ANTIGENS	ROUTE	COUNTRY (AS INDICATED)	MANUFACTURERS: PROPRIETARY NAMES
L	IN	USA	INTERVET: *PROTEX-Bb*
L	IN	Other countries	INTERVET: *NobivacBb* (Europe)

Leukemia Virus *(includes combination products; see also Chapter 13 and Table 100-11 for individual products)*

ANTIGENS	ROUTE	COUNTRY (AS INDICATED)	MANUFACTURERS: PROPRIETARY NAMES
I	SC, IM	USA, Canada	FORT DODGE: *Fel-O-Vax Lv-K, Fel-O-Guard Plus Lv-K;* PFIZER: *Leukocell 2;* SCHERING-PLOUGH: *Fevaxyn, Eclipse/FeLV*
I	SC, IM	Other countries	FORT DODGE: *Fevaxyn FeLV* (Europe, Japan, Latin America), *Fel-O-Vax* (Asia, Europe, Latin America, New Zealand), *Pentofel, Dohycat; Katavac, Fortvax* (Europe), *Eclipse* (Latin America); INTERVET: *Nobivac FeLV* (United Kingdom); PFIZER: *Leukocell 2* (Asia, Europe, Latin America, New Zealand, South Africa); SCHERING-PLOUGH: *Quantum Cat FeLV* (many)
VR	TD	USA	MERIAL: *PUREVAX Recombinant Leukemia*
VR	SC	Other countries	MERIAL: *Eurifel FeLV* (Europe)
SR	SC	Other countries	VIRBAC: *Leucogen* (many)

Giardia

ANTIGENS	ROUTE	COUNTRY (AS INDICATED)	MANUFACTURERS: PROPRIETARY NAMES
I	SC, IM	USA	FORT DODGE: *Fel-O-Vax Giardia*

Feline Immunodeficiency Virus *(see also Chapter 14)*

ANTIGENS	ROUTE	COUNTRY (AS INDICATED)	MANUFACTURERS: PROPRIETARY NAMES
I	SC, IM	USA	FORT DODGE: *Fel-O-Vax FIV; Fel-O-Vax Lv-K/FIV*

L, Live, attenuated; *I,* inactivated; *PS,* purified subunit; *SR,* noninfectious subunit recombinant; *VR,* live vector recombinant; *TD,* transdermal; *A,* annual; *T,* triennial; *Ab,* antibody-containing sera

Monovalent and polyvalent products and brand names are listed together based upon the antigen under consideration.

[a]Potentiated canine parvovirus vaccines generally have a higher infectious dose titer and lower culture passage making them more protective than conventional products in breaking through maternally acquireda immunity.

[b]Sometimes recommended intraocularly, with certain brands, and in young kittens..

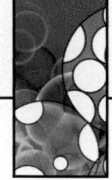

APPENDIX • 4

Compendium of Animal Rabies Prevention and Control, 2006*

National Association of State Public Health Veterinarians, Inc. (NASPHV)

Rabies is a fatal viral zoonosis and a serious public health problem (1). The recommendations in this compendium serve as a basis for animal rabies prevention and control programs throughout the United States and facilitate standardization of procedures among jurisdictions, thereby contributing to an effective national rabies control program. This document is reviewed annually and revised as necessary. These recommendations do not supersede state and local laws or requirements. Principles of rabies prevention and control are detailed in Part I; Part II contains recommendations for parenteral vaccination procedures; all animal rabies vaccines licensed by the United States Department of Agriculture (USDA) and marketed in the United States are listed in Part III.

PART 1: RABIES PREVENTION AND CONTROL

A. Principles of Rabies Prevention and Control

1. **Rabies Exposure.** Rabies is transmitted only when the virus is introduced into bite wounds, open cuts in skin, or onto mucous membranes from saliva or other potentially infectious material such as neural tissue (2). Questions about possible exposures should be directed to state or local public health authorities.

2. **Human Rabies Prevention.** Rabies in humans can be prevented either by eliminating exposures to rabid animals or by providing exposed persons with prompt local treatment of wounds combined with the administration of human rabies immune globulin and vaccine. The rationale for recommending preexposure and postexposure rabies prophylaxis and details of their administration can be found in the current recommendations of the Advisory Committee on Immunization Practices (ACIP) (2). These recommendations, along with information concerning the current local and regional epidemiology of animal rabies and the availability of human rabies biologics, are available from state health departments.

3. **Domestic Animals.** Local governments should initiate and maintain effective programs to ensure vaccination of all dogs, cats, and ferrets and to remove strays and unwanted animals. Such procedures in the United States have reduced laboratory-confirmed cases of rabies in dogs from 6,949 in 1947 to 94 in 2004 (3). Because more rabies cases are reported annually involving cats (281 in 2004) than dogs, vaccination of cats should be required. Animal shelters and animal control authorities should establish policies to ensure that adopted animals are vaccinated against rabies. The recommended vaccination procedures and the licensed animal vaccines are specified in Parts II and III of the compendium respectively.

4. **Rabies in Vaccinated Animals.** Rabies is rare in vaccinated animals (4). If such an event is suspected, it should be reported to state public health officials, the vaccine manufacturer, and USDA, Animal and Plant Health Inspection Service, Center for Veterinary Biologics (Internet: http://www.aphis.usda.gov/vs/cvb/ic/adverseeventreport. htm; telephone: 800-752-6255; or e-mail: CVB@usda.gov). The laboratory diagnosis should be confirmed and the virus characterized by a rabies reference laboratory. A thorough epidemiologic investigation should be conducted.

5. **Rabies in Wildlife.** The control of rabies among wildlife reservoirs is difficult (5). Vaccination of free-ranging wildlife or selective population reduction might be useful in some situations, but the success of such procedures depends on the circumstances surrounding each rabies outbreak (see Part I. C. Control Methods in Wildlife). Because of the risk of rabies in wild animals (especially raccoons, skunks, coyotes, foxes, and bats), AVMA, NASPHV, and CSTE strongly recommend the enactment and enforcement of state laws prohibiting their importation, distribution, and relocation.

6. **Rabies Surveillance.** Laboratory-based rabies surveillance is an essential component of rabies prevention and control programs. Accurate and timely information is necessary to guide human postexposure prophylaxis decisions, determine the management of potentially exposed animals, aid in emerging pathogen discovery, describe the epidemiology of the disease, and assess the need for and effectiveness of oral vaccination programs for wildlife.

7. **Rabies Diagnosis.** Rabies testing should be performed by a qualified laboratory that has been designated by the local or state health department (6) in accordance with the established national standardized protocol for rabies testing (http://www.cdc.gov/ncidod/dvrd/rabies/ Professional/publications/DFA_diagnosis/DFA_ protocol-b.htm). Euthanasia (7) should be accomplished in such a way as to maintain the integrity of the brain so that the laboratory can recognize the anatomical parts. Except in the case of very small animals, such as bats, only the head or brain (including brain stem) should be submitted to the laboratory. Any animal or animal specimen being submitted for testing should preferably be stored and shipped under refrigeration rather than frozen to prevent a delay in testing and to facilitate laboratory processing. Chemical fixation of tissues should be avoided to prevent significant testing delays and

*From the National Association of State Public Health Veterinarians, Inc. (NASPHV). You can visit the NASPHV website at http://www.nasphv.org/4436.html or download the Compendium directly from www.nasphv.org/83416/83301.html.

because it may preclude reliable testing. Questions about testing of fixed tissues should be directed to the local rabies laboratory or public health department.

8. **Rabies Serology.** Some "rabies-free" jurisdictions may require evidence of vaccination and rabies antibodies for importation purposes. Rabies antibody titers are indicative of an animal's response to vaccine or infection. Titers do not directly correlate with protection because other immunologic factors also play a role in preventing rabies, and our abilities to measure and interpret those other factors are not well developed. Therefore, evidence of circulating rabies virus antibodies should not be used as a substitute for current vaccination in managing rabies exposures or determining the need for booster vaccinations in animals (8-10).

B. Prevention and Control Methods in Domestic and Confined Animals

1. **Preexposure Vaccination and Management.** Parenteral animal rabies vaccines should be administered only by or under the direct supervision of a veterinarian. Rabies vaccinations may also be administered under the supervision of a veterinarian to animals held in animal control shelters prior to release. Any veterinarian signing a rabies certificate must ensure that the person administering vaccine is identified on the certificate and is appropriately trained in vaccine storage, handling, and administration and in the management of adverse events. This practice assures that a qualified and responsible person can be held accountable to ensure that the animal has been properly vaccinated.

   Within 28 days after primary vaccination, a peak rabies antibody titer is reached and the animal can be considered immunized. An animal is currently vaccinated and is considered immunized if the primary vaccination was administered at least 28 days previously and vaccinations have been administered in accordance with this compendium.

   Regardless of the age of the animal at initial vaccination, a booster vaccination should be administered 1 year later (see Parts II and III for vaccines and procedures). No laboratory or epidemiologic data exist to support the annual or biennial administration of 3-year vaccines following the initial series. Because a rapid anamnestic response is expected, an animal is considered currently vaccinated immediately after a booster vaccination.

   a. **Dogs, Cats, and Ferrets.** All dogs, cats, and ferrets should be vaccinated against rabies and revaccinated in accordance with Part III of this compendium. If a previously vaccinated animal is overdue for a booster, it should be revaccinated. Immediately following the booster, the animal is considered currently vaccinated and should be placed on an annual or triennial schedule depending on the type of vaccine used.

   b. **Livestock.** Consideration should be given to vaccinating livestock that are particularly valuable or that might have frequent contact with humans (e.g., in petting zoos, fairs, and other public exhibitions) (11,12). Horses traveling interstate should be currently vaccinated against rabies.

   c. **Confined Animals.**
   1) **Wild.** No parenteral rabies vaccines are licensed for use in wild animals or hybrids (the offspring of wild animals crossbred to domestic animals). Wild animals or hybrids should not be kept as pets (13-16).
   2) **Maintained in Exhibits and in Zoological Parks.** Captive mammals that are not completely excluded from all contact with rabies vectors can become infected. Moreover, wild animals might be incubating rabies when initially captured; therefore, wild-caught animals susceptible to rabies should be quarantined for a minimum of 6 months before being exhibited. Employees who work with animals at such facilities should receive preexposure rabies vaccination. The use of pre- or postexposure rabies vaccinations for employees who work with animals at such facilities might reduce the need for euthanasia of captive animals. Carnivores and bats should be housed in a manner that precludes direct contact with the public.

2. **Stray Animals.** Stray dogs, cats, and ferrets should be removed from the community. Local health departments and animal control officials can enforce the removal of strays more effectively if owned animals have identification and are confined or kept on leash. Strays should be impounded for at least 3 business days to determine if human exposure has occurred and to give owners sufficient time to reclaim animals.

3. **Importation and Interstate Movement of Animals.**
   a. **International.** CDC regulates the importation of dogs and cats into the United States. Importers of dogs must comply with rabies vaccination requirements (42 CFR, Part 71.51[c] [http://www.cdc.gov/ncidod/dq/animal.htm]) and complete CDC form 75.37 (http://www.cdc.gov/ncidod/dq/pdf/cdc7537-05-24-04.pdf). The appropriate health official of the state of destination should be notified within 72 hours of the arrival into his or her jurisdiction of any imported dog required to be placed in confinement under the CDC regulation. Failure to comply with these confinement requirements should be promptly reported to the Division of Global Migration and Quarantine, CDC (telephone: 404-639-3441).

   Federal regulations alone are insufficient to prevent the introduction of rabid animals into the country (17, 18). All imported dogs and cats are subject to state and local laws governing rabies and should be currently vaccinated against rabies in accordance with this compendium. Failure to comply with state or local requirements should be referred to the appropriate state or local official.

   b. **Interstate.** Before interstate movement (including commonwealths and territories) dogs, cats, ferrets, and horses should be currently vaccinated against rabies in accordance with the compendium's recommendations (see Part I. B.1. Preexposure Vaccination and Management). Animals in transit should be accompanied by a currently valid NASPHV Form 51, Rabies Vaccination Certificate (http://www.nasphv.org/83416/106001.html). When an interstate health certificate or certificate of veterinary inspection is required, it should contain the same rabies vaccination information as Form 51.

   c. **Areas with Dog-to-Dog Rabies Transmission.** The movement of dogs from areas with dog-to-dog rabies transmission for the purpose of adoption or sale should be prohibited. Rabid dogs have been introduced into the continental United States from areas with dog-to-dog rabies transmission (17,18). This practice poses the risk of introducing canine-transmitted rabies to areas where it does not currently exist.

4. **Adjunct Procedures.** Methods or procedures which enhance rabies control include the following:
   a. **Identification.** Dogs, cats, and ferrets should be identified (e.g., metal or plastic tags or microchips) to allow for verification of rabies vaccination status.
   b. **Licensure.** Registration or licensure of all dogs, cats, and ferrets may be used to aid in rabies control. A fee is frequently charged for such licensure, and revenues collected are used to maintain rabies- or animal-

control programs. Evidence of current vaccination is an essential prerequisite to licensure.

c. **Canvassing.** House-to-house canvassing by animal control officials facilitates enforcement of vaccination and licensure requirements.

d. **Citations.** Citations are legal summonses issued to owners for violations, including the failure to vaccinate or license their animals. The authority for officers to issue citations should be an integral part of each animal-control program.

e. **Animal Control.** All communities should incorporate stray animal control, leash laws, and training of personnel in their programs.

5. **Postexposure Management.** Any animal potentially exposed to rabies virus (see Part I. A.1. Rabies Exposure) by a wild, carnivorous mammal or a bat that is not available for testing should be regarded as having been exposed to rabies.

a. **Dogs, Cats, and Ferrets.** Unvaccinated dogs, cats, and ferrets exposed to a rabid animal should be euthanized immediately. If the owner is unwilling to have this done, the animal should be placed in strict isolation for 6 months. Rabies vaccine should be administered upon entry into isolation or 1 month prior to release to comply with preexposure vaccination recommendations (see Part I.B.1.a.). There are currently no USDA licensed biologics for postexposure prophylaxis of previously unvaccinated domestic animals, and there is evidence that the use of vaccine alone will not reliably prevent the disease (*19*). Animals with expired vaccinations need to be evaluated on a case-by-case basis. Dogs, cats, and ferrets that are currently vaccinated should be revaccinated immediately, kept under the owner's control, and observed for 45 days. Any illness in an isolated or confined animal should be reported immediately to the local health department.

b. **Livestock.** All species of livestock are susceptible to rabies; cattle and horses are among the most frequently infected. Livestock exposed to a rabid animal and currently vaccinated with a vaccine approved by USDA for that species should be revaccinated immediately and observed for 45 days. Unvaccinated livestock should be slaughtered immediately. If the owner is unwilling to have this done, the animal should be kept under close observation for 6 months. Any illness in an animal under observation should be reported immediately to the local health department.

The following are recommendations for owners of livestock exposed to rabid animals:

1) If the animal is slaughtered within 7 days of being bitten, its tissues may be eaten without risk of infection, provided that liberal portions of the exposed area are discarded. Federal guidelines for meat inspectors require that any animal known to have been exposed to rabies within 8 months be rejected for slaughter.

2) Neither tissues nor milk from a rabid animal should be used for human or animal consumption (*20*). Pasteurization temperatures will inactivate rabies virus; therefore, drinking pasteurized milk or eating cooked meat does not constitute a rabies exposure.

3) Having more than one rabid animal in a herd or having herbivore-to-herbivore transmission is uncommon; therefore, restricting the rest of the herd if a single animal has been exposed to or infected by rabies might not be necessary.

c. **Other Animals.** Other mammals bitten by a rabid animal should be euthanized immediately. Animals

maintained in USDA-licensed research facilities or accredited zoological parks should be evaluated on a case-by-case basis.

6. **Management of Animals that Bite Humans.**

a. **Dogs, Cats, and Ferrets.** Rabies virus may be excreted in the saliva of infected dogs, cats, and ferrets during illness and/or for only a few days prior to illness or death (*21-23*). A healthy dog, cat, or ferret that bites a person should be confined and observed daily for 10 days (*24*); administration of rabies vaccine to the animal is not recommended during the observation period to avoid confusing signs of rabies with possible side effects of vaccine administration. Such animals should be evaluated by a veterinarian at the first sign of illness during confinement. Any illness in the animal should be reported immediately to the local health department. If signs suggestive of rabies develop, the animal should be euthanized and the head shipped for testing as described in Part I.A.7. Any stray or unwanted dog, cat, or ferret that bites a person may be euthanized immediately and the head submitted for rabies examination.

b. **Other Biting Animals.** Other biting animals which might have exposed a person to rabies should be reported immediately to the local health department. Management of animals other than dogs, cats, and ferrets depends on the species, the circumstances of the bite, the epidemiology of rabies in the area, the biting animal's history, current health status, and potential for exposure to rabies. Prior vaccination of these animals may not preclude the necessity for euthanasia and testing.

7. **Outbreak Prevention and Control.** The emergence of new rabies virus variants or the introduction of non indigenous viruses poses a significant risk to humans, domestic animals and wildlife (*25-31*). A rapid and comprehensive response should include all or some of the following measures:

a. Characterize the virus at a national or regional reference laboratory.

b. Identify and control the source of the introduction.

c. Enhance laboratory-based surveillance in wild and domestic animals.

d. Increase animal rabies vaccination rates.

e. Restrict the movement of animals.

f. Evaluate the need for vector population reduction.

g. Coordinate a multi-agency response.

h. Provide public and professional outreach and education.

8. **Disaster Response.** Animals may be displaced during and after manmade or natural disasters and require emergency sheltering (http://www.bt.cdc.gov/disasters/hurricanes/katrina/petshelters.asp). Animal rabies vaccination and exposure histories are often not available for displaced animals and disaster response creates situations where animal caretakers may lack appropriate training and previous vaccination. For these situations it is critical to implement and coordinate rabies prevention and control measures to reduce the risk of rabies transmission and the need for human post exposure prophylaxis.

a. Coordinate relief efforts of individuals and organizations with the local emergency operations center prior to deployment.

b. Examine each animal at a triage site for signs of rabies.

c. Isolate animals exhibiting signs of rabies pending evaluation by a veterinarian.

d. Ensure that all animals have a unique identifier.

e. Administer a rabies vaccination to all dogs, cats and ferrets unless reliable proof of vaccination exists.

f. Adopt minimum standards for animal caretakers that include personal protective equipment, previous rabies vaccination, and appropriate training in animal handling (see Part 1.C.).

g. Maintain documentation of animal disposition and location e.g. returned to owner, died or euthanized, adopted, relocated to another shelter, address of new location.

h. Provide facilities to confine and observe animals involved in exposures (see Part 1.A.1.).

i. Report human exposures to appropriate public health authorities (see Part 1.B.6).

C. Prevention and Control Methods Related to Wildlife

The public should be warned not to handle or feed wild mammals. Wild mammals and hybrids that bite or otherwise expose persons, pets, or livestock should be considered for euthanasia and rabies examination. A person bitten by any wild mammal should immediately report the incident to a physician who can evaluate the need for postexposure prophylaxis (2). State-regulated wildlife rehabilitators may play a role in a comprehensive rabies control program. Minimum standards for persons who rehabilitate wild mammals should include rabies vaccination, appropriate training, and continuing education. Translocation of infected wildlife has contributed to the spread of rabies (26-30); therefore, the translocation of known terrestrial rabies reservoir species should be prohibited.

1. **Carnivores.** The use of licensed oral vaccines for the mass vaccination of free-ranging wildlife should be considered in selected situations, with the approval of the state agency responsible for animal rabies control (5). The distribution of oral rabies vaccine should be based on scientific assessments of the target species and followed by timely and appropriate analysis of surveillance data; such results should be provided to all stakeholders. In addition, parenteral vaccination (trap-vaccinate-release) of wildlife rabies reservoirs may be integrated into coordinated oral rabies vaccination programs to enhance their effectiveness. Continuous and persistent programs for trapping or poisoning wildlife are not effective in reducing wildlife rabies reservoirs on a statewide basis. However, limited population control in high-contact areas (e.g., picnic grounds, camps, suburban areas) may be indicated for the removal of selected high-risk species of wildlife (5). State agriculture, public health, and wildlife agencies should be consulted for planning, coordination, and evaluation of vaccination or population-reduction programs.

2. **Bats.** Indigenous rabid bats have been reported from every state except Hawaii and have caused rabies in more than 40 humans in the United States (32-37). Bats should be excluded from houses, public buildings, and adjacent structures to prevent direct association with humans (38,39). Such structures should then be made bat-proof by sealing entrances used by bats. Controlling rabies in bats through programs designed to reduce bat populations is neither feasible nor desirable.

PART II: RECOMMENDATIONS FOR PARENTERAL RABIES VACCINATION PROCEDURES

A. **Vaccine Administration.** All animal rabies vaccines should be restricted to use by, or under the direct supervision of a veterinarian (40) except as recommended in Part I.B.1. All vaccines must be administered in accordance with the specifications of the product label or package insert.

B. **Vaccine Selection.** Part III lists all vaccines licensed by USDA and marketed in the United States at the time of publication. New vaccine approvals or changes in label specifications made subsequent to publication should be considered as part of this list. Any of the listed vaccines can be used for revaccination, even if the product is not the same brand previously administered. Vaccines used in state and local rabies control programs should have a 3-year duration of immunity. This constitutes the most effective method of increasing the proportion of immunized dogs and cats in any population (41). No laboratory or epidemiologic data exist to support the annual or biennial administration of 3-year vaccines following the initial series.

C. **Adverse Events.** Currently, no epidemiologic association exists between a particular licensed vaccine product and adverse events, including vaccine failure (42,43). Adverse events should be reported to the vaccine manufacturer and to USDA, Animal and Plant Health Inspection Service, Center for Veterinary Biologics (Internet: http://www.aphis.usda.gov/vs/cvb/ic/adverseeventreport. htm; telephone: 800-752-6255; or e-mail: CVB@usda.gov).

D. **Wildlife and Hybrid Animal Vaccination.** The safety and efficacy of parenteral rabies vaccination of wildlife and hybrids have not been established, and no rabies vaccines are licensed for these animals. Parenteral vaccination (trap-vaccinate-release) of wildlife rabies reservoirs may be integrated into coordinated oral rabies vaccination programs as described in Part I. C.1. to enhance their effectiveness. Zoos or research institutions may establish vaccination programs, which attempt to protect valuable animals, but these should not replace appropriate public health activities that protect humans (9).

E. **Accidental Human Exposure to Vaccine.** Human exposure to parenteral animal rabies vaccines listed in Part III does not constitute a risk for rabies infection. However, human exposure to vaccinia-vectored oral rabies vaccines should be reported to state health officials (44).

F. **Rabies Certificate.** All agencies and veterinarians should use NASPHV Form 51, Rabies Vaccination Certificate, or equivalent which can be obtained from vaccine manufacturers or from NASPHV (http://www.nasphv.org) or CDC (http://www.cdc.gov/ncidod/dvrd/rabies/professional/prof essi.htm). The form must be completed in full and signed by the administering or supervising veterinarian. Computer-generated forms containing the same information are also acceptable.

REFERENCES

1. Rabies. In: Heymann D, ed. Control of communicable diseases manual. 18th ed. Washington, DC: American Public Health Association; 2004:438-47.

2. CDC. Human rabies prevention—United States, 1999. Recommendations of the Advisory Committee on Immunization Practices (ACIP). MMWR 1999;48: (No. RR-1).

3. Krebs JW, Mandel EJ, Swerdlow DL, Rupprecht CE. Rabies surveillance in the United States during 2004. J Am Vet Med Assoc 2005;227:1912-25.

4. McQuiston J, Yager PA, Smith JS, Rupprecht CE. Epidemiologic characteristics of rabies virus variants in dogs and cats in the United States, 1999. J Am Vet Med Assoc 2001;218:1939-42.

5. Hanlon CA, Childs JE, Nettles VF, et al. Recommendations of the Working Group on Rabies. Article III: Rabies in wildlife. J Am Vet Med Assoc 1999;215:1612-18.

6. Hanlon CA, Smith JS, Anderson GR, et al. Recommendations of the Working Group on Rabies. Article II: Laboratory diagnosis of rabies. J Am Vet Med Assoc 1999;215:1444-6.

7. American Veterinary Medical Association. 2000 Report of the AVMA Panel on Euthanasia. J Am Vet Med Assoc 2001;218:669-96.

8. Tizard I, Ni Y. Use of serologic testing to assess immune status of companion animals. J Am Vet Med Assoc 1998;213:54-60.

9. Rabies and Other Lyssavirus Infections. In: Greene CE Infectious Diseases of the Dog and Cat. 3rd ed. Saunders Elsevier; 2006;167-83.

10. Rupprecht CE, Gilbert J, Pitts R, Marshall K, Koprowski H. Evaluation of an inactivated rabies virus vaccine in domestic ferrets. J Am Vet Med Assoc 1990;196:1614-16.

11. National Association of State Public Health Veterinarians. Compendium of measures to prevent disease and injury associated with animals in public settings. Available at http://www.nasphv.org/83416/84501.html.

12. Bender J, Schulman S. Reports of zoonotic disease outbreaks associated with animal exhibits and availability of recommendations for preventing zoonotic disease transmission from animals to people in such settings. J Am Vet Med Assoc 2004;224:1105-9.

13. Wild animals as pets. In: Directory and resource manual. Schaumburg, IL: American Veterinary Medical Association; 2002:126.

14. Position on canine hybrids. In: Directory and resource manual. Schaumburg, IL: American Veterinary Medical Association; 2002:88-9.

15. Siino BS. Crossing the line. American Society for the Prevention of Cruelty to Animals, Animal Watch 2000;Winter:22-9.

16. Jay MT, Reilly KF, DeBess EE, Haynes EH, Bader DR, Barrett LR. Rabies in a vaccinated wolf-dog hybrid. J Am Vet Med Assoc 1994;205:1729-32.

17. CDC. An imported case of rabies in an immunized dog. MMWR 1987;36:94-6, 101.

18. CDC. Imported dog and cat rabies—New Hampshire, California. MMWR 1988;37:559-60.

19. Hanlon CA, Niezgoda MN, Rupprecht CE. Postexposure prophylaxis for prevention of rabies in dogs. Am J Vet Res 2002;63:1096-100.

20. CDC. Mass treatment of humans who drank unpasteurized milk from rabid cows—Massachusetts, 1996-1998. MMWR 1999;48:228-9.

21. Vaughn JB, Gerhardt P, Paterson J. Excretion of street rabies virus in saliva of cats. J Am Med Assoc 1963;184:705.

22. Vaughn JB, Gerhardt P, Newell KW. Excretion of street rabies virus in saliva of dogs. J Am Med Assoc 1965;193:363-8.

23. Niezgoda M, Briggs DJ, Shaddock J, Rupprecht CE. Viral excretion in domestic ferrets (Mustela putorius furo) inoculated with a raccoon rabies isolate. Am J Vet Res 1998;59:1629-32.

24. Tepsumethanon V, Lumlertdacha B, Mitmoonpitak C, Sitprija V, Meslin FX, Wilde H. Survival of naturally infected rabid dogs and cats. Clin Infect Dis 2004;39:278-80.

25. Jenkins SR, Perry BD, Winkler WG. Ecology and epidemiology of raccoon rabies. Rev Infect Dis 1988;10: Suppl 4:S620-5.

26. CDC. Translocation of coyote rabies—Florida, 1994. MMWR 1995;44:580-7.

27. Rupprecht CE, Smith JS, Fekadu M, Childs JE. The ascension of wildlife rabies: a cause for public health concern or intervention? Emerg Infect Dis 1995;1:107-14.

28. Constantine DG. Geographic translocation of bats: known and potential problems. Emerg Infect Dis 2003;9(1):17-21.

29. Krebs JW, Strine TW, Smith JS, Rupprecht CE, Childs JE. Rabies surveillance in the United States during 1993. J Am Vet Med Assoc 1994;205:1695-709.

30. Nettles VF, Shaddock JH, Sikes RK, Reyes CR. Rabies in translocated raccoons. Am J Public Health 69:601-2.

31. Engeman RM, Christensen KL, Pipas MJ, Bergman DL. Population monitoring in support of a rabies vaccination program for skunks in Arizona J Wildl Dis 2003;39:746-50.

32. Messenger SL, Smith JS, Rupprecht CE. Emerging epidemiology of bat-associated cryptic cases of rabies in humans in the United States. Clin Infect Dis 2002;35:738-47.

33. CDC. Human rabies—California, 2002. MMWR 2002;51:686-8.

34. CDC. Human rabies—Tennessee, 2002. MMWR 2002;51:828-9.

35. CDC. Human rabies—Iowa, 2002. MMWR 2003;52:47-8.

36. CDC. Human death associated with bat rabies—California, 2003. MMWR 2003;53:33-5.

37. CDC. Recovery of a patient from clinical rabies, Wisconsin, 2004. MMWR 2004;53;1171-3.

38. Frantz SC, Trimarchi CV. Bats in human dwellings: health concerns and management. In: Decker DF, ed. Proceedings of the first eastern wildlife damage control conference. Ithaca, NY: Cornell University Press; 1983:299-308.

39. Greenhall AM. House bat management. US Fish and Wildlife Service, Resource Publication 143;1982.

40. Model rabies control ordinance. In: Directory and resource manual. Schaumburg, IL: American Veterinary Medical Association; 2002:114-16.

41. Bunn TO. Canine and feline vaccines, past and present. In Baer GM, ed. The natural history of rabies. 2nd ed. Boca Raton, FL: CRC Press; 1991:415-25.

42. Gobar GM, Kass PH. World wide web-based survey of vaccination practices, postvaccinal reactions, and vaccine site-associated sarcomas in cats. J Am Vet Med Assoc 2002;220:1477-82.

43. Macy DW, Hendrick MJ. The potential role of inflammation in the development of postvaccinal sarcomas in cats. Vet Clin North Am Small Anim Pract 1996;26: 103-9.

44. Rupprecht CE, Blass L, Smith K, et al. Human infection due to recombinant vaccinia-rabies glycoprotein virus. N Engl J Med 2001;345:582-6.

*The NASPHV Committee: Mira J. Leslie, DVM, MPH, Chair; Michael Auslander, DVM, MSPH; Lisa Conti, DVM, MPH; Paul Ettestad, DVM, MS; Faye E. Sorhage, VMD, MPH; Ben Sun, DVM, MPVM. Consultants to the Committee: Carl Armstrong, MD, Council of State and Territorial Epidemiologists (CSTE); Donna M. Gatewood, DVM, MS, Center for Veterinary Biologics, U.S. Department of Agriculture (USDA); Suzanne R. Jenkins, VMD, MPH; Lorraine Moule, National Animal Control Association (NACA); Charles E. Rupprecht, VMD, MS, PhD, CDC; John Schlitz, DVM, American Veterinary Medical Association (AVMA); Dennis Slate, PhD, Wildlife Services, USDA; Chalres V. Trimarchi, MS, New York State Health Department; Burton Wilcke, Jr., PhD, American Public Health Association (APHA).

This compendium has been endorsed by AVMA, CDC, CSTE, NACA, and APHA. Corresponding author: Mira J. Leslie, DVM, MPH, Washington Department of Health, Communicable Disease Epidemiology, 1610 NE 150th Street, MS K17-9, Shoreline, WA 98155-9701.

PART • III

Rabies Vaccines Licensed and Marketed in the United States, 2006

PRODUCT NAME	PRODUCED BY	MARKETED BY	FOR USE IN	DOSAGE (ml)	AGE AT PRIMARY VACCINATION[a]	BOOSTER RECOMMENDED	ROUTE OF INOCULATION
A) MONOVALENT (Inactivated)							
DEFENSOR 1	Pfizer, Inc. License No. 189	Pfizer, Inc.	Dogs	1	3 mos[b]	Annually	IM[c] or SC[d]
			Cats	1	3 mos	Annually	SC
DEFENSOR 3	Pfizer, Inc. License No. 189	Pfizer, Inc.	Dogs	1	3 mos	1 year later and triennially	IM or SC
			Cats	1	3 mos	1 year later and triennially	SC
			Sheep	2	3 mos	Annually	IM
			Cattle	2	3 mos	Annually	IM
RABDOMUN	Pfizer, Inc. License No. 189	Schering-Plough	Dogs	1	3 mos	1 year later and triennially	IM or SC
			Cats	1	3 mos	1 year later and triennially	SC
			Sheep	2	3 mos	Annually	IM
			Cattle	2	3 mos	Annually	IM
RABDOMUN 1	Pfizer, Inc. License No. 189	Schering-Plough	Dogs	1	3 mos	Annually	IM or SC
			Cats	1	3 mos	Annually	SC
RABVAC 1	Fort Dodge Animal Health License No. 112	Fort Dodge Animal	Dogs	1	3 mos	Annually	IM or SC
			Cats	1	3 mos	Annually	IM or SC
RABVAC 3	Fort Dodge Animal Health License No. 112	Fort Dodge Animal Health	Dogs	1	3 mos	1 year later and triennially	IM or SC
			Cats	1	3 mos	1 year later and triennially	IM or SC
			Horses	2	3 mos	Annually	IM
RABVAC 3 TF	Fort Dodge Animal Health License No. 112	Fort Dodge Animal Health	Dogs	1	3 mos	1 year later and triennially	IM or SC
			Cats	1	3 mos	1 year later and triennially	IM or SC
			Horses	2	3 mos	Annually	IM
PRORAB-1	Intervet, Inc. License No. 286	Intervet, Inc.	Dogs	1	3 mos	Annually	IM or SC
			Cats	1	3 mos	Annually	IM or SC
			Sheep	2	3 mos	Annually	IM
IMRAB 3	Merial, Inc. License No. 298	Merial, Inc.	Dogs	1	3 mos	1 year later and triennially	IM or SC
			Cats	1	3 mos	1 year later and triennially	IM or SC
			Sheep	2	3 mos	1 year later and triennially	IM or SC
			Cattle	2	3 mos	Annually	IM or SC
			Horses	2	3 mos	Annually	IM or SC
			Ferrets	1	3 mos	Annually	SC
IMRAB 3 TF	Merial, Inc. License No. 298	Merial, Inc.	Dogs	1	3 mos	1 year later and triennially	IM or SC
			Cats	1	3 mos	1 year later and triennially	IM or SC
			Ferrets	1	3 mos	Annually	SC
IMRAB Large Animal	Merial, Inc. License No. 298	Merial, Inc.	Cattle	2	3 mos	Annually	IM or SC
			Horses	2	3 mos	Annually	IM or SC
			Sheep	2	3 mos	1 year later and triennially	IM or SC
IMRAB 1	Merial, Inc. License No. 298	Merial, Inc.	Dogs	1	3 mos	Annually	SC
			Cats	1	3 mos	Annually	SC
IMRAB 1 TF	Merial, Inc. License No. 298	Merial, Inc.	Dogs	1	3 mos	Annually	SC
			Cats	1	3 mos	Annually	SC
B) MONOVALENT (Rabies glycoprotein, live canary pox vector)							
PUREVAX Feline Rabies	Merial, Inc. License No. 298	Merial, Inc.	Cats	1	8 wks	Annually	SC

PART • III

Continued

PRODUCT NAME	PRODUCED BY	MARKETED BY	FOR USE IN	DOSAGE (ml)	AGE AT PRIMARY VACCINATION[a]	BOOSTER RECOMMENDED	ROUTE OF INOCULATION
C) COMBINATION (Inactivated rabies)							
Equine POTOMAVAC + IMRAB	Merial, Inc. License No. 298	Merial, Inc.	Horses	1	3 mos	Annually	IM
MYSTIQUE II	Intervet, Inc. License No. 286	Intervet, Inc.	Horses	1	3 mos	Annually	IM
D) COMBINATION (Rabies glycoprotein, live canary pox vector)							
PUREVAX Feline 3/ Rabies	Merial, Inc. License No. 298	Merial, Inc.	Cats	1	8 wks	Annually	SC
PUREVAX Feline 4/ Rabies	Merial, Inc. License No. 298	Merial, Inc.	Cats	1	8 wks	Annually	SC
E) ORAL (Rabies glycoprotein, live vaccinia vector)—RESTRICTED TO USE IN STATE AND FEDERAL RABIES-CONTROL PROGRAMS							
RABORAL V-RG	Merial, Inc. License No. 298	Merial, Inc.	Raccoons Coyotes	N/A	N/A	As determined by local authorities	Oral

[a]Minimum age (or older) and revaccinated one year later.
[b]One month = 28 days.
[c]Intramuscularly.
[d]Subcutaneously.

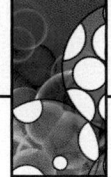

APPENDIX • 5

Laboratory Testing for Infectious Diseases of Dogs and Cats

Geoff Houser, Ashley Ayoob, and Craig E. Greene

Part A: Laboratories Performing Commercial Assays for Infectious Diseases

STATE/ COUNTRY	LAB #	LABORATORY	POSTAL ADDRESS/ INTERNET/E-MAIL ADDRESS	TELEPHONE (P)/ FAX (F) NUMBERS
Many, USA	ANT	Antech Diagnostics	13633 N. Cave Creek Rd., Phoenix, AZ 85022	P: 602-971-4110 800-745-4725
			17672-A Cowan Ave., Suite 200, Irvine, CA 92614	P: 949-752-5612 800-745-4725
			1304 Saratoga Ave., San Jose, CA 95129	P: 408-345-9050 800-745-4725
			3550 S. Jason St., Englewood, CO 80110	P: 949-752-5612 800-745-4725
			10222 N.W. 47th St., Sunrise, FL 33351	P: 954-742-3514 800-872-1001

Continued

STATE/ COUNTRY	LAB #	LABORATORY	POSTAL ADDRESS/ INTERNET/E-MAIL ADDRESS	TELEPHONE (P)/ FAX (F) NUMBERS
		Antech Diagnostics (cont.)	1501 A Belcher Rd., South Largo, FL 33771	P: 727-531-8788 800-872-1001
			4895 S. Atlanta, Suite A, Smyrna, GA 30080	P: 404-367-8344 800-872-1001
			45-608 Kamehameha Way, Kaneohe, HI 96744	P: 949-752-5612 800-745-4725
			5701 W. 120th St., Alsip, IL 60803	P: 708-371-9909 800-745-4725
			11837 Technology Dr., Fishers, IN 46038	P: 317-579-6353 800-745-4725
			11950 W. 110th St., Overland Park, KS 66210	P: 913-529-4391 800-745-4725
			11021 Plantside Dr., Louisville, KY 40299	P: 502-261-0304 800-745-4725
			214 N. Main St., Suite 90, Natick, MA 01760	P: 508-655-8950 800-872-1001
			1390 East Gude St., Rockville, MD 20850	P: 301-251-6142 800-872-1001
			21540 W. Eleven Mile, Southfield, MI 48076	P: 708-371-9909 800-745-4725
			9066 Lacey Dr., Southaven, MS 38671	P: 662-280-2972 800-872-1001
			1111 Marcus Ave., Suite M28, Lake Success, NY 11042	P: 516-326-3900 800-872-1001
			305 E. Ashville Ave., Cary, NC 27511	P: 919-859-0122 800-872-1001
			12616 Southeast Stark, Portland, OR 97233	P: 503-256-1222 800-745-4725
			8432 Sterling St., Suite 102, Irving, TX 75063	P: 972-621-8618 800-745-4725
			1111 W. Loop South, Suite 180, Houston, TX 77027	P: 713-627-9263 800-745-4725
			6360 S. Highland Dr., Salt Lake City, UT 84121	P: 800-745-4725 800-745-4725
			15707 1st Ave. South, Seattle, WA 98148 www.antechdiagnostics.com	P: 206-244-2736 800-745-4725
Many, USA	IDX	IDEXX Laboratories	2320 W. Peoria, Suite B148, Phoenix, AZ 85029	P: 800-444-4210
			1370 Reynolds Ave., Suite 109, Irvine, CA 92614	P: 800-444-4210
			2825 KOVR Dr., Sacramento, CA 95605	P: 800-444-4210
			1245 Reamwood Ave., Sunnyvale, CA 94089-2226	P: 800-444-4210
			1020 W. 124th Ave., Suite 800, Westminster, CO 80234	P: 888-433-9987
			6300 Jimmy Carter Blvd. NW, Norcross, GA 30071	P: 770-903-3430
			501 West Lake St., Suite 208, Elmhurst, IL 60126	P: 888-433-9987
			3 Centennial Dr., Suite One, North Grafton, MA 01536	P: 888-433-9987
			2300 Congress St., Portland, ME 04102	P: 207-856-0929 207-856-8191
			806 Cromwell Park Dr., Suite X, Baltimore, MD 21061	P: 410-242-3540
			80 Commerce Way, Units F-H, Totowa, NJ 07512	P: 888-433-9987

STATE/ COUNTRY	LAB #	LABORATORY	POSTAL ADDRESS/ INTERNET/E-MAIL ADDRESS	TELEPHONE (P)/ FAX (F) NUMBERS
		IDEXX Laboratories (cont.)	48 Notch Rd., Little Falls, NJ 07424 (telemedicine; formerly Cardiopet)	P: 800-726-1212
			12015 N.E. Sumner St., Portland, OR 97220	P: 800-444-4210
			4444 Trinity Mills Rd., Suite 300, Dallas, TX 75287 www.idexx.com	P: 888-433-9987
AL, USA	AL1	Alabama State Veterinary Diagnostic Lab	Wire Rd, Auburn 36830 weblink via AL2 webpage	P: 334-844-4987
AL, USA	AL2	Auburn University	College of Veterinary Medicine, Dept. of Pathobiology, 166 Greene Hall, Auburn University 36849-5519 www.vetmed.auburn.edu/patho/	P: 334-844-4539 F: 334-844-2652
AZ, USA	AZ1	ProtaTek Reference Laboratory	574 East Alamo St., Suite #90, Chandler 85225 www.protatek.com	P: 480-545-8499 F: 480-545-8409
AZ, USA	AZ2	Glen Songer	Dept. of Veterinary Science, University of Arizona, 1117 E. Lowell St., Tucson 85721 gsonger@u.arizona.edu	P: 520-621-2745 or 520-621-2962
AZ, USA	AZ5	Arizona Veterinary Diagnostic Lab	2831 N. Freeway, Tucson 85705 http://microvet.arizona.edu/ AzVDL/index.shtml	P: 520-621-2356 F: 520-626-8696
CA, USA	CA1	Clinical Pathology Laboratory	Veterinary Medical Teaching Hospital, University of California-Davis, Davis, 95616 www.vmth.ucdavis.edu/vmth/ services/clinpath/clinlab.html	P: 530-752-1393 F: 530-752-7373
CA, USA	CA2	California Animal Health and Food Safety Laboratory System (CAHFS)	CAHFS Laboratory (formerly the CA Veterinary Diagnostic Lab System), PO Box 1770, University of California-Davis, Davis 95617 http://cahfs.ucdavis.edu/	P: 530-752-8700 F: 530-752-6253
CO, USA	CO1	Veterinary Diagnostic Laboratory	Colorado State University, 300 West Drake, Fort Collins 80523 www.cvmbs.colostate.edu/dlab/	P: 970-491-1281 F: 970-491-0320
CO, USA	CO2	Plague Branch, Division of Vector-Borne Infectious Diseases	Centers for Disease Control and Prevention, PO Box 2087, Fort Collins 80522 http://www.cdc.gov/ncidod/ dvbid.htm	P: 970-221-6465
CO, USA	CO3	Heska Veterinary Diagnostic Lab	1615 Prospect Parkway, Fort Collins 80505 www.heska.com	P: 800-464-3752
CT, USA	CT1	University of Connecticut	Dept. of Pathobiology, 61 N. Eagleville Rd., Unit 3089, Storrs 06269-3089 www.canr.uconn.edu/patho/	P: 860-486-3738 F: 860-486-3136
FL, USA	FL1	Live Oak Diagnostic Laboratory	Florida State of Agriculture and Consumer Services Dept., Division of Animal Industry, 912 Nobles Ferry Rd., Live Oak 32060 http://www.doacs.state.fl.us/ai/ diag_labs_main.htm	P: 386-362-1216 F: 386-364-3615

Continued

STATE/ COUNTRY	LAB #	LABORATORY	POSTAL ADDRESS/ INTERNET/E-MAIL ADDRESS	TELEPHONE (P)/ FAX (F) NUMBERS
FL, USA	FL2	Kissimmee Diagnostic Laboratory	2700 N. John Young Parkway, Kissimmee 34741 http://www.doacs.state.fl.us/ai/ diag_labs_main.htm	P: 407-846-5200 F: 407-846-5204
FL, USA	FL3	University of Florida	University of Florida, VMTH, Attention Clinical Microbiology, 2015 SW 16th Ave., PO Box 100103, Gainesville 32610 http://www.vetmed.ufl.edu/ path/service/micro/service.htm	P: 352-392-4700 Ext. 4450 F: 352-846-0531
GA, USA	GA1	Diagnostic Assistance Laboratory	College of Veterinary Medicine, The University of Georgia, Athens 30602 http://www.vet.uga.edu/erc/ diagnostic/	P: 706-542-5568 F: 706-542-5977
GA, USA	GA2	Tifton Veterinary Diagnostic Laboratory	PO Box 1389, 43 Brighton Rd., Tifton 31793 http://www.vet.uga.edu/erc/ diagnostic/	P: 229-386-3340 F: 229-386-7128
GA, USA	GA3	Infectious Disease Laboratory	Dept. of Infectious Diseases College of Veterinary Medicine, The University of Georgia, Athens 30602	P: 706-542-5812 F: 706-542-5233
GA, USA	GA4	Centers for Disease Control and Prevention (CDC), National Center for Infectious Diseases (NCID)	Centers for Disease Control and Prevention, Mailstop C-14, 1600 Clifton Rd., Atlanta 30333 http://www.cdc.gov/ncidod/	P: 404-639-3311
GA, USA	GA5	Division of Parasitic Diseases CDC, NCID	Centers for Disease Control and Prevention, Mailstop C-14, 1600 Clifton Rd, Atlanta 30333 http://www.cdc.gov/ncidod/dpd/	P: 770-488-4475
IL, USA	IL1	University of Illinois Veterinary Diagnostic Laboratory	Dept. of Veterinary Pathobiology, 2001 South Lincoln Ave., PO Box U, Urbana 61802 http://www.cvm.uiuc.edu/ ~lamiller/vdl/	P: 217-333-1620 217-344-7630 F: 217-244-2439
IL, USA	IL2	Animal Disease Laboratory	Illinois Department of Agriculture 9732 Shattuc Rd., Centralia 62801-5858 http://www.agr.state.il.us/Animal HW/labs/index.html	P: 618-532-6701 F: 618-532-1195
IL, USA	IL3	Animal Disease Laboratory	Illinois Department of Agriculture 2100 South Lake Storey Rd., Galesburg 61402-2100 http://www.agr.state.il.us/ AnimalHW/labs/index.html	P: 309-344-2451 F: 309-344-7358
IN, USA	IN1	Purdue University	ADDL-West Lafayette, 406 S. University, West Lafayette 47907-1175 www.addl.purdue.edu/	P: 765-474-7440 F: 765-494-9181
IN, USA	IN2	Purdue University	ADDL-SIPAC, 11367 E. Purdue Farm Rd., Dubois 47527 www.addl.purdue.edu/	P: 812-678-3401 F: 812-678-3412
IN, USA	IN3	Mira Vista Diagnostics/ Joe Wheat	4444 Decatur Blvd., Suite 300, Indianapolis 46241 www.miravistalabs.com	P: 866-647-2847 317-856-2681 F: 317-856-3685
IA, USA	IA1	Veterinary Diagnostic Laboratory	College of Veterinary Medicine, Iowa State University, 1600 South 16th St., Ames 50011 www.vetmed.iastate.edu/ departments/vdpam/vdl	P: 515-294-1950 F: 515-294-6961

STATE/ COUNTRY	LAB #	LABORATORY	POSTAL ADDRESS/ INTERNET/E-MAIL ADDRESS	TELEPHONE (P)/ FAX (F) NUMBERS
KS, USA	KS1	Veterinary Diagnostic Laboratory	1800 Denison, Kansas State University, Manhattan 66506 http://www.vet.ksu.edu/depts/dmp/service/index.htm	P: 785-532-5650 F: 785-532-4481
KY, USA	KY1	Veterinary Diagnostic and Research Center	Murray State University, PO Box 2000, 715 North Dr., Hopkinsville 42241-2000 www.murraystate.edu/cit/bvc	P: 270-886-3959 800-745-4725 F: 270-886-4295
KY, USA	KY2	Livestock Disease Diagnostic Center	University of Kentucky, PO Box 14125, Lexington 40512 http://fp1.ca.uky.edu/lddc/	P: 859-253-0571 F: 859-255-1624
LA, USA	LA1	Louisiana Veterinary Medical Diagnostic Laboratory	School of Veterinary Medicine, Louisiana State University, 1909 Skip Bertman Dr., Room 1519, Baton Rouge 70803 www.vetmed.lsu.edu/lavmdl/	P: 225-578-9777 F: 225-578-9784
LA, USA	LA2	Pythium Laboratory, Louisiana State University	Veterinary Clinical Sciences, Louisiana State University, Baton Rouge 70803	P: 225-578-9600 P: 225-578-9526 F: 225-578-9559
MA, USA	MA1	Division of Diagnostic Laboratories	Tufts University, 200 Westboro Rd., North Grafton 01536 www.tvdl.tufts.edu	P: 508-839-7900
ME, USA	ME1	Animal Disease Diagnostic Laboratory	University of Maine, 5735 Hitchner Hall, Room 102, Orono 04469-5735 www.umaine.edu/livestock/diagnost.htm	P: 207-581-2771 F: 207-581-4430
MD, USA	MD1	Quest Diagnostics (formerly Maryland Medical Laboratory, Inc.)	1901 Sulfur Spring Rd., Baltimore 21227 www.questdiagnostics.com	P: 410-247-9100 410-536-1324
MI, USA	MI1	Animal Health Diagnostic Lab	MSU, Diagnostic Ctr for Population and Animal Health PO Box 30076 Lansing 48909-7576 (US Postal); 4125 Beaumont Rd., Rm 122, Lansing 48910-8104 (Courier deliveries)	P: 517-353-0635
MN, USA	MN1	University of Minnesota	College of Veterinary Medicine, Veterinary Diagnostic Laboratory, 1333 Gortner Ave., St. Paul 55108 www.mvdl.umn.edu/	P: 612-625-8787 800-605-8787 F: 612-624-8707
MN, USA	MN2	Wolff Laboratories, Inc.	9025 Penn. Ave. S, Bloomington 55431 www.wolfflaboratories.com	P: 888-642-9085 952-884-3113 F: 952-758-4476
MS, USA	MS1	Mississippi Board of Animal Health and Veterinary Diagnostic Laboratory	PO Box 3889, Jackson 39207 www.mbah.state.ms.us/	P: 888-646-8731 F: 601-359-1177
MO, USA	MO1	Veterinary Medical Diagnostic Lab	University of Missouri-Columbia, PO Box 6023, Columbia 65205 www.cvm.missouri.edu/vmdl/	P: 573-882-6811 F: 573-882-1411
MT, USA	MT1	Montana Veterinary Diagnostic Diagnostic (formerly State of Montana Animal Health Division)	Box 997, Bozeman 59771 http://www.discoveringmontana.com/liv/lab/index.asp South 19th and Lincoln, Bozeman 59718 www.liv.state.mt.us/dolorg/animalhealth/anmlhlth.htm	P: 406-994-4885 F: 406-994-6344

Continued

STATE/ COUNTRY	LAB #	LABORATORY	POSTAL ADDRESS/ INTERNET/E-MAIL ADDRESS	TELEPHONE (P)/ FAX (F) NUMBERS
NE, USA	NE1	Lincoln Diagnostic Laboratories	University of Nebraska, Institute of Agriculture, and Natural Resources, Dept. of Veterinary and Biomedical Sciences, PO Box 830905, Lincoln 68583 http://vbms.unl.edu/nvdls.shtml	P: 402-472-2952 F: 402-472-9690
NH, USA	NH1	New Hampshire Veterinary Diagnostic Lab	Kendall Hall, 129 Main St., University of New Hampshire, Durham 03824 www.unh.edu/nhvdl/	P: 603-862-2726 F: 603-862-0179
NM, USA	NM1	New Mexico Dept. of Agriculture and NM Dept. of Health	Veterinary Diagnostic Services, 700 Camino de Salud, NE, Albuquerque 87196-4700 http://sld.state.nm.us/lab/ default.htm	P: 505-841-2500 F: 505-841-2543
NY, USA	NY1	Diagnostic Laboratory	College of Veterinary Medicine, Cornell University, PO Box 5786, Upper Tower Rd, Ithaca 14353 http://diaglab.vet.cornell.edu/ DL_home.html	P: 607-253-3333 F: 607-253-3943
NY, USA	NY2	Dr. Steve Barr (prior arrangement needed)	New York State College of Veterinary Medicine, Cornell University, Ithaca 14852 email: scb6@cornell.edu	P: 607-253-3043
NY, USA	NY3	Vita-Tech	2316 Delaware Ave #333, Buffalo 14216-2606 www.vita-tech.com	P: 416-798-4988 800-667-3411 F: 905-475-7309
NC, USA	NC1	North Carolina State University	School of Veterinary Medicine, 4700 Hillsborough St., Raleigh 27605 www.cvm.ncsu.edu	P: 919-513-6363 919-513-6357
NC, USA	NC2	Rollins Animal Disease Diagnostic Laboratory	NC Dept. of Agriculture and Consumer Science, Lab.: 2101 Blue Ridge Rd., Raleigh 27607 Mailing: 1031 Mail Service Center, Raleigh 27699-1031 www.ncagr.com/vet/lab/index. htm	P: 919-733-3986
ND, USA	ND1	North Dakota Veterinary Diagnostic Laboratory	North Dakota State University of Agriculture & Applied Science, Van Es Hall, PO Box 5406, Fargo 58105 http://www.vdl.ndsu.edu/	P: 701-231-8307 F: 701-231-7514
OH, USA	OH1	Ohio State University	College of Veterinary Medicine, Veterinary Biosciences, 1925 Coffey Rd., Columbus 43210-1089 http://www.vet.ohio-state.edu/ docs/biosci/services/services. html	P: 614-292-7955 F: 614-292-4688
OH, USA	OH2	ODA-Animal Disease Diagnostic Laboratory	Division of Animal Health, 8995 E. Main St., Bldg 6, Reynoldsburg 43068-3399 www.state.oh.us/agr/addl/	P: 614-728-6220 F: 614-728-6310
OK, USA	OK1	Oklahoma Animal Disease Diagnostic Laboratory	Oklahoma State University, Box 7001, Stillwater 74076 www.cvm.okstate.edu/Depts/ ADL/oaddl/oaddl.htm	P: 405-744-6623

STATE/ COUNTRY	LAB #	LABORATORY	POSTAL ADDRESS/ INTERNET/E-MAIL ADDRESS	TELEPHONE (P)/ FAX (F) NUMBERS
OR, USA	OR1	Oregon State University Veterinary Diagnostic Lab	Oregon State University, College of Veterinary Medicine, Veterinary Diagnostic Lab, PO Box 429, Corvallis 97339-0429 www.vet.orst.edu/biomed/ biomed.htm	P: 541-737-3261 F: 541-737-6817
PA, USA	PA1	Dept. of Pathobiology	3800 Spruce St., School of Veterinary Medicine, University of Pennsylvania, Philadelphia 19104-4192 http://www.vet.upenn.edu/ departments/pathobiology/ microbiology/	P: 215-898-9793 F: 215-573-7023
PA, USA	PA2	Immunology Service Center	VHUP, Room 2016, 3850 Spruce St., Philadelphia 19104-6010	P: 215-898-6882
PA, USA	PA3	PA Animal Diagnostic Lab System (PADLS)	Animal Health & Diagnostic Com, 2301 N Camaron St., Harrisburg 17110-9408 http://www.agriculture.state.pa. us/agriculture/site/default.asp	
PA, USA	PA4	Animal Diagnostic Laboratory	Penn State, Dept. of Veterinary Science, Orchard Rd., University Park 16802 http://adl.cas.psu.edu/default. htm	P: 814-863-0837 F: 814-865-3907
SD, USA	SD1	Animal Disease Research and Diagnostic Laboratory	Department of Veterinary Science, South Dakota State University, PO Box 2175, North Campus Dr., Brookings 57007-1396 http://vetsci.sdstate.edu/	P: 605-688-5171 F: 605-688-6003
TN, USA	TN1	C.E. Kord Animal Disease Laboratory	PO Box 40627, Melrose Station, Nashville 37204-0627 http://www.state.tn.us/ agriculture/regulate/labs/ manual.pdf	P: 615-837-5125 F: 615-837-5250
TN, USA	TN2	University of Tennessee-College of Veterinary Medicine	Dept. of Comparative Medicine, Clinical Immunology Service, RM A -239, 2407 River Dr., Knoxville 37996-4500 http://www.vet.utk.edu	P: 865-974-5643
TX, USA	TX1	Texas Veterinary Medical Diagnostic Laboratory	P.O. Drawer 3040/1 Sippel Rd., College Station 77841-3040/ 77843 http://tvmdlweb.tamu.edu/	P: 979-845-3414 888-646-5623 F: 979-845-1749
TX, USA	TX2	Veterinary Medical Diagnostic Laboratory	Texas A&M University, PO Box 3200/6610 Amarillo Blvd, West, Amarillo 79106-3200 http://tvmdlweb.tamu.edu/	P: 806-353-7478 888-646-5624 F: 806-359-0636
UT, USA	UT1	Utah State University, Dept. of Animal, Dairy, and Veterinary Sciences	950 E. 1440 N, North Logan 84341 www.advs.usu.edu/facilities/ diaglab	P: 435-797-1895

Continued

STATE/ COUNTRY	LAB #	LABORATORY	POSTAL ADDRESS/ INTERNET/E-MAIL ADDRESS	TELEPHONE (P)/ FAX (F) NUMBERS
WA, USA	WA1	Washington Animal Disease Diagnostic Laboratory	College of Veterinary Medicine, Washington State University, 155N Bustad Hall, Pullman 99164-7010 www.vetmed.wsu.edu/depts_ waddl/index.htm	P: 509-335-9696 F: 509-335-7424
WA, USA	WA2	VMRD, Inc.	4641 Pullman-Albion Rd., PO Box 502, Pullman 99163 www.vmrd.com/	P: 509-334-5815 F: 509-332-5356
WI, USA	WI1	Wisconsin Veterinary Diagnostic Lab	WVDL Laboratory—Madison, 6101 Mineral Point Rd., Madison 53705-4494 http://www.wvdl.wisc.edu/ Locations.asp	P: 608-262-5432 800-608-8387 F: 608-262-5005
WI, USA	WI2	Wisconsin Veterinary Diagnostic Lab, Wisconsin Dept. of Agriculture, Trade, and Consumer Protection	WVDL—Barron (Regional Lab), 1521 East Guy Ave., Barron 54812-1207 http://www.wvdl.wisc.edu/ Locations.asp	P: 715-637-3151 800-771-8387 F: 715-637-9220
WY, USA	WY1	Wyoming State Veterinary Laboratory	1174 Snowy Range Rd., Laramie 82070 http://wyovet.uwyo.edu	P: 307-742-6638 800-442-8331 F: 307-721-2051
BC, CAN	BC1	Ministry of Agriculture, Food, and Fisheries	PO Box 9058, STN PROV GOVT, Victoria, BC V8W 9E2 http://www.gov.bc.ca/agf/	P: 250-387-5121
ON, CAN	ON1	Guelph, Ontario, Ministry of Agriculture & Food	Veterinary Laboratory Services, Guelph www.gov.on.ca/OMAFRA/ english/research/labs/index. html	P: 519-826-3535
ON, CAN	ON2	Animal Health Laboratory	University of Guelph, Building 49, McIntosh Lane, Guelph N1G2W1 www.uoguelph.ca/ahl/	P: 519-824-4120
ON, CAN	ON3	Vita-Tech	1345 Denison St. Markham, ON L3R 5V2 www.vita-tech.com	P: 416-798-4988 800-667-3411 F: 905-475-7309
Australia	iAus1	Australian Animal Health Laboratory	5 Port alington Rd., East Geelong Vic, Australia 3220	P: 613 5227 5414 F: 613 5227 5555
Austria	iA1	Bundesanstalt für Virusseuchen-bekämpfung bei Haustieren	Robert Koch gasse 17, Mödling A-2340	P: 43-2236 23 103-0 F: 43-2236 24 716
Austria	iA2	Clinical Virology Group, University of Veterinary Medicine	Veterinärplatz 1, AA, 3rd floor, Vienna A-1210 www.vu-wien.ac.at/kv/seite_ 2.htm	P: 43-1-25077-6094 F: 43-1-25077-2790
Belgium	iB1	Institut Pasteur	Rue Engeland 642, Brüssel B-1180	P: 32-2 3733-158 F: 32-2 3733-174
Belgium	iB2	Laboratory of Immunology	Ghent University, Salisburylaan 133, 9820 Merelbeke http://allserv.UGent.be/ ddmeulen/VPI.html	P: 32-9-2647-387 F: 32-9-2647496
Denmark	iD1	Danmarks Veterinær Institut	Hangøvej 2, Århus DK-8200 www.vetinst.dk	P: 45 35 30 01 00 F: 45 35 30 01 20
Denmark	iD2	Danmarks Veterinær Institut	Lindholm, Kalvhave DK-4771 www.vetinst.dk	P: 45 35 30 01 00 F: 45 55 86 97 00
Denmark	iD3	Danmarks Veterinær Institut	Bülowsvej 27, Copenhagen V DK-1790 www.vetinst.dk	P: 45 35 30 01 00 F: 45 35 30 01 20

STATE/ COUNTRY	LAB #	LABORATORY	POSTAL ADDRESS/ INTERNET/E-MAIL ADDRESS	TELEPHONE (P)/ FAX (F) NUMBERS
Denmark	iD4	Centrallaboratoriet, KVL	GrønnegÅrdsvej 3, Stuen, Frederiksberg C DK-1870 http://www.klin.kvl.dk/Clab	P: 45 35282907 F: 45 35282947
Finland	iFi1	Anstalten för Veterinärmedicin och Livsmedel	Box 368, Helsinki SF-00231	P: 35 8 97 08 51 F: 35 8 97 08 49 799
France	iFr2	CNEVA LERPAS	Domaine de Pixérécourt, B.P.9, Malzeville F-54220	P: 33-383 29 89 50 F: 33-383 29 89 59
Germany	iGer1	Landesuntersuchungsanstalt für das Gesundheits und Veterinärwesen	Sachsen (LUA) Institut Chemnitz Abteilung 4 Zschopauer Strasse 186, Chemnitz D-09126	P: 49-37-15391016 F: 49-37-15391099
Germany	iGer2	Institut für Virologie	Justus-Liebig-Universität Giessen, Frankfurter Strasse 107, Giessen D-35392 http://www.vetmed.uni-giessen. de/viro/homepage.html	P: 49-64-19938350 F: 49-37-15391099
Germany	iGer3	Vet med Lab	Veterinary Laboratory, Institut für klinische Prüfung Ludwigsbürg GmbH Mörikstrasse 28/3, Ludwigsbürg D-71636 www.vetmedlabor.de	P: 49-7141/9 66 38 F: 49-7141/9 66 155
Germany	iGer4	Institutes für Medizinische Mikrobiologie, Infektions- und Seuchenlehre der Ludwig-Maximilians- Universität München	Dienstleistungen/Diagnostik http://www.vetmed.uni- muenchen.de/micro/allgemei. html	P: 089 2180 2528 F: 089 2180 2597
Great Britain (England)	iGB1	Langford Feline Diagnostic Service	Dept. Of Clinical Veterinary Service, University of Bristol, Langford House, Langford, Bristol BS40 5DU http://bris.ac.uk/lvd/lvd.htm	P: 44-117 928 9412 F: 44-117 928 9613
Great Britain (England)	iGB2	The Acarus Laboratory	Dept. Of Clinical Veterinary Service, University Of Bristol, Langford House, Langford, Bristol BS40 5DU http://bris.ac.uk/acarus/ welcome.htm	P: 44-117 928 9287 F: 44-117 928 9505
Great Britain (Scotland)	iGB3	Glasgow University	Dept. of Veterinary Pathology, University of Glasgow Veterinary School, Bearsden Rd, Glasgow G61 1QH www.gla.ac.uk/faculties/vet/ diagnostics/index.htm	P: 0141-330-5773
Italy	iIt1	Laboratorio de Medicina VeterinariaInstituto Superiore di Sanita	Viale Regina Elena 299, Rome I-00161 http://www.iss.it/	P: 39-64 99 02 673 F: 39-64 93 87 077
Italy	iIt2	Instituto Zooprofilattico Sperimentale delle Venezie	Via Romea 14/A, Legnaro (PD) I-35020	P: 39-49-80 70 306 88 30 380 F: 39-49 80 70 570 88 30 046
Italy	iIt3	Clinica Veterinaria Privata, "SanMarco"	Via Sorio 114/c, Padova I-35141 www.sanmarcovet.it	P: 39 049 8561098 F: 39 02 700408367
Netherlands	iN2	Koninklijk Institut de Tropen	Mauritskade 63, 1092 AD Amsterdam www.kit.nl	P: 31 (0)20 568 8711 F: 31 (0)20 668 4579
South Africa	iSA1	Onderstepoort Veterinary Institute (OVI)	The Director, Private Bag X5, Onderstepoort 0110 http://www.onderstepoort.com/ main/intro.htm/	P: 27 (0) 2 529-9111 F: 27 (0) 2 565-6573

Continued

STATE/ COUNTRY	LAB #	LABORATORY	POSTAL ADDRESS/ INTERNET/E-MAIL ADDRESS	TELEPHONE (P)/ FAX (F) NUMBERS
Spain	iSp1	Ministero de Agricultura, Pesca y Alimentacion	Direccion General de Sanidad de la Produccion Agraria Laboratorio de Sanidad dei Estado, Grenada	P: 34-958 44 03 75 F: 34-958 44 12 00
Sweden	iSw1	Statens Veterinärmedisinska Anstalt	751 89, Uppsala www.sva.se	P: 46-18-674000 F: 48-18-309162
Switzerland	iSwi1	Institute of Virology	Faculty of Veterinary Medicine, Wintherthurerstr.266a/CH, Zurich8057 www.vetvir.unizh.ch/frame.html	P: 41-1 635 87 01 F: 41-1 635 89 11
Switzerland	iSwi2	Institut für Veterinär-Bakterilogie	Universität Bern, Längass-Str. 122 Postfach, Bern CH-3001 www.vetmed.unibe.ch/vbi/	P: 41-031 631 26 38 F: 41 031 631 26 34
Switzerland	iSwi3	Diavet Labor AG	Postfach43, Bäch SZ CH-8806 www.diavet.ch	P: 41 1 786 9020 F: 41 1 786 9030

Part B: Laboratory Tests and Interpretation

AGENT (CHAPTER)	INTER-NATIONAL	USA	DETECTION: TEST TYPE	SAMPLE (AMOUNT OR HANDLING)	COMMENTS
			VIRAL, RICKETTSIAL, CHLAMYDIAL, AND MYCOPLASMAL INFECTIONS (1)		
Canine Distemper Virus (3)					
Antemortem	iD4, iSw1	Many	Ag: FA	Blood or buffy coat smear, conjunctival scraping, CSF, transtracheal wash (cytologic smears are air dried and refrigerated, alcohol- or acetone-fixed)	Positive result confirms infection with proper technique; false-negative in chronic (>1 wk) CNS infections; false-positives due to poor lab technique
	iA2, iGer3, iSw1, iSwi3	AL2, CO1, LA1	Genome: PCR	Serum, whole blood, CSF, urine (refrigerated)	Positive result confirms infection if clinical signs are present. False-positive results can occur within several wks following MLV vaccination
	iA2, iD2, iGer3, Sw1	Many	Ab: VN (SN)	Serum: paired samples taken 10-14 days apart (2-3 ml) (refrigerated)	Paired samples: rising (4-fold) titer IgG or high IgM confirms active infection; >1 : 100 single VN (SN) titer indicates relative immune protection against disease
	iA2, iD2, iGer3, Sw1	Many, CA1 NY1, WA1	Ab: FA Ab: VN	As above CSF (1-3 ml) (refrigerated)	As above Positive titer confirms CNS infection if serum contamination is excluded or if CSF titer is high relative to serum titer and titer to another infectious agent; some inconsistencies have been noted. SN titers take such high antibody levels to be detected such that CSF levels may not be measurable
		WA1, TN2, AL2, CA1, IDX	Ab: FA	As above	As above

AGENT (CHAPTER)	INTER-NATIONAL	USA	DETECTION: TEST TYPE	SAMPLE (AMOUNT OR HANDLING)	COMMENTS
Postmortem or tissue biopsy	iD1, iD4, iSw1	Many	Ag: FA	Lung, bladder, cerebellum, or conjunctival smear (refrigerated)	Positive result confirms infection
		Many	Virus: VI	As above	As above
		Many	Lesion: histology	Lung, bladder, brain, liver, stomach (formalin-fixed)	Inclusion body detection with compatible histologic changes indicates infection; some false-positive and false-negative results
	iA2, iSwi3	AL2, MO1, AZ3, TX2, CA1, TX1, LA1	Genome: PCR	Tissues (refrigerated) or in paraffin blocks	Positive result confirms infection
		WA1, NY1, MN1, MI1	Ag: IHC	As above	Specific antigen staining confirms virus in tissues

Infectious Canine Hepatitis (4)

AGENT (CHAPTER)	INTER-NATIONAL	USA	DETECTION: TEST TYPE	SAMPLE (AMOUNT OR HANDLING)	COMMENTS
Antemortem	iSw1	Many	Virus: VI	Oropharyngeal swabs, urine, feces (refrigerated)	Positive result confirms infection
	iA2	CO1, AZ3	Genome: PCR	EDTA blood, urine, liver (refrigerated)	As above
	iSw1	AL2, TX2, NY1, GA2, KS1	Ab: VN (SN)	Serum: paired samples taken 10-14 days apart (2-3 ml) (refrigerated)	Paired samples: rising (4-fold) titer IgG or high IgM confirms active infection; high single VN titer indicates relative immune protection against disease
	iD2		Ab: CF	As above	As above
		CO1	Ab: HA-I	As above	As above
	iGer3	Many	Ab: FA	As above	As above
Postmortem	iD1	Many	Inclusions: cytol	Liver-fresh impression smear (fresh or refrigerated)	Presence of intranuclear inclusions supportive of diagnosis
	iD1		Ag: IHC	Liver	Positive result confirms infection
		Many	Ag: FA	Spleen, liver, brain (refrigerated)	Positive result confirms infection
	iD1, iSw1	Many	Lesions: histol	Liver, gallbladder, kidney, lung, stomach, brain (formalin-fixed)	Compatible histologic changes and intranuclear inclusions indicate infection
		MN1	IHC	Liver, gallbladder, kidney, lung, stomach, brain (fresh or frozen)	Positive result indicates presence of disease

Canine Herpesvirus Infection (5)

AGENT (CHAPTER)	INTER-NATIONAL	USA	DETECTION: TEST TYPE	SAMPLE (AMOUNT OR HANDLING)	COMMENTS
Antemortem	iA1, iSw1	Many	Virus: VI	Nasal swab, vaginal swab (refrigerated)	Positive result confirms infection
	ilt3	Many	Ag: FA	As above	As above
	iA1, iA2, iD2, iGer3, iSwi1, iSw1	KS1, AL2, NY1, IA1, TX2, KY2, ANT	Ab: VN	Serum: paired samples taken 10-14 days apart (2-3 ml) (refrigerated)	Paired samples: rising (4-fold) titer confirms active infection; single titer interpretation only determines prior exposure
	iD2		Ab: IPT	As above	As above
Postmortem	iSwi1, iSw1	Many	Virus: VI	Neonates: lung, liver, kidney, CNS (refrigerated)	Positive result confirms infection

Continued

AGENT (CHAPTER)	INTER- NATIONAL	USA	DETECTION: TEST TYPE	SAMPLE (AMOUNT OR HANDLING)	COMMENTS
	iA2, iGer3	TX2, CO1, MO1, AZ3, TX1	Genome: PCR	Puppy/fetus, tissue (fresh or fixed)	As above
		IN1, IN2, LA1	Ag: FA	Brain, lymph node, liver, adrenal, kidney, spleen, lung (refrigerated)	As above
Canine Parainfluenza Infection (6)					
		Many	Virus: VI	Transtracheal washing, oropharyngeal swab, CSF (refrigerated)	Positive result confirms infection
		IN1, IN2, LA1	Ag: FA	Respiratory washing or tissue section (acetone fixed smears)	As above
		NY1, IA1	Ab: VN	Serum or CSF (2-3 ml) (refrigerated)	Paired serum samples: rising (4-fold) titer confirms active infection; CSF- must show higher relative titer with antibody indexing
	iSw1	OH2, IA1, CO1, IL1, GA1, GA2	Ab: HA-I Ab: FA	As above As above	As above As above
Canine Calicivirus Infection (6)					
		Many	Virus: VI	Oropharyngeal swab, fecal swab, trachea, lung, kidney, intestine (refrigerated)	Positive result confirms infection
Canine Parvovirus Infection (8)					
Antemortem	iA2, iGer3	Many	Ab: HA-I	Serum: paired samples taken 10-14 days apart (2-3 ml) (refrigerated)	Positive titers (level varies with lab) indicate protection; paired samples: rising (4-fold) titer confirms active infection; IgG titer usually increased by the time clinical signs are observed. As a single specimen, high serum IgM titer or fecal Ag examination is more diagnostic of active infection. HA-I and VN titers are considered protective above defined levels
		Many	Ab: VN	As above	As above
		Many	Ab: FA	As above	As above
	iD2	Many	Ab: ELISA	As above	As above
		Many	Ag: HA	Feces or intestinal mucosa (refrigerated)	Positive result confirms infection; clinical disease associated with shedding of large quantities of virus; some shedders are subclinical; false-negative result after 5-7 days clinical illness
	iA2, iGer4, iSA1, iSw1, iSwi3	Many	Virus: EM	As above	As above

AGENT (CHAPTER)	INTER-NATIONAL	USA	DETECTION: TEST TYPE	SAMPLE (AMOUNT OR HANDLING)	COMMENTS
	Many	Many	Ag: FA	As above	As above
	iA2, iD1, iD4, ilt3, iGer3, iSwi1, iSw1	Many	Ag: ELISA	As above	As above
	iA2	CO1, ANT, MO1, AZ3, NY3, MI1, ON3	Genome: PCR	As above	As above
Postmortem		Many	Ag: FA	Small intestine, heart (neonatal) (refrigerated)	Positive result confirms infection
		Many	Virus: VI	As above	As above
	iD1, iGer4	WA1	Lesions: histol	Intestines (formalin-fixed)	As above
		MN1	IHC	Intestines, heart (fresh or frozen)	As above

Canine Coronavirus Infection (8)

AGENT (CHAPTER)	INTER-NATIONAL	USA	DETECTION: TEST TYPE	SAMPLE (AMOUNT OR HANDLING)	COMMENTS
Antemortem		NY1, KS1	Ab: VN	Serum: paired samples taken 10-14 days apart (2-3 ml) (refrigerated)	Single high titer indicates exposure only; serum titer does not reflect degree of protection against infection. Paired samples: rising (4-fold) titer confirms infection
	iD2		Ab: IPT	As above	As above
	iA2	Many	Ab: FA	As above	As above
	iD2	AZ3	Ag: ELISA	Feces (refrigerated)	Positive result confirms infection
	iSwi3	NY1	Virus: VI	As above	As above
	iGer4	IA1, OH2, WA1, IN1, IN2, LA1	Virus: EM	As above	As above
	iA2	MO1, NY3, MI1, ON3	Genome: PCR	As above	As above
Postmortem		Many	Ag: FA	Intestine (refrigerated)	As above
	iD2	Many	Ag: ELISA	As above	As above
		Many	Virus: VI	As above	As above
		Many	Lesions: histol	Intestine (formalin-fixed)	Positive result confirms infection

Canine and Feline Rotavirus Infection (8, 12)

AGENT (CHAPTER)	INTER-NATIONAL	USA	DETECTION: TEST TYPE	SAMPLE (AMOUNT OR HANDLING)	COMMENTS
Antemortem	iSwi3		Virus: VI	Feces (fresh) (refrigerate)	Positive result confirms infection; some shedders may be subclinical carriers
	iA2, iGer4	IA1, OH2, IN1, IN2, LA1	Virus: EM	As above	As above
	iGer3, iSw1	IA1, PA3, SD1, IL2, IL3, KY1, LA1	Ag: ELISA	As above	As above
		Many	Ag: LA	As above	As above
Postmortem		OH2, TX2, IN1, IN2	Ag: FA	Intestine (refrigerated)	Positive result confirms infection
		LA1	Virus: EM	Intestine (glutaraldehyde-fixed)	As above

Canine Papillomatosis (9)

AGENT (CHAPTER)	INTER-NATIONAL	USA	DETECTION: TEST TYPE	SAMPLE (AMOUNT OR HANDLING)	COMMENTS
		Many	Lesion: histol	Oral tissue (formalin-fixed, glutaraldehyde-fixed)	Positive result suggests infection
	iGer4	Many	Virus: EM	As above	Positive indicates viral-induced tumor

Continued

AGENT (CHAPTER)	INTER- NATIONAL	USA	DETECTION: TEST TYPE	SAMPLE (AMOUNT OR HANDLING)	COMMENTS
Feline Panleukopenia (10)					
Antemortem	iGB1, iGB3	Many	Ab: FA, VN	Serum: paired samples taken 10-14 days apart (2-3 ml) (refrigerated)	Paired samples: rising (4-fold) titer confirms active infection. HA-I and VN titers are considered protective above defined levels
	iD2	CO1	Ab: ELISA	As above	As above
	iGer3	KS1, NY1, IL1, TX2, IDX	Ab: HA-I	As above	As above
	iGB1, iGB3, iGer4, iSwi3	IA1, CO1, IL1, IN1, IN2, TN1, WA1	Virus: VI	Feces (fresh) (refrigerated)	Positive result confirms infection; some shedders (usually lower levels) are subclinical carriers
	iD1, iGer3, ilt3, iSwi1, iSw1	Many	Ag: ELISA	As above	As above
	iGer3	GA1, GA2, OH2, LA1	Virus: EM	As above	As above
	iA2	CO1, MI1	Genome: PCR	As above	As above
Postmortem	iD1	WA1	Lesions: histol	Intestine, mesenteric lymph nodes, lung, pharyngeal swab (fresh or refrigerated)	Positive result confirms infection
	iGer4	Many	Virus: VI	As above (fresh or refrigerated)	As above
	iA2	MO1, AZ3, NY3, ON3	Genome: PCR	As above (fresh or refrigerated)	As above
	iGer3	LA1	Virus: EM	As above (glutaraldehyde fixation)	As above
		MN1	IHC	(fresh or frozen)	As above
Feline Infectious Peritonitis (11)					
Antemortem	iA2, ilt3	Many	Ab: FA	Serum, fluid effusion (1-2 ml) (refrigerated)	Positive serum titer at lowest level of reactivity suggests exposure to FCoV; interpretation of higher titer values or high cut-off value must be based upon level of titer with knowledge of exposure of population of cats in environment. Titers vary between labs such that sequential titers should always be done at the same laboratory. The FA titers have the most specificity
		NY1, LA1	Ab: kinELISA	As above	Positive serum titer suggests exposure to FCoV; higher titer levels and knowledge of exposure population can help with diagnosis as with antibody testing by FA
	iGer3, iSw1	Many	Ab: ELISA	As above	Positive serum titer at lowest level of reactivity suggests exposure to FCoV; interpretation of higher titer values or high cut-off value must be based upon level of

AGENT (CHAPTER)	INTER-NATIONAL	USA	DETECTION: TEST TYPE	SAMPLE (AMOUNT OR HANDLING)	COMMENTS
					titer with knowledge of exposure of population of cats in environment. Less specific than with FA methods
	iD3	Many	Ab: PE	As above	High absolute level of globulin and increase compared to albumin is highly suggestive of FIP
		ANT	Ab : 7b (gene): ELISA	Serum (0.5 ml) (refrigerated)	Positive titers range from 1 : 40 to 1 : 640 and indicate exposure to virus; positive cats should be isolated and retested in 4 wks to determine if titer is declining, stable, or rising; vaccination will not interfere with results. Specificity of this titer and its ability to distinguish enteric coronaviral from FIP viral infections is controversial
Postmortem		Many	Ag: FA	Liver, small intestine, kidney (refrigerated)	Positive result confirms infection with virus in extra-intestinal tissues making this test very specific for FIP
	iD1	Many	Lesions: histol	Kidney, liver, small intestine (formalin-fixed)	Compatible histologic changes indicate infection. Can do IHC to detect intralesional virus making this test very specific for FIP
		WA1, MN1	Ag: IHC	Effusion fluid, lymphoid tissue, tissue sample, plasma, CSF (fresh, refrigerated, fixed, or embedded)	Positive result confirms lesions associated with this virus
	iA2, iGer3 iSA1, iSw1	CO2, AL2, MO1, ANT, CO1, NY3, MI1, IDX, ON3	Genome: PCR	Effusion fluid, lymphoid tissue, tissue sample, plasma, CSF (fresh, refrigerated, fixed, or embedded)	Positive result can be seen with enteric coronavirus infection via viral translocation from the gut. Therefore a positive result is nonspecific for FIP

Feline Leukemia Virus Infection (13)

AGENT (CHAPTER)	INTER-NATIONAL	USA	DETECTION: TEST TYPE	SAMPLE (AMOUNT OR HANDLING)	COMMENTS
Antemortem		Many	Ag: FA	Blood film or buffy coat or bone marrow smear (air dried)	Positive result confirms infection and high virus titers that make this test result positive are usually seen in persistently viremic cats. Because of lower test sensitivity, this test is more specific for established bone marrow infections than ELISA methods
	iD2, iGer3, iGB1, iGB3, ilt3	Many	Ag: ELISA	Serum or anticoagulated whole blood (1-2 ml) (fresh or refrigerated)	Positive result confirms infection; ELISA on blood or serum is more sensitive than direct FA; with saliva, false negative results have been reported

Continued

AGENT (CHAPTER)	INTER-NATIONAL	USA	DETECTION: TEST TYPE	SAMPLE (AMOUNT OR HANDLING)	COMMENTS
			Ag: Kits (Appendix 6)	Saliva (fresh or refrigerated)	As above
	iSw1		Ag: Rapid immuno-migration	Blood or serum (fresh or refrigerated)	Positive result confirms infection as with ELISA method
	iGB1, iGB3		Ag: VI	Blood (EDTA) (fresh or refrigerated)	Positive result confirms infection
Postmortem or antemortem		Many	Ag: FA	Blood (heparinized) or tissue, marrow (fresh or refrigerated)	Positive result confirms infection
		ANT, MO1, NY3, GA3, MI1, ON3	Viral genome: PCR	Lymphoid tissue or bone marrow, anticoagulated blood (refrigerated)	As above

Feline Immunodeficiency Virus Infection (14)

AGENT (CHAPTER)	INTER-NATIONAL	USA	DETECTION: TEST TYPE	SAMPLE (AMOUNT OR HANDLING)	COMMENTS
Antemortem or postmortem	iD2, iGer3, iGB1, iGB3, iIt3	Many	Ab: ELISA	Serum, anticoagulated whole blood (1-2 ml) (refrigerated)	Positive result confirms exposure and probable infection with virus
		NY1	Ab: kinELISA	As above	As above
	iSw1		Ab:	As above	As above
		TN1, LA1, IDX	Ab: IgG IFA	As above	As above
		NY1, IDX, NY3, ANT, IDX	Ab: immunoblot	As above	Used for confirmation of nonspecific reactions to the other test methods
	iGB1, iGB3, iGer3	CO1, TN2, NY3, ON3	Virus: PCR	Lymphoid tissue, anticoagulated whole blood, bone marrow (refrigerated)	Positive result confirms infection

Rhinotracheitis Virus Infection (16)

AGENT (CHAPTER)	INTER-NATIONAL	USA	DETECTION: TEST TYPE	SAMPLE (AMOUNT OR HANDLING)	COMMENTS
		KS1	Ab: ELISA	Serum, anticoagulated whole blood (1-2 ml) (refrigerated)	Positive result confirms exposure and probable infection with virus; may be subclinical carriers
		TN1, TN2, IA1, KS1, WA1, NY3, LA1	Ab: FA	As above	Paired samples: rising (4-fold) titer confirms active infection
	iD2, iGer3, iSw1	Many	Ab: VN	As above	Paired samples: rising (4-fold) titer confirms active infection
	iGB1, iGB3, iGer4	Many	Virus: VI	Tissue or exudates (refrigerated)	Positive result indicates infection
	iGB1, iGB3	Many	Virus: VI	Respiratory washing or tissues (refrigerated)	As above
	iGer4	IL1, GA1, GA2	Virus: EM	Lung, trachea, conjunctival smears, feces, CSF, whole blood, body fluids (glutaraldehyde fixation)	As above
	iGer3, iSwi1, iSwi3	AL5, CO1, MO1, LA1, IDX	Viral genome: PCR	As above (refrigerated, not fixed)	As above
		Many	Ag: FA	Smears of lung, liver, kidney, trachea (acetone fixed smears)	As above
		MN1	Ag: IHC	Lung, liver, kidney, trachea (fresh or frozen tissue)	As above

AGENT (CHAPTER)	INTER-NATIONAL	USA	DETECTION: TEST TYPE	SAMPLE (AMOUNT OR HANDLING)	COMMENTS
Feline Calicivirus Infection (16)					
Antemortem		IA1, KS1, TN1, TN2, NY3	Ab: FA	Serum: paired samples taken 10-14 days apart (2-3 ml) (refrigerated)	Paired samples: rising (4-fold) titer confirms active infection. A single high VN titer indicates protection
	iGB1, iGB3, iGer3, Sw1	Many	Ab: VN	As above	As above
	iGB1, iGB3, Sw1	Many	Virus: VI	Oropharyngeal swabs, intestinal and fecal swabs (refrigerated)	Positive result indicates infection
		TN2, ANT	Ag: FA	As above	As above
	iGer4		Virus: EM	As above	As above
Postmortem	iGB1, iGB3	Many	Virus: VI	Trachea, lung, kidney, intestine (refrigerated)	As above
		CO1, CA1, NY3, MI1, ON3	Viral genome: PCR	As above	As above
Feline Foamy (Syncytium-Forming) Virus Infection (17)					
		NY1	SN: Titer	Serum: paired sampled taken 10-14 days apart (2-3 ml) (refrigerated)	Paired samples: rising (4-fold) titer IgG or high IgM confirms active infection; >1 : 100 single VN titer indicates relative immune protection against disease
Feline Cowpox Infection (19)					
Antemortem	iSw1	Many	Virus: EM	Scabs or lesions (dry, sterile vial), fluid (refrigerated)	Positive result confirms infection with Poxvirus
	iGB1, iGB3		Virus: VI	As above	As above
	iGB1, iGB3		Ab: VN	Serum (2-3 ml) (refrigerated)	Positive titer confirms exposure but not necessarily active infection
Feline Papillomavirus Infections (20)					
Antemortem		Many	Lesions: histol	Skin biopsies (formalin-fixed)	A histologic diagnosis suggestive
		CA2, LA1	FA or IHC	Skin biopsies (fixed or embedded)	Positive staining indicates lesions due to papillomavirus infection
Rabies (22)					
	iAus1, iA1, iB1, iD2, iFr2, iGer1, iGer2, iIt1, iIt2, iSp1, iSw1	AL2, KS1, NY3, IDX, ON3	Ab: RFFIT	Serum (refrigerated)	Sufficient titer implies postvaccination immunization *MICROCHIP NUMBER AND VAX HISTORY REQUIRED AT TIME OF SUBMISSION
		KS1	Ab: FAVN	Serum (refrigerated)	Sufficient titer implies postvaccination immunization *MICROCHIP NUMBER AND VAX HISTORY REQUIRED AT TIME OF SUBMISSION
	iSA1	Many	Ab: VN	CSF (2-3 ml) (refrigerated)	High titer means CNS is infected (vaccine or virulent virus); takes 1-2 wks to develop a titer and must compare to serum value

Continued

AGENT (CHAPTER)	INTER-NATIONAL	USA	DETECTION: TEST TYPE	SAMPLE (AMOUNT OR HANDLING)	COMMENTS
Postmortem	iA1, iB1, iD2,iFi1, iFr2, iGer1, iGer2, ilt1, ilt2, iSA1, iSp1, iSw1	Many	Ag: FA	Brain (refrigerated)	Positive result confirms infection; more sensitive than Negri body detection
	Research iFi1, iSA1	Many	Ag: IHC Lesions: histol	As above Brain (formalin-fixed)	As above Negri bodies not present in all cases; false-positive and false-negative results can occur, IHC makes testing more specific and sensitive

Pseudorabies (23)

Antemortem	iD2	Many	Ab: VN	Serum: paired samples taken 10-14 days apart (2-3 ml) (refrigerated)	Positive result indicates exposure; paired samples; rising (4-fold) titer confirms active infection
	iD2, iSw1		Ab: ELISA	As above	As above
		LA1	Ab: LA	As above	As above
Postmortem		Many	Ag: FA	Brain, tonsils, lung, cervical lymph nodes, salivary glands, spleen (refrigerated)	Positive result indicates infection
	iD2	Many	Virus: VI	As above	As above
		Many	Lesions: histol	Brain (formalin-fixed)	Compatible histologic changes and intranuclear inclusions suggest infection

Tick-Borne Encephalitis (26)

Antemortem or postmortem	iA2, iGer3		Genome: PCR	CSF, brain tissue (acute cases only)	Positive result confirms infection

Ehrlichiosis, Anaplasmosis, and Neorickettsiosis (28)

	iGer3	Many	Cells: cytol	Blood films, bone marrow smears (alcohol-fixed or refrigerated)	Positive result confirms infection; many false-negatives due to low numbers of organisms
		Many	Ab: PE	Serum (2-3 ml) (refrigerated)	Nonspecific polyclonal hyperglobulinemia (occasional monoclonal) seen with *Ehrlichia canis* infection and other persistent intracellular infections
	iAus1, iD3, iGer3, ilt3, iSwi2, iSwi3	ANT, AL2, MO1, TN2, TX2, GA3, TN1, TX1, FL3, PA1, MI1, LA1, NC1, IDX	Ab: FA *E. canis*	As above	Positive titer confirms active infection with *E. canis*; however, animal must be infected for at least 30 days to have positive titer. Cross-reactivity with *E. chaffeensis* exists. See Chapter 28 and Table 28-3
		NY3, GA3, ON3	Ab: ELISA *E. canis*	As above	Positive titer indicates exposure or infection, must correlate with clinical signs. Cross-reactivity within genus members is possible. See Chapter 28 and Table 28-3

AGENT (CHAPTER)	INTER- NATIONAL	USA	DETECTION: TEST TYPE	SAMPLE (AMOUNT OR HANDLING)	COMMENTS
	iGer3	LA1, IDX	Ab: *Anaplasma platys*	As above	As above
		MI1, LA1, IDX	Ab: *Neorick-ettsia risticii*	As above	As above
	iD3, iGer3, ilt3, iSw1	LA1, IDX	Ab: *Anaplasma phagocy-tophilum*	As above	As above
	iGB5, iGer3, iSwi3	NY1, AZ3, NY3, ANT, MI1, LA1, NC1, IDX	PCR: *E. canis*	Blood, EDTA anticoagulated (2-3 ml) (sterile, refrigerated)	Positive result indicates active infection with specific *Rickettsia*
	iGB5, iGer3, iSwi3	ANT, LA1, NC1	PCR: *A. platys*	As above	As above
		TN2, NY1, CO1, IL1, MO1, FL3, ANT, LA1, IDX	PCR: *N. risticii*	As above	As above
	iGB5, iGer3, iSwi3	IL1, NY1, TN2, TX2, ANT, LA1, IDX	PCR: *A. phagocy-tophilum*	As above	As above
		KS1, NC1	PCR: *E. chaffeensis*	As above	As above
		KS1, NC1	PCR: *Ehrlichia ewingi*	As above	As above

Rocky Mountain Spotted Fever (29)

AGENT (CHAPTER)	INTER- NATIONAL	USA	DETECTION: TEST TYPE	SAMPLE (AMOUNT OR HANDLING)	COMMENTS
Postmortem or Antemortem	ilt3	AL2, NC1, TN2, TX2, ANT, TX1, FL3, NY3, GA3, PA1, MI1, LA1	Ab: FA-IgG	Serum paired samples (refrigerated)	Paired samples: rising (4-fold) IgG titer confirms active infection; species-specific testing required
	ilt3	AL2, NC1, TN2, TX2, ANT, TX1, FL3, GA3, PA1, MI1, LA1	Ab: FA-IgM	Serum: single sample taken 10-14 days apart (1-2 ml) (refrigerated)	Single positive IgM titer indicates active infection; a second titer may be needed to clarify some low titers
		Many	Ab: LA	Serum: single sample (1-2 ml) (refrigerated)	Single positive latex titer indicates active infection since measures IgM
		MO1, MI1, NC1, ANT	Genome: PCR	Anticoagulated whole blood, tissue	Positive result confirms active infection

Q Fever (29)

AGENT (CHAPTER)	INTER- NATIONAL	USA	DETECTION: TEST TYPE	SAMPLE (AMOUNT OR HANDLING)	COMMENTS
Postmortem or Antemortem		TX2	Ab: FA	Serum (2-3 ml) (refrigerated)	Acute: high phase II antibodies
	iGer3, iSA1	IA1, TX2, TX1, WI1	Ab: CF	As above	Chronic: high phase I lipopolysaccharide antibodies
		NY1	Genome: PCR	Tissues (fresh or frozen)	Positive result confirms infection
		WA1, CA2	Ag: IHC	As above	As above

Continued

AGENT (CHAPTER)	INTER-NATIONAL	USA	DETECTION: TEST TYPE	SAMPLE (AMOUNT OR HANDLING)	COMMENTS
Chlamydial Infection (30)					
	iD3, iGer3, iSA1	NY1, IA1, WI1	Ab: CF	Serum (2-3 ml) (refrigerated)	Paired samples: rising (4-fold) titer confirms active infection, single positive titer indicates exposure
		TX2, PA3, SD3, TN1, TN2, TX1, LA1	Ab: FA	As above	As above
	iSwi2	MO1, OR1, TN2, ANT	Ab: ELISA	As above	As above
	iGB1, iGB3, iSA1	NY1, FL3, OH2, TX2, MN1	*Chlamydia:* cult	Nasal and ocular swabs, lung (refrigerated)	Positive result confirms infection
		IA1, WA1, MN1, NY3, IDX	Ag: ELISA	As above	Positive result confirms infection; large numbers of organisms more indicative of active infection
	iD3	CA2, AL2, TN1, GA1, GA2, LA1, TN2, KY2, OH2	Ag: FA	Conjunctival or tissue smear (refrigerated or air-dried in sterile container)	Positive result confirms infection; large numbers of organisms more indicative of active infection
		NE1, CA2	Ag: IHC	Tissue (formalin-fixed)	Positive result confirms infection
	iGer3	NE1, NY1, MO1, IN1, IN2, CO1, KS1, TX2, AZ3, NY3, WY1, LA1, IDX, ON3	Genome: PCR	Blood or tissue sample (fresh, formalin-fixed or refrigerated)	As above
Hemotrophic Mycoplasmosis (Hemobartonellosis) (31)					
	iD1, iGer3	Many	Organism: cytol	Blood films (unstained and unfixed)	Positive result confirms infection; stained artifacts must be viewed cautiously
		AL2, CO1, IL1, KS1, MO1, NE1, TX2, CO3, MI1, PA1, NY3, IDX	Ag: FA	As above	Positive result confirms infection without risk of false-positives due to stain artifact
	iGB1, iGB3, iGer3	CO1, CO3, ON3	Genome: PCR	Blood, EDTA anticoagulated, (refrigerated)	Positive result confirms active infection and determines which strain is involved
Mycoplasmal Infection (32)					
	iD3, iSA1, iSw1	Many	Mycoplasma: cult	Nasal swab, trachea (refrigerated)	Positive result confirms infection; many infections are subclinical since part of resident microflora
		NY3, TX1, ON3	Genome: PCR	1 ml serum or sterile swab (refrigerated)	Positive result confirms infection

AGENT (CHAPTER)	INTER-NATIONAL	USA	DETECTION: TEST TYPE	SAMPLE (AMOUNT OR HANDLING)	COMMENTS
			BACTERIAL INFECTIONS (33)		
Gram-Negative Bacterial Infections (37)					
Antemortem		Many	Verotoxin (Shiga-like toxins): for enterohem-orrhagic strains	Feces: fresh fecal material (refrigerated)	Positive result with specific antisera neutralization of toxin confirms pathogenic strain
		SD1	LT toxin: enterotoxi-genic strains	As above	As above
	iD3, iSA1	NY1, TX2, TX1, WY1, NY3	Bacteria (O157: A7): cult, PCR	Feces, foods, tissues	Positive result confirms pathogenic strain
		KY2, FL3, SD1, MN1	Pili Ag: FA	Fecal smears (refrigerated)	Positive result with fluorescence
		KS1	PCR: Pillus Ag and toxin ID	Feces, tissues (refrigerated)	Positive result confirms infection with pathogenic strain
		KS1	Pili Ag: ELISA	As above	As above
		NY1, IL1, KS1, NE1, PA3, IN1, IN2	Culture and Genotyping: DNA Probe	As above	As above
Postmortem		Many	Lesions: histol for attaching an effacing strain	Intestinal sections (fresh (refrigerated) or formalin fixed)	Bacterial attachment with associated pathologic changes characteristic for a presumptive diagnosis
Salmonellosis (39)					
	iD3, iSA1, iSwi3	Many	Bacteria: cult	Feces or fecal swab (3 g) (fresh or refrigerated)	Positive result confirms active infection; may be subclinical carrier
	iD3, iSA1, iSwi3	Many	Bacteria: cult	Blood (1-2 ml), internal tissues (collect sterilely, transport blood in blood culture broth media)	Positive result confirms clinically significant bacteremic or systemic infection
	iD3, iSA1, iSwi3	Many	Bacteria: cult	Intestinal lymph nodes, spleen, many internal organs other then intestine (refrigerated)	Positive result confirms active systemic infection
	iD1	Many	Bacteria: cult	Entire animal (fresh or refrigerated)	As above
		IN1, IN2, MO1, KS1, TX2, IL1, CO1, FL3, GA1, NY3, TX1, LA1	Genome: PCR	Intestine, colon, lymph node, lung, spleen (fresh or frozen)	Positive result confirms infection
		MN1	IHC	As above	As above

Continued

AGENT (CHAPTER)	INTER-NATIONAL	USA	DETECTION: TEST TYPE	SAMPLE (AMOUNT OR HANDLING)	COMMENTS
Campylobacteriosis/Helicobacteriosis (39)					
	iSA1, iSwi3	Many	Bacteria: cult	Gastric biopsy material in sterile screw cap with saline or feces (2-3 g, fresh, in sterile airtight container; add thioglycolate medium) (see sample needed)	Positive result confirms infection; may be subclinical carrier
		Many	Lesions: histol	Intestine, colon, lymph node, lung, spleen (formalin fixed)	Compatible histologic changes indicate infection
		IL1, TX1, NY3	Genome: PCR	1 ml EDTA whole blood or feces (refrigerated)	Positive result indicates infection
***Clostridium perfringens* Infection (39)**					
		OR1, AZ2, NY3, ON3	Toxin: RPLA toxin A assay	Feces or loops of intestine (2-3 ml) (refrigerated)	Positive result confirms organism is producing toxins associated with clinical illnesses
	iSA1	IN1, IN2, TX2, IA1, CO1, NY1, TX1	Genome: PCR	Isolated organism (culture material)	Positive result confirms species of organisms
		IL1, PA3, WY1, WI1, MN1, AZ2	Toxin Typing: PCR	Feces or intestine (refrigerated)	Positive result confirms organism is producing toxins associated with clinical illnesses
		NY1, CO1	Toxin: LA	As above	As above
		SD1, NE1	Toxin Typing: cult	As above	As above
		IDX	Toxin Typing: ELISA	As above	As above
Brucellosis (40)					
Antemortem or postmortem	iAus1, iD3, iGer3, iIt3, iSA1, iSwi2	Many	Ab: SAT	Serum: single sample (2-3 ml) (refrigerated until sent)	Screening test for infection, false positive with other bacterial infection. Follow a positive result with serologic testing
	iSwi2	Many	Ab: TAT	As above	Titer of >1:50 suspicious; >1:100 positive; >1:200 usually bacteremic; some false-negative and false-positive results; do AGID or culture (if positive) for confirmation
		TX2, GA1, LA1, IDX	Ab: FA	As above	Has been used for screening to substitute for agglutination testing (see previously). Positive result may be confirmed by AGID and culture
		KS1, NY1, GA2, ANT, IDX	Ab: AGID	As above	May detect rare seronegatives, more specific test; use to check SAT and TAT positives
		IA1, ND1	Ab: ELISA	As above	More sensitive and less specific than agglutination tests
	iSA1, iSwi2	TN1, LA1	Bacteria: cult	Anticoagulated blood (5-10 ml) (heparinized, refrigerated)	Positive result confirms bacteremia; negative is uncertain

AGENT (CHAPTER)	INTER-NATIONAL	USA	DETECTION: TEST TYPE	SAMPLE (AMOUNT OR HANDLING)	COMMENTS
	iD3, iSA1, iSwi2	TN1, LA1	Bacteria: cult	Tissue, fetus, testicles, placenta, semen, genital swabs (refrigerated)	Positive result confirms infection; negative is uncertain
		NY3, ON3	Genome: PCR	Tissue, fetus, testicles, placenta, semen, genital swabs (refrigerated)	Positive result confirms infection
Anaerobic Infections (41)					
		Many	Bacteria: cult	Lesion exudates (refrigerated in airtight or anaerobic transport system)	Positive result confirms infection but usually are contaminants of wounds from penetrating tissue injuries
Botulism (42)					
	iD3, iSA1		Toxin analysis	Feces, blood, serum, intestinal contents (5 ml) (refrigerated)	Test performed with and without specific antisera for confirmation of toxin type involved
Leptospirosis (44)					
Antemortem	iAus1, iD3, iGer3, iSA1, iSwi2	Many	Ab: MA	Serum: paired samples taken 2-3 wks apart (2-3 ml) (refrigerated)	Paired samples: rising (4-fold) titer confirms active infection; single positive titer ≥1:400 confirms past exposure in nonvaccinate; lower or equivalent titers associated with vaccination; titer ≥1:800 by itself, or changing 4-fold titers over 2-3 wks, suggests recent or active infection
		ANT	Ab: LA	Serum (refrigerated)	Titer ≥1 : 250 suggests recent or current infection; negative result does not rule out disease, vaccination can cause positive titers
	iSA1	Many	Spirochetes	Urine (1-2 ml) (refrigerated)	Positive result suggests infection; nonpathogenic spirochetes and artifacts make unreliable
	iSA1	Many	Spirochetes: cult	1 ml serum (refrigerated)	Positive result confirms infection
		Many	Ag: FA	Tissue or body fluids (In transport media)	As above
		Many	Spirochetes: histol	Tissue: kidney, fetal fluid, placenta, or urine (refrigerated)	As above
	iGer3, iSA1	NE1, KS1, MO1, TX2, IN1, IN2, NY3, TX1, ON3	Genome: PCR	Tissue (kidney), urine (refrigerated)	Positive result suggests infection; nonpathogenic spirochetes and artifacts make unreliable
		NE1, WA1, WI1, MN1	Ag: IHC	Tissue (formalin fixed)	Positive result confirms infection
Lyme Borreliosis (45)					
Antemortem	iD1, iIt3, iSw1, iSwi2	Many	Ab: FA	Serum: paired samples taken 10-14 days apart (2-3 ml) (refrigerated)	Paired samples: rising (4-fold) IgG titer confirms active infection with *Borrelia* spp.
	iGer3	Many	Ab: ELISA-IgG	As above	As above

Continued

AGENT (CHAPTER)	INTER-NATIONAL	USA	DETECTION: TEST TYPE	SAMPLE (AMOUNT OR HANDLING)	COMMENTS
	iGer3	NY1, TN2, CT1, MI1, NY3, IDX, ON3	Ab: Immunoblot IgG	As above	Helps distinguish other spirochetal infections and vaccine responses from tissue exposure or infection
	iGer3		Ab: ELISA-IgM	As above	Single high IgM titer confirms recent or active infection with *Borrelia* spp., although IgM from other spirochetal infections such as *Leptospira* may cause some cross-reactivity
	iGer3	NY1	Ab: immunoblot IgM	As above	Specific reactivity can help determine whether natural infection, vaccine exposure, or cross-reactive antibodies exist
	iGB5, iGer3, iSwi3	NY1, MO1, PA3, MI1, NY3, MN1	Genome: PCR	Blood, anticoagulated, tissue, joint fluid (2-3 ml) (refrigerated)	Positive result confirms infection
Postmortem		Many	Ag; IHC, FA	Tissue (formalin fixed)	Positive result confirms infection
Feline Lyme Borreliosis (45)					
Antemortem	LA1		Ab: FA	Serum taken 10-14 days apart (0.5 ml) (refrigerated)	Paired samples: rising (4-fold) IgG titer suggests active infection with *Borrelia* spp
	iGer3		Ab: immunoblot	Serum (0.5 ml) (refrigerated)	Positive result helps distinguish true seroreactivity to *B. burgdorferi* from that with other spirochetes
	iGB5, iGer3, iSwi3		Genome: PCR	Blood, anticoagulated, or body fluid (0.5 ml), or tissue (refrigerated)	Positive result confirms infection
	ANT		Ab: ELISA (IgG)	1 ml serum (refrigerated)	titer ≥1 : 64 suggest exposure or active infection; borderline results should be retested in 3-4 wks, vaccination can cause positive titer
Postmortem		Many	Ag: IHC, FA	Tissue (formalin-fixed, embedded)	Positive result confirms infection
Plague (47)					
Postmortem or antemortem		WY1, NM1	Ab: passive HA	Serum (2-3 ml) (refrigerated)	Positive result confirms exposure; rising (4-fold) titer confirms active infection
		Many	Ag: FA	Blood, sputum, fluid, or tissue smears, exudates (2-3 ml) (shipped with biohazard precautions, refrigerated)	Positive result confirms infection
		Many	Bacteria: cult	Exudates (swabs, sputum, fluid) tissue, blood (shipped with biohazard precautions, refrigerated)	As above
		WY1	Genome: PCR	Tissues or body fluids (refrigerated)	As above
Tularemia (48)					
Antemortem		IA1, KY1, WY1, NM1	Ab: MA	Serum: paired specimens taken 2-3 wks apart (2-3 ml) (refrigerated)	Positive result confirms exposure; rising (4-fold) titer confirms active infection

AGENT (CHAPTER)	INTER-NATIONAL	USA	DETECTION: TEST TYPE	SAMPLE (AMOUNT OR HANDLING)	COMMENTS
		LA1	Bacteria: cult	Swab or exudate (on ice) or tissue (exudate on ice)	Positive result confirms infection
		WY1	Genome: PCR	As above	As above
Nocardiosis (49)					
Antemortem	iSw1	Many	Bacteria: cult	Peritoneal, pleural, and pericardial fluid (refrigerated)	Positive result confirms infection
Mycobacteriosis (50)					
	iD3, iSA1, iSw1	Many	Bacteria: cult	Tissue specimen or exudates (fresh or frozen)	Positive result confirms infection
	iD3	Many	Lesions: histol	Tissue (formalin fixed)	Finding acid-fast bacteria must be combined with bacterial culture for determining organism involved
Feline Bartonellosis (54)					
Antemortem	Many	Many	Bacteria: cult	Blood, EDTA, anticoagulated (aseptically collected)	Positive result confirms infection
	iGB5, iSwi3	IN1, IN2, AL2, NY3, ANT, LA1, ON3	Genome: PCR	As above	As above
		NC1, TX2, CA3, TX1, LA1, IDX	Ab: FA	Serum, free of hemolysis (refrigerated)	Positive result indicates present or past exposure, useful for epidemiologic monitoring. Some bacteremic animals can be seronegative
Canine Bartonellosis (54)					
		NC1	Ab: FA	Blood or serum (refrigerated)	Positive result indicates exposure
		Many	Bacteria: cult	Blood, EDTA, anticoagulated or material from culture plate (aseptically collected)	Positive result conrimss infection
	iGB5	AL2, ANT, LA1, NC1, CO3	Genome PCR	As above	As above
			FUNGAL INFECTIONS (56)		
Fungal Identification and Susceptibility Testing (56)					
	iSA1, iSwi3	Many	Fungus: cult	Tissue, exudate, or body fluid (refrigerated)	Confirms infection
		NY1, IL1, KS1	Susceptibility: antifungal susceptibility testing	Organism from animal is isolated on fungal medium	Determines susceptibility to drugs, which may not always correlate with in vivo efficacy
		ANT	Drug: antifungal drug concentrations	Serum, body fluids, or tissues (refrigerated)	Determines achieved concentrations of antifungal drug

Continued

AGENT (CHAPTER)	INTER- NATIONAL	USA	DETECTION: TEST TYPE	SAMPLE (AMOUNT OR HANDLING)	COMMENTS
Dermatophytosis (58)					
	iD1, iD3, iSA1, iSw1, iSwi3	Many	Fungus: cult	Lesion (scabs or plucked hairs) (sterile, dry tubes)	Positive result confirms infection; some cats may be subclinical carriers
Blastomycosis (59) or Histoplasmosis (60)					
Antemortem or postmortem		Many	Ab: CF	Serum: single sample (2-3 ml) (refrigerated)	Positive result confirms exposure but not necessarily active infection
		Many	Ab: AGID	As above	As above
		Many	Fungus: cult	Tissues or fluid aspirates (1-2 ml) (sterile container)	Positive result confirms infection
		Many	Fungus: cytol	As above	As above
		Many	Lesions: histol	Tissue biopsy (formalin fixed)	As above
		IN3	Ag: ELISA	2 ml serum, separated from clot; urine, plasma, CSF, bronchial fluid, sterile body fludis (ambient temp or refrigerated)	Positive result confirms disease, some cross reaction with other fungal antigens
Cryptococcosis (61)					
Antemortem or postmortem		ANT, TN2, LA1	Ag: ELISA	Serum or CSF: single sample (1-2 ml) (sterile, container refrigerated)	Positive result confirms active infection. Level can be used to monitor treatment
		TX2, MO1, CO1, KS1, GA1, TN1, PA1, GA3, FL3, LA1, IDX	Ag: LA	As above	As above
	iSw1	Many	Fungus: cult	Tissue or fluid aspirate (sterile container, refrigerated)	Positive result confirms infection
	iSw1	Many	Fungus: cytol	Tissue or fluid aspirate on smear	As above
			Ag: FA	Tissue (sterile container, refrigerated)	As above
Coccidioidomycosis (62)					
Antemortem or postmortem		Many	Ab: ELISA	Serum: single or paired samples (2-3 ml) (refrigerated)	See Table 62-1 for interpretation
		Many	Ab: AGID	As above	As above
		TX2, CA1	Ab: CF	As above	As above
		CA1	Ab: FA	As above	As above
		Many	Fungus: cult	Tissue or fluid aspirate (1-2 ml) (refrigerated)	Positive result confirms infection
		Many	Fungus: cytol	Tissue (refrigerated)	As above
Sporotrichosis (63)					
		Many	Fungus: cytol	Exudate from lymphatics (1-2 ml) (refrigerated)	Positive result confirms infection
		IN1, IN2, LA1	Fungus: cult	As above	As above

AGENT (CHAPTER)	INTER-NATIONAL	USA	DETECTION: TEST TYPE	SAMPLE (AMOUNT OR HANDLING)	COMMENTS
Aspergillosis (64)					
		PA1	Ab: ELISA	Serum: single sample (2-3 ml) (refrigerated)	Positive result confirms exposure but not necessarily active infection
		Many	Ab: AGID	As above	As above
		Many	Ab: CF	As above	As above
	iSw1, iGer3	Many	Fungus: cult	Tissue or exudates (refrigerated)	Positive result confirms infection; can be a contaminant. Histopathologic lesions in association with fungus help with confirmation
		IN3	Ag: ELISA	2 ml serum, separated from clot (refrigerated)	Positive result confirms disease
Candidiasis (65)					
	iSw1	Many	Fungus: cult	Blood or tissue (refrigerated)	Positive result of deeper tissues or body fluids confirms disseminated infection in association with microscopic lesions
***Pythium, Lagenidium*, and Zygomycete Infections (67)**					
		LA2	ELISA or WB	Serum (fresh or refrigerated)	Positive result indicates exposure or infection
		LA2	Culture	Tissue (fresh or refrigerated [<36 hr])	Positive result confirms infection
		LA2	IHC	Tissue (paraffin blocks)	As above
		LA2	Genome: PCR	Cultured organisms (In media at ambient temp.)	As above
Pneumocystosis (68)					
		Many	Protozoa: cytol	Sputum, lung aspirates (refrigerated)	Positive result suggest infection; difficult-to-find and numerous artifacts make visualization difficult
		Many	Ag: FA	As above	Positive result confirms infection
Protothecosis (see Diagnosis, Chapter 69)					
			PROTOZOAL INFECTIONS (70)		
Trypanosomiasis (72)					
		TX2	Ab: FA	Serum (refrigerated)	Positive result makes infection likely in animal with compatible signs; infection usually persists
		Many	Protozoa: cytol	Blood film (thick and thin)	Positive result confirms infection
Leishmaniasis (73)					
	iGer3, ilt3, iSwi3	NC1, CO3, TX2, TX1, MI1	Ab: FA	Serum or dried blood spots (on filter paper)	Positive result makes infection likely in animal with compatible signs; infection usually persists
	iN2		Ab: ELISA (Dog-Cat)	Serum (refrigerated)	As above
	iGer3	Many	Protozoa: cytol	Lymph node aspirate (fixed in methanol, stained with Giemsa)	Amastigote I smear confirms infection

Continued

AGENT (CHAPTER)	INTER-NATIONAL	USA	DETECTION: TEST TYPE	SAMPLE (AMOUNT OR HANDLING)	COMMENTS
		NY1, NY3, ON3	Ag: ELISA	Serum (refrigerated)	Positive titer seen with moderate or heavy infections
	iGB5, iGer3	NC1	Genome: PCR	EDTA blood, tissue (refrigerated)	Positive result confirms infection
		NY1	Western Blot	Serum (refrigerated)	As above
Hepatozoonosis (74)					
		Many	Protozoa: cytol	Blood film (air dried smear)	Positive result confirms infection
		Many	Protozoa: histol	Tissues; muscle biopsy (refrigerated or formalin fixed)	As above
Microsporidiosis (Encephalitozoonosis) (see Diagnosis, Chapter 5)					
Cytauxzoonosis (76)					
		Many	Protozoa: cytol	Blood films, bone marrow (air dried smear)	Positive result confirms infection; may be uncommon in peripheral blood films
Babesiosis (77)					
	iSA1, iGer3	Many	Protozoa: cytol	Blood film (air dried smear)	Positive result confirms infection; may be uncommon in peripheral blood films
	iGB5, iGer3	AL2, NC1, NY3, ON3	Genome: PCR	EDTA-whole blood and ticks	Positive result confirms infection; also may be used to determine infecting species
	iGer3, ilt3, iSwi3	TN2, IL1, IA1, NC1, TX2, TX1, NY3, FL3, PA1, MI1, ANT, LA1, IDX, ON3	Ab: FA	Serum: single sample (2-3 ml) (refrigerated)	Positive titer >1 : 40 indicates active or very recent infection. Some variation in titers exists among laboratories
		IA1	Ab: CF	As above	As above
Enteric Protozoal Infections (78)					
	Many	Many	Protozoa: flotation, sedimentation	Feces (refrigerated)	Positive result indicates infection; may be subclinical carrier
		Many	Protozoa: fecal smears, wet mounts	As above	As above
	Many	ANT, CO1, NY1, SD1, TN2, NY3, MT1, MT2, WY1, UT1, LA1, IDX, ON3	*Giardia* Ag: ELISA	Feces (refrigerated)	Positive result confirms infection
	Many	Many	*Giardia* Ag: FA	As above	As above
		NC1, NY3, ON3	Genome: PCR *Trittichomonas foetus*	Feces (2-3 ml) (refrigerated)	Positive result confirms infection when fecal exam has detected suspicious organism

AGENT (CHAPTER)	INTER-NATIONAL	USA	DETECTION: TEST TYPE	SAMPLE (AMOUNT OR HANDLING)	COMMENTS
Toxoplasmosis (80)					
		Many	Ab: HA-I	Serum: paired samples taken 10-14 days apart (2-3 ml) (refrigerated)	Paired samples: rising (4-fold) IgG titer confirms active infection; single positive titer is nonspecific
	iGer3, ilt3	Many	Ab: IFA-IgG	As above	As above
			Ab: CF	As above	As above
		Many	Ab: ELISA-IgG	As above	As above
		NY1	Ab: kinELISA	As above	As above
		Many	Ab: ELISA-IgM	Serum: single sample (2-3 ml) (refrigerated)	A single high IgM or agglutination (LA) titer indicates active or recent infection; evaluation of IgG and IgM simultaneously is more informative
	iGer3, ilt3	TN2, TX2, FL3, MI1, LA1, IDX	Ab: FA-IgM	As above	As above
	iSw1	IA1, KS1, GA1, CA2, MN1, WI1, WY1, LA1	Ab: LA	As above	As above
	iGer3, iSw1	Many	Oocysts: flotatiom	Feces (cat only) (refrigerated)	Oocyst identification is positive, although inoculation into intermediate host is often needed to confirm exact species
		Many	Histol	Tissue biopsy (lung, brain, lymphoid, liver, kidney) (formalin fixed)	Positive for infection; if detected, clinical significance must be determined
	iSw1	IA1, OH2, PA3, WA1, CA2, ND1, MN1	IHC	As above	As above
		MO1, ANT	Genome: PCR	Tissue or body fluids (refrigerated)	Positive result indicates infection; may be subclinical carrier
Neosporosis (80)					
	iD3, ilt3, iGer3, iSw1	TN1, TN2, OH2, OR1, PA3, SD1, TX2, WI1, MI1	Ab: IFA	Serum: paired samples taken 10-14 days apart (2-3 ml) (refrigerated)	Paired samples: rising (4-fold) IgG titer confirms active infection; single high positive titer, as defined by the respective laboratory, indicates previous exposure
	iSw1	CA2, MO1, CO, IL1, OH2, TX2, WI1, ND1, NY3, UT1, ON3	Ab: ELISA	As above	As above
	iSw1	OH2, GA1, GA2, TN1, WY1, LA1	Ag: FA	Tissue biopsy (brain, kidney, liver, muscle, skin) (formalin fixed or refrigerated)	Positive result confirms infection
	iSw1	CA2, OH2, CO1, IA1, PA3, WA1, ND1, MN1	IHC	Tissue (formalin fixed)	As above
	iSw1	IN1, IN2, UT1	PCR	Tissue	As above

Continued

AGENT (CHAPTER)	INTER-NATIONAL	USA	DETECTION: TEST TYPE	SAMPLE (AMOUNT OR HANDLING)	COMMENTS
Coccidiosis (81)					
	Many	Many	Oocysts: flotation	Feces (refrigerated)	Oocyst identification is positive
Cryptosporidiosis (82)					
	iD3	Many	Oocysts: float	Feces (refrigerated)	Oocyst identification is positive
		ANT, AZ3, OH2, TN2, TX2, CT1, IL2, IL3, NC2, MN2, MN1	Ag: FA	Feces (2-3 g) (in 10% formalin)	Positive result confirms infection
	Many	NY1, IL2, IL3, NY3, IDX, ON3	Ag: ELISA	As above	As above
		MI1	Genome: PCR	Feces or intestine (refrigerated)	As above
Immunodeficiency Testing (95)					
		ANT, NY1, TX2, IL1, CA1, CO1, WA2, PA2, TN2, IN1, TX1, IDX	IgG: radial diffusion	Serum (3-5 ml) (refrigerated)	Low immunoglobulin concentration reflects humoral immunodeficiency
		ANT, NY1, TX2, IL1, CA1, CO1, WA2, PA2, TX1, IDX	IgM: radial diffusion	As above	As above
		ANT, NY1, TX2, IL1, CA1, CO1, WA2, PA2, TN2, TX1, IDX	IgA: radial diffusion	As above	As above
	Leukocyte adhesion deficiency (LAD)				
	iB2		PCR	EDTA sample (refrigerated)	Neutrophil adhesion defect in cell culture

Ab, Antibody; *Ag*, antigen; *AGID*, agar gel immunodiffusion; *CF*, complement fixation; *CNS*, central nervous system; *CSF*, cerebrospinal fluid; *Cult*, culture; *Cytol*, cytology; *EDTA*, ethylenediaminetetraacetic acid; *ELISA*, enzyme-linked immunosorbent assay; *EM*, electron microscopy; *FA*, fluorescent antibody; *FAVN*, fluorescent antibody virus neutralization; *FCoV*, feline coronavirus; *FIP*, feline infectious peritonitis; *HA*, hemagglutination; *HA-I*, hemagglutination inhibition; *histol*, histopathology; *IHC*, immunohistochemistry; *IPT*, immunoprecipitin test; *kinELISA*, kinetic ELISA; *LA*, latex agglutination; *LT*, heat labile; *MA*, microscopic agglutination; *PCR*, polymerase chain reaction; *PE*, protein electrophoresis (serum); *RFFIT*, rapid fluorescent focus inhibition test; *RPLA*, reverse passive latex agglutination; *SAT*, slide agglutination test; *SN*, serum neutralization; *TAT*, tube agglutination test; *VI*, viral inhibition; *VN*, viral neutralization; *WB*, western blot.

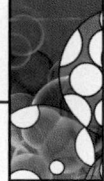
Manufacturers of Diagnostic Test Kits and Their Products

Deborah Joiner and Craig E. Greene

Part A: Manufacturers of Commercially Available Test Kits

KIT NUMBER	MANUFACTURERS	MAILING ADDRESS/WEBSITE/E-MAIL	TELEPHONE (P)/FAX (F) NUMBERS
K1	AGEN Biomedical CY	11 Durbell St, Acacia Ridge QLD 4110, Brisbane, Australia www.agen.com.au/ info@agen.com.au	P: 61-73370-6300 F: 61-73370-6370
K2	Biogal-Galed Labs	Kibbutz Galed, 19240 Israel www.biogal.co.il info@biogal.co.il	P: 972-49898605 F: 972-49898690
K3	Biomed Diagnostics, Inc.	1388 Antelope Rd, White City, OR 97503-1619 USA www.biomed1.com info@biomed1.com	P: 800-964-6466 or 541-830-3000 F: 541-830-3001
K4	CeLLabs	PO Box 421, Brookvale, NSW, 2100, Australia www.cellabs.com.au enquiries@cellabs.com.au	P: 61 2 9905 0133 F: 61 2 9905 6426
K5	Cypress Diagnostics	Langdorpsesteenweg 160 B-3201Langdorp, Belgium www.diagnostics.be/index.html cypress@diagnostics.be	P: 321 644-6389 F: 321 644-7762
K6	EVL (European Vet Lab)	PO Box 198 3440 AD Woerden, Netherlands http://www.evlonline.nl/News/Profile.htm	P: 31 (0) 348 412549 F: 31 (0) 348 414626
K7	Fuller Laboratories	1135 E. Truslow Ave, Fullerton, CA 92831 USA www.fullerlabs.com orders@fullerlabs.com	P: 714-525-7660 or 888-826-7660 F: 714-525-7614
K8	HDC Corporation	628 Gibraltar Ct, Milpitas, CA 95035 USA http://www.hdccorp.com/ service@hdccorp.com	P: 800-227-8162 or 408-942-7340 F: 408-586-8680
K9	Helica BioSystems, Inc.	223 E. Imperial Way, Suite 165, Fullerton, CA 92835 USA www.helica.com info@helica.com	P: 877-9 HELICA or 714-578-7830 F: 714-578-7831
K10	IDEXX Corp.	One IDEXX Dr, Westbrook, ME 04092 USA http://www.idexx.com/animalhealth/	P: 207-856-0300 or 800-248-2483 F: 207-856-0346
K11	Immunetics, Inc.	27 Drydock Ave, 6th Floor, Boston, MA 02210 USA http://www.immunetics.com/c6/ info@immunetics.com	P: 800-227-4765 or 617-896-9100 F: 617-896-9110
K12	ImmunoMycologics, Inc. (IMMY)	PO Box 1151, Norman, OK 73070 USA http://www.immy.com/ info@immy.com	P: 800-654-3639 or 405-288-2383 F: 405-288-2228
K13	Kimberly-Clark	12050 Lone Peak Pkwy, Draper, UT 84020 USA www.kchealthcare.com	P: 801-572-6800 F: 801-572-6999
K14	MegaCor GmbH, Lochauer Straße 2	Lochauer Straße 2, A-6912 Hörbranz, Austria www.megacor.at/ info@megacor.at	P: 43-5573-85400 F: 43-5573-85402

Continued

KIT NUMBER	MANUFACTURERS	MAILING ADDRESS/WEBSITE/E-MAIL	TELEPHONE (P)/FAX (F) NUMBERS
K15	Meridian Bioscience Europe	3471 River Hills Dr, Cincinnati, OH 45244 USA www.mdeur.com mbi@meridianbioscience.com	P: 800-543-1980 or 513-271-3700 F: 513-271-3762
K16	RapiGEN Inc.	3F, 693-11, Geumjung Gunpo Gyengoggi435-862 South Korea www.rapigen-inc.com info@rapigen-inc.com	P: +82-31-427-4677 F: +82-31-427-4678
K17	Remel	12076 Santa Fe Dr, Lenexa, KS 66215 USA www.remel.com remel@remel.com	P: 800-255-6730 F: 800-621-8251
K18	Safepath Laboratories	5909 Sea Lion Pl, Suite D, Carlsbad, CA 92008 USA http://www.safepath.com info@safepath.com	P: 760-929-7744 F: 760-431-7759
K19	SA Scientific	4919 Golden Quail, San Antonio, TX 78240 USA www.sascientific.com info@sascientific.com	P: 210-699-8800 or 800-272-2710 F: 210-699-6545
K20	Svanova Biotech AB	Uppsala Science Park, Glunten, Sweden SE-751 83 http://www.svanova.com info@svanova.com	P: +46-18 65 49 00 F: +46-18 65 49 99
K21	Synbiotics Corp.	11011 Via Frontera, San Diego, CA 92127 USA www.synbiotics.com	P: 800-228-4305 F: 858-451-5719
K22	TechLab	2001 Kraft Dr, Blackburg, VA 24060-6358 USA http://www.techlabinc.com/ techlab@techlab.com	P: 540-953-1664 F: 540-953-1665
K23	Wampole Laboratories	2 Princeton Way, Princeton, NJ 08540 USA http://www.wampolelabs.com/	P: 800-257-9525 or 609-627-8000 F: 800-532-0295 or 609-627-8013

Part B: Test Kits Commercially Available for Infectious Diseases

DISEASE (CHAPTER)	KIT NUMBER	NAME OF TEST AND ORGANISM	SPECIES	SPECIMEN TESTED	TYPE OF TEST
		VIRAL INFECTIONS (SEE ALSO CHAPTER 1)			
Canine Distemper					
3	K2	ImmunoComb Canine Distemper (IgM and IgG Kits)	D	Serum, blood, CSF	Ab: ELISA
3	K21	TiterCHECK CDV/CPV	D	Serum, plasma	Ab: ELISA
3	K7	Canine Distemper Virus	D	Serum	Ab: FA
3	K16	RapiGEN Distempter Ag TEST	D	Serum, plasma	Ag: Lateral flow assay
3	K14	FASTest DISTEMPER Strip	D	Body fluids	Ag: comp to RT-PCR
Canine and Feline Enteric Viral Infections					
8	K2	ImmunoComb Canine Parvovirus	D	Serum	Ab: ELISA
8, 10	K5	Rapid PARVO Dipstick	D, C, M	Feces	Ag: Latex One Step
8	K14	FASTest CPV Ab	D	feces	Ab: H-I
8,10	K14	FASTest PARVO Card	D, C, M	Feces	Ag: ELISA
	K14	FASTest PARVO Pen	D, C,M	Feces	Ag: ELISA
	K14	FASTest PARVO Strip	D, C, M	Feces	Ag: ELISA
8	K7	Canine Parvovirus	D	Feces	Ag: ELISA
8	K10	SNAP Parvo	D	Feces	Ag: ELISA
8, 10	K20	Svanodip	D, C	Feces	Ag: ELISA
10	K19	Parvovirus	C	Feces	Ag: ELISA
8	K21	Assure Parvovirus	D	Feces	Ag: ELISA

DISEASE (CHAPTER)	KIT NUMBER	NAME OF TEST AND ORGANISM	SPECIES	SPECIMEN TESTED	TYPE OF TEST
8, 10	K6	Canine/Feline Parvo One Step	D, C	Feces	Ag: ELISA
8	K21	Witness CPV	D	Feces	Ag: Rapid immunomigration-stat
8	K1	AGEN Parvo Ag Test	D	Feces	Ag: RIM (Rapid Immunomigration)
8	K2	ImmunoComb Canine Distemper & Parvovirus (IgM & IgG Kits)	D	Serum, blood	Ab: ELISA
10	K21	TiterCHECK CDV/CPV	C	Serum, plasma	Ab: ELISA
8, 10	K14	FASTest Rota Strip	D, C	Feces	Ag: ELISA
8, 10	K15	Immunocard STAT! Rotavirus	H (D, C)[a]	Feces	Ag: ELISA
8, 10	K17	ProSpecT Rotavirus	H (D, C)	Feces	Ag: ELISA; available outside US only
8, 10	K15	MERITEC-Rotavirus	H (D, C)	Feces	Ag: LA
8, 10	K23	Virogen Rotatest	H (D, C)	Feces	Ag: LA
8, 10	K17	Rotavirus (REF 30950401)	H (D, C)	Feces	Ag: Rapid latex agglutination
8, 10	K15	Immunocard STAT Rotavirus	H (D, C)	Feces	Ag: Immunochromatography

Feline Panleukopenia

10	K7	Feline Panleukopenia	C	Serum	Ag: ELISA

Feline Infectious Peritonitis

11	K21	ViraChek CV	C	Serum, plasma	Ab: ELISA
11	K2	ImmunoComb Feline Coronavirus Antibody test (FIP)	C	Serum, blood	Ab: ELISA
11	K7	Feline Infectious Peritonitis	C	Serum	Ab: FA
11	K14	FASTest FIP	C	Blood, plasma, serum	Ab: Immunoassay

Feline Retroviral Infections

13	K1	AGEN FeLV test	C	Serum, plasma, whole blood	Ab: Immunochromatography
13	K14	FASTest FeLV	C	Serum, plasma (anticoagulated whole blood for screening only)	Ag: ELISA
13	K21	ViraCheck FeLV	C	Serum, plasma, anticoagulated whole blood	Ag: ELISA
13	K10	SNAP FeLV	C	Serum, plasma, whole blood	Ag: ELISA
13	K21	Assure FeLV	C	Saliva, whole blood, anticoagulated plasma, serum	Ag: ELISA
13	K21	Witness FeLV	C	Serum, plasma, anticoagulated whole blood	Ag: Rapid immunomigration-stat
13	K5	FeLV Dipstick	C	Serum, plasma, whole blood	Ag: Immunochromatogrphy
13, 14	K10	Snap FeLV/FIV	C	Serum, plasma, whole blood	Ag-Ab: ELISA
13, 14	K5	Combo FIV/FeLV Dipstick	C	Serum, plasma, whole blood	Ag-Ab: Immunochromatography
13, 14	K21	Witness FeLV/FIV	C	Serum, plasma, anticoagulated whole blood	Ag: Rapid immunomigration-stat
14	K5	FIV Dipstick	C	Serum, plasma, whole blood	Ab: Immunochromatography

Continued

DISEASE (CHAPTER)	KIT NUMBER	NAME OF TEST AND ORGANISM	SPECIES	SPECIMEN TESTED	TYPE OF TEST
14	K21	Witness FIV	C	Serum, plasma, anticoagulated whole blooe	Ag: Rapid immunomigration-stat
14	K14	FASTest FIV Labcard	C	Serum, plasma, whole blood	Ab: Immunochromatography
14	K1	AGEN FIV test	C	Serum, plasma, whole blood	Ab: Immunochromatography
14	K14	FASTest FIV	C	Serum, plasma, whole blood	Ab: Immunochromatography
14	K21	ViraChek FIV	C	Serum, plasma	Ab: ELISA

Feline Calicivirus Infection

16	K7	Calicivirus	C	Serum	Ab: FA

RICKETTSIAL, CHLAMYDIAL AND MYCOPLASMAL INFECTIONS (SEE ALSO CHAPTER 1)

28	K9	*Ehrlichia canis*	D	Serum	Ab: ELISA
28	K2	Immunocomb *Ehrlichia canis* (Immunocomb Ab test for Canine Ehrlichiosis)	D	Serum, blood	Ab: ELISA
28	K7	*Ehrlichia*	D	Serum	Ab: FA
28	K14	FasTest Canine *Ehrlichia canis*	D	Serum, plasma, whole blood	Ab: Immunoassay
29	K9	*Rickettsia rickettsii*	D	Serum	Ab: ELISA
29	K7	*Rickettsia rickettsii*	D	Serum	Ab: FA
29	K9	*Rickettsia conori*	D	Serum	Ab: ELISA
29	K7	*Rickettsia conorii*	D	Serum	Ab: FA
29	K7	*Rickettsia akari*	C	Serum	Ab: FA
29	K7	*Rickettsia felis*	C	Serum	Ab: FA
29	K7	*Coxiella burnetii* (Q-fever)	D	Serum	Ab: FA
31	K2	ImmunoComb Feline Toxo & *Chlamydophila*	C	Serum, blood	Ab: ELISA
31	K7	*Chlamydophila psittaci*	C	Serum	Ab: FA
31	K4	*Chlamydia* CELISA	D, C	Feces	Ag: ELISA
31	K23	Clearview *Chlamydia*	H (D, C)	Secretions	Ag: ELISA
31	K15	Premier *Chlamydia*	H (D, C)	Secretions	Ag: ELISA
31	K15	Meriflour *Chlamydia*	H (D, C)	Secretions	Ag: FA
28, 45	K10	Canine Snap 3DX Test Heartworm, Lyme, *Ehrlichia canis*	D	Serum, plasma	Ab: Immunoassay for *E. canis*, Ab: ELISA for Lyme; Ag: heartworm

BACTERIAL INFECTIONS (SEE ALSO CHAPTER 33)

39	K13	CLOtest		Tissue biopsy	Colorimetric
	K9	C-Reactive Protein	D	Serum	Protein: ELISA
40	K21	D-TEC-CB (*Brucella canis*)	D	Serum	Ab: RSAT
40	K7	Canine *Brucella*	D	Serum	Ab: FA
44	K7	*Leptospira* IFA	D	Serum	Ab: FA
44	K2	Immunocomb Antibody test for canine leptosporosis	D	Serum, blood	Ab: Enzyme immunoassay
45, 28	K10	Canine Snap 3DX Test Heartworm, Lyme, *Ehrlichia canis*	D	Serum, plasma	Ag for heartworm, Ab for *E. canis* (immunoassay), Ab: ELISA for Lyme
45	K7	*Borrelia burgdorfei*	D	Serum	Ab: FA
45	K14	FASTestLyme	D	Serum, plasma, blood	Ab: Immunoassay
45	K11	Quali Code Canine Lyme Disease	H (D)	Serum	Ab: Immunoblot

DISEASE (CHAPTER)	KIT NUMBER	NAME OF TEST AND ORGANISM	SPECIES	SPECIMEN TESTED	TYPE OF TEST
FUNGAL INFECTIONS (SEE ALSO CHAPTER 56)					
58	K3	Diagnostics In-Tray DM	D	Hair	Organism: color test
58	K16	RapiGEN Ready-DTM Test	D, C	Hair	Organism: color test
58	K21	Fungassay	D, C	Hair	Organism: color test
61	K15	Premier Cryptococcal Antigen	H (D, C)	Serum, CSF	Ag: ELISA
61	K23	Crypto-LA	H (D, C)	Body fluids	Ag: LA
61	K23	"Calas"-Cryptococcal Latex	H (D, C)	Serum, CSF	Ag: LA
61	K12	Latex-*Cryptococcus*	H (D, C)	Body fluids	Ag: LA
61	K17	*Cryptococcus* Antigen	H (D, C)	Serum, CSF	Ag: LA
62	K15	Coccidioides Latex	H (D, C)	Serum	Ag: LA
66	K12	*Candida ID Antigen*	H (D, C)	Serum	Ag: AGID
68	K4	Pneumo Cel IFA	H (D, C)	Respiratory secretions	Ag: FA
68	K15	Meriflour Pneumocystis	H (D, C)	Respiratory secretions	Ag: FA
PROTOZOAL INFECTIONS (SEE ALSO CHAPTER 70)					
73	K9	*Leishmania donovani*	D	Serum	Ab: ELISA
73	K7	*Leishmania*	D	Serum	Ab: FA
73	K7	*Leishmania* IFA	D	Serum	Ab: FA
73	K14	FASTest Leish	D	Serum, plasma, blood	Ab: Immunoassay
73	K5	Canine *Leishmania*	D	Serum	Ab: Enzyme immunoassay
73	K5	Visceral *Leishmania* Dipstick	D	Serum	Ab: Immunochromatographic
78	K17	ProSpecT *Entamoeba histolytica*	H (D, C)	Feces	Ag: ELISA
78	K4	*Entamoeba* CELISA Path	H (D, C)	Feces	Ag: ELISA
78	K8	Enterotest	H (D, C)	Duodenal Fluid	Nylon string in capsule
78	K4	*Giardia* CELISA	D, C	Feces	Ag: ELISA
78	K18	*Giardia lamblia* Immunoassay	D, C	Feces	Ag: ELISA
78	K10	SNAP *Giardia*	D	Feces	Ag: ELISA
78	K15	Premier *Giardia*	D, C	Feces	Ag: ELISA
78	K14	FASTest *Giardia*	D, C	Feces	Ag: ELISA
78	K22	Giardia	H (D, C)	Feces	Cyst detection: MAB-ELISA
78	K17	ProSpecT/*Giardia* rapid assay	H (D, C)	Feces	Ag: ELISA
78	K17	ProSpecT/*Giardia* and *Cryptosporidium*	H (D, C)	Feces	Ag: ELISA
78, 82	K15	Meriflour Crypto & *Giardia*	H (D, C)	Feces	Ag: FA
82	K23	*Cryptosporidium* Test	H (D, C)	Feces	Ag (oocysts): ELISA
80	K2	Immunocomb *Toxoplasma* and *Chlamydia*	C	Serum, blood	Ab: ELISA
80	K4	Toxo CEL IFA	H (D)	Serum	Ag: FA
80	K23	TPM-Toxotest	H (C)	Serum	Ab: HA-I
80	K7	*Neospora caninum*	D	Serum	Ab: FA
82	K15	Premier *Cryptosporidium*	H (D, C)	Feces	Ag: ELISA
82	K18	*Cryptosporidium* Immunoassay Kit	D	Feces	Ag: ELISA
82	K22	*Cryptosporidium* Test	H (D, C)	Feces	Ag: ELISA
82	K4	Crypto Celisa	H (D, C)	Feces	Ag: ELISA
82	K17	ProSpecT Giardia Rapid	H (D, C)	Feces	Ag: ELISA
82	K4	CryptoCEL IFA	D, C	Feces	Ag: FA
82	K17	Xpect Crypto	H (D, C)	Feces	Ag: Rapid immunochromatography
82, 78	K4	Crypto/*Giardia* Cel	D, C	Feces	Ag: FA

D, Dog; *C*, cat; *M*, mink; *H*, human; *CSF*, cerebrospinal fluid; *Ab*, antibody; *Ag*, antigen; *ELISA*, enzyme-linked immunosorbent assay; *CDV*, canine distemper virus; *CPV*, canine parvovirus; *FA*, fluorescent antibody; *FIP*, feline infectious peritonitis; *FeLV*, feline leukemia virus; *FIV*, feline immunodeficiency virus; *RSAT*, rapid slide agglutination test; *PCR*, polymerase chain reaction; *LA*, latex agglutination; *AGID*, ager-gel immunodiffusion; *HA-I*, hemagglutination-inhibition.
[a]Kit is marketed as a human diagnostic test but have been used for small animals.

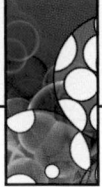

APPENDIX • 7

Disease Rule-Outs for Medical Problems

Craig E. Greene and Christie Mayo

INTEGUMENTAL PROBLEMS

Ulcers or Fistulas

Canine parvovirus-2 infection (8)
Feline poxvirus infection (19)
Pseudorabies (23)
Anaerobic infections (41)
Plague (47)
Actinomycosis (49)
Feline leprosy (50)

Mycobacterial infections (50)
Dermatophilosis (51)
Abscesses and pyogranulomas (52)
Blastomycosis (59)
Histoplasmosis (60)
Cryptococcosis (61)
Coccidioidomycosis (62)

Eumycotic mycetoma (67)
Lagenidiosis (67)
Phaeohyphomycosis (67)
Pythiosis (67)
Bacterial infections of skin (85)

Nodules

Canine viral papillomatosis (9)
Poxvirus infections (19)
Melioidosis (46)
Feline leprosy (50)
Mycobacterial infections (50)
Dermatophytosis (58)
Blastomycosis (59)

Histoplasmosis (60)
Cryptococcosis (61)
Coccidioidomycosis (62)
Sporotrichosis (63)
Eumycotic mycetoma (67)
Lagenidiosis (67)
Hyalohyphomycosis (67)

Pythiosis (67)
Zygomycosis (67)
Protothecosis (69)
Caryosporosis (81)
Sarcocystosis (81)
Bacterial infections of skin (85)

Pruritus

Rabies (22)
Pseudorabies (23)
Dermatophytosis (58)

Mallassezia infections (58)
Candidiasis (65)
Bacterial infections of skin (85)

Otitis externa (85)

Pustules or Vesicles

Distemper (3)
Canine herpesvirus infection (5)
Feline immunodeficiency virus infection (14)

Feline adenovirus infection (15)
Anthrax (35)
Staphylococcal infection (36)

Chryseomonas infection (46)
Dermatophytosis (58)
Bacterial infections of skin (85)

Edema

Infectious canine hepatitis (4)
Feline calicivirus infection (16)
Arthropod-borne viral infections (26)
Canine granulocytotropic ehrlichiosis (28)
Ehrlichiosis (28)
Rocky Mountain spotted fever (29)

Typhus (29)
Q Fever (29)
Anthrax (35)
Endotoxemia (38)
Botulism (42)
Canine aspergillosis-penicilliosis (64)

Miscellaneous fungal infections (67)
Zygomycosis (67)
African trypanosomiasis (72)
Babesiosis (77)
Bacteremia and endocarditis (87)
Inflammatory bowel disease (89)

Abscesses

Mycoplasmal infections (32)
L-form infections (32)
Rhodococcus equi infections (35)
Streptococcal infections (35)

Staphylococcal infections (36)
Salmonellosis (39)
Anaerobic infections (41)
Melioidosis (46)

Plague (47)
Nocardiosis (49)

MUSCULOSKELETAL PROBLEMS

Muscle Inflammation

Canine monocytotropic ehrlichiosis (28)	Feline abscesses (52)	Toxoplasmosis (80)
Rhodococcus equi infection (35)	Candidiasis (65)	Bacterial endocarditis (87)
Anaerobic infections (41, 86)	Trypanosomiasis (72)	
Dermatophilosis (51)	Hepatozoonosis (74)	

Joint Inflammation
Infectious or Immune-Mediated

Feline leukemia virus infection (13)	L-form infections (32)	Bartonellosis (54)
Feline calicivirus infection (16)	Mycoplasmal infections (32)	Coccidioidomycosis (62)
Feline foamy virus infection (17)	Streptococcal infections (35)	Aspergillosis, disseminated (64)
Mumps (25)	Enterococcal infections (35)	Leishmaniasis (73)
Canine ehrlichiosis (28)	Endotoxemia (38)	Bacterial skin infections (85)
Feline ehrlichiosis (28)	Lyme borreliosis (45)	Bacteremia (87)
Rocky Mountain spotted fever (29)	Actinomycosis (49)	Complement (C3) deficiency (95)
Chlamydial infections (30)	Feline abscesses (52)	Immunodeficiencies in Weimaraners (95)

Diskospondylitis

Streptococcal infections (35)	Mycobacterial infections (50)	Hyalohyphomycosis (67)
Staphylococcal Infections (36)	Abscesses and pyogranulomas (52)	Bacteremia (87)
Canine brucellosis (40)	Aspergillosis, disseminated (64)	Pyelonephritis (91)

Bone Inflammation
Osteomyelitis

L-form infections (32)	Anaerobic infections (41)	Phaeohyphomycosis (67)
Rhodococcus equi infections (35)	Nocardiosis (49)	Bacteremia (87)
Streptococcal infections (35)	Actinomycosis (49)	Cyclic hematopoiesis (95)
Proteus mirabilis infection (37)	Abscesses and pyogranulomas (52)	Immunodeficiencies in Weimaraners (95)
Pseudomonas aeruginosa infections (37)	Blastomycosis (59)	Hereditary neutropenia in border collies (95)
Salmonellosis (39)	Candidiasis (65)	

Hypertrophic Pulmonary Osteopathy

Anaerobic infections, pulmonary abscess (41)	Mycobacterial infection, pulmonary granulomas (50)

CARDIOVASCULAR PROBLEMS

Heart Muscle
Cardiomyopathy, Myocarditis

Distemper (3)	Rocky Mountain spotted fever (29)	Borreliosis (45)
Canine parvovirus-1 infections (8)	Q fever (29)	Bartonellosis (54)
Canine parvovirus-2 infections(8)	Streptococcal infections (35)	American trypanosomiasis (72)
Pseudorabies (23)	Campylobacteriosis (39)	Neosporosis (80)
Arthropod-borne viral infections (26)	Yersiniosis (39)	

Endocarditis

Streptococcal infections (35)	*Escherichia coli* infections (37)	Feline bartonellosis (54)
Enterococcal infections (35)	Canine bartonellosis (54)	Bacteremia (87)
Erysipelothrix infections (35)		

Pericarditis

Feline calicivirus infection (16)	Staphylococcal infections (36)	Canine disseminated aspergillosis (64)
Streptococcal infections (35)		

RESPIRATORY PROBLEMS

Upper Respiratory Tract
Rhinitis, Sinusitis

Canine herpesvirus infection (5)
Canine infectious tracheobronchitis (6)
Feline leukemia virus infection (13)
Feline rhinotracheitis (16)

Pseudomonas aeruginosa infections (37)
Leptospirosis (44)
Abscesses and pyogranulomas (52)
Bartonellosis (54)

Canine aspergillosis-penicilliosis (64)
Ciliary dyskinesia (95)
Bacterial rhinitis/bronchopneumonia of Irish wolfhounds (85)

Tracheobronchitis

Distemper (3)
Infectious canine hepatitis (4)
Canine herpesvirus infection (5)
Bordetellosis, canine (6)
Canine parainfluenza virus infection (6)

Feline immunodeficiency virus infection (14)
Influenza (25)

Chlamydial infections (30)
Mycoplasmal infections (32)
Staphylococcal infections (36)
Basidiobolus infection (67)

Lower Respiratory Tract
Alveolar-Interstitial Pneumonia

Distemper (3)
Infectious canine hepatitis (4)
Canine infectious tracheobronchitis (6)
Canine parainfluenza virus infection (6)
Feline enteric viral infections (12)
Bordetellosis (16)

Feline calicivirus infection (16)
Mycoplasmal infections (32)
Streptococcal infections (35)
Endotoxemia (38)
Plague (47)
Nocardiosis (49)

Mycobacterial infections (50)
Acanthamebiasis (79)
Toxoplasmosis (80)
Pneumocystosis (83)
Bacterial respiratory infections (88)
Aspiration pneumonia (88)

Interstitial Pneumonia

Infectious canine hepatitis (4)
Canine herpesviral infection (5)
Canine infectious tracheobronchitis (6)
Feline calicivirus infection (16)
Salmon poisoning disease (27)

Canine monocytotropic ehrlichiosis (28)
Feline monocytotropic ehrlichiosis (28)
Rocky Mountain spotted fever (29)
Mycoplasmal infections (32)

Leishmaniasis (73)
Aspiration pneumonia (88)

Interstitial-Nodular Pneumonia

Glanders (46)
Melioidosis (46)
Mycobacterial infections (50)

Blastomycosis (59)
Histoplasmosis (60)
Cryptococcosis (61)

Coccidioidomycosis (62)
Acanthamebiasis (79)

Pleural Effusion

Feline infectious peritonitis (11)
Feline leukemia virus infection (13)
Equine morbillivirus infection (18)
Anaerobic infections (41)
Actinomycosis (49)

Nocardiosis (49)
Mycobacterial infections (50)
Feline abscesses (52)
Blastomycosis (59)
Coccidioidomycosis (62)

Candidiasis (65)
American trypanosomiasis (72)
Toxoplasmosis (80)
Bacterial respiratory infections (88)

GASTROINTESTINAL PROBLEMS

Oral Inflammation (Stomatitis)

Canine herpesvirus infection (5)
Canine parvoviral-2 infection (8)
Feline parvoviral infections (10)
Feline immunodeficiency virus infection (14)

Feline calicivirus infection (16)
Feline rhinotracheitis (16)
Anaerobic infections (41)
Plague (47)

Feline bartonellosis (54) (controversial)
Candidiasis (65)
Immunodeficiencies in Weimaraners (95)

Dental Enamel Hypoplasia

Canine distemper (3)	Feline panleukopenia (10)

Hepatomegaly/Hepatic Inflammation and/or Infiltration

Infectious canine hepatitis (4)	Anaerobic infections (41)	Babesiosis (77)
Canine herpesvirus infection (5)	Borreliosis (45)	Toxoplasmosis (80)
Feline leukemia virus infection (13)	Melioidosis (46)	Neosporosis (80)
Feline calicivirus (16)	Tularemia (48)	Inflammatory bowel disease (89)
Canine granulocytotropic anaplasmosis (28)	Nocardiosis (49)	Cholecystitis/extrahepatic bile duct occlusion (90)
Rhodococcus equi infections (35)	Mycobacterial infections (50)	Hepatobiliary infections (90)
Intestinal helicobacteriosis (39)	Histoplasmosis (60)	Nonsuppurative cholangitis (90)
Tyzzer's disease (39)	American trypanosomiasis (72)	Pyogenic abscess (90)

Vomiting

Infectious canine hepatitis (4)	Campylobacteriosis (39)	Bacteremia (87)
Canine herpesvirus infection, neonate (5)	*Clostridium difficile*—associated diarrhea (39)	Tonsillitis and pharyngitis (88)
Coronavirus infection (8)	Gastric helicobacteriosis (39)	*Anaerobiospirillum* ileocolitis (89)
Canine parvovirus-1 infection (8)	Salmonellosis (39)	Chronic colitis (89)
Canine parvovirus-2 infection (8)	Anaerobic infections (41)	Hemorrhagic gastroenteritis (89)
Feline parvoviral infections (10)	Leptospirosis (44)	Intraabdominal infections (89)
Feline coronavirus infection (11)	Borreliosis (45)	Bile peritonitis (90)
Feline enteric viral infections (12)	Plague (47)	Nonsuppurative cholangitis (90)
Feline leukemia virus infection (13)	Mycobacterial infections (50)	Emphysematous cholecystitis (90)
Pseudorabies (23)	Canine aspergillosis-penicilliosis, disseminated (64)	Cholecystitis/extrahepatic bile duct occlusion (90)
Salmon poisoning disease (27)	Pythiosis (67)	Hepatic abscess (90)
Canine monocytotropic ehrlichiosis (28)	Zygomycosis (67)	Mastitis (91)
Canine granulocytotropic anaplasmosis (28)	Pneumocystosis (68)	Pyelonephritis (91)
Feline monocytotropic ehrlichiosis (28)	Babesiosis (77)	Pyometra (91)
Rocky Mountain spotted fever (29)	Amebiasis (78)	Immunodeficiencies in Shar-Peis (95)
Enterococcal infections (35)	Toxoplasmosis (80)	Immunodeficiencies in Weimaraners (95)
Listeriosis (35)	Enteric coccidiosis (81)	
Endotoxemia (38)	Intrahepatic biliary coccidiosis (81)	

Diarrhea

Distemper (3)	Chlamydial infections (30)	American trypanosomiasis (72)
Infectious canine hepatitis (4)	Enterococcal infections (35)	Leishmaniasis (73)
Nonrespiratory parainfluenza viral infection (7)	Listeriosis (35)	Hepatozoonosis (74)
Canine parvovirus-1 infection (8)	*Escherichia coli* infection (37)	Amebiasis (78)
Canine parvovirus-2 infection (8)	Endotoxemia (38)	Balantidiasis (78)
Coronavirus infection (8)	Campylobacteriosis (39)	Giardiasis (78)
Rotavirus infection (8)	*Clostridium perfringens* infection (39)	Trichomoniasis (78)
Feline panleukopenia (10)	*Clostridium difficile*—associated diarrhea (39)	Toxoplasmosis (80)
Feline parvoviral infections (10)	Gastric helicobacteriosis (39)	Enteric coccidiosis (81)
Feline coronavirus infection (11)	Salmonellosis (39)	Cryptosporidiosis (82)
Feline enteric viral infections (12)	Yersiniosis (39)	Bacteremia (87)
Feline leukemia virus infection (13)	Anaerobic infections (41)	*Anaerobiospirillum*/ileocolitis (89)
Feline immunodeficiency virus infection (14)	Leptospirosis (44)	Inflammatory bowel disease (89)
Poxvirus infections (19)	Plague (47)	Intraabdominal bacterial infections (89)
Pseudorabies (23)	Nocardiosis (49)	Chronic colitis (89)
Human enterovirus infections (24)	Mycobacterial infections (50)	Nonsuppurative cholangitis (90)
Elokomin fluke fever (27)	Histoplasmosis (60)	Pyogenic abscess (90)
Salmon poisoning disease (27)	Pythiosis (67)	Hereditary neutropenia in border collies (95)
Canine granulocytotropic anaplasmosis (28)	Pneumocystosis (68)	Immunodeficiencies in Shar-Peis (95)
Feline monocytotropic ehrlichiosis (28)	Protothecosis (69)	Immunodeficiencies in Weimaraners (95)

Abdominal Pain

Infectious canine hepatitis (4)	Endotoxemia (38)	Chronic colitis (89)
Canine herpesvirus infection (5)	Salmonellosis (39)	Bile peritonitis (90)
Feline panleukopenia (10)	Tyzzer's disease (39)	Cholecystitis/extrahepatic bile duct
Feline infectious peritonitis (11)	Yersiniosis (39)	occlusion (90)
Rocky Mountain spotted fever (29)	Leptospirosis (44)	Emphysematous cholecystitis (90)
Rhodococcus equi infection (35)	Intraabdominal infections (89)	Pyogenic abscess (90)

Abdominal Effusion

Infectious canine hepatitis (4)	Actinomycosis (49)	Infectious pericardial effusion (87)
Feline infectious peritonitis (11)	Bartonellosis (54)	Inflammatory bowel disease (89)
Feline leukemia virus infection (13)	Histoplasmosis (60)	Intraabdominal infections (89)
Streptococcal infections (35)	*Basidiobolus* infection (67)	Pyogenic abscess (90)
Anaerobic infections (41)	American trypanosomiasis (72)	
Nocardiosis (49)	Toxoplasmosis (80)	

Abdominal Mass

Feline infectious peritonitis (11)	Blastomycosis (59)	Pythiosis (67)
Feline leukemia virus infection (13)	Histoplasmosis (60)	Zygomycosis (67)
Actinomycosis (49)	Coccidioidomycosis (62)	Toxoplasmosis (80)
Nocardiosis (49)	Eumycotic mycetoma (67)	Intraabdominal infections (89)
Mycobacterial infections (50)	Miscellaneous fungal infections (67)	Hepatobiliary infections (90)

URINARY PROBLEMS

Renal Failure

Arthropod-borne viral infections (26)	Protothecosis (69)	Hepatobiliary infections (90)
Rocky Mountain spotted fever (29)	Microsporidiosis (75)	Pyelonephritis (91)
Escherichia coli infection (37)	Babesiosis (77)	Pyometra (91)
Leptospirosis (44)	Bacteremia (87)	Complement C3 deficiency (95)
Surgical and traumatic wound infections (55)	Infective endocarditis (87)	
Cryptococcosis (61)	Sepsis (87)	

GENITAL PROBLEMS

Scrotal Enlargement or Drainage

Feline infectious peritonitis (11)	Rocky Mountain spotted fever (29)	Rhodotorulosis (65)
Feline infectious peritonitis (11)	Canine brucellosis (40)	African trypanosomiasis (72)
Canine ehrlichiosis (28)	Blastomycosis (59)	Genitourinary infections (91)

Reproductive Failure, Infertility, Abortion

Distemper (3)	Arthropod-borne viral infections (26)	Salmonellosis (39)
Canine herpesvirus infection (5)	Q-fever (29)	Canine brucellosis (40)
Canine parvovirus-1 infection (8)	Chlamydial infections (30)	Feline bartonellosis (54)
Feline panleukopenia (10)	Streptococcal infections (35)	Toxoplasmosis (80)
Feline leukemia virus infection (13)	Campylobacteriosis (39)	Neosporosis (80)

Birth of Ill (Fading) Neonates

Canine parvovirus-1 infection (8)	Feline leukemia virus infection (13)	Toxoplasmosis (80)
Feline panleukopenia (10)		

HEMOLYMPHATIC PROBLEMS

Lymphadenomegaly

Distemper (3)
Infectious canine hepatitis (4)
Canine viral papillomatosis (9)
Feline parvoviral infections (10)
Feline infectious peritonitis (11)
Feline leukemia virus infection (13)
Feline immunodeficiency virus infection (14)
Feline foamy virus infection (17)
Mumps (25)
Salmon poisoning disease (27)
Canine granulocytotropic anaplasmosis (28)
Canine monocytotropic ehrlichiosis (28)
Feline monocytotropic ehrlichiosis (28)
Q-fever (29)
Rocky Mountain spotted fever (29)
Chlamydial infections (30)
L-form infections (32)
Rhodococcus equi infections (35)
Streptococcal infections (35)
Salmonellosis (39)
Canine brucellosis (40)

Borreliosis (45)
Glanders (46)
Melioidosis (46)
Plague (47)
Tularemia (48)
Actinomycosis (49)
Nocardiosis (49)
Mycobacterial infections (50)
Dermatophilosis (51)
Abscesses and pyogranulomas (52)
Feline abscesses (52)
Bite wound infections (53)
Feline bartonellosis (54)
Blastomycosis (59)
Histoplasmosis (60)
Cryptococcosis (61)
Coccidioidomycosis (62)
Sporotrichosis (63)
Canine aspergillosis-penicilliosis (64)
Canine disseminated aspergillosis (64)
Candidiasis (65)

Trichosporonosis (66)
Lagenidiosis (67)
Miscellaneous fungal infections (67)
Phaeohyphomycosis (67)
Pythiosis (67)
Zygomycosis (67)
Protothecosis (69)
African trypanosomiasis (72)
American trypanosomiasis (72)
Leishmaniasis (73)
Feline hepatozoonosis (74)
Hepatozoon americanum infection (74)
Encephalitozoonosis (75)
Cytauxzoonosis (76)
Babesiosis (77)
Toxoplasmosis (80)
Bacteremia and endocarditis (87)
Cyclic hematopoiesis (95)
Immunodeficiencies in Weimaraners (95)
Rhinitis/bronchopneumonia in Irish Wolfhounds (95)

Splenomegaly

Feline leukemia virus infection (13)
Feline immunodeficiency virus infection (14)
Canine granulocytotropic anaplasmosis (28)
Canine monocytotropic ehrlichiosis (28)
Feline monocytotropic ehrlichiosis (28)
Q-fever (29)
Hemotrophic mycoplasmosis (hemobartonellosis) (31)
Endotoxemia (38)

Canine brucellosis (40)
Borreliosis (45)
Melioidosis (46)
Plague (47)
Tularemia (48)
Nocardiosis (49)
Mycobacterial infections (50)
Histoplasmosis (60)

African trypanosomiasis (72)
American trypanosomiasis (72)
Leishmaniasis (73)
Cytauxzoonosis (76)
Babesiosis (77)
Bacteremia (87)
Infective endocarditis (87)
Hepatobiliary infections (90)

Immunodeficiency: See Table 95-4

Anemia
Regenerative

Hemotrophic mycoplasmosis (hemobartonellosis) (31)
Bartonellosis (54)

Hepatozoon canis infection (74)

Babesiosis (77)

Nonregenerative

Feline infectious peritonitis (11)
Feline leukemia virus infection (13)
Feline immunodeficiency virus infection (14)
Canine monocytotropic ehrlichiosis (28)
Feline monocytotropic ehrlichiosis (28)
Endotoxemia (38)
Salmonellosis (39)
Actinomycosis (49)

Nocardiosis (49)
Mycobacterial infections (50)
Abscesses and pyogranulomas (52)
Histoplasmosis (60)
Coccidioidomycosis (62)
Leishmaniasis (73)
Hepatozoon americanum infection (74)
Feline hepatozoonosis (74)

Hepatozoon canis infection (74)
Cytauxzoonosis (76)
Toxoplasmosis (80)
Pulmonary abscess (88)
Hepatobiliary infections (90)
Nonsuppurative cholangitis (90)

Circulating Cellular Inclusions

Canine distemper (3)
Feline infectious peritonitis (11)
Elokomin fluke fever (27)
Feline granulocytotropic anaplasmosis (28)
Canine granulocytotropic ehrlichiosis (28)
Canine monocytotropic ehrlichiosis (28)

Feline monocytotropic ehrlichiosis (28)
Thrombocytotropic anaplasmosis (28)
Haemobartonellosis (31)
Histoplasmosis (60)
American trypanosomiasis (72)
Leishmaniasis (73)
Hepatozoonosis (74)

Cytauxzoonosis (76)
Babesiosis (77)
Toxoplasmosis (80)
Bacteremia (87)

Lymphopenia

Distemper (3)
Canine parvovirus-1 infection (8)
Feline infectious peritonitis (11)
Feline leukemia virus infection (13)
Feline immunodeficiency virus infection (14)

Salmon poisoning disease (27)
Feline granulocytotropic anaplasmosis (28)
Salmonellosis (39)
Mycobacterial infections (50)
Blastomycosis (59)

African trypanosomiasis (72)
Acanthamebiasis (79)
Bacteremia and endocarditis (87)

Leukocytosis

Canine herpesvirus infection (5)
Feline infectious peritonitis (11)
Feline viral neoplasia (13)
Salmon poisoning disease (27)
Feline monocytotropic ehrlichiosis (28)
Rocky Mountain spotted fever (29)
L-form infections (32)
Rhodococcus equi infections (35)
Staphylococcal infections (36)
Endotoxemia (38)
Campylobacteriosis (39)
Canine brucellosis (40)
Anaerobic infections (41)
Tetanus (43)
Leptospirosis (44)

Plague (47)
Tularemia (48)
Actinomycosis (49)
Nocardiosis (49)
Mycobacterial infections (50)
Feline abscesses (52)
Bartonellosis (54)
Surgical and traumatic wound infections (55)
Systemic postsurgical infections (55)
Blastomycosis (59)
Histoplasmosis (60)
Coccidioidomycosis (62)
Canine aspergillosis-penicilliosis (64)
Candidiasis (65)
Pneumocystosis (68)

African trypanosomiasis (72)
Leishmaniasis (73)
Hepatozoon americanum infection (74)
Hepatozoon canis infection (74)
Encephalitozoonosis (75)
Microsporidiosis (75)
Babesiosis (77)
Acanthamebiasis (79)
Toxoplasmosis (80)
Pneumocystosis (83)
Bacteremia and endocarditis (87)
Infective endocarditis (87)
Pulmonary abscess (88)
Pyelonephritis (91)

Neutropenia

Canine parvovirus-1 infection (8)
Canine parvovirus-2 infection (8)
Feline panleukopenia (10)
Feline leukemia virus infection (13)
Feline viral neoplasia (13)
Feline immunodeficiency virus (14)

Salmon poisoning disease (27)
Canine granulocytotropic ehrlichiosis (28)
Feline monocytotropic ehrlichiosis (28)
Endotoxemia (38)
Salmonellosis (39)
African trypanosomiasis (72)

Cytauxzoonosis (76)
Babesiosis (77)
Bacteremia and endocarditis (87)
Cyclic hematopoiesis (95)
Hereditary neutropenia in border collies (95)
Selective cobalamin malabsorption (95)

Thrombocytopenia

Infectious canine hepatitis (4)
Canine herpesvirus infection (5)
Canine parvovirus-1 or -2 infections (8)
Feline parvoviral infections (10)
Feline infectious peritonitis (11)
Feline leukemia virus infection (13)
Feline viral neoplasia (13)
Feline adenovirus infection (15)
Elokomin fluke fever (27)
Salmon poisoning disease (27)

Feline granulocytotropic anaplasmosis (28)
Feline monocytotropic ehrlichiosis (28)
Thrombocytotropic anaplasmosis (28)
Rocky Mountain spotted fever (29)
Escherichia coli infection (37)
Endotoxemia (38)
Salmonellosis (39)

Histoplasmosis (60)
Candidiasis (65)
Pneumocystosis (68)
African trypanosomiasis (72)
Feline hepatozoonosis (74)
Hepatozoon canis infection (74)
Cytauxzoonosis (76)
Babesiosis (77)
Bacteremia (87)
Infective endocarditis (87)

Canine granulocytotropic ehrlichiosis (28)	Leptospirosis (44)	Inflammatory bowel disease (89)
Canine monocytotropic ehrlichiosis (28)	Plague (47)	
	Tularemia (48)	
	Bartonella vinsonii infection (54)	
	Surgical and traumatic wound infections (55)	

MISCELLANEOUS LABORATORY PROBLEMS

Increased Liver Enzymes

Infectious canine hepatitis (4)	Tyzzer's disease (39)	*Hepatozoon canis* infection (74)
Canine herpesvirus infection (5)	Anaerobic infections (41)	Microsporidiosis (75)
Feline panleukopenia (10)	Leptospirosis (44)	Cytauxzoonosis (76)
Feline infectious peritonitis (11)	Tularemia (48)	Babesiosis (77)
Feline viral neoplasia (13)	Mycobacterial infections (50)	Neosporosis (80)
Salmon poisoning disease (27)	*Bartonella vinsonii* infection (54)	Toxoplasmosis (80)
Canine granulocytptropic anaplasmosis (28)	Histoplasmosis (60)	Infective endocarditis (87)
Canine monocytotropic ehrlichiosis (28)	Canine aspergillosis-penicilliosis (64)	Inflammatory bowel disease (89)
Rocky Mountain spotted fever (29)	Canine disseminated aspergillosis (64)	Emphysematous cholecystitis (90)
Hemotrophic mycoplasmosis (hemobartonellosis) (31)	Candidiasis (65)	Hepatobiliary infections (90)
Escherichia coli infection (37)	American trypanosomiasis (72)	Nonsuppurative cholangitis (90)
Endotoxemia (38)	*Hepatozoon americanum* infection (74)	Prostatic abscess (91)

Positive Coombs' Testing

Feline viral neoplasia (13)	Hemotrophic mycoplasmosis (hemobartonellosis) (31)	Leishmaniasis (73)
Ehrlichiosis (28)	Canine brucellosis (40)	Babesiosis (77)

Azotemia

Canine herpesvirus infection (5)	Salmonellosis (39)	Microsporidiosis (75)
Feline viral neoplasia (13)	Leptospirosis (44)	Babesiosis (77)
Feline immunodeficiency virus infection (14)	Borreliosis (45)	Infective endocarditis (87)
Ehrlichiosis (28)	*Bartonella vinsonii* infection (54)	Emphysematous cholecystitis (90)
Rocky Mountain spotted fever (29)	Coccidioidomycosis (62)	Nonsuppurative cholangitis (90)
Escherichia coli infection (37)	Leishmaniasis (73)	Genitourinary infections (91)
Endotoxemia (38)	Encephalitozoonosis (75)	

Icterus

Infectious canine hepatitis (4)	Tyzzer's disease (39)	Zygomycosis (67)
Feline parvoviral infection (10)	Leptospirosis (44)	Feline hepatozoonosis (74)
Feline infectious peritonitis (11)	Tularemia (48)	Cytauxzoonosis (76)
Feline viral neoplasia (13)	Mycobacterial infections (50)	Babesiosis (77)
Feline calicivirus infection (16)	*Bartonella vinsonii* infection (54)	Toxoplasmosis (80)
Endotoxemia (38)	Surgical and traumatic wound infections (55)	Sarcocystosis (81)
Salmonellosis (39)	Histoplasmosis (60)	Intrahepatic biliary coccidiosis (81)
Campylobacteriosis (39)	Mucormycosis (67)	Cholangiohepatitis (90)

Proteinuria with an Acellular Sediment

Infectious canine hepatitis (4)	*Escherichia coli* infection (37)	Babesiosis (77)
Feline infectious peritonitis (11)	Endotoxemia (38)	Toxoplasmosis (80)
Feline viral neoplasia (13)	Leptospirosis (44)	Bacteremia (87)
Arthropod-borne viral infections (26)	Borreliosis (45)	Infective endocarditis (87)
Canine granulocytotropic anaplasmosis (28)	*Bartonella vinsonii* infection (54)	
Canine monocytotropic ehrlichiosis (28)	Coccidioidomycosis (62)	
Rocky Mountain spotted fever (29)	Leishmaniasis (73)	

Hyperfibrinogenemia

Feline infectious peritonitis (11)	Leptospirosis (44)	Hepatobiliary infections (90)
L-form Infections (32)	Bacteremia and endocarditis (87)	

Hyperglobulinemia

Feline infectious peritonitis (11)	Actinomycosis (49)	Coccidioidomycosis (62)
Feline viral neoplasia (13)	Mycobacterial infections (50)	Leishmaniasis (73)
Feline immunodeficiency viral infection (14)	*Bartonella vinsonii* infection (54)	*Hepatozoon americanum* infection (74)
Salmon poisoning disease (27)	Blastomycosis (59)	*Hepatozoon canis* infection (74)
Canine monocytotropic ehrlichiosis (28)	Histoplasmosis (60)	
Canine brucellosis (40)		

CENTRAL NERVOUS SYSTEM PROBLEMS

Primary Meningitis or Vasculitis, Secondary Encephalitis

Ehrlichiosis (28)	Cryptococcosis (61)	Acanthamebiasis (79)
Feline infectious peritonitis (11)	Coccidioidomycosis (62)	Granulomatous meningoencephalitis (84)
Rocky Mountain spotted fever (29)	Hyalohyphomycosis (67)	Hydrocephalus with perventricular encephalitis (84)
Listeriosis (35)	Mucormycosis (67)	Pug and Maltese encephalitis (84)
Canine brucellosis (40)	Phaeohyphomycosis (67)	Steroid-responsive meningitis-arteritis (84)
Anaerobic bacterial infections (41)	Zygomycosis (67)	Yorkshire terrier encephalitis (84)
Actinomycosis (49)	Protothecosis (69)	Bacterial meningitis (92)
Feline abscesses (52)	American trypanosomiasis (72)	Brain Abscess (92)
Blastomycosis (59)	Encephalitozoonosis (75)	
Histoplasmosis (60)	Babesiosis (77)	

Primary Encephalitis, Secondary Meningitis

Distemper (3)	Pseudorabies (23)	Toxoplasmosis (80)
Infectious canine hepatitis (4)	Arboviral infections (26)	*Sarcocystis neurona* infection (81)
Neonatal and prenatal parvoviral infections (8, 10)	Louping-Ill (26)	Feline poliomyelitis (84)
Feline paramyxovirus infections (18)	Babesiosis (77)	Feline spongiform encephalopathy (84)
Rabies (22)	Neosporosis (80)	

Cerebrospinal Fluid (CSF) Results (see also Table 92-2)
CSF Protein Increase and Mononuclear Cells

Distemper (3)	Arboviral infections (26)	Hydrocephalus with perventricular encephalitis (84)
Feline paramyxovirus infections (18)	Ehrlichiosis (28)	Pug encephalitis (84)
Rabies (22)	Feline poliomyelitis (84)	
Pseudorabies (23)	Granulomatous meningoencephalitis (84)	

CSF Protein Increase and Neutrophils

Feline infectious peritonitis (11)	Canine brucellosis (40)	Listeriosis (35)
Rocky Mountain spotted fever (29)	Leptospirosis (44)	Phaeohyphomycosis (67)

CSF Protein Increase and Mixed (Mononuclear and Neutrophils) Cells

Blastomycosis (59)	Encephalitozoonosis (75)	Granulomatous meningoencephalitis (84)
Cryptococcosis (61)	Neosporosis (80)	Yorkshire terrier encephalitis (84)
Protothecosis (69)	Toxoplasmosis (80)	

Epidural or Extrdural Compression of Spinal Cord, Diskospondylitis

Feline viral neoplasia (13)	Actinomycosis (49)	Hyalohyphomycosis (67)
Staphylococcal infections (36)	Feline abscesses (52)	Paecilomycosis (67)
Canine brucellosis (40)	Canine aspergillosis-penicilliosis (64)	

Hydrocephalus

Nonrespiratory parainfluenza infection (7)	Periventricular encephalitis (84)	Ciliary dyskinesia (95)
Feline infectious peritonitis (11)		

OCULAR PROBLEMS
CONJUNCTIVA

Conjunctivitis

Distemper (3)	Rocky Mountain spotted fever (29)	Leptospirosis (44)
Canine herpesvirus infection, adult (5)	Chlamydial infections (30)	Tularemia (48)
Feline immunodeficiency virus infection (14)	Mycoplasmal infections (32)	Blastomycosis (59)
Feline calicivirus infection (16)	Staphylococcal infections (36)	Histoplasmosis (60)
Feline herpesvirus infection (16)	*Proteus mirabilis* infection (37)	African trypanosomiasis (72)
Feline rhinotracheitis (16)	Salmonellosis (39)	Leishmaniasis (73)
Influenza (25)	Botulism (42)	Toxoplasmosis (80)

Symplepharon

Feline herpesvirus infection (16)

Prolapsed Third Eyelid

Tetanus (43)

Hemorrhage

Feline leukemia virus infection (13)	Rocky Mountain spotted fever (29)	Leptospirosis (44)
Canine ehrlichiosis (28)		

LACRIMAL SYSTEM

Mucopurulent Secretions

Distemper (3)

CORNEA

Keratitis

Infectious canine hepatitis virus infection (4)	Rocky Mountain spotted fever (29)	Leishmaniasis (73)
Canine herpesvirus infection, neonate (5)	Brucellosis (40)	Bacterial septicemia (87)
Feline leukemia virus infection (13)	Mycobacterial infection (50)	
Feline herpesvirus infection (16)	Botulism (42)	

Edema

Infectious canine hepatitis virus infection (4)

Symplepharon

Feline herpesvirus infection (16)

ANTERIOR CHAMBER

Glaucoma

Infectious canine hepatitis virus infection (4)	Leishmaniasis (73)	Bacterial septicemia (87)
Feline leukemia virus infection (13)	Prototheocosis (69)	

Tumor Mass

Feline leukemia virus infection (13)

Hyphema

Feline leukemia virus infection (13)	Canine ehrlichiosis (28)

ANTERIOR UVEA

Uveitis

Feline infectious peritonitis (11)	Tularemia (48)	Eumycotic mycetoma (67)
Feline immunodeficiency virus infection (secondary infection) (14)	Feline bartonellosis (54)	African trypanosomiasis (72)
Feline leukemia virus infection (13)	Blastomycosis (59)	*Hepatozoon americanum* infection (74)
Feline rhinotracheitis (16)	Coccidioidomycosis (62)	Toxoplasmosis (80)
Thrombocytotropic anaplasmosis (28)	Canine disseminated aspergillosis (64)	Bacteremia (87)
Leptospirosis (44)	Candidiasis (65)	

Paradoxical Pupil Size

Feline leukemia virus infection (13)

LENS

Cataract

Canine herpesvirus infection, adult (5)	Feline leukemia virus infection (13)	Brucellosis (40)
Feline infectious peritonitis (11)		

VITREOUS

Hemorrhage

Canine ehrlichiosis (28)

Hyalitis

Brucellosis (40)	Leishmaniasis (73)	Toxoplasmosis (80)
Prototheocosis (69)		

RETINA/CHOROID

Chorioretinitis

Distemper (3)	Rabies (22)	Prototheocosis (69)
Canine herpesvirus infection, neonate (5)	Brucellosis (40)	Toxoplasmosis (80)
Feline infectious peritonitis (11)	Mycobacterial infections (50)	Bacterial septicemia (87)

Dysplasia

Canine herpesvirus infection, neonate (5)	Feline panleukopenia (10)

Atrophy

Feline panleukopenia (10)

Infiltrates

Canine ehrlichiosis (28)	Hemotrophic mycoplasmosis (hemobartonellosis) (31)

Hemorrhages

Feline leukemia virus infection (13) Rocky Mountain spotted fever (29)	Hemotrophic mycoplasmosis (hemobartonellosis) (31)	Bacterial septicemia (87)

Pale Vessels

Feline leukemia virus infection (13)

Detachment

Feline leukemia virus infection (13) Canine ehrlichiosis (28)	Mycobacterial infections (50)	Protothecosis (69)

Vascular Engorgement

Canine ehrlichiosis (28)

Vasculitis

Rocky Mountain spotted fever (29)

OPTIC NERVE

Neuritis

Distemper (3) Canine herpesvirus infection, Neonate (5)	Feline infectious peritonitis (11) Feline herpesvirus infection (16)	Protothecosis (69) Toxoplasmosis (80)

Hypoplasia

Feline panleukopenia (10)

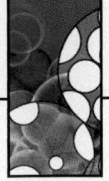

Antimicrobial Drug Formulary

Craig E. Greene, Katrin Hartmann, and Janet Calpin

PROFESSIONAL FLEXIBLE LABELING

This practice of customized dosing of veterinary drugs has been adopted by the Food and Drug Administration in the United States. The concept of individualized dosing of an animal based on the animal and disease being treated is new to veterinary drugs where fixed-dosage regimens have been customary. Dosages given on antimicrobial labels in the past have often been based on licensing data obtained by using the antimicrobial on the most susceptible infection for the organ system under consideration. Thus, dosage information was the lowest level and was ineffective for managing infections involving resistant organisms or other body systems. Future veterinary labels will provide the veterinarian with pharmacokinetic and pharmacodynamic information concerning each drug and its microbiologic susceptibility data. Dosage ranges and specific dosage indications will also be provided.

The information in this formulary is intended to support the concept of flexible labeling. Information is provided on each drug to enable veterinarians to adjust dosages on the bases of clinical and toxicologic data. Recommendations for dosing with each drug are variable depending on the type and location of infection. The reader is referred to other dosage tables in their respective disease chapters for specific dosage regimens. An attempt has been made to include the majority of drugs available internationally to treat animal infections. Many of these drugs are approved for human use, but limited studies have been performed on dogs and cats. References to newer information are cited on the basis of information in the respective chapters on antiviral drugs (Chapter 2), antibacterial drugs (Chapter 34), antifungal drugs (Chapter 57), and antiprotozoal drugs (Chapter 71). References appear with the chapter number followed by the specific citation number.

Additional references used in completion of this work are as follows:

Compendium of Veterinary Products: Port Huron, MI, North American Compendium Inc, 1995.
Facts and Comparisons Staff: *Facts and Comparison: Loose-Leaf Drug Information Series.* St. Louis, MO, Facts and Comparisons Staff, 1997.
Physicians' Desk Reference: Montvale, NJ, Medical Economics Co., 1997.
Plumb DC: *Veterinary Drug Handbook*, ed 2. Ames, IA, Iowa State University Press, 1995.

Reynolds JEF, editor. *Martindale, The Extra Pharmacopoeia.* London, Royal Pharmaceutical Society, 1996.
Micromedex Drug Information on Line 1997: www.micromedex.com.

Numbered references cited in this appendix include:
1. Eddlestone SM, Neer MT, Gaunt SD, et al. 2005. Failure of imidocarb dipropionate to clear experimentally induced *Ehrlichia canis* infection in dogs, Abstract # 134, 23rd Meeting ACVIM, Baltimore, Md., *J Vet Intern Med* 19:436-437.
2. Jacobs LD, Beck RW, Simon JH, et al. 2000. Intramuscular interferon beta-1a therapy initiated during a first demyelinating event in multiple sclerosis, *N Engl J Med* 343:898-904.
3. McCaw DL. Advances in therapy for retroviral infections, pp 21-25. In August J, editior: *Consultations in feline internal medicine*, ed 2. Philadelphia, WB Saunders, 1991.
4. Northsworthy GD. 1996. Interferon-alpha as an immunostimulant, *Vet Forum* October:27.
5. Tasker S, Chaney SMA, Day MJ, et al. 2005a. Effect of chronic FIV infection and efficacy of marbofloxacin treatment on 'Candidatus Mycoplasma haemominutum' infection Abstract # 129, 23rd Meeting ACVIM, Baltimore, Md., *J Vet Intern Med* 19:435.
6. Tasker S, Chaney SMA, Day MJ, et al. 2005b. Effect of chronic FIV infection and efficacy of marbofloxacin treatment on *Mycoplasma haemofelis* infection, Abstract # 130, 23rd Meeting ACVIM, Baltimore, Md., *J Vet Intern Med* 19:435.
7. Weiss RC. 1991. Feline infectious peritonitis: advances in therapy and control, pp 3-12. In Wolf AM, August JD, editors: *Consultations in Feline Internal Medicine*, ed 2, Philadelphia, WB Saunders.
8. Woods JE, Brewer M, Radecki SV, et al. 2004. Treatment of Mycoplasma haemofelis infected cats with imidocarb dipropionate, Abstract # 192, 22nd Meeting ACVIM, Minneapolis, Minn.
9. Zeidner N. 1990. Alpha interferon 2b in combination with zidovudine for treatment of presymptomatic feline leukemia virus-induced immunodeficiency syndrome, *Antimicrob Agents Chemother* 34:1749-1756.

MANUFACTURERS/DISTRIBUTORS	ADDRESS	CITY	STATE/COUNTRY	POSTAL CODE	TELEPHONE	WEBSITE
3M Pharmaceutical	3M Center, Building 275-5W-05	St. Paul	MN	55133	651-773-1110	www.mmm.com
Abbott Laboratories	100 Abbott Park Rd.	Abbott Park	IL	60064-6154	800-633-9110	www.abbott.com
Allen and Hansburys—	See GlaxoSmithKline Pharm.					
Allergan, Inc.	2525 DuPont Dr.	Irvine	CA	9262-9534	714-246-4500	www.allergan.com
American Pharmaceuticals Partners, Inc.	10866 Wilshire Blvd., Ste. 1270	Los Angeles	CA	90024	310-826-8505	www.appdrugs.com
Amgen	1 Amgen Center Dr.	Thousand Oaks	CA	91320	800-282-6436	www.amgen.com
Anthony Products Co.	5600 Peck Rd.	Arcadia	CA	91006	626-357-8711	
Apothecon, Inc.	PO Box 4500	Princeton	NJ	08540	609-897-2000	www.bms.com
Astra Zeneca LP.	1800 Concord Pike	Wilmington	DE	19850	800-456-3669	www.AstraZeneca-us.com
Bayer B.V.	Energieweg 1	3641 RT Mijdrecht	NL		02979-80666	
Bayer Corporation	400 Morgan Ln.	West Haven	CT	06516	203-937-2000	www.bayer.com
Bayer Animal Health	PO Box 390	Shawnee	KS	66201-0390	800-633-3796	www.bayer-ah.com
Bayer Vet Ltd.	Eastern Way	Bury St. Edmunds, Suffolk	UK	IP32 7AH	01284-63200	
Berlex Laboratories, Inc.	6 West Belt	Wayne	NJ	07470-2095	973-694-4100	www.berlex.com
Biocraft Laboratories, Inc.	See Teva Pharmaceuticals					
Bioniche Animal Health USA, Inc.	1551 Jennings Mill Rd., Ste. 300A	Bogard	GA	306222	706-549-4503	www.bioniche.com
Boehringer Ingelheim Pharmaceuticals	900 Ridgebury Rd., PO Box 368	Ridgefield	CT	06877	203-798-9988	Us.boehringer-ingelheim.com
Boots Pharmaceuticals, Inc.	See Abbott Laboratories					www.boots.co.uk/frontpage.html
Bristol Laboratories	See Bristol-Myers Squibb					
Bristol-Myers Squibb	PO Box 4000	Princeton	NJ	08543-4000	800-468-7746	www.bms.com
Burroughs Wellcome Co.	See GlaxoSmithKline Pharm.					
The Butler Company	5600 Blazer Pkwy.	Dublin	OH	43017	614-761-9095	www.AccessButler.com
Carrington Laboratories, Inc.	2001 Walnut Hill Ln.	Irving	TX	75038	972-518-1300	www.carringtonlabs.com
Ciba Agriculture	540 White Plains Rd., PO Box 2005	Tarrytown	NY	10591-9005	914-785-2000	www.cibasc.com
Ciba-Geigy Pharmaceuticals	See Novartis Pharmaceuticals					
Delmont Laboratories, Inc.	PO Box 269	Swarthmore	PA	19081	610-543-3365	www.delmont.com
Dista Products Co.	See Eli Lilly and Co.					
DuPont Pharmaceuticals Co.	See Bristol-Myers Squibb					
Elan Pharmaceuticals	7475 Lusk Blvd.	San Diego	CA	92121	858-457-2553	www.elan.com
Elanco Animal Health USA	Div. of Eli Lilly & Co., Lilly Corp. Center	Indianapolis	IN	46240-3733	317-276-1262	www.elanco.com
Elanco Animal Health	500 East 96th St., Ste. 125-INT	Indianapolis	IN	46240	800-428-4441	www.elanco.com
Elanco Animal Health	Divisie van Eli Lilly B.V., 4872 XL Etten-Leur1	City Kantoren/Raadstede 15	NL		03402-79722	
Elkins-Sinn, Inc.	See Wyeth-Ayerst					
Enzon, Inc.	685 Rt. 202/206	Bridgewater	NJ	08854	908-541-8600	www.enzon.com

Continued

MANUFACTURERS/ DISTRIBUTORS	ADDRESS	CITY	STATE/ COUNTRY	POSTAL CODE	TELEPHONE	WEBSITE
Faro Pharmaceuticals, Inc.	See Prometheus Laboratories, Inc.					
Fermenta Animal Health Co.	See also Boehinger Ingelheim Pharmaceuticals, Inc.					
Fleming & Co.	1733 Gilsinn Ln.	Fenton	MO	63026-2918	636-343-5206	www.flemingcompany.com
Fleming Laboratories, Inc.	PO BOX 34384	Charlotte	NC	28234	704-372-5613	www.forestpharm.com
Forest Pharmaceutical, Inc.	13600 Shoreline	St. Louis	MO	63045	314-493-7000	www.wyeth.com/divisions/ for_dodge.asp
Fort Dodge Laboratories	800-5th St., NW, PO Box 518	Fort Dodge	IA	50501	515-955-4600	www.fujisawa.com
Fujisawa Healthcare, Inc.	3 Parkway North Center	Deerfield	IL	60015-2548	847-317-8800	
Geigy Pharmaceuticals	See Novartis Pharmaceuticals					
Genentech, Inc.	1 DNA Way	S. San Francisco	CA	94080-4990	650-225-1000	www.gene.com
GlaxoSmithKline Pharm.	Five Moore Dr.	Research Triangle Park	NC	27709	919-248-2100	www.gsk.com
Glaxo Wellcome	See GlaxoSmihKline Pharm					
Glenwood, Inc.	111 Cedar Ln.	Englewood	NJ	07631	201-569-0050	www.glenwood-llc.com
Hoechst Marion-Roussel Agri-Vet Co.	See Aventis Pharmaceuticals					
Hoechst Marion-Roussel, Inc.	See Aventis Pharmaceuticals					
ICN Pharmaceuticals, Inc.	3300 Hyland Ave.	Costa Mesa	CA	92626	714-545-0100	www.icnpharm.com
Immunovet (Vetoquinol)	5910-G Breckenridge Pkwy.	Tampa	FL	33610	800-627-9447	www.immvac.com
Imvac Inc.	RR 1, 6080 Bass Ln.	Columbia	MO	65201	573-443-5363	www.interferonsciences.com
Interferon Sciences	783 Jersey Ave.	New Brunswick	NJ	08901	732-249-3250	www.intermune.com
InterMune Pharmaceuticals, Inc.	3280 Bayside Rd.	Bayshore	CA	94005	415-466-2200	www.intervet.com
Intervet Nederland B.V.	Kleine Broekstraat 1	5831 AP Boxmeer	NL		0485-587-600	www.intervetuk.com
Intervet UK Ltd.	Walton Mano, Milton Keynes	Bucks	UK	Mk7 7AJ	44-1908-685-685	www.intervetusa.com
Intervet Inc.	405 State St.	Millsboro	DE	19966	800-992-8051	www.janssen.com
Jacobus Pharmaceutical Co.	37 Cleveland Ln, PO Box 5920	Princeton	NJ	08540	609-921-7447	
Janssen Pharmaceutical, Inc.	1125 Trenton-Harbourton Rd., PO Box 200	Titusville	NJ	08560-0200	609-730-2000	
Knoll Pharmaceuticals	See Abbott Laboratories					
Lannett Co., Inc.	900 State Rd.	Philadelphia	PA	19136	215-333-9000	www.lannett.com
Lederle Laboratories	401 N. Middleton Rd.	Pearl River	NY	10965	914-732-5000	
Lemmon Co.	See Teva Pharmaceuticals USA					
Leo Pharm.	Cashel Rd.	Dublin 12	IRL		+353 1 490 8924	www.leo.ie
Lextron, Inc.	620 "O" St., PO Box 790	Greeley	CO	80632	970-353-6044	www.lextron-inc.com
Eli Lilly and Co.	Lilly Corp. Center	Indianapolis	IN	46285	317-276-2000	www.lilly.com
Lipsome Co.	See Elan Pharmaceuticals					
Lymphomed	See Fujisawa USA, Inc.					
Mallinckrodt Medical, Inc.	675 McDonnell Blvd.	Hazelwood	MO	63042	314-654-2000	www.mallinckrodt.com
Mallinckrodt Veterinary, Inc.	(see Schering-Plough, Inc.)					

Company	Address	City	State	Zip	Phone	Website
Marion Merrell Dow	9300 Ward Pkwy.	Kansas City	MO	64114	816-966-4000	
Mead Johnson Pharm.	See Bristol-Myers Squibb					
Merck AgVet Division	Merck & Co., PO Box 2000	Rahway	NJ	07065-0912	908-855-3800	
Merck & Co.	1 Merck Dr.	White House Station	NJ	08889	908-423-1000	www.merck.com
Merial	3239 Satellite Blvd.	Duluth	GA	30096	678-638-3000	www.merial.com
Miles, Inc.	See Bayer Corp.					
Monarch Pharmaceuticals	501 5th St.	Bristol	TN	37620	423-989-8000	www.monarchpharm.com
Mycofarm Nederland B.V.	Ambachtstraat 2	3732 CN De Bilt	NL		030-2212800	
Mycofarm UK Ltd.	Science Park, Milton Rd.	Cambridge	UK	CB4 4FP	0223-423971	
Neogen Corporation	628 Winchester Rd.	Lexington	KY	40505	859-254-1221	www.neogen.com
NeXstar Pharmaceuticals, Inc.	2860 Wilderness Place	Boulder	CO	80301	303-444-5893	
North American Region, Animal Health Group	Pfizer Inc., Whiteland Business Park, 912 Springdale Dr.	Exton	PA	19341	610-363-3100	
Novartis Animal Health US, Inc.	3200 Northline Ave, Ste. 300	Greensboro	NC	27408	800-332-2761	www.ah.novartis.com
Ora-Pharma, Inc.	732 Louis Dr.	Warminster	PA	18974	215-956-2200	www.orapharma.com
Ortho-McNeil Pharmaceutical	1000 Rt. 202	Raritan	NJ	08869	908-218-6000	www.ortho-mcneil.com
Osborn	11 West Central	Miami	OK	74354	918-542-4444	www.osborndrugs.com
Parke-Davis	201 Tabor Rd.	Morris Plains	NJ	07950	973-385-2000	
Parke-Davis Veterinary	See Pfizer Animal Health					
Pfizer Animal Health Ltd.	235 E. 42ND St.	New York	NY	10017	800-366-5288	www.pfizer.com/ah
Pfizer B.V.	Animal Health Division, Roer 266	2908 MC Capelle a/d IJssel	NL		31-010-4064200	www.pfizer.com
Pharmacia Biotech	800 Centennial Ave., PO Box 1327	Piscataway	NJ	08855-1327	800-526-3593	www.biotech.pharmacia.se/
Pharmacia and Upjohn	700 Portage Rd	Kalamazoo	MI	49001	269-833-9599	
Phoenix Scientific, Inc.	3915 S. 48th St. Terr, PO Box 8039 (64508)	St. Joseph	MO	64503	816-364-3777	
Presutti Laboratories	1685 Winnetka Circle	Rolling Meadows	IL	60008-1272	888-405-7800	www.presuttilabs.com
Procter & Gamble Pharm.	11450 Grroms Rd.	Cincinnati	OH	45242	513-335-3321	www.pg.com
Prolabs Ltd., c/o Agri Laboratories, Ltd.	PO Box 3103	St. Joseph	MO	64503	816-233-9533	www.agrilabs.com
Prometheus Laboratories, Inc.	5739 Pacific Center Blvd.	San Diego	CA	92121-4203	888-423-5227	www.prometheus.com
Pulpdent Corp.	80 Oakland St.	Watertown	MA	02471-0780	800-343-4342	www.pulpdent.com
Purdue Frederick Co.	201 Tressor Blvd.	Stanford	CT	06091-3431	203-588-8000	www.purduepharma.com
Rachelle Laboratories, Inc.	PO Box 187	Culver	IN	46511	219-842-3305	
Reid Rowell	See Solvay Pharmaceuticals					
Rhône Merieux B.V.	Bovenkerkerweg 6-8	1185 XE Amstelveen	NL		020-5473933	
Rhône-Merieux Ltd.	Pinnacles West, Spire Greene Centre	Harlow, Essex	UK	CM19 5TS	0279-439444	
Rhône-Poulenc Rorer Pharmaceuticals, Inc.	See Aventis Pharmaceuticals					

Continued

MANUFACTURERS/ DISTRIBUTORS	ADDRESS	CITY	STATE/ COUNTRY	POSTAL CODE	TELEPHONE	WEBSITE
Roberts Pharmaceutical Corp.	Meridian Center II, 4 Industrial Way West	Eatontown	NJ	07724		www.robertspharm.com
Roche Laboratories	340 Kingsland St.	Nutley	NJ	07110-1199	973-235-5000	www.rocheusa.com
Roche Animal Health	45 Waterview Blvd.	Parsippany	NJ	07054-1290	800-526-0189	
Roerig	See Pfizer					
Ross Laboratories, Inc.	625 Cleveland	Columbus	OH	43215	800-986-8510	www.rosslabs.com
Roussel-Uclaf	95 Chestnut Ridge Rd.	Montvale	NJ	07645	201-307-0378	
RXV	See Walco International					
Sandoz Pharmaceuticals	See Novartis Pharmaceuticals Corp.					
Sanofi Animal Health	7101 College Blvd.	Overland Park	KS	66210	913-451-3434	
Sanofi Animal Health Ltd.	PO Box 209 Rhodes Way	Watford, Herts	UK	WD2 4QE	0923-235022	
Sanofi Sante B.V.	Govert van Wijnkade 48	3144 EG Maassluis	NL		01899-31399	
Sanofi Synthelabo, Inc.	90 Park Ave.	New York	NY	10016	212-551-4000	www.sanofi-synthelabous.com
Schering-Plough Animal Health	1095 Morris Ave.	Union	NJ	07083	908-629-3490	www.sp-animalhealth.com
Schiapparelli Searle	See SCS Pharmaceuticals					
SCS Pharmaceuticals	PO Box 5110	Chicago	IL	60680	800-323-1603	
Searle	See Pharmacia Corp.					
Sequus Pharmaceuticals, Inc.	960 Hamilton Court	Menlo	CA	94025	650-323-9011	
SmithKline Beecham Consumer Healthcare	1500 Littleton Rd.	Parsippany	NJ	07084	973-889-2100	www.sb.com
Solvay Pharmaceuticals	901 Sawyer Rd.	Marietta	GA	30062-2224	404-578-9000	www.solvaypharmaceuticals. com
Solvay Duphar Animal Health Benelux B.V.	Van Houten Industriepark 36, PO Box 900	1381 MZ Weesp	NL		02940-65907	
Solvay-Duphar Veterinary Ltd.	Solvay House, Flanders Rd., Hedge End	Southampton, Hants	UK	SO3 4QH	01489-781711	

Company	Address	City	State	Zip	Phone	Website
E.R. Squibb & Sons, Inc.	See Bristol-Myers Squibb					
Stuart Pharmaceuticals	See Astra Zeneca L.P.					
Syntex Animal Health	4800 Westown Pkwy., Ste. 200	W. Des Moines	IA	50266-6711	515-224-2400	
Teva Pharmaceuticals USA	1090 Horsham Rd., PO Box 1090	North Wales	PA	19454-1090	215-591-3000	www.tevausa.com
UpJohn Co. Animal Health	See Pharmacia Corp.					
Upjohn Limited	Fleming Way	Crawley, West Sussex	UK	RH10 2LZ	0293-531133	
Upjohn Nederland	Rubensstraat 167	6717 VE Ede	NL		08380-36802	
Upsher-Smith Labs, Inc.	14905 23rd Ave. North	Minneapolis	MN	55447-4709	612-473-4412	www.upsher-smith.com
US Bioscience	100 Front St., Ste. 400	W. Conshohocken	PA	19428	215-832-4553	www.usbio.com
Vedco, Inc.	5503 Corporate Dr.	St. Joseph	MO	64507	816-238-8840	www.vedco.com/dvmonly
Vet Tek, Inc.	100 S.E. Magellan Dr., PO Box 279	Blue Springs	MO	64014	816-229-9101	www.durvet.com
Veterinary Pharm. Co.	Div. of Nylos Trading Co. Inc., PO Box D 3700	Pomona	NY	10970	845-354-8787	
Vetico Farma B.V.	Bovenheigraaf 101	8095 PB Wezep	NL		05253-3335	
Vetoquinol B.V.	Postbus 3191	5203 DD's Hertogenbosch	NL		01834-1782	
Vetoquinol USA	5910-G Breckenridge Pkwy.	Tampa	FL	33610-4253	800-627-9447	www.vetsolutions.com
Vetrepharm Res., Inc.	PO Box 210037	Bedford	TX	76095	817-285-8500	
Vetrepharm of Canada	383 Soverign Rd.	London, Ontario	Canada	N6M 1A3	519-453-3384	
Virbac SA	L.I.D. 1 ere Ave.- 2065 m	Carros	France	F-06516		www.virbac.fr.com
Walco	520 South Main St.	Grapevine	TX	76051	817-601-6000	www.walcointl.com
Warner Chilcott Laboratories	100 Enerprise Dr., Ste. 280	Rockaway	NJ	07866	800-521-8813	www.wclabs.com
Willows-Francis Vet. Ltd.	3 Charlwood Court, County Oak Way	Crawley, West Sussex	UK	RH11 7XA	0293-61441	
Winthrop Pharmaceuticals	See Sanofi Synthelabo Pharmaceuticals					
Wyeth-Ayerst Laboratories	PO Box 8299	Philadelphia	PA	19101	610-688-4400	www.wyeth.com
Zeneca Pharmaceuticals	1800 Concord Pike	Wilmington	DE	19897	302-886-3000	
See Astra-Zeneca L.P.						

ACEMANNAN

CLASS. Complex carbohydrate (polymannose) extracted from *Aloe vera*.

ACTION. Immunostimulant and antiviral. Stimulates mononuclear phagocytes and T cells; interferes with viral glycosylation. In murine tissue culture, it induces macrophages to produce tumor necrosis factor-α and interleukin-1.

MORE INFORMATION. See Antivirals, Chapter 2, Table 2-3, and Immunotherapy, Chapter 100; References: Ch 2, ref. 36; 72; 133; 51; 178; 69a; 70a; 98a; 144a.

PHARMACOKINETICS. Uncertain.

SPECTRUM. Interferon inducer; has antitumor activity. Direct antiviral effect as it inhibits growth of HIV, Newcastle disease virus, and influenza virus in vivo.

INDICATIONS. Treatment of clinically affected, symptomatic FeLV-positive or FIV-positive cats (Ch 2, ref. 178). Intralesional injection into vaccine-induced fibrosarcomas. Prospective controlled studies on efficacy not available. Has been used in combination with surgery and radiation therapy for fibrosarcomas in dogs and cats (Ch 2, ref. 72). It may also accelerate wound healing.

APPROVED USES. Veterinary-adjunctive treatment for fibrosarcoma, nonspecific immunostimulant.

CONTRAINDICATIONS. Previous hypersensitivity reaction to the drug.

ADVERSE REACTIONS. IV causes tachypnea, tachycardia, salivation, weakness, collapse, pale mucosae. Avoid by using slow IV drip infusion rather than bolus infusion. Very high (80 mg/kg) IP doses in dogs cause transient abdominal discomfort, vomiting, and diarrhea (Ch 2, ref. 36). Histologic findings of mononuclear phagocyte infiltrates in liver, spleen, and peritoneal surfaces (atypical microgranulomatous peritonitis) when treated IP. When treated IV, mononuclear phagocytes accumulate in lungs (Ch 2, ref. 36). SC injection rarely causes hypersensitivity reactions. Increased WBC counts during treatments. Intralesional injections may cause discomfort and bleeding from injection sites. Necrosis can occur at the injection site (Ch 2, ref. 36). Sedation or anesthesia is recommended. Tumors will become enlarged and painful before regression, if any, is noted.

INTERACTIONS. Unknown.

AVAILABILITY	TYPE	SIZES	PREPARATIONS (COMPANY)
Veterinary	Lyophilized powder for injection	10-mg vial	*Acemannan Immunostimulant, Carrisyn* (Carrington)

HANDLING. Reconstitute to 1 mg/ml with 10 ml of 0.9% NaCl (supplied). Higher concentrations are insoluble and become gelatinous. Discard unused solution within 4 hr of reconstitution.

ADMINISTRATION. Intralesional and/or IP weekly injection given concurrently. Continue injections until necrosis and/or edema evident in mass (usually 4th-7th week). Then use surgery to remove mass by wide excision. May also consider radiotherapy using cobalt 60 teletherapy, immediately after surgery (Ch 2, ref. 72).

Dosage

INDICATIONS (*Dogs & Cats*)	DOSE	ROUTE	INTERVAL	DURATION
Immunostimulant	2 mg/kg	IP, SC	Weekly	6 week
Fibrosarcoma				
Preoperative[a]	1 mg/kg	IP	Weekly	4 week (weeks 1-4)
	2 mg	Intralesional	Weekly	4 week (weeks 1-4)
Surgical removal, week 5	1 mg	IP	Weekly	2 week (weeks 5, 6)
Postoperative	1 mg/kg	IP	Monthly	6 mo-1 yr (thereafter)

[a]The intralesional dose can be used in treatment of papillomatosis.

ADDITIONAL DOSAGES. None.

DISPENSING INFORMATION. IP: animal may have abdominal tenderness; observe for allergic reactions. Intralesional: may cause bleeding or necrosis of lesion with some exudation for days afterward.

ACTIVATED PROTEIN C (SEE DROTRECOGIN ALFA ACTIVATED)

ACYCLOVIR

CLASS. Nucleoside (guanosine) analog.

ACTION. Antiviral; interferes with DNA replication in herpesviruses types 1, 2, and some others. Converted in cell to triphosphate derivative, only in cells with virus since uses viral thymidine kinase making it very selective. Accumulates and activates only in herpesvirus-infected cells, therefore has low toxicity, and high therapeutic index. Viral DNA polymerase is 10 times more sensitive to drug than host enzyme. Affects only replicating and not latent virus. Best therapeutic index (efficacy/toxicity) of available antiviral drugs. Unfortunately, in vitro activity of acyclovir against FHV-1 is 1000-fold less than against human herpes simplex virus (Ch 2, ref. 21; 129). Thymidine kinase activity is lower in FHV-1 than HSV (Ch 2, ref. 28). Activity of deoxycytidine kinase can influence sensitivity to acyclovir (Ch 2, ref. 170). Many animal herpesviruses such as FHV-1 and pseudorabies virus lack this latter enzyme.

MORE INFORMATION. See Acyclovir, Chapter 2. See elsewhere GANCICLOVIR (*Cytovene*, Syntex); Famciclovir (*Famvir*, SmithKline Beecham); Valacyclovir (*Valtrex*, Glaxo Wellcome). See Table 2-2; references: Ch 2, ref. 61; Ch 2, ref. 141; 172. (Ch 2, ref. 117; 112.)

PHARMACOKINETICS. IV gives good bioavailability; with PO use, bioavailability is only 15%-30% of levels of those after the same parenteral dosage (Ch 2, ref. 117). Penetrates into most body tissues, including CNS. CSF concentrations are 50% of plasma. Minimal metabolism and from 45% to 85% excreted unchanged in urine (Ch 2, ref. 117). Excretion is delayed in renal failure. Valacyclovir, a prodrug, has higher bioavailability (see Chapter 2).

SPECTRUM. Herpesvirus infections. Some resistance has developed with extensive use.

INDICATIONS. In humans, for systemic, CNS, respiratory, or genital herpesvirus infections. Suppresses respiratory tract infections and mucosal eruptions. Does not prevent subclinical viral shedding. Should not be used in mild or self-limiting disease.

CONTRAINDICATIONS. Reduce dosage in renal failure. Use with caution in pregnant animals because it crosses placenta. High doses are fetotoxic.

ADVERSE REACTIONS. Nephrotoxic if given rapidly IV, transient renal tubular obstruction by crystals. CNS signs after IV infusion. IV can cause phlebitis and local irritation. Oral use may cause vomiting and diarrhea. Must evaluate initial hemogram prior to treatment and periodically thereafter during drug administration. Leukopenia and mild nonregenerative anemia can occur. Accidental oral ingestion by dogs occurs (see Acyclovir, Chapter 2).

INTERACTIONS. If coadministered with zidovudine, may cause mental drowsiness and depression.

AVAILABILITY	TYPE	SIZES	PREPARATIONS (COMPANY)
Human	Topical (ophthalmic ointment)	5% polyethylene glycol ointment	*Zovirax* (Glaxo Wellcome)
	Oral	200-mg capsule, 400- and 800-mg tablets, 200-mg/5 ml suspension	*Zovirax*
	IV solution	500-mg vial	*Zovirax*

INTERNATIONAL PREPARATIONS. *Acicloftal, Aciyiran, Acyvir, Avyclor, Cusiviral, Cycloviran, Geavir, Herpotern, Maynar, Neviran, Vipral, Virmen, Zovir, Zyclir.*

HANDLING. In people, IV preparation is made by dissolving powder in 10-20 ml of sterile preservative-free water. Add to calculated volume of IV solution to be given over 1 hr. Discard unused solution after 12 hr. Do not add to biologic or colloidial fluids. For cats, prepared IV solution should be further diluted in NaCl to avoid irritation.

ADMINISTRATION. For cats SC route is preferred. With this route the drug has been diluted to a concentration of 1 mg/ml with 0.9% NaCl and given SC (Ch 2, ref. 60). Oral and IV have more side effects in cats. IV use preferred to treat systemic infections in people. Must infuse slowly to avoid crystal precipitation in renal tubules. Rates lower than 5 mg/kg/hr have low toxicity. Give any dose over at least 1-hr time period. Monitor renal function and urine sediment for needle-shaped crystals.

Dosage

INDICATIONS[a]	DOSE	ROUTE	INTERVAL (hr)	DURATION (days)
Pups: Systemic herpesvirus	15 mg/kg	SC, IV	8	5-7
Cats: Systemic herpesvirus	10 mg/kg	SC	8	7-21
Systemic herpesvirus	10-25 mg	PO, SC	12	7-21
Ocular herpesvirus	Ointment	Topically	4	prn

[a]Should be combined with human interferon-α or feline interferon-ω. Similar dosages could be tried in pups with herpesvirus infection.

ADDITIONAL DOSAGES. None.

DISPENSING INFORMATION. Animal may become depressed or drowsy or have vomiting and diarrhea. Notify veterinarian if persists.

ALBENDAZOLE

CLASS. Benzimidazole carbamate.

ACTION. Antinematodal, antiprotozoal by inhibiting parasite intestinal cell microtubular function.

MORE INFORMATION. See FENBENDAZOLE, MEBENDAZOLE (elsewhere). See Antiprotozoals, Chapter 71, and Giardiasis, Chapter 78; Table 78-3; references: Ch 71, ref. 7; 86; 89; 60.

PHARMACOKINETICS. Poorly absorbed (<1%) from GI tract and passes through. Any absorbed drug is rapidly metabolized into sulfoxide and sulfone derivatives with antihelminthic activity. Metabolites are predominantly excreted in urine.

SPECTRUM. Various nematodes and cestodes. **Protozoa:** *Encephalitozoon; Pneumocystis; Giardia.* **Fungus:** *Cryptococcus* (in vitro). **More effective:** 50 times more active than metronidazole and 10-40 times more active than quinacrine against *Giardia.*

INDICATIONS. Microsporidiosis (encephalitozoonosis), pneumocystosis. Closely related fenbendazole (50 mg/kg PO once every 24 hr for 3 days) is also effective against giardiasis in dogs (Ch 71, ref. 7).

CONTRAINDICATIONS. Hepatic dysfunction, cholestasis, pregnancy, or lactation. Do not need to alter dosage in renal failure.

ADVERSE REACTIONS. Vomiting, diarrhea, liver enzyme activity increases, cholestatic hepatitis. Weight loss, myelotoxicity, and blood dyscrasias at 30-60 mg/kg daily for 26 weeks. Pancytopenia has been reported at therapeutic dosages (25 mg/kg) for 4 and 10 days in a cat and a dog, respectively (Ch 71, ref. 89; 60). Leukopenias may be associated with sepsis. They can be reversed with supportive antibiotic and fluid therapy. Embryotoxic and teratogenic in lab animals. Low systemic toxicity with short-term usage because poorly absorbed.

INTERACTIONS. Cimetidine increases its biliary excretion; dexamethasone increases its steady-state concentrations; albendazole potentially increases theophylline concentrations.

AVAILABILITY	TYPE	SIZES	PREPARATIONS (COMPANY)
Human	Oral tablets	200 mg, 400 mg	*Alben* (SmithKline Beecham)
Veterinary	Oral liquid suspension (cattle)	113.6 mg/ml	*Valbazen* (Pfizer Animal Health)

INTERNATIONAL PREPARATIONS. *Albenza, Eskazole, Zeben, Zentel.*

HANDLING. Store at controlled room temperature; shake well before using.

ADMINISTRATION. Give with fatty meals to increase (although variable) absorption. Poor absorption is a benefit in treating intestinal-restricted diseases such as giardiasis. For giardiasis, at least four doses must be given to be effective. For encephalitozoonosis in people, has been given concurrently with trimethoprim or pyrimethamine and sulfonamides. For longer (>30 days) therapy, should have blood count checked every 3-4 weeks to detect myelotoxicity.

Dosage

INDICATIONS	DOSE	ROUTE	INTERVAL (hr)	DURATION (days)
Humans				
Encephalitozoonosis	200-400 mg/person	PO	8-12	14-28
Dogs				
Leishmaniasis	10 mg/kg	PO	24	30
Leishmaniasis	5 mg/kg	PO	6	60
Giardiasis	25 mg/kg[a]	PO	12	2
Cats				
Giardiasis	25 mg/kg[a]	PO	12	5

[a]Potentially myelotoxic at this dose (Ch 71, ref. 60).

ADDITIONAL DOSAGES. Enteric protozoal infections, Table 78-3.

DISPENSING INFORMATION. Contact veterinarian if vomiting, diarrhea, abdominal tenderness, yellow mucous membranes, and skin are observed.

ALLOPURINOL

CLASS. Purine analog. Xanthine oxidase inhibitor.

ACTION. Metabolized by *Leishmania* to produce an inactive analog of inosine. This molecule is incorporated into leishmanial RNA, causing faulty protein synthesis. Interferes with purine and subsequent RNA synthesis.

MORE INFORMATION. References: Ch 71, ref. 10; 21; 35; 48; 51; 55; 56; 43; 17; 24; 11; Ch 73, ref. 213.

PHARMACOKINETICS. Absorbed from GI tract after PO administration, converted to oxypurinol in liver. Distributed in tissues and extracellular fluid spaces but less in CSF. Renal excretion of metabolite predominates, with some in feces.

SPECTRUM. Protozoa: *Leishmania, Trypanosoma cruzi.* **Others:** Treatment of gout or urate urolithiasis.

INDICATIONS. Inexpensive, less toxic, PO therapy for leishmaniasis. Also considered for American trypanosomiasis, because nifurtimox is more toxic.

APPROVED USES. For hyperuricemia and gout in people.

CONTRAINDICATIONS. Reduce dosing, increase interval of administration, or avoid in cases involving renal failure or hepatic dysfunction. Safety in breeding or pregnant animals not established.

ADVERSE REACTIONS. Vomiting, diarrhea, dermatologic eruption (pruritus and rash), myelosuppression, xanthine urolith formation (Ch 71, ref. 50). Monitor for hepatic or renal dysfunction as xanthine uroliths can occur, especially in dogs with liver dysfunction.

INTERACTIONS. May continue adjunctive therapy with meglumine antimoniate or sodium stibogluconate in leishmaniasis. Increases myelotoxicity of cyclophosphamide. Urinary acidifiers increase risk of xanthine urolith formation. Increases toxicity of anticoagulant rodenticides and serum aminophylline concentrations. Dermatologic reactions are enhanced with coadministration of cytotoxic drugs and ampicillin.

AVAILABILITY	TYPE	SIZES	PREPARATIONS (COMPANY)
Human	Oral tablets	100 mg, 300 mg	*Zyloprim* (Glaxo Wellcome), generic (various)

INTERNATIONAL PREPARATIONS. *Alloprin, Allopur, Allopurin, Alloremed, Allural, Aloral, Aluline, Apurin, Caplenal, Capurate, Dabroson, Foligan, Jenapurinol, Lysuron, Novopurol, Purinol, Zyloric.*

HANDLING. Store at room temperature (59-77°F) in airtight container protected from light. A 120-ml suspension of 20 mg/ml may be prepared by taking 24 100-mg tablets (*Zyloprim*) crushed and adding glycerin or distilled water to levigate, methylcellulose 40 ml, and a sufficient quantity of a 2 : 1 simple syrup to bring the volume to 120 ml. The mixture should be refrigerated and labeled "shake well"; is stable for 8 weeks in the dark.

ADMINISTRATION. Check blood cell counts and serum hepatic enzymes, urea, and creatinine every 2 weeks. Use in combination with meglumine antimoniate for the first 30 days to improve efficacy.

Dosage

INDICATIONS	DOSE (mg/kg)	ROUTE	INTERVAL (hr)	DURATION (days)
Dogs				
Leishmaniasis (Induction therapy with or without antimony)	15-30	PO	12	30[a]
Maintenance	15	PO	12	240
Extended maintenance of remission	20	PO	24	7 sequential days each month (every 4th week)[b]
Cats				
Leishmaniasis	20	PO	24	15 mo[c]

[a]May treat for an extended period (≥120 days) as needed to control infection. Switch to maintenance after remission achieved.
[b]For further information see Ch 71, ref. 24.
[c]Cat was infected with FIV and had pancytopenia, but therapy for Leishmania kept it from clinical illness with leishmaniasis (Ch 73, ref. 160b).

ADDITIONAL DOSAGES. Antimicrobial therapy for canine leishmaniasis, Table 73-4.

DISPENSING INFORMATION. Give 1-2 hr after feeding.

AMANTADINE

CLASS. Adamantanamine.

ACTION. Antiviral against RNA viruses. Blocks viral penetration into host cells.

MORE INFORMATION. See Rimantidine and Chapter 2, Antivirals; Table 2-2.

PHARMACOKINETICS. Well absorbed from GI tract when given PO, not metabolized, excreted unchanged in urine, also in milk.

SPECTRUM. At achievable concentrations, only affects influenza A viruses. Resistance can develop.

INDICATIONS. Early (within 48 hr of onset of signs) or prophylactic use in influenza. Reduces severity of pulmonary lesions and clinical illness. Also augments dopaminergic activity, used to treat human parkinsonism.

CONTRAINDICATIONS. Reduce dose in renal failure; avoid in pregnancy, lactation, seizure-prone animals, gastric ulceration.

ADVERSE REACTIONS. Allergic reactions, ataxia, CNS manifestations with overdosage.

INTERACTIONS. Synergistic with anticholinergics.

AVAILABILITY	TYPE	SIZES	PREPARATIONS (COMPANY)
Human	Oral capsules	100 mg	*Symadine* (Solvay), *Symmetrel* (DuPont Pharma), generic (various)
	Syrup, raspberry flavor	50 mg/5 ml	*Symmetrel*

HANDLING. Store in airtight container.

ADMINISTRATION. Treat as early in illness as possible.

Dosage

INDICATIONS (*Dogs and Cats*)	DOSE (mg/kg)	ROUTE	INTERVAL (hr)	DURATION (days)
Dosage and toxicity uncertain[a]	4.4-8.8[a]	PO	24	5-7
	2.2-4.4[a]	PO	12	5-7

[a]Do not exceed 150 mg total/day. Extrapolated from human pediatric dose.

ADDITIONAL DOSAGES. None.

DISPENSING INFORMATION. Can be taken with or without food. Store capsules at room temperature, away from moisture and direct sunlight. Store syrup at room temperature.

AMICARBALIDE ISETHIONATE

CLASS. Aromatic diamidine.

ACTION. Antiprotozoal; interferes with nucleic acid metabolism.

MORE INFORMATION. See IMIDOCARB, DIMINAZENE, PHENAMIDINE, PENTAMIDINE; Chapter 71.

PHARMACOKINETICS. Similar to imidocarb.

SPECTRUM. *Babesia, Ehrlichia.*

INDICATIONS. Babesiosis, ehrlichiosis. Licensed to treat bovine anaplasmosis but has been used in dogs. Not available in U.S.

CONTRAINDICATIONS, ADVERSE REACTIONS, INTERACTIONS. See IMIDOCARB.

AVAILABILITY	TYPE	SIZES	PREPARATION (COMPANY)
Veterinary	Parenteral solution	Unknown	*Diampron* (Rhône-Poulenc Rorer)

HANDLING. See IMIDOCARB.

ADMINISTRATION. May repeat injection after 1 week because of relapses that may occur.

Dosage

INDICATIONS (*Dogs*)	DOSE (mg/kg)	ROUTE	INTERVAL (hr)	DURATION (days)
Babesiosis	20	IM	24	1

ADDITIONAL DOSAGES: Ehrlichiosis, Table 28-4.

DISPENSING INFORMATION: Watch for signs of weakness and neurologic dysfunction, and report them immediately to your veterinarian. See also IMIDOCARB and DIMINAZENE.

AMIKACIN

CLASS. Aminoglycoside.

ACTION. Antibacterial.

MORE INFORMATION. See GENTAMICIN, and Aminoglycosides, Chapter 34; Tables 34-5 and 34-6.

PHARMACOKINETICS. Not well absorbed PO; must give parenterally for systemic use. Distribution restricted to extracellular fluid because of low lipid solubility. Enhanced with inflammation. Reaches therapeutic concentrations in peritoneal, pleural, and synovial fluids, bile, and respiratory secretions. Concentrates in kidney tissues and excreted unchanged in urine. See also GENTAMICIN.

SPECTRUM. Gram positive: *Staphylococcus.* **Gram negative:** *Acinetobacter, Citrobacter, Enterobacter, Escherichia, Klebsiella, Proteus, Serratia, Salmonella, Yersinia.* **Others:** *Nocardia, Mycobacterium tuberculosis.* **More effective:** *Pseudomonas:*
more effective than gentamicin. **Ineffective:** Obligate anaerobes.

INDICATIONS. For infections caused by gentamicin-resistant, gram-negative bacilli. Often shows broader antibacterial spectrum than gentamicin.

APPROVED USES. For *Mycobacterium avium-intracellulare-*complex infections in combination with other effective agents.

CONTRAINDICATIONS. Renal failure.

ADVERSE REACTIONS. Nephrotoxic in dogs and cats; the latter are more sensitive. See also GENTAMICIN; thought to be less nephrotoxic than gentamicin. Ototoxic, causing deafness, especially in cats.

INTERACTIONS. See GENTAMICIN.

AVAILABILITY	TYPE	SIZES	PREPARATIONS (COMPANY)
Human	Parenteral solution	250 mg/ml	*Amikin* (Apothecon), generic (various)
	Pediatric injectable solution	50 mg/ml	As above
Veterinary	Parenteral solution	50 mg/ml, 250 mg/ml	*Amiglyde-V* (Fort Dodge)

INTERNATIONAL PREPARATIONS. *Amicasil, Amikan, Amikine, Amiklin, Amukin, Biklin, Chemacin, Kanbine, Lukadin, Pierami.*

HANDLING. Compatible in 5% dextrose, 0.9% sodium chloride, and lactated Ringer's solutions. Stable for 24 hr. Should not premix or add to any other drug solutions. Solutions may
change from colorless to pale yellow but no loss in potency occurs.

ADMINISTRATION. For IV give over a 30-min period in solutions. Maximum treatment duration usually 7-10 days. Important to monitor renal, vestibular, and auditory function. The greater the interval between doses, the less is its nephrotoxicity.

Dosage

INDICATIONS	DOSE (mg/kg)	ROUTE	INTERVAL (hr)	DURATION (days)
Dogs				
Urinary infections	2.3	IM, SC	12	7-10
Soft tissue infections	7.5	IV, IM, SC	12	7-10
	5	IV, IM, SC	8	7
Orthopedic infections	10	IV, IM, SC	8	7
Bacteremia, sepsis	7	IV	8	7
Cats				
Soft tissue infections	15-10	IV, IM, SC	24	7-10
Soft tissue infections	5-10	IM, SC	12	7
Bacteremia	10-12	IV, IM, SC	8-12	7

ADDITIONAL DOSAGES. None.

DISPENSING INFORMATION. Must be given SC; therefore, not advised for home administration. Monitoring for renal toxicity is also needed.

AMOXICILLIN

CLASS. Aminopenicillin.

ACTION. Bactericidal; inhibits bacterial cell wall synthesis.

MORE INFORMATION. See AMPICILLIN; Chapter 34, Aminopenicillins; Table 34-1.

PHARMACOKINETICS. See also AMPICILLIN. Better absorbed from GI tract than ampicillin and less affected by feeding. Rapidly absorbed after IM or SC. Injection site on body does not markedly affect this uptake from SC tissues. Longer serum half-life than ampicillin permits BID dosing. Mainly distributed in extracellular fluid compartment. Enters most tissues and body fluids except brain and CSF. With PO administration, liquid forms slightly better absorbed than tablets (bioavailability of suspension 77%; drops 68%; tablets 64%) (Ch 34, ref. 208). Most drug excreted unchanged in urine. When dogs were given endotoxin, clearance of the drug decreased significantly (Ch 34, ref. 237). Therefore dosage may be reduced when endotoxemia is suspected.

SPECTRUM. Same as ampicillin. **Gram positive:** *Streptococcus,* non–β-lactamase *Staphylococcus.* **Gram negative:** *Escherichia, Proteus, Pasteurella.* See also AMPICILLIN. Anaerobes: some efficacy but less than penicillin G. **Other:** borreliosis, leptospirosis. **Ineffective:** β-lactamase–producing bacteria.

INDICATIONS. Infections of nasopharynx, middle ear, urinary tracts, skin and soft tissue, upper and lower respiratory tracts, prophylaxis during dentistry, genitourinary infections.

CONTRAINDICATIONS. Previous hypersensitivity to penicillins.

ADVERSE REACTIONS. Dogs: diarrhea and vomiting; facial swelling, dermal rash; less diarrhea than with ampicillin; proximal renal tubular dysfunction (glucosuria, proteinuria, aminoaciduria, isosthenuria, hyposthenuria, with electrolyte loss and metabolic acidosis in one dog [Ch 34, ref. 18]). **Cats:** vomiting, diarrhea, depression, anorexia, facial swelling, ocular irritation, polydipsia and polyuria, salivation, personality change (Ch 34, ref. 209).

INTERACTIONS. False-positive glucosuria result with Clinitest (Ames Laboratories, Elkhart, IN). See also AMPICILLIN.

AVAILABILITY	TYPE	SIZES	PREPARATIONS (COMPANY)
Human	Oral tablets	125 mg	*Amoxil* (SmithKline Beecham), generic (various)
	Oral capsules	250 mg, 500 mg	*Polymox* (Apothecon), *Wymoxl* (Wyeth-Ayerst)
	Powder for oral suspension (trihydrate)	125 mg/5 ml, 250 mg/5 ml, 500 mg/5 ml	*Amoxil, Polymox, Wymox*
Veterinary	Oral tablets	50 mg, 100 mg, 150 mg, 200 mg, 400 mg	*Amoxi-Tabs* (Pfizer Animal Health)
		50 mg, 100 mg, 200 mg, 400 mg	*Robamox-V* Tablets (Fort Dodge)
	Powder for oral suspension	50 mg/ml	*Amoxi-Tabs*, *Robamox-V, Qualamox* (Merial)
	Powder for parenteral suspension	3 gm (dilutes to 100 mg/ml or 250 mg/ml)	*Amoxi-Inject* (Pfizer Animal Health)
	Oral paste	20 mg/ml	*Vetrimoxin* (Sanofi)

INTERNATIONAL PREPARATIONS. *Amoxilan, Amoxina, Cilamox, Flemoxin, Helvamox, Polymox, Supramox, Trimox, Wymox.*

HANDLING. Store all tablets, capsules, and powders in airtight containers away from moisture at room temperature. Reconstituted oral suspension is stable for 2 weeks at refrigerated or room temperatures. Once reconstituted, parenteral suspension is stable for 3 mo at room temperature, 12 mo refrigerated.

ADMINISTRATION. Mix well before administering; food can reduce absorption. Continue treatment for 48 hr after all signs of infection are gone.

Dosage

INDICATIONS	DOSE	ROUTE	INTERVAL (hr)	DURATION (days)
Dogs				
Urinary infections	10-20 mg/kg	PO	12	5-7
	10 mg/kg	IM, SC	24	5
Systemic, bacteremia, sepsis	22-30 mg/kg[a]	IV, IM, SC	8	7
Orthopedic infections	22-30 mg/kg	IV, IM, SC, PO	6-8	7-10
Cats				
Urinary and soft tissue infections	50 mg/cat	PO	24	5-7
	11-22 mg/kg	PO	24	5-7
Sepsis	10-20 mg/kg	IV, SC, PO	12	prn

[a]Clearance of drug is reduced in dogs with endotoxemia (Ch 34, ref. 237) so that dosage increases may not be necessary much above those used to treat localized infections. In fact a reduction might be indicated.

ADDITIONAL DOSAGES. Canine distemper, Table 3-5; feline panleukopenia, Table 10-2; streptococcal infections, Table 35-4; enteric bacteria, Table 39-2; leptospirosis, Table 44-7; Lyme borreliosis, Table 45-5; actinomycosis, Table 49-2; dermatophilosis, Table 51-1; feline abscesses, Table 52-3; musculoskeletal infections, Table 86-4; respiratory infections, Table 88-8; oral infections, Table 89-4; intraabdominal infections, Table 89-21; urinary infections, Table 91-10.

DISPENSING INFORMATION. Shake solution well before using. Give to fasted animal and no feeding for 2 hr before or after dosing. Keep refrigerated. Discard unused drug after 2 weeks.

AMOXICILLIN-CLAVULANATE

CLASS. Aminopenicillin and β-lactamase inhibitor in 4 : 1 ratio.

ACTION. Bactericidal; inhibits bacterial cell wall synthesis and bacterial β-lactamase.

MORE INFORMATION. See Chapter 34, Aminopenicillins; Tables 34-1 and 34-2.

PHARMACOKINETICS. Stable in the presence of gastric acid; absorption not influenced by food. Clavulanate does not affect the pharmacokinetics of amoxicillin. The only orally bioavailable-lactamase inhibitor and penicillin group combination. Widely distributed to most tissues *except* the CNS and CSF, where amoxicillin penetrates only with inflammation. Penetration of clavulanate into CNS is uncertain. High urinary levels of unchanged drug.

SPECTRUM. **Gram positive:** *Staphylococcus, some Streptococcus, Erysipelothrix, Corynebacterium.* **Gram negative:** *Escherichia, Klebsiella, Proteus, Enterobacter, Pasteurella, Bordetella.* **Anaerobes:** *Clostridium, Peptococcus, Peptostreptococcus,* others. **More effective:** Clavulanate has minimal antibacterial activity itself but extends the spectrum of amoxicillin to include β-lactamase producers, improving activity against *Escherichia, Salmonella, Klebsiella, Proteus, Staphylococcus,* and *Bacteroides* and other anaerobes. **Ineffective:** *Pseudomonas, Enterobacter.* Oral administration of β-lactamase concurrent with ampicillin reduced the development of resistant fecal flora in dogs (Ch 34, ref. 152a).

INDICATIONS. Otitis media, sinusitis, respiratory infections, urinary tract infections, anal sacculitis, gingivitis, pyoderma, soft tissue infections, osteomyelitis, bite wounds, *Proteus* urinary infections.

CONTRAINDICATIONS. Some dosage reduction in severe renal failure. Avoid with previous allergic reaction to β-lactam.

ADVERSE REACTIONS. Vomiting and diarrhea, depression, anorexia, dermal rash. Polyuria, polydipsia, lameness, personality change (Ch 34, ref. 209).

INTERACTIONS. False-positive glucosuria using Clinitest (Ames Laboratories). *See also* AMOXICILLIN.

AVAILABILITY	TYPE	SIZES	PREPARATIONS (COMPANY)
Human	Tablets	125 mg, 250 mg, 500 mg	*Augmentin, Clamoxyl, Synulox* (SmithKline Beecham)
	Oral suspension	125 mg/5 ml, 250 mg/5 ml	*Augmentin, Clamoxyl, Syrulox*
Veterinary	Tablets	62.5 mg, 125 mg, 250 mg, 375 mg total	*Clavamox* (Pfizer Animal Health)
	Oral solution	62.5 mg/ml	*Clavamox*

INTERNATIONAL PREPARATIONS. *Bimoxi, Ciblor, Clavepen, Clavucid, Clavulin, Duplamox.*

HANDLING. Oral suspension: powder should be stored in airtight container away from moisture at room temperature. Add water and shake to mix. Once reconstituted, must refrigerate; activity lasts 10 days. **Tablets:** supplied in sealed strips in moisture-proof foil wrapping to maintain stability. Store at room temperature away from moisture.

ADMINISTRATION. Usual duration of treatment is extended for at least 21 days for deep pyoderma in dogs and 10-14 days in cats with resistant infections for up to a maximum of 30 days. Treat for at least 48 hr after signs have resolved.

Dosage

INDICATIONS	DOSE	ROUTE	INTERVAL (hr)	DURATION (days)
Dogs				
Urinary	12.5 mg/kg	PO	12	5-7
Skin, soft tissue infections	12.5 mg/kg	PO	12	5-7[a]
Deep pyoderma	12.5 mg/kg	PO	12	14-120
Systemic, bacteremia	22 mg/kg	PO	8-12	7
Cats				
Urinary tract	62.5 mg/cat	PO	12	10-30
Skin, soft tissue infections	62.5 mg/cat	PO	12	5-7
	10-20 mg/kg	PO	12	5-7
Sepsis, pneumonia	10-20 mg/kg	PO	8	7-10

[a]May have to treat 21 days with resistant infections for a maximum of 30 days. Much higher dosages have been recommended for resistant skin infections. See Table 85-3.

ADDITIONAL DOSAGE. Tracheobronchitis, Table 6-2; gram-negative infections, Table 37-3; *Clostridium perfringens* diarrhea, Table 39-10; anaerobic infections, Table 41-12; canine pyoderma, tetanus, Table 43-2; Table 85-3; respiratory disease, Table 88-8; oral infections, Table 89-4; colitis, Table 89-19; hepatobiliary infections, Table 90-5.

DISPENSING INFORMATION. Can be given with or without food; however, advisable to avoid use within 2 hr of mealtime. See AMOXICILLIN.

AMPHOTERICIN B

CLASS. Polyene antifungal. Originally isolated from a soil sample containing *Streptomyces nodosus*.

ACTION. Amphotericin B (AMB) binds to sterols in fungal cell membrane, opens pores allowing leakage of contents. Preference for ergosterol in fungi instead of cholesterol in mammalian cells. Active against *Leishmania* spp which also contain errgosterol.

MORE INFORMATION. Chapter 57. See Tables 57-1. See 57-2 for comparative features of the four formulations. All four preparations have different properties and dosage regimens. References: Ch 57, ref. 106; 1; 31; 32; 48; 52; 54; 57; 60; 61; 73; 78; 83; 97; 109; 114; 131; 145; Ch 71, ref. 46; 67; 47; 61; Ch 73, ref. 114; 150.

PHARMACOKINETICS. Conventional drug is insoluble in water so prepared as a colloidal dispersion with the bile salt deoxycholate (ABD; *Fungizone*). Available in lipid-complex formulations, which include cholesteryl sulfate (ABCD; *Amphocil); encapsulated unilamellar liposomes (L-AMB; AmBisome) or lipid complexed (ABLC; Abelcet)*. ABD is not absorbed from GI tract after PO administration; given parenterally, usually IV. Initial rise in blood concentration in 24 hr is followed by prolonged elimination period over 2-3 weeks. Strongly bound to cell membranes. Use of AMB in lipid-complex formulations may be less nephrotoxic because of selective uptake by the MPS and reduced uptake of the lipid preparations by mammalian cells. Lipid formulations are taken up by macrophages that carry it to the site of fungal-induced inflammation.

ABD. Poor oral absorption. Painful IM, so usually given IV. Widely distributed and penetrates many tissues and inflammatory exudates but is highly protein bound. Poor penetration into bones, brain and CSF (even with inflammation), aqueous and vitreous humor, amniotic fluid, muscle, respiratory secretions, pancreas, and salivary gland, and uninflamed body cavities (pleura, peritoneum, joints, pericardium). Accumulates in liver, kidneys, and lungs. Metabolism is uncertain; small amount of biliary excretion; slow urinary excretion (up to 2 mo) occurs with a small portion (<10%) as active drug. In dogs, up to 20% dose is excreted in bile over time. Does not accumulate to greater extent in renal failure, but is nephrotoxic (Ch 57, ref. 31; 142).

ABCD. Stable in plasma, not dissociating to free AMB; leads to mononuclear phagocyte uptake and lower renal concentrations and toxicity. In animal studies, compared with ABD, ABCD had lower plasma levels, higher liver concentrations, greater volume of distribution, and longer half-life. Highest drug concentration achieved in organs of the MPS (liver, spleen) and in lung, with lower concentrations in kidney, stomach, and small intestine. Lower concentrations in bone marrow and heart muscle, and little in brain and CSF (Ch 57, ref. 31; 142). With this preparation, concentrations are lower in kidneys, lungs, heart, brain, GI tract, and CSF than with deoxycholate. Most of the drug is concentrated in the liver with this formulation. Lower renal concentrations correlate with less nephrotoxicity of the liposomal-encapsulated derivative. Higher hepatic, splenic, and bone marrow concentrations resulting from increased mononuclear phagocyte concentrations were not associated with increased toxicity.

L-AMB. Highest serum and CSF levels are achieved with this formulation, presumably because of its small particle size and lower uptake by the MPS. Greatest concentrations in liver and spleen compared with ABD with similar levels in lung and kidney (Ch 57, ref. 4).

ABLC. Because of large molecular size and rapid uptake by the MPS, serum concentrations are lower than with ABD. Greatest concentration in dogs has been found in liver, spleen, and lung. Kidney concentrations are slightly lower than with ABD.

SPECTRUM. Fungi: *Histoplasma, Cryptococcus, Coccidioides, Paracoccidioides, Blastomyces, Candida, Sporothrix, Mucor, Aspergillus, Rhizopus, Absidia, Basidiobolus, Entomophthora.* **Others:** *Leishmania* (Ch 71, ref. 46). **Ineffective:** dermatophytes.

INDICATIONS. Cryptococcosis, coccidioidomycosis, histoplasmosis, mucormycosis, sporotrichosis, aspergillosis, candidiasis, leishmaniasis. Primary drug for severe overwhelming systemic mycoses. Most effective antifungal for severe life-threatening infections of disseminated aspergillosis and other filamentous fungal infections. Lipid formulations can be given at higher doses to enhance efficacy at a significantly greater cost. They are indicated over ABD when it has been ineffective or has caused nephrotoxicity if pre-existing renal impairment is evident. In rodents, L-AMB was more effective than ABD in CNS penetration in treating fungal meningoencephalitis (Ch 57, ref. 41a) and potentially suppressing CNS infection in a dog with disseminated phaeohyphomycosis (Ch 57, ref. 79). ABD was superior to fluconazole, or a combination of both drugs, in treatment of experimental CNS histoplasmosis in mice (Ch 57, ref. 49). ABD is better excreted in the urine than lipid formulations and it should be used to treat fungal urinary tract infections. In people, lipid formulations of AMB have been shown to be better tolerated, with respect to nephrotoxicity, and more efficacious in treatment of patients with invasive fungal infections (Ch 57, ref. 141a). Indicated in cases of *Leishmaniasis* unresponsive to other forms of treatment or if a cure is desired.

CONTRAINDICATIONS. Renal failure, hepatic failure. Lipid formulations are associated with less nephrotoxicity.

ADVERSE REACTIONS. The use of AMB deoxycholate is complicated by acute infusion-related toxicity and constitutional and chronic renal toxicities. These limit the dose and duration of AMB in clinical practice. During infusion of ABD, animals can develop fever, vomiting, myalgia, muscle tremors, phlebitis, and occasional anaphylaxis. Lipid formulations have a greater tendency to cause these infusion-related reactions, which can be reduced by slowing the infusion rate. The anaphylactic reaction can be variable and only to certain of the formulations available (Ch 57, ref. 65). Lipid formulations, especially ABCD, may be associated with infusion-related reactions. The theoretical advantage of the three lipid formulations is their ability to concentrate in the MPS and to be transported to the sites of infection. Larger doses of lipid formulations drug can be given with lower renal toxicity (Ch 71, ref. 15). AMB preparations are not advised in pregnancy, although there is no known toxicity. Can cause hypokalemia, which may affect cardiac, skeletal muscle, or renal function. Weight loss with long-term treatment. Nonregenerative normochromic normocytic anemia occurs with long-term therapy, presumably caused by nephrotoxicity or interference with erythropoietin. AMB alters renal tubular cell injury, which may result in potassium loss in urine, decreased medullary tonicity, and decreased urinary acidification. AMB increases intracellular calcium in vascular smooth muscle cells, leading to arachidonic acid cascade and subsequent accumulation of vasoconstrictive eicosanoids. Increased renal vascular resistance develops without changes in blood pressure, thereby reducing renal blood flow. To combat toxicity, renal dopamine DA1 receptors may be stimulated. Dopamine infusion has been used to reduce toxicity but has a nonselective effect; however controlled studies in humans showed no statistical benefit in preventing nephrotoxicity (Ch 57, ref. 14a). Fenoldopam (SmithKline Beecham), a specific DA1 agonist for receptors in renal tubules, might be more selective (Ch 57, ref. 97). Loading of isotonic NaCL by parenteral infusion at the time of AMB administration has been the most beneficial

factor in reducing the nephrotoxicity of these preparations. Reduced nephrotoxicity may relate to lipid binding of drug in plasma and its direct uptake into the MPS. Nephrotoxicity is the dose-limiting factor; may have to interrupt therapy, reduce dosage, or use alternative drugs. Gradually increase dose if drug reinstated.

INTERACTIONS. AMB in any formulation increases nephrotoxicity of cyclosporine, aminoglycosides, vancomycin, inhalation anesthetics, and cisplatin. Sometimes used in conjunction with an azole antifungal. Synergistic effects occur with combined use of rifampin against *Histoplasma*, *Aspergillus*, *Candida*, and tetracycline or fluorocytosine against *Candida* and *Cryptococcus*. AMB may alter the fungal cell membrane, allowing these other drugs to disrupt fungal metabolism. Combination therapy with azole antifungals may induce fungal resistance to AMB, although it is often recommended in rapidly advancing systemic mycoses. In experimental studies with combination therapy either concomittant or in succession, FCZ was synergistic while ITZ was inhibitory (see also Azoles, Chapter 57) (Ch 57, ref. 129).

AVAILABILITY		TYPE	SIZES	PREPARATIONS (COMPANY)
Human	**ABD**	Powder for injection (deoxycholate)	50 mg/vial	*Fungizone* (E.R. Squibb)
	ABCD	Powder for injection (colloidal dispersion)	50 mg/vial and 100 mg/vial	*Amphocil, Amphotec* (Sequus)
	L-AMB	Powder for injection (liposomal)	50 mg/vial	*AmBisome* (Fujisawa; Nexstar)
	ABLC	Solution for injection (lipid complex)	100 mg/20 ml vial (5 mg/ml)	*Abelcet* (Liposome Co.)

INTERNATIONAL PREPARATIONS. *Ampho-Moronal, Funganiline, Fungilin, Fungizona.*

HANDLING. ABD: Dilute powder with 10 ml sterile water (electrolyte or preservative free), shake until clear to give 5 mg/ml solution. Dilute further 1 : 50 with 5% dextrose to give final concentration of 10 mg/100 ml. Incompatible with many other fluids, but can use dilute heparin for flush. Precipitates will form if preservatives or saline are used. Stored powder is refrigerated in the dark in unopened vials. If accidentally left unrefrigerated; powder is stable for 2-4 weeks. Prepared 5-mg/ml solutions are stable for 24 hr in the dark at room temperature and for 1 week when refrigerated. When further diluted in 5% dextrose, solution is stable in PVC IV bags for 24 hr. Exposure to light during daily infusions (<8 hr duration) does not affect potency enough to warrant concern. **To reduce toxicity: heating of ABD** to form superaggregation has been noted to reduce toxicity (Ch 57, ref. 35; 104). The powdered drug as supplied is reconstituted with 10 ml of 5% dextrose. Then the ABD is pre-heated for 20 min at 70°C prior to administration. **Mixing of ABD with lipid** for the treatment of canine leishmaniasis (Ch 71, ref. 47) is done by aseptically adding 40 ml sterile H$_2$O and 10 ml of a commercial soya bean solution *(Intralipid)* to 50 mg AMB. After shaking the mixture (1 mg AMB/ml) is stable for 3 weeks (Ch 71, ref. 97). **ABCD:** As dry powder, stable at room temperature for at least 2 years. After reconstitution, vials can be stored refrigerated for 24 hr but not frozen. With further dilution to approximately 1 mg/ml in 5% dextrose, the stability is 24 hr refrigerated. **L-AMB:** Dry powder is stored under refrigeration. It is diluted with sterile water without preservatives to a 4-mg/ml solution. Shaking is necessary until the drug is completely dispersed. Reconstituted drug is stable up to 24 hr refrigerated, if not frozen. For further dilution to 1-2 mg/ml or lower concentrations, the drug is flushed through a 5-μm

filter (provided) into 5% dextrose. Infusion into the patient should be within 6 hr of dilution. An in-line membrane filter may be used if the mean pore diameter is >1 μm. **ABLC:** Shake vial to suspend yellow sediment, withdraw drug via 18-gauge needle into 20-ml syringes and infuse through the supplied 5-μm filter needle into 5% dextrose for infusion to a concentration of 1-2 mg/ml. Refrigerate suspension until used. Stable in 5% dextrose solution for 48 hr refrigerated and 6 hr at room temperature. Aseptic technique must be practiced because no bacteriostatic preservatives are included. Do not dilute with saline solutions or other drugs. Infusion catheters carrying such fluids can be flushed with 5% dextrose first. In-line filters should not be used. It should not be frozen.

ADMINISTRATION. ABD: Animals should be well hydrated before treatment, and pre-existing dehydration must be corrected by fluid therapy. Manufacturer of deoxycholate preparation recommends dose be given over 2-6 hr. When large-volume infusion is used, an IV catheter is placed and the dose (10 mg/100 ml) is given in 300-500 ml of 5% dextrose, depending on size of animal. Administration over this interval may reduce the likelihood or renal damage. However, clinical experience in dogs and cats has shown that more concentrated solutions, with the dose placed in a volume of 10 ml to 60 ml 5% dextrose, can be placed in a syringe and infused through a butterfly or indwelling catheter over a 5- to 10-min period. Ten milliliters of 5% dextrose flush should be infused immediately before and after administration of the drug. Although bolus infusions may have a higher risk of toxicity, this can be overcome by administering an equal or greater volume of lactated Ringer's or 0.9% NaCl (equal to that otherwise given with routine dilution of AMB) by IV or SC administration without the risks associated with extravasated drug. Supplemental fluid diuresis is highly recommended with each dose. For cats, indwelling catheters are preferable because of the difficulties of repeated venipuncture. Often test dose (1 mg) slowly IV to check for immediate systemic reactions. Co-administration of nonsteroidal anti-inflammatories, antihistamines, antiemetics, and/or small doses of IV glucocorticoids or heparin may reduce systemic reaction. Prevent thrombophlebitis by flushing catheters, using larger veins, rotating sites, adding heparin to the solution. The only way to ensure reaching the CNS is by intrathecal use of deoxycholate preparation, which can be irritating.

Renal toxic effects are monitored at least once, if not twice weekly, by checking serum urea concentrations and by examination of the urine for specific gravity, protein, casts, and hematuria. Serum creatinine and electrolytes (including magnesium, which may decrease) determinations are optional but may be required if screening tests or health becomes altered. Urine changes detect toxicity earlier than blood biochemical alterations. Therapy should be temporarily discontinued if anorexia or vomiting occurs or if serum urea increases to >30 mg/dl. Therapy with AMB or alternative drug is reinstituted after signs and laboratory findings of nephrotoxicity disappear. Maintenance therapy with weekly or monthly injections of AMB or daily oral imidazoles has been used to avoid relapses that develop once therapy is discontinued.

Hypokalemia, a problem in people receiving AMB, has been documented in dogs and cats. Any potassium supplements should be given PO, SC, or by alternative IV route, because these solutions will precipitate the colloid.

Fever, nausea, and vomiting that occur during or immediately after treatment may be less severe if a physiologic dose of hydrocortisone sodium succinate (0.5 mg/kg, IV), diphenhydramine (0.5 mg/kg, IV or PO), or aspirin (10 mg/kg, PO) is given before administration of AMB. Anti-inflammatory or immunosuppressive doses of glucocorticoids should be avoided because they may lead to fungal dissemination. Muscular fasciculations and rigors that develop in people during IV infusions have been controlled with dantrolene sodium (10-50 mg, IV) or meperidine.

Attempts to avoid nephrotoxicity with ABD have been made using mannitol (0.5-1 g/kg, IV), sodium bicarbonate (1-2 mmol/kg, IV), and dopamine (3-10 μg/kg/min, IV), but controlled studies have either not been done or have shown no benefit (Ch 57, ref. 14a). Beneficial effects have been obtained when sodium-containing fluids or furosemide (5 mg/kg route) or aminophylline was given to dogs just before administration of AMB. SC administration is less nephrotoxic (see later).

Heparin has been added to ABD to control phlebitis that develops after repeated infusions, but there is no conclusive evidence that its use decreases the reaction. In-line micropore filters used to remove particulate matter and bacteria from IV solutions are less than 0.45 μm and will also remove the drug. Filters of greater than 1 μm can be used but will not remove bacteria.

Alternative Routes. Usual IV therapy requires repeated venous access, often necessitating catheter placement, especially in cats. ABD may be used topically, intra-articularly, or intrathecally or may be flushed in the bladder or renal pelvis if the infection site is accessible by these means. This will help achieve maximal concentrations with lower risk of systemic toxicity. **Intra-articularly,** 5 to 15 mg can be used to infuse one joint. For **bladder infusions,** AMB is mixed to a concentration of 30 to 50 mg in 50-100 ml sterile water and is infused once daily for 5-15 days. The bladder is distended, and the animal is permitted to void spontaneously. Alternatively, a constant-drip infusion of 50 mg/L has been used. For **intrathecal** use, 0.2-0.5 mg is diluted in 5 ml of 10% dextrose or CSF freshly removed from the animal under anesthesia. It is injected in the lumbar or cisternal space, and the head is lowered for a few minutes if signs of intracranial involvement are apparent. Unfortunately, this procedure must be repeated two to three

times each week. **Aerosol** use achieves higher concentration in the respiratory tract than other tissues, thus reducing nephrotoxicity. Conventional AMB is less efficiently nebulized than lipid-based products. For AMB use 50 mg divided into three doses. Generally well tolerated; however, bronchospasm or vomiting has been observed in people. Aerosol AMB has been used long term (3 weeks-2.5 yrs) in people for prophylaxis or treatment of pulmonary fungal infections. **Ocular injection:** Systemic therapy should suffice for early chorioretinitis before vitreitis develops. Although established intraocular mycotic infections are difficult to cure, enophthalmitis in people has been effectively treated by injecting simultaneously intravitreally 5 μg, peribulbar space 125 μg, and episclerally 5 mg. Intravitreal injections were well tolerated in rabbits (5 μg), monkeys (10-20 μg). Liposomal AMB was well tolerated in doses that were at least 4-fold higher. The drug persists in clinically healthy eyes for at least 7-15 days and for shorter periods following vitrectomy and lens extraction. Single doses have been sometimes effective in clearing infection in experimentally infected rabbits. **Subcutaneous:** Route used in dogs and cats with cryptococcosis and potentially for other systemic mycoses. A daily dose of 0.5 to 0.8 mg/kg is added to 400 ml (cats) and 500 ml (dogs) of 0.45% saline/2.5% dextrose (Ch 57, ref. 83). This total fluid volume is given SC two or three times weekly to a cumulative level of 8-26 mg/kg, which is higher than IV regimen. Concentrations of >20 mg/L are irritating, cause SC abscesses, and should be avoided. The method is suited for outpatient treatment and does not require IV catheter maintenance. Blood levels are lower but more sustained, reducing toxicity and allowing for increased efficacy. **Combined with fat emulsion:** This has been done in an attempt to decrease nephrotoxicity. AMB deoxycholate is stable in combination with fat emulsions. A concentration of 0.5 to 2 mg/ml is stable in a 20% fat emulsion for 4 days at 25°C in fluorescent lighting and 7 days at 4-8°C in the dark. In one study (Ch 71, ref. 47) AMB was added to a commercial lipid preparation (see Handling above). The mixture, which was stored for up to 3 weeks, was given over 30-60 min at a starting dose of 1-1.5 mg/kg twice weekly with progressive increases to 1.6-2.5 mg/kg twice weekly and altered by changes in serum urea and creatinine. The infusion was followed by 50 ml/kg of normal saline and then 10 ml/kg of 20% mannitol.

ABCD: Given by IV infusion at a rate of 1 mg/kg/hr. A test dose (10 ml) should be infused first to check for adverse reactions. The rate of infusion can be increased if it is tolerated.

L-AMB: Given by IV infusion over 60 to 120 min or longer with 5% dextrose as a diluent. Solution is diluted to 1-2 mg/ml.

ABLC: Given by IV infusion at 2.5 mg/kg/hr. With infusion times longer than 2 hr, the mixture should be shaken periodically to disperse any sediment.

DOSAGE. ABD: A wide range of systemic dosages has been described in the veterinary literature. The range has been a total (cumulative) dose of 4-12 mg/kg given as alternate day or Mon-Wed-Fri treatments. Dogs usually receive accumulative doses of 8-12 mg/kg and cats 4-6 mg/kg. Lower dosages are used if adjunctive therapy with oral flucytosine or antezole is used. Higher doses are given SC (see prior discussion). For IV use, the drug is given on these days at 0.15-0.5 mg/kg/day, which is continued until the final calculated total dosage is reached (usually 6 weeks) or when toxicity (elevated serum urea concentration) occurs. Daily doses are lower (0.15-0.25 mg/kg) for cats and higher (0.25-0.5 mg/kg) for dogs. The 0.5-mg/kg dose has a high risk of nephrotoxicity. Initial doses of 0.1 mg/kg for cats and 0.25 mg/kg for dogs are often given the first day and are gradually increased to 0.25 mg/kg and 0.5 mg/kg, respectively. Doses up to 1 mg/kg/day given 2-3 times weekly have been used in particularly resistant infections in dogs that tolerate the drug well. Treatment often lasts for 2-3 mo or longer, and early discontinuance can lead to a relapse. Treatment may require 11 mo in aspergillosis and 9 mo in sporotrichosis. A recommended dose for long-term treatment of sporotrichosis is 0.2-0.5 mg/kg IV given every 48 hr (Ch 57, ref. 144). Higher dosages can be used with SC route; see previously under administration. **Lipid formulations–ABCD, L-AMB, ABLC:** Higher dosages are tolerated and used as outlined in the table that follows. Rates of infusion and total doses are individualized to each animal to ensure maximum efficacy while reducing the potential for systemic toxicity or adverse reactions. General

guidelines are to administer lipid formulations at a level of 1 mg/kg given every 48 hr to a minimum cumulative total dosage of 12 mg/kg. In studies of people with invasive aspergillosis, doses of L-AMB of 3 mg/kg were no more effective than 1 mg/kg (Ch 57, ref. 30a). For human leishmaniasis, cumulative dosages of L-AMB which were shown to be curative have been as high as 20 mg/kg (Ch 71, ref. 61).

Lipid AMB mixtures prepared from ABD are dosed similarly to the commercial AMB lipid formulations. A cumulative dose of 10 mg/kg has been effective in one study (Ch 71, ref. 47) but not another (Ch 71, ref. 64). The dosage was higher and follow-up shorter in the former study which may explain this discrepancy.

INDICATIONS	INITIAL TEST DOSAGE[a] (mg/kg)	USUAL DOSE (mg/kg)	ROUTE	INTERVAL (hr)	DURATION
ABD (Fungizone)					
Dogs (mycoses)	0.25	0.25-0.5	IV	48[b]	6 weeks
Cats (mycoses)	0.1	0.1-0.25	IV	48[b]	6 weeks
Dogs and Cats (mycoses)	—	0.5-0.8	SC	48[b]	3-10 weeks
Dogs (leishmaniasis)	—	0.5-0.8	IV	48[b]	See[c]
L-AMB (AmBisome)					
Dogs (leishmaniasis)	0.5	3.0-3.3	IV	72-96	See[d]
Dogs (mycoses)	0.5	1-2.5	IV	48[b]	4 weeks[e]
ABCD (Amphocil)					
Dogs (mycoses)	0.5	1-2.5	IV	48[b]	4 weeks[e]
ABLC (Abelcet)					
Dogs (mycoses)	0.5	1-2.5	IV	48[b]	4 weeks[e]

[a]Only use this dose first to test for potential adverse reactions or azotemia; animals developing azotemia usually tolerate subsequent administration at the usual dosage.
[b]Every 48 hr, or Monday (M), Wednesday (W), and Friday (F) on a weekly basis until the cumulative dosage is reached. For *Leishmania* the total cumulative dose for ABD is 15 mg/kg. Depending on the type and severity of the systemic mycosis, the cumulative dose for ABD ranges between 4 and 10 mg/kg. For lipid-base AMB, the cumujlative dose is 8-12 mg/kg depending on the systemic mycosis.
[c]Every 48 hr, or MWF, until a cumulative dose of 8 to 16 mg/kg is reached (Ch 71, ref. 46).
[d]Every 72-96 hr, until a cumulative dose of 15 mg/kg is reached (Ch 73, ref. 150). May be possible to give the same cumulative dose with a lower level every 48 hr (some regimens suggest days 1,2,3 and 10 or days 1,2,3,4 and 10).
[e]Every 48 hours, or MWF, or until a minimum cumulative dose of 12 mg/kg is reached (Ch 59, ref. 47) by using 1 mg/kg dose for susceptible yeast or systemic (dimorphic) fungal infections. For more resistant filamentous fungal infections, such as pythiosis, use a 2-2.5 mg dose until a cumulative dose of 24-30 mg/kg is reached. In people with invasive aspergillosis, clinical response to dosage increments of 1 mg/kg were comparable to those of 4 mg/kg at a significantly reduced cost (Ch 57, ref. 30a).

ADDITIONAL DOSAGES. Blastomycosis, Table 59-1; histoplasmosis, Table 60-1; cryptococcosis, Table 61-5; coccidioidomycosis, Table 62-3; nasal aspergillosis, Table 64-1; disseminated aspergillosis, Table 64-3; dermal candidiasis and trichosporonosis, Table 65-2; candidiasis, Table 65-4; prototothecosis, Table 69-1.

AMPICILLIN

CLASS. Aminopenicillin.

ACTION. Bactericidal; inhibits bacterial cell wall synthesis.

MORE INFORMATION. See AMOXICILLIN; Aminopenicillins, Chapter 34; Table 34-1.

PHARMACOKINETICS. Orally up to 50% absorbed, but decreased by ingesta. Oral trihydrate form is less efficiently absorbed than anhydrate. In cats, oral suspension has lower bioavailability (18%) than capsules (42%). IM and SC sodium salt better absorbed than trihydrate. Absorption of anhydrate form is comparable between SC and IM sites. Better absorbed from SC tissues in the dorsal neck region than over the thoracic wall (Ch 34, ref. 366). Penetrates body fluids and parenchymal organs (liver, lung). Only enters acutely inflamed

meninges, CNS, eye, and prostate. One of few β-lactams that is metabolized and excreted by liver: biliary concentration is 40 times that in blood. About 50% excreted unchanged in urine.

SPECTRUM. Gram positive: Non–β-lactamase *Staphylococcus, Streptococcus.* **Gram negative:** *Escherichia, Proteus, Pasteurella.* No advantage using this drug in conjunction with trimethoprim-sulfonamide because it adds very little to spectrum. Has better gram negative, but less anaerobic spectrum, than to natural and β-lactamase–resistant penicillins. See also AMOXICILLIN. **Anaerobes:** Not as effective as penicillin. **Ineffective:** Rickettsiae, mycoplasmas, mycobacteria, and fungi. Not effective against β-Lactamase–producing organisms.

INDICATIONS. Gram-negative infections caused by *Proteus* and *Escherichia*. Appropriate first choice for bacterial meningitis in dogs and cats. Dental prophylaxis, septicemia, urinary, respiratory, and soft tissue infections; prophylaxis with GI surgery when combined with gentamicin.

CONTRAINDICATIONS. Avoid in resistant infections caused by *Klebsiella, Pseudomonas, Enterobacter.* β-Lactamase is main cause of resistance. Safe in pregnancy. In hepatic cirrhosis, clearance is increased, and dose may have to be increased. Increase dose interval to 12 hr or reduce dose in severe renal failure.

ADVERSE REACTIONS. Causes seizures with rapid IV administration; upsets normal intestinal microflora causing diarrhea.

INTERACTIONS. Reduces bioavailability of atenolol. Potential antagonism of activity when coadministered with chloramphenicol, tetracyclines, or erythromycin. See AMOXICILLIN.

AVAILABILITY	TYPE	SIZES	PREPARATIONS (COMPANY)
Human	Powder for injection (IV, IM)	125 mg, 250 mg, 500 mg, 1 g, 2 g, 10 g	*Omnipen-N* (Wyeth-Ayerst), *Polycillin-N* (Bristol)
	Oral capsules	250 mg, 500 mg	*Amcill* (Parke-Davis), *Principen* (Bristol-Myers Squibb)
	Powder for oral suspension	125 mg/5 ml, 250 mg/5 ml, 500 mg/5 ml	*Polycillin, Totacillin* (SmithKline Beecham)
Veterinary	Oral capsules (trihydrate) (dogs, cats)	125 mg, 250 mg, 500 mg	*Princillin* (Solvay)
	Oral suspension (trihydrate) (dogs, cats)	125 mg/5 ml	*Intracillin* (Intervet), *Princillin*
	Powder for parenteral (SC, IM) suspension (trihydrate) (dogs, cats, cattle)	10-g, 25-g vials	*Polyflex* (Fort Dodge)
	Powder for parenteral (IV, SC) Injection (sodium salt) (horses)	1-g, 3-g vials	*Amp-Equine* (Pfizer Animal Health)

INTERNATIONAL PREPARATIONS. *Binotal, Jenampin, Novapen, Penbritin, Principen, Rimacillin, Spectracil, Vidopen.*

HANDLING. Reconstituted parenteral ampicillin sodium (30 mg/ml) in sodium chloride (0.9%) or lactated Ringer's is stable for 8 hr at room temperature and for 48 hr when refrigerated. More dilute concentrations (<20 mg/ml, in 5% dextrose) are stable 2-4 hr at room temperature and 8 hr if refrigerated. Whenever possible, use freshly prepared solutions of ampicillin sodium. Parenteral trihydrate suspension is stable for 3 mo at room temperature or 12 mo if refrigerated. Oral suspensions are stable for 1 week at room temperature or 2 weeks when refrigerated and should be discarded thereafter. Capsules and nonreconstituted powders are stored at room temperature. Ampicillin sodium solutions are incompatible with macrolides, aminoglycosides, tetracyclines, phenothiazines, and various other drugs; therefore, mixing with other compounds is not advised.

ADMINISTRATION. Give PO on empty stomach. For IV, administer slowly over 10-15 min or as slower IV drip. IM or IV forms are used for severe infections that require highest dosages or when oral medication is contraindicated.

Dosage

INDICATIONS	DOSE (mg/kg)	ROUTE	INTERVAL (hr)	DURATION (days)
Dogs				
Urinary infections	12.5	PO	12	3-7
	6.6	SC, IM	12	3-7
Soft tissue infections	10-20	PO, IM, SC	8	7
Pneumonia, systemic	22	PO, IV, SC	8	7-14
Meningitis, orthopedics	22	IV, IM, SC, PO	6-8	prn
Bacteremia, sepsis	20-40	IV, IM, SC	6-8	prn
Neonatal sepsis	50	IV, intraosseous	4-6	prn
Cats				
Urinary infections	20	PO	8-12	7-14
Soft tissue infections	20-40	PO	8-12	14
Systemic infections	7-11	IV, IM, SC	8-12	prn

ADDITIONAL DOSAGES. Canine distemper, Table 3-5; canine viral enteritis, Table 8-1; feline panleukopenia, Table 10-2; feline infectious peritonitis, Table 11-4; streptococcal infection, Table 35-4; sepsis, Table 38-6; salmonellosis, Table 39-2; *Clostridium perfringens* diarrhea, Table 39-10; leptospirosis, Table 44-7; actinomycosis, Table 49-2; nocardiosis, Table 49-3; dermatophilosis, Table 51-1; feline abscesses, Table 52-3; musculoskeletal infections, Table 86-4; bacteremia, Table 87-6; respiratory infections, Table 88-8; oral infections, Table 89-4; urinary infections, Table 91-10; CNS infections, Table 92-5.

DISPENSING INFORMATION. Give drugs to fasted (preferably >5 hr) dogs or at least 1 hr before or 2 hr after feeding (Ch 34, ref. 206). Dry food interferes less with absorption than moist food.

AMPICILLIN-SULBACTAM

CLASS. Aminopenicillin and β-lactamase inhibitor in a 2 : 1 ratio.

ACTION. Bactericidal; inhibitor of bacterial cell wall synthesis and β-lactamase inhibitor.

MORE INFORMATION. Chapter 34; Table 34-2; reference: Ch 34, ref. 225.

PHARMACOKINETICS. Therapeutic levels attained within 15 min of IV or IM dose. Good tissue levels and penetrates peritoneal and interstitial fluids. Up to 85% excreted in urine within 8 hr (Ch 39, ref. 313). Both drugs eliminated at similar rate in dogs. Sulbactam has no intrinsic antibacterial activity but extends spectrum of ampicillin.

SPECTRUM. Gram positive: *Staphylococcus, Streptococcus, Bacillus anthracis, Listeria monocytogenes.* **Gram negative:** *Escherichia, Klebsiella, Proteus, Salmonella, Enterobacter, Pasteurella, Acinetobacter.* **Anaerobes:** *Clostridium, Peptococcus,* *Peptostreptococcus, Bacteroides, Fusobacterium.* **Ineffective:** *Pseudomonas.*

INDICATIONS. Skin and soft tissue, intraabdominal, orthopedic, and genitourinary infections caused by susceptible bacteria. Can substitute wherever amoxicillin-clavulanate is indicated and a parenteral formulation is desired.

CONTRAINDICATIONS. Reduce dose in renal failure. Animals with known penicillin hypersensitivity.

ADVERSE REACTIONS. Local pain with IM; thrombophlebitis or systemic allergic reactions with IV; diarrhea; vomiting; seizures with rapid IV infusions; increased hepatic transaminases. See also AMPICILLIN.

INTERACTIONS. Coadministration of ampicillin and sulbactam to dogs has no effect on the pharmacokinetics of either drug (Ch 34, ref. 225). Do not mix with aminoglycosides during administration.

AVAILABILITY	TYPE	SIZES	PREPARATION (COMPANY)
Human	Powder for injection (sodium)	1.5 g (total), 3.0 g (total)	*UnaSyn* (Pfizer)

Dosage

INDICATIONS	DOSE	ROUTE	INTERVAL (hr)	DURATION (days)
Adult human	1.5-3 g	IV	6	prn
Dog and cat	50 mg/kg	IV	6-8	prn

HANDLING. Dilute in sterile water, 0.9% NaCl, 5% dextrose or lactated Ringer's. Stability of drug is shortest for dextrose (2 hr at room temperature and 4 hr when refrigerated) and 8 or 48 hr, respectively, for both NaCl or sterile water. Maximum storage time for lactated Ringer's is 24 hr refrigerated. Do not mix with aminoglycosides. For IM, can be reconstituted with 2% lidocaine (without epinephrine).

ADMINISTRATION. IV or IM. For IV dose, give slowly over 10-15 min or give with 50-100-ml infusion fluid over 15-30 min. For IM, give deep.

ADDITIONAL DOSAGES: Intrabdominal infections, Table 89-21.

AMPROLIUM

CLASS. Thiamine analogue.

ACTION. Antiprotozoal; inhibits parasite's thiamine utilization (first-generation schizont).

MORE INFORMATION. Chapter 81; Table 81-2; reference: Ch 71, ref. 49.

PHARMACOKINETICS. Unavailable.

SPECTRUM. Coccidia.

INDICATIONS. Coccidiosis; especially convenient for treating litters of animals.

APPROVED USES. Veterinary: coccidiosis in lambs, calves, and poultry.

CONTRAINDICATIONS. Limit duration of therapy for 2 weeks.

ADVERSE REACTIONS. Anorexia, diarrhea, depression. Unpalatable as undiluted liquid or paste. Anorexia may develop in puppies that eat more than 300 mg of amprolium on a daily basis. Prolonged high dosages can cause neurologic signs of thiamine deficiency, characterized by cervical ventroflexion, anisocoria, seizures. Should these develop, stop treatment and administer thiamine 1-10 mg/day IM or IV immediately.

INTERACTIONS. Excess dietary thiamine can interfere with drug effectiveness.

AVAILABILITY	TYPE	SIZES	PREPARATIONS (COMPANY)
Veterinary	Oral crumbles	1.25%	*Corid* (Merck AgVet; Merial)
	Oral solution	9.6%	*Corid*
	Soluble powder	20%	*Corid*

HANDLING. Store all products at room temperature.

ADMINISTRATION. Can add soluble powder in food or water. Use only food or water additives, not both! If given in drinking water, offer this as the sole source of liquids to drink. For animals refusing food or water additive, place in gelatin capsules containing 20% powder. Can treat pups 6 weeks of age and older.

Dosage

INDICATIONS	DOSE	ROUTE	INTERVAL (hr)	DURATION (days)
Dogs				
Coccidiosis (in capsules)				
Small pups (<10 kg adult wt)	100 mg total dose, 20% powder	PO, gelatin capsules	24	7-12
Large pups (≥10 kg adult wt)	200 mg total dose, 20% powder	PO, gelatin capsules	24	7-12
Coccidiosis (in food): pups or bitches	250-300 mg total dose, 20% powder, on food	PO, on food	24	7-12
Coccidiosis (in water): pups or bitches	30 ml of 9.6% solution, 3.8 L (1 gal) of water; no other drinking water provided	PO, in water	24	7-10
Cats				
Coccidiosis (on food)	300-400 mg/kg	PO	24	5
	110-220 mg/kg	PO	24	7-12
Coccidiosis (in water)	1.5 teaspoon/gallon H_2O	PO	24	10
Coccidiosis (in combination)				
Amprolium	150 mg/kg	PO	24	14
and				
Sulfadimethoxine	25 mg/kg	PO	24	14

ADDITIONAL DOSAGES: coccidiosis, Table 81-2.

DISPENSING INFORMATION. Report signs of diarrhea or neurologic problems immediately to your veterinarian.

ATOVAQUONE

CLASS. Hydroxynaphthoquinone.

ACTION. Antiprotozoal; blocks cytochromes, resulting in inhibited nucleic acid and adenosine triphosphate synthesis.

MORE INFORMATION. See Chapter 68; Antiprotozoal Chemotherapy, Chapter 71; Table 71-1; Chapter 77; Table 77-3; reference: Ch 71, ref. 38; 44; 10b.

PHARMACOKINETICS. Highly lipid soluble. Low absorption from GI tract. Bioavailability is increased three times with food and especially fatty meals. Little or no metabolism. Very low CSF penetration. Enterohepatic cycling with prolonged fecal elimination. Minimal urinary excretion.

SPECTRUM. *Pneumocystis:* slightly lower efficacy than trimethoprim-sulfonamide (TMS). May add azithromycin for some *Babesia (B. gibsoni)* infections. Effective against *Toxoplasma* bradyzoites experimentally. Not very effective against *Cryptosporidium.*

INDICATIONS. Pneumocystosis when resistance or toxicity to TMS has occurred. TMS is often used first because of lower toxicity. Used in combination with azithromycin for treatment of *Babesia gibsoni* infection in dogs.

APPROVED USES. Human: *Pneumocystis* pneumonia, malaria.

CONTRAINDICATIONS. Avoid in pregnancy, lactation. If cannot be taken with food owing to GI upsets, then use another drug.

ADVERSE REACTIONS. Nausea, vomiting, diarrhea, dermal hypersensitivity, fetotoxic, hypoglycemia, anemia, neutropenia.

INTERACTIONS. Competes for plasma protein binding with many drugs, but others such as diphenylhydantoin are not affected. Rifampin decreases activity. Rifampin and metoclopramide reduce its plasma concentrations.

AVAILABILITY	TYPE	SIZES	PREPARATIONS (COMPANY)
Human	Oral tablets	250 mg (discontinued in U.S.)	*Mepron* (Glaxo Wellcome)
	Oral solution	150 mg/ml	*Mepron*

INTERNATIONAL PREPARATIONS. *Wellvone.*

HANDLING. Store in airtight containers at controlled room temperature.

ADMINISTRATION. Absorption improved when given with meals (especially fatty). In people, >23 g of fat per meal is recommended.

Dosage[a]

INDICATIONS (Dogs)	DOSE	ROUTE	INTERVAL (hr)	DURATION (days)
Pneumocystosis	13.3 mg/kg[b]	PO	8	21
Babesia gibsoni	30 mg/kg	PO	12	7[c]
	13.3 mg/kg	PO	8	10[d]

[a]Maximum dose per administration is 750 mg. To facilitate absorption, administer with a fatty meal each time dose is given.
[b]Extrapolated from human dose.
[c]Parasite disappeared from blood after treatment; however PCR was still positive and the parasite was visible again after 30 days (Ch 71, ref. 56a).
[d]Ch 71, ref. 10b. In combination with azithromycin, this drug eliminated the infection or suppressed the parasitemia below the level of detection of organisms by PCR when dogs were monitored for up to 120 days posttreatment. Many dogs had been treated previously with either diminazene or imidocarb without success.

ADDITIONAL DOSAGES. Pneumocystosis, Table 68-2; babesiosis, Table 77-3.

DISPENSING INFORMATION. Administer tablet with fat such as butter, tuna oil, ice cream, or meat fat.

AZITHROMYCIN

CLASS. Macrolide. More stable and better absorbed than the parent drug erythromycin.

ACTION. Bacteriostatic; inhibits bacterial RNA-dependent protein synthesis by binding to 50s subunit.

MORE INFORMATION. CLARITHROMYCIN; references: Ch 34, ref. 175; Ch 34, ref. 344.

PHARMACOKINETICS. Better absorption and tissue penetration than erythromycin; more stable in gastric acid than erythromycin. Food decreases bioavailability by up to 50%; however, with fasting, 97% absorbed in dog (Ch 34, ref. 344); 58% absorbed PO in cats (Ch 34, ref. 175) compared with 37% to 52% absorbed in people. Reaches higher concentrations in tissues, phagocytes, and macrophages than in blood, with slow release and antibacterial activity up to 4 days after single dose. Enters tissue fibroblasts and lysosomes of phagocytes. Successive doses increase tissue saturation. Tissue concentrations generally exceed those in plasma by 10-100 times. Transported by neutrophils to sites of inflammation. Concentrations up to 150 times blood levels in sputum, lung, liver, tonsils, nasal sinuses, stomach, kidney, female genital tract, prostate. Crosses the placenta and excreted in milk. Levels in brain and eye are lower than in other tissues but exceed those in blood. High tissue concentrations (5-100 times plasma) are sustained for a period after serum concentrations have declined. Biliary excretion (>50%) of unchanged drug is major route of elimination and metabolites are inactive. Only 6% urinary excretion.

SPECTRUM. Gram positive: Some *Streptococcus*, variable *Staphylococcus*. **Gram negative:** *Salmonella, Bordetella, Heli-* cobacter, Bartonella. **Anaerobes:** *Propionibacterium, Clostridium,* and *Bacteroides.* **Others:** *Mycoplasma, Mycoplasma haemofelis, Chlamydia, Borrelia, Toxoplasma, Isospora, Cryptosporidium, Babesia, Mycobacterium avium-intracellulare* complex but less active than clarithromycin. **More Effective:** Most active macrolide against *Toxoplasma,* in vitro activity against *Cryptosporidium* and *Pneumocystis.* **Ineffective:** Less active than erythromycin against *Staphylococcus* and *Streptococcus* but more active against gram-negative bacteria and some anaerobes.

INDICATIONS. Cryptosporidiosis, toxoplasmosis (with pyrimethamine), Lyme borreliosis; *Mycobacterium leprae* and *Mycobacterium avium-intracellulare* infections. Lower respiratory tract infections, enteropathogenic bacterial infections. Substitute for erythromycin with less GI irritation, lower dosing, but higher cost. Used in combination with atovaquone to treat *Babesia gibsoni* infection in dogs (Ch 71, ref. 10b). Used to treat *Mycoplasma haemofelis* and *Bartonella henselae* infections in cats. Not effective for *Chlamydophila felis* infection in cats (Ch 34, ref. 288a).

CONTRAINDICATIONS. Some reduction in dosage with hepatic and/or biliary dysfunction. Less of a concern with renal failure. Avoid with previous macrolide hypersensitivity.

ADVERSE REACTIONS. GI irritation (vomiting, diarrhea, abdominal pain), hepatomegaly, cholestatic hepatitis, increased liver enzymes.

INTERACTIONS. Some reduction in serum concentration with oral antacids. See ERYTHROMYCIN.

AVAILABILITY	TYPE	SIZES	PREPARATIONS (COMPANY)
Human	Capsules (dihydrate)	250 mg	*Zithromax* (Pfizer)
	Oral suspension	100 mg/5 ml, 200 mg/5 ml	*Zithromax*
Dog and cat	Capsules	M7 200 mg	*Aziplus (Labyes)*

INTERNATIONAL PREPARATIONS. *Azithrocin, Azitromax, Ribotrex, Trozocina.*

HANDLING. Store capsules at controlled room temperature (<30°C). Reconstituted solution should be stored between 5-30°C.

ADMINISTRATION. Do not mix with food or give oral antacids concurrently.

Dosage

INDICATIONS	DOSE (mg/kg)	ROUTE	INTERVAL (hr)	DURATION (days)
Dogs				
Pyoderma, Systemic infections	5-10	PO	12	5-7
Skin infections	10	PO	12-24	10-20
Lyme borreliosis	5	PO, IV	12	10-20
Babesia gibsoni infection	10-11.6	PO	24	10[a]
Cats				
Mycoplasmosis	5-15	PO	24	5[b]
Bacterial infections	7-15	PO	12	5-7[c]
Dogs and Cats				
Coccidiosis and Cryptosporidiosis	15	PO	12	7

[a]Ch 71, ref. 10b. The drug was crushed and reformulated in gelatin capsules for proper dosing.
[b]Then every 48-72 hr (Ch 34, ref. 187).
[c]A dosage of 15 mg/kg, given daily for 3 days and then twice weekly, was not effective in clearing chronically infected cats of *Chlamydophila* infection (Ch 34, ref. 288a).

ADDITIONAL DOSAGES. Lyme borreliosis, Table 45-5; babesiosis, Table 77-3; cryptosporidiosis, Table 82-2.

DISPENSING INFORMATION. Administer without food; give 1 hr before or 2 hr after a meal.

AZTREONAM

CLASS. Monobactam.

ACTION. Bactericidal; interferes with cell wall synthesis, especially gram-negative bacteria resistant to β-lactamases.

MORE INFORMATION. See Chapter 34; Table 34-1.

PHARMACOKINETICS. Poor GI absorption and must be given parenterally (IV or IM). Enters most body fluids, including CSF. Penetrates and effective in abscesses. Primarily renally excreted as unchanged drug. Widely distributed in body tissues, including gallbladder, liver, lungs, kidneys, heart, intestine, prostate. Reaches saliva, bronchial secretions, bile, pericardial, pleural, peritoneal, synovial fluids. Reaches CNS at therapeutic concentration. Eliminated by kidney with 60%-70% as active drug. Hepatic dysfunction does not alter excretion.

SPECTRUM. Gram positive: poor. **Gram negative:** *Pseudomonas, Escherichia, Enterobacter, Klebsiella, Proteus, Serratia, Citrobacter.* Wide activity against *only* gram-negative organisms. Synergistic with aminoglycosides in vitro against most strains of Enterobacteriaceae and other gram-negative aerobic and facultative bacilli. Little or no activity on gram-positive or anaerobic bacteria and intestinal microflora. **Anaerobes:** poor. **More effective:** gram negative. **Ineffective:** most other bacteria.

INDICATIONS. Serious gram-negative infections of the urinary and lower respiratory tracts, meningitis, septicemia, skin, soft tissue, intraabdominal, genital infections. Could be considered as an alternative to aminoglycosides to avoid nephrotoxicity or to fluoroquinolones in young animals. Often as a single agent for resistant gram-negative pathogens such as *Escherichia, Klebsiella, Serratia, Pseudomonas.* Examples are nosocomial pneumonia and aspiration pneumonia (the latter use, in combination with clindamycin). With mixed infections, it should be used in combination with drugs against anaerobic and gram-positive bacteria. Can also combine with erythromycin, metronidazole, penicillins, vancomycin as a substitute for aminoglycosides.

CONTRAINDICATIONS. Must reduce dosages in renal dysfunction. No significant interactions with gentamicin, nafcillin, cephradine, clindamycin, metronidazole. Concurrent therapy needed if gram-positive aerobe or an anaerobe is suspected. Certain antibiotics (e.g., cefoxitin or imipenem) may induce β-lactamases in some gram-negative organisms making concurrent therapy with β-lactams such as aztreonam ineffective.

ADVERSE REACTIONS. Dermal hypersensitivity reactions, local phlebitis with IV, and swelling at injection site with IM. Nausea, vomiting, diarrhea, dermatologic eruptions, pancytopenia, seizures. Transient increase in hepatic transaminases; icterus from hepatotoxicity.

INTERACTIONS. Add to ampicillin for urinary tract infection caused by *Escherichia.* Use with clindamycin and metronidazole for intraabdominal abscesses. Combination therapy with metronidazole for anaerobes and combine with vancomycin for gram positives.

AVAILABILITY	TYPE	SIZES	PREPARATION (COMPANY)
Human	Powder for injection	500 mg; 1 g, or 2 g/vial	*Azactam* (Bristol-Myers Squibb)

INTERNATIONAL PREPARATIONS. *Primbactam.*

HANDLING. IV solutions of 2% (wt/vol) or less can be prepared with 0.9% NaCl or 5% dextrose. Can also add clindamycin phosphate, gentamicin, tobramycin sulfate, or cefazolin sodium. Stable for 48 hr at room temperature or 7 days when refrigerated. May be stored frozen at 20°C for 3 mo. Once thawed, should be used within 24-72 hr. Should not be refrozen. Incompatible in solution with AMB, nafcillin, cephradine, metronidazole.

ADMINISTRATION. For IM use, give deep in large muscle. It is well tolerated and need not be mixed with local anesthetics. IV use recommended for animals with bacteremia, abscesses, severe overwhelming infections. Give IV infusion slowly over 20-60 min.

Dosage

INDICATIONS	DOSE	ROUTE	INTERVAL (hr)	DURATION (days)
Human[a]	1-2 g total	IV, IM	8-12	prn

[a]For dogs and cats, an established dose is not available; the pediatric human dose has not been established, but the drug has a wide margin of safety.

ADDITIONAL DOSAGES. None.

BACILLE CALMETTE-GUÉRIN (BCG): SEE CHAPTER 2

BAQUILOPRIM-SULFONAMIDE

CLASS. Sulfonamide and diaminopyridine in 1 : 5 ratio.

ACTION. Bactericidal, antibacterial, also antiprotozoal; folic acid synthesis inhibitors affecting two steps.

MORE INFORMATION. See TRIMETHOPRIM-SULFONAMIDE, ORMETOPRIM-SULFONAMIDE and Chapter 34.

PHARMACOKINETICS. Similar to trimethoprim-sulfonamide but longer half-life in dogs (15 hr baquiloprim; 13.2 hr sulfadimethoxine). Rapid and complete absorption; maintains antibacterial inhibitory effectiveness in plasma for up to 48 hr after a single dose. Both drugs are metabolized by the liver and are excreted in bile. Dogs do not acetylate sulfonamides, which reduces their nephrotoxicity. Unchanged drug is also excreted in the urine.

SPECTRUM. See ORMETOPRIM-SULFONAMIDE, TRIMETHOPRIM-SULFONAMIDE. **Aerobes:** Synergistic against *Staphylococcus intermedius, Streptococcus canis, E. coli,* and *Proteus mirabilis.* **Anaerobes:** in vitro, but not in vivo; therefore, not recommended for anaerobic infections. **Others:** *Coccidia.* **Ineffective:** anaerobic infections.

INDICATIONS. For coccidiosis, canine pyoderma and urinary tract infections.

CONTRAINDICATIONS. Not for use in dogs with sulfonamide hypersensitivity, hepatic dysfunction, blood dyscrasias, or pregnancy. Not for use in cats.

ADVERSE REACTIONS. Similar to TRIMETHOPRIM-SULFONAMIDE.

INTERACTIONS. See TRIMETHOPRIM-SULFONAMIDE.

AVAILABILITY	TYPE	SIZES	PREPARATIONS (COMPANY)
Human	Oral tablets[a]	600 mg (100 mg baquiloprim and 500 mg sulphamethoxine or sulphadimidine)	*Dazokan* (Merial)
		60 mg (10 mg baquiloprim and 50 mg sulphamethoxine or sulphadimidine)	*Zaquilan C* (Schering-Plough Animal Health)

[a]Not available in the U.S.

HANDLING. Store in airtight, light-proof containers at room temperature.

ADMINISTRATION. Can be given with food. Supply plenty of water at all times.

Dosage

INDICATIONS *(Dogs)*	DOSE (mg/kg)	ROUTE (hr)	INTERVAL (days)	DURATION
Coccidiosis	30	PO	48	4
Urinary infections	30	PO	48	10
Pyoderma	30	PO	48	21[a]

[a]Give drug every 24 hr for the first 2 days.

ADDITIONAL DOSAGES. None.

DISPENSING INFORMATION. This drug can be given with food. Make sure the animal has unlimited access to drinking water while on this medication.

CARBENICILLIN

CLASS. Carboxypenicillin.

ACTION. Bactericidal; inhibits bacterial cell wall synthesis.

MORE INFORMATION. See Penicillins, Chapter 34; Table 34-1.

PHARMACOKINETICS. Carbenicillin is destroyed by gastric acid, resulting in poor GI absorption. Indanyl carbenicillin is more stable, being partially (30%-50%) absorbed. When given parenterally, enters many tissues and body fluids in therapeutic concentration but only in the CSF with meningeal inflammation. Primarily (80%) renal excretion of unchanged drug. Low biliary excretion. Difficult to achieve sufficient blood concentration when given PO so reserved for treatment of urinary tract infection. Carindacillin, the indanyl ester, is better absorbed from the GI tract and is hydrolyzed to the active drug after absorption. Its use is limited to treatment of urinary tract infections caused by *Pseudomonas* and other susceptible gram-negative organisms.

SPECTRUM. Gram positive: *Staphylococcus.* **Gram negative:** *Escherichia, Proteus, Salmonella, Enterobacter, Citrobacter,* *Pseudomonas, Serratia.* **Anaerobes:** *Clostridium, Peptococcus, Peptostreptococcus, Bacteroides, Fusobacterium.*

INDICATIONS. Parenteral formulation for treating systemic infections. Acute and chronic upper and lower urinary tract infection, including prostatitis and cystitis. Oral use should be restricted in treating urinary infections caused by gram-negative bacteria or *Pseudomonas* strains resistant to other drugs, but high dosages are needed for effective therapy. Ticarcillin or piperacillin are sometimes preferred over this drug.

CONTRAINDICATIONS. Dosage reduction in renal failure.

ADVERSE REACTIONS. GI side effects. Occasional hypersensitivity reactions, reversible neutropenia, occasional eosinophilia, hypokalemia. Neurotoxicity at high doses, with impaired renal excretion. In people, platelet malfunction can result in prolonged bleeding times.

INTERACTIONS. Inactivates aminoglycosides in vitro. Can be given with aminoglycosides by alternative route to enhance activity against *Pseudomonas.*

AVAILABILITY	TYPE	SIZES	PREPARATIONS (COMPANY)
Human	Film-coated oral tablets (indanyl sodium)	500 mg total containing 382 mg, carbenicillin	*Geocillin* (Roerig)
	Parenteral powder (sodium)ᵃ	1-g, 2-g, 5-g, 10-g vials	*Geopen* (Roerig), *Pyopen* (SmithKline Beecham)

ᵃNo longer available in U.S.

INTERNATIONAL PREPARATIONS. *Carbapen, Carindapen.*

HANDLING. Oral tablets should be stored in dry, airtight containers at room temperature and are stable indefinitely. A suspension can be prepared by crushing six, 382-mg tablets and adding sufficient water to bring the volume to 60 ml. Shaken and refrigerated, the 38.2 mg/ml solution is stable for 3 days. Because of the bitter taste, the solution or crushed tablets can be added to a syrup before administration. The powder for parenteral injection is stored at room temperature and once reconstituted is stable for 24 hr at room temperature, 72 hr if refrigerated and 1 mo if frozen. With IV solution, up to 15% of solution activity is reduced in 4 hr at 25°F and NaCl but up to 8 hr in dextrose solutions. IV solution is incompatible with AMB, chloramphenicol, gentamicin, kanamycin, carbenicillin, oxytetracycline.

ADMINISTRATION. Parenteral solution can be given IM and can be reconstituted with lidocaine (0.5% without epinephrine) or IV as a slow infusion. Minimum dilution is 1 g/7 ml given over a minimum of 15 min.

Dosage

INDICATIONS (*Dogs and Cats*)	DOSE (mg/kg)	ROUTE	INTERVAL (hr)	DURATION (days)
Urinary	22-33	PO	8	7-10
Systemic infections	22-33	IV	6-8	prn

ADDITIONAL DOSAGES. Gram-negative bacteria, Table 37-3; bacteremia and endocarditis, Table 87-6; respiratory disease, Table 88-8.

CASPOFUNGIN

CLASS. Echindocandin. Water soluble derivative of pnemocandin B

ACTION. Cyclic hexapeptide that interferes with cell wall biosynthesis by noncompetititve inhibition of 1,3-β-D-glucan synthase, an enzyme involved in fungal but not mammalian cell wall synthesis. Inhibits hyphal tip and branch point growth converting mycelium to small clumps. Generally fungicidal in vitro but fungistatic against *Aspergillus*. Antifungal and fungicidal against hyphal organisms such as dermatophytes, *Aspergillus*, and *Sporothrix*. Also effective against yeasts such as a variety of *Candida* spp. Fungal growth required for effectiveness.

MORE INFORMATION. Reference Ch 57, ref. 126; 29.

PHARMACOKINETICS. Poorly absorbed from the GI tract and must be given parenterally. Liver metabolizes drug; however not via the cytochrome P-450 enzyme system, so has less interaction with other hepatically metabolized drugs. Only small amounts of unchanged drug appear in the urine. Daily IV administration leads to drug accumulation with a steady state by 2-3 weeks.

SPECTRUM. Activity against mold (filamentous), dimorphic, and yeast fungi. It has been effective against mouse infections with *Pneumocystis carinii* (Ch 57, ref. 29).

INDICATIONS. Has been used in AMB and azole-resistant aspergillosis or candidiasis in people. Only approved for the treatment of invasive aspergillosis for people who are refractory to, or do not tolerate, conventional antifungals.

CONTRAINDICATIONS. Reduce dosage in hepatic dysfunction.

ADVERSE REACTIONS. Histamine-mediated reactions, observed in people, are characterized by urticaria and pruritus. Injection-site irritation, vomiting, diarrhea, and increased serum ALP have also been observed.

INTERACTIONS. Clearance of the drug is reduced by concurrent cyclosporin treatment. Dexamethasone, phenytoin, and rifampicin reduce caspofungin concentrations in people.

AVAILABILITY	TYPE	SIZES	PREPARATIONS (COMPANY)
Human	IV solution	50 mg, 70 mg vials	*Cancidas* (Merck)

INTERNATIONAL PREPARATION. *Same.*

HANDLING. The vial, which is stored refrigerated, is equilibrated to room temperature. Normal saline is added to the final designated concentration, and the solution is mixed until it is clear. The concentration is 5-7 mg/ml final concentration.

The calculated dose is added to a 250-ml or greater bag of normal saline.

ADMINISTRATION. Infused over 1 hr. Should not be mixed or co-infused with other medications. Average duration of therapy is 1 mo.

Dosage

INDICATIONS (*Dogs*)	DOSE (mg/kg)	ROUTE	INTERVAL (hr)	DURATION (days)
Invasive aspergillosis	50 mg[a]	IV	24	56-84

[a]Extrapolated total human daily dose. This might be suitable for very large dogs; however it is likely that a lower dose will be indicated. A daily dose of 70 mg is generally used for loading the first day in treatment of human infections.

ADDITIONAL DOSAGES. None.

DISPENSING INFORMATION. Reconstituted vials of drug are stable for 1 hr refrigerated. The diluted drug in infusion bag is stable for 24 hr.

CEFACLOR

CLASS. Second-generation cephalosporin.

ACTION. Bactericidal; inhibits bacterial cell wall synthesis.

MORE INFORMATION. See Cephalosporins, Chapter 34; Table 34-4.

PHARMACOKINETICS. Well absorbed after oral administration to fasting animals, but absorption is delayed with feeding. The majority of drug is excreted in the urine unchanged.

SPECTRUM. Gram positive: *Staphylococcus, Streptococcus.* **Gram negative:** *Escherichia, Salmonella, Klebsiella, Proteus mirabilis.* **Anaerobes:** gram negatives, including *Bacteroides.*

Ineffective: *Pseudomonas, Acinetobacter, Enterococcus, Serratia*, other *Proteus.*

INDICATIONS. Otitis media, sinusitis caused by β-lactamase–resistant organisms, lower respiratory tract infections, pyoderma, urinary infections. More active than first-generation drugs against gram-negative bacteria.

CONTRAINDICATIONS. Known cephalosporin or penicillin hypersensitivity. Reduce dosages in renal failure.

ADVERSE REACTIONS. Systemic allergy, previous hypersensitivity, vomiting, diarrhea, increased liver enzymes, mild eosinophilia.

INTERACTIONS. Potentiates anticoagulant rodenticides.

AVAILABILITY	TYPE	SIZES	PREPARATIONS (COMPANY)
Human	Oral capsules	250 mg, 500 mg	*Ceclor* (Eli Lilly), generic (various)
	Powder for oral suspension	125 or 325 mg/5 ml	*Ceclor;* generic

INTERNATIONAL PREPARATIONS. *Alfatil, Cefabiocin, Cef-Diolan, Distaclor, Kefolor, Pancef.*

HANDLING. Refrigerate suspension after reconstituting; stable for 2 weeks. No definitive data exist for freezing and thawing of oral suspension, but it is thought to be unstable after a similar time period after thawing. Store capsules at controlled room temperature (15-30°C).

ADMINISTRATION. Administer to fasting animal because food in stomach interferes with absorption. Maximum daily dose is 1 g. Twice-daily dosing has not been as effective as three-times daily dosing in human clinical studies.

Dosage

INDICATIONS (*Dogs and Cats*)	DOSE (mg/kg)	ROUTE	INTERVAL (hr)	DURATION (days)
Skin, soft tissue infections	7	PO	8	21-30
Systemic, lower respiratory infections	10-13	PO	8	14

ADDITIONAL DOSAGES. None.

DISPENSING INFORMATION. Store liquid in refrigerator and shake well before using. Discard unused portions after 2 weeks. Give at least 1 hr before or 2 hr after meals.

CEFADROXIL

CLASS. First-generation cephalosporin (longer acting derivative of cephalexin).

ACTION. Bactericidal; inhibits bacterial cell wall synthesis.

MORE INFORMATION. See Cephalosporins, Chapter 34; Tables 34-3 and 34-4.

PHARMACOKINETICS. Rapidly absorbed after oral administration even in presence of food. Feeding may slow the onset of peak absorption and maintain higher serum levels of drug for longer periods in dogs (Ch 34, ref. 57). Stable in the presence of gastric acid. More than 90% excreted unchanged in the urine within 24 hr. Slower absorption and longer excretion period than cephalexin or cephradine, allowing for 12-hr dosing and higher serum levels.

SPECTRUM. Gram positive: β-hemolytic *Streptococcus, Staphylococcus,* and others. **Gram negative:** *Escherichia, Proteus mirabilis, Klebsiella, Pasteurella.* **Anaerobes:** poor activity. **Ineffective:** most *Enterococcus, Enterobacter,* other *Proteus, Acinetobacter.*

INDICATIONS. Urinary tract infections caused by susceptible gram-negative bacteria. Skin (pyoderma), respiratory, orthopedic, or systemic infections caused by *Staphylococcus* or *Streptococcus.* Good absorption and decreased frequency of administration are advantages over other first-generation cephalosporins.

CONTRAINDICATIONS. Known cephalosporin or penicillin hypersensitivity; reduce dose in renal failure.

ADVERSE REACTIONS. Vomiting, diarrhea, depression, anorexia, polydipsia, polyuria, salivation (Ch 34, ref. 209). Hypersensitivity reactions. No teratogenic or infertility problems have been seen in laboratory animals receiving high doses.

INTERACTIONS. False-positive Coombs' test results in people. False-positive urine glucose with copper reduction (Clinitest) methods.

AVAILABILITY	TYPE	SIZES	PREPARATIONS (COMPANY)
Human	Oral suspension (monohydrate)	125 mg, 250 mg, 500 mg/5 ml	*Duricef* (Mead-Johnson), *Ultracef* (Bristol), generics (various)
	Capsules (monohydrate)	50 mg, 100 mg, 200 mg, 500 mg	*Duricef, Utracef,* generics
	Tablets	1 g	*Duricef,* generics
Veterinary	Oral tablets	50 mg, 100 mg, 200 mg, 1 g	*Cefa-tabs* (Fort Dodge, Willows Francis Vet), *Cefa-cure* (Mycofarm)
	Oral liquid	50 mg/ml in 15-ml and 50-ml dropper bottles	*Cefa-drops* (Fort Dodge)

INTERNATIONAL PREPARATIONS. *Bidocef, Cefadril, Ceoxil, Cephos, Crenodyn, Duracef, Kefroxil, Moxacef, Oracéfal, Sedral.*

HANDLING. Shake suspension before use; keep container tightly closed in refrigerator; discard unused portion after 14 days. Store tablets in airtight, moisture-proof containers at room temperature.

ADMINISTRATION. Food does not reduce or delay absorption. Liquid has orange-pineapple flavor.

Dosage

INDICATIONS (*Dogs and Cats*)	DOSE (mg/kg)	ROUTE	INTERVAL (hr)	DURATION (days)
Urinary tract infections				
Cat	22	PO	24	≥21
Dog	11-22	PO	12	7-30
Skin, pyoderma	22-35	PO	12	3-30
Systemic, orthopedic infections	22	PO	8-12	30

ADDITIONAL DOSAGES. Canine pyoderma, Table 85-3.

DISPENSING INFORMATION. Can be given without regard to meals. Giving with food may help reduce GI side effects.

CEFAZOLIN

CLASS. First-generation cephalosporin.

ACTION. Bactericidal; inhibits bacterial cell wall synthesis.

MORE INFORMATION. See Cephalosporins, Chapter 34; Table 34-4; references: Ch 34, ref. 235; 318.

PHARMACOKINETICS. Not absorbed from GI tract. Given parenterally, it enters many tissues and body fluids. Primarily excreted by kidneys unchanged in urine. Some is excreted in bile to achieve therapeutic concentrations. Longer half-life and ability to reach higher tissue concentrations gives advantage for surgical prophylaxis over cephalothin and cephapirin in which aerobic infections are anticipated. Good levels achieved in bone, especially with inflammation. Does not penetrate CSF, even with inflamed meninges.

SPECTRUM. Gram positive: *Staphylococcus*, β-hemolytic *Streptococcus*. **Gram negative:** some *Enterobacter*, *Escherichia*, *Klebsiella*, *Proteus mirabilis*. **Anaerobes:** poor activity.

Ineffective: *Proteus vulgaris, Enterobacter cloacae, Serratia, Pseudomonas.*

INDICATIONS. Surgical prophylaxis, for prolonged orthopedic procedures, for reducing postoperative infections of surgical wounds and intraabdominal or biliary surgery. Greatest activity against *Escherichia* and *Klebsiella* compared with others in its class. Respiratory, genitourinary, biliary tract, bone, and joint infections, sepsis.

CONTRAINDICATIONS. Previous penicillin or cephalosporin hypersensitivity. Reduce dose in renal failure.

ADVERSE REACTIONS. Few; hypersensitivity to cephalosporins, diarrhea, neutropenia, leukopenia, eosinophilia, thrombocytopenia, increased liver enzymes, phlebitis with IV, pain on IM injection.

INTERACTIONS. False-positive urine glucose measurements with nonenzymatic methods.

AVAILABILITY	TYPE	SIZES	PREPARATIONS (COMPANY)
Human	Powder for injection	500 mg, 1 g, 5 g, 10 g, 20 g	*Ancef* (SmithKline Beecham), *Kefzol* (Eli Lilly)

HANDLING. Reconstitute in sterile water for IV; can also use 0.9% NaCl for IM; however, not advised because crystals may form in NaCl solution. Stable for 24 hr at room temperature and 96 hr when refrigerated; up to 12 weeks if frozen. Can be mixed with 5% dextrose, lactated Ringer's, 0.9% NaCl for infusion. Avoid admixture with many other drugs, including aminoglycosides, tetracyclines, macrolides, barbiturates.

Powder has been mixed in acrylic bone cement for prophylaxis with surgical implants.

ADMINISTRATION. Inject IM in large muscle mass. Inject IV slowly into vein or through IV tubing access over 3-5 min. For surgical prophylaxis, give IV dose once immediately before surgical incision and repeat SC 6 hr later (Ch 34, ref. 318).

Dosage

INDICATIONS	DOSE (mg/kg)	ROUTE	INTERVAL (hr)	DURATION (days)
Dogs				
Surgical prophylaxis	8	IV	1	a
	20-22	IV	2	a
Systemic infections	5-25	IM, IV	6-8	prn
Orthopedic infections	22	IV, IM, SC	6-8	≥7
Sepsis, bacteremic	15-25	IV, IM, SC	4-8	≥7
Cats				
Systemic infections	33	IM, IV	8-12	prn

aJust before and during surgery (Ch 86, ref. 131). If surgery lasts >90 min then a second dose is given.

ADDITIONAL DOSAGES. Parvoviral enteritis, Table 8-1; endotoxemia, Table 38-6; musculoskeletal infections, Table 86-4; bacteremia and endocarditis, Table 87-6; respiratory infections, Table 88-8; topical intraocular use, Table 93-4.

CEFEPIME

CLASS. Fourth-generation cephalosporin.

ACTION. Bactericidal; has enhanced ability to penetrate outer cell membrane of gram-negative bacteria. Has better gram-positive coverage than third-generation cephalosporins.

MORE INFORMATION. See Cephalosphorins, Chapter 34; Table 34-4.

PHARMACOKINETICS. Poor oral bioavailability. Higher blood levels after IV than IM use. Penetrates blood-CSF barrier. Renal excretion with minimal metabolism.

SPECTRUM. Gram positive: many, including *Staphylococcus*. **Gram negative:** many Enterobacteriaceae. **Anaerobes:** variable activity. **Others:** *M. avium-intracellulare* complex. **Most effective:** resistant gram-negative bacteria. Similar to third-generation drugs; however, good antipseudomonal activity similar to ceftazidine. Good β-lactamase stability and good gram-positive activity. Has activity against some Enterobacteriaceae that are resistant to cefotaxime and ceftazidine. **Ineffective:** not active against methicillin-resistant strains of *Staphylococcus, Enterobacter, Clostridium, Bacteroides*.

INDICATIONS. Severe infections of lower respiratory, urinary, and female reproductive tracts; skin and soft tissue infections; pneumonia; meningitis. For treatment of infections caused by bacteria resistant to other antibiotics.

APPROVED USES. Gram-negative pneumonia.

CONTRAINDICATIONS. Reduced dosage in renal failure. Previous hypersensitivity to cephalosporins.

ADVERSE REACTIONS. Eosinophilia, leukopenia, phlebitis, increased serum hepatic enzyme activities, gastrointestinal signs.

INTERACTIONS. In vitro synergy with quinolones, aminoglycosides, β-lactamase inhibitors. Antagonistic activity with imipenem or polymyxin B. Combine with metronidazole or clindamycin in intraabdominal infections. Should closely monitor renal function in animals receiving cefepime with aminoglycosides.

AVAILABILITY	TYPE	SIZES	PREPARATION (COMPANY)
Human	Powder for injection (as hydrochloride)	500 mg, 1 g, 2 g	*Maxipime* (Bristol-Myers Squibb)

INTERNATIONAL PREPARATIONS. *Axépim*.

HANDLING. Reconstitute powder with 0.9% NaCl, 5% dextrose, 0.5%-1% lidocaine, or bacteriostatic water.

ADMINISTRATION. IV; give slowly over 30 min. Can add to 0.9% NaCl, 5% dextrose, and lactated Ringer's.

Dosage

INDICATIONS	DOSE	ROUTE	INTERVAL (HR)	DURATION (days)
Dogs and Cats[a]	40 mg/kg	IV, IM	6	prn

[a]This is the IV dose for treating sensitive bacteria as determined by pharmacokinetic data in dogs (Ch 34, ref. 122). This dosage will maintain plasma concentrations >2 μg/ml for the entire period.

ADDITIONAL DOSAGES. None.

DISPENSING INFORMATION. Diarrhea may develop during use of this drug.

CEFIXIME

CLASS. Third-generation cephalosporin for oral administration.

ACTION. Bactericidal; inhibits bacterial cell wall synthesis. Very stable to β-lactamase.

MORE INFORMATION. See CEFPODOXIME; references: Ch 34, ref. 26; 215

PHARMACOKINETICS. First licensed third-generation *oral* cephalosporin: rapid oral absorption in absence of food; food impairs its bioavailability in dogs; bioavailability is 40%-55%; suspension achieves higher blood concentrations than tablet; high serum protein binding; lower concentrations in tissues (uterus, ovaries) and fat; tissue concentration may increase with repeated dosing; very high levels in urinary tract. Eliminated in urine by glomerular filtration but reabsorbed by tubules to prolong activity (Ch 34, ref. 26). The long half-life (7 hr) of cefixime in dogs compared to other cephalosporins relates to this renal reabsorption.

SPECTRUM. Gram positive: *Streptococcus, Rhodococcus*. **Gram negative:** *Escherichia, Proteus, Klebsiella*. **Anaerobes:** minimal activity (unlike other third-generation drugs). **Ineffective:** *Pseudomonas, Enterococcus, Staphylococcus, Actinomyces, Bordetella, Listeria, Enterobacter, Clostridium, Bacteroides*.

INDICATIONS. Urinary and upper respiratory tract infections (pharyngitis, bronchitis) caused by susceptible organisms and resistant to more commonly used drugs. One of few orally administered third-generation cephalosporins. Quinolones and aminoglycosides are often more effective against gram-negatives than cefixime. In addition susceptibility, of *E. coli* isolated from dogs to cefixime, has decreased over the last decade (Ch 34, ref. 285).

CONTRAINDICATIONS. Reduce dosage in renal failure.

ADVERSE REACTIONS. GI disturbances, abdominal pain, vomiting, dermal hypersensitivity (fever, urticaria, pruritus).

INTERACTIONS. False-positive results with nonenzymatic test results for urine glucose. False-positive urine ketone test results using nitroprusside.

AVAILABILITY	TYPE	SIZES	PREPARATIONS (COMPANY)
Human	Oral tablets (film coated as trihydrate)	200 mg, 400 mg	*Supran* (Teva Pharm), *Suprax* (Lederle)
	Oral suspension (strawberry flavor)	100 mg/5 ml	*Suprax*

INTERNATIONAL PREPARATIONS. *Aerocef, Cefspan, Cephoral, Denvar, Fixim, Necopen, Oroken, Tricef, Unixime.*

HANDLING. Store capsules in airtight containers at room temperature.

ADMINISTRATION. Possibly give once daily in urinary infections as a result of long half-life.

Dosage

INDICATIONS (*Dogs and Cats*)	DOSE, (mg/kg)	ROUTE	INTERVAL (hr)	DURATION (days)
Urinary infections	5.0	PO	12-24	7-14[a]
Respiratory, systemic infections	12.5	PO	12	7-14[a]

[a]Duration may vary according to chronicity of infection.

ADDITIONAL DOSAGES. None.

DISPENSING INFORMATION. Give on an empty stomach.

CEFOPERAZONE SODIUM

CLASS. Third-generation cephalosporin.

ACTION. Bactericidal; inhibits bacterial cell wall synthesis.

MORE INFORMATION. See Cephalosporins, Chapter 34; Table 34-4.

PHARMACOKINETICS. Longer half-life than others in its class permitting 12-hr dose interval. Not absorbed from the GI tract. After parenteral injection, distributed widely in tissues and body fluids. Erratic penetration of the CNS and CSF, better if meningitis present. Primarily (70%) excreted in bile; remainder unchanged in urine.

SPECTRUM. Gram positive: *Staphylococcus* spp, *Streptococcus,* but less active against these than other cephalosporins. **Gram negative:** *Escherichia, Klebsiella, Enterobacter, Proteus, Serratia, Pseudomonas.* Second most active cephalosporin

against *Pseudomonas.* **Anaerobes:** *Peptococcus, Peptostreptococcus, Clostridium, Bacteroides.*

INDICATIONS. Severe infections, resistant to other drugs, in the lower respiratory tract, peritoneal cavity, skin, genital and urinary tracts, and septicemia. *Pseudomonas* infections.

CONTRAINDICATIONS. Avoid or reduce dosage with hepatic failure or biliary obstruction. Normal dosage in renal failure.

ADVERSE REACTIONS. Local or systemic hypersensitivity; vitamin K deficiency and hemorrhage or neutropenia with prolonged administration; transient diarrhea; azotemia or serum hepatic enzyme increases.

INTERACTIONS. Do not mix directly with an aminoglycoside, and if both are given through the same IV set, use this drug first and flush in between.

AVAILABILITY	TYPE	SIZES	PREPARATIONS (COMPANY)
Human	Sterile crystalline powder for injection or premixed iso-osmotic solution	1-g, 2-g vials	*Cefobid* (Pfizer, Roerig)

INTERNATIONAL PREPARATIONS. *Bioperazone, Cefazone, Céfobis, Cefogram, Cefoneg, Dardum, Ipazone, Mediper, Perocef, Zoncef.*

HANDLING. Protect sterile powder from light before reconstitution. Reconstitute with 5% dextrose or lactated Ringer's. Can dilute with epinephrine-free lidocaine for IM use. Stable for 24 hr at room temperature, 5 days if refrigerated, or 3-5 weeks when frozen. IM or IV solution is stable for 48 hr at room temperature and 5 days in refrigeration (5°C) and 3 weeks if frozen (–20°C). Do not refreeze once thawed.

ADMINISTRATION. Intermittent infusions should be given over 15-30 min. Continuous infusions should be given at a concentration of 2-25 mg/ml.

Dosage

INDICATIONS (*Dogs and Cats*)	DOSE (mg/kg)	ROUTE	INTERVAL (hr)	DURATION (days)
Soft tissue infections	22[a]	IV, IM	12	7-14
Bacteremia, sepsis	22[a]	IV, IM	6-8	prn

[a]Human dose extrapolation.

ADDITIONAL DOSAGES. None.

CEFOTAXIME SODIUM

CLASS. Third-generation cephalosporin.

ACTION. Bactericidal; inhibits bacterial cell wall synthesis.

MORE INFORMATION. See Chapter 34, Cephalosporins; Table 34-4; Reference Ch 34, ref. 361a.

PHARMACOKINETICS. Not absorbed from GI tract. Well absorbed after IM administration. When given parenterally, attains therapeutic concentration in many tissues, including prostate, bone, and both pleural and peritoneal fluids. Enters the aqueous humor and CSF. Relatively rapid clearance of the drug in septicemic dogs given 10 mg/kg or 20 mg/kg doses requires a dosage interval of ≤12 hr, as the half-life at 10 mg/kg was 0.8, 1.48, and 1.52 hr for the IV, SC, and IM routes, respectively (Ch 34, ref. 361a). Metabolized by hepatic esterases to a biologically active form, desacetylcefotaxime, which prolongs the drug's clinical effect. Attains therapeutic levels in meninges with or without inflammation. Primarily renal excretion.

SPECTRUM. Gram positive: *Streptococcus* and *Staphylococcus* (with and without β-lactamase). More active than other third-generation drugs. **Gram negative:** most Enterobacteriaceae: *Acinetobacter, Citrobacter, Escherichia, Klebsiella, Proteus, Ser-* *ratia,* some *Pseudomonas.* Synergistic with aminoglycosides. **Anaerobes:** variable activity against *Bacteroides, Clostridium, Fusobacterium, Peptococcus, Peptostreptococcus.* **Others:** *Borrelia.* **More effective:** most active third-generation drug against *Staphylococcus, Leptospira.* **Ineffective:** *Listeria.*

INDICATIONS. Initial empiric therapy in bacterial sepsis. Also good for problematic or recurrent lower respiratory tract, genitourinary, soft tissue, skin, and intraabdominal infections, bone and joint and CNS infections, and surgical prophylaxis. Inconsistent against *Pseudomonas.*

CONTRAINDICATIONS. Reduce dose in renal failure.

ADVERSE REACTIONS. Local irritation, systemic hypersensitivity, GI signs. Altered bowel flora with diarrhea. Occasional granulocytopenia, increased nephrotoxicity when combined with aminoglycosides or other cephalosporins. Cardiac arrhythmias if infused too rapidly IV.

INTERACTIONS. Possibly synergistic with aminoglycosides but should not be mixed together for simultaneous administration.

INTERNATIONAL PREPARATIONS. *Cefacron, Zariviz.*

AVAILABILITY	TYPE	SIZES	PREPARATIONS (COMPANY)
Human	Powder for injection	1 g, 2 g	*Claforan* (Hoechst-Roussel)
	Frozen, premixed in 5% dextrose in plastic containers	1 g, 2 g	*Claforan*

HANDLING. Store powder at room temperature, reconstitute with sterile water. Stable for 24 hr at room temperature, 10 days when refrigerated, and 13 weeks if frozen. When further diluted in IV fluids, only stable for 5 days if refrigerated. Unstable in alkaline solutions. Stable in 0.9 NaCl, 5% dextrose, lactated Ringer's. Powder and solutions darken with storage without affecting activity.

ADMINISTRATION. IV or IM, dosing interval shortens with increasing severity of infection. Never mix directly with aminoglycosides; can combine as separate infusions. Solution of 1 g Claforan in 14 ml of sterile water is isotonic. For IM give deep into large muscle and aspirate before injection. Use multiple sites with dose greater than 1 g. For IV infusion, 1 or 2 g may be reconstituted in 50 or 100 ml of 0.9% saline or 5% dextrose and be given over 30 min. IV preferred for septicemia, peritonitis, meningitis, or immunocompromised animals. Administer IV, 1 or 2 g in 10 ml sterile water over 3-5 min but not concurrently with other solutions. For surgical prophylaxis, give dose 30-90 min before operative incision. Maximum dose: 1 g for medium-size dogs, 2 g for large dogs.

Dosage

INDICATIONS	DOSE (mg/kg)	ROUTE	INTERVAL (hr)	DURATION (days)
Dogs				
Soft tissue infections	10-20	IV, IM, SC	8	≤7
Orthopedic infections	20-40	IV, IM, SC	8-12	≤7
Severe bacteremia[a]	20-80	IV	6-8	prn
Cats				
Severe bacteremia	20-80	IV, IM	6	prn

[a]IN septicemic dogs given 10-20 mg/kg IV, SC, or IM the drug was rapidly cleared with a maximum allowable dosage interval of 12 hours (Ch 34, ref. 361a).

ADDITIONAL DOSAGES. Gram-negative infections, Table 37-3; Lyme borreliosis, Table 45-5; nocardiosis, Table 49-3; bacteremia and endocarditis, Table 87-6; respiratory infections, Table 88-8; intraabdominal infections, Table 89-21; CNS infections, Table 92-5.

CEFOTETAN DISODIUM

CLASS. Cephamycin, like CEFOXITIN, with similar properties to second-generation cephalosporin.

ACTION. Bactericidal; inhibits bacterial cell wall synthesis inhibitor.

MORE INFORMATION. See CEFOXITIN; Chapter 34; reference: Ch 34, ref. 297.

SPECTRUM. See CEFOXITIN.

INDICATIONS. Cost-effective replacement for cefoxitin. See CEFOXITIN.

CONTRAINDICATIONS. See CEFOXITIN; prior penicillin or cephalosporin hypersensitivity. Reduce dose in renal failure.

ADVERSE REACTIONS. Vomiting after IV bolus infusion. Cutaneous eruptions, angioedema. Coagulation disturbances with vitamin K antagonism. Neutropenia, anemia, eosinophilia.

INTERACTIONS. Potentiate aminoglycoside nephrotoxicity. Unpredictable synergism with penicillins.

AVAILABILITY	TYPE	SIZES	PREPARATION (COMPANY)
Human	Powder for injection	1 g, 2 g	*Cefotan* (Stuart Pharmaceuticals)

INTERNATIONAL PREPARATIONS. *Apacef, Ceftenon, Cepan, Darvilen, Yamatetan.*

HANDLING. Reconstitute with sterile water; for IM use can add lidocaine. For IV infusion, can add to 5% dextrose or 0.9% NaCl. Stable for 24 hr at room temperature, 96 hr if refrigerated, and at least 1 week if frozen. In dextrose 10% or Ringer's, with cefotetan 0.5 to 30 mg/ml, can freeze at −20°C for 30 weeks and thaw in microwave oven before use. Do not mix in solutions containing aminoglycosides.

ADMINISTRATION. IV route preferred for bacteremia or severe infections. Bolus administration via IV catheter over 3-5 min. Flush catheter with heparinized saline (10 U/ml) after injection. Do not coadminister with other drugs. For surgical prophylaxis, begin infusion of 1 g 30-60 min before surgery.

ADDITIONAL DOSAGES. Musculoskeletal infections, Table 86-4; respiratory infections, Table 88-8.

Dosage

INDICATIONS (Dogs)	DOSE (mg/kg)	ROUTE	INTERVAL (hr)	DURATION (days)
Soft tissue infections	30	SC	12	≤7
Bacteremia, sepsis	30	IV, SC	8	prn

CEFOXITIN

CLASS. Cephamycin, like CEFOTETAN, with similar properties to second-generation cephalosporins.

ACTION. Bactericidal; bacterial cell wall synthesis inhibitor.

MORE INFORMATION. See CEFOTETAN; Chapter 34, cephalosporins, Table 34-4; surgical infections, Table 55-5; reference: Ch 34, ref. 297.

PHARMACOKINETICS. Not absorbed from the GI tract. Must use parenteral administration. Reaches therapeutic concentrations in many tissues, including kidney and lung. Little penetration of CSF, even with inflamed meninges. Primarily excreted unchanged in the urine.

SPECTRUM. Gram positive: *Staphylococcus*, hemolytic *Streptococcus*. **Gram negative:** *Escherichia, Klebsiella, Proteus*. **Anaerobes:** *Bacteroides, Clostridium, Peptococcus, Peptostreptococcus*. **Ineffective:** *Salmonella, Pseudomonas, Enterococcus*. Has a similar spectrum to cefotetan.

INDICATIONS. Gram-negative sepsis, gingivitis, pyothorax, polymicrobial infections with renal impairment, surgical prophylaxis, intraabdominal bowel rupture, osteomyelitis. Especially effective for surgical prophylaxis when anaerobic infections (e.g., *Bacteroides fragilis*) are expected (colon surgery).

CONTRAINDICATIONS. Reduce dosage in renal failure.

ADVERSE REACTIONS. Local tissue irritation when given IM or SC. Vomiting after IV bolus injection, cutaneous eruptions, angioedema. Can cause hemolytic anemia, thrombocytopenia, granulocytopenia, increased hepatic enzymes, azotemia.

INTERACTIONS. Increased nephrotoxicity has been observed when combined therapy with aminoglycosides has been used.

AVAILABILITY	TYPE	SIZES	PREPARATION (COMPANY)
Human	Powder for injection	1-g, 2-g vials	*Mefoxin* (Merck)

INTERNATIONAL PREPARATIONS. *Betacef, Cefaxicina, Cefociclin, Mefoxitin, Stovaren, Tifox*.

HANDLING. Store powder at room temperature. IV, reconstitute with 9.7 ml bacteriostatic water to 100 mg/ml solution; stable for 24 hr at room temperature, 1 week if refrigerated, 30 weeks when frozen. Times vary with other diluents.

Powder and solutions darken with storage, but this does not affect potency. SC and IM, can dilute in 0.5% lidocaine (without epinephrine) to minimize irritation after injection.

ADMINISTRATION. Bolus administration via IV catheter over 3-5 min. Flush catheter with heparinized saline (10 U/ml) after injection.

Dosage

INDICATIONS	DOSE (mg/kg)	ROUTE	INTERVAL (hr)	DURATION (days)
Dogs				
Soft tissue infections	30	SC	8	prn[a]
	30	IV	5	prn[a]
Bacteremia	15-30	IV, IM, SC	6-8	prn[a]
Orthopedic infections	22	IV, IM	6-8	prn[a]
Cats				
Systemic infection	25-30	IV, IM	8	prn[a]

[a]Use to control initial infection, then switch to orally administered drugs for longer therapy.

ADDITIONAL DOSAGES. Anaerobic infections, Table 41-12; musculoskeletal infections, Table 86-4; bacteremia and endocarditis, Table 87-6; respiratory infections, Table 88-8.

CEFPODOXIME PROXETIL

CLASS. Third-generation cephalosporin. A pro-drug; active metabolite is cefpodoxime.

ACTION. Bactericidal; inhibits bacterial cell wall synthesis. Stable in the presence of many β-lactamases.

MORE INFORMATION. See CEFIXIME; Chapter 34, cephalosporins; Table 34-4.

PHARMACOKINETICS. One of few oral drugs of its class. The oral form is given as the proxetil ester, which is hydrolyzed by the intestinal epithelium to active drug at the time of absorption. Oral bioavailability in fasting beagle dogs was 63.1 ± 5.3%, according to the supplied product information. Excreted primarily unchanged in urine, with an elimination half-life of approximately 5 hr after PO administration. In dogs, 5 mg/kg or 10 mg/kg dose increases maximum plasma concentration to ~8 μg/ml or ~16 μg/ml, respectively.

SPECTRUM. Gram positive: *Streptococcus, Staphylococcus*. **Gram negative:** *Escherichia, Klebsiella, Pasteurella, Proteus*. **Not active** against most obligate anaerobes, *Pseudomonas* spp, or enterococci. Activity is generally not as broad as the parenterally administered third-generation drugs, partially because of lower achieved concentrations.

INDICATIONS. Upper respiratory and urinary tract infections, pyoderma, otitis media not responding to other drugs.

CONTRAINDICATIONS. Reduce dose in renal failure; no adjustment needed with hepatic dysfunction. Safe in pups over 18 days of age. Avoid in patients with hypersensititivy to penicillin or cephalosporin. Safety in lactating or pregnant animals or breeding males has not been established.

ADVERSE REACTIONS. Low prevalence. Diarrhea, vomiting, eosinophilia, allergic reactions. The drug was given at up to 40 times the typical daily oral dose for 13 weeks in adults and 28 days in pups of 18-23 days of age. Blood dyscrasias, including neutropenia, may be observed with high doses, and if observed, the drug should be discontinued.

INTERACTIONS. Drugs that increase gastric pH interfere with absorption. As with other cephalosporins, may cause a positive Coombs' test.

AVAILABILITY	TYPE	SIZES	PREPARATIONS (COMPANY)
Veterinary	Oral tablets	100 mg, 200 mg	*Simplicef* (Pharmacia & Upjohn, division of Pfizer Animal Health)
Human	Oral tablets	100 mg, 200 mg	*Vantin* (Pharmacia & Upjohn)
	Granules for oral suspension; lemon cream flavored	500 mg/5 ml, 100 mg/5 ml	*Vantin*

INTERNATIONAL PREPARATIONS. *Banan, Biocef, Céfodox, Orelox, Ortreton, Podomexef.*

HANDLING. Store tablets in air-tight vials at controlled room temperature 20-25°C (68-77°F). Mix granules in distilled water, store in refrigerator for up to 2 weeks.

ADMINISTRATION. Food increases absorption. Drug can be given with or without food.

Dosage

INDICATIONS (*Dogs and Cats*)	DOSE (mg/kg)	ROUTE	INTERVAL (hr)	DURATION (days)
Skin, soft tissue infections	5-10	PO	24	5-7[a]

[a]Treatment of acute infection should be for at least 5-7 days or for 2-3 days beyond the cessation of clinical signs. Recommended maximum interval is to 28 days.

ADDITIONAL DOSAGES. None.

DISPENSING INFORMATION. Give drug with meals.

CEFTAZIDIME

CLASS. Third-generation cephalosporin.

ACTION. Bactericidal; inhibits bacterial cell wall synthesis.

MORE INFORMATION. See Chapter 34, cephalosporins, Table 34-4; CNS infections, Table 92-3.

PHARMACOKINETICS. Not absorbed PO; given parenterally. Highest levels in myocardium, bone, skeletal muscle. Good penetration into CSF and synovial, peritoneal, aqueous, lymphatic, and blister fluids. Primarily (80%-90%) excreted renally as unchanged drug.

SPECTRUM. Variable activity against gram-positive bacteria and anaerobes. See CEFTRIAXONE. **More effective:** most active cephalosporin against *Pseudomonas*. Ninety-six percent of isolates of *Pseudomonas* from dogs had susceptible MICs (≤4 ug/ml) while they had 77%, 92%, and 90% susceptibility to gentamicin, amikacin, and ciprofloxacin, respectively (Ch 34, ref. 265).

INDICATIONS. In people, primarily for *Pseudomonas* sepsis; also gram-negative sepsis, meningitis, osteomyelitis, peritonitis, pneumonia. Used in immunosuppressed states (neutropenia) with fever of unknown origin and suspected bacteremia. Has been used in treating nosocomial gram-negative bacterial infections alone and in combination with other drugs. May use with aminoglycosides or clindamycin for severe infections or when antimicrobial resistance is anticipated.

CONTRAINDICATIONS. Renal failure must reduce dosage. No adjustments for hepatic dysfunction.

ADVERSE REACTIONS. See CEFTRIAXONE. GI signs, which are generally mild in dogs, may develop even with parenteral administration (Ch 34, ref. 265).

INTERACTIONS. May increase risk of nephrotoxicity with coadministered aminoglycosides.

AVAILABILITY	TYPE	SIZES	PREPARATIONS (COMPANY)
Human	Powder for injection	500 g, 1-g, 2-g vials	*Fortaz* (Glaxo Wellcome), *Tazicef* (SmithKlineBeecham), *Tazidime* (Lilly)

INTERNATIONAL PREPARATIONS. *Ceftim, Ceptaz, Fortam, Fortum, Glazidim, Kefadim, Kefamin, Kefazim, Kefzim, Panzid, Potendal, Spectrum, Starcef.*

HANDLING. Reconstitute with sterile water, stable for 24 hr at room temperature and 7-10 days if refrigerated. Stable in 0.9% NaCl, Ringer's, or 5% dextrose. Less stable in bicar-bonate. Not recommended to mix with aminoglycosides or metronidazole.

ADMINISTRATION. IV inject over 3-5 min. Administer separately from aminoglycosides. Can mix with 1% lidocaine (without epinephrine) for IM use.

Dosage

INDICATIONS	DOSE (mg/kg)	ROUTE	INTERVAL (hr)	DURATION (days)
Dogs				
Orthopedic infections	25	IV, IM, SC	8-12	prn[a]
Soft tissue infections	20-40	IV, IM, SC	12	prn[a]
Sepsis, bacteremia	30	IV, IM, SC	4-8[b]	prn[a]
Cats				
Systemic infections	25-30	IV, IM, intraosseous	8-12	prn[a]

[a]Use for initial control of infection, then switch to an orally administered drug with similar spectrum of activity.
[b]At 30 mg/kg, serum concentration exceeded effective MIC for 4 hr (Ch 34, ref. 265). The 4-hr interval of administration should be used to maintain efficacy against systemic *Pseudomonas* infections. Continuous IV infusion is another effective alternative.

ADDITIONAL DOSAGES. Gram-negative bacteria, Table 37-3.

CEFTIOFUR

CLASS. Third-generation cephalosporin.

ACTION. Bactericidal; inhibits bacterial cell wall synthesis.

MORE INFORMATION. See Chapter 34, Cephalosporins, Table 34-4; reference: Ch 34, ref. 47.

PHARMACOKINETICS. Rapid blood levels after SC dose, approximately 50% of urinary excretion is metabolites (primarily desfuroylceftiofur) and 50% active drug. Half-life in dog is 6-7 hr.

SPECTRUM. Gram positive: some *Streptococcus, Staphylococcus.* **Gram negative:** *Escherichia, Proteus, Klebsiella, Salmonella,* *Pasteurella.* **Anaerobes:** some but inconsistent; in vitro effective against *Fusobacterium* but poor for *Bacteroides.* **Ineffective:** *Pseudomonas, Enterococcus, Bordetella.*

INDICATIONS. Urinary tract infections.

CONTRAINDICATIONS. Recommendations uncertain with previous hypersensitivity reaction, breeding, or pregnancy.

ADVERSE REACTIONS. Dose and duration related myelosuppression with anemia, leukopenia, and thrombocytopenia, especially at dosages of 6.6 mg/kg once daily.

INTERACTIONS. May expect synergistic antibacterial activity, but nephrotoxic potential is increased when used in combination with aminoglycosides.

AVAILABILITY	TYPE	SIZES	PREPARATIONS (COMPANY)
Veterinary			
Dogs, cattle	Sterile powder for injection	1-g, 4-g vials of 20 and 80 ml, respectively	*Naxcel* (Pharmacia & Upjohn)
Swine	Oil suspension as HCl	5 g	*Excenel* (Pharmacia & Upjohn)

HANDLING. Unreconstituted powder: stable if refrigerated for extended periods, avoid light. Reconstitute with sterile water for injection. Reconstituted solution: refrigerate for 7 days or room temperature for 12 hr; can be aliquoted in syringes and frozen (−20°C) for 8 weeks but thaw at room temperature (never warmer). Never use a single multidose vial more than 20 times.

ADMINISTRATION. Preferably, administer at least twice daily for other than urinary tract infections. At a single 2.2-mg/kg dose, plasma concentrations meet or exceed minimal inhibitory concentrations (MICs) for some organisms such as *Klebsiella, Proteus,* various *Streptococcus, Pseudomonas,* and *Escherichia* at 18-24 hr. With twice-daily dosing, MICs for *S. intermedius* might be adequate but insufficient for some *Streptococcus, Pseudomonas, Bordetella,* and *Klebsiella.* Higher than recommended dosages to affect these organisms may be myelotoxic.

Dosage

INDICATIONS (*Dogs and Cats*)	DOSE (mg/kg)	ROUTE	INTERVAL (hr)	DURATION (days)
Urinary infections	2.2	SC	24	5-14
Systemic, soft tissue infections	2.2	SC	12	5-14
	4.4	SC	24	5-14
Sepsis, bacteremia	4.4	SC	12	2-5

ADDITIONAL DOSAGES. Respiratory disease, Table 88-8.

DISPENSING INFORMATION. Return for recheck CBC count weekly.

CEFTIZOXIME

CLASS. Third-generation cephalosporin.

ACTION. Bactericidal; inhibits bacterial cell wall synthesis.

MORE INFORMATION. See Chapter 34, cephalosporins; CNS infections, Table 92-3.

PHARMACOKINETICS. Not absorbed by PO route. Penetrates many tissues and has therapeutic concentrations in virtually all body fluids. Penetrates meninges with and without inflammation. Not metabolized and primarily renal excretion of unchanged drug.

SPECTRUM. Similar to CEFOTAXIME. **Gram positive:** *Streptococcus, Staphylococcus* (methicillin susceptible). **Gram negative:** *Escherichia, Klebsiella, Proteus, Enterobacter;* low activity against *Pseudomonas.* **Anaerobes:** *Bacteroides.* **More effective:** most active cephalosporin against *Bacteroides.* **Ineffective:** *Enterococcus,* some *Pseudomonas.*

INDICATIONS. Primarily lower respiratory tract infections; urinary, intraabdominal, skin, bone and joint infections; septicemia, meningitis.

CONTRAINDICATIONS. Allergies to this class. Reduce dose in renal failure.

ADVERSE REACTIONS. Hypersensitivities, local and systemic. Transient elevation in serum hepatic enzymes, anemia, leukopenia, thrombocytopenia.

INTERACTIONS. Although not reported, increased nephrotoxicity is expected with concurrent therapy with cephalosporins and aminoglycosides.

AVAILABILITY	TYPE	SIZES	PREPARATION (COMPANY)
Human	Powder or frozen solution for injection	1 g, 2 g	*Cefizox* (Fujisawa)

INTERNATIONAL PREPARATIONS. *Ceftix, Epocelin, Eposerin.*

HANDLING. Thaw plastic container at room temperature and squeeze bag to check for leaks. No additives should be introduced. After thawing, stable for 24 hr at room temperature or 10 days if refrigerated.

ADMINISTRATION. IM in a large muscle, 2-g doses should be divided at different sites. IV bolus infusion over 3-5 min or infusion in 50-100 ml of 0.9% NaCl, 5% or 10% dextrose, lactated Ringer's, or Ringer's. Stable for 24 hr at room temperature or 96 hr if refrigerated.

Dosage

INDICATIONS (*Dogs*)	DOSE (mg/kg)	ROUTE	INTERVAL (hr)	DURATION (days)
Urinary infections	50ᵃ	IV, IM	12	prn
Respiratory, systemic infections	25-50ᵃ	IV, IM	8	prn

ᵃExtrapolated human dosage.

ADDITIONAL DOSAGES. None.

CEFTRIAXONE

CLASS. Third-generation cephalosporin.

ACTION. Bactericidal; inhibits bacterial cell wall synthesis.

MORE INFORMATION. See Chapter 34, cephalosporins, Table 34-4; CNS infections, Table 92-3.

PHARMACOKINETICS. Inactivated in stomach and must be given parenterally. Very soluble and can be given IV or IM. Highly protein bound. Achieves high levels in the CSF. Dual elimination, with 40% excreted in bile, 60% in urine. Longest half-life of third-generation drugs, making once-daily dosing possible.

SPECTRUM. Gram positive: some *Staphylococcus* (some β-lactamase–producing but not methicillin-resistant strains), some *Streptococcus*. **Gram negative:** *Enterobacter, Escherichia, Klebsiella, Proteus, Serratia, Citrobacter, Providencia, Shigella, Acinetobacter,* some *Salmonella* and *Pseudomonas*. **Anaerobes:** variable against *Bacteroides* and *Clostridium*. **Others:** *Borrelia.* **More effective:** *Borrelia.* **Ineffective:** *Enterococcus.*

INDICATIONS. Lower respiratory tract, skin and soft tissue, urinary tract, bone, joint, intraabdominal, genital infections. It has been used to treat meningitis caused by susceptible strains (often gram negatives); gram-negative sepsis. Treatment of severe multisystemic gram-negative bacterial infections when toxicity of aminoglycosides or resistance to quinolones is of concern. Best option for treating systemic manifestations (meningitis, arthritis) of Lyme borreliosis. Used for surgical prophylaxis as a preoperative and interoperative infusion for abdominal contamination by bowel, genital, or biliary sources.

CONTRAINDICATIONS. Avoid with icterus. Reduce doses in renal failure. Previous cephalosporin or penicillin hypersensitivity.

ADVERSE REACTIONS. Diarrhea. Local pain on injection, systemic hypersensitivity, blood dyscrasias, diarrhea, rise in serum liver enzyme activity. Biliary crystal deposition and sludging, vitamin K antagonism, mild or transient azotemia, and hypercreatininemia.

INTERACTIONS. Incompatible with many other antimicrobials in solution.

AVAILABILITY	TYPE	SIZES	PREPARATIONS (COMPANY)
Human	Powder for injection in vials or infusion bottles	250 mg, 500 mg, 1 g, 2 g	*Rocephin* (Roche)

INTERNATIONAL PREPARATIONS. *Hosbocin, Rocephalin, Rocefalin, Rocefin, Rocephine.*

HANDLING. Store powder for injection away from light at controlled room temperature. Diluents can include sterile water, 0.9% NaCl, 5% dextrose. Solutions are stable for 1-3 days at room temperature, 3-10 days if refrigerated; concentrations at or below 100 mg/ml have the longest stability. Lower concentration (10-40 mg/ml) can be stored frozen (–20°C) for 36 weeks.

ADMINISTRATION. Avoid infusion or mixing with any other drugs. IV or IM administration for up to 14 days as necessary. For IM, may be diluted with lidocaine 1% without epinephrine. Available as IM convenience kit containing proper diluent. Use 0.9-ml diluent/250-mg drug. For IV, use 10-40 mg/ml and give by infusion over 30 min.

Dosage

INDICATIONS	DOSE (mg/kg)	ROUTE	INTERVAL (hr)	DURATION (days)
Dogs				
Meningitis, borreliosis	15-50[a]	IM, IV	12	4-14
Preoperative, intraoperative	25[a]	IM, IV	24	1
Skin, genitourinary infections	25[a]	IM	24	7-14
Cats				
Systemic infections	25-50	IV, IM, intraosseous	12	prn

[a]Maximum dose per administration is 1 g for humans.

ADDITIONAL DOSAGES. Lyme borreliosis, Table 45-5.

CEFUROXIME AXETIL OR SODIUM

CLASS. Second-generation cephalosporin.

ACTION. Bactericidal; inhibits bacterial cell wall synthesis.

MORE INFORMATION. See Chapter 34, cephalosporins; Table 34-4.

PHARMACOKINETICS. Oral axetil ester: a prodrug that is hydrolyzed releasing cefuroxime by esterases in intestinal mucosa and blood. Better absorption with food. Parenteral sodium salt: only drug among the first- and second-generation classes to enter the CSF in absence of meningitis and good therapeutic levels with meningeal inflammation. Longer half-life than cefaclor allows twice-daily dosing. Excreted unchanged in urine.

SPECTRUM. Gram positive: *Staphylococcus* and *Streptococcus*. Gram negative: *Escherichia, Klebsiella, Enterobacter*. Ineffective: high-resistance β-lactamase–producing organisms.

Ineffective against *Enterococcus* and methicillin-resistant *Staphylococcus*.

INDICATIONS. Oral, for penicillin-resistant gram-positive infections of skin and upper respiratory tract. Parenteral, also used to treat lower respiratory tract, CNS, and orthopedic infections.

CONTRAINDICATIONS. Reduce dose in renal failure. Previous hypersensitivity to penicillin or cephalosporin.

ADVERSE REACTIONS. Very bitter taste if tablet is bitten or ground up for administration. Adding to dairy products (milk or chocolate milk) may improve absorption and palatability. Some GI upsets may occur with oral axetil preparation. Neutropenia, leukopenia, and eosinophilia have been observed with parenteral sodium drug.

INTERACTIONS. Increased risk of nephrotoxicity when combined with aminoglycoside.

AVAILABILITY	TYPE	SIZES	PREPARATIONS (COMPANY)
Human	Oral tablets (as axetil)	125 mg, 250 mg, 500 mg	*Ceftin* (Glaxo Wellcome)
	Oral suspension (as axetil)	125 mg/5 ml	*Ceftin*
	Powder for injection (as sodium salt)	750 mg, 1.5 g, 7.5 g	*Kefurox* (Lilly), *Zinacef* (Glaxo Wellcome)

NTERNATIONAL PREPARATIONS. *Biociclin, Biofurex, Bioxima, Cefamar, Cefoprim, Cefumax, Cefur, Cefurex, Cefurin, Cepazine, Ceurocef, Colifossim, Curoxim, Deltacef, Duxima, Elobact, Kefox, Nivador, Selan, Zinnat, Zoref.*

HANDLING. Powder and solutions should be stored protected from light; they darken with storage, but potency is unaffected. When reconstituted, stock solutions of parenteral drug are stable for 24 hr at room temperature and for 48 hr when refrigerated. Dilutions of stock for administration, can be added to 0.9% NaCl or 5% or 10% dextrose. These solutions (1-30 mg/ml) are stable for 7 days when refrigerated;

when frozen (–20°C), the solution is stable for 6 mo and should be thawed slowly but not with a microwave, which destroys 85% of activity. Should not add to aminoglycoside-containing solutions, although these can be given separately.

ADMINISTRATION. Oral; advantage over cefaclor is that food enhances absorption and bioavailability. Tablets should be administered whole because of bitter taste, if dose needs are less, use oral suspension. Parenteral; IV is preferred route for systemic infections. IM; can give in large muscle mass; should aspirate first to avoid inadvertent IV inoculation.

Dosage

INDICATIONS (Dogs)	DOSE (mg/kg)	ROUTE	INTERVAL (hr)	DURATION (days)
Prophlyaxis for surgery	20	IV	30 min prior and every 2 hr	During surgery
Soft tissue infections	10[a]	PO	12	10
Systemic infections	15[a]	IV	8	prn
Meningitis	30[a]	IV	8	prn

[a]Extrapolated human dosage.

ADDITIONAL DOSAGES. None.

DISPENSING INFORMATION. Give tablets whole; do not break or crush if put on food. Give with meals.

CEPHALEXIN

CLASS. First-generation cephalosporin.

ACTION. Bactericidal; inhibits bacterial cell wall synthesis.

MORE INFORMATION. See Chapter 34, cephalosporins; Table 34-4; references: Ch 34, ref. 196; 197.

PHARMACOKINETICS. Well absorbed orally (57%-75% bioavailable). Distributed to most tissues, with highest concentrations in kidney, lung, trachea, and skin of dogs. Also penetrates muscle and bone in therapeutic concentrations.

Excreted unchanged in urine and bile. Does not penetrate CNS or CSF.

SPECTRUM. Gram positive: *Staphylococcus, Streptococcus*. Gram negative: *Escherichia, Klebsiella, Proteus mirabilis, Pasteurella multocida*. Ineffective: *Pseudomonas, Aerobacter,* some *Proteus, Bacteroides, Enterococcus*.

INDICATIONS. Skin infections, chronic canine staphylococcal pyoderma; urinary tract infections, pneumonia, localized soft tissue infections, upper respiratory tract infections.

CONTRAINDICATIONS. Previous hypersensitivity to cephalosporins or penicillins. Some reduction in frequency of administration to every 12-24 hr in animals with renal failure.

ADVERSE REACTIONS. Dogs: vomiting, diarrhea, excitement or depression, anorexia, salivation (Ch 34, ref. 209).

Cats: vomiting, diarrhea, pyrexia, salivation, occasional hypersensitivity reactions, cholestatic jaundice.

INTERACTIONS. Positive Coombs' tests have been seen in people treated with cephalosporins. False-positive urine glucose results have been observed in dogs with nonenzymatic test methods (Ch 34, ref. 306c).

AVAILABILITY	TYPE	SIZES	PREPARATIONS (COMPANY)
Human	Powder for oral suspension	125 mg/5 ml, 250 mg/5 ml, 500 mg/5 ml	*Keflex* (Dista), generic (many)
	Capsules, tablets	250 mg, 500 mg, 1 g	*Keflex*
Veterinary	Oral tablets	50 mg, 250 mg	*Ceporex* (Mallinckrodt)
	Oral drops	100 mg/ml	*Ceporex*
	Injectable solution	18 mg/ml	*Ceporex*

INTERNATIONAL PREPARATIONS. *Abiocef, Biocef, Bioporina, Bioscefal, Cefact, Cefadina, Cefadine, Cefadros, Cefalorex, Cefanex, Ceferran, Cepexin, Cephalobene, Cepo, Ceporexin, Ceporexine, Cerexin, Cilicef, Coliceflor; Defaxina, Domucef, Efemida, Fexin, Ibilex, Janocilin, Keflet, Keforal, Keftab, Lafarin, Latoral, Lenocef, Lorexina, Novo-Lexin, Nu-Cephalex, Oracef, Ospexin, Talinsul, Ultralexin, Zartan, Zetacef.*

HANDLING. Oral suspension: refrigerate once reconstituted and discard after 14 days. Capsules: store away from moisture in airtight containers at room temperature.

ADMINISTRATION. Generally given orally with little or no side effects other than occasional diarrhea. Injectable for IM use: localized tissue reaction may occur, massage injection site. Food delays absorption and elimination to a minor degree.

Dosage

INDICATIONS	DOSE (mg/kg)	ROUTE	INTERVAL (hr)	DURATION (days)
Dogs				
Pyoderma	30-35	PO	12	21-42[a]
Respiratory infections	20-40	PO	8	7-14[a]
Systemic infections	25-45	PO	8	14-28[a]
Orthopedic infections	22-30	PO	6-8	28[a]
Cats				
Soft tissue infections	30-50	PO	12	14-28[a]
Systemic infections	35	PO	6-8	14-28[a]

[a]Guideline: treat for 5-7 days beyond resolution of clinical disease or preferably negative culture. For susceptible staphylococci, dosing every 12 hr may be adequate for most tissues; however, infection with more cephalosporin-resistant organisms such as *E. coli*, outside the urinary tract, may require higher levels of dosing on the 8-hr interval (Ch 34, ref. 57).

ADDITIONAL DOSAGES. Streptococcal infections, Table 35-2; anaerobic infections, Table 41-12; canine pyoderma, Table 85-3; musculoskeletal infections, Table 86-4; respiratory disease, Table 88-8; urinary infections, Table 91-10.

DISPENSING INFORMATION. Food may be given with medication to prevent vomiting. Absorption, as a result peak serum concentration, may be reduced slightly after feeding of dogs (Ch 34, ref. 57). The duration of activity is minimally changed by feeding. Oral suspension should be shaken well before using.

CEPHAPIRIN

CLASS. First-generation cephalosporin.

ACTION. Bactericidal; inhibits bacterial cell wall synthesis.

MORE INFORMATION. See Chapter 34, Cephalosporins, Table 34-4.

PHARMACOKINETICS. Not absorbed from the GI tract after PO administration. Widely distributed into some body fluids (synovial, pleural, peritoneal) but poorly into aqueous humor and CSF. Penetrates many tissues, including bone but not prostate.

SPECTRUM. **Gram positive:** *Staphylococcus*, hemolytic *Streptococcus*. **Gram negative:** *Escherichia, Klebsiella, Proteus*.

INDICATIONS. Perioperative surgical prophylaxis, septicemia, pneumonia, osteomyelitis.

CONTRAINDICATIONS. Reduce dose in renal failure.

ADVERSE REACTIONS. Pain on injection, phlebitis.

INTERACTIONS. Use cautiously with nephrotoxic drugs such as aminoglycosides.

AVAILABILITY	TYPE	SIZES	PREPARATIONS (COMPANY)
Human	Powder for injection	500 mg, 1 g, 2 g, 1 g, 2 g,	*Cefadyl* (Bristol), generics (many)

HANDLING. Powder stored at room temperature is stable for 2 yrs. Reconstitute with sterile water. Stable at room temperature for 24 hr or 10 days if refrigerated and 14 days if frozen. Compatible with 0.9% NaCl, dextrose, Ringer's, lactated Ringer's.

ADMINISTRATION. Infuse IV slowly over 3-5 min or give with IV fluids.

Dosage

INDICATIONS (*Dogs and Cats*)	DOSE (mg/kg)	ROUTE	INTERVAL (hr)	DURATION (days)
Soft tissue infections	10-20	IV, IM, SC	6-8	prn
Bacteremia, endotexemia	11-30	IV	4-8	prn

ADDITIONAL DOSAGES. Canine distemper, Table 3-5; feline panleukopenia, Table 10-2; bacteremia or endocarditis, Table 87-6; oral infections, Table 89-4; CNS infections, Table 92-5.

CEPHAZOLIN

CLASS. First-generation cephalosporin.

ACTION. Bactericidal; inhibits bacterial cell wall synthesis.

MORE INFORMATION. See CEPHAPIRIN; Chapter 34, cephalosporins, Table 34-4.

PHARMACOKINETICS. Poorly absorbed from GI tract. After IM or IV injection, enters many tissues and body fluids, including bone and peritoneal, pleural, and synovial fluids. Does not enter CSF appreciably. Predominantly excreted unchanged in urine.

SPECTRUM. See CEPHALEXIN, PENICILLIN G, or CEPHAPIRIN.

INDICATIONS. Surgical prophylaxis, biliary tract, and intraabdominal infections and bacteremia.

CONTRAINDICATIONS. See CEPHALEXIN.

ADVERSE REACTIONS. IM injections are painful and IV can cause thrombophlebitis. See also CEPHALEXIN.

INTERACTIONS. See CEPHRADINE.

AVAILABILITY	TYPE	SIZES	PREPARATIONS (COMPANY)
Human	Powder for injection (as sodium)	1 g	*Ancef* (Smith Kline Beecham), *Kefzol* (Lilly)

INTERNATIONAL PREPARATIONS. *Acef, Areuzolin, Baktozil, Biazolina, Brizolina, Caricef, Cefabiozim, Cefacidal, Cefadrex, Cefamezin, Cefazil, Cilicef, Elzogram, Fazoplex, Firmacef, Gramaxin, Izacef, Kefol, Recef, Sicef, Tasep, Totacef, Zolicef, Zolin, Zolival.*

HANDLING. Should reconstitute in sterile water. Store in light-proof containers. Incompatible with aminoglycosides and basic solutions in which hydrolysis occurs, and at pH < 4.5, the drug precipitates. Crystal formation occurs if reconstituted with 0.9% NaCl and should be avoided.

ADMINISTRATION. Give by deep IM injection or slow (3-5 min) IV infusion.

Dosage

INDICATIONS	DOSE (mg/kg)	ROUTE	INTERVAL (hr)	DURATION (days)
Soft tissue infections	22	IM, IV	8	prn
Surgical infections	22	IV	a	1

ªJust before or during surgical procedure.

ADDITIONAL DOSAGES. None.

CEPHRADINE

CLASS. First-generation cephalosporin.

ACTION. Bactericidal; inhibits bacterial cell wall synthesis.

MORE INFORMATION. See Chapter 34, cephalosporins; Table 34-4.

PHARMACOKINETICS. See CEPHALEXIN. Better absorbed orally (90% bioavailable).

SPECTRUM. Gram positive: *Staphylococcus*, hemolytic *Streptococcus*. **Gram negative:** *Escherichia*, *Klebsiella*, *Proteus*.

INDICATIONS. Oral treatment of respiratory, skin, and urinary tract infections; parenteral treatment for septicemia, osteomyelitis, and perioperative prophylaxis.

CONTRAINDICATIONS. See CEPHALEXIN.

ADVERSE REACTIONS. Dogs: vomiting, diarrhea, anorexia, polydipsia, polyuria.

INTERACTIONS. False-positive results on urine protein tests using sulfosalicylic acid. Monitor renal function if used in combination with aminoglycosides.

AVAILABILITY	TYPE	SIZES	PREPARATIONS (COMPANY)
Human	Oral capsules	250 mg, 500 mg	*Velosef* (Apothecon), generics (many)
	Powder for oral suspension (fruit-flavored)	125 mg/5 ml, 250 mg/5 ml	*Anspor* (SmithKline Beecham)
	Powder for injection	250 mg, 500 mg, 1 g, 2 g	*Velosef*

INTERNATIONAL PREPARATIONS. *Cefamid, Cefrasol, Cefril, Cefral, Celex, Cesporan, Ecosporina, Kelsef, Lisacef, Sefril, Septasef.*

HANDLING. Store powders and capsules below 86°F, and keep bottle closed tight away from light. Oral suspension stable 7 days at room temperature, 14 days if refrigerated. Compatible with most IV solutions except Ringer's or lactated Ringer's or calcium-containing solutions. Do not mix with other antibiotics given concurrently. Reconstituted solutions of less than 50 mg/ml are stable for 10 hr at room temperature and 48 hr if refrigerated. Solutions for injection can be stored frozen for 6 weeks.

ADMINISTRATION. Can be given orally without regard to meals. Food delays absorption but does not affect its extent.

Dosage

INDICATIONS *(Dogs)*	DOSE (mg/kg)	ROUTE	INTERVAL (hr)	DURATION (days)
Skin, pyoderma	22	PO	8	14-28[a]
Systemic, orthopedic infections	22	IV, IM, SC, PO	6-8	28[a]

[a]Treatment duration varies, usually 5-7 days beyond resolution of infection by culture testing.

ADDITIONAL DOSAGES. Respiratory infections, Table 88-8.

DISPENSING INFORMATION. Keep reconstituted oral suspension in refrigerator, discard unused portions after 2 weeks.

CHLORAMPHENICOL

CLASS. Acetamide.

ACTION. Bacterostatic; binds to 50s ribosomes of bacteria, inhibiting protein synthesis.

MORE INFORMATION. See FLORFENICOL, see elsewhere THIAMFENICOL. See Chapter 34, chloramphenicol; references: Ch 34, ref. 289; Ch 34, ref. 407.

PHARMACOKINETICS. GI absorption dependent on formulation. Crystalline salt is better, may cause salivation in cats but has good bioavailability with rapid absorption. Oral palmitate is better tolerated but gives poor systemic drug availability in anorectic cats (Ch 34, ref. 407). In dogs, drug availability with the palmitate is similar to tablets. The inactive palmitate is hydrolyzed in small intestine to release active absorbable drug. Sodium succinate ester can be given IV, SC, IM. Systemic availability is similar with each route, but IM injection is more painful. The succinate ester lacks antimicrobial activity but is hydrolyzed in liver, lung, and kidney to release active drug. It produces better bioavailability than chloramphenicol in aqueous suspensions or dissolved in organic solvents. Chloramphenicol is lipid soluble and distributed well to all tissues, including skeleton, prostate, CNS. Order of decreasing tissue concentrations is as follows: lymph node, spleen, pancreas, liver, kidney, lung, muscle, brain (Ch 34, ref. 407). Penetrates pleural, ascitic, and synovial fluids, saliva, milk, prostatic and amniotic fluids. Tissue concentrations often exceed those in plasma, but the drug is slower (3-4 hr) to penetrate the intact brain and CSF barriers. Compared with plasma, concentrations are 23% in aqueous and 77% in CSF (Ch 34, ref. 407). Concentrations are not altered appreciably by inflammation.

Metabolized in liver by glucuronyl transferase; in dogs 90% of drug is metabolized and metabolites are excreted in urine. Only 5%-10% of a dose in adult dogs and 25% in cats and neonatal dogs is excreted unchanged in urine. Urine concentrations are 10-20 times blood concentrations and are therapeutic. Optimum activity at a urine pH of 7.5-8.0.

SPECTRUM. Gram positive: *Streptococcus, Staphylococcus.* **Gram negative:** *Salmonella, Shigella, Escherichia, Proteus, Bordetella.* **Anaerobes:** *Clostridium, Fusobacterium, Bacteroides.* Resistance can develop during use. **Others:** *Chlamydia, Rickettsia, Mycoplasma, Ehrlichia, Leptospira, Borrelia.* **Most effective:** anaerobic infections, rickettsial infections. **Ineffective:** *Mycobacterium, Pseudomonas, Enterobacter, Serratia, Klebsiella* may be resistant or develop it during treatment.

INDICATIONS. Cats: chronic rhinitis-sinusitis, pneumonia, pyothorax, periodontitis-gingivitis, bacterial enteritis, biliary infections, intraabdominal sepsis, lower urinary infection, hemotropic mycoplasmosis (hemobartonellosis), bordetellosis, rickettsiosis, anaerobic infections (abscesses). **Dogs:** tetracycline-resistant *Ehrlichia canis* infections without myelosuppression; respiratory, urinary, and soft tissue infections.

CONTRAINDICATIONS. Pre-existing leukopenia or anemia; hepatic dysfunction requires reducing dose to lower risk of marrow suppression. Avoid in pregnancy, neonates, hepatic insufficiency, cats with renal failure. Avoid IV use in animals with cardiac failure because it depresses myocardium. Do not use in breeding animals because it may affect gonadal function. No reduction in dosage needed in dogs with mild renal insufficiency, but a 10% reduction is recommended in uremia as a result of protein catabolic effects of the drug.

ADVERSE REACTIONS. Protein synthesis inhibitor; theoretically, might delay wound healing or immunoglobulin synthesis. High plasma concentrations can be toxic for prenatal or neonatal animals owing to immature hepatic metabolism. Inhibits ferrochelatase, an enzyme in hemoglobin synthesis, resulting in reversible nonregenerative anemia. Reversible myelosuppression affecting the maturation of granulocytes occurs in dogs and cats. This should be differentiated from severe, often fatal irreversible idiosyncratic pancytopenia that occurs in some people (Ch 34, ref. 289). Dogs: with >2-3 weeks of treatment at >175 mg/kg/day may develop depression, anorexia; at >225 mg/kg/day, myelosuppression, reticulocytopenia. No morphologic bone marrow effects are found in treated dogs. Erythropoietic response is suppressed at therapeutic dosages in dogs with pre-existing or concurrent blood loss when therapy commences. Regeneration occurs when therapy is discontinued. Cats: at 25-40 mg/kg/day for 3 weeks or 120 mg/kg/day for 1 week develop depression, dehydration, anorexia, weight loss, diarrhea, vomiting, myelotoxicity. Reversible erythroid maturation arrest, vacuolation of marrow elements, and pancytopenia occur.

INTERACTIONS. Avoid prescribing it with other drugs metabolized in the liver, especially to cats. Inhibits cytochrome P-450 activity and resultant hepatic biotransformation of drugs, which may potentiate by prolonging action of pentobarbital, phenobarbital, primidone, warfarin, salicylates, inhalation anesthetics, diphenylhydantoin, digoxin (Ch 34, ref. 174). Action of cyclophosphamide is inhibited because its metabolites are active. Effect on P-450 activity has even been noted with topical ophthalmic preparations. Does not alter the effects or duration of ketamine-xylazine anesthesia. Prolongs propofol anesthesia in dogs (Ch 34, ref. 233; 278). Decreases effectiveness of iron, B_{12} aminoglycosides, penicillins. Rifampin and phenobarbital decrease the effectiveness of chloramphenicol. Oral coadministration of calcium lactate, kaolin-pectin, aluminum hydroxide preparations may increase bioavailability. May cause a spurious positive test result for glucose using glucose oxidase strips.

AVAILABILITY	TYPE	SIZES	PREPARATIONS (COMPANY)
Human	Oral capsules	250 mg, 500 mg	*Chloromycetin* (Parke-Davis)[a]
	Oral liquid (palmitate)	50 mg/ml	*Chloromycetin* Palmitate (Parke-Davis)[a]
	Powder for injection (sodium succinate)	1-g, 10-g vials (100 mg/ml)	*Chloromycetin*
Veterinary	Oral tablets, film coated	100 mg, 250 mg, 500 mg, 1 g	*Amphicol* (Butler)[a], generic (Phoenix)
	Capsules	100 mg, 250 mg, 500 mg	*Chloromycetin*, generic (many)[a]

[a]No longer available in US

INTERNATIONAL PREPARATIONS. *Aquamycetin, Biophenicol, Chemicetina, Chlorcol, Cloranfe, Dispaphenicol, Globenicol, Fenicol, Hortfenicol, Kemicetin, Septicol, Sificetina, Troymycetin.*

HANDLING. Oral palmitate suspension, tablets, capsules should be stored at room temperature away from light. Stable for several years at room temperature. The sodium succinate powder should be kept at controlled room temperatures. Once reconstituted, is stable for 1 mo at room temperature or 6 mo if frozen.

ADMINISTRATION. Oral administration is generally satisfactory. Sodium succinate can be given IV, IM, SC, although pain or irritation may result at extravascular sites. SC or IM for fractious, unconscious animals or animals with GI disturbance; IV for high rapid levels in severe systemic infections. If no response to therapy in 3-5 days, reconsider diagnosis and treatment. Should recheck CBC for myelotoxicity at 1-week and 2-week intervals in cats and dogs, respectively.

Dosage

INDICATIONS	DOSE	ROUTE	INTERVAL (hr)	DURATION (days)
Dogs				
Urinary, rickettsial, localized soft tissue infections	25-50 mg/kg	PO	8	7
Systemic infection	50 mg/kg	IV, IM, SC, PO	6-8	3-5
Severe bacteremia, sepsis	50 mg/kg	IV, IM, SC	4-6	3
Cats				
Urinary, localized soft tissue infections	50 mg/cat	PO	12	14
Systemic infections	25-50 mg/kg	IV, IM, SC, PO	12	≤14
Bacteremia, sepsis	50 mg/cat	IV, IM, SC, PO	6-8	≤5

ADDITIONAL DOSAGES. Canine distemper, Table 3-5; ehrlichiosis, Table 28-4; Rocky Mountain spotted fever, Table 29-4; streptococcal infections, Table 35-2; enteric bacterial infections, Table 39-2; anaerobic infections, Table 41-12; Lyme borreliosis, Table 45-5; plague, Table 47-1; actinomycosis, Table 49-2; feline abscesses, Table 52-3; musculoskeletal infections, Table 86-4; bacteremia, Table 87-6; respiratory disease, Table 88-8; oral infections, Table 89-4; colitis, Table 89-19; intraabdominal infections, Table 89-21; hepatobiliary infections, Table 90-5; urinary infections, Table 91-10; CNS infections, Table 92-5.

DISPENSING INFORMATION. This drug is potentially toxic to people. Wear latex gloves when handling and administering to pets. Return animal every 2 weeks for hematologic testing. Can be administered with food. Tablets or capsules may be bitter if crushed. Shake suspensions well before use.

CIPROFLOXACIN HYDROCHLORIDE

CLASS. Fluoroquinolone.

ACTION. Bactericidal; interferes with DNA gyrase and synthesis of bacterial DNA.

MORE INFORMATION. See ENROFLOXACIN; Chapter 34, quinolones, Table 34-11.

PHARMACOKINETICS. See also ENROFLOXACIN. More variable and slower absorption than enrofloxacin. Well absorbed in dogs (70%) after PO administration. Absorption was lower in cats (Ch 34, ref. 4); however, the drug was given in gelatin capsules. Food may delay rate but not degree of absorption. Approximately 40%-50% excreted unchanged in urine. Urinary metabolites have lower antibacterial activity. Wide tissue distribution. Concentrations in genital tissues of both sexes are high. Present in active form in saliva, nasal and bronchial secretions, sputum, skin blister fluid, lymph, peritoneal fluid, bile and prostatic secretions. Lower concentrations in lung, skin, fat, muscle, cartilage, bone. In people, concentrations in CSF are 40%-90% of serum with inflammation and less than 10% if uninflamed. Concentrations in aqueous humor are 4%-25% of serum, with low concentrations in vitreous.

SPECTRUM. See also ENROFLOXACIN. **Gram positive:** Staphylococcus (including methicillin-resistant strains), most Streptococcus are moderately susceptible. **Gram negative:** Escherichia, Klebsiella, Enterobacter, Citrobacter, Salmonella, Campylobacter, Brucella, Pasteurella, some Pseudomonas develop resistance. **Anaerobes:** most are resistant. **Others:** Mycoplasma, Leptospira, Borrelia, Chlamydia, Mycobacterium tuberculosis, some opportunistic mycobacteria, but not Mycobacterium avium-intracellulare complex. Increased activity and spectrum may occur in combined therapy with metronidazole, clindamycin, β-lactam drugs, or aminoglycosides. **More effective:** gram-negative bacteria. **Ineffective:** Enterococcus, Actinomyces, Nocardia, Ehrlichia, obligate anaerobes, M. avium-intracellulare complex.

INDICATIONS. See also ENROFLOXACIN. Complicated or chronic urinary tract infections or prostatitis caused by Escherichia, Klebsiella, Enterobacter, Serratia, Proteus, Citrobacter, Pseudomonas, Staphylococcus. Infectious diarrhea caused by pathogenic gram-negative bacteria such as enterotoxigenic Escherichia, Campylobacter, and Salmonella. Lower respiratory, skin, bone, and joint infections with very susceptible organisms. Gram-negative bacterial meningitis.

CONTRAINDICATIONS. See also ENROFLOXACIN. In reduced renal function, there is slight prolongation of ciprofloxacin elimination: reduce dose (once daily) in renal failure. Owing to arthropathy, should not be used in growing animals or in pregnant or lactating animals. Avoid in animals with previously documented adverse reaction.

ADVERSE REACTIONS. See also ENROFLOXACIN. Nausea, anorexia, vomiting, diarrhea are most frequent side effects. Malaise and inappetence occurs in cats. May cause CNS stimulation with tremors or seizures in predisposed animals. Permanent cartilage damage and lameness develop in growing animals. Dermal hypersensitivity reactions have occurred. High overdosages in dogs have resulted in nephrotoxicity from crystal deposition in kidneys (especially alkaline urine), cataracts, reduced spermatogenesis. These have not been seen with therapeutic dosages. Tendon ruptures have been observed in people. This drug is the most likely quinolone to cause hepatic necrosis and inflammation (Ch 34, ref. 394).

INTERACTIONS. Concurrent use with theophylline results in elevated theophylline concentrations and increased risk of CNS stimulation.

AVAILABILITY	TYPE	SIZES	PREPARATIONS (COMPANY)
Human	Film coated oral tablets	250 mg, 500 mg, 750 mg	Cipro (Miles-Bayer)
	Parenteral (IV) solution	200 mg, 400 mg	Cipro

INTERNATIONAL PREPARATIONS. *Baycip, Belmacina, Catex, Ceprimax, Ciflox, Ciloxan, Ciprobay, Ciproxin, Cunesin, Flociprin, Quipro.*

HANDLING. Add parenteral solution of 0.9% NaCl or 5% dextrose. Stable for 14 days if refrigerated, but protect from light. Do not mix with clindamycin or clavulanate. Can be formulated for smaller tablet size by compounding pharmacies.

ADMINISTRATION. For IV, dilute in saline before administration and give slowly over 1 hr using large veins. Orally, food slows or reduces absorption of the drug. Preferred dosing is 2 hr after meal. Concurrent administration of antacids containing magnesium or aluminum hydroxide may reduce bioavailability to 90%. Sucralfate given within 2 hr of oral dosing similarly reduces absorption.

Dosage

INDICATIONS (Dogs)	DOSE (mg/kg)	ROUTE	INTERVAL (hr)	DURATION (days)
Urinary tract infections	10	PO	24	7-14
Skin, local soft tissue infections	10-15	PO	24	7-14
Bone, and systemic infections, bacteremia and more resistant pathogens (e.g., *Enterobacter*)	20	PO	24	7-14
Pseudomonas otitis externa[a]				

[a]Ch 85, ref. 42

ADDITIONAL DOSAGES. Gram-negative bacterial infections, Table 37-3; musculoskeletal infections, Table 86-4; bacteremia and endocarditis, Table 87-6. In people, *Pseudomonas* meningitis was successfully treated with high dose IV ciprofloxacin every 8 hr for 1 week (Ch 34, ref. 221).

DISPENSING INFORMATION. Administer at least 1 hr before or 2 hr after meals and do not give concurrently with antacids or sucralfate.

CLARITHROMYCIN

CLASS. Macrolide, methylerythromycin derivative.

ACTION. Bacteriostatic; inhibits bacterial RNA-dependent protein synthesis by binding to 50s subunit of ribosome.

MORE INFORMATION. See AZITHROMYCIN; Chapter 34, Macrolides.

PHARMACOKINETICS. Best absorbed macrolide with or without ingesta (55% bioavailable) because stable in gastric acid. Better absorption and tissue penetration than erythromycin with prolonged elimination half-life. Concentrated in and transported by phagocytes. Lipophilic and distributed widely throughout the body. High concentration reached in sputum, lung, tonsil, nasal sinus, stomach, uterus, ovary, cervix, and prostate. Accumulates in pulmonary tissue. Penetrates and concentrates intracellularly in macrophages and neutrophils, facilitating killing of intracellular pathogens. Does not penetrate well into CNS. Metabolized in liver by hydroxylation and methylation, forming a very biologically active hydroxymetabolite and inactive demethylated compound, which are excreted predominantly in the bile. Metabolites are excreted in urine. From 20%-40% of dose may appear in urine as unchanged drug, depending on the formulation (tablets or powder, respectively).

SPECTRUM. See ERYTHROMYCIN for gram-positive and gram-negative aerobic bacteria. **Anaerobes:** *Bacteroides, Clostridium, Peptococcus,* and *Propionibacterium*. Best activity against gram-positive aerobes and anaerobes. **Others:** opportunistic mycobacteria, *M. avium-intracellulare complex (MAC), Borrelia, Bartonella, Toxoplasma, Chlamydia*. **More effective:** than erythromycin against *Streptococcus, Staphylococcus, Campylobacter, Helicobacter,* and obligate anaerobes.

INDICATIONS. Lower respiratory tract and skin infections, enteropathogenic bacterial infections, nasal sinusitis, *Toxoplasma* (combined with pyrimethamine), many cutaneous opportunistic mycobacterial infections, including those caused by MAC (recommend combining with other effective agents). Used in Lyme borreliosis and gastric helicobacteriosis. A substitute for erythromycin with less GI irritation, lower dose but higher cost.

CONTRAINDICATIONS. Previous erythromycin hypersensitivity. Reduce dose for renal or severe hepatic failure. Active urinary metabolite will not be produced with hepatic dysfunction. Avoid in pregnancy; has adverse effects on fetal development in experimental animals.

ADVERSE REACTIONS. Nausea, diarrhea, abdominal pain, cholestatic hepatitis, increased liver enzymes, thrombocytopenia, rare eosinophilia, allergic skin reactions. Should hepatic enzyme elevations occur, use lower dosage range. May be less likely than erythromycin to cause GI disturbances.

INTERACTIONS. See ERYTHROMYCIN; interferes with metabolism of drugs by cytochrome P-450 system. May inhibit benzodiazepine or digoxin metabolism.

AVAILABILITY	TYPE	SIZES	PREPARATIONS (COMPANY)
Human	Tablets	250 mg, 500 mg	*Biaxin* (Abbott), *Klacid* (many countries)
	Granules for oral suspension	125 mg/5 ml, 250 mg/5 ml	*Biaxin*

INTERNATIONAL PREPARATIONS. *Biclar, Cyllind, Klacid, Klaciped, Klariced, Macladin, Mavid, Veclam.*

HANDLING. Do not refrigerate suspension because it develops a bitter taste; keep at room temperature and use within 14 days.

ADMINISTRATION. Can be given with or without fasting, but food delays absorption.

Dosage

INDICATIONS	DOSE (mg/kg)	ROUTE	INTERVAL (hr)	DURATION (days)
Dogs	5-10	PO	12	prn
Cats	7.5	PO	12	prn

ADDITIONAL DOSAGES. Helicobacteriosis, Table 39-6; mycobacterial infections, Tables 50-4, 50-6, 50-7, and 50-9.

DISPENSING INFORMATION. Can be given with food. Shake suspension before administration. May cause diarrhea or vomiting.

CLINDAMYCIN

CLASS. Lincosamide; semisynthetic derivative of lincomycin.

ACTION. Bacteriostatic and antiprotozoal activity; binds to 50s subunit of bacterial and protozoal ribosome inhibiting protein synthesis. Potentiates opsonization and phagocytosis.

MORE INFORMATION. See LINCOMYCIN; Chapter 34, Lincosamides; references: Ch 34, ref. 47; 150; 156; Ch 71, ref. 34.

PHARMACOKINETICS. After oral administration, GI absorption approached 90%. For oral suspension, palmitate ester is hydrolyzed to active base while aqueous drops are readily absorbed. Absorption is delayed but not prevented by food. Better absorbed than lincomycin. Widely distributed to most tissues, including skin, muscle, bone, body fluids (pleural, peritoneal, synovial) to therapeutic levels. Active transport into phagocytic cells and abscess fluids, killing susceptible intracellular bacteria. Lowest levels reached are in intact CNS and CSF. Levels in inflamed meninges are 40% of blood concentration. Crosses placenta and enters milk. Hepatic metabolism to active and inactive moieties with excretion in bile, feces, urine. Prolonged enterohepatic circulation and excretion in stool for up to 2 weeks after last dose. It is predominantly (80%-90%) excreted in bile with 10%-20% renally excreted. Dogs and cats with periodontitis, treated with 11 mg/kg once daily for 5 days, had mean concentrations of 8.18 μg/g in dogs (range, 3.16 to 24.08 μg/g) and 17.43 μg/g in cats (range, 2.45 to 51.60 μg/g) (Ch 34, ref. 438).

SPECTRUM. Gram positive: Aerobic cocci, including *Streptococcus* (not enterococci) and more susceptible *Staphylococcus*, *Nocardia*, and few *Corynebacterium*. **Gram negative:** *Campylobacter, Helicobacter.* **Anaerobes:** *Peptostreptococcus, Peptococcus, Actinomyces, Propionibacterium, Eubacterium, Clostridium* (except *C. difficile*), *Bacteroides, Fusobacterium.* **Others:** *Chlamydia*; protozoa *Toxoplasma, Neospora, Babesia, Pneumocystis.* **Ineffective:** most gram-negative aerobic bacteria, *Mycobacterium*, and *Mycoplasma*. Whenever resistance to lincomycin or erythromycin exists. Bacterial resistance may develop during treatment and usually also involves lincomycin.

INDICATIONS. Bacteria: For gram-positive aerobic and in anaerobic infections. Intraabdominal or GI abscesses and infections (perforating ulcers, penetrating injuries, biliary infections, ischemic bowel, colitis, hepatic or biliary abscesses, soft tissue or subcutaneous abscesses, pelvic genital infections, or prostatitis caused by anaerobes, chronic sinusitis or otitis, bacterial pharyngitis, stomatitis, bite wounds, dental infections, periodontal disease, dental plaque prevention); for oral, dental, or upper respiratory tract procedures, pleuropulmonary infections (pyothorax, aspiration pneumonia, pleuritis, pulmonary abscesses). Skin and soft tissue infections (staphylococcal pyoderma); osteomyelitis; diskospondylitis; prophylaxis for head, neck, and open bowel surgery (for the latter, combine with aminoglycosides); endocarditis prophylaxis (after amoxicillin and erythromycin), streptococcal or staphylococcal septicemia. Very effective in treating anaerobic infections and could be preferred over chloramphenicol or metronidazole because of less toxicity. Usually combined with an aminoglycoside or quinolone to treat gram-negative aerobic bacterial infections. Clindamycin resistance has been increasing in recent years. It is most common among anaerobes in the *Bacteroides fragilis* group and among anaerobes, *C. difficile* is the most resistant to this drug (Ch 41, ref. 26a). **Protozoa:** Toxoplasmosis and neosporosis: can be used in combination with pyrimethamine. Systemic toxoplasmosis in dogs and cats and enteroepithelial toxoplasmosis in cats. Pneumocystosis: combined with primaquine. Babesiosis: combined with quinine.

CONTRAINDICATIONS. Bacterial resistance to lincomycin. Reduce dose with hepatic dysfunction and biliary obstruction from any cause. Reduce dose with severe renal failure. Safety in reproductively active animals or pregnancy is uncertain.

ADVERSE REACTIONS. GI signs; generally less vomiting than with lincomycin, transient diarrhea when dose is reduced or temporarily discontinued. Pseudomembranous colitis, documented for other species, not a substantiated complication in dogs and cats. Local or systemic or dermal hypersensitivity reactions occur rarely. Local pain and sterile abscesses can form after IM and phlebitis after IV. Oral clindamycin may cause lip smacking and hypersalivation in some cats. Anorexia, vomiting, diarrhea owing to GI irritation can be overcome by parenteral rather than PO use and dosage reductions. May cause diarrhea in pups or kittens of dams receiving therapy. Can produce neuromuscular blockade. May cause leukopenia or increased serum hepatic enzyme activity. Cardiac arrhythmias may develop with bolus infusions of undiluted drug.

INTERACTIONS. Neuromuscular blockade compounded by other similar-acting agents such as aminoglycosides. Erythromycin and chloramphenicol interfere with the action of clindamycin in vivo. Do not use with macrolides.

AVAILABILITY	TYPE	SIZES	PREPARATIONS (COMPANY)
Human	Oral suspension (palmitate)	15 mg/ml	*Cleocin* (Pharmacia & Upjohn)
	Solution for injection (phosphate)	150 mg/ml	*Cleocin*
	Oral capsules	75 mg, 150 mg, 300 mg	*Cleocin*
Veterinary	Oral capsules	25 mg, 75 mg, 150 mg	*Antirobe* (Pharmacia & Upjohn)
	Oral solution (hydrochloride)	25 mg/ml	*Antirobe Aquadrops*

INTERNATIONAL PREPARATIONS. *Clindatech, Dalacin.*

HANDLING. Parenteral phosphate solution can be stored at room temperature, compatible with most isotonic IV solutions. Contains no preservatives, and if refrigerated, crystals will form that dissolve on rewarming. Oral hydrochloride is stable at room temperature for extended periods. Once reconstituted, palmitate stable for 2 weeks at room temperature but congeals if refrigerated. Parenteral solution of 300-900 mg diluted in 20 ml of 10% dextrose solution, is stable in frozen storage for 30 days. Parenteral solution is incompatible in nfusions with aminophylline, calcium gluconate, ceftriaxone, barbiturates, ampicillin.

ADMINISTRATION. Oral preparations can be given with food, which does not modify the normal absorption of drug.

For IV use, always dilute or administer parenteral solution in 0.9% sodium chloride, 5% dextrose, or lactated Ringer's. IV preparation can be added to solutions containing aminoglycosides (some), penicillins, cephalosporins, glucocorticoids, potassium chloride, sodium bicarbonate. Each dose can be given IV over 4-6 hr or slow IV bolus over 20-min period. Never give greater than 15 mg/min. Pain at IM or SC injection site. The SC route using a clindamycin hydrochloride parenteral solution was superior to the IM route in terms of local tolerance and serum drug level (Ch 34, ref. 216). Manufacturer recommends a treatment interval of 5-28 days. Monitor hepatic, renal function, and hematologic test results during prolonged (≥30 day) therapy.

Dosage

INDICATIONS	DOSE (mg/kg)	ROUTE	INTERVAL (hr)	DURATION (days)
Dogs				
Staphylococcal pyoderma	10-11	SC, PO	24[a]	7-28
Anaerobic wounds, abscesses, dental infections, stomatitis	5-11	IV, SC, PO	12	7-28
Dental prophylaxis, reduce plaque and pockets	5	PO	12	5-8[b]
Neosporosis, toxoplasmosis	5-20	IV, SC, PO	12	15
Neosporosis	13.5	PO	8	21
Staphylococcal osteomyelitis	11	PO	12	28-42
Anaerobic osteomyelitis	11	PO	8	28-42
Systemic, bacteremia	3-10	IV, SC, PO	8	prn
Cats				
Skin and soft tissue infections	11-24	PO, SC	24	7-28
Skin and soft tissue infections, stomatitis	5-11	PO, SC	12	7-28
Enteroepithelial toxoplasmosis	25-50	PO	24	7-14
Systemic toxoplasmosis	8-16	PO, SC	8	14-28
	12.5-25	PO, SC	12	14-28

[a]Ch 85, ref. 13. Has also been used at 5.5 (Ch 85, ref. 83). At this dosage level is only moderately effective, so higher levels 10 mg/kg every 12 hr has been more effective against resistant staphylococcal pyoderma (Ch 85, ref. 63).
[b]Ch 34, ref. 274; 405.

ADDITIONAL DOSAGES. FIV stomatitis, Table 14-6; endotoxemia, Table 38-6; *Clostridium perfringens* diarrhea, Table 39-10; anaerobic infections; Table 41-12; tetanus, Table 43-2; actinomycosis, Table 49-2; feline abscesses, Table 52-3; pneumocystosis, Table 68-2; hepatozoon, Table 74-2; babesiosis, Table 77-3; toxoplasmosis, Table 80-3; neosporosis, Table 80-7; musculoskeletal infections, Table 86-4; oral infections, Table 89-4; intraabdominal infections, Table 89-21; hepato-

biliary infections, Table 90-5; local use for ocular infections, Table 93-4.

DISPENSING INFORMATION. Shake oral suspension before each administration. Give liquid or capsules with small amount of food if vomiting occurs; otherwise give on an empty stomach. Cats may salivate when treated with PO preparations. Report any persistent or bloody vomiting or diarrhea to the veterinarian.

CLOFAZIMINE

CLASS. Iminophenazine dye.

ACTION. Antimycobacterial; binds preferentially to mycobacterial DNA. Some antiprotozoal and antifungal activity.

MORE INFORMATION. See Chapters 34 and 50; reference: Ch 34, ref. 189.

PHARMACOKINETICS. Good absorption (45%-60%) from GI tract. Highly lipophilic, taken up in adipose and mononuclear phagocytes. Retained in tissues for long periods and can be excreted via bile into feces for months. Small amounts present in other body secretions.

SPECTRUM. *Mycobacterium avium-intracellulare* complex (MAC), opportunistic rapid-growing mycobacteria. Weak activity against *Mycobacterium leprae*. Resistance rarely develops during treatment.

INDICATIONS. MAC infections, leprosy, opportunistic mycobacteriosis. Combination therapy with other drugs (see Chapter 50) overcomes resistance and increases efficacy in treating mycobacteriosis. Combined with dapsone to treat leprosy. On a limited basis has been used to treat human leishmaniasis and topical mycoses. Has anti-inflammatory activity. Has some antileishmanial activity.

CONTRAINDICATIONS. During pregnancy can cause fetotoxicity and should be avoided in pre-existing gastrointestinal illness. Consider doxycycline or quinolones as alternatives.

ADVERSE REACTIONS. GI pain resulting from crystalline deposits of drug in viscera (nausea, vomiting, abdominal pain). Pitting corneal lesions may develop. Reduce or discontinue drug use if signs occur. Skin and body fluid discoloration (pink to brown) especially when exposed to sunlight (photosensitivity). CNS signs, high serum hepatic transaminases.

INTERACTIONS. Interactions with dapsone are uncertain but combined therapy may be necessary.

AVAILABILITY[a]	TYPE	SIZES	PREPARATION (COMPANY)
Human	Oral capsules	50 mg, 100 mg	*Lamprene* (Geigy)

[a]Drug availability is becoming limited for general use in many countries. See Tables 50-4, 50-6, and 50-9. The "off label" use of clofazamine for other than leprosy is discouraged by the World Health Organizatin and Norvaritis. See www.fda.gov/cder/drug/shortages/lamprene_Doctor_ltr.pdf.

INTERNATIONAL PREPARATIONS. *Lampren.*

HANDLING. Store at room temperature in moisture-proof containers. Capsules contain micronized drug in an oil-wax base, making it difficult to give partial amounts. Clofazimine 'capsules' (which contain 50 mg of the dye) can be cut into halves using a scalpel blade while wearing disposable gloves and the 2 portions placed into gelatin capsules to facilitate dosing.

ADMINISTRATION. When given with food, absorption improved.

Dosage

INDICATIONS	DOSE	ROUTE	INTERVAL (hr)	DURATION (Weeks)
Dogs	4-8 mg/kg	PO	24	4
Cats	8 mg/kg	PO	24	4
	50 mg/cat	PO	24	4

ADDITIONAL DOSAGES. Mycobacterial infections, Tables 50-4 and 50-6.

DISPENSING INFORMATION. Administer with meals. Medicine may turn animal's skin pink and its excretions a brownish-black color.

CLOTRIMAZOLE

CLASS. Imidazole-antifungal.

ACTION. Fungistatic; inhibits ergosterol formation in fungal cell wall.

MORE INFORMATION. See ENILCONAZOLE; Topical Antifungal Therapy, Chapter 57, Aspergillosis, Chapter 64, and Candidiasis, Chapter 65, and Tables 57-4, 58-7, 64-3, and references Ch 64, ref. 29; Ch 57, ref. 34; 133.

PHARMACOKINETICS. Minimally (3%) not absorbed when used topically in mucosa and 0.5% through intact skin. Any absorbed is metabolized and excreted in bile with low concentrations of active drug and predominantly metabolites appearing in urine.

SPECTRUM. Dermatophytes, yeasts *(Candida, Malassezia)*, and *Aspergillus*.

INDICATIONS. Topically used to treat dermatophytosis, yeast-induced otitis externa, and nasal aspergillosis. Used as an intravesicular flush to treat refractory *Candida* urinary infections.

CONTRAINDICATIONS. Previous hypersensitivity, avoid ocular contact.

ADVERSE REACTIONS. Irritating, burning sensation, erythema, nasal discharge when used in nasal passages. Use of commercial preparations containing propylene glycol or isopropyl alcohol may cause severe airway obstruction. Clotrimazole may prolong barbiturate anesthesia.

AVAILABILITY	TYPE	SIZES	PREPARATIONS (COMPANY)
Human	Topical solution 1% (also cream, lotion)	10 ml, 30 ml	*Lotrimin* (Schering-Plough Animal Health), *Mycelex* (Miles)
	Vaginal tablets	100 mg, 500 mg	*Lotrimin*

INTERNATIONAL PREPARATIONS. *Antifungol, Candibene, Canesten, Trimysten.*

HANDLING. Flush for nasal aspergillosis: crush 1 g (two 500-mg tablets) of clotrimazole. Add to 100 ml of polyethylene glycol 400 (PEG-400) and stir on a hot plate until mixed. Keep suspension warm until used.

ADMINISTRATION. Intranasal: surgically place indwelling tubes in nasal passage and frontal sinuses, or alternatively (noninvasively) anesthetize animal and flush retrograde in nostrils. The surgical invasive technique has shown better clinical response than the noninvasive method. For more details on tube placements, see procedure under ENILCONAZOLE and in Chapter 64. The 1% clotrimazole is sufficiently viscous to pass through the tubes yet remain in the passages. Two 60-ml dose syringes containing the drug are attached to tubes. Initially 30 ml of the solution is flushed into each cavity. Then the remainder is flushed slowly over 60 min while the animal remains anesthetized (see Figure 64-5). **Topical:** apply to dermatophyte lesions twice daily for 3 to 4 weeks. **Bladder infusion:** In a dog, the 1% topical solution was infused via ultrasonographically-guided cystocentesis with no or minimal sedation, every other day for three treatments, then one last treatment 2 weeks after the first infusion. Ultrasound observation minimized the chance of extraluminal infusion. Bladder volume is estimated and approximately the same volume of clotrimazole is infused. If the bladder volume is ≥30 ml, then an amount is removed so that a maximum of 30 ml remains. Infusion is done slowly through a 22-gauge 1.5 inch needle attached to a stopcock and catheter extension tube. After the needle is removed the animal is monitored for 1 hr, the solution often remains in the bladder at least 5 min before it is voided by urination. (Ch 57, ref. 34) In a cat, the infusion was performed once weekly for 3 treatments (Ch 57, ref. 133).

ADDITIONAL DOSAGES. See Chapter 64 and Tables 85-6 and 85-8 for topical usages and formulations.

CLOXACILLIN

CLASS. Isoxazolyl penicillin.

ACTION. Bactericidal; inhibits bacterial cell wall synthesis.

MORE INFORMATION. See DICLOXACILLIN, OXACILLIN; Chapter 34, Penicillins; Table 34-1.

PHARMACOKINETICS. Only partially absorbed (40%-50%) from the GI tract after PO administration, and food reduces this further. Distributed to most tissues and body fluids with the exception of CNS and CSF. Metabolized by the liver to active and inactive moieties, predominantly excreted in the urine and minor amounts in bile and feces.

SPECTRUM. *Staphyloccocus,* including β-lactamase producers, other gram-positive aerobic cocci, some gram-positive anaerobes.

INDICATIONS. Staphylococcal infections, especially pyoderma in dogs.

CONTRAINDICATIONS. Hypersensitivity, hepatotoxicity.

ADVERSE REACTIONS. See OXACILLIN.

INTERACTIONS. See OXACILLIN.

AVAILABILITY	TYPE	SIZES	PREPARATIONS (COMPANY)
Human	Oral capsules (as sodium)	250 mg, 500 mg	*Cloxapen* (SmithKline Beecham), *Tegopen* (Bristol), generic (various)
	Oral powder (as sodium)	125 mg/5 ml	*Tegopen*

INTERNATIONAL PREPARATIONS. *Alclox, Anaclosil, Bactopen, Cloxypen, Ekvacillin, Orbenin, Rivoclox.*

HANDLING. Store oral powder and capsules at room temperature. Reconstituted oral solution is stable for 14 days if refrigerated, 3 days at room temperature.

ADMINISTRATION. Give without food.

Dosage

INDICATIONS (*Dogs and Cats*)	DOSE (mg/kg)	ROUTE	INTERVAL (hr)	DURATION (days)
Localized soft tissue infections, staphylococcal pyoderma, diskospondylitis, osteomyelitis	10-15	PO	6	14-84
Systemic infection, bacteremia	20-40	PO	6-8	7-14

ADDITIONAL DOSAGES. Musculoskeletal infections, Table 86-4.

DISPENSING INFORMATION. Give 1 hr before or 2 hr after feeding.

DAPSONE

CLASS. Sulfone, 4-4'-diaminodiphenylsulfone.

ACTION. Antimycobacterial, antiprotozoal. Analog of para-aminobenzoic acid, acts as folic acid synthesis inhibitor. Inhibits dihydropteroate synthetase.

MORE INFORMATION. See Chapter 34, Antituberculous Drugs, and Chapter 50.

PHARMACOKINETICS. Soluble at acidic gastric pH; however concomitantly administered alkalinizing drugs may paradoxically increase absorption. Well absorbed (70%-80%) from GI tract after PO administration. Enters all body tissues and fluids, being retained in skin, muscle, liver, and kidney. Achieves steady state after 1 week. Metabolized in liver and undergoes enterohepatic circulation. Metabolites are excreted in urine for an extended period after drug is stopped.

SPECTRUM. *Mycobacterium leprae, M. lepraemurium, Leishmania, Pneumocystis.*

INDICATIONS. Leprosy, leishmaniasis, *Pneumocystis* pneumonia. Has been used to prevent systemic toxoplasmosis in immunosuppressed people. Recommended in combination with trimethoprim for prophylaxis in pneumocystosis (Ch 68, ref. 29). Has some anti-inflammatory activity at therapeutic dosages.

APPROVED USES. Humans: leprosy and dermatitis herpetiformis.

CONTRAINDICATIONS. Previous hypersensitivity, anemia, pregnancy, lactation. Reduce dosage in renal failure.

ADVERSE REACTIONS. Dermatologic eruption, vomiting, diarrhea, anorexia, sulfone syndrome (dose-related hemolytic anemia, resulting from methemoglobinemia; especially with glucose-6-phosphate dehydrogenase deficiency), CNS signs, motor weakness, myelotoxicity with agranulocytosis, carcinogenic.

INTERACTIONS. Toxicity of dapsone and folate antagonists is increased when used in combination perhaps because of increased concentrations. Rifampin accelerates metabolism and removal of dapsone. Increased levels of both drugs occur when coadministered with trimethoprim. Dapsone should be combined with rifampin or clofazimine or another drug to treat mycobacterial infections and avoid resistance. It should be combined with pyrimethamine or trimethoprim to treat or prevent *Pneumocystis* pneumonia (Ch 68, ref. 29).

AVAILABILITY	TYPE	SIZES	PREPARATION (COMPANY)
Human	Oral tablets	25 mg, 100 mg	*Dapsone* (Jacobus)

INTERNATIONAL PREPARATIONS. *Aulosulfon, Disulone, Isoprodian, Maloprim.*

HANDLING. Tablets should be stored at room temperature away from light.

ADMINISTRATION. An oral suspension can be prepared by grinding tablets, putting in a sweet syrup, and adjusting pH to <5. Stable for 2 weeks if refrigerated. A proprietary liquid form is available (Jacobus) for investigational use.

Dosage

INDICATIONS (MYCOBACTERIOSIS)[a]	DOSE (mg/kg)	ROUTE	INTERVAL (hr)	DURATION (days)
Dogs				
Initial	1.1	PO	6	Until remission
Maintenance	0.3	PO	8-12	After recovery
Cats	8.0	PO	24	6 weeks

[a]Dose for pneumocystosis has not been determined for dogs or cats.

ADDITIONAL DOSAGES. None.

DISPENSING INFORMATION. Avoid prolonged exposure of treated animals to sunlight because photosensitivity may develop.

DECOQUINATE

CLASS. 4-hydroxyquinolone

ACTION. Antiprotozoal. Coccidiostatic drug. Interferes with life cycle of Apicomplexa protozoans. It acts by inhibiting electron transport in the parasite mitochondria, thus interfering with the development of sporozoite stages. Arrests development of *Hepatozoon* merozoites after release from meronts.

MORE INFORMATION. See Chapter 71, Antiprotozoal Drugs, and Chapter 74 (Hepatozoonosis); Reference Ch 71, ref. 54.

PHARMACOKINETICS. Not available.

SPECTRUM. Active against *Hepatozoon* spp, *Sarcocystis* spp, *Toxoplasma gondii, Neospora caninum.*

INDICATIONS. For the treatment of *Hepatozoon americanum* infection in dogs.

APPROVED USES. For use in coccidiosis affecting food-producing animals. Available is a powdered feed additive. Comes as a tan to brown powder composed of drug mixed with corn meal, soybean oil and lecithin.

CONTRAINDICATIONS. Vomiting or anorexia, since given as a food additive.

ADVERSE REACTIONS. The compound has been studied by the manufacturer in a variety of food-producing domestic animals. It has a wide margin of safety. Multiple studies in dogs including two year toxicity studies have shown no adverse effects on body functions including reproduction. No toxic effects were observed in dogs given 15 or 1000 mg/kg for 13 weeks; or 200 µg/g or 1000 µg/g in the diet for 2 yrs.

INTERACTIONS. None known, given with a variety of folate synthesis antagonists and clindamycin as combined therapy for Hepatozoonosis (see Chapter 74).

AVAILABILITY	TYPE	SIZES	PREPARATION (COMPANY)
Cattle, Sheep, Goats, Broiler Chickens	Powder 6%	27.2 gm active compound/lb	Deccox (Alpharma)

INTERNATIONAL PREPARATIONS. Same worldwide.

HANDLING. Powder is stable in the dry form at ambient temperature (25°C) with a 48-mo expiration. Powder is hydroscopic and should be stored in airtight containers.

ADMINISTRATION. Oral powder is mixed with food. Drug therapy must be given continuously on a daily basis to inhibit development of the protozoans. During treatment, organisms have been found to persist for up to 18 mo or more in some cases. It is likely that the infection is never eliminated in treated dogs.

Dosage

INDICATIONS	DOSE (mg/kg)	ROUTE	INTERVAL (hr)	DURATION (days)
Dogs				
Hepatozoonosis	10-20	PO	12	365 to 730[a]
Hepatozoonosis	50	PO	24	730

[a]Given initially with trimethoprim-sulfonamide, clindamycin and pyrimethamine for 14 days (see Table 74-2). Then decoquinate is continued alone. These three drugs are reinstituted if animal relapses. At the end of the treatment period, a muscle biopsy should be examined and if the parasite is eliminated, then therapy can be discontinued.

ADDITIONAL DOSAGES. Could be used at a shorter interval in dogs to control coccidiosis as in food-producing animals; however, not approved for this use.

DISPENSING INFORMATION. Mix measured amount of powder granules to food and twice each day.

DICLAZURIL

CLASS. Benzeneacetonitrile.

ACTION. Antiprotozoal, anticoccidial (coccidiostat).

MORE INFORMATION. Chapter 71. See also similar drugs, TOLTAZURIL and PONAZURIL.

SPECTRUM. Coccidia, *Hepatozoon*.

INDICATIONS. Coccidiosis. Has been used extralabel to treat *Sarcocystis neurona* infection in horses.

APPROVED USES. Coccidiosis in broiler chickens as a feed additive.

AVAILABILITY	TYPE	SIZES	PREPARATION (COMPANY)
Veterinary	Powder 0.5% (5 g/kg)	20 kg bag	Vecoxan, Clinicoxt (Janssen[a])

[a]Supplier in some countries is Pharmacia Upjohn or Schering Canada.

Dosage

INDICATIONS (*Dogs and Cats*)	DOSE (mg/kg)	ROUTE	INTERVAL (hr)	DURATION (days)
Coccidiosis	25	PO	24	1

ADDITIONAL DOSAGES. Coccidiosis, Table 81-2. Reference Ch 71, ref. 52.

DICLOXACILLIN

CLASS. Isoxazolyl penicillin.

ACTION. Bactericidal; inhibits bacterial cell wall synthesis.

MORE INFORMATION. See OXACILLIN, CLOXACILLIN; Chapter 34 and Table 34-1.

PHARMACOKINETICS. Similar in dogs and cats (Ch 34, ref. 95) Following IM dosing, concentrations >4 µg/ml in serum for at least 8 hr. IV levels peak higher but remain lower through duration of elimination. Peak levels and time duration is lower with PO administration. Partially absorbed (35%-70%) from GI tract after PO administration, which is reduced by ingesta. Well distributed to tissues and body fluids with exception of CNS and CSF. This relates to high degree of plasma protein binding (90%) in dogs.

SPECTRUM. *Staphylococcus*, including β-lactamase producers, other gram-positive aerobic cocci, some gram-positive anaerobes.

INDICATIONS. Staphylococcal infections, pyoderma.

CONTRAINDICATIONS. See OXACILLIN.

ADVERSE REACTIONS. See OXACILLIN.

INTERACTIONS. See OXACILLIN.

AVAILABILITY	TYPE	SIZES	PREPARATIONS (COMPANY)
Human	Oral capsules (as sodium)	125 mg, 250 mg, 500 mg	*Pathocil* (Wyeth), *Tegopen* (Bristol), generic (various)
	Oral powder for suspension (as sodium)	125 mg/5 ml	*Pathocil, Tegopen*

INTERNATIONAL PREPARATIONS. *Diclocil, Dicloxan, Diclocillin, Dynapen, Novapen.*

HANDLING. Store capsules and powder at controlled room temperature. Once reconstituted, oral solution is stable for 14 days when refrigerated, 7 days at room temperature.

ADMINISTRATION. Food interferes with absorption.

Dosage

INDICATIONS (*Dogs and Cats*)	DOSE (mg/kg)	ROUTE	INTERVAL (hr)	DURATION (days)
Localized soft tissue or skin infections caused by susceptible (non-β-lactamase producers) bacteria	25	PO	6	14-84
Problematic (resistant) staphylococci, systemic infections	25	IM, IV	6-8	prn

ADDITIONAL DOSAGES. None.

DISPENSING INFORMATION. Give at least 1 hr before or 2 hr after feeding. Store oral suspension in refrigerator.

DIETHYLCARBAMAZINE: SEE IMMUNOMODULATORS, CHAPTER 2.

DIFLOXACIN

CLASS. Fluoroquinolone.

ACTION. Bactericidal, inhibits bacterial DNA gyrase.

MORE INFORMATION. See ENROFLOXACIN, MARBOFLOXACIN, ORBIFLOXACIN; Chapter 34; Table 34-11.

PHARMACOKINETICS. Bioavailability exceeds 80%. Active drug comprises 90% of plasma levels following oral or IV administration. Low plasma protein binding of 46% to 52%. Readily diffuses into tissues. Lipophilic with most (80%) elimination in biliary tract as glucuronide and only 5% excreted in urine. Undergoes enterohepatic circulation. Does not accumulate when a 24-hr interval of administration is used.

BODY FLUID/TISSUE DISTRIBUTION IN DOGS. After a single dose of 10 mg/kg PO (expressed as µg/ml or µg/g).

BODY SYSTEM	2 HOURS (n = 2)	6 HOURS (n = 1)	24 HOURS (n – 1)
Hematopoietic			
Whole Blood	2.3	1.1	0.6
Plasma	2.6	1.2	0.8
Bone	6.5	7.2	6.5
Lymph Node	3.1	2.5	1.7
Liver	10.7	7.8	4.6
Spleen	3.5	1.1	1.1
Urogenital			
Urine[a]	22.6	21.0	10.7
Kidney	5.0	2.8	1.5
Bladder Wall	3.0	1.8	1.7
Testes	3.1	1.6	0.8
Prostate	3.4	1.5	1.4
Gastrointestinal			
Stomach	66.7	8.5	9.9
Small intestine	18.3	38.7	16.4
Cardiopulmonary			
Lung	3.2	0.9	0.8
Heart	3.8	1.6	1.1
Other Tissues			
Muscle	4.1	1.2	1.1
Fat	0.7	0.8	0.8

[a]Based on percent of dose with urine output at 50 ml/kg/day.

SPECTRUM. Gram positive: *Staphylococcus intermedius.* **Gram negative:** *Escherichia, Pasteurella, Enterobacter, Pseudomonas, Proteus, Klebsiella.* **Anaerobes:** Not effective. **Others:** *Mycoplasma, Chlamydia, Rickettsia,* some opportunistic mycobacteria. **Most Effective:** Anaerobic and facultative gram-negative organisms. Intermediate Effective: *Proteus* spp, *Staphylococcus* spp, *Streptococcus canis,* other streptococci. **Ineffective:** *Enterococcus, Actinomyces, Nocardia, M. avium-intracellulare, Leptospira, Ehrlichia,* and obligate anaerobes.

INDICATIONS. Skin, soft tissue, and acute uncomplicated urinary infections. Effective against many gram negative bacteria such as *E. coli* and *Staphyloccus* spp. Alternative to aminoglycosides in presence of renal failure or when oral therapy is desired. See also ENROFLOXACIN.

APPROVED USES. Skin, soft tissue, and urinary infections in dogs.

CONTRAINDICATIONS. Not for growing dogs or dogs with a history of seizures. Not for use in pregnant or lactating bitches or male stud dogs. See also ENROFLOXACIN.

ADVERSE REACTIONS. Generally self limiting, anorexia, vomiting, diarrhea, and anal irritation. See also ENROFLOXACIN. Transient erythema/edema on the facial area, diarrhea, decreased appetite have been seen, especially at higher than therapeutic dosages in dogs.

INTERACTIONS. See ENROFLOXACIN. Compounds (e.g. sucralfate, antacids) containing divalent and trivalent cations may interfere with the absorption of these drugs from the GI tract.

AVAILABILITY	TYPE	SIZES	PREPARATION (COMPANY)
Veterinary (dogs)	Oral tablets (as hydrochloride)	11.4 mg, 45.4 mg, 136 mg (USA) 15, 50, 150 mg (Europe)	*Dicural* (Fort Dodge)
	Solution	50 mg/ml (Europe)	

HANDLING. Store tablets between 15-25°C away from moisture.

ADMINISTRATION. See ENROFLOXACIN.

Dosage

INDICATIONS	DOSE (mg/kg)	ROUTE	INTERVAL (hr)	DURATION (days)
Skin and urinary infections	5	PO	24	Maximum 21 days[a]

[a]Give for 2 to 3 days beyond resolution of clinical signs to a maximum of 30 days.

ADDITIONAL DOSAGES. None.

DISPENSING INFORMATION. See ENROFLOXACIN.

DIIODOHYDROXYQUIN

(See IODOQUINOL)

CLASS. 8-hydroxyquinoline.

ACTION. Antiprotozoal.

MORE INFORMATION. See IODOQUINOL.

DIMINAZENE ACETURATE

CLASS. Aromatic diamidine.

ACTION. See PENTAMIDINE.

MORE INFORMATION. See PENTAMIDINE, IMIDOCARB, AMICARBALIDE; Chapter 71 and Table 71-1; references: Ch 71, ref. 19; 53; 68; 69; 71; 72; 62.

PHARMACOKINETICS. Not well absorbed orally. Rapid uptake after IV or IM administration, distributed extensively in tissues. Some hepatic metabolism with gradual urinary excretion of metabolites and active drug. Residues may persist for weeks in liver and kidneys, with lower amounts in GI tract, lungs, muscle, brain, fat, milk (Ch 71, ref. 69).

SPECTRUM. African *Trypanosoma, Babesia, Leishmania, Hepatozoon, Cytauxzoon;* some resistance may develop with repeated use.

INDICATIONS. African trypanosomiasis, babesiosis, cytauxzoonosis.

APPROVED USES. African trypanosomiasis in cattle.

CONTRAINDICATIONS. Pre-existing cardiomyopathy or heart failure.

ADVERSE REACTIONS. Vomiting may occur. Less likely to produce acute anaphylaxis than other drugs in this class.

Dosages up to 12 mg/kg are more effective in eliminating the organism but are more toxic. In general doses >10 mg/kg should be avoided. Like other diamidines may produce CNS signs, including behavioral changes, nystagmus, ataxia, extensor rigidity, opisthotonus, sometimes death. Although signs have been attributed to parasympathomimetic signs related to cholinesterase inhibition, this was not documented in treated dogs with babesiosis (Ch 71, ref. 62). Acute hemorrhagic gastroenteritis and cardiomyopathy have been reported. Delayed onset (1 week later) of CNS signs may relate to intracerebral killing of *Babesia.* Cats become anorectic, febrile, and depressed after initial treatment for *Cytauxzoon.* Hypotension occurs during treatment of canine babesiosis; however it does not develop as a direct effect of the drug in healthy dogs (Ch 71, ref. 40).

INTERACTIONS. For *T. congolense,* best response when combined with the experimental drug, difluoromethylornithine (DFMO), Hoechst Marion Roussel, Cincinnati, Ohio, (513)-948-7003 (Ch 71, ref. 68). Synergism against trypanosomes has also been observed with suramin. To prevent adverse reactions, antihistamines or nonsteroidal anti-inflammatory drugs (respectively, mepyramine maleate or piroxicam) have been used (Ch 71, ref. 72).

AVAILABILITY	TYPE	SIZES	PREPARATION (COMPANY)
Veterinary	Parenteral injection	Diluted to 70 mg/ml	*Berenil* (Bayer); not available in U.S.

INTERNATIONAL PREPARATIONS. *Azidine, Ganaseg, Ganasegur, Veriben.*

HANDLING. To ensure stability, should be kept refrigerated in sealed glass light-proof containers. At room temperature, solution is stable for at least 10-15 days. Lyophilized powder has an extended shelf-life for months at room temperature.

ADMINISTRATION. For *Babesia,* more effective treatment to eliminate resistant infections has been achieved by 3.5 mg/kg diminazene followed in 24 hr by 5 mg/kg imido-

carb (Ch 71, ref. 71). Trypanosomes may disappear from the blood within 24 hr of treatment, but hematologic changes take at least 3 weeks to correct. CBC should be performed weekly. May have to repeat as needed if parasitemia recurs. Some suggest one or two additional daily treatments for resistant infections, but toxicity increases. Has been used topically to treat cutaneous leishmaniasis. Cats become more depressed, febrile, and anorectic after one injection presumably related to parasite death. A second injection is given after these signs subside. Inflammatory reactions in muscles or skin, causing lameness or dermatitis, respectively, can be prevented by deep IM injection in lumbar muscles.

Dosage

INDICATIONS	DOSE (mg/kg)	ROUTE	INTERVAL (hr)	DURATION (days)
Dogs				
African trypanosomiasis (*T. brucei brucei, T. congolense*)	7.0	IM	24	1
Babesiosis				
Babesia canis	3.5-5.0	IM, SC	24	1
Babesia gibsoni	7.5-10	IM, SC	24	1
Cats				
Cytauxzoonosis	2.0	IM, SC	96	a

[a]A second dose is given at an interval of 72-96 hr after the first injection or when adverse signs of the first injection subside (Ch 76, ref. 14).

ADDITIONAL DOSAGES. African trypanosomiasis, Table 72-1; cytauxzoonosis, Table 76-1, babesiosis, Table 77-3.

DOXYCYCLINE

CLASS. Tetracycline.

ACTION. Bacteriostatic; inhibits bacterial protein synthesis by binding 3 ribosomal units.

MORE INFORMATION. MINOCYCLINE; TETRACYCLINE; Chapter 34; Table 34-7; references: Ch 34, ref. 309; 332.

PHARMACOKINETICS. In presence of food, 93% absorption of PO dose; blood concentration after PO dose is equivalent to IV dose. More lipid soluble (five times) than tetracycline, allowing better GI absorption and good penetration into most tissues and body fluids, including difficult areas such as prostate, female reproductive tract, eye, CNS, lung, sputum, bile. Persists in respiratory and prostatic secretions. Crosses placenta to accumulate in fetal bone, teeth and enters milk. Penetrates well into nasal sinuses. Extensively bound to plasma proteins (>90%) as compared to other tetracyclines, giving it half-life of 10 hr in dogs. Long half-life for a tetracycline, making once- or twice-daily dosing feasible. Primary elimination into digestive tract by nonbiliary secretion as inactive compounds with up to 90% eliminated in feces. Therefore, can be given without concern in animals with renal failure. Has some biliary elimination with enterohepatic circulation. Approximately 20% appears in urine via glomerular filtration. Higher plasma protein binding in cats makes it less well distributed, and plasma concentrations are approximately twice those of dogs given the same dose (Ch 34, ref. 310).

SPECTRUM. Gram positive: few *Streptococcus*, few *Staphylococcus*, *Nocardia*, *Listeria*, *Bacillus*. **Gram negative:** *Bartonella*, *Brucella*, *Francisella*, *Pasteurella*, *Campylobacter*, *Helicobacter*, *Yersinia*, *Enterobacter*, *Klebsiella*, *Bordetella*. **Anaerobes:** *Clostridium*, *Fusobacterium*, *Actinomyces*. **Others:** *Haemobartonella*, *Chlamydia*, *Mycoplasma*, *Rickettsiae* (*Coxiella*, *Rickettsia*, *Ehrlichia*), Spirochetes (*Leptospira*, *Borrelia*), opportunistic rapid-growing mycobacteria, *M. avium-intracellulare* complex, *Entamoeba*, *Balantidium*, Coccidia, *Toxoplasma*. **More effective:** *Borrelia*, *Rickettsia*, *Leptospira*. **Ineffective:** *Proteus*, *Enterobacter*, *Klebsiella*, *Escherichia*, *Pseudomonas*. Gram-negative bacteria frequently develop resistance. Cross-resistance between other tetracyclines occurs.

INDICATIONS. Acute urinary infections, chronic prostatitis, respiratory tract infections, nasal and sinus infections, periodontal disease, rickettsial diseases, borreliosis, chlamydial and mycoplasma infections, hemotropic mycoplasmosis (hemobartonellosis), tularemia, actinomycosis, nocardiosis, mycobacteriosis, canine ehrlichiosis, borreliosis, Rocky Mountain spotted fever, leptospirosis, bartonellosis, intestinal amebiasis. Combined with aminoglycosides in treatment of brucellosis. In leptospirosis, has been used to clear the carrier state. Reduces severity of articular cartilage breakdown in various animal models of noninfectious arthritis (Ch 34, ref. 42; 184), which questions the assumption that all doxycycline-responsive polyarthritis is infectious. Has been used in conjunction with niacinamide to treat immune mediated dermatoses such as pyogranulomatous dermatitis or pemphigus. It has been effective in treating lymphocytic/plasmacytic pododermatitis in cats.

CONTRAINDICATIONS. Pregnancy, (embryotoxic). Minimal dose adjustment needed with hepatic or renal failure. Unlike other tetracyclines, doxycycline does not accumulate in renal failure in dogs because it diffuses passively into the intestinal lumen (Ch 34, ref. 310). Therefore, it is the best tetracycline for use in an azotemic animal. Less of a problem with dental staining so can be used in younger (<6-mo old animals).

ADVERSE REACTIONS. Esophageal irritation and strictures (Ch 34, ref. 126a; 249; 254). Vomiting and GI irritation, especially from esophagitis, can be reduced by administering with food. Esophagitis and esophageal ulcers that form can be reduced by giving liquids or food after dosing and not giving to recumbent animals. May relate to formulation because capsules are more irritating than tablets or enteric coated preparations. The monohydrate salt is less acidic and ulcerogenic than the hydrochloride or hyclate formulations. Gastroenteritis can develop, especially in cats, but this drug is better tolerated than other tetracyclines in this species, causing less fever, anorexia, and vomiting compared with other tetracyclines. Because of more complete absorption, microfloral alterations and diarrhea are less frequent with other tetracyclines. Hypotension or vomiting may be observed with rapid IV infusion of doxycycline hyclate. Photosensitivity and skin eruptions may develop. Teeth and bone deposition and discoloration occur in young, but of all tetracyclines, doxycycline is least likely to have this effect (Ch 34, ref. 101). Diarrhea from enteric microbial alterations is less common than with tetracycline, presumably because of the better enteric absorption and lower dosage needed with doxycycline. Hepatotoxicity can occur in dogs and cats after oral or parenteral therapy. Dramatic increases in serum alanine transaminase and alkaline phosphatase are noted. Thrombocytopenia, neutropenia, and eosinophilia have been observed in people, and neutropenia has been observed in dogs.

INTERACTIONS. GI absorption reduced by divalent and trivalent cations as found in iron preparations, aluminum hydroxide gels, sodium bicarbonate, bismuth subsalicylate, calcium, and magnesium salts. Having a high lipid solubility, it has less affinity for calcium binding as do other tetracyclines. Ingesta has relatively little effect on GI absorption. Half-life of anticonvulsants (phenobarbital, diphenylhydantoin) may be reduced, and these drugs reduce doxycycline serum concentrations. Rifampin may also increase clearance, lowering doxycycline efficacy. Interferes with activity of aminoglycosides, cephalosporins, penicillins. Renal failure can develop owing to calcium oxalate nephrolithiasis after methoxyflurane anesthesia.

AVAILABILITY	TYPE	SIZES	PREPARATIONS (COMPANY)
Human	Oral capsules or tablets (hyclate)	50 mg, 100 mg	Doxychel (Rachelle), Vibramycin (Pfizer), generic (various)
	Oral syrup (calcium)	50 mg/5 ml	Vibramycin
	Powder for oral suspension (monohydrate)	25 mg/5 ml	Vibramycin
	Powder for injection (hyclate)	100 mg, 200 mg	Doxychel, Vibramycin IV
Veterinary	Gingival gel (topical 8.5%, for dogs)	Dispensing syringe	Doxirobe Gel (Pfizer)
	Oral tablets	20 mg, 100 mg	Ronaxan (Rhone Merieux)
	Oral tablets (monohydrate)	50, 100 mg	Vibravet (Pfizer)[a]
	Oral paste (monohydrate)	100 mg/g	Vibravet (Pfizer)[a]

[a]Not available in USA.

INTERNATIONAL PREPARATIONS. *Abadox, Biocyclin, Cyclidox, Diolan, Doxina, Doxydyn, Doxyhexal, Doxymycine, Dumoxin, Gewacyclin, Helvedoclyn, Ronaxan, Rudocycline, Unacil.*

HANDLING. Parenteral hyclate solution is reconstituted with sterile water. Compatible when diluted to 1 mg/ml in 0.9% NaCl, 5% dextrose, Ringer's, and lactated Ringer's. Solutions of infusion fluids are generally stable for at least 12 hr at room temperature to 72 hr if refrigerated. Incompatible with solutions containing lidocaine, penicillin G, and piperacillin-tazobactam. Store tablets and capsules at room temperature in airtight light-proof containers. After reconstitution, the PO suspension is stable at room temperature for 2 weeks. Oral gel should be stored in refrigerator (2-8°C).

ADMINISTRATION. Pareneral: This is the only tetracycline recommended for IV use, because it is less likely to cause thrombophlebitis or hepatic toxicity. For IV use, give as slow infusion over at least 1 hr in diluted form. Do not give IM or SC. **Oral:** Oral fluids, given at the time of medication, will propel the tablets or capsules into the stomach and reduce the effects of esophageal irritation and ulceration (Ch 34, ref. 415). Tablets or capsules can be crushed or opened and mixed with food. Must avoid liquids containing polyvalent cations, which affect absorption. If gastric irritation occurs, give medication with food or milk, because the latter does not affect absorption of doxycycline as much as with other tetracyclines. **Topical:** Teeth should be scaled prior to application. The product is applied under sedation or anesthesia. It is mixed and applied with a canula 1-2 mm below the gingival margin of each tooth. See package insert for complete directions.

Dosage

INDICATIONS[a]	DOSE	ROUTE	INTERVAL (hr)	DURATION (days)
Dogs				
Antiarthritic effect	3-4 mg/kg	PO	24	7-10[b]
General use for infection	3-5 mg/kg	PO	12	7-14
Soft tissue, urinary	4.4-11 mg/kg	PO, IV	12	7-14
Acute *E. canis* infection	5 mg/kg	PO	12	14
Acute *E. canis* infection	10 mg/kg	PO	24	16[c]
Chronic *E. canis* infection	10 mg/kg	PO	24	30-42[d]
Cats[e]				
Hemotropic mycoplasmosis	5-10 mg/kg	PO	24	14[f]
Bartonellosis	50 mg/cat	PO	12	14-28
Systemic infection, bacteremia	5-11 mg/kg	PO, IV	12	prn
Ehrlichiosis or Anaplasmosis	5-10 mg/kg	PO	12	21

[a]For topical use, see under Administration.
[b]Ch 34, ref. 42; 184.
[c]Dogs treated with acute monocytic ehrlichiosis were cleared as tested by PCR of splenic aspirates (Ch 34, ref. 152c)
[d]34:Ch 34, ref. 153 ; 152c.
[e]Because of esophageal irritation from doxycycline, the dosage should be rounded up so that whole capsules or tablets are given, especially to cats.
[f]Effective in reducing quantitative blood PCR gene copy level of *Mycoplasma haemofelis* in treated cats (Ch 34, ref. 365a).

ADDITIONAL DOSAGES. Canine infectious tracheobronchitis, Table 6-1; salmon poisoning, Table 27-2; ehrlichiosis, Table 28-4; Rocky Mountain spotted fever, Table 29-4; hemotropic mycoplasmosis, Table 31-3; canine brucellosis, Table 40-2; leptospirosis, Table 44-7; Lyme borreliosis, Table 45-5; mycobacterial infections, Tables 50-4, 50-7, and 50-9; feline abscesses, Table 52-3; feline bartonellosis, Table 54-3; hepatozoonosis, Table 74-2; babesiosis, Table 77-3; musculoskeletal infections, Tables 86-3 and 86-4; respiratory infections, Table 88-8; hepatobiliary disease, Table 90-5.

DISPENSING INFORMATION. May be given with food if necessary, especially to help reduce vomiting. Do not give with antacids, dairy products (less of a problem), iron supplements. To avoid esophageal irritation, tablets or capsules should not be broken or crushed and water should be given immediately after (by syringe if necessary) to flush the drug into the stomach.

DROTRECOGIN ALFA (RECOMBINANT HUMAN ACTIVATED PROTEIN C, RHAPC)

CLASS. Glycoprotein. Analog of native protein C synthesized and secreted by genetically altered human cells. Activated by thrombin in vitro.

ACTION. Inhibits coagulation, increases fibrinolysis, inhibits synthesis of tumor necrosis factor which has also been incriminated in the pathogenesis of sepsis.

MORE INFORMATION. Chapter 38, Endotoxemia.

PHARMACOKINETICS. In people, reaches a steady state 2 hr after starting an infusion. Is inactivated by plasma protease inhibitors. Drug cannot be detected after infusion is discontinued.

INDICATIONS. Adjunctive treatment of severe sepsis manifested by organ dysfunction.

APPROVED USES. People for treatment of septic shock.

CONTRAINDICATIONS. Patients with active or recent bleeding tendencies or with a risk of bleeding from trauma. Must be avoided where CNS lesions are present that may predispose to bleeding in neural parenchyma.

ADVERSE REACTIONS. GI and intraabdominal bleeding most frequent. Hemorrhage can occur in any other organ.

INTERACTIONS. Bleeding in people was not increased when low-dose SC heparin was used concurrently as prophylaxis for hypercoagulable states. Antibodies to human protein might be expected to develop with repeated use and these might interfere with subsequent effectiveness or produce allergic reactions.

AVAILABILITY	TYPE	SIZE	PREPARATION (COMPANY)
Human	Lyophilized for reconstitution	5- and 20-mg vials	*Xigris* (Lilly)

HANDLING. Once reconstituted, should be used within 12 hr.

ADMINISTRATION. Given as a continuous IV infusion. No change in dose or rate is needed for hepatic or renal failure.

Infusion should be discontinued at least 2 hr prior to surgery or invasive procedures. Can be restarted 12 hr after major surgery or immediately after minor procedures is hemostasis is achieved.

INDICATIONS (NEUTROPENIA)	DOSE[a] (µg/kg/hr)	ROUTE	INTERVAL (hr)	DURATION (hr)
Dogs and Cats				
Severe sepsis	24	IV	Continuous	96

[a]Human dosage regimen.

ADDITIONAL DOSAGES. Doses for dogs and cats have not been established.

DISPENSING INFORMATION. For use in hospitalized patients; coagulation parameters should be monitored during use.

ENDOTOXIN ANTISERA

CLASS. Immunogloblin.

ACTION. Neutralizes gram-negative endotoxin.

MORE INFORMATION. Chapters 8, 38, and 100; references: Ch 100, ref. 122; 429.

PHARMACOKINETICS. Enters systemic circulation at time of infusion.

SPECTRUM. *Salmonella typhimurium* endotoxin antiserum of equine origin.

INDICATIONS. Canine or feline parvoviral diarrhea with signs of bacterial sepsis, gram-negative bacterial infections with endotoxemia.

APPROVED USES. Gram-negative endotoxemia.

CONTRAINDICATIONS. Younger than 8 weeks of age, use only once.

ADVERSE REACTIONS. Anaphylactic reactions likely after repeated administration. If anaphylactoid reaction occurs, administer epinephrine. A second administration is not indicated because the course of illness is limited.

INTERACTIONS. For adjunctive therapy, see Table 38-8.

INDICATIONS. Canine or feline endotoxemia or parvoviral infections with associated endotoxemia.

AVAILABILITY	TYPE	SIZES	PREPARATION (COMPANY)
Veterinary	Equine-origin antisera	50-ml bottles	*SEPTI-serum* (Immvac)

HANDLING. If refrigerated, 36-mo shelf-life. Use or dispose of entire contents once opened.

ADMINISTRATION. Warm refrigerated solution to room (or preferably body) temperature before use. Given IV, diluted 1 : 1 with sterile isotonic saline or lactated Ringer's. Give only once over at least a 30-min period.

Dosage

INDICATIONS	DOSE	ROUTE	INTERVAL (hr)	DURATION (days)
Dogs and Cats	4-8 mg/kg	IV	Once	1

ADDITIONAL DOSAGES. None.

ENILCONAZOLE

CLASS. Triazole (a.k.a., imazalil, ISO 1750).

ACTION. Antifungal. See also KETOCONAZOLE.

MORE INFORMATION. See Chapters 57 and 65; Table 57-4; reference: Ch 57, ref. 118.

PHARMACOKINETICS. Not absorbed from the GI tract after PO administration. Only used topically and not absorbed, even where epithelium is damaged. Creates a vapor phase at the site of local application that may add residual activity.

SPECTRUM. *Microsporum, Trichophyton, Aspergillus, Mallassezia.*

INDICATIONS. Topical for dermatophytosis in dogs and for IN installation in dogs with nasal aspergillosis. Extralabel use with emulsion in treating feline dermatophytosis. For canine nasal aspergillosis, its use in daily nasal flushes via surgically implanted tubes for 14 days is effective.

APPROVED USES. Dermatophytosis in dogs.

CONTRAINDICATIONS. Not recommended for use in cats owing to potential toxicity; however topical use for dermato-phytosis in diluted formulations has been effective at the emulsion concentration of 0.2%.

ADVERSE REACTIONS. Systemic reactions in cats. Oral ingestion during administration can cause salivation, inappe-tence, weight loss, increased hepatic enzymes and itiopathic. However, with topical use, in one study, whole-body applica-tion twice weekly for 8 weeks in cats with dematophytosis failed to reveal any adverse reactions (Ch 57, ref. 26). In another study, Persian cats treated topically with 0.2% solu-tion every 3 days for a total of 8 treatments were monitored for 180 days. (Ch 57, ref. 56). Hypersalivation, idiopathic muscle weakness, and elevated serum ALT were noted. The cats improved clinically and became culture negative by day 28. By day 180 some of the cats developed lesions again and all were culture positive. In general, the solution was effective and well tolerated; however, other measures would be needed to prevent reinfections. The undiluted solution is irritating. However, when it is mixed with water as a diluted emulsion it is nonirritating to the skin or eyes or mucosae. With intranasal solution in conscious dogs with surgically implanted tubes, drooling, sneezing, head shaking may occur for 10-15 min with each flush.

AVAILABILITY	TYPE	SIZES	PREPARATIONS (COMPANY)
Veterinary	Topical solution (for ringworm in cattle, horses, and dogs)	100 mg/ml (10%)	*Imaverol* (Janssen);
	Disinfectant solution (for poultry hatcheries)	750 ml bottle (13.8%)	*Clinifarm EC, Clinifarm SG* (Schering-Plough)

HANDLING. Wear protective rubber gloves when working with solutions. For topical use on skin, the concentrated solution is diluted 1 : 50 with lukewarm water to produce 0.2% (2 mg/ml) emulsion. Higher concentrations diluted 1 : 10 (10 mg/ml) to a strength of 1%, or greater, are used for nasal lavage. Prepare emulsion immediately prior to use. Do not discharge any into streams or untreated water supplies. Store at room temperature protected from light for stability up to 5 yrs.

ADMINISTRATION. Dermatophytosis and dermatomyco-sis: remove crusts on diseased skin. As *Clinifarm EC* solution, dilutions of 50 : 1 with water to produce emulsion have been applied as a sponge dip for topical treatment of dermatophy-tosis, or cutaneous infections with *Malassezia* or *Candida* (Ch 57, ref. 27). For best results, shave long-haired dogs. Unless cats are long-haired with generalized lesions, clip only around visible lesions since shaving spreads fungus and abrades remaining skin. Burn all hair removed. Apply diluted emulsion 3-day intervals for four treatments. Cats can be treated without shaving but by brushing the emulsion through their haircoat. **Environmental control of dermatophytes:** A smoke generator (5 g enilconazole for 50 cubic meter room) or an emulsifiable concentrate (15% solution which is diluted 1 : 100 in tap water) can be used to smoke or spray respec-tively. **Aspergillosis surgical tube placement method:** under anesthesia, holes are drilled in the frontal sinuses and tubes inserted. Combine with turbinectomy initially or later if disease recurs. After anesthetic recovery, infuse 7-10 mg/kg of 10% solution (of *Imaverol*), diluted 50 : 50 with sterile water, through tubes twice daily for 10-14 days. **Nonsurgical method:** see Chapter 64 for tube placement. Various tech-niques have been described. In general, the dog, under general anesthesia, has its nasal passage lavaged with saline, and debris is removed, sometimes via endoscopy. The Foley catheters are positioned in the nasal passages or sinuses, sometimes via endoscopy. The nares and oropharynx are occluded to prevent leakage. The volume, which usually approaches 60-75 ml per nostril for larger breeds, is infused over 1 hr , while the animal is repositioned to bathe all nasal and sinus areas, before anesthetic recovery. **Results of nonsurgical method:** The nonsurgical method has been effective using clotrimazole in polyethylene glycol base (see Clotrimazole). However, treatment failure and mucosal irritation was observed with enilconazole when 1 : 10 diluted Imaverol solution, creating a 1% emulsion (10 mg/ml), was used as a one-hour nasal lavage as a single application under anesthesia (57:Bray et al 1998). These same animals responded to subsequent daily infusion of the same solution via implanted tubes. In a second study (Ch 64, ref. 163), dogs were treated with a nasal lavage under

anesthesia using 1% or 2% enilconazole emulsion (*Imaverol*) with reported success. Dogs having 2% emulsion lavage, followed by subsequent treatment with oral ketoconazole (10 mg/kg every 12 hr for 4-6 weeks), had a better response to treatment. In this study, tubes were endoscopically placed up dorsally in the frontal sinuses. In a third study (Ch 57, ref. 90), dogs were treated by topic intranasal lavage under a single anesthetic procedure using commercial grade enilconazole (*Clinifarm-EC*) diluted to 5% concentration (50 mg/ml) with sterile water. The tubes were placed endoscopically into the caudal nasal passage and the dogs were positioned in dorsal and then ventral recumbency during a 1-hr contact period of intranasal infusion. To minimize mucosal contact with this more concentrated enilconazole solution, cotton plugs were placed in the nares, gauze squares were packed around the endotracheal tube in the oropharynx, and accessible mucosal areas were coated with petrolatum.

Dosage

INDICATIONS	DOSE	ROUTE	INTERVAL (hr)	DURATION (days)
Dogs				
Nasal aspergillosis (*Imaverol*)	10 mg/kg (50 : 50 diluted)	Topically via indwelling tubes	12	7-14
Dermatomycosis (*Clinifarm EC*)	Volume varies (50 : 1 diluted)	Topically via dip, sponge bath or brushing	72-96	21-42[a]

[a]Minimum 21 days for *Malassezia* and 28-42 days for dermatophytes.

ADDITIONAL DOSAGES. Dermatophytosis, Table 58-7.

DISPENSING INFORMATION. Nasal flush: With indwelling tubes, dilute dispensed solution volume for each dose 50 : 50 with provided water immediately prior to use,

and infuse via syringe. **Emulsion:** For dip, emulsion is stable for 4-6 weeks once diluted, if it is protected from light. Manufacturer recommends preparation of a fresh dilution with each use.

ENROFLOXACIN

CLASS. Fluoroquinolone.

ACTION. Bactericidal; inhibits bacterial DNA gyrase.

MORE INFORMATION. See CIPROFLOXACIN, DIFLOXACIN, IBAFLOXACIN, MARBOFLOXACIN, ORBIFLOXACIN; Chapter 34; Table 34-11; references: Ch 34, ref. 3; 14; 15.

PHARMACOKINETICS. This concentration-dependent antimicrobial is well absorbed (80%-100%) from GI tract. Widely distributed in body tissues, including skeleton, CNS, CSF. Highest concentrations in liver, bile, kidney, genital tissues and secretions, urine (Ch 34, ref. 390). Penetrates and concentrates in macrophages, neutrophils. Carried to sites of inflammation and surrounding tissues and fluids. Concentrations in bone, lungs, prostate, kidneys are sufficient to affect aerobic and facultative gram-negative bacteria. Higher than serum concentrations in saliva, genital, nasal, and bronchial secretions. Adequate concentrations in CNS and CSF are only reached at higher doses or with inflamed meninges. Ciprofloxacin, the major metabolite of enrofloxacin, achieves prostatic concentrations 30 times that in blood (Ch 34, ref. 14). Ciprofloxacin also accumulates in leukocytes along with enrofloxacin. Leukocytes likely carry these drugs to sites of infection where the drug may be released after the cells die, or affect intracellular pathogens that survive phagocytosis. Compared with ciprofloxacin, tissue enrofloxacin concentrations are often higher than

in blood owing to less protein binding, high tissue penetration, extended serum half-life. Concentrations in skin exceed those in blood after several days of therapy and may be suitable to treat dermal staphylococcal isolates (Ch 34, ref. 353). Concentrations in inflamed skin (superficial and deep pyoderma) are greater than in healthy skin (Ch 34, ref. 93; 91). Predominate route of excretion in dogs is biliary (70%) via glucuronidation with subsequent enterohepatic circulation. The remainder (30%-40%) is excreted in the urine, with up to 50% unchanged (Ch 34, ref. 194). The remainder is metabolized to less active compounds and to active ciprofloxacin with biliary (fecal) and renal excretion (Ch 34, ref. 208). The amount of ciprofloxacin produced by metabolic elimination varies between and within animal species. Distribution in the body: enrofloxacin penetrates into all canine and feline tissues and body fluids. Concentrations of drug equal to or greater than the minimal inhibitory concentration (MIC) for many pathogens (see following table) are reached in most tissues by 2 hr after dosing at 2.5 mg/kg and are maintained for 8-12 hr after dosing. Particularly high levels of enrofloxacin are found in urine. A summary of the body fluid–tissue drug levels at 2-12 hr after oral dosing at 2.5 mg/kg and at 1-hr or greater intervals after 5 mg/kg is given in following table. High dose (20 mg/kg) IV data is also given for the dog. The drug levels are higher than indicated after multiple dosing as accumulation occurs.

Body Fluid–Tissue Distribution of Enrofloxacin (Post-Treatment) in Dogs and Cats for use with MIC Data from Isolated Organisms (Single Dose)[a]

	CANINE				FELINE		
	2 hr		8 hr				
Dose (mg/kg); Route Time After (hr)	2.5; PO 2	2.5; PO 8	5; PO (hr)	20; IV 2 (hr)	2.5; PO 2	2.5; PO 12	5; PO (hr)
Body Fluids (µg/ml)							
Bile	...	...	30 (1)	22.01	2.13	1.97	39 (1)
Cerebrospinal fluid	...	...	0.9 (1)	5.26	0.37	0.10	0.9 (1)
Urine	43.05	55.35	34.5 (6)	33.54	12.81	26.41	31 (1)
Eye fluids	0.53	0.66	...	2.55	0.45	0.65	...
Whole blood	1.01	0.36	...	...	...	...	...
Plasma	0.67	0.33	...	...	...	...	1.5 (1)
Serum	...	...	...	10.10 (0.5)	0.48	0.18	...
Tissues (µg/g)							
Hematopoietic System							
Liver	3.02	1.36	5.8 (1)	32.70	1.84	0.37	6.5 (1)
Spleen	1.45	0.85	2.8 (1)	21.20	1.33	0.52	3.0 (1)
Bone marrow	2.10	1.22	...	7.70	1.68	0.64	...
Lymph node	1.32	0.91	...	...	0.49	0.21	...
Urogenital System							
Kidney	1.87	0.99	3.5 (1)	24.98	1.43	0.37	5.4 (1)
Bladder wall	1.36	0.98	...	17.30	1.16	0.55	...
Testes	1.36	1.10	...	...	1.01	0.28	...
Prostate	1.36	2.20	4.4 (6)	23.54	1.88	0.55	...
Ovaries	...	...	...	...	0.78	0.56	...
Uterine wall	1.59	0.29	...	18.97	0.81	1.05	...
Gastrointestinal and Cardiopulmonary Systems							
Lung	1.34	0.82	2.5 (1)	18.66	0.91	0.33	4.5 (1)
—Epithelial lining fluid	...	...	4.79 (4)	...	...	...	...
—Alveolar macrophages	...	...	3.34 (4)	...	...	...	...
Heart	1.88	2.16	3.1 (1)	...	0.84	0.32	5.0 (1)
Stomach	3.24	1.11	...	45.32	3.26	0.27	...
Small intestine	2.10	...	...	...	2.72	0.40	...
Large intestine	...	...	...	...	...	...	...
Other							
Fat	0.52	0.40	1.4 (1)	2.26	0.24	0.11	1.3 (1)
Skin—Healthy	0.66	0.48	1.1 (3)	9.16	0.46	0.17	...
—Superficial Pyoderma	...	...	1.7 (3)	...	...	...	...
—Deep Pyoderma	...	...	3.38 (3)	...	...	...	...
Muscle	1.62	0.77	2.3 (1)	21.66	0.53	0.29	2.8 (1)
Brain	0.25	0.24	0.4 (1)	...	0.22	0.12	1.6 (1)
Mammary gland	0.45	0.21	...	...	0.36	0.30	...
Feces	1.65	9.97	...	...	0.37	4.18	...
Bone—Cortical	0.19	...	4.4 (2)	...	...	...	...

[a]This data does not take into account the amount of the active metabolite ciprofloxacin, which comprises an additional amount of antimicrobial activity. Data provided by product insert for enrofloacin and references Ch 34, ref. 262; 308; 250; 194; 38; 93; 91; 157.

SPECTRUM. Gram positive: *Staphylococcus*, variable *Streptococcus*. **Gram negative:** *Brucella, Pasteurella, Escherichia, Aeromonas, Proteus, Shigella, Salmonella,* and other enteropathogens such as *Campylobacter, Yersinia,* and some *Pseudomonas*. In vivo resistance noted with *Clostridium* spp., *Bacteroides* spp. **Others:** *Mycoplasma, Chlamydia, Rickettsia, Haemobartonella,* some slow-growing, opportunistic mycobacteria (see Chapter 50). **More effective:** aerobic and facultative gram-negative organisms. **Ineffective:** *Enterococcus, Actino-myces, Nocardia, Mycobacterium avium-intracellulare* complex, *Leptospira, Ehrlichia,* and obligate anaerobes. Resistance can develop by chromosomal mutation, although plasmid-mediated resistance does not occur. Resistance is more common with some organisms such as *Pseudomonas aeruginosa, Escherichia coli* and *Staphylococcus aureus.* An increase in the number of enrofloxacin-resistant *E. coli* urinary tract infections has been observed in dogs (Ch 34, ref. 76).

INDICATIONS. Complicated or recurrent urinary tract infections caused by more resistant gram-negative bacteria; prostatitis. Good alternative to aminoglycosides in presence of renal dysfunction. Respiratory infections from resistant gram-negative bacteria (often nosocomial). Osteomyelitis and joint infections because quinolones have good penetration and safety for long-term use in gram-negative infections. With staphylococcal osteomyelitis, additions of rifampin may assist. Complicated SC infections caused by *Staphylococcus*, gram negatives, or opportunistic mycobacteria. Always use in combination for treating brucellosis. For severe otitis externa caused by *Pseudomonas*. For enteropathogenic bacterial gastroenteritis (e.g., salmonellosis or campylobacteriosis; see Chapter 39) (Ch 34, ref. 324). GI infections caused by gram-negative bacteria, urinary tract infections, respiratory tract infections, infections of skin, eyes, and joints (Ch 34, ref. 324) and canine bacterial pyoderma (Ch 34, ref. 176; 293). Beneficial responses have been found in dogs treated with histiocytic ulcerative colitis (Ch 89, ref. 131). Can be used topically (see Handling) for resistant gram-negative otitis externa to avoid aminoglycoside toxicity. Fluoroquinolones in combination have been shown to improve in vivo efficacy of some antifungal azoles.

CONTRAINDICATIONS. During a rapid growth period, young animals should not receive the drug because of the potential of cartilaginous injury. Avoid in small- and medium-breed dogs (>8 mo), large breeds (<12 mo), and giant breeds (<18 mo), and cats younger than 8 weeks. Some reduction in dosage is advised for marked renal failure, but hepatic elimination should compensate in minor renal dysfunction. Caution is advised with quinolones in pregnant animals, although side effects are not documented. Dosages of 15 mg/kg to males and to females of various stages of gestation and during lactation had no adverse effects. Animals being treated must always be adequately hydrated. Use cautiously in animals with seizure histories.

ADVERSE REACTIONS. Vomiting when IM solution is given IV. Intravascular hemolysis has been observed in some cats given parenteral solution IM or undiluted parenteral solution IV. Diarrhea and depression are occasionally seen in dogs (Ch 34, ref. 209), especially with higher dosages. Neurotoxicity or seizures at very high (supratherapeutic) IV dosages or with rapid IV infusion. In animals with seizure history, causes increase in the frequency and intensity of seizures in phenobarbital-treated dogs (Ch 34, ref. 390). Cats receiving 50 mg/kg have had neurologic signs, and some dogs receiving 10 mg/kg enrofloxacin have had seizures. Enrofloxacin, as other quinolones, has the potential to produce retinotoxicity as evidenced by mydriasis, blindness, increased tapetal hyperreflectivity and attenuated retinal vasculature. Cats receiving higher than 5 mg/kg/day or treated with parenteral drug at these levels may develop irreversible damage to their photoreceptor cells (Ch 34, ref. 420). Nonsteroidal antiinflammatory drugs (e.g., fenbufen) may accentuate this problem. Occasional anorexia, vomiting, or diarrhea, especially with higher dosages. Cartilaginous damage to weight-bearing joints of immature growing dogs and cats. IM and SC injections are painful. Focal alopecia may occur over sites of SC injection. Efficacy in treating urinary tract infections can be enhanced by raising the urine pH with bicarbonate, but this may favor nephrotoxicity from renal tubular crystalluria. Because of the potential for renal dysfunction with overdosages, hydration should be maintained. Dogs given 5 mg/kg enrofloxacin IM for 14 days developed increased MCV and serum activity of AST, and increased bilirubin and sodium concentrations (Ch 34, ref. 378). Decreases were observed in serum potassium, bicarbonate, and blood pH and a resultant metabolic acidosis. Generally these biochemical changes were mild. Streptococcal superinfection with necrotizing fasciitis has been observed in dogs receiving prior treatment with enrofloxacin (see Chapter 35). Very high supratherapeutic doses (125 mg/kg PO) have been given to dogs and cats in early toxicity studies. Animals showed vomiting, anorexia, depression, locomotor difficulties, and death. For additional information concerning adverse reactions to quinolones, see section on their toxicity, Chapter 34.

INTERACTIONS. Additive antibacterial effects with doxycycline, minocycline, or aminoglycosides for brucellosis. For nocardiosis, leprosy or opportunistic mycobacteriosis, it may be synergistic with doxycycline, dapsone or clofazimine. The coadministration of clindamycin or amoxicillin with quinolones results in increased serum bactericidal activity against gram-positive bacteria. Use of metronidazole, b-lactams, aminoglycosides, or clindamycin may extend the antimicrobial spectrum while not affecting the pharmacokinetics of quinolones (Ch 34, ref. 31). Reduced GI absorption caused by preparations containing polyvalent cations (Al, Mg, Ca, Fe, Zn). Antacids containing these and sucralfate given within 24 hr can interfere with absorption (Ch 34, ref. 295). Concurrent cimetidine can delay quinolone elimination. May interfere with theophylline elimination, producing CNS stimulation. Enrofloxacin may reduce serum levels of anticonvulsants such as phenytoin. Nephrotoxic effect of cyclosporine may be increased when co-administered with enrofloxacin. May potentiate effects of vitamin K antagonist rodenticides. The effectiveness of quinolones on some bacteria may be reduced by microbial protein-synthesis inhibitors such as chloramphenicol, nitrofurans, rifampin, and erythromycin. Enrofloxacin and digoxin do not alter either drug's metabolism when coadministered to dogs (Ch 34, ref. 279). Antineoplastic agents may reduce serum concentrations of enrofloxacin. Enrofloxacin interferes with some glucose test measurements, resulting in underestimated concentrations of urine glucose. Caution must be used when using urine as a basis for monitoring diabetic dogs (Ch 34, ref. 306c).

AVAILABILITY	TYPE	SIZES	PREPARATIONS (COMPANY)
Veterinary	Tablets	5.7 mg, 22.7 mg, 68 mg, 136 mg	*Baytril* (Bayer)
	Chewable (Taste®) Tablets		
	Parenteral solution for IM use	22.7 mg/ml	*Baytril*

HANDLING. Parenteral solution and oral tablets should be stored away from direct sunlight, at room temperature, and never frozen. For topical otic preparation, take one 22.7-mg tablet and crush it with a mortar and pestle. Add powder to petrolatum and mix well with tongue depressor. Place mixture in syringe and administer in ear canals at least once daily. Person administering drug should avoid contact with hands and skin. If contact with eyes occurs, they should be rinsed with copious amounts of water. Skin should be cleansed with soap and water. Alternatively, a 3 mg/ml topical solution can be prepared by taking 4 ml of 20 mg/ml enrofloxacin injection solution and mixing it with 24 ml of sterile normal saline. This solution is stored in a dropper bottle at room temperature (Ch 85, ref. 42).

ADMINISTRATION. Never crush nonchewable tablets because the active ingredient is bitter. Always pill animals using this preparation. With chewables, these may be hand fed or mixed in food. Allow 4-6 hr prior to, and at least 2 hr after, quinolone administration when giving antacid, multivalent cation-containing preparations, or sucralfate. Ingesta may

delay absorption slightly, but may prevent vomiting that occasionally occurs. Preferably, administer on empty stomach. The manufacturer's suggested maximum duration of treatment was 10 days; however, this has been extended to 30 days. An IV preparation is not available; however, some have given the IM solution IV. Dilute 1 part parenteral solution to 3 to 9 parts sterile water or normal saline before IV infusion and give it over 10-30 min. May precipitate in alkaline or balanced electrolyte solutions. Can give in combination with doxycycline, minocyclines, aminoglycosides, or rifampin to improve efficacy in treating certain persistent intracellular bacterial infections.

Dosage

INFECTION WITH SUSCEPTIBLE ORGANISMS INDICATIONS/SITE (FOR SPECIES)	DOSE	ROUTE	INTERVAL (hr)	DURATION (days)
Urinary, respiratory, soft tissue infections (*cats*)[a]	5 mg/kg	PO	24	7-14
Mycoplasma haemofelis infection (*cats*)	5-10 mg/kg	PO	24	14[b]
Skin, urinary infections (*dogs*)	2.5-5 mg/kg	PO	12	7-14
Deep pyodermas, complicated urinary (*dogs*)	5 mg/kg	PO	24	7-14[c]
Lower respiratory infections (*dogs*)	5-10 mg/kg	PO	24	7-84
Prostate infections	5 mg/kg	PO	12	7-14
Histiocytic ulcerative colitis (*dogs*)	5 mg/kg	PO	12	21-90[d]
Hemotropic mycoplasmosis (*dogs*)	5 mg/kg	PO, IM	12	7-14
Systemic, orthopedic infections (*dogs*)	5-11 mg/kg	PO, IM, IV, SC	12	10
Pseudomonas in soft tissues (*dogs*)	11 mg/kg	PO, IM, SC	12	7-14[e]
	20 mg/kg	PO, IM, SC	12	prn[f]
Bacteremia, sepsis (*dogs*)	11 mg/kg	PO, IM, IV, SC	12	prn

[a]Due to potential retinotoxicity, the manufacturer recommends this maximum daily dose of 5 mg/kg.
[b]Dose of 10 mg/kg was more effective than 5 mg/kg and similar in efficacy to doxycycline; care must be taken if drug is used for this infection because this higher than recommended dosage has the risk of causing retinotoxicity (Ch 34, ref. 105; 365a).
[c]10 to 12 weeks of therapy is required in pyoderma, especially in German shepherds (Ch 34, ref. 178).
[d]Ch 34, ref. 131.
[e]Up to 12 weeks with malignant otitis externa caused by *Pseudomonas*. Dosage from Ch 85, ref. 121.
[f]Ch 85, ref. 42.

FLEXIBLE DOSAGES. Enrofloxacin was originally licensed for use in the United States at a dose of 2.5-5.0 mg/kg, given every 12 hr. Now it has been approved with professional label flexible dosage ranges for up to 24-hr intervals, based upon knowledge of the drug pharmacodynamics, its achievable concentrations at the site of infection, properties of the infecting organism, and host factors. The 24-hr dosage range is 5-20 mg/kg and a rough guideline is presented in the preceding table. The low end of the dosage regimen is generally sufficient for infections caused by susceptible organisms in tissues or fluids where sufficient concentrations can be effectively reached. The high end should only be used to treat highly resistant organisms (MIC $\geq$2 µg/ml) or those such as *Pseudomonas aeruginosa*, *Staphylococcus aureus*, and *Escherichia coli* which have shown tendencies to develop resistance. In general the achievable concentration in the desired tissue or body fluid should be at least 2 to 8 times the MIC$_{90}$ of the offending pathogen. The recommendations for maximum length of use of this drug have been extended to 30 days.

ADDITIONAL DOSAGES. Rocky Mountain spotted fever, Table 29-4; gram-negative infections, Table 37-3; endotoxemia, Table 38-6; enteric pathogenic bacteria, Table 39-2; mycobacteria, Tables 50-4 and 50-9; cytauxzoonosis, Table 76-1; canine pyoderma, Table 85-3; musculoskeletal infections, Table 86-4; bacteremia, endocarditis, Table 87-6; respiratory disease, Table 88-8; oral infections, Table 89-4; gastrointestinal infections, Table 89-16; intraabdominal infections, Table 89-21; hepatobiliary infections, Table 90-5; urinary infections, Table 91-10. This drug accumulates in animals with decreased renal or hepatic function; therefore a reduction in dosage may be necessary.

DISPENSING INFORMATION. Give medication without feeding, unless vomiting occurs. Never give antacids or GI protectants within 2 hr of medication. Always be certain pet has plenty of fresh water to drink.

ERTAPENEM

CLASS. Ertapenem is a β-lactam of the carbapenem group. As with meropenem, another newer carbapenem of this group, it does not require cilastatin coadministration.

ACTION. Bactericidal; ertapenem inhibits synthesis of bacterial cell wall peptidoglycan. As other carbapenems, this drug is relatively resistant to hydrolysis by β-lactamases.

MORE INFORMATION. See Chapter 34.

PHARMACOKINETICS. Poorly absorbed from GI tract, but good systemic availability if given parenterally. It is highly protein bound and as a result has a longer half life in serum in people compared to imipenem and meropenem. This allows for once a day dosing. In people, it is partly metabolized by the liver; however, 80% is excreted by the kidney with 38% as unchanged drug. Approximately 10% appears in the feces.

SPECTRUM. Narrower spectrum than other members of this class, see Imipenem. Resistant to most bacterial β-lactamases. In vitro, ertapenem is more active against anaerobes, and is more active than imipenem against Enterobacteriaceae. It has similar activity as do the other carbapenems against gram-positive organisms; however, it has little or no activity against *Pseudomonas aerugiosa* or *Acinetobacter* spp. Methicillin-resistant staphylococci and enterococci, and β-lactamase-resistant streptococci are usually resistant to ertapenem.

INDICATIONS. For treatment of organisms resistant to other antibiotics and for mixed infections that require a broad spectrum including anaerobes. For treatment of intraabdominal, skin and soft tissue, lower respiratory, urinary, and pelvic infections. See Imipemen for more specific indications.

APPROVED USES. Serious and multiple-resistant bacterial infections when a single agent is needed.

CONTRAINDICATIONS. The dosage should be reduced in renal failure. Dosage adjustments are not likely with hepatic impairment. Cross-hypersensitivity to other β–lactams. No complications have been observed in human or animal pregnancy; however, only clear indications should permit its use during this period.

ADVERSE REACTIONS. Diarrhea, vomiting, increased hepatic aminotransferase activities, and thrombophlebitis. Allergic reactions to vehicle, treat as anaphylaxis. All β-lactams can cause seizures if underlying brain disease or if overdosed related to body size and renal function. As with other β–lactams, monitor renal, hepatic, and hematopoietic systems during treatment. Neutropenia was consistently observed in treated rats; however, studies in rabbits and monkeys were inconclusive. The IM product contains lidocaine hydrochloride, which is contraindicated with known hypersensitivity, with shock, or heart block.

INTERACTIONS. Antagonistic interaction may reduce effectiveness of this drug coadministered with other β-lactam drugs. Addition of aminoglycosides or trimethoprim-sulfonamide may be synergistic against certain organisms.

AVAILABILITY	TYPE	SIZES	PREPARATIONS (COMPANY)
Human	Powder for injection	1 g vial for IV	*Invanz* (Merck)

INTERNATIONAL PREPARATIONS. *Same.*

HANDLING. Supplied as a powder, soluble in water and 0.9% NaCl. Never store powder above 25°C For IM use, the drug is reconstituted with 3.2 ml of 1% lidocaine HCl (without epinephrine). This should never be given IV. For IV injection, the powder is added to 10 ml 0.9% NaCl or bacteriostatic water for injection. The drug should not be mixed with other medications and dextrose-containing solutions should never be used as diluents. Reconstituted solutions can be used within 6 hr at 25°C or 24 hr at 5°C. Solutions should be used within 4 hr after removal from refrigeration and never frozen.

ADMINISTRATION. For IM, use a 21-gauge needle and deep injection. Aspirate before injection to avoid inadvertent IV administration.

Dosage

INDICATIONS (*Human*)[a]	DOSE	ROUTE	INTERVAL (hr)	DURATION (days)
Bacteremia/sepsis	1 g	IV, IM	24	prn

[a]This is a dose for adult people; no studies are available for other age or for gender, and none exist for dogs or cats.

ADDITIONAL DOSAGES. None.

ERYTHROMYCIN

CLASS. Macrolide.

ACTION. Bacteriostatic; binds to 50s ribosomes of bacteria-inhibiting protein synthesis.

MORE INFORMATION. AZITHROMYCIN, CLARITHROMYCIN, ROXITHROMYCIN; Chapter 34, Macrolides; Table 34-8.

PHARMACOKINETICS. Several oral formulations exist. The degree of absorption from the GI tract depends on the formulation, gastric pH, presence of ingesta (see Table 34-8). Erythromycin is absorbed in the proximal small intestine and must withstand effects of gastric acid. Estolate and ethylsuccinate compounds resist degradation in the stomach and release free base for absorption in duodenum. Estolate is better absorbed than ethylsuccinate. Enteric-coated tablets required for free base and stearate formulations to prevent gastric acid inactivation. Unlike estolate and ethylsuccinate esters, absorption of the base and stearate are reduced by ingesta. Absorption of coated base tablets is less affected by food than stearate. Enteric-coated pellets are better absorbed than tablets. Well distributed to most body tissues, especially skin and respiratory tract, enters pleural and ascitic fluids, respiratory secretions but only the inflamed meninges. Enters the prostate and concentrates in leukocytes. Primarily eliminated by hepatic metabolism and biliary excretion. Does not achieve high enough levels in urine for likely therapeutic efficacy (4% of oral and 15% of parenteral dose). Bioavailability is lower by SC (40%) than IM (65%) routes.

SPECTRUM. Gram positive: *Staphylococcus, Streptococcus, Corynebacterium, Listeria, Erysipelothrix, Bacillus.* Predominantly for gram-positive infections. **Gram negative:** *Pasteurella, Campylobacter, Bordetella, Legionella.* Not for most gram-negative infections. Cross-resistance can occur with other macrolides and lincosamides. **Anaerobes:** *Fusobacterium, Clostridium* (limited activity). **Others:** *Chlamydia, Mycoplasma* (susceptibility varies), *Borrelia, Leptospira;* protozoa, e.g., amebae. **More effective:** *Campylobacter, Legionella, Mycoplasma.* **Ineffective:** most Enterobacteriaceae.

INDICATIONS. Gram-positive infections involving the GI tract, skin, respiratory tract, soft tissue infections as an alternative to β-lactams (e.g., penicillins, first-generation cephalosporins) when hypersensitivity exists. Campylobacteriosis.

CONTRAINDICATIONS. Previous hypersensitivity, preexisting hepatic dysfunction, reduce dose in severe liver diseases, minimal dosage adjustment in renal failure.

ADVERSE REACTIONS. Vomiting–specific cholinergic effect. Abdominal discomfort or GI irritability–anorexia, vomiting, diarrhea. Can occur with parenteral preparations because of excretion in the bile. Thrombophlebitis with IV; pain on IM injection; rare ototoxicity; and hepatotoxicity (cholestatic hepatitis). The latter syndrome can be reduced in frequency of occurrence by shorter treatment regimens.

INTERACTIONS. Chloramphenicol and lincosamides (lincomycin, clindamycin) have similar action and should not be used in combination. Increases cyclosporin concentrations with resultant nephrotoxicity. Increases blood digoxin, methylprednisolone, theophylline concentrations, and other hepatic metabolized drugs as a result of cytochrome P-450 interactions.

AVAILABILITY	TYPE	SIZES	PREPARATIONS (COMPANY)
Human	Base oral tablets, enteric coated	250 mg, 333 mg, 500 mg	*E-mycin* (Pharmacia & Upjohn), *Ilotycin* (Dista)
	Estolate oral tablets	500 mg	*Ilosone* (Dista)
	Oral capsules, chewable tablets	125 mg, 250 mg	*Ilosone*
	Oral suspension	125 mg/5 ml, 250 mg/5 ml	*Ilosone*
	Stearate oral tablets, enteric coated	250 mg, 500 mg	*Erpar* (Parke-Davis), *Erythril* (E.R. Squibb), generic (various)
	Ethylsuccinate		
	Oral tablets	200 mg (125 mg base), 400 mg (250 mg base)	E.E.S generic (various), *E-Mycin E* (Pharmacia & Upjohn)
	Oral suspension or powder for suspension	100 mg/5 ml, 62.5 mg/5 ml, 200 mg/5 ml (125 mg/5 ml base), 400 (250 mg/5 ml base)	*Eryped* (Abbott), *Pediamycin* (Ross)
	Gluceptate IV solution	250 mg, 500 mg, 1 g	*Ilotycin Gluceptate* (Dista)
	Lactobionate IV infusion	500 mg, 1 g	*Erythrocin Lactobionate-IV* (Abbott)
Veterinary	Polyethylene injectable solution	100 mg/ml, 200 mg/ml	*Erythro* (Sanofi) *Erythromycin-200* (RXV)

INTERNATIONAL PREPARATIONS. *Abboticine, Aknemycin, Betamycin, Cusimicina, Doranol, Eboren, Erycinum, Erythromid, Erytran, Erytrocina, Meromycin, Primacine, Stiemycin.*

HANDLING. Lactobionate is stable at room temperature in dry form. Parenteral solutions are stable at room temperature. Cold temperature may cause solidification, which can be reversed by immersion in warm water for 15-20 min. Once reconstituted the lactobionate is stable for 24 hr and 2 weeks, and the gluceptate for 24 hr and 1 week, at room and refrigerated temperatures, respectively. Erythromycin solutions are more unstable at acid pH (4.0-6.0). Oral suspensions (estolate, ethylsuccinate) should be refrigerated and generally have 14-day stability.

ADMINISTRATION. Given PO, administer on an empty stomach (base and stearate forms) unless GI upset occurs, then take with food. Estolate, ethylsuccinate, and enteric-coated forms can be taken with food. Capsules containing enteric-coated pellets *ERYC* (Parke-Davis) can be opened and sprinkled on food. Ethylsuccinate is nonirritating, tasteless, and suitable as a PO preparation for puppies and kittens. Dilute IV solutions given over 20-60 min. Give slowly IV by intermittent or continuous infusion using concentrations diluted to 1 to 5 mg/ml. IV route is preferred for very ill animals or those with GI signs. If given IM, must be deep into large muscles. IM preparations contain lidocaine. Should not be given SC or IP.

Dosage

INDICATIONS (*Dogs and Cats*)	DOSE (mg/kg)	ROUTE	INTERVAL (hr)	DURATION (days)
Localized, soft tissue infections	15-25	PO	12	7-10
Localized, soft tissue infections	10-15	PO	8	7-10
Systemic, bacteremia infections	22	PO, IV	8	prn

ADDITIONAL DOSAGES. Streptococcal infections, Table 35-2; *Rhodococcus* infection, Table 35-7; enteric bacterial infections, Table 39-2; actinomycosis, Table 49-2; nocardiosis, Table 49-3; canine pyoderma, Table 85-3; gastrointestinal infections, Table 89-16.

DISPENSING INFORMATION. May cause GI irritation and resultant vomiting and diarrhea. If so, give first few doses with food to reduce irritation but then give to fasted animal.

ERYTHROPOIETIN (RHUEPO, EPO)

CLASS. Cytokine. Synthetic human recombinant protein.

ACTION. This substance naturally produced by the kidney and activated by the liver, stimulates erythroid progenitors in bone marrow. Increases blood hematocrit in clinically healthy or anemic animals, predominantly with an anemia caused by renal failure. It also stimulates megakaropoiesis and thrombopoiesis. The effect may take 2-8 weeks.

MORE INFORMATION. Chapters 2 and 58 references: Ch 2, ref. 37; 37a; 124a.

PHARMACOKINETICS. The drug must be given parenterally as it is not absorbed after oral administration. Its pharmacokinetic data is uncertain; however, elimination is prolonged in people with chronic renal failure. As a human recombinant product, anti-EPO antibodies may develop in 25%-30% of treated animals after use for 6 mo to 1 yr. These antibodies bind to native EPO and recombinant EPO nullifying their actions resulting in non regenerative anemia. Antibodies usually disappear after discontinuation of treatment. The drug may cross the placenta and adversely affect the fetus.

INDICATIONS. For anemia of chronic renal failure. This drug has been used in FIV- or FeLV-infected cats in an attempt to stimulate production of erythrocytes; however, its effects in this regard have generally been disappointing. See Chapter 2 for details on studies involving this drug.

APPROVED USES. People for treatment of anemia associated with chronic renal failure.

CONTRAINDICATIONS. Pregnancy. Development of refractory anemia while being treated with this drug suggests development of antibodies. Under such conditions, a bone marrow examination will reveal suppressed erythrogenesis compared to myelogenesis and the drug should be discontinued.

ADVERSE REACTIONS. Systemic hypertension, seizures and iron depletion occur and result from increased erythrocyte mass.

INTERACTIONS. May have compounding of effects if given concurrently with androgenic hormones.

AVAILABILITY	TYPE	SIZE	PREPARATION (COMPANY)
Human	Solution for injection	2000-40,000 units in 1- to 2-ml vials	*Epogen* (Amgen) *Procrit* (Ortho Biotech)

HANDLING. The solution for injection is stored at refrigerator (4°C) temperature. The vial should not be frozen or exposed to sunlight. Sodium chloride, citrate buffers, and albumin are added to the solution for stability which is 2 yrs with proper storage.

ADMINISTRATION. The drug is given SC on a 3 times weekly basis until the hematocrit is achieved and then dosages are adjusted as needed on a not less than 3-week interval to allow time for dosage adjustments to have effects. The hematocrit and blood pressure must be monitored on a continual basis to avoid anemia or hypertension as potential side-effects. Iron supplementation should be adequate to maintain levels needed for regeneration. If beneficial effects are not noticed after the first month of instituting this therapy then it may not be effective. If the hematocrit increases but later decreases, then formation of antibodies can be suspected. In this case treatment should be discontinued. A bone marrow examination will help to determine if iron stores are adequate and the proportion of progenitor cells.

INDICATIONS (NEUTROPENIA)	DOSE (Units/kg)	ROUTE	INTERVAL (hr)	DURATION (days)
Dogs and Cats				
Anemia in infections	100	SC	48[a]	prn[b]

[a]Three times weekly at a dose ranging from 50-150 Units/kg.
[b]Treat until desired hematocrit is reached, then as needed.

ADDITIONAL DOSAGES. FIV infection, Table 14-6.

DISPENSING INFORMATION. Animal should return for monitoring, initially at least weekly, with a complete blood count.

ETHAMBUTOL

CLASS. Synthetic antimycobacterial.

ACTION. Inhibits intracellular metabolism of mycobacterial cells.

MORE INFORMATION. See Tuberculosis, Chapter 50; Table 50-4.

PHARMACOKINETICS. Readily absorbed from GI tract and 80% bioavailable, unaffected by food. Diffuses into tissues and fluids, including the CSF, with inflamed meninges. A lower percentage is metabolized by liver, and some is excreted in feces; most is excreted in urine as unchanged drug and metabolites.

SPECTRUM. *Mycobacterium tuberculosis, M. bovis, M. avium-intracellulare* complex (MAC).

INDICATIONS. Tuberculosis caused by *M. tuberculosis* or *M. bovis* in combination with other antimycobacterial drugs.

CONTRAINDICATIONS. Reduce dose by extending interval of dose administration in renal insufficiency. Has caused teratogenesis in laboratory animals during pregnancy.

ADVERSE REACTIONS. In people, reduced visual acuity from optic neuritis; anorexia, vomiting, abdominal pain, CNS signs, and thrombocytopenia.

INTERACTIONS. Often combined with isoniazid, rifampin, pyrazinamide, or aminoglycosides for tuberculosis. For MAC infections, may be given in combination with fluoroquinolones, azithromycin or clarithromycin, aminoglycosides, rifampin, or clofazimine.

AVAILABILITY	TYPE	SIZES	PREPARATION (COMPANY)
Human	Oral tablets	100 mg, 400 mg	*Myambutol* (Lederle)

INTERNATIONAL PREPARATIONS. *Afimocil, Cidanbutol, Dexambutol, Etapiam, Servambutol.*

HANDLING. Keep in airtight containers at controlled room temperature, protected from moisture, heat, and light. Can mix with water and heat to 49°C for 10 min to dissolve and then put in suspension, which can be refrigerated for 1 week.

ADMINISTRATION. Aluminum-containing compounds reduce absorption. Administering with food reduces GI irritation. Use only in combination with other antimycobacterial drugs.

Dosage

INDICATIONS	DOSE (mg/kg)	ROUTE	INTERVAL (hr)	DURATION (mo)
Dogs	15	PO	24	3-6
	25	PO	72	3-6[a]

[a]Long-term suppressive therapy may be needed.

ADDITIONAL DOSAGES. Tuberculosis, Table 50-4.

DISPENSING INFORMATION. This medicine can be given with food.

FEBANTEL (COMBINED WITH PRAZIQUANTEL AND PYRANTEL PAMOATE)

CLASS. Pro-benzimidazole.

ACTION. Antihelminthic, antiprotozoal. Binds to tubulin subunit and interferes with microtubule formation. Only the febantel and its metabolite, fenbendazole, are effective against *Giardia.*

MORE INFORMATION. Chapter 71; Table 71-1; Reference: Ch 71, ref. 6; 70.

PHARMACOKINETICS. Rapidly absorbed after oral administration and metabolized into fenbendazole, oxfendazole, and 8 other metabolites. These are predominantly excreted in the bile.

SPECTRUM. *Giardia;* in addition, combination is effective against *Toxocara canis, Toxascaris leonina, Ancylostoma caninum, Uncinaria stenocephala, Trichuris vulpis, Taenia pisiformis, Echinococcus granulosus, E. multilocularis,* and *Dipylidium caninum.*

INDICATIONS. Helminths, *Giardia.*

APPROVED USES. For control of ascarids *(Toxocara canis, Toxascaris leonina),* hookworms *(Ancylostoma caninum, Uncinaria stenocephala),* whipworms *(Trichuris vulpis),* and tapeworms *(Taenia pisiformis, Echinococcus granulosus, E. multilocularis, Dipylidium caninum)* in dogs.

CONTRAINDICATIONS. Not for pregnant or lactating bitches. Praziquantel should not be given to pups <4 weeks, or kittens <6 weeks, of age.

ADVERSE REACTIONS. Unusual at label dose since has a wide margin of safety. When given 5 times the label dose for 3 consecutive days, salivation, anorexia, vomiting, and soft stool are noted (Ch 71, ref. 6).

INTERACTIONS. Synergistic activity with these drugs in combination.

AVAILABILITY	TYPE	SIZES	PREPARATIONS (COMPANY)
Dog	Oral tablets	68 mg praziquantel 68 mg pyrantel pamoate 340.2 mg febantel	*Drontal-Plus* (Bayer)

HANDLING. Product should be stored in airtight containers at contolled (15-30°C) temperature.

ADMINISTRATION. Give with food to increase the bioavailability. At the time the last dose is given, the dogs should be bathed and moved from runs to cages to decrease the risk of reinfection (Ch 71, ref. 70).

Dosage

INDICATIONS	DOSE (mg/kg)[a]	ROUTE	INTERVAL (hr)	DURATION (days)
Dogs				
Helminths, *Giardia*	26.8-35.2	PO	24	3-5
Helminths	10-25	PO	24	3
Cats				
Helminths, *Giardia*	10[b]	PO	24	3

[a]Dosed on basis of febantel, other drugs are at a fixed range in tablets.
[b]Two small dog tablets are given to each cat.

ADDITIONAL DOSAGES. None.

DISPENSING INFORMATION. Place amount indicated in mouth and encourage patient to drink fluids and swallow.

FENBENDAZOLE

CLASS. Benzimidazole.

ACTION. Antihelminthic, antiprotozoal.

MORE INFORMATION. Chapter 71; Table 71-1; Reference: Ch 71, ref. 9; 60; 82; 100.

PHARMACOKINETICS. Minimal amount absorbed following oral administration, and any absorbed drug is rapidly metabolized. Increasing the dose to up to 80 mg/kg in dogs did not significantly increase the amount of drug absorbed. Administration with food, irrespective of fat content, increases its bioavailability. A majority of the drug is excreted unchanged in the feces, and minimal amounts (<1%) of the administered dose appear in the urine.

SPECTRUM. *Giardia;* in addition to approved uses, it is effective against various intestinal helminths and *Capillaria aerophila, Filaroides hirthi,* and *Paragonimus kellicotti.* The nematocidal label dosage is effective for treating *Giardia* in dogs (Ch 71, ref. 100).

INDICATIONS. Helminths, *Giardia.* Because of low toxicity, this is the preferred drug for treatment of giardiasis. Infection was more difficult to clear in cats co-infected with *Cryptosporidium* (Ch 71, ref. 41).

APPROVED USES. For control of ascarids (*Toxocara canis, Toxascaris leonina*), hookworms (*Ancylostoma caninum, Uncinaria stenocephala*), whipworms (*Trichuris vulpis*), and tapeworms *(Taenia pisiformis)* in dogs.

CONTRAINDICATIONS. Unknown. Has been safe when administered to cats and pregnant animals.

ADVERSE REACTIONS. Unusual; vomiting occurs uncommonly when given with food. Other drugs of this class have been reported to cause hepatotoxicity. With large burdens of helminths, allergic reactions to dying tissue forms may be noted. Cats have been given dosages of 250 mg/kg for 9 days, which is five times the level and three times the recommended duration of treatment, with no side effects (Ch 71, ref. 82). Although less common than with albendazole use, fenbendazole administration (50 mg/kg PO every 12 hr, for 11 days) was associated with pancytopenia in a dog (Ch 71, ref. 23a). The pancytopenia gradually resolved by 15 days after discontinuation of therapy.

INTERACTIONS. Myelotoxicity was reported with coadministration of trimethoprim-sulfonamide in one dog (Ch 71, ref. 97a). It was reversible after treatment was discontinued.

AVAILABILITY	TYPE	SIZES	PREPARATIONS (COMPANY)
Dog	Oral granules 22.2%, packets or jar	1-g, 2-g, 4-g, 1-lb jar	*Panacur* (Hoechst Marion Roussel)
Horse	Oral granules 22.2%, packets	5.2-g	*Panacur*
	Paste 10%	25-g syringe	*Panacur*
Cattle and horse	Oral Paste 10%	92-g syringe	*Panacur*
	Oral suspension 10%	1 liter	*Panacur*
Cattle	Oral paste 10%	290-g syringe	*Panacur*
	Oral suspension 10%	1 gallon	*Panacur*

HANDLING. Product should be stored away from moisture at a controlled (15-30°C) temperature.

ADMINISTRATION. For a dose of 50 mg/kg, use 1 g of packet granules for each 10 lb of body weight. Mix the correct amount of granules with a small amount of the usual diet. If dry food is fed, add water to facilitate mixing with the drug. To be effective, the drug must be administered for a minimum of 3 days. Treatment for more resistant protozoa or helminths continues for up to 14 days.

Dosage

INDICATIONS (*Dogs and Cats*)	DOSE (mg/kg)	ROUTE	INTERVAL (hr)	DURATION (days)
Helminths, *Giardia*	50	PO	24	3-5

ADDITIONAL DOSAGES. Giardiasis, Table 78-3.

DISPENSING INFORMATION. Place amount indicated on canned pet food or moistened dry food. Make sure all the drug is taken by withholding other food until it is eaten.

FILGRASTIM (GRANULOCYTE COLONY-STIMULATING OR HEMATOPOIETIC GROWTH FACTOR, G-CSF)

CLASS. Cytokine.

ACTION. Stimulates myeloid progenitors in bone marrow. Increases blood neutrophil counts in clinically healthy or neutropenic animals. May also reduce production of inflammatory mediators, such as IL-1, TNF-α, and IFN-γ, which may be beneficial in preventing too severe an inflammatory reaction. In vitro, pretreatment of neutrophils with G-CSF and/or IFN-γ can attenuate the inhibitory effect of glucocorticoids on neutrophil-induced hyphal damage.

MORE INFORMATION. Chapters 2 and 58 and 100; references: Ch 2, ref. 37; 37a; 125.

PHARMACOKINETICS. Human recombinant product, increases blood neutrophil counts in various animals. In dogs and cats, short-term increases in neutrophil counts are followed by neutropenia with continued use owing to development of neutralizing antibodies to this heterologous protein. Neutrophilia occurs by day 7 and reaches maximal levels from 10-14 days of treatment. Short-term increases are followed by neutropenia (between 10 days-7 weeks) with continued use owing to development of neutralizing antibodies to this heterologous product.

INDICATIONS. To stimulate production and function of neutrophils and monocytes. In dogs, for short-term use in treating neutropenia from whole body irradiation, parvovirus and *Ehrlichia* infections, myelosuppressive drugs. Potential uses in cats are leukopenias associated with FeLV, myeloproliferative disease, lymphoid tumors, aplastic anemias. Best for short-term ($\leq$21 days) use for treatment of neutropenia caused by infectious agents, chemotherapy, or total body irradiation. Has been recommended for neutropenia caused by toxins (e.g., cancer chemotherapeutics, estrogens, chloramphenicol, trimethoprim-sulfonamides) or infections (e.g., ehrlichiosis, parvoviral infections). Studies have shown that effect in parvoviral infections of dogs is minimal as high levels are already circulating. Similar studies in cats with parvovirus have not been rewarding. See Chapter 2 for details on studies involving this drug.

APPROVED USES. People for neutropenia associated with HIV infection, cancer and antiviral chemotherapy, and transplantation.

CONTRAINDICATIONS. Treatment for longer than 3 weeks (Ch 2, ref. 3). Enhanced expression of FIV by infected lymphocytes in cats; therefore not recommended for treatment of this disease.

ADVERSE REACTIONS. Bone discomfort or splenomegaly, allergic reactions (Ch 2, ref. 3). After 10 days to 7 weeks of therapy, persistent antibodies develop against endogenous canine or feline G-CSF, resulting in rebound neutropenia.

INTERACTIONS. Artifactual increased serum lactic dehydrogenase and ALP from bone isoenzyme in people.

AVAILABILITY	TYPE	SIZE	PREPARATION (COMPANY)
Human	Solution for injection	300 µg/ml in 1-ml vial	*Neupogen* (Amgen)

HANDLING. Stock solution can be diluted with sterile physiologic buffered saline and bovine serum albumin. The final dilution is 100 µg/ml, which is stored at 4°C. The vial should not be frozen or exposed to sunlight. Incompatible in solution with amphotericin B, some cephalosporins, clindamycin, furosemide, methylprednisolone sodium succinate, metronidazole, and piperacillin.

ADMINISTRATION. Can be given SC or IV. Should give along with supportive care such as concurrent blood transfusions for concurrent anemia or thrombocytopenia or antibiotics for leukopenia. For IV use, may be further diluted to 5 to 15 µg/ml with addition of 5% dextrose. Albumin is added (12 mg/ml) to prevent absorption to plastics. Infusion rate IV should be over at least 15 min. Should not be given earlier than 24 hr after cytotoxic chemotherapy or 24 hr before. Bone pain can be alleviated by concurrent administration of nonsteroidal antiinflammatory drugs. SC injection should be spaced out at different sites for each injection and may be more effective than IV use.

INDICATIONS (NEUTROPENIA)	DOSE (µg/kg)	ROUTE	INTERVAL (hr)	DURATION (days)
Dogs and Cats				
Acute viral infections	5	SC	24	3-5
Chronic viral infections	5	SC	24	≤21

ADDITIONAL DOSAGES. FIV infection, Table 14-6.
DISPENSING INFORMATION. Animal should return for monitoring at least twice weekly with a complete blood count.

Since antibodies develop within 14-21 days, the drug is discontinued prior to this time.

FLORFENICOL

CLASS. Acetamide.

ACTION. Binds to 50s ribosome of bacteria-inhibiting protein synthesis.

MORE INFORMATION. See CHLORAMPHENICOL; Chapter 34.

PHARMACOKINETICS. Similar to chloramphenicol. In dogs PO and IM bioavailability is good; however, absorption is inconsistent by SC route. In cats well absorbed by PO, IM routes (Ch 34, ref. 291a).

SPECTRUM. See CHLORAMPHENICOL.

INDICATIONS. See CHLORAMPHENICOL.

CONTRAINDICATIONS. Pregnancy.

ADVERSE REACTIONS. Chemical modification of this drug has alleviated the myelotoxic effect, although toxicity studies are not available for dogs and cats. Also not associated with human myelotoxicity. Can be locally irritating to animals when administered or to mucosae of sensitive people inadvertently contacting the drug.

INTERACTIONS. See CHLORAMPHENICOL.

INDICATIONS. Systemic bacterial or rickettsial infections when potential myelotoxicity in animals or people is to be avoided. MIC concentrations of 1.0-8.0 for pathogens from dogs and cats.

AVAILABILITY	TYPE	SIZES	PREPARATION (COMPANY)
Veterinary (cattle)	Parenteral solution 300 mg/ml	100, 250, 500 ml	*Nuflor* (Schering-Plough Aniimal Health)

HANDLING. Can be stored between 2-30°C, although refrigeration is not necessary. Color is pale yellow and does not affect patency.

ADMINISTRATION. Can be given IM or SC; the former may cause pain and irritation.

Dosage

INDICATIONS	DOSE (mg/kg)	ROUTE	INTERVAL (hr)	DURATION (days)
Dogs				
Systemic infections	20	IM	8	3-5
Cats				
System infections	22	IM, PO[a]	12	3-5

[a]Oral product is not available, however solution given orally was well absorbed by experimental cats.

ADDITIONAL DOSAGES. Canine distemper, Table 3-5.

FLUCONAZOLE

CLASS. Bis-triazole.

ACTION. Antifungal; inhibits sterol and cytochrome P-450 synthesis. Higher affinity for fungal enzyme than ketoconazole or itraconazole.

MORE INFORMATION. See KETOCONAZOLE, ITRACONAZOLE; Chapter 57; Table 57-1; references: Ch 57, ref. 21; 50; 62.

PHARMACOKINETICS. Low molecular weight and high water solubility results in high bioavailability (>90% systemic availability) after IV or PO administration. GI absorption is unaffected by food intake or changes in gastric acidity caused by cimetidine or antacids containing magnesium or aluminum (Ch 57, ref. 135). In people, reaches effective tissue concentrations by 5-10 doses, which is 5-10 days with once-daily dosing or by 2 days if loading with twice the recommended dose is used the first day. Not extensively bound, so penetrates all body cavities and tissues, including eye and CNS. Sites having concentrations equal to or exceeding those in blood are skin, urine, skin blister fluids, body cavities, nails, saliva, sputum, reproductive tissues. Elimination half-life in cats after 50 mg was 25 hours (Ch 57, ref. 137). Penetration into CSF is 50%-90% of plasma levels independent of inflammation. Not extensively metabolized; therefore primarily eliminated (80%) by renal excretion of active drug (Ch 57, ref. 21; 62).

SPECTRUM. Excellent for yeast forms such as *Cryptococcus, Candida, Blastomyces, Histoplasma, Coccidioides, Malassezia;* variable efficacy against filamentous fungi such as *Aspergillus,* dermatophytes.

INDICATIONS. Systemic fungal infections involving difficult-to-reach tissues (e.g., CNS). Blastomycosis, coccidioidomycosis, histoplasmosis, cryptococcosis, especially for cryptococcal infections of the brain, spinal cord, or eye (57:O'Toole et al 2003). Nasal aspergillosis. Higher doses, if tolerated, may improve therapeutic efficacy. Excellent for fungal urinary tract infections such as caused by *Candida* or *Torulopsis.*

APPROVED USES. Human: for treatment of esophageal candidiasis and maintenance therapy of cryptococcal meningitis and for treatment failures of candidiasis.

CONTRAINDICATIONS. Reduce dose in renal failure; avoid in pregnancy.

ADVERSE REACTIONS. See also KETOCONAZOLE. Can cause vomiting, diarrhea, abdominal discomfort. Dermal eruptions, hepatotoxicity (elevated transaminases, cholestasis, hepatitis, hepatic failure). Hepatotoxicity is much less frequent than with ketoconazole or itraconazole. Does not suppress adrenal or sex hormones like ketoconazole. Alopecia, dry skin and mucosae, and dizziness have been reported only in people.

INTERACTIONS. Cimetidine interferes with absorption. Fluconazole increases concentrations of thiazide diuretics, rifampin, cyclosporine, glipizide, antihistamines, diphenylhydantoin, and theophylline. Potentiates bleeding caused by anticoagulant rodenticides.

AVAILABILITY	TYPE	SIZES	PREPARATIONS (COMPANY)
Human	Oral tablets	50 mg, 100 mg, 150 mg, 200 mg	*Diflucan* (Pfizer)
	Oral capsule	150 mg	*Diflucan*
	Powder for oral suspension	10 mg/ml, 40 mg/ml reconstituted	*Diflucan*
	Parenteral injection	2 mg/ml	*Diflucan*

INTERNATIONAL PREPARATIONS. *Biozolene, Elazor, Fungata, Lavisa, Loitin, Triflucan.*

HANDLING. Keep tablets at controlled room temperature in airtight containers. PO suspension: store powder at room temperature and dilute in distilled water; shake before using. Store reconstituted suspension between refrigerated and room temperature up to 2 weeks. Parenteral injection should be stored at room or refrigerator temperature. Do not add anything or freeze.

ADMINISTRATION. Give twice calculated daily dose for the first day of treatment. Give for 2-3 days if rapidly advancing or severe disseminated mycosis. IV solution should be given over 1-2 hr. Often treat neurologic or ocular cryptococcosis for at least 12 weeks or for 2 weeks after CSF examination shows resolution of inflammation and antigen test results on serum and CSF are negative. The best therapeutic response in CNS cryptococcosis of cats is with the 200 mg/cat/day dosages (Ch 57, ref. 21). Because of high oral bioavailability, dosages for parenteral administration do not differ.

Dosage

INDICATIONS	DOSE	ROUTE	INTERVAL (hr)	DURATION (days)[a]
Dogs				
Cryptococcosis, candidiasis, systemic mycoses, nasal aspergillosis	2.5-5 mg/kg	PO, IV	12-24	56-84
Meningitis	5.0-8.0 mg/kg	PO, IV	12	56-84
	8.0-12 mg/kg	PO, IV	24	56-84
Cats				
Nasal or dermal cryptococcosis[b]	5 mg/kg	PO	12-24	[c]
	10 mg/kg	PO	24	[c]
CNS, intraocular or multisystemic infection	50 mg/cat	PO	24	[c]
CNS, intraocular, or multisystemic cryptococcosis[b]	50-100 mg/cat	PO, IV	12	[c]
Both				
Urinary candidiasis	5-10 mg/kg	PO	24	21-42
Urinary *Candida glabrata* infection	12	PO	24	21-42

[a]For most infections, treatment duration is a minimum of 42-56 days; however cats with cryptococcosis require minimum treatment duration of 120-180 days to prevent relapse. Animals should be monitored with serologic antigen detection methods to determine treatment efficacy.
[b]For most infections in cats, 50 mg/cat per day achieves adequate therapeutic levels (Ch 57, ref. 137).
[c]Treatment should continue until antigen testing results of blood or CSF (with CNS disease) are negative. This is usually at least 2 mo beyond clinical resolution and a mean time of approximately 8 mo.

ADDITIONAL DOSAGES. Blastomycosis, Table 59-1; cryptococcosis, Table 61-5; coccidioidomycosis, Table 62-3; nasal aspergillosis, Table 64-1; candidiasis, Table 65-4; trichosporonosis, Table 66-1.

DISPENSING INFORMATION. This medication can be given with food.

FLUCYTOSINE

CLASS. Fluorinated pyrimidine.

ACTION. Antifungal; converted by specific enzyme in fungal cells to metabolites like 5-fluorouracil that interfere with fungal thymidylate synthase and resultant DNA and RNA synthesis.

MORE INFORMATION. See Chapter 57; Table 57-1.

PHARMACOKINETICS. Well absorbed from GI tract and widely distributed in tissues and body fluids, including joints, peritoneal fluid, and aqueous humor. CSF concentration is 70%-90% that in serum. Only 4% absorbed drug being metabolized, 80%-90% is excreted unchanged in urine.

SPECTRUM. *Candida, Cryptococcus.* Some effect against *Aspergillus.* Always used in combination with amphotericin B. Resistance may develop during treatment. **Ineffective:** filamentous fungi and dermatophytes.

INDICATIONS. Serious (disseminated) infections with *Candida* or *Cryptococcus* such as sepsis, endocarditis, meningitis.

APPROVED USES. In combination therapy for systemic yeast infections.

CONTRAINDICATIONS. Reduce dose or avoid in renal failure. Avoid with pre-existing myelosuppression, pregnancy, or in neonates.

ADVERSE REACTIONS. Myelosuppression (leukopenia, thrombocytopenia), teratogenic in laboratory animals. Renal failure, crystalluria, dermal eruptions, vomiting, diarrhea, abdominal pain, hepatotoxicity (cholestatic hepatitis, icterus and increased liver enzymes), CNS signs. Converted by GI flora to 5-fluorouracil, which can be toxic when absorbed producing myelosuppression or enterocolitis.

INTERACTIONS. Synergistic with amphotericin B, but renal toxicity of both drugs is enhanced.

AVAILABILITY	TYPE	SIZES	PREPARATION (COMPANY)
Human	Oral capsules	250 mg, 500 mg	*Ancobon* (Roche)

INTERNATIONAL PREPARATIONS. *Alcobon, Ancotil.*

HANDLING. Store capsules in airtight, light-proof containers at controlled room temperature.

ADMINISTRATION. Food may slow but not reduce drug absorption after PO administration. Repeatedly monitor hemogram, renal and hepatic test results every 2 weeks during treatment. Assess renal function at least twice a week if amphotericin B is also used.

Dosage

INDICATIONS (*Dogs and Cats*)	DOSE (mg/kg)	ROUTE	INTERVAL (hr)	DURATION (days)
Cryptococcosis, candidiasis[a]	25-50	PO	6	42
	50-65	PO	8	42
Cryptococcosis[a]	50	PO	6	42

[a]Must give in combination with a polyene or azole antifungal drug.

ADDITIONAL DOSAGES. Cryptococcosis, Table 61-5; CNS infections, Table 92-5.

DISPENSING INFORMATION. Monitor animal for any GI signs or bruising tendencies.

FOSCARNET SODIUM (PHOSPHONOFORMATE)

CLASS. Pyrophosphate analog.

ACTION. Antiviral; inhibits replication of all known herpesviruses. Inhibits virus-specific DNA and RNA polymerases and reverse transcriptases at concentrations that do not affect those in cells. Prevents pyrophosphate exchange in virus to a much greater degree than mammalian cells. Activity against retroviruses is by binding to reverse transcriptase in a noncompetitive and reversible manner distinct from other antivirals and it does not require phosphorylation to be active.

MORE INFORMATION. See Foscarnet, Chapter 2; Table 2-1; references: Ch 2, ref. 127; 146.

PHARMACOKINETICS. PO bioavailability 35% in cats, 10% in dogs. A derivative (thiofoscarnet) has higher PO bioavailability (Ch 2, ref. 143). IV route produces higher concentrations and is preferred for systemic therapy. At physiologic pH, it is ionized and has limited cellular penetration. Penetrates CSF (40% of blood concentration) with some accumulation in bone from where it is eliminated slowly, especially in younger cats (Ch 2, ref. 147). Drug undergoes little metabolism and is excreted mainly unchanged in urine. Clearance from plasma in young cats is quicker than in older cats (Ch 2, ref. 146; 147).

SPECTRUM. DNA viruses and RNA viruses, including retroviruses. Most effective against herpesviruses.

INDICATIONS. Herpesvirus infections, retroviral infections. Acyclovir-resistant herpesvirus infections.

APPROVED USES. Human: cytomegalovirus retinitis in AIDS patients.

CONTRAINDICATIONS. Renal failure. Use caution in pregnant and lactating animals owing to potential for fetotoxicity and damage to bones and teeth of young animals.

ADVERSE REACTIONS. Nephrotoxicity; must monitor renal function during therapy. Renal dysfunction is evident in most people after 2 weeks of therapy. Maintenance of adequate hydration, diuresis, and discontinuation of the drug facilitate reversal of nephrotoxicity. Chelates divalent cations such as calcium, so that hypocalcemia, hyperphosphatemia or hypophosphatemia, hypomagnesemia, and hypokalemia may develop. Ulceration of the genital epithelium may occur with urine contamination. Anemia and granulocytopenia may develop. Young cats given high dosages develop widened growth plates, increased osteoid, mineralization failure.

INTERACTIONS. With concurrent pentamidine, may exacerbate hypocalcemia. Renal toxicity increased with concurrent use of amphotericin B or aminoglycosides. Cannot use with other nephrotoxic drugs such as ganciclovir because of additive effect.

AVAILABILITY	TYPE	SIZES	PREPARATION (COMPANY)
Human	Injectable solution	24 mg/ml in 500-ml and 250-ml bottles for IV infusion	*Foscavir* (Astra)

INTERNATIONAL PREPARATIONS. *Triapten, Virudin.*

HANDLING. Store at room temperature (15-30°C) and not frozen. Should use only if bottle and seal are intact.

ADMINISTRATION. Given IV by continuous infusion because of short half-life. Weakness or paresthesias may occur during infusion. Do not infuse as a bolus. This will increase the risk of toxicity. IV maximum rate of infusion of 1 mg/kg/min. Experimentally, has been given PO to dogs and cats (Ch 2, ref. 127; 146).

Dosage

INDICATIONS	DOSE (mg/kg)	ROUTE	INTERVAL (hr)	DURATION (days)
Dogs	20-30	IV, PO	8	prn
Cats				
Retroviral infection	13.3	IV	8	prn

ADDITIONAL DOSAGES. None.

DISPENSING INFORMATION. This drug can cause oral irritation when given by mouth. Report any decrease in appetite or signs of oral bleeding to your veterinarian.

FUMAGILLIN

CLASS. Alicyclic antibiotic derived from *Aspergillus fumigatus*.

ACTION. Inhibitor of endothelial cell proliferation and angiogenesis. It may inhibit methionine aminopeptidase 2.

MORE INFORMATION. See Table 71-1; Microsporidiosis, Chapter 75 (Ch 75, ref. 42a).

PHARMACOKINETICS. Not well absorbed from epithelial surfaces such as the gut and extraocular tissues.

SPECTRUM. *Entamoeba* and microsoporidia such as *Encephalitozoon* and *Enterocytozoon bieneusi*. Has been used to treat infections with a closely related organism, *Nosema*, in honey bees.

INDICATIONS. Intestinal amebiasis. Microsporidial diarrhea or dissemination. Applied topically to the conjunctiva in the treatment of microsporidial keratoconjunctivitis.

APPROVED USES. Treatment of microsporidiosis in honeybees. Has been investigated for effects on angiogenesis in treatment of solid tumors in people. Once used to treat malaria.

CONTRAINDICATIONS. Preexisting neutropenia or thrombocytopenia.

ADVERSE REACTIONS. Myelosuppression (leukopenia, thrombocytopenia), nausea. The exceptional amount of side effects have made this medication less desirable for treatment of intestinal microsporidiosis in humans.

INTERACTIONS. Caution must be used with other myelo-suppressive drugs.

AVAILABILITY[a]	TYPE	SIZES	PREPARATION (COMPANY)
Human Investigational	Oral capsules	20 mg	Sanofi-Synthelabo Labs
Human Investigational	Topical ocular solution as bicyclohexylammonium salt	70 µg/ml	Sandofi-Synthelabo Labs

[a]Available in the United States only through the manufacturer for research or investigational use, but not for human or drug use. Oral and topical formulations may have to be compounded by pharmacists.

INTERNATIONAL PREPARATIONS. *Fumagilina*.

HANDLING. Store capsules in airtight, light-proof containers at controlled room temperature.

ADMINISTRATION. Food may slow but not reduce drug absorption after PO administration. Give separately from meals.

Dosage

INDICATIONS (Humans)	DOSE	ROUTE	INTERVAL (hr)	DURATION (days)
Enterocytozoon[a]	20 mg total dose	PO	8	14

[a]Extrapolated from human dosages (Ch 75, ref. 42a).

ADDITIONAL DOSAGES. None.

DISPENSING INFORMATION. Take on an empty stomach.

FURAZOLIDONE

CLASS. Nitrofuran.

ACTION. Antibacterial, antiprotozoal by unknown action; potentially interferes with carbohydrate metabolism of microorganism. Drug undergoes reductive activation in protozoa and killing correlates with reduced metabolites which damage cellular DNA.

MORE INFORMATION. NITROFURANTOIN; Chapter 34, Nitrofurans; Table 34-9; Antiprotozoals, Chapter 71; Table 71-1.

PHARMACOKINETICS. Small amounts are absorbed from GI tract, the majority is not absorbed and is active in the intestinal lumen. Absorbed fraction may be responsible for most of adverse reactions. Rapid tissue and hepatic metabolism of any absorbed drug. Colored metabolites are excreted in urine and major amount in feces.

SPECTRUM. **Gram positive:** *Staphylococcus*. **Gram negative:** *Escherichia, Salmonella, Proteus, Aerobacter, Campylobacter,* and *Helicobacter*. **Protozoa:** *Giardia, Trichomonas,* Coccidia.

INDICATIONS. Bacterial or protozoal enteritis caused by susceptible pathogens. Gastric helicobacteriosis.

APPROVED USES. Humans: for bacterial and protozoal enteritis.

CONTRAINDICATIONS. Prior sensitivity. Avoid in pregnant and lactating animals and neonates.

ADVERSE REACTIONS. Vomiting, diarrhea, fever, dermatologic eruption, brown urine, hypoglycemia. Hemolysis in animals with glucose–6-phosphate dehydrogenase deficiency, or potentially in neonatal animals.

INTERACTIONS. Increased vasopressor effects of sympathomimetic drugs.

AVAILABILITY	TYPE	SIZES	PREPARATIONS (COMPANY)
Human	Oral liquid	50 mg/15 ml	*Furoxone* (Procter and Gamble)
	Oral tablets	100 mg	*Furoxone*

INTERNATIONAL PREPARATIONS. *Nifuran.*

HANDLING. Store in airtight, light-proof containers at controlled room temperature. If exposed to light, liquids will darken.

ADMINISTRATION. Oral suspension makes medication of cats convenient and dosing more accurate. Tablets can be crushed and added to corn syrup to improve palatability.

Dosage

INDICATIONS	DOSE	ROUTE	INTERVAL (hr)	DURATION (days)
Human				
Adult giardiasis	100 mg/person	PO	6	7
Child giardiasis	1.25 mg/kg	PO	6	7-10
Dogs				
Coccidiosis	8-20 mg/kg	PO	24	7
Entamebiasis	2.2 mg/kg	PO	8	7
Cats				
Coccidiosis	8-20 mg/kg	PO	24	7
Giardiasis	4 mg/kg	PO	12	5-10
Amebiasis	2.2 mg/kg	PO	8	7

ADDITIONAL DOSAGES. Giardiasis, Table 78-3; coccidiosis, Table 81-2.

DISPENSING INFORMATION. Reduce feeding of tyramine-containing foods to your pet such as aged cheese and smoked or pickled meat while administering drug. This drug may cause gastrointestinal side effects in your pet and brown discoloration of urine.

FUSIDIC ACID

CLASS. Antibiotic obtained from *Fusidium coccineum.*

ACTION. Antibacterial, antiprotozoal by interfering with protein synthesis. Interferes with amino acid transfer from aminoacyl-sRNA to protein on the ribosomes. Effective against staphylococci and streptococci. May be bacteriostatic or bactericidal depending on the inoculum size. Bacterial cells stop dividing within 2 min of contact; however, nucleic acid synthesis continues for up to 2 hr thereafter. It is *only* effective against gram-positive bacteria. The poor activity against gram-negative bacteria and mammalian cells may relate to cell-wall permeability differences. With topical preparations, concentrations are adequate to treat other gram-positive organisms such as corynebacteria, *Neisseria*, clostridia, and *Bacteroides* species.

MORE INFORMATION. NONE.

PHARMACOKINETICS. Able to penetrate intact skin makes them effective in skin infections.

SPECTRUM. Gram positive: *Staphylococcus.* Including β-lactamase resistant strains, and other gram positives. **Protozoa:** *Giardia, Plasmodium.*

INDICATIONS. Bacterial dermatitis caused by susceptible pathogens.

APPROVED USES. Bacterial dermatitis.

CONTRAINDICATIONS. Sensitivity to fusidic acid and it salts or lanolin for topical product. Preexisting hepatic disease for parenteral use. No risk or dosage modification if renal dysfunction exists. No cross-resistance with other antibiotics in clinical use; however, bacteria can develop resistance to this drug in vitro and with clinical use.

ADVERSE REACTIONS. In certain circumstances, may cause hypersensitivity. With topical use, if irritation or sensitization develop, discontinue therapy. May cause irritation if used near the eye because of conjunctival inflammation. With IV use, may get venospasm, thrombophlebitis, hemolysis, vomiting, icterus, hypocalcemia. Liver enzymes should be regularly monitored with prolonged therapy. Not recommended in pregnancy or lactation.

INTERACTIONS. Incompatible with amino acid solutions, acidic solutions or whole blood. Do not mix with aminoglycosides, cephalosporins, or penicillins.

AVAILABILITY	TYPE	SIZES	PREPARATIONS (COMPANY)
Human	Topical ointment or as an intertulle dressing	Cream: 2% in tubes of 15 and 30 gm. Intertulle: ointment-impregnated gauze	*Fucidin* Ointment (Leo Pharma; Fusidic Acid)
	Oral tablets	250 mg	*Fucidin* Tablets
	Oral suspension	50 mg/ml	*Fucidin* Suspension
	IV Solution	580 mg sodium fusidate in 50 ml vial	*Fucidin* for Intravenous Infusion, Sodium fusidate

HANDLING. Store at room temperature (<25°C) and protect from light. Reconstitute the IV solution with the buffered diluent provided before diluting further. The diluent contains phosphate-citrate buffer which is essential for stability. IV solution contains no bacteriostat and must be used within 24 hr of preparation. Compatible with normal saline and 5% dextrose.

ADMINISTRATION. Cream, apply topically to affected areas. **Oral preparations** (tablets and liquid), used to treat GI infections. **IV use,** intermittent infusion at a rate of 1-2 ml/min over 2-6 hr.

Dosage

INDICATIONS	DOSE	ROUTE	INTERVAL (hr)	DURATION (days)
Human[a]				
Gram-positive bacterial dermatitis	Small amount	Topically	8-12	7
	500 mg sodium fusidate[b]	PO	8	7-28
	738 mg fusidic acid suspension	PO	8	7-28
Systemic gram-positive infections	500 mg sodium fusidate[b]	IV	8	7-28

[a]No animal dosage available. This is a human dosage schedule.
[b]Equivalent to 480 mg fusidic acid. No doses are confirmed for dogs and cats. All doses listed are for humans. Due to incomplete absorption, the dose of the suspension is higher than other formulations. The dose has been increased to treat acute severe infections.

ADDITIONAL DOSAGES. None.

DISPENSING INFORMATION. Apply to the affected area 2-3 times daily, for up to 7 days.

GANCICLOVIR (CYTOVENE; SYNTEX). SEE ACYCLOVIR AND CHAPTER 2, ACYCLOVIR.

GENTAMICIN

CLASS. Aminoglycoside.

ACTION. Bactericidal; inhibits bacterial protein synthesis by binding to the 30s ribosomal subunit.

MORE INFORMATION. AMIKACIN, KANAMYCIN, STREPTO-MYCIN; Chapter 34, Aminoglycosides; Table 34-5; references Ch 34, ref. 136; 137.

PHARMACOKINETICS. Poor absorption from the GI tract after PO administration. IM absorption (>90%) is more predictable and rapid than SC. Distribution restricted into extracellular fluids (see AMIKACIN). Therapeutic concentrations achieved in some tissues, including lung, bone, and heart; also distributes in limited extent to bile, synovial, peritoneal, abscess, pleural fluids. Low levels in CNS, CSF, or eyes even with inflammation. Must inject intrathecally to achieve adequate concentrations in CSF. Accumulation in kidneys and inner ear may be responsible for intoxication. Small amounts excreted in bile, most excreted in urine as unchanged drug. Can cross placental barrier, which can be risk for fetus.

SPECTRUM. Gram positive: *Corynebacterium,* some *Streptococcus, Staphylococcus.* **Gram negative:** *Escherichia, Pasteurella, Proteus,* some *Pseudomonas, Klebsiella, Serratia, Aerobacter, Citrobacter, Enterobacter, Salmonella.* No specific advantages over other aminoglycosides except possible synergy with penicillins against *Enterococcus.* **More effective:** gram-negative aerobes. **Ineffective:** obligate anaerobes, some resistance developing in strains of *Klebsiella, Escherichia,* and *Pseudomonas.*

INDICATIONS. Synergism with β-lactams is documented in vivo. Use in combination with β-lactams for high-risk animals requiring treatment or prophylaxis of established bacteremia or potential bacteremia during urologic, genital, digestive manipulations, or surgery. With clindamycin for surgery on open fractures; with metronidazole before digestive surgery; with quinolones before endoscopic or radiologic urinary tract procedures. Aminoglycosides are rarely recommended as single agents or for self-limiting infections when less toxic drugs are available. Genitourinary, respiratory, or skin and soft tissue infections caused by gram-negative bacilli; systemic infections (including bacteremia and endocarditis) caused by *Staphylococcus;* persistent fever in neutropenic animals. In serious infections caused by unknown organisms, usually combined with a penicillin or cephalosporin; combine with parenteral carbenicillin for serious infections caused by *Pseudomonas.* Can use in nebulization chambers (2.2 mg/kg) for aerosol treatment of bacterial pneumonia.

APPROVED USES. Many, human and veterinary.

CONTRAINDICATIONS. Avoid usage or greatly reduce dosage in renal failure; reduce dose in neonates. Can cause fetal intoxication during pregnancy. Nephrotoxicity is increased by dehydration, shock, renal failure, cardiac failure, hypotension, nonsteroidal anti-inflammatory (antiprostaglandin) drugs, metabolic acidosis, diuretics, calcium, or magnesium deficiencies. Should not be used in dogs that require hearing or balance for work or sport.

ADVERSE REACTIONS. See also Chapter 34, Aminoglycosides. Higher (> once daily) frequency and dosage is associated with nephrotoxicity and ototoxicity. Higher protein diets reduce nephrotoxicity in dogs (Ch 34, ref. 136). More ototoxic than amikacin in cats. Topical lavage of open wounds or body cavities with parenteral formulation (50 mg/ml) can lead to significant absorption and nephrotoxicity (Ch 34, ref. 251). Topical application of 3 mg/ml otic solution was not ototoxic in ear canals of dogs with intact or ruptured eardrums (Ch 34, ref. 356). Often added at 3 mg/ml in tris-EDTA lavage solutions for *Pseudomonas* (see Chapter 34, Table 34-15). Neuromuscular blockade can result after lavage of pleural or peritoneal cavities.

INTERACTIONS. Increased nephrotoxicity when administered with some older parenteral first-generation cephalosporins, amphotericin B, osmotic (mannitol) or loop (furosemide) diuretics, vancomycin, or anesthesia with methoxyflurane or enflurane. Can potentiate paralysis by neuromuscular blockers (*d*-tubocurarine, pancuronium, atracurium). Increased ototoxicity with concurrent use of furosemide and with reduced renal function. Effectiveness of gentamicin is reduced with concurrent use of penicillin, ampicillin, or carbenicillin.

AVAILABILITY	TYPE	SIZES	PREPARATIONS (COMPANY)
Human	Injectable solution (sulfate)	40 mg/ml, 10 mg/ml	*Garamycin, Garamycin* Pediatric, (Schering-Plough Animal Health), generic (various)
	Intrathecal solution	2 mg/ml without no preservatives	*Garamycin Intrathecal*
Veterinary	Injectable solution (sulfate)	50 mg/ml (dogs and cats) 100 mg/ml (equine)	*Gentocin* (Schering-Plough Animal Health) *Gentocin*

INTERNATIONAL PREPARATIONS. *Akomicin, Biogen, Cidomycin, Dispagent, Gentalline, Gentamen, Gentax, Genticol, Gentogram, Geomycine, Martigenta, Refobacin, Sulmycin.*

HANDLING. Store at controlled room temperature and never refrigerate or freeze. Never mix aminoglycosides and β-lactams owing to inactivation in vitro but can be coadministered separately. For IV dose, can be diluted in 5% dextrose or 0.9% saline for infusion, or give as IV bolus.

ADMINISTRATION. Can be administered IV or IM, but the former preferred for serious life-threatening bacteremia, animals in shock, those with reduced muscle mass, extensive skin lesions, or heart failure. If dosage frequency is increased to treat systemic infections, toxicity will be greater. Higher peak tissue levels are obtained by a greater dosage per administration (Ch 34, ref. 4). However, to prevent toxicity at higher dosages, the dosage interval must be reduced. For this reason, a 24-hr or longer interval is recommended. Treatment usually lasts for a maximum of 7-10 days. Renal function must be monitored wherever possible. Monitor urine for fixed specific gravity, casts, albumin, glucose or blood. Increasing the interval of administration to at least 24 hr will reduce toxicity. If toxicosis is noted, the drug should be stopped immediately and fluid and osmotic diuresis instituted. Appearance of nephrotoxicity may be delayed for 1-3 weeks after dosage is discontinued. Intrathecal dose is 2-4 mg total dose/day. After lumbar or cisternal puncture, remove 1 ml/10 kg CSF volume. Dilute the gentamicin with an equal volume of sterile saline or aspirated CSF (if clear) before infusing over 3-5 min.

Dosage

INDICATIONS	DOSE (mg/kg)	ROUTE	INTERVAL (hr)	DURATION (days)
Dogs				
Localized, urinary infections	2.2[a]	IM, SC	24	7-10
Orthopedic and soft tissue infections	4.4–6.6	IV, IM, SC	24	<7[b]
Bacteremia, sepsis[c]	6.6	IV, IM, SC	24	<7[b]
Cats[d]				
Urinary, soft tissue infections	2.2	IV, IM, SC	24	<7[b]
Systemic, bacteremia	4.4	IV, IM, SC	24	<7[b]

[a]Recommended to give 4.4 mg/kg for first dose to help establish tissue levels.
[b]Renal function must be closely monitored by urine sediment examination and serum urea nitrogen concentration.
[c]Once-daily administration of gentamicin for up to 5 days may provide adequate serum levels to treat most susceptible gram-negative infections with little or no nephrotoxicity in dogs (Ch 34, ref. 4).
[d]Maximum amount for obese cat is 2.5 mg/kg per dose (Ch 34, ref. 429).

ADDITIONAL DOSAGES. Canine viral enteritis, Table 8-1; feline panleukopenia, Table 10-2; *Rhodococcus equi* infection, Table 35-7; gram-negative infections, Table 37-3; enteric bacterial infections, Table 39-2; canine brucellosis, Table 40-2; plague, Table 47-1; opportunistic mycobacterial infection, Table 50-9; dermatophilosis, Table 51-1; otitis externa, Table 85-6; musculoskeletal infections, Tables 86-2 and 86-3; bacteremia, Table 87-6; respiratory disease, Table 88-8; oral infections, Table 89-4; enteric infections, Table 89-16; intraabdominal infections, Table 89-21; hepatobiliary infections, Table 90-5; local ocular infections, Table 93-4.

DISPENSING INFORMATION. Must be given SC; therefore, not advised for home administration. Monitoring for renal toxicity is also needed.

GRANULOCYTE COLONY-STIMULATING OR HEMATOPOIETIC GROWTH FACTOR (G-CSF; FILGRASTIM) SEE FILGRASTIM

GRANULOCYTE MACROPHAGE COLONY-STIMULATING OR HEMATOPOIETIC GROWTH FACTOR (GM-CSF: SARGRAMOSTIM) SEE SARGRAMSTIM

GRISEOFULVIN

CLASS. Antifungal antibiotic derived from *Penicillium* sp.

ACTION. Fungistatic; binds to keratin and inhibits fungal growth by disrupting mitosis.

MORE INFORMATION. See Chapter 57, Griseofulvin; Table 57-1; reference: Ch 57, ref. 95; 139.

PHARMACOKINETICS. Variable absorption can be increased by feeding a high fat content meal. Ultramicrocrystalline size ($<1\ \mu m$) is better absorbed (>95%) than microsized ($4\ \mu m$) preparation (30%-75%) lowering the equivalent dosage. Concentrated in dermis and appendages. Becomes incorporated in newly formed keratinized epithelium. Metabolized in liver to inactive compounds that are excreted.

SPECTRUM. *Microsporum, Trichophyton.* **Ineffective:** *Actinomyces, Nocardia, Aspergillus, Sporothrix, Blastomyces, Histoplasma, Cryptococcus, Coccidioides, Malassezia,* and *Candida.*

INDICATIONS. "Ringworm," dermatophytosis of hair, nails, and skin. Should not be used in cases that are self-limiting or adequately confined for topical therapies.

APPROVED USES. Dermatophytosis in people and animals.

CONTRAINDICATIONS. Hepatic dysfunction, pregnancy, anemia, leukopenia, or feline retroviral infections, especially with leukopenias.

ADVERSE REACTIONS. Nausea, vomiting, diarrhea are most common. Systemic and dermal hypersensitivity (dermal edema and pruritus), hepatotoxicity. May be teratogenic and interferes with spermatogenesis. Myelotoxicity is idiosyncratic, uncommon, and independent of dosage, causing anemia, leukopenia, and/or thrombocytopenia. Neurotoxicity, usually associated with overdosage; ataxia and disorientation, cerebellar signs; may not resolve and may prove fatal (Ch 57, ref. 81). Teratogenic and can cause birth defects in pregnant animals. Given at 25 mg/kg daily for 30 days did not alter the viability, morphology, or motility of sperm in semen of male dogs (Ch 57, ref. 139).

INTERACTIONS. Interferes with porphyrin metabolism. Reduces effectiveness of barbiturates and warfarin rodenticides. Phenobarbital or other anticonvulsants may reduce griseofulvin's effectiveness.

AVAILABILITY	TYPE	SIZES	PREPARATIONS (COMPANY)
Human	Microsize: oral tablets	250 mg, 500 mg	*Fulvicin-U/F* (Schering-Plough Animal Health), *Grisactin* (Wyeth Ayerst)
	Oral capsules	125 mg, 250 mg	*Grisactin*
	Oral suspension	125 mg/5 ml	*Grifulvin V* (Ortho), *Grisactin*
	Ultramicrosize: tablets	125 mg, 165 mg, 250 mg, 330 mg	*Fulvicin P/G, Grisactin Ultra, Gris-PEG* (Allergan Herbert)
Veterinary	Microsize: oral tablets	250 mg, 500 mg	*Fulvicin-U/F*
		125 mg	*Grisovin* (Schering-Plough Animal Health)

INTERNATIONAL PREPARATIONS. *Biogrisin, Delmofulvina, Fulcin, Fulcine, Fungivin, Gricin, Griséfuline, Griseoderm, Griseomed, Griseostatin, Grisol, Grisovin, Grisovina, Lamoryl, Microcidal.*

HANDLING. Store at controlled room temperature in airtight containers. Protect suspension from light.

ADMINISTRATION. Therapy should continue until fungal cultures are negative or for at least 2 weeks after resolution of signs and for at least 5 mo for onychomycosis. Usually need 4-6 weeks of treatment because of drug incorporation into forming keratin. May combine with adjunctive topical therapy. Give tablet size most convenient by 1/4, 1/2, or whole-tablet increments. Give with a fatty meal or corn oil to enhance absorption and decrease GI irritation. Monitor CBC at least every 2 weeks during treatment.

DOSAGE. The dose recommended by the manufacturer of the microsize veterinary formulation (11-22 mg/kg/day) is much less than currently recommended for use in dogs and cats because it does not account for the more rapid clearance of the drug in dogs and cats.

INDICATIONS	DOSE (mg/kg)	ROUTE	INTERVAL(hr)	DURATION (days)
Dogs				
Dermatophytosis (microsized)	25	PO	12	42-56[a]
Dermatophytosis (ultramicrosized)	5-10	PO	24	42[a]
Cats				
Dermatophytosis (microsized)	50	PO	24	42-70
	25	PO	12	42-70
Dermatophytosis (ultramicrosized)	5-10	PO	24	42

[a]May have to treat longer for *Trichophyton* than for *Microsporum*.

ADDITONAL DOSAGES. Dermatophytosis, Table 58-5.

DISPENSING INFORMATION. Return for CBC weekly or biweekly. Duration of therapy at least 6 weeks for skin infections and 5 mo for onychomycotic lesions. May take up to 2.5 mo for mycologic cure of skin infection in many cases (Ch 57, ref. 95).

HETACILLIN

CLASS. Penicillin.

ACTION. Bactericidal; inhibits bacterial cell wall synthesis.

MORE INFORMATION. See also AMPICILLIN; Chapter 34, Aminopenicillins; Table 34-1.

PHARMACOKINETICS. Hydrolyzed in the stomach to ampicillin. See AMPICILLIN.

SPECTRUM, INDICATIONS, CONTRAINDICATIONS, ADVERSE REACTIONS, AND INTERACTIONS. See AMPICILLIN.

AVAILABILITY	TYPE	SIZES	PREPARATION (COMPANY)
Veterinary	Oral tablets (potassium)	50 mg, 100 mg, 200 mg	*Hetacin-K* (Fort Dodge)

INTERNATIONAL PREPARATIONS. *Etaciland.*

HANDLING AND ADMINISTRATION. See AMPICILLIN.

Dosage

INDICATIONS	DOSE	ROUTE	INTERVAL (hr)	DURATION (days)
Dogs				
Urinary tract	11-22 mg/kg	PO	12	7-14
Systemic infections, difficult organism	22-44 mg/kg	PO	12	14
	11-22 mg/kg	PO	8	14
Cats				
Urinary infections	50 mg/cat	PO	12	7-14
Systemic infections	10-20 mg/kg	PO	8	7-14

ADDITIONAL DOSAGES. None.

DISPENSING INFORMATION. Give 1 hr before or 2 hr after feeding.

IBAFLOXACIN

CLASS. Fluoroquinolone.

ACTION. Bactericidal; inhibits bacterial DNA gyrase. Main metabolite, 8-hydroxy-ibafloxacin is also antimicrobial.

MORE INFORMATION. See ENROFLOXACIN; Chapter 34; Table 34-11.

PHARMACOKINETICS. Rapidly absorbed from GI tract; plama concentrations are maximal by 1-2 hr. The drug is 69%-81% bioavailable (Ch 34, ref. 78b). Food positively increases absorption and bioavailability. Maximum concentration of 6 μ/ml at 15 mg/kg dosing. Widely distributed in tissues. Liver metabolizes a majority of the drug, and most found in the urine or feces or urine are metabolites. After multiple dosages, there is no dosage accumulation in dogs; however, moderate accumulation of drug can occur in cats. Following repeated oral administration to cats, increases in the drug and its less active metabolites were noted between days 1 and 10 of treatment (Ch 34, ref. 78a). When administered to dogs at 75 mg/kg (5 times the recommended dose) for 90 days, it was well tolerated. However doses in a range of 15-75 mg/kg to cats for 30 days produced vomiting and hypersalivation.

SPECTRUM. As for other quinolones. **Gram positive:** *Staphylococcus.* **Gram negative:** *Escherichia, Klebsiella, Pseudomonas, Proteus, Salmonella, Serratia, Shigella, Citrobacter, Enterobacter, Brucella, Pasteurella.* Anaerobes: less effective. Moderate activity against *Bordetella bronchiseptica.* Others: see ENROFLOXACIN. **More effective:** gram-negative aerobes and facultative anaerobes. **Low effectiveness:** *Pseudomonas* spp and streptococci **Ineffective:** obligate anaerobes. See also ENROFLOXACIN.

INDICATIONS. For skin, urinary and respiratory infections. For skin infections such as pyoderma (deep or superficial),

wounds or abscesses caused by susceptible strains of staphylococci, *E. coli* and *Proteus mirabilis.* For acute uncomplicated urinary tract infections caused by susceptible strains of staphylococci, *Proteus* spp. *Enterobacter* spp., *E. coli,* and *Klebsiella* spp. For Upper and lower respiratory infections caused by susceptible strains of staphylococci, *E. coli* and *Klebsiella* spp.

APPROVED USES. Dog, for treatment of pyoderma, wounds and abscesses caused by susceptible organisms. Unlike other veterinary quinolones, has been licensed for treatment up to 90 days. Cats, for dermal, soft tissue, and respiratory infections caused by susceptible organisms.

CONTRAINDICATIONS. Not recommended for use in most dogs before 9 mo of age and up to 18 mo in large and giant breeds. The 7.5% gel should not be used in cats.

ADVERSE REACTIONS. As with other quinolones, see ENROFLOXACIN. GI signs of diarrhea and vomiting.

INTERACTIONS. See ENROFLOXACIN. Avoid concurrent administration of products containing multivalent cations which interfere with absorption. Avoid concurrent treatment with nitrofurans due to antagonism.

AVAILABILITY	TYPE	SIZES	PREPARATIONS (COMPANY)
Veterinary (Dogs and cats)	Oral tablets Double scored Gel for cats or dogs	150 and 300 mg tablets; also 30, 900 mg (USA) 3% or 7.5% (Europe)	*Ibaflin* (Intervet Inc., Intervet Nederland B.V.) *Ibaflin* (Intervet Nederland B.V.)

HANDLING. Store tablets in airtight, moisture-proof containers at room temperature below 25°C. Sold in blister packets.

ADMINISTRATION. See ENROFLOXACIN. Has been approved for use in pregnant bitches.

Dosage

INDICATIONS	DOSE (mg/kg)	ROUTE	INTERVAL (hr)	DURATION[a] (days)
Dogs				
Urinary, skin, soft tissue, respiratory infections	15[b]	PO	24	10-21
Cats				
Urinary, soft tissue	15[c]	PO	24	10

[a]Duration of treatment depends on nature and severity of infection. Ten-day course is often sufficient for self-limiting infections. Pyoderma often requires a minimum of 21 days.
[b]Ch 85, ref. 22; Ch 34, ref. 172a.
[c]Ch 34, ref. 78a.

ADDITIONAL DOSAGES. None.

DISPENSING INFORMATION. Medicine should be given with food to help increase its absorption.

IDOXURIDINE (SEE CHAPTER 2)

IMIDOCARB DIPROPIONATE

CLASS. Aromatic diamidine.

ACTION. Antiprotozoal. Interferes with nucleic acid metabolism.

MORE INFORMATION. See DIMINAZENE, AMICARBALIDE, PHENAMIDINE, PENTAMIDINE; Chapter 71; Table 71-1; references: Ch 71, ref. 42; 57; 71; Ch 77, ref. 78.

PHARMACOKINETICS. Slowly metabolized and excreted after IM injection. Persists for long periods in plasma and tissues and gradually eliminated. Protects dogs from infection for up to 5 weeks.

SPECTRUM. *Ehrlichia, Babesia.* Some variation in species and strain susceptibility (Ch 34, ref. 108a). Not effective against *E. platys* or *Mycoplasma haemofelis* (Ch 34, ref. 427a). See Table 77-3 for efficacy against *Babesia* species.

INDICATIONS. Ehrlichiosis, babesiosis.

APPROVED USES. Babesiosis.

CONTRAINDICATIONS. Use of organophosphates or cholinesterase-inhibiting drugs may increase toxicity. Reduce dose or avoid use with preexisting pulmonary impairment or renal or hepatic failure. Safety and efficacy have not been determined for puppies or for breeding, lactating, or pregnant dogs. Not recommended for IV use.

ADVERSE REACTIONS. Pain swelling, abscess, or ulceration at injection site; periorbital edema, hypersalivation, nasal drip, shivering, lacrimation, diarrhea, vomiting, mental agitation, or depression. Posttreatment vomiting is one of the most consistent side effects. The less toxic dipropionate salt produces hypotension and signs similar to those of organophosphate intoxication when given IV (less with IM), but this reaction can be prevented by prior administration of atropine.

Reversal with atropine is recommended. Occasional renal tubular necrosis develops. Dose range of 7-10 mg/kg has been tolerated by dogs but approached toxic levels. Doses of 10 mg/kg cause mild transient tachycardia, and higher dosages may cause premature ventricular tachycardia. Elevations of serum ALT and AST are observed proportional to dosages used as a result of hepatic necrosis. Hepatic vacuolization occurs at therapeutic IV dosage and consistent at overdosages of 20 mg/kg; massive fatal hepatic necrosis after very high (60 mg/kg) accidental overdosage (Ch 71, ref. 42). Inflammatory reactions in muscle or skin causing lameness or dermatitis, respectively, can be prevented by deep IM injection in lumbar muscle. Oncogenesis at high dosages in rats. To report adverse reaction in the U.S., call 1-800-224-5318.

INTERACTIONS. For *Babesia*, synergistic with one injection of diminazene 24 hr later. Potentiates organophosphate toxicity as a result of inherent anticholinesterase activity. Should not be used simultaneously with exposure to cholinesterase-inhibiting substances.

AVAILABILITY	TYPE	SIZES	PREPARATIONS (COMPANY)
Veterinary	Parenteral solution	12% solution multidose vial (120 mg/ml) in 10-ml sterile vials	*Forray-65* (Hoechst Marion Roussel), *Imizol* (Schering-Plough Animal Health) AgriVet

INTERNATIONAL PREPARATIONS. *Carbesia.*

HANDLING. Store between 2-25°C away from light.

ADMINISTRATION. Follow CBC up to 12-20 weeks to monitor response to therapy.

Dosage

INDICATIONS	DOSE (mg/kg)	ROUTE	REPEAT INOCULATION (days)
Dogs			
Ehrlichiosis	5.0	IM, SC	14-21
	5.0	IM, SC	84
Babesiosis	5.0-6.6[a]	IM, SC	14
	7.5	IM, SC	None
Cats			
Cytauxzoonosis	5.0	IM	7

[a]Higher dose from product insert, Schering-Plough.

ADDITIONAL DOSAGES. Ehrlichiosis, Table 28-4; cytauxzoonosis, Table 76-1; babesiosis, Table 77-3.

IMIPENEM-CILASTATIN SODIUM

CLASS. Imipenem is a β-lactam of the carbapenem group. It is used in a 1 : 1 ratio with cilastatin, an inhibitor of renal dehydropeptidase–1 that degrades cilastatin. Meropenem, a newer carbapenem, does not require cilastatin coadministration.

ACTION. Bactericidal; imipenem inhibits synthesis of bacterial cell wall peptidoglycan.

MORE INFORMATION. See Chapter 34; Table 34-1.

PHARMACOKINETICS. Poorly absorbed from GI tract, but good systemic availability (75% of IV) after IM administra-

tion. Imipenem degradation by renal tubular enzyme is inhibited by cilastatin, which increases urine concentration of active drug and reduces potential nephrotoxicity from metabolites. Most of the drug is renally excreted. Penetrates all tissues and fluid compartments, including aqueous humor. Concentrations in CSF with inflamed and normal meninges are lower than in other tissues and body fluids, with the lowest levels in CSF, vitreous, placenta, milk. In pharmacokinetic studies in dogs, 5 mg/kg IV, IM, and SC had similar area-under-curve values. The MIC for *Escherichia coli* was exceeded for at least 4 hr. Ch 34, ref. 18a.

SPECTRUM. Very broad antibacterial activity. Resistant to most bacterial β-lactamases. **Gram positive:** *Staphylococcus*, some *Streptococcus*, including *S. viridans, Listeria, Nocardia*, some *Enterococcus* (not methicillin-resistant strains). **Gram negative:** most gram-negatives, *Escherichia, Klebsiella, Pseudomonas, Citrobacter, Enterobacter, Serratia*. Resistance to *Pseudomonas* can develop during use. **Anaerobes:** *Bacteroides, Fusobacterium, Peptostreptococcus*. **Others:** *Mycobacterium avium-intracellulare* complex. **More effective:** widest spectrum of any single antibacterial, little if any cross-resistance to penicillins or cephalosporins.

INDICATIONS. Bowel ruptures, skin infections, abscesses, cellulitis, wounds, endometritis, lower respiratory tract infections. Single, mixed, and resistant gram-negative bacterial infections. Intraabdominal and genital infections caused by both gram-negative and anaerobic bacteria. May replace combined therapy with aminoglycoside or cephalosporin plus metronidazole or clindamycin. Good for lower respiratory tract infections, bacterial meningitis, bacteremia, sepsis caused by resistant organisms. IM route for less severe infections in soft tissue.

APPROVED USES. Serious and multiple-resistant bacterial infections when a single agent is needed.

CONTRAINDICATIONS. Severe or life-threatening infections, including bacterial sepsis, endocarditis, or shock. The dosage should be reduced in renal failure. Not determined whether safe for pregnant animals. Cross-hypersensitivity to penicillins.

ADVERSE REACTIONS. Allergic reactions to vehicle, treat as anaphylaxis with epinephrine, oxygen, airway management, glucocorticoids. IV preparation may produce phlebitis, pain, erythema at injection site. In people, systemic signs during infusion have been nausea, diarrhea, vomiting, fever, hypotension, seizures, dizziness, urticaria. All β-lactams can cause seizures if underlying brain disease or if overdosed related to body size and renal function. Laboratory alterations include increased bilirubin, hepatic transaminases, hyponatremia, azotemia, thrombocytosis or thrombocytopenia, eosinophilia. The IM product contains lidocaine hydrochloride, which is contraindicated with known hypersensitivity, with shock, or heart block.

INTERACTIONS. Antagonistic interaction may reduce effectiveness of this drug coadministered with other β-lactam drugs or chloramphenicol. Addition of aminoglycosides or trimethoprim-sulfonamide may be synergistic against certain organisms.

AVAILABILITY	TYPE	SIZES	PREPARATIONS (COMPANY)
Human	Powder for injection as 1:1 combination with cilastatin	250 mg, 500 mg, in vials and bottles for IV	*Primaxin* (Merck)
		500 mg and 750 mg for IM (suspension)	*Primaxin* I.M.

INTERNATIONAL PREPARATIONS. *Tenacid, Tienam, Tracix, Zienam*.

HANDLING. Store powder at refrigerated or controlled room temperature. For IV, dilute contents into at least 100 ml of appropriate infusion solution (0.9% NaCl, 5% dextrose, sodium bicarbonate, mannitol [2.5-10%], and KCl [0.15%]). Maintains potency for 4-10 hr at room temperature 24-48 hr if refrigerated; the longer time periods are with 0.9% NaCl

diluent. Never freeze. Give by intermittent IV infusion over 20-60 min. Do not mix with other drugs. For IM, solutions reconstitute with 1% lidocaine (without epinephrine); should be used within 1 hr.

ADMINISTRATION. For IM, use a 21-gauge needle and deep injection. Aspirate before injection to avoid inadvertent IV administration. Absorption following SC and IM administration is comparable with IV and may be more convenient.

Dosage

INDICATIONS (*Dogs and Cats*)	DOSE (mg/kg)	ROUTE	INTERVAL (hr)	DURATION (days)
Tissue infections	3.0-7.5	IV, IM, SC	4-6	3-5
Sepsis, more resistant organism	5	IV	4[a]	3-5

[a]Multidrug-resistant bacteria may require dosing every 2 hr to achieve and maintain therapeutic concentrations (Ch 34, ref. 18a).

ADDITIONAL DOSAGES. Gram-negative bacterial infections, Table 37-3; endotoxemia, Table 38-6; nocardiosis, Table 49-3; bacteremia and endocarditis, Table 87-6; respiratory infections, Table 88-8; intraabdominal infections, Table 89-21.

INTERFERON-α (IFN-α, HUMAN RECOMBINANT)

CLASS. Cytokine produced by recombinant means to match human protein. The 2a and 2b forms differ in the sequence of two amino acids and purification.

ACTION. Acts on terminal stages of virus production by preventing assembly and budding of mature virions, also immunomodulating influences.

MORE INFORMATION. Chapter 2; Table 2-3; Ch 2, ref. 25,122, 169; Appendix 8, ref. 3, 4, 7, 9. Previously known as leucocytic or lymphoblastoid interferon.

PHARMACOKINETICS. Low-dose oral: (1-30 U) possibly stimulates oropharyngeal tonsils locally, not much absorbed systemically as destroyed by gastric acid. **High-dose parenteral:** SC (1.6×10^6 U/kg) resulted in plasma concentration measurable for 8 hr. Well absorbed after SC or IM injection. After IV injection, the drug is distributed primarily to liver and kidneys, with lesser amounts in thyroid, spleen, and GI mucosae. Filtered at renal glomerulus, catabolized by kidneys, and excreted in urine. At lower dosage concentrations of IFN-α (10^5 U/kg), the neutralizing antibody titers that develop (see later) were proportionally lower than those at the high dosages.

SPECTRUM. Many viruses, immunostimulant.

INDICATIONS. Oral: adjunct to alleviate clinical manifestations of ill FeLV—infected cats suffering from immunosuppressive (not neoplastic) effects of FeLV. It may prolong cat's well-being and associated survival time. Stimulates appetite. Does *not* affect viremia but may have some effect on virus-induced myelosuppression. Use only in ill FeLV-positive cats. Can be tried in cats with FIV or chronic upper respiratory tract disease or dogs with systemic mycotic infections as an adjunct to antifungal therapy. There has been subjective improvement in these situations but no controlled studies.

Parenteral: may decrease retroviral viremia for limited periods. Use of recombinant human IFN parenterally can induce neutralizing antibody, which interferes with activity after several weeks. Cats receiving high doses (10^6 U/cat) for 21 days had neutralizing antibody titers develop and therapeutic refractoriness (Ch 2, ref. 179; 180). Cats receiving high dose (10^6 U/cat) had reduced lymphocyte blastogenesis compared with those receiving 10^4 or 10^2 U/kg, which had enhanced lymphocyte activity (Ch 2, ref. 171). Not routinely recommended for parenteral use in animals for these reasons. Low-dose oral is the preferred method of administration. Low doses (1-30 U/cat) given orally have been used in milder cases of noneffusive FIP, when it may help suppress disease progression (Appendix 8, ref. 7). High doses ($>2 \times 0^4$ U/kg) given IM have been used as an immunomodulator in conjunction with glucocorticoids to treat effusive FIP (Appendix 8, ref. 7). **Intralesional:** for viral papillomatosis in people; might be tried for these lesions in dogs (Chapter 9) and cats (Chapter 20). **Topical:** used in eye in conjunction with topical antiviral drugs in cats with chronic herpesvirus keratitis and conjunctivitis (Ch 2, ref. 141). See Chapter 93.

APPROVED USES. In people for various malignancies and viral diseases.

CONTRAINDICATIONS. Limited efficacy of high-dose parenteral human interferon in cats because of neutralizing antibodies (Ch 2, ref. 180). May become refractory 3-7 weeks after initiating treatment. PO, topical, or intralesional treatment does not induce this refractoriness.

ADVERSE REACTIONS. Parenteral: in cats, allergic reactions, fever, lethargy, myalgia, myelotoxicity; in people, also neurotoxicity, hepatotoxicity. **Oral, intralesional, topical:** none.

INTERACTIONS. Unknown.

AVAILABILITY	TYPE	SIZES	PREPARATION (COMPANY)
Human	Interferon-α$_{2a}$, solution or powder for injection	3, 6, 36 × 10^6 U vials	*Roferon A* (Roche)
	Interferon-α$_{2b}$, powder for injection	3, 5, 10, 18, 25, 50 × 10^6 U vials	*Intron A* (Schering-Plough Animal Health)
	Interferon-α$_{n3}$ solution for injection	5 × 10^6 U vials	*Alferon N* (Purdue Frederick)

HANDLING. For 3-U/ml solution: make 1 : 100 dilution of commercial solution (3×10^6 U/ml) using sterile water giving 3×10^4 U/ml. Take 0.1 ml and add to 1 L of 0.9% NaCl containing 4 ml of 25% serum albumin (albumin is optional but adds stability at low concentrations). Package 3 U/ml solution in 15-ml aliquots in sterile injection vials and store frozen (−70°C desirable). Thaw vials as needed, then store refrigerated for administration. Discard unused portion 60 days after first using refrigerated solution. Discard unused 3×10^4 U/ml solution within 2-3 hr after making initial dilutions. **For 30-U/ml solution:** dilute entire contents of commercial solution (3×10^6 U/ml) into 1 L sterile IV fluid bag containing saline to give a solution of 3000 U/ml. This can be divided in 1- or 10-ml aliquots and frozen. The commercial solution or 3000-U/ml solution can be frozen for years without losing activity. The 3000-U/ml solution (1 ml or 10 ml, respectively) can be added to 100 ml sterile saline or to a 1 L IV fluid bag to produce either 100 or 1000 ml of 30-U/ml solution for administration (Appendix 8, ref. 7). Some have advised aliquoting the diluted solution into 1 ml volumes for freezing up to 1 yr. Then the aliquots are defrosted as needed. Once

they are defrosted, the drug can be kept refrigerated up to 1 week. Freezing the most dilute solutions is associated with loss in activity unless protein such as albumin is added during dilution. To get a concentration of 10^4 IU/ml, dilute a 1×10^6 IU vial of interferon into 99 ml sterile saline and divide into 1-ml doses and freeze. For 10^5 IU/ml, use 9 ml saline and proceed as above.

ADMINISTRATION. Oral: for 3 U/ml solution, remove 0.3 ml (1 U) using sterile needle and 1.0-ml syringe. For 30 U/ml, remove 1-ml solution. Remove needle from hub and squirt dose into the oral cavity once each day of treatment. If syringes are reused, a short reusable rubber or plastic catheter segment may aid in keeping syringe from contacting oral mucosae to help preserve sterility of 15- or 30-ml refrigerated aliquots. **Parenteral:** not recommended because it stimulates antibody formation. **Intralesional:** into papillomas, inject 1×0^6 μ/0.1 ml into up to five warts three times/week until regression occurs. **Topical ocular:** Same diluted preparation for oral use can be used by applying in drops to the eye 3-4 times daily.

Dosage

INDICATIONS	DOSE	UNITS	ROUTE	INTERVAL (hr)	DURATION (days)
Cat					
FeLV and appetite stimulation	1[a]	U/cat	PO	24	7[b]
	30	U/cat	PO	24	7[c]
Viral respiratory disease	10×16^6	U/kg	SC	21	≤21
FIP exudative (wet)	2×10^4	U/kg	IM	24	14-21
FIP nonexudative (dry)	30	U/cat	PO	24	7[c]
Dog					
Immunosuppression	1	U/5 kg	PO	24	7[†]

[a]Although daily doses of 30 U have been recommended (Appendix 8, ref. 7), other studies with FeLV-infected cats have shown 1 U to be superior to 5 U (Ch 2, ref. 25).
[b]Treat alternate weeks or continuously (Ch 2, ref. 25).
[c]Treat alternate weeks (Appendix 8, ref. 7).

ADDITIONAL DOSAGES. FIP, Table 11-4.

DISPENSING INFORMATION. Keep medication refrigerated and discard unused portions after 60 days. Use a short catheter on the end of the syringe to keep it from becoming contaminated with oral bacteria. This treatment will not reverse the FeLV-positive status of the cat but may improve appetite, general attitude, health.

INTERFERON-β_{1B}, -β_{1A} (IFN-β, HUMAN RECOMBINANT)

CLASS. Polypeptide cytokine from fibroblasts. Produced by recombinant DNA methods.

ACTION. Antiviral and immunoregulatory.

MORE INFORMATION. Previously known as fibroblast interferon. See Chapter 2, Antivirals and Immunotherapy. Reference: Appendix 8, ref. 2.

PHARMACOKINETICS. Not detectable in blood or tissues after SC administration. Bioavailability is 50% with SC use. After IV use, reaches low levels in blood with rapid clearance.

INDICATIONS. In people for treatment of multiple sclerosis at time of first demyelinating event. Prevents or suppresses progression of disease. Used in immunosuppressed people with AIDS from HIV infection, myelogenous or metastatic neoplasia, some viral hepatitis. No immediate uses in dogs and cats but might be considered in similar disorders. For dogs, demyelinating canine distemper encephalomyelitis might be a potential use. For cats might consider it in retroviral infections.

CONTRAINDICATIONS. Pregnancy, leukopenia, anemia.

ADVERSE REACTIONS. In people similar to IFN-α: myelosuppression, fever, chills, myalgia, photosensitivity, systemic allergic reactions, abortion.

INTERACTIONS. Decreased clearance of AZT given currently.

AVAILABILITY	TYPE	SIZES	PREPARATIONS (COMPANY)
Human-β_{1b}	Powder for injection	0.3 mg (9.6 MIU) contains human albumin	*Betaseron* (Berlex)
Human-β_{1a}	Powder for injection	44 µg	*Rebif* (Serono)
		6.6 MIU	Avonex (Biogen)

HANDLING. Powder should be stored refrigerated. Inject sterile 0.9% NaCl into vial to dissolve drug. After reconstituting solution is 0.25 mg/ml. Only good for single use once reconstituted. Refrigerate, do not freeze if not used immediately.

ADMINISTRATION. Injected SC.

Dosage

INDICATIONS	DOSE	UNITS	ROUTE	INTERVAL (hr)	DURATION (YEARS)
Antiviral, Immunoregulation					
Human (-β_{1b})	0.25	mg (8 MIU)	SC	48	≤2
Human (-β_{1a})					
Multiple sclerosis	30	µg	IM	168	3

ADDITIONAL DOSAGES. None.

INTERFERON-γ₁ᴮ (IFN-γ, HUMAN RECOMBINANT)

CLASS. Polypeptide lymphokine with antiviral, immunomodulatory, and antiproliferative effects.

ACTION. Biologic response modifier, potent phagocyte-activating effects potentiate killing of intracellular organisms such as virulent *Staphylococcus, Toxoplasma, Leishmania, Listeria, Mycobacterium avium-intracellulare* complex.

MORE INFORMATION. Previously known as immune interferon. Chapter 2; references: Ch 2, ref. 38a.

PHARMACOKINETICS. Absorbed slowly after IM or SC administration. Rapid clearance after IV use. Slower elimination and high bioavailability (89%) makes SC use desirable.

SPECTRUM. Immunostimulating for defense against persistent intracellular organisms. Some dose relationship; higher dosages were associated with improved efficacy. Has been effective in experimental animal infections of toxoplasmosis, *Pneumocystis carinii* pneumonia, cryptosporidiosis (Ch 71, ref. 76). Similar experiments were favorable for fungal infections such as histoplasmosis, coccidioidomycosis, candidasis, aspergillosis, and cryptococcosis. Has been combined with Amphotericin B treatment to treat experimental CNS cryptococcosis.

INDICATIONS. Immunodeficiency caused by neutrophil phagocyte defects. Helps prevent infection.

CONTRAINDICATIONS. Pregnancy, leukopenia, thrombocytopenia.

ADVERSE REACTIONS. In people, CNS signs of mental depression and gait dysfunction, myelosuppression, abortion. Because these compounds are species specific, antibody might develop with chronic use in dogs and cats and limit effectiveness.

INTERACTIONS. May be synergistic with concurrent antimicrobial chemotherapy such as roxithromycin, trimethoprim-sulfonamide, sodium stilbogluconate.

AVAILABILITY	TYPE	SIZES	PREPARATION (COMPANY)
Human	Solution for injection	100 µg (3×10^6 U)/0.5 ml	*Actimmune* (Genentech)

HANDLING. No preservatives in vial; must be for single dose; keep refrigerated 2-8°C. Must be discarded if left unrefrigerated >12 hr.

ADMINISTRATION. Drug is given SC. Liquid should be gently mixed but not shaken and should not be discolored or contain particulate matter.

Dosage

INDICATIONS *(Human)*	DOSE	ROUTE	INTERVAL	DURATION (days)
Body surface >0.5 m²	50 µg/m²	SC	3× weekly	prn
Body surface <0.5 m²	1.5 µg/kg	SC	3× weekly	prn

ADDITIONAL DOSAGES. None.

INTERFERON-ω (IFN-ω, IFN—ω, FELINE RECOMBINANT)

CLASS. Cytokine produced by recombinant means to match the feline protein. It is produced in silkworms by a recombinant baculovirus expression system (Ch 2, ref. 159). Omega interferon is a type I interferon related to alpha interferon.

ACTION. Does not act directly or specifically on the virus, but predominantly on virus-infected cells, by an inhibition of mRNA and translation proteins. May nonspecifically enhance immune defenses. Acts on the cell to inhibit the internal synthesis mechanim of terminal stages of virus production by preventing assembly and budding of mature virions.

MORE INFORMATION. Chapters 2 and 8, References (Ch 8, ref. 15; 66; 44; 60; Ch 13, ref. 49a) www.virbagenomega.com.

PHARMACOKINETICS. Parenteral: Similar to human interferons. After injection it is bound to specific receptors of a large variety of cells. The drug is distributed primarily to liver and kidneys. Filtered at renal glomerulus, catabolized by kidneys, and excreted in urine (Ch 2, ref. 158).

SPECTRUM. Acts to suppress infection by many viruses. May be acting as an immunostimulant.

INDICATIONS. Parenteral: may decrease viremia for limited periods. Use of this recombinant heterologous IFN parenterally in dogs may induce neutralizing antibody, which interferes with activity after several weeks.

APPROVED USES. In dogs for the reduction of mortality and clinical signs from parvovirus infection. Animals should be older than 1 mo. In cats as adjunctive therapy for clinical illness associated with FeLV and or FIV infection. In addition to IFN, other forms of adjunctive therapy should be used for the disease being treated.

CONTRAINDICATIONS. Prior or repeated use may theoretically interfere with activity due to the production of antibody to the heterologous protein. In long-term use, cats do not develop antibodies like dogs, which reduces activity with time. Safety in pregnancy and lactation has not been determined. Animals should not be vaccinated during the course of interferon therapy.

ADVERSE REACTIONS. No severe adverse signs have been reported in dogs or cats given this interferon. In dogs transient fever may be seen 3-6 hr after injection and WBC, erythrocyte, and platelet counts may be suppressed for 1 week. Overdose (10-fold) has caused mild lethargy, increased body temperature, increased respiratory rate, sinus tachycardia, which resolve within 7 days.

INTERACTIONS. Never mix with any other IV preparation except supplied diluent.

AVAILABILITY	TYPE	SIZES	PREPARATION (COMPANY)
Canine and feline	Interferon-ω lyophylized powder for injection with saline diluent	5 and 10×10^6 U vials	*Virbagen Omega* (Virbac)[a]

[a]In the United States, it can be obtained for compassionate use through private vendors overseas (e.g., Abbeyvet.com), after obtaining FDA approval for importation.

HANDLING. The product must be used immediately after reconstitution due to the lack of preservative. Store and transport at 4°C. Do not freeze. Stability is 2 yr. The freeze-dried fraction must be reconstituted with the specific solvent supplied.

ADMINISTRATION. Parenteral: Reconsituted product is injected IV, once daily for 3-5 consecutive days. It should be given in conjunction with other supportive care for the infection being treated.

Dosage

INDICATIONS	DOSE	UNITS	ROUTE	INTERVAL (hr)	DURATION (days)
Dogs and Cats					
Parvoviral or acute viral Infections	2.5	Million U/kg	IV,SC	24	3
Cats					
Feline leukemia or immunodeficiency virus infections, caliciviral gingivostomatitis or chronic viral infections	1	Million U/kg	SC	24	5[a]

[a]For FeLV or FIV is given on day 0-4 and has been repeated on days 14-18 and 60-64 (Ch 13, ref. 49a).

ADDITIONAL DOSAGES. See Chapter 2 for those used in specific studies.

DISPENSING INFORMATION. Product should be reconstituted and administered only with provided solvent. Vaccination of treated dogs is contraindicated until the animal recovers clinically.

IODIDE (POTASSIUM AND SODIUM)

CLASS. Inorganic halogen.

ACTION. Antifungal but exact mechanism uncertain. May facilitate phagocytic killing of fungal cells.

MORE INFORMATION. Chapter 57; Chapter 63.

PHARMACOKINETICS. Unknown.

SPECTRUM. *Sporothrix, Basidiobolus*.

INDICATIONS. Sporotrichosis, some treatment failures occur. Preferred for dogs owing to good clinical response and low toxicity. Has been effective in some cases of subcutaneous phycomycosis in people. Trials are being conducted on rhinosporidiosis.

APPROVED USES. Antithyroidal agent, sporotrichosis, expectorant.

CONTRAINDICATIONS. Hyperthyroidism, iodide hypersensitivity, renal failure, dehydration, pregnancy.

ADVERSE REACTIONS. Cats often develop toxic signs of iodism, including vomiting, anorexia, muscle twitching, cardiomyopathy, heart failure, death. Enteric-coated tablets have caused bowel ulceration in people. Prolonged use has caused hypothyroidism, goiter, thyroid adenomas, and dermatitis in people.

INTERACTIONS. Concurrent use with other potassium-containing medications can cause hyperkalemia.

AVAILABILITY	TYPE	SIZES	PREPARATIONS (COMPANY)
Human KI	Oral solution	1 g KI/ml (300 /ml bottle)	*SSKI* (Upsher-Smith), generic (many)
	Oral syrup (black raspberry flavor)	325 mg/5 ml	*Pima* Syrup (Fleming)
Veterinary, NaI	Parenteral solution	200 mg/ml	Sodium Iodide (ProLabs, Vet Tek, Lextron, RXV

KI, Potassium iodide; *NaI*, sodium iodide.

HANDLING. Can produce saturated solution of KI in lieu of commercial preparations or 20% NaI solutions (200 mg/ml). Parenteral NaI solutions listed contain only water. If commercial KI or NaI solutions are used, they should not contain other ingredients intended as expectorants.

ADMINISTRATION. For accuracy, always aspirate dose in graduated 1-ml syringes. Always administer by placing drops directly on food to decrease GI irritation. Continue for at least 1 mo beyond clinical cure.

Dosage

INDICATIONS	DOSE (mg/kg)	ROUTE	INTERVAL (hr)	DURATION (days)
Dogs				
Sporotrichosis	40	PO	8	≥60
Cats				
Sporotrichosis	20	PO	12-24	≥60

ADDITIONAL DOSAGES. Drug therapy for sporotrichosis, Table 63-1.

DISPENSING INFORMATION. Administer by placing liquid on animal's food or give orally immediately after feeding. Report any loss of appetite or other signs to veterinarian.

IODOQUINOL

CLASS. 8-hydroxyquinoline; also called diiodohydroxyquin.

ACTION. Antibacterial, antifungal, and antiprotozoal.

MORE INFORMATION. See elsewhere, Clioquinol (Moebiquin, Vioform); Chapter 71; Table 71-1.

PHARMACOKINETICS. Poorly absorbed (8%) from GI tract, high concentration in intestinal lumen. Will only treat luminal and not systemic spread.

SPECTRUM. *Entamoeba, Balantidium,* yeasts. Acts strictly in the gut lumen.

INDICATIONS. Intraluminal treatment of intestinal amebiasis and balantidiasis. Topical antifungal.

APPROVED USES. Human amebiasis.

CONTRAINDICATIONS. Not effective with extraintesti-nal (hepatic) amebiasis. Do not use in animals with neurologic, renal, or liver impairment or pre-existing thyroid dysfunction.

ADVERSE REACTIONS. Dermatologic eruption, enlarged thyroids, vomiting, diarrhea; optic nerve or peripheral neuropathy after prolonged use at high dosages. Neurotoxicity found in dogs treated with 5 g of a 3% clioquinol topical preparation for 28 days. Causes discoloration of tongue, urine, feces. Oral use of this drug and Clioquinol is restricted because of neurotoxicity.

INTERACTIONS. Interferes with thyroid testing as a result of iodination.

AVAILABILITY	TYPE	SIZES	PREPARATIONS (COMPANY)
Human	Oral tablets	210 mg, 650 mg	*Yodoxin* (Glenwood)
	Oral powder	25 g	*Yodoxin*

INTERNATIONAL PREPARATIONS. *Diodoquin, Direxiode, Floraquin, Sebaquin.*

HANDLING. Insoluble in water and minimally in alcohol. For smaller doses, tablets must be crushed or powder placed on moist food.

ADMINISTRATION. Topical use of this drug as an antifungal has been toxic to dogs.

DOSAGE. Not recommended for routine use in small animals. Amebiasis is uncommon in dogs and cats.

IPRONIDAZOLE

CLASS. Nitroimidazole.

ACTION. See METRONIDAZOLE.

MORE INFORMATION. See METRONIDAZOLE, TINIDAZOLE.

SPECTRUM. *Giardia, Trichomonas.*

INDICATIONS. Used in veterinary medicine to treat blackhead in turkeys. For giardiasis, when added to drinking water in kennel dogs.

CONTRAINDICATIONS. Pregnancy.

ADVERSE REACTIONS. Not noted, although mutagenesis is possible.

INTERACTIONS. See METRONIDAZOLE.

AVAILABILITY	TYPE	SIZES	PREPARATION (COMPANY)
Veterinary	Available as feed/water additive for turkeys[a]	Unknown	*Ipropran* (Roche)

[a]Not available in the USA.

ADMINISTRATION. Mix desired amount in drinking water. Do not give other sources of water until dose is finished.

Dosage

INDICATIONS	DOSE	ROUTE	INTERVAL (hr)	DURATION (days)
Dogs	126-378 mg/L	In water	24	7-14

ADDITIONAL DOSAGES. None.

ISONIAZID (INH)

CLASS. Hydrazide: isonicotinic acid hydrazide.

ACTION. Interferes with nucleic acid and lipid biosynthesis in bacteria.

MORE INFORMATION. Chapter 34; Chapter 50; Table 50-4; reference: Ch 34, ref. 395.

PHARMACOKINETICS. Rapid and completely absorbed after PO administration. All formulations are well absorbed. Inactivated in liver and 85% of unchanged drug and metabolites are excreted in urine. Portion metabolized by acetylation and excreted in urine; 50%-70% excreted unchanged.

SPECTRUM. *Mycobacterium.*

INDICATIONS. *M. tuberculosis* or *M. bovis* infections.

APPROVED USES. Human mycobacteriosis.

CONTRAINDICATIONS. Reduce dose in hepatic dysfunction and in severe renal failure.

ADVERSE REACTIONS. Vomiting; hepatotoxicity Elevated enzymes, bilirubin, hepatic necrosis; peripheral neuropathy in people. Vitamin B_6 (pyridoxine) deficiency, which in dogs causes recurrent tonic clonic seizures followed by salivation, diarrhea, vomiting, incoordination, cardiac arrhythmias (Ch 34, ref. 395). To treat accidental overdosage, 50 mg/kg or more of pyridoxine hydrochloride at a gram-for-gram dose equal to the amount ingested as a 5%-10% total wt/vol IV infusion over 30-60 min. A bolus if in status epilepticus. Additional anticonvulsants diazepam and phenobarbital as needed.

INTERACTIONS. Reduces levels of ketoconazole. Increases levels of benzodiazepines, diphenylhydantoin, hepatotoxicity enhanced with halothane, rifampin. Glucocorticoids decrease its effectiveness.

AVAILABILITY	TYPE	SIZES	PREPARATIONS (COMPANY)
Human	Oral tablets	50 mg, 100 mg, 300 mg	*Laniazid* (Ciba), generics (various)
	Parenteral injection	100 mg/ml	*Nydrazid* (Apothecon)

INTERNATIONAL PREPARATIONS. *Cemidon, Dipasic, Inapsade, Isotamine, Isozid, Laniazid, Nicazide, Nicotibine, Nydrazid, Pyreazid, Rimifon, Tibinide.*

HANDLING. Store in airtight and light-proof containers. Incompatible with sugars. Sterilize solution by autoclaving.

ADMINISTRATION. A 10-mg/ml suspension can be prepared by using 12 100-mg tablets, distilled water to dissolve, and adding aqueous 50% sorbitol to bring the volume to 120 ml. This should be refrigerated and is stable for 3 weeks. Shake well before using. Always use in combination with other antimycobacterial drugs. Aluminum-containing compounds interfere with absorption. Administer on empty stomach.

Dosage

INDICATIONS (*Dogs*)	DOSE	ROUTE	INTERVAL (hr)	DURATION (days)
Tuberculosis	10 mg/kg	PO	24	prn

ADDITIONAL DOSAGES. Mycobacterial Infections, Table 50-4.

DISPENSING INFORMATION. Give for 3-6 mo after cytologic or culture data suggest cure. Usual treatment is at least 6 mo.

ITRACONAZOLE

CLASS. Synthetic triazole antifungal.

ACTION. Inhibits cytochrome P-450 14α-demethylase preventing ergosterol synthesis in fungal cell membrane. It binds weakly to mammalian P-450. Greater potency and less toxicity than ketoconazole, presumably due to its triazole structure.

MORE INFORMATION. See KETOCONAZOLE, FLUCONAZOLE, CLOTRIMAZOLE; Chapter 57, Azoles; Table 57-1; references: Ch 57, ref. 9; 92; 44; 19; 33 Ch 63, ref. 51.

PHARMACOKINETICS. Oral absorption of itraconazole (ITZ) is similar in dogs and people (Ch 57, ref. 148a). **Capsules:** Variable GI absorption of capsules. PO bioavailability 40% with fasting but increases when given with food. Increased stomach acidity (low pH) increases absorption while alkalinity decreases absorption. Capsules can be opened, and a fraction of the dose can be mixed in the food. Variable in some cats requiring higher doses (10 mg/kg) for better efficacy. **Oral suspension** containing cyclodextrin is better (30% greater) absorbed with fasting and may exert some topical oral antifungal effects. Experimentally, oral dose of 5 mg/kg to cats is equivalent to 0.75-1 mg/kg IV or 1.25-1.5 mg/kg of oral solution because of the low bioavailability of oral capsules (Ch 57, ref. 9). Compared to capsules oral solution may be more efficacious on a per milligram basis in cats. Unlike capsules, bioavailability of oral solution is higher under fasted conditions. Drug is highly lipophilic and keratinophilic. Once absorbed, highly (>99%) protein bound to albumin. Extensively distributed into lipophilic tissues: concentrations in liver, kidney, adrenals, lung, and fat at least twice (2-20 times) that in blood. In skin, concentrations may be 3-10 times plasma. Reaches stratum corneum by secretion in sebum. Most of the drug is bound to keratin and persists in skin up to 2-4 weeks after treatment is discontinued. Does not penetrate well into CSF, saliva, aqueous humor. However, it has been used to treat animals with fungal meningitis and ophthalmitis due to inflamed barriers. Fluconazole penetrates better in these areas. Therapeutic concentrations maintained longer in tissues than plasma. Oral formulations require 14-21 days to reach steady state in dogs and cats (Ch 57, ref. 9). Drug concentrations increase after several weeks of therapy. They are three to five times higher compared with single dosing after 2 weeks of treatment of dogs and 21 days in cats.

IV formulation achieves adequate blood levels consistently and more rapidly with a predicted bioavailability. This parenteral formulation achieves steady state within a short time period of 2-7 days in people (Ch 57, ref. 14). Hepatotoxicity may be seen in 10% of dogs owing to inordinately high serum concentrations that develop. Primarily metabolized in liver with predominant biliary and lesser urinary excretion of inactive metabolites. Low activity in the urinary tract makes it unsuitable for treatment of urinary tract infections.

SPECTRUM. *Blastomyces, Histoplasma, Cryptococcus, Coccidioides, Aspergillus.* **Variable activity:** *Trichophyton, Candida, Sporothrix, Acanthamoeba, Malassezia, Microsporum, Pythium.* Broader and more potent in vivo than ketoconazole. **Others:** *Acanthamoeba, Trypanosoma.*

INDICATIONS. Fungal: blastomycosis, histoplasmosis, aspergillosis, coccidioidomycosis, candidiasis, cryptococcosis, sporotrichosis, fungal keratitis, zygomycosis, chromomycosis, onychomycosis. Also effective in some cases of dermatophytosis when griseofulvin was not effective or has caused toxicity. Cutaneous and systemic sporotrichosis least toxic and most effective, although expensive. Nasal, disseminated, and meningeal cryptococcosis. Poor to variable efficacy in nasal and disseminated aspergillosis and no additive effect to that produced by topical enilconazole alone. **Protozoal:** Acanthamebiasis not involving the CNS, cutaneous leishmaniasis. No need to adjust dose in renal insufficiency, unlike fluconazole (Ch 57, ref. 57).

APPROVED USES. Human systemic fungal infections.

CONTRAINDICATIONS. Hepatic disease or insufficiency. Must reduce if used with hepatic disease or dysfunction. Dosage does not need modification in renal failure. Teratogenic and embryotoxic effects have been seen at high dosages in lab animals, so should avoid in pregnancy and lactation.

ADVERSE REACTIONS. Vomiting, diarrhea, abdominal pain, inappetence, increased serum liver enzymes and urea, peripheral edema, fever, hypertension, skin rash and ulcerations (Ch 57, ref. 38). Less hepatotoxic than ketoconazole and unlike ketoconazole, does not affect adrenal or reproductive steroid synthesis. Nausea, anorexia, vomiting, hepatic injury, increased serum ALT are more common in cats; anorexia is associated with increased ALT and serum alkaline phosphatase. ALT decreases after drug is stopped for 1-2 weeks or until appetite returns or serum hepatic enzymes return toward reference levels; then treatment can be restarted at 50% dose or alternate days. Monitor serum hepatic enzyme activity every 2 weeks thereafter. Serious hepatotoxicity leads to icterus and death (Ch 57, ref. 38; 92). Hepatotoxicity and death occurred in one cat given 27.8 mg/kg/day for several weeks. High doses can produce hypokalemia. Ulcerative dermatitis (cutaneous vasculitis) and hepatotoxicity occur more in dogs receiving higher (10 mg/kg) daily dosages. It subsides if dosage is stopped or reduced to 5 mg/kg once daily (see ITZ, Adverse Effects, Chapter 57). Generalized cutaneous drug eruption was observed in one dog (Ch 57, ref. 107)

INTERACTIONS. Do not coadminister with ketoconazole, cisapride, terfenadine; fatal cardiac arrhythmias may occur. Absorption decreased with concurrent antacids (H_2 receptor antagonists, or proton pump blockers) or any disease raising gastric pH. Prolongs effects and increases toxicity of benzodiazepines (midazolam), cyclosporine, glucocorticoids, antihistamines, quinidine, digoxin, vincristine, warfarin, sulfonylureas. H_2-receptor antagonists (cimetidine), diphenylhydantoin, itraconazole, rifampin, or terfenadine. Phenobarbital, which stimulates P-450 metabolism, decreases efficacy of itraconazole. May interfere with the efficacy of AMB when used in combination or succession (Ch 57, ref. 129). For blood levels, send to Fungus Testing Laboratory, University of Texas Health Science Center, 7703 Floyd Curl Dr, San Antonio, TX 78284; (210) 567-4131.

AVAILABILITY. 100-mg bead-containing capsules must be split or formulated for cats and small dogs before use. Expensive, which may limit use. PO suspension available, and injectable solution. Oral suspension has greater bioavailability than capsules.

AVAILABILITY	TYPE	SIZES	PREPARATIONS (COMPANY)
Human	Oral capsules	100 mg	*Sporanox* (Janssen)
	Oral suspension (containing cyclodextrin)	10 mg/ml in 150 ml bottle	*Sporanox* (Janssen)
	IV solution in hydroxy-propyl-β-cyclodextrin	10 mg/ml in 25 ml ampules; 50 ml bags	*Sporanox* (Ortho Biotech)

INTERNATIONAL PREPARATIONS. *Beltop.*

HANDLING. Store capsules at room temperature and protected from light and moisture. Solution should be stored at room temperature and protected from freezing. The compounded preparations should be refrigerated and discarded after 35 days. Before availability of the commercially available solution, compounded liquid preparations were made, as follows, from capsules based on the manufacturer's recommendation. **Oral syrup:** a small amount of oral suspension can be made from capsules for cats and small dogs. Six 100-mg capsules are placed into glass mortar. Add 1.25 ml of 95% ethyl alcohol USP and let it stand 3 min to soften. Grind into a paste and let dry. Add 4 ml of corn syrup and transfer to 15-ml bottle. Continue to add up to 15-ml of syrup to wash the mortar and transfer it to the bottle. The final concentration is 40 mg/ml. It is stable refrigerated for 35 days. Should be shaken well before using and given with food. **Oral liquid:** each capsule can be dissolved in 2 ml of 0.2 N HCl. After 15 min, 20 ml of cranberry juice (pH < 2) is added. The final concentration (mg/ml) is total number of capsules ×100 divided by the total ml of juice used. Stable for 30 days when refrigerated. Shake well before use. **Oral suspension:** Commercially available in lieu of compounding of oral syrup or liquid forms.

ADMINISTRATION. Minimum administration interval for any infection is 4-6 weeks. Minimum treatment interval of blastomycosis often ranges 2-6 months. Treatment of more resistant or "walled-off" systemic mycosis may require 10 mo or more. To achieve a higher steady state in rapidly advancing mycosis, consider initial higher loading dose followed by a lower maintenance level. For sporotrichosis in humans, treatment lasts 3-18 mo. Treatment for dermatophytosis is at least 1 week beyond clinical and mycologic cure (Ch 57, ref. 95). Preadminister amphotericin B with rapidly progressive life-threatening infections. Increasing gastric acid secretion improves absorption. Administration of capsules with or immediately after a meal improves absorption. Note, however, the solution should be administered on an *empty* stomach. Monitor serum ALT monthly since it often increases in cats after 60 days of instituting therapy. Dogs seem less sensitive to the hepatotoxic effects than cats. Anorexia or increased ALT is managed by reducing or discontinuing the dosage. If toxicity develops at any dose, reinstitute dose at 50% after the adverse signs have abated. The capsules containing beads can be emptied and separated to smaller gelatin capsules or placed directly on food. For young kittens with dermatophytosis, can use 10 beads/day placed on food. Some concentration of itraconazole can be measured to ensure therapeutic level (≥2 μg/ml) is being acheived. Measured by Fungus Testing Laboratory, University of Texas, Health Science Center, 7703 Floyd Care Dr, San Antonio, TX 78284; (210) 567-4131.

PULSE DOSING. Because ITZ accumulates in keratin, superficial infections (skin, nails or hair) may be treated with pulse therapy. Pulse doses in cats with dermatophytosis were 1-2 consecutive week treatment periods per month for a 3 month period (Ch 57, ref. 88). Lower dosages than appear in the table below (1.5-3 mg/kg/day, for 15 days) were used in that study, where 50% of the cats improved; however, no control cats were compared to determine if spontaneous recovery was possible. Continuous pulse therapy has also been reported to be successful at doses listed in the table (Ch 57, ref. 19). A dosage of 5 mg/kg/day for 1 week on an alternate week basis during a 6-week period has also been effective for treatment of cutaneous mycoses, according to the manufacturer. In another study, administration of itraconazole for 2 consecutive days each week for 3 weeks was compared to 21-consecutive day administration in the treatment of *Malassezia* dermatitis and otitis in dogs (Ch 57, ref. 105). The pulse dosing was as effective as continuous therapy in reducing yeast numbers. This type of pulse dosing has been recommended for maintenance therapy for long-term treatment of other fungal infections.

Dosage[a]

INDICATIONS	DOSE	ROUTE	INTERVAL (hr)	DURATION (days)
Dogs				
Systemic blastomycosis	5 mg/kg	PO	24[b]	≥60[c]
Ocular or CNS blastomycosis, cryptococcosis, histoplamosis, nasal aspergillosis	5 mg/kg	PO	12	≥60[c]
Sporotrichosis	7.3 mg/kg	PO	24	35[d]
	10 mg/kg	PO	24	≥60[c]
Sporotrichosis, *Malassezia* infections	5-10 mg/kg	PO	12-24	[e]
Cats				
Dermatophytosis	10 mg/kg	PO	24	28-70[f]
Histoplasmosis, Blastomycosis	5-10 mg/kg	PO	12	60-130 days[g]
Phaeohyphomycosis	20 mg/kg	PO	24	120 days[h]
Sporotrichosis	5 mg/kg	PO	12-24	[e]
Cryptococcosis (<3.2 kg weight)	50 mg/cat	PO	24	[i]
Cryptococcosis (≥3.2 kg weight)	100 mg/cat	PO	24	[i]

[a]Dosages listed are for oral capsules. The bioavailability of the oral solution is better (approximately 2 mg solution equals 5 mg capsule) and the dosages may be reduced with the oral solution.
[b]Sometimes a loading dose of 5 mg/kg given every 12 hr, or 10 mg/kg given every 24 hr is used for the first 3-4 days of treatment to achieve a more rapid steady state of drug concentration in tissues.
[c]Continue therapy for at least 60 days after clinical recovery.
[d]Ch 63, ref. 51.
[e]Continue therapy for at least 30 days after clinical recovery.
[f]Some clear in 4-8 weeks; others take 6-10 weeks. One regimen involves this dose daily for 28 days (followed by 1-week on and 1-week off therapy) was reported to cure infected animals in 56-70 days (Ch 57, ref. 94a).
[g]If relapse, may need a second course. Time for treatment may vary; however the usual duration is listed here.
[h]Therapy was effective in treating a cat that did not respond to 10 mg/kg PO for 60 days (Ch 57, ref. 113a).
[i]For 8 weeks after clinical recovery.

ADDITIONAL DOSAGES. Dermatophytosis, Table 58-5; blastomycosis, Table 59-1; histoplasmosis, Table 60-1; cryptococcosis, Table 61-5; coccidioidomycosis, Table 62-3; sporotrichosis, Table 63-1; nasal aspergillosis, Table 64-1; disseminated aspergillosis, Table 64-3; candidiasis, Table 65-4; trichosponosis, Table 66-1; prototheosis, Table 69-1; fungal otitis, Table 85-6.

DISPENSING INFORMATION. Capsules should be given <u>with</u> food to improve absorption and reduce GI side effects. If achlorhydria is present, give drug with an acidic beverage such as carbonated cola. For cats, owners can mix small beads within 100-mg capsule with 1/2 to 1 teaspoon of soft food to a sausage shape on a plate, or aluminum foil, to be placed in freezer. This can be cut into appropriate amount for individual daily dosage. Most cats or dogs will readily eat this. **Oral solution** should be given *without* food, and dosage can be 25%-50% of that listed because of inherently better absorption. The drug should be given 2 hr before drugs are used that reduce gastric acidity. Recheck clinical signs and renal/hepatic tests at 2 weeks, monthly for 3 mo, and every 3 mo thereafter. **IV solution.** The drug is mixed in an IV bag after reconstitution. It should be stored away from light.

KANAMYCIN

CLASS. Aminoglycoside.

ACTION. Bactericidal; inhibits bacterial protein synthesis.

MORE INFORMATION. See GENTAMICIN; Chapter 34; Table 34-5.

PHARMACOKINETICS. See GENTAMICIN. For PO therapy, most of the dose is not absorbed and acts locally.

SPECTRUM. Gram positive: Some *Staphylococcus*, *Listeria*. **Gram negative:** *Escherichia*, *Proteus*, *Salmonella*, *Citrobacter*. Similar to gentamicin except poor against *Pseudomonas*. **Anaerobes:** ineffective. **Ineffective:** *Pseudomonas*, inconsistent against *Staphylococcus*.

INDICATIONS. Skin, soft tissue, and genitourinary infections caused by *Escherichia*, *Proteus*, *Enterobacter*, *Klebsiella*, *Serratia*, *Salmonella*, *Acinetobacter*, *Mycobacterium avium-intracellulare* complex infections.

CONTRAINDICATIONS. See GENTAMICIN; avoid or reduce dosage in renal failure.

ADVERSE REACTIONS. Ototoxicity and nephrotoxicity. See GENTAMICIN. Pain and muscle injury after repeated IM injection.

INTERACTIONS. See GENTAMICIN.

AVAILABILITY	TYPE	SIZES	PREPARATIONS (COMPANY)
Human	Solution for injection	250 mg/ml	*Kantrex* (Bristol-Myers Squibb), generic (various)
Veterinary	Solution for injection	50 mg/ml, 200 mg/ml	*Kantrim* (Fort Dodge)
		50 mg/ml	*Amiglyde-V* (Fort Dodge)
	Oral solution for enteric therapy (with bismuth and absorbent)	100 mg/5 ml	*Amforol* (Fort Dodge)
	Oral tablets for enteric therapy (with bismuth and absorbents)	100 mg	*Amforol*

INTERNATIONAL PREPARATIONS. *Kamycine, Kanamytrex, Kanescin, Kannasyn, Kemicina.*

HANDLING. Can be diluted in 0.9% NaCl or 5% dextrose.

ADMINISTRATION. For IV, do not mix with other antibacterials. Give as dilute solution over 1 hr. For IM, deep injection into large muscle. Can be given as aerosol by nebulization:

add 250 mg to 3 ml 0.9% NaCl and put in nebulizer chamber. Repeat two to four times daily. Monitor for renal dysfunction and neurologic signs. Treat urinary infection until asymptomatic and culture results are negative. After 3 days of no response, re-evaluate treatment. Maximum treatment period is 10 days.

Dosage

INDICATIONS	DOSE (mg/kg)	ROUTE	INTERVAL (hr)	DURATION (days)^a
Dogs				
Skin, soft tissue infection	10-15	SC, IM	24	7
Genitourinary infection	10	SC, IM	24	7-10
Systemic infection	15	SC	24	7
Enteric only infection	5	PO	8	<5
Cats				
Soft tissue, systemic infection	5.5-8	IM, SC	24	<7

^{a}Must closely monitor renal function during treatment.

ADDITIONAL DOSAGES. Plague, Table 47-1; respiratory infections, Table 88-8.

KETOCONAZOLE

CLASS. Imidazole antifungal.

ACTION. Antifungal; impairs ergosterol synthesis in fungal cell wall.

MORE INFORMATION. See ITRACONAZOLE, FLUCONAZOLE, VORICONAZOLE; Chapter 57; Table 57-1.

PHARMACOKINETICS. In fasted dogs ketoconazole (KTZ) tablets have highly variable (4%-89%) absorption from the GI tract. Acid environment, fats, and smaller amounts of food generally enhance absorption. Never give drug with co-administered antacids or H$_2$ blockers. Widely distributed in tissues with highest concentrations of drug reaching the liver, kidney, pituitary, adrenals. Highly protein bound (>84%) but reaches urine, saliva, milk, sweat, ceruminous secretions. CSF concentrations are minimal: dosages of 40 mg/kg/day are required for measurable amounts in CSF, although even then these levels are unpredictable. Higher dosages (>10 mg/kg/day) are similarly needed to reach tissue levels in the testes and intraocular tissues. Metabolized by liver to inactive

metabolites, with majority excreted in bile and feces. Very low (3%-4%) amounts reach the urine unmetabolized. Reaches the stratum corneum by excretion in excretions of sebum. May require 10-14 days of treatment to reach steady state and effective therapeutic tissue concentrations.

SPECTRUM. Fungi: *Blastomyces, Candida, Histoplasma, Paracoccidioides, Coccidioides, Trichophyton, Microsporum, Malassezia, Phialophora.* **Others:** *Leishmania.*

INDICATIONS. Antifungal: Localized or disseminated candidiasis, systemic mycoses: blastomycosis, histoplasmosis, coccidioidomycosis, cryptococcosis. Less effective against aspergillus or sporotrichosis. In rapidly progressing systemic mycoses, treat with amphotericin B first or 1 week of high-dose itraconazole. High (often toxic) doses of KTZ required for CNS mycoses. For dermatophytes resistant to topical therapy; but griseofulvin or itraconazole are preferred for feline dermatophytosis. Not a first choice if CNS or ocular involvement. In more resistant canine nasal aspergillosis, may use KTZ combined with topical enilconazole or clotrimazole, but itraconazole or fluconazole preferred (Ch 57, ref. 118). Although KTZ is less expensive, toxicity and treatment failure rates are higher (Ch 57, ref. 117). For sporotrichosis, but more side effects and less effective than itraconazole. Has been used in treatment of leishmaniasis (see Chapter 73). **Other:** High dosages have been used to suppress steroidogenesis in canine hyperadrenocorticism. It has also been used concurrent with cyclosporine to reduce its clearance and required dosage as a cost-saving measure in treatment of perianal fistulas in dogs (Ch 57, ref. 102).

APPROVED USES. Antifungal for human use. Licensed for dogs in France.

CONTRAINDICATIONS. Pregnancy or lactation since it is embryotoxic and teratogenic; itraconazole or fluconazole a better choice for CNS, intraocular, or testicular infections. Avoid use in lactating animals. The slow response to therapy has made itraconazole preferred for animals with severe or rapidly progressing mycoses. Avoid in patients with hepatic dysfunction since extensively metabolized by that organ. Avoid in patients with thrombocytopenia or previously recognized hypersensitivity to this drug.

ADVERSE REACTIONS. Anorexia may be observed within the first 30 days of therapy in some animals. Fever, depression, vomiting, diarrhea, abdominal pain, weight loss, hepatocellular necrosis, thrombocytopenia, occasional nonregenerative anemia, teratogenic in pregnant and mutagenic in nursing animals. Fetal death causing abortion of mummified fetuses and stillbirths has been found in treated bitches. Hepatotoxicity is associated with increased hepatic enzymes, anorexia, vomiting, and/or icterus. Frequently, adverse effects of GI effects and hepatotoxicity necessitate dosage reduction. Signs may be alleviated by reducing the dose 50%, dividing the dose twice daily or alternate days, or administering each dose with food. At clinical dosages (10-30 mg/kg/day), cats are more sensitive to the hepatotoxic effects than are dogs, although the tolerance is individualistic. Reduced production of cortisol and testosterone in dogs at greater than 10-30 mg/kg/day. Only a transient reduction in testosterone in male cats. In people (and potentially in animals) decreased libido, gynecomastia, azoospermia, impotence in males, and suppressed reproductive cycling in females. Pruritus and alopecia when used at high dosages for extended periods in dogs and cats. Lightening of the haircoat owing to loss of guard hairs and more visible undercoat occurs after 3-4 mo of treatment. It resolves when the drug is discontinued or the dosage is reduced. Months of therapy in dogs induces cataract development. Cats most consistently develop dry haircoats and weight loss from reduced appetite.

INTERACTIONS. Avoid use with mitotane, rifampin, or theophylline owing to KTZ decreasing their activity. Effects of glucocorticoids enhanced due to increased absorption and reduced clearance by enzymatic degradation. Diphenylhydantoin, rifampin, barbiturates, and cyclosporine may increase the metabolism of KTZ. Gastric alkalinizing agents (antacids, H_2 blockers, proton pump inhibitors) and achlorhydria decrease oral absorption. Increases activities of midazolam and diphenylhydantoin and activity and toxicity of cyclosporine. In the case of cyclosporine, KTZ increases the bioavailability and decreases systemic degradation of cyclosporine by decreasing the effective degradative microsomal enzymes in the intestinal cells and liver respectively. Co-administration of KTZ and cyclosporine has been used to lower the dose needed of the latter drug in an attempt to reduce cost of therapy. Midazolam levels were increased in dogs where KTZ was given in combination (Ch 57, ref. 76).

AVAILABILITY	TYPE	SIZES	PREPARATION (COMPANY)
Human	Oral tablets, scored	200 mg	*Nizoral* (Janssen)
	Topical ointment, shampoo, or cream	many	*Ketofungol* (Janssen)

INTERNATIONAL PREPARATIONS. *Panfungal.*

HANDLING. To make suspension: dissolve or crush 200-mg tablet +0.8 ml 1 *N* HCl + 3.1 ml water; gives 50 mg/ml concentration. Add this solution to syrup and 13 mg/ml methylcellulose or 2 g/100 ml DMSO (increases odor and dermal penetration) for topical applications. Stable for 6 mo if refrigerated. Shake well before using. Can be formulated for smaller dosage sizes by compounding pharmacies.

ADMINISTRATION. Monitor serum hepatic enzyme (ALT and ALP) activities, bilirubin, bile acids before and during treatment (at least monthly). Transient subclinical elevations in liver enzymes are tolerated and expected. With significant hepatotoxicity, temporarily discontinue or decrease dosage, go to alternate-day therapy or switch to alternative drugs. Do not give simultaneously with H_2 blockers, anticholinergics, antacids. Space 2 hr between. Treat dermatophyte infections at least 1 mo. Dividing daily dose and giving with small amounts of food help produce an acidic gastric environment favorable to absorption. Higher doses may be used during initial treatment. Once daily therapy may be used because of half life. Once the disease is under control, the dosage can be reduced and therapy continued for months or years if relapse is anticipated.

Dosage

INDICATIONS	DOSE	ROUTE	INTERVAL (hr)	DURATION
Dogs				
Nasal aspergillosis, candidiasis or dermatomycosis	10 mg/kg	PO	24	6 weeks[a,b]
	5 mg/kg	PO	12	2-18 weeks[a,b]
Systemic mycosis	10-20 mg/kg	PO	12	2-9 mo[a]
	15-30 mg/kg	PO	24	2-9 mo[a]
Sporotrichosis	15 mg/kg	PO	12	2-4 mo[a]
Malassezia	5-10 mg/kg	PO	24	3 weeks[c]
Cats				
Dermatomycosis	5-10 mg/kg	PO	24	1-9 mo[a,d]
Coccidioidomycosis	50 mg/cat	PO	24	9-12 mo[a]
	25-75 mg/cat	PO	12-48	9-12 mo[a]
Sporotrichosis	5-10 mg/kg	PO	12-24	2-4 mo[a]

[a]This is an expected range of time. Therapy should continue for at least 1 mo beyond last detection of infection.
[b]Drug is somewhat less effective than itraconazole in treatment of aspergillosis or sporotrichosis.
[c]Ch 57, ref. 6.
[d]Cats almost always require systemic treatment for this infection, while topical therapy is often adequate for localized lesions in dogs.

ADDITIONAL DOSAGES. Dermatophytosis, Table 58-5; histoplasmosis, Table 60-1; cryptococcosis, Table 61-5; coccidioidomycosis, Table 62-3; sporotrichosis, Table 63-1; candidiasis, Table 65-4; trichosponosis, Table 66-1; protozoal infections, Table 71-1; oral infections, Table 89-4.

DISPENSING INFORMATION. Medication should be given with a meal to facilitate absorption. If vomiting occurs give with a small amount of food. Treating every other day may reduce side effects of nausea if they develop.

LACTOFERRIN

CLASS. Protein of bovine origin.

ACTION. Binds iron, reducing its availability for bacteria.

MORE INFORMATION. See Stomatitis, Chapter 89; reference: Ch 14, ref. 552. See Chapter 2. References Ch 2, ref. 2; 131.

PHARMACOKINETICS. Used for its local effects in the oral cavity. Applied in oral cavity.

INDICATIONS. Stomatitis resulting from chronic calicivirus infections, dental disease, secondary to concurrent FeLV and FIV infections.

CONTRAINDICATIONS. None.

ADVERSE REACTIONS. None.

INTERACTIONS. None.

AVAILABILITY. Must be purchased from chemical suppliers.

HANDLING. Powder is mixed in solution. Has also been applied dry by brushing directly to lesions (Ch 2, ref. 2).

ADMINISTRATION. Drug is given by syringe into oral cavity to contact local mucosal surfaces. Soft toothbrush may also be dipped in powder and applied directly to affected areas.

Dosage

INDICATIONS	DOSE	ROUTE	INTERVAL (hr)	DURATION (days)
Stomatitis	40 mg/kg solution	PO topically	24	14
	200 mg powder	PO topically	24	14

ADDITIONAL DOSAGES. FIV Infection, Table 14-6.

DISPENSING INFORMATION. Take specified amount of liquid in syringe and squirt into cat's mouth. Do not mix with food. If applied dry, dip a soft toothbrush in powder and lightly brush on affected areas in the mouth.

LAMIVUDINE (SEE ANTIVIRAL THERAPY, CHAPTER 2)

LEVAMISOLE (SEE IMMUNOMODULATORS, CHAPTER 2)

LINCOMYCIN

CLASS. Lincosamide.

ACTION. Bacteriostatic, binds to 50s bacterial ribosomal subunit inhibiting protein synthesis.

MORE INFORMATION. See CLINDAMYCIN and LINCOMYCIN; Chapter 34.

PHARMACOKINETICS. Absorption from GI tract is incomplete and further impaired by food. IM or IV administration yields higher blood concentrations. Good tissue penetration except for meninges, where concentrations reach 40% of those in blood, even with meningitis. Concentrates in areas of low pH (e.g., abscesses). Metabolized in liver, unchanged drug and metabolites excreted in milk, bile, feces, urine. Most (77%) of PO dose given to a fasting animal is excreted in the bile, only 14% in urine. When given IM, 38% and 49% are excreted in bile and urine, respectively.

SPECTRUM. Gram positive: *Staphylococcus, Streptococcus, Nocardia, Corynebacterium, Erysipelothrix.* **Gram negative:** poor activity. **Anaerobes:** *Bacteroides, Propionibacterium, Fusobacterium, Peptostreptococcus, Peptococcus, Clostridium, Actinomyces.* **Others:** *Mycoplasma, Leptospira.* **More effective:** gram-positive aerobes, obligate anaerobes. Ineffective: most gram-negative aerobes, *Enterococcus, Mycobacterium.* Bacterial resistance may develop during treatment and usually also involves clindamycin.

INDICATIONS. Staphylococcal pyoderma in dogs. Infections caused by gram-positive bacteria involving upper respiratory tract, skin, wound infections, septicemia, abscesses in dogs and cats. Clindamycin is less toxic and better absorbed and may be preferred but is more costly.

APPROVED USES. Oral preparations for dogs and cats. Parenteral solution for dogs and swine.

CONTRAINDICATIONS. *Malassezia* or *Candida* infection or previous hypersensitivity to a lincosamide. Avoid or reduce dose with renal or hepatic dysfunction. In dogs, no problems with breeding performance, during gestation, or with neonates. May cause diarrhea in nursing puppies if dam is being medicated.

ADVERSE REACTIONS. Diarrhea, occasional vomiting (especially cats), anorexia, polydipsia, polyuria. Slight increases in blood hepatic enzyme activities may occur. IM injections cause local pain, and too-rapid IV infusion may cause hypotension and cardiopulmonary arrest.

INTERACTIONS. Reduces activity of coadministered erythromycin, enhanced activity of neuromuscular blockers.

AVAILABILITY	TYPE	SIZES	PREPARATIONS (COMPANY)
Veterinary	Oral tablets	100 mg, 200 mg, 500 mg	*Lincocin* (Pharmacia & Upjohn)
	Oral liquid (hydrochloride)	50 mg/ml	*Lincocin* Aquadrops
	Parenteral solution (licensed for swine)	100 mg/ml	*Lincocin* Sterile Solution

INTERNATIONAL PREPARATIONS. *Albiotic, Lincocine, Cillimicina, Cillimycin.*

HANDLING. Store at controlled room temperature (15-30°C). IV solution stable for at least 24 hr when mixed with IV fluids.

ADMINISTRATION. Ingesta and kaolin-pectin preparations reduce PO absorption. Can be given IM with slight pain or discomfort. For IV, dilute with 5% dextrose or 0.9% saline and give as slow (drip) infusion.

Dosage

INDICATIONS	DOSE (mg/kg)	ROUTE	INTERVAL (hr)	DURATION (days)
Dogs				
Skin, soft tissue infection	15.4	PO	8	21-42,[a] or 56[b]
	22	PO	12	21-42,[a] or 56[b]
Systemic infection	22	IM, SC, IV[c]	24	≤12
	11	IM, SC	12	≤12
Bacteremia, sepsis	11-22	IV	8	≤12
Cats				
Skin and soft tissue infection	11	IM	12	≤12
	22	IM	24	≤12
Systemic infection	15	PO	8	≤12
	22	PO	12	≤12

[a]Superficial pyoderma.
[b]Deep, resistant pyoderma.
[c]Must be diluted; see Administration.

ADDITIONAL DOSAGES. *Rhodococcus equi* infection, Table 35-7; canine pyoderma, Table 85-3.

DISPENSING INFORMATION. Give on empty stomach.

LINEZOLID

CLASS. Synthetic antibiotic of the oxazolidinones.

ACTION. Antibacterial, inhibits initiation process of protein synthesis. Binds to the 23s ribosomal RNA of the 50s subunit, thereby preventing the formation of a functional 70S initiation complex. Works at an earlier and different mechanism from other drugs so that cross-resistance is not a problem. Reversible nonselective inhibition of monamine oxicase.

MORE INFORMATION. LINEZOLID; Chapter 34.

PHARMACOKINETICS. Well absorbed from GI tract (~100%). In people, most of the drug is metabolized by the liver with renal (30%) and fecal (5%) excretion. Can switch from IV to oral therapy with little therapeutic adjustment. In dogs, rapidly absorbed after oral dosing with 95% bioavailability (Ch 34, ref. 346a). Limited protein binding (<35%) and well distributed to most extravascular sites. Circulating and excreted largely unchanged. Renal excretion of parent drug and metabolites is complete by 24-48 hr after a single dose.

SPECTRUM. Gram positive: Including certain drug-resistant enterococci (vancomycin-resistant) and staphylococci (methicillin-resistant). Bacteriostatic for enterococci and staphylococci and bactericidal for most streptococci.

INDICATIONS. Bacterial infections in people with multi-drug resistant gram-positive organisms that are resistant to vancomycin. Since this drug is reserved for restricted treatment in people with highly resistant gram-positive bacterial infections its use in dogs or cats is discouraged.

APPROVED USES. Humans: for multidrug resistant infections with gram-positive bacteria. Use should be limited or avoided in animals to help prevent emerging bacterial resistance.

CONTRAINDICATIONS. High blood pressure.

ADVERSE REACTIONS. Diarrhea, nausea, myelosuppression (leukopenia and thrombocytopenia), neuropathy (Ch 34, ref. 217a). Secondary oral or vaginal candidiasis.

INTERACTIONS. Related to the MAO inhibitors. Avoid use with adrenergic or serotonergic agents such as dopamine, pseudoephedrine, and serotonin reuptake inhibitors. Avoid foods high in tyramine. When used with these drugs dramatic and potentially dangerous increases in blood pressure can occur.

AVAILABILITY	TYPE	SIZES	PREPARATIONS (COMPANY)
Human	Oral suspension, Tablets, Injection	Suspension: 100 mg/5 ml Tablets: 400 mg, 600 mg Injection: 2 mg/ml	*Zyvox* (Pharmacia & Upjohn)

HANDLING. Store in airtight, light-proof containers at controlled room temperature (25°C). Keep away from moisture.

ADMINISTRATION. Oral suspension makes medication of small animals more convenient.

Dosage

INDICATIONS	DOSE	ROUTE	INTERVAL (hr)	DURATION (days)
Human				
Resistant bacterial infections	400-600 mg/person[a]	PO	12	14

[a]Beagle dogs were given 25 mg/kg, IV or PO, had an elimination half-life of 3.9 or 3.6 hr, respectively.[346a]

ADDITIONAL DOSAGES. None.

DISPENSING INFORMATION. The oral liquid should be gently mixed without shaking before each use.

L-LYSINE

CLASS. L-form of an essential amino acid.

ACTION. Interferes with arginine use by FHV-1 through either by substitution, competition, or inducing arginase activity.

MORE INFORMATION. Antivirals, Chapter 2; Feline Respiratory Disease, Chapter 16. References Ch 16, ref. 11; 93; 53.

PHARMACOKINETICS. Serum levels of L-lysine are increased after oral administration; however those of arginine are minimally affected.

SPECTRUM. Viruses: FHV-1.

INDICATIONS. For ocular FHV-1 keratitis and conjunctivitis. Reduces the severity of clinical signs of infection.

APPROVED USES. Available for human use over the counter in drugstores.

CONTRAINDICATIONS. Hepatic insufficiency. Kittens or pups <6 mo old.

ADVERSE REACTIONS. Occasional vomiting, diarrhea or inappetence which is controlled by reducing the dose or discontinuing therapy. Dietary restriction of arginine is recommended for people receiving oral lysine; however this is not advised in cats. Cats fed a diet deficient in arginine develop hyperammonemia, vomiting, neurologic signs and potential fatal complications. Pups <6 mo develop toxicities. Heinz body anemia in cats if propylene glycol containing tablets are used.

INTERACTIONS. Appears safe in addition to regular diet and other medications.

AVAILABILITY	TYPE	SIZES	PREPARATIONS (COMPANY)
Human (Over the counter)	Oral tablets	250, 500 mg tablets	*Many*

FHV-1, Feline herpesvirus, type 1.

HANDLING. Store tablets away from moisture at room temperature (15-30°C). No special precautions for human contact.

ADMINISTRATION. Tablets are large and must be crushed in moist food or broken into small pieces that can be given directly. Arginine should not be restricted from the diet.

Dosage

INDICATIONS	DOSE (mg/kg)	ROUTE	INTERVAL (hr)	DURATION (days)
FHV-1 Ocular Disease	250-500 mg total	PO	12	prn

ADDITIONAL DOSAGES. Feline respiratory disease, Table 16-2.

DISPENSING INFORMATION. Crush tablets and mix into moist food twice daily. If vomiting, anorexia or diarrhea develop discontinue medication and contact your veterinarian.

LUFENURON

CLASS. Benzoylphenyl urea, insect growth regulator, acts by inhibiting chitin synthesis.

ACTION. Interferes with formation of fungal cell wall and insect exoskeleton.

MORE INFORMATION. Coccidioidomycosis, Chapter 62; Dermatophytosis, Chapter Antifungal chemotherapy; Reference (Ch 57, ref. 7).

PHARMACOKINETICS. Rapid and complete absorption from the GI tract after PO administration. Highly lipophilic, it enters the adipose, then redistributes back into the blood for approximately 30 days. Concentrates in the milk of lactating dams.

SPECTRUM. Fungi: *Coccidioides, Candida,* Dermatophytes, perhaps other systemic fungi, fleas.

INDICATIONS. Resistant systemic mycotic infections, alone or in combination with a polyene or azole antifungal drug. Efficacy in treating fungal infections is controversial and has not been shown to be effective in controlled studies. See information under dosage regimens below.

APPROVED USES. Flea control for dogs and cats, when given on a once monthly basis.

CONTRAINDICATIONS. None; appears safe in breeding animals (Ch 57, ref. 125).

ADVERSE REACTIONS. None at recommended concentrations for fungal infections, which are much higher than flea dosages. Mild anorexia, and occasional increase in hepatic transaminases at supratherapeutic doses (Ch 57, ref. 125).

INTERACTIONS. Appears safe in combination with other insecticides and does not alter cholinesterase activity.

AVAILABILITY	TYPE	SIZES	PREPARATIONS (COMPANY)
Veterinary	Oral tablets	Dogs: 45 mg, 90 mg, 204.9 mg, 409.8 mg Cats: 90 mg, 204.9 mg	*Program* (Novartis)
	Tubes	Cats: Tube containing liquid 133 mg	*Program*

HANDLING. Stored at room temperature (15-30°C). No special precautions for human contact.

ADMINISTRATION. Feeding enhances absorption. Suspension for cats is mixed in a palatable diet.

Dosage (see note on questionable efficacy below)[a]

INDICATIONS	MINIMUM DOSE (mg/kg)	ROUTE	INTERVAL (hr)	DURATION (days)
Dermatophytosis and other mycoses				
Dogs	80	PO	24	1
Cats—household	50-80	PO	24	1
Cats—cattery	100	PO	24	1

[a]Efficacy of lufenuron for treatment of fungal infections has not been documented consistently. In uncontrolled studies by one group of investigators (Ch 57, ref. 7; 8), treatment effectiveness was reported; however, the dosage level was found to critical for a favorable response. For dogs, the recommendation was to avoid dividing tablets and to avoid rounding-off to higher dosage. For grouped cats, the entire population was treated at one time and rounding-off to higher dosage was also done by giving entire tube. For treated dogs with dermatophytosis, hair regrowth began 10-11 days after treatment with lesion recovery by 16-25 days. Mycologic recovery preceded this by 6 days. In cats, hair growth occurred after 5-6 days with lesion recovery by 10-15 days. Retreatment was needed after 2 weeks in some cases to prevent reinfection.

A recommended maintenance dose for flea control was suggested for several months.

NOTE: Other investigators have not found this treatment to be effective. In these other controlled studies, a dose as high as 133 mg/kg *was unable to prevent dermatophytosis* in uninfected cats exposed to experimentally infected cats (Ch 57, ref. 23). As with one treatment group in another study, lufenuron given at doses of 60 mg/kg PO given twice at a 1-mo interval in conjunction with topical enilconazole rinses once weekly was not able to control dermatophytosis in a cattery (Ch 57, ref. 47). Fungal cultures became negative in some cats after several weeks and relapses were observed. In another study, cats pretreated with lufenuron at 30-133 mg/kg were no more resistant to challenge with *Microsporum canis* spores than cats given placebo (Ch 57, ref. 95a). This drug is *not* recommended for treatment of fungal infections as efficacy in controlled studies is lacking.

ADDITIONAL DOSAGES. Coccidioidomycosis, Table 62-3; candidiasis, Table 64-4.

DISPENSING INFORMATION. Administer in conjunction with a full meal. Tablets or liquid can be placed in small amount of food to ensure it is eaten. For free-fed cats, food must be temporarily withheld to facilitate eating of an entire meal with medication.

MARBOFLOXACIN

CLASS. Fluoroquinolone.

ACTION. Bactericidal; inhibits bacterial DNA gyrase.

MORE INFORMATION. See ENROFLOXACIN; Chapter 34; Table 34-11.

PHARMACOKINETICS. Well absorbed from GI tract. Widely distributed in tissues. Concentrations in muscle, liver, kidney, lung, skin are ≥ those in blood. Low protein binding occurs. Minimal metabolism (<5% of dose). Renal excretion of 2/3 of dose with therapeutic levels in urine 2-5 days after 4-mg/kg dose. In urine 40% drug excreted unchanged. Liver metabolizes 10%-15% of the drug. Approximately 33% of the dose appears in feces.

TISSUE DISTRIBUTION OF MARBOFLOXACIN IN DOGS (Single Oral Dose)[a]

Time After Dosing (hr)	2		18		24	
Dosage (mg/kg)	2.5	5.0	2.5	5.0	2.5	5.0
Tissue Concentration (µg/ml)						
Urinary Bladder	4.8	12	2.6	6.0	1.11	1.8
Bone Marrow	3.1	4.6	1.5	1.28	0.7	0.9
Feces	15	18	48	52	26	47
Jejunum	3.6	7.8	1.3	2.0	0.7	1.1
Kidney	7.1	12.7	1.4	2.7	0.9	1.6
Lung	3.0	5.48	0.8	1.45	0.57	1.0
Lymph Node	5.5	8.3	1.3	2.3	1.0	2.03
Muscle	4.1	7.5	1.0	1.8	0.7	1.20
Prostate	5.6	11	1.8	2.7	1.1	2.0
Skin	1.9	3.2	0.41	0.71	0.32	0.46

[a]Data provided by product insert for marbofloxacin.

SPECTRUM. Gram positive: *Staphylococcus*, some *Streptococcus*. **Gram negative:** *Escherichia, Klebsiella, Pseudomonas, Proteus, Salmonella, Serratia, Shigella, Citrobacter, Enterobacter, Brucella, Pasteurella*. Anaerobes: poor. Others: see ENROFLOXACIN. **More effective:** gram-negative aerobes and facultative anaerobes. **Ineffective:** obligate anaerobes. See ENROFLOXACIN.

INDICATIONS. See ENROFLOXACIN.

APPROVED USES. Dog and cat, skin and urinary infections.

CONTRAINDICATIONS. Has been given at 6 mg/kg for 3 mo to growing dogs. Do not use in growing dogs (<18 mo for large breeds) or growing cats (<16 weeks). Do not need to adjust dosages in renal failure in dogs as pharmacokinetics are not altered (Ch 34, ref. 218).

ADVERSE REACTIONS. As with other quinolones, See ENROFLOXACIN. Anorexia and vomiting most common; rare reports of polydipsia, diarrhea, tremors, ataxia or seizures in field studies.

INTERACTIONS. See ENROFLOXACIN.

AVAILABILITY	TYPE	SIZES	PREPARATIONS (COMPANY)
Veterinary	Oral tablets	80 mg, 20 mg, 5 mg 25 mg, 50 mg, 100 mg, 200 mg tablets	*Marbocyl* (Vetoquinol, Lure Cedex, France) *Zeniquin* (Pfizer Animal Health, Exton PA)

HANDLING. Store tablets in airtight, moisture-proof containers at room temperature.

ADMINISTRATION. See ENROFLOXACIN.

Dosage

INDICATIONS	DOSE (mg/kg)	ROUTE	INTERVAL (hr)	DURATION (days)
Dogs				
Urinary infections	2	PO	24	10-28
Skin, pyoderma	2-2.5	PO	24	49-213[a]
Systemic infection	2-4	PO	12	<10
Cats				
Urinary, skin infection	2	PO	24	10-28
Mycoplasma haemofelis infection	2	PO	24	43[b]

[a]Ch 85, ref. 22; 115; Ch 34, ref. 172a.
[b]Appendix 8, ref. 5 and 6.

ADDITIONAL DOSAGES. Enteric bacterial infections, Table 39-1; canine pyoderma, Table 85-3.

DISPENSING INFORMATION. Can give medicine with food, especially if vomiting is noted.

MEGLUMINE ANTIMONIATE

CLASS. Pentavalent antimonial, antiprotozoal.

ACTION. Antiprotozoal; interferes with glycolysis of *Leishmania*.

MORE INFORMATION. See STIBOGLUCONATE; Chapter 71; Table 71-1; references: Ch 71, ref. 27; 92; 94; 5; Ch 73, ref. 84; 205.

PHARMACOKINETICS. Bioavailability in dogs is 92% after IM and SC injection because polar molecule has limited tissue distribution (Ch 71, ref. 92). High concentrations are reached in skin, spleen, liver in decreasing order. Rapidly eliminated by renal excretion with 80% of dose excreted within 9 hours. Liposomal-encapsulated formulations are being evaluated to reduce side effects (Ch 71, ref. 93). Even with these preparations, repeated dosing may be needed to achieve effective levels in bone marrow (Ch 71, ref. 81). These formulations have delayed uptake following SC compared with IM. Repetitive dosing at 75 mg/kg every 12 hr produced steady-state peak plasma concentrations after 6 days that exceeded a single 100 mg/kg dose (Ch 71, ref. 94).

SPECTRUM. *Leishmania*. Resistance to drug may develop during treatment of infected dogs (Ch 71, ref. 27). Parasite strains have been developing resistance and dosage regimens have had to be increased in some regions to effectively treat the clinical signs. Twice daily dosing is often indicated to achieve these aims.

INDICATIONS. Leishmaniasis.

APPROVED USES. Humans and dogs for leishmaniasis; not available in U.S.

CONTRAINDICATIONS. Previous hypersensitivity, hepatic or renal insufficiency, cardiac arrhythmias, leukopenia.

ADVERSE REACTIONS. Pain, swelling, lameness with IM injection, SC preferred. Thrombophlebitis with IV use. See also STIBOGLUCONATE.

INTERACTIONS. May combine with allopurinol for increased efficacy.

AVAILABILITY	TYPE	SIZES	PREPARATIONS (COMPANY)
Veterinary	N-methylglucamine antimoniate	300 mg/ml as antimony in 5 ml ampules	*Glucantime* (Merial)[a]

[a]Human preparation is available from Rhone Poulenc, Paris, France.

HANDLING. Store solution in sterile container at room temperature.

ADMINISTRATION. Continue medication until clinical signs or skin lesions have resolved which usually occurs within 1-3 mo. Give by slow IV, deep IM, or by SC or IP. For resist-ant cases, can give alternate dosing with Pentamidine *(Lomidine)*. Treatment involves 10-12 injections in succession if initiated early and 18-20 injections if chronic manifestations (dermatitis) are present. Injections are given 2-3 days apart.

Dosage

INDICATIONS *(Dogs)*	DOSE	ROUTE	INTERVAL (hr)	DURATION (days)
Leishmaniasis	100 mg/kg[a]	SC	24	21-30[b]
	75-100 mg/kg[a]	SC	12	10

[a]Dose has been modified from that on label based on newer clinical information and evidence of drug resistance. Treatment is more effective if meglumine at the above dosages is combined with allopurinol at 15-30 mg/kg every 12 hr. Allopurinol treatment is continued up to 8 mo or longer (Ch 71, ref. 17), see also ALOPURINOL. Meglumine has also been combined with paromomycin where a pharmacokinetic modification of the antimonials delays their excretion allowing for higher blood levels.

[b]Prior regimens have been for 10 days on and off; however, treatment is more effective if meglumine is given for at least 30 days. Treatments with meglumine alone on a 10-day cycle have lasted for 1-8 mo. Steady state is reached after 6 days reaching therapeutic levels (Ch 71, ref. 94).

ADDITIONAL DOSAGES. Leishmaniasis, Table 73-4.

MELARSOPROL

CLASS. Arsenical. It is a melaminophenyl-based organic arsenical initially formed from Melarsen oxide, the trivalent equivalent of Melarsen after incorporation of dimercapol (BAL) and contains 18.8% arsenic. Other names include Mel B, Arsobal, 2-[p-(4,6-diamino-1,3,5-triazin-2ylamino phenyl]-4-hydroxymethyl-1,3,2-dithiarsolan).

ACTION. Antiprotozoal. Initially used as an anti-trypanosomiasis reagent from 1949 (Ch 72, ref. 21a). Melarsoprol is amphipathic and will diffuse across cellular membranes. The drug is, however, rapidly convered to the highly hydrophilic melarsen oxide in plasma (96% clearance within 1 hr) (Ch 72, ref. 33). Melarsen oxide levels peak within 15 min and has a half-life of 3.9 hr. Only limited quantities of the drug up to 1%-2% of maximum plasma levels cross the blood-brain barrier. This information was used in the experimental treatment of dogs at 2.2 mg/kg/ of body weight. Affects *Trypanosoma brucei* parasites after uptake through the P2 transporter (Ch 72, ref. 34). Trypanosomes exposed to arsenicals lyse very rapidly due to a possible loss of ATP due to inhibition of glycolysis caused by the drug in bloodstream forms.

MORE INFORMATION. See Chapter 72; Table 72-1. References: Ch 71, ref. 10d; 21a; 10c.

SPECTRUM. *African trypanosomes.* Drug is reserved for trypanosomiasis control programs.

INDICATIONS. The response to treatment in trypanosomiasis is usually rapid with mental dullness subsiding within days of the initial treatment.

CONTRAINDICATIONS. Cross resistance may result due to similar mode of action at the P2 transporter level.

ADVERSE REACTIONS. The solution is intensely irritating and care should be taken to see that the injections are given strictly IV. Antihistamine (oxomemazine) should be included to counter allergic reactions and irritation at the injection site. A Jarisch-Herxheimer reaction results due to the rapid killing of the parasite. Additional adverse effects relate to the drugs arsenic content. A severe febrile reaction may occur after the first injection in heavily parasitized hosts. The greatest risk is from a reactive encephalopathy and is usually seen between the end of the day 3 or 4 of treatment. Treatment of this encephalopathy involves use of corticosteroids, hypertonic solutions to combat cerebral edema, and anticonvulsants. Other adverse reactions include myelospupression, hypetension, diarrhea, myocardial damage and hepatic inflammation.

INTERACTIONS. Should not be used in otherwise ill animals. Severe hemolytic reactions have occurred in human patients with G6PD deficiency. Patients should be hospitalized during treatment.

AVAILABILITY	TYPE	SIZES	PREPARATION (COMPANY)
Veterinary	Solution for injection in propylene glycol	3.6%, 5 ml vial	*Mel B, Melarsen, Arsobal* (Rhone-Poulenc-Rorer S. Africa) (*Specia*, France)[a]

[a]The drug is no longer marketed actively by the manufacturer.

HANDLING. The drug is presented in ampules as 3.6% solution in propylene glycol. It should be given in a completely dry unused syringe. Glass syringes should be used as the propylene glycol is destructive to plastic. The dry syringe is needed because the solution precipitates in water. When disposable syringes are used the solution should not be prepared in advance.

ADMINISTRATION. Drug can be given at 2.2 mg/kg. body weight using a dry syringe and needle. The dose can be given in one dose or divided in two doses given at a 24-hr interval.

There is a low safety margin as a dosage of 3.6 mg/kg. body weight is lethal.

Dosage

INDICATIONS (Dogs)	DOSE (mg/kg)	ROUTE	INTERVAL (hr)	DURATION (days)
African trypanosomiasis	2.2	IV	24	10

ADDITIONAL DOSAGES. None.

MEROPENEM

CLASS. Meropenem is a β-lactam of the carbapenem group. As with biapenem and ertapenem, other newer carbapenems of this group, it does not require cilastatin coadministration.

ACTION. Bactericidal; ertapenem inhibits synthesis of bacterial cell wall peptidoglycan. As other carbapenems, this drug is relatively resistant to hydrolysis by β-lactamases.

MORE INFORMATION. See penicillins, Chapter 34.

PHARMACOKINETICS. Available for humans. Poorly absorbed from GI tract, but good systemic availability if given parenterally. It is poorly protein bound and, as a result, has a short elimination half-life of approximately 1 hr in people. The drug is generally eliminated from the body by 6 hr after administration. Approximately 60%-80% is excreted in the urine unchanged, the rest as inactive metabolites. Plasma clearance correlates with creatinine clearance. In dogs, plasma elimination half-life was 45 min with >90% being excreted in the urine within 24 hr (Ch 34, ref. 152b).

SPECTRUM. Broad-spectrum carbapenem antibacterial drug. It is bactericidal by interfering with cell-wall synthesis. Readily penetrates the cell wall of most gram-positive and gram-negative bacteria to reach penicillin-binding protein receptors. **Gram positive:** streptococci susceptible to penicillin. **Gram negative:** *Escherichia coli, Klebsiella pneumoniae, Pseudomonas aeruginosa.* **Anaerobes:** *Bacteroides fragilis, Peptostreptococcus* spp. See imipenem-cilastatin for further bacterial susceptibility data for this class of drugs.

INDICATIONS. For treatment of organisms resistant to other antibiotics and for mixed infections that require a broad spectrum including anaerobes. For treatment of intraabdominal or meningeal infections. Restricted use in animals is recommended to avoid bacterial resistance.

APPROVED USES. Serious and multiple drug—resistant bacterial intraabdominal infections and bacterial meningitis.

CONTRAINDICATIONS. The dosage should be reduced in renal failure. Dosage adjustments are not likely with hepatic impairment. Cross-hypersensitivity to other β-lactams. No complications have been observed in human or animal pregnancy; however, only clear indications should permit its use during this period.

ADVERSE REACTIONS. Diarrhea, vomiting, increased hepatic aminotransferase activities, and thrombophlebitis. Allergic reactions to vehicle, treat as anaphylaxis. All β-lactams can cause seizures if underlying brain disease or if overdosed related to body size and renal function. As with other β-lactams, monitor renal, hepatic, and hematopoietic systems during treatment.

INTERACTIONS. Antagonistic interaction may reduce effectiveness of this drug coadministered with other β-lactam drugs. Co-administration of drugs such as probenecid, which competes for active renal excretion, will increase the drug concentrations posing potential toxicity. Dose must be reduced in renal failure.

AVAILABILITY	TYPE	SIZES	PREPARATIONS (COMPANY)
Human	Powder for IV injection	500 mg and 1 gm vials	Merrem IV (Zeneca)

INTERNATIONAL PREPARATIONS. *Same.*

HANDLING. Supplied as a powder, soluble in water and 0.9% NaCl. Stable in this solution for up to 4 hr at 15-25°C. Reduce dosage in renal failure. Give over at least 15-30 min as an infusion. Do not mix with solutions containing any other drugs.

ADMINISTRATION. Administer over 15-30 min ideally or for smaller doses as a bolus injection over 3-5 min.

Dosage

INDICATIONS (Dogs and Cats)[a]	DOSE	ROUTE	INTERVAL (hr)	DURATION (days)
Bacteremia/sepsis	24 mg/kg	IV	24	prn
	12 mg/kg	SC	8	prn
Urinary infections	12 mg/kg	SC	12	prn
CNS infections[a]	40 mg/kg	IV or SC	8	prn

[a]This is an extrapolated dose for children, and maximum dose per administration is 2 gm. To help prevent development of resistant strains that might infect humans, use should be limited or avoided unless ultimately necessary.

ADDITIONAL DOSAGES. None.

METHENAMINE MANDELATE (OR HIPPPURATE)

CLASS. Urinary antiseptic.

ACTION. Produces acid urine, which is bacteriostatic.

MORE INFORMATION. Chapter 34.

PHARMACOKINETICS. Readily absorbed from GI tract but 10%-30% destroyed by gastric acid unless enteric-coated tablets are used. Minimal blood or tissue levels but enters placenta and milk. Excreted (>90%) in urine within 24 hr. In acid urine, methenamine is hydrolyzed to ammonia and formaldehyde. The acid salts (mandelate and hippurate) help lower urine pH. Co-administration of acids (e.g., ascorbate) may help maintain low urine pH.

SPECTRUM. Gram positive: *Staphylococcus, Enterococcus.* **Gram negative:** *Escherichia.* **Ineffective:** in alkaline urine or against *Enterobacter* and other urea-splitting organisms *(Proteus, Pseudomonas)*, which raise urine pH.

INDICATIONS. Chronic or recurrent urinary tract infections for long-term suppression/elimination of infection. Do not use in place of appropriate antimicrobial therapy to eliminate infection. Must eliminate infection by urea-splitting bacteria to allow methenamine to be effective. Only choice in predisposed animals in which anatomic causes cannot be eliminated.

APPROVED USES. Human: urinary infections.

CONTRAINDICATIONS. Pregnancy, lactation, renal or hepatic insufficiency (because of ammonia loading). Use of sulfonamides. Drug itself is not toxic in renal failure; organic acids it produces may be detrimental with mandelate; crystals may form in renal failure.

ADVERSE REACTIONS. Dysuria, bladder irritation, increased serum hepatic transaminases, vomiting, oral irritation.

INTERACTIONS. Urinary alkalinizing agents reduce effectiveness. Co-administration with sulfonamides may induce crystalluria and renal tubular damage in some species, but, because of unique sulfonamide metabolism, dogs are usually not affected. Drug combines with sulfonamides in urine, which results in mutual ineffectiveness of the drugs.

AVAILABILITY	TYPE	SIZES	PREPARATIONS (COMPANY)
Human	Oral tablets	1 g (as hippurate)	*Hiprex* (Marion Merrell Dow), *Urex* (3M Pharmaceuticals)
	Oral tablets	500 mg (as mandelate)	*Mandelamine* (Parke-Davis), Generic (various)
	Oral suspension	500 mg/5 ml (as mandelate)	Generic (various)

HANDLING. Store at room temperature and avoid contact with acids or metallic salts.

ADMINISTRATION. Offer animal free choice water. Give with meals to reduce GI irritation. Also available in combinations with other antimicrobials, pH reducers, urinary analgesics. Feeding diets that decrease urine pH are additive.

Dosage

INDICATIONS	DOSE	ROUTE	INTERVAL (hr)	DURATION (days)
Dogs	16.5 mg/kg	PO	24	prn[a]

[a]Therapy can be extended for months to suppress bacterial growth.

ADDITIONAL DOSAGES. None.

DISPENSING INFORMATION. Report any GI signs to your veterinarian.

METRONIDAZOLE

CLASS. Nitroimidazole.

ACTION. Bactericidal, also antiprotozoal; penetrates cells by diffusion, metabolized in anaerobic organisms to intermediates that prevent DNA synthesis. Has anti-inflammatory activity reducing neutrophil and lymphocyte functions.

MORE INFORMATION. See TINIDAZOLE; Chapters 34 and 71; references: Ch 34, ref. 268; 275; Ch 71, ref. 18; 60; 20; 83.

PHARMACOKINETICS. Virtually 100% GI absorption. Food delays systemic availability in people but not in dogs; also absorbed rectally. Good tissue penetration to all sites, including hard-to-reach areas such as brain, bone, placenta, fetal tissues, fluids (CSF, milk, saliva). Higher concentration in prostate than plasma of dog (Ch 34, ref. 275). Penetrates abscesses and pyothorax well. Metabolized in liver with predominantly active metabolites (60%-80%). Excreted mainly in urine and 10%-15% in feces. PO and IV routes give similar blood drug concentrations, but parenteral route is more expensive.

SPECTRUM. Anaerobic protozoa: *Trichomonas, Giardia, Entamoeba* (trophozoites), *Balantidium*. **Anaerobic bacteria:** *Bacteroides, Veillonella, Fusobacterium, Peptococcus,* most *Clostridium, Eubacterium,* few *Peptostreptococcus*. Alternative choices for anaerobic bacteria are chloramphenicol, clindamycin, cefoxitin. **Others:** *Helicobacter,* oral spirochetes, variable for *Campylobacter*. **More effective:** consistently good against *Bacteroides*. **Ineffective:** *Actinomyces,* yeasts, aerobic bacteria, and aerobic protozoa. Resistance among gram-negative anaerobic bacteria to metronidazole is rare (Ch 41, ref. 26a). Metronidazole resistance is more common among gram-positive anaerobic bacteria, including most *Propionibacterium acnes* and *Actinomyces,* as well as some strains of lactobacilli and anaerobic streptococci.

INDICATIONS. Recurrent or persistent anaerobic infections that fail to respond to penicillins, clindamycin, chloramphenicol. Anaerobic infections: intraabdominal, anaerobic meningitis, intracranial abscesses, bacteremia, osteomyelitis, dermatitis, synovitis, soft tissue infections, chronic colitis, intestinal bacterial overgrowth (Ch 34, ref. 268), stomatitis, oral ulceration, tetanus, *Helicobacter*-associated gastritis, bacterial vaginitis, and prophylaxis (with aminoglycosides) for colorectal surgery. Diagnosis of canine "antibiotic responsive enteropathy" and feline inflammatory bowel disease may be considered by a response to therapy. As antiprotozoal, indicated for trichomoniasis, giardiasis, amebiasis, and balantidiasis.

APPROVED USES. Human: anaerobic infections and abscesses, gastric helicobacteriosis.

CONTRAINDICATIONS. Dose reduction (50%) with liver failure and some reduction with severe renal failure. Reduced dosage for neonates. Avoid in pregnancy because carcinogenic and mutagenic when laboratory rodents given chronic high doses. Benzoate salt must be conjugated in the liver unlike the hydrochloride form; therefore, it should be used with caution in cats, when this pathway is deficient.

ADVERSE REACTIONS. Profuse salivation, anorexia, weight loss with PO administration to cats. The benzoate formulation is less likely to cause this problem. Can discolor urine reddish-brown. Vomiting, diarrhea, glossitis, stomatitis. Peripheral neuropathy with long-term use in people. Rarely pancreatitis, reversible mild leukopenia, thrombocytopenia.

Long-term use may cause *Candida* overgrowth in GI tract. Treatment for 1 mo decreased aerobic and anaerobic bacterial counts and increased the quantity of *Streptococcus* spp and *Corynebacterium* spp in the duodenum of healthy cats (Ch 71, ref. 39). High dosages IV to cats can cause pancreatitis. Neurologic complications are seizures, encephalopathy, cerebellar dysfunction. Generalized ataxia and vertical positional nystagmus. *Never* exceed 30 mg/kg/day for dogs and cats. CNS toxicity in dogs has resulted with high (≥60 mg/kg/day) dosages, often after 7-40 days treatment (Ch 71, ref. 12; 60; 20). Cerebellar and vestibular nuclear injury (Ch 71, ref. 18). Degenerative changes in Purkinje's cells and associated cerebellar and vestibular axons. CNS signs may progress rapidly and develop after acute or chronic overdosage. Signs may take several days to months to resolve, but some dogs develop uncontrollable seizures, fatal encephalopathy, coma. CSF analysis may show increased protein concentration. Treatment of neurotoxicity involves discontinuing the drug and instituting supportive care. Dogs with the toxicosis have recovered quicker when they are treated with diazepam (Ch 71, ref. 20). The range for IV dosing with diazepam is 0.2-0.625 mg/kg, and for oral dosing thereafter is 0.31-0.69 mg/kg. Dogs treated with diazepam respond in an average of 13 hr and recover in an average time of 38.7 hr, compared to 4.25 days response time and 11.6 days recovery time in untreated dogs. Diazepam may competitively reverse the binding of metronidazole to the benzodiazepine site on GABA receptors in the CNS.

INTERACTIONS. Barbiturates may alter metabolism, reducing metronidazole's therapeutic efficacy. Potentiates vitamin K antagonist rodenticides. Cimetidine may increase its concentration and enhance toxicity, whereas phenobarbital and diphenylhydantoin may decrease it. May interfere with measurement of serum triglycerides or some hepatic enzymes. In people, has been given in combination with tetracycline or amoxicillin and bismuth subsalicylate tablets to treat *Helicobacter*-associated gastritis and ulcers (see Chapter 39). Clarithromycin has been substituted for metronidazole when resistance is suspected. In some countries, metronidazole is available combined with spiramycin for treatment of mixed aerobic and anaerobic infections such as stomatitis, abscesses, genital and cutaneous infections. See SPIRAMYCIN.

AVAILABILITY	TYPE	SIZES	PREPARATIONS (COMPANY)
Human	Oral tablets	250 mg, 500 mg	*Flagyl* (Searle), generic (various)
	Oral solution as benzoate	25 mg/ml of base	PCCA, Houston TX
	Powder for injection	500 mg (as HCl)	*Flagyl* IV (SCS Pharmaceuticals)
	Solution for injection	500 mg	*Flagyl* IV, *Metronidazole Redi-Infusion* (Elkins-Sinn)
Veterinary	Solution for injection	5 mg/ml	*Torgyl* (Merial)

In U.S., only HCl salt is approved. It is unpalatable. Benzoate salt, available in Europe and Mexico, is more palatable to animals. Dose of HCl must be multiplied by 1.6 to convert to the benzoate because of the larger molecular weight of the benzoate.

INTERNATIONAL PREPARATIONS. *Abbonidazole, Acuzole, Anabact, Anaerobex, Anaeromet, Arilin, Ascacea, Bemetrazole, Clinazole, Elyzol, Metrazole, Metrogyl, Metrolyl, Metronide, Metrostat, Metrozol, Metryl, Narobic, Nidazol, Oecozol, Pharmaflex, Protostat, Rathimed, Rozex, Trichozole, Trikacide, Zagyl, Stomorgyl* (combined with *Spiramycin*).

HANDLING. Store tablets and powders in airtight, light-resistant containers. IV solution can be diluted with 0.9% NaCl or bacteriostatic water for injection, and further diluted in lactated Ringer's, 0.9% NaCl, or 5% dextrose. The pH is low (0.5-2), so before infusion add 5 mmol sodium bicarbonate for each 500 mg used to raise pH to 6-7. CO_2 bubbles may form during this, and the pressure needs an outlet. The neutralized solution should not be refrigerated, or precipitates may form. It must be used in 24 hr. If not neutralized, it is stable for 96 hr at room temperature. Should not contact aluminum (including needles), or solution may discolor to reddish-brown. Can be mixed in solutions with most aminoglycosides, cephalosporins, and penicillins. Protect from exposure to light. Refrigerated or concentrated (>8 mg/ml) solutions will precipitate.

ADMINISTRATION. When possible, preferably give whole coated tablets to cats to reduce oral contact with bitter drug. Has a metallic taste that is distasteful to cats. Generic tablets can be crushed and powder placed in syrup gum, tragacanth, or melted butter to improve palatability. See administration of ITRACONAZOLE for details on mixing with butter. Can be formulated for smaller doses by compounding pharmacies. This drug is less palatable to cats than furazolidone for giardiasis, and there is risk of neurotoxicity at higher dosages (Ch 71, ref. 18). Can be given with food, and in dogs, absorption is enhanced. When using the drug IV, the lower end of the dosage range should be used and the drug should be infused over 30 min.

Dosage

INDICATIONS	DOSE	ROUTE	INTERVAL (hr)	DURATION (days)
Dogs				
Giardiasis, trichomoniasis	30-50 mg/kg	PO	24	5-7
Stomatitis, colitis, helicobacteriosis	10-15 mg/kg	PO	12	10
	20 mg/kg	PO	24	10
Stomatitis, soft tissue infection	7.5 mg/kg	PO	8	10
Systemic bacteremia, meningitis	10 mg/kg	PO, IV	8	14
Cats				
Giardiasis, trichomoniasis	10-30 mg/kg	PO	24	5
	8-10 mg/kg	PO	12	10
	250 mg/cat	PO	24	5-7
	25 mg/kg[a]	PO	12	7
Helicobacteriosis, bacterial overgrowth	15-20 mg/kg	PO	12	prn
Anaerobic bacteremia or meningitis	10 mg/kg	PO, IV	8	prn
Soft tissue infection	7.5 mg/kg	PO	8-12	prn

[a]Base formulation equivalent to 40 mg benzoate. At this dose, treatment was effective in cats that failed to respond to 50 mg/kg daily PO fenbendazole for 5 days (Ch 71, ref. 83).

ADDITIONAL DOSAGES. FIV infection, Table 14-5; enteric bacterial infections, Table 39-2; gastric helicobacteriosis, Table 39-6; *Clostridium perfringens* diarrhea, Table 39-10; anaerobic infections, Table 41-12; tetanus, Table 43-2; feline abscesses, Table 52-3; enteric protozoal infections, Table 78-3; bacteremia and endocarditis, Table 87-6; oral infections, Table 89-4; gastrointestinal infections, Table 89-16; colitis, Table 89-19; intraabdominal infections, Table 89-21; hepatobiliary infections, Table 90-5; CNS infections, Table 92-5.

DISPENSING INFORMATION. Has an unpleasant metallic taste. May cause excessive salivation if tablets are bitten; do not crush or break. May darken urine color. May cause GI upset; take with food.

MILTEFOSINE (PHOSPHOCHOLINE, OLEYL-PC, HEXADECYLPHOSPHOCHOLINE)

CLASS. Alkyl phosphocholine (ether-lipid) analogue.

ACTION. Antiprotozoal against *Leishmania* and *Trypanosoma*. Closely related miltefosine was developed as an antitumor agent; however, it was ineffective for that purpose. These hemoflagellates have similar lipids on their surfaces and this drug interferes with synthesis of these lipids.

MORE INFORMATION. See Chapter 71, Table 71-1; References Ch 71, ref. 90; 5; 87; 75.

SPECTRUM. *Leishmania, Trypanosoma.*

INDICATIONS. The first oral treatment for leishmaniasis. Possible choice for resistant leishmaniasis, alternative for trypanosomiasis. Should avoid miltefosine and use phosphocholine when it becomes available.

CONTRAINDICATIONS. Pre-existing hepatic or renal failure. For *Leishmania* strains, activity varies depending on strain of the organism.

ADVERSE REACTIONS. Vomiting, diarrhea, increased serum transaminases, increased urea and creatinine, myelospuppression. Miltefosine causes these side effects in people; however, more severe reactions have been observed in dogs; therefore it is not recommended for dogs. Dogs tolerate phosphocholine with less side effects (Ch 71, ref. 5).

INTERACTIONS. Elevates hepatic transaminases so may be interactions with drugs involving hepatic excretion or metabolism.

AVAILABILITY	TYPE	SIZES	PREPARATION (COMPANY)
Human Miltefosine[a]	Oral capsules	50 mg	*Impavido* (Zentaris)

[a]Only miltefosine is available at this time for clinical use.

HANDLING. Store in a dry temperature controlled environment of 22°C.

ADMINISTRATION. Give orally after a meal to increase absorption.

Dosage

INDICATIONS (Dogs)	DOSE (mg/kg)	ROUTE	INTERVAL (hr)	DURATION (days)
Leishmaniasis[a]	2.5	PO	12	30

[a]This dose is for miltefosine as used in people.

ADDITIONAL DOSAGES. None.

MINOCYCLINE

CLASS. Tetracycline.

ACTION. Bacteriostatic; inhibits protein synthesis by binding to 30s ribosomal unit.

MORE INFORMATION. DOXYCYCLINE, TETRACYCLINES; Chapter 34; Table 34-7.

PHARMACOKINETICS. More lipid soluble (10×) than tetracycline; 100% absorbed from GI tract. Penetrates well into most tissues, body fluids, difficult areas such as prostate, female reproductive tract, lung, bronchial secretions, saliva, bile, CSF, CNS. The only tetracycline that penetrates CNS with noninflamed meninges. Crosses the placenta to accumulate in fetal bones and teeth. Clears primarily by extensive hepatic metabolism and biliary elimination. Only small amount excreted in feces in unchanged form; active drug does not accumulate in liver failure. Minimal (4%-9%) urinary excretion; dose reduction not needed for renal failure.

SPECTRUM. See DOXYCYCLINE. **More effective:** than tetracycline against *Staphylococcus* and *Nocardia*. **Ineffective:** see DOXYCYCLINE.

INDICATIONS. Brucellosis (combined with other drugs), borreliosis, nosocomial infections against bacteria resistant to other drugs. Has been unsuccessful as an antipruritic drug for atopic dermatitis (Ch 34, ref. 23).

APPROVED USES. Human: bacterial infections of skin and respiratory and urinary tracts. Has been marketed as a locally-administered (subgingival) paste to treat periodontal disease (Ch 34, ref. 164; 158).

CONTRAINDICATIONS. Pregnancy, lactation, and young (<6 mo). Dosage does not need reducing in renal failure because drug is excreted by biliary tract. However, drug does not accumulate in liver disease.

ADVERSE REACTIONS. Nausea, vomiting, potential yellow dental staining in young animals, increased hepatic enzyme activity, rare ototoxicity. Hypotension, shivering, dyspnea, cardiac arrhythmias, shock, and urticaria have developed in dogs given rapid IV doses that may have been caused by the drug vehicle. Certain vehicles such as propylene glycol in other IV tetracycline preparations may be responsible for acute systemic allergic reactions. In comparison, rapid IV infusions of doxycycline (5 mg/kg) has not produced systemic reactions. Vestibular side effects seen in people are related to a peculiar biotransformation of minocycline that does not occur in dogs and cats. Minocycline, at 10-20 mg/kg daily for 1 mo, decreased erythrocyte mass and increased blood alanine transaminase activity. Daily IV doses of 40 mg/kg produced increased urine calcium and Bromsulphalein retention, decreased food consumption, and weight loss. None of the effects were seen with similar PO dosages. A rare systemic granulomatous reaction has been observed in people.

INTERACTIONS. GI absorption reduced by iron preparations, aluminum hydroxide gels, sodium bicarbonate, calcium, and magnesium salts.

AVAILABILITY	TYPE	SIZES	PREPARATIONS (COMPANY)
Human	Oral capsules	50 mg, 100 mg	*Minocin* (Lederle)
	Oral tablets	50 mg, 100 mg	*Minocin*
	Oral suspension	50 mg/5 ml	*Minocin*
	Powder for injection (IV)	100-mg vial	*Minocin*
	Dental ointment[a]	2%	*PerioCare* (Pulpdent); *Arestin* (OraPharma)

[a]See Doxycycline, Topical Administration, for veterinary use.

INTERNATIONAL PREPARATIONS. *Aknosan, Aknoral, Dynacin, Klinotab, Mestacine, Minoclir, Minogal, Minomycin, Mynocine, Oracyclin.*

HANDLING. Reconstituted IV solution is stable at room temperature for 24 hr; activity declines to 92% after 1 week storage at room temperature and to 98% if refrigerated. Oral capsules should be stored at room temperature away from light. Oral suspension should be stored at room temperature but not frozen.

ADMINISTRATION. For IV, given diluted in 5% dextrose or 0.9% NaCl. Feeding does not affect absorption of oral preparations. Do not administer rapidly IV.

Dosage

INDICATIONS	DOSE (mg/kg)	ROUTE	INTERVAL (hr)	DURATION (days)
Dogs				
Soft tissue, urinary infections	5-12	PO, IV	12	7-14
Brucellosis (in combination)	12.5	PO	12	14-21
Cats				
Hemotropic mycoplasmosis	6-11	PO	12	21

ADDITIONAL DOSAGES. Ehrlichiosis, Table 28-4; canine brucellosis, Table 40-2; actinomycosis, Table 49-2; nocardiosis, Table 49-3; musculoskeletal infections, Table 86-4.

DISPENSING INFORMATION. Can be given with food.

MUPIROCIN

CLASS. Natural product, produced by *Pseudomonas fluorescens*.

ACTION. Bactericidal when used topically; inhibits bacterial protein synthesis. No cross resistance with other antimicrobial agents.

PHARMACOKINETICS. Topical ointment is rapidly inactivated after absorption; systemic levels are undetectable. The drug penetrates and persists in the stratum corneum for up to 72 hr after application. Has been given IV or PO in some countries. Drug is rapidly metabolized into monic acid which is rapidly renally excreted.

SPECTRUM. **Most** strains of staphylococci and streptococci, including methicillin-resistant and multiple-drug resistant organisms. Active against *Listeria monocytogenes* and some gram-negative bacteria.

INDICATIONS. Feline acne, alternative therapies are topical and systemic retinoids, fatty acid supplements, and metronidazole. Has some activity against *Malassezia*.

CONTRAINDICATIONS. Topical application over large infected areas leads to resistant strains. Not for ophthalmic use. Not for use on mucosal surfaces where causes stinging and drying. A paraffin-based formulation ointment is available for intranasal use.

ADVERSE REACTIONS. Irritation, pruritis, urticaria. Hypersensitivity to mupirocin or polyethylene glycol (PEG)-containing ointment.

INTERACTIONS. PEG can be absorbed from open wounds and damaged skin and is excreted by kidneys. Excessive use should be avoided with renal impairment.

AVAILABILITY	TYPE	SIZES	PREPARATION (COMPANY)
Veterinary	Topical ointment, 2%ᵃ	50 mg, 100 mg, 200 mg	*Bactoderm* (Pfizer)

ᵃIn bland water miscible ointment base of PEG.

INTERNATIONAL PREPARATIONS. *Bactroban, Mupirax, Supirocin, T-bact.*

HANDLING AND ADMINISTRATION. Apply cream three times daily for 1-2 weeks. May be covered with a dressing.

Store at room temperature (<25°C), out of the reach of children.

Dosage

INDICATIONS	DOSE	ROUTE	INTERVAL (hr)	DURATION (days)
Dogs and cats				
Burns or open wounds	Small amount	Topical	8-12	<10

ADDITIONAL DOSAGES. None.

DISPENSING INFORMATION. Apply topical to lesions, twice daily, for 3 weeks.

MYCOBACTERIAL CELL WALL EXTRACT

CLASS. Bacterial component.

ACTION. Immunostimulatory. Production of tumor necrosis factor and other cytokines.

MORE INFORMATION. Chapter 2.

PHARMACOKINETICS. From nonpathogenic species and strain of mycobacteria, contains purified mycobacterial cell wall fractions with known immunostimulatory properties. Contains low-level analgesic and a green tracking solution to facilitate location of intra-tumor administration.

SPECTRUM. Stimulates activation of macrophages and thymic lymphocytes in tissue and blood cells. Increases interleukin–1 production.

INDICATIONS. Parenteral nonspecific immunostimulant, vaccine adjuvant, intralesional for antitumor therapy. Canine mammary tumors.

APPROVED USES. Adenocarcinomas in dog and sarcoids in horses.

CONTRAINDICATIONS. Previous allergic reactions to the drug. Pre-existing mycobacterial disease. Concurrent immunosuppression or glucocorticoid therapy.

ADVERSE REACTIONS. Fever, anorexia, systemic inflammatory reaction. Pain at the time of injection.

INTERACTIONS. Increased response of horses to herpesvirus vaccination when given IM, at the same time, but different site.

AVAILABILITY	TYPE	SIZES	PREPARATIONS (COMPANY)
Veterinary	Intratumoral (canine and equine)	10-ml vials	*Regressin-V* (Vetrepharm)
	IV (equine)	1.5-ml syringes	*Equimune I.V.* (Vetrepharm)

HANDLING. Store in a refrigerator (36-45°F [2-7°C]) but do not freeze. Mix the emulsion thoroughly until milky white in color immediately before use. May heat to 65°C to facilitate mixing.

ADMINISTRATION. Using a 20-gauge needle or smaller, mammary tumors are injected intralesionally and perilesionally under sedation or anesthesia once 2-4 weeks before surgery. Without surgery, repeat injections every 1-3 weeks for up to 4 treatments. Tumors that fail to respond after 4 treatments are considered refractory.

Dosage

INDICATIONS	DOSE (ml)	ROUTE	INTERVAL (hr)	DURATION (days)
Equine vaccine adjuvant	1.5	IM (deep)	24	1
Equine respiratory disease	1.5	IV	24	1

Dosages for immunostimulation of dogs and cats would have to be extrapolated.

ADDITIONAL DOSAGES. None.

NEOMYCIN

CLASS. Aminoglycoside.

ACTION. Bactericidal, inhibits protein synthesis.

MORE INFORMATION. See GENTAMICIN; Aminoglycosides, Chapter 34; Tables 34-5, 34-6.

PHARMACOKINETICS. Poorly absorbed (<5%) from intact GI tract. Topical use for ulcerative lesions may allow increased uptake and potential toxicity. Majority of oral dose is excreted unchanged in feces. Any absorbed drug is excreted unchanged in urine. Effects are on intestinal microflora.

SPECTRUM. See GENTAMICIN, less effective than gentamicin against many *Pseudomonas, Klebsiella, Escherichia*.

INDICATIONS. Not used parenterally because more toxic and less effective than other aminoglycosides. Commonly used orally for reduction of enteric flora or pathogens. Effect lasts for 48-72 hr after single dosing. Used orally for prophylaxis before intestinal or colonic surgery and to reduce bacterial ammonia production in hepatic insufficiency or coma.

APPROVED USES. Veterinary, farm animals.

CONTRAINDICATIONS. Pregnancy, because small absorbed amounts are fetotoxic; GI obstruction or ulcerative disease of GI tract suggested by hemoptysis, melena, or hematochezia.

ADVERSE REACTIONS. Diarrhea owing to microflora alterations, nephrotoxicity, ototoxicity, interference with intestinal bacterial vitamin K synthesis and fat malabsorption.

INTERACTIONS. Potentiates vitamin K deficiency and associated coagulopathy. Decreases absorption of digoxin, methotrexate, penicillin V, vitamin K.

AVAILABILITY	TYPE	SIZES	PREPARATIONS (COMPANY)
Human	Oral tablets (as sulfate)	500 mg	Generic (Biocraft)
	Oral solution (as sulfate)	125 mg/5 ml	*Mycifradin* (Pharmacia & Upjohn), generic (various)
Veterinary	Oral liquid (as sulfate)	140 mg/ml	*Biosol* (Pharmacia & Upjohn)
	Oral solution (as sulfate)	50 mg/ml	*Biosol*
	Oral tablets (as sulfate)	100 mg	*Biosol* tablets

INTERNATIONAL PREPARATIONS. *Bykomycin, Francetin, Myciguent, Nebacetin, Neo-fradin, Neointestin.*

HANDLING. Store at room temperature in airtight and light-proof container.

ADMINISTRATION. PO: can give undiluted or diluted with water. Can be added to the sole source of drinking water to be consumed in 24 hr but must be made as fresh solution each day. Can also give by syringe or gavage. Not recommended for parenteral use.

Dosage

INDICATIONS (Dogs and Cats)	DOSE	ROUTE	INTERVAL (hr)	DURATION (days)
Bacterial enteritis, reducing GI flora, hepatic encephalopathy	10-15 mg/kg	PO	6-24	≤14

ADDITIONAL DOSAGES. Endotoxemia, Table 38-6; otitis externa (topical), Tables 85-6 and 85-8.

DISPENSING INFORMATION. If animal shows persistent vomiting or bloody diarrhea, discontinue medication and notify veterinarian immediately.

NIFURTIMOX

CLASS. Nitrofuran derivative.

ACTION. Antiprotozoal; oxidative effects on trypanosomal enzymes, especially involving nucleic acid biosynthesis.

MORE INFORMATION. See Chapters 71, 72; Table 71-1.

PHARMACOKINETICS. Well absorbed from GI tract after PO administration, low plasma concentrations. Undergoes rapid biotransformation in liver to metabolites; little (≤0.5%) of active drug is excreted in urine.

SPECTRUM. *Trypanosoma cruzi.* African trypanosomiasis at higher dosages (second choice).

INDICATIONS. American trypanosomiasis. Some effect on African trypanosomiasis. Reduces severity of acute disease but ineffective in chronic phases; suppresses infection rather than cures. Preexisting seizures or renal or hepatic disease. Alternative drug is benznidazole. Use of allopurinol as adjunctive therapy has not been well studied in this disease.

CONTRAINDICATIONS. Despite toxicity, may be one of few effective drugs for this disease. Preexisting seizures or renal or hepatic disease. Alternative drug is benznidazole.

ADVERSE REACTIONS. Frequent toxicity, including anorexia, vomiting, weight loss, CNS signs, polyneuritis, pulmonary infiltrates, skin eruptions, mitogenic (chromosomal aberrations). Hemolysis with glucose-6 phosphate dehydrogenase deficiency. In people, children tolerate the drug better than adults.

INTERACTIONS. Alcohol ingestion in people enhances adverse reactions.

AVAILABILITY	TYPE	SIZES	PREPARATION (COMPANY)
Human	Investigation drug for human use only in U.S. from CDC, (404) 639-3670; available in other countries.	Oral tablets 120 mg	*Lampit* (Bayer)

HANDLING. Store at room temperature in airtight container.

ADMINISTRATION. Reduce dosage if GI disturbances occur.

Dosage

INDICATIONS (Human)	DOSE (mg/kg)	ROUTE	INTERVAL (hr)	DURATION (days)
Trypanosomiasis (*T. cruzi*)				
Adults	2-2.5	PO	6	90
Children	3-3.5	PO	6	90

ADDITIONAL DOSAGES. Trypanosomiasis, Table 72-1.

DISPENSING INFORMATION. Can be given with food but may cause GI upsets. Food tends to reduce the GI irritation.

NITAZOXANIDE

CLASS. Thiazolide: A nitrothiazolyl-salicylamide derivative.

ACTION. Antiprotozoal. Anaerobic antibacterial, anthelmenthic.

MORE INFORMATION. See Chapter 71 and Reference Ch 71, ref. 1; 4.

PHARMACOKINETICS. In humans is absorbed rapidly with peak levels of its metabolite, tizoxanide, are attained between 2-3 hr after a dosing and are no longer detectable by 24 hr. High degree of protein binding. Excreted as metabolites in the urine, bile, and feces.

SPECTRUM. Active against *Giardia*, *Cryptosporidium*, *Sarcocystis neurona*.

INDICATIONS. For the treatment of drug-resistant *Giardia* and *Cryptosporidium* infections in people. Response is lower in immunocompromised individuals.

APPROVED USES. For use in people with drug-resistant *Giardia* and *Cryptosporidium* infections. Has been used to treat horses with *Sarcocystis neurona* infection. Could be considered for treatment of dogs or cats with these infections; however, data is lacking on effectiveness.

CONTRAINDICATIONS. Generally has a wide margin of safety; however, should be used with caution in animals that are ill or debilitated.

ADVERSE REACTIONS. GI signs such as diarrhea and anorexia caused by effects on the GI microflora.

INTERACTIONS. Since highly protein bound, this drug may displace those bound drugs and increase their activitiy and potential toxicity.

AVAILABILITY	TYPE	SIZES	PREPARATION (COMPANY)
Human	20 mg/ml oral suspension	60 ml bottles	*Alinia* (Romark Laboratories, Tampa FL)
	Oral tablets	500 mg	*Alinia* (*Romark Laboratories*, Tampa FL)
Equine	Oral paste 32%	85 g syringes	*Navigator* (IDEXX)

INTERNATIONAL PREPARATIONS. *Heliton, Daxon, PH-5776.*

HANDLING. Powder for oral suspension for people is stable at 25°C (77°F). with a range of 15-30°C. When mixed the suspension is stable at room temperature for 7 days. The paste for horses should be stored below 30°C and can be refrigerated but not frozen.

ADMINISTRATION. Horse product is dispensed from a prefilled dose syringe with stops to ensure accurate dosage.

Dosage

INDICATIONS	DOSE	ROUTE	INTERVAL (hr)	DURATION (days)
Cryptosporidium **(human)**	100 mg/kg[a]	PO	12	5[b]
	200 mg/kg[a]	PO	12	5-7 days[c]
Horses	25 mg/kg day 1-5	PO	24	28
	50 mg/kg/day day 6-28			

[a]Human dose that is effective for children, higher dose range is needed in immunodeficient people. Dose range has not been established for dogs or cats but a similar regimen could be considered. Doses of 250-500 mg/kg were required to successfully treat C. *parvum* infection in pigs (Ch 71, ref. 91a).
[b]For children 24-47 mo old.
[c]For children 4-11 yr old.

ADDITIONAL DOSAGES. Dosages for dogs and cats would have to be extrapolated.

DISPENSING INFORMATION. Paste or suspension should be given as directed; however, animal should be montored at least once daily for fever, anorexia, lethargy, depression.

NITROFURANTOIN

CLASS. Nitrofuran.

ACTION. Bactericidal or bacteriostatic; inhibits bacterial carbohydrate metabolism and cell wall formation.

MORE INFORMATION. See Nitrofurans, Chapter 34; Table 34-9.

PHARMACOKINETICS. Well absorbed (85%-95%) from GI tract after PO administration. Bioavailability enhanced and irritation reduced by giving with food. The macrocrystalline formulation is less irritating to GI tract but more slowly absorbed. The microcrystals are absorbed faster, reaching higher and more rapid peak urinary bladder levels. Most of the drug is metabolized with 30%-50% excreted unchanged in urine. Concentrations in blood or tissues are too low to be effective but are sufficient to treat urinary tract infections.

SPECTRUM. Gram positive: *Staphylococcus, Streptococcus, Enterococcus.* **Gram negative:** *Escherichia,* some *Klebsiella,* some *Enterobacter, Salmonella.* **Ineffective:** *Proteus, Serratia, Pseudomonas, Acinetobacter.*

INDICATIONS. Urinary tract infections caused by susceptible organisms.

APPROVED USES. Human urinary tract infections.

CONTRAINDICATIONS. Reduce dosage in renal failure, oliguria, pregnancy, breeding males or females.

ADVERSE REACTIONS. Interstitial pneumonitis, hemolysis with glucose–6-phosphate dehydrogenase deficiency, cholestatic hepatitis, LMN paralysis. The latter, (myasthenic-like syndrome) has been noted in a dog by the author (CEG), and by others in personal communications. The weakness resolves after withdrawing the drug. Vomiting is most common side effect in dogs and cats. May discolor urine to dark brown.

INTERACTIONS. Co-administered anticholinergics increase bioavailability while magnesium salts reduce absorption. May interfere with efficacy of fluoroquinolones.

AVAILABILITY	TYPE	SIZES	PREPARATIONS (COMPANY)
Human	Oral suspension	25 mg/ml	*Furadantin* (Proctor & Gamble)
	Oral capsules (microcrystalline)	25 mg, 50 mg, 100 mg	*Macrodantin* (Proctor & Gamble), generics (various)
			Nitrofurantoin generic (various)
	Oral capsules (regular)	50 mg, 100 mg	*Furadantin*

INTERNATIONAL PREPARATIONS. *Chemiofuran, Cistofuran, Cystit, Furabid, Furedan, Macrobid, Microdoïne, Nephronex, Novofuran, Phenurin, Urantoin, Urodid, Urolong.*

HANDLING. Store in airtight, light-proof containers at room temperature. May darken with light exposure. Avoid contact with most metals.

ADMINISTRATION. Bioavailability and GI tolerance is enhanced by giving with food. For long-term prophylaxis, give in evening to maintain nighttime levels in urine. Suspension can be mixed with milk to facilitate administration to animals.

Dosage

INDICATIONS (*Dogs and Cats*)	DOSE (mg/kg)	ROUTE	INTERVAL (hr)	DURATION (days)
Urinary Infections				
Severe or difficult	4	PO	6	14-28
Routine	2.2-4.4	PO	8	7-14
Long-term, prophylaxis, or giardiasis	3-4	PO	24	≥90

ADDITIONAL DOSAGES. Urinary infections, Table 91-10.

DISPENSING INFORMATION. Give with food.

NORFLOXACIN

CLASS. Fluoroquinolone.

ACTION. Inhibits bacterial DNA gyrase.

MORE INFORMATION. See ENROFLOXACIN, MARBOFLOXACIN; Fluoroquinolones, Chapter 34; Table 34-11.

PHARMACOKINETICS. Lower bioavailability (30%-40%) than other quinolones after PO administration. Food reduces absorption. Hepatic metabolism to less active metabolites with biliary and urinary excretion. Penetrates well into genitourinary tract and its secretions.

SPECTRUM. Gram positive: *Staphylococcus.* **Gram negative:** *Escherichia, Proteus, Pseudomonas, Enterobacter.* Activity is lower than with ciprofloxacin and enrofloxacin. **Anerobes:** Minimal activity against obligate anaerobes. Resistance may develop when treating infections caused by *Klebsiella, Pseudomonas, Enterococcus.* **Others:** See ENROFLOXACIN. **More Effective:** aerobic or facultative anaerobic gram-negative bacteria. **Ineffective:** obligate anaerobes.

INDICATIONS. See ENROFLOXACIN.

CONTRAINDICATIONS. See ENROFLOXACIN.

ADVERSE REACTIONS. See ENROFLOXACIN. Interactions: See ENROFLOXACIN.

AVAILABILITY	TYPE	SIZES	PREPARATION (COMPANY)
Human	Oral tablets	400 mg	*Noroxin* (Merck)

HANDLING. Store in airtight, light-proof containers at room temperature.

ADMINISTRATION. Food can delay absorption but not considered to be critical.

Dosage

INDICATIONS (*Dogs and Cats*)	DOSE (mg/kg)	ROUTE	INTERVAL (hr)	DURATION (days)
Skin, urinary infections[a]	5-11	PO	12	14-21
Soft tissues, systemic[b] infections	11-22	PO	12	14-21
Bacteremia	22	PO, IM	12	prn

[a]*Staphylococcus, Escherichia coli, Klebsiella, Serratia.*
[b]*Pseudomonas, Enterobacter.*

ADDITIONAL DOSAGES. None.

DISPENSING INFORMATION. Give medication on empty stomach. Do not give with dairy products or other antacids.

NOVOBIOCIN

CLASS. Coumarin antibiotic.

ACTION. Usually bacteriostatic; interferes with bacterial cell wall synthesis and nucleic acid synthesis.

MORE INFORMATION. See Novobiocin, Chapter 34.

PHARMACOKINETICS. Well absorbed from the GI tract, but food may reduce. High degree of serum protein binding so tissue and body fluid concentrations are low. Little penetration of CSF, even in meningitis. Predominantly excreted in bile and feces with little appearing in urine.

SPECTRUM. Gram positive: some *Streptococcus, Staphylococcus,* few *Enterococcus.* **Gram negative:** most resistant except *Proteus, Pasteurella,* and some *Pseudomonas.* **Anaerobes:** most resistant. **Ineffective:** most *Enterococcus,* and gram negatives.

INDICATIONS. Staphylococcal infections, upper respiratory tract infections in dogs, in combination with tetracycline with or without prednisolone.

CONTRAINDICATIONS. Hepatic insufficiency, biliary obstruction, myelosuppressive diseases.

ADVERSE REACTIONS. Allergic hypersensitivity, dermal eruptions, hepatic dysfunction, vomiting, diarrhea, bone marrow dyscrasia.

INTERACTIONS. May prolong excretion and increase blood concentrations of β-lactam and cephalosporin drugs. May inhibit excretion of bilirubin and bromsulphalein. Often administered in combination with tetracycline or rifampin to prevent resistance.

AVAILABILITY	TYPE	SIZES	PREPARATIONS (COMPANY)
Human	Oral capsules	250 mg	*Albamycin* (Pharmacia & Upjohn)
	Oral syrup	125 mg/5 ml	*Albamycin*
Veterinary	Novobiocin (as sodium) and tetracycline (as HCl)	60 mg each or 180 mg each also with prednisolone (1.5 or 4.5 mg)	*Albaplex* and *Albaplex—3X* (Pharmacia & Upjohn) *Delta Albaplex* and *Delta Albaplex—3X*

HANDLING. Store in airtight containers at room temperature.

ADMINISTRATION. Preferably give on empty stomach. If vomiting occurs, give with small amount of food. Available in combination with tetracycline, with or without prednisolone, for use in dogs. Tetracycline absorption in the combined preparations is more affected by ingesta than is novobiocin.

Dosage

INDICATIONS (*Dogs*)	DOSE (mg/kg)	ROUTE	INTERVAL (hr)	DURATION (days)
Respiratory infections	10	PO	8	5-7
	22[a]	PO	12	5-7

[a]Combined with tetracycline.

ADDITIONAL DOSAGES. None.

DISPENSING INFORMATION. Give at least 1 hr before or 2 hr after feeding. If vomiting occurs, consult veterinarian.

OFLOXACIN

CLASS. Fluoroquinolone.

ACTION. Bactericidal; inhibits bacterial enzyme DNA gyrase.

MORE INFORMATION. See ENROFLOXACIN; Chapter 34, Tables 34-11 and 34-12.

PHARMACOKINETICS. Systemic availability after PO administration, bioavailability is 98% (the highest of the class). Maximum blood concentrations in 1-2 hr. Wide distribution in body tissues and fluids. Detected in blister fluid, genital tissues, lung. CSF concentrations are 40%-90% serum, if inflamed. Human aqueous humor concentration is 44%-88% serum. Minimal metabolism, primarily renally excreted.

SPECTRUM. Gram positive: *Staphylococcus*, some *Streptococcus*, poor activity against *Enterococcus*. **Gram negative:** *Enterobacter, Klebsiella, Pseudomonas, Proteus, Salmonella, Serratia, Yersinia, Campylobacter.* **Anaerobes:** poor activity. *Bacteroides* and *Clostridium* are inhibited in vitro.

INDICATIONS. Complicated urinary tract infections; also lower respiratory tract, skin, and soft tissue infections caused by susceptible gram-negative bacteria.

CONTRAINDICATIONS. Drug clearance reduced with renal failure so must use lower dosages. Avoid in pregnancy or lactation.

ADVERSE REACTIONS. Arthropathies in immature animals. High overdosages have not produced lenticular opacities or crystalluria, although these can occur with other drugs of this class. Nausea, vomiting, diarrhea may occur. All quinolones have potential to cause CNS hyperexcitability and seizures. Phototoxicity has been seen with use of some compounds in this class.

INTERACTIONS. Theophylline concentrations will increase when given concurrently. Should not give orally within 2-4 hr of receiving sucralfate or preparations containing polyvalent cations (Al, Ca, Mg, Fe, Zn). Should not give orally within 2-4 hr of receiving sulcralfate or preparations containing polyvalent cations (Al, Ca, Mg, Fe, Zn).

AVAILABILITY	TYPE	SIZES	PREPARATIONS (COMPANY)
Human	Tablets	200 mg, 300 mg, 400 mg	*Floxin* (Ortho)
	IV solution	200 mg, 400 mg	*Floxin*

INTERNATIONAL PREPARATIONS. *Floxal, Surnox, Tarivid, Trafloxal.*

HANDLING. Store tablets in tightly closed containers below 30°C. Solution can be added to 0.9% NaCl, 5% dextrose, or solutions containing KCl.

ADMINISTRATION. Effect of food on absorption has not been well studied, but it may be better to avoid dosing with food.

Dosage

INDICATIONS (*Dogs and Cats*)	DOSE (mg/kg)	ROUTE	INTERVAL (hr)	DURATION (days)
Uncomplicated urinary infections	2.5	PO	12	7
Complicated urinary, genital infections	5-7.5	PO	12	10
Lower respiratory infections	7.5-10	PO	12	14

ADDITIONAL DOSAGES. None.

DISPENSING INFORMATION. Monitor animal for adequate water intake; avoid sucralfate and vitamin with iron and mineral supplements and antacids within 4 hr of administration.

ORBIFLOXACIN

CLASS. Fluoroquinolone.

ACTION. Bactericidal; inhibits bacterial DNA gyrase.

MORE INFORMATION. See ENROFLOXACIN, MARBOFLOXACIN, DIFLOXACIN; Chapter 34; Tables 34-11 and 34-12.

PHARMACOKINETICS. Well absorbed orally (97% bioavailable) with peak plasma concentrations within 1 hr of administration. Plasma protein binding low (7%-14%). In dogs, after 3 hours of giving 5 mg/kg dose, tissue concentrations are 6.0 µg/ml in prostate and 4.1 µg/ml in lung. It is predominantly (50%) excreted unchanged in urine with concentrations of 100 µg/ml, between 0 and 6 hours after administration of 2.5 mg/kg. After SC injection of 5 mg/kg to cats and dogs, urine recoveries were 28% and 45% and fecal recoveries were 15% and 18% respectively (Ch 34, ref. 241). In the urine, nonmetabloized parent drug comprised 96% and 87% of the amounts recovered, respectively. Following a 7.5 mg/kg daily dose for 4-6 days, mean concentrations in skin of dogs with pyoderma were higher ($9.47 \pm 6.23\,\mu g/g$) than in clinically healthy dogs ($5.43 \pm 1.02\,\mu g/g$) (Ch 34, ref. 191). Skin concentrations were approximately equal to those in plasma for the clinically healthy dogs and 1. 4 times those in plasma for the dogs with pyoderma. At this dose, the mean concentration of orbifloxacin in skin of dogs with pyoderma was approximately 24 times the MIC_{90} for *Staphylococcus intermedius*. Extrapolated mean concentration in the skin of dogs with pyoderma following the 2.5 mg/kg dose was estimated at 8 times this MIC_{90} (Ch 34, ref. 191).

SPECTRUM. Gram-negative and some gram-positive bacteria. Not effective against anaerobes. See ENROFLOXACIN.

INDICATIONS. Skin and soft tissue infections (wounds, abscesses, pyoderma) and urinary tract infections.

CONTRAINDICATIONS. Young growing animals, seizure-prone animals. Safety in pregnancy and breeding dogs has not been established.

ADVERSE REACTIONS. Can cause CNS stimulation and seizures in predisposed animals. Immature animals may develop arthropathy when treated. Avoid in rapid growth phase of 2-8 mo in small and medium breeds and up to 18 mo in giant breeds. Cats receiving higher than recommended dosages (45 or 75 mg/kg PO every 24 hr) developed focal, well-delineated tapetal hyperreflectivity (Ch 34, ref. 420). See also ENROFLOXACIN.

INTERACTIONS. See also ENROFLOXACIN. Compounds such as sucralfate, antacids, and multivitamin that contain divalent and trivalent cations (iron, aluminum, calcium, magnesium or zinc) may interfere with absorption.

AVAILABILITY	TYPE	SIZES	PREPARATION (COMPANY)
Veterinary (dogs and cats)	Oral tablets (scored)	5.7 mg (yellow), 22.7 mg (green), 68 mg (blue)	*Orbax* (Schering-Plough Animal Health)
Veterinary (dogs and cats)	Solution	5% concentration	*Victas* Injection (Dainippon Pharm, Osaka Japan)

HANDLING. Store tablets at controlled temperature between 2-30°C.

ADMINISTRATION. For skin and soft tissue infections, give for 2-3 days beyond cessation of signs for a maximum of 30 days. Effect of feeding on dose has not been determined. Although not clinically available in all countries, the SC route was shown to give similar pharmacokinetic data as compared to oral administration in dogs and cats (Ch 34, ref. 242).

Dosage

INDICATIONS	DOSE[a] (mg/kg)	ROUTE	INTERVAL (hr)	DURATION (days)
Urinary infections	2.5-5.0	PO	24	10[b]
Soft tissue infections	5.0-7.5	PO	24	10[b]
Skin infection with resistant pathogens *(dogs)*	7.5	PO	24	10[b]
Systemic infection, bacteremia	5.0	PO	12	prn

[a]Flexible dosage labeling.
[b]A maximum of 30 days has been evaluated in safety trials.

ADDITIONAL DOSAGES. None.

DISPENSING INFORMATION. Give medication without feeding, unless vomiting occurs. Never give antacids or GI protectants within 2 hr of medication.

ORMETROPRIM-SULFONAMIDE

CLASS. Diaminopyrimidine and sulfonamide.

ACTION. Combination is bactericidal, causes synergistic two-step inhibition of microbial folic acid synthesis. Antibacterial, antiprotozoal.

MORE INFORMATION. Similar to baquiloprim-sulfadimethoxine licensed in Europe. See TRIMETHOPRIM-SULFONAMIDE, BAQUILOPRIM-SULFONAMIDE; Chapter 34; Table 34-10; references: Ch 34, ref. 256; Ch 34, ref. 339.

PHARMACOKINETICS. Sulfadimethoxine and ormetoprim in a 5:1 ratio. Both have an extended blood half-life permitting once-a-day dosing. The sulfadimethoxine is highly protein bound, maintaining high and long-duration blood levels, is slowly excreted by dogs largely unchanged in the urine. Sulfadimethoxine has high solubility in the urine and kidney of dogs precluding precipitation and crystalluria. See also TRIMETHOPRIM-SULFONAMIDE.

SPECTRUM. Gram positive: *Staphylococcus, Nocardia.* **Gram negative:** *Proteus, Escherichia, Salmonella, Klebsiella, Brucella, Bordetella,* coccidiosis. **Anaerobes:** *Clostridium.* **Others:** Coccidia, *Pneumocystis, Neospora.* **Ineffective:** *Pseudomonas.* The combined drugs potentiate activity of each other.

INDICATIONS. Treatment of pyoderma, wounds, abscesses in dogs caused by susceptible strains of *Staphylococcus* and gram-negative organisms like *Escherichia.*

APPROVED USES. Skin and soft tissue infections caused by susceptible organisms in dogs.

CONTRAINDICATIONS. Preexisting hepatic disease, blood dyscrasias, or known previous reaction to sulfonamide. Safety in breeding and pregnant animals is not established; should avoid.

ADVERSE REACTIONS. See also TRIMETHOPRIM-SULFONAMIDE. Keratoconjunctivitis, immune complex–mediated reaction (polyarthritis, urticaria, facial swelling, fever, hemolytic anemia, thrombocytopenia, leukopenia), hepatotoxicity, vomiting, anorexia, diarrhea, polydipsia, polyuria. Rare: generalized anaphylaxis. PO administration of this drug to dogs for 8 weeks at 27.5 mg/kg/day resulted in hypothyroidism (thyroid enlargement, follicular hyperplasia, reduced serum thyroid hormone), reflecting interference with thyroidal hormone synthesis (Ch 34, ref. 146). Very high doses in dogs cause CNS signs, depression, and seizures.

INTERACTIONS. Prolonged use can cause hypothyroidism.

AVAILABILITY	TYPE	SIZES	PREPARATION (COMPANY)
Veterinary	Oral tablet (sulfadimethoxine-ormetoprim in 5 : 1 ratio)	120 mg, 250 mg, 600 mg, 1200 mg	*Primor* (Pfizer Animal Health)

HANDLING. Keep tablets stored in airtight containers at room temperature.

ADMINISTRATION. Not recommended by manufacturer for treatment longer than 21 days; longer periods require careful monitoring. Treatment for infections such as pyoderma requires 3-9 weeks. Continue therapy for at least 2 days after remission of signs. Can be dosed once daily, even in bacterial skin disease (Ch 34, ref. 176). Although soluble in urine, adequate water should be provided at all times. Dehydration and acid urine favor crystal formation.

Dosage

INDICATIONS	DOSE[a] (mg/kg)	ROUTE	INTERVAL (hr)	DURATION (days)
Dogs				
Soft tissue, infection coccidiosis	27.5	PO	24	21
Chronic pyoderma	27.5[b]	PO	24	21-63[c]
Coccidiosis	66[b]	PO	24	23
Cats				
Coccidiosis	66	PO	24	≤23

[a]Dose includes combined sulfadimethoxime-ormetroprim in 5 : 1 ratio.
[b]Use twice this dose on the first day.
[c]Not approved for longer than 21 days, but chronic skin disease often warrants longer treatment.

ADDITIONAL DOSAGES. Coccidiosis, Table 81-2; Canine pyoderma, Table 85-3; otitis externa, Table 85-6.

DISPENSING INFORMATION. Supply animal with unlimited water to drink; notify clinician of any signs of dry eyes, fever, GI upsets, skin eruptions, swelling, lameness, or worsening of clinical condition.

OSELTAMIVIR PHOSPHATE

CLASS. Antiviral.

ACTION. Inhibition of influenza virus neuraminidase. This may alter virus particle aggregation and release from the cell.

MORE INFORMATION. U.S. Food and Drug Administration at http://www.fda.gov/cder/drug/infopage/tamiflu/default.htm, last accessed 04/05/05.

PHARMACOKINETICS. The drug is a pro-drug requiring conversion for its activity. Readily absorbed from the GI tract after oral administration. Extensively converted predominantly by hepatic esterases to oseltamivir carboxylate. Co-administration with food has no significant effect on the peak plasma concentration and the area under the plasma concentration curve. Excreted in the kidney by glomerular filtration and tubular secretion. Less than 20% of an oral radiolabeled dose is eliminated in feces.

SPECTRUM. Parainfluenza virus neuraminidase. There is no evidence for efficacy on any viruses other than influenza A and B.

INDICATIONS. The drug must be given within the first 2 days of onset of clinical illness. Has only been shown to be effective against neuraminidase on the surface of parainfluenza viruses. Although this drug has been suggested for use to treat dogs and cats infected by parvoviruses, there is no valid or logical reason that this should be effective. The parvoviruses are nonenveloped and there is *no* evidence or experimental basis that these viruses would be susceptible. The closest viral infections of dogs and cats would be infection with one of the strains of influenza virus or perhaps canine parainfluenza virus. Use of this drug may help reduce the prevalence of canine infectious tracheobronchitis in a kennel.

APPROVED USES. Humans with influenza beginning the first 2 days after the onset of infection.

CONTRAINDICATIONS. Use during pregnancy or neonates is not recommended.

ADVERSE REACTIONS. Generally well-tolerated. Nausea, vomiting, and diarrhea are most prevalent among the reactions. Taking with food can reverse the potential of side effects. Not recommended for use during pregnancy or nursing.

INTERACTIONS. Clinically significant drug interactions are unlikely.

AVAILABILITY	TYPE	SIZES	PREPARATION (COMPANY)
Human	Oral capsules	75 mg	*Tamiflu* (Roche)
Human	Pediatric suspension	12 mg/ml	*Tamiflu* (Roche)

HANDLING. Store at 25°C (77°F), with limits of 15-30°C (59-86°F). Store constituted suspension under refrigeration at 2°C to 8°C (36-46°F).

ADMINISTRATION. Must be given orally within the first 2 days of infection and never used for longer than 5 days.

Dosage

INDICATIONS	DOSE[a]	ROUTE	INTERVAL (hr)	DURATION (days)
Humans				
Influenza (>40 kg)	75 mg total	PO	12	5
23-40 kg	60 mg total	PO	12	5
15-23 kg	45 mg total	PO	12	5
≤15 kg	30 mg total	PO	12	5

[a]Treatment should begin within 2 days of onset of signs of influenza.

ADDITIONAL DOSAGES. None.

DISPENSING INFORMATION. Administer fasting; however if vomiting or nausea occur then give with food.

OXACILLIN

CLASS. Isoxazolyl penicillin.

ACTION. Bactericidal; inhibits bacterial cell wall synthesis.

MORE INFORMATION. Chapter 34; Table 34-1.

PHARMACOKINETICS. Bioavailability after PO administration is 60%-70%. One of few penicillins that has predominant hepatic inactivation and biliary excretion. Urinary excretion of unchanged drug is 30%-70% of that absorbed.

SPECTRUM. Gram positive: *Staphylococcus* (including β-lactamase producers), other gram-positive aerobic cocci, some gram-positive anaerobes.

INDICATIONS. Staphylococcal pyoderma, staphylococcal infections of the respiratory tract or soft tissues.

CONTRAINDICATIONS. Penicillin hypersensitivity.

ADVERSE REACTIONS. See PENICILLIN. Thrombophlebitis when given IV. Neutropenia in people when given IV for several weeks. Vomiting and diarrhea with oral formulations.

INTERACTIONS. Inactivates aminoglycosides when given in the same parenteral solution. Amikacin is most stable aminoglycoside in the presence of penicillins. Antagonism in activity with tetracyclines or chloramphenicol. Sulfonamides inhibit GI absorption of oxacillin.

AVAILABILITY	TYPE	SIZES	PREPARATIONS (COMPANY)
Human	Capsules	250 mg, 500 mg	*Bactocill* (SmithKline Beecham), *Prostaphlin* (Apothecon)
	Powder for oral solution	250 mg/5 ml	*Bactocill*
	Powder for injection	250 mg, 500 mg, 1 g, 2 g, 4 g, 10 g	*Bactocill*

INTERNATIONAL PREPARATIONS. *Bristopen, Penstapho, Stapenor.*

HANDLING. Reconstitute powder for injection with sterile NaCl or water. For IV, solution stable for 6 hr at room temperature at concentrations of 0.5-40 mg/ml. Compatible with 5% dextrose, Ringer's solution, and 0.9% NaCl. For IM, solution of 250 mg/1.5 ml stable for 3 days at room temperature, 7 days if refrigerated.

ADMINISTRATION. Infuse IV over at least 10 min. Food interferes with PO absorption.

Dosage

INDICATIONS (Dogs)	DOSE (mg/kg)	ROUTE	INTERVAL (hr)	DURATION (days)
Bacterial pyoderma	22	PO	8	14-21
Bacterial pyoderma	15-25	PO	12	14-21
Orthopedic infection	22	IV, IM, SC, PO	6-8	21-42

ADDITIONAL DOSAGES. Canine pyoderma, Table 85-3; musculoskeletal infections, Table 86-4; CNS infections, Table 92-5.

DISPENSING INFORMATION. Administer at least 1 hr before feeding or 2 hr after a meal.

OXYTETRACYCLINE

CLASS. Tetracycline.

ACTION. Bacteriostatic; interferes with bacterial protein synthesis. See TETRACYCLINE.

MORE INFORMATION. TETRACYCLINE; Tetracyclines, Chapter 34; Table 34-7.

PHARMACOKINETICS. See TETRACYCLINE. For long-acting preparation, the elimination half-life and volume of distribution are increased in *Ehrlichia canis*—infected dogs as compared to uninfected dogs (Ch 34, ref. 198).

SPECTRUM. See TETRACYCLINE.

INDICATIONS. See TETRACYCLINE.

APPROVED USES. Equine and food animal.

CONTRAINDICATIONS. See TETRACYCLINE.

ADVERSE REACTIONS. See TETRACYCLINE. Localized pain and allergic or anaphylactic reactions have occurred in dogs after parenteral use. This has been a particular problem with repeated doses of long-acting IM formulations.

INTERACTIONS. See TETRACYCLINE.

AVAILABILITY	TYPE	SIZES	PREPARATIONS (COMPANY)
Human	Capsules	250 mg (as HCl)	*Terramycin* (Pfizer)
	Solution for injection (IV)	500-mg vials	*Terramycin* IV
	Solution for injection (IM) with lidocaine	500 mg/ml, 125 mg/ml	*Terramycin* IM
Veterinary	Solution for injection	50 mg/ml, 100 mg/ml	*Oxytet* (Vedco), *Oxybiotic* 100 (Butler), *Intacycline* (Intervet), *Terramylin* (Pfizer), generic (various)
	Repositol solution for injection (licensed for cattle and pigs in U.S., dogs and cats in U.K.)	200 mg/ml 50 mg/ml, 100 mg/ml	*Liquamycin* LA—200 (Pfizer), *Terramycin LA* (Pfizer) *Engemycin* (Mycofarm)

INTERNATIONAL PREPARATIONS. *Aknin, Imperacin, Innolyre, Oxymycin, Terramycine.*

HANDLING. Store in airtight containers protected from light. Solutions are acidic and incompatible with alkaline solutions and many parenteral antimicrobials and other drugs.

ADMINISTRATION. No more than 1-2 ml should be injected at any one site when using IM route. IM route is painful and produces lower blood concentrations than by oral or IV route. Nonsteroidal analgesics have been given 15 min prior to IM injections to reduce discomfort. Not recommended to use LA—200 by IV route. It is a long acting, less painful formulation developed for use in food-producing animals consisting of a vehicle containing a solvent, 2-pyrrolidone, with a povidone base. Administer PO to fasting animal. Do not give oral formulations with dairy products or substances containing multivalent cations (Fe, Al, Mg, Ca, Bi).

Dosage

INDICATIONS	DOSE (mg/kg)	ROUTE	INTERVAL	DURATION (days)
Dogs				
Systemic infections	22	PO	8 hr	7-14
	20	IM (repositol)	7 days	7[a]
Cats				
Hemotropic mycoplasmosis	10-25	PO, IV	8 hr	5-7

[a]May be repeated every 7 days. For pharmacokinetics, see reference Ch 28, ref. 198.

ADDITIONAL DOSAGES. Salmon poisoning disease, Table 27-2; ehrlichiosis, Table 28-4; hemotropic mycoplasmosis, Table 31-1; bacterial overgrowth, Table 89-16.

DISPENSING INFORMATION. Give PO on an empty stomach.

PARAPOXVIRUS OVIS AND PARAPOXVIRUS OVIS (PIND-AVI/PIND-ORF, BAYPAMUN®): PARAIMMUNITY INDUCER. SEE CHAPTER 2.

PAROMOMYCIN (ANIMOSIDINE)

CLASS. Aminoglycoside.

ACTION. Antiprotozoal, antibacterial, anthelmintic. Inhibits protein synthesis by interfering with the 50S and 30S ribosomal subunits causing misreading of mRNA codons.

MORE INFORMATION. See Chapter 34; Trichomoniasis, Chapter 78; Cryptosporidiosis, Chapter 82; Leishmaniasis, Chapter 73; Table 34-5; Table 71-1; reference: Ch 71, ref. 9.

PHARMACOKINETICS. Minimal absorption from GI tract after PO administration. Most (~100%) excreted unchanged in the feces. Approximately 1%-3% of a dose appears in urine; however this may be higher with disrupted gastrointestinal mucosal barrier.

SPECTRUM. Gram positive: poor. **Gram negative:** *Salmonella, Shigella.* **Protozoa:** *Cryptosporidium, Pentatrichomonas.* Other: some tapeworms. **Less effective:** *Giardia, Leishmania, Entamoeba.*

INDICATIONS. Cryptosporidiosis, amebiasis, hepatic insufficiency, to reduce enteric microflora production of NH$_3$. Second choice for *Entamoeba* and *Leishmania* (Ch 71, ref. 74).

CONTRAINDICATIONS. Intestinal stasis or obstruction, GI ulceration. Not effective in extraintestinal infections (not absorbed when given PO).

ADVERSE REACTIONS. Nephrotoxicity or ototoxicity if absorbed from ulcerative bowel lesions or if given parenterally. Has caused renal failure in cats with infectious enteritis (Ch 34, ref. 133). Overgrowth of resistant bacterial or fungal enteric microflora. Oral use: self-limiting diarrhea, malabsorption at high doses. If given parenterally: ototoxicity, nephrotoxic, pancreatitis. Renal failure may be reversible if it is detected early and the animal is given parenteral fluid diuresis. Drug has been associated with inducing bilateral hypermature cataracts with lens resorption and uveitis during treatment and recovery from drug induced renal failure (Ch 34, ref. 133).

INTERACTIONS. See as for NEOMYCIN (oral).

AVAILABILITY	TYPE	SIZES	PREPARATION (COMPANY)
Human	Oral capsules	250 mg (as sulfate)	*Humatin* (Parke-Davis)

INTERNATIONAL PREPARATIONS. *Gabbroral, Humagel, Sinosid.*

HANDLING. Store in airtight containers.

ADMINISTRATION. Given orally without concern for fasting. Dosage must be reduced or avoided if there is evidence of gastrointestinal hemorrhage. For parenteral use, must be certain animal is not dehydrated and diuresis with fluids may be helpful in averting toxicity. Monitoring of renal function is indicated with any treatment with this drug.

Dosage

INDICATIONS (*Dogs and Cats*)	DOSE (mg/kg)	ROUTE	INTERVAL (hr)	DURATION (days)
Cryptosporidiosis	125-165[a]	PO	12	5
Leishmaniasis (dog)	10-20[b]	IM, SC	24	28
Leishmaniasis (dog)	5.25	SC	12	21
Trichomoniasis (cat)	70	PO	12	5
Amebiasis[c]	70	PO	12	7

[a]Higher oral dosages of the drug have been tolerated in cats treated with cryptosporidiosis, while the same dosages have been nephrotoxic to cats with trichomoniasis. Presumably the damaged integrity of the intestine from trichomoniasis results in increased systemic absorption. Therefore the maximum dose of 125 mg/kg should not be exceeded in these animals or any showing gross evidence of intestinal hemorrhage in their feces. Dosage levels appear to be important in therapeutic studies in experimental animals. For example, 100 mg/kg/day in dairy calves and immunosuppressed mice is effective, whereas 25 mg/kg/day and 50 mg/kg/day is not. In piglets, 500 mg/kg/day is effective, whereas doses of 250 mg/kg/day and 125 mg/kg/day are less or not effective.
[b]Must be given parenterally for *Leishmania* infections and, therefore, has greater risk of toxicity. Doses of 20 mg/kg/day parenterally for leishmaniasis were not as effective as 40 mg/kg/day; however, the higher dosage was associated with greater prevalence of nephrotoxicity (Ch 71, ref. 5). Nephrotoxicity may also be greater if it is co-administered with antimonials. Clinical improvement may occur during treatment period, but relapse may occur 50-100 days after it is discontinued.
[c]For luminal infection only, if disseminated, must also use metronidazole.

ADDITIONAL DOSAGES. Cryptosporidiosis, Table 82-1; *Pentatrichomonas*, Table 78-3.

DISPENSING INFORMATION. Give with meals. Observe pet for vomiting or diarrhea, dizziness, hearing loss.

PENICILLIN G

CLASS. Benzylpenicillin.

ACTION. Bactericidal, inhibits bacterial cell wall synthesis.

MORE INFORMATION. Penicillins, Chapter 34; Table 34-1.

PHARMACOKINETICS. PO: Unpredictable inactivation by gastric acid when given PO. **IV:** rapid high but transient blood levels. **IM:** procaine salt lasts 12-15 hr; benzathine lasts up to 4 weeks but produces very low concentrations. Diffuses readily into liver, lung, heart, skin, kidneys, bone, prostate, spleen, intestines, serosal fluids (synovial, peritoneal, ascitic), bile, urine, wound secretions. Penetration into CSF, brain, or ocular tissues poor unless inflammation present. Crosses placenta but does not enter milk. Excretion occurs unchanged in the urine.

SPECTRUM. Gram positive: *Staphylococcus, Streptococcus, Corynebacterium, Erysipelothrix, Bacillus, Listeria.* **Gram negative:** *Proteus, Salmonella, Enterobacter, Escherichia, Streptobacillus moniliformis, Pasteurella.* **Anaerobes:** *Clostridium, Peptococcus* sp, *Peptostreptococcus, Fusobacterium, Eubacterium, Actinomyces.* **Other:** *Borrelia, Leptospira.* **Ineffective:** *Enterococcus (Streptococcus faecalis),* β-lactamase-producing *Staphylococcus.*

INDICATIONS. PO administration requires higher doses because of gastric acid activation. Generally used parenterally. Penicillin V is an alternative for oral use. Use IV soluble form in presence of severe systemic infections or bacteremia. Recommended for actinomycosis, tetanus, rat bite fever, listeriosis, pasteurellosis, erysipelas, anthrax, streptococcosis, fusospirochetosis of oropharynx, some gram-negative bacteremias, leptospirosis (bacteremic phase), borreliosis.

CONTRAINDICATIONS. Use lower dosages in renal failure.

ADVERSE REACTIONS. IV: thrombophlebitis, convulsions, hyperkalemia with potassium salt. **IM:** peripheral nerve damage.

INTERACTIONS. Penicillins may inactivate aminoglycosides if mixed before administration.

AVAILABILITY	TYPE	SIZES	PREPARATIONS (COMPANY)
Human	Aqueous solutions (potassium or sodium)	2,000,000-20,000,000/U in powder for reconstitution.	Generic (various)
	Oral tablets (as potassium)	200,000-800,000/U	Generic (various)
Veterinary	Procaine suspension for IM injection	300,000-500,000 U/ml	*Crystacillin* (Solvay), *Microcillin* (Anthony)
	Benzathine parenteral	300,000 U/ml	*Crystiben* (Solvay), *Flo-Cillin* (Fort Dodge)
	Procaine and benzathine combined equally	300,000-600,000 units/ml total	*Ambi-Pen* (Butler), *Crystiben* (Solvay), *Duo-Pen* (AgriPharm, RXV, Vet Tek), *DuraPe n* (Vedco)

HANDLING. Dry aqueous powder for injection stable in refrigerator. Dissolve in sterile water, 0.9% sodium chloride, or dextrose. Avoid alkaline dextrose solutions. After reconstitution, keep refrigerated, good for 1 week. Store procaine and benzathine preparations in refrigerator (not frozen). Before use, warm to room temperature and shake well.

ADMINISTRATION. Aqueous sodium or potassium solutions: given IM or by continuous IV infusion; give highest dose IV. For IM, use 100,000 U/ml concentration. For IV, determine daily fluid needs; add required aqueous penicillin and infuse over 24 hr. Local infusion (pleural, peritoneal) prepare as for IM, dilute in 1/4 to 1/2 volume compared with that of fluid aspirated from cavity. **Oral tablets:** administer 1 hr or more before feeding or at least 2 hr or more afterward. Dose for oral use is higher because of gastric acid degradation. **Procaine or benzathine:** administer by deep IM injection. Maximum volume at one site 10 ml.

Dosage

INDICATIONS	DOSE (U/kg)[a]	ROUTE	INTERVAL (hr)	DURATION (days)
Dogs				
Potassium				
Bacteremia, systemic infection	20,000-40,000	IV	4-6	prn
Orthopedic infection	20,000-40,000	IV	6	prn
Prophylaxis for orthopedic surgery	40,000	IV	[b]	[b]
Soft tissue infection	40,000-60,000	PO	8	prn
Procaine	20,000-40,000	IM, SC	12-24	prn
Benzathine	40,000	IM	120	prn
Cats				
Potassium				
Soft tissue, systemic infection	40,000	PO	6-8	prn
Procaine				
Soft tissue infection	20,000	IM, SC	12	prn
Orthopedic infection	20,000-40,000	IM	8	prn
Resistant organisms[c]	50,000-100,000	IM, SC	12	prn
Benzathine	50,000	IM	120	prn

[a]Na penicillin G for injection ≈ 1600 U/mg; procaine penicillin G ≈ 1000 U/mg; benzathine penicillin G ≈ 1200 U/mg.
[b]Given 1 hr prior to surgery, and if surgery lasts greater than 90 min, a second dose is given (Ch 86, ref. 131).
[c]*Actinomyces.*

ADDITIONAL DOSAGES. Streptococcal infections, Table 35-2; anaerobic infections, Table 41-10; tetanus, Table 43-2; leptospirosis, Table 44-4; Lyme borreliosis, Table 45-3; actinomycosis, Table 49-2; feline abscesses, Table 52-3; musculoskeletal infections, Table 86-3; bacteremia and endocarditis, Table 87-6; hepatobiliary infections, Table 90-5; CNS infections, Table 92-5; local ocular infections, Table 93-5.

DISPENSING INFORMATION. Give all PO tablets at least 1 hr before, or 2 hr after feeding.

PENICILLIN V POTASSIUM (PHENOXYMETHYLPENICILLIN)

CLASS. Penicillin.

ACTION. Bactericidal; inhibits bacterial cell wall synthesis.

MORE INFORMATION. PENICILLIN G.

PHARMACOKINETICS. Acid stable with absorption two to five times greater than penicillin G from GI tract after oral administration. For distribution in tissues and body fluids, see PENICILLIN G.

SPECTRUM. See PENICILLIN G. Same as for penicillin G except less active against *Salmonella, Escherichia, Proteus, Fusobacterium, Eubacterium*.

INDICATIONS. Preferred oral therapy when narrow-spectrum penicillin is indicated; borreliosis, streptococcal infections, staphylococcal infections.

CONTRAINDICATIONS. See PENICILLIN G.

ADVERSE REACTIONS. See PENICILLIN G.

INTERACTIONS. See PENICILLIN G.

AVAILABILITY	TYPE	SIZES	PREPARATIONS (COMPANY)
Human	Tablets (potassium)	125 mg, 250 mg, 500 mg	*Pen-Vee K* (Wyeth-Ayerst), *Beepen-VK* (SmithKline Beecham), various others
	Powder for oral suspension (potassium)	125 mg/5 ml, 250 mg/5 ml	

INTERNATIONAL PREPARATIONS. *Abbocillin-VK, Acipen-V, Apocillin, Arcasin, Calciopen, Cilicaine VK, Cliacil, Femepen, Oracilline, Penebene.*

HANDLING. Store products in airtight containers at room temperature. Oral suspension is stable for 2 weeks if refrigerated.

ADMINISTRATION. Food interferes with absorption.

Dosage

INDICATIONS (*Dogs and Cats*)	DOSE[a]	ROUTE	INTERVAL (hr)	DURATION (days)
Soft tissue infection	10 mg/kg	PO	8	7

[a]Equivalency ≈ 1600 U = 1 mg.

ADDITIONAL DOSAGES. Streptococcal infections, Tables 35-2 and 35-4; actinomycosis, Table 49-2; dermatophilosis, Table 51-1; feline abscesses, Table 52-3; musculoskeletal infections, Table 86-4.

DISPENSING INFORMATION. Give at least 1 hr before or 2 hr after feeding pet.

PENTAMIDINE ISETHIONATE

CLASS. Aromatic diamidine.

ACTION. Interferes with nuclear metabolism and inhibits the synthesis of DNA, RNA, proteins and phospholipids.

MORE INFORMATION. Chapter 71; Table 71-1; for inhalation therapy, reference: Ch 71, ref. 36; 85

PHARMACOKINETICS. Not absorbed from GI tract after PO administration. Must be given IV, topical (by inhalation), or IM (well absorbed). Lung tissue levels are lower after parenteral injection than by nebulization. One third excreted unchanged in urine within a few hours, but urinary excretion continues for weeks.

SPECTRUM. *Acanthamoeba, Pneumocystis, Leishmania, Babesia*. Less effective: for treatment of babesiosis, diminazene, imidocarb, or amicarbalide are preferred if available.

INDICATIONS. Invasive acanthamebiasis not involving the CNS. *Pneumocystis carinii* pneumonia by inhalation (nebulization). May add trimethoprim-sulfonamide plus pentamidine for some *Babesia* infections.

APPROVED USES. Humans: aerosolized drug for prophylaxis of *Pneumocystis* pneumonia.

CONTRAINDICATIONS. Renal failure: elimination is impaired but renal elimination is a minor factor in dogs.

ADVERSE REACTIONS. Systemic therapy (IV or IM): hypotension (vasodilation and reduced blood pressure); systemic anaphylaxis, nausea, salivation, vomiting, diarrhea; hypoglycemia (islet cell necrosis and hyperinsulinemia), then diabetes mellitus; myelosuppression; renal failure. Hypocalcemia and hypokalemia are frequent. To avoid allergic reactions, pretreatment with antihistamines just before administration is recommended. IM use causes pain or necrosis at the site of injection. **Inhalation therapy** is associated with lower toxicity. In dogs results in cilia loss, epithelial atrophy, submucosal hemorrhage in the nasal passages.

INTERACTIONS. Concomitant use of potentially nephrotoxic drugs should be avoided.

AVAILABILITY	TYPE	SIZES	PREPARATIONS (COMPANY)
Human	Powder for injection	300 mg/vial	*Pentam* (Lyphomed)
	Powder for aerosolization	300 mg/vial	*NebuPent* (Lyphomed)
Veterinary	Solution for injection	40 mg/ml in 20-ml vial	*Lomidine* (Merial)

INTERNATIONAL PREPARATIONS. *Pentacarinat; Pneumopent.*

HANDLING. Store powders away from light at controlled room temperature. For aerosolization reconstitute with sterile water (6 ml) to 50 mg/ml. For IM dissolve in 3 ml sterile water. For IV dissolve in 3-5 ml sterile water or 5% dextrose; can be further diluted into 50-250 ml of 5% dextrose. Do not dilute with any other solution or precipitate will form. Solution stable for 48 hr at room temperature.

ADMINISTRATION. Aerosol: fit mask over the dog's muzzle. **IV:** give over 60 min to reduce risk of hypotension. Should monitor for azotemia once or twice weekly. Do not give IV or SC. People administering drug in this manner should wear face masks and protective eyewear to prevent exposure to nebulized drug. **IM:** give deep injection in a large muscle or split dose at several sites. Use aseptic technique with a new needle at each site. In dogs, the IP route can be used by diluting product with 10 volumes physiologic saline and using long needles.

Dosage

INDICATIONS	DOSE (mg/kg)	ROUTE	INTERVAL (hr)	DURATION (days)
Human				
Acanthamebiasis	4.0	IV or IM	24	28
Pneumocystis prophylaxis	1.3	Aerosolized	24	7 days every 4th week
Leishmaniasis[a]	4.0	IM, IP	48	30 to 40
Leishmaniasis	4.0	IM	72	24[b]
Babesiosis	4.0	IM	24	1

[a]Alternate with meglumine *(Glucantine)* if resistant to treatment.
[b]This cycle of 8 injections is repeated after a 3-week interval (Ch 71, ref. 77).

ADDITIONAL DOSAGES. Pneumocystosis, Table 68-2; babesiosis, Table 77-3.

PHENAMIDINE ISETHIONATE

CLASS. Aromatic diamidine.

ACTION. Antiprotozoal.

MORE INFORMATION. See PENTAMIDINE as an alternative and closely related drug; Chapter 71; Table 71-1.

SPECTRUM. *Babesia.*

INDICATIONS. Second choice for babesiosis, other aromatic diamidines (e.g., imidocarb) are preferred for dogs and cats.

CONTRAINDICATIONS. See PENTAMIDINE.

ADVERSE REACTIONS. Vomiting, diarrhea, nervous signs, anaphylaxis, urticaria. See PENTAMIDINE, antihistamine (oxomemazine) included to counter allergic reactions and irritation at the injection site.

INTERACTIONS. See PENTAMIDINE.

AVAILABILITY	TYPE	SIZES	PREPARATION (COMPANY)
Veterinary	Solution for injection	15 mg/ml in 10-ml ampules with 1 mg/ml oxememazine	*Oxopirvedine* (Merial)

HANDLING. May be diluted in sterile 5% dextrose solution immediately before injection.

ADMINISTRATION. One 10-ml ampule can be given (SC preferred) for each 8.5 to 12.5 kg body weight. The dose can be given in one dose or divided in two doses given at a 24-hr interval.

Dosage

INDICATIONS (*Dogs*)	DOSE (mg/kg)	ROUTE	INTERVAL (hr)	DURATION (days)
Babesiosis (*B. gibsoni*)	7.5	IM, SC	24	2
	15-20	IM, SC	24	1

ADDITIONAL DOSAGES. Babesiosis, Table 77-3.

PIPERACILLIN SODIUM

CLASS. Semisynthetic penicillin.

ACTION. Bactericidal; inhibits bacterial cell wall synthesis.

MORE INFORMATION. Chapter 34, Penicillins; Table 34-1.

PHARMACOKINETICS. Not absorbed from the GI tract so administered parenterally. Penetrates blood-brain barrier. CSF-serum concentration ratio is 0.06 in noninflamed states and 0.3 in inflammation. Larger volume of distribution and more rapid clearance in pregnancy. Undergoes both biliary and renal excretion; can be used with renal compromise or biliary or hepatic dysfunction and to treat hepatobiliary infections. Majority (60%-80%) of dose is renally excreted.

SPECTRUM. Gram positive: *Enterococcus, Streptococcus,* non β-lactamase–producing *Staphylococcus.* **Gram negative:** *Escherichia, Proteus, Serratia, Klebsiella, Enterobacter, Citrobacter, Salmonella, Shigella, Pseudomonas* (synergistic with aminoglycosides), *Yersinia.* **Anaerobes:** *Actinomyces, Bacteroides, Clostridium, Eubacterium, Fusobacterium, Peptococcus, Peptostreptococcus.* **Others:** against *Pseudomonas,* use in combination with an aminoglycoside. Combine for treatment of bacteremia, endocarditis, osteomyelitis, pneumonia; use alone in treating of meningitis, urinary infection, invasive otitis. Combination with β-lactamase inhibitor, tazobactam, which increases spectrum to include resistant *Escherichia, Enterobacter, Pseudomonas, Enterococcus.* Useful combination to treat skin, soft tissue, respiratory, intraabdominal, gynecologic infections.

INDICATIONS. Serious infections of abdomen, urinary, genital, lower respiratory tracts, skin, soft tissue, bone, joints, septicemia. Prophylaxis for intraabdominal surgery. To treat suspected polymicrobial infections, singly, before isolation of causative organisms.

CONTRAINDICATIONS. Reduce dose in severe renal or hepatic failure.

ADVERSE REACTIONS. Local or systemic allergic reactions such as thrombophlebitis or anaphylaxis. Sudden endotoxin release when treating sepsis. Low toxicity characteristic of the penicillin group. Occasional diarrhea, azotemia, reversible neutropenia, thrombocytopenia, hemorrhagic manifestations.

INTERACTIONS. Prolongs action of some muscle relaxants.

AVAILABILITY	TYPE	SIZES	PREPARATION (COMPANY)
Human	Powder for injection	2 g, 3 g, 4 g, 40 g	*Pipracil* (Lederle)

INTERNATIONAL PREPARATIONS. *Avocin, Ivacin, Picillin, Pipcil, Piperacine, Pipérilline, Piperzam, Pipril.*

HANDLING. Stable in sterile water, 0.9% NaCl, 5% dextrose. Should not be refrigerated or frozen, stable for 24 hr at room temperature. **IV:** can also use Ringer's or lactated Ringer's or additives such as 40 mmol/L KCl; dissolve powder in at least 5 ml diluent, then add to desired infusion. **IM:** dilute to 2 g/5 ml, can use 0.5%-1.0% lidocaine without epinephrine. Do not mix with aminoglycosides or will cause inactivation.

ADMINISTRATION. IV for serious infections: given as a 20- to 30-min infusion every 4-6 hr. IV bolus over 3-5 min is shortest possible duration but risks phlebitis. For surgical prophylaxis, begin IV infusion 30 min before incision and continue no longer than 24 hr afterward. **IM:** limit to 2 g (5 ml) per site, use large muscle, avoid peripheral nerves.

Dosage

INDICATIONS (*Dogs*)	DOSE	ROUTE	INTERVAL (hr)	DURATION (days)
Skin infection, bacteremia	25-50 mg/kg	IV, IM	8-12	prn

ADDITIONAL DOSAGES. Bacteremia and endocarditis, Table 87-6; respiratory infection, Table 88-8.

PIPERACILLIN-TAZOBACTAM

CLASS. Semisynthetic penicillin + β-lactamase inhibitor in 8 : 1 ratio.

ACTION. Bactericidal; inhibits bacterial cell wall synthesis and β-lactamase activity.

MORE INFORMATION. See other β-lactam–β-lactamase inhibitor combinations such as AMPICILLIN-SULBACTAM, TICARCILLIN-CLAVULANATE, AMOXICILLIN-CLAVULANATE; Chapter 34; Tables 34-1 and 34-2.

PHARMACOKINETICS. Tazobactam does not affect pharmacokinetics of piperacillin. High, rapid onset of plasma concentration after IV infusion. Piperacillin is partially metabolized to an active metabolite, whereas tazobactam is metabolized to an inactive form. About 70% of piperacillin and 80% of tazobactam are excreted unchanged in urine, and there is some biliary excretion.

SPECTRUM. Gram positive: see PIPERACILLIN. **Gram negative:** See PIPERACILLIN. *Acinetobacter, Klebsiella.* **Anaerobes:** see PIPERACILLIN. **More effective:** piperacillin alone is active against most *Streptococcus,* some *Pseudomonas,* many Enterobacteriaceae. Adding tazobactam extends the spectrum to include *Staphylococcus,* more anaerobes, and additional gram-negative bacteria, including *Acinetobacter* and *Klebsiella.*

INDICATIONS. Lower respiratory tract, skin, soft tissue, intraabdominal, gynecologic infections. Treatment of bacteremia or life-threatening infections in neutropenic or immunocompromised hosts. For piperacillin-resistant bacteria.

APPROVED USES. For humans with resistant intraabdominal, cutaneous, and lower respiratory tract infections.

CONTRAINDICATIONS. Lower dosage advisable in renal impairment. Previous allergic reaction to penicillins, cephalosporins, or β-lactamase inhibitors.

ADVERSE REACTIONS. Vomiting, diarrhea, systemic allergies, leukopenia, elevated liver enzymes, hyperbilirubinemia.

INTERACTIONS. Not compatible in solution with lactated Ringer's, Ringer's, aminoglycosides but can infuse separately. False-positive urine glucose with copper reduction methods.

AVAILABILITY	TYPE	SIZES	PREPARATION (COMPANY)
Human	Powder for injection	2 g, 3 g, 4 g piperacillin with 0.25 g, 0.375 g, 0.5 g tazobactam, respectively	*Zosyn* (Lederle)

INTERNATIONAL PREPARATIONS. *Fluxapril, Tazobac, Tazobac, Tazocilline, Tazocin.*

HANDLING. Reconstitute powder in at least 5 ml, then place into IV fluid (0.9% NaCl, 5% dextrose). Compatible with 40 milliequivalents of KCl added. Stability of stock solutions is 24 hr at room temperature or 48 hr if refrigerated.

ADMINISTRATION. IV: 30-min infusions every 6 hr, usually treat for 1 week in hospitalized animals.

Dosage

INDICATIONS (*Dogs*)	DOSE (g/dog)	ROUTE	INTERVAL (hr)	DURATION (days)
Bacterial sepsis	3.4	IV	6	7
	4.5	IV	8	7

ADDITIONAL DOSAGES. Intraabdominal infections, Table 89-21.

PONAZURIL

CLASS. Triazinon; toltrazuril-sulfone.

ACTION. Anticoccidial developed for the treatment of equine protozoal myeloencephalitis caused by *Sarcocystis neurona.*

MORE INFORMATION. See TOLTRAZURIL, below and Neosporosis, Chapter 80.

PHARMACOKINETICS. Studies in other animals such as the horse and mouse show good absorption from GI tract following oral administration. Widely distributed in tissues and body fluids including the CSF. Repeated administration at the pharmacologic dose does not lead to drug accumulation in serum or CSF. Serum concentrations are approximately 30 times those in CSF. The drug is a weak acid with high lipid solubility and, as a result, should penetrate many tissues and cross the blood-brain barrier. Inflammation in the CNS associated with treated infections should aid in penetration.

SPECTRUM. Coccidia and members of the Apicomplexa. Concentration to kill *Sarcocystis neurona* in vitro is 0.1 to 1.0 µg/ml.

INDICATIONS. Neosporosis or toxoplasmosis unresponsive to clindamycin or folate synthesis inhibitors such as trimethoprim or pyrimethamine combined with sulfonamides. Has been effective in treatment of experimental *Neospora caninum* infections in calves and mice and *Sarcocystis neurona* infections in horses. Effectiveness in clearing encysted organisms is uncertain.

CONTRAINDICATIONS. Should avoid in pregnant animals.

ADVERSE REACTIONS. In horses, oral blisters, loose stools, and skin rashes were noted. At higher dosages inappetence and weight loss were noted as wa endometrial edema.

INTERACTIONS. See TOLTRAZURIL.

AVAILABILITY	TYPE	SIZES	PREPARATION (COMPANY)
Equine	Oral paste, 15% w/w	127 gram syringesa	*Marquis* (Bayer, USA)

aEach gram of paste contains 150 mg of ponazuril.

INTERNATIONAL PREPARATIONS. *Same.*

HANDLING. Store at controlled room temperature 15-30°C.

ADMINISTRATION. Assemble syringe barrel and plunger which is a multidose tool. Rotate dosage ring to proper amount and insert tip of syringe into animals mouth while depressing the plunger. Lift head to aid in swallowing the paste.

Dosage

INDICATIONS	DOSE (mg/kg)	ROUTE	INTERVAL (hr)	DURATION (days)
Dogs and Cats				
Neosporosis or toxoplasmosis	7.5-15	PO	24	28

ADDITIONAL DOSAGES. Dosage above is extrapolated between that for horses and mice.

DISPENSING INFORMATION. Drug can be given with or without food.

PRIMAQUINE PHOSPHATE

CLASS. 8-aminoquinolone.

ACTION. Antiprotozoal; binds to protozoal DNA and alters mitochondria.

PHARMACOKINETICS. Rapid absorption after PO administration; highest concentrations in liver, brain, lungs, cardiac and skeletal muscle. Metabolizes to compounds with variable activity with small amount (<1%) excreted unchanged in urine.

SPECTRUM. *Hepatozoon, Babesia, Pneumocystis.*

INDICATIONS. Hepatozoonosis.

APPROVED USES. Human malaria. Being evaluated in combination with clindamycin for pneumocystosis.

CONTRAINDICATIONS. Concurrent hemolysis or bone marrow suppression. Concurrent quinacrine or other myelosuppressive drugs, leukopenia, other hemolytic drugs.

ADVERSE REACTIONS. Methemoglobinemia, hemolysis (with glucose–6-phosphate dehydrogenase), myelosuppression.

INTERACTIONS. Quinacrine increases toxicity.

AVAILABILITY	TYPE	SIZES	PREPARATION (COMPANY)
Human	Oral tablets	26.3 mg (15 mg active base)	*Primaquine phosphate* (Sanofi-Winthrop)

HANDLING. Store tablets in airtight container away from heat, light, and moisture.

ADMINISTRATION. Check CBC at least once weekly while being treated. May be given with food to avoid GI side effects.

Dosage

INDICATIONS	DOSEa	ROUTE	INTERVAL (hr)	DURATION (days)
Dogs	0.3 (active base) mg/kg	PO	24	14
Cats (*Babesia*)	0.5 (active base) mg/kg	PO	24	1-3

aHuman dose, extrapolated.

ADDITIONAL DOSAGES. Babesiosis, Table 77-3.

DISPENSING INFORMATION. Give drug with a small amount of food to reduce vomiting if it occurs.

PROPIONIBACTERIUM ACNES (CORYNEBACTERIUM PARVUM)

CLASS. Bacterial product, killed bacterial cells.

ACTION. Stimulates macrophage activation resulting in the release of various cytokines. Immunostimulant.

MORE INFORMATION. Chapter 2; references Ch 2, ref. 80; 10.

SPECTRUM. Antiviral and immunostimulatory. Stimulates mononuclear phagocytes and interleukin (IL-1, IL-6, tumor necrosis factor).

INDICATIONS. Canine staphylococcal pyoderma, FeLV infection, feline herpesvirus infection. Aids in achieving clinical remission or improvement in pyoderma of dogs. May increase hematopoiesis in FeLV-positive cats but does not alter viremic status.

CONTRAINDICATIONS. Canine lymphoma or leukemia with CNS involvement or in animals receiving concurrent glucocorticoids.

ADVERSE REACTIONS. Fever, chills, lethargy involvement within 24 hr after administration. Localized pain and swelling if IV extravasation occurs. Proliferative glomerulonephritis and chronic active hepatitis with cirrhosis was reported in a dog (Ch 2, ref. 79).

INTERACTIONS. Not recommended for animals concurrently receiving glucocorticoids. Concurrent antibacterial therapy recommended.

AVAILABILITY	TYPE	SIZES	PREPARATIONS (COMPANY)
Veterinary[a]	Solution for injection 0.4 mg/ml (in ethanol)	5-ml vials	*ImmunoRegulin* (Immunovet, Vetoquinol)
	0.4 mg/ml (in ethanol)	5-ml and 50-ml vials	Equine product *EqStim* (Immunovet)

[a]Human products *Arthrokehlan "A"*, *Coparvax* (Immunovet).

HANDLING. Unopened vials are stored at room temperature. Keep refrigerated once opened.

ADMINISTRATION. IV or IP. Direct intralesional injection in tumors has also been done. No improvement after 12 weeks indicates that treatment is ineffective and should be discontinued. Some give one injection per month to maintain remission of pyoderma.

Dosage

INDICATIONS/ BODY WEIGHT	DOSE (ml)	ROUTE	INTERVAL	DURATION (weeks)
Dogs				
Pyoderma[a]				
7 kg	0.250	IV, IP	Twice weekly	2[b]
7-20 kg	0.50	IV, IP	Twice weekly	2[b]
20-34 kg	1.00	IV, IP	Twice weekly	2[b]
>34 kg	2.00	IV, IP	Twice weekly	2[b]
Cats				
Antiviral				
5 lb	0.25	IV, IP	Twice weekly	2[b]
10 lb	0.50	IV, IP	Twice weekly	2[c]

[a]Maximum dose in any dog is 2.0 ml. Some protocols suggest a dosage range of 0.1 to 0.8 ml/dog based on weight.
[b]Once weekly thereafter until remission and once monthly after that to maintain clinical improvement.
[c]Once weekly thereafter for 3 weeks and once monthly for 2 mo for a total of nine injections. Some protocols for FeLV suggest follow-up with injections once weekly for 20 weeks or longer as needed. Other protocols suggest follow-up with once weekly until clinical remission, and then once per mo.

ADDITIONAL DOSAGES. None.

PYRIMETHAMINE (AND SULFONAMIDE)

CLASS. Folic acid inhibitor.

ACTION. Inhibits dihydrofolate reductase.

MORE INFORMATION. Toxoplasmosis and neosporosis, Chapter 71; Table 71-1.

PHARMACOKINETICS. After PO administration, well absorbed. Enters many tissues including CNS and CSF. Highly protein bound and suppressive effects of the drug may remain in the plasma for 1-2 weeks. Metabolized by the liver, and metabolites are excreted in urine.

SPECTRUM. Protozoa: *Toxoplasma gondii*, *Neospora caninum*, *Pneumocystis carinii*. **Ineffective:** bacteria (pyrimethamine).

INDICATIONS. Used for treatment of toxoplasmosis, neosporosis, pneumocystosis in combination with sulfonamides.

CONTRAINDICATIONS. Pregnancy because teratogenic. Folate deficiency or previous hypersensitivity. Reduced dose needed with hepatic but not with renal impairment.

ADVERSE REACTIONS. Vomiting, leukopenia, myelosuppression, fetal teratogenesis, myelodysplasia. Folate deficiency can be treated with folinic acid at 5-15 mg/day PO or parenterally.

INTERACTIONS. Use care in dosing with other folate inhibitors (trimethoprim or methotrexate) or other myelosuppressive drugs.

AVAILABILITY	TYPE	SIZES	PREPARATIONS (COMPANY)
Human	Oral tablets	25 mg	*Daraprim* (Burroughs Wellcome)
	Combined product	25 mg pyrimethamine; 500 mg sulfadoxine	*Fansidar* (Roche)

HANDLING. Tablets should be stored in airtight containers away from heat, direct light, and moisture. Formulation of smaller dosage sizes can be done by compounding pharmacies.

ADMINISTRATION. If vomiting occurs, give with meals. Periodically check hemogram.

Dosage

INDICATIONS	DRUG COMBINATION	DOSE	ROUTE	INTERVAL (hr)	DURATION (days)
Dogs					
Neosporosis	Pyrimethamine **plus**	1	PO	24	14
	Sulfonamide	60	PO	24	13
	Pyrimethamine **plus**	1	PO	24	28
	Trimethoprim-sulfonamide	15	PO	12	28
Cat					
Toxoplasmosis	Pyrimethamine **plus**	0.25-1	PO	24	14-28
	Trimethoprim-sulfonamide	15	PO	12	14-28

ADDITIONAL DOSAGES. Hepatozoonosis, Table 74-2; toxoplasmosis, Table 80-3; neosporosis, Table 80-7.

DISPENSING INFORMATION. If GI signs develop, they can be minimized by giving this drug with food.

QUINACRINE (MEPACRINE) HYDROCHLORIDE

CLASS. 9-aminocridine dye.

ACTION. Antiprotozoal.

MORE INFORMATION. Antiprotozoal Chemotherapy, Chapter 71; Table 71-1; Giardiasis, Chapter 78.

PHARMACOKINETICS. Readily absorbed from GI tract and widely distributed in tissues. Accumulates in liver with slow release up to 2 mo after a single dose. Crosses the placenta.

SPECTRUM. Protozoa: Coccidia, *Giardia*, *Leishmania*. **Others:** some tapeworms.

INDICATIONS. Giardiasis, alternative to nitroimidazoles, sometimes cutaneous leishmaniasis (except caused by *Leishmania aethiopica*, *Leishmania braziliensis*).

CONTRAINDICATIONS. Hepatic dysfunction, pregnancy.

ADVERSE REACTIONS. GI upsets, vomiting, diarrhea, CNS signs, fever, blood dyscrasias, dermatologic eruptions, yellow urine, skin, and sclera. Anorexia, lethargy, and pyrexia are common at the prescribed dosage.

INTERACTIONS. Avoid use with other drugs that cause myelodyscrasias.

AVAILABILITY	TYPE	SIZES	PREPARATION (COMPANY)
Human	Oral tablets	100 mg	*Atabrine* HCl (Winthrop); not available in U.S since 1992.

HANDLING. More palatable if administered within gelatin capsules. Can add to liquids but is not stable in solution for more than 6 hr so should be used immediately in this form. Solution for intralesional injections in leishmaniasis is prepared by grinding three 100-mg tablets in a mortar to a fine powder. A solution of 30 ml 0.9% NaCl is added. This is filtered through coarse filter paper and rinsed with 0.9%

saline. The mixture is filtered through a 5-µm filter needle into a sterile empty vial. The final concentration is adjusted to 5%.

ADMINISTRATION. For intralesional injections in leishmaniasis, has been mixed as a 5% solution given at intervals of 3-5 days.

Dosage

INDICATIONS	DOSE	ROUTE	INTERVAL (hr)	DURATION (days)
Dogs				
Giardiasis	50-100 mg/dog	PO	12	3[a]
	6.6 mg/kg	PO	12	5
Cats				
Coccidiosis	10 mg/kg	PO	24	5

[a]Skip 3 days, then repeat again for one more course of therapy.

ADDITIONAL DOSAGES. Enteric protozoal infections, Table 78-2; coccidiosis, Table 81-2.

DISPENSING INFORMATION. Tablets can be crushed and placed in honey or ice cream to increase palatability by masking taste to animals that are difficult to medicate.

QUINUPRISTIN-DALFOPRISTIN

CLASS. Streptogramin. Combined in the ratio 30 : 70 (w/w). The two components act synergistically.

ACTION. Against bacterial 50S ribosomal protein synthesis.

MORE INFORMATION. See QUINUPRISTIN-DALFOPRISTIN; Chapter 34.

PHARMACOKINETICS. After parenteral administration to people and rodents, they are metabolized in the liver and excreted predominantly in the bile into the intestine.

SPECTRUM. Gram positive: Methicillin-resistant staphylococci and vancomycin-resistant enterococci, some penicillin-resistant *streptococci*, poor activity against *Enterococcus faecalis* but good against *Enterococcus faecium*. Differentiating between enterococcal species is important for this reason. **Gram negative:** *Moraxella, Legionella, Neisseria.* **Anaerobes:** *Clostridium perfringens.* **Others:** *Mycoplasma, Toxoplasma gondii.*

INDICATIONS. Bacteremias, nosocomial catheter-related bacteremia, or valvular endocarditis caused by β-lactam or vancomycin-resistant gram-positive bacteria. Complicated cutaneous infections caused by resistant gram-positive organisms. Since this drug is reserved for restricted treatment in people with highly resistant gram-positive bacterial infections, its use in dogs or cats is discouraged.

CONTRAINDICATIONS. Drug clearance reduced with hepatic dysfunction; however, no adjustment for renal impairment.

ADVERSE REACTIONS. Pain, inflammation, swelling and thrombophlebitis at the site of IV infusion can occur. Occasional arthralgia, myalgia, and hyperbilirubinemia.

INTERACTIONS. Metabolized by cytochrome P-450 3A4. Potent inhibitor of CYP3A4 and must be used with caution in patients taking drugs that are substrates of 3A4. Will lead to increased serum concentrations of drugs such as nifedipine, midazolam, and cyclosporine. For broader coverage, can be used simultaneously with antimicrobials with gram-negative spectrum such as zatreonam, cefotaxime, ciprofloxacin, and gentamicin against Enteobacteriaceae and *Pseudomonas.*

AVAILABILITY	TYPE	SIZES	PREPARATIONS (COMPANY)
Human	IV solution	500 mg (150 Q : 350 D)	*Synercid I.V.* (Rhone-Poulenc Rorer) (Aventis Pharmaceuticals)

INTERNATIONAL PREPARATIONS. *Same*

HANDLING. Use caution to ensure drug is given IV. Never mix with normal saline, heparin, or other drugs. Use only 5% dextrose or sterile water for reconstitution and 5% dextrose for dose infusions. Should phlebitis develop, the dose should be further diluted for the next infusion.

ADMINISTRATION. Given IV over 1-hr time period, beginning every 8 hr. Should infuse through a central line to avoid vascular or perivascular irritation.

Dosage

(Human Extrapolation)	DOSE (mg/kg)	ROUTE	INTERVAL (hr)	DURATION (days)
Enterococcal bacteremia	7.5	IV	8	prn
Complicated skin infections	7.5	IV	12	prn

ADDITIONAL DOSAGES. None.

RIBAVIRIN

CLASS. Nucleoside (guanosine) analog.

ACTION. Antiviral; nucleoside analog that interferes with DNA and mRNA synthesis. Inhibits retroviruses; however, unlike other anti retroviral drugs, it allows DNA synthesis to occur but prevents formation of viral proteins by interfering with capping of viral mRNA. It has weak anticellular activity.

MORE INFORMATION. Ribavirin in Chapter 2; references: Ch 2, ref. 165; 166; 167.

PHARMACOKINETICS. Erythrocytes sequester large amounts of drug. Crosses blood-brain barrier, CSF concentration 50%-100% of blood levels.

SPECTRUM. Virostatic against DNA and RNA viruses, including herpes-, orthomyxo-, pox-, paramyxo-, influenza-, arena-, bunya-, hanta-, and immunodeficiency viruses. Also feline infectious peritonitis virus (Ch 2, ref. 9; 170), canine parainfluenza virus, feline calicivirus. Has not been as effective against feline calicivirus in vivo as in vitro studies suggest.

INDICATIONS. Humans: aerosol therapy of infants with respiratory syncytial virus. IV or PO for adults with influenza A or acute viral hemorrhagic fever, for arthropod-borne encephalomyelitis. Not recommended for coronaviral infection in cats because of poor efficacy whether in aqueous or liposomal encapsulated form (Ch 2, ref. 167).

APPROVED USES. Humans for respiratory syncytial virus.

CONTRAINDICATIONS. Preexisting anemia, leukopenia, thrombocytopenia, pregnancy.

ADVERSE REACTIONS. Toxic in cats when used alone at therapeutic dosages or higher (22 or 44 mg/kg) (Ch 2, ref. 166). Diarrhea, myelotoxicity (megakaryocytic hypoplasia, increased myeloid-erythroid ratio, anemia, leukopenia, thrombocytopenia), increased blood alanine transaminase, alkaline phosphatase, creatine kinase activities, enteritis, hepatocellular vacuolation or necrosis, fetotoxic, teratogenic, GI hemorrhage, and ulceration. Treated cats with calicivirus infection have had increased severity of illness, depressed bone marrow, weight loss, increased hepatic enzymes, icterus. Kittens treated for coronaviral infection had pronounced multifocal hemorrhages throughout body tissues (Ch 2, ref. 166). None of these abnormalities have been found in beagle dogs given 60 mg/kg of ribavirin for 2 weeks, although nonregenerative anemia develops in people and other animals given similar dosages.

INTERACTIONS. For cats, use at lower dosages in combination with interferon-α. It antagonizes actions of AZT by inhibition of thymidine kinase such that AZT is not phosphorylated.

AVAILABILITY	TYPE	SIZES	PREPARATION (COMPANY)
Human	Powder for reconstitution for aerosol	6 g	*Virazole* (ICN)

HANDLING. Vials of powder are stored in a dry place at room temperature. Do not mix with any other drug. Solubilize drug with sterile water at final concentration of 20 mg/ml. Reconstituted drug is stable for 24 hr at 20-30°C.

ADMINISTRATION. Aerosol: dilute in reservoir and nebulize by a small particle aerosol generator. Deliver via face mask, ventilator, oxygen hood. Unfortunately, aerosols can leak and be inhaled by health care personnel. **IV:** relative toxicity and dose have been reduced by incorporation of the drug in liposomes but liposome-encapsulated drug was less effective than free ribavirin in treating coronavirus-infected cats (Ch 2, ref. 167).

Dosage

INDICATIONS (*Cats*)	DOSE (mg/kg)	ROUTE	INTERVAL (hr)	DURATION (days)
Systemic infections viral	11	PO, IM, IV	24	7
Children	2.5	PO	6	7

ADDITIONAL DOSAGES. None.

DISPENSING INFORMATION. Can be given orally by placing powder in gelatin capsules.

RIFAMPIN (RIFAMPICIN)

CLASS. Ansamycin.

ACTION. Binds to and inactivates bacterial DNA-dependent RNA polymerase while not affecting mammalian cells.

MORE INFORMATION. Similar to rifabutin (*Mycobutin, Ansatipine*); Chapter 34.

PHARMACOKINETICS. Rapid and almost complete absorption from GI tract. Food reduces rate and extent of absorption. High lipid solubility, penetrates most tissues, including CNS. Penetrates cells, including phagocytes, and organisms in extracellular cavitary spaces or caseous lesions, reaching therapeutic concentrations in abscessed tissues and discharges. Metabolized in liver and active metabolites excreted in urine (30%) and bile (70%), in the former as unchanged and metabolized drug.

SPECTRUM. Gram positive: staphylococci, *Rhodococcus*. **Gram negative:** *Bartonella*, *Brucella*. **Others:** *Neisseria*,

Haemophilus, Mycobacterium. Antiviral (adenoviruses, poxviruses) and antichlamydial at very high doses. Some mycobacteria resistant to rifampin may be susceptible to rifabutin.

INDICATIONS. Resistance develops rapidly. Should always be combined with other drugs to improve efficacy and hinder resistance development. Chronic refractory pyoderma, bacterial abscesses, or granulomas. Resistant staphylococcal infections in difficult sites: osteomyelitis, endocarditis, CNS infections, infection of prosthetic implants. Rhodococcosis, granulomatous, mycobacterial infections, brucellosis, chlamydiosis. Can facilitate penetration of other antimicrobials, such as amphotericin B or flucytosine for fungal infections or isoniazid in tuberculosis. Facilitates metabolism and urinary excretion of bile acids, reducing pruritogenic substances.

APPROVED USES. Human mycobacteriosis and *Neisseria* meningitis.

CONTRAINDICATIONS. Reduce dosage in hepatic dysfunction or biliary obstruction. This drug induces its own accelerated metabolism and excretion. In pregnancy, can cause teratogenesis in laboratory animals.

ADVERSE REACTIONS. Hepatotoxicity: use lower dosages; vomiting, elevated liver enzymes, icterus, hemolytic anemia, thrombocytopenia. Urine, stool, saliva, tears may be discolored orange-red color by drug. CNS disturbances. Higher dosages (30-60 mg/kg PO daily) are more likely to be associated with side effects and should be avoided. Some cats have shown erythema, especially of the pinna, pruritus, dyspnea, and respiratory distress as a result of anaphylaxis, which may require dilute epinephrine and glucocorticoid administration. Pretreatment with antihistamines and reducing the dose has been beneficial in reducing this untoward reaction.

INTERACTIONS. Accelerates metabolism and may reduce effectiveness of drugs metabolized by microsomal enzymes: glucocorticoids, cardiac glycosides, sulfonylureas, benzodiazepines, chloramphenicol, doxycycline, digitoxin, ketoconazole, theophylline, barbiturates, verapamil. Hepatotoxicity increased when used with isoniazid or halothane. Inhibits assays for serum vitamin B_{12} and folate.

AVAILABILITY	TYPE	SIZES	PREPARATIONS (COMPANY)
Human	Oral capsules	150 mg, 300 mg	*Rifadin* (Marion Merrell Dow), *Rimactane* (Geigy)
	Powder for injection	600 mg	*Rifadin* IV

INTERNATIONAL PREPARATIONS. *Diabacil, Eremfat, Fenampicin, Fimizina, Rifa, Rifagen, Rifaldin, Rifapiam, Rifcin, Rifocina, Rifoldin, Rimactan, Rimycin.*

HANDLING. Store at room temperature in moisture and light-resistant containers. Powder for injection reconstituted with sterile water. Stability best in 5% dextrose. After reconstitution can store for 4 weeks at room temperature or refrigerated. To make PO suspension (10 mg/ml), mix contents of four 300-mg caps with simple syrup and bring to 120 ml with syrup. Keep refrigerated, stable for 4 weeks. May have to reformulate into smaller dosage capsules for cats by adding cornstarch and placing it in new capsules. Compounding pharmacists can be used to produce optimal dosage formulations.

ADMINISTRATION. Food interferes with absorption; administer to fasted animal 1 hr before or 2 hr after meals. *Always give in combination* with at least one other drug when treating mycobacteria or other persistent intracellular infections.

Dosage

INDICATIONS	DOSE (mg/kg)	ROUTE	INTERVAL (hr)	DURATION (days)
Dogs				
Pyoderma	10	PO	12	prn
	5-10	PO	8-12	prn
Brucellosis	5-10	PO	24	prn[a]
Systemic bacteremia[b]	10	IV, IM	8-12	prn
Cats				
Bartonellosis, mycobacteriosis[c]	5-10	PO	24	14

[a]For brucellosis, used in combination with doxycycline and a fluoroquinolone (Ch 34, ref. 396a)
[b]Maximum 8 mg/kg/day if hepatic function is impaired.
[c]Use in combination with doxycycline for bartonellosis, see Chapter 54, and for other antimycobacterial drugs, see Chapter 50.

ADDITIONAL DOSAGES. Actinomycosis, Table 49-2; mycobacterial infections, Tables 50-4 and 50-6; *Bartonella*, Table 54-3; CNS infections, Table 92-5.

DISPENSING INFORMATION. Give to fasting animal. May cause harmless reddish-orange discoloration of body excretions and secretions.

RONIDAZOLE

CLASS: Nitroimidazole.

ACTION: See METRONIDAZOLE.

MORE INFORMATION: See TINIDAZOLE, IPRONIDAZOLE.

SPECTRUM: *Tritrichomonas.*

INDICATIONS: Preliminary studies show effectiveness against *Tritrichomonas foetus* infection in cats. At recommended dosages, the drug was effective in clearing infected cats based on PCR and causing clinical resolution of diarrhea. Little or no improvement or clearing was noted in cats treated with lower dosages or placebo, respectively.

CONTRAINDICATIONS: Pregnancy.

ADVERSE REACTIONS: Not noted, although metagenesis is possible.

INTERACTIONS: See METRONIDAZOLE.

AVAILABILITY	TYPE	SIZES	PREPARATIONS (Company)
Veterinary	Feed/water additive for trichomoniasis in birds	200-mg sachets	*TRICHO PLUS* (Oropharma)

HANDLING: Store at room temperature and away from light.

ADMINISTRATION: Mix amount in food or place in gelatin capsules for administration.

Dosage

INDICATIONS (*Cats*)	DOSE (mg/kg)	ROUTE	INTERVAL (hr)	DURATION (days)
Tritrichomonas foetus infection[a]	30-50	PO	12	14

[a]For additional information, see Chapter 78, Trichomoniasis, Therapy; Reference: Ch 78, 49a.

ROXITHROMYCIN

CLASS. Macrolide.

ACTION. Bacteriostatic, interferes with bacteria protein synthesis.

MORE INFORMATION. See ERYTHROMYCIN; reference: Ch 34, ref. 215.

PHARMACOKINETICS. Rapidly absorbed from GI tract after PO administration, and 50% bioavailable. Acid stable in stomach, better absorbed than erythromycin. Feeding increases absorption in dogs. High concentration in pulmonary, prostatic, tonsillar, and pleural fluid. Does not enter saliva, milk, or CSF in absence of inflammation.

SPECTRUM. See ERYTHROMYCIN for bacteria; coccidia.

INDICATIONS. Respiratory, prostatic, urethral infections.

CONTRAINDICATIONS. Reduce dose in renal or hepatic dysfunction.

ADVERSE REACTIONS. See ERYTHROMYCIN.

INTERACTIONS. See ERYTHROMYCIN.

AVAILABILITY	TYPE	SIZES	PREPARATION (COMPANY)
Human	Oral capsules	150 mg	*Rulide* (Roussel-Uclaf)

INTERNATIONAL PREPARATIONS. *Assoral, Claramid, Macrosil, Rossitrol, Rotesan, Rotramin, Rulid, Surlid.*

Dosage

INDICATIONS (*Dogs*)	DOSE	ROUTE	INTERVAL (hr)	DURATION (days)
Soft tissue, respiratory, urinary infections	15 mg/kg	PO	24	prn

ADDITIONAL DOSAGES. Coccidiosis, Table 81-2.

DISPENSING INFORMATION. May be administered with food.

SARGRAMOSTIM (GRANULOCYTE MACROPHAGE COLONY-STIMULATING OR HEMATOPOIETIC GROWTH FACTOR, GM-CSF)

CLASS. Cytokine, Glycoprotein.

ACTION. Stimulates myeloid progenitors in bone marrow and T lymphocyes. Affects both peripheral monocytes and tissue macrophages. Treated macrophages exhibit enhanced conidial phagocytosis and hyphal damage against fungi. GM-CSF given before glucorticoids, blocked the immunosuppressive effect against *Aspergillus* infections in mice. Can act synergistically with TNF-α in experimental murine and clinical human infections.

MORE INFORMATION. Chapters 2 and 58; references: Ch 2, ref. 37; 37a; 124a; 3.

PHARMACOKINETICS: In people, following IV administration, drug is detected in serum from 3-6 hr. With SC injection, was detected up to 6 hr. Clearance was the same regardless of lyophilized or liquid preparations.

INDICATIONS. To stimulate production and function of neutrophils and monocytes. In dogs, for short-term use in treating neutropenia from whole body irradiation, parvovirus and *Ehrlichia* infections, myelosuppressive drugs. Potential uses in cats are leukopenias associated with feline panleukopenia virus, FIV, and FeLV infections, myeloproliferative disease, lymphoid tumors, aplastic anemias. Best for short-term (≤21 days) use for treatment of neutropenia caused by infectious agents, chemotherapy, or total body irradiation. Neutropenia caused by toxins (e.g., cancer chemotherapeutics, estrogens, chloramphenicol, trimethoprim-sulfonamides) or infections (e.g., ehrlichiosis, parvoviral infections).

CONTRAINDICATIONS. Treatment for longer than 3 weeks.

ADVERSE REACTIONS. Bone discomfort or splenomegaly, allergic reactions. High doses of recombinant human GM-CSF in dogs (150 µg/kg) induces antibodies by 10-12 days of treatment that have been thought to blunt the leukocytosis. In cats, a majority of rhGM-CSF treated animals had similar increases in antibodies by 35 days of treatment; however, no blunting of the leukocytosis was observed (Ch 2, ref. 3)

AVAILABILITY	TYPE	SIZE	PREPARATION (COMPANY)
Human	Powder for injection. lyophillized	250 µg vial	*Leukine* (Berlex)
	Liquid	500 µg/ml	*Leukine* (Berlex)

HANDLING. Lyophilized drug is reconstituted with sterile water and used immediately as there are no preservatives. If reconstituted with bacteriostatic water (containing 0.9% benzyl alcohol, can be stored for 20 days. If newly and old stored solutions are mixed, the duration of storage prior to dosage is only 6 hours. The vial should not be frozen or exposed to sunlight. Storage of opened liquid and reconstituted solutions is by refrigeration at 2-8°C for 20 days.

ADMINISTRATION. Can be given SC or IV. Should give along with supportive care such as concurrent blood transfusions for concurrent anemia or thrombocytopenia or antibiotics for leukopenia. For SC use, no further dilution is needed. For IV use, should be further diluted to 5-15 µg/ml with addition of 0.9 % saline. Albumin is added (12 mg/ml) to prevent absorption to plastics when drug is diluted.

Dosage

INDICATIONS *(Neutropenia)*	DOSE (µg/kg)	ROUTE	INTERVAL (hr)	DURATION (days)
Dogs	150	SC	24	≤21
Cats	5	SC	12	≤21

ADDITIONAL DOSAGES. FIV infection, Table 14-5: Reference Ch 2, ref. 3).

SERRATIA MARCESCENS (BESM, IMUVERT®) IMMUNOSTIMULANT. SEE CHAPTER 2

SPECTINOMYCIN

CLASS. Aminocyclitol related to aminoglycoside.

ACTION. Usually bacteriostatic; inhibits bacterial protein synthesis by acting on 30s ribosomal subunit.

MORE INFORMATION. Related to a new derivative trospectomycin, *Spexil* (Pharmacia & Upjohn).

PHARMACOKINETICS. Minor (<8%) absorption from GI tract. When given orally, used to reduce intestinal microflora or treat enteric pathogens. Rapid absorption after IM injection. Tissue concentrations are lower than in blood. Like aminoglycosides, does not enter CSF or ocular tissues and only slightly with inflammation. Majority (70%-80%) excreted in urine as active drug.

SPECTRUM. Gram positive: *Streptococcus.* **Gram negative:** *Proteus, Enterobacter, Salmonella, Escherichia, Klebsiella.* **Anaerobes:** little activity. **Others:** some *Mycoplasma.* **More effective:** most effective single agent for gram-negative bacteria in chemoprophylaxis of open bowel surgery. Used in people to treat gonorrhea. **Less effective:** *Chlamydia,* spirochetes, *Pseudomonas.*

INDICATIONS. Intraabdominal infections or prophylaxis for abdominal surgery. If used orally, for bacterial gastroenteritis or to reduce enteric flora in cases of hepatic encephalopathy.

APPROVED USES. As single injection for penicillin-resistant human gonoccocal infections.

CONTRAINDICATIONS. Pre-existing renal failure, hypersensitivity to this drug.

ADVERSE REACTIONS. Pain or irritation at injection site; elevation in blood hepatic enzymes and urea with repeated doses. Less ototoxic and nephrotoxic than aminoglycosides.

Cholestatic hepatitis in people. Can cause neuromuscular blockade, reversible with IV calcium.

INTERACTIONS. Effectiveness reduced when used with tetracycline or chloramphenicol. Can combine with lincomycin for increased efficacy against *Mycoplasma*.

AVAILABILITY	TYPE	SIZES	PREPARATIONS (COMPANY)
Human	Powder for injection	2 g (as HCl)	*Trobicin* (Pharmacia & Upjohn)
	Powder for oral suppression	2 mg/m, 4 g/ml	
Veterinary	Solution for injection (poultry approval)	100 mg/ml	*Spectam* (Sanofi)

INTERNATIONAL PREPARATIONS. *Kempi, Stanilo, Trobicine.*

HANDLING. Store at room temperature. Mix powder well after diluting. Stable 4 weeks at room temperature, although it is recommended to use reconstituted drug within 24 hr.

ADMINISTRATION. Administer IM in large muscle.

Dosage

INDICATIONS (*Dogs and Cats*)	DOSE	ROUTE	INTERVAL (hr)	DURATION (days)
Prophylactic for bowel surgery, peritonitis	10 mg/kg	IM, SC	8-12	a

[a]Immediately before and during surgery.

ADDITIONAL DOSAGES. None.

SPIRAMYCIN

CLASS. Macrolide.

ACTION. Bacteriostatic; inhibits bacterial protein synthesis; binds to 50 s ribosomal subunits.

MORE INFORMATION. See ERYTHROMYCIN, METRONIDAZOLE (interactions); Antiprotozoals, Chapter 71; Table 71-1.

PHARMACOKINETICS. Incompletely absorbed from GI tract, unaffected by food. Widely distributed except in CSF. Metabolized in liver to active metabolites with a majority excreted in the bile and 10% in urine. Enters milk. Persists in some tissues.

SPECTRUM. Anaerobic bacteria: *Campylobacter, Helicobacter.* Similar antibacterial spectrum as erythromycin but less active. **Others:** *Toxoplasma, Cryptosporidium.*

INDICATIONS. Toxoplasmosis, cryptosporidiosis. Combined with metronidazole for periodontitis and stomatitis.

CONTRAINDICATIONS. Preexisting hepatic disease.

ADVERSE REACTIONS. Irritating after IM injection. Vomiting and diarrhea (similar to erythromycin), allergic reactions, cholestatic hepatitis. Cutaneous irritation to veterinarians exposed to the drug during preparation or administration.

AVAILABILITY	TYPE	SIZES	PREPARATIONS (COMPANY)
Human	Oral tablets	1 g	*Rovamycine* (Rhône-Pôulenc Rorer)
Veterinary	Oral tablets	46.9 mg[a] S, 25 mg M.	*Stomorgyl* (Rhone-Merieux EC) (*Rodogyl* Human drug
		234 mg S, 125 mg M.	counterpart) containing S and M)
		469 mg S, 250 mg M.	

S, Spiramycin; *M*, metronidazole.
[a]46.9 mg spiramycin is 150,000 U.

INTERNATIONAL PREPARATIONS. *Rovamycin, Rovamycina, Selectomycin.*

HANDLING. Store tablets at room temperature in containers away from light and moisture.

ADMINISTRATION. Can give tablets with a meal.

Dosage

INDICATIONS	DOSE (mg/kg)	ROUTE	INTERVAL (hr)	DURATION (days)
Human				
Pediatric toxoplasmosis	50-100	PO	24	21-28
Dogs and Cats				
Periodontal, oral infection	23.4 S 12.5 M	PO	24	5-10
Leishmaniasis	46.9 S 25 M	PO	24	90-120

S, Spiramycin; *M*, metronidazole.

ADDITIONAL DOSAGES. Coccidiosis, Table 81-2; oral infections, Table 89-4.

DISPENSING INFORMATION. Do not break or crush tablets.

STAPHYLOCOCCAL PHAGE LYSATE

CLASS. Immunostimulant.

ACTION. Increases immune response against *Staphylococcus*. Stimulates production of interleukin-γ, interleukin-6, tumor necrosis factor, and γ-interferon.

MORE INFORMATION. Chapter 2; Table 2-3; references: Ch 2, ref. 26a; 78.

FORMULATION. Bacteriologically sterile preparation containing cell wall components of *S. aureus*, a bacteriophage, and some culture media, in solution. Each ml of solution contains 120-180 CFU of *S. aureus* before phage lysis.

INDICATIONS. Chronic or recurrent pyoderma in dogs caused by staphylococci.

CONTRAINDICATIONS. Previous severe hypersensitivity reaction to the product.

ADVERSE REACTIONS. Possible anaphylaxis. Rare fever, chills. Transient swelling, redness, and pruritus at site of inoculation.

AVAILABILITY	TYPE	SIZES	PREPARATION (COMPANY)
Veterinary	Solution for injection	1-ml ampules, 10-ml multidose vials	*Staphage Lysate* (Delmont Labs)

HANDLING. Store refrigerated (2-8°C). Do not freeze. Use entire contents when vial is opened. No preservatives, so must be handled aseptically. Should not use if solution is cloudy.

ADMINISTRATION. Concomitant antibiotic therapy is recommended for the initial 4- to 6-week treatment period. Subcutaneous injection: to test for hypersensitivity, can perform intradermal skin test of 0.05 to 0.1 ml. Should precede initial use. Observe animal and inoculation site for 1 hr for immediate reactions and 48 hr for delayed reactions. Allergic reactions may require epinephrine administration.

Dosage

INDICATIONS	DOSE (ml)	ROUTE	INTERVAL (hr)	DURATION (days)
Canine pyoderma	0.1-0.2	SC	3-7	a
	0.5	SC	Twice weekly	10-12 weeks[b]

[a]*Increase dose in increments every 3-7 days until dose is 1.0 ml. Maximum dose in large dogs is 1.5 ml.
[b]Then 0.5-1.0 ml every 1-2 weeks. The interval may be lengthened to the longest interval that maintains control of the disease.

ADDITIONAL DOSAGES. None.

DISPENSING INFORMATION. Observe the injection site for pain, swelling, or discharge. Should this develop, the dosage can be reduced.

STAPHYLOCOCCAL PROTEIN A

CLASS. Bacterial extract, IgG binding reagent used for its affinity to purify mixtures of Ig.

ACTION. Immunostimulant; activates antibody synthesis, interferon induction, lymphocytes; binds immune complexes. Binds the Fc portion of antibodies (IgG class) by a nonimmune mechanism, without disturbing antigen binding. Reaction is generally not species specific.

MORE INFORMATION. See Chapters 2 and 13, References: Ch 2, ref. 13; 75; 83; 163; 102.

PHARMACOKINETICS. Unknown.

INDICATIONS. FeLV-viremic cats with clinical signs caused by immunosuppression.

APPROVED USES. Reagent grade chemical for experimental purposes.

CONTRAINDICATIONS. Previous hypersensitivity to this compound or closely related compounds.

ADVERSE REACTIONS. Anaphylaxis, low-grade peritonitis.

INTERACTIONS. None.

AVAILABILITY	TYPE	SIZE	PREPARATION (COMPANY)
5 mg	Lyophilized powder (reagent grade)	3 ml volume dilutes	Pharmacia Biotech

HANDLING. Powder (5 mg) is reconstituted according to manufacturer's recommendations in 3 ml sterile water using sterile technique. The resulting solution is filtered through a 0.3 μ filter and added to 500 ml of sterile saline to give 10 μg/ml concentration. This is frozen (−20°C) in 5-ml aliquots, which can be frozen for several years. The solution should not be refrozen after thawing, and self-defrosting freezers with freeze-thaw cycles should be avoided.

ADMINISTRATION. Clip fur from abdominal wall, scrub to remove surface bacteria with detergents. Give injection IP.

Dosage

INDICATIONS	DOSE	ROUTE	INTERVAL	DURATION (weeks)
FeLV	10 μg/kg	IP	twice weekly	10[a]

[a]Then once a month for the life of the animal.

ADDITIONAL DOSAGES. None.

STIBOGLUCONATE (SODIUM)

CLASS. Pentavalent antimonial.

ACTION. Antiprotozoal: interferes with energy metabolism of *Leishmania* amastigotes.

MORE INFORMATION. See MEGLUMINE ANTIMONIATE; Chapter 71, Table 71-1; References Ch 71, ref. 3.

PHARMACOKINETICS. Rapid systemic availability after parenteral administration, attains high serum concentrations, most of drug is excreted in urine within 24 hr. Some accumulation and with delayed excretion occurs after multiple doses.

SPECTRUM. *Leishmania*. Some increased resistance has been noted.

INDICATION. Leishmaniasis.

CONTRAINDICATIONS. Preexisting cardiac arrhythmias or renal dysfunction.

ADVERSE REACTIONS. Musculoskeletal pain or injection, increased hepatic transaminases (usually reversible), pancreatitis, myocardial injury, hemolytic anemia, leukopenia, vomiting, diarrhea, cardiac arrhythmias, renal dysfunction, shock, sudden death. IV use can cause thrombophlebitis. In people, children tolerate the drug better than adults.

INTERACTIONS. Has been combined with paromomycin or pentamidine for resistant leishmaniasis.

AVAILABILITY	TYPE	SIZES	PREPARATIONS (COMPANY)
Human	Solution for parenteral injection. Not available in U.S. for animal use, only for humans through CDC, Atlanta, GA, (404) 639-3670; available in orther countries	100 mg antimony/ml in 100 ml multidose vials	*Pentostam* (Glaxo Wellcome)

HANDLING. Protect from ultraviolet light. Can sterilize solutions by autoclaving.

ADMINISTRATION. Give IV or IM. If adverse reactions occur, can give on alternate days for longer periods. If given IV, should do it slowly (over 5 min) through a fine needle or catheter to avoid thrombophlebitis.

Dosage

INDICATIONS (*Human*)	DOSE[a] (mg/kg)	ROUTE	INTERVAL (hr)	DURATION (days)
Leishmaniasis (cutaneous)	10-20 antimony	IM	24	20
Leishmanasis (visceral)	20 antimony	IM, IV	24	20-28

[a]Doses are expressed as equivalent antimony.

ADDITIONAL DOSAGES. Leishmaniasis, Table 73-4.

STREPTOMYCIN

CLASS. Aminoglycoside.

ACTION. Bactericidal; interferes with bacterial protein synthesis.

MORE INFORMATION. See GENTAMICIN; Aminoglycosides, Chapter 34; Tables 34-5 and 34-6.

PHARMACOKINETICS. See GENTAMICIN.

SPECTRUM. Gram positive: some *Streptococcus.* **Gram negative:** *Escherichia,* some *Pasteurella, Salmonella, Yersinia, Francisella, Brucella.* Bacterial resistance is common with this aminoglycoside. **Others:** *Mycobacterium tuberculosis.*

INDICATIONS. Brucellosis, tularemia, plague, mycobacteriosis. Should always be used in combination.

CONTRAINDICATIONS. Avoid use in cats because of toxicity. Avoid with renal insufficiency, myasthenia gravis.

ADVERSE REACTIONS. Ototoxicity, neuromuscular blockade, renal damage.

INTERACTIONS. Ototoxicity and nephrotoxicity increased with concurrent diuretics (mannitol, furosemide), cephalosporins.

AVAILABILITY	TYPE	SIZES	PREPARATIONS (COMPANY)
Human	Injectable solution	400 mg/ml	*Streptomycin sulfate* (Pfizer); discontinued in U.S.; available only for human use by CDC. Presently for investigational use by veterinarians in U.S. by Roerig, Division of Pfizer; Voice 800-254-4445; Fax 800-251-9445.

INTERNATIONAL PREPARATIONS. *Cidan Est, Novostrep, Solustrep, Streptocol, Strepto-Fatol.*

HANDLING. Stored at refrigerated 2-8°C temperatures. If diluted in fluid for IV use, stable for 24 hr.

ADMINISTRATION. IM use only. If insufficient muscle mass, may give dose in 100 ml of 0.9% NaCl or 5% dextrose and administer it over 30-60 min.

Dosage

INDICATIONS (*Dogs*)	DOSE	ROUTE	INTERVAL (hr)	DURATION (days)
Brucellosis	10-20 mg/kg	IM	12	7[a]

[a]Dose given for first and fourth week of treatment along with concurrent doxycycline (see Chapter 40 and Table 40-2).

ADDITIONAL DOSAGES. Canine brucellosis, Table 40-2; plague, Table 47-1; musculoskeletal infections, Table 86-4.

SULFADIAZINE

CLASS. Sulfonamide.

ACTION. Bacteriostatic; inhibits bacterial folic acid synthesis.

MORE INFORMATION. TRIMETHOPRIM-SULFONAMIDE; Chapter 34, Sulfonamides; Table 34-10.

PHARMACOKINETICS. Rapid absorption after PO administration, 70%-100% absorbed, distributed through body tissues and fluids. Therapeutic levels achieved in eye, CNS, pleura, synovia. Enters placental and fetal tissues. Hepatic metabolism by acetylation. Pantothenic acid deficiency or "slow acetylating" animals may have increased risk of toxicity or accumulation of drug. Metabolites and active drug excreted in urine. Crystals are less soluble in acid urine and with restricted fluid intake.

SPECTRUM. Gram positive: *Streptococcus, Staphylococcus, Nocardia.* **Gram negative:** *Klebsiella, Proteus, Escherichia, Shigella, Salmonella.* **Anaerobes:** poor in vivo. **Others:** *Pneumocystis,* coccidia, *Toxoplasma.*

INDICATIONS. Urinary tract infections, meningitis, nocardiosis, otitis media-interna, toxoplasmosis (with pyrimethamine).

CONTRAINDICATIONS. Hypersensitivity to sulfonamides, thiazide diuretics, or local anesthetics that have similar chemical structure. Avoid with blood dyscrasias, renal or hepatic insufficiency.

ADVERSE REACTIONS. High or overdoses can cause CNS signs or acute vomiting and abdominal pain. Hypersensitivity reactions (see TRIMETHOPRIM-SULFONAMIDE). GI irritation, dermatologic eruptions, polydipsia and polyuria, keratoconjunctivitis sicca. Resembles: goitrogens inhibiting T_4 production; diuretics causing polydipsia, polyuria; sulfonureas causing hypoglycemia.

INTERACTIONS. Chronic administration results in reduced thyroid hormone synthesis. It may increase warfarin activity, phentoin concentrations, thiopental activity, sulfonurea concentrations in treated animals. Increases toxicity of methotrexate, which also affects folate metabolism.

AVAILABILITY	TYPE	SIZES	PREPARATION (COMPANY)
Veterinary	Tablets	500 mg	Generic (various)

HANDLING. Store in airtight containers at room temperature.

ADMINISTRATION. Once daily suitable for urinary tract infections, but twice daily needed to maintain blood and tissue levels. Maintain hydration and adequate fluid therapy, especially in cats.

Dosage

INDICATIONS	DOSE (mg/kg)	ROUTE	INTERVAL (hr)	DURATION (days)
Dogs				
Soft tissue, urinary infections	30	PO	24	7-14
Cats				
Soft tissue, urinary infections	15	PO	12	7-14

ADDITIONAL DOSAGES. Nocardiosis, Table 49-3; hepatozoon (with trimethoprim), Table 74-2; see also TRIMETHOPRIM-SULFONAMIDE for combined use in other infections.

DISPENSING INFORMATION. Watch for vomiting, diarrhea, systemic illness, or reduced tear production.

SULFADIMETHOXINE

CLASS. Sulfonamide.

ACTION. Bacteriostatic; inhibits bacterial synthesis of folic acid from para-aminobenzoic acid. Antiprotozoal.

MORE INFORMATION. See SULFADIAZINE; the SULFONAMIDES; Chapter 34; Table 34-10.

PHARMACOKINETICS. See also SULFADIAZINE. Rapidly absorbed from GI tract. High plasma protein binding allows for sustained blood levels, prolonged excretion, longer dosing intervals. Diffuses especially into tissues that are less acid and in those having high leukocyte concentrations. In the dog, because the drug is excreted unchanged, the potential for drug-induced nephrotoxicity is low.

SPECTRUM. Gram positive: *Streptococcus, Staphylococcus.* Gram negative: *Klebsiella, Proteus, Escherichia, Shigella, Salmonella.* Anaerobes: poor in vivo. Others: coccidia, some activity against *Cryptosporidium.* Ineffective: viruses and *Rickettsia, Pseudomonas.*

INDICATIONS. Treatment of bacterial respiratory, enteric, genitourinary tract, soft tissue infections. Coccidiosis.

CONTRAINDICATIONS. Dehydration. See SULFADIAZINE.

ADVERSE REACTIONS. Few in dogs, diarrhea at higher than therapeutic dosages. IM injections are too painful to be practical.

INTERACTIONS. Reduced thyroid hormone synthesis with chronic (6 weeks) treatment. See SULFADIAZINE.

AVAILABILITY	TYPE	SIZES	PREPARATIONS (COMPANY)
Veterinary	Oral tablets (approved dogs and cats)	125 mg, 250 mg, 500 mg	*Albon* (Pfizer), *Bactrovet* (Schering-Plough)
	Liquid for injection (approved cats, dogs, horses, cows)	400 mg/ml	*Albon*
	Oral suspension (approved dogs, cats)	250 mg/5 ml 125 mg/ml	*Albon* *Bactrovet*

HANDLING. Store injectable liquid at room temperature. If crystals form, dissolve by warming slightly.

ADMINISTRATION. Parenteral liquid: IV or SC to obtain rapid blood levels or to treat anorectic, vomiting, fractious animal. IM route is very painful and should be avoided. PO suspension is custard flavored. Animals should maintain adequate water intake.

Dosage

INDICATIONS	DOSE (mg/kg)	ROUTE	INTERVAL (hr)	DURATION (days)
Dogs and Cats				
Systemic infections, coccidiosis	27.5[a]	IV, IM, PO	24	3-5
Cats				
Coccidiosis	50	PO	24	10
	27[a]	PO	24	prn[b]

[a]Give twice this dose the first day.
[b]Or 48 hr after signs resolve; usual course for coccidiosis may be 14-29 days.

ADDITIONAL DOSAGES. Coccidiosis, Table 81-2; pyoderma (with ormetroprim), Table 85-3. For combination therapy, see also TRIMETHOPRIM-SULFONAMIDE, ORMETROPRIM-SULFONAMIDE, and BAQUILOPRIM-SULFONAMIDE for treatment of other infections.

DISPENSING INFORMATION. Make sure animal has access to water at all times.

SULFASALAZINE (SALICYLAZOSULFAPYRIDINE)

CLASS. Sulfonamide.

ACTION. Inhibits bacterial folic acid synthesis combined to salicylic acid. The salicylate component is believed to be the active moiety, mainly antiinflammatory.

MORE INFORMATION. See Chapter 34, Sulfonamides; Table 34-10.

PHARMACOKINETICS. After PO administration, one third of dose is absorbed from small intestine. The remaining two thirds pass to the colon, where it is hydrolyzed by resident microflora to 5-aminosalicylic acid and sulfapyridine; most of the latter is absorbed and metabolized. Within 3 days, 91% of drug and metabolites is recovered in the urine.

INDICATIONS. Inflammatory large bowel diseases of dogs and cats.

CONTRAINDICATIONS. Previous hypersensitivity to sulfonamides, intestinal, or urinary obstruction. Use caution in treating cats because of salicylate content.

ADVERSE REACTIONS. Anorexia, vomiting, hypersensitivity reactions. Use of enteric-coated tablet may alleviate GI side effects in cats. CNS signs (ataxia, depression), polydipsia, polyuria may inhibit thyroid hormone and produce thyroid enlargement (goiter). Orange-yellow discoloration of urine or skin, reduced spermatogenesis; keratoconjunctivitis sicca. Folate-deficiency anemia, especially in cats on long-term treatment. See TRIMETHOPRIM-SULFONAMIDE.

INTERACTIONS. Reduced thyroid hormone synthesis with chronic (5-6 weeks treatment).

AVAILABILITY	TYPE	SIZES	PREPARATIONS (COMPANY)
Human	Oral tablets ± enteric coating	500 mg	*Azulfidine* (Pharmacia & Upjohn), generic (various)
	Oral suspension	250 mg/5 ml	*Azulfidine*

INTERNATIONAL PREPARATIONS. *Colo-Pleon, Gastroprotetto, Salazopyrin, Salisulf, Sulazine, Sulfazine.*

HANDLING. Tablets should be stored at room temperature. Shake PO suspension before using and refrigerate after use; do not store longer than 14 days after reconstitution.

ADMINISTRATION. Give with food if causes vomiting. Subdividing the dose or using enteric-coated tablets helps avoid GI irritation.

Dosage

INDICATIONS	DOSE (mg/kg)	ROUTE	INTERVAL (hr)	DURATION (days)
Dogs				
Colitis	10-15[a]	PO	6-8	2-4[b]
Cats				
Inflammatory bowel disease	10-20	PO	12	14-42
	25[c]	PO	24	14-42

[a]Maximum of 1 g daily.
[b]Then re-evaluate treatment response. After 4-5 weeks may reduce dose to 12- to 24-hr interval for 2-3 weeks before discontinuing.
[c]Maximum of 250 mg total dose (1/2 tablet) can be given every 24 hr.

ADDITIONAL DOSAGES. Gastroenteric infections, Table 89-16; colitis, Table 89-19.

DISPENSING INFORMATION. See SULFADIAZINE; watch for reduced tear production.

SURAMIN

CLASS. Purine receptor antagonist that is a hexasulfonated naphthyurea.

ACTION. Antiprotozoal, inhibits angiogenesis, and antitumor agent.

MORE INFORMATION. See SURAMIN; Chapter 2, Table 2-2.

PHARMACOKINETICS. Not absorbed from GI tract. Highly bound to serum proteins; therefore minimal penetration of the blood-brain barrier. Excreted slowly in the urine following each dose.

SPECTRUM. *Trypanosoma brucei, Trypanosoma gambiense, Trypanosoma b. rhodesiense.*

INDICATIONS. Treatment of African trypanosomiasis. Active against early stages (see Chapter 72). Has been used to treat FeLV infections without controlled studies (see Chapter 2).

CONTRAINDICATIONS. Renal pathology as determined by the presence of urine casts or biochemical features. Avoid in pregnancy.

ADVERSE REACTIONS. In people, cloudy urine, transient albuminuria, dermal paresthesias from peripheral neuritis, diarrhea, hypoglycemia, anorexia. Collapse and nephrotoxicity.

INTERACTIONS. None reported.

AVAILABILITY	TYPE	SIZES	PREPARATION (COMPANY)
Human (Germany and South Africa)	Powder for injection	1 g vials	*Metaret* (Bayer) Not available in U.S. or Canada

INTERNATIONAL PREPARATIONS. *Bayer 205, Germanin, Moranyl, Fourneau 309, Belganyl, Naphuride, Antrypol.*

HANDLING. Store in tightly capped container away from moisture at 4°C. Drug is a loose powder that dissolves in water and physiologic saline. Diluted to a 10% concentration. IV therapy is preferred as it can be irritating after IM use.

ADMINISTRATION. Best to give a test dose of 100-200 mg first time over 20-30 min and evaluated for any side effects.

Dosage

INDICATIONS	DOSE	ROUTE	INTERVAL (hr)	DURATION
Human infant dose for trypanosomiasis	10-15 mg/kg	IV	24[a]	[b]

[a] 24-hr interval is used for 2-3 days and then subsequent injections are at weekly intervals until a total dose is reached.
[b] Administer until a total dose is up to 5 g for adults. A second course cannot be repeated until at least 3 mo later.

ADDITIONAL DOSAGES. None.

TEICOPLANIN

CLASS. Glycopeptide.

ACTION. Bactericidal; binds to bacterial cell wall peptidoglycan.

MORE INFORMATION. See VANCOMYCIN; Chapter 34.

PHARMACOKINETICS. Not absorbed from GI tract. Usually given IV or IM and 90% bioavailable. After parenteral administration, enters liver, pancreas, bone, mucosal tissues, and peritoneal, biliary, and blister fluids. Poor entry into CNS or CSF with noninflamed meninges. Longer plasma half-life than vancomycin, can give once daily. Little metabolism, most renally excreted unchanged. Slow elimination phase.

SPECTRUM. Gram positive: Only against gram-positive aerobes and gram-positive obigate anaerobes; more activity and less resistance than with vancomycin.

INDICATIONS. β-lactam–resistant gram-positive infections as a result of *Staphylococcus, Streptococcus, Enterococcus, Listeria, Corynebacterium, Clostridium.* Should be combined with aminoglycoside to treat staphylococcal endocarditis, septicemia, endocarditis, skin, soft tissue, and lower respiratory infections, osteomyelitis. For catheter-induced infections; has also been impregnated on IV catheters for prophylaxis. Orally is not absorbed but is given to treat enterococcal and clostridial enterocolitis.

CONTRAINDICATIONS. Renal failure. Should monitor function during therapy.

ADVERSE REACTIONS. Injection site pain (IM) or phlebitis (IV), urticarial rash, eosinophilia, neutropenia, thrombocytopenia, vomiting, diarrhea.

INTERACTIONS. Synergistic with aminoglycosides, imipenem, and rifampin.

AVAILABILITY	TYPE	SIZES	PREPARATION (COMPANY)
Human	Powder for injection	200 mg, 400 mg	*Targocid* (Marion Merrell Dow)

INTERNATIONAL PREPARATIONS. *Targocid.*

HANDLING. Do not mix with other drugs in solution. See VANCOMYCIN.

ADMINISTRATION. Can give over 5-min period compared with 60-min duration required for vancomycin.

Dosage

INDICATIONS (*Dogs*)	DOSE (mg/kg)	ROUTE	INTERVAL (hr)[a]	DURATION (days)
Skin, urinary, soft tissue infections	3	IV, IM	24	prn
Systemic infections	6	IV, IM	24	prn
Bacteremia with resistant organisms	12	IV, IM	24	prn

[a]Often give twice the dose the first day.

ADDITIONAL DOSAGES. None.

TERBINAFINE

CLASS. Allylamine.

ACTION. Inhibits fungal sterol synthesis via enzyme squalene epoxidase. Antifungal and fungicidal against hyphal organisms such as dermatophytes, *Aspergillus, Sporothrix* and less effective against yeast or dimorphic fungi. Has activity against superficial yeasts that cause infections such as *Malassezia* (Ch 57, ref. 45).

MORE INFORMATION. Reference Ch 57, ref. 37; 124, 45; Ch 63, ref. 46.

PHARMACOKINETICS. In people, well absorbed (>70%) from the GI tract. Highly lipophilic and absorption increased when taken with fat; however can be given fasting. Remains in plasma for extended periods of several weeks. Distributed in high concentrations in tissues, skin, sweat, sebum, nail bed, hair. Low amounts in lung tissue which may preclude its use in pulmonary infections. Excreted into milk. Liver metabolizes drug. A majority of the drug (70%) eliminated in the urine. Topical preparations are minimally ($\leq$ 5%) absorbed.

SPECTRUM. Dermatophytes, some activity against *Sporothrix* and systemic fungi. In combination with itraconazole was somewhat successful in treatment of cellulitis caused by *Pythium insidiosum.* Low effectiveness against yeasts. Three species of dermatophytes from dogs and cats were highly susceptible in vitro to terbinafine (Ch 57, ref. 58).

Terbinafine had greater cidal activity than griseofulvin, and oral treatment of animals for up to 39 weeks had no effect on MIC values.

INDICATIONS. Onychomycosis, dermatophytosis, sporotrichosis, aspergillosis. Reduced treatment time, improved cure rates, and lower relapse rate compared with griseofulvin. Has been used in AMB and azole-resistant asperillosis in people. Poor activity against yeasts and systemic (dimorphic) fungal infections. Generally used in combination with azoles, especially for sporotrichosis.

CONTRAINDICATIONS. Reduce dosage in renal failure or hepatic dysfunction. Does not have teratogenic effects and can be used in pregnancy.

ADVERSE REACTIONS. GI disturbances, vomiting, abdominal pain, diarrhea. Hepatotoxicity, intrahepatic biliary stasis, increase hepatic enzyme activities, neutropenia, pancytopenia. In people, alopecia and loss of taste sensation. In one evaluation, some of the dogs receiving 30 mg/kg once daily had mild to moderate elevations in serum ALT and ALP when treated for 3-18 weeks.

INTERACTIONS. Cimetidine increases blood concentrations while rifampin decreases it. There are very few interactions of this drug compared to those with the azole antifungal agents.

AVAILABILITY	TYPE	SIZES	PREPARATIONS (COMPANY)
Human	Oral tablets (as hydrochloride)	125 mg, 250 mg	*Lamisil* (Sandoz)
	Topical cream (as hydrochloride)	1%	*Lamisil* (Sandoz)

INTERNATIONAL PREPARATION. *Daskil.*

HANDLING. Store tablets at room temperature in an airtight, light-proof container. May have to crush tablets and recompound the drug in gelatin capsules to achieve low dose needed.

ADMINISTRATION. Some increase in absorption is noted with administration of food. Must treat for extended periods in onychomycosis to become incorporated into nail surface.

Dosage

INDICATIONS	DOSE (mg/kg)	ROUTE	INTERVAL (hr)	DURATION (days)
Dogs				
Onychomycosis, dermatophytosis	10[a]	PO	24	42-84
Nasal aspergillosis	5-10	PO	12	42-84
Malassezia Infection	30	PO	24	218[b]
Cat				
Dermatophytosis	30-40[c]	PO	24-48	14-42[d]
Dermatophytosis carrier[e]	8.25	PO	24	21
Sporotrichosis	30	PO	24	42-84

[a]Extrapolated human dose. Tablets may have to be reformulated to achieve this dose.
[b]Given with food it reducing levels of dermal yeasts (Ch 57, ref. 45).
[c]Begin on daily regimen. Must use at least 30 mg/kg. Use 40 mg/kg in resistant cases. Lower dosages of 10-20 mg/kg were not different from untreated controls (Ch 57, ref. 72).
[d]Treatment may be effective after 14 days (Ch 57, ref. 87). Higher doses ≥20 mg/kg were needed for a mycologic cure but this took 21 to 126 days (Ch 57, ref. 94a).
[e]Effective for eradication of *Microsporum canis* spores from haircoat of carrier cats (Ch 57, ref. 16).

ADDITIONAL DOSAGES. None.

DISPENSING INFORMATION. This drug may cause GI upsets manifested by anorexia, vomiting, diarrhea.

TETRACYCLINE

CLASS. Tetracycline.

ACTION. Bacteriostatic; inhibits bacterial protein synthesis by binding to 30s ribosomal subunit. Has anti-inflammatory effects by suppression of leukocyte chemotaxis.

MORE INFORMATION. OXYTETRACYCLINE; Tetracyclines, Chapter 34; Antiprotozoals; Table 34-7; Chapter 71; Table 71-1.

PHARMACOKINETICS. 77%-80% absorption from GI tract (fasting). Unabsorbed drug appears in feces and may alter GI flora. Readily enters most body fluids and tissues. Crosses the placenta to accumulate in fetal bones and teeth. Reaches highest concentration in CSF than other tetracyclines except minocycline or doxycycline. Levels in the CNS and CSF may be therapeutic. Primarily (50%-70%) renal excretion by glomerular filtration. Highest concentrations reached in liver, kidney, urine.

SPECTRUM. Gram positive: *Streptococcus*, some *Staphylococcus*, *Bacillus*. **Gram negative:** *Escherichia*, *Pasteurella*, *Klebsiella*, *Enterobacter*, *Brucella*, *Bordetella*, *Aerobacter*, some *Salmonella*. **Anaerobes:** Clostridia, *Actinomyces*. **Others:** Rickettsiae *(Rickettsia, Ehrlichia, Mycoplasma* (formerly *Haemobartonella*), *Chlamydia, Mycoplasma, Balantidium*. **Ineffective:** *Mycobacterium, Proteus, Pseudomonas*.

INDICATIONS. Tick-borne diseases (Rocky Mountain spotted fever [RMSF], ehrlichiosis, borreliosis), leptospirosis, oral spirochetosis, gram-negative bacterial gastroenteritis, yersiniosis, pasteurellosis, campylobacteriosis, brucellosis, chlamydiosis, intestinal amebiasis. Urinary tract infections caused by *Staphylococcus* and *Escherichia*. Intrapleural administration of tetracycline as a sclerosing agent to treat recurrent spontaneous pneumothorax and lymphatic leakage (Ch 34, ref. 220). Intense chest pain is an undesirable side effect of this therapy. Has been used for other uses as an antiinflammatory agent and for treatment of autoimmune skin disease (Ch 34, ref. 418).

CONTRAINDICATIONS. Pregnancy, lactation, and young (<6 mo); renal or hepatic insufficiency. Reduce dose or avoid in renal failure.

ADVERSE REACTIONS. Fewer GI upsets than other tetracyclines. GI side effects are increased when coadministered with theophylline. Sometimes diarrhea from altered GI microflora. Yellow dental staining in young animals. Catabolic effect may exacerbate azotemia in renal failure. Esophagitis, anorexia, nausea, vomiting, occasional anaphylaxis, Fanconi-like syndrome if outdated drug given. Fever (≤41.1°C [106°F]) that resolves when treatment is discontinued. Cats very susceptible to these toxicities. Signs of GI irritation include depression, fever, anorexia, vomiting, diarrhea. Hepatotoxicity, hepatic necrosis, fever in cats (Ch 34, ref. 189). Nephrotoxicity has been associated with concurrent use of methoxyflurane anesthesia. Rapid IV injection may cause cardiac arrhythmias, presumably owing to chelation of calcium.

INTERACTIONS. GI absorption reduced by iron, bismuth, aluminum hydroxide, sodium bicarbonate, cimetidine, calcium, magnesium, kaolin and pectin, milk products. May interfere with penicillin activity when coadministered.

AVAILABILITY	TYPE	SIZES	PREPARATIONS (COMPANY)
Human	Oral suspension	125 mg/5 ml	*Achromycin-V* (Lederle), *Sumycin* (Squibb)
	Oral capsules, tablets	100 mg, 250 mg, 500 mg	*Achromycin*, generic (various), *Panmycin* (Pharmacia & Upjohn), *Sumycin*
Veterinary	Powder for IV injection, also IM	100 mg, 250 mg, 500 mg vials	*Achromycin*
	Oral liquid (chocolate-mint flavor)	100 mg/ml	*Panmycin* Aquadrops; *Actinomycin*, *Sumycin*, *Tetra-Vet*
	Oral capsules	250 mg	Generic (various)

INTERNATIONAL PREPARATIONS. *Acromicina, Austramycin, Hostacyclin, Latycin.*

HANDLING. Store capsules and tablets at room temperature in airtight, dry, light-resistant containers. PO suspension is stable at room temperature. Shake PO liquid well before administering. IV and IM products are stable at 12 and 24 hr, respectively, after reconstitution.

ADMINISTRATION. Administer to fasting animal. Do not mix with dairy products or substances containing multivalent cations (e.g., Fe, Al, Mg, Ca). Usually does not cause vomiting but can be given with a *small* amount of food if necessary.

Dosage

INDICATIONS	DOSE	ROUTE	INTERVAL (hr)	DURATION
Dogs				
Urinary infections	16 mg/kg	PO	8	7-14 days
Rickettsiosis, borreliosis	22 mg/kg	PO	8	14 days
Systemic bacteremia, brucellosis	22-50 mg/kg	PO	8	28 days
Cats				
Soft tissue infections	20 mg/kg	PO	8	21 days
Hemotropic mycoplasmosis	10-25 mg/kg	PO	8-12	21 days
Bacteremia, systemic infections	7 mg/kg	IV, IM	12	prn

ADDITIONAL DOSAGES. Canine distemper, Table 3-5; salmon poisoning, Table 27-2; ehrlichiosis, Table 28-4; RMSF, Table 29-3; haemobartonellosis, Table 31-1; salmonellosis and other enteric bacterial infections, Table 39-2; helicobacteriosis (in combination), Table 39-6; *Clostridium perfringens*-diarrhea, Table 39-10; brucellosis (in combination), Table 40-2; tetanus, Table 43-2; leptospirosis, Table 44-7; plague, Table 47-1; enteric protozoa, Table 78-3; musculoskeletal infections, Tables 86-3 and 86-3; respiratory infections, Table 88-8; oral infections, Table 89-4; gastrointestinal infections; Table 89-16; hepatobiliary infections, Table 90-5; urinary tract infection, Table 91-10.

DISPENSING INFORMATION. Give on an empty stomach.

THIAMPHENICOL

CLASS. Acetamide, an antibacterial analogue of chloramphenicol.

ACTION. Bacteriostatic. Binds to 50s ribosome of bacteria-inhibiting protein synthesis.

MORE INFORMATION. See CHLORAMPHENICOL; Chapter 34. Synonyms are vicemycetin, dextrosulfenidol, thiamphenicol, thiophenicol.

PHARMACOKINETICS. Similar to chloramphenicol. High (90%) bioavailable after oral administration. Bioavailability after IM administration is 96% but absorption from the muscle is delayed (Ch 34, ref. 65). Well absorbed orally, enters most tissues, with lowest concentrations in the CNS. High penetration with greater than serum concentrations in lung, kidneys, and mammary tissues. This drug has a sulpho-group instead of a nitro-group; consequently its metabolism is different than chloramphenicol. It is not a substrate for glucuronyl transferase in the liver so that 95% of the drug is excreted unchanged in the urine and feces (Ch 34, ref. 64). In laboratory animals, 65% of the dose is eliminated in the urine by glomerular filtration, with the remainder in the feces.

SPECTRUM. See CHLORAMPHENICOL. Gram-positive anaerobic bacteria such as *Actinomyces, Propionibacterium,* and *Fusobacterium,* are particularly susceptible. For most aerobic species, the MIC is >32 µg/g indicating ineffectiveness.

INDICATIONS. See CHLORAMPHENICOL. Particularly indicated and highest therapeutic efficacy for treatment of anaerobic infections. Intermediate activity against *Escherichia coli, Streptotcoccus,* and *Bordetella.* Cross resistance between chloramphenicol has been observed. Consider for infections, such as pneumonia, urinary tract infections, mastitis and enterocolitis, caused by susceptible bacteria.

CONTRAINDICATIONS. Pregnancy. Low fetal weights observed at high-dose ranges in rats and rabbits, possibly related to altered enteric microbial flora in the dam and not a direct toxic effect.

ADVERSE REACTIONS. The idiosyncratic irreversible aplastic anemia in people associated with chloramphenicol exposure or treatment has *not* been seen with thiamphenicol. In a 6-mo study on beagle dogs being treated daily, lethargy, tremors, and weight gain was observed at 60 mg/kg/day. Doses as low as 30 mg/kg/day were associated with decreased erythrocyte counts and hematocrits, reduced bone marrow cellularity, and testicular atrophy. These findings were reversible with withdrawal of the drug.

INTERACTIONS. See CHLORAMPHENICOL.

INDICATIONS. Systemic or localized anaerobic infections. Theoretically this drug offers a safety advantage over chloramphenicol with regard to human health risks.

AVAILABILITY	TYPE	SIZES	PREPARATION (COMPANY)
Veterinary (pigs, cattle, sheep, poultry, fin fish)	Parenteral solution	750 mg	*Urfamycin, Urfamucil* (Sanofi Pharma)
	Capsules	250mg, 500 mg	

INTERNATIONAL PREPARATIONS. Acobiotic, Ervin, Fluimicil, Fultrexin, Glitisol, Thiamcin, Thiophenicol, Tiofeniclin, Urfamycin, Urfamycine.

HANDLING. Can be stored between 2-30°C, although refrigeration is not necessary.

ADMINISTRATION. Can be given PO, IV, IM or SC; the IM injection may cause pain and irritation.

Dosage

INDICATIONS	DOSE (mg/kg)	ROUTE	INTERVAL (hr)	DURATION (days)
Dogs				
Systemic infections	15-20[a]	PO, IM, SC	12	3-5

[a]Extrapolated from dosages for food-producing animals and toxicity data in dogs.

ADDITIONAL DOSAGES. None.

TICARCILLIN

CLASS. Carboxypenicillin.

ACTION. Bactericidal, inhibits bacterial cell wall synthesis.

MORE INFORMATION. See CARBENICILLIN; Penicillins, Chapter 34; Table 34-1.

PHARMACOKINETICS. Not absorbed after PO administration, so given parenterally. Reaches many extracellular fluids, soft tissues, and bone. Crosses blood-brain barrier, primarily with inflammation. CSF-serum ratio is 0.06 : 1 with noninflamed meninges and 0.4 : 1 with meningitis. Eliminated primarily by renal excretion.

SPECTRUM. Gram positive: *Staphylococcus* (non β-lactamase producers), some *Streptococcus*, some *Enterococcus*. **Gram negative:** *Escherichia, Proteus, Salmonella, Enterobacter, Pseudomonas, Citrobacter, Serratia*. **Anaerobes:** *Clostridium, Peptococcus, Peptostreptococcus, Bacteroides, Fusobacterium*. **More effective:** more potent than carbenicillin against *Pseudomonas*. Because of low toxicity, can cause large doses to have activity against some resistant strains of *Pseudomonas*.

INDICATIONS. Bone, joint infections, bacterial sepsis, skin, soft tissue infections, acute, chronic respiratory infections, genitourinary infections, intraabdominal, pelvic infections. Infections of these areas involving *Pseudomonas* or anaerobes. Has been used topically to treat otitis externa caused by *Pseudomonas*; see Handling below and under Dosage section of ticarcillin-clavulanate below for details.

CONTRAINDICATIONS. Reduce dosage in renal failure.

ADVERSE REACTIONS. See CARBENICILLIN.

INTERACTIONS. Often combined with β-lactamase inhibitor, clavulanate (see TICARCILLIN-CLAVULANATE). May also use with aminoglycoside (administered separately) for additional activity against gram-negative aerobes and facultative anaerobes in severe infections.

AVAILABILITY	TYPE	SIZES	PREPARATION (COMPANY)
Human	Powder for injection	1 g, 3 g, 6 g, 20 g, 30 g	*Ticar* (SmithKline Beecham)

INTERNATIONAL PREPARATIONS. *Aerugipen, Tarcil, Ticarpen, Ticillin, Triacilline.*

HANDLING. Store powder at room temperature. **IM:** dilute with sterile water, 0.9% NaCl or 1% lidocaine solution. **IV:** dilute to 1 g/4 ml in 0.9% NaCl or 5% dextrose. Should refrigerate if not used within 1 hr because precipitation may occur. Stable for 24 hr at room temperature and 72 hr if refrigerated. Continuous drip required or intermittent pulse administration over 30 min to 2 hr. Never mix solutions with aminoglycosides because they become inactivated; however, they can be given separately at different sites. **For topical use in ears:** use the following protocol (Ch 85, ref. 42): First make a concentrated solution by reconstituting a 6-gm vial of ticarcillin with 12 ml of sterile water. Divide equally into 2-ml portions in syringes and freeze. This will remain stable for 3 mo. To make the final ear solution, thaw and mix a 2-ml aliquot of concentrate with 40 ml of normal saline. Divide this into four 10-ml aliquots and freeze. Clients should thaw one aliquot at a time and keep it refrigerated. This should be used over a week period and any remainder discarded.

ADMINISTRATION. Often given IV for bacterial sepsis, in combination with an aminoglycoside.

Dosage

INDICATIONS	DOSE (mg/kg)	ROUTE	INTERVAL (hr)	DURATION (days)
Dogs				
Soft tissue, systemic infections	15-25	IV, IM, SC	6-8	prn
Septicemia	40-50	IV, IM	4-6	prn
Difficult, severe systemic infections	100	IV	6-8	prn
Cats (Pseudomonas)				
Soft tissue, systemic infections	15-24	IV, IM, SC	8	prn
Systemic, bacteremia	40-50	IV	6	prn

ADDITIONAL DOSAGES. Gram-negative bacterial infection, Table 37-3; otitis externa, topical, Table 85-6; bacteremia and endocarditis, Table 87-6; respiratory infections, Table 88-8; hepatobiliary infections, Table 90-5.

TICARCILLIN-CLAVULANATE

CLASS. Carboxypenicillin and β-lactamase inhibitor in 30 : 1 ratio.

ACTION. Bactericidal; ticarcillin interferes with bacterial cell wall synthesis; clavulanate inactivates plasmid-mediated β-lactamases; that cause resistance to penicillins and cephalosporins.

MORE INFORMATION. See TICARCILLIN; Penicillins, Chapter 34; Tables 34-1 and 34-2.

PHARMACOKINETICS. See also TICARCILLIN. Ticarcillin is not systemically available after PO administration. Parenteral dosages produces good concentration in tissues, bile, pleural and interstitial fluids; CSF in inflamed meninges. Mainly renal elimination, with 60%-70% ticarcillin and 35%-45% clavulanate excreted unchanged in urine. Dogs excrete clavulanate more rapidly than ticarcillin.

SPECTRUM. Gram positive: *Staphylococcus, Streptococcus, Enterococcus.* **Gram-negative:** *Pseudomonas, Proteus, Enterobacter, Salmonella, Klebsiella, Escherichia, Citrobacter, Serratia, Acinetobacter, Pasteurella, Bordetella.* **Anaerobes:** *Bacteroides, Clostridium, Fusobacterium, Peptostreptococcus, Eubacterium, Peptococcus.*

INDICATIONS. Nosocomial pneumonia, severe skin, soft tissue infections; septicemia; bone, joint, urinary tract, intraabdominal, gynecologic infections. Synergistic with aminoglycosides against some strains of *Pseudomonas.*

CONTRAINDICATIONS. Reduce dose in renal failure.

ADVERSE REACTIONS. Platelet dysfunction, hypersensitivity reactions, seizures, vomiting, diarrhea, myelotoxicity. Rarely hepatotoxicity in people.

INTERACTIONS. Synergistic with aminoglycoside for severe infections.

AVAILABILITY	TYPE	SIZES	PREPARATION (COMPANY)
Human	Powder for injection	3.1 g (3.0 g ticarcillin, 0.1 g clavulanate)	*Timentin* (SmithKline Beecham)

INTERNATIONAL PREPARATIONS. *Betabactyl, Claventin, Clavucar, Timenten.*

HANDLING. Concentrated reconstituted solution (200 mg/ml) stable up to 6 hr at room temperature or 72 hr if refrigerated. Can be diluted to 10-100 mg/ml with 5% dextrose, 0.9% NaCl, lactated Ringer's, and is stable for 24 hr at room temperature 7 days refrigerated, and 30 days frozen. For 5% dextrose solution, storage is only 7 days at frozen temperatures. Incompatible with bicarbonate in solution.

ADMINISTRATION. IV slowly over 30 min. Administer any concurrent aminoglycosides separately. IM administration is effective but painful, therefore IV route is recommended for most uses.

Dosage

INDICATIONS	DOSE (mg/kg)	ROUTE	INTERVAL (hr)	DURATION (days)
Dogs				
Bacteremia, *Pseudomonas* sepsis	20-50	IV	6-8	prn
Pseudomonas Otitis externa	3-4 drops	topical	6-8	prn[a]
Pseudomonas Otitis externa	15-25	IV	8	prn[a]
Cats				
Bacteremia, *Pseudomonas* sepsis	40	IV	6	prn

[a]For *Pseudomonas* otitis use the following regimen (Ch 34, ref. 280). Treatment with 1-2 mg/kg prednisolone PO, every 24 hr, and ear cleaning, every 8 hr, followed by 3-4 drops of topical reconstituted ticarcillin-clavulanate solution. If the ear drum is perforated, concurrent IV treatment is given until the ear drum heals. A new vial of drug is reconstituted each day. The prednisolone is tapered over 2 weeks. Topical treatment is continued for 14 days beyond clinical cure. The duration of treatment has been 14-36 days.

ADDITIONAL DOSAGES. Gram-negative bacterial infections, Table 37-3; respiratory disease, Table 88-8; intraabdominal infections, Table 89-21.

TINIDAZOLE

CLASS. Nitroimidazole.

ACTION. Bactericidal, antibacterial, also antiprotozoal; see METRONIDAZOLE, IPRONIDAZOLE.

MORE INFORMATION. See METRONIDAZOLE; Chapter 71; Table 71-1; references: Ch 71, ref. 79a; 79b; 79c; 79d.

PHARMACOKINETICS. Almost complete absorption (≥90%) from GI tract. Widely distributed in tissues and body fluids. Therapeutic concentrations also in gingival crevice fluid. Metabolized in liver to active metabolites. Repeated administration at the pharmacologic dose does not lead to drug accumulation. Elimination half-life 8.4 hr in cats, 4.4 hr in dogs (Ch 71, ref. 79c). Unchanged drug and metabolites are excreted in urine and to lesser extent in feces. In people, half-life of tinidazole is longer than metronidazole, but there is no difference in dogs (Ch 71, ref. 79c).

SPECTRUM. See METRONIDAZOLE. **Anaerobes:** Excellent activity against *Porphyromonas* spp in canine gingival crevice and most obligate anaerobes including β-lactamase–producing *Bacteroides*. **Others:** anaerobic protozoaa *Giardia, Entamoeba,*

Trichomonas. **Ineffective:** aerobic and facultative anaerobic bacteria. **More effective:** anaerobic bacteria and anaerobic protozoa. The MIC for most anaerobes is 2µg/ml.

INDICATIONS. Gingivitis, oral ulceration, periodontitis, abscesses, anal sacculitis, chronic diarrhea of bacterial or protozoal (giardiasis, amebiasis, balantidiasis) association, osteomyelitis, peritonitis, hepatic abscess, pyothorax, pyometra, animal bite wounds. Invasive amebiasis. Used like metronidazole but has a longer duration of action. See also METRONIDAZOLE.

CONTRAINDICATIONS. No dosage modification in renal failure. Avoid in pregnant or lactating animals. Use with caution in animals with hepatic dysfunction as it is metabolized and eliminated by the liver.

ADVERSE REACTIONS. Vomiting and diarrhea, cutaneous reactions, thrombophlebitis after IV use, stomatitis, glossitis, dry mucous membranes, neutropenia, neurologic signs (vestibular), metallic taste, urine discoloration.

INTERACTIONS. See METRONIDAZOLE.

AVAILABILITY	TYPE	SIZES	PREPARATION (COMPANY)
Human	Oral tablets	500 mg	*Fasigyn* (Pfizer, Europe)
	Oral tablets	250 mg, 500 mg	*Tindamax* (Presutti Laboratoris)
	Parenteral solution	5 mg/ml	

INTERNATIONAL PREPARATIONS. *Amebysol, Ametricid, Aplium, Asiazole, Cartrax, Colpolase, Doxifen, Duozol, Dyzole, Estovyn-T, Famidal, Fasigyne, Fundia, Ginec, Idazole, Pletil, Simplotan, Sorquetan, Tinazole, Tinoral, Tonid, Tricolam, Trimonase.*

HANDLING. See METRONIDAZOLE.

ADMINISTRATION. Advisable to give with food to minimize GI side effects. Food does not affect absorption. Often given as a single daily PO dose with or after feeding. It can also be given IV.

Dosage

INDICATIONS	DOSE (mg/kg)[a]	ROUTE	INTERVAL (hr)	DURATION (days)
Dogs				
Stomatitis, anaerobic bacterial infections	15-25	PO	12	7
Cats				
Stomatitis, anarobic bacterial infections	15	PO	24	7

[a]A dose of 15 mg/kg achieved therapeutic levels in plasma for 12 hr in dogs and 24 hr in cats (Ch 71, ref. 79c).

ADDITIONAL DOSAGES. Enteric protozoal infections (e.g., *Giardia*), Table 78-3.

DISPENSING INFORMATION. Drug can be given with or without food.

TOBRAMYCIN

CLASS. Aminoglycoside.

ACTION. Bactericidal; inhibits bacterial protein synthesis.

MORE INFORMATION. GENTAMICIN, Chapter 34, Aminoglycosides; Table 34-5.

PHARMACOKINETICS. See GENTAMICIN.

SPECTRUM. See GENTAMICIN. Similar to gentamicin but more active against *Pseudomonas*.

INDICATIONS. Classically used to treat severe infections caused by *Pseudomonas, Proteus, Klebsiella, Enterobacter,* and *Escherichia.*

CONTRAINDICATIONS. See GENTAMICIN. Reduce dose in renal failure.

ADVERSE REACTIONS. Ototoxicity and nephrotoxicity, see GENTAMICIN. May be more nephrotoxic to cats than gentamicin or amikacin.

INTERACTIONS. See GENTAMICIN.

AVAILABILITY	TYPE	SIZES	PREPARATION (COMPANY)
Human	Solution for injection	10 mg/ml, 40 mg/ml	*Nebcin* (Eli Lilly)

INTERNATIONAL PREPARATIONS. *Brulamycin, Gernebcin, Mytobrin, Nebcina, Obracin, Tobral, Tobralex, Tobramaxin, Tobrex.*

HANDLING. Do not mix with other drugs before infusion. Store at room temperature. Do not use if becomes discolored.

ADMINISTRATION. IM: inject deep into large muscle. **IV:** dilute in 0.9% NaCl or 5% dextrose; administer slowly over 30-60 min.

Dosage

INDICATIONS	DOSE (mg/kg)	ROUTE	INTERVAL (hr)[a]	DURATION (days)
Dogs				
Soft tissue, systemic infections	1-1.7	IV	8	<7
Systemic infections	2	SC	8-12	<7
Persistent bacteremia	3-5	IV, IM, SC	8	<7
Cats				
Soft tissue, systemic infections	2	IV, IM, SC	12	<5
Persistent bacteremia	2	IV, IM, SC	8	<5

[a]There is evidence that administration of higher dosages less frequently may reduce the toxic potential of aminoglycosides and increase therapeutic efficacy by giving higher peak concentrations. Thus with this regimen, the total daily dose calculated can be administered once every 24 hr.

ADDITIONAL DOSAGES. Otitis externa topical, Table 85-6; respiratory infections, Table 88-8, local ocular treatment, Table 93-4.

TOLTRAZURIL

CLASS. Triazinon.
ACTION. Antiprotozoal, anticoccidial.

MORE INFORMATION. Chapter 71; Table 71-1. See also Ponazuril. Related drug available in some countries is Diclazuril (*Clinicox*), Janssen.
SPECTRUM. Coccidia, *Hepatozoon*.

AVAILABILITY	TYPE	SIZES	PREPARATION (COMPANY)
Veterinary	Oral solution 2.5%, 5%	100 ml, 1 L bottle	*Baycox, Baycox Vet* (Bayer)

Dosage

INDICATIONS	DOSE (mg/kg)	ROUTE	INTERVAL (hr)	DURATION (days)
Coccidiosis (**Dog**)	5-20	PO	24	2-3
Coccidiosis (**Cat**)	30	PO	24	2-3

ADDITIONAL DOSAGES. Toxoplasmosis, Table 80-3; coccidiosis, Table 81-2. Reference Ch 71, ref. 52.

TRIFLURIDINE (SEE CHAPTER 2)

TRIMETHOPRIM-SULFONAMIDE

CLASS. Pyrimidine and sulfonamide in 1 : 5 ratio.
ACTION. Bactericidal, antiprotozoal; synergistic blockade of microbial synthesis of folinic acid.
MORE INFORMATION. See ormetroprim-sulfonamide above, and trimethoprim-sulfonamide, Chapter 34; Table 34-10.

PHARMACOKINETICS. Well absorbed orally, rapid and complete. Wide distribution in body tissues. Most (60%-80%) excreted in urine of dogs as unchanged drug. Small amount metabolized by liver and renally excreted. Acetylated metabolites do not accumulate in dogs, which reduces risk of nephrotoxicity compared with cats and people.

SPECTRUM. Gram positive: some *Staphylococcus* (coagulase negative). **Gram negative:** *Escherichia, Proteus, Klebsiella, Enterobacter, Bordetella, Salmonella, Pasteurella; Nocardia* and *Brucella* at high doses. **Anaerobes:** *Fusobacterium, Clostridium.* Despite in vitro efficacy, in vivo effectiveness against anaerobes is poor. **Others:** *Pneumocystis;* weak against *Toxoplasma* (pyrimethamine-sulfonamide better); enteric coccidia; *Cyclospora, Acanthamoeba.* **Ineffective:** many *Pseudomonas, Mycobacterium, Leptospira, Erysipelothrix,* many anaerobes, including *Bacteroides, Mycoplasma.*

INDICATIONS. Uncomplicated urinary tract infection as a result of susceptible bacteria. *Pneumocystis* pneumonia, acute and chronic prostatitis, antimicrobial prophylaxis for immunocompromised host; bacterial CNS infections/meningitis in dogs and cats. Long-term, low-dose therapy for chronic urinary infections. Microsporidiosis.

CONTRAINDICATIONS. Reduce dose with renal dysfunction. Pregnancy: teratogenic at high doses to laboratory animals but safe at therapeutic dosages in dogs. Avoid use in dogs with reduced Schirmer Tear test values. Doberman pinschers have a decreased ability to detoxify sulfonamide hydroxylamine metabolites resulting in increased susceptibility to toxicity (Ch 34, ref. 83). Avoid use in dogs with congenital bleeding disorders because they have an increased potential risk of hemorrhage should thrombocytopenia develop (Ch 34, ref. 97; 98). Avoid in animals with preexisting hepatic parenchymal disease, anemia, or leukopenia.

ADVERSE REACTIONS

1. Dogs: keratoconjunctivitis sicca (KCS), dogs weighing <12 kg appear more at risk. KCS can develop within 1 week of treatment and up to 7 mo after discontinuation (Ch 34, ref. 24; 94).

2. Hepatotoxicity—cholestatic hepatitis: anorexia, depression, icterus, hepatic necrosis, especially with pre-existing hepatobiliary disease (Ch 34, ref. 321; 370; 387). Dogs that develop persistent increases in ALT have a poorer prognosis (Ch 34, ref. 379).

3. Megaloblastic—folate acid deficiency anemia; more dramatic in cats after several weeks; large doses and longer treatment will affect dogs. Dietary supplement with folinic acid (Leukovorin) at 2.5 mg/kg/day can overcome the folate deficiency. Folic acid supplementation should not be used because its activation to folinic acid is blocked by trimethoprim. With folinic supplements, effectiveness against enterococci and some protozoa is reduced.

4. Immune-mediated polyarthritis, retinitis, glomerulitis, vasculitis, serum sickness, urticaria, erythema multiforme, toxic epidermal necrolysis, facial swelling, conjunctivitis and meningitis (Ch 34, ref. 361; 379). For skin reactions see

cutaneous drug eruption, next. Seems more common in large-breed dogs; Doberman pinschers have shown a predilection for immune-complex complications. Samoyeds and miniature schnauzers were also prevalent in one study (Ch 34, ref. 379), signs usually develop 1-3 weeks (range 5-36 days) after first use of the drug or within 1 hr to 10 days after repeated usage. Laboratory abnormalities include hemolytic anemia, neutropenia, thrombocytopenia, and proteinuria. Reaction begins to subside within 24-48 hr of withdrawal of the drug and commencement of glucocorticoid therapy. Dogs with increased ALT or thrombocytopenia had a poorer prognosis for recovery (Ch 34, ref. 379).

5. Cutaneous drug eruption—erythema multiforme, erythroderma, exfoliative dermatitis, urticaria, toxic epidermal necrolysis, vesiculobullous disease, otitis externa, pemphigus, and pemphigoid-like disease (Ch 34, ref. 90; 248; 252; 239). Large-breed dogs, particularly Doberman pinschers and golden and Labrador retrievers, have been most affected (Ch 34, ref. 139). Although early observations suggested that sulfamethoxazole-induced immune reactions were less prevalent in causing cutaneous drug eruption than sulfadiazine-containing combinations, hypersensitivity risk was found to be equal in later reports (Ch 34, ref. 379).

6. Renal failure—sulfonamide nephromicrolithiasis, polydipsia, and polyuria primarily seen in cats.

7. Salivation, diarrhea, and vomiting—especially in cats given crushed or broken tablets. Cats may show consistent vomiting after PO dosing, which may necessitate parenteral therapy. Parenteral therapy can cause local irritation.

8. Ataxia has been observed in dogs and cats given higher therapeutic dosages. Signs usually disappear within 24-48 hr after therapy is discontinued.

9. Prolonged treatment with trimethoprim-sulfonamides interferes with thyroid hormone synthesis because of the sulfonamide (see ORMETROPRIM-SULFONAMIDE). Chronic (6 weeks-dosing) to euthyroid dogs results in decreased serum T_3, T_4 (Ch 34, ref. 146). Effect is dosage- and duration-dependent. Dosages of 60 mg/kg/day for 4-6 weeks, or 48 mg/kg/day for 10 weeks are in the ranges that could produce clinical hypothyroidism (Ch 34, ref. 134). Dogs given 26.5-31.3 mg/kg PO, every 12 hr developed neutropenia, reduced T4, and increased TSH, concentrations after 1 to 4 weeks of treatment (Ch 34, ref. 422).

10. Hyperkalemia—interferes with renal potassium excretion. It can exacerbate hyperkalemia in animals with hypoadrenocorticism (Ch 34, ref. 323). This effect can be reversed by normal saline diuresis.

INTERACTIONS. Prolongs effects of anticoagulants, diphenylhydantoin, increased blood levels or activity of dapsone, sulfonylureas.

AVAILABILITY	TYPE	SIZES	PREPARATIONS (COMPANY)
Human	Trimethoprim-sulfamethoxazole (1:5 ratio)		
	Oral tablets	480 mg, 960 mg	*Bactrim* (Roche), *Cotrim* (Lemmon), *Septra* (Burroughs Wellcome), generic (various)
	Oral suspension	240 mg/5 ml	*Bactrim, Septra,* generic (various)
	IV solution	480 mg/5 ml	*Bactrim* IV, *Septra* V
Veterinary	Trimethoprim-sulfadiazine (1:5 ratio)		
	Oral tablets (approved for dogs)	30 mg, 120 mg, 480 mg, 960 mg	*Delvoprim* (Mycofarm, UK), *Di-Trim* (Syntex), *Duphatrim* (Solvay-Duphar), *Tribrissen* (Schering-Plough Animal Health)
	Oral suspension (approved for dogs)	60 mg	*Tribrissen*

INTERNATONAL PREPARATIONS. *Abactrim, Antrima, Chemitrim, Comox, Coptin, Cotribene, Eusaprim, Fectrim, Isotrim, Polytrim, Resprim, Septrin, Sulfatrim, Sulfotrim, Trimatrim, Ultrasept.*

HANDLING. Store all products at room temperature in airtight containers. Cats should be given whole tablets or PO suspension to avoid hypersalivation. Crushing tablets or putting them on food has little influence on the absorptive process. Once-daily dosing should only be used for treatment of chronic urinary and skin infections, and prophylaxis for urinary infections. Twice-daily dosing is more effective in eliminating established infection.

ADMINISTRATION. Concurrent treatment with folinic and (2.5 mg/kg/day) will reduce the potential of megaloblastic anemia in cats. Hemogram should be done weekly for the first 2 weeks to check for myelotoxic effects. Hematologic studies should be performed at least once a month thereafter if treatment is extended. Always provide plenty of drinking water. Parenteral solutions are used to treat severe infections and for use in comatose or vomiting animals.

Dosage

INDICATIONS	DOSE (mg/kg)	ROUTE	INTERVAL (hr)	DURATION (days)
Dogs				
Urinary, pyoderma	30	PO	24	14
Urinary, pyoderma, soft tissue infection	15	PO	12	14
Chronic pyoderma, acanthamebiasis	30	PO	12	21-42
Systemic, bacteremia	30-45	PO	12	3-5
Cats				
Urinary infections	30	PO	24	7-14
Urinary, soft tissue infections	15	PO	12	7-14
Coccidiosis (weight ≤ 4 kg)	30-60	PO	24	6
(weight > 4 kg)	15-30	PO	24	6

ADDITIONAL DOSAGES. Canine infectious tracheobronchitis, Table 6-2; enteric bacterial infections, Table 39-2; plague, Table 47-1, opportunistic mycobacterial infections, Table 50-9; pneumocystosis, Table 68-2; hepatozoonosis, Table 74-2; toxoplasmosis, Table 80-3; neosporosis, Table 80-7; coccidial infections, Table 81-2; canine pyoderma, Table 85-3; bacteremia, endocarditis, Table 87-6; respiratory infections, Table 88-8; gastrointestinal infections, Table 89-16; hepatobiliary infections, Table 90-5; urinary infections, Table 91-10; CNS infections, Table 92-5.

DISPENSING INFORMATION. Watch for systemic signs such as fever, lameness, vomiting, yellowing of mucosae, or lack of tear production.

TRIMETREXATE GLUCURONATE

CLASS. Diaminoquinazoline.

ACTION. Bacteriostatic, antibacterial, and antiprotozoal; inhibitor of enzyme dihydrofolate reductase.

MORE INFORMATION. Reference: Ch 71, ref. 99.

PHARMACOKINETICS. Not absorbed well orally, must be given by IV route. Metabolized by liver and excreted in bile. Metabolites and some (10%-30%) unchanged drug excreted in urine.

SPECTRUM. *Pneumocystis, Toxoplasma.*

INDICATIONS. *Pneumocystis* pneumonia refractory or resistant to trimethoprim-sulfonamides or pentamidine. As an adjunct or second choice to clindamycin in treatment of toxoplasmosis.

APPROVED USES. Human: *Pneumocystis* pneumonia refractory or resistant to trimethoprim-sulfas or pentamidine.

CONTRAINDICATIONS. Previous sensitivity. Pregnancy.

ADVERSE REACTIONS. Dermatologic eruption, myelosuppression, stomatitis, increased hepatic serum transaminases, vomiting or diarrhea, folic acid deficiency anemia or leukopenia. Fetotoxic and teratogenic.

INTERACTIONS. Co-administer with folinic acid (leucovorin) to minimize mammalian cell toxicity.

AVAILABILITY	TYPE	SIZES	PREPARATION (COMPANY)
Human	Powder for injection	25 mg vials	*Neutrexin* (US Bioscience)

HANDLING. Store powder at controlled room temperatures away from light. Wear gloves while handling. Just before use, reconstitute by adding 2 ml of 5% dextrose or sterile water until powder is completely dissolved without opacity. Further dilute with 5% dextrose to 0.5-2 mg/ml. Solution stable for 24 hr at room temperature or refrigerated. Discard unused drug after 24 hr.

ADMINISTRATION. Must be given concurrently with folinic acid for 3 days after last dose of trimetrexate. Give IV separately from the folinic acid through a flushed IV catheter. Give over 60 min every 6 hr. IV catheters must be flushed with 10 ml of 5% dextrose before and after administering drug.

Dosage

INDICATIONS	DOSE	ROUTE	INTERVAL (hr)	DURATION (days)
(Human) Pneumocystosis or Toxoplasmosis				
Trimetrexate with folinic acid	45 mg/m²	IV	24	21
	20 mg/m²	IV	6	24
Dog				
Trimetrexate	10 mg/kg	IV	24	21

ADDITIONAL DOSAGES. Pneumocystosis, Table 68-2.

DISPENSING INFORMATION. Recheck hemogram and biochemical tests every 2 weeks.

TYLOSIN

CLASS. Macrolide.

ACTION. Bacteriostatic, antibacterial, similar to erythromycin.

MORE INFORMATION. Chapter 34; reference: Ch 34, ref. 337.

PHARMACOKINETICS. Absorbed primarily in the small intestine. Excreted in urine and bile.

SPECTRUM. Gram positive: *Streptococcus, Staphylococcus, Chlamydia, Mycoplasma.* **Gram negative:** *Campylobacter, Helicobacter.*

INDICATIONS. Campylobacteriosis, helicobacteriosis, inflammatory bowel disease, chronic colitis, upper respiratory tract infections in cats owing to *Mycoplasma, Chlamydia.* Bacterial sensitivity often follows that of erythromycin.

APPROVED USES. Food-producing animals.

CONTRAINDICATIONS. Preexisting cardiac arrhythmia, cardiomyopathy, myocarditis.

ADVERSE REACTIONS. Pain and irritation with IM injection. Inject no more than 1-2 ml/site. Nausea and vomiting with PO administration. Wide safety margin. High dosages (200-400 mg/kg/day, given for a 2-yr period) tolerated by clinically healthy dogs with no apparent side effects. Dosages as low as 5 mg/kg have increased the tendency of dogs to develop ventricular tachycardia after experimental myocardial ischemia. Contact dermatitis has developed in some veterinarians who handled the drug.

INTERACTIONS. Erythromycin, chloramphenicol, lincomycin, clindamycin have similar action and should not be used together.

AVAILABILITY	TYPE	SIZES	PREPARATIONS (COMPANY)
Veterinary	Soluble powder astartrate	100 g containers (~3 g/teaspoon)	*Tylan* Soluble (Elanco)
	Injection	50 mg/ml, 200 mg/ml	*Tylan* Injection (Elanco), generic (Fermenta, Lextron)

HANDLING. Should not mix injectable product with other drugs. Store in airtight containers. Unstable at low pH forming an inactive degradation product, desmycosin.

ADMINISTRATION. PO powder: measured amounts placed on food or in gelatin capsules, or diluted with water and given by gavage. Wear gloves when handling, especially when applying the powder to food. Powder can be mixed with dextrose or cornstarch in a 1:9 ratio to make it ~300 mg/teaspoon for more convenient dosing amounts in small animals.

Dosage

INDICATIONS (*Dogs and Cats*)	DOSE (mg/kg)	ROUTE	INTERVAL (hr)	DURATION (days)
Staphylococcal pyoderma	20	PO	12	15-35
	10	PO	12	17-35
Upper respiratory disease,	6.5-12.5	IM	12	prn
inflammatory bowel disease	5-10	PO	12	prn
Clostridium perfringens diarrhea	20-40	PO	12-24	5-7

ADDITIONAL DOSAGES. Enteric bacterial infections, Table 39-2; *Clostridium perfringens*-associated diarrhea, Table 39-10; gastrointestinal infections, Table 89-16; colitis, Table 89-19.

DISPENSING INFORMATION. Use gloves when administering capsules or placing on food.

VALACYCLOVIR (VALTREX, SMITHKLINE): SEE CHAPTER 2

VANCOMYCIN

CLASS. Glycopeptide.

ACTION. Bactericidal; interferes with peptidoglycan biosynthesis in cell walls of replicating gram-positive bacteria. Less effect on cytoplasmic RNA synthesis.

MORE INFORMATION. See also TEICOPLANIN. Chapter 34; references: Ch 34, ref. 182.

PHARMACOKINETICS. Not well absorbed orally. Given PO for treatment of bacterial enterocolitis. For systemic infections it is given parenterally (IV) because IM is painful After IV injection, fair penetration into body tissues. Clinically useful concentrations in tissues such as heart, lung, kidney, bone, synovial and peritoneal fluids. Primarily eliminated by kidneys via glomerular filtration. Concentration in inflamed meninges may be too low for therapeutic effects so that intrathecal administration would be needed. Similar low concentrations in pleural and pericardial fluids and bile.

SPECTRUM. Gram positive: some *Staphylococcus*, most *Streptococcus*, some *Enterococcus*, *Corynebacterium*. Some resistance to *Enterococcus* and *Staphylococcus* occurs. Combination with aminoglycoside increases activity against these organisms. Those with low-level resistance are still susceptible to teicoplanin; however, some *Enterococcus* have high-level resistance, but development of resistance during treatment is unknown. **Anaerobes:** *Clostridium difficile*, other *Clostridium*, *Bacillus anthracis*, *Actinomyces*. **Others:** *Entamoeba*. **More effective:** Gram positive. **Ineffective:** most gram negative bacteria except *Neisseria*, *Mycobacterium*.

INDICATIONS. Bacterial cholangiohepatitis in cats (Ch 34, ref. 182). Prophylaxis or treatment of staphylococcal or streptococcal septicemia or endocarditis, for clostridial enterocolitis, and for resistant of gram-positive bacterial infections. Resistant *Enterococcus* urinary infections. Prophylaxis for orthopedic surgery combined with aminoglycoside. Orally used to treat *Clostridium difficile*–associated diarrhea in people, a rare condition in animals; enterococcal or clostridial enterocolitis is more likely in dogs and cats that might require vancomycin.

CONTRAINDICATIONS. Reduce dosage in renal failure.

ADVERSE REACTIONS. If too rapid IV inoculation, anaphylaxis-like or urticarial reaction may occur. Preadministered antihistamine (H_1 antagonists) prevents the problem. In toxicity studies, dogs receiving bolus IV infusion developed hypotension and bradycardia. Reversible neutropenia and thrombocytopenia. Nephrotoxicity (hematuria, proteinuria, urine casts, azotemia) is infrequent and rare. May cause auditory ototoxicity.

INTERACTIONS. Concurrent administration of an aminoglycoside and sometimes rifampin potentiates the activity of vancomycin. Use with aminoglycosides may potentiate nephrotoxicity.

AVAILABILITY	TYPE	SIZES	PREPARATIONS (COMPANY)
Human	Powder for injection	500 mg; 1 g; 5 g	*Vancocin* (Lilly), *Lyphocin* (Lymphomed)
	Oral solution and capsules (*Pulvules*)	125-mg, 250-mg capsules; 1-g, 10-g solution bottles	*Vancocin*

INTERNATIONAL PREPARATIONS. *Vancocine, Vancoled, Vancor.*

HANDLING. Incompatible in IV solutions with chloramphenicol, glucocorticoids, aminophylline, methicillin, barbiturates, sodium bicarbonate, heparin. Parenteral solutions stable for 14 days if refrigerated as concentrated stock solution. In infusion bottles is only stable for 24 hr at room temperature but 60 days if refrigerated. The oral solution is reconstituted with distilled water and is stable in refrigerator for 2 weeks.

ADMINISTRATION. IV slowly over 30-60 min in 5% dextrose or 0.9% saline or lactated Ringer's. Rate should be less than 15 mg/min. For CNS infections, 5 mg is placed in CSF by intrathecal injection to provide a concentration of about 25 µg/ml. Given orally, it is not absorbed and reaches high intraluminal concentrations for treatment of enteric bacterial infections.

Dosage

INDICATIONS (*Dogs*)	DOSE (mg/kg)	ROUTE	INTERVAL (hr)	DURATION (days)
C. difficle enterocolitis	10-20	PO	6	5-7
Skin, urinary, soft tissue infections	10-20	IV	12	7-10
Systemic infection, bacteremia	15	IV	6	10

ADDITIONAL DOSAGES. Hepatobiliary infections, Table 90-4; local treatment ocular infections, Table 93-4.

DISPENSING INFORMATION. The oral solution may be given with small amounts of food or both. Keep refrigerated.

VIDARABINE (SEE CHAPTER 2)

VORICONAZOLE

CLASS. Broad spectrum triazole (UK-109,496). Synthetic derivative of fluconazole.

ACTION. Antifungal; inhibits sterol and cytochrome P-450 synthesis. Inhibits 24—methylene dehydrolanosterol demethylation explaining why it is more active against molds such as *Aspergillus* while fluconazole is not. More potent than fluconazole in this effect.

MORE INFORMATION. See Chapter 57; references: Ch 57, ref. 53; 103; 63.

PHARMACOKINETICS. Relatively high bioavailability (>90% systemic availability in people) after IV or PO administration. Food reduces absorption. Accumulates up to 8-fold in tissues following multiple dosing as a result of saturating its own metabolism. In dogs, repeated once-daily administration results in twofold clearance of the drug from 3.4 hr to a shorter interval. This is caused by autoinduction of cytochrome P-450 (Ch 57, ref. 113). Distributes rapidly and extensively through tissues after IV use. Plasma protein binding in most species, including dogs ranges from 51%-67%. In dogs, 61% of the drug is excreted in the urine, the remainder is excreted in feces. Of the 61% of excreted drug, 7% is unmetabolized. The drug is extensively metabolized in the liver to up to 9 different inactive compounds.

SPECTRUM. Active against a broad range of yeasts and filamentous fungi including *Candida*, *Cryptococcus*, *Blastomyces*, *Histoplasma*, *Scedosporium*, *Pseudallescheria*, *Fusarium*, and *Aspergillus*. High activity against *Aspergillus* spp. is seen by the geometric mean MIC of 0.4 mg/L which is similar to that of AMB. In experimental animal models of aspergillosis, even in immunocompromized animals, drug is highly fungicidal in sterilizing tissues.

INDICATIONS. Systemic fungal infections with filamentous, yeast, or dimorphic fungi. Has been used alone in people as the first choice with invasive aspergillosis, scedosporiosis, and fusariosis. These filamentous fungal infections have previously only been responsive to treatment with AMB.

APPROVED USES. Human: for treatment of invasive aspergillosis and infections with *Fusarium* spp and *Scedosporium apiospermum*, the asexual form of *Pseudoallescheria boydii*.

CONTRAINDICATIONS. Teratogenic in rats, avoid in pregnancy. IV formation should be avoided in patients with impaired renal function because the solubilizing agent, a cyclodextrin, can accumulate in the body.

ADVERSE REACTIONS. Dose-related photosensitization, visual disturbances, and photophobia have been observed in people. Also noted are hallucinations, increased ALT activity, and rare fulminant hepatic failure. With IV infusion, anaphylactoid reactions can occur.

INTERACTIONS. Drugs that induce cytochrome P-450 enzymes such as rifampin, phenytoin, and phenobarbial will accelerate voriconazole metabolism. Drugs that inhibit these enzymes, such as quinidine, may increase serum levels of the drug. Grapefruit juice, a known cytochrome P-450 enzyme inhibitor, increases concentration and duration of the drug during treatment of experimental infections of mice (Ch 57, ref. 130).

AVAILABILITY	TYPE	SIZES	PREPARATIONS (COMPANY)
Human	Oral tablets	50 mg, 200 mg	*Vfend* (Pfizer)
	Parenteral injection	200 mg single use vials	*Vfend I.V.*

INTERNATIONAL PREPARATIONS. None.

HANDLING. Keep tablets at controlled room temperature in airtight containers. Parenteral injection should be stored at room or refrigerator temperature.

ADMINISTRATION. In people, loading dose is used initially and this is followed by maintenance dose, which is often switched to oral tablets. Give without food. High fat meals reduce the bioavailability of this drug.

Dosages

INDICATIONS	DOSE	ROUTE	INTERVAL (hr)	DURATION (days)
Dogs[a] —For fungal infections				
Loading dose	6 mg/kg	IV, PO	12	2
Maintenance dose	3-4 mg/kg	PO	12	prn

[a]Extrapolated from human dose.

ADDITIONAL DOSAGES. In people <40 kg, 100 mg every 12 hr; >40 kg, 200 mg every 12 hr.

DISPENSING INFORMATION. This medication must be given either 1 hr before or after a meal. Dosage should be reduced in half with liver insufficiency.

ZALCITABINE: SEE ANTIVIRAL THERAPY, CHAPTER 2

ZIDOVUDINE

Formerly AZIDOTHYMIDINE, AZT.

CLASS. Nucleoside (thymidine) analog. Missing OH group at 3′–position.

ACTION. Antiviral; inhibits viral reverse transcriptase. Converted to triphosphate intracellularly; however conversion to the di- and tri-phosphate is slow and thus competitively inhibits enzyme leading to depletion of nucleoside pool for DNA production (anti-herpesvirus activity). Blocks retroviral reverse transcriptase by similarity to thymidine triphosphate. Becomes incorporated into DNA but missing OH causes strand termination. Prevents infection of new cells but virus replication may continue when existing cells are already infected.

MORE INFORMATION. Chapter 2, Zidobudine; Table 2-2; references: Ch 2, ref. 31; 53; 54.

PHARMACOKINETICS. Absorbed rapidly and completely from GI tract, unaffected by presence of food. Has a short half-life. Widely distributed and penetrates well into CNS and CSF, crosses placenta. Metabolized in liver to inactive metabolites, and rapidly excreted in urine.

SPECTRUM. Retroviruses, FeLV, FIV, some herpesviruses. Some resistance by FIV strains has been noted in vitro (Ch 2, ref. 124). Some antibacterial activity against Enterobacteriaceae and synergistic with trimethoprim-sulfonamide.

INDICATIONS. Clinically affected cats with FIV. Has been used in combination with investigational drug PMEA (Ch 2, ref. 31). Reduces viral replication and delays onset of immunodeficiency when given prophylactically to FIV infected cats (Ch 2, ref. 60). Higher doses (30 mg/kg day) did not affect viremia in FeLV-infected cats but reduced FOCMA antibody titers (Ch 2, ref. 59). Does not cure retroviral infections but reduces the risk of opportunistic infections.

APPROVED USES. Human use: for clinically affected people with HIV infection. Use in human pregnancy to protect unborn child from HIV infection.

CONTRAINDICATIONS. Dose must be reduced or dosage interval increased with hepatic insufficiency.

ADVERSE REACTIONS. Myelosuppression, megaloblastic anemia at high dosages (30 mg/kg/day) in cats (Ch 2, ref. 59; 136). Hematocrit of treated cats declines within 3 weeks of initiating treatment to 60% of baseline (Ch 2, ref. 179; 180). Effectiveness at 50 mg/kg/day was greatest in suppressing viral replication but most toxic in causing myelosuppression and anemia. At 5 mg/kg every 8 hr, was effectively reduced clinical signs of FIV infection and less toxic (Ch 2, ref. 52). Neutropenia is less frequent than anemia. In people, fever, malaise, GI signs, myalgia, rash also reported.

INTERACTIONS. Additive effect on FeLV, FIV if given concurrently with PMEA. Delayed metabolism of drug if coadministered with sulfonamides, narcotics, nonsteroidal antiinflammatory drugs.

AVAILABILITY	TYPE	SIZES	PREPARATIONS (COMPANY)
Human	Oral gelatin capsules	100 mg	*Retrovir* (Glaxo Wellcome)
	Oral raspberry syrup	50 mg/5 ml	*Retrovir*
	Solution for injection	10 mg/ml	*Retrovir*

HANDLING. Store capsules and syrup away from moisture and light. Store vials at 15-25°C away from light. Injection: remove calculated dose from vial and add to 5% dextrose for IV use in humans. For SC use in cats should add to 5 ml NaCl instead. Should not add to biologic fluids (plasma or blood). Stable after reconstitution for 24 hr at room temperature, 48 hr if refrigerated.

ADMINISTRATION. Oral capsules or syrup must be individually compounded to proper dose for each cat. Can begin with IV infusions over 1 hr, given every 4 hr. Switch from IV to PO when able to tolerate it. Doses 30 mg/kg/day are more effective in suppressing virus, but are more myelotoxic to cats.

Dosage

INDICATIONS (*Cats*)	DOSE (mg/kg)	ROUTE	INTERVAL (hr)	DURATION (days)
FIV	5-10[a]	SC, PO	12	prn
FeLV	5[a]	SC, PO	12	prn

[a]At higher dosages, cats have more chance for myelotoxicity. Lower dosages are recommended for cats with FeLV infection as they are often already having myelosuppression. See Zidovudine, Chapter 2, for details on monitoring and duration of treatment.

ADDITIONAL DOSAGES. FIV Infection, Table 14-5; FeLV, under Antivirals and Immunotherapy, Chapter 13.

DISPENSING INFORMATION. Return once weekly for physical examination and blood count evaluation.

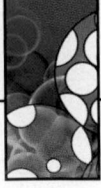

Concentrations and Dosages of Locally Used Ocular Antibacterial Agents[a]

Jean Stiles

AGENT	TOPICAL	SUBCONJUNCTIVAL	INTRAVITREAL
Ampicillin	—	50-250 mg	500 μg
Bacitracin	10,000 U/ml	10,000 U	—
Carbenicillin	4 mg/ml	100 mg	250 μg-2 mg
Cefazolin	50 mg/ml	100 mg	2.25 mg
Cephalothin	50 mg/ml	50-100 mg	2 mg
Chloramphenicol	5 mg/ml	1-2 mg	2 mg
Clindamycin	—	15-40 mg	1 mg
Colistin	5-10 mg/ml	15-37.5 mg	—
Erythromycin	50 mg/ml	100 mg	500 μg
Gentamicin	8-15 mg/ml	10-20 mg	100-400 μg
Lincomycin	—	150 mg	1.5 mg
Methicillin	—	20-100 mg	2 mg
Neomycin	5-8 mg/ml	250-500 mg	—
Penicillin G	100,000 U/ml	0.5-1 million U	—
Polymyxin B	16,250 U/ml	10 mg	—
Streptomycin	—	50-100 mg	—
Sulfacetamide	100-300 mg/ml	—	—
Tobramycin	3 mg/ml	—	0.2-0.4 mg
Vancomycin	50 mg/ml	25 mg	1 mg

[a]For dosage recommendations for systemic administration, see Drug Formulary, Appendix 8.
Adapted from Copyright © *Physician's Desk Reference For Ophthalmology*, 1989 Edition. Published by Medical Economics Co, Inc, Oradell, NJ 07649. With permission.

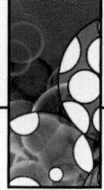

Index

Page numbers followed by f indicate figures; t, tables.

W